Obstetrics

Normal and Problem Pregnancies

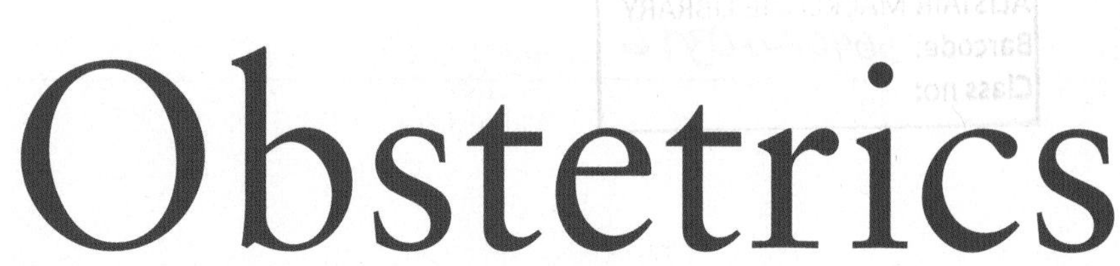

Obstetrics

Normal and Problem Pregnancies

SIXTH EDITION

STEVEN G. GABBE, MD
Senior Vice President for Health Sciences
and Chief Executive Officer
Wexner Medical Center at The Ohio State University
Professor of Obstetrics and Gynecology
The Ohio State University College of Medicine
Columbus, Ohio

JENNIFER R. NIEBYL, MD
Professor
Department of Obstetrics and Gynecology
University of Iowa Carver College of Medicine
University of Iowa Hospitals and Clinics
Iowa City, Iowa

JOE LEIGH SIMPSON, MD
Senior Vice President for Research
and Global Programs
March of Dimes Foundation
White Plains, New York;
Professor of Obstetrics and Gynecology
and Human and Molecular Genetics
Formerly Executive Associate Dean
for Academic Affairs
Herbert Wertheim College of Medicine
Florida International University
Miami, Florida

MARK B. LANDON, MD
Richard L. Melling Professor and Chairman
Department of Obstetrics and Gynecology
The Ohio State University College of Medicine;
Clinical Chief of Obstetrics and Gynecology
Wexner Medical Center at The Ohio State University
Columbus, Ohio

HENRY L. GALAN, MD
Professor and Chief of Maternal-Fetal Medicine
Department of Obstetrics and Gynecology
University of Colorado at Denver Health Sciences Center
Aurora, Colorado

ERIC R. M. JAUNIAUX, MD, PHD
Professor in Obstetrics and Fetal Medicine
Institute for Women's Health
University College London
London, United Kingdom

DEBORAH A. DRISCOLL, MD
Luigi Mastroianni, Jr., Professor and Chair
Department of Obstetrics and Gynecology
Perelman School of Medicine
University of Pennsylvania
Hospital of the University of Pennsylvania
Philadelphia, Pennsylvania

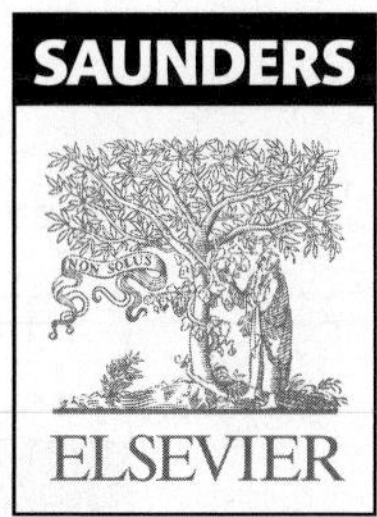

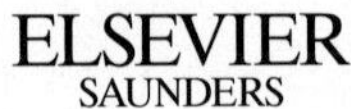

ALISTAIR MACKENZIE LIBRARY
Barcode: 3690240396
Class no: WQ 100 GAB

1600 John F. Kennedy Blvd.
Ste 1800
Philadelphia, PA 19103-2899

OBSTETRICS: NORMAL AND PROBLEM PREGNANCIES, SIXTH EDITION

ISBN: 978-1-4377-1935-2

Copyright © 2012 by Saunders, an imprint of Elsevier Inc. All rights reserved.
Copyright © 2007, 2002, 1996, 1991, 1986 by Churchill Livingstone, an imprint of Elsevier Inc.

No part of this publication may be reproduced or transmitted in any form or by any means, electronic or mechanical, including photocopying, recording, or any information storage and retrieval system, without permission in writing from the publisher. Details on how to seek permission, further information about the Publisher's permissions policies, and our arrangements with organizations such as the Copyright Clearance Center and the Copyright Licensing Agency, can be found at our website: www.elsevier.com/permissions.

This book and the individual contributions contained in it are protected under copyright by the Publisher (other than as may be noted herein).

Notices

Knowledge and best practice in this field are constantly changing. As new research and experience broaden our understanding, changes in research methods, professional practices, or medical treatment may become necessary.

Practitioners and researchers must always rely on their own experience and knowledge in evaluating and using any information, methods, compounds, or experiments described herein. In using such information or methods they should be mindful of their own safety and the safety of others, including parties for whom they have a professional responsibility.

With respect to any drug or pharmaceutical products identified, readers are advised to check the most current information provided (i) on procedures featured or (ii) by the manufacturer of each product to be administered, to verify the recommended dose or formula, the method and duration of administration, and contraindications. It is the responsibility of practitioners, relying on their own experience and knowledge of their patients, to make diagnoses, to determine dosages and the best treatment for each individual patient, and to take all appropriate safety precautions.

To the fullest extent of the law, neither the Publisher nor the authors, contributors, or editors, assume any liability for any injury and/or damage to persons or property as a matter of products liability, negligence or otherwise, or from any use or operation of any methods, products, instructions, or ideas contained in the material herein.

Library of Congress Cataloging-in-Publication Data
Obstetrics : normal and problem pregnancies / [edited by] Steven G. Gabbe [et al.].—6th ed.
p. ; cm.
Includes bibliographical references and index.
ISBN 978-1-4377-1935-2 (hardcover : alk. paper)
I. Gabbe, Steven G.
[DNLM: 1. Obstetrics—methods. 2. Pregnancy Complications. 3. Pregnancy. WQ 100]
618.2—dc23

2012010069

Senior Content Strategist: Stefanie Jewell-Thomas
Content Development Specialist: Lora Sickora
Content Developmental Manager: Lucia Gunzel
Publishing Services Manager: Pat Joiner-Myers
Senior Project Manager: Joy Moore
Designer: Steven Stave

Printed in Canada

Last digit is the print number: 9 8 7 6 5 4 3 2 1

Working together to grow libraries in developing countries
www.elsevier.com | www.bookaid.org | www.sabre.org
ELSEVIER BOOK AID International Sabre Foundation

To Dr. Edward J. Quilligan and Dr. Frederick P. Zuspan, our teachers and mentors, colleagues and friends. "Q" and "Z" trained together as medical students and residents at The Ohio State University and went on to distinguished careers as leaders in obstetrics and gynecology and pioneers in developing the subspecialty of maternal-fetal medicine.*

Steven G. Gabbe, MD
Jennifer R. Niebyl, MD
Joe Leigh Simpson, MD
Mark B. Landon, MD
Henry L. Galan, MD
Eric R. M. Jauniaux, MD, PhD
Deborah A. Driscoll, MD

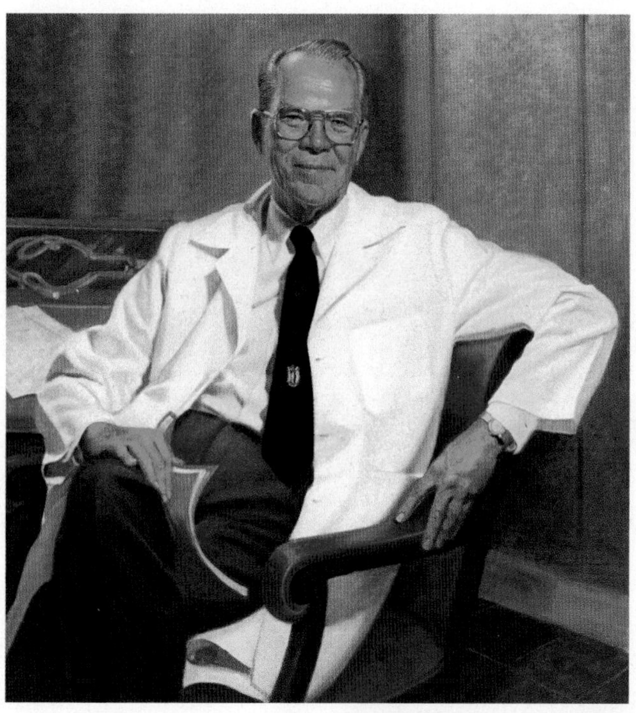

Edward J. Quilligan

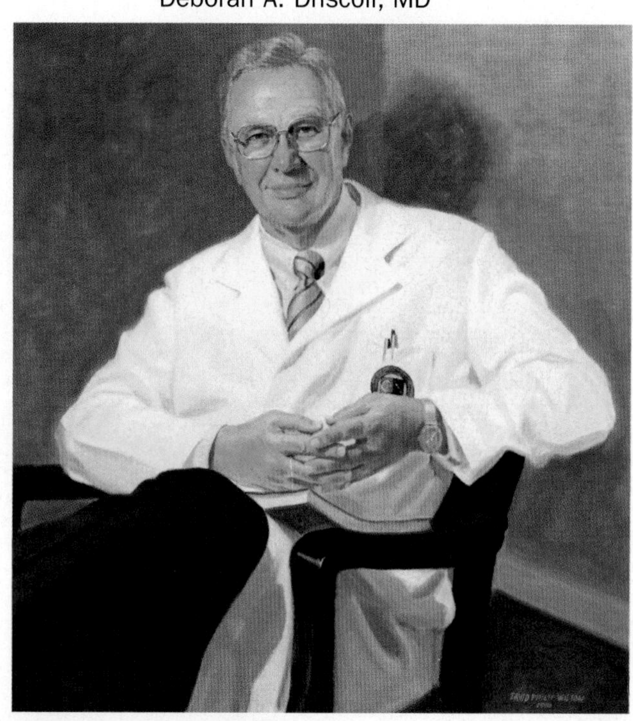

Frederick P. Zuspan

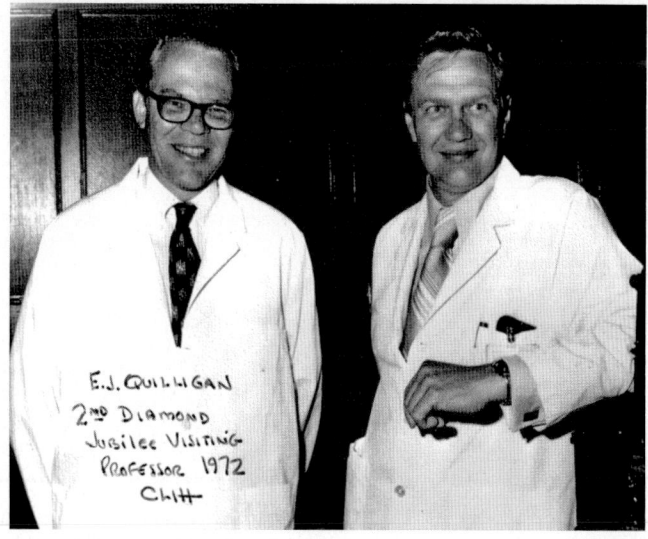

*Dr. Zuspan passed away on June 7, 2009.

Alistair Mackenzie Library
Wishaw General Hospital
50 Netherton Street
Wishaw
ML2 0DP

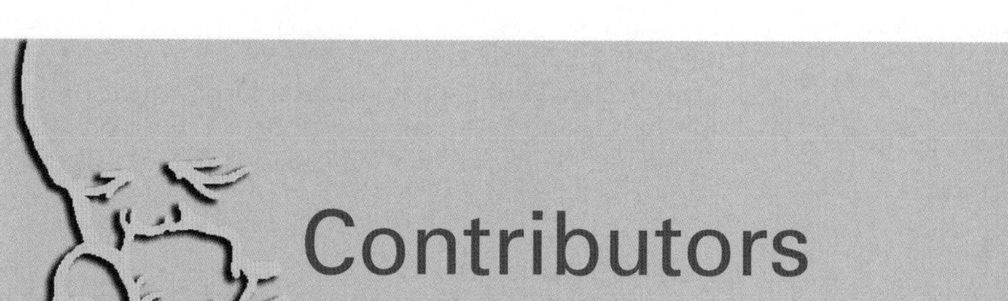

Contributors

Joanna Adamczak, MD
Clinical Fellow, Division of Maternal-Fetal Medicine, Obstetrics and Gynecology, University of Pennsylvania, Philadelphia, Pennsylvania
Surgery During Pregnancy

Kristina M. Adams Waldorf, MD
Assistant Professor, Obstetrics and Gynecology, University of Washington, Seattle, Washington
Maternal-Fetal Immunology

Margaret Altemus, MD
Associate Professor of Psychiatry, Weill Cornell Medical College; Associate Professor of Psychiatry in Complementary and Integrative Medicine, Weill Cornell Medical College; Associate Attending Psychiatrist, New York-Presbyterian Hospital, New York, New York
Mental Health and Behavioral Disorders in Pregnancy

George J. Annas, AB, JD, MPH
Professor of Law; William Fairfield Warren Distinguished Professor and Chairman, Health Law, Bioethics, and Human Rights Department, Boston University School of Public Health, Boston, Massachusetts
Legal and Ethical Issues in Obstetrical Practice

Jennifer L. Bailit, MD, MPH
Department of Obstetrics and Gynecology, MetroHealth Medical Center and the Center for Health Care Research and Policy, Case Western Reserve University, Cleveland, Ohio
Patient Safety and Quality Measurement in Obstetrical Care

Ahmet Alexander Baschat, MD, MB, BCh, BAO
Professor of Obstetrics, Gynecology, and Reproductive Sciences, University of Maryland School of Medicine, Baltimore, Maryland
Intrauterine Growth Restriction

Vincenzo Berghella, MD
Professor, Department of Obstetrics and Gynecology; Director, Division of Maternal-Fetal Medicine; Director, MFM Fellowship Program, Jefferson Medical College, Thomas Jefferson University, Philadelphia, Pennsylvania
Cesarean Delivery

Helene B. Bernstein, MD, PhD
Associate Professor of Reproductive Biology, Molecular Biology, and Microbiology, Case Western Reserve University, Cleveland, Ohio
Maternal and Perinatal Infection—Viral

Debra L. Bogen, MD
Associate Professor of Pediatrics and Psychiatry, University of Pittsburgh School of Medicine, Pittsburgh, Pennsylvania
Mental Health and Behavioral Disorders in Pregnancy

D. Ware Branch, MD
Professor of Obstetrics and Gynecology, University of Utah Health Sciences Center; Medical Director, Women and Newborns Clinical Program, Intermountain Healthcare, Salt Lake City, Utah
Collagen Vascular Diseases

Brenda A. Bucklin, MD
Professor of Anesthesiology and Assistant Dean, Clinical Core Curriculum, Department of Anesthesiology, University of Colorado School of Medicine, Denver, Colorado
Obstetrical Anesthesia

Graham J. Burton, F Med Sci
Centre for Trophoblast Research, University of Cambridge, Cambridge, United Kingdom
Placental Anatomy and Physiology

Mitchell S. Cappell, MD, PhD, FACG
Chief, Division of Gastroenterology and Hepatology, William Beaumont Hospital, Royal Oak, Michigan
Hepatic and Gastrointestinal Diseases

Patrick M. Catalano, MD
Professor and Chair, Department of Reproductive Biology, Case Western Reserve University at MetroHealth Medical Center, Cleveland, Ohio
Nutritional Management During Pregnancy; Diabetes Mellitus Complicating Pregnancy

Jeanette R. Chin, MD
Visiting Instructor, Department of Obstetrics and Gynecology, University of Utah Health Sciences Center; Fellow, Maternal-Fetal Medicine, University of Utah Health Sciences Center, Salt Lake City, Utah
Collagen Vascular Diseases

DAVID F. COLOMBO, MD
Assistant Professor of Maternal-Fetal Medicine, Wexner Medical Center at The Ohio State University, Columbus, Ohio
Renal Disease

LARRY J. COPELAND, MD
Professor, Department of Obstetrics and Gynecology, Division of Gynecologic Oncology, Wexner Medical Center at The Ohio State University, Columbus, Ohio
Malignant Diseases and Pregnancy

MINA DESAI, PHD
Associate Professor, Department of Obstetrics and Gynecology, David Geffen School of Medicine at UCLA; Director of Perinatal Research, Los Angeles Biomedical Center, Harbor-UCLA Medical Center, Torrence, California
Developmental Origins of Adult Health and Disease

MITCHELL P. DOMBROWSKI, MD
Professor and Chief, Department of Obstetrics and Gynecology, St. John Hospital, Detroit, Michigan
Respiratory Diseases in Pregnancy

DEBORAH A. DRISCOLL, MD
Luigi Mastroianni, Jr., Professor and Chair, Department of Obstetrics and Gynecology, Perelman School of Medicine, University of Pennsylvania, Hospital of the University of Pennsylvania, Philadelphia, Pennsylvania
Genetic Counseling and Genetic Screening; Prenatal Genetic Diagnosis

MAURICE L. DRUZIN, MD
Professor and Vice Chair, Department of Obstetrics and Gynecology, Stanford University School of Medicine, Stanford, California
Antepartum Fetal Evaluation

PATRICK DUFF, MD
Professor, Residency Program Director, and Associate Dean for Student Affairs, Department of Obstetrics and Gynecology, University of Florida, Gainesville, Florida
Maternal and Perinatal Infection—Bacterial

THOMAS R. EASTERLING, MD
Professor of Obstetrics and Gynecology, University of Washington, Seattle, Washington
Heart Disease

ERIC L. EISENHAUER, MD
Assistant Professor, Department of Obstetrics and Gynecology, Division of Gynecologic Oncology, Wexner Medical Center at The Ohio State University, Columbus, Ohio
Malignant Diseases and Pregnancy

SHERMAN ELIAS, MD
John J. Sciarra Professor and Chair, Department of Obstetrics and Gynecology, Feinberg School of Medicine, Northwestern University, Chicago, Illinois
Legal and Ethical Issues in Obstetrical Practice

M. GORE ERVIN, PHD
Professor, Department of Biology, Middle Tennessee State University, Murfreesboro, Tennessee
Placental and Fetal Physiology

CHRISTOPHER S. FAMY, MD
Seattle Neuropsychiatric Treatment Center, Seattle, Washington
Mental Health and Behavioral Disorders in Pregnancy

CHRISTINE K. FARINELLI, MD
Clinical Instructor, Maternal-Fetal Medicine, Department of Obstetrics and Gynecology, University of California, Irvine, Orange, California
Abnormal Labor and Induction of Labor

MICHAEL R. FOLEY, MD
Clinical Professor of Obstetrics and Gynecology, University of Arizona School of Medicine, Tucson, Arizona; Chief Medical Officer, Scottsdale Healthcare System, Scottsdale, Arizona
Antepartum and Postpartum Hemorrhage

KARRIE E. FRANCOIS, MD
Clinical Assistant Professor, Department of Obstetrics and Gynecology, University of Arizona, Tucson, Arizona; Perinatal Medical Director, Obstetrics and Gynecology, Scottsdale Healthcare; Partner/Owner, AMOMI Pregnancy Wellness Spa, Scottsdale, Arizona
Antepartum and Postpartum Hemmorhage

STEVEN G. GABBE, MD
Senior Vice President for Health Sciences and Chief Executive Officer, Wexner Medical Center at The Ohio State University; Professor of Obstetrics and Gynecology, The Ohio State University College of Medicine, Columbus, Ohio
Antepartum Fetal Evaluation; Intrauterine Growth Restriction; Diabetes Mellitus Complicating Pregnancy; Appendix II: Anatomy of the Pelvis

HENRY L. GALAN, MD
Professor and Chief of Maternal-Fetal Medicine, Department of Obstetrics and Gynecology, University of Colorado at Denver Health Sciences Center, Aurora, Colorado
Operative Vaginal Delivery; Intrauterine Growth Restriction; Appendix I: Normal Values in Pregnancy

HILARY S. GAMMILL, MD
Assistant Professor, Department of Obstetrics and Gynecology, University of Washington, Seattle, Washington
Maternal-Fetal Immunology

THOMAS J. GARITE, MD
Professor Emeritus, Obstetrics and Gynecology, University of California, Irvine, Orange, California; Director of Research and Education, Obstetrix/Pediatrix Medical Group, Sunrise, Florida
Intrapartum Fetal Evaluation

ETOI GARRISON, MD, PHD
Assistant Professor, Division of Maternal-Fetal Medicine, Department of Obstetrics and Gynecology, Vanderbilt University College of Medicine, Nashville, Tennessee
Normal Labor and Delivery

WILLIAM M. GILBERT, MD
Regional Medical Director, Women's Services, Department of Obstetrics and Gynecology, Sutter Medical Center Sacramento, Sacramento, California
Amniotic Fluid Disorders

LAURA GOETZL, MD, MPH
Associate Professor of Obstetrics and Gynecology, Medical University of South Carolina, Charleston, South Carolina
Appendix I: Normal Values in Pregnancy

MICHAEL C. GORDON, MD
Staff, Maternal-Fetal Medicine, Center for Maternal-Fetal Care, San Antonio, Texas
Maternal Physiology

MARA B. GREENBERG, MD
Clinical Fellow, Obstetrics and Gynecology, Stanford University, Stanford, California
Antepartum Fetal Evaluation

KIMBERLY D. GREGORY, MD, MPH
Professor, David Geffen School of Medicine and UCLA School of Public Health; Vice Chair, Women's Healthcare Quality and Performance Improvement, Department of Obstetrics and Gynecology, Cedars-Sinai Medical Center, Los Angeles, California
Preconception and Prenatal Care: Part of the Continuum

WILLIAM A. GROBMAN, MD, MBA
Department of Obstetrics and Gynecology and the Institute for Healthcare Studies, Feinberg School of Medicine, Northwestern University, Chicago, Illinois
Patient Safety and Quality Measurement in Obstetrical Care

LISA HARK, PHD, RD
Associate Professor of Ophthalmology, Jefferson Medical College; Director, Department of Research, Wills Eye Institute, Philadelphia, Pennsylvania
Nutritional Management During Pregnancy

JOY L. HAWKINS, MD
Professor of Anesthesiology, University of Colorado School of Medicine; Director of Obstetric Anesthesia, University of Colorado Hospital, Aurora, Colorado
Obstetrical Anesthesia

WOLFGANG HOLZGREVE, MD
Professor of Obstetrics and Gynecology; Medical Director and Chair of the Board of Directors, University of Bonn Medical Center, Bonn, Germany
Genetic Counseling and Genetic Screening

JAY D. IAMS, MD
Frederick P. Zuspan Professor and Endowed Chair, Division of Maternal-Fetal Medicine, Department of Obstetrics and Gynecology, Wexner Medical Center at The Ohio State University, Columbus, Ohio
Preterm Birth

ERIC R. M. JAUNIAUX, MD, PHD
Professor in Obstetrics and Fetal Medicine, Institute for Women's Health, University College London, London, United Kingdom
Placental Anatomy and Physiology; Pregnancy Loss

TIMOTHY R. B. JOHNSON, MD
Department Chair of Obstetrics and Gynecology, University of Michigan, Ann Arbor, Michigan
Preconception and Prenatal Care: Part of the Continuum

VERN L. KATZ, MD
Clinical Professor of Obstetrics and Gynecology, Oregon Health Science Center, Portland, Oregon; Adjunct Professor of Human Physiology, University of Oregon, Eugene, Oregon
Postpartum Care

SARAH KILPATRICK, MD, PHD
Head and Vice Dean, Department of Obstetrics and Gynecology, University of Illinois at Chicago College of Medicine, Chicago, Illinois
Normal Labor and Delivery

GEORGE KROUMPOUZOS, MD, PHD, FAAD
Clinical Assistant Professor of Dermatology, Department of Dermatology, Brown Medical School, Providence, Rhode Island
Skin Disease in Pregnancy and Puerperium

DANIEL V. LANDERS, MD
Professor and Vice Chair, Department of Obstetrics and Gynecology; Director, Division of Maternal-Fetal Medicine, University of Minnesota, Minneapolis, Minnesota
Maternal and Perinatal Infection: The Sexually Transmitted Diseases Chlamydia, Gonorrhea, and Syphilis

MARK B. LANDON, MD
Richard L. Meiling Professor and Chairman, Department of Obstetrics and Gynecology, The Ohio State University College of Medicine; Clinical Chief of Obstetrics and Gynecololgy, Wexner Medical Center at The Ohio State University, Columbus, Ohio
Cesarean Delivery; Diabetes Mellitus Complicating Pregnancy

SUSAN M. LANNI, MD
Department of Obstetrics and Gynecology, Virginia Commonwealth University Medical Center, Richmond, Virginia
Malpresentations and Shoulder Dystocia

CHARLES J. LOCKWOOD, MD
Dean, The Ohio State University College of Medicine; Professor of Obstetrics and Gynecology, Wexner Medical Center at The Ohio State University, Columbus, Ohio
Thromboembolic Disorders

JACK LUDMIR, MD
Professor of Obstetrics and Gynecology, Perelman School of Medicine, University of Pennsylvania, Philadelphia, Pennsylvania; Chair, Obstetrics and Gynecology, Pennsylvania Hospital, Philadelphia, Pennsylvania
Surgery During Pregnancy; Cervical Insufficiency

GEORGE A. MACONES, MD, MSCE
Mitchell and Elaine Yanow Professor and Chair, Chair, Department of Obstetrics and Gynecology, Washington University, St. Louis, Missouri
Prolonged and Postterm Pregnancy

BRIAN M. MERCER, BA, MD, FRCSC, FACOG
Professor of Reproductive Biology, Case Western Reserve University; Director, Obstetrics and Gynecology and Maternal-Fetal Medicine, MetroHealth Medical Center, Cleveland, Ohio
Premature Rupture of the Membranes

JORGE H. MESTMAN, MD
Professor of Medicine and Obstetrics and Gynecology, Director of the USC Center for Diabetes and Metabolic Diseases, Department of Medicine, Department of Obstetrics and Gynecology, Keck Hospital of USC and USC Norris Comprehensive Cancer Center and Hospital, Los Angeles, California
Thyroid and Parathyroid Diseases in Pregnancy

DAWN P. MISRA, PHD
Associate Professor and Associate Chair for Research, Department of Family Medicine and Public Health Sciences, Wayne State University, Detroit, Michigan
Mental Health and Behavioral Disorders in Pregnancy

KENNETH J. MOISE, JR., MD
Professor, Department of Obstetrics, Gynecology, and Reproductive Sciences and Department of Pediatric Surgery, University of Texas School of Medicine at Houston; Member, The Texas Fetal Center, Children's Memorial Hermann Hospital, Houston, Texas
Red Cell Alloimmunization

MARK E. MOLITCH, MD
Professor of Medicine, Northwestern University Feinberg School of Medicine; Attending Physician, Northwestern Memorial Hospital, Chicago, Illinois
Pituitary and Adrenal Disorders in Pregnancy

ELLEN L. MOZURKEWICH, MD, MS
Department of Obstetrics and Gynecology, University of Michigan, Ann Arbor, Michigan
Trauma and Related Surgery in Pregnancy

ROGER NEWMAN, MD
Maas Chair for Reproductive Sciences and Professor of Obstetrics and Gynecology, Medical University of South Carolina, Charleston, South Carolina
Multiple Gestations

EDWARD R. NEWTON, MD
Professor and Chair, Department of Obstetrics and Gynecology, Brody School of Medicine, East Carolina University, Greenville, North Carolina
Lactation and Breastfeeding

JENNIFER R. NIEBYL, MD
Professor, Department of Obstetrics and Gynecology, University of Iowa Carver College of Medicine, University of Iowa Hospitals and Clinics, Iowa City, Iowa
Preconception and Prenatal Care: Part of the Continuum; Drugs and Environmental Agents in Pregnancy and Lactation: Embryology, Teratology, Epidemiology; Neurologic Disorders

PETER E. NIELSEN, MD
Clinical Associate Professor of Obstetrics and Gynecology, University of Washington School of Medicine, Seattle, Washington; Adjunct Associate Professor of Obstetrics and Gynecology, Uniformed Services University of the Health Sciences, Bethesda, Maryland; Chairman and Consultant to The Surgeon General, Obstetrics and Gynecology, Madigan Army Medical Center, Tacoma, Washington
Operative Vaginal Delivery

DONALD NOVAK, MD
Professor, Department of Pediatrics, Gastroenterology Division, University of Florida, Gainesville, Florida
Placental and Fetal Physiology

LUCAS OTAÑO, MD
Hospital Italiano de Buenos Aires, Buenos Aires, Argentina
Prenatal Genetic Diagnosis

JOHN OWEN, MD, MSPH
Bruce A. Harris, Jr., Endowed Professor of Obstetrics and Gynecology, University of Alabama at Birmingham, Birmingham, Alabama
Cervical Insufficiency

MARK D. PEARLMAN, MD
Professor of Obstetrics and Gynecology, University of Michigan Von Voigtlander Women's Hospital, Ann Arbor, Michigan
Trauma and Related Surgery in Pregnancy

TERI B. PEARLSTEIN, MD
Associate Professor of Psychiatry and Human Behavior, Department of Psychiatry and Human Behavior, Brown University, Providence, Rhode Island
Mental Health and Behavioral Disorders in Pregnancy

JAMES M. PEREL, PHD
Professor Emeritus of Psychiatry and Pharmacology/Chemical Biology, University of Pittsburgh; Director Emeritus of Clinical Pharmacology, Department of Psychiatry, Western Psychiatric Institute and Clinic, Pittsburgh, Pennsylvania
Mental Health and Behavioral Disorders in Pregnancy

CHRISTIAN M. PETTKER, MD
Assistant Professor of Obstetrics, Gynecology, and Reproductive Sciences, Yale University School of Medicine, New Haven, Connecticut
Thromboembolic Disorders

KIRK D. RAMIN, MD
Associate Professor of Obstetrics, Gynecology, and Women's Health, University of Minnesota, Minneapolis, Minnesota
Maternal and Perinatal Infection: The Sexually Transmitted Diseases Chlamydia, Gonorrhea, and Syphilis

ROXANE RAMPERSAD, MD
Assistant Professor, Department of Obstetrics and Gynecology, Washington University School of Medicine, St. Louis, Missouri
Prolonged and Postterm Pregnancy

SARAH K. REYNOLDS, PHD
Adjunct Assistant Professor, Columbia University School of Social Work, New York, New York; Cognitive & Behavioral Consultants of Westchester, White Plains, New York
Mental Health and Behavioral Disorders in Pregnancy

DOUGLAS S. RICHARDS, MD
Clinical Professor, Division of Maternal-Fetal Medicine, Intermountain Health Care and the University of Utah, Salt Lake City, Utah
Obstetrical Ultrasound: Imaging, Dating, and Growth; Prenatal Genetic Diagnosis

ROBERTO ROMERO, MD
Professor of Molecular Obstetrics, Gynecology, and Genetics, Wayne State University School of Medicine; Chief, Perinatology Research Branch, The Eunice Kennedy Shriver National Institute of Child Health and Development, National Institutes of Health, Department of Health and Human Services, Detroit, Michigan
Preterm Birth

ADAM A. ROSENBERG, MD
Professor of Pediatrics, University of Colorado School of Medicine, Aurora, Colorado
The Neonate

MICHAEL G. ROSS, MD, MPH
Professor of Obstetrics and Gynecology, David Geffen School of Medicine at UCLA; Professor of Public Health, UCLA School of Public Health, Los Angeles, California; Perinatologist, Harbor-UCLA Medical Center, Torrance, California
Placental and Fetal Physiology; Developmental Origins of Adult Health and Disease

PAUL J. ROZANCE, MD
Assistant Professor of Pediatrics, University of Colorado at Denver, Aurora, Colorado
The Neonate

RITU SALANI, MD, MBA
Assistant Professor, Department of Obstetrics and Gynecology, Division of Gynecologic Oncology, Wexner Medical Center at The Ohio State University, Columbus, Ohio
Malignant Diseases and Pregnancy

PHILIP SAMUELS, MD
Associate Professor, Department of Obstetrics and Gynecology; Director, Residency Program in Obstetrics and Gynecology; Director of Fellowship Program, Maternal-Fetal Medicine, Wexner Medical Center at The Ohio State University, Columbus, Ohio
Hematologic Complications of Pregnancy; Neurologic Disorders

NADAV SCHWARTZ, MD
Assistant Professor, Department of Obstetrics and Gynecology, Hospital of the University of Pennsylvania, Philadelphia, Pennsylvania
Surgery During Pregnancy

JOHN W. SEEDS, MD
Department of Obstetrics and Gynecology, Virginia Commonwealth University Medical Center, Richmond, Virginia
Malpresentations and Shoulder Dystocia

LAURENCE E. SHIELDS, MD
California Maternal Quality Care Collaborative, Stanford, California
Maternal-Fetal Immunology

BAHA M. SIBAI, MD
Professor and Principal Investigator, University of Cincinnati, Cincinnati, Ohio
Hypertension

COLIN P. SIBLEY, BSC, PHD
Department of Child Health, University of Manchester, Manchester, United Kingdom
Placental Anatomy and Physiology

HYAGRIV N. SIMHAN, MD, MS
Associate Professor and Chief, Division of Maternal-Fetal Medicine; Vice Chair, Obstetrical Services, Department of Obstetrics, Gynecology, and Reproductive Sciences, University of Pittsburgh School of Medicine, Pittsburgh, Pennsylvania
Preterm Birth

JOE LEIGH SIMPSON, MD
Senior Vice President for Research and Global Programs, March of Dimes Foundation, White Plains, New York; Professor of Obstetrics and Gynecology and Human and Molecular Genetics; Formerly Executive Associate Dean for Academic Affairs, Herbert Wertheim College of Medicine, Florida International University, Miami, Florida
Drugs and Environmental Agents in Pregnancy and Lactation: Embryology, Teratology, Epidemiology; Genetic Counseling and Genetic Screening; Prenatal Genetic Diagnosis; Pregnancy Loss

DOROTHY K. Y. SIT, MD
Assistant Professor of Psychiatry, University of Pittsburgh, Western Psychiatric Institute and Clinic, Pittsburgh, Pennsylvania
Mental Health and Behavioral Disorders in Pregnancy

KAREN STOUT, MD
Associate Professor and Director of Adult Congenital Heart Disease Program and Attending Physician, University of Washington Medical Center, Seattle, Washington
Heart Disease

E. RAMSEY UNAL, MD
Fellow, Obstetrics and Gynecology, Medical University of South Carolina, Charleston, South Carolina
Multiple Gestations

JANICE E. WHITTY, MD
Professor, Director of Maternal-Fetal Medicine, and Chief of Obstetrics, Department of Obstetrics and Gynecology, Meharry Medical College; Adjunct Professor of Maternal-Fetal Medicine, Department of Obstetrics and Gynecology, Vanderbilt University, Nashville, Tennessee
Respiratory Diseases in Pregnancy

DEBORAH A. WING, MD
Professor of Maternal-Fetal Medicine, Department of Obstetrics and Gynecology, University of California, Irvine, Orange, California
Abnormal Labor and Induction of Labor

KATHERINE L. WISNER, MD, MS
Professor of Psychiatry, Obstetrics and Gynecology, Reproductive Sciences, Epidemiology, and Women's Studies; Investigator, Magee Women's Research Institute; Women's Behavioral HealthCARE, University of Pittsburgh, Pittsburgh, Pennsylvania
Mental Health and Behavioral Disorders in Pregnancy

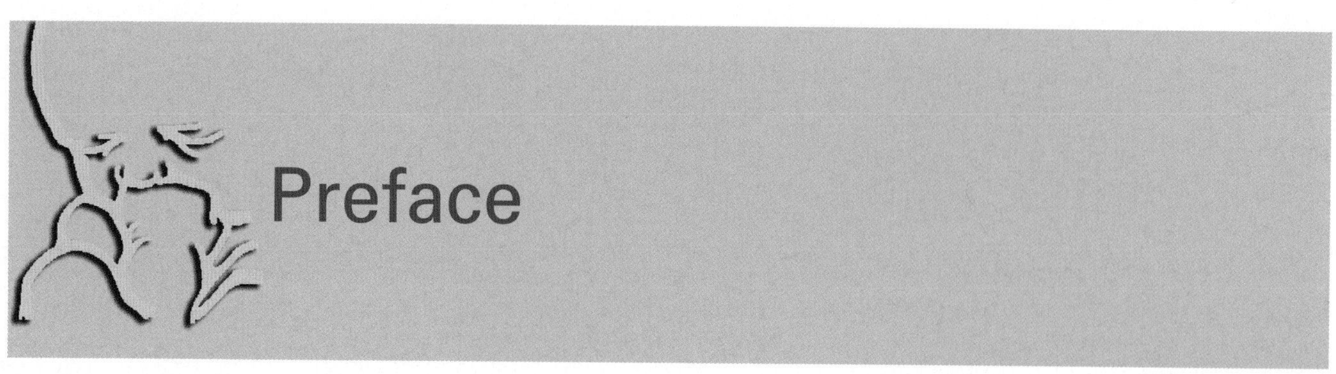

Preface

We're pleased to welcome you to the sixth edition of *Obstetrics: Normal and Problem Pregnancies!* Our book, first published in 1986, now enters its fourth decade. Today, medical information is available in so many different formats and from so many different sources. We are honored that you have turned to (or have returned to) *Obstetrics: Normal and Problem Pregnancies* as a companion in your important work. For many readers this textbook has served as a trusted resource through their years of practice. For newer readers who were introduced to our textbook during medical school or residency training, we hope that you too will find it a valuable companion as you develop your knowledge base and apply what you have learned to patient care.

As in our earlier editions, our book begins with chapters devoted to the basic science and physiology of normal and complicated pregnancies, followed by chapters describing how best to manage first normal and then high-risk patients. In each chapter, we have provided the latest information and used evidence-based studies to justify our recommendations. As you will see on the cover of our textbook and in the list of contributors, we no longer list three senior editors and four associate editors. Rather, we now have an integrated team of seven editors, representing not only a broad range of expertise but each region of our country and Europe.

We believe you will find this edition of our textbook to be the best ever! Our planning process for the sixth edition included surveys conducted of our readers in order that we could assess what you liked best, what topics needed to be expanded, and what we needed to change. Accordingly, we have added four new chapters: Developmental Origins of Adult Health and Disease, Nutritional Management During Pregnancy, Trauma and Related Surgery in Pregnancy, and Patient Safety and Quality Measurement in Obstetrical Care. These new chapters reflect important changes in our field and the way we care for our patients. Every chapter now includes bolded statements our authors have highlighted to emphasize what they want you to learn. These bolded statements, as well as the key points that conclude each chapter, should make review easier. We have also focused more on complementary tables and figures to facilitate learning. We have asked our authors to provide for the printed text a list of approximately 100 key references for you at the end of each chapter. By limiting the number of printed references, we have created more pages for new information in the textbook. As in the past, however, our textbook will be fully available online, where you will find a more extensive bibliography that you can turn to for further exploration of each topic. We have also placed the illustrations for Appendix II, Anatomy of the Pelvis, online for easy access. Appendix I, Normal Values in Pregnancy, has been updated and is available both in the printed textbook and online.

The sixth edition could not have been created without the dedication of our authors. This sixth edition again features the work of nine leaders in our specialty who have contributed to *every* edition: Drs. George J. Annas, D. Ware Branch, Sherman Elias, Timothy R. B. Johnson, Mark B. Landon, Adam A. Rosenberg, Philip Samuels, John W. Seeds, and Baha M. Sibai. We thank each of them! Joining this group of dedicated contributors are 26 new authors, and we thank them as well.

We have received outstanding support from our publisher, Elsevier, and the team of dedicated staff including Judy Fletcher, Melissa Dudlick, Lora Sickora, Stefanie Jewell-Thomas, Joy Moore, and Mike Ederer. Each of the editors wishes to recognize those members of our own team who have provided invaluable editorial and secretarial support, including Joan Lorenz, Beth Mastin, and Susan Dupont (Columbus, Ohio); Martha Altman and Jane Berg (Denver, Colorado); Nancy Schaapveld (Iowa City, Iowa); Elaine Singh (London, United Kingdom); Susan Dent and Esther Lopez (Miami, Florida); and Nancy Bernard (Philadelphia, Pennsylvania).

This sixth edition, like the first published in 1986, has been prepared by our editors, authors, and editorial staff to provide an in-depth understanding of obstetrics, of both normal and problem pregnancies, for the interdisciplinary teams caring for our patients and their families. We hope not only that our readers will find our book a valuable introduction to obstetrics as they begin their careers, but also that they will return to our textbook in the years ahead to review a subject or to share information with their own students and colleagues.

Steven G. Gabbe, MD
Jennifer R. Niebyl, MD
Joe Leigh Simpson, MD
Mark B. Landon, MD
Henry L. Galan, MD
Eric R. M. Jauniaux, MD, PhD
Deborah A. Driscoll, MD

Contents

Section I
Physiology

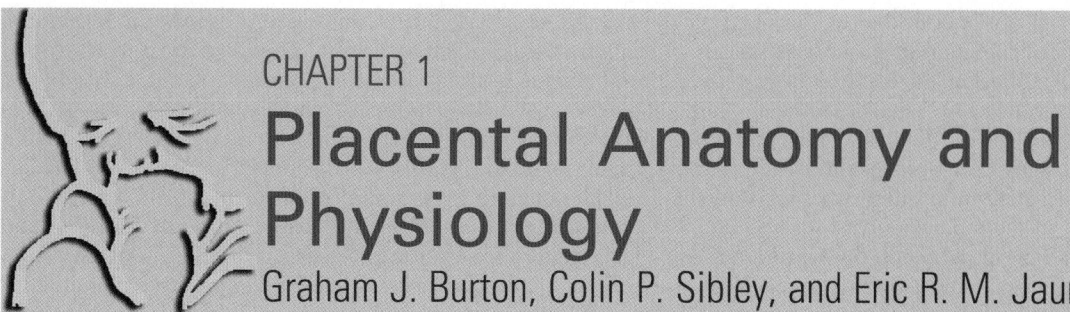

CHAPTER 1

Placental Anatomy and Physiology

Graham J. Burton, Colin P. Sibley, and Eric R. M. Jauniaux

KEY ABBREVIATIONS	
Alpha-fetoprotein	AFP
Adenosine Monophosphate	AMP
Adenosine Triphosphate	ATP
Cytochrome P450scc	P450scc
Dehydroepiandrosterone	DHA
Dehydroepiandrosterone Sulphate	DHAS
Exocoelomic Cavity	ECC
Epidermal Growth Factor	EGF
Glucose Transporter 1	GLUT1
Guanosine Monophosphate	GMP
Human Chorionic Gonadotropin	hCG
Human Immunodeficiency Virus	HIV
Human Placental Lactogen	hPL
Insulin-like Growth Factor	IGF
Immunoglobulin G	IgG
Intervillous Space	IVS
Intrauterine Growth Restriction	IUGR
Kilodaltons	kDA
Killer-cell Immunoglobulin-like Receptor	KIR
Luteinizing Hormone	LH
Major Histocompatibility Complex, Class I, C Antigen	HLA-C
Millivolts	mV
P450 Cytochrome Aromatase	P450arom
Potential Difference	PD
Placental Growth Hormone	PGH
Secondary Yolk Sac	SYS
Type 1 3β-hydroxysteroid Dehydrogenase	3β-HSD

The placenta is a remarkable organ. During a relatively short life span it undergoes rapid growth, differentiation, and maturation. At the same time it performs diverse functions, including the transport of gases and metabolites, immunologic protection, and the production of steroid and protein hormones. As the interface between the mother and her fetus, the placenta plays a key role in ensuring a successful pregnancy. In this chapter, we review the structure of the human placenta and relate this to the contrasting functional demands placed on the organ at different stages of gestation. Because many of the morphologic features are best understood through an understanding of the organ's development, and because many complications of pregnancy arise through aberrations in this process, we approach the subject from this perspective. First, however, for the purposes of orientation and to introduce some basic terminology we provide a brief description of the macroscopic appearance of the delivered organ, with which readers are most likely to be familiar.

OVERVIEW OF THE DELIVERED PLACENTA

At term, the human placenta is usually a discoid organ, 15 to 20 cm in diameter, approximately 3 cm thick at the center, and weighing on average 500 g. These data show considerable individual variation and are also influenced strongly by the mode of delivery.[1] Macroscopically, the organ consists of two surfaces or plates: the chorionic plate to which the umbilical cord is attached, and the basal plate that abuts the maternal endometrium. Between the two plates is a cavity that is filled with maternal blood, delivered from the endometrial spiral arteries through openings in the basal plate. This cavity is bounded at the margins of the disk by the fusion of the chorionic and basal plates, and the smooth chorion, or chorion laeve, extends from the rim to complete the chorionic sac. The placenta is incompletely divided into between 10 and 40 lobes by the presence of septae created by invaginations of the basal plate. The septae are thought to arise from differential resistance of the maternal tissues to trophoblast invasion, and may help to compartmentalize maternal blood flow through the organ. The fetal component of the placenta comprises a series of elaborately branched villous trees that arise from the inner surface of the chorionic plate and project into the cavity of the placenta. This arrangement is somewhat reminiscent of the fronds of a sea anemone wafting in the seawater of a rock pool. Most commonly, each villous tree originates from a single-stem villus that undergoes several generations of branching until the functional units of the placenta, the terminal villi, are created. These consist of an epithelial covering of trophoblast, and a mesodermal core containing branches of the umbilical arteries and tributaries of the umbilical vein. Because of this repeated branching the tree takes on the topology of an inverted wine glass, often referred to as a lobule, and there may be two to three within a single placental lobe (Figure 1-1). As will be seen later, each lobule represents an individual maternal-fetal exchange unit. Toward term the continual elaboration of the villous trees almost fills the cavity of the placenta, which is reduced to a network of narrow spaces collectively referred to as the intervillous space (IVS). The maternal blood percolates through this network of channels, exchanging gases and nutrients with the fetal blood circulating within the villi, before draining through the basal plate into openings of the uterine veins. **The human placenta is therefore classified in comparative mammalian terms as being of the villous hemochorial type,** although as we shall see this arrangement really only pertains to the second and third trimesters of pregnancy.[2] Before that the maternal-fetal relationship is best described as deciduo-chorial.

PLACENTAL DEVELOPMENT

Development of the placenta is initiated morphologically at the time of implantation, when the embryonic pole of the blastocyst establishes contact with the uterine epithelium. At this stage the wall of the blastocyst comprises an outer layer of unicellular epithelial cells, the trophoblast, and an inner layer of extraembryonic mesodermal cells

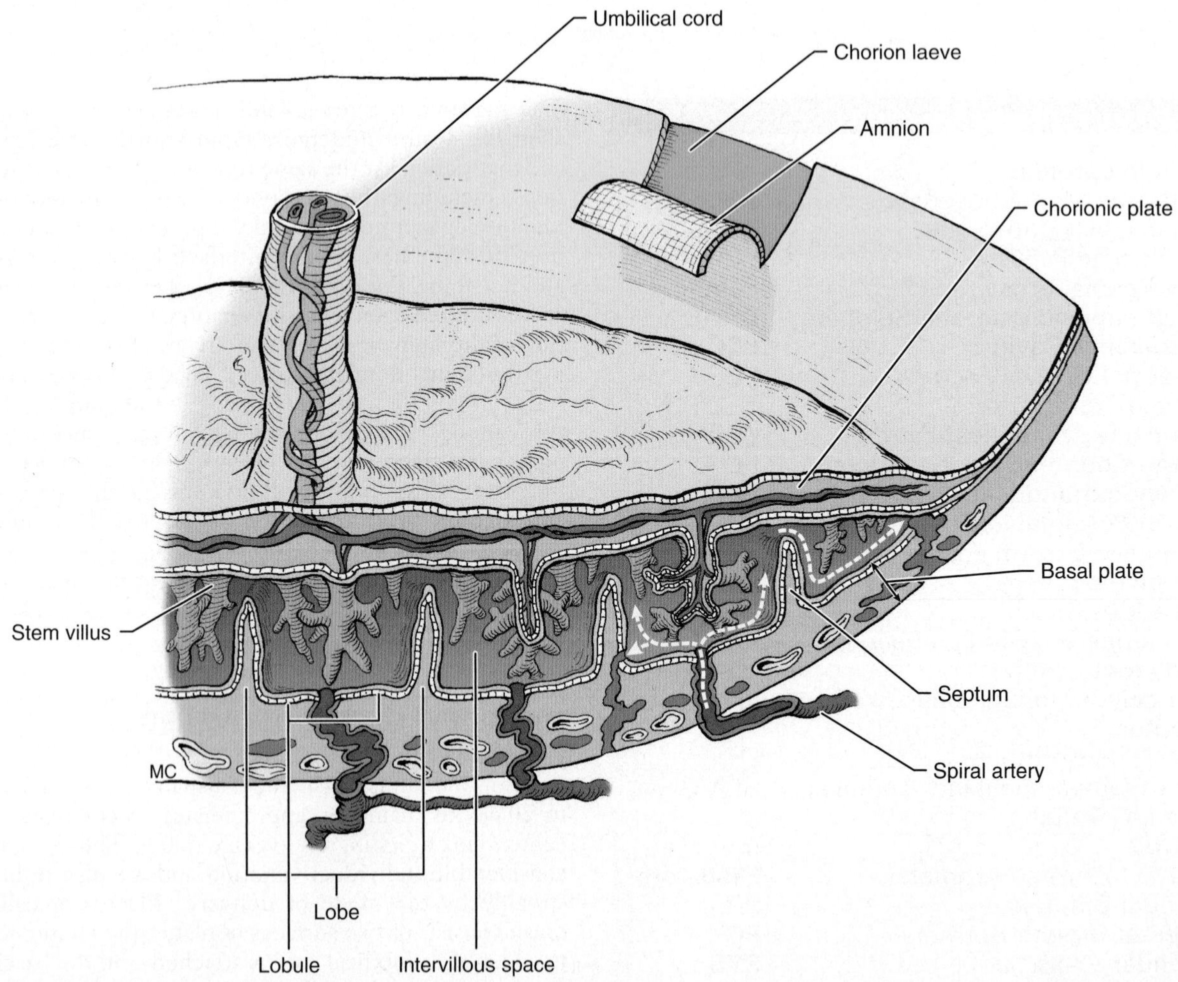

FIGURE 1-1. Diagrammatic cross section through a mature placenta showing the chorionic and basal plates bounding the intervillous space. The villous trees arise from stem villi attached to the chorionic plate, and are arranged as lobules centered over the openings of the maternal spiral arteries.

derived from the inner cell mass.[3] Together, these layers constitute the chorion. The earliest events have never been observed in vivo for obvious ethical reasons, but are thought to be equivalent to those that take place in the rhesus monkey. Attempts have also been made to replicate the situation in vitro by culturing in vitro fertilized human blastocysts on monolayers of endometrial cells. Although such reductionist systems cannot take into account the possibility of paracrine signals emanating from the underlying endometrial stroma, the profound differences in trophoblast invasiveness displayed by various species are maintained. In the case of the human, the trophoblast in contact with the endometrium undergoes a syncytial transformation, and tongues of syncytiotrophoblast begin to penetrate between the endometrial cells. There is no evidence of cell death being induced as part of this process, but gradually the conceptus embeds into the stratum compactum of the endometrium. The earliest ex vivo specimens available for study are estimated to be around 7 days after conception, and in these the conceptus is almost entirely embedded. A plug of fibrin initially seals the defect in the uterine surface, but by days10 to 12 the epithelium is restored.

By the time implantation is complete the conceptus is surrounded entirely by a mantle of syncytiotrophoblast (Figure 1-2). This multinucleated mantle tends to be thicker beneath the conceptus, in association with the embryonic pole, and rests on a layer of uninucleate cytotrophoblast cells derived from the original wall of the blastocyst. Vacuolar spaces begin to appear within the mantle and gradually coalesce to form larger lacunae, the forerunners of the intervillous space. As the lacunae enlarge the intervening syncytiotrophoblast is reduced in thickness, and forms a complex lattice of trabeculae (see Figure 1-2). Soon after, starting around day 12 after fertilization, the cytotrophoblast cells proliferate and penetrate into the

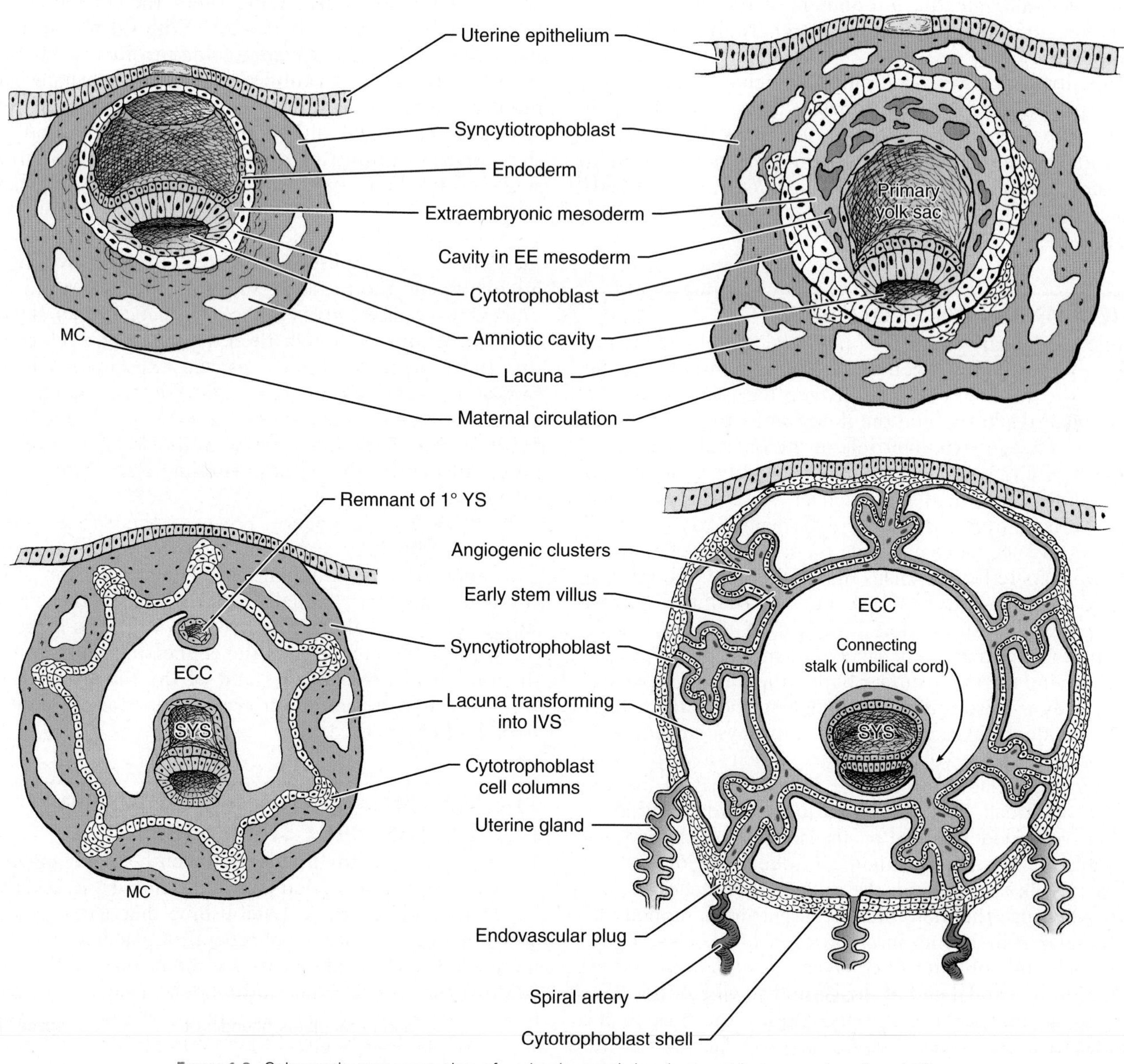

FIGURE 1-2. Schematic representation of early placental development between days 9 and 16.

trabeculae. On reaching their tips, approximately 2 days later, the cells spread laterally, establishing contact with those from other trabeculae to form a new layer interposed between the mantle and the endometrium, the cytotrophoblastic shell (see Figure 1-2). Finally, at the start of the third week of development mesodermal cells derived from the extraembryonic mesoderm invade the trabeculae, bringing with them the hemangioblasts from which the fetal vasculature differentiates. The mesoderm cells do not penetrate right to the tips of the trabeculae, and these remain as an aggregation of cytotrophoblast cells, the cytotrophoblast cell columns, which may or may not have a covering of syncytiotrophoblast (see Figure 1-2). Proliferation of the cells at the proximal ends of the columns, and their subsequent differentiation, contributes to expansion of the cytotrophoblastic shell. Toward the end of the third week the rudiments of the placenta are therefore in place. **The original wall of the blastocyst becomes the chorionic plate, the cytotrophoblastic shell is the precursor of the basal plate, and the lacunae form the intervillous space.** The trabeculae are the forerunners of the villous trees, and repeated lateral branching gradually increases their complexity.

Initially, villi form over the entire chorionic sac, but toward the end of the first trimester they regress from all except the deep pole, where they remain as the definitive discoid placenta. Abnormalities in this process may account for the persistence of villi at abnormal sites on the chorionic sac, and hence the presence of accessory or succenturiate lobes.

THE AMNION AND YOLK SAC

While these early stages of placental development are taking place the inner cell mass also differentiates, giving rise to the amnion, the yolk sac, and the germ disk. The amnion and yolk sac, and the fluid compartment in which they lie, play an important role in the physiology of early pregnancy and so their development will be described at this point. The initial formation of these sacs has been controversial over the years, due mainly to the small number of specimens available for study. However, there now appears to be consensus that at the time of implantation, the amnion extends from the margins of the epiblast layer over the future dorsal surface of the germ disk, whereas the primary yolk sac extends from the hypoblast layer around the inner surface of the trophoblast, separated from it by a loose reticulum thought to be derived from the endoderm.[3] Over the next few days considerable remodeling of the yolk sac occurs, which involves three closely interrelated processes. First, formation of the primitive streak, and the subsequent differentiation of definitive endoderm, lead to displacement of the original hypoblast cells into the more peripheral regions of the primary yolk sac. Second, the sac greatly reduces in size, either because the more peripheral portion is nipped off[3] or because it breaks up into a number of vesicles. Third, the reticulum splits into two layers of mesoderm, except at the future caudal end of the germ disk where it persists as a mass, the connecting stalk, linking the disk to the trophoblast. One layer lines the inner surface of the trophoblast, so contributing to formation of the chorion, and the other covers the outer surfaces of the amnion and yolk sac. In between these layers is a large fluid-filled space, the exocoelomic cavity (ECC). The net result of this remodeling is the formation of a smaller secondary yolk sac (SYS), which is connected to the embryo by the vitelline duct and floats within the exocoelomic cavity (see Figure 1-2).

The exocoelomic cavity is a conspicuous feature ultrasonographically and can be clearly visualized using a transvaginal probe toward the end of the third week after fertilization (fifth week of menstrual age). Between 5 and 9 weeks of pregnancy it represents the largest anatomic space within the chorionic sac. The SYS is the first structure that can be detected ultrasonographically within that space, and its diameter increases slightly between 6 and 10 weeks of gestation, reaching a maximum of 6 to 7 mm, and then decreases slightly. Histologically, the SYS consists of an inner layer of endodermal cells linked by tight junctions at their apical surface and bearing a few short microvilli.[4] Their cytoplasm contains numerous mitochondria, whorls of rough endoplasmic reticulum, Golgi bodies, and secretory droplets, giving them the appearance of being highly active synthetic cells. With further development the epithelium becomes folded to form a series of cystlike structures or tubules, only some of which communicate with the central cavity. The function of these spaces is not known, although it has been proposed that they serve as a primitive circulatory network in the earliest stages of development as they may contain non-nucleated erythrocytes.[5] On its outer surface the yolk sac is lined by a layer of mesothelium derived from the extraembryonic mesoderm. This epithelium bears a dense covering of microvilli, and the presence of numerous coated pits and pinocytotic vesicles gives it the appearance of an absorptive epithelium. Although there is no direct evidence of this function in the human as yet, experiments in the rhesus monkey have revealed that the mesothelial layer readily engulfs horseradish peroxidase. Immediately beneath this epithelium lies a well-developed capillary plexus that drains through the vitelline veins to the developing liver.

By week 9 of pregnancy, however, the SYS begins to exhibit morphologic evidence of a decline in function. This appears to be independent of the expansion of the amnion, which is gradually drawn around the ventral surface of the developing embryo. As it does so it presses the yolk sac remnant against the connecting stalk, forming the umbilical cord. **By the end of the third month the amnion abuts the inner surface of the chorion, and the ECC is obliterated.**

THE MATERNAL-FETAL RELATIONSHIP DURING THE FIRST TRIMESTER

For the placenta to function efficiently as an organ of exchange it requires adequate and dependable access to the maternal circulation. Establishing that access is arguably one of the most critical aspects of placental development, and over recent years has been one of the most controversial. As the syncytiotrophoblastic mantle enlarges it soon comes into close proximity with superficial veins within the endometrium. These undergo dilation, forming sinusoids, which are subsequently tapped into by the syncytium.[6] As a result, maternal erythrocytes come to lie within the lacunae. Although Hertig and colleagues[6] commented that surprisingly few erythrocytes were visible within the lacunae, their presence has been taken by modern embryologists as indicating the onset of the maternal circulation to the placenta. If this is a circulation, however, it is entirely one of venous ebb and flow, possibly influenced by uterine contractions and other forces. Numerous traditional histologic studies have demonstrated that arterial connections are not established with the lacunae until much later in pregnancy,[7,8] although the exact timing was not known for many years. The advent of high-resolution ultrasound and Doppler imaging appeared to answer this question, for most observers agree that moving echoes indicative of significant fluid flow cannot be detected within the IVS until 10 to 12 weeks in normal pregnancies.

It is now well accepted on the basis of evidence from a variety of techniques that a major change in the maternal circulation to the placenta takes place at the end of the first trimester. First, direct vision into the IVS during the first trimester with a hysteroscope reveals the cavity to be filled with a clear fluid rather than maternal blood.[9] Second, perfusion of pregnant hysterectomy specimens with radiopaque and other media demonstrates that there is little flow into the IVS during the first trimester, except perhaps at the margins of the placental disk.[1,7] Third, the oxygen concentration within the IVS is low (<20 mm Hg) before 10 weeks of pregnancy, and rises threefold between weeks 10 and 12.[10] This rise is matched by increases in the activities of, and concentrations of mRNA encoding, the principal antioxidant enzymes in the placental tissues, confirming a change in oxygenation at the cellular level.[10]

The mechanism underlying this change in placental perfusion relates to the phenomenon of extravillous trophoblast invasion.

EXTRAVILLOUS TROPHOBLAST INVASION AND PHYSIOLOGIC CONVERSION OF THE SPIRAL ARTERIES

During the early weeks of pregnancy, a subpopulation of trophoblast cells migrate from the deep surface of the cytotrophoblastic shell into the endometrium. Because these cells do not take part in the development of the definitive placenta, they are referred to as extravillous trophoblast. **Their activities are, however, fundamental to the successful functioning of the placenta, for their presence in the endometrium is associated with the physiologic conversion of the maternal spiral arteries.** The cell biologic basis of this phenomenon is still not understood, but the net effect is the loss of the smooth muscle cells and elastic fibers from the media of the endometrial segments of the arteries and their replacement by fibrinoid.[11-13] There is some evidence to suggest that this is a two-stage process. Very early in pregnancy the arteries display endothelial basophilia and vacuolation, disorganization of the smooth muscle cells, and dilation. Because these changes are observed equally in both the decidua basalis and parietalis, and also within the uterus in cases of ectopic pregnancies, it seems to be independent of local trophoblast invasion. Instead, it has been proposed that it results from activation of decidual renin-angiotensin signaling. Slightly later, during the first few weeks of pregnancy, the invading extravillous trophoblasts become closely associated with the arteries, and infiltrate their walls. Further dilation ensues, and as a result the arteries are converted from small-caliber vasoreactive vessels into funnel-shaped flaccid conduits.

The extravillous trophoblast population can itself be separated into two subgroups: the endovascular trophoblast, which migrate in a retrograde fashion down the lumens of the spiral arteries replacing the endothelium, and the interstitial trophoblast, which migrate through the endometrial stroma. In early pregnancy, the volume of the migrating endovascular cells is sufficient to occlude, or plug, the terminal portions of the spiral arteries as they approach the basal plate[7,8] (Figure 1-3). **It is the dissipation of these plugs toward the end of the first trimester that establishes the maternal circulation to the placenta.** Trophoblast invasion is not equal across the implantation site, being greatest in the central region, where it has presumably been established the longest.[14] It is to be expected, therefore, that the plugging of the spiral arteries will be most extensive in this region, and this may account for the fact that maternal arterial blood flow is most often first detectable ultrasonographically in the peripheral regions of the placental disk.[15] Associated with this blood flow is a high local level of oxidative stress, which can be considered physiologic as it occurs in all normal pregnancies. It has recently been proposed that this stress induces regression of the villi over the superficial pole of the chorionic sac, so forming the chorion laeve (Figure 1-4).[15]

Under normal conditions, the interstitial trophoblast cells invade as far as the inner third of the myometrium, where they appear to fuse and form multinucleated giant cells.[1] It is essential that the process is correctly regulated, for excessive invasion can result in complete erosion of the endometrium and the condition of placenta accreta, which is associated with a high risk of postpartum hemorrhage. As they migrate, the trophoblast cells must interact with cells of the maternal immune system present within the decidua, in particular macrophages and uterine Natural Killer cells.[16] These interactions may play a physiologic role in regulating the depth of invasion, or in the conversion of the spiral arteries. Extravillous trophoblast cells express the polymorphic antigen HLA-C that binds to KIR on the Natural Killer cells. Recent evidence indicates that certain combinations of HLA-C antigen and receptor subtypes are associated with a high risk of pregnancy complications,[17] emphasizing the importance of immunologic interactions to reproductive success.

Physiologic conversion of the spiral arteries is often attributed with ensuring an adequate maternal blood flow to the placenta, but such comments generally oversimplify the phenomenon. By itself, the process cannot increase the volume of blood flow to the placenta as it only affects the most distal portion of the spiral arteries. **The most proximal part of the arteries, where they arise from the uterine arcuate arteries, always remains unconverted and so will act as the rate-limiting segment.** These segments gradually dilate in conjunction with the rest of the uterine vasculature during early pregnancy, most probably under the effects of estrogen and as a result the resistance of the uterine circulation

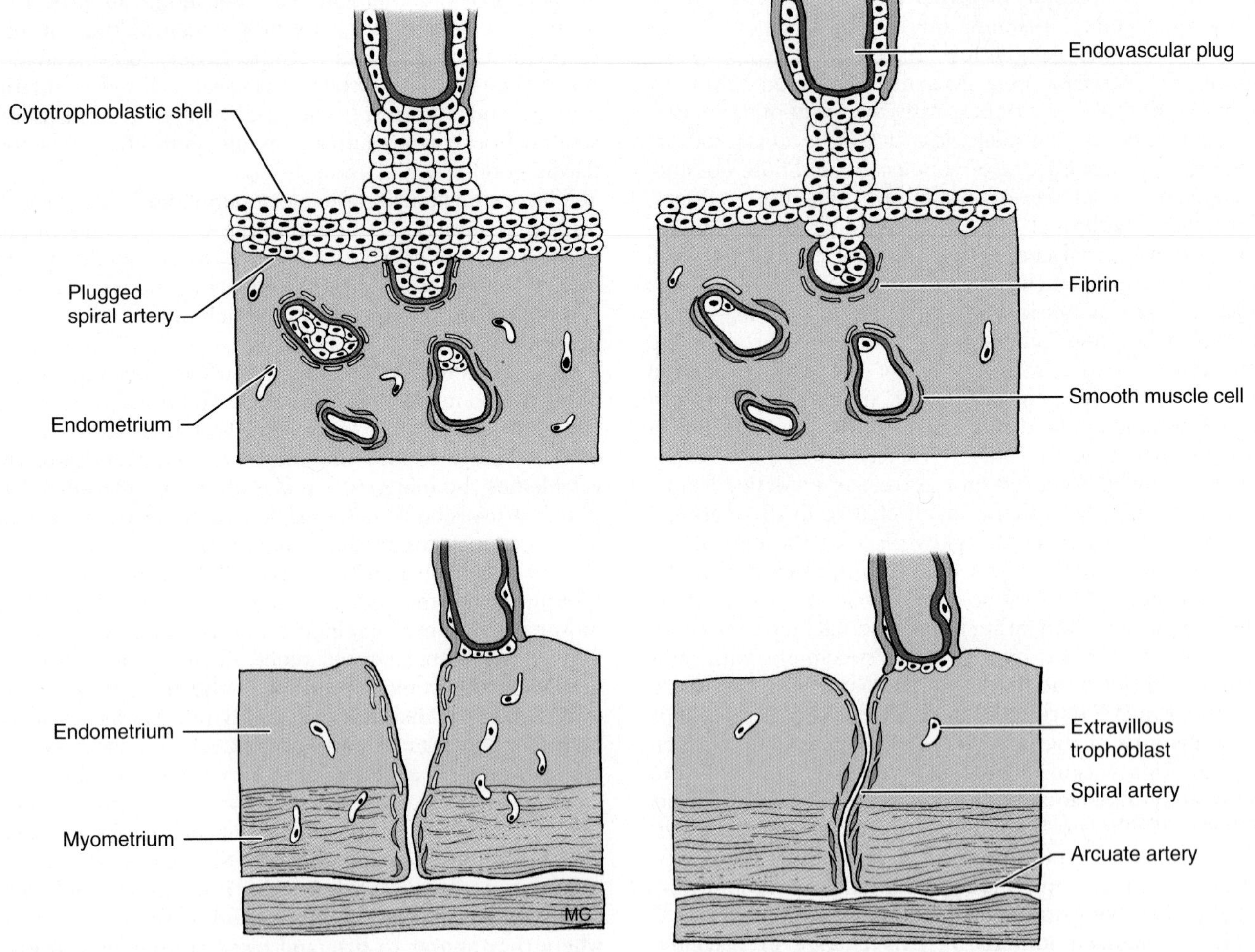

FIGURE 1-3. During early pregnancy the tips of the maternal spiral arteries are occluded by invading endovascular trophoblast cells, impeding flow into the IVS. The combination of endovascular and interstitial trophoblast invasion is associated with physiologic conversion of the spiral arteries. Both processes are deficient in preeclampsia, and the retention of vascular smooth muscle may increase the risk of spontaneous vasoconstriction, and hence an ischemia-reperfusion type injury to the placenta.

falls and uterine blood flow increases from approximately 45 mL/minute during the menstrual cycle to around 750 mL/minute at term. By contrast, the terminal dilation of the arteries will substantially reduce both the rate and pressure with which that maternal blood flows into the IVS.

Mathematic modeling has demonstrated that physiologic conversion is associated with a reduction in velocity from 2 to 3 m/s^{-1} in the nondilated section of a spiral artery to approximately 10 cm/s^{-1} at its mouth.[18] This reduction in the velocity will ensure that the delicate villous trees are not damaged by the momentum of the inflowing blood. Slowing the rate of maternal blood flow across the villous trees will also facilitate diffusional exchange, whereas lowering the pressure in the IVS is important to prevent collapse of the fetal capillary network within the villi.[19] Measurements taken in the rhesus indicate that the pressure at the mouth of a spiral artery is only 15 mm Hg, and within the IVS is on average 10 mm Hg.[20] The pressure within the fetal villous capillaries is estimated to be approximately 20 mm Hg, providing a pressure differential favoring their distention of 10 mm Hg.

Many complications of pregnancy are associated with defects in extravillous trophoblast invasion and failure to establish the maternal circulation correctly. In the most severe cases the cytotrophoblastic shell is thin and fragmented, and this situation is observed in approximately two thirds of spontaneous miscarriages.[21] Reduced invasion may reflect defects inherent in the conceptus, such as chromosomal aberrations, or thrombophilia, endometrial dysfunction, or other problems in the mother. The net result is that onset of the maternal circulation is both precocious and widespread throughout the developing placenta, consequent on absent or incomplete plugging of the maternal arteries.[15] Hemodynamic forces, coupled with excessive oxidative stress within the placental tissues,[22] are likely to be major factors contributing to loss of these pregnancies.

In milder cases the pregnancy may continue, but is complicated by preeclampsia, intrauterine growth restriction, or a combination of the two. The physiologic changes are either restricted in extent to only the superficial endometrial parts of the spiral arteries, or absent all together.[23] In

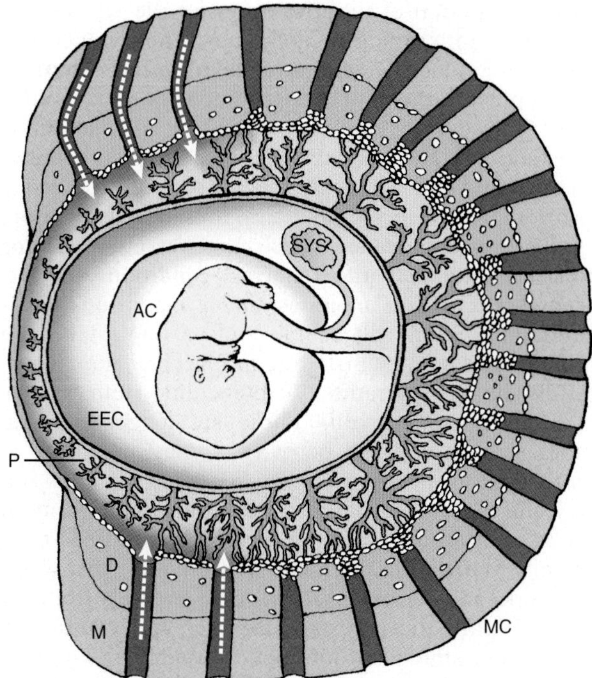

FIGURE 1-4. Onset of the maternal circulation starts in the periphery of the placenta *(arrows)*, where trophoblast invasion, and hence plugging of the spiral arteries, is least developed. The high local levels of oxidative stress induced are thought to induce villous regression and formation of the chorion leave. (Redrawn from Jauniaux E, Cindrova-Davies T, Johns J, et al: Distribution and transfer pathways of antioxidant molecules inside the first trimester human gestational sac. J Clin Endocrinol Metab 89:1452, 2004.)

the most severe cases of preeclampsia associated with major fetal growth restriction only 10% of the arteries may be fully converted, compared to 96% in normal pregnancies.[14] There is still debate as to whether this is due to an inability of the interstitial trophoblast to invade the endometrium successfully, or whether having invaded sufficiently deeply the trophoblast cells fail to penetrate the walls of the arteries. These two possibilities are not mutually exclusive and may reflect different etiologies. Whatever the causation, there are several potential consequences to incomplete conversion of the arteries. First, due to absence of the distal dilation maternal blood will enter the IVS with greater velocity than normal, forming jetlike spurts that can be detected ultrasonographically. The villous trees are often disrupted opposite these spurts, leading to the formation of intervillous blood-lakes, and the altered hemodynamics within the IVS result in thrombosis and excessive fibrin deposition.[24] Second, incomplete conversion will allow the spiral arteries to maintain greater vasoreactivity than normal. There is evidence from the rhesus monkey and the human that spiral arteries are not continuously patent, but that they undergo periodic constriction independent of uterine contractions.[15,25] It has recently been proposed that exaggeration of this phenomenon due to the retention of smooth muscle in the arterial walls may lead to a hypoxia-reoxygenation type of injury in the placenta, culminating in the development of oxidative stress. Placental oxidative stress is a key factor in the pathogenesis of preeclampsia, and clinical evidence suggests that hypoxia-reoxygenation is a more physiologic stimulus for its generation than simply reduced uterine perfusion.[26] The third consequence of incomplete conversion is that the distal segments of the arteries are frequently the site of acute atherotic changes.[23] These are likely to be secondary changes, possibly induced by the involvement of these segments in the hypoxia-reoxygenation process, but if the lesions become occlusive they will further impair blood flow within the IVS, contributing to the growth restriction.

THE ROLE OF THE ENDOMETRIUM DURING THE FIRST TRIMESTER

Signals from the uterine epithelium and secretions from the endometrial glands play a major role in regulating receptivity at the time of implantation, but the potential contribution of the glands to fetal development once implantation is complete has largely been ignored. This has been due to the general assumption that once the conceptus is embedded within the uterine wall it no longer has access to the secretions in the uterine lumen. **However, a review of archival placenta-in-situ hysterectomy specimens has revealed that the glands discharge their secretions into the IVS through openings in the basal plate throughout the first trimester[27] (see Figure 1-2).** The secretions are a heterogenous mix of maternal proteins, carbohydrates (including glycogen), and lipid droplets, and are phagocytosed by the syncytiotrophoblast. Recently, it has been demonstrated that the pattern of sialylation of the secretions changes between the late secretory phase of the nonpregnant cycle and early pregnancy.[28] There is a loss of terminal sialylic acid caps, which will render the secretions more easily degradable by the trophoblast following their phagocytic uptake. The fact that glycodelin, formerly referred to as PP14 or α_2-PEG, is derived from the glands and yet accumulates within the amniotic fluid, with concentrations peaking at around 10 weeks, indicates that the placenta must be exposed to glandular secretions extensively throughout the first trimester.

Ultrasonographic measurements suggest that an endometrial thickness of 8 mm or more is necessary for successful implantation, although not all studies have found such an association.[29] Nonetheless these measurements are in line with observations based on placenta-in-situ specimens, in which an endometrial thickness of over 5 mm was reported beneath the conceptus at 6 weeks of pregnancy.[30] Gradually, over the remainder of the first trimester the endometrium regresses, so that by 14 weeks the thickness is reduced to 1 mm. Histologically, there is also a transformation in the glandular epithelial cells over this period. At 6 weeks they closely resemble those of the secretory phase of the menstrual cycle, being tall and columnar in shape, and their cytoplasm containing abundant organelles and large accumulations of glycogen.[27,30] By the end of the first trimester the cells are more cuboidal and secretory organelles are much less prominent, although the lumens of the glands are still filled with secretions.

The overall picture is that the glands are most prolific and active during the early weeks of pregnancy, with their contribution gradually waning during the first trimester.

This would be consistent with a progressive switch from histiotrophic to hemotrophic nutrition as the maternal arterial circulation to the placenta is established. The glands should not be considered solely as a source of nutrients, however, for their secretions are also rich in growth factors such as leukemia inhibitory factor, vascular endothelial growth factor, epidermal growth factor, and transforming growth factor beta.[30] Receptors for these factors are present on the villous tissues, and so the glands may play an important role in modulating placental proliferation and differentiation during early pregnancy, as in other species. The change in sialylation in early pregnancy will ensure that any of the secretions that gain access to the maternal circulation via the uterine veins will be rapidly cleared in her liver. Hence, a proliferative microenvironment can be created within the intervillous space of the early placenta without placing the mother's tissues at risk of excessive stimulation. Attempts to correlate the functional activity of the glands with pregnancy outcome have met with mixed success. Thus, reduced concentrations of mucin 1, glycodelin, and leukemia inhibitory factor have been reported in uterine flushings from women suffering repeated miscarriages.[31] However, one study has shown no significant association between the expression of these markers within the endometrium and outcome.[32] This difference may reflect impairment in the secretory rather than the synthetic machinery of the gland cells, although further work is required to confirm this point.

From the evidence available it would therefore appear that the functional importance of the endometrial glands to a successful pregnancy extends well beyond the time of implantation.

THE TOPOLOGY OF THE VILLOUS TREES

One of the principal functions of the placenta is diffusional exchange, and the physical requirements for this impose the greatest influence on the structure of the organ. The rate of diffusion of an inert molecule is governed by Fick's law, and so is proportional to the surface area for exchange divided by the thickness of the tissue barrier. **A large surface area will therefore facilitate exchange, and this is achieved by repeated branching of the villous trees.**

The villous trees arise from the trabeculae interposed between the lacunae (see Figure 1-2) through a gradual process of remodeling and lateral branching. Initially, the different branches have an almost uniform composition, and the villi can be separated only by their relative size and position in the hierarchic branching pattern. At this stage the mesodermal core is loosely packed, and at the proximal end of the trees it blends with the extraembryonic mesoderm lining the exocoelomic cavity. The stromal cells possess sail-like processes that often link together to form fluid-filled channels that are orientated parallel to the long axis of the villi. Macrophages are often seen within these channels, and so it is possible they function as a primitive circulatory system prior to vasculogenesis. In this way proteins derived from the uterine glands could freely diffuse into the coelomic fluid, and it is notable that the macrophages within the channels are strongly immunoreactive for maternal glycodelin.[27]

Toward the end of the first trimester the villi begin to differentiate into their principal types. The connections to the chorionic plate become remodeled to form stem villi, which represent the supporting framework of each villous tree.[1,33] These progressively develop a compact fibrous stroma and contain branches of the chorionic arteries and accompanying veins. The arteries are centrally located and are surrounded by a cuff of smooth muscle cells. **Although these have the appearance of resistance vessels, physiologic studies indicate that under normal conditions the fetal-placental circulation operates under conditions of full vasodilation.** Stem villi contain only a few small-caliber capillaries and so play little role in placental exchange.

After several generations of branching, stem villi give rise to intermediate villi. These are longer and more slender in form and can be of two types: immature and mature. The former are seen predominantly in early pregnancy, and represent a persistence of the nondifferentiated form, as indicated by the presence of fluid-filled stromal channels. Mature intermediate villi provide a distributing framework, and terminal villi arise at intervals from their surface. Within the core are arterioles and venules, but there is also a significant number of capillaries, suggesting a capacity for exchange.

The main functional units of the villous tree are, however, the terminal villi. There is no strict definition as to where a terminal villus starts, but they are most often short stubby branches, up to 100 μm in length and approximately 80 μm in diameter, arising from the intermediate villi.[33] They are highly vascularized, but by capillaries alone, and are highly adapted for diffusional exchange, as will be seen later.

This differentiation of the villi coincides temporally with the development of the lobular architecture, and the two processes are most likely interlinked. Lobules can be first identified during the early second trimester, following onset of the maternal circulation when it is thought that hemodynamic forces may shape the villous tree. There is convincing radiographic and morphologic evidence that maternal blood is delivered into the center of the lobule, and that it then disperses peripherally, as in the rhesus monkey placenta[34] (see Figure 1-1). Consequently, it is to be expected that an oxygen gradient will exist across the lobule, and differences in the activities and expression of antioxidant enzymes within the villous tissues suggest strongly that this is the case.[35] Other metabolic gradients, for example glucose concentration, may also exist, and together these may exert powerful influences on villous differentiation. Villi in the center of the lobule, where the oxygen concentration will be highest, display morphologic and enzymatic evidence of relative immaturity, and so this is considered to be the germinative zone. By contrast, villi in the periphery of the lobule are better adapted for diffusional exchange.

Elaboration of the villous tree is a progressive event that continues at a steady pace throughout pregnancy, and **by term the villi present a surface area of 10 to 14 m^2.** This may be significantly reduced in cases of intrauterine growth restriction, although this principally reflects an overall reduction in placental volume rather than maldevelopment of the villous tree.[36] In cases of preeclampsia alone the villous surface area is normal and is only compromised if there is associated growth restriction.[36] Attempts have recently been made to monitor placental growth longitudinally during pregnancy using ultrasound.[37] Although the data show considerable individual variability, they indicate that in cases of growth restriction placental volume is significantly reduced at 12 to 14 weeks, and that thereafter placental development continues at a lower trajectory than normal. These findings suggest that the pathology restricting placental growth has its origins firmly in the first trimester.

PLACENTAL HISTOLOGY

The epithelial covering of the villous trees is formed by the syncytiotrophoblast. As its name indicates this is a true multinucleated syncytium that extends without lateral intercellular clefts over the entire villous surface. **In essence, therefore, the syncytiotrophoblast acts as the endothelium of the IVS, and everything passing across the placenta must pass through this layer, either actively or passively.** This tissue also performs all hormone synthesis in the placenta, and so a number of potentially conflicting demands are placed on it.

The syncytiotrophoblast is highly polarized, and one of its most conspicuous features is the presence of a dense covering of microvilli on the apical surface.[1] In the first trimester the microvilli are relatively long (approximately 0.75 to 1.25 μm in length and 0.12 to 0.17 μm in diameter), but as pregnancy advances they become shorter and more slender, being approximately 0.5 to 0.7 μm in length and 0.08 to 0.14 μm in diameter at term. The microvillous covering is even over the villous surface, and measurements of the amplification factor provided vary from 5.2 to 7.7. Many receptors and transport proteins have been localized to the microvillous surface by molecular biologic and immunohistochemical techniques as will be discussed later. The receptors are thought to reside in lipid rafts, and once bound to their ligand they migrate to the base of the microvilli where clathrin-coated pits are present.[38] Receptor-ligand complexes are concentrated in the pits, which are then internalized. Disassociation of ligands such as cholesterol may occur in the syncytioplasm, whereas other ligands, such as immunoglobulin G, are exocytosed at the basal surface.

Support for the microvillous architecture is provided by a substantial network of actin filaments and microtubules lying just beneath the apical surface. Also present within the syncytioplasm are numerous pinocytotic vesicles, phagosomes, lysosomes, mitochondria, secretory droplets, strands of endoplasmic reticulum, Golgi bodies, and lipid droplets.[38] The overall impression is of a highly active epithelium engaged in absorptive, secretory, and synthetic functions. It is not surprising therefore that the syncytiotrophoblast should have such a high rate of consumption of oxygen.[39,40]

The syncytiotrophoblast is a terminally differentiated tissue, and consequently mitotic figures are never observed within its nuclei. It has been suggested that this condition, which is frequently observed in the fetal cells at the maternal-fetal interface in other species, reduces the risk of malignant transformation in the trophoblast and so protects the mother. Whatever the reason, **the syncytiotrophoblast is generated by the recruitment of progenitor cytotrophoblast cells.** Cytotrophoblast cells are uninucleate, and lie on a well-developed basement membrane immediately beneath the syncytium. A proportion represents stem cells that undergo proliferation, with daughter cells undergoing progressive differentiation.[41] Consequently, a range of morphologic appearances are seen, from cuboidal resting cells with a general paucity of organelles to fully differentiated cells that closely resemble the overlying syncytium.[38,42] Ultimately, membrane fusion takes place between the two, and the nucleus and cytoplasm are incorporated into the syncytiotrophoblast. Early in pregnancy the cytotrophoblast cells form a complete layer beneath the syncytium, but as pregnancy advances the cells become separated and are seen less frequently in histologic sections. In the past this observation was interpreted as indicative of a reduction in the number of cytotrophoblast cells and so a reduction in the proliferative potential of the trophoblast layers. More recent stereologic estimates have revealed a different picture, however, for the total number of these cells increases until term.[43] The apparent decline results from the fact that villous surface area increases at a greater rate, and so cytotrophoblast cell profiles are seen less often in any individual histologic section.

The stimuli regulating cytotrophoblast cell proliferation are not fully understood. In early pregnancy (before 6 weeks) epidermal growth factor (EGF) may play an important role, for expression of both the factor and its receptor are localized principally to these cells. EGF is also strongly expressed in the epithelium of the uterine glands,[30] and in the horse a tight spatial and temporal correlation exists between glandular expression and proliferation in the overlying trophoblast. Later during the first trimester, insulin-like growth factor II can be immunolocalized to the cytotrophoblast cells, as can the receptor for hepatocyte growth factor. Hepatocyte growth factor is a powerful mitogen that is expressed by the mesenchymal cells, providing the possibility of paracrine control. Environmental stimuli may also be important, for hypoxia has long been known to stimulate cytotrophoblast proliferation in vitro. A greater number of cell profiles is also observed in placentas from high altitudes where they are exposed to hypobaric hypoxia and conditions associated with poor placental perfusion.[44] Whether this represents increased proliferation or decreased fusion with the syncytiotrophoblast is, however, uncertain.

The factors regulating and mediating fusion are equally uncertain. Growth factors such as EGF, granulocyte macrophage colony-stimulating factor, and vascular endothelial growth factor are able to stimulate fusion in vitro, as are the hormones estradiol and human chorionic gonadotropin (hCG). By contrast, transforming growth factor ß, leukemia inhibitory factor, and endothelin inhibit the process, suggesting that the outcome in vivo depends on a balance between these opposing influences. One of the actions of hCG at the molecular level is to promote the formation of gap junctions between cells, and there is strong experimental evidence that communication via gap junctions is an essential prerequisite in the fusion process.[45] Whether membrane fusion is initiated at the sites of gap junctions is not known at present, but there has been much interest recently in other potential mechanisms of fusion.

One such is the externalization of phosphatidylserine on the outer leaflet of the cell membrane, although whether this represents part of an apoptotic cascade that is only completed in the syncytiotrophoblast[46] or is inherent to cytotrophoblastic differentiation[47] remains controversial. Another is the expression of the human endogenous retroviral envelope protein HERV-W, commonly referred to as syncytin. Expression of syncytin appears to be necessary for syncytial transformation of trophoblast cells in vitro, and ectopic expression in other cell types renders them fusigenic.[48] Syncytin interacts with the amino acid transporter protein ASCT2, and the expression of both is influenced by hypoxia in trophoblast cell lines in vitro. This could provide an explanation for the increased number of cytotrophoblast cells observed in placentas from hypoxic pregnancies.

Although it is clear that the cascade of events controlling cytotrophoblastic proliferation and fusion has yet to be fully elucidated, it appears to be tightly regulated in vivo. Thus, the ratio of cytotrophoblastic to syncytial nuclei remains at approximately 1:9 throughout pregnancy,[43] although it may be perturbed in pathologic cases.

Early reports suggested that there is little or no transcription within the syncytiotrophoblast and that the tissue relies on the continual fusion of cytotrophoblast cells to bring in the required mRNAs. This has been linked to the hypothesis that the syncytial nuclei undergo a progression of apoptotic changes, culminating in their extrusion into the maternal circulation.[49] More recent evidence from immunohistochemistry and the incorporation of fluorouridine suggests that a proportion of the nuclei are transcriptionally active.[50] Furthermore, analysis of the pattern of chromatin condensation displayed by the nuclei does not support the concept of continual syncytial turnover.[51]

THE INTEGRITY OF THE VILLOUS MEMBRANE

One situation that may alter the balance of the two populations of nuclei is damage to the trophoblast layers and the requirement for repair. Isolated areas of syncytial damage, often referred to as sites of focal syncytial necrosis, are a feature of all placentas, although they are more common in those from pathologic pregnancies. Their origin remains obscure, but they could potentially arise from altered hemodynamics within the IVS or physical interactions between villi. One striking example of the latter is the rupture of syncytial bridges that form between adjacent villi, leading to circular defects on the surface 20 to 40 μm in diameter. Disruption of the microvillous surface leads to the activation of platelets and the deposition of a fibrin plaque on the trophoblastic basement membrane. Apoptosis of syncytial nuclei has been reported in the immediate vicinity of such plaques, but whether this reflects cause or effect has yet to be determined. With time, cytotrophoblast cells migrate over the plaque, differentiate, and fuse to form a new syncytiotrophoblastic layer. As a result, the plaque is internalized, and the integrity of the villous surface is restored. In the interim, however, these sites are nonselectively permeable to creatinine.[52]

More widespread apoptosis has been reported in the syncytiotrophoblast layer in pregnancies complicated by preeclampsia, where it may reflect increased turnover of the trophoblast.[53] Placental oxidative stress is considered a key factor in the pathogenesis of preeclampsia,[26] and hypoxia-reoxygenation is a powerful inducer of apoptosis in the syncytiotrophoblast in vitro. The deportation of apoptotic fragments arising from the villous surface has been put forward as one cause of the maternal endothelial activation that characterizes this syndrome.[54]

An even greater degree of trophoblast oxidative stress and damage is seen in cases of missed miscarriage, where complete degeneration and sloughing of the syncytiotrophoblast layer occurs.[15,22] Although there is increased apoptosis and necrosis among the cytotrophoblast cells, the remaining cells differentiate and fuse to form a new and functional syncytial layer. A similar effect is observed when villi from either first trimester or term placentas are maintained under ambient conditions in vitro.

Thus, it is likely that there is considerable turnover of the syncytiotrophoblast over the course of a pregnancy, although in the absence of longitudinal studies it is impossible to determine how extensive this process is. Nonetheless, it is clear that the villous membrane cannot be considered as an intact physical barrier, and that other elements of the villous trees may play an important role in regulating maternal-fetal transfer.

PLACENTAL VASCULATURE

The development of the fetal vasculature begins during the third week after conception (week 5 of pregnancy) with the de novo formation of capillaries within the villous stromal core. Hemangioblastic cell cords differentiate under the influence of growth factors such as basic fibroblast growth factor and vascular endothelial growth factor.[55,56] By the beginning of the fourth week the cords have developed lumens and the endothelial cells become flattened. Surrounding mesenchymal cells become closely apposed to the tubes and differentiate to form pericytes. During the next few days connections form between neighboring tubes to form a plexus, and this ultimately unites with the allantoic vessels developing in the connecting stalk to establish the fetal circulation to the placenta.

Exactly when an effective circulation is established through these vessels is difficult to determine, however. First, the connection between the corporeal and extracorporeal fetal circulations is particularly narrow, suggesting there can be little flow initially. Second, the narrow caliber of the villous capillaries, coupled with the fact that the fetal erythrocytes are nucleated during the first trimester and hence not readily deformable, will ensure that the circulation presents a high resistance to flow. This is reflected in the Doppler waveform obtained during the first trimester, and the resistance gradually falls as the vessels enlarge over the ensuing weeks.

Early in pregnancy the capillary network is labile and undergoes considerable remodeling. Angiogenesis continues until term and results in the formation of capillary sprouts and loops. Both of these processes contribute to the elaboration of terminal villi.[57,58] The caliber of the fetal capillaries is not constant within intermediate and terminal villi, and frequently on the apex of a tight bend the capillaries become greatly dilated, forming sinusoids. These

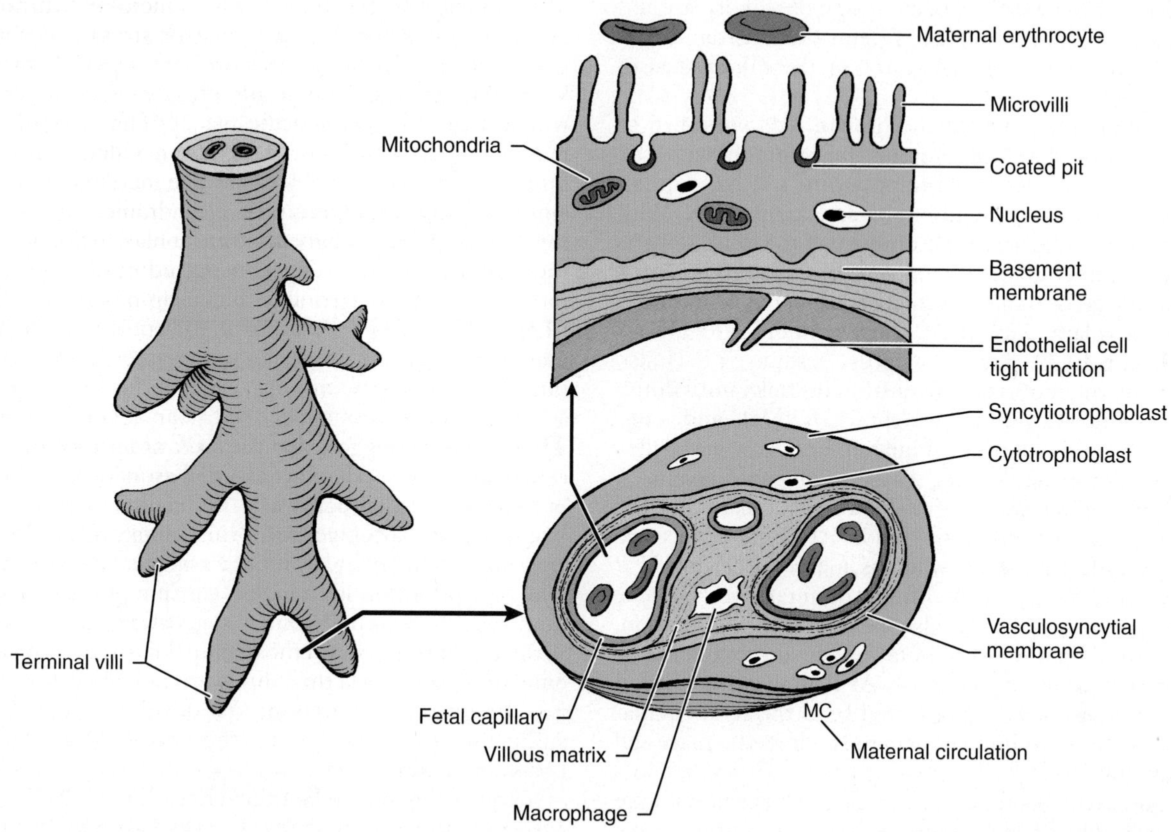

FIGURE 1-5. Diagrammatic representation of an intermediate villus with terminal villi arising from the lateral surface.

regions may help to reduce vascular resistance and so facilitate distribution of fetal blood flow through the villous trees.[57] Equally important is the fact that the dilations bring the outer wall of the capillaries into close juxtaposition with the overlying trophoblast. **The trophoblast is locally thinned, and as a result the diffusion distance between the maternal and fetal circulations is reduced to a minimum (Figure 1-5).** Because of their morphologic configuration these specializations are referred to as vasculosyncytial membranes, and are considered the principal sites of gaseous and other diffusional exchange. The arrangement can be considered analogous to that in the alveoli of the lung where the pulmonary capillaries indent into the alveolar epithelium in order to reduce the thickness of the air-blood diffusion barrier. Thinning of the syncytial layer will not only increase the rate of diffusion into the fetal capillaries, it will also reduce the amount of oxygen extracted by the trophoblast en route. The syncytiotrophoblast is highly active metabolically due to the high rates of protein synthesis and ionic pumping, but by having an uneven distribution of the tissue around the villous surface the oxygen demands of the fetus and the placenta can be separated to a large extent.

It is notable that development of vasculosyncytial membranes is seen to its greatest extent in the peripheral regions of a placental lobule where the oxygen concentration is lowest, and also in placentas from high altitude. In both instances it is associated with enlargement of the capillary sinusoids, and may be viewed as an adaptive response aimed at increasing the diffusing capacity of the placental tissues. Conversely, an increase in the thickness of the villous membrane is often seen in cases of intrauterine growth retardation, and in placentas from cigarette smokers. As mentioned earlier, the hydrostatic pressure differential across the villous membrane is an important determinant of the diameter of the capillary dilatations, and hence of the villous membrane thickness.[19] Raising the pressure in the IVS not only compresses the capillaries, but also increases the resistance within the umbilical circulation. Both effects will impair diffusional exchange, highlighting the importance of full conversion of the spiral arteries.

Vascular changes are observed in many complications of pregnancy,[59] where they may underpin changes in the topology of the villous tree. Thus, increased branching of the vascular network is observed in placentas from high altitude, causing the terminal villi to be shorter and more clustered than normal. At present there are no experimental data indicating that this has any impact on placental exchange, but in theory shortening the arteriovenous pathway may lead to increased efficiency.

PHYSIOLOGY OF THE SECONDARY YOLK SAC AND EXOCOELOMIC CAVITY

Now that development of the placenta and the extraembryonic membranes has been covered we turn to their physiologic roles during pregnancy. Phylogenetically, the oldest membrane is the yolk sac, and the SYS plays a major role in the embryonic development of all mammals. The function of the yolk sac has been most extensively studied in laboratory rodents, and it has been demonstrated that the extraembryonic yolk sac is one of the initial sites of hematopoiesis.[60]

The endodermal layer of the human SYS is known to synthesize several serum proteins in common with the fetal liver, such as alpha-fetoprotein (AFP), alpha$_1$-antitrypsin, albumin, prealbumin, and transferrin. With rare exceptions, the secretion of most of these proteins is confined to the embryonic compartments, and the contribution of the SYS to the maternal protein pool is limited.[61] This can explain why their concentrations are always higher in the ECC than in maternal serum. AFP is also produced by the embryonic liver from 6 weeks until delivery, has a high molecular weight (±70 kDa), and, conversely to hCG, is found in similar amounts on both sides of the amniotic membrane. Analysis of concanavalin A affinity molecular variants of AFP have demonstrated that both coelomic and amniotic fluids AFP molecules are mainly of yolk sac origin, whereas maternal serum AFP molecules are mainly derived from the fetal liver.[62] These results suggest that the SYS also has an excretory function, and secretes AFP toward the embryonic and extraembryonic compartments. By contrast, AFP molecules of fetal liver origin are probably transferred from the fetal circulation to the maternal circulation, mainly across the placental villous membrane.

The potential absorptive role of the yolk sac membrane has been evaluated by examining the distribution of proteins and enzymes between the ECC and SYS fluids, and by comparing the synthesizing capacity of SYS, fetal liver, and placenta for hCG and AFP.[63] The distribution of the trophoblast-specific protein, hCG, in yolk sac and coelomic fluid, together with the absence of hCG mRNA expression in yolk sac tissues, provided the first biologic evidence of its absorptive function. Similarities in the composition of the SYS and coelomic fluids suggest that there is a free transfer for most molecules between the two corresponding compartments. Conversely, an important concentration gradient exists for most proteins between the ECC and amniotic cavity, indicating that transfer of molecules is limited at the level of the amniotic membrane that separates the corresponding fluids.

These findings suggest that the yolk sac membrane is an important zone of transfer between the extraembryonic and embryonic compartments, and that the main flux of molecules occurs from outside the yolk sac (i.e., from the ECC), in the direction to its lumen and subsequently to the embryonic gut and circulation. The identification of specific transfer proteins on the mesothelial covering[64] lends further support to this concept. When after 10 weeks of gestation the cellular components of the wall of the SYS start to degenerate, this route of transfer is no longer functional, and most exchanges between the ECC and the fetal circulation must then take place at the level of the chorionic plate.

The development and physiologic roles of the ECC are intimately linked with that of the SYS, for which it provides a stable environment. The higher concentrations of hCG, estriol, and progesterone in the coelomic fluid than in maternal serum[61] strongly suggest the presence of a direct pathway between the trophoblast and the ECC. Morphologically, this may be via the villous stromal channels and the loose mesenchymal tissue of the chorionic plate. Protein electrophoresis has also shown that the coelomic fluid results from an ultrafiltrate of maternal serum with the addition of specific placental and SYS bioproducts. For the duration of the first trimester, the coelomic fluid remains straw colored and more viscous than the amniotic fluid, which is always clear. This is mainly due to the higher protein concentration in the coelomic than in the amniotic cavity. The concentration of almost every protein is higher in coelomic than in amniotic fluid, ranging from 2 to 50 times depending on the corresponding molecular weight of the protein investigated.[61] The coelomic fluid has a very slow turnover, and so the ECC may act as a reservoir for nutrients needed by the developing embryo. **These findings suggest that the ECC is a physiologic liquid extension of the early placenta, and an important interface in fetal nutritional pathways.** Molecules such as vitamin B_{12}, prolactin, and glycodelin (placental protein 14, PP14) are known to be mainly produced by the uterine decidua.[61] They are often found in higher concentrations in coelomic fluid than in maternal serum, suggesting that preferential pathways exist between the decidual tissue and the embryonic fluid cavities via the villous trophoblast. This pathway may be pivotal in providing the developing embryo with sufficient nutrients before the intervillous circulation becomes established.[27]

Some analogies can be drawn between the ECC and the antrum within a developing Graafian follicle. It has been suggested that the evolution of the latter was necessary to overcome the problem of oxygen delivery to an increasing large mass of avascular cells. As the contained fluid has no oxygen consumption it will permit diffusion more freely than an equivalent thickness of cells. However, as neither follicular nor coelomic fluids contain an oxygen carrier, the total oxygen content must be low. An oxygen gradient will inevitably exist between the source and the target, whether it be an oocyte or an embryo. Measurements in human patients undergoing in vitro fertilization have demonstrated that the oxygen tension in follicular fluid falls as follicle diameter, assessed by ultrasound, increases. Thus, diffusion across the ECC may be an important route of oxygen supply to the embryo before the development of a functional placental circulation, but it will maintain the early fetus in a low-oxygen environment. This may serve to protect the fetal tissues from damage by O_2 free radicals and prevent disruption of signaling pathways during the crucial stages of embryogenesis and organogenesis. The presence in the ECC of molecules with a well-established antioxidant role as such as taurine, transferrin, vitamins A and E, and selenium supports this hypothesis.

PLACENTAL TRANSPORT

For the bulk of pregnancy, the chorioallantoic placenta is the major site of exchange of nutrients (including oxygen) and of waste products of fetal metabolism (including carbon dioxide) between mother and fetus. As described earlier, histiotrophic nutrition most likely occurs in early pregnancy and the yolk sac placenta probably contributes to this. However, once blood flow to the intervillous space begins at around 10 weeks' gestation, exchange across the barrier between maternal and fetal circulations within the villi will be predominant, although there may be some limited transfer between maternal blood in the endometrium and the fluid of the amniotic sac. As discussed later in this chapter, many of the transport mechanisms required to effect exchange are present in the placenta by 10 weeks and these may be up- or down-regulated throughout the rest of pregnancy to meet the requirements of fetal growth and homeostasis.

For a molecule to reach the fetal plasma from the maternal plasma, and vice versa, it must cross the syncytiotrophoblast, the matrix of the villous core, and the endothelium of the fetal capillary. The syncytiotrophoblast is the transporting epithelium and is considered to be the major locus of exchange selectivity and regulation. However, both the matrix and endothelium will contribute to the properties of the placenta as an organ of exchange, both because they contribute to the thickness of the barrier and because they may act as a size filter: the finite width of the space between the endothelial cells is likely to restrict the diffusion of larger molecules.

The fact that the syncytiotrophoblast is a true syncytium, with no obvious intercellular or extracellular water-filled spaces, suggests that it forms a "tight" barrier. However, physiologic data, discussed later, suggest that this is not the case. Nevertheless, exchange most likely occurs predominantly across the two opposing plasma membranes, microvillous (maternal facing) and basal (fetal facing) (see Figure 1-5).

OVERVIEW OF THE EXCHANGE PHYSIOLOGY OF THE PLACENTA AND ITS DEVELOPMENT OVER GESTATION

Maternal-fetal exchange across the placenta may occur, broadly, by one of four mechanisms: bulk flow/solvent drag, diffusion, transporter-mediated mechanisms, and endocytosis/exocytosis.

Bulk Flow/Solvent Drag

Differences in hydrostatic and osmotic pressures between the maternal and fetal circulations within the exchange barrier will drive water transfer by bulk flow, dragging with it dissolved solutes. These dissolved solutes will be filtered as they move through the components of the barrier. Water movement may be via paracellular channels (see later discussion) or across the plasma membranes. The latter may be enhanced by the presence of aquaporins, integral membrane proteins forming water "pores" in the plasma membrane.

Hydrostatic pressure gradients will be created by differences in maternal and fetal blood pressure and vascular resistances on the maternal and fetal sides of the placenta. Although the actual pressures are impossible to measure in vivo at this time, evidence suggests that it is lower in the intervillous space than in the fetal capillaries.[19] As this would drive water from fetus to mother, incompatible with fetal growth, there is clearly a deficit here in our knowledge and understanding. The assumptions involved in assessing the hydrostatic pressures could be simply wrong. On the other hand, fetal-maternal water transfer driven by hydrostatic pressures may be opposed and exceeded by maternal-fetal water transfer driven by osmotic pressure gradients created by the active transport of solute to the fetus across the syncytiotrophoblast.[65] These forces may well be altered as gestation proceeds. Altogether, this is an important area in which further research is required.

Diffusion

Diffusion of any molecule occurs in both directions across any barrier. When there is a concentration gradient and/or, for charged species, an electrical gradient, one of these unidirectional fluxes (rates of transfer) is greater in one direction than it is in the other, so that there is a net flux in one direction. Net flux (Jnet) of solute across the placenta for an uncharged molecule may be described by an adaptation of Fick's Law of Diffusion[66]:

$$\text{Jnet} = (\text{AD} / \text{l})\,(\text{Cm-Cf}) \text{ moles/unit time}$$

where A is the surface area of the barrier available for exchange, D is the diffusion coefficient in water of the molecule (smaller molecules will have larger D), l is the thickness of the exchange barrier across which diffusion is occurring, Cm is the mean concentration of the molecule in maternal plasma, and Cf is the mean concentration of solute in the fetal circulation.

Small, relatively hydrophobic molecules such as O_2 and CO_2 will diffuse rapidly across the plasma membranes of the barrier, so that their flux is dependent much more on the concentration gradients than on A or l. As this concentration gradient is affected predominantly by the blood flows in both circulations, the diffusion of such molecules is said to be flow limited. This explains why reductions in uterine and or umbilical flow may result in fetal asphyxia and, consequently, growth restriction.

By contrast, hydrophilic molecules (glucose, amino acids) will not diffuse across plasma membranes easily; their concentration gradients are maintained and flux will be determined predominantly by barrier surface area and thickness. Flux of such membrane-limited molecules will not be affected by blood flow unless this is dramatically reduced but will be altered if abnormal placental development results in reduced A or increased l; there is evidence that this occurs in idiopathic IUGR.[36]

The term (AD/l) in Fick's Law is equivalent to what is described as the permeability of a molecule. Measurements of the passive permeability of the placenta have been made in vivo[67] and in vitro[68] utilizing hydrophilic molecules, which would be unlikely to be affected by blood flow and which are not substrates for transporter proteins. These measurements show that there is an indirect relationship between permeability and the molecular size of the hydrophilic tracer. Such a relationship is explained, most simply, by the presence of extracellular water-filled channels or pores across the exchange barrier through which the molecules can diffuse. The existence of this "paracellular permeability" pathway has been controversial because of the syncytiotrophoblast being syncytial with no obvious paracellular channels. However, there may be transtrophoblastic channels that are not normally visible by electron microscopy. Furthermore, the areas of syncytial denudation that occur in every placenta may themselves provide a route through which molecules may diffuse.[68]

Rates of transfer of hydrophobic molecules by flow-limited diffusion may change over gestation because, as described in previous sections, both uteroplacental and fetoplacental blood flow changes over gestation. Changes in concentration and, for charged molecules, electrical gradients between maternal and fetal plasma will also affect rates of transfer. Gestational changes do occur in the maternal and fetal plasma concentrations of solutes, affecting driving forces. For example, glucose and amino acid concentrations in maternal plasma increase over gestation, at least partly due to the effects of insulin resistance in pregnancy and of hormones such as human placental lactogen. A maternal-fetal electrical potential difference (PD), if expressed across the placental exchange barrier, will have an effect on the exchange of ions. In the human there is a small but significant PD between maternal and fetal circulations (PD_{mf}), being −2.7 ± 0.4 mV fetus negative in midgestation[69] and zero or close to it at term.[70] A PD between the mother and coelomic cavity was measured in first trimester pregnancies.[71] There was no apparent change in the value of this PD (8.7 ± 1 mV fetus negative) between 9 and 13 weeks of gestation, which was somewhat higher than the PD across the syncytiotrophoblast (3 mV) measured using microelectrodes in term placental villi in vitro. The in vitro PD across the microvillous membrane of human syncytiotrophoblast decreases between early (median −32 mV) and late first trimester (median −24 mV), with a small subsequent fall to term (−21 mV). This suggests that the driving force for cation flux into the syncytiotrophoblast decreases and for anions increases as pregnancy progresses.

Transporter-Protein Mediated Processes

Transporter proteins are integral membrane proteins that catalyze transfer of solutes across plasma membranes at faster rates than they would occur by diffusion. Transporter proteins are a large and diverse group of molecules but are generally characterized by showing substrate specificity (i.e., one transporter or class of transporter will predominantly transfer one substrate or class of substrate, e.g., amino acids), by having saturation kinetics (i.e., raising the concentration of a substrate solute will not infinitely increase the rate at which it is transferred on transporters), and by being competitively inhibitable (i.e., two structurally similar molecules will compete for transfer by a particular transporter protein). Transporter proteins are found most abundantly in the placenta in the microvillous and basal plasma membranes of the syncytiotrophoblast. A detailed description of all these is beyond the scope of this chapter but may be found in Atkinson and colleagues.[66] In overview, there are channel proteins that form pores in the plasma membrane allowing diffusion of ions such as K^+ and Ca^{2+}. There are transporters allowing facilitated diffusion down concentration gradients such as the GLUT1 glucose transporter. Exchange transporters, such as the Na^+/H^+ exchanger (involved in pH homeostasis of the syncytiotrophoblast and fetus), and co-transporters such as the system A amino acid transporter (which co-transports small hydrophilic amino acids including alanine, glycine, and serine with Na^+) require the maintenance of an ion gradient through secondary input of energy, often via the Na^+/K^+ATPase. Finally, there are active transporters that transfer against concentration gradients directly utilizing ATP; these include the Na^+/K^+ATPase and the Ca^{2+}ATPase, which pumps Ca^{2+} across the basal plasma membrane from syncytiotrophoblast cytosol toward the fetal circulation.

Gestational changes in the flux of solutes through transporter proteins could result from changes in the number of transporters in each plasma membrane, their turnover (i.e., rate of binding to and release from the transporter), or their affinity for solute, as well as from changes in the driving forces acting on them such as electrochemical gradients and ATP availability. There is a variety of evidence that such developmental changes do occur. Using the technique of isolating and purifying microvillous plasma membrane and radioisotopic tracers to measure transport rates in vesicles formed from these membranes, it has been shown that the V_{max} of the Na^+-dependent system A amino acid transporter increases by about fourfold, per milligram membrane protein, between first trimester and term. The activity of the system y^+ cationic amino acid (e.g., arginine, lysine) transporter increases over gestation, whereas the activity of the system y^+L transporter decreases.[72] This decrease in system y^+L activity is due to a decrease in the affinity of the transporter for substrate and is accompanied by an increased expression of 4F2hc monomer of the dimer protein.[72] The reason for this decline is not known but could well be associated with a specific fetal need. Glucose transporter, GLUT1, expression in microvillous membrane increases between first trimester and term.[73] Na^+/H^+ exchanger activity is lower in first trimester microvillous membrane vesicles as compared to term,[74] a result borne out by studies on the intrasyncytiotrophoblast pH of isolated placental villi from the two stages in gestation.[75] Interestingly, the expression of the NHE1 isoform of this exchanger in the microvillous membrane does not change across gestation, but the expression of both of its NHE2 and NHE3 isoforms increases between weeks 14 to 18 and term.[74] In contrast there is no difference in Cl^-/HCO_3^- exchanger activity or, by Western blotting, expression of its AE1 isoform, between first trimester and term. Understanding of how these gestational changes are regulated is currently sparse; studies in knockout mice suggest that hormones such as IGF-II from the fetus, signaling demand for the nutrients required for growth, are important,[76] but much further work is needed in this area.

Endocytosis/Exocytosis

Endocytosis is the process by which molecules become entrapped in invaginations of the microvillous plasma membrane of the syncytiotrophoblast, which eventually pinch off and form vesicles within the cytosol. Such vesicles may diffuse through the intracellular compartment and, if they avoid fusion with lysosomes, eventually fuse with the basal plasma membrane and undergo exocytosis, releasing their contents into the fetal milieu. **Evidence suggests that immunoglobulin G (IgG) and other large proteins may cross the placenta by this mechanism.**[66,77] Specificity and the ability to avoid lysosomal degradation during the endocytosis phase may be provided by the presence of receptors for IgG in the microvillous membrane invaginations and vesicles. However, this mechanism of transfer and its gestational regulation, if any, is still not well understood.

TABLE 1-1 CHANGES IN ACTIVITY OF TRANSPORTER PROTEINS IN THE MICROVILLOUS (MVM) AND BASAL (BM) PLASMA MEMBRANE OF PLACENTAS FROM IUGR PREGNANCIES AS COMPARED TO NORMAL PREGNANCIES

TRANSPORTER	MVM	BM	REFERENCE
System A	Decreased	No change	93
System L (leucine)	Decreased	Decreased	94
System y^+/y^+L (arginine/lysine)	No change	Decreased	72, 94
System β	Decreased	No change	95
Na^+-independent taurine	No change	Decreased	95, 96
GLUT1	No change	No change	73
Na^+/K^+ATPase	Decreased	No change	97
Ca^{2+}ATPase	Not present	Increased	98
Na^+/H^+ exchanger	Decreased	Activity not present	99
H^+/lactate	No change	Decreased	100

Placental Nutrient Supply and Intrauterine Growth Restriction

The term *placental insufficiency* as a cause of intrauterine growth restriction (IUGR) has been much quoted but little understood until recently. It is often taken as being synonymous with reduced uteroplacental and/or umbilical blood flow. Doppler measurements of such blood flows have been of assistance in diagnosing and assessing the severity of IUGR but are limited in value.[78] It is now clear that other variables determining the capacity of the placenta to supply nutrients may also contribute to IUGR. **For example, the surface area of the exchange barrier is decreased and its thickness increased in IUGR**[36]; such changes are likely to markedly decrease the passive permeability of the placenta. Furthermore, there is now considerable evidence that the activity and expression of transporter proteins in the syncytiotrophoblast is altered in IUGR.[78] The reported data are summarized in Table 1-1. As can be seen activity of several transporters decrease, at least one increases, and others show no change at all. This variation in response could reflect whether a change in the placenta is causative in IUGR (e.g., the decrease in system A amino acid transporter activity), or is compensatory (e.g., the increase in Ca^{2+} ATPase activity) as well as differential regulation of the transporters. Understanding these placental phenotypes of IUGR may well give clues to novel means of diagnosing and even treating the condition.[78]

PLACENTAL ENDOCRINOLOGY

The human placenta is an important endocrine organ, signaling the presence of the conceptus to the mother in early pregnancy and optimizing the intrauterine environment and maternal physiology for the benefit of fetal growth. **Two major groups of hormones are produced: the steroid hormones, progesterone and the estrogens, and peptide hormones, such as hCG and human placental lactogen (hPL).** All are predominantly synthesized in the syncytiotrophoblast, and although the synthetic pathways have been generally elucidated, the factors regulating secretion are still largely unknown.

Progesterone

During the first few weeks of pregnancy progesterone is mainly derived from the corpus luteum, but gradually as the placental mass increases this organ's contribution becomes dominant, with the production of around 250 mg per day. The corpus luteum regresses at around 9 weeks, and at that stage it is no longer essential for the maintenance of a pregnancy.

Placental synthesis of progesterone begins with the conversion of cholesterol to pregnenolone, as in other steroid-secreting tissues. Placental tissues are poor at synthesizing cholesterol and so utilize maternal cholesterol derived from low-density lipoproteins taken up in coated pits on the surface of the syncytiotrophoblast. Conversion of the cholesterol to pregnenolone occurs on the inner aspect of the inner mitochondrial membrane, catalyzed by cytochrome P450scc (CYP11A1), and in other steroidogenic tissues the delivery of cholesterol to this site is the principal rate-limiting step in progesterone synthesis. There delivery is facilitated by the steroidogenic acute regulatory (StAR) protein, which binds and transports cholesterol, but this protein is not present in the human placenta.[79] Instead, a homologue, MLN64, may carry out a similar function, as freshly isolated cytotrophoblast cells appear to contain concentrations of cholesterol that are near-saturating for progesterone synthesis, indicating that supply of the precursor is not rate-limiting.[80] Side-chain cleavage requires molecular oxygen, but it is unclear whether the conditions that prevail during the first trimester are rate-limiting. The rate of production of pregnenolone from radiolabeled cholesterol by placental homogenates in vitro increases across the first trimester, and both the concentration and activity of P450scc increase in placental mitochondria from the first trimester to term. These changes, coupled with the expansion of the syncytiotrophoblast, most likely account for the increase in progesterone synthesis observed.

Side-chain cleavage also requires a supply of electrons, and this is provided by NADPH through a short electron transport chain in the mitochondrial matrix involving adrenodoxin reductase and its redox partner adrenodoxin. Preliminary studies in Tuckey's laboratory suggest that the transport of electrons to P450scc is rate-limiting for the enzyme's activity at mid pregnancy,[79] and so further research on the factors regulating expression and activity of adrenodoxin reductase during gestation is clearly needed.

The resultant pregnenolone is then converted to progesterone by the enzyme type 1 3β-hydroxysteroid dehydrogenase (3β-HSD), principally in the mitochondria. The activity of 3β-HSD in placental tissues is significantly higher than that of cytochrome P450scc, and so this step is unlikely ever to be rate-limiting for the production of progesterone. Once secreted the principal actions of the hormone are to maintain quiescence of the myometrium, although it may have an immunomodulatory role as well. In addition, our new data on the importance of histiotrophic nutrition during the first few weeks of pregnancy suggest that progesterone may be essential to maintain the secretory activity of the endometrial glands.

Estrogens

The human placenta lacks the enzymes required to synthesize estrogens directly from acetate or cholesterol, and so uses the precursor dehydroepiandrosterone sulphate (DHAS) supplied by the maternal and fetal adrenal glands in approximately equal proportions near term. Following uptake by the syncytiotrophoblast DHAS is hydrolyzed by placental sulphatase to dehydroepiandrosterone (DHA), which is further converted to androstenedione by 3β-HSD. Final conversion to estradiol and estrone is achieved by the action of P450 cytochrome aromatase (P450arom) (CYP19), which has been immunolocalized to the endoplasmic reticulum. The syncytiotrophoblast can also utilize 16-OH DHAS produced by the fetal liver, converting this to 16α-OH androstenedione through the action of 3β-HSD, and then to estriol through the action of P450arom. Since approximately 90% of placental estriol production is reliant on fetal synthesis of the precursor 16-OH DHAS, maternal estriol concentrations have in the past been taken clinically as an index of fetal well-being.

Although the synthesis of estrogens can be detected in placental tissues during the early weeks of gestation, secretion significantly increases toward the end of the first trimester. By 7 weeks of gestation more than 50% of maternal circulating estrogens are of placental origin. Analysis of the transcriptional regulation of the P450arom gene has shown it to be oxygen responsive through a novel pathway involving the basic helix-loop-helix transcription factor Mash-2.[81] Production of Mash-2 is increased under physiologically low oxygen conditions, and leads to repression of P450arom gene expression. Hence the change in oxygenation that occurs at the end of the first trimester[10] may stimulate placental production of estrogens.

Human Chorionic Gonadotropin

hCG is secreted by the trophoblast at the blastocyst stage, and can be detected in the maternal blood and urine approximately 8 to 10 days after fertilization. Its principal function is to maintain the corpus luteum until the placenta is sufficiently developed to take over production of progesterone. It is a heterodimeric glycoprotein (approximately 38,000 Da) consisting of α and β subunits that is principally derived from the syncytiotrophoblast. **The α subunit is common to that of thyroid stimulating hormone, luteinizing hormone (LH) and follicle stimulating hormone, and is encoded by a single gene located at chromosome 6q12-21. It is the β subunit that determines the biologic specificity of hCG, and this evolved by a duplication event at the LHβ gene locus.**[82] Mapping has revealed that in the human there are six copies of the hCGβ gene located together with a single copy of the LHβ gene at chromosome 19p13.3. Polymerase chain reaction–based techniques have revealed that at least five, possibly all six, of the genes are transcribed in vivo during normal pregnancy. Most of the steady-state hCGβ mRNAs are transcribed from hCGβ genes 5, 3, and 8, however, with the levels of expression being β5 > β3 = β8 > β7, β1/2.[83] The β subunits of LH and hCG share 85% amino acid sequence homology, and are functionally interchangeable. One of the principal differences between the two is the presence of a 31-amino acid carboxyl-terminal extension in hCGβ compared to a shorter 7-amino acid stretch in LHβ. This extension is hydrophilic, contains four *O*-glycosylated serine residues, and is thought to act as a secretory routing signal targeting release of hCG from the apical membrane of the syncytiotrophoblast.

Assembly of hCG involves a complex process of folding in which a strand of 20 residues of the β subunit is wrapped around the α subunit, and the two are secured by a disulphide bond. Combination of the subunits occurs in the syncytiotrophoblast before the release of intact hCG, and as there is only limited storage in cytoplasmic granules secretion is largely thought to reflect de novo synthesis. Oxidizing conditions promote combination of the subunits in vitro most probably through their effects on the disulphide bond, and so the wave of physiologic oxidative stress observed in placental tissues at the transition from the first to second trimesters[10] may influence the pattern of secretion in vivo.

Concentrations of the hCG dimer in maternal blood rise rapidly during early pregnancy, peak at 9 to 10 weeks, and subsequently decline to a nadir at approximately 20 weeks. The physiologic role of the hCG peak is unknown, for the serum concentration far exceeds that required to stimulate LH receptors in the corpus luteum. In any case the corpus luteum is coming to the end of its extended life, and so the peak may therefore merely reflect other physiologic events. Production of the β subunit follows the same pattern, whereas the maternal serum concentration of the α subunit continues to rise during the first and second trimesters. Synthesis of the β subunit is therefore considered to be the rate-limiting step. Early experiments using primary placental cultures revealed that cyclic AMP plays a key role in the biosynthesis of both subunits, and subsequent work showed it to increase both the transcription and the stability of the α and β mRNAs. The kinetics were different for the two subunits, however, suggesting that the effect occurs through separate pathways or transcription factors. Possible regulatory elements within the α and β genes were extensively reviewed by Jameson and Hollenberg.[84]

Another theory that has been proposed is that intact hCG may modulate its own secretion in an autocrine/paracrine fashion through the LH/hCG receptor.[85] This G protein–coupled receptor has been identified on the syncytiotrophoblast of the mature placenta and contains a large extracellular domain that binds intact hCG with high affinity and specificity. However, during early pregnancy the receptors in the placenta are truncated and probably functionless until 9 weeks.[86] Hence, in the absence of self-regulation maternal serum concentrations of hCG may rise steeply, until the expression of functional LH/hCG receptors on the syncytiotrophoblast toward the end of the first trimester brings it under control. Reduced synthesis of the functional receptor may underlie the raised serum concentrations of hCG that characterize cases of Down syndrome (trisomy 21).[87]

In addition to changes in the rate of secretion the hormone also exhibits molecular heterogeneity in both its protein and carbohydrate moieties, and the ratio of the different isoforms secreted changes with gestational age. For the first 5 to 6 weeks of gestation hyperglycosylated isoforms of the β subunit predominate, resembling the pattern seen in choriocarcinoma.[88] In normal pregnancies these isoforms then decline and are replaced by those that predominate for the remainder of pregnancy. The rate of decline is greater in pregnancies that go on to spontaneous miscarriage,[88] suggesting there may be some underlying defect in trophoblast differentiation in these cases.

Midtrimester maternal concentrations of hCG were also found to be raised in a retrospective study of early-onset preeclampsia,[89] and a link between the serum concentration and the severity of the maternal oxidative stress has been reported.[90] These data reinforce the putative link between secretion of hCG and the redox status of the trophoblast.

Placental Lactogen

hPL, also known as chorionic sommatotropin, is a single-chain glycoprotein (22,300 Da) that has a high degree of amino acid sequence homology with both human growth hormone (96%) and prolactin (67%). It has been suggested therefore that the genes encoding all three hormones arose from a common ancestral gene through repeated gene duplication. hPL thus has both growth promoting and lactogenic effects, although the former are of rather low activity. The hormone is synthesized exclusively in the syncytiotrophoblast, and is secreted predominantly into the maternal circulation, where it can be detected from the third week of gestation onward. Concentrations rise steadily until they plateau at around 36 weeks of gestation, at which time the daily production rate is approximately 1 g. The magnitude of this effort is reflected by the fact that at term production of hPL accounts for 5% to 10% of total protein synthesis by placental ribosomes, and the encoding mRNA represents 20% of the total placental mRNA.

Little is known regarding the control of hPL secretion in vivo, and maternal concentrations correlate most closely with placental mass. There is evidence that calcium influx into the syncytiotrophoblast or an increase in the external concentration in albumin can cause the release of hPL from placental explants in vitro, and this does not appear to be mediated by activation of the inositol phosphate, cAMP, or cGMP pathways.

The hormone has well-defined actions on maternal metabolism, promoting lipolysis and so increasing circulating free fatty acid levels, and acting as an insulin antagonist and so raising her blood glucose concentrations. It also promotes growth and differentiation of the mammary glandular tissue within the breasts in anticipation of lactation.

Placental Growth Hormone

Placental growth hormone (PGH) is expressed from the same gene cluster as hPL, and differs from pituitary growth hormone by only 13 amino acids.[91] It is secreted predominantly by the syncytiotrophoblast into the maternal circulation in a nonpulsatile manner and cannot be detected in the fetal circulation. Between 10 and 20 weeks of gestation it gradually replaces pituitary growth hormone, which then becomes undetectable until term.[92] In contrast to hPL, PGH has high growth-promoting but low-lactogenic activities.

Secretion on PGH is not modulated by growth-hormone releasing hormone, but appears to be rapidly suppressed by raised glucose concentrations both in vivo and in vitro.[91] Through its actions on maternal metabolism PGH increases nutrient availability for the fetal-placental unit, promoting lipolysis and also gluconeogenesis. It is also one of the key regulators of maternal insulin-like growth factor 1 (IGF1) concentrations, and circulating levels of PGH are reduced in cases of intrauterine growth restriction.[91]

KEY POINTS

- The mature human placenta is a discoid organ consisting of an elaborately branched fetal villous tree that is bathed directly by maternal blood, the villous hemochorial type.
- Continual development throughout pregnancy leads to progressive enlargement of the surface area for exchange (12 to 14 m^2 at term) and reduction in the mean diffusion distance between the maternal and fetal circulations (approximately 5 to 6 μm at term).
- The maternal circulation to the placenta is not fully established until the end of the first trimester; hence organogenesis takes place in a low-oxygen environment of approximately 20 mm Hg that may protect against free radical–mediated teratogenesis.
- During the first trimester the uterine glands discharge their secretions into the placental intervillous space and represent an important supply of nutrients, cytokines, and growth factors before onset of the maternal circulation.
- The exocoelomic cavity acts as an important reservoir of nutrients during early pregnancy, and the secondary yolk sac is important in the uptake of nutrients and their transfer to the fetus.
- Oxygen is a powerful mediator of trophoblast proliferation and invasion, villous remodeling, and placental angiogenesis.
- Ensuring an adequate maternal blood supply to the placenta during the second and third trimesters is an essential aspect of placentation and is dependent on physiologic conversion of the spiral arteries induced by invasion of the endometrium by extravillous trophoblast during early pregnancy. Many complications of pregnancy, such as preeclampsia, appear to be secondary to deficient invasion.
- All transport across the placenta must take place across the syncytial covering of the villous tree, the syncytiotrophoblast, the villous matrix, and the fetal endothelium, each of which may impose its own restriction and selectivity. Exchange will

occur via one of four basic processes: bulk flow/solvent drag, diffusion, transporter-mediated mechanisms, and endocytosis/exocytosis.

- The rate of transplacental exchange depends on many factors, such as the surface area available, the concentration gradient, the rates of maternal and fetal blood flows, and the density of transporter proteins. Changes in villous surface area, diffusion distance, and transporter expression have been linked with intrauterine growth restriction.
- The placenta is an important endocrine gland, producing both steroid and peptide hormones principally from the syncytiotrophoblast. Concentrations of some hormones are altered in pathologic conditions, for example, human chorionic gonadotropin in trisomy 21, but in general little is known regarding control of endocrine activity.

REFERENCES

1. Boyd JD, Hamilton WJ: The Human Placenta. Cambridge, Heffer and Sons, 1970, p 365.
2. Jauniaux E, Gulbis B, Burton GJ: The human first trimester gestational sac limits rather than facilitates oxygen transfer to the fetus—a review. Placenta 24:S86, 2003.
3. Luckett WP: Origin and differentiation of the yolk sac and extraembryonic mesoderm in presomite human and rhesus monkey embryos. Am J Anat 152:59, 1978.
4. Jones CJP: The life and death of the embryonic yolk sac. In Jauniaux E, Barnea ER, Edwards RG (eds): The Life and Death of the Embryonic Yolk Sac. Oxford, Oxford University Press, 1997, p 180.
5. Pereda J, Monge JI, Niimi G: Two different pathways for the transport of primitive and definitive blood cells from the yolk sac to the embryo in humans. Microsc Res Tech 73:803, 2010.
6. Hertig AT, Rock J, Adams EC: A description of 34 human ova within the first 17 days of development. Am J Anat 98:435, 1956.
7. Hustin J, Schaaps JP: Echographic and anatomic studies of the maternotrophoblastic border during the first trimester of pregnancy. Am J Obstet Gynecol 157:162, 1987.
8. Burton GJ, Jauniaux E, Watson AL: Maternal arterial connections to the placental intervillous space during the first trimester of human pregnancy; the Boyd Collection revisited. Am J Obstet Gynecol 181:718, 1999.
9. Schaaps JP, Hustin J: In vivo aspect of the maternal-trophoblastic border during the first trimester of gestation. Troph Res 3:39, 1988.
10. Jauniaux E, Watson AL, Hempstock J, et al: Onset of maternal arterial bloodflow and placental oxidative stress; a possible factor in human early pregnancy failure. Am J Pathol 157:2111, 2000.
11. Pijnenborg R, Vercruysse L, Hanssens M: The uterine spiral arteries in human pregnancy: facts and controversies. Placenta 27:939, 2006.
12. Whitley GS, Cartwright JE: Cellular and molecular regulation of spiral artery remodelling: lessons from the cardiovascular field. Placenta 31:465, 2010.
13. Harris LK: Trophoblast-vascular cell interactions in early pregnancy: how to remodel a vessel (review). Placenta 31:S93, 2010.
14. Brosens IA: The utero-placental vessels at term—the distribution and extent of physiological changes. Troph Res 3:61, 1988.
15. Jauniaux E, Hempstock J, Greenwold N, et al: Trophoblastic oxidative stress in relation to temporal and regional differences in maternal placental blood flow in normal and abnormal early pregnancies. Am J Pathol 162:115, 2003.
16. Moffett A, Loke C: Immunology of placentation in eutherian mammals. Nat Rev Immunol 6:584, 2006.
17. Hiby SE, Apps R, Sharkey AM, et al: Maternal activating KIRs protect against human reproductive failure mediated by fetal HLA-C2. J Clin Invest 120:4102, 2010.
18. Burton GJ, Woods AW, Jauniaux E, et al: Rheological and physiological consequences of conversion of the maternal spiral arteries for uteroplacental blood flow during human pregnancy. Placenta 30:473, 2009.
19. Karimu AL, Burton GJ: The effects of maternal vascular pressure on the dimensions of the placental capillaries. Br J Obstet Gynaecol 101:57, 1994.
20. Moll W, Künzel W, Herberger J: Hemodynamic implications of hemochorial placentation. Eur J Obstet Gynecol Reprod Biol 5:67, 1975.
21. Hustin J, Jauniaux E, Schaaps JP: Histological study of the materno-embryonic interface in spontaneous abortion. Placenta 11:477, 1990.
22. Hempstock J, Jauniaux E, Greenwold N, et al: The contribution of placental oxidative stress to early pregnancy failure. Hum Pathol 34:1265, 2003.
23. Meekins JW, Pijnenborg R, Hanssens M, et al: A study of placental bed spiral arteries and trophoblast invasion in normal and severe pre-eclamptic pregnancies. Br J Obstet Gynaecol 101:669, 1994.
24. Jauniaux E, Nicolaides KH: Placental lakes, absent umbilical artery diastolic flow and poor fetal growth in early pregnancy. Ultrasound Obstet Gynecol 7:141, 1996.
25. Martin CB, McGaughey HS, Kaiser IH, et al: Intermittent functioning of the uteroplacental arteries. Am J Obstet Gynecol 90:819, 1964.
26. Burton GJ, Yung HW, Cindrova-Davies T, et al: Placental endoplasmic reticulum stress and oxidative stress in the pathophysiology of unexplained intrauterine growth restriction and early onset pre-eclampsia. Placenta 30:S43, 2009.
27. Burton GJ, Watson AL, Hempstock J, et al: Uterine glands provide histiotrophic nutrition for the human fetus during the first trimester of pregnancy. J Clin Endocrinol Metab 87:2954, 2002.
28. Jones CJ, Aplin JD, Burton GJ: First trimester histiotrophe shows altered sialylation compared with secretory phase glycoconjugates in human endometrium. Placenta 31:576, 2010.
29. Kolibianakis EM, Zikopoulos KA, Fatemi HM, et al: Endometrial thickness cannot predict ongoing pregnancy achievement in cycles stimulated with clomiphene citrate for intrauterine insemination. Reprod Biomed Online 8:115, 2004.
30. Hempstock J, Cindrova-Davies T, Jauniaux E, et al: Endometrial glands as a source of nutrients, growth factors and cytokines during the first trimester of human pregnancy; a morphological and immunohistochemical study. Reprod Biol Endocrinol 2:58, 2004.
31. Mikolajczyk M, Skrzypczak J, Szymanowski K, et al: The assessment of LIF in uterine flushing—a possible new diagnostic tool in states of impaired infertility. Reprod Biol 3:259, 2003.
32. Tuckerman E, Laird SM, Stewart R, et al: Markers of endometrial function in women with unexplained recurrent pregnancy loss: a comparison between morphologically normal and retarded endometrium. Hum Reprod 19:196, 2004.
33. Kaufmann P, Sen DK, Schweikhert G: Classification of human placental villi. 1. Histology. Cell Tissue Res 200:409, 1979.
34. Ramsey EM, Donner MW: Placental Vasculature and Circulation. Anatomy, Physiology, Radiology, Clinical Aspects, Atlas and Textbook. Stuttgart, Georg Thieme, 1980, p 101.
35. Hempstock J, Bao Y-P, Bar-Issac M, et al: Intralobular differences in antioxidant enzyme expression and activity reflect oxygen gradients within the human placenta. Placenta 24:517, 2003.
36. Mayhew TM, Ohadike C, Baker PN, et al: Stereological investigation of placental morphology in pregnancies complicated by pre-eclampsia with and without intrauterine growth restriction. Placenta 24:219, 2003.
37. Hafner E, Metzenbauer M, Hofinger D, et al: Placental growth from the first to the second trimester of pregnancy in SGA-foetuses and pre-eclamptic pregnancies compared to normal foetuses. Placenta 24:336, 2003.
38. Jones CJP, Fox H: Ultrastructure of the normal human placenta. Elect Microsc Rev 4:129, 1991.
39. Carter AM: Placental oxygen consumption. Part I: in vivo studies—a review. Placenta 21:S31, 2000.
40. Schneider H: Placental oxygen consumption. Part II: in vitro studies—a review. Placenta 21:S38, 2000.
41. Hemberger M, Udayashankar R, Tesar P, et al: ELF5-enforced transcriptonal networks define an epigentically regulated trophoblast stem cell compartment in the human placenta. Mol Hum Genet 19:2456, 2010.
42. Burton GJ, Skepper JN, Hempstock J, et al: A reappraisal of the contrasting morphological appearances of villous cytotrophoblast

cells during early human pregnancy; evidence for both apoptosis and primary necrosis. Placenta 24:297, 2003.
43. Mayhew TM, Leach L, McGee R, et al: Proliferation, differentiation and apoptosis in villous trophoblast at 13-41 weeks of gestation (including observations on annulate lamellae and nuclear pore complexes). Placenta 20:407, 1999.
44. Kingdom JCP, Kaufmann P: Oxygen and placental villous development: origins of fetal hypoxia. Placenta 18:613, 1997.
45. Frendo JL, Cronier L, Bertin G, et al: Involvement of connexin 43 in human trophoblast cell fusion and differentiation. J Cell Sci 116:3413, 2003.
46. Gauster M, Huppertz B: The paradox of caspase 8 in human villous trophoblast fusion. Placenta 31:82, 2010.
47. Rote NS, Wei BR, Xu C, et al: Caspase 8 and human villous cytotrophoblast differentiation. Placenta 31:89, 2010.
48. Frendo JL, Olivier D, Cheynet V, et al: Direct involvement of HERV-W Env glycoprotein in human trophoblast cell fusion and differentiation. Mol Cell Biol 23:3566, 2003.
49. Huppertz B, Kingdom J: Apoptosis in the trophoblast—role of apoptosis in placental morphogenesis. J Soc Gynecol Investig 11:353, 2004.
50. Ellery PM, Cindrova-Davies T, Jauniaux E, et al: Evidence for transcriptional activity in the syncytiotrophoblast of the human placenta. Placenta 30:329, 2009.
51. Burton GJ, Jones CJ: Syncytial knots, sprouts, apoptosis, and trophoblast deportation from the human placenta. Taiwan J Obstet Gynecol 48:28, 2009.
52. Brownbill P, Mahendran D, Owen D, et al: Denudations as paracellular routes for alphafetoprotein and creatinine across the human syncytiotrophoblast. Am J Physiol Regul Integr Comp Physiol 278:R677, 2000.
53. Huppertz B, Kaufmann P, Kingdom J: Trophoblast turnover in health and disease. Fetal Maternal Med Rev 13:103, 2002.
54. Redman CWG, Sargent IL: Placental debris, oxidative stress and pre-eclampsia. Placenta 21:597, 2000.
55. Charnock Jones DS, Kaufmann P, Mayhew TM: Aspects of human fetoplacental vasculogenesis and angiogenesis. I. Molecular recognition. Placenta 25:103, 2004.
56. Burton GJ, Charnock-Jones DS, Jauniaux E: Regulation of vascular growth and function in human placenta. Reproduction 138:895, 2009.
57. Kaufmann P, Bruns U, Leiser R, et al: The fetal vascularisation of term placental villi. II. Intermediate and terminal villi. Anat Embryol 173:203, 1985.
58. Jirkovska M, Janacek J, Kalab J, et al: Three-dimensional arrangement of the capillary bed and its relationship to microrheology in the terminal villi of normal term placenta. Placenta 29:892, 2008.
59. Mayhew TM, Charnock Jones DS, Kaufmann P: Aspects of human fetoplacental vasculogenesis and angiogenesis. III. Changes in complicated pregnancies. Placenta 25:127, 2004.
60. Pereda J, Niimi G: Embryonic erythropoiesis in human yolk sac: two different compartments for two different processes. Microsc Res Tech 71:856, 2008.
61. Jauniaux E, Gulbis B: Fluid compartments of the embryonic environment. Hum Reprod Update 6:268, 2000.
62. Jauniaux E, Gulbis B, Jurkovic D, et al: Protein and steroid levels in embryonic cavities in early human pregnancy. Hum Reprod 8: 782, 1993.
63. Gulbis B, Jauniaux E, Cotton F, et al: Protein and enzyme patterns in the fluid cavities of the first trimester gestational sac: relevance to the absorptive role of the secondary yolk sac. Mol Hum Reprod 4:857, 1998.
64. Jauniaux E, Cindrova-Davies T, Johns J, et al: Distribution and transfer pathways of antioxidant molecules inside the first trimester human gestational sac. J Clin Endocrinol Metab 89:1452, 2004.
65. Stulc J, Stulcova B: Effect of NaCl load administered to the fetus on the bidirectional movement of 51Cr-EDTA across rat placenta. Am J Physiol 270:R984, 1996.
66. Atkinson DE, Boyd RDH, Sibley CP: Placental Transfer. In Neill JD (ed): Knobil and Neill's Physiology of Reproduction, 3rd ed. Amsterdam, Elsevier, 2005, p 2787.
67. Bain MD, Copas DK, Taylor A, et al: Permeability of the human placenta in vivo to four non-metabolized hydrophilic molecules. J Physiol 431:505, 1990.
68. Brownbill P, Edwards D, Jones C, et al: Mechanisms of alphafetoprotein transfer in the perfused human placental cotyledon from uncomplicated pregnancy. J Clin Invest 96:2220, 1995.
69. Stulc J, Svihovec J, Drabkova J, et al: Electrical potential difference across the mid-term human placenta. Acta Obstet Gynecol Scand 57:125, 1978.
70. Mellor DJ, Cockburn F, Lees MM, et al: Distribution of ions and electrical potential differences between mother and fetus in the human at term. J Obstet Gynaecol Br Commonw 76:993, 1969.
71. Ward S, Jauniaux E, Shannon C, et al: Electrical potential difference between exocelomic fluid and maternal blood in early pregnancy. Am J Physiol 274:R1492, 1998.
72. Ayuk PT, Theophanous D, D'Souza SW, et al: L-arginine transport by the microvillous plasma membrane of the syncytiotrophoblast from human placenta in relation to nitric oxide production: effects of gestation, preeclampsia, and intrauterine growth restriction. J Clin Endocrinol Metab 87:747, 2002.
73. Jansson T, Wennergren M, Illsley NP: Glucose transporter protein expression in human placenta throughout gestation and in intrauterine growth retardation. J Clin Endocrinol Metab 77:1554, 1993.
74. Hughes JL, Doughty IM, Glazier JD, et al: Activity and expression of the Na(+)/H(+) exchanger in the microvillous plasma membrane of the syncytiotrophoblast in relation to gestation and small for gestational age birth. Pediatr Res 48:652, 2000.
75. Powell TL, Illsley NP: A novel technique for studying cellular function in human placenta: gestational changes in intracellular pH regulation. Placenta 17:661, 1996.
76. Reik W, Constancia M, Fowden A, et al: Regulation of supply and demand for maternal nutrients in mammals by imprinted genes. J Physiol 547:35, 2003.
77. Sibley CP, Boyd RDH: Mechanisms of transfer across the human placenta. In Polin RA, Fox WW, Abman SH (eds): Mechanisms of Transfer across the Human Placenta. Philadelphia, Saunders, 2004, p 111.
78. Sibley CP, Turner MA, Cetin I, et al: Placental phenotypes of intrauterine growth. Pediatr Res 58:827, 2005.
79. Tuckey RC: Progesterone synthesis by the human placenta. Placenta 26:273, 2005.
80. Tuckey RC, Kostadinovic Z, Cameron KJ: Cytochrome P-450scc activity and substrate supply in human placental trophoblasts. Mol Cell Endocrinol 105:103, 1994.
81. Mendelson CR, Jiang B, Shelton JM, et al: Transcriptional regulation of aromatase in placenta and ovary. J Steroid Biochem Mol Biol 95:25, 2005.
82. Maston GA, Ruvolo M: Chorionic gonadotropin has a recent origin within primates and an evolutionary history of selection. Mol Biol Evol 19:320, 2002.
83. Bo M, Boime I: Identification of the transcriptionally active genes of the chorionic gonadotropin beta gene cluster in vivo. J Biol Chem 267:3179, 1992.
84. Jameson JL, Hollenberg AN: Regulation of chorionic gonadotropin gene expression. Endocrine Rev 14:203, 1993.
85. Licht P, Losch A, Dittrich R, et al: Novel insights into human endometrial paracrinology and embryo-maternal communication by intrauterine microdialysis. Hum Reprod Update 4:532, 1998.
86. Rao CV: The beginning of a new era in reproductive biology and medicine: expression of low levels of functional luteinizing hormone/human chorionic gonadotropin receptors in nongonadal tissues. J Physiol Pharmacol 47:41, 1996.
87. Banerjee S, Smallwood A, Chambers AE, et al: A link between high serum levels of human chorionic gonadotrophin and chorionic expression of its mature functional receptor (LHCGR) in Down's syndrome pregnancies. Reprod Biol Endocrinol 3:25, 2005.
88. Cole LA: Hyperglycosylated hCG, a review. Placenta 31:653, 2010.
89. Shenhav S, Gemer O, Sassoon E, et al: Mid-trimester triple test levels in early and late onset severe pre-eclampsia. Prenatal Diagnosis 22:579, 2002.
90. Kharfi A, Giguere Y, De Grandpre P, et al: Human chorionic gonadotropin (hCG) may be a marker of systemic oxidative stress in normotensive and preeclamptic term pregnancies. Clin Biochem 38:717, 2005.
91. Lacroix MC, Guibourdenche J, Frendo JL, et al: Human placental growth hormone—a review. Placenta 23:S87, 2002.
92. Mirlesse V, Frankenne F, Alsat E, et al: Placental growth hormone levels in normal pregnancy and in pregnancies with intrauterine growth retardation. Pediatr Res 34:439, 1993.

93. Jansson T, Ylven K, Wennergren M, et al: Glucose transport and system A activity in syncytiotrophoblast microvillous and basal plasma membranes in intrauterine growth restriction. Placenta 23: 392, 2002.
94. Jansson T, Scholtbach V, Powell TL: Placental transport of leucine and lysine is reduced in intrauterine growth restriction. Pediatr Res 44:532, 1998.
95. Norberg S, Powell TL, Jansson T: Intrauterine growth restriction is associated with a reduced activity of placental taurine transporters. Pediatr Res 44:233, 1998.
96. Roos S, Powell TL, Jansson T: Human placental taurine transporter in uncomplicated and IUGR pregnancies: cellular localization, protein expression and regulation. Am J Physiol Regul Integr Comp Physiol 287:R886, 2004.
97. Johansson M, Karlsson L, Wennergren M, et al: Activity and protein expression of Na^+/K^+ ATPase are reduced in microvillous syncytiotrophoblast plasma membranes isolated from pregnancies complicated by intrauterine growth restriction. J Clin Endocrinol Metab 88:2831, 2003.
98. Strid H, Bucht E, Jansson T, et al: ATP dependent Ca^{2+} transport across basal membrane of human syncytiotrophoblast in pregnancies complicated by intrauterine growth restriction or diabetes. Placenta 24:445, 2003.
99. Johansson M, Glazier JD, Sibley CP, et al: Activity and protein expression of the Na^+/H^+ exchanger is reduced in syncytiotrophoblast microvillous plasma membranes isolated from preterm intrauterine growth restriction pregnancies. J Clin Endocrinol Metab 87:5686, 2002.
100. Settle P, Mynett K, Speake P, et al: Polarized lactate transporter activity and expression in the syncytiotrophoblast of the term human placenta. Placenta 25:496, 2004.

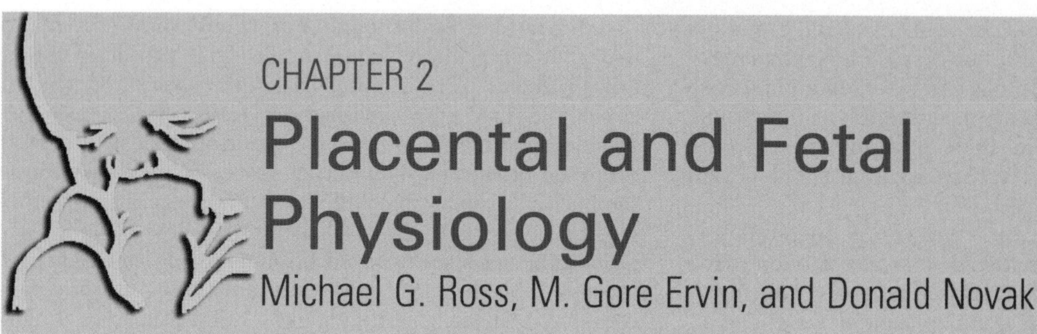

CHAPTER 2

Placental and Fetal Physiology

Michael G. Ross, M. Gore Ervin, and Donald Novak

KEY ABBREVIATIONS	
2,3-Diphosphoglycerate	2,3-DPG
α-Melanocyte-stimulating Hormone	α-MSH
Adenosine Triphosphate	ATP
Adrenocorticotropic Hormone	ACTH
Angiotension-converting Enzyme	ACE
Angiotension II	AII
Arginine Vasopressin	AVP
Atrial Natriuretic Factor	ANF
Carbon Dioxide	CO_2
Corticotropin-like Intermediate Lobe Peptide	CLIP
Epidermal Growth Factor	EGF
Epidermal Growth Factor Receptor	EGF-R
Glomerular Filtration Rate	GFR
Glucose Transporter	GLUT
Human Leukocyte Antigens	HLAs
Immunoglobulin G	IgG
Insulin-like Growth Factor	IGF
Killer Cell Immunoglobulin-like Receptors	KIRs
Low-density Lipoproteins	LDLs
Oxygen	O_2
T-helper Type 1	Th1
Thyrotropin-releasing Hormone	TRH
Thyroid-stimulating Hormone	TSH
Thyroxine	T_4
Triiodothyronine	T_3
Uterine Natural Killer Cells	uNK
Vascular Endothelial Growth Factor	VEGF

In obstetrical practice, recognition of normal fetal growth, development, and behavior often suggests a nonintervention management plan. However, abnormalities may require clinical strategies for fetal assessment and/or intervention. The basic concepts of placental and fetal physiology provide the building blocks necessary for understanding pathophysiology and thus mechanisms of disease. Throughout this chapter, we have reviewed the essential tenets of placental and fetal physiology, while relating this information to normal and abnormal clinical conditions.

Much of our knowledge of placental and fetal physiology derives from observations made in mammals other than humans. We have attempted to include only those observations reasonably applicable to the human placenta and fetus, and in most instances have not detailed the species from which the data were obtained. Should questions arise regarding the species studied, the reader is referred to the extensive bibliography.

PLACENTAL PHYSIOLOGY

The placenta provides the fetus with essential nutrients, water and oxygen, and a route for clearance of fetal excretory products, and produces a vast array of protein and steroid hormones and factors essential to the maintenance of pregnancy. As a result, it has become increasingly clear that the placenta, far from being a passive conduit, plays a key role in the control of fetal growth.

Placental Metabolism and Growth

Anatomic and histologic aspects of placental growth are detailed in Chapter 1. This section focuses on the physiology of placental metabolism and growth, and its influence on the fetus.

The critical function of the placenta is illustrated by its high metabolic demands. For example, placental oxygen consumption equals that of the fetus, and exceeds the fetal rate when expressed on a weight basis (10 mL/min/kg).[1] Between 22 and 36 weeks of gestation, the number of trophoblast nuclei increases fourfold to fivefold, placing increased metabolic demands on the placenta. Glucose is the principal substrate for oxidative metabolism by placental tissue. Of the total glucose leaving the maternal compartment to nourish the uterus and its contents, placental consumption may represent up to 70%.[2] In addition, a significant fraction of placental glucose uptake derives from the fetal circulation, and reflects placental oxidative metabolism. Although one third of placental glucose may be converted to the three-carbon sugar lactate, placental metabolism is not anaerobic. Instead, placental lactate is thought to be a fetal energetic substrate. The factors regulating short-term changes in placental oxygen and glucose consumption are at present incompletely understood, although in pregnancies at high altitude, the placenta appears to spare oxygen for fetal use, at the cost of increased placental utilization of glucose.

The regulation of placental growth is incompletely understood, although dramatic advances have been made in the study of genes as they contribute to placental growth and differentiation. Normal term placental weight averages 450 g, representing approximately one seventh (one sixth with cord and membranes) of fetal weight. Large placentas, either ultrasonographically or at delivery, may prompt investigation into possible etiologies. Clinical observations suggest a link between decreased tissue oxygen content and increased placental growth. Thus, increased placental size is associated with maternal anemia, fetal anemia associated with erythrocyte isoimmunization, and hydrops fetalis secondary to fetal α-thalassemia with Bart's hemoglobin. The association of a large placenta with maternal diabetes also has been recognized, possibly a result of insulin-stimulated mitogenic activity or enhanced angiogenesis. Enlarged placentas are also found in cloned animals, presumably because of defects in the expression of specific imprinted genes, as well as in the placentas of animals in whom specific gene products have been deleted. In humans, increased ratio of placental size to fetal weight is associated with increased morbidity, both in the neonatal period and subsequently.[3]

An array of growth-promoting peptide hormones (factors) have been characterized in placental tissue at the protein and/or receptor levels. These include the insulin receptor, insulin-like growth factors I and II (IGF-I, IGF-II), epidermal growth factor (EGF), leptin, placental growth factor, placental growth hormone, placental lactogen, and a variety of cytokines and chemokines, each of which has been shown to play an important role in fetal/placental development. **IGF-I and IGF-II are polypeptides with a high degree of homology to human proinsulin. Both IGF-I and IGF-II circulate bound to carrier proteins, and are 50 times more potent than insulin in stimulating cell growth. Both are produced within the placenta, as well as in the fetus and mother.** EGF increases RNA and DNA synthesis and cell multiplication in a wide variety of cell types. The integrated physiological role of these and other potential placental growth factors in regulating placental growth remains to be fully defined; however, the development of null-mutation mouse models for IGF-1, IGF-II, IGF-1r, and IGF-IIr, as well as for the EGF receptor, have provided evidence in this regard.[4] Specifically, the EGF receptor appears important in placental development, as does IGF-II. Knockout of IGF-II results in diminished placental size, whereas deletion of the IGF-II receptor results in an increase in placental size. IGF-I does not appear to affect placental growth. Chronic exposure to exogenous corticosteroid may also result in diminished placental size.

Placental Transfer

General Considerations

In the hemochorial human placenta, maternal blood and solutes are separated from fetal blood by trophoblastic tissue and fetal endothelial cells. Thus, transit from the maternal intervillous space to the fetal capillary lumen takes place across a number of cellular structures (Figure 2-1). The first step is transport across the microvillus plasma membrane of the syncytiotrophoblast. Because there are no lateral intercellular spaces in the syncytiotrophoblast, all solutes first interact with the placenta at this plasma membrane. The basal (fetal) syncytiotrophoblast membrane represents an additional step in the transport process. The discontinuous nature of the cytotrophoblast cell layer in later gestation suggests that this layer should not limit maternal-to-fetal transfer. The fetal capillary endothelial cell imposes two additional plasma membrane surfaces.

A number of specific mechanisms allow transit of the placental membranes, including passive diffusion, facilitated diffusion, active transport, and endocytosis/exocytosis. Solutes lacking specialized transport mechanisms cross by extracellular or transcellular diffusional transport pathways with permeability determined by size,

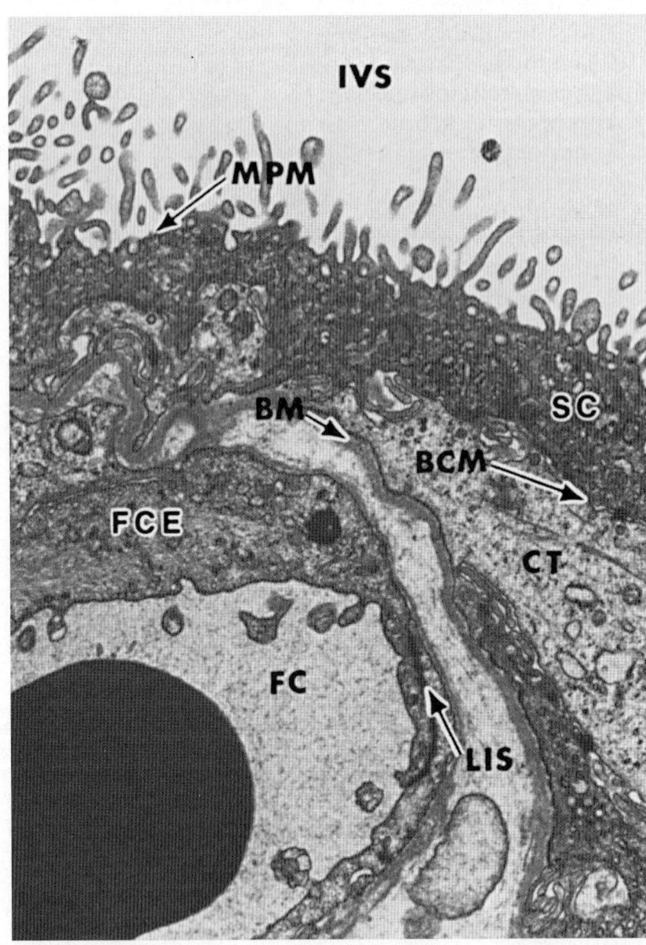

FIGURE 2-1. Electron micrograph of human placenta demonstrating the cellular and extracellular components with which solutes most interact in moving from the maternal intervillous space *(IVS)* to the lumen of the fetal capillary *(FC)*. *MPM,* Microvillous plasma membrane of the syncytiotrophoblast; *SC,* syncytiotrophoblast; *BCM,* basal cell membrane of the syncytiotrophoblast; *BM,* basement membrane; *CT,* cytotrophoblast cell; *FCE,* fetal capillary endothelial cell; *LIS,* lateral intercellular space of fetal endothelial cell. (Courtesy Kent L. Thornburg, Ph.D., Department of Physiology, Oregon Health Sciences University, Portland, OR.)

lipid solubility, ionic charge, and maternal serum protein binding. **Lipid-insoluble (hydrophilic) substances, which cross the trophoblast via extracellular pores, are restricted by molecular size in relation to the extracellular pore size. Up to a molecular weight (MW) of at least 5000 daltons, placental permeability is proportional to the free diffusion of a molecule in water.**[5] For example, urea (MW = 60) is at least 1000 times more permeable than inulin (MW = 5000).[5] Thus, transfer of small solutes will be governed primarily by the maternal-fetal concentration gradient. Because transfer is relatively slow, and the extracellular pore surface area is limited, transfer of these molecules is referred to as *diffusion limited.* In animal models, food restriction enhances the barrier to diffusion, as does placental IGF-II deficiency.[6] **Conversely, highly lipid-soluble (lipophilic) substances diffuse readily through the trophoblastic membrane. Thus, molecular weight is relatively less important in restricting diffusion.** Ethanol, a molecule similar in size to urea, is 500 times more lipid soluble and 10 times more permeable. Because the entire trophoblast surface is available for diffusion and the permeability is high, transfer rates for lipophilic substances to the fetus are limited primarily by placental intervillous and umbilical blood flows (flow limited). **Both facilitated diffusion and active transport utilize carrier-mediated transport systems, with the latter requiring energy, either directly or indirectly linked with ionic pump mechanisms.** Carrier transport systems are specifically limited to unique classes of molecules (i.e., neutral amino acids). In addition, substances may traverse the placenta via endocytosis (invagination of the cell membrane to form an intracellular vesicle containing extracellular fluids) and exocytosis (release of the vesicle to the extracellular space).

Transfer of Individual Solutes

Respiratory Gases

The exchange or transfer of the primary respiratory gases, oxygen and carbon dioxide, is likely flow limited. Thus, the driving force for placental gas exchange is the partial pressure gradient between the maternal and fetal circulations. **Early in gestation, the human embryo develops in a low oxygen environment. Such an environment appears to be necessary, and is associated with the presence of oxygen sensitive regulatory genes and gene products.** After approximately gestation week 10, the placenta becomes important as a respiratory organ. Indeed, estimates of human placental diffusing capacities would predict that placental efficiency as an organ of respiratory gas exchange will allow equilibrium of oxygen and carbon dioxide tensions at the maternal intervillous space and fetal capillary. However, this prediction varies from the observed 10 mm Hg difference in oxygen tension between the umbilical and uterine veins and between the umbilical vein and intervillous space. In contrast, the P_{CO2} difference from umbilical to uterine vein is small (3 mm Hg). P_{O2} differences could be explained by areas of uneven distribution of maternal to fetal blood flows or shunting, limiting fetal and maternal blood exchange, a process that, as in other respiratory organs (i.e., lungs) may be an active one.[7] The most important contribution, however, is likely the high metabolic rate of the placental tissues themselves. Thus, trophoblast cell O_2 consumption and CO_2 production lower umbilical vein O_2 tension and increase uterine vein CO_2 tension to a greater degree than could be explained by an inert barrier for respiratory gas transfer.

The arteriovenous difference in the uterine circulation (and venoarterial difference in the umbilical circulation) widens during periods of lowered blood flow. **Proportionate O_2 uptake increases and O_2 consumption remains unchanged over a fairly wide range of blood flows. Thus, both uterine and umbilical blood flows can fall significantly without decreasing fetal O_2 consumption.**[8] Conversely, unilateral umbilical artery occlusion is associated with significant fetal effects.

Carbon dioxide is carried in the fetal blood both as dissolved CO_2 and as bicarbonate. Because of its charged nature, fetal to maternal bicarbonate transfer is limited. However, CO_2 likely diffuses from fetus to mother in its molecular form, and $[HCO_3^-]$ does not contribute significantly to fetal CO_2 elimination.

Glucose

Placental permeability for D-glucose is at least 50 times the value predicted on the basis of size and lipid solubility.[9] **Thus, specialized transport mechanisms must be available on both the microvillous and basal membranes. Membrane proteins facilitating the translocation of molecules across cell membranes are termed *transporters.* The primary human placental glucose transporter is GLUT1,**[10] **a sodium-independent transporter, as compared to the sodium-dependent transporters found in adult kidney and intestine. This transporter, in contrast to that found in human adipocytes (GLUT4), is not insulin sensitive.** The placental D-glucose transporter is saturable at high substrate concentrations; 50% saturation is observed at glucose levels of approximately 5 mM (90 mg/dL). Thus, glucose transfer from mother to fetus is not linear, and transfer rates decrease as maternal glucose concentration increases. This effect is reflected in fetal blood glucose levels following maternal sugar loading. **Modification of transporter expression within the placenta also occurs in response to maternal diabetes.** In this setting, GLUT1 expression is thought to increase on the basolateral membrane, while holding constant on the maternal-facing microvillous membrane.[11] Alterations in transporter expression may also depend on gestational stage (e.g., early in pregnancy, GLUT4 may be present within the placenta), as well as maternal nutrition/placental blood flow. A second transporter, GLUT3, has also been noted in the fetal-facing placental endothelium. Its presence within the syncytiotrophoblast remains controversial.

Amino Acids

Amino acid concentrations are higher in fetal umbilical cord blood than in maternal blood.[12] Like monosaccharides, amino acids enter and exit the syncytiotrophoblast via specific membrane transport proteins. These proteins allow amino acids to be transported against a concentration gradient into the placenta, and subsequently, if not directly, into the fetal circulation.

Multiple transport proteins mediate neutral, anionic, and cationic amino acid transport into the syncytiotrophoblast. These include both sodium-dependent and sodium-independent transporters. Amino acid entry is, in many cases, coupled to sodium in co-transport systems located at the microvillous membrane facing the maternal intervillous space. As long as an inwardly directed sodium gradient is maintained, trophoblast cell amino acid concentrations will exceed maternal blood levels. **The sodium gradient is maintained by Na^+-K^+ATPase located on the basal or fetal side of the syncytiotrophoblast. In addition, high trophoblast levels of amino acids transported by sodium-dependent transporters can "drive" uptake of other amino acids via transporters that function as "exchangers."** Examples of these include ASCT1 and y^+LAT/4F2HC. Still other transporters function in sodium-independent fashion. Individual amino acids may be transported by single or multiple transport proteins. Transport systems have been defined in human placenta (a general schema may be found in Figure 2-2).

SNAT 1 and 2, responsible for the transport of neutral amino acids with short polar or linear side chains, are sodium-dependent transporters with activity localized on both the microvillous and basolateral membranes of the human placenta. SNAT 4, with similar substrate specificity, is present early in gestation. Other sodium-dependent transport activities localized to the microvillous membrane include that for β-amino acids such as taurine (TauT), as well as perhaps glycine transport via System GLY. Sodium-independent transporters mediating neutral amino acid transfer on the microvillous membrane include System L (LAT-1, 2/4F2HC), which exhibits a high affinity for amino acids with bulky side chains such as leucine, and y^+LAT/4F2HC, capable of transporting both neutral and cationic amino acids such as lysine and arginine. The aforementioned transporters are heterodimeric, requiring the combination of two distinct proteins with the cell membrane for transport to occur. Cationic amino acids may also be transported by the sodium-independent transport protein CAT1, whereas anionic amino acids (glutamate, aspartate) are transported by the sodium-dependent transport proteins EAAT 1-4. Basolateral membrane transport activities are similar; however, a predominance of sodium-independent transport and exchange (e.g., ASCT1) allows flow of amino acids down their concentration gradients into the fetal endothelium/fetal blood space. Although less is known regarding transfer into and out of the fetal endothelium, which, for the most part, abuts the syncytiotrophoblast basolateral membrane, available studies have verified that these cells too have a complement of amino acid transport proteins. Recent reviews of placental nutrient transfer and its impact are available.[13,14]

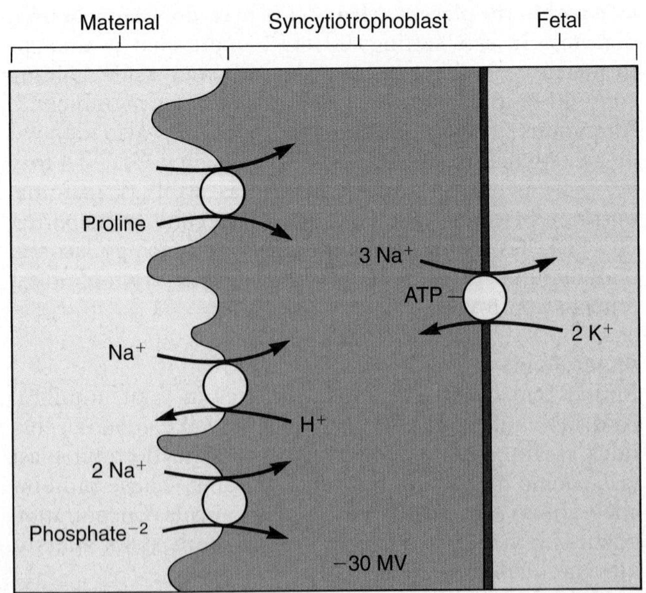

FIGURE 2-2. Pathways for sodium entry into syncytiotrophoblast and exit to the fetal circulation. (Data from online references: Boyd et al., 1981; Whitsett and Wallick, 1980; Lajeunesse and Brunette, 1988; Balkovets et al., 1986; and Bara et al., 1988.)

As implied earlier, more than one protein may mediate each transport activity within a single tissue. Examples include EAAT 1-5, associated with sodium-dependent anionic amino acid transfer; CAT 1, 2, 2a, associated with System y+ activity; and SNAT1, 2, and 4, associated with sodium-dependent transfer of small neutral amino acids. The reasons underlying this duplication within the placenta, more pronounced than in any other organ with the possible exception of the central nervous system, is unclear. Certainly, as is the case for the anionic amino acid transporters EAAT 1-5, differential distribution within different tissue elements plays a role. Differential regulation within single cell types is another likely reason. In isolated trophoblast cells, System A activity (sodium-dependent transfer of small neutral amino acids) is upregulated by the absence of amino acids partially due to an increase in carrier affinity. Conversely, increases in trophoblast amino acid concentrations may suppress uptake (transinhibition). These mechanisms serve to maintain trophoblast cell amino acid levels constant during fluctuations in maternal plasma concentrations. Insulin has also been shown to upregulate this transport activity as has insulin-like growth factor 1. **Placental System A activity is downregulated in intrauterine growth restriction, both in humans and in animal models. It is also downregulated in the placentas of obese mothers.**[15] **Conversely, System A activity is upregulated in the placentas of diabetic mothers, perhaps contributing to the accelerated growth noted in these fetuses. Mechanisms underlying these changes are as of yet unclear.**

The coordination between placental/fetal metabolism and amino acid transfer is illustrated by the anionic amino acids glutamate and aspartate, which are poorly transported from mother to fetus.[16] **Glutamate, however, is produced by the fetal liver from glutamine and then taken up across the basolateral membrane of the placenta. Within the placenta, the majority of glutamate is metabolized and utilized as an energy source.** As a result, sodium-dependent anionic amino acid transfer activity is of particular importance on the basolateral membrane, as is System ASC (ASCT1) activity, responsible for the uptake of serine, also produced by the fetal liver, into the placenta.

Lipids

Esterified fatty acids (triglycerides) are present in maternal serum as components of chylomicrons and very-low-density lipoproteins (VLDLs). Before transfer across the placenta, lipoprotein lipase interacts with these particles, releasing free fatty acids, which, due to their hydrophobic nature, are relatively insoluble in plasma and circulate bound to albumin. As a result, fatty acid transfer involves dissociation from maternal protein, subsequent association with placental proteins, first at the plasma membrane (FABPpm), then after transfer into the cell (thought to be via FAT/CD36 and FATP) with intracytoplasmic binding proteins. Transfer out of the syncytiotrophoblast is less well worked out, but is thought to occur via interaction with FAT/CD36 and FATP, which are present at both the microvillous and basolateral placental membrane surfaces. Subsequently, interaction with fetal plasma proteins occurs. Placental fatty acid uptake is in part regulated by PPARγ and RXR. In turn, long-chain polyunsaturated fatty acids taken up by the placenta can be metabolized into PPAR ligands, thus affecting the expression of an array of placental genes, including those influencing fatty acid metabolism and transfer. **Fatty acids may also be oxidized within the placenta, as a source of energy.** Although precise interactions and mechanisms remain uncertain, it is clear that lipid uptake is of profound importance to fetal development. Targeted deletion of FATP4, found within the placenta, results in fetal lethality.[17]

Early studies documented that placental fatty acid transfer increases logarithmically with decreasing chain length (C16 to C8) and then declines somewhat for C6 and C4. More recent work, however, has clarified the fact that essential fatty acids are, in general, transferred more efficiently than are nonessential fatty acids.[18] Of these, docosahexananoic acid seems to be transferred more efficiently than arachidonic acid; oleic acid is transferred least efficiently. As in the case of amino acids discussed earlier, the fetus is significantly enriched in long chain polyunsaturated fatty acids as compared to the mother. Such selectivity may also relate to the composition of triglycerides in maternal serum, as lipoprotein lipase preferentially cleaves fatty acids in the two positions. In general, fatty acids transferred to the fetus reflect maternal serum lipids and diet. Placental fatty transfer has been recently reviewed.[18] **There is also evidence that the placental secretion of leptin, a hormone generally secreted by adipocytes, may promote maternal lipolysis, thus providing both placenta and fetus the means by which to ensure an adequate lipid supply.** Another possible mechanism by which lipids may be excreted from the placenta involves the synthesis and secretion of apolipoprotein (apo) B–containing lipoproteins. The relative importance of this pathway in the human placenta is at present unclear. Placental uptake and excretion of cholesterol is discussed in the section on receptor-mediated endocytosis.

Water and Ions

Although water transfer across the placenta does not limit fetal water uptake during growth, the factors regulating fetal water acquisition are poorly understood. **Water transfer from mother to fetus is determined by a balance of osmotic, hydrostatic, and colloid osmotic forces at the placental interface.** Calculation of osmotic pressure from individual solute concentrations is unreliable because osmotic pressure forces depend on the membrane permeability to each solute. Thus, sodium and chloride, the principal plasma solutes, are relatively permeable across the placenta[19] and would not be expected to contribute important osmotic effects.[20] As a result, although human fetal plasma osmolality is equal to or greater than maternal plasma osmolality, these measured values do not reflect the actual osmotic force on either side of the membranes.[19] Coupled with findings that hydrostatic pressure may be greater in the umbilical vein than the intervillous space, these data do not explain mechanisms for fetal water accumulation. Alternatively, colloid osmotic pressure differences and active solute transport probably represent the main determinants of net water fluxes—approximately 20 mL/day. It is likely, however, given the large (3.6 L/hr) flux of water between mother and fetus, that more active mechanisms, including perhaps controlled changes in end-vessel resistance, play a significant role. In fact, water flux occurs through both transcellular and paracellular pathways. Water channels (aquaporins 1, 3, 8, and 9) have been identified within the placenta, but their roles relative to water flux within the fetal placental unit have not been discerned.[21]

In comparison to other epithelia the specialized placental mechanisms for ion transport are incompletely understood. Multiple mechanisms for sodium transport in syncytiotrophoblast membranes exist. The maternal-facing microvillous membrane contains, at a minimum, multiple amino acid co-transporters, a sodium phosphate co-transporter in which two sodium ions are transported with each phosphate radical, a sodium-hydrogen ion antiport that exchanges one proton for each sodium ion entering the cell, and other nutrient transporters. In addition, both sodium and potassium channels have been described. A membrane potential with the inside negative (−30 MV) would promote sodium entry from the intervillous space. The fetal directed basal side of the cell contains the Na,K-ATPase. The microvillous or maternal facing trophoblast membrane has an anion exchanger (AE1) that mediates chloride transit across this membrane, in association with Cl^- conductance pathways (channels), present in both the microvillous and basolateral membranes.[22] Paracellular pathways also play an important role. The integration and regulation of these various mechanisms for sodium and chloride transport from mother to fetus is not completely understood; there is accumulating evidence that mineralocorticoids may regulate placental sodium transfer. Further, sodium/hydrogen exchange, mediated by multiple members of the NHE family (NHE1-3), is regulated both over gestation and in response to intrauterine growth restriction as is expression of the sodium-potassium ATPase.

Calcium

Calcium is an essential nutrient for the developing fetus. Ionized calcium levels are higher in fetal than in maternal blood. Higher fetal calcium levels are due to a syncytiotrophoblast basal membrane ATP-dependent Ca^{++} transport system exhibiting high affinity (nanomolar range) for calcium. Indeed, analogous to amino acid and sodium/hydrogen exchange proteins, multiple isoforms of the plasma membrane calcium ATPase (PMCA 1 to 4) are expressed within the placenta[23]; the placental expression of PMCA3 has been linked to intrauterine bone accrual. Sodium/calcium exchange proteins (NCX) may also play a role in extrusion of calcium from the trophoblast—again, multiple isoforms are expressed within the placenta. A variety of calcium channels have been identified in both the apical and basal membranes; TRPV6 plays a significant role in calcium uptake into the syncytiotrophoblast.[23] Intracellular calcium is bound by multiple calcium binding proteins, which have been identified within the placenta; these include CaBP9k, CaBP28k, CaBP57k, oncomodulin, S-100P, S-100alpha, and S-100beta. CaBP9K in particular is thought to have a regulatory and perhaps rate-limiting role. Calcium transport across the placenta is increased by the calcium-dependent regulatory protein calmodulin regulated by 1,25 dihydroxycholecalciferol, calcitonin, parathyroid hormone–related protein, and parathyroid hormone.

Receptor-Mediated Endocytosis/Exocytosis

Endocytosis, via the clatharin-dependent endocytosis pathway, has long been known to occur within the placenta. Placental endocytosis plays a critical role in cell signaling; examples include insulin and EGF receptors, protein recycling (receptors, transporters), substrate transfer (LDL receptor), and transcytosis (immunoglobulin, taken up by endocytosis, and transferred from the maternal to the fetal circulation). The general mechanisms underlying these processes include postligand binding, cell entry, and processing. Following ligand binding, the receptors aggregate on the cell surface and collect in specialized membrane structures termed *clatharin-coated pits* (Figure 2-3). These coated pits invaginate, pinch off, and enter the cell to form vesicles, which fuse to form endosomes. The endosomes move deeper into the cytoplasm where the lower endosome pH facilitates ligand separation from its receptor.

The fate of ligand and receptor differs depending on the specific substrate: Although insulin receptor is probably recycled to the cell surface, maternal insulin does not reach the fetal circulation due to lysosomal degradation. Cholesterol enters the syncytiotrophoblast via the LDL- or HDL-binding scavenger receptors, among others, and may be used for trophoblast pregnenolone/progesterone synthesis and/or transferred across the basal membrane, in part via the ATP-binding cassette transporter.[24] The cholesterol is subsequently transferred across the fetal endothelium into the fetal circulation via ATP-binding cassette transporters ABCA1 and ABCG1. **IgG remains complexed to its receptor (the neonatal Fc receptor [FcRn]) and is transferred to the fetus intact via exocytosis at the basal trophoblast membrane. Immunoglobulin that cannot bind to this receptor is degraded within the placenta.[25] Ferrotransferrin carries two ferric ions per molecule and is unique in that it does not separate from the transferrin receptor. Rather, the iron dissociates and binds to ferritin, a cytoplasmic iron-storing protein.** Iron is thought to then escape the trophoblast via ferroportin, to be picked up at the basal side of the cell by fetal apotransferrin, while the maternal apotransferrin/transferrin receptor complex is recycled to the syncytiotrophoblast microvillous membrane.[26,27]

Endocytosis may also occur via caveolin-dependent and lipid-raft associated mechanisms. The mechanisms are not well understood within the placenta; however, the norepinephrine transporter is recycled by the latter mechanism in trophoblast cells.[28]

Placental Blood Flow

The transport characteristics of the placenta allow respiratory gases and many solutes to reach equal concentration

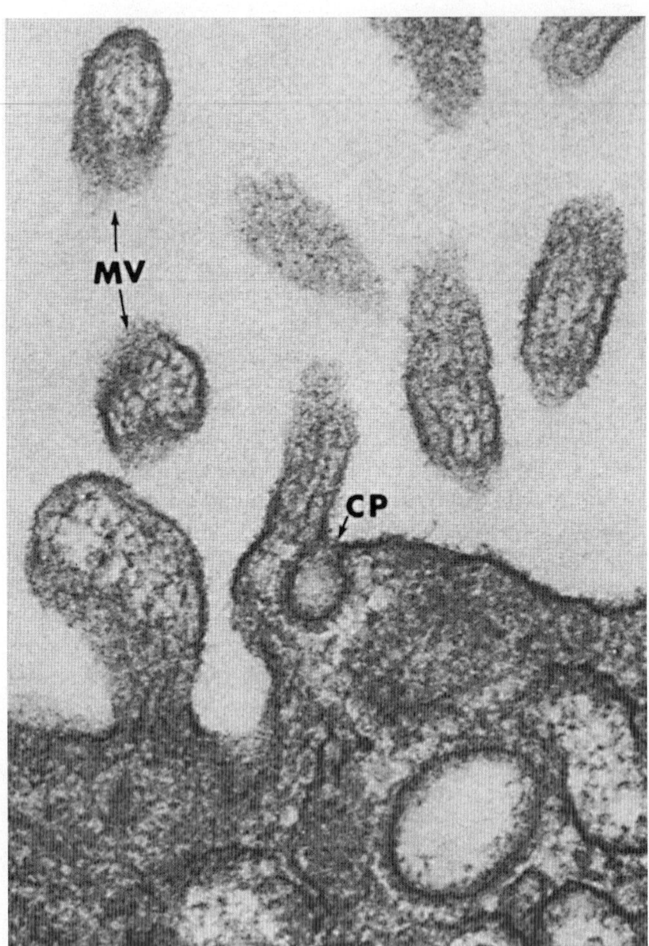

FIGURE 2-3. Electron micrograph of human placental microvillous plasma membrane demonstrating presence of a coated pit *(CP)*. Note the presence of cytoskeletal components extending into the microvillous space *(MV)*. (Courtesy of Kent L. Thornburg, Ph.D., Department of Physiology, Oregon Health Sciences University, Portland, OR.)

between the maternal intervillous space blood (derived from uterine blood flow) and fetal capillary blood (derived from umbilical blood flow). Thus, the rate of blood flow in these two circulations is an important determinant of fetal oxygen and nutrient supply.

Uterine Blood Flow

Uterine blood flow during pregnancy supplies the myometrium, endometrium, and placenta, with the latter receiving nearly 90% of total uterine blood flow near term. Thus, interest has focused primarily on regulation of uteroplacental blood flow. Over the course of a normal singleton ovine gestation, uterine blood flow increases more than 50-fold above nonpregnant values. This long-term increase in uterine blood flow is accompanied by a doubling of maternal cardiac output and a 40% increase in blood volume. **Two primary factors contribute to this dramatic increase in uterine blood flow: placental growth and maternal arterial vasodilation.** Along with fetal and placental growth, placental intervillous space volume almost triples between weeks 22 and 36 of gestation. Thus, the marked growth of the maternal placental vascular bed is consistent with the increase in placental diffusing capacity. **Second, the increase in blood flow is due in part to a direct**

estrogen-induced vasodilation of the uterine vasculature. This effect is mediated through the release of nitric oxide.[29] These combined effects provide uterine blood flow rates at term of at least 750 mL/min, or 10% to 15% of maternal cardiac output. The uterine artery behaves as a nearly maximally dilated system; a number of local vasodilatory agents contribute to this effect including prostanoids (PGI_2), nitric oxide, and kinins.[30] Still, uterine blood flow is subject to short-term regulatory influences. Systemically administered vasodilator agents preferentially dilate systemic vessels, reducing uterine blood flow. Thus, concerns regarding administration of antihypertensive agents or regional anesthesia with sympathetic blockade are well founded. **Although pregnant women display a refractoriness to infused pressor agents,[31] including angiotensin, pressor agent–induced increases in uterine vascular resistance may exceed increases in systemic vascular resistance, reducing uteroplacental blood flow. Thus, increased maternal plasma catecholamine levels during preeclampsia or pressor agents administered for treatment of maternal hypotension may have adverse effects on uterine blood flow.** Although respiratory gases are important regulators of blood flow in a number of organs, there is no indication that either oxygen or carbon dioxide are responsible for short-term changes in uterine blood flow. During uterine contractions the relationship between uterine arterial and venous pressures and blood flow no longer holds. Since intrauterine pressures are directly transmitted to the intervillous space, increases in intrauterine pressure are reflected by decreases in placental blood flow. Calcitonin gene–related peptide produces uterine artery relaxation and enhances uterine artery blood flow and improved fetal growth. **Phosphodiesterase 5–specific inhibitors, including sildenafil, tadalafil, and vardenafil, enhance nitric oxide's vasodilatory effect by inhibition of cGMP (second messenger in the nitric oxide cascade) breakdown, with resultant relaxation of vascular smooth muscle.[32]** Evidence in animal models suggests that fetal outcomes may be improved by these agents.[33] Conversely, it is not surprising that diminished uterine artery blood flow is associated with diminished fetal growth, presumably because of diminished substrate transfer (nutrient, ions, oxygen, etc.) from mother to fetus.

Umbilical Blood Flow

Fetal blood flow to the umbilical circulation represents approximately 40% of the combined output of both fetal ventricles.[34] Over the last third of gestation, increases in umbilical blood flow are proportional to fetal growth, so that umbilical blood flow remains constant when normalized to fetal weight. Human umbilical venous flow can be estimated through the use of triplex mode ultrasonography. Although increases in villous capillary number represent the primary contributor to gestation-dependent increases in umbilical blood flow, the factors that regulate this change are not known. A number of important angiogenic peptides and factors, including VEGF, have been identified.[35] Short-term changes in umbilical blood flow are primarily regulated by perfusion pressure. The relationship between flow and perfusion pressure is linear in the umbilical circulation. As a result, small (2 to 3 mm Hg) increases in umbilical vein pressure evoke proportional decreases in umbilical blood flow. Because both the umbilical artery and vein are enclosed in the amniotic cavity, pressure changes caused by increases in uterine tone are transmitted equally to these vessels without changes in umbilical blood flow. Relative to the uteroplacental bed, the fetoplacental circulation is resistant to vasoconstrictive effects of infused pressor agents, and umbilical blood flow is preserved unless cardiac output decreases. Thus, despite catecholamine-induced changes in blood flow distribution, and increases in blood pressure during acute hypoxia, umbilical blood flow is maintained over a relatively wide range of oxygen tensions. Endogenous vasoactive autacoids have been identified; nitric oxide may also be important. Endothelin-1, in particular, is associated with diminished fetoplacental blood flow.[36]

Immunologic Properties of the Placenta

The syncytiotrophoblast in contact with maternal blood in the intervillous space and the amniochorion in contact with maternal decidua represent the fetal tissues most prone to immunologic reactions from maternal factors. Maternal tolerance of fetal tissue is an area of active, if as yet incomplete, investigation. A variety of immunoregulatory cells are present within the placental bed; these include uterine natural killer cells, macrophages, dendritic cells, T regulatory cells,T lymphocytes, and natural killer T cells. These cells may vary both numerically and functionally throughout gestation.[37] The manner in which immunoregulatory cells interact with fetal derived tissues to allow tolerance remains an area of intense investigation, but as yet consensus has not been reached. It is likely, however, that they participate in not only the development of fetal tolerance, but also in the establishment of placental vasculature, and in limitation of extravillous trophoblast migration once the vascular bed has been sufficiently established.

Trophoblast cells contain a unique complement of histocompatibility antigens, which are integral to the host's recognition of self and non-self. Neither beta-2-microglobulin (which is tightly associated with HLA antigens) nor the HLA antigens A, B, DR, or DC can be demonstrated on the surface of syncytiotrophoblast. This is thought to be the result of the epigenetic silencing of the Class II transactivator gene within the trophoblast. Invasive human cytotrophoblasts (extravillous trophoblast) express a trophoblast-specific, nonclassical class 1b antigen, HLA-G (reviewed in reference 38), in addition to the more widely disseminated HLA-C and HLA-E, each of which serves as a ligand for uterine natural killer (uNK) cells, the predominant leukocyte type found within the maternal-fetal junction in early gestation.[38] These ligands interact with specific killer-cell immunoglobulin-like receptors (KIRs) on uNK cells. Postulated roles for HLA-G include protection of invasive cytotrophoblast from uNK cells, as well as containment of placental infection. HLA-G is also coexpressed with HLA-E, allowing it to be recognized by KIRs, which then induce inhibition of uNK cells. The interaction of uNK cells and HLA-C appears to be more complex, in that, depending on the combinatorial pattern of KIRs and HLA-C alleles present, uterine invasion by extravillous trophoblast can be either facilitated of inhibited, leading, perhaps, to the development of preeclampsia.[39] Trophoblasts also express HLA-F, but the function and interactions of this antigen remain uncertain.

Other postulated "protective" mechanisms include the presence of proteins that "deactivate" the local complement system, alteration of lymphocytes from a Th1 to a Th2 secretory phenotype, associated with a cytokine profile more conducive to fetal survival, as well as a mechanism by which the fetal membranes may facilitate the apoptosis of specific maternal immunoregulatory cells. Others have shown that indoleamine 2,3-dioxygenase (IDO), which breaks down tryptophan, may be important in the control of maternal lymphocytes; blocking this enzyme activity was associated with a high rate of fetal abortion.[39] In summary, immunologic aspects of the placenta are difficult to separate out from those of the maternal uterus and the mixed deciduas. It is now clear, however, that multiple, elegant, overlapping mechanisms ensure the survival of the placenta, and thus the fetus, in an immunologically hostile environment. For a detailed review of immunology in pregnancy, see Chapter 4.

Amniotic Fluid Volume

Mean amniotic fluid volume increases from 250 to 800 mL between 16 and 32 weeks' gestation. Despite considerable variability, the average volume remains stable up to 39 weeks and then declines to about 500 mL at 42 weeks. The origin of amniotic fluid during the first trimester of pregnancy is uncertain. Possible sources include a transudate of maternal plasma through the chorioamnion or a transudate of fetal plasma through the highly permeable fetal skin, before keratinization. The origin and dynamics of amniotic fluid are better understood beginning in the second trimester, when the fetus becomes the primary determinant. **Amniotic fluid volume is maintained by a balance of fetal fluid production (lung liquid and urine) and fluid resorption (fetal swallowing and flow across the amniotic and/or chorionic membranes to the fetus or maternal uterus).**[40]

The fetal lung secretes fluid at a rate of 300 to 400 mL/day near term. Chloride is actively transferred from alveolar capillaries to the lung lumen, and water follows the chloride gradient. Thus, lung fluid represents a nearly protein-free transudate with an osmolarity similar to that of fetal plasma. Fetal lung fluid does not appear to regulate fetal body fluid homeostasis, as fetal intravenous volume loading does not increase lung fluid secretion. Rather, lung fluid likely serves to maintain lung expansion and facilitate pulmonary growth. **Lung fluid must decrease at parturition to provide for the transition to respiratory ventilation.** Notably, several hormones that increase in fetal plasma during labor (i.e., catecholamines, arginine vasopressin [AVP]) also decrease lung fluid production. With the reduction of fluid secretion, the colloid osmotic gradient between fetal plasma and lung fluid results in lung fluid resorption across the pulmonary epithelium, and clearance via lymphatics. **The absence of this process explains the increased incidence of transient tachypnea of the newborn, or "wet lung," in infants delivered by cesarean section in the absence of labor.**

Fetal urine is the primary source of amniotic fluid, with outputs at term varying from 400 to 1200 mL/day. Between 20 and 40 weeks' gestation, fetal urine production increases about tenfold, in the presence of marked renal maturation. The urine is normally hypotonic and the low osmolarity of fetal urine accounts for the hypotonicity of amniotic fluid in late gestation relative to maternal and fetal plasma. Numerous fetal endocrine factors, including AVP, atrial natriuretic factor (ANF), angiotensin II (AII), aldosterone, and prostaglandins, alter fetal renal blood flow, glomerular filtration rate, or urine flow rates.[41] In response to fetal stress, endocrine-mediated reductions in fetal urine flow may explain the association between fetal hypoxia and oligohydramnios. The regulation of fetal urine production is discussed further under Fetal Kidney later in this chapter.

Fetal swallowing is believed to be a major route of amniotic fluid resorption although swallowed fluid contains a mixture of amniotic and tracheal fluids. Human fetal swallowing has been demonstrated by 18 weeks' gestation,[42] with daily swallowed volumes of 200 to 500 mL near term. Similar to fetal urine flow, daily fetal swallowed volumes (per body weight) are markedly greater than adult values. With the development of fetal neurobehavioral states, fetal swallowing occurs primarily during active sleep states associated with respiratory and eye movements.[43] Moderate increases in fetal plasma osmolality increase the number of swallowing episodes and volume swallowed, indicating the presence of an intact thirst mechanism in the near-term fetus.

Because amniotic fluid is hypotonic with respect to maternal plasma, there is a potential for bulk water removal at the amniotic-chorionic interface with maternal or fetal plasma. Although fluid resorption to the maternal plasma is likely minimal, intramembranous flow from amniotic fluid to fetal placental vessels may contribute importantly to amniotic fluid resorption. Thus, intramembranous flow may balance fetal urine and lung liquid production with fetal swallowing to maintain normal amniotic fluid volumes.

The mechanisms by which water is transferred across the amnion into fetal vessels remains uncertain, but evidence implicates the presence of water channels within the amnion, and, as discussed previously, the placental trophoblast and fetal endothelium. Aquaporins 1, 3, 8, and 9 are found within the placenta and fetal membranes. Mice deficient in aquaporin 1 develop polyhydramnios, suggesting an important role for this protein in intramembranous water transfer.[44] Aquaporins 1 and 3 (important in transplacental water flow) are regulated by AVP and by cAMP, as well as showing changes in expression throughout gestation.[45]

FETAL PHYSIOLOGY

Growth and Metabolism

Substrates

Nutrients are utilized by the fetus for two primary purposes: oxidation for energy and tissue accretion. Under normal conditions, glucose is an important substrate for fetal oxidative metabolism. The glucose utilized by the fetus derives from the placenta rather than from endogenous glucose production. However, based on umbilical vein–to–umbilical artery glucose and oxygen concentration differences, glucose alone cannot account for fetal oxidative metabolism. In fact, glucose oxidation accounts for only two thirds of fetal carbon dioxide production.[46] Thus, fetal oxidative metabolism depends on substrates in addition to glucose. A large portion of the amino acids taken up by the umbilical circulation are used by the fetus for aerobic metabolism instead of protein synthesis. Fetal uptake for a number of amino acids actually exceeds their accretion into fetal tissues. In addition, other amino acids, notably glutamate, are taken up by the placenta from the fetal circulation and metabolized within the placenta.[47] **In fetal sheep and likely the human fetus as well, lactate also is a substrate for fetal oxygen consumption.**[46] **Thus, the combined substrates glucose, amino acids, and lactate essentially provide the approximately 87 kcal/kg/day required by the growing fetus.**

Metabolic requirements for new tissue accretion depend on the growth rate and the type of tissue acquired. Although the newborn infant has relatively increased body fat, fetal fat content is low at 26 weeks. Fat acquisition increases gradually up to 32 weeks and rapidly thereafter (about 82 g [dry weight] of fat per week). Because many of the necessary enzymes for carbohydrate to lipid conversion are present in the fetus, fat acquisition reflects glucose utilization in addition to placental fatty acid uptake. In contrast, fetal acquisition of nonfat tissue is linear from 32 to 39 weeks, and may decrease to only 30% of the fat-acquisition rate in late gestation (about 43 g [dry weight] per week).

Hormones

The role of select hormones in the regulation of placental growth was discussed previously under Placental Metabolism and Growth. Fetal hormones influence fetal growth through both metabolic and mitogenic effects. **Although growth hormone and growth hormone receptors are present early in fetal life, and growth hormone is essential to postnatal growth, growth hormone appears to have little role in regulating fetal growth.** Instead, changes in IGF, IGF-binding proteins, or IGF receptors explain the apparent reduced role of growth hormone on fetal growth. Most if not all tissues of the body produce IGF-I and IGF-II and both IGF-I and IGF-II are present in human fetal tissue extracts after 12 weeks' gestation. Fetal plasma IGF-I and IGF-II levels begin to increase by 32 to 34 weeks' gestation. **The increase in IGF-I levels directly correlates with increase in fetal size, and a reduction in IGF-I levels is associated with growth restriction.**[48] **In contrast, there is no correlation between serum IGF-II levels and fetal growth.** However, there is a correlation between small offspring and genetic manipulations resulting in decreased IGF-II messenger RNA production. IGF-II knockout mice are small, and knockout of the IGF-IIr results in fetal overgrowth.[49] Thus, tissue IGF-II concentrations and localized IGF-II release may be more important than circulating levels in supporting fetal growth.

IGF binding proteins (IGFBPs) modulate IGF-I and II concentrations in serum, with IGFBP1 having an inhibitory and IGFBP3 a comparatively stimulatory effect. As such, diminished fetal concentrations of IGFBP3 and enhanced concentrations of IGFBP1 have been associated with smaller fetal size.[50]

A role for insulin in fetal growth is suggested from the increases in body weight, and heart and liver weights, in infants of diabetic mothers. Insulin levels within the high physiologic range increase fetal body weight, and increases in endogenous fetal insulin significantly increase fetal glucose uptake. In addition, fetal insulin secretion increases in response to elevations in blood glucose, although the normal rapid insulin response phase is absent.[51] Plasma insulin levels sufficient to increase fetal growth also may exert mitogenic effects perhaps through insulin-induced IGF-II receptor binding. Separate receptors for insulin and IGF-II are expressed in fetal liver cells by the end of the first trimester. Hepatic insulin receptor numbers (per gram tissue) triple by 28 weeks, while IGF-II receptor numbers remain constant. Thus, although children conceived of diabetic mothers are at increased risk of cardiac defects, the growth patterns of these infants indicate insulin levels may be most important in late gestation. Though less common, equally dramatically low birth weights are associated with the absence of fetal insulin. Experimentally induced hypoinsulinemia causes a 30% decrease in fetal glucose utilization and decreases fetal growth.

As in the adult, β-adrenergic receptor activation increases fetal insulin secretion, whereas β-adrenergic activation inhibits insulin secretion. Fetal glucagon secretion also is modulated by the β-adrenergic system. However, the fetal glycemic response to glucagon is blunted, probably caused by a relative reduction in hepatic glucagon receptors.

Corticosteroids are essential for fetal growth and maturation. Corticosteroid levels within the fetus rise near partuition, in step with maturation of fetal organs such as the lung, liver, kidneys, and thymus, and slowing of fetal growth. Exogenous maternal steroid administration during pregnancy also has the potential to diminish fetal growth in humans, as well as in a variety of other species, perhaps via suppression of the IGF axis.[50] In addition to the insulin-like growth factors, a number of other factors, including epidermal growth factor, transforming growth factor, fibroblast growth factor, and nerve growth factor, are expressed during embryonic development and appear to exert specific effects during morphogenesis; for example, epidermal growth factor has specific effects on lung growth and growth and differentiation of the secondary palate, and normal sympathetic adrenergic system development is dependent on nerve growth factor. However, a specific role of these factors in regulating fetal growth remains to be defined. **Similarly, the fetal thyroid also is not important for overall fetal growth, but is important for central nervous system development.**

Substantial evidence now exists to support the view that several cell-specific growth factors and their cognate receptors play an essential role in placental growth and function in a number of species. Growth factors identified to date include family members of epidermal growth factor, transforming growth factor beta, nerve growth factor, insulin-like growth factor, hematopoietic growth factors, vascular endothelial growth factor, and fibroblast growth factor. A number of cytokines also play a role in normal placental development. The expression, ontogeny, and regulation of most but not all of these growth factors have been explored. In vitro placental cell culture studies support the concept that growth factors and cytokines exert their functions locally promoting proliferation and differentiation through their autocrine and/or paracrine mode of actions. For example, epidermal growth factor (EGF) promotes cell proliferation, invasion, or differentiation depending on the gestational age. Hepatocyte growth factor and vascular endothelial growth factor stimulate trophoblast DNA replication whereas transforming growth factor beta suppresses cytoplast invasion and endocrine differentiation. In support of local actions, functional receptors for various growth factors have been demonstrated on trophoblast and other cells. Various intracellular signal proteins and transcription factors that respond to growth factors are also expressed in placenta. A number of elegant studies have identified alterations in growth factors and growth factor receptors in association with placental and fetal growth restriction. Placental defects in growth factor(s) and receptor(s) pathways, explored through the use of transgenic and mutant mice, have provided potential mechanisms for explaining complications of human placental development.[52] **An illustrative example is EGF, a potent mitogen for epidermal and mesodermal cells that is expressed in human placenta. EGF is involved in embryonal implantation, stimulates syncytiotrophoblast differentiation in vitro, and modulates production and secretion of human chorionic gonadotrophin and placental lactogen.** The effects of EGF are mediated by EGF-receptor (EGF-R), a transmembrane glycoprotein with intrinsic tyrosine kinase activity. EGF-R is expressed on the apical microvillus plasma membrane fractions from early, middle, and term whole placentas. Placental EGF-R expression is regulated by locally expressed parathyroid hormone–related protein, itself important in placental differentiation and maternal-fetal calcium flux.[53,54] Decreased EGF-R expression has been demonstrated in association with intrauterine growth restriction. **Targeted disruption of EGF-R has shown to result in fetal death due to placental defects.**[55] **Overexpression of EGF-R activity results in placental enlargement.**[56]

The EGF family now consists of at least 15 members, many of which have been identified in human placenta. Future studies should reveal whether EGF family members play distinct or overlapping functions in mediating placental growth.

Control of fetal growth may occur via the impact of growth factors/hormones on the placenta or may occur as a direct result of action in and on the fetus. It is clear that nutrition may play a role in these processes. However, the number of genes/gene products known to control or affect fetal growth continues to increase. **Imprinted genes (expressed primarily from maternally or paternally acquired allele) play a particularly important role in controlling fetal growth.**[57] **Abnormalities in the expression of these genes often result in fetal overgrowth or undergrowth.** Environmental influences, such as alterations in gene methylation, or in modification of histones associated with genes, may further alter gene expression, and thus fetal growth, making this a rich area for further exploration.

Fetal Cardiovascular System

Development

The heart and the vascular system develop from splanchnic mesoderm during the third week after fertilization. The two primordial heart tubes fuse, forming a simple contractile tube early in the fourth week, and the cardiovascular system becomes the first functional organ system. **During weeks 5 to 8 this single-lumen tube is converted into the definitive four-chambered heart through a process of cardiac looping (folding), remodeling, and partitioning.** However, an opening in the interatrial septum, the foramen ovale, is present and serves as an important right-to-left shunt during fetal life.

During the fourth embryonic week three primary circulations characterize the vascular system. The aortic/cardinal circulation serves the embryo proper and is the basis for much of the fetal circulatory system. Of note the left sixth aortic (pulmonary) arch forms a connection between the left pulmonary artery and the aorta as the ductus arteriosus. **The ductus arteriosus also functions as a right-to-left shunt by redistributing right ventricular output from the lungs to the aorta and fetal and placental circulations.** The vitelline circulation develops in association with the yolk sac, and though it plays a minor role in providing nutrients to the embryo, its rearrangement ultimately provides the circulatory system for the gastrointestinal tract, spleen, pancreas, and liver. The allantoic circulation develops in association with the chorion and the developing chorionic villi, and forms the placental circulation, comprised of two umbilical arteries and two umbilical veins. **In humans, the venous pathways are rearranged during embryonic weeks 4 to 8 and only the left umbilical vein is retained. Subsequent rearrangement of the vascular plexus associated with the developing liver forms the ductus venosus, a venous shunt that allows at least half of the estimated umbilical blood flow (70 to 130 mL/min/kg fetal weight after 30 weeks' gestation) to bypass the liver and enter the inferior vena cava.**[58]

Placental gas exchange provides well-oxygenated blood that leaves the placenta (Figure 2-4) via the umbilical vein. In addition to the ductus venosus, small branches into the left lobe of the liver and a major branch to the right lobe account for the remainder of umbilical venous flow. Left hepatic vein blood combines with the well-oxygenated ductus venosus flow as it enters the inferior vena cava. Because right hepatic vein blood combines with the portal vein (only a small fraction of portal vein blood passes through the ductus venosus), right hepatic vein blood is less oxygenated than its counterpart on the left,[58] and

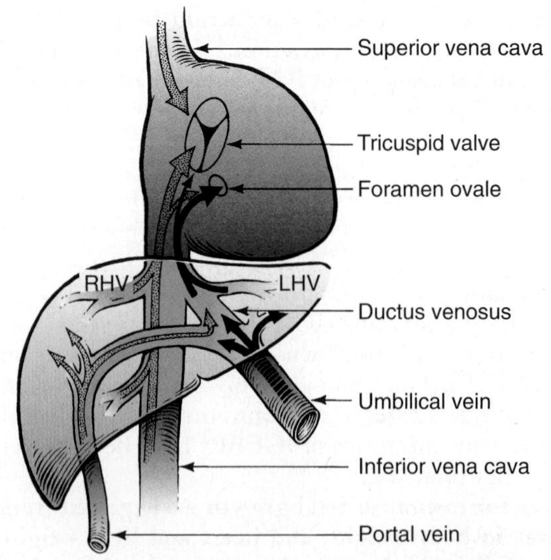

Figure 2-4. Anatomy of the umbilical and hepatic circulation. *Dark arrows* represent nutrient-rich and oxygen-rich blood. *LHV,* Left hepatic vein; *RHV,* right hepatic vein. (From Rudolph AM: Hepatic and ductus venosus blood flows during fetal life. Hepatology 3:254, 1983.)

combination of right hepatic/portal drainage with blood returning from the lower trunk and limbs further decreases the oxygen content. Although both ductus venosus blood and hepatic portal/fetal trunk bloods enter the inferior vena cava and the right atrium, little mixing occurs. **This stream of well-oxygenated ductus venosus blood is preferentially directed into the foramen ovale by the valve of the inferior vena cava and the crista dividens on the wall of the right atrium. This shunts a portion of the most highly oxygenated ductus venosus blood through the foramen ovale with little opportunity for mixing with superior vena cava/coronary sinus venous return** (Figures 2-4 and 2-5). **As a result, left atrial filling results primarily from umbilical vein–ductus venosus blood, with a small contribution from pulmonary venous flow. Thus, blood with the highest oxygen content is delivered to the left atrium and left ventricle, and ultimately supplies blood to the upper body and limbs, carotid and vertebral circulations, and the brain.** Inferior vena cava flow is larger than the volume that can cross the foramen ovale. The remainder of the oxygenated inferior vena cava blood is directed through the tricuspid valve (see Figure 2-4) into the right ventricle (see Figure 2-5) and is accompanied by venous return from the superior vena cava and coronary sinus. However, the very high vascular resistance in the pulmonary circulation maintains mean pulmonary artery pressure 2 to 3 mm Hg above aortic pressure and directs most of the right ventricular output through the ductus arteriosus and into the aorta and the fetal and placental circulations.[58]

Fetal Heart

The adult cardiovascular system includes a high-pressure (95 mm Hg) system and a low-pressure pulmonary circuit (15 mm Hg) driven by the left and right ventricles working in series. Although the ejection velocity is greater in the left ventricle than in the right, equal volumes of blood are delivered into the systemic and pulmonary circulations with contraction of each ventricle. The stroke volume is the volume of blood ejected by the left ventricle with each contraction, and cardiac output is a function of the stroke volume and heart rate (70 mL/beat × 72 beats/min = 5040 mL/min). For a 70-kg adult man, cardiac output averages 72 mL/min/kg. In addition to heart rate, cardiac output varies with changes in stroke volume, which in turn is determined by venous return (preload), pulmonary artery and aortic pressures (afterload), and contractility.

In contrast to the adult heart, where the two ventricles pump blood in a series circuit, the unique fetal shunts provide an unequal distribution of venous return to the respective atria, and ventricular output represents a mixture of oxygenated and deoxygenated blood. **Thus, the fetal right and left ventricles function as two pumps operating in parallel rather than in series, and cardiac output is described as the combined ventricular output. Right ventricular output exceeds 60% of biventricular output[59] and is primarily directed through the ductus arteriosus to the descending aorta (see Figure 2-5). As a result, placental blood flow, which represents over 50% of the combined ventricular output, primarily reflects right ventricular output. Because of the high pulmonary vascular resistance,[59] the pulmonary circulation receives only 5% to 10% of the combined ventricular output.** Instead, left ventricular output is primarily directed through the ductus arteriosus to the upper body and head. Estimates of fetal left ventricular output average 120 mL/min/kg body weight. If left ventricular output is less than 40% of the combined biventricular output,[59] total fetal cardiac output would be above 300 mL/min/kg. The distribution of the cardiac output to fetal organs is summarized in Table 2-1,[34] with fetal hepatic distribution reflecting only the portion supplied by the hepatic artery. In fact, hepatic blood flow derives principally from the umbilical vein and to a lesser extent the portal vein,[60] and represents about 25% of the total venous return to the heart.

The placenta receives approximately 50% of the combined ventricular output, which means the single umbilical vein also conducts 50% of the combined ventricular output. At least half of the umbilical venous blood bypasses the liver via the ductus venosus, and the remainder traverses

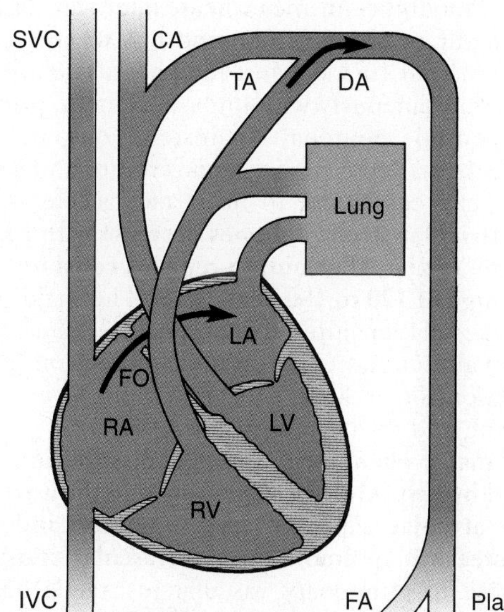

FIGURE 2-5. Anatomy of fetal heart and central shunts. *SVC*, superior vena cava; *CA*, Carotid artery; *TA*, thoracic aorta; *DA*, ductus arteriosus; *RA*, right atrium; *FO*, foramen ovale; *LA*, left atrium; *RV*, right ventricle; *LV*, left ventricle; *IVC*, inferior vena cava; *FA*, femoral artery. (From Anderson DF, Bissonnette JM, Faber JJ, Thornburg KL: Central shunt flows and pressures in the mature fetal lamb. Am J Physiol 241:H60, 1981.)

TABLE 2-1 GASTROINTESTINAL TRACT PERCENTAGE OF BIVENTRICULAR 40.5 (HEPATIC ARTERY)

ORGAN	PERCENTAGE OF BIVENTRICULAR CARDIAC OUTPUT
Placenta	40
Brain	13
Heart	3.5
Lung	7
Liver	2.5 (hepatic artery)
Gastrointestinal tract	5
Adrenal glands	0.5
Kidney	2.5
Spleen	1
Body	25

Data from Rudolph AM, Heymann MA: Circulatory changes during growth in the fetal lamb. Circ Res 26(3):289, 1970.

the hepatic circulation. The combination of umbilical vein blood, hepatic portal blood, and blood returning from the lower body contributes approximately 69% of the cardiac output that enters the right atrium from the inferior vena cava. Flow across the foramen ovale accounts for approximately one third (27%) of the combined cardiac output.[59] Pulmonary venous return to the left atrium is low and represents approximately 7% of combined ventricular output. Thus, the left atrium accounts for only about 34% (27% + 7%) of the combined ventricular output. Because a volume of inferior vena cava venous return equivalent to 27% of the combined ventricular output is shunted across the foramen ovale, 42% remains in the right atrium and contributes to right ventricular output. With another 21% from the superior vena cava and 3% from the coronary circulation, right ventricular output accounts for 66% of the combined ventricular output. However, only 7% of right ventricular output enters the pulmonary circulation, leaving 59% entering the aorta via the ductus arteriosus. Similarly, 24% of the combined ventricular output derived from the left ventricle is distributed to the upper body and brain, with approximately 10% combining with right ventricular output in the aorta. Thus, 69% of the combined ventricular output reaches the descending aorta and 50% of this accounts for placental flow, with the remainder distributed to the fetal abdominal organs and lower body.

Consistent with the greater contribution of the right ventricle to combined ventricular output, coronary blood flow to the myocardium reflects the greater stroke volume of the right side, and right ventricular free wall and septal blood flows are higher than in the left ventricle.[61] It is not surprising then that fetal ventricular wall thickness is greater on the right side relative to the left. As in the adult, fetal ventricular output depends on heart rate, pulmonary artery and aortic pressures, and contractility. The relationship between mean right atrial pressure (the index often used for ventricular volume at the end of diastole) and stroke volume is depicted in Figure 2-6. The steep ascending limb represents the length–active tension relationship for cardiac muscle in the right ventricle.[62] Under normal conditions, fetal right atrial pressure resides at the break point

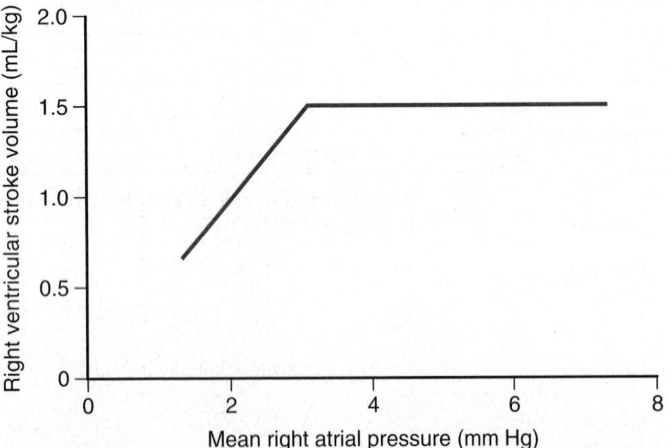

FIGURE 2-6. Stroke volume of the fetal right ventricle as a function of mean right atrial pressure. (From Thornburg KL, Morton MJ: Filling and arterial pressures as determinants of RV stroke volume in the sheep fetus. Am J Physiol 244:H656, 1983.)

in this ascending limb and increases in pressure do not increase stroke volume. Thus, the contribution of Starling mechanisms to increasing right heart output in the fetus is limited. In contrast, decreases in venous return and right atrial pressure decrease stroke volume. Compared to the left ventricle, the fetal right ventricle has a greater anteroposterior dimension, increasing both volume and circumferential radius of curvature. This anatomic difference increases the radius/wall thickness ratio for the right ventricle, producing increased wall stress in systole and a decrease in stroke volume when afterload increases.[61] Because the right ventricle is sensitive to afterload, a linear inverse relationship exists between stroke volume and pulmonary artery pressure.[62]

The relationship between atrial pressure and stroke volume in the left ventricle is similar to that shown in Figure 2-6 for the right ventricle. Although the break point occurs near the normal value for left atrial pressure, there is a small amount of preload reserve.[61] In distinction to the fetal right ventricle, the left side is not sensitive to aortic pressure increases. Thus, postnatal increases in systemic blood pressure do not decrease left ventricular stroke volume, and left ventricular output increases to meet the needs of the postnatal systemic circulation. Although Starling mechanism–related increases in stroke volume are limited, especially in the right side of the heart, late-gestation fetal heart β-adrenergic receptor numbers are similar to those in the adult, and circulating catecholamine induced increases in contractility may increase stroke volume by 50%.

Although fetal heart rate decreases during the last half of gestation, particularly between 20 and 30 weeks, fetal heart rate averages more than twofold above resting adult heart rates. If analysis is confined to episodes of low heart rate variability, mean heart rate decreases from 30 weeks to term. However, if all heart rate data are analyzed, mean heart rate is stable at 142 beats/min over the last 10 weeks of gestation. Variability in mean heart rate over 24 hours includes a nadir between 2 A.M. and 6 A.M. and a peak between 8 A.M. and 10 A.M. Most fetal heart rate accelerations occur simultaneously with limb movement, primarily reflecting central neuronal brainstem output. Also, movement-related decreases in venous return and a reflex tachycardia may contribute to heart rate accelerations.[63] **Because ventricular stroke volumes decrease with increasing heart rate, fetal cardiac output remains constant over a heart rate range of 120 to 180 beats/min.** The major effect of this inverse relationship between heart rate and stroke volume is an alteration in end-diastolic dimension. If end-diastolic dimension is kept constant, there is no fall in stroke volume and cardiac output increases.

At birth major changes in vascular distribution occur with the first breath. Alveolar expansion and the associated increase in alveolar capillary oxygen tension induces a marked decrease in pulmonary microvascular resistance. This decrease in pulmonary vascular resistance has two effects. First, there is an accompanying decrease in right atrial afterload and right atrial pressure. Second, the increase in pulmonary flow increases venous return into the left atrium and therefore left atrial pressure. The combined effect of these two events is to increase left atrial pressure above right atrial pressure and provides a physiologic closure of the foramen ovale. The return of the highly oxygenated blood from the lungs to the left atrium, left ventricle, and aorta and the decrease in pulmonary vascular resistance and hence pulmonary trunk pressure allow backflow of the oxygen-rich blood into the ductus arteriosus. **This local increase in ductus arteriosus oxygen tension alters the ductus response to prostaglandins and causes a marked localized vasoconstriction. Concurrent spontaneous constriction (or clamping) of the umbilical cord stops placental blood flow, reducing venous return and perhaps augmenting the decrease in right atrial pressure.**

Autonomic Regulation of Cardiovascular Function

Through reflex stimulation of peripheral baroreceptors, chemoreceptors, and central mechanisms, the sympathetic and parasympathetic systems have important roles in the regulation of fetal heart rate, cardiac contractility, and vascular tone. The fetal sympathetic system develops early, whereas the parasympathetic system develops somewhat later.[64] Nevertheless, in the third trimester, increasing parasympathetic tone accounts for the characteristic decrease in fetal heart rate with periods of reduced fetal heart rate reactivity. As evidence, fetal heart rate increases in the presence of parasympathetic blockade with atropine. Opposing sympathetic and parasympathetic inputs to the fetal heart contribute to R-R interval variability from one heart cycle to the next, and to basal heart rate variability over periods of a few minutes. However, even when sympathetic and parasympathetic inputs are removed, a level of variability remains.

Fetal sympathetic innervation is not essential for blood pressure maintenance when circulating catecholamines are present. Nevertheless, fine control of blood pressure and fetal heart rate requires an intact sympathetic system. In the absence of functional adrenergic innervation, hypoxia-induced increases in peripheral, renal, and splanchnic bed vascular resistances and blood pressure are not seen.[65] However, hypoxia-related changes in pulmonary, myocardial, adrenal, and brain blood flows occur in the absence of sympathetic innervation, indicating that both local and endocrine effects contribute to regulation of blood flow in these organs.

Receptors in the carotid body and arch of the aorta respond to pressor or respiratory gas stimulation with afferent modulation of heart rate and vascular tone. Fetal baroreflex sensitivity, in terms of the magnitude of decreases in heart rate per millimeter of mercury increase in blood pressure, is blunted relative to the adult.[66] However, fetal baroreflex sensitivity more than doubles in late gestation. Although the set-point for fetal heart rate is not believed to depend on intact baroreceptors, fetal heart rate variability increases when functional arterial baroreceptors are absent.[67] The same observation has been made for fetal blood pressure. Thus, fetal arterial baroreceptors buffer variations in fetal blood pressure during body or breathing movements.[67] Changes in baroreceptor tone likely account for the increase in mean fetal blood pressure normally observed in late gestation. In the absence of functional chemoreceptors, mean arterial pressure is maintained[67] while peripheral blood flow increases. Thus, peripheral arterial chemoreceptors may be important to maintenance of resting peripheral vascular tone. Peripheral arterial chemoreceptors also are important components in fetal reflex responses to hypoxia; the initial bradycardia is not seen without functional chemoreceptors.

Hormonal Regulation of Cardiovascular Function

Adrenocorticotropic hormone (ACTH) and catecholamines are discussed under Fetal Adrenal and Thyroid later in this chapter.

Arginine Vasopressin

Significant quantities of AVP are present in the human fetal neurohypophysis by completion of the first trimester. Ovine fetal plasma AVP levels increase appropriately in response to changes in fetal plasma osmolality induced directly in the fetus[68] or via changes in maternal osmolality.[69] Because of functional high- and low-pressure baroreceptors and chemoreceptor afferents, decreases in fetal intravascular volume or systemic blood pressure[70,71] also increase fetal AVP secretion. Thus, in the late-gestation fetus as in the adult, AVP secretion is regulated by both osmoreceptor and volume/baroreceptor pathways. Hypoxia-induced AVP secretion has been demonstrated beyond mid-pregnancy of ovine gestation, and reductions in fetal PO_2 of 10 mm Hg (50%) evoke profound increases in fetal plasma AVP levels (about 2 pg/mL to 200 to 400 pg/mL or more). Thus, because fetal AVP responsiveness to hypoxia is augmented relative to the adult (as much as 40-fold), and fetal responsiveness appears to increase during the last half of gestation, hypoxemia is the most potent stimulus known for fetal AVP secretion.

The cardiovascular response pattern to AVP infusion includes dose-dependent increases in fetal mean blood pressure and decreases in heart rate at plasma levels well below those required for similar effects in the adult. Receptors (V1) distinct from those mediating AVP antidiuretic effects in the kidney (V2) account for AVP contributions to fetal circulatory adjustments during hemorrhage, hypotension, and hypoxia.[72] Corticotropin-releasing factor (CRF) effects of AVP may contribute to hypoxia-induced increases in plasma ACTH and cortisol levels. In addition to effects on fetal heart rate, cardiac output, and arterial blood pressure, AVP-induced changes in peripheral, placental, myocardial, and cerebral blood flows directly parallel the cardiovascular changes associated with acute hypoxia. Because many of these responses are attenuated during AVP receptor blockade, AVP effects on cardiac output distribution may serve to facilitate O_2 availability to the fetus during hypoxic challenges. However, other hypoxia-related responses, including decreases in renal and pulmonary blood flows, and increased adrenal blood flow are not seen in response to AVP infusions.

Renin–Angiotensin II

Fetal plasma renin levels are typically elevated during late gestation.[73] A variety of stimuli including changes in tubular sodium concentration, reductions in blood volume, vascular pressure or renal perfusion pressure, and hypoxemia all increase fetal plasma renin activity. The relationship between fetal renal perfusion pressure and log plasma renin activity is similar to that of adults. Consistent with the effects of renal nerve activity on renin release in adults, fetal renin gene expression is directly modulated by renal sympathetic nerve activity.

Although fetal plasma AII levels increase in response to small changes in blood volume and hypoxemia, fetal AII and aldosterone levels do not increase in proportion to changes in plasma renin activity. This apparent uncoupling of the fetal renin-angiotensin-aldosterone system and the increase in newborn AII levels may relate to the significant contribution of the placenta to plasma AII clearance in the fetus relative to the adult. Also, limited angiotensin-converting enzyme (ACE) availability due to reduced pulmonary blood flow and direct inhibition of aldosterone secretion by the normally high circulating ANF levels may contribute. Thus, reductions in AII production and aldosterone responses to AII, augmented AII and aldosterone clearances, and the resulting reductions in AII and aldosterone levels and feedback inhibition of renin may account for the elevated renin and reduced AII and aldosterone levels typically observed during fetal life.

Angiotensin II infusion increases fetal mean arterial blood pressure. In contrast to AVP-induced bradycardia, fetal AII infusion increases heat rate (after an initial reflex bradycardia) through both a direct effect on the heart, and decreased baroreflex responsiveness. Both hormones increase fetal blood pressure similar to the levels seen with hypoxemia. However, AII does not reduce peripheral blood flow, perhaps because circulation to muscle, skin, and bone is always under maximum response to AII, thereby limiting increases in resting tone. Angiotensin II infusions also decrease renal blood flow and increase umbilical vascular resistance, although absolute placental blood flow does not change. Whereas the adult kidney contains both AII receptor subtypes (AT_1 and AT_2), the AT_2 subtype is the only form present in the human fetal kidney. Maturational differences in the AII receptor subtype expressed would be consistent with earlier studies demonstrating differing AII effects on fetal renal and peripheral vascular beds. Thus, the receptors mediating AII responses in the renal and peripheral vascular beds differ during fetal life.

Fetal Hemoglobin

The fetus exists in a state of aerobic metabolism, with arterial blood PO_2 values in the 20 to 35 mm Hg range. However, there is no evidence of metabolic acidosis. Adequate fetal tissue oxygenation is achieved by several mechanisms. Of major importance are the higher fetal cardiac output and organ blood flows. A higher hemoglobin concentration (relative to the adult) and an increase in oxygen-carrying capacity of fetal hemoglobin also contribute. The resulting leftward shift in the fetal oxygen dissociation curve relative to the adult (Figure 2-7) increases fetal blood oxygen saturation for any given oxygen tension. For example, at a partial pressure of 26.5 mm Hg, adult blood oxygen saturation is 50%, whereas fetal oxygen saturation is 70%. Thus, at a normal fetal PO_2 of 20 mm Hg, fetal whole blood oxygen saturation may be 50%.

The basis for increased oxygen affinity of fetal whole blood resides in the interaction of fetal hemoglobin with intracellular organic phosphate 2,3-diphosphoglycerate (2,3-DPG). The fetal hemoglobin (HgbF) tetramer is comprised of two α-chains (identical to adult) and two γ-chains. The latter differ from the γ-chain of adult hemoglobin (HgbA) in 39 of 146 amino acid residues. Among

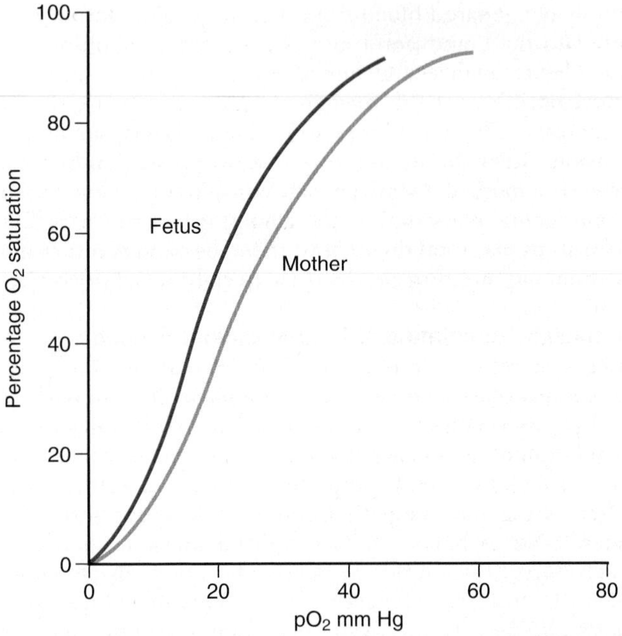

FIGURE 2-7. Oxyhemoglobin dissociation curves of maternal and fetal human blood at pH 7.4 and 37°C. (Modified from Hellegers AE, Schruefer JJP: Normograms and empirical equations relating oxygen tension, percentage saturation, and pH in maternal and fetal blood. Am J Obstet Gynecol 81:377, 1961.)

these differences is the substitution of serine in the γ-chain of HgbF for histidine at the β-143 position of HgbA, which is located at the entrance to the central cavity of the hemoglobin tetramer. Due to a positively charged imidazole group, histidine can bind with the negatively charged 2,3-DPG. Binding of 2,3-DPG to deoxyhemoglobin stabilizes the tetramer in the reduced form. Because serine is nonionized and does not interact with 2,3-DPG to the same extent as histidine, the oxygen affinity of HgbF is increased and the dissociation curve is shifted to the left. If HgbA or HgbF is removed from the erythrocyte and stripped of organic phosphates, the oxygen affinity for both hemoglobins is similar. However, addition of equal amounts of 2,3-DPG to the hemoglobins decreases HgbA oxygen affinity (dissociation curve shifts to the right) to a greater extent than for HgbF. Thus, even though overall oxygen affinities are similar, differences in 2,3-DPG interaction result in a higher oxygen affinity for HgbF.

The proportion of HgbF to HgbA changes between 26 and 40 weeks' gestation. HgbF decreases linearly from 100% to about 70% so that HgbA accounts for 30% of fetal hemoglobin at term. This change in expression from γ- to β-globulin synthesis takes place in erythroid progenitor cells. Although the basis for this switching is not yet known, our understanding of human globin gene regulation has provided important insights into several fetal hemoglobin disorders such as the thalassemias and sickle cell anemia. Duplication of the α-genes on chromosome 16 provides the normal fetus with four gene loci. The genes for the remaining globins are located on chromosome 11 and consist of ${}^{G}\gamma$, ${}^{A}\gamma$, δ and β. The two γ-genes differ in the amino acid in position 36; glycine versus alanine. Hemoglobin A synthesis is dictated by the γ- and β-genes, HgbF by α and γ, and $HgbA_2$ by α and δ. Sequences in the δ region may be responsible for the relative expression of the γ-gene, such that fetal hemoglobin persists when these are absent.

Fetal Kidney

Overall fetal water and electrolyte homeostasis is primarily mediated by fetal–maternal exchange across the placenta. However, urine production by the fetal kidney is essential to maintenance of amniotic fluid volume and composition. Although absolute glomerular filtration rate (GFR) increases during the third trimester, GFR per gram kidney weight does not change because GFR and fetal kidney weight increase in parallel. The genesis of new glomeruli is complete by about 36 weeks. Subsequent increases in GFR reflect increases in glomerular surface area for filtration, effective filtration pressure, and capillary filtration coefficient. Although glomerular filtration is related to hydrostatic pressure, and fetal blood pressure increases in the third trimester, both renal blood flow per gram kidney weight and filtration fraction (GFR/renal plasma flow) remain constant.[74] Newborn increases in filtration fraction parallel increases in arterial pressure, suggesting the lower hydrostatic pressure within the glomerulus contributes to the relatively low filtration fraction and GFR of the intrauterine kidney.[74] A mild glomerulotubular imbalance may describe the early gestation fetus. However, renal tubular sodium and chloride reabsorptions increase in late gestation, such that glomerulotubular balance is maintained in the third-trimester fetus.[74]

Although fetal GFR is low, the daily urine production rate is large (equaling 60% to 80% of the amniotic fluid volume). The large urine output results from the large portion of the filtered water (20%) that is excreted in the form of hypotonic urine. The positive free water clearance characterizing fetal renal function originally led to the hypothesis that the fetal kidney lacked AVP receptors. However, ovine fetal renal collecting duct responses to AVP can be demonstrated in the second trimester, indicating diminished urine-concentrating ability is not caused by AVP receptor absence. Fetal renal V_2 receptors mediate AVP-induced tubular water reabsorption, and functional V_2 receptors are present in the fetal kidney by the beginning of the last third of gestation.[72] In addition, AVP-induced cyclic adenosine monophosphate (cAMP) production is not different from the adult, and AVP-induced apical tubular water channels (aquaporin II) are expressed in the fetal kidney. In fact, the selective AVP V_2 receptor agonist [deamino^1,D-Arg^8]-vasopressin (dDAVP) appropriately increases fetal renal water reabsorption without affecting blood pressure or heart rate.[72] Thus, V_2 receptors mediate AVP effects on fetal urine production and amniotic fluid volume.[72] Instead, the reduced concentrating ability of the fetal kidney primarily reflects reductions in proximal tubular sodium reabsorption, short juxtamedullary nephron loops of Henle, and limited medullary interstitial urea concentrations.

Although fetal plasma renin activity levels are high, effective uncoupling of AII production from plasma renin activity and a high placental clearance rate for AII serve to minimize increases in fetal plasma AII levels. Limiting fluctuations in fetal plasma AII levels may be advantageous for fetal renal function regulation. For example, fetal AII infusion increases fetal mean arterial pressure, and renal and placental vascular resistances. In contrast, fetal treatment with the ACE inhibitor captopril increases plasma renin activity and decreases arterial blood pressure, renal vascular resistance, and filtration fraction, and urine flow effectively ceases. Given the potential for AII to decrease placental blood flow, uncoupling of renin-induced angiotensin I production, limited ACE activity, and augmented placental AII clearance may protect the fetal cardiovascular system from large increases in plasma AII levels. Collectively, plasma AII levels appear to be regulated within a very narrow range, and this regulation may be important to overall fetal homeostasis.

Atrial natriuretic factor (ANF) granules are present in the fetal heart, and fetal plasma ANF levels are elevated relative to the adult. Fetal plasma ANF levels increase in response to volume expansion, and ANF infusion evokes limited increases in ovine fetal renal sodium excretion. Fetal ANF infusion also decreases fetal plasma volume, with minimal effect on blood pressure. These observations suggest that ANF actions in the fetus are primarily directed at volume homeostasis, with minimal cardiovascular effects.

The ability of the fetal kidney to excrete titratable acid and ammonia is limited relative to the adult. In addition, the threshold for fetal renal bicarbonate excretion (defined as the excretion of a determined amount of bicarbonate per unit GFR) is much lower than in the adult. That is, fetal urine tends to be alkaline at relatively low plasma bicarbonate levels, despite the high fetal arterial P_{CO_2}. Because fetal renal tubular mechanisms for glucose reabsorption are qualitatively similar to those in the adult, fetal renal glucose excretion is limited. In fact, the maximum ability of the fetal kidney to reabsorb glucose exceeds that of the adult when expressed as a function of GFR.

Fetal Gastrointestinal System

Gastrointestinal Tract

Amniotic fluid contains measurable glucose, lactate, and amino acid concentrations, raising the possibility that fetal swallowing could serve as a source of nutrient uptake. Fetal swallowing contributes importantly to somatic growth and gastrointestinal development as a result of the large volume of ingested fluid. **About 10% to 15% of fetal nitrogen requirements may result from swallowing of amniotic fluid protein.[75] Amino acids and glucose are absorbed and utilized by the fetus if they are administered into the fetal gastrointestinal tract.[76] Furthermore, intragastric ovine fetal nutrient administration partially ameliorates fetal growth restriction induced by maternal malnutrition.[77]** Further evidence for the role of swallowing in fetal growth results from studies demonstrating that impairment of fetal rabbit swallowing at 24 days' gestation (term = 31 days) induces an 8% weight decrease (compared to controls) by 28 days.[78] The fetal gastrointestinal tract is directly affected, as esophageal ligation of fetal rabbit pups results in marked reductions in gastric and intestinal tissue weight and gastric acidity.[79] Reductions in gastrointestinal and somatic growth were reversed by fetal intragastric infusion of amniotic fluid.[79] Similarly, esophageal ligation of 90-day ovine fetuses (term = 145 to 150 days) induces a 30% decrease of small intestine villus height[80] and a reduction in liver, pancreas, and intestinal weight.[81] Although ingestion of amniotic fluid nutrients may be necessary for optimal fetal growth, trophic growth factors within the amniotic fluid also importantly contribute. Thus, the reduction in fetal rabbit weight induced by esophageal ligation is reversed by gastric infusion of epidermal growth factor.[82] Studies in human infants support the association of fetal swallowing and gastrointestinal growth as upper gastrointestinal tract obstructions are associated with a significantly greater rate of human fetal growth restriction as compared to fetuses with lower gastrointestinal obstructions.[83]

Blood flow to the fetal intestine does not increase during moderate levels of hypoxemia. The artery–mesenteric vein difference in oxygen content is also unchanged so that at a constant blood flow intestinal oxygen consumption can remain the same during moderate hypoxemia. **However, with more pronounced hypoxemia, fetal intestinal oxygen consumption falls as blood flow decreases and the oxygen content difference across the intestine fails to widen. The result is a metabolic acidosis in the blood draining the mesenteric system.**

Liver

Near term, the placenta is the major route for bilirubin elimination. Less than 10% of an administered bilirubin load is excreted in the fetal biliary tree over a 10-hour period; about 20% remains in plasma. Thus, the fetal metabolic pathways for bilirubin and bile salts remain underdeveloped at term. The cholate pool size (normalized to body surface area) is one third and the synthetic rate one half adult levels. In premature infants, cholate pool size and synthesis rates represent less than half and one third, respectively, of term infant values. In fact, premature infant intraluminal duodenal bile acid concentrations are near or below the level required to form lipid micelles.[84] The unique attributes of the fetal hepatic circulation were detailed during the earlier discussion of fetal circulatory anatomy. Notably, the fetal hepatic blood supply primarily derives from the umbilical vein. The left lobe receives its blood supply almost exclusively from the umbilical vein (there is a small contribution from the hepatic artery), whereas the right lobe receives blood from the portal vein as well. **The fetal liver under normal conditions accounts for about 20% of total fetal oxygen consumption.** Because hepatic glucose uptake and release are balanced, net glucose removal by the liver under normal conditions is minimal. During episodes of hypoxemia, β-adrenergic receptor–mediated increases in hepatic glucose release account for the hyperglycemia characteristic of short-term fetal hypoxemia.[85] **Hypoxia severe enough to decrease fetal oxygen consumption selectively reduces right hepatic lobe oxygen uptake, which exceeds that of the fetus as a whole. In contrast, oxygen uptake by the left lobe of the liver is unchanged.**

Fetal Adrenal and Thyroid

Adrenal

The fetal anterior pituitary secretes ACTH in response to "stress," including hypoxemia. The associated increase in cortisol exerts feedback inhibition of the continued ACTH response.[86] In the fetus and adult, pro-opiomelanocortin posttranslational processing gives rise to ACTH, corticotropin-like intermediate lobe peptide (CLIP), and α-melanocyte–stimulating hormone (α-MSH). The precursor peptide preproenkephalin is a distinct gene product giving rise to the enkephalins. Fetal pro-opiomelanocortin processing differs from the adult. For example, although ACTH is present in appreciable amounts, the fetal pituitary contains large amounts of CLIP and α-MSH. The fetal ratio of CLIP plus α-MSH to ACTH decreases from the end of the first trimester to term. Because pituitary corticotropin-releasing hormone (CRH) expression is relatively low until late gestation, AVP serves as the major CRF in early gestation. With increasing gestational age, fetal cortisol levels progressively increase secondary to hypothalamic-pituitary axis maturation. Cortisol is important to pituitary maturation because it shifts corticotrophs from the fetal to the adult type and to adrenal maturation through regulation of ACTH receptor numbers.[87]

On a body weight basis, the fetal adrenal gland is an order of magnitude larger than in the adult. This increase in size is due to the presence of an adrenal cortical definitive zone and a so-called fetal zone that constitutes 85% of the adrenal at birth. Cortisol and mineralocorticoids are the major products of the fetal definitive zone, and fetal cortisol secretion is regulated by ACTH but not human chorionic gonadotrophin (hCG). Low-density lipoprotein–bound cholesterol (see Receptor Mediated Endocytosis/Exocytosis earlier in this chapter) is the major source of steroid precursor in the fetal adrenal. Because the enzyme 3α-hydroxysteroid dehydrogenase is lacking in the fetal adrenal, dehydroepiandrosterone sulfate (DHEAS) is the major product of the fetal zone. At midgestation, DHEAS secretion is determined by both ACTH and hCG. Both fetal ACTH and cortisol levels are relatively low during most of gestation, and there is not a clear correlation between plasma ACTH levels and cortisol production. This apparent dissociation between fetal ACTH levels and cortisol secretion may be explained by (1) differences in ACTH processing and the presence of the large-molecular-weight pro-opiomelanocortin processing products (CLIP and α-MSH) may suppress ACTH action on the adrenal until late gestation (when ACTH becomes the primary product), (2) fetal adrenal definitive zone ACTH responsiveness may increase, or (3) placental ACTH and/or posttranslational processing intermediates may affect the adrenal response to ACTH.

Resting fetal plasma norepinephrine levels exceed epinephrine levels approximately tenfold. The fetal plasma levels of both catecholamines increase in response to hypoxemia, with norepinephrine levels invariably higher than epinephrine levels. Under basal conditions, norepinephrine is secreted at a higher rate than epinephrine, and this relationship persists during a hypoxemic stimulus. Plasma norepinephrine levels increase in response to acute hypoxemia, but decline to remain above basal levels with persistent (greater than 5 minutes) hypoxemia. In contrast, adrenal epinephrine secretion begins gradually, but persists during 30 minutes of hypoxemia. These observations are consistent with independent sites of synthesis and regulation of the two catecholamines.[88] Although the initial fetal blood pressure elevation during hypoxemia correlates with increases in norepinephrine, afterward the correlation between plasma norepinephrine and hypertension is lost.

Thyroid

The normal placenta is impermeable to thyroid-stimulating hormone (TSH), and triiodothyronine (T_3) transfer is minimal.[89] However, appreciable levels of maternal thyroxine (T_4) are seen in infants with congenital hypothyroidism. **By week 12 of gestation, thyrotropin-releasing hormone (TRH) is present in the fetal hypothalamus, and TRH secretion and/or pituitary sensitivity to TRH increases progressively during gestation. Extrahypothalamic sites including the pancreas also may contribute to the high TRH levels observed in the fetus. Measurable TSH is present in the fetal pituitary and serum, and T_4 is measurable in fetal blood by week 12 of gestation.** Thyroid function is low until about 20 weeks, when T_4 levels increase gradually to term. TSH levels increase markedly between 20 and 24 weeks, then slowly decrease until delivery. **Fetal liver T_4 metabolism is immature, characterized by low T_3 levels until week 30. In contrast, reverse T_3 levels are high until 30 weeks, thereafter declining steadily until term.**

Fetal Central Nervous System

Clinically relevant indicators of fetal central nervous system function are body movements and breathing movements. Fetal activity periods in late gestation are often termed *active* or *reactive* and *quiet* or *nonreactive*. The active cycle is characterized by clustering of gross fetal body movements, a high heart rate variability, heart rate accelerations (often followed by decelerations), and fetal breathing movements. The quiet cycle is noted by absence of fetal body movements and a low variability in the fetal heart period. Fetal heart period variability in this context refers to deviations about the model heart rate period averaged over short (seconds) periods,[90] and is distinct from beat-to-beat variability. **In the last 6 weeks of gestation, the fetus is in an active state 60% to 70% of total time. The average duration of quiet periods ranges from 15 to 23 minutes (see Table IV in Visser and colleagues[90] for a review).**

The fetal electrocorticogram shows two predominant patterns. Low-voltage (high-frequency) electrocortical activity is associated with bursts of rapid eye movements and fetal breathing movements. Similar to rapid eye movement sleep in the adult, inhibition of skeletal muscle movement is most pronounced in muscle groups having a high percentage of spindles. Thus, the diaphragm, which is relatively spindle free, is not affected. Fetal body movements during low-voltage electrocortical activity are reduced relative to the activity seen during high-voltage (low-frequency) electrocortical activity.[91] Polysynaptic reflexes elicited by stimulation of afferents from limb muscles are relatively suppressed when the fetus is in the low-voltage state.[92] Short-term hypoxia[91] or hypoxemia inhibit reflex limb movements, with the inhibitory neural activity arising in the midbrain area.[92] Fetal cardiovascular and behavioral responses to maternal cocaine use previously have been attributed to reductions in uteroplacental blood flow and resulting fetal hypoxia. However, fetal sheep studies indicate acute fetal cocaine exposure evokes catecholamine, cardiovascular, and neurobehavioral effects in the absence of fetal oxygenation changes.[93] It is not yet clear whether cocaine-induced reductions in fetal low-voltage electrocortical activity reflect changes in cerebral blood flow or a direct cocaine effect on norepinephrine stimulation of central regulatory centers. However, these observations are consistent with the significant neurologic consequences of cocaine use during pregnancy.

Fetal breathing patterns are rapid and irregular in nature, and are not associated with significant fluid movement into the lung.[94] The central medullary respiratory chemoreceptors are stimulated by carbon dioxide,[95] and fetal breathing is maintained only if central hydrogen ion concentrations remain in the physiologic range. That is, central (medullary cerebrospinal fluid) acidosis stimulates respiratory incidence and depth and alkalosis results in apnea. Paradoxically, hypoxemia markedly decreases breathing activity, possibly due to inhibitory input from centers above the medulla.[96]

Glucose is the principal substrate for oxidative metabolism in the fetal brain under normal conditions. During low-voltage electrocortical activity, cerebral blood flow and oxygen consumption are increased relative to high-voltage values, with an efflux of lactate. During high voltage the fetal brain shows a net uptake of lactate.[97] The fetal cerebral circulation is sensitive to changes in arterial oxygen content. Despite marked hypoxia-induced increases in cerebral blood flow, cerebral oxygen consumption is maintained without widening of the arterial-venous oxygen content difference across the brain.[98] Increases in carbon dioxide also cause cerebral vasodilation. However, the response to hypercarbia is reduced relative to the adult.

SUMMARY

The fetus and placenta depend on unique physiologic systems to provide an environment supporting fetal growth and development, in preparation for transition to extrauterine life. Because specific functions of the various physiologic systems are often gestation specific, differences between the fetus and adult of one species are often larger than the differences between systems. Thus, the clinician or investigator concerned with fetal life or neonatal transition must fully appreciate these aspects of fetal physiology and their application to their area of study or treatment.

KEY POINTS

- Pregnancy-associated cardiovascular changes include a doubling of maternal cardiac output and a 40% increase in blood volume.
- Uterine blood flow at term averages 750 mL/min, or 10% to 15% of maternal cardiac output.
- Normal term placental weight averages 450 g, representing approximately one seventh (one sixth with cord and membranes) of fetal weight.
- Mean amniotic fluid volume increases from 250 to 800 mL between 16 and 32 weeks, and decreases to 500 mL at term.
- Fetal urine production ranges from 400 to 1200 mL/day and is the primary source of amniotic fluid.

- The fetal umbilical circulation receives approximately 40% of fetal combined ventricular output (300 mL/mg/min).
- Umbilical blood flow is 70 to 130 mL/min after 30 weeks' gestation.
- Fetal cardiac output is constant over a heart rate range of 120 to 180 beats/min.
- The fetus exists in a state of aerobic metabolism, with arterial PO_2 values in the 20 to 25 mm Hg range.
- Approximately 20% of the fetal oxygen consumption of 8 mL/kg/min is required in the acquisition of new tissue.

REFERENCES

1. Hauguel S, Chalier J-C, Cedard L, Olive G: Metabolism of the human placenta perfused in vitro: glucose transfer and utilization, O_2 consumption, lactate and ammonia production. Pediatr Res 17:729, 1983.
2. Hay WW Jr, Sparks JW, Wilkening RB, et al: Partition of maternal glucose production between conceptus and maternal tissues in sheep. Am J Physiol 245:E347, 1983.
3. Barker DJ: The long-term outcome of retarded fetal growth. Schweiz Med Wochenschr 129:189, 1999.
4. Fowden AL, Sibley C, Reik W, Constancia M: Imprinted genes, placental development and fetal growth. Horm Res 65:50, 2006.
5. Thornburg KL, Faber JJ: Transfer of hydrophilic molecules by placenta and yolk sac of the guinea pig. Am J Physiol 233:C111, 1977.
6. Sibley CP, Coan PM, Ferguson-Smith AC, et al: Placental-specific insulin-like growth factor 2 (IgF2) regulates the diffusional exchange characteristics of the mouse placenta. Proc Natl Acad Sci U S A 101:8204, 2004.
7. Talbert D, Sebire NJ: The dynamic placenta: I. Hypothetical model of a placental mechanism matching local fetal blood flow to local intervillus oxygen delivery. Med Hypotheses 62:511, 2004.
8. Wilkening RB, Meschia G: Fetal oxygen uptake, oxygenations, and acid-base balance as a function of uterine blood flow. Am J Physiol 244:H749, 1983.
9. Bissonnette JM: Studies in vivo of glucose transfer across the guinea-pig placenta. In Young M, Boyd RDH, Longo LD, Telegdy G (eds): Placental Transfer: Methods and Interpretations. Philadelphia, Saunders, 1981, p 155.
10. Illsley NP, Sellers MC, Wright RL: Glycaemic regulation of glucose transporter expression and activity in the human placenta. Placenta 19:517, 1998.
11. Baumann MU, Deborde S, Illsley NP: Placental glucose transfer and fetal growth. Endocrine 19:13, 2002.
12. Regnault TR, de VB, Battaglia FC: Transport and metabolism of amino acids in placenta. Endocrine 19:23, 2002.
13. Desforges M, Sibley CP: Placental nutrient supply and fetal growth. Int J Dev Biol 54:377, 2010.
14. Jansson T, Myatt L, Powell TL: The role of trophoblast nutrient and ion transporters in the development of pregnancy complications and adult disease. Curr Vasc Pharmacol 7:521, 2009.
15. Farley DM, Choi J, Dudley DJ, et al: Placental amino acid transport and placental leptin resistance in pregnancies complicated by maternal obesity. Placenta 31:718, 2010.
16. Vaughn PR, Lobo C, Battaglia FC, et al: Glutamine-glutamate exchange between placenta and fetal liver. Am J Physiol 268:E705, 1995.
17. Gimeno RE, Hirsch DJ, Punreddy S, et al: Targeted deletion of fatty acid transport protein-4 results in early embryonic lethality. J Biol Chem 278:49512, 2003.
18. Duttaroy AK: Transport of fatty acids across the human placenta: a review. Prog Lipid Res 48:52, 2009.
19. Dancis J, Kammerman BS, Jansen V, et al: Transfer of urea, sodium, and chloride across the perfused human placenta. Am J Obstet Gynecol 141:677, 1981.
20. Faber JJ, Thornburg KL: Placental Physiology: Structure and Function of Fetomaternal Exchange. New York, Raven Press, 1983, p 95.
21. Zhu X, Jiang S, Hu Y, et al: The expression of aquaporin 8 and aquaporin 9 in fetal membranes and placenta in term pregnancies complicated by idiopathic polyhydramnios. Early Hum Dev 86:657, 2010.
22. Riquelme G: Placental chloride channels: a review. Placenta 30:659, 2009.
23. Belkacemi L, Bedard I, Simoneau L, Lafond J: Calcium channels, transporters and exchangers in placenta: a review. Cell Calcium 37:1, 2005.
24. Bhattacharjee J, Ietta F, Giacomello E, et al: Expression and localization of ATP binding cassette transporter A1 (ABCA1) in first trimester and term human placenta. Placenta 31:423, 2010.
25. Radulescu L, Antohe F, Jinga V, et al: Neonatal Fc receptors discriminates and monitors the pathway of native and modified immunoglobulin G in placental endothelial cells. Hum Immunol 65:578, 2004.
26. Fuchs R, Ellinger I: Endocytic and transcytotic processes in villous syncytiotrophoblast: role in nutrient transport to the human fetus. Traffic 5:725, 2004.
27. McArdle HJ, Andersen HS, Jones H, Gambling L: Copper and iron transport across the placenta: regulation and interactions. J Neuroendocrinol 20:427, 2008.
28. Jayanthi LD, Samuvel DJ, Ramamoorthy S: Regulated internalization and phosphorylation of the native norepinephrine transporter in response to phorbol esters. Evidence for localization in lipid rafts and lipid raft-mediated internalization. J Biol Chem 279:19315, 2004.
29. Rosenfeld CR, Cox BE, Roy T, Magness RR: Nitric oxide contributes to estrogen-induced vasodilation of the ovine uterine circulation. J Clin Invest 98:2158, 1996.
30. Valdes G, Kaufmann P, Corthorn J, et al: Vasodilator factors in the systemic and local adaptations to pregnancy. Reprod Biol Endocrinol 7:79, 2009.
31. Rosenfeld CR, Naden RP: Responses of uterine and nonuterine tissues to angiotensin II in ovine pregnancy. Am J Physiol 257:H17, 1995.
32. Reynolds LP, Borowicz PP, Caton JS, et al: Uteroplacental vascular development and placental function: an update. Int J Dev Biol 54:355, 2010.
33. Ramesar SV, Mackraj I, Gathiram P, Moodley J: Sildenafil citrate improves fetal outcomes in pregnant, L-NAME treated, Sprague-Dawley rats, Eur J Obstet Gynecol Reprod Biol 149:22, 2010.
34. Rudolph AM, Heymann MA: Circulatory changes during growth in the fetal lamb. Circ Res 26:289, 1970.
35. Cheung CY, Brace RA: Developmental expression of vascular endothelial growth factor and its receptors in ovine placenta and fetal membranes. J Soc Gynecol Investig 6:179, 1999.
36. Thaete LG, Dewey ER, Neerhof MG: Endothelin and the regulation of uterine and placental perfusion in hypoxia-induced fetal growth restriction. J Soc Gynecol Investig 11:16, 2004.
37. Bulmer JN, Williams PJ, Lash GE: Immune cells in the placental bed. Int J Dev Biol 54:281, 2010.
38. Hunt JS, Langat DL: HLA-G: a human pregnancy-related immunomodulator. Curr Opin Pharmacol 9:462, 2009.
39. Parham P: NK cells and trophoblasts: partners in pregnancy. J Exp Med 200:951, 2004.
40. Beall MH, van den Wijngaard JP, van Gemert MJ, Ross MG: Amniotic fluid water dynamics. Placenta 28:816, 2007.
41. Robillard JE, Ramberg E, Sessions C, et al: Role of aldosterone on renal sodium and potassium excretion during fetal life and newborn period. Dev Pharmacol Ther 1:201, 1980.
42. Abramovich DR: Fetal factors influencing the volume and composition of liquor amnii. J Obstet Gynaecol Br Commonw 77:865, 1970.
43. Harding R, Sigger JN, Poore ER, Johnson P: Ingestion in fetal sheep and its relation to sleep states and breathing movements. Q J Exp Physiol 69:477, 1984.
44. Mann SE, Ricke EA, Torres EA, Taylor RN: A novel model of polyhydramnios: amniotic fluid volume is increased in aquaporin 1 knockout mice. Am J Obstet Gynecol 192:2041, 2005.
45. Beall MH, Wang S, Yang B, et al: Placental and membrane aquaporin water channels: correlation with amniotic fluid volume and composition. Placenta 28:421, 2007.

46. Hay WW Jr, Myers SA, Sparks JW, et al: Glucose and lactate oxidation rates in the fetal lamb. Proc Soc Exp Biol Med 173:553, 1983.
47. Battaglia FC: Glutamine and glutamate exchange between the fetal liver and the placenta. J Nutr 130:974S, 2000.
48. Forbes K, Westwood M: The IGF axis and placental function. a mini review. Horm Res 69:129, 2008.
49. Constancia M, Hemberger M, Hughes J, et al: Placental-specific IGF-II is a major modulator of placental and fetal growth. Nature 417:945, 2002.
50. Murphy VE, Smith R, Giles WB, Clifton VL: Endocrine regulation of human fetal growth: the role of the mother, placenta, and fetus. Endocr Rev 27:141, 2006.
51. Hay WW, Meznarich HK, Sparks JW, et al: Effect of insulin on glucose uptake in near-term fetal lambs. Proc Soc Exp Biol Med 178:557, 1985.
52. Fowden AL: The insulin-like growth factors and feto-placental growth. Placenta 24:803, 2003.
53. El-Hashash AH, Esbrit P, Kimber SJ: PTHrP promotes murine secondary trophoblast giant cell differentiation through induction of endocycle, upregulation of giant-cell-promoting transcription factors and suppression of other trophoblast cell types. Differentiation 73:154, 2005.
54. Bond H, Dilworth MR, Baker B, et al: Increased maternofetal calcium flux in parathyroid hormone-related protein-null mice. J Physiol 586:2015, 2008.
55. Threadgill DW, Dlugosz AA, Hansen LA, et al: Targeted disruption of mouse EGF receptor: effect of genetic background on mutant phenotype. Science 269:230, 1995.
56. Dackor J, Li M, Threadgill DW: Placental overgrowth and fertility defects in mice with a hypermorphic allele of epidermal growth factor receptor. Mamm Genome 20:339, 2009.
57. Frost JM, Moore GE: The importance of imprinting in the human placenta. PLoS Genet 6:e1001015, 2010.
58. Rudolph AM: Hepatic and ductus venosus blood flows during fetal life. Hepatology 3:254, 1983.
59. Anderson DF, Bissonnette JM, Faber JJ, Thornburg KL: Central shunt flows and pressures in the mature fetal lamb. Am J Physiol 241:H60, 1981.
60. Edelstone DI, Rudolph AM, Heymann MA: Liver and ductus venosus blood flows in fetal lambs in utero. Circ Res 42:426, 1978.
61. Thornburg KL, Morton MG: Filling and arterial pressures as determinants of left ventricular stroke volume in fetal lambs. Am J Physiol 251:H961, 1986.
62. Thornburg KL, Morton MJ: Filling and arterial pressures as determinants of RV stroke volume in the sheep fetus. Am J Physiol 244:H656, 1983.
63. Bocking AD, Harding R, Wickham PJ: Relationship between accelerations and decelerations in heart rate and skeletal muscle activity in fetal sheep. J Develop Physiol 7:47, 1985.
64. Assali NS, Brinkman CR III, Woods JR Jr, et al: Development of neurohumoral control of fetal, neonatal, and adult cardiovascular functions. Am J Obstet Gynecol 129:748, 1977.
65. Iwamoto HS, Rudolph AM, Miskin BL, Keil LC. Circulatory and humoral responses of sympathectomized fetal sheep to hypoxemia. Am J Physiol 245:H767, 1983.
66. Dawes GS, Johnston BM, Walker DW: Relationship of arterial pressure and heart rate in fetal, newborn and adult sheep. J Physiol 309:405, 1980.
67. Itskovitz J, LaGamma EF, Rudolph AM: Baroreflex control of the circulation in chronically instrumented fetal lambs. Circ Res 52:589, 1983.
68. Weitzman RE, Fisher DA, Robillard J, et al: Arginine vasopressin response to an osmotic stimulus in the fetal sheep. Pediatr Res 12:35, 1978.
69. Ervin MG, Ross MG, Youssef A, et al: Renal effects of ovine fetal arginine vasopressin secretion in response to maternal hyperosmolality. Am J Obstet Gynecol 155:1341, 1986.
70. Rose JC, Meis PJ, Morris M: Ontogeny of endocrine (ACTH, vasopressin, cortisol) responses to hypotension in lamb fetuses. Am J Physiol 240:E656, 1981.
71. Ross MG, Ervin MG, Leake RD, et al: Isovolemic hypotension in ovine fetus: plasma arginine vasopressin response and urinary effects. Am J Physiol 250:E564, 1986.
72. Ervin MG, Ross MG, Leake RD, Fisher DA: V1- and V2-receptor contributions to ovine fetal renal and cardiovascular responses to vasopressin. Am J Physiol 262:R636, 1992.
73. Robillard JR, Nakamura KT: Neurohormonal regulation of renal function during development. Am J Physiol 254:F771, 1988.
74. Lumbers ER: A brief review of fetal renal function. J Dev Physiol 6:1, 1984.
75. Pitkin RM, Reynolds WA: Fetal ingestion and metabolism of amniotic fluid protein. Am J Obstet Gynecol 123:356, 1975.
76. Charlton VE, Reis BL: Effects of gastric nutritional supplementation on fetal umbilical uptake of nutrients. Am J Physiol 241:E178, 1981.
77. Charlton V, Johengen M: Effects of intrauterine nutritional supplementation on fetal growth retardation. Biol Neonate 48:125, 1985.
78. Wesson DE, Muraji T, Kent G, et al: The effect of intrauterine esophageal ligation on growth of fetal rabbits. J Pediatr Surg 19:398, 1984.
79. Challier JC, Schneider H, Dancis J: In vitro perfusion of human placenta. V. Oxygen consumption. Am J Obstet Gynecol 126:261, 1976.
80. Trahair JF, Harding R, Bocking AD, et al: The role of ingestion in the development of the small intestine in fetal sheep. Q J Exp Physiol 71:99, 1986.
81. Avila C, Harding R, Robinson P: The effects of preventing ingestion on the development of the digestive system in the sheep fetus. Q J Exp Physiol 71:99, 1986.
82. Cohn HE, Sacks EJ, Heymann MA, Rudolph AM: Cardiovascular responses to hypoxemia and acidemia in fetal lambs. Am J Obstet Gynecol 120:817, 1974.
83. Pierro A, Cozzi F, Colarossi G, et al: Does fetal gut obstruction cause hydramnios and growth retardation? J Pediatr Surg 22:454, 1987.
84. Lester R, Jackson BT, Smallwood RA, et al: Fetal and neonatal hepatic function. II. Birth defects 12:307, 1976.
85. Jones CT, Ritchie JWK, Walker D: The effects of hypoxia on glucose turnover in the fetal sheep. J Dev Physiol 5:223, 1983.
86. Wood CE, Rudolph AM: Negative feedback regulation of adrenocorticotropin secretion by cortisol in ovine fetuses. Endocrinology 112:1930, 1983.
87. Challis JR, Brooks AN: Maturation and activation of hypothalamic-pituitary adrenal function in fetal sheep. Endocrinol Rev 10:182, 1989.
88. Padbury J, Agata Y, Ludlow J, et al: Effect of fetal adrenalectomy on cathecholamine release and physiological adaptation at birth in sheep. J Clin Invest 80:1096, 1987.
89. Fisher DA: Maternal-fetal thyroid function in pregnancy. Clin Perinatol 10:615, 1983.
90. Visser GHA, Goodman JDS, Levine DH, Dawes GS: Diurnal and other cyclic variations in human fetal heart rate near term. Am J Obstet Gynecol 142:535, 1982.
91. Natale R, Clewlow F, Dawes GS: Measurement of fetal forelimb movements in the lamb in utero. Am J Obstet Gynecol 140:545, 1981.
92. Blanco CE, Dawes GS, Walker DW: Effect of hypoxia on polysynaptic hindlimb reflexes of unanesthetized foetal and newborn lambs. J Physiol 339:453, 1983.
93. Chan K, Dodd PA, Day L, et al: Fetal catecholamine, cardiovascular, and neurobehavioral responses to cocaine. Am J Obstet Gynecol 167:1616, 1992.
94. Dawes GS, Fox HE, Leduc BM, et al: Respiratory movements and rapid eye movement sleep in the foetal lamb. J Physiol 220:119, 1972.
95. Connors G, Hunse C, Carmichal L, et al: Control of fetal breathing in human fetus between 24 and 34 weeks gestation. Am J Obstet Gynecol 160:932, 1989.
96. Dawes GS, Gardner WN, Johnson BM, Walker DW: Breathing activity in fetal lambs: the effect of brain stem section. J Physiol 335:535, 1983.
97. Chao CR, Hohimer AR, Bissonnette JM: The effect of electrocortical state on cerebral carbohydrate metabolism in fetal sheep. Brain Res Dev Brain Res 49:1, 1989.
98. Jones MD, Sheldon RE, Peeters LL, et al: Fetal cerebral oxygen consumption at different levels of oxygenation. J Appl Physiol: Respirat Envorion Exercise Physiol 43:1080, 1977.

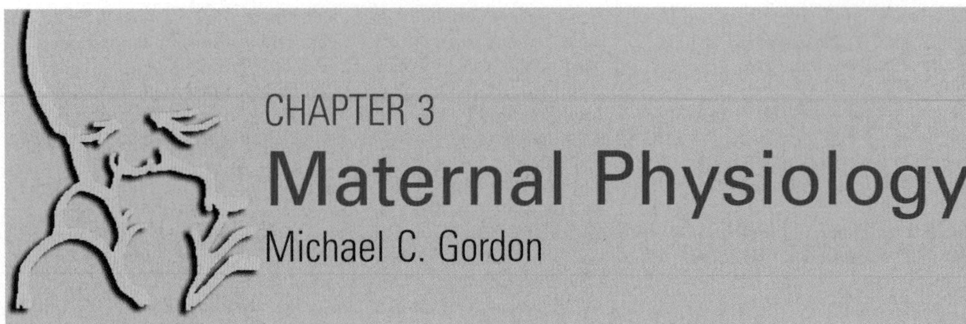

CHAPTER 3

Maternal Physiology

Michael C. Gordon

KEY ABBREVIATIONS	
Adrenocorticotropic Hormone	ACTH
Arginine Vasopressin	AVP
Blood Urea Nitrogen	BUN
Brain Natriuretic Peptide	BNP
Carbon Dioxide	CO_2
Cardiac Output	CO
Colloidal Oncotic Pressure	COP
Corticotropin-Releasing Hormone	CRH
Forced Expiratory Volume in 1 Second	FEV_1
Functional Residual Capacity	FRC
Glomerular Filtration Rate	GFR
Human Chorionic Gonadotropin	hCG
Human Placenta Lactogen	hPL
Mean Arterial Pressure	MAP
Parathyroid Hormone	PTH
Pulmonary Capillary Wedge Pressures	PCWPs
Rapid Eye Movement	REM
Renin-Angiotensin-Aldosterone System	RAAS
Stroke Volume	SV
Systemic Vascular Resistance	SVR
Thyroid-Stimulating Hormone	TSH
Thyroxine-Binding Globulin	TBG
Total Thyroxine	TT_4
Total Triiodothyronine	TT_3

Major adaptations in maternal anatomy, physiology, and metabolism are required for a successful pregnancy. Hormonal changes, initiated before conception, significantly alter maternal physiology and persist through both pregnancy and the initial postpartum period. Although these adaptations are profound and affect nearly every organ system, women return to the nongravid state with minimal residual changes.[1] A full understanding of physiologic changes is necessary to differentiate between normal alternations and those that are abnormal. This chapter describes maternal adaptations in pregnancy and gives specific examples of how they may affect care. Finally, although women may tire of repetitive reassurance that "it is simply normal and of no concern," a complete understanding of physiologic changes allows each obstetrician to provide a more thorough explanation for various changes and symptoms.

Many of the changes to routine laboratory values caused by pregnancy are described in the following text. For a comprehensive review of normal reference ranges for common laboratory tests by trimester, the reader is encouraged to refer to Appendix A1.

BODY WATER METABOLISM

The increase in total body water of 6.5 to 8.5 L by the end of gestation represents one of the most significant adaptations of pregnancy. The water content of the fetus, placenta, and amniotic fluid at term accounts for about 3.5 L. **Additional water is accounted for by expansion of the**

maternal blood volume by 1500 to 1600 mL, plasma volume by 1200 to 1300 mL, and red blood cells by 300 to 400 mL. The remainder is attributed to extravascular fluid, intracellular fluid in the uterus and breasts, and expanded adipose tissue. As a result, pregnancy is a condition of chronic volume overload with active sodium and water retention secondary to changes in osmoregulation and the renin-angiotensin system. Increase in body water content contributes to maternal weight gain, hemodilution, physiologic anemia of pregnancy, and the elevation in maternal cardiac output (CO). Inadequate plasma volume expansion has been associated with increased risks for preeclampsia and fetal growth restriction.

Osmoregulation

Expansion in plasma volume begins shortly after conception, partially mediated by a change in maternal osmoregulation through altered secretion of arginine vasopressin (AVP) by the posterior pituitary. Water retention exceeds sodium retention; even though an additional 900 mEq of sodium is retained during pregnancy, **serum levels of sodium decrease by 3 to 4 mmol/L.** This is mirrored by decreases in overall plasma osmolality of 8 to 10 mOsm/kg, a change that is in place by 10 weeks' gestation and continues through 1 to 2 weeks postpartum[2] (Figure 3-1). Similarly, the threshold for thirst and vasopressin release changes early in pregnancy; during gestational weeks 5 to 8, an increase in water intake occurs and results in a transient increase in urinary volume but a net increase in total body water. Initial changes in AVP regulation may be due to placental signals involving nitric oxide (NO) and the hormone relaxin.[3] After 8 weeks' gestation, the new steady state for osmolality has been established with little subsequent change in water turnover, resulting in decreased polyuria. **Pregnant women perceive fluid challenges or dehydration normally with changes in thirst and AVP secretion, but at a new, lower "osmostat."**[3]

Plasma levels of AVP remain relatively unchanged despite heightened production, owing to a threefold to fourfold increase in the metabolic clearance. Increased clearance results from a circulating vasopressinase synthesized by the placenta that rapidly inactivates both AVP and oxytocin. This enzyme increases about 300-fold to 1000-fold over the course of gestation proportional to fetal weight, with the highest concentrations occurring in multiple gestations. **Increased AVP clearance can unmask subclinical forms of diabetes insipidus, presumably because of an insufficient pituitary AVP reserve, and causes transient diabetes insipidus with an incidence of 2 to 6 per 1000.** Typically presenting with both polydipsia and polyuria, hyperosmolality is usually mild unless the thirst mechanism is abnormal or access to water is limited.[4]

Salt Metabolism

Sodium metabolism is delicately balanced, facilitating a net accumulation of about 900 mEq of sodium. Sixty percent of the additional sodium is contained within the fetoplacental unit (including amniotic fluid) and is lost at birth. By 2 months postpartum, the serum sodium returns to preconceptional levels. Pregnancy increases the preference for sodium intake, but the primary mechanism is enhanced tubular sodium reabsorption. Increased glomerular filtration raises the total filtered sodium load from 20,000 to about 30,000 mmol/day; sodium reabsorption must increase to prevent sodium loss. However, the adaptive rise in tubular reabsorption surpasses the increase in filtered load, resulting in an additional 2 to 6 mEq of sodium reabsorption per day. Alterations in sodium handling represent the largest renal adjustment that occurs in gestation.[5] Hormonal control of sodium balance is under the opposing actions of the renin-angiotensin-aldosterone system (RAAS) and the natriuretic peptides, and both are modified during pregnancy.

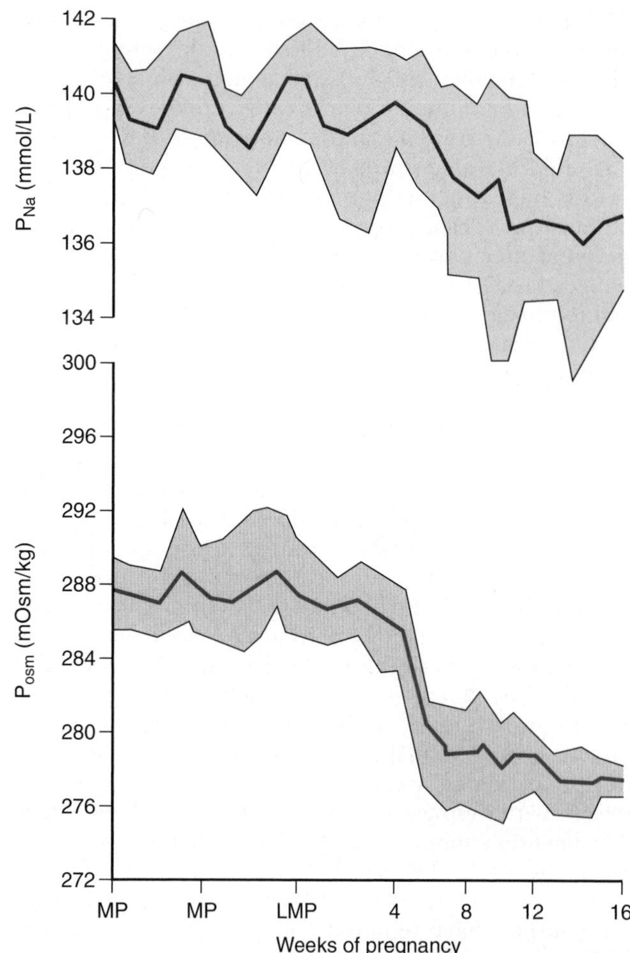

FIGURE 3-1. Plasma osmolality and plasma sodium during human gestation (*n* = 9: mean values ± SD). *LMP,* Last menstrual period; *MP,* menstrual period. (From Davison JM, Vallotton MB, Lindheimer MD: Plasma osmolality and urinary concentration and dilution during and after pregnancy: Evidence that the lateral recumbency inhibits maximal urinary concentration ability. Br J Obstet Gynecol 88:472, 1981.)

Renin-Angiotensin-Aldosterone System

Normal pregnancy is characterized by a marked increase in all components of the RAAS system. In early pregnancy, reduced systemic vascular tone (attributed to gestational hormones and increased NO production) results in decreased mean arterial pressure (MAP). In turn, decreased

MAP activates adaptations to preserve intravascular volume through sodium retention.[6] Plasma renin activity, renin substrate (angiotensinogen), and angiotensin levels are all increased a minimum of fourfold to fivefold over nonpregnant levels. Activation of these components of RAAS leads to twofold elevated levels of aldosterone by the third trimester, increasing sodium reabsorption and preventing sodium loss. Despite the elevated aldosterone levels in late pregnancy, normal homeostatic responses still occur to changes in salt balance, fluid loss, and postural stimuli. In addition to aldosterone, other hormones that may contribute to increased tubular sodium retention include deoxycorticosterone and estrogen.

Atrial and Brain Natriuretic Peptide

The myocardium releases neuropeptides that serve to maintain circulatory homeostasis. Atrial natriuretic peptide (ANP) is secreted primarily by the atrial myocytes in response to dilation, and in response to end-diastolic pressure and volume, the ventricles secrete brain natriuretic peptide (BNP). Both peptides have similar physiologic actions, acting as diuretics, natriuretics, vasorelaxants, and overall antagonists to the RAAS. Elevated levels of ANP and BNP are found in both physiologic and pathologic conditions of volume overload and can be used to screen for congestive heart failure outside of pregnancy in symptomatic patients. Because pregnant women frequently present with dyspnea and many of the physiologic effects of conception mimic heart disease, whether pregnancy affects the levels of these hormones is clinically important. Gestational alterations in ANP are controversial because some authors have reported higher plasma levels during different stages of pregnancy, whereas others have reported no change. In a meta-analysis by Castro and colleagues,[7] ANP levels were 40% higher during gestation and 150% higher during the first postpartum week.

The circulating concentration of BNP is 20% less than that of ANP in normal individuals and has been found to be more useful in the diagnosis of congestive heart failure. Levels of BNP are reported to increase largely in the third trimester of pregnancy compared with first-trimester levels (21.5 ± 8 pg/mL versus 15.2 ± 5 pg/mL) and are highest in pregnancies complicated by preeclampsia (37.1 ± 10 pg/mL). The levels throughout pregnancy have been found to be higher than in nonpregnant controls. In pregnancies with preeclampsia, higher levels of BNP are associated with echocardiographic evidence of left ventricular enlargement.[8] **Although the levels of BNP are increased during pregnancy and with preeclampsia, the mean values are still lower than the levels used to screen for cardiac dysfunction (>75 to 100 pg/mL) and, therefore, can be used to screen for congestive heart failure.**[9]

CARDIOVASCULAR SYSTEM

Pregnancy causes profound physiologic changes in the cardiovascular system. A series of adaptive mechanisms are activated as early as 5 weeks' gestation to maximize oxygen delivery to maternal and fetal tissues.[6] In most women, these physiologic demands are well tolerated. However, in certain cardiac diseases, maternal morbidity and even mortality may occur.

Heart

The combination of displacement of the diaphragm and the effect of pregnancy on the shape of the rib cage (described in the respiratory section below) displaces the heart upward and to the left. In addition, the heart rotates on its long axis, moving the apex somewhat laterally, resulting in an increased cardiac silhouette on radiographic studies, without a true change in the cardiothoracic ratio. Associated radiographic findings include an apparent straightening of the border of the left side of the heart and increased prominence of the pulmonary conus. **Therefore, the diagnosis of cardiomegaly by simple radiography should be confirmed by echocardiogram if clinically appropriate.**[10]

Although true cardiomegaly is rare, physiologic myocardial hypertrophy of the heart is consistently observed as a result of expanded blood volume in the first half of the pregnancy and progressively increasing afterload in later gestation. **These structural changes in the heart are similar to those found in response to exercise and result in eccentric hypertrophy as opposed to concentric hypertrophy that is seen with disease states such as hypertension or aortic stenosis.** The eccentric hypertrophy enables the heart to enhance its pumping capacity in response to increased demand, making the pregnant heart mechanically more efficient.[11,12] Most changes begin early in the first trimester and peak by 30 to 34 weeks' gestation. Left ventricular end-diastolic dimension increases 12% over preconceptional values by M-mode echocardiography. Concurrently, left ventricular wall mass increases by 52% (mild myocardial hypertrophy), and atrial diameters increase bilaterally, peaking at 40% above nonpregnant values.[12] Pulmonary capillary wedge pressures (PCWPs) are stable, reflecting a combination of decreased pulmonary vascular resistance and increased blood volume. Twin pregnancies increase myocardial hypertrophy, atrial dilation, and end-diastolic ventricular measurements even further.[13] Unlike the heart of an athlete that regresses rapidly with inactivity, the pregnant heart regresses in size less rapidly and takes up to 6 months to return to normal.[14]

Evaluation of left ventricular function (contractility) is difficult in pregnancy because it is strongly influenced by changes in heart rate (HR), preload, and afterload. Despite the increase in stroke volume (SV) and CO, normal pregnancy is not associated with hyperdynamic left ventricular function during the third trimester, as measured by ejection fraction, left ventricular stroke work index, or fractional shortening of the left ventricle. However, some studies have shown that contractility might be slightly increased in the first two trimesters, whereas other articles report no change throughout the pregnancy, and some report a decline toward term.[12] One recent study showed that in the third trimester the cardiac systolic function declines as evidenced by a decrease in the ejection fraction and the systolic myocardial velocities compared with the first trimester. The results of this study are consistent with impaired contraction and relaxation of the left ventricle at the end of pregnancy and suggest that a decline in cardiac function at term is a feature of normal pregnancy and that an exaggeration of this decline may explain the etiology for peripartum cardiomyopathy.[15]

Within the past decade, clinicians and researchers have focused on abnormalities of diastolic function as important contributors to cardiac disease and symptom severity, especially in the setting of normal or near-normal systolic function.[16] In a review, diastolic dysfunction was pinpointed as a leading cause of cardiac failure in pregnancy.[17] During the past 5 years, the effects of pregnancy on diastolic function have been thoroughly investigated by using pulsed-wave Doppler echocardiography.[12] In young healthy women, the left ventricle is elastic; therefore, diastolic relaxation is swift, and ventricular filling occurs almost completely by early diastole with minimal contribution from the atrial kick. The E/A ratio compares the peak mitral flow velocity in early diastole (E) to the peak atrial kick velocity (A); although both velocities increase in pregnancy, the overall ratio falls because of a greater rise in the A-wave velocity. **The rise in the A value, which begins in the second trimester and increases throughout the third trimester, indicates the increased importance of the atrial contraction in left ventricular filling during pregnancy.**[12] Veille and associates determined that in healthy women, pregnancy did not adversely affect baseline diastolic function, but that at maximal exercise, diastolic function was impaired. The reason for the impairment was attributed to increased left ventricular wall stiffness. The authors further speculated that this change may be the limiting factor for exercise in pregnancy.[18]

Cardiac Output

One of the most remarkable changes in pregnancy is the tremendous increase in CO. Van Oppen and coworkers reviewed 33 cross-sectional and 19 longitudinal studies and found greatly divergent results on when CO peaked, the magnitude of the rise in CO before labor, and the effect of the third trimester on CO.[19] **However, all of the studies agreed that CO increased significantly beginning in early pregnancy, peaking at an average of 30% to 50% above preconceptional values.** In a longitudinal study by Robson and associates using Doppler echocardiography, CO increased by 50% at 34 weeks from a prepregnancy value of 4.88 L/min to 7.34 L/min[19,20] (Figure 3-2). In twin gestations, CO incrementally increases an additional 20% above that of singleton pregnancies.[13] Robson and associates demonstrated that, by 5 weeks' gestation, CO has already risen by more than 10%. By 12 weeks, the rise in output is 34% to 39% above nongravid levels, accounting for about 75% of the total increase in CO during pregnancy. **Although the literature is not clear regarding the exact gestation when CO peaks, most studies point to a range between 25 and 30 weeks.**[20] The data on whether the CO continues to increase in the third trimester are very divergent, with equal numbers of good longitudinal studies showing a mild decrease, a slight increase, or no change.[19] The differences in these studies cannot be explained by differences in investigative techniques, position of the women during measurements, or study design. This apparent discrepancy appears to be explained by the small number of individuals in each study and the probability that the course of CO during the third trimester is determined by factors specific to the individual.[19] In a recent study, Desai and coworkers reported that CO in the third trimester is significantly correlated with fetal birthweight and maternal height and weight.[21]

Most of the increase in CO is directed to the uterus, placenta, and breasts. In the first trimester, as in the nongravid state, the uterus receives 2% to 3% of CO and the breasts 1%. The percentage of CO going to the kidneys (20%), skin (10%), brain (10%), and coronary arteries (5%) remains at similar nonpregnant percentages, but because of the overall increase in CO, this results in an increase in absolute blood flow of about 50%.[22] By term, the uterus receives 17% (450 to 650 mL/min) and the breasts 2%, mostly at the expense of a reduction of the fraction of the CO going to the splanchnic bed and skeletal muscle. The absolute blood flow to the liver is not changed, but the overall percentage of CO is significantly decreased.

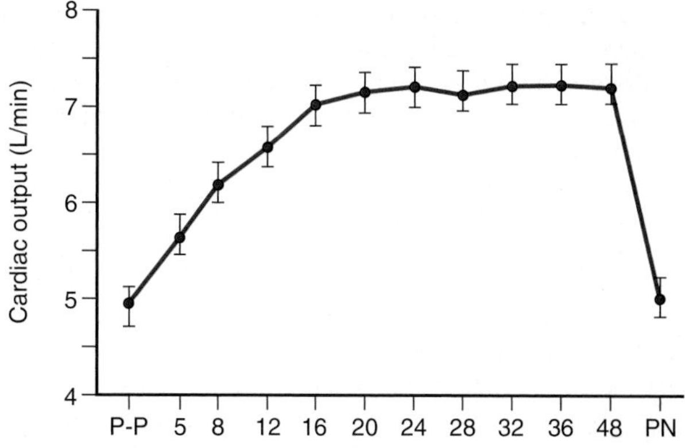

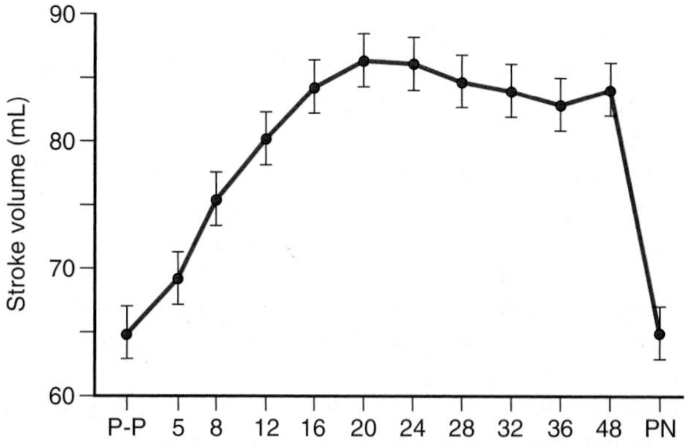

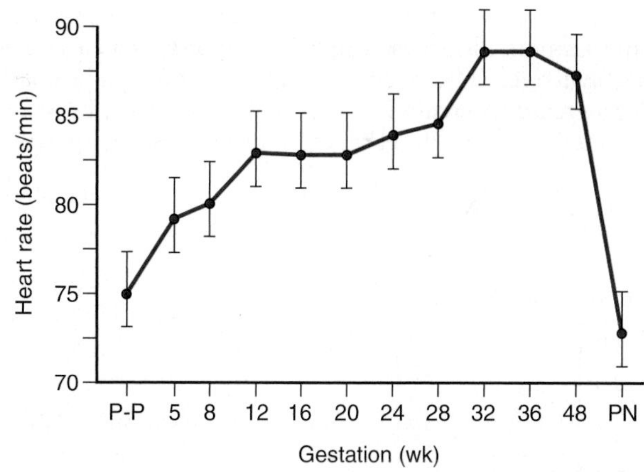

FIGURE 3-2. Increase in cardiac output, stroke volume, and heart rate from the nonpregnant state throughout pregnancy. *PN*, Postnatal; *P-P*, prepregnancy. (From Hunter S, Robson S: Adaptation of the maternal heart in pregnancy. Br Heart J 68:540, 1992.)

CO is the product of SV and HR (CO = SV × HR), both of which increase during pregnancy and contribute to the overall rise in CO. An initial rise in the HR occurs by 5 weeks' gestation and continues until it peaks at 32 weeks' gestation at 15 to 20 beats above the nongravid rate, an increase of 17%. The SV begins to rise by 8 weeks' gestation and reaches its maximum at about 20 weeks, 20% to 30% above nonpregnant values. In the third trimester, it is primarily variations in the SV that determine whether CO increases, decreases, or remains stable, as described earlier.

CO in pregnancy depends on maternal position. In a study in 10 normal gravid women in the third trimester, using pulmonary artery catheterization, CO was noted to be highest in the knee-chest position and lateral recumbent position at 6.6 to 6.9 L/min. CO decreased by 22% to 5.4 L/min in the standing position (Figure 3-3). The decrease in CO in the supine position compared with the lateral recumbent position is 10% to 30%. In both the standing and the supine positions, decreased CO results from a fall in SV secondary to decreased blood return to the heart. In the supine position, the enlarged uterus compresses the inferior vena cava, reducing venous return; before 24 weeks, this effect is not observed. Of note, in late pregnancy, the inferior vena cava is completely occluded in the supine position, with venous return from the lower extremities occurring through the dilated paravertebral collateral circulation.[23]

Despite decreased CO, most supine women are not hypotensive or symptomatic because of the compensated rise in systemic vascular resistance (SVR). **However, 5% to 10% of gravidas manifest supine hypotension with symptoms of dizziness, lightheadedness, nausea, and even syncope.** The women who become symptomatic have a greater decrease in CO and blood pressure (BP) and a greater increase in HR when in the supine position than do asymptomatic women.[24] Some investigators have proposed that the determination of whether women become symptomatic depends on the development of an adequate paravertebral collateral circulation. Interestingly, with engagement of the fetal head, less of an effect on CO is seen.[23] **The ability to maintain a normal BP in the supine position may be lost during epidural or spinal anesthesia because of an inability to increase SVR. Clinically, the effects of maternal position on CO are especially important when the mother is clinically hypotensive or in the setting of a non-reassuring fetal heart rate tracing.** The finding of a decreased CO in the standing position may give a physiologic basis for the finding of decreased birthweight and placental infarctions in working women who stand for prolonged periods.

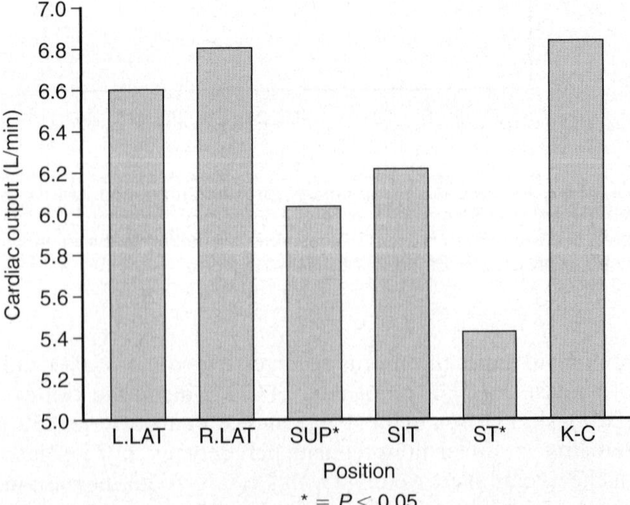

FIGURE 3-3. Effect of position change on cardiac output during pregnancy. *K-C,* Knee-chest; *L.LAT,* left lateral; *R.LAT,* right lateral; *SIT,* sitting; *ST,* standing; *SUP,* supine. (From Clark S, Cotton D, Pivarnik J, et al: Position change and central hemodynamic profile during normal third-trimester pregnancy and postpartum. Am J Obstet Gynecol 164:883, 1991.)

Arterial Blood Pressure and Systemic Vascular Resistance

BP is the product of CO and resistance (BP = CO × SVR). **Despite the large increase in CO, the maternal BP is decreased until later in pregnancy as a result of a decrease in SVR that nadirs midpregnancy and is followed by a gradual rise until term.** Even at full term, SVR remains 21% lower than prepregnancy values in pregnancies not affected by gestational hypertension or preeclampsia. The most obvious cause for the decreased SVR is progesterone-mediated smooth muscle relaxation; however, the exact mechanism for the fall in SVR is poorly understood. Earlier theories that uteroplacental circulation acts as an arteriovenous shunt are unlikely. Increased NO also contributes to decreased vascular resistance by direct actions and by blunting the vascular responsiveness to vasoconstrictors such as angiotensin II and norepinephrine. During conception, the expression and activity of NO synthase is elevated and the plasma level of cyclic guanosine monophosphate, a second messenger of NO and a mediator of vascular smooth muscle relaxation, is also increased.[25] **As a result, despite the overall increase in the RAAS, the normal gravida is refractory to the vasoconstrictive effects of angiotensin II. Gant and colleagues showed that nulliparous women who later become preeclamptic retain their response to angiotensin II before the appearance of clinical signs of preeclampsia.**[26]

Decreases in maternal BP parallel the falling SVR, with initial decreased BP manifesting at 8 weeks' gestation or earlier. Current studies did not include preconception BP or frequent first-trimester BP sampling and, therefore, cannot determine the exact time course of hemodynamic alterations. Because BP fluctuates with menstruation and is decreased in the luteal phase, it seems reasonable that BP drops immediately in early pregnancy. The diastolic BP and the mean arterial pressure [MAP = (2 × diastolic BP + systolic BP)/3] decrease more than the systolic BP, which changes minimally. The overall decrease in diastolic BP and MAP is 5 to 10 mm Hg (Figure 3-4). **The diastolic BP and the MAP nadir at midpregnancy and return to prepregnancy levels by term, and in most studies rarely exceed prepregnancy or postpartum values. However, some investigators have reported that at term, the BP is greater than in matched nonpregnant controls and believe that in the third trimester, the BP is higher than prepregnant values.** Current studies are very limited by the absence of preconceptional values for comparison within individual patients.

The position when the BP is taken and what Korotkoff sound is used to determine the diastolic BP are important. BP is lowest in the lateral recumbent position, and the BP of the superior arm in this position is 10 to 12 mm Hg lower than the inferior arm. In the clinic, BP should be measured in the sitting position and the Korotkoff 5 sound should be used. This is the diastolic BP when the sound disappears as opposed to the Korotkoff 4, when there is a muffling of the sound. In a study of 250 gravidas, the Korotkoff 4 sound could only be identified in 48% of patients, whereas the Korotkoff 5 sound could always be determined. The Korotkoff 4 should only be used when the Korotkoff 5 occurs at 0 mm Hg.[27] Automated BP monitors have been compared with mercury sphygmomanometry during pregnancy, and although they tended to overestimate the diastolic BP, the overall results were similar in normotensive women. Of note in patients with suspected preeclampsia, automated monitors appear increasingly inaccurate at higher BPs.

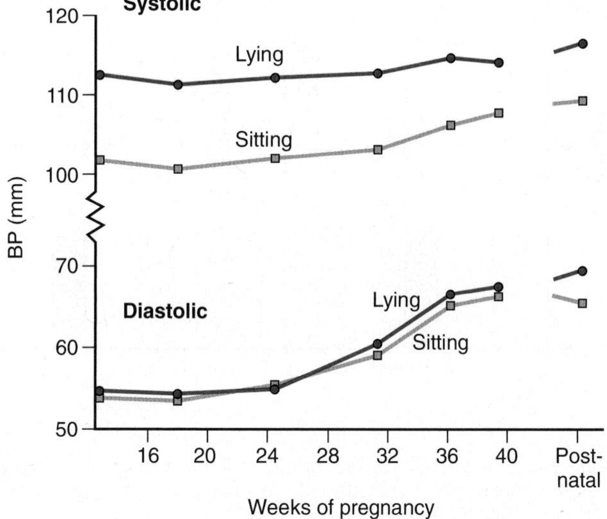

Figure 3-4. Blood pressure trends (sitting and lying) during pregnancy. Postnatal measures performed 6 weeks postpartum. (From MacGillivray I, Rose G, Rowe B: Blood pressure survey in pregnancy. Clin Sci 37:395, 1969.)

Venous Pressure

Venous pressure in the upper extremities remains unchanged in pregnancy but rises progressively in the lower extremities. Femoral venous pressure increases from values near 10 cm H_2O at 10 weeks' gestation to 25 cm H_2O near term.[28] From a clinical standpoint, this increase in pressure, in addition to the obstruction of the inferior vena cava by the expanding uterus, leads to the development of edema, varicose veins, and hemorrhoids, and an increased risk for deep venous thrombosis.

Central Hemodynamic Assessment

Clark and colleagues studied 10 carefully selected normal women at 36 to 38 weeks' gestation and again at 11 to 13 weeks postpartum with arterial lines and Swan-Ganz catheterization to characterize the central hemodynamics of term pregnancy (Table 3-1). As described earlier, CO, HR, SVR, and pulmonary vascular resistance change significantly with pregnancy. **In addition, clinically significant decreases were noted in colloidal oncotic pressure (COP) and the COP-PCWP difference, explaining why gravid women have a greater propensity for developing pulmonary edema with changes in capillary permeability or elevations in cardiac preload. The COP can fall even further after delivery to 17 mm Hg and, if the pregnancy is complicated by preeclampsia, can reach levels as low as 14 mm Hg.[29] When the PCWP is more than 4 mm Hg above the COP, the risk for pulmonary edema increases; therefore, pregnant women can experience pulmonary edema at PCWPs of 18 to 20 mm Hg, which is significantly lower than the typical nonpregnant threshold of 24 mm Hg.**

Normal Changes That Mimic Heart Disease

The physiologic adaptations of pregnancy lead to a number of changes in maternal signs and symptoms that can mimic cardiac disease and make it difficult to determine whether true disease is present. Dyspnea is common to both cardiac disease and pregnancy, but certain distinguishing features should be considered. First, the onset of pregnancy-related

Table 3-1 Central Hemodynamic Changes

	11-12 WEEKS POSTPARTUM	36-38 WEEKS' GESTATION	CHANGE FROM NONPREGNANT STATE
Cardiac output (L/min)	4.3 ± 0.9	6.2 ± 1.0	+43%*
Heart rate (beats/min)	71 ± 10.0	83 ± 10.0	+17%*
Systemic vascular resistance (dyne·cm·sec^{-5})	1530 ± 520	1210 ± 266	–21%*
Pulmonary vascular resistance (dyne·cm·sec^{-5})	119 ± 47.0	78 ± 22	–34%*
Colloid oncotic pressure (mm Hg)	20.8 ± 1.0	18 ± 1.5	–14%*
Mean arterial pressure (mm Hg)	86.4 ± 7.5	90.3 ± 5.8	NS
Pulmonary capillary wedge pressure (mm Hg)	3.7 ± 2.6	3.6 ± 2.5	NS
Central venous pressure (mm Hg)	3.7 ± 2.6	3.6 ± 2.5	NS
Left ventricular stroke work index (g·m·m^{-2})	41 ± 8	48 ± 6	NS

Modified from Clark S, Cotton D, Lee W, et al: Central hemodynamic assessment of normal term pregnancy. Am J Obstet Gynecol 161:1439, 1989.

Data are presented as mean ± standard deviation.

*$P < .05$.

NS, Not significant. Although data are not presented, the pulmonary artery pressures were not significantly different.

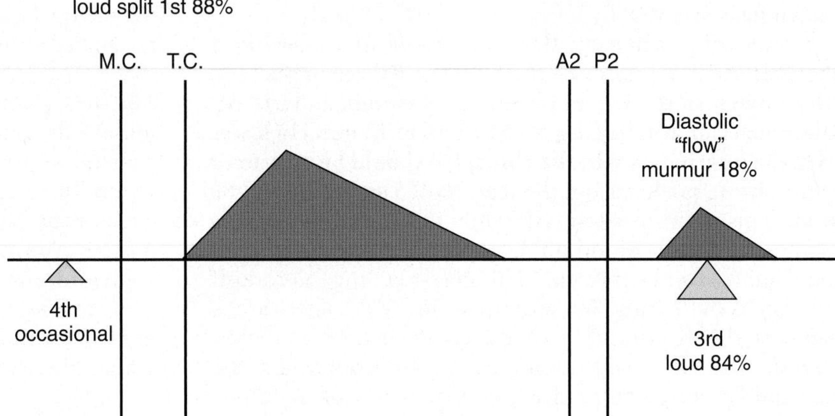

FIGURE 3-5. Summarization of the findings on auscultation of the heart in pregnancy. *M.C.*, Mitral closure; *T.C.*, tricuspid closure; *A2* and *P2*, aortic and pulmonary elements of the second sound. (From Cutforth R, MacDonald C: Heart sounds and murmurs in pregnancy. Am Heart J 71:741, 1966.)

dyspnea usually occurs before 20 weeks, and 75% of women experience it by the third trimester. **Unlike cardiac dyspnea, pregnancy-related dyspnea does not worsen significantly with advancing gestation. Second, physiologic dyspnea is usually mild, does not stop women from performing normal daily activities, and does not occur at rest.**[30] Other normal symptoms that can mimic cardiac disease include decreased exercise tolerance, fatigue, occasional orthopnea, syncope, and chest discomfort. The reason for this increase in cardiac symptoms is not an increase in catecholamine levels, because these levels are either unchanged or decreased in pregnancy. **Symptoms that should not be attributed to pregnancy and need a more thorough investigation include hemoptysis, syncope or chest pain with exertion, progressive orthopnea, or paroxysmal nocturnal dyspnea.** Normal physical findings that could be mistaken as evidence of cardiac disease include peripheral edema, mild tachycardia, jugular venous distention after midpregnancy, and lateral displacement of the left ventricular apex.

Pregnancy also alters normal heart sounds. At the end of the first trimester, both components of the first heart sound become louder, and there is exaggerated splitting. The second heart sound usually remains normal with only minimal changes. Up to 80% to 90% of gravidas demonstrate a third heart sound (S_3) after midpregnancy because of rapid diastolic filling. Rarely, a fourth heart sound may be auscultated, but typically phonocardiography is needed to detect this. Systolic ejection murmurs along the left sternal border develop in 96% of pregnancies, and increased blood flow across the pulmonic and aortic valves is thought to be the cause. Most commonly, these are midsystolic and less than grade 3. Diastolic murmurs have been found in up to 18% of gravidas, but their presence is uncommon enough to warrant further evaluation. A continuous murmur in the second to fourth intercostal space may be heard in the second or third trimester owing to the so-called mammary souffle caused by increased blood flow in the breast (Figure 3-5).

Troponin 1 and creatinine kinase-MB levels are tests used to assess for acute myocardial infarction. **Uterine contractions can lead to significant increases in the creatinine kinase-MB level, but troponin levels are not affected by pregnancy or labor.**[31]

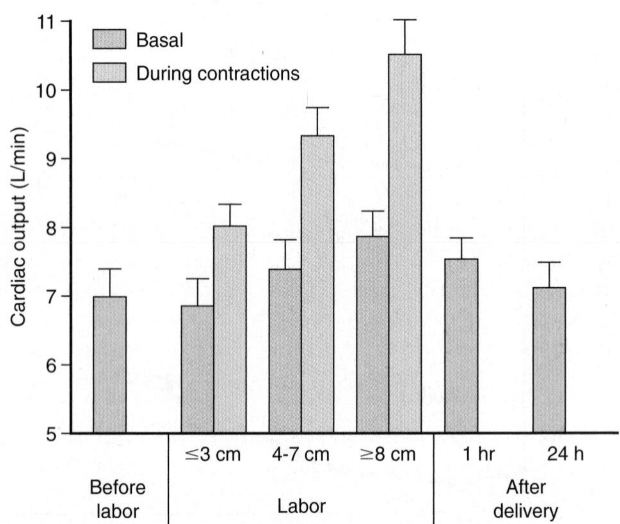

FIGURE 3-6. Changes in cardiac output during normal labor. (From Hunter S, Robson S: Adaptation of the maternal heart in pregnancy. Br Heart J 68:540, 1992.)

Effect of Labor and the Immediate Puerperium

The profound anatomic and functional changes on cardiac function reach a crescendo during the labor process. In addition to the dramatic rise in CO with normal pregnancy, even greater increases in CO occur with labor and in the immediate puerperium. In a Doppler echocardiography study by Robson and associates of 15 uncomplicated women without epidural anesthesia, the CO between contractions increased 12% during the first stage of labor[20] (Figure 3-6). This increase in CO is caused primarily by an increased SV, but HR may also increase. By the end of the first stage of labor, the CO during contractions is 51% above baseline term pregnancy values (6.99 to 10.57 L/min).

Increased CO is in part secondary to increased venous return from the 300- to 500-mL autotransfusion that occurs at the onset of each contraction as blood is expressed from the uterus.[32,33] Paralleling increases in CO, the MAP also rises in the first stage of labor, from 82 to 91 mm Hg in early labor to 102 mm Hg by the beginning of the second stage. MAP also increases with uterine contractions.

Much of the increase in CO and MAP is due to pain and anxiety. With epidural anesthesia, the baseline increase in CO is reduced, but the rise observed with contractions persists.[34] Maternal posture also influences hemodynamics during labor. **Changing position from supine to lateral recumbent increases CO. This change is greater than the increase seen before labor and suggests that during labor, CO may be more dependent on preload. Therefore, it is important to avoid the supine position in laboring women and to give a sufficient fluid bolus before an epidural to maintain an adequate preload.**

In the immediate postpartum period (10 to 30 minutes after delivery), CO reaches its maximum, with a further rise of 10% to 20%. This increase is accompanied by a fall in the maternal HR that is likely secondary to increased SV. Traditionally, this rise was thought to be the result of uterine autotransfusion as described earlier with contractions, but the validity of this concept is uncertain. **In both vaginal and elective cesarean deliveries, the maximal increase in the CO occurs 10 to 30 minutes after delivery and returns to prelabor baseline 1 hour after delivery.** The increase was 37% with epidural anesthesia and 28% with general anesthesia. Over the next 2 to 4 postpartum weeks, the cardiac hemodynamic parameters return to near-preconceptional levels.[35]

The effect of pregnancy on cardiac rhythm is limited to an increase in HR and a significant increase in isolated atrial and ventricular contractions. In a Holter monitor study by Shotan and coworkers, 110 pregnant women referred for evaluation of symptoms of palpitations, dizziness, or syncope were compared with 52 healthy pregnant women.[36] Symptomatic women had similar rates of isolated sinus tachycardia (9%), isolated premature atrial complexes (56%), and premature ventricular contractions (PVCs) (49%), but increased rates of frequent PVCs greater than 10/hour (20% versus 2%, $P = 0.03$). A subset of patients with frequent premature atrial complexes or PVCs had comparative Holter studies performed postpartum that revealed an 85% decrease in arrhythmia frequency ($P < .05$). This dramatic decline, with patients acting as their own controls, supports the arrhythmogenic effect of pregnancy. In a study of 30 healthy women placed on Holter monitors during labor, a similarly high incidence of benign arrhythmias was found (93%). Reassuringly, the prevalence of concerning arrhythmias was no higher than expected. An unexpected finding was a 35% rate of asymptomatic bradycardia, defined as a HR of less than 60 beats/minute, in the immediate postpartum period.[37] In addition, other studies have shown that women with preexisting tachyarrhythmias have an increased incidence of these rate abnormalities during pregnancy.[38] Whether labor increases the rate of arrhythmias in women with cardiac disease has not been thoroughly studied, but multiple case reports suggest labor may increase arrhythmias in these women.

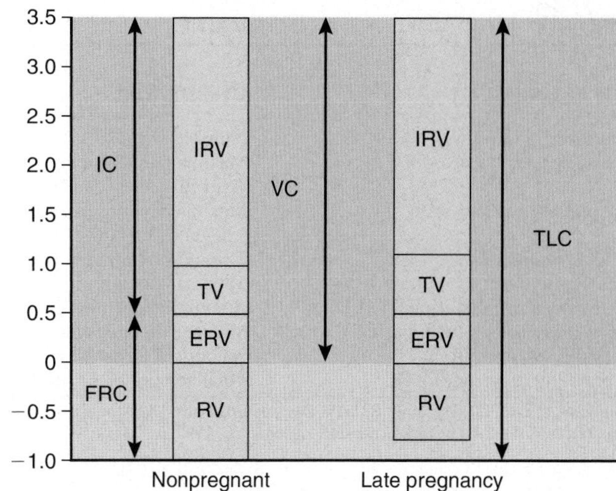

FIGURE 3-7. Lung volumes in nonpregnant and pregnant women. *ERV,* Expiratory reserve; *FRC,* functional residual capacity; *IC,* inspiratory capacity; *IRV,* inspiratory reserve; *RV,* residual volume; *TLC,* total lung capacity; *TV,* tidal volume; *VC,* vital capacity. (From Cruickshank DP, Wigton TR, Hays PM: Maternal physiology in pregnancy. *In* Gabbe SG, Niebyl JR, Simpson JL [eds]: Obstetrics: Normal and Problem Pregnancies, 3rd ed. New York, Churchill Livingstone, 1996, p 94.)

RESPIRATORY SYSTEM

Upper Respiratory Tract

During pregnancy, the mucosa of the nasopharynx becomes hyperemic and edematous with hypersecretion of mucus due to increased estrogen. These changes often lead to marked nasal stuffiness; epistaxis is also common. Placement of nasogastric tubes may cause excessive bleeding if adequate lubrication is not used.[30] Polyposis of the nose and nasal sinuses develops in some individuals but regresses postpartum. **Because of these changes, many gravid women complain of chronic cold symptoms. However, the temptation to use nasal decongestants should be avoided because of risk for hypertension and rebound congestion.**

Mechanical Changes

The configuration of the thoracic cage changes early in pregnancy, much earlier than can be accounted for by mechanical pressure from the enlarging uterus. Relaxation of the ligamentous attachments between the ribs and sternum may be responsible. The subcostal angle increases from 68 to 103 degrees, the transverse diameter of the chest expands by 2 cm, and the chest circumference expands by 5 to 7 cm. As gestation progresses, the level of the diaphragm rises 4 cm; however, diaphragmatic excursion is not impeded and actually increases 1 to 2 cm. Respiratory muscle function is not affected by pregnancy, and maximal inspiratory and expiratory pressures are unchanged.[39]

Lung Volume and Pulmonary Function

The described alterations in chest wall configuration and the diaphragm lead to changes in static lung volumes. In a review of studies with at least 15 subjects compared with nonpregnant controls, Crapo found significant changes (Figure 3-7 and Table 3-2).[30] The elevation of the

TABLE 3-2 LUNG VOLUMES AND CAPACITIES IN PREGNANCY

MEASUREMENT	DEFINITION	CHANGE IN PREGNANCY
Respiratory rate (RR)	Number of breaths per minute	Unchanged
Vital capacity (VC)	Maximal amount of air that can be forcibly expired after maximal inspiration (IC + ERV)	Unchanged
Inspiratory capacity (IC)	Maximal amount of air that can be inspired from resting expiratory level (TV + IRV)	Increased 5% to 10%
Tidal volume (TV)	Amount of air inspired and expired with a normal breath	Increased 30% to 40%
Inspiratory reserve volume (IRV)	Maximal amount of air that can be inspired at end of normal inspiration	Unchanged
Functional residual capacity (FRC)	Amount of air in lungs at resting expiratory level (ERV + RV)	Decreased 20%
Expiratory reserve volume (ERV)	Maximal amount of air that can be expired from resting expiratory level	Decreased 15% to 20%
Residual volume (RV)	Amount of air in lungs after maximal expiration	Decreased 20% to 25%
Total lung capacity (TLC)	Total amount of air in lungs at maximal inspiration (VC + RV)	Decreased 5%

From Cruickshank DP, Wigton TR, Hays PM: Maternal physiology in pregnancy. *In* Gabbe SG, Niebyl JR, Simpson JL (eds): Obstetrics: Normal and Problem Pregnancies, 3rd ed. New York, Churchill Livingstone, 1996, p 95.

diaphragm decreases the volume of the lungs in the resting state, thereby reducing total lung capacity and the functional residual capacity (FRC). The FRC can be subdivided into expiratory reserve volume and residual volume, and both decrease.

Spirometric measurements assessing bronchial flow are unaltered in pregnancy. The forced expiratory volume in 1 second (FEV_1) and the ratio of FEV_1 to forced vital capacity are both unchanged, suggesting that airway function remains stable. In addition, peak expiratory flow rates measured using a peak flow meter seem to be unaltered in pregnancy at rates of 450 ± 16 L/min.[40] Harirah and associates performed a longitudinal study of the peak flow in 38 women from the first trimester until 6 weeks postpartum.[41] They reported that the peak flows had a statistically significant decrease as the gestation progressed, but the amount of the decrease was minimal enough to be of questionable clinical significance. Likewise a small decrease in the peak flow was found in the supine position versus the standing or sitting position. **Therefore, during gestation, both spirometry and peak flow meters can be used in diagnosing and managing respiratory illnesses, but the clinician should ensure that measurements are performed in the same maternal position.**[41]

Gas Exchange

Increasing progesterone levels drive a state of chronic hyperventilation, as reflected by a 30% to 50% increase in tidal volume by 8 weeks' gestation. In turn, increased tidal volume results in an overall parallel rise in minute ventilation, despite a stable respiratory rate (minute ventilation = tidal volume × respiratory rate). The rise in minute ventilation, combined with a decrease in FRC, leads to a larger than expected increase in alveolar ventilation (50% to 70%). **Chronic mild hyperventilation results in increased alveolar oxygen (PAO_2) and decreased arterial carbon dioxide ($PaCO_2$) from normal levels** (Table 3-3). The drop in the $PaCO_2$ is especially critical because it drives a more favorable carbon dioxide (CO_2) gradient between the fetus and mother, facilitating CO_2 transfer. **The low maternal $PaCO_2$ results in a chronic respiratory alkalosis.** Partial renal compensation occurs through increased excretion of bicarbonate, which helps maintain the pH between 7.4 and 7.45 and lowers the serum bicarbonate levels. Early in pregnancy, the arterial oxygen (PaO_2) increases (106 to 108 mm Hg) as the $PaCO_2$ decreases, but by the third trimester, a slight decrease in the PaO_2 (101 to 104 mm Hg) occurs as a result of the enlarging uterus. This decrease in the PaO_2 late in pregnancy is even more pronounced in the supine position, with a further drop of 5 to 10 mm Hg and an increase in the alveolar-to-arterial gradient to 26 mm Hg, and up to 25% of women exhibit a PaO_2 of less than 90 mm Hg.[30,42]

TABLE 3-3 BLOOD GAS VALUES IN THIRD TRIMESTER OF PREGNANCY

	PREGNANT	NONPREGNANT
PaO_2 (mm Hg)*	101.8 ± 1	93.4 ± 2.04
Arterial Hgb saturation (%)†	98.5 ± 0.7%	98 ± 0.8%
$PaCO_2$ (mm hg)*	30.4 ± 0.6	40 ± 2.5
pH*	7.43 ± 0.006	7.43 ± 0.02
Serum bicarbonate (HCO_3) (mmol/L)	21.7 ± 1.6	25.3 ± 1.2
Base deficit (mmol/L)*	3.1 ± 0.2	1.06 ± 0.6
Alveolar-arterial gradient [$P(A\text{-}a)O_2$ (mm Hg)]*	16.1 ± 0.9	15.7 ± 0.6

*Data from Templeton A, Kelman G: Maternal blood-gases, (PAO_2-PaO_2), physiological shunt and *VD/VT* in normal pregnancy. Br J Anaesth 48:1001, 1976. Data presented as mean ± SEM.

†Data from McAuliffe F, Kametas N, Krampl E: Blood gases in prepregnancy at sea level and at high altitude. Br J Obstet Gynaecol 108:980, 2001. Data presented as mean ± SD.

As the minute ventilation increases, a simultaneous but smaller increase in oxygen uptake and consumption occurs. Most investigators have found maternal oxygen consumption to be 20% to 40% above nonpregnant levels. This increase occurs as a result of the oxygen requirements of the fetus, the placenta, and the increased oxygen requirement of maternal organs. With exercise or during labor, an even greater rise in both minute ventilation and oxygen consumption takes place.[30] During a contraction, oxygen consumption can triple. **As a result of the increased oxygen consumption and because the functional residual capacity is decreased, there is a lowering of the maternal oxygen reserve. Therefore, the pregnant patient is more susceptible to the effects of apnea, such as during intubation when a more rapid onset of hypoxia, hypercapnia, and respiratory acidosis is seen.**

TABLE 3-4 CHARACTERISTICS OF SLEEP IN PREGNANCY

STAGE OF PREGNANCY	SUBJECTIVE SYMPTOMS	OBJECTIVE (POLYSOMNOGRAPHY)*
First trimester	Increased total sleep time: ↑ naps Increased daytime sleepiness Increased nocturnal insomnia	Increased total sleep time Decreased stages 3 and 4 non-REM sleep
Second trimester	Normalization of total sleep time Increased awakenings	Normal total sleep time Decreased stages 3 and 4 non-REM sleep Decreased REM sleep
Third trimester	Decreased total sleep time Increased insomnia Increased nocturnal awakenings Increased daytime sleepiness	Decreased total sleep time Increased awakenings after sleep onset Increased stage 1 non-REM sleep Decreased stages 3 and 4 non-REM sleep Decreased REM sleep

Modified from Santiago J, Nolledo M, Kinzler W: Sleep and sleep disorders in pregnancy. Ann Intern Med 134:396, 2001.
*Rapid eye movement (REM) sleep is important for cognitive sleep, 20% to 25% of sleep. Stages 1 and 2 non-REM sleep: light sleep, 55% of sleep. Stages 3 and 4 non-REM sleep: deep sleep, important for rest, 20% of sleep.

Sleep

Pregnancy causes both an increase in sleep disorders and significant changes in sleep profile and pattern that persist into the postpartum period.[43] Pregnancy causes such significant changes that the American Sleep Disorder Association has proposed the existence of a new term: *pregnancy-associated sleep disorder*. Emerging evidence indicates that sleep disturbances are associated with poor health outcomes in the general population and that sleep disturbances in pregnancy may contribute to certain complications of pregnancy. It is well known that hormones and physical discomforts affect sleep (Table 3-4). With the dramatic change in hormone levels and the significant mechanical effects that make women more uncomfortable, it is not difficult to understand why sleep is profoundly affected. Multiple authors have investigated the changes in sleep during pregnancy using questionnaires, sleep logs, and polysomnographic studies. From these studies, investigators have shown that most women (66% to 94%) report alterations in sleep that lead to the subjective perception of poor sleep quality. The disturbances in sleep begin as early as the first trimester and worsen as the pregnancy progresses.[44] During the third trimester, multiple discomforts occur that can impair sleep: urinary frequency, backache, general abdominal discomfort and contractions, leg cramps, restless leg syndrome, heartburn, and fetal movement. Interestingly, no changes are seen in melatonin levels, which modulate the body's circadian pacemaker.

In general, pregnancy is associated with a decrease in rapid eye movement (REM) sleep and a decrease in stages 3 and 4 non-REM sleep. REM sleep is important for cognitive thinking, and stages 3 and 4 non-REM sleep is the so-called deep sleep and is important for rest. In addition, with advancing gestational age, there is a decrease in sleeping efficiency and sleep continuity and an increase in awake time and daytime somnolence. By 3 months postpartum, the amount of non-REM and REM sleep recovers, but a persistent decrease in sleeping efficiency and nocturnal awakenings occur, presumably because of the newborn.[43] Although pregnancy causes changes in sleep, it is important for the clinician to consider other primary sleep disorders unrelated to pregnancy such as sleep apnea. The physiologic changes of pregnancy also increase the incidence of sleep-disordered breathing, which includes snoring (in up to 16% of women), upper airway obstruction, and potentially obstructive sleep apnea. The prevalence of sleep apnea in pregnancy is unknown, but it appears to increase the risk for intrauterine growth restriction and gestational hypertension if it is associated with hypoxemia. **Women with excessive daytime sleepiness, loud excessive snoring, and witnessed apneas should be evaluated for obstructive sleep apnea with overnight polysomnography.**[45] **In addition, individuals with known sleep apnea may need repeat sleep studies to determine whether changes in treatment are necessary to prevent intermittent hypoxia.**

Although the majority of gravidas have sleep problems, most do not complain to their providers or ask for treatment. Treatment options include improving sleep habits by avoiding fluids after dinner, establishing regular sleep hours, avoiding naps and caffeine, minimizing bedroom noises, and using pillow support. Other options include relaxation techniques, managing back pain, and use of sleep medications such as diphenhydramine (Benadryl) and zolpidem (Ambien).

Another potential cause of sleep disturbances in pregnancy is the development of restless leg syndrome and periodic leg movements during sleep. Restless leg syndrome is a neurosensory disorder that typically begins in the evening and can prevent women from falling asleep. Pregnancy can be a cause of this syndrome, and in one study up to 23% of gravidas developed some component of this syndrome in the third trimester, although the true prevalence of this disorder during pregnancy is unknown. Although typically this syndrome is not severe enough to warrant treatment, occasionally it is a source of great discomfort to the gravid woman. Treatment options include improving sleep habits, use of an electric vibrator to the calves, and use of a benzodiazepine such as clonazepam or a dopaminergic agent such as L-dopa or carbidopa.

HEMATOLOGIC CHANGES

Plasma Volume and Red Blood Cell Mass

Maternal blood volume begins to increase at about 6 weeks' gestation. Thereafter, it increases progressively until 30 to 34 weeks and then plateaus until delivery. The average expansion of blood volume is 40% to 50%, although individual increases range from 20% to 100%. Women with multiple pregnancies have a larger increase in blood

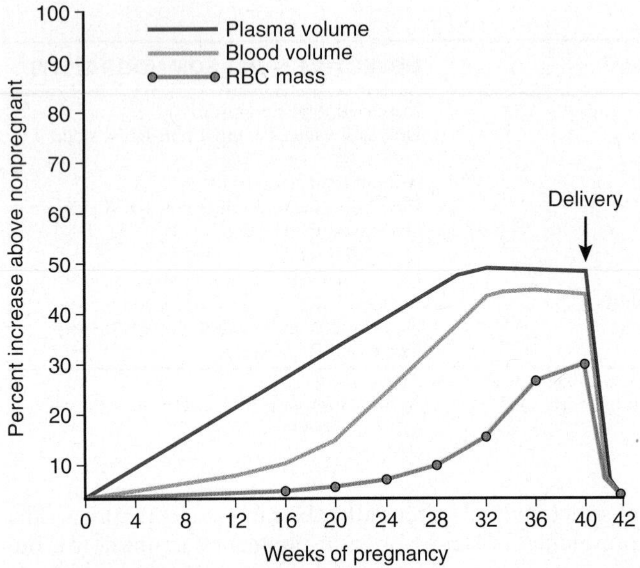

FIGURE 3-8. Blood volume changes during pregnancy. *RBC*, Red blood cell. (From Scott D: Anemia during pregnancy. Obstet Gynecol Ann 1:219, 1972.)

volume than those with singletons.[46] Likewise, volume expansion correlates with infant birthweight, but it is not clear whether this is a cause or an effect. The increase in blood volume results from a combined expansion of both plasma volume and red blood cell (RBC) mass. **The plasma volume begins to increase by 6 weeks and expands at a steady pace until it plateaus at 30 weeks' gestation; the overall increase is about 50% (1200 to 1300 mL).** The exact etiology of the expansion of the blood volume is unknown, but the hormonal changes of gestation and the increase in NO play important roles.

Erythrocyte mass also begins to increase at about 10 weeks' gestation. Although the initial slope of this increase is slower than that of the plasma volume, erythrocyte mass continues to increase progressively until term without plateauing. Without iron supplementation, RBC mass increases about 18% by term, from a mean nonpregnant level of 1400 mL up to 1650 mL. **Supplemental iron increases RBC mass accumulation to 400 to 450 mL, or 30%.[46] Because plasma volume increases more than the RBC mass, maternal hematocrit falls. This so-called physiologic anemia of pregnancy reaches a nadir at 30 to 34 weeks. Because the RBC mass continues to increase after 30 weeks when the plasma volume expansion has plateaued, the hematocrit may rise somewhat after 30 weeks** (Figure 3-8). The mean and fifth percentile hemoglobin concentrations for normal iron-supplemented pregnant women are outlined (Table 3-5). In pregnancy, erythropoietin levels increase twofold to threefold, starting at 16 weeks, and may be responsible for the moderate erythroid hyperplasia found in the bone marrow and mild elevations in the reticulocyte count. The increased blood volume is protective given the possibility of hemorrhage during pregnancy or at delivery. The larger blood volume also helps fill the expanded vascular system created by vasodilation and the large low-resistance vascular pool within the uteroplacental unit preventing hypotension.[30]

TABLE 3-5 HEMOGLOBIN VALUES IN PREGNANCY

WEEKS' GESTATION	MEAN HEMOGLOBIN (g/dL)	FIFTH PERCENTILE HEMOGLOBIN (g/dL)
12	12.2	11.0
16	11.8	10.6
20	11.6	10.5
24	11.6	10.5
28	11.8	10.7
32	12.1	11.0
36	12.5	11.4
40	12.9	11.9

From U.S. Department of Health and Human Services: Recommendations to prevent and control iron deficiency in the United States. MMWR Morb Mortal Wkly Rep 47:1, 1998.

Vaginal delivery of a singleton infant at term is associated with a mean blood loss of 500 mL; an uncomplicated cesarean birth, about 1000 mL; and a cesarean hysterectomy, 1500 mL.[46,47] In a normal delivery, almost all of the blood loss occurs in the first hour. Pritchard and colleagues found that over the subsequent 72 hours, only 80 mL of blood is lost.[47] In the nonpregnant state, blood loss results in an immediate fall in blood volume with a slow re-expansion through volume redistribution; by 24 hours, the blood volume approaches the prehemorrhage level. Isovolemia is maintained with a drop in hematocrit proportional to the blood loss. Gravid women respond to blood loss in a different fashion. **In pregnancy, the blood volume drops after postpartum bleeding, but there is no re-expansion to the prelabor level, and there is less of a change in the hematocrit. Indeed, instead of volume redistribution, an overall diuresis of the expanded water volume occurs postpartum.** After delivery with average blood loss, the hematocrit drops moderately for 3 to 4 days, followed by an increase. By days 5 to 7, the postpartum hematocrit is similar to the prelabor hematocrit. **If the postpartum hematocrit is lower than the prelabor hematocrit, either that the blood loss was larger than appreciated, or the hypervolemia of pregnancy was less than normal, as in preeclampsia.[47]**

Iron Metabolism in Pregnancy

Iron absorption from the duodenum is limited to its ferrous (divalent) state, the form found in iron supplements. Ferric (trivalent) iron from vegetable food sources must first be converted to the divalent state by the enzyme ferric reductase. If body iron stores are normal, only about 10% of ingested iron is absorbed, most of which remains in the mucosal cells or enterocytes until sloughing leads to excretion in the feces (1 mg/day). Under conditions of increased iron needs, the fraction of iron absorbed increases. After absorption, iron is released from the enterocytes into the circulation, where it is carried bound to transferrin to the liver, spleen, muscle, and bone marrow. In those sites, iron is freed from transferrin and incorporated into hemoglobin (75% of iron) and myoglobin or stored as ferritin and hemosiderin. Menstruating women have about half the iron stores of men, with total body iron of 2 to 2.5 g and iron stores of only 300 mg. Before pregnancy, 8% to 10% of women in Western nations have iron deficiency.

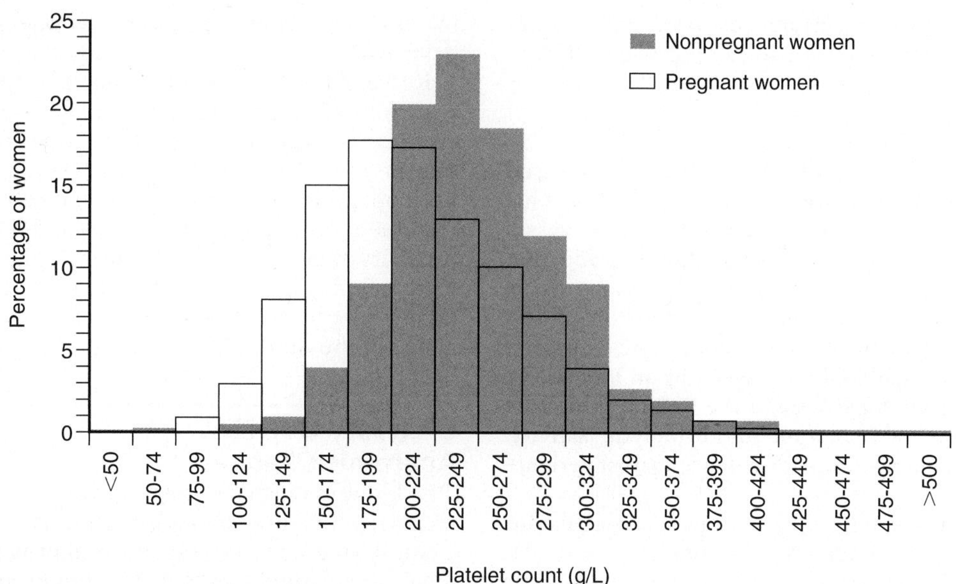

FIGURE 3-9. Histogram of platelet count of pregnant women in the third trimester (n = 6770) compared with nonpregnant women (n = 287). (From Boehlen F, Hohlfield P, Extermann P: Platelet count at term pregnancy: a reappraisal of the threshold. Obstet Gynecol 95:29, 2000.)

The iron requirements of gestation are about 1000 mg. This includes 500 mg used to increase the maternal RBC mass (1 mL of erythrocytes contains 1.1 mg iron), 300 mg transported to the fetus, and 200 mg to compensate for the normal daily iron losses by the mother.[48] Thus, the normal expectant woman needs to absorb an average of 3.5 mg/day of iron. In actuality, the iron requirements are not constant but increase remarkably during the pregnancy from 0.8 mg/day in the first trimester to 6 to 7 mg/day in the third trimester. The fetus receives its iron through active transport, primarily during the last trimester. Adequate iron transport to the fetus is maintained despite severe maternal iron deficiency. Thus, there is no correlation between maternal and fetal hemoglobin concentrations. For a review on use of supplemental iron in pregnancy, see Chapter 42.

Platelets

Before the introduction of automated analyzers, studies of platelet counts during pregnancy reported conflicting results, with some showing a decrease, an increase, or no change with gestation. Unfortunately, even with the availability of automated cell counters, the data on the change in platelet count during pregnancy are still somewhat unclear. Two studies have used true longitudinal methods with serial measurements in the same women. Pitkin and colleagues measured platelet counts in 23 women every 4 weeks and found that the counts dropped from $322 \pm 75 \times 10^3/mm^3$ in the first trimester to $278 \pm 75 \times 10^3/mm^3$ in the third trimester.[49] Similarly, O'Brien, in a study of 30 women, found a progressive decline in platelet counts.[50] Therefore, most recent studies show a decline in the platelet count during gestation possibly caused by increased destruction or hemodilution. **In addition to the mild decrease in the mean platelet count, Burrows and Kelton have demonstrated that in the third trimester, about 8% of gravidas develop gestational thrombocytopenia, with platelet counts between 70,000 and 150,000/mm³.**[51] **Gestational thrombocytopenia is not associated with an increase in pregnancy complications, and platelet counts return to normal by 1 to 2 weeks postpartum.** Gestational thrombocytopenia is thought to be due to accelerated platelet consumption similar to that seen in normal pregnancy, but more marked in this subset of women.[51] Consistent with these findings, Boehlen and associates compared platelet counts during the third trimester of pregnancy with those in nonpregnant controls. They showed a shift to a lower mean platelet count and an overall shift to the left of the "platelet curve" in the pregnant women (Figure 3-9). This study found that only 2.5% of nonpregnant women have platelet counts less than 150,000/mm³ (the traditional value used outside of pregnancy as the cut-off for normal) versus 11.5% of gravid women. **A platelet count of less than 116,000/mm³ occurred in 2.5% of gravid women; therefore, these investigators recommended using this value as the lower limit for normal in the third trimester.** In addition, they suggested that workups for the etiology of decreased platelet count were unneeded at values above this level.

Leukocytes

The peripheral white blood cell (WBC) count rises progressively during pregnancy. During the first trimester, the mean WBC count is 8000/mm³, with a normal range of 5110 to 9900/mm³. During the second and third trimesters, the mean is 8500/mm³, with a range of 5600 to 12,200/mm³.[49] In labor, the count may rise to 20,000 to 30,000/mm³, and counts are highly correlated with labor progression as determined by cervical dilation.[52] Because of the normal increase of WBCs in labor, the WBC count should not be used clinically in determining the presence of infection. The increase in the WBC count is largely due to increases in circulating segmented neutrophils and granulocytes whose absolute number is nearly doubled at term. The reason for the increased leukocytosis is unclear, but it may be caused by the elevated estrogen and cortisol levels. Leukocyte levels return to normal within 1 to 2 weeks of delivery.

Coagulation System

Pregnancy places women at a fivefold to sixfold increased risk for thromboembolic disease (see Chapter 43). This greater risk is caused by increased venous stasis, vessel wall injury, and changes in the coagulation cascade that lead to hypercoagulability. The increase in venous status in the lower extremities is due to compression of the inferior vena cava and the pelvic veins by the enlarging uterus. **The hypercoagulability is caused by an increase in several procoagulants, a decrease in the natural inhibitors of coagulation, and a reduction in fibrinolytic activity. These physiologic changes provide defense against peripartum hemorrhage.**

Most of the procoagulant factors from the coagulation cascade are markedly increased, including factors I, VII, VIII, IX, and X. Factors II, V, and XII are unchanged or mildly increased, and levels of factors XI and XIII decline.[1,53] Plasma fibrinogen (factor I) levels begin to increase in the first trimester and peak in the third trimester at levels 50% higher than before pregnancy. The rise in fibrinogen is associated with an increase in the erythrocyte sedimentation rate. In addition, pregnancy causes a decrease in the fibrinolytic system with reduced levels of available circulating plasminogen activator, a twofold to threefold increase in plasminogen activator inhibitor-1 (PAI-1), and a 25-fold increase in PAI-2.[1] The placenta produces PAI-1 and is the primary source of PAI-2.

Pregnancy has been shown to cause a progressive and significant decrease in the levels of total and free protein S from early in pregnancy but to have no effect on the levels of protein C and antithrombin III.[54,55] The activated protein C (APC)-to-sensitivity (S) ratio, the ratio of the clotting time in the presence and the absence of APC, declines during pregnancy. The APC/S ratio is considered abnormal if less than 2.6. In a study of 239 women,[54] the APC/S ratio decreased from a mean of 3.12 in the first trimester to 2.63 by the third trimester. By the third trimester, 38% of women were found to have an acquired APC resistance, with APC/S ratio values below 2.6.[54] Whether the changes in the protein S level and the APC/S ratio are responsible for some of the hypercoagulability of pregnancy is unknown. **If a workup for thrombophilias is performed during gestation, the clinician should use caution when attempting to interpret these levels if they are abnormal. Ideally the clinician should order DNA testing for the Leiden mutation instead of testing for APC. For protein S screening during pregnancy, the free protein S antigen level should be tested with normal levels in the second and third trimesters being identified as greater than 30% and 24%.**[56]

Most coagulation testing is unaffected by pregnancy. The prothrombin time, activated partial thromboplastin time, and thrombin time all fall slightly but remain within the limits of normal nonpregnant values, whereas the bleeding time and whole blood clotting times are unchanged. Testing for von Willebrand disease is affected in pregnancy because levels of factor VIII, von Willebrand factor activity and antigen, and ristocetin cofactor all increase. Levels of coagulation factors normalize 2 weeks postpartum.

Researchers have found evidence to support the theory that, during pregnancy, a state of low-level intravascular coagulation occurs. Low concentrations of fibrin degradation products (markers of fibrinolysis), elevated levels of fibrinopeptide A (a marker for increased clotting), and increased levels of platelet factor-4 and β-thromboglobulin (markers of increased platelet activity) have been found in maternal blood.[57] The most likely cause for these findings involves localized physiologic changes needed for maintenance of the uterine-placental interface.

URINARY SYSTEM

Anatomic Changes

The kidneys enlarge during pregnancy, with the length as measured by intravenous pyelography increasing about 1 cm. This growth in size and weight is due to increased renal vasculature, interstitial volume, and urinary dead space. **The increase in urinary dead space is attributed to dilation of the renal pelvis, calyces, and ureters. Pelvicaliceal dilation by term averages 15 mm (range, 5 to 25 mm) on the right and 5 mm (range, 3 to 8 mm) on the left.**[58]

The well-known dilation of the ureters and renal pelves begins by the second month of pregnancy and is maximal by the middle of the second trimester, when ureteric diameter may be as much as 2 cm. The right ureter is almost invariably dilated more than the left, and the dilation usually cannot be demonstrated below the pelvic brim. These findings have led some investigators to argue that the dilation is caused entirely by mechanical compression of the ureters by the enlarging uterus and ovarian venous plexus. However, the early onset of ureteral dilation suggests that smooth muscle relaxation caused by progesterone plays an additional role. Also supporting the role of progesterone is the finding of ureteral dilation in women with renal transplant and pelvic kidney.[59] By 6 weeks postpartum, ureteral dilation resolves.[58] A clinical consequence of ureterocalyceal dilation is an increased incidence of pyelonephritis among gravidas with asymptomatic bacteriuria. **In addition, the ureterocalyceal dilation makes interpretation of urinary radiographs more difficult when evaluating possible urinary tract obstruction or nephrolithiasis.**

Anatomic changes are also observed in the bladder. From midpregnancy on, an elevation in the bladder trigone occurs, with increased vascular tortuosity throughout the bladder. This can cause an increased incidence of microhematuria. Three percent of gravidas have idiopathic hematuria, defined as greater than 1+ on a urine dipstick, and up to 16% have microscopic hematuria. Because of the increasing size of the pregnancy, a decrease in bladder capacity develops with an increase in urinary frequency, urgency, and incontinence.

Renal Hemodynamics

Renal plasma flow (RPF) increases markedly from early in gestation and may actually initially begin to increase during the luteal phase before implantation.[60] Dunlop showed convincingly that the effective RPF rises 75% over nonpregnant levels by 16 weeks' gestation (Table 3-6). The increase is maintained until 34 weeks' gestation, when a

TABLE 3-6 SERIAL CHANGES IN RENAL HEMODYNAMICS

		SEATED POSITION (n = 25)*			LEFT LATERAL RECUMBENT POSITION (n = 17)†	
	Nonpregnant	16 wk	26 wk	36 wk	29 wk	37 wk
Effective renal plasma flow (mL/min)	480 ± 72	840 ± 145	891 ± 279	771 ± 175	748 ± 85	677 ± 82
Glomerular filtration rate (mL/min)	99 ± 18	149 ± 17	152 ± 18	150 ± 32	145 ± 19	138 ± 22
Filtration fraction	0.21	0.18	0.18	0.20	0.19	0.21

*Data from Dunlop W: Serial changes in renal haemodynamics during normal pregnancy. Br J Obstet Gynaecol 88:1, 1981.

†Data from Ezimokhai M, Davison J, Philips P, et al: Nonpostural serial changes in renal function during the third trimester of normal human pregnancy. Br J Obstet Gynaecol 88:465, 1981.

decline in RPF of about 25% occurs. The fall in RPF has been demonstrated in subjects studied serially in the sitting and the left lateral recumbent positions. Like RPF, glomerular filtration rate (GFR), as measured by inulin clearance, increases by 5 to 7 weeks. **By the end of the first trimester, GFR is 50% higher than in the nonpregnant state, and this is maintained until the end of pregnancy.** Three months postpartum, GFR values have declined to normal levels.[61] This renal hyperfiltration seen in pregnancy is a result of the increase in the RPF. Because the RPF increases more than the GFR early in pregnancy, the filtration fraction falls from nonpregnant levels until the late third trimester. At this time, because of the decline in RPF, the filtration fraction returns to preconceptional values.

Clinically, GFR is not determined by measuring the clearance of infused inulin (inulin is filtered by the glomerulus and is unaffected by the tubules), but rather by measuring endogenous creatinine clearance. This test gives a less precise measure of GFR because creatinine is secreted by the tubules to a variable extent. Therefore, endogenous creatinine clearance is usually higher than the actual GFR. **The creatinine clearance in pregnancy is greatly increased to values of 150 to 200 mL/min (normal, 120 mL/min).** As with GFR, the increase in creatinine clearance occurs by 5 to 7 weeks' gestation and normally is maintained until the third trimester. GFR is best estimated in pregnancy using a 24-hour urine collection for creatinine clearance. **Formulas that are used in patients with renal disease that estimate the GFR using serum collections and clinical parameters (which avoid a 24-hour urine collection) are inaccurate in pregnancy and underestimate the GFR.**

The increase in the RPF and GFR precede the increase in blood volume and may be induced by a reduction in the preglomerular and postglomerular arteriolar resistance. Importantly, the increase in hyperfiltration occurs without an increase in glomerular pressure, which if it occurred, could have the potential for injury to a women's kidney with long-term consequences.[60] Recently, the mechanisms underlying the marked increase in RPF and GFR has been carefully studied. Although numerous factors are involved in this process, NO has been demonstrated to play a critical role in the decrease in renal resistance and the subsequent renal hyperemia. During pregnancy, the activation and expression of the NO synthase is enhanced in the kidneys, and inhibition of NO synthase isoforms has been shown to attenuate the hemodynamic changes within the gravid kidney.[25] Finally, the hormone relaxin appears to be important by initiating or activating some of the effects of NO on the kidney. Failure of this crucial adaptation to occur is associated with adverse outcomes such as preeclampsia and fetal growth restriction.[7]

The clinical consequences of glomerular hyperfiltration are a reduction in maternal plasma levels of creatinine, blood urea nitrogen (BUN), and uric acid. Serum creatinine decreases from a nonpregnant level of 0.8 mg/dL to 0.5 mg/dL by term. Likewise, BUN falls from nonpregnant levels of 13 to 9 mg/dL by term.[5] Serum uric acid declines in early pregnancy because of the rise in GFR, reaching a nadir by 24 weeks with levels of 2 to 3 mg/dL.[62] After 24 weeks, the uric acid level begins to rise, and by the end of pregnancy, the levels in most women are essentially the same as before conception. The rise in uric acid levels is caused by increased renal tubular absorption of urate and increased fetal uric acid production. **Patients with preeclampsia have elevated uric acid level concentrations; however, because uric acid levels normally rise during the third trimester, over-reliance on this test should be avoided in the diagnosis and management of preeclampsia.**[62]

During pregnancy, urine volume is increased, and nocturia is more common. In the standing position, sodium and water are retained, and therefore, during the daytime, gravidas tend to retain an increased amount of water. At night while in the lateral recumbent position, this added water is excreted, resulting in nocturia. Later in gestation, the renal function is affected by position, and the GFR and renal hemodynamics are decreased with changes from lateral recumbency to supine or standing.[63]

Renal Tubular Function/Excretion of Nutrients

Despite high levels of aldosterone, which would be expected to result in enhanced urinary excretion of potassium, gravid women retain about 350 mmol of potassium. Most of the excess potassium is stored in the fetus and placenta. The mean potassium concentrations in maternal blood are just slightly below nonpregnant levels. The kidney's ability to conserve potassium has been attributed to increased progesterone levels.[64] For information on the changes of sodium, see the section on body water metabolism earlier in this chapter.

Glucose excretion increases in almost all pregnant women, and glycosuria is common. Nonpregnant urinary excretion of glucose is less than 100 mg/day, but 90% of gravidas with normal blood glucose levels excrete 1 to 10 g

TABLE 3-7 COMPARISON OF 24-HOUR URINARY VOLUME PROTEIN AND ALBUMIN EXCRETION

	20 WEEKS (n = 95)	20 WEEKS (n = 175)	SIGNIFICANCE
Protein (mg/24 hr)	98.1 ± 62.3	121.8 ± 71	P = .007
Albumin (mg/24 hr)	9.7 ± 6.2	12.2 ± 8.5	P = .012

From Higby K, Suiter C, Phelps J, et al: Normal values of urinary albumin and total protein excretion during pregnancy. Am J Obstet Gynecol 171:984, 1994.
Values are expressed as mean ± SD.

of glucose per day.[65] This glycosuria is intermittent and not necessarily related to blood glucose levels or the stage of gestation. Glucose is freely filtered by the glomerulus, and with the 50% increase in GFR, a greater load of glucose is presented to the proximal tubules. There may be a change in the reabsorptive capability of the proximal tubules themselves, but the old concept of pregnancy leading to an overwhelming of the maximal tubular reabsorptive capacity for glucose is misleading and oversimplified.[65] The exact mechanisms underlying the altered handling of glucose by the proximal tubules remains obscure. **Even though glycosuria is common, gravidas with repetitive glycosuria should be screened for diabetes mellitus if not already tested.**

Urinary protein and albumin excretion increases during pregnancy, with an upper limit of 300 mg of proteinuria and 30 mg of albuminuria in a 24-hour period.[63] The amount of proteinuria and albuminuria increases both when compared with nonpregnant levels and as the pregnancy advances. Higby and associates collected 24-hour urine samples from 270 women over the course of pregnancy and determined the amount of proteinuria and albuminuria. These investigators found that the amount of protein and albumin excreted in urine did not increase significantly by trimester but did increase significantly when compared between the first and second half of pregnancy (Table 3-7). **They observed that in women without preeclampsia, underlying renal disease, or urinary tract infections, the mean 24-hour urine protein across pregnancy is 116.9 mg, with a 95% upper confidence limit of 260 mg. They also noted that patients do not normally have microalbuminuria, defined as urinary albumin excretion greater than 30 mg/dL. In women with preexisting proteinuria, the amount of proteinuria increases in both the second and third trimesters, and potentially in the first trimester.** In a study of women with diabetic nephropathy, the amount of proteinuria increased from a mean of 1.74 ± 1.33 g per 24 hours in the first trimester to a mean of 4.82 ± 4.7 g per 24 hours in the third trimester, even in the absence of preeclampsia.[66] The increase in the renal excretion of proteins is due to a physiologic impairment of the proximal tubular function within the kidney and the increase in the GFR.[63]

Other changes in tubular function include an increase in the excretion of amino acids in the urine and an increase in calcium excretion (see Chapter 40). Also, the kidney responds to the respiratory alkalosis of pregnancy by enhanced excretion of bicarbonate; however, renal handling of acid excretion is unchanged.

ALIMENTARY TRACT

Appetite

Most women experience an increase in appetite throughout pregnancy. In the absence of nausea or "morning sickness," women eating according to appetite will increase food intake by about 200 kcal/day by the end of the first trimester. The recommended dietary allowance calls for an additional 300 kcal/day, although in reality most women make up for this with decreased activity. Energy requirements vary depending on the population studied, and a greater increase may be necessary for pregnant teenagers and women with high levels of physical activity. Extensive folklore exists about dietary cravings and aversions during gestation. Many of these are undoubtedly due to an individual's perception of which foods aggravate or ameliorate such symptoms as nausea and heartburn. The sense of taste may be blunted in some women, leading to an increased desire for highly seasoned food. Pica, a bizarre craving for strange foods, is relatively common among gravidas, and a history of pica should be sought in those with poor weight gain or refractory anemia. Examples of pica include the consumption of clay, starch, toothpaste, and ice.

Mouth

The pH and the production of saliva are probably unchanged during pregnancy. Ptyalism, an unusual complication of pregnancy, most often occurs in women suffering from nausea and may be associated with the loss of 1 to 2 L of saliva per day. Most authorities believe ptyalism actually represents inability of the nauseated woman to swallow normal amounts of saliva rather than a true increase in the production of saliva. A decrease in the ingestion of starchy foods may help decrease the amount of saliva. No evidence exists that pregnancy causes or accelerates the course of dental caries. However, the gums swell and may bleed after tooth brushing, giving rise to the so-called gingivitis of pregnancy. At times, a tumorous gingivitis may occur, presenting as a violaceous pedunculated lesion at the gum line that may bleed profusely. Called epulis gravidarum or pyogenic granulomas, these lesions consist of granulation tissue and an inflammatory infiltrate (see Chapter 48).

Stomach

The tone and motility of the stomach are decreased, probably because of the smooth muscle–relaxing effects of progesterone and estrogen. Nevertheless, scientific evidence regarding delayed gastric emptying is inconclusive.[67] Macfie and colleagues, using acetaminophen absorption as an indirect measure of gastric emptying, failed to demonstrate a delay in gastric emptying when comparing 15 nonpregnant controls with 15 women in each trimester.[67] In addition, a recent study showed no delay in gastric emptying in parturients at term who ingested 300 mL of water following an overnight fast.[68] However, an increased delay is seen in labor, with the etiology ascribed to the pain and stress of labor.

Pregnancy causes a decreased risk for peptic ulcer disease but, at the same time, causes an increase in gastroesophageal reflux disease and dyspepsia in 30% to 50% of

individuals.[69] This apparent paradox can be partially explained by physiologic changes of the stomach and lower esophagus. The increase in gastroesophageal reflux disease is multifactorial and is attributed to esophageal dysmotility caused by gestational hormones, gastric compression from the enlarged uterus, and a decrease in the pressure of the gastroesophageal sphincter. The decrease in the tone of the gastroesophageal sphincter is caused by progesterone, and estrogen may lead to increased reflux of stomach acids into the esophagus and may be the predominant cause of reflux symptoms. Theories proposed to explain the decreased incidence of peptic ulcer disease include increased placental histaminase synthesis with lower maternal histamine levels; increased gastric mucin production leading to protection of the gastric mucosa; reduced gastric acid secretion; and enhanced immunologic tolerance of *Helicobacter pylori*, the infectious agent that causes peptic ulcer disease[69] (see Chapter 45).

Intestines

Perturbations in the motility of the small intestines and colon are common in pregnancy, resulting in an increased incidence of constipation in some and diarrhea in others. Up to 34% of women in one study noted an increased frequency of bowel movements, perhaps related to increased prostaglandin synthesis.[70] The prevalence of constipation appears to be higher in early pregnancy, with 35% to 39% of women having constipation in the first and second trimester and only 21% in the last trimester.[71] The motility of the small intestines is reduced in pregnancy, with increased oral-cecal transit times. No studies on the colonic transit time have been performed, but limited information suggests reduced colonic motility.[70] Although progesterone has been thought to be the primary cause of the decrease in gastrointestinal motility, newer studies show the actual etiology may be due to estrogen. Estrogen causes an increased release of NO from nerves that innervate the gastrointestinal tract that then results in relaxation of the gastrointestinal tract musculature. Absorption of nutrients from the small bowel (with the exception of increased iron and calcium absorption) is unchanged, but the increased transit time allows for more efficient absorption. Parry and colleagues demonstrated an increase in both water and sodium absorption in the colon.[72]

The enlarging uterus displaces the intestines and, most importantly, moves the position of the appendix. Thus, the presentation, physical signs, and type of surgical incision are affected in the management of appendicitis. Portal venous pressure is increased, leading to dilation wherever there is portosystemic venous anastomosis. This includes the gastroesophageal junction and the hemorrhoidal veins, which results in the common complaint of hemorrhoids.

Gallbladder

The function of the gallbladder is markedly altered because of the effects of progesterone. After the first trimester, the fasting and residual volumes are twice as great, and the rate at which the gallbladder empties is much slower. In addition, the biliary cholesterol saturation is increased, and the chenodeoxycholic acid level is decreased.[73] This change in the composition of the bile fluid favors the formation of cholesterol crystals, and with incomplete emptying of the gallbladder, the crystals are retained, and gallstone formation is enhanced. **During pregnancy, biliary sludge develops in about one third of women, and by the time of delivery 10% to 12% of women have gallstones on ultrasonographic examination. Postpartum, biliary sludge disappears in virtually all women, but only about one third of small stones disappear.**

Liver

The size and histology of the liver are unchanged in pregnancy. However, many clinical and laboratory signs usually associated with liver disease are present. Spider angiomas and palmar erythema, caused by elevated estrogen levels, are normal and disappear soon after delivery. **The serum albumin and total protein levels fall progressively during gestation. By term, albumin levels are 25% lower than nonpregnant levels.** Despite an overall increase in total body protein, decreases in total protein and albumin concentrations occur as a result of hemodilution. **In addition, serum alkaline phosphatase activity rises during the third trimester to levels two to four times those of nongravid women.** Most of this increase is caused by placental production of the heat-stable isoenzyme and not from the liver.[1] The serum concentrations of many proteins produced by the liver increase. These include elevations in fibrinogen, ceruloplasmin, transferrin, and the binding proteins for corticosteroids, sex steroids, and thyroid hormones.[1]

With the exception of alkaline phosphatase, the other "liver function tests" are unaffected by pregnancy, including serum levels of bilirubin, aspartate aminotransferase (AST), alanine aminotransferase (ALT), γ-glutamyltransferase, 5′-nucleotidase, creatinine phosphokinase, and lactate dehydrogenase. In some studies, the mean levels of ALT and AST are mildly elevated but still within normal values.[74] Levels of creatinine phosphokinase and lactate dehydrogenase can increase with labor. Finally, pregnancy may cause some changes in bile acid production and secretion. Pregnancy may be associated with mild subclinical cholestasis resulting from the high concentrations of estrogen. Reports on serum bile acid concentrations are conflicting, with some studies showing an increase and others no change. **The fasting levels are unchanged, and the measurement of a fasting level appears to be the best test for diagnosing cholestasis of pregnancy.**[74] Cholestasis results from elevated levels of bile acids and is associated with significant pruritus, usually mild increases of ALT/AST, and an increased risk for poor fetal outcomes (see Chapter 45).

Nausea and Vomiting of Pregnancy

Nausea and vomiting, or "morning sickness," complicate up to 70% of pregnancies. Typical onset is between 4 and 8 weeks' gestation, with improvement before 16 weeks; however, 10% to 25% of women still experience symptoms at 20 to 22 weeks' gestation, and some women experience symptoms throughout the gestation.[75] Although the symptoms are often distressing, simple morning sickness seldom leads to significant weight loss, ketonemia, or electrolyte disturbances. The cause is not well understood, although relaxation of the smooth muscle of the stomach probably plays a role. Elevated levels of human chorionic gonadotropin (hCG) may be involved, although a good correlation between maternal hCG concentrations and the degree of nausea and vomiting has not been observed. Similarly, minimal data exist to show the etiology is associated with higher levels of estrogen or progesterone. Interestingly, pregnancies complicated by nausea and vomiting generally have a more favorable outcome than do those without such symptoms.[75] Treatment is largely supportive, consisting of reassurance, avoidance of foods found to trigger nausea, and frequent small meals. Eating dry toast or crackers before getting out of bed may be beneficial. **Recently, the American College of Obstetricians and Gynecologists (ACOG) stated that the use of either vitamin B_6 alone or in combination with doxylamine (Unisom) is safe and effective and should be considered a first line of medical treatment.** A recent review of alternative therapies to antiemetic drugs found that acupressure, wristbands, or treatment with ginger root may be helpful.

Hyperemesis gravidarum is a more pernicious form of nausea and vomiting associated with weight loss, ketonemia, electrolyte imbalance, and dehydration. It occurs in 1% to 3% of women, with persistence often throughout pregnancy, and rarely can result in significant complications, including Wernicke encephalopathy, rhabdomyolysis, acute renal failure, and esophageal rupture. For these patients, the clinician must rule out other diseases such as pancreatitis, cholecystitis, hepatitis, and psychiatric disease. **Hospitalization with intravenous replacement of fluids and electrolytes is often needed. Options of antiemetics include the phenothiazines: promethazine (Phenergan), chlorpromazine (Thorazine), and prochlorperazine (Compazine) or metoclopramide (Reglan), or ondansetron (Zofran).**[76] **On admission to the hospital, the patient should be given intravenous hydration and tried on one of the above-mentioned medications (intravenously or intramuscularly initially).** Care must be taken not to combine the phenothiazines with metoclopramide because of the additive risks for causing extrapyramidal reactions. Chlorpromazine given rectally (25 to 50 mg every 8 hours) may be highly effective in the more refractory cases. **Recently, use of oral methylprednisolone, 16 mg three times daily for 3 days and then tapered over 2 weeks, has been shown to be more effective than promethazine, but multiple subsequent studies failed to demonstrate benefit from the use of steroids.**[76] Unfortunately, no single therapy works in all women, and occasionally, multiple different medications must be tried before finding the one that is effective. **Because of potential risks, parenteral caloric replacement should only be used after failure of multiple antiemetic treatments and attempts at enteral tube feedings.**

SKELETON

Calcium Metabolism

Pregnancy was initially thought to be a state of "physiologic hyperparathyroidism" with maternal skeletal calcium loss needed to supply the fetus with calcium. It was thought that this could result in long-term maternal bone loss. **It is now evident that most fetal calcium needs are met through a series of physiologic changes in calcium metabolism without long-term consequences to the maternal skeleton.**[77] This allows the fetus to accumulate 21 g (range, 13 to 33 g) of calcium, 80% of this amount during the third trimester, when fetal skeletal mineralization is at its peak. Calcium is actively transported across the placenta. Surprisingly, calcium is excreted in greater amounts by the maternal kidneys so that, by term, calciuria is doubled.

Maternal total calcium levels decline throughout pregnancy. The fall in total calcium is caused by the reduced serum albumin levels that result in a decrease in the albumin-bound fraction of calcium. However, the physiologically important fraction, serum ionized calcium, is unchanged and constant[77] (Figure 3-10). **Therefore, the actual maternal serum calcium levels are maintained and the fetal calcium needs are met mainly through increased intestinal calcium absorption.** Calcium is absorbed through the small intestines, and its absorption is doubled by 12 weeks' gestation, with maximal absorption in the third trimester.[77,78] The early increase in absorption may allow the maternal skeleton to store calcium in advance of the

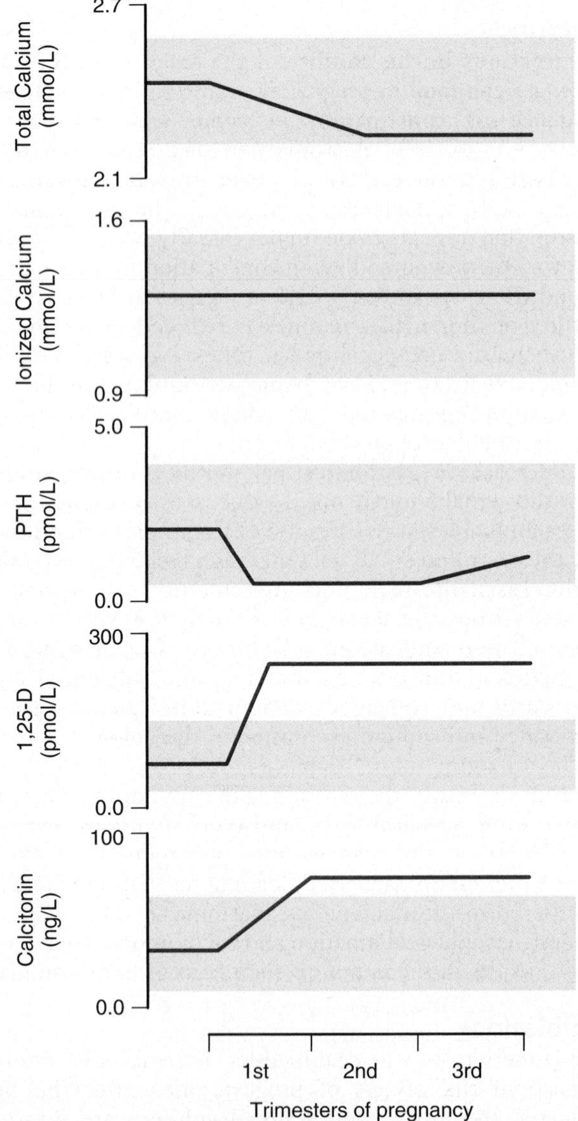

FIGURE 3-10. The longitudinal changes in calcium and calcitropic hormone levels that occur during human pregnancy. Normal adult ranges are indicated by the *shaded areas. 1,25-D,* 1,25-dihydroxyvitamin D; *PTH,* parathyroid hormone. (From Kovacs C, Kronenberg H: Maternal-fetal calcium and bone metabolism during pregnancy, puerperium, and lactation. Endocr Rev 18:832, 1997.)

peak third-trimester fetal demands. Although most fetal calcium needs are met by increased absorption of calcium, accumulating data confirm that at least some calcium resorption from maternal bone occurs to help meet the increased fetal demands in the third trimester. These data are compatible with the hypothesis that physiologic mechanisms exist to ensure an adequate supply of calcium for fetal growth and milk production without sole reliance on the maternal diet.[78] Maternal serum phosphate levels are similarly unchanged.[77]

Older studies showed an increase in maternal parathyroid hormone (PTH) levels. These studies used less sensitive PTH assays that measured multiple different fragments of PTH, most of which are biologically inactive. In five recent prospective studies, all using newer assays, maternal levels of PTH were not elevated and actually remained in the low-normal range throughout gestation.[77] Therefore, pregnancy is not associated with relative hyperparathyroidism (see Chapter 40).

Vitamin D is a prohormone that is derived from cholesterol and occurs in two main nutritional forms: D_3 (cholecalciferol), which is generated in the skin, and D_2 (ergocalciferol), which is derived from plants and absorbed in the gut. **Serum levels of 25-hydroxyvitamin D (25[OH]D) increase in proportion to vitamin D synthesis and intake. Levels of 25[OH]D represent the best indicator of vitamin D status.**[79] 25[OH]D is furthered metabolized to 1,25-dihydroxyvitamin D or active vitamin D. Levels of 1,25-dihydroxyvitamin D increase overall in pregnancy, with prepregnancy levels doubling in the first trimester and peaking in the third trimester. Levels of 25[OH]D do not change in pregnancy unless vitamin D intake or synthesis is changed. The increase in 1,25-dihydroxyvitamin D is secondary to increased production by the maternal kidneys and potentially the fetoplacental unit and is independent of PTH control. The increase in 1,25-dihydroxyvitamin D is directly responsible for most of the increase in intestinal calcium absorption.[77] **Recently, a great deal of interest in vitamin D deficiency in pregnancy has occurred, with estimated prevalence of 5% to 50% in the United States. Controversy exists over the recommendations to institute universal screening during pregnancy by measuring serum levels of 25[OH]D. Levels less than 32 ng/mL indicate vitamin D deficiency, with recommendations to increase vitamin D supplementation if such a deficiency is diagnosed.**[79] Calcitonin levels also rise by 20% and may help protect the maternal skeleton from excess bone loss.[77]

Skeletal and Postural Changes

The effect of pregnancy on bone metabolism is complex, and evidence of maternal bone loss during pregnancy has been inconsistent, with various studies reporting bone loss, no change, and even gain. Whether pregnancy causes bone loss is not the important question; instead, the critical question is whether pregnancy and lactation have a long-term risk for causing osteoporosis later in life.[80] **In a recent review of 23 studies, Ensom and colleagues[80] concluded that pregnancy is a period of high bone turnover and remodeling. Both pregnancy and lactation cause reversible bone loss, and this loss is increased in women who breastfeed for longer intervals. Studies do not support an association between parity and osteoporosis later in life.** Additionally, in a comparison of female twins discordant for parity, pregnancy and lactation were found to have no detrimental effect on long-term bone loss.

Bone turnover appears to be low in the first half of gestation and then increases in the third trimester, corresponding to the peak rate of fetal calcium needs, and may represent turnover of previously stored skeletal calcium.[77] Markers of both bone resorption (hydroxyproline and tartrate-resistant acid phosphatase) and bone formation (alkaline phosphatase and procollagen peptides) are increased during gestation.[78] In the only study of bone biopsies performed in pregnancy, Shahtaheri and associates observed a change in the microarchitectural pattern of bone, but no change in overall bone mass was found. This change in the microarchitectural pattern seems to result in a framework more resistant to the bending forces and biomechanical stresses needed to carry a growing fetus.[81] In support of this study, multiple recent studies have shown that bone loss occurs only in the trabecular bone and not cortical bone. Promislow and coworkers measured bone mineral density twice during pregnancies using dual-energy x-ray absorptiometry and showed the mean loss of trabecular bone was 1.9% per 20 weeks' gestation.[82] However, women placed on bedrest had significantly greater bone loss. In comparison, the mean bone loss in postmenopausal women rarely exceeds 2% per year. Older studies indicate that the cortical bone thickness of long bones may even increase with pregnancy.

Although bone loss occurs in pregnancy, the occurrence of osteoporosis during or soon after pregnancy is rare. Whether additional calcium intake during pregnancy and lactation prevents bone loss is controversial. Most current studies indicate that calcium supplementation does not decrease the amount of bone loss, but Promislow and coworkers[82] found that maternal intake of 2 g per day or greater was modestly protective. This is greater than the recommended dietary allowance of 1000 to 1300 mg/day during pregnancy and lactation.[78]

Pregnancy results in a progressively increasing anterior convexity of the lumbar spine (lordosis). This compensatory mechanism keeps the woman's center of gravity over her legs and prevents the enlarging uterus from shifting the center of gravity anteriorly. The unfortunate side effect of this necessary alteration is low back pain in two thirds of women, with the pain described as severe in one third. The ligaments of the pubic symphysis and sacroiliac joints loosen, probably from the effects of the hormone relaxin, the levels of which increase 10-fold in pregnancy. Marked widening of the pubic symphysis occurs by 28 to 32 weeks' gestation, with the width increasing from 3 to 4 mm to 7.7 to 7.9 mm. This commonly results in pain near the symphysis that is referred down the inner thigh with standing and may result in a maternal sensation of snapping or movement of the bones with walking.

ENDOCRINE CHANGES

Thyroid

Thyroid diseases are common in women of childbearing age (see Chapter 40). However, normal pregnancy symptoms mirror those of thyroid disease, making it difficult to know when screening for thyroid disease is appropriate. In

addition, the physiologic effects of pregnancy frequently make the interpretation of thyroid tests difficult. Therefore, it is important for the obstetrician to be familiar with the normal changes in thyroid function that occur. Recent data have shown that the correct and timely diagnosis and treatment of thyroid disease is important to prevent both maternal and fetal complications.

Despite alterations in thyroid morphology, histology, and laboratory indices, pregnant women remain euthyroid. The thyroid gland increases in size, but not as much as was commonly believed. **If adequate iodine intake is maintained, the size of the thyroid gland remains unchanged or undergoes a small increase in size that can be detected only by ultrasound.**[83] The World Health Organization recommends that iodine intake be increased in pregnancy from 100 mg/day to 150 to 200 mg/day. In an iodine-deficient state, the thyroid gland is up to 25% larger, and goiters occur in 10% of women.[84] Histologically, during pregnancy an increase in thyroid vascularity occurs with evidence of follicular hyperplasia. **The development of a clinically apparent goiter during pregnancy is abnormal and should be evaluated.**

During pregnancy, serum iodide levels fall because of increased renal loss. In addition, in the latter half of pregnancy, iodine is also transferred to the fetus, further decreasing maternal levels.[84] However, at least one investigator has reported that in iodine-sufficient regions, the concentration of iodide does not decrease.[85] These alterations cause the thyroid to synthesize and secrete thyroid hormone actively.[84] Although there is increased uptake of iodine by the thyroid, pregnant women remain euthyroid by laboratory evaluation.

Total thyroxine (TT_4) and total triiodothyronine (TT_3) levels begin to increase in the first trimester and peak at midgestation as a result of increased production of thyroid-binding globulin (TBG). The increase in TBG is seen in the first trimester and plateaus at 12 to 14 weeks. The concentration of TT_4 increases in parallel with the TBG from a normal range of 5 to 12 mg/dL in nonpregnant women to 9 to 16 mg/dL during pregnancy (increases by a factor of about 1.5). **Only a small amount of TT_4 and TT_3 is unbound, but these free fractions (normally about 0.04% for T_4 and 0.5% for T_3) are the major determinants of whether an individual is euthyroid.** The extent of change in free T_4 and T_3 levels during pregnancy has been controversial, and the discrepancies in past studies have been attributed to the techniques used to measure the free hormone levels. **The current best evidence is that the free T_4 levels rise slightly in the first trimester and then decrease so that by delivery, the free T_4 levels are 10% to 15% lower than in nonpregnant women. However, these changes are small, and in most gravidas, free T_4 concentrations remain within the normal nonpregnant range**[84] (Figure 3-11). In clinical practice, the free T_4 level can be measured using either the free thyroxine index (FTI) or estimates of free T_4. These tests use immunoassays that do not measure the free T_4 directly and may be less accurate in pregnancy because they are TBG dependent. **Lee and colleagues showed that the FTI is a more accurate method for measuring free T_4 and that the currently used estimates for free T_4 may incorrectly diagnose women as hypothyroid in the second and third trimesters; however, other authors have shown that these free T_4 estimates are accurate.**[86,87] Free T_3 levels follow a similar pattern as free T_4 levels.

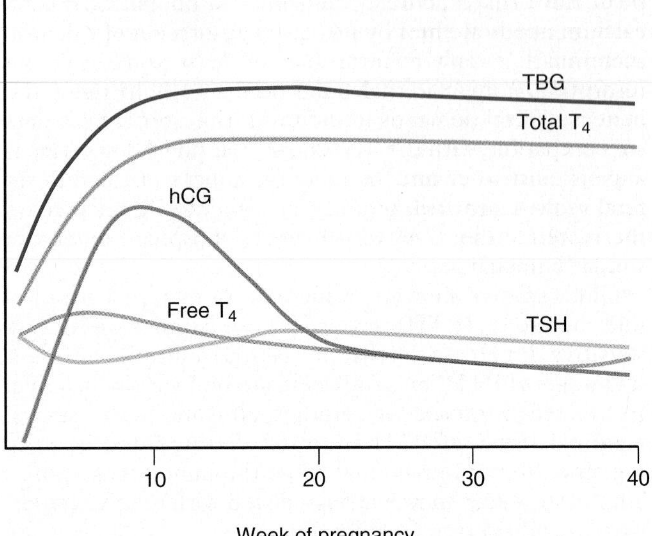

FIGURE 3-11. Relative changes in maternal thyroid function during pregnancy. *hCG,* Human chorionic gonadotropin; *T_4,* thyroxine; *TBG,* thyroxine-binding globulin; *TSH,* thyroid-stimulating hormone. (From Burrow G, Fisher D, Larsen P: Maternal and fetal thyroid function. N Engl J Med 331:1072, 1994.)

Thyroid-stimulating hormone (TSH) concentrations decrease transiently in the first trimester and then rise to prepregnant levels by the end of this trimester. TSH levels then remain stable throughout the remainder of gestation.[84] **The transient decrease in TSH coincides with the first-trimester increase in free T_4 levels, and both appear to be caused by the thyrotropic effects of hCG.** Women with higher peak hCG levels have more TSH suppression. TSH and hCG are structurally very similar, and they share a common α-subunit and have a similar β-unit. **Glinoer and colleagues estimated that a 10,000-IU/L increment in circulating hCG corresponds to a mean free T_4 increment of 0.6 pmol/L (0.1 ng/dL) and, in turn, lowers TSH by 0.1 mIU/L.**[84,88] **These investigators measured TSH levels during successive trimesters of pregnancy in a large group of women and found that TSH was suppressed below normal in 18% in the first trimester, 5% during the second trimester, and 2% in the third trimester.** In the first two trimesters, the mean hCG level was higher in women with suppressed TSH levels.[88] It appears that hCG has some thyrotropic activity, but conflicting data on the exact role of hCG in maternal thyroid function remain.[84] **In some women, the thyrotropic effects of hCG can cause a transient form of hyperthyroidism called gestational transient thyrotoxicosis.**

The influence of maternal thyroid physiology on the fetus appears much more complex than was previously thought. Whereas the maternal thyroid does not directly control fetal thyroid function, the systems interact by means of the placenta, which regulates the transfer of iodine and a small but important amount of thyroxine to the fetus. It was previously thought that little if any transplacental passage of T_4 and T_3 occurred. **It is now**

recognized that T_4 crosses the placenta and that, in fact, in early pregnancy, the fetus is critically dependent on the maternal T_4 supply for normal neurologic development.[89] However, as a result of the deiodinase activity of the placenta, a large percentage of T_4 is broken down before transfer to the fetus. **The human fetus cannot synthesize thyroid hormones until after 12 weeks' gestation, and any fetal requirement before this time is totally dependent on maternal transfer.** Even after the fetal thyroid is functional, the fetus continues to rely to some extent on a maternal supply of thyroxine.

Neonates with thyroid agenesis or a total defect in thyroid hormone synthesis have umbilical cord thyroxine levels between 20% and 50% of those in normal infants, demonstrating that the placenta is not impermeable to T_4. Further evidence that the fetus is dependent on the maternal thyroid for normal development has been published. In women living in iodine-deficient areas, maternal hypothyroidism is associated with neonatal hypothyroidism and defects in long-term neurologic function and mental retardation termed *endemic cretinism*. These abnormalities can be prevented if maternal iodine intake is initiated at the beginning of the second trimester.[90] **Haddow and coworkers[91] have found that maternal hypothyroidism during pregnancy results in slightly lower IQ scores in children tested at ages 7 to 9 years. These findings have resulted in controversy over whether all pregnant women should be screened for subclinical hypothyroidism, which has an incidence of 2% to 5%. Position statements from various organizations are currently contradictory. The Endocrine Society recommends universal screening. ACOG opposes routine screening in pregnancy (Committee Opinion No. 381).** Like T_4, thyrotropin-releasing hormone crosses the placenta; TSH does not.

Because iodine is actively transported across the placenta and the concentration of iodide in the fetal blood is 75% that of the maternal blood, the fetus is susceptible to iodine-induced goiters when the mother is given pharmacologic amounts of iodine. **Similarly, radioactive iodine crosses the placenta and, if given after 12 weeks' gestation when the fetal thyroid is able to concentrate iodine, profound adverse effects can occur.** These include fetal hypothyroidism, mental retardation, attention deficit disorder, and a 1% to 2% increase in the lifetime cancer risk.

Adrenal Glands

Increased steroid production is essential in pregnancy to meet the need for an increase in maternal production of estrogen and cortisol and the fetal need for reproductive and somatic growth development. **Pregnancy is associated with marked changes in adrenocortical function, with increased serum levels of aldosterone, deoxycorticosterone, corticosteroid-binding globulin (CBG), adrenocorticotropic hormone (ACTH), cortisol, and free cortisol and causes a state of "physiologic" hypercorticolism**[92,93] (see Chapter 41 and Appendix A1). Although the combined weight of the adrenal glands does not increase significantly, expansion of the zona fasciculata, which primarily produces glucocorticoids, is observed. The plasma concentration of CBG doubles (because of hepatic stimulation by estrogen) by the end of the sixth month of gestation compared with nonpregnant values, resulting in elevated levels of total plasma cortisol. **The levels of total cortisol rise after the first trimester and by the end of pregnancy are nearly three times higher than nonpregnant values and reach values that are in the range seen in Cushing syndrome.** The diurnal variations in cortisol levels may be partly blunted but are maintained, with the highest values in the morning.

Only free cortisol, the fraction of cortisol not bound to CBG, is metabolically active, but direct measurements are difficult to perform. However, urinary free cortisol concentrations, the free cortisol index, and salivary cortisol concentrations, all of which reflect active free cortisol levels, are elevated after the first trimester.[93,94] In a study of 21 uncomplicated pregnancies, Goland and associates found that the urinary free cortisol concentration doubled from the first to the third trimester.[93] Although the increase in total cortisol concentrations can be explained by the increase in CBG, this does not explain the higher free cortisol levels. The elevation in free cortisol levels seems to be caused in part by a marked increase in corticotropin-releasing hormone (CRH) during pregnancy, which, in turn, stimulates the production of ACTH in the pituitary and from the placenta. Outside of pregnancy, CRH is mainly secreted from the hypothalamus. During pregnancy, CRH is also produced by the placenta and fetal membranes and is secreted into the maternal circulation. First-trimester values of CRH are similar to prepregnant levels, followed by an exponential rise in CRH during the third trimester predominantly as a result of the placental production.[93] Goland and associates have shown that CRH and ACTH concentrations continue to rise in the third trimester despite the increased levels of total and free cortisol levels, supporting the theory that an increase in CRH drives the increased levels of cortisol seen in pregnancy. Furthermore, significant correlation is observed between the rise in CRH levels and maternal ACTH and urinary free cortisol concentrations.[93] Other possible causes for the hypercortisolism include delayed plasma clearance of cortisol as a result of changes in renal clearance, pituitary desensitization to cortisol feedback, or enhanced pituitary responses to corticotropin-releasing factors such as vasopressin and CRH.[92,95]

Although the levels of cortisol are increased to concentrations observed in Cushing's syndrome, little clinical evidence is present for hypercortisolism during pregnancy with the exception of weight gain, striae, hyperglycemia, and tiredness. **However, the diagnosis of Cushing syndrome during pregnancy is difficult because of these changes. The hypothalamic-pituitary axis response to exogenous glucocorticoids is blunted during normal pregnancy and makes interpretations of dexamethasone suppression tests for adrenal excess problematic.**[95] **In addition, pregnancy causes an enhanced adrenal responsiveness to higher-dose ACTH stimulation tests using 250 mcg of cosyntropin, making the diagnosis of adrenal insufficiency also difficult.**

Deoxycorticosterone (DOC), like aldosterone, is a potent mineralocorticoid. Marked elevations in the maternal concentrations of DOC are present by midgestation, reaching peak levels in the third trimester. In contrast to the nonpregnant state, plasma DOC levels in the third trimester do not respond to ACTH stimulation, dexamethasone suppression, or salt intake.[92] These findings suggest that an autonomous source of DOC, specifically the fetoplacental unit, may be responsible for the increased levels. Dehydroepiandrosterone sulfate levels are decreased in gestation because of a marked rise in the metabolic clearance of this adrenal androgenic steroid. Maternal concentrations of testosterone and androstenedione are slightly higher; testosterone is increased because of an elevation in sex hormone-binding protein, and androstenedione is increased because of an increase in its synthesis.

Pituitary Gland

The pituitary gland enlarges in pregnancy, principally because of proliferation of prolactin-producing cells in the anterior pituitary (see Chapter 41). Gonzalez and colleagues demonstrated that the mean pituitary volume increased by 36% at term.[96] **The enlargement of the pituitary gland makes it more susceptible to alterations in blood supply and increases the risk for postpartum infarction (Sheehan syndrome) should a large maternal blood loss occur.** Anterior pituitary hormone levels are significantly affected by pregnancy. Serum prolactin levels begin to rise at 5 to 8 weeks' gestation and by term are 10 times higher. Consistent with this, the number of lactotroph (prolactin-producing) cells increases dramatically within the anterior lobe of the pituitary from 20% of the cells in nongravid women to 60% in the third trimester. In the second and third trimesters, the decidua is a source of much of the increased prolactin production. Despite the increase, prolactin levels remain suppressible by bromocriptine therapy.[97] The principal function of prolactin in pregnancy is to prepare the breast for lactation. In nonlactating women, the prolactin levels return to normal by 3 months postpartum. In lactating women, the return to baseline levels takes several months, with intermittent episodes of hyperprolactinemia in conjunction with nursing. **Maternal follicle-stimulating hormone and luteinizing hormone are decreased to undetectable levels as a result of feedback inhibition from the elevated levels of estrogen, progesterone, and inhibin.**[97] Maternal pituitary growth hormone production is also suppressed because of the action of placental growth hormone variant on the hypothalamus and pituitary; however, the serum levels of growth hormone increase as a result of the production of growth hormone from the placenta.[97]

The hormones produced by the posterior pituitary are also changed. The changes in AVP were discussed earlier in this chapter. Oxytocin levels increase from 10 pg/mL in the first trimester to 30 pg/mL in the third trimester. At term, an increase is noted to about 75 pg/mL, and during labor, these levels dramatically rise and peak in the second stage of labor.[98]

PANCREAS AND FUEL METABOLISM

Glucose

Pregnancy is associated with significant physiologic changes in carbohydrate metabolism. This allows for the continuous transport of energy, in the form of glucose, from the gravid woman to the developing fetus and placenta. Pregnancy taxes maternal insulin and carbohydrate physiology, and in all pregnancies, some deterioration in glucose tolerance occurs. In most women, only mild changes take place. In others, pregnancy is sufficiently diabetogenic **to result in gestational diabetes mellitus. Overall, pregnancy results in fasting hypoglycemia, postprandial hyperglycemia, and hyperinsulinemia.**[99] To accommodate the increased demand for insulin, hypertrophy and hyperplasia of the β cells (insulin producing) occur within the islets of Langerhans in the maternal pancreas. For a complete review of the physiologic changes in glucose metabolism, refer to Chapter 39.

Proteins and Fats/Lipids

Amino acids are actively transported across the placenta for the fetus to use for protein synthesis and as an energy source. In late pregnancy, the fetoplacental unit contains about 500 mg of protein. During pregnancy, fat stores are preferentially used as a substrate for fuel metabolism, and thus, protein catabolism is decreased.

Plasma lipids and lipoproteins increase in pregnancy. A gradual twofold to threefold rise in triglyceride levels occurs by term, and levels of 200 to 300 mg/dL are normal. Total cholesterol and low-density lipoprotein levels are also higher so that, by term, a 50% to 60% increase is observed. High-density lipoprotein levels initially rise in the first half of pregnancy and then fall in the second half. By term, high-density lipoprotein concentrations are 15% higher than nonpregnant levels. Triglyceride concentrations return to normal by 8 weeks postpartum even with lactation, but cholesterol and low-density lipoprotein levels remain elevated (Figure 3-12). The mechanisms for the pregnancy-induced changes in lipids are not completely understood but appear to be partly caused by the elevated levels of estrogen, progesterone, and human placenta lactogen. The rise in low-density lipoproteins appears to be necessary for placental steroidogenesis. Despite the increase in cholesterol and lipids, no increase in the long-term risk for atherosclerosis has been found. However, women with preexisting hyperlipidemia can have a transient worsening of their lipid profiles that is accentuated by the necessity for discontinuing medications such as HMG-CoA reductase inhibitors (statins).

EYE

Two consistent and significant ocular changes occur during pregnancy: increased thickness of the cornea and decreased intraocular pressure. Corneal thickening is apparent by 10 weeks' gestation and may cause problems with contact lenses. **Corneal changes persist for several weeks postpartum, and patients should be advised to wait before obtaining a new eyeglass or contact prescription.** Pizzarello found that 14% of women complained of vision changes. All had changes in their visual acuity and refractive error as well as a myopic shift (became more far-sighted) from pregravid levels, with return to baseline vision postpartum.[100] Because of these transient alterations in the eye, pregnancy is considered by most to be a contraindication to photorefractive keratectomy, and it has been recommended that pregnancy be avoided for 1 year after such surgery.

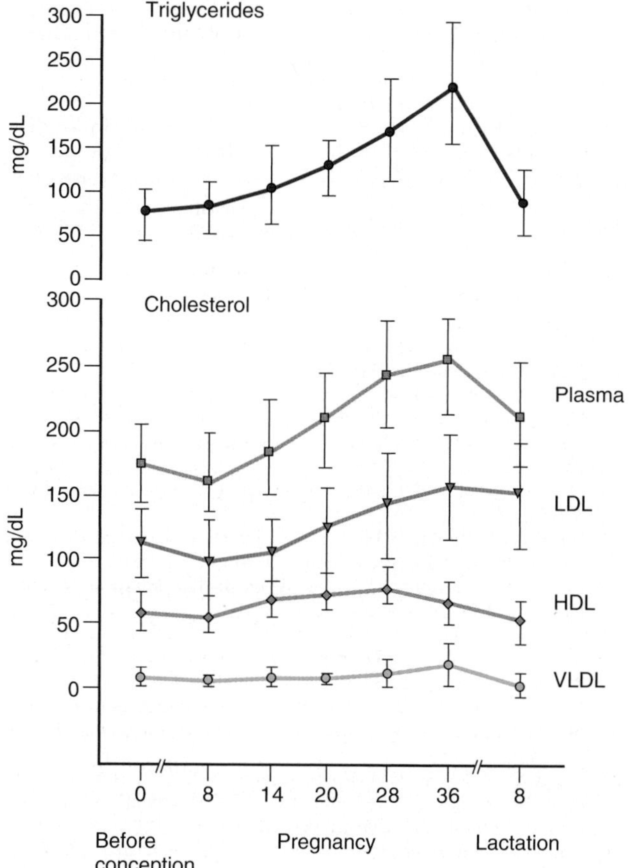

FIGURE 3-12. Triglycerides *(upper panel)* and cholesterol *(lower panel)* in plasma and in lipoprotein fractions before, during, and after pregnancy. *HDL,* High-density lipoprotein; *LDL,* low-density lipoprotein; *VLDL,* very-low-density lipoprotein. (From Salameh W, Mastrogiannis D: Maternal hyperlipidemia in pregnancy. Clin Obstet Gynecol 37:66, 1994.)

Intraocular pressure falls by about 10%, and individuals with preexisting glaucoma typically improve. Pregnancy either does not change or minimally decreases visual fields. Any complaints of visual field changes are atypical and need evaluation.

KEY POINTS

- Plasma osmolality decreases during pregnancy as a result of a reduction in the serum concentration of sodium and associated anions. The osmolality set point for AVP release and thirst is also decreased.
- CO increases 30% to 50% during pregnancy. Supine positioning and standing are both associated with a fall in CO. CO is maximum during labor and the immediate postpartum period.
- As a result of the marked fall in systemic vascular resistance and pulmonary vascular resistance, PCWP does not rise, despite an increase in blood volume.
- Maternal BP decreases early in pregnancy. The diastolic BP and the mean arterial pressure reach a nadir at midpregnancy (16 to 20 weeks) and return to prepregnancy levels by term.
- PaO_2 and $PaCO_2$ fall during pregnancy because of increased minute ventilation. This facilitates transfer of CO_2 from the fetus to the mother and results in a mild respiratory alkalosis.
- Maternal plasma volume increases 50% during pregnancy. RBC volume increases about 18% to 30%, and the hematocrit normally decreases during gestation, but not below 30%.
- Pregnancy is a hypercoagulable state, with increases in the levels of most of the procoagulant factors and decreases in the fibrinolytic system and in some of the natural inhibitors of coagulation.
- BUN and creatinine normally decrease during pregnancy as a result of the increased glomerular filtration rate.
- Despite alterations in thyroid morphology, histology, and laboratory indices, the normal pregnant woman is euthyroid, with levels of free T_4 within nonpregnant norms.
- Pregnancy is associated with a peripheral resistance to insulin, primarily mediated by human placental lactogen. Insulin resistance increases as pregnancy advances; this results in hyperglycemia, hyperinsulinemia, and hyperlipidemia in response to feeding, especially in the third trimester

REFERENCES

1. Lockitch G: Clinical biochemistry of pregnancy. Crit Rev Clin Lab Sci 34:67, 1997.
2. Lindheimer M, Davison J: Osmoregulation, the secretion of arginine vasopressin and its metabolism during pregnancy. Eur J Endocrinol 132:133, 1995.
3. Bernstein I, Ziegler W, Badger G: Plasma volume expansion in early pregnancy. Obstet Gynecol 97:669, 2001.
4. El-Hennawy A, Bassi T, Koradia N, et al: Transient gestational diabetes insipidus: report of two cases and review of pathophysiology and treatment. J Matern Fetal Med 14:349, 2003.
5. Schobel H: Pregnancy-induced alterations in renal function. Kidney Blood Press Res 21:276, 1998.
6. Duvekot J, Cheriex E, Pieters F, et al: Early pregnancy changes in hemodynamics and volume homeostasis are consecutive adjustments triggered by a primary fall in systemic vascular tone. Am J Obstet Gynecol 169:1382, 1993.
7. Castro L, Hobel C, Gornbein J: Plasma levels of atrial natriuretic peptide in normal and hypertensive pregnancies: a meta-analysis. Am J Obstet Gynecol 71:1642, 1994.
8. Borghi C, Esposti D, Immordino V, et al: Relationship of systemic hemodynamics, left ventricular structure and function, and plasma natriuretic peptide concentrations during pregnancy complicated by preeclampsia. Am J Obstet Gynecol 183:140, 2000.
9. Hameed A, Chan K, Ghamsary M, et al: Longitudinal changes in the B-type natriuretic peptide levels in normal pregnancy and the postpartum. Clin Cardiol 32:E60, 2009.
10. Bhagwat A, Engel P: Heart disease and pregnancy. Cardiol Clin 13:163, 1995.
11. Eghbali M, Wang Y, Toro L, et al: Heart hypertrophy during pregnancy: a better functioning heart. Trends Cardiovascul Med 16:285, 2006.
12. Kametas N, McAuliffe F, Hancock J, et al: Maternal left ventricular mass and diastolic function during pregnancy. Ultrasound Obstet Gynecol 18:460, 2001.

13. Kametas N, McAuliffe F, Krampl E, et al: Maternal cardiac function in twin pregnancy. Obstet Gynecol 102:806, 2003.
14. Turan O, De Paco C, Khaw A, et al: Effect of parity on maternal cardiac function during the first trimester of pregnancy. Ultrasound Obstet Gynecol 32:849, 2008.
15. Zenter D, Plessis M, Brennecke S, et al: Deterioration in cardiac systolic and diastolic function late in normal human pregnancy. Clin Sci 116:599, 2009.
16. Labovitz A, Pearson A: Evaluation of left ventricular diastolic function: clinical relevance and recent Doppler echocardiographic insights. Am Heart J 114:836, 1987.
17. Desai D, Moodley J, Naidoo D, et al: Cardiac abnormalities in pulmonary oedema associated with hypertensive crises in pregnancy. Br J Obstet Gynaecol 103:523, 1996.
18. Veille JC, Kitzman D, Millsaps P, et al: Left ventricular diastolic filling response to stationary bicycle exercise during pregnancy and the postpartum period. Am J Obstet Gynecol 185:822, 2001.
19. van Oppen A, Stigter R, Bruinse H: Cardiac output in normal pregnancy: a critical review. Obstet Gynecol 87:310, 1996.
20. Robson S, Hunter S, Boys R, et al: Serial study of factors influencing changes in cardiac output during human pregnancy. Am J Physiol 256:H1061, 1989.
21. Desai K, Moodley J, Naidoo D: Echocardiographic hemodynamics in normal pregnancy. Obstet Gynecol 104:20, 2004.
22. McAnolty J, Metcalfe J, Ueland K: Heart disease and pregnancy. In Hurst JN: The Heart, 6th ed. New York, McGraw-Hill, 1985, p 1383.
23. Kerr M: The mechanical effects of the gravid uterus in late pregnancy. J Obstet Gynaecol Br Commonw 72:513, 1965.
24. Lanni S, Tillinghast J, Silver H: Hemodynamic changes and baroreflex gain in the supine hypotensive syndrome. Am J Obstet Gynecol 187:1636, 2002.
25. Granger J: Maternal and fetal adaptations during pregnancy and integrative physiology. Am J Physiol Regul Integr Comp Physiol 283:R1289, 2002.
26. Gant N, Daley G, Chand S, et al: A study of angiotensin II pressor response throughout primigravid pregnancy. J Clin Invest 52:2682, 1973.
27. de Swiet M, Shennan A: Blood pressure measurement in pregnancy. Br J Obstet Gynaecol 103:862, 1996.
28. McLennan C: Antecubital and femoral venous pressure in normal and toxemia pregnancy. Am J Obstet Gynecol 45:568, 1943.
29. Zinaman M, Rubin J, Lindheimer M: Serial plasma oncotic pressure levels and echoencephalography during and after delivery in severe preeclampsia. Lancet 1:1245, 1985.
30. Crapo R: Normal cardiopulmonary physiology during pregnancy. Clin Obstet Gynecol 39:3, 1996.
31. Roth A, Elkayam U: Acute myocardial infarction associated with pregnancy. J Am Coll Cardiol 52:171, 2008.
32. Robson S, Dunlop W, Boys R, et al: Cardiac output during labour. BMJ 295:1169, 1987.
33. Kerr M: Cardiovascular dynamics in pregnancy and labour. Br Med Bull 24:19, 1968.
34. Ueland K, Hansen J: Maternal cardiovascular dynamics. III. Labor and delivery under local and caudal analgesia. Am J Obstet Gynecol 103:8, 1969.
35. Robson S, Boys R, Hunter S, et al: Maternal hemodynamics after normal delivery and delivery complicated by postpartum hemorrhage. Obstet Gynecol 74:234, 1989.
36. Shotan A, Ostrzega E, Mehra A, et al: Incidence of arrhythmias in normal pregnancy and relation to palpitations, dizziness, and syncope. Am J Cardiol 79:1061, 1997.
37. Romem A, Romem Y, Katz M, et al: Incidence and characteristics of maternal cardiac arrhythmias during labor. Am J Cardiol 93:931, 2004.
38. Silvades C, Harris L, Haberer K, et al: Recurrence rate of arrhythmias during pregnancy in women with previous tachyarrhythmia and impact on fetal and neonatal outcomes. Am J Cardiol 97:1206, 2006.
39. Gilroy R, Mangura B, Lavietes M: Rib cage displacement and abdominal volume displacement during breathing in pregnancy. Am Rev Respir Dis 137:668, 1988.
40. Brancazio L, Laifer S, Schwartz T: Peak expiratory flow rate in normal pregnancy. Obstet Gynecol 89:383, 1997.
41. Harirah H, Donia S, Nasrallah F: Effect of gestational age and position on peak expiratory flow rate: a longitudinal study. Obstet Gynecol 105:372, 2005.
42. Awe R, Nicotra B, Newson T, et al: Arterial oxygenation and alveolar-arterial gradients in term pregnancy. Obstet Gynecol 53:182, 1979.
43. Lee K, Zaffke M, Mcenany G: Parity and sleep patterns during and after pregnancy. Obstet Gynecol 95:14, 2000.
44. Facco F, Kramer J, Ho K, et al: Sleep disturbance in pregnancy. Obstet Gynecol 115:77, 2010.
45. Venkata C, Venkateshiah S: Sleep-disordered breathing during pregnancy. J Am Board Fam Med 22:158, 2009.
46. Pritchard J: Changes in blood volume during pregnancy and delivery. Anesthesiology 26:393, 1965.
47. Pritchard J, Baldwin R, Dickey J, et al: Blood volume changes in pregnancy and the puerperium. II. Red blood cell loss and changes in apparent blood volume during and following vaginal delivery, cesarean section, and cesarean section plus total hysterectomy. Am J Obstet Gynecol 84:1271, 1962.
48. McFee J: Iron metabolism and iron deficiency during pregnancy. Clin Obstet Gynecol 22:799, 1979.
49. Pitkin R, Witte D: Platelet and leukocyte counts in pregnancy. JAMA 242:2696, 1979.
50. O'Brien JR: Platelet count in normal pregnancy. J Clin Pathol 29:174, 1976.
51. Burrows R, Kelton J: Incidentally detected thrombocytopenia in healthy mothers and their infants. N Engl J Med 319:142, 1988.
52. Acker DB, Johnson MP, Sachs BP, et al: The leukocyte count in labor. Am J Obstet Gynecol 153:737, 1985.
53. Johnson RL: Thromboembolic disease complicating pregnancy. In Foley MR, Strong TH: Obstetric Intensive Care: A Practical Manual. Philadelphia, Saunders, 1997, p 91.
54. Clark P, Brennand J, Conkie J, et al: Activated protein C sensitivity, protein C, protein S, and coagulation in normal pregnancy. Thromb Haemost 79:1166, 1998.
55. Goodwin A, Rosendaal F, Kottke-Marchant K, et al: A review of the technical, diagnostic, and epidemiologic considerations for protein S assays. Arch Pathol Lab Med 126:1349, 2002.
56. American College of Obstetricians and Gynecologists: ACOG practice bulletin. Inherited thrombophilias in pregnancy, Number 113, July 2010.
57. Gerbasi F, Bottoms S, Farag A, et al: Increased intravascular coagulation associated with pregnancy. Obstet Gynecol 75:385, 1990.
58. Fried A, Woodring J, Thompson D: Hydronephrosis of pregnancy: a prospective sequential study of the course of dilatation. J Ultrasound Med 2:255, 1983.
59. Davison J: The effect of pregnancy on kidney function in renal allograft recipients. Kidney Int 27:74, 1985.
60. Lindheimer M, Davison J, Katz A: The kidney and hypertension in pregnancy: Twenty exciting years. Semin Nephrol 21:173, 2001.
61. Davison J, Noble F: Glomerular filtration during and after pregnancy. J Obstet Gynaecol Br Commonw 81:588, 1974.
62. Lind T, Godfrey K, Otun H: Changes in serum uric acid concentrations during normal pregnancy. Br J Obstet Gynaecol 91:128, 1984.
63. Conrad K, Bager L, Lindheimer M: The kidney in normal pregnancy and preeclampsia. In Lindheimer M, Roberts J, Cunningham F: Chesley's Hypertensive Disorders in Pregnancy, 3rd ed. San Diego, Elsevier, 2009, p 297.
64. Lindheimer M, Richardson D, Ehrlich E, et al: Potassium homeostasis in pregnancy. J Reprod Med 32:517, 1987.
65. Davison J, Hytten F: The effect of pregnancy on the renal handling of glucose. Br J Obstet Gynaecol 82:374, 1975.
66. Gordon M, London M, Samuels P, et al: Perinatal outcome and long-term follow-up associated with modern management of diabetic nephropathy. Obstet Gynecol 87:401, 1996.
67. Macfie A, Magides A, Richmond M, et al: Gastric emptying in pregnancy. Br J Anaesth 67:54, 1991.
68. Wong C, McCarthy R, Fitzgerald P, et al: Gastric emptying of water in obese pregnant women at term. Anesth Analg 105:751, 2007.
69. Cappell M, Garcia A: Gastric and duodenal ulcers during pregnancy. Gastroenterol Clin North Am 27:169, 1998.
70. Bonapace E, Fisher R: Constipation and diarrhea in pregnancy. Gastroenterol Clin North Am 27:197, 1998.
71. Derbyshire E, Davies J, Costarelli V: Diet, physical inactivity and the prevalence of constipation throughout pregnancy. Matern Child Nutr 2:127, 2006.
72. Parry E, Shields R, Turnbull A: The effect of pregnancy on the colonic absorption of sodium, potassium and water. J Obstet Gynaecol Br Commonw 77:616, 1970.

73. Kern F, Everson G, DeMark B, et al: Biliary lipids, bile acids, and gallbladder function in the human female: effects of pregnancy and the ovulatory cycle. J Clin Invest 68:1229, 1981.
74. Bacq Y, Zarka O, Brechot J-F, et al: Liver function tests in normal pregnancy: a prospective study of 103 pregnant women and 103 matched controls. Hepatology 23:1030, 1996.
75. Furneaux E, Langley-Evans A, Langley-Evans S: Nausea and vomiting of pregnancy: endocrine basis and contribution to pregnancy outcome. Obstet Gynecol Surv 56:775, 2001.
76. Magee L, Mazzotta P, Koren G: Evidence-based view of safety and effectiveness of pharmacologic therapy for nausea and vomiting of pregnancy. Am J Obstet Gynecol 186:S256, 2002.
77. Kovacs C, Kronenberg H: Maternal-fetal calcium and bone metabolism during pregnancy, puerperium, and lactation. Endocr Rev 18:832, 1997.
78. Prentice A: Maternal calcium metabolism and bone mineral status. Ann J Clin Nutr 71:1312S, 2000.
79. Mulligan M, Felton S, Riek A, et al: Implications of vitamin D deficiency in pregnancy and lactation. Am J Obstet Gynecol 202:e1, 2010.
80. Ensom M, Liu P, Stephenson M: Effect of pregnancy on bone mineral density in healthy women. Obstet Gynecol Surv 57:99, 2002.
81. Shahtaheri S, Aaron J, Johnson D, et al: Changes in trabecular bone architecture in women during pregnancy. Br J Obstet Gynaecol 106:432, 1999.
82. Promislow J, Hertz-Picciotto I, Schramm M, et al: Bed rest and other determinants of bone loss during pregnancy. Am J Obstet Gynecol 191:1077, 2004.
83. Berghout A, Endert E, Ross A, et al: Thyroid function and thyroid size in normal pregnant women living in an iodine replete area. Clin Endocrinol 42:375, 1994.
84. Glinoer D: The regulation of thyroid function in pregnancy: pathways of endocrine adaptation from physiology to pathology. Endocr Rev 18:404, 1997.
85. Lieberman C, Fang S, Braverman L, et al: Circulating iodide concentrations during and after pregnancy. J Clin Endocrinol Metab 83:3545, 1998.
86. Lee R, Spencer C, Mestman J, et al: Free T4 immunoassays are flawed during pregnancy. Am J Obstet Gynecol 200:260.e1, 2009.
87. Mandel S, Spencer C, Hollowell J: Are detection and treatment of thyroid insufficiency in pregnancy feasible? Thyroid 15:44, 2005.
88. Glinoer D, De Nayer P, Robyn C, et al: Serum levels of intact human chorionic gonadotropin (hCG) and its free α and β subunits, in relation to maternal thyroid stimulation during normal pregnancy. J Endocrinol Invest 16:881, 1993.
89. Ekins R, Sinha A, Ballabio M, et al: Role of the maternal carrier proteins in the supply of thyroid hormones to the feto-placental unit: evidence of a feto-placental requirement for thyroxine. In Delange F, Fisher DA, Glinoer D: Research in Congenital Hypothyroidism. New York, Plenum Press, 1989, p 45.
90. Utiger R: Maternal hypothyroidism and fetal development. N Engl J Med 341:601, 1999.
91. Haddow J, Palomaki G, Allan W, et al: Maternal thyroid deficiency during pregnancy and subsequent neuropsychological development of the child. N Engl J Med 341:549, 1999.
92. Nolten W, Lindheimer M, Oparil S, et al: Deoxycorticosterone in normal pregnancy. I. Sequential studies of the secretory patterns of deoxycorticosterone, aldosterone, and cortisol. Am J Obstet Gynecol 132:414, 1978.
93. Goland R, Jozak S, Conwell I: Placental corticotrophin-releasing hormone and the hypercortisolism of pregnancy. Am J Obstet Gynecol 171:1287, 1994.
94. Scott E, McGarrigle H, Lachelin G: The increase in plasma and saliva cortisol levels in pregnancy is not due to the increase in corticosteroid-binding globulin levels. J Clin Endocrinol Metab 71:639, 1990.
95. Lindsay J, Nieman L: The hypothalamic-pituitary-adrenal axis in pregnancy: challenges in disease detection and treatment. Endocr Rev 26:775, 2005.
96. Gonzalez J, Elizondo G, Saldivar D, et al: Pituitary gland growth during normal pregnancy: an in vivo study using magnetic resonance imaging. Am J Med 85:217, 1988.
97. Prager D, Braunstein G: Pituitary disorders during pregnancy. Endocrinol Metab Clin North Am 24:1, 1995.
98. Garner P, Burrow G: Pituitary and adrenal disorders of pregnancy. In Burrow G, Duffy T, Copel C: Medical Complications During Pregnancy, 6th ed. Philadelphia, Saunders, 2004, p 163.
99. Kuhl C: Etiology and pathogenesis of gestational diabetes. Diabetes Care 21:19B, 1998.
100. Pizzarello L: Refractive changes in pregnancy. Graefes Arch Clin Exp Ophthalmol 241:484, 2003.

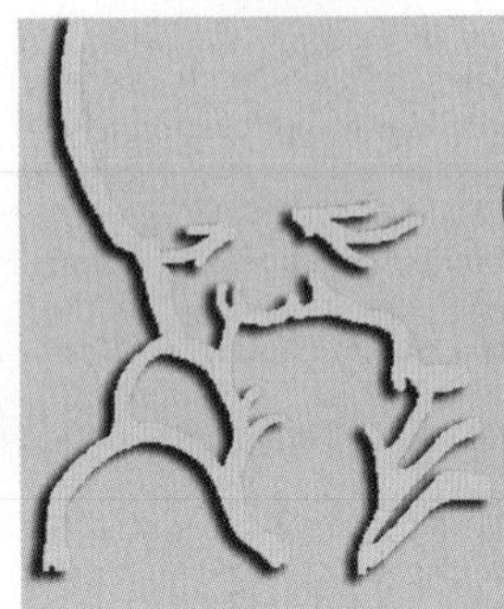

CHAPTER 4

Maternal-Fetal Immunology

Hilary S. Gammill, Laurence E. Shields, and Kristina M. Adams Waldorf

KEY ABBREVIATIONS	
Alpha-fetoprotein	AFP
B-cell Receptor	BCR
CC Receptor	CCR
Class II Transactivator	CIITA
CXC Receptor	CXCR
Fas Ligand	FasL
Graft-versus-host Disease	GVHD
Helper T Cell Type 1	Th1
Helper T Cell Type 2	Th2
Human Immunodeficiency Virus	HIV
Human Leukocyte Antigen	HLA
Indoleamine 2,3 Dioxygenase	IDO
Immunoglobulin	Ig
Interferon-γ	IFN-γ
Interleukin-1	IL-1
Kilodalton	kDa
Killer Cell Immunoglobulin-like Receptor	KIR
Lipopolysaccharide	LPS
LPS Binding Protein	LBP
Major Histocompatibility Complex	MHC
Membrane Attack Complex	MAC
Natural Killer	NK
Pattern-recognition Receptors	PRR
T-cell Receptor	TCR
TNF-related Apoptosis-inducing Ligand/Apo-2L	TRAIL
Toll-like Receptor	TLR
Transforming Growth Factor-β	TGF-β
Tumor Necrosis Factor-α	TNF-α
Uterine NK Cells	u-NK

The study of maternal-fetal immunology was initially driven by a desire to understand how a genetically foreign fetus could develop within the mother without immune rejection. Sir Peter Medawar described the immunologic paradox posed by pregnancy by asking, "How does the pregnant mother contrive to nourish within itself, for many weeks or months, a fetus that is an antigenically foreign body?"[1] He suggested several possibilities for fetal tolerance, including anatomic separation of the fetus and mother, antigenic immaturity of the fetus, and immunologic inertness of the mother. Although it was later discovered that fetal and maternal cells come into direct contact, these ideas became the basis for many early studies of maternal-fetal immunology. In fact, discovery of complex immunologic mechanisms at the maternal-fetal interface suggest that placental immune functions and active maternal-fetal interactions are critical for fetal development and maternal health. The finding of immunologic proteins in blood, amniotic fluid, and vaginal fluid of women with preterm labor and intra-amniotic infection has further led to the rapid investigation of maternal-fetal immune responses.[2-4] Discoveries arising from the study of immune responses in the mother and fetus have improved our understanding of maternal tolerance of the fetus, infection-associated preterm birth, preeclampsia, and pregnancy loss. Understanding concepts in maternal-fetal immunology will allow the clinician to gain a deeper appreciation for pregnancy and many perinatal complications.

IMMUNE SYSTEM OVERVIEW: INNATE AND ADAPTIVE IMMUNITY

The immune system is classically divided into two arms, the innate (Figure 4-1) and adaptive immune systems

INNATE IMMUNITY
- First line of host defense to infection
- Rapid response
- Nonspecific recognition of broad classes of pathogens
- Preexisting effector cell population *(no amplification required)*
- Inability to discriminate self vs. non-self; only recognizes pathogens

A. Cells

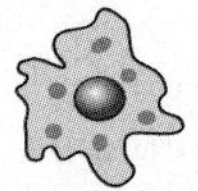
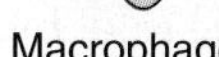

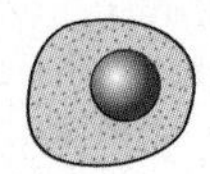

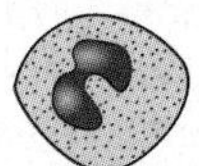

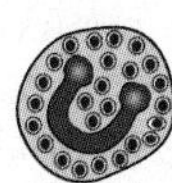

B. Pattern Recognition Receptors: Recognize common microbial patterns and structures

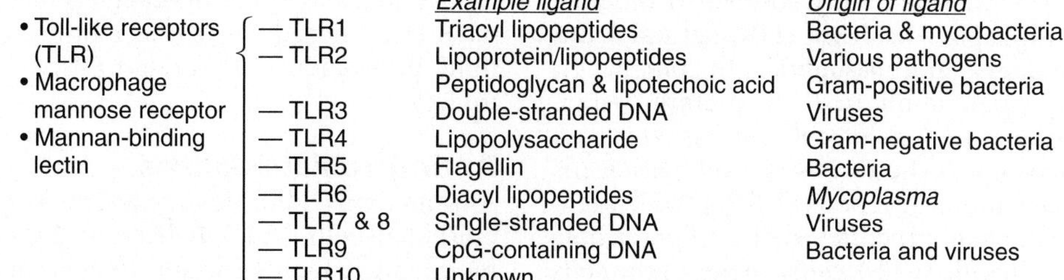

		Example ligand	*Origin of ligand*
• Toll-like receptors (TLR)	— TLR1	Triacyl lipopeptides	Bacteria & mycobacteria
• Macrophage mannose receptor	— TLR2	Lipoprotein/lipopeptides	Various pathogens
• Mannan-binding lectin		Peptidoglycan & lipotechoic acid	Gram-positive bacteria
	— TLR3	Double-stranded DNA	Viruses
	— TLR4	Lipopolysaccharide	Gram-negative bacteria
	— TLR5	Flagellin	Bacteria
	— TLR6	Diacyl lipopeptides	*Mycoplasma*
	— TLR7 & 8	Single-stranded DNA	Viruses
	— TLR9	CpG-containing DNA	Bacteria and viruses
	— TLR10	Unknown	

C. Complement System: Plasma proteins that cooperate to facilitate destruction of pathogens

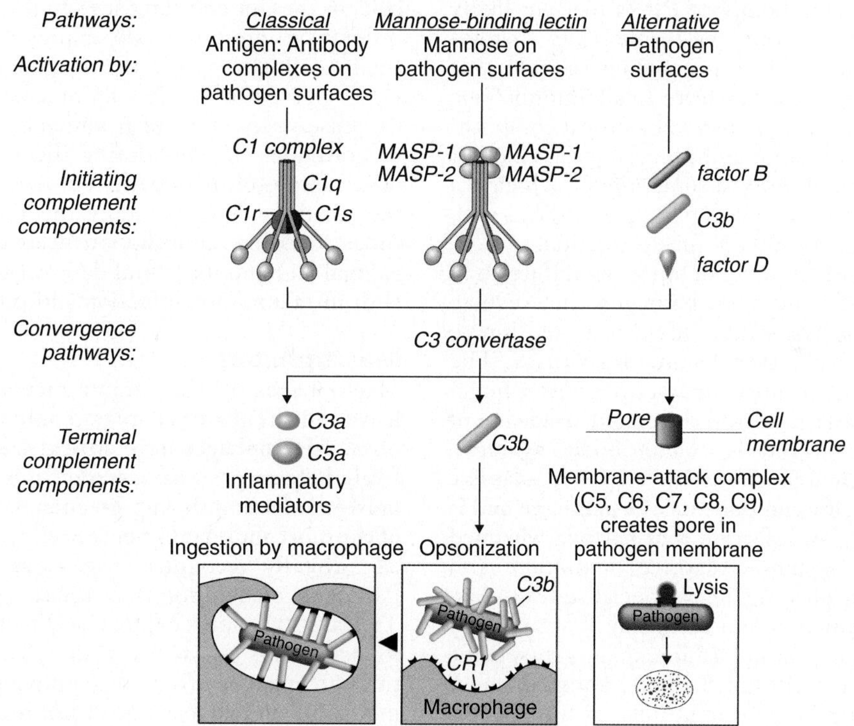

D. Induced Innate Immune Responses

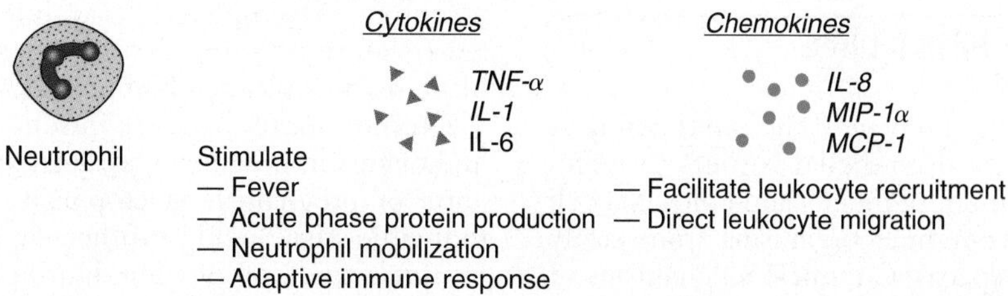

FIGURE 4-1. The innate immune system. The innate immune system acts as the first line of host defense and consists of immune cells **(A)**, the pattern-recognition receptors that target common pathogen structures **(B)**, the complement system **(C)**, and induced innate immune responses **(D)**. The toll-like receptors and their common ligands are listed because they act as the principal immune sensors of pathogens **(B)**. Complement activation may occur through three different initiating pathways, which converge with production of the C3 convertase and generation of the terminal complement proteins **(C)**. As a result of activation of these components of the innate immune system, neutrophils may be recruited to the site of infection and cytokines/chemokines may be produced **(D)**.

(Figure 4-2). Each arm of the immune system fights infection by a slightly different and complementary method. In both systems, there are several important mechanisms to prevent maternal immunity from targeting and killing the fetus. Yet, the immune system must remain competent to overcome an infection to preserve the mother's life. Achieving a balance between controlling normal immune responses and maintaining immune function is one major challenge of pregnancy.

The innate immune system employs fast, nonspecific methods of pathogen detection to prevent and control an initial infection. Innate immunity consists of immune cells such as macrophages, dendritic cells, natural killer (NK) cells, eosinophils, and basophils. In pregnancy, these cells have been implicated in preterm labor, preeclampsia, maternal-fetal tolerance, and intrauterine growth restriction. Many of these cells identify pathogens through pattern-recognition receptors (PRRs), which recognize common pathogen structures such as lipoteichoic acid and lipopolysaccharide (LPS), constituents of the cells walls of gram-positive and gram-negative bacteria. PRRs include the macrophage mannose receptor and toll-like receptors (TLRs), a large family of PRRs that are likely responsible for the earliest immune responses to a pathogen.[5] TLR activation initiates a signaling cascade that leads to release of cytokines, which are small immunologic proteins that are implicated in many obstetrical complications, including preterm labor and preeclampsia. Another component of innate immunity is complement, which is a system of plasma proteins that coat pathogen surfaces with protein fragments, targeting them for destruction.

In many cases, innate immune defenses are effective in combating pathogens. Sometimes pathogens may evolve more rapidly than the hosts they infect or evade innate immune responses, like seasonal influenza viruses. The adaptive immune system must then act to control infection. **Adaptive immunity results in the clonal expansion of lymphocytes (T cells and B cells) and antibodies against a specific antigen. Although slower to respond, adaptive immunity targets specific components of a pathogen and is capable of eradicating an infection that has overwhelmed the innate immune system.** Adaptive immunity also requires presentation of antigen by specialized antigen-presenting cells, production and secretion of stimulatory cytokines, and ultimately, amplification of antigen-specific lymphocyte clones (T cells and B cells). These memory T and B cells provide lifelong immunity to the specific antigen.

INNATE IMMUNITY: FIRST LINE OF HOST DEFENSE

Epithelial surfaces of the body are the first defenses against infection. Mechanical epithelial barriers to infection include ciliary movement of mucus and epithelial cell tight junctions that prevent microorganisms from easily penetrating intercellular spaces. Chemical mechanisms of defense include enzymes (e.g., lysozyme in saliva, pepsin), low pH in the stomach, and antibacterial peptides (e.g., defensins in the vagina) that degrade bacteria.

After a pathogen enters the tissues, it is often recognized and killed by phagocytes, which is a process mediated by macrophages and neutrophils. The presence of TLRs, a family of PRRs, on the surface of macrophages and other innate immune cells, represents the primary mechanism of pathogen detection. TLR activation results in secretion of cytokines, which initiate inflammatory responses. Neutrophils are then recruited to sites of inflammation by small immunologic proteins, called chemokines (i.e., interleukin-8 [IL-8]) released by macrophages. Chemokines and cytokines are small immunologic proteins (e.g., IL-8, IL-6, tumor necrosis factor-α [TNF-α]) that coordinate many immune functions as well as cell activation, replication, and differentiation. Proinflammatory cytokines have been described in the mother, fetus, and amniotic fluid in women with preterm labor and intra-amniotic infection.[2,3]

Antimicrobial Peptides

Antimicrobial peptides are secreted by neutrophils and epithelial cells and kill bacteria by damaging pathogen membranes. Defensins are a major family of antimicrobial peptides that protect against bacterial, fungal, and viral pathogens. Neutrophils secrete α-defensins and epithelial cells in the gut and lung secrete β-defensins. Both α- and β-defensins are temporally expressed by endometrial epithelial cells during the menstrual cycle.[6] Susceptibility to upper genital tract infection may be related in part to the decreased expression of antimicrobial peptides in response to hormonal changes during the menstrual cycle. Many other tissues of the female reproductive tract and placenta secrete defensins, including the vagina, cervix, fallopian tubes, decidua, and chorion. Elevated concentrations of vaginal and amniotic fluid defensins have been associated with intra-amniotic infection and preterm birth.

Macrophages

Macrophages mature from circulating monocytes that leave the circulation to migrate into tissues throughout the body. **Macrophages have critical scavenger functions that likely help to prevent bacteria from establishing an intrauterine infection during pregnancy. Macrophages are one of the most abundant immune cell types in the placenta and can directly recognize, ingest, and destroy pathogens.** Pathogen recognition may occur through PRRs, such as TLRs, scavenger receptors, and mannose receptors. Macrophages also internalize pathogens or pathogen particles through phagocytosis, macropinocytosis, and receptor-mediated endocytosis. Multiple receptors on the macrophage can induce phagocytosis, including the mannose receptor, scavenger receptor, CD14, and complement receptors. Macrophages also release many bactericidal agents after ingesting a pathogen, such as oxygen radicals, nitric oxide, antimicrobial peptides, and lysozyme.

Uterine macrophages represent up to one third of total leukocytes in pregnancy-associated tissue during the later parts of pregnancy. Macrophages are a major source of inducible nitric oxide synthetase, a rate-limiting enzyme for nitric oxide production. During pregnancy, nitric oxide is thought to relax uterine smooth muscle, and uterine nitric oxide synthetase activity and expression decreases before parturition. Uterine macrophages are also a major source of prostaglandins, inflammatory cytokines, and matrix metalloproteinases that are prominent during term

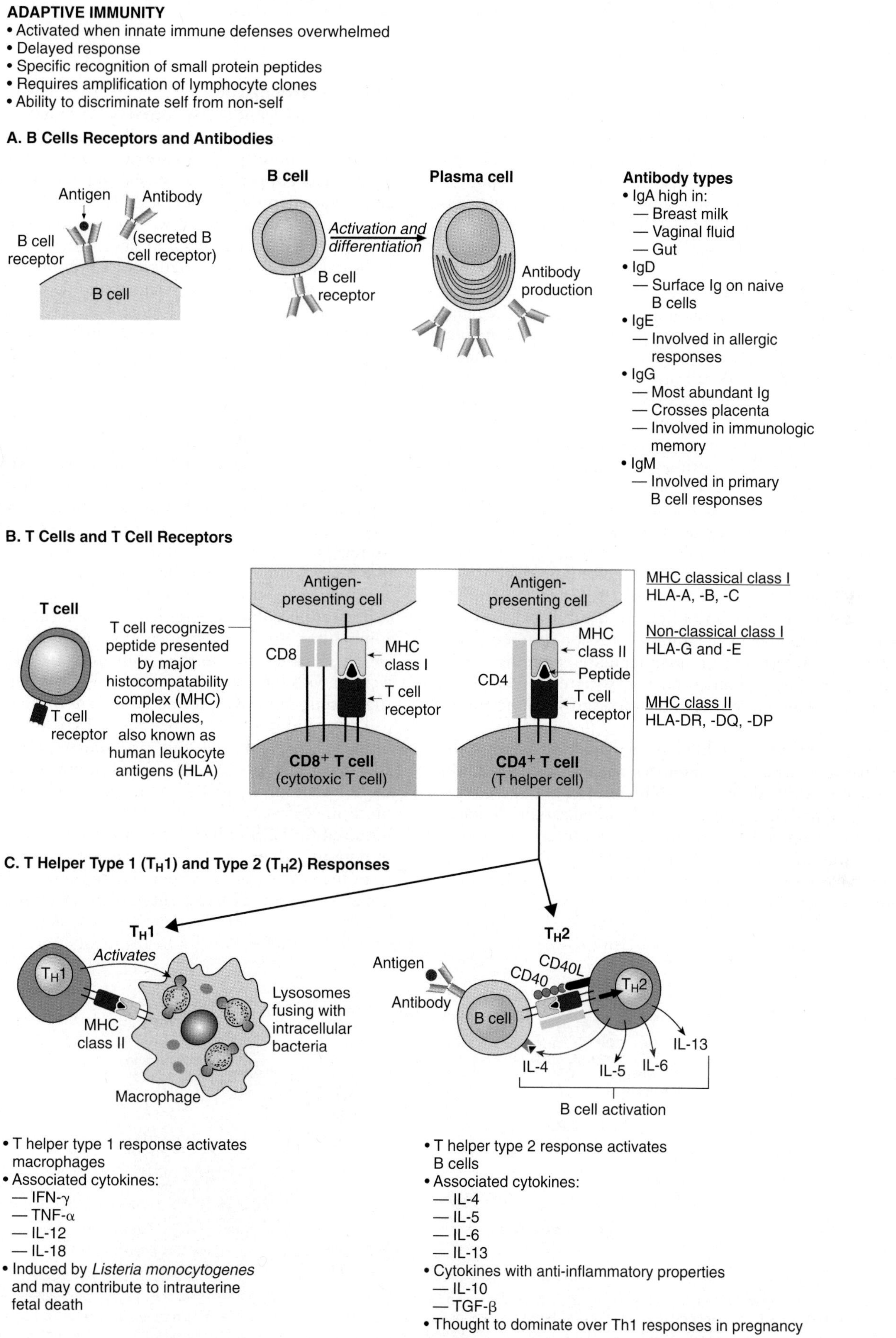

ADAPTIVE IMMUNITY

- Activated when innate immune defenses overwhelmed
- Delayed response
- Specific recognition of small protein peptides
- Requires amplification of lymphocyte clones
- Ability to discriminate self from non-self

A. B Cells Receptors and Antibodies

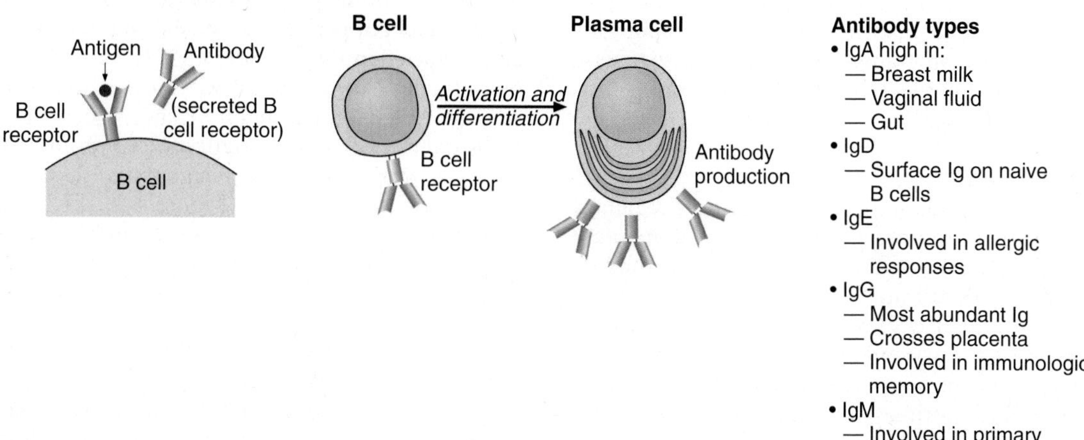

B. T Cells and T Cell Receptors

T cell

T cell receptor

T cell recognizes peptide presented by major histocompatability complex (MHC) molecules, also known as human leukocyte antigens (HLA)

Antigen-presenting cell

CD8

MHC class I

T cell receptor

CD8⁺ T cell (cytotoxic T cell)

Antigen-presenting cell

MHC class II

Peptide

CD4

T cell receptor

CD4⁺ T cell (T helper cell)

<u>MHC classical class I</u>
HLA-A, -B, -C

<u>Non-classical class I</u>
HLA-G and -E

<u>MHC class II</u>
HLA-DR, -DQ, -DP

C. T Helper Type 1 (T_H1) and Type 2 (T_H2) Responses

T_H1

T_H1

Activates

MHC class II

Lysosomes fusing with intracellular bacteria

Macrophage

T_H2

Antigen

Antibody

B cell

CD40

CD40L

T_H2

IL-4

IL-5

IL-6

IL-13

B cell activation

- T helper type 1 response activates macrophages
- Associated cytokines:
  - — IFN-γ
  - — TNF-α
  - — IL-12
  - — IL-18
- Induced by *Listeria monocytogenes* and may contribute to intrauterine fetal death

- T helper type 2 response activates B cells
- Associated cytokines:
  - — IL-4
  - — IL-5
  - — IL-6
  - — IL-13
- Cytokines with anti-inflammatory properties
  - — IL-10
  - — TGF-β
- Thought to dominate over Th1 responses in pregnancy

FIGURE 4-2. The adaptive immune system. The adaptive immune system acts to control infection that has overwhelmed the innate immune system and is also important in transplant rejection and tumor killing. B cells secrete antibodies to protect the extracellular spaces of the body from infection and assist in the activation of helper T ($CD4^+$) cells **(A).** Different classes of antibodies reflect structural variations that allow antibodies to be targeted to different bodily compartments and serve slightly different functions. The first step in T-cell activation occurs when the T-cell receptor recognizes a complex of peptide presented by an MHC molecule **(B).** A $CD4^+$ T cell recognizes peptide presented by MHC class II and a $CD8^+$ T cell interacts with peptides presented by MHC class I. Peptides may be presented by many different types of the listed MHC class I or class II molecules. After activation, the $CD4^+$ T cell (or helper T cell) may either activate macrophages through a helper T-cell type 1 response or activate B cells through the helper T-cell type 2 response **(C).**

and preterm parturition. Throughout pregnancy, macrophages are also in close proximity to invading trophoblasts that establish placentation. Placental growth involves trophoblast remodeling and programmed cell death (apoptosis). Macrophages in the placenta phagocytose apoptotic trophoblast, which also programs the macrophage to release anti-inflammatory cytokines (e.g., IL-10) promoting fetal tolerance.

Natural Killer Cells

The NK cell has important functions during pregnancy and becomes the most abundant leukocyte in the pregnant uterus. NK cells differ from T and B cells in that they do not express clonally distributed receptors for foreign antigens and can lyse target cells without prior sensitization. The phenotype of uterine NK (u-NK) cells is different from that of NK cells in peripheral blood, which seems to correlate with different primary functions. Most (90%) NK cells in blood have low CD56 and high CD16 expression ($CD56^{dim}/CD16^{bright}$); in the uterine decidua, u-NK cells have high CD56 expression ($CD56^{bright}$). The level of CD56 expression determines whether an NK cell has a primary cytolytic ($CD56^{dim}$) or cytokine-producing function ($CD56^{bright}$). Analysis of 10,000 genes from peripheral blood NK cells (dim and bright) and u-NK cells revealed more than 250 genes in which expression differed at least threefold. At least two of the upregulated proteins in u-NK cells, galectin-1 and progestagen-associated protein-14, are known to have immunomodulatory and immunosuppressive functions.

u-NK cells are thought to play a major role in remodeling of the spiral arteries to establish normal placentation. Mice with genetically defective u-NK cells fail to undergo spiral artery remodeling and normal decidualization, which are critical to normal placentation. This defect is corrected with administration of interferon-γ (IFN-γ), a prominent NK cell cytokine, suggesting that u-NK cells may play a role in trophoblast invasion.

Toll-like Receptors

TLRs are a recently discovered large family of PRRs on macrophages and many other cell types that play a key role in innate immunity.[5] **TLRs are now recognized as the principal sensors of pathogens and can activate both the innate and adaptive immune system.** At least 11 mammalian toll homologues have been identified, and they recognize a wide range of pathogen ligands (see Figure 4-1, *B*). TLR4 is a TLR that recognizes LPS from gram-negative bacteria, which triggers a signaling cascade leading to cytokine gene expression (Figure 4-3). TLR4 is expressed on macrophages, dendritic cells, endothelium, and numerous epithelial tissues. TLR2 recognizes motifs from gram-positive bacteria, including lipoteichoic acid and peptidoglycan.

Both TLR2 expression and TLR4 expression have been demonstrated in the placenta, and first-trimester trophoblast expresses both TLR2 and TLR4.[7] Activation of TLR2 triggers Fas-mediated apoptosis, whereas TLR4 activation induces proinflammatory cytokine production. The immunologic capability of first-trimester trophoblast to recognize pathogens and induce apoptosis suggests that innate immunity may be an important placental mechanism for triggering spontaneous abortion. TLR4 is also expressed in villous macrophages, villous and extravillous trophoblast, and the amniochorion. Expression of TLR4 and TLR2 increases in the chorioamniotic membranes of women with intraamniotic infection and also in term labor, suggesting an important role in both of these processes.[8]

Although intrauterine injection of LPS induces preterm birth in many murine and nonhuman primate models, administration of LPS to TLR4 mutant mice or LPS blockade with a TLR4 antagonist does not result in preterm delivery.[9,10] This finding suggests TLR4 is required for LPS-induced preterm birth in mice and is an important driver of the inflammatory cascade resulting from intra-amniotic infection. There is also a distinct progression in the responsiveness of fetal murine tissue to

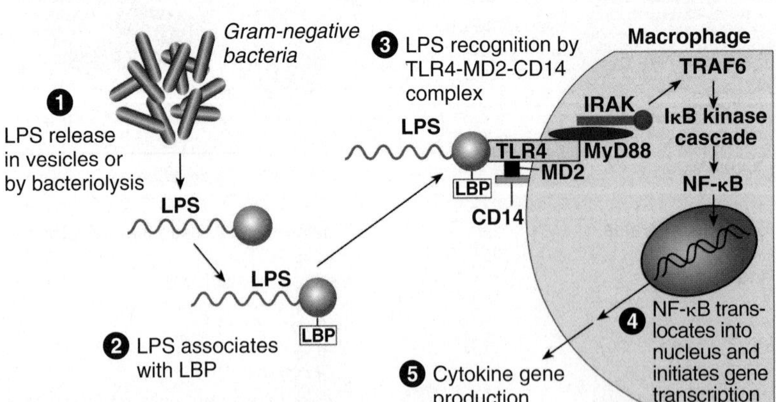

FIGURE 4-3. Toll-like receptor-4 (TLR4) recognition of lipopolysaccharide (LPS). Recognition of LPS by TLR4 occurs through several steps. (1) LPS is released from intact or lysed bacteria. (2) LPS binds to LPS-binding protein (LBP). (3) The LPS-LBP complex is recognized by a cell surface receptor complex TLR4, CD14, and MD-2. Binding of LPS-LBP to the TLR4, CD14, MD-2 receptor recruits the intracellular adaptor molecule, myeloid differentiation factor-88 (MyD88). Binding of MyD88 promotes the association of IL-1 receptor-associated protein kinase-4 (IRAK). Next, tumor necrosis factor receptor–associated kinase-6 (TRAF6) initiates a signaling cascade resulting in degradation of Iκ-B, which releases nuclear factor-κB (NF-κB), a transcription factor, into the cytoplasm. (4) NF-κB translocates into the nucleus and activates cytokine gene expression. Although the figure depicts TLR4 activation in a macrophage, many other immunologic and epithelial cells express TLR4 and induce cytokine production through this mechanism.

LPS as a function of gestational age.[11] When fetal lung is exposed to LPS on fetal day 14 (term is 20 days), both the expression of TLR4 and the acute cytokine response are undetectable. By day 17, TLR4 is expressed and an acute cytokine response occurs in fetal lungs. TLR4 likely controls the magnitude of the LPS-induced cytokine response during the perinatal period, and TLR4 placental expression appears to be dependent on gestational age.

Complement System

An important component of the innate immune system is the complement system, which consists of a large number of plasma proteins that cooperate to destroy and facilitate the removal of pathogens (see Figure 4-1, *C*). Complement proteins are detected in the amniotic fluid during intraamniotic infection, and regulation of complement is necessary to protect placental and fetal tissues from inflammation and destruction. The complement cascade is first activated by the surface antigens of pathogens. The nature of the initial pathogen trigger determines one of three activation pathways: classical, alternate, and lectin-binding pathways. For example, the classical pathway of complement activation is triggered when the complement protein, C1q, binds to antigen-antibody complexes on the surface of pathogens. This binding then results in a series of activation and amplification steps that result in production of the membrane attack complex (MAC), which creates a pore in the pathogen membrane leading to cell lysis. Formation of the MAC is an important mechanism of host defense against *Neisseria* species. Genetic deficiencies in C5-C9 complement proteins have been associated with susceptibility to *Neisseria gonorrhea* and *Neisseria meningitidis*.[12]

Regulatory proteins exist to protect cells from the deleterious effects of complement and are expressed on the placental membranes. Placental tissues at the maternal-fetal interface strongly express several negative regulators of complement activation, including CD59 (MAC antagonist), membrane cofactor protein, and decay accelerating factor (inhibitor of C3 and C5 convertases).[13,14] Whether these regulatory proteins might become overwhelmed during an intra-amniotic infection, leading to weakening of the membranes by complement proteins, is unknown.

Cytokines

The release of cytokines and chemokines by macrophages and other immune cells represents an important induced innate immune response (Table 4-1; see Figure 4-1, *D*) **Activated macrophages secrete cytokines that initiate inflammatory responses to control infections, which include IL-1, IL-6, IL-12, and TNF-α.** These cytokines are often referred to as proinflammatory because they mediate fever, lymphocyte activation, tissue destruction, and shock. Elevations in cytokines may influence the degree of morbidity and mortality associated with maternal influenza infection. Dramatic elevations in IL-6 have been implicated in deaths due to the 1918 influenza virus with an estimated mortality in pregnancy of 27%.[15]

Abnormal cytokine profiles have been associated with both preterm labor and preeclampsia. Proinflammatory cytokines have been identified in the amniotic fluid, maternal and fetal blood, and vaginal fluid of women with intra-amniotic infection.[2-4,16] These cytokines not only serve as a marker of intraamniotic infection but also may induce preterm labor and neonatal complications. The connection between elevated proinflammatory cytokines in fetal blood, preterm labor, and increased adverse fetal outcomes has been described as the "fetal inflammatory response syndrome."[16]

TABLE 4-1 CYTOKINES AND THEIR PRIMARY ACTION

Regulating Immune/Inflammatory Response

CYTOKINE	PRODUCED BY	PRIMARY ACTION
Interferons	Monocytes and macrophages	Produced in response to viruses, bacteria, parasites, and tumor cells Action includes killing tumor cells and inducing secretion of other inflammatory cytokines One of the first cytokines that appear during an inflammatory response
Interleukin-1	Monocytes and macrophages	Induces fever; co-stimulator of CD4+ helper T cells
Interleukin-2		Primary growth factor and activation factor for T cells, NK cells
Interleukin-4	CD4+ helper T cells	B-cell growth factor for antigen activated B cells
Interleukin-6	Monocytes and macrophages	Regulates growth and differentiation of lymphocytes and growth factor for plasma cells, and induces the synthesis of acute phase reactants by the liver
Interleukin-8	Monocytes	Chemoattractant for neutrophils
Interleukin-10	CD4+ helper T cells	Suppresses production of interferon, suppresses cell-mediated immunity, enhances humoral immunity
Transforming growth factor-β	T cells and monocytes	Inhibits the proliferation of lymphocytes

The relative contribution of individual cytokines and chemokines on induction of preterm labor was studied in a unique nonhuman primate model. Preterm labor was induced by intra-amniotic infusions of IL-1β and TNF-α, but not by IL-6 or IL-8. IL-1β stimulated preterm labor in all cases and an intense contraction pattern.[17] TNF-α induced a variable degree of uterine activity among individual animals characterized as either preterm labor or a uterine contraction pattern of moderate intensity. Despite prolonged elevations in amniotic fluid levels, neither IL-6 nor IL-8 induced an increase in uterine contractions until near term. These results suggested a primary role for IL-1β and TNF-α in the induction of infection-associated preterm birth.

Anti-inflammatory cytokines like IL-10 and transforming growth factor-β (TGF-β) act to downregulate inflammatory responses. IL-10 has been tested as a potential therapy for infection-induced preterm labor in a nonhuman primate model.[18] In the model, preterm labor was first induced by intraamniotic administration of IL-1β. IL-10 inhibited IL-1β-induced uterine contractions and elevations in amniotic fluid TNF-α and prostaglandins. However, other proinflammatory cytokines and hormones involved in labor were not suppressed.

Investigation of the individual effect of a single cytokine on pregnancy or complications of pregnancy in humans has proved challenging for several reasons. Many cytokines tend to be functionally redundant, and the absence of one cytokine can be compensated for by another. Second, there are multiple cytokine receptors (i.e., IL-1 receptor antagonist, IL-18 binding protein) that modulate similar cytokine effects. New families of decoy or silent cytokine receptors and suppressors of cytokine signaling have also been discovered in the placenta and amniotic fluid. Finally, molecular variants of cytokines may act as receptor antagonists. Therefore, individual cytokine effects during pregnancy must be interpreted in the context of cytokine receptors, receptor antagonists, silent cytokine receptors, and suppressors of cytokine signaling.

Chemokines

Chemokines are a class of cytokines that act primarily as chemoattractants and direct leukocytes to sites of infection. These chemotactic agents constitute a superfamily of small (8 to 10 kDa) molecules that can be divided into three groups (C, CC, and CXC) based on the position of either one or two cysteine residues located near the amino terminus of the protein. IL-8, macrophage chemoattractant protein-1, and RANTES (CCL5) are a few examples of chemokines. CXC chemokines, like IL-8, bind to CXC receptors (CXCRs) and are important for neutrophil activation and mobilization. IL-8 has been described in the amniotic fluid, maternal blood, and vaginal fluid with infection-associated preterm birth.[19] IL-8 and MCP-1 are also implicated in uterine stretch-induced preterm labor thought to occur in multiple gestation.[20]

Some chemokine receptors are used as a coreceptor for the viral entry of the human immunodeficiency virus (HIV). The two major coreceptors for HIV are CXCR4 and CCR5, both of which are expressed on activated T cells. CCR5 is also expressed on dendritic cells and macrophages, which allows HIV to infect these cell types. Rare resistance to HIV infection was discovered to correlate with homozygosity for a nonfunctional variant of CCR5 caused by a gene deletion in the coding region. The gene frequency for this CCR5 variant is highest in Northern Europeans but has not been detected in many black or Southeast Asian populations, in whom the prevalence of HIV infection is high.[21]

ADAPTIVE IMMUNITY

The function of the adaptive immune system is to eliminate infection as the second line of immune defense and provide increased protection against reinfection through "immunologic memory." Adaptive immunity consists primarily of B cells and T cells (lymphocytes), which differ from innate immune cells in several important respects, including the mechanism for pathogen recognition and lymphocyte activation. Targeting a specific pathogen component in an immune response is a critical feature of the adaptive immune system and necessary, in most cases, for resolution of the infection. However, achieving this specificity requires generation of an incredible diversity of T-cell receptors (TCRs) and B-cell receptors (BCRs). This creates the potential that self-antigens could be mistakenly targeted, resulting in an autoimmune response. Self-reactive T cells and B cells are thought to either undergo apoptosis in the thymus or be regulated in the periphery. A small population of T cells (regulatory T cells) is now known to contribute to peripheral regulatory mechanisms to prevent autoimmune responses and is discussed specifically in reference to mechanisms of fetal tolerance.

Major Histocompatibility Complex

Discriminating cells that are "self" from "nonself" is a critical function of the immune system to determine which cells should be destroyed and which to leave alone. In pregnancy, this process must be carefully regulated to prevent the killing of fetal cells, which express paternal genes that appear foreign to the maternal immune system, in effect expanding the definition of self to include the fetus. The ability of a lymphocyte to recognize self from nonself is based on the expression of unique MHC molecules on a cell's surface, which present small peptides from within the cell. MHC molecules are highly polymorphic proteins produced by a cluster of genes on the short arm of chromosome 6. This gene complex is classically divided into two distinct regions referred to as class I and II. Class I contains classical transplantation human leukocyte antigen (HLA) genes (e.g., HLA-A, -B, and -C) and nonclassical HLA genes that are distinguished by more limited polymorphism (e.g., HLA-G, -E, and -F). Class II contains polymorphic genes that are often matched for transplantation, including HLA-DR, -DQ, and -DP. Reduced HLA matching is associated with graft rejection through activation of T cells. This system is significantly different from the innate immune system, in which recognition of MHC is not necessary for pathogen destruction.

Humoral Immune Response: B Cells and Antibodies

The function of B cells is to protect the extracellular spaces (e.g., plasma, vagina) in the body through which infectious pathogens usually spread (see Figure 4-2, *A*). B cells mainly fight infection by secreting antibodies, also called immunoglobulins. There are many similarities between B and T lymphocytes. B cells also undergo clonal expansion after antigen stimulation and can be identified by a variety of specific cell surface markers (e.g., CD19, CD20, and BCR antigens). Activated B cells may proliferate and differentiate into antibody-secreting plasma cells. Antibodies control infection by several mechanisms, including neutralization, opsonization, and complement activation. Neutralization of a pathogen refers to the process of antibody binding, which prevents the pathogen from binding to a cell surface and internalizing. Alternatively, antibodies coating the pathogen may enhance phagocytosis, also referred to as *opsonization*. Antibodies may also directly activate the classical complement pathway. Activation of the B cell drives the B cell to proliferate and differentiate into an antibody-secreting plasma cell.

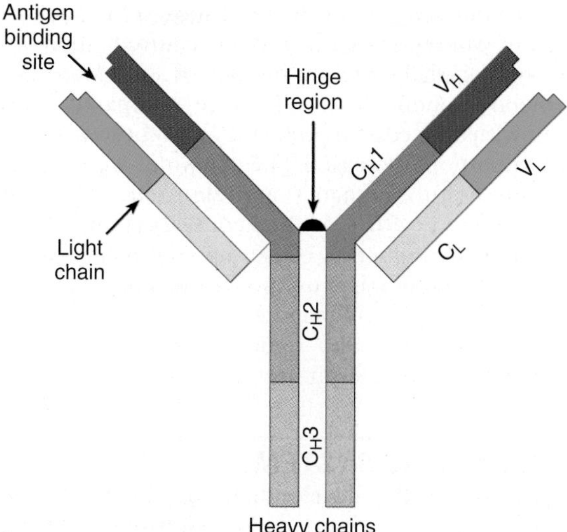

FIGURE 4-4. Structure of immunoglobulin (IgG).

Antibody Isotypes

Antibodies share the same general structure produced by the interaction and binding of four separate polypeptides (Figure 4-4). These include two identical light (L) chains (23 kDa), and two identical heavy (H) chains (55 kDa). The composition of the H chain determines the antibody isotype, function, and distribution in the body. In humans, there are five types of H chains designated mu (M), delta (D), gamma (G), alpha (A), and epsilon (E) that correspond to the five major antibody isotypes (immunoglobulin M [IgM], IgD, IgG, IgA, and IgE). During normal pregnancy, serum concentrations of IgG, IgA, and IgM are unchanged.

To effectively combat extracellular pathogens, antibodies must be specialized to cross epithelia into different bodily compartments. In fact, antibodies are made in several distinct classes or isotypes (i.e., IgM and IgG) that vary in their composition. Naïve B cells express only IgM and IgD. Activated B cells undergo isotype switching, a process that produces different antibody isotypes specialized for different functions and areas of the body.

The first antibody to be produced during an immune response is IgM because IgM is expressed before isotype switching. The serum concentration of IgM is 50 to 400 mg/dL, with a circulation half-life of 5 days. IgM antibodies are low in affinity, but the antibodies form pentamers that compensate by binding at multiple points to the antigen. IgM is highly efficient at activating the complement system, which is critical during the earliest stages of controlling an infection. Other isotypes dominate in the later stages of antibody responses.

IgG represents about 75% of serum immunoglobulin in adults and is further divided into four subclasses (IgG1, IgG2, IgG3, and IgG4). **Two subtypes of IgG, IgG1 and IgG3, are efficiently transported across the placenta and are important in conferring humoral immune protection for the fetus after birth.** The smaller size of IgG and its monomeric structure allows it to easily diffuse into extravascular sites.

IgA is the predominant antibody class in epithelial secretions from the vagina, intestine, and lung. IgA forms dimers and mainly functions as a neutralizing antibody. As a secreted antibody, IgA is not in close contact with either phagocytes or complement and, therefore, is less efficient in opsonization and complement activation. In the vagina, an IgA response mounted against anti–*Gardnerella vaginalis* hemolysin was associated with higher levels of IL-1β.[22] Induction of both innate and adaptive immune responses to lower genital tract infections may be a necessary event in preventing spread to the upper genital tract.

IgA is also the principal antibody in breast milk, which provides the neonate with humoral immunity from the mother. Neonates are particularly susceptible to infectious pathogens through their intestinal mucosa, and IgA is highly effective in neutralizing these bacteria and toxins. Epidemiologic studies indicate that deaths from diarrheal diseases could be reduced between 14-fold and 24-fold by breastfeeding, owing in part to the maternal-infant transmission of IgA.[23]

IgE has the lowest concentration in serum of all the antibodies but is bound efficiently by mast cell receptors. IgE binding of antibody triggers the mast cell to release granules, resulting in an allergic response. Prenatal maternal exposure to allergens may have an effect on IgE in the fetus at birth; concentration of house dust mite allergens has been correlated in a dose-dependent manner, with total IgE measured in heel capillary blood. IgE also plays a prominent role in immune responses to eukaryotic parasites.

T CELLS

When pathogens replicate inside cells (all viruses, some bacteria and parasites), they are inaccessible to antibodies and must be destroyed by T cells. T cells are lymphocytes responsible for the cell-mediated immune responses of adaptive immunity, which require direct interactions between T lymphocytes and cells bearing the antigen that the T cells recognize. Common to all mature T cells is the TCR complex. T cells develop the vast array of antigen specificity through a series of TCR gene rearrangements, and many aspects of TCR rearrangements are similar to those producing antibody specificity. For example, during viral replication inside a host cell, viral antigen is expressed on the surface of the infected cell. These foreign antigens are then recognized by T cells along with HLA. HLA class I molecules present peptides from proteins in the cytosol, which may include degraded host or viral proteins. HLA class II molecules bind peptides derived from proteins in intracellular vesicles, and thus display peptides derived from pathogens in macrophage vesicles, internalized by phagocytic cells, and B cells.

A variety of T cells are recognized based on their expression of different cell surface markers (i.e., CD2, CD3, CD4, CD8). Cytotoxic T cells kill infected cells directly and express a variety of cell surface antigen and specific receptors, including CD8. Helper T cells activate B cells and express CD4. Cytotoxic and helper T cells recognize peptides bound to proteins of two different classes of HLA molecules (see Figure 4-2, *B*). Antigen-presenting cells will present antigen to $CD8^+$ T cells in the context of MHC class I molecules (e.g., HLA-A). In contrast, antigen-presenting cells that present antigens with MHC class II molecules (e.g. HLA-DR) interact with T cells bearing CD4.

HIV employs multiple strategies to disable T-cell responses. Targeting viral infection to the $CD4^+$ T cells allows the virus to control and ultimately destroy this important T-cell subset. HIV destroys $CD4^+$ T cells through direct viral killing, lowering the apoptosis threshold of infected cells, and through $CD8^+$ T cells that recognize viral peptides on the $CD4^+$ T-cell surface. $CD8^+$ T cells likely contain the infection but are unable to eradicate the virus. Viral mutants produced during one of the earliest steps of viral infection may contribute to escape of virus-infected cells from $CD8^+$ T cell killing. The error-prone reverse-transcriptase copies the RNA viral genome into DNA, making "mistakes" that lead to production of these viral variants. The presentation of peptides from HIV variants by $CD4^+$ T cells may also interfere and downregulate the $CD8^+$ T-cell response to the original (wild-type) virus. Finally, the HIV negative-regulation factor gene *(nef)* downregulates expression of MHC class II and CD4, which decreases the presentation of viral antigens on the cell surface.

Helper T Subsets

$CD4^+$ T cells were originally classified into Th1 and Th2 subsets depending on whether their main function involved cell-mediated responses and selective production of IFN-γ (Th1) or humoral-mediated responses with production of IL-4 (Th2). The number of subsets identified continues to expand and now includes regulatory T cells, Th3, Th17, Th9, Th22, and follicular helper T cells (T_{FH}).[24] Helper T cells are also no longer thought to be committed to this function and may exhibit plasticity between some of these subsets. Description of the Th1 and Th2 subsets follows because there is evidence to suggest that they may play a role in pregnancy tolerance.

The Th1 subset is important in the control of intracellular bacterial infections such as *Mycobacterium tuberculosis* and *Chlamydia trachomatis.* Intracellular bacteria survive because the vesicles they occupy do not fuse with intracellular lysosomes, which contain a variety of enzymes and antimicrobial substances. Th1 cells activate macrophages to induce fusion of their lysosomes with vesicles containing the bacteria. Th1 cells also release cytokines and chemokines that attract macrophages to the site of infection, like IFN-γ, TNF-α, IL-12, and IL-18. Activating a Th1 immune response is a common feature of current vaccines targeting *Chlamydia* species.[25]

Th2 immune responses are mainly responsible for activating B cells by providing a critical "second signal" necessary for B-cell activation. Th2 cells produce cytokines, including IL-4, IL-5, IL-6, IL-10, IL-13, and TGF-β. The signals that trigger differentiation down these two pathways are unknown but are thought to be influenced by cytokines produced in response to the infection.

Th2-type and perhaps Th3-type activity may predominate during pregnancy, a theory based on the adverse effects of Th1 cytokines on murine pregnancy and weakened maternal immunity to intracellular infections requiring Th1 cytokine activity.[26-28] IL-10 may be a critical Th2 cytokine in maintaining pregnancy because it downregulates Th1 cytokine production and prevents fetal resorption in mice genetically predisposed to abortion.[29] In a study of women with a history of recurrent spontaneous abortion, maternal cytokine profiles of stimulated peripheral blood mononuclear cells were compared between women with a successful pregnancy and those with a spontaneous abortion. Increased Th2 cytokines were associated with a successful pregnancy, and elevated Th1 cytokines were associated with a spontaneous abortion.[30] Whether Th1 cytokine production causes spontaneous abortion or occurs after fetal death is unknown. Recent evidence suggests that the Th1/Th2 paradigm may be an oversimplification and that cytokine signaling during pregnancy is likely to be a more complicated process.

FETAL IMMUNE SYSTEM

Descriptions of the development of the fetal immune system are relatively limited, but sufficient information exists to determine that the fetus, even very early in gestation, has innate immune capacity.[31-33] **Acquired immunity, particularly the capacity to produce a humoral response, develops more slowly and is not completely functional until well after birth.** Many of the immune protective mechanisms that are present to protect the fetus from both pathogens and maternal immune recognition occur at the maternal-fetal interface.

Fetal hematologic development initiates in the fetal yolk sac and aortic-genital ridge. The exact contribution of these two sites to hematopoietic development is controversial, with many now favoring the initial site of hematopoietic development for the fetus initiating at the aortic-genital ridge. Hematopoietic stem cells migrate from their site of initial production in the fetal liver, and ultimately reside in the fetal bone marrow, which becomes the major site of hematopoiesis at about 28 weeks of gestation.

Fetal thymic development begins from the third and fourth brachial pouches and cleft. A primordial thymus is present at about 7 weeks' gestation. The thymus is first colonized with cells from the fetal liver at 8.5 to 9.5 weeks' gestation. These cells express primitive (CD34) and early T-cell surface antigen, $CD7^+$. Shortly after this, 20% to 50% percent of cells in the fetal thymus express the common T-cell surface phenotypes (CD7, CD2). Between 12 and 13 weeks, cells within the fetal liver and spleen express the TCR. By 16 weeks' gestation, the fetal thymus has distinct cortical and medullary regions, suggesting functional maturity, and this is confirmed by the brisk response to allogeneic and mitogen stimulation. Functionally, fetal T cells show proliferative capacity very early in gestation. In vitro stimulation by phytohemagglutinin can be demonstrated as early as 10 weeks. Allogeneic responses in mixed lymphocyte culture can be detected in cells obtained from fetal liver as early 9.5 weeks and are consistently seen at 12 weeks of gestation.[34]

The ontogeny of fetal B-cell development in many ways parallels the development of T cells, with early pre-B cells (CD19 and CD20) being identified by cell surface markings in the fetal liver by 7 to 8 weeks' gestation.[35] Ultimately, these cells are produced in the fetal bone marrow as the marrow becomes the primary hematopoietic organ in the second trimester. Surface expression of IgM can be

TABLE 4-2 COMMON IMMUNE DEFECTS

COMMON NAME	DEFECT	CELLS AFFECTED	COMMENTS
X-SCID	Common γ chain of IL-2 receptor	T cells and NK cells	X-linked recessive and most common form of SCID accounting for about 45% to 50% of cases
ADA-SCID	Defect in purine metabolism leading to abnormal accumulation of adenosine	T cells, B cells, and NK cells	Autosomal recessive affecting both male and female infants Accounts for about 20% of SCID cases
Jak-3 deficiency	Mutation on chromosome 19 of Janus kinase-3 that is activated by cytokine binding to the common γ chain of the IL-2 receptor	T cells and NK cells	Autosomal recessive affecting both male and female infants Accounts for about 10% of SCID cases
Hyper-IgM syndrome Autosomal recessive	Defect in CD40 ligand (T cell) and CD40 (B cell) signaling resulting in the inability of immunoglobulin class switching	Elevated IgM	X-linked and autosomal recessive

ADA-SCID, Adenosine deaminase severe combined immunodeficiency; *IgG*, immunoglobulin G; *IgM*, immunoglobulin M; *IL-2*, interleukin-2; *NK*, natural killer; *X-SCID*, X-linked severe combined immunodeficiency.

noted as early as 9 to 10 weeks. Cells in the fetal circulation express the common B-cell antigens (CD20) by 14 to 16 weeks' gestation, and secretion of IgM has been noted as early as 15 weeks. The level of IgM continues to increase and reaches normal postnatal levels by 1 year of age. The appearance of surface IgG and IgA is noted in fetal B cells at 13 weeks with secretion of IgG at 20 weeks' gestation. Postnatal levels of immunoglobulin are not reached until about 5 years of age.

NK cells also play an important role in fetal immunity. Expressed as a percentage of the total lymphocytes, the proportion of NK cells in the fetal circulation is high (30% at 13 weeks). Based on their high number, early presence, and the ability to kill cells directly or through antibody-mediated toxicity, it is likely that NK cells play a significant role in the fetal innate immune system.

Fortunately, abnormalities of normal immune development are relatively rare. However, when they do occur, they can have profound effects on newborn and child health. Some of the more common immunodeficiencies are listed in Table 4-2.[36,37]

Cord Blood Transplantation

Fetal blood contains a high frequency of hematopoietic stem cells as well as naïve T cells and NK cells. All these features make fetal blood an ideal source of cells for bone marrow transplantation. In 1988, the first bone marrow transplantation was carried out in a child with Fanconi anemia using a cord blood sample from an HLA-identical sibling.[38] During the ensuing 20 years, more than 20,000 cord blood transplantations have been performed, and obstetricians are frequently requested to collect umbilical cord blood remaining in the placenta after cord clamping. Cord blood is typically collected into closed-system bags or syringes that contain anticoagulation additives. The average volume per collection is about 75 mL of cord blood, which is processed to deplete red blood cells and then cryopreserved for later use. Cord blood samples are processed at either private or public cord blood banks. Specimens banked at private cord blood banks will be reserved for the donor family, with an estimated need for use between 1 per 1000 and 1 per 200,000.[39] Samples donated to public cord blood banks are processed, HLA typed, and entered into the National Marrow Donor Program, where they are made available to any individual requiring bone marrow transplantation. The major advantage of public banks is that samples are available to ethnic groups, which traditionally have difficulty finding a suitable HLA-matched donor (e.g. Native Americans, Asian/Pacific Islanders, and African Americans).[40] The American Congress of Obstetricians and Gynecologists recommends that if a patient requests information regarding collection and banking of umbilical cord blood, balanced and accurate information regarding the advantages and disadvantages of public versus private banking should be provided. Private umbilical cord blood banking seems to be cost-effective only for children with a very high likelihood of needing a stem cell transplant.[41] Physicians or other professionals who recruit pregnant women and their families for for-profit umbilical cord blood banking should disclose any financial interests or other potential conflicts of interest.

Cord blood specimens were initially used only in children because of the reduced number of $CD34^+$ cells that were present in the donor specimen. As use increased, even in the setting of less than ideal HLA matching, engraftment success was accompanied by a reduction in the frequency of severe (grades 3 and 4) graft-versus-host disease (GVHD). Because of the success noted in children, cord blood specimens are now commonly used in adults. The relative immaturity of the donor cells and total number of stem cells in the donor graft often result in delayed engraftment compared with other sources of donor hematopoietic cells. In some settings, in which the donor CD34 count is considered insufficient or less than ideal, more than one donor cord blood specimen is used. After engraftment, usually only one donor source predominates, and the recipient does not develop multisource mixed chimerism. The National Marrow Donor Program estimates that by 2015, more than 10,000 cord blood transplantations will be carried out annually worldwide, suggesting that cord blood collection for public banking will become commonplace in many obstetrical units. At the present time, the need for autologous cord blood cells is limited. In 2006, the World Marrow Donor Association stated that there were, at present, no established protocols for the use of autologous cord blood. Cord blood has been cited as a potential source of stem cells that could ultimately be used

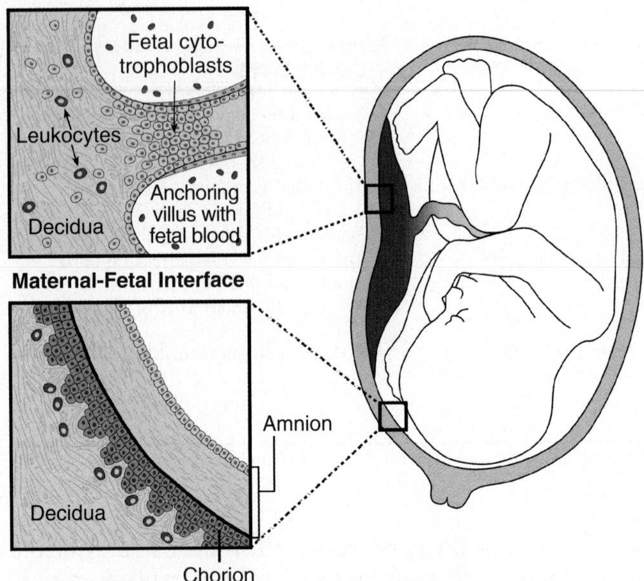

FIGURE 4-5. The maternal-fetal interface and mechanisms of fetal tolerance. Maternal and fetal cells are in close contact in several sites of the placenta, including the decidua and chorion layer of the fetal membranes.

for regenerative medicine and cellular therapy. Currently, the use of cord blood for regenerative cell therapy has not reached a state at which recommendations for autologous cord blood storage can be made.

MATERNAL TOLERANCE OF THE FETUS

Pregnancy is a unique immunologic phenomenon, in which the normal immune rejection of foreign tissues does not occur. The placenta is not a barrier between maternal and fetal cells, and these cells come into direct contact in several locations, which represent the maternal-fetal interface (Figure 4-5). Syncytiotrophoblast, the outermost layer of chorionic villi, is in direct contact with maternal blood in the intervillous space. Extravillous trophoblast in the decidua is in contact with many different maternal cells, including macrophages, u-NK cells, and T cells. Endovascular trophoblast replaces endothelial cells in the maternal spiral arteries and is in direct contact with maternal blood. Fetal and maternal macrophages are also in close contact in the chorion layer of the fetal membranes. A final interface may be considered within the periphery, where shed fetal trophoblast from the placenta and intact fetal cells come into contact with maternal immune cells.[42]

Immunologic mechanisms of fetal tolerance must be acting at the maternal-fetal interface to prevent fetal rejection because the maternal immune system clearly recognizes fetal cells as foreign. About 30% of primiparous and multiparous women develop antibodies against the inherited paternal HLA of the fetus.[43] Persistence of these antibodies does not appear to be harmful to the fetus.[44] Persistent fetal cells in the mother may play a role in the persistence of these antibodies because in some women the antibodies persist, whereas in others they disappear. Formation of IgG antibodies against inherited paternal HLA antigens is associated with the presence of primed cytotoxic T lymphocytes specific for these HLA antigens. Maternal T lymphocytes specific for fetal antigens do exist during pregnancy but appear to be hyporesponsive.[45,46] The normal growth and development of the fetus despite maternal immune recognition requires several maternal and fetal adaptations that, in most women, allow pregnancy to be carried uneventfully to term.

Tolerance Through Human Leukocyte Antigens

Fetal trophoblast and cells in the placental membranes are in direct contact with maternal blood and should be at risk for maternal immunologic rejection. The expression of MHC molecules by these fetal cells may at first appear to be an evolutionary disadvantage that could trigger a graft rejection–type immune response. Of the various forms of placental trophoblast, HLA expression is limited to class I antigens, primarily the class Ib HLA-E, HLA-F, and HLA-G, all of which have limited polymorphisms. The exception to this rule of limited genetic variability is expression of HLA-C, a class Ia molecule that is highly polymorphic and is expressed primarily by extravillous trophoblast. Owing to its unique distribution on fetal trophoblastic tissue, HLA-G is thought to be a significant component of fetal tolerance. Although the exact function of HLA-G is unknown, evidence indicates that HLA-G protects the invasive cytotrophoblast from killing by u-NK cells, as well as containment of placental infection.[47] HLA-G also inhibits macrophage activation through ILT-4, an inhibitory receptor. The presence of a soluble form of HLA-G in high concentration in the amniotic fluid that declines near term suggests a possible role in the initiation of normal labor.[48] **HLA-G, through interactions with u-NK cells, likely contributes to maintaining immune tolerance at the maternal-fetal interface and normal pregnancy.** However, other mechanisms must also contribute to this process because normal pregnancies in women and fetuses lacking a functional HLA-G gene (HLA-G null) have been described.[49]

Tolerance Through Regulation of Maternal T Cells

Maternal T cells acquire a transient state of tolerance for specific paternal alloantigens. This has been elegantly demonstrated in female mice that were sensitized to known paternal antigens before pregnancy.[45,46] The female mice became tolerant to the same paternal antigens expressed by the fetus that were previously recognized and destroyed. Several mechanisms must therefore exist to suppress maternal T-cell responses. This tolerance induction may occur naturally through the generation of paternal-specific regulatory T cells induced after exposure to seminal fluid.[50]

Regulatory T cells suppress antigen-specific immune responses and are elevated in the maternal circulation of women and mice during pregnancy.[51] Outside of pregnancy, regulatory T cells ($CD4^+$, $CD25^+$) act mainly to prevent autoimmune responses from occurring when self-reactive T cells escape from the thymus during normal T-cell development. The mechanism of regulatory T-cell suppression of T-cell responses is unknown but may involve either direct cell contact or production of anti-inflammatory cytokines, like IL-10 and TGF-β. Estrogen has been shown to increase proliferation of regulatory T cells, and the higher levels of estrogen in pregnancy may drive expansion of this cell population during pregnancy.[52] In addition, spontaneous abortion could be prevented in a unique murine model by the transfer of regulatory T cells from mice with a normal pregnancy into mice destined to abort.[53]

Another strategy for suppressing maternal T-cell responses at the maternal-fetal interface involves tryptophan depletion by indoleamine 2,3-dioxygenase (IDO), an enzyme that catabolizes tryptophan.[54] IDO normally functions as an innate antimicrobial defense mechanism by allowing cells to deplete tryptophan from intracellular pools or local microenvironments. IDO is thought to contribute to T-cell hyporesponsiveness during pregnancy because tryptophan is an essential amino acid for T-cell function. IDO-producing cells can be identified in the decidua of human and murine placenta a few days after implantation. At this interface, IDO creates a local tissue microenvironment that precludes maternal T-cell activation to fetal alloantigens. Inhibition of IDO leads to rapid rejection and abortion of murine fetuses a few days after implantation.[55] By contrast, mice pregnant with a genetically identical fetus did not reject their fetuses after exposure to an IDO inhibitor. Regulatory T cells may also stimulate IDO expression, which may link these two mechanisms for downregulating T-cell responses.[56]

Activated maternal T cells may also be killed through interactions with Fas ligand (FasL) and TNF-related apoptosis-inducing ligand/Apo-2L (TRAIL) expressed on placental trophoblast.[57,58] Both TRAIL and FasL may cooperate to control lymphocyte proliferation after activation and induce apoptotic cell death.

Recently, another mechanism for maternal tolerance of the fetus was proposed that takes into account cell trafficking, which occurs between the mother and fetus.[42,59] Fetal cells escape into maternal blood, and how the mother tolerates these cells is poorly understood. The hypothesis describes how a significant impact on maternal immunity is expected as a result of continuous shedding of apoptotic syncytiotrophoblast debris throughout gestation, a process recently appreciated to result in gram quantities of apoptotic fetal debris entering the maternal circulation daily. Maternal dendritic cells are proposed to present fetal HLA derived from apoptotic syncytiotrophoblast under noninflammatory conditions, leading to tolerogenic signals and tolerance of fetal cells. This novel hypothesis was also suggested to explain the beneficial effects of pregnancy on rheumatoid arthritis, an autoimmune disease that remits or improves in nearly three fourths of women during pregnancy. Amelioration of rheumatoid arthritis may occur during pregnancy as a secondary benefit of changes in the maternal peripheral tolerance to fetal cells.

Tolerance Through Regulation of Complement and Cytokines

In the absence of certain autoimmune disorders, serum complement levels are unchanged or elevated during normal pregnancy.[60,61] However, local inhibition of complement in the placenta may be important in preventing certain immunologically mediated complications of pregnancy. In a murine model of antiphospholipid antibody–induced abortion, antagonism of factor B (alternative complement component) protected against immune-mediated fetal loss.[62] Defects of placental formation were also observed in a murine model associated with activation of the alternative complement pathway and maternal C3.[63] **Finally, several negative regulators of complement are expressed by trophoblast, including CD59 (MAC antagonist), membrane cofactor protein, and decay accelerating factor (inhibitors of C3 and C5 convertases).**[14,64] When a negative regulator of murine complement *Crry* was genetically ablated, embryo survival was compromised and placental inflammation observed.[65] C3 activation plays a major role in fetal rejection in this model because the embryos survived when genetically deficient *Crry* mice were mated to C3-deficient mice. Therefore, complement activation at the maternal-fetal interface may contribute significantly to fetal tolerance.

Although it is speculated that uterine or placental leukocytes regulate trophoblast invasion through cytokine production, many studies in transgenic mouse models have not linked defects in cytokine production with abnormal invasion and pregnancy loss.[66] Among the Th2 cytokines thought to be protective for pregnancy, there is a great deal of functional redundancy. Genetic deficiencies in four of these cytokines (IL-4, IL-5, IL-9, IL-13) did not reduce murine fetal or neonatal survival.[67] Other evidence implicates IFN-γ in normal placental vascular development, which was previously thought to be detrimental for pregnancy.[68] Whether Th2 cytokines play a major role in fetal tolerance and pregnancy maintenance is unknown.[69]

IMMUNITY IN INFECTION-ASSOCIATED PRETERM BIRTH

Preterm birth is a complex process with many different etiologies. **A large body of evidence suggests that intra-amniotic infection and inflammation are important causes of early preterm births, particularly before 28 to 30 weeks of gestation.**[70,71] The immunologic response has been implicated in driving preterm labor in women with intra-amniotic infection. Bacteria recovered from the amniotic fluid usually consist of organisms colonizing the lower genital tract, which then induce production of proinflammatory cytokines like IL-1β, IL-6, IL-8, and TNF-α. Many placental tissues and immune cells in the placenta produce cytokines/chemokines in response to bacteria or bacterial products including amniotic epithelium, macrophages, decidual cells, and trophoblasts.

A role for proinflammatory cytokines and chemokines in the development of preterm labor is based on several observations. Amniotic fluid levels of IL-1, IL-6, IL-8, and TNF-α are elevated in humans and rabbits with intra-amniotic infection and preterm labor. Bacterial products stimulate the production of IL-1β, IL-6, and TNF-α by human placental tissues. These cytokines can then stimulate prostaglandin production in decidual explants and amniotic epithelial cell lines in vitro, as well as fetal membrane apoptosis. Finally, the administration of recombinant IL-1β into the amniotic fluid of pregnant nonhuman primates or systemically in mice induces preterm labor. Other cytokines, like IL-6 and IL-8, are unlikely to be required for infection-induced preterm birth based on data in a mouse and nonhuman primate model.[17] Interestingly, progesterone reduces apoptosis in fetal membranes induced by TNF-α in vitro, suggesting a possible immune mechanism by which progesterone might inhibit preterm birth.

Gaps in the scientific knowledge of mechanisms leading to preterm labor and those promoting uterine quiescence are significant, particularly when one considers the many different etiologies of preterm birth.[72] Of the many different factors linked to preterm labor, intrauterine infection remains one of the most important and potentially preventable causes. Several immunomodulators have been successful in inhibiting contractions or delaying infection-induced preterm birth in a nonhuman primate model. Initial studies investigated the efficacy of immunomodulators on preterm labor induced by IL-1β. Dexamethasone (corticosteroid), indomethacin (inhibitor of prostaglandin synthesis), and IL-10 (anti-inflammatory cytokine) were studied.[18] All three inhibited IL-1β-induced uterine contractility but differed in their ability to suppress specific amniotic fluid cytokines and prostaglandins. When dexamethasone and indomethacin were used with antibiotics to treat a group B streptococcal infection in the nonhuman primate model, gestation was significantly longer than in controls treated with antibiotics alone.[73] This evidence suggests that blockade of the immune response, in combination with antibiotics, may delay infection-induced preterm birth. Further, blockade of initial immune responses to LPS with a TLR4 antagonist prevented increases in uterine activity, cytokines, and prostaglandins in a nonhuman primate model.[10] Whether immunomodulators ultimately prove to reduce preterm birth or neonatal morbidity in humans remains to be demonstrated.

Fetal systemic inflammation has been hypothesized to directly contribute to the pathogenesis of preterm birth. The fetal inflammatory response syndrome describes a condition with elevated levels of fetal plasma IL-6 and systemic inflammation, which has been documented in fetuses from women with preterm labor and preterm premature rupture of membranes.[74] **This syndrome is a significant predictor not only of preterm labor but also of neonatal morbidity with multiorgan involvement.** How the fetal inflammatory response might trigger preterm birth is unknown, but it has been associated with elevations in fetal hormones linked to parturition. Specifically, fetal inflammation has been associated with elevations in fetal plasma cortisol and an abnormal fetal plasma cortisol–to–dehydroepiandrosterone sulfate ratio, which in turn are associated with a shorter interval to delivery. The fetal inflammatory response syndrome may play a significant role in the timing of preterm birth.

IMMUNITY IN PREECLAMPSIA

Multiple lines of investigation implicate immune dysfunction in the pathogenesis of preeclampsia, including epidemiologic findings and evidence of abnormalities in both innate and adaptive immunity. Epidemiologic studies have found a higher risk for preeclampsia in women with new partners as well as among couples with a shorter duration of cohabitation and who previously used barrier contraception. The risk is also greater in pregnancies using assisted reproductive technologies, particularly when sperm are surgically obtained and in egg donor pregnancies. These relationships support the hypothesis that exposure to paternal antigens, either through intercourse or a prior pregnancy, decreases the risk for preeclampsia and may represent a "tolerizing" phenomenon.[75] Interestingly, in the 1970s, prior blood transfusion was also found to be protective for preeclampsia,[76] further supporting the idea that prior antigenic exposures influence the maternal response to the immune challenge of pregnancy. Animal studies may help to explain these findings; in mice, mucosal exposure to paternal antigens in semen induces paternal-specific regulatory T cells, which modulate the immune response to specific antigens.[50] Some studies have also suggested an association with maternal HLA homozygosity and with maternal-paternal or maternal-fetal HLA sharing, although other studies have not confirmed these associations.

As a framework for understanding abnormal immune responses linked to preeclampsia, it is important to consider maternal-fetal immune interactions within the placenta and also the periphery. Preeclampsia may be considered to develop in two stages: a preclinical stage characterized by abnormal placentation and spiral artery remodeling, followed by clinically evident maternal disease associated with heightened systemic inflammation. Early in gestation, the primary maternal-fetal interface involves interactions of trophoblast with maternal immune cells within the decidua. For example, HLA-G has a crucial function in implantation and placentation; studies have associated decreased placental HLA-G expression with preeclampsia as opposed to normal pregnancy. Later in gestation, there is an additional maternal-fetal interface in the maternal circulation and tissues. Maternal immune cells in the periphery may interact with necrotic debris shed from the syncytiotrophoblast or intact fetal cells predisposing to preeclampsia through aberrant immune interactions.

Successful placentation depends on extravillous trophoblast acquisition of an invasive phenotype, which allows for remodeling of the maternal spiral arteries, lowering blood flow resistance and vasoreactivity. In preeclampsia, extravillous trophoblast does not acquire an invasive phenotype to the same degree as normal pregnancy, limiting spiral arterial remodeling and resulting in persistent hypoxia-reperfusion cycles. Spiral artery remodeling depends on the interactions of extravillous trophoblast with uterine NK cells, primarily through HLA-C and KIR receptors, respectively. Specific maternal-fetal combinations of KIR and HLA-C genotypes are strongly associated with preeclampsia.[77] In addition, trophoblast interactions with maternal T cells likely play a key role in the establishment of a healthy placenta. Early in normal pregnancy, fetus-specific regulatory T cells are recruited from the maternal periphery to the decidua, and the quantity and function of decidual regulatory T cells is increased in the setting of maternal-fetal HLA-C mismatch.[78]

The clinically evident phase of preeclampsia is characterized by widespread inflammation and endothelial dysfunction. Although it is now understood that inflammation underlies pregnancy normally, a broad range of data show that these responses are further heightened in preeclampsia.[79] This generalized response is characterized by activation of granulocytes and monocytes. Intracellular reactive oxygen species is increased in not only these populations but also lymphocytes. Cytokine abnormalities include higher concentrations of IFN-γ, TNF-α, IL-6, IL-1β, IL-8, and IL-16, and lower concentrations of IL-10 in preeclampsia compared with normal pregnancy. In addition, clotting factor and complement abnormalities are associated with preeclampsia. During this phase, the primary maternal exposure to fetoplacental material occurs through acquisition of syncytiotrophoblast microparticles, but one must also consider the maternal acquisition of intact fetal cells with a more mature HLA expression profile and the ramifications of those interactions within the maternal system.

In addition to the role of T cells in placentation, alterations in T-cell function have also been implicated in clinically evident preeclampsia. Classically, consideration of the adaptive immune response in preeclampsia focused on the paradigm of a Th1/Th2 T-cell dichotomy. Normal pregnancy has been characterized by a shift from Th1 predominance to Th2, and preeclampsia was considered to relate to an insufficient shift. More recently, the complexity of T-cell subpopulations, as well as their interconnectedness and plasticity, has become clear. **Although studies vary by methodology and specific results, most data suggest that regulatory T cells are decreased in number and function in preeclampsia compared with normal pregnancy.** One study has recently shown that the ratio of regulatory T cells (Foxp3$^+$) to IL-17-expressing CD4$^+$ T cells is higher in normal pregnancy than preeclampsia; this suggests that the normal homeostasis in pregnancy between regulatory T cells and IL-17-producing CD4$^+$ T cells compartment was lost in preeclampsia.[80] Whether the proinflammatory Th17 subpopulation is overrepresented in preeclampsia is not yet clear.

Maternal immune dysfunction underlying preeclampsia is an active area of investigation. Additional areas of ongoing study of immune dysfunction include the association of an activating autoantibody against the angiotensin II type I receptor with preeclampsia.[81] The links between the preclinical and clinical stages of disease and between the innate and adaptive immune response also remain a focus, whereby γ/δ T cells have been investigated and found to have increased cytotoxic potential in preeclampsia. IDO, which inhibits proliferation of activated T cells, has been shown to have lower activity in preeclampsia. In addition, the proinflammatory potential of necrotic syncytiotrophoblast microparticles remains a subject of ongoing investigation.

MATERNAL-FETAL HUMAN LEUKOCYTE ANTIGEN COMPATIBILITY AND RECURRENT PREGNANCY LOSS

The hypothesis that maternal-fetal HLA incompatibility is beneficial in mammalian pregnancy was first proposed in the 1960s based on observations of larger placental size with genetically incompatible murine fetuses compared with compatible fetuses.[82] Incompatible murine zygotes were also more likely to implant than compatible zygotes.[83] Several studies began to test the idea that maternal-fetal HLA compatibility in human pregnancy might also result in defective implantation or placentation predisposing to spontaneous abortion. The first studies to evaluate this hypothesis in humans demonstrated significantly more matching at the HLA-A and HLA-B loci among couples with a history of recurrent spontaneous abortion of unknown etiology, compared with fertile control couples.[84,85] **However, more than 30 studies of HLA matching in couples with recurrent miscarriage have yielded conflicting results. There is no clear relationship between HLA matching and fetal loss from these retrospective studies.[86]** Prospective studies in the Hutterites, one of the most inbred human populations, suggest that HLA matching is a significant risk factor for recurrent spontaneous abortion.[87,88] The overall significance of these findings remains unknown. Randomized immunologically based therapeutic trials in couples with HLA compatibility and recurrent pregnancy loss have produced conflicting results likely because they preceded a thorough understanding of this phenomenon and the heterogeneity of the populations tested.[89,90]

MATERNAL-FETAL CELL TRAFFICKING AND MICROCHIMERISM

It was classically thought that the placenta served as an impenetrable barrier between mother and fetus. The application of molecular techniques to the study of human pregnancy has demonstrated that bidirectional cell trafficking occurs routinely between the mother and the fetus. **Thus, in nearly every pregnancy, cells that originate from the fetus can be found in the mother, and conversely, cells that originate from the mother can be found in the fetus. The long-term persistence of fetal cells in the mother and maternal cells in her progeny leads to the coexistence of at least two cell populations in a single person and is referred to as *microchimerism*.**

Fetal microchimerism can be detected in the maternal system as both cell-free fetal DNA and intact fetal cells. Cell-free fetal DNA is detectable throughout gestation, beginning as early as 4 to 5 weeks of gestational age; this material is cleared rapidly from the maternal plasma postpartum.[91] In contrast, cellular fetal microchimerism can also be detected early in gestation but is more commonly detected quite late in pregnancy, and its acquisition may primarily be a peripartum event.[92] The kinetics and prevalence of cell-free fetal DNA in maternal circulation make it an attractive source for performing noninvasive prenatal diagnosis, and active investigation in this area is underway.[93] The amount of cell-free fetal DNA has been found to be greater in pregnancies complicated by obstetrical outcomes such as preeclampsia compared with normal pregnancies. Intact fetal cells, both during pregnancy and in subsequent years, have been shown to occupy many cells types, including CD34$^+$ progenitor cells, and to inhabit many maternal organs, including lymph nodes, liver, thyroid, spleen, heart, and kidneys.[91,94] From an immunologic perspective, the unique characteristics, including HLA expression, of cell-free fetal DNA compared with intact fetal cells raise intriguing questions about mechanisms of maternal tolerance of the fetus and its perturbations.

Fetal acquisition of maternal microchimerism during pregnancy has also been shown to occur physiologically.

Maternal cells have been detected at an early gestational age in many fetal tissues, including liver, lung, heart, thymus, spleen, adrenal, kidney, pancreas, brain, gonads, and lymph nodes.[91] Within fetal lymph nodes, maternal cells are found ubiquitously, and they appear to influence the development of fetal regulatory T cells.[95]

Cells exchanged in pregnancy, persisting as durable maternal or fetal microchimerism, continue to inhabit immunologically competent or pluripotent cell populations. As such, they may play a functional role in health and disease. A role in autoimmune disease has been hypothesized to occur, similar to chronic GVHD in transplantation, when an "auto"-immune response to or by the microchimeric cells becomes generalized.[96] Several autoimmune diseases, including systemic sclerosis, autoimmune thyroid disease, and neonatal lupus syndrome, have been linked to microchimerism.[91,97,98] On the other hand, microchimerism may also serve in a protective, immunosurveillance role. This has been supported by the association of lower levels of fetal microchimerism in women with breast cancer compared with healthy controls.[99] Pregnancy history also seems to influence the type of microchimerism harbored by women because increasing parity, reflecting the acquisition of a greater number of fetal sources of microchimerism, is associated with lower levels of maternal microchimerism.[100]

The long-term consequences of naturally acquired microchimerism derived from pregnancy are not yet clear. It is likely that microchimerism can have an adverse, neutral, or beneficial effect on the host, depending on other factors, with HLA genes and the HLA relationship among cells probably of key importance. Elucidating the mechanisms by which naturally acquired microchimerism is permitted without detriment to the host may lead to novel strategies with application to prevention or treatment of autoimmune diseases.

SUMMARY

During pregnancy, the immunologic adaptations, particularly at the maternal-fetal interface, are remarkable. No other condition in medicine allows foreign tissue to be so readily accepted and tolerated. Although we have gained tremendous insight into how the maternal-fetal interface adapts to the challenge of maintaining the pregnancy and protecting the fetus from immunologic attack, mechanisms that control this aspect of pregnancy are only partially understood. As we gain more knowledge of how pregnancy is maintained in the context of an otherwise normally functioning immune system, we hope to also gain insight into the development and treatment of common complications of pregnancy such as preeclampsia and preterm labor.

KEY POINTS

- The innate immune system employs fast, nonspecific methods of pathogen detection to prevent and control an initial infection. Innate immunity consists of immune cells such as macrophages, dendritic cells, natural killer (NK) cells, eosinophils, and basophils.
- The adaptive immune system targets specific components of a pathogen and is capable of eradicating an infection that has overwhelmed the innate immune system by clonal expansion of lymphocytes (T cells and B cells) and antibodies against a specific antigen.
- The fetal immune system, even very early in gestation, has innate immune capacity. Acquired immunity, particularly the capacity to produce antibodies, develops more slowly and is not completely functional until well after birth.
- Fetal blood contains a high frequency of hematopoietic stem cells, making it an ideal source of cells for hematopoietic stem cell transplantation. The estimated need for use of privately banked cord blood is between 1/1000 and 1/200,000, which is cost-effective only for children with a very high likelihood of needing a transplant.
- HLA-G, through interactions with u-NK cells, likely contributes to maintaining immune tolerance at the maternal-fetal interface and normal pregnancy.
- Several mechanisms exist to suppress maternal T cell responses, including the generation of paternal-specific T-regulatory cells, tryptophan depletion by IDO production, and interactions with FasL and TRAIL.
- Serum complement levels are unchanged or elevated during normal pregnancy but are balanced by trophoblast expression of several negative regulators of complement.
- The proinflammatory cytokine response to an intrauterine infection is thought to drive preterm labor in most cases of early preterm births. Fetal systemic inflammation with elevated plasma IL-6 is a significant predictor of preterm labor and neonatal morbidity with multiorgan involvement.
- The clinically evident phase of preeclampsia is characterized by widespread inflammation and endothelial dysfunction. Specific maternal-fetal combinations of KIR and HLA-C genotypes are strongly associated with preeclampsia. Regulatory T cells are decreased in number and function in preeclampsia compared with normal pregnancy.
- There is no clear relationship between HLA matching and fetal loss from more than 30 retrospective studies.
- In nearly every pregnancy, cells that originate from the fetus can be found in the mother, and conversely, cells that originate from the mother can be found in the fetus. The long-term persistence of fetal cells in the mother and maternal cells in her progeny leads to the coexistence of at least two cell populations in a single person and is referred to as microchimerism.
- It is likely that microchimerism can have an adverse, neutral, or beneficial effect on the host, depending on several factors, with HLA genes and the HLA-relationship among cells probably of key importance.

REFERENCES

1. Medawar PB: Some immunological and endocrinological problems raised by the evolution of viviparity in vertebrates. Symp Soc Exp Biol 7:320, 1954.
2. Romero R, Manogue KR, Mitchell MD, et al: Infection and labor. IV. Cachectin-tumor necrosis factor in the amniotic fluid of women with intraamniotic infection and preterm labor. Am J Obstet Gynecol 161:336, 1989.
3. Romero R, Brody DT, Oyarzun E, et al: Infection and labor. III. Interleukin-1: a signal for the onset of parturition. Am J Obstet Gynecol 160:1117, 1989.
4. Hitti J, Hillier SL, Agnew KJ, et al: Vaginal indicators of amniotic fluid infection in preterm labor. Obstet Gynecol 97:211, 2001.
5. Kawai T, Akira S: The role of pattern-recognition receptors in innate immunity: update on toll-like receptors. Nat Immunol 11:373, 2010.
6. Quayle AJ: The innate and early immune response to pathogen challenge in the female genital tract and the pivotal role of epithelial cells. J Reprod Immunol 57:61, 2002.
7. Abrahams VM, Bole-Aldo P, Kim YM, et al: Divergent trophoblast responses to bacterial products mediated by TLRs. J Immunol 173:4286, 2004.
8. Kim YM, Romero R, Chaiworapongsa T, et al: Toll-like receptor-2 and -4 in the chorioamniotic membranes in spontaneous labor at term and in preterm parturition that are associated with chorioamnionitis. Am J Obstet Gynecol 191:1346, 2004.
9. Elovitz MA, Wang Z, Chien EK, et al: A new model for inflammation-induced preterm birth: the role of platelet-activating factor and Toll-like receptor-4. Am J Pathol 163:2103, 2003.
10. Adams Waldorf KM, Persing D, Novy MJ, et al: Pretreatment with toll-like receptor 4 antagonist inhibits lipopolysaccharide-induced preterm uterine contractility, cytokines, and prostaglandins in rhesus monkeys. Reprod Sci 15:121, 2008.
11. Harju K, Ojaniemi M, Rounioja S, et al: Expression of toll-like receptor 4 and endotoxin responsiveness in mice during perinatal period. Pediatr Res 57:644, 2005.
12. Walport MJ: Complement: second of two parts. N Engl J Med 344:1140, 2001.
13. Vanderpuye OA, Labarrere CA, McIntyre JA: Expression of CD59, a human complement system regulatory protein, in extraembryonic membranes. Int Arch Allergy Immunol 101:376, 1993.
14. Cunningham DS, Tichenor JR Jr: Decay-accelerating factor protects human trophoblast from complement-mediated attack. Clin Immunol Immunopathol 74:156, 1995.
15. Kobasa D, Jones SM, Shinya K, et al: Aberrant innate immune response in lethal infection of macaques with the 1918 influenza virus. Nature 445:319, 2007.
16. Romero R, Gomez R, Ghezzi F, et al: A fetal systemic inflammatory response is followed by the spontaneous onset of preterm parturition. Am J Obstet Gynecol 179:186, 1998.
17. Sadowsky DW, Adams KM, Gravett MG, et al: Preterm labor is induced by intraamniotic infusions of interleukin-1beta and tumor necrosis factor-alpha but not by interleukin-6 or interleukin-8 in a nonhuman primate model. Am J Obstet Gynecol 195:1578, 2006.
18. Sadowsky DW, Novy MJ, Witkin SS, Gravett MG: Dexamethasone or interleukin-10 blocks interleukin-1beta-induced uterine contractions in pregnant rhesus monkeys. Am J Obstet Gynecol 188:252, 2003.
19. Romero R, Ceska M, Avila C, et al: Neutrophil attractant/activating peptide-1/interleukin-8 in term and preterm parturition. Am J Obstet Gynecol 165:813, 1991.
20. Loudon JA, Sooranna SR, Bennett PR, Johnson MR: Mechanical stretch of human uterine smooth muscle cells increases IL-8 mRNA expression and peptide synthesis. Mol Hum Reprod 10:895, 2004.
21. Su B, Sun G, Lu D, et al: Distribution of three HIV-1 resistance-conferring polymorphisms (SDF1-3'A, CCR2-641, and CCR5-delta32) in global populations. Eur J Hum Genet 8:975, 2000.
22. Cauci S, Driussi S, Guaschino S, et al: Correlation of local interleukin-1 beta levels with specific IgA response against *Gardnerella vaginalis* cytolysin in women with bacterial vaginosis. Am J Reprod Immunol 47:257, 2002.
23. Brandtzaeg P: Mucosal immunity: integration between mother and the breast-fed infant. Vaccine 21:3382, 2003.
24. Veldhoen M: The role of T helper subsets in autoimmunity and allergy. Curr Opin Immunol 21:606, 2009.
25. Miyairi I, Ramsey KH, Patton DL: Duration of untreated chlamydial genital infection and factors associated with clearance: review of animal studies. J Infect Dis 201:S96, 2010.
26. Wegmann TG, Lin H, Guilbert L, Mosmann TR: Bidirectional cytokine interactions in the maternal-fetal relationship: is successful pregnancy a TH2 phenomenon? Immunol Today 14:353, 1993.
27. Raghupathy R: Th1-type immunity is incompatible with successful pregnancy. Immunol Today 18:478, 1997.
28. Raghupathy R: Pregnancy: success and failure within the Th1/Th2/Th3 paradigm. Semin Immunol 13:219, 2001.
29. Chaouat G, Assal Meliani A, Martal J, et al: IL-10 prevents naturally occurring fetal loss in the CBA x DBA/2 mating combination, and local defect in IL-10 production in this abortion-prone combination is corrected by in vivo injection of IFN-tau. J Immunol 154:4261, 1995.
30. Makhseed M, Raghupathy R, Azizieh F, et al: Th1 and Th2 cytokine profiles in recurrent aborters with successful pregnancy and with subsequent abortions. Hum Reprod 16:2219, 2001.
31. Westgren M, Shields LE: In utero stem cell transplantation in humans. Ernst Schering Res Found Workshop 33:197, 2001.
32. Shields LE, Lindton B, Andrews RG, Westgren M: Fetal hematopoietic stem cell transplantation: a challenge for the twenty-first century. J Hematother Stem Cell Res 11:617, 2002.
33. Hermann E, Truyens C, Alonso-Vega C, et al: Human fetuses are able to mount an adultlike CD8 T-cell response. Blood 100:2153, 2002.
34. Lindton B, Markling L, Ringden O, et al: Mixed lymphocyte culture of human fetal liver cells. Fetal Diagn Ther 15:71, 2000.
35. Gathings WE, Lawton AR, Cooper MD: Immunofluorescent studies of the development of pre-B cells, B lymphocytes and immunoglobulin isotype diversity in humans. Eur J Immunol 7:804, 1977.
36. Fischer A: Severe combined immunodeficiencies (SCID). Clin Exp Immunol 122:143, 2000.
37. Gulino AV, Notarangelo LD: Hyper IgM syndromes. Curr Opin Rheumatol 15:422, 2003.
38. Gluckman E, Broxmeyer HA, Auerbach AD, et al: Hematopoietic reconstitution in a patient with Fanconi's anemia by means of umbilical-cord blood from an HLA-identical sibling. N Engl J Med 321:1174, 1989.
39. Lubin BH, Shearer WT: Cord blood banking for potential future transplantation. Pediatrics 119:165, 2007.
40. Delaney M, Ballen KK: The role of HLA in umbilical cord blood transplantation. Best Pract Res Clin Haematol 23:179, 2010.
41. Kaimal AJ, Smith CC, Laros RK, et al: Cost-effectiveness of private umbilical cord blood banking. Obstet Gynecol 114:848, 2009.
42. Taglauer ES, Adams Waldorf KM, Petroff MG: The hidden maternal-fetal interface: events involving the lymphoid organs in maternal-fetal tolerance. Int J Dev Biol 54:421, 2010.
43. Van Rood JJ, Eernisse JG, Van Leeuwen A: Leucocyte antibodies in sera from pregnant women. Nature 181:1735, 1958.
44. Regan L, Braude PR, Hill DP: A prospective study of the incidence, time of appearance and significance of anti-paternal lymphocytotoxic antibodies in human pregnancy. Hum Reprod 6:294, 1991.
45. Tafuri A, Alferink J, Moller P, et al: T cell awareness of paternal alloantigens during pregnancy. Science 270:630, 1995.
46. Jiang SP, Vacchio MS: Multiple mechanisms of peripheral T cell tolerance to the fetal "allograft." J Immunol 160:3086, 1998.
47. Rouas-Freiss N, Goncalves RM, Menier C, et al: Direct evidence to support the role of HLA-G in protecting the fetus from maternal uterine natural killer cytolysis. Proc Natl Acad Sci U S A 94:11520, 1997.
48. Hackmon R, Hallak M, Krup M, et al: HLA-G antigen and parturition: maternal serum, fetal serum and amniotic fluid levels during pregnancy. Fetal Diagn Ther 19:404, 2004.
49. Ober C, Aldrich C, Rosinsky B, et al: HLA-G1 protein expression is not essential for fetal survival. Placenta 19:127, 1998.
50. Robertson SA, Guerin LR, Bromfield JJ, et al: Seminal fluid drives expansion of the CD4+CD25+ T regulatory cell pool and induces tolerance to paternal alloantigens in mice. Biol Reprod 80:1036, 2009.
51. Somerset DA, Zheng Y, Kilby MD, et al: Normal human pregnancy is associated with an elevation in the immune suppressive CD25+ CD4+ regulatory T-cell subset. Immunology 112:38, 2004.

52. Polanczyk MJ, Carson BD, Subramanian S, et al: Cutting edge: estrogen drives expansion of the CD4+CD25+ regulatory T cell compartment. J Immunol 2004;173:2227.
53. Zenclussen AC, Gerlof K, Zenclussen ML, et al: Abnormal T-cell reactivity against paternal antigens in spontaneous abortion: adoptive transfer of pregnancy-induced CD4+CD25+ T regulatory cells prevents fetal rejection in a murine abortion model. Am J Pathol 166:811, 2005.
54. Mellor AL, Sivakumar J, Chandler P, et al: Prevention of T cell-driven complement activation and inflammation by tryptophan catabolism during pregnancy. Nat Immunol 2:64, 2001.
55. Mellor AL, Munn DH: Tryptophan catabolism and T-cell tolerance: immunosuppression by starvation? Immunol Today 20:469, 1999.
56. Fallarino F, Grohmann U, Hwang KW, et al: Modulation of tryptophan catabolism by regulatory T cells. Nat Immunol 4:1206, 2003.
57. Hunt JS, Vassmer D, Ferguson TA, Miller L: Fas ligand is positioned in mouse uterus and placenta to prevent trafficking of activated leukocytes between the mother and the conceptus. J Immunol 158:4122, 1997.
58. Phillips TA, Ni J, Pan G, et al: TRAIL (Apo-2L) and TRAIL receptors in human placentas: implications for immune privilege. J Immunol 162:6053, 1999.
59. Adams KM, Yan Z, Stevens AM, Nelson JL: The changing maternal "self" hypothesis: a mechanism for maternal tolerance of the fetus. Placenta 28:378, 2007.
60. Kovar IZ, Riches PG: C3 and C4 complement components and acute phase proteins in late pregnancy and parturition. J Clin Pathol 41:650, 1988.
61. Johnson U, Gustavii B: Complement components in normal pregnancy. Acta Pathol Microbiol Immunol Scand [C] 95:97, 1987.
62. Thurman JM, Kraus DM, Girardi G, et al: A novel inhibitor of the alternative complement pathway prevents antiphospholipid antibody-induced pregnancy loss in mice. Mol Immunol 42:87, 2005.
63. Mao D, Wu X, Deppong C, et al: Negligible role of antibodies and C5 in pregnancy loss associated exclusively with C3-dependent mechanisms through complement alternative pathway. Immunity 19:813, 2003.
64. Holmes CH, Simpson KL, Okada H, et al: Complement regulatory proteins at the feto-maternal interface during human placental development: distribution of CD59 by comparison with membrane cofactor protein (CD46) and decay accelerating factor (CD55). Eur J Immunol 22:1579, 1992.
65. Xu C, Mao D, Holers VM, et al: A critical role for murine complement regulator crry in fetomaternal tolerance. Science 287:498, 2000.
66. Hunt JS, Petroff MG, Burnett TG: Uterine leukocytes: key players in pregnancy. Semin Cell Dev Biol 11:127, 2000.
67. Fallon PG, Jolin HE, Smith P, et al: IL-4 induces characteristic Th2 responses even in the combined absence of IL-5, IL-9, and IL-13. Immunity 17:7, 2002.
68. Croy BA, He H, Esadeg S, et al: Uterine natural killer cells: insights into their cellular and molecular biology from mouse modelling. Reproduction 126:149, 2003.
69. Chaouat G, Ledee-Bataille N, Dubanchet S, et al: TH1/TH2 paradigm in pregnancy: paradigm lost? Cytokines in pregnancy/early abortion: reexamining the TH1/TH2 paradigm. Int Arch Allergy Immunol 134:93, 2004.
70. Preterm Birth: Causes, Consequences, and Prevention. Washington, DC, National Academies Press, 2006.
71. Goldenberg RL, Hauth JC, Andrews WW: Intrauterine infection and preterm delivery. N Engl J Med 342:1500, 2000.
72. Gravett MG, Rubens CE, Nunes TM: Global report on preterm birth and stillbirth (2 of 7): discovery science. BMC Pregn Childbirth 10:S2, 2010.
73. Gravett MG, Adams KM, Sadowsky DW, et al: Immunomodulators plus antibiotics delay preterm delivery after experimental intraamniotic infection in a nonhuman primate model. Am J Obstet Gynecol 197:518.e1, 2007.
74. Gotsch F, Romero R, Kusanovic JP, et al: The fetal inflammatory response syndrome. Clin Obstet Gynecol 50:652, 2007.
75. Dekker G: The partner's role in the etiology of preeclampsia. J Reprod Immunol 57:203, 2002.
76. Feeney JG, Tovey LA, Scott JS: Influence of previous blood-transfusion on incidence of pre-eclampsia. Lancet 1:874, 1977.
77. Hiby SE, Walker JJ, O'Shaughnessy KM, et al: Combinations of maternal KIR and fetal HLA-C genes influence the risk of pre-eclampsia and reproductive success. J Exp Med 200:957, 2004.
78. Tilburgs T, Scherjon SA, van der Mast BJ, et al: Fetal-maternal HLA-C mismatch is associated with decidual T cell activation and induction of functional T regulatory cells. J Reprod Immunol 82:148, 2009.
79. Redman CW, Sacks GP, Sargent IL: Preeclampsia: an excessive maternal inflammatory response to pregnancy. Am J Obstet Gynecol 180:499, 1999.
80. Santner-Nanan B, Peek MJ, Khanam R, et al: Systemic increase in the ratio between Foxp3+ and IL-17-producing CD4+ T cells in healthy pregnancy but not in preeclampsia. J Immunol 183:7023, 2009.
81. Zhou CC, Zhang Y, Irani RA, et al: Angiotensin receptor agonistic autoantibodies induce pre-eclampsia in pregnant mice. Nat Med 14:855, 2008.
82. Billington WD: Influence of immunological dissimilarity of mother and foetus on size of placenta in mice. Nature 202:317, 1964.
83. Kirby DR: The egg and immunology. Proc R Soc Med 63:59, 1970.
84. Komlos L, Zamir R, Joshua H, et al: antigens in couples with repeated abortions. Clin Immunol Immunopathol 7:330, 1977.
85. Schacter B, Muir A, Gyves M, Tasin M: HLA-A,B compatibility in parents of offspring with neural-tube defects or couples experiencing involuntary fetal wastage. Lancet 1:796, 1979.
86. Ober C, Rosinsky B, Grimsley C, et al: Population genetic studies of HLA-G: allele frequencies and linkage disequilibrium with HLA-A1. J Reprod Immunol 32:111, 1996.
87. Ober C, Elias S, O'Brien E, et al: HLA sharing and fertility in Hutterite couples: evidence for prenatal selection against compatible fetuses. Am J Reprod Immunol Microbiol 18:111, 1988.
88. Ober CL, Hauck WW, Kostyu DD, et al: Adverse effects of human leukocyte antigen-DR sharing on fertility: a cohort study in a human isolate. Fertil Steril 44:227, 1985.
89. Coulam CB: Immunotherapy with intravenous immunoglobulin for treatment of recurrent pregnancy loss: American experience. Am J Reprod Immunol 32:286, 1994.
90. Daya S, Gunby J: The effectiveness of allogeneic leukocyte immunization in unexplained primary recurrent spontaneous abortion. Recurrent Miscarriage Immunotherapy Trialists Group. Am J Reprod Immunol 32:294, 1994.
91. Gammill HS, Nelson JL: Naturally acquired microchimerism. Int J Dev Biol 54:531, 2010.
92. Adams Waldorf KM, Gammill HS, et al: Dynamic changes in fetal microchimerism in maternal peripheral blood mononuclear cells, CD4+ and CD8+ cells in normal pregnancy. Placenta 31:589, 2010.
93. Lo YMD, Rossa WKC: Prenatal diagnosis: progress through plasma nucleic acids. Nat Rev Genet 8:71, 2007.
94. Fujiki Y, Johnson KL, Peter I, et al: Fetal cells in the pregnant mouse are diverse and express a variety of progenitor and differentiated cell markers. Biol Reprod 81:26, 2009.
95. Mold JE, Michaelsson J, Burt TD, et al: Maternal alloantigens promote the development of tolerogenic fetal regulatory T cells in utero. Science 322:1562, 2008.
96. Nelson JL: Maternal-fetal immunology and autoimmune disease: is some autoimmune disease auto-alloimmune or allo-autoimmune? Arthritis Rheum 39:191, 1996.
97. Adams KM, Nelson JL: Microchimerism: an investigative frontier in autoimmunity and transplantation. JAMA 291:1127, 2004.
98. Nelson JL: Your cells are my cells. Sci Am 298:64, 2008.
99. Gadi VK, Malone KE, Guthrie KA, et al: Case-control study of fetal microchimerism and breast cancer. PLoS One 3:e1706, 2008.
100. Gammill HS, Guthrie KA, Aydelotte TM, et al: Effect of parity on fetal and maternal microchimerism: interaction of grafts within a host? Blood 116:2706, 2010.

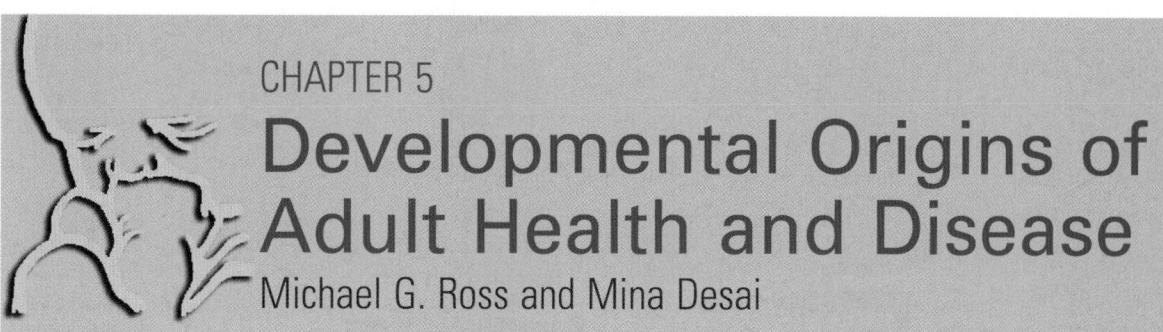

CHAPTER 5

Developmental Origins of Adult Health and Disease

Michael G. Ross and Mina Desai

KEY ABBREVIATIONS

11-β-hydroxysteroid Dehydrogenase Type 2	11β-HSD2
C-reactive Protein	CRP
Diethylstilbestrol	DES
Hypothalamic Pituitary Adrenal	HPA
Large for Gestational Age	LGA
Low Birth Weight	LBW
Neuropeptide-Y	NPY
Nonalcoholic Fatty Liver Disease	NAFLD
Pancreatic Duodenal Homeobox-1	Pdx-1
Peroxisome-proliferator-activated Receptor	PPAR
Polycystic Ovary Syndrome	PCOS
Small for Gestational Age	SGA

Perinatal care has progressed remarkably from an original focus on maternal mortality, which approximated 1% per pregnancy in the early 1900s. Following the tremendous strides in reducing maternal morbidity and mortality rates, obstetrical care has made great advances in regard to optimization of fetal and neonatal health, including the diagnosis, prevention, and treatment of congenital malformations, reduction in infectious disease, and improvements in sequelae of prematurity. It is now commonplace to deliver infants who would not have survived childbirth or the neonatal period in previous eras. For example, low-birth-weight (LBW) premature infants routinely survive beyond 400 to 500 g. Conversely, large-for-gestational-age (LGA) infants are often delivered by cesarean section, avoiding potential trauma of labor. As we now examine the long-term consequences associated with this improved survival, as well as effects of treatment aimed at improving outcomes (e.g., maternal glucocorticoids), we have begun to recognize long-term health effects in the adult. An understanding of the developmental origins of adult health and disease provides an appreciation of the critical role of perinatal care and may ultimately guide our treatment paradigms.

The concept of developmental origins of adult disease should not be surprising to obstetricians. Teratogenesis represents perhaps the most acute consequence of developmental effects. In the late 1950s, thalidomide was marketed as both a sedative and a morning sickness prescription for pregnant women. Although the drug was not actively marketed in the United States (due to lack of Food and Drug Administration [FDA] approval), more than 2.5 million tablets were distributed to private physicians in the United States. Thalidomide was widely used in Europe, and was included in some 50 over-the-counter products for a diversity of indications. Thalidomide-induced limb malformations are now well recognized. Notably, similar to mechanisms of developmental programming discussed later in this chapter, thalidomide may induce its teratogenic effects through epigenetic mechanisms. As described by Stephens and colleagues,[1] thalidomide likely binds to promotor sites of insulin-like growth factor and fibroblast growth factor, as well as downstream signaling genes that regulate angiogenesis. The resulting inhibition of angiogenesis truncates limb development. A diversity of mechanisms may "program" the offspring phenotype via aberrations in cellular signaling or epigenetic function.

Whereas the short-term consequences of thalidomide were rapidly recognized, longer-term programming effects of diethylstilbestrol (DES) were slow to be recognized. Before FDA approval in 1947, DES was used off-label to prevent adverse pregnancy outcomes in women with a history of miscarriage. Despite a double-blind trial in the early 1950s demonstrating no benefit of taking DES during pregnancy,[2] DES continued to be given to pregnant women throughout the 1960s. It was not until 1971, in response to a report demonstrating the link between DES and vaginal clear cell adenocarcinoma in girls and young women, that the FDA advised against the use of DES in pregnant women. Similar to thalidomide, it is now recognized that the oncogenic and teratogenic effects of in utero DES exposure may be mediated via epigenetic mechanisms. As reported by Bromer and colleagues,[3] in utero

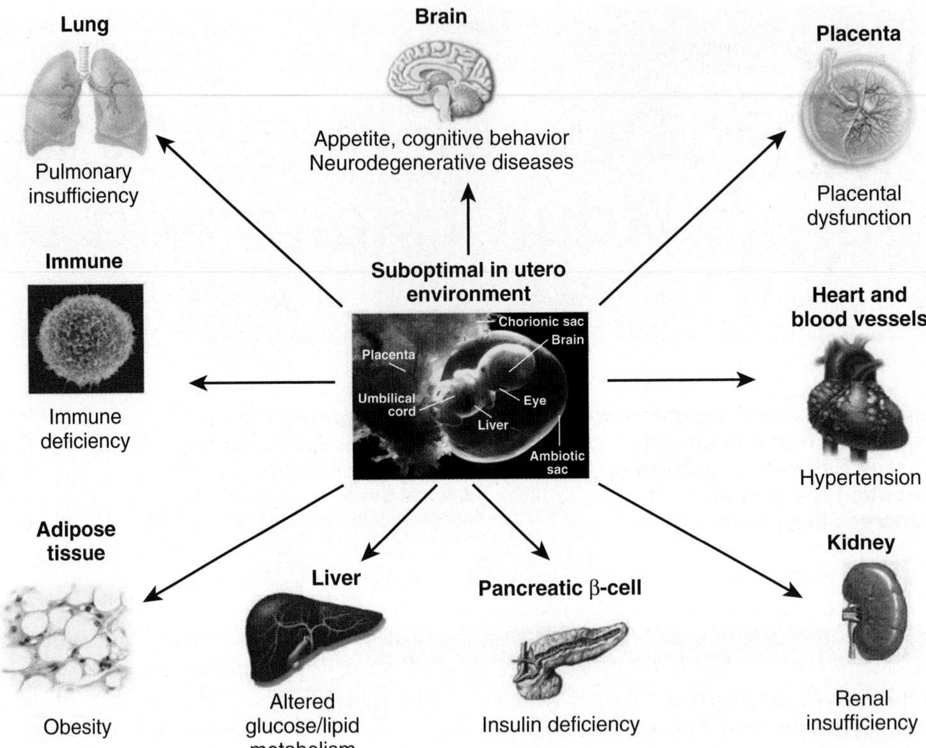

Figure 5-1. Impact of gestational programming on organ systems.

DES exposure results in hypermethylation of the HOXA10 gene, which regulates uterine organogenesis. Thus, both the short-term anatomic defects associated with thalidomide and the delayed oncogenic effects associated with DES are examples of developmental origins of adult disease mediated via epigenetic effects.

EPIGENETICS AND PROGRAMMING

The essential concept of "gestational programming" signifies that the nutritional, hormonal, and metabolic environment provided by the mother permanently alters organ structure, cellular responses, and gene expression that ultimately affect metabolism and physiology of her offspring (Figure 5-1). Further, these effects vary depending on the developmental period, and as such, rapidly growing fetuses and neonates are more vulnerable. The programming events may have immediate effects, for example, impairment of organ growth at a critical stage, whereas other programming effects are deferred until expressed by altered organ function at a later age. In this instance, the question is how the memory of early events is stored and later expressed, despite continuous cellular replication and replacement. This may be mediated through epigenetic control of gene expression, which involves modification of the genome without altering the deoxyribonucleic acid (DNA) sequence itself.

Epigenetic phenomena are a fundamental feature of mammalian development that cause heritable and persistent changes in gene expression without altering DNA sequence. Epigenetic regulation includes changes in the DNA methylation pattern and/or modifications of chromatin packaging via posttranslational histone changes.

DNA methylation represents a primary epigenetic mechanism. The DNA of the early embryo is hypomethylated, and with progressive increases in DNA methylation in response to environmental signals, organogenesis and tissue differentiation occur. DNA methylation typically occurs on cytosine bases that are followed by a guanine, termed *CpG dinucleotides*. The methylation by a DNA methyl-transferase leads to recruitment of methyl-CpG binding proteins, which induce transcriptional silencing both by blocking transcription factor binding and by recruiting transcriptional corepressors or histone-modifying complexes. Anomalous DNA methylation in normally hypomethylated CpG-rich regions of gene promoters is associated with inappropriate gene silencing (e.g., cancer). It is during embryogenesis and early postnatal life that DNA methylation patterns are fundamentally established, and are imperative for silencing of specific gene regions, such as imprinted genes and repetitive nucleic acid sequences. The epigenome is reestablished at specific stages of development and is largely maintained throughout life, making it a prime candidate as the basis for fetal programming. As such, changes in epigenetic marks are associated with multiple human diseases, including many cancers, neurologic disorders, and even inflammation. As methylation involves the supply and enzymatic transfer of methyl groups, it is plausible that in utero nutritional, hormonal, or other metabolic cues alter the timing and direction of methylation patterns during fetal development (Figure 5-2).

Another essential mechanism of gene expression and silencing is the packaging of chromatin into open (euchromatic) or closed (heterochromatic) states, respectively. Chromatin consists of DNA packaged around histones into

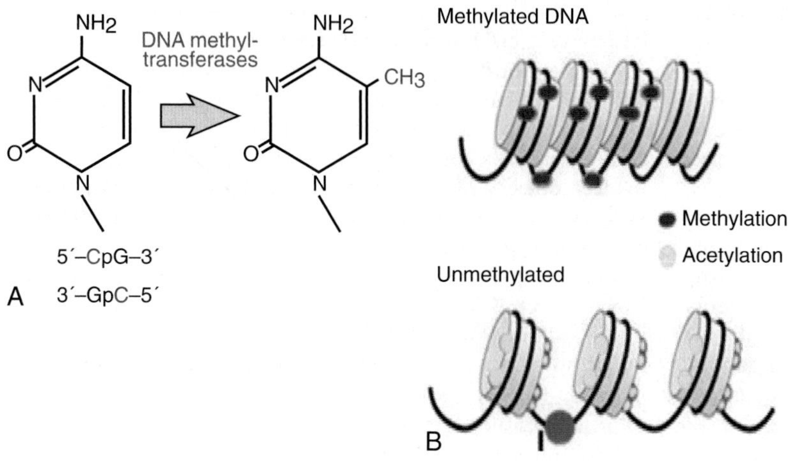

Figure 5-2. DNA methylation. **A,** Methylation by DNA methyltransferases at CpG islands. **B,** DNA demethylation relaxes chromatin structure allowing histone acetylation and the binding of transcriptional complexes.

a nucleo-protein complex. Posttranslational modification of histone tails through acetylation, methylation, phosphorylation, ubiquitination, and sumoylation can alter histone interaction with DNA and recruit proteins (e.g., transcriptional factors) that alter chromatin conformation. Histone tail acetylation by histone acetyl-transferases promotes active gene expression, whereas histone tail deacetylation by histone deacetylases (HDACs) is associated with gene silencing (Figure 5-3). Histone modifications and DNA methylation patterns are not exclusively independent, and thus can reciprocally regulate one another's state.

Finally, microRNAs are emerging as a potential third epigenetic mediator. Although these noncoding RNAs are usually associated with regulation of gene expression at the translational level, recent work suggests they may be involved in DNA methylation as well, thereby further regulating transcription of their targets.

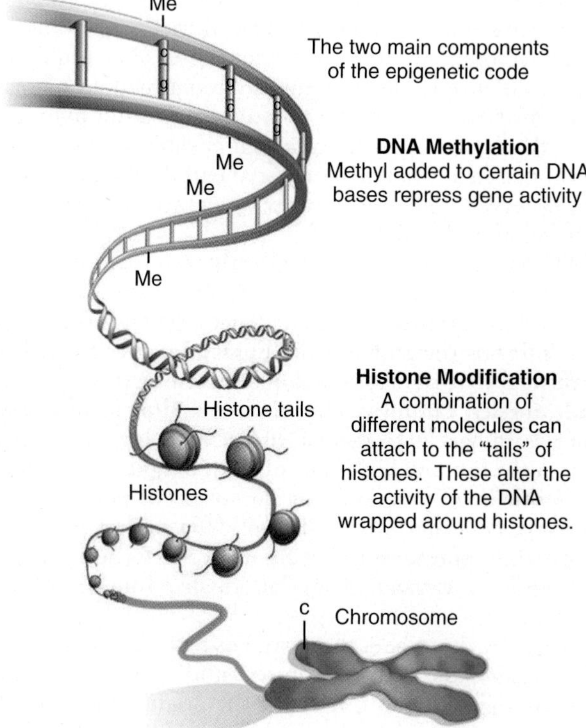

Figure 5-3. DNA methylation and histone modification.

FETAL NUTRITION AND GROWTH

Unquestionably, nutrition is one of the cornerstones of health. More important, there is good evidence that appropriate nutritional supplementation before conception and during pregnancy may reduce the risk of some birth defects. **Perhaps the most convincing argument that can be made for the need to consider maternal nutrition as a critical modulator of embryonic development is the observation that maternal iodine supplementation has eradicated the occurrence of iodine-deficiency-induced cretinism (iodine-deficiency-associated developmental defects).** In addition, adverse maternal nutrition that has an immediate and visible impact on the outcome of pregnancy is seen in the case of folate deficiency and spina bifida. The functional mechanism for folate likely involves epigenetic effects because it generates the principal methyl donor (s-adenosyl methionine) that participates in methylation of DNA and histones.

Animal studies too have irrevocably shown the importance of a mother's diet in shaping the epigenome of her offspring. A classic example is that of permanent hypomethylation of certain regions of the genome as a result of deficient folate or choline (methyl donors) during late fetal or early postnatal life. Specifically, in mice, when the agouti gene is completely unmethylated, the mouse has a yellow coat color, is obese, and is prone to diabetes and cancer. When the agouti gene is methylated (as it is in normal mice), the coat color is brown and the mouse has a low disease risk. Although both the fat yellow and skinny brown mice are genetically identical, the former exhibits an epigenetic "mutation."[4]

Although teratogenesis, structural malformations, and even oncogenic risks can be linked to developmental insults, it is only recently that the epidemic of metabolic syndrome has been attributed, in part, to consequences of fetal and newborn development. **Obesity now represents**

a major public health problem and health epidemic. As recently reported, the adverse consequences of obesity are projected to overwhelm the beneficial effects of reduced smoking in the United States,[5] and have resulted in an actual decline in life expectancy. In the United States, 66% of adults are overweight (body mass index [BMI] 25 to less than 30 kg/m^2) and 33% are obese (BMI ≥30 kg/m^2). Of concern to obstetricians, there is a marked and continuing increase in the prevalence of obesity among pregnant women, a factor associated with both high-birth-weight newborns and a known risk factor for childhood obesity. Whereas the epidemic of obesity in the United States was originally attributed to changes in the work environment, a surplus of high calories, inexpensive food, and a lack of childhood exercise, it is now recognized that the risks of obesity in metabolic syndrome can be markedly influenced by early life events, particularly prenatal and neonatal growth and environmental exposures. Barker and Hales in the early 1990s brought attention to this field with epidemiologic studies demonstrating that nutritional insufficiency during embryonic and fetal development resulted in latent disease in adulthood. A series of studies have demonstrated a marked increase in deaths from coronary heart disease and adult hypertension in association with small-for-gestational-age (SGA) newborns. In addition to coronary heart disease, investigators observed impaired glucose tolerance or diabetes in association with LBW.

Whereas the incidence of growth restriction continues to rise in the United States, there has been an approximately 25% increase in the incidence of high-birth-weight babies during the past decade. **Epidemiologic studies have confirmed that the relationship between birth weight and adult obesity, cardiovascular disease, and/or insulin resistance is in fact a U-shaped curve, with increasing risks at both the low and high ends of birth weight.** Importantly, the sequelae of programming do not occur as a threshold response associated with either very low or very high birth weight, but represents a continuum of risk for adult disease in relation to variance from "an idealized newborn birth weight."

As will be described, these studies have spawned a burst of epidemiologic and mechanistic studies of the developmental origins of adult diseases; the original focus on cardiovascular disease and metabolic syndrome has been extended to a diversity of adult diseases including those affecting kidneys, lung, immunity, learning ability, mental health, aging, cancer, and others. **Thus, the field of developmental origins of adult disease has progressed from short-term toxic or teratogenic effects to long-term adult sequelae of LBW or high birth weight.** In addition to these influences, additional factors, including maternal stress, preterm delivery, and maternal glucocorticoid therapy, among others, may significantly affect adult health and disease. This chapter reviews the consequences and mechanisms of these prenatal/neonatal influences on developmental programming. We will primarily focus on the associations demonstrated in human studies, using evidence from case reports, epidemiologic studies, and meta-analyses. We selectively discuss evidence from animal models that confirms the phenotype or suggest pathogenic pathways and potential mechanisms.

ENERGY BALANCE PROGRAMMING

As noted, epidemiologic studies demonstrate that metabolic syndrome, a cluster of conditions including obesity, hypertension, dyslipidemia, and impaired glucose tolerance, may be a result in part of the effects of LBW. **Ultimately, obesity results from an imbalance in energy intake and expenditure, as regulated by appetite, metabolism, adipogenic propensity, and energy utilization. Hales and Barker proposed the "thrifty phenotype hypothesis"[6] in 1992.** These authors suggested that in response to an impaired nutrient supply in utero, the growing fetus adapts in utero to maximize metabolic efficiency, which will increase survival likelihood in the postnatal environment. This adaptation would be beneficial in response to environmental cycles of famine/drought in which reduced maternal and fetal nutrient supply would likely be replicated in the subsequent extrauterine environment. Numerous studies have demonstrated the increased risk of obesity associated with LBW. In addition to obesity, LBW appears to predispose to excess central adiposity, a phenotype specifically associated with the risk for cardiovascular disease.

Although the long-term effects of LBW are linked to adult obesity, several studies have demonstrated important effects of newborn or childhood catch-up growth among the LBW infants. Those infants that are born small, and yet remain small (in comparison to peers), exhibit a lower risk of obesity and metabolic syndrome than those born small who catch up and exceed normal weights through infancy or early adolescence. These findings, replicated in animal models, have great significance for neonatal and childhood care. For example, a major goal of treatment for premature, LBW infants is the achievement of a weight satisfactory for discharge. Contrary to current practice, it may be advisable to limit the rapid weight gain in the neonatal period. **Importantly, breastfeeding results in a lower obesity risk compared to formula feeding.**[7] Breastfeeding may have advantages to formula feeding both in nutrient and hormone composition and the natural limitation that avoids excessive feeding.

As discussed, programming effects of birth weight simulate a U-shaped curve, as LGA infants also are at an increased risk of adult cardiovascular disease and diabetes.[8] Understandably, LGA infants are often born to obese women, who frequently express glucose intolerance/insulin resistance and who often consume high-fat Western diets before and throughout pregnancy. Studies demonstrate that each of these risks (obesity, glucose intolerance, high-fat diet) and outcomes (LGA) may individually contribute to programming of adult obesity. When combined with variations in maternal feeding and childhood diets, it is understandable that epidemiologic studies have not yet determined which of these factors is paramount in programming mechanisms. Animal models demonstrate programming effects independently associated with each of these risks.

Animal models of LBW, using a variety of methods, such as maternal nutrient restriction (global or specific), placental uterine ligation, or glucocorticoid exposure, among others, have effectively demonstrated increased adult adiposity. Similar to human studies, the propensity to obesity is particularly evident in LBW newborns exhibiting postnatal catch-up growth.[9] Studies primarily on rodents and sheep have provided important insights into the underlying mechanisms of programmed obesity, which include lasting changes in proportions of fat and lean body mass, central nervous system appetite control, adiposity structure and function, adipokine secretion and regulation, and energy expenditure.

The hypothalamic regulation of **appetite** and satiety function develops in utero in precocial species in order to prepare for newborn life. In the rat and humans, although neurons that regulate appetite and satiety become detectable in the fetal hypothalamus early in gestation, the functional neuronal pathways form during the second week of postnatal life in the rat and likely during the third trimester in humans. Notably, the obesity (ob) gene product **leptin,** which is synthesized primarily by adipose tissue and placenta, is a critical neurotrophic factor during development. In the fetus/newborn, leptin promotes the development of satiety pathways. In contrast, in the adult, leptin acts as a satiety factor. In leptin-deficient (ob/ob) mice, satiety pathways are permanently disrupted, demonstrating axonal densities one-third to one-fourth those of controls.[10] Treatment of *adult* ob/ob mice with leptin does not restore satiety projections, but leptin treatment of *newborn* ob/ob mice does rescue the neuronal development,[10] indicating the critical role of leptin during the perinatal period.

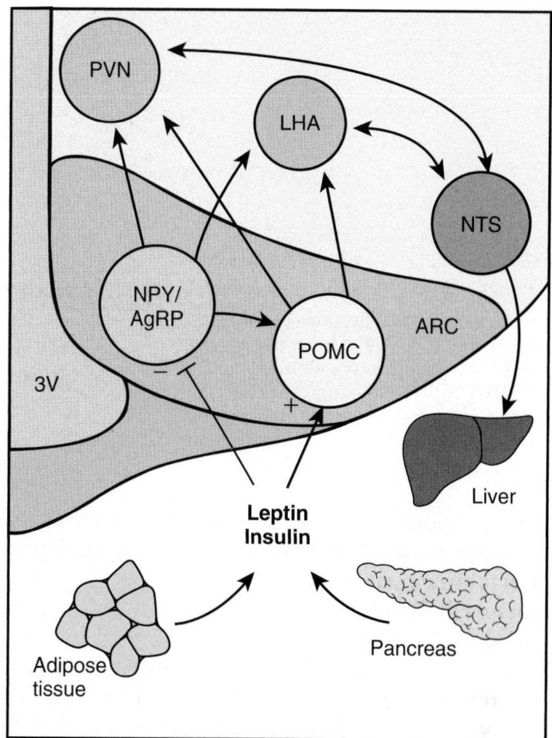

Figure 5-4. Leptin secreted by adipose tissue and insulin by pancreas suppress NPY and increase POMC. *3V,* Third ventricle; *ARC,* arcuate nucleus; *PVN,* paraventricular nucleus; *LHA,* lateral hypothalamic area; nucleus of the solitary tract; orexigenic peptides—*NPY,* neuropeptide Y; *AgRP,* agouti gene-related protein; anorexigenic peptide—*POMC,* pro-opiomelanocortin.

Early life leptin exposure is likely a putative programming mechanism in SGA and LGA human newborns. In LBW human offspring, leptin levels are low at delivery as cord blood levels reflect neonatal fat mass. In contrast to the low serum levels of leptin in SGA newborns, LGA infants have elevated leptin levels. Obese pregnant mothers further have elevated leptin levels related to maternal adiposity, and breast milk leptin levels also reflect maternal fat mass.

Leptin binding to its receptor activates pro-opiomelanocortin neurons and anorexigenic downstream pathways. Obesity is often associated with leptin resistance, resulting in an inability to balance food intake with actual energy needs. The leptin pathway is counterregulated by the orexigenic neuropeptide-Y (NPY) (Figure 5-4). Impaired leptin signaling could result in increased expression of NPY, which would promote increased nutrient intake while decreasing overall physical activity. In LBW newborns, appetite dysregulation has been demonstrated as a key predisposing factor for the obese phenotype.[11] Studies on LBW offspring specifically indicate dysfunction at several aspects of the satiety pathway, as evidenced by reduced satiety and cellular signaling responses to leptin.[12] **Recent studies have demonstrated an up-regulation of the hypothalamic nutrient sensor (SIRT1), a factor that epigenetically regulates gene transcription of factors critical to neural development.** Importantly, neuronal stem cells from rodent SGA fetuses/newborns demonstrate reduced growth and impaired differentiation to neurons and glial cells.[13] **Thus, impaired neuronal development (and ultimately reduced satiety pathways) may be a consequence of a reduction in neural stem cell growth potential and reduced leptin-mediated neurotrophic stimulation during periods of axonal development.**

In addition to appetite/satiety dysfunction, mechanisms regulating adipose tissue development and function (lipogenesis) may be a key factor in the development of programmed obesity. Increase in adipose tissue mass or adipogenesis occurs primarily during the prenatal and postnatal development, though some adipogenesis continues throughout adulthood. The process of adipogenesis requires highly organized and precisely controlled expression of a cascade of transcription factors within the preadipocyte (Figure 5-5). **Of note, LBW offspring show a paradoxical increased expression of principal adipogenic transcription factor (peroxisome-proliferator-activated receptor, [PPARγ]) as a result of upregulated PPARγ co-activators.** As the signaling pathways of adipogenesis and lipogenesis are up-regulated before the development of obesity, they may be among the crucial contributory factors that predispose to programmed obesity. Furthermore, cellular studies indicate that LBW adipocytes at birth have fundamental traits that are identical to those seen with thiazolidine (PPAR agonist) treatment; that is, they are more insulin sensitive and demonstrate increased glucose uptake and thereby facilitate increased lipid storage within the adipocytes. Thus, early activation of PPAR or its downstream targets could promote the storage of lipids, thereby increasing the risk of developing obesity. This concept reverberates with study on maternal exposure to PPAR agonists, which induce fetal mesenchymal stem cells along the adipocyte lineage, and a reduction in the osteogenic potential in these cells, resulting in greater fat mass in adult offspring.[14] The role of stem cell precursor programming in metabolic disease pathways in response to

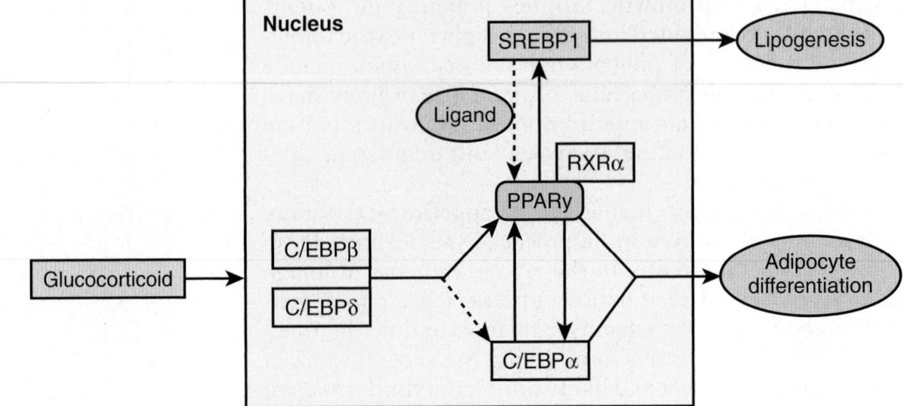

Figure 5-5. Transcriptional regulation of adipogenesis. *C/EBP,* CCAAT/enhancer binding protein; *SREBP,* sterol regulatory element binding proteins; *RXR,* retinoic X receptor; *PPAR,* peroxisome proliferator-activated receptor.

maternal nutrient supply is an intriguing area for understanding developmental plasticity and potential preventive therapeutic strategies.

Akin to LBW, offspring born to obese rat dams fed a high-fat diet also demonstrate increased food intake, adiposity, and circulating leptin levels.[15] The underlying phenotype appears to be similar to that of LBW with altered appetite regulation, enhanced adipogenesis, and reduced energy expenditure. Nonetheless, there are salient mechanistic differences such as increased proliferation of orexigenic neurons in the fetus, inability of elevated leptin to down-regulate NPY, and decreased PPARγ corepressors.

HEPATIC PROGRAMMING

In conjunction with the increased incidence of childhood and adolescent obesity, children and adolescents now have an increased risk of developing nonalcoholic fatty liver disease (NAFLD) and type 2 diabetes. Type 2 diabetes has increased tenfold in regions of the United States during the past decade and the prevalence is particularly high in adolescent North American Indians, approaching rates of 6%. NAFLD (as determined by elevated serum aminotransferase) may occur in up to 10% of obese adolescents in the United States, though studies using ultrasonographic measures of fatty liver have estimated rates of up to 25% to 50% of obese adolescents.[16] As a reflection of the severity of metabolic syndrome, cases of cirrhosis associated with nonalcoholic steatohepatitis in obese children have been described recently. Further evidence suggests that obesity can potentiate additional insults to the liver such as alcohol and hepatitis C infection.

Men and women with reduced abdominal circumference at birth, potentially reflecting reduced hepatic growth during fetal life, have elevated serum cholesterol and plasma fibrinogen. Similarly, poor weight gain in infancy is associated with altered adult liver function, reflected by elevated serum total and low-density lipoprotein cholesterol and increased plasma fibrinogen concentrations.[17] Although human studies have focused on the diagnosis and consequences of NAFLD in obese children and adolescents, animal studies indicate the early expression of fatty liver in fetuses exposed to maternal high-fat diet, though not expressing LGA. Consequently, there may be a heretofore undiagnosed increase in liver adiposity among normal-weight offspring of mothers exposed to Western, high-fat diets.

Animal models of maternal nutrient restriction and excess demonstrate presence of NAFLD, alteration in liver structure, and changes in key metabolic transcription factors and enzymes involved in glucose/lipid homeostasis in the offspring. Specifically, maternal protein restriction during rat pregnancy shifts the enzyme setting of the liver in favor of glucose production rather than utilization, as evident by increased phosphoenolpyruvate carboxykinase and decreased glucokinase enzyme activities in the offspring. Furthermore, these key hepatic enzymes of glucose homeostasis retained the ability to respond to the challenge of a high-fat, high-calorie diet, though with an altered "set point" of regulation. Moreover, as these enzymes are predominantly located in different metabolic zones of the liver (glucokinase in perivenous and phosphoenolpyruvate carboxykinase in periportal zone), the altered activities have been attributed to clonal expansion of periportal and contraction of perivenous cell population.[18]

Five potential mechanisms lead to abnormal hepatic lipid metabolism and NAFLD (Figure 5-6). On a molecular level, PPAR transcription factors are implicated in regulating lipid metabolism. PPARα in particular is predominantly expressed in the liver and regulates genes involved in fatty acid oxidation. Although PPARγ is expressed at very low levels in the liver, PPARγ agonists can ameliorate NAFLD in a rat model.[19] **In addition, PPARα and PPARγ modulate the inflammatory response. PPAR activators have been shown to exert anti-inflammatory activities in various cell types by inhibiting the expression of acute-phase proteins, such as C-reactive protein (CRP).**[20,21] CRP is produced by hepatocytes in response to tissue injury, infection, and inflammation and is moderately elevated in obesity, metabolic syndrome, diabetes, and NAFLD. Rat studies have demonstrated NAFLD and elevated hepatic CRP levels in LBW adult offspring, and this is associated with reduced expression of hepatic PPARγ and PPARα.[22]

PANCREAS PROGRAMMING

Although programmed adult obesity or diet-induced obesity may be attributed to the etiology of insulin resistance, studies in humans and animals indicate that in utero nutrition and environmental exposures directly affect the

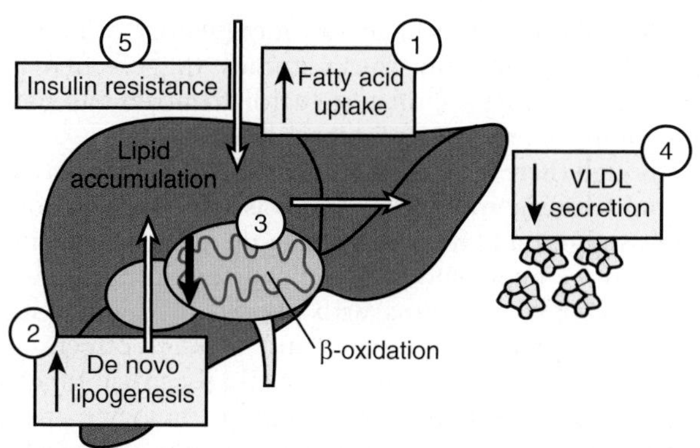

Figure 5-6. Mechanisms for nonalcoholic hepatic steatosis (NAFLD): (1) increased fatty acid uptake by the liver and increased triglyceride synthesis; (2) increased de novo lipogenesis; (3) decreased fatty acid oxidation; (4) decreased VLDL secretion, preventing release of fatty acid from the liver; (5) hepatic insulin resistance (promotes lipogenesis and gluconeogenesis and inhibits lipolysis).

pancreas. **Alterations of pancreatic β-cell mass by maternal malnutrition was demonstrated in the mid-1960s. Whereas LGA human neonates have pancreatic β-cell hyperplasia and increased vascularization, SGA infants have reduced plasma insulin concentrations and pancreatic β-cell numbers.**[23] Consistent with adverse effects of rapid catch-up growth, the greatest insulin resistance is observed in individuals who are LBW but develop adult obesity.[24] In humans, growth in utero is directly associated with fetal insulin levels. **Importantly, beyond the regulation of glucose uptake, insulin has important developmental functions, including skeletal and connective tissues and neural development.**

The extremes of weight are critical, as the risk of insulin resistance in adult life is twofold greater among men who weighed less than 8.2 kg at 1 year of age and those who weighed 12.3 kg or more.[25] There is further a link between reduced early growth and pro-insulin concentrations, suggesting that pancreatic tissue or function may be impaired, and other studies have suggested that fetal programming may alter the structure or function of insulin-sensitive target tissues.

Notably, depending on the prevalence of obesity, approximately 25% of individuals with normal glucose tolerance have similar insulin resistance as those with type 2 diabetes, but compensate for this with enhanced insulin secretion.[26] These individuals are at increased risk of development of overt diabetes. Studies of fetal programming have focused on the finding that birth weight and newborn plasma glucose levels are directly correlated in normal as well as diabetic pregnancies. Far less focus has been paid to levels of amino acids in maternal or fetal blood, although amino acids are major determinants of fetal growth.

In addition to low and high birth weight, studies suggest that antenatal exposure to betamethasone itself may result in insulin resistance in adult offspring. A 30-year follow-up of a double-blind placebo-controlled randomized trial of antenatal betamethasone for the prevention of neonatal respiratory distress syndrome demonstrated no differences among those exposed to betamethasone or placebo in body size, blood lipids, blood pressure, or cardiovascular disease. However, offspring exposed to betamethasone demonstrated higher plasma insulin concentrations at 30 minutes of a 75 g oral glucose tolerance test and lower glucose concentrations at 120 minutes.[27] The authors suggest that antenatal exposure to betamethasone may result in insulin resistance in adult offspring. A study of 20-year-old offspring demonstrated significantly reduced blood pressure in betamethasone-exposed offspring.[28] In view of these findings, the authors recommend that obstetricians use a single course, rather than multiple courses, of antenatal glucocorticoids.

Various animals models of maternal diabetes, nutritional manipulation (undernutrition and overnutrition), and uterine ligation all have reported altered β-cell growth, disturbances in insulin secretion, and long-term effects on insulin sensitivity. Reduced β-cell growth and insulin secretion have been observed in LBW offspring,[29] whereas accelerated β-cell mass and excess insulin secretion were observed in offspring of obese pregnancy.[30] Despite differing nutrition and growth, both lead to β-cell failure, tissue-specific insulin resistance, and development of diabetes in the adult offspring. This phenomenon has been attributed to developmental epigenetic regulation. **The β-cell transcription factor pancreatic duodenal homeobox-1 (Pdx-1) is critical for β-cell development, and progressive silencing of Pdx-1 expression has been observed in β-cells isolated from LBW offspring.** Importantly, this silencing corresponds with persistent altered epigenetic regulation of the Pdx-1 gene. Additionally, increased circulating lipids can induce β-cell apoptosis via endoplasmic reticulum stress pathways. Interestingly, Pdx-1 is protective against pancreatic endoplasmic reticulum stress in response to high-fat feeding in rodents. Although obese pregnancy can increase pancreatic fat deposition in rodent models, whether this in turn leads to permanent changes in gene expression as observed with growth-restricted pregnancies remains unknown.

In a rat model of maternal diabetes, there is evidence of transgeneration diabetogenic effect: female offspring of diabetic mothers develop gestational diabetes and induce the effect in their fetuses and thereby in the next generation. Notably, male offspring have impaired glucose tolerance, but do not transmit the effect to their offspring.[31]

CARDIAC PROGRAMMING

In addition to the aforementioned glucocorticoid effects on insulin resistance, there is evidence that maternal betamethasone treatment of preterm infants is associated with long-term adverse cardiac outcomes, including hypertrophic cardiomyopathy.[32] Animal models confirm the association of fetal cortisol exposure with increased left ventricular cardiomyocyte size. A reduction in cardiomyocyte number through either reduced cellular proliferation or increased apoptosis appears to be a central feature. As cardiomyocytes are highly differentiated and rarely replicate after birth, an inappropriate prenatal reduction of cardiomyocytes is likely to result in a permanent loss of myocardium functioning units and thereby increasing susceptibility to cardiac hypertrophy and ischemic heart disease. Confounding the direct association, left ventricular hypertrophy also has been reported in growth-restricted infants.

Similar to programming of metabolic syndrome, extensive epidemiologic data have demonstrated the association of birth weight with adult coronary heart disease. Slow growth during fetal life and infancy followed by accelerated weight gain in childhood predisposes to adult coronary heart disease in both men and women.[33] The association between LBW and coronary heart disease has been replicated among men and women throughout North America, the Indian subcontinent, and Europe.

As a result of similar pathophysiologic mechanisms, there is a strong interaction of these risk factors with stroke. However, the impact of programming is again evident in the marked differences in adult phenotype depending on the fetal and childhood environment. In a study of over 2000 people within the Helsinki birth cohort, two different paths of early growth preceded the development of hypertension in adult life.[34] Small body size at birth and low weight gain during infancy followed by a rapid gain in BMI during childhood was associated with an increase in coronary heart disease as adults. In contrast, LBW in utero and throughout infancy followed by a persistent small body size at adolescence resulted in an increased risk of a stroke and an atherogenic lipid profile.[35] These two different paths of growth may lead to hypertension via altered biologic processes. Although restriction of rodent weight gain following LBW prevents an obese phenotype, there are significant atherogenic and pancreatic abnormalities. Notably, these offspring exhibit markedly elevated cholesterol levels and insulin deficiency.[36]

In addition to the effect of fetal nutrient exposure on cardiac development, there are significant vasculogenesis mechanisms underlying the programming of hypertension. These may include modifications in arterial stiffness, arterial elastin, and the size of the arterial and capillary bed.[37] Although there is no direct evidence that elastin synthesis is impaired in the developing of large arteries of human fetuses whose growth is restricted, children with a single umbilical artery demonstrate striking asymmetry in the compliance of iliac arteries at 5 to 9 years of age.[38]

Although this chapter does not seek to review all toxic teratogenic exposures, prenatal cocaine exposure has been demonstrated to have significant effects on neonatal and offspring cardiac function. Cocaine exposure results in an increased rate of neonatal arrhythmia and transient ST elevation. Though a blinded cross-sectional study did not demonstrate any significant differences in human left ventricular cardiac function,[39] prenatal cocaine exposure did result in changes in diastolic filling in neonates with the degree of change correlated to the degree of cocaine exposure. Some changes persisted to age 26 months, particularly in those infants exposed to high levels of in utero cocaine.[40] The mechanisms of cocaine effects may relate to the inhibition of dopamine, serotonin, and norepinephrine reuptake. In addition to direct effects, cocaine programming of cardiac function may be mediated via effects on the autonomic nervous system. Some, though not all, studies have demonstrated an alteration in resting heart rate and heart rate variability.[41] A well-performed study further demonstrated a dose-dependent effect of fetal cocaine on neonatal heart rate at 4 to 8 weeks of age, though the duration of this effect is unknown.[42] Further effects on static stress, renal sympathetic activity, and heart rate variability further confirm offspring effects of cardioregulatory systems by cocaine. Taken in sum, these studies suggest that fetal cocaine has at least a short-term cardiac impact and potentially a longer-term cardiac impact in humans.

Although there is no clear epidemiologic evidence to link prenatal hypoxia and adult cardiovascular disease, animal models suggest an effect of hypoxia on adult cardiac function. Chronic hypoxia during the course of pregnancy also results in LBW newborns with altered myocardial structure and heart development. Among other effects, prolonged hypoxia in utero suppresses fetal cardiac function, alters cardiac gene expression, increases myocyte apoptosis, and results in a premature exit of the cell cycle of cardiomyocytes and myocyte hypertrophy.[43]

OSTEOPOROSIS PROGRAMMING

Recent evidence indicates that the fetal and neonatal life may be a critical factor in the development of osteoporosis, a disease typically associated with aging. In considering the major determinants of bone mass in later life, the most critical issues are (1) peak bone mass achieved during the third decade of life and (2) the rate of bone loss following this period. Thus, bone mass in the elderly is largely determined by peak bone mass occurring much earlier in life. Several epidemiologic studies have demonstrated that LBW and weight at 1 year are directly correlated with reduced bone marrow content, as well as bone mineral density.[44] Consistent with these findings, poor childhood growth is associated with an increased risk of hip fracture in elderly adults.[45]

The mechanisms by which the fetal and neonatal period can influence peak bone mineral content include the interaction of vitamin D and calcium, as well as additional factors including fetal and neonatal growth hormone, cortisol, and insulin-like growth factor 1. An undernourished fetus, deprived of calcium, may up-regulate vitamin D activity in an attempt to increase calcium availability.[46] Although more than 60% of peak bone mass is gained during puberty, there is a growing body of evidence suggesting that a substantial proportion of peak bone mass is determined by growth earlier in life. Additional maternal factors may influence neonatal bone mineral content. Low maternal fat stores, maternal smoking or increased physical exercise in late pregnancy, and low maternal birth weight all predict lower whole body bone marrow content in the neonate.[45] In rats, maternal diet modulation or uterine ligation affects offspring bone structure.[47] The adult offspring has lower serum 25-OH vitamin D levels, bone mineral content, and bone area, which is also associated with changes in the growth plates. This is consistent with the nutritional programming of skeletal growth trajectory and complements the epidemiologic evidence for programming of osteoporosis in humans.

BRAIN PROGRAMMING

As complex as is cerebral function and development during the critical fetal/neonatal window, it is understandable that a number of stressors during early life may affect a diversity of cerebral functions, including cognition, behavior, anxiety, and even addictive potential. In utero exposure to cocaine, and perhaps methamphetamine, demonstrates a diversity of cerebral effects.[48] Among children exposed to prenatal cocaine, there are significant effects on behavior (aggression), attention-deficit/hyperactivity disorder (ADHD), offspring substance abuse (e.g., cigarettes), and impaired language (reviewed in reference 48). Additional studies have suggested potential impairment of intelligence quotient (IQ), cognition, motor function, and school performance. Understandably, windows of exposure and dose-dependent responses are difficult to quantify. Nevertheless, a number of studies have suggested that heavy cocaine use is related to worse outcome in regard to behavior, language, and IQ.[48] Studies of neuroimaging have demonstrated significant alterations in brain-region-specific volumes among cocaine-exposed children, when assessed as children, adolescents, or adults.[49] Studies of diffusion tensor imaging and functional magnetic resonance imaging (MRI) demonstrate increased creatine in the frontal white matter, potentially a sign of abnormal energy metabolism.[50] Cocaine-exposed children demonstrate greater activation in the white inferior frontal cortex and the caudate nucleus during response inhibition, suggesting that prenatal cocaine may affect the development of brain systems involved in the regulation of attention and response inhibition.[48]

Considering other substances of abuse, among children exposed to methamphetamine, magnetic resonance spectroscopy demonstrated increases in total creatine in the basal ganglia, again indicative of possible alterations in cellular energy metabolism.[51] Neuroimaging of children exposed to opiates in utero further demonstrate smaller intracranial and brain volumes, including smaller cerebral cortex, amygdala, brain stem, and cerebellum white matter, among other areas.[52] **This is consistent with animal studies that indicate prenatal nicotine or cocaine exposure targets specific neurotransmitter receptors in the fetal brain, eliciting abnormalities in cell proliferation and differentiation, and thus leading to reduced neurogenesis and altered synaptic activity.**[53] The underlying mechanism may involve increased apoptosis of neuronal cells.

Maternal Stress and Anxiety

Although the effects of maternal substance abuse may be a direct effect of the specific drug-receptor interaction, the commonality of offspring behavioral effects suggests that disruption in the fetal neuroendocrine environment, potentially associated with increased fetal ACTH/cortisol, may affect fetal/neonatal brain development. In view of these findings there has been extensive epidemiologic investigation of maternal stress and anxiety. **During the second trimester, increased maternal anxiety has been associated with lower neonatal dopamine and serotonin levels, greater right frontal electroencephalograph (EEG) activation, and lower vagal tone.**[54] In late pregnancy, maternal anxiety has been associated with salivary cortisol levels among 10-year-old children, suggesting that maternal anxiety during pregnancy programs offspring stress responsiveness.[55] In a recent study, neonates of high-anxiety mothers demonstrated altered auditory evoked responses, suggesting differences in attention allocation.[56] In addition to chronic maternal anxiety, acute stress responses during pregnancy may include death of close relatives, natural disasters, and maternal neuropsychiatric conditions. Many of these stress exposures have a significant impact on offspring neurodevelopmental consequences. Children of mothers with posttraumatic stress disorder during pregnancy display altered cortisol levels that are accompanied by signs of behavioral distress during the first 9 months of life.[57]

The role of the maternal hypothalamic-pituitary-adrenal axis (HPA) is recognized as contributing to maternal stress-mediated effects on fetal development. Although the developing fetus is normally protected from high levels of circulating maternal cortisol by the placental enzyme 11-β-hydroxysteroid dehydrogenase type 2 (11β-HSD2), which metabolizes cortisol to inactive cortisone, downregulation of placental 11β-HSD2 may occur in response to drug exposure, maternal diet, and obstetrical conditions, including preeclampsia, preterm birth, and intrauterine growth restriction.[58] A reduction in placental 11β-HSD2 may thus increase fetal exposure to maternal cortisol levels and secondary effects on brain maturation and development. Among pregnant women undergoing amniocentesis, there is a strong correlation between maternal plasma and amniotic fluid cortisol levels (indicative of fetal levels). The correlation with maternal anxiety suggests that measures of amniotic fluid cortisol may serve as an index for fetal hormone exposure.

Offspring psychiatric disorders associated with maternal pregnancy stress may be a consequence of cortisol binding to select brain regions during development. Notably, most fetal tissues express glucocorticoid receptors from midgestation onward. It is well established that steroid hormones in the fetus are involved in organ development and maturation (brain, heart, lungs, gastrointestinal tract, kidneys). Of note, the hippocampus, which is critical for learning and memory, has extensive glucocorticoid receptors. Although not studied in humans, glucocorticoid exposure in rat dams results in a reduction in the volume and number of cells in the nucleus accumbens, a central limbic nucleus critical to reward circuitry.[59] These findings may provide a mechanism by which maternal stress and/or substance abuse contributes to offspring addictive behavior, itself representing a dysfunction of the limbic system.

The effects of maternal stress may extend beyond fetal/neonatal neurologic/behavioral issues. Maternal prenatal anxiety/stress predicts a significant adverse effect on infant illness and antibiotic use,[60] whereas a wide range of prenatal stressors are associated with child morbidity. **Specifically, prenatal anxiety has been associated with childhood asthma, whereas stress-related maternal factors have been associated with increased eczema during early childhood.**[61,62]

A generational effect of fetal programming and the HPA axis is suggested by findings that LBW babies have raised cortisol concentrations in umbilical cord blood and raised urinary cortisol secretion in childhood.[63] Nilsson and colleagues demonstrated that there was a continuous relationship between size at birth and stress susceptibility,[64] whereas other studies have demonstrated that cortisol responses to stress were significantly and inversely related to birth weight.[65] Similarly, in regard to physiologic responses, LBW is associated with increased blood pressure and heart rate responses to psychological stressors in women, though not men.[66]

In corroboration of the human data, findings from experiments with rodent models show that prenatal stress (such as restraint) and administration of exogenous glucocorticoids not only impair cognition, increase anxiety, and increase reactivity to stress but also alter brain development.[67] Furthermore, prenatal stress increases sensitivity to nicotine and other addictive drugs. **Maternal nurturing affects offspring epigenome and behavior.** In rats, maternal nurturing behavior altered the offspring epigenome at a glucocorticoid receptor gene promoter in the hippocampus. As a result, highly nurtured rat pups demonstrated less anxiety than those that received minimal nurturing.[68]

More recent studies on nonhuman primates implicate chronic consumption of a high-fat diet during pregnancy for increased anxiety-like behavior in offspring, thought to be caused by perturbations in the fetal brain serotonergic/melanocortin pathways.[69]

Glucocorticoids and Prematurity

Although glucocorticoid therapy for the preterm infant has made a significant contribution to the reduction of neonatal respiratory distress syndrome, intraventricular hemorrhage, and infant mortality, there has been a tendency for clinicians to use multiple courses of glucocorticoids. **Studies that have examined the impact of human perinatal glucocorticoid exposure have demonstrated that children exposed to dexamethasone during preterm gestation and who were born at term have increased emotionality, general behavioral problems, and impairments in verbal working memory.**[60,70] Further, offspring of women given multiple doses of antenatal glucocorticoids have reduced head circumference and significantly increased aggressive violent behavior and attention deficits.[71] These findings suggest that fetal exposure to pharmacologic glucocorticoid levels during critical developmental periods (before normal high level in the term neonate) may have adverse consequences, including the programming of the offspring HPA. Preterm babies exposed to antenatal betamethasone had a lower salivary cortisol response to heel stick than matched controls at 3 to 6 days after delivery.[72] Additional studies demonstrate that exposure to antenatal corticosteroids is associated with suppressed cortisol responses to corticotropin-releasing factor during the immediate neonatal period.[73] Salivary cortisol responses to immunization at 4 months of age are significantly correlated with the mean plasma cortisol in the first 4 weeks, independent of maternal glucocorticoid exposure. It is notable that preterm infants have a similar spectrum of developmental and behavioral problems as do babies whose mothers have experienced extreme stress or anxiety during pregnancy, with both groups demonstrating increased levels of attention deficit, hyperactivity, anxiety, and depression.

Although there are consequences of premature exogenous glucocorticoid exposure (via maternal administration), it should be recognized that if actually delivered preterm, infants are exposed to increased endogenous cortisol before that which they would normally experience at term. Several studies demonstrate that LBW is associated with increased resting heart rate and fasting plasma cortisol concentrations in adulthood. Among preterm babies born at less than 32 weeks, newborn plasma cortisol levels are 4 to 7 times higher than would be fetal levels at the same gestational age. As the elevated levels persist through 4 weeks of age, they likely result from a combination of the acute antenatal steroids and postnatal endogenous glucocorticoids. Whether a consequence of prematurity itself, or perhaps premature cortisol exposure, preterm infants (especially born before 28 weeks' gestational age) have significant neurologic impairments, including visual-motor coordination (when measured at 8 years of age). In view of these consequences of exogenous and endogenous glucocorticoids, maternal glucocorticoid use should be directed only at those infants most likely to benefit and those most likely to deliver preterm.

Whereas the effects of glucocorticoids on programming brain development and organ maturation is well accepted, it is less well recognized that glycyrrhiza (a natural constituent of licorice) may also affect fetal programming via a cortisol mechanism. Glycyrrhiza inhibits placental 11β-HSD2, resulting in a potential increased transmission of maternal cortisol to the fetal compartment. In a study of Finnish children 8 years of age, those with high exposure to glycyrrhiza from maternal licorice ingestion had significant detriments in verbal and visual-spatial abilities and in narrative memory, and significant increases in externalizing symptoms and in aggression-related problems. These effects on cognitive performance appear to be related to the degree of licorice consumption.[74] In addition to licorice, glycyrrhiza is often used as flavoring in candies, chewing gum, herbal teas, alcoholic and nonalcoholic drinks, and herbal medications. Although these results suggest that exposure to glycyrrhiza be limited during pregnancy, it more importantly indicates the diversity of foods and drugs that may affect fetal development and programming, perhaps through effects on fetal cortisol exposure.

Prematurely born infants also display abnormalities of insulin resistance, elevated blood pressure, and abnormal retinal vasculature as adults.[75,76] Although much attention has been focused on the effects of LBW on the programming of metabolic syndrome, a study of 49-year-old Swedish men demonstrated that systolic and diastolic blood pressures were inversely correlated with gestational age rather than birth weight, independent of current body mass index.[76] Similar results have been demonstrated in women born preterm.[75] An intergenerational effect may occur, as consequences of elevated blood pressure and abnormal vascularization among women may have a subsequent impact on future pregnancies. Thus, women born before 37 weeks of age demonstrate a 2.5-fold increased risk of developing gestational hypertension.[77]

In a recent study from western North Carolina, boys and girls aged 9 to 16 were tested for depression in relation to birth weight and additional prenatal and perinatal factors. Low birth weight predicted depression in adolescent girls (38.1% versus 8.4% among girls with normal birth weight), though not boys. In addition, LBW was associated with an increased risk of social phobia, posttraumatic stress symptoms, and generalized anxiety disorder, all of which were far more common in girls than in boys.[78] Further studies have demonstrated that LBW is associated with an increased risk of schizophrenia, ADHD, and eating disorders. These findings are consistent with those of animal studies indicating gender-specific effects of developmental programming.

Immune Function

As noted, prenatal stress may influence the developing immune system, particularly asthma and atopic diseases. Maternal nervousness during gestation correlates with elevated IgE levels in cord blood and may predict atopic diseases in early childhood.[79] **Importantly, pregnant women with prenatal stress have elevated pro-inflammatory cytokine levels,[80] and these levels may affect the risk of allergy in childhood offspring. Although these findings suggest that *enhanced* immunologic responses may occur following maternal stress, LBW may be associated with *reduced* inflammatory responses contributing to increased morbidity.** Young adults born during seasonal famine (and likely growth restricted) are more likely to die from infectious disease.[81] These infants demonstrated reduced thymic size and altered patterns of T-cell subsets with a lower CD4-CD8 ratio, suggestive of lower thymic output. Postpartum maternal influences also may contribute as mothers of these infants express lower levels of maternal breast milk IL7, a putative thymic trophic factor.[82] In support of the impaired inflammation response among LBW infants, antibody responses to typhoid vaccination are positively related to birth weight.[83] These findings suggest that atopy-related immune function may be enhanced in either LBW offspring or offspring associated with maternal prenatal stress, though LBW may well have significant impairment in offspring infectious disease–related immune function. The consequences of LBW and reduced immune function may be a critical factor predisposing to infant mortality in the developing world.

Much as perinatal factors can influence offspring immunity, mothers who are allergic have lower interferon γ responses during pregnancy, which has been postulated to influence the cytokine milieu of the fetus.[84] Similarly, maternal asthma during pregnancy is associated with fetal growth retardation and preterm birth,[85] and placental expression of pro-inflammatory placental cytokines is significantly increased in pregnancies complicated by mild asthma, though only in the presence of a female fetus.[86] There is significant evidence that both the maternal allergic phenotype and maternal environmental exposures during pregnancy affect the risk of subsequent infant allergic disease. Evidence indicates that maternal allergy is a recognized risk factor for infant allergic disease. In regard to maternal environmental exposure, a number of factors may influence fetal immune development and allergic outcomes. Although evidence is inconsistent and mechanisms are unclear, several studies have demonstrated that a Mediterranean diet may protect against early childhood wheezing.[87] Other studies have explored the effects of folate supplementation, polyunsaturated fatty acids, antioxidants, and a range of vitamins and micronutrients, though again with a lack of consistency.

Interestingly, recent evidence suggests that maternal exposure to microbials may influence fetal immune competence. In utero exposure to a farming environment has been demonstrated to protect against the development of childhood asthma and eczema.[88] Similar results have demonstrated that farming environments alter the expression of innate immune genes and modify umbilical cord IgE levels.[89] **In contrast to the potential beneficial effect of microbial exposure, maternal cigarette smoking increases the risk of offspring asthma.** This likely occurs via an allergic sensitization, rather than classic direct pulmonary effects of cigarette smoke. Animal studies also support the premise that innate immune function can be programmed as a result of perinatal challenge to the immune system during development. In rats, neonatal bacterial endotoxin, lipopolysaccharide (LPS) administration influences the adult neuroimmune response to a second LPS challenge through the HPA axis.[90] In addition, undernutrition, particularly during prenatal and postnatal periods, affects offspring immune competence by increasing basal inflammation while reducing cytokine induction to inflammatory stimuli.[91]

Potentially confounding the association of cigarette smoking is a finding that children with a smaller head circumference at 10 to 15 days of age had a markedly increased odds ratio for wheezing at 7 years of age.[92] Thus, factors that determine fetal growth may be associated with wheezing in childhood. Children with both small and large head circumferences at birth (consistent with both undernutrition and overnutrition) have increased atopic sensitization and elevated serum IgE at age 5 to 7.[93] Large head circumference at birth has previously been reported to be associated with elevated IgG in adulthood and with risk of asthma in adolescents.[94] The association of developmental origins with childhood asthma is complex as there are several asthma phenotypes, including those that are associated with atopy as compared to those associated with acute childhood viral infection. Although both these diseases exhibit childhood wheezing and/or are immune modulated, they likely have significant alterations in predisposition. As asthma is associated with an exaggerated T-helper type 2 (TH2) response to both allergic and nonallergic stimuli, it has been proposed that genes involved in IgE synthesis and airway remodeling have failed to be silenced during early infancy. In utero programming of these genes may result in the predisposition to allergic responses.

ENDOCRINE PROGRAMMING

Low birth weight may also be associated with additional endocrine disorders affecting gonadal and adrenal axes. Reduced fetal growth may be associated with exaggerated adrenarche, early puberty, and small ovarian size with the subsequent development of ovarian hyperandrogenism.[95] Children born SGA may have puberty at a normal age or even earlier, but appear to exhibit a more rapid progression, compromising adult ovarian function.[96] SGA as compared to AGA girls displayed increased baseline estradiol, stimulated estradiol, and 17-hydroxyprogesterone at the beginning of puberty,[97] whereas LBW is associated with precocious puberty in girls.[95] Among LBW girls, those who demonstrate postnatal catch-up growth have greater fat mass and central fat. Whether this suggests that early puberty is a consequence of hyperandrogenism or hyperinsulinism associated with the central adiposity is uncertain. **Importantly, children with precocious puberty, particularly those with a history of LBW, have an increased risk of developing ovarian hyperandrogenism and other**

features of polycystic ovary syndrome (PCOS) during early post menarche.[95] Growth restriction may thus program adrenal function, inducing permanent changes in ovarian morphology and function in utero, contributing to PCOS in adult life.

Despite the association with PCOS, women born during famine do not appear to have differences in fertility rates as measured by age at first pregnancy, completed family size, and interpregnancy interval.[98] Recent studies have suggested that the Dutch famine offspring cohort may even have an increased fertility as compared to controls.[99] Furthermore, despite the impact on puberty, LBW does not appear to advance the age of menopause in women.[100] There is evidence, however, of an increased prevalence of anovulation in adolescent girls born SGA as compared with controls (40% vs. 4%),[101] though this may be a consequence of obesity-associated endocrine perturbations. These findings suggest that there are relatively small effects of maternal nutritional status during pregnancy on reproductive performance of offspring.

In the female rat, pubertal timing and subsequent ovarian function is influenced by the animal's nutritional status in utero, with both maternal caloric restriction and maternal high-fat nutrition resulting in early pubertal onset. However, the former leads to a reduction in progesterone levels whereas the latter causes elevated progesterone concentrations in adult offspring.[102] In sheep, reduced lifetime reproductive capacity has been demonstrated in ewes born to mothers undernourished during late pregnancy or the first months of life.[103] Prenatal exposure to testosterone impairs female reproductive capacity in sheep,[104] whereas prepubertal administration of estradiol disrupts ovarian cyclicity in adult rats.[105] Furthermore, exposure of animals to an excess of thyroxine during the neonatal period changes the pituitary-hypothalamic responses linked to the secretion of thyroid-stimulating hormone in later life.[106]

SEXUALITY PROGRAMMING

The following discussion is not meant to imply disease states or opine on issues of normalcy of sexuality, but rather to discuss the developmental processes that result in adult sexual orientation. Among males, sexual orientation is largely dichotomous (heterosexual, homosexual), though there is likely increased bisexual orientation among women. A genetic component for sexual orientation is evident from studies demonstrating increased rates of homosexuality among relatives of homosexuals.[107] Twin studies report moderate hereditability of sexual orientation,[108] though there have been limited advances in the identification of specific genetic loci responsible for sexual orientation. **However, significant research demonstrates a major role for gonadal steroidal androgens in regulating sexual dimorphism in the brain and subsequent behavior.**[109] Animal studies confirm that hormonal signals operating during critical periods may have programming effects on sexuality. The classic example of such a phenomenon is the exposure of female rats at a critical period of fetal life to a single exogenous dose of testosterone, which permanently reoriented sexual behavior. A similar dose of testosterone in 20-day-old females had no effect. Thus, there is a critical time at which the animal's sexual physiology is sensitive and can be permanently changed.[110] Based on early animal models, initial studies resulted in what is likely an oversimplified theory: relative overexposure of females to androgens may contribute to female homosexuality, whereas underexposure to prenatal androgens in men may contribute to male homosexuality. Using proxy markers of prenatal hormonal androgen exposure (ratio of second to fourth finger lengths), several studies have demonstrated that homosexual women have significantly masculine measurements compared to heterosexual women,[111] though one study reported no difference.[112] A further proxy marker is oto-acoustic emissions (OAEs), which represent sounds emitted by the cochlea that are more numerous in females than in males. There is significant evidence that OAEs are influenced by prenatal androgen exposure, with evidence that females with male co-twins have a masculinized OAE pattern.[113] Despite the tendency for homosexual women to be exposed to more prenatal androgens than heterosexual women, there is considerable overlap between the two female groups, indicating that prenatal androgens do not act in isolation.[114] Reports among heterosexual and homosexual men are inconclusive in regard to proxy markers.

In contrast to the stronger correlation of female versus male homosexuality with measures of prenatal androgen exposure, birth order has a more significant effect among males. The paternal birth order effect indicates that homosexual men have a greater number of older brothers than heterosexual men do, with the estimated odds of being homosexual increasing by 33% with each older brother.[114] Of note, homosexual males with older brothers have significantly lower birth weights compared to heterosexual males from older brothers.[115] These findings may suggest an interaction of birth weight and additional developmental factors. Several investigators have suggested a role of immunization of mothers to male-linked androgens, resulting in maternal Y-chromosome linked antibodies that may act on male differentiating receptors within the fetal brain.[114] Further studies demonstrate sexual orientation–related neuronal variation, including hypothalamic and selected cortical regions. Despite these associations, there is little conclusive understanding of specific neurodevelopmental mechanisms that produce homosexuality or heterosexuality.

RENAL PROGRAMMING

In humans, the total number of nephrons ranges between approximately 600,000 and slightly over 1 million, although the factors that determine an individual's glomerular number are unknown. **Nephrogenesis occurs up to approximately 36 weeks of gestation, and both genetic and environmental effects alter or regulate the number of nephrons.** From a genetic perspective, select genes regulating renal signaling and transcription permutation have been associated with renal hypoplasia. Thus, most congenital renal anomalies have an inheritable component.

Environmental exposures/stresses are well demonstrated to alter nephron number. Autopsies of newborn and children have demonstrated a marked association between LBW and reduced nephron number.[116] Importantly, low glomerular number and high glomerular size have been associated with the development of hypertension, cardiovascular diseases, and an increased susceptibility to renal disease in later life. Reduced nephron number as a result of developmental programming may result in single-nephron glomerular hyperfiltration. The compensatory glomerular hypertrophy that maintains normal glomerular filtration rate (GFR) ultimately may cause glomerular sclerosis, nephron loss, and contribute to later hypertension and chronic renal disease.

Reduced nephron number beginning in the fetal/neonatal period may have effects different from those of adult nephrectomy. In sheep, fetal unilateral nephrectomy at 110 days' gestation leads to offspring hypertension.[117] Similarly, unilateral nephrectomy in the neonatal rat results in adult hypertension and impaired renal function. These findings differ from those of human nephrectomy performed in adults (e.g., renal transplant donors) in which hypertension generally does not develop. The mechanisms that contribute to hypertension resulting from reduced glomerular number occurring during fetal and neonatal life are unclear, but indicate that developmental impact on nephron number may have significant impact on programmed hypertension. These include role of specific genes and growth factors involved in this process (Pax2 and GDNF), as well as apoptotic markers and signaling pathways.

In view of the contribution of renal disease to hypertension, it is notable that very LBW infants exhibit a high rate of hypertension during adolescence.[118] Preterm children also exhibit a higher prevalence of hypertension, occurring in both AGA and SGA offspring.[119] Among both African Americans in the southeastern United States and Australian Aboriginals, LBW is associated with adult-onset renal disease.[116,120,121] As a marker of impending renal disease, microalbuminuria is more than twofold greater in SGA offspring at a young adult age than that occurring in AGA offspring, though not all studies demonstrate this effect. Nutritional insults associated with SGA, LBW, and prematurity are perhaps associated with excess glucocorticoid exposure and secondarily reduced glomerular number.

Pregnant patients are also exposed to a variety of nephrotoxic drugs, including nonsteroidal anti-inflammatories, ampicillin/penicillin, and aminoglycosides. Nonsteroidal anti-inflammatories may lead to renal hypoperfusion during critical nephrogenic periods, resulting in cystic changes in developing nephrons[122] and acute or chronic renal failure in preterm newborns.[123] The impairment in renal development resulting from angiotensin-converting enzyme inhibitors is well documented, likely a result of the critical role of angiotensin in nephrogenesis.

Although less is known regarding offspring of diabetic pregnancies, exposure to transiently high blood glucose concentrations may reduce nephron development in rat pups.[124] In humans, increased urinary albumin excretion has been demonstrated in adult offspring of Pima Indian mothers with diabetes, suggesting an early glomerular injury.[125] Notably, individuals with a history of hypertension contained only 50% as many nephrons as those without hypertension.[126] Nephron number in adult kidneys is correlated to birth weight, with each kilogram increase in birth weight associated with an additional 250,000 nephrons.[116] However, these studies could not differentiate age- or disease-related loss of nephrons as compared to developmental origins. Reduced nephron number has been demonstrated in the absence of hypertension, indicating that additional processes of programmed hypertension may occur independently of a reduction in nephron number. Whether a reduced nephron number is etiologic of hypertension, a consequence of hypertension, or a coincident finding may depend on the individual.

CONCLUSION

As we are beginning to learn of the significance and mechanisms of developmental programming of adult health and disease, the critical consequences of developmental windows are increasingly recognized. Programming effects may have an impact on development by altering organ size, structure, or function. Cellular signaling mechanisms and/or epigenetic consequences may be highly dependent on the magnitude of the exposure and the window of exposure during embryogenesis or organogenesis. Most important, we are only beginning to recognize how consequences of prophylactic treatments may alter programmed phenotypes. Certainly, it appears there is no one single mechanism, nor one single developmental window that affects each organ or system development. Consequently, the ultimate management of fetuses and newborns is likely to be individualized rather than universal. We hope to achieve a greater understanding of the relative risks and benefits of current-day obstetrical decisions, including repeated doses of maternal glucocorticoids, advantages versus disadvantages of early delivery of SGA fetuses, and use of oral hypoglycemic agents that cross the placenta, as well as many other management dilemmas.

KEY POINTS

- Maternal in utero environment (nutrition, hormonal, metabolic, stress, and drugs) is a critical determinant of fetal growth and influences a wide variety of metabolic, developmental, and pathologic processes in adulthood.
- Both ends of growth spectrum (i.e., low and high birth weight newborns) are associated with increased risk of adult obesity, metabolic syndrome, cardiovascular disease, insulin resistance, and neuroendocrine disorders.
- The mechanisms linking early developmental events to later manifestation of disease states involve "programmed" changes in organ structure, cellular responses, gene expression, and epigenome.
- Prenatal care is evolving to reach essential goals of optimizing maternal, fetal, and neonatal health to prevent or reduce adult-onset diseases.
- Guiding policy regarding optimal pregnancy nutrition and weight gain, management of low and high fetal weight pregnancies, use of maternal glucocorticoids, and newborn feeding strategies, among others, has yet to comprehensively integrate long-term consequences on adult health.

REFERENCES

1. Stephens TD, Bunde CJ, Fillmore BJ: Mechanism of action in thalidomide teratogenesis. Biochem Pharmacol 59:1489, 2000.
2. Dieckmann WJ, Davis ME, Rynkiewicz LM, Pottinger RE: Does the administration of diethylstilbestrol during pregnancy have therapeutic value? Am J Obstet Gynecol 66:1062, 1953.
3. Bromer JG, Wu J, Zhou Y, Taylor HS: Hypermethylation of homeobox A10 by in utero diethylstilbestrol exposure: an epigenetic mechanism for altered developmental programming. Endocrinology 150:3376, 2009.
4. Waterland RA: Is epigenetics an important link between early life events and adult disease? Horm Res 71:13, 2009.
5. Stewart ST, Cutler DM, Rosen AB: Forecasting the effects of obesity and smoking on U.S. life expectancy. N Engl J Med 361: 2252, 2009.
6. Hales CN, Barker DJ: The thrifty phenotype hypothesis. Br Med Bull 60:5, 2001.
7. Dewey KG: Is breastfeeding protective against child obesity? J Hum Lact 19:9, 2003.
8. McCance DR, Pettitt DJ, Hanson RL, et al: Glucose, insulin concentrations and obesity in childhood and adolescence as predictors of NIDDM. Diabetologia 37:617, 1994.
9. Desai M, Gayle D, Babu J, Ross MG: Programmed obesity in intrauterine growth-restricted newborns: modulation by newborn nutrition. Am J Physiol Regul Integr Comp Physiol 288:R91, 2005.
10. Bouret SG, Draper SJ, Simerly RB: Trophic action of leptin on hypothalamic neurons that regulate feeding. Science 304:108, 2004.
11. Yousheng J, Nguyen T, Desai M, Ross MG: Programmed alterations in hypothalamic neuronal orexigenic responses to ghrelin following gestational nutrient restriction. Reprod Sci 15:702, 2008.
12. Desai M, Gayle D, Han G, Ross MG: Programmed hyperphagia due to reduced anorexigenic mechanisms in intrauterine growth-restricted offspring. Reprod Sci 14:329, 2007.
13. Desai M, Li T, Ross MG: Hypothalamic neurosphere progenitor cells in low birth weight rat newborns: neurotrophic effects of leptin and insulin. Brain Res 1378:29, 2011.
14. Kirchner S, Kieu T, Chow C, et al: Prenatal exposure to the environmental obesogen tributyltin predisposes multipotent stem cells to become adipocytes. Mol Endocrinol 24:526, 2010.
15. Levin BE. Epigenetic influences on food intake and physical activity level: review of animal studies. Obesity (Silver Spring) 16:S51, 2008.
16. Kinugasa A, Tsunamoto K, Furukawa N, et al: Fatty liver and its fibrous changes found in simple obesity of children. J Pediatr Gastroenterol Nutr 3:408, 1984.
17. Barker DJ, Meade TW, Fall CH, et al: Relation of fetal and infant growth to plasma fibrinogen and factor VII concentrations in adult life. BMJ 304:148, 1992.
18. Burns SP, Desai M, Cohen RD, et al: Gluconeogenesis, glucose handling, and structural changes in livers of the adult offspring of rats partially deprived of protein during pregnancy and lactation. J Clin Invest 100:1768, 1997.
19. Seo YS, Kim JH, Jo NY, et al: PPAR agonists treatment is effective in a nonalcoholic fatty liver disease animal model by modulating fatty-acid metabolic enzymes. J Gastroenterol Hepatol 23:102, 2008.
20. Watkins SM, Reifsnyder PR, Pan HJ, et al: Lipid metabolome-wide effects of the PPARgamma agonist rosiglitazone. J Lipid Res 43: 1809, 2002.
21. Kleemann R, Verschuren L, de Rooij BJ, et al: Evidence for anti-inflammatory activity of statins and PPARalpha activators in human C-reactive protein transgenic mice in vivo and in cultured human hepatocytes in vitro. Blood 103:4188, 2004.
22. Magee TR, Han G, Cherian B, et al: Down-regulation of transcription factor peroxisome proliferator-activated receptor in programmed hepatic lipid dysregulation and inflammation in intrauterine growth-restricted offspring. Am J Obstet Gynecol 199:271, 2008.
23. Economides DL, Proudler A, Nicolaides KH: Plasma insulin in appropriate- and small-for-gestational-age fetuses. Am J Obstet Gynecol 160:1091, 1989.
24. Phillips DI, Barker DJ, Hales CN, et al: Thinness at birth and insulin resistance in adult life. Diabetologia 37:150, 1994.
25. Hales CN, Barker DJ, Clark PM, et al: Fetal and infant growth and impaired glucose tolerance at age 64. BMJ 303:1019, 1991.
26. Hellerstrom C: The life story of the pancreatic B cell. Diabetologia 26:393, 1984.
27. Dalziel SR, Walker NK, Parag V, et al: Cardiovascular risk factors after antenatal exposure to betamethasone: 30-year follow-up of a randomised controlled trial. Lancet 365:1856, 2005.
28. Dessens AB, Haas HS, Koppe JG: Twenty-year follow-up of antenatal corticosteroid treatment. Pediatrics 105:E77, 2000.
29. Reusens B, Remacle C: Programming of the endocrine pancreas by the early nutritional environment. Int J Biochem Cell Biol 38:913, 2006.
30. Ford SP, Zhang L, Zhu M, et al: Maternal obesity accelerates fetal pancreatic beta-cell but not alpha-cell development in sheep: prenatal consequences. Am J Physiol Regul Integr Comp Physiol 297: R835, 2009.
31. Aerts L, Van Assche FA: Animal evidence for the transgenerational development of diabetes mellitus. Int J Biochem Cell Biol 38:894, 2006.
32. Werner JC, Sicard RE, Hansen TW, et al: Hypertrophic cardiomyopathy associated with dexamethasone therapy for bronchopulmonary dysplasia. J Pediatr 120:286, 1992.
33. Barker DJ: Fetal programming of coronary heart disease. Trends Endocrinol Metab 13:364, 2002.
34. Eriksson JG, Forsen TJ, Kajantie E, et al: Childhood growth and hypertension in later life. Hypertension 49:1415, 2007.
35. Eriksson JG, Forsen T, Tuomilehto J, et al: Early growth, adult income, and risk of stroke. Stroke 31:869, 2000.
36. Desai M, Gayle D, Babu J, Ross MG: The timing of nutrient restriction during rat pregnancy/lactation alters metabolic syndrome phenotype. Am J Obstet Gynecol 196:555, 2007.
37. Khorram O, Momeni M, Ferrini M, et al: In utero undernutrition in rats induces increased vascular smooth muscle content in the offspring. Am J Obstet Gynecol 196:486, 2007.
38. Berry CL, Gosling RG, Laogun AA, Bryan E: Anomalous iliac compliance in children with a single umbilical artery. Br Heart J 38:510, 1976.
39. Tuboku-Metzger AJ, O'Shea JS, Campbell RM, et al: Cardiovascular effects of cocaine in neonates exposed prenatally. Am J Perinatol 13:1, 1996.
40. Mehta SK, Super DM, Connuck D, et al: Diastolic alterations in infants exposed to intrauterine cocaine: a follow-up study by color kinesis. J Am Soc Echocardiogr 15:1361, 2002.
41. Mehta SK, Super DM, Connuck D, et al: Autonomic alterations in cocaine-exposed infants. Am Heart J 144:1109, 2002.
42. Schuetze P, Eiden RD: The association between maternal cocaine use during pregnancy and physiological regulation in 4- to 8-week-old infants: an examination of possible mediators and moderators. J Pediatr Psychol 31:15, 2006.
43. Patterson AJ, Zhang L: Hypoxia and fetal heart development. Curr Mol Med 10:653, 2010.
44. Cooper C, Eriksson JG, Forsen T, et al: Maternal height, childhood growth and risk of hip fracture in later life: a longitudinal study. Osteoporos Int 12:623, 2001.
45. Godfrey K, Walker-Bone K, Robinson S, et al: Neonatal bone mass: influence of parental birthweight, maternal smoking, body composition, and activity during pregnancy. J Bone Miner Res 16:1694, 2001.
46. Harvey N, Cooper C: The developmental origins of osteoporotic fracture. J Br Menopause Soc 10:14, 2004.
47. Mehta G, Roach HI, Langley-Evans S, et al: Intrauterine exposure to a maternal low protein diet reduces adult bone mass and alters growth plate morphology in rats. Calcif Tissue Int 71:493, 2002.
48. Lester BM, Lagasse LL: Children of addicted women. J Addict Dis 29:259, 2010.
49. Dow-Edwards DL, Benveniste H, Behnke M, et al: Neuroimaging of prenatal drug exposure. Neurotoxicol Teratol 28:386, 2006.
50. Smith LM, Chang L, Yonekura ML, et al: Brain proton magnetic resonance spectroscopy and imaging in children exposed to cocaine in utero. Pediatrics 107:227, 2001.
51. Smith LM, Chang L, Yonekura ML, et al: Brain proton magnetic resonance spectroscopy in children exposed to methamphetamine in utero. Neurology 57:255, 2001.
52. Walhovd KB, Moe V, Slinning K, et al: Volumetric cerebral characteristics of children exposed to opiates and other substances in utero. Neuroimage 36:1331, 2007.
53. Slotkin TA: Fetal nicotine or cocaine exposure: which one is worse? J Pharmacol Exp Ther 285:931, 1998.
54. Field T, Diego M, Hernandez-Reif M, et al: Pregnancy anxiety and comorbid depression and anger: effects on the fetus and neonate. Depress Anxiety 17:140, 2003.

55. O'Connor TG, Ben-Shlomo Y, Heron J, et al: Prenatal anxiety predicts individual differences in cortisol in pre-adolescent children. Biol Psychiatry 58:211, 2005.
56. Harvison KW, Molfese DL, Woodruff-Borden J, Weigel RA: Neonatal auditory evoked responses are related to perinatal maternal anxiety. Brain Cogn 71:369, 2009.
57. Yehuda R, Teicher MH, Seckl JR, et al: Parental posttraumatic stress disorder as a vulnerability factor for low cortisol trait in offspring of holocaust survivors. Arch Gen Psychiatry 64:1040, 2007.
58. Dy J, Guan H, Sampath-Kumar R, et al: Placental 11beta-hydroxysteroid dehydrogenase type 2 is reduced in pregnancies complicated with idiopathic intrauterine growth restriction: evidence that this is associated with an attenuated ratio of cortisone to cortisol in the umbilical artery. Placenta 29:193, 2008.
59. Mesquita AR, Wegerich Y, Patchev AV, et al: Glucocorticoids and neuro- and behavioural development. Semin Fetal Neonatal Med 14:130, 2009.
60. Hirvikoski T, Nordenstrom A, Lindholm T, et al: Cognitive functions in children at risk for congenital adrenal hyperplasia treated prenatally with dexamethasone. J Clin Endocrinol Metab 92:542, 2007.
61. Cookson H, Granell R, Joinson C, et al: Mothers' anxiety during pregnancy is associated with asthma in their children. J Allergy Clin Immunol 123:847, 2009.
62. Sausenthaler S, Rzehak P, Chen CM, et al: Stress-related maternal factors during pregnancy in relation to childhood eczema: results from the LISA Study. J Investig Allergol Clin Immunol 19:481, 2009.
63. Clark PM, Hindmarsh PC, Shiell AW, et al: Size at birth and adrenocortical function in childhood. Clin Endocrinol (Oxf) 45:721, 1996.
64. Nilsson PM, Nyberg P, Ostergren PO: Increased susceptibility to stress at a psychological assessment of stress tolerance is associated with impaired fetal growth. Int J Epidemiol 30:75, 2001.
65. Wust S, Entringer S, Federenko IS, et al: Birth weight is associated with salivary cortisol responses to psychosocial stress in adult life. Psychoneuroendocrinology 30:591, 2005.
66. Ward AM, Moore VM, Steptoe A, et al: Size at birth and cardiovascular responses to psychological stressors: evidence for prenatal programming in women. J Hypertens 22:2295, 2004.
67. McCormick CM, Mathews IZ, Thomas C, Waters P: Investigations of HPA function and the enduring consequences of stressors in adolescence in animal models. Brain Cogn 72:73, 2010.
68. Weaver IC, Cervoni N, Champagne FA, et al: Epigenetic programming by maternal behavior. Nat Neurosci 7:847, 2004.
69. Sullivan EL, Grayson B, Takahashi D, et al: Chronic consumption of a high-fat diet during pregnancy causes perturbations in the serotonergic system and increased anxiety-like behavior in nonhuman primate offspring. J Neurosci 30:3826, 2010.
70. Trautman PD, Meyer-Bahlburg HF, Postelnek J, New MI: Effects of early prenatal dexamethasone on the cognitive and behavioral development of young children: results of a pilot study. Psychoneuroendocrinology 20:439, 1995.
71. French NP, Hagan R, Evans SF, et al: Repeated antenatal corticosteroids: effects on cerebral palsy and childhood behavior. Am J Obstet Gynecol 190:588, 2004.
72. Davis EP, Townsend EL, Gunnar MR, et al: Effects of prenatal betamethasone exposure on regulation of stress physiology in healthy premature infants. Psychoneuroendocrinology 29:1028, 2004.
73. Ng PC, Lam CW, Lee CH, et al: Reference ranges and factors affecting the human corticotropin-releasing hormone test in preterm, very low birth weight infants. J Clin Endocrinol Metab 87:4621, 2002.
74. Raikkonen K, Pesonen AK, Heinonen K, et al: Maternal licorice consumption and detrimental cognitive and psychiatric outcomes in children. Am J Epidemiol 170:1137, 2009.
75. Kistner A, Jacobson L, Jacobson SH, et al: Low gestational age associated with abnormal retinal vascularization and increased blood pressure in adult women. Pediatr Res 51:675, 2002.
76. Siewert-Delle A, Ljungman S: The impact of birth weight and gestational age on blood pressure in adult life: a population-based study of 49-year-old men. Am J Hypertens 11:946, 1998.
77. Pouta A, Hartikainen AL, Sovio U, et al: Manifestations of metabolic syndrome after hypertensive pregnancy. Hypertension 43:825, 2004.
78. Costello EJ, Worthman C, Erkanli A, Angold A: Prediction from low birth weight to female adolescent depression: a test of competing hypotheses. Arch Gen Psychiatry 64:338, 2007.
79. Lin YC, Wen HJ, Lee YL, Guo YL: Are maternal psychosocial factors associated with cord immunoglobulin E in addition to family atopic history and mother immunoglobulin E? Clin Exp Allergy 34:548, 2004.
80. Coussons-Read ME, Okun ML, Nettles CD: Psychosocial stress increases inflammatory markers and alters cytokine production across pregnancy. Brain Behav Immun 21:343, 2007.
81. Moore SE, Cole TJ, Collinson AC, et al: Prenatal or early postnatal events predict infectious deaths in young adulthood in rural Africa. Int J Epidemiol 28:1088, 1999.
82. Prentice AM, Moore SE: Early programming of adult diseases in resource poor countries. Arch Dis Child 90:429, 2005.
83. Chen JC, Turiak G, Galler J, Volicer L: Postnatal changes of brain monoamine levels in prenatally malnourished and control rats. Int J Dev Neurosci 15:257, 1997.
84. Breckler LA, Hale J, Taylor A, et al: Pregnancy IFN-gamma responses to foetal alloantigens are altered by maternal allergy and gravidity status. Allergy 63:1473, 2008.
85. Breton MC, Beauchesne MF, Lemiere C, et al: Risk of perinatal mortality associated with asthma during pregnancy. Thorax 64:101, 2009.
86. Scott NM, Hodyl NA, Murphy VE, et al: Placental cytokine expression covaries with maternal asthma severity and fetal sex. J Immunol 182:1411, 2009.
87. Shaheen SO, Northstone K, Newson RB, et al: Dietary patterns in pregnancy and respiratory and atopic outcomes in childhood. Thorax 64:411, 2009.
88. Douwes J, Cheng S, Travier N, et al: Farm exposure in utero may protect against asthma, hay fever and eczema. Eur Respir J 32:603, 2008.
89. Ege MJ, Herzum I, Buchele G, et al: Specific IgE to allergens in cord blood is associated with maternal immunity to *Toxoplasma gondii* and rubella virus. Allergy 63:1505, 2008.
90. Spencer SJ, Galic MA, Pittman QJ: Neonatal programming of innate immune function. Am J Physiol Endocrinol Metab 300:E11, 2011.
91. Desai M, Gayle DA, Casillas E, et al: Early undernutrition attenuates the inflammatory response in adult rat offspring. J Matern Fetal Neonatal Med 22:571, 2009.
92. Carrington LJ, Langley-Evans SC: Wheezing and eczema in relation to infant anthropometry: evidence of developmental programming of disease in childhood. Matern Child Nutr 2:51, 2006.
93. Bolte G, Schmidt M, Maziak W, et al: The relation of markers of fetal growth with asthma, allergies and serum immunoglobulin E levels in children at age 5-7 years. Clin Exp Allergy 34:381, 2004.
94. Gregory A, Doull I, Pearce N, et al: The relationship between anthropometric measurements at birth: asthma and atopy in childhood. Clin Exp Allergy 29:330, 1999.
95. Ibanez L, Potau N, Francois I, et al: Precocious pubarche, hyperinsulinism, and ovarian hyperandrogenism in girls: relation to reduced fetal growth. J Clin Endocrinol Metab 83:3558, 1998.
96. Lazar L, Pollak U, Kalter-Leibovici O, et al: Pubertal course of persistently short children born small for gestational age (SGA) compared with idiopathic short children born appropriate for gestational age (AGA). Eur J Endocrinol 149:425, 2003.
97. Mericq V: Low birth weight and endocrine dysfunction in postnatal life. Pediatr Endocrinol Rev 4:3, 2006.
98. Lumey LH: Reproductive outcomes in women prenatally exposed to undernutrition: a review of findings from the Dutch famine birth cohort. Proc Nutr Soc 57:129, 1998.
99. Painter RC, Westendorp RG, de Rooij SR, et al: Increased reproductive success of women after prenatal undernutrition. Hum Reprod 23:2591, 2008.
100. Cresswell JL, Egger P, Fall CH, et al: Is the age of menopause determined in-utero? Early Hum Dev 49:143, 1997.
101. Ibanez L, Potau N, Ferrer A, et al: Reduced ovulation rate in adolescent girls born small for gestational age. J Clin Endocrinol Metab 87:3391, 2002.
102. Sloboda DM, Howie GJ, Pleasants A, et al: Pre- and postnatal nutritional histories influence reproductive maturation and ovarian function in the rat. PLoS ONE 4:e6744, 2009.
103. Rhind SM, McNeilly AS: Effects of level of food intake on ovarian follicle number, size and steroidogenic capacity in the ewe. Anim Reprod Sci 52:131, 1998.

104. Guzman C, Cabrera R, Cardenas M, et al: Protein restriction during fetal and neonatal development in the rat alters reproductive function and accelerates reproductive ageing in female progeny. J Physiol 572:97, 2006.
105. Rosa-E-Silva A, Guimaraes MA, Padmanabhan V, Lara HE: Prepubertal administration of estradiol valerate disrupts cyclicity and leads to cystic ovarian morphology during adult life in the rat: role of sympathetic innervation. Endocrinology 144:4289, 2003.
106. Besa ME, Pascual-Leone AM: Effect of neonatal hyperthyroidism upon the regulation of TSH secretion in rats. Acta Endocrinol (Copenh) 105:31, 1984.
107. Bailey JM, Pillard RC: Genetics of human sexual orientation. Ann Rev Sex Res 60:126, 1995.
108. Kirk KM, Bailey JM, Dunne MP, Martin NG: Measurement models for sexual orientation in a community twin sample. Behav Genet 30:345, 2000.
109. Morris JA, Jordan CL, Breedlove SM: Sexual differentiation of the vertebrate nervous system. Nat Neurosci 7:1034, 2004.
110. Angelbeck JH, DuBrul EF: The effect of neonatal testosterone on specific male and female patterns of phosphorylated cytosolic proteins in the rat preoptic-hypothalamus, cortex and amygdala. Brain Res 264:277, 1983.
111. Williams TJ, Pepitone ME, Christensen SE, et al: Finger-length ratios and sexual orientation. Nature 404:455, 2000.
112. Lippa RA: Are 2D:4D finger-length ratios related to sexual orientation? Yes for men, no for women. J Pers Soc Psychol 85:179, 2003.
113. McFadden D: A masculinizing effect on the auditory systems of human females having male co-twins. Proc Natl Acad Sci U S A 90:11900, 1993.
114. Rahman Q: The neurodevelopment of human sexual orientation. Neurosci Biobehav Rev 29:1057, 2005.
115. Blanchard R, Zucker KJ, Cavacas A, et al: Fraternal birth order and birth weight in probably prehomosexual feminine boys. Horm Behav 41:321, 2002.
116. Hughson M, Farris AB III, Douglas-Denton R, et al: Glomerular number and size in autopsy kidneys: the relationship to birth weight. Kidney Int 63:2113, 2003.
117. Moritz KM, Wintour EM, Dodic M: Fetal uninephrectomy leads to postnatal hypertension and compromised renal function. Hypertension 39:1071, 2002.
118. Rodriguez-Soriano J, Aguirre M, Oliveros R, Vallo A: Long-term renal follow-up of extremely low birth weight infants. Pediatr Nephrol 20:579, 2005.
119. Puddu M, Podda MF, Mussap M, et al: Early detection of microalbuminuria and hypertension in children of very low birthweight. J Matern Fetal Neonatal Med 22:83, 2009.
120. Lackland DT, Bendall HE, Osmond C, et al: Low birth weights contribute to high rates of early-onset chronic renal failure in the southeastern United States. Arch Intern Med 160:1472, 2000.
121. Hoy WE, Rees M, Kile E, et al: A new dimension to the Barker hypothesis: low birthweight and susceptibility to renal disease. Kidney Int 56:1072, 1999.
122. van der Heijden BJ, Carlus C, Narcy F, et al: Persistent anuria, neonatal death, and renal microcystic lesions after prenatal exposure to indomethacin. Am J Obstet Gynecol 171:617, 1994.
123. Norton ME, Merrill J, Cooper BA, et al: Neonatal complications after the administration of indomethacin for preterm labor. N Engl J Med 329:1602, 1993.
124. Amri K, Freund N, Vilar J, et al: Adverse effects of hyperglycemia on kidney development in rats: in vivo and in vitro studies. Diabetes 48:2240, 1999.
125. Nelson RG, Morgenstern H, Bennett PH: Intrauterine diabetes exposure and the risk of renal disease in diabetic Pima Indians. Diabetes 47:1489, 1998.
126. Keller G, Zimmer G, Mall G, et al: Nephron number in patients with primary hypertension. N Engl J Med 348:101, 2003.

Section II

Prenatal Care

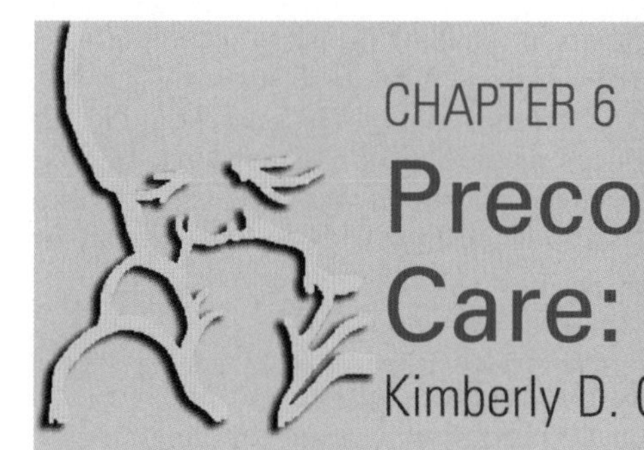

CHAPTER 6

Preconception and Prenatal Care: Part of the Continuum

Kimberly D. Gregory, Jennifer R. Niebyl, and Timothy R. B. Johnson

KEY ABBREVIATIONS	
American Academy of Pediatrics	AAP
American Congress of Obstetricians and Gynecologists	ACOG
Azidothymidine	AZT
Centers for Disease Control and Prevention	CDC
Computed Tomography	CT
Cytomegalovirus	CMV
Diethylstilbestrol	DES
Electronic Medical Record	EMR
Group B Streptococcus	GBS
Human Chorionic Gonadotropin	hCG
Human Immunodeficiency Virus	HIV
Last Menstrual Period	LMP
Magnetic Resonance Imaging	MRI
National Institutes of Health	NIH
Neural Tube Defect	NTD
Nuchal Translucency	NT
Pregnancy-Associated Placental Protein	PAPP-A
Rapid Plasma Reagin Test	RPR
Recommended Dietary Allowances	RDA
Restless Legs Syndrome	RLS
Rhesus Immune Globulin	RhIG
Routine Antenatal Diagnostic Imaging with Ultrasound Study	RADIUS
Vaginal Birth after Cesarean Delivery	VBAC
Women, Infants, and Children Program	WIC

Pregnancy and childbirth are major life events. **Preconception and prenatal care are not only part of the pregnancy continuum that culminates in delivery, the postpartum period, and parenthood, but they should also be considered in the context of women's health throughout the life span.[1,2]** This chapter reviews pertinent considerations for prenatal care using the broader definitions espoused by the U.S. Public Health Service and the American College of Obstetrician Gynecologists.[3] Specifically, prenatal care should consist of a series of interactions defined as visits and contacts with caretakers that includes three components: (1) early and continuing risk assessment; (2) health promotion; and (3) medical and psychosocial interventions and follow-up.[4] The overarching objective of prenatal care is to promote the health and well-being not only of the pregnant woman, fetus, and newborn, but also the family. Hence, the breadth of prenatal care does not end with delivery but rather includes preconception care, postpartum care, and up to 1 year after the infant's birth.[3] Importantly, this introduces the concept of interconception care, and the notion that almost all health care interactions with reproductive-age women are opportunities to assess risk, promote healthy lifestyle behaviors, and identify, treat, and optimize medical and psychosocial issues that could affect pregnancy.

Prenatal care is an excellent example of preventive medicine. In 1929, the Ministry of Health of Great Britain issued a memorandum on the conduct of prenatal clinics. In 1942, vitamin tablets were provided for all British women in the last 6 months of pregnancy. United Kingdom maternal mortality rate declined from 319 per 100,000 live births in 1936 to 15 per 100,000 live births in 1985. In the United States, the maternal mortality rate was 13.2 per

100,000 live births in 1999.[4] The decline in maternal mortality rate was partly attributed to prenatal care and partly to medical and public policy advances such as maternal mortality reviews with attention to preventable causes of maternal death, shift to hospital births, improvements in anesthesia, widespread availability of blood transfusions, antibiotics, and access to safe and legal abortion services. Recent guidelines addressing the content and efficacy of prenatal care have focused on the medical, psychosocial, and educational aspects of the prenatal care system. Prenatal care satisfies the definition of primary care from the Institute of Medicine as "integrated, accessible health care services by clinicians who are accountable for addressing a large majority of personal health care needs, developing a sustained partnership with patients, and practicing in the context of family and community." In fact, prenatal care services can be used by obstetricians/gynecologists and other primary care providers as a general model for primary care. Prenatal care satisfies other criteria for primary care in that it is comprehensive and continuous, and provides coordinated health care. Preconception care—planning to ensure the healthiest possible pregnancy outcome—is consistent with this model. We will further argue that the preconception and prenatal care periods—just as labor, delivery, the puerperium, and postgestation and interconceptional periods—must be seen as episodes in a woman's life and that they provide important opportunities to advance wellness and prevention. It must be recognized that for pregnant women all these events are part of a life continuum with birth leading to the multiple challenges of parenting. They are opportunities to introduce and reinforce habits, knowledge, and life-long skills in self-care, health education, and wellness, to inculcate principles of routine screening, immunization, and regular assessment for psychological, behavioral, and medical risk factors.[1,5] Phelan argues that clinicians are not taking advantage of pregnancy as a "teachable moment"—a naturally occurring life transition that motivates people to spontaneously adopt risk-reducing behaviors.[6] Pregnancy qualifies as a teachable moment because it meets the following criteria proposed by McBride and colleagues[7]:

- There is increased perception of personal risk and outcome expectancies.
- The perceptions are associated with strong affective or emotional responses.
- The event is associated with a redefinition of self-concept or social role.

The goal of prenatal care is to help the mother maintain her well-being and achieve a healthy outcome for herself and her infant. Education about pregnancy, childbearing, and childrearing is an important part of prenatal care, as are detection and treatment of abnormalities. This process is best realized when begun even before pregnancy. Many services provided traditionally during the intrapartum hospital stay will be provided at prenatal and postpartum outpatient visits.[8] Too often, hospitalization for childbirth has been seen as an opportunity for education about self-care, child care and parenthood rather than as a time to ensure safe passage. Educational interventions have been targeted for the intrapartum stay, when they can better and more cheaply be performed in the preconceptional, antenatal, or home care environment.[8-10] However, more recently, contemporary models of prenatal and childbirth education have been criticized because research has not shown a strong association between class attendance and childbirth experiences or parenting expectations. In fact, among first-time mothers, there has been a decline in childbirth class attendance from 70% in 2002 to 56% in 2005.[11,12]

MATERNAL MORTALITY

Maternal and neonatal mortality rates are the most widely used indicators of the health of a nation. Maternal death is the demise of any woman from any pregnancy-related cause while pregnant or within 42 days of termination of pregnancy, irrespective of the duration and the site of pregnancy. A direct maternal death is an obstetrical death resulting from obstetrical complications of the pregnancy state, labor, or puerperium. An indirect maternal death is an obstetrical death resulting from a disease previously existing or developing during the pregnancy, labor, or puerperium; death is not directly due to obstetrical causes but may be aggravated by the physiologic effects of pregnancy. A nonmaternal death is an obstetrical death resulting from accidental or incidental causes unrelated to the pregnancy or its management.

The maternal mortality rate is the number of maternal deaths (direct, indirect, or nonmaternal) per 100,000 women of reproductive age but, since this denominator is difficult to determine precisely, most clinical and research entities use the maternal mortality ratio defined as the number of maternal deaths (indirect and direct) per 100,000 live births.

Direct obstetrical deaths have six major causes: hypertensive diseases of pregnancy, hemorrhage, infections/sepsis, thromboembolism, and, in developing countries, obstructed labor and complications from illegal abortion. There are other direct causes of death, such as ectopic pregnancy, complications of anesthesia, and amniotic fluid embolism. The main causes of indirect obstetrical deaths are asthma, heart disease, type 1 diabetes, systemic lupus erythematosus, and other conditions that are aggravated by pregnancy to the point of death.

Maternal mortality has been an underrecognized issue worldwide despite an estimated 600,000 maternal deaths per year from pregnancy-related causes.[13] Put in numerical perspective, this is equivalent to six jumbo jet crashes per day with the deaths of all 250 passengers on board, all of them women in the reproductive years of life. Or, put in a time perspective, every minute of every day a woman dies from pregnancy-related causes.[14] There is also a marked inequity in geographic distribution, because 95% of these deaths occur in developing countries (Figure 6-1). Maternal mortality is the health indicator with the greatest disparity between wealthy and poor countries (and wealthy and poor women in developed countries). Maternal mortality is highest in Africa, Asia, Latin America, and the Caribbean.[15] The World Health Organization estimates that over 80% of maternal deaths could be prevented through actions that have been proven to be effective and affordable. Specifically, providing maternal health services defined as trained birth attendants, aseptic birth environments, identification

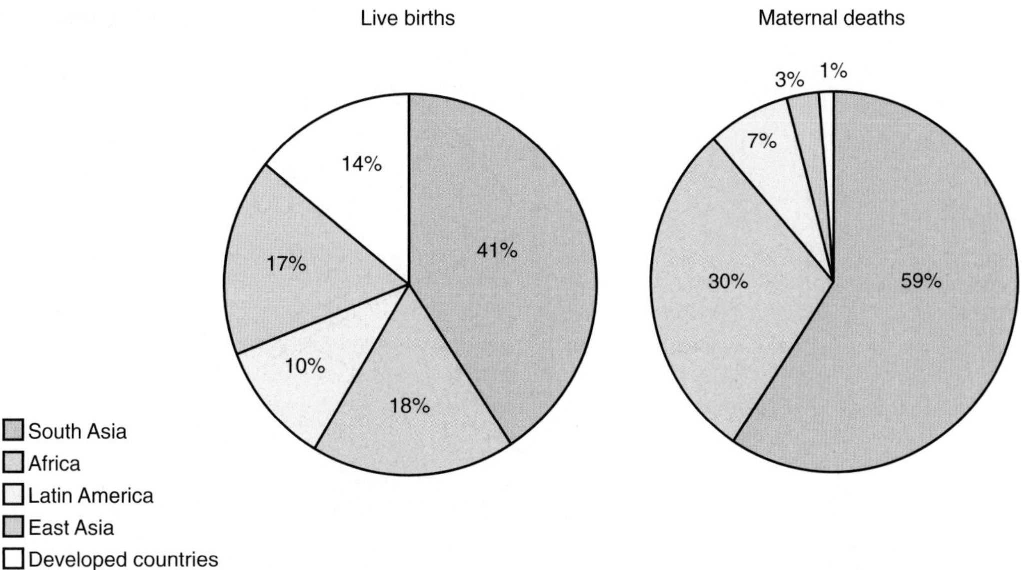

FIGURE 6-1. Worldwide distribution of live births and maternal deaths by region. (From WHO 861663.)

of maternal/fetal/neonatal complications, and transport to a higher level of care when indicated.[14,16] Even in developed countries, the changing demographic profile of childbearing women (e.g., older women and/or women with chronic medical conditions) has contributed to an increase in maternal mortality, and many argue that these too are preventable—requiring rapid recognition and response to treatable emergency conditions.[14] Worldwide, we are far from achieving the international Safe Motherhood goal of reducing maternal mortality by 50%.[16] **Similarly, nationwide, the Centers for Disease Control and Prevention (CDC) reported a maternal mortality rate of 12.1 per 100,000, indicating we have not achieved the *Healthy People 2010* goal of 3.3 per 100,000 and emphasizing that it will take an integrated, multifaceted, multidisciplinary public health approach to achieve these goals for 2020.**[17,18]

The CDC and the American Congress of Obstetricians and Gynecologists (ACOG) have introduced the concept that *pregnancy-associated mortality* is defined as death of a woman, from any cause, while pregnant, or within 1 year of termination of pregnancy.[19] Unfortunately, the United States is seeing an increase in nonmaternal deaths of pregnant women resulting from trauma and violence, many of these related to illegal drugs (Figure 6-2).

In North Carolina from 1992 to 1994, 167 deaths of pregnant and postpartum women were identified through an enhanced surveillance system. When all deaths of pregnant women were categorized, direct and indirect obstetrical deaths (classically defined maternal deaths) accounted for only 37% of deaths of pregnant and postpartum women. Injuries accounted for 38% of deaths with homicide being the most common (36%), followed by motor vehicle accidents (32%), drug-related death (13%), other (11%), and suicide (8%). Acceptance of pregnancy-associated mortality as the appropriate measure will lead to increased recognition of these important problems. The prenatal care provider can play a role in preventing these common causes of death in women by advocating use of seat belts and screening for alcohol use, drug use, depression, and violence.

Significant disparities exist between the maternal mortality rates of white and black women. In the United States, maternal mortality occurs four times more often in black women than in white women. In a *Morbidity and Mortality Weekly Report* review of maternal deaths from 1991 to 1999, the pregnancy-related mortality rate for white women was 8.1; for black women it was 30. On a state-by-state basis, maternal mortality rates for black women were higher in every state.[20,21] Many of the tenets espoused to bring about safe motherhood internationally could arguably be applicable to help understand and eradicate the maternal health disparities seen in poor urban and rural environments in the United States. Specifically, they are health education and promotion, identification of maternal/fetal/neonatal complications, transport to a higher level of care, and rapid responses to acute obstetrical emergencies. For example, one study demonstrated an inverse relationship between the maternal mortality rate and the state density of maternal-fetal medicine specialists after controlling for state-level measures of maternal poverty, education, race, age, and interactions.[22] Similarly, regionalization of perinatal services has been a cornerstone for improved neonatal outcomes.[23]

Last, although much attention has been focused nationally and internationally on maternal mortality, perhaps of greater concern is the less well documented prevalence of maternal morbidity, or "near misses," defined as "pregnant women with severe life-threatening conditions who nearly die but, with good luck or good care, survive." Wen and colleagues found that the overall rate of severe maternal morbidity was 4.4 per 1000 deliveries, but many believe it is significantly underreported.[24] Severe morbidity was defined as thromboembolism, eclampsia, pulmonary, cardiac or central nervous system complications of anesthesia, cerebrovascular disorders, uterine rupture, acute respiratory distress syndrome, pulmonary edema, myocardial

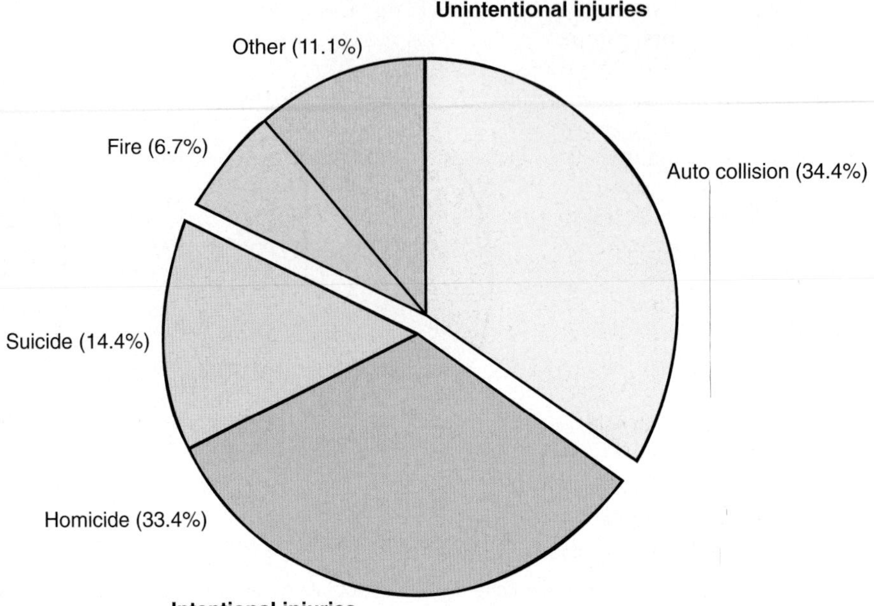

FIGURE 6-2. Distribution of deaths due to injury in the United States, 1980-1985 ($N = 90$). (From MMWR Morb Mortal Wkly Rep 37[SS5]:26, 1988.)

infarction, acute renal failure associated with delivery, cardiac arrest, severe postpartum hemorrhage requiring hysterectomy, and assisted ventilation. Rates of venous thromboembolism, uterine rupture, acute respiratory distress syndrome, pulmonary edema, myocardial infarction, severe postpartum hemorrhage requiring hysterectomy, and assisted ventilation all appear to be increasing in incidence since 1991.[24] The concept of "near misses" and rates of adverse pregnancy-related complications have taken on new significance as payers and providers look for ways to demonstrate safety and quality in health care systems.

Finally, presence of preexisting chronic conditions (e.g., systemic lupus, cystic fibrosis, chronic renal disease, hypertension, diabetes, pulmonary hypertension, and congenital, rheumatic, and ischemic heart disease) also appears to be increasing among pregnant women, and this is significant since the presence of preexisting conditions increases the risk of both maternal morbidity (sixfold increase) and mortality (158-fold increase).[24-27]

NEONATAL MORTALITY AND MORBIDITY

Historically, in developed countries, when decreased maternal mortality was achieved, attention was then turned to infant mortality, and then neonatal mortality and later fetal mortality. The stillbirth rate (fetal death rate) is the number of stillborn infants per 1000 infants born. The neonatal mortality rate is the number of neonatal deaths (deaths in the first 28 days of life) per 1000 live births. The perinatal mortality combines these two—the number of fetal deaths (stillbirths) plus neonatal deaths per 1000 total births.

In 1990, the U.S. infant mortality rate was 9.2 per 1000 live births, ranking the United States 19th internationally.[13] However, there are international differences in the way live births are classified, as some countries exclude infants weighing less than 1 kg and those with fatal anomalies. Final vital statistics data for 2005 indicate that the United States met the *Healthy People 2000* goal of decreasing the infant mortality rate to 7 per 1000 live births, but has not met the 2010/2020 goal of 4.5 per 1000 live births.[17,28] Infant mortality varies by maternal demographic and health characteristics. Rates are higher in the extreme reproductive ages (teens and over 40 years old). Other maternal characteristics associated with increased risk for infant mortality include unmarried, poorly educated, little or no prenatal care, smoking, or illicit substance use. Pregnancy-related complications include but are not limited to multiple births and preterm delivery. There are significant racial differences in infant mortality, with African Americans having a 2.5-fold increased risk.[28] Infant mortality rates in Hispanics are comparable to those of Caucasians; however, variation exists between country of origin and amount of acculturation.

PRENATAL CARE

Historically, the primary goal of prenatal care was to minimize maternal and neonatal mortality. During the past 40 years, new technology has been introduced to assess the fetus antepartum, including electronic fetal monitoring, sonography, amniocentesis, and other in utero interventions, with the fetus emerging as a patient in utero. Prevention of morbidity as well as mortality is now the goal. This has made the task of the prenatal care more complex, since mother and fetus now require an increasingly sophisticated level of care. At the same time, pregnancy is basically a physiologic process, and the normal pregnant patient may not benefit from application of advanced technology.

Prenatal care is provided at a variety of sites, ranging from the private office, to the public health and county hospital clinics, to the patient's home. Obstetricians must optimize their efforts by resourceful use of other professionals and support groups, including nutritionists, childbirth educators, public health nurses, nurse practitioners, family physicians, nurse-midwives, and specialty medical consultants. Most pregnant women are healthy, with normal pregnancies, and can be followed by an obstetrical team including nurses, nurse practitioners, and nurse-midwives, with an obstetrician available for consultation. These women can be followed by practitioners who have adequate time to spend on patient education and parenting preparation, while physicians can appropriately concentrate on complicated problems requiring their medical skills. This also provides for improved continuity of care, which is recognized as extremely important for patient satisfaction.[29,30]

There have been no prospective controlled trials demonstrating efficacy of prenatal care overall. Two documents addressing the content and efficacy of prenatal care have suggested changes in the current prenatal care system.[2,29-34] Since publication of these recommendations, several well-designed randomized clinical trials and cost-benefit analyses have been reported using alternative visit schedules[33,34] (Table 6-1). There was no difference in outcomes for patients undergoing reduced frequency of visits as measured by rates of preterm birth and low birth weight, and the reduced frequency model has been shown to be cost-effective. However, fewer visits have been associated with decreased maternal satisfaction with care, as well as increased maternal anxiety.[33,34] Some studies support the concept of reduced antenatal visits for selected women.[10,33,34]

Efficacy of prenatal care also depends on the quality of care provided by the caretaker. If a blood pressure is recorded as elevated and no therapeutic maneuvers are recommended, this will not change the outcome. Recommendations must be made and must be carried out by the patient, whose compliance is essential to alter outcome. Kogan and colleagues,[35] using national survey data, reported that women received only 56% of the procedures and 32% of the advice recommended as part of prenatal care content, and that poor women and African American women received fewer of the recommended interventions. Site of care was also an important determinant, suggesting that infrastructure must be geared to address population-specific needs.[35]

RISK ASSESSMENT

The concept of risk in obstetrics can be examined at many levels. All the problems that arise in pregnancy, whether common complaints or more hazardous diseases, convey some risk to the pregnancy, depending on how they are managed by the patient and her care provider. Risk assessment has received detailed attention in the past. It has been shown that most women and infants suffering morbidity and mortality will come from a small segment of women with high-risk factors; by reassessing risk factors before pregnancy, during pregnancy, and again in labor, our ability to identify those at highest risk increases. Most of the emphasis for screening, risk assessment, and associated trials for therapeutic interventions have focused primarily on preeclampsia and preterm birth prevention; Table 6-2 lists representative examples of other clinical conditions that have been proposed to be included as part of routine screening and/or risk assessment during the antepartum period since 1989. Many of these conditions are part of current routine screening programs, but few were implemented as routine care as a result of evidence-based criteria. Most have been implemented as a result of expert or consensus opinion, cost/benefit, and/or risk management decisions. Still others have yet to be commonly accepted and await definitive research trials demonstrating efficacy as a screening test, or more importantly, effective treatment options. For example, cervical length assessment and fetal fibronectin evaluation have been proposed to assess risk of prematurity (see Chapter 28), yet definitive trials proving effectiveness of screening and efficacy of treatment have yet to be done.

TABLE 6-1 COMPARISON OF DIFFERENT RECOMMENDATIONS REGARDING VISIT FREQUENCY AND PROPOSED CLINICAL INTERVENTIONS FOR PRENATAL CARE FOR LOW-RISK WOMEN

WEEKS' GESTATION	ACOG 1997	EXPERT PANEL NULLIPAROUS WOMAN	EXPERT PANEL MULTIPAROUS WOMAN	CLINICAL INTERVENTION
1-4		X	X	Preconception Dating
5-8	X	X	X	Dating
9-12	X	X		*
13-16	X	X	X	*
17-20	X			AFP/multiple marker screening*
21-24	X			
25-28	X	X	X	Glucose tolerance test
31-32	X	X	X	Childbirth education Risk assessment
35-36	X	X	X	Risk assessment Growth
37	X	X		Risk assessment
38	X	X		Risk assessment
39	X			
40	X	X		Risk assessment
41	X	X	X	Post term evaluation

Modified from Gregory KD, Davidson E: Prenatal care: who needs it and why? Clin Obstet Gynecol 42(4):725, 1999.

*Current standard of care would likely include offering first trimester screening and/or some multiple marker screening strategy (integrated or sequential) in the second trimester.

TABLE 6-2 EXAMPLES OF CLINICAL CONDITIONS AMENABLE TO ANTENATAL SCREENING AND/OR RISK ASSESSMENT

Clinical Condition SCREENING/DIAGNOSTIC TEST	COMMENT	REFERENCE
Postdates/Multiple Gestation/IUGR		
Early ultrasound	Increased precision of dating; "routine" use unclear benefit yet widely used over 80% of pregnancies	85, 87, 89
IUGR		
Fundal height	Increased identification of small and large infants; fewer ultrasounds, economic benefit	84, 86
Smoking history	Smoking has demonstrated dose-response association with poor fetal growth; smoking cessation/ reduction reverses growth disturbance; likelihood of cessation increased during pregnancy	29, 31, 32, 100-103
Fetal Structural Malformation		
Ultrasound Maternal serum AFP Drug exposure	Ultrasound, MSAFP standard of care for screening for neural tube defects. See text re: prenatal genetic test	104
Fetal Chromosomal Aberrations		
Multiple marker screening	Combination of specific maternal serum analytes used to screen for Down syndrome, trisomies 13 and 18, with potential detection rate of 60%-90% when used with targeted ultrasound, see text	23, 105
Genetic Conditions		
Cystic fibrosis	Recommended by ACOG	24
Canavan's disease, "Jewish panel"	Recommended by ACOG	106
Preterm Birth (PTB)		
Cervical length	No benefit from routine screening; unclear "best practice" and/or benefit of treatment once identified "at risk"	17, 18, 107, 108
Fetal fibronectin	No clear benefit as screening test to predict PTB (poor sensitivity and specificity); potential benefit from high negative predictive value	107, 109
Periodontal disease	May be independent risk factor for PTB; treatment reduced risk	19
Bacterial vaginosis	Independent risk factor for PTB; inconclusive if treatment alters risk but shown to be beneficial in selected populations	110-116
Preeclampsia		
Uterine Doppler	No effective prevention	15, 85
Serum markers	Nonspecific; no effective prevention	16, 94, 117
Thromboembolic Disease		
Pregnancy history Clinical history Laboratory evaluation for hereditary thrombophilias	Clinically relevant topic due to association with adverse pregnancy outcome; potential for life-threatening thromboembolic event; disseminating into practice; inconclusive data re: treatment efficacy	78
Infections		
Group B streptococcus	Screening and treatment prevents neonatal disease	118
HIV	Routine screening and treatment recommended by ACOG; treatment significantly decreases rate of perinatal transmission	119, 120
Bacterial vaginosis	See PTB	121
Psychosocial Risk		
Demographics	Socioeconomic status, race/ethnicity related to PTB, adverse pregnancy outcomes; not mutable	122-124
Cocaine use	Associated with structural malformations, PTB, abruptions, preeclampsia; comprehensive care deters use	30
Depression		
Screening instruments	Risk/benefit decision re: treatment—not contraindicated; increased likelihood of relapse in postpartum period; related to infection, child development	125
Domestic Abuse		
Screening instruments	Increased likelihood of abuse during pregnancy in women in abusive environment	126

It is important to individualize patient care and to be thorough. The initial visit will include a detailed history and physical and laboratory examinations. The initial history requires that the patient be seen in an office setting. Ideally, she should not be first seen undressed sitting on an examining table.

PRECONCEPTIONAL EDUCATION

We have reached a level of awareness about prenatal care at which the optimal time to assess, manage, and treat many pregnancy conditions and complications is before pregnancy occurs.[36,37] Recognizing that half of pregnancies are unplanned, all reproductive-age women should be asked about their plans for pregnancy at routine gynecologic visits or health maintenance examinations. At that time, much of the risk assessment described later in this chapter can be performed, as well as the basic physical and laboratory evaluations. If there are questions about the history, such as family history of fetal anomaly, or previous cesarean delivery, further details can be obtained from family members or the appropriate medical facility. This is the time to draw a rubella titer and immunize the susceptible patient. Hepatitis B immunization can be given to appropriate patients and human immunodeficiency virus (HIV) testing offered. Varicella titers or immunization is recommended in women with no history of chickenpox. Patients need to use contraception for up to 3 months following immunizations (see Chapter 50). Toxoplasmosis screening based on risk factors may be indicated at this time because approximately one fourth of the U.S. population is infected.[37] Patients who have negative screens are at risk for congenital toxoplasmosis and should be counseled to avoid risks such as contact with wild felines and ingestion of raw or undercooked meat. Immunocompetent patients who screen positive can be reassured of lack of risk with regard to fetal loss or stillbirth, although rare reports of congenital infection after previous infection have been described. A prospective analysis of the population risks and benefits to substantiate routine screening for and/or education about toxoplasmosis has not been done in the United States. However, proponents argue a theoretical benefit based on treatment availability, extrapolated epidemiologic data from European countries where screening is widespread, and the prevalence of congenital infection that is comparable to other congenital diseases that we currently screen for by mandate (e.g., phenylketonuria, congenital hypothyroidism).

Before pregnancy is the time to screen appropriate populations for genetic disease carrier states such as Tay-Sachs disease, Canavan's disease, cystic fibrosis, or hemoglobinopathies. Resolution of these issues is much easier and less hurried without the time limits placed by an advancing pregnancy. Medical conditions such as anemia, hypothyroidism, hypertension, and diabetes can be fully evaluated and medical treatment can be optimized before pregnancy. If the patient is obese, weight reduction should be attempted before pregnancy. The value of prepregnancy counseling needs to be emphasized to all those who treat women at significant risk for pregnancy problems. Women who are followed by other physicians (family physicians, pediatricians, general internists) for such problems as diabetes, hypertension, or systemic lupus erythematosus should be seen, evaluated, and counseled before pregnancy. Patients in whom risks are very serious are potentially at risk for progressive disease, end-organ damage, or death and should be so counseled, and every attempt should be made to let them make a fully informed decision about pregnancy. Often, significant risk factors can be treated or managed so as to reduce risk during pregnancy.

There is evidence that for some conditions, such as diabetes mellitus and phenylketonuria, medical disease management before conception can positively influence pregnancy outcome. Medical management to normalize the biochemical environment should be discussed with the patient and appropriate management plans outlined before conception. This is also the time to review drug usage and other practices such as alcohol ingestion and smoking (see Chapter 8). Advice can be given about avoiding specific medications in the first trimester (e.g., isotretinoin), and general advice can be given concerning diet, exercise, and occupational exposures.

Periconceptional supplements with folic acid can reduce the incidence of neural tube defects (NTDs) and the use of therapeutic doses to decrease the risk of recurrence has been repeatedly demonstrated. This has resulted in national regulatory mandates for food supplements and national media campaigns to increase public awareness about the importance of this practice. **The CDC recommends that all women of childbearing age who are capable of becoming pregnant should consume 0.4 mg of folic acid daily, which is most easily achieved by taking a supplement. For women with a previously affected child, the recommendation is that the patient take 4 mg daily from 4 weeks before conception through the first 3 months of pregnancy.** The benefits of folic acid supplementation are being investigated with regard to the prevention of other complications of pregnancy, as well as chronic maternal disease states (e.g., preterm birth, cardiac disease), further emphasizing the appropriateness of prenatal care as both a model for primary care and a model for the provision of care in the context of a life span approach. Care provided at each visit affects not only pregnancy outcome, but ultimately long-term health outcomes for the woman and her family.

The importance of seeking care early for confirmation of pregnancy and gestational age dating can be discussed with the patient. Great precision can be achieved with an accurate menstrual calendar predating pregnancy and provide an opportunity for access to first trimester screening for aneuploidy and to prevent ambiguity about postdatism.

THE INITIAL PRECONCEPTIONAL OR PRENATAL VISIT

Social and Demographic Risks

Extremes of age are obstetrical risk factors. The pregnant teenager has particular nutritional and emotional needs. She is at special risk for sexually transmitted diseases; it has been shown that she benefits particularly from education in areas of childbearing and contraception. The pregnant woman over age 35 is at increased risk for a chromosomally abnormal child. Patients should be asked about family histories of Down syndrome, NTDs, hemophilia, hemoglobinopathies, and other birth defects, as well as mental retardation (see Chapter 10). Consultation for genetic counseling and genetic testing, if desired, may be appropriate. Women over 35 are at increased risk for almost all pregnancy-related morbidities, maternal mortality, and neonatal complications, including miscarriage, stillbirth, preterm birth, and neonatal mortality. The age of the father is also important, as there may be genetic risks to the fetus when the father is older than 55 years. Certain diseases may be related to race/ethnicity or geographic origin. Patients of African, Asian, or Mediterranean descent should be screened for the various heritable hemoglobinopathies (sickle cell disease, alpha and beta thalassemia). Patients of Jewish and French Canadian heritage should be screened for Tay-Sachs disease, Canavan's disease, and cystic fibrosis. More recently, it has been suggested that cystic fibrosis screening be offered to all couples planning a pregnancy or seeking prenatal testing.

Low socioeconomic status should be identified and attempts to improve nutritional and hygienic measures undertaken. Appropriate referral to federal programs, such as that for women, infants, and children (WIC), and to public health nurses can have real benefits. If a patient has a history of previous neonatal death, stillbirth, or preterm birth, records should be carefully reviewed so that the correct diagnosis is made and recurrence risk appropriately assessed. A history of drug abuse or recent blood transfusion should be elicited. The history of medical illnesses should be detailed and records obtained if possible. A rapid procedure for diagnosing mental disorders in primary care may be useful in pregnancy.[38] If appropriate, patients should be screened and treated for depression.

Occupational hazards should be identified. If a patient works in a laboratory with chemicals, for example, she should be advised to identify potential reproductive toxins and limit her exposure. This is an active area of research and there are several online resources for information about potential environmental and occupational teratogens.[39] Patients whose occupations require heavy physical exercise or excess stress should be informed that they may need to decrease such activity later in pregnancy as both have been associated with increased risk of preterm birth and reduced fetal growth in observational studies.[40]

Tobacco, alcohol, and recreational drug use can all adversely affect pregnancy and questions regarding information about their use are a critical part of the history. Specific questions concerning smoking, alcohol, and drugs (prescriptive, over-the-counter, and illicit) should be asked. Regular screening for alcohol and substance use should be carried out using such tools as the T-ACE questionnaire (see Chapter 8) or other simple screening tools, and appropriate directed therapy should be made available to those women who screen positive. Women should be urged to stop smoking before pregnancy and to drink not at all or minimally once they are pregnant. Studies show that smoking cessation counseling by the health care provider works. Pregnancy is an ideal time to initiate this intervention.[41] Drug addiction confers a particularly high risk, and addicted mothers require specialized care throughout pregnancy (see Chapter 8). Discussions about caffeine use should also be addressed, as caffeine is addictive, associated with withdrawal symptoms, and relatively ubiquitous. It is present in coffee, tea, cocoa, cola drinks and other carbonated sodas, chocolate, "energy drinks," and many over-the-counter headache, cold, and flu treatments, as well as diet pills and prescription medications. The average cup of instant or brewed coffee contains 90 to 130 mg of caffeine. High-end coffee from select coffee houses can approach 250 mg.[42] A recent study sponsored by the ACOG suggests that there is considerable variation in assessment and advice related to caffeine consumption in pregnant or reproductive-age women. In a self-reported survey, Anderson and colleagues[42] found that most clinicians did not know the caffeine content of common beverages and were not familiar with scientific data suggesting adverse reproductive consequence. Due to hormonal influences, caffeine metabolism slows during second and third trimester of pregnancy. It crosses the placenta and is distributed to all fetal tissues. Due to immature liver systems, caffeine metabolism is slow in fetuses and neonates, with an extremely long reported half-life ranging from 80 to 100 hours.[43] ACOG[44] concluded that moderate caffeine consumption (less than 200 mg/day) does not appear to be a major contributing factor in miscarriage or preterm birth although a conclusion cannot be made regarding a correlation between higher caffeine intake and miscarriage. The relationship of caffeine to growth restriction is undetermined. **Hence, practice guidelines suggest that pregnant women should be advised to limit their caffeine consumption to 200 mg/day** (2 cups of coffee or cola drinks per day)[43-46] (see Chapter 8).

Violence against women is increasingly recognized as a problem that should be addressed, with reports suggesting that abuse occurs during 3% to 8% of pregnancies. Questions addressing personal safety and violence should be included during the prenatal period, and such tools as the Abuse Assessment Score are recommended.[47] It consists of five questions that assess the pregnant woman's history of abuse (emotional, physical, and sexual). It asks if a woman has ever experienced abuse in her lifetime by a partner or someone close to her and then focuses on questions regarding abuse during the current pregnancy. For example, in cases in which women did experience abuse during their pregnancy, they are asked to "score" each incident according to a scale provided, ranging from mild threats to the dangerous use of a weapon or wound from a weapon.

Medical Risk

Family history of diabetes, hypertension, tuberculosis, seizures, hematologic disorders, multiple pregnancies, congenital abnormalities, and reproductive wastage should be elicited. Often, a family history of mental retardation, birth defect, or genetic trait is difficult to elicit without formal genetic counseling or questionnaires; nonetheless, these areas should be emphasized at the initial history. A better history may be obtained if patients are asked to fill out a preinterview questionnaire or history form. Any significant maternal cardiovascular, renal, or metabolic disease should be defined. Infectious diseases such as urinary tract disease, syphilis, tuberculosis, or herpes genitalis should be identified. Surgical history with special attention to any abdominal or pelvic operations should be noted. A history of previous cesarean birth should include indication, type of uterine incision, and any complications. A copy of the surgical report may be informative. Allergies, particularly drug allergies, should be prominent on the problem list.

Hyperthyroidism

Neonatal hyperthyroidism is rare, with an incidence of 1:4000 to 1:40,000 live births. Fetal thyrotoxic goiter is usually secondary to maternal autoimmune disease, most commonly Graves disease or Hashimoto's thyroiditis (see Chapter 40). As many as 12% of infants of mothers with a known history of Graves disease are affected with neonatal thyrotoxicosis. This can occur even if the mother is euthyroid. The underlying mechanism is transplacental passage of maternal IgG antibodies. These antibodies, known as thyroid-stimulating antibody or thyroid-stimulating immunoglobulin, are predominantly directed against the thyroid-stimulating hormone (TSH) receptor. Often fetal goiter is diagnosed on ultrasound in pregnancies in which the mother has elevated thyroid-stimulating antibodies. In some cases, fetal goiters are incidentally detected on routine ultrasonography. In still others, detection follows scan for polyhydramnios. Untreated fetal hyperthyroidism may be associated with a mortality rate of 12% to 25% owing to high-output cardiac failure.

Hypothyroidism

Congenital hypothyroidism is relatively rare, affecting about 1:3000 to 1:4000 infants. About 85% of the cases are the result of thyroid dysgenesis, a heterogenous group of developmental defects characterized by inadequate thyroid tissue. Congenital hypothyroidism is only rarely associated with errors of thyroid hormone synthesis, TSH insensitivity, or absence of the pituitary gland. Congenital hypothyroidism presenting with a goiter is observed in only about 10% to 15% of cases.

Fetal goiterous hypothyroidism also follows maternal exposure to thyrostatic agents such as propylthiouracil and radioactive iodine-131 used to treat maternal hyperthyroidism. Maternal ingestion of amiodarone or lithium may also cause hypothyroidism in the fetus. Fetal hypothyroidism may also follow transplacental passage of maternal blocking antibodies (known as TBIAb or TBII). Rarely, defects in fetal thyroid hormone biosynthesis may exist.

An enlarged fetal goiter may cause esophageal obstruction and polyhydramnios, leading to preterm delivery or premature rupture of membranes. A goiter may even lead to high-output fetal heart failure. A large fetal goiter can also cause extension of the fetal neck, leading to dystocia. Fetal hypothyroidism itself may be devastating, and without treatment, postnatal growth delay and severe mental retardation ensue. Even with immediate diagnosis and treatment at birth, children with congenital hypothyroidism demonstrate lower scores on long-term perceptual-motor, visuospatial, and language tests.

Obstetrical Risk

Previous obstetrical and reproductive history is essential to optimizing care in subsequent pregnancies. The gravidity and parity should be noted and the outcome for each prior pregnancy recorded in detail. Previous miscarriages (and documentation about the gestational age at the time of the loss) not only confer risk and anxiety for another pregnancy loss but can be associated with an increased risk for genetic disease, as well as preterm delivery.

Previous preterm delivery is strongly associated with recurrence; it is important to delineate the events surrounding the preterm birth. Did the membranes rupture before labor? Were there painful uterine contractions? Was there bleeding? Were there fetal abnormalities? What was the neonatal outcome? All these questions are vital in determining the etiology and prognosis of the condition, although specific recommendations will vary and the efficacy of routine prevention programs is not clear. In patients with a previous premature delivery, after preterm labor or premature rupture of membranes, progesterone administration reduces the recurrence risk.[48,49] Diethylstilbestrol (DES) exposure, incompetent cervix, and uterine anomalies are all conditions that may be known from a previous pregnancy. Previous fetal macrosomia makes glucose screening essential.

After all the specific questions, it is recommended to ask the patient a few simple questions: What important items haven't I asked? What else about you and your pregnancy do I need to know? What problems and questions do you have? Leaving time for open-ended questions is the best way to complete the initial visit.

Physical and Laboratory Evaluation

Physical examination should include a general physical examination, as well as a pelvic examination. Baseline height and weight and prepregnancy weight are recorded. Special attention should be given to the initial vital signs and cardiac examination, because many healthy young women have not had a physical examination immediately before becoming pregnant. Any physical finding that might have an impact on pregnancy or that might be affected by pregnancy should be defined. It is particularly important to perform and record a complete physical examination at this initial visit, because less emphasis will be placed on nonobstetrical portions of the examination as pregnancy progresses in the absence of specific problems or complaints.

The pelvic examination should focus on the uterine size. Before 12 to 14 weeks, size can give a fairly accurate estimate of gestational age in a thin patient. Papanicolaou smear and culture for gonorrhea and chlamydia are done. Bacterial vaginosis should be recognized. The cervix should be carefully palpated, and any deviation from normal should be noted. Clinical pelvimetry should be performed and the clinical impression of adequacy noted. The pelvic examination is limited by examiner and patient variation, as well as by obesity. If there is difficulty in examining the uterus, an ultrasound study is indicated.

Basic laboratory studies are routinely performed (see Table 6-2). Some studies need not be repeated if recent normal values have been obtained, such as at a preconceptional visit or a recent gynecologic or infertility examination. Blood studies should include Rh type and screening for irregular antibodies, hemoglobin level, or hematocrit and serologic tests for syphilis and rubella. A urine sample should be obtained and tested for abnormal protein and glucose levels. Screening for asymptomatic bacteriuria has been traditionally done by urine culture, but screening may be simplified by testing for nitrites and leukocyte esterase.[50] Tuberculosis screening should also be performed in areas of disease prevalence.

First trimester screening, a multiple marker screen, uses sonographic evaluation of nuchal translucency and biochemical markers (PAPP-A and free βhCG) to allow earlier screening for chromosomal aberrations. It is offered between 11 and 14 weeks.[51] The QUAD test (α-fetoprotein, human chorionic gonadotropin [hCG], estriol, and inhibin A) or maternal serum α-fetoprotein screening is offered from 15 to 20 weeks' gestation to screen for NTDs and aneuploidy[52] (see Chapter 10). Patients who undergo first trimester screening require a maternal serum α-fetoprotein level after 15 weeks for NTDs screening. The integrated screen combines first and second trimester screening and gives the result only after the second trimester evaluation is completed.

The laboratory evaluations outlined above are the minimum standard tests. Specific conditions will require further evaluation. A history of thyroid disease will lead to thyroid function testing. Anticonvulsant therapy requires blood level studies to determine adequacy of medication. The importance of compliance with dosing and serial evaluation of serum blood levels should be emphasized as both thyroid medications and anticonvulsant levels are sensitive to the physiologic changes in blood volume that occur during pregnancy. Adequacy of replacement and/or blood levels will need to be monitored throughout pregnancy. Identification of problems on screening (e.g., anemia, abnormal glucose screen) will mandate further testing. Screening for varicella has been suggested for women with no known history of chickenpox. The ACOG has recommended routine screening of all pregnant women for hepatitis B.[53] HIV screening should also be offered, because maternal therapy with antiretroviral agents can reduce vertical transmission (see Chapter 50).[53] Hepatitis C and CMV screening should be considered for at-risk populations. Recommendations for the content of prenatal care are summarized in Table 6-3. Note that these recommendations are drawn from various sources, most are based on expert opinion, and although similar are not entirely in agreement with regard to all recommendations.[54-58]

ASSESSMENT OF GESTATIONAL AGE

During the course of the prenatal interview, assessment of gestational age begins with the question, "What was the first day of the last menstrual period?" From that point, the establishment of an estimated date of delivery and confirmation of that date by accumulation of supportive information remains one of the most important tasks of good prenatal care.

Human pregnancy has a duration of 280 days, measured from the first day of the last menstrual period (LMP) until delivery. The standard deviation is 14 days. It is important to remember that clinicians are measuring menstrual weeks (not conceptional weeks) with an assumption of ovulation and conception based on day 14 of a 28-day cycle. This gives pregnancy the 40-week gestational period in common clinical use. Much confusion exists among patients who try to measure pregnancy in terms of 9 months, when in fact, it is 10 (40/4 = 10), or who try to measure in conceptional weeks. Another problem exists in women whose menstrual cycles do not follow a 28-day cycle and who therefore do not conceive on day 14 of the menstrual cycle. The commonly used term "4 months' pregnant" has no meaning (one does not know whether this is 16 or 20 weeks) and has no place on a contemporary prenatal record. It is often helpful to explain to patients and their families that their pregnancy will be described in terms of weeks, rather than months, and that the pregnancy can be broken into three trimesters lasting 1 to 14 weeks, 14 to 28 weeks, and 28 weeks to delivery. Every effort should be made to be consistent in usage to prevent

TABLE 6-3 RECOMMENDATIONS FOR ALL WOMEN FOR PRENATAL CARE

PRECONCEPTION OR FIRST VISIT		WEEKS								
		6-8*	14-16	24-28	32	36	38	39	40	41
History										
Medical, including genetic	X									
Psychosocial	X									
Update medical and psychosocial		X	X	X	X	X	X	X	X	X
Physical examination										
General	X									
Blood pressure	X	X	X	X	X	X	X	X	X	X
Height	X									
Weight	X	X	X	X	X	X	X	X	X	X
Height and weight profile	X									
Pelvic examination and pelvimetry	X	X								
Breast examination	X	X								
Fundal height			X	X	X	X	X	X	X	X
Fetal position and heart rate			X	X	X	X	X	X	X	X
Cervical examination	X									
Laboratory tests										
Hemoglobin or hematocrit	X	X		X		X				
Rh factor, type blood	X									
Antibody screen	X			X						
Pap smear	X									
Diabetic screen				X						
MSAFP			X							
Urine										
• Dipstick	X									
• Protein	X									
• Sugar	X									
• Culture		X								
Infections										
Rubella titer	X									
Syphilis test	X									
Gonococcal culture	X	X				X				
Hepatitis B	X									
HIV (offered)	X	X								
Toxoplasmosis	X									
Illicit drug screen (offered)	X									
Genetic screen	X									

*If preconception care has preceded.
HIV, Human immunodeficiency virus; *MSAFP*, maternal serum α-fetoprotein.

confusion among patients and among clinicians who may assume care of the pregnancy.

Knowledge of gestational age is critical for obstetrical decision making. Generally, in a normal pregnancy, we can extrapolate from gestational age to estimate fetal weight. Throughout pregnancy, these are the two most important determinants of fetal viability and survival. Without accurate knowledge of gestational age, diagnosis of such conditions as postterm pregnancy and intrauterine growth restriction is often impossible. Multiple gestation is most often detected early when the size of the uterine fundus is greater than expected for gestation. Appropriate management of preterm labor or a medically complicated pregnancy depends on an accurate estimate of fetal age and weight. Within regional perinatal systems, records of gestational age are important for flow of information, and rapid access to consistent, clear data is vital. In such situations, and during prolonged hospitalization, it is sometimes helpful to define gestational age further by using the notation of fractional weeks ($27^4/_7$ weeks). It must be remembered, however, that we are describing a biologic system and that such precision is being used more for ease of communication and organization than for any ability to date the pregnancy with such a degree of accuracy.

Clinical Dating

Historically, the most reliable clinical estimator of gestational age is an accurate LMP. Using Naegele's rule, the estimated date of delivery is calculated by subtracting 3 months and adding 1 week from the first day of the LMP. A careful history must be taken from the patient verifying that the date given is the first day of the period, as well as whether the period was normal, heavy, or light. The date of the previous menstrual period will help ascertain the length of the cycle. History should also be taken about previous use of oral contraceptives, which might influence ovulation.

Other clinical tools can be used to confirm and support LMP data and, in cases in which the LMP is inaccurate or unknown, it has been shown that accumulated clinical information from early pregnancy can predict gestational age with an accuracy approaching that of menstrual dating.

The size of the uterus on early pelvic examination, or by direct measurement of the abdomen from the pubic symphysis to the top of the uterine fundus (over the curve), provides useful information. Experienced practitioners can assess the early pregnancy with reproducibility before 12 to 14 weeks. Fundal height measurement in centimeters using the over-the-curve technique approximates the gestational age from 16 to 38 weeks within 3 cm in non-obese patients.

The uterus also tends to reach the umbilicus at about 20 weeks, and this too can be assessed when uterine fundal measurements are made. The uterus may be elevated in early pregnancy in a patient with a previous cesarean delivery or with uterine myomas, making the fundal height appear abnormally high. Considerable variations in the level of the umbilicus and in the height of patients make this clinical marker variable. Quickening, the first perception of fetal movement by the mother, occurs at predictable times in gestation. In the first pregnancy, quickening is usually noted at about 19 weeks; in subsequent pregnancies, probably because of the experience of the observer, it tends to occur about 2 weeks earlier. It is helpful to ask the woman to mark on a calendar the first time she feels the baby move and to report this date.

Audible fetal heart tones, in addition to being absolute evidence of pregnancy, are another marker of gestational age. Using an unamplified Hillis-DeLee fetoscope, they are generally audible at 19 to 20 weeks. Observer experience, acuity, and the time spent listening can all affect this number, so this guideline may need to be adapted individually.

Use of the electronic Doppler device is widespread and permits detection of the fetal heart by 11 to 12 weeks. Practitioners can set a standard individualized to their own equipment, which can be used as a gestational age marker. If fetal heart tones are not heard at the expected time, a sonogram is appropriate to look for date/examination discrepancy, fetal viability, twins, or polyhydramnios.

The conversion of a negative urinary pregnancy test to a positive one may be helpful in assessing gestational age, but the sensitivity of the test used must be known in order to interpret the data accurately. These tests may be negative if they are performed too early.

Comparison of the various clinical estimators shows a known LMP date to be the most precise predictor. The clinical estimators can be ranked according to decreasing order of accuracy as follows: (1) last menstrual period; (2) the uterus reaching umbilicus; and (3) fetal heart tone documentation, fundal height measurements, and quickening. Because of inherent biologic variability and differences in the examiner acuity, the estimated date of confinement can be predicted with 90% certainty only within ±3 weeks by even the best single estimator.

Ultrasound

Ultrasound plays a major role in assessment of size and duration of pregnancy. The National Institutes of Health (NIH) consensus conference in 1984 concluded that in a low-risk pregnancy followed from the first trimester, routine ultrasound examination was not justified for determining gestational age. However, a long list of indications justify an ultrasound examination and studies on resource utilization indicate that at least 70% of women receive an ultrasound at some point in their pregnancy, and, importantly, women have come to expect an ultrasound as part of standard prenatal care. **With the advent of first trimester screening including nuchal translucency measurement, many women are receiving first trimester ultrasounds, and ultrasound is an accurate means of estimating gestational age in the first half of pregnancy.** The crown-rump length, biparietal diameter, and femur length in the first half of pregnancy correlate closely with age. As pregnancy progresses, fetal size varies considerably, and measurement of the fetus is a less reliable tool for estimation of gestational age, especially in the third trimester.

Recognizing that most women are receiving ultrasounds at some time in their pregnancy, the following question arises: What should be done if there is a discrepancy in the clinical dates (based on LMP) and the ultrasound dates? If ultrasound differs more than 7 days from LMP during the first trimester, or more than 10 days between 12 and 20 weeks' gestation, change the estimated due date to the ultrasound date.[59] Issues arise when the patient is late to care and there is a size/date discrepancy. In general, one can assume an 8% margin of error in the ultrasound (measured in days).[60] Hunter[61] advocates using the "rule of 8's" in this special circumstance. Calculate the difference in dates using days based on LMP and ultrasound. Then multiply the LMP days by 0.08 (margin of error). If the difference is greater than 0.08, use the ultrasound date; if it is less than 0.08, use the LMP dates.[61] It would be prudent to follow up with an interval growth scan to evaluate for growth abnormalities.

Although the benefits of routine ultrasound are widely debated, a randomized trial has shown that the risk of being called overdue was reduced from 8% to 2% for patients who received early ultrasound.[62] Also, twins were detected more often and perinatal mortality was reduced in the ultrasound group. The Routine Antenatal Diagnostic Imaging with Ultrasound (RADIUS) study reported no improvement in perinatal outcome with use of routine ultrasound in normal, low-risk women.[63] However, 61% of women were excluded for many reasons such as an uncertain menstrual history, and only 35% of anomalies were detected in the ultrasound-screened group (only 17% before 24 weeks). The meta-analysis by Bucher and Schmidt indicated that routine scanning can detect many more anomalies. The authors' practice is to perform ultrasound in the first trimester for women requesting integrated serum marker screening or if heart tones are not heard by Doppler by 11 weeks. We screen for fetal abnormality or multiple gestation at 18 to 20 weeks. If ultrasound is not done routinely, the caregiver must be vigilant in detecting problems that are indications for a scan.

REPEAT PRENATAL VISITS

A plan of visits is outlined to the patient. Traditionally, this has been every 4 weeks for the first 28 weeks of pregnancy, every 2 to 3 weeks until 36 weeks, and weekly thereafter, if the pregnancy progresses normally. The Public Health Service suggested that this number of visits can be decreased, especially in parous, healthy women, and studies suggest that this can be done safely[64] (see Table 6-1). If there are any complications, the intervals can be increased appropriately. For example, patients with hypertensive disease or at risk for preterm delivery may require weekly visits. Fetal heart tones can be documented before the 12th week by Doppler devices, and this information can be used for gestational dating purposes.

At regular visits, the patient is weighed, the blood pressure is recorded, and the presence of edema is evaluated (see Intercurrent Problems, following). Fundal height is regularly measured with a tape measure, fetal heart tones are recorded, and fetal position is noted. The goal of subsequent pregnancy visits is to assess fetal growth and maternal well-being. In addition, at each prenatal visit, time should be allowed for the following questions: Do you have any problems? Do you have any questions? Family members should be encouraged to come to prenatal visits, ask questions, and participate to the degree that the patient wishes.

A pelvic examination is usually only performed on the first visit. In patients at risk of prematurity or in those with a history of DES exposure, however, frequent cervical checks or sonographic evaluation of cervical length may reveal premature dilation or effacement.

Further laboratory evaluations are routinely performed at 28 weeks, when the hemoglobin or hematocrit and Rh type and the screen for antibodies, as well as the serologic test for syphilis and possibly HIV testing, can be repeated. If the patient is Rh negative and unsensitized, she should receive Rhesus immune globulin (RhIG) prophylaxis at this time. A glucose screening test for diabetes is also appropriately performed at this time (see Chapter 39), and routine fetal movement counting can begin using an organized system. At 36 weeks, a repeat hematocrit, especially in those women with anemia or at risk for peripartum hemorrhage (multipara, repeat cesarean), may be performed. GBS screening should be done at 35 to 37 weeks and results made available for possible intrapartum prophylaxis. Also, appropriate cultures for sexually transmitted disease (gonorrhea, chlamydia) should be obtained as indicated in the third trimester based on geographic prevalence rates and demographic risk factors.

After 41 weeks from the last menstrual period, the patient should be entered into a screening program for fetal well-being, including electronic monitoring tests and ultrasound evaluation, or offered induction of labor if the dating is accurate (see Chapter 34).

INTERCURRENT PROBLEMS

It is the practice in prenatal care to evaluate the pregnant patient for the development of certain complications. Inherent in these checks is surveillance for intervening problems, an important one being preeclampsia. If a patient shows a blood pressure elevation at 28 weeks, for example, she should be seen again in a week, not a month. Blood pressure will change physiologically in response to pregnancy, but development of hypertension must be recognized and evaluation and hospitalization appropriately instituted.

Weight gain and obesity in pregnancy have been shown to be important predictors of pregnancy outcome. Weight gain is an important correlate of fetal weight gain and is therefore closely monitored. Too little weight gain should lead to an evaluation of nutritional factors and an assessment of associated fetal growth. Excess weight gain is one of the first signs of fluid retention, but it may also reflect increased dietary intake or decreased activity. Sixty-five percent of Americans are overweight (body mass index [BMI] $\geq$25 kg/m^2) or obese (BMI $\geq$30 kg/m^2).[65] Compared to women with normal weight, pregnant obese women are at increased risk of miscarriage, gestational diabetes, preeclampsia, venous thromboembolism, induced labor, cesarean delivery, anesthetic complication, and wound infections. Obese women are less likely to initiate or maintain breastfeeding. Babies of obese mothers are at increased risk of stillbirth, congenital anomalies, prematurity, macrosomia, and neonatal death.[66] Furthermore, weight gain, and weight retention after pregnancy, is a risk factor for subsequent obesity.[6,67] Thus, postpartum weight loss should be encouraged. A study by Rooney and Schauberger[68] demonstrated that women who resumed their prepregnancy weight by 6 months postpartum gained only

2.4 kg over the next 10 years as compared 8.3 kg for women who retained weight after delivery. Whereas clinicians have been inundated with teaching women that appropriate weight gain is important for pregnancy, the concomitant importance of postpartum weight loss has not been given equal attention.[6,12,69] Likewise, interventions and public education based on this knowledge have been poorly addressed. In fact, studies suggest that prenatal care providers are not addressing diet, weight gain, or physical activity, or are giving incorrect advice.[70] Factors that contribute to excessive weight gain during pregnancy include high fat, low fiber intake, high carbohydrate or sugar intake, and decreased physical activity during pregnancy.[71] Several small studies suggest that monitoring weight gain, quantity of food intake, and physical activity, combined with behavioral counseling, can limit weight gain during pregnancy and promote postpartum weight loss. However, larger randomized trials are needed to demonstrate long-term effectiveness.[66,67]

Dependent edema is physiologic in pregnancy, but generalized or facial edema can be a first sign of disease. It is critical here, as in all areas, for the practitioner to understand the normal changes associated with pregnancy not only to accept and explain the normal changes, but also to manage aggressively any abnormal changes.

Proteinuria reflects urinary tract disease, generally either infection or glomerular dysfunction, possibly the result of preeclampsia. Urinary tract infection should be looked for, and the degree of protein quantitated in a 24-hour urine collection.

Glycosuria is common because of increased glucose filtered through the kidney in pregnancy, but warrants evaluation for diabetes with a measurement of capillary glucose when clinical suspicion exists.

Fetal abnormalities are often first detected by deviation from the clinical expectation. In some conditions, risk of fetal anomaly will be so high as to prompt some kind of baseline screening or testing (e.g., amniocentesis, sonography, fetal echocardiography). At other times, risk only becomes evident during the course of prenatal care. Growth restriction and macrosomia can often be suspected clinically, usually on the basis of an abnormality in fundal growth. For the patient who has a history of these conditions or other predisposing factors, such as hypertension, renal disease, or diabetes, particular vigilance is in order. Excess amniotic fluid is another condition that can be clinically detected, and an etiology for the hydramnios should be sought. In addition to maternal conditions, hydramnios may be caused by fetal disease that can also be defined using sonography and that may alter management of the pregnancy.

THE PRENATAL RECORD

The prenatal care record describes in a consistent fashion the comprehensive care that is provided and allows for documentation of coordinated services. Prenatal care should be documented by a prenatal record of good quality designed to systematically capture important clinical and psychosocial information over time. One such example is the antepartum record designed by ACOG. Many of the advances in risk assessment and in regionalization result directly from an improvement in this record and electronic medical records (EMRs) are being developed.[72] Technology allows sophisticated recording, display, and retrieval (often computer-based) of prenatal care records, but quality relies on accurate, consistent compiling and concurrent recording of the information. The record must be complete, yet simple; directive, but flexible; and transmittable, legible, and able to display necessary data rapidly. European nations often have one record for uniform care; many states and regions have adopted records to permit internal consistency.

The commonly used records accurately reflect the following:

1. Demographic data, obstetrical history
2. Medical and family history, including genetic screening
3. Baseline physical examination, with emphasis on gynecologic examination
4. Menstrual history, especially last normal menstrual period with documentation of established due date and reference criteria for dating if other than LMP
5. Record of individual visits
6. Routine laboratory data (e.g., Rh, GBS, rapid plasma reagin (RPR), rubella, hepatitis, and HIV)
7. Problem list
8. Space for special notations and plans (e.g., planned VBAC or repeat cesarean, tubal ligation)

These records must be made available to consultants, and they should be available at the facility where delivery is planned. If transfer is expected, a copy of the prenatal record should accompany the patient.

PRENATAL EDUCATION

Patient education leads to better self-care. As maternal and neonatal outcomes improve, efforts become more sophisticated to improve understanding, involvement, and satisfaction with pregnancy and the perinatal period. In this area, more than any other, the options for paramedical support have expanded. Practitioners and patients have access to a vast array of support persons and groups to assist and advise in the pregnancy and subsequent parenthood. Group prenatal care has recently been proposed and evaluated. The wise practitioner stays abreast of these advances and integrates them into practice. Patients should be educated about care options and participate in decision making. Although not exhaustive, the following section includes common issues or concerns that practitioners should address at some point during successive prenatal visits as part of their health education, promotion, and prevention goals with each patient.

Informed Consent and VBAC

During the educational components of prenatal care there is significant opportunity to accomplish most if not all the informed consent required for the delivery process. There are also advantages to securing documentation of appropriate informed consent for management of labor and associated obstetrical procedures, possible interventions, and risks and benefits when they can be thoroughly reviewed and discussed rather than in the throes of labor. It is our practice to obtain consent, whenever possible, in the third trimester for "delivery and related procedures including IV fluids, fetal monitoring, labor augmentation, episiotomy, operative vaginal delivery including forceps and vacuum, and cesarean delivery," and this is documented on institutional consent forms and signed by the patient. Consent for anesthesia can also be obtained before admission. Risks such as third- and fourth-degree lacerations with episiotomy and operative delivery are appropriate to discuss, as well as the benefits of birth spacing and contraceptive options. Maternal, newborn, and familial benefits have been associated with optimal birth spacing—estimated to be approximately 2 to 5 years. Short pregnancy intervals are associated with increased low birth weight, preterm birth, and other adverse pregnancy outcomes attributed to decreased maternal reserves, whereas prolonged birth spacing has been associated with increased risk of breast cancer, preeclampsia, and stillbirths. The benefits of intermediate birth spacing needs to be emphasized by health care practitioners and more widely disseminated. It is associated with improved maternal health (decreased risk of uterine rupture, endometritis, antepartum bleeding, anemia, depression), improved child health (decreased childhood illnesses, injuries, death, improved education), and improved family health, functioning, and socioeconomic status.[73,74] Although contraceptive options are numerous, tubal ligation is the most common method in the United States. If tubal ligation is offered, the risks, benefits, and alternatives of postpartum versus interval ligation should be discussed.

The special benefits and risks of vaginal birth after cesarean section are particularly important to discuss before labor, and it is common to document both the components of the informed consent process and the patient's choice with respect to route of delivery.

Smoking Cessation

Smoking has a demonstrated dose-response relationship to impaired fetal growth. Smoking cessation or reduction can reverse this growth disturbance. The likelihood of interventions to stop or reduce smoking are increased during pregnancy. Every effort should be made to identify prepregnancy and pregnant smokers and provide both pharmacologic and psychosocial interventions and programs to maximize likelihood of smoking cessation (see Chapter 8).

Drugs and Teratogens

At the preconceptional or first prenatal visit, recommendations for nonpharmacologic remedies for common ailments can be given. This can often be integrated into a discussion of the common side effects of pregnancy. Because of widespread use of over-the-counter drugs, the patient should be warned to take only those drugs specifically approved or prescribed by her practitioner (see Chapter 8). Likewise, the patient should be advised to inform her practitioner about all natural or herbal supplements that are being used. Practitioners should be aware of current studies estimating that roughly 40% to 87% of women have used complementary and alternative medicines (including herbal therapy).[75]

Radiologic Studies

Elective radiologic studies can safely be delayed until completion of the pregnancy; however, dental and radiologic diagnostic procedures should be performed during pregnancy when they are indicated with proper shielding of the abdomen. Tests to evaluate life-threatening events such as thromboembolic phenomenon, or as needed for trauma evaluation, particularly should not be deferred as this could put the mother's health at undue risk. Judicious use of pulmonary perfusion scans, spiral computed tomography (CT), and magnetic resonance imaging (MRI) have been life-saving for pregnant women with minimal radiation exposure risks. Dental restorative work especially should be performed to allow optimal maternal nutrition (see Chapter 8).

Nutrition

One of the earliest purposes of prenatal care was to counsel and ensure that women received adequate nutrition for pregnancy. The health care provider may be influential in correcting inappropriate dietary habits. Strict vegetarians may need supplemental vitamin B_{12}. Occasionally, consultation with a registered dietitian may be necessary when there is poor compliance or a special medical need such as diabetes mellitus.

Dietary allowances for most substances increase during pregnancy. According to the 1989 recommended dietary allowances (RDAs), only the recommendations for iron, folic acid, and vitamin D double during gestation.[76] The RDA for calcium and phosphorus increase by half; the RDA for pyridoxine and thiamine increase by about one third. The RDA for protein, zinc, and riboflavin increase by about one fourth. The RDA for all other nutrients except vitamin A increase by less than 20% (Tables 6-4 and 6-5) and vitamin A not at all, as that is believed to be stored adequately. All of these nutrients, with the exception of iron, are supplied by a well-balanced diet.

The National Academy of Sciences currently recommends that 30 mg of ferrous iron supplements be given to pregnant women daily, because the iron content of the habitual American diet and the iron stores of many women are not sufficient to provide the increased iron required during pregnancy. For those at high nutritional risk, such as some adolescents, those with multiple gestation, heavy cigarette smokers, and drug and alcohol abusers, a vitamin/mineral supplement should be given. Increased iron is needed both for the fetal needs and for the increased maternal blood volume. Thus, iron-containing foods should also be encouraged. Iron is found in liver, red meats, eggs, dried beans, leafy green vegetables, whole-grain enriched bread and cereal, and dried fruits. The 30-mg iron supplement is contained in approximately 150 mg of ferrous sulfate, 300 mg of ferrous gluconate, or 100 mg of ferrous fumarate. Taking iron between meals on an empty stomach will facilitate its absorption.

Because women of higher socioeconomic status have better reproductive performance and fewer low-birth-weight babies than do women of lower socioeconomic status, and because they also consume more protein, it is probably prudent to continue to recommend a generous amount of dietary protein. However, protein supplementation does not improve pregnancy outcome. Acute caloric restriction in a well-nourished population such as occurred during the Dutch famine of 1944 to 1945 caused the average birth weight to drop about 250 g, yet no adverse effect on long-term outcome was observed. These mothers

TABLE 6-4 RECOMMENDED DIETARY ALLOWANCES

	NONPREGNANT WOMEN				LACTATION (MONTHS)	
	15-18	**19-24**	**25-50**	**PREGNANCY**	**1-6**	**7-12**
Calories (kcal)						
Protein (g)	1244	1246	250	1260	1265	1262
Vitamin A (mcg RE)	1800	1800	800	1800	1300	1200
Vitamin D (mcg)	1210	1205	1, 25	1210	1210	1210
Vitamin E (mg TE)	1208	1208	1, 28	1210	1212	1211
Vitamin C (mg)	1260	1260	1, 60	1270	1295	1290
Thiamin (mg)	1201.1	1201.1	1, 21.1	1201.5	1201.6	1201.6
Riboflavin (mg)	1201.3	1201.3	1, 21.3	1201.6	1201.8	1201.7
Niacin (mg NE)	1215	1215	1, 15	1217	1220	1220
Vitamin B_6 (mg)	1201.5	1201.6	1, 21.6	1212.2	1202.1	1202.1
Folate (mcg)	1180	1180	180	1400	1280	1260
Vitamin B_{12} (mcg)	1202.0	1202.0	1, 22.0	1202.2	1202.6	1202.6
Calcium (mg)	1200	1200	800	1200	1200	1200
Phosphorus (mg)	1200	1200	800	1200	1200	1200
Magnesium (mg)	1300	1280	280	1320	1355	1340
Iron (mg)	1215	1215	1, 15	1230	1215	1215
Zinc (mg)	1212	1212	1, 12	1215	1219	1216
Iodine (mcg)	1150	1150	150	1175	1200	1200
Selenium (mcg)	1250	1255	1, 55	1265	1275	1275

Data from Spitzer RL, Williams JBW, Kroenke K, et al: Utility of a new procedure for diagnosing mental disorders in primary care. JAMA 272:1749, 1994.

TABLE 6-5 SUMMARY OF RECOMMENDED DIETARY ALLOWANCES FOR WOMEN AGED ≥25-50 YEARS, CHANGES FROM NONPREGNANT TO PREGNANT, AND FOOD SOURCES

NUTRIENT	NONPREGNANT	PREGNANT	PERCENT INCREASE	DIETARY SOURCES
Energy (kcal)	2200.6	2500.6	+13.6	Proteins, carbohydrates, fats
Protein (g)	2250.6	2560.6	+20.6	Meats, fish, poultry, dairy
Calcium (mg)	2800.6	1200.6	+50.6	Dairy products
Phosphorus (mg)	2800.6	1200.6	+50.6	Meats
Magnesium (mg)	2280.6	1320.6	+14.3	Seafood, legumes, grains
Iron (mg)	2215.6	1230.6	+100.6	Meats, eggs, grains
Zinc (mg)	2212.6	2515.6	+25.6	Meats, seafood, eggs
Iodine (mcg)	1150.6	1175.6	+16.7	Iodized salt, seafood
Vitamin A (mcg RE)	1800.6	1800.6	+100.6	Dark green, yellow, or orange fruits and vegetables, liver
Vitamin D (IU)	1200.6	1400.6	+100.6	Fortified dairy products
Thiamin (mg)	1201.2	1201.5	+36.3	Enriched grains, pork
Riboflavin (mg)	1201.3	1201.6	+23.2	Meats, liver, enriched grains
Pyridoxine (mg)	1201.6	1202.2	+37.5	Meats, liver, enriched grains
Niacin (mg NE)	1215.2	1217.2	+13.3	Meats, nuts, legumes
Vitamin B_{12} (mcg)	2202.0	2202.2	+10.2	Meats
Folic acid (mcg)	2180.2	2400.2	+122.2	Leafy vegetables, liver
Vitamin C (mg)	2260.2	2270.2	+16.7	Citrus fruits, tomatoes
Selenium (mcg)	2255.2	2265.2	+18.2	

From National Academy of Sciences: Recommended Dietary Allowances, ed 10. Washington, DC, National Academy Press, 1989.

ate a calorie-restricted, balanced diet in their second and third trimesters.

Weight Gain

The total weight gain recommended in pregnancy is 25 to 35 lb for normal women.[77] **Underweight women may gain up to 40 lb, and overweight women should limit weight gain to 15 lb, although they do not need to gain any weight if they are morbidly obese.**[78] About 2 to 3 lb are from increased fluid volume, 3 to 4 lb from increased blood volume, 1 to 2 lb from breast enlargement, 2 lb from enlargement of the uterus, and 2 lb from amniotic fluid. At term, the infant weighs approximately 6 to 8 lb and the placenta 1 to 2 lb. A 4- to 6-lb increase in maternal stores of fat and protein is important for lactation. Usually, 3 to 6 lb are gained in the first trimester and ½ to 1 lb per week in the last two trimesters of pregnancy.

If the patient does not show a 10-lb weight gain by midpregnancy, her nutritional status should be reviewed, unless she is obese. Inadequate weight gain is associated with an increased risk of a low-birth-weight infant (Figure 6-3). Inadequate weight gain seems to have its greatest effect in women who are low or normal weight before pregnancy. Underweight mothers must gain more weight during pregnancy to produce infants of normal weight. Patients should be cautioned against weight loss during pregnancy.

When excess weight gain is noted, patients should be counseled to avoid high fat, high carbohydrate, or sugar intake, and to increase their physical activity. Rapid weight

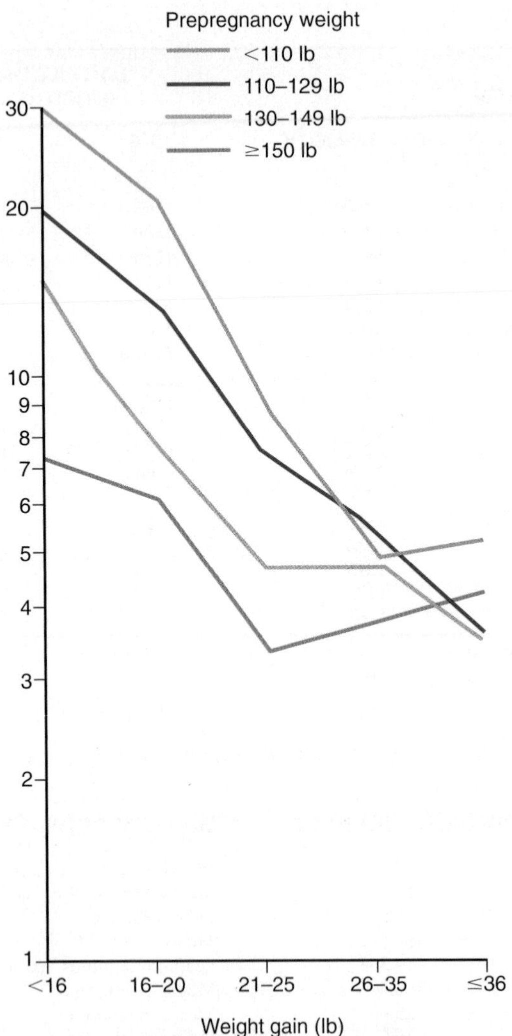

FIGURE 6-3. Percentage of live-born infants of low birth weight by maternal weight gain during pregnancy according to the mother's prepregnancy weight. *Low birth weight* is defined as birth weight of less than 2500 g or 5 lb, 8 oz. (From the National Natality Survey—United States. DHHS Pub No. [PHS] 86-1922, 1980.)

gain requires an assessment for fluid retention. In the assessment of edema, some dependent edema in the legs is normal as pregnancy advances because of venous compression by the weight of the uterus. Elevation of the feet and bedrest on the left side will help correct this problem. Turning the patient from her back to her left side increases venous return from the legs as the pressure on the vena cava is relieved. This maneuver increases the effective circulating blood volume, cardiac output, and thus the blood flow to the kidney. A diuresis will follow, as well as increased blood flow to the uterus.

Limitation of fluids will neither prevent nor correct fluid retention. Salt is not restricted, although patients with hypertension may be advised to decrease salt load.

Activity and Employment

Most patients are able to maintain their normal activity levels in pregnancy. Mothers tolerate pregnancy with considerable physical activity, such as looking after small children, but heavy lifting and excessive physical activity should be avoided. Modification of activity level as the pregnancy progresses is seldom needed, except if the job involves physical danger. Recreational exercises should be encouraged, such as those available in prenatal exercise classes. Unfortunately, many women are routinely told to decrease their physical activity, but research on moderate aerobic activity shows no negative impact on pregnancy outcomes. In the absence of medical or obstetrical complications, current ACOG recommendations advocate for 30 minutes (or more) of moderate exercise daily.[79] A Cochrane review of aerobic exercise in pregnancy indicated improved maternal fitness, but insufficient evidence to determine if there are maternal or neonatal risks or benefits.[40]

Previously sedentary women with no medical contraindications can start with 15 minutes of continuous exercise three times per week and work toward a goal of 30 minutes four times per week. With regard to exercise intensity, a good rule of thumb is the "talk test." If a pregnant, exercising woman cannot maintain a conversation (perceived moderate intensity), she is probably overexercising. Studies suggest that women who engage in regular recreational activity have less gestational diabetes, less preeclampsia, and less low back pain/pelvic pain.[79] The patient should be counseled to discontinue activity whenever she experiences discomfort.

Healthy pregnant women may work until their delivery, if the job presents hazards no greater than those encountered in daily life. Strenuous physical exercise, standing for prolonged periods, and work on industrial machines, as well as other adverse environmental factors, may be associated with increased risk of poor pregnancy outcome, and these should be modified as necessary.[79]

Travel

A pregnant woman should be advised against prolonged sitting during car or airplane travel because of the risk of venous stasis and possible thromboembolism. The usual recommendation is a maximum of 6 hours per day driving, stopping at least every 2 hours for 10 minutes to allow the patient to walk around and increase venous return from the legs. Hydration and support stockings are also recommended.

The patient should be instructed to wear her seat belt during car travel, but under the abdomen as pregnancy advances. It may also be helpful to take pillows along in a car to increase comfort. If the patient is traveling a significant distance, it might be helpful for her to carry a copy of her medical record with her in case an emergency arises in a strange environment. She should also become familiar with the medical facilities in the area or perhaps obtain the name of an obstetrician in the event of a problem.

Immunizations

Because of a theoretical risk to the fetus, pregnant women or women likely to become pregnant should not be given live, attenuated-virus vaccines. Influenza vaccination should be given during flu season.[80] Yellow fever and oral polio may be given to women exposed to these infections. Despite theoretical risks, no evidence of congenital rubella syndrome in infants born to mothers inadvertently given rubella vaccine has been reported. Measles, mumps, and rubella viruses are not transmitted by those immunized and can be given to children of pregnant women. There is no evidence of fetal risk from inactivated virus vaccines, bacterial vaccines, toxoids, or tetanus immunoglobulin, which should be administered if appropriate. Postdelivery rubella and varicella vaccinations should be encouraged as this remains a substantial missed opportunity. Tdap is given postpartum if the patient has not received it previously, regardless of the interval since the last Td (see Chapter 22).

Nausea and Vomiting in Pregnancy

Nausea and vomiting is a common symptom of pregnancy affecting approximately 75% of pregnancies.[81,82] Hyperemesis gravidarum is an extreme form characterized by unexplained vomiting, dehydration, and weight loss and frequently results in hospitalization.[81] The exact etiology of hyperemesis gravidarum is unknown, but is believed to be related to a product of the placenta, and its occurrence is correlated with human chorionic gonadotropin (hCG) and estradiol concentration. Twin and sibling studies suggest there may be a genetic component.[81] Epidemiologic risk factors include younger age, low prepregnancy body mass, female fetus, and a history of motion sickness or migraines.[81,82] Smoking and obesity are associated with decreased risk of hyperemesis.[81,83] If hyperemesis gravidarum occurs in a first pregnancy, the recurrence risk is approximately 15%, although this can be reduced by a change in paternity.[81,82]

Women with hyperemesis gravidarum can have transient laboratory abnormalities including suppressed TSH or elevated free thyroxine. They can also have elevated liver enzymes, bilirubin, amylase, lipase, and altered electrolytes (loss of sodium, potassium, and chloride).[84] Women with severe hyperemesis can develop rare, severe complications such as Wernicke's encephalopathy, beriberi, central pontine myelinolysis, peripheral neuropathy, hepatic failure, or renal failure. Similarly, severe retching has been associated with Mallory-Weiss tears, esophageal rupture, pneumomediastinum, and retinal detachment.[81]

Fetal effects of hyperemesis gravidarum are unclear. In general, if the problem is corrected or resolves and the patient is able to gain weight, there are no consequences. However, if the woman has poor weight gain (fewer than 15 lb), the fetus is at increased risk for low birth weight and preterm birth.[85]

Treatment of hyperemesis gravidarum is primarily symptomatic. There is no evidence to support an ideal diet in these cases, but women are frequently advised to eat small meals that favor protein over carbohydrates and liquids over solids.[86] **Women admitted to the hospital typically require IV hydration, and most recommend initial supplementation with thiamine (100 mg) for 3 days to prevent the possibility of Wernicke's encephalopathy.**[81,82] Three randomized controlled trials suggest a benefit of vitamin B_6 in reducing nausea.[87] If symptoms persist, adding an antihistamine may be beneficial.[88] In additional to antihistamines, benzamides, phenothiazines, butyrophenones, type 3 serotonin receptor antagonists, and corticosteroids have all been used in the treatment of hyperemesis. Although anecdotally successful, the evidence of efficacy from randomized trials is inconclusive.[81,82] This is important to consider given that some of the agents can cause adverse reactions including but not limited to extrapyramidal symptoms, anxiety, and depression. Alternative therapies that have been described with variable success include acupuncture and acupressure.[81,82] Ginger has been shown in two randomized placebo-controlled trials to be effective.[89,90]

In rare instances, patients do not respond to treatment, are unable to tolerate oral intake, and are unable to maintain or continue to lose weight. These patients may benefit from enteral or parenteral nutrition although significant complications have been described with parenteral nutrition, including infection, thrombophlebitis, and death from infection or pericardial tamponade.[81] A recent study by Holmgren and colleagues[91] described maternal and neonatal outcomes from 94 patients admitted with hyperemesis gravidarum and treated with medication only as compared to nasogastric tube or peripherally inserted central catheter (PICC). They found no difference in neonatal gestational age, mean birth weight, or Apgar scores, but found an increased risk of NICU admission in the PICC line group (9.1% vs. 4.1% or 0%). Of patients managed with medication, 7% (3/42) had an adverse reaction from the medication that resolved after treatment, whereas 11% (2/19) of patients had the nasogastric tube dislodged, and 66% (21/33) of patients with a PICC line required treatment for infection, thromboembolism, or both. Based on their findings, and those of others, the authors suggested that PICC lines should be avoided.[91]

Finally, there are patients who fail treatment and opt to terminate pregnancy. The exact incidence is unknown. However, a Web-based survey of over 800 women who agreed to be part of a hyperemesis gravidarum registry noted that 15% had at least one termination and 6% had more than one termination as a direct or indirect result of severe hyperemesis gravidarum. These women felt they were too sick to care for their family or themselves or they were concerned about the potential adverse consequences of hyperemesis gravidarum on their baby. Further, these women indicated that health care providers were uncaring or did not appear to understand or acknowledge how sick they were, suggesting that further education within the medical community about the physical and psychological burden of hyperemesis gravidarum is needed.[92]

Heartburn

Heartburn is a common complaint in pregnancy because of relaxation of the esophageal sphincter. Overeating contributes to this problem. The patient should be advised to save part of her meal for later if she is experiencing postprandial heartburn and also not to eat immediately before lying down. Pillows at bedtime may help. If necessary, antacids may be prescribed. Liquid antacids coat the esophageal lining more effectively than do tablets. In a subset of patients, H-2 blockers may be helpful (see Chapter 8).

Restless Legs Syndrome

About 1 in 10 women will develop restless legs syndrome (RLS) during the second half of pregnancy. RLS usually occurs as women fall asleep and is characterized by tingling or other uncomfortable sensations in the lower legs, resulting in the overwhelming urge to move the legs. Unfortunately, movement, walking around, or other measures do not relieve RLS. Iron deficiency anemia has been associated with an increased chance of RLS, and in anemic women, iron supplementation may reduce leg restlessness. Avoiding caffeine-containing drinks such as coffee, tea, or sodas in the last half of the day should also be recommended, as caffeine may increase symptoms.

Sciatica

Sciatica refers to nerve pain that shoots rapidly down from the buttocks and unilaterally down one leg, usually ending in the foot. True sciatica is rare in pregnancy, affecting only about 1% of pregnancies. True sciatica is caused either by a herniated disc or, less commonly, by uterine pressure on the sciatic nerve. In addition to pain, other signs of nerve compression include numbness in the affected leg. True sciatica should prompt referral to a neurologist or an orthopedic surgeon for further evaluation.

Carpal Tunnel Syndrome

The extra fluid retention of pregnancy can exacerbate carpal tunnel syndrome; higher weight gain during pregnancy is also a risk factor. The most common symptoms of carpal tunnel syndrome are pain and numbness in the thumb, index, and middle fingers and weakness in the muscle that moves the thumb. Between 25% and 50% of pregnant women will notice some symptoms of carpal tunnel syndrome. Treatment during pregnancy is usually limited to supportive measures such as nighttime splinting that may help reduce increased pressure on the nerve that occurs when the wrist is bent; about 80% of women will notice reduction in symptoms with splinting alone. Severe cases of carpal tunnel syndrome can be treated with steroid injections into the area around the carpal tunnel to reduce swelling and inflammation. After delivery, symptoms generally resolve within 4 weeks (see Chapter 46).

Hemorrhoids

Hemorrhoids are varicose veins of the rectum. Because straining during bowel movements contributes to their aggravation, avoidance of constipation is preventive, and prolonged sitting should also be avoided. Hemorrhoids will often regress after delivery but usually will not disappear completely.

Constipation

Constipation is physiologic during pregnancy with decreased bowel transit time, and the stool may be hardened. Dietary modification with increased bulk such as with fresh fruit and vegetables and plenty of water can usually help this problem. Constipation is aggravated by the addition of iron supplementation; if dietary measures are inadequate, patients may require stool softeners. Additional dietary fibers such as Metamucil (psyllium hydrophilic muciloid) or surface-active agents such as Colace (docusate) can be used, if indicated. Laxatives are rarely necessary.

Urinary Frequency and Incontinence

Often during the first 3 months of pregnancy, the growing uterus places increased pressure on the bladder. Urinary frequency usually will improve as the uterus rises out of the pelvis by the second trimester. However, as the head engages near the time of delivery, urinary frequency may return as the head presses against the bladder. About 40% to 50% of women will experience urinary incontinence during their pregnancy. The risk of incontinence of urine is highest in the third trimester. The chances of experiencing incontinence are increased in multiparous women, especially those with a history of incontinence. Incontinence during pregnancy is a risk factor for persistent incontinence. If the patient experiences pain with urination or new-onset incontinence, it is appropriate to check for infection.

Round Ligament Pain

Frequently, patients will notice sharp groin pains caused by spasm of the round ligaments associated with movement. This is more frequently felt on the right side as a result of the usual dextrorotation of the uterus. The pain may be helped by application of local heat such as with hot soaks or a heating pad. Patients may awaken at night with this pain after having suddenly rolled over in their sleep without realizing it. During the daytime, however, modification of activity with gradual rising and sitting down, as well as avoidance of sudden movement, will decrease problems with this type of pain. An elastic four-way stretch can minimize movement of the uterus. Analgesics are rarely necessary.

Syncope

Compression of the veins in the legs from the advancing size of the uterus places patients at risk of venous pooling associated with prolonged standing. This may lead to syncope. Measures to avoid this possibility include wearing support stockings and exercising the calves to increase venous return. In later pregnancy, patients may have problems with supine hypotension, a distinct problem when undergoing a medical evaluation or an ultrasound examination. A left lateral tilt position with wedging below the right hip will help keep the weight of the uterus and fetus off the inferior vena cava.

Backache

Back pain is a common complaint in pregnancy affecting over 50% of women. Numerous physiologic changes of pregnancy likely contribute to the development of back pain, including ligament laxity related to relaxin and estrogen, weight gain, hyperlordosis, and anterior tilt of the pelvis. These altered biomechanics lead to mechanical strain on the lower back. Backache can be prevented to a large degree by avoidance of excessive weight gain, and a regular exercise program before pregnancy. Exercises to strengthen back muscles can also be helpful. Posture is important, and sensible shoes, not high heels, should be worn. Scheduled rest periods with elevation of the feet to flex the hips may be helpful. Other successful treatment modalities that have been described include nonelastic maternity support binders, acupuncture, aquatic exercises, and pharmacologic regimens incorporating acetaminophen, narcotics, prednisone, and rarely antiprostaglandins (if remote from term).

Sexual Activity

No restriction need generally be placed on sexual intercourse. However, the patient should be advised that pregnancy may cause changes in comfort and sexual desire.

Frequently, increased uterine activity is noted after sexual intercourse; it is unclear whether this is due to breast stimulation, female orgasm, or prostaglandins in male ejaculate. Fox and colleagues,[93] in a survey of 425 primiparous women, reported that over 60% of women reported sexual activity in the third trimester and up to one third engaged in sexual activity within 2 days of delivery. Studies suggest that sexual activity during pregnancy is rarely discussed, although most women feel the need to receive more information.[94] For women at risk for preterm labor or with a history of previous pregnancy loss and who note increased uterine activity after sex, use of a condom or avoidance of sexual activity may be recommended.

Circumcision

Newborn circumcision is a widely practiced elective procedure with significant variation by race/ethnicity, geographic region, education level, and religious belief. Although the medical benefits have been widely debated, recent studies suggest that circumcision offers protection against urinary tract infections, some sexually transmitted diseases, HIV transmission, cervical cancer, penile cancer, and phimosis. Despite these findings, the American Academy of Pediatrics (AAP) does not recommend routine neonatal circumcision.[95] Education in good personal foreskin hygiene offers many of the advantages of circumcision without the risks.

Circumcision in the newborn is an elective procedure and should be performed only if the infant is stable and healthy. If performed, the AAP recommends a multifaceted approach to pain management in order to reduce the observed physiologic response to the newborn's pain.[95]

Breastfeeding

Breastfeeding as a public policy has been widely endorsed and supported by the Department of Health and Human Services. *Healthy People 2000 and 2010* called for 50% of mothers to breastfeed for at least 6 months. Hence, during prenatal visits, the patient should be encouraged to breastfeed her infant (see Chapter 23). Human milk is the most appropriate nutrient for human infants and also provides significant immunologic protection against infection. Infants who are breastfed have a lower incidence of infection and require fewer sick child office visits and hospitalizations than do infants who are fed formula exclusively. A myriad of other infant benefits have been reported, including but not limited to decreased incidence of sudden infant death syndrome, diabetes, otitis media, respiratory tract disease, tonsillitis, dental caries, and a host of immunologic-mediated conditions such as rheumatoid arthritis, Crohn's disease, multiple sclerosis, eczema, and allergic reactions. These benefits are greatest if the infant is exclusively breastfed for 6 months and the protection decreases in proportion to the amount of supplementation.

Maternal advantages of lactation include economy, convenience, more rapid involution of the uterus, and natural child spacing. Breastfeeding protects the mother from infections, cancer (breast, endometrial, and ovarian), osteoporosis, diabetes, and rheumatoid arthritis. The reasons a woman decides to bottle-feed should be explored, as they may be based on a misconception. For example, preterm birth and medical problems are usually not contraindications for breastfeeding. Practitioner encouragement, liberal use of lactation consultants, and spouse and peer support will sometimes convince a hesitant mother who may then be able to nurse successfully. The American Dietetic Association recommends exclusive breastfeeding for the first 6 months and breastfeeding with complementary foods for at least 12 months as the ideal feeding pattern for infants. Studies on incidence and duration of breastfeeding indicate that U.S. women fall far short of that. Based on survey data, the United States cites initiation rates ranging from 27% to 70% and only 19% to 33% of women reporting duration of breastfeeding for at least 6 months. Initiation and duration of breastfeeding are widely influenced by age, race/ethnicity, cultural, and peer influences.

Working outside the home need not be a contraindication to breastfeeding. Many women who previously would not have considered nursing an option, such as those with careers, are now finding time to breastfeed their infants. Employer-based lactation support programs have demonstrated prolonged breastfeeding duration, as well as specific employer benefits—mothers of breastfed infants were more productive at work, missed fewer days, and used fewer health care benefits because of child care issues. Women should be aware that alternative ways of breastfeeding can be used to correspond with their work schedules. They can decrease the frequency of lactation to a few times a day in most cases and still continue to nurse. Other women may pump their breasts at work, leaving milk for the child's caretaker during the day and thus providing breast milk to the infant even more frequently. The milk may be collected in containers and, if refrigerated, is safe to use for 24 hours. For a longer duration, the milk should be frozen. Because freezing and thawing destroy the cellular content, fresh milk is preferred.

There is no need for specific nipple preparation during pregnancy. In one study, women prepared one nipple and not the other with a variety of techniques, including massage and breast creams, and found no difference in the two. Soap and drying agents should not be used on the nipples, which should be washed only with water.

Preparation for Childbirth

The introduction of childbirth education and consumerism has had significant impact on the practice of obstetrics. Studies have shown that prepared childbirth education can have a beneficial effect on labor and delivery. Although the education can be transmitted by the obstetrician at the initial visit or over a series of shorter return visits, patients have come to expect more personal involvement than to be given a book or handout to read. The appropriate place for such education has evolved to be a series of planned, structured prenatal education classes taught by informed, qualified individuals. These classes can be given in the physician's office, at the hospital, or in free-standing classes. National organizations such as the Childbirth Education Association and the American Society for Psychoprophylaxis in Obstetrics have recognized the need for such instruction and teach prepared childbirth. There are also advantages to office- and hospital-based programs, if the patient volume permits it, since specifics of management and alternatives offered by that practice or hospital can be discussed in these programs. On the other hand, free-standing classes offer the advantage of open-endedness and of presenting many options to the patient, who can then discuss them with her care provider. Group prenatal care also can apparently serve an important education function. However, attendance at traditional childbirth classes has been waning.[11,12] This has been attributed to various factors such as a growing preference for medicated birth including scheduled inductions and epidurals, increased elective cesareans, and a perception that the content and philosophy of childbirth education classes are not consistent with the changing needs of childbearing women.[11,96] Many advances in family-centered practice (e.g., allowing fathers in the delivery room and operating room) have come from consumer requests and demands. Additional research is needed to understand how clinicians and educators might help inform women and their partners in the current childbirth climate. The prenatal period should be one in which the patient is exposed to information about pregnancy, normal labor and delivery, anesthesia and analgesia, obstetrical complications, and obstetrical operations (e.g., episiotomy, cesarean delivery, and forceps or vacuum delivery). Although the physician, midwife, or childbirth educator is the ideal person to transmit this information, patients have ready access to Internet, media, and peers, all of which can propagate both information and misinformation. Of concern is that many younger women enter pregnancy believing that all technology and medical interventions increase the safety and outcome for both mother and baby.[11]

The primary purpose of childbirth education is to provide the mother with information regarding the range of interventions that could be encountered during childbirth and to empower the patient to participate in shared decision making. Late third trimester is an ideal time to obtain informed consent from the patient for her intrapartum care and management, and to discuss her concerns and preferences about childbirth. A pregnant patient often makes a list of what she would like to discuss with her practitioner in the peripartum period. Thus, the care provider can understand her needs and desires, better address these needs and desires if labor and delivery do not proceed normally or as planned, and explain why certain requests are not possible or reasonable.

Signs of Labor

It is important to instruct the patient about certain warning signs that should trigger a call to her care provider or a visit to the hospital. All women should be informed of what to do if contractions become regular, if rupture of membranes is suspected, or if vaginal bleeding occurs. Patients should be given a number to call where assistance is available 24 hours a day.

Prepared Parenthood and Support Groups

Routine classes on newborn child care and parenting should be part of the prenatal care program. Many parents are completely unprepared for the myriad of changes in their lives, and some idea of what to expect is beneficial. As pregnancy progresses, special needs can arise. Support groups for families with genetic or medical conditions such as Down syndrome, skeletal dysplasias, preterm infants, or maternal support groups for mothers of twins or triplets, and for women who have had cesarean delivery, have all shown that they can meet the special needs of these parents. Unsuccessful pregnancies lead to special problems and needs, for which social workers, clergy, and specialized support groups can be invaluable. Miscarriage, stillbirth, and infant death are particularly devastating events, best managed by a team approach, with special attention to the grieving process. Referral to such groups as Compassionate Friends of Miscarriage, Infant Death, and Stillbirth is recommended. Careful evaluation and follow-up for depression should be part of the routine pregnancy postpartum care.

Postpartum Visit

Most patients should be seen approximately 6 weeks postpartum, sooner for complicated deliveries and/or cesarean deliveries. **The goal of this visit is to evaluate the physical and psychosocial and mental well-being of the mother, provide support and referral for breastfeeding, initiate or encourage compliance with the preferred family planning option, and to initiate preconception care for the next pregnancy.** Current estimates suggest that 82% and 58.5% of commercial and Medicaid enrollees, respectively, obtain a postpartum visit. Data suggest that maternal health after pregnancy is associated with improved child health, and so increasing compliance with postpartum visits has been identified as both a national and an international public health priority.[97-99] Specific attention should be directed toward counseling about weight loss and follow-up for medical complications including heart disease, hypertension, and diabetes (conditions that may have been exacerbated by pregnancy), as well as thyroid disease and epilepsy (conditions in which medication adjustments may be required).

SUMMARY

Prenatal care is effective, if incompletely understood and studied. It provides a model for primary care services for both obstetricians/gynecologists and other primary care providers. It satisfies the Institute of Medicine criteria for primary care, as it is comprehensive and continuous, and provides coordinated services. Preconceptional care has the potential to improve pregnancy outcome if key conditions are recognized and treatment is optimal. Risk assessment, with subsequent elimination or management of risks, health education, advocacy, and disease prevention, as well as appropriate medical management of complications, remain the core of the process. Changes in number of visits and improved understanding of the successful components of prenatal care will improve services and efficiency without altering the substance of what has been developed and achieved. Prenatal care should reinforce the importance of lifelong disease surveillance and prevention, as well as active participation in personal wellness behavior for women and their families. Care providers and patients should embrace pregnancy as a teachable moment and capitalize on the potential to directly improve the health and well-being of the mother, and indirectly improve the health and well-being of the child and family.

KEY POINTS

- Preconception and prenatal care are not only part of the pregnancy continuum that culminates in delivery, the postpartum period, and parenthood, but they should also be considered in the context of women's health throughout the life span. Importantly, this introduces the concept of interconception care—almost all health care interactions with reproductive-age women are opportunities to assess risk, promote healthy lifestyle behaviors, and identify, treat, and optimize medical and psychosocial issues that could affect pregnancy.
- Maternal mortality is the demise of any woman from any pregnancy-related cause while pregnant or within 42 days of termination of a pregnancy. The United States has not met its *Healthy People 2010* goal of 3.3 per 100,000. The current maternal mortality rate is 12.1 per 100,000 and appears to be rising, with significant ethnic disparity.
- Preconception evaluation should include rubella, hepatitis B, and HIV testing. In selected situations, screening should be extended to varicella, toxoplasmosis, tuberculosis, and hepatitis C. Further tests may be indicated depending on historical genetic risk factors identified.
- Preconception supplementation with folic acid can reduce the incidence of NTDs and other defects. All women of childbearing age should consume 0.4 mg of folic acid daily. Women who have had a child previously affected by an NTD should take 4 mg daily from 4 weeks before conception through the first 3 months of pregnancy.
- Tobacco, alcohol, recreational drugs, and even caffeine have been associated with adverse pregnancy outcomes. Women should be urged to stop smoking, avoid alcohol, and limit caffeine to 2 cups of coffee or cola drinks per day (200 mg/day)
- Accurate dating of pregnancy is essential to optimize screening and to minimize unnecessary interventions for management of postdate pregnancies. Ultrasound evaluation between 16 and 20 weeks allows accurate assessment of gestational age and survey for fetal abnormality and multiple gestation.
- A number of multiple marker tests are available for screening for aneuploidy in the first trimester and/or second trimester. Practitioners should be familiar with the various options and offer them to their patients irrespective of maternal age.
- The total weight gain recommended for healthy women is 25 to 35 lb. Underweight women may gain up to 40 lb, and overweight women should limit weight gain to 15 lb. Women should be monitored on overall weight gain and actively encouraged to return to prepregnancy weight during the postpartum period to minimize long-term risk of subsequent obesity.
- Most patients are able to maintain their normal activity levels in pregnancy. Mothers tolerate pregnancy with considerable physical activity, but heavy lifting and excessive physical activity should be avoided.
- The pregnant woman should be advised against prolonged sitting during car or airplane travel because of the risk of venous stasis and possible thromboembolism.
- Women with hyperemesis gravidarum can have transient laboratory abnormalities including suppressed TSH, elevated liver enzymes, bilirubin, amylase, lipase, and altered electrolytes. Treatment of hyperemesis gravidarum is primarily symptomatic. Recent studies suggest increased risks associated with rare cases requiring parenteral treatment.
- Prenatal care should include information on labor, delivery, possible operative procedures, obstetrical analgesia, breastfeeding, postpartum recovery, and contraception.
- For infant nutrition, "breast is best." The Department of Health and Human Services and *Healthy People 2000 and 2010* called for 50% of mothers to breastfeed for at least 6 months. Human milk is the most appropriate nutrient for human infants, providing significant immunologic protection. Infants who are breastfed have a lower incidence of infection and require fewer office visits and hospitalizations than do infants who are fed formula exclusively. Other reported infant benefits include decreased incidence of sudden infant death syndrome, diabetes, otitis media, respiratory tract disease, tonsillitis, dental caries, rheumatoid arthritis, Crohn's disease, multiple sclerosis, eczema, and allergic reactions. Maternal advantages include economy, convenience, more rapid involution of the uterus, and natural child spacing. Breastfeeding protects the mother from infections, cancer (breast, endometrial, and ovarian), osteoporosis, diabetes, and rheumatoid arthritis.
- Postpartum visits and interconception visits are valuable times for ongoing risk assessment, health promotion, and screening about factors likely to affect the health of women and their families (e.g., diet, exercise, breastfeeding, family planning, substance use, depression, violence and injury prevention). Practitioners should develop the infrastructure within their practices to provide opportunities for patient education about these issues and referral as appropriate.
- Pregnancy is a "teachable moment" (naturally occurring life transition) that motivates people to adopt risk-reducing behaviors. Health care providers should capitalize on this opportunity to educate and facilitate healthy lifestyle changes and primary prevention strategies that may benefit women and their families.

REFERENCES

1. Misra DP, Guyer B, Allston A: Integrated perinatal health framework. A multiple determinants model with a life span approach. Am J Prev Med 25:65, 2003.
2. Public Health Service: Caring for Our Future: The Content of Prenatal Care—A Report of the Public Health Service Expert Panel on the Content of Prenatal Care. Washington, DC, PHS-DHRS, 1989.
3. American Academy of Pediatrics, American College of Obstetricians and Gynecologists: Guidelines for Perinatal Care, 4th ed. Elk Grove Village, IL, American Academy Pediatrics, 1997.
4. Chang J, Elam-Evans LD, Berg CJ, et al: Pregnancy-related mortality surveillance—United States, 1991-1999. MMWR Morb Mortal Wkly Rep 52:1, 2003.
5. Lu MC, Kotelchuck M, Culhane JF, et al: Preconception care between pregnancies: the content of internatal care. Matern Child Health J 10:S10, 2006.
6. Phelan S: Pregnancy: a "teachable moment" for weight control and obesity prevention. Am J Obstet Gynecol 202:135e1, 2010.
7. McBride CM, Emmons KM, Lipkus IM: Understanding the potential of teachable moments: the case of smoking cessation. Health Educ Res 8:156, 2003.
8. Johnson TRB, Zettelmaier MA, Warner PA, et al: A competency based approach to comprehensive pregnancy care. Women's Health Issues 10:240, 2000.
9. Johansen KS, Hod M: Quality development in perinatal care—the OBSQID project. Int J Gynecol Obstet 64:167, 1999.
10. Binstock MA, Wolde-Tsadik G: Alternative prenatal care. Impact of reduced visit frequency, focused visits and continuity of care. J Reprod Med 40:507, 1995.
11. Hanson L, VandeVusse L, Roberts J, et al: A critical appraisal of guidelines for antenatal care: Components of care and priorities in prenatal education. J Midwifery Womens Health 54:458, 2009.
12. Walker DA, Wisger JM, Rossie D: Contemporary childbirth education models. J Midwifery Womens Health 54:469, 2009.
13. Revised 1990 Estimates of Maternal Mortality. A New Approach by WHO and UNICEF, World Health Organization, April 1996.
14. Callister LC: Global maternal mortality: contributing factors and strategies for change. MCN Am J Matern Child Nurs 30:184, 2005.
15. World Health Organization: Maternal Mortality in 2000. Estimates Developed by WHO, UNICEF, and UNFPA. Geneva, 2001.
16. www.safemotherhood.org/facts. Accessed Jan 6, 2006.
17. www.healthypeople.gov/hp2020/. Accessed Nov 8, 2010.
18. Hoyert DL: Maternal mortality and related concepts. National Center for Health Statistics. Vital Health Stat 3, 2007.
19. Berg CJ, Danel I, Atrash H, et al (eds): Strategies to Reduce Pregnancy-Related Deaths: from Identification and Review to Action. Centers for Disease Control and Prevention 1-214, 2002.
20. Pregnancy related mortality surveillance in the United States, 52:1, 2003. www.cdc.gov/mmwr/pdf/ss/ss5202.pdf.
21. Centers for Disease Control and Prevention (CDC): Differences in maternal mortality among black and white women—United States, 1987–1996. MMWR Morb Mortal Wkly Rep 48:492, 1999.
22. Sullivan SA, Hill EG, Newman RB, et al: Maternal-fetal medicine specialist density is inversely associated with maternal mortality ratios. Am J Obstet Gynecol 193:1083, 2005.
23. Yeast JD, Poskin M, Stockbauer JW, et al: Changing patterns in regionalization of perinatal care and the impact on neonatal mortality. Am J Obstet Gynecol 178:131, 1998.
24. Wen SW, Huang L, Liston R, et al, the Maternal Health Study Group, Canadian Perinatal Surveillance System: Severe maternal morbidity in Canada, 1991-2001. CMAJ 173:759, 2005.
25. Berg CJ, Berg CJ, Chang J, et al: Pregnancy-related mortality in the United States, 1991-1997. Obstet Gynecol 101:289, 2003.
26. Danel I, Berg C, Johnson CH, et al: Magnitude of maternal morbidity during labor and delivery: United States, 1993-1997. Am J Pub Health 93:631, 2003.
27. Geller SE, Rosenberg E, Cox SM, et al: The continuum of maternal morbidity and mortality. Am J Obstet Gynecol 191:939, 2004.
28. Kung HC, Hoert DL, Xu J, et al: Deaths: final data for 2005. Natl Vital Stat Rep 56, 2008.
29. Stone PW, Zwanziger J, Hinton Walker P, et al: Economic analysis of two models of low-risk maternity care: a freestanding birth center compared to traditional care. Res Nurs Health 23:279, 2000.
30. Tucker JS, Hall MH, Howie PW, et al: Should obstetricians see women with normal pregnancies? A multicentre randomised controlled trial of routine antenatal care by general practitioners and midwives compared with shared care led by obstetricians. BMJ 312:554, 1996.
31. Kogan MD, Martin JA, Alexander GR, et al: The changing pattern of prenatal care utilization in the United States, 1981-1995, using different prenatal care indices. JAMA 279:1623, 1998.
32. Misra DP, Guyer B: Benefits and limitations on prenatal care from counting visits to measuring content. JAMA 279:1661, 1998.
33. Jewell D, Sharp D, Sanders J, et al: A randomised controlled trial of flexibility in routine antenatal care. Br J Obstet Gynaecol 107:1241, 2000.
34. Villar J, Ba'aqeel H, Piaggio G, et al: WHO antenatal care randomised trial for the evaluation of a new model of routine antenatal care. Lancet 357:1551, 2001.
35. Kogan MD, Alexander GR, Kotelchuck M, et al: Comparing mothers' reports on the content of prenatal care received with recommended national guidelines for care. Pub Health Rep 109:637, 1994.
36. Moos MK, Cefalo RC: Preconceptional health promotion: a focus for obstetric care. Am J Perinatol 4:63, 1987.
37. Adams EM, Bruce C, Shulman MS, et al: The PRAMS Working Group: pregnancy planning and pre-conceptional counseling. Obstet Gynecol 82:955, 1993.
38. Spitzer RL, Williams JBW, Kroenke K, et al: Utility of a new procedure for diagnosing mental disorders in primary care. JAMA 272:1749, 1994.
39. www.osha.gov/SLTC/reproductivehazards/index.html. Accessed Nov 8, 2010.
40. Kramer MS, McDonald SW: Aerobic exercise for women during pregnancy (review). Cochrane Syst Rev 2010.
41. Gregory KD, Johnson CT, Johnson TRB, et al: Content of prenatal care: update 2005. Womens Health Issues 16:198, 2006.
42. Anderson BL, Juliano LM, Schulkin J: Caffeine's implications for women's health and survey of obstetrician-gynecologists' caffeine knowledge and assessment practices. J Women's Health 18:1457, 2009.
43. Parsons WD, Neims AH: Prolonged half-life of caffeine in healthy term newborn infants. J Pediatr 98:640, 1981.
44. American College of Obstetricians and Gynecologists, ACOG Committee on Obstetric Practice: Moderate caffeine consumption during pregnancy. Obstet Gynecol 116:467, 2010.
45. http://cot.food.gov.uk/pdfs/cotstatementcaffeine200804.pdf. Accessed Nov 1, 2010.
46. Health Canada: Caffeine and your health. www.hc-sc.gc.ca/hl-vs/iyh-vsv/food-aliment/caffeine-eng.php#th. Accessed Nov 1, 2010.
47. Wiist WH, McFarlane J: The effectiveness of an abuse assessment protocol in public health prenatal clinics. Am J Public Health 89:1217, 1999.
48. Meis PJ, Klebanoff M, Thom E, et al: Prevention of recurrent preterm delivery by 17α-hydroxyprogesterone caproate. N Engl J Med 348:2379, 2003.
49. da Fonseca EB, Bittar RE, Carvalho MHB, et al: Prophylactic administration of progesterone by vaginal suppository to reduce the incidence of spontaneous preterm birth in women at increased risk: a randomized placebo-controlled double-blind study. Am J Obstet Gynecol 188:419, 2003.
50. Abbasi IA, Hess LW, Johnson TRB Jr, et al: Leukocyte esterase activity in the rapid detection of urinary tract and lower genital tract infection in pregnancy. Am J Perinatol 2:311, 1985.
51. American College Obstetrician and Gynecologists Committee Opinion: Number 296, July 2004. First trimester screening for fetal aneuploidy. ACOG Compendium of Selected Publications, 2005, p 43.
52. American College Obstetrician and Gynecologists Practice Bulletin: Number 44, July 2003. Neural Tube Defects. ACOG Compendium of Selected Publications, 2005, p 614.
53. ACOG Committee on Obstetric Practice: Scheduled cesarean delivery and the prevention of vertical transmission of HIV infection. ACOG 234:158, 2000.
54. US Department of Veterans Affairs and the Department of Defense: VA/DoD clinical practice guideline: management of pregnancy 2009. http://healthquality.va.gov/pregnancy.asp. Accessed Nov 8, 2010.

55. Institute for Clinical Systems Improvement: Health care guideline. Routine prenatal care. www.icsi.org/prenatal_care_4/prenatal_care_routine_ful_version_2.html. Accessed Nov 8, 2010.
56. American Academy of Pediatrics & American College of Obstetricians and Gynecologists: Guidelines for Perinatal Care, ed 6. Washington, DC, American Academy of Pediatrics, 2007.
57. Kirkham C, Harris S, Grzybowski S: Evidence-based prenatal care: I. General prenatal care and counseling issues. Am Fam Physician 71:1307, 2005.
58. Kirkham C, Harris S, Grzybowski S: Evidence-based prenatal care: II. Third trimester care and prevention of infectious diseases. Am Fam Physician 71:1555, 2005.
59. ACOG Practice Bulletin: Clinical management guidelines for obstetricians-gynecologists. No 98, October 2008. Ultrasonography in pregnancy. Obstet Gynecol 112:951, 2008.
60. Hadlock F: Sonographic estimation of fetal age and weight. Radiol Clin North Am 28:39, 1990.
61. Hunter LA: Issues in pregnancy dating: revisiting the evidence. J Midwifery Womens Health 54:184, 2009.
62. Eik-Nes SH, Okland O, Aure JC: Ultrasound screening in pregnancy: a randomized controlled trial. Lancet 1:1347, 1984.
63. Ewigman BG, Crane JP, Frigoletto FD, et al: Effect of prenatal ultrasound screening on perinatal outcome. N Engl J Med 329:821, 1993.
64. Gregory KD, Davidson E: Prenatal care: who needs it and why? Clin Obstet Gynecol 42:725, 1999.
65. Hedly AA, Ogden, CL, Johnson CL, et al: Prevalence of overweight and obesity among US children, adolescents, and adults, 1992-2002. JAMA 291:2847, 2004.
66. Fitzsimons KJ, Modder J: Setting maternity care standards for women with obesity in pregnancy. Semin Fetal Neonatal Med 15:100, 2010.
67. Linne Y, Dye L, Barkeling B, et al: Long-term weight development in women: a 15 year follow up of the effects of pregnancy. Obes Res 12:1166, 2004.
68. Rooney BL, Schauberger CW: Excess pregnancy weight gain and long term obesity: one decade later. Obstet Gynecol 100:245, 2002.
69. Institute of Medicine (US): Subcommittee on Nutritional Status and Weight Gain during Pregnancy. Institute of Medicine (US) Subcommittee on Dietary Intake and Nutrient Supplements during Pregnancy. Nutrition During Pregnancy: Part I, Weight Gain; Part II, Nutritional Supplements. Washington, DC, National Academy Press, 1990.
70. Institute of Medicine (US) & National Research Council (US) Committee to Reexamine IOM Pregnancy Weight Guidelines; Rasmussen KM, Yaktine AL, Committee to Reexamine IOM Pregnancy Weight Guidelines, Food and Nutrition Board and Board on Children, Youth, and Families: Weight Gain during Pregnancy: Reexamining the Guidelines. Washington, DC, Institute of Medicine, 2009.
71. Clapp JF 3rd, American College of Obstetricians and Gynecologists: Exercise during Pregnancy and the Postpartum Period: Technical Bulletin No. 189. Washington, DC, American College of Obstetricians and Gynecologists, 1994.
72. Miller DW Jr: Prenatal care: a strategic first step toward EMR acceptance. J Healthc Inf Manag 17:47, 2003.
73. Zhu BP: Effect of interpregnancy interval on birth outcomes: findings from three recent US studies. Int J Gynecol Obstet 89:S25, 2005.
74. Gold R, Connell FA, Heagerty P, et al: Income inequality and pregnancy spacing. Soc Sci Med 59:1117, 2004.
75. Adams J, Lui C, Sibbritt D, et al: Women's use of complementary and alternative medicine during pregnancy: a critical review of the literature. Birth 36:237, 2009.
76. National Academy of Sciences: Recommended Dietary Allowances, 10th ed. Washington, DC, National Academy Press, 1989.
77. Food and Nutrition Board, Institute of Medicine, National Academy of Sciences: Nutrition during Pregnancy. Washington, DC, National Academy Press, 1990, p 10.
78. Bianco AT, Smilen SW, Davis Y, et al: Pregnancy outcome and weight gain recommendations for the morbidly obese woman. Obstet Gynecol 91:97, 1998.
79. American College Obstetricians and Gynecologists: Committee opinion #267. Exercise during Pregnancy and the Postpartum Period. Washington, DC, ACOG, 2002.
80. American Academy of Pediatrics, American College of Obstetricians and Gynecologists, Committee on Fetus and Newborn, Committee on Obstetric Practice: Guidelines for Perinatal Care, 4th ed. Elk Grove Village, IL, 1997.
81. Goodwin TM: Hyperemesis gravidarum. Obstet Gynecol Clin North Am 35:401, 2008.
82. Ismail SK, Kenny L: Review on hyperemesis gravidarum. Best Pract Res Clin Gastroenterol 21:755, 2007.
83. Cedergren M, Bryhildsen J, Josefsson A, et al: Hyperemesis gravidarum that requires hospitalization and the use of antiemetic drugs in relation to maternal body mass. Am J Obstet Gynecol 198:412.e1, 2008.
84. Goodwin TM, Montoro M, Mestman JH: Transient hyperthyroidism and hyperemesis gravidarum: clinical aspects. Am J Obstet Gynecol 167:648, 1992.
85. Dodds L, Fell DB, Joseph KS, et al: Outcome of pregnancies complicated by hyperemesis gravidarum. Obstet Gynecol 107:285, 2006.
86. Jednak MA, Shadigian EM, et al: Protein meals reduce nausea and gastric slow wave dysrhythmic activity in first trimester pregnancy. Am J Physiol 27:G855, 1999.
87. Jewell D, Young G: Interventions for nausea and vomiting in early pregnancy. Cochrane Database Syst Rev CV000145, 2003.
88. Seto A, Einarson T, Koren G: Pregnancy outcome following first trimester exposure to antihistamines: meta-analysis. Am J Perinatol 14:119, 1997.
89. Niebyl JR, Goodwin TM: Overview of nausea and vomiting of pregnancy with an emphasis on vitamins and ginger. Am J Obstet Gynecol 186:253, 2002.
90. Anderson FWJ, Johnson CT: Complementary and alternative medicine in obstetrics. IJGO 91:116, 2005.
91. Holmgren C, Aagaard-Tillery KM, Silver RM, et al: Hyperemesis in pregnancy: an evaluation of treatment strategies with maternal and neonatal outcomes. Am J Obstet Gynecol 198:56.e1, 2008.
92. Poursharif B, Korst LM, MacGibbon KW, et al: Elective pregnancy termination in a large cohort of women with hyperemesis gravidarum. Contraception 76:451, 2007.
93. Fox NS, Gelber SE, Chasen ST: Physical and sexual activity during pregnancy and near delivery. J Womens Health 17:1431, 2008.
94. Shojaa M, Jouybari L, Sanagoo A: The sexual activity during pregnancy among a group of Iranian women. Arch Gynecol Obstet 279:353, 2009.
95. American Academy of Pediatrics: Circumcision policy statement (RE9850). Pediatrics 103:686, 1999.
96. Morton CH, Hsu C: Contemporary dilemmas in American childbirth education: findings from a comparative ethnographic study. J Perinat Educ 16:25, 2007.
97. Lu MC, Prentice J: The postpartum visit: risk factors for nonuse and association with breast-feeding. Am J Obstet Gynecol 187:1329, 2002.
98. Technical Working Group, World Health Organization: Postpartum care of the mother and newborn: a practical guide. Birth 26:255, 1999.
99. Kahn RS, Zuckerman B, Bauchner H, et al: Women's health after pregnancy and child outcomes at age 3 years: a prospective cohort study. Am J Public Health 92:1312, 2002.
100. Arias E, MacDorman MF, Strobino DM, Guyer B: Annual summary of vital statistics—2002. Pediatrics 112(6 Pt 1):1215, 2003.
101. National Center for Health Statistics: Healthy United States, 2003. Hyattsville, MD: NCHS, 2003.
102. Martin JA, Hamilton BE, Ventura SJ, et al: Births: Final data for 2000. National Vital Statistics Reports, vol 50, issue 5. Hyattsville, MD, NCHS, 2002.
103. Singh GK, Miller BA: Health, life expectancy, and mortality patterns among immigrant populations in the United States. Canadian Journal of Public Health. Revue Canadienne de Sante Publique 95:I14, 2004.
104. Dermer A: Overcoming medical and social barriers to breast feeding. Am Family Physician 51:755, 1995.
105. Grugliania ERJ, Calatta WT, Vogelhut J: Effect of breastfeeding support form different sources on mothers' decisions to breastfeed. Journal of Human Lactation 10:157, 1994.
106. Pattinson RC, Hall M: Near misses: a useful adjunct to maternal death enquiries. Br Med Bull 67:231, 2003.

107. Horon IL: Underreporting of maternal deaths on death certificates and the magnitude of the problem of maternal mortality. Am J Pub Health 95:478, 2005.
108. Minkoff H: Maternal mortality in America: lessons from the developing world. J Am Womens Assoc 57:171, 2002.
109. Widman K, Bouvier-Colle MH, the MOMS Group: Maternal mortality as an indicator of obstetric care in Europe. BJOG 111:164, 2004.
110. Frautschi S, Cerulli A, Maine D: Suicide during pregnancy and its neglect as a component of maternal mortality. Int J Gynecol Obstet 47:275, 1994.
111. Centers for Disease Control and Prevention: Enhanced maternal mortality surveillance—North Carolina, 1988 and 1989. MMWR Morb Mortal Wkly Rep 40:469, 1996.
112. Harper M, Parsons L: Maternal death due to homicide and other injuries in North Carolina: 1992-1994. Obstet Gynecol 90:920, 1997.
113. Dannenberg AL, Carter DM, Lawson HW, et al: Homicide and other injuries as causes of maternal death in New York City, 1987 through 1991. Am J Obstet Gynecol 172:1557, 1995.
114. Mamelle N, Laumon B, Lazar P: Prematurity and occupational activity during pregnancy. Am J Epidemiol 119:309, 1984.
115. Luke B, Mamelle N, Keith L, et al: The association between occupational factors and preterm birth: a U.S. nurses' study. Am J Obstet Gynecol 173:849, 1995.
116. Mozurkewich E, Luke B, Avni M, Wolf FM: Working conditions and adverse pregnancy outcome: a meta-analysis. Obstet Gynecol 95:623, 2000.
117. James DC, Dobson B: Position of the American Dietetic Association: Promoting and supporting breastfeeding. J Am Dietetic Assoc 105:810, 2005.
118. Callen J, Pinelli J: Incidence and duration of breastfeeding for term infants in Canada, United States, Europe, and Australia: A literature review. Birth 31:285, 2004.
119. Shadigian EM, Bauer ST: Pregnancy-associated death: a qualitative systematic review of homicide and suicide. Obstet Gynecol Survey 60:183, 2005.
120. Deneux-Tharaux C, Berg C, Bouvier-Colle MH, et al: Underreporting of pregnancy-related mortality in the United States and Europe. Obstet Gynecol 106:684, 2005.
121. Brown MS, Hurloch JT: Preparation of the breast for breast feeding. Nurs Res 24:449, 1975.
122. Cochrane A: In Effective Care in Pregnancy and Childbirt, eds. Chalmers, Enkin & Keirse, Oxford University Press, 1989.
123. Alanis MC, Lucidi RS: Neonatal circumcision: a review of the world's oldest and most controversial operation. Obstet Gynecol Surv 59:379, 2004.
124. Dermer A: Overcoming medical and social barriers to breast feeding. Am Fam Physician 51:755, 1995.
125. American Academy of Pediatrics: Circumcision Policy Statement (RE9850) 103:686, 1999.
126. Mullen P: Smoking Cessation Counseling in Prenatal Care. In Merkatz IR, Thompson JE, Mullen PD, Goldenberg RL, eds. New Perspectives in Prenatal Care. New York, Elsevier, 1990, p 161.

Additional references and figures for this chapter can be found online at www.expertconsult.com.

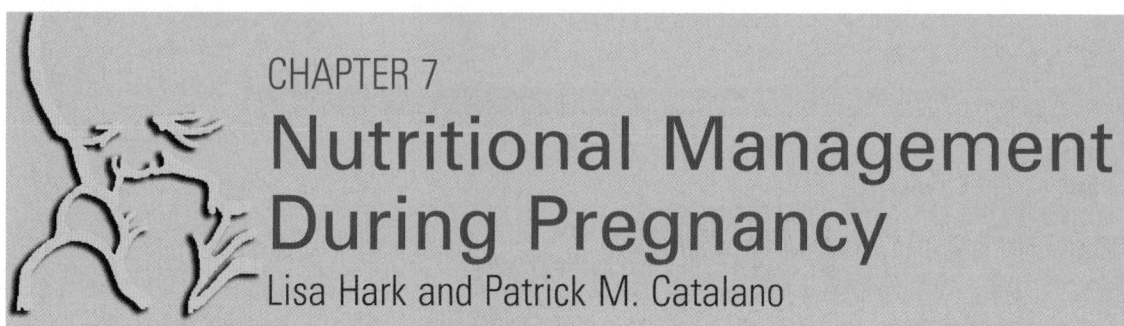

CHAPTER 7 Nutritional Management During Pregnancy

Lisa Hark and Patrick M. Catalano

KEY ABBREVIATIONS	
American College of Obstetricians and Gynecologists	ACOG
Biliopancreatic Diversion	BPD
Body Mass Index	BMI
Centers for Disease Control and Prevention	CDC
Dietary Reference Index	DRI
Docosahexenoic Acid	DHA
Elcosapentaenoic Acid	EPA
Institute of Medicine	IOM
Neural Tube Defect	NTD
Polyunsaturated Fatty Acid	PUFA
Recommended Daily Allowance	RDA
Resting Metabolic Rate	RMR
Small for Gestational Age	SGA
Thermic Effect of Energy	TEE
Thermic Effect of Food	TEF
World Health Organization	WHO

The concept of eating for two when pregnant, along with many other myths of pregnancy, has come under greater scrutiny in the past decade. This is because of the changes in population demographics, as well as alterations in women's lifestyles. In the past 50 years, the number of women of reproductive age who are overweight (body mass index [BMI] greater than 25.0 [kg/m^2] to 29.9) has remained stable at approximately 30%.[1] More concerning is the twofold increase in obesity (BMI ≥30) from 13% to 35% (Figure 7-1).[2] This increase in obesity has occurred disproportionately in minority populations such as Hispanics and African Americans.[1] The increase in obesity in the population has been ascribed to our increased consumption of non-nutritious foods and decreased physical activity. Obstetricians need to assume an important role in preventing the progression of obesity in women.

Excessive weight gain in pregnancy significantly increases the risk of postpartum weight retention[3] and contributes to the accretion of excess adipose tissue in the fetus.[4] Weight management, however, is not the only issue. The importance of specific nutrients is also a critical issue which needs to be considered during gestation, as deficiencies and/or excess of various nutrients can have both short- and long-term consequences in the mother and her fetus. In this chapter, we address the specific nutrient requirements in pregnancy, energy requirements, recommendations for weight gain, and special conditions such as bariatric surgery.

INTEGRATING NUTRITION INTO THE OBSTETRICAL HISTORY

Every woman should have the opportunity to meet with a health care provider for a prepregnancy history and physical examination that includes a nutrition assessment. The purpose of a nutrition assessment is to identify a woman's nutritional risk factors that could jeopardize her health or the health of her fetus and to determine the quality and quantity of nutrients in the mother's diet. Adequate intake of nutrients positively influences the quality of nutritional support for the developing fetus and may reduce fetal risk and improve pregnancy outcome.[5] A thorough evaluation of a woman's nutritional status before and during pregnancy encompasses medical history and weight status, dietary intake, and laboratory data. Pertinent dietary information includes appetite, meal patterns, dieting regimens, cultural or religious dietary practices, vegetarianism, food allergies, and cravings and/or aversions. Information about abnormal eating practices, such as following fad

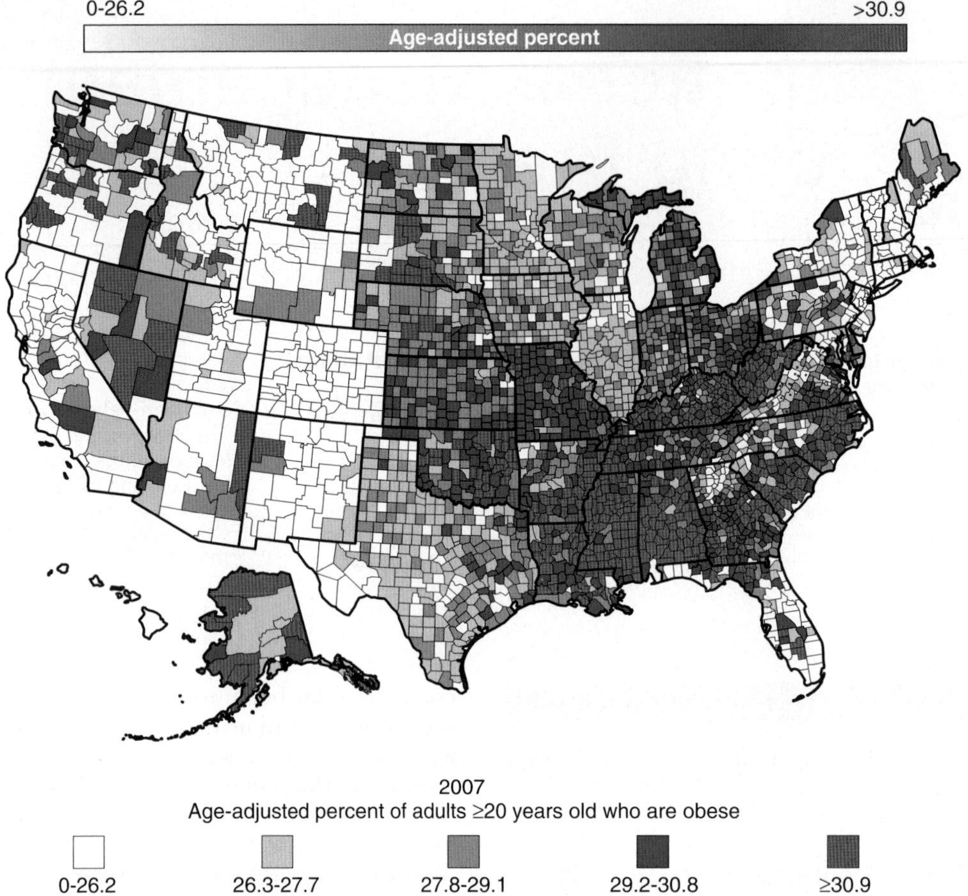

FIGURE 7-1. Adult obesity in the United States 2007, by county. (Modified from CDC Division of Diabetes Translation, National Diabetes Surveillance System. www.cdc.gov/diabetes/statistics)

diets, bingeing, purging, laxative or diuretic use, or pica (eating nonfood items, e.g., ice, detergent, starch, chalk, clay, or rocks), should be ascertained.

Other relevant information includes the habitual use of caffeine-containing beverages, tobacco, alcohol, recreational drug consumption, and any vitamin or herbal supplementation or alternative pharmacologic therapies the woman may be consuming. Dietary supplements may not be volunteered and their use may be inappropriate or dangerous during pregnancy, such as high levels of vitamin A. A woman's current dietary intake can be assessed using the 24-hour recall method, asking her to describe what she ate and drank the day before, or she could complete a diet history questionnaire.

Obtaining a history of previous weight gain patterns during pregnancy; prior history of nausea, vomiting, or hyperemesis during pregnancy; gestational diabetes; eclampsia; anemia; pica; and weight status (BMI) should be determined. The medical history also identifies maternal risk factors for nutritional deficiencies and chronic diseases with nutritional implications (e.g., absorption disorders, cystic fibrosis, eating disorders, metabolic disorders, infections, diabetes mellitus, phenylketonuria, sickle cell trait, or renal disease). Women who have had closely spaced pregnancies (i.e., less than a year between pregnancies) are at increased risk of having depleted nutrient reserves. Maternal nutrient depletion may be associated with an increased incidence of preterm birth, intrauterine growth restriction (IUGR), and maternal mortality/morbidity.

In addition to the medical history, questions regarding professional, social, economic, and emotional stresses and specific religious practices (including dietary restrictions and fasting) that may affect a woman's nutritional status should be asked. Some work environments adversely affect dietary intake, as they may not provide adequate time during the day to eat proper meals or allow access to only nutritionally marginal food. For this reason, it is important to ask pregnant woman about the conditions of their employment, and identify limitations and potential solutions. Women with lower socioeconomic status often need support to obtain nutritious food, and referral to food assistance programs may be appropriate (e.g., Women, Infants and Children Program [WIC]).

Many women are receptive to nutrition counseling just before or during pregnancy, making this an opportune time to encourage the development of good nutritional and physical activity practices aimed at preventing future medical problems such as obesity, diabetes, hypertension, and osteoporosis.[5] Pregnant women with nutritional risk factors may benefit from a referral to a registered dietitian as shown in the accompanying box, Medical Conditions in Which Consultation with a Registered Dietitian Is Advisable.

MEDICAL CONDITIONS WHERE CONSULTATION WITH A REGISTERED DIETITIAN IS ADVISABLE

- Multiple gestation (twins, triplets)
- Frequent gestations (less than a 3-month interpregnancy interval)
- Tobacco, alcohol, or chronic medicinal or illicit drug use
- Severe nausea and vomiting (hyperemesis gravidarum)
- Eating disorders (anorexia, bulimia, and compulsive eating)
- Inadequate weight gain during pregnancy
- Adolescence
- Restricted eating (vegetarianism, macrobiotic, raw food, vegan)
- Food allergies or food intolerances
- Gestational diabetes mellitus (GDM) or prior history of GDM
- Prior history of low-birth-weight babies or other obstetrical complications
- Social factors that may limit appropriate intake (e.g., religion, poverty)

Source: Lisa Hark, PhD, RD. Used with permission.

MATERNAL WEIGHT GAIN RECOMMENDATIONS

In 1990 the Institute of Medicine (IOM) published weight gain recommendations during pregnancy.[6] The guidelines were first proposed to address many issues regarding the role of nutrition in pregnancy, including the prevention of small-for-gestational-age (SGA) and growth-restricted neonates. In view of the recent obesity epidemic, the IOM convened a workshop conference in 2006 to evaluate the available data and reexamine the 1990 IOM guidelines. Shortly thereafter the IOM, at the behest of various federal agencies, organized a committee to evaluate the currently available information regarding weight gain recommendations in pregnancy. These guidelines considered both the short- and long-term outcome for the pregnant woman, as well as her child. Additionally, because of the great importance of achieving appropriate pregravid weight, the 2009 guidelines recommend that women begin pregnancy at a healthy weight. Last, the guidelines call for individualized preconceptual, prenatal, and postpartum care to help women attain a healthy weight gain, within the guidelines, and return to a healthy pregravid weight after delivery. The interested reader is encouraged to access the online report at www.iom.edu/Reports/2009/Weight-Gain-During-Pregnancy-Reexamining-the-Guidelines.aspx in order to understand the complexity of these issues and ensuing recommendations.[7]

Low or Underweight Preconception BMI

The 2009 IOM guidelines use the World Health Organization (WHO) criteria established in 1995 and subsequently adopted by the National Heart, Lung and Blood Institute to characterize pregravid BMI. An underweight BMI is classified as a BMI less than 18.5 kg/m^2. Based on the available data women with low pregnancy BMI and low weight gain during pregnancy appear to be at increased risk for having a small-for-gestational-age infant (less than 10th percentile), preterm birth, and perinatal mortality.[7] In contrast, excessive weight gain in low pregravid BMI women is associated with increased risk for large-for-gestational-age neonates,[7] as well as increased maternal weight retention postpartum[3] (Figure 7-2). The recommended weight gain guidelines and rate of weight gain in the second and third trimesters are provided in Table 7-1.

TABLE 7-1 New Recommendations for Total and Rate of Weight Gain During Pregnancy, by Prepregnancy BMI*

PREGNANCY BMI	BMI (kg/m^2)	TOTAL WEIGHT GAIN (lb)	RATES OF WEIGHT GAIN† 2ND AND 3RD TRIMESTER (lb/week)
Underweight	<18.5	28-40	1 (1-1.3)
Normal weight	18.5-24.9	25-35	1 (0.8-1)
Overweight	25.0-29.9	15-25	0.6 (0.5-0.7)
Obese (all classes)	≥30.0	11-20	0.5 (0.4-0.6)

From Rasmussin KM, Yaktin AL (eds): Weight Gain during Pregnancy: Reexamining the Guidelines. Institute of Medicine of the National Academies. Washington, DC, National Academy Press, 2009, Chapter 3, Composition and compound of gestational weight gain: physiology and metabolism, pp 77-83.
*To calculate BMI go to www.nhlbisupport/com/bmi/.
†Calculations assume a 0.5 to 2 kg (1.1 to 4.4 lb) weight gain in the first trimester (IOM, 2009).

Overweight and Obese Preconception BMI

Approximately 60% of women of reproductive age are overweight (BMI >25 kg/m^2) and of these, 50% are obese (BMI >30 kg/m^2). Additionally, 8% meet the criteria for class III obesity, or a BMI greater than 40 kg/m^2. Women who are overweight or obese generally have lower gestational weight gain as compared with a normal-weight population.[8] Data from the Centers for Disease Control and Prevention (CDC) found that 30% of obese women gained within, 46% exceeded, and 24% gained less than the 1990 IOM gestational weight gain guidelines.[6] In obese women, high gestational weight gain during pregnancy was associated with an increased risk for cesarean delivery. High gestational weight gain was also weakly associated with preterm birth, but this may have been related to a possible increased risk of hypertensive disorders such as preeclampsia; however, the evidence again was not sufficient to make definitive conclusions. There was moderate evidence for low gestational weight gain to be associated with failure to initiate breastfeeding. Weight gain in excess of 15 kg was associated with increased postpartum weight retention.[7,9]

The 2009 IOM guidelines recommend a gestational weight gain of between 11 and 20 lb. These recommendations were based primarily on Class 1 obesity. There was a paucity of data regarding the weight gain recommendations for all of the specific classes of obesity. The 11 to 20 lb gestational weight gain primarily represents the obligatory weight gain of pregnancy. This includes approximately 1.0 kg of protein, 7 to 8 kg of water, and a variable amount of adipose tissue (Table 7-2). The potential effects

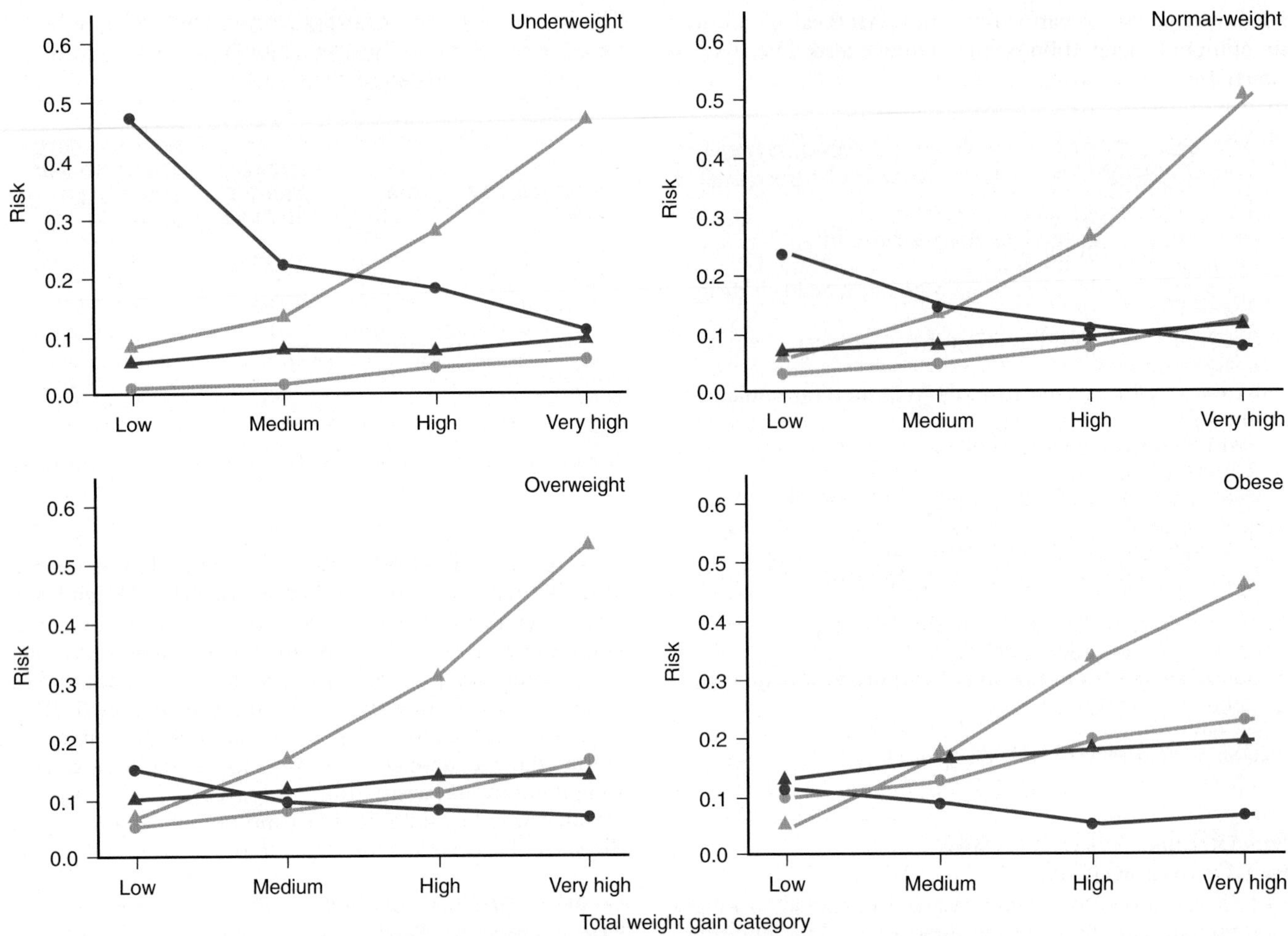

FIGURE 7-2. Adjusted absolute risks for small-for-gestational-age *(red circle),* large-for-gestational-age *(blue circle),* emergency cesarean section *(red triangle),* and postpartum weight retention of ≥5 kg *(blue triangle)* according to prepregnancy BMI (in kg/m^2) and gestational weight gain categories of the World Health Organization. (Modified from Nohr EA, Vaeth M, Baker JL, et al: Combined associations of prepregnancy body mass index and gestational weight gain with the outcome of pregnancy. Am J Clin Nutr 87:1750, 2008.)

TABLE 7-2 OBLIGATORY COMPONENTS OF WEIGHT GAIN

PROTEIN	GRAMS
Fetus	420
Uterus	170
Blood	140
Placenta	100
Breast	80
Total	900-1000
WATER	
Fetus	2400
Placenta	500
Amniotic fluid	500
Uterus	800
Breast	300
Maternal blood	1300
Extracellular fluid	1500
Total	7000-8000 g
Variable Components of Weight Gain	
OTHER	
CHO	NIL
Lipids	0-6 kg

From Rasmussin KM, Yaktin AL (eds): Weight Gain during Pregnancy: Reexamining the Guidelines. Institute of Medicine of the National Academies. Washington, DC, National Academy Press, 2009, Chapter 3, Composition and compound of gestational weight gain: physiology and metabolism, pp 77-83.

of lack of gestational weight gain or weight loss during pregnancy on maternal metabolism, physiologic function, and long-term effects on the developing fetus were insufficient for the committee to make any recommendations on less gestational weight gain. Epidemiologic data suggest that less weight gain in pregnancy is associated with a decreased risk of preeclampsia.[10,11] Finally, it is recognized that a healthy pregnancy outcome is often achieved by obese women gaining less than the recommended minimal gestational weight gain. However, arbitrary minimal weight gain recommendations in obese women should not be advised. Rather, focus should be on ensuring adequate nutrient intake, avoidance of urinary ketones, and appropriate fetal growth. Further research is needed regarding these issues.

Maternal Weight Gain Recommendations for Special Populations

Multiple Gestation

There is limited evidence-based literature to make specific recommendations regarding weight gain in women who are pregnant with multiple fetuses. However, similar to what is observed in singleton pregnancies, neonatal outcome appears to vary with gestational weight gain as a function of pregravid BMI.[7] The committee offered provisional gestational weight gain guidelines for women with twin pregnancies based on the work of Luke and others (Table 7-3).[12] These data are based on women delivering beyond 37 weeks and having fetuses greater than 2500 g. There was insufficient data to make recommendations for underweight women with twins or women carrying triplet or higher-order multiples.

Adolescents

Pregnancy in adolescents is associated with an increased risk of preterm delivery and low birth weight,[13] and hence the 1990 IOM report recommended that adolescents gain at the upper end of the gestational weight gain guidelines according to their prepregnancy BMI.[6] The rationale for these recommendations was based on the fact that these young women themselves were growing and there would be a potential competition between the mother and her fetus for nutrients. However, a study by Howie and colleagues reported that adolescents have an increased likelihood of excessive gestational weight gain compared with older women.[14] In addition, adolescents who exceeded the 1990 IOM weight gain recommendations were more likely to become obese 9 years after delivery as compared to those who gained within the guidelines.[15] Based on these data, the 2009 IOM report recommends adolescents gain within the guidelines based on their pregravid BMI.[7]

Other Groups

Based on the available evidence, there were no specific recommendations for gestational weight gain guidelines in women of short stature, various racial or ethnic groups, parity, or smoking status. The IOM report recognized that each of these special groups might possibly benefit from specific gestational weight gain guidelines, but the available evidence was again insufficient to make recommendations.[7]

LABORATORY EVALUATION OF NUTRITIONAL STATUS

The evaluation of nutritional status during pregnancy requires an understanding of the physiologic changes during pregnancy. In particular, the alterations in plasma volume in early gestation may result in hemodilution of various measures but not reflect the total body concentration. Furthermore, the effect of estrogen on hepatic production of certain proteins requires careful interpretation of plasma concentrations. Circulating concentrations of albumin are an example of the potential effects of these physiologic processes on assessment of nutrient status. Reference values for most laboratory measures in pregnancy should be assessed relative to normative pregnancy values and, if available, gestational age or trimester, and are available in a review by Abbassi-Ghanavati and colleagues.[16]

TABLE 7-3 PROVISIONAL GUIDELINES FOR WEIGHT GAIN FOR WOMEN WITH TWIN PREGNANCIES

PREPREGNANCY BMI	BMI (kg/m²)	TOTAL WEIGHT GAIN (lb)
Normal weight	18.5-24.9	37-54
Overweight	25.0-29.9	31-50
Obese	≥30.0	25-42

From Rasmussin KM, Yaktin AL (eds): Weight Gain during Pregnancy: Reexamining the Guidelines. Institute of Medicine of the National Academies. Washington, DC, National Academy Press, 2009, Chapter 3, Composition and compound of gestational weight gain: physiology and metabolism, pp 77-83.

MATERNAL NUTRIENT NEEDS: CURRENT RECOMMENDATIONS

Energy

Energy expenditure consists of four basic components: resting metabolic rate (RMR), the thermic effect of food (TEF) or dietary-induced thermogenesis, the thermic effect of exercise (TEE), and adaptive or facultative thermogenesis. RMR is the amount of energy or calories used at rest and accounts for approximately 60% of total energy expenditure in normal healthy people. TEF is the caloric cost of eating, digesting, absorbing, resynthesizing, and storing food. The TEF accounts for 5% to 10% of total energy expenditure. TEE is quite variable and in sedentary individuals may account for only 15% to 20% of total energy expenditure. Adaptive or facultative thermogenesis refers to adaptations by an organism to adjust to environmental changes, such as overfeeding, underfeeding, and alterations in ambient temperature. Adaptive thermogenesis accounts for no more that 10% of RMR and varies in individuals (Figure 7-3).[17]

The classic teaching is that the total maternal energy requirement for a full-term pregnancy is estimated at 80,000 kilocalories (kcal). This accounts for the increased metabolic activity of the maternal and fetal tissues, as well as the growth of the fetus and placenta. Maternal energy needs to be increased to move a heavier body and thus provide extra work on the maternal cardiovascular, renal, and respiratory systems. Basal requirements can be determined based on maternal age, stature, activity level, preconception weight, BMI, and gestational weight gain goals.[18] Daily caloric requirements have been estimated by the WHO by dividing the gross energy cost (80,000 kcal) by the approximate duration of pregnancy (250 days after the first month), producing an average additional

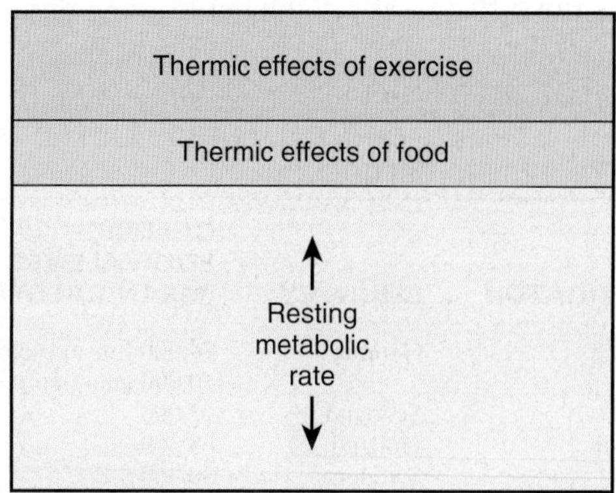

FIGURE 7-3. Components of energy expenditure. (Modified from Catalano PM, Hollenbeck C: Energy requirements in pregnancy. Obstet Gynecol Surv 47:368, 1992.)

300 kcal/day for the entire pregnancy. During the first trimester, total energy expenditure does not change greatly and weight gain is minimal assuming the woman began her pregnancy without depleted body reserves. Therefore, additional energy intake is recommended primarily in the second and third trimesters. Current recommendations are an additional 340 kcal/day above the nonpregnant energy requirements during the second trimester and 452 kcal/day during the third trimester.[19]

A series of prospective studies were conducted in the late 1980s and 1990s in various countries to assess energy expenditure in pregnancy. Many of these studies obtained baseline data before a planned pregnancy and incorporated measurements such as estimates of body composition, energy intake in the diet, RMR, standard measures of exercise, and activity diaries. The conclusion of this research was that the energy cost of pregnancy was much lower than previously estimated (Table 7-4).[20-24]

The introduction of the doubly labeled water method made it possible to estimate total energy expenditure in the free living state. In well-nourished women, RMR usually begins to rise soon after conception and continues to rise until delivery. However, there is considerable interindividual variation and cumulative increases in RMR are positively correlated with prepregnancy weight and the percent body fat.[25] In healthy well-nourished women the average increases in RMR above prepregnancy values were 4.5%, 10.8%, and 24.0% for the first, second, and third trimesters, respectively. Using a room calorimeter, 24-hour energy expenditure averaged 1%, 4%, and 20% above prepregnancy values for the first, second, and third trimesters, respectively. Estimates of total energy expenditure using doubly labeled water increased by 1%, 6%, and 9% and weight increased by 2%, 8%, and 18% over baseline measures in the first, second, and third trimesters, respectively. The TEE averaged −2%, 3%, and 6% relative to baseline. Because of the larger increments in RMR and changes in behavior, physical activity level declined from the time before conception to later in gestation.

Pregnancy also induces changes in fuel utilization. Butte and colleagues reported an increased contribution of carbohydrate to oxidative metabolism in later pregnancy.[26] Using respiratory calorimetry, the 24-hour nonprotein respiratory quotient (NPRQ) was significantly higher in late pregnancy compared with postpartum measures, such that carbohydrate oxidation as a percentage of nonprotein energy expenditure decreased from 66% to 58%. As a consequence the NPRQ was also higher during pregnancy. In summary, there is a large interindividual variability in the energy requirements of pregnancy. These are related to an individual's pregravid metabolic status, her diet, and physical activity. Therefore, these factors should be considered as well as the growth of the fetus when counseling pregnant women about their individualized dietary and nutritional needs.

TABLE 7-4 ESTIMATE OF TOTAL ENERGY EXPENDITURE DURING PREGNANCY

INVESTIGATOR	COUNTRY	CALORIC EQUIVALENTS (MEAN CALORIES)
Lawrence	Gambia	24,000 (unsupplemented) 10,000 (supplemented)
Durnin	Scotland	67,000
Van Raaij	Holland	68,300
Forsum	Sweden	50,300
Goldberg	England	variable

Data from references 20 through 24.

Protein

Additional protein is required during pregnancy for fetal, placental, and maternal tissue development. Maternal protein synthesis increases in order to support expansion of the blood volume, uterus, and breasts. Fetal and placental proteins are also synthesized from amino acids supplied by the mother. The amount of protein deposited during pregnancy for the fetus, placenta, and maternal tissues has been used to determine the increased requirements.[19] Protein retention increases fivefold from the first to the second trimester and about 80% from the second to the third trimester; a total of approximately 925 g of protein are retained during pregnancy.[19] Protein recommendations are therefore increased from 46 g/day for an adult, nonpregnant woman to 71 g/day during pregnancy.[19] This represents a change in protein recommendation from 0.8 g/kg/day for nonpregnant women to 1.1 g/kg/day during pregnancy.

Omega-3 Fatty Acids

The structural and metabolic functions of the body require utilization of polyunsaturated fatty acids (PUFAs). The human body cannot synthesize fatty acids with double bonds three (n-3) or six (n-6) from the n terminus and must be obtained from the diet as either linoleic (18:2 n-6) or alpha linolenic (18:3 n-3). The long-chain PUFA derivatives (LCPUFA) eicosapentaenoic acid (20:6 n-3, EPA) and docosahexaenoic acid (22:6 n-3, DHA) are the most important. Because n-3 PUFAs are essential fatty acids, they can only be obtained through the diet as alpha linoleic acid and converted to DHA and EPA at a rate of between 1% and 4%. The availability of the PUFA/LCPUFA to the fetus depends on maternal dietary intake, as well as placental function.

Although the U.S. expert panel recommends that pregnant women consume at least 300 mg/day of DHA, the mean intake of DHA for pregnant and lactating women was only 52 mg/day and 20 mg/day for EPA.[27] This may in part be explained by the decrease in fish consumption after the Food and Drug Administration (FDA) issued an advisory aimed at pregnant women to avoid consuming fish due to its high levels of mercury, and raw fish, which may contain food-borne illness.[28] With n-3 PUFA supplementation, there is a positive relationship between maternal intake and maternal plasma concentration,[29] as well as between maternal plasma and cord concentrations.[30] Two human studies reported increased plasma levels of DHA in maternal[31] as well as maternal/cord samples in randomized placebo-controlled trials.[32]

There are numerous studies reporting that n-3 PUFA supplementation, especially those derived from fish oils, have beneficial effects on lipid levels, cardiovascular function, and immune function. For example, in rats fed a high-sucrose diet, fish oil protects against visceral fat hypertrophy, hypertriglyceridemia, and hyperglycemia.[27]

In another rodent study, n-3 PUFAs have a protective effect against a high-fat diet inducing insulin resistance. In human studies, Meydani and colleagues reported that 2.4 g of n-3 PUFA supplementation reduced IL-6 and TNF-alpha synthesis between 30% and 58% in young women.[33] In a longitudinal observational study, intake of n-3 PUFA was associated with a reduced risk of islet cell autoimmunity in children at risk for type 1 diabetes.[34]

During pregnancy, Dunstan and colleagues reported that in a randomized controlled trial n-3 PUFA supplementation from the midtrimester resulted in a significant decrease in IL-10 and IL-13.[35,36] Dietary supplementation with n-3 PUFA has been promoted as a means to prolong gestation and prevent prematurity. However, a Maternal Fetal Medicine Network trial did not find any evidence that PUFA supplementation (fish oil) had any beneficial effect in decreasing the risk of preterm delivery in women at risk.[37] Although older trials of n-3 PUFA supplementation purported an increase in birth weight because of a prolongation of gestational age,[38] more recent trials have reported a decrease in birth weight, after adjusting for gestational age.[39,40] Similarly, Groh-Wargo and colleagues reported decreased fat but not lean body mass in infants at 1 year of age whose formulas were supplemented with n-3 PUFA.[41] In summary, although there appears to be a decrease in n-3 PUFA concentrations in pregnant women, the information available regarding the beneficial metabolic effects of supplementation in pregnancy require further evaluation in controlled trials.

VITAMIN AND MINERAL SUPPLEMENTATION GUIDELINES

Dietary Reference Intake

To address the changing nutritional needs of the American population, the Food and Nutrition Board of the IOM established the first Dietary Reference Intakes (DRIs) in 1997. The DRIs moved beyond the traditional Recommended Daily Allowances (RDAs) to focus on the prevention of chronic disease. The DRIs provide a range of safe and appropriate intakes, as well as tolerable upper limits, based on the available research. DRI is a collective term that includes four nutrient-based dietary reference values for every life-stage and gender group. These include estimated average requirement, recommended dietary allowance, adequate intake, and tolerable upper intake level. The tolerable upper intake level is the highest level of daily nutrient intake that is unlikely to pose risks of adverse health effects to the majority (97% to 98%) of individuals in a specified life-stage and gender group. At present, DRIs have been established for vitamin A, carotenoids, the B vitamins, vitamin C, vitamin D, vitamin K, folate, calcium, choline, chromium, copper, fluoride, iodine, iron, magnesium, manganese, molybdenum, phosphorus, biotin, pantothenic acid, selenium, and zinc (Table 7-5).[19,42-45] Recommendations regarding the intake of other nutrients will be available over the next decade as the scientific evidence is evaluated.

Routine vitamin/mineral supplementation for women reporting appropriate dietary intake and demonstrating adequate weight gain (without edema) is not mandatory. However, most health care providers prescribe a prenatal vitamin and mineral supplement because many women do not consume an adequate diet to meet their increased nutritional requirements during the first trimester of pregnancy, especially with regard to folic acid and iron.

Vitamins

Vitamin A

Vitamin A is a fat-soluble vitamin and refers to compounds or mixtures of compounds having vitamin A activity. In animals, vitamin A usually exists as a retinal, retinyl esters, retinol, and retinoic acid. Retinoic acid is the most active form of vitamin A. Retinol is referred to as preformed vitamin A. In plants, vitamin A exists in its precursor form, provitamin A, carotinoids (e.g., beta-carotene), and cryptoxanthin. **Vitamin A is required for cell differentiation and proliferation for the development of the vertebrae, spinal cord, limbs, heart, eyes, and ears, as well as regulation of gene expression.**

Severe vitamin A deficiency is rare in the United States and an adequate intake of vitamin A is readily available in a healthy diet. Women with lower socioeconomic status, however, may consume diets with inadequate amounts of vitamin A. Vitamin A deficiency during pregnancy weakens the immune system, increases risk of infections, and has been linked with night blindness. However, increasing dietary intake of vitamin A, rather than supplements, is advised because excess retinal intake in the first trimester is teratogenic and causes abnormalities of the cranial neural crest cells such as craniofacial and cardiac defects. The DRI for vitamin A during pregnancy is 770 mcg/day, and the tolerable upper intake has been established at 3000 mcg/day.[45] Over-the-counter multivitamin supplements may contain excessive doses of vitamin A and therefore should be discontinued during pregnancy.

Vitamin D

Vitamin D intake is essential for proper absorption of calcium and normal bone health. During pregnancy, vitamin D is also critically important for fetal growth and development, as well as regulation of genes associated with normal implantation and angiogenesis. Low maternal vitamin D status has been associated with reduced intrauterine long bone growth, shorter gestation, reduced childhood bone-mineral accrual, and decreased birth weight. Low maternal vitamin D status may also have consequences for fetal "imprinting" that may affect neurodevelopment, immune function, and chronic disease susceptibility later in life, as well as soon after birth.

Maternal vitamin D status may also be an independent risk factor for preeclampsia; supplementation may be helpful in promoting neonatal well-being and preventing preeclampsia.[46] Vitamin D deficiency is also associated with increased odds of having a primary cesarean section. One study showed that women who were severely vitamin D deficient (25[OH]D ≤37.5 nmol/L) at the time of delivery had almost four times the odds of cesarean birth compared to women who were not deficient.[47] One large study showed an inverse relationship between vitamin D supplementation and spontaneous preterm birth. Higher doses of vitamin D supplementation were associated with decrease in spontaneous preterm birth.

TABLE 7-5 DIETARY REFERENCE INTAKE (DRI): RECOMMENDED INTAKES FOR INDIVIDUALS

VITAMIN/MINERAL	AGE	NONPREGNANT	PREGNANT	UPPER INTAKE LEVELS
Vitamin A (mcg/day)	<18 y/o	700	750	2800
	19-30 y/o	700	770	3000
	31-50 y/o	700	770	3000
Vitamin C (mg/day)	<18 y/o	65	80	1800
	19-30 y/o	75	85	2000
	31-50 y/o	75	85	2000
Vitamin D (mcg/day)	<18 y/o	5	5	50
	19-30 y/o	5	5	50
	31-50 y/o	5	5	50
Vitamin E (mg/day)	<18 y/o	15	15	800
	19-30 y/o	15	15	1000
	31-50 y/o	15	15	1000
Vitamin K (mcg/day)	<18 y/o	75	75	ND
	19-30 y/o	90	90	ND
	31-50 y/o	90	90	ND
Thiamin (mg/day)	<18 y/o	1.1	1.4	ND
	19-30 y/o	1.1	1.4	ND
	31-50 y/o	1.1	1.4	ND
Riboflavin (mg/day)	<18 y/o	1.1	1.4	ND
	19-30 y/o	1.1	1.4	ND
	31-50 y/o	1.1	1.4	ND
Niacin (mg/day)	<18 y/o	14	18	30
	19-30 y/o	14	18	35
	31-50 y/o	14	18	35
Vitamin B_6 (mg/day)	<18 y/o	1.2	1.9	80
	19-30 y/o	1.3	1.9	100
	31-50 y/o	1.3	1.9	100
Folate (mcg/day)	<18 y/o	400	600	800
	19-30 y/o	400	600	1000
	31-50 y/o	400	600	1000
Vitamin B_{12} (mcg/day)	<18 y/o	2.4	2.6	ND
	19-30 y/o	2.4	2.6	ND
	31-50 y/o	2.4	2.6	ND
Pantothenic acid (mg/day)	<18 y/o	5	6	ND
	19-30 y/o	5	6	ND
	31-50 y/o	5	6	ND
Biotin (mcg/day)	<18 y/o	25	30	ND
	19-30 y/o	30	30	ND
	31-50 y/o	30	30	ND
Choline (mg/day)	<18 y/o	400	450	3
	19-30 y/o	425	450	3.5
	31-50 y/o	425	450	3.5
Calcium (mg/day)	<18 y/o	1300	1300	2500
	19-30 y/o	1000	1000	2500
	31-50 y/o	1000	1000	2500
Chromium (mcg/day)	<18 y/o	24	29	ND
	19-30 y/o	25	30	ND
	31-50 y/o	25	30	ND
Copper (mcg/day)	<18 y/o	890	1000	8000
	19-30 y/o	900	1000	10000
	31-50 y/o	900	1000	10000
Flouride (mg/day)	<18 y/o	3	3	10
	19-30 y/o	3	3	10
	31-50 y/o	3	3	10
Iodine (mcg/day)	<18 y/o	150	220	900
	19-30 y/o	150	220	1100
	31-50 y/o	150	220	1100
Iron (mg/day)	<18 y/o	15	27	45
	19-30 y/o	18	27	45
	31-50 y/o	18	27	45
Magnesium (mg/day)	<18 y/o	360	400	350
	19-30 y/o	310	350	350
	31-50 y/o	320	360	350
Phosphorous (mg/day)	<18 y/o	1250	1250	3.5
	19-30 y/o	700	700	3.5
	31-50 y/o	700	700	3.5
Selenium (mcg/day)	<18 y/o	55	60	400
	19-30 y/o	55	60	400
	31-50 y/o	55	60	400
Zinc (mg/day)	<18 y/o	9	12	34
	19-30 y/o	8	11	40
	31-50 y/o	8	11	40

ND, Not determined.

Modified from references 19 and 42-45.

The DRI for vitamin D for nonpregnant, pregnant, and, lactating women is 5 mcg/day, and the tolerable upper intake has been established at 50 mcg/day.[42] Recent studies, in the United States and other countries, have shown that low maternal vitamin D status is common during pregnancy. Lee and colleagues found that 50% of mothers and 65% of newborns were significantly vitamin D deficient at the time of birth despite mothers taking a prenatal vitamin containing 400 IU of vitamin D and drinking two glasses of vitamin D–fortified milk.[48] In addition, poor vitamin D status has been shown to be significantly more common among African American pregnant women.[49,50]

Vitamin D supplementation is advised for women who are strict vegetarians or for those who avoid sunlight or dairy foods. To evaluate vitamin D levels before and during pregnancy, check serum 25(OH)D levels and aim for vitamin D levels greater than 20 nmol/L and prescribe 1000 to 5000 mg/day of vitamin D_3 depending on the level of deficiency.

Vitamin C

Vitamin C, also known as ascorbic acid, is a water-soluble vitamin with numerous functions, including reducing free radicals and assisting in procollagen formation. Adequate vitamin C is also needed for iron uptake. Women who smoke have an increased need for vitamin C. Current recommendations indicate that pregnant women should consume 85 mg/day, rather than the 75 mg/day recommended for nonpregnant adult women, in order to protect against depleted plasma vitamin C levels and to ensure that adequate vitamin C is transported to the developing fetus. The tolerable upper intake for vitamin C has been established at 2000 mg/day. However, because vitamin C is actively transported from the maternal to the fetal circulation, and no human studies have examined the effects of large doses of vitamin C on fetal growth and development, a tolerable upper intake has been set at 1800 to 2000 mg/day.[44]

Vitamin B_6

Vitamin B_6, also known as pyridoxine, is a water-soluble B-complex vitamin required for protein, carbohydrate, and lipid metabolism. Vitamin B_6 is involved in the synthesis of heme compounds and helps form maternal and fetal red blood cells, antibodies, and neurotransmitters. Research shows that extra vitamin B_6 may be effective at relieving nausea or vomiting for some women during pregnancy.[51] The DRI during pregnancy is 1.9 mg/day. The dose commonly recommended to reduce nausea and vomiting is 10 to 25 mg, three times a day. Because excessive amounts of vitamin B_6 can cause numbness and nerve damage, the tolerable upper intake level for vitamin B_6 is set at 100 mg/day for pregnant women.[43]

Vitamin K

Vitamin K, a fat-soluble vitamin, is required for synthesis of clotting factors VII, IX, and X. Transportation of vitamin K from mother to fetus is limited; nevertheless, significant bleeding problems in the fetus are rare. **However, newborn infants are often functionally deficient in vitamin K and receive parenteral supplementation at birth.** The DRI for vitamin K is 90 mg for pregnant and nonpregnant women, and the tolerable upper intake has not been established.[45]

Folate

Folate and its metabolically active form tetrahydrofolate function as coenzymes involved in one-carbon transfer reactions that include the synthesis of nucleic acids and several amino acids. **Adequate levels of dietary folate are important during pregnancy to support rapid cell growth, replication, cell division, and nucleotide synthesis for fetal and placental development.**[52] Therefore, it is crucial that pregnant women consume adequate folate before and during the first 4 weeks of pregnancy.[43,52] The increased demand for folate during pregnancy is also needed for maternal erythropoiesis, mainly during the second and third trimesters.

Unfortunately, folate deficiency is the most prevalent vitamin deficiency during pregnancy, with well-known associations with birth defects, in particular, neural tube defects (NTDs).[53,54] Folate deficiency in humans is attributed to suboptimal dietary intake, behavioral and environmental factors, and genetic defects. Humans cannot synthesize folate from other sources and are therefore entirely dependent on dietary sources or supplements to meet their requirements. In 1992, the U.S. CDC recommended that all women of childbearing age take 400 mcg/day of supplemental folate, in order to ensure adequate folate levels are present when pregnancy occurs, whether intended or not.[55] The DRI for folate in women of childbearing age is currently 400 mcg/day, and for pregnant women is 600 mcg/day. The tolerable upper intake for folate has been established at 1000 mcg/day.[43] Additionally, evidence suggests that the long-term use of oral contraceptives inhibits folate absorption and enhances folate degradation in the liver.[56] Therefore, folate stores may be more rapidly depleted in women who have used oral contraceptives, which may lead to a higher incidence of folate deficiency in such women if they become pregnant.[43]

Folate and Neural Tube Defects

Spina bifida and anencephaly, the two most common types of NTDs, occur in approximately 3000 pregnancies each year in the United States (0.76 per 1000 births).[55] Prevalence varies according to race and ethnicity, with Hispanic women having the highest rates, while the lowest rates are found among African American and Asian women.[57] Women who have had a previous pregnancy with an NTD or who are personally affected by an NTD are at a higher risk (2% to 3%) for having an offspring with an NTD in a subsequent pregnancy. Other risk factors include a sibling with an NTD, maternal diabetes, and antiseizure medications such as valproic acid or carbamazepine. A higher risk of NTDs is also associated with increased maternal weight.[54] However, 95% of children with NTDs are born to couples without any family history of NTDs.

The etiology of NTDs has been associated with an increased folate demand during pregnancy, combined with a decreased dietary intake of folate. A genetic defect in the production of enzymes involved in folate metabolism has also been linked to NTDs.[53] The neural tube is formed very early in pregnancy, between 18 and 30 days after conception; defects in the formation of the neural tube can include the absence of formation of most of the brain (anencephaly) and defects in the closure of the lower tube (spina bifida, meningomyeloceles). The early formation and detrimental effects of folate deficiency on neural tube formation form the basis for the recommendation that **folate supplementation should be begun before conception and continued at least through the first trimester of pregnancy.**[52]

FOLATE SUPPLEMENTATION

In women with a history of a previous pregnancy with an NTD, it has been shown that supplementation with 4000 mcg/day (4 mg/day) of folate per day, initiated 1 month before attempting to conceive and continued throughout the first trimester of pregnancy, reduced the risk of a repeat NTD by 72%.[52] Although there is not yet definitive evidence that other high-risk groups (i.e., women with diabetes, women on antiseizure medications) will benefit from higher levels of supplementation, many experts recommend a higher dose of folate, at least 1000 mcg/day, before conception and in early pregnancy.[53,55] For these women, separate folate supplementation should be prescribed; additional doses of multivitamins should not be used. Additional daily multivitamin consumption could lead to toxicity of other vitamins, particularly vitamin A, which is teratogenic to the developing fetus.[5]

Several controlled and observational trials have shown that periconceptional and early pregnancy consumption of folate supplements can reduce a woman's risk for having an infant with an NTD by as much as 50% to 70%.[53] Since the U.S. government began the Folate Fortification Program in 1998, whereby cereals, pastas, rice, and breads are fortified with folate, NTD rates have declined.[55,57] Using data from eight population-based birth-defect surveillance systems with prenatal diagnosis of NTDs, the CDC reported that the prevalence of NTDs in the United States declined by an estimated 1000 cases from 4000 cases (1995-1996) to 3000 cases (1999-2000).[58] This 26% decrease in pregnancies with NTDs highlights the success of this public health policy. A Canadian study, where the level of folate fortification is similar, showed a 46% reduction in the prevalence of NTDs.[59] The higher baseline rate of NTDs compared to the United States might explain the greater risk reduction.

Minerals

Iron

Iron is an essential component of hemoglobin production and requirements increase significantly during pregnancy. Additional iron is needed to expand maternal red cell mass by 20% to 30%, as well as for fetal and placental tissue production. Throughout pregnancy, an additional 450 mg of iron is delivered to the maternal marrow and 250 mg is lost in blood during delivery. Therefore, approximately 1000 mg is required during pregnancy and the DRI has been established at 27 g/day compared to 18 mg/day for nonpregnant women. The tolerable upper intake for iron has been established at 45 mg/day.[45] Maintaining adequate iron stores is important, but difficult for many women during pregnancy.

According to the CDC, screening for anemia should take place before pregnancy, as well as during the first, second, and third trimesters in high-risk individuals. Iron deficiency anemia increases the risk of maternal and infant death, preterm delivery, and low neonatal birth weight, and has negative consequences for normal infant brain development and function.[60] The prevalence of iron deficiency in pregnancy is higher in African American women, low-income women, teenagers, women with less than a high school education, and women with multiple parity.[61]

TABLE 7-6 DIAGNOSIS OF ANEMIA IN PREGNANCY

LABORATORY TEST	FIRST TRIMESTER	SECOND TRIMESTER	THIRD TRIMESTER
Hemoglobin (g/dL)	11	10.5	11
Hematocrit (%)	33	32	<33

From Centers for Disease Control and Prevention (www.cdc.gov).

As shown in Table 7-6, hemoglobin less than 11 g/dL or hematocrit below 33% in the first or third trimester indicates anemia. Hemoglobin less than 10.5 g/dL or hematocrit below 33% in the second trimester also indicates anemia. As the significant increase in maternal blood volume during pregnancy typically reduces hemoglobin levels, serum ferritin and mean corpuscular volume should also be used as a diagnostic criteria because these measures are not affected by the increased blood volume. Serum ferritin is also useful in the assessment of the post–gastric bypass pregnant patient. A serum ferritin level of less than 15 ng/mL warrants aggressive treatment and may require intramuscular injection rather than oral supplementation.

Prenatal care providers generally recommend iron supplementation in the form of a daily supplement of 30 mg of elemental iron in the form of simple salts, beginning around the twelfth week of pregnancy for women who have normal preconception hemoglobin measurements. For women who are pregnant with multiple fetuses or have low preconception hemoglobin measurements, a supplement of between 60 and 100 mg/day of elemental iron is recommended until hemoglobin levels are normal. Once hemoglobin levels become normal, they may decrease their supplemental iron intake to 27 mg/day. Iron supplementation can have gastrointestinal side effects specific to pregnancy, which should be taken into account when prescribing the course of treatment. During the first trimester, nausea is a common problem and can be exacerbated by oral iron supplements. Deferring supplementation until the second trimester, when iron requirements increase and nausea has waned, may be necessary. Nausea resulting from iron supplements can be minimized by taking the supplement following a meal; however, iron absorption may be inhibited if the supplement is ingested immediately following a meal. Oral iron supplements can also cause constipation, which can be effectively treated with bulk laxatives, stool softeners, and increased fiber.

Antacids impair iron absorption and should not be taken concurrently; this is of particular importance during the third trimester, when gastroesophageal reflux is common. Iron is better absorbed if the maternal diet contains adequate amounts of vitamin C. Occasionally, pregnant women develop pica, a craving for nonfood substances such as clay, dirt, or ice. Iron deficiency has been postulated to cause pica but there are also cultural beliefs that lead to these practices. Pregnant women with iron deficiency should be questioned about pica (the ingestion of nonfood substances), and women experiencing pica should be tested for iron deficiency. Pica is mostly of concern if it prevents the mother from consuming nutrient-rich foods.[62]

Calcium

Large quantities of calcium are essential for the development of the fetal skeleton, fetal tissues, and hormonal adaptations during pregnancy. These include changes in calcium regulatory hormones affecting intestinal absorption, renal reabsorption of calcium, and bone turnover of calcium.[42] The presence of $1,25(OH)_2D_3$ stimulates increased intestinal absorption of calcium during the second and third trimesters, protecting maternal bone, while meeting fetal calcium requirements. In contrast to maternal iron and folate stores, which are relatively small and easily depleted, maternal calcium stores are large and are mostly stored skeletally, allowing for easy mobilization. Fetal calcium needs are highest during the third trimester, when the fetus absorbs an average of 300 mg/day in response to the increased maternal $1,25(OH)_2D_3$.[2] Studies suggest that inadequate calcium during pregnancy is associated with gestational hypertension, preterm delivery, and preeclampsia.[63,64]

The DRI for calcium in women 19 to 50 years old is 1000 mg/day; it is 1300 mg/day for females age 9 to 19.[42] Adolescents may need additional calcium during pregnancy since their own bones still require calcium deposition to ensure adequate bone density as an adult.[65] The tolerable upper intake for calcium during pregnancy is 2500 mg/day.[42] Obtaining adequate dietary calcium is difficult for many women before and during pregnancy and supplementations may be needed, especially for African Americans, Hispanics, and American Indians.[42] Consuming at least three servings of dairy foods every day, including calcium-fortified juices and soy beverages, can help meet these requirements.[5] Women who limit their intake of dairy foods because of lactose intolerance seem to be able to tolerate yogurt and cheese on a daily basis, but may also require a supplement. Calcium carbonate, gluconate, lactate, or citrate may provide 500 to 600 mg/day of calcium to account for the difference between the amount of calcium required and that consumed. The standard prenatal vitamin typically contains 150 to 300 mg/serving. Multivitamins marketed to the nonpregnant population generally have less than 200 mg/serving. Calcium is thought to be absorbed in doses of 600 mg at one time, making it unlikely that pregnant women would reach the tolerable upper intake level.

The data concerning the role of calcium in controlling pregnancy-induced hypertension or preeclampsia remain controversial. Although calcium supplementation has been shown to decrease blood pressure and preeclampsia in smaller studies, larger trials have failed to show an effect.[64,66] Evidence has shown that calcium supplementation reduces the risk of developing hypertension during pregnancy, but only in women who did not have adequate calcium intake before supplementation.[63,64] It is prudent to make sure women are meeting their calcium requirements for their age and to stress the importance of adequate calcium intake before and during pregnancy.

Zinc

Zinc is involved in catalytic, structural, and regulatory functions for nucleic acid and protein metabolism and requirements increase during pregnancy. More than 100 enzymes require zinc and maternal zinc deficiency can lead to prolonged labor, intrauterine growth retardation, teratogenesis, and embryonic or fetal death.[45] The DRI for pregnant women is 11 mg/day and may be higher for vegetarians or vegans because phytates from whole grains and beans bind with zinc and may reduce absorption. The tolerable upper intake for zinc has been established at 40 mg/day for both pregnant and nonpregnant women. Pregnant women eating well-balanced diets do not typically require zinc supplementation. However, if a woman is prescribed elemental iron greater than 60 mg/day, zinc supplementation is recommended, because both iron and copper compete with zinc for absorption. In addition, zinc supplementation should be combined with copper supplement to prevent deficiency.[45] Prenatal vitamin formulations vary and usually include copper and zinc.

NUTRITION-RELATED PROBLEMS IN PREGNANCY

Nausea and Vomiting

Nausea and vomiting during pregnancy commonly occurs between 5 and 18 weeks of gestation and typically improves by 16 to 18 weeks.[67] From 15% to 20% of women may experience these symptoms until the third trimester and 5% of women up until delivery.[68] Between 50% to 90% of women have some degree of nausea, with or without vomiting, but only a small percentage of these women require hospitalization for severe hyperemesis gravidarum.[69] Women with hyperemesis may vomit multiple times throughout the day, lose more than 5% of their prepregnancy body weight, and usually require hospitalization for dehydration.

The causes of pregnancy-related nausea and vomiting are unclear, but may be related to increased levels of human chorionic gonadotropin, which peaks at about 12 weeks' gestation.[68] Studies show that women are more likely to have nausea or vomiting during pregnancy if they have the following:

- Multiple gestation
- Nausea and vomiting in a previous pregnancy
- Nausea or vomiting as a side effect of taking birth control pills
- History of motion sickness
- A relative (mother or sister) who had morning sickness during pregnancy
- History of migraine headaches

Strategies for managing nausea and vomiting during pregnancy are shown in the accompanying box, Strategies for Managing Nausea, Vomiting, Heartburn, and Indigestion in Pregnancy. Vitamin B_6 supplements (10 to 25 mg three times a day) have been used to treat nausea and vomiting during pregnancy. Ginger and acupuncture may also be helpful.[70,71]

Heartburn and Indigestion

Heartburn and indigestion affects two thirds of pregnant women and is usually caused by gastric content reflux that results from both lower esophageal pressure and decreased

Strategies for Managing Nausea, Vomiting, Heartburn, and Indigestion in Pregnancy

- Eat small, low-fat meals and snacks (fruits, pretzels, crackers, nonfat yogurt).
- Eat slowly and frequently.
- Avoid strong food odors by eating room temperature or cold foods and using good ventilation while cooking.
- Drink fluids between meals, rather than with meals.
- Avoid foods that may cause stomach irritation such as spearmint, peppermint, caffeine, citrus fruits, spicy foods, high-fat foods, or tomato products.
- Wait 1 to 2 hours after eating a meal before lying down.
- Take a walk after meals.
- Wear loose-fitting clothes.
- Brush teeth after eating to prevent symptoms.

Source: Lisa Hark, PhD, RD. Used with permission.

motility secondary to increased progesterone.[70] Limited gastric capacity, due to a shift of organs to accommodate the growing fetus, contributes to these symptoms in the third trimester of pregnancy. Strategies for managing heartburn or indigestion are shown in the accompanying box, Strategies for Managing Nausea, Vomiting, Heartburn, and Indigestion in Pregnancy.[59,72]

Constipation

Constipation rates during pregnancy range from 16% to 26%.[73] Fifty percent of pregnant women experience constipation at some point during their pregnancy, which is often associated with symptoms of straining, hard stools, and incomplete evacuation, rather than infrequent defecation.[73] Constipation during pregnancy is associated with an increase in water reabsorption from the large intestine, smooth muscle relaxation, and slower gastrointestinal motility. The pregnant woman often notes overall gastrointestinal discomfort, a bloated sensation, an increase in hemorrhoids and heartburn, and decreased appetite. Constipation can also be aggravated by iron supplements. Constipation management strategies are shown in the accompanying box, Strategies for Managing Constipation in Pregnancy.

Food Contamination

Pregnant women have an increased risk of developing food-borne infections secondary to the hormonal changes associated with pregnancy.[74] Pathogens that are a growing concern during pregnancy include *Listeria monocytogenes*, *Toxoplasma gondii*, *Brucella* species, *Salmonella* species, and *Campylobacter jejuni*. Many of these organisms can cross the placenta and therefore increase the fetus's risk of becoming infected.[75]

Strategies for Managing Constipation in Pregnancy

- Increase fluid intake to 2 or 3 quarts per day (water, herbal teas, noncaffeinated beverages).
- Increase daily fiber intake (high-fiber cereals, whole grains, legumes, bran).
- Use psyllium fiber supplement (Metamucil).
- Increase consumptions of fruits and vegetables (fresh, frozen, and dried).
- Participate in moderate physical activity (walking, swimming, yoga).
- Take stool softeners if prescribed iron supplements.

Source: Lisa Hark, PhD, RD. Used with permission.

Listeria monocytogenes results from food poisoning during pregnancy and an estimated 14-fold increase in the incidence of listeriosis among pregnant women compared to nonpregnant women has been seen in recent years.[75] In addition, pregnant women make up an estimated 27% of all reported cases of listeriosis.[75] Listeriosis can be found in soil, ground water, plants, and animals.[76] In pregnancy, however, listeriosis can develop into a blood-borne, transplacental infection that can cause chorioamnionitis, premature labor, spontaneous abortion, or fetal demise.[77] Symptoms include fever, chills, headache, muscle and back aches, and gastrointestinal symptoms, which may appear 2 to 3 days after exposure. Blood tests can confirm the diagnosis and women should be treated with antibiotics. To avoid listeriosis, pregnant women should be advised to wash vegetables and fruits well, cook all meats, avoid processed, precooked meats (cold cuts), soft cheeses (brie, blue cheese, Camembert, and Mexican caso-blanco), and only consume pasteurized dairy products.[75] All foods should be handled in a sanitary and appropriate manner to prevent bacterial contamination.[75]

Toxoplasmosis can be passed to humans by water, dust, soil, and eating contaminated foods. Cats are the main host of *T. gondii*. Toxoplasmosis most often results from eating raw or uncooked meat, eating unwashed fruits and vegetables, cleaning the litter box, or handling contaminated soil. Most individuals will not experience any recognizable symptoms and will develop a protective resistance to the parasite. However, if a pregnant woman is exposed during the first few months of gestation, she can pass the parasite on to the fetus. This could result in stillbirth, early prenatal death, or other serious health problems.[76,78]

Salmonellosis infection results in a similar infection, and symptoms include headache, diarrhea, abdominal pain, nausea, chills, fever, and vomiting and usually appear 12 to 36 hours after contamination. *Campylobacter* can cause diarrhea accompanied by fever. These organisms thrive in reduced-oxygen environments. Fetal exposure to *Salmonella* and *Campylobacter* is associated with abortion, stillbirth, and premature labor.[75] Foods that contain these pathogens include raw unpasteurized milk, raw or undercooked meat, poultry, eggs, salads, cream deserts, filling, and untreated water. To avoid these infections, pregnant women should wash their hands often, especially after handling animals or working in the garden, and avoid undercooked food and unpasteurized juices. All surfaces that come into contact with raw meat, fish, or poultry should also be washed with hot soapy water.[75]

Food thought to be contaminated with heavy metals can also produce devastating neurotoxic and teratogenic effects on the developing fetus, which may result in miscarriage, stillbirth, premature labor, or other fetal complications.[79,80] In particular, case reports of teratogenicity or embryotoxicity have been reported with exposure to methyl mercury, lead, cadmium, nickel, and selenium.[81] Consumption of raw fish products and highly carnivorous fish (including tuna, shark, tilefish, swordfish, and mackerel) should be limited or avoided during pregnancy.[82,83] Mercury can be removed from vegetables by peeling or washing well with soap and water. All dairy foods and juices consumed during pregnancy should be pasteurized.[80]

Pregnancy Following Bariatric Surgery

Because of the increase in obesity in women of reproductive age, obstetricians are seeing many more women who have undergone bariatric surgery. It is estimated that approximately 50,000 women of reproductive age undergo inpatient bariatric surgery per year.[84] Most likely, many more women are undergoing outpatient procedures. How many of these women then go on to become pregnant is not known.

Bariatric surgery may be considered in patients with class III obesity (BMI greater than 40 kg/m^2) or class II (BMI greater than 35 kg/m^2 with comorbid conditions and failure of nonsurgical treatment). There are two major types of bariatric surgical procedures: (1) malabsorptive procedures such as the Roux-en-Y gastric bypass and biliopancreatic diversion (BPD) and (2) restrictive procedures such as laparoscopic adjustable gastric banding (LAGB).

Complications have been associated with both types during pregnancy, including small bowel ischemia[85] and nutritional (folate, vitamin B_{12}) deficiencies.[86] There have also been reported cases of fetal anomalies, SGA neonates, and preterm births.[87,88] Scheiner and colleagues reported malabsorptive and restrictive procedures in a series of 298 pregnant patients after bariatric surgery.[89] Compared with a general population, there was a significant increase in premature rupture of the membranes, labor induction, and macrosomia. Bariatric surgery was also an independent risk factor for cesarean delivery but was not associated with adverse neonatal outcome.

There are no prospective randomized trials of pregnancy outcome in obese women treated by conventional means or bariatric surgery. However, there have been reports using the patient as her own control (i.e., a pregnancy outcome before bariatric surgery and a subsequent pregnancy outcome after having a bariatric procedure)[90-92] or retrospective case-controlled studies.[93] Three of the studies reported a decrease in weight gain during pregnancy in the women who had undergone bariatric surgery; Ducarme and colleagues (5.5 vs. 7.1 kg, $P < 0.05$),[93] Skull and colleagues (3.7 vs. 15.6 kg, $P < 0.0001$),[92] and Dixon and colleagues (9.6 vs. 14.4 kg, $P < 0.001$).[90] Gestational diabetes and hypertensive disorders were also decreased in the bariatric surgery groups. Last, the effect of bariatric surgery on the risk of fetal macrosomia and birth weight are inconclusive. Only two of the four studies reported a decreased risk of macrosomia in women after having bariatric surgery from 14.6% to 7.7% ($P < 0.05$) and 34.8% to 7.7%, respectively.[91,93] Care must be taken in the interpretation of these studies because of their retrospective nature and use of various definitions of outcome measures.

The long-term effects of biliopancreatic diversion (BPD) surgery on the offspring have been addressed in follow-up studies by Kral and colleagues.[94] After maternal bariatric surgery the prevalence of obesity in the offspring decreased by 52% and severe obesity by 45%, with no increase in underweight. The reduction in obesity in the offspring was greater in the male as compared with female offspring. A follow-up study of this same cohort assessing metabolic function was recently published by Smith and colleagues.[95] The offspring of the women who were born after their mothers had BPD had a threefold lower prevalence of severe obesity, greater insulin sensitivity, improved lipid profile, lower C-reactive protein and leptin, and increased ghrelin as compared with their siblings born before maternal BPD surgery. The authors caution in the interpretation of the results as these data do not prove causality but need to be confirmed in other populations with further understanding of potential mechanisms.

ACOG published a Committee Opinion on Obesity and Pregnancy addressing the issue of bariatric surgery and pregnancy.[96] ACOG recommends that obese women who have undergone bariatric surgery receive the following counseling before and during pregnancy:

1. Patients with adjustable gastric banding should be advised that they are at risk of becoming pregnant unexpectedly after weight loss following surgery.
2. All patients are advised to delay pregnancy for 12 to 18 months after surgery to avoid pregnancy during the rapid weight loss phase.
3. Women with gastric banding should be monitored by their general surgeons during pregnancy because adjustments of the band may be necessary.
4. Patients should be evaluated for nutritional deficiencies, including iron, vitamin B_{12}, folate, vitamin D, and calcium, and supplemented with vitamins as necessary.

KEY POINTS

- Pregnant women may need as much as an additional 300 kcal/day for the entire pregnancy, but requirements may be significantly less and vary among individuals and ethnic groups.
- The IOM recommendations for total weight gain during pregnancy are as follows: underweight (BMI <18.5; 28 to 40 lb), normal weight (BMI 18.5 to 24.9; 25 to 35 lb), overweight (BMI 25.0 to 29.9; 15 to 25 lb), and obese (BMI ≥30; 11 to 20 lb) women.
- Protein requirements during pregnancy increase from 0.8 g/kg/day for nonpregnant women to 1.1 g/kg/day during pregnancy.
- Women at high risk of a neural tube defect should be prescribed a higher dose of folate, at least 1000 mcg/day, before conception and in early pregnancy.
- Iron supplementation can have gastrointestinal side effects specific to pregnancy, which should be taken into account when prescribing treatment.
- To evaluate vitamin D levels before and during pregnancy, check serum 25(OH)D levels and aim for vitamin D levels greater than 20 nmol/L. The dietary reference intake (DRI) for vitamin D is 600 IU/day.
- The DRI for calcium in nonpregnant and pregnant women 19 to 50 years old is 1000 mg/day; it is 1300 mg/day for females age 9 to 19.
- Women who have undergone previous bariatric surgery should be evaluated for nutritional deficiencies including iron, vitamin B_{12}, folate, vitamin D, and calcium and supplemented as necessary.

REFERENCES

1. Ogden CL, Carroll MD, Curtin LR, et al: Prevalence of overweight and obesity in the US 1999-2004. JAMA 295:1549, 2006.
2. Flegal KM, Carroll MD, Ogden CL, Curtin LR: Prevalence and trends in obesity among US adults, 1999-2008. JAMA 303:235, 2010.
3. Nohr EA, Vaeth M, Baker JL, et al: Combined associations of prepregnancy body mass index and gestational weight gain with the outcome of pregnancy. Am J Clin Nutr 87:1750, 2008.
4. Sewell MF, Huston-Presley L, Super DM, Catalano PM: Increased neonatal fat mass not lean body mass, is associated with maternal obesity. Am J Obstet Gynecol 195:1100, 2006.
5. Hark LA, Deen DD: Nutrition in Pregnancy and Lactation. In Medical Nutrition and Disease, 4th ed. Malden, MA, Wiley-Blackwell, 2009.
6. Subcommittee on Nutritional Status and Weight Gain during Pregnancy. Subcommittee on Dietary Intake and Nutrient Supplements during Pregnancy Committee on Nutritional Status during Pregnancy and Lactation, Food and Nutrition Board. Institute of Medicine, National Academy of Sciences. In Nutrition during Pregnancy, Part I, Weight Gain, Part II, Nutrient Supplements. Washington, DC, National Academy Press, Part 1, 1990, pp 1-222.
7. Rasmussin KM, Yaktin AL (eds): Weight Gain during Pregnancy: Reexamining the Guidelines. Institute of Medicine of the National Academies. Washington, DC, National Academy Press, 2009, pp 77-83.
8. Chu SY, Callaghan WM, Bisch CC, D'Angelo D: Gestational weight gain by body mass index among US women delivering live births, 2004-2005: fueling future obesity. Am J Obstet Gynecol 200:271, 2009.
9. Viswanathan M, Siega-Riz AM, Moos M-K, et al: Outcomes of maternal weight gain, evidence report/technology assessment no. 168. (Prepared by RTI International-University of North Carolina Evidence-based Practice Center under contract No. 290-02-0016.) AHRQ Publication No. 08-E-0-09. Rockville, MD, Agency for Healthcare Research and Quality, 2008.
10. Oken E, Rifas-Shimar SL, Field AE, et al: Maternal gestational weight gain and offspring weight in adolescence. Obstet Gynecol 112:999, 2008.
11. Kiel DW, Dodson EA, Artal R, et al: Gestational weight gain and pregnancy outcomes in obese women: how much is enough? Obstet Gynecol 110:752, 2007.
12. Luke B, Hediger ML, Nugent C, et al: Body mass index—specific weight gains associated with optimal birth weights in twin pregnancies. J Reprod Med 48:217, 2003.
13. Chen XK, Wen SW, Fleming N, et al: Teen-age pregnancy and adverse birth outcomes: a large population based retrospective cohort study. Int J Epidemiol 35:368, 2007.
14. Howie LD, Parker JD, Schoendorf KC: Excessive maternal weight gain patterns in adolescents. J Am Diabetes Assoc 103:1653, 2003.
15. McAnarney ER, Stevens-Simon C: First, do no harm. Low-birth-weight and adolescent obesity. Am J Dis Child 147:983, 1993.
16. Abbassi-Ghanavati M, Green LG, Cunningham FG: Pregnancy and laboratory studies: a reference table for clinicians. Obstet Gynecol 114:1326, 2009.
17. Catalano PM, Hollenbeck C: Energy requirements in pregnancy. Obstet Gynecol Surv 47:368, 1992.
18. Forsum E, Löf M: Energy metabolism during human pregnancy. Ann Rev Nutr 27:277, 2007.
19. Trumbo P, Schlicker S, Yates AA, Poos M, Food and Nutrition Board, Institute of Medicine: Dietary Reference Intakes for Energy, Carbohydrate, Fiber, Fat, Fatty Acids, Cholesterol, Protein, and Amino Acids. Washington, DC, National Academies Press, 2002.
20. Forsum E, Kabir N, Sadurskis A, Westerterp K: Total energy expenditure of healthy Swedish women during pregnancy and lactation. Am J Clin Nutr 56:334, 1992.
21. Durnin JVGA, McKillop FM, Grant S, et al: Energy requirements of pregnancy in Scotland. Lancet 2:897, 1987.
22. Lawrence M, Lawrence F, Coward WA, et al: Energy requirements of pregnancy in the Gambia. Lancet 2:1072, 1987.
23. Van Raaij JMA, Vermat-Miedema SH, Schonk CM, et al: Energy requirements of pregnancy in the Netherlands. Lancet 2:953, 1987.
24. Goldberg GR, Prentice AM, Coward WA, et al: Longitudinal assessment of energy expenditure in pregnancy by the doubly labeled water method. Am J Clin Nutr 57:94, 1993.
25. Prentice A, Goldbert G: Maternal obesity increases congenital malformations. Nutr Rev 54:146, 1996.
26. Butte NF, Hopkinson JM, Mehta N, Moon JK, et al: Adjustments in energy expenditure and substrate utilization during late pregnancy and lactation. Am J Clin Nutr 69:299, 1999.
27. Peyron-Caso E, Quignard-Boulange A, Laromiguiere M, et al: Dietary fish oil increase lipid mobilization but does not decrease lipid storage-related enzyme activities in adipose tissue of insulin-resistant, sucrose-fed rats. J Nutr 133:2239, 2003.
28. Oken E, Kleinman KP, Berland WE, et al: Decline in fish consumption among pregnant women after a national mercury advisory. Obstet Gynecol 102:346, 2003.
29. Innes SM, Elias SL: Intakes of essential n-6 and n-polyunsaturated fatty acids among pregnant Canadian women. Am J Clin Nutr 77:73, 2003.
30. Elias SL, Innes SM: Infant plasma trans, n-6 and n-3 fatty acids and conjugated linoleic acids are related to maternal plasma fatty acids, length of gestation and birth weight and length. Am J Clin Nutr 73: 807, 2001.
31. Montgomery C, Speake BK, Cameron A, et al: Maternal docosahexaenoic acid supplementation and fetal accretion. Br J Nutr 90:135, 2003.
32. Haggarty P: Effect of placental function on fatty acid requirements during pregnancy. Eur J Clin Nutr 58:1559, 2004.
33. Meydani SN, Endres S, Woods MM, et al: Oral (n-3) fatty acid supplementation suppresses cytokine production and lymphocyte proliferation: comparison between young and older women. J Nutr 121:547, 1991.
34. Norris JM, Yin X, Lamb MM, et al: Omega-3 polyunsaturated fatty acid intake and islet autoimmunity in children at increased risk for type 1 diabetes. JAMA 298:1420, 2007.
35. Dunstan JA, Mori TA, Barden A, et al: Fish oil supplementation in pregnancy modifies neonatal allergen-specific immune responses and clinical outcomes in infants at high risk of atopy: a randomized, controlled trial. J Allergy Clin Immunol 112:1178, 2003.
36. Dunstan JA, Mon TA, Barden A, et al: Maternal fish oil supplementation in pregnancy reduces interleukin-13 levels in cord blood of infants at high risk of atopy. Clin Exp Allergy 33:442, 2003.
37. Harper M, Thom E, Klebanoff MA, et al: Omega-3 fatty acid supplementation to prevent recurrent preterm birth: a randomized controlled trial. Obstet Gynecol 115:234, 2010.
38. Simopoulos A, Leaf A, Salem N: US Expert Panel: essentiality of and recommended diet intakes for omega-6 and omega-3 fatty acids. Ann Nutr Metab 43:127, 1999.
39. Oken E, Kleinman KP, Olsen SF, et al: Associations of seafood and elongated n-3 fatty acid intake with fetal growth and length of gestation: results from a US pregnancy cohort. Am J Epidemiol 160:774, 2004.
40. Grandjean P, Bjerve KS, Weihe P, Steuerwald U: Birth weight in a fishing community: significance of essential fatty acids and marine food contaminants. Int J Epidemiol 30:1272, 2001.
41. Groh-Wargo S, Jacobs J, Auestad N, et al: Body composition in preterm infants who are fed long-chain polyunsaturated fatty acids: a prospective, randomized, controlled trial. Pediatr Res 57:712, 2005.
42. Bergman C, Gray-Scott D, Chen JJ, Meacham S: Food and Nutrition Board, Institute of Medicine. Dietary Reference Intakes for Calcium, Phosphorous, Magnesium, Vitamin D, and Fluoride. Washington, DC, National Academy Press, 1997.
43. Food and Nutrition Board, Institute of Medicine: Dietary Reference Intakes for Thiamin, Riboflavin, Niacin, Vitamin B_6, Folate, Vitamin B_{12}, Pantothenic Acid, Biotin, and Choline. Washington, DC, National Academy Press, 1998.
44. Food and Nutrition Board, Institute of Medicine: Dietary Reference Intakes: Vitamin C, Vitamin E, Selenium, and Carotenoids. Washington, DC, National Academy Press, 2000.
45. Trumbo P, Yates AA, Schlicker S, Poos M: Food and Nutrition Board, Institute of Medicine. Dietary Reference Intakes for Vitamin A, Vitamin K, Arsenic, Boron, Chromium, Copper, Iodine, Iron, Manganese, Molybdenum, Nickel, Silicon, Vanadium, and Zinc. Washington, DC, National Academy Press, 2001.
46. Bodnar LM, Catov JM, Simhan HN, et al: Maternal vitamin D deficiency increases the risk of preeclampsia. J Clin Endocrinol Metab 92:3517, 2007.
47. Merewood A et al: Association between vitamin D deficiency and primary cesarean section. J Clin Endocrinol Metab 94:940, 2008.

48. Lee JM, Smith JR, Philipp BL, et al: Vitamin D deficiency in a healthy group of mothers and newborn infants. Clin Pediatr 46:42, 2007.
49. Looker A et al: Serum 25-hydroxyvitamin D status of the US population: 1988-1994 compared with 2000-2004. Am J Clin Nutr 88:1519, 2008.
50. Bodnar LM, Simhan HN: Vitamin D may be a link to black-white disparities in adverse birth outcomes. Obstet Gynecol Surv 65:273, 2010.
51. Chittumma P, Kaewkiattikun K, Wiriyasiriwach B: Comparison of the effectiveness of ginger and vitamin B_6 for treatment of nausea and vomiting in early pregnancy: a randomized double-blind controlled trial. J Med Assoc Thai 90:15, 2007.
52. Molloy AM, Kirke PN, Brody LC, et al: Effects of folate and vitamin B_{12} deficiencies during pregnancy on fetal, infant, and child development. Food Nutr Bull 29:S101, 2008.
53. Blencowe H, Cousens S, Modell B, et al: Folic acid to reduce neonatal mortality from neural tube disorders. Int J Epidemiol 39:110, 2010.
54. Black M: Effects of vitamin B_{12} and folate deficiency on brain development in children. Food Nutr Bull 29:126, 2008.
55. US Preventive Services Task Force, Agency for Healthcare Research and Quality: Folic acid for the prevention of neural tube defects: US Preventive Services Task Force recommendation statement. Ann Intern Med 150:626, 2009.
56. Burau KD, Cech I: Serological differences in folate/vitamin B_{12} in pregnancies affected by neural tube defects. South Med J 103:419, 2010.
57. Bentley TG, Willett WC, Weinstein MC, Kuntz KM: Population-level changes in folate intake by age, gender, and race/ethnicity after folic acid fortification. Am J Public Health 96:2040, 2006.
58. Pfeiffer CM, Caudill SP, Gunter EW, et al: Biochemical indicators of B vitamin status in the US population after folic acid fortification: results from the National Health and Nutrition Examination Survey 1999-2000. Am J Clin Nutr 82:442, 2005.
59. De Wals P, Tairou F, Van Allen MI, et al: Reduction in neural-neural tube defects after folic acid fortification in Canada. N Engl J Med 357:135, 2007.
60. Georgieff MK: The role of iron in neurodevelopment: fetal iron deficiency and the developing hippocampus. Biochem Soc Trans 36:1267, 2008.
61. Belfort M, Rifas-ShimanSL, Rich-Edwards JW, et al: Maternal iron intake and iron status during pregnancy and child blood pressure at age 3 years. Int J Epidemiol 37:301, 2008.
62. Beyan C, Kaptan K, Infran A, Beyan E: Pica: a frequent symptom in iron deficiency anemia. Arch Med Sci 5:471, 2009.
63. Atallah AN, Hofmeyer GJ, Duley L: Calcium supplementation during pregnancy for preventing hypertensive disorders and related problems. Cochrane Database Syst Rev 2006.
64. Solomon CG, Seely EW: Hypertension in pregnancy. Endocrinol Metab Clin North Am 35:157, 2006.
65. Chan G, McElligott K, McNaught T, Gill G: Effects of dietary calcium intervention on adolescent mothers and newborns: a randomized controlled trial. Obstet Gyneol 108:565, 2006.
66. Levine RJ, Hauth JC, Curet LB, et al: Trial of calcium to prevent preeclampsia. N Engl J Med 337:69, 1997.
67. Holmgren C, Aagaard-Tillery KM, Silver RM, et al: Hyperemesis in pregnancy: an evaluation of treatment strategies with maternal and neonatal outcomes. Am J Obstet Gynecol 56:1, 2008.
68. Fejzoa MS, Inglesb SA, Wilsonab M, et al: High prevalence of severe nausea and vomiting of pregnancy and hyperemesis gravidarum among relatives of affected individuals. Eur J Ob Gyn Repr Biol 141:13, 2008.
69. Dodds L, Fell DB, Joseph KS, et al: Outcomes of pregnancies complicated by hyperemesis gravidarum. Obstet Gynecol 107:285, 2006.
70. Jewell D, Young G: Interventions for nausea and vomiting in early pregnancy. Cochrane Database Syst Rev CD000145, 2003.
71. Chittumma P, Kaewkiattikun K, Wiriyasiriwach B: Comparison of the effectiveness of ginger and vitamin B_6 for treatment of nausea and vomiting in early pregnancy: a randomized double-blind controlled trial. J Med Assoc Thai 90:15, 2007.
72. King T, Murphy PA: Evidence-based approaches to managing nausea and vomiting in early pregnancy. J Midwifery Womans Health 54:430, 2009.
73. Bradley CS, Kennedy CM, Turcea AM, et al: Constipation in pregnancy: prevalence, symptoms, and risk factors. Obstet Gynecol 110:1351, 2007.
74. American Congress of Obstetricians and Gynecologists: Your Pregnancy and Birth, 4th ed. Washington, DC, ACOG, 2005.
75. Dean J, Kendall P: Food safety during pregnancy. Colorado State University Cooperative Extension. www.ext.colostate.edu. Accessed Oct 1, 2010.
76. Delgado A: Listeriosis in pregnancy. J Midwifery Womens Health 53:255, 2008.
77. Posfay-Barbe KM, Wald ER: Listeriosis. Semin Fetal Neonatal Med 14:228, 2009.
78. Centers for Disease Control and Prevention: Preventing congenital toxoplasmosis. Morb Mortal Wkly Rep 49:RR02, 2000.
79. Olsen SF, Østerdal ML, Salvig JD, et al: Duration of pregnancy in relation to seafood intake during early and mid pregnancy: prospective cohort. Eur J Epidemiol 21:749, 2006.
80. Hibbein JR, Davis JM, Steer C, et al: Maternal seafood consumption in pregnancy and neurodevelopmental outcomes in childhood (ALSPAC Study): an observational cohort study. Lancet 269:578, 2007.
81. Brender JD, Suarez L, Felkner M, et al: Maternal exposure to arsenic, cadmium, lead, and mercury and neural tube defects in offspring. Environ Res 101:132, 2006.
82. Fei X, Holzman C, Rahbar MH, et al: Maternal fish consumption, mercury levels, and risk of preterm delivery. Environ Health Perspect 115:42, 2007.
83. US Department of Health and Human Services & US Environmental Protection Agency: What you need to know about mercury in fish and shellfish. 2005. www.epa.gov. Accessed Oct 1, 2010.
84. Kulick D, Hark L, Deen D: The bariatric surgery patient, a growing role for registered dietitians. J Am Diet Assoc 110:593, 2010.
85. Charles A, Domingo S, Goldfadden A, et al: Small bowel ischemia after Roux-en-y gastric bypass complicated by pregnancy: a case report. Am Surg 71:231, 2005.
86. Gurewitsch ED, Smith-Levitin M, Mack J: Pregnancy following gastric bypass surgery for morbid obesity. Obstet Gynecol 88:658, 1996.
87. Ingardia CJ, Fischer JR: Pregnancy after jejunoileal bypass and SGA infant. Obstet Gynecol 52:215, 1978.
88. Knudsen LB, Kallen B: Intestinal bypass operation and pregnancy outcome. ACTA Obstet Gynecol Scand 65:831, 1986.
89. Sheiner E, Levy A, Silverberg D, et al: Pregnancy after bariatric surgery is not associated with adverse perinatal outcome. Am J Obstet Gynecol 190:1335, 2004.
90. Dixon JB, Dixon ME, O'Brien PE: Birth outcomes in obese women after laparoscopic adjustable gastric banding. Obstet Gynecol 106: 965, 2005.
91. Marceau P, Kaufman D, Biron S, et al: Outcome of pregnancies after biliopancreatic diversion. Obes Surg 14:318, 2004.
92. Skull AJ, Slater GH, Duncombe JE, Fielding GA: Laparoscopic adjustable banding in pregnancy: safety, patient tolerance and effect on obesity-related pregnancy outcomes. Obes Surg 14:230, 2007.
93. Ducarme G, Revaux A, Rodrigues A, et al: Obstetric outcome following laparoscopic adjustable gastric banding. Int J Gynecol Obstet 98:244, 2007.
94. Kral JG, Biron S, Simard S, et al: Large maternal weight loss from obesity surgery prevents transmission of obesity to children who were followed for 2 to 18 years. Pediatrics 118:e1644, 2006.
95. Smith J, Cianflone K, Biron S, et al: Effects of maternal surgical weight loss in mothers on intergenerational transmission of obesity. J Clin Endocrinol Metab 94:4275, 2009.
96. American Congress of Obstetricians and Gynecologists Committee Opinion Number 315: Obesity in pregnancy. Am Col Obstet Gynecol 106:1, 2005.

For full reference list, log onto www.expertconsult.com.

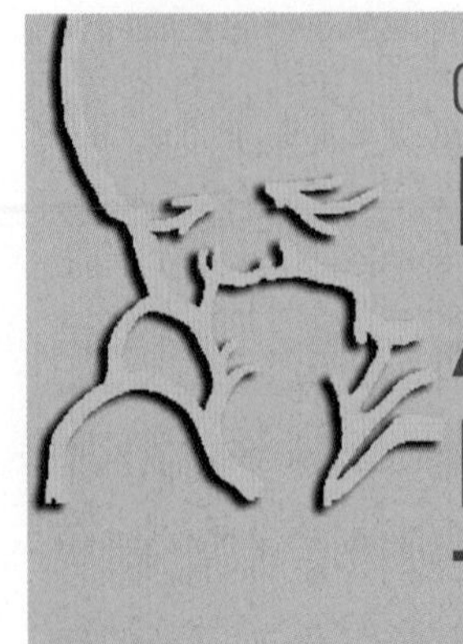

CHAPTER 8

Drugs and Environmental Agents in Pregnancy and Lactation: Embryology, Teratology, Epidemiology

Jennifer R. Niebyl and Joe Leigh Simpson

KEY ABBREVIATIONS	
Angiotensin-converting Enzyme	ACE
Birth Defect Surveillance Monitoring System	BDMS
Diethylstilbestrol	DES
Electroencephalogram	EEG
Fetal Alcohol Syndrome	FAS
Glucose-6-phosphate Dehydrogenase	G6PD
Neural Tube Defect	NTD
Propylthiouracil	PTU
Sudden Infant Death Syndrome	SIDS
Saturated Solution of Potassium Iodide	SSKI
Thyroid-stimulating Hormone	TSH
U.S. Food and Drug Administration	FDA
Zidovudine	ZDV

The placenta allows for the transfer of many drugs and dietary substances. Lipid-soluble compounds readily cross the placenta, and water-soluble substances pass less well the greater their molecular weight. The degree to which a drug is bound to plasma protein also influences the amount of drug that is free to cross the placenta. **Virtually all drugs cross the placenta to some degree, with the exception of large molecules such as heparin and insulin.**

Developmental defects in humans may result from genetic, environmental, or unknown causes. About 25% are unequivocally genetic in origin; drug exposure accounts for only 2% to 3% of birth defects. About 65% of defects are of unknown etiology but may be from combinations of genetic and environmental factors.

The incidence of major malformations in the general population is 2% to 3%.[1] A major malformation is defined as one that is incompatible with survival, such as anencephaly; one requiring major surgery for correction, such as cleft palate or congenital heart disease; or one producing major dysfunction, such as mental retardation. If minor malformations are also included, such as ear tags or extra digits, the rate may be as high as 7% to 10%. The risk for malformation after exposure to a drug must be compared with this background rate.

There is a marked species specificity in drug teratogenesis. For example, thalidomide was not found to be teratogenic in rats and mice but is a potent human teratogen. Thus, extrapolating from animal studies to humans is hazardous and of limited applicability clinically.

The U.S. Food and Drug Administration (FDA) lists five categories of labeling for drug use in pregnancy. The rating system weighs the degree to which available information has ruled out risk to the fetus against the drug's potential benefit to the patient. The ratings, and their interpretation, are as follows:

A. *Controlled studies show no risk.* Adequate, well-controlled studies in pregnant women have failed to demonstrate a risk to the fetus in any trimester of pregnancy.
B. *No evidence of risk in humans.* Adequate, well-controlled studies in pregnant women have not shown increased risk for fetal abnormalities despite adverse findings in animals; or in the absence of adequate human studies, animal studies show no fetal risk. The chance of fetal harm is remote but remains a possibility.
C. *Risk cannot be ruled out.* Adequate, well-controlled human studies are lacking, and animal studies have shown a risk to the fetus or are lacking as well. There is a chance of fetal harm if the drug is administered during pregnancy, but the potential benefits may outweigh the potential risk.
D. *Positive evidence of risk.* Studies in humans, or investigational or postmarketing data, have demonstrated fetal risk. Nevertheless, potential benefits from the use of the drug may outweigh the potential risk. For example, the drug may be acceptable if needed in a life-threatening situation or serious disease for which safer drugs cannot be used or are ineffective.
X. *Contraindicated in pregnancy.* Studies in animals or humans, or investigational or postmarketing reports, have demonstrated positive evidence of fetal abnormalities or risk that clearly outweighs any possible benefit to the patient.

The Teratology Society has suggested abandoning the FDA classification,[2] and 15 years later this is still being considered. The categories imply that risk increases from category A to X. However, the drugs in different categories may pose similar risks but be in different categories based on risk and benefit considerations. Second, the categories create the impression that drugs within a category present similar risks, whereas the category definition permits inclusion in the same category drugs that vary in type, degree, or extent of risk, depending on potential benefit.

The categories were designed for prescribing physicians and not to address inadvertent exposure. For example, isotretinoin (Accutane) and oral contraceptives are both category X based on lack of benefit for oral contraceptives during pregnancy, yet oral contraceptives do not have any teratogenic risk with inadvertent exposure. When counseling patients or responding to queries from physicians, we recommend using specific descriptions in teratogen information databases (Table 8-1).

The classic teratogenic period is from day 31 after the last menstrual period in a 28-day cycle to 71 days from the last period (Figure 8-1). **During this critical period, organs are forming, and teratogens may cause malformations that are usually overt at birth.** Timing of exposure is important. Administration of drugs early in the period of organogenesis affects the organs developing at that time, such as the heart or neural tube. Closer to the end of the classic teratogenic period, the ear and palate are forming and may be affected by a teratogen.

Before day 31, exposure to a teratogen produces an all-or-none effect. With exposure around conception, the conceptus usually either does not survive or survives without anomalies. Because so few cells exist in the early stages, irreparable damage to some may be lethal to the entire organism. If the organism remains viable, however, organ-specific anomalies are not manifested because either repair or replacement will occur to permit normal development. A similar insult at a later stage may produce organ-specific defects.

TABLE 8-1 TERATOGEN INFORMATION DATABASES

- **MICROMEDEX, Inc.** 6200 South Syracuse Way, Suite 300, Greenwood Village, Colorado 80111-4740, Telephone #800-525-9083 (in United States and Canada), http://www.micromedex.com
- Reproductive Toxicology Center, **REPROTOX.** 7831 Woodmont Avenue, Suite 375, Bethesda, MD 20814, Telephone #301-514-3081, http://www.reprotox.org
- **ORGANIZATION OF TERATOLOGY INFORMATION SERVICES (OTIS),** Medical Center, 200 W. Arbor Drive, #8446, San Diego, CA 92103-9981, Telephone #886-626-6847, http://www.otispregnancy.org

EMBRYOLOGY

During the first 3 days after ovulation, development takes place in the fallopian tube. At the time of fertilization, a pronuclear stage exists during which the nuclei from the egg and the sperm retain their integrity within the egg cytoplasm. After the pronuclei fuse, the fertilized egg begins a series of mitotic cell divisions (cleavage). The two-cell stage is reached about 30 hours after fertilization. With continued division, the cells develop into a solid ball of cells (morula), which reaches the endometrial cavity about 3 days after fertilization. Thereafter, a fluid-filled cavity forms within the cell mass, at which time the conceptus is called a *blastocyst.* The number of cells increases from about 12 to 32 by the end of the third day to 250 by the sixth day.

Until about 3 days after conception, any cell is totipotential, that is, capable of initiating development of any organ system. For this reason, separation of cells during this period gives rise to monozygotic twins, usually each normal. At the blastocyst stage, cells first begin to differentiate. By this stage of development, the embryo is located in the uterus, where implantation occurs 6 to 7 days after conception.

One group of cells forms the inner cell mass that will ultimately develop into the fetus. Different tissues arise from each of the three cell layers. Brain, nerves, and skin develop from the ectoderm, the lining of the digestive tract, respiratory tract, and part of the bladder, as well as the liver and pancreas from the endoderm, and connective tissue, cartilage, muscle, blood vessels, the heart, kidneys, and gonads develop from the mesoderm. The group of cells forming the periphery of the blastocyst is termed the *trophoblast.* The placenta and the fetal membranes develop from this outer cell layer.

The trophoblast continues to grow, and lacunae form within the previously solid syncytiotrophoblast. The lacunae are the precursors of the intervillous spaces of the placenta, and by 2 weeks after conception, maternal blood is found within them. Meanwhile, the cytotrophoblast is forming cell masses that become chorionic villi.

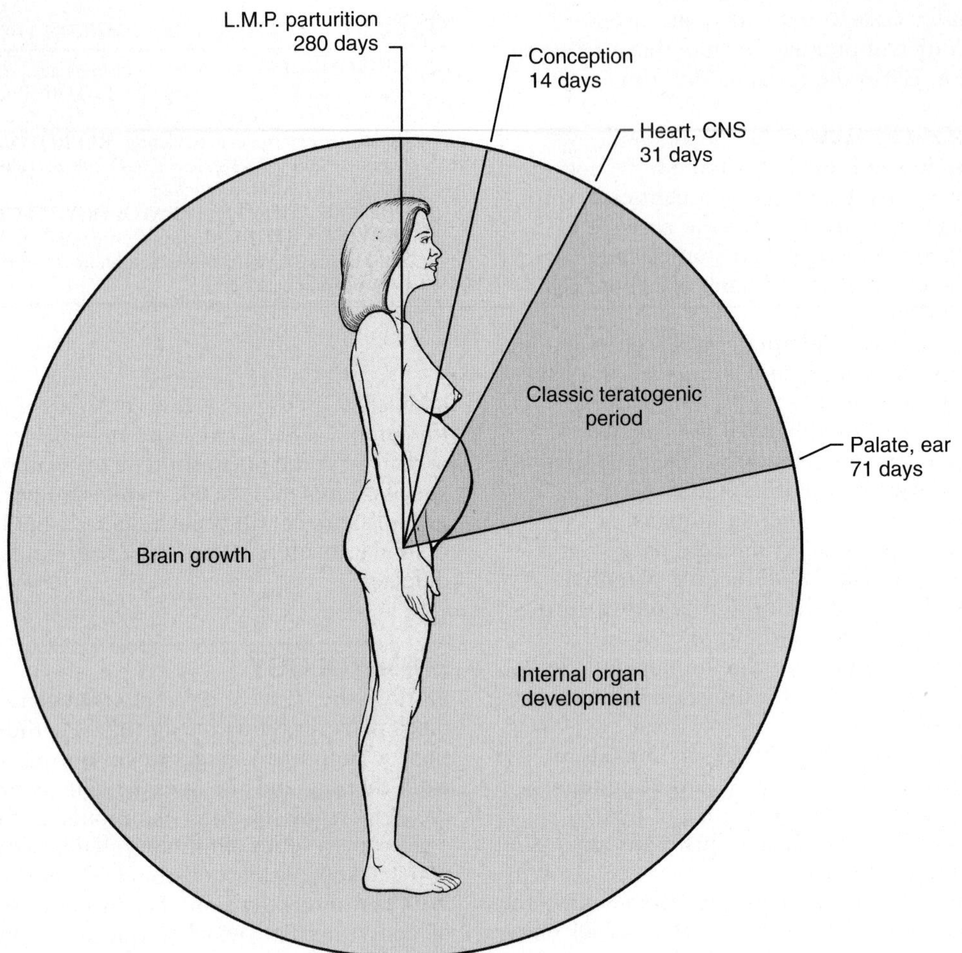

FIGURE 8-1. Gestational clock showing the classic teratogenic period. (From Blake DA, Niebyl JR: Requirements and limitations in reproductive and teratogenic risk assessment. *In* Niebyl JR [ed]: Drug Use in Pregnancy, 2nd ed. Philadelphia, Lea & Febiger, 1988, p 2.)

From the third to the eighth week after conception, the embryonic disk undergoes major developments that lay the foundation for all organ systems. By 4 weeks after conception, the fertilized ovum has progressed from one cell to millions of cells. The rudiments of all major systems have differentiated. The embryo has been transformed into a curved tube about 6 mm long and isolated from the extraembryonic membranes.

Five weeks after conception, the embryo first begins to assume features of human appearance. The face is recognizable, with the formation of discernible eyes, nose, and ears. Limbs emerge from protruding buds; digits, cartilage, and muscles develop. The cerebral hemispheres begin to fill the brain area, and the optic stalk becomes apparent. Nerve connections are established between the retina and the brain. The digestive tract rotates from its prior tubular structure, and the liver starts to produce blood cells and bile. Two tubes emerge from the pharynx to become bronchi, and the lungs have lobes and bronchioles. The heart is beating at 5 weeks and is almost completely developed by 8 weeks after conception. The diaphragm begins to divide the heart and lungs from the abdominal cavity. The kidneys approach their final form at this time. The urogenital and rectal passages separate, and germ cells migrate toward the genital ridges for future transformation into ovaries or testes. Differentiation of internal ducts begins, with persistence of either müllerian or wolffian ducts. Virilization of external genitalia occurs in male embryos. The embryo increases from about 6 to 33 mm in length and increases 50 times in weight.

Structurally, the fetus has become straighter, and the tubular neural canal along which the spinal cord develops becomes filled with nerve cells. Ears remain low on the sides of the head. Teeth are forming, and the two bony plates of the palate fuse in the midline. Disruptions during the latter part of the embryonic period lead to various forms of cleft lip and palate. **By 10 weeks after the last menstrual period, all major organ systems have become established and integrated.**

Development of other organs continues in the second and third trimesters of pregnancy. Therefore, we still need to be concerned about drug use at this time in pregnancy, although the effects may not be recognized until later in life. Some of the uterine anomalies resulting from diethylstilbestrol (DES) occurred with exposure as late as 20 weeks but were not recognized until after puberty. The brain continues to develop throughout pregnancy and the neonatal period. Fetal alcohol syndrome (FAS) may occur with chronic exposure to alcohol in the later stages of pregnancy.

BASIC PRINCIPLES OF TERATOLOGY

To understand the etiology of birth defects, it is important to enumerate the principles of abnormal development (teratogenesis). **Wilson's six general principles of teratogenesis[3] provide a framework for understanding how structural or functional teratogens may act.**

Genotype and Interaction with Environmental Factors

The first principle is that susceptibility to a teratogen depends on the *genotype of the conceptus* and on the manner in which the genotype interacts with environmental factors. This is perhaps most clearly shown by experiments in which different genetic strains of mice have varied greatly in their susceptibility to teratogens that lead to oral clefts. Some of the variability in responses to human teratogens, such as to anticonvulsant drugs like valproic acid and hydantoin, probably relates to genotype of the embryo. The increasing complexity of these potential interactions is illustrated by a series of elegant studies by Musselman and colleagues.[4]

Timing of Exposure

The second principle is that susceptibility of the conceptus to teratogenic agents varies with the developmental stage at the time of exposure. This concept of *critical stages of development* is particularly applicable to alterations in structure. **It is during the second to the eighth weeks of development after conception—the embryonic period—that most structural defects occur.** For such defects, it is believed that there is a critical stage in the developmental process, after which abnormal embryogenesis cannot be initiated. For example, neural tube defects result from the failure of the neural tube to close. Given that this process occurs between 22 and 28 days postconception, any exogenous effect on development must be present at or before this time. The neural tube has five distinct closure sites that may respond differentially to agents and may respond differently in timing. Investigations of thalidomide teratogenicity have clearly shown that the effects of the drug differ as a function of the developmental stage at which the pregnant woman took it.

Mechanisms of Teratogenesis

The third principle is that teratogenic agents act in specific ways *(mechanisms)* on developing cells and tissues in initiating abnormal embryogenesis (pathogenesis). Teratogenic mechanisms are considered separately later.

Manifestation

The fourth principle is that irrespective of the specific deleterious agent, the final manifestations of abnormal development are death, malformation, growth restriction, and functional disorder. The manifestation is thought to depend largely on the stage of development at which exposure occurs; a teratogen may have one effect if exposure occurs during embryogenesis and another if the exposure is during the fetal period. Embryonic exposure is likely to lead to structural abnormalities or embryonic death; fetal exposure is likely to lead to functional deficits or growth restriction.

Despite the importance of teratogen timing on specificity of anomalies, a general pattern usually emerges with respect to any given teratogen. This will be evident throughout this chapter as we consider various agents. If no pattern is evident for a purported teratogen, it increases the suspicion that any purported association is spurious, the observation reflecting confounding variables not recognized and, hence, not taken into account.

Agent

The fifth principle is that access of adverse environmental influences to developing tissues depends on the nature of the influence *(agent)*. This principle relates to such pharmacologic factors as maternal metabolism and placental passage. Although most clearly understood for chemical agents or drugs, the principle also applies to physical agents such as radiation or heat. For an adverse effect to occur, an agent must reach the conceptus, either transmitted indirectly through maternal tissues or directly traversing the maternal body.

Dose Effect

The final principle is that manifestations of abnormal development increase in degree from the no-effect level to the lethal level as *dosage* increases. This means that the response (e.g., malformation, growth restriction) may be expected to vary according to the dose, duration, or amount of exposure. For most human teratogens, this dose-response relationship is not clearly understood, but along with the principle of critical stages of development, these concepts are important in supporting causal inferences about human reproductive hazards. Data regarding in utero exposure to ionizing radiation clearly show the importance of dose on observed effects. The potential complexity of relationships between dose and observed effects for teratogens has been noted.

EPIDEMIOLOGIC APPROACHES TO BIRTH DEFECTS

Teratogens and reproductive toxicants have been identified and are being sought in various ways. Here we enumerate most common approaches, their strengths, and their pitfalls.

Case Reports

Many known teratogens and reproductive toxicants were identified initially through case reports of an unusual number of cases or a constellation of abnormalities. These have often come from astute clinicians, who observed something out of the ordinary. Although the importance of astute observations of abnormal aggregations of cases or patterns of malformations must be recognized, we cannot rely on such methods for identifying health hazards. Furthermore, etiologic speculations based on case reports or case series usually do not lead to a causal agent and are often false-positive speculations. **Whereas case reports may identify a new teratogen, they can never provide an estimate of the risk for disease after exposure.**

Descriptive Studies

Descriptive epidemiologic studies provide information about the distribution and frequency of some outcome of interest, resulting in rates of occurrence that can be compared among populations, places, or times. Defining the population at risk is the first step. The population at risk can be defined geographically, such as residents within a state, or medically, such as being a patient at a particular hospital. Definition of the population at risk includes the time period under consideration. The population at risk constitutes the *denominator* for calculating rates of the occurrence of outcomes of interest.

The second step in a descriptive study is to determine the *numerator* for calculating rates for comparison. This involves two important concepts: (1) case definition (what defines a case to be counted) and (2) case ascertainment (how are cases to be identified).

Relevant examples of descriptive studies are surveillance programs. An at-risk population is identified and then followed over time to detect outcomes of interest. Cases are included in the database. Surveillance programs can develop baseline data and subsequently permit early recognition of potential problems, based on ongoing data collection and analysis. **Birth defect surveillance (monitoring) systems (BDMSs) are designed to identify cases occurring in a defined population, usually by reviewing vital records or hospital record abstracts or charts.** In the past 20 years, there has been a dramatic increase in the number of state-based birth defect surveillance systems. About half the states now have some type of birth defect surveillance system. These programs conduct routine reviews of occurrence rates of specific malformations and attempt to identify increases in rates or clusters of cases.

Case-Control Studies

In a case-control study design, groups of individuals with some outcome or disease of interest (cases) (e.g., a congenital malformation) are compared with controls with regard to a history of one or more exposures. This is the most widely used approach in reproductive outcomes research. Controls are ideally as similar as possible to the cases, except of course lacking the outcome of interest. After cases and controls have been identified, the hypothesis to be tested is whether these two groups differ in exposure as well as outcome. How accurately exposure and its timing are determined may vary greatly among studies, but in any study the same methods must be used to establish the exposure of both cases and controls.

Case-control studies are advantageous in testing outcomes of infrequent occurrence. This can be conducted relatively rapidly and inexpensively. A disadvantage is the potential for several important types of bias, including bias in recalling exposure, in selecting appropriate controls, and in ascertaining cases.

These problems can be addressed in part by use of two control groups, one "normal" and the second "abnormal." Any of several abnormal controls seem equally useful, for example, infants with mendelian or chromosomal disorders as well as infants with no specific malformation.[5] In the former, mothers have incentive to recall, but teratogenesis is not the etiology. Ideally, case-control studies of potential teratogens should follow descriptive studies. After suspecting on the basis of case observations that thalidomide was teratogenic, Lenz[6] conducted a case-control study. **The association between valproic acid use and spina bifida was verified by case-control studies.[7]**

Cohort Studies

In cohort studies, groups are defined by the presence or absence of exposure to a given factor and then are followed over time and compared for rates of occurrence (i.e., incidence rates) of the outcome of interest. Cohort studies have three advantages: (1) the cohort is classified by exposure before the outcome is determined, thereby eliminating exposure recall bias; (2) incidence rates can be calculated among those exposed; and (3) multiple outcomes can be observed simultaneously.

Cohort studies, often called *prospective studies,* require that groups differing in exposure be followed through time, with outcomes observed. Therefore, these studies tend to be time consuming and expensive. In addition, occurrence rates for many adverse reproductive outcomes, such as congenital malformations, are low; thus, large samples must be followed for a considerable period of time. Two main types of cohort studies have been developed: (1) those that identify a cohort and follow it into the future (concurrent cohort study), and (2) those that identify a cohort at some time in the past and follow it to the present (nonconcurrent or historical cohort study). In both cases, risks for adverse outcomes are compared between groups. **Cohort studies enable investigators to calculate incidence rates that provide a measure of risk for an outcome after the exposure.** Risk in the exposed group can be compared with risk in an unexposed group. Most frequently, ratio of the incidence rate among the exposed to the rate among the unexposed is determined. This ratio, referred to as *relative risk,* is a measure of how much the presence of exposure increases the risk for the outcome.

In *historical prospective studies,* one begins by identifying groups that differ in terms of some past exposure and follow them to the present and determine outcomes; exposure groups are defined before outcomes are known. A major advantage is that although the time frame is prospective, investigators do not have to follow the cohort into the future, waiting for events to occur. A disadvantage is that these studies require the ability to determine exposure status retrospectively.

Clinical Trials

Ideally, analytical studies (case control or cohort) are followed by a randomized clinical trial, in which the efficiency of a prevention or treatment regimen is evaluated. That is, subjects are randomly assigned to different treatment groups. The individuals should be as similar as possible in terms of unknown factors that may affect the response before they are randomly assigned to the treatment groups and receive the different regimens.

Clinical trials of both neural tube defect (NTD) recurrence[8] and occurrence[9] have shown a protective effect of periconceptional folic acid supplementation, findings that have led to key public health recommendations regarding the use of folic acid to reduce the risk of these often devastating defects.

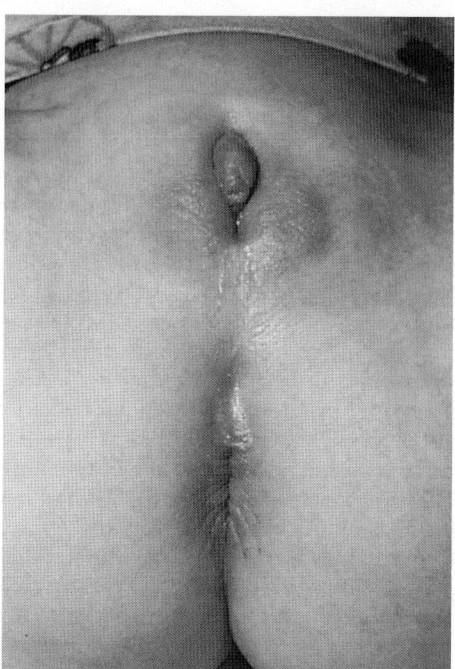

FIGURE 8-2. Perineum of a female fetus exposed to danazol in utero. (From Duck SC, Katayama KP: Danazol may cause female pseudohermaphroditism. Fertil Steril 35:230, 1981.)

MEDICAL DRUG USE

Patients should be educated about avenues other than the use of drugs to cope with tension, aches and pains, and viral illnesses during pregnancy. Drugs should be used only when necessary. The risk-to-benefit ratio should justify the use of a particular drug, and the minimal effective dose should be employed. Because long-term effects of drug exposure in utero may not be revealed for many years, caution with regard to the use of any drug in pregnancy is warranted. Also, some drug doses may have a significant effect on the concentrations of analytes routinely used in serum screening for aneuploidy and NTDs.[10] Methadone has been reported to increase screen positive results for trisomy 18. Screen-positive rates for NTDs were higher for those on corticosteroids, antibiotics, and antidepressants.[10]

Effects of Specific Drugs

Estrogens and Progestins

Studies have not confirmed any teratogenic risk for oral contraceptives or progestins. A meta-analysis of first-trimester sex hormone exposure revealed no association between exposure and fetal genital malformations. However, because of the medicolegal climate and the conflicting past literature, it is wise to exclude pregnancy before giving progestins to an amenorrheic patient.

Androgenic Steroids

Androgens may masculinize a developing female fetus. Danazol (Danocrine) has been reported to produce clitoral enlargement and labial fusion after being given inadvertently for the first 9 to 12 weeks after conception (Figure 8-2) in 23 of 57 female infants exposed.

Spermicides

The once-touted increased risk for abnormal offspring in mothers who had used spermicides for contraception has not been confirmed. **A meta-analysis of reports of spermicide exposure concludes that there is no increased risk for birth defects.**[11]

Anticonvulsants

Epileptic women taking anticonvulsants during pregnancy have about double the general population risk for malformations. Compared with the general risk of 2% to 3%, the risk for major malformations in epileptic women on anticonvulsants is about 5%, especially cleft lip with or without cleft palate and congenital heart disease. **Valproic acid (Depakene) and carbamazepine (Tegretol) each carry about a 1% risk for NTDs and other anomalies.** Valproic acid monotherapy significantly increases risk for spina bifida (odds ratio [OR], 12.7), atrial septal defect (2.5), cleft palate (5.2), hypospadias (4.8), polydactyly (2.2), and craniosynostosis (6.8).[12] A high daily dose or a combination of two or three drugs increases the chance of malformations.

Holmes and associates[13] screened 128,049 pregnant women at delivery to identify three groups of infants: those exposed to anticonvulsant drugs, those unexposed to anticonvulsant drugs but with a maternal history of seizures, and those unexposed to anticonvulsant drugs with no maternal history of seizures (control group). The infants were examined systematically for the presence of malformations. The combined frequency of anticonvulsant embryopathy was higher in 223 infants exposed to one anticonvulsant drug than in 508 control infants (20.6% vs. 8.5%; OR, 2.8; 95% confidence interval [CI], 1.1 to 9.7). The frequency was also higher in 93 infants exposed to two or more anticonvulsant drugs than in the controls (28.0% vs. 8.5%; OR, 4.2; 95% CI, 1.1 to 5.1). The greater the number of anticonvulsants, the higher the risk for malformation. The 98 infants whose mothers had a history of epilepsy but took no anticonvulsant drugs during the pregnancy did not have a higher frequency of abnormalities than the control infants.

Phenytoin (Dilantin) decreases folate absorption and lowers the serum folate, which has been implicated in birth defects. Therefore, folic acid supplementation should be given to these mothers, but this may require adjustment of the anticonvulsant dose. Although epileptic women were not included in the Medical Research Council study, most authorities would recommend 4 mg/day folic acid for high-risk women. One study suggested that folic acid at doses of 2.5 to 5 mg daily could reduce birth defects in women on anticonvulsant drugs.[14]

Fewer than 10% of offspring show the fetal hydantoin syndrome,[15] **which consists of microcephaly, growth deficiency, developmental delays, mental retardation, and dysmorphic craniofacial features** (Figure 8-3). In fact, the risk may be as low as 1% to 2% above background. Although several of these features are also found in other syndromes, such as FAS, more common in the fetal hydantoin syndrome are hypoplasia of the nails and distal phalanges (Figure 8-4) and hypertelorism. Carbamazepine (Tegretol) is also associated with an increased risk for a dysmorphic syndrome.[15] A genetically determined metabolic defect

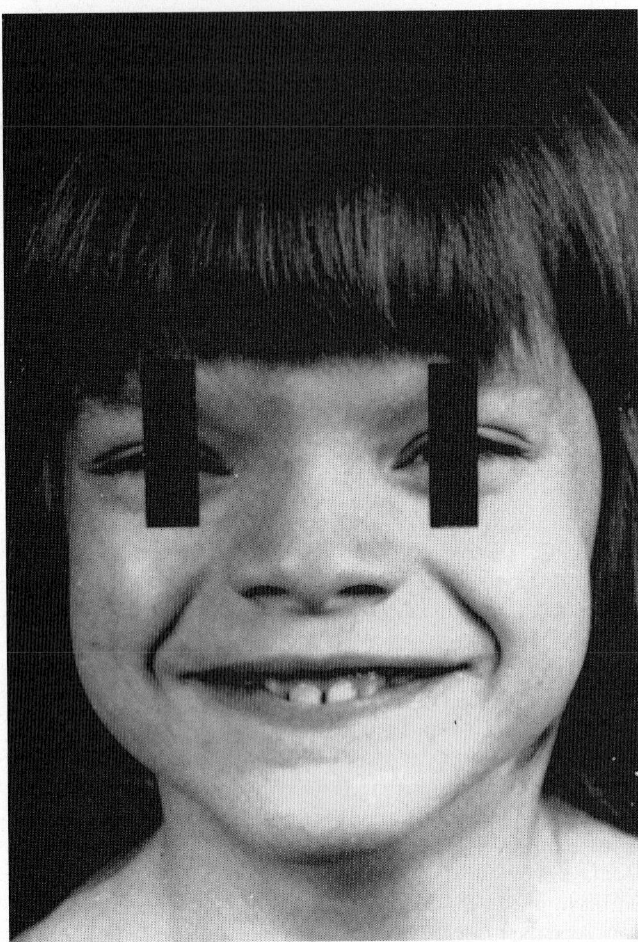

FIGURE 8-3. Facial features of the fetal hydantoin syndrome. Note broad, flat nasal ridge, epicanthic folds, mild hypertelorism, and wide mouth with prominent upper lip. (Courtesy Dr. Thaddeus Kelly, Charlottesville, VA.)

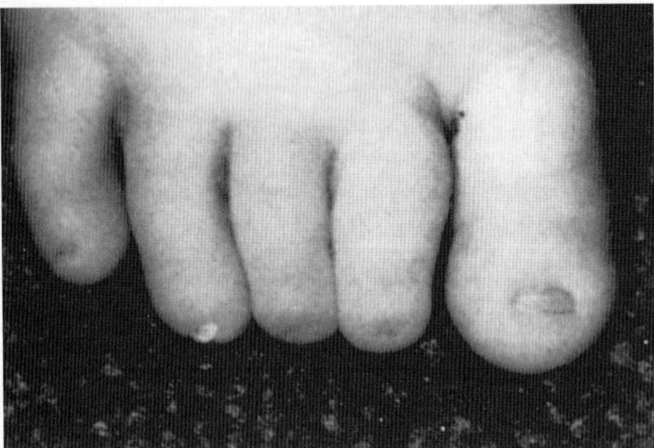

FIGURE 8-4. Hypoplasia of toenails and distal phalanges. (From Hanson JWM: Fetal hydantoin syndrome. Teratology 13:186, 1976.)

in arene oxide detoxification in the infant may increase the risk for a major birth defect. Epoxide hydrolase deficiency may indicate susceptibility to fetal hydantoin syndrome.[16]

In a follow-up study of long-term effects of antenatal exposure to phenobarbital and carbamazepine, there were no neurologic or behavioral differences between the two groups. However, children exposed in utero to phenytoin scored 10 points lower on IQ tests than children exposed to carbamazepine and nonexposed controls. At 3 years of age, children who had been exposed to valproate in utero had significantly lower IQ scores than those exposed to other antiepileptic drugs.[17] **Valproate should not be used as a first choice drug in women of reproductive age.**[17] Also, prenatal exposure to phenobarbital decreased verbal IQ scores in adult men.

Lamotrigine exposures have been compiled in a voluntary registry established by the manufacturer, GlaxoSmithKline. After 1558 exposures in the first trimester, no increased risk for birth defects overall has been observed.[18] Monitoring the risk for specific birth defects will continue. **Of 1532 infant exposures to newer-generation antiepileptic drugs, 1019 were to lamotrigine, and 3.7% had major birth defects. Of 393 infants exposed to oxcarbazepine, the rate was 2.8%, and for 108 exposed to topiramate, the rate was 4.6%. None of these differences was statistically different from controls.** Gabapentin and levetiracetam were used infrequently.

Some women may have taken anticonvulsant drugs for a long period without reevaluation of the need for continuation of the drugs. For patients with idiopathic epilepsy who have been seizure free for 2 years and who have a normal electroencephalogram (EEG), it may be safe to attempt a trial of withdrawal of the drug before pregnancy.

Most authorities agree that the benefits of anticonvulsant therapy during pregnancy outweigh the risks of discontinuation of the drug if the patient is first seen during pregnancy. The blood level of drug should be monitored to ensure a therapeutic level but minimize the dosage. If the patient has not been taking her drug regularly, a low blood level may demonstrate her lack of compliance, and she may not need the drug. Because the albumin concentration falls in pregnancy, the total amount of phenytoin measured is decreased because it is highly protein bound. However, the level of free phenytoin, which is the pharmacologically active portion, is unchanged.

Pediatric care providers need to be notified at birth when a patient has been on anticonvulsants, because this therapy can affect vitamin K–dependent clotting factors in the newborn. Some have recommended vitamin K supplementation at 10 mg daily for these mothers for the last month of pregnancy, but this is not common practice in the United States.

Isotretinoin

Isotretinoin (Accutane) is a significant human teratogen. This drug is marketed for treatment of cystic acne and unfortunately has been taken inadvertently by women who were not planning pregnancy.[19] It is labeled as contraindicated in pregnancy (FDA category X) with appropriate warnings that a negative pregnancy test is required before therapy. Of 154 exposed human pregnancies, there have been 21 reported cases of birth defects, 12 spontaneous abortions, 95 elective abortions, and 26 normal infants in women who took isotretinoin during early pregnancy. **The risk for structural anomalies in patients studied prospectively is now estimated to be about 25%. An additional 25%**

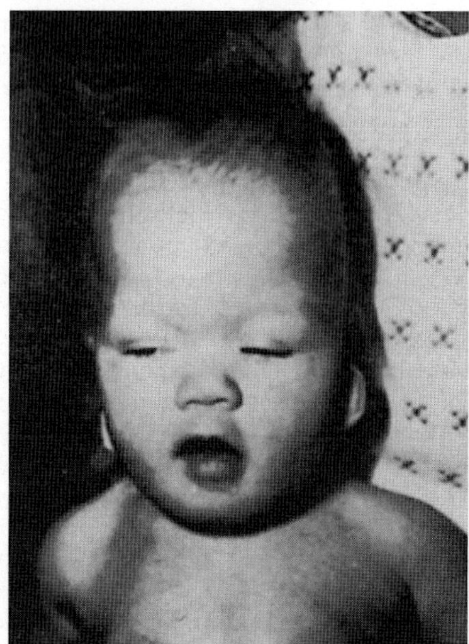
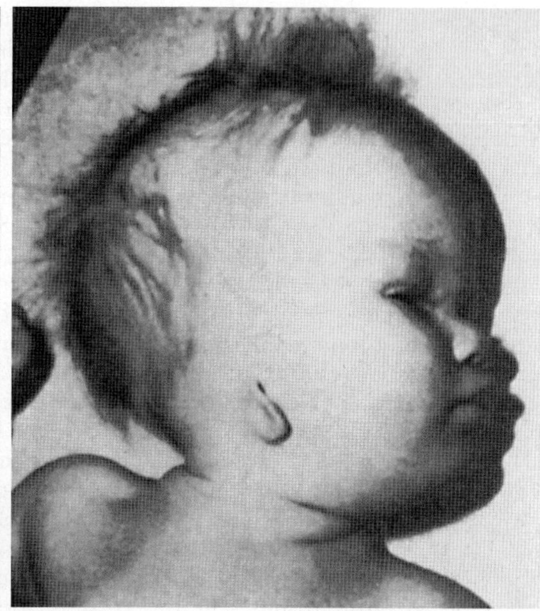

FIGURE 8-5. Infant exposed to Accutane in utero. Note high forehead, hypoplastic nasal bridge, and abnormal ears. (From Lot IT, Bocian M, Pribam HW, Leitner M: Fetal hydrocephalus and ear anomalies associated with use of isotretinoin. J Pediatr 105:598, 1984.)

have mental retardation alone. The malformed infants have a characteristic pattern of craniofacial, cardiac, thymic, and central nervous system anomalies. They include microtia/anotia (small/absent ears) (Figure 8-5), micrognathia, cleft palate, heart defects, thymic defects, retinal or optic nerve anomalies, and central nervous system malformations, including hydrocephalus.[19] Microtia is rare as an isolated anomaly yet appears commonly as part of the retinoic acid embryopathy. Cardiovascular defects include great vessel transposition and ventricular septal defects.

Unlike vitamin A, isotretinoin is not stored in tissue. Therefore, a pregnancy after discontinuation of isotretinoin is not at risk because the drug is no longer detectable in serum 5 days after its ingestion. **In 88 pregnancies prospectively ascertained after discontinuation of isotretinoin, no increased risk for anomalies was noted.** Topical tretinoin (Retin-A) has not been associated with any teratogenic risk.

Vitamin A

There is no evidence that vitamin A itself in normal doses is teratogenic, nor is β-carotene. The levels in prenatal vitamins (5000 IU/day orally) have not been associated with any documented risk. **Eighteen cases of birth defects have been reported after exposure to levels of 25,000 IU of vitamin A or greater during pregnancy.** Vitamin A in doses greater than 10,000 IU/day was shown to increase the risk for malformations in one study but not in another.

Psychoactive Drugs

There is no clear risk documented for most psychoactive drugs with respect to overt birth defects. However, effects of chronic use of these agents on the developing brain in humans is difficult to study, and so a conservative attitude is appropriate. Lack of overt defects does not exclude the possibility of behavioral teratogenesis, and neonatal withdrawal may occur.

Tranquilizers

Conflicting reports of the possible teratogenicity of the various tranquilizers, including meprobamate (Miltown) and chlordiazepoxide (Librium), have appeared, but in prospective studies, no increased risk for anomalies has been shown.

A fetal benzodiazepine syndrome has been reported in seven infants of 36 mothers who regularly took benzodiazepines during pregnancy. However, the high rate of abnormality occurred with concomitant alcohol and substance abuse and may not be caused by the benzodiazepine exposure. In most clinical situations, however, the risk-to-benefit ratio does not justify the use of benzodiazepines in pregnancy. Use of diazepam (Valium) in labor has been associated with neonatal hypotonia, hypothermia, and respiratory depression.

Lithium (Eskalith, Lithobid)

In the International Register of Lithium Babies, 217 infants were listed as exposed at least during the first trimester of pregnancy, and 25 (11.5%) were malformed. Eighteen had cardiovascular anomalies, including six cases of the rare Ebstein anomaly, which occurs in only 1 in 20,000 of the nonexposed population. Of 60 unaffected infants who were followed to age 5 years, no increased mental or physical abnormalities were noted compared with unexposed siblings.

However, two other reports suggest bias of ascertainment in the registry and a risk for anomalies much lower than previously thought. A case-control study of 59 patients with Ebstein anomaly showed no difference in the rate of lithium exposure in pregnancy from a control group of 168 children with neuroblastoma.[20] **A prospective study of 148 women exposed to lithium in the first trimester showed no difference in the incidence of major anomalies compared with controls.**[21] One fetus in the lithium-exposed group had Ebstein anomaly, and one infant in the control group had a ventricular septal defect. The authors concluded that lithium is not a major human teratogen. **Nevertheless, we recommend that women exposed to lithium be offered ultrasound and fetal echocardiography.**

Lithium is excreted more rapidly during pregnancy; thus, serum lithium levels should be monitored. Perinatal effects of lithium have been noted, including hypotonia, lethargy, and poor feeding in the infant. Also, complications similar to those seen in adults on lithium have been noted in newborns, including goiter and hypothyroidism.

Two cases of polyhydramnios associated with maternal lithium treatment have been reported. Because nephrogenic diabetes insipidus has been reported in adults taking lithium, the presumed mechanism of this polyhydramnios is fetal diabetes insipidus. **Polyhydramnios may be a sign of fetal lithium toxicity.**

It is usually recommended that drug therapy be changed in pregnant women on lithium to avoid fetal drug exposure. Tapering over 10 days delays the risk for relapse. However, discontinuing lithium is associated with a 70% chance of relapse of the affective disorder in 1 year as opposed to 20% in those who remain on lithium. **Discontinuation of lithium may pose an unacceptable risk for increased morbidity in women who have had multiple episodes of affective instability. These women should be offered appropriate prenatal diagnosis with ultrasound, including fetal echocardiography.**

Antidepressants

Imipramine (Tofranil) was the original tricyclic antidepressant claimed to be associated with cardiovascular defects, but the number of patients studied remains small. Of 75 newborns exposed in the first trimester, six major defects were observed, three being cardiovascular, and neonatal withdrawal has been observed.

Amitriptyline (Elavil) has been more widely used, and most of the evidence supports its safety. In the Michigan Medicaid study, 467 newborns had been exposed during the first trimester, with no increased risk for birth defects.

No increased risk for major malformations has been found after first-trimester exposure to fluoxetine (Prozac) in several studies.[22] However, one recent study showed a twofold increased risk for ventricular septal defects.[23] Chambers and associates found more minor malformations and perinatal complications among infants exposed to fluoxetine throughout pregnancy, but this study is difficult to interpret because the authors did not control for depression. When a group whose mothers received tricyclic agents was used as a control for depression, infants exposed to fluoxetine in utero did not appear to have more minor malformations or perinatal complications. One study suggested an increased risk for low-birthweight infants with higher doses of fluoxetine (40 to 80 mg) throughout pregnancy.

Nulman and colleagues evaluated the neurobehavioral effects of long-term fluoxetine exposure during pregnancy and found no abnormalities among 228 children aged 16 to 86 months (average age, 3 years). Theoretically, some psychiatric or neurobehavioral abnormality might occur as a result of exposure, but it would be very difficult to ascertain because of all of the confounding variables.

Current data on other selective serotonin reuptake inhibitor (SSRI) exposures show no consistent teratogenic risk.[24] **However, two studies found an increased risk for cardiac defects after exposure to paroxetine (Paxil),[23,25] and the FDA reclassified the agent as pregnancy category D.** One study showed a twofold increased risk for neural tube defects after citalopram (Celexa).[23]

Studies have described neonatal withdrawal in the first 2 days after in utero exposure to these drugs.[26] Infants exposed during pregnancy exhibited more tremulousness and sleep changes at 1 to 2 days of age. However, no abnormalities were found when children were examined at age 16 to 86 months after prolonged exposure during pregnancy.

A sixfold increased risk for persistent pulmonary hypertension (PPH) in the newborn has been reported in infants exposed to SSRIs after 20 weeks of pregnancy,[27] raising the absolute risk from 1 to 2 per 1000 in unexposed infants to 6 to 12 per 1000 in exposed infants. Another study did not confirm this finding, but confirmed a fivefold increased risk for PPH with cesarean delivery before labor.[28]

No major malformations have occurred in 133 infants exposed to bupropion (Zyban, Wellbutrin).[29]

When considering the use of antidepressant drugs during pregnancy, it should be noted that among women who maintained their medication throughout pregnancy, 26% relapsed, compared with 68% who discontinued medication.[30] Also, fetal alcohol spectrum disorders were 10 times more common in SSRI-exposed offspring than in unexposed.[23]

Anticoagulants

Warfarin (Coumadin) has been associated with chondrodysplasia punctata, which is similar to the genetically determined Conradi-Hünermann syndrome. **Warfarin embryopathy occurs in about 5% of exposed pregnancies and includes nasal hypoplasia, bone stippling seen on radiologic examination, ophthalmologic abnormalities including bilateral optic atrophy, and mental retardation** (Figure 8-6). Ophthalmologic abnormalities and mental retardation may occur even with use only beyond the first trimester. **The risk for pregnancy complications is higher when the mean daily dose of warfarin is more than 5 mg.**

The alternative drug, heparin, does not cross the placenta because it is a large molecule with a strong negative charge. **Because heparin does not have an adverse effect on the fetus when given in pregnancy, it should be the drug of choice for patients requiring anticoagulation, except in women with artificial heart valves.[31]** However, therapy with 20,000 units/day for more than 20 weeks has been associated with bone demineralization. Thirty-six percent of patients had more than a 10% decrease from baseline bone density to postpartum values. The risk for spine fractures was 0.7% with low-dose heparin and 3% with a high-dose regimen.[32] Heparin can also cause thrombocytopenia.

Low-molecular-weight heparins may have substantial benefits over standard unfractionated heparin. The molecules are still relatively large and do not cross the placenta. The half-life is longer, allowing for once-daily administration. **However, enoxaparin (Lovenox) is cleared more rapidly during pregnancy, so twice-daily dosing is advised.**

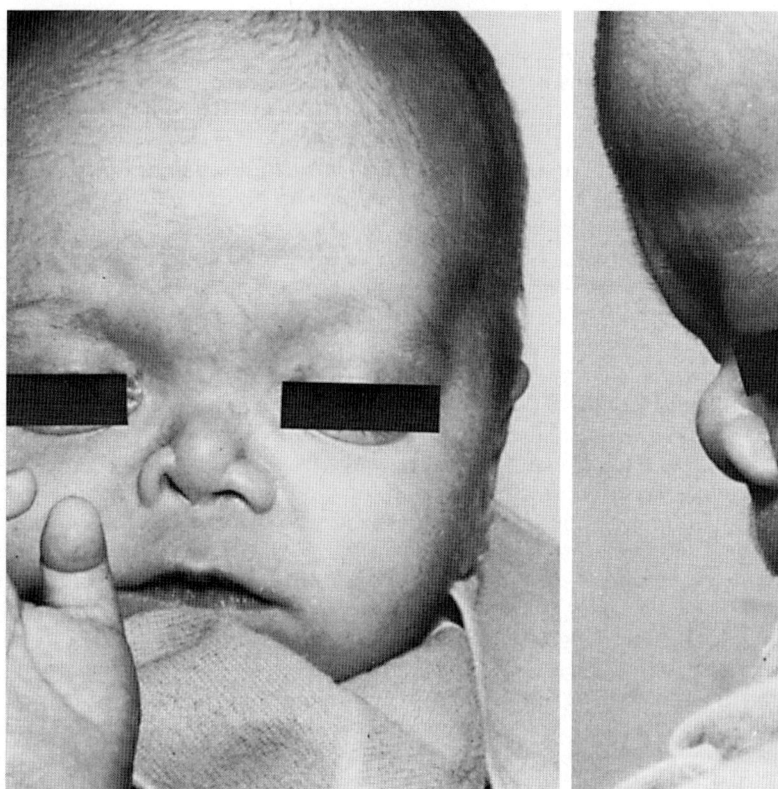
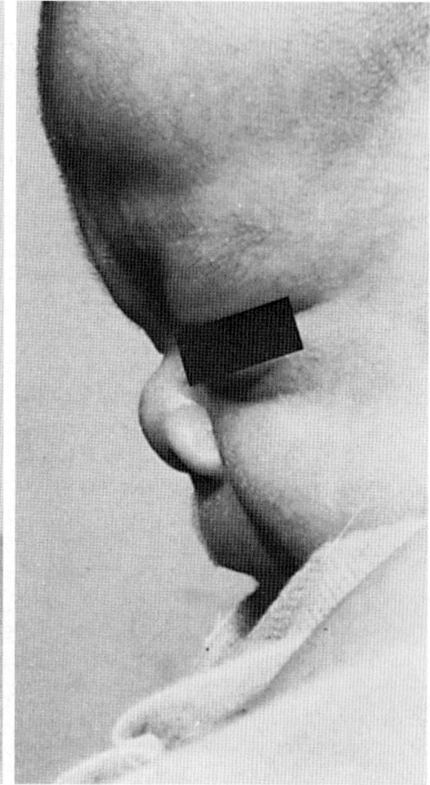

FIGURE 8-6. Warfarin embryopathy. Note small nose with hypoplastic bridge. (From Shaul W, Hall JG: Multiple congenital anomalies associated with oral anticoagulants. Am J Obstet Gynecol 127:191, 1977.)

Low-molecular-weight heparins have a much more predictable dose-response relationship, obviating the need for monitoring of partial thromboplastin time. There is less risk for heparin-induced thrombocytopenia and clinical bleeding at delivery, but studies suggesting less risk for osteoporosis are preliminary.

Women with mechanical heart valves, especially the first-generation valves, require warfarin anticoagulation because heparin is not safe or effective.[33] Heparin treatment is associated with more thromboembolic complications and more bleeding complications than warfarin therapy.[31]

The risks of heparin during pregnancy may not be justified in patients with only a single remote episode of thrombosis in the past. Certainly, conservative measures should be recommended, such as elastic stockings and avoidance of prolonged sitting or standing.

Thyroid and Antithyroid Drugs

Propylthiouracil (PTU) and methimazole (Tapazole) both cross the placenta and may cause some degree of fetal goiter. In contrast, the thyroid hormones triiodothyronine and thyroxine cross the placenta poorly, so fetal hypothyroidism produced by antithyroid drugs cannot be corrected satisfactorily by administration of thyroid hormone to the mother. Thus, the goal of such therapy during pregnancy is to keep the mother slightly hyperthyroid to minimize fetal drug exposure. By the third trimester, 30% of women no longer need antithyroid medication.[34]

Methimazole has been associated with scalp defects in infants and choanal or esophageal atresia,[34] as well as a higher incidence of maternal side effects. However, PTU and methimazole are equally effective and safe for therapy of hyperthyroidism. **However, in 2009, the FDA released a black box warning highlighting serious liver injury with PTU treatment, to a greater extent than methimazole. Some authors are now advocating treatment with PTU only during the first trimester, and switching to methimazole for the remainder of the pregnancy.**[35]

Radioactive iodine (^{131}I or ^{125}I) administered for thyroid ablation or for diagnostic studies is not concentrated by the fetal thyroid until after 12 weeks of pregnancy. Thus, with inadvertent exposure before 12 weeks, there is no specific risk to the fetal thyroid from ^{131}I or ^{125}I administration.

The need for thyroxine increases in many women with primary hypothyroidism when they are pregnant, as reflected by an increase in serum thyroid-stimulating hormone (TSH) concentrations.[36] Because hypothyroidism in pregnancy may adversely affect the fetus, possibly by increasing prematurity,[37] it is prudent to monitor thyroid function throughout pregnancy and to adjust the thyroid dose to maintain a normal TSH level. **It is recommended that women with hypothyroidism increase their levothyroxine dose by about 30% as soon as pregnancy is confirmed (two extra doses each week) and then have dosing adjustments based on TSH levels.**[36]

Topical iodine preparations are readily absorbed through the vagina during pregnancy, and transient hypothyroidism has been demonstrated in the newborn after exposure during labor.

Digoxin (Lanoxin)

In 194 exposures, no teratogenicity of digoxin was noted. Blood levels should be monitored in pregnancy to ensure adequate therapeutic maternal levels.

Digoxin-like immunoreactive substances may be mistaken in assays for fetal concentrations of digoxin. In one study of fetuses with cardiac anomalies, there was no difference in the immunoreactive digoxin levels whether or not the mother had received digoxin. In hydropic fetuses, digoxin may not easily cross the placenta.

Antihypertensive Drugs

α-Methyldopa (Aldomet) has been widely used for the treatment of chronic hypertension in pregnancy. Although postural hypotension may occur, no unusual fetal effects have been noted. Hydralazine (Apresoline) is used frequently in pregnancy, and no teratogenic effect has been observed. (See also Chapter 35.)

Sympathetic Blocking Agents

Propranolol (Inderal) is a β-adrenergic blocking agent in widespread use for various indications. Theoretically, propranolol might increase uterine contractility. However, this has not been reported, presumably because the drug is not specific for uterine β_2-receptors. No evidence of teratogenicity has been found. Bradycardia has been reported in the newborn as a direct effect of a dose of the drug given to the mother within 2 hours of delivery.[38]

Several studies of propranolol use in pregnancy show an increased risk for intrauterine growth restriction or at least a skewing of the birthweight distribution toward the lower range. Ultrasound monitoring of exposed patients is prudent. Studies from Scotland suggest improved outcome with the use of atenolol (Tenormin) to treat chronic hypertension during pregnancy.

Calcium channel blockers (e.g., nifedipine [Procardia]) have been widely used for chronic hypertension in pregnancy, without evidence of teratogenicity. Magnesium sulfate should be used with caution in women taking these agents.

Angiotensin-Converting Enzyme Inhibitors and Angiotensin Receptor Blockers

Angiotensin-converting enzyme (ACE) inhibitors (e.g., enalapril [Vasotec], captopril [Capoten]) and angiotensin II receptor antagonists (e.g., valsartan [Diovan]) can cause fetal renal tubular dysplasia in the second and third trimesters, leading to oligohydramnios, fetal limb contractures, craniofacial deformities, and hypoplastic lung development.[39] Fetal skull ossification defects have also been described. Fetal exposure in the first trimester is also associated with an increased risk for birth defects. **For these reasons, women taking these medications who plan pregnancy should be switched to other agents.**

Antineoplastic Drugs and Immunosuppressants

Mycophenolate mofetil [CellCept] carries a moderate teratogenic risk.[40] Frequent features include microtia or anotia, cleft lip, cleft palate, heart defects, and dysmorphic facial features. The numbers are too small to determine the actual rate of malformations.

Methotrexate, a folic acid antagonist, appears to be a human teratogen, although experience is limited. Infants of three women known to receive methotrexate in the first trimester of pregnancy had multiple congenital anomalies, including cranial defects and malformed extremities. Two had Tetralogy of Fallot. Eight normal infants were delivered to seven women treated with methotrexate in combination with other agents after the first trimester. When low-dose oral methotrexate (7.5 mg/week) was used for rheumatoid disease in the first trimester, five full-term infants were normal and three patients experienced spontaneous abortions.

Azathioprine (Imuran) has been used by patients with renal transplants or systemic lupus erythematosus. The frequency of anomalies in 375 total women treated in the first trimester was not increased. Some infants had leukopenia, some were small for gestational age, and the others were normal.

No increased risk for anomalies in fetuses exposed to cyclosporine (Sandimmune) in utero has been reported. An increased rate of prematurity and growth restriction has been noted, but it is difficult to separate the contributions of the underlying disease and the drugs given to these transplant patients. The B-cell line may be depleted more than the T-cell line, and one author recommends that infants exposed to immunosuppressive agents be followed for possible immunodeficiency.

Eight malformed infants have resulted from first-trimester exposure to cyclophosphamide (Cytoxan), but these infants were also exposed to other drugs or radiation. Low birthweight may be associated with use after the first trimester, but this may also reflect the underlying medical problem.

Chloroquine (Aralen) is safe in doses used for malarial prophylaxis, and there was no increased incidence of birth defects among 169 infants exposed to 300 mg once weekly.[41] However, after exposure to larger anti-inflammatory doses (250 to 500 mg/day), two cases of cochleovestibular paresis were reported.[42] No abnormalities were noted in 114 other infants.

When cancer chemotherapy must be used during embryogenesis, there is an increased rate of spontaneous abortion and major birth defects. Later in pregnancy, there is a greater risk for stillbirth and intrauterine growth restriction, and myelosuppression is often present in the infant.

Antiasthmatics

Terbutaline (Brethine)

Terbutaline has been widely used in the treatment of preterm labor. It is more rapid in onset, has a longer duration of action than epinephrine, and is preferred for asthma in the pregnant patient. No risk for birth defects has been reported. Long-term use has been associated with an increased risk for glucose intolerance.

Cromolyn Sodium (Intal)

Cromolyn sodium may be administered in pregnancy, and the systemic absorption is minimal. Teratogenicity has not been reported in humans.

Isoproterenol (Isuprel) and Metaproterenol (Alupent)

When isoproterenol and metaproterenol are given as topical aerosols for the treatment of asthma, the total dose absorbed is usually not significant. With oral or intravenous doses, however, the cardiovascular effects of the agents may decrease uterine blood flow. For this reason, they should be used with caution. No teratogenicity has been reported.

CORTICOSTEROIDS

All steroids cross the placenta to some degree, but prednisone (Deltasone) and prednisolone are inactivated by the placenta. When prednisone or prednisolone is maternally administered, the concentration of active compound in the fetus is less than 10% of that in the mother. Therefore, these agents are the drugs of choice for treating medical diseases such as asthma. Inhaled corticosteroids are also effective therapy, and very little drug is absorbed. When steroid effects are desired in the fetus to accelerate lung maturity, betamethasone (Celestone) and dexamethasone (Decadron) are preferred because these are minimally inactivated by the placenta. **A meta-analysis of exposure to corticosteroids showed an OR of 3 for cleft lip and/or cleft palate.**[43]

IODIDE

Iodide such as found in a saturated solution of potassium iodide (SSKI) expectorant crosses the placenta and may produce a fetal goiter large enough to produce respiratory obstruction in the newborn (Figure 8-7). Before a pregnant patient is advised to take a cough medicine, one should be sure to ascertain that it does not contain iodide.

Antiemetics

Remedies suggested to help nausea and vomiting in pregnancy without pharmacologic intervention include eating crackers at the bedside on first awakening in the morning (before getting out of bed), getting up very slowly, omitting iron tablets, consuming frequent small meals, and eating protein snacks at night. **None of the medications used to treat nausea and vomiting have been found to be teratogenic, except possibly methylprednisolone (Medrol) used before 10 weeks of gestation.**[44]

VITAMIN B_6

Vitamin B_6 (pyridoxine), 10 to 25 mg three times a day, has been reported in two randomized placebo-controlled trials to be effective for treating the nausea and vomiting of pregnancy. In several other controlled trials, there was no evidence of teratogenicity.

DOXYLAMINE

Doxylamine (Unisom SleepTabs) is an effective antihistamine for nausea in pregnancy and can be combined with vitamin B_6 to produce a therapy similar to the former preparation Bendectin. Vitamin B_6 (50 mg) and doxylamine (25 mg) at bedtime, and half of each tablet in the morning and afternoon, is an effective combination. The Canadian formulation Diclectin, delayed-release doxylamine 10 mg + pyridoxine 10 mg, is effective and well tolerated.[45]

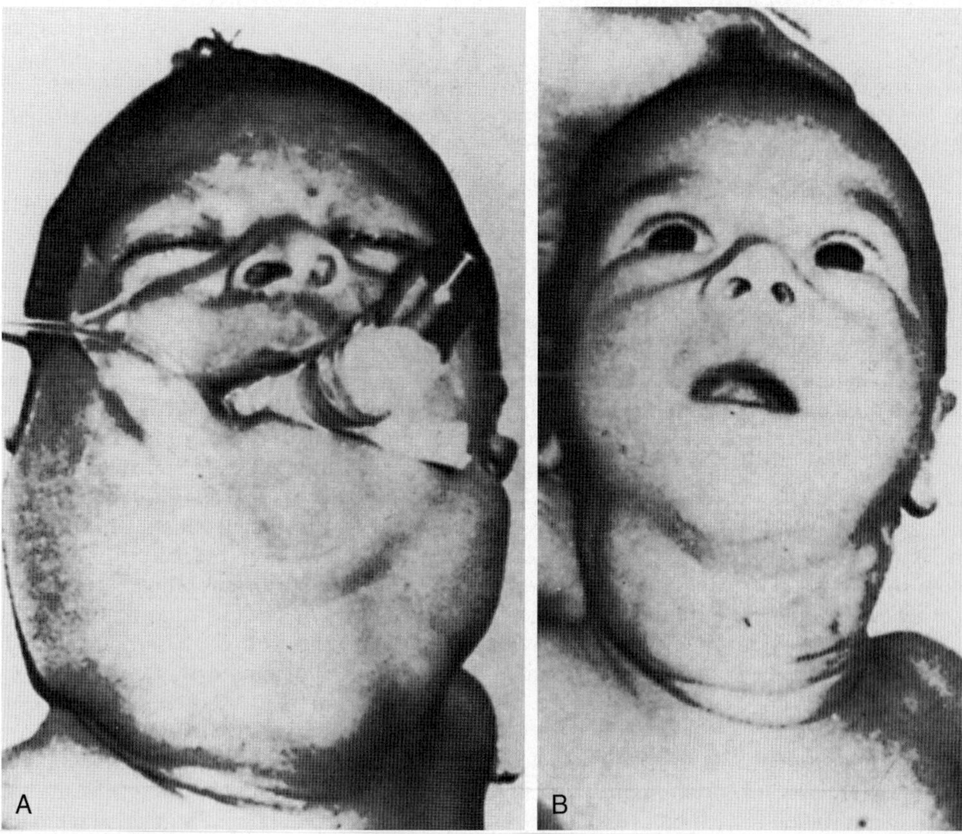

FIGURE 8-7. Iodide-induced neonatal goiter. **A,** Appearance on the first day of life. **B,** Appearance at 2 months of age. (From Senior B, Chernoff HL: Iodide goiter in the newborn. Pediatrics 47:510, 1971.)

MECLIZINE (BONINE)

In one randomized, placebo-controlled study, meclizine gave significantly better results than placebo. Prospective clinical studies have provided no evidence that meclizine is teratogenic in humans. In 1014 patients in the Collaborative Perinatal Project and an additional 613 patients from the Kaiser Health Plan, no teratogenic risk was found.

DIMENHYDRINATE (DRAMAMINE)

No teratogenicity has been noted with dimenhydrinate, but a 29% failure rate and a significant incidence of side effects, especially drowsiness, have been reported.

DIPHENHYDRAMINE (BENADRYL)

In 595 patients treated in the Collaborative Perinatal Project, no teratogenicity was noted with diphenhydramine. Drowsiness can be a problem.

PHENOTHIAZINES

Teratogenicity does not appear to be a problem with the phenothiazines when evaluated as a group. In the Kaiser Health Plan Study, 976 patients were treated, and in the Collaborative Perinatal Project, 1309 patients were treated; in both studies, no evidence of association between these drugs and malformations was noted. In 114 mothers treated with promethazine (Phenergan) and in 877 mothers given prochlorperazine (Compazine), no increased risk for malformations was found.

METOCLOPRAMIDE

Of 3458 infants exposed to metoclopramide (Reglan) during the first trimester, there was no increased risk for malformations, low birthweight, or preterm delivery.[46]

ONDANSETRON (ZOFRAN)

Ondansetron is no more effective than promethazine (Phenergan), but less sedating.[47] Ondansetron has not been evaluated in large numbers of patients for teratogenicity.

METHYLPREDNISOLONE

Forty patients with hyperemesis who were admitted to the hospital were randomized to oral methylprednisolone or oral promethazine, and methylprednisolone was more effective.[48] In a larger study in which all patients received promethazine and metoclopramide as well, methylprednisolone did not reduce the need for rehospitalization. The drug should be used only after 10 weeks of pregnancy because of the potential risk for cleft lip and cleft palate.[43]

GINGER

Ginger has been used with success for treating hyperemesis, and nausea and vomiting in the outpatient setting. A significantly greater relief of symptoms was found after ginger treatment than with placebo. Patients took 250-mg capsules containing ginger as powdered root four times a day.

Acid-Suppressing Drugs

The use of cimetidine, omeprazole, and ranitidine has not been found to be associated with any teratogenic risk in 2261 exposures.[49] Of an additional 3651 infants exposed to proton-pump inhibitors in the first trimester, there was no increased risk for birth defects.[50] Drugs taken were mostly omeprazole but also included lansoprazole, esomeprazole, and pantoprazole.

Antihistamines and Decongestants

No increased risk for anomalies has been associated with most of the commonly used antihistamines, such as chlorpheniramine (Chlor-Trimeton). However, several reports of note are presented in the following section.

Terfenadine (Seldane) has been associated in one study with an increased risk for polydactyly. Astemizole (Hismanal) did not increase the risk for birth defects in 114 infants exposed in the first trimester.

An association between exposure to antihistamines during the last 2 weeks of pregnancy and retrolental fibroplasia in premature infants has been reported.

In the Collaborative Perinatal Project, an increased risk for birth defects was noted with phenylpropanolamine (Entex LA) exposure in the first trimester. In one retrospective study, an increased risk for gastroschisis was associated with first-trimester pseudoephedrine (Sudafed) use. Although these findings have not been confirmed, use of these drugs for trivial indications should be discouraged because long-term effects are unknown. If decongestion is necessary, topical nasal sprays will result in a lower dose to the fetus than systemic medication.

Patients should be educated that antihistamines and decongestants are only symptomatic therapy for the common cold and have no influence on the course of the disease. Other remedies should be recommended, such as use of a humidifier, rest, and fluids. If medications are necessary, combinations with two drugs should not be used if only one drug is necessary. If the diagnosis is truly an allergy, an antihistamine alone will suffice.

Antibiotics and Anti-infective Agents

Because pregnant patients are particularly susceptible to vaginal yeast infections, antibiotics should be used only when clearly indicated. Therapy with antifungal agents may be necessary during or after the course of therapy.

PENICILLINS

Penicillin, ampicillin, and amoxicillin (Amoxil) are safe in pregnancy. In the Collaborative Perinatal Project, 3546 mothers took penicillin derivatives in the first trimester of pregnancy, with no increased risk for anomalies. Of 86 infants exposed to dicloxacillin in the first trimester, there was no increase in birth defects.

Clavulanate is added to penicillin derivatives to broaden their antibacterial spectrum. Of 556 infants exposed in the first trimester, no increased risk for birth defects was observed. Amoxicillin-clavulanate (Augmentin) was studied in randomized controlled trials as potential therapy for chorioamnionitis in women with preterm premature rupture of membranes.[51] During this trial, amoxicillin-clavulanate was compared with both placebo and erythromycin. An increased incidence of necrotizing enterocolitis was found in the amoxicillin-clavulanate group compared with both the placebo and erythromycin groups. It has been suggested that amoxicillin-clavulanate selects for specific pathogens, which leads to abnormal microbial colonization of the gastrointestinal tract and ultimately initiation of necrotizing enterocolitis. **Therefore, amoxicillin-clavulanate should be avoided in women at risk for preterm delivery.**[52]

Cephalosporins

In a study of 5000 Michigan Medicaid recipients, there was a suggestion of possible teratogenicity (25% increased birth defects) with cefaclor, cephalexin, and cephradine, but not other cephalosporins. However, another study of 308 women exposed in the first trimester showed no increase in malformations. The consensus is that these drugs are safe.

Sulfonamides

Among 1455 human infants exposed to sulfonamides during the first trimester, no teratogenic effects were noted. However, the administration of sulfonamides should be avoided in women deficient in glucose-6-phosphate dehydrogenase (G6PD) because dose-related hemolysis may occur.

Sulfonamides cause no known damage to the fetus in utero because the fetus can clear free bilirubin through the placenta. These drugs might theoretically have deleterious effects if they are present in the blood of the neonate after birth, however. Sulfonamides compete with bilirubin for binding sites on albumin, thus raising the levels of free bilirubin in the serum and increasing the risk for hyperbilirubinemia in the neonate.[53] Although this toxicity occurs with direct administration to the neonate, kernicterus in the newborn following in utero exposure has not been reported.

Sulfamethoxazole with Trimethoprim (Bactrim, Septra)

Trimethoprim is often given with sulfa to treat urinary tract infections. However, one unpublished study of 2296 Michigan Medicaid recipients suggested an increased risk for cardiovascular defects after exposure in the first trimester. **In one retrospective study of trimethoprim with sulfamethoxazole, the OR for birth defects was 2.3, whereas in another study, it was 2.5 to 3.4.**[54]

Nitrofurantoin (Macrodantin)

Nitrofurantoin is used in the treatment of acute uncomplicated lower urinary tract infections as well as for long-term suppression in patients with chronic bacteriuria. Nitrofurantoin is capable of inducing hemolytic anemia in patients deficient in G6PD. However, hemolytic anemia in the newborn as a result of in utero exposure to nitrofurantoin has not been reported.

No reports have associated nitrofurantoins with congenital defects. In the Collaborative Perinatal Project, 590 infants were exposed, 83 in the first trimester, with no increased risk for adverse effects. Other studies have confirmed these findings.

Tetracyclines

Tetracyclines readily cross the placenta and are firmly bound by chelation to calcium in developing bone and tooth structures. This produces brown discoloration of the deciduous teeth, hypoplasia of the enamel, and inhibition of bone growth.[55] **The staining of the teeth takes place in the second or third trimesters of pregnancy, whereas bone incorporation can occur earlier.** Depression of skeletal growth was particularly common among premature infants treated with tetracycline. First-trimester exposure to doxycycline is not known to carry any risk. **First-trimester exposure to tetracyclines has not been found to have any teratogenic risk in 341 women in the Collaborative Perinatal Project or in 174 women in another study. Alternative antibiotics are currently recommended during pregnancy.**

Aminoglycosides

Streptomycin and kanamycin have been associated with congenital deafness in the offspring of mothers who took these drugs during pregnancy. Ototoxicity was reported with doses as low as 1 g of streptomycin twice a week for 8 weeks during the first trimester. Of 391 mothers who had received 50 mg/kg of kanamycin for prolonged periods during pregnancy, nine children (2.3%) were found to have hearing loss.

Nephrotoxicity may be greater when aminoglycosides are combined with cephalosporins. Neuromuscular blockade may be potentiated by the combined use of aminoglycosides and curariform drugs. Potentiation of magnesium sulfate–induced neuromuscular weakness has also been reported in a neonate exposed to magnesium sulfate and gentamicin. Gentamicin has not been as well studied as the other aminoglycosides.

No known teratogenic effect other than ototoxicity has been associated with aminoglycosides in the first trimester. In 135 infants exposed to streptomycin in the Collaborative Perinatal Project, no teratogenic effects were observed. Among 1619 newborns whose mothers were treated for tuberculosis with multiple drugs, including streptomycin, the incidence of congenital defects was the same as in a healthy control group.

Antituberculosis Drugs

There is no evidence of any teratogenic effect of isoniazid, para-aminosalicylic acid, rifampin (Rifadin), or ethambutol (Myambutol).

Erythromycin

No teratogenic risk for erythromycin has been reported. In 79 patients in the Collaborative Perinatal Project and 260 in another study, no increase in birth defects was noted.

Clarithromycin

Of 122 first-trimester exposures, there was no significant risk for birth defects.

Fluoroquinolones

The quinolones (e.g., ciprofloxacin [Cipro], norfloxacin [Noroxin]) have a high affinity for bone tissue and cartilage and may cause arthralgia in children. However, no malformations or musculoskeletal problems were noted in 38 infants exposed in utero in the first trimester, in 132 newborns exposed in the first trimester in the Michigan Medicaid data, or in 200 other first-trimester exposures.

Metronidazole (Flagyl)

Studies have failed to show any increase in the incidence of congenital defects among the newborns of mothers treated with metronidazole during early or late gestation. Among

1387 prescriptions filled, no increase in birth defects could be determined. A meta-analysis confirmed lack of teratogenic risk.[56]

Antiviral Agents

The Acyclovir Registry has recorded 756 first-trimester exposures, with no increased risk for abnormalities in the infants.[57] Among 1561 pregnancies exposed to acyclovir, 229 exposed to valacyclovir, and 26 exposed to famciclovir, all in the first trimester, there was no increased risk for birth defects.[58] The Centers for Disease Control and Prevention recommend that pregnant women with disseminated infection (e.g., herpetic encephalitis or hepatitis or varicella pneumonia) be treated with acyclovir.

Lindane (Kwell)

After application of lindane to the skin, about 10% of the dose used can be recovered in the urine. Toxicity in humans after use of topical 1% lindane has been observed almost exclusively after misuse and overexposure to the agent. Although no evidence of specific fetal damage is attributable to lindane, the agent is a potent neurotoxin, and its use during pregnancy should be limited. Pregnant women should be cautioned about shampooing their children's hair because absorption could easily occur across the skin of the hands. An alternative drug for lice is usually recommended, such as pyrethrins with piperonyl butoxide (RID).

Antiretroviral Agents

Zidovudine (ZDV) should be included as a component in the antiretroviral regimen whenever possible because of its record of safety and efficacy. In a prospective cohort study, children exposed to ZDV in the perinatal period through Pediatric AIDS Clinical Trials Group Protocol 076 were studied up to a median age of 4.2 years. No adverse effects were observed in these children. The International Antiretroviral Registry was established in 1989 to detect any major teratogenic effect of the antiretroviral drugs. Through January 2004, more than 1000 pregnancies had first-trimester exposures to ZDV and lamivudine, and no teratogenicity was reported.

Concerns have been raised regarding use of other antiretroviral therapies. Efavirenz is not recommended during pregnancy due to reports of significant malformations in monkeys receiving efavirenz during the first trimester and also three case reports of fetal NTDs in women who received the drug.[59] In 2001, Bristol-Myers Squibb issued a warning advising against the use of didanosine and stavudine in pregnant women due to case reports of lactic acidosis, some of which were fatal. These two drugs should only be used if no other alternatives are available.

Antifungal Agents

Nystatin (Mycostatin) is poorly absorbed from intact skin and mucous membranes, and topical use has not been associated with teratogenesis. Clotrimazole (Lotrimin) or miconazole (Monistat) in pregnancy is not known to be associated with congenital malformations. However, in one study, a statistically significantly increased risk for first-trimester abortion was noted after use of these drugs, but these findings were considered not to be definitive evidence of risk. Of 2092 newborns exposed in the first trimester in the Michigan Medicaid data, there was no increased risk for anomalies.

Limb deformities were reported in three infants exposed to 400 to 800 mg/day of fluconazole in the first trimester. However, in systematic studies of 460 patients who received a single 150-mg dose of fluconazole, no increased risk for defects was observed.[60]

Drugs for Induction of Ovulation

In more than 2000 exposures, no evidence of teratogenic risk of clomiphene (Clomid) has been noted, and the percentage of spontaneous abortions is close to the expected rate. Although infants are often exposed to bromocriptine (Parlodel) in early pregnancy, no teratogenic effects have been observed in more than 1400 pregnancies.

Mild Analgesics

Some pains during pregnancy justify the use of a mild analgesic. Pregnant patients should be encouraged to use nonpharmacologic remedies, such as local heat and rest.

Aspirin

There is no evidence of any teratogenic effect of aspirin taken in the first trimester. **Aspirin does have significant perinatal effects, however, because it inhibits prostaglandin synthesis. Uterine contractility is decreased, and patients taking aspirin in analgesic doses have delayed onset of labor, longer duration of labor, and an increased risk for a prolonged pregnancy.**

Aspirin also decreases platelet aggregation, which can increase the risk for bleeding before as well as at delivery. Platelet dysfunction has been described in newborns within 5 days of ingestion of aspirin by the mother. Because aspirin causes permanent inhibition of prostaglandin synthetase in platelets, the only way for adequate clotting to occur is for more platelets to be produced.

Multiple organs may be affected by chronic aspirin use. Of note, prostaglandins mediate the neonatal closure of the ductus arteriosus. In one case report, maternal ingestion of aspirin close to the time of delivery was related to closure of the ductus arteriosus in utero.

Acetaminophen (Tylenol, Datril)

Acetaminophen has also shown no evidence of teratogenicity.[61] With acetaminophen, inhibition of prostaglandin synthesis is reversible; thus, once the drug has cleared, platelet aggregation returns to normal. **Bleeding time is not prolonged with acetaminophen in contrast to aspirin,** and the drug is not toxic to the newborn. Thus, if a mild analgesic or antipyretic is indicated, acetaminophen is preferred over aspirin.

Other Nonsteroidal Anti-inflammatory Agents

No evidence of teratogenicity has been reported for other nonsteroidal anti-inflammatory drugs (e.g., ibuprofen [Motrin,Advil], naproxen [Naprosyn]), but limited information is available. Chronic use may lead to oligohydramnios, and constriction of the fetal ductus arteriosus or neonatal pulmonary hypertension as has been reported with indomethacin might occur.

CODEINE

In the Collaborative Perinatal Project, no increased relative risk for malformations was observed in 563 codeine users. In one recent study, maternal treatment with opioid analgesics was associated with an increased risk for heart defects, spina bifida, and gastroschisis. **Codeine can cause addiction and newborn withdrawal symptoms if used to excess perinatally.**

SUMATRIPTAN

Of 479 exposures to sumatriptan (Imitrex) in the first trimester,[62] 4.6% of infants had birth defects. This percentage is not significantly different from the nonexposed population. **For women whose severe headaches do not respond to other therapy, sumatriptan may be used during pregnancy.**[63]

DRUGS OF ABUSE

Smoking

It is not simple to sort out potential confounding factors when comparing smokers with nonsmokers. However, smoking is associated with a fourfold increase in small size for gestational age as well as an increased prematurity rate.[64] **The higher perinatal mortality rate associated with smoking is attributable to an increased risk for abruptio placentae, placenta previa, premature and prolonged rupture of membranes, and intrauterine growth restriction.** The risks for complications and the associated perinatal loss rise with the number of cigarettes smoked. Discontinuation of smoking during pregnancy can reduce the risk for both pregnancy complications and perinatal mortality, especially in women at high risk for other reasons. Maternal passive smoking was also associated with a twofold risk for low birthweight at term in one study.

There is also a positive association between smoking and sudden infant death syndrome (SIDS) and increased respiratory illnesses in children. In such reports, it is not possible to distinguish between apparent effects of maternal smoking during pregnancy and smoking after pregnancy, but both may play a role.

The spontaneous abortion rate may be up to twice that of nonsmokers, and abortions associated with maternal smoking tend to have a higher percentage of normal karyotypes and occur later than those with chromosomal aberrations.[65]

Smoking Cessation During Pregnancy

Tobacco smoke contains nicotine, carbon monoxide, and thousands of other compounds. Although nicotine is the mechanism of addiction to cigarettes, other chemicals may contribute to adverse pregnancy outcomes. For example, carbon monoxide decreases oxygen delivery to the fetus, whereas nicotine decreases uterine blood flow.

Nicotine withdrawal may first be attempted with nicotine fading, switching to brands of cigarettes with progressively less nicotine over a 3-week period. Exercise may also improve quitting success rates. **Nicotine medications are indicated for patients with nicotine dependence.** This is defined as smoking greater than one pack per day, smoking within 30 minutes of getting up in the morning, or prior withdrawal symptoms. Nicotine medications are available as patches, gum, or inhalers. **Although one might question the propriety of prescribing nicotine during pregnancy, cessation of smoking eliminates many other toxins, including carbon monoxide; nicotine blood levels are not increased over those of smokers.**

Congenital anomalies occurred in 5 of 188 infants of women treated with bupropion (Zyban) during the first trimester of pregnancy, not a significant difference from the number expected. There is no knowledge of the safety of varenicline (Chantix) use in pregnancy.[66] However, both of these medications have recently had product warnings mandated by the FDA about the risk for psychiatric symptoms and suicide associated with their use.

Alcohol

Fetal alcohol syndrome (FAS) has been reported in the offspring of alcoholic mothers and includes the features of gross physical retardation with onset prenatally and continuing after birth (Figure 8-8).

In 1980, the Fetal Alcohol Study Group of the Research Society on Alcoholism proposed criteria for the diagnosis of FAS.[67] At least one characteristic from each of the following three categories had to be present for a valid diagnosis of the syndrome:

1. Growth retardation before and/or after birth
2. Facial anomalies, including small palpebral fissures, indistinct or absent philtrum, epicanthic folds, flattened nasal bridge, short length of nose, thin upper lip, low-set and unparallel ears, and retarded midfacial development
3. Central nervous system dysfunction, including microcephaly, varying degrees of mental retardation, or other evidence of abnormal neurobehavioral development, such as attention deficit disorder with hyperactivity

The full FAS occurs in 6% of infants of heavy drinkers, and less severe birth defects and neurocognitive deficits occur in a larger proportion of children whose mothers drink heavily during pregnancy.

Jones and associates compared 23 chronically alcoholic women with 46 controls and compared the pregnancy outcomes of the two groups. Among the alcoholic mothers, perinatal deaths were about eight times more frequent. Growth restriction, microcephaly, and IQ below 80 were considerably more frequent than among the controls. Overall outcome was abnormal in 43% of the offspring of the alcoholic mothers compared with 2% of the controls.

Ouellette and colleagues addressed the risks of smaller amounts of alcohol. Nine percent of infants of abstinent or rare drinkers and 14% of infants of moderate drinkers were abnormal, not a significant difference. **In heavy drinkers (average daily intake of 3 oz of 100-proof liquor or more), 32% of the infants had anomalies.** The aggregate pool of anomalies, growth restriction, and an abnormal neurologic examination were found in 71% of the children of heavy drinkers, twice the frequency in the moderate and rarely drinking groups. In this study, an increased frequency of abnormality was not found until 45 mL of ethanol (equivalent to three drinks) daily were exceeded. The study of Mills and Graubard also showed that total malformation rates were not significantly higher among offspring of women who had an average of less than one drink per day or one to two drinks per day, than among nondrinkers.

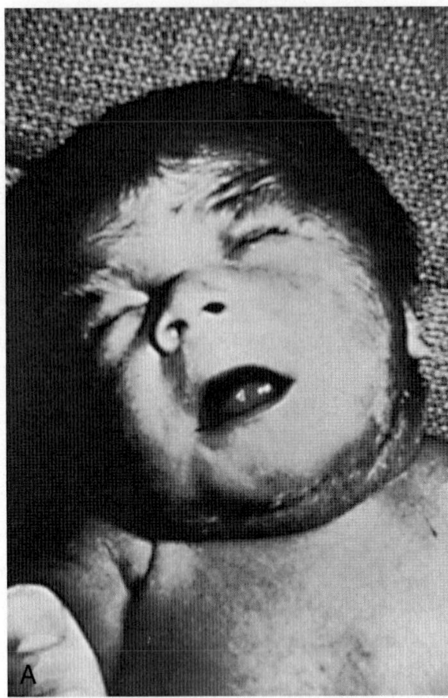

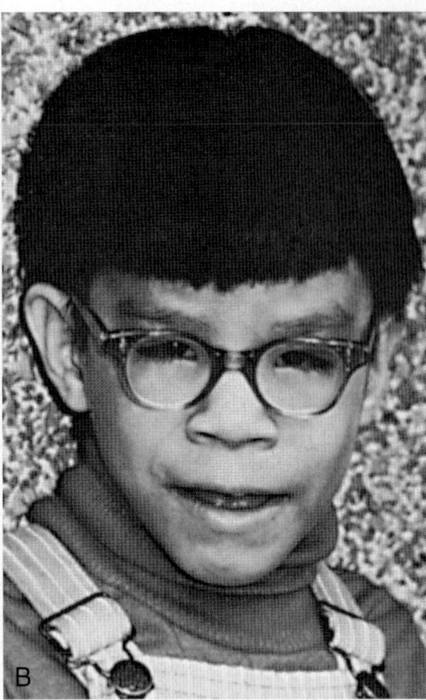

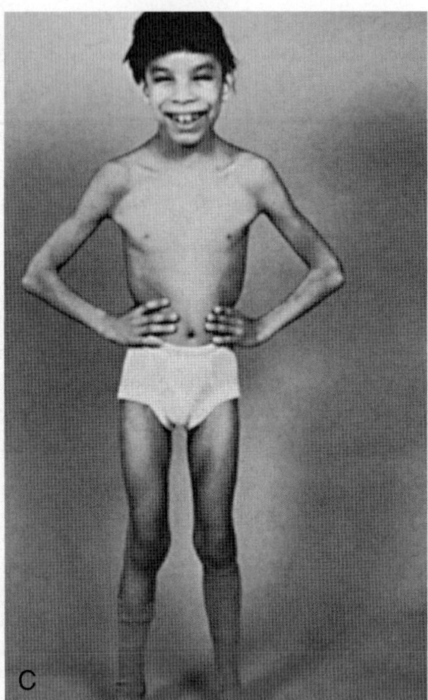

FIGURE 8-8. Fetal alcohol syndrome. Patient photographed at birth **(A)**, 5 years **(B)**, and 8 years **(C)**. Note short palpebral fissures, short nose, hypoplastic philtrum, thinned upper lip vermilion, and flattened midface. (From Streissguth AP: CIBA Foundation Monograph 105. London, Pitman, 1984.)

TABLE 8-2 T-ACE QUESTIONS FOUND TO IDENTIFY WOMEN DRINKING SUFFICIENTLY TO POTENTIALLY DAMAGE THE FETUS*

T	How many drinks does it take to make you feel high (can you hold) *(tolerance)*?
A	Have people *annoyed* you by criticizing your drinking?
C	Have you felt you ought to *cut down* on your drinking?
E	Have you ever had to drink first thing in the morning to steady your nerves or to get rid of a hangover *(eye-opener)*?

From Sokol RJ, Martier SS, Ager JW: The T-ACE questions: practical prenatal detection of risk-drinking. Am J Obstet Gynecol 160:863, 1989.

*Two points are scored as a positive answer to the tolerance question and one each for the other three. A score of 2 or more correctly identified 69% of risk drinkers.

Genitourinary malformations increased with increasing alcohol consumption, however, so the possibility remains that for some malformations, no safe drinking level exists.

Heavy drinking remains a major risk to the fetus, and reduction even in midpregnancy can benefit the infant. An occasional drink during pregnancy carries no documentable risk, but no level of drinking is known to be safe.

Sokol and associates have addressed history taking for prenatal detection of risk drinking. Four questions help differentiate patients drinking sufficiently to potentially damage the fetus (Table 8-2). The patient is considered at risk if more than two drinks are required to make her feel "high." The probability of "risk drinking" increases to 63% for those responding positively to all four questions.

Marijuana

No significant teratogenic effect of marijuana has been documented, but the data are insufficient to say that there is no risk. One study finding a mean 73-g decrease in birthweight associated with marijuana use validated exposure with urine assays rather than relying on self-reporting. Other studies have not shown an effect on birthweight or length. Behavioral and developmental alterations have been observed in some studies but not in others.

Cocaine

A serious difficulty in defining the effects of cocaine on the infant is the frequent presence of many confounding variables in the population using cocaine. These mothers often abuse other drugs, smoke, have poor nutrition, fail to seek prenatal care, and live under poor socioeconomic conditions. All of these factors are difficult to take into account in comparison groups. Another difficulty is the choice of outcome measures for infants exposed in utero. The neural systems likely to be affected by cocaine are involved in neurologic and behavioral functions that are not easily quantitated by standard infant development tests.

Cocaine-using women have a higher rate of spontaneous abortion than controls. **Three other studies suggested an increased risk for congenital anomalies after first-trimester cocaine use, most frequently cardiac and central nervous system.** In the study of Bingol and colleagues, the malformation rate was 10% in cocaine users, 4.5% in polydrug users, and 2% in controls. MacGregor and coworkers reported a 6% anomaly rate compared with 1% for controls.

Cocaine is a central nervous system stimulant and has local anesthetic and marked vasoconstrictive effects. Not surprisingly, **abruptio placentae has been reported to occur immediately after nasal or intravenous administration.**[67] Several studies have also noted increased stillbirths, preterm labor, premature birth, and small-for-gestational-age infants with cocaine use.

The most common brain abnormality in infants exposed to cocaine in utero is impairment of intrauterine brain growth as manifested by microcephaly.[68] In one study, 16% of newborns had microcephaly compared with 6% of controls. Somatic growth is also impaired, and the growth restriction may be symmetrical or characterized by a relatively low head-to-abdominal circumference ratio. Multiple other neurologic problems have been reported after cocaine exposure, as well as dysmorphic features and neurobehavioral abnormalities.

Aside from causing congenital anomalies in the first trimester, cocaine has been reported to cause fetal disruption, presumably due to interruption of blood flow to various organs. Bowel infarction has been noted with unusual ileal atresia and bowel perforation. Limb infarction has resulted in missing fingers in a distribution different from the usual congenital limb anomalies. Central nervous system bleeding in utero may result in porencephalic cysts.

Narcotics and Methadone

Menstrual abnormalities, especially amenorrhea, are common in heroin abusers, although they are not associated with the use of methadone. Medical intervention is more likely to involve methadone maintenance, with the goal being a dose of about 20 to 40 mg/day. The dose should be individualized at a level sufficient to minimize the use of supplemental illicit drugs, which represent greater risk to the fetus than even the higher doses of methadone required by some patients. Manipulation of the dose in women maintained on methadone should be avoided in the last trimester because of an association with increased fetal complications and deaths attributed to fetal withdrawal in utero. Because management of narcotic addiction during pregnancy requires a host of social, nutritional, educational, and psychiatric interventions, these patients are best managed in specialized programs. Buprenorphine (Subutex) is also an acceptable treatment, and infants exposed to this drug required less morphine, had shorter hospital stays, and had shorter duration of treatment for neonatal abstinence syndrome than infants exposed to methadone. However, women on buprenorphine were more likely to discontinue treatment.

The pregnancy of the narcotic addict is at increased risk for abortion, prematurity, and growth restriction. Withdrawal should be watched for carefully in the neonatal period.[69]

Caffeine

There is no evidence of teratogenic effects of caffeine in humans.[70] The Collaborative Perinatal Project showed no increased incidence of congenital defects in 5773 women taking caffeine in pregnancy, usually in a fixed-dose analgesic medication. The average cup of coffee contains about 100 mg, and a 12 oz can of soda contains about 50 mg of caffeine. Some conflicting evidence exists concerning the association between heavy ingestion of caffeine and increased pregnancy complications. Early studies suggested that the intake of greater than seven to eight cups of coffee per day was associated with low birthweight infants, spontaneous abortions, prematurity, and stillbirths. However, these studies were not controlled for the concomitant use of tobacco and alcohol. **In one report that controlled for smoking, other habits, demographic characteristics, and medical history, no relationship was found between malformations, low birthweight, or short gestation and heavy coffee consumption.** When pregnant women consumed more than 300 mg of caffeine per day, one study suggested an increase in term low-birthweight infants,[71] less than 2500 g at greater than 36 weeks.

Concomitant consumption of caffeine with cigarette smoking may increase the risk for low birthweight. Maternal coffee intake decreases iron absorption and may contribute to maternal anemia.

Two other studies have shown conflicting results. One retrospective investigation reporting a higher risk for fetal loss was biased by ascertainment of the patients at the time of fetal loss because these patients typically have less nausea and would be expected to drink more coffee. A prospective cohort study found no evidence that moderate caffeine use increased the risk for spontaneous abortion or growth restriction.[72] Measurement of serum paraxanthine, a caffeine metabolite, revealed that only extremely high levels are associated with spontaneous abortions.

The American College of Obstetricians and Gynecologists (ACOG) concluded that moderate caffeine consumption (<200 mg/day) does not appear to be a major contributing factor in miscarriage or preterm birth, but the relationship to growth restriction remains undetermined.[73] High caffeine intake may or may not be related to miscarriage, so limiting intake to 200 mg/day seems prudent.[73]

Aspartame (NutraSweet)

The major metabolite of aspartame is phenylalanine,[74] which is concentrated in the fetus by active placental transport. Sustained high blood levels of phenylalanine in the fetus as seen in maternal phenylketonuria are associated with mental retardation in the infant. However, within the usual range of aspartame ingestion in normal individuals, peak phenylalanine levels do not exceed normal postprandial levels, and even with high doses, phenylalanine concentrations are still very far below those associated with mental retardation. These responses have also been studied in women who are obligate carriers of PKU, and their levels are still normal. **Thus, it seems unlikely that aspartame during pregnancy would cause any fetal toxicity.**

DRUGS IN BREAST MILK

Many drugs can be detected in breast milk at low levels that are not usually of clinical significance to the infant. The rate of transfer into milk depends on the lipid solubility, molecular weight, degree of protein binding, degree of ionization of the drug, and the presence or absence of active secretion. Nonionized molecules of low molecular weight such as ethanol cross easily.[75] If the mother has unusually high blood concentrations such as with increased dosage or decreased renal function, drugs may appear in higher concentrations in the milk.

The amount of drug in breast milk is a variable fraction of the maternal blood level, which itself is proportional to the maternal oral dose. Thus, the dose to the infant is usually subtherapeutic, about 1% to 2% of the maternal dose on the average. This amount is usually so trivial that no adverse effects are noted. In the case of toxic drugs, however, any exposure may be inappropriate. Allergy may also exist or be initiated. Long-term effects of even small doses of drugs may yet be discovered. Also, drugs are eliminated more slowly in the infant with immature enzyme systems. Short-term effects of most maternal medications on breastfed infants are mild and pose little risk to the infants. The benefits of breastfeeding are well known, and the risk of drug exposure must be weighed against these benefits.

With drug administration in the immediate few days postpartum before lactation is fully established, the infant receives only a small volume of colostrum; thus, little drug is excreted into the milk. It is also helpful to allay fears of patients undergoing cesarean deliveries that analgesics or other drugs administered at this time have no known adverse effects on the infant. For drugs requiring daily dosing during lactation, knowledge of pharmacokinetics in breast milk may minimize the dose to the infant. For example, dosing immediately after nursing decreases the neonatal exposure because the blood level will be at its nadir just before the next dose.

Short-term effects, if any, of most maternal medications on breastfed infants are mild and pose little risk to the infants.[76] Of 838 breastfeeding women, 11.2% reported minor adverse reactions in the infants, but these reactions did not require medical attention. In 19%, antibiotics caused diarrhea; in 11%, narcotics caused drowsiness; in 9%, antihistamines caused irritability; and in 10%, sedatives, antidepressants, or antiepileptics caused drowsiness.[76]

The American Academy of Pediatrics has reviewed drugs in lactation[77] and categorized the drugs as listed below in six categories:

Drugs Commonly Listed as Contraindicated During Breastfeeding

Cytotoxic Drugs That May Interfere with Cellular Metabolism of the Nursing Infant

Cyclosporine (Sandimmune), doxorubicin (Adriamycin), and cyclophosphamide (Cytoxan) might cause immune suppression in the infant, although data are limited with respect to these drugs. In general, the potential risks of these drugs would outweigh the benefits of continuing nursing.[77]

After oral administration to a lactating patient with choriocarcinoma, methotrexate was found in milk in low but detectable levels. Most individuals would elect to avoid any exposure of the infant to this drug. However, in environments in which bottle feeding is rarely practiced or presents practical and cultural difficulties, therapy with this drug would not in itself appear to constitute a contraindication to breastfeeding.

Drugs of Abuse for Which Adverse Effects on the Infant During Breastfeeding Have Been Reported

Drugs of abuse, such as amphetamines, cocaine, heroin, marijuana, and phencyclidine, are all contraindicated during breastfeeding because they are hazardous to the nursing infant and to the health of the mother.[77]

Radioactive Compounds That Require Temporary Cessation of Breastfeeding

The American Academy of Pediatrics[77] suggests consultation with a nuclear medicine physician so that the radionuclide with the shortest excretion time in breast milk can be used. The mother can attempt to store breast milk before the study. She should continue to pump to maintain milk production but discard the milk during therapy. **Radiopharmaceuticals require variable intervals of interruption of nursing.** Recommended intervals are as follows:

1. Gallium-67, 2 weeks
2. ^{131}I, 2 to 14 days
3. Radioactive sodium, 4 days
4. Technetium-99m, 15 hours to 3 days

The physician may reassure the patient by counting the radioactivity of the milk before nursing is resumed.

Drugs for Which the Effect on Nursing Infants Is Unknown but May Be of Concern

The category includes several classes of psychotropic drugs, amiodarone (associated with hypothyroidism), lamotrigine (potential for therapeutic serum concentration in the infant), metoclopramide (potential dopaminergic blocking, but no reported detrimental effects), and metronidazole.[77]

Antianxiety, antidepressant, and antipsychotic agents are sometimes given to nursing mothers. Although there are no data about adverse effects in infants exposed to these drugs through breast milk, they could theoretically alter central nervous system function.[77] Fluoxetine (Prozac) is excreted in breast milk at low levels, so the infant receives about 6.7% of the maternal dose.[78] The level in the breastfed newborn is certainly lower than the level during pregnancy.

Sertraline causes a decline in 5-hydroxytryptamine levels in mothers, but not in their breastfed infants.[79] **This implies that the small amount of drug the infant ingests in breast milk is not enough to have a pharmacologic effect** (Figure 8-9). **Infants of mothers on psychotropic drugs should be monitored for sedation during use and withdrawal after cessation of the drug.**

A bigger problem is postpartum depression, exacerbated by fatigue. **The benefits of breastfeeding should be weighed against the negative effect on bonding resulting from untreated postpartum depression.**

Temporary cessation of breastfeeding after a single dose of metronidazole (Flagyl) may be considered. Its half-life is such that interruption of lactation for 12 to 24 hours after single-dose therapy usually results in negligible exposure to the infant. However, no adverse effects in infants have been reported.

Drugs That Have Been Associated with Significant Effects in Some Nursing Infants and Should Be Given to Nursing Mothers with Caution

Bromocriptine

Bromocriptine is an ergot alkaloid derivative. Because it has an inhibitory effect on lactation, it should be avoided unless the mother has taken it during the pregnancy.

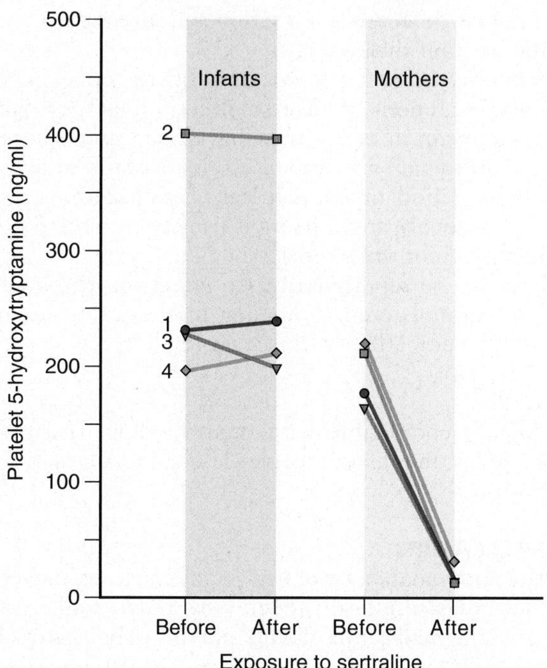

Figure 8-9. Effect of sertraline on platelet 5-hydroxytryptamine levels in four breast-fed infants and their mothers. (From Epperson CN, Anderson GM, McDougle CJ: Sertraline and breast-feeding. N Engl J Med 336:1189, 1997. Copyright 1997 Massachusetts Medical Society.)

Ergotamine

Ergotamine, as used by those with migraine headache, has been associated with vomiting, diarrhea, and convulsions in the infant. Administration of an ergot alkaloid for the treatment of uterine atony does not contraindicate lactation.

Lithium

Breast milk levels of lithium are one-third to one-half maternal serum levels, and the infant's serum levels while nursing are much lower than the fetal levels that occur when the mother takes lithium during pregnancy. The benefits of breastfeeding must be weighed against the theoretical effects of small amounts of the drug on the developing brain.[77] (See comment above about the need to minimize fatigue in order to mitigate against postpartum psychoses.)

Maternal Medication Usually Compatible with Breastfeeding

Narcotics, Sedatives, and Anticonvulsants

In general, no evidence of adverse effect is noted with most of the sedatives, narcotic analgesics, and anticonvulsants. Patients may be reassured that, in normal doses, carbamazepine (Tegretol), phenytoin (Dilantin), magnesium sulfate, codeine, morphine, and meperidine (Demerol) do not cause any obvious adverse effects in the infants because the dose detectable in the breast milk is about 1% to 2% of the mother's dose, which is sufficiently low to have no significant pharmacologic activity.

With diazepam (Valium), the milk-to-plasma ratio at peak dose is 0.68, with only small amounts detected in the breast milk. In two patients who took carbamazepine (Tegretol) while nursing, the concentration of the drug in breast milk at 4 and 5 weeks postpartum was similar, about 60% of the maternal serum level. Accumulation does not seem to occur, and no adverse effects were noted in either infant.

Cold Preparations

No harmful effects of acetaminophen (Tylenol, Datril) have been noted. Although studies are not extensive, no harmful effects have been noted from antihistamines or decongestants. Less than 1% of a pseudoephedrine dose or triprolidine dose ingested by the mother is excreted in the breast milk.

Antihypertensives

Thiazides

After a single 500-mg oral dose of chlorothiazide (Diuril), no drug was detected in breast milk. In one mother taking 50 mg of hydrochlorothiazide (Hydrodiuril) daily, the drug was not detectable in the nursing infant's serum, and the infant's electrolytes were normal. Thiazide diuretics may decrease milk production in the first month of lactation.[77]

β-Blockers

Propranolol (Inderal) is excreted in breast milk, with milk concentrations after a single 40-mg dose less than 40% of peak plasma concentrations. Thus, an infant consuming 500 mL/day of milk would ingest an amount representing about 1% of a therapeutic dose, which is unlikely to cause any adverse effect.

Atenolol (Tenormin) is concentrated in breast milk to about three times the plasma level. One case has been reported in which a 5-day-old term infant had signs of β-adrenergic blockade with bradycardia (80 beats/minute) with the breast milk dose calculated to be 9% of the maternal dose. Adverse effects in other infants have not been reported. Because milk accumulation occurs with atenolol, infants must be monitored closely for bradycardia. Propranolol is a safer alternative.

Clonidine (Catapres) concentrations in milk are almost twice maternal serum levels. Neurologic and laboratory parameters in the infants of treated mothers are similar to those of controls.

Angiotensin-Converting Enzyme Inhibitors

Captopril (Capoten) is excreted into breast milk in low levels, and no effects on nursing infants have been observed.

Calcium Channel Blockers

Nifedipine is excreted into breast milk at a concentration of less than 5% of the maternal dose, and verapamil at an even lower level. Neither have caused adverse effects in the infant.

Anticoagulants

Most mothers requiring anticoagulation may continue to nurse their infants with no problems. Heparin does not cross into milk and is not active orally.

At a maternal dose of warfarin (Coumadin) of 5 to 12 mg/day in seven patients, no warfarin was detected in breast milk or infant plasma. This low concentration is probably because warfarin is 98% protein bound, and the milk would contain insignificant drug to exert an anticoagulant effect.[80] Another report confirmed that warfarin appears only in insignificant quantities in breast milk.[81] The oral anticoagulant bishydroxycoumarin (Dicumarol) has been given to 125 nursing mothers with no effect on the infants' prothrombin times and no hemorrhages. **Thus, with careful monitoring of maternal prothrombin time so that the dosage is minimized and of neonatal prothrombin times to ensure lack of drug accumulation, warfarin may be safely administered to nursing mothers.**

Corticosteroids

Prednisone enters breast milk in an amount not likely to have any deleterious effect. In a study of seven patients, 0.14% of a sample was secreted in the milk in the subsequent 60 hours, a negligible quantity. Even at 80 mg/day, the nursing infant would ingest less than 0.1% of the dose, less than 10% of its endogenous cortisol.

Digoxin (Lanoxin)

Digoxin enters breast milk in a small amount due to significant maternal protein binding. In 24 hours, an infant would receive about 1% of the maternal dose. No adverse effects in nursing infants have been reported.

Antibiotics

Penicillin derivatives are safe in nursing mothers. With the usual therapeutic doses of penicillin or ampicillin, no adverse effects are noted in the infants. In susceptible individuals or with prolonged therapy, diarrhea and candidiasis are concerns.

Dicloxacillin is 98% protein bound. If this drug is used to treat breast infections, very little will get into the breast milk, and nursing may be continued.

Cephalosporins appear only in trace amounts in milk. In one study after cefazolin 500 mg intramuscularly three times a day (Ancef, Kefzol), no drug was detected in breast milk. After 2 g of cefazolin intravenously, the infant was exposed to less than 1% of the maternal dose.

Tooth staining or delayed bone growth from tetracyclines has not been reported after the drug was taken by a breastfeeding mother. This finding is probably because of the high binding of the drug to calcium and protein, limiting its absorption from the milk. The amount of free tetracycline available is too small to be significant.

Sulfonamides only appear in small amounts in breast milk and are ordinarily not contraindicated during nursing. However, the drug is best avoided in premature, ill, or stressed infants in whom hyperbilirubinemia may be a problem because the drug may displace bilirubin from binding sites on albumin. On the other hand, sulfasalazine was not detected in the breast milk of a mother taking this drug.[82]

Gentamicin (Garamycin) is transferred into breast milk, and half of nursing newborn infants have the drug detectable in their serum. The low levels detected would not be expected to cause clinical effects.

Nitrofurantoin (Macrodantin) is excreted into breast milk in very low concentrations. In one study, the drug could not be detected in 20 samples from mothers receiving 100 mg four times a day.

Erythromycin is excreted into breast milk in small amounts. No reports of adverse effects on infants exposed to erythromycin in breast milk have been noted. Azithromycin (Zithromax) also appears in breast milk in low concentrations. Clindamycin (Cleocin) is excreted into breast milk in low levels, and nursing is usually continued during administration of this drug.

There are no reported adverse effects on the infant of isoniazid administered to nursing mothers, and its use is considered compatible with breast-feeding.[77]

Acyclovir

Acyclovir is compatible with breastfeeding. If a mother takes 1 g/day, the infant receives less than 1 mg/day, a very low dose.

Antifungal Agents

No data are available with nystatin, miconazole, or clotrimazole in breast milk. However, with only small amounts absorbed vaginally, this would not be expected to be a clinical problem. Infant exposure to ketoconazole in human milk was 0.4% of the therapeutic dose, again unlikely to cause adverse effects.

Oral Contraceptives

Estrogen and progestin combination oral contraceptives cause dose-related suppression of milk production. Oral contraceptives containing 50 mcg and more of estrogen during lactation have been associated with shortened duration of lactation, decreased milk production, decreased infant weight gain, and decreased protein content of the milk. Lactation is inhibited to a lesser degree if the pill is started about 3 weeks postpartum and with doses of estrogen lower than 50 mcg. Although the magnitude of the changes is low, the changes may be of nutritional importance, particularly in malnourished mothers.

An infant consuming 600 mL of breast milk daily from a mother using an oral contraceptive containing 50 mcg of the ethinylestradiol receives a daily dose in the range of 10 ng of the estrogen. The amount of natural estradiol received by infants who consume a similar volume of milk from mothers not using oral contraceptives is estimated at 3 to 6 ng during anovulatory cycles and 6 to 12 ng during ovulatory cycles. No consistent long-term adverse effects on growth and development have been described.

Evidence indicates that norgestrel (Ovrette) is metabolized rather than accumulated by the infants, and to date, no adverse effects have been identified as a result of progestational agents taken by the mother. ACOG recommends placement of the etonogestrel contraceptive implant 4 weeks or more after childbirth. Progestin-only contraceptives do not cause alteration of breast milk composition or volume, making them ideal in the breastfeeding mother. When the infant is weaned, the mother should be switched to combined oral contraceptives for maximal contraceptive efficacy.

Alcohol

Alcohol levels in breast milk are similar to those in maternal blood. If a moderate social drinker had two cocktails and had a blood alcohol concentration of 50 mg/dL, the nursing infant would receive about 82 mg of alcohol, which would produce insignificant blood concentrations. There is no evidence that occasional ingestion of alcohol by a mother is harmful to the infant. However, one study showed that ethanol ingested chronically through breast milk might have a detrimental effect on motor development, but not mental development.[83] Also, alcohol in breast milk has an immediate effect on the odor of the milk, and this may decrease the amount of milk the infant consumes.[84]

Propylthiouracil

PTU is found in breast milk in small amounts. If the mother takes 200 mg PTU three times a day, the child would receive 149 mcg daily, or the equivalent of a 70-kg adult receiving 3 mg/day. Several infants studied up to 5 months of age show no changes in thyroid parameters. **Lactating mothers on PTU can thus continue nursing with close supervision of the infant.** PTU is preferred over methimazole (Tapazole) because of its high protein-binding (80%) and lower breast milk concentrations.

Histamine-2 Receptor Blockers

In theory, histamine-2 (H_2) receptor antagonists (e.g., ranitidine, cimetidine) might suppress gastric acidity and cause central nervous system stimulation in the infant, but these effects have not been confirmed. The American Academy of Pediatrics now considers H_2 receptor antagonists to be compatible with breastfeeding.[77] Famotidine, nizatidine, and roxatidine are less concentrated in breast milk and may be preferable in nursing mothers.

Caffeine

Caffeine has been reported to have no adverse effects on the nursing infant, even after the mother consumes several cups of strong coffee. In one study, the milk level contained 1% of the total dose 6 hours after coffee ingestion, which is not enough to affect the infant. In another report, no significant difference in 24-hour heart rate or sleep time was observed in nursing infants when their mothers drank coffee for 5 days or abstained for 5 days.[85]

Smoking

Nicotine and its metabolite cotinine enter breast milk. Infants of smoking mothers achieve significant serum concentrations of nicotine even if they are not exposed to passive smoking; exposure to passive smoking further raises the levels of nicotine. Women who smoke should be encouraged to stop during lactation as well as during pregnancy.

OCCUPATIONAL AND ENVIRONMENTAL HAZARDS

Ionizing Radiation

The general hazards of radiation exposure are well known. To provide counseling in specific clinical situations, key variables are dose, timing, and temporal sequence.

Acute Exposure

Systematic studies of atomic bomb survivors in Japan showed conclusively that in utero exposure to high-dose radiation increased the risk for microcephaly and mental retardation and growth restriction in the offspring.

Distance from the hypocenter—the area directly beneath the detonated bomb—and gestational age at the time of exposure were directly related to microcephaly and mental retardation and growth restriction in the infant. **The greatest number of children with microcephaly, mental retardation, and growth restriction were in the group exposed at 15 weeks' gestation or earlier.** Exposures were calculated by the distance of the victims from the epicenter. Microcephaly and mental retardation were associated with ionizing radiation at doses of 50 cGy or greater, with 20 cGy being the lowest dose in which microcephaly was observed. It is of note that radiation from the atomic bomb blast differs from the low linear transfer of filtered radiation that is used in diagnostic studies.

Although teratogenic effects have been found in several organ systems of animals exposed to acute, high-dose radiation, the only structural malformations reported among humans exposed prenatally are those mentioned earlier. Using data from animals and from outcomes of reported human exposures at various times during pregnancy, DeKaban[86] constructed a timetable for extrapolating acute, high-dose radiation (>250 cGy) to various reproductive outcomes in humans. Similarities between animal and known human effects support DeKaban's proposal.

Effects of chronic low-dose radiation on reproduction have not been identified in animals or humans. Increased risk of adverse outcomes was not detected among animals with continuous low-dose exposure (<5 rad) throughout pregnancy. The National Council for Radiation Protection[87] concluded that exposures less than 5 rads were not associated with increased risk of malformations.

Exposures are expressed as Gray (Gy): 1 Gy equals 1000 mGy equals 100 cGy (rad) (Table 8-3). Thus 10 mGy equals 1 rad. **Fortunately, virtually no single diagnostic test produces a substantive risk.** Table 8-3 shows mean and maximal fetal exposure. Only multiple computed tomography scans and fluoroscopies would lead to cumulate

TABLE 8-3 Approximate Fetal Doses from Common Diagnostic Procedures

EXAMINATION	MEAN (mGy)	MAXIMUM (mGy)
Conventional Radiographic Examinations		
Abdomen	1.4	4.2
Chest	<0.01	<0.01
Intravenous urogram	1.7	10
Lumbar spine	1.7	10
Pelvis	1.1	4
Skull	<0.01	<0.01
Thoracic spine	<0.01	<0.01
Fluoroscopic Examinations		
Barium meal (upper gastrointestinal)	1.1	5.8
Barium enema	6.8	24
Computed Tomography		
Abdomen	8.0	49
Chest	0.06	0.96
Head	<0.005	<0.005
Lumbar spine	2.4	8.6
Pelvis	25	79

From Lowe SA: Diagnostic radiography in pregnancy: risks and reality. Aust N Z J Obstet Gynaecol 44:191, 2004.

exposures of 100 mGy or 10 cGy (rad). Internal exposures are 50% less than maternal surface doses.

Female frequent flyers or crew members may be exposed to radiation during frequent long, high-altitude flights. The Federal Aviation Administration recommends limiting exposure to 1 mSv (0.1 cGy) during the pregnancy.[88]

Therapeutic exposures for maternal thyroid ablation with I^{131} are rare but can cause fetal thyroid damage after 12 weeks of pregnancy.

Mutagenesis

Mutagenic effects in the offspring of irradiated women may be manifested years after the birth of the infant. Mutagenic effects presumably explain the 50% increased risk for leukemia in children exposed in utero to radiation during maternal pelvimetry examinations compared with nonirradiated controls. However, clinical consequence is almost nil. The absolute risk is about 1 in 2000 for exposed versus 1 in 3000 for unexposed children.

Lowe[87] estimates one additional cancer death per 1700 10 mGy (1 rad) exposures. If one were to recommend that pregnancies be terminated whenever exposure from diagnostic radiation occurred because of the increased probability of leukemia in the offspring, 1699 exposed pregnancies would have to be terminated to prevent a single case of leukemia. Radiation exposures should be minimized, but fear of radiation should never preclude one from necessary diagnostic procedures. A consent form has been developed for use with pregnant women.[89]

Questions have also been raised about potential risks to children associated with parental (paternal) occupational exposure to low-dose radiation. A case-control study by Gardner and colleagues in the area around the Sellafield Nuclear Facility in the United Kingdom found a statistically significant association between paternal preconception radiation dose and childhood leukemia risk. A similar association had been observed between paternal preconception radiation and risk in workers at the Hanford Nuclear Facility in the United States. The finding regarding childhood leukemia risk is a particularly contentious issue, contradicting studies of the children born to atomic bomb survivors who do not show genetic effects, such as increased risks for childhood cancers. A study in the vicinity of nuclear facilities in Ontario also failed to demonstrate an association between childhood leukemia risk and paternal preconceptional radiation exposure.

Video Display Terminals

Concern about video display terminals linked to adverse reproductive outcomes now seems unwarranted. Early concern grew out of reports of spontaneous abortion clusters among groups of women who used video display terminals at work; some reported clusters included birth defects. Since then, numerous reassuring papers have been published on this topic, along with a number of reviews.[90] **VDT use does not increase the risk for adverse reproductive outcomes.**

Lead

Twenty-five years of public health efforts have produced a striking reduction in lead exposure in the United States. The average blood lead level has decreased to less than 20% of levels measured in the 1970s. However, elevated blood lead (>20 mcg/dL) has a higher incidence among immigrants to Southern California. In Los Angeles, 25 of the 30 cases of elevated blood lead occurred in immigrants.

High lead concentration in maternal blood is associated with an increased risk for delivery of a small-for-gestational-age infant. The frequency of preterm birth was also almost three times higher among women who had umbilical cord levels greater than or equal to 5.1 mcg/dL, compared with those who had levels below that cutoff. One study in Norway found an increased risk for low birthweight and also NTDs.[91]

Lead poisoning has been reported after a pregnant woman ingested Garbhpal ras, an Asian Indian health supplement which contained extremely high levels of lead.[92]

Asking pregnant women about risk factors for lead exposure can aid in assessing prenatal exposure risk. A questionnaire that gathered information on housing conditions, smoking status, and consumption of canned foods had a sensitivity of 89.2% and a negative predictive value of 96.4%.[93] Consumption of calcium and avoidance of the use of lead-glazed ceramics resulted in lowering of blood lead, especially in pregnant women of low socioeconomic status in Mexico City.

Because the nervous system may be more susceptible to the toxic effects during the embryonic and fetal periods than at any other time of life and because maternal and cord blood lead concentrations are directly correlated, lead concentrations in blood should not exceed 25 mcg/dL in women of reproductive age.[94]

Ideally, the maternal blood lead level should be less than 10 mcg/dL to ensure that a child begins life with minimal lead exposure. A dose-response relationship is strongly supported by numerous epidemiologic studies of children showing a reduction in IQ with increasing blood lead concentrations above 10 mcg/dL. Of note, these studies measured blood lead concentrations over time (often 2 years or more) and reported averaged values. **Other neurologic impairments associated with increased blood lead concentrations include attention deficit disorder ("hyperactivity"), hearing deficits, learning disabilities, and shorter stature.** Thus, for public health purposes, childhood lead poisoning has been defined as a blood lead level of 10 mcg/dL or higher.

In occupational settings, federal standards mandate that women should not work in areas where air lead concentrations can reach 50 mcg/cm, because this may result in blood concentrations above 25 to 30 mcg/dL.[95] Subtle but permanent neurologic impairment in children may occur at lower blood lead concentrations.

Mercury

Fish and shellfish are an important part of a healthy diet, but some large fish contain significant amounts of mercury. **Mercury in high levels may harm the unborn baby or young child's developing nervous system.[96]**

Women who may become pregnant, pregnant women, and nursing mothers should avoid shark, swordfish, king mackerel, and tile fish because they contain high levels of

mercury.[97] They may eat up to 12 oz a week of shrimp, canned light tuna, salmon, pollock, and catfish, all of which are very low in mercury. Albacore (white) tuna and tuna steaks have more mercury than canned light tuna, but 6 oz per week is allowed.

THE OBSTETRICIAN'S ROLE IN EVALUATING DRUG AND REPRODUCTIVE RISKS IN AND BEYOND THE WORKPLACE

Clinical questions about adverse reproductive outcomes of potential drug teratogens or environmental or occupational exposures are difficult to answer. Answers are seldom as clearcut as the obstetrician would like. Even if the exposure were known, there is often not a study of similar exposure with a sufficient sample size. Without this, a physician cannot give a reliable estimate of risk.

For drugs and other exposures discussed in this chapter, the threshold is unknown below which no adverse reproductive outcome can be expected. Except for ionizing radiation, maximal recommended exposure levels are difficult to quantify. Epidemiologic studies, when available, often have limitations in design, execution, analysis, or interpretation. Thus, often the questions must be answered on the basis of reasoned judgments in the face of inadequate data.

In addition to traditional genetic referral sources, a variety of teratology information services and computer databases are available to physicians who counsel pregnant women (see Table 8-1). The options include personal computer software (Grateful Med, commercial services) and CD-ROM copies in medical libraries or leased from commercial versions. Information is available from a TOXNET representative, National Library of Medicine, Specialized Information Services, 8600 Rockville Pike, Bethesda, MD 20894, 301-496-6531.

The National Library of Medicine in Bethesda, Maryland, maintains several files on the TOXNET database system, including reproductive and developmental toxicology information in bibliographic or text form. Examples include Developmental and Reproductive Toxicology, GEN-TOX (genetic toxicology), and Environmental Mutagen Information Center. Other very useful sources are Reprotox [http://reprotox.org] and TERIS [depts.washington.edu/%7Eterisweb/teris/index.html].

SUMMARY

Many medical conditions during pregnancy and lactation are best treated initially with nonpharmacologic remedies. Before a drug is administered in pregnancy, the indications should be clear, and the risk-to-benefit ratio should justify drug use. If possible, therapy should be postponed until after the first trimester. In addition, patients should be cautioned about the risks of social drug use such as smoking, alcohol, and cocaine during pregnancy. Most drug therapy does not require cessation of lactation because the amount excreted into breast milk is sufficiently small to be pharmacologically insignificant.

KEY POINTS

- The critical period of organ development extends from day 31 to day 71 after the first day of the last menstrual period.
- Infants of epileptic women taking anticonvulsants have double the rate of malformations of unexposed infants; the risk for fetal hydantoin syndrome is less than 10%.
- The risk for malformations after in utero exposure to isotretinoin is 25%, and an additional 25% of infants have mental retardation.
- Heparin is the drug of choice for anticoagulation during pregnancy except for women with artificial heart valves, who should receive Coumadin despite the 5% risk for warfarin embryopathy.
- Angiotensin-converting enzyme inhibitors and angiotensin receptor blockers can cause fetal renal failure in the second and third trimesters, leading to oligohydramnios and hypoplastic lungs.
- Vitamin B_6, 25 mg three times per day, is a safe and effective therapy for first-trimester nausea and vomiting; doxylamine (Unisom), 12.5 mg three times per day, is also effective in combination with B_6.
- Most antibiotics are generally safe in pregnancy. Trimethoprim may carry an increased risk in the first trimester, and tetracyclines taken in the second and third trimesters may cause tooth discoloration. Aminoglycosides can cause fetal ototoxicity.
- Aspirin in analgesic doses inhibits platelet function and prolongs bleeding time, increasing the risk for peripartum hemorrhage.
- Fetal alcohol syndrome occurs in infants of mothers drinking heavily during pregnancy. A safe level of alcohol intake during pregnancy has not been determined.
- Cocaine has been associated with increased risk for spontaneous abortions, abruptio placentae, and congenital malformations, in particular, microcephaly.
- Most drugs are safe during lactation because subtherapeutic amounts appear in breast milk, about 1% to 2% of the maternal dose.
- Only a small amount of prednisone crosses the placenta, so it is the preferred corticosteroid for most medical illnesses. In contrast, betamethasone and dexamethasone readily cross the placenta and are preferred for acceleration of fetal lung maturity.
- Exposure to high-dose ionizing irradiation during gestation causes microcephaly and mental retardation; however, diagnostic exposures of less than 5 cGy do not pose increased teratogenic risks. Mutagenic effects presumably are responsible for the 50% increased risk for leukemia in children exposed in utero to radiation during maternal pelvimetry; the absolute risk is very low.
- Lead levels in blood have decreased in recent years in all except immigrant populations, making

it easier to achieve blood levels less than 25 mcg/dL in women of reproductive age; this low level minimizes fetal growth restriction.

- Mercury in high levels deleteriously affects the fetal nervous system. For this reason pregnant and nursing women should avoid shark, swordfish, king mackerel, and tile fish; exposures to mercury can further be limited by restricting ingestion of certain other seafood (shrimp, canned tuna, salmon, pollock, catfish) to 12 oz/week.

REFERENCES

1. Wilson JG, Fraser FC: Handbook of Teratology. New York, Plenum, 1979.
2. Teratology Society Public Affairs Committee: FDA Classification of drugs for teratogenic risk. Teratology 49:446, 1994.
3. Wilson JG: Current status of teratology-general principles and mechanisms derived from animal studies. In Wilson JG, Fraser FC: Handbook of Teratology. New York, Plenum, 1977, p 47.
4. Musselman AC, Bennett GD, Greer KA, et al: Preliminary evidence of phenytoin-induced alterations in embryonic gene expression in a mouse model. Reprod Toxicol 8:383, 1994.
5. Lieff S, Olshan AF, Werler M, et al: Selection bias and the use of controls with malformations in case-control studies of birth defects. Epidemiology 10:238, 1999.
6. Lenz W: Thalidomide and congenital abnormalities. Lancet 1:45, 1962.
7. Lammer EJ, Sever LE, Oakley GP Jr: Teratogen update: valproic acid. Teratology 35:465, 1987.
8. MRC Vitamin Study Research Group: Prevention of neural tube defects: results of the Medical Research Council Vitamin Study. Lancet 338:131, 1991.
9. Czeizel AE, Dudas I: Prevention of the first occurrence of neural-tube defects by periconceptional vitamin supplementation. N Engl J Med 327:1832, 1992.
10. Pekarek DM, Chapman VR, Neely CL, et al: Medication effects on midtrimester maternal serum screening. Am J Obstet Gynecol 201:622, e1-e5, 2009.
11. Einarson TR, Koren G, Mattice D, et al: Maternal spermicide use and adverse reproductive outcome: a meta-analysis. Am J Obstet Gynecol 162:665, 1990.
12. Jentink J, Loane MA, Dolk H, et al: Valproic acid monotherapy in pregnancy and major congenital malformations. N Engl J Med 362:2185, 2010.
13. Holmes LB, Harvey EA, Coull BA, et al: The teratogenicity of anticonvulsant drugs. N Engl J Med 344:1132, 2001.
14. Biale Y, Lewenthal H: Effect of folic acid supplementation on congenital malformations due to anticonvulsive drugs. Eur J Obstet Gynecol Reprod Biol 18:211, 1984.
15. Jones KL, Lacro RV, Johnson KA, et al: Pattern of malformations in the children of women treated with carbamazepine during pregnancy. N Engl J Med 320:1661, 1989.
16. Buehler BA, Delimont D, VanWaes M, et al: Prenatal prediction of risk of the fetal hydantoin syndrome. N Engl J Med 322:1567, 1990.
17. Meador KJ, Baker GA, Browning N, et al: Cognitive function at 3 years of age after fetal exposure to antiepileptic drugs. N Engl J Med 360:1597, 2009.
18. GlaxoSmithKline International, Lamotrigine Pregnancy Registry, Interim Report, 1/2005.
19. Lammer EJ, Chen DT, Hoar RM, et al: Retinoic acid embryopathy. N Engl J Med 313:837, 1985.
20. Zalzstein E, Koren G, Einarson T, et al: A case-control study on the association between first trimester exposure to lithium and Ebstein's anomaly. Am J Cardiol 65:817, 1990.
21. Jacobson SJ, Jones K, Johnson K, et al: Prospective multi-centre study of pregnancy outcome after lithium exposure during first trimester. Lancet 339:530, 1992.
22. Way CM: Safety of newer antidepressants in pregnancy. Pharmacotherapy 27:546, 2007.
23. Malm H, Artama M, Gissler M, et al: Selective serotonin reuptake inhibitors and risk for major congenital anomalies. Obstet Gynecol 118:111, 2011.
24. Yonkers KA, Wisner KL, Stewart DE, et al: The management of depression during pregnancy: a report from the American Psychiatric Association and the American College of Obstetricians and Gynecologists. Obstet Gynecol 114:703, 2009.
25. Kallen B, Olaussan PO: Antidepressant drugs during pregnancy and infant congenital heart defect. Reprod Toxicol 21:221, 2006.
26. Zeskind PS, Stephens LE: Maternal selective serotonin reuptake inhibitor use during pregnancy and newborn neurobehavior. Pediatrics 113:368, 2004.
27. Chambers CD, Hernandez-Diaz S, Von Marter LJ, et al: Selective serotonin-reuptake inhibitors and risk of persistent pulmonary hypertension of the newborn. N Engl J Med 354:579, 2006.
28. Wilson KL, Zelig CM, Harvey JP, et al: Persistent pulmonary hypertension of the newborn is associated with mode of delivery and not with maternal use of selective serotonin reuptake inhibitors. Am J Perinatol 28:19, 2011.
29. Chun-Fai-Chan B, Koren G, Fayez I, et al: Pregnancy outcome of women exposed to bupropion during pregnancy: a prospective comparative study. Am J Obstet Gynecol 192:932, 2005.
30. Cohen LS, Altshuler LL, Harlow BL, et al: Relapse of major depression during pregnancy in women who maintain or discontinue antidepressant treatment. JAMA 295:499, 2006.
31. Sbarouni E, Oakley CM: Outcome of pregnancy in women with valve prostheses. Br Heart J 71:196, 1994.
32. Dahlman TC: Osteoporotic fractures and the recurrence of thromboembolism during pregnancy and the puerperium in 184 women undergoing thromboprophylaxis with heparin. Am J Obstet Gynecol 168:1265, 1993.
33. Vitale N, De Feo M, De Santo LS, et al: Dose-dependent fetal complications of warfarin in pregnant women with mechanical heart valves. J Am Coll Cardiol 33:1637, 1999.
34. Cooper DS: Antithyroid drugs. N Engl J Med 352:905, 2005.
35. Cooper DS, Rivkees SA: Putting propylthiouracil in perspective. J Clin Endocrinol Metab 94:1881, 2009.
36. Alexander EK, Marqusee E, Lawrence J, et al: Timing and magnitude of increases in levothyroxine requirements during pregnancy in women with hypothyroidism. N Engl J Med 351:241, 2004.
37. Casey BM, Dashe JS, Wells CE, et al: Subclinical hypothyroidism and pregnancy outcomes. Obstet Gynecol 105:239, 2005.
38. Pruyn SC, Phelan JP, Buchanan GC: Long-term propranolol therapy in pregnancy: maternal and fetal outcome. Am J Obstet Gynecol 135:485, 1979.
39. Hanssens M, Keirse MJNC, Vankelecom F, et al: Fetal and neonatal effects of treatment with angiotensin-converting enzyme inhibitors in pregnancy. Obstet Gynecol 78:128, 1991.
40. Velinov M, Zellers N: The fetal mycophenolate mofetil syndrome. Clin Dysmorphol 17:77, 2008.
41. Wolfe MS, Cordero JF: Safety of chloroquine in chemosuppression of malaria during pregnancy. Br Med J 290:1466, 1985.
42. Hart CW, Naunton RF: The ototoxicity of chloroquine phosphate. Arch Otolaryngol 80:407, 1964.
43. Park-Wyllie L, Mazzotta P, Pastuszak A, et al: Birth defects after maternal exposure to corticosteroids: Prospective cohort study and meta-analysis of epidemiological studies. Teratology 62:385, 2000.
44. Niebyl JR: Nausea and vomiting in pregnancy. N Engl J Med 363:1544, 2010.
45. Koren G, Clark S, Hankins GD, et al: Effectiveness of delayed-release doxylamine and pyridoxine for nausea and vomiting of pregnancy: a randomized placebo controlled trial. Am J Obstet Gynecol 203:571, e1-e7, 2010.
46. Matok I, Gorodischer R, Koren G, et al: The safety of metoclopramide use in the first trimester of pregnancy. N Engl J Med 360:2528, 2009.
47. Sullivan CA, Johnson CA, Roach H, et al: A pilot study of intravenous ondansetron for hyperemesis gravidarum. Am J Obstet Gynecol 174:2565, 1996.
48. Safari HR, Fassett MJ, Souter IC, et al: The efficacy of methylprednisolone in the treatment of hyperemesis gravidarum: a randomized, double-blind, controlled study. Am J Obstet Gynecol 179:921, 1998.
49. Ruigomez A, Garcia Rodriguez LA, Cattaruzzi C, et al: Use of cimetidine, omeprazole, and ranitidine in pregnant women and pregnancy outcomes. Am J Epidemiol 150:476, 1999.

50. Pasternak B, Hviid A: Use of proton pump inhibitors in early pregnancy and the risk of birth defects. N Engl J Med 363:2114, 2010.
51. Kenyon S, Boulvain M, Neilson J: Antibiotics for preterm rupture of the membranes: a systematic review. Obstet Gynecol 104:1051, 2004.
52. Kenyon SL, Taylor DJ, Tarnow-Mordi W: Broad-spectrum antibiotics for preterm, prelabour rupture of fetal membranes: the ORICLE I randomized trial. ORACLE Collaborative Group. Lancet 357:979, 2001.
53. Harris RC, Lucey JF, MacLean JR: Kernicterus in premature infants associated with low concentration of bilirubin in the plasma. Pediatrics 23:878, 1950.
54. Hernandez-Diaz S, Werler MM, Walker AM, et al: Folic acid antagonists during pregnancy and the risk of birth defects. N Engl J Med 343:1608, 2000.
55. Cohlan SQU, Bevelander G, Tiamsic T: Growth inhibition of prematures receiving tetracycline. Am J Dis Child 105:453, 1963.
56. Burtin P, Taddio A, Ariburnu O, et al: Safety of metronidazole in pregnancy: a meta-analysis. Am J Obstet Gynecol 172:525, 1995.
57. Stone KM, Reiff-Eldridge R, White AD, et al: Pregnancy outcomes following systemic prenatal acyclovir exposure: conclusions from the international acyclovir pregnancy registry, 1984-1999. Birth Defects Res Part A. Clin Mol Teratol 70:201, 2004.
58. Pasternak B, Hviid A: Use of acyclovir, valacyclovir and famciclovir in the first trimester of pregnancy and the risk of birth defects. JAMA 304:859, 2010.
59. Perinatal HIV Guidelines Working Group: Public Health Service Task Force. Recommendations for use of antiretroviral drugs in pregnant HIV-1-infected women for maternal health and interventions to reduce perinatal HIV-1 transmission in the United States. June 23, 2004, Available from AIDS info website: http://AIDSinfo.nih.gov.
60. Mastroiacovo P, Mazzone T, Botto LD, et al: Prospective assessment of pregnancy outcomes after first-trimester exposure to fluconazole. Am J Obstet Gynecol 175:1645, 1996.
61. Feldkamp M, Meyer RE, Krikov S, et al: Acetaminophen use in pregnancy and risk of birth defects: findings from the National Birth Defects Prevention Study. Obstet Gynecol 115:109, 2010.
62. Cunnington M, Ephross S, Churcill P: The safety of sumatriptan and naratriptan in pregnancy: what have we learned? Headache 49:1414, 2009.
63. Loder E: Triptan therapy in migraine. N Engl J Med 363:63, 2010.
64. Shah NR, Bracken MB: A systematic review and meta-analysis of prospective studies on the association between interval cigarette smoking and preterm delivery. Am J Obstet Gynecol 182:465, 2000.
65. Alberman E, Creasy M, Elliott M, et al: Maternal factors associated with fetal chromosomal anomalies in spontaneous abortions. J Obstet Gynecol 83:621, 1976.
66. American College of Obstetricians and Gynecologists: ACOG Committee Opinion: smoking cessation during pregnancy. Obstet Gynecol 116:1241, 2010.
67. Acker D, Sachs BP, Tracey KJ, et al: Abruptio placentae associated with cocaine use. Am J Obstet Gynecol 146:220, 1983.
68. Volpe JJ: Effect of cocaine use on the fetus. N Engl J Med 327:399, 1992.
69. Brown HL, Britton KA, Mahaffey D, et al: Methadone maintenance in pregnancy: a reappraisal. Am J Obstet Gynecol 179:459, 1998.
70. Linn S, Schoenbaum SC, Monson RR, et al: No association between coffee consumption and adverse outcomes of pregnancy. N Engl J Med 306:141, 1982.
71. Martin TR, Bracken MB: The association between low birth weight and caffeine consumption during pregnancy. Am J Epidemiol 126:813, 1987.
72. Mills JL, Holmes LB, Aarons JH, et al: Moderate caffeine use and the risk of spontaneous abortion and intrauterine growth retardation. JAMA 269:593, 1993.
73. American College of Obstetricians and Gynecologists: ACOG Committee Opinion: moderate caffeine consumption during pregnancy. Obstet Gynecol 116:467, 2010.
74. Sturtevant FM: Use of aspartame in pregnancy. Int J Fertil 30:85, 1985.
75. Wilson JT, Brown RD, Cherek DR, et al: Drug excretion in human breast milk: principles of pharmacokinetics and projected consequences. Clin Pharmacokinet 5:1, 1980.
76. Ito S, Blajchman A, Stephenson M, et al: Prospective follow-up of adverse reactions in breast-fed infants exposed to maternal medication. Am J Obstet Gynecol 168:1393, 1993.
77. American Academy of Pediatrics Committee on Drugs: the transfer of drugs and other chemicals into human milk. Pediatrics 108:776, 2001.
78. Nulman I, Koren G: The safety of fluoxetine during pregnancy and lactation. Teratology 53:304, 1996.
79. Epperson CN, Anderson GM, McDougle CJ: Sertraline and breastfeeding. N Engl J Med 336:1189, 1997.
80. Orme ME, Lewis PJ, deSwiet M, et al: May mothers given warfarin breastfeed their infants? Br Med J 1:1564, 1977.
81. deSwiet M, Lewis PJ: Excretion of anticoagulants in human milk. N Engl J Med 297:1471, 1977.
82. Berlin CM Jr, Yaffe SJ: Disposition of salicylazosulfapyridine (Azulfidine) and metabolites in human breast milk. Dev Pharmacol Ther 1:31, 1980.
83. Little RE, Anderson KW, Ervin CH, et al: Maternal alcohol use during breastfeeding and infant mental and motor development at one year. N Engl J Med 321:425, 1989.
84. Mennella JA, Beauchamp GK: The transfer of alcohol to human milk: effects on flavor and the infant's behavior. N Engl J Med 325:981, 1991.
85. Ryu JE: Effect of maternal caffeine consumption on heart rate and sleep time of breast-fed infants. Dev Pharmacol Ther 8:355, 1985.
86. Dekaban AS: Abnormalities in children exposed to x-radiation during various stages of gestation: tentative timetable of radiation injury to the human fetus. J Nucl Med 9:471, 1968.
87. Lowe SA: Diagnostic radiography in pregnancy: risks and reality. Aust N Z J Obstet Gynaecol 44:191, 2004.
88. Barish RJ: In-flight radiation exposure during pregnancy. Obstet Gynecol 103:1326, 2004.
89. El-Khoury GY, Madsen MT, Blake ME, et al: A new pregnancy policy for a new era. Am J Roentgenol 181:335, 2003.
90. Blackwell R, Chang A: Video display terminals and pregnancy: a review. Br J Obstet Gynaecol 95:446, 1988.
91. Irgens A, Kruger K, Skorve AH, et al: Reproductive outcome in offspring of parents occupationally exposed to lead in Norway. Am J Ind Med 34:431, 1998.
92. Shamshirsaz AA, Yankowitz J, Rijhsinghani A, et al: Severe lead poisoning caused by use of health supplements presenting as acute abdominal pain during pregnancy. Obstet Gynecol 114:448, 2009.
93. Stefanak MA, Bourguet CC, Benzies-Styka T: Use of the Centers for Disease Control and Prevention childhood lead poisoning risk questionnaire to predict blood lead elevations in pregnant women. Obstet Gynecol 87:209, 1996.
94. Centers for Disease Control: Preventing lead poisoning in young children. Atlanta, Department of Health and Human Services. Atlanta, Public Health Service, Centers for Disease Control, 1991, p 7.
95. Needleman HL, Schell A, Bellinger D, et al: The long-term effects of exposure to low doses of lead in childhood: an 11-year follow-up report. N Engl J Med 322:83, 1990.
96. Harada M: Congenital Minamata disease: intrauterine methylmercury poisoning. Teratology 18:285, 1978.
97. Food and Drug Administration and the U.S. Environmental Protection Agency: What you need to know about mercury in fish and shellfish. Available at: www.epa.gov/fishadvisories/advice/factsheet.html. Accessed December 7, 2009.

For full reference list, log onto www.expertconsult.com.

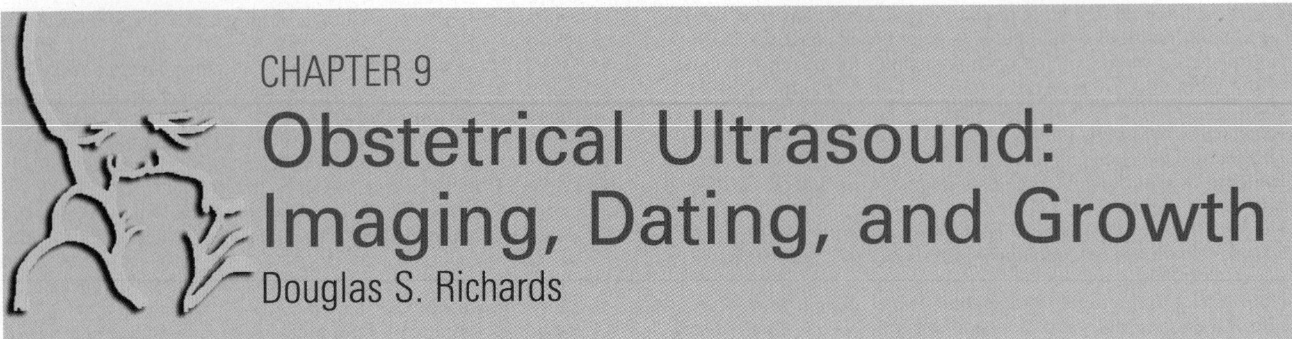

CHAPTER 9

Obstetrical Ultrasound: Imaging, Dating, and Growth

Douglas S. Richards

KEY ABBREVIATIONS	
Abdominal Circumference	AC
American College of Obstetricians and Gynecologists	ACOG
Amniotic Fluid Index	AFI
American Institute of Ultrasound in Medicine	AIUM
As Low as Reasonably Achievable	ALARA
Biparietal Diameter	BPD
Crown-Rump Length	CRL
Estimated Fetal Weight	EFW
Expected Date of Confinement	EDC
Femur Length	FL
Food and Drug Administration	FDA
Head Circumference	HC
Intrauterine Growth Restriction	IUGR
Kilohertz, 1000 Cycles Per Second	KHz
Last Menstrual Period	LMP
Megahertz, 1,000,000 Cycles Per Second	MHz
Spatial-Peak Temporal-Average	SPTA
Thermal Index for Bone	TIb
Thermal Index for Soft Tissues	TIs
Three Dimensional	3-D
Time-Gain Compensation	TGC

Over the past several decades, the clinical use of ultrasound imaging in obstetrics has expanded remarkably. It is now considered by many to be the most valuable diagnostic tool in the field. Ultrasound was first used clinically in pregnancy in the early 1960s to measure the biparietal diameter—the distance between spikes on an oscilloscope screen. Since then, the technology has progressed to the point that even relatively inexpensive ultrasound machines yield detailed real-time images of the fetus. This chapter addresses general aspects of ultrasound use in pregnancy. More detailed discussions of the use of ultrasound to evaluate specific pregnancy problems, such as multiple gestation, third-trimester bleeding, and incompetent cervix, are covered in other chapters.

BIOPHYSICS OF ULTRASOUND

The underlying basis of ultrasound image production is the piezoelectric effect. When electrical impulses are applied to certain ceramic crystals, mechanical oscillations are induced. Conversely, induced vibrations of piezoelectric crystals generate a detectable electric current. In diagnostic ultrasound applications, the ultrasound machine sends an electric signal of the desired frequency to piezoelectric crystals embedded in the ultrasound probe. When the probe is placed in contact with a patient's skin, the skin and underlying tissues begin to vibrate, generating a sound or pressure wave. As this pulse of energy encounters an interface between materials of different impedance, a small amount of the energy is reflected as an echo. The pulses returning to the patient's skin cause the crystals in the probe to vibrate, generating an electric current that is passed back to the ultrasound machine. The pulses of energy that are emitted are very brief—about 1 microsecond. The number of pressure peaks produced in 1 second is the frequency of the sound waves. Ultrasound machines used in obstetrics operate at frequencies of between about 2 and 9 MHz. Sound frequencies above 20 KHz cannot be detected by the human ear, hence the term *ultrasound.*

Between each emitted sound pulse, the probe "listens" for an echo. Because of this alternating send-receive function, the piezoelectric crystal serves as both the transmitter and receiver of the ultrasonic waves.

To produce an image, the ultrasound machine needs to sense the intensity and the time elapsed from send to receive of returning echoes. Highly reflective tissues (e.g., bone) generate relatively more intense echoes. The deeper an object lies, the longer it will take for the return echo to be registered. Because the velocity of sound in tissues is known, the return time can be used to calculate the distance of the object from the transducer. Intensity and depth characteristics are registered in the machine's computer memory, and this information is then used by the computer to activate pixels on the monitor with the appropriate location and intensity.

Modern ultrasound transducers used in obstetrics have a curved face, within which are embedded a row of crystals. The linear arrangement of the crystals on the transducer allows the mechanical oscillations generated by each crystal to be combined into to a wedge-shaped beam. The shape of the transducer face and the resultant beam is depicted on the ultrasound monitor display. In older machines, an unwieldy flat-faced transducer was used to mount this linear array of crystals, but the curved face of current transducers provides a more convenient "footprint" for optimal contact with the patient's skin across the entire transducer. With endovaginal probes, the crystals are mounted on a smaller surface with a tighter curvature. This is apparent on the display as well.

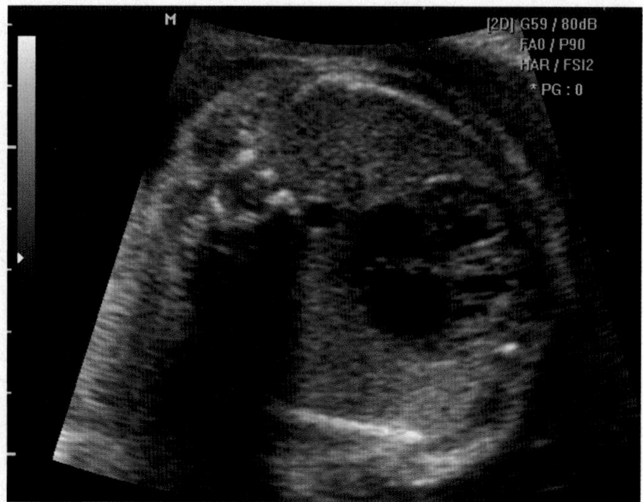

FIGURE 9-1. Transverse four-chamber view of the fetal heart showing appropriate gain settings. The image has a uniform brightness from top to bottom and is neither too light nor too dark.

OPTIMIZING THE ULTRASOUND IMAGE

Power

Ultrasound machines have the capability of delivering varying amounts of voltage to the transducer elements. Increasing the power output increases the amplitude of energy waves in the ultrasound beam and results in stronger returning echoes. This can be advantageous in that it can improve the signal-to-noise ratio and improve imaging capabilities. However, energy is required to create oscillations in the molecules of insonated tissues. Because this energy is absorbed into the tissues, delivering an unnecessarily high energy dose raises safety concerns. The safety of diagnostic ultrasound will be discussed later in this chapter. Suffice it to say that it is good practice to operate at as low power as is consistent with adequate ultrasound penetration. Current ultrasound machines have a preset power level that is sufficient for most situations, and a higher power setting is usually not needed.

Gain

Signals from the weak echoes returning to the transducer elements must be amplified before being used for display. This amplification process is referred to as *gain*. Because of attenuation, echoes returning from deeper within the body have a lower intensity, and the machine must boost the amplification from these echoes. This built-in processing feature is known as *time-gain compensation* (TGC), meaning that echoes with a greater time delay automatically have greater amplification. The amount of amplification, or gain, can be controlled by the sonographer in two ways. Machines come with a gain control knob that adjusts the overall gain up or down. The brightness level of the image can be changed to optimize visualization of anatomic details. When an image is too bright or too dark, much diagnostic information is lost (Figures 9-1 and 9-2). Because tissue characteristics vary from patient to patient, penetration of sound waves at different depths may vary, so the gain at different depths may be adjusted. This is done using the TGC controls—a set of sliders on the instrument control panel (Figures 9-3 and 9-4). A uniform scale across the brightness values should be sought.

Attenuation

Attenuation of ultrasound waves is affected by the medium through which the sound waves pass. Virtually no pulses pass through gas. This is why there must be a coupling agent applied between the transducer face and the patient's skin. For several reasons, ultrasound waves lose intensity as they pass through tissues. The pressure waves gradually diverge from the central beam, they are scattered by reflection from small structures within the tissue, and part of the sound energy is absorbed within tissues. Some tissues, such as bone, strongly attenuate sound waves. The thicker the tissues through which sound waves must pass before arriving at the target, the more the attenuation, and the greater the difficultly in retrieving good information from the echoes. Because of attenuation, obstetrical ultrasound imaging is greatly affected by patient obesity. In patients with a thick, dense abdominal wall, image quality is greatly reduced. In such patients, attention to equipment controls and scanning technique is essential.

Focus

As stated, a linear array transducer makes an ultrasound beam by firing a row of crystals placed along the surface of the probe. When adjacent crystals fire, the pressure waves reinforce one another by a process called *constructive*

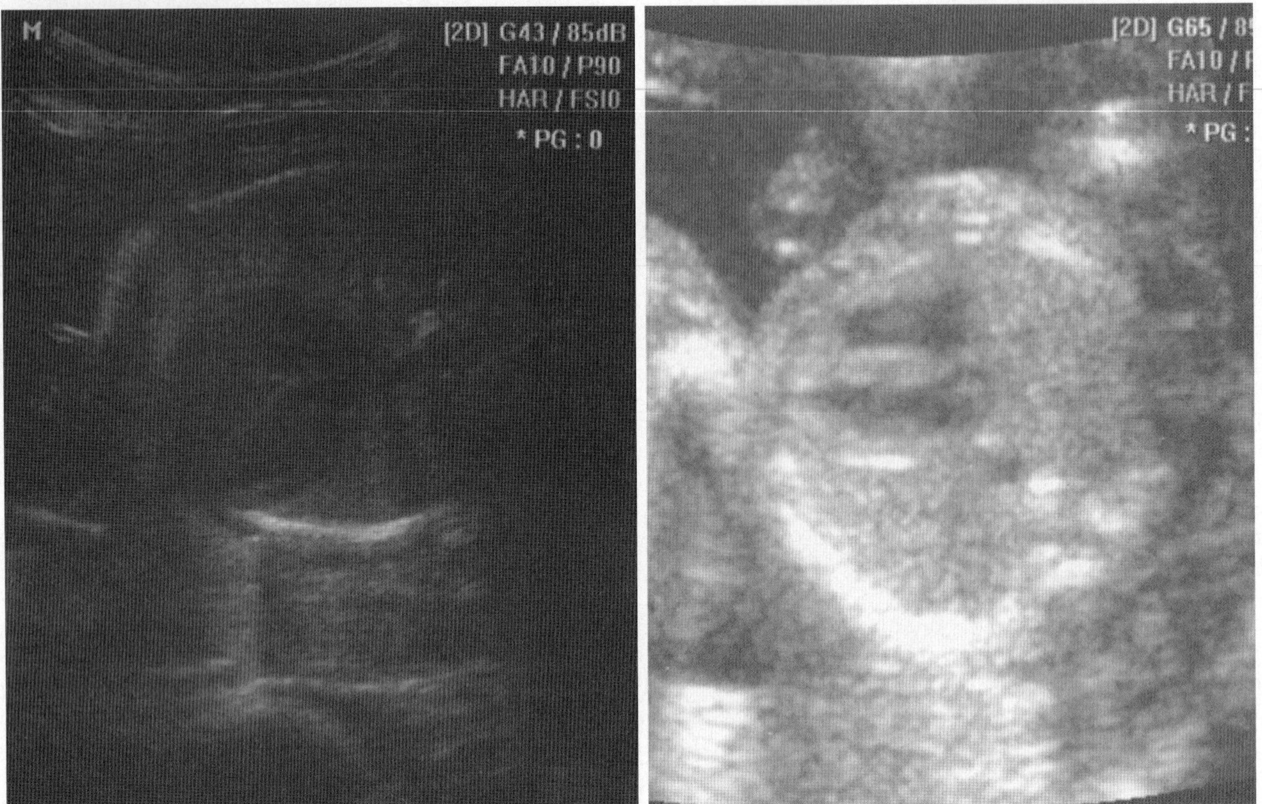

FIGURE 9-2. In the image on the left, the overall gain is too low, yielding a dark image. The image on the right has too much gain. In both cases, diagnostic detail is lost.

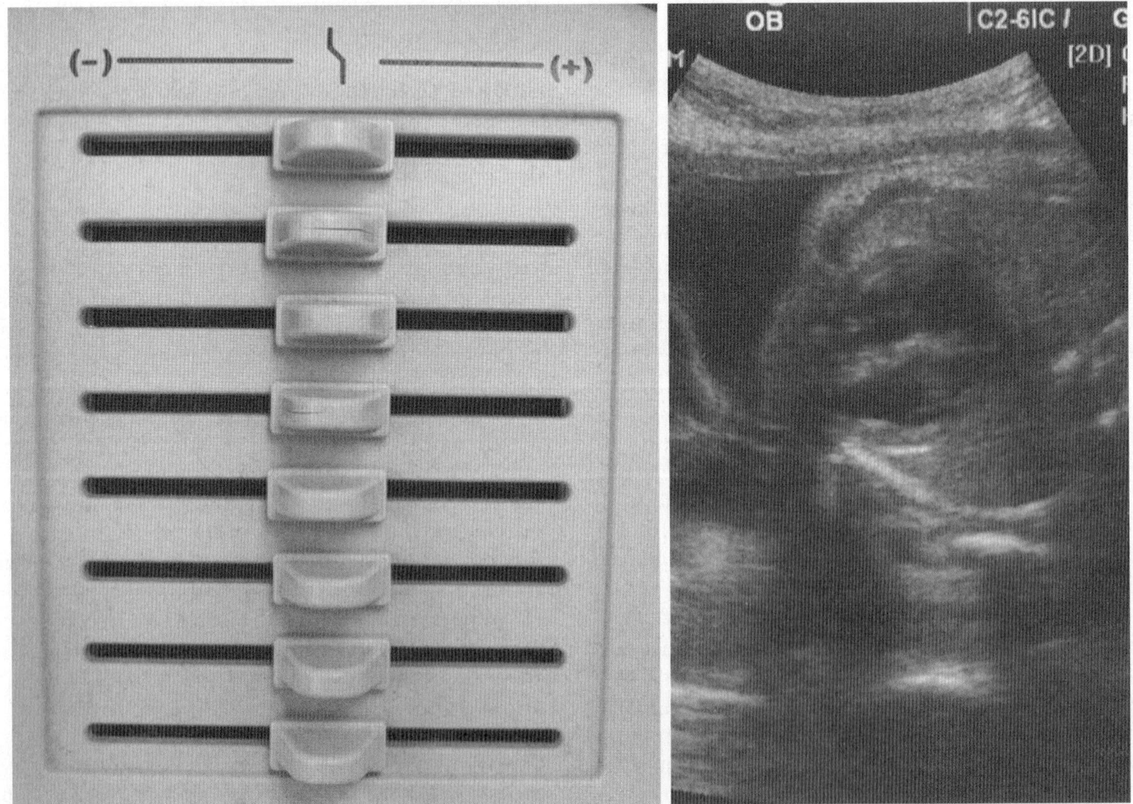

FIGURE 9-3. The photograph on the left shows the slide bars comprising the time-gain compensation controls. In this case, the fact they are lined up in the center indicates that no adjustment for different depths was needed.

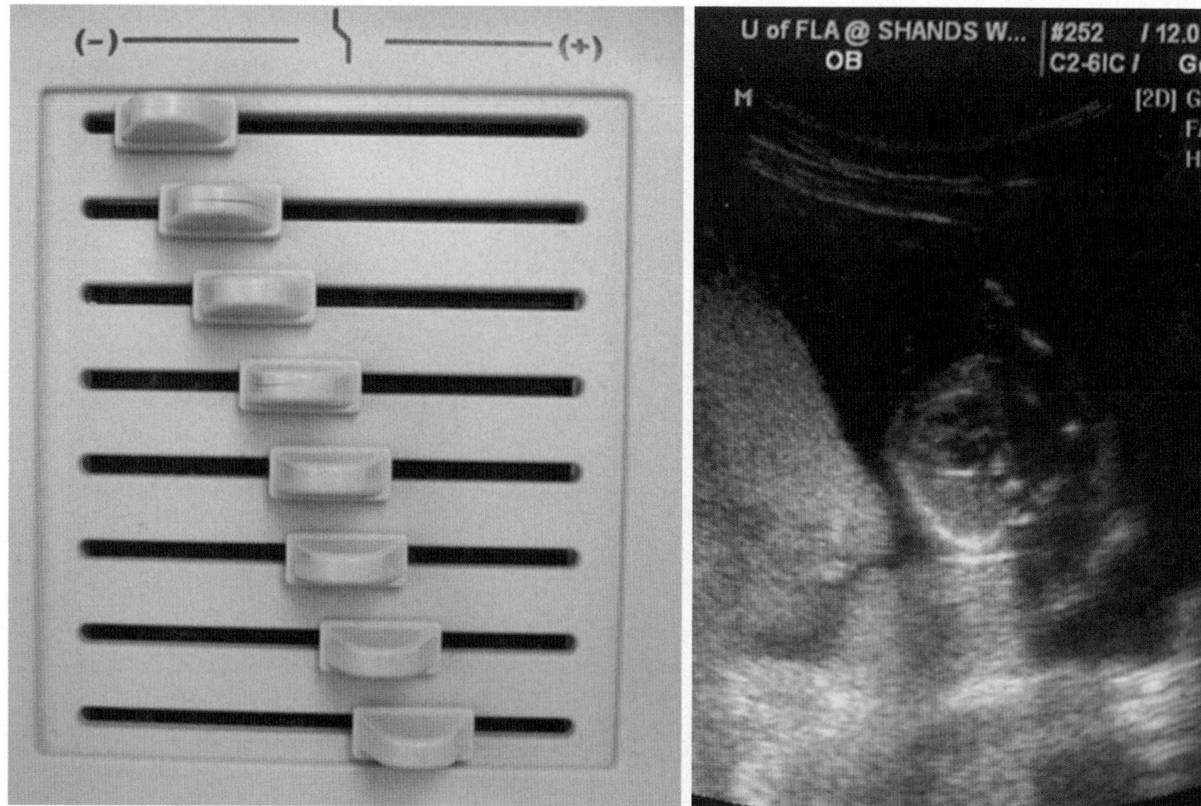

FIGURE 9-4. Incorrect time-gain compensation settings. The slide bars are inappropriately shifted to the left in the near field, making the corresponding area of the image too dark.

interference. This phenomenon creates the central ultrasound beam that extends out from the probe. Electronic control of the timing and order that crystals are activated can work to focus this beam at a certain depth within the tissues. Image resolution is optimal when the structure of interest lies within this zone of optimal focus (Figure 9-5). Using the focus control on the machine console, the user can adjust the depth of this zone for best focus. Many machines allow the operator to set multiple focal zones. With this setting, the computer successively focuses at different depths. It then stores echo information from each zone in turn while filtering echoes from outside the zone, finally displaying the collated information. This can improve clarity over a wider depth range, but at the cost of higher sound exposure, and, more importantly, an appreciably slower frame rate. The focal depths are indicated by small triangles or arrows at the edge of the screen (Figure 9-6). Many sonographers fail to note and adjust the focal depth—an oversight that significantly decreases the quality of images.

Depth and Zoom

Structures of interest vary in depth from the skin surface. When scanning, you should strive to demonstrate important structures without filling the screen with irrelevant material. Extraneous structures at the bottom of the image can be deleted by simply adjusting the depth of insonation. The zoom control is a little more sophisticated because it magnifies a box within the image rather than just removing information from the bottom of the image (Figures 9-7 and 9-8).

Proper depth and zoom are important for several reasons. First, eliminating unnecessary clutter draws the sonographer's attention to important detail within the scanned area. It also makes pertinent detail stand out in the stored images. Decreasing the size of the scanned area allows a higher frame rate and resolution.

Harmonic Imaging

Many high-quality ultrasound machines now have a feature that is called *tissue harmonic imaging.* With this modality, a standard frequency (e.g., 3 MHz) is transmitted and propagated in the usual manner. Because a relatively low frequency wave is emitted, good penetration is preserved. However, in the receive part of the cycle, the ultrasound machine listens for the reflection of the first harmonic wave (e.g., 6 MHz). This higher frequency wave only has to travel one direction; thus, some of the resolution benefit of high-frequency scanning is retained. This process also reduces noise in the image by removing various forms of artifact, making cystic structures appear free of echoes (Figure 9-9). Harmonic imaging often significantly improves image quality and should be used liberally when it is available.

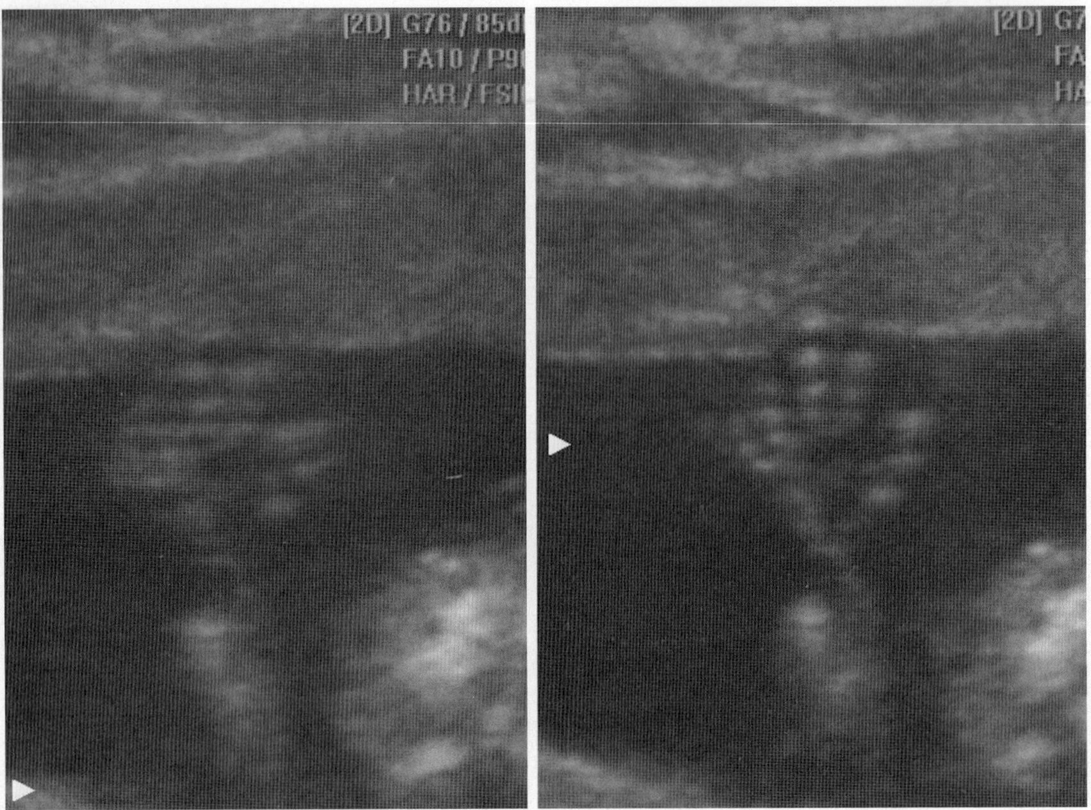

FIGURE 9-5. In the image on the left, the focus was set too low (indicated by the *triangle* on the left), whereas it is at the appropriate level in the image on the right.

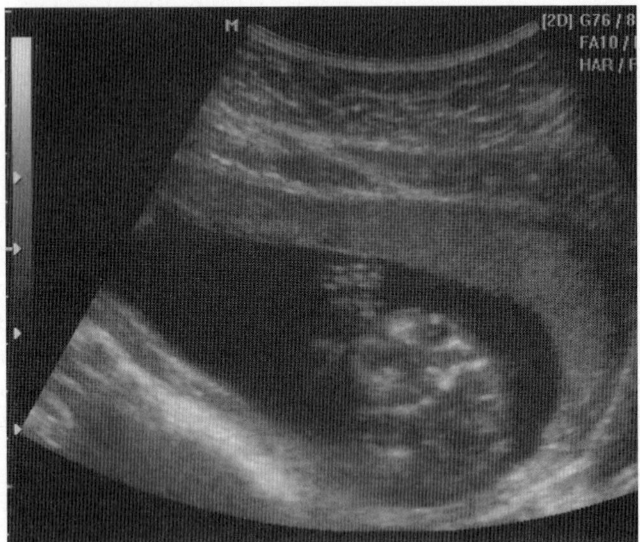

FIGURE 9-6. For this illustration, four focal zones were selected (*triangles* on the left of the image). This setting slowed the frame rate from 35 frames per second with one focal zone to a very noticeable 9 frames per second.

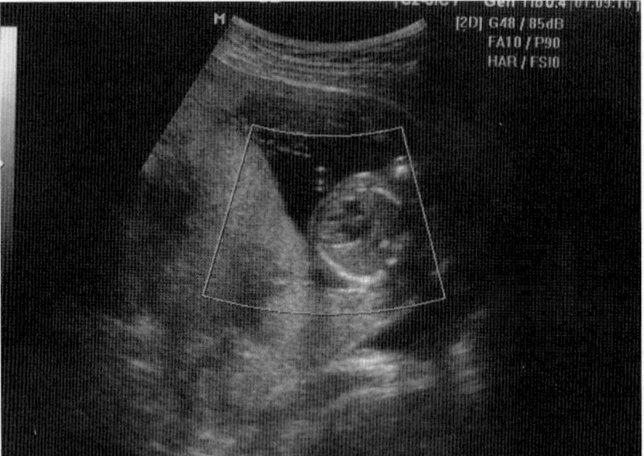

FIGURE 9-7. Ultrasound image before zoom is applied. The area within the box will be expanded to fill the entire screen.

SPECIAL ULTRASOUND MODALIES

M-Mode

For most obstetrical applications, the familiar two-dimensional (2-D) gray-scale real-time ultrasound is used. This is formally known as B-mode ultrasound. Another ultrasound modality that is available on most machines is referred to as *M-mode* (meaning "motion mode"). M-mode ultrasound shows changes along a single ultrasound beam over time. The depth of the echo-producing structures is shown on the y-axis, and time is shown on the x-axis. It is useful for documenting the presence of fetal cardiac activity (Figure 9-10) and can be valuable for specialized echocardiography applications.

Color and Pulse-Wave Doppler

Over the past 15 years, Doppler ultrasound imaging has assumed a key role in obstetrics. With this modality, the ultrasound machine detects shifts in the frequency of echoes returning from a specific location in the image. This frequency shift—the Doppler shift—is caused by motion of the insonated material toward or away from the transducer. Doppler ultrasound is primarily used to demonstrate the presence, direction, and velocity of blood flow.

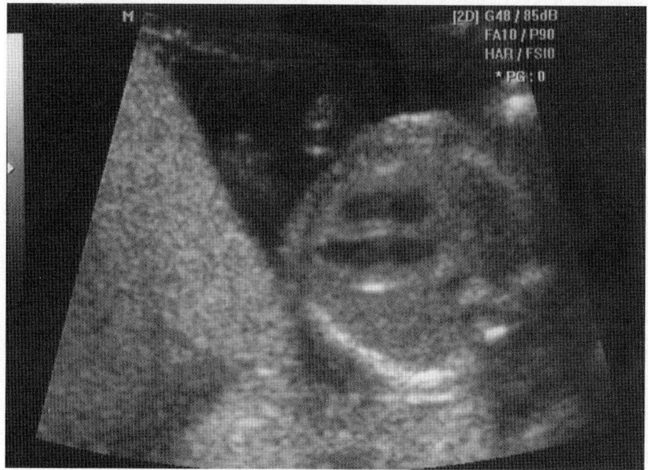

FIGURE 9-8. Appearance after zoom is applied. Compared with Figure 9-7, the cardiac structures are more easily seen. Additionally, because a smaller area is being scanned, the frame rate increased from 25 to 58 frames per second.

The machine displays moving blood as color superimposed on the 2-D gray-scale image. By convention, flow toward the ultrasound transducer is displayed in red and flow away in blue. Pulse-wave Doppler measures the relative velocity of flow within a designated gate inside a vessel. For most obstetrical applications, absolute blood flow velocity is not required. Rather, pulse-wave Doppler is used to generate a waveform showing relative flow velocity over a cardiac cycle. These flow velocity waveforms are primarily used to assess downstream resistance in the vessel being interrogated. This technique has many uses in obstetrics—most importantly as a way to assess placental function. This is done by interrogating the flow within the umbilical artery (Figure 9-11). For some applications, such as fetal echocardiography, the absolute velocity is measured. To do this, the angle of insonation must be very nearly in line with the direction of blood flow. In screening for fetal anemia, the absolute velocity of flow in the middle cerebral artery of the fetus is measured with pulse-wave Doppler ultrasound. To give meaningful results, it is absolutely essential that the Doppler angle (theta) is zero (Figure 9-12).

Three-Dimensional Ultrasound

High-performance computers have allowed the development of ultrasound machines and probes that can acquire, process, and display a three-dimensional (3-D) volume, as opposed to the single plane that is displayed with 2-D ultrasound. To obtain this volume, the transducer uses an internal mechanical sweep mechanism that summates contiguous 2-D planes. This volume data can either be stored

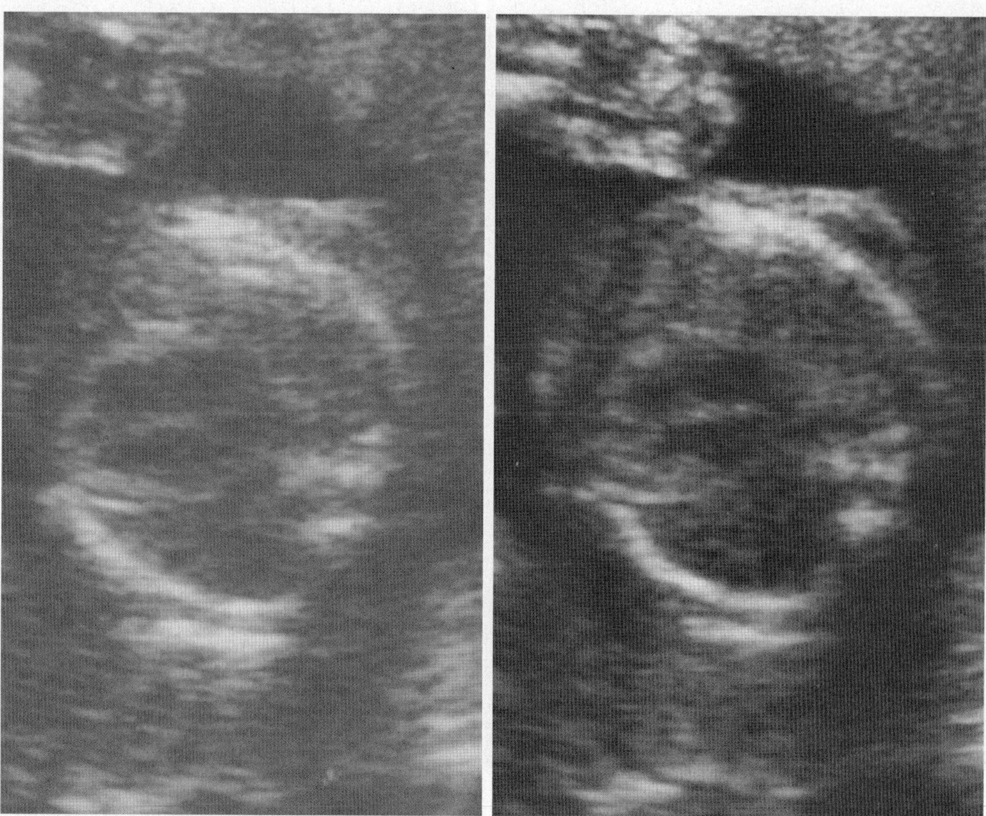

FIGURE 9-9. These figures show the difference that harmonic imaging can have in an obese patient.

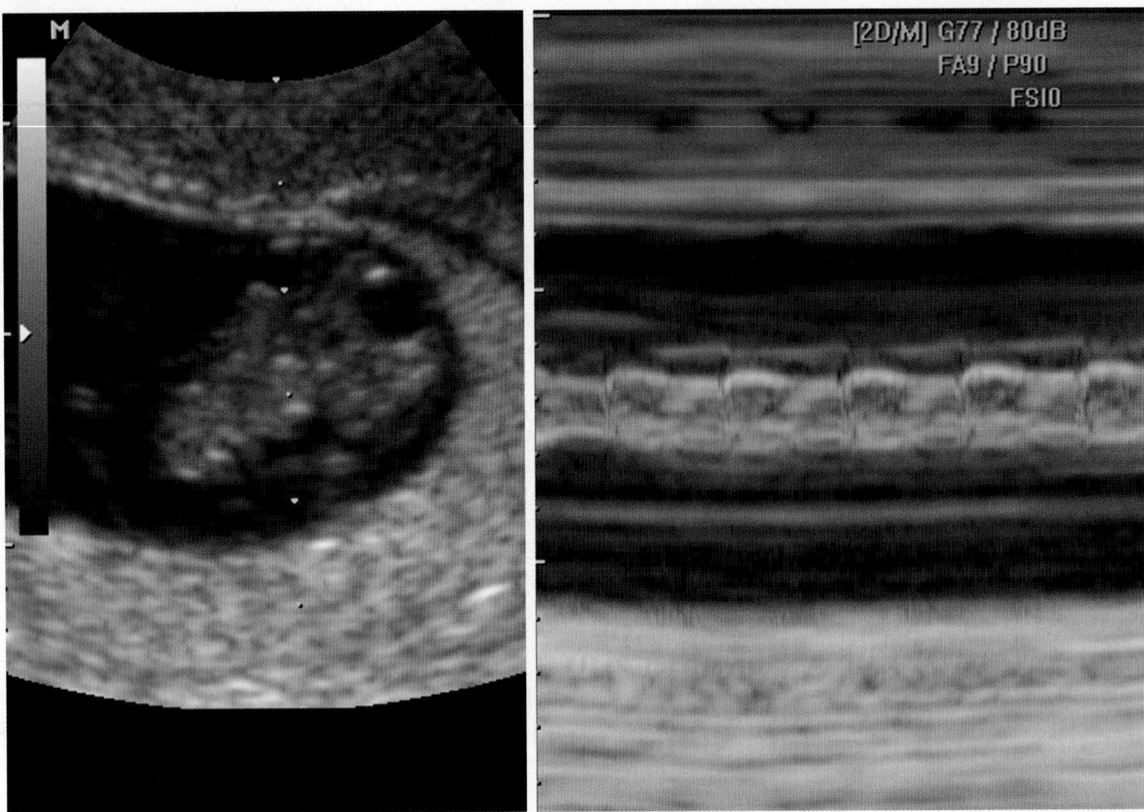

FIGURE 9-10. M-mode application in an 8-week fetus. The *row of dots* in the left panel indicates the line of information (in this case cardiac pulsations) that is being displayed over time in the right panel. Note the prominent brain vesicle in the fetal head.

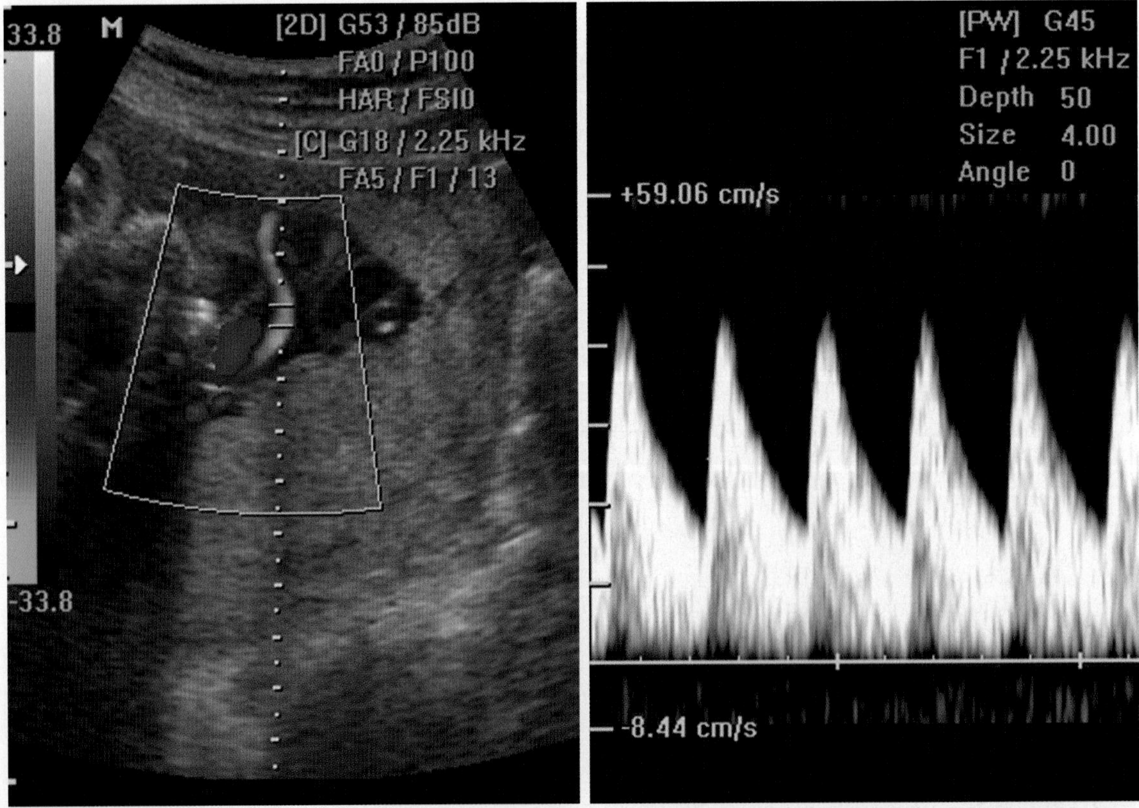

FIGURE 9-11. Color and spectral Doppler evaluation of the umbilical artery. In the left panel, the coiling arteries and vein are shown. Red indicates flow toward the transducer and blue is flow away. The sample gate for the pulse Doppler is superimposed. On the right is the result of the pulse Doppler, depicting a normal flow velocity waveform.

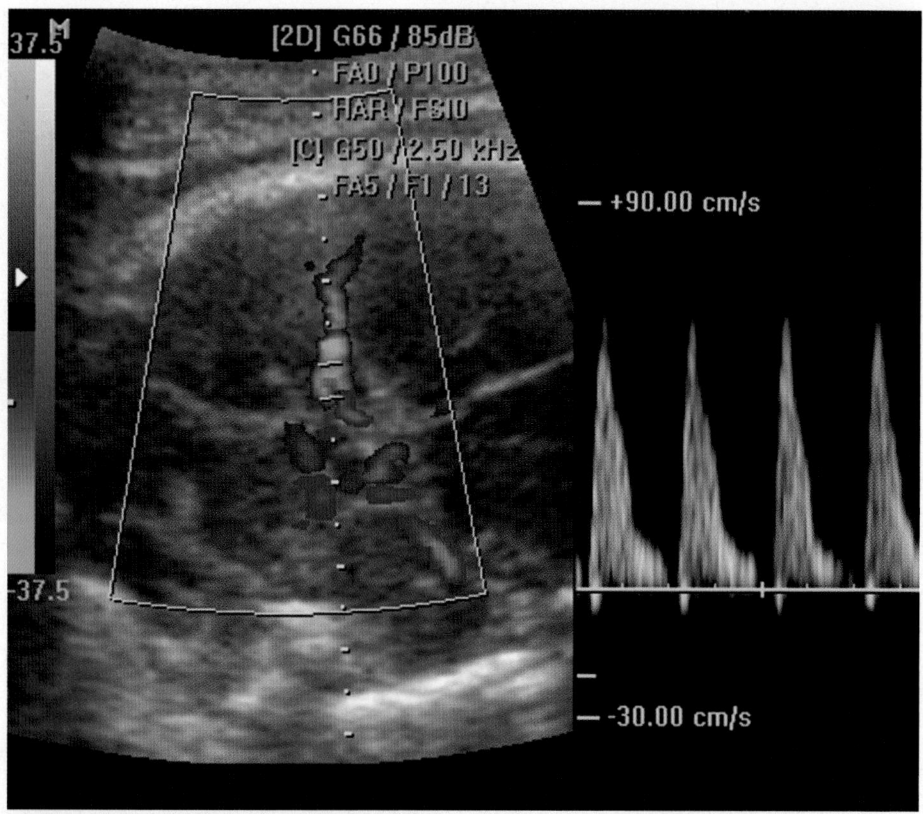

FIGURE 9-12. Color and spectral Doppler interrogation of the middle cerebral artery. Abnormally high peak velocity is an indicator of moderate to severe fetal anemia. Because the actual velocity is being measured, the angle of insonation has to line up with the vessel.

for analysis or updated and displayed on a continuous basis. Adding a real-time updating of a rendered image is commonly referred to as four-dimensional ultrasound.

Three-dimensional ultrasound may be useful for diagnosing certain birth defects. Information from an acquired volume may be processed in such a way that the fetal surface is displayed in a lifelike manner. Surface abnormalities, such as facial cleft, can be well demonstrated with this approach.[1] In addition to being a possible aid in the diagnosis of these and other abnormalities that distort the surface of the fetus, 3-D images may be more readily understood by patients and other professionals who will participate in care of the baby. Software in 3-D ultrasound machines can be used to manipulate stored volume data off-line to show any desired plane through the scanned area. Some of these planes may be very difficult to obtain with standard 2-D imaging. For example, manipulating the 3-D ultrasound volume data can generate an ideal plane for measuring the first-trimester nuchal translucency or for visualizing the nasal bone.[2] Despite these demonstrated capabilities of 3-D ultrasound, there is no proof of an advantage of this technology over standard 2-D imaging for prenatal diagnosis. A 2009 American College of Obstetricians and Gynecologists (ACOG) practice bulletin states that **"three dimensional ultrasonography may be helpful in diagnosis as an adjunct to, but not a replacement for, two dimensional ultrasonography."**[3]

Another suggested use of a stored 3-D volume data set is that it could allow evaluation of a fetus by an expert who is not physically present at the time and place in which the scan is performed.[4] Presumably, the initial volume data set could be obtained by a less-expert examiner, who would perhaps not have sufficient skill to obtain images of the 2-D planes that are required. The potential for this remote approach to ultrasound interpretation has yet to be realized.

Another promising feature of 3-D ultrasound is its ability to calculate tissue and fluid volumes. For example, lung volume measurements have been used to try to better predict pulmonary hypoplasia.[5] In a novel application, Lee and colleagues added measurement of the fetal thigh volume to an equation to improve fetal weight estimation.[6] Although they raise intriguing possibilities, these and similar uses of 3-D ultrasound have not yet found their way into widespread clinical use.

SCANNING TECHNIQUE

Orientation

Every effort should be made to perform the scan with the sonographer and the patient in a standard position. In most settings, the ultrasound machine and the sonographer are on the patient's right, with the sonographer comfortably seated facing the head of the patient. The probe is held in such a way that the image on the screen is properly oriented. By convention, the probe surface is shown at the top of the screen. For sagittal views, the right of the screen corresponds to the inferior aspect of the patient (Figure

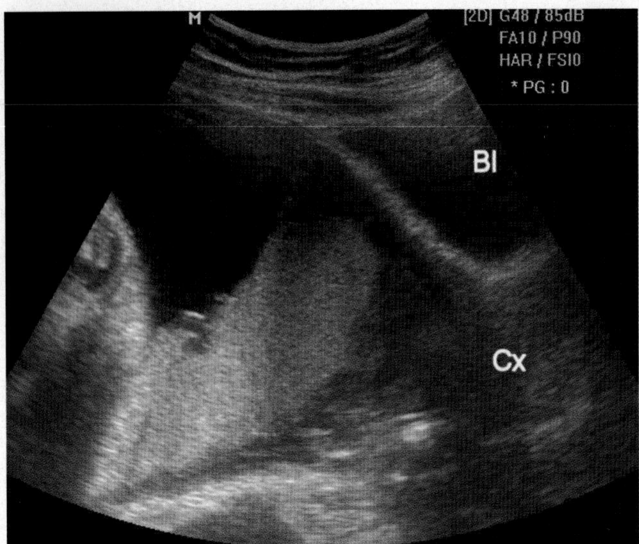

FIGURE 9-13. Transabdominal sagittal view of the lower uterus. The maternal bladder *(Bl)* and location of the cervix *(Cx)* are labeled. By convention, the right side of the ultrasound screen corresponds to the inferior aspect of the patient. Note that placenta previa is present.

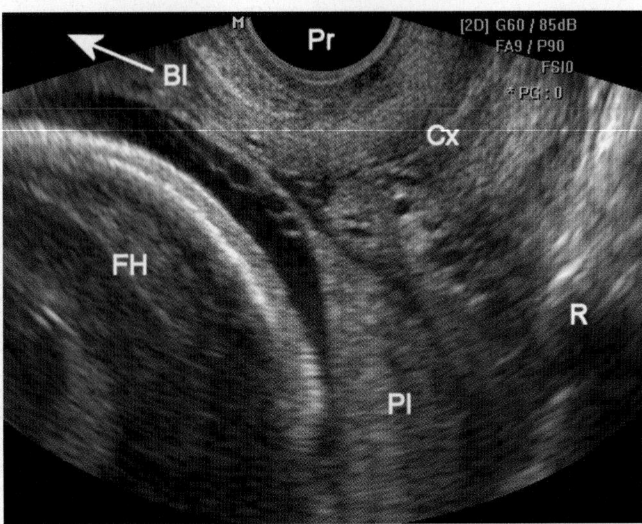

FIGURE 9-14. Transvaginal sagittal view showing proper orientation. The left of the screen is "up" on the patient, that is, toward the bladder *(Bl)*. The probe tip *(Pr)*, fetal head *(FH)*, cervix *(Cx)*, placenta *(Pl)*, and rectum *(R)* are labeled. Note how transvaginal ultrasound provides the ultimate "window," showing very clear views of structures that are close to the vaginal apex. Also note the presence of vasa previa.

9-13). For transverse views, the patient's right is shown on the left of the screen. With transvaginal ultrasound, transverse views also show the patient's right side to the left of the screen. In transvaginal sagittal views, "up" is to the left of the screen (i.e., toward the bladder), and "down" (toward the sacrum) is to the right of the screen (Figure 9-14). Ultrasound transducers have a notch or mark of some type that demarcates the side of the probe that will correspond to the left side of the monitor. Thus, with transabdominal work, this mark would be toward the patient's head for sagittal views and toward the patient's right for transverse views. With transvaginal scanning, the mark is up for sagittal views and to the patient's right for transverse views. Thus, in going from sagittal to transverse, the probe is always rotated counterclockwise, and clockwise to move from transverse to sagittal.

If the sonographer sits or stands on the wrong side of the patient or holds the probe backward, standard orientation of the images cannot be maintained. This is clearly unacceptable for diagnostic and documentation purposes and for performance of invasive procedures. Also, a casual approach to probe orientation will prevent the sonographer from developing the hand-eye coordination needed to quickly steer the probe. With improper probe orientation, the principle probe movements—sliding, rotation, and angulation—will not give predictable results as the sonographer tries to produce the desired image. If the sonographer must scan from the patient's left side, the same considerations for a standardized approach should be maintained, especially with regard to the orientation of the image on the ultrasound screen.

To establish the position of the fetus, the orientation of the probe must obviously be correct. This is important not only when deciding whether the fetus is cephalic or breech, but also when determining the right and left side of the fetus. For example, when the image shows the fetal spine to the right side of the uterus, the fetal left will be up in a cephalic presentation and down with a breech. It is important to mentally go through this orienting exercise at the start of each fetal examination, and not to "cheat" and define left as the side of the stomach or apex of the heart, which could result in missing disorders of sidedness, such as situs inversus (Figure 9-15).

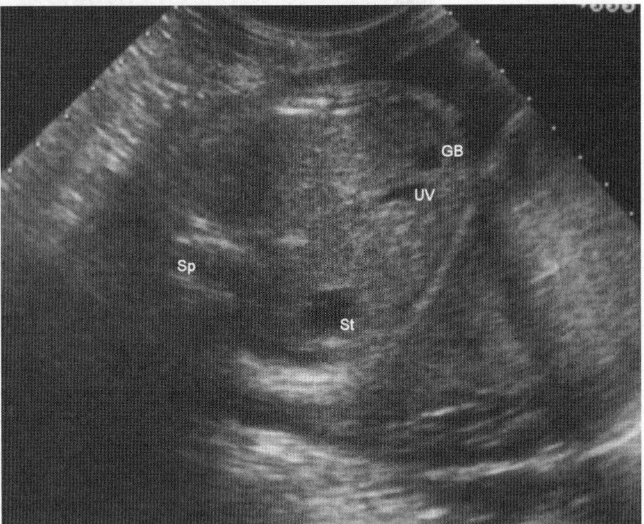

FIGURE 9-15. This view would be normal if the fetus were in a breech presentation. Because the fetus is in a cephalic presentation, with the spine *(Sp)* to the maternal right, the right side of the fetus is down on the image. This indicates that situs inversus is present. You cannot decide which side is right or left based on the sidedness of the viscera. The stomach *(St)*, umbilical vein *(UV)*, and gallbladder *(GB)* are also labeled.

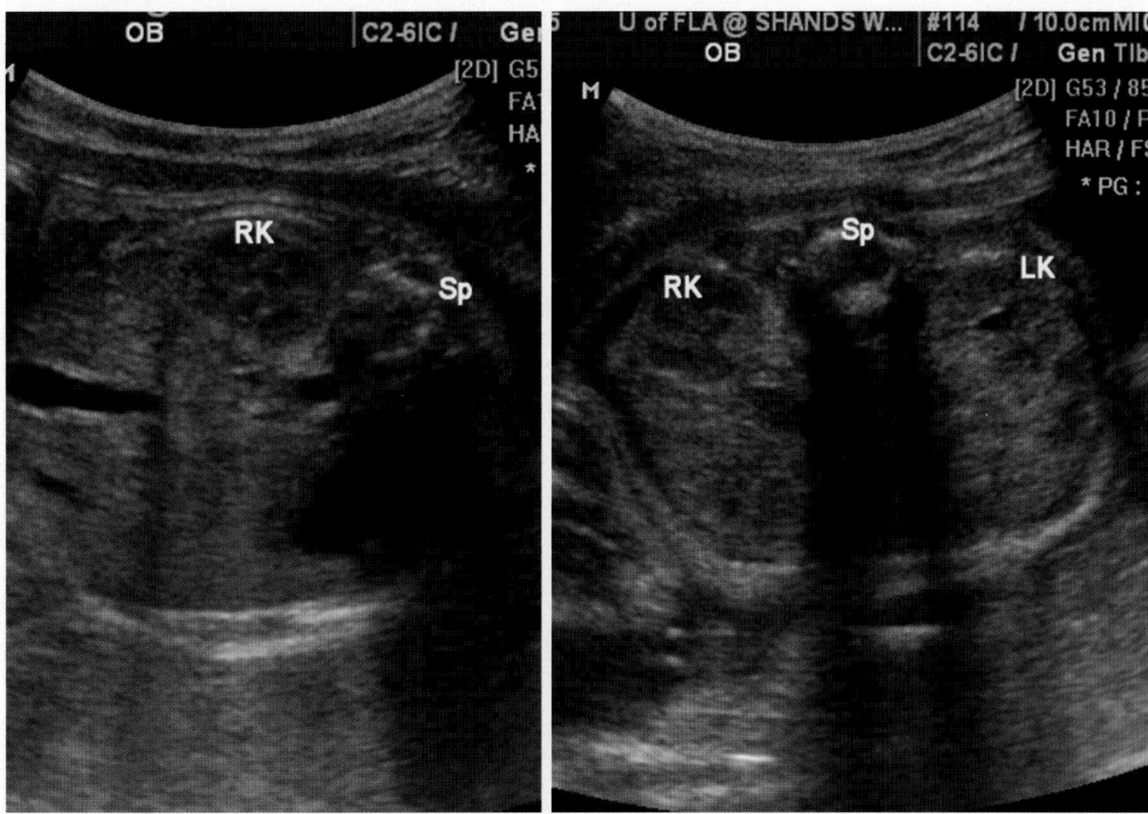

FIGURE 9-16. In the image to the left, shadowing by the spine precludes visualization of the left kidney. By sliding the transducer to a different location on the maternal abdominal wall, a more favorable angle of insonation is possible. The spine *(Sp)*, right kidney *(RK)*, and left kidney *(LK)* are denoted.

Angle of Insonation

Novice sonographers often try to look straight down on a structure to be visualized, as if looking down into a room from a skylight. Actually, the uterus can be thought of as a glass house, and the fetus can be looked at from a wide variety of angles. For many structures, there is a best angle with which to view the structure. For example, a lateral view of the fetus may result in shadowing of one kidney by the spine (Figure 9-16). Sliding the transducer across the mother's abdomen to change the angle of insonation by 90 degrees allows a posterior-anterior view that avoids the spine and shows the kidneys much more clearly. Sometimes, significant pressure with the transducer is needed to get the probe into position for optimal visualization. If the fetal position precludes clear visualization of a structure, a good strategy is to move forward with the examination, then come back to the troublesome area. The fetus will often have moved in such a way that adequate views can be obtained.

Using Natural Windows

As previously noted, increasing the power of ultrasound impulses can overcome some of the effects of attenuation in maternal tissues. Although it is tempting to use higher-power settings for obese patients, other methods should be attempted first. As a starting point, the proper probe frequency and gain setting should be employed. **Even more effective, however, is to avoid attenuation altogether by scanning though one of the natural "windows" in the maternal abdominal wall.** The abdominal wall thickness in obese women is substantially less near the umbilicus and in the suprapubic area. To a lesser extent, thickness is also decreased lateral to the central pannus. Using these windows can often improve the quality of images dramatically (Figure 9-17). Of course, in early pregnancy, or when structures of interest are low in the pelvis, the problem of attenuation is reduced considerably by the use of an endovaginal probe (see Figure 9-14). The reduction of attenuation with transvaginal ultrasound allows the use of a higher frequency probe, resulting in significantly improved resolution. Another natural window is amniotic fluid. Scanning through amniotic fluid improves the image quality below or deep to the amniotic fluid. This is especially true for imaging the surface of the fetus.

FIRST-TRIMESTER ULTRASOUND

Transvaginal ultrasound is almost always superior to transabdominal ultrasound for evaluation of the very early pregnancy and fetus. The fact that the uterus is still within the pelvis makes the developing pregnancy accessible to visualization with the vaginal probe. Because the distance between the probe and pregnancy structures is often just a few centimeters, there is very little attenuation of sound waves, and high-frequency probes may be used. As previously noted, this allows better resolution of detail. Although basic information can be obtained transabdominally (e.g., the presence and size of a gestational sac and presence of

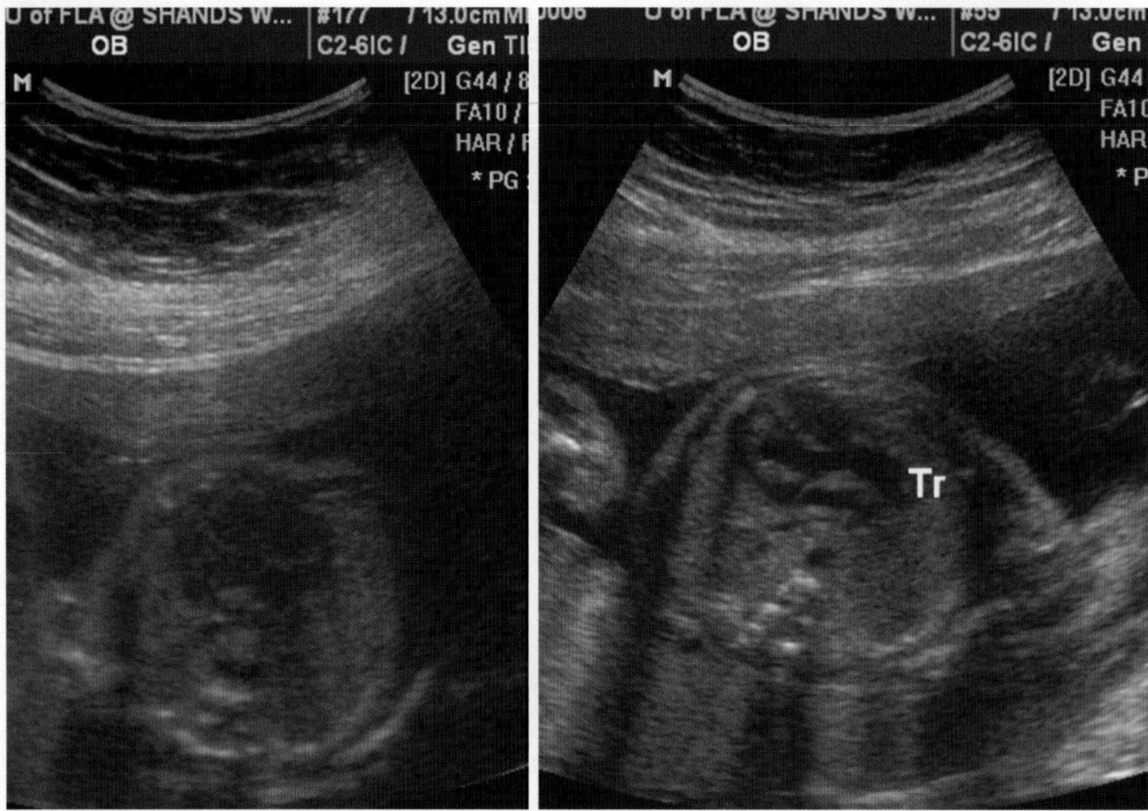

FIGURE 9-17. In the panel on the left, the scan is through the pannus of the woman's abdominal wall. By moving the probe into the thinner area near the maternal umbilicus, the resolution improved dramatically. A similar result can be obtained when scanning below the pannus, in the suprapubic area. Of course, when an object of interest is in the maternal pelvis, transvaginal ultrasound provides an even better window (see Figure 9-14). This fetus has truncus arteriosus *(Tr)*.

fetal cardiac activity), important findings may be missed if transvaginal ultrasound is not performed. In general, structures are visible 1 week earlier with transvaginal ultrasound. At about 12 weeks' gestation, the uterus has grown enough, and the fetus is far enough away from the transducer, that images through the desired fetal plane may be difficult to obtain with transvaginal ultrasound. In these cases, transabdominal ultrasound may give better views, so it should be used instead of or in conjunction with transvaginal ultrasound. The transvaginal probe can be rotated, and there is quite a lot of freedom to angulate up and down, but the tip of the probe is essentially fixed at the apex of the vagina. For this reason, not all scan planes of the fetus and uterine contents are possible. Because of the need for a precise midsagittal plane for the nuchal translucency measurement as part of the first-trimester aneuploidy screen, this scan is usually done transabdominally.

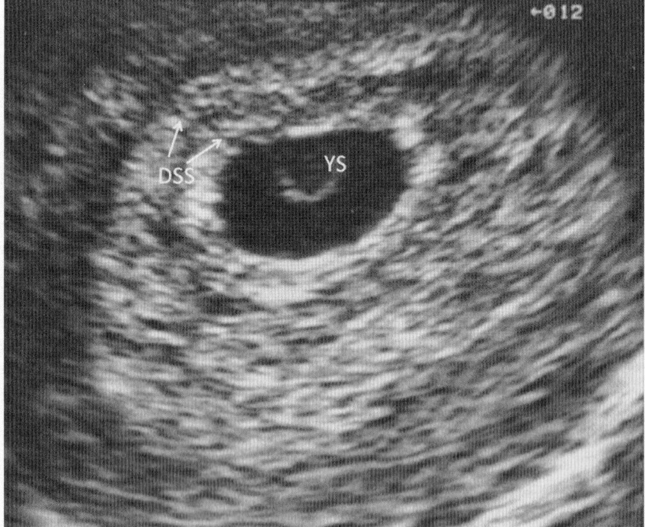

FIGURE 9-18. This image shows a normal yolk sac *(YS)* and the double sac sign *(DSS)*.

First-Trimester Normal Findings

Knowledge of the time at which embryonic structures normally appear is important for identifying pathologic pregnancies. For the reasons noted earlier, it will be assumed that transvaginal ultrasound is being used for this discussion.

The gestational sac can usually be seen at 4 weeks, the yolk sac at 5 weeks (Figure 9-18), and the fetal pole with cardiac activity by 6 weeks. Cardiac activity can be seen simultaneously with the appearance of a fetal pole as a pulsation at the lateral aspect of the yolk sac. Starting at 7 weeks, the embryo has grown to the point that recognizable features, such as a cephalic pole, can be seen. After this time, a prominent midline brain vesicle, the earliest sonographic manifestation of the five vesicles from which arise the parts of the brain (prosencephalon, mesencephalon, rhombencephalon, telencephalon, and diencephalon) can be seen (see Figure 9-10). The cerebral falx can be seen at 9 weeks, and the appearance and disappearance of physiologic gut herniation are noted between 8 and 11 weeks (Figure 9-19). Normally, the bowel is seen to lie within the umbilical cord and does not float freely. Obviously, the diagnosis of an abdominal wall defect should be made with great caution at this age. The stomach can consistently be seen by 11 weeks. If conditions are favorable, it is often possible to also visualize the bladder and kidneys at 11 weeks. Using color Doppler, the two umbilical arteries can often be identified at about 12 weeks as they course around the bladder. The fetal heart rate is initially quite slow, averaging 100 beats per minute at 5 to 6 weeks,[7] then it increases steadily to a mean peak of 175 beats per minute at 9 weeks.[8] When the fetal position is favorable, transvaginal ultrasound has the potential for giving good views of the fetal cardiac anatomy in most patients at 13 weeks.[9] Until 13 to 16 weeks' gestation, the amnion has not fused to the chorion and is seen as a separate membrane (see Figure 9-19). Until 12 weeks, the crown-rump length (CRL) should be measured. Care should be taken to measure the full length of the fetus. The gestational age can be significantly underestimated if an oblique plane is taken (Figure 9-20) or if the fetus is in a flexed position.

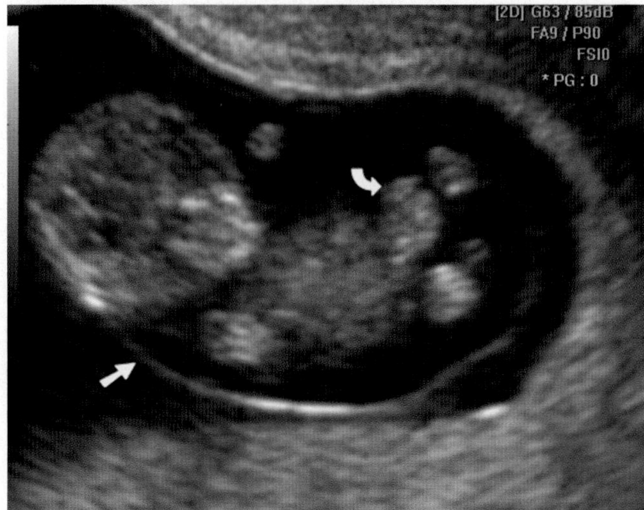

FIGURE 9-19. Nine-week fetus showing the physiologic gut herniation *(curved arrow)*. Note also how the amnion *(straight arrow)* has not yet fused to the chorion at the uterine wall.

First-Trimester Abnormal Findings

Spontaneous abortion occurs in 15% of clinically established pregnancies. **When cardiac activity has been demonstrated, the miscarriage rate is reduced to 2% to 3% in asymptomatic low-risk women.**[10] It is important to note, however, that in some groups at very high risk for miscarriage, such as women over the age of 35 years who are undergoing infertility treatments, early visualization of cardiac activity does not provide quite as much

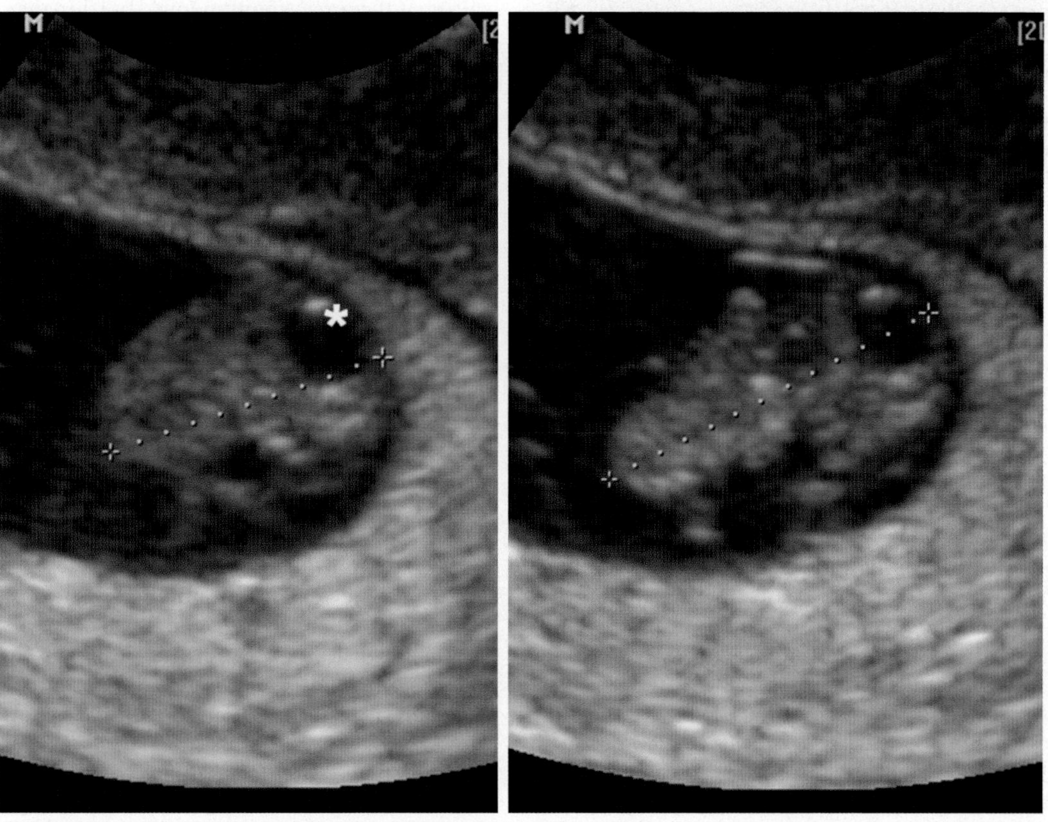

FIGURE 9-20. In the image on the left, the fetus is cut obliquely, and the CRL is inappropriately short. It is measured correctly on the right. There was a difference of 5 days in the calculated gestational age from these two measurements. The normal brain vesicle *(*)* is again denoted.

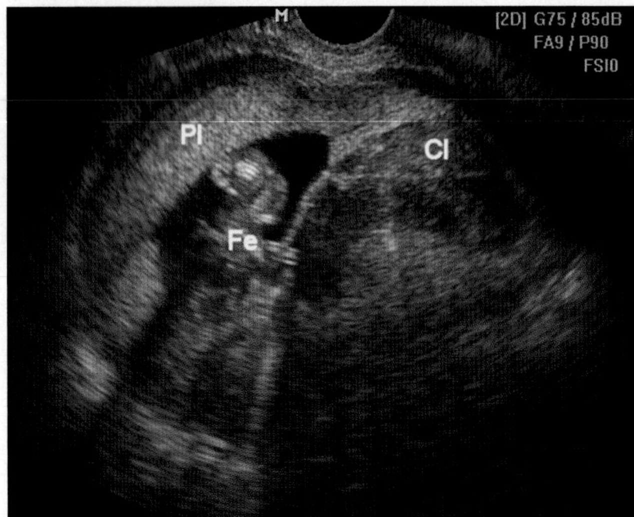

FIGURE 9-21. This patient presented with vaginal bleeding. A subchorionic clot *(Cl)* was present in the lower uterine segment. This patient carried the pregnancy successfully. The fetus *(Fe)* and placenta *(Pl)* are shown.

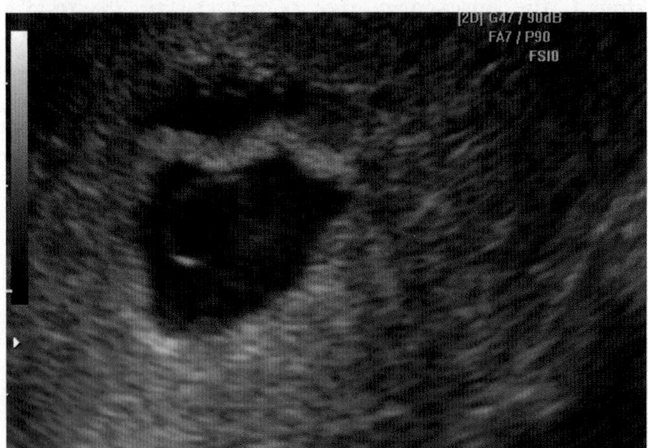

FIGURE 9-22. Irregular gestational sac from an anembryonic gestation.

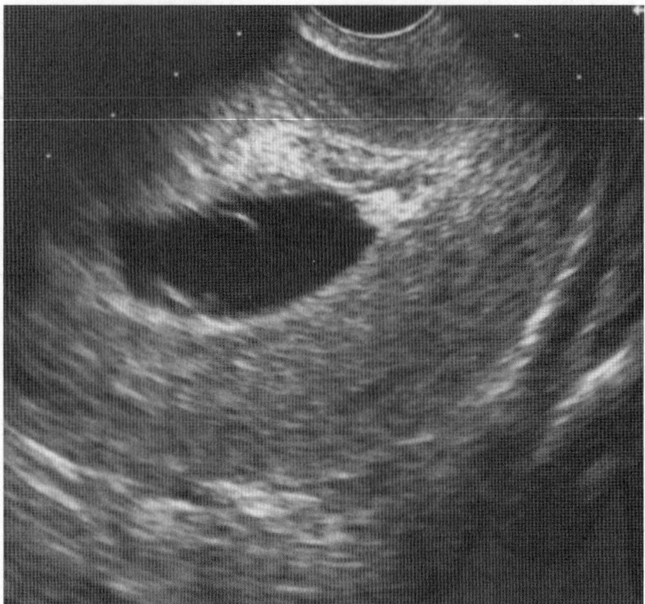

FIGURE 9-23. Compared with Figure 9-18, the yolk sac in this image is relatively large for gestational age. An embryo was never seen with this pregnancy.

reassurance. In one study involving such women, the miscarriage rate in asymptomatic women was still 16% after a heartbeat was documented.[11] In younger women who present with bleeding, only 5% miscarry if the ultrasound is normal and shows a live embryo.[12] If there is an intrauterine clot present (Figure 9-21), coexistent with an otherwise normal appearing pregnancy, the miscarriage rate is 15%.[12]

In most pregnancies destined to abort, the embryo does not develop, and ultrasound shows an empty gestational sac (Figure 9-22). Such a pregnancy is termed an *anembryonic gestation*. When there is no yolk sac seen and the mean sac diameter is at least 13 mm or there is no embryo seen with mean sac diameter of at least 20 mm, it is almost certain that the pregnancy is nonviable.[3,13] The absence of cardiac activity when the fetal pole measures greater than 5 mm reliably diagnoses embryonic death.[14] Other findings that are somewhat predictive of spontaneous abortion include a yolk sac that is unusually large or small for gestational age[15] (Figure 9-23), a relatively small gestational sac (mean sac diameter/CRL difference <5 mm),[16] or fetal bradycardia.[7] **If there are borderline findings and uterine evacuation is being considered, it is prudent to repeat the ultrasound in 1 week to be absolutely sure that a viable pregnancy is not interrupted.**[16] Although this is a trying time for the patient, there is no significant medical risk in waiting. Of course, spontaneous abortion may occur during this time. Although a quantitative human chorionic gonadotropin value that does not show an appropriate rise indicates a likely abnormal pregnancy, a decision to terminate a pregnancy is most often based on the failure of development of normal findings by ultrasound.

First-trimester ultrasound findings including thick nuchal translucency, absent nasal bone, abnormally fast or slow fetal heart rate, and some structural malformations, can be very useful for predicting the risk for a chromosome abnormality.[17] The use of ultrasound for aneuploidy screening is discussed in detail in Chapter 11.

SECOND- AND THIRD-TRIMESTER ULTRASOUND

Types of Examinations

The American Institute of Ultrasound in Medicine (AIUM), in conjunction with the ACOG and the American College of Radiology, have defined a set of criteria for standard obstetrical ultrasound examinations performed in the second and third trimesters.[18] Components of a standard obstetrical examination are shown in Table 9-1. Components of the fetal anatomic survey are listed in Chapter 11. A complete description of the AIUM guidelines can be found in the listed reference.

These guidelines recognize that not all ultrasound examinations have the same purpose. For this reason, types of fetal sonographic evaluations have been defined. Components of the first-trimester ultrasound examination

TABLE 9-1 IMAGING PARAMETERS FOR A STANDARD FETAL EXAMINATION

1. Fetal cardiac activity
2. Fetal number
   a. Chorionicity, amnionicity
   b. Comparison of fetal sizes
   c. Estimation of amniotic fluid volume
   d. Fetal genitalia
3. Presentation
4. Qualitative or semiquantitative estimate of amniotic fluid volume
5. Placental location, appearance, and relationship to the internal os
6. Umbilical cord visualized and number of vessels determined, if possible
7. Gestational age assessment
8. Fetal measurements
   a. Crown-rump length in the first trimester
   b. Biparietal diameter
   c. Head circumference
   d. Abdominal circumference
   e. Femur length
9. Fetal weight estimation
10. Maternal anatomy
    a. Uterus
    b. Adnexal structures
    c. Cervix
11. Fetal anatomic survey

From American Institute of Ultrasound in Medicine. AIUM Practice Guideline for the performance of an antepartum obstetric ultrasound examination. J Ultrasound Med 22:1116, 2003.

were described previously. A *standard* second- or third-trimester examination, as defined in Table 9-1, can be performed by any appropriately qualified sonographer. It is recognized that certain scans should be performed by individuals with special training in the recognition and management of unusual or serious fetal conditions. These scans are referred as *specialized* examinations. This category of examination is considered more complex than the complete standard examinations performed in the course of routine pregnancy care. This designation (and the appropriate billing code) is intended to be used for referral practices with special expertise in the identification of, and counseling about, fetal anomalies.

Another examination category is the *limited* examination. Limited ultrasound examinations are appropriate when needed to obtain specific information about the pregnancy, but only when performed by a trained examiner, and when a complete standard examination has been previously performed. The importance of restricting limited examinations to those cases in which a complete examination has previously been performed should be self-evident. Consider the consequences if a brief ultrasound is performed to answer a question such as "what is the fetal presentation?" or "is placenta previa present?" and critically important information, such as the fact that the fetus has a severe malformation, is missed. Unfortunately, it is all too common for practitioners to perform limited examinations in a manner that is not consistent with good medical practice. For example, in some clinics, practitioners perform an ultrasound at the first prenatal visit to document viability, but without measuring the fetus or recording the results of the examination. Such a practice can create problems later in pregnancy when the gestational age is in doubt.

All the aspects of the standard obstetrical examination listed in Table 9-1 are important for clinical management and should not be neglected. For example, it is obvious that there could be serious consequences if an ultrasound fails to reveal the presence of placenta previa, multiple gestation, or an ovarian tumor. The diagnosis and management of these and other conditions are discussed in detail elsewhere in this book, but a brief description of the importance of the components of the standard ultrasound examination to screen for these conditions will be given here.

Qualifications for Interpreting Diagnostic Ultrasound Examinations

The AIUM recently published guidelines on the training and experience needed for physicians to perform or interpret ultrasound examinations. In brief, these guidelines recommend that licensed physicians have completed an equivalent of 3 months training dedicated to ultrasound in the context of an approved residency, fellowship, or other postgraduate training. In the absence of a formal training program, physicians can qualify through having 100 American Medical Association Category I credits dedicated to diagnostic ultrasound. Along with participation in either a formal training program or by taking postgraduate courses, physicians should have been involved with the performance, evaluation, and interpretation of at least 300 appropriately supervised sonograms.[19] The full text of the guidelines are in the referenced document.

COMPONENTS OF THE EXAMINATION

Cardiac Activity

Obviously, the presence of absence of cardiac activity should be documented. As noted previously, after about 6 weeks' gestation, the diagnosis of fetal life is rarely difficult. Even though fetal death may be obvious with B-mode imaging, confirming the absence of a heart beat with color or pulse-wave Doppler is recommended. Absence of color signal in the fetal chest, contrasted with demonstration of flow in the surrounding uterine tissues, can increase the confidence that fetal death has indeed occurred. Throughout pregnancy, an abnormally fast, slow, or irregular heartbeat can be detected by visual inspection with gray-scale ultrasonography. The abnormal rate can be quantified and documented with M-mode or pulse-wave Doppler ultrasound.

Number of Fetuses

When a multiple pregnancy is diagnosed, the number of amnions and chorions should always be determined. Determination of chorionicity is most easily accomplished in early pregnancy. The presence of unlike sex twins, separate placentas, or a thick membrane dividing the sacs with a "lambda sign" all indicate the presence of two chorions. It is well-recognized that the level of fetal risk is much higher when fetuses share chorions.[20] The risk is extremely high if there is a single amnion. Monochorionic pregnancies require early referral for a specialized ultrasound. In all twin pregnancies, periodic ultrasound examinations should be performed to assess fetal growth. Twins are at significantly increased risk for growth abnormalities, and it is not possible to assess the growth of the twins individually by abdominal palpation.

Presentation

The assessment of presentation is not merely a matter of determining whether the fetus is head down or breech. A more precise ultrasound analysis of presentation is important in certain circumstances. If a transverse lie is diagnosed, it is important to diagnose whether the fetus is back down (i.e., back toward the cervix) because this may require a vertical incision for cesarean delivery. If the patient has preterm labor or ruptured membranes, a back-up transverse lie indicates a high risk for cord prolapse. The attitude of the fetal head, especially the presence of a face presentation, can be important in assessing progress in labor. In cases in which a breech vaginal delivery is contemplated, ultrasound can show the position of the legs and feet as well as the degree of flexion of the head—all factors that can predict the safety of vaginal birth. In cases in which there is marked caput or molding in late labor, it is often difficult to determine the position of the fetal head by palpation of the cranial sutures. Under these circumstances, ultrasound can be used to readily identify fetal cranial landmarks to clarify the position of the fetal head.[21]

Amniotic Fluid Volume

Every ultrasound examination should include an assessment of the amniotic fluid volume. It is acceptable for an experienced examiner to make this determination subjectively.[18] However, to aid in communication and to provide criteria for management protocols, several semiquantitative methods have been devised. A popular method is the amniotic fluid index (AFI)—the sum of the measurements of the deepest vertical pocket of fluid in each of the uterine quadrants. The limits of the quadrants are the maternal midline and a horizontal line through the maternal umbilicus. The line between the calipers should not cross through loops of cord or fetal parts. Polyhydramnios and oligohydramnios can be defined either by an AFI outside of a fixed range (usually >25 cm and <5 cm)[22] or a value that is greater or less than the 95th or 5th percentile for gestational age.[23] A simpler semiquantitative method is to diagnose polyhydramnios when the single deepest pool measures greater than 8 cm, and oligohydramnios when the shallowest pool measures less than 2 cm.[24]

The actual volume of amniotic fluid can be determined by dye-dilution techniques performed at the time of amniocentesis. The semiquantitative ultrasound methods described previously correlate somewhat with actual fluid volume, but their accuracy for predicting abnormal fluid volume is limited.[24] **Although there are some differences in the predictive ability of the different ultrasound methods, no system has been clearly shown to be superior to another.** However, when the ultrasound amniotic fluid assessment is to be used to guide clinical management, it seems reasonable to employ methods that have been used in studies that correlate outcomes with ultrasound assessment. Most of the studies correlating ultrasound-diagnosed oligohydramnios with clinical outcomes have used an AFI of less than 5 or, for specific use as part of the biophysical profile, a deepest single pocket measuring less than 2 cm. It is less critical to have a standard definition of polyhydramnios because clinical decision making is only affected by the presence of moderate to severe polyhydramnios, when the excess fluid would be recognized by any of the commonly used systems or cut-offs.

Severe polyhydramnios is usually indicative of a fetal problem and requires a specialized ultrasound to determine the cause. It is often caused by malformations that can greatly affect neonatal management or prognosis. For many of these conditions, the excess amniotic fluid is a result of poor fetal swallowing—from neurologic abnormalities, genetic syndromes, or gastrointestinal malformations. Other serious causes of severe polyhydramnios include twin-to-twin transfusion syndrome and fetal hydrops. Mild polyhydramnios may simply be a variant of normal, but may be associated with maternal diabetes or fetal macrosomia.

The absence of amniotic fluid before labor is never normal and can indicate fetal malformations, rupture of membranes, or placental insufficiency. Malformations causing absence of fluid usually involve the urinary tract. This may be from complete bladder outlet obstruction or from bilateral renal anomalies in which no urine is produced. Examples include bilateral renal agenesis, bilateral multicystic dysplastic kidneys, or autosomal recessive polycystic kidney disease. **The outcome with anhydramnios is generally poor but depends on the cause and the gestational age at which it is first present.** Onset of anhydramnios before the middle of the second trimester usually results in lethal pulmonary hypoplasia.[25]

For many years, it has been recognized that less extreme alterations of amniotic fluid volume can be important. Chamberlain and associates found that when there was less than a 1-cm pocket of fluid, there was a 40-fold increase in perinatal mortality.[26] The incidence of intrauterine growth restriction (IUGR) was also much higher when this degree of oligohydramnios was found. These findings led to the inclusion of the amniotic fluid volume assessment as part of the biophysical profile. More recently, researchers have shown that isolated ultrasound-diagnosed oligohydramnios is not as predictive of perinatal outcome as was previously thought. In a review of the available literature, Ott found that **although polyhydramnios helped diagnose macrosomia and anomalies, oligohydramnios was a weak predictor of poor outcome.**[27] Chauhan and coworkers performed a meta-analysis that showed an AFI of less than 5 was linked to an increased risk for cesarean delivery for distress and low Apgar scores, but argued against using a low AFI as the sole criterion for delivery.[28]

Placenta and Umbilical Cord

One of the principal advantages of routine ultrasound is that serious problems of placentation, such as placenta previa, placenta accreta, and vasa previa, can be diagnosed in a timely manner. At the time of a screening ultrasound, it should be definitely determined whether the placenta covers the internal cervical os. **If the placenta and the cervix are not seen clearly, or if it appears that the edge of the placenta is close to the cervix, vaginal ultrasound should be used liberally to clarify this relationship.**[29] The terms "complete" and "partial" placenta previa date from the pre-ultrasound era, when the relationship of the placenta to the partially dilated cervix was determined by digital examination. A preferred method for use with ultrasound is to measure and report the distance from the edge of the placenta to the internal os. Positive numbers are used to denote an overlap, whereas negative numbers describe a placenta edge that ends short of the cervix.[30]

It is common for placenta previa that is diagnosed early in pregnancy to resolve as pregnancy progresses. In a 1998 study by Taipale and associates, the edge of the placenta extended to or over the internal os of the cervix in 1.5% of patients between 18 and 23 weeks' gestation.[31] The rate of persistence of placenta previa depended on the degree of overlap. When the degree of overlap was 15 mm or greater, 19% persisted, whereas when the overlap was 25 mm or greater, 40% covered the cervix at term. Dashe and colleagues found that when placenta previa was present at 15 to 19 weeks, only 12% persisted. The rate of persistence gradually increased as the gestational age advanced; up to 73% persistence if placenta previa was present at 32 to 35 weeks. This study also showed that the degree of overlap was helpful in predicting persistence.[32] These results suggest that repeated ultrasound examinations should be performed until the placenta moves well away from the cervix or it becomes clear that the previa will persist. If the placenta previa persists, ultrasound can be very valuable in planning delivery.

The diagnosis of vasa previa is critical because the recognition of this finding at the time of a screening ultrasound greatly affects the chance of fetal survival (see Figure 9-14).[33] There is a high fetal mortality rate when vasa previa is not diagnosed before labor. Conversely, early diagnosis and aggressive obstetrical management of patients with vasa previa almost always result in a live baby, born in good condition. The fetal vessels covering the cervix may not be readily apparent with a routine transabdominal screening examination. Therefore, a high index of suspicion should be maintained, and transvaginal color Doppler ultrasound should be strongly considered in any case in which there is a velamentous cord insertion, when there is a succenturiate lobe, or when portions of umbilical cord are noted to be low in the uterus. The sonographer should also be aware that when placenta previa "resolves," branches of the umbilical vessels on the chorionic plate may still course over the cervix as placental villi degenerate beneath them, resulting in vasa previa. Identifying the cord insertion onto the placenta eliminates the possibility of velamentous cord insertion, but it does not exclude vasa previa from the other placentation abnormalities. Documentation of the cord insertion onto the placenta can be difficult, especially with a posterior placenta, and is not listed by the AIUM statement as a required element of a standard examination.[18]

In addition to determining the placenta's location, its appearance should be assessed. Many changes observed in the placenta are related to calcification, fibrosis, and infarction. There is a general trend for these changes to become more apparent as pregnancy progresses, but their clinical significance is unclear. It has recently been recognized that a "globular" placenta, with a narrow base compared with height, is associated with an increased rate of adverse perinatal events.[34]

An attempt should be made to confirm that there are two arteries and a vein in the umbilical cord. In late pregnancy, this can be easily ascertained by looking at a transverse cut of the cord in a free loop (Figure 9-24). In the second trimester, two umbilical arteries are most easily confirmed by identifying the vessels as they course around the fetal bladder. These can be seen with gray-scale ultrasound but are made much more obvious with color Doppler ultrasound. A single umbilical artery is present in 1% of all newborns. Because of the increased incidence of associated malformations, especially involving the kidneys and heart, this finding should prompt a detailed fetal survey. Fetuses with a single umbilical artery are at increased risk for growth restriction as well.[35]

Uterus and Adnexa

With any obstetrical ultrasound, including those performed in the first trimester, the adnexal and uterine morphology should be evaluated. Many women enter pregnancy without being aware that they have fibroids or a Müllerian malformation. Fibroids are usually readily apparent with transvaginal or transabdominal ultrasound. **A common pitfall is to confuse uterine contractions, which are commonly present in the second trimester, with fibroids** (Figure 9-25). Contractions have a more lenticular shape and blend with the surrounding myometrium, whereas fibroids usually are spherical, have distinct borders, and have a whorled internal echo texture. Pedunculated fibroids, even large ones, can be missed if the sonographer does not examine areas around the periphery of the uterus. Most studies have shown a higher rate of pregnancy complications when fibroids are present. A recent large study reported by Stout showed a statistically significantly increase of a wide variety of pregnancy complications when fibroids were present. However, the odds ratios were modest and differences were of limited clinical importance.[36] It is difficult to predict how fibroids will affect an individual patient's pregnancy because the number, size, and location can vary markedly. Ultrasound mapping of fibroids can help in making a delivery plan. Although large fibroids that fill the pelvis may preclude vaginal birth, it is usually prudent to not predict early in the pregnancy the need for cesarean delivery. Fibroids can rise out of the pelvis, leaving a relatively clear lower uterine segment. Because multiple fibroids in the lower uterus can greatly complicate the performance of a low transverse cesarean delivery, ultrasound may help predict the need for a classic incision. **There is conflicting evidence regarding the growth of fibroids during pregnancy.** Using serial ultrasound measurements, Rosati and associates showed that they tend to grow,[37] whereas a more recent study by Neiger and colleagues did not demonstrate significant growth during pregnancy.[38]

Obviously, it is important for a complete obstetrical ultrasound to include an assessment of the adnexa. Normal-sized ovaries may be difficult or impossible to see in the second or third trimester because of shielding by bowel. In a study of sonographic visualization of normal ovaries, Shalev and coworkers found that although both ovaries were visible in almost all first-trimester scans, both ovaries were visible in only 16% of second- and third trimester scans, and in 60% of these, neither ovary was seen.[39]

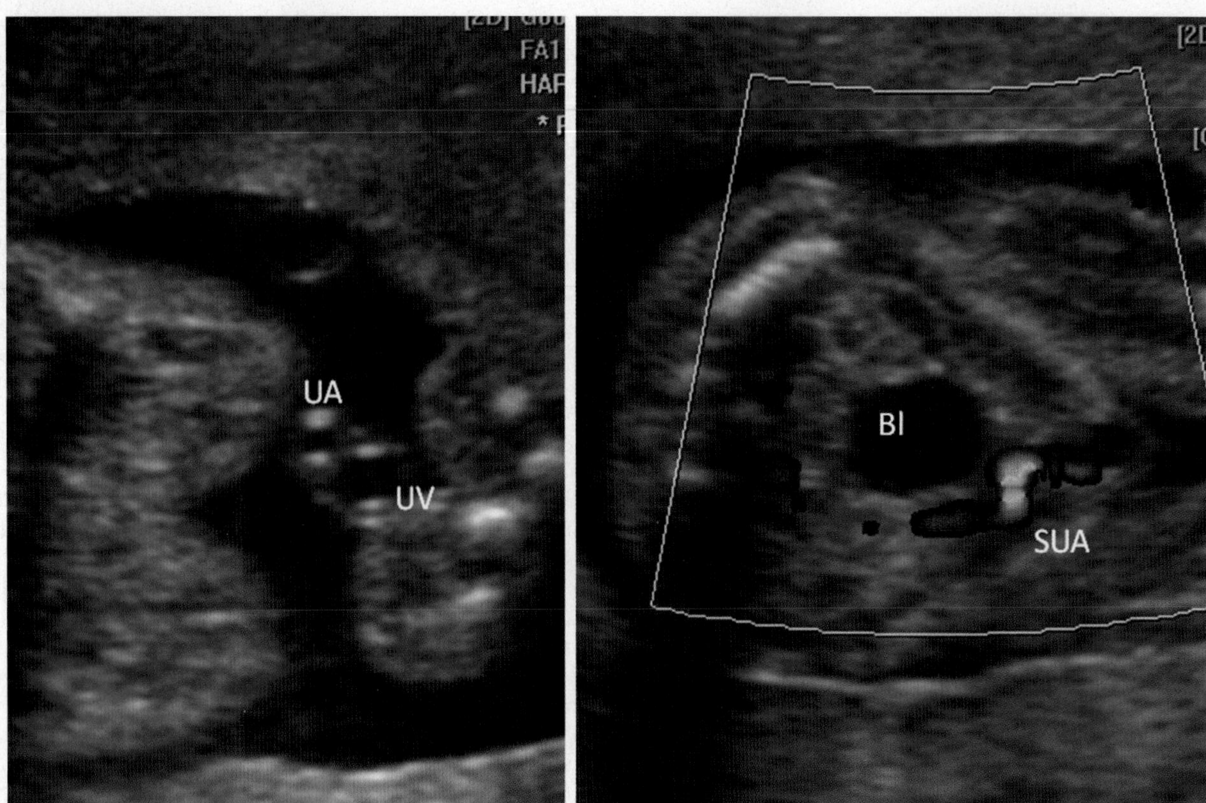

FIGURE 9-24. Two views documenting a single umbilical artery. The view on the left shows the single umbilical artery *(UA)* and the umbilical vein *(UV)* in a transverse section of a free loop of cord. On the right, a transverse view of the fetal pelvis shows a single artery *(SUA)* coursing around the bladder *(Bl)*. Note the absence of a paired artery on the other side. It is easier to document the umbilical arteries in early pregnancy with this color Doppler method.

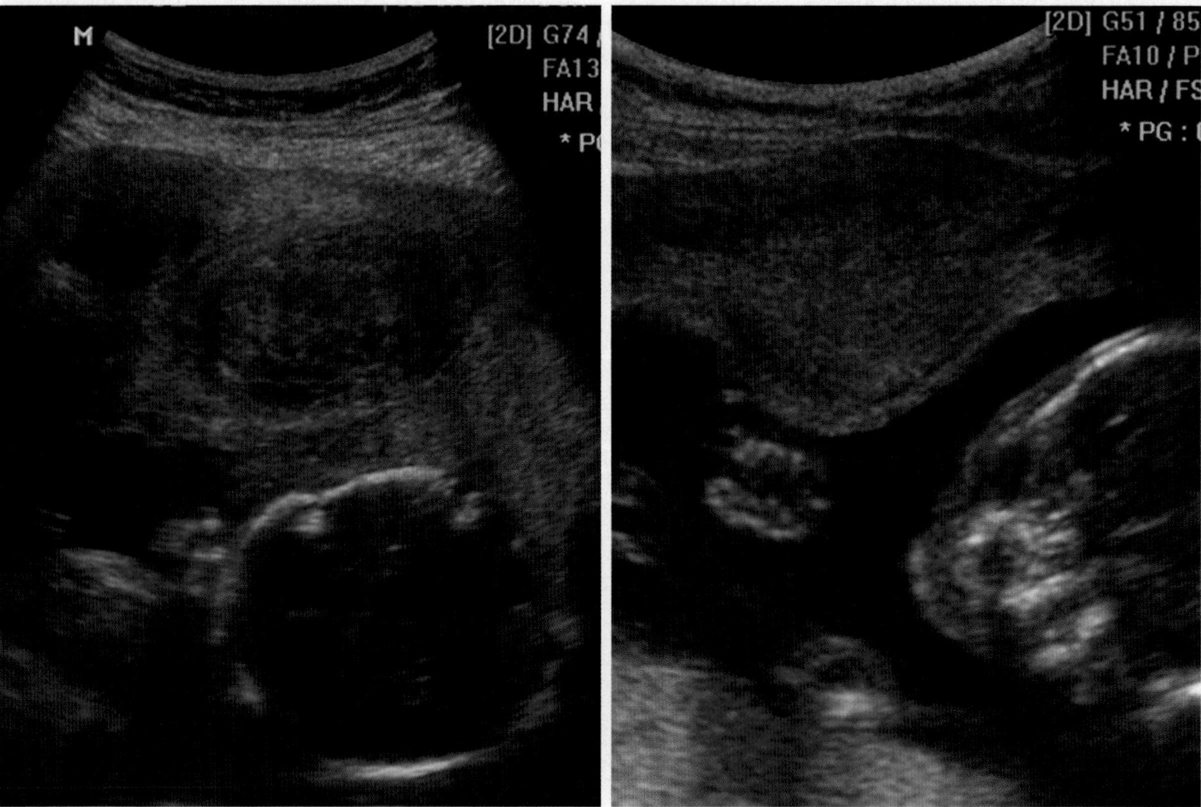

FIGURE 9-25. Two fibroids are seen in the image on the left. They are round and well circumscribed. On the right, a uterine contraction is shown. It is lenticular in shape and does not have a clear border. Contractions such as this are very common in the second trimester.

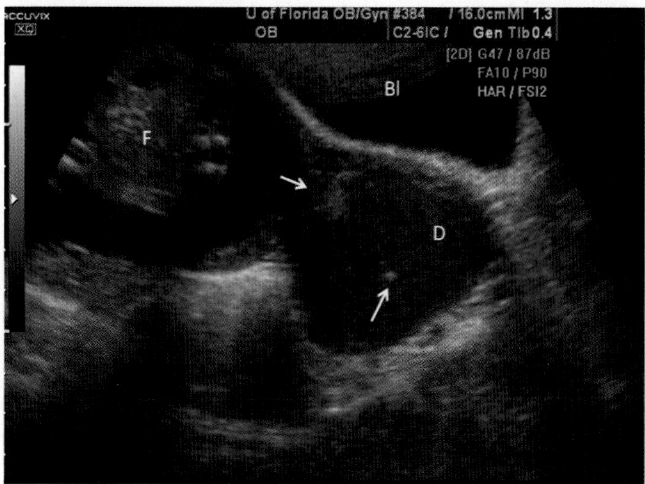

FIGURE 9-26. Transverse view of the maternal uterus and left adnexa in the early second trimester, showing a left ovarian dermoid *(D)*. Note the mixture of homogeneous material with low level echoes and the scattered areas of more echogenic material *(arrows)*. The fetus *(F)* and maternal bladder *(Bl)* are also labeled.

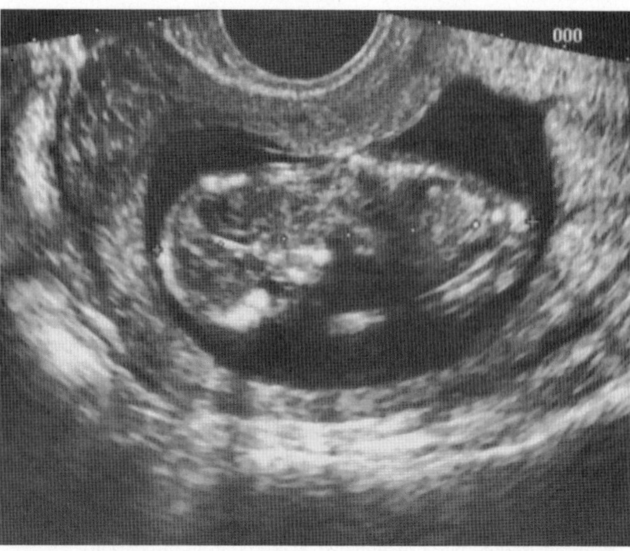

FIGURE 9-27. Measurement of the CRL. This is a sagittal view of the fetus with the crown (the head) to the left and the rump to the right. Errors that could lead to an incorrect CRL measurement would be to obtain an oblique view through the fetus, to measure when the fetus is in a flexed position, or to include the yolk sac with the fetal pole.

However, significant tumors should be visible in most cases. The sonographic appearance of an adnexal mass discovered during pregnancy guides decision making regarding the need for surgical removal. Masses consisting of simple cysts usually represent benign processes and do not require surgical removal during pregnancy. Masses with features of malignancy (large size, multiple cystic cavities, thick septae, internal papillae, or solid areas) require careful evaluation and may require operative removal. The most common neoplasm in pregnancy is a benign cystic teratoma (Figure 9-26). These can usually be identified by their sonographic characteristics.

Anatomic Survey

Systematic evaluation of fetal anatomy is critical. It is a good idea to proceed with an examination in a consistent order so that important parts are not forgotten. **Although there are many well-recognized maternal risk factors for congenital anomalies, most birth defects occur in fetuses of low-risk women.**[40] For this reason, it is important that anyone who performs obstetrical ultrasound have familiarity with the appearance of normal fetal anatomy in order to recognize deviations from normal. **As mentioned previously, although more advanced detailed sonograms (specialized examinations) are appropriate for patients with identified risk factors, all standard examinations should include a full anatomic survey.**

Documentation

Documentation of ultrasound findings is important not only for good patient care but also for quality review and legal defense. AIUM guidelines regarding record keeping state: **"Adequate documentation of the study is essential for high-quality patient care.** This should include a permanent record of the sonographic images, incorporating whenever possible … measurement parameters and anatomic findings."[18] Additionally, it is considered standard practice to include a written report in the patient's medical record.

ULTRASOUND FOR DETERMINING GESTATIONAL AGE

Determination of the correct gestational age is one of the most important aspects of prenatal care. Making correct management decisions for conditions such as preterm labor, postdates pregnancy, and preeclampsia depends heavily on knowledge of the gestational age of the fetus. Without early confirmation of the expected date of confinement (EDC), it is very difficult to diagnose growth disorders in the fetus. Biochemical screening for open fetal defects and chromosomal anomalies likewise requires accurate dating. For these and other reasons, it has become routine in developed countries to offer at least one ultrasound examination in the first half of pregnancy to accurately establish the gestational age.

Standard Measurements

Ian Donald first demonstrated the clinical use of ultrasound in obstetrics in the early 1960s with the measurement of the biparietal diameter BPD.[41] Since that time, a large number of publications have correlated this parameter with gestational age. The BPD can be measured from 12 to 13 weeks' gestation, when the skull has become ossified.

In the early 1970s, static scanners had advanced to the point that the gestational age could be determined in the first trimester by measuring the CRL.[42] With modern transvaginal ultrasound, the embryo can be measured when it is only a few millimeters long, between 5 and 6 weeks' gestation.[43] From 6 to 10 weeks' gestation, the maximal length of the embryo is measured. After about 10 weeks, the head, trunk, and extremities are visible, and the measurement is literally from the well-visualized "crown" to the "rump." Views of the CRL such as those shown in Figure 9-27 are obtained. Measurement of the

TABLE 9-2 DESCRIPTION OF IMAGES FOR FETAL BIOMETRY

Head
- Imaged from side, not front or back
- Head oval rather than round
- Midline structures centered, not displaced to the side
- Measured at level of thalamus and cavum septum pellucidum
- Should not include the top of orbits or any part of the brainstem or cerebellum
- Measured outer edge of the proximal skull to the inner edge of the distal skull
- Head circumference measured at the same level as the biparietal diameter, around the outer perimeter of the skull

Abdomen
- Abdomen nearly round, not oval or squashed
- True transverse image (not oblique)
- Images of ribs should be symmetrical on both sides
- Measured at the level where the umbilical vein joins the portal sinus
- Calipers all the way to the skin surface; not rib, liver, or spine edge

Femur
- Femur should be perpendicular to direction of insonation
- Ends should be sharply visible, not tapered or fuzzy
- Measurement should exclude the distal epiphysis

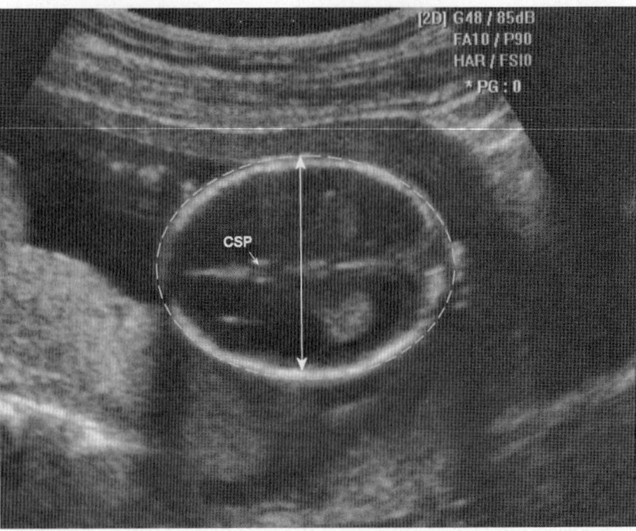

FIGURE 9-28. Image of fetal head for biparietal diameter and head circumference measurements. The cavum septum pellucidum *(CSP)* is indicated. Criteria for an appropriate image are listed in Table 9-2.

femur length (FL) for growth assessment was first described by Queenan and coworkers in 1980 and was enabled by the development of real-time ultrasound.[44] Using real-time linear array transducers, measurement of the FL is straightforward after the first trimester. It is possible to measure virtually any body part on a fetus. However, a standard set of measurements has been accepted as being the most useful for gestational age prediction. In addition to the BPD, CRL, and FL, the standard set now includes the head circumference (HC) and abdominal circumference (AC). Unless these are measured according to standard criteria (Table 9-2), their value in defining the age or growth of a fetus is limited. Optimal views for obtaining measurements are shown in Figures 9-28 to 9-32. Common errors to be avoided are also shown. With experience, a sonographer learns to slide the transducer to the proper position on the maternal abdominal wall, then angulate and rotate the transducer until the precise plane for biometry or anatomic assessment is obtained. Making these adjustments becomes second nature with practice.

Gestational Age Determination

An intrauterine pregnancy can first be identified with transvaginal ultrasound at 4 weeks from the last menstrual period. From this time until the embryo can be seen and measured at 5½ to 6 weeks, formulas using the sac diameter can give a fairly close approximation of the gestational age.[45] The mean sac diameter increases by about 1 mm per day during this interval, and the gestational age (in days) can be figured by adding 30 to the mean sac diameter (in millimeters).[46] **Because the range of error in age prediction from sac measurement is significantly greater than for the CRL and other standard measurements, the sac size should not be used as the final gestational age determinant.**[47] The measurement of the early embryo, either as the maximal embryo length or CRL, is commonly accepted as the best sonographic method for gestational age determination. Using a static scanner in pregnancies dated by "good" menstrual dates, Robinson found that the 95% confidence intervals for gestational age prediction using the CRL was ±4.7 days.[42] Later studies, in which gestational age was determined by in vitro fertilization, showed an even smaller random error.[48] The small random dating error found in early embryos is explained by their high weekly percentage change in size and the fact that there is very little variation among early embryos in their growth rates. However, in the late first trimester, flexion and extension of the fetus can significantly alter the CRL, making it less accurate for dating purposes. MacGregor and colleagues found in a study of patients with known ovulation dates that the 95% confidence intervals for CRL gestational age determination reached ±9.1 days at 14 weeks' gestation.[49] In comparison, Hadlock and others have shown that the 95% confidence intervals for gestational age prediction using the BPD as a single parameter between 14 and 21 weeks is ±7 days.[50,51] In a study of pregnancies dated by in vitro fertilization, Chervenak and colleagues found that in this period of pregnancy, all of the single parameters considered (BPD, HC, FL) performed quite well, with 95% confidence intervals for the gestational age ranging between ±7.5 days for the HC and ±8.7 days for the FL.[52] These studies demonstrate that a dating ultrasound performed between 14 and 22 weeks is comparable to one performed in the first trimester, and that the obstetrician need not refer a patient for ultrasound in the first trimester for the sole purpose of obtaining optimal dates.

Before the mid-1980s, second- or third-trimester gestational age assignment at the time of ultrasound was typically done by consulting a chart that had BPD or FL as the independent variable and gestational age as the dependent variable. This method did not allow for incorporation of multiple measurements in the gestational age assessment, unless ad hoc averaging of the age from different parameters was done. Starting in the late 1980s, computer programs that calculated a composite gestational age from multiple

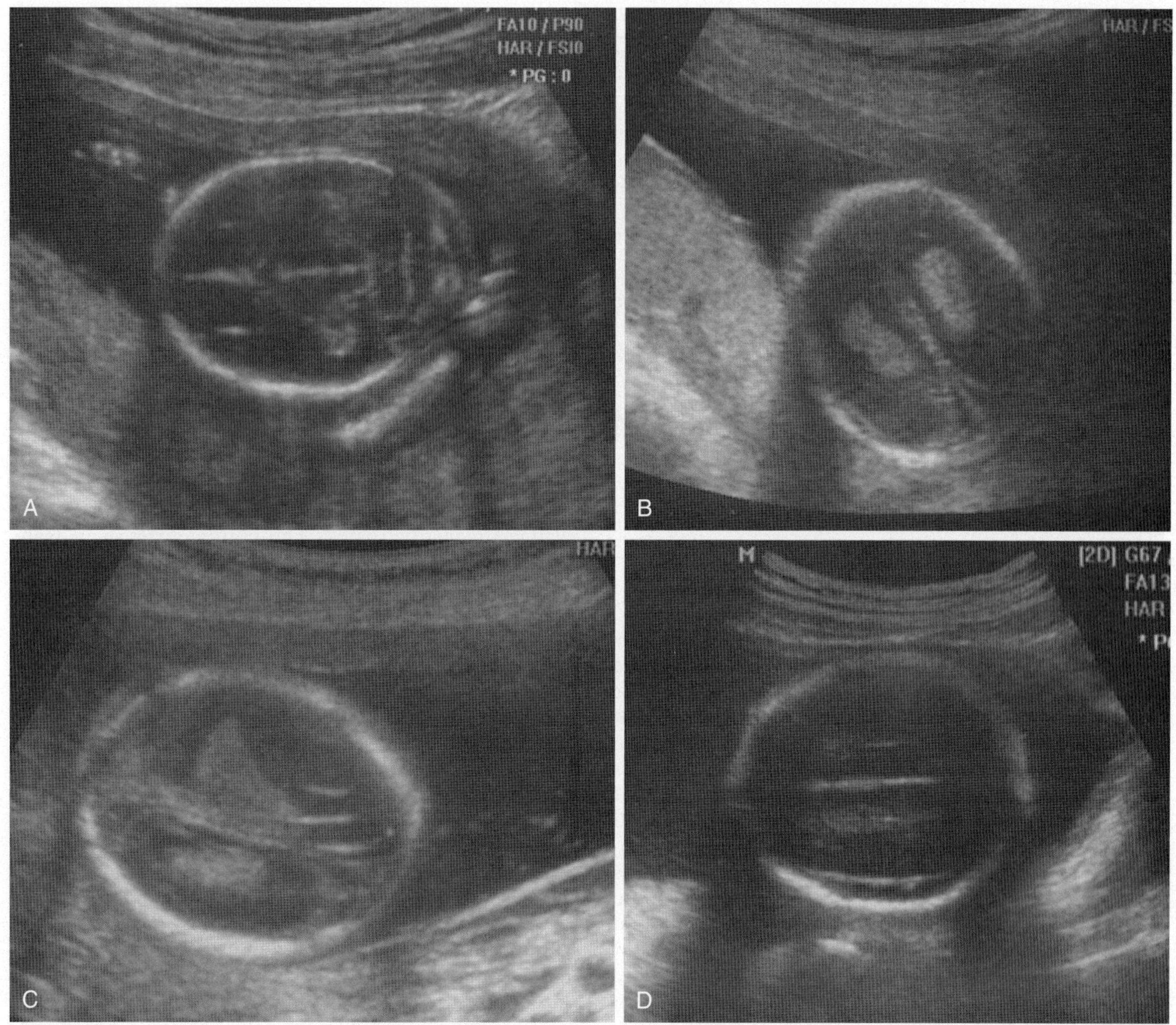

FIGURE 9-29. Examples of head views that are inappropriate for biparietal diameter and head circumference measurements. **A,** The transducer is rotated in such a way that the image includes the cerebellum. **B,** The head is imaged from the back and not from the side. **C,** The scan plane goes though the head obliquely. Note how the brain structures are asymmetrical. **D,** This true axial image is too high on the head. The cavum septum pellucidum is not seen.

measurements became available. These are now routinely used by ultrasound reporting software. Several studies have shown a significant reduction in variability of gestational age estimates when mathematical modeling from multiple parameters (BPD, HC, AC, and FL) is employed.[50,52] This technique reduces the impact of technical errors in measurement and smooths out effects from body part variations. Composite gestational age assessment using mathematical modeling from multiple parameters is now the most accepted method of ultrasound dating after the first trimester. The studies previously cited show that **gestational age calculation using a combination of standard parameters before 22 weeks is accurate to within ±7 days and is comparable to CRL measurement in the first trimester. As pregnancy progress beyond this range, variability in fetal size grows considerably, and ultrasound prediction of gestational age becomes progressively less accurate.**[50] **In one study, the composite gestational age assessment has a variability (±2 standard deviations) of 1.8 weeks at 24 to 30 weeks, and 2 to 3 weeks beyond 30 weeks.**[50]

These variability figures represent a statistical description of the variability of the gestational age calculations in the studied population. Assuming a normally growing fetus, it is likely that the gestational age of a pregnancy falls within the bounds described. However, there is no guarantee that the gestational age of a particular fetus is "at least" or "not more than" the lower or upper limit of the variability estimate. In the third trimester, growth disorders in fetuses are relatively common and can bring about marked size variation. For this reason, the obstetrician must exercise caution when basing management decisions on third-trimester ultrasound dates.

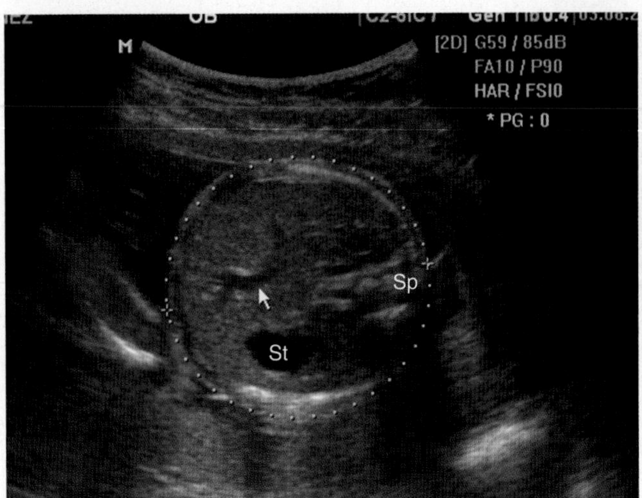

FIGURE 9-30. Proper image for measuring the abdominal circumference. Criteria for an appropriate image are listed in Table 9-2. The *arrow* shows the junction between the umbilical vein and portal sinus. The stomach *(St)* and spine *(Sp)* are labeled.

When to Use Ultrasound Dating

Since the time of Nägele in the early 1800s, obstetricians have routinely used menstrual dates for determining the EDC. In pregnancies in which the menstrual dates are unsure or thought to be unreliable because of a history of irregular cycles, recent hormonal contraception use, or an abnormally light last menstrual period (LMP), dates derived from ultrasound biometry are always preferred. It is now common practice in many countries for ultrasound to be performed routinely in the first half of all pregnancies, even those with good menstrual dates. In these cases in which both menstrual dates and ultrasound dates are available, which should be used? Possible strategies would be to always retain the menstrual dates, to use the menstrual dates unless the ultrasound size is out of the expected size range and thus "contradicts" the menstrual dates, or to ignore the menstrual dates altogether and use the ultrasound dates. A common practice is for ultrasound dates to take precedence over the menstrual dates if an ultrasound performed before about 22 weeks' gestation shows a gestational age more than 1 week different from the menstrual dates.[53]

Changing the dates in favor of the ultrasound dates can lead to an incorrect age assignment if the fetus has an early-onset significant growth disorder that accounts for the discrepancy. In the absence of maternal risk factors for early growth restriction or ultrasound signs suggesting a genetic syndrome or placental insufficiency, most sonographers feel safe in changing to ultrasound dates when a discrepancy exists. Delayed ovulation and incorrect recall of the LMP are common, whereas early-onset severe growth disorder is rare; thus, this is usually a good policy. However, **in the third trimester, aberrant growth is relatively common, so changing certain menstrual dates in favor of a late ultrasound date risks masking the presence of a significant growth disorder.** Uncertainties are best avoided by a policy that encourages routine early prenatal care so that firm dates can be established and risk factors for altered fetal growth can be recognized.

There is growing evidence that a dating ultrasound performed before 22 weeks should be used in preference to menstrual dates, regardless of the reliability or closeness of fit with menstrual dates. In 1996, Mongelli and associates evaluated 34,249 patients who had both "certain" menstrual dates and an ultrasound performed in the first half of pregnancy.[53] Using ultrasound exclusively led to a 70% reduction in the number of pregnancies considered postterm and more accurately predicted the onset of spontaneous labor. A policy of changing dates only when there was a significant discrepancy between menstrual dates and ultrasound gave inferior results compared with the exclusive use of ultrasound dates. Other studies using the same end points have similarly shown that there is no advantage of taking menstrual dates into account if a relatively early dating sonogram is available.[54] Exclusive use of ultrasound dating has also been shown to improve the predictive accuracy of serum screening for Down syndrome.[55] In first-trimester nuchal translucency assessment, measurements are correlated with the CRL, with no consideration of the claimed menstrual dates. The current practice in many developed countries of performing ultrasound in the first half of almost all pregnancies and the apparent superiority of ultrasound dating make it likely that in the future menstrual dating will become obsolete in these settings.

ASSESSING FETAL GROWTH

The first ultrasound examination is generally considered to be a dating examination; that is, the measurements are used to determine the gestational age. An accurate knowledge of gestational age determined by or confirmed by the first ultrasound examination forms the basis for subsequent clinical and sonographic assessment of fetal growth. Because insufficient or excessive growth can be associated with significant fetal morbidity, recognition of growth abnormalities is one of the primary aims of prenatal care and is an important aspect of ultrasound examinations. In most obstetrical practices, growth ultrasound examinations are obtained when abdominal palpation and fundal height measurement raise the suspicion of abnormal growth.[56] A lagging fundal height, combined with the knowledge of clinical risk factors for IUGR, is commonly used as a "screening test" for insufficient fetal growth, whereas ultrasound is considered the "diagnostic test." This scheme for the prenatal detection of growth-restricted fetuses has met with mixed results. In 1987, Pearce and Campbell showed that fundal height measurement in the third trimester had a sensitivity of 76% for detecting small-for-gestational-age births, with a specificity of 79% and positive predictive value of 36%.[57] In contrast, other studies in low- and high-risk pregnancies showed the sensitivity of this stepwise screening for IUGR (defined as birthweight lower than the 10th percentile) to be only 15% to 26%, whereas the positive predictive value was only in the range of 50%.[58,59] The sensitivity of schemes for the antenatal diagnosis of small fetuses is significantly better if clinical risk factors are taken into account.[59]

Serial ultrasound examinations have been shown to be superior to physical examination for diagnosing insufficient growth.[60] For this reason, some European countries have established formal policies requiring a third-trimester

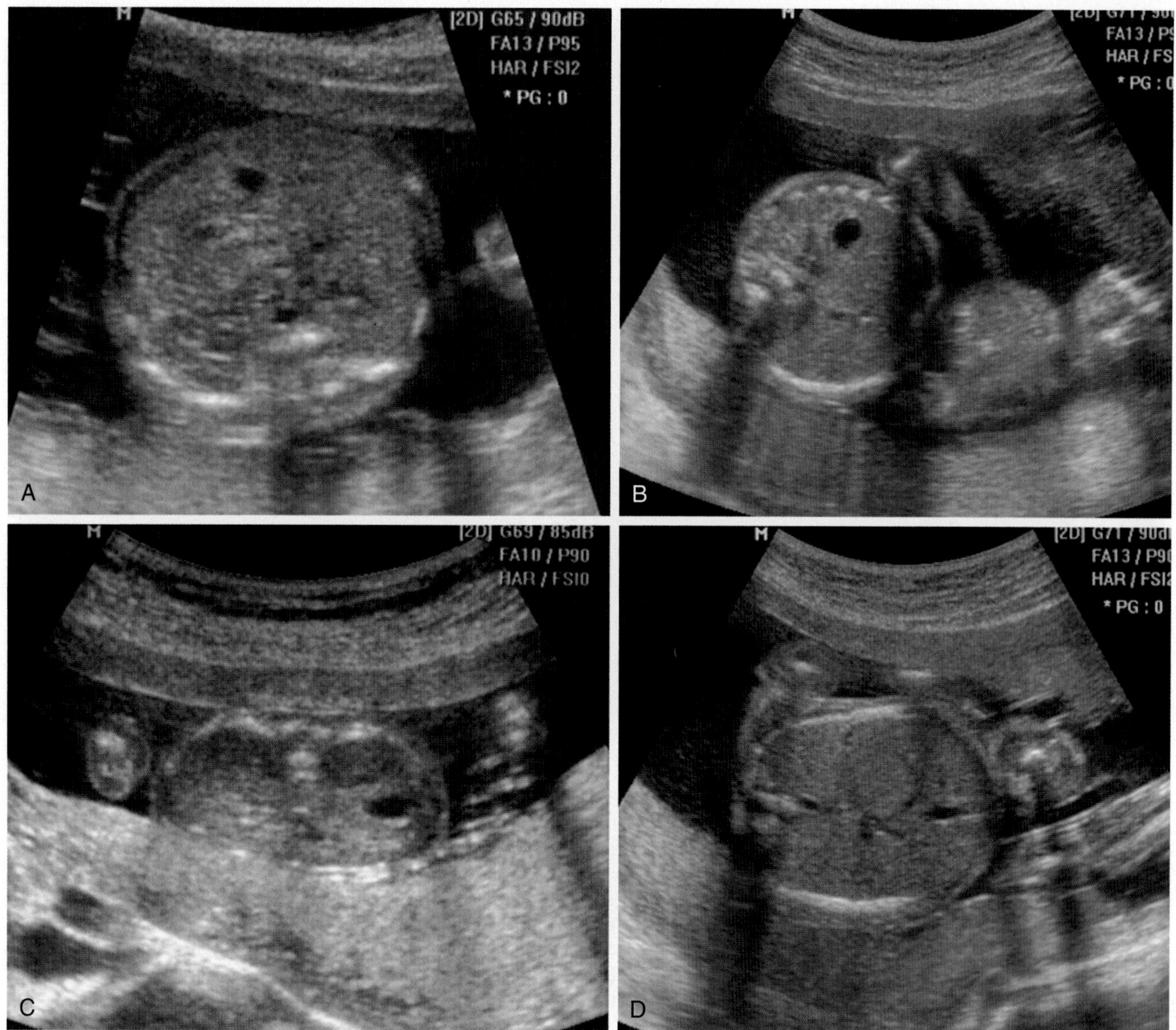

FIGURE 9-31. Examples of abdominal views that are inappropriate for abdominal circumference measurements. **A,** This true axial image is too low on the abdomen. The umbilical vein is seen close to the anterior abdominal wall. **B,** This is an oblique cut through the abdomen. Note the asymmetrical appearance of the ribs. **C,** The abdomen is squashed because the sonographer has applied too much pressure to the maternal abdominal wall. **D,** The transducer is rotated in such as way that an oblong view of the abdomen is obtained. This gives an artificially elongated anterior-posterior dimension.

ultrasound examinations to screen for growth abnormalities, even in low-risk pregnancies. Studies have shown, however, that this policy has little or no impact on perinatal morbidity and mortality.[61,62] **Because of the high cost and unproven benefit of such a screening program, routine ultrasound examinations for growth are generally not a part of prenatal care in the United States.** Because of the high rates of morbidity associated with growth restriction, it is still accepted that **ultrasound should be ordered when clinical examination is suspicious and when there are significant risk factors for a growth abnormality.** Such risk factors include diabetes, maternal hypertension, previous small or large baby, multiple gestation, or poor maternal weight gain. A risk-based approach is particularly appropriate in cases such as multiple gestation or marked maternal obesity, in which clinical evaluation of fetal size is difficult or impossible.

Estimating Fetal Weight

A large number of formulas for calculating the estimated fetal weight (EFW) have been proposed. The most popular of these have been compiled in a review by Nyberg and colleagues.[63] All incorporate the abdominal circumference because this is the standard measurement most susceptible to the variations in fetal soft tissue mass. Although the abdominal circumference alone is a fairly good marker for detecting abnormal fetal growth, the addition of other standard measurements to estimated weight formulas increases their accuracy.[64] It has been shown that the addition of measurements beyond the standard set (BPD, HC,

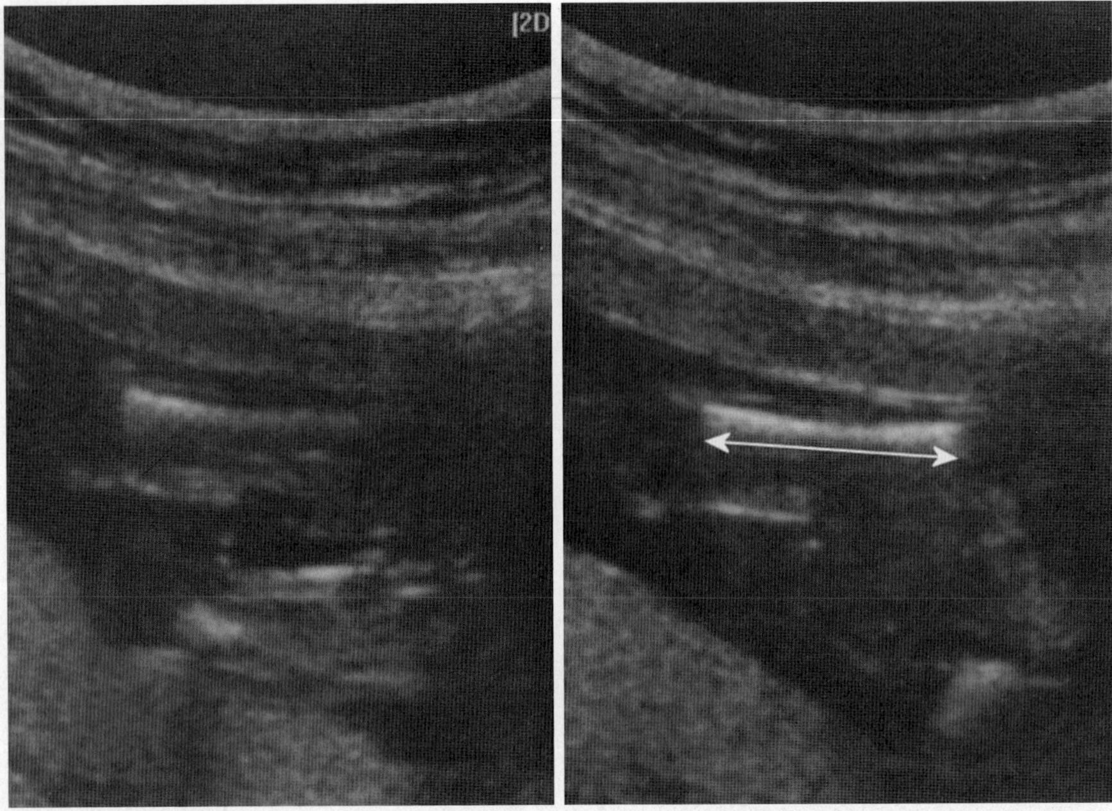

FIGURE 9-32. In the left image, the entire diaphysis of the femur is not clearly shown. This will give an inappropriately short measurement. The ends should be distinct, as shown in the image on the right.

AC, and FL) does not significantly improve weight estimations. It appears that the error inherent in obtaining the basic measurements (especially the AC) is great enough to obscure any refinement in accuracy that might be gained from additional measurements.

Because procedures for standard biometry are well defined, and formulas using these measurements yield seemingly precise weight predictions, some clinicians place more confidence in ultrasound weight estimates than is warranted. There have been a large number of studies in which the accuracy of ultrasound for predicting birthweight has been evaluated.[63,65] It has been claimed in some publications that one formula is better than another when statistically significant differences in accuracy are seen. **However, the differences in accuracy are usually of limited clinical significance, and no formula has been consistently shown to be superior to another.**[65] When scans are done by well-trained sonographers, most studies show a mean absolute error in birthweight prediction of about 8% to 10% of the birthweight. Perhaps a more telling statistic is that in about 30% of cases, the absolute error in estimated weight is greater than 10% of the birthweight. In most of the remaining cases, the error is less than 20% of the birthweight. The rate of clinically significant errors is greater if an inexperienced person performs the ultrasound examination.[66]

It is often assumed that ultrasound is more objective than clinical examination and therefore that ultrasound estimates of fetal weight are more reliable. Most studies have not shown this to be true. In a review by Sherman of 12 studies in which ultrasound was compared with clinical examination for weight estimation, ultrasound was shown to be clearly superior in only one; this involved a subgroup of patients in which the birthweight was less than 2500 g. In three studies, clinical estimates were superior, and in the remaining eight, the two methods either were equivalent or had mixed results depending on the specific formula used.[65] One small study showed that the estimate by the patient was only marginally less accurate than an ultrasound estimate.[66]

There have been several strategies aimed at improving the performance of ultrasound for estimating fetal weight. One is to develop formulas based on subpopulations of fetuses, such as those who are preterm or are thought to be small or large for gestational age. Although this approach seems reasonable, most studies have not shown an improvement in the accuracy of weight estimates compared with traditional "one-size-fits-all" formulas.[67]

Diagnosing Abnormal Growth

The most accepted way of diagnosing abnormal growth in a fetus is to calculate the EFW using standard ultrasound measurements, then to compare the estimated weight with an accepted standard. Some tables still in use were based on the birthweight distribution at different gestational ages of children born in the 1960s or 1970s.[68] Kramer questioned the reliability of these and many subsequent studies. Problems he identified were that patients often had an unconfirmed gestational age, infants were included with implausible birthweight, there was insufficient sample size at low gestational ages, the samples were not population based, and the studies used inadequate statistical modeling techniques. He and his colleagues published sex-specific growth standards that avoided these problems.[69]

If the EFW is less than the 10th or greater than the 90th percentile, the fetus is said to be small or large for the gestational age. Defining abnormal growth using these percentile cut-offs includes many babies who are healthy and are constitutionally large or small. Using a more restrictive definition such as a birthweight less than the 3rd or greater than the 97th percentile is much more predictive of a poor neonatal outcome. Of course, with this approach, many less severely affected fetuses are not detected. Additionally, some infants have a birthweight within the normal range but have not grown to their genetic potential. For this reason, some have argued that individual birthweight percentile limits that incorporate such characteristics as maternal weight, height, ethnic group, parity, and fetal sex should be used.[70] Claussen and colleagues found that about one fourth of fetuses judged to be abnormally small using conventional limits were within normal limits with adjusted percentiles. Conversely, one fourth of babies identified as small or large with adjusted percentiles would have been missed by conventional assessment. In another study from the same institution, it was demonstrated that the risk for stillbirth, neonatal death, and low Apgar scores can be better predicted by the customized weight percentiles.[71]

In 1977, Campbell and colleagues described the HC/AC ratio as a useful marker for detecting fetal growth restriction.[72] This is based on the observation that growth of the soft tissues in the fetal abdomen is more likely to be compromised than the head when there is nutritional deprivation. This understanding led to the concept that asymmetrical growth restriction is virtually pathognomonic for nutritional deprivation, whereas symmetrical growth restriction signifies an underlying condition such as aneuploidy. This categorization has some utility, but it should be recognized that **there is a great deal of overlap between body ratios of fetuses that are growth restricted from either nutritional or intrinsic factors.** However, because a very high HC/AC ratio is uncommon in normal fetuses, a **high HC/AC ratio points away from constitutional smallness.**[73] Additionally, it has been shown in newborns that a low weight-to-length ratio is associated with an increase in several markers of morbidity even if the birthweight is greater than the 10th percentile; perhaps indicating these infants also experienced growth restriction.[74] Currently, there is no consensus concerning the level of surveillance appropriate for a fetus with a high HC/AC ratio but normal estimated weight.

When a patient presents late for prenatal care and the gestational age is uncertain, diagnosis of a growth disorder is particularly difficult. In these cases, a high or low HC/AC ratio can raise the suspicion of a growth disorder. Other ultrasound findings may be useful to help confirm the suspicion. For example, IUGR is often associated with oligohydramnios, abnormal Doppler flow studies, or an abnormal-appearing placenta. Macrosomic fetuses may demonstrate obviously thickened subcutaneous fat pads. In suspected cases, as long as the fetus is stable, serial ultrasound examinations to evaluate growth are appropriate. The rate of growth can be valuable for predicting adverse outcome. Formulas defining rates of normal growth have been published, but most clinicians rely on an observation of progressively increasing or decreasing weight percentiles to evaluate the severity of an ongoing growth disorder.

It has been hoped by many that ultrasound could aid in the difficult decisions faced by obstetricians when macrosomia is suspected. One of the most feared complications in obstetrics is shoulder dystocia because it can lead to permanent neurologic injury in the fetus. **Unfortunately, ultrasound for fetal weight estimation has proved to be of limited usefulness for the prevention of shoulder dystocia and other complications associated with fetal macrosomia.** A study by Gonen and colleagues demonstrated several explanations for this.[75] In a review of 4480 deliveries, only 17% of infants weighing over 4500 grams were detected by an ultrasound ordered because of a clinical suspicion of macrosomia. Only 1 of the 23 infants who weighed over 4500 grams had a brachial plexus injury. Additionally, 93% of infants who had shoulder dystocia weighed less than 4500 grams. For these reasons, these and other authors have concluded that most cases of injury resulting from shoulder dystocia cannot be predicted by ultrasound, and that if cesarean delivery were routinely performed when macrosomia was suspected, the cesarean rate would be increased with very little benefit.

SAFETY OF ULTRASOUND

Ever since diagnostic ultrasound was introduced for clinical use, attention has appropriately been given to ensuring its safety. It has been recognized that the energy from sound waves is converted into heat as sound waves are attenuated. Mechanical energy from the sound waves can cause the formation of microbubbles, resulting in a phenomenon called *cavitation*. Because cavitation occurs only under high ultrasound intensities in areas in which air is present, it is not of significant concern with diagnostic ultrasound of the fetus.

Quantifying Machine Power Output

As of 1976, trials had indicated that there were no clinically significant biologic effects from diagnostic ultrasound. It was subsequently recognized that it would be impractical to repeat safety studies for each new generation of ultrasound machines, operating with different modalities and power outputs. The U.S. Food and Drug Administration (FDA) decided that approval for equipment marketed after 1976 would require acoustic outputs less than that of equipment that existed at that time, which was 94 mW/cm^2 spatial-peak temporal-average (SPTA). However, it has become apparent that improvements in ultrasound imaging could be obtained with higher power levels than was allowed under this regulation. The FDA agreed to relax this standard if machines provided users with real-time information that indicated the potential for fetal harm from the higher power outputs now allowed. An *output display standard* was adopted, which showed the required information on the ultrasound monitor. The numbers that are pertinent to users of obstetrical ultrasound are the TIs and TIb values, which are the thermal indices for ultrasound in soft tissues and bone, respectively. The thermal index denotes the potential for increasing the temperature of tissue that is being insonated with that power output. It is determined by the settings and ultrasound modalities that are being used. A TI of 1.0 indicates that the temperature of the tissue may be increased by 1° C. Because there is little bone formation in the first trimester, the TIs is more relevant. Later in pregnancy, as ossification occurs, sounds waves have a greater impact on bone, so the TIb becomes more important. If the output display standard is followed, the new regulations allow the ultrasound intensity to be as high as 720 mW/cm^2. Machines that do not have the output display still must operate with a maximal sound intensity of less than 94 mW/cm^2.[76]

A 2008 official statement from the AIUM on ultrasound bioeffects states that no effects have been observed from unfocused beam SPTA intensities below 100 mW/cm^2, or thermal index values of less than 2.[77] In 2009, the World Health Organization sponsored a systematic review and meta-analysis to evaluate the safety of human exposure to ultrasonography in pregnancy. This study showed no adverse maternal or perinatal effects, impaired physical or neurologic development, increased risk for malignancy in childhood, subnormal intellectual performance, or mental diseases. **This analysis concluded that according to the available evidence, exposure to diagnostic ultrasonography during pregnancy appears to be safe.**[78] Taking into account the many studies that have been done to date, an official statement from the AIUM on prudent use and clinical safety states, "No independently confirmed adverse effects caused by exposure from present diagnostic ultrasound instruments have been reported in human patients in the absence of contrast agents."[79] **Nevertheless, researchers in the field caution about the possibility that unrecognized harm exists. For this reason, the AIUM position remains that ultrasound should be used by qualified health professionals to provide medical benefit to the patient. In another official statement, the AIUM propounds the ALARA principle (as low as reasonably achievable).**[80] This means that the potential benefits and risks of each examination should be considered, and equipment controls should be adjusted to reduce as much as the possible the acoustical output from the transducer.

In general, ultrasound energy and the potential for temperature elevation become progressively greater from B-mode to color Doppler to spectral Doppler. For this reason, M-mode ultrasound is preferred for documenting fetal viability in the first trimester[81] (see Figure 9-10). However, Doppler modes should be used liberally to confirm fetal death.

"Entertainment" Ultrasound Examinations

It has been proposed that natural-appearing 3-D ultrasound images of the fetus could improve patient-fetal bonding. Given the recognized importance of maternal-child bonding immediately postpartum, it seems reasonable that extending this bonding experience into the fetal period could be beneficial. However, **a psychological benefit of viewing fetal photos has not been proven, and obtaining such images largely remains in the realm of "entertainment."**

The use of ultrasound for nondiagnostic purposes has been condemned by the AIUM and the ACOG.[79,81,82] Concerns that were raised in their policy statements include possible adverse bioeffects of ultrasound energy, the possibility that an examination could give false reassurance to women, and the fact that abnormalities may be detected in settings where personnel are not prepared to discuss and provide follow-up for concerning findings. The 2007 statement by the AIUM regarding the prudent use of ultrasound in obstetrics states: **"The AIUM advocates the responsible use of diagnostic ultrasound and strongly discourages the non-medical use of ultrasound for entertainment purposes.** The use of ultrasound without a medical indication to view the fetus, obtain a picture of the fetus or determine the fetal gender is inappropriate and contrary to responsible medical practice. Ultrasound should be used by qualified health professionals to provide medical benefit to the patient."[79]

KEY POINTS

- Sonographers should become familiar with basic physics of ultrasound, equipment controls, and scanning techniques to optimize ultrasound images.
- All of the elements of the standard obstetrical ultrasound examination are important for clinical management and should not be neglected.
- Because most birth defects occur in fetuses of low-risk women, all standard examinations should include a full anatomic survey.
- Limited obstetrical ultrasound examinations are only appropriate when a complete standard examination has previously been performed.
- Physicians performing and interpreting obstetrical ultrasound examinations should have appropriate training and experience.
- Appropriate documentation of ultrasound studies is important for good medical care.
- There is evidence that a dating ultrasound performed before 22 weeks' gestation may be more accurate than menstrual dates. Beyond this time, variability in fetal size grows considerably, and ultrasound prediction of gestational age becomes progressively less accurate.
- Clinical estimate of fetal weight is as accurate as an ultrasound estimate. Ultrasound for fetal weight estimation is of limited usefulness for the prevention of shoulder dystocia and other complications associated with fetal macrosomia.
- Exposure to diagnostic ultrasonography during pregnancy appears to be safe for the fetus.
- Ultrasound should be used by qualified health professionals to provide medical benefit to the patient. Because of the possibility of unrecognized harm, exposing the fetus to ultrasound should follow the ALARA (as low as reasonably achievable) principle.
- The AIUM and ACOG strongly discourage the non-medical use of ultrasound for entertainment purposes.

REFERENCES

1. Ramos GA, Ylagan MV, Romine LE, et al: Diagnostic evaluation of the fetal face using 3-dimensional ultrasound. Ultrasound Q 24:215, 2008.
2. Clementschitsch G, Hasenöhrl G, Schaffer H, et al: Comparison between two- and three-dimensional ultrasound measurements of nuchal translucency. Ultrasound Obstet Gynecol 18:475, 2001.
3. American College of Obstetricians and Gynecologists. ACOG Practice Bulletin No. 101: ultrasonography in pregnancy. Obstet Gynecol 113:451, 2009.
4. Michailidis GD, Simpson JM, Karidas C, et al: Detailed three-dimensional fetal echocardiography facilitated by an Internet link. Ultrasound Obstet Gynecol 18:325, 2001.
5. Ruano R, Aubry MC, Barthe B, et al: Ipsilateral lung volumes assessed by three-dimensional ultrasonography in fetuses with isolated congenital diaphragmatic hernia. Fetal Diagn Ther 24:389, 2008.
6. Lee W, Deter RL, Ebersole JD, et al: Birth weight prediction by three-dimensional ultrasonography: fractional limb volume. J Ultrasound Med 20:1283, 2001.
7. Laboda LA, Estroff JA, Benacerraf BR: First trimester bradycardia: a sign of impending fetal loss. J Ultrasound Med 8:561, 1989.
8. Blaas HG, Eik-Nes SH, Kiserud T, et al: Early development of the abdominal wall, stomach and heart from 7 to 12 weeks of gestation: a longitudinal ultrasound study. Ultrasound Obstet Gynecol 6:240, 1995.
9. Haak MC, Twisk JW, Van Vugt JM: How successful is fetal echocardiographic examination in the first trimester of pregnancy? Ultrasound Obstet Gynecol 20:9, 2002.
10. Tongsong T, Srisomboon J, Wanapirak C, et al: Pregnancy outcome of threatened abortion with demonstrable fetal cardiac activity: a cohort study. J Obstet Gynaecol 21:331, 1995.
11. Smith KE, Buyalos RP: The profound impact of patient age on pregnancy outcome after early detection of fetal cardiac activity. Fertil Steril 65:35, 1996.
12. Maso G, D'Ottavio G, De Seta F, et al: First-trimester intrauterine hematoma and outcome of pregnancy. Obstet Gynecol 105:339, 2005.
13. Tongsong T, Wanapirak C, Srisomboon J, et al: Transvaginal ultrasound in threatened abortions with empty gestational sacs. Int J Gynaecol Obstet 46:297, 1994.
14. Pennell RG, Needleman L, Pajak T, et al: Prospective comparison of vaginal and abdominal sonography in normal early pregnancy. J Ultrasound Med 10:63, 1991.
15. Stampone C, Nicotra M, Muttinelli C, et al: Transvaginal sonography of the yolk sac in normal and abnormal pregnancy. J Clin Ultrasound 24:3, 1996.
16. Rowling SE, Coleman BG, Langer JE, et al: First-trimester US parameters of failed pregnancy. Radiology 203:211, 1997.
17. Nicolaides KH: Nuchal translucency and other first-trimester sonographic markers of chromosomal abnormalities. Am J Obstet Gynecol 191:45, 2004.
18. American Institute of Ultrasound in Medicine: AIUM Practice Guideline for the performance of an antepartum obstetric ultrasound examination. J Ultrasound Med 22:1116, 2003.
19. American Institute of Ultrasound in Medicine: AIUM Training Guidelines for Physicians Who Evaluate and Interpret Diagnostic Ultrasound Examinations. Approved November 6, 2010.
20. Hack KE, Derks JB, Elias SG, et al: Increased perinatal mortality and morbidity in monochorionic versus dichorionic twin pregnancies: clinical implications of a large Dutch cohort study. BJOG 115:58, 2008.
21. Rozenberg P, Porcher R, Salomon LJ, et al: Comparison of the learning curves of digital examination and transabdominal sonography for the determination of fetal head position during labor. Ultrasound Obstet Gynecol 31:332, 2008.
22. Rutherford SE, Phelan JP, Smith CV, Jacobs N: The four-quadrant assessment of amniotic fluid volume: an adjunct to antepartum fetal heart rate testing. Obstet Gynecol 70:353, 1987.
23. Moore TR, Cayle JE: The amniotic fluid index in normal human pregnancy. Am J Obstet Gynecol 162:1168, 1990.
24. Magann EF, Perry KG Jr, Chauhan SP, et al: The accuracy of ultrasound evaluation of amniotic fluid volume in singleton pregnancies: the effect of operator experience and ultrasound interpretative technique. J Clin Ultrasound 25:249, 1997.
25. Thomas IT, Smith DW: Oligohydramnios, cause of the nonrenal features of Potter's syndrome, including pulmonary hypoplasia. J Pediatr 84:811, 1974.
26. Chamberlain PF, Manning FA, Morrison I, et al: Ultrasound evaluation of amniotic fluid volume. I. The relationship of marginal and decreased amniotic fluid volumes to perinatal outcome. Am J Obstet Gynecol 150:245, 1984.
27. Ott WJ: Reevaluation of the relationship between amniotic fluid volume and perinatal outcome. Am J Obstet Gynecol 192:1803, 2005.
28. Chauhan SP, Sanderson M, Hendrix NW, et al: Perinatal outcome and amniotic fluid index in the antepartum and intrapartum periods: a meta-analysis. Am J Obstet Gynecol 181:1473, 1999.
29. Leerentveld RA, Gilberts EC, Arnold MJ, et al: Accuracy and safety of transvaginal sonographic placental localization. Obstet Gynecol 76:759, 1990.
30. Oppenheimer LW, Farine D, Ritchie JW, et al: What is a low-lying placenta? Am J Obstet Gynecol 165:1036, 1991.
31. Taipale P, Hiilesmaa V, Ylöstalo P: Transvaginal ultrasonography at 18-23 weeks in predicting placenta previa at delivery. Ultrasound Obstet Gynecol 12:422, 1998.
32. Dashe JS, McIntire DD, Ramus RM, et al: Persistence of placenta previa according to gestational age at ultrasound detection. Obstet Gynecol 99:692, 2002.
33. Oyelese Y, Catanzarite V, Prefumo F, et al: Vasa previa: the impact of prenatal diagnosis on outcomes. Obstet Gynecol 103:937, 2004.
34. Fisteag-Kiprono L, Neiger R, Sonek JD, et al: Perinatal outcome associated with sonographically detected globular placenta. J Reprod Med 51:563, 2006.
35. Hua M, Odibo AO, Macones GA, et al: Single umbilical artery and its associated findings. Obstet Gynecol 115:930,2010.
36. Stout MJ, Odibo AO, Graseck AS, et al: Leiomyomas at routine second-trimester ultrasound examination and adverse obstetric outcomes. Obstet Gynecol 116:1056, 2010.
37. Rosati P, Exacoustòs C, Mancuso S: Longitudinal evaluation of uterine myoma growth during pregnancy: a sonographic study. J Ultrasound Med 11:511, 1992.
38. Neiger R, Sonek JD, Croom CS, Ventolini G: Pregnancy-related changes in the size of uterine leiomyomas. J Reprod Med 51:671, 2006.
39. Shalev J, Blankstein J, Mashiach R, et al: Sonographic visualization of normal-size ovaries during pregnancy. Ultrasound Obstet Gynecol 15:523, 2000.
40. VanDorsten JP, Hulsey TC, Newman RB, et al: Fetal anomaly detection by second-trimester ultrasonography in a tertiary center. Am J Obstet Gynecol 178:742, 1998.
41. Donald I, Abdulla U: Ultrasonics in obstetrics and gynaecology. Br J Radiol 40:604, 1967.
42. Robinson HP, Fleming JEE: A critical evaluation of sonar "crown-rump length" measurements. Br J Obstet Gynecol 82:702, 1975.
43. Hadlock FP, Shah YP, Kanon DJ, et al: Fetal crown rump length: reevaluation of relation to menstrual age (5-18 weeks) with high-resolution real-time US. Radiology 182:501, 1992.
44. Queenan JT, O'Brien GD, Campbell S: Ultrasound measurement of fetal limb bones. Am J Obstet Gynecol 138:297, 1980.
45. Hellman LM, Koboyashi M, Fillisti L, et al: Growth and development of the human fetus prior to the twentieth week of gestation. Am J Obstet Gynecol 103:789, 1969.
46. Nyberg DA, Abuhamad A, Ville Y: Ultrasound assessment of abnormal fetal growth. Semin Perinatol 28:3, 2004.
47. Robinson HP: Gestational age determination: first trimester. In Chervenak FA, Isaacson GC, Campbell S: Ultrasound in Obstetrics and Gynecology, Boston, Little, Brown, 1993, p 295.
48. Schats R, Van Os HC, Jansen CA, et al: The crown-rump length in early human pregnancy: a reappraisal. BJOG 98:460, 1991.
49. MacGregor SN, Tamura RK, Sabbagha RE, et al: Underestimation of gestational age by conventional crown rump length dating curves. Obstet Gynecol 70:344, 1987.
50. Hadlock FP, Harrist RB, Martinez-Poyer J: How accurate is second trimester fetal dating? J Ultrasound Med 10:557, 1991.
51. Degani S: Fetal biometry: clinical, pathological, and technical considerations. Obstet Gynecol Surv 56:159, 2001.
52. Chervenak FA, Skupski DW, Romero R, et al: How accurate is fetal biometry in the assessment of fetal age? Am J Obstet Gynecol 178:678, 1998.

53. Mongelli M, Wilcox M, Gardosi J: Estimating the date of confinement: ultrasonographic biometry versus certain menstrual dates. Am J Obstet Gynecol 174:278, 1996.
54. Savitz DA, Terry JW Jr, Dole N, et al: Comparison of pregnancy dating by last menstrual period, ultrasound scanning, and their combination. Am J Obstet Gynecol 187:1660, 2002.
55. Rahim RR, Cuckle HS, Sehmi IK, et al: Compromise ultrasound dating policy in maternal serum screening for Down syndrome. Prenat Diagn 22:1181, 2002.
56. Bergsjo P, Villar J: Scientific basis for the content of routine antenatal care. II. Power to eliminate or alleviate adverse newborn outcomes: some special conditions and examinations. Acta Obstet Gynecol Scand 76:15, 1997.
57. Pearce JM, Campbell S: A comparison of symphysis-fundal height and ultrasound as screening tests for light-for-gestational age infants. Br J Obstet Gynaecol 94:100, 1987.
58. Hepburn M, Rosenberg K: An audit of the detection and management of small-for-gestational age babies. BJOG 93:212, 1986.
59. Bais JM, Eskes M, Pel M, et al: Effectiveness of detection of intrauterine growth retardation by abdominal palpation as screening test in a low risk population: an observational study. Eur J Obstet Gynecol Reprod Biol 116:164, 2004.
60. Harding K, Evans S, Newnham J: Screening for the small fetus: a study of the relative efficacies of ultrasound biometry and symphysiofundal height. Aust N Z J Obstet Gynaecol 35:160, 1995.
61. Jahn A, Razum O, Berle P: Routine screening for intrauterine growth retardation in Germany: low sensitivity and questionable benefit for diagnosed cases. Acta Obstet Gynecol Scand 77:643, 1998.
62. Bricker L, Neilson JP: Routine ultrasound in late pregnancy (after 24 weeks gestation). Cochrane Database Syst Rev 2:CD001451, 2000.
63. Nyberg DA, Abuhamad A, Ville Y: Ultrasound assessment of abnormal fetal growth. Semin Perinatol 23:3, 2004.
64. Hadlock F: Evaluation of fetal weight estimation procedures. In Deter R, Harist R, Birnholz J, et al: Quantitative Obstetrical Ultrasonography, New York, Wiley, 1986, p 113.
65. Sherman DJ, Arieli S, Tovbin J, et al: A comparison of clinical and ultrasound estimation of fetal weight. Obstet Gynecol 91:212, 1998.
66. Baum JD, Gussman D, Wirth JC 3rd: Clinical and patient estimation of fetal weight vs. ultrasound estimation. J Reprod Med 47:194, 2002.
67. Robson SC, Gallivan S, Walkinshaw SA, et al: Ultrasonic estimation of fetal weight: use of targeted formulas in small for gestational age fetuses. Obstet Gynecol 82:359, 1993.
68. Brenner WE, Edelman DA, Hendricks CH: A standard of fetal growth for the United States of America. Am J Obstet Gynecol 126:555, 1976.
69. Kramer MS, Platt RW, Wen SW, et al: A new and improved population-based Canadian reference for birth weight for gestational age. Fetal/Infant Health Study Group of the Canadian Perinatal Surveillance System. Pediatrics 108:E35, 2001.
70. Gardosi J, Chang A, Kalyan B, et al: Customised antenatal growth charts. Lancet 339:283, 1992.
71. Clausson B, Gardosi J, Francis A, et al: Perinatal outcome in SGA births defined by customised versus population-based birthweight standards. Br J Obstet Gynecol 108:830, 2001.
72. Campbell S, Thoms A: Ultrasound measurement of fetal head to abdomen circumference ratio in the assessment of growth retardation. BJOG 84:165, 1977.
73. David C, Gabrielli S, Pilu G, et al: The head-to-abdomen circumference ratio: a reappraisal. Ultrasound Obstet Gynecol 5:256, 1995.
74. Williams MC, O'Brien WF: A comparison of birth weight and weight/length ratio for gestation as correlates of perinatal morbidity. J Perinatol 17:346, 1997.
75. Gonen R, Spiegel D, Abend M: Is macrosomia predictable, and are shoulder dystocia and birth trauma preventable? Obstet Gynecol 88:526, 1996.
76. Nyborg WL: History of the American Institute of Ultrasound in Medicine's efforts to keep ultrasound safe. J Ultrasound Med 22:1293, 2003.
77. American Institute of Ultrasound Medicine: Official Statement, Mammalian In Vivo Ultrasonic Biological Effects. Approved November 8, 2008.
78. Torloni MR, Vedmedovska N, Merialdi M, et al, for the ISUOG-WHO Fetal Growth Study Group: Safety of ultrasonography in pregnancy: WHO systematic review of the literature and meta-analysis. Ultrasound Obstet Gynecol 33:599, 2009.
79. American Institute of Ultrasound in Medicine: Official Statement, Prudent Use and Clinical Safety, American Institute of Ultrasound in Medicine, March 2007.
80. American Institute of Ultrasound in Medicine. Official Statement, As Low As Reasonably Achievable (ALARA) Principle. Approved March 16, 2008.
81. Fowlkes JB, for the Bioeffects Committee of the American Institute of Ultrasound in Medicine: American Institute of Ultrasound in Medicine consensus report on potential bioeffects of diagnostic ultrasound: executive summary. J Ultrasound Med 27:503, 2008.
82. American College of Obstetricians and Gynecologists: Nonmedical use of obstetric ultrasound. ACOG Committee Opinion No. 297. Obstet Gynecol 104:423, 2004.

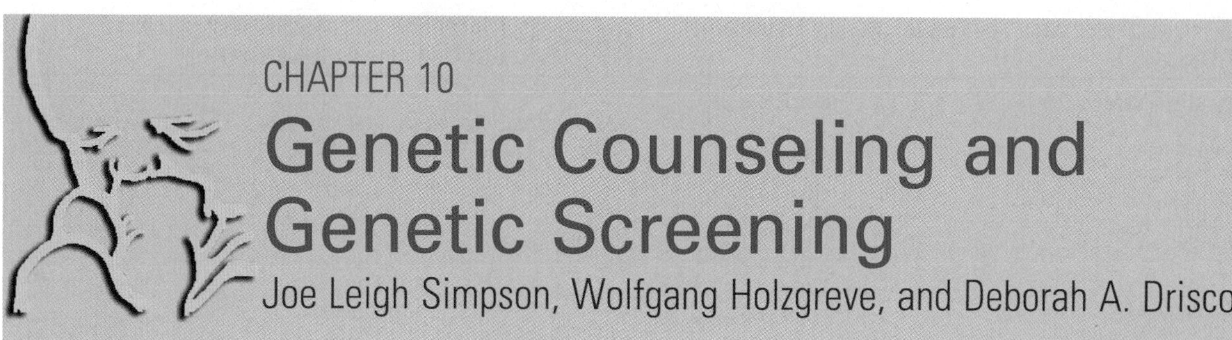

CHAPTER 10

Genetic Counseling and Genetic Screening

Joe Leigh Simpson, Wolfgang Holzgreve, and Deborah A. Driscoll

KEY ABBREVIATIONS	
Alpha-Fetoprotein	AFP
American College of Medical Genetics	ACMG
American College of Obstetricians and Gynecologists	ACOG
Biochemistry, Ultrasound, Nuchal Translucency	BUN
Congenital Bilateral Absence of the Vas Deferens	CBAVD
Cystic Fibrosis	CF
Cystic Fibrosis Transmembrane Conductance Regulator	CFTR
Deoxyribonucleic Acid	DNA
First and Second Trimester Evaluation of Risk	FASTER
Gap Junction B	GJB
Health Resources and Services Administration	HRSA
Intelligence Quotient	IQ
International Standards for Cytogenomic Array	ISCA
Mean Corpuscular Volume	MCV
Nasal Bone	NB
Nuchal Translucency	NT
Unconjugated Estriol	uE_3
Uniparental Disomy	UPD

Genetic counseling and screening for common inherited conditions, chromosomal abnormalities, and congenital defects are an integral part of routine obstetrical care. Approximately 3% of liveborn infants have a major congenital anomaly. About one half of these anomalies are detected at birth; the remainder become evident later during childhood or, less often, during adult life. Although nongenetic factors may cause malformations, genetic factors are usually responsible. In addition, more than 50% of first trimester spontaneous abortions and at least 5% of stillborn infants exhibit chromosomal abnormalities (see Chapter 26). In this chapter we focus on identifying pregnancies in which the couple is at increased risk for abnormal offspring compared to the general population. We review the principles of genetic counseling, common chromosome abnormalities including aneuploidy, and the value of screening for selected single-gene disorders and neural tube defects. Screening the general population to identify at-risk individuals can be followed by definitive diagnosis, using genetic approaches and ultrasound examination covered in Chapter 11.

FREQUENCY AND ETIOLOGY OF GENETIC DISEASE

Phenotypic variation—normal or abnormal—may be considered in terms of several etiologic categories: (1) chromosomal abnormalities, numeric or structural; (2) single-gene or mendelian disorders; (3) polygenic and multifactorial disorders, polygenic implying an etiology resulting from cumulative effects of more than one gene and multifactorial implying interaction as well with environmental factors; and (4) teratogenic disorders, caused by exposure to exogenous factors (e.g., drugs) that deleteriously affect an embryo otherwise destined to develop normally. Principles of these mechanisms are reviewed elsewhere in detail.[1]

Chromosomal Abnormalities

The incidence of chromosomal aberrations is 1 in 160 newborns. Table 10-1 shows the incidence of individual abnormalities.[2] The chromosomal abnormalities that generate the greatest attention are the autosomal trisomies. Autosomal trisomy usually arises as a result of abnormalities of

TABLE 10-1 Chromosomal Abnormalities in Newborn Infants

TYPE OF ABNORMALITY	INCIDENCE
Numeric aberrations	
Sex chromosomes	
• 47,XYY	1/1000 MB
• 47,XXY	1/1000 MB
• Other (men)	1/1350 MB
• 47,X	1/10,000 FB
• 47,XXX	1/1000 FB
• Other (females)	1/2700 FB
Autosomes	
Trisomies	
• 13-15 (D group)	1/20,000 LB
• 16-18 (E group)	1/8000 LB
• 21-22 (G group)	1/800 LB
• Other	1/50,000 LB
Structural aberrations	
Balanced	
Robertsonian	
• T(Dq; Dq)	1/1500 LB
• T(Dq; Gq)	1/5000 LB
Reciprocal translocations and insertional inversions	1/7000 LB
Unbalanced	
Robertsonian	1/14,000 LB
Reciprocal translocations and insertional inversions	1/8000 LB
Inversions	1/50,000 LB
Deletions	1/10,000 LB
Supernumeraries	1/5000 LB
Other	1/8000 LB
Total	1/160 LB

Data from Hook EB, Hamerton JL: The frequency of chromosome abnormalities detected in consecutive newborn studies: differences between studies-results by sex and by severity of phenotype involvement. *In* Hook EB, Porter IH (eds): Population Cytogenetic Studies in Humans. New York, Academic Press, 1977, p 63.

FB, Female births; *LB*, live births; *MB*, male births.

TABLE 10-2 Maternal Age and Chromosomal Abnormalities (Live Births)*

MATERNAL AGE	RISK FOR DOWN SYNDROME	RISK FOR ANY CHROMOSOME ABNORMALITIES
20	1/1667	1/526†
21	1/1667	1/526†
22	1/1429	1/500†
23	1/1429	1/500†
24	1/1250	1/476†
25	1/1250	1/476†
26	1/1176	1/476†
27	1/1111	1/455†
28	1/1053	1/435†
29	1/1100	1/417†
30	1/952	1/384†
31	1/909	1/385†
32	1/769	1/322†
33	1/625	1/317†
34	1/500	1/260
35	1/385	1/204
36	1/294	1/164
37	1/227	1/130
38	1/175	1/103
39	1/137	1/82
40	1/106	1/65
41	1/82	1/51
42	1/64	1/40
43	1/50	1/32
44	1/38	1/25
45	1/30	1/20
46	1/23	1/15
47	1/18	1/12
48	1/14	1/10
49	1/11	1/7

Data from Hook EB: Rates of chromosome abnormalities at different maternal ages. Obstet Gynecol 58:282, 1981; and Hook EB, Cross PK, Schreinemachers DM: Chromosomal abnormality rates at amniocentesis and in live-born infants. JAMA 249:2034, 1983.

*Because sample size for some intervals is relatively small, confidence limits are sometimes relatively large. Nonetheless, these figures are suitable for genetic counseling.

†47,XXX excluded for ages 20 to 32 (data not available).

meiosis, nondisjunction producing a gamete with 24 rather than the expected 23 chromosomes. This results in a zygote having 47 chromosomes. **This error most commonly occurs during maternal meiosis, and is associated with the well-known maternal age effect.** Table 10-2 shows the year-to-year (maternal age) increase in frequency of Down syndrome and other aneuploidies.[3] Another calculation has shown that the progressive increase with advancing maternal age plateaus around age 45, but this is of relatively little clinical significance.[4] The frequency is about 30% higher in midpregnancy than at term, reflecting lethality throughout pregnancy.[5] Some trisomies, for example, trisomy 16, arise almost exclusively in maternal meiosis, usually maternal meiosis I. For a few chromosomes, there is a relatively higher frequency of errors in meiosis II (e.g., trisomy 18), and in yet others, errors in paternal meiosis are not uncommon (e.g., trisomy 2). Autosomal trisomy can also recur, the recurrence risk being approximately 1% following either trisomy 18 or 21. This suggests that genetic factors perturb meiosis, a phenomenon that serves as justification for offering prenatal genetic screening or testing after one aneuploid conception.

In addition to numeric abnormalities, structural chromosomal abnormalities occur. In a balanced interchange (translocation) between two or more chromosomes, individuals are phenotypically normal. However, such individuals are at increased risk for offspring with unbalanced gametes. This topic is also discussed in Chapter 26 in the context of repeated pregnancy loss. Small, often submicroscopic, deletions and duplications of chromosomal material occur that can result in recognizable syndromes such as the 22q11.2 deletion syndrome.

Single-Gene Disorders

Approximately 1% of liveborn infants are phenotypically abnormal as result of a single-gene mutation. Mendelian or single-gene disorders thus account for 40% of the congenital defects seen in liveborn infants.

The human genome has now been sequenced and shown to contain approximately 22,000 human genes. In addition, posttranscriptional modifications result in perhaps three times as many proteins (gene products). Perturbation of each gene (deoxyribonucleic acid [DNA] sequence) or protein should theoretically result in a mendelian disorder. However, function is known for only a few thousand genes. Moreover, even the most common single-gene disorder is individually rare except in its predominant ethnic group: cystic fibrosis (CF) in whites of European or Ashkenazi Jewish origin; sickle cell anemia in blacks; β-thalassemia in Greeks and Italians; α-thalassemia in Southeast Asians; and Tay-Sachs disease, Canavan disease, and familial dysautonomia in Ashkenazi Jews. Carrier screening for these disorders is discussed later in this chapter.

Polygenic/Multifactorial Disorders

Approximately 1% of neonates are abnormal but have an apparently normal chromosomal complement and have not ostensibly undergone mutation at a *single* genetic locus. It is postulated that several different genes are responsible (polygenic/multifactorial inheritance) and possibly gene-environmental interactions.[1]

Disorders in this etiologic category include most common malformations limited to a single organ system. These include hydrocephaly, anencephaly, and spina bifida (neural tube defects); facial clefts (cleft lip and palate); cardiac defects; pyloric stenosis; omphalocele; hip dislocation; uterine fusion defects; and club foot (Table 10-3). **After the birth of one child with a birth defect involving only one organ system, the recurrence risk in subsequent progeny is 1% to 5%.**[1] This frequency is less than would be expected if only a single gene were responsible but greater than that for the general population. The recurrence risks for malformations are also 1% to 5% for offspring of affected parents. Recurrence risks are similar for both siblings and offspring, which diminishes the likelihood that environmental causes are the exclusive etiologic factor because it is highly unlikely that households in different generations would be exposed to the same teratogen. Further excluding environmental factors as exclusive etiologic agents are observations that monozygotic twins are much more often concordant (similarly affected) than dizygotic twins, despite the fact that both types of twins share a common intrauterine environment.

Teratogenic Disorders

The perhaps 20 proved teratogens are reviewed in Chapter 8. Although many other agents are suspected teratogens, the quantitative contribution of known teratogens to the incidence of anomalies is thought to be relatively small (with the possible exception of alcohol).

TABLE 10-3 POLYGENIC/MULTIFACTORIAL TRAITS*

Hydrocephaly (excepting some forms of aqueductal stenosis and Dandy Walker syndrome)
Neural tube defects (anencephaly, spina bifida, encephalocele)
Cleft lift, with or without cleft plate
Cleft lip (alone)
Cardiac anomalies (most types)
Diaphragmatic hernia
Pyloric stenosis
Omphalocele
Renal agenesis (unilateral or bilateral)
Ureteral anomalies
Posterior urethral values
Hypospadias
Müllerian fusion effects
Müllerian aplasia
Limb reduction defects
Talipes equinovarus (clubfoot)

*Relatively common traits considered to be inherited in polygenic/multifactorial fashion. For each, normal parents have recurrence risks of 1% to 5% after one affected child. After two affected offspring, the risk is higher.

CLINICAL SPECTRUM OF CHROMOSOMAL ABNORMALITIES

A basic fund of knowledge about common chromosomal disorders may be helpful to the obstetrician, who may encounter abnormal fetuses or infants during prenatal genetic studies or at delivery. In this section, we briefly review the clinical and cytogenetic features characteristic of the common numeric chromosomal abnormalities. Standard genetic texts, some geared for the obstetrician-gynecologist,[1] cover the broader spectrum of rare (often mosaic) trisomies and autosomal duplication or deficiency syndromes.

Autosomal Trisomy

Trisomy 21

Trisomy 21 (Down syndrome) is the most frequent autosomal chromosomal syndrome, occurring in 1 of every 800 liveborn infants (see Table 10-1). The relationship of Down syndrome to advanced maternal age is well known (see Table 10-2). Consistent with this maternal age effect, approximately 95% of cases arise in maternal meiosis, usually meiosis I. Characteristic craniofacial features include brachycephaly, oblique palpebral fissures, epicanthal folds, broad nasal bridge, a protruding tongue, and small, low-set ears with an overlapping helix and a prominent antihelix (Figure 10-1). The mean birth weight in Down syndrome, 2900 g, is decreased compared to normal infants but less so than in other autosomal trisomies. At birth, Down syndrome infants are usually hypotonic. Other features include iridial Brushfield spots, broad short fingers (brachymesophalangia), clinodactyly (incurving deflections resulting from an abnormality of the middle phalanx), a single flexion crease on the fifth digit, and an

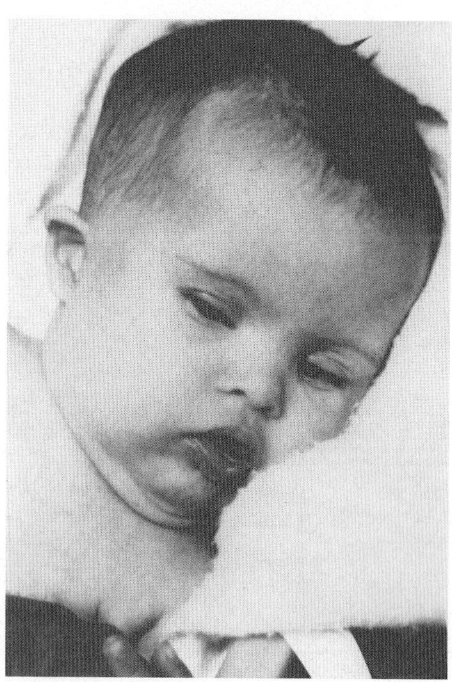

FIGURE 10-1. An infant with trisomy 21. (From Simpson JL, Elias S: Genetics in Obstetrics and Gynecology, ed 3. Philadelphia, WB Saunders, p 24, 2003.)

unusually wide space between the first two toes. A single palmar crease (simian line) is not pathognomonic, being present in only 30% of individuals with trisomy 21 and in 5% of normal individuals. Relatively common anomalies include cardiac defects and duodenal atresia. Cardiac anomalies and increased susceptibility to both respiratory infections and leukemia contribute to reduced life expectancy. However, mean survival extends into the fifth decade.

Individuals with Down syndrome who survive beyond infancy invariably exhibit mental retardation. Mean intelligence quotient (IQ) ranges approximately from 25 to 70. Mosaicism for chromosome 21 should be suspected in Down syndrome individuals with IQs in the 70 to 80 range. Women with Down syndrome are fertile. Although relatively few trisomic mothers have reproduced, about 30% of their offspring are also trisomic. Men are not considered fertile.

Several cytogenetic mechanisms may be associated with Down syndrome. **The cause of Down syndrome is triplication of a small portion of chromosome 21, namely, band q22.** Triplication may be caused either by the presence of an entire additional chromosome 21 or the addition of only band q22. Of all cases of Down syndrome, 95% have primary trisomy (47 instead of the normal 46 chromosomes) (Figure 10-2). It is these cases that show the well-known relationship to both maternal age effect and to errors in maternal meiosis.

Structural chromosomal abnormalities—translocations—show no association to parental age. They may be either sporadic or familial. The translocation most commonly associated with Down syndrome involves chromosomes 14 and 21. With translocation Down syndrome, one parent may have the same translocation (rearrangement), that is, 45,t(14q;21q), referred to as a Robertsonian translocation. Empiric risks are approximately 10% for offspring of female Robertsonian translocation carriers and 2% for offspring of male translocation carriers. A potential concern is that diploid (46,XX or 46,XY) cases actually show uniparental disomy (UPD), both chromosomes originating from the same parent. In 65 Robertsonian translocation carriers [44 t(13q;14q), 11 t(14q;21q), 4 t(14q;22q), 6 others], only 1 UPD case was observed (0.6%).[6] The authors also surveyed 357 inherited and 102 de novo published cases, and concluded overall UPD risk for UPD 14 or 15 was 3%.

Other structural rearrangements resulting in Down syndrome include t(21q;21q), t(21q;21q), and translocations involving chromosome 21 and other acrocentric chromosomes (13 to 15) or G (21 to 22). In t(21q;21q)carriers, normal gametes do not ordinarily form. Thus, only trisomic or monosomic zygotes are produced, the latter presumably appearing as preclinical embryonic losses. Parents having the other translocations have a low empiric risk of having offspring with Down syndrome.

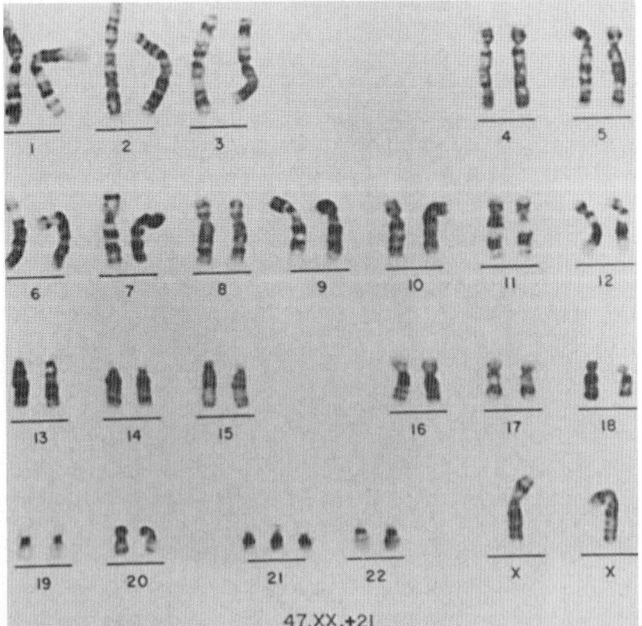

FIGURE 10-2. Karyotype of a trisomy 21 cell. Trypsin-Giemsa (GTG) banding. (From Simpson JL, Elias S: Genetics in Obstetrics and Gynecology, ed 3. Philadelphia, WB Saunders, 2003.)

Trisomy 13

Trisomy 13 occurs in about 1 per 20,000 live births. Intrauterine and postnatal growth restrictions are pronounced, and developmental retardation is severe. Nearly 50% of affected children die in the first month, and relatively few survive past 3 years of age. Characteristic anomalies include holoprosencephaly, eye anomalies (microphthalmia, anophthalmia, or coloboma), cleft lip and palate, polydactyly, cardiac defects, and low birth weight. Other relatively common features include cutaneous scalp defects, hemangiomata on the face or neck, low-set ears with an abnormal helix, and rocker-bottom feet (convex soles and protruding heels).

Trisomy 13 is usually associated with nondisjunctional (primary) trisomy (47,XX,+13 or 47,XY,+13). As in trisomy 21, a maternal age effect exists, and most cases are maternal in origin. Translocations are responsible for less than 20% of cases, invariably associated with two group D (13 to 15) chromosomes joining at their centromeric regions (Robertsonian translocation). If neither parent has a rearrangement, the risk for subsequent affected progeny is not increased. If either parent has a balanced 13q;14q translocation, the recurrence risk for an affected offspring is increased but only to 1% to 2%. The exception is a 13q;13q parental translocation, which carries the same dire prognosis as a 21q;21q translocation.

Trisomy 18

Trisomy 18 occurs in 1 per 8000 live births. Among liveborn infants, girls are affected more often than boys (3:1). Among stillborns and abortuses, however, the sex distribution is more equal.

Facial anomalies characteristic of trisomy 18 include microcephaly, prominent occiput, low-set and pointed "fawn-like" ears, and micrognathia. Skeletal anomalies include overlapping fingers (V over IV, II over III), short sternum, shield chest, narrow pelvis, limited thigh abduction or congenital hip dislocation, rocker-bottom feet with protrusion of the calcaneum, and a short dorsiflexed hallux ("hammer toe"). Cardiac and renal anomalies are common.

Mean birth weight is 2240 g. Fetal movement is feeble, and approximately 50% develop fetal distress during labor.

The mean survival is months. Liveborn infants show pronounced developmental and growth retardation. Trisomy 18 is not uncommonly detected among stillborn infants.

Approximately 80% of trisomy 18 cases are caused by primary nondisjunction (47,XX,+18 or 47,XY,+18). Errors usually arise in maternal meiosis, frequently meiosis II. Recurrence risk is about 1%.

Other Autosomal Trisomies

All autosomes show trisomies, but usually these end in abortuses. In addition to numbers 13, 18, and 21, only a few other trisomies are detected in liveborns (8, 9, 14, 16, and 22), and often in mosaic forms. All cases show mental retardation, various somatic anomalies, and intrauterine growth restriction. The extent of retardation and the spectrum of anomalies vary.

Monosomy has been claimed for trisomy 21,[7] although undetected mosaicism is always difficult to exclude.

Autosomal Deletions or Duplications

Deletions or duplications of portions of autosomal chromosomes also exist. Well-described genetic disorders have been associated with deletions or duplications of chromosomes 4p, 5p, 16q, 17p, 15q, 16p, 20p, and 22q. Specific clinical features vary, but may include learning difficulties, mental retardation, neurologic and behavioral disorders, psychiatric disorders, and various congenital anomalies.

If a chromosomal deletion or duplication is detected, a parental chromosomal rearrangement should be suspected. If a parent has a balanced translocation, duplication or inversion risks are increased in subsequent pregnancies as discussed in Chapter 11.

Availability of chromosomal microarrays (CMAs) (see Chapter 11) enable detection of duplication or deletions (copy number variants) far smaller than the 5Mb (5,000,000 base pairs) possible by conventional karyotypes. A major problem is determining clinical significance, especially in a prenatal setting. A CMA finding that can de deduced logically (if not certainly) as clinically significant in the postnatal setting cannot be so readily implicated in the prenatal state. In a postnatal setting one can compare frequency of microduplication or microdeletion in an abnormal (case) group versus a control group. A collaborative registry, the International Standards for Cytogenetic Array (ISCA) consortium, is compiling data on postnatal cases. However, changes associated involve anomalies less than conditions such as autism. Case and control groups in ISCA have not yet been stratified by de novo versus familial CMA status. For a de novo change in chorionic villi or amniotic fluid cells, clinical significance is more likely, especially if of sufficient size (e.g., 1Mb). If genes are known to be present in the region in question, the likelihood of clinical significance is reinforced. If a normal parent has the same duplication or deletion as a fetus, however, a CMA finding is not typically considered clinically significant. This complex topic is being evaluated in a large NICHD study with results expected in 2012. Thereafter, guidelines can be expected. At present regions that seem most likely to be implicated with phenotypic change, especially if de novo deletions, include 1q21.1, 15q13.2-q13.3, 16p11.2, 17q11.2-q13, and 22q11.2.;[8] all data have been derived from postnatal ascertainment.[8]

Sex Chromosomal Abnormalities

Monosomy X (45,X)

The incidence of 45,X in liveborn girls is about 1 in 10,000. Because monosomy X accounts for 10% of all first trimester abortions, it can be calculated that more than 99% of 45,X conceptuses must end in early pregnancy loss. The error usually (80%) involves loss of a paternal sex chromosome.

A common feature is primary ovarian failure due to gonadal dysgenesis. Structural abnormalities of the X chromosome may also result in premature ovarian failure. Mosaicism is frequent, usually involving a coexisting 45,X cell line. Both the long arm and the short arm of the X chromosome contain determinants necessary for ovarian differentiation and for normal stature, as discussed in detail elsewhere.[1]

45,X individuals not only have streak gonads and absent pubertal development but invariably are short (less than 150 cm). Growth hormone treatment increases the final adult height 6 to 8 cm. Low-dose estrogen therapy is needed to induce puberty, and long-term hormone replacement is needed in adulthood. Pregnancy may be achieved with the use of donor egg but requires careful monitoring of cardiovascular status before and throughout pregnancy and in the postpartum period. Various somatic anomalies including renal and cardiac defects, skeletal abnormalities such as cubitus valgus and clinodactyly, vertebral anomalies, pigmented nevi, nail hypoplasia, and a low posterior hairline. Performance IQ is lower than verbal IQ, but overall IQ is considered normal. Adult-onset diseases include hypertension, coronary artery disease, hypothyroidism, and type 2 diabetes mellitus. Comprehensive guidelines for evaluation and clinical management of Turner syndrome are available.[9,10]

Klinefelter Syndrome

About 1 in 1000 males are born with Klinefelter syndrome, the result of two or more X chromosomes. Characteristic features include small testes, azoospermia, elevated follicle-stimulating hormone and luteinizing hormone levels, and decreased testosterone. The most common chromosomal complement associated with this phenotype is 47,XXY; 48,XXXY and 49,XXXXY are less common.

Mental retardation is uncommon in 47,XXY Klinefelter syndrome, but behavioral problems and receptive language difficulties are common. Mental retardation is invariably associated with 48,XXXY and 49,XXXXY. Skeletal, trunk, and craniofacial anomalies occur infrequently in 47,XXY but are commonly observed in 48,XXXY and 49,XXXXY. Regardless of the specific chromosomal complement, patients with Klinefelter syndrome all have unquestioned male phenotypes. The penis may be hypoplastic, but hypospadias is uncommon. With intracytoplasmic sperm injection and other assisted reproductive technologies, siring a pregnancy is now possible. Simpson and colleagues[11] and Graham and colleagues[12] provide guidelines on evaluation and clinical management.

Polysomy X in Girls (47,XXX; 48,XXXX; 49,XXXXX)

About 1 in 800 liveborn girls has a 47,XXX complement. The IQ of 47,XXX individuals is 10 to 15 points lower than that of their siblings. The absolute risk for mental retardation does not exceed 5% to 10%, and even then, IQ is usually 60 to 80. Most 47,XXX patients have a normal reproductive system. The theoretical risk of 47,XXX women delivering an infant with an abnormal chromosomal complement is 50%, given half of the maternal gametes carry 24 chromosomes (24,XX). Empiric risks are much less. Somatic anomalies are not common in 47,XXX individuals but anomalies may occur and have been observed in some prenatally detected cases.[13] However, 48,XXXX and 49,XXXXX individuals are invariably retarded and more likely to have somatic malformations than 47,XXX individuals.

Polysomy Y in Boys (47,XYY and 48,XXYY)

Presence of more than one Y chromosome is another frequent chromosomal abnormality in liveborn boys (1 in 1000). 47,XYY are more likely than 46,XY boys to be tall and are at increased risk for learning disabilities, speech and language delay, and behavioral and emotional difficulties. These males have normal male phenotype and sexual development.

GENETIC HISTORY

Obstetricians/gynecologists should attempt to take a thorough personal and family history to determine whether a woman, her partner, or a relative has a heritable disorder, birth defect, mental retardation, or psychiatric disorder that may increase their risk of having an affected offspring. To address this question, some obstetricians find it helpful to elicit genetic information through the use of questionnaires or checklists (Figure 10-3).

One should inquire into the health status of first-degree relatives (siblings, parents, offspring), second-degree relatives (nephews, nieces, aunts, uncles, grandparents), and third-degree relatives (first cousins, especially maternal). A positive family history of a genetic disorder may warrant referral to a clinical geneticist or genetic counselor who can accurately assess the risk of having an affected offspring and review genetic screening and testing options. In some cases, it may be straightforward enough for the well-informed obstetrician to manage. For example, if a birth defect (e.g., cleft lip and palate or neural tube defect) exists in a second- or third-degree relative, the risk for that anomaly will usually not prove substantially increased over that in the general population. In contrast, identification of a second-degree relative with an autosomal recessive disorder such as cystic fibrosis increases the risk for an affected offspring. Adverse reproductive outcomes such as repetitive spontaneous abortions, stillbirths, and anomalous liveborn infants should be pursued. Couples having such histories should undergo chromosomal studies in order to exclude balanced translocations (see Chapter 26).

Parental ages should also be recorded. Advanced maternal age confers an increased risk for aneuploidy (see Table 10-2). A few studies indicate an increased frequency of aneuploidy in sperm in the sixth and seventh decades. However, risks are only marginally increased above background, and there remains no indication that a liveborn pregnancy risk is increased. **A paternal age effect is associated with a small increased risk (0.3% to 0.5% or less in men over 40 years of age) for sporadic gene mutations** for some autosomal dominant conditions such as achondroplasia and craniosynostosis. There are no specific screening tests for advanced paternal age, although some of these conditions may be detected by ultrasonography (see Chapter 11). The American College of Medical Genetics (ACMG) recommends that a pregnancy sired by an older father be treated in no special way, save anatomic ultrasound scan.[14] This can detect certain autosomal dominant disorders (e.g., achondoplasia) that may often arise as de novo mutations.

Ethnic origin should also be recorded because certain genetic diseases are increased in selected ethnic groups (see Genetic Screening, later in this chapter). Such queries also apply to gamete donors.

GENETIC COUNSELING

Although situations exist in which referral to a clinical geneticist or genetic counselor is indicated, it is impractical for obstetricians to refer all patients with genetic inquiries. Obstetricians should be able to counsel patients before performing screening tests for aneuploidy and neural tube defects, carrier screening, and diagnostic procedures such as amniocentesis. Therefore, salient principles of the genetic counseling process are described.

Communication

Pivotal to counseling is communicating in terms that are readily understood by most patients. It is useful to preface remarks with a few sentences recounting the major causes of genetic abnormalities, such as cytogenetic, single-gene, polygenic/multifactorial ("complex"), and environmental (teratogens) causes. Writing unfamiliar words and using tables or diagrams to reinforce important concepts is helpful. Repetition is essential. Allow the couple not only to ask questions but to talk with one another to formulate their concerns.

Written information (letters or brochures) can serve as a couple's permanent record, allaying misunderstanding and assisting in dealing with relatives. Preprinted forms describing common problems (e.g., advanced maternal age) have the additional advantage of emphasizing that the couple's problem is not unique. More complicated scenarios require a detailed letter.

Irrespective of how obvious a diagnosis may seem, confirmation is always obligatory. Accepting a patient's verbal recollection does not suffice, nor would accepting a diagnosis made by a physician not highly knowledgeable about the condition. Medical records should be requested and reviewed. It may be necessary for an appropriate specialist to examine the affected individual and order confirmatory diagnostic tests; examining first-degree relatives may be required as well to detect subtle findings. This is particularly applicable for autosomal dominant disorders such as neurofibromatosis or Marfan syndrome, for which variable expressivity is expected. If a definitive diagnosis cannot be established, the physician should not hesitate to acknowledge this. Accurate counseling requires a definitive diagnosis.

Nondirective Counseling

In genetic counseling, one should provide accurate genetic information yet ideally dictate no particular course of

Prenatal Genetic Screen

Name ______________________ Patient# ______________ Date __________

1. Will you be 35 years or older when the baby is due? Yes ___ No ___
2. Have you, the baby's father, or anyone in either of your families ever had any of the following disorders?
   Down syndrome (mongolism) Yes ___ No ___
   Other chromosomal abnormality Yes ___ No ___
   Neural tube defect, i.e., spina bifida (meningomyelocele or open spine), anencephaly Yes ___ No ___
   Hemophilia Yes ___ No ___
   Muscular dystrophy Yes ___ No ___
   Cystic fibrosis Yes ___ No ___
   If yes, indicate the relationship of the affected person to you or to the baby's father:
   ____
3. Do you or the baby's father have a birth defect? Yes ___ No ___
   If yes, who has the defect and what is it? ______________________
4. In any previous marriages, have you or the baby's father had a child born, dead or alive, with a birth defect not listed in question 2 above? Yes ___ No ___
5. Do you or the baby's father have any close relatives with mental retardation? Yes ___ No ___
   If yes, indicate the relationship of the affected person to you or to the baby's father:
   ____
   Indicate the cause, if known: ______________________
6. Do you, the baby's father, or a close relative in either of your families have a birth defect, any familial disorder, or a chromosomal abnormality not listed above? Yes ___ No ___
   If yes, indicate the condition and the relationship of the affected person to you or to the baby's father:
   ____
7. In any previous marriage, have you or the baby's father had a stillborn child or three or more first-trimester spontaneous pregnancy losses? Yes ___ No ___
   Have either of you had a chromosomal study? Yes ___ No ___
8. If you or the baby's father is of Jewish ancestry, have either of you been screened for Tay-Sachs disease, Canavan disease, or cystic fibrosis? Yes ___ No ___
   If yes, indicate who and the results: ______________________
9. If you or the baby's father is black, have either of you been screened for sickle cell trait? Yes ___ No ___
   If yes, indicate who and the results: ______________________
10. If you or the baby's father is of Italian, Greek, or Mediterranean background, have either of you been tested for β–thalassemia? Yes ___ No ___
    If yes, indicate who and the results: ______________________
11. If you or the baby's father is of Philippine or Southeast Asian ancestry, have either of you been tested for α–thalassemia? Yes ___ No ___
    If yes, indicate who and the results: ______________________
12. Irrespective of ethnic group, have you or the baby's father been screened for cystic fibrosis? Yes ___ No ___
13. Excluding iron and vitamins, have you taken any medications or recreational drugs since becoming pregnant or since your last menstrual period? (include nonprescription drugs)
    If yes, give name of medication and time taken during pregnancy: ______________________
    ____
14. Have you currently been taking folic acid supplements? Yes ___ No ___

FIGURE 10-3. Questionnaire for identifying couples having increased risk for offspring with genetic disorders. (Modified from a form recommended by the American College of Obstetricians and Gynecologists: Antenatal Diagnosis of Genetic Disorders. Technical Bulletin No. 108. Washington, DC, ACOG, 1987.)

action. Of course, completely nondirective counseling may be considered unrealistic. For example, a counselor's unwitting facial expressions may expose his or her unstated opinions. Merely offering antenatal diagnostic services implies approval. Despite the difficulties of remaining truly objective, one should attempt to provide information in a nondirective manner and then support the couple's decision.

Psychological Defenses

If not appreciated, psychological defenses can impede the entire counseling process. Anxiety is low in couples counseled for advanced maternal age or for an abnormality in a distant relative. So long as anxiety remains low, comprehension of information is usually not impeded. However, couples who have experienced a stillborn infant, an anomalous child, or multiple repetitive abortions are inherently more anxious. Their ability to retain information may be hindered.

Couples experiencing abnormal pregnancy outcomes manifest the same grief reactions that occur after the death of a loved one: denial, anger, guilt, bargaining, and resolution. One should pay deference to this sequence by not attempting definitive counseling immediately after the

TABLE 10-4 GENETIC SCREENING IN VARIOUS ETHNIC GROUPS

ETHNIC GROUP	DISORDER	SCREENING TEST
All ethnic groups	Cystic fibrosis	DNA analysis of selected panel of 23 CFTR mutations (alleles present in 0.1% of the general U.S. population)
Black	Sickle cell anemia	Mean corpuscular volume (MCV) <80%, followed by hemoglobin electrophoresis
Ashkenazi Jewish	Tay-Sachs disease	Decreased serum Hexosaminidase-a or DNA analysis for selected alleles
	Canavan disease	DNA analysis for selected alleles
	Familial dysautonomia	DNA analysis for selected alleles
Cajuns	Tay-Sachs disease	DNA analysis for selected alleles
French-Canadians	Tay-Sachs disease	DNA analysis for selected alleles
Mediterranean people (Italians, Greek)	β-thalassemia	MCV <80%, followed by hemoglobin electrophoresis if iron deficiency excluded
Southeast Asians (Filipinos, Chinese, African, Vietnamese, Laotian, Cambodian, Filipino)	α-thalassemia	MCV <80%, followed by hemoglobin electrophoresis if iron deficiency excluded

CFTR, Cystic fibrosis transmembrane conductance regulator.

birth of an abnormal neonate. The obstetrician should avoid discussing specific recurrence risks for fear of adding to the immediate burden. By 4 to 6 weeks, the couple has begun to cope and is often more receptive to counseling.

An additional psychological consideration is that of parental guilt. One naturally searches for exogenous factors that might have caused an abnormal outcome. In the process of such a search, guilt may arise. Conversely, a tendency to blame the spouse may be seen. Usually, guilt or blame is not justified, but occasionally the "blame" is realistic (e.g., in autosomal dominant traits). Fortunately, most couples can be assured that nothing could have prevented a given abnormality in their offspring.

Appreciating the psychological defenses helps one to understand the failure of ostensibly intelligent and well-counseled couples to comprehend genetic information.

GENETIC SCREENING

The goal of genetic screening is to identify individuals or couples at risk for having a child with an inherited condition, chromosomal abnormality, or birth defect. Ideally, screening to identify individuals who are carriers of genetic disorders based on ethnicity or family history should take place before conception, to ensure that couples are fully informed of their reproductive options, or as early as possible in pregnancy to allow couples the opportunity to have prenatal diagnostic testing (see Chapter 11). Screening is now offered routinely to all individuals of certain ethnic groups to identify those individuals heterozygous for a given autosomal recessive disorder (see Table 10-3). Noninvasive screening during pregnancy for aneuploidy and neural tube defects is offered to all women, regardless of age. Ultrasound screening for fetal abnormalities during pregnancy is reviewed in Chapter 11.

Carrier Screening for Heritable Conditions

Carrier screening is performed to determine if an individual has a mutation in one of two copies (heterozygous carrier) of the gene of interest. Screening is voluntary and informed consent is recommended. Ideally, individuals should be provided with information about the condition, prevalence, severity, and treatment options in addition to information about the test, including detection rates and the limitations. When the detection rate is less than 100%, it is important to explain that a negative screening test reduces the likelihood that an individual is a carrier and at risk for having an affected offspring but does not eliminate the possibility. Individuals should also be assured that their test results are confidential. For some individuals, genetic counseling may assist with the decision-making process. It may be helpful to provide individuals with disease-specific educational material. Further, it is prudent to document in the medical record that screening tests were offered and the individual's decision.

A cost-effective approach to carrier screening begins with testing the partner at risk (e.g., family history of the disease of interest) or the mother. However, it is also acceptable to test both concurrently. If one member of the couple has a mutation for an autosomal recessive disorder, the next step is to test the partner. When both parents are carriers for an autosomal recessive disorder, the risk of having an affected offspring is 25%. Genetic counseling is recommended, and the couple is informed of the availability of prenatal diagnostic testing, preimplantation genetic diagnosis, donor gametes (eggs or sperm), and adoption to avoid the risk for having an affected child (see Chapter 11). In addition, the parents should be informed that their relatives are at risk and also informed of the availability of carrier screening. Infrequently, a screening test may identify an individual with two mutations who is so mildly affected that the mutations escaped medical attention. In this situation, the individual may benefit from a referral to a specialist for further evaluation.

ACOG recommends population carrier screening for selected disorders in families in which no previously affected individual has been born.[15-19] These autosomal recessive disorders are amenable to prenatal diagnosis and are listed in Table 10-4. DNA-based tests also exist for fragile X mental retardation; however, ACOG and ACMG do not recommend screening the normal population for these conditions, save at the patient's request.[20] Fragile X testing is recommended with a family history of unexplained mental retardation, autism, a motor movement disorder,[21] premature ovarian failure, and, of course, fragile X syndrome itself.

TABLE 10-5 GENETIC SCREENING FOR SELECTED DISORDERS IN THE ASHKENAZI JEWISH POPULATION

DISORDERS	HETEROZYGOTE FREQUENCY	HETEROZYGOTE DETECTION RATE (%)
Tay-Sachs	1/25	99
Canavan	1/40	97
Familial dysautonomia	1/35	99.5
Cystic fibrosis	1/25	96
Niemann-Pick	1/70	95
Fanconi anemia, type C	1/90	95
Bloom syndrome	1/100	95
Mucolipidosis type IV	1/125	96
Gaucher disease, type I	1/19	95

ACOG also does not recommend population screening for spinal muscular atrophy (SMA), formerly called Werdnig-Hoffman disease.[22] On the other hand, the American College of Medical Genetics (ACMG) recommends SMA screening, reasoning that 95% of carriers can be detected for a disorder in which the pan-ethnic population incidence is comparable to systemic fibrosis.[23]

Ashkenazi Jewish Genetic Diseases

A number of genetic conditions are very prevalent among individuals of Ashkenazi Jewish ancestry (Table 10-5). Heterozygote or carrier detection rates for each condition are 95% to 99%, the sensitivity reflecting only a few mutations being responsible for each disorder. In aggregate, the likelihood of an Ashkenazi Jewish individual being heterozygous for one of the autosomal recessive disorders listed in this section is 1 in 4.[16] In the United States, Jewish individuals may be uncertain whether they are of Ashkenazic or Sephardic descent (90% are Ashkenazi); thus, obstetricians should offer screening to all Jewish couples. Applying criteria long in place for screening for Tay-Sachs disease, **ACOG also recommends that screening "be offered" for Ashkenazi couples for cystic fibrosis, Canavan disease, and familial dysautonomia.**[16] **For less common diseases prevalent in this ethnic group, ACOG**[16] **notes that carrier screening is available and that couples may inquire.**[16] It is recommended by ACOG that educational material should be available and couples could benefit from genetic counseling. These disorders include mucolipidosis IV, Niemann-Pick disease type A, Fanconi anemia type C, Bloom syndrome, and Gaucher disease.[16] The Genetic Disease Foundation recommends inquiring about screening for a total of 18 disorders for those of Ashkenazi Jewish ancestry (www.geneticdiseasefoundation.org).

Screening usually involves molecular testing for common selected mutations. In all the disorders listed in Table 10-4, screening only a few mutations (alleles for the mutant gene) will detect a very high percentage of heterozygotes. In Tay-Sachs disease, for example, molecular testing in Ashkenazi Jews detects 94% of heterozygotes; screening by the more laborious biochemical methods (based on ratio of hexosaminidase A to total hexosaminidase—A plus B) detects 98%.[15] If only one partner is Ashkenazi, ACOG[15,16] suggests screening that individual first. In low-risk populations (e.g., non-Ashkenazi Europeans), carrier frequency is only 1 in 300.[15] Given molecular heterogeneity being so prevalent, biochemical testing is often necessary in testing individuals who are not Ashkenazi Jews.

With the exception of Tay-Sachs disease and CF, the carrier rate and the detection rate applicable for the non-Jewish partner has not been established and, hence, screening is of limited value. It may thus not be possible to provide the couple with an accurate assessment of their risk to have an affected child.

Hemoglobinopathies

Sickle cell disease occurs most commonly among individuals of African origin but is also found in high frequency in Greeks, Italians (Sicilians), Turks, Arabs, Southern Iranians, and Asian Indians. Classic sickle cell disease is caused by homozygosity for a single base pair mutation in the β-globin gene (hemoglobin S) (see Chapter 42). **Approximately 1 in 12 African Americans are carriers of a single copy (heterozygous) of the mutation and have sickle cell trait.** Hemoglobin electrophoresis is the recommended[17] screening test because it can detect other abnormal forms of hemoglobin and thalassemia.

Thalassemia is caused by the reduced synthesis of either α- or β-globin (see Chapter 42) and is more common among individuals of Southeast Asian, African, or West Indian and Mediterranean (Greek, Italian), Asian, and Middle Eastern origin. Initial screening relies on mean corpuscular volume (MCV).[17] MCV of greater than 80% excludes heterozygosity for α- or β-thalassemia. Values less than 80% are more likely to reflect iron deficiency anemia than thalassemia heterozygosity; thus, tests to exclude the former are indicated. If iron deficiency is not found, hemoglobin electrophoresis showing elevated hemoglobin A_2 and hemoglobin F will confirm β-thalassemia. DNA-based testing is necessary to detect α-globin deletions, which cause α-thalassemia.[17] **ACOG recommends a complete blood count (MCV) and hemoglobin electrophoresis to detect thalassemia.**[17]

Cystic Fibrosis

Since 2001, screening for CF has been recommended by ACOG and ACMG.[18,19,24] CF caused by homozygosity or compound heterozygosity for mutations in the CF gene is more common in whites of Northern European and Ashkenazi Jewish ancestry. **Classic CF affects pulmonary and pancreatic function. The disorder usually is manifested early in childhood; 10% to 20% are detected at birth because of meconium ileus.** Increasing accumulation of viscous secretions progressively leads to chronic respiratory obstruction. Malnutrition and poor postnatal growth arise secondary to blockage of pancreatic ducts, producing insufficient pancreatic enzymes that interfere with intestinal absorption. Almost all men with CF have azoospermia, the result of congenital bilateral absence of the vas deferens (CBAVD). Sometimes CBAVD is the only manifestation of CF. In these cases, the mutant alleles are less deleterious than those causing severe CF. Individuals without pancreatic involvement have a milder course and longer survival (median survival 56 years compared to 30 years).[25] **CF may be diagnosed by the chloride sweat test or suspected on a newborn screening test, but mutation testing or DNA sequencing is used to confirm the diagnosis.** Once a mutation is identified in a given family, genetic studies are indicated to detect other carriers (heterozygotes) and affected relatives.

The CF gene is relatively large (27 exons), and its gene product is a chloride channel. Since the initial report localizing the CFTR gene[26] and its value recognized for screening, ACOG provided educational material for providers caring for couples both of whom are carriers.[27] Over 1300 disease-causing mutations have been identified, but one mutation (del F 508) deletion phenylalanine [F] at codon 508 accounts for about 75% of CF mutations in non-Ashkenazi Jewish whites and 97% in the Ashkenazim.[28] **ACOG and ACMG recommend using a pan-ethnic panel of 23 mutations (Table 10-6)[29] as a screening test to identify CF carriers.** Detection rates vary depending on ethnic origin. Screening for other alleles is optional because there is only minimal increase in sensitivity. Vendors offer expanded panels of up to nearly 100 mutations and even sequencing of the entire gene. Neither approach is recommended for routine carrier screening. However, an expanded panel or sequencing may be considered if a family member is affected and routine panels have failed to reveal molecular basis. Even if the entire gene is sequenced, not all CF mutations will be identified. Those not identified presumably act in promoter regions or perturb posttranslational modification.

Although the initial ACOG/ACMG recommendation was to offer CF carrier screening to non-Jewish whites and Ashkenazi Jews, obstetricians usually offer screening regardless of ethnicity because it can be unwieldy to assign a single ethnicity to a given patient.[19,29,30] The carrier frequency and detection rates in various ethnic groups and under varying scenarios are shown in Tables 10-7 and 10-8, respectively. Individuals without a family history of CF, an affected partner, or a male partner with CBAVD may benefit from genetic counseling, expanded screening, and, possibly, gene sequencing.

Newborn Screening

Newborn screening is mandated by each state; ACMG and the March of Dimes have recommended screening for a core panel of 29 to 30 conditions, including inborn errors of metabolism amenable to treatment such as phenylketonuria, galactosemia, homocystinuria; endocrine conditions such as hypothyroidism and 21-hydroxylase deficiency; and sickle cell anemia. Information by state is available at www.marchofdimes.com/professionals/580.asp

TABLE 10-6 RECOMMENDED PANEL OF 23 MUTATIONS IN THE CYSTIC FIBROSIS TRANSMEMBRANE CONDUCTANCE REGULATOR (CFTR) GENE THAT SHOULD BE SOUGHT IN CARRIER DETECTION PROGRAMS[29]*

DF508	DI507 N1303K	G542X	G551D	W1282Z
R533X	621 + 1G > T	R117H	1717 – 1G > A	A455E
	R560T			
R1162X	G85E	R334W	R347P	711 + 1G > T
	1898 + 1G > A			
2184delA	3120 + 1G > A	3849 + 10kbC > T	2789 + 5G > A	3659delC

*The panel is applicable in all ethnic groups. If R117H is detected, status of the 5T-7T-9T polymorphism should be determined reflexly. After originally consisting of 25 mutations,[24] two mutations were removed. 1078delT was removed because of its rarity, whereas I148T was removed because the causative gene was actually a second mutation (3199del6) in linkage disequibrium. However, this mutation (3199del6) is alone too rare to justify screening.

TABLE 10-7 DETECTING CYSTIC FIBROSIS (CF) HETEROZYGOTES (23 MUTATION PANEL)[19]

ETHNIC GROUP	HETEROZYGOTE CARRIER FREQUENCY	PERCENT OF HETEROZYGOTES DETECTABLE (%)	LIKELIHOOD OF BEING HETEROZYGOUS DESPITE NEGATIVE SCREEN
Ashkenazi Jewish	1/24	94	1/380
European non-Hispanic white	1/25	88	1/200
Hispanic-white	1/58	72	1/200
African American	1/61	64	1/170
Asian American	1/94	49	1/180

Data of ACOG Committee Opinion 486 (2011). The current panel encompasses 23 mutations,[29] rather than the original 25.[24]

TABLE 10-8 LIKELIHOOD OF AFFECTED FETUS AFTER CONCURRENT (FATHER AND MOTHER) VERSUS SEQUENTIAL (SINGLE PARTNER INITIALLY) SCREENING FOR CYSTIC FIBROSIS

	NON-HISPANIC EUROPEAN WHITES	ASHKENAZI JEWISH
No screening	1/2500	1/2304
Both partners negative (concurrent)	1/173,056	1/640,000
One partner negative, one untested (sequential)	1/20,800	1/38,400
One partner positive, one negative (concurrent)	1/832	1/1600
One partner positive, other untested	1/100	1/96
Both partners positive	1/4	1/4

These calculations are based on the frequencies shown in Table 10-6.

or at the National Newborn Screening and Genetics Resource Center's website at genes-r-us.uthsca.edu.

Considerable recent attention is being given to newborn screening for hearing loss. More than 70 genes related to hearing are already known. Mutations in gap junction B *(GJB2)*, the gene that codes connexin 26, and the neighboring gene *GJB6* (connexin 30) account for 50% of deafness in the newborn.[31] The heterozygote frequency for *GJB2* alone is 3% in North American whites.[32] Screening the neonate is standard of care but parents may decline testing and in some states need to consent. These screening tests may also identify couples who are carriers and may benefit from genetic counseling to learn about their options in subsequent pregnancies.

Screening for Aneuploidy

Noninvasive screening for chromosomal disorders such as trisomy 21 and 18 is routinely offered to women during pregnancy regardless of maternal age. Currently available noninvasive screening tests have high detection rates and can decrease the need for diagnostic testing and potential loss of a normal pregnancy; however, there are also limitations to screening, namely false-negative and false-positive results. This section focuses on first and second trimester screening tests; Chapter 11 discusses invasive diagnostic tests and prenatal ultrasonography as a screening and diagnostic tool. The strategy underlying currently employed aneuploidy screening involves deriving likelihood ratios. Likelihood risks for multiple informative markers are taken into account to yield an overall ratio, which is multiplied by the a priori age-related risk. If a marker reveals a likelihood ratio for having a fetus with Down syndrome of 2.6 for MSAFP (a second trimester aneuploidy marker) (Figure 10-4) and the a priori (age-specific) risk was 1 in 581, the recalculated risk after taking into account PAPPA becomes 1 in 148. One calculates likelihood ratio for each analyte tested, each value contributing to an overall likelihood that can be translated into the specific aneuploidy risk for a given patient.

First Trimester Screening

First trimester screening is best performed between 11 and 14 weeks. **The most effective first trimester biochemical markers are PAPP-A and free β-hCG, and the ultrasound measurement of nuchal translucency (NT), a sonolucent space present in all fetuses behind the fetal neck.** PAPP-A levels are reduced, hCG increased, and the NT measurement increased in trisomy 21. NT measurement alone has about a 70% detection rate with a false-positive rate of about 5%.[33] A critical necessity is the requirement for a robust quality NT assurance program. In combination with biochemical markers, the detection rate is greater than 80% with a false-positive rate of 5%. **First trimester screening is comparable or superior to second trimester screening alone and, more important, provides women with the option of earlier diagnostic testing in the event the screen indicates that the fetus is at high risk for aneuploidy.**

Several large collaborative, prospective studies have validated the clinical application of first trimester screening. In the first U.S. large-scale prospective study, 10,251 women of all ages were screened with PAPP-A and free β-hCG using a dried blood spot method; 5809 also had an NT measurement.[34] **Using both ultrasound (NT) and serum analytes (PAPP-A, free β-hCG), the detection rate for trisomy 21 was 87.5% (7 of 8 cases) in women younger than 35 years of age; in women older than 35 years, the detection rate was 92%** (23 of 25), albeit with a higher false-positive or invasive procedure rate. For trisomy 18, detection rates were 100% in both age groups. These impressive results validated the application of first trimester screening for aneuploidy.

In 2003, an NICHD multicenter cohort study, the Blood Ultrasound Nuchal (BUN) Study, reported results in 8514 women screened between 74 and 97 days' gestation[35] (Table 10-9). Applying the traditional midtrimester screen positive cutoff of 1 in 270, 85.2% of trisomy 21 pregnancies were identified at a false-positive rate of 9.4%. The high false-positive rate was predictable, given the higher mean maternal age of the sample. Stratifying by age, the detection rate for trisomy 21 was 66.7% for patients younger than age 35 years at a 3.7% false-positive rate and 89.8% in patients older than age 35 years with a 15.2% false-positive rate. The detection rate for trisomy 18 was 90.9%. Modeling for the general population (with a lower mean age) and setting a false-positive procedures rate of 5%, sensitivity for trisomy 21 would still be 78.7%; at a false-positive rate of 1%, the sensitivity would be 63.9%. These findings were consistent with other studies.

Two other large collaborative studies have also provided results comparable to the NICHD BUN Study. SURUSS (*S*erum *UR*ine and *U*ltrasound *S*creening *S*tudy) was a 25-center European trial[36] in which 47,000 patients were evaluated in both the first and second trimester. Results of

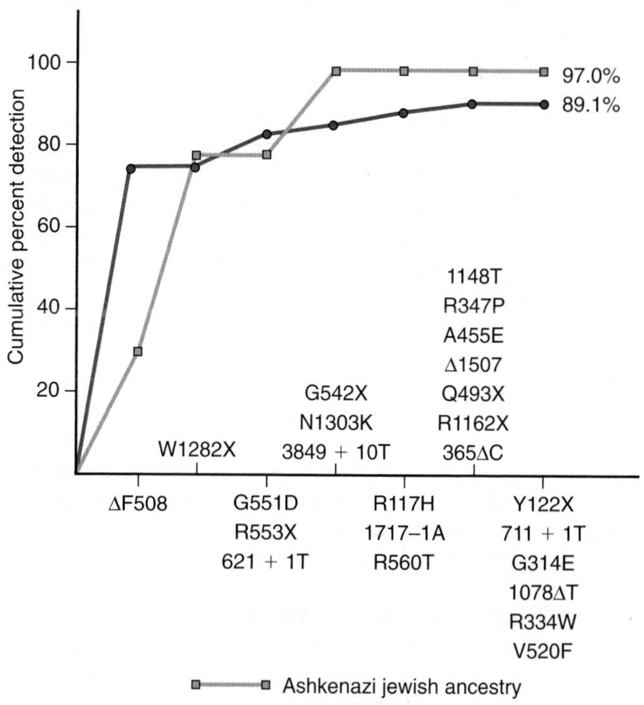

FIGURE 10-4. Increasing detection rate in northern European white and Ashkenazi Jewish populations as increasing numbers of CF-causing alleles are sought. (From Cystic Fibrosis Foundation Annual Report. New York, 1996.)

TABLE 10-9 DETECTION RATES IN THE NICHD BUN STUDY OF WAPNER AND COLLEAGUES[35]*

MATERNAL AGE	DETECTION TRISOMY 21 RATE (%)	FALSE-POSITIVE (PROCEDURE) (%)
<35 yr	66.7	3.7
≥35 yr	89.8	15.2
Total	**85.2**	**9.4**
Modeling for U.S.		
Population (mean)	78.7	5
(Maternal age 27 yr)	63.9	1

*The NICHD first trimester only screening (NT, PAPP-A, free β-hCG) cohort of Wapner and colleagues.[35] The sample of 8515 pregnancies prospectively applied a cut off of 1/270. Detection rate increases with prevalence (increased maternal age), albeit at the cost of more procedures. Because the mean maternal age was 34.5 years, data were then modeled to apply to the U.S. population (whose mean maternal age is 27) at a 5% to 1% false-positive rate.
BUN, Blood ultrasound nuchal translucency; *NICHD*, U.S. National Institute of Child Health and Human Development.

TABLE 10-10 DETECTION RATES IN THE NICHD FASTER TRIAL OF MALONE AND COLLEAGUES[37]

TESTS*	TRISOMY 21 DETECTION (%)
First Trimester (free β-hCG, PAPP-A, NT)	
11 wk	87
12 wk	85
13 wk	82
Second Trimester (15-18 wk)	
AFP, uE_3, total hCG ("triple test")	69
AFP, uE_3, total hCG, inhibin A ("quad test")	81
First Plus Second Trimester (PAPP-A, NT, AFP, uE_3, hCG, inhibin A)	
Disclosure of first trimester results	95
Nondisclosure of first trimester results	96
Serum screening only	88

*If first trimester ultrasound revealed septated cystic hygromas, intervention was taken (CVS offered). Otherwise results were not disclosed until after second trimester screening. Compiled data were then used to compare detection rates that would have occurred given various approaches, all at 5% false-positive (procedure) rates for each.
AFP, Alpha-fetoprotein; *CVS*, chorionic villus sampling; *FASTER*, First and Second Trimester Evaluation of Risk; *hCG*, human chorionic gonadotropin; *NICHD*, U.S. National Institute of Child Health and Human Development; *NT*, nuchal translucency; *PAPP-A*, pregnancy-associated placental protein; *uE_3*, unconjugated estriol.

first trimester assays were not disclosed to patients; thus, there could be no intervention. Nonetheless, setting the detection rate at 85% and using first trimester PAPP-A, hCG, and NT would have required procedures in 5.6% of women screened. Using a similar design, Malone and colleagues[37] studied 38,167 women in 15 U.S. centers in the NICHD FASTER trial. Detection rates were 87% for Down syndrome at 11 weeks and 85% at 12 weeks (Table 10-10). In this study, 134 women having a fetus with a septated cystic hygroma were removed from the cohort; 51% had a chromosomal abnormality and 34% had other major abnormalities.[38] The group[31] later stratified their data and found that NT greater than 4 mm was never associated with a normal noninvasive screen and, therefore, women should be offered diagnostic testing. In fact, only 8% of pregnancies with NT greater than 3 mm had a screen negative value.

Nicolaides[33] tabulated that NT, PAPP-A, and hCG detected 87% of 215 trisomy fetuses at a false-positive rate of 5%. Later results of Avgidou and colleagues[40] reported superior results from the same U.K. group. This group screened 30,564 women with NT, PAPP-A, and hCG, providing results the same day and detecting 93% of trisomy 21 cases. The incorporation of the other sonographic markers such as the presence of a nasal bone have been proposed to increase the detection rates further. However, at present these are not routinely employed.

When an increased NT measurement is associated with a normal karyotype, fetal loss rates are increased, and other fetal anomalies and genetic syndromes are observed, in particular, congenital heart defects.[41] **A targeted ultrasound examination during the second trimester and fetal echocardiography are recommended when the NT measurement is 3.5 mm or greater and the fetal karyotype is normal.**

Second Trimester Serum Screening

Multiple marker serum screening is used between 15 and 22 weeks' gestation to screen for both aneuploidy and open neural tube defects. **The most widely used second trimester aneuploidy screening test is the "quad screen," which utilizes four biochemical analytes—alpha-fetoprotein (AFP), hCG, unconjugated estriol (uE_3), and dimeric inhibin-A. The detection for trisomy 21 is about 75% in women who are less than 35 years of age and over 80% in women 35 years of older, with a false-positive rate of 5%.** For trisomy 18, using only the first three markers the detection rate is about 70%. Screening does not detect other age-related forms of aneuploidy such as Klinefelter syndrome, 47,XXY. Women with a positive screening test or a risk equal to or greater than a 35-year-old woman (e.g., 1 in 270) are referred for genetic counseling and offered diagnostic testing (see Chapter 11).

Use of all four analytes increases the second trimester detection rate for trisomy 21. The most informative single second trimester analyte is human chorionic gonadotropin (hCG). Levels of hCG rise from implantation to 8 weeks' gestation, plateau between 8 and 12 weeks' gestation, decrease from 12 to 18 weeks, and then plateau again until term. Serum hCG levels are increased in women carrying fetuses with Down syndrome.[42] Controversy exists as to whether the free β subunit of hCG is preferable to total hCG in Down syndrome screening, especially in the second trimester. The analyte unconjugated estriol (uE_3) is synthesized from dehydroepiandrosterone sulfate following conversion to 16 alpha-hydroxydehydroepiandrostenedione sulfate in the fetal liver and then to uE_3 in the placenta. Levels of uE_3 in maternal serum are lower (25%) in pregnancies affected with Down syndrome compared with those in unaffected pregnancies.[43] Like hCG, inhibin A (INHA) is elevated in Down syndrome pregnancies. This dimeric glycoprotein has an α-subunit and a βA-subunit linked by a disulfide bond. During pregnancy, inhibin is produced by the corpus luteum and then the placenta. Serum inhibin A levels from women carrying fetuses with Down syndrome have a median multiples of the median (MoM) of about 1.8[44] and do not change significantly with gestational age, unlike most other serum markers.

Typically, levels of AFP, uE_3, and hCG are reduced in trisomy 18. A simple approach to detect trisomy 18 is to offer invasive prenatal diagnostic testing whenever serum screening for each of these three markers falls below certain thresholds (MSAFP 0.6 MoM; hCG 0.55 MoM; uE_3 0.5 MoM).[45] Using these thresholds would detect 60% to 80% of trisomy 18 fetuses, with a 0.4% amniocentesis rate. Calculating individual risk estimation on the basis of three markers and maternal age, Palomaki and colleagues[46] reported that 60% of trisomy 18 pregnancies can be detected with a low false-positive rate of 0.2%. The value of individual risk estimates is that one in nine pregnancies identified as being at increased risk for trisomy 18 by serum screening would actually be affected.

First and Second Trimester Screening

Several different approaches have been proposed to use both first and second trimester screening to increase the detection rate over that achieved by screening in either trimester alone, with detection rates of 88% to 96% with false-positive rates of 5% reported. A caveat is that independent screening (i.e., using both first and second trimester screening tests to assess separately and independently the risk) is not recommended because of the unacceptably high false-positive rates. The best screening approaches combine first and second trimester approaches.

Sequential screening begins with first trimester screening. A woman is informed of the adjusted risk for aneuploidy based on the first trimester results. If her risk is high (greater than 1 in 50), she is offered genetic counseling and diagnostic testing (see Chapter 11). If the risk is low or moderate, a second trimester screening test is performed with results of both the first and second trimester screening tests used to generate a final adjusted risk for trisomy 21 and 18. This is called the stepwise approach. With contingency screening not all women will even proceed to second trimester screening. This occurs only with an intermediate risk; if the risk is low after the first trimester screen, no further testing is indicated. The detection rates are about 90% with low positive screening rates (2% to 3%). Malone and colleagues[47] compared several different first plus second trimester contingent sequential approaches (see Table 10-9). They concluded that the optimal method was contingency screening in which patients were divided into three groups: women whose calculated (NT, PAPP-A, hCG) first trimester risk was greater than 1/30 would undergo CVS; women whose risk was less than 1/1500 would undergo no further testing; all other women would undergo second trimester serum testing. Using this approach, only 21.8% of the cohort would need second trimester testing in order to detect 93% of trisomy 21 cases at a 4.3% false-positive rate; 65% would be detected in the first trimester with only 1.5% of patients having CVS procedures.

Integrated screening has the highest theoretical (modeling) detection rate (93% to 96%), but with this approach the first trimester screening results are withheld until the second trimester screen is completed. The individual receives only a single adjusted risk for trisomy 21 and trisomy 18 based on the results of both the first and second trimester screen. The obvious disadvantage with this approach is that the individual does not have an option of early diagnostic testing in the event that the first trimester screen would have indicated a high risk for trisomy 21 or 18. Another is that patients may not return for their second trimester screen. In the SURUSS trial, one third of patients failed to return for second trimester testing, despite being requested to do so and part of a study protocol.[25] Fortunately, integrated screening is not necessary; Cuckle and colleagues[48,49] showed that disclosure of first trimester results could be made with very little loss in sensitivity. Conversely, detection rates need not be diminished at all if procedure rates were increased only slightly (1% to 2%).

Lastly, serum integrated screening is useful when an NT measurement cannot be obtained or in communities where NT measurement is not available. With this approach, the first trimester PAPP-A and the second trimester analytes are used to adjust the risk for trisomy 21 and the individual receives one adjusted risk after the second trimester screen is completed. With this approach, sensitivity was 88% in the FASTER trial.[37]

In conclusion, **sequential (first plus second trimester) screening increases the detection rates over first trimester screening alone, but by no more than perhaps 5%.** This difference may shrink if other sonographic markers such as nasal bone are incorporated into the screening process (see Chapter 11). Both ACOG and ACMG recommend that women be offered either first trimester screening alone; sequential (stepwise or contingency) or integrated first and second trimester screening; or second trimester screening alone. **The only screening option not recommended by ACOG is second trimester screening independent of first trimester screening; both first and second trimester screening, should, if pursued, be done in the context of the integrated test, stepwise sequential test, or contingent sequential test.**[50]

Factors Confounding Detection Rates

Maternal Age

Detection rates vary according to sample characteristics, an important caveat in comparing studies. In particular, sensitivity for noninvasive screening is age dependent. Software is constructed such that the proportion of cases detected at a given age is greater for older women than for younger women; the "false-positive" (procedure) rate also increases with maternal age. **More than 90% of cases of Down syndrome will be identified by noninvasive screening in women aged 35 or older, whereas a considerably lower proportion will be identified in much younger women. Therefore, women should be given precise answers as to proportion of trisomy 21 cases excluded by screening.** In particular, one should not counsel a 25-year-old to expect the same proportion of trisomy 21 fetuses to be detected as in the general population (70% or 80%). Although the proportion of cases detected in younger women is lower, the absolute risk remains very low in the screen-negative 25-year-old. Detection rates also depend on *week* (not just trimester) of gestation and on the arbitrarily set procedure rate (false-positive rate). If one accepts more procedures (higher false-positive rate), detection rates increases. The converse is also true.

Maternal Weight and Ethnicity

Confounding factors influence serum screening, and adjustments may be necessary. **Adjustments for maternal weight and ethnic group are routinely employed.** The initial MSAFP assay should be performed at 15 to 20 weeks' gestation. When MSAFP is used for aneuploidy screening, corrections for gestational age, maternal weight, diabetes, ethnicity, and number of fetuses are necessary. Weight adjustment is needed because without adjustment, dilutional effects would result in heavier women having a spuriously low value, whereas thinner women would have a spuriously elevated value. In women with type 1 diabetes mellitus, a population at increased risk for a neural tube defect (NTD), the median MSAFP is 15% lower than in nondiabetic women. In women of black ethnicity, who have a lower risk for a fetal NTD, the median MSAFP is higher than in other ethnic groups.

With increased maternal weight, decreased levels of AFP, uE_3, and hCG levels all occur. Type 1 diabetes mellitus is associated with decreased uE_3 and hCG. Maternal smoking increases MSAFP by 3% but decreases maternal serum uE_3 and hCG levels by 3% and 23%, respectively.[51] Maternal serum hCG is higher and MSAFP lower in pregnancies conceived in vitro, compared with pregnancies conceived spontaneously.[51] A claim has been made that adjustments should be made for prior aneuploidy; β-hCG is reported to be 10% higher in a pregnancy after aneuploidy, whereas pregnancy-associated placental protein A (PAPP-A) is increased 15% in the first trimester.[52]

Multiple Gestation

Down syndrome occurs 20% more often in twin pregnancies than in singleton pregnancies, as expected given the known positive correlation between twinning and maternal age. Unfortunately, Down syndrome screening using multiple serum markers is less sensitive in twin pregnancies than in singleton pregnancies. **Using singleton cutoffs**, one study showed that 73% of monozygotic twin pregnancies were detected but **only 43% of dizygotic twin pregnancies with Down syndrome, given a 5% false-positive rate.**[53] Decreased sensitivity in detecting trisomy 21 in dizygotic twins reflects the blunting effect of the concomitant presence of one normal and one aneuploid fetus. Thus, patients with twins should be informed that the detection rate by serum screening is less than in singleton pregnancies. First trimester screening identifies about 70% of Down syndrome pregnancies; NT measurement alone has been shown to be as effective as a screening test for higher-order multiple gestation. Addition of the nasal bone assessment increased the detection rate to 87% to 89% in a retrospective study of twin pregnancies. First trimester screening provides the option of early diagnostic testing if the risk is increased and if selective reduction is an option.

MATERNAL SERUM ALPHA-FETOPROTEIN SCREENING FOR NEURAL TUBE DEFECTS

Screening for NTDs was the first application of maternal serum analyte to screening. Because relatively few (5%) NTDs occur in families who have had previously affected offspring, a method other than a positive family history was needed to identify couples in the general population at risk for offspring with an NTD. MSAFP and ultrasound examination (see Chapter 11) are now both useful screening tests.

MSAFP screening for NTD detection should be performed at 15 to 20 weeks' gestation. As with aneuploidy screening, corrections must be made for gestational age, multiple gestations, presence of diabetes mellitus, and maternal age. However, correction for maternal age is not necessary. Maternal serum values above either 2.0 or 2.5 MoM are usually considered elevated with respect to NTD, but exact values are less important than maintaining a consistent policy in the screening program. Values above 2.0 MoM are considered elevated in women with type 1 diabetes, whereas in twin gestations MSAFP is considered abnormal only at 4.5 to 5.0 MoM or greater. Irrespective, threshold values are used for NTD detection in contrast to likelihood ratios derived for aneuploidy screening.

Approximately 3% to 5% of women have an elevated MSAFP depending on threshold set and accuracy of pregnancy dating, and these are mostly false-positive results. If gestational age assessment is determined accurately (e.g., by first trimester sonogram), the number of women having an abnormal serum value is relatively lower. If MSAFP is elevated, a repeat sample may or may not be necessary according to the established protocol, usually based on the accessibility of ultrasound evaluation. In our opinion, there is value in repeating the MSAFP if the value lies between 2.50 and 2.99 MoM and if gestational age is 18 weeks or less.

MSAFP is greater than 2.5 MoM in 80% to 90% of pregnancies in which the fetus has an NTD: 90% in anencephaly and 80% in open spina bifida.[54] With ultrasound alone, one should be able to achieve very high detection rates for anencephaly, but there may be limitations to the detection of small spinal defects and ultrasound examination can confirm gestational age, confirm multiple gestation, and detect other anomalies. In some cases, amniocentesis to measure the amniotic fluid AFP and acetylcholinesterase levels may be necessary (see Chapter 11).

MSAFP may be spuriously elevated (with respect to NTD) in other circumstances, such as (1) underestimated gestational age, inasmuch as MSAFP increases as gestation progresses; (2) unrecognized multiple gestation (60% of twins and almost all triplets having MSAFP values that would be elevated if judged on the basis of singleton values); (3) fetal demise, presumably reflecting fetal blood extravasating into the maternal circulation; (4) Rh isoimmunization, cystic hygroma, and other conditions associated with fetal edema; and (5) other anomalies, mainly abdominal wall defects such as gastroschisis and omphalocele. Follow-up for the conditions cited is obviously necessary.

Absent ultrasound, approximately 1 in 15 women having an unexplained elevated serum AFP will have a fetus with a NTD. The sensitivity for detection of an NTD in twin gestations is predictably lower than in singleton gestations, being only about 30% for spina bifida given a threshold of 4.5 MoM. The lower sensitivity exists because twins are usually discordant for an NTD. Liberal use of ultrasound is recommended in twin gestations.

If aneuploidy screening is performed in the second trimester, an MSAFP value will already be available as part of three (triple) or four (quad) analyte screening for aneuploidy. First trimester MSAFP is, however, not a sensitive method for detecting NTDs. If first trimester aneuploidy screening alone is performed, second trimester MSAFP screening or ultrasound is still necessary to detect NTDs.

Obstetrical Significance of Unexplained Elevated Maternal Serum Alpha-Fetoprotein

Often, no evident cause is detected after a comprehensive assessment of a patient with an elevated MSAFP. This group of patients has been consistently described to be at higher risk of adverse perinatal outcome: spontaneous abortion, preterm birth, small for gestational age, low birth weight, and infant death. On the other hand, extremely low MSAFP values (less than 0.25 MoM) have also been associated with an increased morbidity: spontaneous abortion, preterm birth, stillbirth, and infant death.[55,56]

Interestingly, in a large prenatal screening database in western Scotland a direct association between MSAFP and the risk of sudden infant death syndrome (SIDS) has been observed.[57]

KEY POINTS

- The frequency of major birth defects is 2% to 3%, based on the definition of a defect causing death, a severe dysfunction, or a structural malformation requiring surgery.
- Major etiologic categories include chromosomal abnormalities (1 in 160 live births), single-gene or mendelian disorders, polygenic/multifactorial disorders, and disorders caused by exogenous factors (teratogens).
- The frequency of autosomal trisomies is higher in midtrimester (30% for Down syndrome) than at term, and many trisomies are so lethal that they are found only in abortuses.
- Single-gene disorders in aggregate result in major defects in 1% of neonates, with additional disorders manifested later in life. However, individual disorders are uncommon, rarely exceeding 1 per 4000.
- Genetic counseling requires adequate communication, appreciation of psychological defenses, and adherence to the principle of nondirective counseling.
- Genetic screening to detect heterozygotes in the nonpregnant and, if not already evaluated, in the pregnant population is appropriate for the following autosomal recessive disorders: Tay-Sachs disease, Canavan disease, familial dysautonomia in Jewish populations; Tay-Sachs disease in Cajun and French-Canadian populations; cystic fibrosis in all populations; α-thalassemia in Asians; β-thalassemia in Mediterranean populations (Greek and Italians); and sickle cell disease in blacks. ACOG does not currently recommend screening for spinal muscular atrophy (SMA), although the American College of Medical Genetics (ACMG) does.
- Carriers for β-thalassemia and α-thalassemia can be inexpensively detected on the basis of MCV less than 80% followed by hemoglobin electrophoresis, once iron deficiency is excluded. Alternatively, ACOG recommends hemoglobin electrophoresis for screening.
- Cystic fibrosis is found in all ethnic groups, but the heterozygote frequency is higher in non-Hispanic whites of northern European (1 in 25) or Ashkenazi Jewish origin (1 in 24) than in other ethnic groups (black 1/61, Hispanic 1/58, Asian 1/94). In the former two groups incidence is approximately 1 in 3600. ACOG and the ACMG originally recommended that CF screening be offered to whites and "made available" to other groups. In 2005, the ACOG acknowledged the difficulty in assigning a single ethnicity and stated that it was reasonable to offer screening to all pregnant women.
- The cystic fibrosis transmembrane regulatory (CFTR) gene is large (27 exons), and more than 1500 disease-causing mutations have been recognized. Screening is obligatory only for a specified panel of 23 mutations. In northern European white and Ashkenazi Jewish individuals, the heterozygote detection rate using the specified panel is 88% and 94%, respectively. In other ethnic groups detection rates are lower (64% blacks, 72% Hispanics, 49% Asian Americans).
- Noninvasive screening for trisomies can be offered at any age, providing patient-specific aneuploidy risks (trisomy 21; trisomy 18). If the calculated risk is greater than a given threshold risk (that of a 35-year-old in midgestation), an invasive procedure is offered. Comparing different methods is usually done by assuming a given number of procedures (false-positive rates) (5%). Detection rates vary if a different false-positive rate is applied.
- First trimester noninvasive screening uses serum free hCG, PAPP-A, and nuchal translucency (NT) measurements. The detection rate is at least 87% at 11 weeks and 85% at 12 weeks at a false-positive (procedure) rate of 5%.
- Second trimester noninvasive screening with three analytes (hCG, AFP, uE3) has a 70% detection rate, whereas screening with four analytes (hCG, AFP, uE3,inhibin A) has an 80% detection rate. Thus, second trimester screening has a lower detection rate than first trimester screening.
- In sequential screening, one performs first followed by second trimester screening. In contingency screening, one discloses first trimester results, offering CVS to high-risk women, and performing second trimester screening only on low-risk women. Alternatively, first trimester results can be withheld (nondisclosure or integrated), with only a single result provided in the second trimester. The two approaches show almost identical detection rates (95% and 96%); thus, offering nondisclosure is usually unnecessary. If pursued, nondisclosure screening necessitates rigorous patient follow-up to ensure compliance.

REFERENCES

1. Simpson JL, Elias S: Genetics in Obstetrics and Gynecology, 3rd ed. Philadelphia, WB Saunders, 2003.
2. Hook EB, Hamerton JL: The frequency of chromosome abnormalities detected in consecutive newborn studies: differences between studies—results by sex and by severity of phenotype involvement. In Hook EB, Porter IH (eds): Population Cytogenetic Studies in Humans. New York, Academic Press, 1977, p 63.
3. Hook EB: Rates of chromosome abnormalities at different maternal ages. Obstet Gynecol 58:282, 1981.
4. Morris JK, Mutton DE, Alberman E: Revised estimates of the maternal age specific live birth prevalence of Down's syndrome. J Med Screen 9:2, 2002.
5. Hook EB, Cross PK, Schreinemachers DM: Chromosomal abnormality rates at amniocentesis and in live-born infants. JAMA 249:2034, 1983.
6. Ruggeri A, Dulcetti F, Miozzo M, et al: Prenatal search for UPD 14 and UPD 15 in 83 cases of familial and de novo heterologous robertsonian translocations. Prenat Diagn 24:997, 2004.
7. Mori MA, Lapunzina P, Delicado A, et al: A prenatally diagnosed patient with full monosomy 21: ultrasound, cytogenetic, clinical, molecular, and necropsy findings. Am J Med Genet A 127:69, 2004.
8. Slavotinek AM: Novel microdeletion syndromes detected by chromosome microarrays. Hum Genet 124:1-17, 2008.
9. Bondy CA, Turner Syndrome Study Group: Care of girls and women with Turner syndrome: a guideline of the Turner Syndrome Study Group. J Clin Endocrinol Metab 92:10, 2007.
10. Sybert VP: Turner syndrome. In Cassidy SB, Allanson J (eds): Management of Genetic Syndromes, 2nd ed. Hoboken, NJ, John Wiley & Sons, 2005, p 589.
11. Simpson JL, de La Cruz F, Swerdloff RS, et al: Klinefelter syndrome: expanding the phenotype and identifying new research directions. Genet Med 5:460, 2003.
12. Graham JM, Simpson JL, Samango-Sprouse C: Klinefelter syndrome. In Cassidy SB, Allanson J (eds): Management of Genetic Syndromes, 2nd ed. Hoboken, NJ, John Wiley & Sons, 2005, p 323.
13. Haverty CE, Lin AE, Simpson E, et al: 47,XXX associated with malformations. Am J Med Genet A 125:108, 2004.
14. Toriello HV, Meck JM, Professional Practice and Guidelines Committee: ACMG Practice Guidelines Statement on guidance counseling in advanced paternal age. Genet Med 10:457, 2008.
15. ACOG Committee Opinion: Screening for Tay-Sachs Disease. Report 318. Washington, DC, American College of Obstetricians and Gynecologists, 2005.
16. ACOG Committee Opinion: Prenatal and Preconceptional Carrier Screening for Genetic Diseases in Individuals of Eastern European Jewish Descent. Number 442. Washington, DC, American College of Obstetricians and Gynecologists, 2009.
17. ACOG Practice Bulletin: Hemoglobinopathies in Pregnancy. Number 78. Washington, DC, American College of Obstetrician and Gynecologists, 2007.
18. ACOG: Preconception and Prenatal Carrier Screening for Cystic Fibrosis. Clinical and Laboratory Guidelines. Washington, DC, Bethesda, MD, ACMG, 2001.
19. ACOG Committee Opinion: Update on carrier screening for cystic fibrosis. Number 486. Washington, DC, American College of Obstetricians and Gynecologists, 2011.
20. American College of Obstetricians and Gynecologists Committee on Genetics: ACOG Committee Opinion: carrier screening for fragile X syndrome. Obstet Gynecol 116:1008, 2010.
21. Sherman S, Pletcher B, Driscoll D: Fragile X syndrome: diagnostic and carrier testing. Genet Med 7:584, 2005.
22. ACOG Committee on Genetics: ACOG Committee Opinion no. 432: spinal muscular atrophy. Obstet Gynecol 113:1194, 2009.
23. Prior TW: Carrier screening for spinal muscular atrophy. Genet Med 10:840, 2008.
24. Grody WW, Cutting GR, Klinger KW, et al: Laboratory standards and guidelines for population-based cystic fibrosis carrier screening. Genet Med 3:149, 2001.
25. Cutting GR: Cystic fibrosis. In Rimoin DL, Connor JM, Pyeritz RE (eds): Principles and Practices of Medical Genetics, 5th ed. Edinburgh, Churchill-Livingstone, 2007, p 1354.
26. Riordan JR, Rommens JM, Kerem B, et al: Identification of the cystic fibrosis gene: cloning and characterization of complementary DNA. Science 245:1066, 1989.
27. ACOG/ACMG: Cystic fibrosis testing—what happens if both my partner and I are carriers? Washington, DC, American College of Obstetricians and Gynecologists, 2001.
28. Abeliovich D, Lavon IP, Lerer I, et al: Screening for five mutations detects 97% of cystic fibrosis (CF) chromosomes and predicts a carrier frequency of 1:29 in the Jewish Ashkenazi population. Am J Hum Genet 51:951, 1992.
29. Watson MS, Cutting GR, Desnik RJ, et al: Cystic fibrosis population carrier screening: 2004 revision of American College of Medical Genetics mutation panel. Genet Med 6:387, 2004.
30. Morgan MA, Driscoll DA, Mennuti MT, et al: Practice patterns of obstetrician-gynecologists regarding preconception and prenatal screening for cystic fibrosis. Genet Med 6:450, 2004.
31. Prasad S, Cucci RA, Green GE, et al: Genetic testing for hereditary hearing loss: connexin 26 (GJB2) allele variants and two novel deafness-causing mutations (R32C and 645-648delTAGA). Hum Mutat 16:502, 2000.
32. Green GE, Scott DA, McDonald JM, et al: Carrier rates in the midwestern United States for GJB2 mutations causing inherited deafness. JAMA 281:2211, 1999.
33. Nicolaides KH: Nuchal transparency and other first trimester sonographic markers of chromosomal abnormalities. Am J Obstet Gynecol 191:45, 2004.
34. Krantz DA, Hallahan TW, Orlandi F, et al: First-trimester Down syndrome screening using dried blood biochemistry and nuchal translucency. Obstet Gynecol 96:207, 2000.
35. Wapner R, Thom E, Simpson JL, et al: First trimester screening for trisomies 21 and 18. N Engl J Med 349:1405, 2003.
36. Wald NJ, Rodeck C, Hackshaw AK, et al: First and second trimester antenatal screening for Down's syndrome: the results of the serum, urine and ultrasound screening study (SURUSS). J Med Screen 10:56, 2003.
37. Malone FD, Canick JA, Ball RH, et al: First-trimester or second trimester screening or both for Down's syndrome. N Engl J Med 353:2001, 2005.
38. Malone FD, Ball RH, Nyberg DA, et al: First-trimester septated cystic hygroma: prevalence, natural history and pediatric outcome. Obstet Gynecol 106:288, 2005.
39. Comstock CH, Malone FD, Ball RH, et al: Is there a nuchal translucency millimeter measurement above which there is no added benefit from first trimester serum screening? Am J Obstet Gynecol 195:843, 2006.
40. Avgidou K, Papageorghiou A, Bindra R, et al: Prospective first-trimester screening for trisomy 21 in 30,564 pregnancies. Am J Obstet Gynecol 192:1761, 2005.
41. Souka AP, Krampl E, Bakalis S, et al: Outcome of pregnancy in chromosomally normal fetus with increased nuchal translucency in the first trimester. Ultrasound Obstet Gynecol 18:9, 2001.
42. Bogart MH, Pandian MR, Jones OW: Abnormal maternal serum chorionic gonadotropin levels in pregnancies with fetal chromosome abnormalities. Prenat Diagn 7:623, 1987.
43. Canik JA, Knight GI, Palomaki GE, et al: Low second trimester maternal serum unconjugated oestriol in pregnancies with Down's syndrome. Br J Obstet Gynaecol 95:330, 1988.
44. Wald NJ, Densem JW, George L, et al: Prenatal screening for Down's syndrome using inhibin-A as a serum market. Prenat Diagn 16:143, 1996.
45. Palomaki GE, Knight GJ, Haddow JE, et al: Prospective intervention trial of a screening protocol to identify fetal trisomy 18 using maternal serum alpha-fetoprotein, unconjugated oestrial and human chorionic gonadotropin. Prenat Diagn 12:925, 1992.
46. Palomaki GE, Haddow JE, Knight GJ, et al: Risk-based prenatal screening for trisomy 18 using alpha-fetoprotein, unconjugated oestriol and human chorionic gonadotrophin. Prenat Diagn 15:713, 1995.
47. Malone FD, Cuckle H, Ball RH, et al: Contingent screening for trisomy 21 results from a general population screening trial. Am J Obstet Gynecol 193:S29, 2005.
48. Cuckle H: Integrating antenatal Down's syndrome screening. Curr Opin Obstet Gynecol 13:175, 2001.
49. Cuckle H, Arbuzova S: Multimarkers maternal serum screening for chromosomal abnormalities. In Milunsky A (ed): Genetic Disorders and the Fetus, 5th ed. Baltimore, Johns Hopkins University Press, 2004, p 795.
50. ACOG Committee on Practice Bulletins: ACOG screening for fetal chromosomal abnormalities, ACOG Practice Bulletin 77 (Jan 2007). Obstet Gynecol 109:217, 2007.

51. Palomaki GE, Knight GJ, Haddow JE, et al: Cigarette smoking and levels of maternal serum alpha-fetoprotein, unconjugated estriol, and hCG: impact on Down syndrome screening. Obstet Gynecol 81:675, 1993.
52. Cuckle HS, Spenser K, Nicolaides KH: Down syndrome screening marker levels in women with a previous aneuploidy pregnancy. Prenat Diagn 25:47, 2005.
53. Nicolaides KH, Brizot ML, Snijders RJ: Fetal nuchal translucency: ultrasound screening for fetal trisomy in the first trimester of pregnancy. Br J Obstet Gynaecol 101:782, 1994.
54. ACOG Practice Bulletin: Neural tube defects. Number 44. Washington, DC, American College of Obstetricians and Gynecologists, 2003.
55. Simpson JL, Palomaki GE, Mercer B, et al: Associations between adverse perinatal outcome and serially obtained serum. Am J Obstet Gynecol 173:1742, 1995.
56. Krause TG, Christens P, Wohlfahrt J, et al: Second-trimester maternal serum alpha-fetoprotein and risk of adverse pregnancy outcome (1). Obstet Gynecol 97:277, 2001.
57. Smith GC, Wood AM, Pell JP, et al: Second-trimester maternal serum levels of alpha-fetoprotein and the subsequent risk of sudden infant death syndrome. N Engl J Med 351:978, 2004.

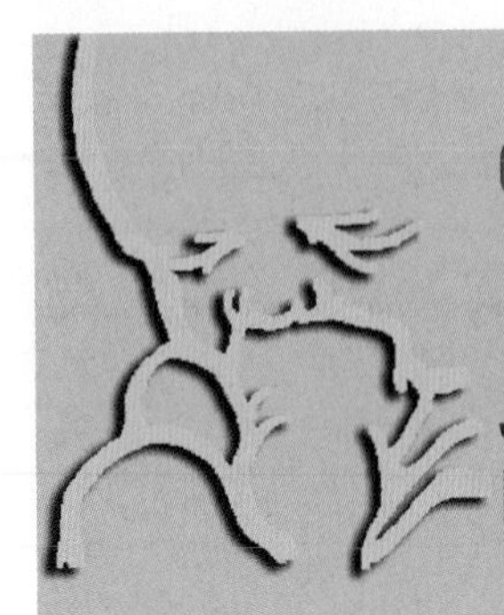

CHAPTER 11

Prenatal Genetic Diagnosis

Joe Leigh Simpson, Douglas S. Richards, Lucas Otaño, and Deborah A. Driscoll

KEY ABBREVIATIONS

Acetylcholinesterase	AchE
American Institute of Ultrasound in Medicine	AIUM
Allele Dropout	ADO
α-Fetoprotein	AFP
American College of Obstetricians and Gynecologists	ACOG
Assisted Reproduction Technology	ART
Cell Free Fetal DNA	CffDNA
Comparative Genomic Hybridization	CGH
Confidence Interval	CI
Congenital Pulmonary Adenomatoid Malformation	CPAM
Confined Placental Mosaicism	CPM
Chorionic Villus Sampling	CVS
Chromosomal Microarray	CMA
Deoxyribonucleic Acid	DNA
Early Amniocentesis	EA
European Society of Human Reproduction and Embryology	ESHRE
Familial Adenomatous Polyposis	FAP
First- and Second-Trimester Evaluation of Risk	FASTER
Fluorescence in Situ Hybridization	FISH
Human Chorionic Gonadotropin	hCG
Human Leukocyte Antigen	HLA
Intrauterine Growth Restriction	IUGR
Intracytoplasmic Sperm Injection	ICSI
Limb Reduction Deformity	LRD
Maternal Serum α-Fetoprotein	MSAFP
Nasal Bone	NB
Neural Tube Defects	NTDs
Nuchal Translucency	NT
Odds Ratio	OR
Percutaneous Umbilical Blood Sampling	PUBS
Polymerase Chain Reaction	PCR
Preimplantation Genetic Diagnosis	PGD
Qualitative Polymerase Chain Reaction	QPCR
Routine Antenatal Diagnostic Imaging with Ultrasound Study	RADIUS
Reproductive Genetics Institute	RGI
Single Nucleotide Polymorphism	SNP
Spinal Muscular Atrophy	SMA
Talipes Equinovarus	TE
Transabdominal Chorionic Villus Sampling	TA-CVS
Transcervical Chorionic Villus Sampling	TC-CVS
Uniparental Disomy	UPD
U.S. National Institute of Child Health and Human Development	NICHD
Ventricular Septal Defect	VSD
Von Hippel-Lindau Syndrome	VHL
World Health Organization	WHO

Prenatal genetic diagnosis is an important process used to evaluate the fetus at risk for a chromosomal abnormality, genetic disorder, or a congenital anomaly. Amniotic fluid, placental tissue, and cord blood can be readily obtained and analyzed during the first and second trimester. It is also possible to diagnose chromosomal abnormalities and genetic disorders from fetal cells or DNA recovered from the maternal blood and cells from embryos obtained through in vitro fertilization. The detection of many congenital malformations is possible using ultrasonography and fetal echocardiography.

In this chapter, we review the indications for prenatal diagnosis and specifically discuss the procedures used to obtain fetal tissue and cells for prenatal diagnosis and to visualize congenital anomalies. This chapter complements Chapter 10 on genetic counseling, which discusses noninvasive screening for aneuploidy and neural tube defects.

DIAGNOSTIC PROCEDURES FOR PRENATAL GENETIC DIAGNOSIS

Prenatal detection of chromosomal abnormalities and many genetic conditions requires an invasive procedure such as amniocentesis or chorionic villus sampling (CVS) to obtain fetal or placental tissue for chromosomal and genetic testing. Less frequently, cordocentesis is performed to obtain fetal blood. In this section, we review these techniques and their safety.

As a common feature of any prenatal invasive procedure, the patient should receive genetic counseling and be fully informed about the nature of the procedure. It is essential in clinical practice to obtain formal consent before an invasive procedure. Written or oral information should include nature, accuracy, and possible results; how, when, and by whom it is performed; safety of the procedure; culture failure rates; reporting time; and postprocedure recommendations.

Amniocentesis

Genetic amniocentesis was first performed in the 1950s. Analytes such as α-fetoprotein (AFP) can be measured in the amniotic fluid, and amniocytes can be cultured for cytogenetic and molecular analyses. Amniocentesis is probably the most widely used prenatal diagnostic invasive procedure.

Technique

Genetic amniocentesis is usually performed after 15 weeks' gestation. A 20- or 22-gauge spinal needle with the stylet is introduced percutaneously into the amniotic cavity under continuous ultrasound guidance taking care to avoid the fetus, cord, and whenever possible, the placenta. A local anesthetic in the site of puncture may be given, but a randomized trial showed that local anesthetic did not reduce pain scores reported by women undergoing amniocentesis.[1] Approximately 20 to 30 mL of amniotic fluid is aspirated and the first 1 or 2 mL usually discarded in order to avoid maternal cell contamination. Rh immune globulin should be administered to the Rh-negative, Du-negative, unsensitized patient who has an Rh-positive fetus (or if fetal Rh status is not known, through cell free fetal DNA studies).

Continuous visualization of the needle by ultrasound significantly reduces the incidence of bloody amniotic fluid, dry taps, and the need for multiple insertions. Bloody amniotic fluid is occasionally aspirated; however, the blood is almost always maternal in origin and does not adversely affect amniotic cell growth. Brown, dark red, or wine-colored amniotic fluid indicates that intra-amniotic bleeding has occurred earlier in pregnancy and hemoglobin breakdown products are persistent in the fluid. Pregnancy loss eventually occurs in about one third of such cases. If the abnormally colored fluid is associated with an elevated AFP level, then the outcome is almost always unfavorable (fetal demise or fetal abnormality). Greenish amniotic fluid is the result of meconium staining and is apparently not associated with poor pregnancy outcome.

After amniocentesis, the patient may resume all normal activities. Common sense dictates that strenuous exercise such as jogging or aerobic exercise is deferred for a day or so. Deferring sexual activity for 24 to 48 hours seems prudent. The patient should report persistent uterine cramping, vaginal bleeding, leakage of amniotic fluid, or fever; however, physician intervention is almost never required, unless of course overt abortion occurs.

Amniocentesis in Twin Pregnancies

In multiple gestations, amniocentesis can usually be performed on all fetuses. It is important to assess and record chorionicity, placental location, fetal viability, anatomy, and gender and to carefully identify each sac should selective termination be desired at a later date. A simple and reliable technique to ensure that the same sac is not sampled twice is to inject 2 to 3 mL of indigo carmine following aspiration of amniotic fluid from the first sac, before the needle is withdrawn. A second amniocentesis is then performed at a site determined after visualizing the membranes separating the two sacs. Aspiration of clear fluid confirms that the second (new) sac was entered. Gestations greater than two can be managed similarly, sequentially injecting dye into successive sacs. Cross-contamination of fetal cells in multiple gestations appears rare, but confusion may sometimes arise in interpreting amniotic fluid acetylcholinesterase (AchE) or AFP results. Some obstetricians aspirate the second sac without dye injection, use a single-puncture technique, or perform simultaneous visualization of the two inserted needles in each sac.[2,3]

If only one fetus in a multiple gestation is abnormal, parents should be prepared to choose between aborting all fetuses or continuing the pregnancy with one or more normal fetuses and one abnormal fetus. Selective termination in the second trimester is possible but is associated with a higher rate of complications (fetal loss and prematurity); therefore, CVS should be considered the preferred test for multiple gestations.

Safety

Any procedure that involves entering the pregnant uterus carries some risk to the fetus. **However, the risk for amniocentesis is very low in experienced hands, approximately 1 in 400 procedure-related losses, or less.**[4] The risk for pregnancy loss has decreased since the large collaborative studies to assess safety were first done in the 1970s.[5,6] In none of these early collaborative studies, nor others of that era, was high-quality ultrasonography as defined by today's standards available, nor was concurrent ultrasonography ever universally applied.[3] By contrast, studies conducted within the past decade universally employ high-quality ultrasound and have shown no statistical difference between outcomes following amniocentesis groups and controls. Increased risks logically should be increased even further when amniocentesis is performed in twins. However, even this is difficult to prove.

Maternal risks are low, with symptomatic amnionitis occurring only rarely (0.1%). Minor maternal complications such as transient vaginal spotting or minimal amniotic fluid leakage occur in 1% or less of cases, but these complications are almost always self-limited in nature. Other complications include intra-abdominal viscus injury or hemorrhage. The most serious is fulminant sepsis (*Escherichia coli* or clostridia) resulting in maternal mortality, but this is extraordinarily rare.[7]

Early Amniocentesis

The American College of Obstetricians and Gynecologists (ACOG) states that amniocentesis before 14 weeks' gestation, especially before 13 weeks' gestation, should not be performed for genetic indications.[8] The basis for this strong statement is four large studies all showing untoward results including higher rates of pregnancy loss, talipes equinovarus (TE), and amniotic fluid leakage.

Amniocentesis in Women with Hepatitis B, Hepatitis C, and Human Immunodeficiency Virus

Blood-borne viruses constitute a risk factor for maternal-fetal transmission. Available evidence is limited, but the risk for transmission for hepatitis B seems to be very low.[9] Knowledge of the maternal hepatitis B "e" antigen status is valuable in the counseling of risks associated with amniocentesis. There is less information about hepatitis C, but to date there is no evidence that transmission is increased following amniocentesis.[10] **Invasive prenatal testing can be carried out in women who carry hepatitis B or C; however, the patient should be informed of the limited data on transmission.**

In HIV-positive women, noninvasive testing is preferable, and invasive testing should be avoided, particularly in the third trimester when the relative risk for transmission is 4 when an invasive procedure is performed.[10,11] Some authors have suggested that procedures early in pregnancy would carry a very low risk provided that antiretroviral therapy is administered and the maternal viral load is low.[12]

The Society of Obstetricians and Gynaecologists of Canada states that for women infected with hepatitis B, hepatitis C, or HIV, the use of noninvasive methods for prenatal screening, (e.g., nuchal translucency [NT] measurement, maternal serum screening, and anatomic ultrasound) may help reduce that age-related risk to a level below the threshold for genetic amniocentesis. For those who insist on amniocentesis, every effort should be made to avoid traversing the placenta.

Chorionic Villus Sampling

CVS allows diagnosis in the first trimester of pregnancy. If desired, pregnancy termination can be performed earlier, when it is much safer for the mother. For example, the maternal death rate is 1 per 100,000 early in pregnancy compared with 7 to 10 per 100,000 in midpregnancy.[13] Early diagnosis also makes it feasible to perform selective fetal reduction in multiple gestations, a relatively safe procedure in the first trimester but decidedly less so in the second trimester. Early termination also protects patient privacy. Both chorionic villi analysis and amniotic fluid cell analysis offer the same information concerning chromosomal status, enzyme levels, and gene mutations. CVS is not useful for the few assays requiring amniotic fluid liquor, such as AFP for neural tube defects.

Technique

CVS is performed between 10 and 13 weeks' gestation. Before performing a CVS, an ultrasound evaluation is necessary to determine gestational age, uterine anatomy, placental location, chorionicity, number of fetuses, fetal status, and potential aneuploidy markers, such as cystic hygroma and increased NT measurement. When abnormal ultrasound findings are detected, it is useful to reevaluate the indication and to discuss it with the patient before performing the CVS.

CVS can be performed by either a transcervical or transabdominal approach. Transcervical CVS (TC-CVS) is usually performed with a flexible polyethylene catheter with a metal obturator, which is introduced through the cervical canal toward the placenta under direct ultrasonographic visualization (Figure 11-1). After withdrawal of the obturator, 10 to 25 mg of villi is aspirated by negative pressure into a 20- or 30-mL syringe containing tissue culture media.

TA-CVS is performed by introducing an 18- or 20- gauge spinal needle percutaneously into the long axis of the placenta (Figure 11-2), under ultrasound guidance. After removal of the stylet, villi are aspirated into a 20-mL syringe containing about 5 mL of tissue culture media,

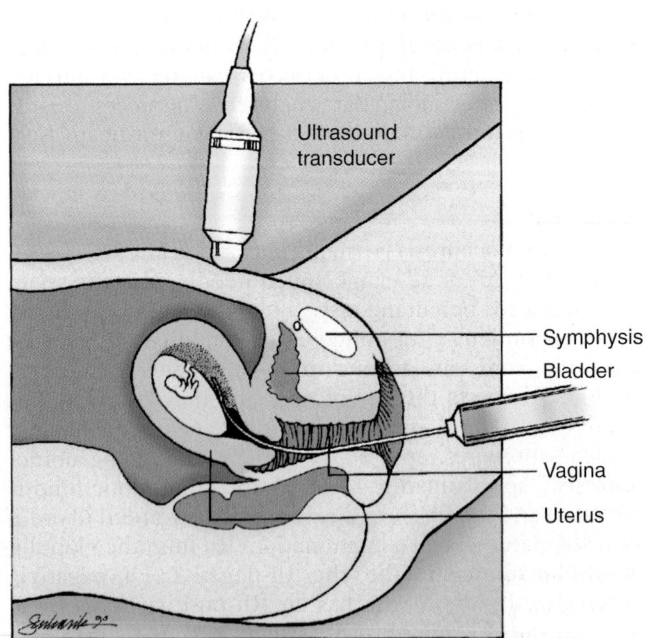

FIGURE 11-1. Transcervical chorionic villus sampling.

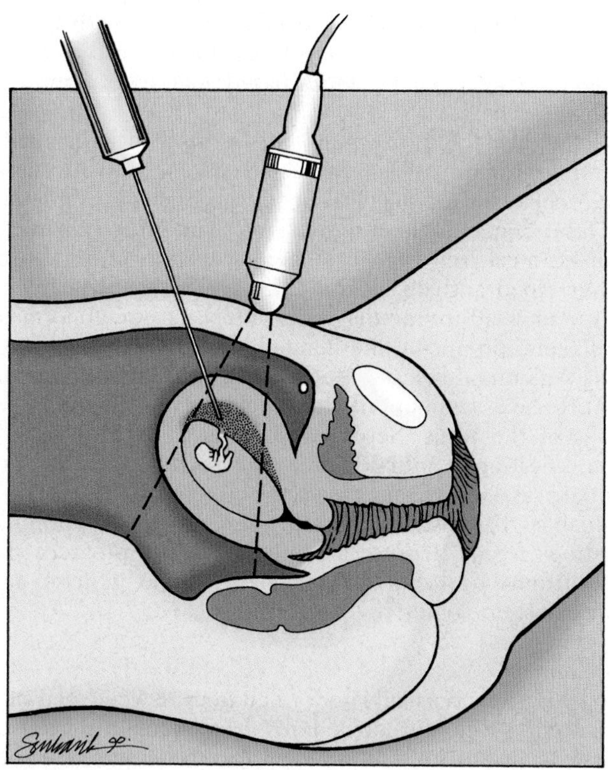

FIGURE 11-2. Transabdominal chorionic villus sampling.

keeping negative pressure and performing a gentle, longitudinal, back-and-forth movement of the needle. TA-CVS is typically performed at 10 to 13 weeks' gestation but can be performed later in gestation for rapid fetal karyotyping or when there is severe oligohydramnios. After the first trimester, this procedure is better known as *late CVS* or *placental biopsy*. Placental biopsy has now replaced cordocentesis for rapid fetal karyotyping during the second and third trimesters in many centers, given that it carries a lower risk, is technically easier, and can yield cytogenetic results within 24 to 48 hours.[14]

In many cases, either TA-CVS or TC-CVS is acceptable. However, there are situations in which one approach may be preferable. For example, cervical myomas or sharply angulated uteri may preclude transcervical passage of the catheter, whereas TA-CVS would permit sampling. The transabdominal approach is preferable in the presence of genital herpes, cervicitis, or bicornuate uteri.

With either approach, Rh immune globulin should be administered to the Rh-negative, Du-negative, unsensitized patient unless the fetus is known (cell free fetal DNA studies) to be Rh-negative. Sampling women sensitized to Rh(D) should probably be deferred until later in gestation.

Safety

CVS is a relatively safe procedure. In experienced hands, the risk for pregnancy loss is similar to second trimester amniocentesis. The prevalence of intrauterine growth restriction, placental abruption, and premature delivery is no higher in women undergoing CVS than expected in the general population.[15]

The U.S. Cooperative Clinical Comparison of Chorionic Villus Sampling and Amniocentesis study[16] and the Canadian Collaborative CVS-Amniocentesis Trial Group study[17] reported that pregnancy losses after CVS were no different than loss rates after second-trimester amniocentesis. A systematic review assessing comparative safety between TA-CVS and TC-CVS, and EA and second-trimester amniocentesis concluded that second-trimester amniocentesis and TA-CVS are safer than TC-CVS and EA.[18] Randomized studies in the United States and in Italy found no difference between TC-CVS and TA-CVS. In the second phase of the U.S. National Institute of Child Health and Human Development (NICHD) collaborative study, 1194 patients were randomized to TC-CVS and 1929 patients to TA-CVS. Loss rates in cytogenetically normal pregnancies through 28 weeks were 2.5% and 2.3%, respectively.[19] Of interest, the overall loss rate (i.e., background plus procedure related) during the randomized trial was 0.8% lower than rates observed during the mid-1980s, probably reflecting increasing operator experience as well as availability of both transcervical and transabdominal approaches.

In contrast, a multicenter randomized study in the United Kingdom compared second-trimester amniocentesis and CVS, as performed in any fashion deemed suitable by the obstetrician. The outcome assessed was completed pregnancies. The 4.4% fewer completed pregnancies in the U.K. CVS cohort reflected both unintended and intended pregnancy terminations.[17] The operators in this study were also considerably less experienced than in the U.S. trials. The only requirement for participation in the U.K. study was 30 "practice" CVS procedures. Greater experience is clearly necessary to become facile with CVS.

Another important factor in assessing safety is the indication for CVS. If CVS is performed because of an increased NT measurement, a cystic hygroma, or any other anomaly, the risk for miscarriage is increased. Thus, simple comparison to amniocentesis is not always valid.

In the early 1990s, controversy about the safety of CVS focused on the risk for limb reduction defects. Severe limb reduction deformity (LRD), transverse limb defects, and oromandibular-limb hypogenesis following transcervical CVS were reported in the United Kingdom, United States, and Taiwan. The U.S. Centers for Disease Control and Prevention conducted a case-control study of 131 infants with nonsyndromic limb deficiency, identified in seven population-based birth defects surveillance programs, compared with 131 controls with other birth defects matched to cases by the infant year of birth, mother's age, race, and state of residence.[20] The odds ratio (OR) for all limb deficiencies after CVS during 8 to 12 weeks' gestation was only 1.7, not significantly increased given the 95% confidence interval (CI) of 0.4 to 6.3. However, the authors found a significant association for transverse digital deficiency (OR, 6.4; 95% CI, 1.1 to 38.6) when stratified by anatomic subtypes.

The consensus of other studies is, however, that LRD is not a major concern when CVS is performed by experienced individuals at 10 to 13 weeks of gestation.[21,22] The types of limb defects and calculation of overall incidences have failed to reveal a difference between the

CVS and background populations. Nonetheless, teratogenic mechanisms by which CVS might cause LRDs can be hypothesized. These include (1) decreased blood flow caused by fetomaternal hemorrhage or pressor substances released by disturbing villi or chorion and (2) embolization of chorionic villus material or maternal clots into the fetal circulation. It has been suggested that at least some of the LRDs associated with CVS could result from disruption of the amniotic membrane due to incorrect sampling.[23]

A possible association between late first-trimester CVS (13 to 14 weeks) and a higher risk for hypertension and preeclampsia was reported,[24] but other reports have not confirmed this.[25] It could be hypothesized that focal placental disruption is the involved mechanism, supporting the theory that disturbances of early placentation lead to maternal hypertension.[24]

In summary, patients should be informed that in experienced hands, the fetal loss rates are comparable in CVS and second-trimester amniocentesis. When the CVS procedure is performed after 9 completed weeks, the risk for limb reduction problems is low, and no higher than the general population risk of 6 per 10,000.

Chorionic Villus Sampling in Twin Pregnancies

In experienced hands, CVS is safe in multiple gestations. In a U.S. study, the total loss rate of chromosomally normal fetuses (spontaneous abortions, stillborns, neonatal deaths) was 5%,[26] only slightly higher than the 4% absolute rate observed in singleton pregnancies.[16] A critical issue in counseling twin pregnancies for prenatal diagnosis is to establish chorionicity. In providing genetic risk figures and considering technical issues, monochorionic or dichorionic twin pregnancies may imply significant differences. Monochorionic twins are monozygotic and, therefore, carry the same genetic constitution, with a few exceptions. Thus, if there are not any significant sonographic differences in both fetuses, only one sample need be obtained. For dichorionic twin pregnancies, both placentas must be sampled. When the placentas appear to be fused, it can be helpful to identify the cord insertion sites to avoid the cross-contamination of chorionic tissue, leading to either false-positive or false-negative results. Alternatively, amniocentesis may be the preferred test.

CVS is widely used before selective reduction in multiple gestations. Here, it is especially desirable to sample the inferiorly lying fetus (usually retained to minimize risk for ascending infection) as well as at least two or three of the other fetuses potentially slated to be retained.

Fetal Blood Sampling

Ultrasound-directed percutaneous umbilical blood sampling (PUBS), also termed *cordocentesis* or *funipuncture*, can be used to obtain fetal blood for cytogenetic or molecular analyses. One of the most common indications for PUBS is a fetal malformation detected during the second and third trimesters. However, as previously described, placental biopsy is a safer, easier, and faster alternative and has replaced fetal blood sampling in many centers. Further, improvements in cytogenetic and molecular diagnostic testing have decreased the need for fetal blood sampling. For instance, fetal blood sampling was once frequently performed for diagnostic reasons in regions with a high prevalence of hemoglobinopathies. Now, most of those diagnoses are made by DNA-based analysis of chorionic villi.

Fetal blood samples may still be used to help clarify chromosome mosaicism detected in cultured amniotic fluid cells or chorionic villi or for the prenatal evaluation of fetal hematologic abnormalities. The fetal hematocrit can be measured to assess anemia resulting from Rh or other blood antigen isoimmunization states. Fetal blood has been used for the diagnosis of blood factor abnormalities (gene products) like hemophilia A, hemophilia B, or von Willebrand disease. Recovery of fetal blood is important in the assessment of viral, bacterial, or parasitic infections of the fetus. Serum studies of fetal blood permit quantification of antibody titers, and serum can be used to initiate viral, bacterial, or parasitic cultures. PUBS is also a valuable diagnostic approach in cases of nonimmune hydrops fetalis because a single procedure provides the opportunity to assess different hematologic, genetic, and infectious etiologies.

Technique

Cordocentesis is usually performed from 18 weeks onward, although successful procedures have been reported as early as 12 weeks. Ultrasonographic examination before the procedure is necessary to assess fetal viability, placental and umbilical cord location, fetal position, and presence or absence of fetal or placental anomalies. Color-flow Doppler imaging is an important tool in evaluating the cord and placenta. Maternal sedation is not usually required, but oral benzodiazepine before the procedure may be of benefit. Although there is no good evidence, many centers use prophylactic antibiotics.

Under continuous ultrasound guidance, a 21- or 22-gauge spinal needle with stylet is inserted percutaneously and directed into the umbilical vein. The needle may be inserted using a freehand technique or using a needle-guiding device fixed to the transducer. Most experienced maternal-fetal medicine specialists use the freehand technique.[27] The umbilical vein is preferred over the artery because the former is larger and less likely to be associated with fetal bradycardia and significant hemorrhage when punctured. Puncture of the umbilical cord at the placental insertion site is technically easier but is associated with a higher rate of maternal blood contamination. Free loops of cord and the intrahepatic vein are alternatives.[28] Cardiocentesis has also been described for fetal blood sampling, but obviously it carries a higher risk for fetal loss, about 6%.[29]

Once the needle is positioned in the umbilical vein, the stylet is removed, and a small amount of blood is aspirated into a heparin-coated syringe. It is crucial to confirm that the sample is fetal in origin; thus, a small amount is used for a complete blood count to assess the mean corpuscular volume. Fetal blood cells (140 fL) are larger than maternal cells (80 fL). The mean corpuscular volume of a sample of fetal blood should be higher than 100. A useful alternative when a complete blood analysis cannot be performed at once is the "Apt test" or hemoglobin alkaline denaturation test, especially before 28 weeks of gestation. Based on the ability of fetal hemoglobin to resist denaturation in alkaline conditions, the Apt test is a rapid, inexpensive, and simple bedside alternative.

Fetal movements can interfere with the procedure and sometimes can dislodge the needle, with the risk for complications (bleeding, cord hematoma) and the necessity of further cord punctures. In some situations, it may be helpful to perform a fetal neuromuscular blockade as is done in therapeutic cordocentesis. An intravascular injection as part of the cordocentesis or intramuscular administration of pancuronium bromide (0.1 to 0.3 mg/kg of estimated fetal weight) can achieve fetal paralysis.[30]

In at least 1% of pregnancies, a single umbilical artery (usually having a larger diameter than normal umbilical cord arteries) is present. The fetal loss risk associated with puncture of a single umbilical artery (two vessel cord) appears to be no different from that with a normal three-vessel cord.[31] Nevertheless, the use of Doppler color-flow mapping to guide the procedure and an experienced operator is recommended.

Safety

Loss rates for patients undergoing PUBS vary greatly by indication and by operator experience, more so than with amniocentesis or CVS. No randomized clinical trial has been reported. The ACOG[8] suggests "less than 2%" as the procedure-related loss risk, citing Ghidini and colleagues.[32] Data from several large perinatal centers similarly estimate the risk for in utero death or spontaneous abortion to be 3% or less following PUBS.[33] Collaborative data from 14 North American centers sampling 1600 patients at varying gestational ages for a variety of indications found an uncorrected fetal loss rate of 1.6%.[34] Tongsong and associates[34] compared a cohort of 1281 women with a singleton gestation without a fetal anomaly and undergoing cordocentesis between 16 and 24 weeks of gestational age with a control group matched for maternal and gestational age; the fetal loss rate was 3.2% in the study group compared with 1.8% in the controls. In another series of 2010 cordocentesis procedures in singleton pregnancies, the procedure-related fetal loss rates within 2 weeks were 1% when performed before 24 weeks and 0.8% after 24 weeks.[35] Cordocentesis can be successfully performed in multifetal gestation; limited data suggest a higher overall fetal loss rates (10.5%) with no increase in the procedure-related loss rates.[36] **Cordocentesis is thus a relatively safe procedure, although fetal loss rates vary with indication (preexisting fetal status) and operator experience.**

Other complications associated with cordocentesis include cord hematomas, bleeding from the puncture site in the umbilical cord, transient fetal bradycardia, and fetomaternal hemorrhage. Bleeding from the cord puncture is the most common complication and may be seen in 30% to 41% of cases.[37] Duration of bleeding is significantly longer after arterial than umbilical vein puncture. However, usually the blood loss is not clinically significant in either case. Van Kamp and coworkers[38] also describe bleeding from the puncture site significantly more often and of longer duration after transamniotic cord puncture than after transplacental puncture. Transient fetal bradycardia occurs in approximately 10% of procedures. Both umbilical artery puncture and severe, early-onset growth restriction were associated with increased rates of bradycardia. Finally, the extent of fetomaternal hemorrhage or transfusion depends on the duration of the procedure, bleeding time, puncture site, and use of a transplacental approach.[39]

Maternal complications are rare but include amnionitis (>1%) and transplacental hemorrhage.[38] In general, these complications do not significantly compromise maternal health status. However, there are case reports of severe sepsis.[38,40]

INDICATIONS FOR PRENATAL GENETIC STUDIES

Indications for prenatal genetic studies arise from those clinical situations associated with an increased risk for a diagnosable prenatal genetic condition. Some of these risk factors are present preconceptionally and are discussed in Chapter 10. These include maternal age, parental chromosome rearrangements, and parents both heterozygous for the same mendelian disorders. Other risk factors become evident only during the pregnancy. These include positive results for aneuploidy screening, unexpected ultrasound detection of fetal structural anomalies, and intrauterine growth restriction (IUGR).

Cytogenetic Disorders

Every chromosomal disorder is potentially detectable in utero. Thus, any pregnant woman could if desired undergo an invasive procedure to exclude these conditions, with near 100% certainty. However, for most couples, the risk for an invasive procedure outweighs the diagnostic benefits, as discussed earlier in this chapter. The most common indications that justify prenatal cytogenetic diagnosis are the following:

- Advanced maternal age, resulting in increased risk for autosomal trisomy
- Parental chromosome rearrangements
- Previous pregnancy with autosomal trisomy
- Abnormal ultrasound findings during the current pregnancy: fetal structural anomalies, IUGR, amniotic fluid volume abnormalities
- Increased risk, as calculated from noninvasive screening results: nuchal translucency and maternal serum analytes (see Chapter 10)

Advanced Maternal Age

Antenatal prenatal cytogenetic studies (screening or invasive procedures) are most commonly pursued because of advanced maternal age. A procedure may be requested at any age, as stated by ACOG.[41] The incidence of trisomy 21 is 1 per 800 live births in the United States. A commonly used table showing age-specific risks is provided in Table 11-1.[42] Other calculations exist. Trisomy 13, trisomy 18, 47,XXX, and 47,XXY also increase with advanced age.

Risk figures shown in Table 11-1 are applicable for liveborn infants. The prevalence of chromosomal abnormalities when amniocentesis is performed is higher than that at birth by approximately 30%.[43] It follows that the risk at the time of noninvasive screening (10 to 15 weeks) is higher. In using noninvasive screening protocols, the likelihood of Down syndrome is usually set at 1 per 270 (screen positivity), the midtrimester risk for a 35-year-old woman

TABLE 11-1 MATERNAL AGE AND CHROMOSOMAL ABNORMALITIES (LIVE BIRTHS)*

MATERNAL AGE (yr)†	RISK FOR DOWN SYNDROME AT BIRTH	RISK FOR ANY CHROMOSOME ABNORMALITY AT BIRTH†
20	1:1667	1:526
21	1:1667	1:526
22	1:1429	1:500
23	1:1429	1:500
24	1:1250	1:476
25	1:1250	1:476
26	1:1176	1:476
27	1:1111	1:455
28	1:1053	1:435
29	1:1000	1:417
30	1:952	1:385
31	1:909	1:385
32	1:769	1:323
33	1:602	1:312
34	1:482	1:253
35	1:375	1:202
36	1:289	1:163
37	1:224	1:129
38	1:173	1:103
39	1:136	1:82
40	1:106	1:65
41	1:82	1:51
42	1:63	1:40
43	1:49	1:32
44	1:38	1:25
45	1:30	1:20
46	1:23	1:16
47	1:18	1:12
48	1:14	1:10
49	1:11	1:8

Data from Hook EB, Cross PK, Schreinemachers DM: Chromosomal abnormality rates at amniocentesis and in live-born infants. JAMA 249:2034, 1983; and Schreinemachers DM, Cross PK, Hook EB: Rates of trisomies 21, 18, 13 and other chromosome abnormalities in about 20,000 prenatal studies compared with estimated rates in live births. Hum Genet 61:318, 1982.

*Because sample size for some intervals is relatively small, confidence limits are sometimes relatively large. Nonetheless, these figures are suitable for genetic counseling.

†47,XXX excluded for ages 20 to 32 yr (data not available).

(Chapter 10). There is a further increase (50%) in prevalence at CVS compared with amniocentesis.[43,44] The frequency of aneuploidy in the first trimester is 5% higher than in the second trimester. That the frequency of chromosomal abnormalities is lower in liveborn infants than in first- or second-trimester fetuses reflects the disproportionate likelihood that fetuses lost spontaneously will have chromosomal abnormalities. Some abnormal fetuses would have died spontaneously in utero had iatrogenic intervention not occurred in the second trimester. In fact, 8% to 13% of stillborn infants show chromosomal abnormalities (see Chapter 26), more if the stillborn has overt malformations.

In January 2007, ACOG published new recommendations concerning prenatal cytogenetic screening.[41] Before this, it was standard medical practice in the United States to offer invasive chromosomal diagnosis to all women who at their expected delivery date will be 35 years or older and have singleton pregnancies, but not necessarily to those younger. The cutoff of age 35 years was, however, always largely arbitrary, chosen at a time when risk figures were available only in 5-year intervals (i.e., 30 to 34 years, 35 to 39 years, 40 to 44 years) (see Simpson[45]). In twin gestations, it had been recommended that an invasive procedure be offered at age 32 or 33 years.[46,47] The rationale was that most twins being dizygotic, the likelihood that either one of the two would be aneuploid is the sum of the individual risks. At age 33, this combined risk for either liveborn infant being trisomic was 1 in 347, comparable to the singleton risk at age 35 (1 in 375) (see Table 11-1). The same reasoning applies to all chromosomal aneuploidies: 1 in 176 versus 1 in 202.

The 2007 ACOG[41] guidelines state unequivocally that neither age 35 years nor any specific age should be used as a threshold for invasive or noninvasive screening. ACOG stated: "All women, regardless of age, should have the option of invasive testing." ACOG[41] specifically elaborates that "patients informed of the risks, especially those at increased risk for having an aneuploid fetus, may elect to have diagnostic testing without first having screening." Relatively younger women who elect an invasive procedure directly may do so because of the ability to detect not only trisomies but also microdeletions and microduplication syndromes. This is possible through chromosomal microarrays based on comparative genome hybridization (CGH), a topic discussed later.

If an invasive procedure is not selected initially, first- or second-trimester noninvasive screening is now considered by ACOG[41] as appropriate to offer all women who present before 20 weeks of gestation, irrespective of age. As discussed in Chapter 10, only those who are "screen positive" are offered an invasive procedure. If a noninvasive screening program has been instituted in a population in which women older than maternal age 34 years were previously offered an invasive procedure, potential litigious hazard exists if counseling is not lucid. Detection rates for Down syndrome are good (80% to 93%) with noninvasive screening but less than the near 100% achieved with an invasive diagnostic test. Noninvasive screening is most likely to be applicable to women ages 33 to 37 years, after which most women will be screen positive and still require a procedure.

Previous Child with Chromosomal Abnormality

After the occurrence of one child, stillborn fetus, or abortus with autosomal trisomy, the likelihood that subsequent progeny will have autosomal trisomy is increased, even if parental chromosomal complements are normal. Recurrence risks are approximately 1%.[48] Invasive antenatal chromosomal studies should be offered for couples with a prior trisomic pregnancy. Recurrence risk data following trisomy 18 are comparable.[48] Describing a risk of 1% for either the same or a different chromosomal abnormality seems appropriate in women younger than 40 years. Risk for recurrence applies also if the trisomy was detected in a spontaneous abortion.

Parental Chromosomal Rearrangements

An uncommon but important indication for prenatal cytogenetic studies is presence of a parental chromosomal abnormality. A balanced translocation is the most common indication, but inversions and other chromosomal rearrangements exist. See Chapter 10 for a more detailed discussion and figures. A mother or father having a balanced translocation is at risk for offspring with an unbalanced translocation and, hence, abnormal offspring. Fortunately, empirical data show that theoretical risks for abnormal (unbalanced) offspring are greater than empirical risks, but miscarriages are common. It is for this reason that preimplantation genetic diagnosis (see later) can be especially helpful; otherwise, time to achieve pregnancy could be delayed beyond that realistic for an older woman. The risk for having a liveborn infant with an unbalanced chromosomal complement varies by rearrangement, sex of the carrier, and method of ascertainment.[49] Pooled empirical risks tabulated at CVS or amniocentesis approximate 12% risk for clinically abnormal offspring of either male or female translocation carriers with reciprocal translocations.[49] For Robertsonian (centric fusion) translocations, risks vary according to the chromosomes involved. For t(14q;21q), risks are 10% for offspring of heterozygous mothers and 2% for offspring of heterozygous fathers.[50] For other nonhomologous Robertsonian translocations, empirical risks for liveborn infants are less than 1%. Later in this chapter, we discuss the different percentages observed at preimplantation genetic diagnosis (PGD).

For homologous translocations (e.g., 21q;21q), all liveborn offspring should have trisomy 21. For other homologous Robertsonian translocations (13q;13q or 22q;22q), almost all pregnancies result in abortions.

In Robertsonian translocations, risk also exists for uniparental disomy (UPD). In UPD, both homologous chromosomes are derived from a single parent. UPD has been observed in offspring of a carrier having a balanced robertsonian translocation. Excluding UPD is most appropriately performed in prenatal cases in which a chromosome with known UPD clinical effect is involved (e.g., chromosomes 7, 11, 14, 15).

Assisted Reproduction through Intracytoplasmic Sperm Injection

Intracytoplasmic sperm injection (ICSI) is used in assisted reproduction technology (ART) when the male partner is subfertile. Empirical data have showed an increased frequency of aneuploidies, mainly sex chromosome anomalies (1% to 2%).[51] The excess risk appears not related to the ICSI technique but rather to the underlying male infertility that necessitated ICSI.

Accuracy of Prenatal Cytogenetic Diagnosis

The obstetrician-gynecologist should be aware of the common pitfalls associated with analysis of chorionic villi or amniotic fluid cells and may be called on to interpret or explain these findings to patients. One obvious problem is that cells may not grow, or growth may be insufficient for proper analysis. Analysis of maternal rather than fetal cells is another problem, fortunately uncommon. In amniocentesis, maternal cell contamination can be minimized by discarding the first 1 to 2 mL of aspirated amniotic fluid. In CVS, examination under a dissecting microscope allows one to distinguish villi from maternal decidua.

A more vexing concern is that chromosomal abnormalities detected in villi or amniotic fluid may not reflect fetal status. Chromosomal aberrations may arise in culture (in vitro) or may be confined to placental tissue. This possibility should be suspected when mosaicism (more than one cell line) is restricted to only one of the several culture flasks or clones initiated from a single amniotic fluid or CVS specimen, or when an abnormal karyotype with a known severely anomalous phenotype does not correlate with a normal ultrasound. Although the reference laboratory and clinical geneticists are naturally expected to have requisite expertise, the obstetrician should be prepared to discuss certain common dilemmas with the patient.

Numerical

Cells containing at least one additional structurally normal chromosome are not uncommonly detected (1% to 2%) in amniotic fluid or CVS specimens.[52] If these abnormal cells are found in a single culture or clone, the phenomenon is termed *pseudomosaicism*. Usually no clinical significance is attached. Defined by the presence of the same abnormality in more than one clone or culture flask, true fetal mosaicism is rarer but more significant. True mosaicism is confirmed by studies of the abortus or liveborn infant in 70% to 80% of cases[53] and actually can never truly be excluded because the abnormality could be restricted to a tissue not readily accessible.

Numerical problems are more frequent in short-term cultures, which can be performed on chorionic villi but not on amniotic fluid cells. However, array CGH (chromosomal microarrays), discussed later, can be performed on uncultured DNA from either villi or amniotic fluid cells). Metaphases from the trophoblasts or villi can accumulate within hours of sampling, allowing rapid answers. In CVS, discrepancies may arise between short-term trophoblast cultures and long-term cultures, which are initiated from the mesenchymal core of villi.[54] Discrepancies may further exist between CVS preparations and the embryo. If CVS results seem at odds with clinical findings, it is reasonable to track interval growth and, if normal, perform a follow-up amniocentesis. Several rare trisomies (+16, +22, +7)[54] in particular may not be confirmed. Sometimes mosaicism is present in the placenta but not in the embryo; this is called *confined placental mosaicism* (CPM). In this circumstance, the likelihood of anomalies is considered low.[55] However, the U.S. NICHD Collaborative CVS Trial observed increased late loss rates (8.6%) in pregnancies showing CPM compared with pregnancies without mosaicism (3.4%). Although CPM usually does not have clinical significance,[54] two potential adverse effects associated with CPM should be considered: IUGR and UPD. UPD, the inheritance of both homologous chromosomes from a single parent, may result from a reduction to disomy from a trisomic embryo rescue.[57] The phenotypic effect of UPD depends on the chromosome involved.[58] Imprinted genes that have phenotypic effects with regard to UPD include chromosomes 7 (Russell-Silver syndrome), 11 (Beckwith-Wiedemann syndrome), 14 (mental retardation and multiple anomalies), and 15 (Prader-Willi and Angelman syndromes).

Potential technical problems notwithstanding, amniotic fluid analysis and chorionic villi analysis are highly accurate. The U.S. NICHD Collaborative CVS Trial evaluated 11,473 chorionic villus samples by direct methods, long-term culture, or both. There were no incorrect sex predictions.[54] No diagnostic errors occurred among 148 common autosomal trisomies (+13, +18, +21), 16 sex chromosomal aneuploidies, and 13 structural aberrations; no normal cytogenetic diagnosis with CVS has ever been followed by birth of a trisomic infant. Overall, accuracy of CVS is comparable to that of amniocentesis.

Structural

If an ostensibly balanced inversion or translocation is detected in the fetus but not found in either parent, the rearrangement arose de novo. In this situation, there is increased likelihood that the neonate will be phenotypically abnormal at birth. The inversion or translocation may not actually be balanced; there may be genes around breakpoints deleted and unappreciated by cytogenetic analysis whose resolution is 5 million base pairs (5 Mb). The risk for the fetus being abnormal has been tabulated at 6% for a de novo reciprocal inversion and 10% to 15% for a de novo translocation.[59] Risks are not chromosome specific but represent pooled data involving many chromosomes. These risks also apply only to anatomic or developmental abnormalities evident at birth, not taking into account abnormalities that become evident only later in life. In ostensibly balanced de novo translocations, more subtle changes responsible for risks may be detected by chromosomal microarrays (array CGH), whose resolution is much better than standard karyotypes. Thus, more precise counseling is now possible, but normalcy cannot be promised even if array CGH shows no abnormality.

Marker chromosomes, also called *supernumerary chromosomes,* by definition cannot be fully characterized on the basis of standard cytogenetic analyses. These small chromosomes usually contain a centromere, a high proportion derived from the short arms of acrocentric chromosomes (13, 14, 15, 21, and 22). Marker chromosomes are observed in approximately 0.06% of the population.[60] Analogous to translocations and inversions, the risk for phenotypic abnormality in a fetus with a marker chromosome then depends on whether the marker is de novo or familial. Risk is higher when de novo markers are encountered. With FISH or chromosomal microarrays, the chromosome from which the marker chromosomes originated can now usually be established.

In reviewing 15,522 prenatal diagnostic procedures, Hume and colleagues[61] ascertained 19 marker chromosomes, 5 from CVS specimens and 14 from amniotic fluid samples. Monitoring these pregnancies with high-resolution ultrasonography revealed an association between de novo marker chromosomes and anomalies. When ultrasound examination was normal, the likelihood of a phenotypically normal offspring was high. Analogous to de novo translocations, array CGH can characterize the marker and elucidate whether gain or loss of genetic material exists.

Newer Cytogenetic Approaches

A plethora of cytogenetic advances has become available within the past decade, and the obstetrician may encounter patients whose diagnostic studies have used these technologies. A brief summary of those tests, some alluded to already, is therefore provided. Standard genetic texts provide additional information.

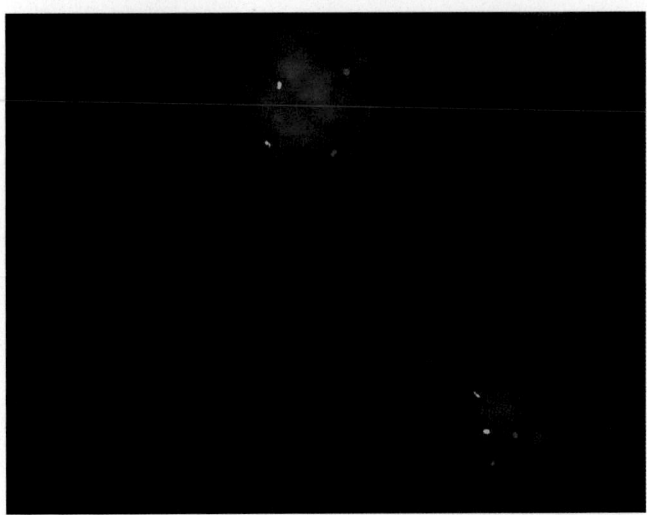

FIGURE 11-3. Fluorescence in situ hybridization *(FISH)* performed on interphase nuclei obtained from peripheral blood lymphocytes. Dual-color FISH has been performed using Vysis (Abbot Molecular, Abbott Park, IL) locus-specific probes *(LSI)* for chromosome 13 (green) and chromosome 21 (red). Chromosomal DNA is stained with DAPI (blue). Two signals for each indicates disomy (normal numbers) for these two chromosomes. (Courtesy Helen Tempest, Florida International University, Miami, FL.)

Fluorescence in Situ Hybridization

Available for 20 years now, fluorescence in situ hybridization (FISH) merges molecular genetics with cytogenetics. Using DNA sequences unique to the chromosome in question, chromosome-specific probes (e.g., chromosomes 13, 18, 21, the X, or the Y) can be created (Figure 11-3). The probe is then labeled with a fluorochrome and used to challenge unknown DNA that is denatured. Now single-stranded, this DNA becomes amenable to hybridization to its complementary sequence, whether from the same individual or reference (normal) DNA. Disomic cells (metaphase or interphase) should show two separate signals; trisomic cells show three signals. Because of geometric vicissitudes (e.g., one chromosome overlying another and unappreciated in a two-dimensional scan), not every trisomic cell shows three signals; however, the modal count is readily indicated. A single cell can be interrogated for up to five chromosomes. FISH uses interphase cells, thus permitting rapid or same-day diagnosis of aneuploidy. This becomes particularly important when a rapid diagnosis is needed to aid in the management of a fetus at high risk, such as one with multiple anomalies detected by ultrasound. FISH can also be used on preserved tissue (e.g., paraffin blocks), when culture for metaphase analysis is obviously not possible.

Quantitative Fluorescent Polymerase Chain Reaction

Polymerase chain reaction (PCR) is a widely used test that permits a small amount of DNA (e.g., one cell) to be amplified to generate an amount sufficient for a diagnostic test. In quantitative PCR (QPCR), the rapidity with which the exponential increase in DNA occurs allows rapid and accurate detection of major numerical chromosomal disorders in CVS.[62] This technique can be a powerful adjunct to conventional cytogenetics and in some venues (Europe) has replaced the traditional karyotype in prenatal diagnosis.

Comparative Genomic Hybridization and Chromosomal Microarrays

Comparative genomic hybridization (CGH) is an exciting molecular cytogenetic technique that, as alluded to already, allows comprehensive analysis of the entire genome at a finer resolution than banded karyotypes. The principle is based on single-stranded DNA annealing (hybridizing) with a complementary single-stranded DNA. Hybridization occurs whether from the same individual or from different individuals. Initially, normal (control) DNA in the form of a metaphase was labeled with a fluorochrome of one color (e.g., green), whereas test (patient) DNA was labeled with a fluorochrome of a different color (e.g., red). When both test and control DNA are denatured (single stranded), the test DNA hybridizes to the control metaphase. If equal amounts of control and test DNA are present, one would expect the color of the hybridized mixture to be yellow. If the test DNA were in excess (e.g., trisomy), the mixture for the relevant chromosome region would be relatively more of the color used to connote test (patient) DNA. This would be red in the previous example. For trisomy, this would apply to the entire chromosome. For duplications or deficiencies of chromosomal regions, only a portion of the chromosome would be red or green. The converse would apply for deletions or monosomy. Metaphase CGH has evolved into more sensitive chromosome microarrays, but the same principle applies.

The principles discussed earlier can be applied to smaller portions of DNA, even several thousand bases. Small amounts of single-stranded DNA (cDNA) of known sequence are placed by photolithography onto a platform (array) in ordered fashion. The amount of DNA in each spot is small (i.e., micro). Compared with karyotypes, the ability to detect deletions or duplications is greatly increased. Conventional karyotypes can only detect abnormalities of 5 to 10 Mb, whereas chromosomal microarrays easily detect abnormalities 200 kilobases (200,000) in size and if desired, 20 to 50 bases. The number of sequences is set in advance but is expected to encompass the entire genome, one sequence overlaying the adjacent one ("tiling"). The "control" DNA embedded by photolithography is labeled with a fluorochrome of one color (e.g., green). Exposure is then made to single-stranded test DNA (e.g., patient), now labeled with a fluorochrome of different color (e.g., red). If control and test DNA are quantitatively equal for a given sequence, the color is yellow. If test DNA is excess (trisomy), the color is more red; if test DNA is deficient, the color is more green. One thus detects deletion or excess (gain) of DNA, de facto generating a "molecular karyotype" (Figure 11-4).

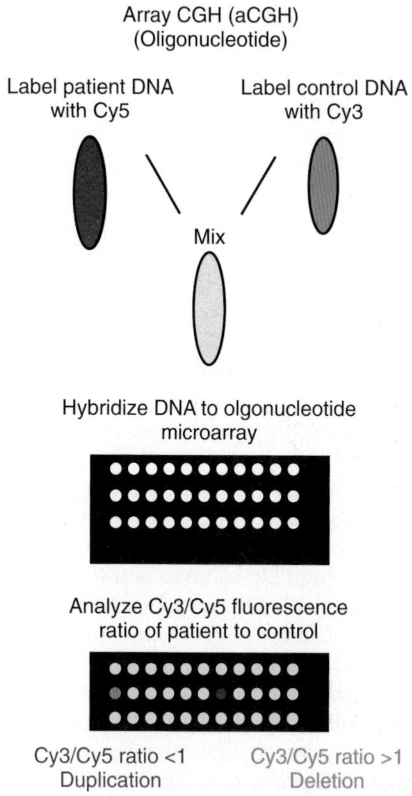

Several different commercial platforms are available, but all interrogate sequences of DNA along every chromosome. "Coverage" varies slightly based on sensitivity sought, and in all there is redundancy, that is, a given region is interrogated more than once to ensure replicability before making a diagnosis. The smaller the copy number variants (CNVs) the less likely a pathogenic effect, but even small CNVs can be significant. At the 50- to 200-base level, CNVs (duplications or deletions) are often polymorphisms, inherited from a clinically normal parent and without clinical significance. Some 70 CNVs can be confidentially predicted to have pathogenic consequences and readily detected by CMAs but not by traditional karyotype. In aggregate these occur in perhaps 1 per 1500 births in the general population, but this number is higher in selected populations. An estimated 5% to 7% of children with developmental delay have CNVs, and array CGH is now considered a standard part of evaluation in such cases.[63]

In prenatal studies, determining case and effort is more arguable. In postnatal cases, array CGH is usually requested only if a clinical abnormality is obvious in a liveborn child. This is not so in prenatal cases, and even if so (e.g., ultrasound), the extent of abnormalities is never clear. It is thus more difficult to predict the significance of a CNV detected in villi or amniotic fluid cells. Several principles are,

FIGURE 11-4. Schematic diagram illustrating principles of array comparative genome hybridization *(CGH)*. Patient DNA is labeled in red *(CY5)*, whereas references (normal control) are labeled in green *(Cy3)*. When denatured into single-stranded DNA, patient DNA and control DNA hybridize with DNA of the same type that is embedded on a platform *(circles)*. The diagram shows only 33 "spots" of similar sequence, whereas in actual practice, a diagnostic platform would consist of thousands of embedded sequences. If the region being interrogated shows equal amounts of patient DNA and control DNA, the signal is yellow. A green signal indicates deficiency of test DNA (deletion or mosaicism), whereas a red signal indicates excess of test DNA (duplication or trisomy). Array CGH detects trisomies just like a karyotype; smaller deletions or duplications (<5,000,000 base pairs) are detected only by array CGH. (Courtesy Ron J. Wapner, Columbia University, New York).

however, applicable. A large CNV present in a fetus but in neither parent (de novo) warrants the most attention, and a deletion is more consequential than a duplication. The region involved is also important; some sequences of DNA are relatively "gene poor," whereas others contain genes known to be deleterious if perturbed. Familial heritable transmission of CNVs may be clinically significant. Exceptions exist because CNVs may display incomplete penetrance with respect to phenotypic effect.

The recently reported NICHD prenatal cytogenetic array study involved 4401 women having varying indications (46% maternal age; 26% ultrasound anomaly) All trisomies and sex chromosome aneuploidies detected by karyotypes were also detected by array CGH.[64] All microdeletions and microduplications predicted to be detected (e.g., DiGeorge syndrome) were in fact detected. A difficulty is that additional CNVs of uncertain clinical significance were also detected. A Clinical Advisory Committee independent of laboratory directions considered one third of CNVs to be benign based on extant data, not warranting disclosure to parents.[65] Of the remaining, 1.6% were considered to be potentially significant and for a variety of reasons required disclosure. Sometimes disclosure was considered on the basis of potential termination, sometimes because follow-up ultrasound seemed warranted and would otherwise not have been pursued, and sometimes on the basis of relevance to a family history of abnormalities. The manner in which disclosure and counseling are conveyed is thus crucial.[65,66]

In summary, prenatal array CGH promises to be a major addition to the diagnostic armamentarium, but providers need to be prepared for anxiety in deciding when to disclose variants of uncertain clinical significance.

One disadvantage of array CGH compared with the traditional karyotype is that chromosomal microarrays cannot distinguish between balanced translocations and normal; unbalanced (duplication, deficiency) rearrangements are readily detected. Another is difficulty in detecting low-level mosaicism in which one of the two cell lines is infrequent. In some platforms, triploidy cannot be excluded. On the other hand, array CGH can be performed on uncultured DNA, including circumstances (e.g., stillborn fetuses) in which cell cultures for chromosomal abnormalities are not often successful.

MENDELIAN DISORDERS

The combination of sequencing the human genome (2001) and subsequently developing molecular diagnostics has completely changed the approach to prenatal genetic diagnosis for single gene disorders. Previously, many different approaches had to be applied, as recounted in earlier editions of this text. This reflected the reality that for a very few disorders was the actual molecular basis (e.g., missense or nonsense mutations) known. Rarely was the gene's location even known. Only a relatively small proportion of at-risk couples could thus be tested for a disorder of interest. The prototype exception was sickle cell anemia, in which virtually almost all cases result from a point mutation in codon 6 of β-globin. Prenatal diagnosis more often required measuring the presence or absence of the deficient gene product (proteins), an accumulated substrate (e.g., inborn errors of metabolism) in chorionic villus of amniotic fluid cells. Although this was readily possible for inborn errors of metabolism (e.g., galactosemia), it was not for disorders lacking a known metabolic basis. Imaging (ultrasound or radiographic) was the preferred approach for mendelian disorders like skeletal dysplasias. Cytogenetic studies could be used for chromosomal breakage syndromes like Bloom syndrome and Fanconi anemia. Fetal skin biopsy for histologic studies was required for epidermolysis bullosa and genodermatosis, and fetal muscle biopsy for Duchenne muscular dystrophy. With sequencing of the human genome, the paradigm has completely changed. Indirect approaches like those enumerated above are used less frequently for definitive diagnosis, and theoretically not at all if the location of the causative gene is known.

Molecular Approach to Diagnosis

Sequencing the human genome has revealed approximately 22,000 genes (based on certain established sequencing criteria defining a gene). The function of many genes is still unknown, but increasingly, mendelian disorders of potential prenatal genetic diagnosis interest are being identified and their molecular perturbations known. The illustration of cystic fibrosis discussed in Chapter 10 is paradigmatic. Molecular basis of recognized single gene disorders varies—point mutations leading to a single nucleotide and hence a single amino acid change (e.g., sickle cell anemia), premature stop codon truncating the protein gene product, deletions of three nucleotides leading to loss of an entire amino acid, deletion of one or two nucleotides leading to a frame shift that results in an altered reading frame with all subsequent amino acids being coded erroneously.

In a given disorder, it is exceptional for a single molecular perturbation to be responsible, as is the case in sickle cell anemia and achondroplasia. One or more perturbations may account for a significant proportion, at least within a given ethnic group; however, the molecular basis is typically heterogeneous. In the near future, we can expect panels to be available for genes likely to result in, say, the most common forms of skeletal dysplasia. An array of mutations or targeted sequencing of such genes can be constructed. If the cost of sequencing the entire genome decreases as expected, diagnosis may become conceptually straightforward for the obstetrician (albeit with considerable pitfalls for the interpreting geneticist). Still, the molecular basis may not always be evident for every affected individual, even in well-studied disorders like cystic fibrosis. If sequencing the coding regions of the gene in question does not reveal a perturbation, the assumption is that pathogenesis involves the promoter region or post-transcriptional processes (e.g., translation). However, diagnosis is still possible by linkage analysis.

The general approach for detecting single gene disorders involves directly determining presence of a known molecular perturbation. Alternatively, if the actual mutation is not known, linkage analysis can still be used to identify affected cases if the chromosomal location has been determined. Suppose a couple is at risk for a known disorder, but the molecular basis in their family is unknown. Recall that the chromosomal location may still be known, even if no perturbation is evident. In linkage analysis, one relies on polymorphic markers upstream and downstream from the mutation site. These polymorphisms are without clinical significance but can serve as markers (short tandem repeats of nucleotides; single nucleotide polymorphisms). At every locus (polymorphic or mutant), one marker allele is of paternal origin and one is maternal. A panel of markers can be identified that coexist (in phase) with the chromosome having the mutation, said to be *cis* and in contrast to those markers on the chromosome having the normal allele (*trans*). That is, given two chromosomes, one set of markers will be on the chromosome containing the mutant allele for the disorder in question (dominant or recessive), whereas the other will lie on the "normal" chromosome. Studying affected and unaffected family members will allow one to determine the "phase" of markers unique to that family. If there are no surviving affected family members, one may still be able to deduce phase (*cis* versus *trans*) by analyzing individual sperm, should the disorder have arisen de novo in a male. Regardless, the principle is that a diagnosis can be deduced without knowledge of the precise nucleotide perturbations.

A molecularly based diagnosis can thus be readily achieved for patients at risk for hundreds of disorders. Any nucleated fetal cell (chorionic villus, amniotic fluid cell, blastomere from an embryo) will suffice. Technical details are beyond the purview of this text, save appreciation that molecular diagnosis is highly accurate in good laboratories, and none is perfect.

Mendelian Disorders Without Known Molecular Basis

There remain disorders whose genetic basis is not yet elucidated. If the causative gene is not known, linkage analysis is not applicable. Whether the concern originates in a previously affected child or the current pregnancy, one may have to resort to imaging, assuming cytogenetic findings (including microarrays) are normal in the previously affected child and structural anomalies are present. The spectrum of disorders detectable by imaging studies is discussed later in this chapter, including sensitivity at varying stages of gestation.

MULTIFACTORIAL DISORDERS

Although some progress has been made, the genetic basis of isolated birth defects involving a single organ system remains elusive. These are listed in Chapter 10 (see Table 10-1). Thus, even with a history of a prior affected offspring, no specific genetic tests are available. Prenatal diagnosis depends on ultrasound (see later), although for disorders in which fetal skin is discontinuous (e.g., myelomeningocele, omphalocele), nonspecific measures like amniotic fluid AFP are useful.

ULTRASOUND DIAGNOSIS OF FETAL MALFORMATIONS

Over the past few decades, many publications have described the ultrasound diagnosis of fetal malformations. A catalog of the diseases that are now considered detectable with prenatal ultrasound is beyond the scope of this chapter. In this section, we discuss the use of ultrasound as a screening test, outline the role of ultrasound in aneuploidy screening, and describe the relatively common birth defects that may be diagnosed with a standard ultrasound examination.

Ultrasound as a Screening Test for Birth Defects

With improvements of ultrasound equipment in the past few decades, many patients and clinicians have come to assume an ultrasound examination will likely detect all serious fetal anomalies. Indeed, in the 1980s and early 1990s, several individual centers reported detection rates of greater than 75% in referral[65] and low-risk[66] patients. However, serious questions regarding the sensitivity of routine ultrasound examinations in more general settings were raised by a large multicenter trial published in 1993.[67] The Routine Antenatal Diagnostic Imaging with Ultrasound Study (RADIUS)[67] was a randomized trial that included standardized ultrasound examinations of more than 15,000 women between 16 and 20 weeks of gestation, then again at 31 to 33 weeks. Patients were selected to be at low risk for pregnancy complications. In this study, only 17% of major anomalies were diagnosed by ultrasound before 24 weeks' gestation, and only 35% were detected overall. The study's authors concluded that routine ultrasound to screen for birth defects in low-risk women was not efficacious. A subsequent large study of ultrasound screening for birth defects, the "Eurofetus" study, included more than 200,000 women screened with routine ultrasound in 61 hospital units in 14 European countries.[68] In contrast to the low rate of detection of anomalies in the RADIUS trial, 61% of malformed fetuses were detected; sensitivity was much higher for major malformations (74%), albeit with a significant difference in detection rates according to the particular malformation or organ system involved. Defects of the central nervous system and urinary tract were detected 88% of the time, whereas only 18% of cases of cleft lip and palate were diagnosed. Eighteen percent of minor musculoskeletal malformations and 21% of minor cardiac malformations were detected, whereas sensitivities were 74% and 39%, respectively, for major anomalies of these two organ systems.

In the hands of a well-trained examiner, the detection rate of some anomalies should approach 100%. For example, anencephaly, abdominal wall defects, and anomalies involving an abnormal accumulation of fluid within a body cavity (i.e., hydronephrosis, hydrocephalus) will rarely be missed. Spina bifida, which itself may be difficult to see, is almost always accompanied by easily recognized intracranial findings, making the detection rate of this defect quite high. The growing awareness that **a screening ultrasound should include not only the four-chamber view of the heart** (Figure 11-5) **but also views of the outflow tracts** (Figures. 11-6 and 11-7**)** has resulted in a significant increase in detection rate of heart defects. DeVore reviewed three studies from the 1990s in which only the four-chamber view was obtained as a part of a screening ultrasound in low-risk populations.[69] In that 1998 report, only 8 of 151 cases were detected with the four-chamber screening, a detection rate of 5%. In contrast, a 2006 Norwegian study of more than 30,000 unselected patients screened

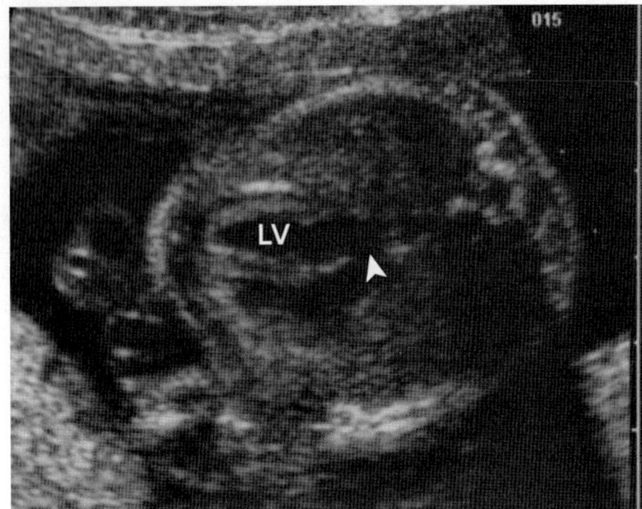

Figure 11-5. Normal four-chamber view of the heart. Note that the heart's position is central in the chest, and the axis is about 45 degrees to the left of the midline. The ventricles are approximately equal in size, while the left ventricle *(LV)* extends further into the apex. The intraventricular septum is intact, and the foramen ovale *(arrowhead)* is seen.

using not only the four chamber but also the great vessel views achieved a 57% detection rate.[70] Because of studies such as this that show the importance of outflow tract visualization for the detection of many heart defects, the American Institute of Ultrasound in Medicine (AIUM) recommends that attempts should be made to obtain these views in all second- and third-trimester scans.[71]

It is well recognized **that adequate training is essential to the proper performance and interpretation of obstetric ultrasound examinations.** In the RADIUS trial,[67] the detection rate for anomalies was almost three times higher when the examinations were performed at a tertiary center compared with a general practice setting (13% versus 35%), presumably because of greater experience of sonographers at the tertiary centers. Although qualifications for those performing ultrasound examinations to screen for birth defects have not been standardized, the AIUM has made recommendations regarding the training and experience needed for physicians to perform obstetrical ultrasound. These include the completion of an approved training program with the equivalent of 3 months of ultrasound experience and the involvement in the performance of at least 300 examinations, continuing education in the field (at least 30 hours every 3 years), and ongoing practice consisting of at least 170 obstetrical or gynecologic ultrasound examinations performed annually.[72]

The nature of the population being screened and the thoroughness of postnatal ascertainment of birth defects also affect the sensitivity of ultrasound for detecting defects. The detection rate has been shown to be higher in high-risk populations screened at centers with extensive experience at diagnosing birth defects. In studies that did not include rigorous prospective neonatal evaluation, subtle anomalies may not have been noted, and a sonographic "miss" of these defects would not be counted. This would give a falsely optimistic detection rate. The

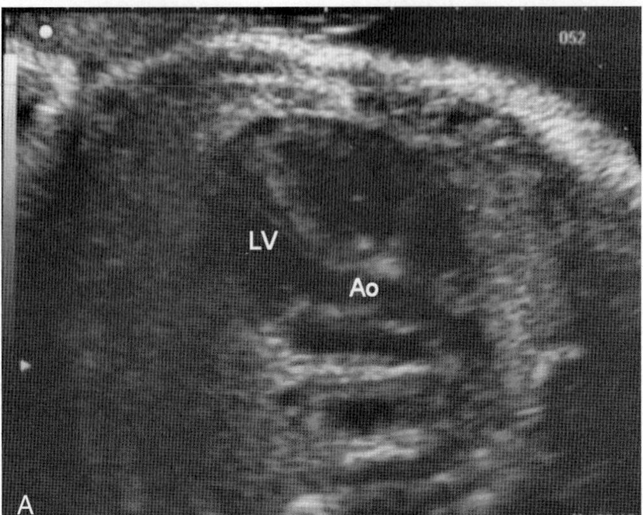

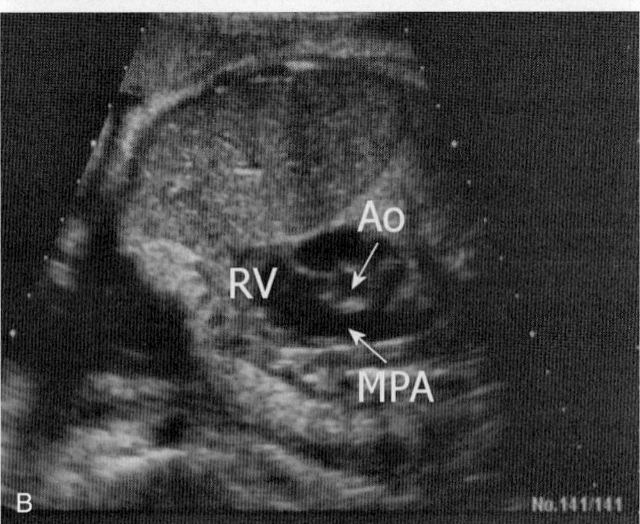

Figure 11-6. A, Left ventricular outflow tract. A normal aorta *(Ao)* is seen arising from the left ventricle *(LV)*. **B,** Right ventricular outflow tract. The main pulmonary artery *(MPA)* arises from the right ventricle *(RV)* and crosses anterior to the ascending aorta *(Ao)*.

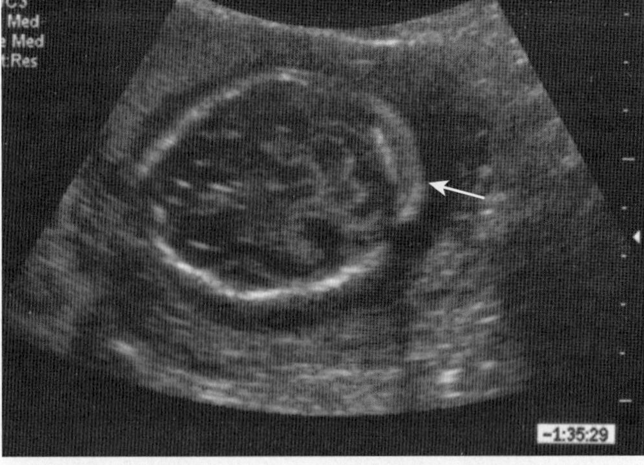

Figure 11-7. An 18-week fetus with trisomy 21, showing a thick nuchal fold *(arrow)*.

gestational age at which ultrasound is performed can influence the sensitivity of anomaly screening. Although many defects can now be recognized in the late first trimester (i.e., anencephaly and large abdominal wall defects), many are not visible until later. Some defects may become more readily apparent late in pregnancy. Although multiple examinations in each pregnancy would undoubtedly increase the pick-up rate of malformations, resource and financial constraints make this impractical. **It is generally agreed that the most cost-effective approach for screening low-risk pregnancies is to perform a standard examination between 18 and 20 weeks.** At this gestational age, adequate visualization of major organs is possible for most women.

False-positive results must be taken into account when considering the effectiveness of ultrasound screening for birth defects. Falsely abnormal results can cause patients and families considerable anguish and result in unnecessary follow-up tests. Fortunately, in both the RADIUS[67] and the Eurofetus[68] trials, fewer than 1 in 500 women was erroneously told that her healthy fetus had a malformation. However, of the nearly 3000 suspected malformations in the Eurofetus study, 10% were false-positive diagnoses, and 6% involved fetuses in which an initial concern was resolved on a subsequent ultrasound examination.[68]

Ultrasound Screening for Aneuploidy

Second Trimester

As discussed earlier in this chapter, well-established diagnostic tests for fetal aneuploidy include amniocentesis and CVS. In the past two decades, it has increasingly been possible to diagnose with ultrasound specific birth defects that are associated with aneuploidy, such as duodenal atresia and certain heart defects. In 1985, Benacerraf showed that there was **a significant association between the thickness of the fetal skinfold (see Figure 11-7) and the presence of trisomy 21.**[73] For the first time, a "marker," as opposed to an actual birth defect, could be used to assess the likelihood that Down syndrome was present. **Other markers that are now commonly used in the genetic sonogram include the nasal bone length, short femur or humerus, echogenic intracardiac focus, echogenic bowel, and pyelectasis.** The use of these markers has gradually become common clinical practice. Most of the markers perform poorly as individual predictors of Down syndrome, with a very low sensitivity and a high rate of false-positive results.[74] However, as markers were studied in larger numbers of women, it became possible to assign likelihood ratios to each marker and to do a formal risk adjustment from the a priori risk to an ultrasound-adjusted risk.[75] Most women undergoing a genetic sonogram have no markers. Therefore, most who are initially considered to be at high risk because of maternal age, a family history, or serum screening have an ultrasound-adjusted risk that places them in the low-risk category, such as a trisomy 21 risk less than that of a 35-year-old woman. **With patients increasingly relying on ultrasound and serum screening methods, the rate of women choosing invasive testing has decreased considerably.**[76]

There are problems with the use of these soft markers. First, some women may assume that the genetic sonogram is a diagnostic test that accurately identifies fetuses with aneuploidy. Women should be made to understand that although a genetic sonogram may reduce the chance that her fetus is affected, **the absence of markers does not rule out the possibility of Down syndrome or other chromosome abnormalities.** Second, it is difficult to assign a definite detection rate for the genetic sonogram because the test performs differently in the hands of different sonographers. Possible reasons include different skill levels of examiners and the subjective assessment required for several markers, particularly echogenic intracardiac focus and echogenic bowel.

The incidental finding of soft markers in otherwise low-risk pregnancies can cause a great deal of anxiety in the expectant parents. Opinions vary as to what to do when so-called minor markers, such as, echogenic intracardiac focus or pyelectasis, are noted in a low-risk patient. A reasonable approach is to refer such a patient for a consultation by an expert to evaluate for the presence of other markers. This individual can then use published likelihood ratios to adjust the patient's prior risk. In most cases, the patient's ultrasound-adjusted risk will be less than that of a 35-year-old woman. She can then be reassured that the finding is probably a variant of normal and that she remains in a low-risk category.

First Trimester

As discussed in detail in Chapter 10, ultrasound assessment is an important part of first-trimester aneuploidy screening. Discussion of the role of ultrasound for this application is much more straightforward because there is good standardization of the imaging and measurement techniques. The most important sonographic component of first-trimester screening is the nuchal translucency measurement. The presence or absence of a visible nasal bone is another important ultrasound finding (Figure 11-8). Other ultrasound findings have been described, such as reverse ductus venosus flow and tricuspid regurgitation,

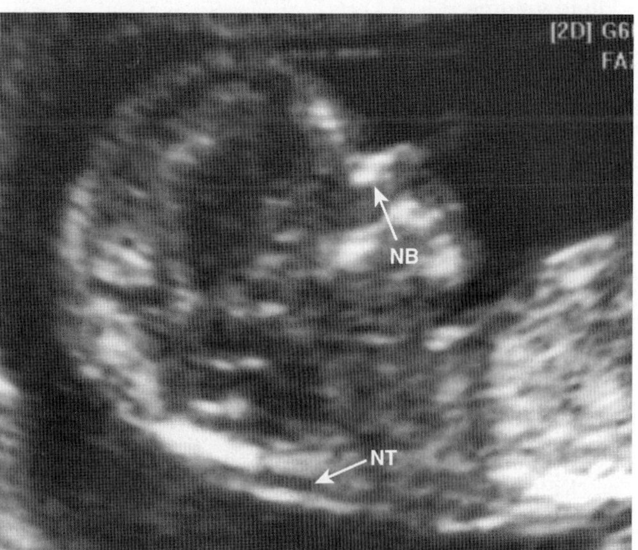

FIGURE 11-8. Midsagittal view of a 12-week fetus showing the nuchal translucency *(NT)* and nasal bone *(NB)*.

but they are not in general use.[77] There are rigorous criteria for appropriate nuchal translucency and nasal bone images. **Individuals who wish to perform the ultrasound component of the first-trimester screen must be trained and certified.** The standardization that comes through certification allows much greater confidence in the risk estimates for aneuploidy than is possible with the second-trimester genetic sonogram.

Screening for Anomalies with the Standard Ultrasound Examination

The AIUM has published specific components of a standard ultrasound examination performed in the second or third trimester (see box, Suggested Components of the Standard Obstetrical Ultrasound Performed in the Second and Third Trimesters). Careful attention to each of these components will allow detection of many, if not most, serious birth defects. In the following sections, normal structures will be demonstrated, and the alterations expected with different birth defects will be shown. The conditions described are those for which the general obstetrician should have familiarity, and that might reasonably be detected with a standard screening ultrasound examination. **Most of the associated images with these conditions are found in the on-line version of this book.**

Suggested Components of the Standard Obstetrical Ultrasound Performed in the Second and Third Trimesters

- Standard biometry
- Fetal cardiac activity (present or absent, normal or abnormal)
- Number of fetuses (if multiples, document chorionicity, amnionicity, comparison of fetal sizes, estimation of amniotic fluid normality in each sac, fetal genitalia)
- Presentation
- Qualitative or semiquantitative estimate of amniotic fluid volume
- Placental location, especially its relationship to the internal os
- Evaluation of the uterus (including fibroids) and adnexal structures
- Anatomic survey to include:
  - Head and neck
    Cerebellum
    Choroid plexus
    Cisterna magna
    Lateral cerebral ventricles
    Midline falx
    Cavum septum pellucidum
  - Chest
    Four-chamber view of the heart
    Outflow tracts (if possible)
  - Abdomen
    Stomach (presence, size, and situs)
    Kidneys
    Bladder
    Umbilical cord insertion into the abdomen
    Number of umbilical cord vessels
  - Spine
  - Extremities (presence or absence of legs and arms)

Head and Neck

General Appearance

On axial views the head should have an oval appearance. Elongation of the head (termed *dolichocephaly*) is often caused by lateral compressive forces associated with oligohydramnios, especially if the fetus is in a breech presentation. An abnormally round shape (termed *brachycephaly*) can be an important indicator of fetal abnormalities, especially holoprosencephaly and aneuploidies.

Neural Tube Defects

Anencephaly is often first suspected when a proper image for measuring the biparietal diameter cannot be obtained. The absence of the cranial vault can be diagnosed after 10 weeks' gestation. Although the skull is missing, lobulated disorganized brain tissue can be prominent between 9 and 11 weeks. This tissue degenerates by 15 weeks, leaving the characteristic appearance in which there is there is no cortex or cranium and the fetal eyes appear at the top of an intact lower face. Meningomyelocele extending varying distances from the base of the skull down the neck and body may be present with the anencephaly. Fetuses with anencephaly do not swallow normally, so polyhydramnios usually develops in pregnancies that are allowed to continue.

Whenever anencephaly is seen, especially if there are additional clefts or amputations in the fetus, a careful search should be made for strands of membranes attached to the fetus, which are diagnostic of the amniotic band sequence. When there are major skull deficits caused by amniotic bands, there is typically some remaining cerebral cortex, although this is not the case with anencephaly.

Encephalocele is the least common type of neural tube defect and is manifested by a protrusion of the meninges and sometimes brain tissue through a midline defect in the cranium. Ultrasound shows a midline sac protruding though the skull, most often in the occiput. The outcome is very poor if there is brain tissue within the encephalocele sac or there are other significant associated anomalies. When there is an isolated defect with no brain involvement, most children have a good neurologic outcome.

The sensitivity of ultrasound for diagnosing spina bifida increased dramatically in the 1980s when it was discovered that fetuses with this condition have readily apparent secondary changes in the brain and skull.[78] These include frontal narrowing of the skull (the *lemon sign*), ventriculomegaly, and an abnormal cerebellum and posterior fossa. The cerebellum is deformed and drawn backward to obliterate the posterior fossa. This finding, the Chiari type II malformation, is referred to as the *banana sign*.

Cystic Hygroma

A cystic hygroma is a loculated accumulation of fluid in the skin of the posterior neck. In fetuses with this finding, edema may be widespread and is often associated with full-blown hydrops. These fetuses do not survive into the third trimester. When a cystic hygroma is present, there is more than a 60% chance that the fetus has a chromosome abnormality, most commonly Turner syndrome.[79]

Cleft Lip and Palate

While not specifically listed as an AIUM required component of the standard exam, a coronal view of the fetal face is usually readily obtainable. This view shows the presence of cleft lip. Approximately two-thirds of those with cleft lip also have cleft palate. Cleft palate may be demonstrated with oblique views showing a defect in the maxillary ridge. An isolated cleft palate is rarely diagnosed with prenatal ultrasound.

Micrognathia

A midsagittal view of the face is the best in which to detect micrognathia. Micrognathia may be an important marker for genetic syndromes, such as trisomy 18. Severe hypoplasia of the mandible, such as is seen with Pierre Robin sequence, can cause breathing difficulties at birth; therefore, prenatal diagnosis is invaluable in planning neonatal management.

Cerebellum and Cisterna Magna

The cerebellum and posterior fossa should always be visualized in order to diagnose spina bifida, as described previously, and the Dandy-Walker malformation. In the latter condition, there is a posterior fossa cyst continuous with the fourth ventricle, complete or partial absence of the cerebellar vermis, and varying degrees of hydrocephalus. About 50% of affected fetuses have other intracranial malformations, 35% have extracranial abnormalities, and 15% to 30% have aneuploidy.[80] Many infants with the Dandy-Walker syndrome die after birth, usually as a result of associated malformations. Most survivors have some degree of mental handicap.

Choroid Plexus

Cysts within the choroid plexus are noted in about 1% of normal fetuses.[81] They generally are benign and resolve before 26 weeks without sequelae. Because their presence indicates a seven-fold increase in risk that the fetus has trisomy 18, referral to a specialty center or ultrasonographer is indicated.[82]

Lateral Ventricles

Hydrocephalus is a general term used to describe a head in which the cerebral ventricles are dilated. There are many causes, including spina bifida, stenosis of the aqueduct of Sylvius, normal pressure hydrocephalus, agenesis of the corpus callosum, fetal TORCH (*t*oxoplasmosis, *o*ther infections, *r*ubella, *c*ytomegalovirus, and *h*erpes simplex) infections, and other serious developmental malformations of the brain. In some cases, particularly those caused by aqueductal stenosis, the head can be markedly enlarged. The lateral and third ventricles may be very dilated with marked thinning of the cerebral cortex. With atraumatic delivery and appropriate neurosurgical treatment, more than half of infants with aqueductal stenosis survive, but about 75% of survivors have moderate to severe developmental delay.[83] The degree of hydrocephalus and the thickness of the remaining cerebral cortex are weak predictors of the neurologic outcome.

The appearance of the choroid plexus can assist in the diagnosis of less obvious hydrocephalus. With hydrocephalus, this structure, which usually fills this portion of the lateral ventricle from side to side, is compressed and "dangles." The accepted upper limit of the transverse diameter of the lateral ventricles at the atrium is 10 mm. When the ventricles measure between 10 and 12 mm, there is a 96% chance of a normal neurologic outcome, and an 86% chance with a measurement between 12 and 15 mm.[84] Whenever any degree of hydrocephalus is seen, a careful search for other malformations is essential because their presence strongly influences the prognosis. Agenesis of the corpus callosum should be considered when there is modest ventricular dilation that is primarily confined to posterior horns. Although fetuses with spina bifida usually have dilation of the lateral ventricles, the head size is usually not increased.[85]

A unilateral cystic lesion adjacent to the cerebral cortex most likely represents an arachnoid cyst. These generally are associated with a good prognosis but can reach considerable size, causing symptoms such as seizures or hydrocephalus. Porencephalic cysts are unilateral cystic lesions in the brain that have a much worse outcome. These arise from intracerebral infarcts or hemorrhages with subsequent liquefaction of the brain tissue or clot. The resultant cystic cavity within the brain parenchyma may be in communication with the subarachnoid space or a cerebral ventricle.

Midline Falx

Absence or abnormality of midline structures of the brain should point to a diagnosis of holoprosencephaly. This condition results from incomplete division of the cerebral hemispheres. With the "alobar" form of holoprosencephaly, the head is usually small and brachycephalic. There is no midline echo dividing the cerebral cortex, and there is a single crescent-shaped ventricle anterior to the bulbous-appearing thalamus. Many fetuses with holoprosencephaly have facial abnormalities as well, which may include hypotelorism or cyclopia, facial clefts, absent nose or single nostril, and presence of a proboscis above the eye or between the eyes. Chromosome abnormalities (especially trisomy 13) and other malformations are present in one third of cases. Regardless of the karyotype or presence of other malformations, alobar holoprosencephaly is associated with a dismal neurologic prognosis; death almost always occurs either before or shortly after birth. When there is partial division of the brain, the fetus may have "semilobar" or "lobar" holoprosencephaly, both of which have a somewhat more favorable prognosis.

Chest

Chest Masses

Displacement of the heart away from the midline is often a sign of a diaphragmatic hernia or a lung mass such as congenital pulmonary adenomatoid malformation (CPAM) or pulmonary sequestration. The presence of these conditions can be life-threatening to the fetus because vital chest structures are compressed or displaced. Space-occupying chest lesions can severely impair lung growth. Compression of the esophagus by a lung mass may cause symptomatic polyhydramnios. Similar pressure on the central veins and lymphatics may cause fetal death from generalized hydrops.

With diaphragmatic hernia, the heart is displaced to the side opposite the location of the defect, which is on the left in 75% of cases. The condition can be distinguished from other chest masses by the appearance of bowel, stomach, and other abdominal organs in the chest at the level of the four-chamber view of the heart. In the midabdominal view, the stomach is typically not seen with left-sided hernias and is shifted toward the right in right-sided lesions. The intrahepatic umbilical vein is usually shifted toward the side of the defect, and variable amounts of liver will sometimes be seen prolapsed into the chest. Ultrasound does not usually demonstrate significant lung tissue on the affected side. The contralateral lung can be very small. Displacement of the gastrointestinal tract often results in swallowing abnormalities, and half of cases develop polyhydramnios.

CPAM appears as a solid or cystic lung mass that is almost always unilateral and confined to one lobe. Frequently, there is a shift in the mediastinum with compression of the contralateral lung. Nonimmune hydrops can develop, and this finding is associated with a poor prognosis. Because an apparently very large CPAM can appear to regress as a pregnancy advances the clinician should be cautious about predicting a poor outcome.[86] Most affected children require nonemergent surgical resection.

Pulmonary sequestration is a congenital anomaly in which a mass of lung tissue arises from the foregut independently of the normal lung. It does not communicate with the tracheobronchial tree, and it receives its blood supply directly from the aorta. Ultrasound shows an echogenic intrathoracic or intra-abdominal mass, usually just above or just below the diaphragm. Color Doppler ultrasound can sometimes show the aberrant blood supply, thus distinguishing a pulmonary sequestration from CPAM. A pulmonary sequestration usually must be removed in childhood but rarely causes prenatal complications.[87]

Four-Chamber View of the Heart

In addition to the position of the heart within the chest, the axis should be carefully noted. The sonographer must identify the fetal right and left side based on the position of the fetus, not the position of the organs. Otherwise, abnormalities of sidedness, such as situs inversus, would be missed.

The starting place for diagnosing congenital heart defects is the four-chamber view (see Figure 11-5). Examples of defects that present with an abnormal four-chamber view include many septal defects and hypoplastic left heart syndrome. Ventricular septal defects account for 20% to 30% of congenital heart defects. Although large defects can often be seen in the four-chamber view, small defects are commonly missed, even by experienced examiners. Some significant defects are in the anterior, membranous portion and are not visible with the four-chamber view. The most obvious septal defect visible with prenatal ultrasound consists of an atrioventricular canal defect. With this, there is a large defect in the atrial and ventricular septum and a common atrioventricular valve. This particular lesion has a strong association with Down syndrome, which is present in about half of cases. In about half of the cases of ventricular septal defects there are other, more complex malformations. It is difficult to distinguish an atrial septal defect from a normal patent foramen ovale.

Hypoplastic left heart syndrome is suspected when the left ventricle, which should be similar in size to the right ventricle, appears very small with a four-chamber view. To better characterize such defects, visualizing the outflow tracts is critical (see Figure 11-6). In hypoplastic left heart syndrome, the ascending aorta and aortic arch are very narrow in comparison with the pulmonary artery and ductus arteriosus.

Outflow Tracts

Many relatively common serious congenital heart defects may be missed entirely unless the outflow tracts are assessed. One example of such a condition is tetralogy of Fallot, which consists of a ventricular septal defect (VSD), pulmonary stenosis, and aorta that overrides the VSD. The fourth finding is hypertrophy of the right ventricle, which develops postnatally. Transposition of the great arteries may also present with a completely normal four-chamber view. This disorder is recognized with the outflow tract views when the aorta and pulmonary artery run parallel to each other instead of crossing. The aorta, which can be recognized from the shape of the arch, arises from the right ventricle and runs anterior to the main pulmonary, which arises posteriorly from the left ventricle. A ventricular septal defect is found in 40% of cases.

Abdomen

The fetal stomach should always be visualized after the first trimester. If the stomach is small or absent and does not fill after 30 to 60 minutes of observation, esophageal atresia should be suspected. In most cases, polyhydramnios will also be present, resulting from an inability of the fetus to swallow amniotic fluid normally. An empty stomach in a fetus with anhydramnios is not suggestive of gastrointestinal pathology but simply reflects that absence of fluid available for the fetus to swallow.

Duodenal atresia is usually easily diagnosed by third trimester fetal ultrasound. The diagnosis is based on the demonstration of the double-bubble sign in which adjacent fluid filled structures are seen, representing the fluid-filled dilated stomach and proximal duodenum. Polyhydramnios is a consistent feature in these cases; trisomy 21 is found in about 30%. Small bowel obstruction further along the intestinal tract is less common than duodenal atresia. Ultrasound in these cases shows multiple actively peristalsing loops of distended small bowel. The degree of polyhydramnios depends on the proximity of the obstruction.

Kidneys

Bilateral renal agenesis is usually first suspected when there is absent amniotic fluid and nonvisualization of the fetal bladder. The diagnosis is confirmed by the absence of kidneys in the renal fossae. The diagnosis is sometimes difficult because the absent amniotic fluid makes adequate visualization of the fetal anatomy difficult and because the discoid-shaped adrenals can be confused with fetal kidneys. Transvaginal scanning can be very helpful because with absent amniotic fluid the fetus is often close to the upper vagina. Bilateral agenesis is invariably associated with pulmonary hypoplasia, which is the cause of death in liveborn infants. In this setting, ultrasound shows a small, bell-shaped chest.

Infantile polycystic kidney disease is an autosomal recessive disorder characterized by bilateral symmetrical enlargement of the kidneys. In this condition, normal parenchyma is replaced by dilated collecting tubules, which measure less than 2 mm in diameter. These cysts are not seen macroscopically with ultrasound but rather give the kidneys a markedly echogenic appearance. In most cases, these kidneys are nonfunctioning in the fetus, and there is no bladder filling or amniotic fluid production. Neonates die of pulmonary hypoplasia.

Multicystic dysplasia is a disorder with sporadic occurrence characterized by noncommunicating cysts of various sizes scattered randomly through the kidneys. The renal parenchyma between the cyst has an echogenic appearance. The disorder can be bilateral, unilateral, or segmental. Affected kidneys may become quite large. This condition should be differentiated from hydronephrosis, in which the parenchyma is normal, and a dilated renal pelvis communicates with dilated calyces. In bilateral multicystic dysplasia, there is nonproduction of urine, so the bladder is not visualized and there is no amniotic fluid. As with renal agenesis, unilateral disease is associated with normal bladder filling and amniotic fluid volume and has an excellent prognosis.

With hydronephrosis, there are varying degrees of dilation of the renal pelvis and calices. The degree of dilation is recorded as the anteroposterior diameter of the renal pelvis. If this measurement is greater than 4 mm up to 32 weeks or greater than 7 mm beyond 32 weeks, follow-up ultrasound is indicated.[88] These cut-offs were set to ensure a sensitivity of nearly 100% for detecting any postnatal compromise or the need for surgery. Using these cut-offs, 20% to 50% of cases have normal kidneys at postnatal evaluation. Persistent hydronephrosis is most often caused by ureteropelvic junction obstruction or vesicoureteral reflux. Dilated ureters signify the presence of severe vesicoureteral reflux, bladder outlet obstruction, or ureterovesical junction obstruction. The latter condition is often associated with a duplicated collecting system. A ureterocele may form at the point of ureteral implantation into the bladder.

Bladder

Bladder outlet obstruction is most commonly seen in male fetuses and is usually caused by posterior urethral valves. These are membrane-like structures in the posterior urethra that cause varying grades of urethral obstruction. More complex malformations involving the urogenital tract may also cause bladder outlet obstruction and are more common when the affected fetus is a female. Sonographically, bladder outlet obstruction is diagnosed when the bladder is abnormally enlarged, and normal emptying is not seen. When the obstruction is severe, other findings include oligohydramnios, dilated ureters, hydronephrosis, and cystic dysplasia of the kidneys. When complete urethral obstruction has been present from early in pregnancy, anhydramnios causes lethal pulmonary hypoplasia, and ureteral reflux results in irreversible damage to the kidneys. Prune-belly syndrome occurs in male fetuses and has the same sonographic appearance as bladder outlet obstruction. With this condition, however, the impairment of bladder emptying is thought to result from a neuromuscular defect in the bladder and not physical obstruction of the urethra.

Umbilical Cord Insertion into the Abdomen

Omphalocele is a ventral wall defect characterized by a membrane-covered herniation of the intra-abdominal contents into the base of the umbilical cord. Bowel loops, stomach, and liver are the most frequently herniated organs. With omphalocele, there is a 75% likelihood of associated birth defects; the karyotype is abnormal in 20%.[89] These associated problems account for most of the mortality associated with this condition.

Gastroschisis is a right paraumbilical defect of the anterior abdominal wall associated with evisceration of the abdominal organs. Gastroschisis is distinguished from omphalocele by the fact that the umbilical cord inserts normally into the abdominal wall and there is no membrane covering the herniated viscera. Most commonly, only bowel loops are involved, but liver, stomach, and bladder may be outside the abdomen. Because of associated atresias or obstruction at the small abdominal wall ring, bowel loops and the stomach may be dilated inside or outside the abdomen. Gastroschisis is rarely associated with chromosome abnormalities and usually does not involve abnormalities outside of the gastrointestinal tract.[90]

Number of Umbilical Cord Vessels

An attempt should be made to confirm that there are two arteries and a vein in the umbilical cord. In late pregnancy, this can be easily ascertained by looking at a transverse cut of the cord in a free loop. In the second trimester, two umbilical arteries are most easily confirmed by identifying the vessels as they course around the fetal bladder. These can be seen with gray-scale ultrasound but are made much more obvious with color Doppler ultrasound. A single umbilical artery (two-vessel cord) is present in 1% of all newborns. Because of the 20% incidence of associated malformations, this finding should prompt a detailed fetal survey.

Spine

With spina bifida, transverse views of the spine show widening of the lateral echocenters. In longitudinal images, the ossification centers, which usually run a parallel course down the back, are widened in the area of the defect. A meningomyelocele sac is usually present. The presence of clubfoot and absence of movement of the lower extremities signify a poor prognosis for motor function of the lower extremities.

Extremities

In most cases of confirmed skeletal dysplasia, the long bones are obviously abnormal, with measurements far below the normal range. Concern sometimes arises when routine measurement of the femur gives a result several weeks less than expected for the gestational age. For most long bone nomograms, the lower confidence limit corresponds to "2 weeks behind" up to 28 weeks, and "3 weeks behind" beyond 28 weeks. For this reason, when the femur is more than 2 or 3 weeks less than expected, a detailed survey of fetal anatomy, especially the long bones, is advisable. A femur-to-foot ratio close to 1 usually implies that the fetus is normal or merely constitutionally small.

Achondroplasia is the most common form of skeletal dysplasia and is associated with a normal life span. Ultrasound shows severe shortening of the long bones, a relatively large head with a protruding forehead, and polyhydramnios. Although this condition exhibits autosomal dominant inheritance, 80% of cases result from new mutations.

Thanatophoric dysplasia is the most common lethal skeletal dysplasia. In this condition, there is extreme shortening of the long bones. The femur is often bowed, resembling an old-fashioned telephone receiver. The fetus has a small, narrow chest that results in lethal pulmonary hypoplasia. The abdomen and head appear relatively enlarged. In about one of six cases, the head has a cloverleaf shape. Hydrocephalus and polyhydramnios are common.

There are more than a dozen discrete forms of osteogenesis imperfecta, all characterized by abnormalities of the biochemical composition of the bone matrix. The more severe forms are lethal, manifesting very short limbs and the prenatal occurrence of multiple fractures. More mild forms may show few or no fractures, bowing of the femurs, and limb lengths close to the normal range.

Clubfoot is best diagnosed with a coronal view of the lower leg, with the tibia and fibula both seen in a lengthwise section. A normal foot is perpendicular to this plane, but a clubfoot is turned down and in and is seen falling within the coronal plane. It may be very difficult to diagnose clubfoot in the third trimester or in the presence of oligohydramnios.

Hydrops

The term *hydrops* refers to generalized edema in the neonate, manifested by skin edema and accumulations of fluid in body cavities, including the pleural spaces, pericardium, and peritoneal cavity. Before the introduction of Rh immune prophylaxis, most hydrops resulted from erythroblastosis fetalis. Currently, most cases of hydrops are from nonimmune causes. With improvement in diagnostic methods, the etiology of most cases of nonimmune hydrops can be determined. See the box, Causes of Hydrops Fetalis, for the more common causes of nonimmune hydrops. In recent years, it has become apparent that parvovirus infection is responsible for many of the cases of hydrops, which were previously classified as idiopathic.

CAUSES OF HYDROPS FETALIS

- Twin-to-twin transfusion
- Chromosomal abnormalities
- Structural cardiac defects
- Cardiac arrhythmia (especially tachyarrhythmia)
- Cardiac tumor
- High-output failure from vascular malformation or tumor
- Sacrococcygeal teratoma
- Vein of Galen malformation
- Placenta chorangioma
- Twin reverse arterial perfusion sequence
- Fetal anemia
  - Parvovirus infection
  - α-Thalassemia
  - Fetomaternal hemorrhage
- Other infections
  - TORCH infection
  - Syphilis
- Chest mass
  - Congenital cystic adenomatoid malformation
  - Pulmonary sequestration

Effect of Prenatal Ultrasound on Neonatal Outcome

It is initially surprisingly difficult to prove that prenatal ultrasound reduces morbidity or mortality in newborns with birth defects. The RADIUS trial demonstrated similar outcomes in the control group and the group with routine screening.[67] A randomized trial of routine ultrasound conducted in Finland demonstrated a decrease in perinatal mortality when routine ultrasound was used, but this was because most pregnancies with serious malformations were terminated, not because offspring from continued pregnancies did better.[91] However, more **recent studies have shown improved outcome when congenital heart defects were diagnosed with prenatal ultrasound.** This has been shown for hypoplastic left heart syndrome[92] and transposition of the great arteries.[93] Although less critical, the prenatal diagnosis of urinary tract malformations can also lead to proper postnatal evaluation and treatment, presumably leading to improved long-term prognosis.[94]

Although definitive proof remains scarce for most conditions, it seems self-evident that there are advantages to prenatal diagnosis. For one, it gives parents the option of pregnancy termination when serious malformations are diagnosed. Another advantage is that it allows families and caregivers time to gather complete information about the fetal problem so that practical and emotional preparations can be made. Plans can be made for delivery at the proper time at a high-risk perinatal center where the newborn can receive optimal care. When the mother delivers at the tertiary care center, there is no need to transport a potentially unstable newborn, and the mother and baby are not separated.

Routine ultrasound to screen for birth defects involves significant costs, but the cost per defect diagnosed are not out of line with other accepted screening tests. It has been shown that the cost-to-benefit ratio is much more favorable when examinations are performed by sonographers with good detection rates.[95] Ideally, in offering a screening ultrasound, the obstetrician should inform the patients in general terms of the sensitivity of this test in the setting in which it is to be performed. **Most importantly, ultrasound to screen for birth defects should always be performed by a well-qualified examiner, following a standardized approach.**

CELL FREE FETAL DNA AND INTACT FETAL CELLS IN MATERNAL BLOOD: DEFINITIVE NONINVASIVE DIAGNOSIS

As currently practiced, noninvasive screening for detecting chromosomal aneuploidy (see Chapter 10) is *not definitive*. A screen-positive result must be followed by an invasive procedure (CVS or amniocentesis) to determine whether fetal aneuploidy is present. In fact, only 1 per 15 to 20 procedures will reveal aneuploidy. Thus, most women undergo procedures unnecessarily.

The holy grail of prenatal genetic diagnosis is *definitive noninvasive prenatal diagnosis*, that is, a blood sample to detect fetal aneuploidy (or other disorders) without a subsequent invasive procedure. CVS or amniocentesis might then be performed only to exclude rare confounding circumstances that would result in false-positive noninvasive results. (An example would be excluding a vanishing twin, which could lead to unrepresentative results.) If a definitive noninvasive test were robust, one would expect that invasive procedures would almost always confirm abnormal findings.

The goal of definitive noninvasive prenatal diagnosis has been pursued for decades, since the first detection of fetal trisomy 18 in 1991 using intact fetal cells (nucleated fetal red blood cells) recovered from maternal blood.[96] Subsequent confirmation detected trisomy 21.[97-99] However, clinical utility is still lacking with respect to detecting fetal trisomy. By contrast, mendelian disorders can be confidentially detected in certain families. Both cell free fetal DNA and intact fetal cells using maternal blood.

Cell Free Fetal DNA in Maternal Blood

Maternal blood contains cell free fetal DNA in plasma and whole blood.[100] Approximately 5% of cell free DNA in maternal blood is fetal. Fetal DNA fragments are smaller (50 to 200 base pairs), providing the basis for separation from the more plentiful maternal cell free DNA. The goal is to isolate and interrogate fetal DNA sequences but not maternal DNA sequences. Confirmation of success is presence of DNA that cannot be of maternal origin. The obvious example is a Y-sequence, connoting presence of a male fetus. The mother has no Y-sequences; thus, Y DNA must be fetal in origin.

Y-Sequences

Detection of Y-sequence in maternal blood is well documented. A meta-analysis of 792 reports research clinical series resulted in 52 publications suitable for analysis.[101] In pregnancies with a male fetus, Y sequences are detected with 95.4% sensitivity and 98.5% specificity. Sensitivity increased with gestational age: 75.8%, less than 7 weeks; 95.1%, 7 to 12 weeks; 95.6%, 13 to 20 weeks; and 99%, after 20 weeks. Sensitivity was comparable using SRY, DYS14, DYS, DA2, and DY23. Reverse-transcriptase PCR outperformed conventional PCR (96.1% vs. 93.7%). Although these studies were not being designed for clinical application and in fact were usually done in research laboratories, scientific consensus is that validity should be achievable for clinical application.

Single Gene Disorders

Certain mendelian disorders can be detected from cell free DNA, usually when the father has a mutation not present in the mother. If the father has a DNA sequence that the mother lacks and that mutant sequence is detected in the mother, it must be of fetal origin. An example is a father with an autosomal dominant disorder (i.e., polycystic kidney disease or Marfan syndrome). Presence of the paternal (mutant) DNA sequence causing the disorder in *maternal* blood indicates the paternal mutant allele must have been transmitted to the fetus. Another example arises when the father is heterozygous (Aa) and the mother homozygous abnormal (aa) for an autosomal recessive trait. If the normal allele is found in mother, it must have come from a heterozygous fetus inheriting the normal paternal allele.

There exist a host of disorders in which noninvasive definitive diagnosis has been made by this method. Case reports amply validate proof of principle, and series concerning selected disorders (i.e., hemophilia) are now accumulating.[101-103]

Rhesus (D)

Analysis of cell free fetal DNA is already used to assess fetal rhesus status (D). By analysis of maternal blood, fetal Rh(D) can be determined without amniocentesis. The molecular basis of Rh(D) negativity (dd) is usually a gene deletion, the *d* allele representing lack of the DNA sequence that if present would encode *D*. One can distinguish Rh(D)-positive (DD or Dd) from Rh(D)-negative (dd) fetuses by molecular techniques. If the mother is Rh negative and the father heterozygous for Rh(D) (Rh positive), the likelihood is only 50% that the fetus would inherit his Rh(D) gene and, hence, place the pregnancy at risk for isoimmunization; the other 50% of pregnancies would not be at risk for Rh isoimmunization and would not require Rh immune globulin. However, if fetal Rh status were not known, Rh immune globulin would need to be administered, in retrospect, unnecessarily. By contrast, if Rh(D) sequences are found in a pregnant Rh-negative woman (dd), their origin must be fetal, meaning the fetus is Dd and that Rh immune globulin is needed. In many European countries, cell free DNA testing for this purpose is available, and interest is increasing in adopting this technology in the United States.

Trisomy 21

Cell free DNA in maternal blood is being actively pursued for detection of fetal aneuploidy, specifically trisomy 21. At present, cell free fetal DNA testing for aneuploidy is not offered clinically, but promising reports presage introduction. The task here is more difficult than for single gene disorders because detecting fetal trisomy must reflect quantitative differences between affected and unaffected pregnancies. Current strategies are based on counting the total number of chromosome 21 transcripts in maternal blood, using techniques called *massive parallel genomic sequencing*. A pregnancy carrying a trisomy 21 fetus will have more chromosome 21 transcripts than one carrying a normal fetus; the trisomic fetus has three chromosomes 21, whereas the latter only two. Assume 5% of cell free DNA in maternal blood is of fetal origin; thus, a trisomy 21 pregnancy should contain 2.5% more fetal chromosome 21 transcripts than a euploid pregnancy. However, the mother contributes 95% of the total cell free DNA. Thus, the task is to distinguish the 2.5% overall difference. Table 11-2 illustrates the underlying principle on the assumption that maternal blood cell free DNA consists of 95% that is her own (maternal) and 5% that is from her fetus. Various biotechnology companies and academic partners are seeking to exploit this small but finite difference, using various approaches but all fundamentally quantitative in nature. Obtaining a relatively enriched portion of fetal DNA is the universal goal, using microfluidic approaches (fetal DNA size) or selected characteristics by which fetal DNA differ from maternal DNA (e.g., methylated genes). The most straightforward approach is simply to compare quantitatively the total number of targeted sequences compared with expectations.[102] Another is to place greatly diluted cell free fetal DNA transcripts in wells. Simply counting (digital PCR) the number of wells with a chromosome

TABLE 11-2 TOTAL CHROMOSOME 21 CELL FREE DNA IN MATERNAL BLOOD: DISOMIC VERSUS TRISOMIC FETUSES

	DISOMIC FETUS	TOTAL 21 TRANSCRIPTS	TRISOMIC FETUS	TOTAL 21 TRANSCRIPTS
Mother	2	95	2	95
Fetus	2	5	3	7.5
		100		102.5
			2.5%	

Assume 95% of cell free DNA in maternal (pregnant) blood is derived from the mother and 5% from the fetus. The 5% of fetal origin will have 50% more 21 transcripts if that fetus is trisomic. Thus, the total (maternal and fetal) 21 transcripts will be 2.5% higher if the fetus is trisomic.

21 signal should reveal a greater number in trisomy 21 pregnancies.[103]

Although the validity of cell free fetal DNA to detect fetal trisomies is proved in principle, a problem is obtaining an answer consistently. For clinical applications, a robust test must be able to provide a definitive answer in a specified percentage of cases. The "call rate" should be high and well defined, but not necessarily 100%. By contrast, false-negative cases must be near zero if analysis of cell free fetal DNA on fetal cues is to be a *test* and not merely another *method of screening.*

Several promising series have been recently reported, and ability to detect fetal trisomy 21 is no longer in doubt.[104] Ehrich and associates[104a] assessed 480 cases (some samples prospective, others archived); 13 had "insufficient volume," and 18 failed quality control parameter. Of the remaining 449, all 39 trisomy 21 samples were correctly identified, but 1 false-positive case was observed. Papageorgiou and colleagues[104] used certain genes that were methylated in the fetus but not in the mother. In 40 "blind" samples, euploid versus trisomy 21 maternal blood samples could be discriminated. Chiu and coworkers[105] studied a mixed sample consisting of prospective pregnant women and archived plasma samples. Of the 576 pregnant women, 1.7% "did not meet recruitment criteria," and 5.6% samples "did not pass the specimen quality requirements." All trisomy 21 cases were detected with 97.9% specificity when a two-plex approach was applied, meaning two cases were sequenced and analyzed concurrently. On the other hand, testing eight samples concurrently (eight-plex) resulted in unacceptable (79.1%) sensitivity. The rationale for an eight-plex approach is to decrease the cost of a given diagnostic test. The same research team has detected trisomy 13 and trisomy 18, but only after a complex bioinformatics approach applying statistical correction.[106] An additional salutary report (39 trisomy 21 cases detected with one false positive) was reported in early 2012.[107]

Intact Fetal Cells

Intact fetal cells are rare but present in 1 per million to 10 million maternal cells. Original efforts toward definitive noninvasive prenatal diagnosis involved recovering intact fetal cells from maternal blood.

Given the rarity of fetal cells in maternal blood (one fetal cell per 10^7 nucleated maternal cells), it has long been accepted that one must enrich the sample for these rare fetal cells. This process first requires targeting a specific fetal cell type: fetal trophoblasts, lymphocytes, granulocytes, or nucleated red blood cells.

Analyzing interphase cells by FISH with chromosome-specific probes, Elias, Simpson, and colleagues were the first to detect fetal aneuploidy (trisomy 18)[96] in maternal blood. This 1991 advance was soon followed by noninvasive detection of trisomy 21.[97,98] Diagnosis was made on the basis of one to three trisomic and, hence, fetal cells recovered from a 20- to 30-mL maternal specimen and studied by FISH with chromosome-specific probes. The major problem was that the expected number of fetal cells were not recovered, presumably lost in processing and thus impeding sensitivity. An NICHD collaborative study toward this goal assessed the accuracy of intact fetal cell recovery in four centers, using two different methods. Overall, 74% of aneuploidies were detected (32 of 43) cases.[108] This approach was, however, laborious and hindered by lack of consistent recovery. Subsequent attempts focused on recovering *intact* fetal cells using microelectronic mechanism devices or analyzing cells for FISH signals through automated microscopy. Neither has provided consistent results to date.

The most promising current approach appears to involve recovery of fetal trophoblasts in maternal blood. Paterlini-Brechot and colleagues demonstrated proof of principle for recovery and diagnosis of both cystic fibrosis (ΔF508)[109] and spinal muscular atrophy (SMA).[110] Individual trophoblasts can be recovered on a filter, with individual trophoblasts laser-microdissected and analyzed molecularly to confirm first fetal origin (based on parental polymorphisms) and then fetal genotype. Fetal cells can thus be distinguished from maternal cells. All pregnancies having a fetus affected with cystic fibrosis or SMA were correctly detected; results were identical to those obtained by CVS, the study that was performed concurrently in "blind" fashion. In a recent report from this group, 63 consecutive cases of cystic fibrosis and SMA impressively showed 100% cellular and clinical sensitivity and specificity,[109] a sine que non typically lacking in studies involving either intact fetal cells or cell free fetal DNA.

Intact fetal cells retain considerable advantages over cell free fetal DNA. Recovery of intact fetal cells would allow ready diagnosis of not only aneuploidy but also many other conditions concurrently. This approach would be analogous to that already routinely performed on blastomeres or polar bodies in PGD (see later). Analyzing intact fetal cells rather than cell free fetal DNA should facilitate provision of information on not only trisomy 21 but also all chromosomes and selective mendelian traits.

PREIMPLANTATION GENETIC DIAGNOSIS

Preimplantation genetic diagnosis (PGD) is not simply "earlier" prenatal genetic diagnosis but rather a technology also with novel application. PGD requires access to embryonic DNA—gametes or embryos before 6 days of conception, when implantation occurs. **There are three potential approaches for obtaining embryonic DNA for PGD: (1) polar body biopsy, (2) blastomere biopsy (aspiration) from the 3-day six- to eight-cell cleaving embryo, and (3) trophectoderm biopsy from the 5- to 6-day blastocyst.**

Obtaining Embryonic and Gamete DNA

Initial work in most centers involved blastomere biopsy, the zona pellucida being traversed by mechanical, laser, or chemical means to extract a cell. This is not without risk: removal of cell is believed to reduce embryo survival by 10%; removal of two cells reduces the pregnancy rate further and is generally not performed.[110]

Initially, PGD predominantly used blastomeres from the cleavage stage embryo. Polar body biopsy has recently become accepted as the most accurate method for chromosomal analysis. A polar body is extruded at both first and second meiotic divisions as the number of chromosomes is first reduced (46 to 23), and then each chromosome is divided into single chromatids. The underlying principle is illustrated by considering a heterozygous individual. Absent recombination, a mutant maternal allele in the first polar body should be complemented by a primary oocyte having the normal allele. Oocytes deduced to be genetically normal can be allowed to fertilize in vitro and be transferred for potential implantation. Conversely, a normal polar body indicates an abnormal oocyte; thus, fertilization would not be allowed. If the first polar body fails to show chromosome 21, the oocyte is presumed to have two 21 chromosomes and, hence, once fertilized, leads to a trisomic zygote. Maternal meiotic error is actually now recognized to involve chromatids in both meiotic I and II, the result of premature chromatid separation. Thus, segregation patterns are more complex; however, the general principle holds, deducing oocyte status as the complement of the second polar body. Polar body biopsy has special value in detecting chromosomal abnormalities because maternal meiotic errors account for 95% of numerical chromosomal abnormalities. Surprisingly, polar body biopsy detects maternal meiotic errors more robustly than blastomeres of the actual embryo because polar body biopsy correlates with greater fidelity to embryonic status. The explanation is that a single abnormal blastomere in a cleavage stage embryo may merely reflect a mitotic error that will not persist; thus, one would erroneously deduce the entire embryo to be aneuploidy and lose the opportunity to transfer a normal embryo.

The obvious disadvantage of polar body biopsy is inability to assess paternal genotype, precluding application if the father has an autosomal dominant disorder and making analysis less efficient in managing couples at risk for autosomal recessive traits. See Simpson[111] for additional details, in particular concerning how to handle recombination observed in the first polar body.

Biopsy of the trophectoderm is the third approach. In the 5- to 6-day blastocyst, there are 120 or more cells. The greater number of cells potentially facilitates diagnosis. Another advantage is that the trophectoderm forms the placenta; thus, cells detained to produce the embryo are not removed, an advantage shared with polar body biopsy. The additional 2 to 3 days in culture for blastocysts beyond that required for an eight-cell embryo further allows self-selection against nonthriving embryos. Approximately one third of embryos with chromosomal abnormalities are selected against (lost) between days 3 and 5; however, PGD remains necessary to exclude the remaining aneuploidies. The value of trophectoderm biopsy has been enhanced by the recent development of new techniques (vitrification) by which cryopreservation of biopsied embryos has become possible. Cryopreservation has long been routine to generate ART pregnancies using nonbiopsied embryos, but not until recently was it possible to do so using cryopreserved biopsied embryos. Thought to minimize formation of intracellular ice crystals, vitrification can be used following blastocyst biopsy, thawing available embryo at a later time for transfer. In the intervening period, CGH based on single nucleotide polymorphisms (SNPs)[112] or array CGH can be performed.

Chromosomal Indications

The most common indication for PGD is detection of chromosomal abnormalities, most often selected aneuploidies. It is not possible to obtain a karyotype on a single cell reliably, for which reason preimplantation cytogenetic analysis (numerical or structural) traditionally relied on FISH using chromosome-specific probes.[111,112] PGD for detecting unbalanced translocations is also applicable, also using FISH. In Chapter 26, we describe how most translocations predispose to unbalanced genetics. This unavoidably delays the time needed to achieve a normal pregnancy, for some women beyond the age realistic to achieve pregnancy.

Sensitivity for detecting aneuploidy naturally increases as the number of chromosomes tested increases. Usually 5 to 9 chromosomes were studied. Approximately 70% to 80% of aneuploidy embryos can be detected using 9 to 12 chromosomes (e.g., X, Y, 13, 18, 21, 16, 17, 15, 22).[113] A single cell can be interrogated over two to three hybridization cycles to reach that number. The current preference is, however, to obtain information on all 24 chromosomes. One approach is simply to perform additional hybridization cycles, eventually covering all chromosomes. Actually, 90% of aneuploidy can be detected by studying only 10 to 12 chromosomes because rarer trisomies are often found to be trisomic concomitant with another trisomy (double trisomy). Thus, screening for 10 chromosomes predicts correctly 89% (382 of 427) of embryos to be either normal or abnormal[114]; testing 12 chromosomes predicts 91% (389 of 427).

FISH for PGD aneuploidy testing is now being replaced by genome-wide molecular approaches, namely SNPs from all chromosomes[112] or array CGH (chromosomal microarrays).[114] The microarrays used in PGD are different from those used in prenatal array CGH on amniocentesis or chronic villi. In PGD, bacterial artificial chromosomes are used, producing large sequences that in aggregate detect only major abnormalities like aneuploidy, in either chromosomes (blastomeres) or polar bodies (chromatids). Thus, the dilemma of disclosing or not disclosing polymorphic CNVs of uncertain clinical significance does not arise.

Single Gene Disorders

Approximately one fourth of PGD cases are performed for disorders caused by a single mutant gene.[111,115] Like other forms of single gene prenatal genetic diagnosis, PGD can be performed whenever the chromosomal location is known, even if the causative mutation is not. Linkage analysis can still be performed and, in fact, is routinely employed in PGD. The Reproductive Genetics Institute has tested more than 220 different conditions, the most frequent being hemoglobinopathies, cystic fibrosis, fragile X syndrome, and Duchenne muscular dystrophy. See Verlinsky and Kuliev[115] for a list of disorders tested. The implantation rate per embryo in their series of more than 2000 cases was 27.1% (gestational sacs per embryos transferred). A pitfall is that amplification rates do not exceed 90% to 95% per allele, even in experienced hands.[116] This phenomenon—allele dropout (ADO)—probably reflects stochastic phenomena (failure of probes to locate patient DNA) or in turn perhaps exacerbated by embryo damage that has resulted in loss of embryonic DNA. Linkage data are obligatory in single gene PGD for mitigating against erroneous or noninformative results in ADO that involves the mutant allele itself. The Reproductive Genetics Institute has observed only three errors in 2300 single gene PGD cycles, which resulted in more than 500 babies.[111,115] In Brussels, Liebaers and colleagues[117] reported 0.6% misdiagnosis in 581 PGD pregnancies studied in Brussels. That the rate of diagnostic accuracy is so high, despite 5% to 10% unavoidable ADO, probably reflects the policy in experienced PGD centers of transferring only the most diagnostically robust and morphologically normal embryos, which presumably are less likely to have ADO.

Novel Indications

Preimplantation genetic diagnosis is not simply early prenatal genetic diagnosis. PGD allows unique applications not possible using traditional prenatal diagnosis (CVS or amniocentesis).

Avoiding Clinical Termination

Couples may wish to avoid an abnormal fetus yet are opposed to pregnancy termination for religious or other reasons. The considerable disquiet of any couple undergoing pregnancy termination becomes exacerbated when repeated pregnancy terminations are necessary because of consecutively affected offspring. Moreover, the first polar body is present before fertilization; thus, its analysis offers the unique possibility of *preconceptional* diagnosis. The second polar body is, however, not extruded until the mature oocyte is fertilized; thus, its analysis would not truly be preconceptional.

Nondisclosure of Parental Genotype

PGD is the only practical prenatal diagnostic approach when a person at risk for an adult-onset disorder wishes to remain unaware of his or her genotype, yet not transmit the mutation to his or her offspring. Prototypic indications involve Huntington disease and autosomal dominant Alzheimer disease. Using PGD, multiple embryos can be screened with only unaffected embryos transferred; the patient can remain oblivious to diagnostic methods underway. A caveat is that the scenario must be repeated in subsequent cycles, even if the (undisclosed) patient proves unaffected. Otherwise, all at-risk patients could readily deduce his or her genotype.

Cancer and Other Adult-Onset Disorders

Performing prenatal genetic diagnosis for adult-onset mendelian conditions had been considered arguable before application through PGD. In the United States, relatively little controversy now exists. However, there remains reticence in Europe (see Chapter 54). The first case of PGD performed for adult-onset cancer involved Li-Fraumeni syndrome, a disorder caused by a *p53* perturbation.[118] *BRCA1*, multiple endocrine neoplasia, familial adenomatous polyposis (FAP), retinoblastoma, and von Hippel-Lindau syndrome are other common indications.[119]

HLA-Compatible Embryos

Having a human leukocyte antigen (HLA) compatible sibling is invaluable if an older, moribund sibling with a lethal disease requires stem cell transplantation to repopulate his or her bone marrow. The ideal source of stem cells is an HLA-matched sibling because among siblings, one in four is HLA compatible (identical). Sufficient cells can be obtained from its umbilical cord blood. Stem cell transplantation using cord blood is very successful (95%) if the cord blood is HLA compatible, but much less so (65%) if not HLA compatible. Given the risk for a single gene disorder usually coexisting when HLA matching is requested, the couple can not only avoid another genetically abnormal child but also take advantage of the possibility of a normal offspring who is HLA compatible with the affected child. **HLA-compatible umbilical cord blood contains stem cells that if transplanted could allow their older, moribund offspring to survive.** Success rates using HLA-compatible stem cells are more than 90% compared with much less (60% to 65%) if not HLA compatible. If the pregnancy is at risk for an autosomal recessive disorder, the likelihood of a genetically normal, HLA-compatible embryo is 3 in 16 (1 in 4 for the desired HLA-compatible embryo multiplied by the 3 in 4 likelihood of also being unaffected = 3/16).

PGD for the purpose of transferring HLA-compatible embryos was first performed by Verlinsky and colleagues in a couple at risk for Fanconi anemia.[120] By 2004, 45 cycles for HLA typing had been performed[121]; 17.5% embryos were genetically suitable for transfer, very near the expected 18.7% (3/16). The most common genetic indication worldwide for HLA testing is β-thalassemia.[111,115]

In the United States and Turkey, testing for HLA-compatible embryos *without* risk for genetic disease[121] is well accepted. A prime indication is an older sibling with leukemia. In the United States, approximately one third of HLA PGD cases are performed for this purpose; this indication is uncommon in the United Kingdom.[111]

Aneuploidy Testing to Improve Pregnancy Rates

In addition to excluding aneuploidy in couples at increased risk who wish to avoid clinical pregnancy termination or must undergo ART for other reasons, PGD has been pursued to improve the low (30 to 40%) pregnancy rates in ART. The success rate for ART declines precipitously beginning late in the fourth decade. The primary reason is the high embryonic loss due to aneuploidy; endometrial factors are not paramount, as witnessed by successful pregnancies following use of donor oocytes for women in their fifth decade or beyond. Not only does aneuploidy increase with increasing maternal age, but so, too, do miscarriage rates. This is logical given most early pregnancy losses resulting from aneuploidy (Chapter 26), and a maternal age effect existing for aneuploidy. Thus, an obvious strategy is to perform PGD, transfer euploid embryos and increase the proportion of potentially viable pregnancies.

By 2000, larger PGD and ART centers in the United Stated and Europe increasingly were offering PGD to improve pregnancy rates in older women. However, these centers were not able to conduct a randomized clinical trial (RCT). RCTs in smaller centers, mostly in Europe, were conducted and did not show salutary benefits. These RCTs have methodologic flaws, however, and PGD aneuploidy testing is still pursued. Still, lack of a RCT providing benefit has understandably impeded acceptance. This controversy, discussed elsewhere,[122] is ongoing and unresolved.

The current recommendation worldwide largely mirrors that of the European Society of Human Reproduction and Embryology (ESHRE) Consortium.[123] In PGD aneuploidy testing one should interrogate embryonic tissues *other* than blastomeres (the traditional method), namely polar body biopsy. One should also use methods other than FISH, namely array CGH. A RCT to test this approach is underway in Europe. While awaiting results, the following seems appropriate counsel for couples considering PGD aneuploidy testing: (1) Pursue PGD only in women of relatively advanced maternal age, perhaps >37 years old. (2) Proceed only if there are at least 6 morphologically normal embryos; two to three chromosomally normal embryos can thus be reasonably expected. If fewer embryos exist, PGD should not be pursued without parental consent. (3) Use only highly skilled embryologists, and if unavailable do not proceed. (4) Interrogate at least 8 and preferably 10 to 12 chromosomes by FISH, or preferably all 24 chromosomes either by FISH or array CGH.

Safety of Preimplantation Genetic Diagnosis

Removal of any embryonic cell logically might decrease survival or implantation and, hence, reduce pregnancy rates. This appears true at least with respect to removal of blastomeres.[110] If viability is reduced by 10% when a single blastomere is removed, PGD aneuploidy must first overcome this 10% decrease and then generate another 10% or more improvement in pregnancy rate in order to show clinical utility.

Viability aside, the totipotential nature of embryonic cells confers safety against organ-specific anomalies in resulting liveborn infants. Loss of one or more cells prior to irrevocable differentiation into a specific embryologic developmental pathway is obviated if another cell has capacity to accomplish the same purpose. In determining safety of PGD in liveborn infants, it is relevant that the birth defects rate in ART is 30% over background.[124] A **30% increase in birth defects associated with ART is not likely the result of ART per se but rather a reflection of the underlying infertility that necessitated ART. This can be deduced because the frequency of birth defects is above background not only in ART pregnancies but in pregnancies spontaneously conceived but only after 12 months of trying to conceive (the traditional definition of infertility).**[125] Irrespective, available data indicate no increased rate of birth defects in liveborn infants previously subjected to PGD. Liebaers et al.[117] conducted a thorough, systematic study of PGD offspring assessed by physical examination 2 months after birth. Frequencies of anomalies in 563 PGD liveborn infants, 18 stillborn fetuses, and 9 neonatal deaths were compared to those in a previously reported cohort study of ICSI offspring not undergoing PGD.[126] Approximately half the PGD cases were at risk for a single gene disorder, whereas the others underwent aneuploidy testing. Structural malformations were found in 2.13% for PGD alone and 3.38% for ICSI.[117] There were no differences between offspring resulting from single gene PGD versus PGD aneuploidy testing. The anomaly rate observed in PGD cases in Brussels[117] was also similar to that tabulated by the Reproductive Genetics Institute in the U.S.[111] PGD appears safe for resulting liveborns.[127]

Current Utility

Single embryonic cells can be transported to referral centers; thus, PGD is widely available. The many different testable conditions have shown high accuracy. The obstetrician should be aware that PGD has certain unique indications, foremost being HLA testing to identify a compatible embryo whose umbilical cord blood can be used for stem cell transplantation for an older, moribund sibling. Other indications applicable only by PGD include nondisclosure testing and avoidance of clinical pregnancy terminations. PGD can be applied for any mendelian disorder whose location is known, using linkage analysis even when the causative mutation is not known.

PGD for translocations is also well accepted, and PGD to avoid repeated pregnancy losses in couples having recurrent aneuploidy is known to be efficacious. Controversy exists concerning whether PGD aneuploidy testing improves pregnancy rates.

KEY POINTS

- All invasive prenatal diagnostic procedures are accurate but carry risks. Amniocentesis at 15 weeks and later carries a procedure-related risk of 1 in 400 to 500. Amniocentesis before 13 weeks is not recommended because of an unacceptable risk for clubfoot (talipes equinovarus).
- Chorionic villus sampling (CVS) is, in experienced hands, equal to amniocentesis in safety (loss rates) and diagnostic accuracy. Transcervical and transabdominal CVS are equivalent in safety and accuracy.
- Newer molecular diagnostic methods (array CGH) provide greater sensitivity for detecting gains or losses of chromosomal regions than the traditional karyotype.
- The precise complication rate associated with fetal blood sampling is undefined, but the loss rate is considered to be 1% to 2%. Rates depend greatly on the associated fetal status.
- Most single-gene disorders can now be detected by molecular methods if fetal tissue is available, given location of the causative mutant gene being known for most disorders. Linkage analysis can be

applied if the gene has been localized but not yet sequenced or if the mutation responsible for the disorder in a given family remains unknown despite sequencing. This option represents a transformational improvement over previous methods, which relied on a number of different indirect approaches.

- Multifactorial disorders most often use ultrasound for detection, but many single gene disorders (e.g., skeletal dysplasias) can be detected as well and then confirmed by molecular tests. Sensitivity of ultrasound for the detection of birth defects depends on the level of training of examiners and the maintenance of a structured approach to the fetal examination.
- In experienced hands, the use of the "genetic sonogram" is a noninvasive way to adjust the likelihood that a fetus has trisomy 21. However, patients should understand that the genetic sonogram is used only to *adjust* risk estimates and cannot definitively diagnose aneuploidy. Sensitivity is never 100%.
- Cell free fetal DNA can be recovered from maternal blood and has allowed *definitive* noninvasive diagnosis for fetal Rh(D), fetal sex, and certain paternally transmitted single gene disorders. Screening ror aneuploidy is possible.
- Definitive noninvasive prenatal diagnosis using intact fetal cells (nucleated red blood cells) was the initial approach for detecting fetal disorders, and more recently fetal trophoblasts have been recovered to make diagnosis. However, detection of fetal trisomy by analysis of maternal blood is not yet available or able to yield the near 100% detection following an invasive procedure (amniocentesis or CVS). Promising results are being achieved using cell-free DNA.
- Preimplantation genetic diagnosis (PGD) requires removal of one or more cells (polar body blastomere, trophectoderm) from the embryo. Diagnosis uses molecular techniques to detect single gene disorders and either FISH or chromosomal array CGH to detect chromosomal abnormalities (trisomy). Safety does not seem to be a major concern among resulting live born infants.
- PGD has certain unique indications not possible with traditional prenatal diagnosis. These include avoidance of clinical pregnancy termination, fetal (embryonic) diagnosis without disclosure of parental genotype (e.g., Huntington disease), and desire to select HLA-compatible unaffected embryos. In the latter, cord blood of resulting HLA compatible babies can be used for stem cell transplantation in an older, moribund sibling who has a bone marrow infiltrative condition.

REFERENCES

1. van den Berg C, Braat AP, Van Opstal D, et al: Amniocentesis or chorionic villus sampling in multiple gestations? Experience with 500 cases. Prenat Diagn 19:234, 1999.
2. Bahado-Singh R, Schmitt R, Hobbins JC: New technique for genetic amniocentesis in twins. Obstet Gynecol 79:304, 1992.
3. Elias S: Amniocentesis and fetal blood sampling. In Milunsky A (ed): Genetic Disorders and the Fetus: Diagnosis, Prevention and Treatment, 6th ed. Baltimore, The John Hopkins University Press, 2004.
4. Simpson JL: Choosing the best prenatal screening protocol. N Engl J Med 353:2068, 2005.
5. Midtrimester amniocentesis for prenatal diagnosis: safety and accuracy. JAMA 236:1471, 1976.
6. Simpson NE, Daillarie L, Miller JR: Prenatal diagnosis of genetic disease in Canada: report of a collaborative study. CMAJ 115:739, 1976.
7. Elchalal U, Shachar IB, Peleg D, Schenker JG: Maternal mortality following diagnostic 2nd-trimester amniocentesis. Fetal Diagn Ther 19:195, 2004.
8. ACOG Practice Bulletin No. 27: Clinical Management Guidelines for Obstetrician-Gynecologists. Prenatal diagnosis of fetal chromosomal abnormalities. Obstet Gynecol 97:1, 2001.
9. Alexander JM, Ramus R, Jackson G, et al: Risk of hepatitis B transmission after amniocentesis in chronic hepatitis B carriers. Infect Dis Obstet Gynecol 7:283, 1999.
10. Davies G, Wilson RD, Desilets V, et al: Amniocentesis and women with hepatitis B, hepatitis C, or human immunodeficiency virus. JOGC 25:145, 2003.
11. Mandelbrot L, Mayaux MJ, Bongain A, et al: Obstetric factors and mother-to-child transmission of human immunodeficiency virus type 1: the French perinatal cohorts. SEROGEST French Pediatric HIV Infection Study Group. Am J Obstet Gynecol 175:661, 1996.
12. Maiques V, Garcia-Tejedor A, Perales A, et al: HIV detection in amniotic fluid samples: Amniocentesis can be performed in HIV pregnant women? Eur J Obstet Gynaecol 108:137, 2003.
13. Lawson HW, Frye A, Atrash HK, et al: Abortion mortality, United States, 1972 through 1987. Am J Obstet Gynecol 171:1365, 1994.
14. Carroll SG, Davies T, Kyle PM, et al: Fetal karyotyping by chorionic villus sampling after the first trimester. BJOG 106:1035, 1999.
15. Golbus MS, Simpson JL, Fowler SE, et al: Risk factors associated with transcervical CVS losses. Prenat Diagn 12:373, 1992.
16. Rhoads GG, Jackson LG, Schlesselman SE, et al: The safety and efficacy of chorionic villus sampling for early prenatal diagnosis of cytogenetic abnormalities. N Engl J Med 320:609, 1989.
17. Medical Research Council European trial of chorion villus sampling. MRC working party on the evaluation of chorion villus sampling. Lancet 337:1491, 1991.
18. Alfirevic Z, Sundberg K, Brigham S: Amniocentesis and chorionic villus sampling for prenatal diagnosis. Cochrane Database Syst Rev CD003252, 2003.
19. Jackson LG, Zachary JM, Fowler SE, et al: A randomized comparison of transcervical and transabdominal chorionic-villus sampling. The U.S. National Institute of Child Health and Human Development Chorionic-Villus Sampling and Amniocentesis Study Group. N Engl J Med 327:594, 1992.
20. Olney RS, Khoury MJ, Alo CJ, et al: Increased risk for transverse digital deficiency after chorionic villus sampling: results of the United States Multistate Case-Control Study, 1988-1992. Teratology 51:20, 1995.
21. Simpson JL, Elias S: Techniques for Prenatal Diagnosis. Philadelphia, Saunders, 2003.
22. Brambati B, Tului L: Prenatal genetic diagnosis through chorionic villus sampling. In Milunsky A (ed): Genetic Disorders and the Fetus, Diagnosis, Prevention and Treatment, 6th ed. Baltimore, Johns Hopkins University Press, 2010.
23. Brambati B, Tului L: Chorionic villus sampling and amniocentesis. Curr Opin Obstet Gynecol 17:197, 2005.
24. Silver RK, Wilson RD, Philip J, et al: Late first-trimester placental disruption and subsequent gestational hypertension/preeclampsia. Obstet Gynecol 105:587, 2005.
25. Khalil A, Akolekar R, Pandya P, et al: Chorionic villus sampling at 11 to 13 weeks of gestation and hypertensive disorders in pregnancy. Obstet Gynecol 116:374, 2010.
26. Pergament E, Schulman JD, Copeland K, et al: The risk and efficacy of chorionic villus sampling in multiple gestations. Prenat Diagn 12:377, 1992.
27. Evans MI: Teaching new procedures. Ultrasound Obstet Gynecol 19:436, 2002.

28. Tangshewinsirikul C, Wanapirak C, Piyamongkol W, et al: Effect of cord puncture site in cordocentesis at mid-pregnancy on pregnancy outcomes. Prenat Diagn 2011 Jun 27 [Epub ahead of print].
29. Antsaklis AI, Papantoniou NE, Mesogitis SA, et al: Cardiocentesis: an alternative method of fetal blood sampling for the prenatal diagnosis of hemoglobinopathies. Obstet Gynecol 79:630, 1992.
30. Copel JA, Grannum PA, Harrison D, Hobbins JC: The use of intravenous pancuronium bromide to produce fetal paralysis during intravascular transfusion. Am J Obstet Gynecol 158:170, 1988.
31. Abdel-Fattah SA, Bartha JL, Kyle PM, et al: Safety of fetal blood sampling by cordocentesis in fetuses with single umbilical arteries. Prenat Diagn 24:605, 2004.
32. Ghidini A, Sepulveda W, Lockwood CJ, Romero R: Complications of fetal blood sampling. Am J Obstet Gynecol 168:1339, 1993.
33. Weiner CP, Okamura K: Diagnostic fetal blood sampling-technique related losses. Fetal Diagn Ther 11:169, 1996.
34. Tongsong T, Wanapirak C, Kunavikatikul C, et al: Fetal loss rate associated with cordocentesis at midgestation. Am J Obstet Gynecol 184:719, 2001.
35. Liao C, Wei J, Li Q, et al: Efficacy and safety of cordocentesis for prenatal diagnosis. Int J Gynaecol Obstet 93:13, 2006.
36. Tongprasert F, Tongsong T, Wanapirak C, et al: Cordocentesis in multifetal pregnancies. Prenat Diagn 27:1100, 2007.
37. Weiner CP, Wenstrom KD, Sipes SL, Williamson RA: Risk factors for cordocentesis and fetal intravascular transfusion. Am J Obstet Gynecol 165:1020, 1991.
38. Van Kamp IL, Klumper FJ, Oepkes D, et al: Complications of intrauterine intravascular transfusion for fetal anemia due to maternal red-cell alloimmunization. Am J Obstet Gynecol 192:171, 2005.
39. Li Kim Mui SV, Chitrit Y, Boulanger MC, et al: Sepsis due to Clostridium perfringens after pregnancy termination with feticide by cordocentesis: a case report. Fetal Diagn Ther 17:124, 2002.
40. Plachouras N, Sotiriadis A, Dalkalitsis N, et al: Fulminant sepsis after invasive prenatal diagnosis. Obstet Gynecol 104:1244, 2004.
41. ACOG Practice Bulletin No. 77: Screening for fetal chromosomal abnormalities. Obstet Gynecol 109:217, 2007.
42. Hook EB, Cross PK, Schreinemachers DM: Chromosomal abnormality rates at amniocentesis and in live-born infants. 249:2034, 1983.
43. Hook EB, Cross PK, Jackson L, et al: Maternal age-specific rates of 47, +21 and other cytogenetic abnormalities diagnosed in the first trimester of pregnancy in chorionic villus biopsy specimens: comparison with rates expected from observations at amniocentesis. Am J Hum Genet 42:797, 1988.
44. Hook EB, Cross PK: Maternal age-specific rates of chromosome abnormalities at chorionic villus study: a revision. Am J Hum Genet 45:474, 1989.
45. Simpson JL: Maternal serum screening in the United States: current perspective (1996). In Grudzinskas JG, Ward RH (eds): Screening for Down Syndrome in the First Trimester. London, Royal College of Obstetricians and Gynaecologists, 1997, p 97.
46. ACOG Practice Bulletin: Multiple Gestation complicated twin, triplet, and high-order multifetal pregnancy. Washington, DC, ACOG, 2005.
47. Rodis JF, Egan JF, Craffey A, et al: Calculated risk of chromosomal abnormalities in twin gestations. Obstet Gynecol 76:1037, 1990.
48. Stene J, Stene E, Mikkelsen M: Risk for chromosome abnormality at amniocentesis following a child with a non-inherited chromosome aberration. A European Collaborative Study on Prenatal Diagnoses 1981. Prenat Diagn 4:81, 1984.
49. Boue A, Gallano P: A collaborative study of the segregation of inherited chromosome structural rearrangements in 1356 prenatal diagnoses. Prenat Diagn 4:45, 1984.
50. Daniel A, Hook EB, Wulf G: Risks of unbalanced progeny at amniocentesis to carriers of chromosome rearrangements: data from United States and Canadian laboratories. Am J Med Genet 33:14, 1989.
51. Simpson JL, Lamb DJ: Genetic effects of intracytoplasmic sperm injection. Semin Reprod Med 19:239, 2001.
52. Benn P: Prenatal diagnosis of chromosomal abnormalities through amniocentesis. In Milunsky A, Milunsky JM (eds): Genetic Disorders and the Fetus, 6th ed. Oxford, UK, Wiley-Blackwell, 2010.
53. Hsu LY: Prenatal diagnosis of chromosome abnormalities through amniocentesis. In Milunsky A (ed): Genetic Disorders and the Fetus, 3rd ed. Baltimore, The Johns Hopkins University Press, 1986, p 155.
54. Ledbetter DH, Zachary JM, Simpson JL, et al: Cytogenetic results from the U.S. Collaborative Study on CVS. Prenat Diagn 12:317, 1992.
55. Stetten G, Escallon CS, South ST, et al: Reevaluating confined placental mosaicism. Am J Med Genet A 131:232, 2004.
56. Wolstenholme J, Rooney DE, Davison EV: Confined placental mosaicism, IUGR, and adverse pregnancy outcome: a controlled retrospective U.K. collaborative survey. Prenat Diagn 14:345, 1994.
57. Hahnemann JM, Vejerslev LO: European collaborative research on mosaicism in CVS (EUCROMIC): fetal and extrafetal cell lineages in 192 gestations with CVS mosaicism involving single autosomal trisomy. Am J Med Genet 70:179, 1997.
58. Kotzot D: Abnormal phenotypes in uniparental disomy (UPD): fundamental aspects and a critical review with bibliography of UPD other than 15. Am J Med Genet 82:265, 1999.
59. Warburton D: De novo balanced chromosome rearrangements and extra marker chromosomes identified at prenatal diagnosis: clinical significance and distribution of breakpoints. Am J Med Genet 49:995, 1991.
60. Sachs ES, Van Hemel JO, Den Hollander JC, Jahoda MG: Marker chromosomes in a series of 10,000 prenatal diagnoses: cytogenetic and follow-up studies. Prenat Diagn 7:81, 1987.
61. Hume RF Jr, Drugan A, Ebrahim SA, et al: Role of ultrasonography in pregnancies with marker chromosome aneuploidy. Fetal Diagn Ther 10:182, 1995.
62. Pertl B, Kopp S, Kroisel PM, et al: Rapid detection of chromosome aneuploidies by quantitative fluorescence PCR: first application on 247 chorionic villus samples. J Med Genet 36:300, 1999.
63. Kearney HM, Thorland EC, Brown KK, et al: American College of Medical Genetics standards and guidelines for interpretation and reporting of postnatal constitutional copy number variants. Genet Med 13:680, 2011.
64. Wapner R: A multicenter, prospective, masked comparison of chromosomal microarray with standard karyotyping for routine and high risk prenatal diagnosis. Abstracts; 32nd Annual Meeting Society for Maternal-Fetal Medicine, Dallas, 2012. American Journal of Obstetrics & Gynecology 206 Suppl. 52, 2012.
65. Simpson JL: Interpreting uncertain findings in prenatal array copy number analysis (aCNA): Results from the NICHD Prenatal Microarray Study. Annual meeting of American College of Medical Genetics, Abstract 64, Charlotte, 2012.
66. Chitty LS, Hunt GH, Moore J, Lobb MO: Effectiveness of routine ultrasonography in detecting fetal structural abnormalities in a low risk population. BMJ 303:1165, 1991.
67. Ewigman BG, Crane JP, Frigoletto FD, et al: Effect of prenatal ultrasound screening on perinatal outcome. RADIUS Study Group. N Engl J Med 329:821, 1993.
68. Grandjean H, Larroque D, Levi S: The performance of routine ultrasonographic screening of pregnancies in the Eurofetus Study. Am J Obstet Gynecol 181:446, 1999.
69. DeVore GR: Influence of prenatal diagnosis on congenital heart defects. Ann N Y Acad Sci 847:46, 1998.
70. Tegnander E, Williams W, Johansen OJ, et al: Prenatal detection of heart defects in a non-selected population of 30,149 fetuses: detection rates and outcome. Ultrasound Obstet Gynecol 27:252, 2006.
71. AIUM Practice Guideline for the performance of an antepartum obstetric ultrasound examination. J Ultrasound Med 22:1116, 2003.
72. Commission AUPA: Application for practice accreditation. Laurel, MD, American Institute of Ultrasound in Medicine.
73. Benacerraf BR, Barss VA, Laboda LA: A sonographic sign for the detection in the second trimester of the fetus with Down's syndrome. Am J Obstet Gynecol 151:1078, 1985.
74. Smith-Bindman R, Hosmer W, Feldstein VA, et al: Second-trimester ultrasound to detect fetuses with Down syndrome: a meta-analysis. JAMA 285:1044, 2001.
75. Aagaard-Tillery KM, Malone FD, Nyberg DA, et al: Role of second-trimester genetic sonography after Down syndrome screening. Obstet Gynecol 114:1189, 2009.
76. Benn PA, Egan JF, Fang M, Smith-Bindman R: Changes in the utilization of prenatal diagnosis. Obstet Gynecol 103:1255, 2004.
77. Borrell A: Promises and pitfalls of first trimester sonographic markers in the detection of fetal aneuploidy. Prenat Diagn 29:62, 2009.
78. Nicolaides KH, Campbell S, Gabbe SG, Guidetti R: Ultrasound screening for spina bifida: cranial and cerebellar signs. Lancet 2:72, 1986.

79. Descamps P, Jourdain O, Paillet C, et al: Etiology, prognosis and management of nuchal cystic hygroma: 25 new cases and literature review. Eur J Obstet Gyneacol 71:3, 1997.
80. Ulm B, Ulm MR, Deutinger J, Bernaschek G: Dandy-Walker malformation diagnosed before 21 weeks of gestation: associated malformations and chromosomal abnormalities. Ultrasound Obstet Gynecol 10:167, 1997.
81. Peleg D, Yankowitz J: Choroid plexus cysts and aneuploidy. J Med Genet 35:554, 1998.
82. Ghidini A, Strobelt N, Locatelli A, et al: Isolated fetal choroid plexus cysts: role of ultrasonography in establishment of the risk of trisomy 18. Am J Obstet Gynecol 182:972, 2000.
83. Levitsky DB, Mack LA, Nyberg DA, et al: Fetal aqueductal stenosis diagnosed sonographically: how grave is the prognosis? AJR Am J Roentgenol 164:725, 1995.
84. Pilu G, Falco P, Gabrielli S, et al: The clinical significance of fetal isolated cerebral borderline ventriculomegaly: report of 31 cases and review of the literature. Ultrasound Obstet Gynecol 14:320, 1999.
85. Van den Hof MC, Nicolaides KH, Campbell J, Campbell S: Evaluation of the lemon and banana signs in one hundred thirty fetuses with open spina bifida. Am J Obstet Gynecol 162:322, 1990.
86. Roggin KK, Breuer CK, Carr SR, et al: The unpredictable character of congenital cystic lung lesions. J Pediatr Surg 35:801, 2000.
87. Lopoo JB, Goldstein RB, Lipshutz GS, et al: Fetal pulmonary sequestration: a favorable congenital lung lesion. Obstet Gynecol 94:567, 1999.
88. Corteville JE, Gray DL, Crane JP: Congenital hydronephrosis: correlation of fetal ultrasonographic findings with infant outcome. Am J Obstet Gynecol 165:384, 1991.
89. Hwang PJ, Kousseff BG: Omphalocele and gastroschisis: an 18-year review study. Genet Med 6:232, 2004.
90. Barisic I, Clementi M, Hausler M, et al: Evaluation of prenatal ultrasound diagnosis of fetal abdominal wall defects by 19 European registries. Ultrasound Obstet Gynecol 18:309, 2001.
91. Saari-Kemppainen A, Karjalainen O, Ylostalo P, Heinonen OP: Fetal anomalies in a controlled one-stage ultrasound screening trial: a report from the Helsinki Ultrasound Trial. J Perinat Med 22:279, 1994.
92. Tworetzky W, McElhinney DB, Reddy VM, et al: Improved surgical outcome after fetal diagnosis of hypoplastic left heart syndrome. Circulation 103:1269, 2001.
93. Bonnet D, Coltri A, Butera G, et al: Detection of transposition of the great arteries in fetuses reduces neonatal morbidity and mortality. Circulation 99:916, 1999.
94. Persutte WH, Koyle M, Lenke RR, et al: Mild pyelectasis ascertained with prenatal ultrasonography is pediatrically significant. Ultrasound Obstet Gynecol 10:12, 1997.
95. DeVore GR: The Routine Antenatal Diagnostic Imaging with Ultrasound Study: another perspective. Obstet Gynecol 84:622, 1994.
96. Price JO, Elias S, Wachtel SS, et al: Prenatal diagnosis with fetal cells isolated from maternal blood by multiparameter flow cytometry. Am J Obstet Gynecol 165:1731, 1991.
97. Elias S, Price J, Dockter M, et al: First trimester prenatal diagnosis of trisomy 21 in fetal cells from maternal blood. Lancet 340:1033, 1992.
98. Bianchi DW, Mahr A, Zickwolf GK, et al: Detection of fetal cells with 47, XY, +21 karyotype in maternal peripheral blood. Hum Genet 90:368, 1992.
99. Simpson JL, Elias S: Isolating fetal cells from maternal blood: advances in prenatal diagnosis through molecular technology. JAMA 270:2357, 1993.
100. Lo YM, Corbetta N, Chamberlain PF, et al: Presence of fetal DNA in maternal plasma and serum. Lancet 350:485, 1997.
101. Devance SA, Palomaki GE, Scott JA, Bianchi DW: Noninvasive fetal sex determination using cell-free fetal DNA: a systematic review and meta-analysis. JAMA 306:627, 2011.
102. Fan HC, Blumenfeld YJ, Chitkara U, et al: Noninvasive diagnosis of fetal aneuploidy by shotgun sequencing DNA from maternal blood. Proc Natl Sci USA 105:16266, 2008.
103. Lo YM, Lun FM, Chan KC, et al: Digital PCR for the molecular detection of fetal chromosomal aneuploidy. Proc Natl Acad Sci USA 104:13166, 2007.
104. Simpson JL: Is cell-free fetal DNA from maternal blood finally ready for prime time? Obst Gynecol 119: [Epub ahead of print] 2012.
104a. Ehrich M, Deciu C, Zwiefelhofer T, et al: Noninvasive detection of fetal trisomy 21 by sequencing of DNA in maternal blood: a study in a clinical setting. Am J Obst Gynecol 204:205e1, 2011.
105. Chiu RW, Akolekar R, Zheng YW, et al: Non-invasive prenatal assessment of trisomy 21 by multiplexed maternal plasma DNA sequencing: large scale validity study. BMJ 342:d7401, 2011.
106. Rava R, Bianchi D, Platt L, Goldberg J, et al: Genome-wide fetal aneuploidy detection by maternal plasma DNA sequencing. Obst Gynecol 119: [Epub ahead of print] 2012.
107. Chen EZ, Chiu RW, Sun H, et al: Noninvasive prenatal diagnosis of fetal trisomy 18 and trisomy 13 by maternal plasma DNA sequencing. PloS One 6:e21791, 2011.
108. Bianchi DW, Simpson JL, Jackson LG, et al: Fetal gender and aneuploidy detection using fetal cells in maternal blood: analysis of NIFTY I data. National Institute of Child Health and Development Fetal Cell Isolation Study. Prenatal Diagnosis 22:609,2002.
109. Saker A, Benachi A, Bonnefont JP, et al: Genetic characterisation of circulating fetal cells allows non-invasive prenatal diagnosis of cystic fibrosis. Prenatal Diagnosis 26:906, 2006.
110. Beroud C, Karliova M, Bonnefont JP, et al: Prenatal diagnosis of spinal muscular atrophy by genetic analysis of circulating fetal cells. Lancet 361:1013, 2003.
111. Simpson JL. Preimplantation genetic diagnosis at 20 years. Prenatal diagnosis 30:682, 2010
112. Handyside AH, Harton GL, Mariani B, et al: Karyomapping: a universal method for genome wide analysis of genetic disease based on mapping crossovers between parental haplotypes. J Med Genet 47:651, 2010.
113. Munne S, Lee A, Rosenwaks Z, et al: Diagnosis of major chromosome aneuploidies in human preimplantation embryos. Hum Reprod 8:2185, 1993.
114. Munne S, Fragouli E, Colls P, et al: Improved detection of aneuploid blastocysts using a new 12-chromosome FISH test. Reprod Biomed Online 20:92, 2010.
115. Verlinsky Y, Kuliev A: Preimplantation genetic diagnosis. In Milunsky A, Milunsky JM (eds): Genetic Disorders and the Fetus, 6th ed. Sussex, UK, Blackwell Publishing, 2010, pp 950-977.
116. Guidelines for good practice in PGD: programme requirements and laboratory quality assurance. Reprod Biomed Online 16:134, 2008.
117. Liebaers I, Desmyttere S, Verpoest W, et al: Report on a consecutive series of 581 children born after blastomere biopsy for preimplantation genetic diagnosis. Hum Reprod 25:275, 2010.
118. Verlinsky Y, Rechitsky S, Verlinsky O, et al: Preimplantation diagnosis for p53 tumour suppressor gene mutations. Reprod Biomed Online 2:102, 2001.
119. Rechitsky S, Verlinsky O, Chistokhina A, et al: Preimplantation genetic diagnosis for cancer predisposition. Reprod Biomed Online 5:148, 2002.
120. Verlinsky Y, Rechitsky S, Schoolcraft W, et al: Preimplantation diagnosis for Fanconi anemia combined with HLA matching. JAMA 285:3130, 2001.
121. Verlinsky Y, Rechitsky S, Sharapova T, et al: Preimplantation HLA testing. JAMA 291:2079, 2004.
122. Simpson JL: What next for preimplantation genetic screening? Randomized clinical trial in assessing PGS: necessary but not sufficient. Hum Reprod 23:2179, 2008.
123. Geraedts J, Collins J, Gianaroli L, et al: What next for preimplantation genetic screening? A polar body approach! Hum Reprod 25:575, 2010.
124. Hansen M, Bower C, Milne E, et al: Assisted reproductive technologies and the risk of birth defects: a systematic review. Hum Reprod 20:328, 2005.
125. Zhu JL, Basso O, Obel C, et al: Infertility, infertility treatment, and congenital malformations: Danish national birth cohort. BMJ 333:679, 2006.
126. Bonduelle M, Ponjaert I, Steirteghem AV, et al: Developmental outcome at 2 years of age for children born after ICSI compared with children born after IVF. Hum Reprod 18:342, 2003.
127. Simpson JL: Children born after preimplantation genetic diagnosis show no increase in congenital anomalies. Hum Reprod 25:6, 2010.

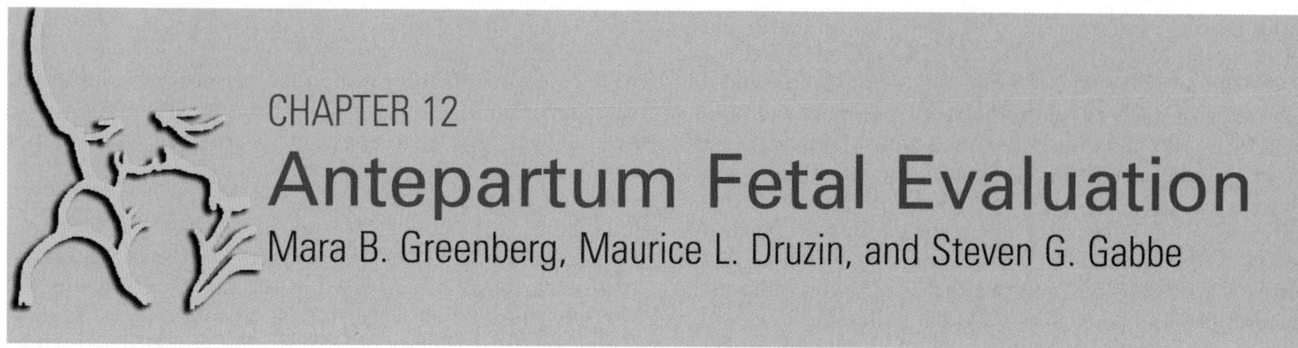

CHAPTER 12

Antepartum Fetal Evaluation

Mara B. Greenberg, Maurice L. Druzin, and Steven G. Gabbe

KEY ABBREVIATIONS	
American College of Obstetricians and Gynecologist	ACOG
Amniotic Fluid Index	AFI
Antiphospholipid Antibody Syndrome	APLAS
Assisted Reproductive Technologies	ART
Biophysical Profile	BPP
Body Mass Index	BMI
Central Nervous System	CNS
Contraction Stress Test	CST
Deepest Vertical Pocket	DVP
Fetal Breathing Movement	FBM
Fetal Movement Counting	FMC
Human Chorionic Gonadotropin	hCG
Foam Stability Index	FSI
Intrauterine Growth Restriction	IUGR
Lecithin-to-Sphingomyelin Ratio	L/S ratio
Modified Biophysical Profile	mBPP
Multiples of the Median	MoM
National Center for Health Statistics	NCHS
National Institute for Child Health and Development	NICHD
Nonstress Test	NST
Perinatal Mortality Rate	PMR
Phosphatidylglycerol	PG
Pregnancy-Associated Plasma Protein A	PAPP-A
Rapid Eye Movement	REM
Respiratory Distress Syndrome	RDS
Systemic Lupus Erythematosus	SLE
Vibroacoustic Stimulation	VAS
World Health Organization	WHO

Antepartum fetal evaluation is an ever-growing and changing science. **The goal of evidence-based antepartum fetal evaluation is to decrease perinatal mortality and permanent neurologic injury through judicious use of reliable and valid methods of fetal assessment, without acting prematurely to modify an otherwise-healthy pregnancy or providing a false sense of well-being in cases of impending morbidity.** The opportunity for obstetrical care providers to participate in this delicate balance has been made possible by continued advances in our ability to assess the physiologic well-being of the fetus, concurrent with great improvement in neonatal care and survival.[1] However, despite these advances in antepartum fetal surveillance and the widespread use of antepartum testing programs, the ability of these techniques to prevent intrauterine injury or death remains unproved in many cases.[2] The focus of this chapter is on antepartum evaluation in the United States and similarly technologically advanced and resource-rich countries, noting that the worldwide problem of stillbirth is a vast and compelling area of international interest.[3]

DEFINING THE PROBLEM OF PERINATAL MORTALITY

Identification of fetuses at risk for perinatal mortality has historically been the goal of antepartum fetal assessment. Our emerging understanding that long-term neurologic disability is an integrally related and often competing entity to perinatal mortality makes this goal more complex.[2]

The National Center for Health Statistics (NCHS) provides two different definitions for perinatal mortality, acknowledging that variation in definitions and reporting rates both among states in the United States and throughout different countries worldwide makes comparisons difficult; an agenda to develop a classification consensus has been the focus of a number of international committees, including the National Institute for Child Health and Development (NICHD).[3] The NCHS National Vital Statistics Report (NVSR) on fetal and perinatal mortality describes two different definitions for perinatal mortality rate (PMR). PMR definition I includes infant deaths of less than 7 days of age and fetal deaths of 28 weeks of gestation or more per 1000 live births plus fetal deaths, whereas PMR definition II is more comprehensive, including infant deaths of less than 28 days of age and fetal deaths of 20 weeks or more per the same denominator.[4,5] The definitions of PMR provided by the World Health Organization (WHO) and the American College of Obstetricians and Gynecologists (ACOG) differ slightly, including the number of fetuses and live births weighing at least 500 g rather than using a gestational age cut-off.[6,7] According to the NCHS, "Fetal death means death prior to the complete expulsion or extraction from its mother of a product of human conception, irrespective of the duration of pregnancy and which is not an induced termination of pregnancy. The death is indicated by the fact that after such expulsion or extraction, the fetus does not breathe or show any other evidence of life such as beating of the heart, pulsation of the umbilical cord, or definite movement of voluntary muscles."[4] The term *fetal death* is used in these definitions and hereafter rather than stillbirth, spontaneous abortion, or miscarriage.

In 2005, there were about 26,000 fetal deaths in the United States. **Although the PMR has fallen steadily in the United States since 1965, the number of fetal deaths has not changed substantially in the past decade** (Figure 12-1).[4,5,8] Using NCHS definition I, the PMR reported in 2005 was 6.6 per 1000, with fetal deaths accounting for about 50% of all perinatal mortality in the United States.[4] The PMR varies greatly by maternal race and ethnicity (Figure 12-2). In 2005, rates (per 1000) were lowest for Asian/Pacific Islander women (4.96), followed by non-Hispanic white (5.36), Hispanic (5.89), and American Indian/Alaskan Native women (6.29). The rate for non-Hispanic black women (12.19) was the highest among the racial and ethnic groups and was 2.3 times the rate for non-Hispanic white women. The significantly greater PMR in blacks results from higher rates of *both* neonatal and fetal deaths.[4]

Characteristics of Fetal Death

Another way to consider the contribution of fetal events on PMR is to look at the infant mortality rate (Figure 12-3).[8] Although the infant mortality rate includes all deaths of infants younger than 1 year of age, 50% of all infant deaths occur in the first week of life, and 50% of these losses result during the first day of life.[7] The infant mortality rate has fallen progressively and even more steeply over time than the fetal death rate, from 47 per 1000 in 1940 to 6.8 per 1000 in 2005, although the rate has remained largely unchanged from 2000 to 2005.[6,9,10] In 2005 there were about 28,000 infant deaths (7 per 1000 live births), including 19,000 (4.7 per 1000 live births) neonatal deaths, 15,000 of which were in the first week of life.[6,9,10] In 2005, the leading causes of infant mortality were congenital malformations (19.5%); disorders relating to short gestation and low birthweight, not elsewhere classified (16.5%); sudden infant death syndrome (7.4%); newborn affected by maternal complications of pregnancy (maternal complications) (6.3%); and newborn affected by complication of placenta, cord, and membranes (4%).[10] Clearly, **perinatal events play an important role in infant mortality.**

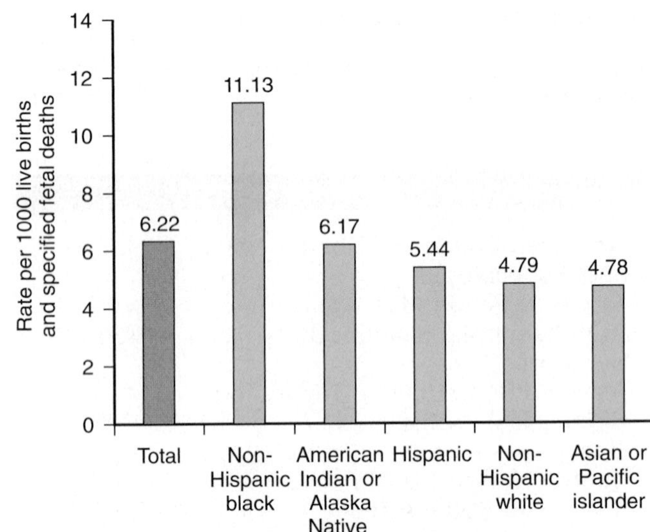

FIGURE 12-2. Fetal mortality rates by maternal race and ethnicity, United States 2005. (Data from the CDC/NCHS, National Vital Statistics System, as presented in NCHS Data Brief No. 16, April 2009, McDorman and Kirmeyer.)

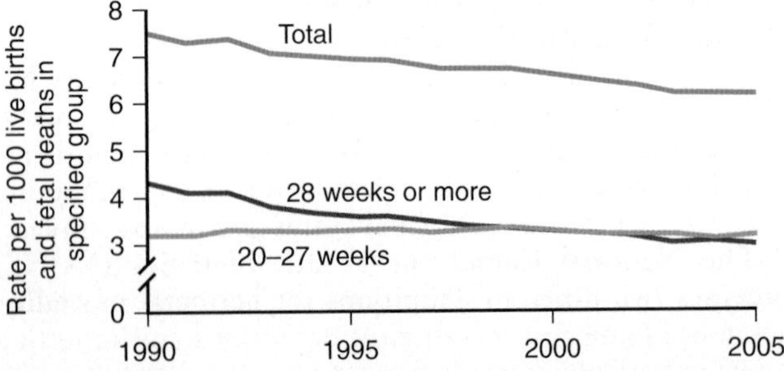

FIGURE 12-1. Trends in fetal mortality rates over time, by period of gestation, United States 1990-2005. (Data from the CDC/NCHS, National Vital Statistics System, as presented in NCHS Data Brief No. 16, April 2009, McDorman and Kirmeyer.)

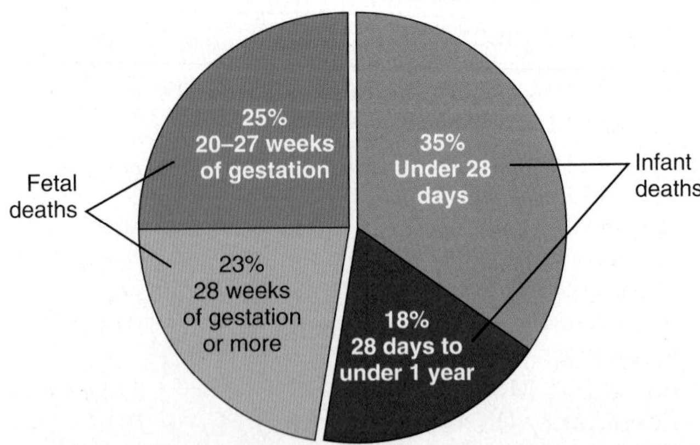

FIGURE 12-3. Relative magnitude of components of fetal and infant mortality, United States 2005. (Data from the CDC/NCHS, National Vital Statistics System, as presented in NCHS Data Brief No. 16, April 2009, McDorman and Kirmeyer.)

Causes of Fetal Deaths

In addition to declining frequency in PMR over time, the overall pattern of perinatal deaths in the United States has changed considerably during the past 40 years. Manning and associates[11] suggest that antepartum deaths may be divided into four broad categories: (1) chronic asphyxia of diverse origin; (2) congenital malformations; (3) superimposed complications of pregnancy, such as Rh isoimmunization, placental abruption, and fetal infection; and (4) deaths of unexplained cause. Fretts and colleagues[12,13] analyzed the causes of deaths, confirmed by autopsy, in fetuses weighing more than 500 g in 94,346 births at the Royal Victoria Hospital in Montreal from 1961 to 1993. The population studied was predominantly white, participated in prenatal care, and included patients from all socioeconomic groups. Overall, the fetal death rate in this group declined by 70%, from 11.5 per 1000 in the 1960s to 3.2 per 1000 during 1990 to 1993.[13] The decline in the fetal death rate in this cohort was attributed to the prevention of Rh sensitization, antepartum and intrapartum fetal surveillance, improved detection of intrauterine growth restriction (IUGR) and fetal anomalies with ultrasound, and improved care of maternal diabetes mellitus and preeclampsia. The role of antenatal diagnosis and management of congenital malformations and aneuploidy is obviously critical to a goal of reducing perinatal morbidity and mortality and will be discussed separately (see Chapters 9, 10, and 11).

Fretts and colleagues[12,13] noted that most of the deaths in the Canadian cohort occurred between 28 and 36 weeks' gestation and that the diagnosis of IUGR was rarely identified before death. In addition to IUGR, leading causes of fetal death after 28 weeks' gestation included abruptio placentae and unexplained antepartum losses. Despite a marked fall in unexplained fetal deaths, from 38.1 to 13.6 per 1000, this category was used for more than 25% of all stillbirths. Fetal-maternal hemorrhage may occur in 10% to 15% of cases of unexplained fetal deaths. Fetal deaths caused by infection, most often associated with premature rupture of the membranes before 28 weeks' gestation, did not decline over the 30 years of the study and accounted for about 19% of fetal deaths. Further population-based analyses of the causes of fetal death have confirmed these findings.

In summary, based on available data, about 30% of antepartum fetal deaths may be attributed to asphyxia (IUGR, prolonged gestation), 30% to maternal complications (placental abruption, hypertension, preeclampsia, and diabetes mellitus), 15% to congenital malformations and chromosomal abnormalities, and 5% to infection. **At least 20% of fetal deaths have no obvious fetal, placental, maternal, or obstetrical etiology, and this percentage increases with advancing gestational age.** Late-gestation stillbirths are more likely to have no identifiable etiology.[6] The ability of our current methods of surveillance to make an impact on the perinatal mortality will depend on the ability of available tests to predict and predate injury and on use of obstetrical interventions to prevent adverse outcomes. In one British series, obstetrical and pediatric assessors reviewed the circumstances surrounding each case of perinatal death to identify any *avoidable* factors contributing to the death.[14] Of the 309 perinatal deaths in this population (half fetal and half in the first week of life), 59% were considered to have had avoidable factors, including 74% of normal-birthweight infants with no fetal abnormalities and no maternal complications. Most avoidable factors were found to be obstetrical rather than pediatric or maternal and social. The failure to respond appropriately to abnormalities during pregnancy and labor, including results from the monitoring of fetal growth or intrapartum fetal well-being, significant maternal weight loss, or reported reductions in fetal movement, constituted the largest groups of avoidable factors. This characterization of avoidable factors contributing to perinatal death has been confirmed in additional studies.

Timing of Fetal Death

Another way to classify fetal deaths may be to differentiate those that occur during the antepartum period and those that occur during labor, or intrapartum deaths. **Antepartum fetal death is much more common than intrapartum fetal death,[15] and unexplained fetal death occurs far more commonly than unexplained infant death.**[4,10] In a population-based study in the United States in 2007, the antepartum fetal death rate was 3.7 per 1000, compared with 0.6 per 1000 intrapartum fetal deaths.[15] Although most fetal deaths occur before 32 weeks' gestation, in planning a strategy for antepartum fetal monitoring, one must examine the risk for fetal death in the population of women who are still pregnant at that point in pregnancy.[16] When this approach is taken, the data would suggest that fetuses at 40 to 41 weeks are at a threefold greater risk and those at 42 or more weeks are at a 12-fold greater risk for intrauterine death than fetuses at 28 to 31 weeks. The risks are even higher in multiple gestations, as pregnancy progresses. For twin gestations, the optimal time for delivery to prevent late gestation perinatal deaths is by 39 weeks, and for triplets, 36 weeks.[17]

Identifying Those at Risk

Some risk factors have a clear etiologic relationship to fetal compromise and death, such as exposures to teratogens or maternal conditions that alter the fetal environment or blood supply or content. Other risk factors, such as epidemiologic factors including maternal age, race, and body habitus, have a perhaps more complex and less well-understood link to fetal death risk (Figure 12-4).[3] Common risk factors for fetal death in the United States are listed in Table 12-1.[2,18] Many of these conditions may coexist in individual patients, making assessment of the contribution of each factor to perinatal mortality a challenge. Additionally, the contribution of these conditions to fetal injury resulting in liveborn children with permanent neurologic compromise has yet to be determined but is an important alternative outcome to perinatal mortality that, as mentioned previously, deserves further study.[2]

DETAILS ON SELECT MATERNAL CONDITIONS

Obesity: Prepregnancy obesity is associated with increased perinatal mortality, especially in late gestation. This has been demonstrated in several large series, including a meta-analysis of nine studies that included

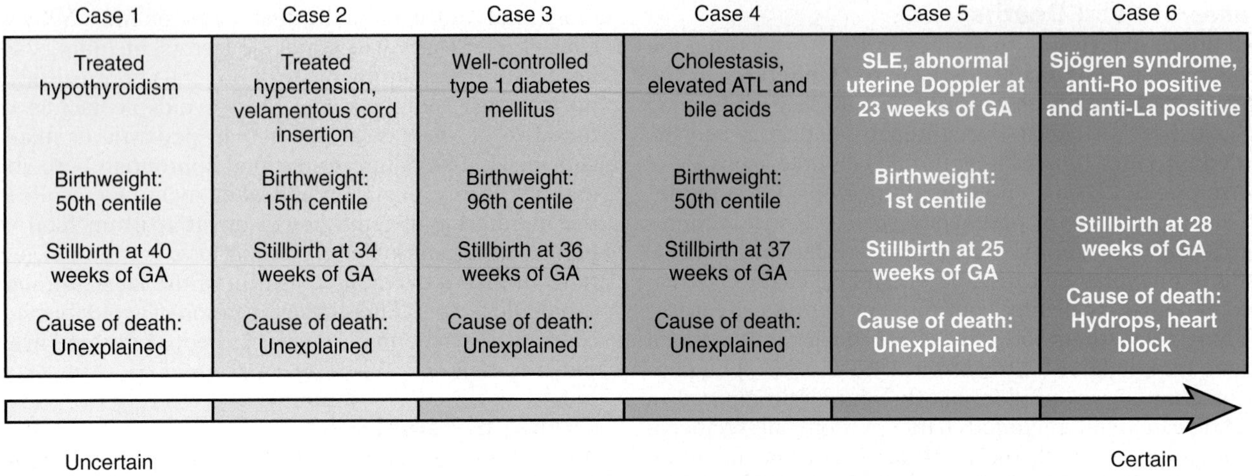

Case 1	Case 2	Case 3	Case 4	Case 5	Case 6
Treated hypothyroidism	Treated hypertension, velamentous cord insertion	Well-controlled type 1 diabetes mellitus	Cholestasis, elevated ATL and bile acids	SLE, abnormal uterine Doppler at 23 weeks of GA	Sjögren syndrome, anti-Ro positive and anti-La positive
Birthweight: 50th centile	Birthweight: 15th centile	Birthweight: 96th centile	Birthweight: 50th centile	Birthweight: 1st centile	
Stillbirth at 40 weeks of GA	Stillbirth at 34 weeks of GA	Stillbirth at 36 weeks of GA	Stillbirth at 37 weeks of GA	Stillbirth at 25 weeks of GA	Stillbirth at 28 weeks of GA
Cause of death: Unexplained	Cause of death: Unexplained	Cause of death: Unexplained	Cause of death: Unexplained	Cause of death: Unexplained	Cause of death: Hydrops, heart block

Uncertain → Certain

FIGURE 12-4. Continuum of certainty in pathophysiology of cause of fetal death. As one progresses from left to right on the continuum, there are increasing levels of certainty as to the role of the pathophysiology of a particular condition in causing the fetal death. *ALT,* Alanine aminotransferase; *GA,* gestational age. (Courtesy Professor Gordon Smith. Modified from Reddy UM, Goldenberg R, Silver R, et al: Stillbirth classification: developing an international consensus for research. Executive summary of a National Institute of Child Health and Human Development workshop. Stillbirth Classification of Cause of Death. Obstet Gynecol 114:901-914, 2009.)

more than 325,000 women.[19] The connection between obesity and fetal death is still under investigation and is made more complex by the frequent comorbidities encountered in patients with prepregnancy obesity. Theoretical contributors to adverse perinatal outcomes in this group include placental dysfunction, sleep apnea, metabolic abnormalities, and difficulty in clinical assessment of fetal growth.[18]

Parity: Nulliparity and high parity have both been associated with fetal death, in contrast to women having their second child. This association has not been fully explored and may be subject to significant confounding influences, including advanced maternal age, related conditions in nulliparous women with delayed childbearing in developed nations, and other medical and socioeconomic comorbidities in women with high parity.[8,18]

Maternal age: Fretts and coworkers and others[2,13,20] have found that, after controlling for risk factors such as multiple gestation, hypertension, diabetes mellitus, placenta previa and abruption, previous abortion, and prior fetal death, women 35 years of age or older have a greater risk for fetal death than women younger than 30 years, and women 40 years or older have an even further increased risk. **Data from other countries and other investigators have confirmed a J-shaped curve relationship between maternal age and fetal deaths, with the highest rates in teenagers and women older than 35 years of age** (Figure 12-5). The interplay of fetal death, maternal age, and gestational age was demonstrated in a population-based 2006 study in the United States of almost 5.5 million births.[21] In this cohort, compared with their counterparts aged 30 to 34 years at 41 weeks of gestation, women older than 35 to 39 years had the same risk for fetal death at 40 weeks, and women older than 40 years had the same risk at 39 weeks of gestation. Only 10% of the women older than 35 years had medical comorbidities, and the results of this study did not change when those women were excluded, highlighting the point that the increase in fetal death risk exists in otherwise healthy older gravidas compared with younger women.

Multiple gestation: **The higher rate of perinatal mortality in multiple gestations compared with singletons is related both to complications unique to multiple gestations (such as twin-to-twin transfusion syndrome) and to more general complications such as fetal abnormalities and growth restriction.**[18,22] Additionally, many women carrying more than one fetus have maternal risk factors for increased perinatal mortality, including advanced maternal age and use of assisted reproductive technologies (ART), and are subject to development of complications such as preeclampsia and preterm delivery.[2,23] Optimal timing of delivery between 37 and 38 weeks has been considered for twins, compared with 39 to 40 weeks among singletons, because of increased rate of late fetal death in this group. Chorionicity is of paramount importance in determining fetal risk, with higher rates of adverse outcomes among monochorionic twins.[2,23]

Diabetes mellitus: **Although historically insulin-dependent diabetes has been a major risk factor for fetal death, the fetal death rate in women with optimal glycemic control now approaches that of women without diabetes.**[2,24] However, the relationship between glycemic control and fetal death remains uncertain. Poor glycemic control remains associated with increased perinatal mortality, in large part as a result of congenital anomalies, indicated preterm deliveries, and sudden unexplained fetal death. There is no evidence that gestational diabetes controlled by diet alone is associated with increased rates of adverse perinatal outcomes.[2,25]

Serum markers: First- and second-trimester serum markers for aneuploidy, when abnormally low or elevated, have been associated to varying degrees with adverse perinatal outcomes even in the absence of aneuploidy. Regarding fetal death after 24 weeks,

TABLE 12-1 COMMON RISK FACTORS FOR FETAL DEATH IN THE UNITED STATES

RISK FACTOR	PREVALENCE (%)	ODDS RATIO
All pregnancies	—	1.0
Low-risk pregnancies	80	0.86
Obesity		
BMI 25-29.9	21-24	1.4-2.7
BMI >30	20-34	2.1-2.8
Nulliparity compared with second pregnancy	40	1.2-1.6
Fourth child or greater compared with second	11	2.2-2.3
Maternal age (reference <35 yr)		
35-39 yr	15-18	1.8-2.2
≥40 yr	2	1.8-3.3
Multiple gestation		
Twins	2.7	1.0-2.2
Triplets or greater	0.14	2.8-3.7
Oligohydramnios	2	4.5
Assisted reproductive technologies (all)	1-3	1.2-3.0
Abnormal serum markers		
First-trimester PAPP-A <5%	5	2.2-4.0
Two or more second-trimester markers	0.1-2	4.2-9.2
Intrahepatic cholestasis	<0.1	1.8-4.4
Renal disease	<1	2.2-30
Systemic lupus erythematosus	<1	6-20
Smoking	10-20	1.7-3.0
Alcohol use (any)	6-10	1.2-1.7
Illicit drug use	2-4	1.2-3.0
Low education and socioeconomic status	30	2.0-7.0
Antenatal visits <4*	6	2.7
Black (reference white)	15	2.0-2.2
Hypertension	6-10	1.5-4.4
Diabetes	2-5	1.5-7.0
Large for gestational age (>97% without diabetes)	12	2.4
Fetal growth restriction (%)		
<3	3.0	4.8
3-10	7.5	2.8
Previous growth-restricted infant	6.7	2.0-4.6
Previous preterm birth with growth restriction	2	4.0-8.0
Decreased fetal movement	4-8	4.0-12.0
Previous stillbirth	0.5	2.0-10.0
Previous cesarean section	22-25	1.0-1.5
Postterm pregnancy compared with 38-40 wk		2.0-3.0
41 wk	9	1.5
42 wk	5	2.0-3.0

Modified from Signore C, Freeman RK, Spong CY: Antenatal testing: a reevaluation. Executive Summary of a Eunice Kennedy Shriver National Institute of Child Health and Human Development Workshop. Obstet Gynecol 113:687-701, 2009; and Fretts RC: Stillbirth epidemiology, risk factors, and opportunities for stillbirth prevention. Clin Obstet Gynecol 53:588-596, 2010.

*For stillbirths 37 weeks' gestation.

BMI, Body mass index; PAPP-A, pregnancy associated plasma protein A.

markers of interest include first-trimester levels of pregnancy-associated plasma protein A (PAPP-A) of less than the 5th percentile (0.415 multiples of the median [MoM]), and second trimester free β-human chorionic gonadotropin (free β-hCG), α-fetoprotein (AFP), and inhibin A of more than 2 MoM. The sensitivity and positive predictive value of these markers for fetal death have yet to be determined. The pathophysiologic link between these markers and adverse outcomes is under investigation but most plausibly involves abnormal placental attachment or function.[26]

Thrombophilia: In general, there has been no demonstrable link between inherited thrombophilia and risk for fetal death.[3,27] Although initial reports seemed to support an association between thrombophilias, such as factor V Leiden mutation and prothrombin gene mutation, and fetal death, large prospective trials have failed to substantiate this association. The presence of circulating maternal antiphospholipid antibodies, in particular lupus anticoagulant, anticardiolipin antibodies, and anti-β_2-glycoprotein-I antibodies, in the antiphospholipid antibody syndrome (APLAS) has been associated with a variety of adverse pregnancy outcomes, including fetal loss. The mechanism of these adverse outcomes remains unclear but likely includes inflammation, thrombosis, and placental infarction.[3] However, the link between these antibodies or presence of APLAS and fetal death in particular is still under investigation, with insufficient evidence to conclude that there is an increased risk for fetal death.[28]

Maternal race: The variation in fetal death risk in the United States by maternal race is complex, making ascertainment of biologic risk factors related to race difficult.[18] Factors contributing to increased rates of fetal death among black women compared with white women include disparities in socioeconomic status, access to health care, and preexisting medical conditions. A 2009 population-based study of more than 5 million U.S. births demonstrated that the greatest black and white disparity is in preterm perinatal death, with a hazard ratio at 20 to 23 weeks of 2.75, which decreases to 1.57 at 39 to 40 weeks. Lower education levels and higher rates of medical, pregnancy, and labor complications contributed more to the adverse outcomes in blacks compared with whites, with congenital anomalies more contributory in whites.[29]

Hypertensive disorders: Studies have shown conflicting evidence regarding whether fetal death rates with well-controlled preexisting hypertension are comparable to those in the general population, or increased. The increased risk for perinatal mortality associated with hypertension is most often related to complicated hypertension, with sequelae of placental insufficiency including IUGR and oligohydramnios. Proteinuric hypertension, including especially severe preeclampsia or eclampsia, may be associated with fetal death through placental and coagulation-related pathways, including placental abruption.[3,30]

Fetal growth restriction (IUGR): IUGR is a well-known risk factor for perinatal death but historically has been under-recognized before fetal death. Placental dysfunction is commonly implicated in nonmalformed and chromosomally normal IUGR fetuses. This topic is reviewed in further detail in Chapter 31.

Amniotic fluid abnormalities: The predictive value of either oligohydramnios or polyhydramnios for adverse pregnancy outcomes, in particular fetal death, typically lies in their association with other abnormal conditions,

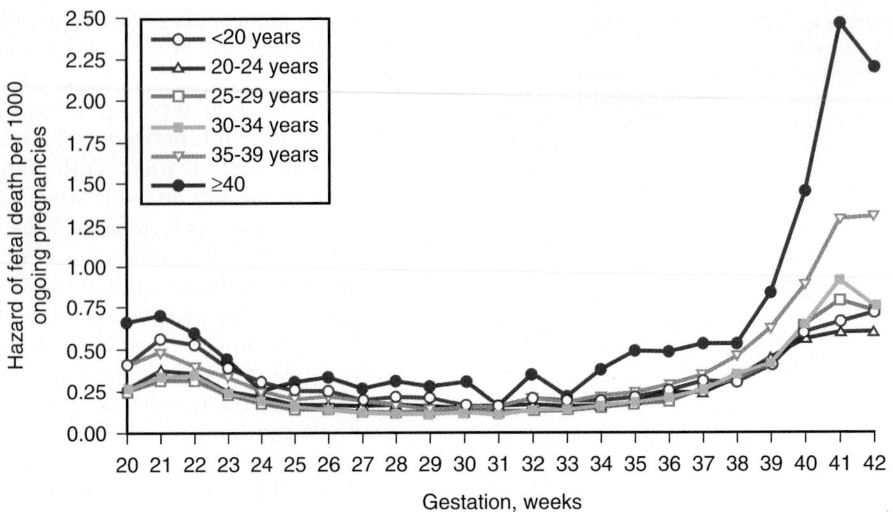

FIGURE 12-5. Relationship of fetal death and maternal age across gestation. (From Reddy UM, Ko CW, Willinger M: Maternal age and the risk of stillbirth throughout pregnancy in the United States. Am J Obstet Gynecol 195:764-770, 2006.)

such as maternal diabetes mellitus, hypertensive disorders, rupture of membranes, fetal growth restriction, or fetal anomalies. Isolated oligohydramnios and polyhydramnios have not been conclusively linked to increased risk for fetal death; nevertheless, evaluation of amniotic fluid volume as a marker of long-term fetal health status is a mainstay of antepartum fetal evaluation.[2,31]

Prior obstetrical and fertility history ART: Multiple aspects of a woman's obstetrical and fertility history may contribute to risk for fetal death in a current pregnancy, including parity, use of assisted reproductive technologies, and history of prior adverse obstetrical outcomes. Both nulliparity and high parity are associated with an increased risk for fetal death compared with "low multiparity" (one, two, or three prior births).[32] This association is likely mediated through a variety of sociodemographic risk factors related to overall health and interconception health status, although studies have confirmed the association between parity and fetal death after controlling for several social and medical comorbidities. History of prior adverse pregnancy outcomes, including fetal growth restriction, preterm birth, and fetal death marks a current pregnancy at risk for fetal death. However, the association with preventable recurrent fetal death is complex and is modified by coexistence of other high-risk conditions. Recurrence risk for fetal death in particular has received recent scrutiny because rates vary dramatically by study population and presence of other risk factors. Given that many fetal deaths occur in pregnancies with no identifiable risk factors and that well-designed studies with appropriate comparison groups (i.e., low-risk women without identifiable risk factors) are lacking, clinician and patient perception of increased risk in a pregnancy subsequent to a fetal death will likely continue to drive management of these patients.[33] Regarding use of ART and risk for fetal death, several systematic reviews have confirmed an independent association between the use of in vitro fertilization in particular and fetal death. However, whether the association is mediated through the technologies themselves or the underlying infertility or through other undetermined mechanisms remains unclear.[34]

Postdates: The definition of postterm pregnancy has been reevaluated in the past decade, based on reappraisal of the peak time of fetal risk in relation to the 40-week mark. The pathophysiology of increased fetal death risk in the postterm pregnancy is thought to be mediated by impaired placental gas exchange and is often associated with oligohydramnios. Traditionally oligohydramnios has been as a marker for increased risk in the postterm pregnancy for which intervention in the form of delivery is thought to be necessary, although as described previously, whether oligohydramnios is independently associated with fetal death in pregnancies after 40 weeks' gestation is unclear.[35]

Socioeconomic factors, prenatal care, and substance use: Poor access to prenatal care and poor underlying health and nutrition have been linked to increase risk for fetal death both in developing and in developed nations. As with other sociodemographic risk factors, these potential influences on fetal death risk are difficult to quantify and may be additive to other high-risk conditions.[36] Smoking and use of alcohol and other substances, along with obesity, represent potentially modifiable risk factors for fetal death. Although these behaviors are attractive candidates for fetal death prevention through counseling and modification of intake, prospective trials of behavioral modification strategies have generally been underpowered to detect a difference in fetal death with these interventions.[18]

Intrahepatic cholestasis: **The cause of fetal death in women with gestational cholestasis remains unknown, and timing and predictive features of impending fetal death remain unpredictable.** Fetal deaths in these pregnancies are not preceded by signs of placental insufficiency such as growth restriction or abnormal placental pathology, and normal fetal heart rate tracings proximal to fetal death (i.e., within 24 hours) have often been reported. It has also not been established whether maternal serum levels of bile acids, liver enzymes, or pharmacologic therapy modify or predict fetal death risk.[37]

Renal disease, systemic lupus erythematosus (SLE): With chronic maternal renal disease, perinatal outcome is largely associated with degree of renal dysfunction and presence of coexisting hypertension or diabetes. Although data are limited by lack of prospective studies with appropriate control groups, the greatest risk for fetal death appears to be in those with severe renal impairment (i.e., serum creatinine levels >2.4 to 2.8 mg/dL).[38] As with maternal renal disease, the prognosis for fetal outcome in women with SLE is dependent on disease state and comorbid conditions, including hypertension, circulating autoantibodies, and renal involvement.[39] Prognosis for fetal survival in pregnancies complicated by both maternal renal disease and maternal SLE has improved over time, with advances in therapies promoting disease quiescence for both of these conditions.

The best use of available antenatal testing modalities may vary according to the risk profile of each individual pregnancy. Discussion of condition-specific testing will be undertaken after review of the individual testing modalities described later.

POTENTIAL UTILITY OF ANTEPARTUM FETAL TESTING

Can antepartum fetal deaths and injury be prevented? Before using antepartum fetal testing, the obstetrician must ask several important questions:

1. Does the test provide information not already known by the patient's clinical status?
2. Can the information be helpful in managing the patient?
3. If an abnormality is detected, is there a treatment available for the problem?
4. Could an abnormal test result lead to increased risk for the mother or fetus?
5. Will the test ultimately decrease perinatal morbidity and mortality?

A large body of clinical and research experience suggests that antepartum fetal assessment can have a significant impact on the frequency and causes of antenatal fetal deaths.[1] However, according to several recent reviews of the benefits and costs of antenatal testing, "strong evidence for the efficacy of antepartum testing is lacking."[40] **Unfortunately, few of the antepartum tests commonly employed in clinical practice today have been subjected to large-scale prospective and randomized evaluations that can speak to the true efficacy of testing.**[27,41] In most cases, when the test has been applied and good perinatal outcomes observed, the test has gained further acceptance and has been used more widely. In such cases, one cannot be sure whether it is actually the information provided by the test that has led to the improved outcomes or the total program of care that has made the difference. When prospective randomized investigations are conducted, large numbers of patients must be studied because many adverse outcomes, such as intrauterine death, are uncommon even in high-risk populations. For example, although several controlled trials have failed to demonstrate improved outcomes with nonstress testing, the study populations ranged from only 300 to 530 subjects.

To determine the clinical application of antepartum diagnostic testing, the predictive value of the tests must be considered. The sensitivity of the test is the probability that the test will be positive or abnormal when the disease is present. The specificity of the test is the probability that the test result will be negative when the disease is not present. Note that the sensitivity and specificity refer not to the actual numbers of patients with a positive or abnormal result but to the proportion or probability of these test results. The predictive value of an abnormal test would be that fraction of patients with an abnormal test result who have the abnormal condition, and the predictive value of a normal test would be the fraction of patients with a normal test result who are normal.

Antepartum fetal tests may be used to screen a large obstetrical population to detect fetal disease. In this setting, a test of high sensitivity is preferable because one would not want to miss patients whose fetus might be compromised. One would be willing to overdiagnose the problem, that is, accept some false-positive diagnoses. In further evaluating the patient whose fetus may be at risk and when attempting to confirm the presence of disease, one would want a test of high specificity. One would not want to intervene unnecessarily and deliver a fetus that was doing well. In this setting, multiple tests may be helpful. When multiple test results are normal, they tend to exclude disease. When all are abnormal, however, they tend to support the diagnosis of fetal disease.

The prevalence of the abnormal condition has great impact on the predictive value of antenatal fetal tests and the number needed to evaluate with testing and to treat with interventions (delivery) to presumably prevent fetal death. The impact of these parameters on the utility of testing was illustrated in a decision analysis of the risks and benefits of antepartum testing late in pregnancy for women 35 years or older using the McGill Obstetrical Neonatal Database to obtain risk estimates.[42] In this model, as in practice, the relative benefit of antenatal testing lies in the balance of number of fetal deaths prevented with number and type of interventions required to prevent them. At an estimated risk for unexplained fetal death of 5.2 per 1000 pregnancies (nulliparas ≥35 years of age in the McGill cohort), 863 additional antenatal tests, 71 additional inductions of labor, and 14 additional cesarean deliveries would be required to prevent one additional fetal death using this model. Comparatively, using the same model, at an estimated risk for 1 to 2 per 1000 pregnancies, 2862 additional antenatal tests, 233 additional inductions, and 44 additional cesarean deliveries would be required to prevent one additional fetal death. Thus, the number needed to evaluate and treat to prevent one fetal death decreases as risk for fetal death increases in the population being tested.

In interpreting the results of studies of antepartum testing, the obstetrician must consider the application of that test to his or her own population. If the study has been done in a population of patients at great risk, it is more likely that an abnormal test will be associated with an abnormal fetus. If the obstetrician is practicing in a community with patients who are, in general, at low risk, an abnormal test result would more likely be associated with a false-positive diagnosis.

For most antepartum diagnostic tests, a cut-off point used to define an abnormal result must be arbitrarily established. The cut-off point is selected to maximize the separation between the normal and diseased populations (Figure 12-6). Changing the cut-off will have a great impact on the predictive value of the test. For example, suppose that 10 accelerations in 10 minutes were required for a fetus to have a reactive nonstress test (NST) (threshold A). The fetus who fulfilled this rigid definition would almost certainly be in good condition. However, many fetuses who failed to achieve 10 accelerations in 10 minutes would also be in good condition, but would be judged to be abnormal by this cut-off. In this instance, the test would have many abnormal results. It would be highly sensitive and capture all of the abnormal fetuses, but it would have a low specificity. If the number of accelerations required to pass an NST were lowered to 1 in 10 minutes, it would decrease the sensitivity of the test (threshold C). That is, one might miss a truly sick fetus. At the same time, however, one would improve the specificity of the test or its ability to predict that percentage of the patients who are normal. Using the criterion of two accelerations of the fetal heart rate in 20 minutes for a reactive NST (threshold B), one hopes to have a test with both high sensitivity and high specificity.

WHAT DO THESE TESTS TELL US ABOUT THE FETUS?

Fetal State

To be able to diagnose suspected fetal compromise using tests of fetal biophysical state, blood flow, and heart rate, we must be able to appreciate how these parameters appear under normal conditions and in response to suboptimal conditions.

Regarding fetal biophysical characteristics, one must appreciate that, during the third trimester, the normal fetus may exhibit marked changes in its neurologic state.[43] Four fetal states have been identified. The near-term fetus spends about 25% of its time in a quiet sleep state (state 1F) and 60% to 70% in an active sleep state (state 2F). Active sleep is associated with rapid eye movement (REM). In fetal lambs, electrocortical activity during REM sleep is characterized by low-voltage, high-frequency waves. The fetus exhibits regular breathing movements and intermittent abrupt movements of its head, limbs, and trunk. The fetal heart rate in active sleep (state 2F) exhibits increased variability and frequent accelerations with movement. During quiet, or non-REM, sleep, the fetal heart rate slows, and heart rate variability is reduced. The fetus may make infrequent breathing movements and startled movements. Electrocortical activity recordings at this time reveal high-voltage, low-frequency waves. Near term, periods of quiet sleep may last 20 minutes, and those of active sleep about 40 minutes.[43] The mechanisms that control these periods of rest and activity in the fetus are not well established. External factors such as the mother's activity, her ingestion of drugs, and her nutrition may play a role. Specific factors that may decrease fetal movement in the third trimester include fetal anomalies, particularly central nervous system (CNS) anomalies; maternal exposures, including corticosteroids, sedatives, and smoking; low amniotic fluid volume; and decreased placental blood flow due to placental insufficiency.[44]

When evaluating fetal condition using the NST or the biophysical profile (BPP), one must ask whether a fetus that is not making breathing movements or shows no accelerations of its baseline heart rate is in a quiet sleep state or is neurologically compromised. In such circumstances, prolonging the period of evaluation usually allows a change in fetal state, and more normal parameters of fetal well-being appear.

Regarding regulation of fetal heart rate and blood flow, **fetal adaptation to hypoxemia is mediated through changes in heart rate and redistribution of cardiac output.** However, changes in fetal cardiac output are generally observed during hypoxemia only when there is coexisting acidemia. In response to sudden hypoxemia, one can initially observe fetal heart rate slowing and increased variability, through vagally mediated chemoreceptor responses. With prolonged hypoxemia (30 to 60 minutes), increasing levels of circulating adrenergic agonists and modulation of vagal activity by endogenous opiates lead to a fetal heart rate return to or rise from the previous baseline.[45] Development of acidemia on top of hypoxemia can accelerate the rate of fetal deterioration and amplify the hypoxemia, by a shift of the oxyhemoglobin dissociation curve to the right, further reducing oxygen carrying capacity of fetal blood and eventually leading to redistribution of cardiac output that can be appreciated as a "brain-sparing" effect in evaluation of fetal blood flow. Redistribution of blood flow in the compromised fetus preferentially preserves perfusion to not only the brain but also the heart and adrenal glands.[45]

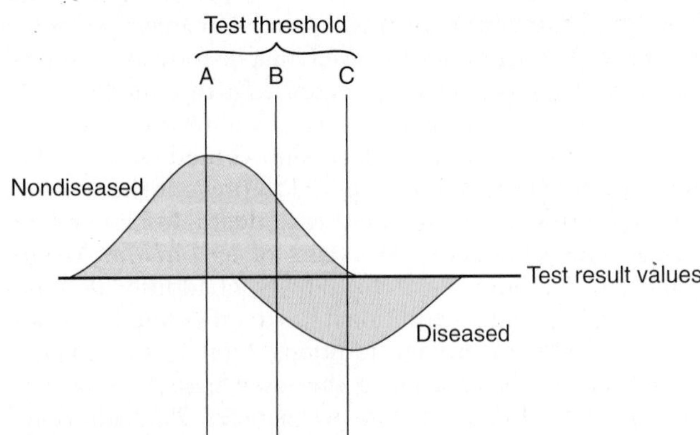

FIGURE 12-6. Hypothetical distribution of test results in a normal and diseased population, demonstrating the differences in test sensitivity and specificity with a change in test threshold. Making it more difficult for the fetus to pass the test by raising the test threshold *(A)* will increase the sensitivity but decrease the specificity, of the test. On the other hand, making the test easier to pass by decreasing the test threshold *(C)* will increase the specificity of the test but decrease the sensitivity. (Modified from Carpenter M, Coustan D: Criteria for screening tests for gestational diabetes. Am J Obstet Gynecol 144:768, 1982.)

Fetal movement is a more indirect indicator of fetal oxygen status and CNS function, with decreased fetal

movements in response to hypoxemia.[2] However, gestational development of fetal movement must be considered when evaluating fetal well-being as marked by fetal activity. Periods of absent fetal movement become more prolonged as gestation advances, with normal fetuses progressively exhibiting longer periods of quiescence as the late second and third trimesters advance. Up to and perhaps longer than 40 minutes of fetal inactivity at 40 weeks may be a normal finding, compared with less than 10 minutes at 20 weeks and less than 20 minutes at 32 weeks.[45] Keeping these trends in mind, abnormal degree or absence of fetal movement can be an appropriate marker for fetal hypoxemia. Fetal activity levels have been seen in animal studies to adapt to inducement of hypoxemia, however, with a resumption of fetal breathing and body movements after a prolonged period of hypoxemia, especially if induced gradually. Therefore, observation of these fetal states during antenatal testing does not guarantee a normoxic fetus.

BIOPHYSICAL TECHNIQUES OF FETAL EVALUATION

Description of the predictive value of several commonly performed antenatal tests of fetal well-being is presented in Table 12-2,[2] with detail on each methodology in the following sections.

Maternal Assessment of Fetal Activity

Studies performed using real-time ultrasonography have demonstrated that during the third trimester, the human fetus spends 10% of its time making gross fetal body movements and that 30 such movements are made each hour.[46] Periods of active fetal body movement last about 40 minutes, whereas quiet periods last about 20 minutes. Patrick and colleagues[46] noted that the longest period without fetal movements in a normal fetus was about 75 minutes. The mother is able to appreciate about 70% to 80% of gross fetal movements. The fetus does make fine body movements such as limb flexion and extension, hand grasping, and sucking, which probably reflect more coordinated CNS function. However, the mother is generally unable to perceive these fine movements. Fetal movement appears to peak between 9:00 PM and 1:00 AM, a time when maternal glucose levels are falling.[43,46] In a study in which maternal glucose levels were carefully controlled with an artificial pancreas, Holden and coworkers[47] found that hypoglycemia was associated with increased fetal movement. Fetal activity does not increase after meals or after maternal glucose administration.[48]

The decrease in fetal movement with hypoxemia makes maternal assessment of fetal activity a potentially simple and widely applicable method of monitoring fetal well-being. However, prospective trials of this method for prevention of perinatal mortality have failed to conclusively show benefit.[2] Neldam demonstrated a 73% reduction in avoidable fetal deaths in a prospective trial of more than 1500 women instructed to count fetal movements.[49] In contrast, a subsequent international trial of more than 68,000 women randomized to routine fetal movement assessment versus no formal assessment of fetal activity failed to show a significant reduction in fetal deaths in the group randomized to routine movement counting (weighted mean difference between groups, 0.23; 95% confidence interval [CI], 0.61 to 1.07).[50] There were significant differences in method of fetal movement counting, definition of abnormal fetal movements, patient compliance with the intervention, and provider response to patients who presented to care as a result of an abnormal fetal movement count in the latter compared with the former trial, as well as throughout the literature on this topic. This illustrates the difficulties in validating and reproducing the results of these trials and the uncertain clinical benefit that may be derived from introducing maternal assessment of fetal movement into routine clinical practice. A 2007 Cochrane review of four trials involving more than 71,000 women in 2007 concluded that there is insufficient evidence to recommend routine fetal movement counting to prevent fetal death.[51]

Despite these results, there may be some advantages to this type of fetal assessment. Although there will be a wide but normal range in fetal activity, with fetal movement counting, each mother and her fetus serve as their own control.[16] Factors affecting maternal perception of fetal movement are not well understood. Fetal and placental factors that may contribute include placental location, the length and type of fetal movements, and amniotic fluid volume (AFV), although whether AFV affects maternal perception or actual fetal movement is not clear.[44] Maternal factors that may influence the evaluation of fetal movement include maternal activity, parity, obesity, medications, and psychological factors, including anxiety. Studies of these associations have demonstrated conflicting results.[44] **About 80% of all mothers are able to comply with a program of counting fetal activity.**[16]

Several methods have been used to monitor fetal activity in research and clinical practice. These methods include fetal movement counting over a prescribed time period, such as 30 to 60 minutes one to three times daily, or conversely a target number of fetal movements to be counted over a variable time range. A variety of "normal" and "abnormal" fetal movement count results or thresholds have been proposed, to which the patient should be instructed to respond by presenting for further evaluation of fetal condition (Figure 12-7). These potential triggers for further evaluation include fewer than three movements in 1 hour or no movements for 12 hours, Sadovsky's "movement alarm signal"[52]; fewer than three movements an hour for 2 consecutive days[53]; or inability to

TABLE 12-2 COMPARISON OF SELECTED ANTENATAL TESTS

TEST	FALSE-NEGATIVE RATE (%)	FALSE-POSITIVE RATE (%)
Contraction stress test (CST)	0.04	35-65
Nonstress test (NST)	0.2-0.8	55-90
Biophysical profile (BPP)	0.07-0.08	40-50
Modified biophysical profile (mBPP)	0.08	60

Modified from Signore C, Freeman RK, Spong CY: Antenatal testing: a reevaluation. Executive Summary of a Eunice Kennedy Shriver National Institute of Child Health and Human Development Workshop. Obstet Gynecol 113:687-701, 2009.

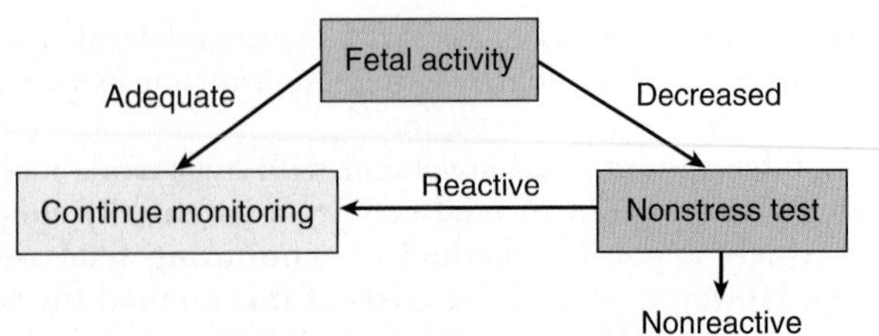

FIGURE 12-7. Maternal assessment of fetal activity is a valuable screening test for fetal condition. Should the mother report decreased fetal activity, an NST is performed. In this situation, most NSTs are reactive.

count 10 movements in a 12-hour period, the Cardiff count-to-10 method advocated by Pearson and Weaver.[54] Although the count-to-10 method has received wide scrutiny and is used perhaps most frequently in clinical practice, the use of this technique as a screening tool has most recently been reexamined by Froen and associates, who found in a cohort of 1200 women instructed to start their fetal movement count at the first convenient time of the day that the mean time to count to 10 was less than 10 minutes, compared with significantly longer and more variable average times reported in previous investigations.[55] Noting the variation in defining normal and abnormal patterns and maternal perception of fetal movement as mentioned previously, Froen and associates concluded that significant research is needed to better define the changes in fetal activity patterns and perception that are associated with good and adverse perinatal outcomes.

Potential negative impacts of maternal assessment of fetal activity include maternal anxiety as well as potential increase in utility of other testing modalities and antepartum admissions.[56] However, given the likely low impact of false-positive fetal movement count results, and the fact that this has been the only form of antenatal testing to be compared with no testing and found to have a favorable impact on fetal death, it seems reasonable to continue to prescribe some form of maternal assessment of fetal movement to patients until more conclusive evidence can be generated. As stated by Froen and associates in a 2008 review, "the fact that FMC versus no counting seems to be beneficial irrespective of the chosen definition of Decreased Fetal Movement (DFM) would support the hypothesis that benefit was derived from increased maternal vigilance regarding FM. When awareness, vigilance, and fetal movement counting is to be promoted, we have suggested that a maternal perception of significant and sustained reduction in fetal activity should remain the main definition of DFM. Any alarm limits, as '10 FM in 2 hours,'[57] should only be for guidance as a 'rule of thumb.' "[55]

Contraction Stress Test

The contraction stress test (CST), also known as the oxytocin challenge test (OCT), was the first biophysical technique widely applied for antepartum fetal surveillance. It was well known that uterine contractions produced a reduction in blood flow to the intervillous space. Analyses of intrapartum fetal heart rate monitoring had shown that a fetus with inadequate placental respiratory reserve would demonstrate recurrent late decelerations in response to hypoxia, in particular a fetal arterial oxygen pressure below 20 mm Hg (see Chapter 16). This drop in fetal heart rate in response to transient hypoxia is mediated, as noted earlier, by a vagal response to transient systemic fetal vascular reactivity provoked by hypoxia. The CST extended these observations to the antepartum period. The response of the fetus at risk for uteroplacental insufficiency to uterine contractions formed the basis for this test.

To perform the CST, the patient is placed in the semi-Fowler's position at a 30- to 45-degree angle with a slight left tilt to avoid the supine hypotensive syndrome. Continuous external fetal heart rate and uterine contraction monitoring is recorded, obtaining a baseline before stimulating uterine activity. Maternal blood pressure is determined every 5 to 10 minutes to detect maternal hypotension. In some cases, adequate uterine activity occurs spontaneously, and additional uterine stimulation is not necessary. An adequate CST requires uterine contractions of moderate intensity lasting about 40 to 60 seconds with a frequency of three in 10 minutes. These criteria were selected to approximate the stress experienced by the fetus during the first stage of labor. If uterine activity is absent or inadequate, intravenous oxytocin is begun to initiate contractions and increased until adequate uterine contractions have been achieved.[27] Several methods of nipple stimulation have been used to induce adequate uterine activity, and the success rate at achieving adequate contractions and test results is comparable to that of oxytocin infusion.[23,27] After the CST has been completed, the patient should be observed until uterine activity has returned to its baseline level. Contraindications to the test include a high risk for premature labor, such as in patients with premature rupture of the membranes, multiple gestation, and cervical incompetence, although the CST has not been associated with an increased incidence of premature labor.[58] The CST should also be avoided in conditions in which uterine contractions may be dangerous, such as placenta previa and a previous classic cesarean delivery or uterine surgery.

Most clinicians use the definitions proposed by Freeman and colleagues to interpret the CST[58,59] (detail in Table 12-3):

Negative: No late or significant variable decelerations
Positive: Late decelerations with at least 50% of contractions
Suspicious: Intermittent late or variable decelerations
Hyperstimulation: Decelerations with contractions longer than 90 seconds' duration or 2-minute frequency
Unsatisfactory: Fewer than three contractions per 10 minutes or an uninterpretable tracing

Predictive Value of the Contraction Stress Test

A negative CST has been consistently associated with good fetal outcome. Studies have shown the incidence of perinatal death within 1 week of a negative CST (i.e., the false-negative rate) to be less than 1 per 1000.[2,23,60,61] Many of these deaths, however, can be attributed to cord accidents, malformations, placental abruption, and acute deterioration of glucose control in patients with diabetes. Thus, the CST, like most methods of antepartum fetal surveillance, cannot predict acute fetal compromise. If the CST is negative and reactive, a repeat study is usually scheduled in 1 week (Figure 12-8). A negative but nonreactive

TABLE 12-3 INTERPRETATION OF THE CONTRACTION STRESS TEST

INTERPRETATION	DESCRIPTION	INCIDENCE (%)
Negative	No late decelerations appearing anywhere on the tracing with adequate uterine contractions (three in 10 min)	80
Positive	Late decelerations that are consistent and persistent, present with the majority (>50%) of contractions without excessive uterine activity; if persistent late decelerations seen before the frequency of contractions is adequate, test interpreted as positive	3-5
Suspicious	Inconsistent late decelerations	5
Hyperstimulation	Uterine contractions closer than every 2 min or lasting >90 sec, or five uterine contractions in 10 min; if no late decelerations seen, test interpreted as negative	5
Unsatisfactory	Quality of the tracing inadequate for interpretation, or adequate uterine activity cannot be achieved	5

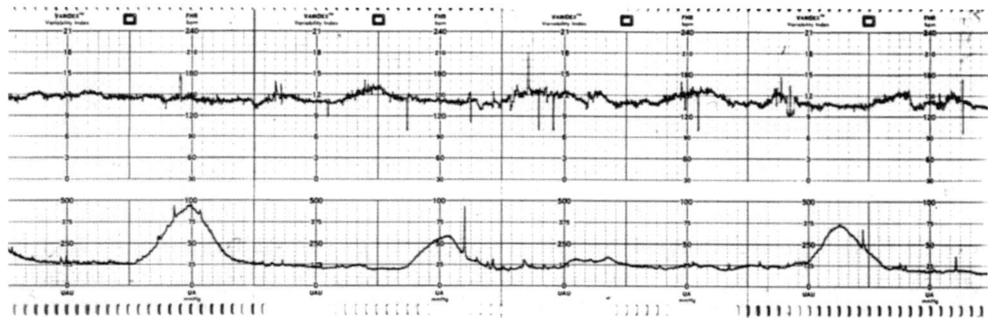

FIGURE 12-8. A reactive and negative CST. With this result, the CST would ordinarily be repeated in 1 week.

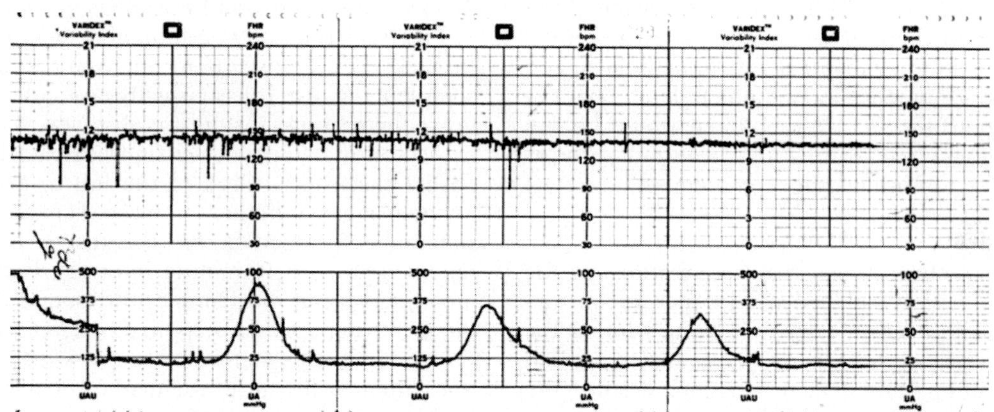

FIGURE 12-9. A nonreactive and negative CST. After this result, the test would ordinarily be repeated in 24 hours.

CST is not suggestive of acute fetal compromise, but cannot be seen as constituting the same low false-negative rate over the course of 1 week as a negative reactive CST. A negative nonreactive CST is usually repeated in 24 hours (Figure 12-9). Changes in the patient's clinical condition may warrant more frequent studies. A positive CST has been associated with an increased incidence of intrauterine death, late decelerations in labor, low 5-minute Apgar scores, IUGR, and meconium-stained amniotic fluid (Figure 12-10),[60] with an overall likelihood of perinatal death after a positive CST ranging from 7% to 15%. On the other hand, there has been a significant incidence of false-positive CSTs that, depending on the end point used, can be between 35% and 65%.[2,61] The positive CST is more likely to be associated with fetal compromise if the baseline heart rate lacks accelerations and the latency period between the onset of the uterine contractions and the onset of the late deceleration is less than 45 seconds.

The high incidence of false-positive CSTs is one of the greatest limitations of this test because such results could lead to unnecessary premature intervention. False-positive CSTs may be attributable to misinterpretation of the tracing; supine hypotension, which decreases uterine perfusion; uterine hyperstimulation, which is not appreciated using the tocodynamometer; or an improvement in fetal condition after the CST has been performed. The high false-positive rate also indicates that a patient with a positive CST need not necessarily require an elective cesarean delivery. If a trial of labor is to be undertaken after a positive CST, the cervix should be favorable for induction so that direct fetal heart rate monitoring and careful assessment of uterine contractility with an intrauterine pressure

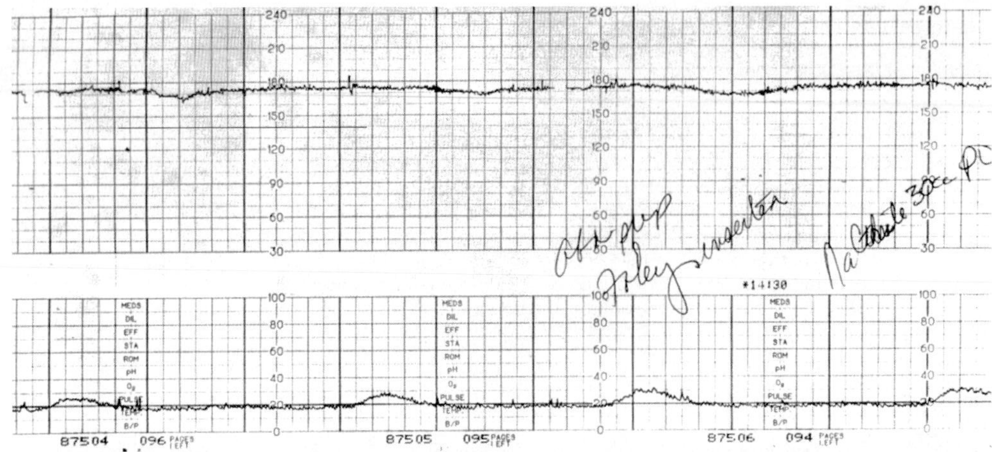

FIGURE 12-10. A nonreactive and positive CST with fetal tachycardia. At 34 weeks, a poorly compliant patient with type 1 diabetes mellitus reported decreased fetal activity. The NST revealed a fetal tachycardia of 170 beats/minute and was nonreactive. The CST was positive, and a BPP score was 2. The patient's cervix was unfavorable for induction. The patient underwent a low transverse cesarean delivery of a 2200-g male infant with Apgar scores of 1 and 3. The umbilical arterial pH was 7.21.

catheter can be performed. False-positive results are not increased when the CST is used early in the third trimester, between 28 and 33 weeks' gestation. A suspicious or equivocal CST or one that is unsatisfactory or shows hyperstimulation should be repeated in 24 hours. In one series, 7.5% of patients with an initially suspicious CST exhibited positive tests on further evaluation, 53.7% became negative, and 38.8% remained suspicious.[62] In follow-up studies of children who demonstrated a positive CST, few have exhibited abnormalities in neurologic and psychological development.[63] An important determinant in the long-term outcome for these children would be the early recognition of nonreassuring fetal heart rate patterns and the prevention of intrapartum compromise.

Nonstress Test

Mid-20th-century observations that **accelerations of the fetal heart rate in response to fetal activity, uterine contractions, or stimulation reflect fetal well-being formed the basis for the NST.** The NST is the most widely applied technique for antepartum fetal evaluation, despite the uncertainty regarding its reliability and reproducibility as a test of fetal assessment and that the basic technology that underlies its performance and application has changed little since its introduction and wide acceptance into antenatal practice.[64]

In late gestation, the healthy fetus exhibits an average of 34 accelerations above the baseline fetal heart rate each hour.[65] These accelerations, which average 20 to 25 beats/minute in amplitude and about 40 seconds in duration, require intact neurologic coupling between the fetal CNS and the fetal heart.[65] Fetal hypoxia disrupts this pathway. At term, fetal accelerations are associated with fetal movement more than 85% of the time, and more than 90% of gross movements are accompanied by accelerations. Fetal heart rate accelerations may be absent during periods of quiet fetal sleep. Studies by Patrick and associates[65] demonstrated that the longest time between successive accelerations in the healthy term fetus is about 40 minutes. However, the fetus may fail to exhibit heart rate accelerations for up to 80 minutes and still be normal.

Although an absence of fetal heart rate accelerations is most often attributable to a quiet fetal sleep state, CNS depressants such as narcotics and phenobarbital, as well as the β-blocker propranolol, can reduce heart rate reactivity.[66,67] Chronic smoking is known to decrease fetal oxygenation through an increase in fetal carboxyhemoglobin and a decrease in uterine blood flow. Fetal heart rate accelerations are also decreased in smokers.[68]

The NST is usually performed in an outpatient setting. In most cases, only 10 to 15 minutes are required to complete the test. It has virtually no contraindications, and few equivocal test results are observed. The patient may be seated in a reclining chair, with care being taken to ensure that she is tilted to the left to avoid the supine hypotensive syndrome.[27] The patient's blood pressure should be recorded before the test is begun and then repeated at 5- to 10-minute intervals. Fetal heart rate is monitored using the Doppler ultrasound transducer, and the tocodynamometer is applied to detect uterine contractions or fetal movement. Fetal activity may be recorded by the patient using an event marker or noted by the staff performing the test.

Fetal Heart Rate Patterns Observable on the Nonstress Test

Reactive

The most widely applied definition of a reactive test requires that at least two accelerations of the fetal heart rate, each with a peak amplitude of 15 beat/minute and total duration of 15 seconds, be observed in 20 minutes of monitoring (Figure 12-11).[69] Gestational age affects reactivity criteria because sympathetic and parasympathetic influences on fetal heart rate change with advancing gestational age. Increased frequency and amplitude of fetal heart rate accelerations are seen after 30 weeks of gestation compared with early third trimester; although half of normal fetuses demonstrate accelerations with fetal movements at 24 weeks, nearly all fetuses will do so after 30 weeks. Similarly, before 30 to 32 weeks' gestation, acceptable criteria for a reactive fetal heart rate tracing include accelerations with a peak of only 10 beats/minute

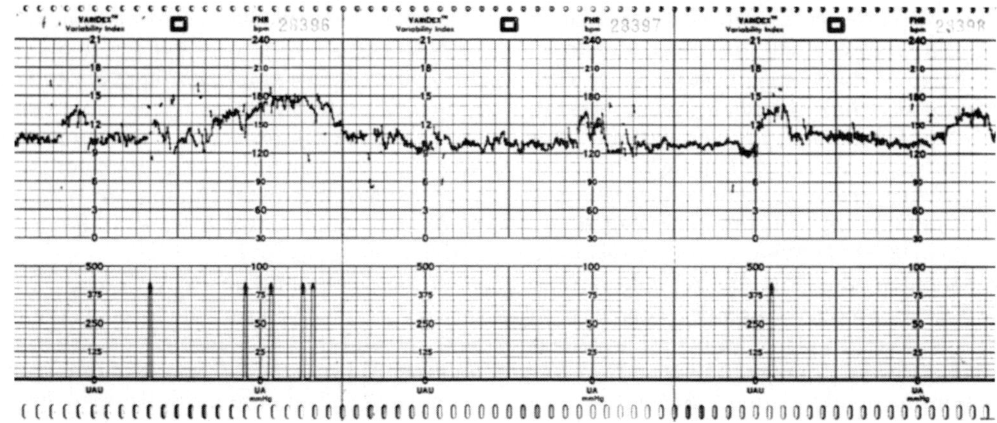

FIGURE 12-11. A reactive NST. Accelerations of the fetal heart that are greater than 15 beats/minute and last longer than 15 seconds can be identified. When the patient appreciates a fetal movement, she presses an event marker on the monitor, creating the *arrows* on the lower portion of the tracing.

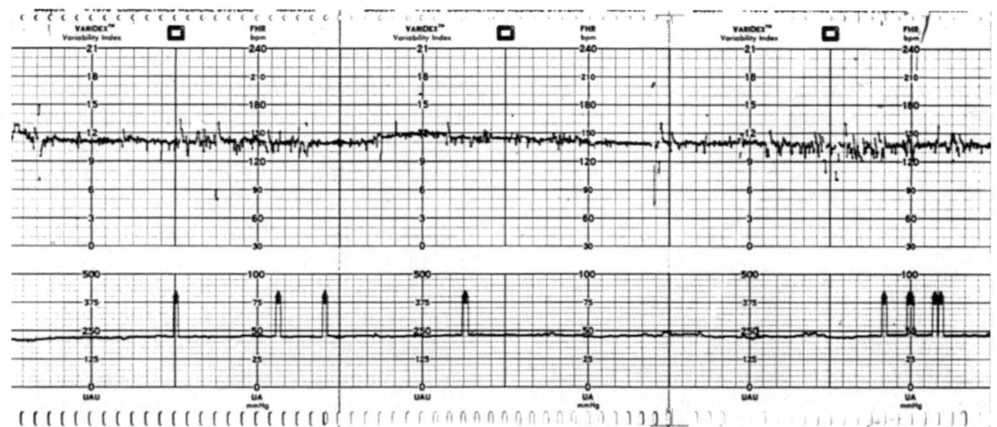

FIGURE 12-12. An NST. No accelerations of the fetal heart rate are observed. The patient has perceived fetal activity as indicated by the *arrows* in the lower portion of the tracing.

amplitude and 10 seconds' duration rather than the 15 and 15 mentioned previously.[69]

NONREACTIVE

If the criteria for reactivity are not met, the test is considered nonreactive (Figure 12-12). The most common cause for a nonreactive test is a period of fetal inactivity or quiet sleep. Therefore, the test may be extended for an additional 20 minutes with the expectation that fetal state will change and reactivity will appear. Keegan and colleagues[70] noted that about 80% of tests that were nonreactive in the morning became reactive when repeated later the same day. In an effort to change fetal state, some clinicians have manually stimulated the fetus or attempted to increase fetal glucose levels by giving the mother orange juice. There is no evidence that such efforts will increase fetal activity.[71,72] If the test has been extended for 40 minutes, and reactivity has not been seen, a BPP or CST should be performed. Of those fetuses that exhibit a nonreactive NST, about 25% will a positive CST on further evaluation.[73-75] Reactivity that occurs during preparations for the CST has proved to be a reliable index of fetal well-being.

Overall, on initial testing, 85% of NSTs are reactive, and 15% are nonreactive (Figure 12-13).[73] Fewer than 1% of NSTs prove unsatisfactory because of inadequately recorded fetal heart rate data.

The likelihood of a nonreactive test is substantially increased early in the third trimester. Between 24 and 28 weeks' gestation, about 50% of NSTs are nonreactive. Fifteen percent of NSTs remain nonreactive between 28 and 32 weeks.[76] After 32 weeks, the incidences of reactive and nonreactive tests is comparable to that seen at term. **In summary, when accelerations of the baseline heart rate are seen during monitoring in the late second and early third trimesters, the NST has been associated with fetal well-being.**

When nonreactive, the NST is extended in an attempt to separate the fetus in a period of prolonged quiet sleep from those who are hypoxemic or asphyxiated. Most fetuses exhibiting a nonreactive NST are not compromised but simply fail to exhibit heart rate reactivity during the 40-minute period of testing. Malformed fetuses also exhibit a significantly higher incidence of nonreactive NSTs.[77] Vibroacoustic stimulation (VAS) may be used to change fetal state from quiet to active sleep (Figure 12-14).

Auditory brainstem response appears to be functional in the fetus at 26 to 28 weeks' gestation. Thus, VAS may significantly increase the incidence of reactive NSTs after 26 weeks' gestation and reduce the testing time, making this a potentially useful adjunct to antepartum fetal testing.[76,78] Most studies of VAS have employed an electronic artificial larynx that generates sound pressure levels measured at 1 m in air of 82 dB with a frequency of 80 Hz and a harmonic of 20 to 9000 Hz. Whether it is the acoustic or vibratory component of this stimulus that alters fetal state is unclear. VAS may produce a significant increase in the mean duration and amplitude of heart rate accelerations, fetal heart rate variability, and gross fetal body movements, within 3 minutes of stimulation.[79] Several studies using VAS have shown a decreased incidence of nonreactive NSTs from 13% to 14% down to 6% to 9%. A reactive NST after VAS stimulation appears to be as reliable an index of fetal well-being as spontaneous reactivity. However, those fetuses that remain nonreactive even after VAS may be at increased risk for poor perinatal outcome with increased rates of intrapartum fetal distress, growth restriction, and low Apgar scores in fetuses that are nonreactive after acoustic stimulation.

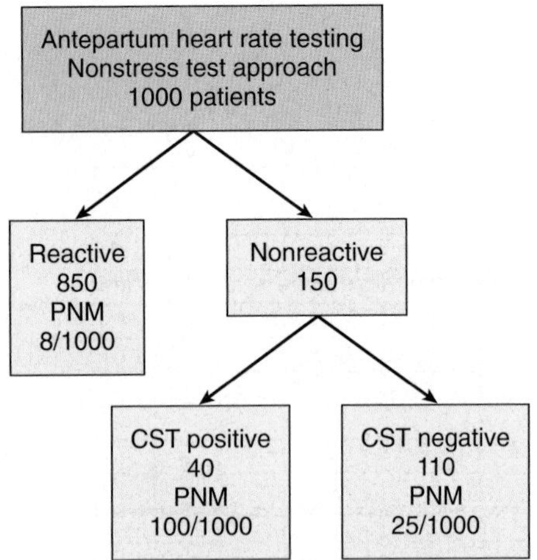

FIGURE 12-13. Results of NST in 1000 high-risk patients. In general, 85% of the NSTs are reactive, and 15% are nonreactive. Of those patients with a nonreactive NST, about 25% have a positive CST on further evaluation. The highest perinatal mortality (PNM) is observed in patients with a nonreactive NST and positive CST. Patients with a nonreactive NST and negative CST have a perinatal mortality rate higher than that found in patients whose NST is initially reactive. (PNM rates based on data from Evertson L, Gauthier R, Schifrin B, et al: Antepartum fetal heart rate testing. I. Evolution of the nonstress test. Am J Obstet Gynecol 133:29, 1979.)

In most centers that use VAS, the baseline fetal heart rate is first observed for 5 minutes. If the pattern is nonreactive, a stimulus of 3 seconds or less is applied near the fetal head. If the NST remains nonreactive, the stimulus is repeated at 1-minute intervals up to three times. If there continues to be no response to VAS, further evaluation should be carried out with a BPP or CST. **In summary, VAS may be helpful in shortening the time required to perform an NST and may be especially useful in centers where large numbers of NSTs are done.**

Could the sound generated by an electronic artificial larynx damage the fetal ear? Using intrauterine microphones, Smith and colleagues[80] documented baseline intrauterine sound levels of up to 88 dB during labor. Transabdominal stimulation with an electronic artificial larynx increased these levels minimally, up to 91 to 111 dB. Sound vibrations and intensity are attenuated by amniotic fluid.[81] Therefore, a 90-dB sound pressure produced by VAS in air results in exposure of the fetal ear to the equivalent of 40 dB, the level of normal conversation at about 3 feet. Arulkumaran and associates[81] concluded that intrauterine sound levels from VAS were not hazardous to the fetal ear. Studies have confirmed the safety of VAS use during pregnancy, with no long-term evidence of hearing loss in children followed in the neonatal period and up to 4 years of age.[82]

Other Nonstress Test Patterns or Findings

SINUSOIDAL

On rare occasions, a sinusoidal heart rate pattern may be observed, as described in Chapter 16. This undulating heart rate pattern with virtually absent variability has been

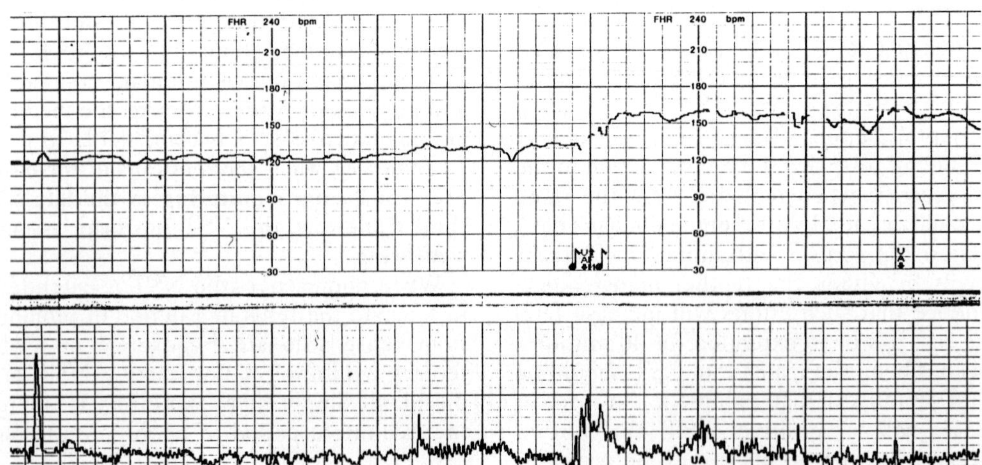

FIGURE 12-14. Reactive NST after VAS. The stimulus was applied in panel 54042, at the point marked by the musical notes. A sustained fetal heart rate acceleration was produced.

associated with fetal anemia, fetal asphyxia, congenital malformations, and medications such as narcotics. In one of the earliest reports on the use of the NST, Rochard and coworkers[83] described a sinusoidal pattern in 20 of 50 pregnancies complicated by Rh isoimmunization. One half of these pregnancies ended in a perinatal death, and 40% of the surviving infants required prolonged hospitalization. Only 10% of the babies with a sinusoidal pattern had an uncomplicated course.

Bradycardia

Before 27 weeks' gestation, the normal fetal heart rate response to fetal movement may in fact be a bradycardia. However, in some settings such as IUGR associated with antiphospholipid syndrome, bradycardia at a gestational age of 26 to 28 weeks may be a predictor of fetal compromise and impending fetal death. Druzin and associates[84] reported three cases in which antenatal steroid administration and elective premature delivery led to good perinatal outcome. In these challenging cases, the entire clinical situation needs to be evaluated, and a full discussion with the patient, including neonatal consultation, should be initiated before intervention and delivery of the very preterm fetus exhibiting fetal heart rate decelerations.

Significant fetal heart rate bradycardias have been observed in 1% to 2% of all NSTs, defined as a fetal heart rate of 90 beats/minute or a fall in the fetal heart rate of 40 beats/minute below the baseline for 1 minute or longer (Figure 12-15). In a review of 121 cases, bradycardia was associated with increased perinatal morbidity and mortality, particularly antepartum fetal death, cord compression, IUGR, and fetal malformations.[85] Although about one half of the NSTs associated with bradycardia were reactive, the incidence of a nonreassuring fetal heart rate pattern in labor leading to emergency delivery in this group was identical to that of patients exhibiting nonreactive NSTs. Clinical management decisions should be based on the finding of bradycardia, *not* on the presence or absence of reactivity. Bradycardia has a higher positive predictive value for fetal compromise (fetal death or fetal intolerance of labor) than does the nonreactive NST. In this setting, antepartum fetal death is most likely due to a cord accident.

If a bradycardia is observed, an ultrasound examination should be performed to assess amniotic fluid volume and to detect the presence of anomalies such as renal agenesis. Expectant management in the setting of a bradycardia has been associated with a PMR of 25%. Therefore, several reports have recommended that delivery be undertaken if the fetus is mature. When the fetus is premature, one might elect to administer corticosteroids to accelerate fetal lung maturation before delivery. Continuous fetal heart rate monitoring is necessary if expectant management is followed.

Tachycardia

Fetal heart rate baseline evaluation must also take gestational age into account, as with fetal heart rate reactivity. Vagal activity has a greater influence on fetal heart rate at baseline as gestation advances; thus, baseline fetal heart rate will decrease from an average of 155 beats/minute at 20 weeks to 145 beats/minute at 30 weeks. The most common etiology of fetal tachycardia is maternal-fetal fever, secondary to maternal-fetal infection such as chorioamnionitis. Other causes include chronic hypoxemia, maternal hyperthyroidism, and fetal tachyarrhythmia. Fetal heart rates above 200 beats/minute, and certainly above 220 beats/minute, should increase the index of suspicion of fetal tachyarrhythmia and lead to further fetal cardiac evaluation with a targeted fetal echocardiogram. For fetal heart rates between 160 and 180 beats/minute, the presence or absence of baseline variability is an important indicator of fetal acid-base status. Fetal acidosis is more likely if baseline variability is absent.[69]

Arrhythmia

Among fetal arrhythmias, most (about 90%) are tachyarrhythmias. Fetal tachyarrhythmia is most often diagnosed when the fetal ventricular heart rate is faster than 180 beats/minute. Common causes of fetal tachyarrhythmias are paroxysmal supraventricular tachycardia and atrial flutter. The administration of antiarrhythmic therapy to the pregnant mothers of fetuses with sustained supraventricular tachycardia represented the first examples of successful prenatal cardiac therapy. Multiple publications

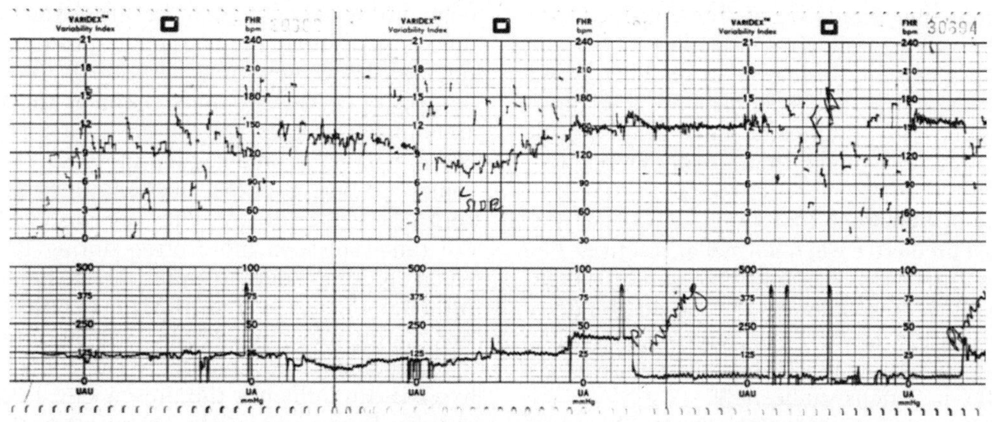

FIGURE 12-15. An NST in this primigravid patient of 43 weeks' gestation reveals a spontaneous bradycardia (panel 30692). The fetal heart rate has fallen from a baseline of 150 to 100 beats/minute. Upon induction of labor, the patient required cesarean delivery for fetal distress associated with severe variable decelerations. The amniotic fluid was decreased in amount and was meconium stained.

described treatment protocols for this arrhythmia. Characteristics of fetuses needing treatment include hydrops fetalis in the face of a sustained arrhythmia and a gestational age too early to preclude safe delivery and postnatal treatment. In such cases, therapy is best initiated with medications that have a relatively broad therapeutic margin and a low risk for proarrhythmia (unwanted precipitation or exacerbation of the arrhythmia) for fetus or mother.[86,87] Digoxin is the most commonly used first-line agent but is rarely effective in the presence of fetal hydrops, for which sotalol or flecainide are typical first-line choices.[88]

Fetal bradyarrhythmia is diagnosed when the fetal ventricular heart rate is slower than 100 beats/minute, mainly due to atrioventricular block. About half of all cases are caused by fetal cardiac anomalies, and of the remaining cases with normal cardiac structure, many are related to maternal antibodies. These antibodies, which include SS-A and SS-B, may directly target the fetal atrioventricular node or the myocardium, resulting in heart block and myocarditis. Fetuses with bradyarrhythmia may develop hydrops fetalis, particularly with sustained bradycardia at a rate less than 55 beats/minute. In utero heart failure with congenital heart block, with or without congenital heart disease, represents an absolute indication for electrical pacemaker therapy in surviving neonates.[87] This condition is less often successfully treated antenatally than fetal tachyarrhythmia. Available therapies include maternal administration of β-agonists, which have been shown to increase fetal ventricular rate by 10% to 20%, and steroid or immunoglobulin administration, which may be effective in cases of fetal heart block caused by maternal antibodies. Potential improved fetal outcome includes reversal of hydrops in several reports.[88]

Deceleration

In most cases, mild variable decelerations are not associated with poor perinatal outcome. Meis and associates[89] reported that variable decelerations of 20 beats/minute or more below the baseline heart rate but lasting less than 10 seconds were noted in 50.7% of patients undergoing an NST. Whereas these decelerations were more often associated with a nuchal cord, they were not predictive of IUGR or a nonreassuring fetal heart rate pattern, or more severe variable decelerations during labor. When mild variable decelerations are observed, even if the NST is reactive, an ultrasound examination should be performed to rule out oligohydramnios. A low amniotic fluid index (AFI) and mild variable decelerations increase the likelihood of a cord accident. If late decelerations in response to contractions are observed in the performance of an NST, criteria for interpretation of CST should then be implemented.

Predictive Value of Nonstress Test

The NST is most predictive when normal or reactive. The reported false-negative rate over multiple studies ranges from 0.2% to 0.8%, corresponding to a fetal death rate of 3 to 8 per 1000 within 1 week of a reactive NST. The false-positive rate is considerably higher, ranging from 50% to more than 90% in various studies.[2,23]

A 2010 Cochrane review integrated the results of six randomized controlled trials including 2105 women; four studies with 1636 women compared NST (or NST with results revealed) to no NST (or NST with results concealed), and two studies with 469 women compared NST with computerized analysis to traditional (visually analyzed) NST.[64] The six included studies only recruited high-risk women, and none provided information about singleton and multiple pregnancies. Of note, all four of the studies comparing NST with no NST were performed in the 1980s. In the studies comparing NST with no NST, there were no significant differences identified in the risk for perinatal mortality (risk ratio [RR], 2.05; 95% CI, 0.95 to 4.42; 2.3% versus 1.1%). There were also no differences identified in rates of cesarean delivery, "potentially preventable perinatal mortality," Apgar scores, neonatal intensive care admissions, gestational age at birth, or neonatal seizures. However, in the two studies comparing computerized analysis to visual analysis, there was a significant reduction in perinatal mortality with computerized analysis (RR, 0.20; 95% CI, 0.04 to 0.88; 0.9% versus 4.2%).[64] The authors concluded that the analysis was underpowered to detect possible important differences in perinatal mortality and pointed out that many aspects of antenatal and postnatal care may have changed since the included trials were performed. They called for new studies to assess the effects of traditional and computer-analyzed NST in order to assess the true impact on perinatal mortality and other outcomes.

In selected high-risk pregnancies, the false-negative rate associated with a weekly NST may be unacceptably high, in particular those pregnancies complicated by diabetes mellitus, IUGR, and prolonged gestation. In these cases, increasing frequency of the NST to twice weekly may be considered.[90,91]

Fetal Biophysical Profile

The use of real-time ultrasonography to assess antepartum fetal condition has enabled the obstetrician to perform an in utero physical examination and evaluate dynamic functions reflecting the integrity of the fetal CNS.[92] As emphasized by Manning and colleagues,[93] "fetal biophysical scoring rests on the principle that the more complete the examination of the fetus, its activities, and its environment, the more accurate may be the differentiation of fetal health from disease states."

Fetal breathing movements (FBMs) were the first biophysical parameter to be assessed using real-time ultrasonography. It is thought that the fetus exercises its breathing muscles in utero in preparation for postdelivery respiratory function. With real-time ultrasonography, FBM is evidenced by downward movement of the diaphragm and abdominal contents and by an inward collapsing of the chest. FBMs become regular at 20 to 21 weeks and are controlled by centers on the ventral surface of the fourth ventricle of the fetus.[94] They are observed about 30% of the time, are seen more often during REM sleep, and, when present, demonstrate intact neurologic control. Although the absence of FBMs may reflect fetal asphyxia, this finding may also indicate that the fetus is in a period of quiet sleep.[43] Several factors other than fetal state and hypoxia can influence the presence of FBM. As maternal glucose levels rise, FBM becomes more frequent, and during periods of maternal hypoglycemia, FBM decreases. Maternal smoking reduces FBM, probably as a result of fetal hypoxemia.[95] Narcotics that depress the fetal CNS also decrease FBM.

Regarding other observable fetal states as markers of fetal oxygen status and well-being, Vintzileos and coworkers[94] stressed that **those fetal biophysical activities that are present earliest in fetal development are the last to disappear with fetal hypoxia.** The fetal tone center in the cortex begins to function at 7.5 to 8.5 weeks. Therefore, fetal tone would be the last fetal parameter to be lost with worsening fetal condition. The fetal movement center in the cortex-nuclei is functional at 9 weeks and would be more sensitive than fetal tone. As noted earlier, FBM becomes regular at 20 to 21 weeks. Finally, fetal heart rate control, residing within the posterior hypothalamus and medulla, becomes functional at the end of the second trimester and early in the third trimester. An alteration in fetal heart rate would theoretically be the earliest sign of fetal compromise.

Using these principles, Manning and colleagues[96] developed the concept of the fetal BPP score. These workers elected to combine the NST with four parameters that could be assessed using real-time ultrasonography: FBM, fetal movement, fetal tone, and AFV. FBM, fetal movement, and fetal tone are mediated by complex neurologic pathways and should reflect the function of the fetal CNS at the time of the examination. On the other hand, AFV should provide information about the presence of chronic fetal asphyxia. Finally, the ultrasound examination performed for the BPP has the added advantage of detecting previously unrecognized major fetal anomalies. A BPP score was developed that is similar to the Apgar score used to assess the condition of the newborn.[96] The presence of a normal parameter, such as a reactive NST, was awarded 2 points, whereas the absence of that parameter was scored as 0. The highest score a fetus can receive is 10, and the lowest score is 0. The BPP may be used as early as 26 to 28 weeks' gestation. The time required for the fetus to achieve a satisfactory BPP score is closely related to fetal state, with an average of only 5 minutes if the fetus is in a 2F state but over 25 minutes if it is in a 1F state.[97]

The criteria proposed by Manning and colleagues,[96] and the clinical actions recommended in response to these scores, are presented in Tables 12-4 and 12-5. Regardless of a low score on the BPP, Manning and colleagues have emphasized that vaginal delivery is attempted if other obstetrical factors are favorable.

In a prospective blinded study of 216 high-risk patients, Manning and colleagues[96] found no perinatal deaths when all five variables described earlier were normal, but a PMR of 60% in fetuses with a score of zero. Fetal deaths were increased 14-fold with the absence of fetal movement, and the PMR was increased 18-fold if FBM was absent. Any single test was associated with a significant false-positive rate ranging from 50% to 79%. However, combining abnormal variables significantly decreased the false-positive rate to as low as 20%. The false-negative rate, that is, the incidence of babies who were compromised but who had normal testing, was low, ranging from a PMR of 6.9 per

TABLE 12-4 TECHNIQUE OF BIOPHYSICAL PROFILE SCORING

BIOPHYSICAL VARIABLE (SCORE = 0)	NORMAL (SCORE = 2)	ABNORMAL
Fetal breathing movements	At least one episode of ≥30 sec duration in 30-min observation	Absent or no episode of ≥30 sec duration in 30 min
Gross body/limb movement	At least three discrete body/limb movements in 30 min (episodes of active continuous movement considered a single movement)	Up to two episodes of movements in 30 min
Fetal tone	At least one episode of active extension with return to flexion of fetal limb or trunk; opening and closing of hand considered normal tone	Either slow extension with return to partial flexion, or movement of limb in full extension, or absent fetal movement
Reactive fetal heart rate	At least two episodes of acceleration of ≥15 beats/min and 15 sec duration associated with fetal movement in 20 min*	Fewer than two accelerations or acceleration <15 beats/min in 20 min
Amniotic fluid volume	At least one pocket of amniotic fluid measuring ≥2 cm in two perpendicular planes	Either no amniotic fluid pockets or a pocket <2 cm in two perpendicular planes

Modified from Manning FA: Biophysical profile scoring. *In* Nijhuis J (ed): Fetal Behaviour. New York, Oxford University Press, 1992, p 241.
*For gestational age >30 weeks.

TABLE 12-5 MANAGEMENT BASED ON BIOPHYSICAL PROFILE

SCORE	INTERPRETATION	MANAGEMENT
10	Normal; low risk for chronic asphyxia	Repeat testing at weekly to twice-weekly intervals
8	Normal; low risk for chronic asphyxia	Repeat testing at weekly to twice-weekly intervals
6	Suspect chronic asphyxia	If ≥36-37 wk gestation or <36 wk with positive testing for fetal pulmonary maturity, consider delivery; if <36 wk and/or fetal pulmonary maturity testing negative, repeat biophysical profile in 4 to 6 hr; deliver if oligohydramnios is present
4	Suspect chronic asphyxia	If ≥36 wk gestation, deliver; if <32 wk gestation, repeat score
0-2	Strongly suspect chronic asphyxia	Extend testing time to 120 min; if persistent score ≤4, deliver, regardless of gestational age

Modified from Manning FA, Harman CR, Morrison I, et al: Fetal assessment based on fetal biophysical profile scoring. Am J Obstet Gynecol 162:703, 1990; and Manning FA: Biophysical profile scoring. *In* Nijhuis J (ed): Fetal Behaviour. New York, Oxford University Press, 1992, p 241.

1000 for infants with normal amniotic fluid volume to 12.8 per 1000 for fetuses demonstrating a reactive NST. These investigators found that, in most cases, the ultrasound-derived BPP parameters and NST could be completed within a relatively short time, each requiring about 10 minutes.

Manning and colleagues presented their experience with 26,780 high-risk pregnancies followed with the BPP. In their protocol, a routine NST is not performed if all of the ultrasound parameters are found to be normal for a score of 8.[98] An NST is performed when one ultrasound finding is abnormal. The corrected PMR in this series was 1.9 per 1000, with fewer than 1 fetal death per 1000 patients within 1 week of a normal profile. Of all patients tested, almost 97% had a score of 8, which means that only 3% required further evaluation for scores of 6 or less. In a study of 525 patients with scores of 6 or less, poor perinatal outcome was most often associated with either a nonreactive NST and absent fetal tone or a nonreactive NST and absent FBM.[99] A significant inverse linear relationship was observed between the last BPP score and both perinatal morbidity and mortality (Figures 12-16 and 12-17).[100] The false-positive rate, depending on the end point used, ranges from 75% for a score of 6 to less than 20% for a score of 0. Manning has summarized the data reported in eight investigations using the BPP for fetal evaluation. Overall, 23,780 patients and 54,337 tests were reviewed. The corrected PMR, excluding lethal anomalies, was 0.77 per 1,000.

The BPP correlates well with fetal acid-base status. Vintzileos and associates[94] studied 124 patients undergoing cesarean birth *before* the onset of labor. Deliveries were undertaken for severe preeclampsia, elective repeat cesarean delivery, growth restriction, breech presentation, placenta previa, and fetal macrosomia. Acidosis was defined as an umbilical cord arterial pH less than 7.20. The earliest manifestations of fetal acidosis were a nonreactive NST and loss of FBM. With scores of 8 or more, the mean arterial pH was 7.28, and only 2 of 102 fetuses were acidotic. Nine fetuses with scores of 4 or less had a mean pH of 6.99, and all were acidotic.

Some studies have demonstrated that antenatal corticosteroid administration may have an effect on the BPP, decreasing the profile score. Because corticosteroids are used in cases of anticipated premature delivery (24 to 34

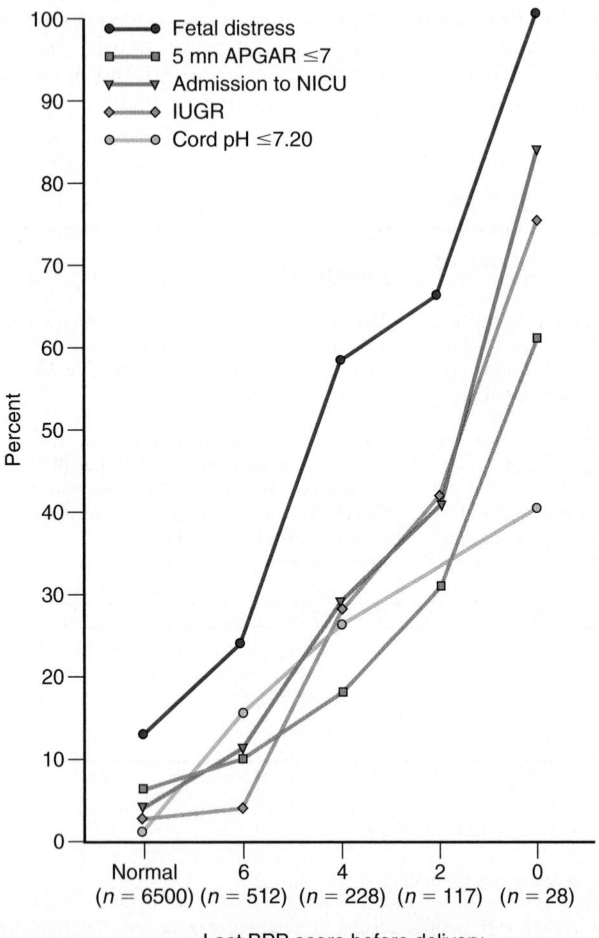

FIGURE 12-16. The relationship between five indices of perinatal morbidity and last BPP score before delivery. A significant inverse linear correlation is observed for each variable. (From Manning FA, Harman CR, Morrison I, et al: Fetal assessment based on fetal biophysical profile scoring. Am J Obstet Gynecol 162:703, 1990.)

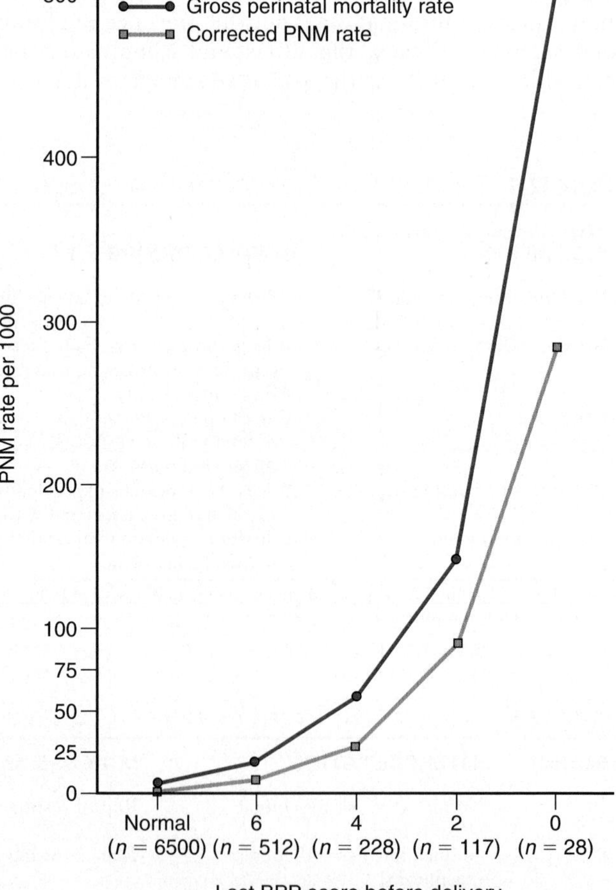

FIGURE 12-17. The relationship between perinatal mortality, both total and corrected for major anomalies, and the last BPP score before delivery. A highly significant inverse and exponential relationship is observed. (From Manning FA, Harman CR, Morrison I, et al: Fetal assessment based on fetal biophysical profile scoring. Am J Obstet Gynecol 162:703, 1990.)

weeks), any false-positive results on biophysical testing may lead to inappropriate intervention and delivery. Kelly and coworkers reported that BPP scores were decreased in more than one third of the fetuses tested at 28 to 34 weeks' gestation. This effect was seen within 48 hours of corticosteroid administration. Neonatal outcome was not affected. Repeat BPPs within 24 to 48 hours were normal in cases in which the BPP score had decreased by 4 points. The most commonly affected variables were FBM and the NST. Other investigators have reported transient suppression of FBM and heart rate reactivity after corticosteroid administration at less than 34 weeks' gestation, with return of these parameters to normal by 48 to 96 hours after corticosteroid treatment. This effect must be considered at institutions where daily BPPs are used to evaluate the fetus in cases of preterm labor or preterm premature rupture of the membranes.

There has been some controversy concerning the utility of the BPP in predicting chorioamnionitis in pregnancies complicated by preterm labor or preterm premature rupture of the membranes. Sherer and colleagues reported that the absence of FBM is associated with histologic evidence of fetal inflammation and intrauterine infection in patients with preterm labor and intact membranes before 32 weeks' gestation. However, they recommend that this finding not be used to guide clinical management because of the low positive predictive value of absent FBM. Lewis and associates performed a randomized trial of daily NSTs versus BPP in the management of preterm premature rupture of the membranes. They concluded that neither daily NSTs nor BPPs had high sensitivity in predicting infectious complications in these patients. Daily BPPs increased cost without apparent benefit.

Manning and colleagues have described the correlation between biophysical scoring and the incidence of cerebral palsy in Manitoba. In patients referred for a BPP, there was an inverse, exponential, and highly significant relationship between last BPP score and the incidence of cerebral palsy. Scores of 6 or less had a sensitivity of 49%. The more abnormal the last BPP, the greater the risk for cerebral palsy. Gestational age, birthweight, or assumed timing of the injury were not related to the incidence of cerebral palsy. The incidence of cerebral palsy ranged from 0.7 per 1000 live births, for a normal BPP score; to 13.1 per 1000 live births, for a score of 6; and 333 per 1000 live births, for a score of 0.

Is an NST needed if all ultrasound parameters of the BPP are normal? Prospective and blinded studies by and Manning and others using both the BPP and NST have demonstrated that each of these tests is a valuable predictor of normal outcome. In the experience of Manning and colleagues, an NST was needed in less than 5% of tests. As emphasized by Eden and associates, however, the NST allows the detection of fetal heart rate decelerations. In the presence of reduced amniotic fluid, these decelerations may be associated with a cord accident. Eden and associates reported that when spontaneous fetal heart rate decelerations lasting at least 30 seconds with a decrease of at least 15 beats/minute are seen in the presence of normal amniotic fluid, there is an increased likelihood of late decelerations in labor and cesarean delivery for fetal distress.

Several drawbacks of the BPP should be considered. Unlike the NST and CST, an ultrasound machine is required, and unless the BPP is videotaped, it cannot be reviewed. If the fetus is in a quiet sleep state, the BPP can require a long period of observation. The present scoring system does not consider the impact of hydramnios. In a pregnancy complicated by diabetes mellitus, the presence of excessive amniotic fluid is of great concern.

Predictive Value of Biophysical Profile

To summarize the results of multiple studies, the false-negative rate of a normal BPP is less than 0.1%, or fewer than 1 fetal death per 1000 within 1 week of a normal BPP.[2]

The false-positive rate of a particular test has always been of concern because of the possibility of unnecessary intervention (usually delivery) and subsequent iatrogenic complications. The BPP was developed in part to address the issue of the high false-positive rate of the CST and the NST. There has been little attention paid to the possible false-positive rate of the abnormal or equivocal BPP. This is particularly relevant because the BPP is most commonly used as the final backup test in the NST and CST sequence of testing and is critically important when dealing with the premature fetus. As noted earlier, the false-positive rate of a score of 0 is less than 20%, but for a score of 6, it is up to 75%. Inglis and coworkers used VAS to define fetal condition with BPP scores of 6 or less in 81 patients at 28 to 42 weeks. Obstetrical and neonatal outcomes of 41 patients whose score improved to normal after VAS were compared with those of 238 patients who had normal scores without VAS. The obstetrical and neonatal outcomes were not significantly different between the two groups. VAS improved the BPP in about 80% of cases. Use of VAS for an equivocal BPP did not increase the false-negative rate and may reduce the likelihood of unnecessary obstetrical intervention.

A 2008 Cochrane review included evaluation of 2829 women randomized to BPP versus NST. The majority were term pregnancies. No differences were found in perinatal mortality, cesarean delivery rate, Apgar scores, or admission to the neonatal intensive care unit. As with the 2010 Cochrane review of NST, mentioned earlier, this analysis was underpowered to detect a significant difference in perinatal mortality between BPP and other modalities. The authors also note that, "It is regrettable that since the introduction of the BPP in the 1980s, and following reports of observational studies of tens of thousands of pregnancies, less than 3000 women have been enrolled into randomised trials."

Modified Biophysical Profile

A variety of modifications of the full BPP have been evaluated, in an attempt to simplify and reduce the time necessary to complete testing, by focusing on the components of the BPP that are most predictive of perinatal outcome. The NST, an indicator of present fetal condition, may be combined with the AFI (see Chapter 33), a marker of long-term status, in a modified BPP (mBPP). In this setting, an AFI greater than 5 cm is usually considered normal, although different criteria have been applied. VAS may be used to shorten the time required to achieve a reactive NST. **Multiple investigators**, including a trial by

Miller of 56,617 antepartum tests in 15,482 women, **have demonstrated comparable results of the mBPP to the full BPP, namely a false-negative rate (or rate of fetal death within 1 week of a normal mBPP) of 0.8 per 1000.** Nageotte and associates demonstrated that the mBPP was as good a predictor of adverse fetal outcome as a negative CST. Additional evaluation for abnormal mBPP is required in about 10% of patients. If the NST is nonreactive despite VAS or extended monitoring, or if the AFI is abnormal, either a full BPP or CST is performed. The CST as a backup test is associated with a higher rate of intervention for an abnormal test than the use of a complete BPP as a backup test. Overall, the modified BPP has a false-positive rate comparable to the NST but higher than the CST and full BPP. The low false-negative rate and ease of performance of the modified BPP make it an excellent approach for the evaluation of large numbers of high-risk patients. As such, although potentially still a useful test, the CST has becoming less frequently used in current practice.

Whether to use a full AFI for AFV assessment, or an abbreviated measure, the single deepest vertical pocket (DVP), has been under investigation. Trends have varied over time, without substantial evidence to reliably link either method to perinatal outcomes. Chauhan and colleagues performed a randomized trial of more than 1000 women and found that the AFI led to more diagnoses of oligohydramnios and a higher rate of intervention, including iatrogenic prematurity, but offered no advantage in detecting or preventing adverse outcomes. Similarly, a 2009 Cochrane review of five trials including more than 3200 women concluded that there were no differences in perinatal outcomes. However, the use of AFI did result in increased rate of diagnosis of oligohydramnios and rate of induction of labor compared with DVP. This review could not comment on the relative ability of AFI compared with DVP for prevention of perinatal death because there were no deaths reported in the included trials. Clearly, further study of these modalities is warranted with regard to their utility in preventing perinatal mortality.

Doppler Ultrasound

The advent of Doppler ultrasound has permitted noninvasive assessment of the fetal, maternal, and placental circulations. With Doppler ultrasound, we can obtain information about uteroplacental blood flow and resistance, which may be markers of fetal adaptation and reserve. This method of fetal assessment has only been demonstrated to be of value in reducing perinatal mortality and unnecessary obstetrical interventions in fetuses with suspected IUGR and possibly other disorders of uteroplacental blood flow.[2] A detailed description of the underlying principles and use of Doppler ultrasound for fetal assessment is available in Chapter 31 on IUGR. For the purposes of this chapter on antenatal fetal assessment, Doppler interrogation of fetal vascular flow and resistance can be conceptualized as a follow-up test to determine fetal reserve in cases of suspected IUGR, and not as a primary method of antenatal fetal surveillance for either high-risk or low-risk pregnancies.

Perhaps ironically, however, Doppler ultrasound has been more stringently evaluated in randomized trials than other antenatal testing methods, as has been summarized in an editorial by Divon and Ferber. The most recent summary of the available evidence comes from a 2010 Cochrane review of 18 randomized trials including more than 10,000 high-risk women, in which the use of Doppler ultrasound was associated with decreased perinatal deaths (RR, 0.71; 95% CI, 0.52 to 0.98) as well as significantly fewer inductions of labor and cesarean deliveries. Studies of low-risk pregnancies have not shown a benefit from the use of Doppler ultrasound, as has been most recently described in a 2010 systematic review of five studies including more than 14,000 women.

CLINICAL APPLICATION OF TESTS OF FETAL WELL-BEING

Our ability to detect and prevent impending fetal death or injury depends not only on the predictive value of the tests employed and the population selected for testing, but also on our ability to respond to abnormal test results. In order to have an impact on testing outcomes and the overall fetal death rate, we must consider available strategies to deal with abnormal test results. These strategies would ideally include a series of antenatal evaluations and interventions short of premature delivery, with premature delivery ultimately reserved for cases when it is ascertained that intrauterine injury or death can no longer be delayed or prevented. Figure 12-18 presents a practical testing scheme that has been used successfully by several centers.[92] This strategy would include using combinations of antepartum tests in an organized sequence to evaluate the fetus further; administration of antenatal steroids; potentially modified maternal activity level; and correction of maternal metabolic, cardiopulmonary, or other medical disorders. In some cases, fetal therapy may be indicated, such as intrauterine transfusion for anemia, removal of fluid from body cavities, diagnostic procedures, and direct administration of medication to the fetus.

Testing can be initiated at early gestational ages in high-risk pregnancies (25 to 26 weeks) to identify the fetus at risk. Maternal and fetal interventions can then be considered. Obviously, safe prolongation of intrauterine life is the primary goal, and better understanding of the pathophysiology of the premature fetus and the use of combinations of tests will allow this to be accomplished.

The question of routine antepartum fetal surveillance must be carefully examined. Antepartum fetal testing can more accurately predict fetal outcome than antenatal risk assessment using an established scoring system. Patients judged to be at high risk based on known medical factors but whose fetuses demonstrated normal antepartum fetal evaluation had a lower PMR than did patients considered at low risk, whose fetuses had abnormal antepartum testing results. Routine antepartum fetal evaluation would be necessary to detect the considerable proportion of fetuses destined for fetal death or injury with no identifiable risk factors. It would seem reasonable, therefore, to consider extending some form of antepartum fetal surveillance to all obstetrical patients, such as maternal assessment of fetal activity as described previously.

How, therefore, to combine antenatal tests in clinical practice, and in which patients? **The approach to**

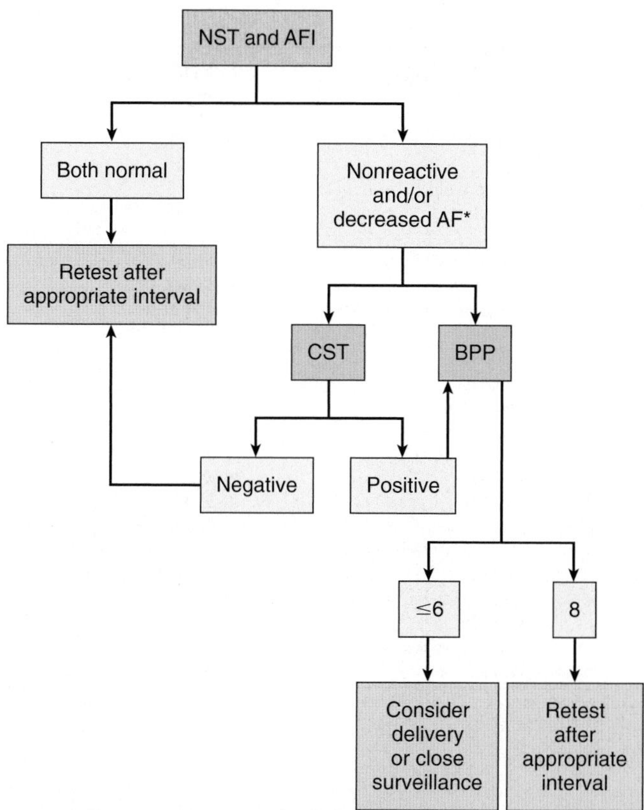

Figure 12-18. Flow chart for antepartum fetal surveillance in which the NST and AFI are used as the primary methods for fetal evaluation. A nonreactive NST and decreased AFI are further evaluated using either the CST or the BPP. Further details regarding the use of the BPP are provided in Table 12-6.
*If the fetus is mature and amniotic fluid volume is reduced, delivery should be considered before further testing is undertaken. (Modified from Finberg HJ, Kurtz AB, Johnson RL, et al: The biophysical profile: a literature review and reassessment of its usefulness in the evaluation of fetal well-being. J Ultrasound Med 9:583, 1990.)

prescribing testing modalities must take into account gestational age, medical comorbidities, and sociodemographic risk factors described in this chapter, in order to prevent fetal injury or death without causing iatrogenic prematurity or an excess of testing and worry. According to a summary by Fretts and Duru in 2008, "The best opportunity for stillbirth reduction is to identify patients who have an increased risk of stillbirth, late in pregnancy, where the downside of antepartum testing and early delivery, if warranted, can be minimized."[20]

The condition-specific use of antenatal testing may be illustrated by the following examples. In a prolonged pregnancy, one would use a parallel testing scheme. In this situation, the obstetrician is not concerned with fetal maturity but rather with fetal well-being. Several tests are performed at the same time, such as antepartum fetal heart rate testing and the BPP. It is acceptable in this high-risk situation to intervene when a single test is abnormal. One is willing to accept a false-positive test result to avoid the intrauterine death of a mature and otherwise healthy fetus. In most other high-risk pregnancies, such as those complicated by diabetes mellitus or hypertension, it is preferable to allow the fetus to remain in utero as long as possible. In these situations, a branched testing scheme is used. To decrease the likelihood of unnecessary premature intervention, the obstetrician uses a series of tests and, under most circumstances, would only deliver a premature infant when all parameters suggest fetal compromise. In this situation, one must consider the likelihood of neonatal respiratory distress syndrome (RDS) as predicted by the evaluation of AFIs and review these risks with colleagues in neonatology.

The comparable performance of the various available antenatal tests, along with their utility in series, has been illustrated by numerous investigators (see Table 12-2).[2] Maternal assessment of fetal activity would appear to be a reasonable first-line screening test for both high-risk and low-risk patients. The use of this approach may decrease the number of unexpected intrauterine deaths in so-called normal pregnancies. The NST and mBPP remain the primary methods used for antepartum fetal evaluation in high-risk patients at most centers, with full BPP and CST to assess fetal condition in patients exhibiting a persistently nonreactive NST or abnormal mBPP. This sequential approach may be particularly valuable in avoiding unnecessary premature intervention. The NST and mBPP can be quickly performed in an outpatient setting and are easily interpreted. In contrast, the CST is usually performed near the labor and delivery suite, may require an intravenous infusion of oxytocin, and may be more difficult to interpret. However, the ability of the CST to stress the fetus and evaluate its response to intermittent interruptions in intervillous blood flow may provide an earlier warning of fetal compromise than the NST or mBPP.

The frequency with which to employ specific tests will depend on a number of features, including the predictive value of the test and the underlying condition prompting the test. Most tests described previously have relatively reliable risk profiles over the course of a week when normal, with decreased intervals between tests recommended for abnormal results. Regarding the underlying condition contributing to risk for adverse outcomes, consideration must be given to whether that condition is stable, worsening, or improving. The gestational age at which to initiate testing has not been clearly defined for most high-risk conditions. Initiating testing at 32 to 34 weeks of gestation has historically been prescribed for most high-risk pregnancies, with earlier testing recommended for cases with multiple comorbidities or particularly worrisome features.

Signore and coworkers, on behalf of the Eunice Kennedy Shriver National Institute of Child Health and Human Development Workshop, have proposed a series of guidelines for condition-specific antenatal testing, based on the available evidence (Table 12-6).[2] In their 2009 publication, they stress that **"the basis for antepartum testing relies on the premise that the fetus whose oxygenation in utero is challenged will respond with a series of detectable physiologic adaptive or decompensatory signs as hypoxemia or frank metabolic academia develop"**—hence the recommendation for the use of antenatal tests in series to follow the changes in observable measures of fetal response to a suboptimal intrauterine environment. Although this proposed strategy is certainly not comprehensive, future

TABLE 12-6 PROPOSED INITIAL TESTING STRATEGY BY SELECTED ANTENATAL CONDITION

RISK FACTOR	TEST	FREQUENCY	START
All pregnancies	FMC	Daily	24-28 wk
Low-risk pregnancies	FMC	Daily	24-28 wk
Insulin-treated diabetes			
Uncomplicated pregestational, or A2	mBPP	Twice weekly	32 wk
with hypertension, renal disease, or IUGR	Above, plus consider CST	Weekly	26-28 wk
Hypertensive disorders			
Uncomplicated	mBPP	Twice weekly	32 wk
With comorbidities	mBPP	Twice weekly	26-28 wk
IUGR	mBPP/Doppler	Once or twice weekly	At diagnosis
Multiple gestation			
Twins			
Concordant growth	mBPP	Weekly	32 wk
Discordant growth or AFV	mBPP	Twice weekly	At diagnosis
Triplets or greater	mBPP	Twice weekly	28 wk
Oligohydramnios	mBPP	Twice weekly	At diagnosis
Intrahepatic cholestasis	mBPP	Weekly	34 wk
Renal disease	mBPP	Weekly	30-32 wk
Decreased fetal movement	mBPP	PRN	At diagnosis
Previous fetal death	mBPP Alternative: BPP or CST	Once or twice weekly Weekly	32-34 wk, or 1 wk before previous fetal death
Postterm pregnancy	mBPP	Once or twice weekly	≥41 wk
SLE	mBPP	Weekly	26 wk
Renal disease	mBPP	Once or twice weekly	30-32 wk
Intrahepatic cholestasis	mBPP	Weekly	34 wk

Modified from Signore C, Freeman RK, Spong CY: Antenatal testing: a reevaluation. Executive Summary of a Eunice Kennedy Shriver National Institute of Child Health and Human Development Workshop. Obstet Gynecol 113:687-701, 2009.

See Key Abbreviations box at beginning of chapter for definition of abbreviations used.

research into specific testing strategies stratified by risk category will hopefully enhance our ability to prescribe these tests effectively and safely.

Evidence for Condition-Specific Testing Strategies

For most of the conditions identified as constituting an increased risk for fetal death, insufficient studies exist to permit an evidence-based recommendation for a particular testing scheme. In addition to this limitation, condition-specific testing is problematic as a general strategy for prevention of fetal death, given the many fetal deaths that occur in pregnancies otherwise categorized as low risk, or without identifiable risk factors.[2] However, it is incumbent on care providers to consider all conditions associated with an increased risk for fetal death or other adverse outcomes as a potential indication for some form of antenatal surveillance[2,27] and perhaps to individualize antenatal testing plans based on specific underlying conditions. This strategy is outlined in an excellent 2004 summary by Kontopoulos and Vintzileos, in which several pathophysiologic mechanisms are explored as potentially distinct etiologies for risk of fetal death in different populations. **The authors acknowledge that there is no ideal single test or testing strategy for all high-risk pregnancies but that clinician judgement and logic, as well as evidence from observational trials, should guide testing strategies for each patient.**

Difficulty in generating evidence-based recommendations for condition-specific testing schemes in cases of identified risk factors can be illustrated by considering the example of hypertensive disorders. Well-designed prospective trials providing evidence for any specific testing strategy are not available, despite the very frequent use of a variety of antenatal testing schemes employed in clinical practice for hypertensive disorders. The heterogeneity of pathophysiologic mechanisms at play in the general category of hypertensive disorders contributes to the difficulty in generating specific recommendations. Freeman summarized the situation in a 2008 review.[30] He noted that despite previous testing guidelines recommending a more wide application of antenatal testing in women with varying degrees of hypertension, the most recent expert recommendations do not support antepartum fetal testing for mild to moderate blood pressure abnormalities and in the absence of preeclampsia or IUGR. However, for many practitioners, the evidence that all forms of chronic hypertension constitute an increased risk for fetal death and adverse outcomes prompts broad use of testing modalities for these patients.

ASSESSMENT OF FETAL PULMONARY MATURATION

This section reviews those techniques that enable the obstetrician to predict accurately the risks of RDS for the infant requiring premature delivery and to avoid the unnecessary complications of iatrogenic prematurity. It is the risk of iatrogenic prematurity for the neonate, balanced against the risk of continued antepartum assessment of the potentially compromised fetus, that determines ultimate management strategies. As such, incorporation of the discussion of assessment of fetal pulmonary maturity with that of antepartum assessment is critical.

RDS is caused by a deficiency of pulmonary surfactant, an antiatelectasis factor that is able to maintain a low stable surface tension at the air-water interface within alveoli. Surfactant decreases the pressure needed to distend the lung and prevents alveolar collapse (see Chapter 21). The type II alveolar cell is the major site of surfactant synthesis. Surfactant is packaged in lamellar bodies, discharged into the alveoli, and carried into the amniotic cavity with pulmonary fluid.

Phospholipids account for more than 80% of the surface active material within the lung, and more than 50% of this phospholipid is dipalmitoyl lecithin. The latter is a derivative of glycerol phosphate and contains two fatty acids as well as the nitrogenous base choline. Other phospholipids contained in the surfactant complex include phosphatidylglycerol (PG), phosphatidylinositol, phosphatidylserine, phosphatidylethanolamine, sphingomyelin, and lysolecithin. PG is the second most abundant lipid in surfactant and significantly improves its properties.

Important differences in neonatal adaptation, including development of RDS, have been demonstrated not only between preterm and term neonates but also with each advancing gestational week from 37 to 39 weeks. This places even more responsibility on the physician to judiciously assess indications for and timing of delivery before 39 weeks. In weighing the risks and benefits of effecting delivery as a result of antenatal testing results before 39 weeks, assessment of fetal pulmonary maturity may in some cases be indicated. At the same time, it is important to recognize that many perinatal processes contribute to the prognosis for neonatal respiratory function, including surfactant deficiency, immaturity, and intrapartum complications, which are prime factors in determining the pathogenesis of RDS and may not be predicted by fetal pulmonary maturity testing.

Tests of Fetal Pulmonary Maturity

Available methods for evaluating fetal pulmonary maturity rely generally on either presence or quantitation of components of pulmonary surfactant, or measurement of surfactant function. The former category has become the most common and reliable in current practice, although no data show that one method is preferable to the others with regard to prediction of pulmonary maturity. In general, a test that is positive for fetal pulmonary maturity will much more accurately predict the absence of RDS than a negative test will predict the presence of RDS.

With the exception of amniotic fluid specimens obtained from the vaginal pool, the evaluation of fetal pulmonary maturation requires that a sample of amniotic fluid be obtained by amniocentesis. This is generally a low-risk procedure, with few potential adverse outcomes, including unsuccessful amniocentesis (1.6% to 4.4%) and complications requiring same-day delivery (0.7% to 3.3%).

Quantitation of Pulmonary Surfactant

The lecithin-to-sphingomyelin (L/S) ratio was the first reliable assay for the assessment of fetal pulmonary maturity. The amniotic fluid concentration of lecithin increases markedly at about 35 weeks' gestation, whereas sphingomyelin levels remain stable or decrease. Thus, by comparing the ratio of these two components, rather than measuring them, variations in amniotic fluid volume will not affect the outcome of the test. Amniotic fluid sphingomyelin exceeds lecithin until 31 to 32 weeks, when the L/S ratio reaches 1. Lecithin then rises rapidly, and an L/S ratio of 2 is observed at about 35 weeks. Wide variation in the L/S ratio at each gestational age has been noted. Nevertheless, a ratio of 2 or greater has repeatedly been associated with pulmonary maturity. In more than 2100 cases, a mature L/S ratio predicted the absence of RDS in 98% of neonates. With a ratio of 1.5 to 1.9, about 50% of infants will develop RDS. Below 1.5, the risk for subsequent RDS increases to 73%. Thus, the L/S ratio, like most indices of fetal pulmonary maturation, rarely errs when predicting fetal pulmonary maturity but is frequently incorrect when predicting subsequent RDS. Many neonates with an immature L/S ratio do not develop RDS.

Several important variables must be considered in interpreting the predictive accuracy of the L/S ratio, including presence of blood or meconium. Blood has been reported both to increase and decrease the ratio, and meconium can produce falsely mature results. The presence of PG in a bloody or meconium-stained amniotic fluid sample remains a reliable indicator of pulmonary maturity. PG is not normally found in blood, and meconium generally does not interfere with the identification of PG. PG, which does not appear until 35 weeks' gestation and increases rapidly between 37 and 40 weeks, is a marker of completed pulmonary maturation. Most infants who lack PG but who have a mature L/S ratio fail to develop RDS. However, PG may provide further insurance against the onset of RDS despite intrapartum complications. A rapid immunologic semiquantitative agglutination test (AmnioStat-FLM) can be used to determine the presence of PG. This assay can detect PG at a concentration greater than 0.5 mcg/mL of amniotic fluid. The test takes 20 to 30 minutes to perform and requires only 1.5 mL of amniotic fluid.

Visual inspection of amniotic fluid can give some information about the presence of pulmonary surfactant components. During the first and second trimesters, amniotic fluid is yellow and clear. It becomes colorless in the third trimester. By 33 to 34 weeks' gestation, cloudiness and flocculation are noted, and as term approaches, vernix appears. Amniotic fluid with obvious vernix or fluid so turbid it does not permit the reading of newsprint through it will usually have a mature L/S ratio.

The TDx analyzer is an automated fluorescence polarimeter that is used to detect the ratio of surfactant to albumin in amniotic fluid. The test requires 1 mL of amniotic fluid and can be run in less than 1 hour. The surfactant-to-albumin ratio is determined with amniotic fluid albumin used as an internal reference. With the newer FLM-II test, 55 mg/g is the mature cut-off. A mature value reliably predicts the absence of RDS requiring intubation in infants of diabetic mothers. The TDx test correlates well with the L/S ratio and has few falsely mature results, making it an excellent screening test. The TDx assay proved to be reliable in predicting fetal lung maturity in vaginal pool specimens from patients with preterm premature rupture of the membranes at 30 to 36 weeks. About 50% of infants with an immature TDx result develop RDS. The test has gained wide popularity because of its ease, low cost, and reproducibility and is commonly available in practice.

Measurements of Surfactant Function

Lamellar bodies are the storage form of surfactant released by fetal type II pneumocytes into the amniotic fluid. Because they are the same size as platelets, the amniotic fluid concentration of lamellar bodies may be determined using a commercial cell counter. The test requires less than 1 mL of amniotic fluid and takes only 15 minutes to perform. A lamellar body count greater than 30,000 to 55,000/μL is highly predictive of pulmonary maturity, whereas a count below 10,000/μL suggests a significant risk for RDS. Lewis and associates have reported that a lamellar body count of less than 8000 predicted an immature L/S and PG assay in all cases, whereas a value greater than 32,000 predicted a mature L/S or PG assay in 99% of cases. The cut-off used to predict fetal pulmonary status depends on the type of cell counter used and the speed of centrifugation of the amniotic fluid specimen. Neither meconium nor lysed blood has a significant effect on the lamellar body count. The ease and relatively low cost of this test have contributed to its popularity, although poor concordance among various instruments for the assay of lamellar body counts has been noted.

The manual foam stability index (FSI) is a variation of the shake test. The kit currently available contains test wells with a predispensed volume of ethanol. The addition of 0.5 mL of amniotic fluid to each test well in the kit produces final ethanol volumes of 44% to 50%. A control well contains sufficient surfactant in 50% ethanol to produce an example of the stable foam end point. The amniotic fluid and ethanol mixture is first shaken, and the FSI value is read as the highest value well in which a ring of stable foam persists.

This test appears to be a reliable predictor of fetal lung maturity. Subsequent RDS is very unlikely with an FSI value of 47 or higher. The methodology is simple, and the test can be performed at any time of day by persons who have had only minimal instruction. The assay appears to be extremely sensitive, with a high proportion of immature results being associated with RDS, as well as moderately specific, with a high proportion of mature results predicting the absence of RDS. Contamination of the amniotic fluid specimen by blood or meconium invalidates the FSI results. The FSI can function well as a screening test, but has lost popularity in current practice to other more reliable and convenient tests.

Determination of Fetal Pulmonary Maturation in Clinical Practice

A large number of techniques are now available to assess fetal pulmonary maturation. Several rapid screening tests, including the TDx test and lamellar body count, appear to be highly reliable when mature. In an uncomplicated pregnancy, when a screening test such as the TDx demonstrates fetal pulmonary maturation, one can safely proceed with delivery. The more complicated, expensive, and timely L/S ratio may be reserved for those borderline TDx or lamellar body count results in the clinical circumstance of a fetus that may benefit from delivery if maturity is ultimately confirmed with advanced testing. This sequential approach is also extremely cost-effective. When the screening test is immature, the L/S ratio and PG assessment should be considered.

As data have been assimilated in recent years related to lung maturity assessment and its role in high-risk pregnancy management, new important paradigms are emerging. Traditionally, lung maturity tests have been interpreted in categorical fashion, usually as either "positive," indicating lung maturity and a low risk for RDS, or "negative," indicating the absence of maturity and a higher risk for RDS. However, the presence of RDS in neonates is associated with both gestational age and lung maturity assessments. As further information has been gathered, it is now possible to stratify risk for RDS based on both gestational age and lung maturity assessment. This represents a more appropriate use of the lung maturity tests. For instance, the risk for RDS given an FLM result of 30 to 40 mg/g is about 50% at 28 weeks, about 25% at 32 weeks, and only about 10% at 36 weeks. **In assessing the risk for RDS complicating subsequent delivery, results from fetal lung maturity testing are most appropriately correlated with the gestational age at the time of fluid retrieval.**

CONCLUSIONS AND FUTURE DIRECTIONS

We must be aware of our limited understanding of the pathophysiology of fetal death and injury in many occasions and attempt judicious use of antenatal testing measures with the hope of preventing some adverse outcomes and the goal of doing no harm. As Scifres and Macones state in a 2008 review of costs and benefits of antenatal testing, although we assume that by testing and intervening with delivery for abnormal test results we are contributing to a good outcome, "in the absence of data we cannot be assured that our interventions, even if they prevent stillbirth, may not involve a tradeoff between long term neurologic dysfunction and fetal death."[40] Additionally, aside from potential unknown medical sequelae of antenatal testing and interventions, monetary, time, and psychological costs must also be considered, but these are difficult to quantify in both research settings and in practice.

As clinicians aim to implement evidence-based strategies to screen for and prevent fetal injury and death, the limitations of existing research must be considered. Because it is in many ways impractical and perhaps unethical to carry out placebo-controlled trials of antenatal testing methodologies in high-risk pregnancies, we must acknowledge that this type of rigorous evidence is not likely to be imminently forthcoming.[2] Nevertheless, we propose that biologic plausibility and clinician judgment prevail over therapeutic nihilism in clinical practice, and that future research efforts embrace a creative approach to both condition-specific and apparently unpredictable fetal death and injury.

KEY POINTS

- Although the PMR has fallen steadily in the United States since 1965, the number of fetal deaths has not changed substantially in the past decade.
- Perinatal events play an important role in infant mortality and long-term disability of survivors, in addition to their contribution to fetal death.
- At least 20% of fetal deaths have no obvious fetal, placental, maternal, or obstetrical etiology, and this percentage increases with advancing gestational age.

- The prevalence of an abnormal condition (i.e., fetal death) has great impact on the predictive value of antepartum fetal tests.
- Few of the antepartum tests commonly employed in clinical practice today have been subjected to large-scale prospective and randomized evaluations that can speak to the true efficacy of testing.
- Fetal adaptation to hypoxemia is mediated by changes in heart rate and redistribution of cardiac output.
- The decrease in fetal movement with hypoxemia makes maternal assessment of fetal activity a potentially simple and widely applicable method of monitoring fetal well-being. However, prospective trials of this method for prevention of perinatal mortality have failed to conclusively show benefit.
- The CST has a low false-negative rate but a high false-positive rate and is cumbersome to perform and thus is used less frequently in common practice than other testing modalities.
- The observation that accelerations of the fetal heart rate in response to fetal activity, uterine contractions, or stimulation reflect fetal well-being is the basis for the NST.
- Use of VAS for a nonreactive NST or equivocal BPP does not increase the false-negative rate and may reduce the likelihood of unnecessary obstetrical intervention.
- The NST has a low false-negative rate, although higher than that of CST, and a high false-positive rate.
- Fetal biophysical activities can be evaluated with real-time ultrasonography by BPP, and those fetal biophysical activities that are present earliest in fetal development are the last to disappear with fetal hypoxia.
- The modified BPP performs comparably to the full BPP. Both modalities have a false-negative rate, or rate of fetal death within 1 week of a normal test, of 0.8 per 1000.
- Most amniotic fluid tests of fetal pulmonary maturation accurately predict maturity, but improved accuracy in predicting subsequent RDS is noted when the indices are correlated with gestational age.
- Condition-specific testing involves modifying the frequency, type, and initiation of antenatal tests according to maternal high-risk conditions.

REFERENCES

1. Manning FA: Antepartum fetal testing: a critical appraisal. Curr Opin Obstet Gynecol 21:348, 2009.
2. Signore C, Freeman RK, Spong CY: Antenatal testing: a reevaluation. Executive Summary of a Eunice Kennedy Shriver National Institute of Child Health and Human Development Workshop. Obstet Gynecol 113:687, 2009.
3. Reddy UM, Goldenberg R, Silver R, et al: Stillbirth classification: developing an international consensus for research. Executive Summary of a National Institute of Child Health and Human Development Workshop. Obstet Gynecol 114:901, 2009.
4. MacDorman MF, Kirmeyer S: Fetal and perinatal mortality, United States, 2005. In National Vital Statistics Reports, vol. 57, no, 8. Hyattsville, MD, National Center for Health Statistics, 2009.
5. Fretts RC: Etiology and prevention of stillbirth. Am J Obstet Gyncecol 193:1923, 2005.
6. World Health Organization: The OBSQUID Project: quality development in perinatal care, final report. Publ Eur Surv 1995.
7. American College of Obstetricians and Gynecologists: Perinatal and infant mortality statistics. Committee Opinion 167, December 1995.
8. MacDorman M, Kirmeyer S: *The challenge of fetal mortality*. In NCHS Data Brief, no. 16. Hyattsville, MD, National Center for Health Statistics, 2009.
9. MacDorman MF, Mathews TJ: Recent trends in infant mortality in the United States. In NCHS Data Brief, no. 9. Hyattsville, MD, National Center for Health Statistics, 2008.
10. Martin JA, Hsiang-Ching K, Mathews TJ, et al: Annual summary of vital statistics: 2006. Pediatrics 121:788, 2008.
11. Manning FA, Lange IR, Morrison I, Harman CR: Determination of fetal health: methods for antepartum and intrapartum fetal assessment. In Leventhal J: *Current Problems in Obstetrics and Gynecology*. Chicago, Year Book Medical Publishers, 1983.
12. Fretts RC, Boyd ME, Usher RH, Usher H: The changing pattern of fetal death, 1961-1988. Obstet Gynecol 79:35, 1992.
13. Fretts RC, Schmittdiel J, McLean FH, et al: Increased maternal age and the risk of fetal death. N Engl J Med 333:953, 1995.
14. Mersey Region Working Party on Perinatal Mortality: Perinatal health. Lancet 1:491, 1982.
15. Getahun D, Ananth CV, Kinzler WL: Risk factors for antepartum and intrapartum stillbirth: a population-based study. Am J Obstet Gynecol 196:499, 2007.
16. Grant A, Elbourne D: Fetal movement counting to assess fetal wellbeing. In Chalmers I, Enkin M, Keirse MJNC: *Effective Care in Pregnancy and Childbirth*. Oxford, Oxford University Press, 1989, p 440.
17. Kahn B, Lumey LH, Zybert PA, et al: Prospective risk of fetal death in singleton, twin, and triplet gestations: implications for practice. Obstet Gynecol 102:685, 2003.
18. Fretts RC: Stillbirth epidemiology, risk factors, and opportunities for stillbirth prevention. Clin Obstet Gynecol 53:588, 2010.
19. Chu SY, Kim SY, Lau J, et al: Maternal obesity and risk of stillbirth: a metaanalysis. Am J Obstet Gynecol 197:223, 2007.
20. Fretts RC, Duru UA: New indications for antepartum testing: making the case for antepartum surveillance or timed delivery for women of advanced maternal age. Semin Perinatol 32:312, 2008.
21. Reddy UM, Chia-Wen K, Willinger M: Maternal age and the risk of stillbirth throughout pregnancy in the United States. Am J Obstet Gynecol 195:764, 2006.
22. Salihu HS, Aliyu MH, Rouse DJ, et al: Potentially preventable excess mortality among higher-order multiples. Obstet Gynecol 102:679, 2003.
23. Devoe LD: Antenatal fetal assessment: contraction stress test, nonstress test, vibroacoustic stimulation, amniotic fluid volume, biophysical profile, and modified biophysical profile: an overview. Semin Perinatol 32:247, 2008.
24. Lagrew DC, Pircon RA, Towers CV, et al: Antepartum fetal surveillance in patients with diabetes: when to start? Am J Obstet Gynecol 168:1820, 1993.
25. Nageotte MP: Antenatal testing: diabetes mellitus. Semin Perinatol 32:269, 2008.
26. Dugoff L, for the Society for Maternal-Fetal Medicine: First- and second-trimester maternal serum markers for aneuploidy and adverse obstetric outcomes. Obstet Gynecol 115:1052, 2010.
27. ACOG: Practice bulletin: antepartum fetal surveillance. Number 9, October 1999, Reaffirmed 2009 (replaces Technical Bulletin Number 188, January 1994). Clinical management guidelines for obstetrician-gynecologists. Int J Gynaecol Obstet 68:175, 2000.
28. Werner EF, Lockwood CJ: Thrombophilias and stillbirth. Clin Obstet Gynecol 53:617, 2010.
29. Willinger M, Chia-Wen K, Reddy UM: Racial disparities in stillbirth across gestation in the United States. Am J Obstet Gynecol 201:469. e1, 2009.
30. Freeman RK: Antepartum testing in patients with hypertensive disorders in pregnancy. Semin Perinatol 32:271, 2008.

31. Harman CR: Amniotic fluid abnormalities. Semin Perinatol 32:288, 2008.
32. Bai J, Wong FW, Bauman A, et al: Parity and pregnancy outcomes. Am J Obstet Gynecol 186:274, 2002.
33. Weeks JW: Antepartum testing for women with previous stillbirth. Semin Perinatol 32:301, 2008.
34. Allen VM, Wilson RD, Cheung A, for the Genetics Committee of the Society of Obstetricians and Gynaecologists of Canada (SOGC) and the Reproductive Endocrinology Infertility Committee of the Society of Obstetricians and Gynaecologists of Canada (SOGC): Pregnancy outcomes after assisted reproductive technology. J Obstet Gynaecol Can 28:220, 2006.
35. Divon MY, Feldman-Leidner N: Postdates and antenatal testing. Semin Perinatol 32:295, 2008.
36. Smith GCS, Fretts RC: Stillbirth. Lancet 370:1715, 2007.
37. Williamson C, Hems LM, Goulis DG, et al: Clinical outcome in a series of cases of obstetric cholestasis identified via a patient support group. BJOG 111:676, 2004.
38. Vidaeff AC, Yeomans ER, Ramin SM: Pregnancy in women with renal disease. I. General principles. Am J Perinatol 25:385, 2008.
39. Adams D, Druzin ML, Edersheim T, et al: Condition specific antepartum testing: systemic lupus erythematosus and associated serologic abnormalities. Am J Reprod Immunol 28:159, 1992.
40. Scifres CM, Macones GA: Antenatal testing: benefits and costs. Semin Perinatol 32:318, 2008.
41. Divon MY, Ferber A: Evidence-based antepartum fetal testing. In *Prenatal and Neonatal Medicine*. New York, Parthenon, 2000.
42. Fretts RC, Elkin EB, Myers ER, Heffner LJ: Should older women have antepartum testing to prevent unexplained stillbirth? Obstet Gynecol 104:56, 2004.
43. Van Woerden EE, VanGeijn HP: Heart-rate patterns and fetal movements. In Nijhuis J: *Fetal Behaviour*. New York, Oxford University Press, 1992, p 41.
44. Hijazi ZR, East CE: Factors affecting maternal perception of fetal movement. Obstet Gynecol Surv 64:489, 2009.
45. Martin CB: Normal fetal physiology and behavior, and adaptive responses with hypoxemia. Semin Perinatol 32:239, 2008.
46. Patrick J, Campbell K, Carmichael L, et al: Patterns of gross fetal body movements over 24-hour observation intervals during the last 10 weeks of pregnancy. Am J Obstet Gynecol 142:363, 1982.
47. Holden K, Jovanovic L, Druzin M, Peterson C: Increased fetal activity with low maternal blood glucose levels in pregnancies complicated by diabetes. Am J Perinatol 1:161, 1984.
48. Druzin ML, Foodim J: Effect of maternal glucose ingestion compared with maternal water ingestion on the nonstress test. Obstet Gynecol 67:4, 1982.
49. Neldam S: Fetal movements as an indicator of fetal well being. Dan Med Bull 30:274, 1983.
50. Grant A, Valentin L, Elbourne D, Alexander S: Routine formal fetal movement counting and risk of antepartum late death in normally formed singletons. Lancet 2:345, 1989.
51. Mangesi L, Hofmeyr GJ: Fetal movement counting for assessment of fetal wellbeing. Cochrane Database Syst Rev 24:CD004909, 2007.
52. Sadovsky E, Yaffe H, Polishuk W: Fetal movement monitoring in normal and pathologic pregnancy. Int J Gynaecol Obstet 12:75, 1974.
53. Rayburn W, Zuspan F, Motley M, Donaldson M: An alternative to antepartum fetal heart rate testing. Am J Obstet Gynecol 138:223, 1980.
54. Pearson J, Weaver J: Fetal activity and fetal well being: an evaluation. BMJ 1:1305, 1976.
55. Froen JF, Heazell AEP, Holm Tveit JP, et al: Fetal movement assessment. Semin Perinatol 32:243, 2008.
56. Mikhail MS, Freda MC, Merkatz RB, et al: The effect of fetal movement counting on maternal attachment to fetus. Am J Obstet Gynecol 165:988, 1991.
57. Moore TR, Piacquadio K: Study results vary in count-to-10 method of fetal movement screening. Am J Obstet Gynecol 163:264, 1990.
58. Braly P, Freeman R, Garite T, et al: Incidence of premature delivery following the oxytocin challenge test. Am J Obstet Gynecol 141:5, 1981.
59. Freeman R: The use of the oxytocin challenge test for antepartum clinical evaluation of uteroplacental respiratory function. Am J Obstet Gynecol 121:481, 1975.
60. Freeman R, Anderson G, Dorchester W: A prospective multi-institutional study of antepartum fetal heart rate monitoring. I. Risk of perinatal mortality and morbidity according to antepartum fetal heart rate test results. Am J Obstet Gynecol 143:771, 1982.
61. Freeman R, Anderson G, Dorchester W: A prospective multi-institutional study of antepartum fetal heart rate monitoring. II. CST vs NST for primary surveillance. Am J Obstet Gynecol 143:778, 1982.
62. Bruce S, Petrie R, Yeh S-Y: The suspicious contraction stress test. Obstet Gynecol 51:415, 1978.
63. Beischer N, Drew J, Ashton P, et al: Quality of survival of infants with critical fetal reserve detected by antenatal cardiotocography. Am J Obstet Gynecol 146:662, 1983.
64. Grivell RM, Alfirevic Z, Gyte GM, et al. Antenatal cardiotocography for fetal assessment. Cochrane Database Syst Rev 20:CD007863, 2010.
65. Patrick J, Carmichael L, Chess L, Staples C: Accelerations of the human fetal heart rate at 38 to 40 weeks' gestational age. Am J Obstet Gynecol 148:35, 1984.
66. Margulis E, Binder D, Cohen A: The effect of propranolol on the nonstress test. Am J Obstet Gynecol 148:340, 1984.
67. Keegan K, Paul R, Broussard P, et al: Antepartum fetal heart rate testing. III. The effect of phenobarbital on the nonstress test. Am J Obstet Gynecol 133:579, 1979.
68. Phelan J: Diminished fetal reactivity with smoking. Am J Obstet Gynecol 136:230, 1980.
69. Macones GA, Hankins GD, Spong CY, et al: The 2008 National Institute of Child Health and Human Development workshop report on electronic fetal monitoring: update on definitions, interpretation, and research guidelines. Obstet Gynecol 112:661, 2008.
70. Keegan K, Paul R, Broussard P, et al: Antepartum fetal heart rate testing. V. The nonstress test: an outpatient approach. Am J Obstet Gynecol 136:81, 1980.
71. Tan KH, Sabapathy A: Maternal glucose administration for facilitating tests of fetal wellbeing. Cochrane Database Syst Rev 4:CD003397, 2001.
72. Tan KH, Sabapathy A: Fetal manipulation for facilitating tests of fetal wellbeing. Cochrane Database Syst Rev 4:CD003396, 2001.
73. Lavery J: Nonstress fetal heart rate testing. Clin Obstet Gynecol 25:689, 1982.
74. Keegan K, Paul R: Antepartum fetal heart rate testing. IV. The nonstress test as a primary approach. Am J Obstet Gynecol 136:75, 1980.
75. Evertson L, Gauthier R, Schifrin B, et al: Antepartum fetal heart rate testing. I. Evolution of the nonstress test. Am J Obstet Gynecol 133:29, 1979.
76. Druzin ML, Edersheim TG, Hutson JM, et al: The effect of vibroacoustic stimulation on the nonstress test at gestational ages of thirty-two weeks or less. Am J Obstet Gynecol 1661:1476, 1989.
77. Phillips W, Towell M: Abnormal fetal heart rate associated with congenital abnormalities. Br J Obstet Gynaecol 87:270, 1980.
78. Gagnon R, Hunse C, Foreman J: Human fetal behavioral states after vibratory stimulation. Am J Obstet Gynecol 161:1470, 1989.
79. Tan KH, Smyth R: Fetal vibroacoustic stimulation for facilitation of tests of fetal wellbeing. Cochrane Database Syst Rev 1:CD002963, 2001.
80. Smith CV, Satt B, Phelan JP, et al: Intrauterine sound levels: intrapartum assessment with an intrauterine microphone. Am J Perinatol 7:312, 1990.
81. Arulkumaran S, Talbert D, Hsu TS, et al: In-utero sound levels when vibroacoustic stimulation is applied to the maternal abdomen: an assessment of the possibility of cochlea damage in the fetus. Br J Obstet Gynaecol 99:43, 1992.
82. Arulkumaran S, Skurr B, Tong H, et al: No evidence of hearing loss due to fetal acoustic stimulation test. Obstet Gynecol 78:2, 1991.
83. Rochard F, Schifrin B, Goupil F, et al: Nonstressed fetal heart rate monitoring in the antepartum period. Am J Obstet Gynecol 126:699, 1976.
84. Druzin ML, Lockshin M, Edersheim T, et al: Second trimester fetal monitoring and preterm delivery in pregnancies with systematic lupus erythematosus and/or circulating anticoagulant. Am J Obstet Gynecol 157:1503, 1987.
85. Druzin ML: Fetal bradycardia during antepartum testing, further observations. J Reprod Med 34:47, 1989.
86. Michaelsson M, Engle MA: Congenital complete heart block: an international study of the natural history. Cardiovascular Clin 4:85, 1972.

87. Anandakumar C, Biswas A, Chew SS, et al: Direct fetal therapy for hydrops secondary to congenital atrioventricular heart block. Obstet Gynecol 87:835, 1996.
88. Maeno J: Fetal arrhythmia: prenatal diagnosis and perinatal management. Obstet Gynaecol Res 35:623, 2009.
89. Meis P, Ureda J, Swain M, et al: Variable decelerations during nonstress tests are not a sign of fetal compromise? Am J Obstet Gynecol 154:586, 1994.
90. Boehm FH, Salyer S, Shah DM, et al: Improved outcome of twice weekly nonstress testing. Obstet Gynecol 67:566, 1986.
91. Barss V, Frigoletto F, Diamond F: Stillbirth after nonstress testing. Obstet Gynecol 65:541, 1985.
92. Finberg HJ, Kurtz AB, Johnson RL, et al: The biophysical profile: a literature review and reassessment of its usefulness in the evaluation of fetal well-being. J Ultrasound Med 9:583, 1990.
93. Manning FA, Morrison I, Lange IR, et al: Fetal assessment based on fetal biophysical profile scoring: experience in 12,620 referred high-risk pregnancies. Am J Obstet Gynecol 151:343, 1985.
94. Vintzileos AM, Gaffney SE, Salinger LM, et al: The relationship between fetal biophysical profile and cord pH in patients undergoing cesarean section before the onset of labor. Obstet Gynecol 70:196, 1987.
95. Gennser G, Marsal K, Brantmark B: Maternal smoking and fetal breathing movements. Am J Obstet Gynecol 123:861, 1975.
96. Manning F, Platt L, Sipos L: Antepartum fetal evaluation: development of a fetal biophysical profile. Am J Obstet Gynecol 136:787, 1980.
97. Pillai M, James D: The importance of behavioral state in biophysical assessment of the term human fetus. BJOG 97:1130, 1990.
98. Manning FA, Morrison I, Lange IR, et al: Fetal biophysical profile scoring: selective use of the nonstress test. Am J Obstet Gynecol 156:709, 1987.
99. Manning FA, Morrison I, Harman CR, et al: The abnormal fetal biophysical profile score. V. Predictive accuracy according to score composition. Am J Obstet Gynecol 162:918, 1990.
100. Manning FA, Harman CR, Morrison I, et al: Fetal assessment based on fetal biophysical profile scoring. Am J Obstet Gynecol 162:703, 1990.

For full reference list, log onto www.expertconsult.com.

Section III
Intrapartum Care

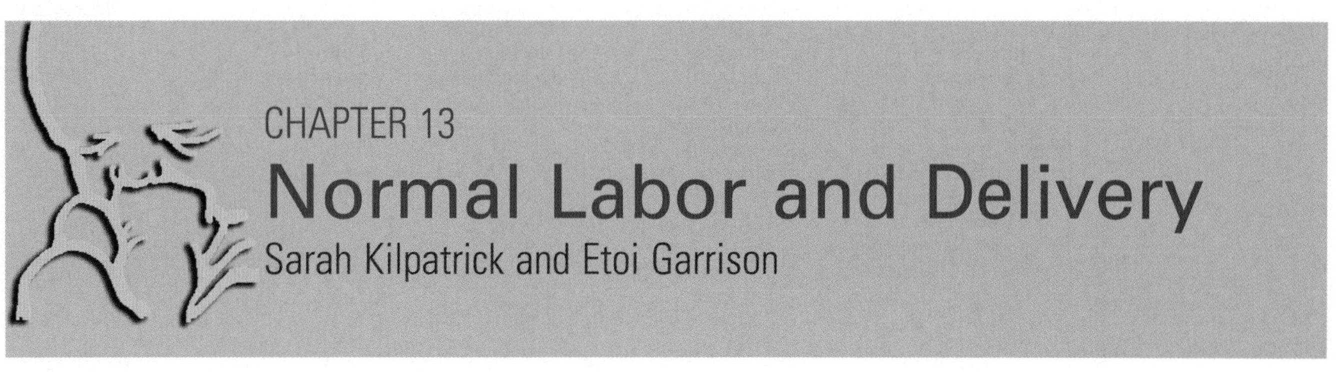

CHAPTER 13

Normal Labor and Delivery

Sarah Kilpatrick and Etoi Garrison

KEY ABBREVIATIONS

American College of Obstetricians and Gynecologists	ACOG
Cephalopelvic Disproportion	CPD
Left Occiput Anterior	LOA
Occiput Anterior	OA
Occiput Posterior	OP
Occiput Transverse	OT
Prostaglandins	PGs
Randomized Controlled Trial	RCT
Right Occiput Anterior	ROA

LABOR: DEFINITION AND PHYSIOLOGY

Labor is defined as the process by which the fetus is expelled from the uterus. **More specifically, labor requires regular, effective contractions that lead to dilation and effacement of the cervix.** This chapter describes the physiology and normal characteristics of term labor and delivery.

The physiology of labor initiation has not been completely elucidated, but the putative mechanisms have been well reviewed by Liao and colleagues.[1] Labor initiation is species-specific, and the mechanisms in human labor are unique. The four phases of labor from quiescence to involution are outlined in Figure 13-1.[2] The first phase is quiescence and represents that time in utero before labor begins when uterine activity is suppressed by the action of progesterone, prostacyclin, relaxin, nitric oxide, parathyroid hormone–related peptide, and possibly other hormones. During the activation phase, estrogen begins to facilitate expression of myometrial receptors for prostaglandins (PGs) and oxytocin, which results in ion channel activation and increased gap junctions. This increase in the gap junctions between myometrial cells facilitates effective contractions.[3] In essence, the activation phase readies the uterus for the subsequent stimulation phase, when uterotonics, particularly PGs and oxytocin, stimulate regular contractions. In the human, this process at term may be protracted, occurring over days to weeks. The final phase, uterine involution, occurs after delivery and is mediated primarily by oxytocin. The first three phases of labor require endocrine, paracrine, and autocrine interaction between the fetus, membranes, placenta, and mother.

The fetus has a central role in the initiation of term labor in nonhuman mammals; in humans, the fetal role is not completely understood (Figure 13-2).[2-5] In sheep, term labor is initiated through activation of the fetal hypothalamic-pituitary-adrenal axis, with a resultant increase in fetal adrenocorticotrophic hormone and cortisol.[4,5] Fetal cortisol increases production of estradiol and decreases production of progesterone by a shift in placental metabolism of cortisol dependent on placental 17α-hydroxylase. The change in the progesterone/estradiol ratio stimulates placental production of oxytocin and PG, particularly $PGF_{2\alpha}$.[4] If this increase in fetal adrenocorticotrophic hormone and cortisol is blocked, parturition is delayed.[5] In contrast, humans lack placental 17α-hydroxylase and there is no increase in fetal cortisol near term. Rather, in humans, uterine activation may be potentiated in part by increased fetal adrenal production of dehydroepiandrostenedione, which is converted in the placenta to estradiol and estriol. Placental estriol stimulates an increase in maternal (likely decidual) $PGF_{2\alpha}$, PG receptors, oxytocin receptors, and gap junctions. In humans, there is no documented decrease in progesterone near term and a fall in progesterone is not necessary for labor initiation. However, some research suggests the possibility of a "functional progesterone withdrawal" in humans: Labor is accompanied by a decrease in the concentration of progesterone receptors, as well as a change in the ratio of progesterone receptor isoforms A and B in both the myometrium[6,7] and membranes.[8] More research is needed to elucidate the precise mechanism through which the human parturition cascade is activated. Fetal maturation may play an important role, as well as maternal

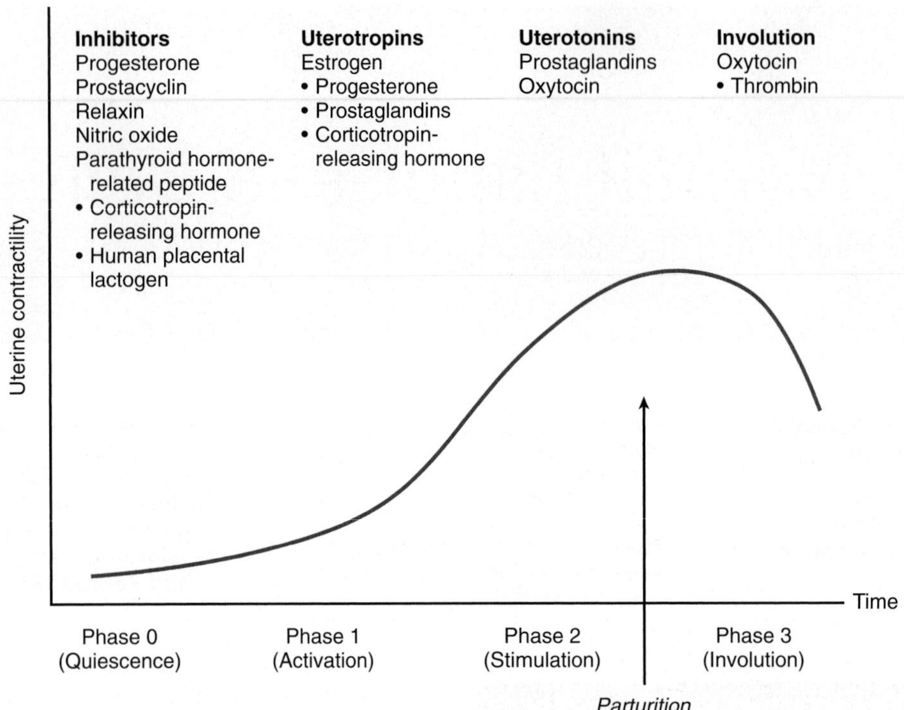

FIGURE 13-1. Regulation of uterine activity during pregnancy and labor. (Modified from Challis JRG, Gibb W: Control of parturition. Prenat Neonat Med 1:283, 1996.)

cues that affect circadian cycling. There are distinct diurnal patterns of contractions and delivery in most species, and in humans, the majority of contractions occur at night.[2,9]

Oxytocin is used commonly for labor induction and augmentation; a full understanding of the mechanism of oxytocin action is helpful. **Oxytocin is a peptide hormone synthesized in the hypothalamus and released from the posterior pituitary in a pulsatile fashion. At term, oxytocin is a potent uterotonic agent that is capable of stimulating uterine contractions at intravenous infusion rates of 1 to 2 mIU/min.**[10] **Oxytocin is inactivated largely in the liver and kidney, and during pregnancy, it is degraded primarily by placental oxytocinase. Its biologic half-life is approximately 3 to 4 minutes, but appears to be shorter when higher doses are infused.** Concentrations of oxytocin in the maternal circulation do not change significantly during pregnancy or before the onset of labor, but they do rise late in the second stage of labor.[10,11] Studies of fetal pituitary oxytocin production and the umbilical arteriovenous differences in plasma oxytocin strongly suggest that the fetus secretes oxytocin that reaches the maternal side of the placenta.[10,12] The calculated rate of active oxytocin secretion from the fetus increases from a baseline of 1 mIU/min before labor to around 3 mIU/min after spontaneous labor.

Significant differences in myometrial oxytocin receptor distribution have been reported, with large numbers of fundal receptors and fewer receptors in the lower uterine segment and cervix.[13] Myometrial oxytocin receptors increase on average by 100- to 200-fold during pregnancy, reaching a maximum during early labor.[10,11,14,15] This rise in receptor concentration is paralleled by an increase in uterine sensitivity to circulating oxytocin. Specific high-affinity oxytocin receptors have also been isolated from human amnion and decidua parietalis but not decidua vera.[10,13] **It has been suggested that oxytocin plays a dual role in parturition.** First, through its receptor, oxytocin directly stimulates uterine contractions. Second, oxytocin may act indirectly by stimulating the amnion and decidua to produce PG.[13,16,17] Indeed, even when uterine contractions are adequate, induction of labor at term is successful only when oxytocin infusion is associated with an increase in PGF production.[13]

Oxytocin binding to its receptor activates phospolipase C. In turn, phospholipase C increases intracellular calcium both by stimulating the release of intracellular calcium and by promoting the influx of extracellular calcium. Oxytocin stimulation of phospholipase C can be blocked by increased levels of cyclic adenosine monophosphate. Increased calcium levels stimulate the calmodulin-mediated activation of myosin light-chain kinase. Oxytocin may also stimulate uterine contractions via a calcium-independent pathway by inhibiting myosin phosphatase, which in turn increases myosin phosphorylation. **These pathways ($PGF_{2\alpha}$ and intracellular calcium) have been the target of multiple tocolytic agents: indomethacin, calcium channel blockers, beta mimetics (through stimulation of cyclic adenosine monophosphate), and magnesium.**

MECHANICS OF LABOR

Labor and delivery are not passive processes in which uterine contractions push a rigid object through a fixed aperture. The ability of the fetus to successfully negotiate the pelvis during labor and delivery depends on the complex interactions of three variables: uterine activity,

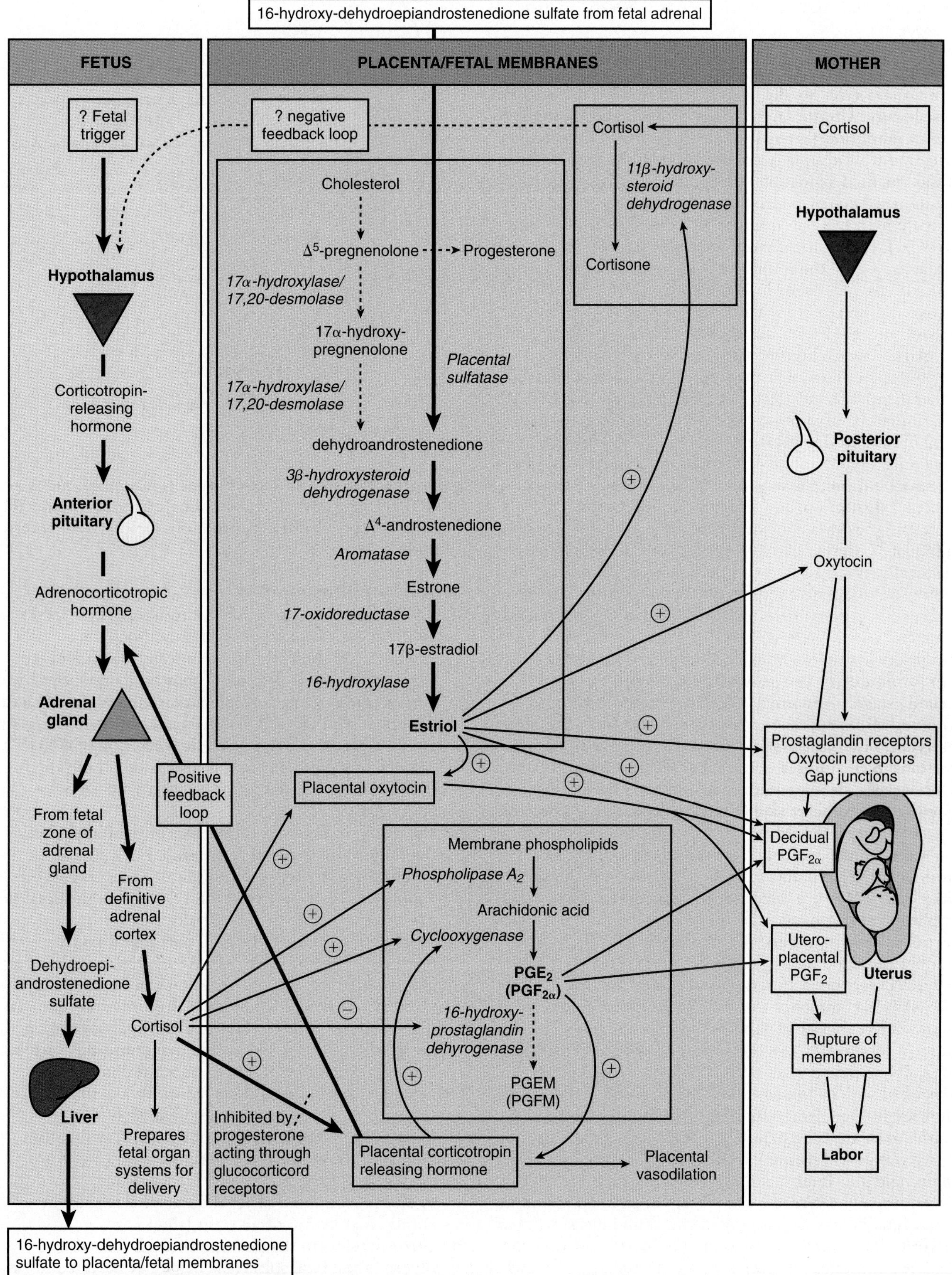

FIGURE 13-2. Proposed "parturition cascade" for labor induction at term. The spontaneous induction of labor at term in the human is regulated by a series of paracrine/autocrine hormones acting in an integrated parturition cascade responsible for promoting uterine contractions. *PGE₂*, Prostaglandin E_2; *PGEM*, 13, 14-dihydro-15-keto-PGE_2; *$PGF_{2\alpha}$*, prostaglandin $F_{2\alpha}$; *PGFM*, 13, 14-dihydro-15keto-$PGF_{2\alpha}$. (Modified from Norwitz ER, Robinson JN, Repke JT: The initiation of parturition: a comparative analysis across the species. Curr Prob Obstet Gynecol Fertil 22:41, 1999.)

the fetus, and the maternal pelvis (*Powers, Passenger, Passage*).

Uterine Activity (Powers)

The powers refer to the forces generated by the uterine musculature. Uterine activity is characterized by the frequency, amplitude (intensity), and duration of contractions. Assessment of uterine activity may include simple observation, manual palpation, external objective assessment techniques (such as external tocodynamometry), and direct measurement via an internal uterine pressure catheter (IUPC). External tocodynamometry measures the change in shape of the abdominal wall as a function of uterine contractions and, as such, is qualitative rather than quantitative. Although it permits graphic display of uterine activity and allows for accurate correlation of fetal heart rate patterns with uterine activity, external tocodynamometry does not allow measurement of contraction intensity or basal intrauterine tone. The most precise method for determination of uterine activity is the direct measurement of intrauterine pressure with an IUPC. However, this procedure should not be performed unless indicated given the small but finite associated risks of uterine perforation, placental disruption, and intrauterine infection.

Despite technologic improvements, the definition of "adequate" uterine activity during labor remains unclear. Classically, three to five contractions per 10 minutes has been used to define adequate labor; this pattern has been observed in approximately 95% of women in spontaneous labor. In labor, patients usually contract every 2 to 5 minutes, with contractions becoming as frequent as every 2 to 3 minutes in late active labor, as well as during the second stage. Abnormal uterine activity can also be observed either spontaneously or resulting from iatrogenic interventions. ***Tachysystole* is defined as more than five contractions in 10 minutes, averaged over 30 minutes. If tachysytole occurs, documentation should note the presence or absence of fetal heart rate (FHR) decelerations. The term *hyperstimulation* should no longer be used.**[18]

Various units have been devised to objectively measure uterine activity, the most common of which is the *Montevideo unit* (MVU), a measure of average frequency and amplitude above basal tone (the average strength of contractions in millimeters of mercury multiplied by the number of contractions per 10 minutes). Although 150 to 350 MVU has been described for adequate labor, 200 to 250 MVU is commonly accepted to define adequate labor in the active phase of labor.[19,20] There are no data that identify adequate forces during latent labor. Although it is generally believed that optimal uterine contractions are associated with an increased likelihood of vaginal delivery, there are limited data to support this assumption. If uterine contractions are "adequate" to effect vaginal delivery, one of two things will happen: either the cervix will efface and dilate, and the fetal head will descend, or there will be worsening caput succedaneum (scalp edema) and molding of the fetal head (overlapping of the skull bones) without cervical effacement and dilation. The latter situation suggests the presence of cephalopelvic disproportion (CPD), which can be either absolute (in which a given fetus is simply too large to negotiate a given pelvis) or relative (in which delivery of a given fetus through a given pelvis would be possible under optimal conditions, but is precluded by malposition or abnormal attitude of the fetal head), or pelvic outlet obstruction such as with uterine fibroids.

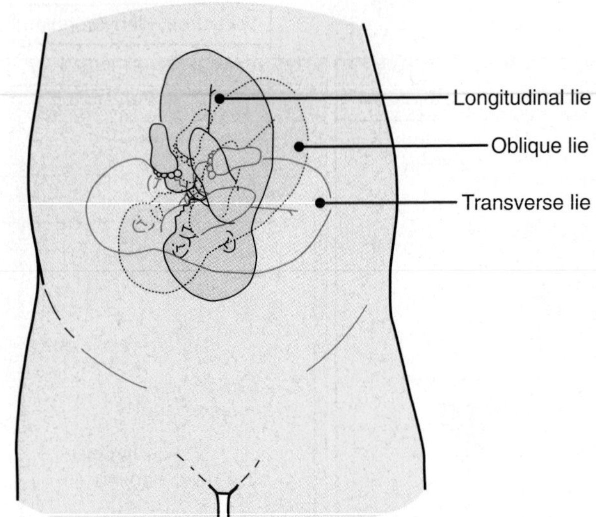

Figure 13-3. Examples of different fetal lie.

The Fetus (Passenger)

The passenger, of course, is the fetus. Several fetal variables influence the course of labor and delivery.

1. Fetal *size* can be estimated clinically by abdominal palpation or with ultrasound, but both are subject to a large degree of error. **Fetal macrosomia (defined by the American College of Obstetricians and Gynecologists [ACOG] as actual birth weight greater than 4500 g**[21]**)** is associated with an increased likelihood of failed trial of labor and may be associated with labor abnormalities.[22]
2. ***Lie* refers to the longitudinal axis of the fetus relative to the longitudinal axis of the uterus**. Fetal lie can be longitudinal, transverse, or oblique (Figure 13-3). In a singleton pregnancy, only fetuses in a longitudinal lie can be safely delivered vaginally.
3. ***Presentation* refers to the fetal part that directly overlies the pelvic inlet.** In a fetus presenting in the longitudinal lie, the presentation can be cephalic (vertex) or breech. Compound presentation refers to the presence of more than one fetal part overlying the pelvic inlet, such as a fetal hand and the vertex. Funic presentation refers to presentation of the umbilical cord and is rare at term. In a cephalic fetus, the presentation is classified according to the leading bony landmark of the skull, which can be either the occiput (vertex), the chin (mentum), or the brow (Figure 13-4). *Malpresentation*, referring to any presentation other than vertex, is seen in approximately 5% of all term labors.
4. ***Attitude* refers to the position of the head with regard to the fetal spine (the degree of flexion and/or extension of the fetal head).** Flexion of the head is important to facilitate *engagement* of the head in the maternal pelvis. When the fetal chin is optimally

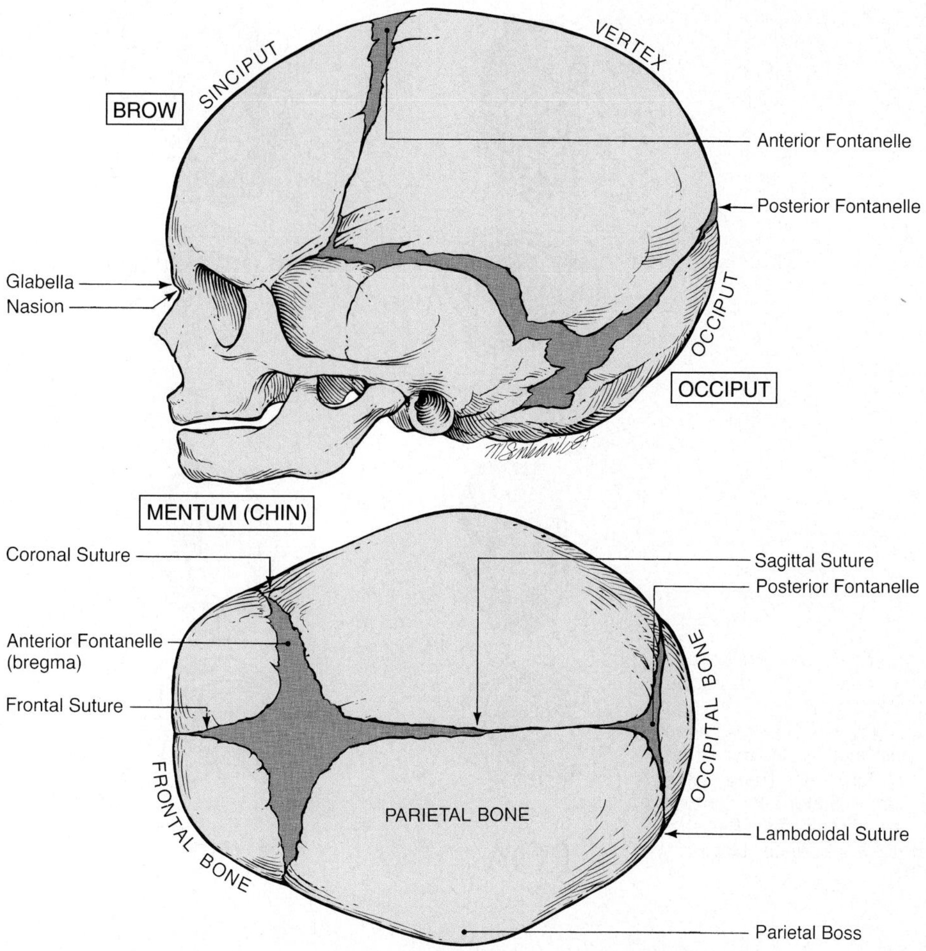

FIGURE 13-4. Landmarks of fetal skull for determination of fetal position.

flexed onto the chest, the suboccipitobregmatic diameter (9.5 cm) presents at the pelvic inlet (Figure 13-5). This is the smallest possible presenting diameter in the cephalic presentation. As the head deflexes (extends), the diameter presenting to the pelvic inlet progressively increases even before the malpresentations of brow and face are encountered (see Figure 13-5), and may contribute to failure to progress in labor. The architecture of the pelvic floor along with increased uterine activity may correct deflexion in the early stages of labor.

5. ***Position*** **of the fetus refers to the relationship of the fetal presenting part to the maternal pelvis, and it can be assessed most accurately on vaginal examination.** For cephalic presentations, the fetal occiput is the reference. If the occiput is directly anterior, the position is occiput anterior (OA). If the occiput is turned toward the mother's right side, the position is right occiput anterior (ROA). In the breech presentation, the sacrum is the reference (right sacrum anterior). The various positions of a cephalic presentation are illustrated in Figure 13-6. In a vertex presentation, position can be determined by palpation of the fetal sutures. The sagittal suture is the easiest to palpate. Palpation of the distinctive lamdoid sutures should identify the position of the fetal occiput. The frontal suture can also be used to determine the position of the front of the vertex. Most commonly, the fetal head enters the pelvis in a transverse position and, then as a normal part of labor, rotates to an OA position. Most fetuses deliver in the OA, LOA, or ROA position. In the past, less than 10% of presentations were occiput posterior (OP) at delivery.[23] However, epidural analgesia is associated with an increased risk of OP presentation (observed in 12.9% of women with epidural analgesia).[24]

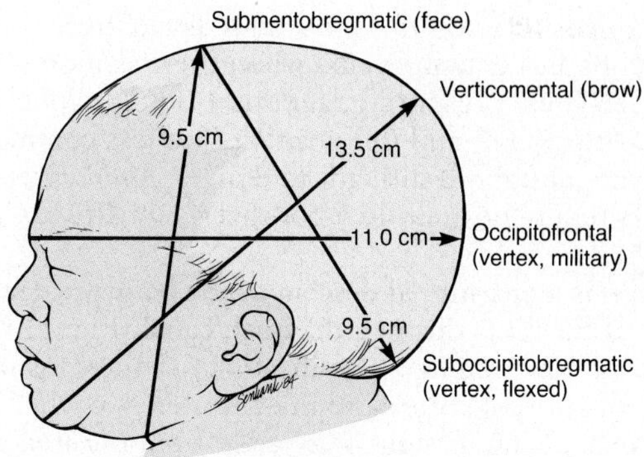

FIGURE 13-5. Presenting diameters of the average term fetal skull.

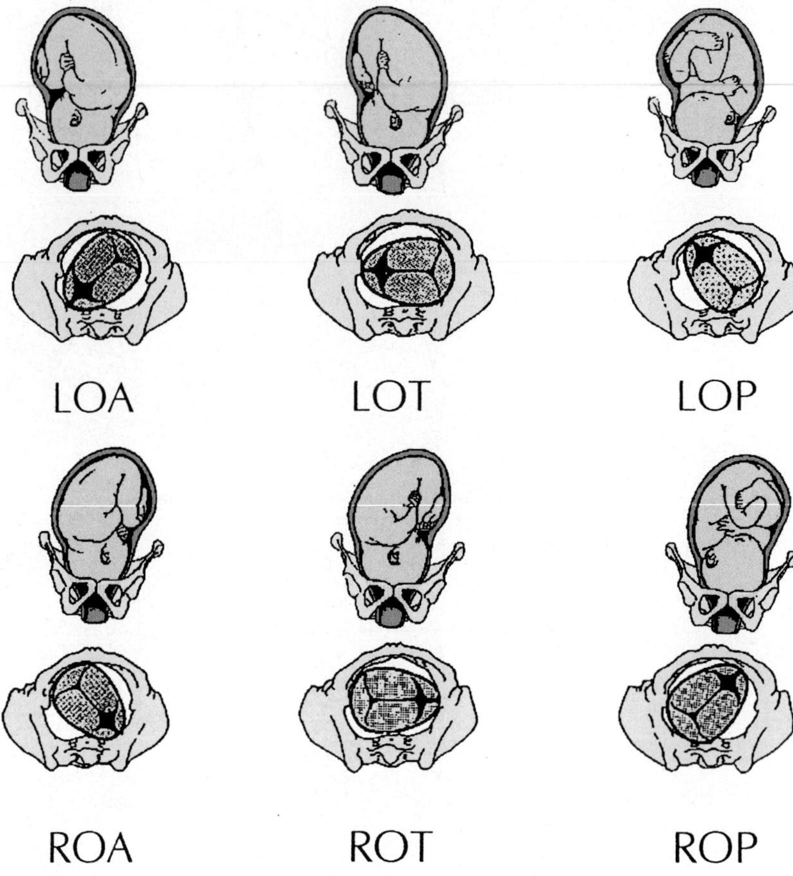

FIGURE 13-6. Fetal presentations and positions in labor. *LOA*, Left occiput anterior; *LOP*, left occiput posterior; *LOT*, left occiput transverse; *ROA*, right occiput anterior; *ROT*, right occiput transverse; *ROP*, right occiput posterior. (Modified from Norwitz ER, Robinson J, Repke JT: The initiation and management of labor. *In* Seifer DB, Samuels P, Kniss DA [eds]: The Physiologic Basis of Gynecology and Obstetrics. Philadelphia, Lippincott Williams & Wilkins, 2001.)

Asynclitism occurs when the sagittal suture is not directly central relative to the maternal pelvis. If the fetal head is turned such that more parietal bone is present posteriorly, the sagittal suture is more anterior and this is referred to as posterior asynclitism. Anterior asynclitism occurs when there is more parietal bone presenting anteriorly. The occiput transverse (OT) and OP positions are less common at delivery and more difficult to deliver. *Malposition* refers to any position in labor that is not ROA, OA, or LOA.

6. ***Station* is a measure of descent of the bony presenting part of the fetus through the birth canal** (Figure 13-7). The current standard classification (–5 to +5) is based on a quantitative measure in centimeters of the distance of the leading bony edge from the ischial spines. The midpoint (0 station) is defined as the plane of the maternal ischial spines. The ischial spines can be palpated on vaginal examination at approximately 8 o'clock and 4 o'clock. For the right-handed person, they are most easily felt on the maternal right.

An abnormality in any of these fetal variables may affect both the course of labor and the likelihood of vaginal delivery. For example, OP presentation is well known to be associated with longer labor.[25]

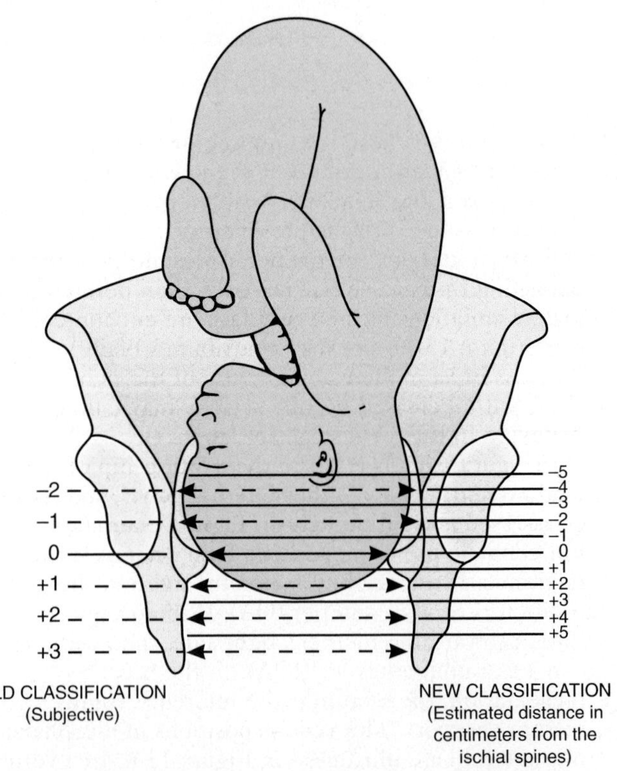

FIGURE 13-7. The relationship of the leading edge of the presenting part of the fetus to the plane of the maternal ischial spines determines the station. Station +1/+3 (old classification) or +2/+5 (new classification) is illustrated.

The Maternal Pelvis (Passage)

The passage consists of the bony pelvis (composed of the sacrum, ilium, ischium, and pubis) and the resistance

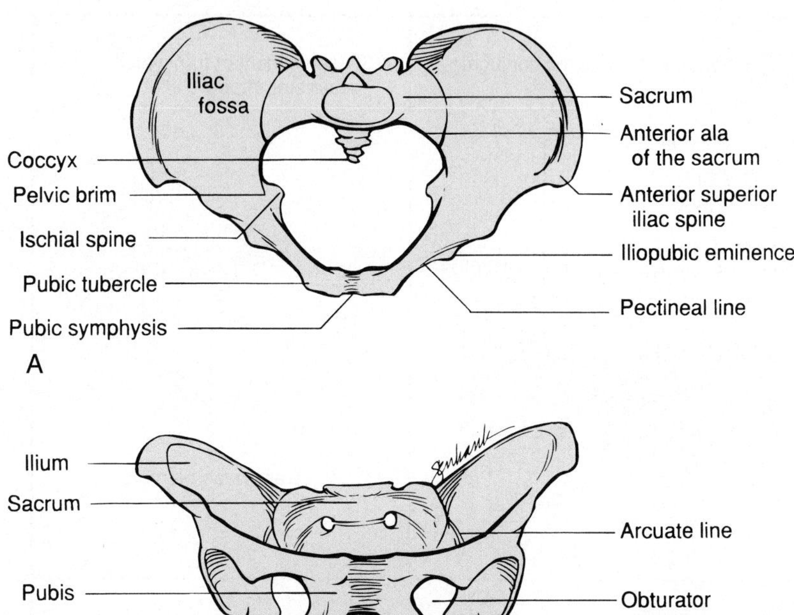

FIGURE 13-8. Superior **(A)** and anterior **(B)** view of the female pelvis. (From Repke JT: Intrapartum Obstetrics. New York, Churchill Livingstone, 1996, p 68.)

provided by the soft tissues. The bony pelvis is divided into the false (greater) and true (lesser) pelvis by the pelvic brim, which is demarcated by the sacral promontory, the anterior ala of the sacrum, the arcuate line of the ilium, the pectineal line of the pubis, and the pubic crest culminating in the symphysis (Figure 13-8). Measurements of the various parameters of the bony female pelvis have been made with great precision, directly in cadavers and using radiographic imaging in living women. Such measurements have divided the true pelvis into a series of planes that must be negotiated by the fetus during passage through the birth canal, which can be broadly classified into the pelvic inlet, midpelvis, and pelvic outlet. X-ray pelvimetry and computed tomography (CT) have been used to define average and critical limit values for the various parameters of the bony pelvis (Table 13-1).[26,27] Critical limit values are measurements that are associated with a significant probability of CPD.[26] **However, CT and x-ray pelvimetry are rarely used, having been replaced by a clinical trial of the pelvis (labor).** The remaining indications for x-ray or CT pelvimetry are evaluation for vaginal breech delivery or evaluation of a woman who has suffered a significant pelvic fracture.[28]

Clinical pelvimetry is currently the only method of assessing the shape and dimensions of the bony pelvis in labor. A useful protocol for clinical pelvimetry is detailed in Figure 13-9 and involves the assessment of the pelvic inlet, midpelvis, and pelvic outlet. The inlet of the true pelvis is largest in its transverse diameter (usually greater than 12.0 cm). The *diagonal conjugate* (the distance from the sacral promontory to the inferior margin of the symphysis pubis as assessed on vaginal examination) is a clinical representation of the anteroposterior diameter of the pelvic inlet. The *true conjugate* (or *obstetric conjugate*) of the pelvic inlet is the distance from the sacral promontory to the superior aspect of the symphysis pubis. This measurement cannot be made clinically but can be estimated by subtracting 1.5 to 2.0 cm from the diagonal conjugate. This is the smallest diameter of the inlet, and it usually measures approximately 10 to 11 cm. The limiting factor in the midpelvis is the interspinous diameter (the measurement between the ischial spines), which is usually the smallest diameter of the pelvis but should be greater than 10 cm. The pelvic outlet is rarely of clinical significance. The anteroposterior diameter from the coccyx to the symphysis pubis is approximately 13 cm in most cases, and the transverse diameter between the ischial tuberosities is approximately 8 cm.

TABLE 13-1 AVERAGE AND CRITICAL LIMIT VALUES FOR PELVIC MEASUREMENTS BY X-RAY PELVIMETRY

DIAMETER	AVERAGE VALUE	CRITICAL LIMIT*
Pelvic Inlet		
Anteroposterior (cm)	12.5	10.0
Transverse (cm)	13.0	12.0
Sum (cm)	25.5	22.0
Area (cm^2)	145.0	123.0
Pelvic Midcavity		
Anteroposterior (cm)	11.5	10.0
Transverse (cm)	10.5	9.5
Sum (cm)	22.0	19.5
Area (cm^2)	125.0	106.0

Modified from O'Brien WF, Cefalo RC: Labor and delivery. *In* Gabbe SG, Niebyl JR, Simpson JL (eds): Obstetrics: Normal and Problem Pregnancies, ed 3. New York, Churchill Livingstone, 1996, p 377.
*The critical limit values cited imply a high likelihood of cephalopelvic disproportion.

The shape of the female bony pelvis can be classified into four broad categories: gynecoid, anthropoid, android, and platypelloid (Figure 13-10). This classification, based

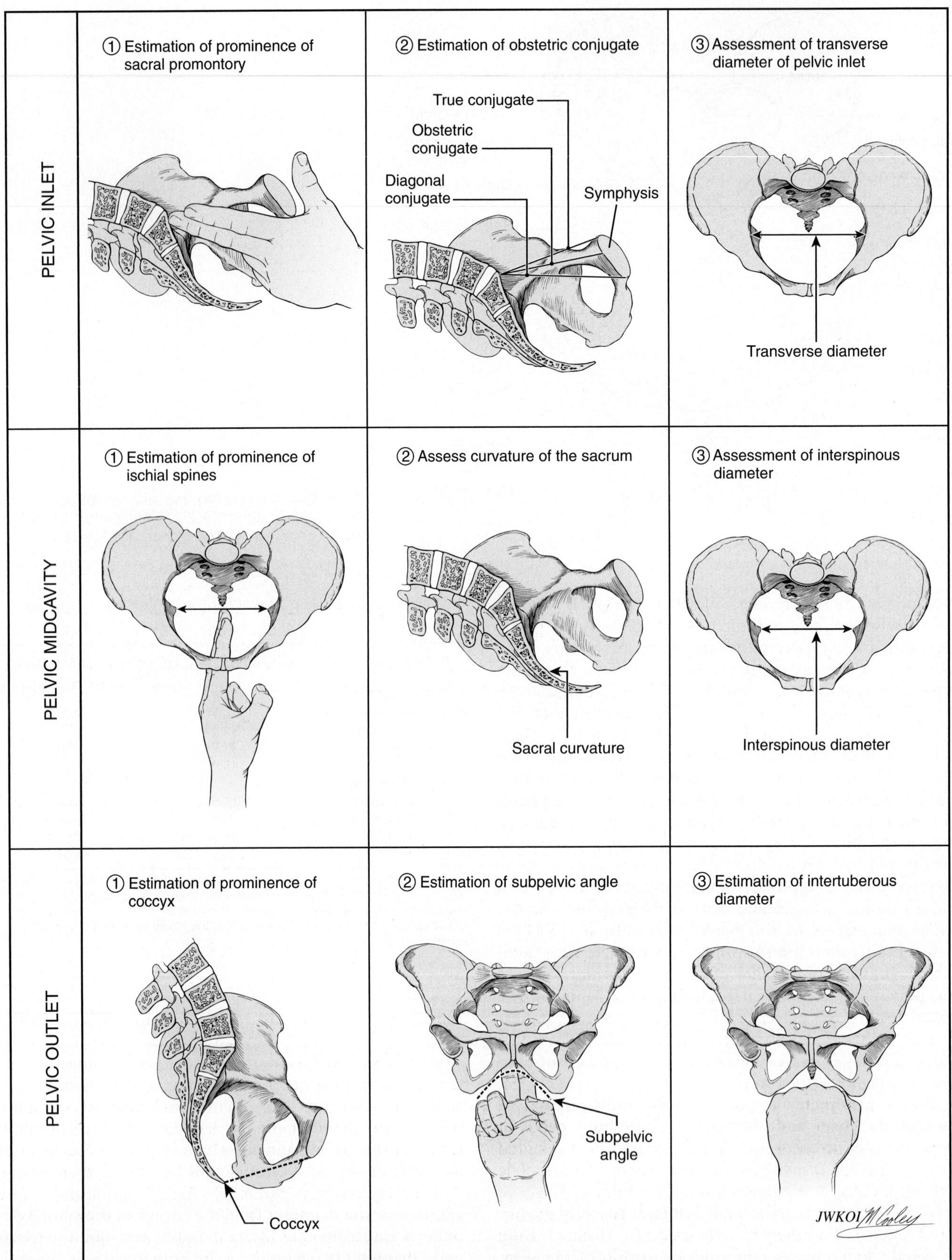
PELVIC INLET
① Estimation of prominence of sacral promontory
② Estimation of obstetric conjugate
True conjugate
Obstetric conjugate
Diagonal conjugate
Symphysis
③ Assessment of transverse diameter of pelvic inlet
Transverse diameter
PELVIC MIDCAVITY
① Estimation of prominence of ischial spines
② Assess curvature of the sacrum
Sacral curvature
③ Assessment of interspinous diameter
Interspinous diameter
PELVIC OUTLET
① Estimation of prominence of coccyx
Coccyx
② Estimation of subpelvic angle
Subpelvic angle
③ Estimation of intertuberous diameter
JWKOI M Cooley

FIGURE 13-9. A protocol for clinical pelvimetry.

		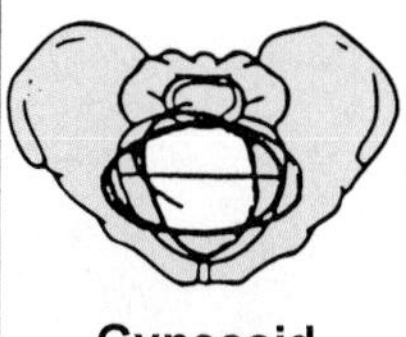 Gynecoid	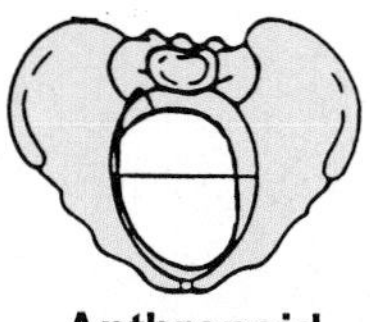 Anthropoid	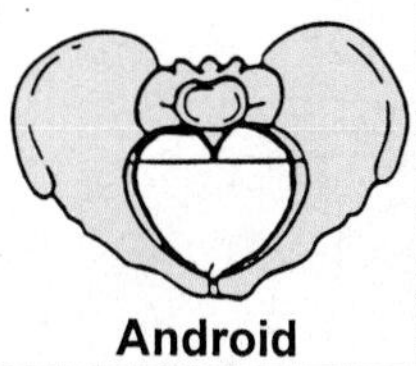 Android	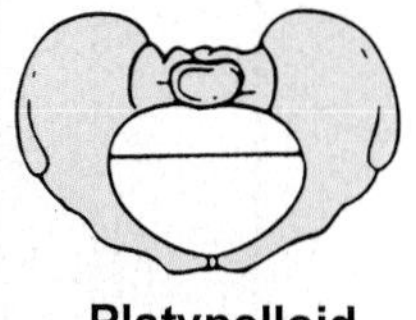 Platypelloid
Pelvic inlet					
	Widest transverse diameter of inlet	12 cm	<12 cm	12 cm	12 cm
	Anteroposterior diameter of inlet	11 cm	>12 cm	11 cm	10 cm
	Forepelvis	Wide	Divergent	Narrow	Straight
Pelvic midcavity					
	Side walls	Straight	Narrow	Convergent	Wide
	Sacrosciatic notch	Medium	Backward	Narrow	Forward
	Inclination of sacrum	Medium	Wide	Forward (lower third)	Narrow
	Ischial spines	Not prominent	Not prominent	Not prominent	Not prominent
Pelvic outlet					
	Subpubic arch	Wide	Medium	Narrow	Wide
	Transverse diameter of outlet	10 cm	10 cm	<10 cm	10 cm

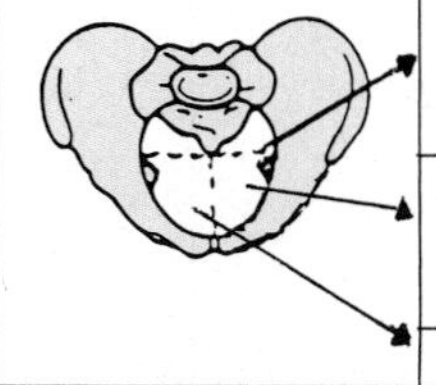

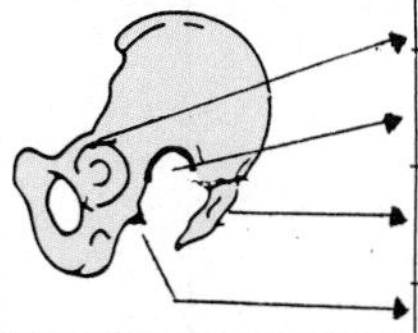

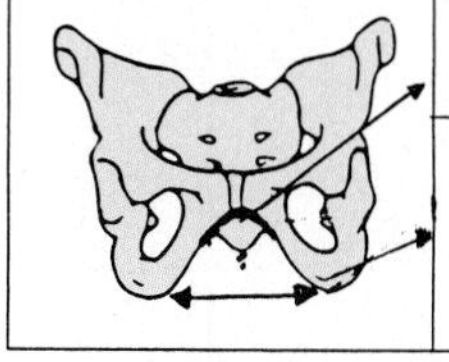

FIGURE 13-10. Characteristics of the four types of female bony pelvis. (Modified from Callahan TL, Caughey AB, Heffner LJ [eds]: Blueprints in Obstetrics and Gynecology. Malden, MA, Blackwell Science, 1998, p 45.)

on the radiographic studies of Caldwell and Moloy, separates those with more favorable characteristics (gynecoid, anthropoid) from those that are less favorable for vaginal delivery (android, platypelloid).[29] In reality, however, many women fall into intermediate classes, and the distinctions become arbitrary. The gynecoid pelvis is the classic female shape. The anthropoid pelvis with its exaggerated oval shape of the inlet, largest anterioposterior diameter, and limited anterior capacity is more often associated with delivery in the OP position. The android pelvis is male in pattern and theoretically has an increased risk of CPD, and the platypelloid pelvis with its broad, flat pelvis theoretically predisposes to a transverse arrest. Although the assessment of fetal size along with pelvic shape and capacity is still of clinical utility, it is a very inexact science. An adequate trial of labor is the only definitive method to determine whether a given fetus will be able to safely negotiate a given pelvis.

Pelvic soft tissues may provide resistance in both the first and second stages of labor. In the first stage, resistance is offered primarily by the cervix, whereas in the second stage, it is offered by the muscles of the pelvic floor. In the second stage of labor, the resistance of the pelvic musculature is believed to play an important role in the rotation and movement of the presenting part through the pelvis.

CARDINAL MOVEMENTS IN LABOR

The mechanisms of labor, also known as the cardinal movements, refer to the changes in position of fetal head during its passage through the birth canal. Because of the asymmetry of the shape of both the fetal head and the maternal bony pelvis, such rotations are required for the fetus to successfully negotiate the birth canal. **Although labor and birth comprise a continuous process, seven discrete cardinal movements of the fetus are described: engagement, descent, flexion, internal rotation, extension, external rotation or restitution, and expulsion** (Figure 13-11).

Engagement

Engagement refers to passage of the widest diameter of the presenting part to a level below the plane of the pelvic inlet (Figure 13-12). In the cephalic presentation with a well-flexed head, the largest transverse diameter of the fetal head is the biparietal diameter (9.5 cm). In the breech, the widest diameter is the bitrochanteric diameter. Clinically, engagement can be confirmed by palpation of the presenting part both abdominally and vaginally. With a cephalic presentation, engagement is achieved when the presenting part is at 0 station on vaginal examination. Engagement is considered an important clinical prognostic sign because it demonstrates that, at least at the level of the pelvic inlet,

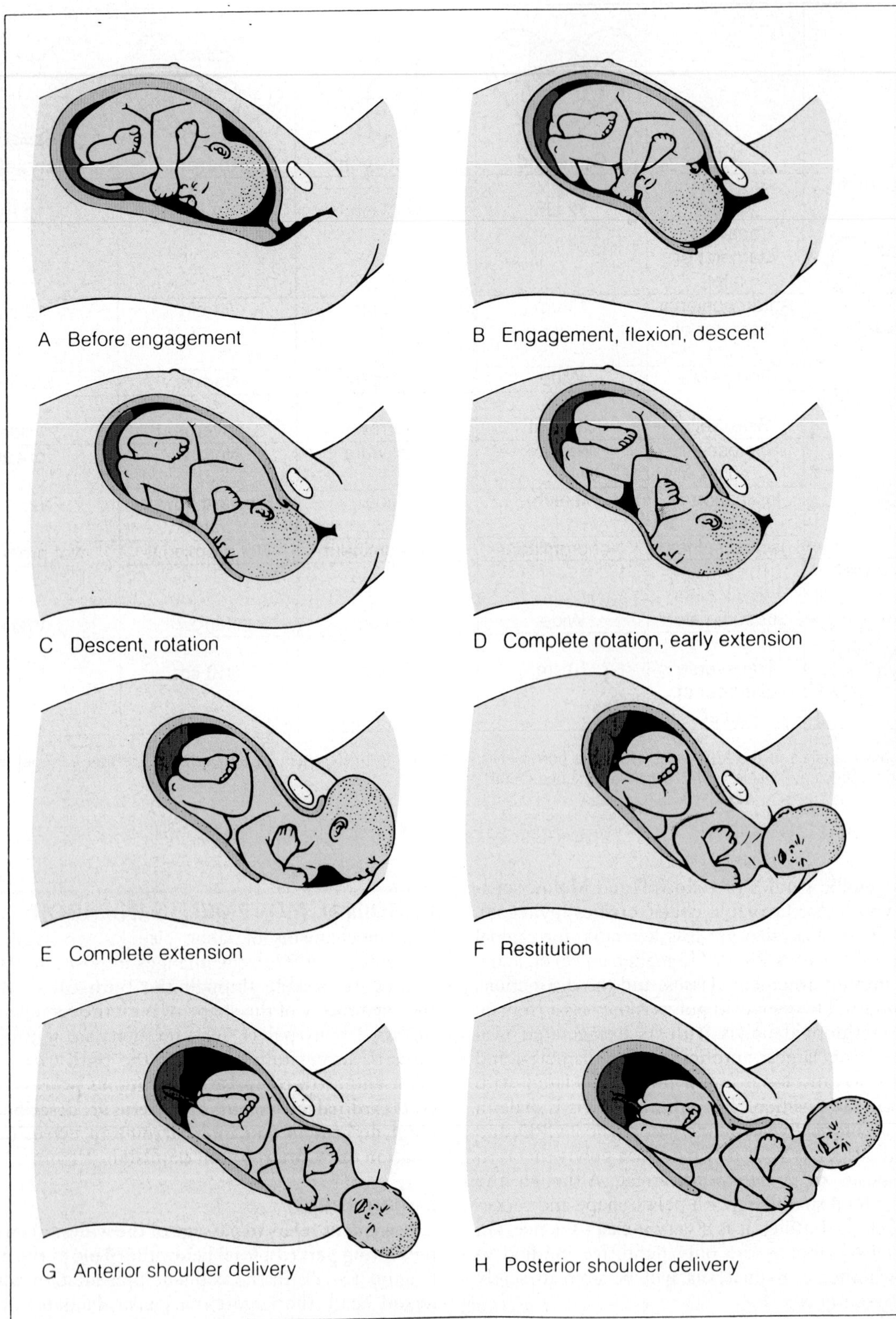

FIGURE 13-11. Cardinal movements of labor.

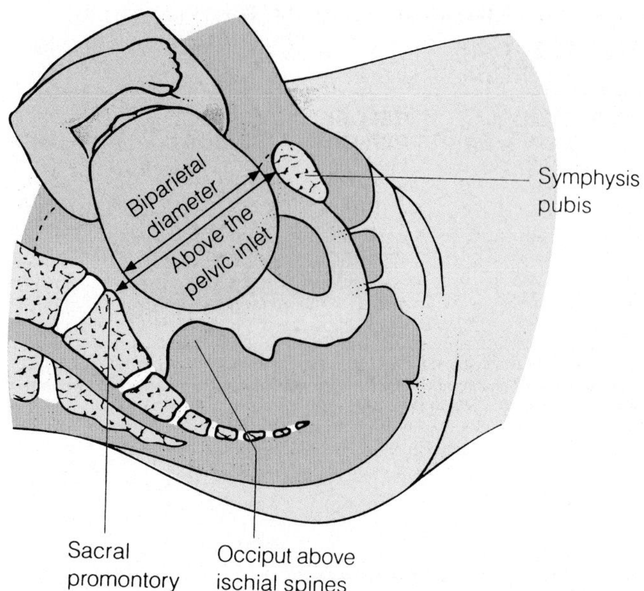

FIGURE 13-12. Engagement of the fetal head.

the maternal bony pelvis is sufficiently large to allow descent of the fetal head. In nulliparas, engagement of the fetal head usually occurs by 36 weeks' gestation. In multiparas, however, engagement can occur later in gestation or even during the course of labor.

Descent

Descent refers to the downward passage of the presenting part through the pelvis. Descent of the fetus is not continuous; the greatest rates of descent occur during the deceleration phase of the first stage of labor and during the second stage of labor.

Flexion

Flexion of the fetal head occurs passively as the head descends owing to the shape of the bony pelvis and the resistance offered by the soft tissues of the pelvic floor. Although flexion of the fetal head onto the chest is present to some degree in most fetuses before labor, complete flexion usually occurs only during the course of labor. The result of complete flexion is to present the smallest diameter of the fetal head (the suboccipitobregmatic diameter) for optimal passage through the pelvis.

Internal Rotation

Internal rotation refers to rotation of the presenting part from its original position as it enters the pelvic inlet (usually OT) to the anteroposterior position as it passes through the pelvis. As with flexion, internal rotation is a passive movement resulting from the shape of the pelvis and the pelvic floor musculature. The pelvic floor musculature, including the coccygeus and ileococcygeus muscles, forms a V-shaped hammock that diverges anteriorly. As the head descends, the occiput of the fetus rotates toward the symphysis pubis (or, less commonly, toward the hollow of the sacrum), thereby allowing the widest portion of the fetus to negotiate the pelvis at its widest dimension. Owing to the angle of inclination between the maternal lumbar spine and pelvic inlet, the fetal head engages in an asynclitic fashion (i.e., with one parietal eminence lower than the other). With uterine contractions, the leading parietal eminence descends and is first to engage the pelvic floor. As the uterus relaxes, the pelvic floor musculature causes the fetal head to rotate until it is no longer asynclitic.

Extension

Extension occurs once the fetus has descended to the level of the introitus. This descent brings the base of the occiput into contact with the inferior margin at the symphysis pubis. At this point, the birth canal curves upward. The fetal head is delivered by extension and rotates around the symphysis pubis. The forces responsible for this motion are the downward force exerted on the fetus by the uterine contractions along with the upward forces exerted by the muscles of the pelvic floor.

External Rotation

External rotation, also known as restitution, refers to the return of the fetal head to the correct anatomic position in relation to the fetal torso. This can occur to either side depending on the orientation of the fetus. This is again a passive movement resulting from a release of the forces exerted on the fetal head by the maternal bony pelvis and its musculature and mediated by the basal tone of the fetal musculature.

Expulsion

Expulsion refers to delivery of the rest of the fetus. After delivery of the head and external rotation, further descent brings the anterior shoulder to the level of the symphysis pubis. The anterior shoulder is delivered in much the same manner as the head, with rotation of the shoulder under the symphysis pubis. After the shoulder, the rest of the body is usually delivered without difficulty.

NORMAL PROGRESS OF LABOR

Progress of labor is measured with multiple variables. With the onset of regular contractions, the fetus descends in the pelvis as the cervix both effaces and dilates. The clinician must assess not only cervical effacement and dilation but fetal station and position with each vaginal examination to judge labor progress. This assessment depends on skilled digital palpation of the maternal cervix and the presenting part. In labor, the cervix shortens (becomes more effaced). Cervical effacement refers to the length of the remaining cervix and can be reported in length or as a percentage. If percentage is used, 0% effacement refers to at least a 2 cm long or a very thick cervix, and 100% effacement refers to no length remaining or a very thin cervix. Most clinicians use percentage to follow cervical effacement during labor. Generally, 80% or greater effacement is required for the diagnosis of active labor. Dilation, perhaps the easiest assessment to master, ranges from closed (no dilation) to complete (10 cm dilated). For most people, a cervical dilation that accommodates a single index finger is equal to 1 cm and 2 index fingers dilation is equal to 3 cm. If no cervix can be palpated around the presenting part, the cervix is 10 cm or completely dilated. The assessment of station (see earlier) is important for documentation

TABLE 13-2 SUMMARY OF MEANS AND 95TH PERCENTILES FOR DURATION OF FIRST- AND SECOND-STAGE LABOR

PARAMETER	MEAN	95th PERCENTILE
Nulliparas		
Latent labor	7.3-8.6 hr	17-21 hr
First stage	7.7-13.3 hr	16.6-19.4 hr
First stage, epidural	10.2 hr	19 hr
Second stage	53-57 min	122-147 min
Second stage, epidural	79 min	185 min
Multiparas		
Latent labor	4.1-5.3 hr	12-14 hr
First stage	5.7-7.5 hr	12.5-13.7 hr
First stage, epidural	7.4 hr	14.9 hr
Second stage, F2	17-19 min	57-61 min
Second stage, epidural	45 min	131 min

Data from references 30, 31, 32, 35, 38.

TABLE 13-3 MEDIAN DURATION OF TIME ELAPSED IN HOURS* FOR EACH CENTIMETER OF DILATION DURING LABOR

CERVICAL DILATION (cm)	BEFORE PERIOD	AFTER PERIOD	*p* VALUE
3-4	2.03	2.30	.36
4-5	1.29	2.17	<.01
5-6	0.66	0.67	.84
6-7	0.62	0.54	.32
7-8	0.44	0.51	.25
8-9	0.41	0.52	.05
9-10	0.44	0.50	.27

From Vahratian A, Zhang J, Hasling J, et al: The effect of early epidural versus early intravenous analgesia use on labor progression: a natural experiment. Am J Obstet Gynecol 191:259, 2004.

*An interval-censored regression model with a log normal distribution was fitted to adjust for maternal age, prepregnancy BMI, and gravidity.

of progress, but it is also critical when determining if an operative vaginal delivery is feasible. Fetal head position should be regularly determined once the woman is in active labor and ideally before significant caput has developed, obscuring the sutures. Like station, knowledge of the fetal position is critical before performing an operative vaginal delivery.

Labor has two categorizations: phases and stages. Phases are divided into latent and active. The *latent phase* of labor is defined as the period between the onset of labor and the point when labor becomes active. The onset of labor is difficult to identify objectively. Usually, it is defined by the initiation of regular painful contractions. Women are frequently at home at this time; therefore, the identification of labor onset depends on patient memory, and hence the length of latent labor is difficult to truly quantify. The beginning of active labor is a retrospective diagnosis because the definition of the active phase of labor is when the slope of cervical dilation accelerates. **In general, active labor requires ≥80% effacement and ≥4 cm dilation of the cervix, but the dilation at which active labor begins is particularly variable.**

In addition, there are three stages of labor. The first stage is from labor onset until full dilation. The second stage is from full dilation until delivery of the baby, and the third stage is from the delivery of the baby until the delivery of the placenta.

The work of Dr. Emanuel Friedman in the 1950s and 1960s was seminal to the current knowledge of labor progress. He analyzed labor progress in 500 nulliparous and multiparous women, and reported normative data that are still useful today.[30,31] Of note, Friedman's second-stage lengths are somewhat artificial because most nulliparous women in that era had a forceps delivery once the duration of the second stage reached 2 hours. More recent data evaluating women in spontaneous labor without augmentation or operative delivery from multiple countries are amazingly similar in the means, suggesting that these normative data are reliable and useful (Table 13-2).[32-35] Of interest, epidural use appears to add about 2 hours to the first stage and about 20 minutes to the second stage in both multiparous and nulliparous women.[35] Friedman's data popularized the use of the labor graph, first depicting only cervical dilation and then modified to include descent and dilation.[37] **Rates of 1.5 cm and 1.2 cm dilation per hour in the active phase for multiparous and nulliparous women, respectively, represent the 5th percentile for rates of dilation[31] and have led to the general concept that in active labor, dilation of at least 1 cm per hour should occur** (Table 13-3). More recent analysis of data from the National Collaborative Perinatal Project, the same data evaluated by Friedman, suggested that progress in active labor in women who ultimately have a vaginal delivery is in fact faster but that these women enter active labor later than initially described.[36] Specifically, most nulliparous women were not in active labor until approximately 5-6 cm and the slope of labor progress did not really increase until after 6 cm. This is an important finding and suggests that clinicians may be diagnosing active phase arrest too early, which could result in unnecessary cesarean deliveries[36,37] (see Chapter 14). The time when an individual patient enters the active phase becomes obvious only retrospectively, as noted earlier, and is more difficult to recognize in nulliparous women.[36]

A more practical approach to following labor progress was introduced by Schulman and Ledger, when they published a modified labor graph that evaluated labor progress focused on latent and active phase only, and this is the graph most commonly used today (Figure 13-13).[38] When evaluating labor progress, it is extremely important to understand that progress in latent phase is slower and less predictable both in multiparas and nulliparas. Factors affecting the duration of labor include parity, maternal body mass index, fetal position, maternal age, and fetal size. Longer labors are associated with increased maternal body mass index,[39] fetal position other than OA,[40] and older maternal age.[41,42] **Factors significantly associated with a prolonged second stage included induced labor, chorioamnionitis, older maternal age, non–African American ethnicity, and parity ≥5.**[41,43] Limits of lengths of first and second stages incorporating the effect of epidural use are helpful in identifying those women who may benefit from interventions (see Table 13-2).[32,34,35]

Mean lengths of the third stage of labor are not affected by parity. In a case series of nearly 13,000 singleton vaginal deliveries greater than 20 weeks' gestation, the median

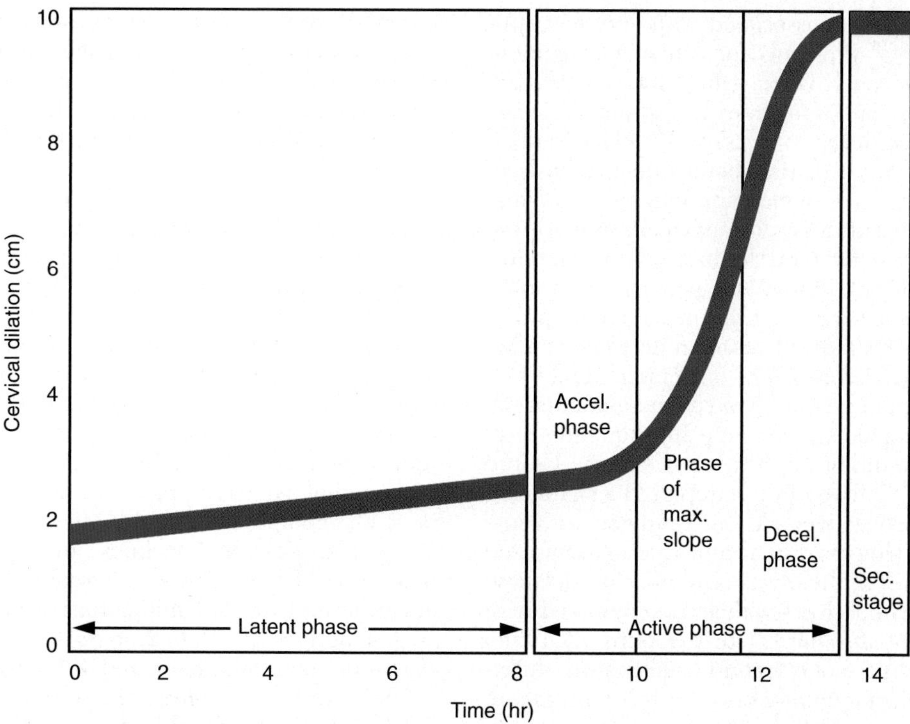

FIGURE 13-13. Modern labor graph. Characteristics of the average cervical dilation curve for nulliparous labor. (Modified from Friedman EA: Labor: Clinical Evaluation and Management, ed 2. Norwalk, CT, Appleton-Century-Crofts, 1978.)

third stage duration was 6 minutes and exceeded 30 minutes in only 3% of women.[44] A threshold of 30 minutes was associated with a significantly increased risk of a greater than 500 mL blood loss, a drop in postdelivery hematocrit by greater than or equal to 10%, or a need for dilation and curettage.[44] This suggests that manual removal and/or extraction of the placenta is indicated after 30 minutes.

Interventions Affecting Normal Labor Outcomes

Various interventions have been suggested to promote normal labor progress, including maternal ambulation during active labor (Figure 13-14). However, a well-designed randomized trial of over 1000 women in active labor comparing ambulation with usual care found no differences in the duration of the first stage, need for oxytocin, use of analgesia, or route of delivery.[45] In contrast, upright rather than recumbent positioning during labor was associated with significantly shorter first stage of labor and less epidural use.[46] In addition, the presence of a labor doula compared with no support was associated with a significant reduction in use of analgesia, oxytocin, and operative or cesarean delivery and an increase in satisfaction by the woman.[47] These data were compelling enough for doula support in labor to receive an A rating, meaning that it should be recommended for use during labor.[48] **In a randomized trial of nulliparas in active labor, IV administration at 125 mL/min of D_5NS was associated with a significant reduction in labor length and in second stage length compared to NS.**[49]

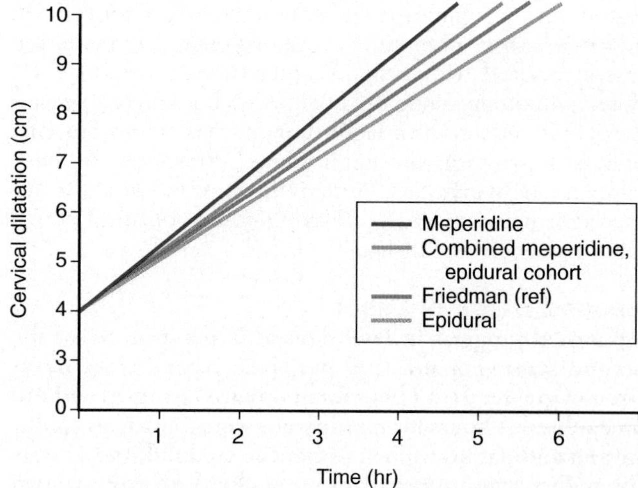

FIGURE 13-14. Comparison of the rates of cervical dilation during the active phase of labor originally reported by Friedman and now reported for the women who received patient-controlled intravenous meperidine, patient-controlled epidural analgesia, and the combined cohort. (From Alexander JM, Sharma SK, McIntire DD, Leveno KJ: Epidural analgesia lengthens the Friedman active phase of labor. Obstet Gynecol 100:46, 2002.)

Active Management of Labor

Dystocia is lack of progress of labor for any reason and is the second most common indication for cesarean delivery, following previous cesarean delivery. In the late 1980s, in an effort to reduce the rapidly rising cesarean delivery rate, active management of labor was popularized in the United States based on findings in Ireland, where the routine use of active management was associated with very low rates of cesarean delivery.[50] Protocols for active management included admission only when labor was established (painful contractions and spontaneous rupture of membranes, 100% effacement, or passage of blood-stained mucus); artificial rupture of membranes on diagnosis of labor; aggressive oxytocin augmentation for labor progress of less than 1 cm/hr with high-dose oxytocin (6 mIU/min initial dose, increased by 6 mIU/min every 15 minutes to a maximum of 40 mIU/min); and patient education.[50] Observational data suggested that this management protocol was associated with rates of cesarean delivery of 5.5% and delivery within 12 hours in 98% of women.[50] Only 41% of the nulliparas actually required oxytocin augmentation. Multiple nonrandomized studies were subsequently published attempting to duplicate these results in the United States and Canada.[51-54] Two of these reported a significant reduction in cesarean delivery when compared with historical controls.[51,53] However, in two of three randomized controlled trials (RCTs), there was no significant decrease in the rate of cesarean delivery with active compared with routine management of labor.[55,56] In the third RCT, the overall cesarean delivery rate was not significantly different; however, when confounding variables were controlled, cesarean delivery was significantly lower in the actively managed group.[54] In all randomized trials, labor duration was significantly decreased by a range of 1.7 to 2.7 hours, and neonatal morbidity was not different between groups. A recent Cochrane review concluded that early oxytocin augmentation in women with spontaneous labor was associated with a significant decrease in cesarean delivery. In addition, early amniotomy with oxytocin augmentation was associated with a significantly shortened labor.[57] Of note, amniotomy alone did not affect labor length or cesarean. This reduction in labor duration has significant cost and bed management implications, especially for busy labor and delivery units. Perhaps the most important factor in active management is delaying admission until active labor has been established.

Second Stage of Labor

Abnormal progress in fetal descent is the dystocia of the second stage. For practical purposes, second-stage durations of greater than 1 hour for multiparous women without an epidural, 2 hours for multiparous women with an epidural and nulliparous women without an epidural, and 3 hours for nulliparous women with an epidural identify women who are outliers, representing only 5% of women in these categories (see Table 13-2).[35] In nulliparous women vaginal delivery decreased, and chorioamnionitis, severe tears, and uterine atony increased significantly with second stages longer than 3 hours. However, neonatal outcome was not altered.[58] Although there is no indication that these limits should be used arbitrarily to justify ending the second stage, they identify a subset of women who require further evaluation.[58]

Other models include prospectively determined second-stage partograms in which the median second-stage lengths are similar to those outlined in Table 13-2.[59] Women with a prolonged second stage by these criteria should be evaluated for potential interventions. As with active labor, poor progress may be related to inadequate contractions; initiating oxytocin in the second stage may be effective if contraction frequency is diminished. If malposition is diagnosed, rotation to OA (either manually or by forceps) may be indicated in the second stage. If neither uterine forces nor fetal position are abnormal, the default diagnosis is cephalopelvic disproportion. No excess neonatal morbidity has been reported in association with a prolonged second stage in the absence of nonreassuring fetal heart rate tracings. Therefore, if steady progress is observed, there is no need for arbitrary time cut-offs.[60-64] In contrast, maternal morbidity, including perineal trauma, postpartum hemorrhage, and chorioamnionitis, is significantly higher in women with a second stage lasting longer than 2 or 3 hours.[58,64] However, it is important to note that performing an instrument-assisted vaginal delivery is unlikely to reduce perineal trauma and morbidity. If the fetal heart rate tracing is reassuring, continuing the second stage beyond 3 hours is reasonable. After 4 hours, the likelihood of vaginal delivery declines and maternal morbidity increases. The incidence of a vaginal delivery, including operative delivery, in nulliparous women with a second stage length of less than 2 hours, 2 to 4 hours, and longer than 4 hours is 98%, 81%, and 45%, respectively.[58]

Multiple factors influence the duration of the second stage, including epidural analgesia, nulliparity, older maternal age, longer active phase, larger birth weight, and excess maternal weight gain.[58,59] Modifiable factors that have been evaluated in the management of the second stage include maternal position, decreasing epidural analgesia (see Chapter 17), and delayed pushing. Two of three RCTs of decreased second-stage epidural analgesia found no difference in outcome or second-stage length.[65-67] One reported a decrease in second-stage length and operative delivery in the group that was randomized to reduced levels of epidural analgesia.[65] Epidural analgesia is clearly associated with an increased rate of operative delivery and associated perineal injury.[67,68] Delayed pushing has also been studied in nulliparas with epidural analgesia to determine if this strategy reduces the need for operative delivery, but little benefit has been demonstrated.[68-71] Only one trial reported a significant decrease in operative deliveries, and that was limited to midpelvic deliveries.[69] Conversely, the risk of delayed pushing appears to be negligible. Finally, the effect of maternal position has been evaluated.[72,73] Randomization to squatting using a birth cushion was associated with a significant reduction in operative deliveries and a significantly shorter second stage in nulliparas compared with delivery in the lithotomy position.[72] In a second trial randomizing women to either a routine delivery position or any upright position (squatting, kneeling, sitting, or standing per patient choice), no difference in operative deliveries was noted between groups but a significant increase in the percent of women with an intact perineum was noted in the upright group.[73] Therefore, allowing women to choose alternative positions during the second stage may be beneficial, especially in nulliparas.

SPONTANEOUS VAGINAL DELIVERY

Preparation for delivery should take into account the patient's parity, the progression of labor, fetal presentation, and any labor complications. Among women for whom delivery complications are anticipated (shoulder dystocia risk factors or multiple gestation), transfer to a larger and better equipped delivery room, removal of the foot of the bed, and delivery in the lithotomy position may be appropriate. If no complications are anticipated, delivery can be accomplished with the mother in her preferred position. Common positions include the lateral (Sims) position or the partial sitting position.

The goals of clinical assistance at spontaneous delivery are the reduction of maternal trauma, prevention of fetal injury, and initial support of the newborn, if required. When the fetal head crowns and delivery is imminent, gentle pressure should be used to maintain flexion of the fetal head and to control delivery, potentially protecting against perineal injury. Once the fetal head is delivered, external rotation (restitution) is allowed. If a shoulder dystocia is anticipated, it is appropriate to proceed directly with gentle downward traction of the fetal head before restitution occurs. During restitution, nuchal umbilical cords should be identified and reduced; in rare cases in which simple reduction is not possible, the cord can be doubly clamped and transected. **There is no evidence that DeLee suction reduces the risk of meconium aspiration syndrome in the presence of meconium; thus this should not be performed.**[74] The anterior shoulder should then be delivered by gentle downward traction in concert with maternal expulsive efforts. The posterior shoulder is delivered by upward traction. These movements should be performed with the minimal force possible to avoid perineal injury and traction injuries to the brachial plexus. The timing of cord clamping is usually dictated by convenience and commonly performed immediately after delivery. However, an ongoing debate exists about the benefits and risks of late cord clamping to the newborn. One meta-analysis of trials comparing late (greater than 2 minutes) to immediate cord clamping in term babies showed a significant increase in infant hematocrit, ferrintin, and stored iron levels at 2 to 6 months.[75] However, there was also a significant increase in neonatal polycythemia in the delayed group. After delivery, the infant should be wiped dry and kept warm while any mucus remaining in the airway is suctioned. Keeping the infant warm is particularly important, and, because heat is lost quickly from the head, placing a hat on the infant is appropriate. If possible all of these steps can best be done with the infant on the mother's abdomen.

DELIVERY OF THE PLACENTA AND FETAL MEMBRANES

The third stage of labor can be managed either passively or actively. Passive management is characterized by patiently waiting for the classic signs of placental separation: (1) lengthening of the umbilical cord, and (2) a gush of blood from the vagina signifying separation of the placenta from the uterine wall. In addition, two techniques of controlled cord traction are commonly used to facilitate separation and delivery of the placenta: the *Brandt-Andrews maneuver* (in which an abdominal hand secures the uterine fundus to prevent uterine inversion while the other hand exerts sustained downward traction on the umbilical cord) or the *Crède maneuver* (in which the cord is fixed with the lower hand while the uterine fundus is secured and sustained upward traction is applied using the abdominal hand). Care should be taken to avoid avulsion of the cord. Active management with uterotonic agents such as oxytocin administered at delivery hasten delivery of the placenta and may reduce the incidence of postpartum hemorrhage and total blood loss.[76] Conversely, other studies have shown no benefit to active management in the second stage.[77]

After delivery, the placenta, umbilical cord, and fetal membranes should be examined. Placental weight (excluding membranes and cord) varies with fetal weight, with a ratio of approximately 1:6. Abnormally large placentae are associated with such conditions as hydrops fetalis and congenital syphilis. **Inspection and palpation of the placenta should include the fetal and maternal surfaces and may reveal areas of fibrosis, infarction, or calcification.** Although each of these conditions may be seen in the normal term placenta, extensive lesions should prompt histologic examination. Adherent clots on the maternal placental surface may indicate recent placental abruption; however, their absence does not exclude the diagnosis. A missing placental cotyledon or a membrane defect (suggesting a missing succenturiate lobe) suggests retention of a portion of placenta and should prompt further clinical evaluation. There is no need for routine manual exploration of the uterus after delivery unless there is suspicion of retained products of conception or a postpartum hemorrhage.

The site of insertion of the umbilical cord into the placenta should be noted. Abnormal insertions include marginal insertion (in which the cord inserts into the edge of the placenta) and membranous insertion (in which the vessels of the umbilical cord course through the membranes before attachment to the placental disk). The cord itself should be inspected for length, the correct number of umbilical vessels (normally two arteries and one vein), true knots, hematomas, and strictures. The average cord length is 50 to 60 cm. A single umbilical artery discovered on pathologic examination is associated with other fetal structural anomalies in 27% of cases.[78,79] Therefore, this finding should be relayed to the attending neonatologist or pediatrician. Any abnormalities of the placenta or cord should be noted in the mother's chart.

EPISIOTOMY, PERINEAL INJURY, AND PERINEAL REPAIR

Following delivery of the placenta, the vagina and perineum should be carefully examined for evidence of injury. If a laceration is seen, its length and position should be noted and repair initiated. Adequate analgesia (either regional or local) is essential for repair. Special attention should be paid to repair of the perineal body, the external anal sphincter, and the rectal mucosa. Failure to recognize and repair rectal injury can lead to serious long-term morbidity, most notably fecal incontinence. The cervix should be inspected for lacerations if an operative delivery was performed or if there is significant bleeding with or after the delivery.

Perineal injuries, either spontaneous or with episiotomy, are the most common complications of spontaneous or operative vaginal deliveries. **A first-degree tear is defined as a superficial tear confined to the epithelial layer and may**

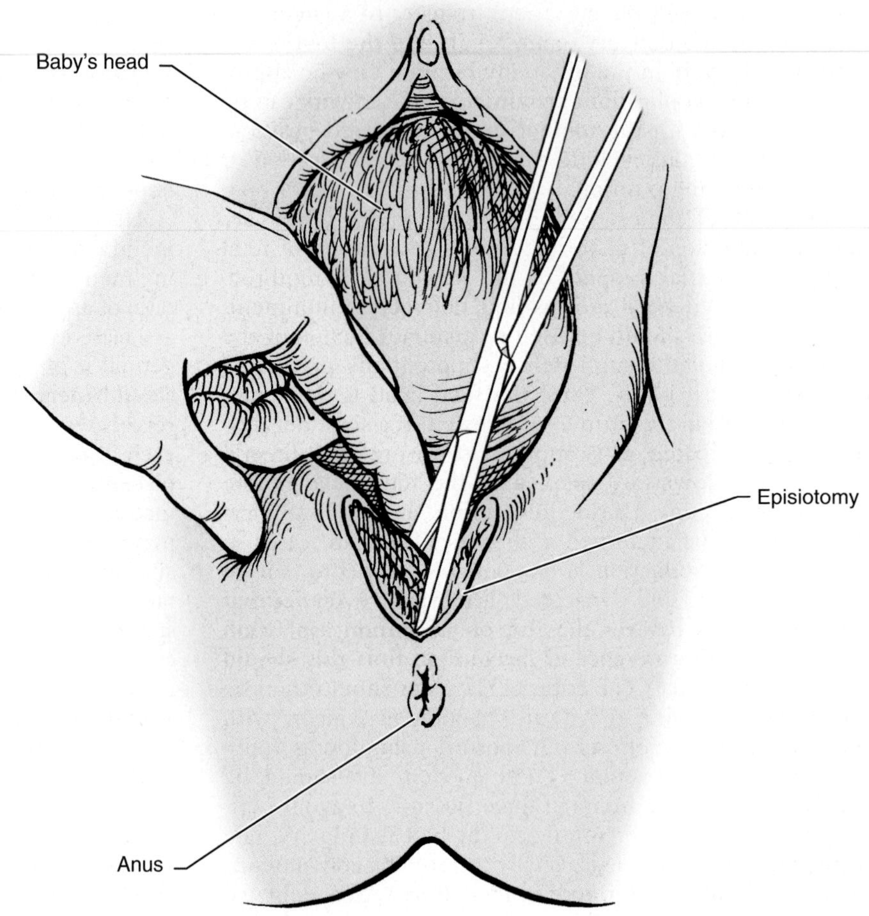

FIGURE 13-15. Cutting a midline episiotomy.

or may not need to be repaired generally depending on amount of bleeding. Second-degree tears extend into the perineal body, but not into the external anal sphincter. Third-degree tears involve superficial or deep injury to the external anal sphincter, whereas a fourth-degree tear extends completely through the sphincter and the rectal mucosa. All second-, third-, and fourth-degree tears should be repaired. Significant morbidity is associated with third- and fourth-degree tears, including risk of flatus and stool incontinence, rectovaginal fistula, infection, and pain. Primary approximation of perineal lacerations affords the best opportunity for functional repair, especially if there is evidence of rectal sphincter injury. The external anal sphincter should be repaired by direct apposition or overlapping the cut ends and securing them using interrupted sutures.

Episiotomy is an incision into the perineal body made during the second stage of labor to facilitate delivery. It is by definition a second-degree tear. Episiotomy can be classified into two broad categories: median (midline) and mediolateral. Median episiotomy refers to a vertical midline incision from the posterior forchette toward the rectum (Figure 13-15). After adequate analgesia, either local or regional, has been achieved, straight Mayo scissors are generally used to perform the episiotomy. Care should be taken to displace the perineum from the fetal head. The size of the incision depends on the length of the perineum but is generally approximately half of the length of the perineum and should be extended vertically up the vaginal mucosa for a distance of 2 to 3 cm. Every effort should be made to avoid direct injury to the anal sphincter. **Complications of median episiotomy include increased blood loss (especially if the incision is made too early), fetal injury, and localized pain.** With a mediolateral episiotomy, the incision is made at a 45-degree angle from the inferior portion of the hymeneal ring (Figure 13-16). The length of the incision is less critical than with median episiotomy, but longer incisions require lengthier repair. The side to which the episiotomy is performed is usually dictated by the dominant hand of the practitioner. Because such incisions appear to be moderately protective against severe perineal trauma, they are the procedure of choice for women with inflammatory bowel disease, if an episiotomy is needed, because of the critical need to prevent rectal injury. Historically, it was believed that episiotomy improved outcome by reducing pressure on the fetal head, protecting the maternal perineum from extensive tearing, and subsequent pelvic relaxation. However, consistent data since the late 1980s confirm that midline episiotomy does not protect the perineum from further tearing and data do not show that episiotomy improves neonatal outcome.[64,80,81] Midline episiotomy was associated with a significant increase of third- and fourth-degree lacerations in spontaneous vaginal

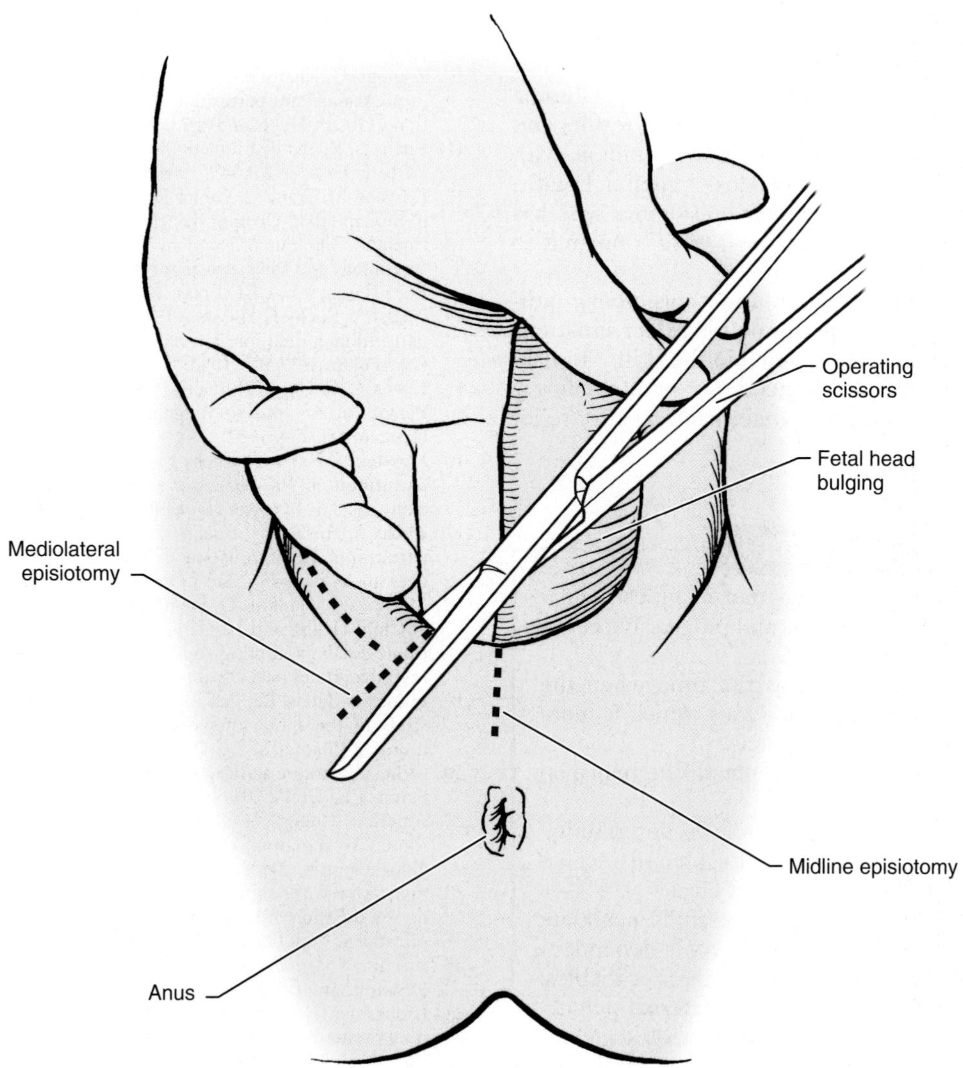

FIGURE 13-16. Cutting a mediolateral episiotomy.

delivery in nulliparous women with both spontaneous and operative vaginal delivery.[81-87] Episiotomy had the highest odds ratio (OR 3.2; CI 2.73-3.80) for anal sphincter laceration in a large study of nulliparous women when compared to other risk factors, including forceps delivery.[88] Fewer papers reported that midline episiotomy was associated with no difference in fourth-degree tears compared to no episiotomy.[89] **Based on the lack of consistent evidence that episiotomy is of benefit, there is no role for routine episiotomy in modern obstetrics.**[80,81,90,91] In fact, a recent evidence-based review recommended that episiotomy should be avoided if possible, based on U.S. Preventive Task Force quality of evidence.[48] Based on these data and ACOG recommendations,[91] rates of midline episiotomy have decreased, although episiotomies are performed in 10% to 17% of deliveries, suggesting that elective episiotomy continues to be performed.[83,92] Decreasing episiotomy rates from 87% in 1976 to 10% in 1994 were associated with a parallel decrease in the rates of third- or fourth-degree lacerations (9% to 4%) and an increase in the incidence of an intact perineum (10% to 26%).[83] Randomized trials comparing routine to indicated use of episiotomy report a 23% reduction in perineal lacerations requiring repair in the indicated group (11% to 35%).[92] Finally, a recent Cochrane review of eight randomized trials comparing restrictive to routine use of episiotomy showed a significant reduction of severe perineal tears, suturing, and healing complications in the restrictive group.[93] Although the restrictive episiotomy group had a significantly higher incidence of anterior tears, there was no difference in pain measures between the groups. All of these findings were similar whether median or mediolateral episiotomy was used.

The relationship of episiotomy to subsequent pelvic relaxation and incontinence has been evaluated, with no studies suggesting that episiotomy reduces risk of incontinence. Clearly, fourth-degree tears are associated with future incontinence.[94] Neither midline nor mediolateral episiotomy was associated with a reduction in incontinence.[95] **Therefore, there are no data to suggest that episiotomy protects the woman from later incontinence and avoidance of fourth-degree tear should be a priority.**

If an episiotomy is deemed indicated, the decision of which type to perform rests on their individual risks. It does appear that mediolateral episiotomy is associated with fewer fourth-degree tears compared to median episiotomy.[96-98] However, other studies do not show benefit of mediolateral over median for future prolapse.[95] Chronic complications such as unsatisfactory cosmetic results and inclusions within the scar may be more common with mediolateral episiotomies, and blood loss is greater. Finally, it must be remembered that neither episiotomy type has been shown to reduce severe perineal tears compared to no episiotomy.

Although there is no role for routine episiotomy, indicated episiotomy should be performed in select situations and providers should receive training in the skill.[89] Indications for episiotomy include the need to expedite delivery in the setting of fetal heart rate abnormalities or for relief of shoulder dystocia.

KEY POINTS

- ◆ Labor is a clinical diagnosis that includes regular painful uterine contractions and progressive cervical effacement and dilation.
- ◆ Active labor is diagnosed as the time when the slope of cervical change increases, which is more difficult to identify in nulliparas.
- ◆ Active labor and latent labor should be managed differently.
- ◆ The fetus likely plays a key role in determining the onset of labor, although the precise mechanism by which this occurs is not clear.
- ◆ The ability of the fetus to successfully negotiate the pelvis during labor and delivery is dependent on the complex interaction of three variables: uterine force, the fetus, and the maternal pelvis.
- ◆ Labor length is affected by many variables, including parity, epidural use, fetal position, fetal size, and BMI.
- ◆ Routine median episiotomy is associated with a significant increase in the incidence of severe perineal trauma and should be avoided.

REFERENCES

1. Liao J, Buhimschi C, Norwitz E: Normal labor: mechanism and duration. Obstet Gynecol Clin North Am 32:145, 2005.
2. Challis J, Gibb W: Control of parturition. Prenat Neonat Med 1:283, 1996.
3. Garfield R, Blennerhassett M, Miller S: Control of myometrial contractility: role and regulation of gap junctions. Oxford Rev Reprod Biol 10:436, 1988.
4. Liggins G: Initiation of labour. Neonatology 55:366, 1989.
5. Nathanielsz P: Comparative studies on the initiation of labor. Eur J Obstet Gynecol Reprod Biol 78:127, 1998.
6. Pieber D, Allport V, Hills F, et al: Interactions between progesterone receptor isoforms in myometrial cells in human labour. Molec Hum Reprod 7:875, 2001.
7. Mesiano S, Chan E, Fitter J, et al: Progesterone withdrawal and estrogen activation in human parturition are coordinated by progesterone receptor A expression in the myometrium. J Clin Endocrinol Metab 87:2924, 2002.
8. Oh S, Kim C, Park I, et al: Progesterone receptor isoform (A/B) ratio of human fetal membranes increases during term parturition. Am J Obstet Gynecol 193:1156, 2005.
9. Honnebier M, Nathanielsz P: Primate parturition and the role of the maternal circadian system. Eur J Obstet Gynecol Reprod Biol 55:193, 1994.
10. Zeeman G, Khan-Dawood F, Dawood M: Oxytocin and its receptor in pregnancy and parturition: current concepts and clinical implications. Obstet Gynecol 89:873, 1997.
11. Fuchs A, Fuchs F: Endocrinology of human parturition: a review. Br J Obstet Gynaecol 9:948, 1984.
12. Dawood M, Wang C, Gupta R, et al: Fetal contribution to oxytocin in human labor. Obstet Gynecol 52:205, 1978.
13. Fuchs A: The role of oxytocin in parturition. In Huszar G (ed): The Physiology and Biochemistry of the Uterus in Pregnancy and Labour. Boca Raton, FL, CRC Press, 1986, p 163.
14. Fuchs A, Fuchs F, Husslein P, et al: Oxytocin receptors and human parturition: a dual role for oxytocin in the initiation of labor. Obstet Gynecol Surv 37:567, 1982.
15. Fuchs A, Fuchs F, Husslein P, Soloff M: Oxytocin receptors in the human uterus during pregnancy and parturition. Am J Obstet Gynecol 150:734, 1984.
16. Husslein P, Fuchs A, Fuchs F: Oxytocin and the initiation of human parturition. I. Prostaglandin release during induction of labor by oxytocin. Am J Obstet Gynecol 141:688, 1981.
17. Fuchs A, Husslein P, Fuchs F: Oxytocin and the initiation of human parturition. II. Stimulation of prostaglandin production in human decidua by oxytocin. Am J Obstet Gynecol 141:694, 1981.
18. Macones G, Hankins G, Spong C, et al: The 2008 National Institute of Child Health and Human Development workshop report on electronic fetal monitoring: update on definitions, interpretation, and research guidelines. Obstet Gynecol 112:661, 2008.
19. Caldeyro-Barcia R, Sica-Blanco Y, Poseiro J, et al: A quantitative study of the action of synthetic oxytocin on the pregnant human uterus. J Pharmacol Exp Ther 121:18, 1957.
20. Miller F: Uterine activity, labor management, and perinatal outcome. Semin Perinatol 2:181, 1978.
21. American College of Obstetricians and Gynecologists: Fetal Macrosomia. Washington, DC, American College of Obstetricians and Gynecologists, 2000.
22. Siggelkow W, Boehm D, Skala C, et al: The influence of macrosomia on the duration of labor, the mode of delivery and intrapartum complications. Arch Gynecol Obstet 278:547, 2008.
23. Friedman E, Kroll B: Computer analysis of labor progression. II. Distribution of data and limits of normal. J Reprod Med 6:20, 1971.
24. Lieberman E, Davidson K, Lee-Parritz A, Shearer E: Changes in fetal position during labor and their association with epidural analgesia. Obstet Gynecol 105:974, 2005.
25. Piper J, Bolling D, Newton E: The second stage of labor: factors influencing duration. Am J Obstet Gynecol 165:976, 1991.
26. Joyce D, Giwa-Osagie F, Stevenson G: Role of pelvimetry in active management of labour. BMJ 4:505, 1975.
27. Morris C, Heggie J, Acton C: Computed tomography pelvimetry: accuracy and radiation dose compared with conventional pelvimetry. Aust Radiol 37:186, 1993.
28. Jeyabalan A, Larkin R, Landers D: Vaginal breech deliveries selected using computed tomographic pelvimetry may be associated with fewer adverse outcomes. J Maternal Fetal Neonatal Med 17:381, 2005.
29. Caldwell W, Moloy H: Anatomical variations in the female pelvis and their effect in labor, with a suggested classification. Am J Obstet Gynecol 26:479, 1933.
30. Friedman E: Primigravid labor. Obstet Gynecol 6:567, 1955.
31. Friedman E: Labor in multiparas; a graphicostatistical analysis. Obstet Gynecol 8:691, 1956.
32. Albers L, Schiff M, Gorwoda J: The length of active labor in normal pregnancies. Obstet Gynecol 87:355, 1996.
33. Bergsjo P, Halle C: Duration of the second stage of labor. Acta Obstet Gynecol Scand 59:193, 1980.
34. Duignan N, Studd J, Hughes A: Characteristics of normal labour in different racial groups. Br J Obstet Gynaecol 82:593,1975.
35. Kilpatrick S, Laros R Jr: Characteristics of normal labor. Obstet Gynecol 74:85, 1989.
36. Zhang J, Troendle J, Mikolajczyk R, et al: The natural history of the normal first stage of labor. Obstet Gynecol 115:705, 2010.
37. Rouse D, Owen J, Savage K, Hauth J: Active phase labor arrest: revisiting the 2-hour minimum. Obstet Gynecol 98:550, 2001.
38. Schulman H, Ledger W: Practical applications of the graphic portrayal of labor. Obstet Gynecol 23:442, 1964.

39. Vahratian A, Zhang J, Troendle J, et al: Maternal prepregnancy overweight and obesity and the pattern of labor progression in term nulliparous women. Obstet Gynecol 104:943, 2004.
40. Sheiner E, Levy A, Feinstein U, et al: Risk factors and outcome of failure to progress during the first stage of labor: a population based study. Acta Obstet Gynecol Scand 81:222, 2002.
41. Greenberg MB, Cheng YW, Sullivan M, et al: Does length of labor vary by maternal age? Am J Obstet Gynecol 197:428, 2007.
42. Dencker A, Berg M, Bergqvist L, Lilja H: Identification of latent phase factors associated with active labor duration in low-risk nulliparous women with spontaneous contractions. Acta Obstet Gynecol Scand 89:1034, 2010.
43. Greenberg MB, Cheng YW, Hopkins LM, et al: Are there ethnic differences in the length of labor? Am J Obstet Gynecol 195:743, 2006.
44. Combs C, Laros R Jr: Prolonged third stage of labor: morbidity and risk factors. Obstet Gynecol 77:863, 1991.
45. Bloom S, McIntire D, Kelly M, et al: Lack of effect of walking on labor and delivery. N Engl J Med 339:76, 1998.
46. Lawrence A, Lewis L, Hofmeyr G, et al: Maternal positions and mobility during first stage labour. Cochrane Database Syst Rev, 2009.
47. Hodnett E, Gates S, Hofmeyr G, Sakala C: Continuous support for women during childbirth. Cochrane Database Syst Rev CD003766, 2007.
48. Berghella V, Baxter JK, Chauhan SP: Evidence-based labor and delivery management. Am J Obstet Gynecol 199:445, 2008.
49. Shrivastava VK, Garite TJ, Jenkins SM, et al: A randomized, double-blinded, controlled trial comparing parenteral normal saline with and without dextrose on the course of labor in nulliparas. Am J Obstet Gynecol 200:379, 2009.
50. O'Driscoll K, Foley M, MacDonald D: Active management of labor as an alternative to cesarean section for dystocia. Obstet Gynecol 63:485, 1984.
51. Akoury H, Brodie G, Caddick R, et al: Active management of labor and operative delivery in nulliparous women. Am J Obstet Gynecol 158:255, 1988.
52. Akoury H, MacDonald F, Brodie G, et al: Oxytocin augmentation of labor and perinatal outcome in nulliparas. Obstet Gynecol 78:227, 1991.
53. Boylan P, Frankowski R, Rountree R, et al: Effect of active management of labor on the incidence of cesarean section for dystocia in nulliparas. Am J Perinatol 375:389, 1991.
54. López-Zeno J, Peaceman A, Adashek J, Socol M: A controlled trial of a program for the active management of labor. N Engl J Med 326:450, 1992.
55. Frigoletto F, Lieberman E, Lang J, et al: A clinical trial of active management of labor. N Engl J Med 333:745, 1995.
56. Rogers R, Gilson G, Miller A, et al: Active management of labor: does it make a difference? Am J Obstet Gynecol 177:599, 1997.
57. Wei S, Wo B, Xu H, et al: Early amniotomy and early oxytocin for prevention of, or therapy for, delay in first stage spontaneous labour compared with routine care. Cochrane Database Syst Rev 2009.
58. Rouse D, Weiner S, Bloom S, et al: Second-stage labor duration in nulliparous women: relationship to maternal and perinatal outcomes. Am J Obstet Gynecol 201:357, 2009.
59. Sizer A, Evans J, Bailey S, Wiener J: A second-stage partogram. Obstet Gynecol 96:678, 2000.
60. Cohen W: Influence of the duration of second stage labor on perinatal outcome and puerperal morbidity. Obstet Gynecol 49:266, 1977.
61. Deiham R, Crowhurst J, Crowther C: The second stage of labour: durational dilemmas. Aust N Z J Obstet Gynaecol 31:31, 1991.
62. Menticoglou S, Manning F, Harman C, Morrison I: Perinatal outcome in relation to second-stage duration. Am J Obstet Gynecol 173:906, 1995.
63. Moon J, Smith C, Rayburn W: Perinatal outcome after a prolonged second stage of labor. J Reprod Med 35:229, 1990.
64. Myles T, Santolaya J: Maternal and neonatal outcomes in patients with a prolonged second stage of labor. Obstet Gynecol 102:52, 2003.
65. Chestnut D, Bates J, Choi W: Continuous infusion epidural analgesia with lidocaine: efficacy and influence during the second stage of labor. Obstet Gynecol 69:323, 1987.
66. Chestnut D, Laszewski L, Pollack K, et al: Continuous epidural infusion of 0.0625% bupivacaine-0.0002% fentanyl during the second stage of labor. Anesthesiology 72:613, 1990.
67. Chestnut D, Vandewalker G, Owen C, et al: The influence of continuous epidural bupivacaine analgesia on the second stage of labor and method of delivery in nulliparous women. Anesthesiology 66:774, 1987.
68. Manyonda I, Shaw D, Drife J: The effect of delayed pushing in the second stage of labor with continuous lumbar epidural analgesia. Acta Obstet Gynecol Scand 69:291, 1990.
69. Fraser W, Marcoux S, Krauss I, et al: Multicenter, randomized, controlled trial of delayed pushing for nulliparous women in the second stage of labor with continuous epidural analgesia. Am J Obstet Gynecol 182:1165, 2000.
70. Hansen S, Clark S, Foster J: Active pushing versus passive fetal descent in the second stage of labor: a randomized controlled trial. Obstet Gynecol 99:29, 2002.
71. Plunkett B, Lin A, Wong C, et al: Management of the second stage of labor in nulliparas with continuous epidural analgesia. Obstet Gynecol 102:109, 2003.
72. Gardosi J, Hutson N: Randomised, controlled trial of squatting in the second stage of labour. Lancet 334:74, 1989.
73. Gardosi J, Sylvester S, B-Lynch C: Alternative positions in the second stage of labour: a randomized controlled trial. Br J Obstet Gynaecol 96:1290, 1989.
74. ACOG Committee Obstetric Practice ACOG Committee No. 346: Amnioinfusion does not prevent meconium aspiration syndrome. Obstet Gynecol 108:1053, 2006.
75. Hutton E, Hassan E: Late vs early clamping of the umbilical cord in full-term neonates: systematic review and meta-analysis of controlled trials. JAMA 297:1241, 2007.
76. Rogers J, Wood J, McCandlish R, et al: Active versus expectant management of third stage of labour: the Hinchingbrooke randomised controlled trial. Lancet 351:693, 1998.
77. Jackson K: A randomized controlled trial comparing oxytocin administration before and after placental delivery in the prevention of postpartum hemorrhage. Am J Obstet Gynecol 185:873, 2001.
78. Prucka S, Clemens M, Craven C, McPherson E: Single umbilical artery: what does it mean for the fetus? A case-control analysis of pathologically ascertained cases. Genet Med 6:54, 2004.
79. Thummala M, Raju T, Langenberg P: Isolated single umbilical artery anomaly and the risk for congenital malformations: a meta-analysis. J Pediatr Surg 33:580, 1998.
80. Thorp J, Bowes W: Episiotomy: can its routine use be defended? Am J Obstet Gynecol 160:1027, 1989.
81. Shiono P, Klebanof M, Carey J: Midline episiotomies: more harm than good? Obstet Gynecol 75:765, 1990.
82. Angioli R, Gómez-Marín O, Cantuaria G, O'Sullivan M: Severe perineal lacerations during vaginal delivery: the University of Miami experience. Am J Obstet Gynecol 182:1083, 2000.
83. Bansal R, Tan W, Ecker J, et al: Is there a benefit to episiotomy at spontaneous vaginal delivery? A natural experiment. Am J Obstet Gynecol 175:897, 1996.
84. Robinson J, Norwitz E, Cohen A, et al: Epidural analgesia and the occurrence of third and fourth degree obstetric laceration in nulliparas. Obstet Gynecol 94:259, 1999.
85. Helwig J, Thorp J Jr, Bowes W Jr: Does midline episiotomy increase the risk of third- and fourth-degree lacerations in operative vaginal deliveries? Obstet Gynecol 82:276, 1993.
86. Ecker J, Tan W, Bansal R, et al: Is there a benefit to episiotomy at operative vaginal delivery? Observations over ten years in a stable population. Am J Obstet Gynecol 176:411, 1997.
87. Robinson J, Norwitz E, Cohen A, et al: Episiotomy, operative vaginal delivery, and significant perineal trauma in nulliparous women. Am J Obstet Gynecol 181:1180, 1999.
88. Baumann P, Hammoud AO, McNeeley SG, et al: Factors associated with anal sphincter laceration in 40,923 primiparous women. Int Urogynecol J 18:985, 2007.
89. Eason E, Labrecque M, Wells G, Feldman P: Preventing perineal trauma during childbirth: a systematic review. Obstet Gynecol 95:464, 2000.
90. Hartmann K, Viswanathan M, Palmieri R, et al: Outcomes of routine episiotomy: a systematic review. JAMA 293:2141, 2005.
91. American College of Obstetricians and Gynecologists: ACOG Practice Guidelines on Episiotomy. Washington, DC, American College of Obstetricians and Gynecologists, 2006.
92. Clemons J, Towers G, McClure G, O'Boyle A: Decreased anal sphincter lacerations associated with restrictive episiotomy use. Am J Obstet Gynecol 192:1620, 2005.

93. Carroli G, Belizan J: Episiotomy for vaginal birth. Cochrane Database Syst Rev 1: CD000081, 2009.
94. Fenner D, Genberg B, Brahma P, et al: Fecal and urinary incontinence after vaginal delivery with anal sphincter disruption in an obstetrics unit in the United States. Am J Obstet Gynecol 189:1543, 2003.
95. Sartore A, De Seta F, Maso G, et al: The effects of mediolateral episiotomy on pelvic floor function after vaginal delivery. Obstet Gynecol 103:669, 2004.
96. Riskin-Mashiah S, O'Brian Smith E, Wilkins I: Risk factors for severe perineal tear: can we do better? Am J Perinatol 19:225, 2002.
97. Signorello L, Harlow B, Chekos A, Repke J: Midline episiotomy and anal incontinence: retrospective cohort study. BMJ 320:86, 2000.
98. De Leeuw J, Vierhout M, Struijk P, et al: Anal sphincter damage after vaginal delivery: functional outcome and risk factors for fecal incontinence. Acta Obstet Gynecol Scand 80:830, 2001.

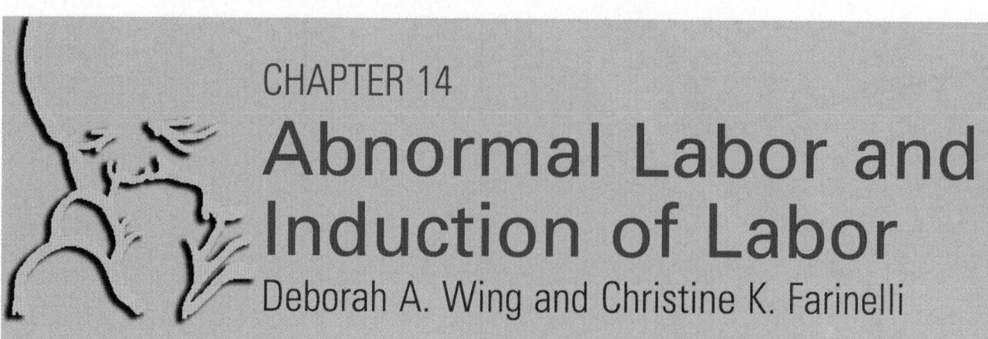

CHAPTER 14

Abnormal Labor and Induction of Labor

Deborah A. Wing and Christine K. Farinelli

KEY ABBREVIATIONS	
American College of Obstetricians and Gynecologists	ACOG
Active Management of Risk in Pregnancy at Term	AMOR-IPAT
Cephalopelvic Disproportion	CPD
Confidence Interval	CI
Electronic Fetal Monitoring	EFM
Extra-amniotic Saline Infusion	EASI
Food and Drug Administration	FDA
Group B Streptococcus	GBS
Intrauterine Pressure Catheter	IUPC
National Institute of Child Health and Human Development	NICHD
Occiput Posterior	OP
Odds Ratio	OR
Premature Rupture of Membranes	PROM
Prostaglandin	PG
Prostaglandin E_1 Misoprostol	PGE_1
Prostaglandin E_2 Dinoprostone	PGE_2
Relative Risk	RR

Labor is the physiologic process by which a fetus is expelled from the uterus to the outside world. A switch from contractures (long-lasting, low-frequency activity) to contractions (frequent, high-intensity, high-frequency activity) occurs before progressive cervical effacement and dilation of the cervix and regular uterine contractions. The timing of the switch varies from patient to patient. The exact trigger for the onset of labor is unknown, but there is considerable evidence to suggest that the fetus provides the stimulus through complex neuronal-hormonal signaling (see Chapter 13).

The mean duration of a human singleton pregnancy is 280 days or 40 weeks from the first day of the last menstrual period assuming a normal 28-day menstrual cycle. *Term* is defined as the period from 36 completed ($37^{0/7}$) to 42 weeks of gestation. *Preterm* labor refers to the onset of labor before 36 completed weeks of gestation. Prolonged or *postterm pregnancy* refers to gestation continuing beyond 42 completed weeks.

DIAGNOSIS

Labor is a clinical diagnosis defined as uterine contractions resulting in progressive cervical effacement and dilation, often accompanied by a bloody discharge referred to as *bloody show,* which results in birth of the baby. The diagnosis of bona fide labor is often elusive. There are wide variations in the clinical spectrum of normal labor, as well as many opinions of the definitions for normal and abnormal labor progress. To gain an understanding of abnormal labor progress and induction of labor, a fundamental understanding of normal spontaneous labor is needed.

ABNORMAL LABOR AT TERM

Most guidelines for normal human labor progress are derived from Friedman's clinical observations of women in labor.[1] Friedman characterized a sigmoid pattern for labor when graphing cervical dilation against time (Figure 14-1). He divided labor into three functional divisions: the *preparatory division, dilation division,* and *pelvic division.* The preparatory division is better known as the *latent phase,* during which little cervical dilation occurs but considerable changes are taking place in the connective tissue components of the cervix. The dilation division or *active phase* is the period when dilation proceeds at its most rapid rate to complete cervical dilation. These two phases together make up the *first stage of labor.* The *pelvic division* or *second stage of labor* refers to the time of full cervical

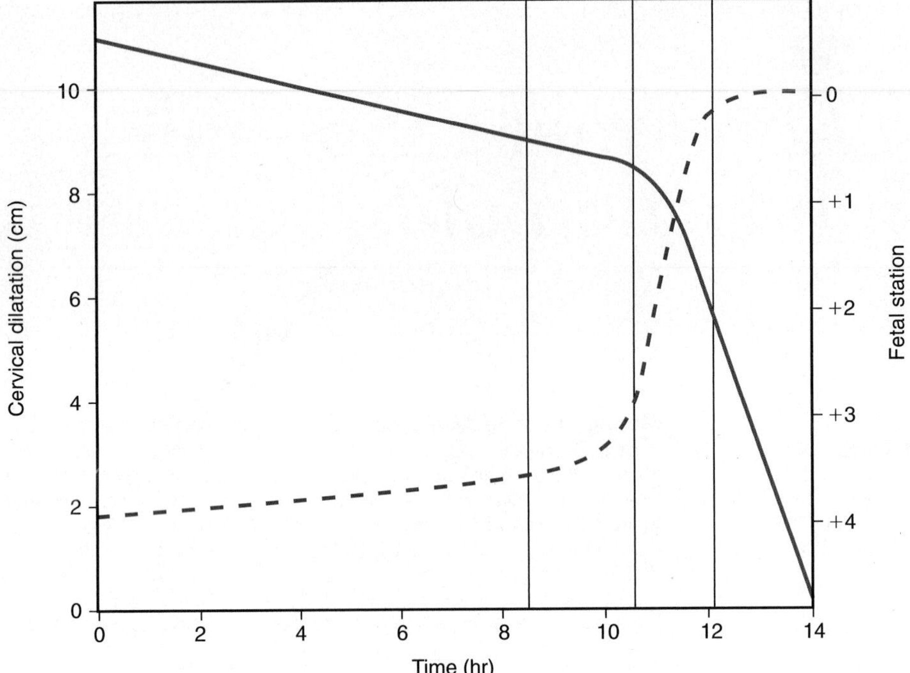

FIGURE 14-1. Characteristics of the average cervical dilation curve for nulliparous labor. (Modified from Friedman EA: Labor: Clinical Evaluation and Management, 2nd ed. Norwalk, CT, Appleton-Century-Crofts, 1978.)

dilation to the delivery of the infant. The *third stage of labor* refers to the time from the delivery of the infant to expulsion of the placenta.

Subsequent observations challenge Friedman's original labor curves. Between 1959 and 1966, the National Collaborative Perinatal Project prospectively observed labor progression, as well as several other factors possibly associated with cerebral palsy. This large multicenter project gathered data at a time when natural labor progress could be evaluated more easily than current obstetrical practices allow. Using these data, Zhang and colleagues for the Consortium for Safe Labor[2] determined that the active phase of labor as described by Friedman may not actually begin until 5 cm dilation in multiparas and even later in nulliparas. As well, before 6 cm of dilation, a 2-hour threshold for diagnosing labor arrest may be too brief whereas a 4-hour threshold may be too lengthy after 6 cm of dilation. Although cervical dilation does accelerate as labor advances, a precipitous dilation as described by Friedman may not necessarily occur, especially in nulliparas. Additional analyses regarding contemporary labor progress are expected from this project. Regardless of those results, a **graduated approach for diagnosis of labor protraction and arrest should be considered, based on the level of cervical dilation** (Table 14-1).

TABLE 14-1 PROGRESSION OF SPONTANEOUS LABOR AT TERM (ZHANG)

CERVICAL DILATION (cm)	PARITY 0	PARITY 1	PARITY 2+
From 3 to 4	1.2 (6.6)		
From 4 to 5	0.9 (4.5)	0.7 (3.3)	0.7 (3.5)
From 5 to 6	0.6 (2.6)	0.4 (1.6)	0.4 (1.6)
From 6 to 7	0.5 (1.8)	0.4 (1.2)	0.3 (1.2)
From 7 to 8	0.4 (1.4)	0.3 (0.8)	0.3 (0.7)
From 8 to 9	0.4 (1.3)	0.3 (0.7)	0.2 (0.6)
From 9 to 10	0.4 (1.2)	0.2 (0.5)	0.2 (0.5)
From 4 to 10	3.7 (16.7)	2.4 (13.8)	2.2 (14.2)

Data presented in hours as median (95th percentile). Data from Zhang J, Troendle J, Mikolajczyk R, et al: The natural history of the normal first stage of labor. Obstet Gynecol 115:705, 2010.

Disorders of the Latent Phase

The onset of latent labor is considered to be the point at which regular uterine contractions are perceived. Friedman found that the mean duration of latent labor was 6.4 hours for nulliparas and 4.8 hours for multiparas. The 95th percentiles for maximum length in latent labor was 20 hours for nulliparous women and 14 hours for multiparous women. These are considered the upper limits for time spent in latent labor (Table 14-2).[1]

Latent phase arrest implies that labor has not truly begun. Prolonged latent phase refers to a latent phase lasting longer than the 95th percentiles.[1] **Because the duration of latent labor is highly variable, expectant management is most appropriate.** Some women can spend days in latent labor; provided there is no indication for delivery, awaiting active labor is appropriate. If expeditious delivery is indicated, augmentation of labor may be initiated with a pharmacologic agent such as oxytocin. Another option is to administer "therapeutic rest," especially if contractions are painful or the patient is exhausted, with an analgesic agent such as morphine. A recommended dosing regimen is a single administration of 15 to 20 mg of morphine subcutaneously or intramuscularly. Often this will help abate or alleviate painful contractions and allow the patient to rest comfortably until active labor begins. The onset of regular contractions is often unpredictable after amniotomy and, therefore, such therapy is not recommended in nulliparas with prolonged latent phase. Early amniotomy may increase the risk of prolonged membrane rupture and its associated infectious morbidity.

TABLE 14-2 PROGRESSION OF SPONTANEOUS LABOR AT TERM (FRIEDMAN)

PARAMETER	MEDIAN	5th PERCENTILE
Nulliparas		
Total duration	10.1 hr	25.8 hr
Stages		
First	9.7 hr	24.7 hr
Second	33.0 min	117.5 min
Third	5.0 min	30 min
Latent phase (duration)	6.4 hr	20.6 hr
Maximal dilation (rate)	3.0 cm/hr	1.2 cm/hr
Descent (rate)	3.3 cm/hr	1.0 cm/hr
Multiparas		
Total duration	6.2 hr	19.5 hr
Stages		
First	8.0 hr	18.8 hr
Second	8.5 min	46.5 min
Third	5.0 min	30 min
Latent phase (duration)	4.8 hr	13.6 hr
Maximal dilation (rate)	5.7 cm/hr	1.5 cm/hr
Descent (rate)	6.6 cm/hr	2.1 cm/hr

Data from Friedman EA: Primigravid labor: a graphicostatistical analysis. Obstet Gynecol 6:567, 1955; Friedman EA: Labor in multiparas: a graphicostatistical analysis. Obstet Gynecol 8:691, 1956; and Cohen W, Friedman EA (eds): Management of Labor. Baltimore, University Park Press, 1983.

Disorders of the Active Phase

Active labor demarcates a rapid change in cervical dilation. The change to active phase usually occurs when the cervix is dilated between 3 and 5 cm, but the most accurate diagnosis is retrospective. Friedman observed that the mean duration of active phase labor in nulliparas was 4.9 hours, with a standard deviation of 3.4 hours. The active phase begins once cervical dilation progresses at a minimum rate of 1.2 cm/hr for nulliparous women and 1.5 cm/hr for multiparous women, with a maximum duration of active phase reported to be 11.7 hours. Rates of cervical dilation varied greatly, ranging from 1.2 to 6.8 cm/hr.

Active-phase disorders may be divided into *protraction* and *arrest* disorders.[1] *Protraction* is defined as a slow rate of cervical change less than 1.2 cm/hr for the nullipara and less than 1.5 cm/hr for the multipara. These rates represent less than the 5th percentile for most gravidas (Figure 14-2). Whereas protraction disorders reflect slower than normal progress, arrest disorders consist of complete cessation of progress.

The most common cause of a protraction disorder is inadequate uterine activity. External tocodynamometry is used to evaluate the duration of and time interval between contractions but cannot be used to evaluate the strength of uterine contractions. The external monitor is held against the abdominal wall and records a relative measurement of uterine contraction intensity, reflecting the monitor's movement as the uterine shape changes. More precise measurements of uterine activity must be obtained with an intrauterine pressure catheter (IUPC). After amniotomy, an IUPC can be placed into the uterus to measure

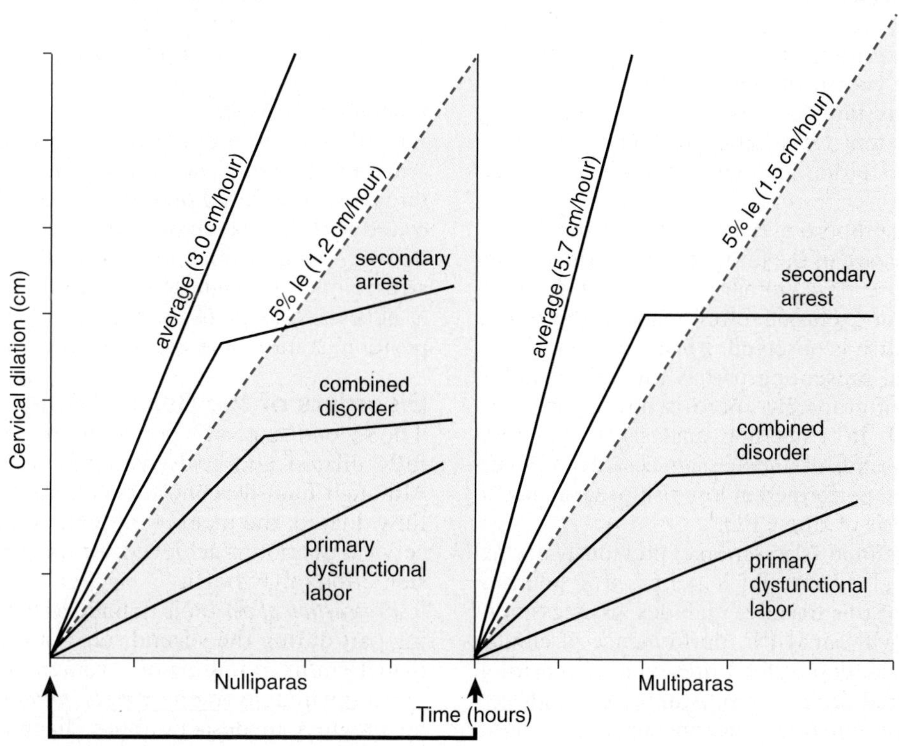

FIGURE 14-2. Disorders of the first stage of labor. Combined disorder implies an arrest in a gravida previously exhibiting primary dysfunctional labor.

the pressure generated during a uterine contraction. **An IUPC is frequently used when inadequate uterine activity is suspected owing to a protraction or arrest disorder. It can also be used to monitor and titrate oxytocin augmentation of labor to desired uterine effect.** The lower limit of contraction pressure required to dilate the cervix is observed to be 15 mm Hg over baseline. Normal spontaneous contractions often exert pressures up to 60 mm Hg.

Once inadequate uterine activity is diagnosed with an IUPC, oxytocin is usually administered. Typically, the dose is increased until there is normal progression of labor, resulting in strong contractions occurring at 2- to 3-minute intervals lasting 60 to 90 seconds, with a peak intrauterine pressure of 50 to 60 mm Hg and a resting tone of 10 to 15 mm Hg, or uterine activity equal to 150 to 350 Montevideo units. Montevideo units are calculated by subtracting the baseline uterine pressure from the peak contraction pressure of each contraction in a 10-minute window and adding the pressures generated by each contraction.

Another common cause of protraction disorders is abnormal positioning of the fetal presenting part. Some examples of malpresentation are an extended (rather than flexed) fetal head, brow or face presentation, and occiput posterior (OP) position. When persistent OP position is present, labor is reported to be prolonged an average 1 hour in multiparous women and 2 hours in nulliparous women. In one series, sonography showed OP position in 35% of women in early active labor, indicating that this may contribute to prolongation of labor in many women. In another investigation, the prevalence of persistent OP position at the time of vaginal delivery regardless of parity was 5.5% (7.2% in nulliparas and 4.0% in multiparas).[3] The OP position was found to be associated with longer first and second stages, and a lower rate of vaginal delivery (26% for nulliparas and 57% for multiparas) when compared with the occiput anterior (OA) position. Most fetuses in the OP position undergo spontaneous anterior rotation during the course of labor, and expectant management is generally indicated. However, approximately 5% remain in persistent OP position or transverse arrest, which often requires either an operative vaginal or cesarean delivery.

Cephalopelvic disproportion (CPD) refers to the disproportion between the size of the fetus relative to the mother and can be the cause of a protraction or arrest disorder. This is a diagnosis of exclusion, often made at the time a protracted labor course is observed. Most frequently, malposition of the fetal presenting part is the culprit rather than true CPD. Unfortunately, there is no way to accurately predict CPD. In a decision analysis, it has been estimated that thousands of unnecessary cesarean deliveries would need to be performed in low-risk pregnancies to prevent one diagnosis of true CPD.[4]

Arrest of labor is defined as cessation of previously normal active phase cervical dilation for a period of 2 hours or more.[1] Evaluation of this disorder includes an assessment of uterine activity with an IUPC, performance of clinical pelvimetry, and evaluation of fetal presentation, position, station, and estimated fetal weight. Amniotomy and oxytocin therapy can be initiated if uterine activity is found to be inadequate. The majority of gravidas respond to this intervention, and resume progression of cervical dilation and achieve vaginal delivery. Although the definition reflects a 2-hour window before diagnosis of arrest, Rouse and colleagues[5] found that at least 4 hours of observation can be undertaken without oxytocin augmentation before making this diagnosis without incurring additional maternal or fetal compromise.

Electromechanical Classification

An alternative classification system for disorders of the active phase of labor is based on the electromechanical state of the uterus regarding uterine tone. This classification reflects an understanding of the propagation of electrical signals through the myometrium. In normal labor, a gradient of myometrial activity sweeps from the fundus and, through the excitation of cellular gap junctions, propagates toward the cervix. *Hypotonic dysfunction* reflects an inefficient generation and propagation of these action potentials through the myometrium or a lack of contractile response of myometrial cells to the initial stimulus. Hypotonic uterine contractions are infrequent, of low amplitude, and accompanied by low or normal baseline intrauterine pressures. Maternal discomfort is minimal. Oxytocin augmentation is usually applied in this clinical situation if active labor has already begun.

Hypertonic dysfunction is primarily a condition of primiparas and usually occurs in early labor. It is characterized by the presence of regular uterine contractions that fail to effect cervical effacement and dilation. Frequent contractions of low amplitude are often associated with an elevated basal intrauterine pressure. Maternal discomfort is usually significant. Therapeutic rest or expectant management can be initiated in this clinical situation if the patient is in latent labor. When diagnosed, the most likely scenario is that the patient will soon enter active labor. If the patient is in active labor and found to have hypertonic dysfunction, amniotomy can be performed with or without concomitant oxytocin administration.

Combined Disorder

A combined disorder of active phase dilation is defined as arrest of dilation or descent occurring when a patient has previously exhibited protracted labor. This pattern is associated with less favorable outcomes with regard to vaginal delivery when compared with patients with secondary arrest alone.[1] If diagnosed, an evaluation of uterine activity is necessary, as is an assessment of pelvic capacity, fetal position, station, and estimated fetal weight.

Disorders of the Second Stage

The second stage of labor begins once the cervix becomes fully dilated and ends with the delivery of the infant. Although fetal descent begins before the cervix becomes fully dilated, the majority of fetal descent occurs once full cervical dilation is achieved. At this time, maternal expulsion efforts may begin.

Protraction of descent is defined as descent of the presenting part during the second stage of labor occurring at less than 1 cm/hr in nulliparous women and less than 2 cm/hr in multiparous women.[1] *Arrest (failure) of descent* refers to no progress in descent. Both diagnoses require prompt evaluation of uterine activity, maternal expulsive efforts, fetal heart rate status, fetal position, clinical pelvimetry, and a reevaluation of estimated fetal weight. Decisions then may be made regarding interventions, such as increasing or initiating oxytocin infusion to improve maternal expulsion efforts, or proceeding with operative vaginal or cesarean delivery. Management of the second stage of labor can be difficult, and decisions regarding intervention must be individualized.

The median duration of the second stage is 50 to 60 minutes for nulliparas and 20 to 30 minutes for multiparas, but this is highly variable.[6,7] In classic obstetrical teaching, the upper limit for the duration of the second stage of labor was considered to be 2 hours. Factors influencing the length of the second stage include parity, maternal size, birth weight, OP position, fetal station at complete dilation, and, potentially, conduction anesthesia.[8] Currently, the American College of Obstetricians and Gynecologists' (ACOG's) guidelines[9] for the definition of prolonged second stage, provided the fetal heart rate tracing is normal and there is some degree of labor progress, are as follows: For nulliparous women, the diagnosis should be considered when the second stage exceeds 3 hours if regional anesthesia has been administered or 2 hours if no regional anesthesia is used, and in multiparous women, the diagnosis can be made when the second stage exceeds 2 hours with regional anesthesia or 1 hour without. Janakiraman and colleagues compared the second stage in 3139 induced women to that of 11,588 women in spontaneous labor.[10] No differences in the length of second stage or the risk of a prolonged second stage were noted between the groups, although the induced nulliparas appeared to be at increased risk of postpartum hemorrhage and cesarean delivery (4.2% vs. 2.0%, OR 1.62, 95% CI 1.02 to 2.58; 10.9% vs. 7.2%, OR 1.32, 95% CI 1.01 to 1.71, respectively).

Many authors have studied the perinatal and maternal effects of a prolonged second stage. Several studies found no increase in infant morbidity or mortality with a second stage lasting longer than 2 hours,[11] although the rate of vaginal delivery precipitously decreases after 3 hours in the second stage. However, a recent population-based cohort study by Allen and colleagues examined 63,404 nulliparous women and found increased risks of low 5-minute Apgar score, birth depression, and admission to the neonatal intensive care unit (NICU) with increasing duration of the second stage greater than 3 hours.[7] This study is the largest thus far evaluating neonatal and maternal outcomes with prolonged second stage. **In this study, as well as others, there is evidence that maternal morbidities including perineal trauma, chorioamnionitis, instrumental delivery, and postpartum hemorrhage increase with prolonged second stages lasting greater than 2 hours.** Effective management of the second stage should be individualized.

Disorders of the Third Stage

The third stage of labor refers to the period from delivery of the infant to the expulsion of the placenta. Separation of the placenta is the consequence of continued uterine contractions. Signs of placental separation include a gush of blood, lengthening of the umbilical cord, and change in shape of the uterine fundus from discoid to globular with elevation of the fundal height. The interval between delivery of the infant and delivery of the placenta and fetal membranes is usually less than 10 minutes and is complete within 15 minutes in 95% of deliveries.[12] The most important risk associated with a prolonged third stage is hemorrhage; this risk increases proportionally with increased duration.[13] Because of the associated increased incidence of hemorrhage after 30 minutes, most practitioners diagnose retained placenta after this time interval has elapsed. Interventions to expedite placental delivery are usually undertaken at this time.

Management of the third stage of labor may be expectant or active. Expectant management refers to the delivery of the placenta without cord clamping, cord traction, or the administration of uterotonic agents such as oxytocin. Active management consists of early cord clamping, controlled cord traction, and administration of a uterotonic agent. Oxytocin is the usual uterotonic agent given, but others have been used, such as misoprostol or other prostaglandin compounds. **Comparing active to expectant management of the third stage, there appears to be a reduced risk of postpartum hemorrhage when active management is used.**[14] Cochrane reviewers evaluated five studies (6486 women) that compared active and expectant management. They confirmed that active management reduced the average risk of maternal hemorrhage (RR 0.34, 95% CI 0.14 to 0.87), but that significant increases in maternal diastolic blood pressure, afterpains, and analgesia use occurred as well. These adverse events may reflect the side effects of the various uterotonic medications used in different countries.

There is some debate regarding the timing of oxytocin administration when the active management of the third stage is practiced: after the placenta has delivered versus after the anterior shoulder of the fetus has delivered. A randomized controlled trial including 1486 women comparing the effects of oxytocin administration on delivery of the anterior shoulder to administration after delivery of the placenta showed no significant differences in blood loss or retained placenta between the groups.[15]

Retained placenta can usually be treated with measures such as manual removal or sharp curettage. Attempting manual removal can be performed under regional anesthesia or conscious sedation. If this is not successful, a sharp curettage can be performed under sonographic guidance. Prophylactic broad-spectrum antimicrobial agents are often administered when manual removal of the placenta is performed, although there is little evidence to support or refute their use.[16]

Precipitous Labor

Precipitous labor refers to delivery of the infant in less than 3 hours. This occurs in approximately 2% of all deliveries in the United States. Precipitous labor and delivery alone is not usually associated with significant maternal or infant morbidity and mortality. Short labors can be associated with placental abruption, uterine tachysystole, and recent maternal cocaine use—all of which are major contributors to poor outcomes for mothers and infants. Other investigators have looked at intrapartum risk factors associated with permanent brachial plexus injury and found that a precipitous second stage is the most common labor abnormality associated with shoulder dystocia, although the rates of permanent injury did not increase.[17]

Anesthesia Effects on Labor Progress

Conduction regional anesthesia's effects on the rate of cervical change remains controversial. In a recent meta-analysis,[18] 15 randomized controlled trials including 4619 patients compared the effects of epidural anesthesia to parenteral opioid. The incidence of cesarean section was the same between the groups, although the incidence of operative vaginal delivery was increased in the conduction anesthesia group (OR 1.92; 95% CI 1.52 to 1.22). It has been difficult to establish whether this increase in operative vaginal delivery was due to a direct effect of the epidural analgesia on the rate of labor or an indirect effect, such as resident training. No difference in the duration of the first stage was noted; however, the second stage was prolonged by approximately 16 minutes (95% CI 10 to 23 minutes). This statistically significant finding lacks clinical relevance.[18]

It has also been suggested that receiving regional anesthesia during latent labor, as opposed to during the active phase, results in prolongation of the labor, such that many practitioners refrain from administering regional analgesia until the patient reaches 4 cm or more dilation. An investigation including 12,693 nulliparas randomized subjects to receive early epidural analgesia (at first request if cervical dilation was at least 1 cm) compared with late epidural analgesia (parenteral meperidine until cervical dilation of 4 cm was achieved). The median cervical dilation at the time of epidural placement was 1.6 cm for the early group and 5.1 for the late group. These researchers found no difference in the incidence of cesarean birth, operative vaginal delivery, or length of first or second stages of labor.

MANAGEMENT OF ABNORMAL LABOR AND DELIVERY

Pharmacologic Augmentation

When the first stage of labor is protracted or an arrest disorder is diagnosed, an evaluation of uterine activity, clinical pelvimetry, and fetal position, station, and estimated weight should be performed. If uterine activity is found to be suboptimal, the most common remedy is oxytocin augmentation, because once labor is initiated, the uterus becomes more sensitive to oxytocin stimulation. Various oxytocin dosing regimens have been described in the obstetrical literature. Local protocols for oxytocin administration should specify the dose of oxytocin being delivered (milliunits per minute) as opposed to the volume of fluid being infused (milliliters per minute), initial dose, incremental increases with periodicity, and maximum dose. Although oxytocin currently is used in a majority of labors in the United States, it is important for clinicians to recognize that it is also the medication implicated in approximately half of all paid obstetrical litigation claims and is the medication most commonly associated with preventable adverse events during childbirth.[19]

Recently, attention has been turned to misoprostol solution as an alternative augmentation agent. Ho and colleagues[20] evaluated a solution of 200 mcg misoprostol dissolved in 200 mL tap water randomized against intravenous oxytocin in 231 women. This small study yielded promising results with similar rates of vaginal delivery between the two groups and no difference noted in side effects of neonatal outcomes. As well, a recent study by Bleich and colleages compared oral misoprostol tablets (25 mcg) versus intravenous oxytocin for labor augmentation in 350 women, with no differences in maternal or neonatal outcomes. Further research is ongoing in this area.

Side Effects

Uterine Overactivity

The most frequently encountered complication of oxytocin or prostaglandin administration is *uterine overactivity*. Historically, the most commonly used terms to describe this activity were *hyperstimulation*, *tachysystole*, *hypercontractility*, and *hypertonus*. However, there were no uniform definitions for these terms until a recent National Institutes of Child Health and Human Development (NICHD) workshop attempted to provide standardized nomenclature for uterine activity, as well as electronic fetal heart monitoring.[21] These guidelines quantify the number of uterine contractions present in a 10-minute window, averaged over 30 minutes. A *normal* contraction pattern is considered five contractions or less in 10 minutes, averaged over 30 minutes, accounting as well for frequency, intensity, duration, and relaxation time when described. *Tachysystole* is defined as more than five contractions in 10 minutes, averaged over a 30-minute window. Tachysystole can occur in spontaneous or stimulated labor and can be associated with fetal heart rate changes or not. The NICHD guidelines recommend abandoning the terms *hyperstimulation* and *hypercontractility*.[21]

One of the advantages of oxytocin administration is that if uterine overactivity is encountered, the infusion can quickly be stopped. The half-life of oxytocin is approximately 3 minutes; therefore, stopping the infusion usually results in the resolution of such uterine overactivity. In addition, placing the woman in the left lateral position, administering oxygen, and increasing intravenous fluids may be of benefit. If fetal heart rate tracing abnormalities persist and uterine tachysystole is ongoing, the use of a tocolytic, such as terbutaline, may be considered. Oxytocin may then be reinitiated, if appropriate, once uterine tone has returned to baseline and fetal status is reassuring.

Water Intoxication

Oxytocin is structurally and functionally related to vasopressin, or antidiuretic hormone. It binds to vasopressin and oxytocin receptors in the kidney and the brain. Oxytocin can have an antidiuretic effect at high doses and can, in extreme situations, result in water intoxication. Severe symptomatic hyponatremia can result if oxytocin is administered at high concentrations (e.g., 40 mU/min) in large quantities of hypotonic solutions (>3 liters) for prolonged periods of time. Symptoms of severe acute hyponatremia include headache, anorexia, nausea, vomiting, abdominal pain, lethargy, drowsiness, unconsciousness, grand mal seizures, and potentially irreversible neurologic injury. Fortunately, this side effect is extremely rare even with high-dose oxytocin regimens.

If water intoxication occurs, oxytocin and any hypotonic solutions should be stopped. Correction of hyponatremia must be performed carefully and consists of restricting water intake and careful administration of hypertonic saline. Correction of hyponatremia must occur

TABLE 14-3 MATERNAL COMPLICATIONS ASSOCIATED WITH TRIAL OF LABOR AFTER PREVIOUS CESAREAN BIRTH

COMPLICATION	TRIAL OF LABOR (n = 17,898)	ELECTIVE REPEAT CESAREAN DELIVERY (n = 15,801)	ODDS RATIO (95% CI)	p VALUE
Uterine rupture	124 (0.7%)	0	—	<0.001
Uterine dehiscence	119 (0.7%)	76 (0.5%)	1.38 (1.04-1.85)	0.03
Hysterectomy	41 (0.2%)	47 (0.3%)	0.77 (0.51-1.17)	0.22
Thromboembolic disease (DVT, PE)	7 (0.04%)	10 (0.1%)	0.62 (0.24-1.62)	0.32
Transfusion	304 (1.7%)	158 (1.0%)	1.71 (1.41-2.08)	<0.001
Endometritis	517 (2.9%)	285 (1.8%)	1.62 (1.40-1.87)	<0.001
Maternal death	3 (0.02%)	7 (0.04%)	0.38 (0.10-1.46)	0.21
Other maternal adverse events*	64 (0.4%)	52 (0.3%)	1.09 (0.75-1.57)	0.66
One or more of the above	978 (5.5%)	563 (3.6%)	1.56 (1.41-1.74)	<0.001

Landon MB, Hauth JC, Leveno KJ, et al for the NICHD MFMU Network: Maternal and perinatal outcomes associated with a trial of labor after prior cesarean delivery. N Engl J Med 351:2581, 2004.

*Other adverse events include broad-ligament hematoma, cystotomy, bowel injury, ureteral injury.

DVT, Deep vein thrombosis; *PE,* pulmonary embolism.

slowly and cautiously because overly rapid correction can be deleterious.

Hypotension

Historically, bolus injections of oxytocin were thought to cause hypotension. Current practice for labor management is administration by infusion pump or slow drip. Mean arterial blood pressure and peripheral vascular resistance have been noted to decrease 30% and 50%, respectively, after oxytocin bolus injection of 5 to 10 units. This caused increases of 30% in heart rate, 25% in stroke volume, and 50% in cardiac output when compared with patients receiving slow dilute infusions. Fewer cardiovascular side effects are observed when oxytocin is given as a slow intravenous infusion or intramuscularly, as may be needed for third-stage labor management. However, a report by Davies and colleagues[22] revealed that a 10-IU bolus of oxytocin given in the third stage of labor was not associated with adverse hemodynamic responses compared with oxytocin given as an infusion. Although multiple boluses during labor are not recommended, consideration may be given to its use in the third stage of labor as a single bolus.

Uterine Rupture

Uterine rupture is rare and in most instances occurs in women with prior uterine surgery such as cesarean delivery or myomectomy. Other risk factors for uterine rupture are grand multiparity; marked uterine overdistention either with a macrosomic fetus, multiple gestation, or polyhydramnios; and fetal malpresentation. Although there is no association between maximum dose of oxytocin and risk of uterine rupture, it is likely that some cases of uterine rupture can be avoided by using the lowest dose of oxytocin possible that produces regular contractions and cervical change.

Recent investigations have shed light on the question of labor augmentation and induction for women attempting trials of labor after previous cesarean deliveries. Although randomized trials currently do not exist, a large prospective investigation evaluated more than 17,000 women attempting trials of labor after previous cesarean deliveries.[23] The incidence of uterine rupture was 0.4% for those subjects who spontaneously labored versus 0.9% for those who received augmentation and 1.0% for subjects undergoing induction. The highest risk of rupture was in those patients who received a combination of prostaglandins and oxytocin. Other complications of attempting a trial of labor after a previous cesarean section can be seen in Table 14-3. The ACOG currently recommends the use of oxytocin in augmentation and induction of women undergoing a trial of labor after previous cesarean deliveries, although caution is encouraged in women with unfavorable cervices.[24]

Use of intrauterine pressure catheters does not appear to be helpful in diagnosis of uterine rupture, because the ruptures usually evolve gradually in labor and are often heralded by abnormal fetal heart rate patterns. There is no evidence that amnioinfusion increases the risk of uterine rupture; however, studies to date have been small and retrospective.

Anaphylaxis of Pregnancy (Amniotic Fluid Embolism)

A population-based retrospective cohort study including 3 million deliveries reported that medical induction of labor was associated with an increased risk of amniotic fluid embolism (adjusted OR 1.8; 95% CI 1.2 to 2.7).[25] However, the absolute risk was small: 10.3 per 100,000 births with medical induction versus 5.2 per 100,000 births without medical induction. Moreover, given that these women were induced for medical indications, not inducing labor could potentially result in greater maternal-fetal morbidity and mortality than inducing labor. These findings should be confirmed by others before changes in management of induction are considered.

INDUCTION OF LABOR

Induction of labor is one of the most commonly performed obstetrical procedures in the United States. Induction of labor refers to the iatrogenic stimulation of uterine contractions before the onset of spontaneous labor to accomplish vaginal delivery. Augmentation of labor refers to increasing the frequency and improving the intensity of existing uterine contractions in a patient who is in labor and not progressing adequately, in order to accomplish vaginal delivery.

Indications and Contraindications

Induction of labor should be undertaken when the benefits of prompt delivery to either mother or fetus outweigh the risks of pregnancy continuation.[26] Many accepted medical and obstetrical indications for labor induction and several relative indications for labor induction exist (Table 14-4). Contraindications are those that preclude vaginal delivery, among others (Table 14-5). "Impending" macrosomia, a favorable cervix, or patients considered to be at increased risk of preeclampsia (such as having a prior history of preeclampsia) or at risk for intrauterine growth restriction (e.g., a fetus with an estimated weight of 19th percentile) are not considered indications for induction.

Careful examination of the maternal and fetal condition is required before undertaking labor induction (Table 14-6). Indications and contraindications for induction should be reviewed, as well as the alternatives. Risks and benefits of labor induction should be discussed with the patient, including the risk of cesarean delivery (to be discussed later). Confirmation of gestational age is critical, and evaluation of fetal lung maturity status should be performed if indicated (Table 14-7).[26] Fetal weight should be estimated and clinical pelvimetry performed. Fetal presentation and position should be confirmed. A cervical examination should be performed and documented as well. In addition, labor induction should be performed at a location where personnel are available who are familiar with the process and its potential complications. Uterine activity and electronic fetal monitoring (EFM) are recommended for any gravida receiving uterotonic medications.

Prolonged Pregnancy

Postterm pregnancy (>41 completed weeks) is associated with significant risks to the fetus and mother. Antepartum stillbirths account for more perinatal deaths than either complications of prematurity or sudden infant death syndrome. According to a large epidemiologic study by Hilder and colleagues,[27] the perinatal mortality rate (stillbirths plus early neonatal deaths) at greater than 42 weeks of gestation is approximately twice that at term (4 to 7 deaths vs. 2 to 3 deaths per 1000 deliveries) and increases sixfold

TABLE 14-4 INDICATIONS FOR LABOR INDUCTION

ACCEPTED ABSOLUTE INDICATIONS	RELATIVE INDICATIONS
Hypertensive disorders	**Hypertensive disorders**
• Preeclampsia/eclampsia	• Chronic hypertension
Maternal medical conditions	**Maternal medical conditions**
• Diabetes mellitus	• Systemic lupus erythematosus
• Renal disease	• Gestational diabetes
• Chronic pulmonary disease	• Hypercoagulable disorders
	• Cholestasis of pregnancy
Prelabor rupture of membranes	Polyhydramnios
Chorioamnionitis	Fetal anomalies requiring specialized neonatal care
Fetal compromise	**Logistic factors**
• Fetal growth restriction	• Risk of rapid labor
• Isoimmunization	• Distance from hospital
• Nonreassuring antepartum fetal testing	• Psychosocial indications
	• Advanced cervical dilation
• Oligohydramnios	
Fetal demise	Previous stillbirth
Postdates pregnancy (>42 weeks)	Postterm pregnancy (>41 weeks)

TABLE 14-5 CONTRAINDICATIONS TO LABOR INDUCTION

ACCEPTED ABSOLUTE CONTRAINDICATIONS	RELATIVE CONTRAINDICATIONS
Prior classical uterine incision or transfundal uterine surgery	Cervical carcinoma
Active genital herpes infection	Funic presentation
Placenta or vasa previa	Malpresentation (breech)
Umbilical cord prolapse	
Transverse or oblique fetal lie	
Absolute cephalopelvic disproportion (as in women with pelvic deformities)	

TABLE 14-6 EVALUATION BEFORE INDUCTION OF LABOR

PARAMETER	CRITERIA
Maternal	Confirm indication for induction Review contraindications to labor and/or vaginal delivery Perform clinical pelvimetry to assess pelvic shape and adequacy of bony pelvis Assess cervical condition (assign Bishop score) Review risks, benefits, and alternatives of induction of labor with patient
Fetal/neonatal	Confirm gestational age Assess need to document fetal lung maturity status Estimate fetal weight (either by clinical or ultrasound examination) Determine fetal presentation and lie Confirm fetal well-being

TABLE 14-7 CRITERIA FOR CONFIRMATION OF GESTATIONAL AGE AND/OR FETAL PULMONARY MATURITY

	PARAMETERS
Confirmation of Gestational Age	Fetal heart tones have been documented as present for ≥30 weeks by Doppler ultrasound. ≥36 weeks have elapsed since a positive serum or urine human chorionic gonadotropin pregnancy test. Ultrasound measurement at less than 20 weeks of gestation supports gestational age of 39 weeks or greater.
Fetal Pulmonary Maturity	If term gestation cannot be confirmed by two or more of the above obstetrical clinical or laboratory criteria, amniotic fluid analyses can be used to provide evidence of fetal lung maturity. A variety of tests are available. The parameters for evidence of fetal pulmonary maturity are as follows: 1. Lecithin/sphingomyelin (L/S) ratio >2.1 2. Presence of phosphatidylglycerol (PG) 3. TDxFLM assay ≥70 mg surfactant per 1 g albumin present 4. Presence of saturated phosphatidylcholine (SPC) ≥500 ng/mL in nondiabetic patients (≥1000 ng/mL for pregestational diabetic patients) 5. Lamellar body count exceeding 30,000/mcL

Modified data from Induction of Labor. ACOG Practice Bulletin No 107. American College of Obstetricians and Gynecologists. Obstet Gynecol 2009:114, 386; and Fetal Lung Maturity. ACOG Practice Bulletin No. 97. American College of Obstetricians and Gynecologists. Obstet Gynecol 112:717, 2008.

and higher at 43 weeks of gestation and beyond. However, several other epidemiologic studies suggested that other risk factors (such as congenital malformations and intrauterine growth restriction) outweighed prolonged pregnancy as the cause of neonatal mortality. Weaknesses of these studies overall included a lack of recording of the actual cause of death for many of the infants, as well as pregnancy dating by last menstrual period rather than early ultrasounds, and possible inequality or poor access to care of the populations evaluated.

Two more recent studies consisted of prospective cohort evaluations of singleton pregnancies based on ultrasound dating.[28,29] Nakling and colleagues[28] found an incidence of postterm pregnancies to be 7.6% in their cohort, with 0.3% of pregnancies progressing to 301 days (43 weeks' gestation) if inductions were not permitted before 43 weeks. This investigation found a significantly increased rate of perinatal mortality after 41 weeks' gestation, although whether the prolonged pregnancy or intrauterine growth restriction was the actual culprit is difficult to ascertain in this study. In contrast, Heimstad and colleagues[29] found an increased trend toward intrauterine fetal demise at 42 weeks' gestation compared to 38 weeks, but this study allowed inductions before 43 weeks and did not calculate the perinatal mortality rates. Factors that may contribute to the increased rate of perinatal deaths are uteroplacental insufficiency, meconium aspiration, intrauterine growth restriction, and intrauterine infection.[30] For these reasons, the tendency has been to deliver by 41 completed weeks of gestation (42 weeks, 294 days, EDD + 14 days).

Postterm pregnancy is also associated with significant risks to the pregnant woman, including an increase in labor dystocia (9% to 12% vs. 2% to 7% at term), which is denoted by an increase in severe perineal injury related to macrosomia (3.3% vs. 2.6% at term), and a doubling in the rate of cesarean delivery.[29,31-35] Cesarean delivery is associated with higher risks of complications, such as hemorrhage, endometritis, and thromboembolic disease. In a recent randomized, controlled trial of women at 41 weeks of gestation, those who were induced would desire the same management 74% of the time, whereas women with serial antenatal monitoring desired the same management only 38% of the time.

Management of low-risk postterm pregnancy is controversial. A recent meta-analysis included 19 studies that compared induction and expectant management for uncomplicated, singleton pregnancies of at least 41 weeks' gestation.[36] There was no difference in cesarean delivery rates (RR 0.92; 95% CI 0.76 to 1.12; RR 0.97; 95% CI 0.72 to 1.31) for women induced at 41 and 42 completed weeks, respectively. There was a small and statistically significant reduction in perinatal mortality rates, but none in neonatal intensive care admission rates, meconium aspiration, or abnormal Apgar scores. In this subset of women, elective labor induction may be justified.

Because delivery cannot always be brought about readily, maternal risks from cesarean delivery resulting from failed inductions or other dystocia, and the impact on future pregnancies from cesarean delivery, need to be considered. Some studies have demonstrated the risks of abnormal placentation from multiple cesarean deliveries.[37] Also, with the declining rates of vaginal birth after cesarean, once the first cesarean has occurred, there is a less than 10% chance that future pregnancies will be delivered vaginally.

In 1954, approximately 20% of postterm fetuses were diagnosed with dysmaturity syndrome, with characteristics resembling chronic intrauterine growth restriction from uteroplacental deficiency. These pregnancies were considered at increased risk of umbilical cord compression from oligohydramnios, meconium aspiration, and short-term neonatal complications (such as hypoglycemia, seizures, and respiratory insufficiency) and had an increased incidence of nonreassuring fetal testing, both antepartum and intrapartum. Whether such infants also are at risk of long-term neurologic sequelae was not apparent. In a large, prospective, follow-up study of children from 1 to 2 years of age, the general physical milestones, intelligence quotient, and frequency of intercurrent illnesses were not significantly different between normal infants born at term and those born postterm. Again, these infants might have increased neonatal complications secondary to intrauterine growth restriction and uteroplacental insufficiency, rather than from prolonged pregnancy itself.

Elective Induction of Labor

Elective induction of labor refers to the initiation of labor for convenience in an individual with a term pregnancy who is free of medical or obstetrical indications. The rate of elective induction in the United States has increased dramatically from 9.5% to 19.4% from 1989 to 1998.[38] Factors associated with higher induction rates are white race, higher education, and early initiation of prenatal care. Although elective induction is not recommended or encouraged, it may be appropriate in specific instances such as a history of very short labors or for patients who live a great distance from the hospital.[26] Also, a patient who has experienced a prior stillbirth at or near term may require labor induction to ease anxiety and fears about the loss of a subsequent pregnancy. In addition, there are certain maternal medical conditions that require multispecialty participation in which the benefit of a planned delivery to have experienced personnel readily available is most appropriate. Examples of such cases are pregnancies with maternal cardiac disease that may require invasive monitoring during labor or those complicated by chronic renal disease in which considerations for hemodialysis may dictate a scheduled birth.

The major risks of elective induction of labor at term are thought to be increased rates of cesarean delivery (especially in nulliparas), increased neonatal morbidity, and cost. The risk of cesarean delivery following elective induction, especially for the nullipara with an unfavorable cervix, was clearly established in the literature with several cohort and case-control studies.[39] These studies revealed an increased risk of cesarean of at least twice the risk of spontaneously laboring patients. Seyb and colleagues also noted in their investigation that the mean time spent on labor and delivery was almost twice as long, and postpartum stays were prolonged if labor induction was undertaken. The total cost associated with hospitalization for elective induction was 17.4% higher than for spontaneous labor, including costs for labor and delivery, pharmacy, and postpartum care. These findings were confirmed by the investigations undertaken by Maslow, Sweeney, and Cammu and colleagues.[39] These data reinforced the finding that labor induction was a significant predictor of cesarean delivery for both nulliparous and multiparous women and contributed to rising health care costs.

Following these cohort and case-control studies, several randomized controlled trials were undertaken. In a meta-analysis by Caughey and colleagues,[40] nine randomized controlled trials were evaluated. These trials utilized patients undergoing expectant management (rather than spontaneous labor) as the comparison group for the patients being electively induced. The rationale for this change of perspective consists of examining the actual decision made by the clinician when a patient at 38 or 39 weeks' gestation is seen at the office. The clinician and patient do not make a decision at that time between spontaneous labor and induction, but rather, between expectant management and induction. In contrast to the previous reports of the cohort studies, the meta-analysis of randomized controlled trials actually revealed a decreased risk of cesarean in the induction group compared to the expectantly managed group (RR 1.17, 95% CI 1.05 to 1.29). As well, Cochrane reviewers examined 19 trials including 7984 women and found that the women induced at 37 to 40 completed weeks were more likely to have a cesarean with expectant management than those in the labor induction group (RR 0.58, 95% CI 0.34 to 0.99).[36]

Caughey and colleagues[41] also examined the risk of cesarean delivery for each week of gestational age ranging from 38 to 41 weeks. In their retrospective study, again comparing induction to expectant management, cesarean delivery was decreased in the induction groups.

In contrast to these studies, the Consortium of Safe Labor, consisting of 10 U.S. institutions throughout the nation, reviewed their electronic medical record data from 2002 to 2008.[42] In this large study of 115,528 deliveries, the outcomes of mothers and neonates undergoing either spontaneous labor, elective induction, medically indicated induction, or cesarean without labor were evaluated. The incidence of cesarean delivery in this study was again increased in the group undergoing elective induction compared to the spontaneous laboring group, particularly at 37 to 38 completed weeks' gestation and at 41 weeks' gestation. When the outcomes were adjusted for race, maternal age, parity, preeclampsia, eclampsia, chronic hypertension, diabetes, and GBS status, the odds ratio for electively induced patients from 37 to 42 weeks' gestation to undergo cesarean was 1.58 compared to spontaneously laboring patients (95% CI 1.48 to 1.69).

Neonatal respiratory problems, sepsis, and asphyxia are the major pediatric concerns when mothers undergo elective delivery. Respiratory problems can result from inadvertent delivery of a premature infant or transient tachypnea related to cesarean delivery after failed induction. This is counterbalanced by observations that fewer electively induced infants have meconium passage when compared to spontaneously labored infants, and, therefore, likely have reduced incidence of meconium aspiration syndrome.[40] Macrosomia also may be reduced, as noted in an ecological study performed by Zhang and colleagues.[43] This study revealed that the increased induction rate between 1992 and 2003 (14% to 27%) was significantly associated with reduced mean fetal birth weight ($r = -0.54$, 95% CI −0.71 to −0.29) and rate of macrosomia ($r = -0.55$, 95% CI −0.74 to −0.32).

TABLE 14-8 NEONATAL RESPIRATORY MORBIDITY

GESTATIONAL AGE (WEEKS)	FREQUENCY OF NICU ADMISSION PER 1000 DELIVERIES	ODDS RATIO (95% CI)
Following Vaginal Delivery		
37 0/7 to 37 6/7	12.6 (7.6-19.6)	2.5 (1.5-4.2)
38 0/7 to 38 6/7	7.0 (4.6-10.2)	1.4 (0.8-2.2)
39 0/7 to 39 6/7	3.2 (1.8-4.5)	0.6 (0.4-1.0)
Following Cesarean Delivery		
37 0/7 to 37 6/7	57.7 (26.7-107.1)	11.2 (5.4-13.1)
38 0/7 to 38 6/7	9.4 (1.9-27.2)	1.8 (0.6-5.9)
39 0/7 to 39 6/7	16.2 (5.9-35.5)	3.2 (1.4-7.4)

Morrison JJ, Rennie JM, Milton PJ: Neonatal respiratory morbidity and mode of delivery at term: influence of timing of elective caesarean section. Br J Obstet Gynaecol 102:101, 1995.

The risk of respiratory morbidity was illustrated in a retrospective review of infants admitted to the neonatal intensive care unit following elective delivery at term.[44] These results support delaying elective delivery until 39 weeks' gestation (Table 14-8). In further support of these findings, Clark and colleagues[45] performed a prospective observational study of 27 hospitals, including 17,794 deliveries. Of these deliveries, 44% were planned, and 73% of those deliveries were considered elective. The percentage of the electively induced infants admitted to the NICU at 37 weeks was 15.2% ($n = 112$), at 38 weeks 7.0% ($n = 678$), and at 39 weeks 6.0% ($n = 2004$). These studies reiterate the importance of considering neonatal morbidity with elective induction before 40 weeks' gestation. However, examining the results of the Consortium of Safe Labor provides a conflicting result for neonatal morbidity in elective inductions. In this study, infants of electively induced mothers were less likely to receive ventilatory support, become septic, or be admitted to the NICU.[42]

On one risk of elective induction, the scientific evidence agrees: Costs with elective induction are increased. Kaufman and colleagues[46] studied the economic consequences of elective induction of labor at term. Using decision analysis, these researchers examined a hypothetical cohort of 100,000 pregnant patients for whom an initial decision was made to either induce labor at 39 weeks' gestation or to follow the patient expectantly through the remainder of pregnancy. All patients in this model underwent elective induction at 42 weeks' gestation. Clinical outcomes of patients undergoing expectant management were evaluated. Using baseline estimates, the investigators concluded that elective induction would result in more than 12,000 excess cesarean deliveries and impose an annual cost to the medical system of nearly $100 million. A policy of induction at any gestational age, regardless of parity or cervical ripeness, required economic expenditures by the medical system. Although never cost saving, inductions were less expensive at later gestational ages, for multiparous patients, and for those women with a favorable cervix. The inductions most costly to the health care system were those performed in nulliparas with unfavorable cervices at 39 weeks. When nulliparous women with favorable cervices undergo labor induction, the estimated cost is approximately halved, but is still considerably higher than allowing spontaneous labor.

One approach called the Active Management of Risk in Pregnancy at Term (AMOR-IPAT) provides promise for reducing the risk of cesarean delivery following induction of labor.[47] Using a retrospective cohort design, delivery outcomes of 100 women with a tailored approach to prenatal care and individualization of risk of cesarean delivery were compared with 300 nonexposed women. Consideration was given to the most common indications for nonelective cesarean delivery: cephalopelvic disproportion and uteroplacental insufficiency. A hypothetical ceiling for gestational age at delivery, always ≤41 weeks and ≥38 weeks, was set for each subject. Cervical ripening was used for all women with Bishop scores less than 5. Despite an increase in the labor induction rate in the women exposed to AMOR-IPAT (63% vs. 26%, $P<0.001$), there was a significant reduction in the cesarean births in this same group (4% vs. 17%, $P<0.001$). In a similar retrospective cohort study from the same authors, a protocol of risk-guided prostaglandin-assisted preventive labor induction with differing intensity was applied. Compared with nonexposed subjects, the exposed group ($n = 794$) had a significantly higher rate of labor induction (31.4% vs. 20.4%), and use of prostaglandin E_2 (23.3% vs. 15.7%), and a significantly lower cesarean delivery rate (5.3% vs. 11.8%). A small prospective trial of AMOR-IPAT, however, failed to confirm these promising results. Lack of a difference in the cesarean delivery rates (10.3% in the AMOR-IPAT group vs. 14.9% in the conventional management group; $p = 0.25$) may have been because the sample size was too small to reveal a true difference between treatment groups.[48] Larger randomized controlled multicenter investigations are planned.

Prediction of Labor Induction Success

In observational studies, characteristics associated with successful induction include multiparity, tall stature (over 5 feet 5 inches), increasing gestational age, nonobese maternal weight or body mass index, and infant birth weight less than 3.5 kg.[49,50] However, these characteristics are predictive of success even in spontaneous labors, which suggests they are more predictive of the route of delivery than the likelihood that the patient will reach the active phase of labor.

Because of the risk of cesarean delivery and the rising costs of health care associated with labor induction, some researchers have tried to identify, with varying success, biochemical and biophysical assays to predict the probability of vaginal delivery following labor induction.[51] These measures include digital evaluation of the cervix, ultrasonographic cervical length measurements, and use of fetal fibronectin before labor induction.

The modified Bishop score is the system most commonly used in clinical practice in the United States to evaluate the cervix before induction. This system tabulates a score based on the station of the presenting part and four characteristics of the cervix: dilation, effacement, consistency, and position (Table 14-9).[52] If the Bishop score is high (variously defined as ≥5 or ≥8), the likelihood of vaginal delivery is similar whether labor is spontaneous or induced.[53] In contrast, a low Bishop score is predictive that induction will fail and result in cesarean delivery. These relationships are particularly strong in nulliparous women who undergo induction.[54,55] Of note, the relationship between a low Bishop score and failed induction, prolonged labor, and a high cesarean birth rate was first described before widespread use of cervical ripening agents.[56]

TABLE 14-9 MODIFIED BISHOP SCORE

Score Parameter	0	1	2	3
Dilation (cm)	Closed	1-2	3-4	5 or more
Effacement (%)	0-30	40-50	60-70	80 or more
Length (cm)*	*>4*	*2-4*	*1-2*	*1-2*
Station	−3	−2	−1 or 0	+1 or +2
Consistency	Firm	Medium	Soft	
Cervical position	Posterior	Midposition	Anterior	

Bishop EH: Pelvic scoring for elective induction. Obstet Gynecol 24:266, 1964.
*Modification by Calder AA, Brennand JE: Labor and normal delivery: induction of labor. Curr Opin Obstet Gynecol 3:764, 1991. This modification replaces percent effacement as one of the parameters of the Bishop score.

Cervical length is also predictive of the likelihood of spontaneous onset of labor postterm. Sonographic assessment of cervical length for predicting the outcome of labor induction has been evaluated in numerous studies. A systematic review of 20 prospective studies found that cervical length was predictive of successful induction (likelihood ratio of a positive test, 1.66; 95% CI 1.20 to 2.31) and failed induction (likelihood ratio of a negative test, 0.51; 95% CI 0.39 to 0.67).[57] However, sonographic cervical length performed poorly for predicting vaginal delivery within 24 hours (sensitivity 59%, specificity 65%), vaginal delivery (sensitivity 67%, specificity 58%), achieving active labor (sensitivity 57%, specificity 60%), and delivery within 24 hours (sensitivity 56%, specificity 47%), and did not perform significantly better than the Bishop score for predicting a successful induction. These data are limited by substantial heterogeneity among the studies. The role of ultrasound examination as a tool for selecting women likely to have a successful induction is uncertain.

Two studies examined the use of magnetic resonance imaging (MRI) as a tool for assessing cervical readiness for labor, the idea behind this being that MRI delineates the internal signal changes as well as morphologic alterations of the cervix during pregnancy. Studies have evaluated the cervical hydration status and signal intensities. The largest study published thus far was by Pates and colleagues and examined 93 women undergoing labor induction at term. No correlation was found between MRI T2 relaxation time estimates (measuring cervical hydration) and clinical indicators of ripening (Bishop score) or obstetrical outcome. Practicality and cost concerns abound with any radiographic predictions of labor induction success.

The presence of an elevated fetal fibronectin (fFN) concentration in cervicovaginal secretions has also been used to predict uterine readiness for induction. Elevated fFN is thought to represent a disruption or inflammation of the chorionic-decidual interface. In several studies, women with a positive fFN result had a significantly shorter interval until delivery than those with a negative fFN result and there was reduction in the frequency of cesarean delivery.[58] Positive fFN results were predictive of a shorter interval to delivery, even in nulliparas with low (<5) Bishop scores. However, other investigations have not confirmed these findings.[59]

Bailit and colleagues[60] used a decision analysis to determine if the vaginal delivery rate is increased in nulliparous women undergoing elective labor induction following fFN testing. In this model, three management strategies were evaluated presuming fFN testing was performed in select groups at 39 weeks of pregnancy: (1) no elective induction of labor for any candidate until 41 weeks' gestation (spontaneous labor), (2) induction only of those patients with a positive fFN result at 39 weeks, and (3) elective induction for every woman at no less than 39 weeks' gestation without performance of a fFN test. The investigators based estimates and assumptions for their statistical model on previous published clinical studies regarding rates of cesarean delivery for women in spontaneous labor, rates of cesarean delivery after an induction for a prolonged pregnancy, distribution of fFN results at 39 weeks' gestation, and percentage of pregnancies beyond 41 weeks. Investigators found that the spontaneous labor strategy had the highest rate of vaginal delivery (90%) and the elective induction strategy had the lowest rate (79%). When fFN test results were used to screen candidates for elective induction, the rate of vaginal delivery was higher than the induction strategy but lower than the spontaneous labor strategy (83%). These investigators concluded that the best approach to improve vaginal delivery rates was to avoid elective induction in nulliparous women. fFN may, however, improve chances of vaginal delivery over nonselective induction. Larger trials are needed to further clarify the role of fFN in predicting the success of labor induction in the nulliparous patient and the cost-effectiveness of this approach.

Cervical Ripening

As discussed earlier, the condition of the cervix greatly influences the success of inducing labor. Cervical ripening is a complex process that results in physical softening and distensibility of the cervix, ultimately leading to partial cervical effacement and dilation.[61] Remodeling of the cervix involves enzymatic dissolution of collagen fibrils, increase in water content, and chemical changes. These changes are induced by hormones (estrogen, progesterone, relaxin), as well as cytokines, prostaglandin, and nitric oxide synthesis enzymes.[61] **Cervical ripening methods fall into two main categories: pharmacologic and mechanical (Table 14-10). Because the state of the cervix plays such a crucial role in labor induction, a cervical examination is essential before determining which method to use for labor induction.**

Although Bishop originally used his scoring system to prevent iatrogenic prematurity in an era before the widespread use of sonography, it is now widely used to assess the state of the cervix before induction, as well as to predict the success of labor induction. The higher the Bishop score, the more "ripe" or "favorable" the cervix is for labor induction. A low Bishop score, usually considered 5 or less, is "unripened" or "unfavorable" and will benefit from cervical ripening. For example, the likelihood of a vaginal delivery after labor induction is similar to that after spontaneous onset of labor if the Bishop score is 8 or higher in multiparous patients. A low Bishop score is particularly predictive of failure in nulliparous women who undergo induction of labor at term. The high risk of cesarean delivery associated with failure of induction in nulliparous women at term with low Bishop scores is well established in the literature.[53,56] The rates of cesarean delivery were compared in 4635 nulliparas women in spontaneous labor with 2647 nulliparas women who underwent induction of labor.[54] Cesarean delivery was performed in 11.5% of the spontaneous labor group and 23.7% of the labor induction group. The most important variable in predicting the risk of cesarean delivery was a Bishop score at the initiation of labor induction, with a 31.5% cesarean section rate among patients with a Bishop score less than 5 versus 18.1% for patients with a Bishop score greater than 5.

TABLE 14-10 METHODS OF CERVICAL RIPENING

PHARMACOLOGIC METHODS	MECHANICAL METHODS
Oxytocin	Membrane stripping
Prostaglandins	Amniotomy
• E_2 (dinoprostone, Prepidil gel and Cervidil time-released vaginal insert)	Mechanical dilators
• E_1 (misoprostol, Cytotec)	• Laminaria tents
Estrogen	• Dilapan
Relaxin	• Lamicel
Hyaluronic acid	• Transcervical balloon catheters
Progesterone receptor antagonists	• With extra-amniotic saline infusion
	• With concomitant oxytocin administration

Failed Induction

Vaginal delivery is the goal of the induction process; however, this occurs less often than when women labor spontaneously. **There are currently no standards of what constitutes a failed induction. It is important for the clinician to recall that cervical ripening itself can take some time, and that the development of an active labor pattern should be achieved before the determination that the induction has failed.** The definitions and durations of labor described by Friedman in the 1950s were in regard to spontaneous labor, not inductions of labor. The importance of allowing enough time to progress from the latent phase of labor to the active phase is illustrated by the following studies.

In one large prospective study, the mean duration of the latent phase of labor (defined as the interval from initiation of induction with either prostaglandins or oxytocin to a cervical dilation of 4 cm) in women with a Bishop score of 0 to 3 was 12 hours in multiparas and 16 hours in nulliparas.[53] In another study, requiring a minimum of 12 hours of oxytocin administration after membrane rupture before diagnosing failed labor induction led to vaginal deliveries in 75% of nulliparas and eliminated failed labor induction as an indication for cesarean birth in parous women.[62] A third series found that 73% of women who ultimately delivered vaginally had a latent phase of up to 18 hours.[63] Latent phase was defined as the interval from initiation of oxytocin or amniotomy to the beginning of the active phase (i.e., cervical dilation of 4 cm with 80% effacement or 5 cm dilation).

The definition of failed induction should be derived from what is known about the pattern of labor progression in women undergoing induced labor who ultimately achieve vaginal delivery. The goal is to minimize the number of cesarean deliveries performed for failed induction in patients who are progressing slowly because they are still in the latent phase of labor.[53,62,63] Once induced women enter active labor, progression should be comparable to progression in women with spontaneous active labor, or faster.[64]

One group proposed that failed induction be defined as the inability to achieve cervical dilation of 4 cm and 80% effacement or 5 cm (regardless of effacement) after a minimum of 12 to 18 hours of both oxytocin administration and membrane rupture.[65] They also specified that uterine contractile activity should reach five contractions per 10 minutes or 250 Montevideo units, which is the minimum level achieved by most women whose labor is progressing normally. The cervical criteria were based on the observation that most women have entered the active phase when dilation reached 4 to 5 cm; thus, intervention before this dilation is likely to represent a latent phase abnormality rather than a protracted or arrested active phase. The duration of oxytocin administration was based on the observational studies cited previously, which described the maximum duration of latent phase in over 70% of induced women who went on to deliver vaginally. The membrane rupture requirement established a clear time point for "starting the clock," removed the time required for preinduction cervical ripening from the latent phase, and acknowledged the contribution of amniotomy as a method of induction.

An Australian researcher evaluated a group of 978 nulliparous women after either artificial or spontaneous rupture of membranes to determine factors that could predict failed induction.[66] There was a direct correlation between increasing duration of the latent phase and the probability of cesarean birth. After 10 hours of oxytocin administration, the 8% of women not in the active phase of labor had an approximately 75% chance of being delivered by cesarean for failed induction; after 12 hours of oxytocin administration, the chance of cesarean was almost 90%. Multivariable analysis showed that short maternal stature and use of pharmacologic or mechanical methods of cervical ripening contributed to an increased probability of cesarean delivery. Similarly, there was a linear relationship between lack of cervical dilation and cesarean birth. The authors concluded that the continuation of oxytocin after amniotomy for women who had not yet reached at least 4 cm dilation was not unreasonable, but that beyond 12 hours, the benefit was unclear.

TECHNIQUES FOR CERVICAL RIPENING AND LABOR INDUCTION

Oxytocin

Oxytocin is a polypeptide hormone produced in the hypothalamus and secreted from the posterior lobe of the pituitary gland in a pulsatile fashion. It is identical to its synthetic analog, which is among the most potent uterotonic agents known. Synthetic oxytocin is an effective means of labor induction.[67] Exogenous oxytocin administration produces periodic uterine contractions first demonstrable at approximately 20 weeks' gestation, with increasing responsiveness with advancing gestational age primarily due to an increase in myometrial oxytocin binding sites. There is little change in myometrial sensitivity to oxytocin from 34 weeks to term; however, once spontaneous labor begins, the uterine sensitivity to oxytocin increases rapidly. This physiologic mechanism makes oxytocin more effective in augmenting labor than in inducing labor, and even less successful as a cervical ripening agent.

Oxytocin is most often given intravenously. It cannot be given orally because the polypeptide is degraded to small, inactive forms by gastrointestinal enzymes. The plasma half-life is short, estimated at 3 to 6 minutes, and steady-state concentrations are reached within 30 to 40 minutes of initiation or dose change. Synthetic oxytocin is generally diluted by placing 10 units in 1000 mL of an isotonic solution, such as normal saline, yielding an oxytocin concentration of 10 mU/mL. It is given by infusion pump to allow continuous, precise control of the dose administered. A common practice is to make a solution of 60 units in 1000 mL crystalloid to allow the infusion pump setting to match the dose administered (e.g., 1 mU/min equals a pump infusion rate of 1 mL/hr).

Although oxytocin is an effective means of labor induction in women with a favorable cervix as noted earlier, it is less effective as a cervical ripening agent. Many randomized controlled trials comparing oxytocin with various prostaglandin (PG) formulations and other methods of cervical ripening confirm this observation. Lyndrup and colleagues compared the efficacy of labor induction with vaginal PGE_2 with continuous oxytocin infusion in 91 women with an unfavorable cervix (Bishop score <6). They found PGE_2 more efficacious for labor induction in 12 to 24 hours, with fewer women undelivered at 24 hours. However, by allowing the inductions to proceed for 48 hours, they found no difference in vaginal delivery rates after 48 hours between the two groups. In a larger study involving 200 women with an unfavorable cervix undergoing labor induction, vaginally applied prostaglandin E_2 was compared with continuous oxytocin infusion. These investigators found a shorter time interval to active labor, a significantly greater change in Bishop score, fewer failed inductions, and fewer multiple-day inductions with PGE_2 compared with oxytocin. No difference in the rate of cesarean delivery was found between the groups overall. In a Cochrane review of 110 trials including more than 11,000 women comparing oxytocin with any vaginal prostaglandin formulation for labor induction, oxytocin alone was associated with an increase in unsuccessful vaginal delivery within 24 hours (52 vs. 28%, RR 1.85, 95% CI 1.41 to 2.43). There was no difference in the rate of cesarean delivery between groups. When intracervical prostaglandins were compared with oxytocin alone for labor induction, oxytocin alone was associated with an increase in unsuccessful vaginal delivery within 24 hours (51 vs. 35%, RR 1.49, 95% CI 1.12 to 1.99) and an increase in cesarean delivery (19% vs. 13%, RR 1.42, 95% CI 1.11 to 1.82).[67]

In the setting of premature rupture of membranes (PROM) at term (defined as rupture of membranes before

TABLE 14-11 LABOR STIMULATION WITH OXYTOCIN: EXAMPLES OF LOW- AND HIGH-DOSE OXYTOCIN DOSING REGIMENS

REGIMEN	STARTING DOSE (mU/MIN)	INCREMENTAL INCREASE (mU/MIN)	DOSAGE INTERVAL (MIN)
Low-dose	0.5-2.0	1-2	15-40
High-dose	6	3-6*	15-40

Induction of Labor. ACOG Practice Bulletin No 107. American College of Obstetricians and Gynecologists. Obstet Gynecol 114:386, 2009.
*The incremental increase is reduced to 3 mU/min in the presence of hyperstimulation and reduced to 1 mU/min with recurrent hyperstimulation.

the onset of labor), labor induction is recommended if spontaneous labor does not ensue within a reasonable amount of time because, as the time between rupture of membranes and the onset of labor increases, so may the risk of maternal and fetal infection.[68] A series of systematic reviews examined the outcomes of pregnancies with PROM at or near term.[68] One trial accounts for most of the patients included in the analysis. Hannah and colleagues studied 5041 women with PROM at term. Subjects were randomly assigned to receive intravenous oxytocin, vaginal prostaglandin E_2 gel, or expectant management for up to 4 days, with labor induced with either intravenous oxytocin or vaginal prostaglandin E_2 gel. Those randomized to the expectant management group were induced if complications such as chorioamnionitis developed. The rates of neonatal infection and cesarean delivery were not statistically different between the groups. Rates of clinical chorioamnionitis were less in the group receiving intravenous oxytocin. When oxytocin alone was compared with vaginal prostaglandins in 14 trials for labor induction after PROM by Cochrane reviewers, both medications were found to be equally efficacious.[67] Thus, both can be used in this clinical setting. Because the majority of women with PROM enter labor spontaneously, a policy of expectant management for up to 96 hours is not unreasonable. However, active management of PROM does not increase the risk of cesarean delivery and significantly shortens the time until delivery. Therefore, patients should be offered a choice between active and expectant management, although more prefer active management.

The optimal regimen for oxytocin administration is debatable, although success rates for varying protocols are similar. Protocols differ as to the initial dose, incremental time period, and steady state dose (Table 14-11).[26] A maximum oxytocin dose has not been established, but most protocols do not exceed 42 mU/min.

Low-Dose Versus High-Dose Oxytocin

Low-dose protocols mimic endogenous maternal physiology and are associated with lower rates of uterine tachysystole. Low-dose oxytocin is initiated at 0.5 to 1 mU and increased by 1 mU per minute at 40- to 60-minute intervals. Slightly higher doses beginning at 1 to 2 mU/min increased by 1 to 2 mU/min, with shorter incremental time intervals of 15 to 30 minutes, have also been recommended. Pulsatile oxytocin administration, which truly mimics endogenous oxytocin release from the posterior pituitary, at 8- to 10-minute intervals, is considered a variant of low-dose oxytocin administration. It has the advantage of reducing total oxytocin requirements by 20% to 50%.[69] Proponents of low-dose oxytocin administration maintain that a slow rate of oxytocin administration is as effective for inducing labor and labor augmentation as faster rates of increase, while at the same time minimizing oxytocin requirements with lower rates of uterine overactivity.

High-dose oxytocin regimens are often employed in active management of labor protocols. These regimens are largely used for labor augmentation, rather than for labor induction. Examples of these protocols start with an initial oxytocin dose of 6 mU/min increased by 6 mU/min at 20 minute intervals, with a maximum dose of 40 mU/min[69] or start at 4 mU/min with 4 mU/min incremental increases (no maximum dose described).[53] A prospective study involving nearly 5000 women at Parkland Hospital comparing low-dose with high-dose oxytocin regimens for labor induction and augmentation was undertaken.[70] The high-dose protocol allowed for reduction of the dosage to 3 mU/min in the presence of uterine tachysystole. The results indicated that subjects given the high-dose regimen had a significantly shorter mean admission to delivery time, fewer failed inductions, fewer forceps deliveries, fewer cesarean deliveries for failure to progress, less chorioamnionitis, and less neonatal sepsis than subjects given the low-dose regimen. Notably, these subjects had a higher rate of cesarean delivery performed for "fetal distress," but no difference in neonatal outcomes was observed. Merrill and Zlatnik[71] conducted a randomized, double-masked trial including 1307 patients, comparing high-dose (4.5 mU/min initially increased by 4.5 mU/min every 30 minutes) with low-dose (1.5 mU/min initially, increased by 1.5 mU/min every 30 minutes) oxytocin for augmentation and induction of labor. Oxytocin solutions were prepared by a central pharmacy, and infusion volumes were identical to ensure double masking. In the group receiving high-dose oxytocin, labor was significantly shortened when used for induction (8.5 vs. 10.5 hours, $p < 0.001$), and augmentation (4.4 vs. 5.1 hours, $p = 0.3$). There was no significant difference in cesarean section rates between the two regimens (15% vs. 11.3%, $p = 0.17$). There were, however, more decreases or discontinuations of oxytocin in the high-dose group both for uterine tachysystole and fetal heart rate abnormalities. Discontinuation of oxytocin did not appear to have an adverse impact on cesarean section rates or lengthening of labor. Neonatal outcomes were observed to be similar in both groups.

In contemporary obstetrical practice, based on the aforementioned evidence, oxytocin is most often used to augment labor in patients with inadequate uterine activity or to induce labor in a patient with a favorable cervical status. One of many dosing regimens may be used depending on the standard practice in the community or the preference of the individual practitioner. Satin and colleagues[70] studied the differences in outcomes when oxytocin was used to augment as opposed to induce labor. These investigators prospectively studied 2788 consecutive women with singleton pregnancies. Indications for oxytocin stimulation were divided into augmentation ($n = 1676$) and induction ($n = 1112$). The low-dose regimen consisted of a starting dose of 1 mU/min with incremental increases of 1 mU/min at 20-minute intervals until 8 mU/min, then 2 mU/min increases up to a maximum of 20 mU/min, and was used first for 5 months in 1251 pregnancies. The high-dose regimen consisted of a starting dose of 6 mU/min, with increases of 6 mU/min at 20-minute intervals up to a maximum dose of 42 mU/min, and was used for the subsequent 5 months in 1537 pregnancies. Labor augmentation was more than 3 hours shorter in the high-dose group compared with that of the low-dose group. High-dose augmentation resulted in fewer cesarean deliveries for labor dystocia and fewer failed inductions when compared with the low-dose regimen, although cesarean deliveries for fetal distress were performed more frequently. A literature review of randomized clinical trials of high- versus low-dose oxytocin regimens published from 1966 to 2003 concluded that high-dose oxytocin decreased the time from admission to vaginal delivery, but did not decrease the incidence of cesarean delivery compared with low-dose therapy.[72] Only one double-blinded randomized trial has been published, and had the same findings.[71] High-dose regimens are associated with a higher rate of tachysystole than low-dose regimes, and in some studies this has resulted in a higher rate of cesarean delivery for fetal distress,[70] but no significant difference in neonatal outcomes. When making decisions regarding which oxytocin regimen to use, the risks and benefits need to be carefully considered depending on the ultimate outcome desired.

Oxytocin Dosing Intervals

Varying dosing intervals have also been studied and, in contemporary practice, vary from 15 to 40 minutes. One comparison of the efficacy and outcomes with differing oxytocin dosing intervals included 1801 consecutive pregnancies receiving high-dose oxytocin (starting dose of 6 mU/min with incremental increases of 6 mU/min) at 20- and 40-minute intervals. In this study, 949 women received oxytocin at 20-minute intervals (n = 603 labor augmentations and n = 346 labor inductions) and 852 women received oxytocin at 40-minute dosing intervals (n = 564 labor augmentations and n = 288 labor inductions). The rates of cesarean delivery for dystocia or fetal distress were not statistically different between groups; however, the 20-minute regimen for augmentation was associated with a significant reduction in cesareans for dystocia (8% vs. 12%, $p = 0.05$). The incidence of uterine tachysystole was greater with the 20-minute regimen compared to the 40-minute regimen (40% vs. 31%; $P = 0.02$). Neonatal outcomes were unaffected by the dosing interval. The authors concluded that the 40-minute dosing interval offered no clear advantage over the 20-minute interval and that both were safe and efficacious.

Oxytocin Dosing Protocols

Several experts have suggested that implementation of a standardized protocol is desirable to minimize errors in oxytocin administration.[73-75] Clark and colleagues[75] implemented an oxytocin checklist-based protocol at a tertiary facility and evaluated outcomes in 100 women before utilization of the protocol versus another 100 women after the protocol was put into practice. In the checklist-managed group, the maximum dose of oxytocin used to achieve delivery was significantly lower. No differences were noted preprotocol or postprotocol in the length of labor, total time of oxytocin administration, or rate of operative vaginal or abdominal delivery. When the protocol was then implemented throughout the Hospital Corporation of American system (125 obstetrical facilities in 20 states), the rate of cesarean birth was notably decreased from 23.6% to 21.0% and newborn complications requiring NICU admission or Apgar scores less than 8 were improved. Hayes and Weinstein[73] describe a standardized protocol for oxytocin administration based on a literature review, as well as the specific pharmacokinetics of oxytocin (see box, Standardized Oxytocin Regimen). However, at this time, no protocol has been subjected to the scientific scrutiny necessary to demonstrate its superiority in both efficacy and safety over another.

Standardized Oxytocin Regimen

1. Dilution: 10 U oxytocin in 1000 mL normal saline for resultant concentration of 10 mU oxytocin/mL
2. Infusion rate: 2 mU/min or 12 mL/hr
3. Incremental increase: 2 mU/min or 12 mL/hr every 45 minutes until contraction frequency adequate
4. Maximum dose: 16 mU/min or 96 mL/hr

Hayes EJ, Weinstein L: Improving patient safety and uniformity of care by a standardized regimen for the use of oxytocin. Am J Obstet Gynecol 198:622.e1, 2008. Epub Mar 20, 2008.

Prostaglandins

Administration of PG results in dissolution of collagen bundles and an increase in submucosal water content of the cervix. These changes in cervical connective tissue at term are similar to those observed in early labor. PGs are endogenous compounds found in the myometrium, deciduas, and fetal membranes during pregnancy. The chemical precursor is arachidonic acid. PG formulations have been used since they were first synthesized in the laboratory in 1968. Prostaglandin analogs were originally given by intravenous and oral routes. Later, local administration of prostaglandins in the vagina or the endocervix became the route of choice because of fewer side effects and acceptable clinical response. Side effects of all PG formulations and routes may include fever, chills, vomiting, and diarrhea.

The efficacy of locally applied PG (vaginal or intracervical) for cervical ripening and labor induction as compared with oxytocin (alone or in combination with amniotomy) has been demonstrated in a Cochrane review involving more than 10,000 women. Vaginal prostaglandin E_2 compared with placebo reduced the likelihood of vaginal delivery not being achieved within 24 hours, the risk of the cervix remaining unfavorable or unchanged, and the need for oxytocin. There was no difference between cesarean section rates, although there was a trade-off with prostaglandin E_2 use as the risk of uterine tachysystole with fetal heart rate changes was increased. The various administration vehicles (tablet, gel, and timed-release pessary) appear to be equally efficacious. The optimal route, frequency, and dose of prostaglandins of all types and formulations for cervical ripening and labor induction have not been determined. Also, prostaglandin formulations of any kind should be avoided in women with a prior uterine scar such as a prior cesarean delivery or myomectomy because their use appears to increase the risk for uterine rupture.[76] Uterine activity and fetal heart rate monitoring are indicated for 0.5 to 2 hours after administration of prostaglandins for cervical ripening, and should be maintained as long as regular uterine activity is present.[26]

Prostaglandin E_2

One of the first randomized controlled trials using intravaginal PG was conducted in 1979 by Liggins and colleagues. Eighty-four term women with singleton pregnancies were randomly assigned to three groups receiving placebo, 0.2 mg, or 0.4 mg PGE_2 compound. Labor was established in 48 hours in 9.3% of placebo women, 65.4% of women receiving 0.2 mg PGE_2, and 85.7% of women receiving 0.4 mg PGE_2. Rayburn summarized the experience with more than 3313 pregnancies representing 59 prospective clinical trials in which either intracervical or intravaginal PGE_2 was used for cervical ripening before the induction of labor. He concluded that local administration of PGE_2 is effective in enhancing cervical effacement and dilation, reducing the failed induction rate, shortening the induction to delivery interval, and reducing oxytocin use and cesarean delivery for failure to progress. These findings were confirmed in a meta-analysis of 44 controlled trials performed worldwide using various PG compounds and dosing regimens. Because there appears to be no difference in clinical outcomes when comparing intravaginal or intracervical PGE_2 preparations, and for ease of administration and patient satisfaction, vaginal administration is recommended.[77] A sustained-release vaginal pessary for PGE_2 has been developed. Its use eliminates the need for repeated dosing. Although data are limited, when comparing the efficacy of the intravaginally applied PGE_2 to the sustained-release suppository, there appears to be no difference in rates of vaginal delivery, fetal heart rate abnormalities, or uterine tachysystole.

Currently, there are two PGE_2 preparations approved by the U.S. Food and Drug Administration (FDA) for cervical ripening. There are a variety of other PGE_2 compounds such as suppositories available in the United States and tablets available in Europe, although these latter formulations are not approved for use by the FDA for cervical ripening. Many clinicians and pharmacists may prepare their own formulations of PGE_2 gel by thawing and resuspending 20 mg PGE_2 suppositories in small amounts of methylcellulose gel. The resulting gel preparation is then frozen in plastic syringes in various doses ranging from 1 to 6 mg.

Prepidil (Upjohn Pharmaceuticals, Kalamazoo, Michigan) contains 0.5 mg of dinoprostone in 2.5 mL of gel for intracervical administration. The dose can be repeated in 6 to 12 hours if there is inadequate cervical change and minimal uterine activity following the first dose. The manufacturer recommends that the maximum cumulative dose of dinoprostone not exceed 1.5 mg (three doses) within a 24-hour period. Oxytocin should not be initiated until 6 to 12 hours after the last dose because of the potential for uterine tachysystole with concurrent oxytocin and prostaglandin administration.

Cervidil (Forest Pharmaceuticals, St. Louis, Missouri) is a vaginal insert containing 10 mg of dinoprostone in a timed-release formulation. The vaginal insert administers the medication at 0.3 mg/hr and may be left in place for up to 12 hours. An advantage of the vaginal insert over the gel formulation is that the insert may be removed with the onset of active labor, rupture of membranes, or the development of uterine overactivity. This abnormality of uterine contractions is more often defined as six or more contractions in 10 minutes for a total of 20 minutes with concurrent fetal heart rate tracing abnormalities. Per the manufacturer's recommendations, oxytocin may be initiated 30 to 60 minutes after removal of the insert.

These two preparations are relatively expensive, require refrigerated storage, and become unstable at room temperature.

Prostaglandin E_1

Misoprostol (Cytotec, Searle Pharmaceuticals, Chicago, Illinois) is a synthetic prostaglandin E_1 analog available as 100 mcg and 200 mcg tablets. The current FDA-approved use for misoprostol is for the treatment and prevention of peptic ulcer disease related to chronic nonsteroidal anti-inflammatory use. Administration of misoprostol for preinduction cervical ripening is considered a safe and effective "off-label" use by the College.[78] Misoprostol is inexpensive and is also stable at room temperature. Misoprostol can be administered orally or placed vaginally with few systemic side effects. Although not scored, the tablets are usually divided to provide 25 or 50 mcg doses.

Multiple studies suggest that misoprostol tablets placed vaginally are either superior to or equivalent in efficacy compared with intracervical PGE_2 gel.[79] More recently a meta-analysis of 70 trials revealed the following points regarding the use of misoprostol compared with other methods of cervical ripening and labor induction.[80] Misoprostol improved cervical ripening compared with placebo and was associated with a reduced failure to achieve vaginal delivery within 24 hours (RR 0.36; 95% CI 0.19 to 0.68). There was a trend toward fewer cesarean deliveries that did not reach statistical significance. Compared with other vaginal prostaglandins for labor induction, vaginal misoprostol was more effective in achieving vaginal delivery within 24 hours (RR 0.80; 95% CI 0.73 to 0.87). Compared with vaginal or intracervical PGE_2, oxytocin augmentation was also less common with misoprostol (RR 0.65; 95% CI 0.57 to 0.73). However, uterine tachysystole with fetal heart rate changes (RR 2.04; 95% CI 1.49 to 2.80) and meconium-stained amniotic fluid (RR 1.42; 95% CI 1.11 to 1.81) was more common. Most studies suggested that restricting the dose of misoprostol to 25 mcg every 4 hours significantly reduced the risk of uterine tachysystole with and without fetal heart rate changes and meconium passage. Most important, regardless of misoprostol dose, there were no significant differences in immediate neonatal outcomes.

Although the ACOG, based on its review of the existing evidence, recommends 25 mcg dosing every 3 to 6 hours with vaginally applied misoprostol, the optimal dose and timing interval is not known.[26] Oxytocin may be initiated, if necessary, 4 hours after the final misoprostol dose. A meta-analysis comparing 25 mcg with 50 mcg dosing reported that 50 mcg dosing resulted in a higher rate of vaginal delivery within 24 hours with higher rates of uterine tachysystole and meconium passage but without compromising in neonatal outcomes.[81] A statistically significant difference in fetal acidosis defined as a umbilical arterial pH of less than 7.16 was found in infants born to mothers given 50 mcg of intravaginally applied misoprostol every 3 hours compared with those born to mothers given 25 mcg every 3 hours. In their Committee Opinions on the use of misoprostol for labor induction, the College concludes that safety using the higher 50 mcg dosing could not be adequately evaluated and suggests the higher dose could be used only in select circumstances. A time-released misoprostol vaginal insert [MVI] is under development. In a three-arm Phase III investigation, an MVI dose of 100 mcg did not have appreciably better clinical outcomes than Cervidil.

Oral administration of misoprostol for cervical ripening has also been studied. Oral administration has the promise for offering more patient comfort, satisfaction, and convenience of administration. Most of these studies compared lower oral doses of misoprostol such as 50 mcg given every 3 to 6 hours and compared them to similar vaginal misoprostol dosing regimens such as 25 to 50 mcg given every 3 to 6 hours. This oral regimen of dosing appears to be no more effective than vaginal administration for achieving vaginal delivery or affecting cesarean rates, but may be associated with less uterine overactivity. There is a clear positive dose-response relationship seen between the dosage of oral misoprostol and rate of tachysystole. With the 25- and 50-mcg dosages, there is a lower tachysystole rate; it is higher in those given 200 mcg.[82] In this meta-analysis, oral misoprostol use was clearly superior to placebo, as women administered oral misoprostol were more likely to deliver vaginally within 24 hours, needed less oxytocin, and had a lower cesarean rate.

Some investigators have described titrating oral misoprostol to its desired effect.[83] This method appears to achieve vaginal delivery rates similar to vaginally administered misoprostol with less uterine overactivity. Low doses of oral misoprostol were achieved by making a solution (e.g., dissolving a 200 mcg tablet in 200 mL tap water), as this was believed to provide more accurate dosing than simply cutting the tablet into pieces. Because oral dosing has a short (2 hours) duration of action, administration was repeated at 2-hour intervals. The authors of this Cochrane review recommend that if clinicians choose to use oral misoprostol, a dose of 20 to 25 mcg in solution is preferred for safety considerations and addresses concerns regarding imprecision of dividing misoprostol tablets for recommended dosages. There are concerns, however, that the pharmacy and nursing administration needed for dose titration is complex.[82] More data are needed to shed light on the optimal dosing, safety, and cost considerations of oral misoprostol for cervical ripening and labor induction.

Other novel approaches include buccal and sublingual misoprostol administration. The theory is that avoiding first-pass hepatic circulation from oral administration will lead to bioavailability similar to that achieved with vaginal administration. This hypothesis has been substantiated by pharmacokinetic studies that have shown that the buccal and sublingual routes of administration are associated with rapid onset of action and greater bioavailability than other routes.[84] In a randomized controlled trial including 250 women admitted for labor induction, 50 mcg of sublingual misoprostol was compared to 100 mcg of orally administered misoprostol given every 4 hours to a maximum of five doses. Sublingual misoprostol appeared to have the same efficacy as orally administered misoprostol to achieve vaginal delivery within 24 hours with no increase in uterine tachysystole. However, the 100 mcg oral dose had higher rates of uterine overactivity than 25 mcg administered vaginally. A randomized controlled trial including 152 women received either 200 mcg of buccal misoprostol every 6 hours or 50 mcg of misoprostol administered vaginally every 6 hours. There was no statistically significant difference in time interval to vaginal delivery, the rate of vaginal delivery, or the rate of uterine tachysystole between the two groups. The buccal route was associated with a trend toward fewer cesarean sections than with the vaginal route. Based on only three small trials included in the Cochrane meta-analysis, sublingual misoprostol appears to be at least as effective as when the same dose is administered orally. There are inadequate data to comment on the relative complications and side effects. More data are needed to clarify not only safety but the efficacy of buccal and sublingual misoprostol use as well.[85] Optimal dosing regimens are yet to be defined, and concern exists because of greater bioavailability associated with these routes of administration when compared to vaginal use.

Outpatient or ambulatory approaches to cervical ripening and labor induction for elective or marginal indications could be useful in reducing the duration of hospitalization and the staffing requirements of labor and delivery. The body of evidence to support this approach, however, is limited.[86-89] Relevant published studies reflect a variety of different approaches to cervical ripening, including local applications of prostaglandin compounds and placement of Foley balloon catheters to the lower uterine segment with or without immediate hospitalization for further labor management. To adequately address safety of any outpatient cervical ripening and labor induction technique, large numbers of subjects will be necessary. For this reason, outpatient cervical ripening and labor induction is not recommended at this time, other than in a research setting.

Alternative Pharmacologic Methods

Researchers have evaluated several other compounds as alternatives for cervical ripening and labor induction in term pregnancies, including RU-486 (mifepristone), estrogen, relaxin, and hyaluronic acid.

RU-486 (mifepristone) is a competitive steroid receptor antagonist and, because of its antiprogestational action, it has been used for early pregnancy termination. It has also been studied as a potential alternative for cervical ripening and labor induction in term pregnancies. Although these studies demonstrate that mifepristone is more effective than placebo, there are no studies to date comparing mifepristone to other agents for cervical ripening and labor induction.[90] At this time, access to this medication limits widespread research and use.

Seminal parturition studies in sheep showed that there is a prelabor rise in estrogen associated with a decrease in progesterone. These changes stimulate prostaglandin production and may help initiate labor. Through this mechanism, estrogen has been suggested and studied as a cervical ripening agent and labor induction agent. At this time, estrogen is not currently used in common practice as an induction agent, and there is insufficient evidence to draw any conclusions regarding its efficacy.

Relaxin, produced by the corpus luteum in pregnancy, is a protein hormone thought to have a promoting effect on cervical ripening through connective tissue remodeling. Its use was thought to have advantages over other agents that promoted uterine activity by potentially decreasing the risk of uterine tachsystole. Two studies totaling 113 women who received human recombinant relaxin for induction of labor compared with placebo showed no effect on cervical ripening or labor induction. The place of relaxin as an induction or cervical priming agent is unclear, and further trials are needed to determine its place in current clinical practice.

The cervix is a fibrous organ composed principally of hyaluronic acid, collagen, and proteoglycan. Hyaluronic acid increases as pregnancy progresses, peaks after the onset of labor, and decreases rapidly after birth of the infant. The increase in the level of hyaluronic acid is associated with an increase in tissue water content of the cervix, which is one of the mechanisms involved in cervical ripening. In the past, investigators postulated that cervical injection of hyaluronic acid would lead to cervical ripening. Although there is a theoretical physiologic mechanism for hyaluronic acid as a cervical ripening agent, there are no published studies using this agent for this indication.

Mechanical Methods

Mechanical methods are among the oldest approaches used to promote cervical ripening. Advantages of these techniques compared to pharmacologic methods include their low cost, low risk of tachysystole, few systemic side effects, and convenient storage requirements (no refrigeration or expiration).[91] Comparing mechanical methods with placebo or no treatment, tachysystole with fetal heart rate changes was not reported. The risk of cesarean birth was similar between groups (34%; RR 1.00; 95% CI 0.76 to 1.30, n = 416, six studies). There were no reported cases of severe neonatal and maternal morbidity among them. The risk of tachysystole was reduced when compared with all prostaglandins (intracervical, intravaginal, or misoprostol). Compared with oxytocin in women with unfavorable cervix, mechanical methods reduce the risk of cesarean delivery. Disadvantages of mechanical methods include a small increase in the risk of maternal and neonatal infection from introduction of a foreign body,[92] the potential for disruption of a low-lying placenta, and some maternal discomfort on manipulation of the cervix. The most common mechanical methods are stripping (or sweeping) of the fetal membranes, amniotomy, placement of hygroscopic dilators within the endocervical canal, and insertion of a balloon catheter above the internal cervical os (with or without infusion of extra-amniotic saline). All of these methods likely work, at least in part, by causing the release of prostaglandin $F_{2\text{-alpha}}$ from the decidua and adjacent membranes or prostaglandin E_2 from the cervix. The latter two methods physically cause gradual cervical dilation with minimal discomfort to the patient.

Membrane Stripping

Stripping or sweeping of the fetal membranes refers to digital separation of the chorioamniotic membrane from the wall of the cervix and lower uterine segment by inserting the examiner's finger beyond the internal cervical os and then rotating the finger circumferentially along the lower uterine segment. This procedure was first reported for induction of labor at term in 1810 by Hamilton in England. For membrane stripping, the fetal vertex should be well applied to the cervix, and the cervix should be dilated sufficiently to allow introduction of the examiner's finger.

Many investigations have been conducted using routine membrane stripping at 38 or 39 weeks to either prevent prolonged pregnancies or decrease the frequency of more formal inductions occurring after 41 weeks.[93] Two randomized trials compared outcomes of women who underwent membrane stripping or no membrane stripping at initiation of labor induction with oxytocin. The results of these trials suggested that membrane stripping increased the rate of spontaneous vaginal delivery and shortened the induction to delivery interval. However, differences in study design and management of induction preclude definitive conclusions. As an example, in one trial, these benefits were only observed in nulliparas, and, in the other trial, induction was performed using amniotomy or dinoprostone pessary.

Other randomized trials have tried to assess whether membrane stripping hastens the onset of spontaneous labor. In one randomized trial, women assigned to membrane stripping had a significant reduction in the subsequent duration of pregnancy (2 days compared to 5 days in controls) and frequency of induction (8.1% vs. 18.8% in controls), whereas two other randomized trials found no beneficial effects from membrane sweeping. None of these trials reported harmful side effects that could be attributed to the procedure.

Routine membrane stripping is not recommended given that there is no evidence this practice results in an improvement in maternal or neonatal outcome. However, **weekly membrane stripping at term shortens the interval of time to onset of spontaneous labor and reduces the need for formal induction.** For this reason, we offer membrane stripping after 39 weeks of gestation to patients who wish to hasten the onset of spontaneous labor.

Although the existing meta-analysis on the use of membrane stripping[94] was not associated with an increase in either maternal or neonatal infection, it is unclear if the included studies involved carriers of group B streptococcus (GBS). There are no studies currently in the literature specifically designed to address the safety of membrane stripping in known carriers of GBS and, as a result, this is not considered a contraindication to membrane stripping.[95]

Complications that can result from membrane stripping include rupture of membranes, hemorrhage from disruption of an occult placenta previa, and the development of chorioamnionitis. **Most commonly, however, membrane stripping is associated with maternal discomfort and clinically insignificant vaginal bleeding.**

Amniotomy

Amniotomy, artificial rupture of membranes, is a technique involving the perforation of the chorioamniotic membranes. It is an effective method of labor induction performed in multiparous women with favorable cervices. Before amniotomy is performed, confirmation is essential that the fetal vertex, and not the umbilical cord or other fetal part, is presenting and is well applied to the cervix. These precautions are taken to prevent umbilical cord prolapse, which often necessitates emergent cesarean delivery. The amniotomy procedure usually involves a toothed clamp such as an Allis clamp, or more commonly, a plastic hook that is applied to the membranes and manipulated so as to puncture the membranes. The fetal heart rate status before and after the procedure should be monitored, and the amniotic fluid character and color should be recorded.

Although trials evaluating amniotomy alone versus placebo or no treatment are lacking,[96] combined use of amniotomy and intravenous oxytocin is more effective than amniotomy alone with fewer women undelivered vaginally after 24 hours.[97] In the meta-analysis of amniotomy, 17 trials involving 2566 women were included. Amniotomy and intravenous oxytocin were found to result in (1) fewer women being undelivered vaginally at 24 hours than amniotomy alone (RR 0.03; 95% CI 0.001 to 0.49, $n = 100$, one study); (2) significantly fewer instrumental vaginal deliveries than placebo (RR 0.18; CI 0.05 to 0.58); and (3) more postpartum hemorrhage than vaginal prostaglandins (RR 5.5; CI 1.26 to 24.07). There is also more dissatisfaction with amniotomy and intravenous oxytocin when compared with vaginal prostaglandins (RR 53.0; CI 3.32 to 846.51).[97]

Hygroscopic Dilators

Mechanical dilators placed in the lower uterine segment release endogenous prostaglandins from the fetal membranes and maternal decidua. In addition, the osmotic properties of hygroscopic dilators promote cervical ripening. These hygroscopic dilators absorb endocervical and local tissue fluids that cause swelling and allow for controlled dilation by mechanical pressure. There are two types of hygroscopic dilators: one is made from natural seaweed *(Laminaria japonicum)* and the other is a synthetic product (e.g., Lamicel). Hygroscopic dilators are safe and effective for dilating the cervix, although they are used primarily during pregnancy termination rather than for preinduction cervical ripening of term pregnancies. They function by disrupting the chorioamniotic decidual interface, causing lysosomal destruction and prostaglandin release. These events lead to active stretching of the cervix beyond the passive mechanical stretching provided by the dilator itself.

A meta-analysis of randomized trials comparing hygroscopic dilators to placebo/no treatment found that pregnant women in both groups had similar rates of not achieving a vaginal delivery by 24 hours (RR 0.90; 95% CI 0.64 to 1.26), cesarean deliveries (RR 0.98; 95% CI 0.74 to 1.30), and infection.[91] These data suggest that although hygroscopic dilators can dilate the cervix, they are inadequate for improving the outcome of induction. However, no large trials have been performed and there are no well-designed comparative studies evaluating the optimal use of hygroscopic dilators with other modalities, such as amniotomy, to improve the rate of successful induction. A significant disadvantage of the use of laminaria for cervical ripening is patient discomfort both at the time of insertion and with progressive cervical dilation. With other equally effective agents available, there is no obvious benefit to support their routine use for labor induction at term. In specific clinical circumstances in which prostaglandins should be avoided or are unavailable because of supply or cost, laminaria can be used both safely and effectively.

Transcervical Balloon Catheters

A deflated Foley catheter, usually a 16-French 30-mL balloon, can be passed through an undilated cervix into the extra-amniotic space and then inflated. The balloon is then retracted to rest against the internal os. Some clinicians remove the top of the catheter before insertion although there are no data to suggest that this is necessary. To add more traction, pressure may be applied by attaching a weight such as a liter of intravenous fluid to the end of the catheter and suspending it with the force of gravity or by taping the catheter under tension to the patient's inner thigh. The benefit of traction has not been proven.

Transcervical balloon catheters appear to be as effective for preinduction cervical ripening as prostaglandin E_2 gel and intravaginal misoprostol in most studies. The combination of a balloon catheter plus administration of a prostaglandin does not appear to be more effective than prostaglandins alone. Although the risk of infection may theoretically be associated with the insertion of a foreign object in the cervix, existing meta-analysis data did not show evidence of an increased risk of infectious morbidity. This technique is a superior method of preinduction cervical ripening when compared with intravenous oxytocin and has been associated with a lower rate of cesarean delivery in one investigation.[91] Some studies show more rapid cervical ripening, a shortened induction to delivery interval, and reduced frequency of patients undelivered in 24 hours when combining a transcervical balloon catheter with a pharmacologic method of cervical ripening such as a prostaglandin, whereas others do not. No increased risk of preterm delivery in subsequent pregnancies following the placement of balloon catheters in the lower uterine segment was found by Sciscione and colleagues in 126 women.

The use of the Atad double-balloon device has also been described in a limited group of studies. One investigation included 95 women with Bishop scores no more than 4 and randomly assigned them to vaginally administered PGE_2, Atad balloon dilator technique, or continuous oxytocin for labor induction. They found a significant mean change in Bishop score after 12 hours in the PGE_2 group and Atad balloon dilator group of 5 compared with 2.5 in the oxytocin group. In addition they found a higher rate of failed induction in the oxytocin group (58%) compared with 20% in the PGE_2 and 5.7% in the Atad balloon dilator groups. Vaginal delivery rates in the oxytocin group were 26.7% compared with 77% and 70% in the Atad balloon dilator and PGE_2 groups, respectively.

Extra-Amniotic Saline Infusion

Infusion of isotonic fluid into the extra-amniotic space has been employed as an adjunct to transcervical balloon catheter placement in the lower uterine segment. The hypothesis for this approach is that this disruption of the fetal-maternal interface will result in added release of endogenous prostaglandins and other parturition-related hormones to facilitate the onset of spontaneous uterine activity. Most commonly, isotonic saline is used (hence the name extra-amniotic saline infusion [EASI]) and is infused continuously at rates of 20 to 40 mL/hr. The use of EASI with a transcervical Foley balloon catheter appears to be effective for cervical ripening when compared with intravaginal prostaglandins, although EASI does not appear to improve induction outcomes over those observed with the use of Foley catheter alone. In three randomized trials, both techniques resulted in similar rates of delivery less than 24 hours, cesarean delivery, and complications, although one small trial reported a shorter induction-to-vaginal-delivery time with the combined method.

A Cochrane review comparing EASI to any prostaglandin for cervical ripening showed that EASI infusion was significantly less likely to result in vaginal delivery within 24 hours (43% vs. 58%, RR 1.33; 95% CI 1.02 to 1.75), had a higher risk of cesarean delivery (31% vs. 22%, RR 1.48; 95% CI 1.14 to 1.90), and did not reduce the risk of tachysystole.[91] From these data, there is little support for the use of EASI as an adjunct to transcervical balloon catheter placement.

The only trials using the transcervical Foley catheter with simultaneous oxytocin infusion compared with vaginally administered misoprostol incorporated EASI along with the transcervical catheter. The largest trial by Buccellato and colleagues included 250 women undergoing labor induction with an unfavorable cervix who were randomly assigned to receive either a transcervical Foley catheter with concomitant oxytocin infusion or vaginally administered misoprostol 50 mcg every 4 hours for a maximum of three doses. There were no significant differences in the rate of cesarean delivery, rate of uterine tachysystole, or time intervals to vaginal delivery, indicating that both methods of labor induction appear to be equally effective. Mullin and colleagues studied 200 women undergoing labor induction with an unfavorable cervix. Subjects were randomized to receive a transcervical Foley catheter with EASI and concomitant oxytocin infusion or vaginally administered misoprostol 25 mcg every 4 hours for a maximum of six doses. They found that subjects receiving misoprostol had a longer average interval from labor induction to delivery of 1323 minutes compared with 970 minutes for subjects receiving the transcervical Foley catheter. There were no differences in cesarean births between the two groups. These data indicate that the transcervical Foley catheter with simultaneous oxytocin infusion may be just as efficacious as the usual dosing regimen for vaginally administered misoprostol for preinduction cervical ripening, and may, in fact, result in shorter induction to delivery time intervals.

MIDTRIMESTER INDUCTION

In particular circumstances, such as when a fetus has died in utero or in cases of termination of pregnancy in which a fetus would not survive or would survive but with significant handicaps, a woman may need to give birth before spontaneous labor. Several delivery options are available for these women, and the decision as to which option is chosen depends on physician expertise, gestational age, clinical circumstances, and the patient's preferences. Many women will desire immediate delivery secondary to the emotional difficulties of continuing to carry a nonviable fetus; however, some would prefer expectant management in order to avoid an induction of labor. In most cases, there is no medical urgency for immediate delivery. Expectant management raises concerns regarding consumptive coagulopathy and intrauterine infection, but these are rarely associated with prolonged expectant management. Some studies report that 80% to 90% of women will spontaneously labor within 2 weeks of a fetal demise, but the latency period may be longer.[98]

TABLE 14-12 SECOND TRIMESTER TERMINATION METHODS

SURGICAL TECHNIQUES	MEDICAL TECHNIQUES
Dilation and evacuation	Intravenous oxytocin
Laparotomy	Intra-amniotic hyperosmotic fluid
Hysterotomy	20% saline
Hysterectomy	30% urea
	Prostaglandins E_2, $F_{2\alpha}$, E_1, and analogs
	RU-486 (mifepristone)
	Various combinations of above

Options of delivery include induction of labor and dilation and evacuation (D&E), among others (Table 14-12). Again, the decision for which mode of delivery to choose must be individualized by practitioner experience, gestational age, and the patient's desires. The emotional and psychological factors vary with each patient, with one advantage of induction being the delivery of an intact fetus whereas an advantage of D&E may be avoiding a prolonged induction.

Most of the research available regarding modes of delivery for midtrimester delivery are extrapolated from the investigations performed regarding second trimester elective abortions. One study evaluated patients undergoing surgical termination between 14 and 24 weeks of gestation and women undergoing labor induction, which revealed an overall lower rate of complications in those undergoing D&E (4% vs. 29%). The groups were similar, however, in their need for blood transfusion, infection, cervical laceration, maternal organ damage, and hospital readmission. Cochrane reviewers recently concluded that D&E is superior to intra-amniotic instillation of prostaglandin $F_{2\text{-alpha}}$ and may be favored over mifepristone and misoprostol, but larger randomized studies are necessary to confirm these latter findings.[99] At this time, both methods of delivery are considered reasonably safe.

Several methods of labor induction have been used, with no standard protocol currently accepted. In the 1940s, physicians attempted to "salt out" the fetus by injecting hypertonic agents into the amniotic cavity. Hypertonic saline thus became the mainstay of second trimester medical abortion through the 1970s. However, significant risks associated with this method included hypernatremia, coagulopathy, and massive hemorrhage requiring blood transfusions. Instillation regimens using hyperosmolar urea were associated with less coagulopathy and hypernatremia than saline. However, the urea regimens have not

TABLE 14-13 SUGGESTED PROTOCOLS FOR STILLBIRTH DELIVERY

D&E FOR UTERUS BETWEEN 13 AND 22 WK SIZE	INDUCTION OF LABOR
• Admit to hospital, day operating room, or clinic • Obtain hematocrit and type and screen • Give doxycycline 100 mg orally 1 hr before procedure and 200 mg after procedure or postoperative metronidozole 500 mg orally twice a day for 5 days	• Admit to labor and delivery • Obtain complete blood count and type and screen; consider fibrinogen if fetus has been dead for >4 wk
To Facilitate Cervical Dilation • Administer misoprostol 200 mcg in the posterior fornix 4 hr before procedure (may be placed by patient) • Place laminaria in cervix (usually carried out in office on the afternoon before the procedure)	**Induction Protocols** • For uterus <28 wk: misoprostol 200-400 mcg vaginally or orally every 4 hr until delivery of fetus • For uterus >28 wk: misoprostol 25-50 mcg vaginally or orally every 4 hr or oxytocin infusion per usual protocol • Consider transcervical Foley catheter or laminaria for cervical ripening
Operative • Perform D&E under ultrasound guidance	**Intrapartum** • To minimize risk of retained placenta, allow for spontaneous placental delivery, avoid pulling on umbilical cord, consider further doses of misoprostol or high-dose oxytocin • Monitor vital signs as per routine for labor and delivery • Pain management includes epidural, intravenous narcotics via patient-controlled analgesia or intermittent doses • Parents should be encouraged to spend time with the infant and offered keepsake items (pictures, handprints/footprints, etc.)
Postprocedure Instructions • Discharge home after anesthesia has worn off and vaginal bleeding is minimal • Administer RhD immune globulin if patient is Rh negative • Schedule a follow-up visit in 2 wk • Prescribe NSAIDs or mild narcotics • Offer bereavement services	**Postprocedure Instructions** • Discharge home in 6 to 24 hr if vital signs are stable and bleeding is appropriate • Consider postpartum care on a nonmaternity ward • Administer RhD immune globulin if patient is Rh negative • Follow-up visit in 2-6 wk • Offer bereavement services

Modified from Silver RM, Heuser CC: Stillbirth workup and delivery management. Clin Obstet Gynecol 53:681, 2010.
D&E, Dilation and evacuation; *NSAIDs*, nonsteroidal anti-inflammatory drugs.

been compared to more recent induction protocols. Hyperosmolar regimens often require concomitant use of medical induction agents, such as oxytocin, to stimulate contractions and delivery.

More recent protocols have implemented regimens with gemeprost or misoprostol, both PGE_1 analogs; however, a meta-analysis of randomized trials comparing the two medications reported that misoprostol suppositories were associated with a reduced need for narcotic analgesia and surgical evacuation of the uterus. The application of gemeprost is limited secondary to its expense, instability at room temperature, and narrow routes of administration. It is also not currently available in the United States. At this time, the World Health Organization also recommends the use of mifepristone before PGE_1 analogs for expeditious and safe second trimester abortions. Mifepristone, as an antiprogestin, increases uterine sensitivity to prostaglandins, permitting lower doses and minimizing side effects. However, current studies do not reveal any advantage of pretreatment with mifepristone for induction in second trimester fetal demise.[100]

When planning an induction of labor, gestational age plays a significant role regarding the methods of induction. When the gestational age is less than 28 weeks, the uterus is less sensitive to oxytocin and, therefore, prostaglandins or mechanical devices may be required to commence labor. Current induction protocols vary by dose, route, and gestational age (Table 14-13). It is important to keep in mind that although side effects (uterine tachysystole, nausea, vomiting, diarrhea) and safety remain important considerations for the patient in these circumstances, the fetal well-being is no longer an issue.

Women with a prior cesarean section are candidates for induction of labor in these circumstances as well. A recent review by Berghella and colleagues reported an incidence of uterine rupture of 0.4%, hysterectomy 0%, and transfusion 0.2% for women undergoing second trimester misoprostol terminations. Patients may elect for a repeat cesarean delivery, but the risks and benefits should be carefully considered.

SUMMARY

Induction of labor is one of the most commonly performed procedures in obstetrical medicine, and can be undertaken for a variety of medical and obstetrical indications. The prediction of labor induction success has been studied with focus on a number of clinical, biochemical, and radiographic approaches. Cervical dilation at the time of initiation is the best independent predictor of induction success. A variety of pharmacologic and mechanical methods exist for cervical ripening. The most commonly used approaches include use of prostaglandins such as dinoprostone and misoprostol, as well as transcervical Foley balloon catheter placement. Augmentation of labor is usually accomplished with intravenous oxytocin, which can be administered using either low- or high-dose infusion protocols. In the case of a midtrimester induction, either induction of labor or dilation and evacuation is considered a safe approach.

KEY POINTS

- Labor is a clinical diagnosis defined as uterine contractions resulting in progressive cervical effacement and dilation, often accompanied by a bloody discharge referred to as bloody show, which results in birth of the baby.
- A graduated approach for diagnosis of labor protraction and arrest should be considered, based on the level of cervical dilation.
- Because the duration of latent labor is highly variable, expectant management is most appropriate.
- The most common causes of protraction or arrest disorders are inadequate uterine activity and abnormal positioning of the fetal presenting part.
- An intrauterine pressure catheter is frequently used when inadequate uterine activity is suspected owing to a protraction or arrest disorder. It can also be used to monitor and titrate oxytocin administration.
- There is evidence that maternal morbidities including perineal trauma, chorioamnionitis, instrumental delivery, and postpartum hemorrhage increase with prolonged second stages lasting greater than 2 hours.
- Comparing active to expectant management of the third stage, there is a reduced risk of postpartum hemorrhage when active management is used.
- Complications of oxytocin administration include water intoxication, uterine tachysystole, and uterine rupture. These complications are most commonly seen with high-dose, prolonged infusions. The condition of the cervix at the start of labor induction is critical to the success of the induction attempt. Both pharmacologic and mechanical methods of cervical ripening are available.
- Induction of labor should be undertaken when the benefits of prompt delivery to either mother or fetus outweigh the risks of pregnancy continuation.
- Recent studies have demonstrated that routine induction of labor at 41 weeks' gestation is not associated with an increased risk of cesarean delivery regardless of parity, state of the cervix, or method of induction. This indicates that some target populations may be appropriate for elective induction without incurring the added risks of cesarean delivery.
- The three major potential complications of elective induction of labor are increased neonatal morbidity, increased cost, and increased cesarean delivery resulting from failed induction. However, elective induction between 37 and 39 weeks' gestational age may be associated with a decreased risk of cesarean birth compared to expectant management.
- Cervical ripening methods fall into two main categories: pharmacologic and mechanical. Because the state of the cervix plays such a crucial role in labor induction, a cervical examination is essential before determining which method to use for labor induction.
- There are currently no standards of what constitutes a failed induction. It is important for the clinician to recall that cervical ripening itself can take some time, and that the development of an active labor pattern should be achieved before the determination that the induction has failed.
- Membrane sweeping is effective in reducing the interval to spontaneous onset of labor and the overall duration of pregnancy when performed at term. It is not associated with increased maternal or neonatal infection, but can cause maternal discomfort and vaginal bleeding.
- In women with intact membranes, combined use of amniotomy and intravenous oxytocin is more effective than amniotomy alone, with fewer women undelivered vaginally after 24 hours.
- Induction of labor with intravenous oxytocin, intravaginal prostaglandin compounds, and expectant management (with defined time limits) are all reasonable options for women and their infants in the face of PROM at term, because they result in similar rates of neonatal infection and cesarean delivery.
- There are a variety of different dosing protocols and dosing intervals for the administration of oxytocin for labor induction and augmentation. In general, higher doses are associated with shorter times to delivery, but more uterine tachysystole than are lower doses. Lower doses of oxytocin do not increase operative delivery rates or prolong delivery intervals.
- Options of delivery for midtrimester stillbirth or induction for lethal fetal anomalies include induction of labor and dilation and evacuation (D&E), among others. The decision for which mode of delivery to choose must be individualized by practitioner experience, gestational age, and the patient's desires.

REFERENCES

1. Friedman E: An objective approach to the diagnosis and management of abnormal labor. Bull N Y Acad Med 48:842, 1972.
2. Zhang J, Troendle J, Mikolajczyk R, et al: The natural history of the normal first stage of labor. Obstet Gynecol 115:705, 2010.
3. Ponkey SE, Cohen AP, Heffner LJ, Lieberman E: Persistent fetal occiput posterior position: obstetric outcomes. Obstet Gynecol 101:915, 2003.
4. Rouse DJ, Owen J, Goldenberg RL, Cliver SP: The effectiveness and costs of elective cesarean delivery for fetal macrosomia diagnosed by ultrasound. JAMA 276:1480, 1996.
5. Rouse DJ, Owen J, Hauth JC: Active-phase labor arrest: oxytocin augmentation for at least 4 hours. Obstet Gynecol 93:323, 1999.
6. Kilpatrick SJ, Laros RK: Characteristics of normal labor. Obstet Gynecol 74:85, 1989.
7. Allen VM, Baskett TF, O'Connell CM, et al: Maternal and perinatal outcomes with increasing duration of the second stage of labor. Obstet Gynecol 113:1248, 2009.
8. Piper JM, Bolling DR, Newton ER: The second stage of labor: factors influencing duration. Am J Obstet Gynecol 165:976, 1991.

9. American College of Obstetricians and Gynecologists: Dystocia and augmentation of labor. ACOG Practice Bulletin No. 49. Obstet Gynecol 102:1445, 2004.
10. Janakiraman V, Ecker J, Kaimal AJ: Comparing the second stage in induced and spontaneous labor. Obstet Gynecol 116:606, 2010.
11. Myles TD, Santolaya J: Maternal and neonatal outcomes in patients with a prolonged second stage of labor. Obstet Gynecol 102:52, 2003.
12. Dombrowski MP, Bottoms SF, Saleh AA, et al: Third stage of labor: analysis of duration and clinical practice. Am J Obstet Gynecol 172:1279, 1995.
13. Magann EF, Evans S, Chauhan SP, et al: The length of the third stage of labor and the risk of postpartum hemorrhage. Obstet Gynecol 105:290, 2005.
14. Begley CM, Gyte GML, Murphy DJ, et al: Active versus expectant management for women in the third stage of labour. Cochrane Database Syst Rev CD007412, 2010.
15. Jackson KW, Allbert JR, Schemmer GK, et al: A randomized controlled trial comparing oxytocin administration before and after placental delivery in the prevention of postpartum hemorrhage. Am J Obstet Gynecol 185:873, 2001.
16. American College of Obstetricians and Gynecologists: Prophylactic antibiotics in labor and delivery. Obstet Gynecol 102:875, 2003.
17. Poggi SH, Stallings SP, Ghidini A, et al: Intrapartum risk factors for permanent brachial plexus injury. Am J Obstet Gynecol 189:725, 2003.
18. Halpern SH, Abdallah FW: Effect of labor analgesia on labor outcome. Curr Opin Anaesthesiol 23:317, 2010.
19. Clark S, Simpson KR, Knox GE, Garite TJ: Oxytocin: new perspectives on an old drug. Am J Obstet Gynecol 200:35.e1, 2009.
20. Ho M, Cheng SY, Tsai-Chung L: Titrated oral misoprostol solution compared with intravenous oxytocin for labor augmentation. Obstet Gynecol 116:612, 2010.
21. Robinson B, Nelson L: A review of the proceedings from the 2008 NICHD workshop on standardized nomenclature for cardiotocography. Rev Obstet Gynecol 1:186, 2008.
22. Davies GA, Tessier JL, Woodman MC, et al: Maternal hemodynamics after oxytocin bolus compared with infusion in the third stage of labor: a randomized controlled trial. Obstet Gynecol 105:294, 2005.
23. Landon MB, Hauth JC, Leveno KJ, et al: Maternal and perinatal outcomes associated with a trial of labor after prior cesarean delivery. For the NICHD Maternal Fetal Medicine Unit Network. N Engl J Med 351:2581, 2004.
24. American College of Obstetricians and Gynecologists: Vaginal birth after previous cesarean delivery. ACOG Practice Bulletin No. 115. Obstet Gynecol 116:450, 2010.
25. Kramer MS, Rouleau J, Baskett TF, Joseph KS: Amniotic fluid embolism and medical induction of labor: a retrospective, population-based cohort study. Lancet 368:1444, 2006.
26. ACOG Committee on Practice Bulletins: Obstetrics. Induction of labor. ACOG Practice Bulletin No. 107. American College of Obstetricians and Gynecologists. Obstet Gynecol 114:386, 2009.
27. Hilder L, Costeloe K, Thilaganathan B: Prolonged pregnancy: evaluating gestation-specific risks of fetal and infant mortality. Br J Obstet Gynecol 105:169, 1998.
28. Nakling J, Backe B: Pregnancy risk increases from 41 weeks gestation. Acta Obstet Gynecol Scand 85:663, 2006.
29. Heimstad R, Romundstad PR, Eik-Nes SH, Salvesen KA: Outcomes of pregnancy beyond 37 weeks gestation. Obstet Gynecol 108:500, 2006.
30. Hannah ME: Postterm pregnancy: should all women have labour induced? A review of the literature. Fetal Maternal Med Rev 5:3, 1993.
31. Alexander JM, McIntire DD, Leveno KJ: Forty weeks and beyond: pregnancy outcomes by week of gestation. Obstet Gynecol 96:291, 2000.
32. Alexander JM, McIntire DD, Leveno KJ: Prolonged pregnancy: induction of labor and cesarean births. Obstet Gynecol 97:911, 2001.
33. Caughey AB, Musci TJ: Complications of term pregnancies beyond 37 weeks gestation. Obstet Gynecol 103:57, 2004.
34. Caughey AB, Stotland NE, Washington AE, et al: Maternal obstetric complications of pregnancy are associated with increasing gestational age at term. Am J Obstet Gynecol 196:155:e1, 2007.
35. Caughey AB, Bishop J: Maternal complications of pregnancy increase beyond 40 weeks of gestation in low risk women. J Perinatol 26:540, 2006.
36. Gulmezoglu AM, Crowther CA, Middleton P: Induction of labour for improving birth outcomes for women at or beyond term. Cochrane Database Syst Rev CD004945, 2006.
37. Silver RM, Landon MB, Rouse DJ, et al: Maternal morbidity associated with multiple repeat cesarean deliveries. Obstet Gynecol 107:1226, 2006.
38. Zhang J, Yancey MK, Henderson CE: US national trends in labor induction, 1989-1998. J Reprod Med 47:120, 2002.
39. Cammu H, Martens G, Ruyssinck G, Amy JJ: Outcome after elective labor induction in nulliparous women: a matched cohort study. Am J Obstet Gynecol 186:240, 2002.
40. Caughey AB, Sundaram V, Kaimal AJ, et al: Systematic review: elective induction of labor versus expectant management of pregnancy. Ann Intern Med 151:252, 2009.
41. Caughey AB, Nicholson JM, Cheng YW, et al: Induction of labor and cesarean delivery by gestational age. Am J Obstet Gynecol 195:700, 2006.
42. Bailit JL, Gregory KD, Reddy UM, et al: Maternal and neonatal outcomes by labor onset type and gestational age. Am J Obstet Gynecol 202:245.e1, 2010.
43. Zhang X, Joseph KS, Kramer MS: Decreased term and postterm birthweight in the US: impact of labor induction. Am J Obstet Gynecol 124:e1, 2010.
44. Morrison JJ, Rennie JM, Milton PJ: Neonatal respiratory morbidity and mode of delivery at term: influence of timing of elective caesarean section. Br J Obstet Gynecol 102:101, 1995.
45. Clark SL, Miller DD, Belfort MA, et al: Neonatal and maternal outcomes associated with elective term delivery. Am J Obstet Gynecol 200:156.e1, 2009.
46. Kaufman KE, Bailit JL, Grobman W: Elective induction: an analysis of economic and health consequences. Am J Obstet Gynecol 187:858, 2002.
47. Nicholson JM, Kellar LC, Cronholm PF, Macones GA: Active management of risk in pregnancy at term in an urban population: an association between a higher induction of labor rate and a lower cesarean delivery rate. Am J Obstet Gynecol 191:1516, 2004.
48. Nicholson JM, Parry S, Caughey AB, et al: The impact of the active management of risk in pregnancy at term on birth outcomes: a randomized clinical trial. Am J Obstet Gynecol 198:511, 2008.
49. Pevzner L, Rayburn WF, Rumney P, Wing DA: Factors predicting successful labor induction with dinoprostone and misoprostol vaginal inserts. Obstet Gynecol 114:261, 2009.
50. Crane JM: Factors predicting labor induction success: a critical analysis. Clin Obstet Gynecol 49:573, 2006.
51. Chandra S, Crane JM, Hutchens D, Young DC: Transvaginal ultrasound and digital examination in predicting successful labor induction. Obstet Gynecol 98:2, 2001.
52. Calder AA, Brennand JE: Labor and normal delivery: induction of labor. Curr Opin Obstet Gynecol 3:764, 1991.
53. Xenakis EM, Piper JM, Conway DL, Langer O: Induction of labor in the nineties: conquering the unfavorable cervix. Obstet Gynecol 90:235, 1997.
54. Johnson DP, Davis NR, Brown AJ: Risk of cesarean delivery after induction at term in nulliparous women with an unfavorable cervix. Am J Obstet Gynecol 188:1565, 2003.
55. Vrouenraets FP, Roumen FJ, Dehing CJ, et al: Bishop score and risk of cesarean delivery after induction of labor in nulliparous women. Obstet Gynecol 105:690, 2005.
56. Arulkumaran S, Gibb DM, TambyRaja RL, et al: Failed induction of labour. Aust N Z J Obstet Gynaecol 25:190, 1985.
57. Hatfield AS, Sanchez-Ramos L, Kaunitz AM: Sonographic cervical assessment to predict the success of labor induction: a systematic review with meta-analysis. Am J Obstet Gynecol 197:186, 2007.
58. Sciscione A, Hoffman MK, Deluca S, et al: Fetal fibronectin as a predictor of vaginal birth in nulliparas undergoing preinduction cervical ripening. Obstet Gynecol 106:980, 2005.
59. Reis FM, Gervasi MT, Florio P, et al: Prediction of successful induction of labor at term: role of clinical history, digital examination, ultrasound assessment of the cervix, and fetal fibronectin assay. Am J Obstet Gynecol 189:1361, 2003.
60. Bailit JL, Downs SM, Thorp JM: Reducing the caesarean delivery risk in elective inductions of labour: a decision analysis. Paediatr Perinat Epidemiol 16:90, 2002.
61. Maul H, Mackay L, Garfield RE: Cervical ripening: biochemical, molecular, and clinical considerations. Clin Obstet Gynecol 49:551, 2006.

62. Rouse DJ, Owen J, Hauth JC: Criteria for failed labor induction: prospective evaluation of a standardized protocol. Obstet Gynecol 96:671, 2000.
63. Simon CE, Grobman WA: When has an induction failed? Obstet Gynecol 105:705, 2005.
64. Hoffman MK, Vahratian A, Sciscione AC, et al: Comparison of labor progression between induced and noninduced multiparous women. Obstet Gynecol 107:1029, 2006.
65. Lin MG, Rouse DJ: What is a failed labor induction? Clin Obstet Gynecol 49:585, 2006.
66. Beckmann M: Predicting a failed induction. Aust N Z J Obstet Gynaecol 47:394, 2007.
67. Kelly AJ, Tan B: Intravenous oxytocin alone for cervical ripening and induction of labour. Cochrane Databae Syst Rev CD003246, 2001.
68. Tan BP, Hannah ME: Oxytocin for preterm labor rupture of membranes at or near term. Cochrane Database Syst Rev CD000157, 2000.
69. O'Driscoll K, Foley M, MacDonald D: Active management of labor as an alternative to cesarean section for dystocia. Obstet Gynecol 63:485, 1984.
70. Satin AJ, Leveno KJ, Sherman ML, et al: High- versus low-dose oxytocin for labor stimulation. Obstet Gynecol 80:111, 1992.
71. Merrill DC, Zlatnik FJ: Randomized double-masked comparison of oxytocin dosage in induction and augmentation of labor. Obstet Gynecol 94:455, 1999.
72. Patka JH, Lodolce AE, Johnston AK: High- versus low-dose oxytocin for augmentation or induction of labor. Ann Pharmacother 39:95, 2005.
73. Hayes EJ, Weinstein L: Improving patient safety and uniformity of care by a standardized regimen for the use of oxytocin. Am J Obstet Gynecol 198:622, 2008.
74. Freeman RK, Nageotte M: A protocol for use of oxytocin. Am J Obstet Gynecol 197:445, 2007.
75. Clark S, Belfort M, Saade G, et al: Implementation of a conservative checklist-based protocol for oxytocin administration: maternal and newborn outcomes. Am J Obstet Gynecol 197:480, 2007.
76. Lydon-Rochelle M, Holt VL, Easterling TR, Martin DP: Risk of uterine rupture during labor among women with a prior cesarean delivery. N Engl J Med 345:3, 2001.
77. Kelly AJ, Kavanagh J, Thomas J: Vaginal prostaglandin (PGE_2 and PGF_{2a}) for induction of labour at term. Cochrane Database Syst Rev CD003101, 2003.
78. American College of Obstetricians and Gynecologists: New US Food and Drug Administration labeling on Cytotec (misoprostol) use and pregnancy. ACOG Committee Opinion No. 283. Obstet Gynecol 101:1049, 2003.
79. Wing DA, Rahall A, Jones MM, et al: Misoprostol: an effective agent for cervical ripening and labor induction. Am Obstet Gynecol 172: 1811, 1995.
80. Hofmeyr GJ, Gulmezoglu AM: Vaginal misoprostol for cervical ripening and induction of labour. Cochrane Database Syst Rev CD000941, 2003.
81. Sanchez-Ramos L, Kaunitz AM, Wears RL, et al: Misoprostol for cervical ripening and labor induction: a meta-analysis. Obstet Gynecol 89:633, 1997.
82. Alfirevic Z, Weeks A: Oral misoprostol for induction of labour. Cochrane Database Syst Rev CD001338, 2006.
83. Hofmeyr GJ, Alfirevic Z, Matonhodze B, et al: Titrated oral misoprostol solution for induction of labour: a multi-centre, randomised trial. Br J Obstet Gynecol 108:952, 2001.
84. Tang OS, Schweer H, Seyberth HW, et al: Pharmacokinetics of different routes of administration of misoprostol. Hum Reprod 17:332, 2002.
85. Muzonzin IG, Hofmeyr GJ: Buccal or sublingual misoprostol for cervical ripening and induction of labour. Cochrane Database Syst Rev CD004221, 2004.
86. Sawai SK, O'Brien WF: Outpatient cervical ripening. Clin Obstet Gynecol 38:301, 1995.
87. McKenna DS, Duke JM: Effectiveness and infectious morbidity of outpatient cervical ripening with a Foley catheter. J Reprod Med 49:28, 2004.
88. McKenna DS, Ester JB, Proffitt M, Waddell KR: Misoprostol outpatient cervical ripening without subsequent induction of labor: a randomized trial. Obstet Gynecol 104:579, 2004.
89. Kelly AJ, Alfirevic Z, Dowswell T: Outpatient versus inpatient induction of labour for improving birth outcomes. Cochrane Database Syst Rev CD007372, 2009.
90. Neilson JP: Mifepristone for induction of labour. Cochrane Database Syst Rev CD002865, 2000.
91. Boulvain M, Kelly AJ, Lohse C, et al: Mechanical methods for induction of labour. Cochrane Database Syst Rev CD001233, 2001.
92. Heinemann J, Gillen G, Sanchez-Ramos L, Kaunitz AM: Do mechanical methods of cervical ripening increase infectious morbidity? A systematic review. Am J Obstet Gynecol 199:177, 2008.
93. Cammu H, Haitsma V: Sweeping of the membranes at 39 weeks in nulliparous women: a randomised controlled trial. Br J Obstet Gynaecol 105:41, 1998.
94. Boulvain M, Stan C, Irion O: Membrane sweeping for induction of labour. Cochrane Database Syst Rev CD000451, 2005.
95. Centers for Disease Control and Prevention: Prevention of perinatal group B streptococcal disease. MMWR 59 (No. RR-10):1, 2010.
96. Booth JH, Kurdyak VB: Amniotomy alone for induction of labour. Cochrane Database Syst Rev CD002862, 2000.
97. Howarth G, Botha DJ: Amniotomy plus intravenous oxytocin for induction of labour. Cochrane Library, Cochrane Review 1, 2010.
98. Silver RM, Heuser CC: Stillbirth workup and delivery management. Clin Obstet Gynecol 53:681, 2010.
99. Lohr PA, Hayes JL, Gemzell-Danielsson K: Surgical versus medical methods for second trimester induced abortion. Cochrane Database Syst Rev CD006714, 2008.
100. Wagaarachchi PT, Ashok PW, Narvekar NN, et al: A medical management of late intrauterine death using a combination of mifepristone and misoprostol. Br J Obstet Gynaecol 109:443, 2002.

For full reference list, log onto www.expertconsult.com.

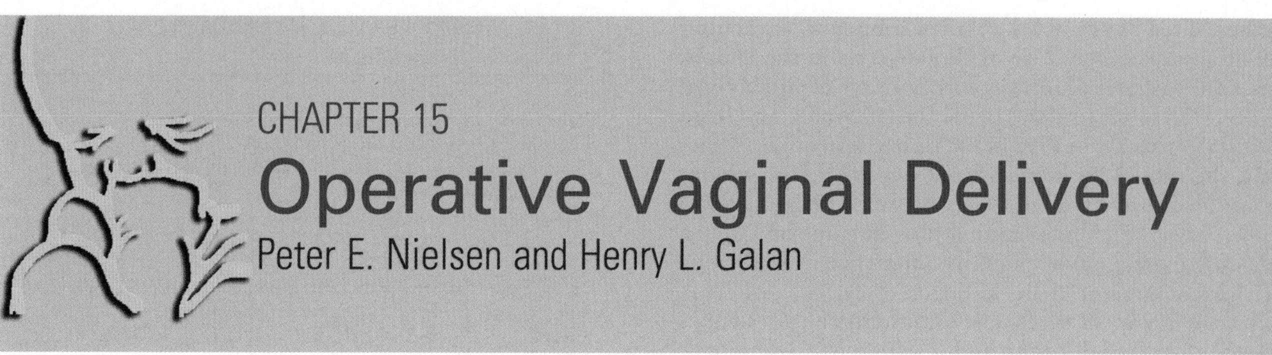

CHAPTER 15

Operative Vaginal Delivery

Peter E. Nielsen and Henry L. Galan

KEY ABBREVIATIONS	
American College of Obstetricians and Gynecologists	ACOG
Biparietal Diameter	BPD
Confidence Interval	CI
Food and Drug Administration	FDA
Intracranial Hemorrhage	ICH
Intelligence Quotient	IQ
Left Occiput Anterior	LOA
Left Occiput Posterior	LOP
Maternal Fetal	MF
Neonatal Intensive Care Unit	NICU
Occiput Anterior	OA
Occiput Posterior	OP
Occiput Transverse	OT
Odds Ratio	OR
Relative Risk	RR
Right Occiput Anterior	ROA

Obstetrical forceps are the one instrument that makes the practice of obstetrical care unique to obstetricians. The proper use of these instruments has afforded safe and timely vaginal delivery to those whose abnormal labor course and/or urgent need for delivery required their use. Following the introduction of forceps by Chamberlin during the 1600s, much discussion about the proper use and timing of forceps application ensued. Following Smellie's retirement from practice in 1760, forceps began to be used very frequently, resulting in an increase in both maternal and neonatal injury owing to the application techniques used at the time. In his 1788 text entitled "An Introduction to the Practice of Midwifery," Thomas Denman stated that "the head of the child shall have rested for 6 hours as low as the perineum before the forceps are applied though the pains should have ceased during that time."[1] Denman's Law then became widely accepted as the standard of this time. However, after the news of Princess Charlotte's death following the birth of a stillborn Prince on November 6, 1817, a review of Denman's Law ensued with much public discussion regarding the timely use of forceps. Princess Charlotte's labor had been managed by one of Denman's students and son-in-law, Sir Richard Croft, whose second-stage labor management during this delivery came into question. Croft had permitted the second stage to last 24 hours, including 6 hours on the perineum, as Denman's Law had advised. However, the Princess delivered a 9 lb stillborn male heir, and within 24 hours of delivery the Princess herself died of a massive postpartum hemorrhage. Disturbed with depression and despair at the blame for the death of both the Princess and the heir to the British throne, Croft shot himself 3 months later. During a lecture delivered at the Royal College of Obstetricians and Gynaecologists on September 28, 1951, Sir Eardley Holland named his lecture on these events "A Triple Obstetric Tragedy" in which he described a mother, baby, and accoucheur all dead, victims of a mistaken system.[2] In a subsequent text in 1817, Denman wrote: "Care is also to be taken that we do not, through an aversion to the use of instruments, too long delay that assistance we have the power of affording them."[3] The debate regarding the use of these instruments continued into the twentieth century with prophylactic forceps delivery advocated by DeLee in 1920.[4] This clinical management strategy resulted in forceps delivery rates in excess of 65% by 1950.

With these lessons in mind, a review of operative vaginal delivery in modern obstetrical practice is extremely important and timely. **Rates of cesarean delivery have risen in**

both the United States and the United Kingdom,[5,6] reaching a rate of approximately 25% of all deliveries in the United States, whereas rates of forceps delivery have declined from 17.7% in 1980 to 4% in 2000[5] in the United States, and from 8.6% in 1989 to 6.2% in 1993 in the United Kingdom.[7] Conversely, the rate of vacuum-assisted vaginal delivery more than doubled in the United States between 1980 and 2000 to 8.4%.[4] Most residency training programs in the United States still expect proficiency in outlet and low forceps (less than or greater than 45-degree rotation), whereas less than 40% expect proficiency in midforceps delivery.[8] **However, to make education and teaching of these procedures even more challenging, new resident work hour restrictions have resulted in a decline in resident experience with both primary cesarean delivery and vacuum-assisted vaginal delivery, despite increased institutional volumes of these procedures.** In a study by Blanchard and colleagues,[9] the decrease in experience with these procedures has been dramatic, noting a 54% decline in experience with primary cesarean delivery and a 56% decline in vacuum-assisted vaginal delivery. Because both forceps and vacuum extractors are acceptable and safe instruments for operative vaginal delivery, operator experience is the determining factor in which instrument should be used in a specific clinical situation.[10] Declining use and resident experience may make it difficult to provide the level of operator experience required for proficiency of this obstetrical art. However, because most women prefer a vaginal delivery, focused experience with the use of these instruments during residency training is crucial to ensure safe, timely, and effective vaginal delivery because women are more likely to achieve a spontaneous vaginal delivery in a subsequent pregnancy after forceps delivery than after cesarean delivery (78% vs. 31%).[11-14] The challenge, therefore, is to ensure that women who experience second-stage labor abnormalities are afforded options for safe and timely delivery.

OPERATIVE VAGINAL DELIVERY

Classification, Prerequisites, and Indications

The use of a well-defined and consistent classification system for operative vaginal deliveries makes comparison of maternal and neonatal outcomes among spontaneous delivery, cesarean delivery, and operative vaginal delivery as well as instruction in these techniques easier. It is intuitive that not all operative vaginal deliveries are the same with respect to degree of difficulty or maternal and fetal risk. Therefore, classification systems have been developed and modified over time. In 1949, Titus created a classification system that permitted general practitioners to perform operative vaginal delivery without consultation from a specialist.[15] This system divided the pelvis into thirds from the ischial spines to the inlet and, in the opposite direction, in thirds to the outlet. Dennen proposed an alternative classification system in 1952 that was based on the four major obstetrical planes of the pelvis with the following definitions: high forceps as the biparietal diameter (BPD) in the plane of the inlet, but above the ischial spines; midforceps as the BPD just at or below the ischial spines and the sacral hollow not filled; low-midforceps as the BPD below the ischial spines, the leading bony part within a fingerbreadth of the perineum between contractions and the hollow of the sacrum filled; and outlet as the BPD below the level of the ischial spines, the sagittal suture in the anteroposterior diameter and the head visible at the perineum during a contraction.[15]

TABLE 15-1 1988 OPERATIVE VAGINAL DELIVERY CLASSIFICATION

Outlet
- Scalp visible at introitus without separating labia
- Fetal skull has reached the pelvic floor
- Sagittal suture is in the AP diameter, or left or right occiput anterior or posterior position
- Fetal head is at or on the perineum
- Rotation does not exceed 45°

Low Forceps
- Leading point of fetal skull is at ≥+2 cm and not on the pelvic floor
  - Rotation ≤45° (to LOA /ROA to OA, or LOP/ROP to OP), or
  - Rotation ≥45°

Midforceps
- Station above +2 cm, but head engaged

High
- Not included in classification

Modified from American College of Obstetricians and Gynecologists, Committee on Obstetrics, Maternal and Fetal Medicine: Obstetric Forceps. Technical Bulletin No. 59, February 1988.

In 1965, the American College of Obstetricians and Gynecologists (ACOG) created a classification system that defined midforceps extremely broadly (from the ischial spines to the pelvic floor and any rotation). This category clearly included many forceps operations that ranged from delivery of a straightforward anteroposterior position of the fetal vertex to complex rotations.[16] The broad category for these operations lead many practicing clinicians to question whether the classification should be narrowed to reflect the clinically significant differences between deliveries such as these. **Therefore, in 1988, ACOG revised the classification of forceps operations to address two significant shortcomings of the previous system, that midforceps was too widely defined and outlet forceps too narrowly defined.**[17] This system was validated in 1991 by Hagadorn-Freathy and colleagues,[18] demonstrating that 25% of deliveries in this study that would have been previously classified as midforceps (but were reclassified into the low-forceps [greater than 45-degree] rotation and midforceps categories) were associated with 41% of episiotomy extensions and 50% of the lacerations in the cohort. Clearly, the outcomes of these operations confounded the relatively low-risk group of low-forceps operations with up to 45-degree rotation (which would also have been classified as midforceps by the previous system). **In short, these investigators validated the 1988 ACOG classification scheme by demonstrating that the higher station and more complex deliveries carried a greater risk of maternal and fetal injury compared with those that were more straightforward.** This differentiation was lost in the 1965 classification scheme owing to the broad definition of low forceps. It is extremely important to appropriately classify operative vaginal delivery based on this system, including accurate determination of fetal station and position. The 1988 classification scheme for operative vaginal delivery is shown in Table 15-1.

TABLE 15-2 PREREQUISITES FOR FORCEPS OR VACUUM EXTRACTOR APPLICATION

Engaged fetal vertex
Ruptured membranes
Fully dilated cervix
Position is precisely known
Assessment of maternal pelvis reveals adequacy for the estimated fetal weight
Adequate maternal analgesia is available
Bladder drained
Knowledgeable operator
Willingness to abandon the procedure, if necessary
Informed consent has been obtained
Necessary support personnel and equipment are present

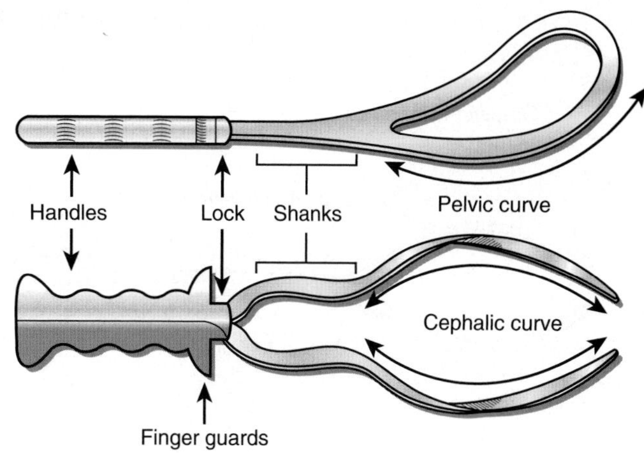

FIGURE 15-1. Anatomy of the forceps.

With respect to operative vaginal delivery of the vertex, station is defined as the relationship of the estimated distance, in centimeters, between the leading bony portion of the fetal head and the level of the maternal ischial spines, and position refers to the relationship of the occiput to a denominating location on the maternal pelvis. Operative vaginal delivery with a fetus in the left occiput anterior (LOA) position, with the leading bony portion of the vertex 3 cm below the ischial spines (+3 station) would be classified as a low forceps, less than 45-degree rotation delivery. It is also important to note that this classification system applies to both forceps and vacuum extraction instruments, and that the precise position and station must be known before the placement of either instrument.

In addition to precise evaluation of the position and station, several other extremely important data are necessary before performing operative vaginal delivery. **The prerequisites for application of either forceps or vacuum extractor are listed in Table 15-2. When these prerequisites have been met, the following indications are appropriate for consideration of either forceps delivery or vacuum extraction:**

- Prolonged second stage
- Nulliparous women: lack of continuing progress for 3 hours with regional analgesia or 2 hours without regional analgesia
- Multiparous women: lack of continuing progress for 2 hours with regional analgesia or 1 hour without regional analgesia
- Suspicion of immediate or potential fetal compromise
- Nonreassuring fetal heart rate tracing
- Shortening of the second stage of labor for maternal benefit (i.e., maternal exhaustion, maternal cardiopulmonary or cerebrovascular disease)

OPERATIVE VAGINAL DELIVERY INSTRUMENTS

Forceps Instruments

Invention and modification have led to a description and use of more than 700 varieties of forceps instruments. Most of them are of historic interest only, but many common features remain among those still in use. **Forceps are paired instruments, except when used at cesarean delivery and are broadly categorized according to their intended use: "classic" forceps, rotational forceps, and specialized forceps designed to assist vaginal breech deliveries.** Each forceps type consists of two halves joined by a lock, which may be sliding or fixed. The key structures of forceps include the blade, shank, lock, finger guards, and handle (Figure 15-1). The toe refers to the tip of the blade and the heel to the end of the blade that is attached to the shank at the posterior lip of the fenestration (if present). The cephalic curve is defined by the radius of the two blades when in opposition and the pelvic curve by the upward (or reverse as in the case of Kielland and Piper forceps) curve of the blades from the shank. The handles transmit the applied force, the screw or lock represent the fulcrum, and the blades transmit the load (Figure 15-2).[19]

The pelvic curve permits ease of application along the maternal pelvic axis (Figure 15-3). Forceps have two functions, traction and rotation, both of which can only be accomplished by some degree of compression on the fetal head. The cephalic curvature of the blade is designed to aid in the even distribution of force about the fetal parietal bone and fetal malar eminence. Blades may be solid (Tucker-McLane), fenestrated (Simpson), or pseudofenestrated (Luikart-Simpson). The pseudofenestration modification can be applied to the design of any type of forceps and is known as the Luikart modification. In general, use of solid or pseudofenestrated blades results in less risk of maternal soft tissue injury, especially during rotation, but fenestrated blades provide improved traction in comparison to solid blades.

"Classic" Forceps

Classic forceps instruments are typically used when rotation of the vertex is not required for delivery. However, they may be used for rotations such as the Scanzoni-Smellie maneuver. All classic forceps have a cephalic curve, a pelvic curve, and an English lock, in which the articulation is fixed in a slot into which the shank of the opposite blade fits. The type of classic forceps instrument is determined by its shank, whether overlapping or parallel. Examples of classic forceps with parallel shanks include Simpson, DeLee, Irving, and Hawks-Dennen forceps. Classic forceps with overlapping shanks include Elliott and Tucker-McLane. Because these instruments have a more rounded cephalic curve than the Simpson forceps, they are often used for assisting delivery of the unmolded head, such as that commonly encountered in the multiparous patient. In addition,

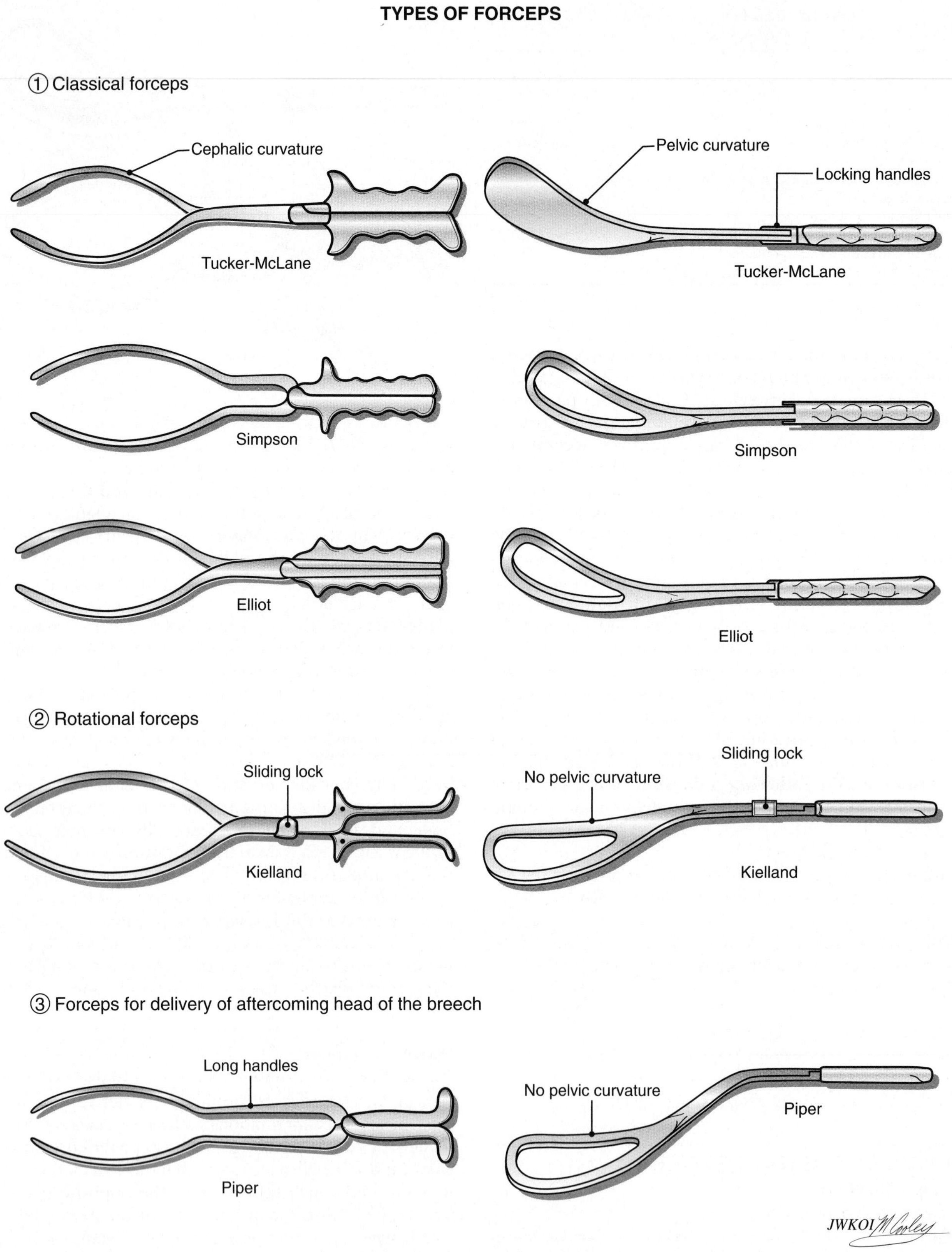

TYPES OF FORCEPS
① Classical forceps
Cephalic curvature
Tucker-McLane
Pelvic curvature
Locking handles
Tucker-McLane
Simpson
Simpson
Elliot
Elliot
② Rotational forceps
Sliding lock
Kielland
No pelvic curvature
Sliding lock
Kielland
③ Forceps for delivery of aftercoming head of the breech
Long handles
Piper
No pelvic curvature
Piper
JWKOI M Cooley

FIGURE 15-2. Classification of forceps.

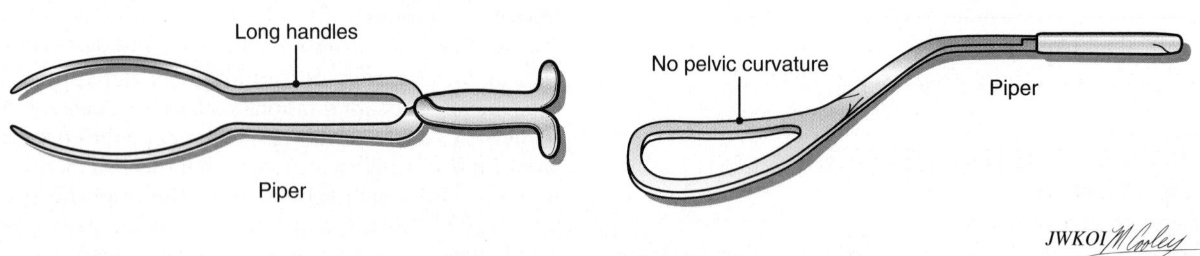

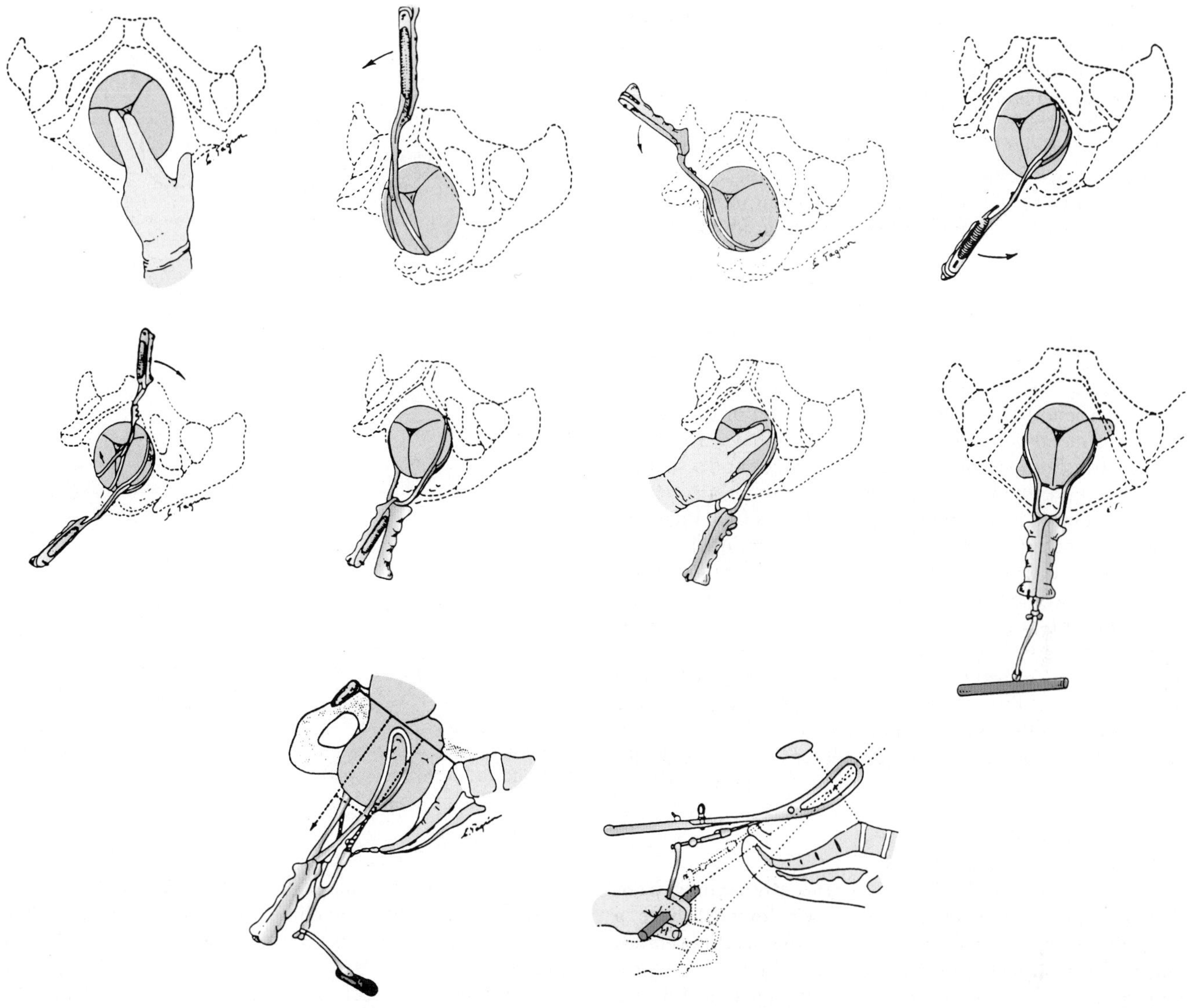

FIGURE 15-3. Stepwise approach to application of obstetrical forceps.

because the Tucker-McLane forceps have a shorter, solid blade and overlapping shanks, they are more often used for rotations than other classic instruments.

Rotational Forceps

Forceps instruments used for rotation are characterized as having a cephalic curve amenable to application to the molded vertex, and either only a slight pelvic curve or none at all. **The absence of a pelvic curve in these instruments facilitates rotation of the vertex without moving the handles of the instrument through a wide arch, as is necessary when using one of the classic instruments to accomplish rotation.** Forceps that may be used for rotation include some of the classic instruments (e.g., Tucker-McLane) and those with minimal pelvic curvature (e.g., Kielland and Leff). In 1916, Christian Kielland of Norway described the rationale for the introduction of his new forceps:

> When the head is high it has to be pulled through a greater length of the birth canal, which is incompletely prepared. The child's head is in such a position that it cannot be grasped by the blades of the forceps in the way which is possible when the head is low and completely rotated. The forceps do not hold the head in the biparietal diameter, but over the occipital and frontal areas which cannot withstand much pressure. These factors are responsible for the difficulties which occur in such a delivery, but they do not entirely explain the amount of force required nor the resistance which is encountered. In the search for an explanation of the chief cause for the remarkable amount of force, which had to be used, it was thought that traction might be in the wrong direction, because the blade of the ordinary forceps is curved to correspond with the birth canal. This type of forceps cannot be depressed sufficiently low against the perineum without the risk of damaging it or losing the good position on the fetal head when an attempt is made to exert traction in the pelvic axis.[20]

Following their introduction, Kielland's forceps have become a frequently used instrument for rotation of the vertex (see Figure 15-1). These forceps have a slightly backward pelvic curve with overlapping shanks and a sliding lock. The advantages of the Kielland's forceps compared with the classic instruments for rotation include the following:

- A straight design that places the handle and shanks in the same plane as the long axis of the fetal head, permitting the toe to travel through a very small arch during rotation.
- The distance between the heel and the intersecting point of the shanks is long, which accommodates heads of various shapes and sizes associated with unusual molding.
- A slight degree of axis traction is produced by the reverse pelvic curve.
- The sliding lock permits placement of the handles at any level on the shank to accommodate the asynclitic head and subsequent correction of asynclitism.

In 1955, another forceps used for rotation of the vertex was introduced by Leff.[21] These forceps have a locking shank with short, straight, and narrow blades and a smaller cephalic curve than the Kielland's forceps. In a series of 104 consecutive rotational forceps deliveries (>90 degrees) using Leff forceps compared with 163 nonrotational forceps deliveries with traditional instruments, Feldman demonstrated a lower episiotomy (66% vs. 82%) and perineal laceration rate (16% vs. 23%) with the Leff forceps compared with the nonrotational forceps group, attributed to a 40% spontaneous vaginal delivery rate after Leff forceps rotation.[22] In addition, there was no difference in the low incidence of fetal bruising between the groups (3% in each). They concluded that Leff forceps were also a safe option for rotation of the persistent occipitoposterior fetal position.

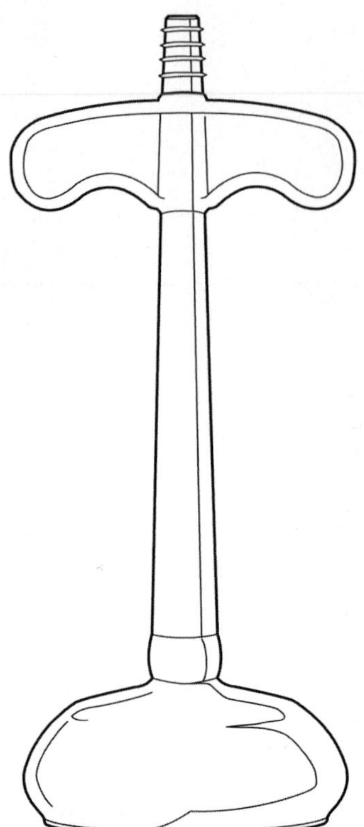

FIGURE 15-4. "M"-style mushroom vacuum extractor cup with a centrally located stem and handle.

Other Specialized Instruments

Forceps to assist with delivery of the aftercoming head during vaginal breech delivery (Piper forceps) have a cephalic curve, a reverse pelvic curve, long parallel shanks, and an English lock (see Figure 15-2). This design provides easy application to the aftercoming head, stabilizing and protecting the fetal head and neck during delivery. The long shanks permit the body of the breech to rest against it during delivery of the head.

Vacuum Extraction Devices

Swedish obstetrician Tage Malmstrom was credited with the introduction of the first successful vacuum cup into the field of modern obstetrics in 1953. It consisted of a metal cup, suction tubing, and a traction chain.[23] Vacuum devices are classified by the material used to make the cup: either stainless steel or plastic (silicone). Plastic ("soft") cups are used much more commonly in the United States than the stainless steel cups owing to the lower rates of scalp trauma associated with these devices.[24] These devices consist of the cup, which is connected to a handle grip and tubing that connects them both to a vacuum source (Figure 15-4). The vacuum generated through this tubing attaches the fetal scalp to the cup and allows traction on the vertex. The vacuum force can be generated either from wall suction or by a hand-held device with a pumping mechanism.

Stainless Steel Devices

The Malmstrom device is the most commonly used instrument for vacuum extraction in the world.[25] This device consists of a mushroom-shaped stainless steel cup, two vacuum hoses, a traction chain and attached metallic disk, a traction handle, and a vacuum source. The cup is available in 40, 50, and 60 mm diameter sizes and is designed such that the diameter of the opening is smaller than the internal diameter of the cup. Therefore, when vacuum is established, the fetal scalp fills the internal dimension of the cup and an artificial caput succedaneum is formed (the "chignon"). This allows for appropriate traction force to be applied to the vertex without a "pop-off" or detachment.

Soft Cup Devices

These devices may be classified into three groups by the shape of the cup: funnel shaped, bell shaped, and mushroom shaped (Figures 15-5 and 15-6). The Kobayashi style funnel-shaped Silastic cup is the prototype and the largest cup available (65 mm). It was designed to fit over the fetal occiput without requiring formation of a chignon. This feature results in a lower rate of scalp trauma and more rapid time to effect delivery compared with the stainless steel devices, but with a slightly higher failure rate owing to pop-off.[24] Bell-shaped cups are available from a number of vendors and include the following brands: Mityvac (Prism Enterprises, San Antonio, Texas), Kiwi (Clinical Innovations, Murray, Utah) and CMI (Utah Medical, Midvale, Utah). The mushroom-shaped cups are a hybrid of the stainless steel and plastic devices. Examples of these devices include the M-cup (Mityvac, Prism Enterprises, San Antonio, Texas), the Flex Cup (CMI,

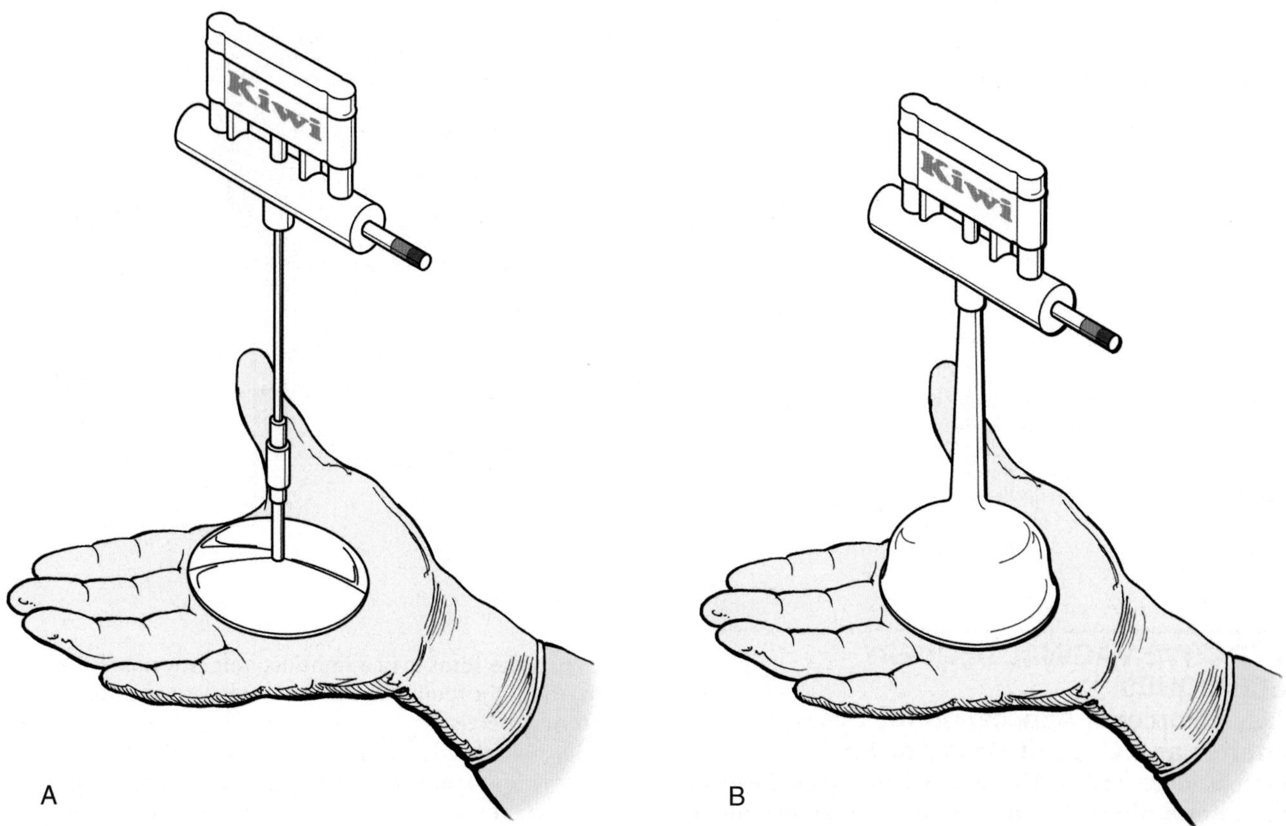

FIGURE 15-5. Depicted are two Kiwi vacuum devices demonstrating the hand-held pump and pressure gauge device. Unlike the cup in **B,** the stem on the cup in **A,** OmniCup is flexible and can be laid flat against the cup. (From Vacca A: Handbook of Vacuum Delivery in Obstetric Practice. Albion, Australia, Vacca Research Pty. Ltd., 2003.)

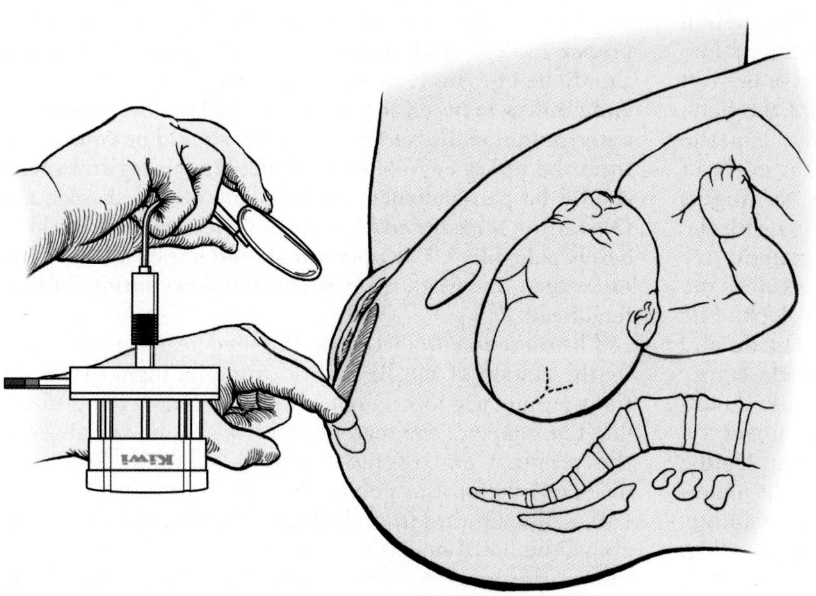

FIGURE 15-6. Placement of the OmniCup with flexible stem at the point of flexion of a fetal head in the occiput posterior position, which is otherwise difficult to accomplish with the traditional vacuum devices. (From Vacca A: Handbook of Vacuum Delivery in Obstetric Practice. Albion, Australia, Vacca Research Pty, Ltd., 2003.)

Utah Medical, Midvale, Utah) and the Omni-cup (Kiwi, Clinical Innovations, Murray, Utah). The maneuverability of these devices is superior to either the funnel-shaped or bell-shaped devices owing to their smaller size and increased flexibility of the traction stem relative to the cup. However, they (like other vacuum devices) are still limited in their use for either occiput posterior (OP) or occiput transverse (OT) positions owing to an inability to achieve the proper median flexing application. Advances to the Kiwi product have resulted in a style of cup in which the stem is completely collapsible against the cup (see Figure 15-5), thus allowing placement of the vacuum on the point of flexion of the head that is asynclitic or in the OP position.

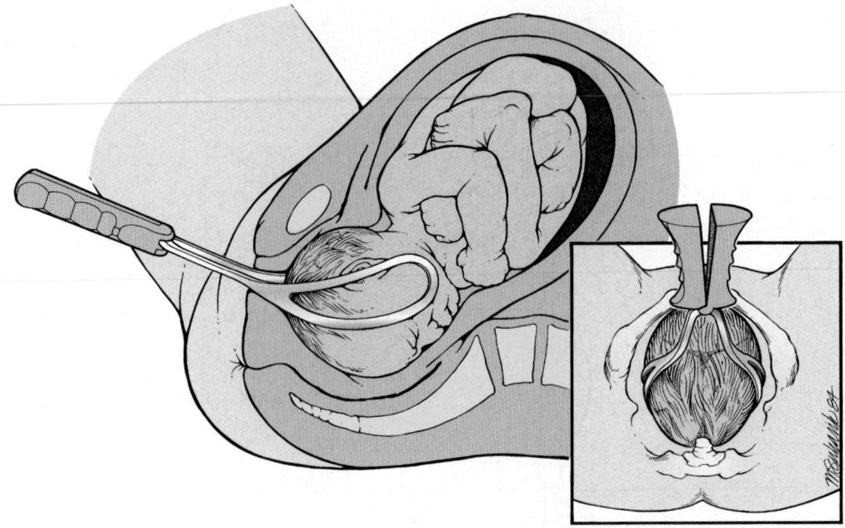

FIGURE 15-7. Proper application of obstetrical forceps. (From O'Brien WF, Cefalo RC: Labor and delivery. *In* Gabbe SG, Niebyl JR, Simpson JL [eds]: Obstetrics: Normal and Problem Pregnancies, ed 3. New York, Churchill Livingstone, 1996, p 377.)

OPERATIVE VAGINAL DELIVERY TECHNIQUES

Classic Forceps: Application for Occiput Anterior and Occiput Posterior Positions

Forcep blades are labeled left and right based on the maternal side into which they are placed. For example, the left blade refers to the maternal left side and its handle is held in the operator's left hand for placement (see Figure 15-3).[26] The posterior blade is conventionally placed first because it provides a splint for the fetal head to prevent rotation from the occiput anterior (OA) position to a more OP position when the second blade is applied. Therefore, when the fetus is OA to LOA, the left blade is placed first. The operator holds the handle of the left blade in his or her left hand, with the toe of the blade directed toward the floor. With the plane of the shank perpendicular to the floor, the cephalic curve of the blade is to be applied to the curve of the fetal head. To protect the vaginal sidewalls, the fingers of the right hand are placed within the left vagina with the palm of the hand facing the fetal skull. The cephalic curve of the blade should lie evenly against the fetal skull as the toe of the blade is placed at approximately 6 o'clock. The operator's right thumb guides the heel of the blade and the right index finger guides the toe of the blade gently over the left parietal bone. The handle of the blade should be held lightly with the left thumb and index finger. As the blade is inserted into the pelvis, its shank and handle are to be rotated counterclockwise toward the right maternal thigh and then inward toward the maternal midline. This movement will guide the toe of the blade over the left parietal bone and onto the left malar eminence. The force applied by the left thumb and index finger on the handle should be minimal as the blade enters the maternal pelvis. If there is anything more than very light or slight resistance to blade entry into the maternal pelvis, the blade should be removed and the application technique reevaluated. Once the blade has been applied, an assistant may hold it in place. To place the right blade, this process is repeated with opposite hands doing the maneuvers described earlier.

When the fetus is in a right occiput anterior (ROA) position, the right fetal parietal bone is located in the posterior maternal pelvis so the posterior blade will be the right blade, and this is placed first. Once both blades are in place, if the handles do not lock easily, the application is incorrect. The blades should have a bimalar, biparietal placement when applied properly (Figure 15-7). Once the handles are locked, proper blade location must be confirmed. Identification of the posterior fontanel, sagittal suture, lamdoid sutures, and blade fenestrations, if present, enable the operator to confirm proper forceps blade placement before their use. **The three criteria needed to confirm proper forceps application are (1) the posterior fontanel should be one finger breath above the plane of the shanks and midway between the blades or the lamdoid sutures (or anterior fontanelle for the OP fetus) should be equidistant from the upper edge of each blade; (2) the sagittal suture should be perpendicular to the plane of the shanks; and (3) if using fenestrated blades, the fenestrations should be barely palpable.[26] The operator should not be able to place more than one fingertip between the fenestration and the fetal head.**

The direction of traction on the fetal head is determined by the station of the BPD. For example, higher fetal stations require a steeper angle of traction below the horizontal. The shape of the maternal pelvis may be visualized as the terminal end of the letter "J." As the fetal head descends within the pelvis, the axis of traction follows a curved line upward from the floor. The axis of traction rises above the horizontal as the fetal head crowns and extends just as the head does in a spontaneous vaginal delivery. With the axis traction principle, force is directed in two vectors—downward and out. One hand holds the shanks and exerts downward traction while the operator's other hand holds the handles and exerts traction outward. An alternative method may be employed by the use of an axis traction instrument. This attachment may be joined to the handle to facilitate traction below the handles in the line of the pelvic axis (see Figure 15-2). Forceps traction should begin with the uterine contraction and coincide with maternal pushing efforts until the contraction ends. Fetal heart tones should be monitored. Descent should occur with each pull, and if no descent occurs after two to three pulls, the operative delivery should be halted and measures should be taken to proceed with cesarean delivery. Switching to a vacuum should be done very cautiously (see Sequential Use of Vacuum and Forceps later in this chapter).

Forceps may also be appropriate for OP, left occiput posterior (LOP), or right occiput posterior (ROP) positions if the station of the bony part of the head is truly at least +2 station. Infants in persistent OP presentation present a unique challenge. With a deflexed or extended head, a wider diameter presents through the pelvic outlet. This requires more force for descent of the fetal head. Proper assessment of fetal station can be made complex by extension and molding of the fetal head.[26] With fetal molding, the widest diameter of the fetal head may be at a much higher station than the leading bony part, thus making traction within the proper pelvic axis difficult to ascertain. There is a tendency to overestimate station in OP presentations, so the operator must be confident in their station assessment.

Rotational Forceps: Application for Occiput Transverse Positions

Rotation must be accomplished from the OT position before delivery of the fetal head. This may happen spontaneously, with manual assistance, or with use of forceps, when appropriate. The reader is referred to *Dennen's Forceps Deliveries* for more extensive review of forceps rotation techniques.[26] Forcep rotations should be attempted only with an experienced operator.

Classic Forceps

For LOT presentations, the posterior left blade should be applied first. The toe of the blade is placed at 6 o'clock, and the cephalic curve is applied to the fetal head. The handle is lowered to facilitate blade entry into the posterior pelvis and rests below the horizontal, the degree of which will be determined by fetal station. The anterior right blade is labeled the wandering blade. The right blade is inserted with the right hand posteriorly at approximately 7 o'clock. Upward pressure on the blade is exerted with the fingers of the left hand as the right hand moves the handle in a clockwise arc across the left thigh toward the floor. The toe of the blade "wanders" from posterior to anterior, around the frontal bone, to rest anterior to the right ear. Elevation of the handle of the right blade permits movement of the blade further into the pelvis beyond the symphysis and articulation at the handles. The proper attitude of flexion is created by moving the handles toward the pelvic midline. Rotation of the fetal head is accomplished by counterclockwise rotation of the handles in a wide arc across the left thigh toward 12 o'clock. With classic forceps a wide rotational arc at the handles produces the desired smaller arc of rotation at the toe of the blades. Once the OA position is reached, the blades may be readjusted before the generation of traction. This same procedure may be employed for the right OT presentation with classic forceps. In this instance, however, the right blade is posterior and should be applied first.

Keilland's Forceps

Keilland's forceps were originally designed for delivery of the fetal head in deep transverse arrest.[20] They are now also used for rotation of the fetal head from OP or OT positions. The advantage of Keilland's forceps lies in the reverse pelvic curve, which permits placement of the blades in the direct OT position without elevation of the fetal head and loss of station. Unlike classic forceps, with Keilland's forceps the anterior blade is applied first. Three methods of Keilland's forceps application have been described: (1) the inversion method ("classic application"), (2) the wandering method, and (3) the direct method of application.[26]

The inversion method may be used in OT and LOP or ROP presentations. In left OT presentation, the right anterior blade is gently guided below the symphysis with assistance from the operator's left hand. With this application, the cephalic curve is facing up and beyond the symphysis, the handle is dropped below the horizontal, and the blade is rotated 180 degrees toward the midline until the cephalic curve rests on the parietal bone and malar eminence. If resistance is met with the inversion technique, the wandering technique may be used.

The wandering method for Keilland's forceps is similar to that used for classic forceps. The wandering method requires initial placement of the anterior blade onto the posterior parietal bone, with the cephalic curve directly applied to the fetus. The blade is then gently advanced around the face and frontal bone until it rests above the anterior fetal ear.

The direct method of application is preferred when the head is at low fetal station near the pelvic outlet. If the anterior ear is palpable beyond the symphysis, the forceps may be directly applied, often with less difficulty than the other two methods. With the cephalic curve facing the fetus, the blade is applied by lowering the handle toward the floor. The toe is then gently advanced with guidance from the operator's opposite hand. The posterior blade is then inserted at 6 o'clock, with the cephalic curve facing the fetal skull. The operator's free hand is inserted into posterior pelvis palm side up, and the blade is gently guided into position over the posterior ear. The sliding lock will permit closure of the blades and correction of asynclitism. Unlike rotation with classic forceps, the reverse pelvic curve of Keilland's forceps permits rotation directly on the axis of the shanks.[26] The shanks and handles are rotated around the midline point of application and should be held during rotation in a plane perpendicular to the plane of the fetal BPD. In some instances, the fetal head may need to be elevated and even disengaged to accomplish the rotation. This is performed by keeping the handles of the Keilland's forceps well below the horizontal plane pushing the forceps in an anterior-cephalad direction with respect to the maternal pelvis (e.g., toward the maternal umbilicus). Failure to angle in such a direction will result in the forceps making contact with the sacral promontory with an inability to achieve the room needed for rotation. During the rotation, one figure should follow the sutures to ensure that the forceps and fetal head move as a single unit. Generally speaking, use of one hand should provide sufficient force to complete the rotation and is a good guide for avoiding excess force. After successful rotation, proper forceps placement should be confirmed before downward traction is applied. Alternatively, Keilland's forceps could be removed, and classic forceps placed before traction.

Forceps Rotation: Application for the Occiput Posterior Position

The fetal head may be rotated from OP to OA by use of the Scanzoni-Smellie technique using classic forceps.[27] The posterior blade should be applied first and then appropriate placement of forceps confirmed. Minimal elevation of the fetal head upward within the pelvis will facilitate rotation. Movement of the handles in a wide arc toward the fetal back will enable rotation from the LOP position to OA. After rotation of the handles in a wide arc, the toe of the blades will be upside down with respect to the fetal malar eminence. They must then be removed and replaced properly before traction on the fetal head. Rotation from OP may also be accomplished with Keilland's forceps. After successful rotation, traction can be applied for delivery of the fetal head.

Vacuum Extraction

As with forceps, successful use of the vacuum extractor is determined by (1) proper application on the fetal head and (2) traction within the pelvic axis.[28] **The leading point of the fetal head is the ideal position for vacuum cup placement.** It is labeled the flexion point or pivot point and is located on the sagittal suture 2 to 3 cm below the posterior fontanel for the OA presentation and 2 to 3 cm above the posterior fontanel for the OP presentation.[28] Placement of the vacuum cup over the pivot point maintains the attitude of flexion for a well-flexed head and creates flexion in a deflexed head if traction is applied correctly. Incorrect placement on an asynclitic head results in unequal distribution of force and increase the risk of neonatal intracranial injury and scalp lacerations.[28,29] Therefore, knowledge of exact fetal position is important for efficacious vacuum placement. The force generated by vacuum suction is substantial, with recommended pressures ranging from 550 to 600 mm Hg (11.6 psi).[30] After initial placement of the cup, correct application must be confirmed, including determining that there is no vaginal tissue caught underneath the vacuum cup, before the vacuum pressure is raised to the desired level. Just as with forceps, traction should begin with each contraction and coincide with maternal pushing efforts. Routine traction between contractions should be avoided. In the absence of maternal pushing, traction alone increases the force required for fetal descent and increases the risk of cup detachment.[28] Twisting or rocking of the vacuum cup to facilitate descent of the fetal head is not recommended because there is an increased risk of scalp laceration and intracranial hemorrhage (ICH).[28,31]

With correct application, however, traction in the pelvic axis often results in flexion and autorotation, depending on fetal station and the vacuum cup selected.[29]

Detachment of the vacuum cup during traction should be viewed as an indication for reevaluation of the site of application, direction of axis traction, and fetal maternal pelvic dimensions. The rapid decompression resulting from cup detachment for the soft and rigid vacuum cups has been associated with scalp injury, and it should not be viewed as a safety mechanism that is without potential for fetal risk.[29,32] There are limited data to provide evidence-based support for the maximum duration of safe vacuum application, maximum number of pulls required before delivery of the fetal head, and the maximum number of pop-offs or cup detachments before abandonment of the procedure.[28,29,33,34] There is a general consensus, however, that descent of the fetal bony vertex should occur with each pull, and if no descent occurs after three pulls, the operative attempt should be stopped. Most authorities have recommended that the maximum number of cup detachments (e.g., pop-offs) be limited to two or three and the duration of vacuum application before abandonment of the procedure a maximum of 20 to 30 minutes.[34,35] A randomized controlled trial (RCT) compared maintenance of suction of 600 mm Hg throughout the operative delivery to reduction of suction to 100 mm Hg between contractions and found no differences in duration of operative delivery or in neonatal outcome.[36] Finally, vacuum cup selection may play a role in the likelihood of successful vaginal delivery. The soft cup instruments used in modern practice are associated with less scalp trauma but have a higher failure rate than rigid metal vacuum cups.[35] A meta-analysis of nine RCTs of soft versus rigid vacuum extractor cups determined that the average failure rates were 16% and 9% for the soft and metal cups, respectively. The detachment rates were 22% and 10% for the soft and metal cups, respectively. Higher failure rates with the soft cup may be secondary to difficulties associated with proper placement and traction, particularly if the fetus is deflexed, malpositioned, or at higher station.[27,35]

RISKS AND BENEFITS OF OPERATIVE VAGINAL DELIVERY

Benefits of Operative Vaginal Delivery

Most women desire a vaginal delivery.[14] **As such, the safe and effective application of instrumental delivery during the second stage of labor is crucial. In addition, acknowledging the benefits of operative vaginal delivery and the maternal views following these interventions is an important component to enhance counseling.** In a cohort study of 393 women who had either a "difficult" operative vaginal delivery performed in the operating suite or a cesarean delivery for an arrest disorder in the second stage of labor, an equal proportion of patients in both groups desired future pregnancy (51% vs. 54%) when asked before hospital discharge. However, women who had an operative vaginal delivery were much more likely to desire a subsequent vaginal delivery compared with women delivered by cesarean section when asked immediately postpartum (79% vs. 39%)[11] and when asked again 3 years later (87% vs. 33%).[12] In addition, of those patients who achieved pregnancy within 3 years of the index delivery in this cohort, substantially more women who had an operative vaginal delivery achieved subsequent vaginal delivery compared with those who had a prior cesarean delivery (78% vs. 31%).[12] Johanson and colleagues followed patients 5 years after a randomized trial comparing forceps with vacuum extraction and demonstrated that more than 75% achieved a spontaneous vaginal delivery with a larger fetus in their second pregnancy.[37]

Because women report fear of childbirth as a common reason for avoiding future pregnancies,[12] patients who had an operative delivery were asked about their views on this procedure including preparation for this type of delivery. Most women felt that their birth plan or antenatal classes had not properly prepared them for the possibility of an operative delivery in the second stage of labor.[13] In addition, most had difficulty understanding the need for the intervention despite a review of the indications by the medical staff before discharge. These patients desired more focused antenatal information on operative delivery and a postdelivery debriefing by their delivering physician or midwife focusing on the reasons for the intervention and their future pregnancy and delivery implications.[13]

Maternal Risks

The focus of recent attention regarding operative vaginal delivery has been the risk of perineal trauma and subsequent pelvic floor dysfunction. The principle risks appear to be those of urinary and fecal incontinence. However, the difficulty in establishing the precise risks of this dysfunction in patients who have had an operative vaginal delivery compared with those who have not is confounded by many factors, including the indication for the operative delivery, number of deliveries, maternal weight, neonatal birth weight and head circumference, perineal body length, episiotomy, and the effects of maternal aging.[38] We will examine three aspects of maternal risk associated with operative vaginal delivery: significant perineal trauma (third- and fourth-degree laceration), urinary incontinence, and fecal incontinence.

Perineal Trauma

Significant perineal trauma is generally defined as a third-degree laceration, involving the anal sphincter, or fourth-degree laceration, involving the rectal mucosa. Estimated frequencies of these injuries vary based on multiple maternal factors, including parity, birth weight, type of delivery, and use of episiotomy. In a large, population-based retrospective study of more than 2 million vaginal deliveries, the frequency of severe perineal injury was noted to be 11.5% in nulliparous patients, 13.8% in patients with a successful vaginal birth after cesarean delivery, and 1.8% in multiparous patients.[39] Increased risks of anal sphincter injuries were found to be associated with primiparity, macrosomia, shoulder dystocia, maternal diabetes mellitus, prolonged pregnancy, nonreassuring fetal heart rate patterns, and operative vaginal delivery. In contrast to other studies demonstrating a much larger risk of severe perineal injury due to forceps and vacuum delivery (sevenfold to eightfold), the study by Handa and colleagues observed an odds ratio (OR) of only 1.4 for forceps delivery and 2.3 for vacuum delivery, suggesting that operative vaginal delivery may be associated with a much lower risk of third- and fourth-degree lacerations than was previously thought.[39] In addition, Handa and colleagues found that episiotomy was associated with a 10% decrease in anal sphincter laceration. Other studies have also observed that episiotomy associated with forceps use either did not increase the risk of third- or fourth-degree lacerations[40] or reduced their risk.[41] However, other investigations have noted an increased risk of severe perineal injury with episiotomy use.[42] Finally, in a retrospective review of more than 2000 consecutive deliveries, reduction in episiotomy use was found to be associated with an increased rate of vaginal lacerations, a decreased rate of fourth-degree lacerations, and no change in the rate of third-degree lacerations over a 10-year period from one institution.[43] Whether more liberal use of episiotomy affects the rate of severe perineal lacerations remains to be evaluated in a prospective randomized trial.

Urinary Incontinence

Stress urinary incontinence is defined as the involuntary leakage of urine during effort or exertion and occurs at least once weekly in one third of adult women.[44] **Both pregnancy and the interval time following pregnancy predispose women to urinary incontinence.** Viktrup and colleagues observed that 32% of nulliparous women developed urinary incontinence during pregnancy and 7% after delivery. One year following delivery, only 3% reported incontinence; however, 5 years later, 19% of women asymptomatic following delivery had incontinence.[45] The Norwegian EPINCONT study, with an 80% response rate to a survey of more than 11,000 nulliparous patients, observed a 24% prevalence of urinary incontinence and increased urinary incontinence symptoms with increasing age, body mass index (BMI), and number of years since their delivery.[46] In addition, incontinence was significantly associated with birthweight greater than 4000 g and fetal head circumference greater than 38 cm. Having at least one vacuum or forceps delivery in this cohort did not affect the risk of developing urinary incontinence. In a prospective study of the short- and long-term effects of forceps delivery compared with spontaneous vaginal delivery, which included both patient survey and clinical examination data, Meyer and colleagues observed a similar incidence of urinary incontinence at both 9 weeks (32% vs. 21%) and 10 months (20% vs. 15%).[47] In addition, bladder neck behavior, urethral sphincter function, and intravaginal pressures were similar between the groups. The only difference noted was an increased incidence of a weak pelvic floor in the forceps group (20% vs. 6%) at the 10-month examination. In a 5-year follow-up study of patients randomized to either forceps or vacuum delivery, Johanson and colleagues observed no difference in the incidence of urinary dysfunction between these groups.[48] However, Arya and colleagues in a prospective observational study using patient survey data reported that urinary incontinence after forceps delivery was more likely to persist at 1 year compared with spontaneous vaginal delivery or vacuum delivery (11% vs. 3%).[49] **The only prospective randomized trial to assess urinary incontinence symptoms after planned elective cesarean delivery compared with planned vaginal delivery is the Term Breech Trial.**[50] At 3 months postpartum, women randomized to cesarean delivery reported less urinary incontinence compared with those in the planned vaginal delivery group (4.5% vs. 7.3%; relative risk 0.62, 95% confidence interval [CI] 0.41 to 0.93). Finally, in a long-term (34-year) follow-up study of patients following either forceps, spontaneous vaginal delivery, or an elective cesarean delivery without labor, urinary incontinence was found more frequently in those women who had a spontaneous vaginal delivery compared with those who had a forceps delivery (19% vs. 7%). In addition, the total number of vaginal deliveries was the only risk factor attributed to urinary incontinence in this cohort (OR 19.5; 95% CI, 4.01 to 34.8; $P = 0.001$).[51] **The precise association between mode of vaginal delivery (spontaneous, forceps, or vacuum) and urinary incontinence remains unclear at this time in light of the many other factors that appear to contribute to this condition. However, there appears to be little if any effect of forceps delivery on the subsequent development of urinary incontinence.** Therefore, it is reasonable to counsel patients that the use of forceps or vacuum for an appropriate obstetrical indication likely has no increased long-term affect on urinary incontinence compared with spontaneous vaginal delivery.

Fecal Incontinence

Overall rates of anal sphincter injury noted at the time of vaginal delivery in nulliparous patients are reported to be between 7% and 11.5%.[39,52,53] Operative vaginal delivery has been associated with an increased risk of perineal injury, specifically third- and fourth-degree lacerations.[39,40] However, what is not clear is the precise incidence of occult anal sphincter injury in patients delivering vaginally and the resulting effect on fecal incontinence. In the largest prospective study evaluating the prevalence of anal sphincter injury after forceps delivery in nulliparous women using endoanal ultrasound, de Parades and colleagues examined 93 patients 6 weeks after delivery and found a 13% prevalence of anal sphincter injury.[54] These findings are in contrast to other studies that have evaluated fewer patients each, but found a higher prevalence of anal sphincter injury shortly following forceps delivery[54-59] (Table 15-3).

The difficulty with many of the studies noted in Table 15-3 is the extremely low number of patients that return for the endoanal ultrasound following delivery. For example, even though Sultan recruited patients from a previous RCT of forceps and vacuum delivery, only 44 of the original 313 patients (14%) were assessed.[58] Because not all patients were evaluated, it is possible that significant selection bias occurred and that the actual prevalence of anal sphincter injury was lower because those patients most symptomatic would be likeliest to return for endoanal ultrasound. Indeed, in the largest randomized trial to date evaluating anal sphincter function following forceps or vacuum extraction, Fitzpatrick and colleagues was able to follow up on all 61 patients randomized to forceps delivery and demonstrated a much lower rate of anal sphincter injury than previously reported (56%). Even though more patients who delivered by forceps compared with vacuum delivery in this study described altered fecal continence (59% vs. 33%), there were no differences seen in endoanal ultrasound defects or in anal manometry results. In addition, there were no differences in symptom scores between the groups and the degree of disturbance to continence was low in both groups, with the most common symptom being occasional flatal incontinence.[59]

However, de Parades and colleagues found lower rates of anal sphincter injury (13%) and complaints of altered fecal continence (30%) following forceps delivery. Most symptomatic patients complained of persistence of incontinence of flatus (17/28), as noted in the study by Fitzpatrick. In addition, a significant increase in the daily number of stools was associated with anal sphincter defects visible on endoanal ultrasound, but the development of altered fecal continence symptoms was not.[54]

Even though it appears that immediate complaints of altered fecal continence and evidence of anal sphincter injury may be as high as 60% immediately following operative vaginal delivery, data from long-term follow-up does not bear this figure out. For example, Johanson and colleagues followed patients 5 years after randomization to either forceps or vacuum delivery and found no significant difference in complaints of altered fecal continence between the groups (15% vs. 26%).[48] In addition, most patients in the forceps and vacuum groups who noted altered fecal continence had occasional incontinence of flatus or diarrhea as their only symptom (70% and 68%, respectively). In addition, 34-year follow-up data on 42 patients delivered by forceps compared with 41 patients delivered by spontaneous vaginal delivery demonstrated a higher rate of anal sphincter injury on ultrasonography in the forceps group (44% vs. 22%), but no difference in the rate of altered fecal continence (14% vs. 10%).[51] **These data suggest that forceps delivery is a risk for sphincter injury but not for long-term fecal incontinence. In fact, logistic regression revealed that the largest neonatal birth weight, and not forceps delivery, was the contributing risk for significant fecal incontinence in this study.**[51] Therefore, based on these data, the anal sphincter injury rate in women who deliver by forceps may be higher; however, long-term rates of fecal incontinence appear to be no different than in women who deliver spontaneously. These findings could reflect the body's ability to heal and compensate for anal sphincter injury over time and may also be the basis for questioning the importance and validity of early outcome assessments of anal incontinence.

Fetal Risks

The focus of possible fetal injury associated with operative vaginal delivery includes craniofacial/intracranial injury and neurologic/cognitive effects. The risks of fetal injury

TABLE 15-3 PREVALENCE OF ANAL SPHINCTER INJURY FOLLOWING FORCEPS DELIVERY

STUDY SPHINCTER	FORCEPS DELIVERIES (*N*)	IAS INJURY (*N*)	EAS INJURY (*N*)	IAS AND EAS INJURY (*N*)	TOTAL ANAL INJURY (%)
Sultan[55]	26	7	3	11	81
Sultan[58]	19	MD	MD	MD	79
Abramowitz[56]	35	MD	MD	MD	63
Belmonte-Montes[57]	17	0	11	2	76
Fitzpatrick[59]	61	0	34	0	56
De Parades[54]	93	0	11	1	13

EAS, External anal sphincter; *IAS*, internal anal sphincter; *MD*, missing data.

are generally instrument specific, with vacuum deliveries accounting for statistically significantly higher rates of cephalohematoma, and subgaleal and retinal hemorrhages, and forceps deliveries accounting for a nonsignificantly higher rate of scalp/facial injuries.[60] In addition, the sequential use of vacuum and forceps requires particular attention because use in this manner is associated with a maternal and neonatal risk, which is greater than the sum of the individual risks of these instruments.[53]

Craniofacial and Intracranial Injury

Cephalohematoma and Subgaleal Hemorrhage

Rates of subperiosteal cephalohematoma in vacuum-assisted vaginal deliveries are higher than rates for either forceps or spontaneous vaginal delivery (112/1000, 63/1000, and 17/1000, respectively).[61,62] However, the most clinically significant and potentially life-threatening injury in this category is a subgaleal hemorrhage (see Chapter 21). This "false cephalohematoma" was first described by Naegele in 1819 to differentiate it from a true subperiosteal cephalohematoma.[63] Subgaleal hemorrhage occurs when blood collects in the loose areolar tissue in the space between the galea aponeurotica and the periosteum. If the veins that connect the dural sinus and the scalp rupture in this layer due to shear forces, the potential space within this loosely applied connective tissue in the subgaleal space may expand with blood well beyond the limits of the suture lines (unlike a subperiosteal cephalohematoma, which is limited to blood and fluid collections within the margins of the suture lines). This space has the potential volume of several hundred milliliters of blood, which may produce profound neonatal hypovolemia, leading to hypoxia, disseminated intravascular coagulation (DIC), end-organ injury, and death.[64] Older literature cites several causes of subgaleal hemorrhage with the source as follows: vacuum extraction, 48%; spontaneous vaginal delivery, 28%; forceps, 14%; and cesarean delivery, 9%.[63] Although this is older literature reporting in an era when a "low-forceps" delivery was broadly defined by the 1965 ACOG Classification scheme, it is most important to note that these potentially life-threatening bleeds can also occur with spontaneous vaginal deliveries. **More recent data suggest that subgaleal hemorrhage occurs nearly exclusively with the vacuum device**[65-67] with an incidence of subgaleal bleeding of 26 to 45 per 1000.[68] Benaron[69] reported an incidence of 1 per 200 with soft silicone vacuum cups.

Subgaleal hemorrhage has an estimated incidence of approximately 4 per 10,000 spontaneous vaginal deliveries.[63] In a 30-month prospective study, Boo[70] evaluated more than 64,000 neonates and found that the incidence per live birth was much higher for vacuum extraction than other modes of delivery (41 per 1000 vs. 1 per 1000). Both the type of cup and the duration of its use are predictors of scalp injury. Soft cups are more likely to be associated with a decreased incidence of scalp injuries, but may not be less likely to result in a subgaleal hemorrhage.[4] In one study, vacuum application duration of more than 10 minutes was the best predictor of scalp injury.[71] **In May 1998, the Food and Drug Administration (FDA) issued a public health advisory regarding the use of vacuum-assisted delivery devices. The advisory cited a fivefold increase in the rate of deaths and serious morbidity during the previous 4 years compared with the past 11 years and recommended use of these devices only when a specific obstetrical indication is present.** Other recommendations included the following:

- Persons who use vacuum devices for assisted delivery are versed in their use, and that they are aware of the indications, contraindications, and precautions as supported in the accepted literature and current device labeling.
- The recommended use for all these products is to apply steady traction in the line of the birth canal. Rocking movements or applying torque to the device may be dangerous. Because the instructions may be different for each device type or style, it is important to use the instructions provided by the manufacturer of the particular product being used.
- Alert those who will be responsible for the infant's care that a vacuum-assisted delivery device has been used, so that they can monitor the infant for signs of complications.
- Educate the neonatal care staff about the complications of vacuum-assisted delivery devices that have been reported to the FDA and in the literature. They should watch for the signs of these complications in any infant in whom a vacuum-assisted delivery device was used.
- Report reactions associated with the use of vacuum-assisted delivery devices to the FDA.[31]

Despite the fact that many recommend allowing no more than three pop-offs before successful delivery, there is no clear evidence that three applications are safe because if the cup slips during traction without descent of the vertex, neonatal scalp injury may still occur.[71] For example, Benaron[69] demonstrated that the risk of injury and bleeding is increased in nulliparous patients and in those with severe dystocia, malposition, and forceful, prolonged vacuum extractor use. Therefore, caution must be taken with the use of vacuum extractor devices to avoid prolonged (greater than 30 minutes) or forceful use.

Intracranial Hemorrhage

Rates of clinically significant ICH for vacuum, forceps and cesarean delivery during labor are similar (1/860, 1/664, and 1/907, respectively) but are higher than for cesarean delivery without labor (1/2750) or spontaneous vaginal delivery (1/1900).[72] Because cesarean delivery following abnormal labor was associated with the same rate of ICH as forceps and vacuum in this study, it is likely that the common risk factor for any increased risk of ICH is abnormal labor and not the type of operative vaginal delivery performed. In fact, because the prevalence of clinically silent subdural hemorrhages is approximately 6% following uncomplicated spontaneous vaginal delivery, the presence of this hemorrhage in an otherwise asymptomatic neonate does not necessarily indicate excessive birth trauma and again reflects the natural history of labor and delivery.[73] In these neonates with silent subdural hemorrhages, all resolved within 4 weeks of delivery.

Neurologic and Cognitive Effects

Vacuum-assisted vaginal deliveries increase the risk of neonatal retinal hemorrhages by approximately twofold compared with forceps deliveries.[60] Despite this finding, data on the long-term consequences of these hemorrhages do not demonstrate any significant effect. Johanson and colleagues followed a cohort of children 5 years following an RCT of forceps versus vacuum extraction and found a 13% rate of visual problems in the group. However, there was no difference between those delivered by forceps compared with those delivered by vacuum extraction (12.8% vs. 12.5%).[48] Seidman and colleagues were also unable to detect any increased risk of vision abnormalities in a cohort of 1747 individuals delivered by vacuum extraction compared with more than 47,000 individuals delivered by spontaneous vaginal delivery and examined at age 17 years by the Israeli Defense Forces draft board.[74] There also does not appear to be any long-term effect of operative vaginal delivery on cognitive development. Seidman and colleagues demonstrated that mean intelligence scores at age 17 years were no different between those delivered by forceps or vacuum extraction compared to those delivered by spontaneous vaginal delivery. However, the mean intelligence scores for those delivered by cesarean delivery were significantly lower than those of the spontaneous delivery group.[74] Similarly, in a 1993 report from patients within the Kaiser system in Oakland, CA, Wesley and colleagues were unable to detect a difference in cognitive development by measuring intelligence quotient (IQ) in 1192 children delivered by forceps compared with 1499 who delivered spontaneously and were examined at age 5 years. Furthermore, of the 1192 forceps deliveries, there were 114 midforceps, and no differences in IQ were seen at age 5 compared with 1500 controls.[75] Finally, there also appears to be no association between forceps delivery and epilepsy in adulthood. Murphy and colleagues evaluated a cohort of more than 21,000 individuals and found forceps delivery was not associated with an increased risk of epilepsy or anticonvulsant therapy when compared with other methods of delivery.[76]

Dierker and colleagues[77] followed 110 infants for 5 years delivered by midforceps and matched with infants born by cesarean delivery for the same indications and found no differences in IQ or neurologic abnormalities.

Finally, in a similar 5-year follow-up of a prospective cohort of 264 women with term, singleton, cephalic pregnancies that required a second-stage operative delivery from 1999 to 2000, neonates delivered by forceps were found to have no significant differences in neurodevelopmental outcome compared to those delivered by cesarean section.[78]

Complex Operative Vaginal Delivery Procedures

Rotations Greater Than 45 Degrees

The correct application and delivery technique using forceps is critical to the safe performance of this procedure. The outcomes of forceps delivery are often directly compared to and contrasted with those of spontaneous vaginal delivery. When these comparisons are made, forceps deliveries are associated with a higher rate of maternal injury than spontaneous vaginal delivery. However, the comparison of these two modes of delivery is not appropriate because forceps applications require an indication for use that confounds the clinical outcome when compared with spontaneous vaginal delivery. A more appropriate comparison to forceps delivery (or operative vaginal delivery in general) is cesarean delivery for second-stage arrest disorder. Unfortunately, there are no prospective, randomized trials directly comparing these two modes of delivery. However, numerous retrospective studies comparing midcavity and rotational forceps delivery with cesarean delivery demonstrate no increased risk of fetal/neonatal adverse outcomes including Apgar score, umbilical cord blood gas values, birth trauma, and neonatal intensive care unit (NICU) admission.[79-82] Specifically, the rates of neonatal morbidity associated with Kielland's forceps rotation are similar to cesarean delivery, including rates of cephalohematoma (9% to 17%), facial bruising (13% to 18%), facial nerve injury (1% to 5%) and brachial plexus injury (less than 1%).[83,84] Interestingly, rates of maternal morbidity (intraoperative and postoperative complications, blood loss, and length of stay) have been found to be higher in patients delivered by cesarean delivery compared with those delivered by midcavity forceps delivery.[79,80]

The outcomes of rotational forceps deliveries have also been evaluated and compared with nonrotational forceps delivery. Healy and colleagues evaluated 552 Kielland's forceps rotations, 95 Scanzoni-Smellie maneuvers with classic instruments, and 160 manual rotations followed by delivery with a classic instrument and found no difference in neonatal outcomes between the groups.[85] Krivac and colleagues[86] compared 55 Kielland's forceps rotations with 213 nonrotational forceps deliveries. Fifteen of the rotations were greater than 90 degrees, and 40 were less than 90 degrees but greater than 45 degrees. They found that the Kielland's forceps rotation group had both a longer labor and longer second stage than the nonrotational group and a higher rate of 1-minute Apgar scores less than 6 and meconium at delivery. However, the nonrotational forceps group had a greater incidence of postpartum hemorrhage (14% vs. 7%) and a higher rate of third- and fourth-degree lacerations (24% vs. 14%). No other differences in maternal or neonatal morbidity were noted, including no difference in rates of nerve compromise (less than 1%), facial bruising (7%), shoulder dystocia (1%), or NICU admissions. Hankins and colleagues[87] performed a retrospective case-controlled study comparing 113 forceps deliveries greater than 90 degrees compared with 167 forceps deliveries less than 45 degrees. No differences in major fetal injury were demonstrated between these two groups. Major fetal injury was defined as skull fracture, subdural hematoma and brachial plexus or facial nerve injury, and fetal acidemia (pH less than 7.0). Finally, Feldman and colleagues compared 104 rotational forceps deliveries using Leff forceps for persistent OP position with 163 nonrotational forceps deliveries and found lower rates of episiotomy (66% vs. 82%) and perineal lacerations (16% vs. 23%) in the forceps rotation group and no differences in the rates of neonatal morbidity between the groups.[88] **These data suggest that when properly applied and used, forceps deliveries requiring greater than 45 degree rotation may be safely accomplished without increased risk of maternal or neonatal morbidity and, therefore, should remain a management option for women with second-stage labor abnormalities.**

Midpelvic Cavity Delivery

Like rotational forceps deliveries, delivery of the fetus from a 0 or +1 station (midpelvic or midforceps) requires a specific set of skills and precautions. In 1988, ACOG reported on required conditions for a midforceps delivery that included the following: (1) an experienced person performing or supervising the procedure, (2) adequate anesthesia, (3) assessment of maternal-fetal size, and (4) willingness to abandon the attempt at delivery. This information should be taken together with the prerequisites set forth by Richardson and colleagues[89]: the midforceps procedure (1) must rationally be needed as an alternative method of delivery to cesarean delivery, (2) must be associated with demonstrably less maternal morbidity than cesarean section, and (3) should not result in fetal harm. Several studies that compare cesarean delivery to midforceps procedures show that midforceps delivery is not associated with more adverse neonatal outcomes including cord blood gases, Apgar scores, NICU admissions, and birth trauma.[79,80,90] In 1997, Revah and colleagues[90] reported their findings of a retrospective chart review of 401 cesarean deliveries over a 7-year period in which a trial of operative delivery (forceps or vacuum) was conducted in 75 cases. There were no differences between cesarean delivery with a trial of operative delivery versus without an operative delivery attempt for any maternal or fetal outcome. **Although the outcomes of these studies are reassuring, because of the technical skills required, it is most reasonable to abide by the guidance set forth in the ACOG practice bulletin published in 2000, which states, "Unless the preoperative assessment is highly suggestive of successful outcome, trial of operative vaginal delivery is best avoided."**[68] In short, following the ACOG statement and the previously stated prerequisites provides the skilled practitioner with guidelines and support for attempting a safe midpelvic cavity delivery.

Sequential Use of Vacuum and Forceps

The sequential use of these instruments appears to increase the likelihood of adverse maternal and neonatal outcomes more than the sum of the relative risks of each instrument.[53,62] Compared with spontaneous vaginal delivery, deliveries by sequential use of vacuum and forceps are associated with significantly higher rates of ICH (RR, 3.9; 95% CI, 1.5 to 10.1), brachial plexus injury (RR, 3.2; 95% CI, 1.6 to 6.4), facial nerve injury (RR, 3.0; 95% CI, 4.7 to 37.7), neonatal seizures (RR, 13.7; 95% CI, 2.1 to 88.0), requirement for mechanical ventilation of the neonate (RR, 4.8; 95% CI, 2.1 to 11.0), severe perineal lacerations (RR, 6.2; 95% CI, 6.4 to 20.1), and postpartum hemorrhage (RR, 1.6; 95% CI, 1.3 to 2.0).[53] Therefore, care should be taken to avoid the sequential use of these instruments to reduce maternal and neonatal morbidity. Such switching of instruments should be limited to situations in which there is failure of application of one type of instrument and be performed by individuals skilled and experienced with operative vaginal delivery procedures.

Trial of Operative Vaginal Delivery

Historically, an unsuccessful operative vaginal delivery has been associated with a high maternal and neonatal morbidity and up to a 38% fetal mortality rate and 2% maternal mortality rate.[91] Reports of increased morbidity and mortality in these cases led to the development of the concept of a trial of forceps in which immediate cesarean delivery was performed if, following correction of malposition and gentle traction, further decent of the fetal vertex was not noted.[92] These attempts were often performed in the operating room instead of the delivery room, permitting rapid transition to cesarean delivery. Following implementation of this concept, rates of morbidity and mortality have fallen, documenting no difference in neonatal or maternal outcomes associated with a failed forceps or vacuum attempt in the absence of a nonreassuring fetal heart rate tracing.[93]

Vacuum Delivery and the Preterm Fetus

There are no quality data for firm recommendations regarding a gestational age limit below which the vacuum extractor should not be used. There are two studies reporting the use of soft cups without adverse outcomes in preterm fetuses. However, these studies were small and lacked power to demonstrate significance. There are no RCTs comparing forceps versus vacuums or comparing different vacuum types to pass judgment on a gestational age cut-off. **ACOG reports that most experts in operative vaginal delivery limit the vacuum procedure to fetuses greater than 34 weeks' gestation.**[68] This is a reasonable cut-off, given that the premature head is likely at greater risk for compression-decompression injuries simply due to the pliability of the preterm skull and the more fragile soft tissues of the scalp.

COUNSELING: FORCEPS, VACUUM, OR CESAREAN DELIVERY

The increasing use of vacuum extraction over forceps has resulted in numerous publications comparing efficacy and morbidity between methods. Table 15-4 provides a summary of the disadvantages associated with both methods. In a Cochrane meta-analysis including 10 RCTs of vacuum and forceps use, vacuum extraction had a greater failure rate than that of forceps.[94] Vacuum extraction was associated with less maternal trauma, including third- and fourth-degree extensions, and vaginal lacerations, than forceps use.[94] Less maternal regional and general anesthesia was used for vacuum extractions. There

TABLE 15-4 COMPARATIVE MORBIDITIES ASSOCIATED WITH FORCEPS DELIVERY AND VACUUM EXTRACTION

FORCEPS	VACUUM EXTRACTION
Greater third- and fourth-degree and vaginal lacerations	Higher failure rate than forceps Increased risk of neonatal injury:
Greater maternal discomfort postpartum	Minor: cephalohematoma, retinal hemorrhage
Greater duration of training needed	Major: subarachnoid hemorrhage, subgaleal hemorrhage
Increased risk of neonatal facial nerve injury	Less need for maternal anesthesia

Modified from Johanson RB, Menon BK: Vacuum extraction versus forceps for assisted vaginal delivery. Cochrane Database Syst Rev (2):CD000224, 2000.

were no differences in significant neonatal injury between the two groups. Despite small sample sizes, vacuum extraction was associated with an increased risk of cephalohematoma and retinal hemorrhage when compared with forceps use. Cephalohematoma formation with vacuum extraction was reported to have a mean incidence of 6%, with no difference between soft or rigid vacuum cups, and is considered to be a finding of little significance.[29,94]

Unless a patient is willing to undergo cesarean delivery before the onset of advanced labor, there does not appear to be any advantage to avoiding operative vaginal delivery in an attempt to reduce the long-term risks of incontinence. The effects of both forceps and vacuum delivery on the risk of developing urinary incontinence appear to be the same as those of spontaneous vaginal delivery with between 5% and 20% of women developing long-term persistent urinary incontinence regardless of vaginal delivery method. In addition, despite evidence that the anal sphincter injury rate in women who deliver by forceps is higher, it is not clear that the long-term rates of fecal incontinence in these women is any different than in those who deliver spontaneously. Approximately 10% to 30% of women develop some degree of altered fecal continence following vaginal delivery, with cesarean delivery before the onset of labor as the only reliable means of reducing this risk.

The greatest risk for urinary incontinence appears to be the total number of vaginal deliveries, and the greatest risk for subsequent development of fecal incontinence appears to be related to the effect of the largest neonate delivered vaginally, irrespective of mode of delivery. Regarding fetal risks, vacuum deliveries appear to increase the incidence of cephalohematoma, and subgaleal and retinal hemorrhages compared with forceps or spontaneous vaginal deliveries. Forceps deliveries increase the risk of facial bruising and transient facial nerve palsies compared with vacuum or spontaneous vaginal deliveries. However, there is no evidence that these immediate neonatal morbidities result in any long-term visual, neurologic, or cognitive developmental abnormalities. Finally, patients delivered by cesarean delivery in the second stage have a higher risk of intraoperative and postoperative complications, higher rates of blood loss, and longer hospital stays than those delivered by operative vaginal delivery.

Patients should also be informed that substantially more women who have an operative vaginal delivery achieve subsequent vaginal delivery in the next pregnancy compared with those who have a cesarean delivery (78% vs. 31%). Therefore, it is reasonable to counsel patients that the options for second-stage assisted delivery include both forceps and vacuum when appropriate, because the proper application of these instruments and execution of these deliveries can avoid the maternal morbidity associated with cesarean delivery and increase the likelihood of a subsequent vaginal delivery for the next pregnancy without additional long-term maternal or neonatal risk.

In a Cochrane review of 10 randomized studies comparing the use of forceps to vacuum extraction for assisted vaginal delivery, vacuum devices were found more likely to fail than forceps.[61] However, vacuum use was also more likely to result in vaginal delivery, probably because failed vacuum extraction led to the use of forceps and subsequent vaginal delivery due to a lower forceps failure rate. A lower failure rate is not the only reason to consider forceps. Forceps may be the only acceptable instrument to effect an operative vaginal delivery in some circumstances. Some examples of these clinical situations include delivery of the head at assisted breech delivery, assisted delivery of a preterm infant younger than 34 weeks' gestation, delivery with a face presentation, suspected coagulopathy or thrombocytopenia in the fetus, and instrumental delivery for maternal medical conditions that preclude pushing.[14] Because the specific clinical situation and operator experience are the key factors that contribute to the choice of instrument, it is critical that students of obstetrics be thoroughly familiar with the use of both instruments. Finally, an attempt at counseling patients on the risks, benefits, and alternatives of operative vaginal delivery should take place during prenatal visits. This is because it is not ideal to counsel patients in the second stage of labor when they are generally experiencing pain, exhaustion, and/or are under the influence of narcotics. This counseling should also be documented in the medical record.

SIMULATION AND RESIDENCY TRAINING IN OPERATIVE VAGINAL DELIVERY

The overall incidence of operative vaginal delivery has remained stable over the past 15 years. Interestingly, over this same time span, vacuum extraction procedures have overtaken forceps procedures as the instrument of choice (Figure 15-8). In a review of operative vaginal delivery, Yeomans strongly advocates that residency training programs incorporate detailed instructions in forceps techniques and that simulation training precede clinical work to enhance understanding of the mechanics.[95] Bahl and colleagues reviewed video recordings to establish critical components of nonrotational vacuum deliveries, defining key technical skills required for evaluating clinical competence of trainees in this technique.[96] Further detailed studies are needed to ensure that both vacuum and forceps techniques can be taught and evaluated first with the use of simulation and then in the clinical setting.

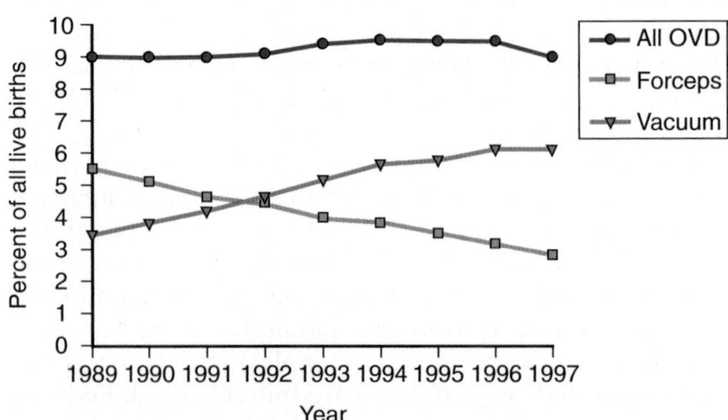

FIGURE 15-8. The overall incidence of operative vaginal delivery has remained stable over the last 15 years. Interestingly, over this same time span, vacuum extraction procedures have overtaken forceps procedures as the instrument of choice. (Modified from Miksovsky P, Watson WJ: Obstetric vacuum extraction: state of the art in the new millennium. Obstet Gynecol Surv 56:736, 2001.)

A 1992 report of a survey conducted by Ramin and colleagues of U.S. residency training programs reported that most programs use the 1988 classification scheme and that 86% taught midforceps.[97] It should be noted that even though a large percentage of programs teach the complex forceps procedures, the number of such procedures to reach proficiency has not been elucidated. In short, the overall decline in forceps procedures performed, the complexity of midpelvic cavity deliveries, and the shift from complex rotational deliveries to vacuum extraction and cesarean deliveries by younger faculty as shown by Tan and colleagues[83] and Jain and colleagues[98] may make the midforceps procedure obsolete in the near future.[97] In response to these types of concerns, Kim and colleagues[99] conducted a unique study to determine whether the rates of vacuum extraction and forceps procedures could be reversed without an increase in morbidity in a residency program. This retrospective study compared outcomes 2 years before and 2 years after an obstetrics faculty member was dedicated to the labor floor from Monday through Thursday, 7 AM to 5 PM **Table 15-5 depicts how such a dedicated instructor can increase the number of forceps relative to vacuum extractions without increasing third- or fourth-degree lacerations or adverse neonatal outcomes.**

Although the early 1990 report by Ramin and colleagues[97] provided encouraging information regarding the use of the 1988 classification scheme, a more recent study by Carollo and colleagues[100] is unsettling. In this 2004 study, Carollo conducted a survey of several teaching hospitals in the Denver area asking the following important questions: (1) How do you define fetal station? (2) How do you think a majority of your colleagues define fetal station? (3) How do you think the ACOG defines the classification of fetal station? and (4) How important do you think these distinctions are? What makes this study additionally unique is that these questions were asked of both attendings and residents in obstetrics and gynecology as well as nurses. Approximately 35% of attending physicians still defined station by dividing the pelvis into thirds rather than centimeters, as set forth in the old 1965 ACOG classification scheme. In addition, nearly 15% used the BPD rather than the presenting part as the landmark on the fetus to define station. These percentage numbers were higher for nurses and residents. The percent of correctly used techniques for defining station was highest at the university teaching hospital. These data suggest that, although we do fairly well at teaching proper technique for determining station, we are poor at disseminating the information into practice. Operative vaginal deliveries will be more difficult and dangerous if misunderstandings in defining fetal station persist.

TABLE 15-5 MODES OF DELIVERY AND BIRTH OUTCOMES BEFORE AND AFTER INITIATION OF DEDICATED OBSTETRICS STAFF LOCATED ON LABOR AND DELIVERY

	BEFORE	AFTER	P
Births	3481	4338	0.0001
Cesarean section	888 (26%)	1183 (27%)	NS
Operative vaginal delivery	394 (11%)	461 (11%)	NS
Forceps	172 (5%)	337 (8%)	0.00001
Vacuum	222 (6%)	124 (3%)	0.00001
Third- or fourth-degree lacerations	126 (4%)	134 (3%)	NS
Birth injury	8 (0.2%)	13 (0.3%)	NS
AS <7 at 5 minutes	67 (2%)	104 (2%)	NS

KEY POINTS

- Obstetrical forceps are the one instrument that makes the practice of obstetrical care unique to obstetricians. The proper use of these instruments has afforded safe and timely vaginal delivery to those whose abnormal labor course and urgent need for delivery require their use.
- Rates of cesarean delivery have risen in the United States, reaching a rate of approximately 25% of all deliveries in the United States, whereas rates of forceps deliveries have declined from 17.7% in 1980 to 4% in 2000.
- Resident work hour restrictions have resulted in a decline in resident experience with both primary cesarean delivery and vacuum-assisted vaginal delivery.
- Treat the vacuum extractor with the same respect as the forceps. The prerequisites for application of forceps or vacuum extractor are identical.
- When using vacuum extraction, descent of the fetal head should occur with each pull. If no descent occurs after three pulls, the operative attempt should be stopped.
- There appears to be little if any effect of forceps delivery on the subsequent development of urinary incontinence.
- The rate of anal sphincter injury in women who deliver by forceps may be higher; however, long-term rates of fetal incontinence appear to be no different than in women who deliver spontaneously.
- The risks of fetal injury associated with operative vaginal delivery are generally instrument specific, with vacuum deliveries accounting for higher rates of cephalohematoma and subgaleal and retinal hemorrhages, and forceps deliveries accounting for a nonsignificantly higher rate of scalp and facial injuries.
- Numerous retrospective studies comparing midcavity and rotation forceps delivery with cesarean delivery demonstrate no increased risk of fetal or neonatal adverse outcomes, including Apgar score, umbilical cord blood gas values, trauma, and neonatal intensive care unit admission.
- When properly applied and used, forceps deliveries requiring greater than 45 degrees may be safely accomplished without increased risk of maternal or neonatal morbidity and therefore should remain a management option for women with second-stage labor abnormalities.
- The sequential use of vacuum extraction and forceps increases the likelihood of adverse maternal and neonatal outcomes more than the sum of the relative risks of each instrument.

REFERENCES

1. Denman T: An Introduction to the Practice of Midwifery 1st ed. London, 1788.
2. Holland E: The Princess Charlotte of Wales: a triple obstetric tragedy. J Obstet Gynaecol Br Emp 58:905, 1951.
3. Denman T: Aphorisms on the Application and Use of the Forceps, 6th ed. London, 1817.
4. DeLee JB: The prophylactic forceps operation. Am J Obstet Gynecol 1:34, 1920.
5. Kozak LJ, Weeks JD: US trends in obstetric procedures. 1990-2000. Birth 29:157, 2002.
6. Thomas J, Paranjoth S: National sentinel caesarean section audit report. London, Royal College of Obstetricians and Gynaecologists Clinical Effectiveness Support Unit, 2001.
7. Meniru GI: An analysis of recent trends in vacuum extraction and forceps delivery. Br J Obstet Gynaecol 103:168, 1996.
8. Hankins GD, Uckan E, Rowe TF, Collier S: Forceps and vacuum delivery: expectations of residency and fellowship training program directors. Am J Perinatol 16:23, 1999.
9. Blanchard MH, Amini SB, Frank TM: Impact of work hour restrictions on resident case experience in an obstetrics and gynecology residency program. Am J Obstet Gynecol 191:1746, 2004.
10. American College of Obstetricians and Gynecologists Practice Bulletin Number 17. Operative Vaginal Delivery. June 2000.
11. Murphy DJ, Liebling RE: Cohort study of maternal views on future mode of delivery following operative delivery in the second stage of labor. Am J Obstet Gynecol 188:542, 2003.
12. Bahl R, Strachan B, Murphy DJ: Outcome of subsequent pregnancy three years after previous operative delivery in the second stage of labour: cohort study. BMJ 328:311, 2004.
13. Murphy DJ, Pope C, Frost J, Liebling RE: Women's views on the impact of operative delivery in the second stage of labour—qualitative study. BMJ 327:1132, 2003.
14. Patel RR, Murphy DJ: Forceps delivery in modern practice. BMJ 328:1302, 2004.
15. Dennen EH: A classification of forceps operations according to station of head in pelvis. Am J Obstet Gynecol 63:272, 1952.
16. American College of Obstetricians and Gynecologists: Manual of Standards of Obstetric-Gynecologic Practice: American College of Obstetricians and Gynecologists, 2nd ed. Washington, DC, ACOG, 1965.
17. American College of Obstetricians and Gynecologists, Committee on Obstetrics, Maternal and Fetal Medicine: Obstetric Forceps. Technical Bulletin No. 59, February 1988.
18. Hagadorn-Freathy AS, Yeomans ER, Hankins GDV: Validation of the 1988 ACOG Forceps Classification System. Obstet Gynecol 77:356, 1991.
19. Laube DW: Forceps delivery. Clin Obstet Gynecol 29:286, 1986.
20. Kielland C: The application of forceps to the unrotated head. A description of a new type of forceps and a new method of insertion. Translated from the original article in Monafs schrift fur Geburshilfe und Gynakologie 43:48, 1916.
21. Leff M: An obstetric forceps for rotation of the fetal head. Am J Obstet Gynecol 70:208, 1955.
22. Feldman DM, Borgida AF, Sauer F, Rodis JF: Rotational versus nonrotational forceps: maternal and neonatal outcomes. Am J Obstet Gynecol 181:1185, 1999.
23. Malmstrom T: The vacuum extractor: an obstetrical instrument. Acta Obstet Gynecol Scand 36:5, 1957.
24. Kuit JA, Eppinga HG, Wallenburg HC, Hiukeshoven FJ: A randomized comparison of vacuum extraction delivery with a rigid and a pliable cup. Obstet Gynecol 82:280, 1993.
25. Hillier CEM, Johanson RB: Worldwide survey of assisted vaginal delivery. Int J Gynecol Obstet 47:109, 1994.
26. Hale RW (ed): Dennen's Forceps Deliveries, 4th ed. Washington, DC, American College of Obstetrics and Gynecology, 2001.
27. Scanzoni FW: Lehrbuch der Geburtshulfe, 3rd ed. Vienna, Seidel, 1853, p 838.
28. Mikovsky P, Watson WJ: Obstetric vacuum extraction: state of the art in the new millennium. Obstet Gynecol Surv 56:736, 2001.
29. Vacca A: Vacuum assisted delivery. Best Pract Res Clin Obstet Gynecol 16:17, 2002.
30. Vacca A: Handbook of Vacuum Extraction in Obstetrical Practice. London, Edward Arnold, 1992.
31. Center for Devices and Radiological Health. FDA Public Health Advisory: Need for caution when using vacuum assisted delivery devices. Rockville, MD, Food and Drug Administration. Accessed December 5, 2006. Available at www.fda.gov/cdrh/feta1598.html.
32. Plauche WC: Fetal cranial injuries related to delivery with the Malmstrom vacuum extractor. Obstet Gynecol 53:750, 1979.
33. O'Grady JP, Pope CS, Patel SS: Vacuum extraction in modern obstetric practice: a review and critique. Curr Opin Obstet Gynecol 12:475, 2000.
34. Bofill JA, Rust OA, Schorr SJ, et al: A randomized prospective trial of obstetric forceps versus the m-cup vacuum extractor. Am J Obstet Gynecol 175:1325, 1996.
35. Johanson R, Menon V: Soft vs. rigid vacuum extractor cups for assisted vaginal delivery. Cochrane Database Syst Rev CD000446, 2000.
36. Bofill JA, Rust OA, Schorr SJ, et al: A randomized trial of two vacuum extraction techniques. Obstet Gynecol 89:758, 1997.
37. Johanson RB, Heycock E, Carter J, et al: Maternal and child health after assisted vaginal delivery: five-year follow up of a randomized controlled study comparing forceps and ventouse. Br J Obstet Gynaecol 106:544, 1999.
38. Handa VL, Harris TA, Ostergard DR: Protecting the pelvic floor: obstetric management to prevent incontinence and pelvic organ prolapse. Obstet Gynecol 88:470, 1996.
39. Handa VL, Danielsen BH, Gilbert WM: Obstetric anal sphincter lacerations. Obstet Gynecol 98:225, 2001.
40. Robinson JN, Norwitz ER, Cohen AP, et al: Episiotomy, operative vaginal delivery, and significant perineal trauma in nulliparous women. Am J Obstet Gynecol 181:1180, 1999.
41. Bodner-Alder B, Bodner K, Kimberger O, et al: Management of the perineum during forceps delivery: association of episiotomy with the frequency and severity of perineal trauma in women undergoing forceps delivery. J Reprod Med 48:239, 2003.
42. Christianson LM, Bovbjerg VE, McDavitt EC, Hullfish KL: Risk factors for perineal injury during delivery. Am J Obstet Gynecol 189:255, 2003.
43. Ecker JL, Tan WM, Bansal RK, et al: Is there a benefit to episiotomy at operative vaginal delivery? Observations over ten years in a stable population. Am J Obstet Gynecol 176:411, 1997.
44. Nygaard IE, Heit M: Stress urinary incontinence. Obstet Gynecol 104:607, 2004.
45. Viktrup L, Lose G: The risk of stress incontinence 5 years after first delivery. Am J Obstet Gynecol 185:82, 2001.
46. Rortveit G, Daltveit AK, Hannestad YS, Hunskaar S: Vaginal delivery parameters and urinary incontinence: the Norwegian EPINCONT study. Am J Obstet Gynecol 189:1268, 2003.
47. Meyer S, Hohlfeld P, Achtare C, et al: Birth trauma: short and long term effects of forceps delivery compared with spontaneous delivery on various pelvic floor parameters. Br J Obstet Gynaecol 107: 1360. 2000.
48. Johanson RB, Heycock E, Carter J, et al: Maternal and child health after assisted vaginal delivery: five-year follow up of a randomized controlled study comparing forceps and ventouse. Br J Obstet Gynaecol 106:544, 1999.
49. Arya LA, Jackson ND, Myers DL, Verma A: Risk of new-onset urinary incontinence after forceps and vacuum delivery in primiparous women. Am J Obstet Gynecol 185:1318, 2001.
50. Hannah ME, Hannah WJ, Hodnett ED, et al: Outcomes at 3 months after planned cesarean versus planned vaginal delivery for breech presentation at term: the International Randomized Term Breech Trial. JAMA 287:1822, 2002.
51. Bollard RC, Gardiner A, Duthie GS: Anal sphincter injury, fetal and urinary incontinence: a 34-year follow-up after forceps delivery. Dis Colon Rectum 46:1083, 2003.
52. Richter HE, Brumfield CG, Cliver SP, et al: Risk factors associated with anal sphincter tear: a comparison of primiparous patients, vaginal births after cesarean deliveries and patients with previous vaginal delivery. Am J Obstet Gynecol 187:1194, 2002.
53. Gardella G, Taylor M, Benedetti T, et al: The effect of sequential use of vacuum and forceps for assisted vaginal delivery on neonatal and maternal outcomes. Am J Obstet Gynecol 185:896, 2001.
54. deParades V, Etienney I, Thabut D, et al: Anal sphincter injury after forceps delivery: myth or reality? Dis Colon Rectum 47:24, 2004.
55. Sultan AH, Kamm MA, Bartram CI, Hudson CN: Anal sphincter trauma during instrumental delivery. Int J Gynecol Obstet 43:263, 1993.

56. Abramowitz L, Sobhani I, Ganansia R, et al: Are sphincter defects the cause of anal incontinence after vaginal delivery? Results of a prospective study. Dis Colon Rectum 43:590, 2000.
57. Belmontes-Montes C, Hagerman G, Vega-Yepez PA, et al: Anal sphincter injury after vaginal delivery in primiparous females. Dis Colon Rectum 44:1244, 2001.
58. Sultan AH, Johanson RB, Carter JE: Occult anal sphincter trauma following randomized forceps and vacuum delivery. Int J Gynecol Obstet 61:113, 1998.
59. Fitzpatrick M, Behan M, O'Connell PR, O'Herlihy C: Randomised clinical trial to assess anal sphincter function following forceps or vacuum assisted vaginal delivery. BJOG 110:424, 2003.
60. Johanson RB, Menon V: Vacuum extraction versus forceps for assisted vaginal delivery. [revised 23 Nov 2001]. In The Cochrane Pregnancy and Childbirth Database. The Cochrane Collaboration; Issue 1, Oxford, Update Software; 2002.
61. Johnson JH, Figueroa R, Garry D, et al: Immediate maternal and neonatal effects of forceps and vacuum-assisted deliveries. Obstet Gynecol 103:513, 2004.
62. Demissie K, Rhoads GG, Smulian JC, et al: Operative vaginal delivery and neonatal and infant adverse outcomes: population based retrospective analysis. BMJ 329:24, 2004.
63. Plauche WC: Subgaleal haematoma: a complication of instrumental delivery. JAMA 244:1597, 1980.
64. Eliachar E, Bret AJ, Bardiaux M, et al: Hematome souscutane cranien du nouveau-ne. Arch Fr Pediatr 20:1105, 1963.
65. Govaert P, Defoort P, Wigglesworth JS: Cranial haemorrhage in the term newborn infant. Clin Dev Med 129:1, 1993.
66. Ngan HY, Miu P, Ko L, Ma HK: Long-term neurological sequelae following vacuum extractor delivery. Aust N Z J Obstetr Gynaecol 30:111, 1990.
67. Chadwick LM, Pemberton PJ, Kurinczuk JJ: Neonatal subgaleal haematoma: associated risk factors, complications and outcome. J Paediatr Child Health 32:228, 1996.
68. ACOG Practice Bulletin, No 17, June 2000; or ACOG Compendium of Selected Publications, 2005, p 640.
69. Benaron DA: Subgaleal hematoma causing hypovolemic shock during delivery after failed vacuum extraction: case report. J Perinatol 12:228, 1993.
70. Boo N: Subaponeurotic haemorrhage in Malaysian neonates. Singapore Med J 31:207, 1990.
71. Teng FY, Sayer JW: Vacuum extraction: does duration predict scalp injury? Obstet Gynecol 89:281, 1997.
72. Towner D, Castro MA, Eby-Wilkens E, Gilbert WM: Effect of mode of delivery in nulliparous women on neonatal intracranial injury. N Engl J Med 341:1709, 1999.
73. Whitby EH, Griffiths PD, Rutter S, et al: Frequency and natural history of subdural haemorrhages in babies and relation to obstetric factors. Lancet 363:846, 2004.
74. Seidman DS, Laor A, Gale R, et al: Long-term effects of vacuum and forceps deliveries. Lancet 337:15835, 1991.
75. Wesley BD, van den Berg BJ, Reece EA: The effect of forceps delivery on cognitive development. Am J Obstet Gynecol 169:1091, 1993.
76. Murphy DJ, Libby G, Chien P, et al: Cohort study of forceps delivery and the risk of epilepsy in adulthood. Am J Obstet Gynecol 191:392, 2004.
77. Dierker LJ Jr, Rosen MG, Thompson K, Lynn P: Midforceps deliveries: long-term outcome of infants. Am J Obstet Gynecol 154:764, 1986.
78. Bahl R, Patel RR, Swingler R, et al: Neurodevelopmental outcome at 5 years after operative vaginal delivery in the second stage of labor: a cohort study. Am J Obstet Gynecol 197:147.e1, 2007.
79. Bashore RA, Phillips WH Jr, Brickman CR 3rd: A comparison of the morbidity of midforceps and cesarean delivery. Am J Obstet Gynecol 162:1428, 1990.
80. Traub AI, Morrow RJ, Ritchie JW, et al: A continuing use for Kielland's forceps? Br J Obstet Gynaecol 91:894, 1984.
81. Murphy DJ, Liebling RE, Verity L, et al: Early maternal and neonatal morbidity associated with operative delivery in the second stage of labour: a cohort study. Lancet 358:1203, 2001.
82. Hinton L, Ong S, Danielian PJ: Kiellands forceps delivery—quantification of neonatal and maternal morbidity. Int J Gynecol Obstet 74:289, 2001.
83. Tan KH, Sim R, Yam KL: Kielland's forceps delivery: is it a dying art? Singapore Med J 33:380, 1992.
84. Hankins GDV, Rowe TF: Operative vaginal delivery—year 2000. Am J Obstet Gynecol 175:275, 1996.
85. Healy DL, Quinn MA, Pepperell RJ: Rotational delivery of the fetus: Kielland's forceps and two other methods compared Br J Obstet Gynaecol 89:501, 1982.
86. Krivac TC, Drewes P, Horowitz GM, et al: Kielland vs. nonrotational forceps for the second stage of labor. J Reprod Med 44:511, 1999.
87. Hankins GDV, Leicht T, Van Hook J, Uckan EM: The role of forceps rotation in maternal and neonatal injury. Am J Obstet Gynecol 180:231, 1999.
88. Feldman DM, Borgida AF, Sauer F, Rodis JF: Rotational versus nonrotational forceps: maternal and neonatal outcomes. Am J Obstet Gynecol 181:1185, 1999.
89. Richardson DA, Evans MI, Cibils LA: Midforceps delivery: a critical review. Am J Obstet Gynecol 145:621, 1983.
90. Revah A, Ezra Y, Farine D, Ritchie K: Failed trail of vacuum or forceps-maternal and fetal outcome. Am J Obstet Gynecol 176:200, 1997.
91. Freeth HD: The cause and management of failed forceps cases. BMJ 2:18, 1950.
92. Douglass LH, Kaltreider DF: Trial forceps. Am J Obstet Gynecol 65:889, 1953.
93. Alexander JM, Leveno KJ, Hauth JC, et al: Failed operative vaginal delivery. Obstet Gynecol 114:1017, 2009.
94. Johanson R, Menon V: Vacuum extraction vs. forceps delivery. Cochrane Pregnancy and Childbirth Group. Cochran Database Syst Rev 2, 2005.
95. Yeomans ER: Operative vaginal delivery. Obstet Gynecol 115:645, 2010.
96. Bahl R, Murphy DJ, Strachan B: Qualitative analysis by interviews and video recordings to establish the components of a skilled low-cavity non-rotational vacuum delivery. BJOG 116:319, 2009.
97. Ramin SM, Little BB, Gilstrap LC 3rd: Survey of forceps delivery in North America in 1990. Obstet Gynecol 81:307, 1993.
98. Jain V, Guleria K, Gopalan S, Narang A: Mode of delivery in deep transverse arrest. Int J Gynecol Obstet 43:129, 1993.
99. Kim M, Simpson W, Moore T: Teaching forceps: the impact of proactive faculty. Am J Obstet Gynecol 184:S185, 2001.
100. Carollo TC, Reuter JM, Galan HL, Jones RO: Defining fetal station. Am J Obstet Gynecol 191:1793, 2004.

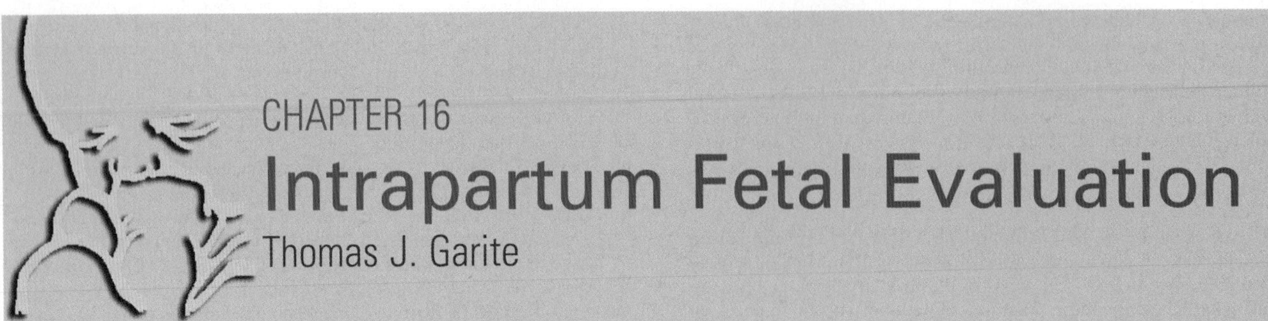

CHAPTER 16

Intrapartum Fetal Evaluation

Thomas J. Garite

KEY TERMS

Acidemia	Increased hydrogen ion concentration in blood
Acidosis	Increased hydrogen ion concentration in tissue
Asphyxia	Hypoxia with metabolic acidosis
Base deficit	Buffer base content below normal (this is calculated from a normogram using pH and P_{CO_2})
Base excess	Buffer base content above normal
Hypoxemia	Decreased oxygen concentration in blood
Hypoxia	Decreased oxygen concentration in tissue
pH	The negative log of hydrogen ion concentration ($7.0 = 1 \times 10^{-7}$)

KEY ABBREVIATIONS

American Congress of Obstetricians and Gynecologists	ACOG
Association of Women's Health, Obstetric and Neonatal Nurses	AWHONN
Cardiotocography	CTG
Central Nervous System	CNS
Electrocardiogram	ECG
Electronic Fetal Heart Rate Monitoring	EFM
Federal Drug Administration	FDA
Fetal Heart Rate	FHR
Human Immunodeficiency Virus	HIV
Magnesium Sulfate	$MgSO_4$
Non-reassuring Fetal Status	NRFS
National Institute of Child Health and Human Development	NICHD
Premature Rupture of the Membranes	PROM

The question being asked by the clinician evaluating the fetus in labor is quite simple: What is the status of fetal oxygenation? If hypoxia is severe enough and lasts long enough, fetal tissue and organ damage will result, which may result in long-term injuries or death. Hypoxia severe enough to cause tissue damage virtually always occurs only in the face of a significant metabolic acidosis, and the term *asphyxia* is used in this situation (Figure 16-1). To clarify the terminology used in these situations, see the Key Terms.

Although there are other, less frequent causes of fetal injury and death in labor (e.g., infection, hemorrhage), hypoxia is by far the most common etiology and the one for which medical and surgical interventions have the potential for preventing injury and death. Before intensive intrapartum fetal heart rate (FHR) monitoring, relatively uniform intrapartum fetal death rates of 3 to 4 per 1000 were reported.[1] Thus, on an obstetrical service of 200 to 300 monthly deliveries, 1 intrapartum death would occur each month; but now such events are extremely rare in monitored fetuses. Fetal hypoxia that is severe and associated with metabolic acidosis, but not sufficient to result in death, may alternatively cause asphyxial injury to the fetus and newborn. The fetal central nervous system (CNS) is the organ system most vulnerable to long-term injury. **However, the fetus destined to have permanent neurologic damage will virtually always have multiorgan dysfunction**

in the newborn period. Usually, complications such as seizures, respiratory distress, pulmonary hypertension with persistent fetal circulation, renal failure, bowel dysfunction, and pulmonary hemorrhage are seen in the baby who will ultimately have permanent neurologic injury.[2] Babies who recover from these complications and survive may be normal or may develop cerebral palsy. Cerebral palsy is defined as a movement disorder, usually spastic in nature, that is present at birth, nonprogressive and often, but not always, associated with varying degrees of mental retardation.[3] Seizures are often seen in children with cerebral palsy. However, mental retardation or seizures, in the absence of spasticity, are rarely the result of peripartum asphyxia. It is still unclear whether other neurologic dysfunction in children, such as learning and behavioral disorders, can be the result of perinatal asphyxia. Cerebral palsy will develop in 0.5% of all births and is prevalent in about 0.1% of all school-aged children.[3,4] Prematurity remains the leading cause of cerebral palsy. It is estimated that peripartum events contribute to no more than 25% of the overall rate of this disease.[5]

Thus, the goal of intrapartum monitoring is to detect hypoxia in labor and allow the clinician to implement non-operative interventions such as positioning and oxygen (O_2) administration to correct or ameliorate the oxygen deficiency. If this is unsuccessful, the monitor should help the clinician to determine the severity and duration of the hypoxia and whether there is a metabolic acidosis. And finally, if there is sufficient hypoxia and metabolic acidosis is present or developing, the monitor should give adequate warning and time to permit the clinician to deliver the baby expeditiously, whether by operative vaginal or cesarean delivery, to prevent damage or death from occurring. Unfortunately, the fetus is quite inaccessible, and until recently we have had crude and limited tools available to determine all the above information necessary to make correct and timely decisions to accomplish these goals.

HISTORY OF FETAL MONITORING

Because of the inaccessible location of the fetus, evaluating fetal well-being, or more specifically, fetal oxygen status, has been an ongoing and difficult challenge. In the 1600s, Kilian first proposed that the FHR might be used to diagnose fetal distress and to indicate when the clinician should intervene on behalf of the fetus. The sound of the fetal heart had first been detected by Marsac of France in the 1600s and described in a poem by his colleague, Philipe LeGaust. This observation went unnoticed until 1818, when Mayor, and subsequently Kergaradec, described the fetal heart sounds by placing an ear on the maternal abdomen. Kergaradec suggested that auscultation of the fetal heart could be used to determine fetal viability and fetal lie. In 1893, Von Winckel described the criteria for fetal distress that were to remain essentially unchanged until the arrival of electronic FHR monitoring. These included tachycardia (FHR >160 beats/minute), bradycardia (FHR <100 beats/minute), irregular heart rate, passage of meconium, and gross alteration of fetal movement.[1]

These criteria went unquestioned until 1968, when Benson and colleagues published the results of the Collaborative Project.[6] These authors reviewed the benefits of auscultation in more than 24,000 deliveries and concluded, "there was no reliable indicator of fetal distress in terms of FHR save in extreme degree." Thus, it became apparent that other, more sophisticated means of intrapartum fetal evaluation were required. In 1906, Cremer described the use of the fetal electrocardiogram (ECG) using abdominal and intravaginal electrical leads.[7] Several investigators made attempts using ECG waveforms to detect fetal hypoxia, but ultimately concluded that there was no consistent fetal electrocardiographic changes with fetal distress.[8] The subsequent history of electronic FHR monitoring (EFM) is a story of technologic development and empirical observations of alterations in FHR associated with various causes of fetal hypoxia and acidosis.

In 1958, Edward Hon (the "father of EFM" in the United States) reported on the instantaneous recording of the fetal ECG from the maternal abdomen.[9] He and his colleagues manually measured R-R intervals from a continuous ECG tracing and mathematically converted these to rate, in beats per minute, and then hand-recorded each interval on graph paper. From these efforts Hon, Caldeyro-Barcia in Uruguay, and Hammacher in Germany began to describe various FHR patterns associated with fetal distress.[10-12] Despite attempts by these and subsequent

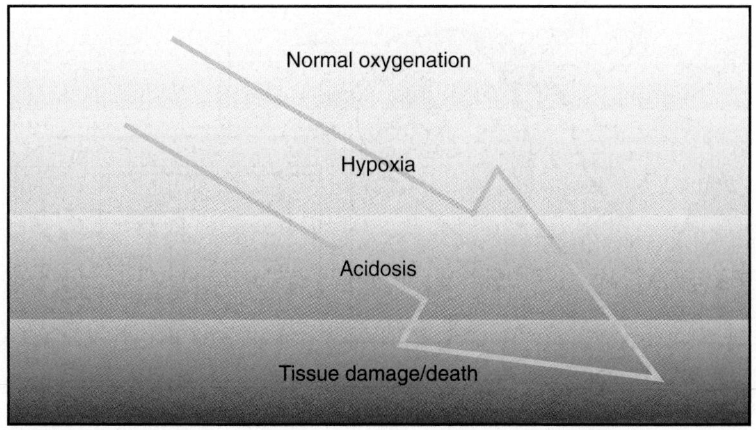

FIGURE 16-1. The purpose of fetal heart rate monitoring is to detect fetal hypoxia and metabolic acidosis. Many intrapartum fetuses develop hypoxia intermittently but never progress to metabolic acidosis. The idea is to avoid intervention for hypoxia, but to intervene in the presence of early metabolic acidosis before it can result in tissue damage or fetal death.

leaders in the field, universal standards for monitoring and terminology were never really established. For example, Europeans tend to refer to electronic fetal heart rate monitoring (EFM in the United States) as "cardiotocography" (CTG) and run their tracings at a paper speed of 1 cm/minute, compared with 3 cm/minute in the United States. **However, in recent years efforts by organizations such as the National Institute of Child Health and Human Development (NICHD) and American College of Obstetricians and Gynecologists (ACOG), *and similar societies in other countries,* have finally set standards for terminology that appear to be gaining widespread acceptance.** The first commercially available electronic fetal monitor was produced in the late 1960s, and by the mid-1970s, EFM was in use in most labor and delivery units in the United States. Today, most women giving birth in the United States have electronic FHR monitoring during labor.

INSTRUMENTATION FOR ELECTRONIC FETAL HEART RATE MONITORING

Many technologic advances have been made since the first monitors were produced. External FHR monitoring using electrocardiography did not work in labor, and phonocardiography was subject to fetal and maternal movement and other external noise. Doppler became the dominant modality for external monitoring. Initially, this modality was difficult to use because the complex Doppler signal made it difficult to determine which point within that signal the computer should use to measure the interval from beat to beat to convert to rate (Figure 16-2). Logic, or computer processing formulas, were used to get apparently good continuous signals, but this process introduced artifact, and the apparent variability and other aspects of the FHR were often inaccurate. Ultimately, better Doppler devices, coupled with autocorrelation formulas for processing the signal, have resulted in excellent external FHR signals that can be relied on clinically. **External monitoring is necessary at all times when the membranes are intact and cannot or should not be ruptured** (Figure 16-3). In addition, certain clinical situations make it unwise to puncture the skin with a fetal electrode for fear of vertical transmission of infection to the fetus. Such conditions include maternal infection with human immunodeficiency virus (HIV), hepatitis C, and herpes simplex.

It is often necessary to apply an internal electrode to obtain a high-quality, accurate, continuous FHR tracing. This is especially true in patients who are obese, in those with a premature fetus, or when the mother or fetus is moving too much to obtain an adequate signal. The original internal electrode was made from a modified skin clip that required a special instrument to place on the fetal scalp. In the mid-1970s, an easier to insert and less traumatic spiral electrode was introduced (Figure 16-4). This is applied to the fetal scalp manually without additional instruments and without the requirement for a speculum to visualize the scalp. The electrical circuit for this electrode includes the spiral electrode for one pole and a small

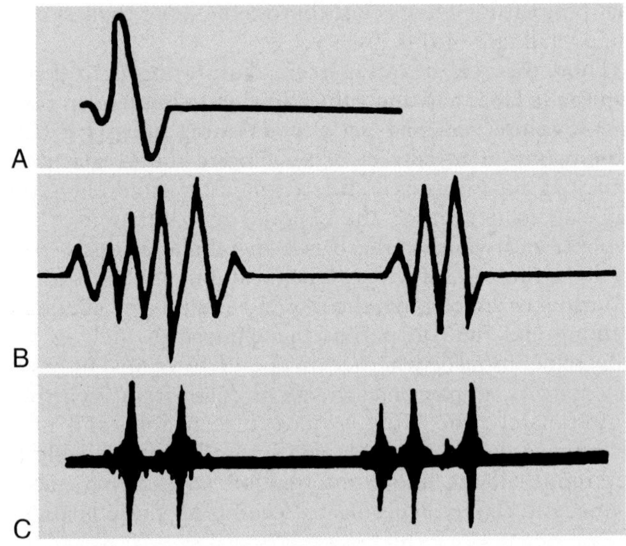

FIGURE 16-2. These complexes represent the types of signals that the fetal heart rate may be required to count. **A,** Electrocardiogram. **B,** Doppler. **C,** Phonocardiogram. Note the complexity of the Doppler signal. To consistently count the same place in the signal complex and avoid artifactually increasing variability, complex signal processing formulas are required.

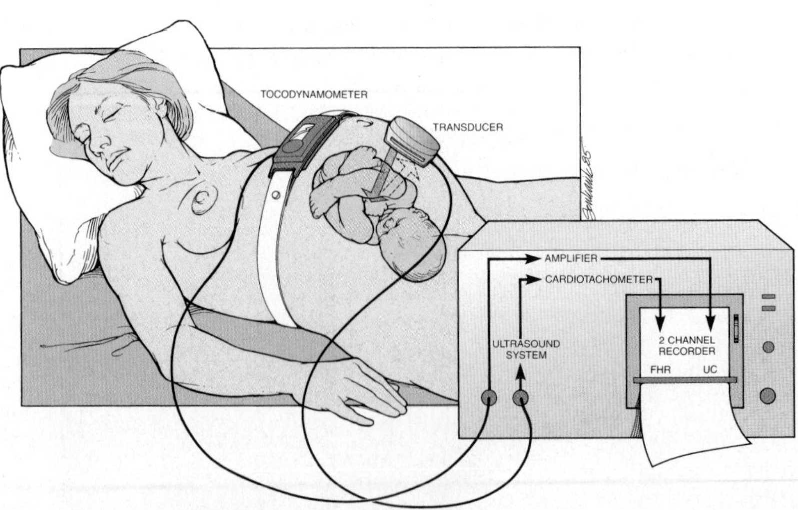

FIGURE 16-3. Instrumentation for external monitoring. Contractions are detected by the pressure-sensitive tocodynamometer, amplified, and then recorded. Fetal heart rate is monitored using the Doppler ultrasound transducer, which both emits and receives the reflected ultrasound signal that is then counted and recorded.

metal bar at the base of the plastic, which, bathed in vaginal secretions, completes the circuit through the mother's body. The spiral electrode has remained in use without substantial change since its introduction. **The FHR tracing results from the signal processor, which counts every R-R interval of the ECG from the scalp electrode, converts this interval to rate, and displays every interval (in rate as beats/minute) on the top channel of the two-channel fetal monitor recording paper.** The signal is amplified by an automatic gain amplifier, which increases the amplitude (gain) until an adequate signal is available to count (Figure 16-5). It must be remembered that when the fetus is dead, the amplifier may increase the gain of the small maternal ECG transmitted through the dead fetus, and this may be easily misinterpreted as a fetal bradycardia (Figure 16-6).

It is clear that the term *electronic fetal monitoring*, unlike the European version *cardiotocography*, undervalues the lower channel of the fetal monitor tracing, which provides information about the uterine contractions in labor. Contractions can also be monitored externally or internally. The external monitoring device, or tocodynamometer, is basically a ring-style pressure transducer attached to the maternal abdomen by a belt that maintains tight continuous contact. When the uterus contracts, the change in shape and rigidity depresses the plunger of the sensor, which changes the voltage of the electrical current. The change in voltage is proportional to the strength of the uterine contractions. **The tocodynamometer depicts the frequency of the contractions accurately, but the strength of the contractions only relatively, because it cannot measure actual intrauterine pressure.** In addition, the apparent duration of the contraction varies with the sensitivity of the monitor, which is negatively affected by variables such as maternal obesity and premature gestational age (Figure 16-7). The advantage of the external monitor is that it can be used when membranes are intact, and it is noninvasive. Its disadvantages, in addition to its inherently limited accuracy, is that it is more uncomfortable for the mother and limits her mobility. Contractions can be more accurately monitored using an intrauterine pressure catheter. The catheters require that the membranes be ruptured and are inserted transcervically beyond and above the fetal presenting part to rest within the uterine cavity. The original pressure catheters were open water-filled systems attached to a pressure transducer adjacent to the fetal monitor. These systems, while accurate, required frequent adjustments and flushing. Newer catheters have closed systems with the strain gauges in the tips or with sensors that relay the signal to a strain gauge at the base of the catheter. Although more expensive, they are easier to use

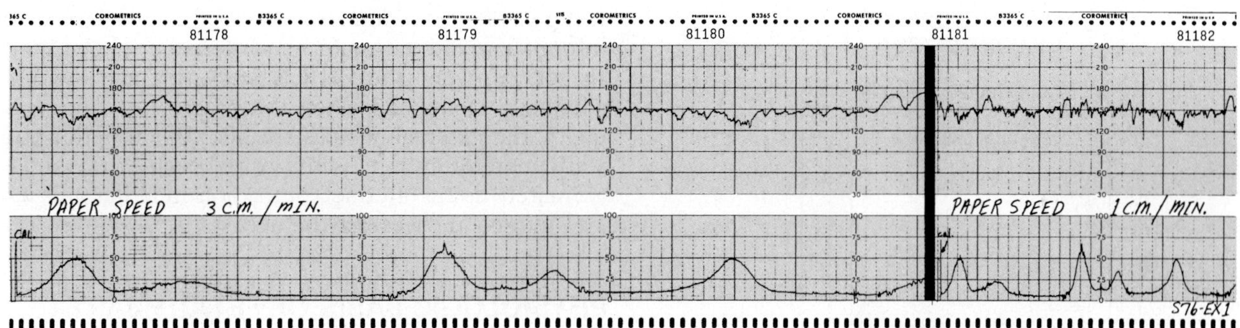

FIGURE 16-4. Internal fetal heart rate data gathered at the standard recording speed of 3 cm/minute for the first portion. The same data are being recorded at a speed of 1 cm/minute in the last segment. Normal long-term and short-term variabilities are present. Note that the uterine activity channel has been calibrated so that the intrauterine pressure readings can be measured correctly.

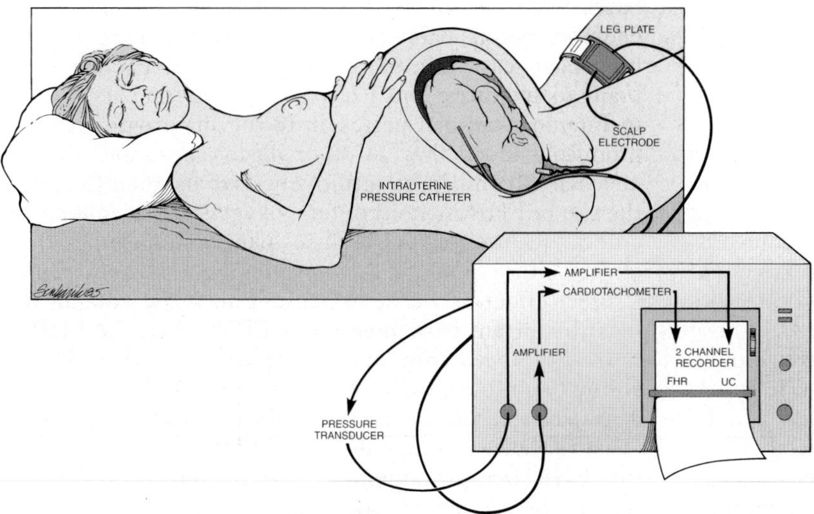

FIGURE 16-5. Techniques used for direct monitoring of fetal heart rate and uterine contractions. Uterine contractions are assessed with an intrauterine pressure catheter connected to a pressure transducer. This signal is then amplified and recorded. The fetal electrocardiogram is obtained by direct application of the scalp electrode, which is then attached to a leg plate on the mother's thigh. The signal is transmitted to the monitor, where it is amplified, counted by the cardiotachometer, and then recorded.

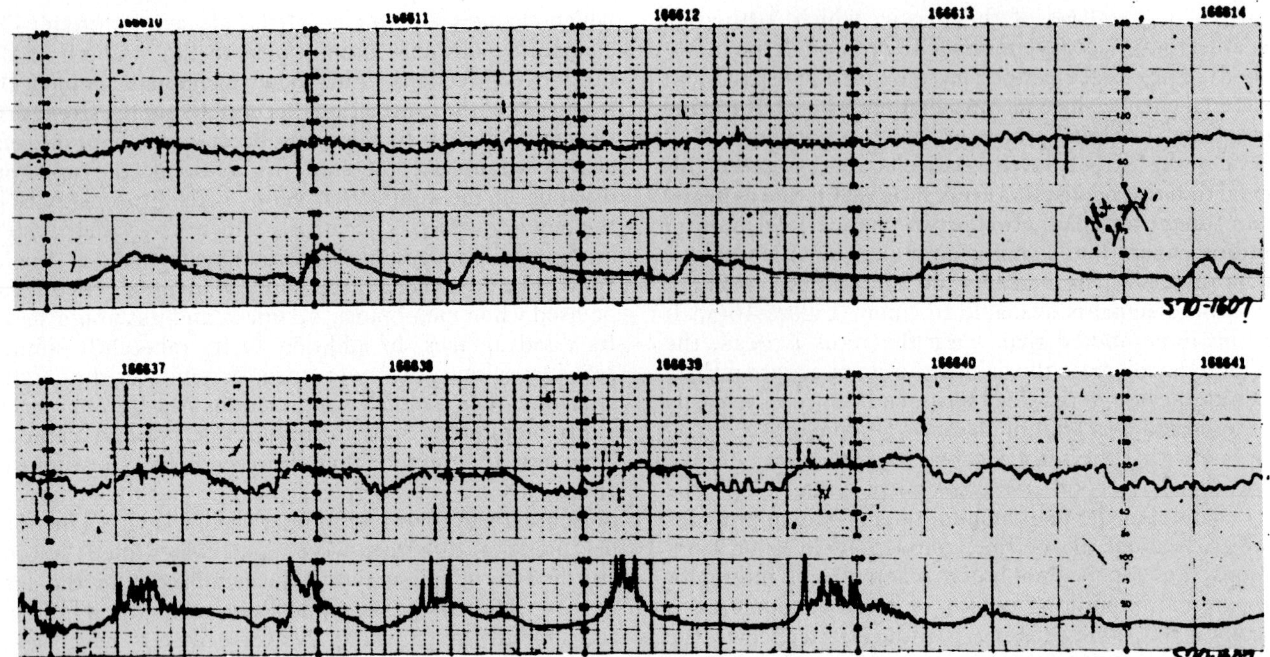

FIGURE 16-6. This is a tracing from an internal electrode demonstrating an apparent bradycardia with a rate of about 90 beats/minute. In actuality, this tracing is from a dead fetus, and the automatic gain amplifier increases the amplitude of the maternal electrocardiogram signal, allowing the monitor to count and display maternal heart rate. Note the accelerations of the maternal heart rate with contractions, typical of a heart rate response to the pain from contractions.

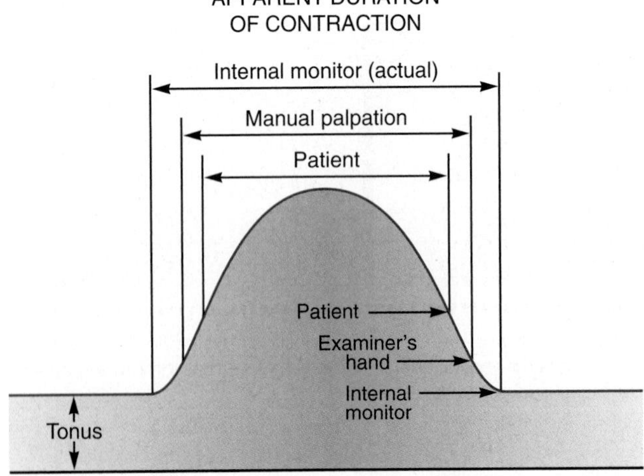

FIGURE 16-7. The sensitivity of the device used to monitor a uterine contraction can affect not only the apparent strength of the contraction but also the apparent duration of the contraction.

and require less nursing attention. Once the catheter is electronically "zeroed" (calibrated), the contractions are accurately recorded in terms of frequency, duration, and intensity on the lower channel of the two-channel recording paper or television monitor. This channel is conveniently calibrated at 0 to 100 mm Hg on its vertical scale, from which contraction amplitude can be read. These catheters also are often made with a second port through which saline can be infused for amnioinfusion (see later).

The goal of monitoring is to maintain adequate, high-quality, continuous FHR and contraction tracings while maintaining maximal maternal comfort and avoiding the risk for trauma and infection in the fetus and mother. External devices minimize risk but often give less accurate information and are more uncomfortable for the mother. In general, when the FHR is reassuring and there is an adequate tracing and when the progress of labor is adequate, the external devices are fine. When better-quality FHR monitoring is required or it becomes important to accurately assess uterine contraction duration and intensity, internal devices may be necessary.

PHYSIOLOGIC BASIS OF FETAL HEART RATE MONITORING

The basis of FHR monitoring is, in a real sense, fetal brain monitoring. The fetal brain is constantly responding to stimuli, both peripheral and central, with signals to the fetal heart that alter the heart rate on a moment-to-moment basis. Such stimuli to which the brain responds include chemoreceptors, baroreceptors, and direct effects of metabolic changes within the brain itself. The benefit for the brain to modulate the FHR is derived from its goal of maintaining optimal perfusion to the brain without compromising blood flow to other organs any more than is necessary. It should be intuitively obvious, therefore, that the use of FHR to monitor fetal oxygenation is inherently crude and nonspecific because many stimuli other than oxygen either cause the brain to alter the FHR or may have a direct effect on the fetal heart. **This really explains the most important basic premise of EFM: when the FHR is normal in appearance, one can be assured with high reliability that the fetus is well oxygenated, but when the FHR is not entirely normal, it may be the result of hypoxia or of other variables that may also affect FHR.** In the past when the FHR became abnormal and the clinician decided intervention was necessary because of concern over fetal hypoxia, the term *fetal distress* was used. More often than not, however, such intervention results in the delivery of a well-oxygenated, nonacidotic, vigorous newborn. This understanding led to an attempt at more accurately reflecting the limitations of interpreting an abnormal FHR. **The term fetal distress was abandoned in favor of the more intellectually honest term, *non-reassuring fetal status* (NRFS).**[13] Even more recently, a further refinement has been recommended as a result of a second workshop sponsored by the NICHD and subsequently adopted by both ACOG and the Association of Women's Health, Obstetric and Neonatal Nurses (AWHONN), **which placed FHR patterns into three categories based on the likelihood of adequate or inadequate oxygenation and acidosis.**[14]

Fetal oxygenation is determined by many factors. **The placenta functions as the fetal lung.** Oxygen transfer across the placenta, as in the lung or any membrane, is proportional to the difference between partial pressures of oxygen between the mother and the fetus, the blood flow to the placenta, a coefficient of diffusion for the gas, and the surface area of the placenta. Transfer is inversely proportional to the thickness of the membrane (placenta). Thus, under normal circumstances during labor, the only variable that alters fetal oxygenation is the temporary interruption in blood flow to the placenta that occurs as a result of the compression of the spiral arteries by the wall of the uterus at the peak of the contraction. The duration that the spiral arteries will be compressed will thus depend on the duration and strength of the contraction (Figure 16-8). Under normal circumstances, the fetus tolerates these periods of stasis well without a significant change in its oxygen content. Contractions that are unusually long or unusually strong may, however, result in transient periods of fetal hypoxemia.

Other variables that have the potential for altering fetal oxygenation most commonly include those that affect uterine perfusion. A laboring woman in the supine position can develop hypotension as a result of vena caval compression from the uterus. Maternal hypotension with redistribution of blood flow away from the placenta occurs not infrequently with regional anesthesia. Maternal hemorrhage, such as in placenta previa or abruptio placentae, may have similar effects. There are several forms of microvascular disease that can impair fetal oxygenation from poor perfusion within the uteroplacental vascular bed. Examples include hypertension, preeclampsia or eclampsia, collagen vascular disease, diabetic vasculopathy, and postmaturity. Abruptio placentae may compromise fetal oxygenation in several ways. These include maternal hypotension, as previously mentioned; a decrease in the surface area of the placenta; and uterine hyperactivity.

Although the placenta functions as the fetal lung, the umbilical cord functions as its trachea, leading oxygen to the baby and carbon dioxide (CO_2) away. Alteration in umbilical cord blood flow is a very common occurrence during labor, either from direct compression or from stretch. Direct compression may occur when the cord becomes impinged between any part of the fetal body and the uterine wall, either with contractions or with fetal movement. This is especially more common when there is oligohydramnios because there is less amniotic fluid to provide a cushion for the cord.[15] Alternatively, cord stretch may occur as the fetus descends into the pelvis. Typically, this is seen just before complete dilation, when descent of the vertex normally occurs. There are three potent stimuli that produce spasm of the umbilical vessels that have evolved to allow cessation of fetal umbilical cord blood flow following birth. These include a lower ambient temperature, a higher oxygen tension as the baby begins breathing, and the stretch of the umbilical cord as the baby falls from the birth canal.[16] Thus, it should not be surprising that transient cessation of cord blood flow will occur with stretching of the cord during descent if the cord is looped around the baby's neck and descent of the vertex occurs.

It becomes important, therefore, to understand the physiologic mechanisms that control the FHR. This is so not only because the FHR may be used to determine the severity of the hypoxia and whether a metabolic acidosis is ensuing but also because the FHR pattern can elucidate the mechanism of the reduction in fetal oxygenation. Thus, by knowing the cause of any hypoxia, the treatment, when possible, can be more specifically directed at the cause. Finally, an understanding of the mechanism and progression of the FHR pattern can often also provide an opportunity to predict how fetal oxygenation will progress over time.

The FHR has many characteristics that we are able to use to accomplish this interpretation. These include the *baseline rate;* the *variability* of the FHR from beat to beat; transient alterations below the baseline, termed *decelerations;* and transient alterations above the baseline, termed *accelerations.* Rate and variability are generally included as *characteristics of the baseline* FHR, and decelerations and accelerations as *periodic changes.* In 1997, the NICHD convened a workshop to standardize terminology in FHR monitoring subsequently accepted and endorsed by most obstetrical organizations, and the subsequent descriptions and definitions in this chapter are consistent with those recommendations, except where explanations are provided to explain potential limitations of this newer system.[14]

Tachycardia

The baseline FHR is typically between 120 and 160 beats/minute. In very early gestation (15 to 20 weeks), the FHR is significantly higher than in the term fetus. The decline in FHR represents a maturation of fetal vagal tone with progressing gestation.[18] If atropine or other vagolytic drugs are administered, the FHR will regress to the higher baseline of 160 beats/minute. Thus, the baseline heart rate is largely a function of vagal activity. Many factors have the potential to alter the fetal baseline. For interpretation of the baseline rate, the minimal duration must be at least 2 minutes of adequate signal in a 10-minute window, or the baseline for that period is indeterminate. Rates above 160 beats/minute are called *tachycardia.* Tachycardia may have great clinical significance. **The two most common causes of tachycardia are maternal fever and drugs that directly raise the FHR.** Maternal fever raises the core temperature of the fetus, which is always about 1° F higher than the maternal temperature. With maternal fever, virtually all fetuses have tachycardia (Figure 16-9). The FHR rises approximately 10 beats/minute for each 1° F increase in

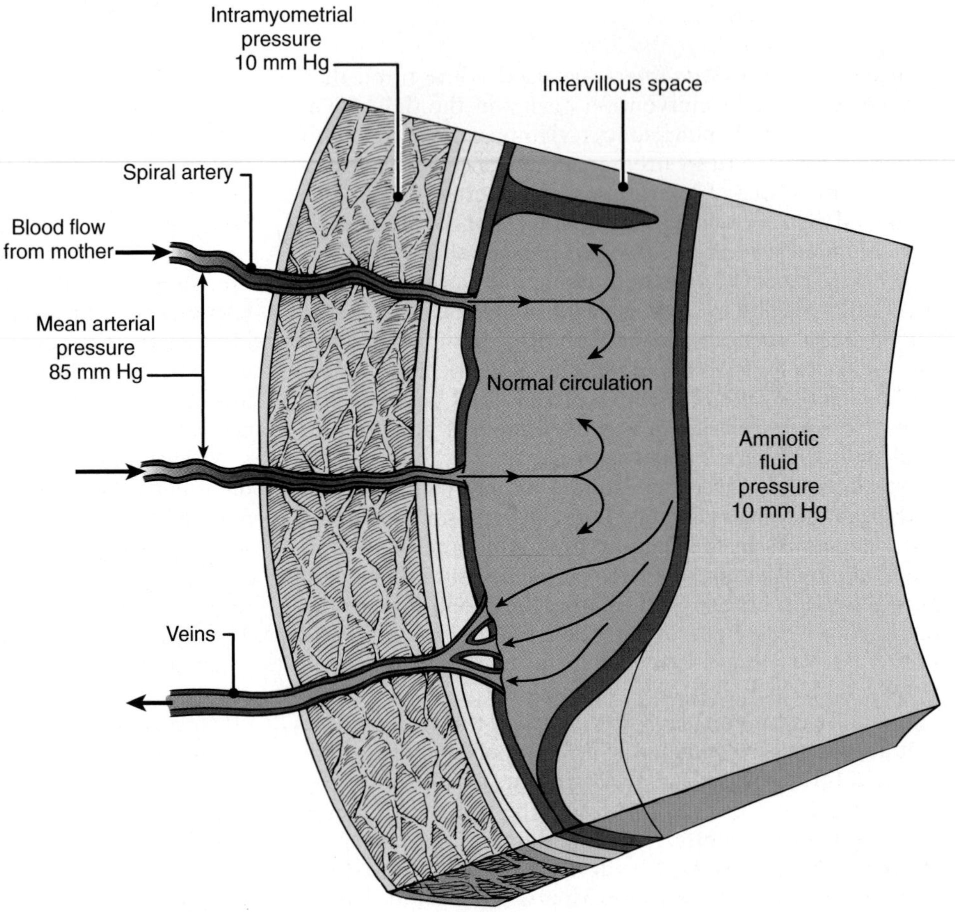

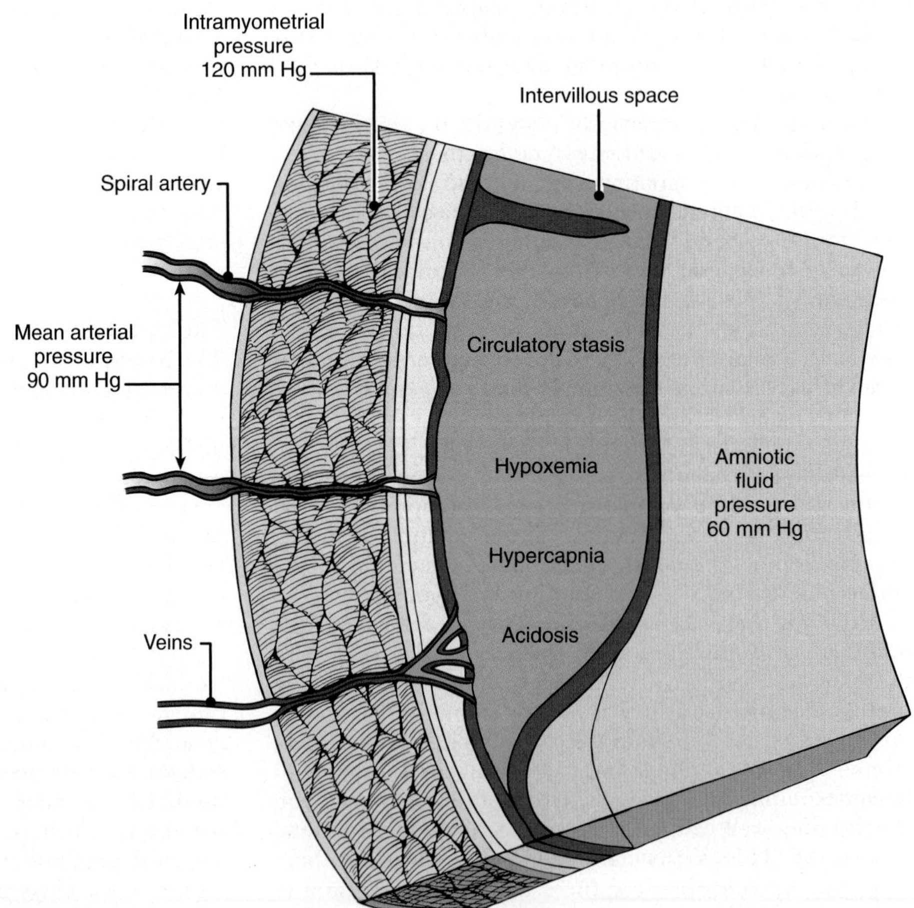

FIGURE 16-8. In the resting state between contractions **(A),** the intraluminal pressure within the spiral arteries exceeds the intramyometrial pressure. Thus, uteroplacental blood flow is sustained. However, at the peak of a uterine contraction **(B),** the myometrial pressure can exceed the arterial pressure, and uterine blood flow will be transiently interrupted, temporarily halting oxygen delivery to the placenta.

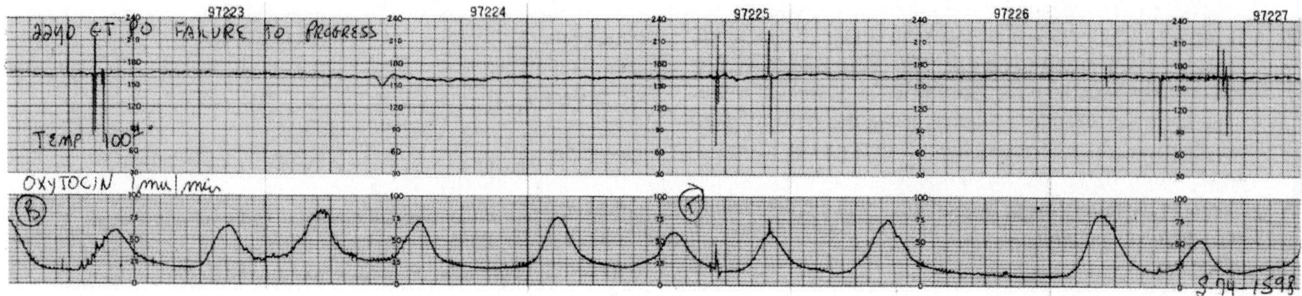

FIGURE 16-9. A tachycardia with a fetal heart rate of 170 beats/minute seen in association with a maternal fever of 38° C (100.4° F).

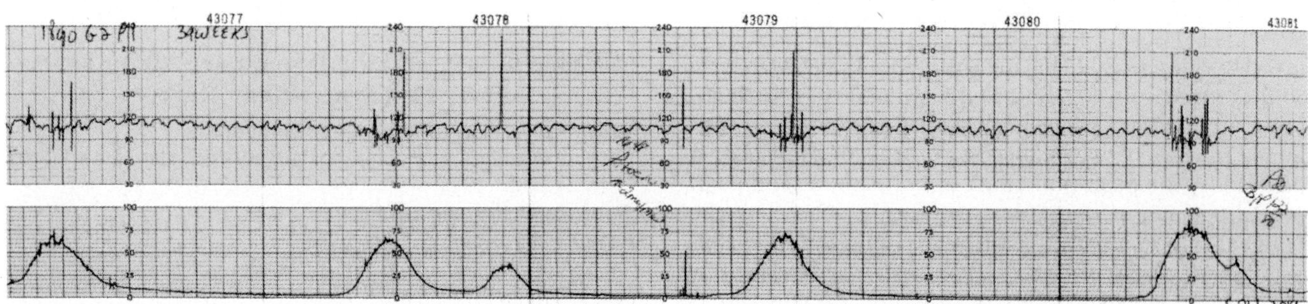

FIGURE 16-10. A bradycardia with a fetal heart rate of 110 beats/minute. This patient is in premature labor at 34 weeks' gestation and is being treated with magnesium sulfate. The fetal bradycardia is probably because of maternal hypothermia, which can be seen with vasodilation caused by the magnesium sulfate.

maternal temperature. Because at term with chorioamnionitis only 1% to 2% of fetuses are septic, the tachycardia is unlikely to indicate fetal sepsis, but rather is probably caused by an increase in fetal metabolic rate associated with the elevated temperature. Drugs that elevate the FHR fall into one of two categories: vagolytic and β-sympathomimetic. Commonly used drugs that are vagolytic include scopolamine, atropine and phenothiazines, and hydroxyzine. These drugs, however, rarely raise the FHR above 160 beats/minute. β-Sympathomimetics include terbutaline and ritodrine, used for preterm labor, and terbutaline and epinephrine, used for bronchospasm. Other, less common causes of fetal tachycardia include fetal hyperthyroidism, fetal anemia, fetal heart failure, and fetal tachyarrhythmias. As fetal hypoxia becomes progressively worse and persists over time, fetal tachycardia often develops. However, when contractions are present, tachycardia is not the first physiologic response to hypoxia and, in the absence of decelerations, in the laboring patient, is rarely if ever caused by hypoxia.[19]

Bradycardia

An FHR less than 110 beats/minute is termed a *bradycardia*. One must distinguish between a baseline FHR less than 110 beats/minute that is an established baseline and one that follows a prolonged deceleration. This is an important issue because an established baseline bradycardia is often innocuous (Figure 16-10), whereas a prolonged deceleration to less than 110 beats/minute lasting more than 60 to 90 seconds may often indicate significant fetal hypoxia (Figure 16-11). When a prolonged deceleration lasts more than 10 minutes it becomes a bradycardia according to the newer NICHD terminology.[17] True established fetal bradycardias occur infrequently and can be due to several possible causes. In the range of 90 to 110 beats/minute, a bradycardia may often be a normal variant, and these fetuses are usually bradycardic after birth, but are otherwise well oxygenated and normal. **As with tachycardia and fever, maternal hypothermia may cause fetal bradycardia.** This is commonly seen with patients on magnesium sulfate ($MgSO_4$) who are vasodilated and has also been described with maternal hypoglycemia and hypothermia.[20,21] Drugs, such as propranolol, may also result in fetal bradycardia. A fetal baseline heart rate in the range of 80 beats/minute or less, especially with minimal or absent variability, may be caused by a complete heart block. Complete heart block may be caused by antibodies associated with maternal lupus erythematosus, may be seen with congenital cardiac anomalies, or is idiopathic.[22] Whereas a heart block is not associated with hypoxia, it makes the FHR uninformative in monitoring fetal oxygenation because the fetal brain is no longer communicating with the ventricle of the heart that is being monitored. When a patient is admitted with a baseline bradycardia, one should also consider the possibility of maternal heart rate being recorded with a dead fetus (whether internal or external monitor) (see Figure 16-6). Real-time ultrasound is used to verify that the bradycardia is fetal in origin.

Variability

The fetal cardiotachometer is unique compared to adult monitors in that it records the interval-to-interval difference in rate for every heart beat. Thus, differences in heart rate from beat to beat are recorded as "variability" reflected visually as a line that fluctuates above and below the baseline. **This variability is a reflection of neuromodulation of the FHR by an intact and active CNS and also reflects normal cardiac responsiveness.** Generally, the variability of

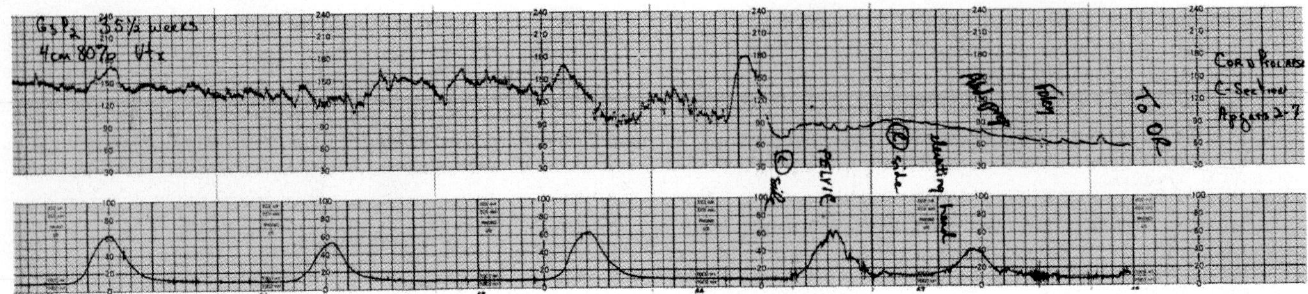

FIGURE 16-11. The prolonged deceleration to 60 beats/minute, in this case caused by umbilical cord prolapse, evolves following a prolonged deceleration from a normal baseline rate. When the prolonged deceleration lasts longer than 10 minutes, it then becomes a bradycardia according to the new NICHD terminology.[17]

the FHR is described as having two components: *short-term* and *long-term variability*. Short-term variability is the beat-to-beat irregularity in the FHR and is caused by the difference in rates between successive beats of the FHR. It is caused by the push-pull effect of sympathetic and parasympathetic nerve input, but the vagus nerve has the dominant role in affecting variability. Long-term variability is the waviness of the FHR tracing, and is generally seen in three to five cycles per minute. Previous texts spent considerable effort in distinguishing between the significance of short- and long-term variability, but in general they are reduced or increased together, and there is no clear evidence that distinguishing between the two is helpful clinically. **The NICHD Research Planning Workshop also concluded that no distinction should be made between short- and long-term variability.**[17]

POTENTIAL CAUSES OF DECREASED VARIABILITY OF THE FETAL HEART RATE

Depression due to hypoxia and acidosis
Fetal anomalies, especially of the central nervous system
Fetal sepsis
Tumors of the central nervous system
Fetal heart block
Tachycardia
Extreme prematurity
Previous neurologic insult
Fetal sleep cycles
Drugs, medications
- Narcotics
- Barbiturates
- Tranquilizers
- Phenothiazines
- Parasympatholytics
- General anesthetics

This characteristic of the fetal baseline can be one of the most useful single parameters in determining the severity of fetal hypoxia if understood correctly. The simplest way to describe the causes of alterations, especially reductions, in FHR variability is to say that this parameter reflects the activity of the fetal brain. When the fetus is alert and active, the FHR variability is normal or increased. When the fetus is obtunded, by whatever cause, the variability is reduced. Because severe hypoxia, especially when it reaches the level of metabolic acidosis, will always depress the CNS, normal variability reliably indicates the absence of severe hypoxia and acidosis (Figure 16-12*A*). Unfortunately, the converse is not true because there are many things that cause the CNS to be depressed (see box, Potential Causes of Decreased Variability of the Fetal Heart Rate); thus, reduced (minimal or absent) variability is a very nonspecific finding and must be interpreted in the context of other indicators of hypoxia, and other causes of reduced variability must be considered (Figure 16-12*B*). **In general, anything that is associated with depressed or reduced brain function will diminish variability.** This includes fetal sleep cycles; drugs, especially CNS depressants; fetal anomalies, especially of the CNS; and previous insults that have damaged the fetal brain. FHR variability is also affected by gestational age, and very immature fetuses of less than 26 weeks' gestation often have reduced variability from an immature CNS, although this varies from fetus to fetus. In addition, as heart rate increases with fetal tachycardia, variability is often reduced from the rate alone because sympathetic dominance overrides the natural influence of the vagus. Increased FHR variability, original referred to as a "saltatory" FHR pattern, in nonlaboring animals has been shown to be associated with very early or minimal hypoxia.[23] This is a rare pattern and difficult to interpret. In labor, late, variable, or prolonged decelerations will virtually always be present with early hypoxia, and increased variability is not consistent with an acidotic fetus; therefore, this finding can be interpreted in context with the entire FHR pattern.

Another problem with variability besides its nonspecificity is that the interpretation of variability is quite subjective. Variability is usually described quantitatively, The NICHD Research Planning Workshop[17] suggested that FHR variability be defined as follows:
Absent: amplitude undetectable
Minimal: amplitude > undetectable and ≤5 beats/minute
Moderate: amplitude 6 to 25 beats/minute
Marked: >25 beats/minute.

Experts given tracings to interpret often disagree on the quantification of variability even using just these four categories. Trying to categorize variability any further is fraught with even more potential for disagreement and does not appear to have predictive value.

PERIODIC CHANGES

Variability, tachycardia, and bradycardia are characteristic alterations of the baseline heart rate. Periodic changes of the FHR include decelerations and accelerations. These

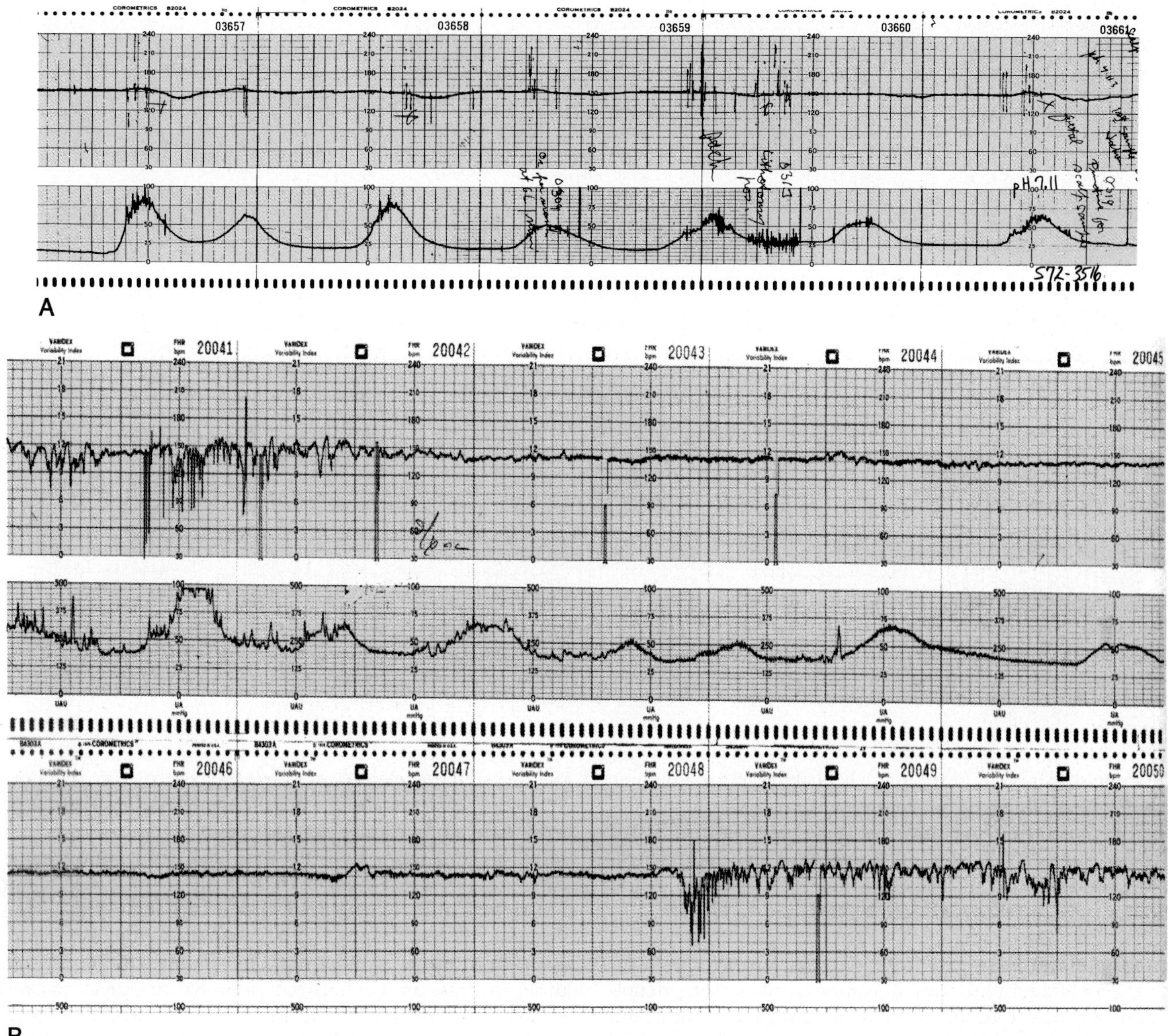

FIGURE 16-12. **A,** The markedly decreased variability seen in this case is in association with persistent late decelerations. A scalp pH of 7.11 confirms that the loss of variability is because of central nervous system depression caused by acidosis. **B,** The abrupt decrease in variability seen here, in contrast to **A,** is not seen in association with any decelerations that might suggest hypoxia. Thus, the decreased variability must be because of another reason, and in this case, given the equally abrupt return to normal variability in **B,** is probably caused by a fetal sleep cycle.

are transient changes in the FHR of relatively brief duration with return to the original baseline FHR. In labor, these usually occur in response to uterine contractions but may also occur with fetal movement.

Decelerations

There are four principal types of decelerations: *early, late, variable,* and *prolonged.* These are named for their timing, relationship to contractions, duration, and shape, but are important distinctions more because they describe the cause of the decelerations.

Early Decelerations

Early decelerations are shallow, symmetrical, uniform decelerations with onset and return that are gradual, resulting in a U-shaped deceleration (Figure 16-13). They begin early in the contraction, have their nadir coincident with the peak of the contraction, and return to the baseline by the time the contraction is over. Early decelerations are not associated with accelerations that precede or follow the deceleration. These decelerations typically do not descend more than 30 to 40 beats/minute below the baseline rate. **They are thought to be caused by compression of the fetal head by the uterine cervix as it overrides the anterior fontanel of the cranium.**[24] This results in altered cerebral blood flow, precipitating a vagal reflex with the resultant slowing of the FHR. More nonspecific head compression can result in decelerations that are indistinguishable from variable decelerations. Because of the similar cause, these latter decelerations have often been called *early decelerations*, but are by definition not so. Because the cervix creates the pressure, typically early decelerations are usually seen

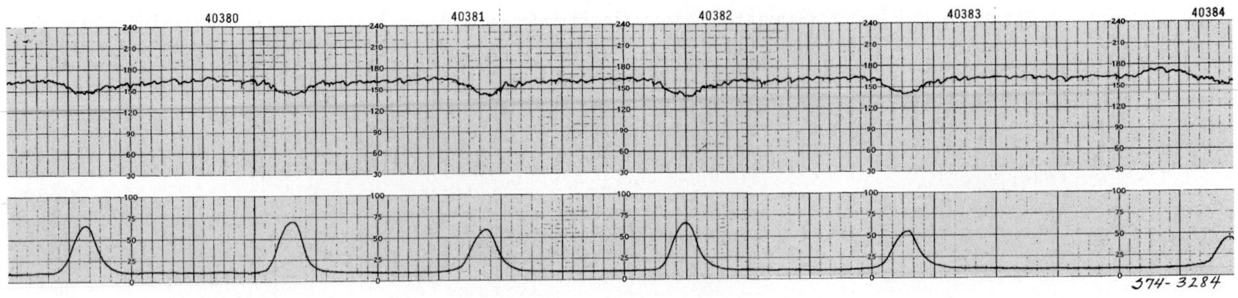

FIGURE 16-13. Early decelerations.

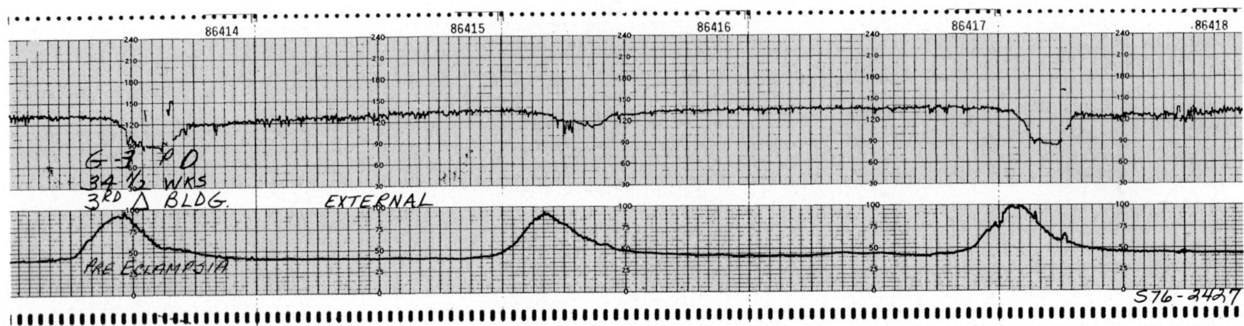

FIGURE 16-14. A case complicated by third-trimester bleeding in which the external heart rate and uterine activity data are collected. Note the presence of persistent late decelerations with only three contractions in 20 minutes as well as the apparent loss of variability of the fetal heart rate. The rise in baseline tone of the uterine activity channel cannot be evaluated with the external system.

between 4 and 6 cm of dilation (E.H. Hon, personal communication). They do not indicate fetal hypoxia and are only significant in that they may be easily confused with late decelerations because of their similar shape and depth. They are the most infrequent of decelerations, occurring in about 5% to 10% of all fetuses in labor.

Late Decelerations

Late decelerations are similar in appearance to early decelerations. They, too, are of gradual onset and return, are U-shaped, and generally descend below the baseline no more than 30 to 40 beats/minute, although there are exceptions. **However, in contrast to early decelerations, late decelerations are delayed in timing relative to the contraction.** They begin usually about 30 seconds after the onset of the contraction or even at or after its peak. Their nadir is after the peak of the contraction. In most cases, the onset, nadir, and recovery of the deceleration occur after the beginning, peak, and ending of the contraction, respectively. FHR variability may be unchanged or even increased during the decelerations. These decelerations are not associated with accelerations immediately preceding or following their onset and return (Figure 16-14).

The physiology of late decelerations is quite complex, but an understanding of the physiology pays dividends in terms of interpreting and managing these important FHR changes. **Late decelerations are generally said to be caused by "uteroplacental insufficiency."** This implies that uteroplacental perfusion is temporarily interrupted during the peak of strong contractions. The fetus that normally will not become hypoxic with this temporary halt in blood flow may do so if there is insufficient perfusion or oxygen exchange, as with, for example, hypotension or microvascular diseases within the uterus or placenta. Whereas this may be a correct idealized description, in reality any compromise of delivery, exchange, or uptake in fetal oxygen, other than by umbilical cord compression, can result in a late deceleration if the insult is sufficient. Physiologically, oxygen sensors within the fetal brain detect a relative drop in fetal oxygen tension in association with the uterine contraction. This change initially results in an increase in sympathetic neuronal response, causing an elevation in fetal blood pressure that, when detected by baroreceptors, produces a protective slowing in the FHR in response to the increase in peripheral vascular resistance. This has been referred to as the "reflex" type of late deceleration. This complex double reflex is probably the reason the deceleration is delayed.[25] During this type of reflex, the depth of the deceleration is proportional to the severity of the hypoxia, and the deceleration moves closer to the contraction as the hypoxia becomes more severe. However, there is also a second type of late deceleration, caused by "myocardial depression." As the hypoxia continues and becomes more severe, late decelerations are no longer vagally mediated and are seen even with interruption of the vagus nerve; thus, they are directly myocardial in origin. These decelerations are *not* proportional in their depth to the severity of the hypoxia and actually may become more shallow as the hypoxia becomes quite severe. Because of this latter type of deceleration, the depth of the late deceleration cannot always be used to judge the severity of the hypoxia. **Because of the mechanisms causing these changes, *late decelerations virtually always indicate fetal hypoxia.*** Only the severity of the hypoxia and the overall duration of the hypoxia will determine whether a metabolic acidosis will occur, and this is highly unpredictable.

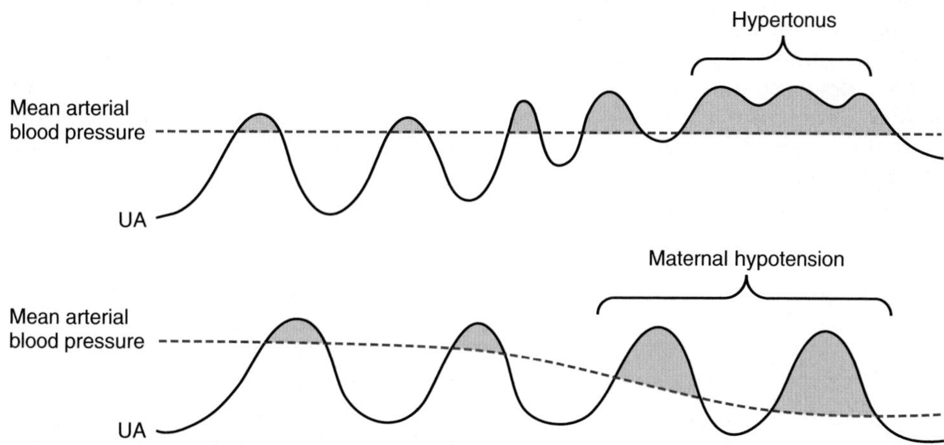

Figure 16-15. The two most common causes of late decelerations in labor are excessive uterine contractions (usually caused by oxytocin) and maternal hypotension. Both result in decrease in uteroplacental perfusion, hypertonus by interrupting the transmyometrial perfusion for a prolonged period, and hypotension by dropping the perfusion pressure, thus increasing the amount of time perfusion is interrupted even with a normal contraction. *UA,* Uterine artery.

One reason this may be so is found in recent data suggesting that the oxygen threshold that triggers the brain to slow the fetal heart in this characteristic way may be more related to the relative drop from baseline oxygenation rather than an absolute number.[26] Thus, the fetus accustomed to higher than average oxygen saturation may have a drop in oxygen at or only slightly below the normal range—a level deep enough to signal a late deceleration, but not low enough to require anaerobic metabolism. Another important point in understanding the results of hypoxia associated with late decelerations is that the placenta's capacity for exchanging oxygen is substantially less than its capacity for exchanging CO_2. In situations in which there are persistent late decelerations and the fetus becomes sufficiently hypoxic to develop a metabolic acidosis, there may be no retention of CO_2. This is quite analogous to the adult with lung but no airway disease in whom hypoxia is often seen without difficulty in eliminating CO_2. Thus, the metabolic acidosis is usually not mixed with a respiratory acidosis. The only common exception to this is with abruptio placentae, in which CO_2 retention is seen with late decelerations.[27]

Causes of late decelerations include any factor that can alter delivery, exchange, or uptake of oxygen at the fetal-maternal interface within the placenta. Most commonly, late decelerations are observed in patients without inherent pathology. Excessive uterine contractions, usually seen with oxytocin, are the single most common cause of late decelerations. In these situations, the duration of interruption of uterine blood flow is prolonged, the hypoxia is more than the normal fetus can endure, and late decelerations are expressed. Conduction anesthesia (spinal or epidural) can cause either systemic or local hypoperfusion or hypotension, and thus the level of contractions required to interrupt uterine blood flow is lower, and again the duration of interruption of uterine blood flow is prolonged (Figure 16-15). The most common pathologic conditions of the placenta associated with late decelerations are those characterized by either microvascular disease in the placenta or local vasospasm compromising blood flow and thus exchange. Common causes include postmaturity, maternal hypertension (chronic hypertension or preeclampsia), collagen vascular diseases, and diabetes mellitus in its more advanced stages. Besides altering perfusion, abruptio placentae is an example of altered placental exchange caused by a combination of reduced placental surface area and increased contractions that typically result in late decelerations when the separation is sufficient to cause fetal hypoxia. Severe maternal anemia or maternal hypoxemia may compromise oxygen delivery and result in late decelerations. Conversely, chronic fetal anemia may diminish fetal oxygen uptake and be associated with late decelerations.

Variable Decelerations

The most common type of decelerations seen in the laboring patient are variable decelerations. Variable decelerations are, in general, synonymous with umbilical cord compression, and anything that results in the interruption of blood flow within the umbilical cord will result in a variable deceleration. The variable deceleration is the most difficult pattern to describe, but the easiest to recognize visually. First and foremost, the term *variable* is by far the best single word to describe this type of deceleration. It is variable in all ways: size, shape, depth, duration, and timing relative to the contraction. The onset is usually abrupt and sharp. The return is similarly abrupt in most situations. The depth and duration are proportional to the severity and duration of interruption of cord blood flow. Variable decelerations are usually seen with accelerations immediately preceding the onset of the deceleration and immediately following the return to baseline. The definitions from the NICHD Research Planning Workshop also include that variable decelerations are those lasting a minimum of 15 seconds and descending 15 beats or more below the baseline and that the duration of a variable deceleration should be limited to 2 minutes, and that beyond 2 minutes, it should be called a prolonged deceleration.[17] More than 50 years ago, Barcroft first described the variable deceleration when he ligated the umbilical cord of a fetal goat[28] (Figure 16-16). In 1975, Lee and Hon externalized the human umbilical cord before cesarean delivery and demonstrated that the reflex involved in the complex pattern of the variable deceleration is one that is caused primarily by changes in systemic blood pressure in the fetus and is mediated through baroreceptors (Figure 16-17).[29] When the umbilical cord is gradually compressed, the thinner-walled umbilical vein collapses first, and blood flow returning to the fetus is interrupted. This results in decreased cardiac return, fetal hypotension, and a baroreceptor reflex that leads the brain to accelerate the heart rate in order to maintain cardiac output. This increase in heart rate is the acceleration that precedes the variable deceleration. With continuing compression, the umbilical artery is compressed, and the fetus detects an increase in systemic vascular resistance because the previously low-resistance placental bed, to which 50% of fetal cardiac output normally flows, is occluded. The baroreceptors detect the increase in resistance, and the heart slows as a protective mechanism. As the cord vessels gradually open, the arteries open first, and the heart rate returns to baseline; but if the flow in the vein is still blocked, an acceleration of the same mechanism of the one that preceded the deceleration occurs. Although this model is idealized, one might surmise that the orderly occlusion of vein, vein and artery, vein does not always occur. This is probably the reason that, with variable decelerations, any combination of deceleration with acceleration preceding, preceding and following, following only, neither, or even acceleration alone may be seen with cord compression, as in Figure 16-18.

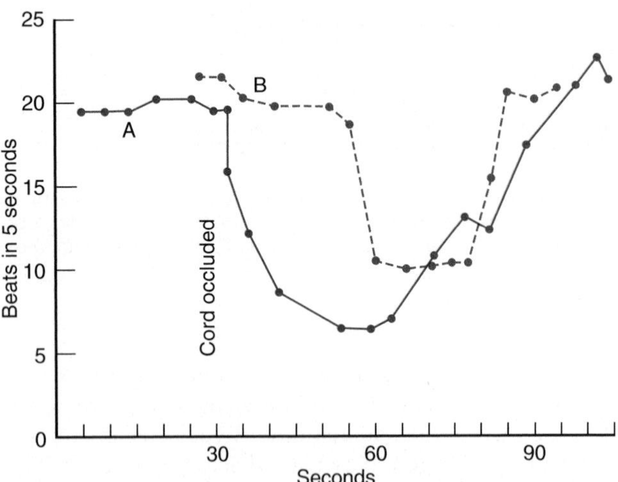

FIGURE 16-16. This is the original description of a variable deceleration in a fetal goat by Barcroft. The *solid line A* represents the fetal heart rate with temporary umbilical cord occlusion and the *dotted line B* is the fetal heart rate with temporary cord occlusion after the vagal nerve has been severed.

In reality, although we refer to umbilical cord compression as the single mechanism for interruption of cord blood flow, there are probably several different mechanisms that may have the same end result. Compression may be the mechanism that occurs when the cord is impinged between a fetal body part and the uterine wall during contractions or with fetal movement. As previously mentioned, cord stretch may be the reason the flow is compromised with

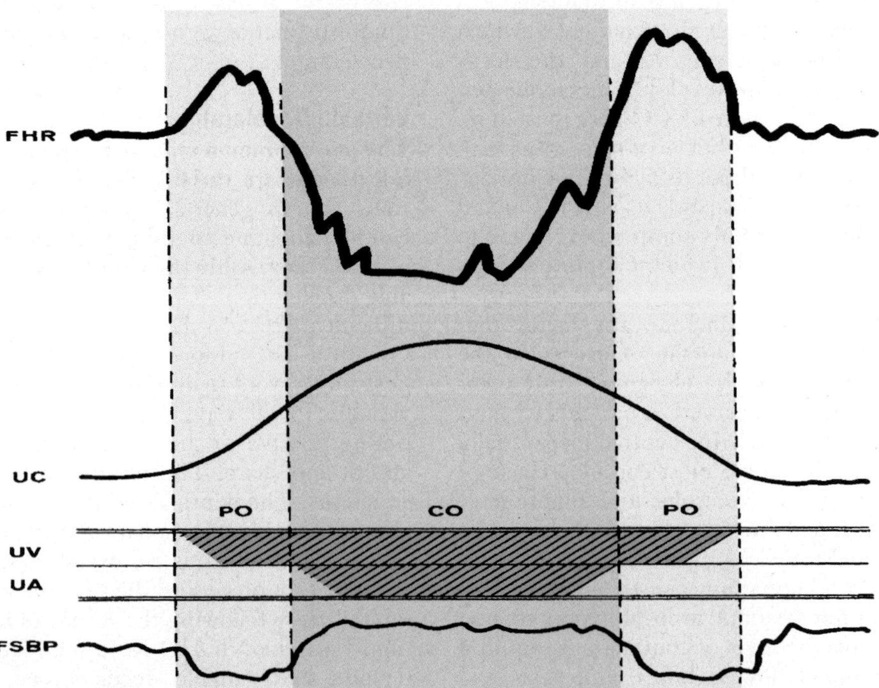

FIGURE 16-17. This figure represents fetal heart rate *(FHR)* and fetal systemic blood pressure *(FSBP)* occurring during compression of the umbilical vein *(UV)* and umbilical artery *(UA)*. Note the acceleration of the FHR as the FSBP is decreased, marking a baroreceptor response to decreased cardiac return, and the deceleration of the FHR when the FSBP is increased, the baroreceptor response to increased peripheral resistance. *UC,* Uterine contraction.

nuchal cords and seen as the baby descends through the pelvis. If cold saline is infused too rapidly with amnioinfusion, the FHR may slow, presumably as a result of cord spasm, the natural fetal reflex to cold stimulus. **Whatever the mechanism, it is most important to realize that variable decelerations are initially caused by a reflex in response to changes in pressure and not hypoxia.** Thus, variable decelerations (even deep and prolonged) can be seen in fetuses with no change in oxygen saturation (Figure 16-19).

Variable decelerations are seen in most labors, and most often these decelerations occur without fetal hypoxemia. It is apparent that additional criteria are needed to separate those benign variable decelerations not likely to be associated with hypoxia from those that are. Kubli and coworkers described a category of mild, moderate, and severe variable decelerations based on depth and duration (see box, Classifications of the Severity of Variable Decelerations).[30] Although there is indeed a correlation between the severity of these decelerations and the likelihood of hypoxia, one can see from Figure 16-19 that it is difficult to pick a specific depth and duration that always predicts oxygen compromise. Therefore, in addition, characteristics of the fetal baseline are also used, including the development of tachycardia and loss of variability (Figure 16-20). When cord compression occurs with each contraction and is sustained for a prolonged period of time, there can be a change from the usual abrupt return to baseline to a slow or delayed return to baseline (Figure 16-21). This is also often called a *late component*, although a combined pattern of late and variable decelerations (Figure 16-22) should be distinguished from progressive, severe variable decelerations that result in slow return to baseline because the etiologies and thus the potential treatments will differ. This particular discriminator of variable decelerations can be one of the most confusing aspects in all of fetal monitoring. Because a slow return to baseline can represent fetal hypoxia from either progressive cord compression or from a coincident late deceleration, the question is, Does this finding always represent hypoxia? Many times this sign appears without significant cord compression preceding its onset; therefore, it is unlikely that a substantial oxygen deficit has developed. Thus, many times these are benign findings and may represent more slow release of the cord or some other unexplained phenomenon. Finally, in extreme situations in which there is profound fetal hypoxia and acidosis, the variable decelerations will appear smoother and rounded or "blunted," rather than having the usual abrupt changes seen with the more common

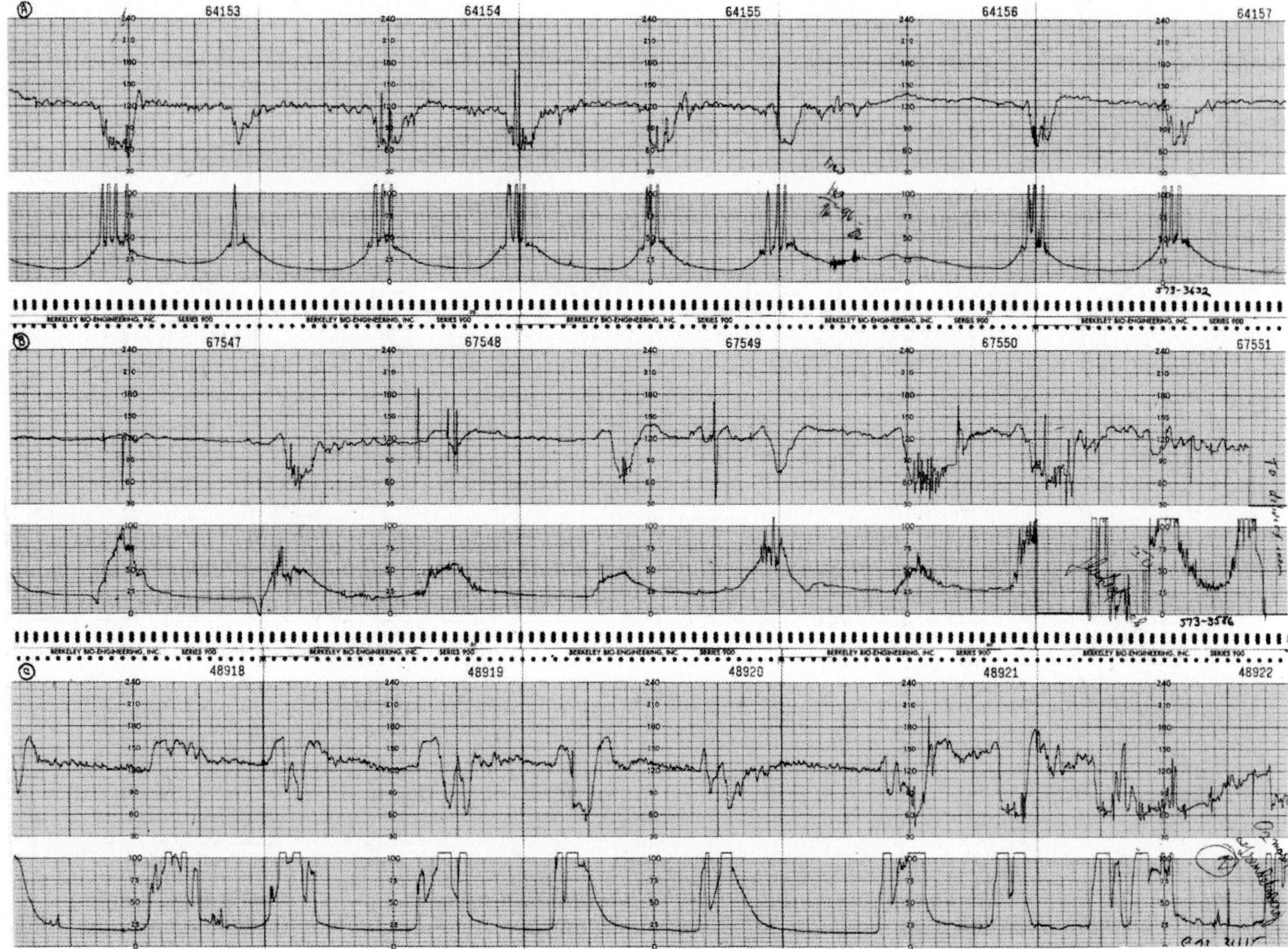

FIGURE 16-18. These are typical variable decelerations. Note that such decelerations are often recognized by the accelerations that precede and follow the decelerations.

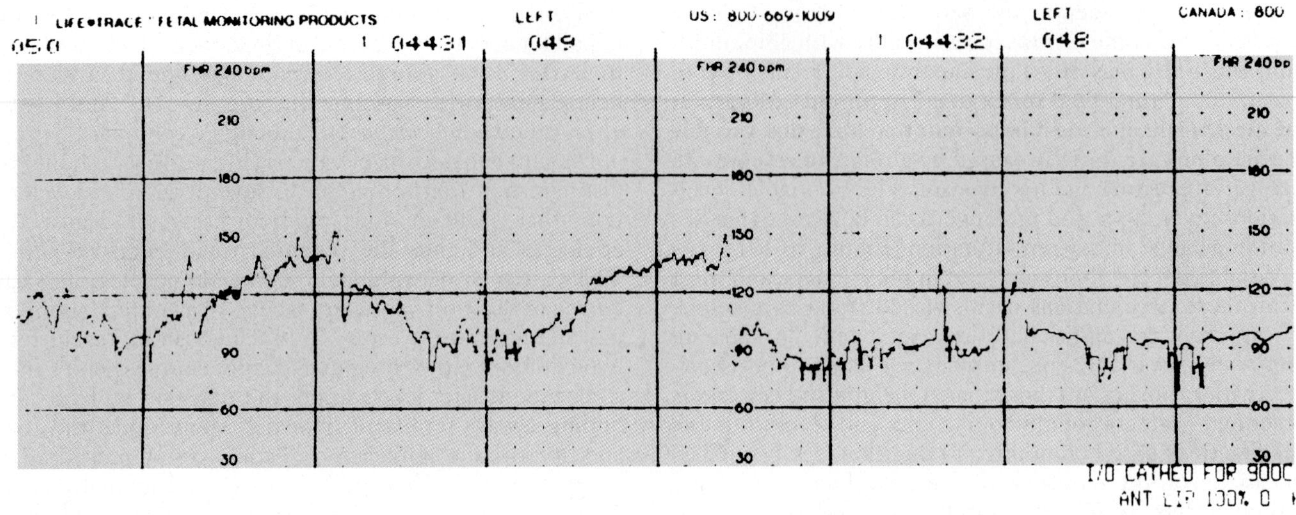

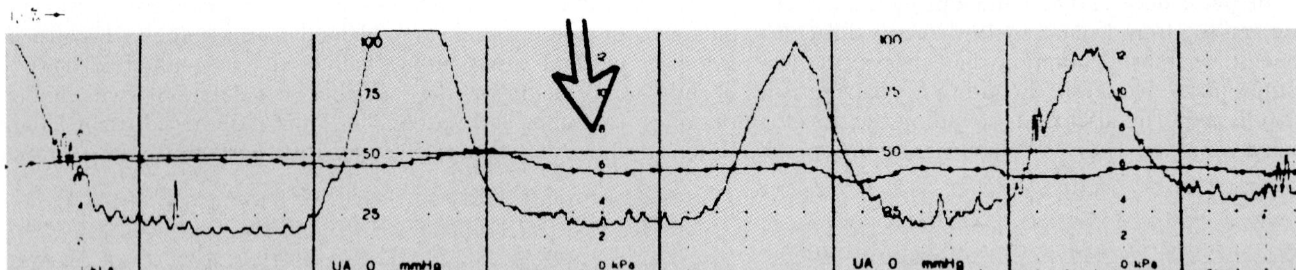

FIGURE 16-19. Superimposed on the contraction monitor tracing is a continuous tracing using a fetal pulse oximeter. The tracing shows an fetal oxygen saturation value ranging from 50% to 40% (normal, 35% to 60%). Note the consistently normal saturation values despite the prolonged fetal heart rate decelerations to 80 beats/minute.

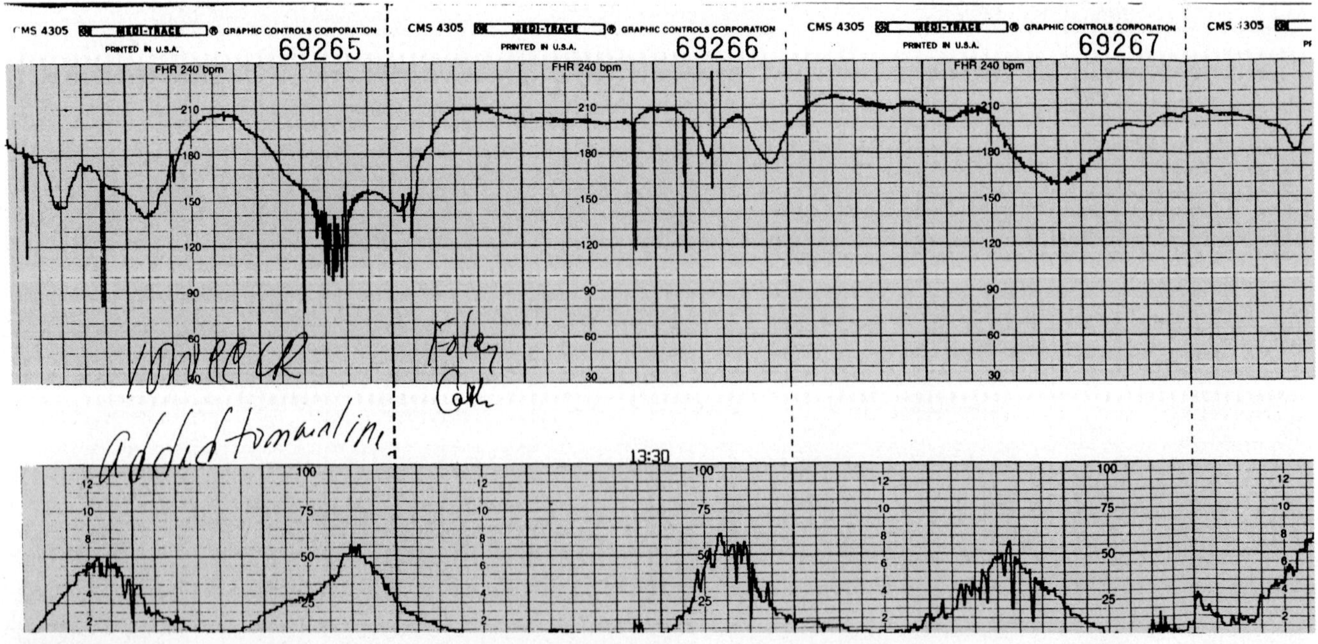

FIGURE 16-20. The loss of variability and tachycardia in association with these variable decelerations makes this a non-reassuring fetal heart rate pattern (NICHD Category III).[17]

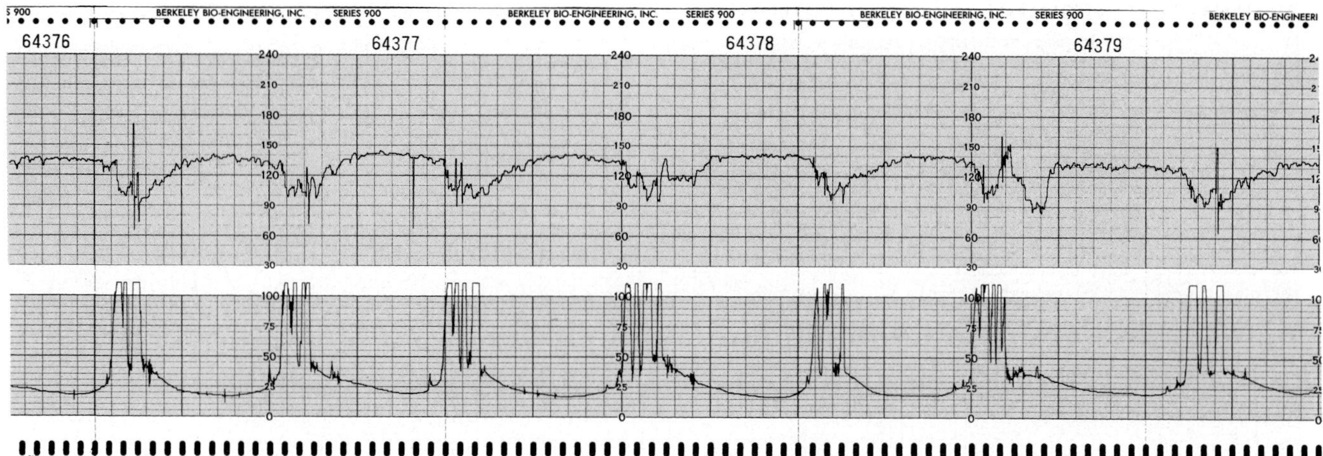

FIGURE 16-21. These variable decelerations, although mild in depth and duration, are associated with a slow, rather than abrupt, return to baseline. This may be a sign of developing hypoxia as a result of repetitive umbilical cord compression with inadequate opportunity to reoxygenate between events. Generally, this finding makes the variable decelerations non-reassuring.

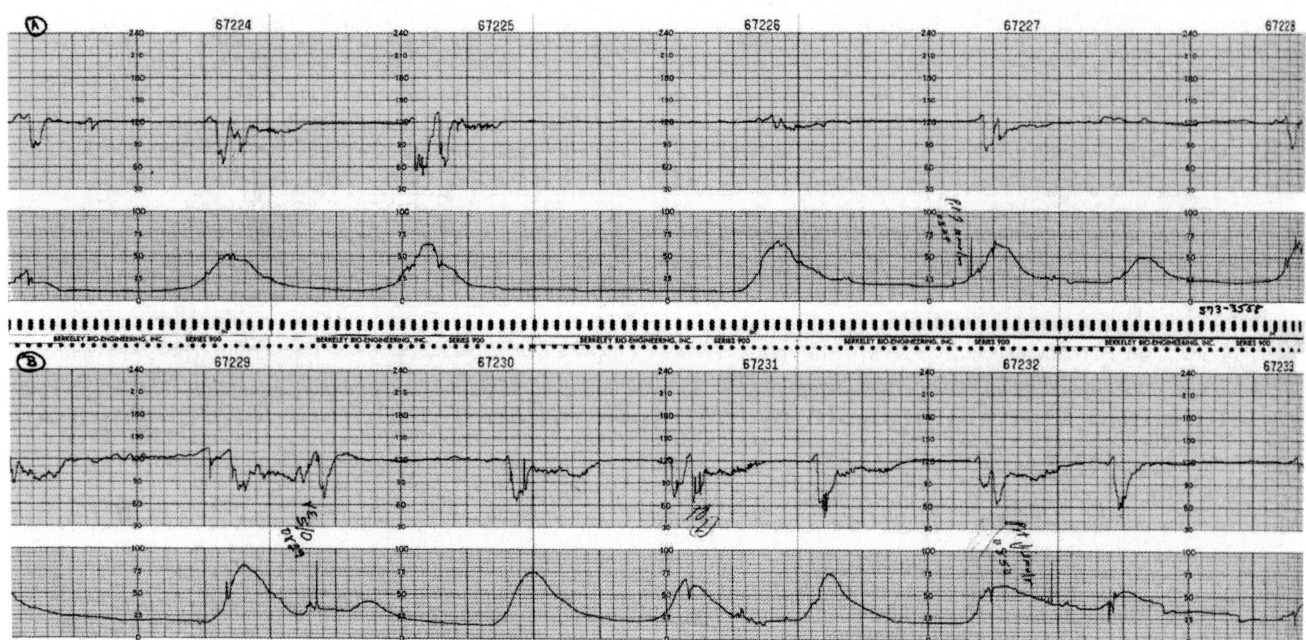

FIGURE 16-22. Here are repetitive variable decelerations with a slow return to baseline. However, the minimal depth and duration of the variable decelerations and the fact that one can see an independent late deceleration with the third contraction would suggest that this pattern is actually a combined one of mild variable and persistent late decelerations.

Classifications of the Severity of Variable Decelerations

Mild

Deceleration of a duration of less than 30 seconds, regardless of depth

Decelerations not below 80 beats/minute, regardless of duration

Moderate

Deceleration with a level below 80 beats/minute

Severe

Deceleration to a level below 70 beats/minute or more than 70 beats/minute below the baseline for more than 60 seconds

Data from Kubli FW, Hon EH, Khazin AE, et al: Observations on heart rate and pH in the human fetus during labor. Am J Obstet Gynecol 104:1190, 1969.

benign decelerations. Such cases are virtually always seen in association with absent FHR variability, and they can also be followed by a blunted acceleration following the return to baseline described by Goodlin and Lowe as "overshoot" (Figure 16-23).[31] This is a rare situation and is only seen when all criteria are met, including absent variability, blunted variable decelerations, no acceleration preceding the variable deceleration, and no other spontaneous accelerations of the FHR.

There are four categories of causes of cord compression patterns that are useful to consider from a management standpoint. Variable decelerations appearing early in labor are often caused by oligohydramnios. Other variable decelerations often first appear when the patient reaches 8 to 9 cm of dilation, the time in labor when the curve for descent of the presenting part becomes steep. This is

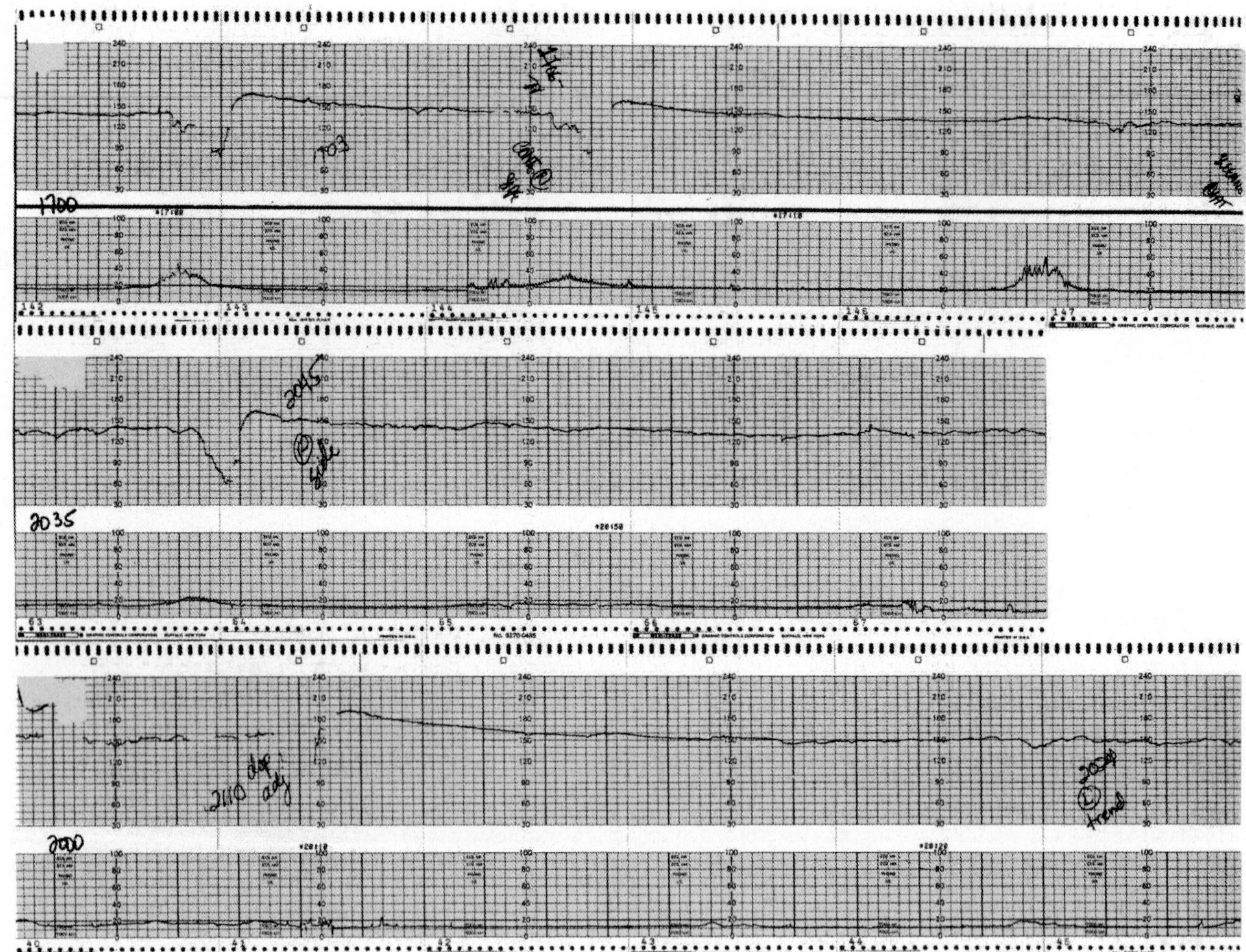

FIGURE 16-23. The accelerations following these variable decelerations, without any acceleration preceding, in association with absent variability fulfill the criteria to describe the accelerations as "overshoot." Such a finding can be ominous and is often associated with marked metabolic acidosis.

probably most often because of nuchal cords, wherein the cord becomes stretched with descent of the fetal head, and as previously described, cord stretch is a profound stimulus for vasospasm in the cord vessels.[16] Unusual types of abnormal umbilical cords, such as short cords, true knots, velamentous cord insertion, cord looped around the extremities, and occult cord prolapse, will produce variable decelerations. And finally, the rarest form of cord compression, and one that usually requires rapid cesarean delivery, is true umbilical cord prolapse.

Because the umbilical cord is most analogous to the adult trachea, interruption in cord flow results in both retention of CO_2 and cessation of O_2 delivery. When this becomes progressive, the intermittent compression often first leads to a progressive increase in fetal CO_2, which results in a respiratory acidosis. If the cord compression continues and also is sufficiently severe to cause insufficient delivery of oxygen, then a metabolic acidosis can also develop. Thus, in a fetal acidosis resulting from cord compression, the acidosis can be respiratory or combined respiratory and metabolic, but should not be metabolic alone.

Prolonged Decelerations

Prolonged decelerations are sporadically occurring decelerations lasting 90 to 120 seconds or more. The NICHD Research Planning Workshop proposed that prolonged decelerations be defined as those lasting 2 to 10 minutes and that beyond 10 minutes this is a baseline change.[17] In most cases, the sudden drop in FHR is the result of some adverse afferent stimulus caused by the brain detecting changes in oxygenation, blood pressure, or even intracranial pressure, as with sustained head compression. Unlike the other three decelerations, in which the type of deceleration defines the pathophysiologic mechanism, prolonged decelerations may be caused by virtually any of the mechanisms previously described, but usually are of a more profound and sustained nature. Prolonged umbilical cord compression, profound placental insufficiency, or even sustained head compression may lead to prolonged decelerations.

The presence of and severity of hypoxia are thought to correlate with the following variables with a prolonged deceleration: the depth and duration of the deceleration, how abruptly it returns to baseline, how much variability is

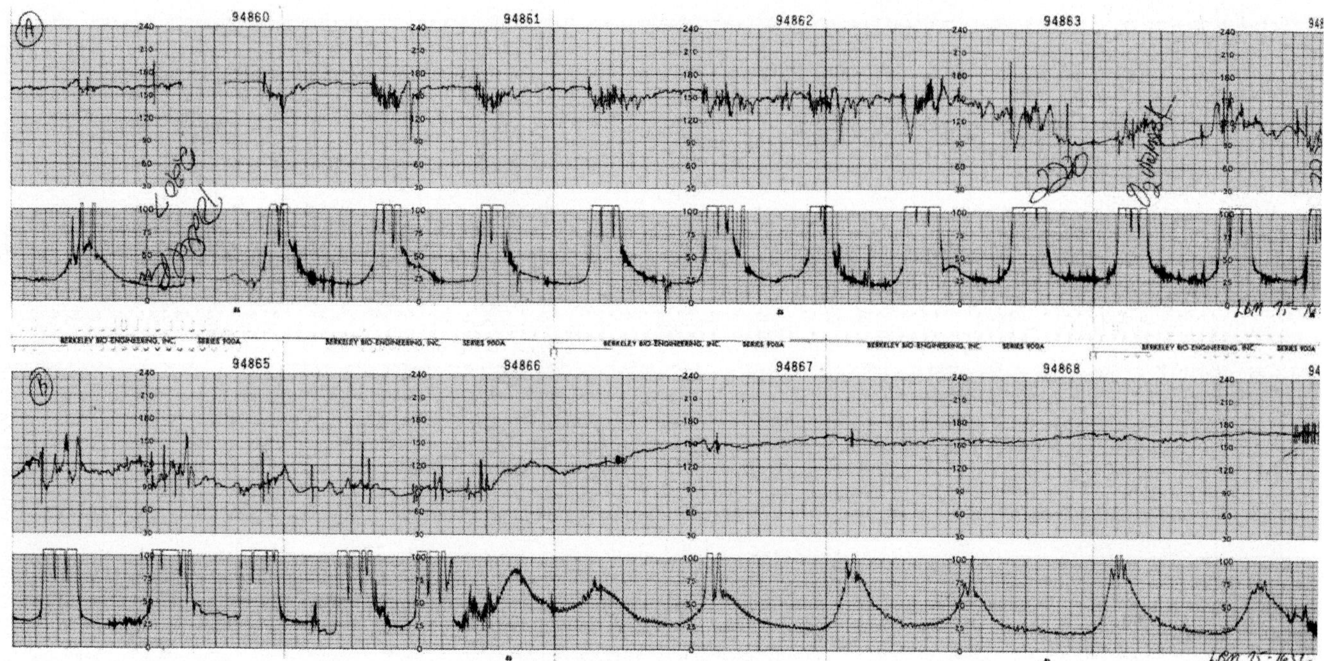

FIGURE 16-24. Often following a prolonged deceleration, as with the one shown in this figure, there is a temporary period of tachycardia and loss of variability. Such a response would suggest that this was a significant hypoxic event. The etiology of this deceleration is not clear but may have been a result of excessive uterine contractions compounded by maternal pushing.

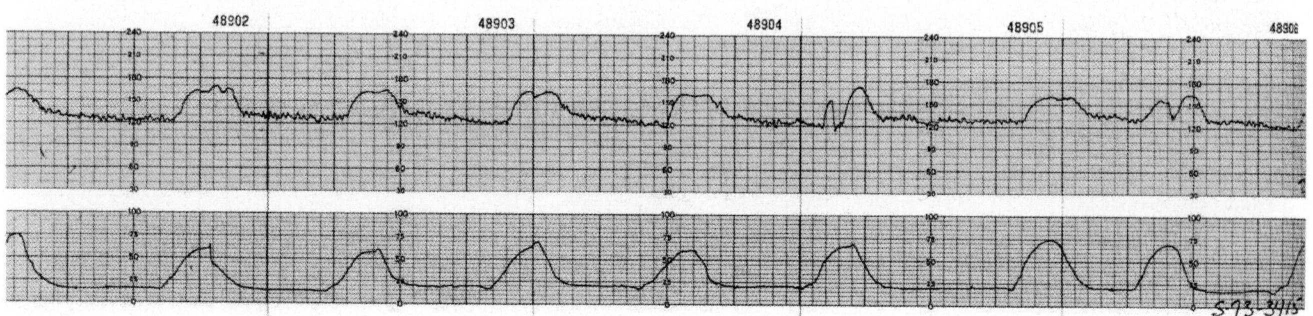

FIGURE 16-25. These are accelerations of the fetal heart. They are usually seen with fetal movement and are often coincident with uterine contractions as well, as in this patient.

lost during the deceleration, and whether there is a rebound tachycardia and loss of variability following the deceleration (Figure 16-24). Examples of the more profound stimuli that may result in this type of deceleration include prolapsed umbilical cord or other forms of prolonged cord compression, prolonged uterine hyperstimulation, hypotension following conduction anesthesia, severe degrees of abruptio placentae, uterine rupture, paracervical anesthesia, an eclamptic seizure, and rapid descent through the birth canal. Occasionally, less severe stimuli such as examination of the fetal head, Valsalva maneuvers, or application of a scalp electrode may cause milder forms of prolonged decelerations.

Accelerations

Accelerations are periodic changes of the FHR above the baseline (Figure 16-25) **defined as an transient increase of the FHR lasting at least 15 seconds and rising 15 beats or more above the baseline.** Because decelerations are of lower amplitude in more premature gestations, the definition of accelerations in the fetus before 32 weeks are those of an amplitude of 10 beats/minute or more lasting 10 or more seconds. They are not classified by type. Except for those accelerations previously described that are associated with variable decelerations, virtually all accelerations are a physiologic response to fetal movement.[32] Accelerations are usually short in duration, lasting no more than 30 to 90 seconds, but in an unusually active fetus, they can be sustained as long as 30 minutes or more. Again, the NICHD Research Planning Workshop disagrees somewhat on this definition, in that they propose that accelerations of more than 10 minutes be defined as a change in baseline.[17] This definition may not always be consistent with the actual fetal physiology because one can on occasion see sustained accelerations (Figure 16-26) that are associated with an actively moving fetus, and when the fetus becomes quiet, the FHR will return to baseline. It is important that this acceleration not be confused with a

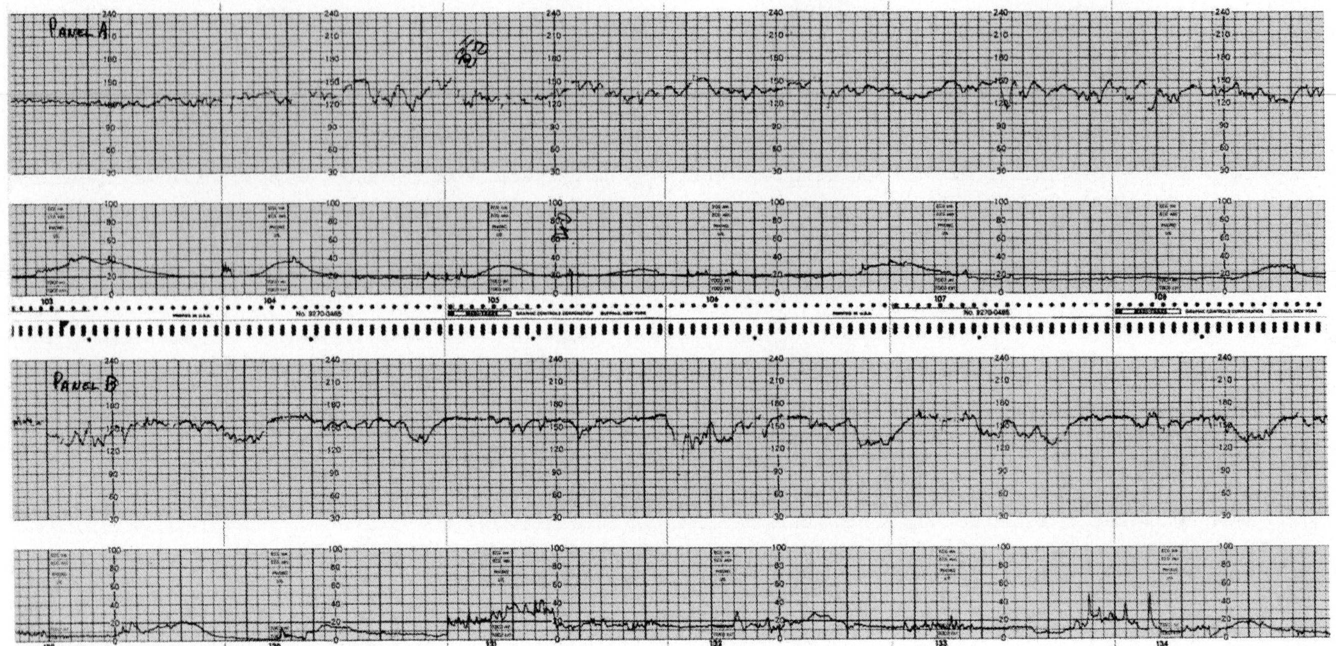

FIGURE 16-26. This figure shows prolonged and repetitive accelerations, especially in the lower panel. Accelerations that are sustained or confluent can be easily confused with a tachycardia, and the return to baseline can be confused with decelerations.

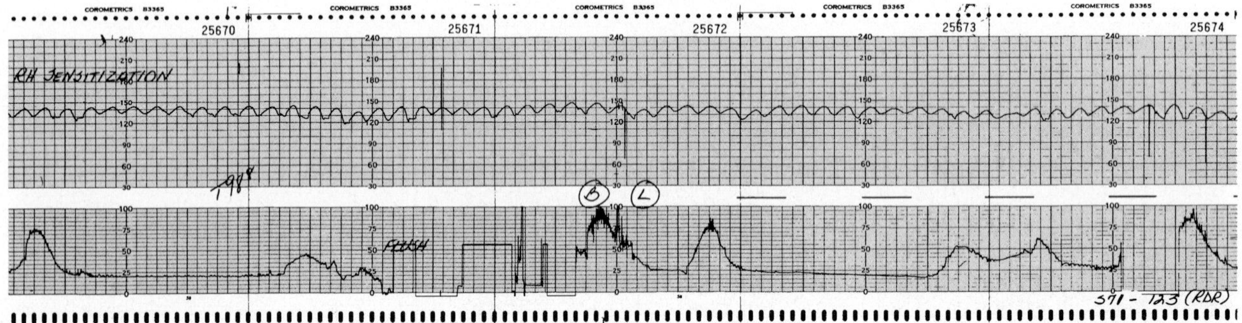

FIGURE 16-27. The sinusoidal heart rate pattern with its even undulations is demonstrated. Internal monitoring shows the absence of beat-to-beat variability characteristic of true sinusoidal patterns.

baseline change because sustained accelerations, which are consistent with a well-oxygenated, vigorous fetus, can be confused visually with fetal tachycardia, and the return of the FHR to the original baseline can be confused with decelerations.

The presence of accelerations has virtually the same meaning as normal FHR variability, but the absence of accelerations means only that the baby is not moving. Because accelerations can be quantified in beats per minute above the baseline and duration, their presence is less subjective than quantifying FHR variability. Clark and coworkers made the observation that in fetuses having otherwise non-reassuring FHR patterns, the presence of accelerations virtually always ruled out a pH less than 7.20 on scalp sampling.[33] Subsequently, these authors and others have confirmed that the presence of spontaneous accelerations or accelerations induced by stimulation of the fetal scalp or acoustic stimulation with a vibroacoustic stimulator has the same reliability.[34,35] If there is no acceleration in the face of an otherwise concerning (category II) FHR, most studies have shown that about 50% of these fetuses have an acidotic pH value on scalp sampling. However, the absence of accelerations in a fetus with a category I or otherwise reassuring pattern rarely indicates fetal acidosis.

Sinusoidal Patterns

This pattern was originally described by Kubli and colleagues in 1972[36] and Shenker in 1973[37] and is rare, but significant. This pattern is strongly associated with fetal hypoxia, most often seen in the presence of severe fetal anemia. Using strict criteria for this pattern, defined by Modanlou and associates, there will be a high correlation with significant fetal acidosis and/or severe anemia.[38] These criteria for identifying a sinusoidal FHR include (1) a stable baseline FHR of 120 to 160 beats/minute with regular sine wave–like oscillations, (2) an amplitude of 5 to 15 beats/minute, (3) a frequency of 2 to 5 cycles/minute, (4) fixed or absent short-term variability, (5) oscillation of the sine wave above and below the baseline, and (6) absence of accelerations (Figure 16-27). **The NICHD has defined the sinusoidal pattern more simply as one "having**

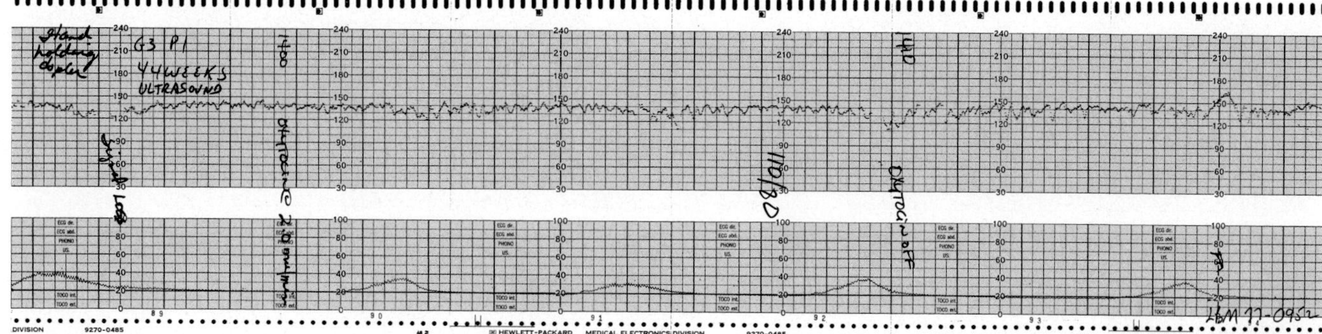

FIGURE 16-28. More common than sinusoidal tracings are those that are actually normal but can easily be confused with a sinusoidal pattern. There are often small accelerations or above-average variability that mimics the sine wave–like pattern. It is important to use the strict criteria defined in the text before interpreting a pattern as sinusoidal.

a visually apparent, smooth, sine wave-like undulating pattern in FHR baseline with a cycle frequency of 3-5 per minute lasting for 20 minutes or more." The pathophysiology of the sinusoidal pattern has been elucidated by Murata and colleagues, who correlated the pattern with levels of fetal arginine vasopressin and subsequently reproduced the pattern with vagotomy and injection of arginine vasopressin.[39] Arginine vasopressin is elevated with hemorrhage or acidosis, and it appears that in such situations with a severely compromised fetus and little vagal activity, the hormone directly affects the fetal heart, and this FHR pattern results. The sinusoidal pattern has also been described after injection of certain narcotics such as butorphanol (Stadol)[40] and meperidine (Demerol).[41] Unfortunately, there are relatively commonly seen FHR patterns that mimic sinusoidal patterns (pseudosinusoidal) and are associated with well-oxygenated and nonanemic fetuses.[38] These can easily be confused with sinusoidal FHR patterns (Figure 16-28); therefore, it is quite important to strictly apply all six criteria before calling a pattern sinusoidal.

Additional Terminology from the NICHD Workshop

In addition to those definitions provided previously, there are some additional points made in the accepted terminology for FHR patterns that are important to include.[17] When describing decelerations, they are termed *recurrent* if they occur with 50% or more of contractions and *intermittent* if they occur with less than 50% of contractions in any 20-minute segment of the tracing.

Uterine contractions are quantified as the number of contractions present in a 10-minute window averaged over 30 minutes. Normal contraction frequency is five or fewer per 10 minutes, and tachysystole is six or more. The Workshop advised abandonment of the terms *hyperstimulation* and *hypercontractility*.

TABLE 16-1 THREE-TIERED FETAL HEART RATE INTERPRETATION SYSTEM

Category I

Category I fetal heart rate (FHR) tracings include all the following:

- Baseline rate: 110-160 beats/min
- Baseline FHR variability: moderate
- Late or variable decelerations: absent
- Early decelerations: present or absent
- Accelerations: present or absent

Category II

Category II FHR tracings include all FHR tracings not categorized as category I or category III. Category II tracings may represent an appreciable fraction of those encountered in clinical care. Examples of category II FHR tracings include any of the following:

Baseline Rate

- Bradycardia not accompanied by absent baseline variability
- Tachycardia

Baseline FHR Variability

- Minimal baseline variability
- Absent baseline variability not accompanied by recurrent decelerations
- Marked baseline variability

Accelerations

- Absence of induced accelerations after fetal stimulation

Periodic or Episodic Decelerations

- Recurrent variable decelerations accompanied by minimal or moderate baseline variability
- Prolonged deceleration: >2 minutes but <10 minutes
- Recurrent late decelerations with moderate baseline variability
- Variable decelerations with other characteristics, such as slow return to baseline, "overshoots," or "shoulders"

Category III

Category III FHR tracings include either:

- Absent baseline FHR variability and any of the following:
  - Recurrent late decelerations
  - Recurrent variable decelerations
  - Bradycardia
- Sinusoidal pattern

From Macones GA, Hankins GD, Spong CY, et al: The 2008 National Institute of Child Health and Human Development Workshop Report on Electronic Fetal Monitoring. Obstet Gynecol 112:661-666, 2008.

Evolution of Fetal Heart Rate Patterns

One of the sources of greatest confusion regarding FHR pattern interpretation and management is that the patterns have very poor specificity in terms of predicting fetal hypoxia and acidosis, newborn depression, or need for resuscitation (Table 16-1). **When patterns are normal or "reassuring"** (category I), there is almost always normal oxygenation, and the baby is born vigorous, with normal pH and Apgar scores. However, when the pattern is non-reassuring (category II), the baby is more often normal than depressed or acidotic.

In addition to the inherent problem we have in trying to use EFM, a nonspecific modality, to determine fetal oxygenation, there is another reason why many studies have demonstrated such poor correlation with adverse

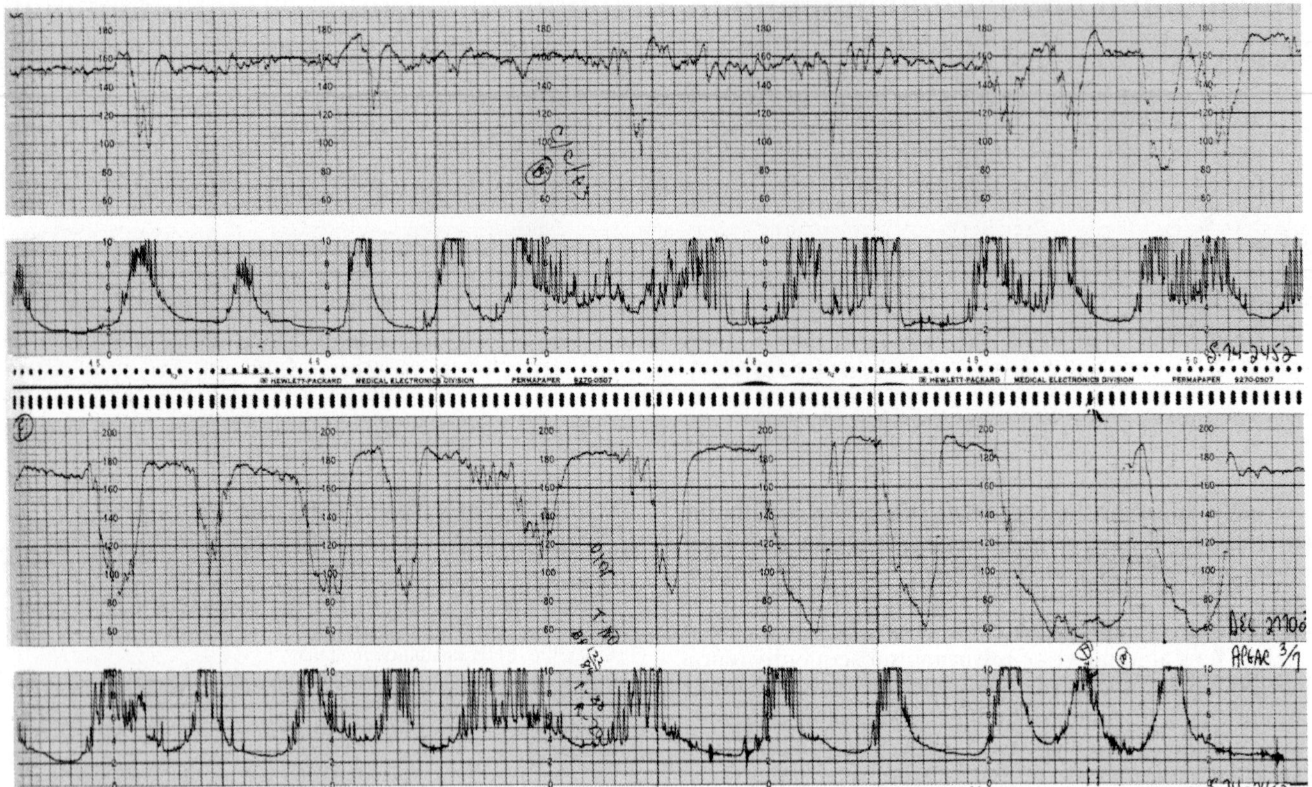

FIGURE 16-29. Loss of variability and tachycardia should only be interpreted as indicative of hypoxia and developing acidosis when they are associated with decelerations that suggest progressive hypoxia as with these variable decelerations, which are becoming deeper and more prolonged.

perinatal outcome. Investigators have tried to correlate specific FHR findings in isolation without taking into account the expected evolution of the FHR patterns.[19,30] For example, if one attempts to correlate FHR variability with acidosis or depression, normal variability will correlate well with a normal pH and normal Apgar scores, but reduced or absent variability will correlate poorly with acidosis or depression. This is partly because of the multiple causes of reduced variability. However, in the fetus with persistent late decelerations who then loses FHR variability, the correlation with acidosis and depression should improve substantially because there was evidence that *hypoxia led to the acidosis*. This is a critical concept in understanding FHR monitoring. Murata and coworkers demonstrated that, in the fetal monkey whose oxygenation was progressively reduced, late decelerations consistently *preceded* the loss of variability and accelerations.[42] **Decelerations are the indicators of hypoxia. If hypoxia is the cause of the reduced variability, then those decelerations indicative of hypoxia should *precede* the development of tachycardia, loss of variability, or disappearance of accelerations** (Figure 16-29). Furthermore, the duration and appearance of the decelerations should be of sufficient magnitude to suggest that CNS depression could have resulted.

Therefore, the fetus who develops one of the latter variables (e.g., loss of accelerations) in the absence of decelerations is not likely to have hypoxia and another cause should be considered (e.g., drugs, sleep cycle). It must be remembered that when the fetus demonstrates one of these baseline changes or absence of accelerations on admission, it is not possible to know whether evidence of hypoxia preceded these changes. In addition, this approach does not apply antepartum, when the nonstress test is used. Contractions are not present, and there will not be an opportunity to assess for the presence or absence of decelerations in response to contractions.

MANAGEMENT OF NON-REASSURING FETAL HEART RATE PATTERNS

Traditionally, a FHR pattern that suggested fetal hypoxia would be called fetal distress if it was sufficiently concerning to warrant immediate operative intervention. But, as previously mentioned, in most cases, when a cesarean or forceps delivery was done for "fetal distress," the fetus was delivered without evidence of significant hypoxia or acidosis. This has led to the recommendation from the ACOG to use the term *NRFS*[13] and subsequently to the *three-tiered system*. This is also descriptive of the approach to the management of the fetus with concerning FHR patterns. That is, when the FHR pattern is suggestive of hypoxia, and therefore non-reassuring, other means of reassurance should be used when possible.

Interventions for Non-reassuring Fetal Status

The ideal intervention for fetal hypoxia is a cause-specific, noninvasive one that permanently reverses the problem. Although not always possible, this should certainly be the goal. Obviously, the first step in achieving this goal is to recognize the cause of the abnormal FHR pattern. A thorough knowledge of the pathophysiology of FHR changes, coupled with a careful clinical patient evaluation and a knowledge of common causes of specific FHR changes, will maximize the opportunity for this goal to succeed. In addition to cause-specific types of interventions, virtually all cases of hypoxia should theoretically also benefit by more generic interventions that have the potential to maximize oxygen delivery and placental exchange.

Nonsurgical Interventions

Oxygen Administration

One of the most obvious ways to maximize oxygen delivery to the fetus is to give additional oxygen to the mother. Whereas diffusion across a membrane is driven by PO_2 as opposed to oxygen content, and whereas maternal PO_2 can be raised substantially with mask O_2, it is not well established that fetal PO_2 is raised substantially by routine maternal oxygen administration. In the classic study by Khazin, Hon, and Hehre,[43] late decelerations were alleviated within a few minutes by administration of oxygen to the mother. Later studies showed beneficial effects with decreased FHR variability and tachycardia.[44,45] In 2003, Fawole and Hofmer[46] reviewed the available studies for the *Cochrane Database of Systematic Reviews* and concluded that there was not sufficient evidence that maternal oxygen administration improved fetal oxygenation and that maternal oxygen administration could not be supported at the time. Recent evidence, from fetuses being monitored with pulse oximetry, demonstrated that fetal oxygen did increase significantly in patients with both a regular face mask and even more so with a non-rebreathing face mask and that fetuses with the lower initial oxygen saturation increased the most.[47,48] Simpson and James[49] found similar results with oxygen administration, showing a 15% increase with normal baseline oxygen saturations and a 26% increase with a baseline oxygen saturation of less than 40%. These studies are physiologically plausible because the larger the difference in oxygen tension between the mother and the fetus, the larger the effect that would be expected to be seen in the fetal oxygen tension and saturation. **Routine oxygen administration by face mask has become such standard practice with non-reassuring FHR patterns that it is difficult to recommend otherwise until further studies are available to substantiate or refute current knowledge.**

Lateral Positioning

Ideally, all patients should labor in the lateral recumbent position, at least from the standpoint of maximizing uterine perfusion. The reasons for this are, at least theoretically, twofold: (1) in being inactive and recumbent, the body is required to deliver the least amount of blood flow to other muscles; and (2) in the lateral position, there is no compression by the uterus on the vena cava or aorta, thus maximizing cardiac return and cardiac output. Several studies have confirmed the beneficial effects of lateral maternal positioning.[50,51] In the study by Simpson and James,[49] patients were randomized to six positions, and fetal oxygen saturation was highest in both right and left lateral recumbent positions compared with the supine position by an average of 29%.

Hydration

Most patients in labor are either restricted or prohibited from taking oral fluids for fear of requiring an urgent operative delivery in the presence of a full stomach. If not fluid restricted, individuals involved in sustained exercise, and possibly by inference in active labor, do not voluntarily ingest adequate amounts of fluid because of a phenomenon called *autodehydration*.[52] In addition, recent evidence would suggest that the usual amount of intravenous fluid of 125 mL/hour is a gross underestimate of the replacement required in labor.[53] Thus, by increasing fluid administration, there is the potential to maximize intravascular volume and thus uterine perfusion.

Oxytocin

In a patient with a non-reassuring pattern, the more time there is between contractions, the more time there is to maximally perfuse the placenta and deliver oxygen. **In patients receiving oxytocin, there is potential to improve oxygenation by decreasing or discontinuing oxytocin.** Often, however, this becomes a difficult situation because many patients will stop progressing in labor in terms of continued dilation and descent if the oxytocin is discontinued. It is often necessary to restart the oxytocin, and this may be appropriate, especially if there are accelerations or other means to document the absence of acidosis. Written documentation explaining the necessity and appropriateness of continuing oxytocin in this situation is especially important. The situation with patients who develop persistently non-reassuring patterns, especially with loss of accelerations or absence of other reassurance, and who require discontinuation of oxytocin, but then fail to progress because adequate contractions cannot be sustained, is often referred to as *fetal intolerance to labor*, although this is not an endorsed term in the newer terminology.

Tocolytics

There are numerous references in the obstetrical literature to the use of tocolytics to maximize oxygen delivery, by essentially the same mechanism described in the earlier paragraph on discontinuing oxytocin.[54-57] Tocolytics are appropriate when patients are having spontaneous excessive contractions leading to non-reassuring FHR patterns, especially prolonged decelerations (Figure 16-30). Different tocolytics have been described, but the most commonly used one, and perhaps the one that provides the most rapid response, is subcutaneous terbutaline, 0.25 mg. Tocolytics have also been used for intrauterine resuscitation after the decision is made to perform an operative delivery while waiting for preparations to be made. Subcutaneous terbutaline in this latter setting has been demonstrated to improve Apgar scores and cord pH values without apparent complications such as postpartum hemorrhage.[58]

Amnioinfusion

In situations in which variable decelerations appear to be caused by oligohydramnios, reestablishing intrauterine fluid volume by a process called *amnioinfusion* has been demonstrated in numerous randomized studies to ameliorate the variable decelerations, improve Apgar scores and

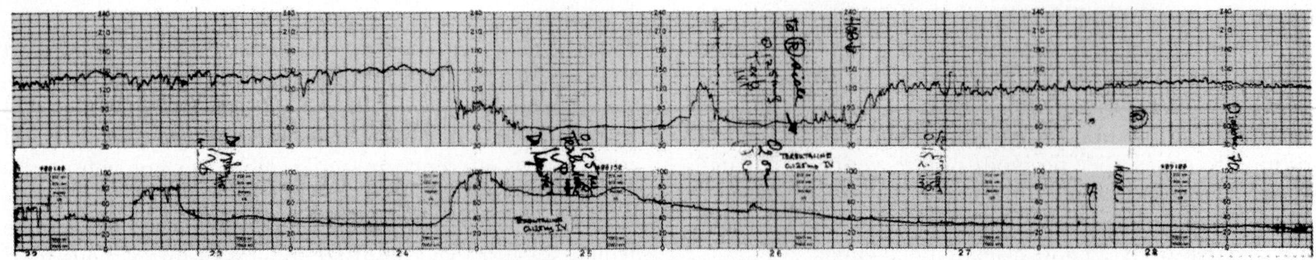

FIGURE 16-30. This prolonged deceleration in a patient with a spontaneous prolonged contraction is treated with subcutaneous terbutaline with apparent resolution of both the contraction and the deceleration.

cord pH values, and even reduce the need for cesarean delivery for NRFS.[59-61] Reference to this idea can be found as far back as 1925,[62] but it was rediscovered and proposed by Miyazaki and Taylor in 1983.[63] Intrauterine pressure catheters are now made with a port that allows the simultaneous administration of saline to accomplish this goal. Thus, in the patient with variable decelerations that suggest progression to more non-reassuring types, and in whom the likely cause is oligohydramnios, the implementation of amnioinfusion is warranted. What has not yet been established is whether in some situations amnioinfusion should be started prophylactically when there is an unusually high risk for the development of variable decelerations from oligohydramnios, such as preterm premature rupture of membranes (PROM).

Theoretically, using amnioinfusion before the onset of the decelerations in certain fetuses, such as very premature ones or those with intrauterine growth restriction that will progress to acidosis and depression much more rapidly with cord compression, will prevent the rapid evolution of hypoxia and acidosis. No studies are available as of yet to compare therapeutic and prophylactic amnioinfusion. Amnioinfusion also has been proposed, in several prospective randomized trials, to be used to avoid the fetal and neonatal pulmonary problems in the presence of meconium.[64] The theory behind this use of amnioinfusion is that (1) it dilutes the meconium by increasing fluid volume, and (2) by avoiding fetal gasping, which can occur with significant hypoxic episodes (i.e., sustained cord compression), the likelihood of meconium aspiration before delivery is reduced. Although initial studies of the benefits of amnioinfusion in the setting of meconium were promising and for a time its use for this indication gained widespread implementation,[65] recent studies have been less supportive. A review of this subject for the Cochrane database[66] including 13 studies of more than 4000 women concluded there was no reduction in meconium aspiration, perinatal death, or severe morbidity, except in an unexplained subgroup of studies done in populations in which "limited peripartum surveillance" was available.

MECONIUM

The presence of meconium is an extremely confusing issue when evaluating the fetus in labor. The quandary arises from the fact that although a hypoxic insult eliciting a significant vagal response from the fetus often results in the passage of meconium from the fetal gut, passage of meconium can also occur in the absence of any significant or sustained hypoxia. Meconium is not only a potential sign of fetal hypoxia but is also a potential toxin if the fetus aspirates this particulate matter with a gasping breath in utero or when it takes its first breaths following birth. **The thickness of the meconium is also a reflection of the amount of amniotic fluid, and thick meconium virtually always reflects some degree of oligohydramnios.** Thus, there may be a vicious cycle in such a situation. Oligohydramnios often leads to cord compression; the vagal response to cord compression may also lead to further passage of meconium, but also when sustained or prolonged, it may lead to fetal gasping, increasing the likelihood that meconium aspiration can occur before birth. Furthermore, because oligohydramnios may be an indicator of failing placental function, meconium may also indicate that the fetus is at risk for placental insufficiency. **In general, meconium should alert the clinician to the potential for oligohydramnios, umbilical cord compression, placental insufficiency, and meconium aspiration.** Fortunately, a reassuring FHR tracing is generally reliable, and patients with meconium can be managed expectantly. But in the presence of meconium, especially thick meconium, the risk factors associated with meconium should be entered in the equation when managing relatively non-reassuring patterns, as should all clinical variables.

Alternatives for Evaluating the Fetus with a Non-reassuring Fetal Heart Rate Pattern

In the fetus with a persistently non-reassuring FHR pattern, when nonsurgical efforts at reversing or improving the pattern fail, the next step is to attempt to find out whether the hypoxia has progressed to metabolic acidosis.

FETAL SCALP pH

Determination of fetal scalp pH is historically the oldest and most well-tested method for determining whether the fetus is acidotic. Technically, a plastic cone is inserted transvaginally against the fetal vertex. The cervix needs to be at least 4 to 5 cm dilated and the vertex at a −1 station or below to accomplish this. Mineral oil or another lubricant is applied to the scalp so that blood will bead, and then using a lancet, the scalp is pricked and blood is then collected in a long capillary tube (Figure 16-31). The tube will hold about 100 μL of blood, and about 30 μL is needed to perform a pH test alone and 70 μL to determine P_{CO_2} as well. To determine whether an acidosis is metabolic or respiratory, the P_{CO_2} is needed. This is an important distinction because the question being asked is whether there

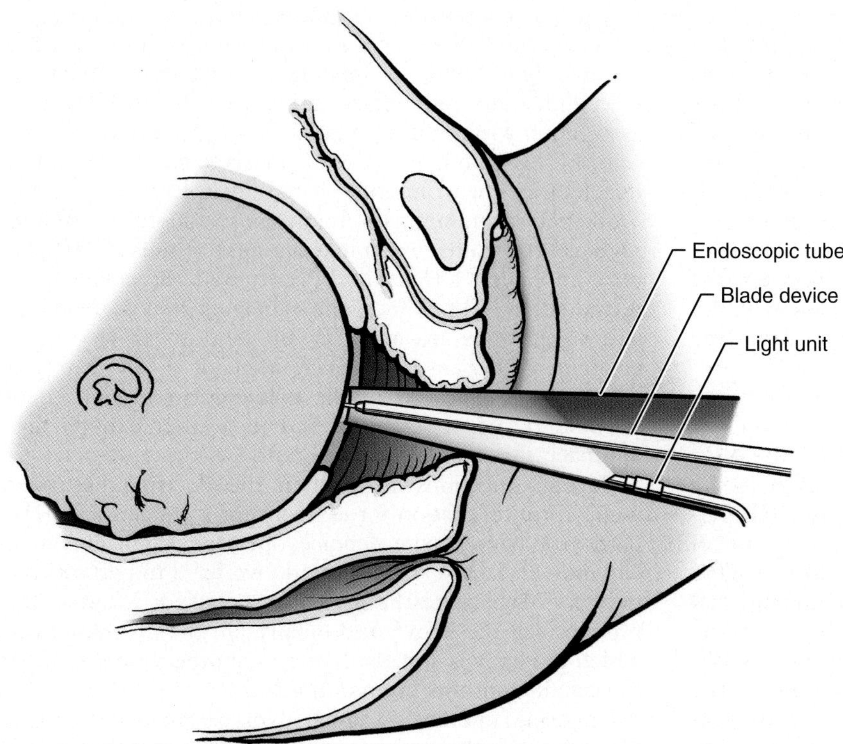

FIGURE 16-31. Technique of fetal scalp blood sampling.

has been sufficient hypoxia to lead to metabolic acidosis. Respiratory acidosis is far less concerning, but without determining PCO_2, this cannot be sorted out. Unfortunately, it is difficult to obtain enough blood for both pH and PCO_2 in most instances. PCO_2 determination is especially important when doing scalp pH for variable decelerations because most acidosis is respiratory in this situation. **A scalp pH less than 7.20 is consistent with fetal acidosis and a pH of 7.20 to 7.25 is borderline and should be repeated immediately.** A reassuring value higher than 7.25 must be repeated every 20 to 30 minutes as long as the pattern persists, and the fetus is not acidotic. In practice, because this technique is cumbersome, fraught with technical inaccuracy, uncomfortable for the patient, and with the requirement to perform repeated samples, scalp pH assessment is used very infrequently.[67] Even in large teaching services accustomed to using this technique, its abandonment, coupled with an appreciation for the utility of accelerations for predicting presence or absence of acidosis, does not appreciably increase the need for operative intervention.[68]

Accelerations and Variability

In the fetus with a non-reassuring pattern, spontaneous accelerations have the same significance as those elicited by scalp or acoustic stimulation. **Thus, any acceleration—spontaneous or induced—indicates the absence of acidosis.** It should be emphasized that the absence of accelerations as well when there is an absence of decelerations or other patterns suggesting hypoxia should not elicit concern. The fetus is often not moving in labor; and from a pathophysiologic perspective, without evidence of hypoxia, the fetus cannot develop a metabolic acidosis. Thus, the application of the interpretation of accelerations should generally be restricted to the fetus with an otherwise non-reassuring FHR pattern, when the question is being asked: Hypoxia is present. Is the fetus now developing a metabolic acidosis? Although moderate variability similarly can also be used to rule out the acidotic fetus, the problem with this choice is that interpretation of variability is not nearly as reliable as it is with accelerations. And although one can reliably wait on a pattern with non-reassuring decelerations such as recurrent late or recurrent severe variable decelerations based on moderate variability alone, one should be sure that there is no question that the FHR variability is at least moderate and that there is consistent agreement of this among the clinicians providing care to the patient.

Fetal Pulse Oximetry

One of the most potentially exciting yet currently disappointing developments in obstetrics was the introduction of fetal pulse oximetry. Because FHR monitoring is specifically intended to monitor fetal oxygenation and because this modality is so nonspecific, it stands to reason that what we should be using ideally is a device that directly monitors fetal oxygenation, pH, or both. Since the mid-1980s, the use of pulse oximetry has revolutionized monitoring of "air-breathing" adults, children, and neonates. Animal studies of this technology validated its accuracy.[69,70] Fetal pulse oximetry when first introduced was approved by the U.S. Food and Drug Administration (FDA) for clinical use. Its value for more accurately assessing fetal oxygenation in labor was promising in initial studies,[71] but not supported in later investigations[72] and ultimately not endorsed by ACOG. As a result, the manufacturer removed the product from the market, and it is no longer in use.

ST Analysis, the STAN Technology

One other promising new technology for improving interpretation of non-reassuring, especially category II, tracings is the introduction of fetal ECG waveform analysis using computerized algorithms detecting changes in the ST waveform which are indicative of fetal metabolic acidosis. Trials in Europe, including several randomized controlled trials usually coupled with scalp pH monitoring, have generally shown a reduction in operative deliveries for concerning FHR patterns and a reduction in the incidence of fetal acidosis.[73-75] An ongoing trial of this technology in the United States by the NICHD Maternal-Fetal Medicine Units Network is currently underway.

Computerized Interpretation of Fetal Heart Rate Patterns

One of the problems with FHR monitoring has been the dismal record of agreement on interpretation of FHR patterns. Intraobserver and interobserver comparisons of interpretation usually achieves only about 30% to 70% agreement.[76] The idea of computer interpretation of FHR patterns has been a goal attempted by many over the history of EFM. Recently, the first FDA-approved EFM computer-based interpretation system has come onto the market. Termed the *PeriCALM EFM system*, this product shows promise in accuracy of assessing which tracings are and are not associated with metabolic acidosis[77] and compares favorably with the agreement of interpretation of FHR patterns with expert interpreters.[78]

Operative Intervention for Non-reassuring Fetal Status

When the fetus is determined to have a persistently non-reassuring FHR pattern and backup methods (e.g., scalp pH, moderate variability, accelerations, ST waveform analysis) cannot provide reassurance that the fetus is not acidotic, operative intervention is indicated to expeditiously deliver the baby to avoid further deterioration. Because the interpretation of FHR patterns has been so inconsistent and the predictability of most non-reassuring patterns has been so poor, the NICHD convened a second Workshop on the Intrapartum Interpretation of EFM.[14] Their proposal, which has since been accepted by ACOG and AWHONN and many hospitals throughout the country, is that FHR patterns be divided into three categories (see Table 16-1). **Category I is strongly predictive of the absence of hypoxia and normal fetal acid-base status, and these patterns require no intervention. Category III patterns are predictive of a fetal metabolic acidosis and require "prompt evaluation."** Moreover, it can easily be stated that if measures at improving category III patterns, such as position change, oxygen administration, fluid boluses, and discontinuing oxytocin, do not improve the pattern, immediate operative delivery is warranted. **Category II includes more than 80% of FHR patterns seen in labor[79] and is said by the Workshop to "require evaluation and continued surveillance and reevaluation taking into account the entire clinical circumstances."** However, there are some substantial limitations of this new system for most patterns in category II. As Parer points out in his editorial on the limitations of this three-tiered system,[79] category II contains a mixture of patterns, some of which are well established to have no association with hypoxia or acidosis (e.g., mild or moderate variable decelerations with moderate variability) and others that have a high association with, or if left unchanged are likely to develop into, a fetus with hypoxia and acidosis (e.g., persistent late decelerations with minimal variability). Furthermore the Workshop recommendations and those adopted by ACOG give us little guidance on management of these FHR patterns in category II beyond "continued surveillance and reevaluation." Therefore, the following issues are raised and suggestions are made in an effort to provide more clearcut guidance on management of FHR patterns, acknowledging fully that the evidence to support these statements may be limited and that other experts may approach these situations differently.

Several questions arise when the decision has been made for intervention for delivery for a concerning FHR pattern. What is the best choice, operative vaginal or cesarean delivery? How much time do we have to perform the delivery? What anesthetic should be used? What is the prognosis of the baby? And, finally, are there situations in which the baby is already damaged or otherwise not likely to benefit from this intervention?

Choosing operative vaginal over cesarean delivery is not difficult if the patient is in early labor. For the patient near or at complete dilation, this becomes a question of judgment. Which route is more likely to create the more rapid delivery while at the same time result in the least complications for mother and baby? When the clinician is unsure whether an attempt at operative vaginal delivery will succeed, the question is even more difficult. This decision will depend not only on the variables that predict success for an operative vaginal delivery (e.g., station, clinical pelvimetry, size of the baby, skill of the clinician), but also on the severity of the FHR pattern and whether there is time to find out whether an operative delivery will succeed. The time for intervention also is a question of judgment. Except for the situation of a prolonged deceleration to less than 70 beats/minute with loss of variability that will not recover and requires the most rapid intervention safely possible, most other situations require judgment and integration of the entire clinical picture of mother and baby.

The question of how much time is available to perform an operative intervention in the face of a non-reassuring FHR pattern is a complex one, muddied not only by the unpredictability of the non-reassuring pattern but also by the medicolegal pressures that have arisen as a result of EFM. **The ACOG recommends that "all hospitals have the capability of performing a cesarean delivery within 30 minutes of the decision to operate,"[80] but that "not all indications for a cesarean delivery will require a 30-minute response time."** The examples given that mandate an expeditious delivery include hemorrhage from placenta previa, abruptio placentae, prolapse of the umbilical cord, and ruptured uterus. In some situations (e.g., sustained prolonged deceleration to <70 beats/minute with loss of variability), 30 minutes may be too long to avoid damage; in others, this may be too restrictive and may result in suboptimal anesthetic choices and compromised preoperative preparation. Thus, a judgment made on the basis of the severity of the FHR pattern and the overall clinical status of mother and baby must be integrated into this difficult decision.

MANAGEMENT OF NON-REASSURING FETAL HEART RATE PATTERNS: A PROPOSED PROTOCOL

The following algorithm for management of non-reassuring (categories II and III) FHR patterns is proposed:

1. When the pattern suggests the beginning development of hypoxia or is already non-reassuring:
   a. Identify, when possible, the cause of the problem (e.g., hypotension from an epidural).
   b. Correct the cause when possible (e.g., fluids and ephedrine to correct the hypotension).
   c. Give measures to maximize placental oxygen delivery and exchange: oxygen by face mask, lateral positioning, hydration, consider decreasing or discontinuing oxytocin.
2. If the pattern becomes or remains non-reassuring and the above measures have been completed:
   a. Attempt to provide other measures to rule out metabolic acidosis.
      - Accelerations—spontaneous or elicited
      - Moderate variability
      - Scalp pH (if used)
   b. If reassurance using one of the above methods can be provided, and the pattern persists, continuous or intermittent (every 30 minutes) evidence of absence of acidosis must be ascertained.
   c. If reassurance of the absence of acidosis cannot be provided, deliver expeditiously by the safest and most reasonable means (operative vaginal or cesarean delivery).

Category II patterns that qualify as non-reassuring and cannot be corrected and therefore warrant evidence of the absence of metabolic acidosis include the following:

1. Recurrent late decelerations (≥50% of contractions)
2. Non-reassuring variable decelerations
   a. Progressively severe in depth and duration
   b. With developing tachycardia and loss of variability
3. Recurrent prolonged decelerations
4. The confusing pattern
   a. A pattern of absent variability but without explanatory decelerations at the time of initiating monitoring
   b. An unusual pattern that does not fit into one of the categories defined previously but does not have elements of a reassuring pattern.

Several of the previous presentations and others warrant additional discussion. Prolonged decelerations proceeding to bradycardia that will not return to baseline are a potentially ominous situation. Causes of these patterns include virtually any substantial insult that can cause severe hypoxia, especially when the FHR goes below 80 beats/minute. Examples include abruptio placentae, ruptured uterus, cord prolapse or sustained cord compression, profound hypotension, maternal seizure or respiratory arrest, and rapid descent and impending delivery of the fetus. Generally, the following approach to these bradycardias should be taken. First, be patient. Often these are noticed on the central monitor, and caregivers unnecessarily run to the room and frighten the patient and family. Because most of these decelerations will spontaneously resolve in 1 to 3 minutes, such action is usually unwarranted. If the deceleration does not resolve, the patient should be examined to rule out cord prolapse and sudden descent. If these are not present, determine whether there is an apparent cause that can be specifically corrected. If the cause cannot be found, the general explanation by process of elimination is sustained cord compression, and repositioning the patient, oxygen administration, and discontinuing oxytocin are done. Should none of these work, operative delivery will be required unless spontaneous delivery is imminent. How long one should wait for the corrective measures or spontaneous recovery to occur is somewhat variable. This will be determined by the depth of the deceleration, the loss of variability during the deceleration, whether evidence of hypoxia preceded the deceleration, and whether the heart rate is intermittently returning toward baseline or is just staying down. Evidence to recommend a precise amount of time wherein intervention must occur is difficult to integrate because the problem is usually relative hypoxia rather than complete anoxia. Complete anoxia in real life probably occurs only with severe degrees of uterine rupture and complete abruption. Even with cord prolapse there is usually some cord blood flow. Windle performed the classic experiment using complete anoxia in fetal monkeys.[81] Monkeys allowed to breathe in 6 minutes or less showed no clinical or pathologic ill effects. Asphyxiation for 7 to 12 minutes resulted in transient motor and behavioral changes, with some scarring in certain specific areas of the brain in some animals. Those anoxic for 12 to 17 minutes, if death did not occur, had the most severe neurologic and clinical effects. Therefore, in the worst case of all, if delivery occurs in less than 12 minutes from the onset of the deceleration, damage will be unlikely, unless there was some hypoxia before the deceleration.

The most difficult pattern to manage is recurrent prolonged decelerations with or without bradycardia that do recover (Figure 16-32). Generally, these can be managed using the same algorithm for non-reassuring patterns described previously. However, even if one can provide reassurance that acidosis does not exist following any of the decelerations, there is a concern that this pattern portends a deceleration that will recur and will not recover, and one will be placed in the situation described in the previous paragraph. Therefore, there will be occasions when the recurrent prolonged decelerations are concerning enough that operative intervention is warranted even if there is no concern about acidosis at the present moment. One must integrate the frequency, severity, and duration of the deceleration; the fetal response in terms of tachycardia and loss of variability; presence or absence of meconium, and how much time is expected before spontaneous delivery will occur to make this difficult decision. Therefore, for example, in the nulliparous patient at 4 cm, having decelerations lasting 4 minutes to 70 beats/minute every 10 minutes, operative delivery may be warranted. However, in the multipara at 8 cm making normal progress with similar or less frequent decelerations, it may be justified to manage these expectantly, but with all preparations

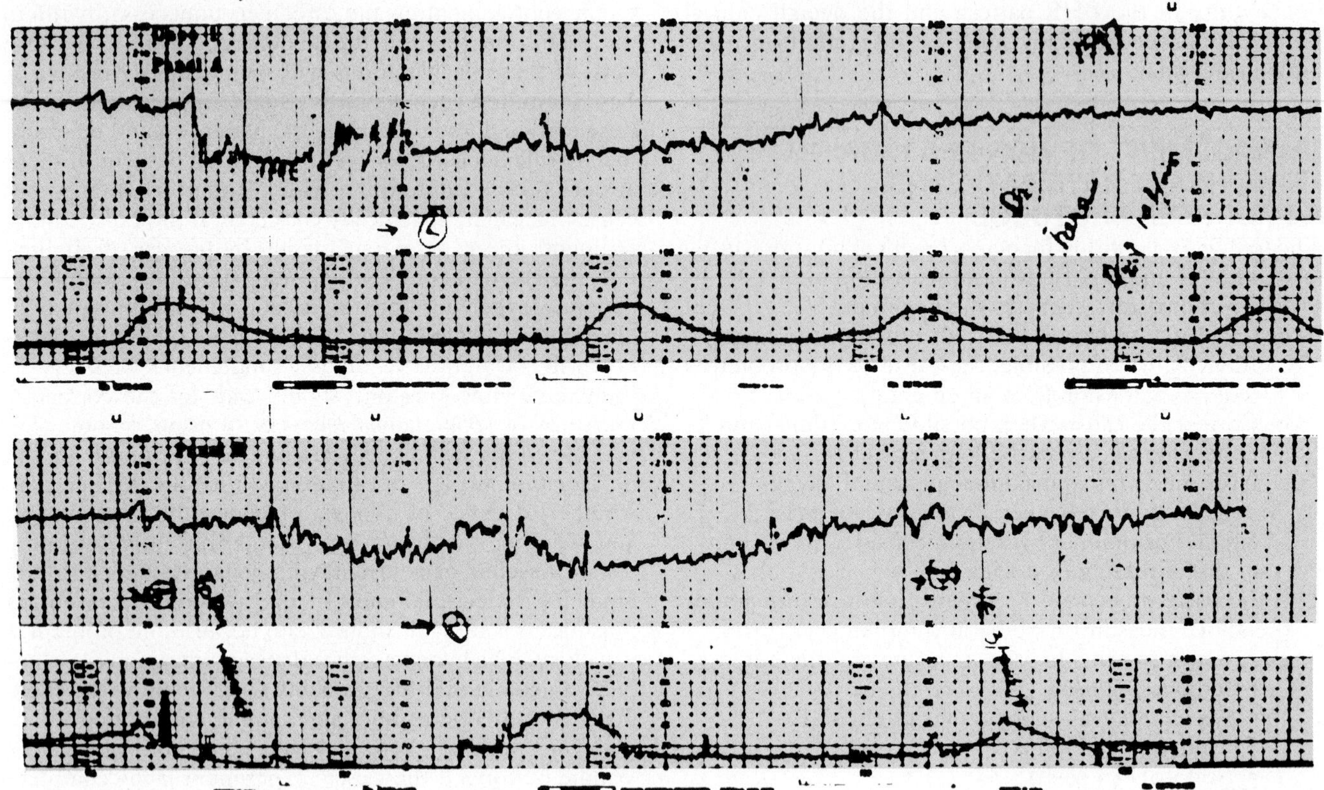

FIGURE 16-32. Recurrent unexplained prolonged decelerations.

made for immediate delivery should one of the decelerations not recover.

Auscultation as an Alternative

Almost all randomized controlled trials have demonstrated that intermittent auscultation is as effective as EFM in detecting fetal hypoxia in labor. There are some limitations to this statement, however. Virtually all these trials compared EFM to intermittent auscultation with one-on-one nursing, in which the auscultation was performed every 15 minutes in the first stage and every 5 minutes in the second stage, and the auscultation was performed for a period of 60 seconds through and following an entire uterine contraction. This is a situation that is difficult to duplicate in everyday practice because of lower nurse-to-patient ratios and because emergencies with other patients often take a nurse away from the bedside for long periods of time. Second, in most of the studies, fetuses who entered labor may have been monitored electronically before randomization, and often very-high-risk patients were excluded from study. Ingemarsson and associates have shown that 50% of patients who develop non-reassuring FHR patterns in labor had a non-reassuring FHR pattern on admission.[82] Finally, in virtually all the studies comparing EFM with auscultation, when the auscultated FHR was abnormal, the patient was then monitored electronically. Furthermore, there are non-reassuring FHR tracings that are quite indicative of hypoxia and acidosis and not likely to be detected with auscultation (Figure 16-33).

Therefore, it is reasonable to conclude that auscultation is an acceptable option for monitoring the fetus in labor when certain conditions are in place. The fetus should have a reassuring FHR on admission monitored electronically. The patient should have one-on-one nursing. The standards for frequency from the ACOG for auscultation are at least every 30 minutes in the first stage and every 15 minutes in the second stage for the low-risk patient and every 15 minutes in the first stage and every 5 minutes in the second stage for the high-risk patient.[83] Fetuses with abnormal FHR patterns on auscultation should have electronic monitoring to define the pattern and monitor for progression to worsening or non-reassuring patterns.

ASSESSMENT OF FETAL CONDITION AT BIRTH

The Apgar score was originally introduced as a tool to be used in guiding the need for neonatal resuscitation. Subsequently, this means of fetal assessment became used routinely for all births. However, the Apgar score has been expected to predict far more than was originally intended. Such expectations have included evaluating acid-base status at birth (i.e., the presence or absence of perinatal asphyxia) and even predicting long-term prognosis. **Unfortunately, the Apgar is a nonspecific measure of these parameters because many other causes of fetal depression may mimic that seen with asphyxia, such as drugs, anomalies, prematurity, suctioning for meconium, and so forth.** In situations in which FHR patterns have been concerning and other backup methods for evaluating fetal oxygenation or fetal acid-base status have been used, or in cases in which the baby is unexpectedly depressed, it is important to

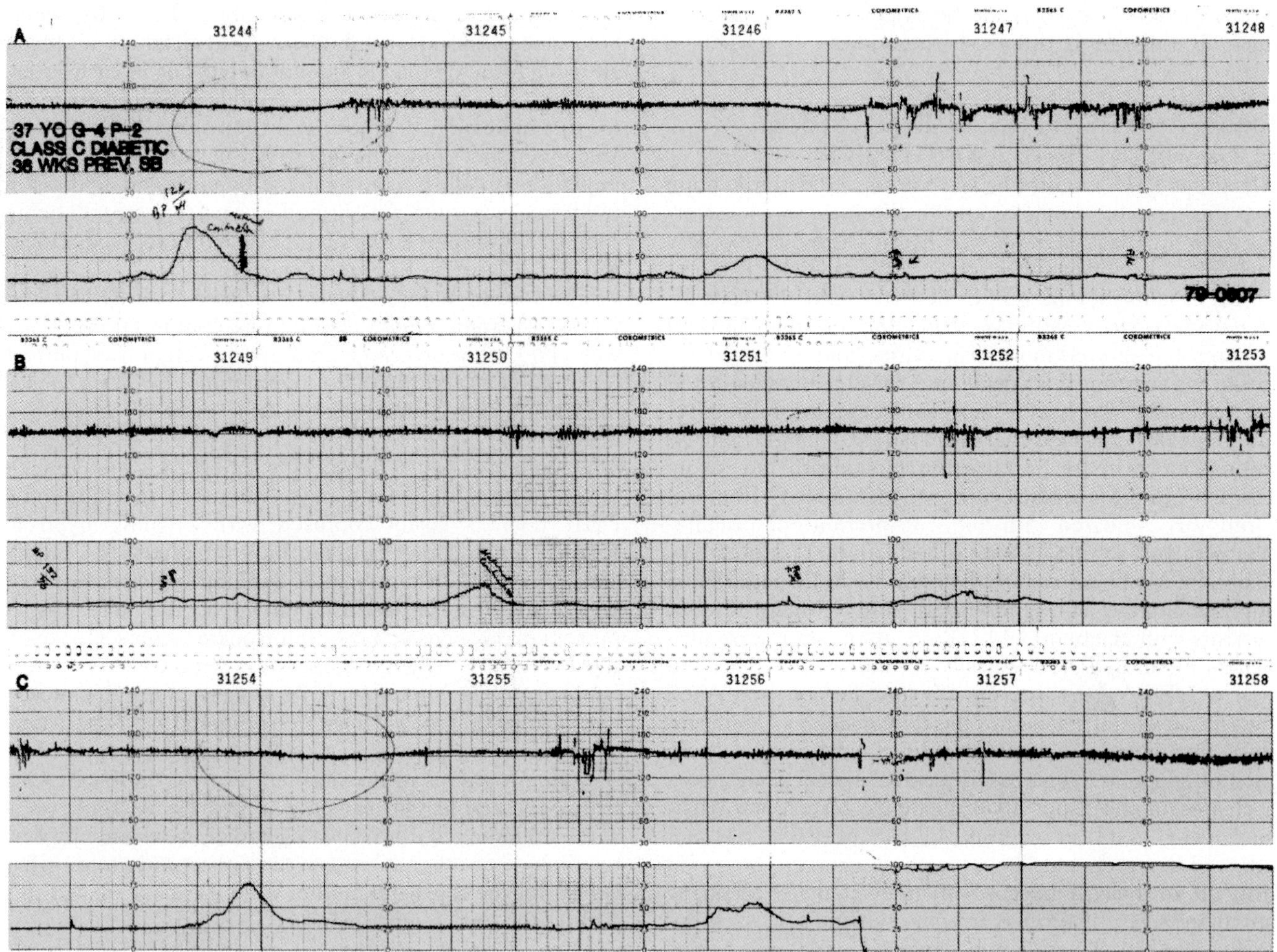

FIGURE 16-33. These persistent late decelerations associated with absent variability are difficult to recognize even with an internal electrode. This is a non-reassuring fetal heart rate pattern, which is often ominous. It is unlikely that such decelerations, associated with a normal baseline rate, would be recognized with intermittent auscultation.

specifically evaluate these parameters at birth, using umbilical cord blood gases. To accomplish this, a doubly clamped 10- to 30-cm section of umbilical cord is taken after the original cord clamping and separation of the baby from the cord. Using heparinized syringes, samples of umbilical artery and vein are separately obtained. These samples are evaluated for respiratory gases. Normal ranges for umbilical cord gases are shown in Table 16-2. Cord blood Po_2 or O_2 saturation is not useful because many normal newborns are initially hypoxemic until normal extrauterine respiration is established. Although cord pH, especially arterial, is the essential value, Pco_2 is also very important because if the pH is low, the Pco_2 is used to determine whether the acidosis is respiratory or metabolic. Respiratory acidosis is not predictive of newborn or long-term injury and should correlate with little or no need for resuscitation. In addition, the cord gases should be used to correlate interpretation of the FHR patterns, as previously described in the sections on their pathophysiology, and to determine the appropriateness of operative intervention or lack of it. These gases can help the pediatrician in determining the etiology of immediate complications and the need for more intense observation of the baby. In addition, these values are often useful if the baby develops any long-term neurologic injury in determining whether any such injury may have been related to peripartum asphyxia.[84] Studies have shown that if such asphyxia is present, in order for it to result in long-term injury, it must have been severe (metabolic acidosis

TABLE 16-2 Normal Blood Gas Values of Umbilical Artery and Vein

	MEAN VALUE	NORMAL RANGE*
Artery		
pH	7.27	7.15 to 7.38
Pco_2	50	–.35 to 70
Bicarbonate	–3.34	–.17 to 28
Base excess	–3.6	–2.0 to –9.0
Vein		
pH	7.34	7.20 to 7.41
Pco_2	40	33 to 50
Bicarbonate	21	15 to 26
Base excess	–2.6	–1.0 to –8.0

Data from Nijland R, Jongsma HW, Nijhuis JG, et al: Arterial oxygen saturation in relation to metabolic acidosis in fetal lambs. Am J Obstet Gynecol 172:810-819, 1994.

*Values are ±2 SD and represent a composite of multiple studies.

with a pH <7.00 to 7.05) and be associated with multiple organ dysfunction in the newborn period.[2]

RISKS AND BENEFITS OF ELECTRONIC FETAL HEART RATE MONITORING

Electronic FHR monitoring was introduced with the hope that this modality would reduce or eliminate the devastating consequences of asphyxia. Enthusiasm for this new technology established the role of continuous FHR monitoring in labor before studies demonstrated its accuracy. Initial retrospective studies evaluated more than 135,000 patients and showed more than a three-fold improvement in the intrapartum fetal death rate for patients monitored electronically.[1] However, most subsequent prospective, randomized, controlled trials have failed to demonstrate an improvement in the intrapartum fetal death rate using EFM.[85-91] In these studies, however, electronic FHR monitoring was compared with frequent intermittent auscultation with one-on-one nursing, a standard that is difficult to maintain. Many patients with abnormal FHR patterns on admission were not randomized, and virtually always, patients with an abnormal FHR on auscultation were ultimately monitored electronically. A randomized controlled trial of EFM versus intermittent auscultation conducted by Vintzileos and colleagues did demonstrate a significant improvement in perinatal mortality in the electronically monitored group.[92] The past three decades have not shown a change in the 2 per 1000 incidence of cerebral palsy, suggesting that the widespread use of EFM has not affected this problem. However, these data are somewhat difficult to analyze because of other changes occurring simultaneously. There has been a dramatic improvement in the survival of very-low-birthweight premature babies during this time period, and prematurity accounts for most cases of cerebral palsy. Second, term babies with asphyxia have had an increase in survival during this time period, allowing for a potential increase in surviving children with brain damage. Any of these factors may obscure an effect that FHR monitoring may have had in reducing the incidence of cerebral palsy. EFM has other potential benefits. These include an ability to understand the mechanism of developing hypoxia and to treat it more specifically. **It provides the ability to accurately monitor uterine contractions so that we can better understand progress or lack of progress in labor as well as monitor the effects of oxytocin-stimulated contractions on fetal oxygenation.** The monitor is ultimately, like all other monitors in intensive care situations, a labor-saving device that allows nurses to perform other tasks simultaneously.

EFM has several disadvantages, however. During the period in which FHR monitoring has risen in popularity, there was a parallel increase in the cesarean delivery rate. Certainly, this was not all caused by EFM because there were many other changes in obstetrical practice during this time period. In virtually all the randomized controlled trials, EFM resulted in an increase in the cesarean delivery rate over intermittent auscultation without a concomitant improvement in outcome.[85-89] There is also, however, a desire to deliver babies before significant hypoxia has any potential to damage the baby, and the nonspecific changes in FHR only fuel this concern, setting up the current environment of excessive intervention. **In reality, metabolic acidosis occurs in only about 2% of all labors, and even allowing for a reasonable amount of latitude in early intervention, cesarean delivery rates should not exceed 4% to 5% for this indication.** Unfortunately, rates of 10% for NRFS are common. Thus, the need for better, more specific modalities to allow us to evaluate hypoxia and acidosis in the fetus with a non-reassuring FHR pattern are still being sought. It was hoped that fetal pulse oximetry would meet this need, but that has not been realized.

The second major problem associated with EFM is the fear of a lawsuit should the child be compromised in any way. The monitor has created an expectation of perfect outcome. The interpretation of abnormal FHR tracings is highly subjective and variable, and "experts" often give diametrically opposite interpretations of the same tracing. The modality itself is nonspecific, and babies with anomalies or preexisting brain damage will often have abnormal FHR tracings easily confused with ongoing hypoxia. Finally, a jury cannot help but be sympathetic to a family and baby with disfiguring and debilitating cerebral palsy, and large financial awards seem to be the only way at present to compensate these unfortunate victims. However, these outcomes are not consistent with what we know about asphyxia. More than 75% of brain-damaged children have causes that are *not* related to perinatal asphyxia. Many cases of asphyxia occur *before* labor or early in labor before the patient arrives in the hospital. Few of these cases are truly preventable. One can only hope that once these pressures are removed from the labor and delivery suite by new technology or other solutions, the opportunity to do what is best for the fetus and mother will be enhanced, and this will be the only motivating force.

SUMMARY

EFM has become the standard means for evaluating fetal oxygenation in labor. Because of fetal inaccessibility and the lack of alternatives to more specifically evaluate fetal oxygenation, this modality has been the only alternative. EFM is highly reliable when reassuring (category I) and most often unreliable with equivocal tracings (category II), except in the extreme (category III), when there is high likelihood of fetal acidosis. Despite or even because of these limitations, it is imperative that the clinician understand as much as possible about the underlying physiologic explanations of normal and abnormal FHR patterns because this allows the only reasonable opportunity to appropriately evaluate and manage these changes. The new terminology proposed by the NICHD Workshop and endorsed by ACOG and AWHONN should be used consistently. The goals of FHR monitoring should be to carefully and thoroughly monitor all patients in active labor; avoid unnecessary operative and nonoperative intervention for benign and innocuous FHR patterns; correct non-reassuring FHR patterns with noninvasive, etiology-specific therapies when possible, or if not possible use appropriate means such as scalp pH, accelerations, or moderate variability to rule out acidosis; and finally, if acidosis cannot be ruled out, operatively intervene in an expeditious manner appropriate for the entire clinical situation.

KEY POINTS

- The goals of intrapartum fetal evaluation by electronic FHR monitoring and available back-up methods are to detect fetal hypoxia, reverse the hypoxia with nonsurgical means, or if unsuccessful, determine whether the hypoxia has progressed to metabolic acidosis, and if so deliver the baby expeditiously to avoid the hypoxia and acidosis from resulting in any damage to the baby.
- New terminology has been proposed by the NICHD Workshop on intrapartum EFM and should be consistently employed in practice.
- EFM is an inherently suboptimal method of determining fetal hypoxia and acidosis because many factors besides these variables may alter the FHR and mimic changes caused by hypoxia and acidosis. When the FHR is normal, its reliability for predicting the absence of fetal compromise is high, but when the FHR is abnormal, its reliability for predicting the presence of asphyxia is poor.
- The three-tiered classification of FHR patterns proposed by the NICHD Workshop on EFM and endorsed by ACOG and AWHONN should be used as a template for evaluation and management of FHR patterns, but the limitations of the guidelines for the frequently occurring category II patterns should be realized and plans made to deal more specifically with different types of FHR patterns within this group.
- Late decelerations are always indicative of relative fetal hypoxia and are caused by inadequate oxygen delivery, exchange, or uptake that is aggravated by the additional hypoperfusion of the placenta caused by contractions. Variable decelerations are caused by a decrease in umbilical cord flow resulting from cord compression or cord stretch. Prolonged decelerations may be caused by any mechanism that decreases fetal oxygenation.
- In labor, loss of variability, loss of accelerations, and tachycardia should only be interpreted as indicative of fetal compromise in the presence of non-reassuring decelerations (late, non-reassuring variable or prolonged decelerations) because signs of hypoxia should always precede signs of neurologic depression secondary to hypoxia.
- In the presence of oligohydramnios and variable decelerations, intrapartum amnioinfusion has been shown to decrease rates of cesarean delivery for NRFS.
- In the presence of an otherwise non-reassuring FHR pattern, the presence of accelerations of the FHR, either spontaneous or elicited by scalp stimulation or vibroacoustic stimulation, indicates the absence of fetal acidosis. The absence of accelerations is associated with a 50% chance of fetal acidosis, but only in the setting of a non-reassuring FHR.
- Umbilical cord blood gases should be obtained and documented in situations in which there is a non-reassuring or confusing FHR pattern during labor, neonatal depression following birth, prematurity, or suctioning for meconium. These values will help clarify the reasons for abnormal FHR patterns or for neonatal depression.
- Although there is correlation between a non-reassuring FHR pattern and neonatal depression, the FHR is a poor predictor of long-term neurologic sequelae. Furthermore, fetuses with previous neurologic insults may have significantly abnormal FHR patterns even when they are well oxygenated in labor.

REFERENCES

1. Freeman RK, Garite TJ, Nageotte MP: Clinical management of fetal distress. In Fetal Heart Rate Monitoring, 2nd ed. Baltimore, Williams & Wilkins, 1991.
2. American College of Obstetricians and Gynecologists: Fetal and Neonatal Neurologic Injury. Technical Bulletin No. 163, January 1992.
3. Eastman NJ, Kohl SG, Maisel JE, et al: The obstetrical background of 753 cases of cerebral palsy. Obstet Gynecol Surv 17:459, 1962.
4. Nelson KB, Ellenberg JH: Epidemiology of cerebral palsy. In Schoenberg BS: Advances in Neurology, Vol. 19. New York, Raven Press, 1979.
5. Wegman M: Annual summary of vital statistics. Pediatrics 70:835, 1982.
6. Benson RC, Shubeck F, Deutschberger J, et al: Fetal heart rate as a predictor of fetal distress: a report from the Collaborative Project. Obstet Gynecol 32:529, 1968.
7. Cremer M: Munch. Med Wochensem 58:811, 1906.
8. Hon EH, Hess OW: The clinical value of fetal electrocardiography. Am J Obstet Gynecol 79:1012, 1960.
9. Hon EH: The electronic evaluation of the fetal heart rate. Am J Obstet Gynecol 75:1215, 1958.
10. Hon EH: Observations on "pathologic" fetal bradycardia. Am J Obstet Gynecol 77:1084, 1959.
11. Caldeyro-Barcia R, Mendez-Bauer C, Poseiro JJ, et al: Control of human fetal heart rate during labor. In Cassels D: The Heart and Circulation in the Newborn Infant. New York, Grune & Stratton, 1966.
12. Hammacher K: In Kaser O, Friedberg V, Oberk K: Gynakologie v Gerburtshilfe BD II. Stutgart, Georg Thieme Verlag, 1967.
13. American College of Obstetricians and Gynecologists: Inappropriate use of the terms fetal distress and birth asphyxia. ACOG Committee Opinion 326, 2005.
14. Macones GA, Hankins GD, Spong CY, et al: The 2008 National Institute of Child Health and Human Development Workshop Report on Electronic Fetal Monitoring. Obstet Gynecol 112:661, 2008.
15. Vintzileos M, Campbell WA, Nochimson DJ, Weinbaum PJ: Degree of oligohydramnios and pregnancy outcome in patients with PROM. Obstet Gynecol 66:162, 1985.
16. Roach MR: The umbilical vessels. In Goodwin JM, Godden DO, Chance GW: Perinatal Medicine. Baltimore, Williams & Wilkins, 1976, p 136.
17. Electronic Fetal Heart Rate Monitoring: Research Guidelines for Interpretation, National Institute of Child Health and Human Development Research Planning Workshop. Am J Obstet Gynecol 177:1385, 1997.
18. Schifferli P, Caldeyro-Barcia R: Effects of atropine and beta adrenergic drugs on the heart rate of the human fetus. In Boreus L: Fetal Pharmacology. New York, Raven Press, 1973, p 259.
19. Bisonette JM: Relationship between continuous fetal heart rate patterns and Apgar score in the newborn. Br J Obstet Gynaecol 82:24, 1975.
20. Langer O, Cohen WR: Persistent fetal bradycardia during maternal hypoglycemia. Am J Obstet Gynecol 149:688, 1984.

21. Parsons MT, Owens CA, Spellacy WN: Thermic effects of tocolytic agents: decreased temperature with magnesium sulfate. Obstet Gynecol 69:88, 1987.
22. Gembruch U, Hansmann M, Redel DA, et al: Fetal complete heart block: antenatal diagnosis, significance and management. Eur J Obstet Gynecol Reprod Biol 31:9, 1989.
23. Druzen M, Ikenoue T, Murata Y, et al: A possible mechanism for the increase in FHR variability following hypoxemia. Presented at the 26th Annual Meeting of the Society for Gynecological Investigation, San Diego, California, March 23, 1979.
24. Paul WM, Quilligan EJ, MacLachlan T: Cardiovascular phenomenon associated with fetal head compression. Am J Obstet Gynecol 90:824, 1964.
25. Martin CB Jr, de Haan J, van der Wildt B, et al: Mechanisms of late deceleration in the fetal heart rate: a study with autonomic blocking agents in fetal lambs. Eur J Obstet Gynecol Reprod Biol 9:361, 1979.
26. Lee R, Moore M, Brewster W, et al: Late decelerations and severe variables are predictive of fetal hypoxia. Poster Presentation at the Annual Meeting of the Society for Maternal Fetal Medicine, New Orleans, LA, January 14-19, 2002.
27. Francis J, Garite T: The association between abruptio placentae and abnormal FHR patterns. (Submitted for publication.)
28. Barcroft J: Researches on Prenatal Life. Oxford, Blackwell Scientific Publications, 1946.
29. Lee ST, Hon EH: Fetal hemodynamic response to umbilical cord compression. Obstet Gynecol 22:554, 1963.
30. Kubli FW, Hon EH, Khazin AE, et al: Observations on heart rate and pH in the human fetus during labor. Am J Obstet Gynecol 104:1190, 1969.
31. Goodlin RC, Lowe EW: A functional umbilical cord occlusion heart rate pattern. The significance of overshoot. Obstet Gynecol 42:22, 1974.
32. Navot D, Yaffe H, Sadovsky E: The ratio of fetal heart rate accelerations to fetal movements according to gestational age. Am J Obstet Gynecol 149:92, 1984.
33. Clark S, Gimovsky M, Miller FC: Fetal heart rate response to scalp blood sampling. Am J Obstet Gynecol 144:706, 1982.
34. Clark S, Gimovsky M, Miller F: The scalp stimulation test: a clinical alternative to fetal scalp blood sampling. Am J Obstet Gynecol 148:274, 1984.
35. Smith C, Hguyen H, Phelan J, Paul R: Intrapartum assessment of fetal well-being: a comparison of fetal acoustic stimulation with acid base determinations. Am J Obstet Gynecol 155:776, 1986.
36. Kubli F, Ruttgers, H, Haller U, et al: Die antepartale fetale Herzfrequenz. II. Verhalten von Grundfrequenz, Fluktuation und Dezerationo bei antepartalem Fruchttod, Z. Gerburtshilfe Perinatol 176:309, 1972.
37. Shenker L: Clinical experience with fetal heart rate monitoring of 1000 patients in labor. Am J Obstet Gynecol 115:1111, 1973.
38. Modanlou H, Freeman RK: Sinusoidal fetal heart rate pattern: its definition and clinical significance. Am J Obstet Gynecol 142:1033, 1982.
39. Murata Y, Miyake Y, Yamamoto T, et al: Experimentally produced sinusoidal fetal heart rate pattern in the chronically instrumented fetal lamb. Am J Obstet Gynecol 153:693, 1985.
40. Angel J, Knuppel R, Lake M: Sinusoidal fetal heart rate patterns associated with intravenous butorphanol administration. Am J Obstet Gynecol 149:465, 1984.
41. Epstein H, Waxman A, Gleicher N, et al: Meperidine induced sinusoidal fetal heart rate pattern and reversal with naloxone. Obstet Gynecol 59:225, 1982.
42. Murata Y, Martin CB, Ikenoue T, et al: Fetal heart rate accelerations and late decelerations during the course of intrauterine death in chronically catheterized rhesus monkeys. Am J Obstet Gynecol 144:218, 1982.
43. Khazin AF, Hon EH, Hehre FW: Effects of maternal hyperoxia on the fetus. I. Oxygen tension. Am J Obstet Gynecol 109:628, 1971.
44. Althabe O Jr, Schwarcz RL, Pose SV, et al: Effects on fetal heart rate and fetal pO2 of oxygen administration to the mother. Am J Obstet Gynecol 98:858, 1967.
45. Bartnicki J, Saling E: Influence of maternal oxygen administration on the computer-analysed fetal heart rate patterns in small-for-gestational-age fetuses. Gynecol Obstet Invest 37:172, 1994.
46. Fawole B, Hofmeyr GJ: Maternal oxygen administration for fetal distress. Cochrane Database Syst Rev 4:CD000136, 2003.
47. Dildy G, Clark S, Loucks C: Intrapartum fetal pulse oximetry: the effects of maternal hyperoxia on fetal oxygen saturation mark. Am J Obstet Gynecol 171:1120, 1994.
48. Haydon ML, Gorenberg DM, Nageotte MP, et al: The effect of maternal oxygen administration on fetal pulse oximetimetry during labor in fetuses with nonreassuring fetal heart rate patterns. Am J Obstet Gynecol 195:735, 2006.
49. Simpson KR, James DC: Efficacy of intrauterine resuscitation techniques in improving fetal oxygen status during labor. Obstet Gynecol 105:1362, 2005.
50. Aldrich CJ, D'Antona D, Spencer JA, et al: The effect of maternal posture on fetal cerebral oxygenation during labour. Br J Obstet Gynaecol 102:14, 1995.
51. Carbonne B, Benachi A, Leveque ML, et al: Maternal position during labor: effects on fetal oxygen saturation measured by pulse oximetry. Obstet Gynecol 88:797, 1996.
52. Noakes TD: Fluid replacement during exercise. Exerc Sport Sci Rev 21:297, 1993.
53. Garite TJ, Weeks J, Peters-Phair K, et al: A randomized controlled trial of the effect of increased intravenous hydration on the course of labor in nulliparas. Am J Obstet Gynecol 183:1544, 2000.
54. Lipshitz J: Use of B2 sympathomimetic drug as a temporizing measure in the treatment of acute fetal distress. Am J Obstet Gynecol 129:31, 1977.
55. Tejani N, Verma UL, Chatterjee S, et al: Terbutaline in the management of acute intrapartum fetal acidosis. J Reprod Med 28:857, 1983.
56. Arias F: Intrauterine resuscitation with terbutaline: a method for the management of acute intrapartum fetal distress. Am J Obstet Gynecol 131:39, 1977.
57. Patriarcho MS, Viechnicki BN, Hutchinson TA: A study on intrauterine fetal resuscitation with terbutaline. Am J Obstet Gynecol 157:383, 1987.
58. Burke MS, Porreco RP, Day D, et al: Intrauterine resuscitation with tocolysis: an alternate month clinical trial. J Perinatol 10:296, 1989.
59. Miyazaki F, Nevarez F: Saline amnioinfusion for relief of repetitive variable decelerations: a prospective randomized study. Am J Obstet Gynecol 153:301, 1985.
60. Nageotte MP, Freeman RK, Garite TJ, et al: Prophylactic intrapartum amnioinfusion in patients with preterm premature rupture of membranes. Am J Obstet Gynecol 153:557, 1985.
61. Owen J, Henson BV, Hauth JC: A prospective randomized study of saline solution amnioinfusion. Am J Obstet Gynecol 162:1146, 1990.
62. Delee JB, Pollack C: Intrauterine injection of saline to replace the amniotic fluid. Obstet Gynecol 1925.
63. Miyazaki F, Taylor N: Saline amnioinfusion for relief of variable or prolonged decelerations. Am J Obstet Gynecol 14:670, 1983.
64. Pierce J, Gaudier FL, Sanchez-Ramos L: Intrapartum amnioinfusion for meconium-stained fluid: meta-analysis of prospective clinical trials. Obstet Gynecol 95:1051, 2000.
65. Wenstrom K, Andrews WW, Maher JE: Amnioinfusion survey: prevalence, protocols and complications. Obstet Gynecol 86:572, 1995.
66. Hofmeyr GJ, Xu H: Amnioinfusion for meconium-stained liquor in labour. Cochrane Database Syst Rev 20:CD000014, 2010.
67. Clark SL, Paul RH: Intrapartum fetal surveillance: the role of fetal scalp blood sampling. Am J Obstet Gynecol 153:717, 1985.
68. Goodwin TM, Milner-Masterson C, Paul R: Elimination of fetal scalp blood sampling on a large clinical service. Obstet Gynecol 83:971, 1994.
69. Nijland R, Jongsma HW, Nijhuis JG, et al: Arterial oxygen saturation in relation to metabolic acidosis in fetal lambs. Am J Obstet Gynecol 172:810, 1994.
70. Richardson B, Carmichael L, Homan J, Patrick J: Cerebral oxidative metabolism in fetal sheep with prolonged, graded hypoxemia. Presented at the 36th Meeting of the Society for Gynecologic Investigation, San Diego, California, March 1989.
71. Garite TJ, Dildy GA, McNamara H, et al: A multicenter controlled trial of fetal pulse oximetry in the intrapartum management of nonreassuring fetal heart rate patterns. Am J Obstet Gynecol 183:1049, 2000.
72. Bloom SL, Spong CY, Thom E, et al: Fetal pulse oximetry and cesarean delivery. N Engl J Med 355:2195, 2006.
73. Amer-Wåhlin I, Hellsten C, Norén H, et al: Cardiotocography only versus cardiotocography plus ST analysis of fetal electrocardiogram for intrapartum fetal monitoring: a Swedish randomised controlled trial. Lancet 358:534, 2001.

74. Westgate J, Harris M, Curnow JSH, Greene KR: Plymouth randomised trial of cardiotocogram only versus ST waveform plus cardiotocogram for intrapartum monitoring: 2,400 cases. Am J Obstet Gynecol 169:1151, 1993.
75. Neilson JP: Fetal electrocardiogram (ECG) for fetal monitoring during labour. Cochrane Database Syst Rev 19:CD000116, 2006.
76. Nielsen PV, Stigsby B, Nickelsen C, Nim J: Intra- and inter-observer variability in the assessment of intrapartum cardiotocograms. Acta Obstet Gynecol Scand 66:421, 1987.
77. Elliott C, Warrick PA, Graham E, Hamilton EF: Graded classification of fetal heart rate tracings: association with neonatal metabolic acidosis and neurologic morbidity. Am J Obstet Gynecol 202:258, 2010.
78. Parer JT, Hamilton EF: Comparison of 5 experts and computer analysis in rule-based fetal heart rate interpretation. Am J Obstet Gynecol 2010 Jul 14. [Epub ahead of print]
79. Parer JT: Fetal heart rate monitoring: the next step? [editorial]. Am J Obstet Gynecol 203:5, 2010.
80. American Academy of Pediatrics and American College of Obstetricians and Gynecologists: Guidelines for Perinatal Care, 4th ed. Washington, DC, ACOG, 1997, p 112.
81. Windle WF: Neuropathology of certain forms of mental retardation. Science 140:1186, 1963.
82. Ingemarsson I, Arulkumaran S, Ingemarsson E, et al: Admission test: a screening test for fetal distress in labor. Obstet Gynecol 68:800, 1986.
83. American College of Obstetricians and Gynecologists: Fetal Heart Rate Patterns: Monitoring, Interpretation and Management. Technical Bulletin No. 207, July 1995.
84. Thorp JA, Rushing RS: Umbilical cord blood gas analysis. Obstet Gynecol Clin North Am 26:695, 1999.
85. Haverkamp AD, Thompson HE, McFee JG, et al: The evaluation of continuous fetal heart rate monitoring in high risk pregnancy. Am J Obstet Gynecol 125:310, 1976.
86. Haverkamp AD, Orleans M, Langendoerfer S, et al: A controlled trial of the differential effects of intrapartum fetal monitoring. Am J Obstet Gynecol 134:399, 1979.
87. Renou P, Chang A, Anderson I, et al: Controlled trial of fetal intensive care. Am J Obstet Gynecol 126:470, 1976.
88. Kelso IM, Parsons RJ, Lawrence GF, et al: An assessment of continuous fetal heart rate monitoring in labor: a randomized trial. Am J Obstet Gynecol 131:526, 1978.
89. Wood C, Renou P, Oates J, et al: A controlled trial of fetal heart rate monitoring in a low-risk population. Am J Obstet Gynecol 141:527, 1981.
90. McDonald D, Grant A, Sheridan-Pereira M, et al: The Dublin randomized control trial of intrapartum fetal heart rate monitoring. Am J Obstet Gynecol 152:524, 1985.
91. Leveno KJ, Cunningham FG, Nelson S, et al: A prospective comparison of selective and universal electronic fetal monitoring in 34,995 pregnancies. N Engl J Med 315:615, 1986.
92. Vintzileos AM, Antsaklis A, Varvarigos I, et al: A randomized trial of intrapartum electronic fetal heart rate monitoring versus intermittent auscultation. Obstet Gynecol 81:899, 1993.

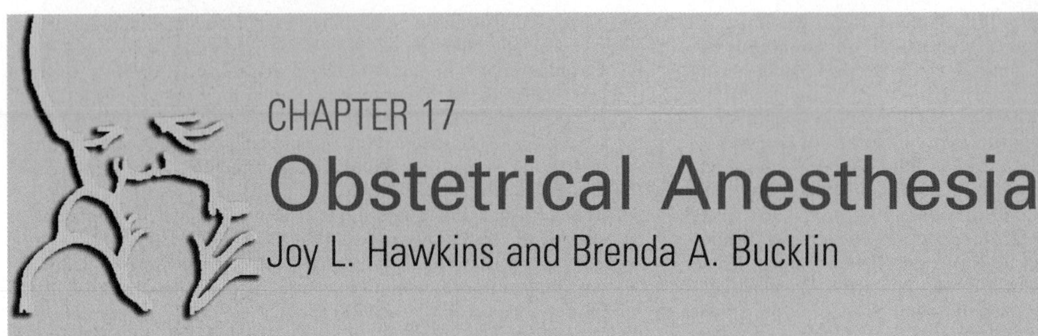

CHAPTER 17 Obstetrical Anesthesia

Joy L. Hawkins and Brenda A. Bucklin

KEY ABBREVIATIONS	
American Society of Anesthesiologists	ASA
Confidence Interval	CI
Central Nervous System	CNS
Combined Spinal-epidural	CSE
Effective Dose	ED
Induction-to-delivery Interval	I-D
Odds Ratio	OR
Patient-controlled Analgesia	PCA
Patient-controlled Epidural Analgesia	PCEA
Patient-controlled Intravenous Analgesia	PCIA
Postdural Puncture Headache	PDPH
Relative Risk	RR
Uterine Incision-to-delivery Interval	U-D

Obstetrical anesthesia encompasses all techniques used by anesthesiologists and obstetricians to alleviate the pain associated with labor and delivery: general anesthesia, neuraxial anesthesia (spinal or epidural), local anesthesia (local infiltration, paracervical block, pudendal block), and parenteral analgesia. **Pain relief during labor and delivery is an essential part of good obstetrical care.** Unique clinical considerations guide anesthesia provision for obstetrical patients; physiologic changes of pregnancy and increases in certain complications must be considered. This chapter reviews the various methods that can be used for obstetrical analgesia and anesthesia, as well as their indications and complications.

PERSONNEL

Anesthesiologists, working either independently or supervising a team of residents or certified nurse anesthetists, provide anesthesia for 98% of obstetrical procedures in larger hospitals in the United States.[1] Nurse anesthetists, independent of anesthesiologists, rarely provide anesthesia for obstetrical cases in larger hospitals but provide anesthesia for 34% of obstetrical procedures in hospitals with fewer than 500 births per year.[1] The American Society of Anesthesiologists (ASA) partnered with the American College of Obstetricians and Gynecologists (ACOG) to issue the Joint Statement on the Optimal Goals for Anesthesia Care in Obstetrics,[2] recommending that a qualified anesthesiologist assume responsibility for anesthetics in every hospital providing obstetrical care. The statement notes: "There are obstetric units where obstetricians or obstetrician-supervised nurse anesthetists administer anesthetics. **The administration of general or regional anesthesia requires both medical judgment and technical skills.** Thus, a physician with privileges in anesthesiology should be readily available."[2] To provide optimal care for the parturient, the ASA also states in their Practice Guidelines for Obstetric Anesthesia that, "**A communication system should be in place to encourage early and ongoing contact between obstetric providers, anesthesiologists, and other members of the multidisciplinary team.**"[3]

PAIN PATHWAYS

Pain during the first stage of labor results from a combination of uterine contractions and cervical dilation. Painful sensations travel from the uterus through visceral afferent (sympathetic) nerves that enter the spinal cord through the posterior segments of thoracic spinal nerves 10, 11, and 12 (Figure 17-1). During the second stage of labor, additional painful stimuli are added as the fetal head distends the pelvic floor, vagina, and perineum. The sensory fibers of sacral nerves 2, 3, and 4 (i.e., the pudendal nerve) transmit painful impulses from the perineum to the spinal cord during second stage and during any perineal repair (see Figure 17-1). **During cesarean delivery, although the incision is usually around thoracic spinal nerve 12 (T12) dermatome, anesthesia is required to a level of thoracic spinal nerve 4 (T4) to completely block peritoneal discomfort,**

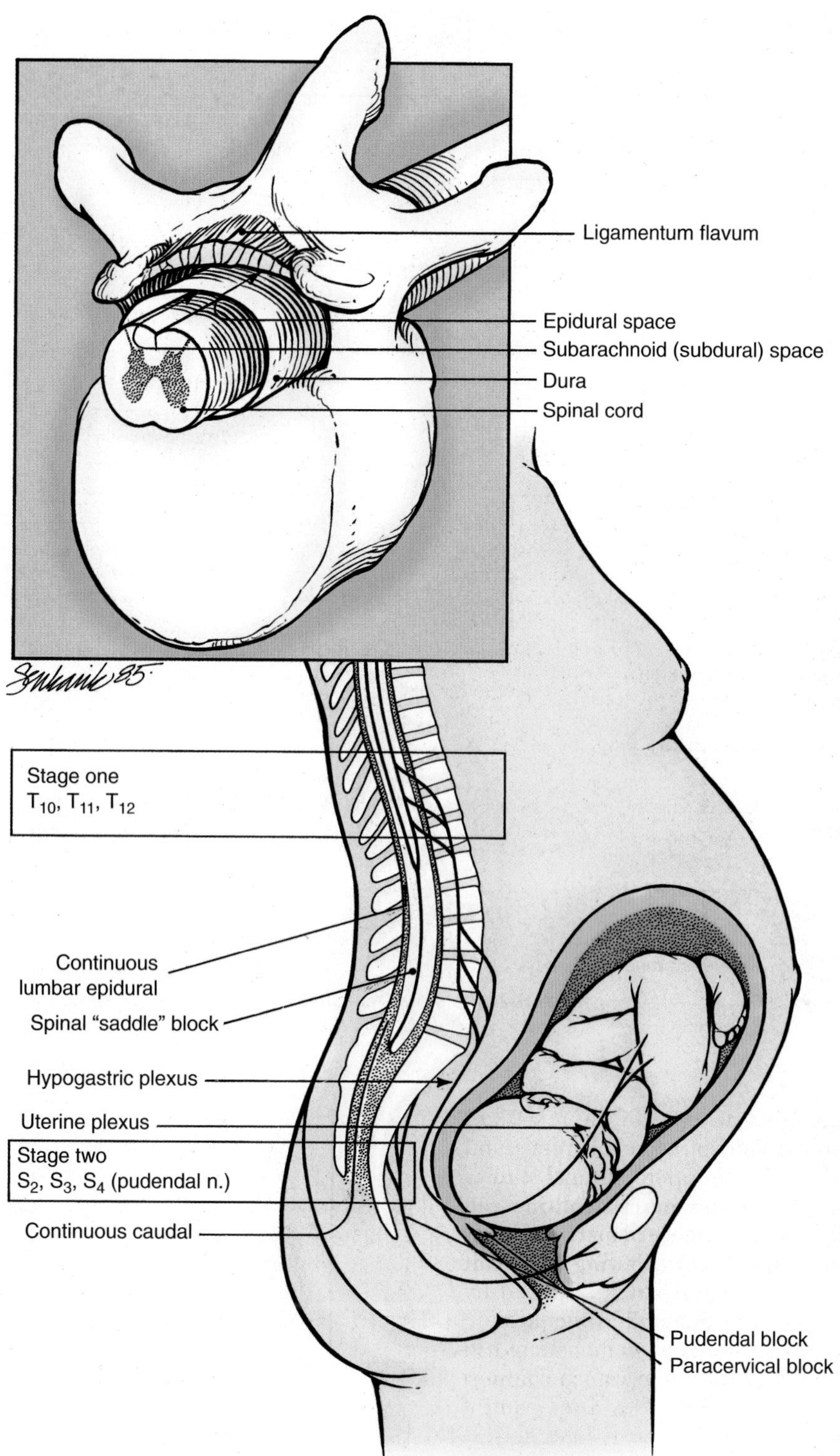

FIGURE 17-1. Pain pathways of labor and delivery and nerves blocked by various anesthetic techniques.

especially during uterine exteriorization. Pain after cesarean delivery is due to both incisional pain and uterine involution.

EFFECTS OF PAIN AND STRESS

The process of labor involves significant pain and stress for most women. Using the McGill Pain Questionnaire, which measures intensity and quality of pain, Melzack and colleagues[4] found that 59% of nulliparous and 43% of parous patients described their labor pain in terms more severe than did those suffering from cancer pain. **The most substantial predictors of pain intensity were ultimately socioeconomic status and prior menstrual difficulties.**

The maternal and fetal stress response to the pain of labor has been difficult to assess. Most investigators have

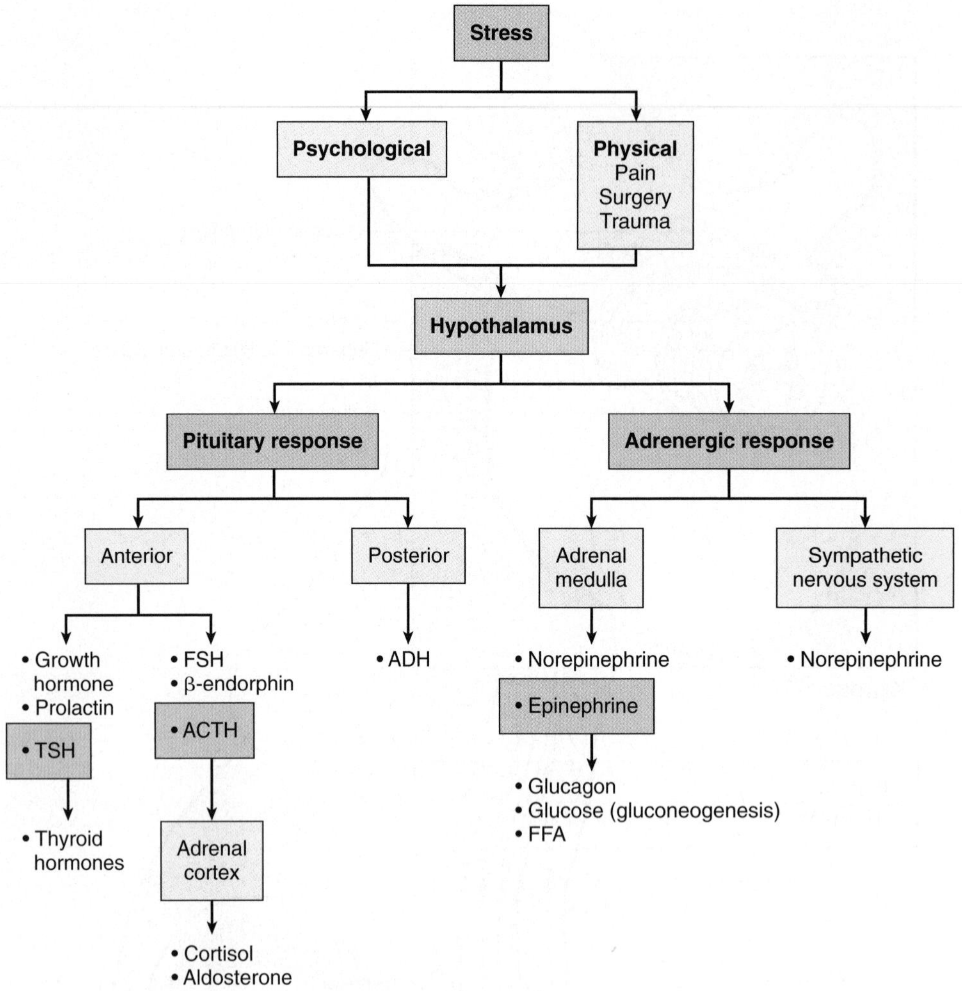

FIGURE 17-2. The stress response.

described and quantified stress in terms of the release of adrenocorticotropic hormone, cortisol, catecholamines, and β-endorphins (Figure 17-2). Furthermore, **animal studies indicate that both epinephrine and norepinephrine can decrease uterine blood flow in the absence of maternal heart rate and blood pressure changes, contributing to occult fetal asphyxia.** Maternal psychological stress (induced by bright lights or toe clamp) can detrimentally affect uterine blood flow and fetal acid-base status as demonstrated in baboons and monkeys.[5] In pregnant sheep, catecholamines increase and uterine blood flow decreases after painful stimuli and after nonpainful stimuli (such as loud noises) that induce fear and anxiety, as evidenced by struggling (Figure 17-3).

Although some of the physiologic stress of labor is unavoidable, analgesia and anesthesia may reduce stress responses that are secondary to pain. Postpartum women suffer objective deficits in cognitive and memory function compared with nonpregnant women.[6] Intrapartum analgesia does not exacerbate, but rather *lessens*, the cognitive defect compared with unmedicated parturients. Analgesia also reduces paternal anxiety and stress, increases the fathers' feelings of helpfulness, and enhances their involvement and satisfaction with the childbirth experience.[7]

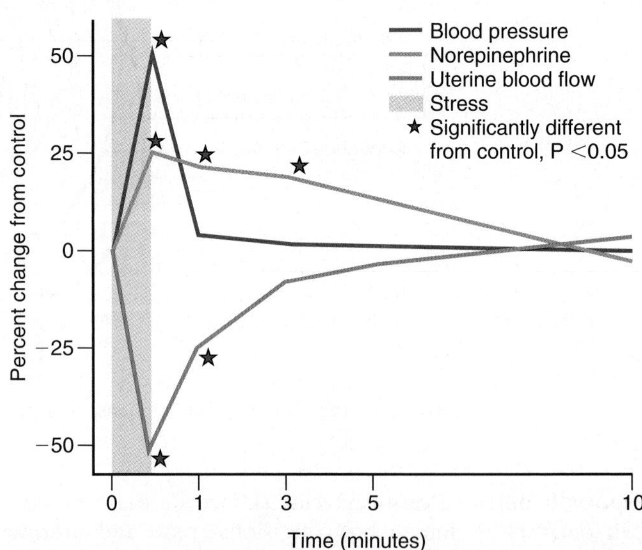

FIGURE 17-3. Effects of electrically induced stress (30 to 60 seconds) on maternal mean arterial blood pressure, plasma norepinephrine levels, and uterine blood flow. (Modified from Shnider SM, Wright RG, Levinson G, et al: Uterine blood flow and plasma norepinephrine changes during maternal stress in the pregnant ewe. Anesthesiology 50:524, 1979.)

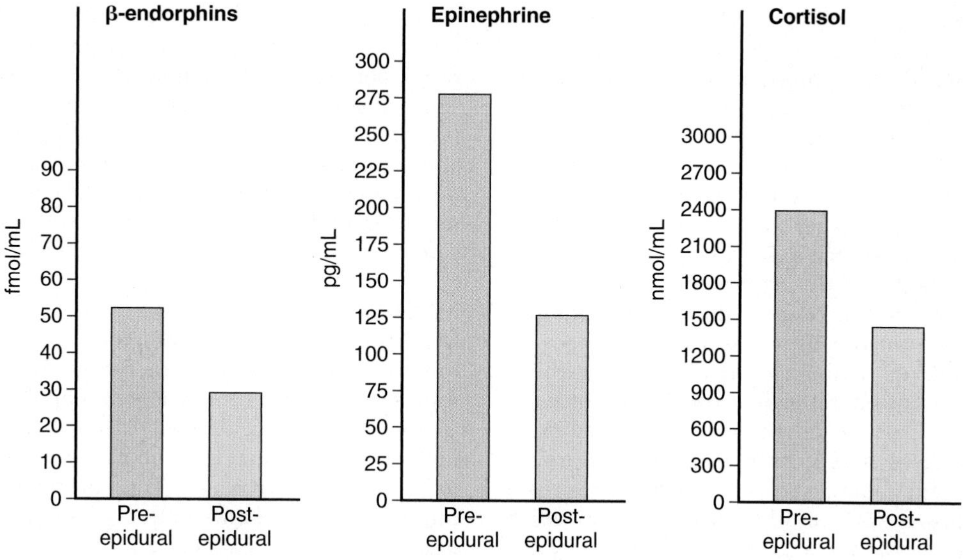

FIGURE 17-4. Effects of epidural analgesia on the response to stress.

TABLE 17-1 ANALGESIC PROCEDURES USED FOR LABOR PAIN RELIEF IN 2001 ACCORDING TO SIZE OF DELIVERY SERVICE

HOSPITAL SIZE (BIRTHS/YEAR)	NO ANESTHESIA (%)	NARCOTICS BARBITURATES TRANQUILIZERS (%)	PARACERVICAL BLOCK (%)	SPINAL OR EPIDURAL BLOCK (%)
<500	12	37	3	57
500-1499	10	42	3	59
>1500	6	34	2	77

Modified from Bucklin BA, Hawkins JL, Anderson JR, Ullrich FA: Obstetric anesthesia workforce survey. Anesthesiology 103:645, 2005.

Epidural analgesia prevents increases in both cortisol and 11-hydroxycorticosteroid levels during labor, but systemically administered opioids do not. Epidural analgesia also attenuates elevations of epinephrine, norepinephrine, and endorphin levels[8] (Figure 17-4). Assuming any hypotension is rapidly treated and perfusion is preserved by uterine displacement, fetal acid-base status (as measured by base deficit) of human infants whose mothers receive epidural anesthesia during the first stage of labor is altered less than that of infants of mothers who receive systemic opioid analgesia.

ANALGESIA FOR LABOR

Table 17-1 presents the frequency with which the various forms of analgesia are used during labor. The data are from a large survey of hospitals in the United States, stratified by the size of their delivery service.[1]

Psychoprophylaxis and Nonpharmacologic Analgesia Techniques

Psychoprophylaxis is any nonpharmacologic method that minimizes the perception of painful uterine contractions. Relaxation, concentration on breathing, gentle massage, and partner or doula participation contribute to effectiveness. One of the method's most valuable contributions is that it is often taught in prepared childbirth classes, where parents tour the labor and delivery suite and learn about the normal processes of labor and delivery, in many instances mitigating their fear of the unknown.

Although psychoprophylactic techniques can be empowering, most women will still ultimately blend them with pharmacologic methods.[1] Because most first-time mothers choose epidural analgesia, teaching that use of drug-induced pain relief represents failure or will harm the child is counterproductive and can heighten fear and anxiety during labor.

Nonpharmacologic techniques for labor analgesia may be used alone or in conjunction with parenteral or regional techniques. A systematic review of acupuncture concluded that the evidence for efficacy is promising but that there is a paucity of data.[9] From the three randomized clinical trials they reviewed, the authors suggest that acupuncture alleviates labor pain and reduces use of both epidural analgesia and parenteral opioids. Acupuncture may be helpful for patients who feel strongly about avoiding epidural analgesia in labor, although arranging to have a qualified and credentialed acupuncture provider available at the time of delivery may be challenging. A randomized controlled trial of laboring in water found no advantage in labor outcome or in reducing the need for analgesia, but the request for epidural analgesia was delayed by about 30 minutes.[10] The American Academy of Pediatrics Committee on Fetus and Newborn has expressed concerns about *delivering* in water because of the lack of trials demonstrating safety and the rare but reported unusual complications such as infection or asphyxia.[11] They state that, "underwater birth should be considered an experimental procedure that should not be performed except within the context of an appropriately designed RCT after informed parental consent." Intracutaneous sterile water injections are simple to perform and have good evidence for efficacy, perhaps by a similar gating mechanism as acupuncture.[12] An intradermal injection of 0.1 mL of sterile water at four sites in the lower back significantly lowers visual analog pain scores during labor. A number of studies have examined transcutaneous electrical nerve stimulation during labor. Patients tend to rate the device as helpful, despite the fact it does not decrease pain scores or the use of additional analgesics. As one study noted, transcutaneous electrical nerve stimulation units do not appear to change the degree of pain, but somehow may have made the pain less disturbing.[13] **Although the efficacy of these techniques is largely unproved because of a lack of randomized clinical trials, there are no serious safety concerns with any of these techniques, which is attractive to patients and their caregivers.** Women expect to have choices and a degree of control during their childbirth, and their caregivers should provide analgesic options for them to choose from, including nonpharmacologic methods.

Systemic Opioid Analgesia

Opioids can be given in intermittent doses by intramuscular or intravenous routes at the patient's request, or through patient-controlled administration. All opioids provide sedation and a sense of euphoria, but their analgesic effect in labor is limited, and their primary mechanism of action is sedation.[14] Opioids can also produce nausea and respiratory depression in the mother, the degree of which is usually comparable for equipotent analgesic doses. Also, all opioids freely cross the placenta to the newborn, decreasing beat-to-beat variability, and can increase the likelihood of significant respiratory depression in the newborn at birth, with subsequent need for treatment. A meta-analysis that aggregates the results of several randomized trials reveals that opioid treatment is associated with an increased risk for an Apgar score of less than 7 at 5 minutes (odds ratio [OR], 2.6; 95% confidence interval [CI], 1.2 to 5.6) and increased need for neonatal naloxone (OR, 4.17; 95% CI, 1.3 to 14.3), although the overall incidence of both was low.[15]

An important and significant disadvantage of opioid analgesia is the prolonged effect of these agents on maternal gastric emptying. When parenteral or epidural opioids are used, gastric emptying is prolonged, and if general anesthesia becomes necessary, the risk for aspiration is increased.[16] The opioids in common use today are meperidine, nalbuphine, butorphanol, and fentanyl. Morphine fell out of favor in the 1960s to 1970s because of a single study reporting increased respiratory depression in the newborn compared with meperidine, but no recent study has compared their relative safety for the newborn in the setting of modern practice.

Patient-Controlled Analgesia

Intravenous patient-controlled analgesia (PCA) is often used for women with a contraindication to neuraxial analgesia (e.g., severe thrombocytopenia). The infusion pump is programmed to give a predetermined dose of drug on patient demand. The physician will program the pump to include a lockout interval to limit the total dose administered per hour. Advantages of this method include the sense of autonomy, which patients appreciate, and elimination of delays in treatment while the patient's nurse obtains and administers the dose. In general, PCA results in a decreased total dose of opioid during labor.[17] Fentanyl, remifentanil,[18] and meperidine are the opioids most commonly employed with this technique.

Meperidine (Demerol)

Meperidine is a synthetic opioid. Meperidine 100 mg is roughly equianalgesic to morphine 10 mg but has been reported to have a somewhat less depressive effect on respiration. Usually, a dose of 25 to 50 mg is administered intravenously; it may also be used intramuscularly or in a PCA pump delivering 15 mg of meperidine every 10 minutes as needed until delivery.[19] Intravenously, the onset of analgesia begins almost immediately and lasts approximately 1.5 to 2 hours. Side effects may include tachycardia, nausea and vomiting, and delayed gastric emptying.

Normeperidine is an active metabolite of meperidine, potentiating meperidine's depressant effects in the newborn. Normeperidine concentrations increase slowly, and therefore, it exerts its effect on the newborn during the second hour after administration. Multiple doses of meperidine result in greater accumulation of both meperidine and normeperidine in fetal tissues[20]; thus, administration of large doses of meperidine in the first stage of labor (rather than during the second stage of labor) leads to high doses accumulated in the fetus. A randomized controlled study using intravenous PCA meperidine for labor analgesia found 3.4% of infants required naloxone at delivery (versus 0.8% with epidural analgesia).[21] Normeperidine accumulation in the fetus can result in prolonged neonatal sedation and neurobehavioral changes.[22] These neurobehavioral changes are evident into day 2 and day 3 of life.

Nalbuphine (Nubain)

Nalbuphine is a synthetic agonist-antagonist opioid, meaning it has opioid blocking properties as well as analgesic properties. Its analgesic potency is similar to that of morphine when compared on a milligram-per-milligram basis, and usual doses are 5 to 10 mg intravenously every 3 hours. A reported advantage of nalbuphine is its ceiling effect for respiratory depression[23]; that is, respiratory depression from multiple doses appears to plateau. One limitation of nalbuphine is that its antagonist activity may also limit the analgesia it can produce, and it may interfere with spinal and epidural opioids given as part of a neuraxial technique. Nalbuphine causes less maternal nausea and vomiting than meperidine, but it tends to produce more maternal sedation, dizziness, and dysphoria, as well as the risk for opioid withdrawal in susceptible patients.

Butorphanol (Stadol)

Butorphanol is also a synthetic agonist-antagonist opioid analgesic drug. The dose of 1 to 2 mg is administered intravenously and compares favorably with 40 to 80 mg of meperidine or 5 to 10 mg morphine.[24] Nausea and vomiting appear to occur less often with butorphanol than with other opioids. Like nalbuphine, the major advantage is a ceiling effect for respiratory depression, and the side effects of the two drugs are similar. Rarely, a pseudosinusoidal fetal heart rate pattern may occur after administration, but this is not unique to butorphanol.

Fentanyl

Fentanyl is a fast-onset, short-acting synthetic opioid with no active metabolites. In a randomized comparison with meperidine, fentanyl 50 to 100 mcg every hour provided equivalent analgesia, with fewer neonatal effects and less maternal sedation and nausea. The main drawback of fentanyl is its short duration of action requiring frequent redosing or the use of a patient-controlled intravenous infusion pump. A sample PCA setting for fentanyl is a 50-mcg incremental dose with a 10-minute lockout and no basal rate.[17]

Sedatives

Sedatives (barbiturates, phenothiazines, and benzodiazepines) do not possess analgesic qualities. All sedatives and hypnotics cross the placenta freely, and except for the benzodiazepines, they have no known antagonists. Sedation is rarely desirable during the childbirth experience.

Promethazine may actually impair the analgesic efficacy of opioids. In a randomized double-blind trial, women received placebo, metoclopramide, or promethazine as an antiemetic with meperidine analgesia.[25] Analgesia after placebo or metoclopramide was significantly better than that after promethazine as measured by pain scores and need for supplemental analgesics. Metoclopramide 10 mg has also been shown to improve PCA analgesia during second-trimester termination of pregnancy.[26] In two randomized double-blind studies, the group receiving metoclopramide (versus saline) used 54% and 66% less intravenous morphine.

Two major disadvantages of benzodiazepines are that they cause undesirable maternal amnesia[27] and may disrupt thermoregulation in newborns, which renders them less able to maintain body temperature.[28] Presumably this can occur with any of the benzodiazepines. As with many drugs, beat-to-beat variability of the fetal heart rate can be reduced even with a single intravenous dose, although these changes do not reflect alterations in the acid-base status of the newborn. Flumazenil, a specific benzodiazepine antagonist, can reliably reverse benzodiazepine-induced sedation and ventilatory depression.

Placental Transfer

Essentially, all analgesic and anesthetic agents except highly ionized muscle relaxants cross the placenta freely (see box, Factors Influencing Placental Transfer from Mother to Fetus).[29] The limited transfer of muscle relaxants such as succinylcholine enables anesthesiologists to use general anesthesia for cesarean delivery without causing fetal paralysis.

Because the placenta has the properties of a lipid membrane, most drugs and all anesthetic agents cross by simple diffusion. Thus, the amount of drug that crosses the placenta increases as concentrations in the maternal circulation and total area of the placenta increase. Diffusion is also affected by the properties of the drug itself, including molecular weight, spatial configuration, degree of ionization, lipid solubility, and protein binding. For example, bupivacaine is highly protein bound, a characteristic that some believe explains why fetal blood concentrations are so much lower than with other local anesthetics. On the other hand, bupivacaine is also highly lipid soluble. The more lipid soluble a drug is, the more freely it passes through a lipid membrane. Furthermore, once in the fetal system, lipid solubility enables the drug to be taken up by fetal tissues rapidly (i.e., redistribution), which again contributes to the lower blood concentration of the agent.

The degree of ionization of a drug is also important. Most drugs exist in both an ionized and nonionized state, with the nonionized form more freely crossing lipid membranes. The degree of ionization is influenced by the pH[30]; this may become relevant in situations in which there is a significant pH gradient between mother (normal pH 7.40) and an acidotic infant (pH <7.2) (Figure 17-5). For example, local anesthetics are more ionized at a lower pH, so the nonionized portion of the drug in the maternal circulation (normal pH) crosses to the acidotic fetus, becomes ionized, and thus remains in the fetus, potentially leading to higher local anesthetic concentrations in the fetus and newborn. Whether this has relevant adverse clinical effects on the fetus is unknown.

Factors Influencing Placental Transfer from Mother to Fetus

- Drug
  - Molecular weight
  - Lipid solubility
  - Ionization, pH of blood
  - Spatial configuration
- Maternal
  - Uptake into bloodstream
  - Distribution via circulation
  - Uterine blood flow: amount, distribution (myometrium versus placenta)
- Placental
  - Circulation: intermittent spurting arterioles
  - Lipid membrane: Fick's law of simple diffusion
- Fetal
  - Circulation: ductus venosus, foramen ovale, ductus arteriosus

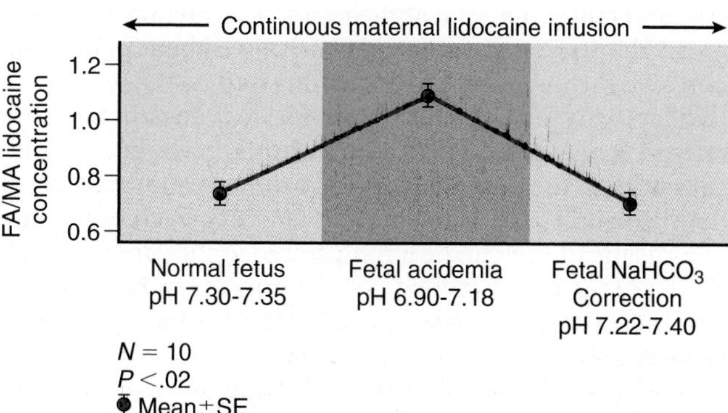

Figure 17-5. Fetal-maternal arterial (FA/MA) lidocaine ratios were significantly higher ($P<.02$) during fetal acidemia than during control or when pH was corrected with bicarbonate ($N = 10$; mean ± SE). (From Biehl D, Shnider SM, Levinson G, Callender K: Placental transfer of lidocaine: effects of fetal acidosis. Anesthesiology 48:409, 1978.)

Neuraxial Analgesic and Anesthetic Techniques

Neuraxial analgesic and anesthetic techniques (spinal, epidural, or a combination) use local anesthetics to provide sensory as well as various degrees of motor blockade over a specific region of the body. In obstetrics, neuraxial and other regional analgesic techniques include major blocks, such as lumbar epidural and spinal, and minor blocks, such as paracervical, pudendal, and local infiltration (see Figure 17-1).

Lumbar Epidural Analgesia and Anesthesia

Epidural blockade is a neuraxial anesthetic used to provide *analgesia* during labor, or surgical *anesthesia* for vaginal or cesarean delivery.[31] Epidural analgesia offers the most effective form of pain relief[32] and is used by most women in the United States.[1] In most obstetrical patients, the primary indication for epidural analgesia is the patient's desire for pain relief. Medical indications for epidural analgesia during labor may include anticipated difficult intubation due to morbid obesity or other causes, a history of malignant hyperthermia, selected forms of cardiovascular and respiratory disease, and prevention or treatment of autonomic hyper-reflexia in parturients with a high spinal cord lesion. The technique uses a large-bore (16-, 17-, or 18-gauge) needle to locate the epidural space. Next, a catheter is inserted through the needle, and the needle is removed over the catheter. After aspirating the catheter, a test dose of local anesthetic with a "marker" such as epinephrine may be given first to be certain the catheter has not been unintentionally placed in the subarachnoid (spinal) space or in a blood vessel. Intravascular placement will lead to maternal tachycardia due to the epinephrine, and rapid onset of sensory and motor block will occur if the local anesthetic is placed in the spinal fluid. Once intravascular and intrathecal placement have been ruled out, local anesthetic is injected through the catheter, which remains taped in place to the mother's back to enable subsequent injections throughout labor (Figure 17-6; see Figure 17-1). Thus, it is often called *continuous epidural analgesia*. Anesthesiologists use a technique described as *segmental epidural analgesia* (Figure 17-7). Low concentrations of local anesthetic[3] (<0.25% bupivacaine) are injected at L2 to L5, affecting the small, easily blocked sympathetic nerves that mediate early labor pain, but sparing the sensation of pressure and motor function of the perineum and lower extremities. The patient should be able to move about in bed and perceive the impact of the presenting part on the perineum. Patients vary in their responses to local anesthetics, and infusions may need to be adjusted to a lower rate or concentration if the patient develops excessive motor block. If perineal anesthesia is needed for delivery, a larger volume of local anesthetic can be administered at that time through the catheter (see Figure 17-7). Alternatively, for perineal anesthesia, the obstetrician can perform a pudendal block or local infiltration of the perineum.

A variant of the epidural technique involves passing a small-gauge pencil-point spinal needle through the epidural needle before catheter placement. This combined spinal-epidural (CSE) technique provides more rapid onset of analgesia using a very small dose of opioid or a local anesthetic and opioid combination. Some practitioners have used an opioid only or opioid plus local anesthetic technique to allow parturients to ambulate during labor (the "walking epidural") because there is little or no interference with motor function. Because the dose of drug used in the subarachnoid space is much smaller than that used for epidural analgesia, the risks for local anesthetic toxicity or high spinal block are avoided. Side effects of spinal opioids are usually mild and easily treated and include pruritus and nausea.

Non-reassuring fetal heart rate changes may occur more often in patients receiving combined spinal-epidural analgesia than epidural analgesia alone.[33] Although the incidence of hypotension is similar between the two techniques, the etiology of fetal bradycardia after spinal analgesia may relate more to uterine hypertonus than hypotension. Rapid onset of spinal analgesia decreases maternal catecholamines, specifically epinephrine, which may cause uterine relaxation through its β-agonist activity. Fortunately, these non-reassuring fetal heart rate changes do not seem to affect labor outcome. In a review of 2380 deliveries in a community hospital, there was no increase in emergency cesarean delivery in the 1240 patients who received regional analgesia for labor (98% of which were CSE) compared with the 1140 patients who received systemic or no medication.[34] A systematic review of randomized comparisons of intrathecal opioid analgesia versus epidural or parenteral opioids in labor found that the use of intrathecal opioids significantly increased the risk for fetal bradycardia (OR, 1.8; 95% CI, 1 to 3.1).[35] However, the risk for cesarean delivery for fetal heart rate abnormalities was similar in the two groups (6% versus 7.8%). Fetal heart rate should be monitored during and after the administration of either epidural or intrathecal medications to allow for timely intrauterine resuscitation.[3]

Complications of Neuraxial Blocks

Side effects of epidural or CSE analgesia include hypotension, local anesthetic toxicity, allergic reaction, high or total spinal anesthesia, neurologic injury, and postdural puncture headache. In addition, epidural analgesia use may increase the rate of intrapartum fever and possibly operative vaginal delivery. The effect of epidural analgesia on labor progression, fetal position, and risk for cesarean delivery is discussed in detail later. Because epidural anesthesia is associated with side effects and complications, some of which are dangerous, those who administer it must be thoroughly familiar not only with the technical aspects of its administration but also with the signs and symptoms of complications and their treatment. Specifically, the ASA and ACOG have stated: "Persons administering or supervising obstetric anesthesia should be qualified to manage the infrequent but occasionally life-threatening complications of major regional anesthesia such as respiratory and cardiovascular failure, convulsions due to toxic levels of local anesthetic, or vomiting and aspiration. Mastering and retaining the skills and knowledge necessary to manage these complications require adequate training and frequent application."[2] The ASA Practice Guidelines also state: "When a neuraxial technique is chosen, appropriate resources for the treatment of complications (e.g., hypotension, systemic toxicity, high spinal anesthesia) should be available."[3]

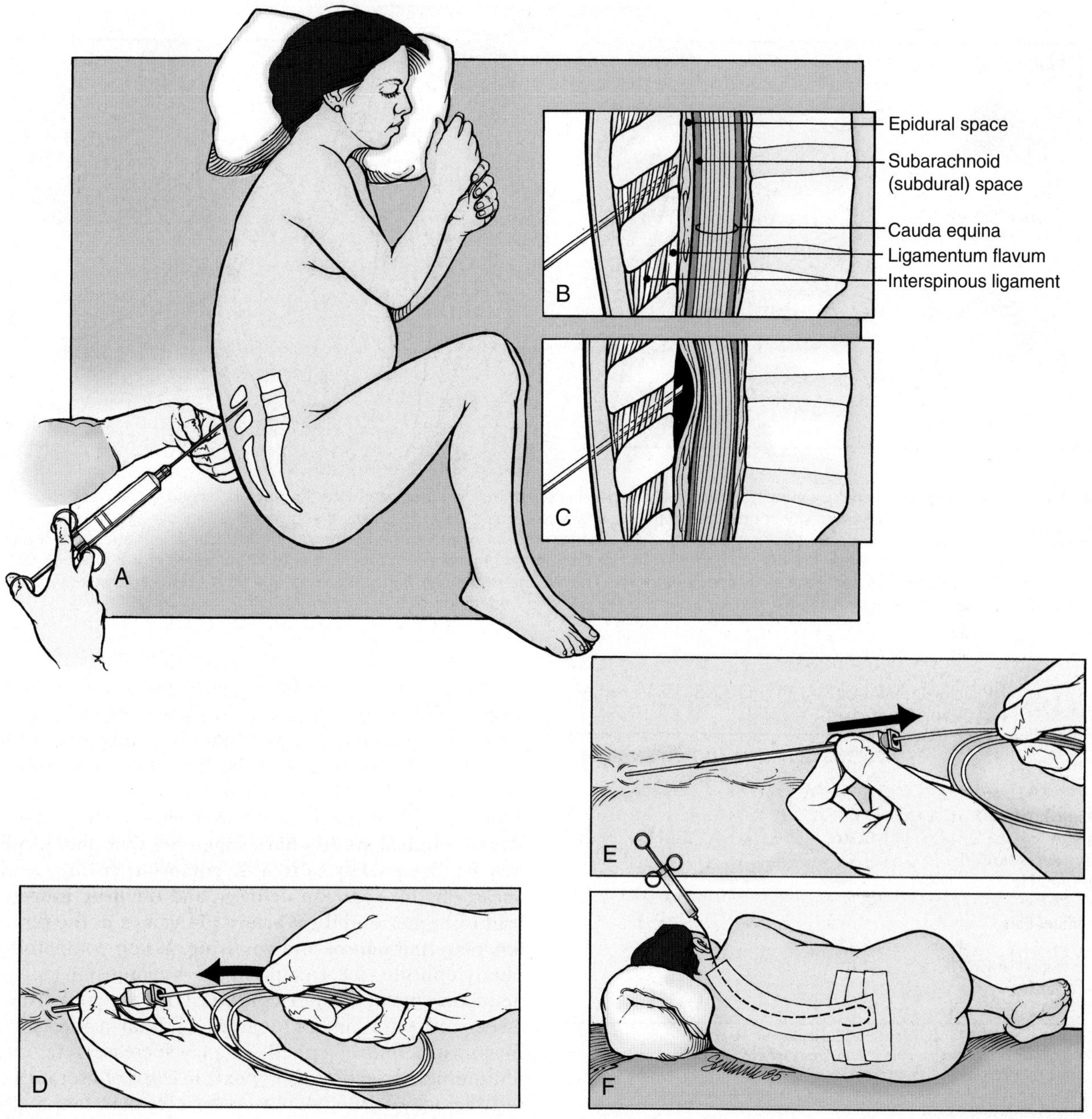

FIGURE 17-6. Technique of lumbar epidural puncture by the midline approach. **A,** This side view shows left hand held against patient's back, with thumb and index finger grasping hub. Attempts to inject solution while point of needle is in the interspinous ligament meet resistance. **B,** Point of needle is in the ligamentum flavum, which offers marked resistance and makes it almost impossible to inject solution. **C,** Entrance of the needle's point into epidural space is discerned by sudden lack of resistance to injection of saline. Force of injected solution pushes dura-arachnoid away from point of needle. **D,** Catheter is introduced through needle. Note that hub of needle is pulled caudad toward the patient, increasing the angle between the shaft of the needle and the epidural space. Also note technique of holding the tubing: It is wound around the right hand. **E,** Needle is withdrawn over tubing and held steady with the right hand. **F,** Catheter is immobilized with adhesive tape. Note the large loop made by the catheter to decrease risk for kinking at the point where the tube exits from the skin. (From Bonica JJ: Obstetric Analgesia and Anesthesia. Amsterdam, World Federation of Societies of Anesthesiologists, 1980.)

HYPOTENSION

Hypotension is defined variably, but most often as a systolic blood pressure of less than 100 mm Hg or a 20% decrease from baseline. It occurs after about 10% of spinal or epidural blocks given during labor.[36] Hypotension occurs primarily as a result of the effects of local anesthetic agents on sympathetic fibers, which normally maintain blood vessel tone. Vasodilation results in decreased venous return of blood to the right side of the heart, with subsequent decreased cardiac output and hypotension. A secondary mechanism may be decreased maternal endogenous catecholamines following pain relief. Hypotension threatens the fetus by decreasing uterine blood flow. However, when recognized promptly and treated effectively, few, if any, untoward effects accrue to either mother or fetus (Table 17-2). Special care should be taken to avoid or promptly

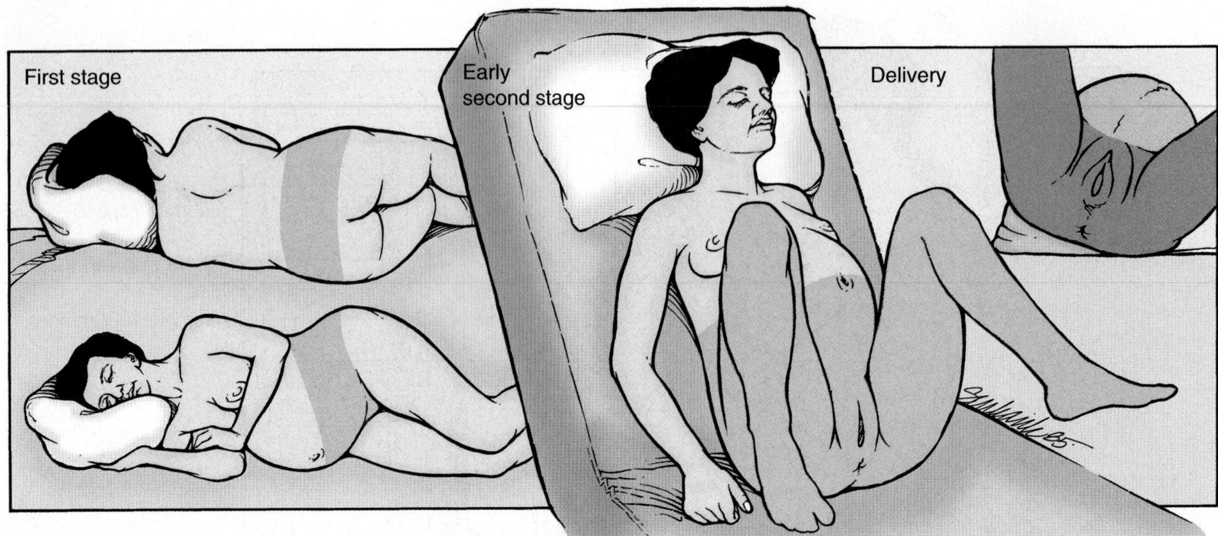

FIGURE 17-7. Segmental epidural analgesia for labor and delivery. A single catheter is introduced into the epidural space and advanced so that its tip is at L2. Initially, small volumes of low concentrations of local anesthetic are used to produce segmental analgesia. For the second stage, the analgesia is extended to the sacral segments by injecting a larger amount of the same concentration of local anesthetic, with the patient in the semirecumbent position. After internal rotation, a higher concentration of local anesthetic is injected to produce motor block of the sacral segments and thus achieve perineal relaxation and anesthesia. The wedge under the right buttock causes the uterus to displace to the left. (From Bonica JJ: Obstetric Analgesia and Anesthesia. Amsterdam, World Federation of Societies of Anesthesiologists, 1980.)

TABLE 17-2 EPIDURAL ANALGESIA: HYPOTENSION VERSUS NO HYPOTENSION*

	HYPOTENSION† (N = 5)	NO HYPOTENSION (N = 20)
Umbilical Artery		
pH	7.269	7.311
Base excess (mEq/L)	1.4	1.3
PO_2 (mm Hg)	23.6	23.2
SaO_2 (%)	48.2	50.2
Umbilical Vein		
pH	7.344	
Base excess (mEq/L)	1.8	1.5
PO_2 (mm Hg)	41	33.7
SvO_2 (%)	84.6	72

Modified from James FM III, Crawford JS, Hopkinson R, et al: A comparison of general anesthesia and lumbar epidural analgesia for elective cesarean section. Anesth Analg 56:228, 1977.

*Values are means; they indicate that properly treated hypotension need not result in a compromised fetus.

†Hypotension was severe enough to be treated with the vasopressor ephedrine.

treat hypotension, especially in situations in which acute or chronic fetal compromise is suspected.

Treatment of hypotension begins with prophylaxis, which includes (1) intravenous access for volume expansion and administration of pressors and (2) left uterine displacement to maintain cardiac preload. Isotonic crystalloid infusion may mitigate the effects of vasodilation. Rapid boluses should not contain dextrose because of the association with subsequent neonatal hypoglycemia. Proper treatment of hypotension depends on immediate diagnosis. Therefore, the individual administering the anesthesia must be present and attentive. **Once diagnosed, hypotension is corrected by increasing the rate of intravenous fluid infusion and exaggerating left uterine displacement. If these simple measures do not suffice, a vasopressor is indicated.**

The vasopressor of choice has evolved from ephedrine, given in 5- to 10-mg doses, to phenylephrine, in 50- to 100-mcg increments. Ephedrine is a mixed α- and β-agonist, and was thought to be less likely to compromise uteroplacental perfusion than the pure α-agonists. Of concern, ephedrine is associated with fetal tachycardia. **Recent clinical studies have suggested that phenylephrine may be given safely to treat hypotension during neuraxial anesthesia for cesarean delivery, and the drug indeed may lead to higher umbilical artery pH values in the fetus and less maternal nausea and vomiting.** When compared with phenylephrine for treatment of hypotension following neuraxial analgesia in a randomized trial, ephedrine was associated with higher degrees of fetal acidosis.[37] The β-agonist action of ephedrine may increase fetal oxygen requirements, leading to hypoxia in cases of uteroplacental insufficiency.[38] Phenylephrine corrects maternal hypotension, apparently without causing clinically significant uterine artery vasoconstriction or decreased placental perfusion, even in extremely high doses. Rather than causing abnormal increases in systemic vascular resistance, these doses may simply return vascular tone to normal after spinal anesthesia. It is also possible that constricting peripheral arteries may preferentially shunt blood to the uterine arteries. The parturient has decreased sensitivity to all vasopressors, and that may also protect the fetus from excessive vasoconstriction. α-Adrenergic agents such as methoxamine and phenylephrine cause reflex bradycardia that may be useful when a parturient is excessively tachycardic in association with hypotension, or if tachycardia associated with ephedrine would be detrimental.

LOCAL ANESTHETIC TOXICITY

The incidence of systemic local anesthetic toxicity (high blood concentrations of local anesthetic) after obstetrical lumbar epidural analgesia is 1 in 5000, or 0.02%.[39] However,

TABLE 17-3 MAXIMAL RECOMMENDED DOSES OF COMMON LOCAL ANESTHETICS

	WITH EPINEPHRINE*		WITHOUT EPINEPHRINE	
Local Anesthetic	**mg/kg**	**Dose (mg/70 kg)**	**mg/kg**	**Dose (mg/70 kg)**
Bupivacaine	3.0	210	2.5	175
Chloroprocaine	14.0	980	11.0	770
Etidocaine	5.5	385	4.0	280
Lidocaine	7.0	490	4.0	280
Mepivacaine	—	—	5.0	350

*All epinephrine concentrations 1:200,000.

cases of local anesthetic toxicity were absent from most recent review of the ASA Closed Claims Project database.[40] In contrast, the Confidential Enquiries into Maternal Deaths in Great Britain reported a maternal death during labor when a bupivacaine epidural infusion was connected to an intravenous line instead of the epidural catheter.[41] Most often, toxicity occurs when the local anesthetic is injected into a blood vessel rather than into the epidural space or when too much is administered even though injected properly. **These reactions can also occur during placement of pudendal or paracervical blocks. All local anesthetics have maximal recommended doses, and these should not be exceeded.** For example, the maximal recommended dose of lidocaine is 4 mg/kg when used without epinephrine and 7 mg/kg when used with epinephrine. Epinephrine delays and decreases the uptake of local anesthetic into the blood stream. Package inserts for all local anesthetics contain appropriate dosing information (Table 17-3).

Local anesthetic reactions have two components: central nervous system (CNS) and cardiovascular. Usually, the CNS component precedes the cardiovascular component. Prodromal symptoms of the CNS reaction include excitation, bizarre behavior, ringing in the ears, and disorientation. These symptoms may culminate in convulsions, which are usually brief. After the convulsions, cognitive depression follows, manifested by the postictal state. The cardiovascular component of the local anesthetic reaction usually begins with hypertension and tachycardia but is soon followed by hypotension, arrhythmias, and in some instances, cardiac arrest. Thus, the cardiovascular component also has excitant and depressant characteristics. One frequently sees the CNS component without the more serious cardiovascular component. Bupivacaine may represent an exception to this principle. **Resuscitation of patients who receive an intravascular injection of bupivacaine is extremely challenging, likely owing to the prolonged blocking effect on sodium channels.**[42] Laboratory evidence supports bupivacaine's increased cardiotoxicity over equianalgesic doses of other amide local anesthetics such as ropivacaine and lidocaine.[43] The manufacturers of bupivacaine have recommended that the 0.75% concentration not be used in obstetrical patients or for paracervical block. However, use of a more dilute concentration does not guarantee safety; bupivacaine and all local anesthetics should be administered by slow, incremental injection.

Adverse events due to local anesthetic toxicity have decreased because of greater emphasis on incremental dosing and use of a test dose, typically containing 15 mcg of epinephrine to exclude unintentional intravenous or subarachnoid catheter placement. Others have questioned the lack of specificity of test doses during labor and the potential harm to the fetus or hypertensive mother.[44] Intravascular injection of 15 mcg of epinephrine produces maternal tachycardia, which may be difficult to differentiate from that seen during a contraction. Non-reassuring fetal heart tones due to decreased uterine blood flow may also occur after intravascular epinephrine, especially when there is fetal compromise.

Treatment of a local anesthetic reaction depends on recognizing the signs and symptoms.[45] Prodromal symptoms should trigger the immediate cessation of the injection of local anesthetic. If convulsions have already occurred, treatment is aimed at maintaining proper oxygenation and preventing the patient from harming herself. Convulsions use considerable amounts of oxygen, which results in hypoxia and acidosis (Table 17-4). Should the convulsions continue for more than a brief period, small intravenous doses of propofol (30 to 50 mg) or a benzodiazepine (2 to 5 mg midazolam) are useful. The depressant effects of these agents add to the depressant phase of the local anesthetic reaction; therefore, appropriate equipment and personnel must be available to maintain oxygenation and a patent airway and to provide cardiovascular support. Rarely, succinylcholine is needed for paralysis to prevent the muscular activity and to facilitate ventilation and perhaps intubation. In cases of complete cardiac collapse, delivery of the infant may facilitate maternal resuscitation. The American Heart Association has stated: "Several authors now recommend that the decision to perform a perimortem cesarean section should be made rapidly, with delivery effected within 4 to 5 minutes of the arrest."[3] **Intravenous lipid emulsion may be an effective therapy for cardiotoxic effects of lipid-soluble local anesthetics such as bupivacaine or ropivacaine.[46] Intralipid should be available wherever regional anesthesia is provided.**

ALLERGY TO LOCAL ANESTHETICS

There are two classes of local anesthetics: amides and esters. **A true allergic reaction to an amide-type local anesthetic (e.g., lidocaine, bupivacaine, ropivacaine) is extremely rare. Allergic reactions to the esters (2-chloroprocaine, procaine, tetracaine) are also uncommon but can occur.** They are often associated with a reaction to para-aminobenzoic acid (PABA) in skin creams or suntan lotions. When a patient reports that she is "allergic" to local anesthetics, she is frequently referring to a normal reaction to the epinephrine that is occasionally added to local anesthetics,

TABLE 17-4 BLOOD GAS DETERMINATIONS DURING AND AFTER LOCAL ANESTHETIC–INDUCED CONVULSIONS

CONVULSION	TIME	OXYGEN	pH	BLOOD GAS VALUES			
				P_{CO_2} (mm Hg)	P_{O_2} (mm Hg)	HCO_3 (mEq/L)	Base Excess (mEq/L)
Patient 1							
1st	19:50:00	10*	—	—	—	—	—
2nd	9:50:30		7.27	48	48	21.5	–14.2
3rd	9:51:00		—	—	—	—	—
4th	9:53:00		7.09	59	33	17.1	–10.2
Cessation	9:54:00		—	—	—	—	—
	9:55:30	6†	7.01	71	210	17.2	–11.2
	10:22:00	Room air	7.25	48	99	20.5	–5.2
			7.56	25	106	22.5	–10.2
Patient 2							
1st	19:47:00	—	—	—	—	—	—
2nd	9:47:30		6.99	76	87	17.4	–10.2
3rd	9:48:00		—	—	—	—	—
Cessation	9:50:00	—	—	—	—	—	—
	10:02:00	10*	7.16	54	140	18.5	–6.9

Modified from Moore DC, Crawford RD, Scurlock JE: Severe hypoxia and acidosis following local anesthetic-induced convulsions. Anesthesiology 53:259, 1980.
*Bag and mask with oral Guedel airway and artificial respiration.
†Nasal prongs.

particularly by dentists. Epinephrine can cause increased heart rate, pounding in the ears, and nausea, symptoms that may be interpreted as an allergy. Therefore, it is important to document the situation in which the reaction occurred.

HIGH SPINAL OR "TOTAL SPINAL" ANESTHESIA

This complication occurs when the level of anesthesia rises dangerously high, resulting in paralysis of the respiratory muscles, including the diaphragm (C3 to C5). The incidence of total spinal anesthesia after epidural anesthesia is 1 in 16,200 or 0.006%.[39] Total spinal anesthesia can result from a miscalculated dose of drug or unintentional subarachnoid injection during an epidural block. The ASA Closed Claims Project analysis of obstetrical anesthesia liability claims found that the most common cause of maternal death or brain damage in neuraxial anesthesia claims was high block; 80% were associated with dosing epidural anesthesia, and 20% involved spinal anesthesia.[40] The accessory muscles of respiration are paralyzed earlier, and their paralysis may result in apprehension and anxiety and a feeling of dyspnea. The patient usually can breathe adequately as long as the diaphragm is not paralyzed, but treatment must be individualized. Dyspnea, real or imagined, should always be considered an effect of paralysis until proved otherwise. Cardiovascular effects, including hypotension and even cardiovascular collapse, may accompany total spinal anesthesia.

Treatment of total spinal anesthesia includes rapidly assessing the true level of anesthesia. Therefore, individuals who administer major regional anesthesia should be thoroughly familiar with dermatome charts (Figure 17-8) and should also be able to recognize what a certain sensory level of anesthesia means with regard to innervation of other organs or systems. For example, a T4 sensory level may represent total sympathetic nervous system blockade. **Numbness and weakness of the fingers and hands indicates that the level of anesthesia has reached the cervical level (C6 to C8), which is dangerously close to the innervation of the diaphragm.** If the diaphragm is not paralyzed, the patient is breathing adequately, and cardiovascular stability is maintained, administration of oxygen and reassurance may suffice. If the patient remains anxious or if the level of anesthesia seems to be involving the diaphragm, then assisted ventilation is indicated, and endotracheal intubation will be necessary to protect the airway. In addition, cardiovascular support is provided as necessary. Delay in treatment due to inadequate monitoring, absence of the anesthesia provider, lack of airway equipment or emergency drugs in the labor room, or delay in resuscitation during transfer of the patient to the operating room for delivery will worsen outcome.[47] With prompt and adequate treatment, serious sequelae should be extremely rare.

NERVE INJURY

Paralysis after either epidural or spinal anesthesia is extremely rare; even minor injuries such as footdrop and segmental loss of sensation are uncommon. **However, the ASA Closed Claim Project analysis of liability claims notes that the incidence of claims for nerve injury has increased in their most recent review and is now the most common cause of liability in obstetrical anesthesia.**[40] Nerve injury occurs in 0.06% of spinal anesthetics and 0.02% of epidural anesthetics.[48] With commercially prepared drugs, ampules, and disposable needles, infection and caustic injury rarely occur. When nerve damage follows regional analgesia during obstetrical or surgical procedures, the anesthetic technique must be suspected, although causation is rare. Other potential etiologies include incorrectly positioned stirrups, difficult forceps applications, or abnormal fetal presentations. During abdominal procedures, overzealous or prolonged application of pressure with retractors on sensitive nerve tissues may also result in injury. Fortunately, most neurologic deficits after labor and delivery are minor and transient; however, consultation with a neurologist or neurosurgeon should be considered.

A systematic review of serious adverse events among 1.37 million women receiving epidural analgesia during labor

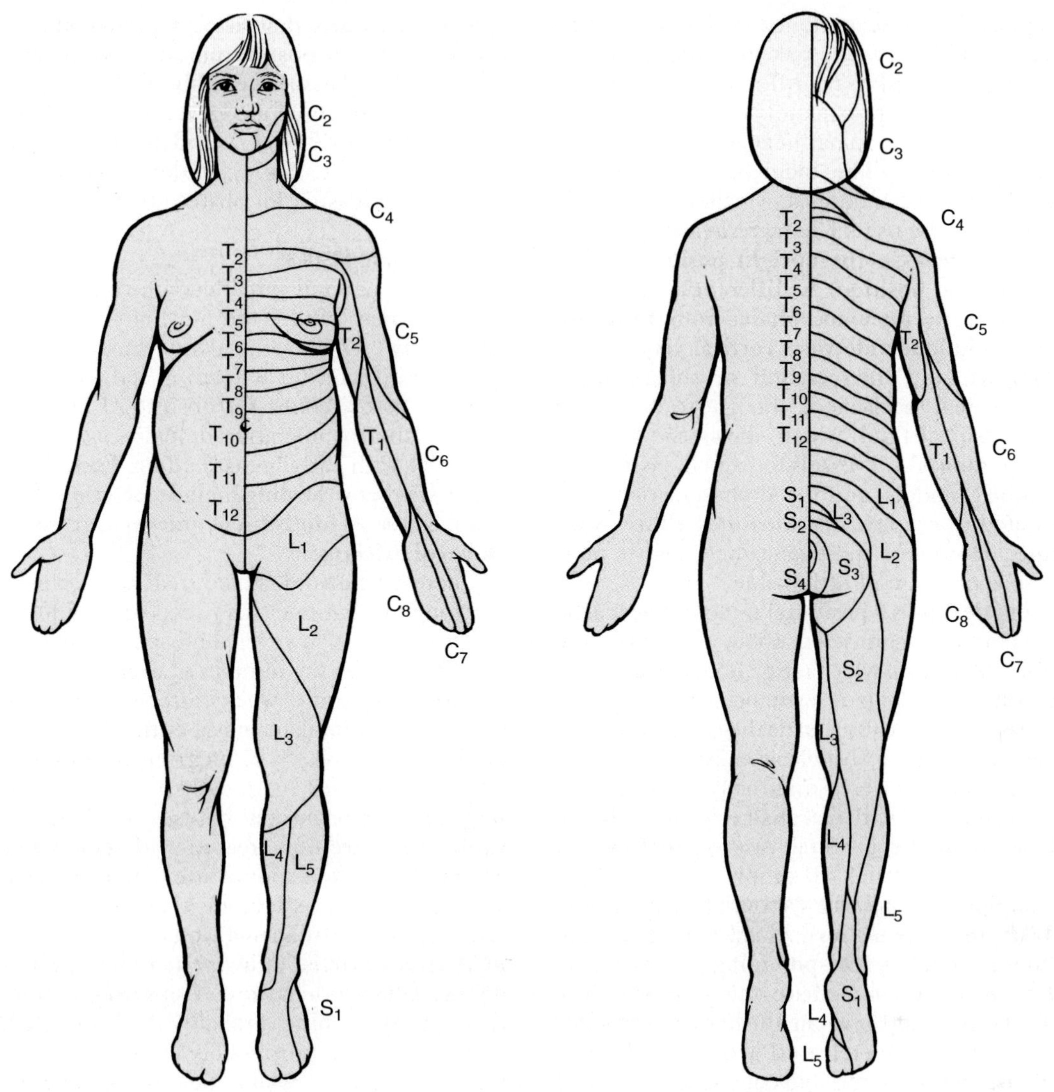

FIGURE 17-8. Dermatome chart. (Modified from Haymaker L, Woodhall B: Peripheral Nerve Injuries. Philadelphia, WB Saunders, 1945.)

found the risks for epidural hematoma and epidural abscess were 1 case per 168,000 women and 1 per 145,000, respectively.[49] The risk for persistent neurologic injury was 1 case per 240,000 women, and the risk for transient neurologic injury was 1 per 6700. One of the more dramatic and correctable forms of nerve damage follows compression of the spinal cord by a hematoma that has formed during the administration of spinal or epidural anesthesia, presumably from accidental puncture of an epidural vessel. If the condition is diagnosed early, usually with the aid of a neurologist or neurosurgeon, the hematoma can be removed by laminectomy and the problem resolved without permanent damage. Fortunately, this is a rare complication. Nonetheless, spinal and epidural blocks are contraindicated if the patient has a coagulopathy or if the patient is pharmacologically anticoagulated. Hemolysis, elevated liver enzymes, and low platelets (HELLP) syndrome may be a particularly strong risk factor because of multifactorial sources for coagulation defects.[50] Any significant motor or sensory deficit after regional anesthesia should be investigated immediately and thoroughly (Figure 17-8).

Although the incidence of neuraxial infection such as spinal meningitis or epidural abscess is rare, it is an important cause of significant maternal morbidity and mortality. Recently, the Centers for Disease Control and Prevention reviewed five cases of bacterial meningitis linked to intrapartum spinal anesthesia in which one woman died.[51] A common denominator in these cases was that either the anesthesiologist performing the block or visitors in the room were not wearing masks. **Both the American Society of Regional Anesthesia (ASRA) and the ASA have published guidelines on prevention of infection during regional anesthesia that include recommendations to remove jewelry, wash hands, wear a fresh face mask, and disinfect the patient's back using 2% chlorhexidine in alcohol.**[52,53]

Spinal Headache

Spinal headache may follow uncomplicated spinal anesthesia, but it is far more common when, during the process of administering an epidural block, the dura is punctured and spinal fluid leaks out (i.e., "wet tap"). The incidence of this complication varies between 1% and 3%, and its occurrence depends on the experience of the person performing the epidural block.[54] The risk for postdural puncture headache following CSE is no different than that with epidural analgesia alone, approximately 1.5%.

Once a wet tap occurs, a spinal headache results in as many as 70% of patients. The incidence is much less following spinal anesthesia because smaller, atraumatic (pencil-point) needles are used. **Characteristically, a spinal headache is more severe in the upright position and is relieved by the supine position. A differential diagnosis should include migraine, pneumocephalus from the loss of resistance to air technique, infection, cortical vein thrombosis, preeclampsia, and intracerebral or subarachnoid hemorrhage.**[55] A spinal headache is thought to be caused by loss of cerebrospinal fluid, which allows the brain to settle and thus meninges and vessels to stretch. Hydration, bedrest, abdominal binders, and the prone position have all been advocated as prophylactic measures after known dural puncture. However, most anesthesiologists now agree that these actions are of little value.[55]

When a patient develops a postdural puncture headache (PDPH), she should be counseled about the cause and potential treatment options, which range from conservative to aggressive. Close follow-up, reassurance, and treatment if required are important because headache is the third most common cause of a lawsuit in obstetrical anesthesia.[40] If the headache is mild and interferes minimally with activity, treatment may be initiated with oral analgesics and caffeine or theophylline, which are cerebral vasoconstrictors that may provide symptomatic relief.[56] If simple measures prove ineffective, an epidural blood patch should be considered. About 20 mL of the patient's own blood is placed aseptically into the epidural space, providing a tamponade effect that may result in immediate relief. It may also coagulate over the hole and prevent further cerebrospinal fluid leakage. Patients can be released within 1 to 2 hours. Patients should be instructed to avoid coughing or straining for the first day after insertion of the blood patch. **The epidural blood patch has been found to be remarkably effective and nearly complication free, despite the fact that it is an iatrogenic epidural hematoma.** Prophylactic epidural blood patches inserted through the epidural catheter immediately after delivery are not effective in preventing headaches. A preventive measure that may be effective is passing the epidural catheter through the dural hole at the time of wet tap to provide continuous spinal anesthesia, with removal of the catheter 24 hours after delivery.[57] Injecting preservative-free saline through the catheter before removing the spinal catheter may also decrease the incidence of headache, although these data are preliminary.

Back Pain

Back pain is a common peripartum complaint, and a common concern for women considering regional anesthesia for their delivery. An antepartum survey of pregnant patients, before their delivery or any use of regional anesthesia, found that 69% of patients reported back pain, 58% reported sleep disturbances due to back pain, 57% said it impaired activities of daily living, and 30% had stopped at least one daily activity because of pain.[58] Only 32% informed their obstetrical providers they had back pain, and only 25% of those providers recommended treatment. **Despite concerns that using regional anesthesia contributes to back pain, postpartum surveys indicate that the incidence of back pain after childbirth is the same whether women had regional analgesia for their delivery or not—about 40% to 50% at 2 and 6 months postpartum.**[59,60] Despite these reassuring findings, liability for back pain claims is increasing for obstetrical anesthesiologists.[40]

Breastfeeding Issues

Some patients and providers are concerned that regional analgesia may hinder the newborn's ability to breastfeed effectively.[61] Observational studies showing an association between difficult breastfeeding and anesthetic use during labor do not account for obstetrical events such as prolonged labor or operative delivery, factors that can cause difficulty with early breastfeeding. **Factors contributing to successful breastfeeding include lactation consultation services, maternal motivation, and support from obstetricians and pediatricians.**

There are no randomized trials comparing breastfeeding outcomes in patients who received epidural analgesia or no medication. However, a prospective cohort study found no difference in the number of women successfully breastfeeding 1, 4, and 6 weeks after delivery, whether or not they used epidural analgesia during labor.[62] Large doses of epidural fentanyl (>150 mcg) given during the course of labor may interfere with early breastfeeding success; thus, high concentrations and boluses should be avoided.[63] Not surprisingly, women treated with epidural analgesia for postoperative pain control after cesarean delivery are more successful at breastfeeding than those treated with systemic opioids.[64] Infants of women treated with intravenous PCA after cesarean delivery were less alert and had more neonatal neurobehavioral depression after meperidine than after morphine, probably due to meperidine's active metabolites, and presumably intravenous opioids administered during labor would have the same effect.

Effects on Labor and Method of Delivery

In the past there was significant controversy about how to appropriately counsel patients regarding the effect of regional analgesia on their labor course and risk for cesarean delivery. **The most recent opinion on this subject from the ACOG states: "Neuraxial techniques are the most effective and least depressant treatments for labor pain. The ACOG previously recommended that practitioners delay initiating epidural analgesia in nulliparous women until the cervical dilation reached 4 to 5 cm. However, more recent studies have shown that epidural analgesia does not increase the risks for cesarean delivery. The fear of unnecessary cesarean delivery should not influence the method of pain relief that women can choose during labor."**[65] More recent studies,[66,67] as well as a meta-analysis[68] of eight randomized controlled trials and cohort studies ($N = 3320$), of early labor versus late initiation of neuraxial analgesia further support the most recent ACOG Committee Opinion that there is no increase in cesarean delivery rate when epidural analgesia is initiated early in labor (<4 cm dilated).

Study Design

Multiple prospective randomized studies of epidural analgesia have been performed both in nulliparous populations and in mixed populations. However, the poor quality of analgesia provided by systemic opioids typically leads to high rates of crossover of control patients into the epidural analgesia arm. Neither intent-to-treat analysis nor actual-use analysis are entirely satisfactory in this situation. Studies with the lowest crossover rates have accomplished their goal through the use of substantial doses of parenteral opioids, resulting in higher than expected rates of neonatal resuscitation in the opioid groups.[20,22] Nonrandomized studies provide interesting observational data; however, careful analysis of potential confounders is critical because patients who self-select epidural analgesia are clearly different from patients who avoid it. Furthermore, with declining rates of operative vaginal delivery and increasing rates of cesarean delivery, up-to-date studies are needed to examine these outcomes. Of concern, randomized studies are often conducted in academic centers where operative delivery rates in low-risk patients may be significantly lower than in community hospitals. Finally, regional analgesia techniques vary, and modifications in technique occur continuously. More modern techniques use lower concentrations of local anesthetic and titrate the dose to the specific needs of the patient, potentially lowering the risk for operative delivery. Despite these limitations, the published literature offers considerable insight regarding the effects of regional analgesia on the progress of labor and method of delivery.

Progress of Labor and Cesarean Delivery Rate

Management of epidural analgesia and timing of administration should be individualized to the patient's needs and level of pain. Attention should be focused on minimizing local anesthetic concentrations while still providing adequate pain control, and on avoiding routine administration of epidural analgesia in latent labor.

The impact of neuraxial analgesia on cesarean delivery rates has been one of the most important labor and delivery outcomes studied over the past several decades. Multiple studies have evaluated this outcome in an attempt to identify factors associated with cesarean delivery. **Although older observational studies suggested an increased risk for cesarean delivery associated with neuraxial analgesia, the preponderance of recent evidence now supports the use of neuraxial analgesia without a significant increase in cesarean delivery rates.** A recent Cochrane Review assessed the effects of all modalities of neuraxial analgesia (including CSE) on obstetrical outcome when compared with nonepidural or no pain relief during labor.[69] Twenty-one randomized controlled trials involving 6664 women were included. All studies except one compared epidural analgesia with opiates. The authors concluded that epidural analgesia was effective in reducing pain during labor without evidence of a significant difference in the risk for caesarean delivery (relative risk [RR], 1.07; 95% CI, 0.93 to 1.23; 20 trials, 6534 women). Another concern has been a possible dose-response effect; that is, more dense analgesia could result in an increased cesarean delivery rate. Several randomized controlled trials evaluated traditional epidural analgesia with 0.25% bupivacaine compared with low-dose bupivacaine or fentanyl epidural techniques and found no differences in the rate of cesarean delivery.[70] **Although epidural analgesia itself does not increase the risk for cesarean delivery, management of neuraxial analgesia should be individualized to the patient's needs and level of pain, with a focus on minimizing local anesthetic concentrations and motor block while still providing adequate pain control.**

Potential for prolonged labor, increased oxytocin use, and increased risk for instrumental delivery have been additional considerations for clinicians and their patients who receive neuraxial analgesia. Although the relative risk of oxytocin treatment after initiation of epidural analgesia varies considerably depending on obstetrical practice (i.e., rates of induction and active management of labor), systematic reviews[70] evaluating this outcome demonstrate that **epidural analgesia is associated with a significant increase in the use of oxytocin after initiation of epidural analgesia**. Despite aggressive use of oxytocin, there are some effects of epidural analgesia on the length of active labor. **Although neuraxial analgesia may shorten first-stage labor in some women and lengthen it in others, there is little doubt that effective neuraxial analgesia prolongs the second stage of labor by 15 to 30 minutes.** Although few obstetricians in the past would allow the second stage to continue for more than 2 hours, most agree that a delay in the second stage does not adversely affect maternal or neonatal outcome, provided that (1) electronic fetal monitoring confirms reassuring fetal status; (2) maternal hydration and analgesia are adequate; and (3) there is ongoing progress in the descent of the fetal head. ACOG has stated that if progress is being made, the duration of the second stage alone does not mandate intervention. In such cases, **potential strategies for decreasing the risk for instrument-assisted delivery include reducing the density of neuraxial analgesia during the second stage, delaying pushing, and avoiding arbitrary definitions of a prolonged second stage.**

Any analysis of the relationship between neuraxial analgesia and instrument-assisted vaginal delivery is complicated by the strong influence of obstetrical practice and the obstetrician's attitude toward operative vaginal delivery. Also, obstetricians may be more likely to perform elective instrument-assisted delivery in patients with effective analgesia. Three systematic reviews have evaluated the effect of neuraxial analgesia on mode of vaginal delivery.[70-72] These trials included nearly 10,000 patients, and the results suggested that epidural analgesia was associated with an increased risk for instrumental vaginal delivery. However, operator bias is an important consideration. In clinical practice, indications vary widely among obstetricians, and it is often difficult to distinguish between "indicated" and elective instrumental deliveries. Although most obstetricians are more likely to perform such deliveries in women with adequate pain relief, another factor affecting the rate of instrumental vaginal deliveries is whether these deliveries are conducted in teaching institutions. Such deliveries are more likely to be performed in patients with adequate analgesia for the purposes of teaching. Minimizing the risk for instrumental vaginal delivery while maximizing analgesia in such cases requires attention by the anesthesiologist to the individual needs of the patient. Modern neuraxial techniques use lower concentrations of local anesthetic and a titrated dose. These factors likely contribute to lowering the risk for operative delivery in such patients.

In a given population, the risk for cesarean delivery may vary depending on the patient population, obstetrical management, protocols for oxytocin augmentation, obstetrical provider, patient attitudes toward cesarean delivery, and provider comfort with instrument-assisted vaginal delivery, as well as other risk factors. Neuraxial analgesia alone does not increase the risk for cesarean delivery.

FEVER

Epidural analgesia during labor is associated with an increase in maternal temperature compared with women receiving no analgesia or systemic opioids alone.[73] In a well-designed study with a low crossover rate (6%), Sharma and colleagues[72] reported a 33% rate of intrapartum fever greater than 37.5° C in nulliparous patients randomized to epidural analgesia, compared with 7% in those receiving parenteral opioids. The more than fourfold increased risk for fever occurred despite relatively minor prolongations in the mean duration of labor (50 minutes). Similarly, Yancey and associates[74] also described an 18-fold increase in the rate of intrapartum fever in nulliparous patients (from 0.6% to 11%) in a single year following the introduction of an epidural analgesia service in their hospital.

The etiology of this febrile response is not well understood; possible mechanisms include noninfectious inflammatory activation, changes in thermoregulation, and acquired intrapartum infection. Intrapartum fever after epidural analgesia is associated with increased serum levels of inflammatory cytokines in the mother and fetus, but no mechanism in which epidural blockade might cause inflammation has been elucidated.[75] Thermoregulation may be altered because epidural analgesia leads to decreased sweating (by providing sympathetic blockade) and less hyperventilation due to pain in labor. Both sweating and hyperventilation would otherwise provide heat dissipation. Although infants of women randomized to epidural analgesia in one institution had a 1.5-fold increase (95% CI, 1.1 to 2) in neonatal sepsis evaluations, actual sepsis was extremely rare and did not differ between epidural and nonepidural groups.[76] Other institutions have not found an increase in sepsis evaluations, probably reflecting differences in neonatology practice styles and greater awareness of temperature increases associated with epidural analgesia.

Despite the lack of infectious morbidity, intrapartum exposure to hyperthermia may not be benign for the neonate. Animal study indicates that the presence of hyperthermia during an ischemic event increases susceptibility to hypoxic-ischemic insult. In addition, Impey and coworkers[77] reported a 10-fold higher risk for neonatal encephalopathy in term infants exposed to intrapartum fever, defined as an oral temperature greater than 37.5° C (OR, 10.8; 95% CI, 4 to 29.3). The absolute risk for encephalopathy in neonates born to febrile mothers was 2.1%. Finally, although the absolute risk is low, maternal temperature greater than 38° C is associated with 9.3-fold increased risk for cerebral palsy in term infants (95% CI, 2.7 to 31).[78] It is important to clarify that there is no evidence that epidural analgesia is associated with encephalopathy or cerebral palsy. Acetaminophen, the standard therapy used to ameliorate hyperthermia, is not effective in preventing fever secondary to epidural analgesia. High-dose maternal corticosteroids given to parturients with epidural analgesia block the febrile response but also substantially increase the risk for bacteremia in exposed babies.[79]

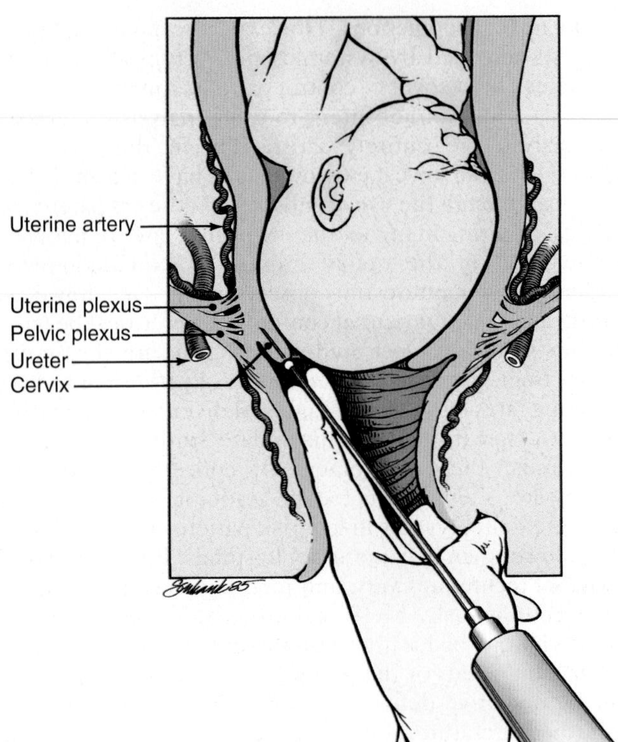

FIGURE 17-9. Technique of paracervical block. Schematic coronal section *(enlarged)* of lower portion of cervix and upper portion of vagina shows relation of needle to paracervical region. (Modified from Bonica JJ: Principles and Practice of Obstetric Analgesia and Anesthesia. Philadelphia, FA Davis, 1967, p 234.)

Paracervical Block

Paracervical block analgesia is a simple and effective procedure when performed properly (see Table 17-1). Commonly, 5 to 6 mL of a dilute solution of local anesthetic without epinephrine (e.g., 1% lidocaine or 1% or 2% 2-chloroprocaine) is injected into the mucosa of the cervix at the 3- and 9-o'clock positions (Figure 17-9). The duration of analgesia depends on the local anesthetic used. This technique has fallen out of favor owing to its association with the fetal bradycardia that follows in 2% to 70% of applications. Occurring within 2 to 10 minutes and persisting from 3 to 30 minutes, these bradycardias are usually benign. However, cases of fetal acidosis and death have been reported. A significant decrease in pH and a rise in base deficit occur only in those fetuses with bradycardia persisting more than 10 minutes.[80] **Paracervical block should be used cautiously at all times and should not be used at all in mothers with fetuses in either acute or chronic distress.**

There is no consensus regarding the mechanism of post-paracervical block bradycardia. High fetal blood concentrations of local anesthetic could occur if local anesthetic injected close to the uterine artery passed to the fetus. This theory is consistent with the finding that infants who suffer bradycardia frequently have higher local anesthetic

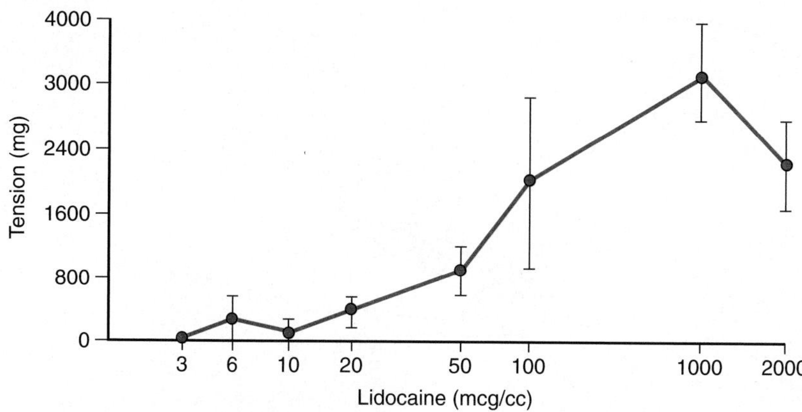

FIGURE 17-10. Dose-response curve of the pregnant human uterine artery to lidocaine hydrochloride (mean ± SEM; N = 9). (From Gibbs CP, Noel SC: Response of arterial segments from gravid human uterus to multiple concentrations of lignocaine. Br J Anaesth 45:409, 1977.)

concentrations than their mothers. Alternatively, bradycardia may result from uterine artery vasoconstriction secondary to a direct effect of the local anesthetic on the uterine artery (Figure 17-10).[81] The fetal electrocardiogram (ECG) pattern during one of these episodes suggests hypoxia, a finding that supports the uterine artery vasoconstriction theory.[81] Furthermore, the high concentrations of local anesthetic required to produce vasoconstriction during the administration of a paracervical block can be achieved close to the uterine artery (see Figure 17-10). A third theory is based on the possibility that local anesthetic injected directly into the uterine musculature increases uterine tone.

ANESTHESIA FOR VAGINAL DELIVERY

The goal of pain relief for vaginal delivery is to match the patient's wishes with the requirements of the delivery without subjecting either mother or fetus to unnecessary risk.

Local Anesthesia

In the form of perineal infiltration, local anesthesia is widely used and very safe. Spontaneous vaginal delivery, episiotomy, and perhaps outlet vacuum deliveries can be accomplished with this simple technique. Local anesthetic toxicity may occur if large amounts of local anesthetic are used or if an inadvertent intravascular injection occurs. Usually, 5 to 15 mL of 1% lidocaine suffices. There is rapid and significant transfer of lidocaine to the fetus after perineal infiltration. In 5 of 15 infants, the concentration of lidocaine at delivery was greater in the umbilical vein than in the mother (Table 17-5).

TABLE 17-5 LIDOCAINE CONCENTRATIONS AT DELIVERY IN MATERNAL PLASMA AND UMBILICAL CORD VEIN AFTER PERINEAL INFILTRATION

SAMPLE (N = 15)	CONCENTRATION (ng/mL)	
	Mean ± SD	**Range**
Maternal Plasma		
Peak concentration	648 ± 666	60-2400
At delivery	548 ± 468	33-1474
Umbilical cord vein	420 ± 406	45-1380
Fetal-to-maternal ratio*	1.32 ± 1.46	0.05-4.66

From Philipson EH, Kuhnert BR, Syracuse CD: Maternal, fetal, and neonatal lidocaine levels following local perineal infiltration. Am J Obstet Gynecol 149:403, 1984.

*Ratio of level in cord vein to level in maternal vein at delivery (mean of individual ratios, not ratio of means).

SD, Standard deviation.

Pudendal Nerve Block

Pudendal nerve block is a minor regional block that also is reasonably effective and very safe. The obstetrician, using an Iowa trumpet and a 20-gauge needle, injects 5 to 10 mL of local anesthetic just below the ischial spine. Because the hemorrhoidal nerve may be aberrant in 50% of patients, some physicians prefer to inject a portion of the local anesthetic somewhat posterior to the spine (Figure 17-11). Although a transperineal approach to the ischial spine is possible, most prefer the transvaginal approach. One percent lidocaine or 2% 2-chloroprocaine can be used.

Pudendal block is generally satisfactory for all spontaneous vaginal deliveries and episiotomies, and for some outlet or low operative vaginal deliveries, but it may not be sufficient for deliveries requiring additional manipulation. **The potential for local anesthetic toxicity is higher with pudendal block compared with perineal infiltration because of large vessels proximal to the injection site** (see Figure 17-11). Therefore, aspiration before injection is particularly important. When perineal and labial infiltration are required in addition to pudendal block, it is critically important to closely monitor the total amount of local anesthetic given.

Monitored Anesthesia Care with Sedation

For urgent or unanticipated instrumental deliveries, an anesthesiologist or nurse anesthetist may administer inhalation or intravenous analgesia while still maintaining protective laryngeal and cough reflexes. The obstetrician should add local infiltration or a pudendal block. The combined effects are additive and satisfactory for most operative vaginal deliveries, shoulder dystocias, and head entrapments. The anesthesiologist frequently questions the patient to determine the level of anesthesia and to ensure that deeper planes of anesthesia are avoided. Such precautions are important because if the patient becomes unconscious, all of the hazards associated with general

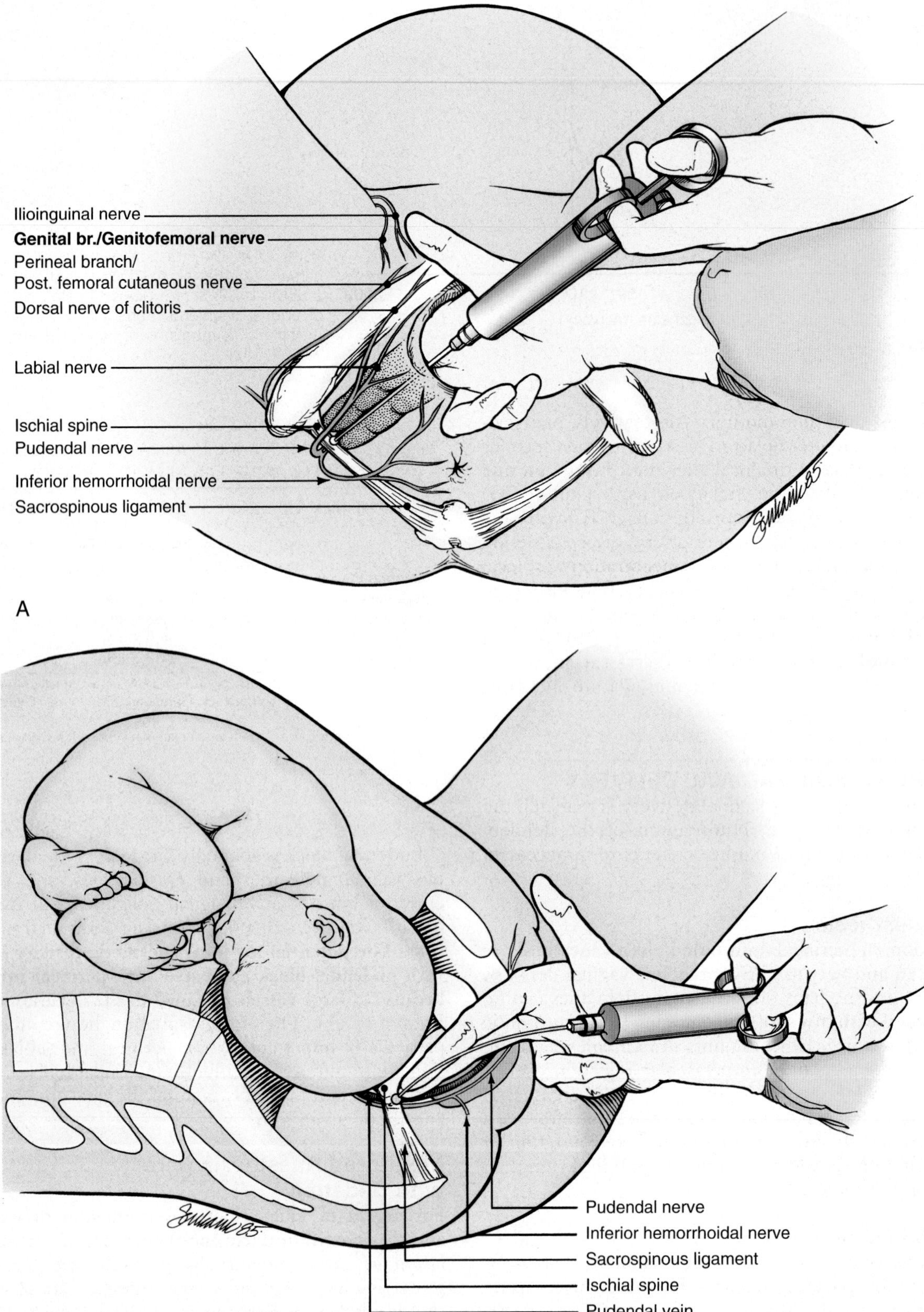

FIGURE 17-11. **A** and **B,** Anatomy of the pudendal nerve and techniques of pudendal block.

TABLE 17-6 ANESTHETIC PROCEDURES USED FOR CESAREAN DELIVERY IN 2001 ACCORDING TO SIZE OF DELIVERY SERVICE

HOSPITAL SIZE (BIRTHS/YEAR)	EPIDURAL BLOCK (%)		SPINAL BLOCK (%)		GENERAL ANESTHESIA (%)	
	Elective	Emergent	Elective	Emergent	Elective	Emergent
<500	14	14	80	59	3	25
500-1499	17	21	75	48	5	30
>1500	22	36	67	45	3	15

Modified from Bucklin BA, Hawkins JL, Anderson JR, Ullrich FA: Obstetric anesthesia workforce survey. Anesthesiology 103:645, 2005.

anesthesia are possible, including inadequate airway, hypoxia, and aspiration. Because continual assessment of the patient's state of consciousness is required and is sometimes difficult, only anesthesiologists or nurse anesthetists should administer inhalation analgesia. Furthermore, in the United States, this technique requires use of the anesthesia machine, misuse of which can prove disastrous. Most frequently, the anesthesiologist uses 50% nitrous oxide or, for intravenous analgesia, ketamine, 0.25 to 0.5 mg/kg. This latter agent may be particularly effective in the labor room when an anesthesia machine is not available, or for the patient who cannot or will not tolerate an anesthetic face mask. Inhalation or intravenous analgesia renders some patients amnesic of the event, a characteristic that may be undesirable.

Spinal (Subarachnoid) Block

A saddle block is a spinal block in which the level of anesthesia is limited to little more than the perineum. Spinal anesthesia is reasonably easy to perform and usually provides total pain relief in the blocked area. Therefore, spontaneous delivery, forceps delivery, perineal repairs, and more complicated deliveries can all be accomplished without pain for the mother. The patient's ability to push may be compromised somewhat by diminished motor strength as well as significant sensory block.

Usually, spinal anesthesia is achieved by injecting 25 to 50 mg hyperbaric lidocaine or 5 to 7.5 mg hyperbaric bupivacaine into the subarachnoid space through a 24- to 27-gauge spinal needle. It is preferable to use a pencil-point needle of the smallest possible gauge because these needles reduce the risk for spinal headache. Fentanyl, 10 to 25 mcg, may also be added to the spinal anesthetic. Because the solution is hyperbaric relative to cerebrospinal fluid, the most important determinant of anesthesia level is gravity. For example, the sitting position causes the level to fall toward the sacral nerve roots for a perineal block. Less controllable factors affecting spread include the Valsalva maneuver, coughing, and straining, any of which may cause the level to rise. Injecting the local anesthetic during a contraction may result in higher than expected levels of anesthesia and should be avoided.

Persons other than anesthesiologists sometimes administer spinal anesthesia, which is technically easy to perform. In such situations, it is important to remember that all hazards associated with major blocks are possible, including hypotension and "total spinal." **The person who administers spinal anesthesia must never leave the patient unattended without ensuring that another competent individual will assume responsibility for monitoring the blood pressure and level of anesthesia.** Usually, the level of the spinal block will be complete and fixed within 5 to 10 minutes, but it may continue to creep upward for 20 minutes or longer. Left uterine displacement should be maintained after the local anesthetic has been injected to maintain venous return and prevent excess hypotension.

Lumbar Epidural Anesthesia

Single-dose epidural anesthesia techniques are rarely used in modern obstetrical anesthesia practice. The relative difficulty, slow onset, and large amounts of local anesthetic required to block sacral nerves are significant disadvantages compared with spinal anesthesia. Usually, when these techniques are used, they are instituted during labor as continuous techniques and maintained or intensified for the delivery.

General Anesthesia

General anesthesia is rarely indicated for vaginal delivery. Airway management engenders risk; therefore, general anesthesia should not be used without a strong indication. An unanticipated breech presentation, shoulder dystocia, internal version, and extraction of a second twin or uterine inversion may represent rare indications for general anesthesia. General anesthesia may rarely be indicated for a difficult forceps delivery in a patient in whom major regional anesthesia is contraindicated. **When general anesthesia is indicated for vaginal delivery, the technique specific for cesarean delivery is used, including administration by experienced and competent personnel, rapid-sequence induction, and endotracheal intubation.** For breech delivery or delivery of a second twin, administration of a high concentration of a volatile halogenated agent (e.g., isoflurane, desflurane, or sevoflurane) may be used to effect uterine and perhaps cervical relaxation. Equipotent doses of any of these three agents will provide equivalent uterine relaxation.[82]

ANESTHESIA FOR CESAREAN DELIVERY

In the United States, general anesthesia is used for about 10% of cesarean births (depending on size of hospital), and spinal and epidural anesthetics are used for about 90% of these deliveries (Table 17-6).[1] Local anesthesia for cesarean delivery is possible, with the mother undergoing general anesthesia after delivery of the infant, but it is rarely used or taught anymore. Although general anesthesia may have increased risk for the mother, regional or general anesthesia results in similar fetal outcomes as ascertained by Apgar scores and blood gas measurements (Table 17-7).

TABLE 17-7 ELECTIVE CESAREAN SECTION—BLOOD GAS AND APGAR SCORES

	GENERAL ANESTHESIA* (N = 20)	EPIDURAL ANESTHESIA* (N = 15)	SPINAL ANESTHESIA† (N = 15)
Umbilical Vein			
pH	–7.38	–7.359	–7.34
PO_2 (mm Hg)	35	36	37
PCO_2 (mm Hg)	38	42	48
Apgar <6			
1	–1	–0	–0
5	–0	–0	–0
Umbilical Artery			
pH	–7.32	–7.28	–7.28
PO_2 (mm Hg)	22	18	18
PCO_2 (mm Hg)	47	55	63
Base excess (mEq/L)	–1.80	–1.60	–1.40

*Data from James FM III, Crawford JS, Hopkinson R, et al: A comparison of general anesthesia and lumbar epidural analgesia for elective cesarean section. Anesth Analg 56:228, 1977.
†Data from Datta S, Brown WU: Acid-base status in diabetic mothers and their infants following general or spinal anesthesia for cesarean section. Anesthesiology 47:272, 1977.

Neurobehavioral testing that quantifies responses to certain stimuli in the early postpartum hours suggests that infants of mothers who receive regional anesthesia achieve somewhat higher scores than those whose mothers receive general anesthesia. The usefulness of neurobehavioral testing has been called into question because of poor interrater reliability. Neurobehavioral considerations do not weigh heavily in the choice of anesthesia or anesthetic agent; the choice can be based on the preferences of the mother, the obstetrician, and the anesthesiologist, as well as on the demands of the particular clinical situation.

Premedication

Premedication using sedative or opioid agents is usually omitted because these agents cross the placenta and can depress the fetus. Sedation should be unnecessary if the procedure is explained well and the patient is reassured.

Antacids

Use of a clear antacid is considered routine for all parturients before surgery. Additional aspiration prophylaxis using an H_2-receptor blocking agent and metoclopramide may be given to parturients with risk factors such as morbid obesity, diabetes mellitus, or a difficult airway, or those who have previously received opioids. As soon as it is known that the patient requires cesarean delivery, whether with regional or general anesthesia, 30 mL of a clear, nonparticulate antacid, such as 0.3 M sodium citrate, Bicitra, or Alka Seltzer, 2 tablets in 30 mL water, is administered to decrease gastric acidity and ameliorate the consequences of aspiration, should it occur. The chalky white particulate antacids are avoided because they can produce lung damage (Figure 17-12).[83]

Left Uterine Displacement

As during labor, the uterus may compress the inferior vena cava and the aorta during cesarean delivery; **aortocaval compression is detrimental to both mother and fetus.** The duration of anesthesia has little effect on neonatal acid-base status when left uterine displacement is practiced; however, when patients remain supine, Apgar scores decrease as time of anesthesia increases.[84]

ADVANTAGES AND DISADVANTAGES OF GENERAL ANESTHESIA FOR CESAREAN DELIVERY

- Advantages
  - Patient does not have to be awake during a major operation.
  - General anesthesia provides total pain relief.
  - Operating conditions are optimal.
  - The mother can be given 100% oxygen if needed.
- Disadvantages
  - Patients will not be awake during childbirth, but there is a small risk for undesirable awareness.
  - There is a slight risk for fetal depression immediately after birth.
  - Intubation causes hypertension and tachycardia, which may be particularly dangerous in severely preeclamptic patients.
  - Intubation can be difficult or impossible.
  - Aspiration of stomach contents is possible.

General Anesthesia

Balanced general anesthesia, referring to a combination of various agents, including barbiturates or other hypnotic agents to induce sleep, inhalation agents, opioids, and muscle relaxants as opposed to high concentrations of potent inhalation agents alone, is preferred for obstetrical applications (see box, Advantages and Disadvantages of General Anesthesia for Cesarean Delivery).

Failure to intubate and aspiration continue to cause anesthesia-related maternal mortality, and as a result, many anesthesiologists, obstetricians, and patients now prefer regional anesthesia over general anesthesia.[1] To understand how these complications may arise, the obstetrician should be aware of the sequence of events during general anesthesia.

Preoxygenation

Preoxygenation is especially important in pregnant patients who have decreased functional residual capacity and are more likely than nonpregnant patients to rapidly become hypoxemic if difficult intubation accompanied by apnea occurs. Before starting induction, 100% oxygen should be

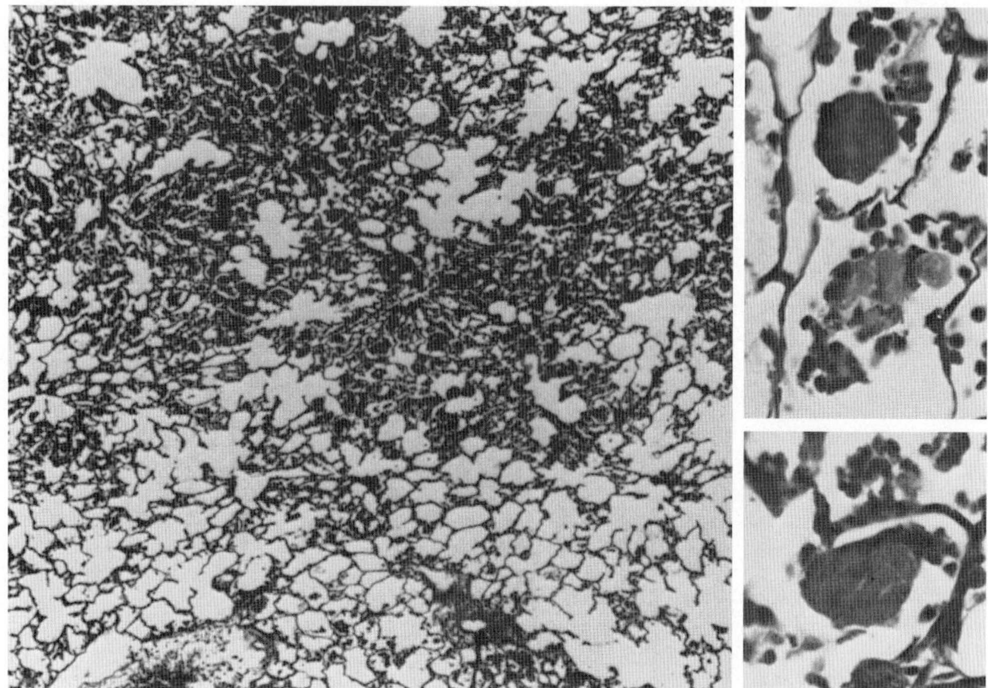

FIGURE 17-12. Lung after aspiration of particulate antacid. Note marked extensive inflammatory reaction. The alveoli are filled with polymorphonuclear leukocytes and macrophages in approximately equal numbers. *Insets at right* show large and small intra-alveolar particles surrounded by inflammatory cells (48 hours). Later, the reaction changed to an intra-alveolar cellular collection of clusters of large macrophages with abundant granular cytoplasm, in some of which were small amphophilic particles similar to those seen in the insets. No fibrosis or other inflammatory reaction was seen (28 days). (From Gibbs CP, Schwartz DJ, Wynne JW, et al: Antacid pulmonary aspiration in the dog. Anesthesiology 51:380, 1979.)

administered through a face mask for 2 to 3 minutes. In situations of dire emergency, four vital capacity breaths of 100% oxygen through a tight circle system will provide similar benefit.[85]

Induction

The anesthesiologist rapidly administers a short-acting induction agent to render the patient unconscious. An appropriate dose has little effect on the fetus. **Induction agents that may be used are thiopental, propofol,[86] etomidate,[87] and ketamine,[88] all of which are rapidly redistributed in the mother and fetus.** Women who receive ketamine for induction require less analgesic medications in the first 24 hours after their cesarean delivery compared with those who received thiopental.[89] Its antagonism of NMDA receptors may prevent central hypersensitization, providing preemptive analgesia.

Although obstetricians are often concerned about the induction-to-delivery interval (I-D) during general anesthesia, uterine incision-to-delivery interval (U-D) is more predictive of neonatal status.[84,90] With a prolonged I-D interval, there is fetal uptake of the inhaled anesthetic and depressed Apgar scores (i.e., sleepy babies), but fetal acid-base status is normal, and effective ventilation is all that is needed. Prolonged U-D intervals greater than 3 minutes lead to depressed Apgar scores with regional or general anesthesia, and they are associated with elevated fetal umbilical artery norepinephrine concentrations and associated fetal acidosis.[90]

Muscle Relaxants

Immediately after the induction agent, the anesthesiologist gives a muscle relaxant to facilitate intubation. Succinylcholine, a rapid-onset, short-acting muscle relaxant, remains the agent of choice in most patients.

Cricoid Pressure

In rapid-sequence induction, as the induction agent begins to take effect and the patient approaches unconsciousness, an assistant applies pressure to the cricoid cartilage, just below the thyroid cartilage, and does not release the pressure until an endotracheal tube is placed, its position verified by end-tidal carbon dioxide measurement, and the cuff on the tube inflated. **Pressure on the cricoid compresses the esophagus and is extremely important in preventing aspiration should regurgitation or vomiting occur.**

Intubation

In most cases, intubation proceeds smoothly. However, in approximately 1 in 238 obstetrical patients, it is difficult, delayed, or impossible. The incidence of failed intubation in obstetrical patients is about seven times more common than in patients in the general operating room (i.e., 1 in 230 to 280 in obstetrical patients versus 1 in 2230 in surgical patients).[91] When the delay is prolonged or the intubation impossible, **the critical factors include delivering oxygen to the now unconscious and paralyzed patient and preventing aspiration.**[92] Delay in intubation is associated with escalating aspiration risk. Therefore, it is particularly important during a difficult intubation that the person applying cricoid pressure not release that pressure until told to do so by the anesthesiologist.

The patient at risk for a difficult or impossible intubation can often be identified before surgery. Examination of the airway is a critical part of the preanesthetic evaluation. The anesthesiologist will assess (1) the ability to visualize

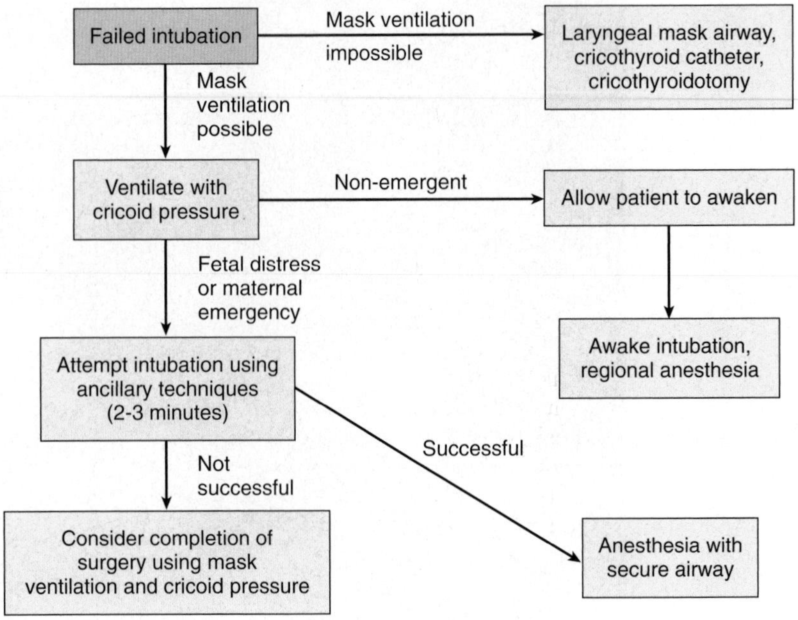

FIGURE 17-13. An algorithm for the management of failed intubation in the obstetrical patient.

oropharyngeal structures (Mallampati classification[93]); (2) range of motion of the neck; (3) presence of a receding mandible, which indicates the depth of the submandibular space; and (4) whether protruding maxillary incisors are present. **Obstetricians should be alert to the presence of obesity, severe edema, anatomic abnormalities of the face, neck, or spine, including trauma or surgery, abnormal dentition, difficulty opening the mouth, extremely short stature, short neck or arthritis of the neck, or goiter. When the obstetrician recognizes airway abnormalities, patients should be referred for an early preoperative evaluation by the anesthesiologist.**

Proper Tube Placement

Before the operation begins, the anesthesiologist must ensure that the endotracheal tube is properly positioned. End-tidal carbon dioxide analysis is the preferred method to confirm that the tube is within the trachea. Of course, the anesthesiologist will also confirm that breath sounds are bilateral and equal. The operation should not proceed until the airway is secure because the patient cannot be allowed to awaken after the abdomen is opened.

When intubation cannot be accomplished and cesarean delivery is not urgent, the decision to delay the operation and allow the mother to awaken is easy. However, if the operation is being done because of rapidly worsening fetal condition or maternal hemorrhage, allowing the mother to awaken may further jeopardize the fetus or mother. Rarely, in situations of dire fetal compromise, the anesthesiologist and obstetrician may jointly decide to proceed with cesarean delivery while the anesthesiologist provides oxygenation, ventilation, and anesthesia by face mask ventilation or laryngeal mask airway, with an additional person maintaining continuous cricoid pressure. In these emergent situations, it may be necessary to have additional trained personnel to provide assistance. After delivery, the obstetrician may need to obtain temporary hemostasis and then halt surgery while the anesthesiologist secures the airway by fiberoptics or other methods.

An algorithm for management of failed intubation in the obstetrical patient is shown in Figure 17-13. Nursing staff should also be familiar with the difficult airway algorithm in case they are called on to assist during an airway emergency. Equipment to manage the difficult airway must be immediately available in the labor and delivery suite.[3,94]

Nitrous Oxide and Oxygen

Once the endotracheal tube is in place, a 50:50 mixture of nitrous oxide and oxygen, which is safe for both mother and fetus, is added to provide analgesia and amnesia.

Volatile Halogenated Agent

In addition to nitrous oxide, a low concentration of a volatile halogenated agent (e.g., isoflurane, sevoflurane, or desflurane) is added to provide maternal amnesia and additional analgesia. These agents, in low concentrations, are not harmful to mother or fetus. **Uterine relaxation does not result from low concentrations of these agents, and bleeding should not be increased secondary to their addition.**[82] **Proceeding without a potent inhalation agent results in an unacceptably high incidence of maternal awareness and recall.** Even with the use of one of these agents, maternal awareness and recall occasionally occur. Therefore, it is important that all operating room personnel use discretion in conversation and conduct themselves as if the patient were awake.

Postdelivery

The concentration of nitrous oxide can usually be increased after delivery. In addition, the volatile halogenated agent is continued at a low concentration, and pain relief is supplemented with an opioid such as fentanyl or morphine. Other intravenous agents such as benzodiazepines may be added to ensure maternal amnesia. Oxytocin, 20 to 80 U/L, is infused intravenously. Large bolus injections of oxytocin are avoided because they can cause a drop in systemic vascular resistance, hypotension, and tachycardia. **Maternal deaths have been reported following intravenous bolus oxytocin in the setting of hypovolemia or pulmonary hypertension.**[95]

Extubation

Because the patient can aspirate while awakening as well as during induction, extubation is not done until the patient is awake and can respond appropriately to commands. Coughing and bucking do not necessarily indicate that the patient is awake, merely that she is in the second stage—the excitement stage—of anesthesia. It is during this period of anesthesia that laryngospasm is most likely to occur should any foreign body, including the endotracheal tube or bits of stomach contents, stimulate the larynx. **The patient must therefore be awake and conscious, not merely active, before extubation.**

Aspiration

Aspiration is a serious and potentially fatal complication of general anesthesia and, therefore, deserves specific attention. In most instances, it can be prevented. When it cannot, the consequences depend in part on the volume and acidity of the aspirate. The conventional wisdom is that patients are at risk when their stomach contents are greater than 25 mL and when the pH of those contents is less than 2.5. Pregnant patients are at higher risk for aspiration. The enlarged uterus increases intra-abdominal pressure and thus intragastric pressure. The gastroesophageal sphincter is distorted by the enlarged uterus, making it less competent, and possibly explaining the high incidence of heartburn that occurs during pregnancy. Increased progesterone levels affect smooth muscle, delaying gastric emptying and relaxing the gastroesophageal sphincter. Gastrin, the hormone that increases both acidity and volume of gastric contents, is increased during pregnancy, and motilin, a hormone that speeds gastric emptying, is decreased during pregnancy. Labor itself delays gastric emptying, primarily when patients have received opioids.[96] Many patients undergo cesarean delivery after a prolonged labor, during which they may have received several doses of opioids.

The severity of lung damage and rates of morbidity after aspiration vary and depend on the type of material aspirated. Less acidic aspirates (pH >2.5) fill the alveoli, decreasing PaO_2 without a significant destructive or inflammatory effect. Aspirates with a pH of less than 2.5 cause hemorrhage, inflammatory exudates, and edema resulting in lower PaO_2. **Aspiration of partially digested food produces the most severe physiologic and histologic alterations.** PaO_2 decreases more than with any other type of aspiration, and lung damage is considerably more destructive (Table 17-8).

Although acidic stomach contents can be neutralized safely and effectively with clear antacids or an H_2-receptor antagonist, antacids cannot ameliorate the risks for aspiration after food intake. Aspiration of partially digested food causes significant hypoxia and lung damage, even at a pH level as high as 5.9. To decrease aspiration risk in cases of unplanned cesarean delivery, oral intake during labor should be limited to modest amounts of clear liquids or ice chips.[3]

TABLE 17-8 ARTERIAL BLOOD GAS TENSIONS AND PH OF DOGS 30 MINUTES AFTER ASPIRATION OF 2 ML/KG OF VARIOUS MATERIALS

ASPIRATE		RESPONSE		
COMPOSITION	pH	Po_2 (mm Hg)	Pco_2 (mm Hg)	pH
Saline	5.9	61	34	7.37
HCl	1.8	41	45	7.29
Food particles	5.9	34	51	7.19
Food particles	1.8	23	56	7.13

From Gibbs CP, Modell JH: Management of aspiration pneumonitis. *In* Miller RD (ed): Anesthesia, 3rd ed. New York, Churchill Livingstone, 1990, p 1293.

Neuraxial Anesthesia

If the fetal status permits and there are no maternal contraindications, regional anesthesia is preferred for cesarean delivery (see box, Advantages and Disadvantages of Regional Anesthesia). Contraindications to regional anesthesia include hemodynamically significant hemorrhage, infection at the site of needle insertion, coagulopathy, increased intracranial pressure caused by a mass lesion, patient refusal, and perhaps some forms of heart disease. Significant ongoing hemorrhage is a firm contraindication to regional anesthesia because the sympathetic blockade overrides compensatory vasoconstriction, potentially precipitating cardiovascular decompensation.

ADVANTAGES AND DISADVANTAGES OF REGIONAL ANESTHESIA

- Advantages
  - The patient is awake and can participate in the birth of her child.
  - There is little risk for drug depression or aspiration and no intubation difficulties.
  - Newborns generally have good neurobehavioral scores.
  - The father is more likely to be allowed in the operating room.
  - Postoperative pain control using neuraxial opioids may be superior to intravenous patient-controlled analgesia.
- Disadvantages
  - Patients may prefer not to be awake during major surgery.
  - A block that provides inadequate anesthesia may result.
  - Hypotension, perhaps the most common complication of regional anesthesia, occurs during 25% to 75% of spinal or epidural anesthetics.
  - Total spinal anesthesia may occur, necessitating airway management.
  - Local anesthetic toxicity may occur.
  - Although extremely rare, permanent neurologic sequelae may occur.
  - There are several contraindications (see text).

The use of regional anesthesia in patients with fetal compromise depends on the severity of fetal condition. **If the situation is severe and acute, do not delay delivery to perform a regional technique de novo. Ongoing acute fetal deterioration is usually an indication for general anesthesia.** However, a history or suspicion of difficult intubation should prompt performance of either awake intubation or regional anesthesia, despite the presence of fetal compromise, because of the risk for maternal death from unsuccessful intubation. Lesser degrees of fetal compromise may permit regional anesthesia. For example, if an epidural catheter has been placed earlier, a partial level of anesthesia already exists, and there is hemodynamic stability, extension of epidural anesthesia may be appropriate for cesarean delivery. The anesthesiologist may give additional local anesthetic while the urethral catheter is inserted and the abdomen is prepared and draped. Often, there will be satisfactory anesthesia when the surgeon is ready to make the skin incision. If not, the fetal heart rate pattern will dictate whether a delay is acceptable. When partial but inadequate epidural anesthesia results, one may consider supplemental local infiltration of local anesthetic, but most often general anesthesia will be indicated.

In cases in which the fetal heart rate tracing is not critical, de novo spinal or epidural anesthesia may be performed for cesarean delivery. In cases in which extension of existing epidural anesthesia is unsuccessful, spinal anesthesia should be placed with caution because the risk for high spinal anesthesia is increased.

In healthy patients, the choice between epidural, spinal, and CSE anesthesia primarily rests with the anesthesiologist. With the recent availability of small-gauge spinal needles with pencil-point tip design, the risk for headache is no different after spinal or epidural anesthesia. Most consider spinal block to be easier and quicker to perform, and most believe that the resulting anesthesia will be more solid and complete.[97] Perhaps the most significant advantage of spinal anesthesia is that it requires considerably less local anesthetic, and therefore, the potential for local anesthetic toxicity is reduced. Either technique is satisfactory, however, and should provide safe, effective anesthesia for mother, newborn, and obstetrician.

Postoperative Care

If spinal or epidural anesthesia is used for cesarean delivery, excellent postoperative analgesia can be obtained by addition of preservative-free morphine to the local anesthetic solution. The more lipid-soluble opioids, such as fentanyl or sufentanil, provide fast onset of analgesia with minimal side effects but have a short duration of 2 to 4 hours. They may be used postoperatively in combination with a local anesthetic in a continuous or patient-controlled epidural infusion to improve the quality of the block. In contrast, morphine is hydrophilic, which gives it a prolonged duration of up to 24 hours, and it can be given as a single dose at the time of cesarean delivery. Unfortunately, its water solubility gives it a long onset time and higher incidence of side effects. The most common side effects of spinal and epidural opioids are itching and nausea. Respiratory depression is a rare but serious complication. **Several studies have shown that spinal or epidural opioids provide superior pain relief compared with parenteral (intramuscular or intravenous PCA) opioids with a trend toward earlier hospital discharge and lower cost.**[3]

If general anesthesia was used or neuraxial opioids provide inadequate pain control, an intravenous PCA can be used for postoperative pain management. Morphine, hydromorphone (Dilaudid), and fentanyl have all been used successfully. When intravenous PCA is used, the pump settings include an incremental dose of 1 to 2 mg morphine, 0.2 to 0.4 mg hydromorphone, or 25 mcg fentanyl; a lockout interval of 6 to 10 minutes; and rarely, a basal or continuous infusion rate. Basal rates are rarely necessary for pain control and only increase maternal sedation and side effects. Using PCA provides better patient satisfaction by allowing her to control her pain medication.

The addition of nonsteroidal anti-inflammatory agents significantly improves pain scores with neuraxial morphine and reduces use of PCA opioids.[98] Intravenous ketorolac, rectal indomethacin, or oral ibuprofen can be used depending on the patient's ability to tolerate oral intake. Contraindications for nonsteroidal use include renal insufficiency or low urine output, use of gentamicin or similar drugs with renal toxicity, coagulopathy, and uterine atony. Although the package insert for ketorolac (Toradol) states that it is contraindicated for use in breastfeeding mothers, the American Academy of Pediatrics approves its use while women are breastfeeding.

In most cases, postoperative care is uneventful in obstetrical patients. However, **recent reports suggest that the postoperative period can be an important time for anesthetic-related maternal mortality.** In a state review of maternal deaths in Michigan from 1985 to 2003, 8 of 855 maternal deaths were anesthesia related and occurred during emergence or recovery from general anesthesia.[99] Hypoventilation or airway obstruction occurred in these cases, and obesity and African American race were factors associated with these deaths. Similar reports of anesthesia-related maternal mortality have emerged from the United Kingdom. During the time period from 2003 to 2005, there were six anesthesia-related maternal deaths.[41] Of those deaths, three were related to postoperative respiratory failure, and four of the patients had a body mass index greater than 35. These cases raise important questions about appropriate postanesthesia care unit management after general anesthesia for cesarean delivery, as well as the need for additional monitoring in obese patients at risk for obstructive sleep apnea. In a recent survey of obstetrical anesthesia recovery practices from obstetrical anesthesiology directors of North American academic institutions, 45% (28 of 62) of institutions had no specific postanesthesia recovery training for nursing staff providing postcesarean care for patients recovering from neuraxial or general anesthesia.[100] In addition, 43% (29 of 67) of respondents rated the recovery care provided to cesarean delivery patients as lower quality than care given to general surgical patients. Results from this survey suggest that in many cases, the level of care provided for postanesthesia recovery from cesarean delivery may not meet guidelines established by the ASA Task Force on Postanesthetic Care and the American Society of PeriAnesthesia Nurses. However, the most recent ASA Practice Guidelines for

Obstetric Anesthesia[3] emphasize that labor and delivery units should have the same staffing and equipment as surgical operating and recovery rooms to reduce risks associated with emergence after general anesthesia for cesarean delivery as well as to reduce the risk associated with obesity and obstructive sleep apnea.

KEY POINTS

- Analgesia during labor can reduce or prevent potentially adverse stress responses to the pain of labor.
- Parenteral opioids for labor analgesia work primarily by sedation and, except at high doses, result in minimal reduction of maternal pain. Side effects include nausea and respiratory depression in both the mother and newborn. The routine use of promethazine (Phenergan) in conjunction with opioids should be avoided.
- Placental transfer of a drug between mother and fetus is governed by the characteristics of the drug (including its size, lipid solubility, and ionization), maternal blood levels and uterine blood flow, placental circulation, and fetal circulation.
- Continuous regional analgesia is the most effective form of intrapartum pain relief currently available and has the flexibility to provide additional anesthesia for spontaneous or instrumental delivery, cesarean delivery, and postoperative pain control.
- Spinal opioids provide excellent analgesia during much of the first stage of labor, while decreasing or avoiding the risks for local anesthetic toxicity, high spinal anesthesia, and motor block. Most patients need additional analgesia later in labor and during the second stage.
- Side effects and complications of regional anesthesia include hypotension, local anesthetic toxicity, total spinal anesthesia, neurologic injury, and spinal headache. Personnel providing anesthesia must be available and competent to treat these problems.
- Epidural analgesia does not increase the rate of cesarean delivery but may increase oxytocin use and the rate of instrument-assisted vaginal deliveries. The duration of the second stage is increased by 15 to 30 minutes. Maternal-fetal factors and obstetrical management are the most important determinants of the cesarean delivery rate.
- Epidural analgesia is associated with an increased rate of maternal fever during labor. This does not alter the rate of documented neonatal sepsis. Other neonatal implications are unclear.
- General anesthesia is used for less than 5% of elective and roughly 25% of emergent cesarean deliveries. Although safe for the newborn, general anesthesia can be associated with failed intubation and aspiration, causes of anesthesia-related maternal mortality.
- Aspiration of gastric contents is most detrimental when food particles are present or the pH is less than 2.5; therefore, patients should be encouraged not to eat during labor, and acid-neutralizing medications should be used before operative deliveries.
- The use of regional anesthesia is not absolutely contraindicated in cases of non-reassuring fetal testing; the method of anesthesia should be chosen based on the degree of fetal compromise and maternal safety.

REFERENCES

1. Bucklin BA, Hawkins JL, Anderson JR, Ullrich FA: Obstetric anesthesia workforce survey. Anesthesiology 103:645, 2005.
2. American Society of Anesthesiologists/American College of Obstetricians and Gynecologists Joint Statement: Optimal goals for anesthesia care in obstetrics. Park Ridge, IL, 2008. Available at: www.asahq.org.
3. American Society of Anesthesiologists Task Force on Obstetric Anesthesia: Practice guidelines for obstetric anesthesia. Anesthesiology 106:843, 2007.
4. Melzack R: The myth of painless childbirth. Pain 19:321, 1984.
5. Morishima HO, Yeh M-N, James LS: Reduced uterine blood flow and fetal hypoxemia with acute maternal stress: experimental observation in the pregnant baboon. Am J Obstet Gynecol 134:270, 1979.
6. Eidelman AI, Hoffmann NW, Kaitz M: Cognitive deficits in women after childbirth. Obstet Gynecol 81:764, 1993.
7. Campogna G, Camorcia M, Stirparo S: Expectant fathers' experience during labor with or without epidural analgesia. Int J Obstet Anesth 16:110, 2007.
8. Reynolds F, Sharma SK, Seed PT: Analgesia in labour and fetal acid-base balance: a meta-analysis comparing epidural with systemic opioid analgesia. Br J Obstet Gynaecol 109:1344, 2002.
9. Lee H, Ernst E: Acupuncture for labor pain management: a systematic review. Am J Obstet Gynecol 191:1573, 2004.
10. Cluett ER, Pickering RM, Getliffe K, St. George Saunders NJ: Randomised controlled trial of labouring in water compared with standard of augmentation for management of dystocia in first stage of labour. BMJ 328:314, 2004.
11. Committee on Fetus and Newborn of the American Academy of Pediatrics: Underwater births. Pediatrics 115:1413, 2005.
12. Huntley AL, Coon JT, Ernst E: Complementary and alternative medicine for labor pain: a systematic review. Am J Obstet Gynecol 191:36, 2004.
13. Harrison RF, Woods T, Shore M, et al: Pain relief in labour using transcutaneous electrical nerve stimulation (TENS). Br J Obstet Gynaecol 93:739, 1989.
14. Olofsson C, Ekblom A, Ekman-Ordeberg G, et al: Lack of analgesic effect systemically administered morphine or pethidine on labour pain. Br J Obstet Gynaecol 103:968, 1996.
15. Halpern SH, Leighton BL, Ohlsson A, et al: Effect of epidural vs parenteral opioid analgesia on the progress of labor: a meta-analysis. JAMA 280:2105, 1998.
16. O'Sullivan GM, Sutton AJ, Thompson SA, et al: Noninvasive measurement of gastric emptying in obstetric patients. Anesth Analg 66:505, 1987.
17. Campbell DC: Parenteral opioids for labor analgesia. Clin Obstet Gynecol 46:616, 2003.
18. Hill D, Van de Velde M: Remifentanil patient-controlled analgesia should be routinely available for use in labour. Int J Obstet Anesth 17:336, 2008.
19. Sharma SK, Alexander JM, Messick G, et al: A randomized trial of epidural analgesia versus intravenous meperidine analgesia during labor in nulliparous women. Anesthesiology 96:546, 2002.
20. Kuhnert BR, Kuhnert PM, Philipson EH, Syracuse CD: Disposition of meperidine and normeperidine following multiple doses during labor. II Fetus and neonate. Am J Obstet Gynecol 151:410, 1985.

21. Sharma SK, Sidawi JE, Ramin SM, et al: A randomized trial of epidural versus patient-controlled meperidine analgesia during labor. Anesthesiology 87:487, 1997.
22. Wittels B, Glosten B, Faure EA, et al: Postcesarean analgesia with both epidural morphine and intravenous patient-controlled analgesia: neurobehavioral outcomes among nursing neonates. Anesth Analg 85:600, 1997.
23. Romagnoli A, Keats AS: Ceiling effect for respiratory depression by nalbuphine. Clin Pharmacol Ther 27:478, 1980.
24. Maduska AL, Hajghassemali M: A double-blind comparison of butorphanol and meperidine in labour: maternal pain relief and effect on the newborn. Can Anaesth Soc J 25:398, 1978.
25. Vella L, Francis D, Houlton P, Reynolds F: Comparison of the antiemetics metoclopramide and promethazine in labour. BMJ 290:1173, 1985.
26. Rosenblatt WH, Cioffi AM, Sinatra R, Silverman DG: Metoclopramide-enhanced analgesia for prostaglandin-induced termination of pregnancy. Anesth Analg 75:760, 1992.
27. Camann W, Cohen MB, Ostheimer GW: Is midazolam desirable for sedation in parturients? Anesthesiology 65:441, 1986.
28. Owen JR, Irani SF, Blair AW: Effect of diazepam administered to mothers during labour on temperature regulation of neonate. Arch Dis Child 47:107, 1972.
29. Zakowski MI, Herman NL: The Placenta: Anatomy, Physiology, and Transfer of Drugs. In Chestnut DH, Polley LS, Tsen LC, Wong CA (eds): Chestnut's Obstetric Anesthesia: Principles and Practice, 4th ed. Philadelphia, Elsevier, 2009, p 55.
30. Johnson RF, Herman NL, Johnson HV, et al: Effects of fetal pH on local anesthetic transfer across the human placenta. Anesthesiology 85:608, 1996.
31. Hawkins JL: Epidural analgesia for labor and delivery. N Engl J Med 362:1503, 2010.
32. American College of Obstetricians and Gynecologists: Obstetric analgesia and anesthesia. ACOG Practice Bulletin No. 36. Obstet Gynecol 100:177, 2002.
33. Abrao KC, Francisco RPV, Miyadahira S, et al: Elevation of uterine basal tone and fetal heart rate abnormalities after labor analgesia. Obstet Gynecol 113:41, 2009.
34. Albright GA, Forster RM: Does combined spinal-epidural analgesia with subarachnoid sufentanil increase the incidence of emergency cesarean delivery? Reg Anesth 22:400, 1997.
35. Mardirosoff C, Dumont L, Boulvain M, Tramer MR: Fetal bradycardia due to intrathecal opioids for labor analgesia: a systematic review. Br J Obstet Gynaecol 109:274, 2002.
36. Simmons SW, Cyna AM, Dennis AT, Hughes D: Combined spinal-epidural versus epidural analgesia in labour. Cochrane Database Syst Rev CD003401, 2007.
37. Ngan Kee WD, Lee A, Khaw KS, et al: A randomized double-blinded comparison of phenylephrine and ephedrine infusion combinations to maintain blood pressure during spinal anesthesia for cesarean delivery: the effects on fetal acid-base status and hemodynamic control. Anesth Analg 107:1295, 2008.
38. Riley ET: Spinal anesthesia for caesarean delivery: keep the pressure up and don't spare the vasoconstrictors [editorial]. Br J Anaesth 92:459, 2004.
39. Jenkins JG: Some immediate serious complications of obstetric epidural analgesia and anaesthesia: a prospective study of 145,550 epidurals. Int J Obstet Anesth 14:37, 2004.
40. Davies JM, Posner KL, Lee LA, et al: Liability associated with obstetric anesthesia. Anesthesiology 110:131, 2009.
41. Cooper GM, McClure JH: Anaesthesia chapter from Saving Mothers' Lives: reviewing maternal deaths to make pregnancy safer. Br J Anaesth 100:17, 2008.
42. Clarkson CW, Hondeghem LM: Mechanism for bupivacaine depression of cardiac conduction: fast block of sodium channels during the action potential with slow recovery from block during diastole. Anesthesiology 62:396, 1985.
43. Groban L, Deal DD, Vernon JC, et al: Cardiac resuscitation after incremental overdosage with lidocaine, bupivacaine, levobupivacaine, and ropivacaine in anesthetized dogs. Anesth Analg 92:37, 2001.
44. Leighton BL, Norris MC, Sosis M, et al: Limitations of epinephrine as a marker of intravascular injection in laboring women. Anesthesiology 66:688, 1987.
45. Weinberg GL: Current concepts in resuscitation of patients with local anesthetic cardiac toxicity. Reg Anesth Pain Med 27:568, 2002.
46. Neal JM, Bernards CM, Butterworth JF, et al: ASRA practice advisory on local anesthetic systemic toxicity. Reg Anesth Pain Med 35:152, 2010.
47. Leighton BL: Why obstetric anesthesiologists get sued. Anesthesiology 110:8, 2009.
48. Wong CA: Neurologic deficits and labor analgesia. Reg Anesth Pain Med 29:341, 2004.
49. Ruppen W, Derry S, McQuay H, Moore RA: Incidence of epidural hematoma, infection and neurologic injury in obstetric patients with epidural analgesia/anesthesia. Anesthesiology 105:394, 2006.
50. Moen V, Dahlgren N, Irestedt L: Severe neurological complications after central neuraxial blockades in Sweden 1990-1999. Anesthesiology 101:950, 2004.
51. de Fijter S, DiOrio M, Carmean J: Bacterial meningitis after intrapartum spinal anesthesia: New York and Ohio, 2008-2009. MMWR Morb Mortal Wkly Rep 59:65, 2010.
52. Hebl JR: The importance and implications of aseptic techniques during regional anesthesia. Reg Anesth Pain Med 31:311, 2006.
53. American Society of Anesthesiologists Task Force on Infectious Complication Associated with Neuraxial Techniques: Practice advisory for the prevention, diagnosis, and management of infectious complications associated with neuraxial techniques. Anesthesiology 112:530, 2010.
54. Turnbull DK, Shepherd DB: Post-dural puncture headache: pathogenesis, prevention and treatment. Br J Anaesth 91:718, 2003.
55. Stella CL, Jodicke CD, How HY, et al: Postpartum headache: is your work-up complete? Am J Obstet Gynecol 196:318.e1, 2007.
56. Benzon HT, Wong CA: Postdural puncture headache: mechanisms, treatment and prevention. Reg Anesth Pain Med 26:293, 2001.
57. Ayad S, Demian Y, Narouze SN, Tetzlaff JE: Subarachnoid catheter placement after wet tap for analgesia in labor: influence on the risk of headache in obstetric patients. Reg Anesth Pain Med 28:512, 2003.
58. Wang SM, Dezinno P, Maranets I, et al: Low back pain during pregnancy: prevalence, risk factors, and outcomes. Obstet Gynecol 104:65, 2004.
59. Howell CJ, Dean T, Lucking L, et al: Randomised study of long term outcome after epidural versus non-epidural analgesia during labour. BMJ 325:357, 2002.
60. Loughnan BA, Carli F, Romney J, et al: Epidural analgesia and backache: a randomized controlled comparison with intramuscular meperidine for analgesia during labour. Br J Anaesth 89:466, 2002.
61. Wiklund I, Norman M, Uvnas-Moberg K, et al: Epidural analgesia: breast-feeding success and related factors. Midwifery 25:e31, 2009.
62. Halpern S, MacDonell J, Levine NT, Wilson D: Does epidural analgesia influence breast-feeding outcomes six weeks postpartum? Birth 26:83, 1999.
63. Beilin Y, Bodian CA, Weiser J, et al: Effect of labor epidural analgesia with and without fentanyl on infant breast-feeding: a prospective, randomized, double-blind study. Anesthesiology 103:1211, 2005.
64. Hirose M, Hara Y, Hosokawa T, Tanaka Y: The effect of postoperative analgesia with continuous epidural bupivacaine after cesarean section on the amount of breast feeding and infant weight gain. Anesth Analg 82:1166, 1996.
65. American College of Obstetricians and Gynecologists Committee on Obstetric Practice: Analgesia and cesarean delivery rates. ACOG Committee Opinion No. 339. Obstet Gynecol 107:1487, 2006.
66. Wong CA, Scavone BM, Peaceman AM, et al: The risk of cesarean delivery with neuraxial analgesia given early versus late in labor. N Engl J Med 352:655, 2005.
67. Ohel G, Gonen R, Vaida S, et al: Early versus late initiation of epidural analgesia in labor: does it increase the risk of cesarean section? A randomized trial. Am J Obstet Gynecol 194:600, 2006.
68. Marucci M, Cinnella G, Perchiazzi G, et al: Patient-requested neuraxial analgesia for labor: impact on rates of cesarean and instrumental vaginal delivery. Anesthesiology 106:1035, 2007.
69. Anim-Somuah M, Smyth RMD, Howell CJ: Epidural versus non-epidural or no analgesia in labour. Cochrane Database Syst Rev CD000331, 2005.
70. Comparative Obstetric Mobile Epidural Trial (COMET) Study Group UK: Effect of low-dose mobile versus traditional epidural techniques on mode of delivery: a randomised controlled trial. Lancet 358:19, 2001.
71. Liu EHC, Sia ATH: Rates of caesarean section and instrumental vaginal delivery in nulliparous women after low concentration

epidural infusions or opioid analgesia: systematic review. BMJ 328:1410, 2004.
72. Sharma SK, McIntire DD, Wiley J, Leveno KJ: Labor analgesia and cesarean delivery. Anesthesiology 100:142, 2004.
73. Goetzl L, Rivers J, Zighelboim I, et al: Intrapartum epidural analgesia and maternal temperature regulation. Obstet Gynecol 109:687, 2007.
74. Yancey MK, Zhang J, Schwarz J, et al: Labor epidural analgesia and intrapartum maternal hyperthermia. Obstet Gynecol 98:763, 2001.
75. Goetzl L, Evans T, Rivers J, et al: Elevated maternal and fetal serum interleukin-6 levels are associated with epidural fever. Am J Obstet Gynecol 187:834, 2002.
76. Lieberman E, Lang JM, Frigoletto F, et al: Epidural analgesia, intrapartum fever, and neonatal sepsis evaluation. Pediatrics 99:415, 1997.
77. Impey L, Greenwood C, MacQuillan K, et al: Fever in labour and neonatal encephalopathy: a prospective cohort study. Br J Obstet Gynecol 108:594, 2001.
78. Wu YW, Escobar GJ, Grether JK, et al: Chorioamnionitis and cerebral palsy in term and near term infants. JAMA 290:2677, 2003.
79. Goetzl L, Zighelboim I, Badell M, et al: Maternal corticosteroids to prevent intrauterine exposure to hyperthermia and inflammation: a randomized, double-blind, placebo-controlled trial. Am J Obstet Gynecol 195:1031, 2006.
80. Freeman RK, Gutierrez NA, Ray ML, et al: Fetal cardiac response to paracervical block anesthesia. Part I. Am J Obstet Gynecol 113:583, 1972.
81. Greiss FC Jr, Still JG, Anderson SG: Effects of local anesthetic agents on the uterine vasculatures and myometrium. Am J Obstet Gynecol 124:889, 1976.
82. Gambling DR, Sharma SK, White PF, et al: Use of sevoflurane during elective cesarean birth: a comparison with isoflurane and spinal anesthesia. Anesth Analg 81:90, 1995.
83. Gibbs CP, Schwartz DJ, Wynne JW, et al: Antacid pulmonary aspiration in the dog. Anesthesiology 51:380, 1979.
84. Datta S, Ostheimer GW, Weiss JB, et al: Neonatal effect of prolonged anesthetic induction for cesarean section. Obstet Gynecol 58:331, 1981.
85. Norris MC, Dewan DM: Preoxygenation for cesarean section: a comparison of two techniques. Anesthesiology 62:827, 1985.
86. Gin T. Propofol during pregnancy. Acta Anaesthesiol Sin 32:127, 1994.
87. Gregory MA, Davidson DG: Plasma etomidate levels in mother and fetus. Anaesthesia 46:716, 1991.
88. Bernstein K, Gisselsson L, Jacobsson T, Ohrlander S: Influence of two different anaesthetic agents on the newborn and the correlation between foetal oxygenation and induction-delivery time in elective caesarean section. Acta Anaesthesiol Scand 29:157, 1985.
89. Kee WDN, Khaw KS, Ma ML, et al: Postoperative analgesic requirement after cesarean section: a comparison of anesthetic induction with ketamine or thiopental. Anesth Analg 85:1294, 1997.
90. Bader AM, Datta S, Arthur GR, et al: Maternal and fetal catecholamines and uterine incision-to-delivery interval during elective cesarean. Obstet Gynecol 75:600, 1990.
91. Samsoon GLT, Young JRB: Difficult tracheal intubation: a retrospective study. Anaesthesia 42:487, 1987.
92. Rahman K, Jenkins JG: Failed tracheal intubation in obstetrics: no more frequent but still managed badly. Anaesthesia 60:168, 2005.
93. Mallampati SR, Gatt SP, Gugino LD, et al: A clinical sign to predict difficult tracheal intubation: a prospective study. Can Anaesth Soc J 32:429, 1985.
94. American Society of Anesthesiologists Task Force on Difficult Airway Management: Practice guidelines for management of the difficult airway: an updated report. Anesthesiology 98:1269, 2003.
95. Thomas TA, Cooper GM: Maternal deaths from anaesthesia. An extract from *Why Mothers Die 1997-1999*, the confidential enquiries into maternal deaths in the United Kingdom. Br J Anaesth 89:499, 2002.
96. O'Sullivan GM, Bullingham RE: Noninvasive assessment by radiotelemetry of antacid effect during labor. Anesth Analg 64:95, 1985.
97. Riley ET, Cohen SE, Macario A, et al: Spinal versus epidural anesthesia for cesarean section: a comparison of time efficiency, costs, charges, and complications. Anesth Analg 80:709, 1995.
98. Lowder JL, Shackelford DP, Holbert D, Beste TM: A randomized, controlled trial to compare ketorolac tromethamine versus placebo after cesarean section to reduce pain and narcotic usage. Am J Obstet Gynecol 189:1559, 2003.
99. Mhyre JM, Riesner MN, Polley LS, Naughton NN: A series of anesthesia-related maternal deaths in Michigan, 1985-2003. Anesthesiology 106:1096, 2007.
100. Wilkins KK, Greenfield MLVH, Polley LS, Mhyre JM: A survey of obstetric perianesthesia care unit standards. Anesth Analg 108:1869, 2009.

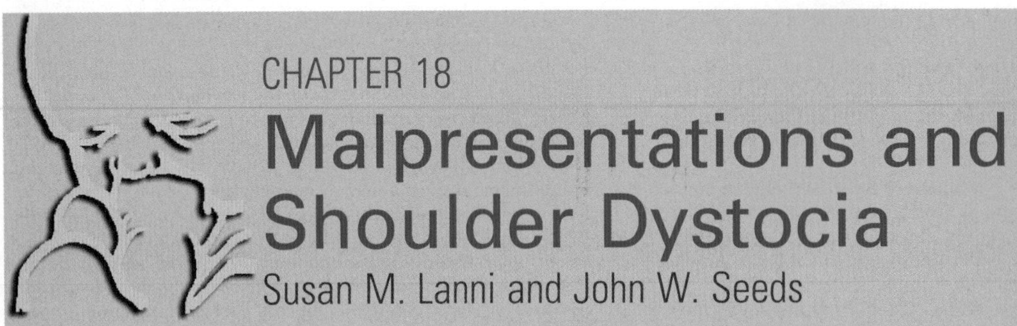

CHAPTER 18

Malpresentations and Shoulder Dystocia

Susan M. Lanni and John W. Seeds

KEY ABBREVIATIONS	
Anteroposterior	AP
Cerebral Palsy	CP
Computed Tomography	CT
Confidence Interval	CI
External Cephalic Version	ECV
Magnetic Resonance Imaging	MRI
Odds Ratio	OR
Perinatal Mortality Rate	PMR
Periventricular Leukomalacia	PVL
Preterm Premature Rupture of the Membranes	PPROM
Relative Risk	RR

Near term or during labor, the fetus normally assumes a vertical orientation or lie and a cephalic presentation, with the flexed fetal vertex presenting to the pelvis (Figure 18-1). In about 5% of cases, however, deviation occurs from this normal lie, presentation, or flexed attitude; such deviation constitutes a fetal malpresentation. **The word "malpresentation" suggests the possibility of adverse consequences, and malpresentation is often associated with increased risk to both the mother and the fetus.** Malpresentation once led to a variety of maneuvers intended to facilitate vaginal delivery, and early in the twentieth century, such interventions included destructive operations leading, predictably, to fetal death. Later, manual or instrumental attempts to convert the malpresenting fetus to a more favorable orientation were devised. Internal podalic version followed by a complete breech extraction was once advocated as a solution to many malpresentation situations. However, internal podalic version along with most manipulative efforts to achieve vaginal delivery were associated with a high fetal or maternal morbidity or mortality rate and have been largely abandoned. **In contemporary practice, cesarean delivery has become the recommended alternative to manipulative vaginal techniques when normal progress toward vaginal delivery is not observed.**

This chapter examines malpresentations, possible etiologies, and the mechanics of labor and vaginal delivery unique to each situation.

CLINICAL CIRCUMSTANCES ASSOCIATED WITH MALPRESENTATION

Generally, factors associated with malpresentation include (1) diminished vertical polarity of the uterine cavity, (2) increased or decreased fetal mobility, (3) obstructed pelvic inlet, and (4) fetal malformation. The association of great parity with malpresentation is presumably related to laxity of maternal abdominal musculature and, therefore, loss of the normal vertical orientation of the uterine cavity. Placentation either high in the fundus or low in the pelvis (Figure 18-2) is another factor that diminishes the likelihood of a fetus assuming a longitudinal axis. Uterine myomata, intrauterine synechiae, and müllerian duct fusion abnormalities such as septate uterus or uterus didelphys are likewise associated with a higher than expected rate of malpresentation. Because both prematurity and polyhydramnios permit increased fetal mobility, there is a greater probability of a noncephalic presentation if labor or rupture of membranes occurs. Furthermore, preterm birth involves a fetus that is small relative to the maternal pelvis and may result in morbidity often secondary to prematurity. Pelvic engagement and descent with labor or rupture of membranes can occur despite malpresentation. In contrast, conditions such as aneuploidies, myotonic dystrophy, joint contractures from various etiologies, arthrogryposis, oligohydramnios, and fetal neurologic dysfunction that result in decreased fetal muscle tone, strength, or activity are also associated with an increased incidence of fetal malpresentation. Finally, the cephalopelvic disproportion associated with severe fetal hydrocephalus or with a contracted maternal pelvis may be

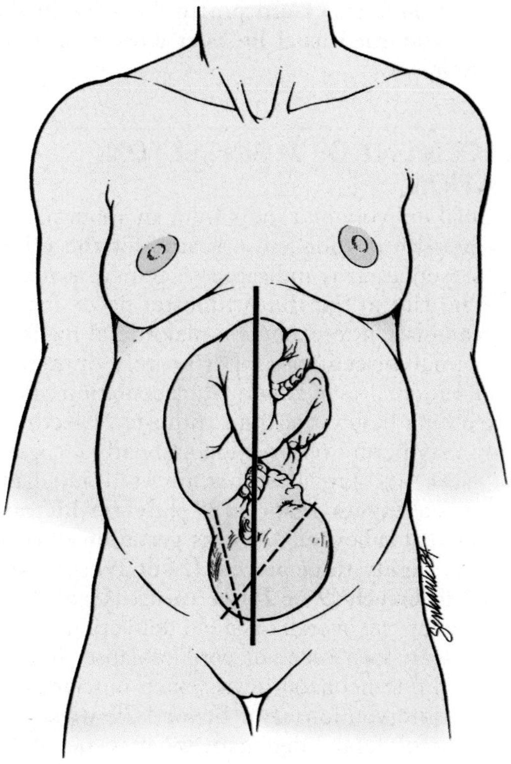

FIGURE 18-1. Frontal view of a fetus in a longitudinal lie with fetal vertex flexed on the neck.

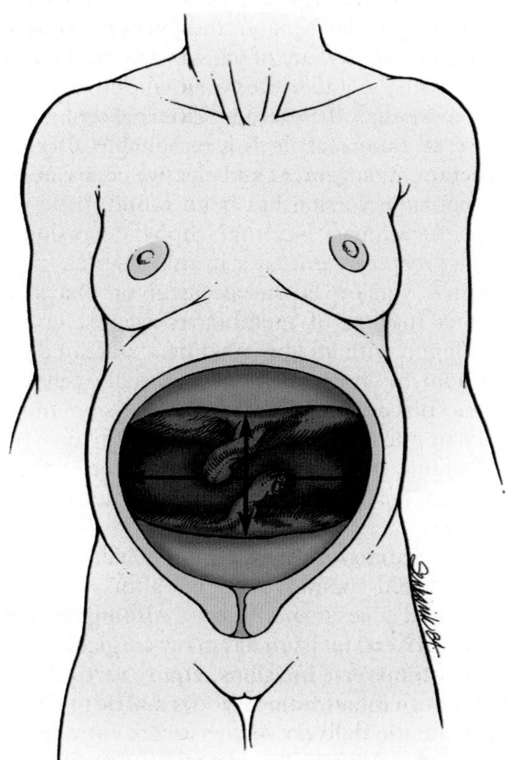

FIGURE 18-2. Either the high fundal or low implantation of the placenta illustrated here would normally be in the vertical orientation of the intrauterine cavity and increase the probability of a malpresentation.

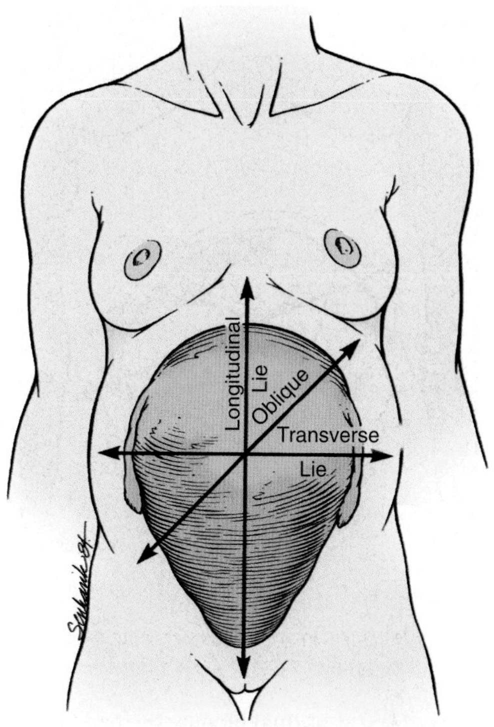

FIGURE 18-3. A fetus may occupy a longitudinal, oblique, or transverse axis, as illustrated by these vectors. The lie does not indicate whether the vertex or the breech is closest to the cervix.

implicated as an etiology of malpresentation because normal engagement of the fetal head is prevented.

ABNORMAL AXIAL LIE

The fetal "lie" indicates the orientation of the fetal spine relative to the spine of the mother. The normal fetal lie is longitudinal and by itself does not indicate whether the presentation is cephalic or breech. If the fetal spine or long axis crosses that of the mother, the fetus may be said to occupy a *transverse* or *oblique lie* (Figure 18-3), which may cause either an arm, a foot, or a shoulder to be the presenting part (Figure 18-4). The lie may be termed *unstable* if the fetal membranes are intact and there is great fetal mobility resulting in frequent changes of lie or presentation.

Abnormal fetal lie is diagnosed in approximately 1 in 300 cases, or 0.33% of pregnancies at term. Prematurity is often a factor, with abnormal lie reported to occur in about 2% of pregnancies at 32 weeks, or six times the rate found at term. Persistence of a transverse, oblique, or unstable lie beyond 37 weeks requires a systematic clinical assessment and a plan for management, because rupture of membranes without a fetal part filling the inlet of the pelvis imposes a high risk of cord prolapse, fetal compromise, and maternal morbidity if neglected.

Great parity, prematurity, contraction or deformity of the maternal pelvis, and abnormal placentation are the most commonly reported clinical factors associated with abnormal lie; however, often, none of these factors is present. In fact, any condition that alters the normal vertical polarity of the intrauterine cavity will predispose to abnormal lie.

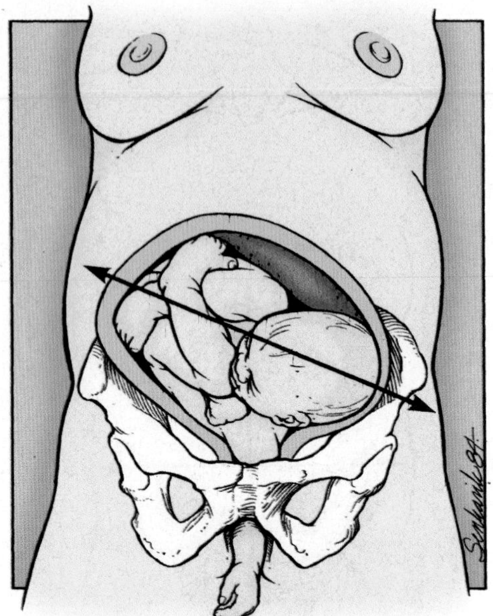

FIGURE 18-4. This fetus lies in an oblique axis with an arm prolapsing.

Diagnosis of the abnormal lie may be made by palpation or vaginal examination and verified by ultrasound. Routine use of Leopold's maneuvers may assist detection, but **Thorp and colleagues[1] found the sensitivity of Leopold's maneuvers for the detection of malpresentation to be only 28% and the positive predictive value only 24% compared with immediate ultrasound verification.** Others have observed prenatal detection in as few as 41% of cases before labor. Recently, adaptations have been made to the Leopold's maneuvers that may improve detection of abnormal lie or presentation. The Sharma modified Leopold's maneuver and the Sharma right and left lateral maneuvers in the original report have demonstrated improved diagnostic accuracy, detecting vertex presenting occipito-anterior (95% vs. 84.4%, $P = 0.04$) and posterior presentations (96.3% vs. 66.6%, $P = 0.00012$) and breech presentation correctly more often than Leopold's maneuvers.[2] These maneuvers employ the use of the forearms in addition to the hands and fingers. As with any abdominal palpation technique, limitations on accuracy are to be expected in the obese patient or a patient with uterine myomata. The ready availability of ultrasound in most clinical settings is of benefit, and its use can obviate the vagaries of the abdominal palpation techniques. In all situations, early diagnosis of malpresentation is of benefit. A reported fetal loss rate of 9.2% with an early diagnosis versus a loss rate of 27.5% with a delayed diagnosis indicates that early diagnosis improves fetal outcome.

Reported perinatal mortality rate for unstable or transverse lie (corrected for lethal malformations and extreme prematurity) varies from 3.9% to 24%, with maternal mortality as high as 10%. Maternal deaths are usually related to infection after premature rupture of membranes, hemorrhage secondary to abnormal placentation, complications of operative intervention for cephalopelvic disproportion, or traumatic delivery. Fetal loss of phenotypically and chromosomally normal gestations at ages considered to be viable is primarily associated with neglect, prolapsed cord, or traumatic delivery. **Cord prolapse occurs 20 times as often with abnormal axial lie as it does with a cephalic presentation.**

MANAGEMENT OF A SINGLETON GESTATION

Safe vaginal delivery of a fetus from an abnormal axial lie is not generally possible, so a search for the etiology of the malpresentation is indicated. A transverse/oblique or unstable lie late in the third trimester necessitates ultrasound examination to exclude a major fetal malformation and abnormal placentation. Fortunately, most cases of major fetal anomalies or abnormal placentation can now be diagnosed long before the third trimester. Elective hospitalization may permit observation and early recognition of cord prolapse, and provides proximity to immediate care. **Phelan and colleagues[3] reported 29 patients with transverse lie diagnosed at or beyond 37 weeks' gestation and managed expectantly. Eighty-three percent (24 of 29) spontaneously converted to breech (9 of 24) or vertex (15 of 24) before labor**; however, the overall cesarean delivery rate was 45%, and there were two cases of cord prolapse, one uterine rupture, and one neonatal death. Such outcomes suggest that active intervention at or beyond 37 weeks or after confirmation of fetal lung maturity may be of benefit. External cephalic version with subsequent induction of labor, if successful, might diminish the risk of adverse outcome.

In cases of an abnormal lie, the risk of fetal death varies with the obstetrical intervention. Fetal mortality should approach zero for cesarean birth but has been reported as high as 10% in older reports and between 25% and 90% when internal podalic version and breech extraction are performed. A mortality rate of 6% was reported for successful external version and vertex vaginal delivery in papers published more than 40 years ago. **External cephalic version in the case of abnormal lie is a reasonable alternative to both expectant management and elective cesarean delivery**. External cephalic version has been found to be safe and relatively efficacious.[4] External cephalic version is discussed to a greater extent later in this chapter.

If external version is unsuccessful or unavailable, if spontaneous rupture of membranes occurs, or if active labor has begun with an abnormal lie, cesarean delivery is the treatment of choice for the potentially viable infant. There is no place for internal podalic version and breech extraction in the management of transverse or oblique lie or unstable presentation in singleton pregnancies because of the unacceptably high rate of fetal and maternal complications.

A persistent abnormal axial lie, particularly if accompanied by ruptured membranes, also alters the choice of uterine incision at cesarean delivery. **Although a low cervical transverse (Kerr) incision has many surgical advantages, up to 25% of transverse incisions require vertical extension for delivery of an infant from an abnormal lie to allow access to and atraumatic delivery of the vertex entrapped in the muscular fundus.** Furthermore, the lower uterine segment is often poorly developed and insufficiently "broad" such that atraumatic delivery of the presenting part is nearly impossible. **Therefore, when managing a transverse or**

oblique lie with ruptured membranes or a poorly developed lower segment, a vertical incision (low vertical or classical) is more prudent. Intraoperative cephalic version may allow the use of a low transverse incision, but ruptured membranes or oligohydramnios makes this difficult. The use of uterine relaxing agents such as inhalational anesthetics or intravenous nitroglycerine may improve success of these maneuvers if the difficulty is attributable to a contracted uterine fundus.

DEFLECTION ATTITUDES

"Attitude" refers to the position of the fetal head in relation to the neck. The normal attitude of the fetal vertex during labor is one of full flexion on the neck, with the fetal chin against the upper chest. Deflexed attitudes include various degrees of deflection or even extension of the fetal head on the neck (Figure 18-5). Spontaneous conversion to a more normal, flexed attitude or further extension of an intermediate deflection to a fully extended position commonly occurs as labor progresses owing to resistance exerted by the bony pelvis and soft tissues. Although safe vaginal delivery is possible in many cases, experience indicates that cesarean delivery is the only appropriate alternative when arrest of progress is observed.

FACE PRESENTATION

A face presentation is characterized by a longitudinal lie and full extension of the fetal head on the neck, with the occiput against the upper back (Figure 18-6). **The fetal chin (mentum) is chosen as the point of designation during vaginal examination.** For example, a fetus presenting by the face whose chin is in the right posterior quadrant of the maternal pelvis would be called a *right mentum posterior* (Figure 18-7). The reported incidence of face presentation ranges from 0.14% to 0.54%, averaging about 0.2%, or 1 in 500 live births overall.[5,6] Reported perinatal mortality rate, corrected for nonviable malformations and extreme prematurity, varies from 0.6% to 5%, averaging about 2% to 3%.

All clinical factors known to increase the general rate of malpresentation (see the accompanying box, Etiologic Factors in Malpresentation) have been implicated in face presentation; many infants with a face presentation have malformations. Anencephaly, for instance, is found in about one third of cases of face presentation. Fetal goiter as well as tumors of the soft tissues of the neck may also cause deflexion of the head. Frequently observed maternal factors include a contracted pelvis or cephalopelvic disproportion in 10% to 40% of cases. In a review of face presentation, Duff found that one of these etiologic factors was found in up to 90% of cases.[6]

Early recognition of the face presentation is important, and the diagnosis can be suspected anytime abdominal palpation finds the fetal cephalic prominence on the same side of the maternal abdomen as the fetal back (Figure 18-8); however, **face presentation is more often discovered by vaginal examination**. In practice, fewer than 1 in 20 infants with face presentation is diagnosed by abdominal examination. In fact, only half of these infants are found to have a face presentation by any means before the second stage of labor, and half of the remaining cases are undiagnosed until delivery. Perinatal mortality may be higher, however, with late diagnosis.

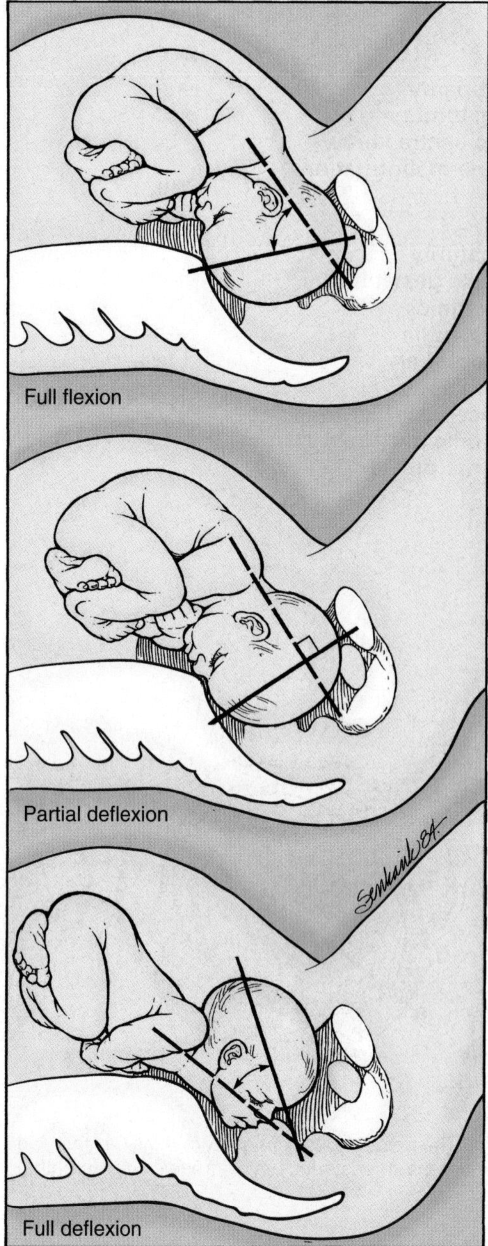

FIGURE 18-5. The normal "attitude" *(top view)* shows the fetal vertex flexed on the neck. Partial deflexion *(middle view)* shows the fetal vertex intermediate between flexion and extension. Full deflexion *(lower view)* shows the fetal vertex completely extended, with the face presenting.

Mechanism of Labor

Knowledge of the early mechanism of labor for face presentation is incomplete. **Many infants with a face presentation probably begin labor in the less extended brow position.** With descent into the pelvis, the forces of labor press the fetus against maternal tissues; either flexion or full extension of the head on the spine then often occurs. **The labor of a face presentation must include engagement, descent,**

ETIOLOGIC FACTORS IN MALPRESENTATION

Maternal

- Great parity
- Pelvic tumors
- Pelvic contracture
- Uterine malformation

Fetal

- Prematurity
- Multiple gestation
- Hydramnios
- Macrosomia
- Hydrocephaly
- Trisomies
- Anencephaly
- Myotonic dystrophy
- Placenta previa

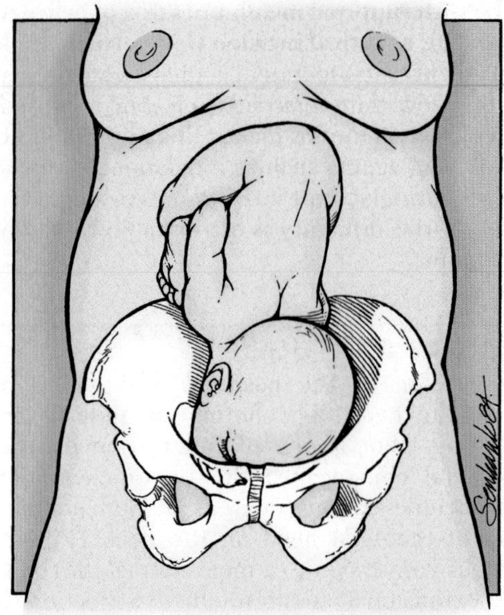

FIGURE 18-6. This fetus with the vertex completely extended on the neck enters the maternal pelvis in a face presentation. The cephalic prominence would be palpable on the same side of the maternal abdomen as the fetal spine.

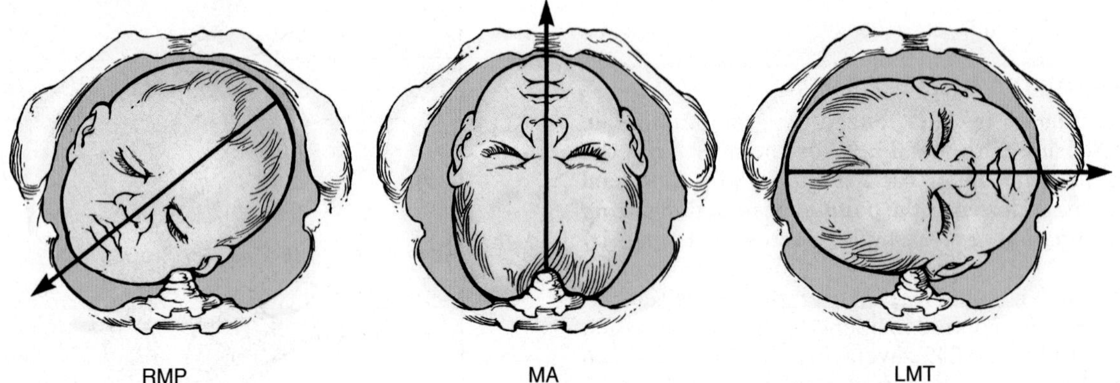

FIGURE 18-7. The point of designation from digital examination in the case of a face presentation is the fetal chin relative to the maternal pelvis. *Left,* Right mentum posterior *(RMP). Middle,* Mentum anterior *(MA). Right,* Left mentum transverse *(LMT).*

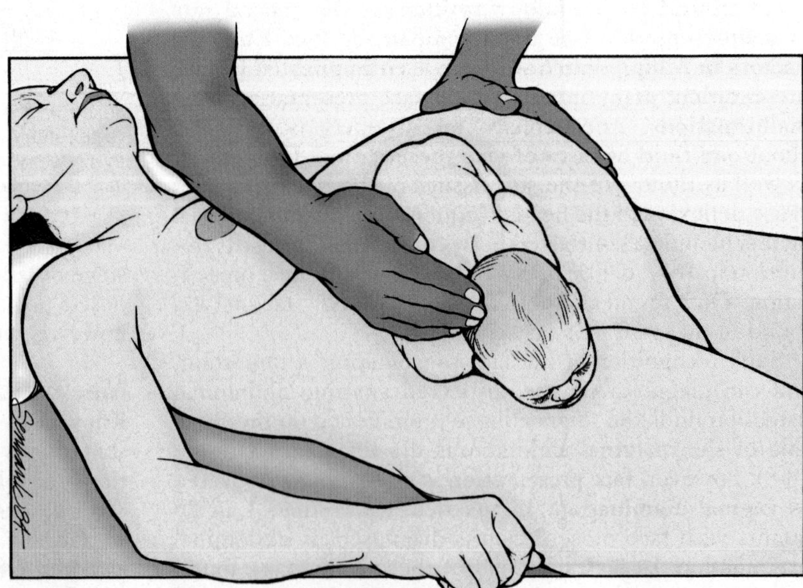

FIGURE 18-8. Palpation of the maternal abdomen in the case of a face presentation should find the fetal cephalic prominence on the side away from the fetal small parts instead of on the same side as in the case of a normally flexed fetal head.

internal rotation generally to a mentum anterior position, and delivery by flexion as the chin passes under the symphysis (Figure 18-9). However, flexion of the occiput may not always occur; delivery in the fully extended attitude may be common.

The prognosis for labor with a face presentation depends on the orientation of the fetal chin. At diagnosis, 60% to 80% of infants with a face presentation are mentum anterior,[6] 10% to 12% are mentum transverse,[7] and 20% to 25% are mentum posterior.[7] Almost all average-sized infants presenting mentum anterior with adequate pelvic dimensions will achieve spontaneous or easily assisted vaginal delivery. Furthermore, most mentum transverse infants will rotate to the mentum anterior position and deliver vaginally, and even 25% to 33% of mentum posterior infants will rotate and deliver vaginally in the mentum anterior position. In a review of 51 cases of persistent face presentation, Schwartz and colleagues[7] found that the mean birth weight of those infants in mentum posterior who did rotate and deliver vaginally was 3425 g, compared with 3792 g for those infants who did not rotate and deliver vaginally. **Persistence of mentum posterior with an infant of normal size, however, makes safe vaginal delivery less likely.** Overall, 70% to 80% of infants with face presentation can be delivered vaginally, either spontaneously or by low forceps, whereas 12% to 30% require cesarean delivery. Manual attempts to convert the face to a flexed attitude or to rotate a posterior position to a more favorable mentum anterior are rarely successful and increase both maternal and fetal risks.[5] Internal podalic version and breech extraction for face presentation historically are associated with unacceptably high fetal loss rates. Maternal deaths from uterine rupture and trauma have also been documented. Thus, contemporary management through spontaneous delivery or cesarean delivery are the preferred routes for maternal and fetal safety.[5]

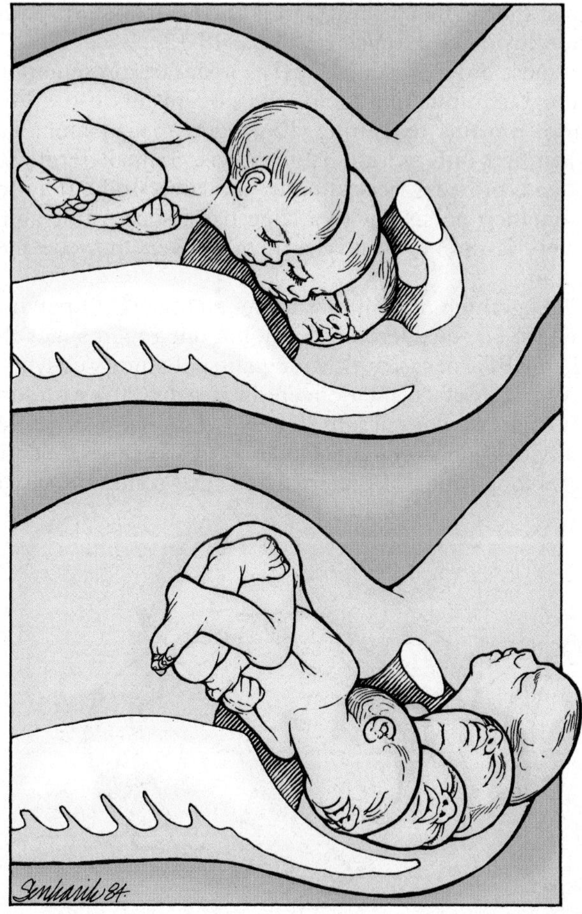

FIGURE 18-9. Engagement, descent, and internal rotation remain cardinal elements of vaginal delivery in the case of a face presentation, but successful vaginal delivery of a term-size fetus presenting a face generally requires delivery by flexion under the symphysis from a mentum anterior position, as illustrated here.

Prolonged labor is a common feature of face presentation and has been associated with an increased number of intrapartum deaths. Therefore, prompt attention to an arrested labor pattern is recommended. In the case of an average or small fetus, adequate pelvis, and hypotonic labor, oxytocin may be considered. No absolute contraindication to oxytocin augmentation of hypotonic labor in face presentations exists, but an arrest of progress despite adequate labor should call for cesarean delivery.

Worsening of the fetal condition in labor is common. **Salzmann and colleagues observed a 10-fold increase in fetal compromise with face presentation.** Several other observers have also found that abnormal fetal heart rate (FHR) patterns occur more often with face presentation.[5,6] Continuous intrapartum electronic FHR monitoring of a fetus with face presentation is considered mandatory, but extreme care must be exercised in the placement of an electrode, because ocular or cosmetic damage is possible. **If external Doppler heart rate monitoring is inadequate and an internal electrode is considered necessary, placement of the electrode on the fetal chin is often recommended.** Cesarean delivery is warranted if a non-reassuring heart rate pattern is identified, even if sufficient progress in labor is occurring.

Safe vaginal delivery may be accomplished in many cases of face presentation, and a trial of labor with careful monitoring of fetal condition and labor progress is not contraindicated unless macrosomia or a small maternal pelvis is identified. However, cesarean delivery has been reported in as many as 60% of cases of face presentation.[6] If cesarean delivery is warranted, care should be taken to flex the head gently both to accomplish elevation of the head through the hysterotomy incision, as well as to avoid potential nerve damage to the neonate. Forced flexion may also result in damage, especially with fetal goiter, or neck tumors.

Laryngeal and tracheal edema resulting from pressures of the birth process might require immediate nasotracheal intubation. Nuchal tumors or simple goiters, fetal anomalies that might have caused the malpresentation, require expert neonatal management.

BROW PRESENTATION

A fetus in a brow presentation occupies a longitudinal axis, with a partially deflexed cephalic attitude, midway between full flexion and full extension (Figure 18-10). **The frontal bones are the point of designation.** If the anterior fontanel is on the mother's left side, with the sagittal suture in the transverse pelvic axis, the fetus would be in a left frontum transverse position (Figure 18-11). **The reported incidence of brow presentation varies widely, from 1 in 670 to 1 in 3433, averaging about 1 in 1500 deliveries.** Brow presentation is detected more often in early labor before flexion occurs to a normal attitude. Less frequently, further extension results in a face presentation.

Perinatal mortality rate corrected for lethal anomalies and very low birth weight varies from 1% to 8%.[8] In a study of 88,988 deliveries, corrected perinatal mortality rates for brow presentations depended on the mode of delivery, and a loss rate of 16%, the highest in this study, was associated with manipulative vaginal birth.

In general, factors that delay engagement are associated with persistent brow presentation. Cephalopelvic disproportion, prematurity, and great parity are often found and have been implicated in more than 60% of cases of persistent brow presentation.

Detection of a brow presentation by abdominal palpation is unusual in practice. More often, a brow presentation is detected on vaginal examination. As in the case of a face presentation, diagnosis in labor is more likely. Fewer than 50% of brow presentations are detected before the second stage of labor, with most of the remainder undiagnosed until delivery. **Frontum anterior is reportedly the most common position at diagnosis,** occurring about twice as often as either transverse or posterior positions. Although the initial position at diagnosis may be of limited prognostic value, the cesarean delivery rate is higher with frontum transverse or frontum posterior than with frontum anterior.

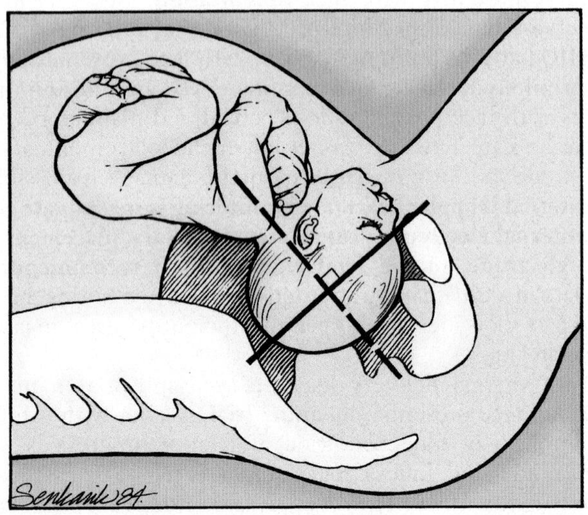

FIGURE 18-10. This fetus is a brow presentation in a frontum anterior position. The head is in an intermediate deflexion attitude.

A persistent brow presentation requires engagement and descent of the largest (mento-occipital) diameter or profile of the fetal head. This process is possible only with a large pelvis or a small infant, or both. However, most brow presentations convert spontaneously by flexion or further extension to either a vertex or a face presentation and are then managed accordingly. The earlier the diagnosis is made, the more likely conversion will occur spontaneously. Fewer than half of fetuses with persistent brow presentations undergo spontaneous vaginal delivery, but in most cases, a trial of labor is not contraindicated.[8]

Prolonged labors have been observed in 33% to 50% of brow presentations, and secondary arrest is not uncommon. Forced conversion of the brow to a more favorable position with forceps is contraindicated, as are attempts at manual conversion. One unexpected cause of persistent brow presentation may be an open fetal mouth pressed against the vaginal wall, splinting the head and preventing either flexion or extension (Figure 18-12).

In most brow presentations, as with face presentations, minimal manipulation yields the best results if the FHR pattern remains reassuring. Expectant management may be justified only with a large pelvis, a small fetus, and adequate progress, according to one large study. If a brow presentation persists with a large baby, successful vaginal delivery is unlikely, and cesarean delivery may be most prudent.

Radiographic or computed tomographic (CT) pelvimetry might be considered helpful, but one report states that although 91% of cases with adequate pelvimetry converted to a vertex or a face and delivered vaginally, 20% with some form of pelvic contracture did also. Therefore, regardless of pelvic dimensions, consideration of a trial of labor with careful monitoring of maternal and fetal condition may be

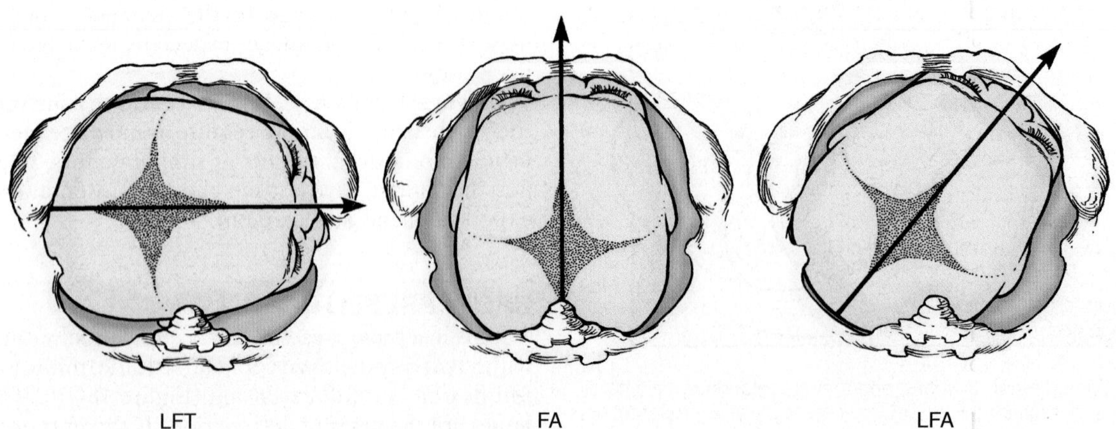

FIGURE 18-11. In brow presentation, the anterior fontanel (frontum) relative to the maternal pelvis is the point of designation. *Left,* Fetus in left frontum transverse *(LFT)*. *Middle,* Frontum anterior *(FA)*. *Right,* Left frontum anterior *(LFA)*.

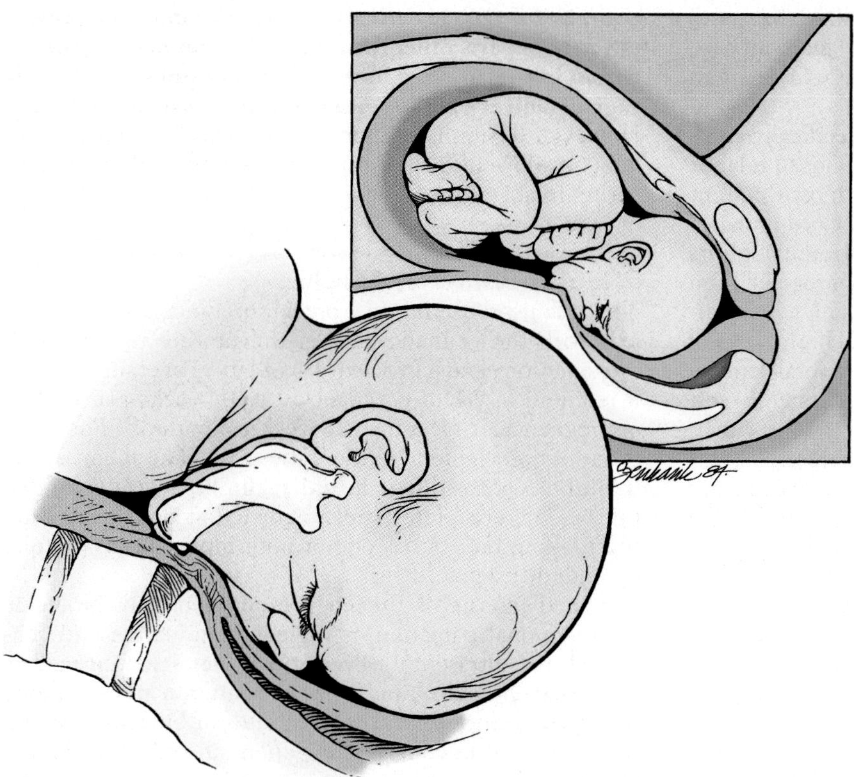

FIGURE 18-12. The open fetal mouth against the vaginal sidewall may brace the head in the intermediate deflexion attitude as shown here.

appropriate. As in the case of a face presentation, oxytocin may be used cautiously to correct hypotonic contractions, but prompt resumption of progress toward delivery should follow.

COMPOUND PRESENTATION

Whenever an extremity is found prolapsed beside the main presenting fetal part, the situation is referred to as a compound presentation (Figure 18-13). The reported incidence ranges from 1 in 377 to 1 in 1213 deliveries.[8] The combination of an upper extremity and the vertex is the most common.

This diagnosis should be suspected with any arrest of labor in the active phase or failure to engage during active labor. Diagnosis is made by vaginal examination by discovery of an irregular mobile tissue mass adjacent to the larger presenting part. Recognition late in labor is common, and as many as 50% of persisting compound presentations are not detected until the second stage. Delay in diagnosis may not be detrimental because it is likely that only the persistent cases require intervention.

Although maternal age, race, parity, and pelvic size have been associated with compound presentation, prematurity is the most consistent clinical finding. The very small premature fetus is at great risk of persistent compound presentation. In late pregnancy, external cephalic version of a fetus in breech position increases the risk of a compound presentation.

Older, uncontrolled studies report elevated perinatal mortality rates with a compound presentation, with an overall rate of 93 per 1000. Higher loss rates of 17% to 19% have been reported when the foot prolapses. As with other malpresentations, fetal risk is directly related to the method of management. A fetal mortality rate of 4.8% has been noted if no intervention is required compared with 14.4% with intervention other than cesarean delivery. A 30% fetal mortality rate has been observed with internal podalic version and breech extraction. These figures may

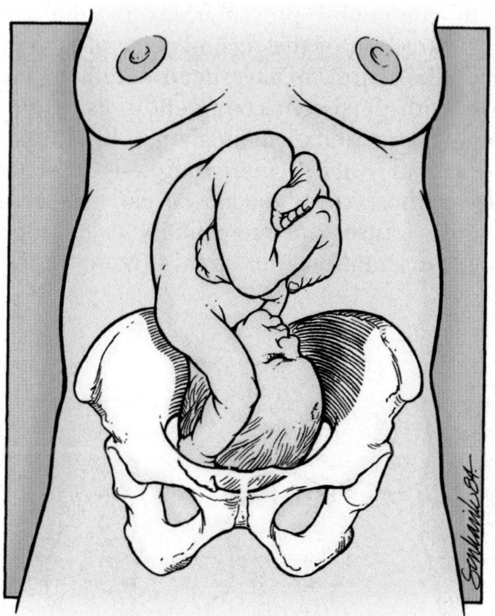

FIGURE 18-13. The compound presentation of an upper extremity and the vertex illustrated here most often spontaneously resolves with further labor and descent.

demonstrate selection bias because it is possible that more often the difficult cases were chosen for manipulative intervention. When intervention is necessary, cesarean delivery appears to be the only safe choice.

Fetal risk in compound presentation is specifically associated with birth trauma and cord prolapse. Cord prolapse occurs in 11% to 20% of cases, and it is the most frequent single complication of this malpresentation. Cord prolapse probably occurs because the compound extremity splints the larger presenting part, resulting in an irregular fetal aggregate that incompletely fills the pelvic inlet. In addition to the hypoxic risk of cord prolapse, common fetal morbidity includes neurologic and musculoskeletal damage to the involved extremity. Maternal risks include soft tissue damage and obstetrical laceration.

Despite these dangers, labor is not necessarily contraindicated with a compound presentation; however, the prolapsed extremity should not be manipulated. The accompanying extremity may retract as the major presenting part descends. Seventy-five percent of vertex/upper extremity combinations deliver spontaneously. Occult or undetected cord prolapse is possible, and, therefore, continuous electronic FHR monitoring is recommended.

The primary indications for surgical intervention are cord prolapse, non-reassuring fetal heart rate (FHR) patterns, and arrest of labor. **Cesarean delivery is the only appropriate clinical intervention for cord prolapse and non-reassuring FHR pattern, because both version extraction and repositioning the prolapsed extremity are associated with adverse outcome and are to be avoided.** From 2% to 25% of compound presentations require abdominal delivery. Protraction of the second stage of labor and dysfunctional labor patterns have been noted to occur more frequently with persistent compound presentation. As in other malpresentations, spontaneous resolution occurs more often and surgical intervention is less frequently necessary in those cases diagnosed early in labor. Small or premature fetuses are more likely to have persistent compound presentations but are also more likely to have a successful vaginal delivery. **Persistent compound presentation with parts other than the vertex and hand in combination in a term-sized infant has a poor prognosis for safe vaginal delivery, and cesarean delivery is usually necessary.** However, a simple compound presentation (e.g., hand) may be allowed to labor if progressing normally with reassuring fetal status.

BREECH PRESENTATION

The infant presenting as a breech occupies a longitudinal axis with the cephalic pole in the uterine fundus. This presentation occurs in 3% to 4% of labors overall, although it is found in 7% of pregnancies at 32 weeks and in 25% of pregnancies of less than 28 weeks' duration.[10] The three types of breech are noted in Table 18-1. The infant in the frank breech position is flexed at the hips with extended knees. The complete breech is flexed at both joints, and the footling breech has one or both hips partially or fully extended (Figure 18-14).

The diagnosis of breech presentation may be made by abdominal palpation or vaginal examination and confirmed by ultrasound. **Prematurity, fetal malformation, müllerian anomalies, and polar placentation are commonly observed causative factors.** High rates of breech presentation are noted in certain fetal genetic disorders, including trisomies 13, 18, and 21; Potter's syndrome; and myotonic dystrophy. Thus, conditions that alter fetal muscular tone

TABLE 18-1 BREECH CATEGORIES

TYPE	OVERALL PERCENT OF BREECHES	RISK (%) PROLAPSE	PREMATURE
Frank breech	48-73[13,14,51]	0.5[15]	38[14]
Complete	4.6-11.5[14,51]	4-6[15]	12[14]
Footling	12-38[14]	15-18[15]	50[14]

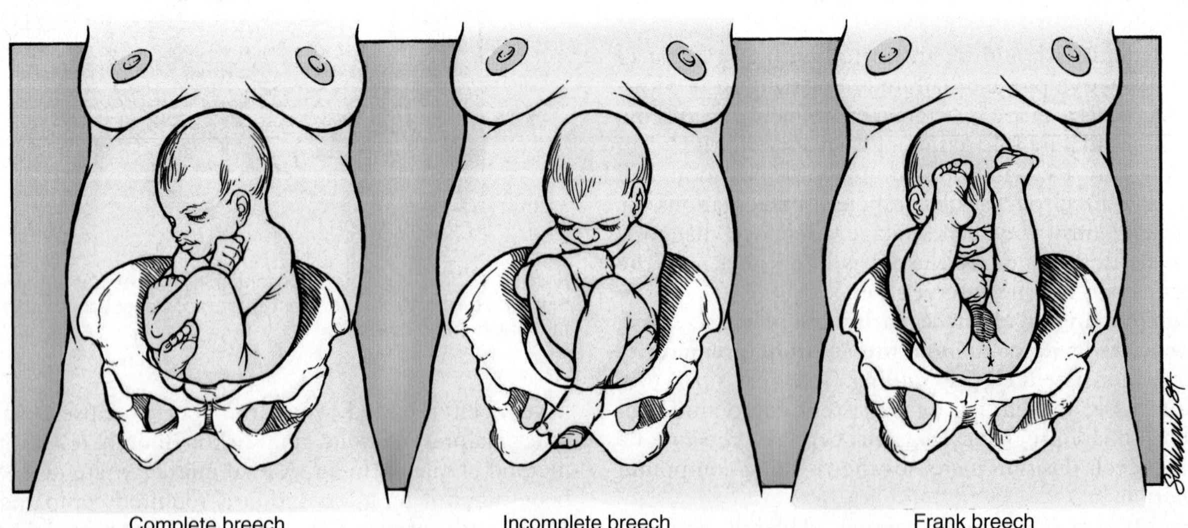

FIGURE 18-14. The complete breech is flexed at the hips and flexed at the knees. The incomplete breech shows incomplete deflexion of one or both knees or hips. The frank breech is flexed at the hips and extended at the knees.

and mobility such as increased and decreased amniotic fluid, for example, also increase the frequency of breech presentation.

Mechanism and Conduct of Labor and Vaginal Delivery

The two most important elements for the safe conduct of vaginal breech delivery are continuous electronic FHR monitoring and noninterference until spontaneous delivery of the breech to the umbilicus has occurred. Early in labor, the capability for immediate cesarean delivery should be established. Anesthesia should be available, the operating room readied, and appropriate informed consent obtained (discussed later). Two obstetricians should be in attendance, as well as a pediatric team. Appropriate training and experience with vaginal breech delivery are fundamental to success. The instrument table should be prepared in the customary manner, with the addition of Piper forceps and extra towels. There is no contraindication to epidural analgesia in labor; many even view epidural anesthesia as an asset in the control and conduct of the second stage.

The infant presenting in the frank breech position usually enters the pelvic inlet in one of the diagonal pelvic diameters (Figure 18-15). **Engagement has occurred when the bitrochanteric diameter of the fetus has progressed beyond the plane of the pelvic inlet, although by vaginal examination, the presenting part may be palpated only at –2 to –4 station (of 5).** As the breech descends and encounters the levator ani muscular sling, internal rotation usually occurs to bring the bitrochanteric diameter into the anteroposterior (AP) axis of the pelvis. **The point of designation in a breech labor is the fetal sacrum,** and, therefore, when the bitrochanteric diameter is in the AP axis of the pelvis, the fetal sacrum will lie in the transverse pelvic diameter (Figure 18-16).

If normal descent occurs, the breech will present at the outlet and begin to emerge, first as a sacrum transverse, then rotating to sacrum anterior. Crowning occurs when the bitrochanteric diameter passes under the pubic symphysis. An episiotomy may facilitate delivery but should be delayed until crowning begins. As the infant emerges, rotation begins, usually toward a sacrum anterior position. This direction of rotation may reflect the greater capacity

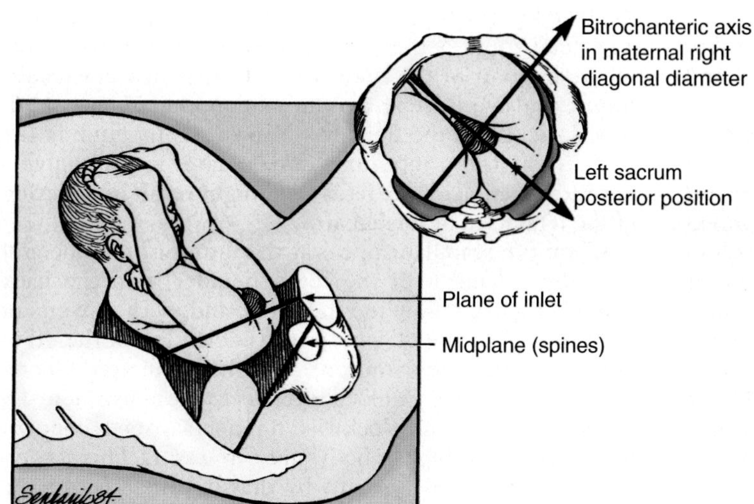

FIGURE 18-15. The breech typically enters the inlet with the bitrochanteric diameter aligned with one of the diagonal diameters, with the sacrum as the point of designation in the other diagonal diameter. This is a case of left sacrum posterior.

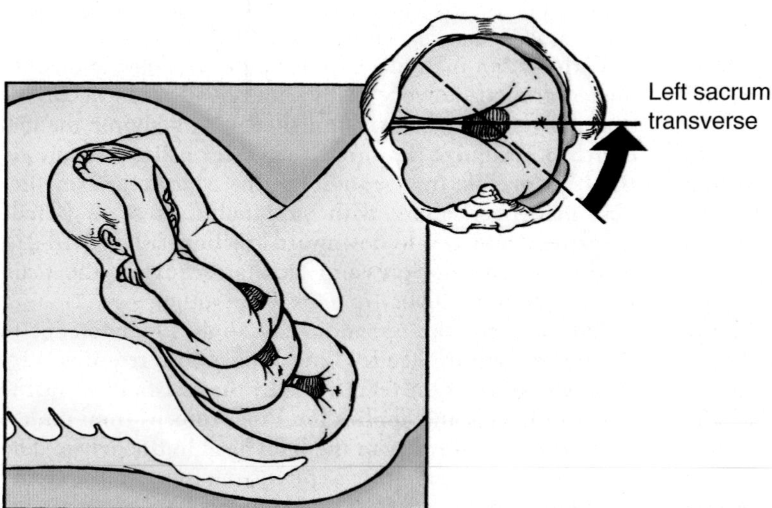

FIGURE 18-16. With labor and descent, the bitrochanteric diameter generally rotates toward the anteroposterior axis and the sacrum toward the transverse.

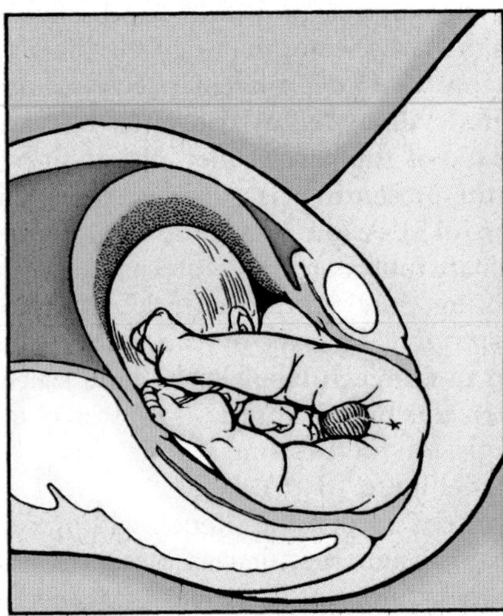

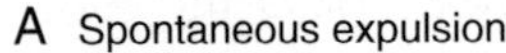

A Spontaneous expulsion

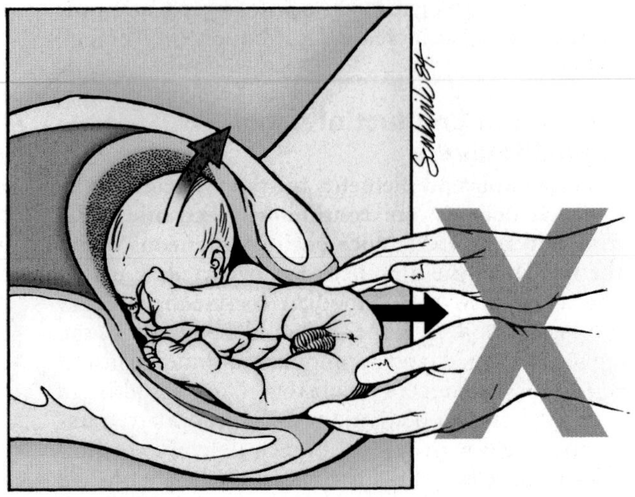

B Undesired deflexion

FIGURE 18-17. The fetus emerges spontaneously **(A)**, whereas uterine contractions maintain cephalic flexion. Premature aggressive traction **(B)** encourages deflexion of the fetal vertex and increases the risk of head entrapment or nuchal arm entrapment.

of the hollow of the posterior pelvis to accept the fetal chest and small parts. It is important to emphasize that operator intervention is not yet needed or helpful other than possibly to perform the episiotomy if indicated and encourage maternal expulsive efforts.

Premature or aggressive assistance may adversely affect the delivery in at least two ways. **First, complete cervical dilation must be sustained for sufficient duration to retard retraction of the cervix and entrapment of the after-coming fetal head. Rushing the delivery of the trunk may result in cervical retraction. Second, the safe descent and delivery of the breech infant must be the result of uterine and maternal expulsive forces only, in order to maintain neck flexion. Any traction by the provider in an effort to speed delivery would encourage deflexion of the neck and result in the presentation of the larger occipitofrontal fetal cranial profile to the pelvic inlet** (Figure 18-17). Such an event could be catastrophic. **Rushed delivery also increases the risk of a nuchal arm,** with one or both arms trapped behind the head above the pelvic inlet. Entrapment of a nuchal arm makes safe vaginal delivery much more difficult, because it dramatically increases the aggregate size of delivering fetal parts that must egress vaginally. Safe breech delivery of an average-sized infant, therefore, depends predominantly on maternal expulsive forces, and patience, not traction, from the provider.

As the frank breech emerges further, the fetal thighs are typically flexed firmly against the fetal abdomen, often splinting and protecting the umbilicus and cord. The Pinard maneuver may be needed to facilitate delivery of the legs in a frank breech presentation. After the umbilicus has been reached, pressure is applied to the medial aspect of the knee, which causes flexion and subsequent delivery of the lower leg. Simultaneous to this, the fetal pelvis is rotated away from that side (Figure 18-18). This results in external rotation of the thigh at the hip, flexion of the knee, and delivery of one leg at a time. The dual movement of counterclockwise rotation of the fetal pelvis as the operator externally rotates the right thigh and clockwise rotation of the fetal pelvis as the operator externally rotates the fetal left thigh, is most effective in facilitating delivery. The fetal trunk is then wrapped with a towel to provide secure support of the body while further descent results from expulsive forces from the mother. The operator primarily facilitates the delivery of the fetus by guiding the body through the introitus. **The operator is not applying outward traction on the fetus that might result in deflexion of the fetal head or nuchal arm.**

When the scapulae appear at the introitus, the operator may slip a hand over the fetal shoulder from the back (Figure 18-19), follow the humerus, and, with movement from medial to lateral, sweep first one and then the other arm across the chest and out over the perineum. Gentle rotation of the fetal trunk counterclockwise assists delivery of the right arm, and clockwise rotation assists delivery of the left arm (turning the body "into" the arm). This accomplishes delivery of the arms by drawing them across the fetal chest in a fashion similar to that used for delivery of the legs (Figure 18-20). Once both arms have been delivered, if the vertex has remained flexed on the neck, the chin and face will appear at the outlet, and the airway may be cleared and suctioned (Figure 18-21).

With further maternal expulsive forces alone, spontaneous controlled delivery of the fetal head often occurs. **If not, delivery may be accomplished with a simple manual effort to maximize flexion of the vertex using pressure on the fetal maxilla (not mandible), the Mauriceau-Smellie-Veit maneuver, along with suprapubic pressure (Credé maneuver) and gentle downward traction** (Figure 18-22). Although maxillary pressure facilitates flexion, the main force effecting delivery remains the mother.

Alternatively, the operator may apply Piper forceps to the after-coming head. **The application requires *very slight* elevation of the fetal trunk by the assistant, while the operator kneels and applies the Piper forceps from underneath the fetus directly to the fetal head in the pelvis.** The position of the operator for applying the forceps is depicted in Figure 18-23, which also demonstrates how *excessive*

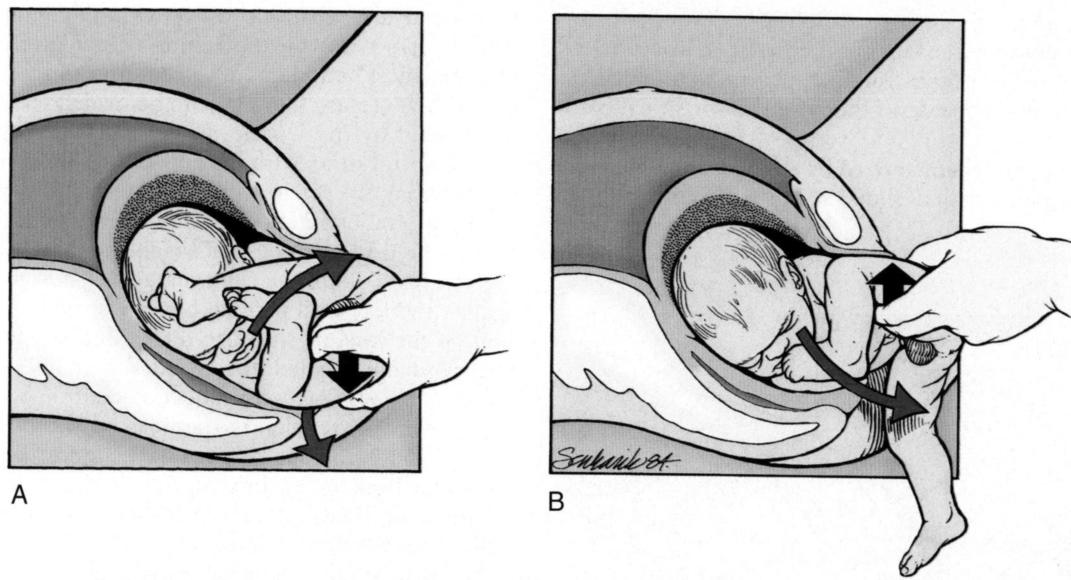

FIGURE 18-18. After spontaneous expulsion to the umbilicus, external rotation of each thigh **(A)** combined with opposite rotation of the fetal pelvis results in flexion of the knee and delivery of each leg **(B)**.

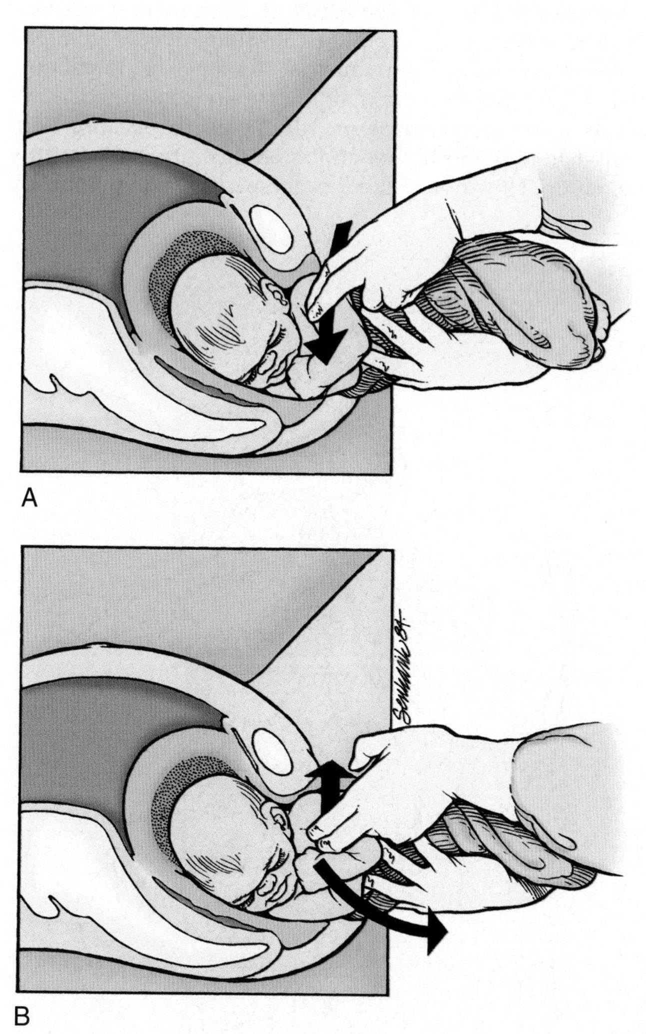

FIGURE 18-19. When the scapulae appear under the symphysis, the operator reaches over the left shoulder, sweeps the arm across the chest **(A)**, and delivers the arm **(B)**.

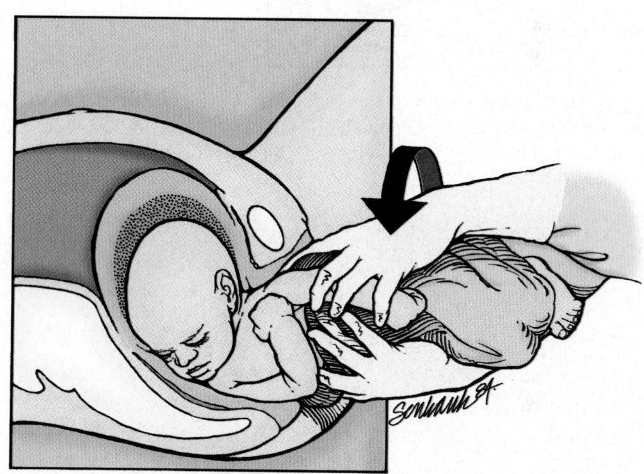

FIGURE 18-20. Gentle rotation of the shoulder girdle facilitates delivery of the right arm.

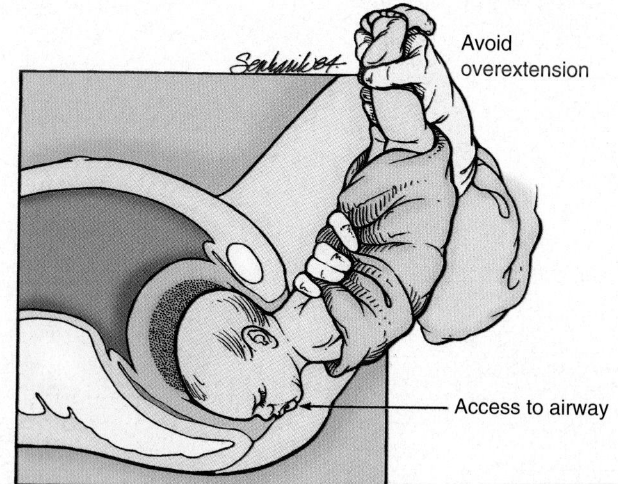

FIGURE 18-21. Following delivery of the arms, the fetus is wrapped in a towel for control and slightly elevated. The fetal face and airway may be visible over the perineum. Excessive elevation of the trunk is avoided.

elevation by the assistant may potentially cause harm to the neonate. Hyperextension of the fetal neck from excessive elevation of the fetal trunk, shown in Figure 18-23, should be avoided because of the potential for spinal cord injury.

Piper forceps are characterized by absence of pelvic curvature. This modification allows *direct* application to the fetal head and avoids conflict with the fetal body that would occur with the application of standard instruments from below. The forceps are inserted into the vagina from beneath the fetus. The blade to be placed on the maternal left is held by the handle in the operator's left hand and the blade inserted with the operator's right hand in the vagina along the left maternal sidewall and placed against the right fetal parietal bone. The handle of the right blade is then held in the operator's right hand and inserted by the left hand along the right maternal sidewall and placed against the left fetal parietal bone. Gentle downward traction on the forceps with the fetal trunk supported on the forceps shanks results in controlled delivery of the vertex (Figure 18-24). Forceps application controls the fetal head and prevents extension of the head on the neck. Application of Piper forceps to the after-coming head may be advisable both to ensure control of the delivery and to maintain optimal operator proficiency in anticipation of deliveries that may require their use.

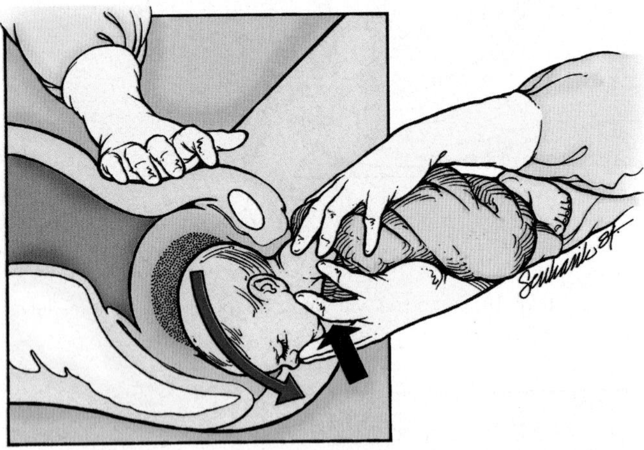

FIGURE 18-22. Cephalic flexion is maintained by pressure *(heavy arrow)* on the fetal maxilla (not mandible!). Often, delivery of the head is easily accomplished with continued expulsive forces from above and gentle downward traction.

Arrest of spontaneous progress in labor with adequate uterine contractions necessitates consideration of cesarean delivery. Any evidence of fetal compromise or sustained cord compression on the basis of continuous electronic fetal monitoring also requires consideration of cesarean delivery. Vaginal interventions directed at facilitating delivery of the breech that is complicated by an arrest of spontaneous progress are discouraged, because fetal and maternal morbidity and mortality are both greatly increased. However, if labor is deemed to be hypotonic by

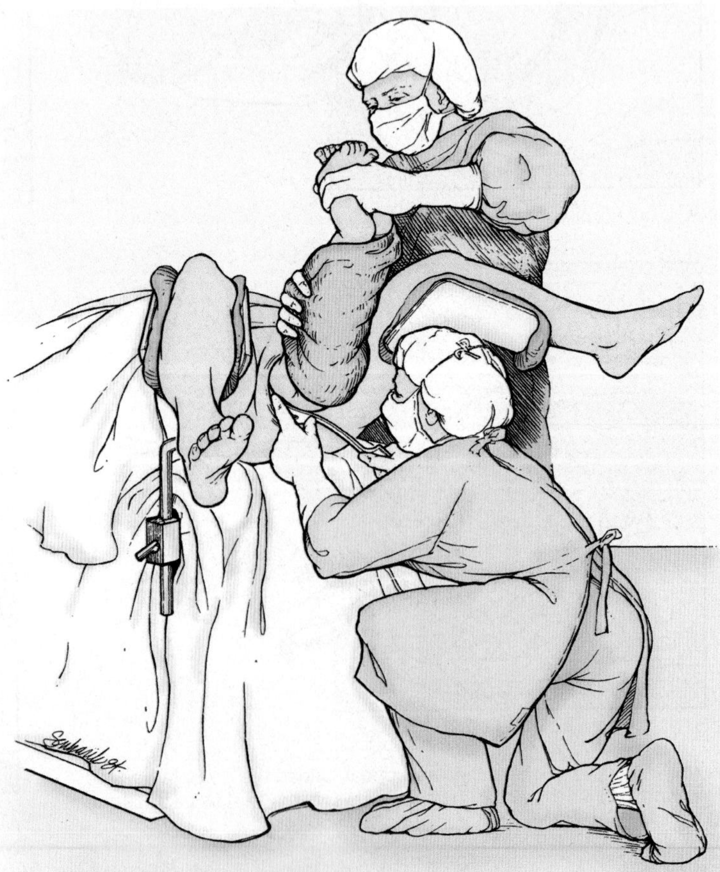

FIGURE 18-23. Demonstration of *incorrect* assistance during the application of Piper forceps; the assistant hyperextends the fetal neck. Positioning as such increases the risk for neurologic injury.

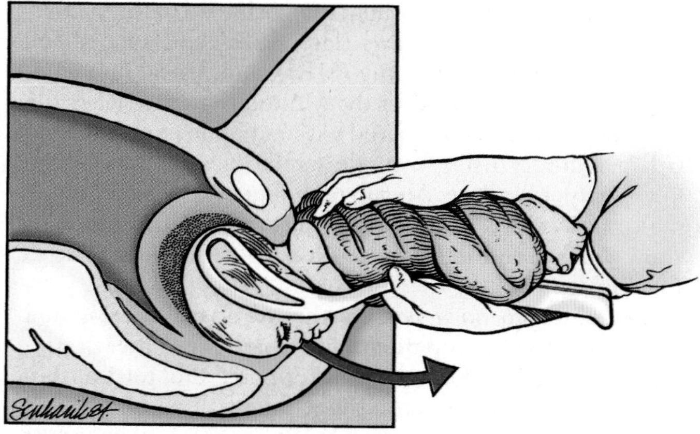

FIGURE 18-24. The fetus may be laid on the forceps and delivered with gentle downward traction, as illustrated here.

TABLE 18-2 INCIDENCE OF COMPLICATIONS SEEN WITH BREECH PRESENTATION

COMPLICATION	INCIDENCE
Intrapartum fetal death	Increased 16-fold[23]
Perinatal mortality	1.3%[20]
Intrapartum asphyxia	Increased 3.8-fold[31]
Cord prolapse	Increased 5- to 20-fold[14,15] 1.3%[20]
Birth trauma	Increased 13-fold[14] 1.4%[20]
Dystocia, difficulty delivering head	4.6%[20] to 8.8%[14]
Spinal cord injuries with extended head	21%
Major anomalies	6%-18%[31]
Prematurity	16%-33%[22,25]
Hyperextension of head	5%
Fetal heart rate abnormalities	15.2%[20]

TABLE 18-3 ZATUCHNI-ANDROS SYSTEM

Factor	0	1	2
Parity	Nullipara	Multipara	Multipara
Gestational age	39	38	37
Estimated fetal weight	8 lb	7-8 lb	7 lb
Previous breech	No	One	Two
Dilation	2	3	4 or more
Station	−3 or greater	−2	−1 or less

From Zatuchni GI, Andros GJ: Prognostic index for vaginal delivery in breech presentation at term. Am J Obstet Gynecol 93:237, 1965.

internally monitored uterine pressures, oxytocin is not contraindicated.[11,12]

Mechanisms of descent and delivery of the incomplete and the complete breech are not unlike those used for the frank breech described earlier; at least one leg may not require attention. The risk of cord prolapse or entanglement is greater, and hence, the possibility of emergency cesarean delivery is increased. Furthermore, incomplete and complete breeches may not be as effective as cervical dilators as either the vertex or the larger aggregate profile of the thighs and buttocks of the frank breech. Thus, the risk of entrapment of the after-coming head is increased, and as a result, primary cesarean delivery is often advocated for nonfrank breech presentations. However, the randomized trial of Gimovsky and colleagues[13] found the vaginal delivery of the nonfrank breech to be reasonably safe as well.

Contemporary Management of the Term Breech

Debate has largely diminished about the proper management of the term breech. Much of the older data were derived from relatively few studies of varied methodologies, patient populations, and multiple retrospective cohort analyses, which are subject to bias. These reports indicated that the perinatal mortality rate for the vaginally delivered breech appears to be greater than for its cephalic counterpart, but much of the reported perinatal mortality rate associated with breech presentation was largely due to lethal anomalies and complications of prematurity, both of which are found more frequently among breech infants. Excluding anomalies and extreme prematurity, the corrected perinatal mortality reported by some investigators approached zero regardless of the method of delivery, whereas others find that even with exclusion of these factors, the term breech infant has been found to be at higher risk for birth trauma and asphyxia.[14] To date, only three randomized trials have been reported.[11,13] Although conclusions regarding safety of breech vaginal delivery from a fetal standpoint may continue to vary, the practical reality today is that intentional vaginal breech deliver is rare. A summary of some of the reported complications is listed in Table 18-2. Overall, consideration of a potential breech vaginal delivery must be mutually agreed on by the patient and the physician after a complete informed consent is obtained.

Further Discussion of Delivery for the Term Frank or Complete Breech

The cesarean delivery rate for breech presentation began to approach 90% in some centers in the mid-1970s without a consequent proportionate drop in perinatal mortality rate. Maternal mortality rate is clearly higher with cesarean delivery, ranging from 0.2% to 0.43%.[10] Maternal morbidity is also higher with abdominal delivery. Some institutions reported a 50% incidence of postcesarean maternal morbidity compared with as little as 5% with vaginal delivery.[10,13] In an attempt to balance both maternal and fetal risks, plans were proposed to select appropriate candidates for a trial of labor.

In 1965, Zatuchni and Andros retrospectively analyzed 182 breech births, of which 25 infants had poor outcomes.[16] Therefore, these investigators devised a score based on six clinical variables at the time of admission (Table 18-3) that identified those patients destined to manifest difficulties in labor for whom prompt and appropriate interventions could be made. The score used parity, gestational age, estimated weight, prior successful breech vaginal delivery, dilation, and station to ascertain likelihood of successful vaginal delivery. However, the parturient herself could increase the score by presenting later in labor; other factors that affect the score are less modifiable. At least three subsequent prospective studies applied the Zatuchni-Andros system and found it to be both sensitive and accurate in selecting candidates for successful vaginal delivery.[17] **A Zatuchni-Andros score of less than 4 in these studies accurately predicted poor outcomes in patients with infants presenting as a breech.** Furthermore, in applying the scoring system, only 21% to 27% of patients failed to qualify for a trial of labor.[17] Previous breech delivery, one of the items scored in the Zatuchni-Andros system, has a significant odds ratio (OR) for recurrence of breech (4.32, 95% confidence interval [CI], 4.08 to 4.59) after one breech delivery, and up to 28.1 (95% CI, 12.2 to 64.8) after three. This study did not, however, control for recurrent causes of breech presentation such as uterine malformations and abnormal placentation.[18]

Because most reports of breech delivery are of level II to III evidence, their validity and, most important, universal applicability may be questioned. Many data were gathered before electronic FHR monitoring became commonplace. Until 2000, only one randomized trial (level I evidence) had examined term frank breech and method of delivery.[11] Improved perinatal survival had been reported for abdominally delivered breeches, and there is some evidence, although inconsistent, that the method of delivery may also have an impact on the quality of survival.[14] Functional neurologic defects were found by 2 years of age in 24% of breech infants born vaginally but only in 2.5% of those breech weight- and age-matched infants born by cesarean delivery.[19] However, in comparing 175 breech infants having a 94% cesarean delivery rate with 595 historical controls having a 22% rate of abdominal delivery, Green and colleagues[20] found no significant differences in outcome. Neurologic outcomes were reviewed for 239 of 348 infants delivered from breech position.[21] Examinations performed at 3 to 10 years of age showed no statistically significant neurologic differences between neonates delivered by vaginal breech versus matched vertex controls. Thus, these authors concluded that breech outcomes relate to degree of prematurity, maternal pregnancy complications, and fetal malformations, as well as birth trauma or asphyxia. A 2009 Norwegian study demonstrated that breech presentation *and* breech delivery are significant risk factors for cerebral palsy and a trend toward increasing risk for cerebral palsy among singletons born at term in breech by vaginal delivery (nearly fourfold). This adds to the body of literature that demonstrates that **breech presenting fetuses are already at increased risk for neurologic adversity, even when controlled for birth order, prematurity, smallness for gestational age, assisted reproduction, and sex, as well as route of delivery.**[22]

Pelvimetry is frequently employed when deciding to allow trial of labor in a breech presenting fetus. Clinical pelvimetry is an acceptable technique and can be used to determine the dimensions of the midpelvis and the outlet, and the inlet by way of surrogate measurement (the obstetrical conjugate). The reader is referred to the Intrapartum Care section in Chapter 13 on normal labor and delivery for discussion and demonstration of clinical pelvimetry. Radiographic pelvimetry has been included in the management of the breech presentation with little objective validation. Regardless, it is expected to predict successful vaginal delivery when adequate pelvic dimensions are present. There are at least four techniques for pelvimetry that are presently in common usage worldwide, including conventional plain film radiography using up to three films, CT with up to three views (lateral, AP, and axial slice), magnetic resonance imaging (MRI), and digital fluorography, not presently used in the United States. MRI is the only technique not associated with radiation exposure, and CT pelvimetry using a single lateral view results in the lowest exposure dose. Air gap technique with conventional radiography will lower the radiation dosage. **Current trends show a move toward the lower-dose CT techniques of up to three images.**

The clinician must possess the necessary training and experience to offer a patient with a persistent breech presentation a trial of labor. Furthermore, the relationship between the patient and the clinician should be well established and the discussions of risks and benefits must be objective and nondirective with accurate documentation of the discussion. If any of these factors are lacking, cesarean delivery becomes the safer choice. **However, even if a clinician has made the choice that he or she will never prospectively offer a patient with breech presentation a trial of labor, the burden of responsibility to know and understand the mechanism and management of a breech delivery is not relieved.** No one active in obstetrics will avoid the occasional emergency breech delivery. Regular review of principles, and practice with simulations using a mannequin and model pelvis with an experienced colleague, can increase the skills and improve the performance of anyone facing such an emergency. **A 2006 study of resident skill before and after simulation training showed universal improvement in technique and performance of key maneuvers required for vaginal delivery of a breech fetus when performed in mock emergency settings using a Noelle pelvic trainer.**[23] Maintenance of skill is particularly important as breech vaginal delivery becomes less frequently encountered in routine obstetrical practice (this is discussed in greater detail in regard to the Term Breech Trial).

Factors that affect the decision to deliver a breech vaginally or by cesarean section are listed in the accompanying box, Management of the Breech. The obvious implication of the dramatically diminished experience in training programs with vaginal breech delivery is that inexperience itself will constitute an indication for cesarean delivery. Certainly, in no case should a woman with an infant presenting as a breech be allowed to labor unless (1) anesthesia coverage is immediately available, (2) cesarean delivery can be undertaken promptly, (3) continuous FHR monitoring is used, and (4) the delivery is attended by a pediatrician and two obstetricians, of whom at least one is experienced with vaginal breech birth.

THE TERM BREECH TRIAL

One of the most influential publications of the last decade was the multicenter prospective study called the Term Breech Trial. The impetus for this investigation was a series of retrospective studies that demonstrated increased morbidity and mortality of neonates after vaginal breech delivery including neonatal intensive care unit admission, hyperbilirubinemia, bone fracture, intracranial hemorrhage, neonatal depression,[15] convulsions, and death.[24] Other studies, however, found that emergent cesarean

MANAGEMENT OF THE BREECH

Trial of labor may be considered if
- Estimated fetal weight (EFW) = 2000 to 3800 g
- Frank breech
- Adequate pelvis
- Flexed fetal head
- Fetal monitoring
- Zatuchni-Andros score ≥4
- Rapid cesarean possible
- Good progress maintained in labor
- Experience and training available
- Informed consent possible

Cesarean delivery may be prudent if
- EFW <1500 or >4000 g
- Footling presentation
- Small pelvis
- Hyperextended fetal head
- Zatuchni-Andros score 4
- Absence of expertise
- Non-reassuring fetal heart rate pattern
- Arrest of progress

delivery was also associated with poor neonatal outcomes. Irion and colleagues[25] reported similarly poor neonatal outcomes from cesarean deliveries of 705 singleton breeches, and concluded that as a result of the increased *maternal* morbidity associated with cesarean birth, delivery of the breech by cesarean section was not firmly indicated. This opinion was supported by Brown and colleagues[12] in their prospective case series, noting that the corrected perinatal mortality rate did not differ for neonates weighing ≥1500 g.

In October 2000, the first results from the Term Breech Trial were published.[14] Overall, 2088 patients from 121 centers in 26 countries with varied national perinatal mortality statistics, according to the World Health Organization, were enrolled in the study, with random assignment of 1041 to the planned cesarean delivery group, and 1042 to the planned vaginal delivery group. The data were analyzed by the intention to treat method, and 941 of 1041 (90.4%) and 591 of 1042 (56.7%) delivered by their intended route of delivery, cesarean section and vaginal birth, respectively. Intrapartum events, including cord prolapse and FHR abnormalities, occurred at rates similar to prior studies. Maternal and fetal/neonatal short-term (immediate, 6 weeks, and 3 months) and long-term (2-year) outcome data were presented in this and subsequent reports. **For both countries with low and high perinatal mortality rates (PMRs), the occurrence of perinatal mortality, or serious neonatal morbidity (defined within the report) was significantly lower in the planned cesarean delivery group than the planned vaginal delivery group (relative risk [RR] = 0.33 [0.19 to 0.56], P <0.0001). In countries with an already low PMR, there was a proportionately greater risk reduction in PMR in the planned cesarean delivery.** The effects of operator experience and prolonged labor did not affect the direction of the risk reduction and marginally affected the amplitude. No differences existed in maternal mortality or serious maternal morbidity between the groups.[14]

The effects on the correlation between labor and delivery factors were assessed in a separate regression analysis, using only delivery mode in one regression, and only labor factors including all other variables, such as fetal monitoring, length of labor, and medications in the other. **Mode of delivery and birth weight were both significantly associated with adverse fetal outcome, without a significant degree of interaction of these variables. Essentially, smaller infants (less than 2800 g) were at greatest risk (OR 2.13 [1.2 to 3.8], p=0.01).** Birth weights greater than 3500 g showed a trend toward more adverse outcomes, but the trend did not reach significance. The analysis of the labor data shows a "dose-response relationship between the progression of labor and the risk of adverse perinatal outcome," such that a prelabor cesarean delivery is associated with the lowest rates of adverse outcome compared with vaginal breech delivery.[26] Maternal outcomes at 3 months showed a reduced rate (RR = 0.62, 0.41 to 0.93) of urinary incontinence in the planned cesarean delivery group,[27] but 2 years after delivery, no differences in urinary incontinence or breastfeeding, medical, sexual, social, pain, or reproductive issues, as outlined in the text, existed.[28] Neonatal outcomes at 2 years showed no difference in mortality rates or neurodevelopmental delay between the planned cesarean section and planned vaginal delivery groups.[29] **Thus, the term breech trial can be summarized as follows: If a trial of labor is attempted and is successful, babies born by planned vaginal delivery have a small but significant risk of dying or sustaining a debilitating insult in the short term. If they survive, there is no difference in the mortality rate or in the presence of developmental delay when compared with those children born by planned cesarean delivery.**

The worldwide repercussions of the Term Breech Trial are still being realized. Eighty of the collaborating centers in 23 of 26 countries responded to a follow-up questionnaire regarding change in practice patterns after the results of the Term Breech Trial were published. A plurality stated that practice had changed (92.5%). Eighty five percent of respondents reported that an analysis of relative costs would not affect the continued implementation of a policy of planned cesarean delivery for the breech at term.[30]

A Dutch study examining the effects on delivery statistics and outcomes following the Term Breech Trial showed an increase in the cesarean delivery rate for the term breech from 50% to 80%, which was associated with a concomitant reduction in perinatal mortality rate from 0.35% to 0.18%.[31]

The total cesarean delivery rate in the United States in 2004 was 29.1% of all deliveries[32] and has increased substantially such that in 2007, the most recent year with complete statistics, the total cesarean rate was 31.8%, with 2008 preliminary data showing a further increase still. In 1978, the rate of cesarean deliveries in the United States was 24.4% of deliveries, with a drastic variation in rates in the intervening years. The 1981 National Institutes of Health Consensus Report found that 12% of cesarean deliveries in 1978 were performed for breech presentation and that this indication contributed 10% to 15% to the overall rise in the rate of cesarean births. At least a portion of the increase in cesarean delivery rates is a response to the perceived risk of morbidity and mortality associated with the breech presentation.[14,20] In the United States, the cesarean delivery rate for breech presentation increased from 11.6% to 79.1% between 1970 and 1985.[20,33]

Comparing the U.S. cesarean delivery rates from 1998 and 2002, before and after the Term Breech Trial's publication, one notes a marked increase in the rates for cesarean section: 21.2% of all live births in 1998, compared to 26.1% in 2002, and 29.1% in 2004. Rates of both primary and repeat cesarean deliveries increased. This may be in part because of the staggering number of multiple births and their related degree of prematurity, the relative reduction in vaginal birth after cesarean section,[34] and the self-fulfilling prophecy of lack of experience owing to increasing trends toward cesarean delivery for breech, leaving a void of experienced operators to perform breech vaginal deliveries (see Chapter 21). **The rates for cesarean delivery for breech presentation showed an increase over this period from 84.2% in 1998 compared with 86.9% in 2002, and remaining relatively stable in 2003 (85.1%).**[34] Although not as large a percentage increase as compared with the Netherlands, these trends are significant. The implications for future pregnancies have not been studied but may be implied by the trend toward decreasing attempts at vaginal birth after cesarean section: maternal morbidity and mortality rates are significantly increased with each subsequent cesarean birth.

Even though greater risks appear to face the breech infant, there remain many who believe that complete abandonment of vaginal delivery for the breech is not yet justified. The Term Breech Trial also has its detractors, who state inclusion of fetuses with estimated weights up to 4 kg and less than 2500 g, and procedural aberrations in labor assessment and adequacy (length of time permitted for first and second stage of labor, liberal use of induction and augmentation of labor), as well as worldwide differences in standards of obstetrical care and its providers make the trial's results not generalizable. No study is perfect in its methodology or results; the Term Breech Trial certainly adds to the body of literature on breech vaginal delivery but may not be the final answer to the question of the safety of vaginal breech delivery.

Special Clinical Circumstances and Risks: Preterm Breech, Hyperextended Head, Footling Breech

The various categories of breech presentation clearly demonstrate dissimilar risks, and management plans might vary among these situations. The premature breech, the breech with a hyperextended head, and the footling breech are categories that have high rates of fetal morbidity or mortality. Complications associated with incomplete dilatation and cephalic entrapment may be more frequent. For these three breech situations, in general, cesarean delivery appears to optimize fetal outcome and, therefore, is recommended.

Low birth weight (less than 2500 g) is a confounding factor in about one third of all breech presentations.[16] **Whereas the benefit of cesarean delivery for the breech infant weighing 1500 to 2500 g remains controversial,[12] some studies showed improved survival with abdominal delivery in the 1000 to 1500 g weight group.**[35] A multicenter study of long-term outcomes of vaginally delivered infants at 26 to 31 weeks' gestation found no differences in rates of death or developmental disability within 2 years of follow-up.[36] Traumatic morbidity is reportedly decreased in both weight groups by the use of cesarean delivery, including a lower rate of both intraventricular and periventricular hemorrhage. Although some advocate a trial of labor in the frank breech infant weighing over 1500 g, others recommend labor only when the infant exceeds 2000 g. There are proportionately fewer frank breech presentations in the low-birth-weight group. In fact, most infants weighing less than 1500 g and presenting as a breech are footling breeches. **Although most deaths in the very-low-birth-weight breech group are due to prematurity or lethal anomalies, cesarean delivery has been shown by some to decrease corrected perinatal mortality in this weight group compared with that in similar-sized vertex presentations.**[37] Other authors suggest that improved survival in these studies relates to improved neonatal care of the premature infant when compared with the outcomes of historical controls. However, when vaginal delivery of the preterm breech is chosen or is unavoidable, older studies demonstrated reduced fetal morbidity and mortality when conduction anesthesia and forceps for the delivery of the after-coming head are employed. Neither are commonplace in modern obstetrics.

Preterm premature rupture of the fetal membranes (PPROM) is associated with prematurity and chorioamnionitis, both of which have been found to be independent risk factors for the development of cerebral palsy (CP). PPROM is associated with a high rate of malpresentations because of prematurity and decreased amniotic fluid. Knowing the association of chorioamnionitis with periventricular leukomalacia (PVL), a lesion found to precede development of CP in the premature neonate, Baud and colleagues[38] correlated the mode of delivery with PVL, and subsequent CP in breech preterm deliveries. **The authors found that in the presence of chorioamnionitis, delivery by elective cesarean section was associated with a dramatic decrease in the incidence of PVL.**

Hyperextension of the fetal head during vaginal breech delivery has been consistently associated with a high (21%) risk of spinal cord injury. It is important to differentiate simple deflexion of the head from clear hyperextension, given that Ballas and colleagues demonstrated that simple deflexion carries no excess risk. Deflexion of the fetal vertex as opposed to hyperextension is similar to the relationships between the occipitofrontal cranial plane and the axis of the fetal cervical spine illustrated in Figure 18-5. Often, as labor progresses, spontaneous flexion will occur in response to fundal forces.

Finally, the footling breech carries a prohibitively high (16% to 19%) risk of cord prolapse during labor. In many cases, cord prolapse is manifest only late in labor, after commitment to vaginal delivery may have been made. Cord prolapse necessitates prompt cesarean delivery. Furthermore, the footling breech is a poor cervical dilator, and cephalic entrapment becomes more likely.

Breech Second Twin

Approximately one third of all twin gestations present as vertex/breech (i.e., first twin is a vertex, and the second is a breech; see also Chapter 30, Multiple Gestations). The management alternatives in the case of the vertex/breech twin pregnancy in labor include cesarean delivery, vaginal delivery of the first twin and attempted external cephalic version of the second twin, or internal podalic version and extraction of the second twin. Blickstein and colleagues compared the obstetrical outcomes of 39 cases of vertex/breech twins with the outcomes of 48 vertex/vertex twins. **Although the breech second twin had a higher incidence of low birth weight and a longer hospital stay, the authors found no basis for elective cesarean delivery in this clinical circumstance.** The outcomes of another study of 136 pairs of vertex/nonvertex twins weighing more than 1500 g allows us to conclude that breech extraction of the second twin appears to be a safe alternative to cesarean delivery.[39] Laros and Dattel[40] studied 206 twin pairs and likewise found no clear advantage to arbitrary cesarean delivery because of a specific presentation. **When comparing outcomes of 390 vaginally delivered second twins (207 delivered vertex; 183 delivered breech), with 95% of the breech deliveries being total breech extractions, it is noted that no significant differences existed between the vertex and breech infants, even when stratified by birth weight.**[41] These outcomes assume the skills and experience required to perform a successful breech extraction. Any clinician uncomfortable with the prospective delivery of a singleton breech, however, would be unwise to consider a breech extraction of a second twin.

Vaginal delivery followed by external version is a viable alternative, using ultrasound in the delivery room to directly visualize the fetus. Often there is a transient decrease in uterine activity after the delivery of the first infant, which can be used to advantage in the performance of a cephalic version. Description of experience with 30 malpositioned second twins (12 transverse and 18 breech) shows that version after birth of the first twin was successful in 11 of the 12 transverse infants and in 16 of the 18 breech infants.[42] These twins were all older than 35 weeks' gestation, with intact membranes of the second twin after delivery of the first, no evidence of anomalies, and normal amniotic fluid volume.

If internal podalic version/extraction of the second twin is to be performed, it can be facilitated by ultrasonic guidance. A hand is inserted into the uterus, both fetal feet are identified and grasped with membranes intact, and traction is applied to bring the feet into the pelvis and out the introitus, with maternal expulsive efforts remaining the major force in effecting descent of the fetus. Membranes are left intact until both feet are at the introitus. Once membranes are ruptured, the delivery is subsequently managed as a footling breech delivery. If the operator has difficulty identifying the fetal feet, intrapartum ultrasound may be of assistance.

During breech extraction, and perhaps more often with a breech extraction of a smaller twin, the fetal head can become entrapped in the cervix. In such cases, the operator's entire hand is placed in the uterus, the fetal head is cradled, and as the hand is withdrawn, the head is protected.[43] This splinting technique has also been used for the safe extraction of the breech head at the time of cesarean delivery. Head entrapment may also occur because of increased uterine tone, or contractions. **In this case, a uterine relaxing agent may be employed, with nitroglycerin (50 to 200 mcg intravenously) being one of the fastest acting, safest agents in appropriately selected patients.** Terbutaline, ritodrine, or inhalational anesthesia may also be used.

A small, prospective trial in the near-term gestation (greater than 35 weeks) found no difference in neonatal morbidity between vaginal delivery and cesarean birth of vertex/nonvertex twins. However, increased maternal morbidity with cesarean delivery was found. Again, safe vaginal delivery of the breech second twin by podalic version and extraction requires specific skills and experience.

External Cephalic Version

External cephalic version (ECV) is a third alternative to vaginal delivery or cesarean delivery for the breech fetus.[4,44] Many have found that ECV significantly reduces the incidence of breech presentation in labor and is associated with few complications such as cord compression or placental abruption.[4] Reported success with ECV varies from 60% to 75%, with a similar percentage of these remaining vertex at the time of labor.[4] Although many infants in breech presentation before 34 weeks will convert spontaneously to a cephalic presentation, the percentage that spontaneously convert decreases as term approaches. Repetitive external version applied weekly after 34 weeks in one report was successful in converting more than two thirds of cases and reducing their breech presentation rate by 50%. **In another randomized trial of ECV in low-risk pregnancies between 37 and 39 weeks, success was achieved in 68% of 25 cases in the version group, whereas only 4 of the 23 controls converted to a vertex spontaneously before labor.**[44] All of those in whom external version was successful presented in labor as a vertex.[44] In another prospective, controlled study of ECV performed weekly between 33 weeks and term, 48% of the study group were vertex in labor compared with only 26% of controls. Another experience with 112 patients demonstrated a 49% success rate with ECV. The cesarean delivery rate was 17% among those patients with successful ECV compared with 78% among those patients with an unsuccessful version attempt.

Outcomes of pregnancies after ECV prove that it is a safe and effective intervention.[4] **The overall success rate among investigators in the United States was 65%, with an average cesarean delivery rate of 37% among those undergoing an attempted version compared with 83% among controls.** Successful version was reported more often in parous than nulliparous women and more often between 37 and 39 weeks than after 40 weeks. Fetal complications include abruption, a non-reassuring FHR pattern, rupture of membranes, cord prolapse, spontaneous conversion back to breech, and fetomaternal hemorrhage. Maternal complications include a high rate of cesarean delivery (up to 64% in one study; twofold to fourfold risk in another), primarily for dystocia, despite successful conversion.[45]

Gentle constant pressure applied in a relaxed patient with frequent FHR assessments are elements of success stressed by all investigators.[44] Methodology varies, although the "forward roll" is more widely supported than the "back flip" (Figure 18-25).[44] The mechanical goal is to squeeze the fetal vertex gently out of the fundal area to the transverse and finally into the lower segment of the uterus.

A number of factors predict success of ECV with reliability. A study by Burgos and colleagues in 2010 demonstrated increased rates of successful ECV at approximately

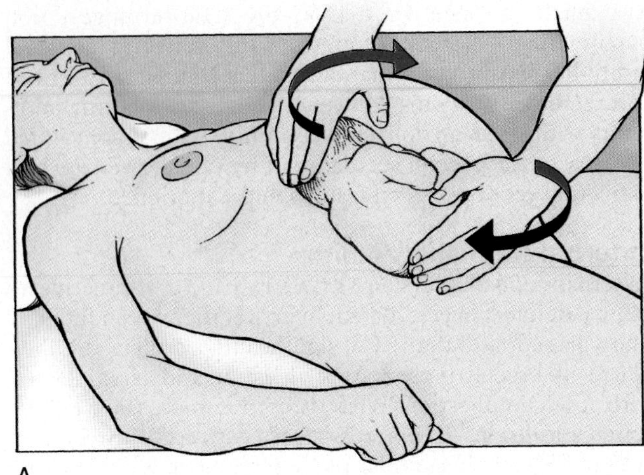

A

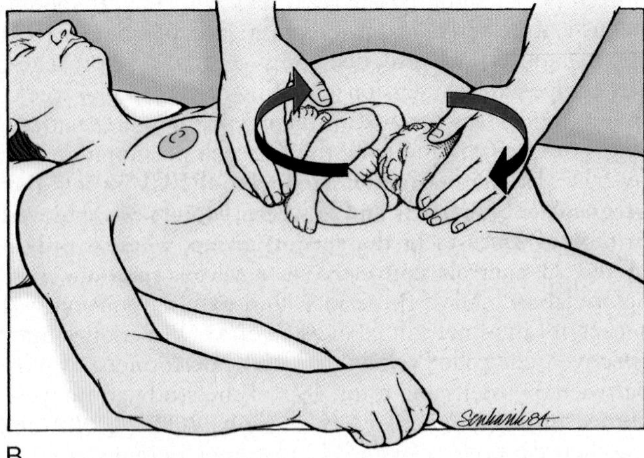

B

FIGURE 18-25. External cephalic version is accomplished by gently "squeezing" the fetus out of one area of the uterus and into another. Here, the "forward roll," often the most popular, is illustrated.

37 weeks' gestation with parity greater than 2 (OR 3.74; 95%CI 2.37 to 5.9), posterior placental location (OR 2.85; 1.87 to 4.36), and double footling breech as opposed to frank breech (2.77; 95%CI 1.16 to 6.62).[46] Complete breech also showed increased odds of success, but not to the extent that double footling did. Relative assessment of amniotic fluid was also made, and both "normal" and "abundant" fluid volumes showed improved successes. This study employed IV ritodrine, which is no longer available in the United States; therefore, these results may not be generalizable to our population, per se. Two recent studies showed improved successes when AFI exceeded 7 cm.[47,48] Tocolysis, regional anesthesia, and ultrasound during the procedure may also be helpful. Use of a number of tocolytics has been reported; however, considerable experience has been reported using intravenous ritodrine, which has been voluntarily pulled from the U.S. market by the manufacturer. Other agents used are hexoprenaline, salbutamol, nitroglycerin, and terbutaline (which now carries an FDA black box warning). A randomized trial of 103 nulliparous patients found success rates with subcutaneous terbutaline were 52% compared with 27% in the control group. No adverse maternal effects resulting from the drug were found.[49] A randomized trial of 58 patients at 37 to 41 weeks' gestation with breech presentation found no benefit from β-mimetic tocolysis, with success rates of approximately two thirds in each group. Factors associated with failure of version included obesity, deep pelvic engagement of the breech, oligohydramnios, and posterior positioning of the fetal back. The use of regional anesthesia for external cephalic version has also been controversial. Many believe that operators might apply excessive pressure to the maternal abdomen when epidural anesthesia is employed, which might make fetal compromise more likely, indicated by FHR decelerations and possibly related to placental abruption. However, a randomized trial of 69 women using epidural anesthesia demonstrated a better than twofold increase in success of the procedure when epidural was employed.[50] Disparate results are demonstrated when combined spinal-epidural analgesia or spinal anesthesia is employed. A randomized study of nulliparas undergoing ECV showed fourfold improvement in ECV success and reduced visual analog pain score when spinal anesthesia was used compared to no anesthetic.[51] Another randomized trial of combined spinal epidural at analgesic doses versus systemic opioids showed no difference in rates of ECV success.[52] This trial had low ECV success rates both overall (39%) and each arm (47% in CSE and 31% in opioid arms, respectively), and the utilization of 47 different physicians suggests the possibility of highly varied skill levels across providers. This trial specifically aimed to determine if analgesia as opposed to anesthesia improves success. It appear that the relationship of ECV success may be dose dependent where neuraxial anesthetic use is concerned, because other trials using anesthetic doses favor improved ECV success rates. A Cochrane database study of the effects of tocolysis, regional anesthesia, vibroacoustic stimulation, and transabdominal amnioinfusion for ECV was performed and reported in 2004. **Tocolysis reduced the failure rate of ECV (RR = 0.74, 95% CI, 0.64 to 0.87); the reduction of noncephalic presentations at birth did not reach significance, but the cesarean delivery rate was reduced (RR = 0.85, 95% CI, 0.72 to 0.99). Regional anesthesia also showed a reduced rate of cesarean sections and noncephalic presentations at birth in two out of five trials included. No other interventions improved success rates of ECV.**[53] Performing the version before term does not appear to significantly affect the likelihood of noncephalic presentations at term (RR = 1.02, 95% CI, 0.89 to 1.17); cesarean delivery (RR = 1.10, 95% CI, 0.78 to 1.54); low Apgar scores (RR = 0.81, 95% CI, 0.44 to 1.49); or perinatal mortality (RR = 1.19, 95% CI, 0.46 to 3.05).[54] Fetomaternal transfusion has been reported to occur in up to 6% of patients undergoing external version,[55] and thus, Rh-negative unsensitized women should receive Rh-immune globulin. Quantitation of fetomaternal hemorrhage with the Kleihauer-Betke or flow cytometry test will determine the number of ampules of Rh immune globulin to be administered.

In the case of the gravida with a previous cesarean delivery, ECV has also been controversial. Studies of limited sample size have concluded that ECV is safe for mother and fetus and results in increased vaginal delivery rates. Success rates of up to 82% in patients with a previous cesarean delivery have been reported.[56] Use of intravenous ritodrine tocolysis in 11 patients with history of previous low cervical transverse cesarean section resulted in no uterine dehiscences found clinically or at the time of cesarean delivery.[57]

A 2009 study by Sela and colleagues that included a review of the world literature (of ≥36-week nonanomalous singleton fetuses; all were retrospective studies) found ECV success rates in multipara ranging between 65.8% and 100% (mean 76.6%) in patients with a single prior cesarean delivery.[58] Prior successful vaginal delivery was predictive of higher success rates for ECV overall, and no excess morbidity/mortality or asymptomatic scar dehiscence was noted in these patients. The largest study of complication rates from ECV included patients with a prior cesarean delivery but neither the success or complication rates for this subgroup was reported; descriptions of overall complications included no case of overt uterine rupture or scar dehiscence.[59] With the liberalization of recommendations for patients with two prior cesarean deliveries to attempt TOLAC (trial of labor after cesarean) with appropriate counseling, it would not be surprising to this author if the next edition of this text includes information on success rates for ECV in patients with two prior cesarean deliveries, given evidence of normal placentation.

Of interest are the recent trials employing moxibustion of acupoint BL 67 (Zhiyin; beside the outer corner of the fifth toenail) to resolve breech presentation, with and without acupuncture or percutaneous low-frequency electrical stimulation, also applied to the same acupoint. Moxibustion is a traditional Chinese method that uses the application of heat generated by the combustion of herbs to provide stimulation to accupoints. The particular herb used, *Artemisia vulgaris* (mugwort), is purported to work by stimulating fetal movements. Of 130 patients in the treatment group of one study, only one required cephalic version, whereas 24 of 130 in the controls group required this procedure. Seventy-five percent of the treatment group and 62% of the control group were cephalic at birth.[60] When acupuncture is used in conjunction with moxibustion, rates of spontaneous conversion approach 54% compared with the observed group (37%, $P = 0.01$).[61] Another study noted significantly higher spontaneous and moxibustion-induced correction rates of breech presentation: 74% versus 92.5%, respectively.[62] This study enrolled patients on average 4 weeks earlier than the prior study. No FHR abnormalities have been noted with the use of acupuncture and moxibustion in combination.[63] **A large meta-analysis from 2009 that included 1087 patients from studies comparing true moxibustion at BL67 alone or in combination with acupuncture, or postural measures to observation or postural methods alone, showed an improvement in the rate of cephalic version among the moxibustion group (72.5% vs. 53.2%; RR 1.36, 95%CI 1.17 to 1.58).** The increasing role of complementary and alternative medicine and traditional techniques in modern practice is only beginning to be realized, and remains to be further examined.

SHOULDER DYSTOCIA

Shoulder dystocia is diagnosed when, after delivery of the fetal head, further expulsion of the infant is prevented by impaction of the fetal shoulders within the maternal pelvis. Specific efforts are necessary to facilitate delivery (Figure 18-26).

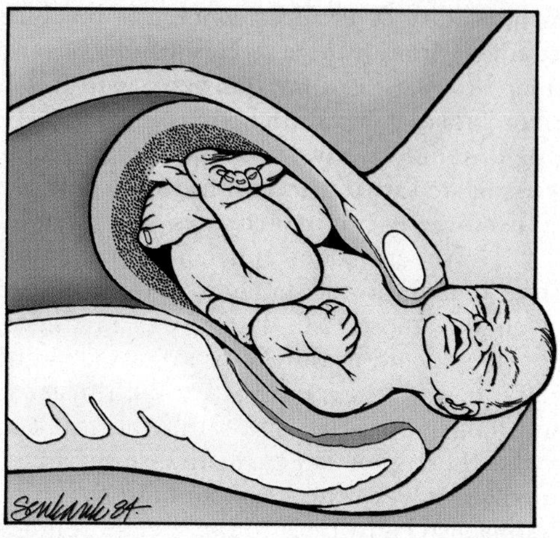

FIGURE 18-26. When delivery of the fetal head is not followed by delivery of the shoulders, the anterior shoulder has often become caught behind the symphysis, as illustrated here. The head may retract toward the perineum. Desperate traction on the fetal head is not likely to facilitate delivery and may lead to trauma.

Although a difficult shoulder dystocia occurs infrequently, one does not soon forget the experience. Often, but not always, at the end of a difficult labor, the fetal head may be delivered spontaneously or by forceps, but progresses no further. The fetal head appears to be drawn back with the chin close to the maternal perineum or thigh, creating difficulty suctioning the infant's mouth. As maternal expulsive efforts are encouraged, the fetal head becomes plethoric, and the danger to the infant is apparent if delivery cannot be promptly accomplished.

Shoulder dystocia has been reported in 0.15% to 1.7% of all vaginal deliveries,[64] but this number is highly variable based on lack of uniformity of definition. **Spong and colleagues have proposed employing the use of a "prolonged head to body delivery time (>60 seconds) and/or the necessitated use of ancillary obstetric measures" designed to facilitate delivery of the obstructed shoulder.**[65] **The >60-second interval is indicative of >2 standard deviations (SDs) above the mean for head to body delivery times in uncomplicated deliveries.** All investigators have documented increased perinatal morbidity and mortality rates with shoulder dystocia.[64] Mortality rate varies from 21 to 290 in 1000 when shoulder girdle impaction occurs, and neonatal morbidity has been reported to be immediately obvious in 20% of infants.[64] In reviewing 131 macrosomic infants, Boyd and colleagues[66] found that only half of all cases of brachial palsy occurring in macrosomic infants also carried a diagnosis of shoulder dystocia. Obviously, brachial palsy was noted in half of these cases without a clinical diagnosis of shoulder dystocia. Severe asphyxia was observed in 143 of 1000 births with shoulder dystocia compared with 14 of 1000 overall.[66] Fetal morbidity is not always immediately apparent. McCall[67] found that 28% of infants born with shoulder dystocia demonstrated some neuropsychiatric dysfunction at 5- to 10-year follow-up. Fewer than one half of these children had immediate morbidity. **The**

neonatal morbidity of greatest concern is brachial plexus injury, resulting from trauma to cervical nerve roots 5 and 6. Fortunately, most cases are transient, with full recovery observed in 90% to 95% of infants.[68]

Although shoulder dystocia has traditionally been strongly associated with macrosomia, up to half of cases of shoulder dystocia occur in neonates weighing less than 4000 g.[69,70] However, Acker and colleagues[68] found that the relative probability of shoulder dystocia in the 7% of infants weighing more than 4000 g was 11 times greater than the average, and in the 2% of infants weighing more than 4500 g it was 22 times greater. With macrosomia or continued fetal growth beyond term, the trunk and particularly the chest grow larger relative to the head. Chest circumference exceeds the head circumference in 80% of cases.[69] Arms also contribute to the greater dimensions of the upper body. **Macrosomia shows the strongest correlation with shoulder dystocia of any clinical factor and occurs more often with gestational diabetes and twice as often in prolonged pregnancies. Macrosomia is also associated with an abnormal 1-hour glucose screen and a nondiagnostic 3-hour glucose tolerance test. Other clinical factors associated with shoulder dystocia appear to be related to macrosomia as well and include maternal obesity,**[66,71] **previous birth of an infant weighing more than 4000 g,**[66,69,71] **diabetes mellitus,**[71] **prolonged second stage of labor,**[70,71] **prolonged deceleration phase (8 to 10 cm), instrumental midpelvic delivery, and previous shoulder dystocia, which has been found to have a recurrence risk of almost 14%.**[72] Increased maternal age and excess maternal weight gain have been found by some but not all investigators[66,71] to increase the risk of macrosomia and shoulder dystocia. Father's birth weight and adult size during young adulthood have also been found to correlate with fetal weight in addition to the traditional determinants.[70,74]

Macrosomia has been variously defined as a birth weight greater than either 4000 g or 4500 g.[64,66] Male predominance is routinely observed, and the condition is associated with the clinical features described earlier. **The two most common complications observed with macrosomia are postpartum hemorrhage and shoulder dystocia.**[71] Golditch and Kirkman[74] observed shoulder dystocia in 3% of deliveries of infants weighing between 4100 and 4500 g and in 8.2% of those weighing more than 4500 g. Benedetti and Gabbe[64] reported that fetal injury occurred in 47% of infants weighing more than 4000 g who were delivered from the midpelvis and had shoulder dystocia.

Clinical efforts to detect macrosomia prenatally could be helpful in anticipating problems with delivery of the shoulders. Such efforts, however, have been disappointing. Numerous sonographic markers have been assessed to determine their usefulness in predicting macrosomia. These include the estimation of fetal weight using a variety of fetal dimensions and the comparison of chest to head circumference. **Most recently, another biometric parameter, the fetal abdominal diameter–biparietal diameter difference (AD-BPD), was evaluated retrospectively both in diabetic and in nondiabetic women.**[75] **A difference of greater than or equal to 2.6 cm was found to predict shoulder dystocia with sensitivity and specificity of 100% and 46%, respectively, with positive and negative predictive values of 30% and 100%, respectively.** A similar study was performed in 2007 by Miller and colleagues.[76] Patients who experienced a dystocia birth were compared to a nondystocia group; all participants had a growth scan within the preceding 2 weeks. The dystocia group had an AD-BPD difference that was greater (2.9 vs. 1.97, $p = 0.0002$), and when the difference was ≥2.6 cm the risk of dystocia was 25% for unselected patients and 38.5% for patients with diabetes. Overall, an OR of 5.88 (95% CI 1.18 to 19.09) for presence of dystocia was noted in all patients and carried a sensitivity of 35.7% and a specificity of 91.4%. For diabetic patients, an OR of 7.19 (95% CI 1.58 to 32.67) and carried SE and SP of 55.5% and 85.2%.[76] **Furthermore, a fetal abdominal circumference of 35 cm or greater has been found to identify more then 90% of macrosomic infants.**[77] Both of these studies are retrospective and limited by difficulty measuring the fetal abdominal outline at advanced gestational age caused by acoustic shadowing. Parks and Ziel[71] found that of 110 macrosomic infants, the diagnosis was made prenatally in only 20%. The clinical estimate of birth weight was more than 3 lb in error in 6% of cases. **Numerous efforts in the literature repeatedly demonstrate the shortcomings of both clinical and ultrasonographic estimations of fetal weight and have concluded that the best estimation is a combination of the two.**

There is a growing trend to consider cesarean delivery of any infant with an estimated weight more than 4500 g or of any infant of a diabetic mother with an estimated weight more than 4000 g[70] to avoid birth trauma, particularly brachial plexus injury. Any consideration of elective abdominal delivery on the basis of estimated fetal weight alone, however, must consider the technical error of the method. **If 90% confidence is desired that the actual fetal weight is at least 4000 g, the sonographic estimate by most current methods must exceed 4600 g. This is a result of the expected methodologic error of ±10% (±1 SD).** Furthermore, the fetal vertex is often too deeply engaged in the pelvis to allow accurate measurement of head circumference. Estimated fetal weight should be only one of several factors considered in the management of the laboring patient. In the obese diabetic patient with an estimated fetal weight more than 4500 g and showing poor progress in labor, cesarean delivery may be the most prudent course. However, in most other cases, the risks of cesarean delivery to the mother, the accuracy of prediction of macrosomia, and the alternative of a carefully monitored trial of labor should be discussed. Gross and colleagues[78] carefully reviewed the clinical characteristics of 394 mothers delivering infants weighing more than 4000 g and concluded that although birth weight, prolonged deceleration phase, and length of second stage were all individually predictive, no prospective model adequately discriminated the infant destined to sustain trauma from shoulder dystocia from the infant not so destined. Taking this one step further, identifying macrosomic fetuses for the ultimate prevention of neurologic injury has been the subject of studies that report a significant increase in annual cost for routine cesarean deliveries for macrosomia in the nondiabetic population but improved ratios of cost per brachial plexus injury prevented per year in the diabetic population. **Ultrasound detection and elective cesarean delivery of the macrosomic infant of the nondiabetic mother has been predicted to result in $4.9 million of expenditure to prevent one**

permanent neurologic injury, whereas one maternal death would result from cesarean delivery for every 3.2 neonatal nerve injuries prevented.[78] Elective cesarean delivery for fetuses of diabetic mothers (both gestational and pregestational) has also been controversial. Langer and colleagues[79] found that 76% of shoulder dystocias could be prevented if a policy of elective cesarean delivery was instituted at an estimated weight of 4250 g, whereas Acker and colleagues[70] found that using a fetal weight threshold of 4000 g, 55% could be prevented in the diabetic population. Although many clinicians perform an elective cesarean delivery in a patient with diabetes mellitus and an estimated fetal weight of 4000 to 4500 g,[79] Keller and colleagues expressed concern about the inaccuracy of ultrasound estimation of fetal weight in the gestational diabetic population, with 50% of shoulder dystocias occurring in fetuses who weighed less than 4000 g.[80]

Using computer modeling, the forces applied to the fetal brachial plexus during dystocia delivery, and also with the addition of release maneuvers, were estimated by Grimm and colleagues[81] **All maneuvers resulted in less stretch to the brachial plexus than with standard lithotomy delivery alone. Delivering the posterior arm showed a 71% reduction in stretch applied to the anterior nerve plexus, and was the maneuver that required the least force to deliver the anterior arm.** In the past, however, it was believed that brachial plexus injury resulted primarily from operator-induced excess traction in the setting of shoulder dystocia. **Evidence now exists that plexus injuries may result from endogenous forces during the second stage of labor. Shoulder dystocia itself places the brachial plexus on stretch. Maternal endogenous forces may actually exceed clinician-applied exogenous forces as well.**[82] The occurrence of brachial plexus injury in the absence of shoulder dystocia has been described and attributed to in utero forces, such as the posterior shoulder impacting on the sacral promontory (although anterior injuries have been described as well), malpresentations,[83] and dysfunctional labor, mostly precipitate labor.[70] Interestingly, in neonates with brachial plexus injury without shoulder dystocia, there was a trend toward lower birth weight, more clavicular fractures, and longer persistence of the condition than their counterparts in the shoulder-dystocia-present group.[84]

The most effective preventive measure is to be familiar with the normal mechanism of labor and to be constantly prepared to deal with shoulder dystocia. Normally, after the delivery of the head, external rotation (restitution) occurs, returning the head to its natural perpendicular relationship to the shoulder girdle. The fetal sagittal suture is usually oblique to the AP diameter of the outlet, and the shoulders occupy the opposite oblique diameter of the inlet (Figure 18-27). As the shoulders descend in response to maternal pushing, the anterior shoulder emerges from its oblique axis under one of the pubic rami. However, if the anterior shoulder descends in the AP diameter of the outlet and the fetus is relatively large for the outlet, impaction behind the symphysis can occur, and further descent is blocked. Shoulder dystocia also occurs with an extremely rapid delivery of the head, as can occur with vacuum extraction or forceps or precipitous labor.

Successful treatment follows anticipation and preparation. Anticipation involves the prenatal suspicion of macrosomia by clinical and sonographic means. One must be aware of the clinical features that have been cited and consider a pregnancy at high risk for macrosomia and, therefore, for shoulder dystocia.

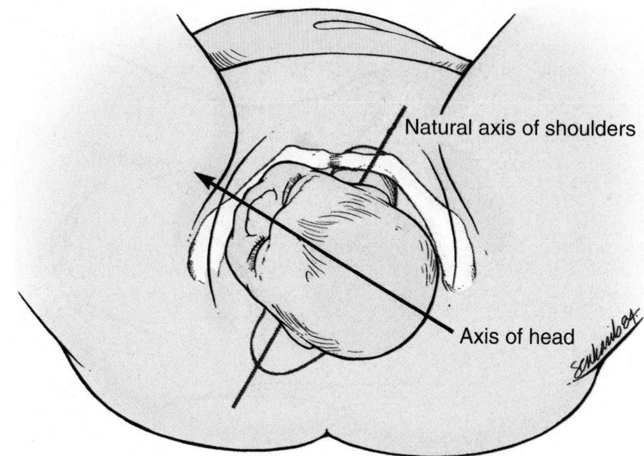

FIGURE 18-27. After delivery of the head, "restitution" results in the long axis of the head reassuming its normal orientation to the shoulders as seen here.

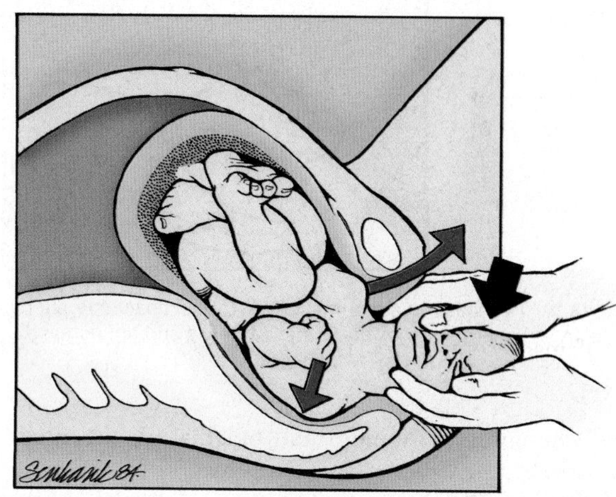

FIGURE 18-28. Gentle, symmetrical pressure on the head will move the posterior shoulder into the hollow of the sacrum and encourage delivery of the anterior shoulder. Care should be taken not to "pry" the anterior shoulder out asymmetrically, because this might lead to trauma to the anterior brachial plexus.

Such deliveries are best managed in a delivery room. Deliveries in bed increase the difficulty of reducing a shoulder dystocia because the bedding precludes fullest use of the posterior pelvis and outlet. Strong consideration for cesarean delivery is recommended when a prolonged second stage occurs in association with macrosomia.

Once a vaginal delivery has begun, the obstetrician must resist the temptation to rotate the head forcibly to a transverse axis. Maternal expulsive efforts should be used rather than traction. Gentle manual pressure on the fetal head inferiorly and posteriorly will push the posterior shoulder into the hollow of the sacrum, increasing the room for the anterior shoulder to pass under the pubis (Figure 18-28). This pressure is not outward traction and must be symmetrical. If the head is pressed asymmetrically, as if to

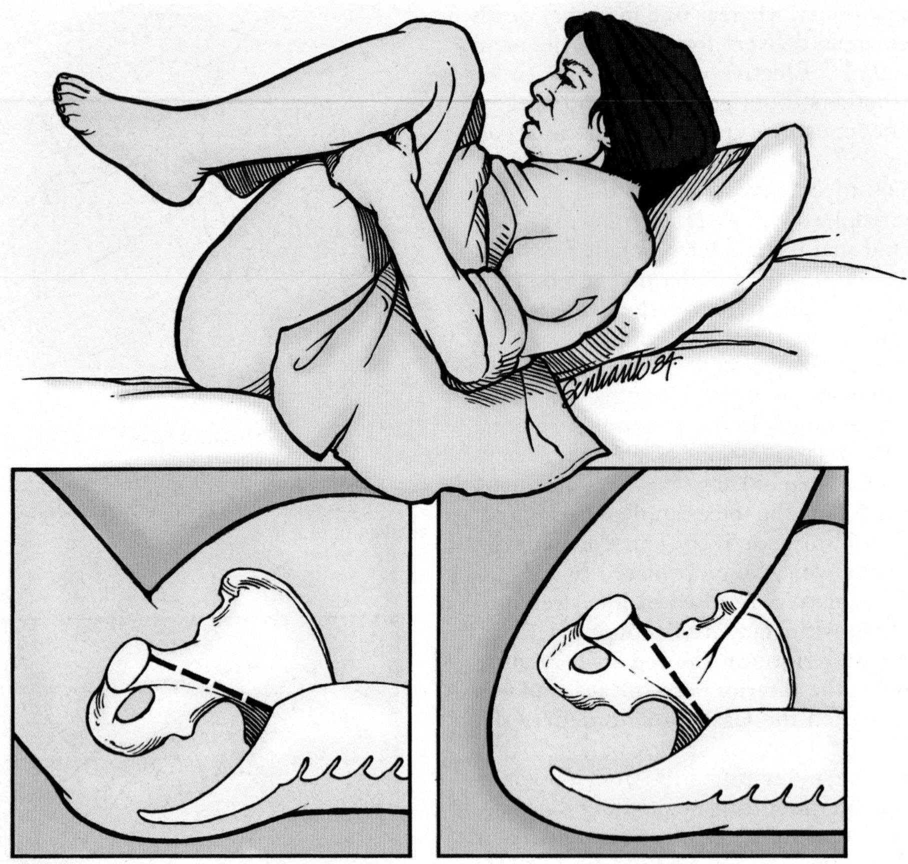

FIGURE 18-29. The least invasive maneuver to disimpact the shoulders is the McRoberts maneuver. Sharp ventral flexion of the maternal hips results in ventral rotation of the maternal pelvis and an increase in the useful size of the outlet.

"pry" the anterior shoulder out, brachial plexus injury is more likely.

If delivery is not accomplished, a deliberate, planned sequence of efforts should then be initiated. Pulling desperately on the fetal head is dangerous and should be avoided, and fundal expulsive efforts, including maternal pushing and fundal pressure, should be discontinued. Fundal pressure applied before disimpaction or rotation of the shoulders will not facilitate delivery and may be counterproductive in that it may increase the degree of impaction of the shoulder.

The McRoberts maneuver[85] is a simple, logical, and usually successful measure to promote delivery of the shoulders. **The McRoberts maneuver involves hyperflexion of maternal legs on the maternal abdomen that results in flattening of the lumbar spine and ventral rotation of the maternal pelvis and symphysis** (Figure 18-29). This maneuver may increase the useful size of the posterior outlet, resulting in easier disimpaction of the anterior shoulder. Gonik and colleagues[86] showed that the McRoberts maneuver significantly reduces shoulder extraction forces, brachial plexus stretching, and likelihood of clavicular fracture. In a retrospective review of shoulder dystocia, Gherman and colleagues[87] found that the McRoberts maneuver was the only step required in 42% of 236 cases. **When shoulder dystocia occurs because of failure of the bisacromial diameter to engage, the Walcher position, which entails dropping the maternal legs down toward the floor with concurrent suprapubic pressure in a dorsal-caudal direction, has been advocated. Only then, while constant suprapubic pressure is being maintained, should the parturient be placed in the McRoberts position; this may allow for the disimpaction of the fetal shoulder from the symphysis by increasing the AP diameter of the inlet before increasing the outlet.** Additionally, the "all fours," or Gaskin maneuver, which differs from the knee-chest position, may relieve the dystocia.[88] Use of this maneuver is reasonable only in the setting of a mobile parturient with no significant motor blockade from regional anesthetic, and a stable and wide surface on which to assume this position in order to avoid the potential for injury during transition to this position.

If the shoulders remain undelivered, often only moderate suprapubic pressure is required to disimpact the anterior shoulder and allow delivery. If this is not effective, **the operator's hand may be passed behind the occiput into the vagina, and the anterior shoulder may be pushed forward to the oblique,** after which, with maternal efforts and gentle posterior pressure, delivery should occur (Figure 18-30). **Alternatively, the posterior shoulder may be rotated forward, through a 180-degree arc, and passed under the pubic ramus as in turning a screw (Wood's screw maneuver). As the posterior shoulder rotates anteriorly, delivery will often occur.**[89]

Many authorities have advocated delivery of the posterior arm (Barnum's maneuver; Jacquemier's maneuver)

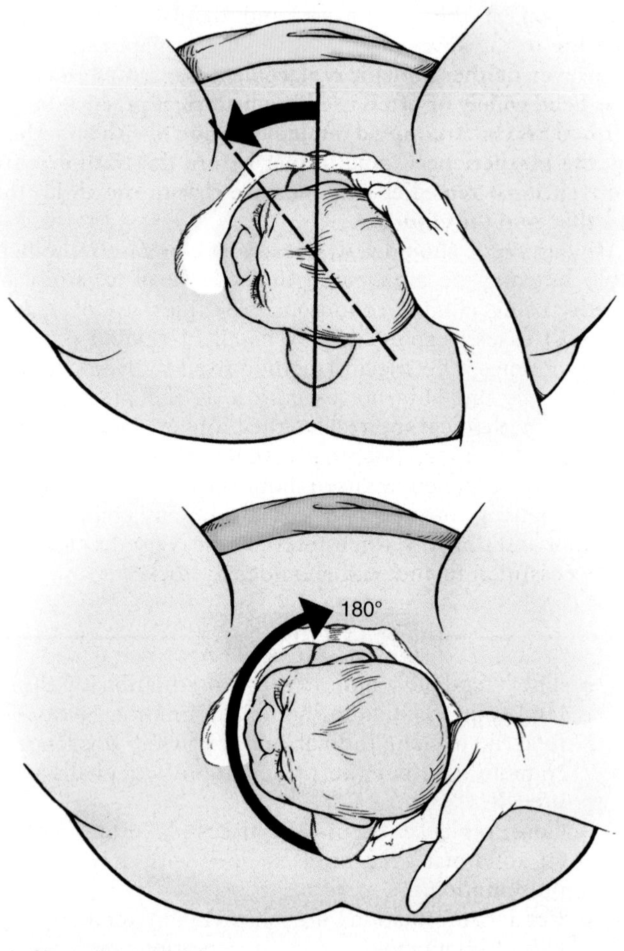

FIGURE 18-30. Rotation of the anterior shoulder forward through a small arc or the posterior shoulder forward through a larger one will often lead to descent and delivery of the shoulders. Forward rotation is preferred, because it tends to compress and diminish the size of the shoulder girdle, whereas backward rotation would open the shoulder girdle and increase the size.

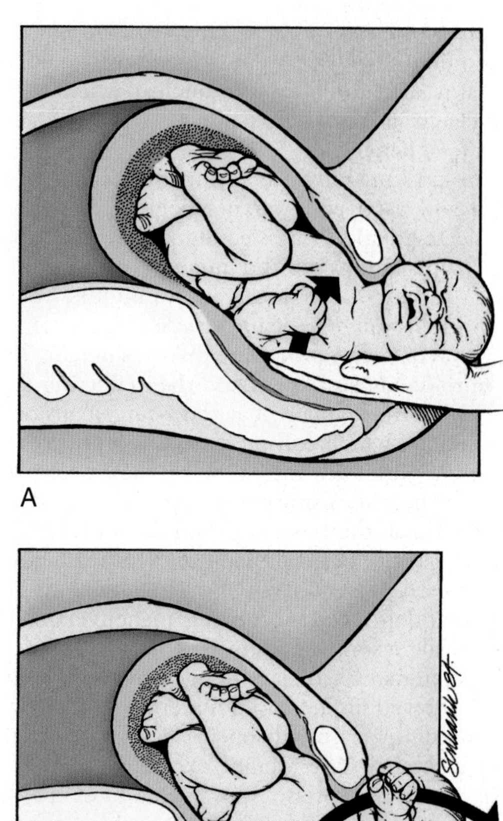

FIGURE 18-31. The operator here inserts a hand and sweeps the posterior arm across the chest and over the perineum. Care should be taken to distribute the pressure evenly across the humerus to avoid unnecessary fracture.

and shoulder should the aforementioned methods fail. The operator's hand is passed into the vagina, following the posterior arm of the fetus to the elbow. The arm is flexed and swept out over the chest and the perineum (Figure 18-31). In some cases, delivery will now occur without further manipulation. In others, rotation of the trunk, bringing the freed posterior arm anteriorly, is required.[69] **These maneuvers are highly likely to fracture the clavicle (up to 25%), humerus (up to 15%), or both, or they may result in transient or permanent nerve injury in up to approximately 9% of cases.**[89] Overall, similar rates of bone fracture were noted when any type of manipulation was performed to accomplish delivery of an impacted fetal shoulder.[90] Deliberate fracture of the clavicle is possible and will facilitate delivery by diminishing the rigidity and size of the shoulder girdle. It is best if the pressure is exerted in a direction away from the lung to avoid puncture. Sharp instrumental transection of the clavicle is not recommended, because lung puncture is common with such a method, and infection of the bone through the open wound is a serious possible complication.

Maneuvers to prevent shoulder dystocia have been evaluated in two separate studies: one compared McRoberts position and suprapubic pressure to no intervention,[91] and the other examined the use of lithotomy versus McRoberts position.[92] In the first study, head to body delivery times did not differ significantly. The "prophylactic" group had greater numbers of subjects who required cesarean delivery, and, when these were included in the analysis, results strongly favored use of prophylactic measures for reducing incidence of shoulder dystocia (RR = 0.33, 95% CI, 0.12 to 0.86). A greater number of patients required additional maneuvers to relieve the shoulder dystocia in the control group. Additionally, no differences were noted in NICU admissions or birth injuries. This study does not support routine use of these maneuvers in cases of suspected shoulder dystocia. The study by Poggi and colleagues[92] compared the traditional lithotomy position to McRoberts position, and additionally evaluated the forces required to release the shoulder with force-sensing gloves. The study concluded that peak forces and force rates did not differ between groups. The head to body delivery time was longer by 4 seconds in the prophylactic group, which was statistically significant. There were similar numbers of actual shoulder dystocias (one per group) encountered in each arm. **In summary, it is unclear whether the use of prophylactic measures in patients at risk for shoulder dystocia are of benefit.**

The Gaskin's maneuver (all-fours maneuver) has been described and used with varying degrees of penetration into physician practice, but is commonly used for shoulder dystocia management in the modern practice of midwifery.[93] A survey of physicians in the middle Tennessee area found that only 8% of practitioners knew of the all-fours maneuver.[94] **The procedure involves moving the parturient onto hands and knees and then effecting delivery.** The purported mechanism of action is an expansion at the sacroiliac joints, which can increase the sagittal diameter of the pelvic outlet by 1 to 2 cm.[95] Change of maternal position may help to disimpact the shoulders, and gravitational forces push the posterior shoulder anteriorly, allowing it to bypass the sacral promontory. This maneuver has not been tested prospectively or comparatively to the traditional shoulder-dystocia-relieving maneuvers, and may be impractical for some patients. Reports of 82 consecutive cases of shoulder dystocia managed with the all-fours maneuver showed no increased maternal or neonatal morbidity or mortality, with only one case of humerus fracture noted in a fetus whose weight exceeded 4500 g. Mean diagnosis to delivery time was 2.3 minutes ±1 minute (SD).[96] Delivery in all fours requires a stable surface, generally, not a narrow OR table, and a fully mobile patient. Fetal monitors and intravenous lines may hinder the patient's mobility and neuraxial anesthesia, with concomitant motor blockade, may reduce strength, making this maneuver unsafe in some situations.

Two techniques rarely used in the United States for the management of shoulder dystocia are vaginal replacement of the fetal head with cesarean delivery (Zavanelli maneuver) and subcutaneous symphysiotomy. Sandberg[97] reviewed the Zavanelli maneuver for both the vertex- and breech-presenting undeliverable fetuses. Cephalic replacement was successful in 84 of 92 vertex-presenting fetuses, and in 11 of 11 breech-presenting fetuses, podalic replacement was successful. Maternal risks included soft tissue trauma and sepsis, but the fetal risks were described as "minimal," with no fetal injuries attributed to the maneuver; this may be misleading because of the presence of a multitude of etiologies for permanent injury or death, likely from attempts at disimpaction, prolonged delivery time, and hypoxia.[97] O'Leary and Cuva[98] described 35 cases, 31 of which were considered successful and one of which needed a hysterotomy incision to allow manual disimpaction of the fetal shoulders and facilitate vaginal delivery when the fetal head could not be replaced into the vagina from below.

Subcutaneous symphysiotomy has been practiced in remote areas of the world for many years as an expedient alternative to cesarean delivery with very good results.[99] In a case series of three symphysiotomies, the procedure was used as a last resort and was associated with the death of all three neonates because of hypoxic complications. The procedure was concluded to be safe and effective as long as attention is paid to the three main points in the procedure: lateral support of the legs, partial sharp dissection of the symphysis, and displacement of the urethra to the side with an indwelling urinary catheter.[100] **However, neither cephalic replacement nor symphysiotomy has been widely or often used in obstetrical practice in the United States. Attempted implementation of either method by the inexperienced practitioner before the trial of more conventional remedies may increase risk to the child, the mother, and the clinician.**

In summary, shoulder dystocia is not precisely predictable but may be anticipated in the case of a variety of predisposing clinical conditions. Shoulder dystocia will, in most cases, respond to any or all of several prudent interventions. The specific method used to disimpact the shoulder is probably not as critical as the practice of a careful, methodical approach to the problem and the avoidance of desperate, potentially traumatic or asymmetric traction. The maneuvers used should be carefully described in the delivery note. There may not be any complication of labor and delivery when forethought is used to achieve a successful outcome with shoulder dystocia.

KEY POINTS

- The "fetal lie" indicates the orientation of the fetal spine relative to that of the mother. Normal fetal lie is longitudinal and by itself does not connote whether the presentation is cephalic or breech.
- Cord prolapse occurs 20 times as often with an abnormal axial lie as it does with a cephalic presentation.
- Fetal malformations are observed in more than half of infants with a face presentation.
- Fetal malpresentation requires timely diagnostic exclusion of major fetal or uterine malformations and/or abnormal placentation.
- With few exceptions, a closely monitored labor and vaginal delivery is a safe possibility with most malpresentations. However, cesarean delivery is the only acceptable alternative if normal progress toward spontaneous vaginal delivery is not observed.
- External cephalic version of the infant in breech presentation near term is a safe and often successful management option. Use of tocolytics and epidural anesthesia may improve success.
- Appropriate training and experience is a prerequisite to the safe vaginal delivery of selected infants in breech presentation.
- Simple compound presentation may be permitted a trial of labor as long as labor progresses normally with reassuring fetal status. Compression or reduction of the fetal part may result in damage, however.
- Shoulder dystocia cannot be precisely predicted or prevented but is often associated with macrosomia, maternal obesity, gestational diabetes, and a prolonged pregnancy.
- The clinician must be prepared to deal with shoulder dystocia at every vaginal delivery with a deliberate, controlled sequence of interventions.

REFERENCES

1. Thorp JM, Jenkins TJ, Watson W: Utility of Leopold maneuvers in screening for malpresentation. Obstet Gynecol 78:394, 1991.
2. Sharma JB: Evaluation of Sharma's modified Leopold's maneuvers: a new method for fetal palpation in late pregnancy. Arch Gynecol Obstet 279:4, 481, 2009.
3. Phelan JP, Boucher M, Mueller E, et al: The nonlaboring transverse lie. J Reprod Med 31:184, 1986.
4. Zhang J, Bowes WA, Fortney JA: Efficacy of external cephalic version: a review. Obstet Gynecol 82:306, 1993.
5. Benedetti TJ, Lowensohn RI, Trluscott AM: Face presentation at term. Obstet Gynecol 55:199, 1980.
6. Duff P: Diagnosis and management of face presentation. Obstet Gynecol 57:105, 1981.
7. Schwartz A, Dgani R, Lancet M, et al: Face presentation. Aust N Z J Obstet Gynaecol 26:172, 1986.
8. Levy DL: Persistent brow presentation—a new approach to management. South Med J 69:191, 1976.
9. Dignam WJ: Difficulties in delivery, including shoulder dystocia and malpresentations of the fetus. Clin Obstet Gynecol 19:577, 1976.
10. Collea JV: Current management of breech presentation. Clin Obstet Gynecol 23:525, 1980.
11. Collea JV, Chein C, Quilligan EJ: The randomized management of term frank breech presentation—a study of 208 cases. Am J Obstet Gynecol 137:235, 1980.
12. Brown L, Karrison T, Cibils L: Mode of delivery and perinatal results in breech presentation. Am J Obstet Gynecol 171:28, 1994.
13. Gimovsky ML, Wallace RL, Schifrin BS, et al: Randomized management of the non-frank breech presentation at term—a preliminary report. Am J Obstet Gynecol 146:34, 1983.
14. Hannah ME, Hannah WJ, Hewson SA, et al: Planned caesarean section versus planned vaginal birth for breech presentation at term: a randomised multicentre trial. Term Breech Trial Collaborative Group. Lancet 356:1375, 2000.
15. Diro M, Puangsricharem A, Royer L, et al: Singleton term breech deliveries in nulliparous and multiparous women: a 5 year experience at the University of Miami/Jackson Memorial Hospital. Am J Obstet Gynecol 181:247, 1999.
16. Zatuchni GI, Andros GJ: Prognostic index for vaginal delivery in breech presentation at term. Am J Obstet Gynecol 93:237, 1965.
17. Bird CC, McElin TW: A six year prospective study of term breech deliveries utilizing the Zatuchni-Andros prognostic scoring index. Am J Obstet Gynecol 121:551, 1975.
18. Albrechtsten S, Rasmussen S, Dalaker K, Irgens L: Reproductive career after breech presentation: subsequent pregnancy rates, interpregnancy interval and recurrence. Obstet Gynecol 92:345, 1998.
19. Westgren M, Ingemarsson I, Svenningsen NW: Long-term follow up of preterm infants in breech presentation delivered by cesarean section. Dan Med Bull 26:141, 1979.
20. Green JE, McLean F, Smitt LP, et al: Has an increased cesarean section rate for term breech delivery reduced the incidence of birth asphyxia, trauma, and death? Am J Obstet Gynecol 142:643, 1982.
21. Faber-Nijholt R, Huisjes JH, Touwen CL, et al: Neurological follow up of 281 children born in breech presentation-a controlled study. BMJ 286:9, 1983.
22. Andersen GL, Irgens LM, Skranes J, et al: Is breech presentation a risk factor for cerebral palsy? A Norwegian birth cohort study. Dev Med Child Neuro 51:860, 2009.
23. Deering, S, Brown J, Hodor J et al: Simulation training and resident performance of singleton vaginal breech delivery. Obstet Gynecol 107:86, 2009.
24. Roman J, Bakos O, Cnattingius S: Pregnancy outcomes by mode of delivery among term breech births: Swedish experience 1987-1993. Obstet Gynecol 92:945, 1998.
25. Irion O, Almagbaly PH, Morabia A: Planned vaginal delivery versus elective cesarean section: a study of 705 singleton term breech presentations. Br J Obstet Gynaecol 105:710, 1998.
26. Su M, McLeod L, Ross S, et al: Term Breech Trial Collaborative Group: factors associated with adverse perinatal outcome in the Term Breech Trial. Am J Obstet Gynecol 189:740, 2003.
27. Hannah ME, Hannah WJ, Hodnett ED, et al: Term Breech Trial 3-Month Follow-up Collaborative Group: outcomes at 3 months after planned cesarean vs planned vaginal delivery for breech presentation at term: the international randomized Term Breech Trial. JAMA 287:1822, 2002.
28. Hannah ME, Whyte H, Hannah WJ, et al: Term Breech Trial Collaborative Group: maternal outcomes at 2 years after planned cesarean section versus planned vaginal birth for breech presentation at term: the international randomized Term Breech Trial. Am J Obstet Gynecol 191:917, 2004.
29. Whyte H, Hannah ME, Saigal S, et al: Term Breech Trial Collaborative Group: outcomes of children at 2 years after planned cesarean birth versus planned vaginal birth for breech presentation at term: the International Randomized Term Breech Trial. Am J Obstet Gynecol 191:864, 2004.
30. Hogle KL, Hewson S, Gafini A, et al: Impact of the international term breech trial on clinical practice and concerns: a survey of center collaborators. J Obstet Gynaecol Can 25:14, 2003.
31. Rietberg CC, Elferick-Stinkens PM, Visser GH: The effect of the Term Breech trial on medical intervention behaviours and neonatal outcome in the Netherlands: an analysis of 35,453 term breech infants. BJOG 112:205, 2005.
32. Martin JA, Hamilton BE, Menacker F, et al: Preliminary births for 2004: infant and maternal health. Health E-stats. Hyattsville, MD, National Center for Health Statistics. Released November 15, 2005.
33. Croughan-Minihane MS, Petitt DB, Gordis L, Golditch I: Morbidity among breech infants according to method of delivery. Obstet Gynecol 75:821, 1990.
34. Lee HC, Yasser YE, Gould JB. Population trends in cesarean delivery for breech presentation in the United States 1997-2003. Am J Obstet Gynecol 199:59.e1, 2008.
35. Ulstein M: Breech delivery. Ann Chir Gynaecol Fenn 69:70, 1980.
36. Wolf H, Schaap HP, Brunise HW, et al: Vaginal delivery compared with cesarean section in early preterm breech delivery: a comparison of long term outcome. Br J Obstet Gynaecol 106:486, 1999.
37. Duenhoelter JH, Wells CE, Reisch JS, et al: A paired controlled study of vaginal and abdominal delivery of the low birth weight breech fetus. Obstet Gynecol 54:310, 1979.
38. Baud O, Ville Y, Zupan V, et al: Are neonatal brain lesions due to infection related to mode of delivery? Br J Obstet Gynaecol 105:121, 1998.
39. Gocke SE, Nageotte MP, Garite T, et al: Management of the nonvertex second twin: primary cesarean section, external version, or primary breech extraction. Am J Obstet Gynecol 161:111, 1989.
40. Laros RK, Dattel BJ: Management of twin pregnancy: the vaginal route is still safe. Am J Obstet Gynecol 158:1330, 1988.
41. Fishman A, Grubb DK, Kovacs BW: Vaginal delivery of the nonvertex second twin. Am J Obstet Gynecol 168:861, 1993.
42. Tchabo JG, Tomai T: Selected intrapartum external cephalic version of the second twin. Obstet Gynecol 79:421, 1992.
43. Druzin ML: Atraumatic delivery in cases of malpresentation of the very low birthweight fetus at cesarean section: the splint technique. Am J Obstet Gynecol 154:941, 1986.
44. Van Dorsten JP, Schifrin BS, Wallace RL: Randomized control trial of external cephalic version with tocolysis in late pregnancy. Am J Obstet Gynecol 141:417, 1981.
45. Vezina Y, Bujold E, Varin J, et al: Cesarean delivery after successful external cephalic version of breech presentation at term: a comparative study. Am J Obstet Gynecol 190:763, 2004.
46. Burgos J, Melchor JC, Pijoan JI, et al: A prospective study of the factors associated with the success rate of external cephalic version for breech presentation at term. Int J Obstet Gynecol 112:48, 2011.
47. Tasnim N, Mahmud G, Khurshid M: External cephalic version with salbutamol—success rate and predictors of success. J Coll Phys Surg Pak 19(2):91, 2009.
48. Assaf BM, Yair E, Hen YS, et al: Prognostic parameters for successful external cephalic version. J Maternal Fetal Neonatal Med 21:660, 2008.
49. Fernandez CO, Bloom SL, Smulian JC, et al: A randomized placebo controlled evaluation of terbutaline for external cephalic version. Obstet Gynecol 90:775, 1997.
50. Schorr SJ, Speights SE, Ross EL, et al: A randomized trial of epidural anesthesia to improve external cephal version success. Am J Obstet Gynecol 177:1133, 1997.
51. Weiniger CF, Ginosar Y, Elchalal U, et al: External cephalic version for breech presentation with or without spinal analgesia in nulliparous women at term. Obstet Gynecol 110:1343, 2007.

52. Sullivan JT, Grobman WA, Bauchat JR, et al: A randomized controlled trial of the effect of combined spinal epidural analgesia on the success rate of external cephalic version for breech presentation. Int J Obstet Anesth 18:328, 2009.
53. Hofmeyr GJ, Gyte G: Interventions to help external cephalic version for breech presentation at term. Cochrane Database Syst Rev 2004, Issue 1.
54. Hofmeyr GJ: External cephalic version for breech presentation before term. Cochrane Database Syst Rev 1996, Issue 1.
55. Marcus RG, Crewe-Brown H, Krawitz S, et al: Fetomaternal hemorrhage following successful and unsuccessful attempts at external cephalic version. Br J Obstet Gynaecol 82:578, 1975.
56. Flamm BL, Fried MW, Lonky NM, Giles SW: External cephalic version after previous cesarean section. Am J Obstet Gynecol 165:370, 1991.
57. Schachter M, Kogan S, Blickstein I: External cephalic version after previous cesarean section—a clinical dilemma. Int J Gynecol Obstet 45:17, 1994.
58. Sela HY, Fiegenberg T, Ben-Meir A, et al: Safety and efficacy of external cephalic version for women with a previous cesarean delivery. Eur J Obstet Gynecol Reprod Biol 142:111, 2009.
59. Collins S, Ellaway P, Harrington D, et al: The complications of external cephalic version: results from 805 consecutive attempts. BJOG 114:636, 2007.
60. Cardini F, Weixin H: Moxibustion for the correction of breech presentation: a randomized controlled trial. JAMA 280:1580, 1998.
61. Neri I, Airola G, Contu G, et al: Acupuncture plus moxibustion to resolve breech presentation: a randomized controlled study. J Matern Fetal Neonatal Med 15:247, 2004.
62. Kanakura Y, Kometani K, Nagata T, et al: Moxibustion treatment of breech presentation. Am J Chin Med 29:37, 2001.
63. Neri I, Fazzio M, Menghini S, et al: Non-stress test changes during acupuncture plus moxibustion on BL 67 point in breech presentations. J Soc Gynecol Investig 9:158, 2002.
64. Benedetti TJ, Gabbe SG: Shoulder dystocia—a complication of fetal macrosomia and prolonged second stage of labor with midpelvic delivery. Obstet Gynecol 52:526, 1978.
65. Spong CY, Beall M, Rodrigues D, et al: An objective definition of shoulder dystocia: prolonged head to body delivery intervals and or the use of ancillary obstetric maneuvers. Obstet Gynecol 86:433, 1995.
66. Boyd ME, Usher RH, McLean FH: Fetal macrosomia—prediction, risks, and proposed management. Obstet Gynecol 61:715, 1983.
67. McCall JO: Shoulder dystocia—a study of aftereffects. Am J Obstet Gynecol 83:1486, 1962.
68. Sandmire HF, DeMott RK: The Green Bay cesarean section study. IV. The physician factor as a determinant of cesarean birth rates for the large fetus. Am J Obstet Gynecol 174:1557, 1996.
69. Seigworth GR: Shoulder dystocia—review of 5 years' experience. Obstet Gynecol 28:764, 1966.
70. Acker DB, Sachs BP, Friedman EA: Risk factors for Erb-Duchenne palsy. Obstet Gynecol 66:764, 1985.
71. Parks DG, Ziel HK: Macrosomia—a proposed indication for primary cesarean section. Obstet Gynecol 52:407, 1978.
72. Lewis DF, Raymond RC, Perkins MB, et al: Recurrence rate of shoulder dystocia. Am J Obstet 172:1369, 1995.
73. Klebanoff MA, Mednick BR, Schulsinger C, et al: Father's effect on infant birthweight. Am J Obstet Gynecol 178:1022, 1998.
74. Golditch IM, Kirkman K: The large fetus—management and outcome. Obstet Gynecol 52:26, 1978.
75. Cohen B, Penning S, Major C, et al: Sonographic prediction of shoulder dystocia in infants of diabetic mothers. Obstet Gynecol 88:10, 1996.
76. Miller RS, Devine PC, Johnson EB. Sonographic fetal asymmetry predicts shoulder dystocia. J Ultrasound Med 26:1523, 2007.
77. Jazayeri A, Heffron JA, Phillips R, Spellacy WN: Macrosomia prediction using ultrasound fetal abdominal circumference of 35 centimeters or more. Obstet Gynecol 93:523, 1999.
78. Gross TL, Sokol RJ, Williams T, et al: Shoulder dystocia: a fetal-physician risk. Am J Obstet Gynecol 156:1408, 1987.
79. Langer O, Berkus MD, Huff RW, Samueloff A: Shoulder dystocia: should the fetus weighing >4000 g be delivered by cesarean section? Am J Obstet Gynecol 165:831, 1991.
80. Keller JD, Lopez-Zano JA, Dooley SL, Socol ML: Shoulder dystocia and birth trauma in gestational diabetes: a five year experience. Am J Obstet Gynecol 165:928, 1991.
81. Grimm MJ, Costello RE, Gonik B: Effect of clinician-applied maneuvers on brachial plexus stretch during a shoulder dystocia event: investigation using a computer simulation model. Am J Obstet Gynecol 203:339, 2010.
82. Gonik B, Zhang N, Grimm M: Prediction of brachial plexus stretching during shoulder dystocia using a computer simulation model. Am J Obstet Gynecol 189:1168, 2003.
83. Gilbert WM, Nesbitt TS, Danielsen B: Associated factors in 1611 cases of brachial plexus injury. Obstet Gynecol 93:536, 1999.
84. Gurewitsch ED, Johnson E, Hamzehzadeh S, Allen RH: Risk factors for brachial plexus injury with and without shoulder dystocia. Am J Obstet Gynecol 194:486, 2006.
85. Gonik B, Stringer CA, Held B: An alternate maneuver for management of shoulder dystocia. Am J Obstet Gynecol 145:882, 1983.
86. Gonik B, Allen R, Sorab J: Objective evaluation of the shoulder dystocia phenomenon: effect of maternal pelvic orientation on force reduction. Obstet Gynecol 74:44, 1989.
87. Gherman RB, Goodwin TM, Souter I, et al: The McRoberts maneuver for the alleviation of shoulder dystocia: how successful is it? Am J Obstet Gynecol 176:656, 1997.
88. Brunner JP, Drummond SB, Meenan AL, Gaskin IM: All fours maneuver for reducing shoulder dystocia during labor. J Reprod Med 43:439, 1998.
89. Gross SJ, Shime J, Farine D: Shoulder dystocia: predictors and outcome. Am J Obstet Gynecol 156:334, 1987.
90. Gherman RB, Ouzounian JG, Goodwin TM: Obstetric maneuvers for shoulder dystocia and associated fetal morbidity. Am J Obstet Gynecol 178:1126, 1998.
91. Beall MH, Spong CY, Ross MG: A randomized controlled trial of prophylactic maneuvers to reduce head-to-body delivery time in patients at risk for shoulder dystocia. Obstet Gynecol 102:31, 2003.
92. Poggi SH, Allen RH, Patel CR, et al: Randomized trial of McRoberts versus lithotomy positioning to decrease the force that is applied to the fetus during delivery. Am J Obstet Gynecol 191:874, 2004.
93. Gaskin IM. Shoulder dystocia: controversies in management. Birth Gazette 5:14, 1988.
94. Drummond SB, Bruner JP, Reed GW: Management of shoulder dystocia. Tenn Med 93:331, 2000.
95. Borell U, Femstrom I: A pelvimetric method for the assessment of pelvic "mouldability." Acta Radiol 47:365, 1957.
96. Bruner JP, Drummond SB, Meenan AL, Gaskin IM: All fours maneuver for reducing shoulder dystocia during labor. J Reprod Med 43:439, 1998.
97. Sandberg EC: The Zavanelli maneuver: 12 years of recorded experience. Obstet Gynecol 93:312, 1999.
98. O'Leary JA, Cuva A: Abdominal rescue after failed cephalic replacement. Obstet Gynecol 80:514, 1992.
99. Hartfield VJ: Symphysiotomy for shoulder dystocia [letter]. Am J Obstet Gynecol 155:228, 1986.
100. Goodwin TM, Banks E, Millar LK, Phelan JP: Catastrophic shoulder dystocia and emergency symphysiotomy. Am J Obstet Gynecol 177:463, 1997.

For full reference list, log onto www.expertconsult.com.

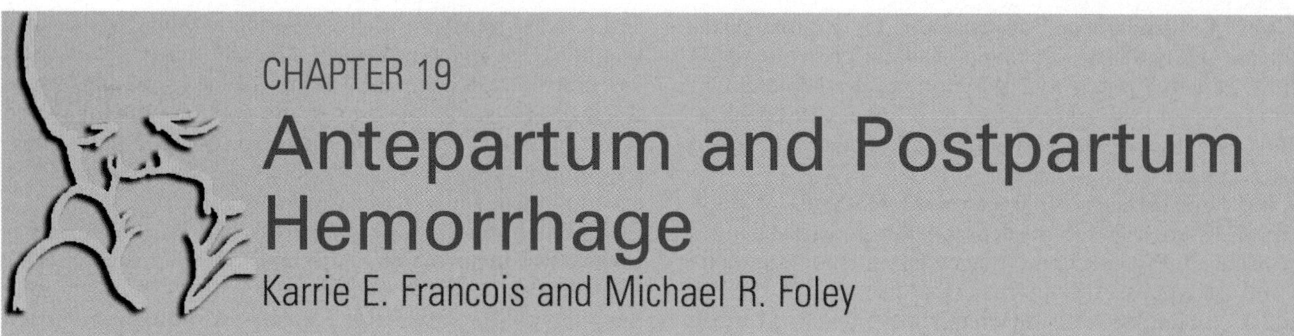

CHAPTER 19

Antepartum and Postpartum Hemorrhage

Karrie E. Francois and Michael R. Foley

KEY ABBREVIATIONS	
Fresh Frozen Plasma	FFP
Packed Red Blood Cells	PRBCs

Obstetrical hemorrhage is one of the leading causes of maternal morbidity and mortality throughout the world. Not only is hemorrhage the leading reason for an obstetrical admission to the intensive care unit, it is responsible for 17% to 25% of all pregnancy-related deaths.[1,2] Because of this significant contribution to maternal morbidity and mortality, it is critical for the obstetrician to have a thorough understanding of the hemodynamic changes that accompany pregnancy and the maternal adaptations that occur with excessive blood loss.

PREGNANCY-RELATED HEMODYNAMIC CHANGES

Pregnancy is associated with four significant hemodynamic changes. The first of these changes is **plasma volume expansion.** The average singleton pregnancy has a 40% to 50% increase in plasma volume by the 30th week of gestation. This increase in plasma volume is accompanied by an **increase in red blood cell mass**. With appropriate substrate availability, red blood cell mass can be expected to increase 20% to 30% by the end of pregnancy. **Maternal cardiac output rises** with normal pregnancy owing to both increased stroke volume and heart rate. Consensus exists that the average rise in cardiac output is 30% to 50% above nonpregnant levels, with the peak occurring in the early third trimester. **Systemic vascular resistance falls** in parallel with this rise in cardiac output and blood volume expansion. Finally, **fibrinogen and the majority of procoagulant blood factors (II, VII, VIII, IX, and X) increase** during pregnancy.[3] These four physiologic changes are protective of maternal hemodynamic status and, thus, allow for further physiologic adaptations that accompany obstetrical hemorrhage.

PHYSIOLOGIC ADAPTATION TO HEMORRHAGE

During pregnancy and the puerperium, a **defined sequence of physiologic adaptations takes place with hemorrhage** (Figure 19-1). When 10% of the circulatory blood volume is lost, vasoconstriction occurs in both the arterial and venous compartments in order to maintain blood pressure and preserve blood flow to essential organs. As blood loss reaches 20% or more of the total blood volume, increases in systemic vascular resistance can no longer compensate for the lost intravascular volume and blood pressure decreases. Cardiac output falls in parallel because of a loss in preload, resulting in poor end-organ perfusion. If the intravascular volume is not appropriately replaced, cardiogenic shock will ensue.

In severe preeclampsia, these physiologic adaptations are altered. Unlike in most pregnant patients, the protective mechanism of blood volume expansion is diminished with severe preeclampsia. It is estimated that plasma volume expansion is 9% lower in preeclamptic patients.[4] In addition, because of the significant vasoconstriction that accompanies preeclampsia, blood loss in these patients may be underestimated because blood pressure is often maintained in the normotensive range despite significant hemorrhage. Finally, with preeclampsia, oliguria may not be as reliable an indicator of poor end-organ perfusion secondary to hemorrhage because reduced urine output is typically a manifestation of the severity of the hypertensive disorder.

CLASSIFICATION OF HEMORRHAGE

A standard classification for acute blood loss is illustrated in Table 19-1. **Understanding the physiologic responses that accompany varying degrees of volume deficit can assist the clinician when caring for hemorrhaging patients.** Determination of the hemorrhage class reflects the volume deficit, which may not be the same as volume loss. **The average 60-kg pregnant woman maintains a blood volume of 6000 mL by 30 weeks of gestation.**

Class 1 hemorrhage corresponds to approximately 1000 mL of blood loss. This blood loss correlates to a **15% volume deficit.** Women with this amount of volume deficit exhibit mild physiologic changes of dizziness and palpitations, owing to the hemodynamic adaptations that accompany pregnancy.

Class 2 hemorrhage is characterized by 1500 mL of blood loss, or a 20% to 25% volume deficit. Early physical changes that occur during this hemorrhage class include **tachycardia and tachypnea.** Although tachycardia is usually recognized as a compensatory mechanism to increase cardiac output, the significance of tachypnea is unclear and often unappreciated clinically. Tachypnea can represent a sign of impending clinical decompensation.

Narrowing of the pulse pressure is another sign of class 2 hemorrhage. The pulse pressure represents the difference between the systolic and diastolic blood pressures. Systolic blood pressure is a good representation of stroke volume and β_1 stimulation. Diastolic blood pressure is a reflection of systemic vasoconstriction. Therefore, the pulse pressure represents the interrelationship between these entities. With a class 2 volume deficit, the sympathoadrenal system is activated, resulting in a diversion of blood away from nonvital organs (skin, muscle, and kidney) and a redistribution of the circulation to vital body organs, including the brain and heart. The end result is increased vasoconstriction, increased diastolic blood pressure, maintenance of systolic blood pressure, and a narrowing of the pulse pressure. With greater narrowing of the pulse pressure, more compensatory vasoconstriction is occurring to accommodate for a loss in stroke volume.

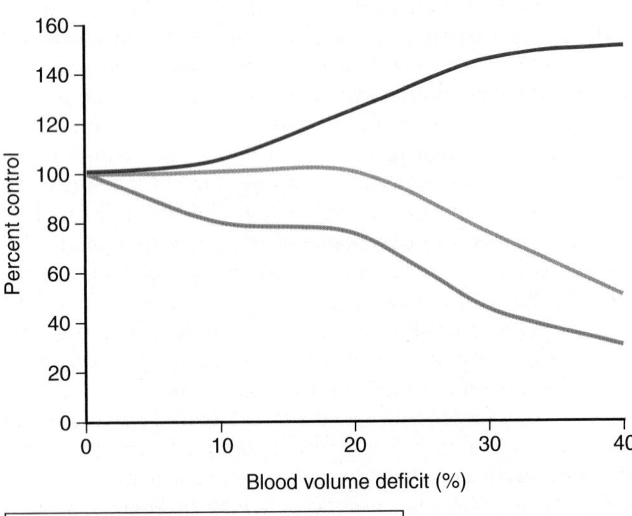

FIGURE 19-1. Relationships among systemic vascular resistance, blood pressure, and cardiac output in the face of progressive blood volume deficit.

A final physiologic response of class 2 hemorrhage is **orthostatic hypotension.** Although blood pressure comparisons can be made in the supine, sitting, and standing positions to document this response, a practical approach is to assess the time needed to refill a blanched hypothenar area on the patient's hand. Typically, a patient with normal volume status can reperfuse this area within 1 to 2 seconds after pressure is applied. A patient with class 2 hemorrhage and orthostatic hypotension will have significant reperfusion delay.

Class 3 hemorrhage is defined as a blood loss of 2000 mL and corresponds to a volume deficit of 30% to 35%. Within this hemorrhage class, the physiologic responses noted in class 2 hemorrhage are exaggerated. Patients demonstrate **significant tachycardia** (120 to 160 beats/minute), **tachypnea** (30 to 50 breaths/minute), **overt hypotension, restlessness, pallor, and cool extremities.**

Class 4 hemorrhage is characterized by more than 2500 mL of blood loss. This amount of blood loss exceeds **40% of the patient's total blood volume.** The clinical manifestations of this volume deficit include **absent distal pulses, cardiogenic shock, air hunger, and oliguria or anuria.** When a large hemorrhage occurs, renal blood flow is reduced and redirected from the outer renal cortex to the juxtamedullary region. In this region, increased water and sodium absorption occur, resulting in less urine volume, lower urinary sodium concentration, and increased urine osmolarity. A urine sodium concentration less than 10 to 20 mEq/L or a urine-to-serum osmolar ratio greater than 2 indicates significantly reduced renal perfusion in the face of hemorrhage.

ANTEPARTUM HEMORRHAGE

Placental Abruption

Definition and Pathogenesis

Placental abruption, or abruptio placenta, refers to the premature separation of a normally implanted placenta from the uterus. Typically, defective maternal vessels in the decidua basalis rupture and cause the separation. On rare occasions, the separation may be caused by a disruption of the fetal-placental vessels.[5] These damaged vessels cause bleeding, which results in a decidual hematoma that may

TABLE 19-1 HEMORRHAGE CLASSIFICATION AND PHYSIOLOGIC RESPONSE

HEMORRHAGE CLASS	ACUTE BLOOD LOSS	PERCENTAGE LOST	PHYSIOLOGIC RESPONSE
1	1000 mL	15	Dizziness, palpitations, minimal blood pressure change
2	1500 mL	20-25	Tachycardia, tachypnea, sweating, weakness, narrowed pulse pressure
3	2000 mL	30-35	Significant tachycardia and tachypnea, restlessness, pallor, cool extremities
4	≥2500 mL	40	Cardiogenic shock, air hunger, oliguria or anuria

Modified from Baker R: Hemorrhage in obstetrics. Obstet Gynecol Annu 6:295, 1977; and Bonnar J: Massive obstetric haemorrhage. Baillieres Best Pract Res Clin Obstet Gynaecol 14:1-18, 2000.

lead to placental separation, destruction of placental tissue, and a loss of maternal-fetal surface area for nutrient and gas exchange.

Placental abruption is often the result of both acute and chronic processes. Thrombin, which is released in response to decidual hemorrhage or hypoxia, appears to play an active role in the pathogenesis of placental abruption.[6] Thrombin acts as a direct uterotonic, enhances the action of matrix metalloproteinases, upregulates apoptosis genes, and increases the expression of inflammatory cytokines.[6,7] These thrombin-mediated events initiate a cyclic pathway of vascular disruption, hemorrhage, inflammation, contractions, and rupture of membranes.[5]

Incidence

The overall incidence of placental abruption is 1 in 100 births; however, a range of 1 in 75 to 1 in 226 deliveries has been reported.[5,8] The range in incidence likely reflects variable criteria for diagnosis as well as an increased recognition in recent years of milder forms of abruption. **About one third of all antepartum bleeding can be attributed to placental abruption.**[8] **Placental abruption peaks at 24 to 26 weeks of gestation.**[5] The incidence has risen in the United States because of increased rates of gestational diabetes mellitus, preterm labor, and umbilical cord abnormalities.[9]

Clinical Manifestations

Several factors determine the clinical manifestations of placental abruption. These factors include the temporal nature of the abruption (acute versus chronic), the clinical presentation (overt versus concealed), and the **severity**.[5] An acute, overt abruption typically presents with vaginal bleeding, abdominal pain, and uterine contractions. As the placental separation worsens, uterine tenderness, tachysystole, non-reassuring fetal heart rate patterns, and fetal death may occur.[10] **The amount of vaginal bleeding correlates poorly with the extent of placental separation and its potential for fetal compromise. In fact, concealed abruption occurs in 10% to 20% of cases.**[11] With severe abruptions, more than 50% of the placental surface area separates.[5] In these scenarios, maternal compromise in the form of consumptive coagulopathy may result from the triggering of the clotting cascade by hemorrhage and extensive thrombin deposition.[10,12]

Chronic abruption may be insidious in its presentation and is often associated with ischemic placental disease.[13] Typically, these cases present with intermittent, light vaginal bleeding and evidence of chronic placental inflammation and dysfunction, such as oligohydramnios, fetal growth restriction, preterm labor, premature preterm rupture of membranes, and preeclampsia.[14]

Risk Factors

Although the exact etiology of placental abruption is unclear, a variety of risk factors have been identified (Table 19-2).

Increasing Parity and Maternal Age

Several studies have noted a **higher incidence of placental abruption with increasing parity.**[15] Among primigravid women, the frequency of placental abruption is less than 1%; however, 2.5% of grand multiparas experience placental abruption. Theories suggest that damaged endometrium, impaired decidualization, and aberrant vasculature may have causal roles with increasing parity or age.

Maternal age is often cited as an associated risk factor for placental abruption. Although a 15-year population-based study in Norway was able to demonstrate a strong relationship between maternal age and placental abruption for all levels of parity, others studies suggest that there is no increased risk for placental abruption among older women when parity and hypertensive disease are excluded.

Cigarette Smoking

Cigarette smoking is associated with a significantly increased incidence of placental abruption and fetal death.[15,16] There appears to be a dose-response relationship with the number of cigarettes smoked and the risks for placental abruption and fetal loss.[17] Compared with nonsmokers, smokers have a 40% increased risk for fetal death from placental abruption with each pack of cigarettes smoked.[15] In addition, smoking and hypertensive disease appear to have an additive effect on placental abruption.[16] Proposed etiologies include placental hypoperfusion with resulting decidual ischemia and necrosis.

Cocaine Abuse

Cocaine abuse in the third trimester has been associated with as high as a 10% placental abruption rate.[18] The pathogenesis appears to be related to cocaine-induced vasospasm with subsequent decidual ischemia, reflex vasodilation, and vascular disruption within the placental bed.[5]

Trauma

Blunt or penetrating trauma to the gravid abdomen has been associated with placental abruption. After a **minor trauma,** the risk for placental abruption is between **1% and 5%,** whereas the risk may be as high as **50% after severe injury.**[19] The two most common causes of maternal trauma are motor vehicle crashes and domestic abuse. With motor vehicle crashes, uterine stretch, direct penetration, and placental shearing from acceleration-deceleration forces are the primary etiologies of trauma-related placental abruption.

Maternal Hypertension

Maternal hypertension is the most consistently identified risk factor for placental abruption.[13,15,16] This relationship

TABLE 19-2 Placental Abruption Risk Factors

Increasing parity and/or maternal age
Cigarette smoking
Cocaine abuse
Trauma
Maternal hypertension
Preterm premature rupture of membranes
Rapid uterine decompression associated with multiple gestation and polyhydramnios
Inherited or acquired thrombophilia
Uterine malformations or fibroids
Placental abnormalities or ischemia
Prior abruption

has been noted with both chronic and pregnancy-related hypertension. Compared with normotensive women, hypertensive women have a fivefold increased risk for placental abruption. This relationship is most strongly associated with fetal death due to placental abruption, in which 40% to 50% of cases have underlying hypertensive disease.[20] Unfortunately, antihypertensive therapy does not reduce the risk for placental abruption in women with chronic hypertension.[21]

Preterm Premature Rupture of Membranes

Placental abruption occurs in 2% to 5% of pregnancies with preterm premature rupture of membranes.[14,22] Intrauterine infection and oligohydramnios significantly increase the risk for placental abruption, and non-reassuring fetal heart rate patterns occur in nearly half of these pregnancies.[14]

It is unclear whether placental abruption is the cause or consequence of preterm premature rupture of membranes.[5] Hemorrhage and associated thrombin generation may stimulate cytokine and protease production, resulting in membrane rupture. Alternatively, the cytokine-protease cascade that follows ruptured membranes may cause damage to the decidual vasculature, predisposing the placenta to an abruption.

Rapid Uterine Decompression Associated with Multiple Gestation and Polyhydramnios

Rapid decompression of an overdistended uterus can cause placental abruption. This may occur in the setting of multiple gestations or with polyhydramnios. Compared with singletons, twins have been reported to have nearly a threefold increased risk for placental abruption.[23] Although the exact timing of placental abruption in multiple gestations is difficult to ascertain, it has been attributed to rapid decompression of the uterus after the delivery of the first twin. Likewise, rapid loss of amniotic fluid in pregnancies complicated by polyhydramnios has been implicated in placental abruption. This can occur with spontaneous rupture of membranes or may follow therapeutic amniocentesis.

Thrombophilia

Inherited and acquired thrombophilias have been implicated as risk factors for placental abruption.[24] The thrombophilias most commonly cited include factor V Leiden mutation, prothrombin G20210A mutation, antithrombin deficiency, protein C deficiency, protein S deficiency, hyperhomocysteinemia due to thermolabile methylene tetrahydrofolate reductase mutation (C677T), hypofibrinogenemia or dysfibrinogenemia, and antiphospholipid antibody syndrome. There appears to be a dose-response increase in the risk for placental abruption with increasing numbers or combinations of thrombophilias.[25]

Uterine and Placental Factors

Placental implantation over a uterine malformation (e.g., septum) **or fibroid can be associated with abruption.**[26] In addition, abnormal placental formation (e.g., circumvallate placenta) or chronic ischemia associated with preeclampsia and fetal growth restriction have been implicated in placental abruption.[16,25]

Prior Abruption

A previous abruption is associated with a risk for recurrence between 5% and 17%. After two consecutive abruptions, the recurrence risk rises to 25%. In the largest series of placental abruption with resultant fetal death, the recurrence rate of repeat placental abruption with fetal demise was 11%.

Diagnosis

Placental abruption is primarily a clinical diagnosis that is supported by radiographic, laboratory, and pathologic studies. Any patient with findings of vaginal bleeding, preterm labor, abdominal pain, or trauma should prompt an investigation of placental abruption.[5]

Radiology

Although early studies evaluating the use of **ultrasound** for the diagnosis of placental abruption identified less than 2% of cases, recent advances in imaging and its interpretation have improved detection rates. Early hemorrhage is typically hyperechoic or isoechoic, whereas resolving hematomas are hypoechoic within 1 week and sonolucent within 2 weeks of the abruption. Acute hemorrhage may be misinterpreted as a thickened placenta or fibroid.

Ultrasound can identify **three predominant locations for placental abruption.** These are **subchorionic** (between the placenta and the membranes), **retroplacental** (between the placenta and the myometrium), and **preplacental** (between the placenta and the amniotic fluid). Figure 19-2 illustrates the classification of hematomas in and around the placenta. Figure 19-3 demonstrates a sonographic representation of a subchorionic abruption.

The location and extent of the placental abruption identified on ultrasound examination is of clinical significance. **Retroplacental hematomas are associated with a worse prognosis for fetal survival than subchorionic hemorrhage.** The size of the hemorrhage is also predictive of fetal survival. Large retroplacental hemorrhages (>60 mL) are associated with a 50% or greater fetal mortality, whereas similarly sized subchorionic hemorrhages are associated with a 10% mortality risk.[26]

Magnetic resonance imaging (MRI) has been used successfully for diagnosing placental abruption when sonography is equivocal.

Laboratory Findings

Few laboratory studies assist in the diagnosis of placental abruption. **Hypofibrinogenemia and evidence of consumptive coagulopathy are supportive of a severe abruption**; however, clinical correlation is necessary.

Abnormal serum markers early in pregnancy, such as an unexplained elevated maternal serum α-fetoprotein (MSAFP) and human chorionic gonadotropin (hCG), have been associated with an increased risk for subsequent placental abruption.[5,27]

Pathologic Studies

Macroscopic inspection of the placenta may demonstrate adherent clot and depression of the placental surface. Fresh or acute placental abruptions may not have any identifiable evidence on pathologic examination.

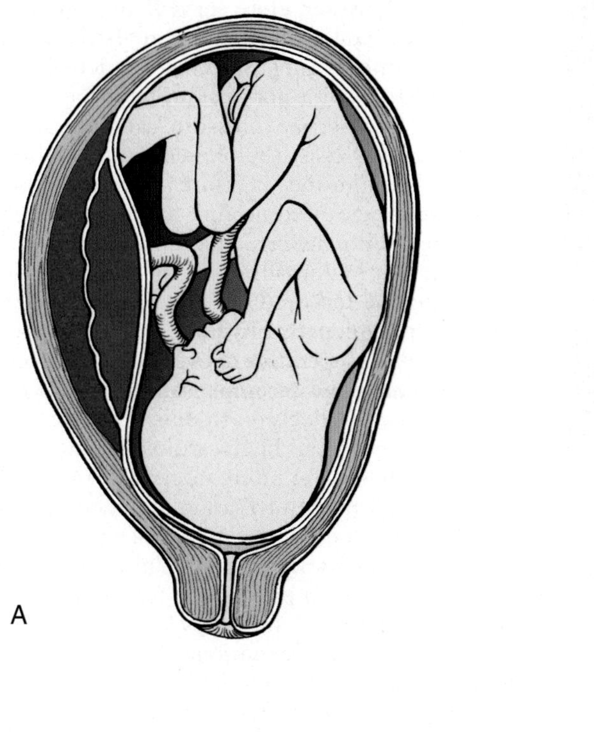

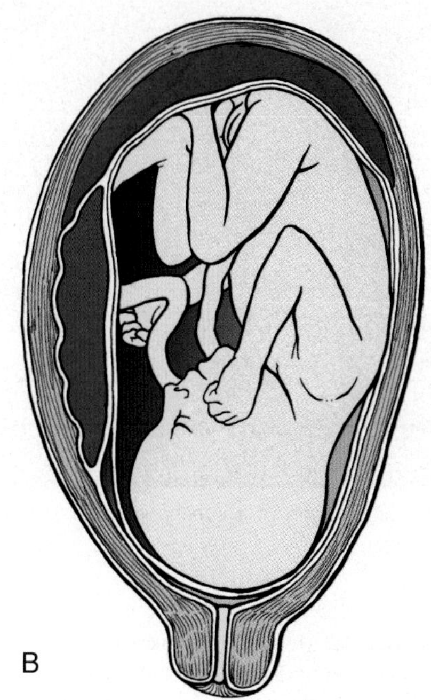

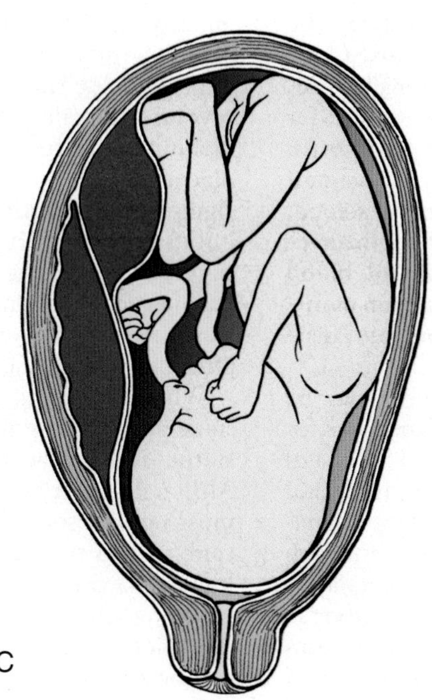

FIGURE 19-2. Drawings demonstrating the classification system of placental abruption. **A,** Retroplacental abruption: the *bright red area* represents a blood collection behind the placenta *(dark red)*. **B,** Subchorionic abruption: the *bright red area* represents subchorionic bleeding, which is observed to dissect along the chorion. **C,** Preplacental abruption: the *bright red area* represents a blood collection anterior to the placenta within the amnion and chorion (subamniotic). (From Trop I, Levine D: Hemorrhage during pregnancy: Sonography and MR imaging. AJR Am J Roentgenol 176:607, 2001. Copyright 2001 American Roentgen Ray Society.)

Management

Both maternal and fetal complications may occur with placental abruption. Maternal complications include blood loss, consumptive coagulopathy, need for transfusion, end-organ damage, and death. Fetal complications include intrauterine growth restriction, oligohydramnios, hypoxemia, prematurity, and death.[12,28] Although maternal complications are related to the severity of the abruption, fetal complications are due to the severity and timing of the hemorrhage.[11] Nearly half of all placental abruptions will result in delivery at less than 37 weeks' gestation. Gestational age at the time of presentation is an important

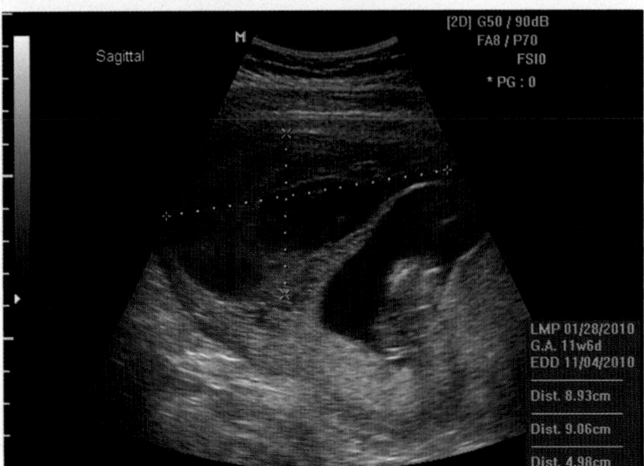

FIGURE 19-3. Ultrasonic image of a subchorionic abruption. (Courtesy K. Francois.)

prognostic factor. In patients presenting at less than 20 weeks, 82% can be expected to have a term delivery despite evidence of placental abruption. However, if the presentation occurs after 20 weeks' gestation, only 27% will deliver at term.

Management of placental abruption depends on the severity, gestational age, and maternal-fetal status. Once the diagnosis of placental abruption has been made, precautions should be taken to anticipate the possible life-threatening consequences for both mother and fetus. These precautions include baseline **laboratory assessment** (hemoglobin, hematocrit, platelet count, type and screen, fibrinogen, and coagulation studies), **appropriate intravenous access** (large-bore catheter), **availability of blood products, continuous fetal heart rate and contraction monitoring, and communication with operating room and neonatal personnel.**

Small placental abruptions remote from term may be managed expectantly in the hospital. A trial of tocolysis for documented preterm labor and administration of antenatal corticosteroid therapy can be considered if maternal-fetal status is stable.[29] Reported series of expectant management in preterm gestations with placental abruption have shown a significant prolongation of the pregnancy (>1 week) in more than 50% of patients without adverse maternal or fetal outcomes.[30] In a large series of preterm patients who presented with placental abruption and received tocolysis, about one third delivered within 48 hours of admission, one third delivered within 7 days, and one third delivered greater than 1 week from initial presentation. There were no cases of intrauterine demise in women presenting with a live fetus.[31] Although these results are encouraging, the clinician must always keep in mind that placental abruption can result in both maternal and fetal morbidity. Any attempt to arrest preterm labor in a known or suspected placental abruption must be weighed against the likelihood of neonatal survival and morbidity, the severity of the abruption, and the safety of the mother.

Women presenting at or near term with a placental abruption should undergo delivery. Induction or augmentation of labor is not contraindicated in the setting of an abruption; however, close surveillance for any evidence of maternal or fetal compromise is advised. Continuous fetal heart rate monitoring is recommended because 60% of fetuses may exhibit non-reassuring intrapartum heart rate patterns. Intrauterine pressure catheters and fetal scalp electrodes can assist the clinician during the intrapartum course. Intrauterine pressure catheter monitoring can demonstrate elevated uterine resting tone, which may be associated with deficits in uterine blood flow and fetal oxygenation. Maternal hemodynamic and clotting parameters must be followed closely in order to detect signs of evolving coagulopathy. **Although vaginal delivery is generally preferable, operative delivery is often necessary owing to fetal or maternal decompensation.** When cesarean delivery is needed, a decision-to-delivery time of less than 20 minutes from a fetal bradycardic episode results in better outcomes than a 30-minute interval.[32] A Couvelaire uterus, characterized by extravasation of blood into the myometrium, may be noted in some cases and is often associated with significant uterine atony. Administration of uterotonic therapy usually improves the condition. Hysterectomy should be reserved for cases of atony and hemorrhage unresponsive to conventional uterotonic therapies and replacement of blood products.

The management of women with consumptive coagulopathy and fetal demise requires a thorough knowledge of the natural history of severe placental abruption. More than four decades ago, Pritchard and Brekken noted several clinically important and relevant observations, including the following: (1) about 40% of patients with placental abruption and fetal demise will demonstrate signs of consumptive coagulopathy; (2) within 8 hours of initial symptoms, hypofibrinogenemia will be present; (3) severe hypofibrinogenemia will not recover without blood product replacement; and (4) the time course for recovery from hypofibrinogenemia is roughly 10 mg/dL per hour after delivery of the fetus and placenta.[33]

When managing patients with severe placental abruptions and fetal demise, maintenance of maternal volume status and replacement of blood products is essential. Although operative delivery may appear to lead to the most rapid resolution of the problem, it may pose significant risk to the patient. Unless the consumptive coagulopathy is corrected, surgery can result in uncontrollable bleeding and increased need for hysterectomy. The uterus does not need to be evacuated before coagulation status can be restored. Blood product replacement and delayed delivery until hematologic parameters have improved are generally associated with good maternal outcomes.

Neonatal Outcome

Placental abruption is associated with increased perinatal morbidity and mortality. When compared with normal pregnancies, pregnancies complicated by abruption have a **tenfold increased risk for perinatal death.**[28] A case-control study has also shown a **greater risk for adverse long-term neurobehavioral outcomes** in infants delivered after placental abruption.[34] Neonates at risk for abnormal outcomes had higher incidences of abnormal fetal heart rate tracings (45%) and emergency cesarean deliveries (53%) compared with controls (10% and 10%, respectively). Finally, **periventricular leukomalacia and sudden infant death syndrome**

are more common in newborns delivered after placental abruptions.[35]

Placenta Previa

Definition and Pathogenesis

Placenta previa is defined as the presence of placental tissue over or adjacent to the cervical os. Traditionally, three variations of placenta previa were recognized: complete, partial, and marginal. Although complete placenta previa referred to the total coverage of the cervical os by placental tissue, the differences between partial (placental edge at the cervical os) and marginal (placental edge near the cervical os) were often subtle and varied by the timing and method of diagnosis. In more recent years, improved ultrasound technology and precision have allowed for more accurate assessments of the placental location in relation to the cervical os. With this in mind, **contemporary classification of placenta previa consists of two variations: *placenta previa,* in which the cervical os is covered by placental tissue, and *marginal placenta previa,* in which the placenta lies within 2 cm of the cervical os but does not cover it.** Low-lying placenta has also been described. Within the literature, a variety of definitions have been ascribed to a low-lying placenta, including an apparent second-trimester placenta previa, a placenta that lies within the lower uterine segment, and a placental edge that lies within 2 to 3 cm of the cervical os. Although not true placenta previa, low-lying placentas are associated with increased risks for bleeding and other adverse pregnancy events.[36]

Incidence

The overall reported incidence of placenta previa at delivery is 4 in 1000 deliveries.[37] **In the second trimester, placenta previa may be found in 4% to 6% of pregnancies.**[38] **The term *placental migration* has been used to explain this "resolution" of placenta previa that is noted near term. Two theories have been suggested to account for this phenomenon.** The first hypothesis proposes that as the pregnancy advances, the stationary lower placental edge relocates away from the cervical os with the development of the lower uterine segment. Indeed the lower uterine segment has been noted to increase from 0.5 cm at 20 weeks to more than 5 cm at term.[39] The second hypothesis suggests that trophotropism, or the growth of trophoblastic tissue away from the cervical os toward the fundus, results in resolution of the placenta previa.

Clinical Manifestations

Placenta previa typically presents as painless vaginal bleeding in the second or third trimester. Between 70% and 80% of patients with placenta previa will have at least one bleeding episode.[38,40] About 10% to 20% of patients present with uterine contractions before bleeding, and fewer than 10% remain asymptomatic.[38,40] Of patients with bleeding, one third will present before 30 weeks' gestation, **one third between 30 and 36 weeks' gestation, and one third after 36 weeks' gestation.**[38,40] Patients with early-onset bleeding (<30 weeks' gestation) have the greatest risk for blood transfusion and associated perinatal morbidity and mortality. The bleeding is believed to occur from disruption of placental blood vessels in association with the development and thinning out of the lower uterine segment.

TABLE 19-3 PLACENTAL PREVIA RISK FACTORS

Increasing parity and/or maternal age
Maternal race
Cigarette smoking
Residence at higher elevation
Multiple gestations
Male fetal gender
Previous placenta previa
Prior curettage
Prior cesarean delivery

Risk Factors

Several risk factors for placenta previa have been noted (Table 19-3). Additionally, some reports have documented a higher association of fetal malpresentation, preterm premature rupture of membranes, intrauterine growth restriction, congenital anomalies, and amniotic fluid embolism with placenta previa.[38,41]

Increasing Parity, Maternal Age, and Maternal Race

Studies have reported **more cases of placenta previa with increasing parity.** Grand multiparas have been reported to have a 5% risk for placenta previa compared with 0.2% among nulliparous women.[39] **Maternal age also seems to influence the occurrence of placenta previa.** Women older than 35 years of age have more than a fourfold increased risk for placenta previa, and women older than 40 years of age have a ninefold greater risk.[42] **Maternal race has been associated with placenta previa.** In a large population-based cohort, the rate of placenta previa among white, black, and other races was 3.3, 3, and 4.5 per 1000 births, respectively.[43] Asian women appear to have the highest rates of placenta previa.

Cigarette Smoking and Residence at Higher Elevation

Cigarette smoking has been associated with as high as a threefold increased risk for previa formation.[44,45] Likewise, **residence at higher elevations may contribute to previa development.**[38] The need for increased placental surface area secondary to decreased uteroplacental oxygenation may contribute to these associations.

Multiple Gestations and Male Fetal Gender

Controversy exists regarding an increased risk for placenta previa with multiple gestations. Although some studies have shown a higher incidence of placenta previa among twins, others have not documented a significantly increased risk.[23,45,46] There is a consistently **higher proportion of male offspring in women with placenta previa.**[44] This association is unexplained; however, two theories suggest larger placental sizes among male fetuses and delayed implantation of the male blastocyst in the lower uterine segment.

Previous Placenta Previa

Having had a previous placenta previa increases the risk for the development of another previa in a subsequent pregnancy. This association has been reported to be as high as an eightfold relative risk.[47] The exact etiology for this increased risk is unclear but may be attributed to a genetic predisposition for the phenomenon.

Prior Curettage and Prior Cesarean Delivery

Prior uterine surgery has been associated with placenta previa formation. Although a history of curettage has a slightly elevated previa risk (1.3 relative risk), prior cesarean delivery is a significant risk factor.[48] **In the pregnancy following a cesarean delivery, the risk for placenta previa has been reported to be between 1% and 4%.**[48,49] There is a **linear increase in placenta previa risk with the number of prior cesarean deliveries.** Placenta previa occurs in 0.9% of women with one prior cesarean delivery, 1.7% of women with two prior cesarean deliveries, and 3% of those with three or more cesarean deliveries.[50] In patients with four or more cesarean deliveries, the risk for placenta previa has been reported as high as 10%.[49] Endometrial scarring is thought to be the etiologic factor for this increased risk.

Diagnosis

The timing of the diagnosis of placenta previa has undergone significant change in the past three decades. Painless third-trimester bleeding was a common presentation for placenta previa in the past, whereas **most cases of placenta previa are now detected antenatally with ultrasound** before the onset of significant bleeding.

Radiology

Transabdominal and transvaginal ultrasound provide the best means for diagnosing placenta previa. Although transabdominal ultrasound can detect at least 95% of placenta previa cases, transvaginal ultrasound has a reported diagnostic accuracy approaching 100%.[51] Typically, a combined approach can be used in which transabdominal ultrasound is employed as the initial diagnostic modality followed by transvaginal ultrasound for uncertain cases. Of note, good images can be obtained using transvaginal ultrasound without the probe contacting the cervix (Figure 19-4). Also, translabial ultrasound can be used to assist in the diagnosis if reservation exists regarding the use of a transvaginal probe.

If placenta previa is diagnosed in the midtrimester, repeat sonography should be obtained in the early third trimester. More than 90% of the cases of placenta previa diagnosed in the midtrimester resolve by term. The potential for placenta previa resolution is dependent on the timing of the diagnosis, the extent over the cervical os, and the location. For example, one study of 714 women with an ultrasound diagnosis of placenta previa noted that the earlier the diagnosis in the pregnancy, the more likely for the previa to resolve by term (Table 19-4).[52] In addition, complete placenta previa diagnosed in the second trimester will persist into the third trimester in 26% of cases, whereas marginal placenta previa will persist in only 2.5% of cases.[53] Finally, anterior placenta previa is less likely to migrate away from the cervical os than posterior locations.

Occasionally, MRI is used to diagnose placenta previa. MRI is particularly helpful with posterior placenta previa identification and assessment of invasive placentation (see later).

Management

General management principles for patients with placenta previa in the third trimester include serial ultrasounds to assess placental location and fetal growth, avoidance of cervical examinations and coitus, activity restrictions, counseling regarding labor symptoms and vaginal bleeding, dietary and nutrient supplementation to avoid maternal anemia, and early medical attention if any vaginal bleeding occurs.[1]

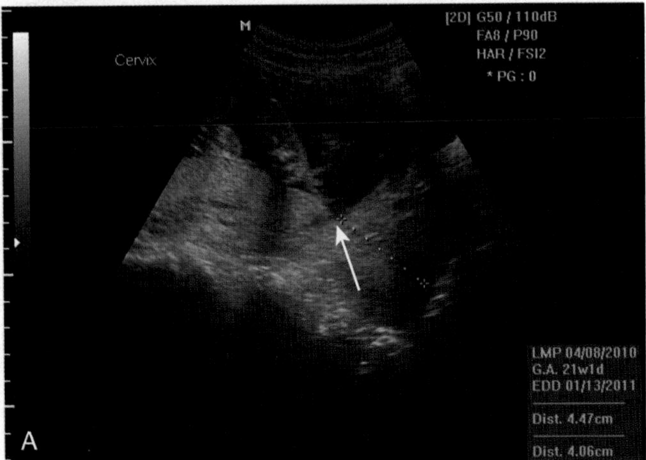

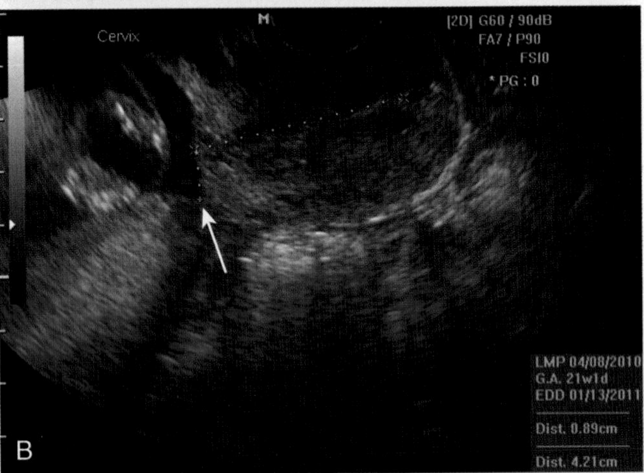

Figure 19-4. Transabdominal and transvaginal ultrasounds of marginal placenta previa. *Arrows* identify placental edge. (Courtesy K. Francois.)

Table 19-4 Potential for Placenta Previa at Term by Gestational Age at Diagnosis

Gestational Age at Diagnosis	Previa at Term (%)
15-19 wk	12
20-23 wk	34
24-27 wk	49
28-31 wk	62
32-35 wk	73

From Dashe JS, McIntire DD, Ramus RM, et al: Persistence of placenta previa according to gestational age at ultrasound detection. Obstet Gynecol 99:692-697, 2002.

Outpatient Management

Asymptomatic patients with placenta previa or patients with a history of a small bleed that has resolved for greater than 7 days are potential candidates for outpatient management. Several studies have documented the safety, efficacy, and cost savings of outpatient versus inpatient management in such cases.[54] **Candidates for outpatient management must be highly compliant, live within 20 minutes from the hospital, have 24-hour emergency transportation to the hospital, and verbalize a thorough understanding of the risks associated with placenta previa and outpatient management.**

Expectant Management of Preterm Patients

Patients with placenta previa who present preterm with vaginal bleeding require hospitalization and immediate evaluation to assess maternal-fetal stability. In at least 50% of women who present with a symptomatic previa, delivery can be delayed for more than 4 weeks, including patients with initial bleeding episodes greater than 500 mL.[38,40,54]

In order to optimize maternal-fetal outcome, **patients should initially be managed in a labor and delivery unit with continuous fetal heart rate and contraction monitoring. Large-bore intravenous access and baseline laboratory studies** (hemoglobin, hematocrit, platelet count, blood type and screen, and coagulation studies) should be obtained. **If the patient is less than 34 weeks' gestation, administration of antenatal corticosteroids should be undertaken** as well as an assessment of the facility's emergency resources for both the mother and the neonate. In some cases, maternal transport and consultation with a maternal-fetal medicine specialist and a neonatologist may be warranted. **Finally, tocolysis can be employed if the vaginal bleeding is preceded by or associated with uterine contractions.** Magnesium sulfate and β-mimetic therapy have both been shown to be efficacious; however, some authorities recommend magnesium sulfate as a first-line agent given its reduced potential for hemodynamic-related side effects.[55]

Once stabilized, patients can be maintained on hospitalized bed rest and expectantly managed. Minimizing maternal anemia by employing blood conservation techniques is recommended. Although some patients may require transfusion, many patients can be supplemented with iron replacement (oral or intravenous), vitamin C to enhance oral iron absorption, and B vitamins. Erythropoietin may be used in selected cases to hasten red cell formation. Lastly, autologous donation may be considered in patients with hemoglobin concentrations greater than 11 g/dL.[56]

Although maternal hemorrhage is of utmost concern, **fetal blood can also be lost during the process of placental separation. Rh immune globulin (RhoGAM) should be given to all Rh-negative, unsensitized women with third-trimester bleeding from placenta previa.** A Kleihauer-Betke preparation of maternal blood should be considered. Occasionally, a fetomaternal hemorrhage of greater than 30 mL occurs, necessitating additional doses of RhoGAM. One study noted that 35% of infants whose mothers received an antepartum transfusion were also anemic and required a transfusion after delivery.[38]

Delivery

Cesarean delivery is indicated for all patients with sonographic evidence of placenta previa. In women with a low-lying placenta in which the placental edge is clearly greater than 2 to 3 cm from the cervical os, vaginal delivery may be considered; however, precautions should be made for the possibility of an emergent cesarean delivery with labor.

The timing of delivery depends on clinical circumstances. Any patient with persistent hemorrhage mandates delivery regardless of gestational age. **For asymptomatic patients with placenta previa, delivery is typically recommended by 37 weeks' gestation** with documented fetal lung maturity or after administration of antenatal corticosteroids.[54]

When performing a cesarean delivery for placenta previa, the surgeon should be aware of the potential for rapid blood loss during the delivery process. Patients should have blood products cross-matched and readily available for delivery, including packed red blood cells and fresh-frozen plasma, with or without pooled platelets. In addition, before incising the lower uterine segment, the surgeon should assess the vascularity of this region. Although a low transverse incision is not contraindicated in patients with placenta previa, performing a vertical uterine incision may be preferable in selected cases. This is particularly true with an anterior placenta previa. Ideally, the placenta should not be disrupted when entering the uterus. If disruption occurs, expedited delivery is essential. Once the fetus has been removed from the uterus, the cord blood should be "milked" to the fetus to avoid immediate neonatal hypovolemia and anemia. Given the potential for invasive placentation, the physician should allow the placenta to spontaneously deliver. If it does not separate easily, precautions should be taken for dealing with a placenta accreta (see below). Once the placenta separates, bleeding is controlled by the contraction of uterine myometrial fibers around the spiral arterioles. Because the lower uterine segment often contracts poorly, significant bleeding can occur from the placental implantation site. Aggressive uterotonic therapy, surgical intervention, or tamponade techniques, or a combination of these, should be undertaken to rapidly control the bleeding.

Associated Conditions

Placenta Accreta

Definition and Pathogenesis

Placenta accreta represents the abnormal attachment of the placenta to the uterine lining due to an absence of the decidua basalis and an incomplete development of the fibrinoid layer. Variations of placenta accreta include placenta increta and placenta percreta, in which the placenta extends to and through the uterine myometrium, respectively (Figure 19-5).

Incidence and Risk Factors

The overall incidence of placenta accreta or one of its variations ranges from 1 in 533 to 1 in 2510 deliveries.[57] Based on histologic diagnosis, placenta accreta is the most common form of invasive placentation (79%) followed by placenta increta (14%) and placenta percreta (7%), respectively.[57] **The two most significant risk factors for placenta accreta are placenta previa and prior cesarean delivery.** The risk for placenta accreta in patients with placenta previa and an unscarred uterus is approximately 3%.[49] This risk dramatically increases with one or more cesarean deliveries (Table 19-5). Even without a placenta previa, placenta accreta is more common with a prior cesarean delivery.[50]

Other risk factors that have been reported include increasing **parity and maternal age, submucosal uterine fibroids, prior uterine surgery, and endometrial defects.**

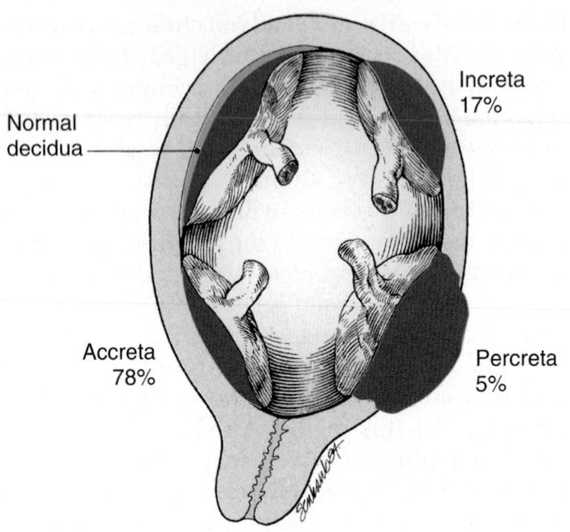

Figure 19-5. Uteroplacental relationships found with invasive placentation.

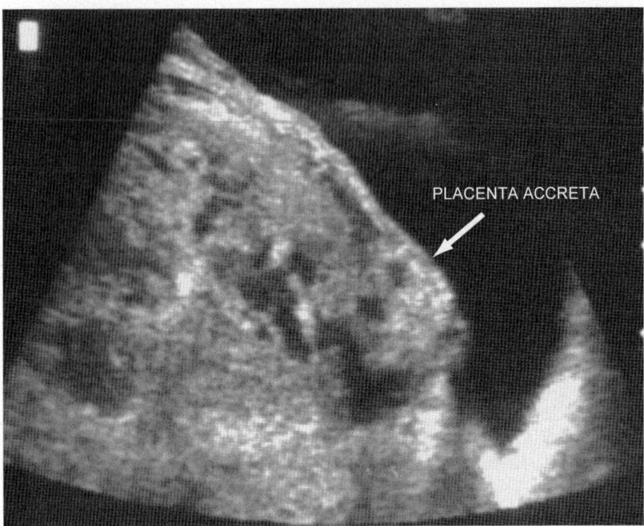

Figure 19-6. Ultrasonic image of focal placenta accreta. *Arrow* identifies an area at the uterine placental interface that demonstrates a loss of the normal hypoechoic zone, thinning and disruption of the uterine serosa-bladder interface, and a focal exophytic mass within the placenta.

Table 19-5 Risk for Placenta Accreta with Placenta Previa and Prior Cesarean Delivery

NUMBER OF PRIOR CESAREAN DELIVERIES	PLACENTA ACCRETA RISK (%)
0	3
1	11
2	40
3	61
≥4	67

From Silver RM, Landon MB, Rouse DJ, et al: Maternal morbidity associated with multiple repeat cesarean deliveries. Obstet Gynecol 107:1226, 2006.

Contrary to placenta previa, **female fetal gender is more common with invasive placentation.**[58]

Clinical Manifestations

The clinical manifestations are similar to those of placenta previa. **Hematuria can be feature of placenta percreta with bladder invasion.**

Diagnosis

In the past, placenta accreta was usually diagnosed intrapartum by the difficult or incomplete removal of the placenta and associated postpartum hemorrhage. Today with advanced **radiographic technology, the diagnosis can be made antenatally.** In fact, prenatal diagnosis has been shown to improve maternal outcomes, resulting in lower blood loss and transfusion requirements.[59]

Radiology

Ultrasound is the best radiographic modality for the diagnosis of placenta accreta. Findings that are suggestive of placenta accreta include a loss of the normal hypoechoic retroplacental-myometrial zone, thinning and disruption of the uterine serosa–bladder interface, focal exophytic masses within the placenta, and numerous intraplacental vascular lacunae (Figure 19-6).[60] With experienced sonographers, the diagnostic sensitivity and specificity approach 85% to 90%.[60] Color Doppler ultrasound is also useful as an adjunctive tool in diagnosing placenta accreta.[61] Specific color Doppler findings that differentiate placenta accreta from normal placentation include diffuse and focal intraparenchymal placental lacunar blood flow, hypervascularity of the bladder and uterine serosa, prominent subplacental venous complexes, and loss of subplacental Doppler vascular signals. Finally, color-flow mapping studies suggest that a myometrial thickness less than 1 mm with large intraplacental venous lakes is highly predictive of invasive placentation (sensitivity, 100%; specificity, 72%; positive predictive value, 72%; and negative predictive value, 100%).[62]

MRI can be used in conjunction with sonography to assess abnormal placental invasion. Situations in which MRI has been particularly helpful include equivocal ultrasound findings, posterior placental location, and determination of the extent of placental invasion within surrounding tissue, such as the parametrium and bladder.[63] In one series of 300 patients with ultrasound-detected placenta accreta, MRI was able to characterize the level and extent of the placenta invasion with an accuracy of greater than 97%.[64]

Laboratory Findings

Placenta accreta has also been associated with unexplained elevations in MSAFP concentration.[65]

Pathologic Studies

Placenta accreta is confirmed by the pathologic evaluation of a hysterectomy specimen. Histologic evaluation demonstrates placental villi within the uterine myometrium. In focal accreta cases in which the uterus is not removed, curettage specimens may show myometrial cells adherent to the placenta.

Management

Because of its associated risk for massive postpartum hemorrhage, **placenta accreta accounts for most peripartum hysterectomies.**[38,66] **A multidisciplinary team approach is the most ideal way to manage these cases.** Preoperative

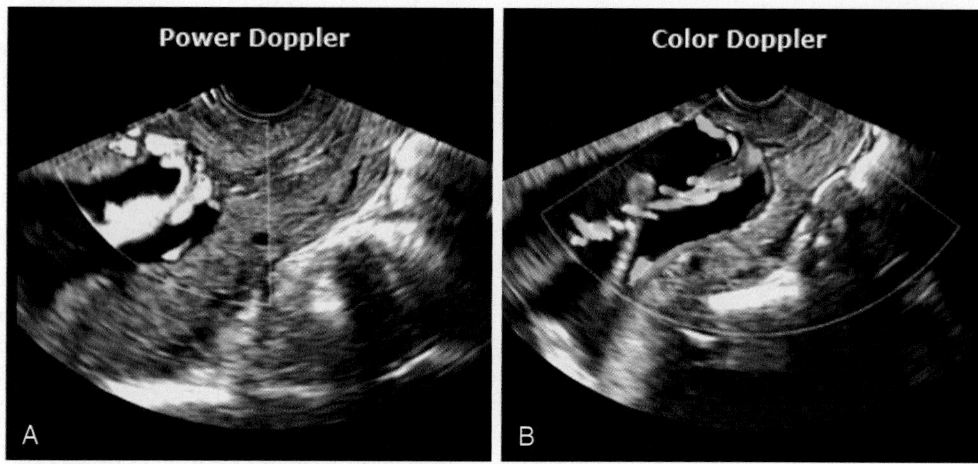

FIGURE 19-7. Transvaginal ultrasound images showing vasa previa and velamentous cord. The placenta is posterior with an anterior succenturiate lobe. (From Lockwood CJ, Russo-Steiglitz K: Vasa previa and velamentous umbilical cord. Available at http://www.uptodate.com. Accessed August 2010.)

assessments by **blood conservation teams, anesthesiologists, advanced pelvic surgeons, and urologists** (especially for a suspected placenta percreta) are recommended. The delivery should occur at a facility that is prepared to manage significant obstetrical hemorrhage. **Adequate intravenous access with two large-bore catheters and ample blood product availability are mandatory.** When performing the surgery, it is recommended that the **uterus be incised above the placental attachment site and the placenta left in situ after clamping the cord because disruption of the implantation site may result in rapid blood loss.** Adjuvant use of aortic or internal iliac artery balloon occlusion catheters, or both, with postsurgical embolization may be considered.[67]

When future fertility is desired, a variety of uterine conservation techniques may be attempted. These techniques include delayed manual removal of the placenta, wedge resection or oversewing of the placental implantation site, tamponade of the lower uterine segment, curettage, uterine artery embolization, and administration of methotrexate. Although each of these techniques has reported success, they are also associated with potential complications, including delayed hemorrhage, infection, fistula formation, subsequent surgery, and uterine necrosis.[68] Data are limited regarding future reproduction in patients treated conservatively for invasive placentation. In a case series of 35 women treated conservatively for placenta accreta, 12 of 14 women desiring future pregnancy were successful in conceiving; however, 5 women had pregnancies that ended in spontaneous abortion, 4 delivered preterm, and 2 had recurrent placenta accreta.[69]

Vasa Previa

Definition and Pathogenesis

Vasa previa is defined as the presence of fetal vessels over the cervical os. Typically, these fetal vessels lack protection from Wharton's jelly and are prone to rupture and compression. When the vessels rupture, the fetus is at high risk for exsanguination. There are **two variations of vasa previa: (1) velamentous cord insertion; and (2) fetal vessels running between a bilobed or succenturiate-lobed placenta.**

Incidence and Risk Factors

The overall incidence of vasa previa is 1 in 2500 deliveries; however, data have shown a range from 1 in 2000 to 1 in 5000 deliveries.[70] **Reported risk factors for vasa previa include bilobed, succenturiate-lobed, and low-lying placentas; pregnancies resulting from assisted reproductive technology; multiple gestations; history of second-trimester placenta previa, and vaginal bleeding.**[70,71]

Clinical Manifestations

Vasa previa usually presents after rupture of membranes with the acute onset of vaginal bleeding from a lacerated fetal vessel. If immediate intervention is not provided, fetal bradycardia and subsequent death occur.

Diagnosis

In the past, vasa previa was usually detected by palpation of the fetal vessels within the membranes during labor or with the acute onset of vaginal bleeding and subsequent fetal bradycardia and/or death after membrane rupture. Today with widespread use of **ultrasound and color-flow Doppler imaging, most cases are diagnosed antenatally.**[72] Transabdominal, transvaginal, and translabial approaches have been used. **The diagnosis is confirmed by documenting umbilical vessels over the cervical os using color-flow Doppler imaging** (Figure 19-7).[73]

Management

When diagnosed antenatally, vasa previa should be managed similarly to placenta previa. Some authorities have recommended hospitalization in the third trimester with administration of antenatal corticosteroids, serial antepartum testing, and cesarean delivery by 36 weeks' gestation.[71,74] If an intrapartum diagnosis of vasa previa is made, expeditious delivery is needed. Immediate neonatal blood transfusion is often required in these circumstances. **The importance of antenatal detection was emphasized in a large series based on data from the Vasa Previa Foundation. The overall perinatal mortality rate was 36%, but the neonatal survival was 97% in cases diagnosed antenatally compared with 44% in those diagnosed intrapartum.**[74]

POSTPARTUM HEMORRHAGE

Postpartum hemorrhage is an obstetrical emergency that complicates between 1 in 100 and 1 in 20 deliveries.[75] It is a major cause of maternal morbidity and mortality. Obstetricians need to have a clear understanding of normal delivery-related blood loss in order to efficiently recognize postpartum hemorrhage.

Normal Blood Loss and Postpartum Hemorrhage

Normal delivery-related blood loss depends on the type of delivery. Based on objective data, the mean blood losses for a vaginal delivery, cesarean delivery, and cesarean hysterectomy are 500 mL, 1000 mL, and 1500 mL, respectively.[76] These values are often underestimated and unappreciated clinically owing to the significant blood volume expansion that accompanies normal pregnancy.

Postpartum hemorrhage has been variably defined in the literature. Definitions have included subjective assessments greater than the standard norms, a 10% decline in hematocrit, and the need for a blood transfusion. A more practical definition is delivery-related blood loss that is excessive in nature and results in a symptomatic patient or signs of hypovolemia.

Postpartum Hemorrhage Etiologies

The etiologies of postpartum hemorrhage can be categorized as primary (or early), those occurring within 24 hours of delivery, and secondary (or late), those occurring from 24 hours until 6 weeks after delivery. Table 19-6 lists the most common causes of primary and secondary postpartum hemorrhage. Because primary postpartum hemorrhage is more common than secondary, the remainder of this discussion focuses on its causes and management (Figure 19-8).

Uterine Atony

Definition and Pathogenesis

Uterine atony, or the inability of the uterine myometrium to contract effectively, is the most common cause of primary postpartum hemorrhage. At term, blood flow through the

TABLE 19-6 ETIOLOGIES OF POSTPARTUM HEMORRHAGE

Early	Uterine atony
	Lower genital tract lacerations (perineal, vaginal, cervical, periclitoral, periurethral, rectal)
	Upper genital tract lacerations (broad ligament)
	Lower urinary tract lacerations (bladder, urethra)
	Retained products of conception (placenta, membranes)
	Invasive placentation (placenta accreta, placenta increta, placenta percreta)
	Uterine rupture
	Uterine inversion
	Coagulopathy
Late	Infection
	Retained products of conception
	Placental site subinvolution
	Coagulopathy

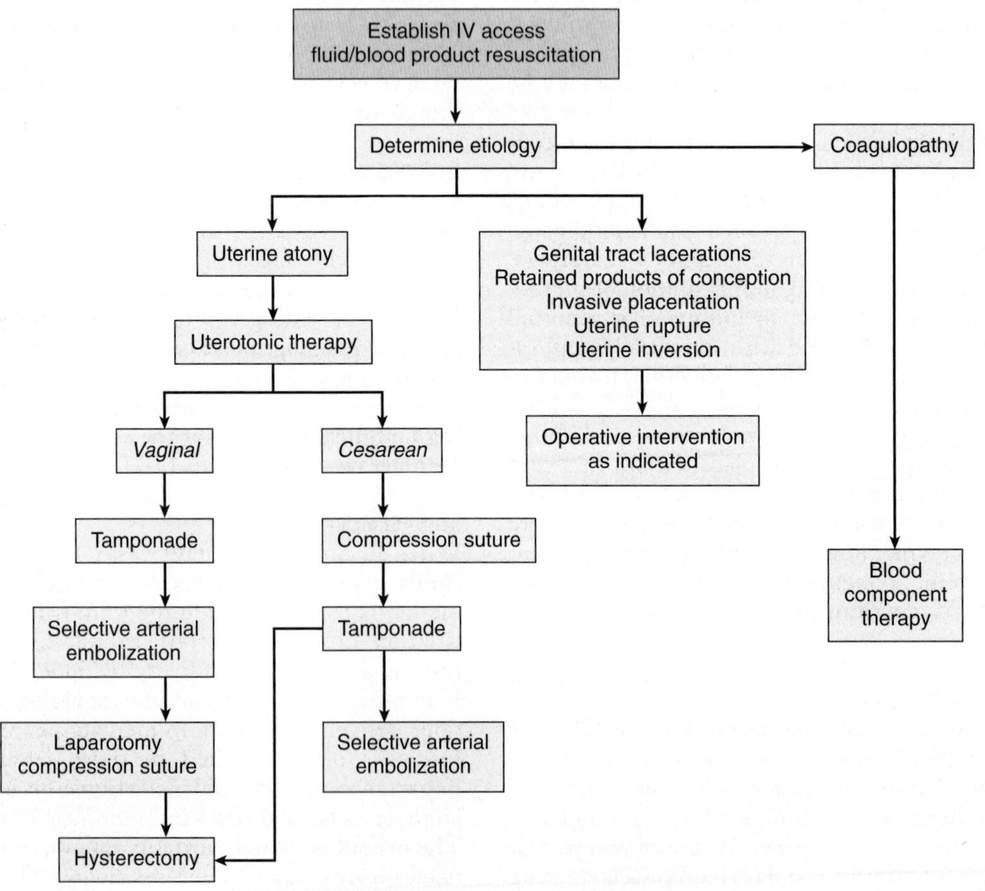

FIGURE 19-8. Management of postpartum hemorrhage.

placental site averages 600 mL/minute. After placental delivery, the uterus controls bleeding by contracting its myometrial fibers in a tourniquet fashion around the spiral arterioles. If inadequate uterine contraction occurs, rapid blood loss can ensue.

Incidence and Risk Factors

Uterine atony complicates 1 in 20 deliveries and is responsible for 80% of postpartum hemorrhages.[77] **Risk factors** for uterine atony include uterine overdistention (multiple gestation, polyhydramnios, fetal macrosomia), **labor induction, rapid or prolonged labor, grand multiparity, uterine infection, uterine inversion, retained products of conception, placenta previa, and use of uterine-relaxing agents** (tocolytic therapy, halogenated anesthetics, nitroglycerin).

Clinical Manifestations and Diagnosis

Uterine atony is diagnosed clinically by rapid uterine bleeding associated with a lack of myometrial tone and an absence of other etiologies for postpartum hemorrhage. Typically, bimanual palpation of the uterus confirms the diagnosis.

Prevention and Management

By recognizing risk factors for uterine atony and quickly initiating a treatment cascade, the clinician can minimize blood loss. Two preventive methods for atonic postpartum hemorrhage are active management of the third stage of labor and spontaneous placental separation after cesarean delivery. Active management of the third stage of labor includes early cord clamping, controlled cord traction, uterine massage, and administration of uterotonic therapy before placental separation. A systematic review of five randomized controlled trials comparing active to expectant management of the third stage of labor showed significant reductions in maternal blood loss, postpartum hemorrhage, prolonged third stage of labor, and the need for additional uterotonic therapies.[78] Controversy exists regarding the timing of uterotonic administration. Although some studies suggest that giving uterotonic therapy before delivery of the placenta results in less blood loss and fewer postpartum transfusions, other trials have found no significant differences in these outcomes.[79] Spontaneous separation of the placenta during cesarean delivery is also associated with reduced blood loss. In one controlled study, spontaneous placental separation reduced blood loss by 30% and postpartum endometritis sevenfold compared with manual removal.[80]

If preventive measures are unsuccessful, medical management for uterine atony should be initiated. This treatment includes bimanual uterine massage and uterotonic therapy.

Bimanual Uterine Massage

Figure 19-9 demonstrates the proper technique for **bimanual uterine massage.** To provide effective massage, the **uterus should be compressed between the external fundally placed hand and the internal intravaginal hand.** Care must be taken to avoid aggressive massage that can injure the large vessels of the broad ligament.

Uterotonic Therapy

Uterotonic medications represent the mainstay of drug therapy for postpartum hemorrhage secondary to uterine atony. Table 19-7 lists available uterotonic agents with

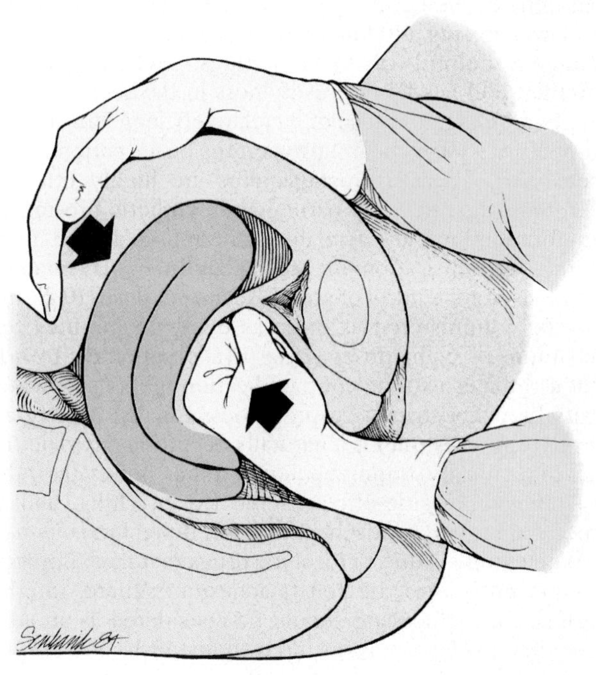

Figure 19-9. Bimanual uterine massage.

Table 19-7 Uterotonic Therapy

AGENT	DOSE	ROUTE	DOSING INTERVAL	SIDE EFFECTS	CONTRAINDICATIONS
Oxytocin (Pitocin)	10-80 U in 1000 mL crystalloid solution	First line: IV Second line: IM or IU	Continuous	Nausea, emesis, water intoxication	None
Misoprostol (Cytotec)	200-1000 mcg	First line: PR Second line: PO or SL	Single dose	Nausea, emesis, diarrhea, fever, chills	None
Methylergonovine (Methergine)	0.2 mg	First line: IM Second line: IU or PO	Every 2 to 4 hr	Hypertension, hypotension, nausea, emesis	Hypertension, preeclampsia
Prostaglandin $F_{2\alpha}$ (Hemabate)	0.25 mg	First line: IM Second line: IU	Every 15 to 90 min (maximum of 8 doses)	Nausea, emesis, diarrhea, flushing, chills	Active cardiac, pulmonary, renal, or hepatic disease
Prostaglandin E_2 (Dinoprostone)	20 mg	PR	Every 2 hr	Nausea, emesis, diarrhea, fever, chills, headache	Hypotension

IM, Intramuscular; *IU*, intrauterine; *IV*, intravenous; *PO*, per oral; *PR*, per rectum; *SL*, sublingual.

their dosages, side effects, and contraindications. **Oxytocin** (Pitocin) is usually given as a first-line agent. Intravenous therapy is the preferred route of administration, but intramuscular and intrauterine dosing is possible. Initial treatment starts with 10 to 20 U of oxytocin in 1000 mL of crystalloid solution. Higher doses (80 units in 1000 mL) have proved safe and efficacious, with a 20% reduction in the need for additional uterotonic therapy compared with standard dosing.[81]

When oxytocin fails to produce adequate uterine tone, second-line therapy must be initiated. Currently, a variety of other uterotonic agents are available for use. The choice of a second-line agent depends on its side-effect profile as well as its contraindications. **Misoprostol (Cytotec), a synthetic prostaglandin E_1 analog,** is a safe, inexpensive, and efficacious uterotonic medication. It has been used for both the prevention and treatment of postpartum hemorrhage.[82] Misoprostol is attractive as a second-line agent in that it has multiple administration routes that can be combined. Although higher doses (600 to 1000 mcg) have traditionally been used rectally, the sublingual route allows for lower dosing (400 mcg) with higher bioavailability.[82] Although helpful in some settings, **methylergonovine (Methergine)** has limited usefulness in the acute postpartum hemorrhage because of its relatively long half-life and its potential for worsening hypertension in patients with preexisting disease. **Prostaglandins** are highly effective uterotonic agents. Both natural and synthetic prostaglandin formulations are available. Intramuscular and intrauterine administration of **prostaglandin $F_{2\alpha}$ (Hemabate)** can be used for control of atony. Recurrent doses (0.25 mg) may be administered as often as every 15 minutes to a maximum of eight doses (2 mg). It is important to note that asthma is a strong contraindication to its use because of its bronchoconstrictive properties. Finally, **prostaglandin E_2 (dinoprostone)** is a naturally occurring oxytocic that can dramatically improve uterine tone; however, it has an unfavorable side-effect profile (fever, chills, nausea, emesis, diarrhea, headaches) that often precludes its use.

When atony is due to tocolytic drugs that have impaired calcium entry into the cell (magnesium sulfate, nifedipine), calcium gluconate should be considered as an adjuvant therapy. Given as an intravenous push, one ampule (1 g) of calcium gluconate can effectively improve uterine tone and resolve bleeding due to atony.

If pharmacologic methods fail to control atony-related hemorrhage, alternative measures must be undertaken. These include uterine tamponade, selective arterial embolization, and surgical intervention.

Uterine Tamponade

Uterine packing is a safe, simple, and effective way to control postpartum hemorrhage by providing tamponade to the bleeding uterine surface.[83] Although packing techniques vary, a few basic principles should be followed. The pack should be made of long, continuous gauze (Kerlix) rather than multiple small sponges. Placement of the gauze within a sterile plastic bag or glove can ease removal of the pack. When packing the uterus, placement should begin at the fundus and progress downward in a side-to-side fashion to avoid dead space for blood accumulation.[77] Transurethral Foley catheter placement and prophylactic antibiotic use should be considered to prevent urinary retention and infection, respectively. Finally, prolonged packing should be avoided (not more than 12 to 24 hours), and close attention to the patient's vital signs and blood indices should be paid while the pack is in place in order to minimize unrecognized ongoing bleeding.

In recent years, **intrauterine tamponade balloons** have replaced traditional uterine packing. Multiple balloon types have been employed, including the **Bakri SOS (Surgical Obstetric Silicone) balloon** and the **BT-Cath balloon**. Both devices were developed specifically for postpartum hemorrhage management. The Bakri SOS balloon (Cook Women's Health, Bloomington, IN; Figure 19-10) consists of a silicone balloon attached to a catheter. The catheter is inserted into the uterus either manually or under ultrasound guidance, and the silicone balloon is subsequently inflated with sterile saline (maximum of 500 mL). Once inflated, the balloon should adapt to the uterine configuration and provide tamponade to the endometrial surface. The intraluminal catheter allows drainage from within the uterus, allowing for ongoing assessment of blood loss.[84] Proper placement of the balloon is essential to provide adequate tamponade (Figure 19-11). The BT-Cath is a silicone balloon shaped like an inverted pear. Similar to the Bakri balloon, this tamponade balloon has a double-lumen catheter that allows saline filling of the balloon as well as drainage of blood from within the uterus.

The Glenveigh *ebb* Complete Tamponade System is a new postpartum tamponade balloon (Figure 19-12). Developed by maternal-fetal specialists, this system incorporates both intrauterine and intravaginal tamponade. Both balloons are made of strong yet malleable polyurethane, allowing for better conformation to the uterine and vaginal shapes. In addition, the uterine balloon can be rapidly inflated from a saline bag to a larger volume of 750 mL for circumstances in which the smaller balloons are inadequate (such as multiple gestations). Finally, like the other balloons, this system has a drainage port to assess for ongoing bleeding; however, unlike the others, it also has an infusion port to irrigate the uterus.

Selective Arterial Embolization

Selective arterial embolization is an increasingly common therapeutic option for hemodynamically stable patients with postpartum hemorrhage. The procedure can be performed alone or after failed surgical intervention.[85] Pelvic angiography is used to visualize bleeding vessels, and Gelfoam (gelatin) pledgets are placed into the vessels for occlusion. **Cumulative success rates of 90% to 95% have been reported.**[85]

Selective arterial embolization has several advantages over surgical intervention. First, it allows for selective occlusion of bleeding vessels. This can be extremely valuable in circumstances of aberrant pelvic vasculature, such as uterine arteriovenous malformations. Second, the uterus and potential future fertility are preserved. Cases series have reported successful pregnancies after pelvic embolization.[85] Finally, the procedure has minimal morbidity, enables the physician to forego or delay surgical intervention, and can be performed in coagulopathic patients, allowing more time for blood and clotting factor replacement. Procedure-related complications occur in 3% to 6%

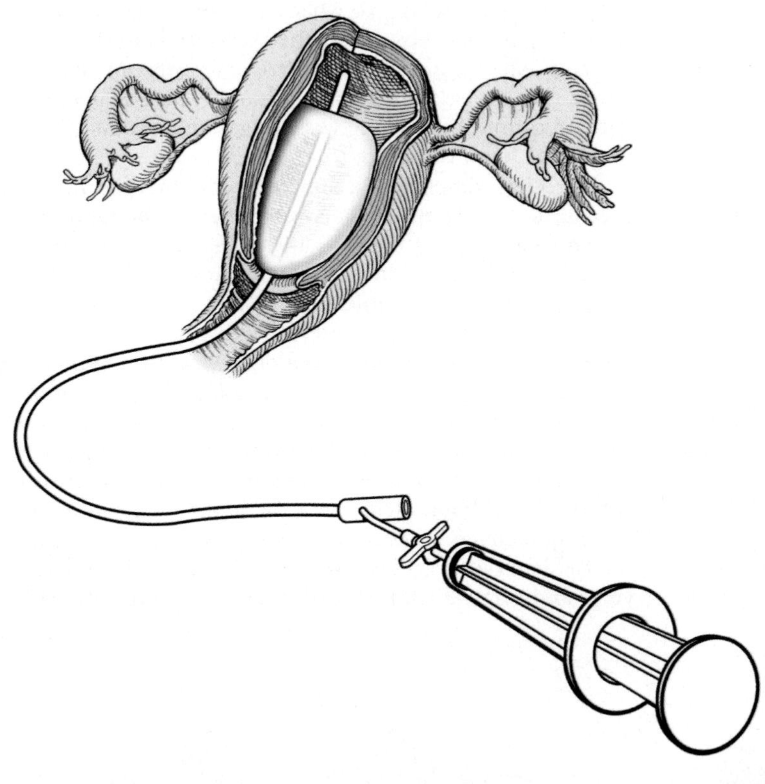

FIGURE 19-10. The Bakri SOS Tamponade Balloon. (Courtesy Cook Women's Health.)

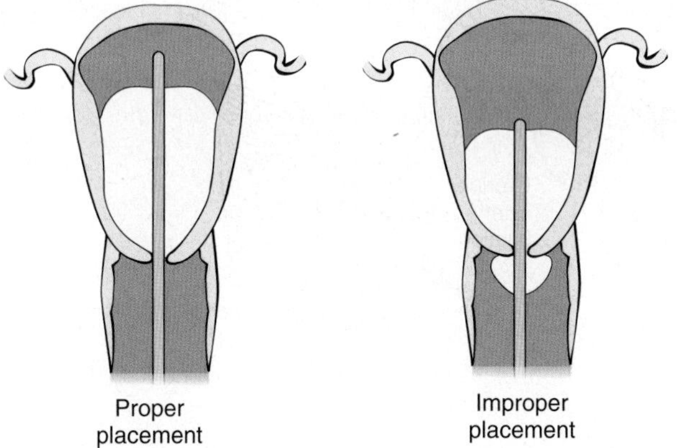

FIGURE 19-11. Proper placement of the Bakri SOS Tamponade Balloon.

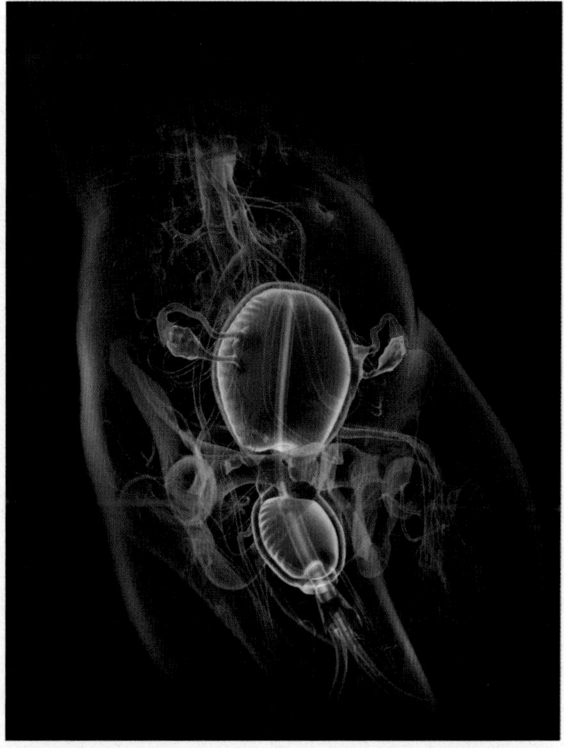

FIGURE 19-12. The Glenveigh *ebb* Complete Tamponade System. (Courtesy Glenveigh Medical, LLC.)

of cases.[85] Reported complications include postembolization fever, infection, ischemic pain, vascular perforation, and tissue necrosis. A relative disadvantage of the procedure is its limited availability. Timely coordination of services between the obstetrical team and interventional radiology is necessary to provide this treatment option.

SURGICAL INTERVENTION

When uterine atony is unresponsive to conservative management, surgical intervention by laparotomy is necessary. Possible interventions include arterial ligation, uterine compression sutures, and hysterectomy.

The goal of arterial ligation is to decrease uterine perfusion and subsequent bleeding. Success rates have varied from 40% to 95% in the literature depending on which vessels are ligated.[86] Arterial ligation may be performed on the ascending uterine arteries, the utero-ovarian arteries, the infundibulopelvic ligament vessels, and the hypogastric arteries. Because hypogastric arterial ligation can be technically challenging and time-consuming, it is not advised as a first-line technique unless the surgeon is extremely skilled in performing the procedure. Instead, a stepwise progression of uterine vessel ligation is recommended.

Nearly 45 years ago, O'Leary described a technique of bilateral uterine artery ligation for control of postpartum hemorrhage.[87] Today, it is still considered the best initial ligation technique given its ease in performance and the accessibility of the uterine artery. To perform the procedure, the ascending uterine artery should be located at the border of the upper and lower uterine segment. Absorbable suture is passed through the uterine myometrium at the level of the lower uterine segment and laterally around the uterine vessels through the broad ligament. The suture is then tied to compress the vessels against the uterine wall (Figure 19-13). Because the suture is placed fairly high in the lower uterine segment, the ureter is not in jeopardy, and the bladder does not need to be mobilized. Unilateral artery ligation will control hemorrhage in 10% to 15% of cases, whereas bilateral ligation will control an additional 75%.[88]

If bleeding persists, the utero-ovarian and infundibulopelvic vessels should be ligated. The utero-ovarian arteries can be ligated similarly to what has been described for the ascending uterine vessels. If this measure is unsuccessful, interruption of the infundibulopelvic vessels can be undertaken. Although the ovarian blood supply may be decreased with an infundibulopelvic vessel ligation, successful pregnancy has been reported.[89]

Bakri has described a newer technique for bilateral uterine artery ligation in combination with tamponade balloon placement (Figure 19-14).[90] The procedure, termed **Bilateral Looped Uterine Vessels Sutures** (B-LUVS), incorporates looped absorbable sutures bilaterally through the myometrium around the uterine vessels from the lower segment up to the corneal region. Once the sutures are tied, a Bakri SOS balloon is placed within the uterine cavity to provide tamponade. A small series has had 100% success with this combined ligation-tamponade approach.[90]

In addition to arterial ligation, **uterine compression sutures** have been described for atony control. Several techniques have evolved over the past decade, including the **B-Lynch suture, Hayman vertical sutures, Pereira transverse and vertical sutures, and multiple square sutures.**[91-93]

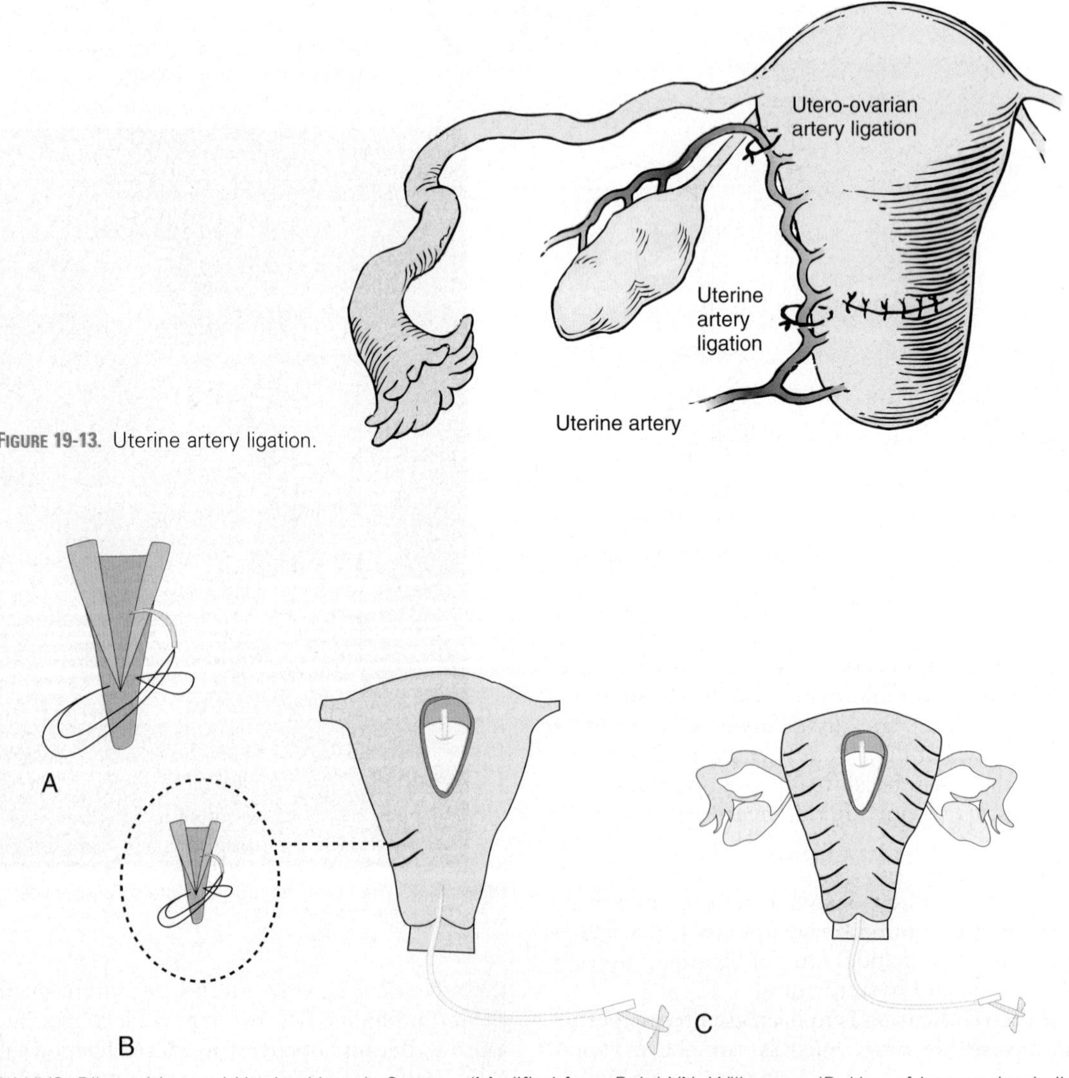

FIGURE 19-13. Uterine artery ligation.

FIGURE 19-14. B-LUVS: Bilateral Looped Uterine Vessels Sutures. (Modified from Bakri YN, Wilkenson JP: Use of intrauterine balloon catheters for control of uterine hemorrhage. Available at http://www.uptodate.com. Accessed September 2010.)

To place a compression suture, the patient should lie in the dorsal lithotomy position so that an assessment of vaginal bleeding can occur. Large absorbable suture is typically anchored within the uterine myometrium both anteriorly and posteriorly. It is passed in a continuous or intermittent fashion around or through the external surface of the uterus and tied firmly so that adequate uterine compression occurs. Figures 19-15 to 19-18 demonstrate proper placements of these sutures. Like arterial ligation, uterine compression sutures can be combined with tamponade balloons for refractory bleeding. The "uterine sandwich" technique refers to placement of a B-Lynch suture followed by a Bakri SOS balloon within the uterine cavity.[94] Typically, the tamponade balloon is inflated to a lesser degree (median volume of 100 mL) in these scenarios. Small series have demonstrated 100% success for this combined approach.[94]

The final surgical intervention for refractory bleeding due to atony is hysterectomy. Hysterectomy provides definitive therapy. Because blood loss may be severe, it is often prudent to modify the surgical approach by using the "clamp-cut-drop" technique or performing a supracervical hysterectomy (Figure 19-19), or both.[95] These considerations are especially important when the patient is hemodynamically unstable.

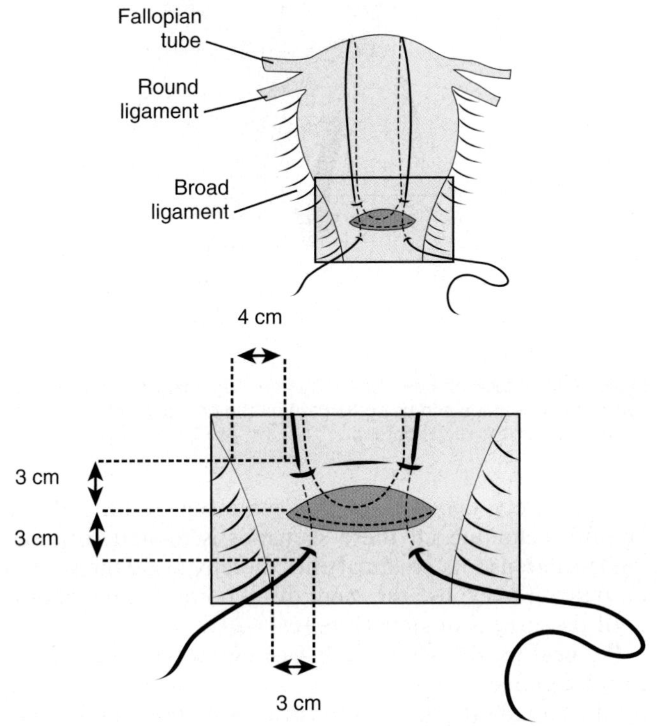

Genital Tract Lacerations

Definition and Pathogenesis

Genital tract lacerations may occur with both vaginal and cesarean deliveries. These lacerations involve the maternal

Figure 19-15. B-Lynch compression suture. (Modified from Jacobs AJ: Management of postpartum hemorrhage at cesarean delivery. Available at http://www.uptodate.com. Accessed September 2010.)

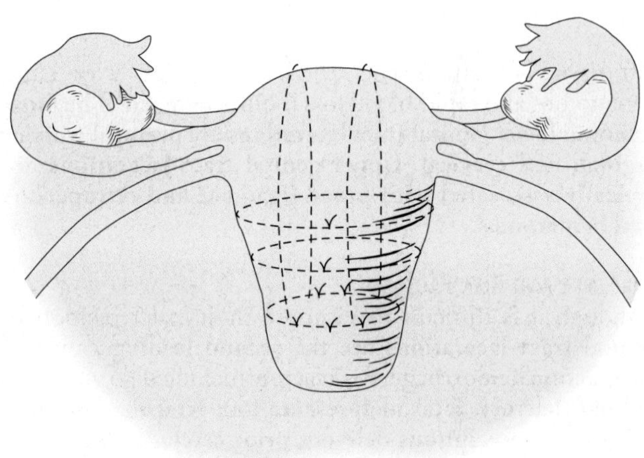

Figure 19-17. Pereira transverse and vertical sutures. (Modified from Jacobs AJ: Management of postpartum hemorrhage at cesarean delivery. Available at http://www.uptodate.com. Accessed September 2010.)

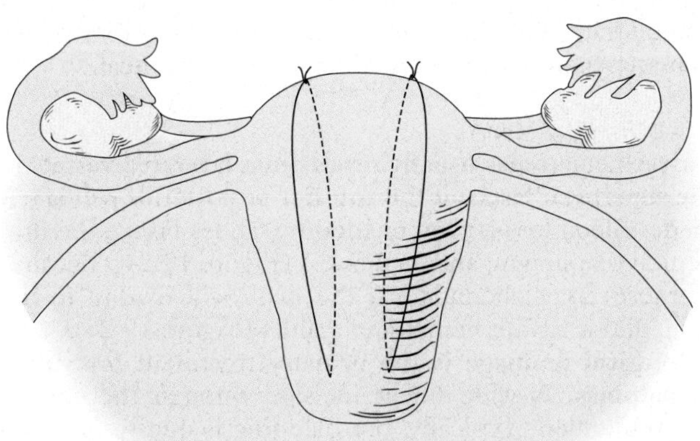

Figure 19-16. Hayman vertical sutures. (Modified from Jacobs AJ: Management of postpartum hemorrhage at cesarean delivery. Available at http://www.uptodate.com. Accessed September 2010.)

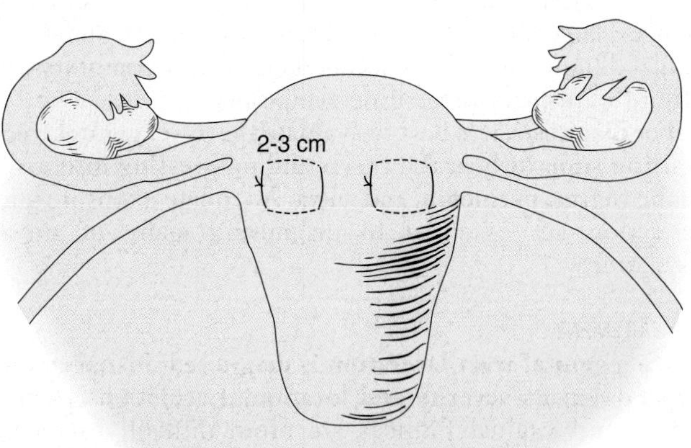

Figure 19-18. Multiple square sutures. (Modified from Jacobs AJ: Management of postpartum hemorrhage at cesarean delivery. Available at http://www.uptodate.com. Accessed September 2010.)

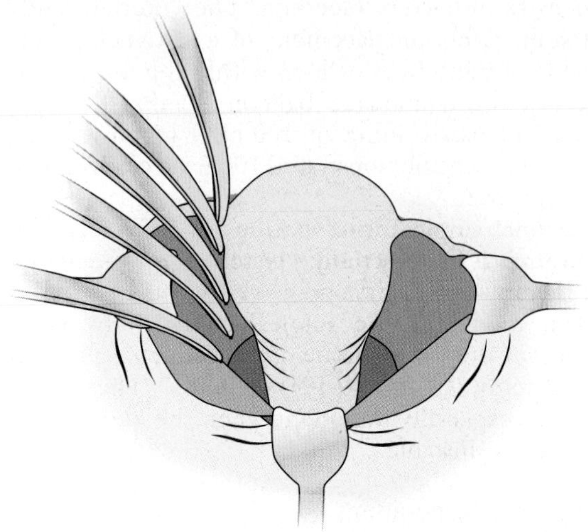

FIGURE 19-19. "Clamp-cut-drop" technique for hysterectomy. The vascular pedicles are clamped and divided. The pedicles are ligated after the hemorrhage is controlled. (Modified from Wright JD, Bonanno C, Shah M, et al: Peripartum hysterectomy. Obstet Gynecol 116:429, 2010.)

soft tissue structures and can be associated with large hematomas and rapid blood loss if unrecognized. **The most common lower genital tract lacerations are perineal, vulvar, vaginal, and cervical. Upper genital tract lacerations are typically associated with broad ligament and retroperitoneal hematomas.**

Incidence and Risk Factors

Although it is difficult to ascertain their exact incidence, **genital tract lacerations are the second leading cause of postpartum hemorrhage. Risk factors** include instrumented **vaginal delivery, fetal malpresentation, fetal macrosomia, episiotomy, precipitous delivery, prior cerclage placement, Dührssen incisions, and shoulder dystocia.**

Clinical Manifestations and Diagnosis

A genitourinary tract laceration should be suspected if bleeding persists after delivery despite adequate uterine tone. Occasionally, the bleeding may be masked because of its location, that is, the broad ligament. In these circumstances, large amounts of blood loss may occur in an unrecognized hematoma. Pain and hemodynamic instability are often the primary presenting symptoms.

For diagnosis, it is best to evaluate the lower genital tract starting superiorly at the cervix and progressing inferiorly to the vagina, perineum, and vulva. Adequate exposure and retraction are essential to diagnosing many of these lacerations.

Management

Once a genital tract laceration is diagnosed, management depends on its severity and location. Lacerations of the cervix and vaginal fornices are often difficult to repair owing to their position. In these circumstances, relocation to an operating room for better pain relief, pelvic relaxation, and visualization are recommended. For cervical lacerations, it is important to secure the apex of the tear because this is often a major source of bleeding.

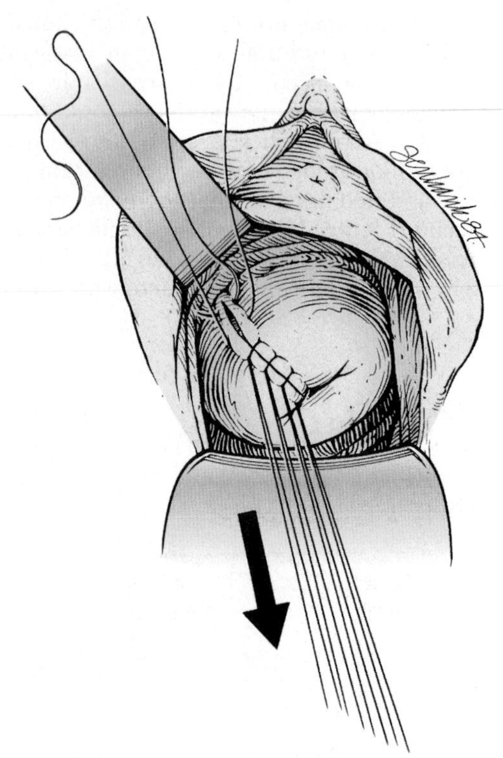

FIGURE 19-20. Repair of a cervical laceration, beginning at the proximal part of the laceration and using traction on the previous sutures to aid in exposure of the distal defect.

Unfortunately, exposure of this angle can be difficult. A helpful technique for these scenarios is to start suturing the laceration at its proximal end, thereby using the suture for traction to expose the more distal portion of the cervix until the apex is in view (Figure 19-20).

Perineal repairs are the most common types of genital tract lacerations. Figures 19-21 to 19-23 illustrate second-, third-, and fourth-degree perineal lacerations and techniques for their repair. If the laceration is adjacent to the urethra or bowel, the use of additional instrumentation (e.g., transurethral catheter) can protect uninjured organs and allow for more efficient repair.

On occasion, a blood vessel laceration may lead to the formation of a pelvic hematoma in the lower or upper genital tract. The three most common locations for a pelvic hematoma are vulvar, vaginal, and retroperitoneal.

Vulvar Hematoma

Vulvar hematomas usually result from lacerated vessels in the superficial fascia of the anterior or posterior pelvic triangle. Blood loss is tamponaded by Colles fascia, the urogenital diaphragm, and anal fascia (Figure 19-24). Because of these fascial boundaries, the mass will extend to the skin, and a visible hematoma results (Figure 19-25).

Surgical drainage is the primary treatment for vulvar hematomas. A wide linear incision through the skin is recommended. Typically, the bleeding is due to multiple small vessels; hence, vessel ligation is not possible. Once the hematoma is evacuated, the dead space should be closed in layers with absorbable suture and a sterile pressure dressing applied. A transurethral Foley catheter should be placed until significant tissue edema subsides.

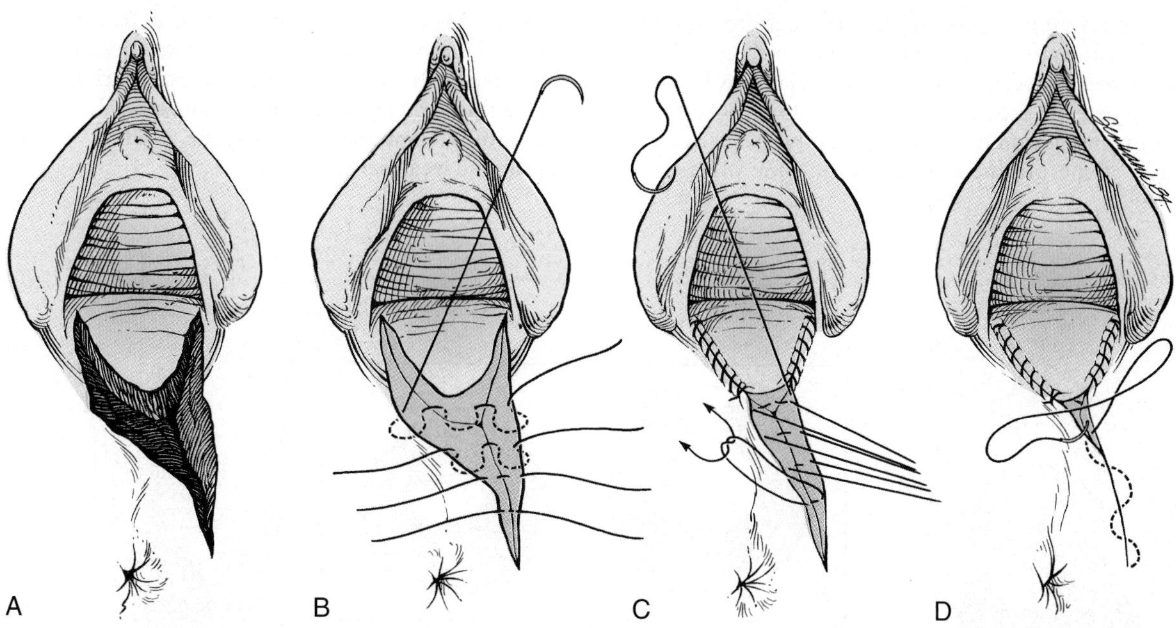

FIGURE 19-21. Repair of a second-degree laceration. A first-degree laceration involves the fourchet, the perineal skin, and the vaginal mucous membrane. A second-degree laceration also includes the muscles of the perineal body. The rectal sphincter remains intact.

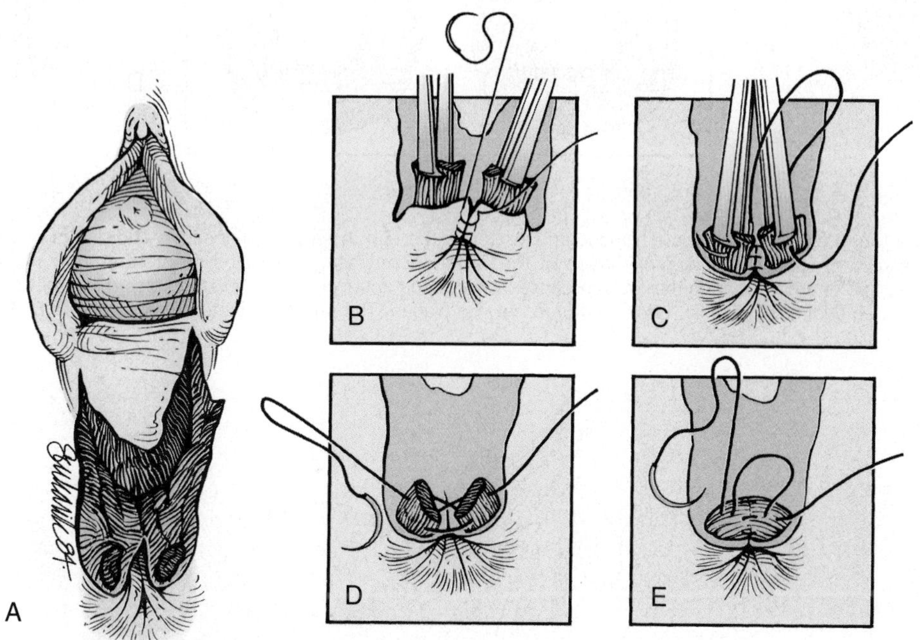

FIGURE 19-22. Repair of the sphincter after a third-degree laceration. A third-degree laceration not only extends through the skin, mucous membrane, and perineal body but also includes the anal sphincter. Interrupted figure-of-eight sutures should be placed in the capsule of the sphincter muscle.

VAGINAL HEMATOMA

Vaginal hematomas result from delivery-related soft tissue damage. These hematomas accumulate above the pelvic diaphragm (Figure 19-26). Occasionally, these hematomas protrude in the vaginal-rectal area. Like vulvar hematomas, vaginal hematomas are due to multiple small vessel lacerations. Depending on the extent of the hemorrhage, **vaginal hematomas may or may not require surgical drainage.** Small, nonexpanding hematomas are often best managed expectantly. Larger, expanding hematomas require surgical intervention. Unlike vulvar hematomas, the incision of a vaginal hematoma does not require closing; rather a vaginal pack or tamponade device should be placed on the raw edges. If bleeding persists, **selective arterial embolization may be considered.**

RETROPERITONEAL HEMATOMA

Although infrequent, **retroperitoneal hematomas are the most serious and life threatening.** The early symptoms of a retroperitoneal hematoma are often subtle, with the hematoma being unrecognized until the patient is hemodynamically unstable from massive hemorrhage. **These hematomas usually occur after a vessel laceration from the hypogastric arterial tree** (Figure 19-27). Such lacerations may result from instrumented vaginal delivery, inadequate hemostasis of the uterine arteries at the time of cesarean delivery, or uterine rupture during a trial of labor after cesarean delivery. **Treatment of a retroperitoneal hematoma typically involves surgical exploration, hematoma evacuation, and arterial ligation. In some situations, selective arterial embolization may be used as a primary or adjunctive treatment.**

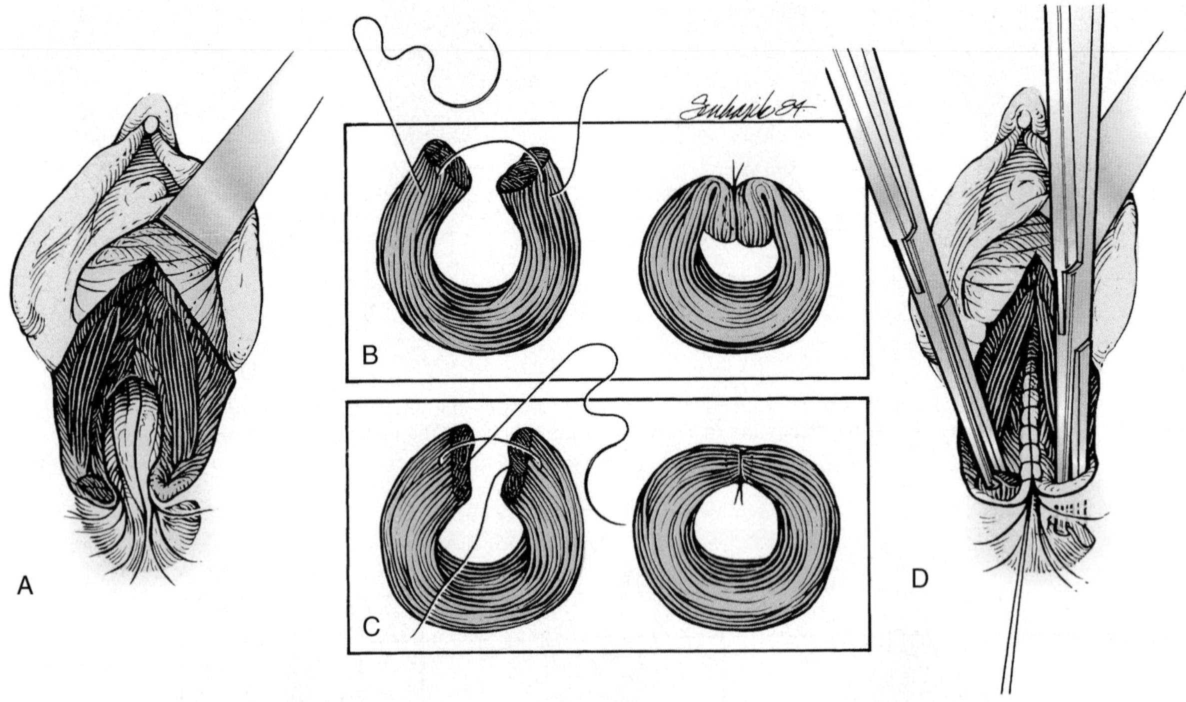

FIGURE 19-23. Repair of a fourth-degree laceration. This laceration extends through the rectal mucosa. **A,** The extent of this laceration is shown, with a segment of the rectum exposed. **B,** Approximation of the rectal submucosa. This is the most commonly recommended method for repair. **C,** Alternative method of approximating the rectal mucosa in which the knots are actually buried inside the rectal lumen. **D,** After closure of the rectal submucosa, an additional layer of running sutures may be placed. The rectal sphincter is then repaired.

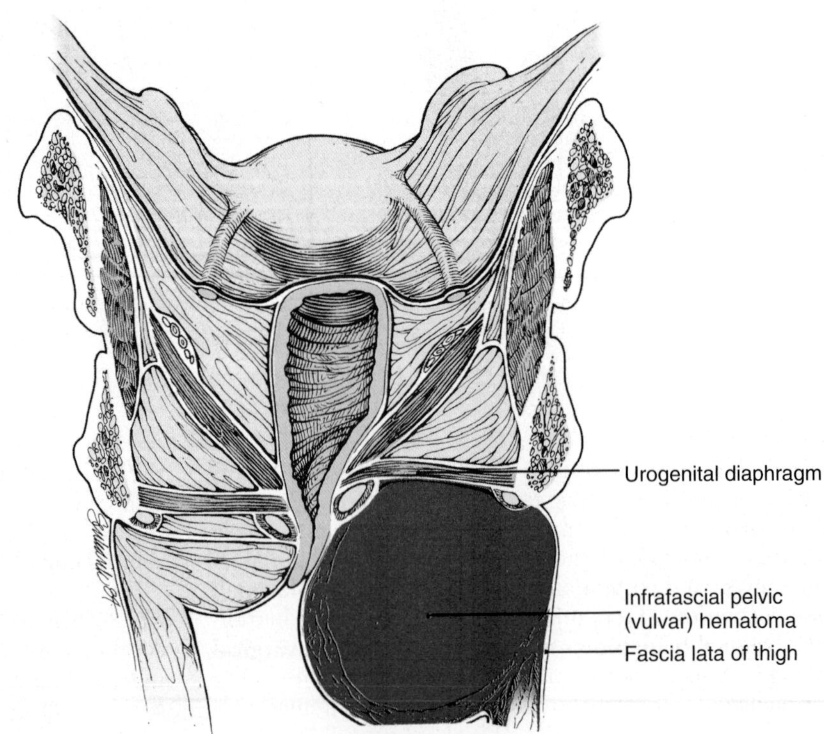

FIGURE 19-24. Vulvar hematoma fascial boundaries.

Retained Products of Conception

Definition and Pathogenesis

Retained products of conception, namely placental tissue and amniotic membranes, can inhibit the uterus from adequate contraction and result in hemorrhage. The diagnosis is made when there has not been spontaneous expulsion of the tissue within 30 to 60 minutes of delivery.[96]

Incidence and Risk Factors

Retained products of conception complicate 1 in 100 to 1 in 200 deliveries. Risk factors include midtrimester delivery, chorioamnionitis, and accessory placental lobes.

Clinical Manifestations and Diagnosis

Retained products of conception typically present with uterine bleeding and associated atony. To assess the uterus for retained products of conception, the uterine cavity needs to be explored. Manual exploration is not only diagnostic but also often therapeutic (Figure 19-28). By wrapping the examination hand with moist gauze, removal of retained placental fragments and amniotic membranes can be facilitated. If manual access to the uterine cavity is difficult or limited owing to maternal body habitus or inadequate pain relief, **transabdominal or transvaginal ultrasound may be used to determine whether retained placental fragments are present.**

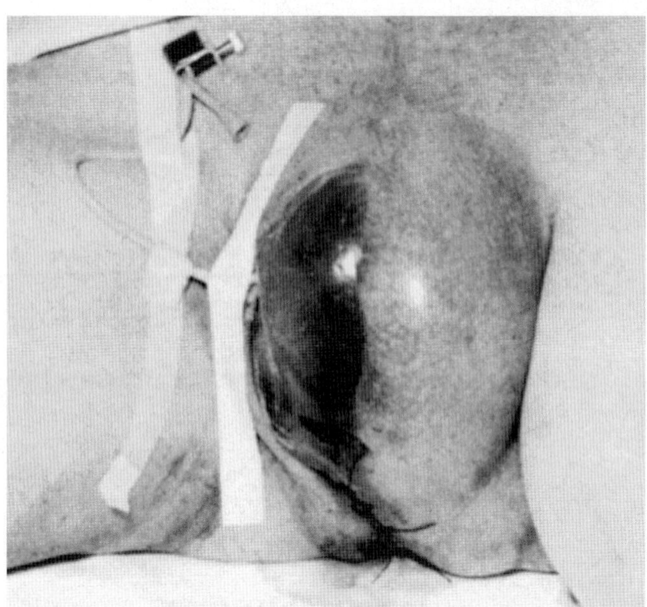

Figure 19-25. Large vulvar hematoma.

Management

Once a diagnosis of retained products of conception is made, removal must be undertaken. Therapeutic options include **manual extraction,** as noted previously, or **uterine curettage.** Nitroglycerin (50 to 200 mcg intravenous) has been used effectively to assist with manual placental extraction.[97] Nitroglycerin provides rapid uterine relaxation to assist with removal of the retained tissue. Uterine curettage may be performed in a delivery room; however, excessive bleeding mandates that an operating room be used for the procedure. Either a large Banjo curette or vacuum suction curette can be employed. Transabdominal ultrasound guidance is helpful in determining that tissue evacuation is complete.

Pharmacologic options for retained products of conception include intraumbilical vein oxytocin injection and Misoprostol (Cytotec). Although initial studies of intraumbilical vein oxytocin injection were promising, larger systematic reviews and meta-analyses have shown no significant reduction in need for manual placental extraction.[98] Misoprostol administration (800 mcg), on the other hand, demonstrated a significant reduction in need for manual placental removal compared with intraumbilical vein oxytocin and saline injections.[99]

Uterine Rupture

Definition and Pathogenesis

Uterine rupture refers to the complete nonsurgical disruption of all uterine layers (endometrium, myometrium, and

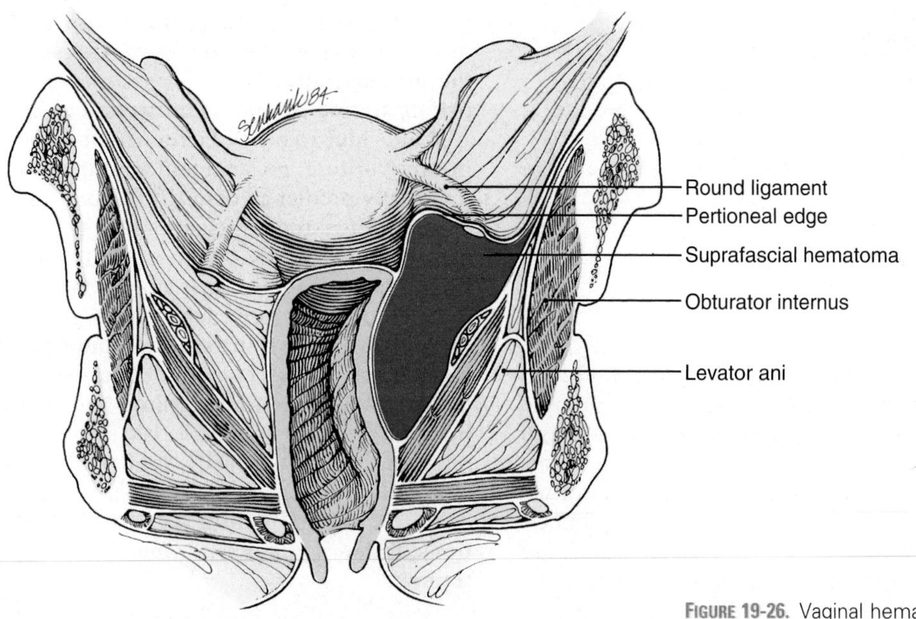

Figure 19-26. Vaginal hematoma.

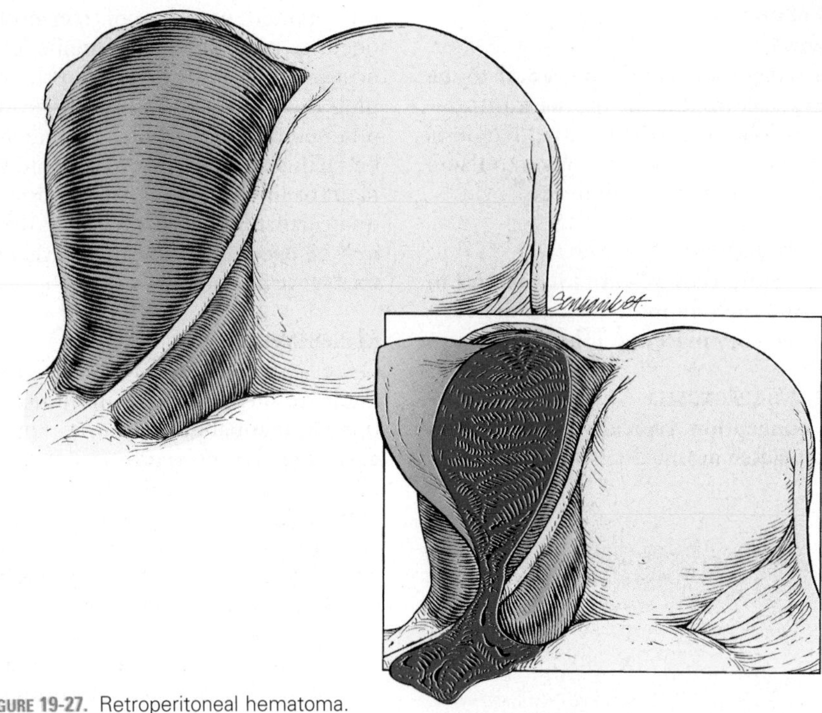

FIGURE 19-27. Retroperitoneal hematoma.

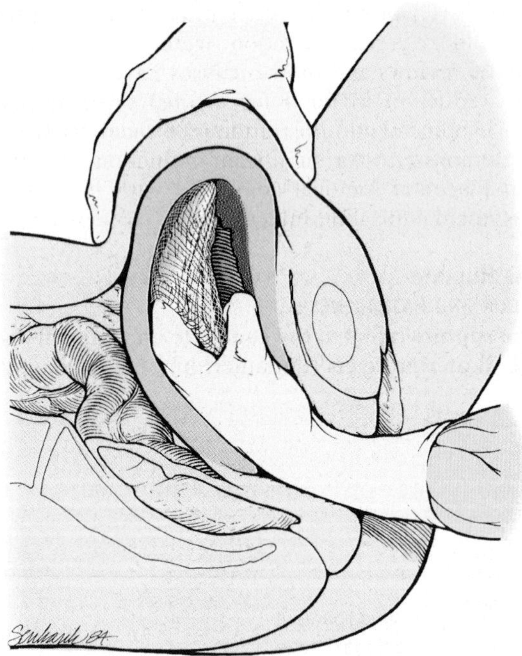

FIGURE 19-28. Manual uterine exploration.

serosa). The severity of hemorrhage and maternal-fetal morbidity depends on the extent of the rupture. A large rupture may be associated with massive hemorrhage and extrusion of the fetus or placenta into the maternal abdomen, whereas a small rupture may have minimal bleeding and insignificant maternal-fetal consequences. The terms *uterine dehiscence* and *incomplete uterine rupture* are often used to describe the latter type of disruption.

TABLE 19-8 RISK FOR UTERINE RUPTURE BASED ON INCISION OF PRIOR CESAREAN DELIVERY

INCISION OF PRIOR CESAREAN DELIVERY	UTERINE RUPTURE RISK (%)
Classical	4-9
T-shaped	4-9
Low vertical	1-7
Low transverse	0.5-2

From Welischar J, Quirk JG: Trail of labor after cesarean delivery. Available at http://www.uptodate.com. Accessed September 2010.

INCIDENCE AND RISK FACTORS

The overall incidence of uterine rupture is 1 in 2000 deliveries. Uterine rupture is most common in women with a scarred uterus, including prior cesarean delivery and myomectomy. The location of the previous hysterotomy affects the uterine rupture risk. For prior cesarean deliveries, the risk of uterine rupture is illustrated in Table 19-8.

While **multiple risk factors** have been associated with uterine rupture, no single or combination of factors is able to reliably predict all cases.[100] Despite this, consistent data demonstrate strong associations for trial of labor after cesarean delivery and one or more of the following: **multiple prior cesarean deliveries, no previous vaginal delivery, induced or augmented labor, term gestation, thin uterine scar identified by ultrasound, multiple gestation, fetal macrosomia, post–cesarean delivery infection, single layer closure of hysterotomy incision, and short interpregnancy interval.**[101] Other reported risk factors include increasing **maternal age, multiparity, fetal malpresentation, uterine manipulation** (e.g., internal podalic version), **mid- to high-operative vaginal delivery, congenital uterine malformations, Ehlers-Danlos syndrome, invasive placentation, and trauma.**[102]

Clinical Manifestations and Diagnosis

Uterine rupture is associated with both fetal and maternal clinical manifestations. Fetal bradycardia with or without preceding variable or late decelerations is the most common clinical manifestation of symptomatic uterine rupture, occurring in 33% to 70% of cases.[103] In some circumstances, a **loss of fetal station in labor** may occur. **Maternal clinical manifestations** are variable and may include **acute vaginal bleeding, constant abdominal pain or uterine tenderness, change in uterine shape, cessation of contractions, hematuria** (if extension into the bladder has occurred), and **signs of hemodynamic instability.**

Uterine rupture is suspected clinically but confirmed surgically. Laparotomy will demonstrate complete disruption of the uterine wall, with bleeding and partial or complete extravasation of the fetus into the maternal abdomen.

Management

Once the fetus and placenta are delivered, the **site of rupture should be assessed to determine whether it can be repaired. If feasible, the rupture can be repaired in multiple layers with absorbable suture.** Hysterectomy should be reserved for cases of massive hemorrhage, irreparable uterine defects, or maternal hemodynamic instability.

Maternal and Neonatal Outcomes

Although maternal mortality is uncommon with a uterine rupture, **significant morbidity** can occur. The most comprehensive review of trial of labor after cesarean delivery found **increased risks for blood transfusion, hysterectomy, and genitourinary injury.**[104] With regard to perinatal outcome, **increased rates of low 5-minute Apgar scores (<5), umbilical artery pH less than 7.0, admission to the neonatal intensive care unit, hypoxic-ischemic encephalopathy, and neonatal death** have been documented.[105]

Uterine Inversion

Definition and Pathogenesis

Uterine inversion refers to the collapse of the fundus into the uterine cavity. Uterine inversion is classified by degree and timing. With regard to degree, uterine inversion may be incomplete, complete, or prolapsed. Incomplete uterine inversion represents a partial extrusion of the fundus into the uterine cavity. With complete uterine inversion, the internal lining of the fundus crosses through the cervical os, forming a rounded mass in the vagina with no palpable fundus abdominally. Prolapsed uterine inversion refers to the entire uterus prolapsing through the cervix with the fundus passing out of the vaginal introitus. Uterine inversion timing is classified as **acute (≤24 hours of delivery), subacute (>24 hours postpartum), or chronic (>1 month postpartum).**

The two most commonly proposed etiologies for uterine inversion include excessive umbilical cord traction with a fundally attached placenta and fundal pressure in the setting of a relaxed uterus. However, a causal relationship between active management of the third stage of labor and uterine inversion remains unproved.[106]

Incidence and Risk Factors

Uterine inversion is a rare event, complicating about 1 in 2000 to 1 in 23,000 deliveries.[107] Proposed **risk factors** for uterine inversion include **uterine overdistention, fetal macrosomia, rapid labor, congenital uterine malformations, invasive placentation, short umbilical cord, use of uterine-relaxing agents, nulliparity, manual placental extraction, and Ehlers-Danlos syndrome.**

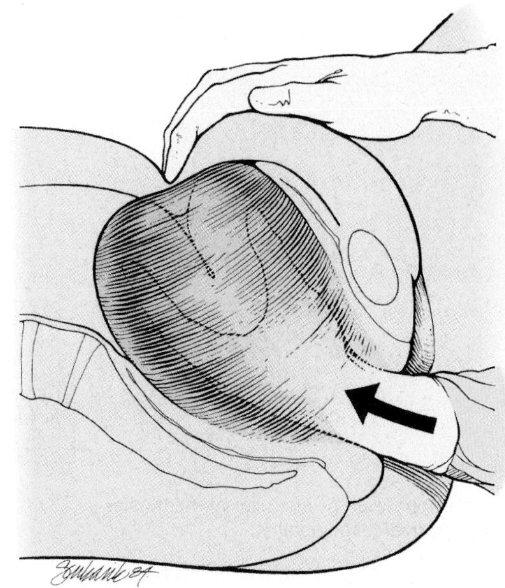

FIGURE 19-29. Manual replacement of uterine inversion.

Clinical Manifestations and Diagnosis

Uterine inversion should be suspected with the **sudden onset of brisk vaginal bleeding in association with the inability to palpate the fundus abdominally and maternal hemodynamic instability.** It may occur before or after placental detachment. The diagnosis is made clinically with bimanual examination, during which the uterine fundus is palpated in the lower uterine segment or within the vagina. Sonography can be used to confirm the diagnosis if the clinical examination is unclear.[108]

Management

Once diagnosed, uterine inversion requires rapid intervention in order to restore maternal hemodynamic stability and control hemorrhage. Maternal fluid resuscitation through a large-bore intravenous catheter is recommended. The uterus must be replaced to its proper orientation to resolve the hemorrhage. This is best accomplished in an operating room with the assistance of an anesthesiologist. The uterus and cervix should initially be relaxed with nitroglycerin (50 to 500 mcg), a tocolytic agent (magnesium sulfate or β-mimetic), or a halogenated anesthetic.[109] Once relaxed, gentle manual pressure is applied to the uterine fundus in order to return it to its proper abdominal location (Figure 19-29). Uterotonic therapy should then be given to assist with uterine contraction and prevent recurrence of the inversion.

If manual repositioning is unsuccessful, other options include hydrostatic reduction and surgical correction. With hydrostatic reduction, warmed sterile saline is infused into the vagina. The physician's hand or a Silastic ventouse cup is used as a fluid retainer in order to generate intravaginal hydrostatic pressure and resultant correction of the

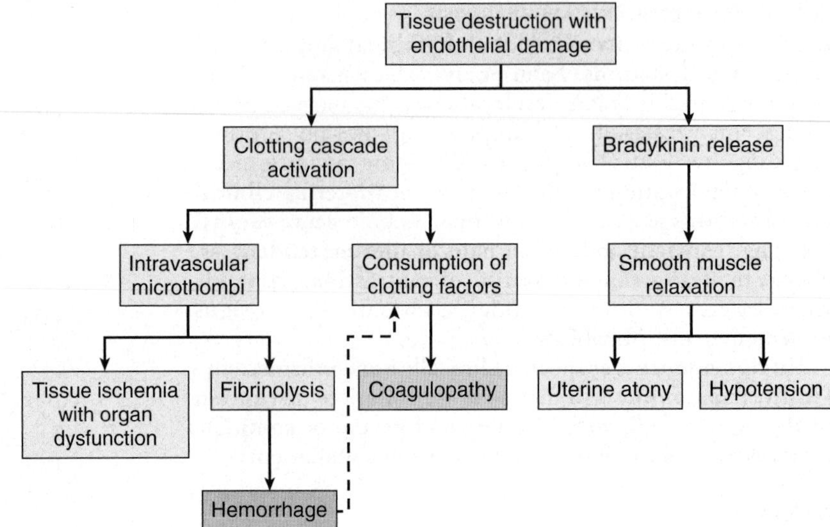

Figure 19-30. Pathophysiology and clinical manifestations of consumptive coagulopathy.

inversion.[110] Surgical options include the Huntington and Haultain procedures, laparoscopic-assisted repositioning, and cervical incisions with manual uterine repositioning.[111] The Huntington procedure involves a laparotomy with serial clamping and upward traction of the round ligaments to restore the uterus to its proper position. If this technique fails, the Haultain procedure, which uses a vertical incision within the inversion and manual repositioning of the fundus, can be attempted. As with manual repositioning, uterotonic therapy should be administered immediately after uterine replacement.

Coagulopathy

Definition and Pathogenesis

Coagulopathy represents an imbalance between the clotting and fibrinolytic systems. This imbalance may be hereditary or acquired in origin. Hereditary coagulopathies are relatively rare and have variable etiologies. Although **acquired coagulopathy** can be due to iatrogenic causes, such as anticoagulant administration, it is **usually the result of clotting factor consumption.** Figure 19-30 demonstrates the pathophysiology of consumptive coagulopathy and its association with hemorrhage.

Incidence and Risk Factors

The overall incidence of coagulopathy in the obstetrical population has not been reported; however, several **risk factors** have been documented. These include **massive antepartum or postpartum hemorrhage, sepsis, severe preeclampsia, HELLP syndrome, amniotic fluid embolism, fetal demise, placental abruption, septic abortion, and acute fatty liver of pregnancy.**

Clinical Manifestations and Diagnosis

The primary clinical manifestations of consumptive coagulopathy include bleeding, hypotension out of proportion to blood loss, microangiopathic hemolytic anemia, acute lung injury, acute renal failure, and ischemic end-organ tissue damage.

Consumptive coagulopathy is a clinical diagnosis that is confirmed with laboratory data, such as thrombocytopenia, hemolytic changes on the peripheral blood smear, decreased fibrinogen, elevated fibrin degradation products, and prolonged prothrombin time (PT) and activated partial thromboplastin time (aPTT). When timely laboratory assessment is unavailable, drawing 5 mL of maternal blood into an empty red-topped tube and observing for clot formation provide the clinician with a rough estimate of the degree of existing coagulopathy. If a clot is not visible within 6 minutes or forms and lyses within 30 minutes, the fibrinogen level is usually less than 150 mg/dL.

Management

The most important factor in the successful treatment of coagulopathy is identifying and correcting the underlying etiology. For most obstetrical causes, **delivery of the fetus initiates resolution of the coagulopathy.** In addition, rapid replacement of blood products and clotting factors should occur simultaneously. The patient should have **two large-bore intravenous catheters for fluid and blood component therapy. Laboratory studies should be drawn serially every 4 hours until resolution** of the coagulopathy is evident. The obstetrician should attempt to achieve a hematocrit greater than 21%, a platelet count greater than 50,000/mm^3, a fibrinogen level greater than 100 mg/dL, and PT and aPTT less than 1.5 times control. It also is important to maintain adequate oxygenation and normothermia. Finally, adjuvant therapies, such as vitamin K, recombinant activated factor VIIa, fibrinogen concentrate, and hemostatic agents, should be considered.

Vitamin K

Factors II, VII, IX, and X are vitamin K–dependent clotting factors. In consumptive coagulopathy, these clotting factors are consumed. Administration of vitamin K (5 to 10 mg) by the subcutaneous, intramuscular, or intravenous routes can assist with endogenous replenishment of these procoagulants.

Recombinant Activated Factor VIIa

Factor VII is a precursor for the extrinsic clotting cascade. When massive procoagulant factor consumption occurs, factor replacement is necessary. **Human recombinant factor VIIa has been used successfully in cases of consumptive**

coagulopathy attributed to postpartum hemorrhage. The dosage of this intravenous therapy has ranged from 16.7 to 120 mcg/kg.[112] Important advantages of this therapy are its rapid bioavailability and reversal of coagulopathy (10 to 40 minutes); however, disadvantages include a relatively short half life (2 hours), cost (approximately $1 per 1 mcg), and thromboembolism risk. Recombinant activated factor VIIa should be considered in cases of refractory coagulopathy or when blood component replacement is delayed.

Fibrinogen Concentrate

Human fibrinogen concentrate (RiaStap) has recently been approved by the U.S. Food and Drug Administration. This intravenous therapy has been used successfully in Europe for the treatment of massive hemorrhage due to consumptive coagulopathy (trauma, surgery, gastrointestinal hemorrhage) and congenital fibrinogen deficiency.[113]

Hemostatic Agents

A variety of topical hemostatic agents are available for control of coagulopathic surface bleeding. These agents have different clotting factors and mechanisms of action. Examples include fibrin sealants (e.g., Tisseal), hemostatic matrices (e.g., Floseal), and Gelfoam. These agents may be used alone or in combination.

Fluid Resuscitation and Transfusion

All obstetricians will encounter antepartum and postpartum hemorrhage. In most instances, **fluid resuscitation and blood component therapy is life-saving.** Therefore, every physician should have a thorough understanding of appropriate volume and transfusion therapy, alternative treatment options, and their risks.

Volume Resuscitation

Initial management of a hemorrhaging patient requires appropriate volume resuscitation. Two large-bore intravenous catheters are recommended. **Warmed crystalloid solution in a 3 : 1 ratio to the estimated blood loss should be rapidly infused.** Goals of therapy are to prevent hypotension (systolic blood pressure >90 mm Hg) and maintain urine output (at least 30 mL/hr). If the hemorrhage is easily controlled, this may be the only volume resuscitation needed. The patient should have serial assessments of her vital signs and hematologic profiles to confirm hemodynamic stability.

Colloid Solutions

Colloid solutions contain larger particles, called *colloids*, which are less permeable across vascular membranes. These solutions provide a greater increase in colloid oncotic pressure and plasma volume; however, they are more expensive than crystalloids and may be associated with anaphylactoid reactions. Examples of colloid solutions include albumin, hetastarch, and dextran.

Blood Component Therapy

Whole Blood

Whole blood contains red cells, clotting factors, and platelets. Whole blood is rarely used in modern obstetrics because of its many disadvantages, including a short storage life (24 hours), large volume (500 mL per unit), and potential for hypercalcemia.

Packed Red Blood Cells

Packed red blood cells (PRBCs) are the most appropriate therapy for patients requiring red blood cell replacement due to hemorrhage. They are the only blood product to provide oxygen-carrying capacity. **Each PRBC unit contains approximately 300 mL of volume: 250 mL red blood cells and 50 mL of plasma. In a 70-kg patient, one unit of PRBCs will raise the hemoglobin by 1 g/dL and the hematocrit by 3%.** Transfusion of PRBCs should be considered in any gravida with hemoglobin less than 8 g/dL or with active hemorrhage and associated coagulopathy.

Platelet Concentrates

Platelets are separated from whole blood and stored in plasma. Because 1 U of platelets provides an increase of only approximately 7500/mm^3, platelet concentrates of 6 to 10 U need to be transfused. Platelet concentrates can be derived from multiple donors or single donors. The single donor concentrates are preferred because they expose the patient to fewer potential antigenic and immunologic risks. Transfusion of a single donor platelet concentrate will increase the circulating platelet count by 30,000 to 60,000/mm^3. Because sensitization can occur, it is important for platelets to be ABO and Rh specific. **Transfusion of platelets should be considered when the platelet count is less than 20,000/mm^3 after a vaginal delivery or less than 50,000/mm^3 after a cesarean delivery, or if there is evidence of coagulopathy.**

Fresh-Frozen Plasma

Fresh-frozen plasma (FFP) is plasma that is extracted from whole blood. FFP primarily contains fibrinogen, antithrombin, and clotting factors V, XI, XII. Transfusing FFP not only assists with coagulation but also provides the patient with volume resuscitation because **each unit contains approximately 250 mL.** Typically, fibrinogen levels are used to monitor a patient's response to FFP. Each unit of **FFP should raise the fibrinogen level by 5 to 10 mg/dL.** FFP does not need to be ABO or Rh compatible. FFP should be considered for hemorrhaging patients with evidence of consumptive coagulopathy, coagulopathic liver disease, or warfarin reversal.

Cryoprecipitate

Cryoprecipitate is the precipitate that results from thawed FFP. It is rich in fibrinogen, von Willebrand factor, factor VIII, and factor XIII. Like FFP, **cryoprecipitate can be measured clinically by the fibrinogen response, which should increase by 5 to 10 mg/dL per unit. Unlike FFP, each unit of cryoprecipitate provides minimal volume (10 to 15 mL),** so it is an ineffective agent for volume resuscitation. Cryoprecipitate is indicated for patients with coagulopathy and concerns of volume overload, hypofibrinogenemia, factor VIII deficiency, and von Willebrand disease.

Table 19-9 contains a summary of the available blood component therapies.

Transfusion Protocols

In the past, no consensus existed regarding the optimal ratio of blood product replacement. Newer data from trauma, military, and hospital-based protocols suggests that more aggressive replacement of coagulation factors with

TABLE 19-9 BLOOD COMPONENT THERAPY

PRODUCT	CONTENTS	VOLUME	ANTICIPATED EFFECT (PER UNIT)
Whole blood	All components	500 mL	*Used only in emergencies*
Packed red blood cells	Red blood cells	300 mL	Increase hemoglobin by 1 g/dL Increase hematocrit by 3%
Platelets (single donor pooled)	Platelets	300 mL (6 U)	Increase platelet count by 30,000-60,000/mm^3
Fresh-frozen plasma	All clotting factors	250 mL	Increase fibrinogen by 5-10 mg/dL
Cryoprecipitate	Fibrinogen, von Willebrand factor, factors VIII and XIII	10-15 mL	Increase fibrinogen by 5-10 mg/dL

PRBCs improves outcomes and survival.[114-116] A variety of protocols have been recommended. **Two of the most common are 1 U of PRBCs to 1 U of FFP to 1 U of platelets (1:1:1) and 6 U of PRBCs to 4 U of FFP to 1 U of pooled platelets (6:4:1).**[114,115]

TRANSFUSION RISKS AND REACTIONS

METABOLIC ABNORMALITIES AND HYPOTHERMIA

When PRBCs are stored, leakage of potassium and ammonia can occur into the plasma. This may result in hyperkalemia and high ammonia concentrations in patients requiring massive transfusion. In addition, because most PRBCs units are stored with a calcium-chelating agent, hypocalcemia may occur. Serial assessments of metabolic profiles and ionized calcium levels can assist the clinician in managing these changes.

In addition to metabolic abnormalities, hypothermia may complicate the clinical course of massive transfusion and result in cardiac arrhythmias. Hypothermia can be prevented by warming PRBC units before transfusion and by providing alternative heating devices to the patient (e.g., "bear-hugger" anesthesia warmer).

IMMUNOLOGIC REACTIONS

Transfusions introduce interactions between inherited or acquired antibodies and the foreign antigens of the transfused blood products. The most common immunologic reactions are febrile nonhemolytic transfusion reactions and urticarial reactions. Transfusion of leukoreduced blood products has been proposed to decrease the frequency of these reactions; however, supportive data have been inconsistent.[117] Rare immunologic complications include acute or delayed hemolytic transfusion reactions, anaphylaxis, posttransfusion purpura, and graft-versus-host disease.

INFECTION RISKS

All blood products have the potential to transmit viral and bacterial infections. Although transmission rates have substantially decreased in the past decade, they are still a potential risk that must be disclosed when a transfusion is needed. Table 19-10 lists current transfusion-related infection risks.[118]

TABLE 19-10 TRANSFUSION-RELATED INFECTIONS RISKS

INFECTION	TRANSMISSION RISK
HIV-1, HIV-2	1 in 1.5-2.1 million
Hepatitis B	1 in 205,000-355,000
Hepatitis C	1 in 1.1-1.9 million
HTLV I and II	1 in 2 million
Bacterial contamination	
• Red blood cells	1 in 30,000
• Platelets	1 in 5000

From Kleinman S: Blood donor medical history. Available at http://www.uptodate.com. Accessed September 2010; and Spelman D, MacLaren G: Transfusion-transmitted bacterial infection. Available at http://www.uptodate.com. Accessed September 2010.

HIV, Human immunodeficiency virus; *HTLV*, human T-cell lymphotropic virus.

ACUTE LUNG INJURY

Acute lung injury complicates 1 in 2000 transfusions.[119] This complication is characterized by acute respiratory distress, hypoxemia, hypotension, fever, and pulmonary edema. Symptoms can be mild or severe, and resolution is usually complete within 96 hours. Three etiologies have been proposed, including antileukocyte antibodies, granulocyte priming, and a combination of the two. Treatment consists of supportive care with oxygen administration and diuresis.

Blood Conservation Approaches

Autologous Donation and Transfusion

Autologous donation and transfusion refers to the collection and reinfusion of the patient's own red blood cells. Although it is unreasonable to have all pregnant individuals consider autologous donation, patients at high risk for transfusion (e.g., placenta previa or accreta) may be good candidates. Guidelines for autologous donation are as follows: minimal predonation hemoglobin of 11 g/dL, first donation within 6 weeks of anticipated delivery due to PRBC storage life of 42 days, weekly interval between donations, and no donation within 2 weeks of anticipated delivery.[120]

Autologous transfusion should be used selectively. Not only is it significantly more expensive than homologous transfusion, but also the risks for bacterial contamination and subsequent homologous transfusion are not completely eliminated.

Acute Normovolemic Hemodilution

Acute normovolemic hemodilution refers to a blood conservation technique in which blood is removed from a patient immediately before surgery, the patient is given crystalloid or colloid solution to maintain normovolemia during surgery, and then the blood is reinfused to the patient after surgery. The goal is for more dilute blood loss at the time of surgery. Acute normovolemic hemodilution can be considered for patients with good initial hemoglobin concentrations who are expected to have a blood loss of at least 1000 mL during surgery (e.g., patients with suspected placenta accreta).

Intraoperative and Postoperative Blood Salvage

***Blood salvage* refers to collecting the patient's blood during or after surgery, filtering the blood, and then reinfusing the red cells back to the patient. Cell Saver technology is the most widely used blood salvage system.** In the past, theoretical concerns regarding the risks for infection and amniotic fluid embolism limited the use of blood salvage technology in obstetrics; however, **several small studies have documented its safety and effectivenes.**[121] Blood salvage has many advantages over homologous transfusion. Not only does it eliminate the risk for infectious disease transmission, alloimmunization, and immunologic transfusion reactions, but it also can rapidly provide the patient with red cells (1 U in a 3-minute interval).

Alternative Oxygen Carriers

Because some patients refuse to accept blood products (e.g., Jehovah's Witness patients) or are unable to be transfused owing to a lack of compatible blood, new oxygen carriers are being developed and have promise as alternatives to transfusion therapy. The two primary products are hemoglobin-based oxygen carriers and perfluorocarbons. Hemoglobin-based oxygen carriers use hemoglobin from animals, outdated human blood, or recombinant technology. The hemoglobin is separated from the red cell stroma and undergoes multiple filtration and polymerization processes before use. Perfluorocarbons are inert compounds that can dissolve gases, including oxygen. Both products have high oxygen-carrying capacities and have been used in phase III trials for elective surgery and in patients with hemorrhagic shock.

Hemorrhage Prevention and Protocols

Because obstetrical hemorrhage is such a widespread problem, it is important for institutions to develop standardized management protocols and conduct hemorrhage drills.[122] The California Maternal Quality Care Collaborative and related efforts in New York have developed best practice approaches that can be adopted by other institutions. The use of obstetrical rapid response teams and massive transfusion protocols is vital to program success.

KEY POINTS

- ◆ Hemorrhage is a major cause of obstetrical morbidity and mortality throughout the world and is the leading reason for obstetrical intensive care unit admissions.
- ◆ Understanding the hemodynamic changes of pregnancy and the physiologic responses that occur with hemorrhage assists in appropriate management. Clinicians should recognize the four classes of hemorrhage in order to allow for intervention.
- ◆ Placental abruption is diagnosed primarily by clinical findings and confirmed by radiographic, laboratory, and pathologic studies. Management of placental abruption is dependent on the severity, gestational age, and maternal-fetal status.
- ◆ Placenta previa is typically diagnosed with sonography. Placenta previa remote from term can be expectantly managed. Outpatient management is possible in selected cases.
- ◆ Placenta previa in association with a prior cesarean delivery is a major risk factor for placenta accreta. Additional radiographic surveillance should be attempted in these cases to provide antenatal diagnosis of placenta accreta.
- ◆ Placenta accreta is best managed with a multidisciplinary approach, including blood conservation teams, anesthesiologists, advanced pelvic surgeons, and urologists.
- ◆ Antenatal detection of vasa previa is possible with sonography and significantly improves perinatal outcomes.
- ◆ Postpartum hemorrhage complicates 1 in 100 to 1 in 20 deliveries. Every obstetrician needs to have a thorough understanding of normal delivery-related blood loss in order to recognize postpartum hemorrhage.
- ◆ Management of uterine atony should follow a rapidly initiated sequenced protocol, including bimanual massage, uterotonic therapy, uterine tamponade, selective arterial embolization, and surgical intervention.
- ◆ Coagulopathy mandates treatment of the initiating event and rapid replacement of consumed blood products. Transfusion of blood components should not be delayed, and replacement protocols should be followed.
- ◆ Blood conservation approaches should be considered if clinically appropriate.
- ◆ Standardized obstetrical hemorrhage management protocols and drills improve outcomes.

REFERENCES

1. Jacobs A: Overview of postpartum hemorrhage. Available at: http://www.uptodate.com Accessed August 2010.
2. World Health Organization, Regional Office for Africa: Available at: http://www.afro.who.int/press/2003. Accessed August 2004.
3. Lochitch G: Clinical biochemistry of pregnancy. Crit Rev Clin Lab Sci 34:67, 1997.
4. Bletka M, Hlavaty V, Trnkova M, et al: Volume of whole blood and absolute amount of serum proteins in the early stage of late toxemia in pregnancy. Am J Obstet Gynecol 106:10, 1970.
5. Ananth CV, Kinzler W: Clinical features and diagnosis of placental abruption. Available at: http://www.uptodate.com. Accessed August 2010.
6. Mackenzie AP, Schatz F, Krikun G, et al: Mechanisms of abruption-induced premature rupture of the fetal membranes: thrombin enhanced decidual matrix metalloproteinase-3 (stromelysin-1) expression. Am J Obstet Gynecol 191:1996, 2004.
7. Lockwood CJ, Toti P, Arcuri F, et al: Mechanisms of abruption-induced premature rupture of the fetal membranes: thrombin-enhanced interleukin-8 expression in term decidua. Am J Pathol 167:1443, 2005.
8. Karegard M, Gennser G: Incidence and recurrence rate of abruption placentae in Sweden. Obstet Gynecol 67:523, 1986.
9. Ananth CV, Oyelese Y, Yeo L, et al: Placental abruption in the United States, 1979 through 2001: temporal trends and potential determinants. Am J Obstet Gynecol 192:191, 2005.
10. Sher G: Pathogenesis and management of uterine inertia complicating abruption placentae with consumption coagulopathy. Am J Obstet Gynecol 129:164, 1977.
11. Oyelese Y, Ananth CV: Placental abruption. Obstet Gynecol 108:1005, 2006.

12. Ananth CV, Berkowitz GS, Savitz DA, et al: Placental abruption and adverse perinatal outcomes. JAMA 282:1646, 1999.
13. Ananth CV, Peltier MR, Kinzler WL, et al: Chronic hypertension and risk of placental abruption: is the association modified by ischemic placental disease? Am J Obstet Gynecol 197:273, 2007.
14. Vintzileos AM, Campbell WA, Nochimson DJ, et al: Preterm premature rupture of membranes: A risk factor for the development of abruptio placentae. Am J Obstet Gynecol 156:1235, 1987.
15. Kramer MS, Usher RH, Pollack R, et al: Etiologic determinants of abruptio placentae. Obstet Gynecol 89:221, 1997.
16. Ananth CV, Savitz DA, Bowes WA Jr, et al: Influence of hypertensive disorders and cigarette smoking on placental abruption and uterine bleeding during pregnancy. Br J Obstet Gynaecol 04:572, 1997.
17. Ananth CV, Smulian JC, Demissie K, et al: Placental abruption among singleton and twin births in the United States: risk factor profiles. Am J Epidemiol 153:177, 2001.
18. Hulse GK, Milne E, English DR, et al: Assessing the relationship between maternal cocaine use and abruptio placentae. Addiction 92:1547, 1997.
19. Harris CM: Trauma and pregnancy. *In* Foley MR, Strong TH Jr, Garite TJ (eds): Obstetric Intensive Care Manual, 2nd ed. New York, McGraw-Hill, 2004, p 239.
20. Naeye R, Harkness WL, Utts J: Abruptio placentae and perinatal death: a prospective study. Am J Obstet Gynecol 128:740, 1977.
21. Sibai BM, Mabie WC, Shamsa F, et al: A comparison of no medication versus methyldopa or labetalol in chronic hypertension during pregnancy. Am J Obstet Gynecol 162:960, 1990.
22. Major CA, deVeciana M, Lewis DF, et al: Preterm premature rupture of membranes and abruptio placentae: Is there an association between these pregnancy complications? Am J Obstet Gynecol 172:672, 1995.
23. Spellacy WN, Handler A, Ferre CD: A case-control study of 1253 twin pregnancies from 1982-1987 perinatal data base. Obstet Gynecol 75:168, 1990.
24. Nurk E, Tell GS, Refsum H, et al: Associations between maternal methylenetetrahydrofolate reductase polymorphisms and adverse outcomes of pregnancy: the Hordaland Homocysteine study. Am J Med 117:26, 2004.
25. Roque H, Paidas MJ, Funal EF, et al: Maternal thrombophilias are not associated with early pregnancy loss. Thromb Haemost 91:290, 2004.
26. Nyberg DA, Mack LA, Benedetti TJ, et al: Placental abruption and placental hemorrhage: correlation of sonographic findings with fetal outcome. Radiology 358:357, 1987.
27. Tikkanen M, Hamalainen E, Nuutila M, et al: Elevated maternal second-trimester serum alpha-fetoprotein as a risk factor for placental abruption. Prenat Diagn 27:240, 2007.
28. Ananth CV, Wilcox AJ: Placental abruption and perinatal mortality in the United States. Am J Epidemiol 153:332, 2001.
29. Towers CV, Pircon RA, Heppard M: Is tocolysis safe in the management of third-trimester bleeding? Am J Obstet Gynecol 180:1572, 1999.
30. Combs C, Nyberg D, Mack L, et al: Expectant management after sonographic diagnosis of placental abruption. Am J Perinatol 9:170, 1992.
31. Saller DJ: Tocolysis in the management of third trimester bleeding. J Perinatol 10:125, 1990.
32. Kayani SI, Walkinshaw SA, Preston C: Pregnancy outcome in severe placental abruption. BJOG 110:679, 2003.
33. Pritchard JA, Brekken AL: Clinical and laboratory studies on severe abruption placenta. Am J Obstet Gynecol 108:22, 1967.
34. Spinillo A, Fazzi E, Stronati E, et al: Severity of abruptio placenta and neurodevelopmental outcome in low birth weight infants. Early Hum Dev 35:44, 1993.
35. Li DK, Wi S: Maternal placental abnormality and the risk of sudden infant death syndrome. Am J Epidemiol 149:608, 1999.
36. Magann EF, Doherty DA, Turner K: Second trimester placental location as a predictor of an adverse pregnancy outcome. J Perinatol 27:9, 2007.
37. Faiz AS, Anath CV: Etiology and risk factors for placenta previa: an overview and metaanalysis of observational studies. J Matern Fetal Neonatal Med 13:175, 2003.
38. Cotton DB, Read JA, Paul RH, et al: The conservative aggressive management of placenta previa. Am J Obstet Gynecol 137:687, 1980.
39. Lavery JP: Placenta previa. Clin Obstet Gynecol 33:414, 1990.
40. Silver R, Depp R, Sabbagha RE, et al: Placenta previa: aggressive expectant management. Am J Obstet Gynecol 150:15, 1984.
41. Abenhaim HA, Azoulay L, Kramer MS: Incidence and risk factors of amniotic fluid embolisms: a population-based study on 3 million births in the United States. Am J Obstet Gynecol 199:49. e1-8, 2008.
42. Ananth CV, Wilcox AJ, Savitz DA, et al: Effect of maternal age and parity on the risk of uteroplacental bleeding disorders in pregnancy. Obstet Gynecol 88:511, 1996.
43. Yang Q, Wu Wen S, Caughey S: Placenta previa: its relationship with race and the country of origin among Asian women. Acta Obstet Gynecol Scand 87:612, 2008.
44. Faiz AS, Ananth CV: Etiology and risk factors for placenta previa: an overview and meta-analysis of observational studies. J Matern Fetal Neonatal Med 13:175, 2003.
45. Ananth CV, Demissie K, Smulian JC: Placenta previa in singleton and twin births in the United States, 1989 through 1998: a comparison of risk factor profiles and associated conditions. Am J Obstet Gynecol 188:275, 2003.
46. Francois K, Johnson J, Harris C: Is placenta previa more common in multiple gestations? Am J Obstet Gynecol 188:1226, 2003.
47. Monica G, Lilja C: Placenta previa, maternal smoking, and recurrence risk. Acta Obstet Gynaecol Scand 74:341, 1995.
48. Taylor VM, Kramer MD, Vaughan TL, et al: Placenta previa and prior cesarean delivery: how strong is the association? Obstet Gynecol 84:55, 1994.
49. Silver RM, Landon MB, Rouse DJ, et al: Maternal morbidity associated with multiple repeat cesarean deliveries. Obstet Gynecol 107:1226, 2006.
50. National Institutes of Health Consensus Development Conference Statement: NIH Consensus Development Conference. Vaginal Birth After Cesarean: New Insights. March 8-10, 2010.
51. Smith RS, Lauria MR, Comstock CM, et al: Transvaginal ultrasonography for all placentas that appear to be low-lying or over the internal cervical os. Ultrasound Obstet Gynecol 9:22, 1997.
52. Dashe JS, McIntire DD, Ramus RM, et al: Persistence of placenta previa according to gestational age at ultrasound detection. Obstet Gynecol 99:692, 2002.
53. Zelop C, Bromley B, Frigoletto FJ, et al: Second trimester sonographically diagnosed placenta previa: prediction of persistent previa at birth. Int J Gynaecol Obstet 44:207, 1994.
54. Wing DA, Paul RH, Millar LK: Management of the symptomatic placenta previa: a randomized, controlled trial of inpatient versus outpatient expectant management. Am J Obstet Gynecol 75:806, 1996.
55. Sharma A, Suri V, Gupta I: Tocolytic therapy in conservative management of symptomatic placenta previa. Int J Gynaecol Obstet 84:109, 2004.
56. Toedt ME: Feasilibity of autologous blood donation in patients with placenta previa. J Fam Pract 48:219, 1999.
57. Wu S, Kocherginsky M, Hibbard JU: Abnormal placentation: twenty-year analysis. Am J Obstet Gynecol 192:1458, 2005.
58. James WH: Sex ratios of offspring and the causes of placental pathology. Hum Reprod 10:1403, 1995.
59. Warshak CR, Ramos GA, Eskander R, et al: Effect of predelivery diagnosis in 99 consecutive cases of placenta accrete. Obstet Gynecol 115:65, 2010.
60. Finberg H, Williams J: Placenta accreta: prospective sonographic diagnosis in patients with placenta previa and prior cesarean section. J Ultrasound Med 11:333, 1992.
61. Chou MM, Ho ES, Lee YH: Prenatal diagnosis of placenta previa accreta by transabdominal color Doppler ultrasound. Ultrasound Obstet Gynecol 15:28, 2000.
62. Twickler DM, Lucas MJ, Balis AB, et al: Color flow mapping for myometrial invasion in women with a prior cesarean delivery. J Matern Fetal Med 9:330, 2000.
63. Maldjian C, Adam R, Pelosi M, et al: MRI appearance of placenta percreta and placenta accreta. Magn Reson Imaging 17:965, 1999.
64. Jaraquemada JM, Bruno CH: Magnetic resonance imaging in 300 cases of placenta accreta: surgical correlation of new findings. Acta Obstet Gynecol Scand 84:716, 2005.
65. Kupferminc MJ, Tamura RK, Wigton TR, et al: Placenta accreta is associated with elevated maternal serum alpha-fetoprotein. Obstet Gynecol 82:266, 1993.
66. Glaze S, Ekwalanga P, Roberts G, et al: Peripartum hysterectomy: 1999 to 2006. Obstet Gynecol 111:732, 2008.

67. Ojala K, Perala J, Kariniemi J, et al: Arterial embolization and prophylactic catheterization for the treatment for severe obstetric hemorrhage. Acta Obstet Gynecol Scand 84:1075, 2005.
68. Sentilhes L, Ambroselli C, Kayem G, et al: Maternal outcome after conservative treatment of placenta accreta. Obstet Gynecol 115:526, 2010.
69. Provansal M, Courbiere B, Agostini A, et al: Fertility and obstetric outcome after conservative management of placenta accreta. Int J Gynaecol Obstet 109:147, 2010.
70. Francois K, Mayer S, Harris, C, et al: Association of vasa previa with a history of second-trimester placenta previa. J Reprod Med 48:771, 2003.
71. Gagnon R, Morin L, Bly S, et al: Guidelines for the management of vasa previa. J Obstet Gynaecol Can 31:748, 2009.
72. Oyelese KO, Turner M, Lees C, et al: Vasa previa: an avoidable obstetric tragedy. Obstet Gynecol Survey 54:138, 1999.
73. Lockwood CJ, Russo-Steiglitz K: Vasa previa and velamentous umbilical cord. Available at: http://www.uptodate.com. Accessed August 2010.
74. Oyelese Y, Catanzarite V, Perfumo F, et al: Vasa previa: the impact of prenatal diagnosis on outcomes. Obstet Gynecol 103:937, 2004.
75. Lu MC, Fridman M, Korst LM: Variations in the incidence of postpartum hemorrhage across hospitals in California. Matern Child Health J 9:297, 2005.
76. Stafford I, Dildy GA, Clark SL: Visually estimated and calculated blood loss in vaginal and cesarean delivery. Am J Obstet Gynecol 199:519. e1-7, 2008.
77. Dildy GA: Postpartum hemorrhage: new management options. Clin Obstet Gynecol 45:330, 2002.
78. Elbourne DR, Prendiville WJ, Carroli G, et al: Prophylactic use of oxytocin in the third stage of labour. Cochrane Database Syst Rev CD001808, 2001.
79. Jackson KW Jr, Allbert JR, Schemmer GK, et al: A randomized controlled trial comparing oxytocin administration before and after placental delivery in prevention of postpartum hemorrhage. Am J Obstet Gynecol 185:873, 2001.
80. McCurdy CM, Magann EF, McCurdy CJ, et al: The effect of placental management at cesarean delivery on operative blood loss. Am J Obstet Gynecol 167:1363, 1993.
81. Munn MB, Owen J, Vincent R, et al: Comparison of two oxytocin regimens to prevent uterine atony at cesarean delivery: a randomized controlled trial. Obstet Gynecol 98:386, 2001.
82. Hofmeyr GJ, Gulmezoglu AM, Novikova N, et al: Misoprostol to prevent and treat postpartum haemorrhage: a systematic review and meta-analysis of maternal deaths and dose-related effects. Bull World Health Org 87:666, 2009.
83. Hsu S, Rodgers B, Lele A, et al: Use of packing in obstetric hemorrhage of uterine origin. J Reprod Med 48:69, 2003.
84. Condous GS, Arulkumaran S, Symonds I, et al: The "tamponade test" in the management of massive postpartum hemorrhage. Obstet Gynecol 101:767, 2003.
85. Sentilhes L, Gromez A, Clavier E, et al: Predictors of failed pelvic arterial embolization for severe postpartum hemorrhage. Obstet Gynecol 113:992, 2009.
86. Mousa HA, Walkinshaw S: Major postpartum haemorrhage. Curr Opin Obstet Gynecol 13:595, 2001.
87. O'Leary JL, O'Leary JA: Uterine artery ligation in the control of intractable postpartum hemorrhage. Am J Obstet Gynecol 94:920, 1966.
88. O'Leary JA: Uterine artery ligation in the control of postcesarean hemorrhage. J Reprod Med 40:189, 1995.
89. Mengert W, Burchell R, Blumstein R, et al: Pregnancy after bilateral ligation of internal iliac and ovarian arteries. Obstet Gynecol 34:664, 1969.
90. Bakri YN, Wilkenson JP: Use of intrauterine balloon catheters for control of uterine hemorrhage. Available at: http://www.uptodate.com. Accessed September 2010.
91. Ferguson JE, Bourgeois FJ, Underwood PB: B-Lynch suture for postpartum hemorrhage. Obstet Gynecol 95:1020, 2000.
92. Ghezzi F, Cromi A, Uccella S, et al: The Hayman technique: a simple method to treat postpartum haemorrhage. BJOG 114:362, 2007.
93. Pereira A, Nunes F, Pedroso S, et al: Compressive uterine sutures to treat postpartum bleeding secondary to uterine atony. Obstet Gynecol 106:569, 2005.
94. Nelson WL, O'Brien JM: The uterine sandwich for persistent uterine atony: combining the B-Lynch compression suture and an intrauterine Bakri balloon. Am J Obstet Gynecol 196:e9, 2007.
95. Wright JD, Bonanno C, Shah M, et al: Peripartum hysterectomy. Obstet Gynecol 116:429, 2010.
96. World Health Organization, Maternal and Child Health and Family Planning: The prevention and management of postpartum haemorrhage. Report of a technical working group. WHO/MCH 90 7:3, 1990.
97. Jha S, Chiu JW, Yeo IS: Intravenous nitro-glycerine versus general anaesthesia for placental extraction: a sequential comparison. Med Sci Monit 9:CS63, 2003.
98. Weeks AD, Alia G, et al. Umbilical vein oxytocin for the treatment of retained placenta (release study): a double-blind randomised controlled trial. Lancet 375:141, 2010.
99. Rogers MS, Yuen PM, Wong S: Avoiding manual removal of placenta: evaluation of intra-umbilical injection of uterotonics using the Pipingas technique for management of adherent placenta. Acta Obstet Gynecol Scand 86:48, 2007.
100. Grobman WA, Lai Y, Landon MB, et al: Prediction of uterine rupture associated with attempted vaginal birth after cesarean delivery. Am J Obstet Gynecol 199:30.e1-5, 2008.
101. Mercer BM, Gilbert S, Landon MB, et al: Labor outcomes with increasing number of prior vaginal births after cesarean delivery. Obstet Gynecol 111:285, 2008.
102. Walsh CA, Baxi LV: Rupture of the primigravid uterus: a review of the literature. Obstet Gynecol Surv 62:327, 2007.
103. Zwart JJ, Richters JM, Ory F, et al: Uterine rupture in the Netherlands: a nationwide population-based cohort study. BJOG 116:1069, 2009.
104. Chauhan SP, Martin JN Jr, Henrichs CE, et al: Maternal and perinatal complications with uterine rupture in 142,075 patients who attempted vaginal birth after cesarean delivery: a review of the literature. Am J Obstet Gynecol 189:408, 2003.
105. Bujold E, Gauthier B: Neonatal morbidity associated with uterine rupture: what are the risk factors? Am J Obstet Gynecol 186:311, 2002.
106. Watson P, Besch N, Bowes WA Jr: Management of acute and subacute puerperal inversion of the uterus. Obstet Gynecol 55:12, 1980.
107. Baskett TF: Acute uterine inversion: a review of 40 cases. J Obstet Gynaecol Can 24:953, 2002.
108. Hseih TT, Lee JD: Sonographic findings in acute puerperal uterine inversion. J Clin Ultrasound 19:306, 1991.
109. Smith GN, Brien JF: Use of nitroglycerin for uterine relaxation. Obstet Gynecol Surv 53:559, 1998.
110. Tan KH, Luddin NS: Hydrostatic reduction of acute uterine inversion. Int J Gynaecol Obstet 91:63, 2005.
111. Sardeshpande NS, Sawant RM, Sardeshpande SN, et al: Laparoscopic correction of chronic uterine inversion. J Minim Invasive Gynecol 16:646, 2009.
112. Alfirevic Z, Elbourne D, Pavord S, et al: Use of recombinant activated factor VII in primary postpartum hemorrhage: the Northern European registry 2000-2004. Obstet Gynecol 110:1270, 2007.
113. Ramin SM, Ramin KD: Emergency delivery in women with disseminated intravascular coagulopathy. Available at: http://www.uptodate.com. Accessed September 2010.
114. Burtelow M, Riley E Druzin M, et al: How we treat: management of life-threatening primary postpartum hemorrhage with a standardized massive transfusion protocol. Transfusion 47:1564, 2007.
115. Holcomb JB, Wade CE, Michalek JE, et al: Increased plasma and platelet to red blood cell ratios improves outcome in 466 massively transfused civilian trauma patients. Ann Surg 24:447, 2008.
116. Shaz BH, Dente CJ, Nicholas J, et al: Increased number of coagulation products in relationship to red blood cell products transfused improves mortality in trauma patients. Transfusion 50:493, 2010.
117. Ibojie J, Greiss MA, Urbaniak SJ: Limited efficacy of universal leucodepletion in reducing the incidence of febrile nonhaemolytic reactions in red cell transfusions. Transfus Med 12:181, 2002.
118. Spelman D, MacLaren G: Transfusion-transmitted bacterial infection. Available at: http://www.uptodate.com. Accessed September 2010.

119. Silliman CC, Paterson AJ, Dickey WO, et al: The association of biologically active lipids with the development of transfusion-related acute lung injury: a retrospective study. Transfusion 37:719, 1997.
120. Martin SR, Strong TH Jr: Transfusion of blood components and derivatives in the obstetric intensive care patient. *In* Foley MR, Strong TH Jr, Garite TJ (eds): Obstetric Intensive Care Manual, 2nd ed. New York, McGraw-Hill, 2004, p 19.
121. Rebarber A, Lonser R, Jackson S, et al: The safety of intraoperative autologous blood collection and autotransfusion during cesarean section. Am J Obstet Gynecol 179:715, 1998.
122. Skupski DW, Lowenwirt IP, Weinbaum FI, et al: Improving hospital systems for the care of women with major obstetric hemorrhage. Obstet Gynecol 107:977, 2006.

For full reference list, log onto www.expertconsult.com.

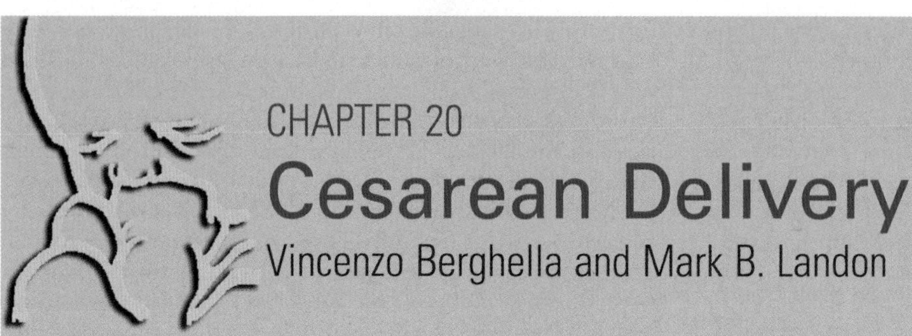

CHAPTER 20

Cesarean Delivery

Vincenzo Berghella and Mark B. Landon

KEY ABBREVIATIONS	
American College of Obstetricians and Gynecologists	ACOG
Cephalopelvic Disproportion	CPD
Computed Tomography	CT
Deep Venous Thrombosis	DVT
Fetal Heart Rate	FHR
Hypoxic-Ischemic Encephalopathy	HIE
Maternal-Fetal Medicine Units	MFMU
National Institute of Child Health and Human Development	NICHD
National Institutes of Health	NIH
Odds Ratio	OR
Pulmonary Embolus	PE
Relative Risk	RR
Trial of Labor After Cesarean	TOLAC
Vaginal Birth After Cesarean Delivery	VBAC

DEFINITIONS

Cesarean section has classically been defined as delivery of a fetus through a surgically created incision in the anterior uterine wall. Because cesarean and section both refer to an incision, some prefer the terms *cesarean delivery* and *cesarean birth* to describe the procedure. *Primary cesarean* is the "first-time" operation, whereas *repeat cesarean* refers to the operation done after a prior cesarean. This chapter reviews the history, incidence, indications, techniques, and complications of cesarean delivery.

HISTORY OF CESAREAN DELIVERY

Cesarean delivery has been described since ancient times, and there is evidence from both early Western and non-Western societies of this surgical procedure being performed. The evolution of the term "cesarean" has been debated over time. Although this term was originally believed to have been derived from the birth of Julius Caesar, it is unlikely that his mother, Aurelia, would have survived the operation. Her knowledge of her son's invasion of Europe many years later indicates that she survived childbirth. In Caesar's time, surgical delivery was reserved for cases when the mother was dead or dying. Roman law under Numa Pompilius first ("Lex Regia"), then renamed after Caesar ("Lex Cesarea"), specified surgical removal of the fetus before burial of deceased pregnant women. Religious edicts required separate burial for the infant and mother. The term cesarean may also refer to being cut open because the Latin verb *caedare* means to cut. Cesarean operation was the preferred term before the 1598 publication of Guillimeau, who introduced the term "section."

Although sporadic reports of heroic life-saving efforts through cesarean childbirth existed for hundreds of years, it was not until the later part of the 19th century that the operation began to be established as part of obstetrical practice. This coincided with the gradual transition of childbirth as primarily a midwife-attended event, often in rural settings, to an urban hospital experience. The wide emergence of hospitals laid the foundation for establishing obstetrics as a hospital-based specialty. As new methods for anesthesia emerged, cesarean delivery for obstructed labor gained popularity over destructive procedures such as craniotomy accompanying difficult vaginal births. Despite the dangers that still existed with cesarean delivery, the operation was viewed as preferable to a difficult high forceps delivery, which was associated with fetal injury and deep pelvic lacerations. Whereas refinements in anesthesia techniques allowed the operation to be performed, mortality rates remained very high, with sepsis and peritonitis as leading causes of postoperative deaths. Primitive surgical techniques and lack of antisepsis clearly contributed to such outcomes. Surgeons attempted to complete the operation without closing the uterus, fearing that the suture material itself would promote infection and that the uterus would best heal by intention. As a result, women were placed at risk for both hemorrhage and infection.

In 1876, Eduardo Porro advocated hysterectomy with cesarean delivery in order to control bleeding and to prevent postoperative infection. Shortly thereafter, surgeons gained experience with internal suturing because silver wire stitches were developed by the gynecologist J. Marion Sims. Sims had perfected the use of these sutures in the treatment of vesicovaginal fistulas resulting from obstructed labors.

As gynecologic surgeons performed more cesarean deliveries and the outcomes improved, greater attention was placed on technique, including the site of uterine incision. Between 1880 and 1925, surgeons began employing transverse incisions of the uterus. It was noted that such incisions reduced the rate of infection and the risk for rupture with subsequent pregnancies. However, owing to the risk for peritonitis, extraperitoneal cesarean was advocated by Frank (1907) and Latzko (1909) and was popularized by Beck (1919) in the United States.

The introduction of penicillin in 1940 dramatically reduced the risks for infection associated with childbirth. As antibiotic therapy emerged, the need for extraperitoneal dissection and incision diminished. The low cervical incision introduced by Munro Kerr (1926) became further established as the technique of choice. As technology, including improved anesthesia, developed and the medical management of pregnancy and childbirth accelerated, cesarean delivery became more commonplace in obstetrics. Given its current safety and effectiveness, a liberalized approach to using cesarean childbirth has emerged in the United States over the past 40 years.

INCIDENCE

Trends in Cesarean Delivery Rates

The cesarean delivery rate describes the proportion of women undergoing cesarean delivery of all women giving birth during a specific time period. The cesarean delivery rate may be further subdivided into the primary and the repeat cesarean delivery rates, both as a proportion of the entire obstetrical population. **Cesarean delivery rates have risen in the United States in a dramatic fashion from less than 5% in the 1960s to 32.8% by 2008. Among the reasons for this increase are (1) continued increase in primary cesarean deliveries for dystocia, failed induction, and abnormal presentation; (2) an increase in the proportion of women with obesity, diabetes mellitus, and multiple gestation, which predispose to cesarean delivery; (3) increased practice of cesarean delivery on request; and (4) limited use of trial of labor after cesarean (TOLAC) delivery owing to both safety and medicolegal concerns** (Table 20-1).

A recent increase in international cesarean delivery rates has also been documented, with some countries with cesarean rates in the 40% (e.g., Italy), or even higher (e.g., Brasil), range.

Given the discrepancy in cesarean delivery rates between the United States and other countries without a perceivable benefit in neonatal outcomes, health policy groups have critically evaluated this issue, including its cause and possible solutions. Twenty-five years ago, the National Institutes of Health (NIH) established a task force on cesarean childbirth and sponsored a consensus development conference on this subject. It was recognized that almost all of the increase in cesarean section rates was due to increased repeat operations and primary cesarean deliveries for dystocia and fetal distress (see Table 20-1). With expanding indications for cesarean delivery, and little enthusiasm for vaginal birth after cesarean delivery (VBAC) before 1980, it was obvious that prior cesarean delivery had emerged as a major indication. Dystocia was also being diagnosed more frequently through the 1970s and 1980s, along with a parallel decline in operative vaginal delivery rates. Not surprisingly, the increased cesarean delivery rates in the United States compared with other countries can be explained almost entirely by cephalopelvic disproportion and repeat cesarean delivery as the dominant indications for the operation.

Fear of litigation is also recognized as liberalizing the indications for cesarean section, particularly with respect to labor management and the diagnosis of non-reassuring fetal heart rate (FHR) patterns. The widespread use of intrapartum electronic FHR monitoring has been cited

TABLE 20-1 FACTORS RESPONSIBLE FOR INCREASED CESAREAN DELIVERY RATES

Obstetrical Factors
Increased primary cesarean delivery rate
Failed induction and increased use of induction of labor
Decreased use of operative vaginal delivery
Increased macrosomia and cesarean delivery for macrosomia
Decline in vaginal breech delivery
Increased repeat cesarean delivery rate
Decreased use of vaginal birth after cesarean delivery
Maternal Factors
Increased proportion of women older than 35 years
Increased proportion of nulliparous women
Increased primary cesarean deliveries on maternal request
Physician Factors
Malpractice litigation concerns

as a factor in increasing the diagnosis of non-reassuring FHR and thus cesarean delivery. The NIH task force recommended that both dystocia and repeat cesarean deliveries clearly required further study and institution of strategies to reduce their contribution to the overall rise in cesarean delivery. This recommendation was appealing in that these two categories contributed greatly to the rise in cesarean section, and they represent indications that would likely be amenable to a reduction since physician practice patterns clearly influence these categories of cesarean delivery.

Cesarean delivery accounts for more than 1 million major operations performed annually in the United States.[1] It is the most common major surgical procedure undertaken today. **Following efforts championed by institutions and payers to reduce the cesarean section rate, between 1988 and 1996, the overall cesarean delivery rate in the United States fell from 24.7% to a nadir of 20.7%. This decline can be largely attributed to the increased practice of TOLAC after prior cesarean birth. However, over the past decade, cesarean rates have steadily climbed and exceed those of the late 1980s. This rise is reflected by an increase in the primary cesarean rate and a steep drop in the rate of vaginal births after previous cesarean deliveries. VBAC rates plummeted from a peak of 28.3% in 1996 to 9.2% in 2004** (Figure 20-1).

The rise in cesarean section rates has prompted increased interest in the indications, complications, and techniques involved with this procedure. Despite clear documentation of the prevalence of cesarean section, there is remarkably little prospectively gathered information concerning a variety of issues related to abdominal delivery. The overwhelming economic burden of cesarean birth on health care delivery continues to focus efforts on strategies aimed at reducing cesarean delivery rates. Because cesarean section carries with it a risk for uncommon complications such as maternal mortality and more often observed infectious complications extending the mother's length of stay in the hospital, cesarean section data continue to be employed as an indicator to reflect overall quality of care for obstetrical services. The appropriate use of a TOLAC

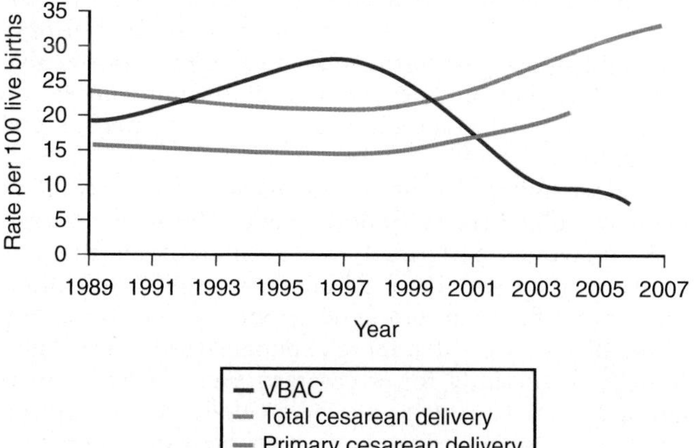

FIGURE 20-1. Total and primary cesarean rate and vaginal birth after previous cesarean (VBAC): United States, 1989 to 2006. (Data from National Center for Health Statistics: Births: final data for 2005. National Vital Statistics Report 57[7], 2009.)

in women with a prior cesarean section has also been a focus for providers and payers of obstetrical care.

Monitoring Cesarean Delivery Rates

It is not possible to determine an optimal cesarean delivery rate because an "ideal" rate must be a function of multiple clinical factors that vary in each population and are influenced by the level of obstetrical care provided. Further complicating this issue is the absence of complete and accurate data that focus on both maternal and infant outcomes. Thus, although cesarean delivery rates can be considered a measure of a specific health care process (mode of delivery), these rates are not outcome measures because they do not indicate whether cesarean or vaginal birth results in optimal perinatal outcomes. Maternal and perinatal morbidity and mortality should be the outcomes most monitored to ensure best quality of care. Higher cesarean delivery rates have been associated with better perinatal outcomes in several studies. So, instead of setting goals or limits for overall cesarean delivery rates, it is most important to monitor maternal and perinatal health outcomes. We would all agree with a 0% or 100% cesarean delivery rate if either of these were associated with the lowest incidences of complications for mother or baby. The optimal cesarean delivery rate in the early 21st century is in between these extremes and depends on the population.

Despite little consensus regarding the best mode of delivery for many complicated pregnancies, third-party payers and institutions continue to rely on expert opinion concerning optimal cesarean delivery rates without the benefit of risk stratification. It follows that institutions involved in tertiary obstetrical care thus managing a large number of preterm deliveries and maternal complications of pregnancy should have higher cesarean rates than primary care facilities. Several models have been developed to provide risk-adjusted cesarean delivery rates. Use of hospital billing information consisting of International Classification of Diseases codes is a common methodology; however, important information such as parity and other demographics are lacking with this approach. In contrast, Leiberman and colleagues employed a case-mix system, which stratified women according to parity, prior cesarean delivery, presentation, gestational age, and the presence of medical conditions precluding a TOLAC. In their study, the crude cesarean delivery rate was higher for hospital-based practice physicians (24.4%) than for community-based practitioners (21.5%). However, the proportion of women falling into categories conferring a high risk for cesarean delivery was twice as high for the hospital-based practice. Standardizing the case mix resulted in an overall cesarean rate of 20.1% for the hospital-based physicians.

In 2000, the American College of Obstetricians and Gynecologists (ACOG) developed a simple formula to help institutions and physicians assess their risk-adjusted cesarean delivery rates.[1] Two populations were targeted that included (1) nulliparous women with a singleton vertex gestation at 37 weeks or greater without other complications; and (2) women with one prior low-transverse cesarean delivery, delivering a single vertex fetus at 37 weeks or greater without other complications. The use of these simple case-mix adjusted rates should make comparative evaluation of cesarean delivery rates and their comparison to maternal and perinatal outcomes more meaningful. As data become more unified and methodologically sound, the quality of obstetrical care can be better assessed.

Using raw and risk-adjusted data, institutions have sought to reduce cesarean birth rates through quality improvement initiatives. Myers and Gleicher successfully reduced overall cesarean rates from 17.5% to 11.9% after developing guidelines in concert with a comprehensive data collection process and intensive feedback to physicians. Outliers were identified and subjected to "one-on-one" reviews of their individual practices. Other successful programs aimed at lowering cesarean rates have also relied on the combination of providing quality data and counseling to physicians who become invested in changing their practice pattern.[1] **The 2000 ACOG report on evaluation of cesarean delivery concludes with two major observations:**

1. **Improved residency or postresidency training in operative (forceps or vacuum-assisted) vaginal delivery is recommended to foster better understanding of the use of these techniques and the normal progression of labor. Surveys show that operative vaginal delivery is less than 15% among ACOG Fellows and residents in the United States, yet safe use of these techniques may help reduce the cesarean delivery rate** (see Chapter 15).
2. **Certain management practices may affect cesarean delivery rates, so institutions and physicians should consider some changes if their cesarean delivery rates are believed to be too high. The continuous presence of nurses or other trained individuals who provide comfort and support to women in labor may lead to lower rates. In addition, 24-hour dedicated in-house obstetrical coverage by hospitals and practice groups may help reduce cesarean delivery rates.**

INDICATIONS FOR CESAREAN DELIVERY

Indications for cesarean delivery can be divided in maternal-fetal, fetal, and maternal. The most common current indications are, in order of frequency, failure to progress (also called *cephalopelvic disproportion*, or *dystocia*) (about 30%), prior cesarean (i.e., repeat cesarean) (30%), non-reassuring FHR patterns (10%), and fetal malpresentation (10%) (Table 20-2).

TABLE 20-2 COMMON INDICATIONS FOR CESAREAN DELIVERY

Maternal-Fetal
Cephalopelvic disproportion
Placental abruption
Placenta previa
Repeat cesarean delivery
Cesarean delivery on maternal request
Maternal
Specific cardiac disease (e.g., Marfan syndrome, unstable coronary artery disease)
Specific respiratory disease (e.g., Guillain-Barré syndrome)
Conditions associated with increased intracranial pressure
Mechanical obstruction of the lower uterine segment (tumors, fibroids)
Mechanical vulvar obstruction (e.g. extensive condylomata)
Fetal
Non-reassuring fetal status
Breech or transverse lie
Maternal herpes
Congenital anomalies

Maternal-Fetal Indications

Most cesarean deliveries are performed for conditions that might pose a threat to both mother and fetus if vaginal delivery occurred. Placenta previa and placental abruption with the potential for hemorrhage are clear examples. Dystocia presents a risk for both direct fetal and maternal trauma. It may also compromise fetal oxygenation and metabolic status. **Cephalopelvic disproportion (CPD) is a diagnosis that is generally made on a relative basis after a trial of sufficient labor, often with oxytocin augmentation. The criteria for CPD remain subjective, and at present, norms for progress during labor have been challenged.** Although failure to make sufficient progress in the active phase of labor has been attributed to deficiencies in uterine activity ("power"), large baby ("passenger"), and unfavorable maternal pelvis ("passage"), the failure to progress may also be the potential of varying physician approaches to the management of labor itself. **The proper length of time for an adequate TOLAC with oxytocin stimulation in protraction disorders is undefined, with most practitioners allowing "a few hours." Because it has been shown that oxytocin has not been employed at all in many cesarean deliveries performed for dystocia, it can be concluded that inadequate trials of oxytocin stimulation may be a significant factor in the performance of some unnecessary cesarean deliveries.**

Blumenthal and colleagues found a large difference between the incidence of dystocia in public and private patients and concluded that the difference probably resulted from differences in criteria used for the two groups. However, they were unable to determine whether the difference resulted from excessive intervention in the private group or from less than optimal intervention in the public groups. Haynes de Regt and colleagues similarly demonstrated an overall cesarean section rate of 17.1% in nonprivate versus 21.4% in private patients. In this study, private patients giving birth to their first child were significantly more likely than clinic patients to undergo cesarean delivery if dystocia, malpresentation, or fetal distress were diagnosed. Unfortunately, this large retrospective study could not provide detailed information concerning criteria used to diagnose both dystocia and suspected fetal compromise.

Understanding that physician characteristics may affect cesarean delivery rates, Berkowitz and colleagues analyzed 6327 deliveries performed by 48 different practitioners between 1983 and 1985. Although no significant differences were found according to gender or practice setting of the physicians, older, more experienced physicians performed significantly fewer cesarean sections for dystocia and a higher percentage of forceps deliveries for breech extractions. This finding is of great interest inasmuch as Frigoletto and coworkers noted that between 30% and 40% of primary cesarean deliveries at both Brigham and Women's Hospital and Northwestern University are performed during the second stage of labor, in contrast to less than 5% at the National Maternity Hospital in Dublin. These findings may provide insight into potential strategies to further reduce cesarean deliveries performed for dystocia.

Fetal Indications

Fetal indications are primarily recognized by non-reassuring FHR testing with the potential for long-term consequences of metabolic acidosis. Somewhere between 1% and 3% of women undergo cesarean section for a non-reassuring FHR pattern. The diagnosis of *fetal distress* (a term ACOG prefers to avoid) has been cited as the third leading cause for the rise in cesarean birth over the past several decades. It is noteworthy that no apparent reduction in the frequency of cerebral palsy has accompanied this rise and has led to challenging the benefit of continuous electronic fetal monitoring and associated increases in the cesarean delivery rate. Haverkamp and colleagues first noted that cesarean delivery is more often performed for labor abnormalities in women who undergo continuous fetal monitoring compared with controls. This finding is of particular interest considering a more recent randomized trial involving the use of continuous fetal pulse oximetry during labor. Whereas women monitored with this device demonstrated a 50% reduction in the number of cesarean deliveries for non-reassuring fetal status compared with continuous FHR monitoring, the overall cesarean delivery rates between study groups was not different. The women monitored with fetal pulse oximetry had an increased rate of cesarean delivery for dystocia.

Other fetal indications for cesarean delivery include risk for transmission of infection or potential for fetal trauma. Examples of these categories would include active maternal herpes infection and breech delivery, in which head entrapment is a possibility. By the mid-1990s, the cesarean delivery rate for breech presentation had reached nearly 85% in the United States, and following current recommendations from ACOG, it will likely rise further. Excessive fetal size or suspected macrosomia has been increasingly designated as an indication for cesarean delivery, yet little data exist to support this approach in the nondiabetic woman. Fetuses with certain birth defects such as hydrocephalus with macrocephaly and neural tube defects have traditionally undergone cesarean delivery, yet insufficient data exist to make this an absolute indication. Similarly, few data exist to suggest a benefit for cesarean delivery with fetal abdominal wall defects, such as omphalocele and gastroschisis.

Maternal Indications

Maternal indications for cesarean delivery are relatively few and can be considered as medical or mechanical in nature (see Table 20-2). Most of these indications are not based on evidence from randomized trials. Although somewhat debatable, certain maternal cardiac conditions such as unstable ischemic coronary artery disease and a dilated aortic root with Marfan syndrome have been considered indications for cesarean section. These diagnoses may pose a risk for deterioration of maternal condition with the stress of labor. Serious respiratory disease requiring assisted ventilation and conditions resulting in altered mental status might also mandate cesarean delivery. Central nervous system abnormalities in which increased intracranial pressure such as accompanies the second stage of labor would be undesirable have also led some to recommend cesarean section.

Alterations in the capacity of the maternal pelvis can be indications for cesarean delivery. Mechanical vaginal obstruction due to pelvic masses such as lower segment myomata or ovarian neoplasm are examples. Finally, women with massive condylomata may require cesarean section as well.

Cesarean Delivery on Maternal Request

As cesarean delivery has become safer, women have occasionally voiced their wish for a cesarean without a medical indication with their obstetrician. This clinical scenario has been recently called "cesarean delivery on maternal request." **The lack of specificity of the term "elective" suggests the most reasonable and prudent course of action is to not use it, but rather to document the specific indication (whether medical or nonmedical) for the intervention or procedure (i.e., cesarean delivery on maternal request).** At times, physicians have also advocated cesarean as the preferred mode of delivery, even in the absence of accepted indications as described previously. We would term this scenario "cesarean delivery on physician request."

Feldman and Freiman first proposed cesarean delivery to prevent fetal morbidity and mortality associated with intrapartum events. In their 1985 publication, the fetal benefits of "elective" cesarean were weighed against the increased risk for maternal mortality with cesarean section. The increasing safety of cesarean delivery over the next 20 years and emergence of improved data concerning benefits and risks has rekindled interest in this subject. In 2000, Harer endorsed cesarean delivery, citing better infant outcomes compared with vaginal birth as well as lower rates of pelvic floor injury.

The decision to plan a cesarean or a vaginal birth should be based on the best literature available comparing these choices. Cases in which cesarean (or vaginal) delivery is indicated for accepted indications as described previously should be excluded from this comparison. The NIH and ACOG have carefully reviewed the literature on this topic.[2,3] NIH and ACOG reported that there is no high-quality evidence to compare planned cesarean to planned vaginal delivery because there are no randomized studies for most women—those with a singleton gestation in vertex presentation at term. Moderate-quality evidence shows that planned cesarean is associated with less postpartum hemorrhage, more mild neonatal respiratory morbidity, longer maternal hospital stay, and possibly greater complications in subsequent pregnancies[2,3] (Table 20-3). **Cesarean delivery on maternal request is not recommended for women desiring several children because there is a direct association with an increasing number of cesarean deliveries and increasing life-threatening complications such as placenta previa, placenta accreta, and the need for cesarean hysterectomy.**[3] Cesarean delivery on maternal request is unfortunately performed at times because of maternal fear of excessive pain. Fear of childbirth is present in about 3% to 8% of women. These women should be reassured of adequate maternal pain

TABLE 20-3 RISKS AND BENEFITS OF CESAREAN DELIVERY ON MATERNAL REQUEST (OR WITHOUT MEDICAL INDICATIONS)

Potential Benefits
Reduction in perinatal morbidity and mortality
Elimination of intrapartum events associated with perinatal asphyxia
Reduction in traumatic birth injuries
Reduction in stillbirth beyond 39 weeks' gestation
Possible protective effect against pelvic floor dysfunction
Less postpartum hemorrhage
Potential Risks
Increased short-term maternal morbidity
Increased endometritis, transfusion, venous thrombosis rates
Increased length of stay and longer recovery time
Increased short-term neonatal morbidity
Increased mild neonatal respiratory morbidity
Increased long-term maternal and neonatal morbidity
Increased risk for placenta accreta, hysterectomy with subsequent cesarean deliveries

relief in labor and directly reassured and counseled regarding TOLAC.

All remaining comparisons, discussed later, are based on weak evidence and should not decisively sway clinical decisions. Perinatal mortality has been reported to be several times lower with a planned cesarean delivery compared with labor and vaginal birth. Additionally, hypoxic-ischemic encephalopathy (HIE) of the newborn related to intrapartum events, including abruption, cord prolapse, and progressive asphyxia, may occur in approximately 1 in 3000 to 5000 births. Many of these cases presumably would be prevented by planned cesarean delivery, as would unexplained stillbirths occurring beyond 39 weeks' gestation. Traumatic birth injuries, including intracranial hemorrhage, fractures, and brachial plexus injury, are reduced with cesarean delivery as well.

Increased maternal risks attributed to vaginal delivery include urinary and fetal incontinence, pelvic prolapse, and sexual dysfunction. The precise contribution of vaginal delivery versus pregnancy and labor to these complications has been difficult to ascertain. In a survey of 2000 women, Wilson and colleagues reported a prevalence of incontinence of 24.5% following vaginal delivery compared with 5.2% after cesarean section. In primiparous women, cesarean delivery significantly reduced the risk for incontinence (relative risk [RR] = 0.2) compared with vaginal birth. However, these authors noted that in women with more than three cesarean deliveries, no difference was noted compared with rates in women delivered vaginally. In a Norwegian study of 15,000 women, Rortveit reported a 10.1% rate of incontinence in nulliparous women, 15.9% in those having cesarean section, and 21% in the vaginal delivery group. These authors concluded that pregnancy itself can cause pelvic floor damage and that cesarean delivery may not be completely protective. MacLennan's survey of 3000 women also supports an increased risk for prolapse with all methods of delivery. The author concluded that pregnancy, more than mode of delivery, appeared to contribute to long-term pelvic floor damage. Nonetheless, Minkoff and Chervenak assert that a policy of prophylactic cesarean delivery might reduce the risk for significant urinary incontinence from 10% to 5%.

The maternal risks of cesarean delivery have been considered marginal compared with those of vaginal delivery. Rates of maternal mortality (excluding indicated cesarean deliveries) are comparable to vaginal delivery. Sachs and colleagues reported a cesarean mortality rate of 22.3 per 100,000 compared with 10.9 per 100,000 for vaginal delivery; however, the rates were comparable excluding medical complications. A British survey reported one death in 78,000 cesarean deliveries, which was lower than the rate for vaginal births. In contrast, a population-based 7-year study (1992 to 1998) revealed cesarean section to be associated with a fourfold increased risk for maternal death, when controlling for various pregnancy complications.

Cesarean delivery does increase maternal morbidity. The rate of endometritis (3.0%) versus vaginal birth (0.4%) is increased, yet one study indicates comparable rates of postpartum hemorrhage, transfusion, and deep venous thrombosis (DVT). Other reports confirm increased risks for these morbidities with cesarean section, including major complication rates as high as 4.5%. **Cesarean delivery also presents a risk for future placental abnormalities, including placenta previa and placenta accreta. These risks increase with the increasing number of cesarean deliveries performed for each woman and are substantial with more than three operations. Thus, the decision to undergo cesarean delivery on request must include thoughtful consideration of future childbearing plans.**

When a cesarean delivery is performed without accepted indications, but for either maternal or physician request, it should be performed at 39 weeks.[2-4] After appropriate counseling, if the woman still insists on cesarean delivery on maternal request, implementing the woman's request is ethically permissible. Less than 10% of women prefer a cesarean delivery based solely on their request.

TECHNIQUE OF CESAREAN SECTION

Because more than 500,000 cesarean deliveries are performed in the United States every year, and about 20 million worldwide, it extremely important to adhere to the safest, most effective technique that is associated with the lowest perinatal and maternal complications. Each aspect of cesarean delivery should be evaluated individually, optimally by randomized trials, because it is impossible to evaluate the benefit of a technical aspect if this is studied together with others. Proper universal surgical precautions aimed at preventing blood loss and infections should be employed. Preferred technical aspects of cesarean delivery are shown in Table 20-4.

Prophylactic Pre-cesarean Interventions, Including Antibiotics and Thromboprophylaxis

Prophylactic antibiotics are of clear benefit in reducing the frequency of postcesarean endomyometritis and wound infection in both laboring and nonlaboring cesarean delivery.[5] Timing, agents, and dose of prophylactic antibiotics have been extensively studied.[6]

Prophylactic antibiotics should be given, if possible, about 30 minutes before skin incision for cesarean.[7] The preferred agent for prophylaxis is either ampicillin or a

TABLE 20-4 EVIDENCE-BASED RECOMMENDATIONS FOR CESAREAN DELIVERY TECHNIQUES

- No preoperative hair removal; or clipping or depilatory creams on the day of surgery or the preceding day (no shaving)
- No specific antiseptic for preoperative bathing
- Antibiotic prophylaxis with ampicillin or a first-generation cephalosporin 30 minutes before skin incision (one dose)
- Spinal and epidural anesthesia preferred to general anesthesia
- Chlorhexidine-alcohol for skin preparation
- Transverse lower abdominal wall opening using Pfannenstiel or Joel-Cohen-based methods
- Mostly blunt dissection of subcutaneous fat layer
- Low-transverse uterine incision initially done with scalpel
- Blunt uterine incision expansion, with cephalad-caudad traction
- Spontaneous placental removal with cord traction
- Extra-abdominal (exteriorization) or intra-abdominal repair of the uterus
- Uterine closure with single-layer continuous locking suture has short-term benefits. However, the evidence from observational studies of an increased risk for scar rupture favors the use of double-layer closure pending evidence on this outcome from randomized trials.
- Nonclosure of both peritoneal layers
- Closure of the subcutaneous tissues when the thickness is ≥2 cm.
- No routine drainage of the subcutaneous tissues
- Closure of skin with staples (leave in at least 4 days) or sutures

(Modified from Berghella V, Baxter JK, Chauhan SP: Evidence-based surgery for cesarean delivery. Am J Obstet Gynecol 193:107, 2005.)

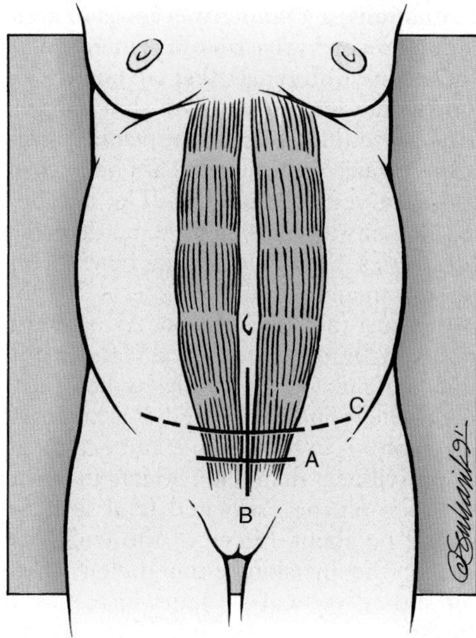

FIGURE 20-2. The obstetrician most commonly uses the Pfannenstiel abdominal incision for cesarean **(A)**. Other, much less common incisions are midline **(B)** and Maylard **(C)** incisions. *Hatched lines* indicate possible extension. (Modified from Baker C, Shingleton HM: Incisions. Clin Obstet Gynecol 31:701, 1988.)

first-generation cephalosporin (e.g., cefazolin).[6] For women with an anaphylactic allergic reaction to penicillin, either metronidazole or clindamycin and gentamicin can be used. There is no apparent advantage to more broad-spectrum antibiotic prophylaxis (e.g., azithromycin or metronidazole[8,9]), except perhaps for women who do not get antibiotic prophylaxis before cesarean delivery, high-risk populations, and use of drugs effective against *Ureaplasma urealiticum*.[10] Single-dose therapy is as effective as multidose therapy[11,12] and is therefore preferred.

For women with clinical chorioamnionitis, treatment with combination antibiotic therapy (e.g., UNASYN, ampicillin sodium/sulbactam sodium) supplants the need for prophylaxis. This therapy should be instituted promptly before delivery and continued until the patient exhibits a clinical response.

Because venous thromboembolism (VTE) is the leading cause of maternal mortality in developed countries, and cesarean delivery increases this risk, thromboprophylaxis should be considered in all cesarean deliveries. There is an insufficient number of women randomized to either heparin or no heparin to assess its safety and efficacy.[13] Mechanical prophylaxis, with graduated compression stockings or a pneumatic compression device during and after cesarean delivery until ambulation is restarted, is suggested. Women with additional risk factors (e.g., morbid obesity, prior VTE, immobility) may benefit from medical thromboprophylaxis (e.g., with prophylactic heparin after cesarean).

Lateral tilt of about 15 degrees elevating the mother's right side; left lateral tilt, head-up, or head-down position; and the use of wedges and cushions, flexion of the table, and a mechanical displacer have been insufficiently studied to provide any strong recommendation for clinical use.[14]

Vaginal irrigation with chlorhexidine has not been associated with a decrease in maternal or neonatal infections.[15]

Site Preparation

Preparation of the skin is performed to reduce the risk for wound infection by decreasing the amount of skin flora and contaminants at the incision site. Hair does not have to be removed from the operative site. Removal with a razor may actually increase the risk for infection by breaks in the skin allowing entry of bacteria. For this reason, some advocate clipping of the hair before surgery.[16] Only enough hair should be removed to allow good approximation of skin edges.

Incision site preparation is accomplished in the operating room through application of a surgical scrub. Cesarean delivery wounds are considered to be clean contaminated. Chlorhexidine-alcohol scrub is the scrub we use because it has been associated with a lower incidence of wound infections compared with povidone-iodine scrub.[17]

Drapes should not be adhesive because adhesive drapes have been associated with higher rate of wound infections compared with nonadhesive drapes.[18,19]

Abdominal Incision Type and Dissection

In general, universally accepted good surgical techniques, aimed at avoiding excessive blood loss and tissue trauma, should be employed.[20] The use of blunt needles during a cesarean delivery is associated with a decrease in rate of surgeon glove perforation, but also a decrease in the surgeon's satisfaction, compared with sharp needles.[21]

The surgeon has a choice of a transverse or vertical skin incision, with the transverse Pfannenstiel being the most common incision type in the United States (Figure 20-2). **Factors that influence the type of incision include the urgency of the delivery, prior incision type, and the potential need to explore the upper abdomen for nonobstetrical pathology. Although some prefer a vertical incision in**

emergent situations, a Pfannenstiel incision actually adds only 1 minute extra operative time in primary and 2 minutes in repeat cesareans, differences that are not associated with improved neonatal outcomes.[22] The skin incision used in the previous procedure is usually repeated in most cesarean deliveries. Transverse incisions are more cosmetic and less painful than vertical incisions. The authors prefer a transverse Pfannenstiel incision for more than 90% of their cesarean deliveries. Studies reporting benefits of the Joel-Cohen incision include multiple aspects of the cesarean technique, not just the skin incision. As stated previously, studies evaluating multiple technical features of the cesarean delivery together are not clinically helpful.[23] When a transverse skin incision is employed, it is made about 3 cm above the symphysis in the midline and extended laterally in a slightly curvilinear manner. The length of the incision should be based on the estimated fetal size. At term, it usually should be about 15 cm, or the length of an Allis clamp. Site of the incision, either below or above the pannus, or either vertical or transverse, has not been sufficiently studied in obese individuals to provide an evidence-based recommendation.

Occasionally, a transverse incision of the rectus sheath and muscles (Maylard incision) is necessary for proper exposure and room to deliver the fetus. In these cases, only the medial half of the muscle is incised to avoid lacerating the deep epigastric vessels. Complete transection of the rectus muscles is the Cherney incision, which requires identification of the epigastric vessels and ligation bilaterally.

The subcutaneous tissue can then be bluntly pushed away to identify the underlying fascia. In repeat operations, sharp dissection of the subcutaneous adipose tissue may be required. The fascia is incised and dissected or bluntly extended in a curvilinear manner bilaterally. It should be tented with the surgeon's forceps to separate it from the underlying muscle and to identify perforating vessels, which require ligation or coagulation. Curvilinear extension is essential because direct transverse extension often leads to inadvertent muscle incisions and bleeding.

Once the fascial incision is completed, the fascia is then grasped in the midline bilaterally and is separated from the underlying rectus muscles superiorly and inferiorly by blunt and sharp dissection from the median raphe.

The rectus muscles can be separated bluntly in the midline to reveal the posterior rectus sheath and peritoneum, which can also be entered bluntly with fingers, to avoid trauma to underlying bowel. The point of entry should be as superior as possible to avoid bladder injury, particularly in repeat operations in which the bladder may be adherent superiorly.

Uterine Incision and Delivery of the Fetus

Following full entry into the peritoneal cavity, the surgeons should palpate the uterus for fetal presentation and alignment, and then place a bladder retractor to expose the lower uterine segment. The uterus is often dextrorotated, and its position must be appreciated to plan the incision site. The safety and efficacy of using special retractors, especially in obese women, has been insufficiently studied.

Creation of a bladder flap versus a direct uterine incision above the bladder fold has been compared in a randomized trial of 102 women. Bladder flap development was associated with a longer incision to delivery interval and total operating time and a greater fall in maternal hemoglobin.[24] Given these findings, we generally do not develop a bladder flap at cesarean delivery. Should the obstetrician elect to create a bladder flap, the vesicouterine serosa is picked up with smooth forceps and is incised in the midline with Metzenbaum scissors. The incision is carried out laterally in a curvilinear manner. The vesicouterine fold is then tented with forceps or a pair of hemostats, which allows direct visualization as the bladder flap is bluntly created using the index and middle fingers of the surgeon's hand. Sharp dissection may be necessary, particularly in repeat operations. The surgeon then bluntly sweeps out laterally on each side to allow just enough room for insertion of the bladder blade. A Richardson retractor is then inserted laterally, and continuous suction is made available for preparation of the uterine incision.

A low-transverse uterine incision is employed in more than 90% of cases (Figure 20-3). **It is preferred to a vertical incision because it is associated with less blood loss, is easier to perform and repair, and provides for the option of subsequent TOLAC because the rate of subsequent rupture is lower than with incisions incorporating the upper uterine segment.**

In cases of a low-transverse incision, the incision is begun at least 2 cm above the bladder margin. Suction is applied. Tamponade with sponges superiorly and inferiorly can be performed if considerable bleeding is encountered. This technique allows better visualization and minimizes the chance of fetal laceration. The incision is extended laterally and superiorly at the angles by blunt spreading using the index fingers. Two randomized trials have compared blunt versus sharp extension of the uterine incision. Sharp extension is associated with increased blood loss and carries with it the potential risk for cutting the umbilical cord or direct fetal injury.[25,26] Blunt uterine incision extension can be done preferably with cephalad-caudad traction because transverse expansion is associated with more unintended extension and blood loss.[27] As per the skin and the fascial incisions, adequate exposure for an easy extraction of the fetus should be obtained. At term, this is usually more than 15 cm.

A vertical uterine incision, now rarely performed (Table 20-5), is either low (involving mostly low uterine segment) or classic (involving upper uterine segment) and should have clear indications. **A vertical uterine incision may need to be performed if the lower uterine segment is poorly developed (e.g., at 24 to 25 weeks), if the fetus is in a back-down transverse lie, in most cases of a complete anterior placenta previa, or if there are leiomyomas obstructing the lower segment.** Other, even less common indications may include certain fetal abnormalities such as massive hydrocephalus or a very large sacrococcygeal teratoma. The disadvantages of a classic incision are its tendency for greater adhesion formation and a greater risk for uterine rupture with subsequent pregnancy. The low-vertical incision depends on the downward displacement of the bladder to confine the incision to the true lower segment (Figure 20-4). The incision is begun as inferiorly as possible and

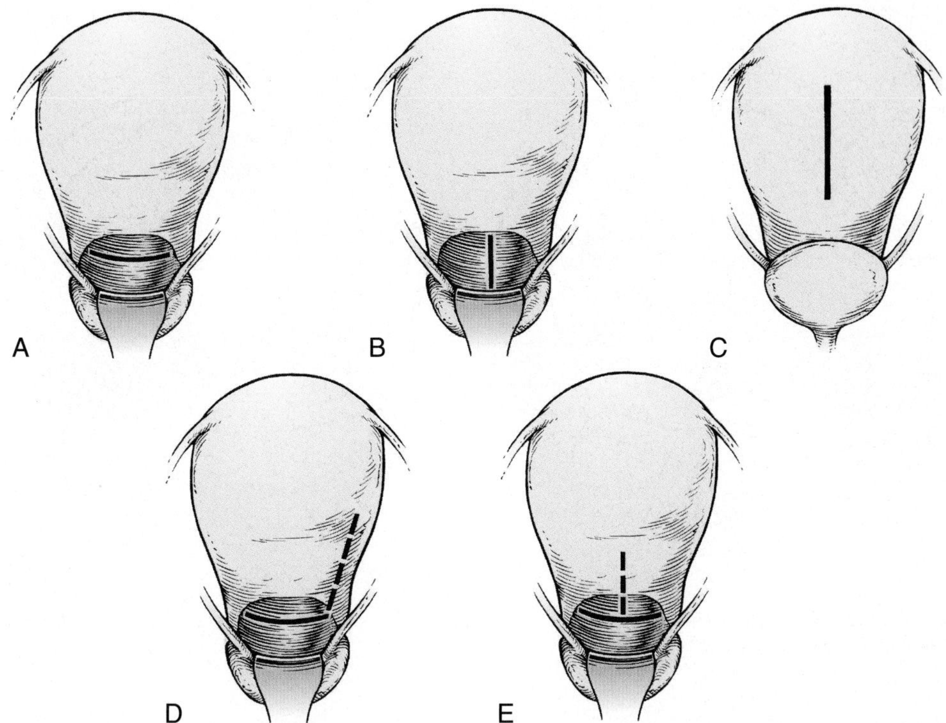

FIGURE 20-3. Uterine incisions for cesarean delivery. **A,** Low transverse incision (performed in >90% of cesarean deliveries). The bladder can be retracted downward as needed, and the incision is made in the lower uterine segment, curving gently upward. If the lower segment is poorly developed, the incision can also curve sharply upward at each end to avoid extending into the ascending branches of the uterine arteries. **B,** Low-vertical incision. The incision is made vertically in the lower uterine segment after reflecting the bladder, avoiding extension into the bladder below. If more room is needed, the incision can be extended upward into the upper uterine segment. **C,** Classic incision. The incision is entirely within the upper uterine segment and can be at the level shown or in the fundus. **D,** J incision. If more room is needed when an initial transverse incision has been made, either end of the incision can be extended upward into the upper uterine segment and parallel to the ascending branch of the uterine artery. **E,** T incision. More room can be obtained in a transverse incision by an upward midline extension into the upper uterine segment.

TABLE 20-5 POTENTIAL INDICATIONS FOR VERTICAL UTERINE INCISION

- Underdeveloped lower uterine segment
- Breech or transverse lie with undeveloped lower uterine segment
- Inability to develop bladder flap with repeat cesarean delivery
- Lower segment anterior myoma
- Anterior placenta previa

extended cephalad with fingers or bandage scissors. If the thick myometrium of the upper segment is incised, the incision becomes a classic one and should be described as such in the operative report.

Extraction of the Fetus

Once an adequate uterine incision has been completed, the fetal head is extracted by elevation and flexion using the operator's hand as a fulcrum. Adequate fundal pressure by the assistant is often critical to obtain delivery. If the head is not easily delivered, the uterine incision (or skin or abdomen incisions) may be extended. Rarely, a T-incision will be made to facilitate delivery. **In cases in which the vertex is wedged in the maternal pelvis, usually in advanced second-stage arrest, reverse breech extraction ("pull" method) has been associated with shorter operating time, less extension of the uterine incision, and postpartum endometritis compared with vaginal displacement of the presenting part upward,**[28] but the evidence is insufficient to make a strong recommendation. Vacuum extraction or short Simpson forceps should in general be avoided because they are rarely necessary if the previously mentioned steps are taken.

Following delivery, the cord is clamped and cut, and the infant is passed from the field to the pediatric team.

Placental Extraction and Uterine Repair

Following delivery of the infant, intravenous oxytocin is started as a drip (at least 20 U/L). One randomized trial has reported benefit from using 80 versus 20 U/L.

Removal of the placenta by spontaneous expulsion with gentle cord traction has been shown by several randomized trials to be associated with less blood loss and a lower rate of endometritis than by manual extraction.[29-31] **Therefore, spontaneous expulsion with gentle cord traction and uterine massage should be performed for delivery of the placenta.**

The uterine repair may be greatly facilitated by lifting the fundus and delivering the uterus through the abdominal incision. Uterine exteriorization facilitates better visualization of the extent of the incision to be repaired as well as the adnexa. There is no significant increased risk for blood loss, infection, hypotension, or nausea and vomiting with exteriorization of the uterus compared with intra-abdominal repair, as shown by a meta-analysis of 11 trials.[32]

Bleeding along the incision line is temporarily controlled by using ring clamps because they are less traumatic than

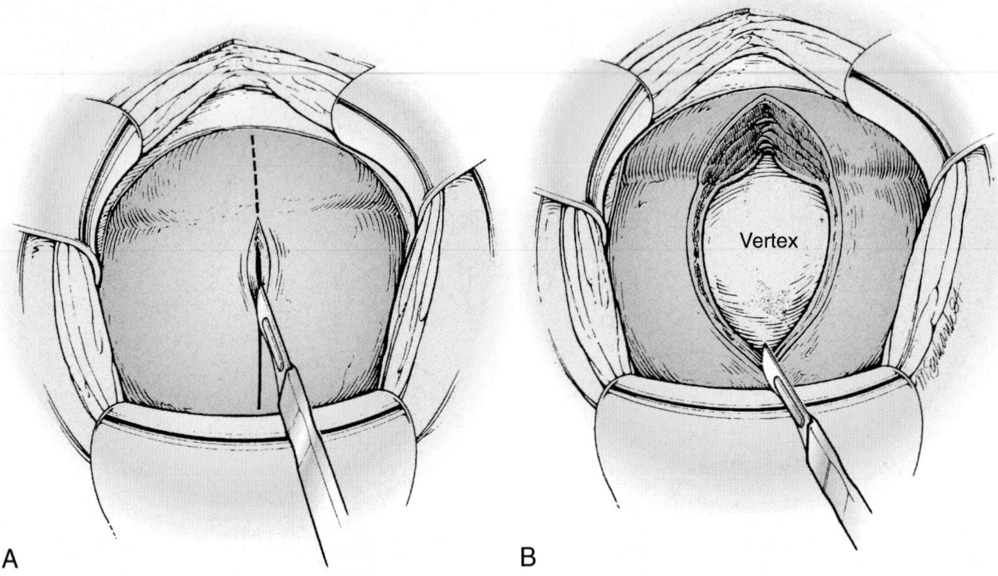

FIGURE 20-4. Low-vertical incision. **A,** Ideally, a vertical incision is contained entirely in the lower uterine segment. **B,** Extension into the upper uterine segment, either inadvertently or by choice, is common.

other instruments. The uterus is then manually curetted with a moistened sponge, and all placental fragments or membranes are teased away from the uterine wall. Routine cervical dilation is not necessary, even if the patient has not labored and the cervix is not dilated, because it is not associated with any benefit.[33]

The uterine incision should be well inspected before closure. Any inferior extensions of the incision should be visualized and repaired separately before closure.

The first layer of uterine closure is always performed. Continuous suturing is associated with less operating time and reduced blood loss compared with interrupted sutures.[34] The locking of the primary layer of closure facilitates hemostasis, but may not be necessary if the incision is fairly hemostatic before closure. Size 1-0 or 0-0 synthetic suture is employed. Full-thickness repair, including the endometrial layer, is associated with improved healing as checked by ultrasound 6 weeks after cesarean.[35,36]

The lower uterine incision may be closed with either a single or a double layer of sutures (Figure 20-5). Single-layer closure is associated with a statistically significant but clinically small reduction in mean blood loss, duration of the operative procedure, and presence of postoperative pain compared with double-layer closure.[36] There is controversy about whether an increased risk for subsequent uterine rupture accompanies the single-layer closure technique. (see later). In women who receive a tubal ligation at the time of cesarean delivery, we perform a single-layer closure. Otherwise, we prefer a double-layer closure; however, this practice is not based on level I evidence.

A vertical uterine incision generally requires at least a double-layer, and often a triple-layer, closure technique (Figure 20-6).

The uterine incision is carefully inspected for hemostasis before returning it to the peritoneal cavity. Individual bleeding points are cauterized or ligated using as little suture material as possible. The adnexa are inspected.

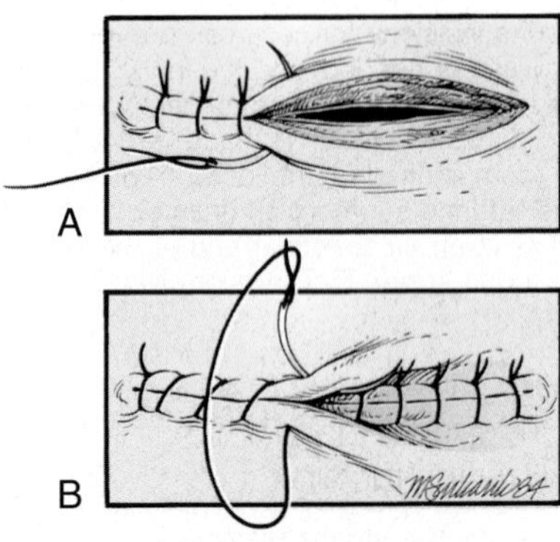

FIGURE 20-5. Closure of low-transverse incision. **A,** The first layer can be either continuous (recommended) or interrupted. A continuous locking suture is less desirable, despite its reputed hemostatic abilities, because it may interfere with incision vasculature and, hence, with healing and scar formation. **B,** A second inverted layer is created by using a continuous Lembert or Cushing stitch. Inclusion of too much tissue produces a bulky mass that may delay involution and interfere with healing.

Tubal ligation is performed, if so desired. Following return of the uterus inside the pelvis, sponge and needle counts are then performed before abdominal closure. Intra-abdominal irrigation does not reduce intrapartum or postpartum maternal morbidity.[37]

Abdominal Closure

The parietal and visceral peritoneum are not reapproximated because spontaneous closure will occur within days, and nonclosure is associated with less operative time, less fever, and less need for analgesia compared with closure.[38]

There are no trials evaluating technical aspects of fascial closure at cesarean. The rectus fascia is usually closed with a continuous nonlocking technique, but some prefer interrupted sutures. A suture with good tensile strength

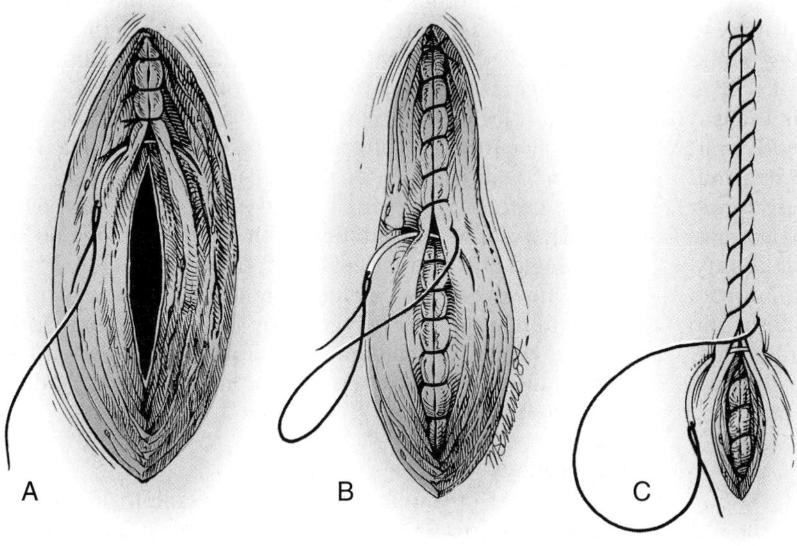

FIGURE 20-6. Repair of a classic incision. Three-layer closure of a classic incision, including inversion of the serosal layer to discourage adhesion formation. The knot at the superior end of the incision of the second layer can be buried by medial to lateral placement of the suture from within the depth of the incision and subsequent lateral to medial reentry on the opposing side with resultant knot placement within the incision.

and relatively delayed absorption is preferred. Synthetic braided or monofilament sutures are best to use. In most instances, a running continuous monofilament propylene suture will suffice for a transverse incision. **In closing the fascia, placement of sutures should be at a minimum 1.5 cm from the margin of the incision. Sutures are placed at about 1-cm intervals. In most cases of wound disruption, the suture remains intact but has cut through the fascia as a result of placement too close to the cut margin.** Patients at risk for wound disruption may benefit from either the Smead-Jones technique or interrupted figure-of-eight suturing, both employing delayed absorption suture material such as monofilament polyglycolic acid. The Smead-Jones closure technique is preferred for vertical incisions in high-risk cases (Figure 20-7). A suture with either far-near or near-far placement that passes through the lateral side of the anterior rectus fascia and adjacent subcutaneous adipose tissue and then crosses the midline of the incision to pick up the medial edge of the rectus fascia, then catches the near side of the opposite rectus sheath before returning to the far margin of the opposite rectus sheath and subcutaneous fat, accomplishes this technique.

The subcutaneous tissue is closed if it will facilitate skin closure or if the fat thickness is at least 2 cm. Closure of the subcutaneous tissue with sutures is associated with less wound complications such as a hematoma, seroma, wound infection, or wound separation compared with no closure.[39]

Closure is more beneficial than drainage in these cases. In fact, routine prophylactic wound drainage is not associated with benefits and should therefore not be performed.[40] When hemostasis is not adequate either intra-abdominally or subcutaneously, drains can be used, but there are no level I data assessing their effectiveness.

The skin is closed with either a staple device or a subcuticular closure for transverse incisions. There is insufficient evidence to recommend one skin closure over the other. Staples, as long as they are left in for at least 4 days, appear to be associated with shorter operating times, with no significant differences in pain or cosmesis.[41-43]

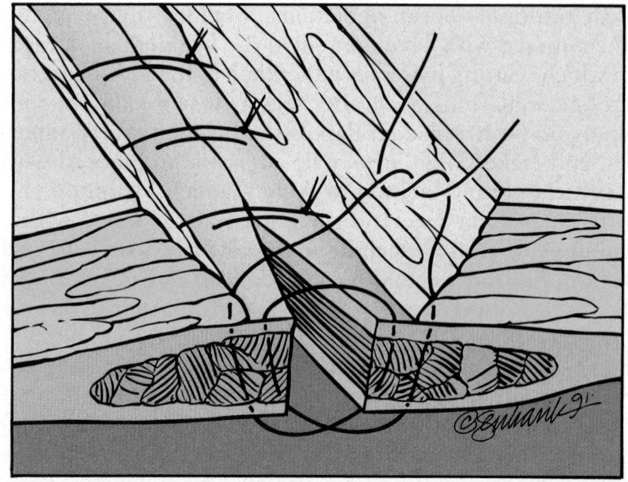

FIGURE 20-7. Modification of far-near, near-far Smead-Jones suture. Suture passes deeply through lateral side of anterior rectus fascia and adjacent fat, crosses the midline of the incision to pick up the medial edge of the rectus fascia, then catches the near side of the opposite rectus sheath, and, finally, returns to the far margin of the opposite rectus sheath and subcutaneous fat. (Modified from American College of Obstetricians and Gynecologists: Prolog. In Gynecologic Oncology and Surgery. Washington, DC, ACOG, 1991, p 187.)

COMPLICATIONS OF CESAREAN DELIVERY

Intraoperative Complications

Women undergoing cesarean delivery are at risk for several intraoperative complications, including hemorrhage and injury to adjacent organs. Injury to the bowel, bladder, and ureters is uncommon; however, the obstetrician must be familiar with management of these problems. The key element is to recognize and define the extent of these injuries and to promptly institute repair. Consultation with a urologist, general surgeon, or gynecologic oncologist may be necessary depending on the skill level of the obstetrician and the complexity of the injury encountered.

Uterine Lacerations

Lacerations of the uterine incision most commonly involve extension of a low-transverse incision following arrest of descent in the second stage or with delivery of a large fetus. **Most lacerations are myometrial extensions and can be closed with a running locking suture independently or in conjunction with closure of the primary uterine incision. High lateral extensions may require unilateral ascending uterine artery branch ligation.** In cases that extend laterally and inferiorly, care must be taken to avoid ureteral injury. On occasion, if the extension involves bleeding into the broad ligament, opening this space and identifying the ureters before suture placement may be helpful. On rare occasions, retrograde ureteral stent placement may be necessary. Opening the dome of the bladder is the preferred technique for retrograde stent placement.

Bladder Injury

Minor injury to the bladder from vigorous retraction and bruising with resultant hematuria is common. More significant injury such as a bladder dome laceration is infrequent but can occur on entering the peritoneum, particularly with multiple repeat operations. Bladder injury is also encountered with development of the bladder flap in cases in which scarring increases adherence to the lower anterior uterine wall. This is another reason that we do not routinely perform a bladder flap. If the bladder is very adherent and tacked high, it may be advisable to proceed with a vertical uterine incision to avoid bladder disruption.

Bladder dome lacerations are generally repaired with a double-layer closure technique employing 2-0 or 3-0 vicryl suture. The mucosa may be avoided with closure, although this is not imperative. If there is any question regarding possible trigone or ureteral injury before repair, intravenous indigo carmine is administered, and the ureteral orifices are visualized for dye spillage. Retrograde filling of the bladder with sterile milk may be useful following closure to ensure its integrity. Continuous Foley drainage should be accomplished for several days following repair of a bladder injury.

Ureteral Injury

Ureteral injury has been reported to occur in about 1 in 1000 cesarean deliveries. The frequency of injury increases with cesarean hysterectomy. **Most ureteral injuries follow attempts to control bleeding from lateral extensions into the broad ligament. As described previously, opening the broad ligament before suture placement may reduce the risk for this complication.** If the integrity of the ureter is in doubt, intravenous indigo carmine can be administered, with visualization of spillage in the bladder by cystoscope (usually performed by a urologic consultant). The ureteral orifices are visualized for dye spillage, signifying ureteral patency. If ureteral injury is recognized postoperatively, cystoscopy with stent placement or nephrostomy with radiologic imaging may define the extent of injury and help in planning appropriate management.

Gastrointestinal Tract Injury

Bowel injury during cesarean section is rare. Most cases involve incidental enterotomy on entering the abdomen for a repeat laparotomy, especially if scissors or scalpel are used. This is another reason why we employ blunt dissection, with fingers, for peritoneal entry. Defects in the bowel serosa are closed with interrupted suture of fine silk using an atraumatic needle. If the lumen of the small bowel is lacerated, closure is accomplished in two layers. A 3-0 absorbable suture is preferred for the mucosa, followed by interrupted silk sutures for the serosa.

Large defects of the small bowel or injuries of the colon generally require consultation with a general surgeon or gynecologic oncologist. Small defects may be closed primarily; however, large defects with fecal contamination may require a temporary colostomy. Broad-spectrum antibiotic coverage is recommended for such cases, which must include administration of an aminoglycoside in addition to metronidazole or clindamycin.

Uterine Atony

A more complete review of the management of uterine atony is found in Chapter 19. Uterine atony can be controlled in most cases by a combination of uterine massage and uterotonic agents. Intravenous oxytocin in dosages up to 80 U/L running wide open is attempted initially. If this fails to result in uterine contraction, either methergonovine maleate (Methergine), 0.2 mg administered intramuscularly, or 0.25 mg of 15-methylprostaglandin F2 alpha (Hemabate), is administered intramuscularly or directly into the myometrium. Several successive doses of Hemabate every 10 to 15 minutes may be tried (up to 1 mg) if necessary. Most individuals respond to one or two doses. Misoprostol, up to 1000 mcg per rectum, can be administered. Packing or use of a uterine balloon is also effective in these cases, if medical management is not fully effective. Medical management is successful, if employed correctly and promptly, in most cases of uterine atony.

In the rare cases in which nonsurgical management does not control bleeding, a surgical approach should be employed. The initial surgical approach is bilateral ascending uterine artery branch ligation, especially if future fertility is desired. If this fails, hypogastric artery ligation or hysterectomy may be undertaken (Figure 20-8). Hypogastric artery ligation is effective in less than 50% of cases.

Placenta Accreta

Placenta accreta has increased in frequency with rising cesarean delivery rates, and in some series of cesarean hysterectomy, placenta accreta is the most common indication. The risk for placenta accreta increases with each repeat cesarean delivery and is substantially increased by the presence of placenta previa (see Chapter 19).[44]

Focal placenta accreta may be managed by oversewing the implantation site with figure-of-eight absorbable sutures. However, hemostasis must be ensured. If the lower segment continues to bleed, it should be packed tightly to reduce blood loss while proceeding with hysterectomy. **In cases of total placenta previa with clinically apparent placenta accreta, it is advisable to leave the placenta attached while proceeding with hysterectomy.** This approach may lower blood loss considerably. Most cases of placenta accreta with previa require total hysterectomy because of placental attachment to the relatively hypocontractile lower uterine segment.

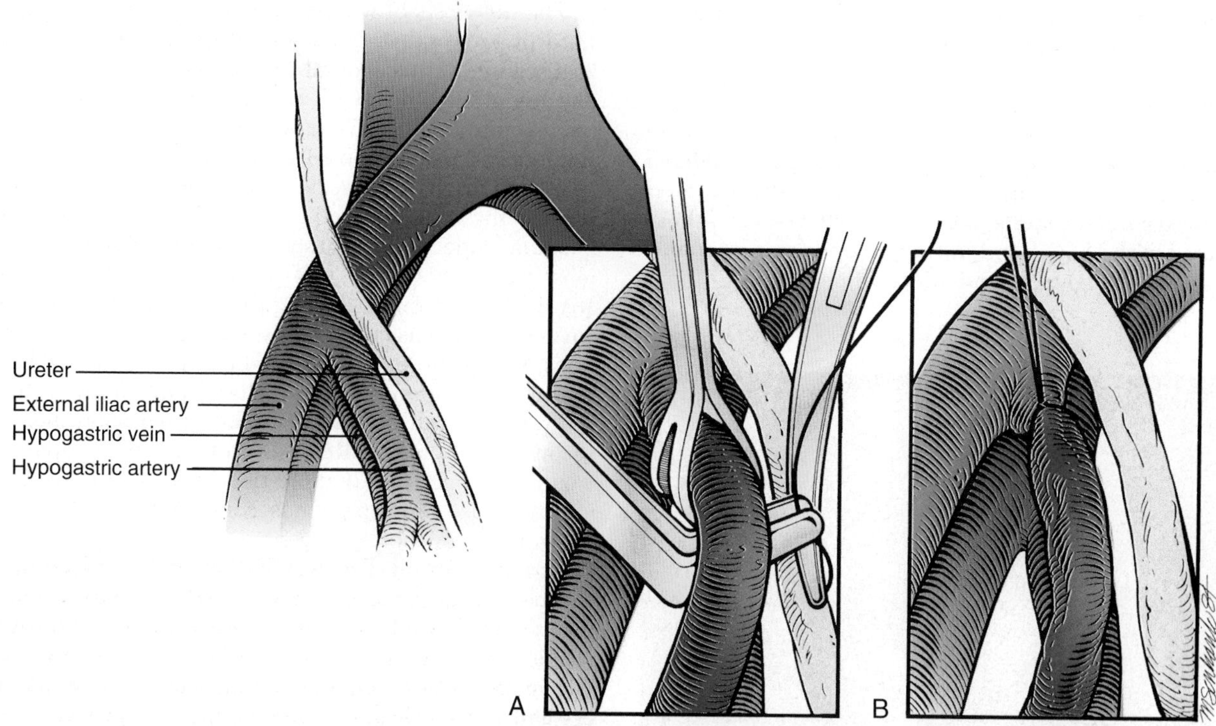

FIGURE 20-8. Hypogastric artery ligation. Approach to the hypogastric artery through the peritoneum, parallel and just lateral to the ovarian vessels, exposing the interior surface of the posterior layer of the broad ligament. The ureter will be found attached to the medial leaf of the broad ligament. The bifurcation of the common iliac artery into its external and internal (hypogastric) branches is exposed by blunt dissection of the loose overlying areolar tissues. Identification of these structures is essential. **A** and **B,** To avoid traumatizing the underlying hypogastric vein, the hypogastric artery is elevated by means of a Babcock clamp before passing an angled clamp to catch a free tie. (Modified from Breen J, Cregori CA, Kindierski JA: Hemorrhage in Gynecologic Surgery. Hagerstown, MD, Harper & Row, 1981, p 438.)

Maternal Mortality

The attributable maternal death rate has ranged from 6 to 22 per 100,000. In a study of 250,000 deliveries, Lilford and colleagues[45] reported the RR for maternal death from cesarean delivery compared with vaginal birth to be about seven-fold higher when preexisting medical conditions were excluded. In contrast, Lydon-Rochelle noted similar rates of maternal death among women delivered by cesarean section versus vaginal birth when adjusting for maternal age and the presence of severe preeclampsia.[46]

Anesthesia-related morbidity and mortality have been substantially reduced through the expanded use of regional anesthesia and the employment of awake intubation for patients requiring general anesthesia who may have a difficult airway for standard intubation.

Maternal Postoperative Morbidity

Endomyometritis

Postcesarean endomyometritis remains the most common complication of cesarean delivery. Its frequency, with the use of appropriate prophylactic antibiotics as described previously, is usually less than 5%,[9,10] much reduced from preantibiotic times. Prolonged labor, rupture of membranes, and lower socioeconomic status appear to be the factors that most influence the rate of this complication.

Most cases of endomyometritis arise from ascending infection from cervicovaginal flora. Infections past the deepest part of the uterine incision may extend to the uterine musculature and, if not adequately treated, may produce peritonitis, abscess, and septic phlebitis. Using antibiotic prophylaxis, pelvic abscesses are rare, developing in 0.47% of cases following the diagnosis of chorioamnionitis compared with only 0.1% if fever was not observed during labor.

The diagnosis of postpartum endomyometritis is based on fever (100.4° F or more) with either fundal tenderness or foul-smelling discharge, in the absence of any other source. The presence of chorioamnionitis, prolonged labor, and ruptured membranes should prompt early treatment in suspected cases. The utility of endometrial cultures is limited owing to contamination with vaginal flora and the fact that therapy is rarely guided by these results. Treatment is primarily based on clinical findings, including uterine tenderness and fever.

Parenteral antibiotics employing a regimen directed against possible anaerobic infection are the preferred therapeutic agents. A regimen of clindamycin and an aminoglycoside such as gentamicin is associated with better safety and efficacy compared with other regimens. An alternative is a single-agent penicillin-based regimen using β-lactamase inhibition to allow for anaerobic coverage (e.g., ampicillin and sulbactam). These antibiotics should be continued until at least 24 hours after the patient has defervesced. Once uncomplicated endometritis has clinically improved with intravenous therapy, oral therapy is not needed.

For women who fail to respond to antibiotic therapy over 2 to 3 days, an alternative source for the fever such as a wound infection, deep abscess, hematoma, or septic pelvic thrombophlebitis should be considered. On occasion, mastitis may produce significant temperature elevations (Figures 20-9 and 20-10).

Wound Infection

Wound infection complicates about 1% to 5% of cesarean deliveries.[5] **Most cesarean section wounds are considered clean contaminated owing to the interface with the lower reproductive tract. Emergent cesarean deliveries and those associated with chorioamnionitis are considered contaminated and have higher wound infection rates.**

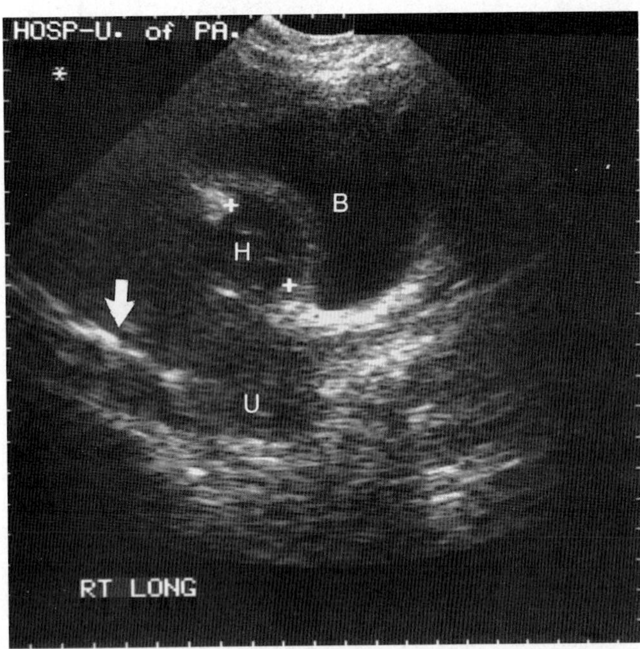

FIGURE 20-9. Ultrasound of infected bladder flap hematoma marked by cursors (+). The patient presented about 1 week after cesarean delivery with fever. She responded to antibiotics. Note that the full bladder *(B)* enhances visualization of the hematoma *(H)*. The *arrow* designates the endometrial cavity of the uterus *(U)*.

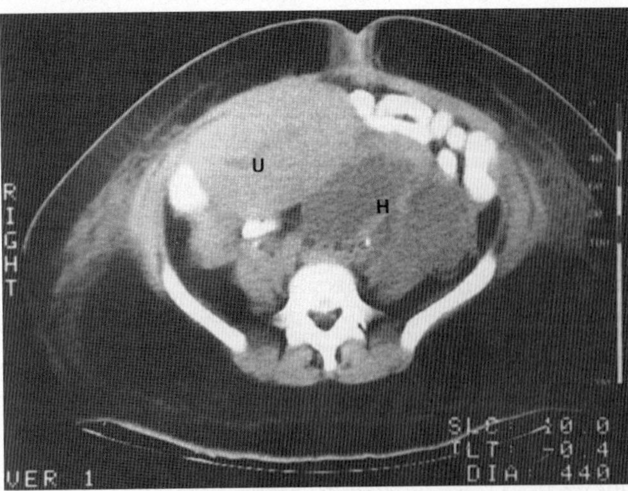

FIGURE 20-10. Computed tomography scan of pelvis 6 days after a cesarean section showing left-sided broad ligament hematoma *(H)*. The uterus *(U)* is displaced to the right. The patient responded to antibiotics. (Courtesy of Dr. Michael Blumenfeld, Department of Obstetrics and Gynecology, Ohio State University, Columbus, OH.)

The diagnosis of wound infection is usually straightforward in patients who present with tenderness, erythema, or discharge. Early wound infection (first 2 postoperative days) is often a result of streptococcal infection, whereas later wound infection is generally caused by overgrowth of staphylococcus or a mixed aerobic-anaerobic infection.

Wound discharge may be sent for culture before instituting therapy. The infected portion of the wound should be opened, inspected, irrigated, and débrided as necessary. In most cases, this alone will suffice for therapy. A wound abscess may require drainage (Figure 20-11). Antibiotic coverage, which is rarely necessary for simple wound infections, should be instituted promptly for advanced serious wound disruptions. Wound closure once the infection has resolved can be accomplished either surgically or by secondary intention. Reclosure of disrupted laparotomy wounds is successful in more than 80% of patients, is safe, and decreases healing times compared with healing by secondary intention.

Extreme wound discoloration, extensive infection, discoloration, gangrene, bullae, or anesthesia of the surrounding tissue should prompt consideration of necrotizing fasciitis. Necrotizing fasciitis has been reported to develop in 1 in 2500 of women undergoing primary cesarean delivery and is a surgical, life-threatening emergency. In these cases, the wound should be débrided under general

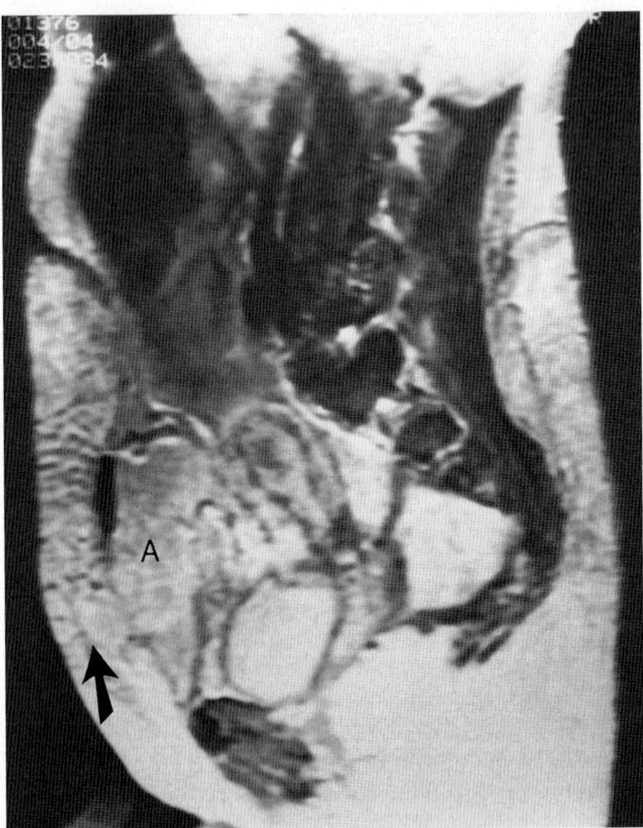

FIGURE 20-11. Magnetic resonance imaging (MRI) scan of abdominal wall abscess. This patient presented 1 week after a cesarean delivery with fever and an abdominal mass. The differential diagnosis included an intraperitoneal infection with extension or a wound abscess. This MRI shows a wound abscess *(A)* above fascia that extended to the abdominal wall *(arrow)*. The abscess responded to drainage and antibiotics.

anesthesia. Examination of histologic specimens may aid in the diagnosis of necrotizing infection. In such cases, all nonviable tissue should be removed, and consultation with an experienced surgeon is recommended. Antibiotic coverage, which is rarely necessary for simple wound infections, should be instituted promptly for advanced serious wound disruptions.

Thromboembolic Disease

VTE occurs more commonly during pregnancy secondary to higher levels of clotting factors and venous stasis (see Chapter 43) and is the leading cause of maternal death in developed countries. Risk factors are also the puerperal period, cesarean delivery, immobility, obesity, advanced age, and parity. The incidence of DVT was reported at 0.17% and that of pulmonary embolism (PE) at 0.12% in women undergoing cesarean birth.

The diagnosis of DVT is suggested by the presence of unilateral leg pain and swelling. A significant difference in the calf or thigh diameter may be present; however, error with this measurement is possible. The presence of Homans sign (pain with foot dorsiflexion) is often observed if the calf is involved. Many cases of DVT present as PE, particularly in the postoperative patient. Tachypnea, dyspnea, tachycardia, and pleuritic pain are the classic symptoms, with cough and specific pulmonary auscultatory findings less common.

If DVT is suggested, Doppler studies may be useful for proximal disease but are less sensitive for calf thrombosis. Impedance plethysmography is also helpful in detecting proximal disease, but it is of limited value in the diagnosis of pelvic thrombosis. If DVT is highly suspected and the previous studies are inconclusive, a venogram should be obtained.

The workup for suspected PE includes an arterial blood gas and chest film followed by a ventilation-perfusion study or spiral computed tomography (CT) study. Oxygen should be administered and heparin begun if a clinical PE appears likely. An indeterminate perfusion scan requires pulmonary angiography to establish or rule out the diagnosis of PE.

Septic Pelvic Thrombophlebitis

Probably less than 1% of women with endomyometritis develop septic pelvic thrombophlebitis; however, accurate figures for the frequency of this condition in current practice are lacking.

Septic pelvic thrombophlebitis is most often a diagnosis of exclusion established in refractory cases of women being treated for endomyometritis. A pelvic CT scan may aid in the diagnosis, although the sensitivity and specificity of this technique are clearly difficult to establish. In practice, a febrile patient who has undergone cesarean delivery and fails to respond to appropriate broad coverage antibiotic therapy for suspected uterine infection for several days, usually more than 5 to 7 days, may be started on full-dose heparin therapy, which is continued for several days following a clinical response. Long-term anticoagulation is not prescribed. Patients with septic pelvic phlebitis may present with spiking nocturnal fever and chills. However, these findings may be absent, and a persistent febrile state may be all that is present. In cases in which there is no response to anticoagulation therapy, imaging studies including pelvic CT are indicated to rule out an abscess or hematoma.

VAGINAL BIRTH AFTER CESAREAN DELIVERY

Trends

In a recent review of contemporary cesarean delivery practice in the United States, Zhang and colleagues concluded that primary emphasis should be placed on reducing cesarean section for dystocia and repeat operations because these two indications have increased the rate of cesarean section far beyond any other indications.[47] The modest decline in cesarean delivery observed to a nadir of 21% in 1996 was largely due to an increased TOLAC rate in women with a prior cesarean section. However, at the present time, only 8.5% of women with a prior cesarean delivery undergo a TOLAC in the United States. **It has been suggested that about two thirds of women with a prior cesarean delivery are actually candidates for a TOLAC. Thus, most repeat operations are influenced by physician discretion and patient choice.** A comparison of TOLAC rates between the United States and several European nations where TOLAC rates vary between 50% and 70% indicates significant underuse of TOLAC in this country. Given this information and the fact that 8% to 10% of the obstetrical population has had a previous cesarean delivery, more widespread use of TOLAC continues to have the potential to decrease the overall cesarean section rate.

The evolution in management of the woman with a prior cesarean delivery can be traced through several ACOG documents and key studies over the past 25 years. In 1988, ACOG published "Guidelines for Vaginal Delivery after a Previous Cesarean Birth," recommending VBAC-TOLAC as it became clear that this procedure was safe and did not appear to be associated with excess perinatal morbidity compared with repeat cesarean delivery. They recommended that each hospital develop its own protocol for the management of VBAC patients and that women with one prior low-transverse cesarean section should be counseled and encouraged to attempt labor in the absence of a contraindication such as a prior classic incision. This recommendation was supported by several large case series attesting to the safety and effectiveness of TOLAC. With this information, VBAC rates reached a peak of 28.3%. Some third-party payers and managed care organizations began to mandate a TOLAC for women with a prior cesarean delivery. Physicians, feeling institutional pressure to lower cesarean section rates, began to offer a TOLAC liberally and likely included less-than-optimal candidates. With the rise in VBAC experience, a number of reports appeared in the literature suggesting a possible increase in uterine rupture and its maternal and fetal consequences. Sachs and colleagues[48] reported a tripling of the incidence of uterine rupture in Massachusetts from 1985 to 1995. Further descriptions of uterine rupture with hysterectomy and adverse perinatal outcomes, including fetal death and neonatal brain injury, set the stage for the precipitous decline in VBAC during the past 15 years.[49,50]

In 1999, ACOG issued a practice bulletin that acknowledged the apparent statistically small but significant risks of uterine rupture with poor outcomes for both women and their infants. It was also recognized that such adverse events during a TOLAC may lead to malpractice suits.[51] ACOG thus recommended that TOLAC be conducted in settings in which a physician capable of performing a cesarean be "immediately available" and institutions be equipped to respond to emergencies such as uterine rupture. The language in the 1999 document also suggested that instead of "encouraging" TOLAC, women with prior low-transverse cesareans should be "offered" TOLAC. A more conservative approach to TOLAC then followed with recognition of the need to reevaluate VBAC recommendations.[52] Nonetheless, the 1999 practice bulletin and the 2004 version consistently conclude that most women with one previous cesarean delivery with a low-transverse incision are candidates for VBAC and should be counseled about VBAC and offered a TOLAC.[52] The 2004 practice bulletin added that insufficient data existed to provide counseling for patients presenting with a prior low-vertical incision, multiple gestation, breech presentation, or an estimated fetal weight greater than 4000 g.

In response to a growing body of evidence indicating restriction to a women's access to VBAC-TOLAC, despite two recent large-scale contemporary multicenter studies attesting to the relative safety of VBAC-TOLAC, the NIH held a consensus development conference concerning VBAC in 2010. The panel concluded that trial of labor is a reasonable birth option for many women with previous cesarean delivery. The panel also found that existing practice guidelines and the medical liability climate were restricting access to VBAC-TOLAC and that these factors need to be addressed.[53] A specific concern raised was the low level of evidence for the requirement for "immediately available" surgical and anesthesia personnel in existing guidelines and the need to reassess this recommendation with reference to other obstetrical complications of comparable risk given limited physician and nursing resources.

Several months later, in 2010, ACOG issued an updated practice bulletin concerning VBAC.[54] The ACOG acknowledged a background of limited access to TOLAC-VBAC evolving over time as well as recommendation by the NIH panel to facilitate access. In doing so, while again recommending that TOLAC-VBAC be undertaken in facilities with staff immediately available to provide emergency care, ACOG recognized that resources for immediate cesarean may not be available in smaller institutions. In such cases, the decision to offer and pursue VBAC-TOLAC should be carefully considered by patients and their health care providers. It is recommended that the best alternative may be to refer patients to a facility with available resources.[54]

Candidates for Trial of Labor After Cesarean

Most women who have had a low-transverse uterine incision with a prior cesarean delivery and have no contraindications to vaginal birth can be considered candidates for a TOLAC. **The following are selection criteria suggested by ACOG[54] for identifying candidates for VBAC:**

- **One or two previous low-transverse cesarean deliveries**
- **Clinically adequate pelvis**
- **No other uterine scars or previous rupture**
- **Physicians immediately available throughout active labor capable of monitoring labor and performing an emergency cesarean delivery**

Additionally, several retrospective studies indicate that it may be reasonable to offer a TOLAC to women in other clinical situations. These would include macrosomia, gestation beyond 40 weeks, previous low-vertical incision, unknown uterine scar type, and twin gestation.

A TOLAC is contraindicated in women at high risk for uterine rupture. **A TOLAC should not be attempted in the following circumstances:**

- **Previous classical or T-shaped incision, or extensive transfundal uterine surgery**
- **Previous uterine rupture**
- **Medical or obstetrical complications that preclude vaginal delivery**

TABLE 20-6 SUCCESS RATES FOR TRIAL OF LABOR AFTER CESAREAN

	VBAC SUCCESS (%)
Prior Indication	
CPD/FTP	63.5
NRFWB	72.6
Malpresentation	83.8
Prior Vaginal Delivery	
Yes	86.6
No	60.9
Labor Type	
Induction	67.4
Augmented	73.9
Spontaneous	80.6

Modified from Landon MB, Leindecker S, Spong CY, et al: Factors affecting the success of trial of labor following prior cesarean delivery. Am J Obstet Gynecol 193:1016, 2005.

CPD, Cephalopelvic disproportion; *FTP*, failure to progress; *NRFWB*, nonreassuring fetal well-being.

Success Rates for Trial of Labor After Cesarean

The overall success rate for VBAC appears to be in the 60% to 80% range according to published reports.[54] At the peak of VBAC experience with high TOLAC rates, success was observed in only 60% of cases. More selective criteria resulting in TOLAC rates in the 30% range have yielded a higher number of vaginal births, 70% to 75%.[55,56] Predictors of successful TOLAC are well described. The prior indication for cesarean delivery clearly affects the likelihood of successful VBAC. A history of prior vaginal birth or a non-recurring condition such as a breech or nonreassuring fetal testing is associated with the highest success rates for VBAC (Table 20-6). Grobman and colleagues[57] have developed a nomogram for predicting VBAC (Figure 20-12). The prediction model is based on a multivariable logistic regression, including the variables of maternal age, body mass index, ethnicity, prior vaginal delivery, the occurrences of a VBAC, and a potential recurrent indication for the cesarean delivery. After analyzing the model with cross-validation techniques, it was found to be accurate and discriminating. Several factors have been studied that influence success, and these are summarized in the following sections.

Maternal Demographics

Race, age, body mass index, and insurance status have all been demonstrated to affect the success of TOLAC.[55] In

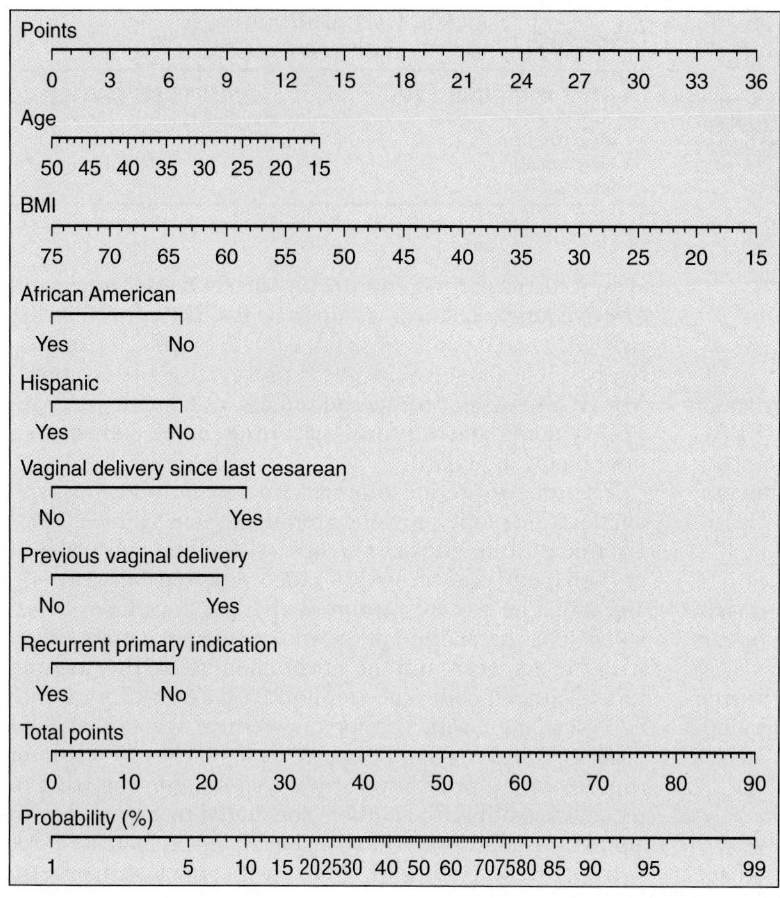

FIGURE 20-12. Graphic nomogram used to predict probability of vaginal birth after cesarean delivery (VBAC). The nomogram is used by locating each patient characteristic and finding the number of points on the upper most scale, to which that characteristic corresponds. The sum of total points predicts the probability of VBAC on the lower scale. (Modified from Grobman WA, Lai Y, Landon MB, et al: For the National Institute of Child Health and Human Development [NICHD] Maternal Fetal Medicine Units Network [MFMU]. Development of a normogram for prediction of vaginal birth after cesarean delivery. Obstet Gynecol 109:806-812, 2007.)

a multicenter study of 14,529 term pregnancies undergoing TOLAC, white women had a 78% success rate compared with 70% in nonwhite women.[55] Obese women are more likely to fail a TOLAC, as are women older than age 40 years.[55] Conflicting data exist with regard to payer status.[55]

Prior Indication for Cesarean Delivery

Success rates for women whose first cesarean delivery was performed for a non-recurring indication (breech, non-reassuring fetal well-being) are similar to vaginal delivery rates for nulliparous women. Prior cesarean delivery for a breech presentation is associated with the highest reported success rate of 89%.[55] In contrast, prior operative delivery for cephalopelvic disproportion or failure to progress is associated with success rates ranging from 50% to 67%.

Prior Vaginal Delivery

Prior vaginal delivery, including prior successful VBAC, can be considered the greatest predictor for successful TOLAC.[55] In one series, prior vaginal delivery had an 87% success rate compared with a 61% success in women without a prior vaginal delivery. Caughey and colleagues reported that for patients with a prior VBAC, the success rate is 93%, compared with 85% in women with a vaginal delivery before their cesarean birth but who had not had a successful VBAC.[58] Mercer and colleagues[59] have noted that success rate increases from 87.6% with one prior vaginal delivery to 90.0% in those with two prior successful attempts.

Birthweight

Increased birthweight is associated with a lower likelihood of a successful VBAC.[56] Birthweight greater than 4000 g in particular is associated with a significantly higher risk for failed VBAC.[56] However, 60% to 70% of women who attempt VBAC with a macrosomic fetus are successful. Peaceman and colleagues[60] reported a 34% success rate when the second pregnancy birthweight exceeded the first by 500 g and the prior indication was dystocia, compared with a 64% success rate with other prior indications.

Labor Status and Cervical Examinations

Both labor status and cervical examination on admission influence the success of a TOLAC. Flamm and colleagues reported an 86% success rate in women presenting with cervical dilation greater than 4 cm. Conversely, the VBAC success rate drops to 67% if the cervical examination is less than 4 cm on admission.[61]

Not surprisingly, women who undergo induction of labor are at higher risk for repeat cesarean delivery compared with those who enter spontaneous labor.[55,62] The National Institute of Child Health and Human Development (NICHD) Maternal-Fetal Medical Units (MFMU) Cesarean Registry reported a 67.4% success rate in women undergoing induction versus 80.5% in those entering spontaneous labor. In a study of 429 women undergoing induction with a prior cesarean delivery, Grinstead and Grobman[63] reported an overall 78% success rate. These authors noted several factors in addition to past obstetrical history, including indication for induction and the need

TABLE 20-7 SUCCESS RATES FOR TRIAL OF LABOR AFTER CESAREAN WITH TWO PRIOR CESAREAN DELIVERIES

STUDY	NO. OF SUBJECTS	SUCCESS RATE (%)
Miller et al., 1994[66]	2936	75.3
Caughey et al., 1999[65]	134	62.0
Macones et al., 2005[68]	1082	74.6
Landon et al., 2006[67]	876	67.0

for cervical ripening as determinants of VBAC success.[63] Grobman and colleagues[62] have also reported a VBAC success rate of 83% in 1208 women with a prior cesarean delivery and prior vaginal delivery undergoing induction of labor.

Previous Incision Type

Previous incision type cannot be ascertained in certain patients, which may challenge the obstetrician. It appears that women with an unknown scar have VBAC success rates similar to those of women with documented prior low-transverse incisions.[55] Similarly, women with previous low-vertical incisions do not appear to have lower VBAC success rates.[64]

Multiple Prior Cesarean Deliveries

Women with more than one prior cesarean delivery have been demonstrated to consistently have a lower likelihood of achieving VBAC[65-67] (Table 20-7). Caughey and colleagues reported a 75% success rate for women with one prior cesarean delivery compared with 62% in women with two prior operations.[65] In contrast, a larger multicenter study of 13,617 women undergoing a TOLAC revealed a 75.5% success rate for women with two prior cesarean deliveries, which was not statistically different from the 75% success rate in women with one prior operation.[68]

RISKS OF VAGINAL BIRTH AFTER CESAREAN DELIVERY–TRIAL OF LABOR

Uterine Rupture

The principal risk associated with VBAC-TOLAC is uterine rupture. This complication is directly attributable to attempted VBAC because symptomatic rupture is rarely observed in planned repeat operations.[69,70] **It is important to differentiate between uterine rupture and uterine scar dehiscence. This distinction is clinically relevant because dehiscence most often represents an occult scar separation observed at laparotomy in women with a prior cesarean section.** The serosa of the uterus is intact, and hemorrhage with its potential for fetal and maternal sequelae is absent. In contrast, uterine rupture is a through-and-through disruption of all uterine layers, with consequences of hemorrhage, non-reassuring fetal status, stillbirth and significant maternal morbidity, and the potential for mortality. Terminology, definitions, and ascertainment for uterine rupture vary significantly in the existing VBAC literature.[71] A review of four observational studies reported the risks of

TABLE 20-8 RISK FOR UTERINE RUPTURE WITH TRIAL OF LABOR AFTER CESAREAN

PRIOR INCISION TYPE	RUPTURE RATE (%)
Low transverse	0.5-1.0
Low-vertical	0.8-1.1
Classic or T	4-9

symptomatic uterine rupture in the TOLAC group and elective repeat cesarean group to be 0.47% (95% CI, 0.28% to 0.77%) and 0.026% (95% CI, 0.009% to 0.082%), respectively.[72] The large multicenter prospective observational MFMU Network Study reported a 0.69% incidence, with 124 symptomatic ruptures occurring in 17,898 women undergoing a TOLAC.[73]

The rate of uterine rupture depends on both the type and location of the previous uterine incision (Table 20-8).[74] Uterine rupture rates are highest with a previous classical or T-shaped incision, with a range reported between 4% and 9%. The risk for rupture with a previous low-vertical incision has been difficult to estimate owing to imprecision with the diagnosis and the uncommon use of this incision type. Naif and colleagues reported a 1.1% risk for rupture in 174 women with a prior low-vertical scar undergoing TOLAC, whereas Shipp reported a 0.8% (3 of 377) risk for rupture with a prior low-vertical incision. On the basis of these two studies, the authors concluded that women with a prior low-vertical uterine incision are not at increased risk for rupture compared with women with prior low-transverse incisions.

Women with an unknown type of scar do not appear to be at increased risk for uterine rupture. Among 3206 women with an unknown scar in the MFMU Network report, uterine rupture occurred in 0.5% of the trials of labor.[73]

The most serious sequelae of uterine rupture include perinatal death, HIE, and hysterectomy. Citing six deaths in 74 uterine ruptures among 11 studies, Guise and colleagues[75] calculated 0.14 additional perinatal deaths per 1000 trials of labor. This figure is remarkably similar to that from the NICHD MFMU Network study, in which there were two neonatal deaths among 124 ruptures, for an overall rate of rupture related perinatal death of 0.11 per 1000 TOLACs.[73] An all-inclusive review of 880 maternal uterine ruptures in studies of varying quality during a 20-year period showed 40 perinatal deaths in 91,039 trials of labor, for a rate of 0.4 per 1000[74] (Table 20-9).

Perinatal hypoxic brain injury is recognized as an underreported adverse outcome related to uterine rupture. Perinatal asphyxia has been poorly defined in VBAC studies, and variables such as cord blood gas levels and Apgar scores are reported in only a fraction of cases. Landon and colleagues[73] found a significant increase in the rate of HIE related to uterine rupture among the offspring of women who underwent a TOLAC at term compared with the children of women who underwent an planned repeat cesarean delivery (0.46 per 1000 trials of labor versus no cases, respectively). In 114 cases of uterine rupture at term, seven (6.2%) infants sustained HIE, and two of these infants died in the neonatal period (Table 20-10).

TABLE 20-9 RISK FOR PERINATAL DEATH RELATED TO UTERINE RUPTURE

STUDY	NO. OF PERINATAL DEATHS/ RUPTURES WITH TRIALS OF LABOR AFTER CESAREAN	
Guise et al., 2004 (pooled data)[75]	74	0.14/1000
Landon et al., 2004[73]	123	0.11/1000
Chauhaun et al., 2003 (pooled date)[74]	880	0.40/1000

TABLE 20-10 PERINATAL OUTCOMES AFTER UTERINE RUPTURE IN TERM PREGNANCIES

OUTCOME	TERM PREGNANCIES WITH UTERINE RUPTURE (*N* = 114)
Intrapartum stillbirth	0
Hypoxic-ischemic encephalopathy	7 (6.2)
Neonatal death	2 (1.8)
Admission to the neonatal intensive care unit	46 (40.4)
5-minute Apgar score ≤5	16 (14.0)
Umbilical artery blood pH ≤7.0	23 (33.3)

Modified from Landon MB, Hauth JC, Leveno KJ, et al, for the National Institute of Child Health and Human Development Maternal-Fetal Medicine Units Network: Maternal and perinatal outcomes associated with a trial of labor after prior cesarean section. N Engl J Med 351:2581, 2004.

Maternal hysterectomy may be a complication of uterine rupture, if the defect cannot be repaired or is associated with uncontrollable hemorrhage. In five studies reporting on hysterectomies related to rupture, seven cases occurred in 60 symptomatic ruptures (13%; range, 4% to 27%), indicating that 3.4 per 10,000 women electing a TOLAC sustain a rupture that necessitates hysterectomy.[71] The NICHD MFMU Network study included 5 of 124 (4%) cases requiring hysterectomy in which the uterus could not be repaired following rupture.[73] Guise and colleagues have reported no significant difference in the risk for hysterectomy in women with a prior cesarean attempting TOLAC compared with those undergoing planned repeat cesareans.[72]

Risk Factors for Uterine Rupture

Rates of uterine rupture vary significantly depending on a variety of associated risk factors. In addition to the type of uterine scar, characteristics of the obstetrical history, including number of prior cesarean deliveries, prior vaginal delivery, interdelivery interval, and uterine closure technique, have been reported to affect the risk for uterine rupture. Similarly, factors related to labor management, including induction and the use of oxytocin augmentation, have been studied.

Number of Prior Cesarean Deliveries

In a large single-center study of more than 1000 women with multiple prior cesarean deliveries undergoing a TOLAC, Miller and colleagues[66] reported uterine rupture in 1.7% of women with two or more previous cesarean deliveries compared with a frequency of 0.6% in those with one prior operation (odds ratio [OR], 3.06; 95% confidence interval [CI], 1.95 to 4.79). Interestingly, the risk for uterine rupture was not increased further for women with three prior cesarean deliveries. Caughey and colleagues[65] conducted a smaller study of 134 women with two prior cesarean deliveries and controlled for labor characteristics as well as obstetrical history. These authors reported a rate of uterine rupture of 3.7% among these 134 women compared to 0.8% in the 3757 women with one previous scar (OR, 4.5; 95% CI, 1.18 to 11.5). The risk was 4.8 times greater for these women after multivariate analysis. Macones and colleagues[68] reported a rate of uterine rupture of 20 of 1082 (1.8%) women with two prior cesarean deliveries compared with 113 of 12,535 (0.9%) women with one prior operation (adjusted OR, 2.3; 95% CI, 1.37 to 3.85). A recently published meta-analysis also suggested a nearly threefold increased risk for uterine rupture with two previous cesarean deliveries.[76] In contrast, Landon's analysis from the MFMU Network Cesarean Registry found no significant difference in rupture rates in women with one prior cesarean (115 of 16,916 [0.7%] versus multiple prior cesareans [9 of 975 (0.9%)].[67] **It thus appears that if multiple prior cesarean section is associated with an increased risk for uterine rupture, the magnitude of any additional risk is fairly small** (Table 20-11). **ACOG considers it reasonable to offer TOLAC to women with two prior cesareans and to counsel such women based on the combination of other factors that affect their probability of achieving a successful VBAC.** There are limited data available concerning the risk for women undergoing TOLAC with more than two previous cesarean deliveries.

TABLE 20-11 RISK FOR UTERINE RUPTURE FOLLOWING MULTIPLE PRIOR CESAREAN DELIVERIES

STUDY	RUPTURE RATE			
	N	Single Prior (%)	Multiple Prior (%)	RR (CI)
Miller et al., 1994[66]	3728	0.6	1.7	3.1 (1.9-4.8)
Caughey et al., 1999[65]	134	0.8	3.7	4.5 (1.2-11.5)
Macones et al., 2005[68]	1082	0.9	1.8	2.3 (1.4-3.9)
Landon et al., 2006[67]	975	0.7	0.9	1.4 (0.7-2.7)

CI, Confidence interval; *N*, number of women with multiple prior cesarean sections attempting vaginal birth after cesarean; *RR*, relative risk.

Prior Vaginal Delivery

Prior vaginal delivery appears to be protective against uterine rupture following TOLAC. In a study of 3783 women undergoing a TOLAC, Zelop and colleagues[77] noted that the rate of uterine rupture among women with a prior vaginal birth was 0.2% (2 of 1021) compared with 1.1% (30 of 2762) among women with no prior vaginal deliveries. After controlling for demographic differences and labor characteristics, women having one or more vaginal deliveries had a rate of uterine rupture that was one fifth that of women without prior vaginal birth (OR, 0.2; 95% CI, 0.04 to 0.8). A similar protective effect of prior vaginal birth has been reported in two large multicenter studies.[67,78] There is currently no information about whether a history of successful VBAC is also protective against uterine rupture.

Uterine Closure Technique

Over the past 15 years, the single-layer closure technique has gained popularity because it has appeared to be associated with shorter operating time and comparable short-term complications compared with the traditional two-layer technique. In a randomized trial, Chapman and colleagues[79] compared the incidence of uterine rupture in 145 women who received either one- or two-layer closure at their primary cesarean delivery. Following TOLAC, no cases of uterine rupture were found in either group; however, the study is underpowered to detect a potential difference. A large observational cohort study identified an approximate fourfold increased rate of rupture following single-closure technique when compared with previous double-layer closure.[80] This study included detailed review of operative reports in which the rate of rupture was 15 of 489 (3.1%) with single-layer closure versus 8 of 1491 (0.5%) with a previous double-layer closure. Finally, in a recent case-control study, the same authors[81] suggested an increased risk for uterine rupture with a single-layer closure (OR, 2.69; 95% CI, 1.57 to 5.28) compared with a two-layer closure. In the absence of randomized controlled studies, it remains unclear whether the single-layer closure technique increases the risk for rupture.

Interpregnancy Interval

Three studies have addressed whether a short interpregnancy interval may be associated with an increased risk for uterine rupture with a TOLAC. Shipp and colleagues reported an incidence of rupture of 2.3% (7 of 311) in women with an interdelivery interval less than 18 months compared with 1.1% (22 of 2098) with a longer interdelivery interval. After controlling for demographic characteristics and oxytocin use, women with a shorter interpregnancy interval were three times more likely to experience uterine rupture. In a study of 1185 women undergoing a TOLAC, Huang and colleagues found no increased risk for uterine rupture with an interdelivery interval of less than 18 months. Using a multivariate approach, Bujold and associates have reported an interdelivery interval of less than 24 months to be associated with an almost threefold increased risk for uterine rupture. In this study, the rate of rupture was 2.8% in women with a short interval versus 0.9% in women with greater than 2 years since the prior cesarean birth.

Induction of Labor

Induction of labor may be associated with an increased risk for uterine rupture.[82,83] In a population-based retrospective cohort analysis, Lydon-Rochelle and colleagues[82] reported a rate of uterine rupture of 24 of 2326 (1.0%) for women undergoing induction compared with 56 of 10,789 (0.5%) in women with the spontaneous onset of labor. In the prospective MFMU Network cohort analysis, Landon and coworkers noted the risk for uterine rupture to be elevated nearly threefold (OR, 2.86; 95% CI, 1.75 to 4.67) with induction in 48 of 4708 (1.0%) versus spontaneous labor in 24 of 6685 (0.4%).[73] A secondary analysis of 11,778 women from this study with one prior low-transverse cesarean showed an increase in uterine rupture in women undergoing induction who had no prior vaginal delivery (1.5% vs 0.8%).[62] In controlling for various potential confounders, Zelop and colleagues[77] compared the risk for uterine rupture in women undergoing labor induction with oxytocin versus spontaneous labor. Induction of labor with oxytocin was found to be associated with a 4.6-fold increased risk for uterine rupture (rupture rate of 2% versus 0.7%). Most recently, Dekker and colleagues reported a risk for rupture with induction using oxytocin alone of 0.54% compared with 0.15% for those women attempting VBAC in spontaneous labor. Compared with spontaneous labor, risks were increased three to five times for any type of induction.[83] Despite these analyses, **it remains unclear whether induction causes uterine rupture or whether an associated risk factor is present** (Table 20-12). **There are also conflicting data concerning whether various induction methods increase the risk for uterine rupture.** Lydon-Rochelle's[82] study suggested an increased risk for uterine rupture with the use of prostaglandins for labor induction. Uterine rupture was noted in 15 of 1960 (0.8%) women induced without prostaglandins compared with 9 of 366 (2.5%) women induced with prostaglandin. Unfortunately, these authors could not determine which specific prostaglandin agent was used. In Dekker's study,[83] the risk for rupture with oxytocin alone was 0.54% compared with 0.68% with prostaglandins and 0.88% when the combined agents were used.

Neither Landon nor Macones confirmed the findings of Lydon-Rochelle of an increased risk for rupture associated with the use of prostaglandin agents alone for induction.[73,78] Macones did report an increased risk for rupture in women undergoing induction only if they received both prostaglandins *and* oxytocin.[78] The methodology in this study did allow the authors to distinguish between induction methods. In contrast, this was not possible in Lydon-Rochelle's report, which relied on procedure codes for the use of prostaglandins that did not exclude the concomitant use of oxytocin. Interestingly, in the MFMU Network Study, there were no cases of uterine rupture when prostaglandin alone was used for induction, including 52 cases

TABLE 20-12 RISK FOR UTERINE RUPTURE AFTER LABOR INDUCTION

	STUDY		
	Lydon-Rochelle et al., 2001[82]	**Landon et al., 2004[73]**	**Dekker et al., 2010[83]**
All inductions	24/2326 (1.0)	48/4708 (1.0)	16/1867 (0.9)
Spontaneous	56/10,789 (0.5)	24/6685 (0.4)	16/8221 (0.2)
Prostaglandins	9/366 (2.5)	0/227 (0.0)	4/586 (0.7)
Prostaglandin + and oxytocin	—	13/926 (1.4)	4/226 (1.8)

in which misoprostol was used.[73] The safety of this medication, which is popular for cervical ripening and labor induction (see Chapter 14), has been challenged for women attempting VBAC. Plaut reported a uterine rupture rate of 5.6% (5 of 89) in women receiving misoprostol for labor induction. However, as in other series, it is unclear whether these women received oxytocin as well. The timing (delay) of uterine rupture in relation to misoprostol administration also calls into question cause and effect. Following several case reports of uterine rupture with misoprostol use, Wing and colleagues[84] conducted a randomized trial of intravaginal misoprostol versus oxytocin in women attempting VBAC. Seventeen women received misoprostol and 21 oxytocin. The study was stopped prematurely because two emergency cesarean deliveries were performed with uterine disruption in patients receiving misoprostol. Unfortunately, many VBAC studies fail to specify the prostaglandin used for labor induction. In the largest report of woman receiving prostaglandins for labor induction attempting VBAC, Smith and colleagues[85] reported a 0.87% risk for uterine rupture among 4475 women receiving unspecified prostaglandins compared with 0.29% in 4429 cases not receiving this class of medication. Although the relative risk associated with prostaglandin use was elevated, clearly the absolute risk for rupture was impressively low in this series. **At present, based on limited data, ACOG suggests avoiding sequential use of prostaglandin E_2 and oxytocin in women undergoing TOLAC.** This recommendation has thus limited options for induction in women undergoing TOLAC to primarily oxytocin or mechanical methods with or without oxytocin. At present, the use of mechanical methods, such as Foley catheters, indicate relative safety.

Labor Augmentation

Excessive use of oxytocin may be associated with uterine rupture, and careful labor augmentation should be practiced in women attempting TOLAC. A meta-analysis concluded that oxytocin use does not appear to influence the risk for a dehiscence or uterine rupture. In a case-control study, Leung and colleagues reported an OR of 2.7 for uterine rupture in women receiving oxytocin augmentation. Dysfunctional labor, including arrest disorders, actually increased the risk sevenfold and, thus, may be the primary factor responsible for rupture. In contrast to Leung's data, Zelop[77] found that labor augmentation with oxytocin did not significantly increase the risk for rupture. **Cahill and colleagues[86] have reported that a dose-response relationship exists between maximal oxytocin dose and the risk for rupture compared with women who attempt VBAC with no oxytocin exposure.** A limitation of this report is that it includes both women undergoing induction and those receiving oxytocin augmentation. At their maximal dose of oxytocin (>20 mU/minute), these authors noted the risk for uterine rupture to be 2.07%. In a follow-up study, these authors considered the association of maximum oxytocin exposure and risk for uterine rupture by estimated time to event in their analysis.[87] Their previous analysis suggested an approximate 1% attributable risk for rupture at higher oxytocin doses; however, the more recent report estimated the attributable risks to be 2.9% and 3.6% for doses greater than 20 and 30 mU/minute, respectively. **From these data, large doses of oxytocin should be used with caution in women undergoing TOLAC, and an upper limit of 20 mU/minute seems reasonable.**

Sonographic Evaluation of the Uterine Scar

To better identify women at risk for uterine rupture undergoing TOLAC, the thickness of the lower uterine segment (LUS) has been assessed with ultrasound. Bujold and colleages[88] conducted a prospective study of 125 women with previous cesarean undergoing TOLAC who received sonographic measurement of the LUS before labor. There were only three cases of uterine rupture; however, receiver operative curve analysis showed that full thickness of less than 2.3 mm was the optimal cutoff for the prediction of uterine rupture (3 of 33 vs. 0 of 92; $P = .02$). The rate of uterine rupture (9.1%) reported is significantly greater than previously cited risk factors and, thus, if confirmed in additional studies, may identify a subgroup of women at sufficiently high risk to advise against TOLAC. Limitations of Bujold's study include the small number of ruptures as well as the fact that most women with an LUS of less than 2 mm did not undergo TOLAC. This later fact suggests that practice patterns have been established that may limit further investigation concerning the utility of ultrasound to predict uterine rupture.[87]

Other Risks Associated with Vaginal Birth After Cesarean Delivery–Trial of Labor

In the absence of randomized controlled trials, there are limited data to inform women and health care providers about adverse outcomes associated with a TOLAC. Meta-analysis of these data have been criticized owing to lack of comparability between women undergoing a TOLAC and those having a planned repeat cesarean delivery.[70]

It has generally been accepted that vaginal delivery is associated with lower morbidity and mortality rates than is cesarean delivery. In contrast to Mozurkevich's meta-analysis of 15 studies, Landon and colleagues found an increased risk for both postpartum endometritis and the need for blood transfusion in women undergoing a TOLAC compared with planned repeat cesarean delivery without labor[70,73] (Table 20-13). However, the exclusion of women who presented in early labor who subsequently underwent repeat operation may have lowered the risk for complications in the planned repeat cesarean group. Nonetheless, most of the excess adverse events accompanying a TOLAC are attributable to the failure group of women who require a repeat cesarean operation[89] (Table 20-14).

An increased risk for maternal mortality accompanying all cases of cesarean delivery has been extrapolated to women undergoing a planned repeat operation versus a planned TOLAC, although the data to support this suggestion are limited. The infrequency of maternal death, confounding variables such as maternal disease, and the classification of a planned or nonplanned procedure, complicate comparisons of mortality. Maternal death attributable to uterine rupture is exceedingly rare.[49] The MFMU Cesarean Registry study found that maternal deaths were not significantly more common with planned

TABLE 20-13 COMPARISON OF MATERNAL COMPLICATIONS IN A TRIAL OF LABOR AFTER CESAREAN VERSUS PLANNED REPEAT CESAREAN DELIVERY

COMPLICATION	TRIAL OF LABOR (*N* = 17,898)	PLANNED REPEAT CESAREAN DELIVERY (*N* = 15,801)	ODDS RATIO (98% CI)
Uterine rupture	124 (0.7)	0	—
Hysterectomy	41 (0.2)	47 (0.3)	0.77 (0.51-1.17)
Thromboembolic disease	7 (0.04)	10 (0.1)	0.62 (0.24-1.62)
Transfusion	304 (1.7)	158 (1.0)	1.71 (1.41-2.08)
Endometritis	517 (2.9)	285 (1.8)	1.62 (1.40-1.87)
Maternal death	3 (0.02)	7 (0.04)	0.38 (1.10-1.46)
One or more of the above	978 (5.5)	563 (3.6)	1.56 (1.41-1.74)

Modified from Landon MB, Hauth JC, Leveno KJ, et al, for the National Institute of Child Health and Human Development Maternal-Fetal Medicine Units Network: Maternal and perinatal outcomes associated with a trial of labor after prior cesarean section. N Engl J Med 351:2581, 2004.

TABLE 20-14 MATERNAL COMPLICATIONS ACCORDING TO THE OUTCOME OF A TRIAL OF LABOR AFTER CESAREAN

COMPLICATION	FAILED VAGINAL DELIVERY (*N* = 4759)	SUCCESSFUL VAGINAL DELIVERY (*N* = 13,139)	ODDS RATIO (95% CI)	*P* VALUE
Uterine rupture	110 (2.3)	14 (0.1)	22.18 (12.70-38.72)	$P < .001$
Uterine dehiscence	100 (2.1)	19 (0.1)	14.82 (9.06-24.23)	$P < .001$
Hysterectomy	22 (0.5)	19 (0.1)	3.21 (1.73-5.93)	$P < .001$
Thromboembolic disease*	4 (0.1)	3 (0.02)	3.69 (0.83-16.51)	$P < .09$
Transfusion	152 (3.2)	152 (1.2)	2.82 (2.25-3.54)	$P < .001$
Endometritis	365 (7.7)	152 (1.2)	7.10 (5.86-8.60)	$P < .001$
Maternal death	2 (0.04)	1 (0.01)	5.52 (0.50-60.92)	$P < .17$
Other maternal adverse events†	63 (1.3)	1 (0.01)	176.24 (24.44-1,271.05)	$P < .001$
One or more of the above	669 (14.1)	309 (2.4)	6.81 (5.93-7.83)	$P < .001$

Modified from Landon MB, Hauth JC, Leveno KJ, et al, for the National Institute of Child Health and Human Development Maternal-Fetal Medicine Units Network: Maternal and perinatal outcomes associated with a trial of labor after prior cesarean section. N Engl J Med 351:2581, 2004.
*Thromboembolic disease includes deep venous thrombosis or pulmonary embolism.
†Other adverse events include broad ligament hematoma, cystotomy, bowel injury, and ureteral injury.
CI, Confidence interval.

repeat cesarean delivery. However, the study was not powered to detect a difference between this group and women attempting VBAC.[73] Guise and colleagues evaluated 24 maternal deaths among 402,833 patients with prior a cesarean delivery and noted the overall risk for maternal death associated with TOLAC is significantly lower (RR, 0.33; 95% CI, 0.13 to 0.88) than with repeat operation.[72]

Management of Vaginal Birth After Cesarean Delivery–Trial of Labor

The management of labor in women undergoing a TOLAC is primarily based on opinion. Women attempting VBAC should be encouraged to contact their health care provider promptly when labor or ruptured membranes occur. Continuous electronic fetal monitoring is prudent, although the need for intrauterine pressure catheter monitoring is controversial. **Studies that have examined FHR patterns before uterine rupture consistently report that non-reassuring signs, particularly significant variable decelerations or bradycardia, are the most common finding accompanying uterine rupture.**[90,91] Leung analyzed FHR and contraction patterns in association with 78 cases of uterine rupture. Prolonged decelerations (FHR <90 beats/minute exceeding 1 minute without return to baseline) occurred in 55 of 78 cases (71%) of uterine rupture. Prolonged deceleration was also noted in 36 of 36 cases (100%) in which the fetus was extruded from the uterus.

Despite the presence of adequate personnel to conduct an emergency cesarean delivery, prompt intervention does not always prevent fetal neurologic injury or death.[92] It appears that a non-reassuring FHR pattern occurring before uterine rupture identified cases in which the amount of time necessary to deliver an intact fetus is limited (Figure 20-13). In Leung's study, significant neonatal morbidity occurred when 18 minutes or longer elapsed between the onset of FHR deceleration and delivery. In cases in which prolonged deceleration was preceded by severe variable or late decelerations, fetal injury was noted as early as 10 minutes from the onset of a prolonged deceleration. In contrast to Leung's findings, Bujold and Gauthier[93] reported that less than 18 minutes elapsed between prolonged decelerations and delivery in two of three neonates diagnosed with HIE in 23 cases of uterine rupture.

TOLAC is not a contraindication to the use of epidural analgesia and does not appear to affect success rates.[55] Epidural analgesia also does not mask the signs and symptoms of uterine rupture. The role of oxytocin augmentation in uterine rupture has been discussed previously. Most studies, again, do not support a marked increased risk for associated uterine rupture with modest doses of oxytocin employed.[94] In a case-control study, Goetzel and colleagues[94] reported no association between uterine rupture and oxytocin-dosing intervals, total dose used, and the mean duration of oxytocin administration.

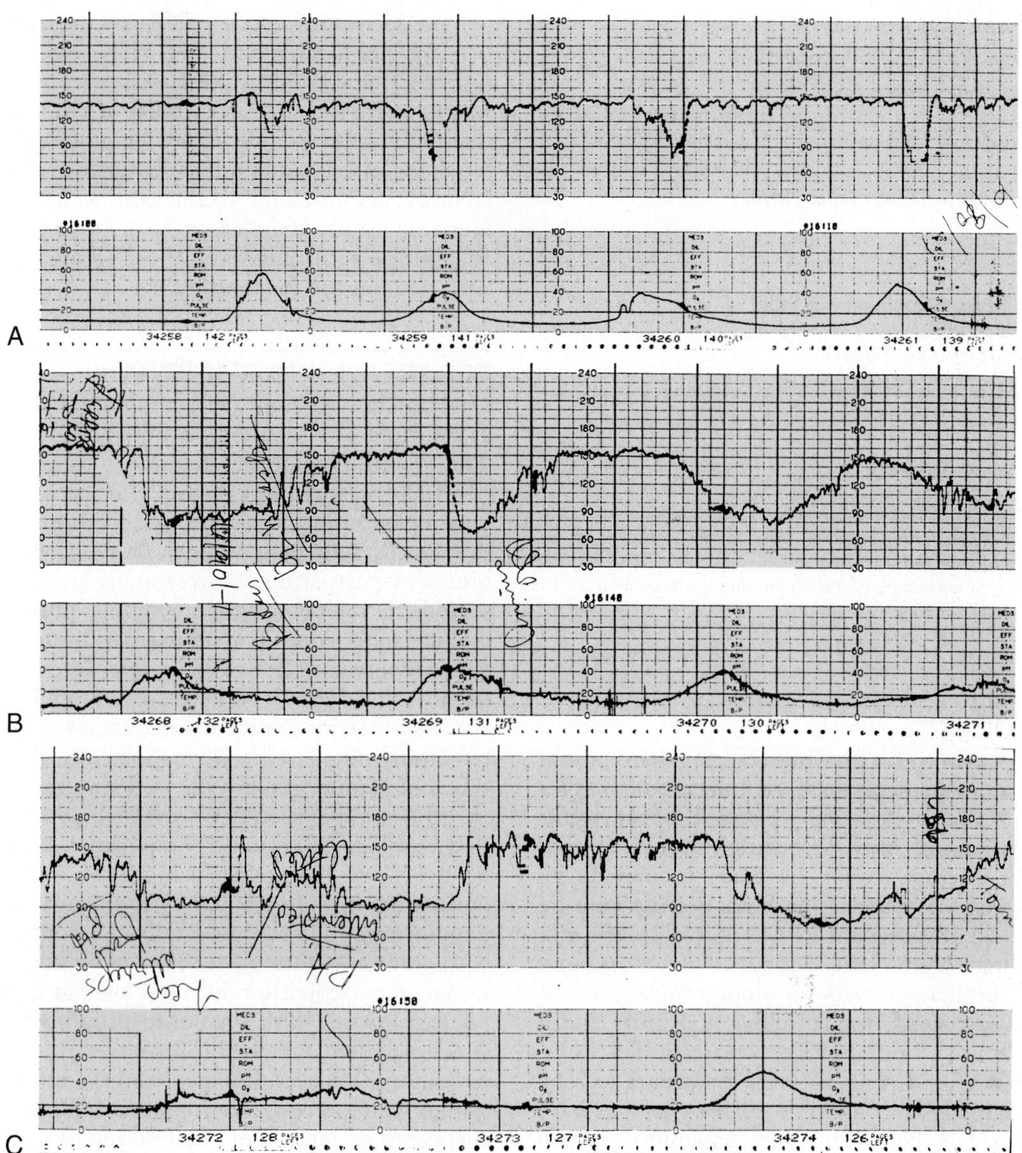

FIGURE 20-13. **A,** The patient is a 37-year-old gravida 7 para 3 Ab3 woman at 41 weeks' gestation who presented for induction of labor. She had had two prior vaginal deliveries, but her last baby was born at 33 weeks by low-transverse cesarean section for nonimmune hydrops caused by a cardiac malformation. The patient's induction was begun with prostaglandin gel. Her cervix changed from fingertip dilated, 50% effaced, to 1-cm dilated, 70% effaced with a cephalic presentation at −2 station. Oxytocin was then begun at 1 mU/minute. The patient progressed well, and epidural anesthesia was administered at 4 to 5 cm dilation, 90% effaced, and 0 station. The patient was at 6 cm dilation with a tracing demonstrating normal heart rate variability and variable decelerations. **B,** Thirty minutes after the above tracing was recorded, the fetal heart rate pattern changed to severe variable decelerations. **C,** The tracing then demonstrated prolonged decelerations at 90 beats/minute. The patient was taken to the operating room for an emergency cesarean delivery. Uterine rupture had occurred along the site of the previous uterine incision. A female fetus weighting 3200 g with Apgar scores of 7 and 8 was delivered. The umbilical arterial pH was 7.17 and the venous pH 7.22. The uterine incision had not extended and was easily closed. The baby did well.

The conduct of vaginal delivery itself is not altered by a history of prior cesarean birth. Most obstetricians do not routinely explore the uterus in order to detect asymptomatic scar dehiscences because these generally heal well. However, excessive vaginal bleeding or maternal hypotension should be promptly evaluated, including assessment for possible uterine rupture. Of 124 cases of uterine rupture accompanying 17,898 trials of labor, 14 (11%) were identified following vaginal delivery.[73]

Counseling for Vaginal Birth After Cesarean Delivery–Trial of Labor

Because uterine rupture may be a catastrophic event, ACOG continues to recommend that VBAC should only be attempted in institutions equipped to respond to emergencies, with physicians immediately available to provide emergency care. Thus, both in-house obstetrical and obstetrical anesthesia coverage are necessary to comply with this recommendation. ACOG recognizes that referral

TABLE 20-15 RISKS ASSOCIATED WITH TRIAL OF LABOR AFTER CESAREAN

Uterine Rupture and Related Morbidity	
Uterine rupture	(0.5-1.0/100 TOLAC)
Perinatal death and/or encephalopathy	(0.5/1000 TOLAC)
Hysterectomy	(0.3/1000 TOLAC)
Increased Maternal Morbidity with Failed TOLAC	
Transfusion	
Endometritis	
Length of stay	
Potential Risk for Perinatal Asphyxia with Labor (Cord Prolapse, Abruption)	
Potential risk for antepartum stillbirth beyond 39 weeks' gestation	

TABLE 20-16 RISKS ASSOCIATED WITH PLANNED REPEAT CESAREAN DELIVERY

- Increased maternal morbidity compared with successful trial of labor
- Increased length of stay and recovery
- Increased risks for abnormal placentation and hemorrhage with successive cesarean operations

may be required if a facility has inadequate resources to offer VBAC-TOLAC.[54]

A pregnant woman with a previous cesarean delivery is at risk for both maternal and perinatal complications whether undergoing TOLAC or choosing a planned repeat operation. Complications of both procedures should be discussed, and an attempt should be made to include an individualized risk assessment for both uterine rupture and the likelihood of successful VBAC (Table 20-15). For example, a woman who might require induction of labor may be at a slight increased risk for uterine rupture and is also less likely to achieve vaginal delivery. Future childbearing and the risks for multiple cesarean deliveries, including the risks for placenta previa and placenta accreta, should be considered as well (Table 20-16).

It is essential to make every effort possible to obtain records of the prior cesarean delivery in order to ascertain previous uterine incision type. This is particularly relevant to cases of prior preterm breech delivery in which a vertical uterine incision or a low-transverse incision in an undeveloped lower uterine segment might preclude a TOLAC. If previous uterine incision type is unknown, the implications of this missing information should be discussed as well.

Following complete informed consent detailing the risks and benefits for the individual woman, the delivery plan should be formulated by both the patient and physician. It is inappropriate to mandate VBAC-TOLAC because many women desire a planned repeat operation after thorough counseling. However, **VBAC-TOLAC should continue to remain an option for most women with a prior cesarean delivery, particularly when one considers the low absolute risks accompanying TOLAC. The attributable risk for a serious adverse perinatal outcome (perinatal death or HIE) at term appears to be about 1 in 2000 trials of labor. Combining an independent risk for hysterectomy attributable to uterine rupture at term with the risk for newborn HIE indicates the chance of one of these adverse events occurring to be about 1 in 1250 cases.**

The decision to elect a TOLAC may also increase the risk for perinatal death and HIE unrelated to uterine rupture. For women awaiting spontaneous labor beyond 39 weeks, there is a small possibility of unexplained stillbirth that might be avoidable with a scheduled repeat operation. A risk for fetal hypoxia and its sequelae may also accompany labor events unrelated to the uterine scar. In the MFMU Network Study, five cases of non-rupture-related HIE occurred in term infants in the TOLAC group compared with none in the planned repeat cesarean population.[73]

CESAREAN HYSTERECTOMY

Cesarean hysterectomy refers to the removal of the uterus at the time of a planned or unplanned cesarean delivery. The reported incidence of cesarean hysterectomy is 5 to 8 per 1000 cesarean deliveries.[95] Postpartum hysterectomy encompasses both cesarean hysterectomy and removal of the uterus following vaginal delivery. Cesarean section precedes postpartum hysterectomy in 73% of cases.[96] A systematic review of 981 emergency postpartum hysterectomies for uncontrolled hemorrhage indicated prior cesarean delivery in 449 cases. In this series, maternal death occurred in 26 (2.6%) of these postpartum hysterectomies.[96]

Substantial morbidity also accompanies peripartum hysterectomy compared with nonobstetrical hysterectomy.[97] Rates of bladder injury (9% vs. 1%), ureteral injury (0.7% vs. 0.1%), reoperation (4% vs. 0.5%), postoperative hemorrhage (5% vs. 2%), wound complications (10% vs. 3%), and VTE (1% vs. 0.7%) are all higher in women undergoing peripartum hysterectomy.[97] Wright and colleagues have demonstrated a lower incidence of perioperative morbidity with intensive care as well as mortality among women undergoing peripartum hysterectomy at high-volume hospitals compared with smaller institutions.[98] These authors concluded that, given the resources required to manage patients with placenta accreta and the improved outcomes at high-volume centers, women at high risk or those with suspected accreta should be referred to tertiary centers for delivery.

In most cases of hysterectomy following vaginal birth, the indication for the procedure is uterine atony with uncontrolled hemorrhage that has failed to respond to conservative measures (see Chapter 19). In contrast, placenta accreta has emerged as the most common indication for postcesarean hysterectomy (Table 20-17). In a series of 186 cesarean hysterectomies, 38% were performed for placenta accreta, whereas 35% had atony as the primary indication. Of the 71 placenta accreta cases, 82% accompanied a repeat cesarean delivery.[95] **There appears to be a trend of increasing cesarean hysterectomy as a result of an increased frequency of prior cesarean birth, itself a risk factor for placenta accreta. Nearly 25% of women with placenta previa and prior cesarean delivery develop placenta accreta, which in most cases requires a hysterectomy to control bleeding.**[99] With two or more prior cesarean deliveries and an existing placenta previa, the risk for cesarean hysterectomy ranges from 30% to 50%. Although placenta accreta itself poses a risk for peripartum hysterectomy, its association with prior uterine scarring, such as a cesarean delivery incision, is responsible for the about 50- to 100-fold increased risk for hysterectomy following cesarean section compared with

TABLE 20-17 INDICATIONS FOR CESAREAN HYSTERECTOMY

INDICATION	OVERALL NUMBER (n = 186)*	PRIMARY CESAREAN DELIVERIES*	REPEAT CESAREAN DELIVERIES (n = 106)
Accreta	71 (38.2)	13 (16.3)	58 (54.7)
Atony	64 (34.4)	42 (52.5)	22 (20.8)
Cervical cancer	13 (7.0)	9 (11.3)	4 (3.8)
Uterine rupture	10 (5.4)	2 (2.5)	8 (7.5)
Leiomyomas	9 (4.8)	6 (7.5)	3 (2.8)
Extension	2 (1.1)	2 (2.5)	0 (0.0)
Other†	17 (9.1)	6 (7.5)	11 (10.4)

Modified from Shellhaas CS, Gilbert S, Landon MB, et al, for the Eunice Kennedy Shriver National Institutes of Health and Human Development Maternal-Fetal Medicine Units Network: The frequency and complication rates of hysterectomy accompanying cesarean delivery. Obstet Gynecol 114:224-229, 2009.

*Data presented as n (%)

†Extensive adhesions, patient desire, uterine artery laceration, inability to close uterus, and diffuse hemorrhage/uncontrolled bleeding.

vaginal delivery. A history of prior cesarean section is now present in 57% to 67% of women undergoing a peripartum hysterectomy.[97]

Most cesarean hysterectomies are emergent procedures performed to control hemorrhage when conservative measures have failed. Occasionally, cesarean hysterectomy is planned for the treatment of cervical cancer or large myomas. The most common indications for emergency cesarean hysterectomy are placenta accreta, uterine atony, and uterine rupture. In Shellhaas and colleagues' series from the MFMU Network, these accounted for more than 75% of the procedures.[95]

Before the introduction of effective oxytocics such as prostaglandin $F_{2\alpha}$, uterine atony was the most common indication for cesarean hysterectomy. Today, improved oxytocics have reduced uterine atony as an indication. However, the rising rate of cesarean delivery has increased the frequency of abnormal placentation that has resulted in placenta accreta becoming the most common indication for cesarean hysterectomy. In two reports from Los Angeles County–University of Southern California Medical Center over an 18-year period, placenta accreta accounted for 30% of peripartum hysterectomies initially and later was associated with 45% of procedures.[99] The frequency of atony associated with peripartum hysterectomy fell from 43% to 20% from 1978 to 1990.[99]

In the previously mentioned series, uterine rupture was responsible for 11% to 13% of peripartum hysterectomies. In most cases of symptomatic rupture, the uterus can be preserved if so desired. The decision to proceed with hysterectomy ultimately depends on the ability to satisfactorily repair the uterus with hemostasis as well as the patients' wishes for future childbearing. Small dehiscences discovered at cesarean delivery or following successful VBAC are generally not indications for cesarean hysterectomy.

Technique and Complications

A peripartum hysterectomy, including cesarean hysterectomy, may be subtotal (supracervical) or total depending on the clinical circumstances. **In most planned procedures, a total hysterectomy is performed, whereas a subtotal hysterectomy may be preferable in cases in which emergency surgery is necessary for life-threatening hemorrhage and dissection of the cervix is difficult. Subtotal hysterectomy is a faster procedure and has been suggested in unstable patients.**

Subtotal hysterectomy is more likely to be performed in cases of atony. In one series of 30 cases of peripartum hysterectomy for atony, a subtotal procedure was accomplished in 77% of patients. Subtotal hysterectomy is less often performed in cases of placenta previa or accreta because lower uterine segment bleeding with these conditions often requires a total hysterectomy to control hemorrhage. In Shellhaas' series of 186 procedures, 66% were total hysterectomies.[95]

The operative technique for cesarean hysterectomy consists of the same general surgical considerations for the procedure performed in the nonpregnant individual. Specific considerations include adequate inferior displacement of the bladder if possible before the hysterectomy because taking the bladder down may be difficult following uterine incision and delivery of the infant. Additionally, care must be taken to avoid bladder and ureteral injury, which appears to be relatively common with peripartum hysterectomy. Cystotomy has been reported to occur in up to 5% to 9% of cases, although many of these represent intentional procedures.[98] Ureteral injury is observed in 1 in 200 operations. The ureter is particularly vulnerable to injury if broad ligament bleeding occurs and lateral clamping is necessary to control this. If ureteral injury is suspected, the dome of the bladder may be incised, and retrograde stenting of the ureter is performed. Intravenous injection of indigo carmine may also be useful in identifying a ureteral injury or detecting a suspected ligature.

The sequence of maneuvers for hysterectomy is not different from the procedure in the nonpregnant state. As mentioned previously, efforts to displace the bladder inferiorly before delivery are advised. Following delivery and removal of the placenta, the uterine incision is frequently reapproximated, or attention is given to securing hemostasis by ligating the uteroovarian anastomosis bilaterally. The bladder should be inspected and mobilized by blunt and sharp dissection. In cases of accreta or percreta with bladder involvement, creation of a bladder flap is not advised. Intentional cystotomy may be performed to determine the extent of placental involvement. In most cesarean hysterectomies, the ovaries are left, although the adnexa in the pregnant state are vulnerable to hematoma formation, which may necessitate salpingo-oophorectomy. The avascular portion of the broad ligaments is incised, and the uterine vessels are identified, clamped, and suture-ligated (Figures 20-14 and 20-15). Clamps are placed tightly along the lateral aspect of the uterus to prevent injury to the ureter and hematoma formation. At this point, the decision is often made whether to proceed with subtotal versus total hysterectomy. In most instances, a total procedure is performed unless the patient is unstable, and bleeding can be adequately controlled by the subtotal approach. If the cervix is amputated, it is closed with figure-of-eight sutures and reperitonealization may or may not be performed (Figure 20-16). If total hysterectomy is to be accomplished, after further consideration, the cervical stump is elevated with traction and is separated from the cardinal and uterosacral ligaments by clamping and

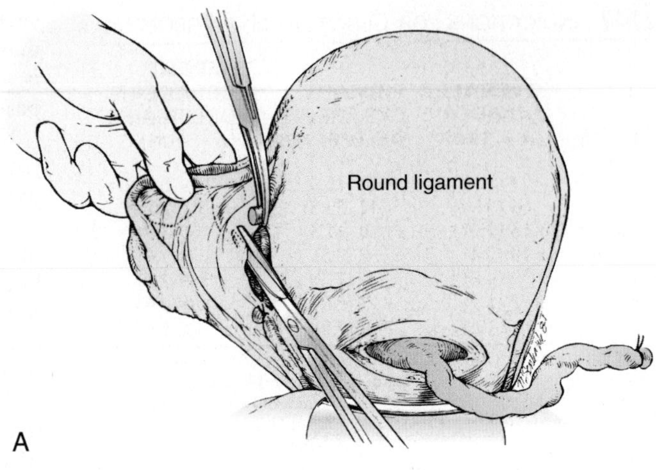

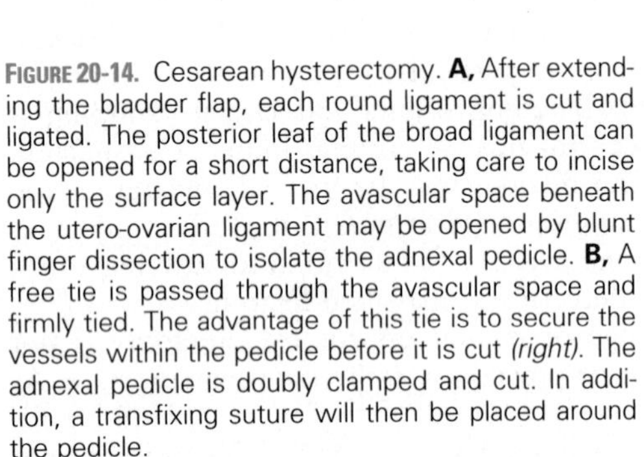
FIGURE 20-14. Cesarean hysterectomy. **A,** After extending the bladder flap, each round ligament is cut and ligated. The posterior leaf of the broad ligament can be opened for a short distance, taking care to incise only the surface layer. The avascular space beneath the utero-ovarian ligament may be opened by blunt finger dissection to isolate the adnexal pedicle. **B,** A free tie is passed through the avascular space and firmly tied. The advantage of this tie is to secure the vessels within the pedicle before it is cut *(right)*. The adnexal pedicle is doubly clamped and cut. In addition, a transfixing suture will then be placed around the pedicle.

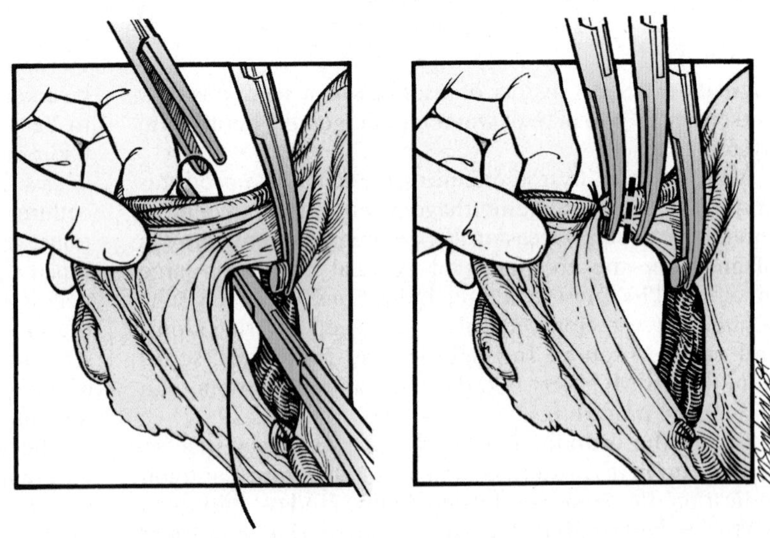

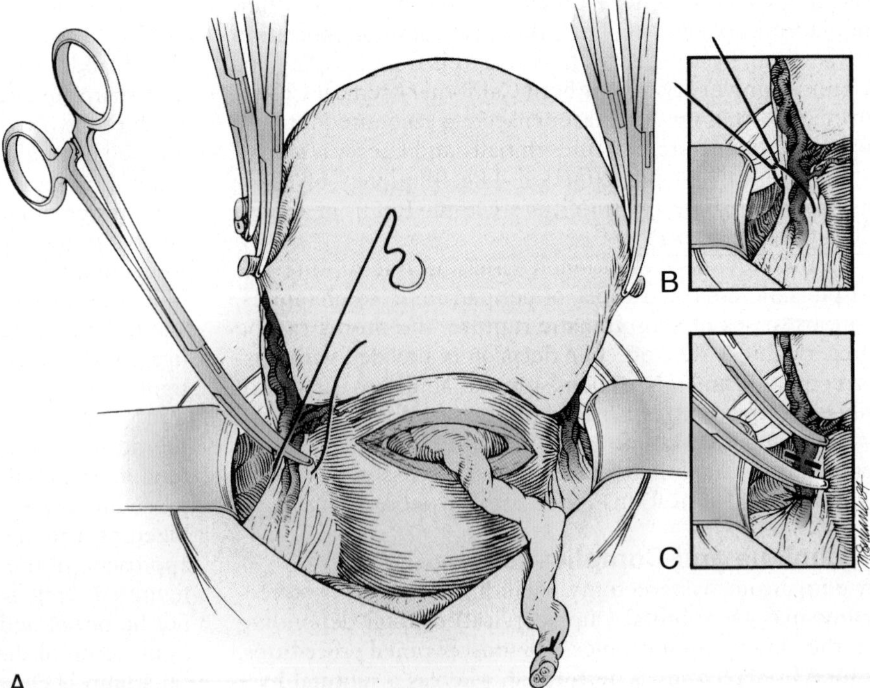

FIGURE 20-15. A, The ascending branches of the uterine artery are clamped and cut, and a suture is placed just below the tip of the clamp and immediately next to the uterine wall. **B,** After removing the clamp, the suture is tied, thus securing the vessels before they are cut. **C,** The pedicle is regrasped just above the tie and then doubly ligated.

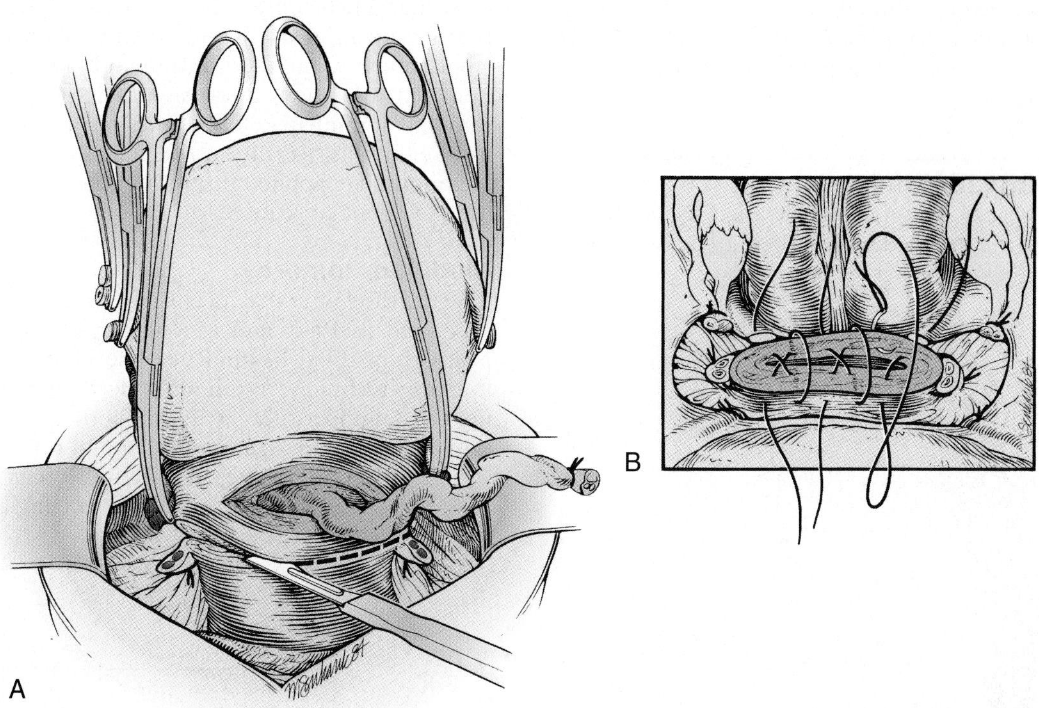

Figure 20-16. Subtotal hysterectomy. **A,** The cervix is incised just below the level of the ligated pedicles of the uterine arteries, amputating the uterine corpus from its cervical stump. **B,** The cervical stump may be closed with several interrupted figure-of-eight sutures; reperitonealization is then accomplished as in a total hysterectomy.

ligature (Figure 20-17). The vagina is then entered anteriorly or at the lateral angle above a curved clamp. An effort should be made to be certain the cervix is completely removed, although in cases following labor, this may be difficult. Similarly, excess portions of the superior vagina should not be excised. In order to minimize these complications, some surgeons prefer to insert a finger through an incision in the lower uterine segment to identify the cervicovaginal junction before excision of the cervix (Figure 20-18). The vaginal cuff is supported by approximation to the cardinal and uterosacral ligament pedicles (Figures 20-19 and 20-20). The cuff may be left open or closed in with interrupted or running locking continuous sutures (Figure 20-21). If significant bleeding is a concern, the cuff is better left open for dependent drainage or placement of a drain. Reperitonealization has become less favored and has been replaced by many with fixation of the ovarian pedicles to the round ligaments, to reduce the chance of adhesion to the vaginal cuff (Figure 20-22).

The principal complications of cesarean hysterectomy are urologic injury, as discussed earlier, and hemorrhage. The average blood loss varies, with an excess of 500 to 1000 mL beyond a routine cesarean delivery. The frequency of transfusion has been reported to be 75%[95] (Table 20-18). In many cases, the indication for hysterectomy is hemorrhage itself with a large preexisting blood loss before commencing the hysterectomy. Febrile morbidity is common, particularly with an unplanned cesarean hysterectomy, with infection rates of 25% to 30% observed, despite prophylactic antibiotic administration.[99] With the friability of pelvic tissues, as well as the indications for

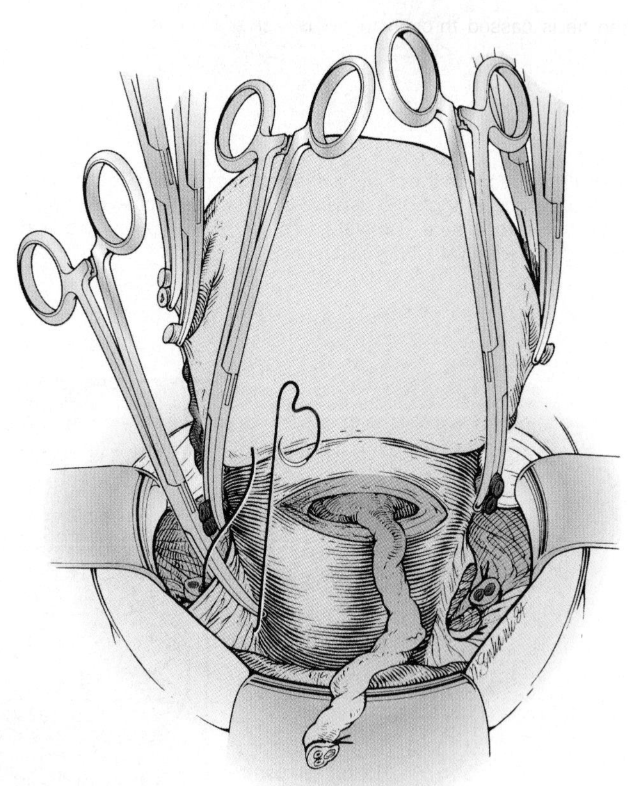

Figure 20-17. The cardinal ligaments are clamped at their point of insertion, cut, and singly ligated. Because these structures are hypertrophied, several bites may be necessary. Some physicians clamp, cut, and ligate the uterosacral ligaments separately.

hysterectomy often resulting in coagulopathy, postsurgical bleeding is observed with increased frequency following peripartum hysterectomy. Reexploration has been reported in 2% to 4% of cases.[95,98]

TUBAL STERILIZATION

Surgical approach to tubal sterilization is influenced by whether the procedure is being performed on a postpartum or on an interval basis. Advantages to the postpartum approach include the use of one anesthesia for labor, delivery, and sterilization and only one hospitalization. Tubal ligations after vaginal delivery are performed through a minilaparotomy incision at the level of the uterine fundus, usually subumbilically. The same surgical techniques are applied if tubal ligation is performed at the time of cesarean section.

Modified Pomeroy

The method of tubal occlusion used by Pomeroy was described in 1930, and it is the most popular means of postpartum tubal ligation because of its simplicity. The Pomeroy technique as originally described included grasping the fallopian tube at its midportion, creating a small knuckle, and then ligating the loop of tube with a double strand of catgut suture. It is critical that the fallopian tube be conclusively identified. Visualizing the fimbriated

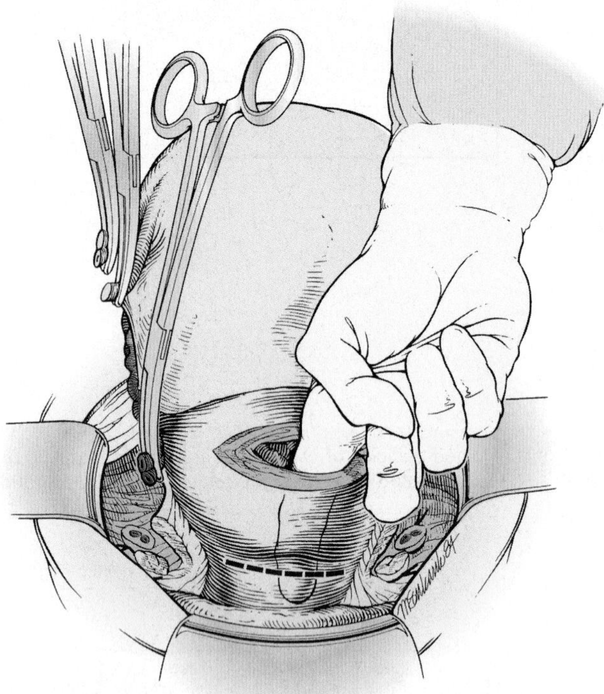

FIGURE 20-18. Because the cervix is elongated, it may be useful to insert an index finger through the cervical canal to demarcate the vaginal incision and to ensure complete removal of the cervix and avoid unnecessary removal of vaginal length.

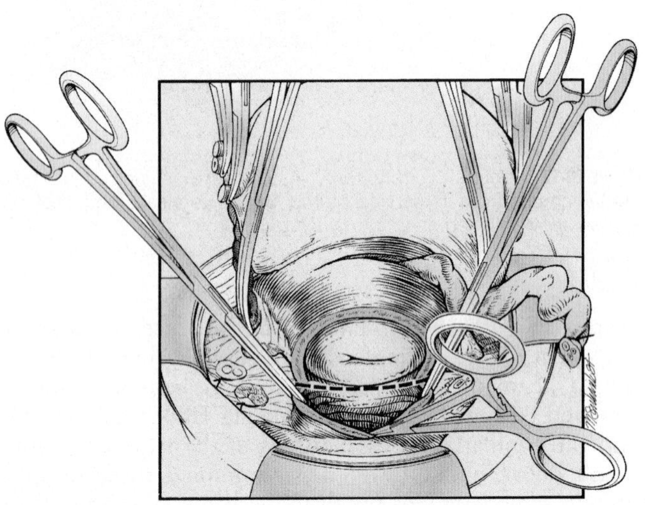

FIGURE 20-19. The vagina is circumferentially incised at its cervical attachment and grasped with four clamps.

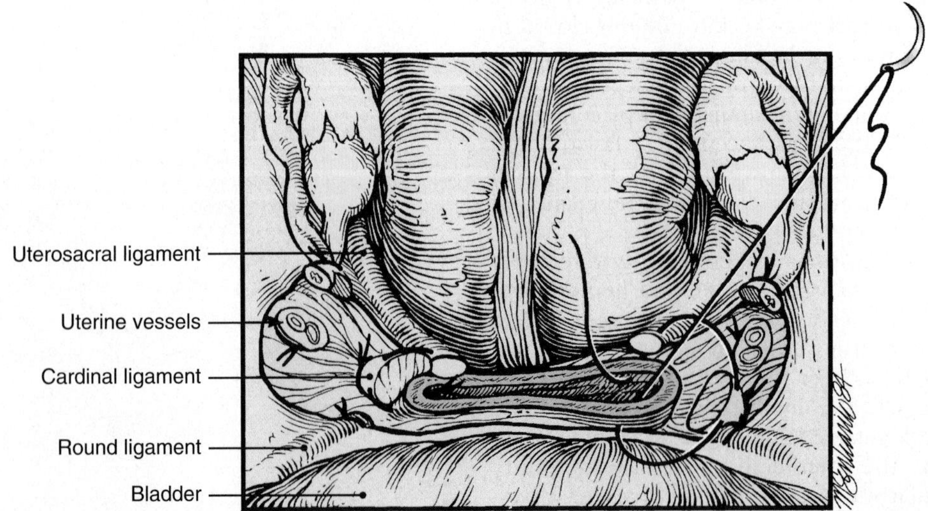

FIGURE 20-20. The angles of the vaginal cuff are closed with sutures to include the cardinal and uterosacral ligaments, thus providing fascial support to the vaginal vault. A simple loop suture is commonly used at this location to reduce the likelihood of breakage during the state of postoperative edema.

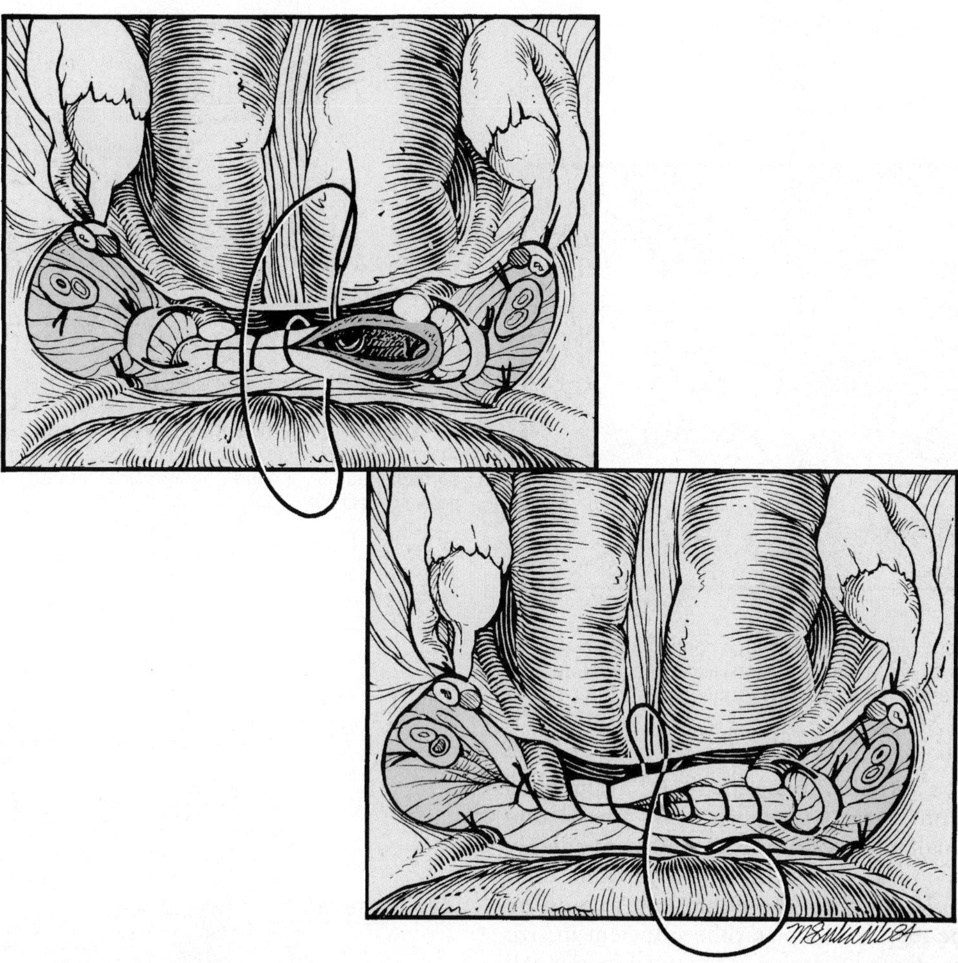

FIGURE 20-21. There are a number of methods of closing the vaginal cuff. Illustrated is a two-layer closure. The first layer closes the vagina, and the second layer closes the endopelvic fascia. Many operators prefer to leave the cuff "open" by using one continuous suture that circles the cuff, approximating the cut edge to its surrounding fascia.

TABLE 20-18 CESAREAN HYSTERECTOMY MORBIDITY AND MORTALITY

	CLARK ET AL. (1978-1982)		STANCO ET AL. (1985-1990)		SHELLHAAS ET AL. (1999-2001)		WRIGHT ET AL. (1999-2001)	
	No.	**%**	**No.**	**%**	**No.**	**%**	**No.**	**%**
Procedures	70		123		186		4967	
Subtotal procedures	38	54	65	53	63	34	1672	33.7
Operative time (mean)	3.1 hr		NA		2.8 hr	NA		
Blood loss (mean)	3575 mL		3000 mL*		—		NA	
Transfused patients	67	96	102	83		80	2284	46.0
Reexplored	—	—	—	—	7	3.8	202	4.1
Infection morbidity	—	—	—	—			614	12.4
Febrile	35	50	NA		21	11	NA	
Urinary tract infection			NA		6	3.2	NA	
Wound infection	8	12	11	9	2	1.1	507	10.2
Urologic injury	3	4	4				539	10.9
Cystotomy		0	12†		18	9.7	458	9.2
Ureteral	3	4	—		0		33	0.7
Maternal death	1‡	1	0		3	1.6	48	1

Data from Clark et al.,[92] Stanco et al.,[99] and Shellhaas et al.[95] include cesarean hysterectomies only. Wright[98] includes all peripartum hysterectomies.

*Median value 50% >3000 mL and 50% <3000 mL.

†Intentional cystotomies for ureteral stent passage.

‡Cardiac arrest secondary to amniotic fluid embolus.

NA, Not applicable.

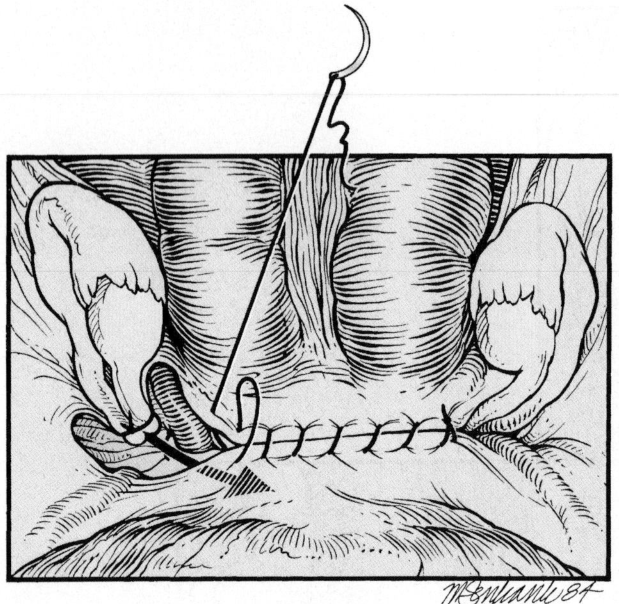

FIGURE 20-22. The bladder flap is closed with a continuous suture that inverts the pedicles of the round ligaments and adnexa. Note that these structures have not been attached to the vaginal cuff.

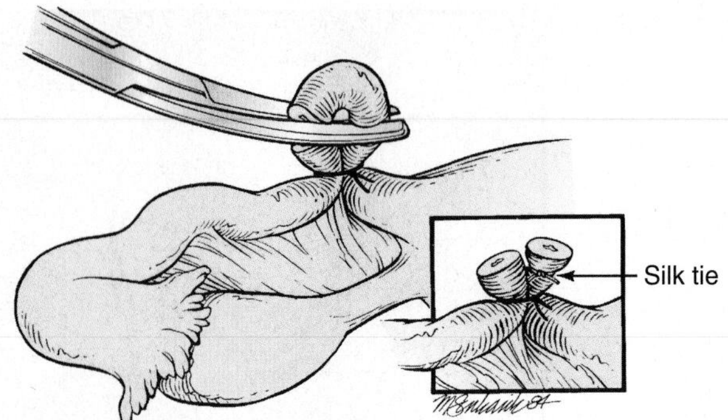

FIGURE 20-23. Pomeroy sterilization. A knuckle of tube is ligated with absorbable suture, and a small segment is being excised. Note that the ligation is performed at a site that will favor reanastomosis, should that become desirable. Some surgeons place an extra tie of nonabsorbable suture around the proximal stump as added protection against recanalization.

portion of the tube and identifying the round ligament as a separate structure can accomplish this. Absorbable sutures are used so that the tubal ends will separate quickly after surgery, leaving a gap between the proximal and distal ends. In performing the procedure, care should be taken to make the loop of fallopian tube sufficient in size to ensure that complete transection of the tubal lumen will occur. After the loop of fallopian tube is ligated, the mesosalpinx of the ligated loop should be perforated using scissors, and the knuckle of the tube is transected (Figure 20-23). It is important not to resect the fallopian tube so close to the suture that the remaining portion of the fallopian tube slips out of the ligature and causes delayed bleeding.

The Parkland Procedure

The Parkland procedure was designed to avoid close approximation of the cut ends of the fallopian tube accompanying the Pomeroy procedure. An avascular segment of midposition mesosalpinx is identified. A hemostat or coagulation can be used to create an opening. The freed fallopian tube is then ligated proximally and distally with the intervening segment being excised and submitted for pathologic examination. The proximal ligated end of the tube may be left free or can be buried in the mesosalpinx (Figure 20-24).

The Irving Procedure

Irving first reported his sterilization technique in 1924, with a modification in 1950. In the modified procedure, a window is created in the mesosalpinx and the fallopian tube is doubly ligated as in the Parkland procedure. The fallopian tube is then transected about 4 cm from the uterotubal portion; the two free ends of the ligation stitch on the proximal tubal segment are held long. The proximal portion of the fallopian tube is dissected free from the

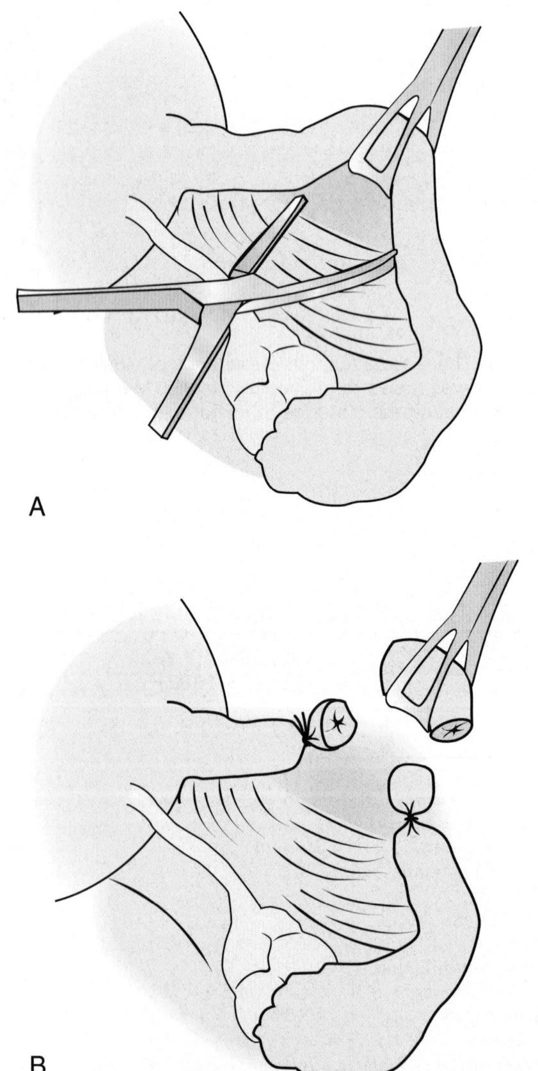

FIGURE 20-24. Parkland tubal ligation. The avascular mesosalpinx is opened by blunt dissection. A 2-cm midsegment of tube is ligated with 0-0 chromic suture and divided between the sutures. (Modified from Cunningham FG, Leveno KJ, Bloom SL, et al [eds]: Williams Obstetrics, 22nd ed. New York, McGraw-Hill, 2005.)

mesosalpinx and then buried into an incision in the myometrium of the posterior uterine wall, near the uterotubal junction. This is accomplished by first creating a tunnel about 2 cm in length with a mosquito clamp in the uterine wall. The two free ends of the ligation stitch on the proximal tubal segment are then brought deep into the myometrial tunnel and are brought out through the uterine serosa. Traction is then placed on the sutures to draw the proximal tubal stump into the myometrial tunnel; tying the free sutures fixes the tube in that location. No treatment of the distal tubal stump is necessary, but some choose to bury the segment in the mesosalpinx (Figure 20-25). Although this technique is slightly more complicated than the others, it has the lowest failure rate.

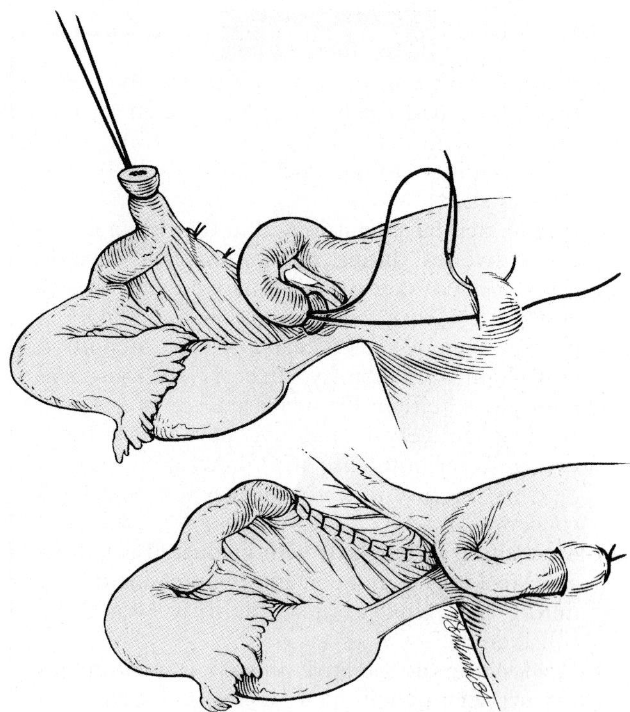

FIGURE 20-25. Irving sterilization. The tube is transected 3 to 4 cm from its insertion, and a short tunnel is created by means of a sharp-nosed hemostat in either the anterior or posterior uterine wall. The cut end of the tube can then be buried in the tunnel and, if necessary, further secured by an interrupted suture at the opening of the tunnel. The distal cut end is buried between the leaves of the broad ligament.

The Uchida Procedure

In this sterilization procedure, the muscular portion of the fallopian tube is separated from its serosal cover and grasped about 6 to 7 cm from the uterotubal junction. Saline solution is injected subserosally, and the serosa is then incised. The muscular portion of the fallopian tube is grasped with a clamp and divided. The serosa over the proximal tubal segment is bluntly dissected toward the uterus, exposing about 5 cm of the proximal tubal segment. The tube is then ligated with chromic suture near the uterotubal junction, and about 5 cm of the tube is resected. The shortened proximal tubal stump is allowed to retract into the mesosalpinx. The serosa around the opening in the mesosalpinx is sutured in a pursestring with a fine absorbable stitch; when the suture is tied, the mesosalpinx is gathered around the distal tubal segment (Figure 20-26). Some surgeons choose to excise only 1 cm of fallopian tube rather than the recommended 5 cm in case the patient wishes to have a tubal reanastomosis in the future.

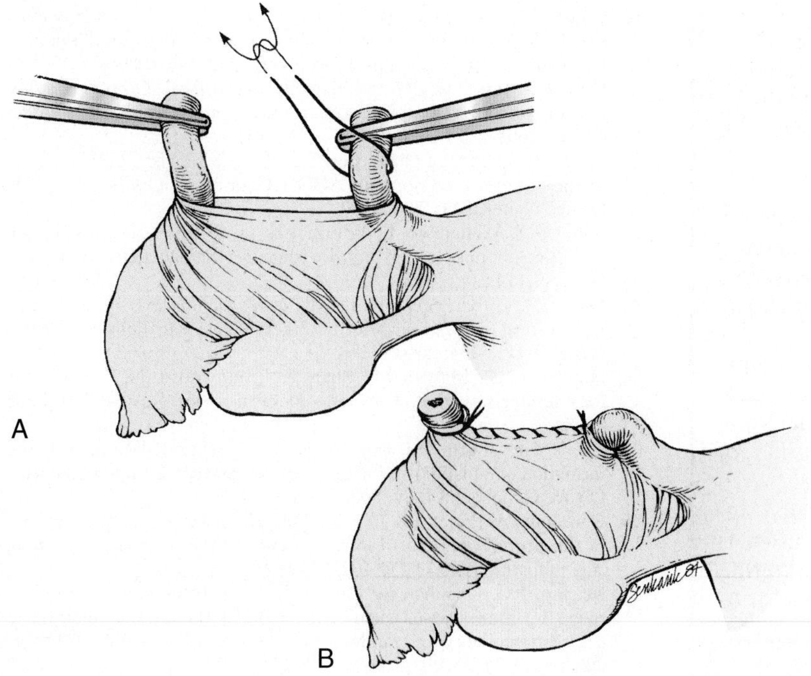

FIGURE 20-26. Uchida sterilization. The leaves of the broad ligament and peritubal peritoneum are infiltrated with saline so that the tube can be easily isolated from these structures, divided **(A)**, and ligated **(B)**. The broad ligament is then closed, burying the proximal stump between the leaves and including the distal stump in the line of closure.

KEY POINTS

- In 1970, the cesarean delivery rate was about 5%. By 2008, it had reached 32.8%, the highest rate ever recorded in the United States. VBAC rates have plummeted from a peak of 28.3% in 1996 to 8.5% in 2008.
- Factors that have contributed to the rise in cesarean deliveries during the past decade include (1) continued increase in primary cesarean deliveries for dystocia, failed induction, and abnormal presentation; (2) an increase in the proportion of women with obesity, diabetes mellitus, and multiple gestation; (3) increased use of planned cesarean delivery to preserve pelvic floor function; and (4) limited use of TOLAC after cesarean delivery because of both safety and medicolegal concerns.
- Mechanical prophylaxis with graduated compression stockings or a pneumatic compression device during and after cesarean delivery should be considered.
- Single-dose, preoperative prophylactic antibiotics are of clear benefit in reducing the frequency of postcesarean endomyometritis and wound infection.
- A low-transverse uterine incision is performed in more than 90% of cesarean deliveries. A vertical uterine incision may rarely be performed for cesarean delivery if the lower uterine segment is poorly developed or if the fetus is in a back-down transverse lie.
- Sharp uterine extension appears to be associated with increased blood loss as well as the potential risk for cutting the umbilical cord or direct fetal injury.
- Several randomized trials have demonstrated greater blood loss and a higher rate of endometritis with manual extraction of the placenta at cesarean delivery. Thus, spontaneous expulsion of the placenta with gentle cord traction is preferred.
- When closing the abdomen after a cesarean delivery, the subcutaneous tissue is closed if its thickness exceeds 2 cm. This approach reduces the risk for wound disruption by 34% in women with excessive subcutaneous fat.
- The risk for uterine rupture in a TOLAC depends greatly on the previous uterine incision, ranging from 0.5% to 1.0% with a prior low-transverse cesarean delivery to 4% to 9% with a prior classic or T-incision.
- Misoprostol should not be used in women attempting VBAC. Oxytocin use may marginally increase the risk for uterine rupture in women undergoing a TOLAC. Therefore, judicious stimulation of labor should be used in these patients.
- A non-reassuring FHR pattern, particularly significant variable decelerations or bradycardia, is the most common finding accompanying uterine rupture.

REFERENCES

1. American College of Obstetricians and Gynecologists: ACOG Executive Summary: Evaluation of Cesarean Delivery. Washington, DC, ACOG, 2000.
2. National Institutes of Health: State-of-the-science conference statement. Obstet Gynecol 107:1386, 2006.
3. American College of Obstetricians and Gynecologists: Cesarean delivery on maternal request. ACOG Committee Opinion No. 386. Obstet Gynecol 110:1209, 2007.
4. Tita ATN, Landon MB, Spong CY, et al: Timing of elective cesarean delivery at term and neonatal outcomes. N Engl J Med 360:111, 2009.
5. Gibbs RS, Sweet RL, Duff WP: Maternal and fetal infectious disorders. *In* Creasy RK, Resnik R (eds): Maternal-Fetal Medicine Principles and Practice. Philadelphia, WB Saunders, 2004, p 752.
6. Small F, Hofmeyr GJ: Antibiotic prophylaxis for cesarean section. Cochrane Database Syst Rev 1, 2005.
7. Hopkins L, Smaill FM. Antibiotics prophylaxis regimens and drugs for cesarean delivery. Cochrane Database Syst Rev 1, 2009.
8. Costantine MM, Rahman M, Ghulmiyah L, et al: Timing of perioperative antibiotics for cesarean delivery: a metaanalysis. Am J Obstet Gynecol 199:301.e1-6, 2008.
9. Tita ATN, Rouse DJ, Blackwell S, et al: Emerging concepts in antibiotic prophylaxis for cesarean delivery. Obstet Gynecol 113:675, 2009.
10. Tita ATN, Hauth JC, Grimes A, et al: Decreasing incidence of postcesarean endometritis with extended-spectrum antibiotic prophylaxis. Obstet Gynecol 111:51, 2008.
11. Hopkins L, Smaill F: Antibiotic prophylaxis regimens and drugs for cesarean section (Cochrane Review). *In* The Cochrane Library, Issue 2. Oxford, Update Software, 2003.
12. Faro S, Martens MG, Hammill HA, et al: Antibiotic prophylaxis: is there a difference? Am J Obstet Gynecol 162:900, 1990.
13. Tooher R, Gates S, Dowswell T, Davis LJ: Prophylaxis for venous thromboembolic disease in pregnancy and the early postnatal period. Cochrane Database Syst Rev 5:CD001689, 2010.
14. Cluver C, Novikova N, Hofmeyr JG, Hall DR: Maternal position during caesarean section for preventing maternal and neonatal complications. Cochrane Database Syst Rev 6:CD007623, 2010.
15. Cutland CL, Madhi SA, Zell ER, et al: Chlorhexidine maternal-vaginal and neonate body wipes in sepsis and vertical transmission of pathogenic bacteria in South-Africa: a randomized, controlled trial. Lancet 374:1909, 2009.
16. Alexander JW, Fischer JE, Bovajian M, et al: The influence of hair removal methods on wound infections. Arch Surg 118:347, 1983.
17. Darouiche RO, Wall MJ Jr, Itani KM, et al: Chlorhexidine-alcohol versus povidone-iodine for surgical-site antisepsis. N Engl J Med 362:18, 2010.
18. Cordtz T, Schouenborg L, Laursen K, et al: The effect of incisional plastic drapes and redisinfection of operation site on wound infection following caesarean section. J Hosp Infect 13:267, 1989.
19. Ward HR, Jennings OG, Potgieter P, Lombard CJ: Do plastic adhesive drapes prevent post caesarean wound infection? J Hosp Infect 47:230, 2001.
20. American College of Obstetricians and Gynecologists: Patient safety in the surgical environment. ACOG Committee Opinion No. 328. Obstet Gynecol 116:786, 2010.
21. Sullivan S, Williamson B, Wilson LK, et al: Blunt needles for the reduction of needlestick injuries during cesarean delivery. Obstet Gynecol 114:211, 2009.
22. Wylie BJ, Gilbert S, Landon MB, et al: Comparison of transverse and vertical skin incision for emergency cesarean delivery. Obstet Gynecol 115:1134, 2010.
23. Hofmeyr JG, Mathai M, Shah AN, Novikova N: Techniques for caesarean section. Cochrane Database Syst Rev 3:CD004662, 2008.
24. Hohlagschwandtner M, Ruecklinger E, Husslein P, Joura EA: Is the formation of a bladder flap at cesarean necessary? A randomized trial. Obstet Gynecol 98:1089, 2001.
25. Rodriguez A, Porter KB, O'Brien WF: Blunt versus sharp expansion of the uterine incision in low-segment transverse cesarean section. Am J Obstet Gynecol 171:1022, 1994.
26. Magann EG, Chauhan SP, Bufkin L, et al: Intraoperative haemorrhage by blunt versus sharp expansion of the uterine incision at cesarean delivery: a randomized clinical trial. BJOG 109:448, 2002.

27. Cromi A, Ghezzi F, DiNaro E, et al: Blunt expansion of the low transverse uterine incision at cesarean delivery: a randomized comparison of 2 techniques. Am J Obstet Gynecol 199:292.e1, 2008.
28. Fasubaa OB, Ezechi OC, Orji EO, et al: Delivery of the impacted head of the fetus at caesarean section after prolonged obstructed labor: a randomized comparative study of two methods. J Obstet Gynecol 22:375, 2002.
29. Magann EF, Dodson MK, Albert JR, et al: Blood loss at time of cesarean section by method of placental removal and exteriorization versus in situ repair of the uterine incision. Surg Gynecol Obstet 177:389, 1993.
30. Atkinson MW, Owen J, Wren A, Hauth JC: The effect of manual removal of the placenta on post-cesarean endometritis. Obstet Gynecol 87:99, 1996.
31. Anorlu RI, Maholwana B, Hofmeyr GJ: Methods of delivering the placenta at caesarean section. Cochrane Database Syst Rev 3: CD004737, 2008.
32. Walsh CA, Walsh SR: Extraabdominal vs intraabdominal uterine repair at cesarean delivery: a metaanalysis. Am J Obstet Gynecol 200:625.e1, 2009.
33. Ahmed B, Nahia FA, Abushama M: Routine cervical dilatation during elective cesarean section and its influence on maternal morbidity: a randomized controlled trial. J Perinat Med 233:510, 2005.
34. Hohlagschwandtner M, Chalubinski K, Nather A, et al: Continuous vs interrupted sutures for single-layer closure of uterine incision at cesarean section. Arch Gynecol Obstet 268:26, 2003.
35. Yazicioglu F, Gokdogan A, Kelekci S, Aygun M: Incomplete healing of the uterine incision after cesarean section: is it preventable? Eur J Obstet Gynecol Reprod Biol 124:32, 2006.
36. Dodd JM, Anderson ER, Gates S: Surgical techniques for uterine incision and uterine closure at the time of caesarean section. Cochrane Database Syst Rev 3:CD004732, 2008.
37. Harrigill K, Miller HS, Haynes DE: The effect of intraabdominal irrigation at cesarean delivery on maternal morbidity: a randomized trial. Obstet Gynecol 101:80, 2003.
38. Bamigboye AA, Hofmeyr JG: Closure versus non-closure of the peritoneum at caesarean section. Cochrane Database Syst Rev 7: CD000163, 2003.
39. Anderson ER, Gates S: Techniques and materials for closure of the abdominal wall in caesarean section. Cochrane Database Syst Rev 4: CD004663, 2004.
40. Gates S, Anderson ER: Wound drainage for caesarean section. Cochrane Database Syst Rev 3:CD004549, 2005.
41. Frishman GN, Schwartz T, Hogan JW. Closure of Pfannenstiel skin incisions: staples vs. subcuticular suture. J Reprod Med 42:627, 1997.
42. Rousseau JA, Girard K, Turcot-Lemay L, Thomas N: A randomized study comparing skin closure in cesarean sections: staples vs subcuticular sutures. Am J Obstet Gynecol 200:265, 2009.
43. Cromi A, Ghezzi F, Gottardi A, et al: Cosmetic outcomes of various skin closure methods following cesarean delivery: a randomized trial. Am J Obstet Gynecol 203:36.e1-8, 2010.
44. Silver RM, Landon MB, Rouse DJ, et al: Maternal morbidity associated with multiple repeat cesarean deliveries. Obstet Gynecol 107:1226, 2006.
45. Lilford RJ, Van Coeverden SC, De Groot HA, et al: The relative risks of cesarean section (intrapartum and elective) and vaginal delivery: a detailed analysis to exclude the effects of medical disorders and other acute pre-existing physiological disturbance. BJOG 97:883, 1990.
46. Lydon-Rochelle M, Holt V, Easterling TR, et al: Cesarean delivery and postpartum mortality among primiparas in Washington State, 1987-1986. Obstet Gynecol 97:169, 2001.
47. Zhang J, Troendle J, Reddy UM, et al, for the Consortium on Safe Labor: Contemporary cesarean delivery practice in the United States. Am J Obstet Gynecol 303:326e1-10, 2010.
48. Sachs BP, Kobelin C, Castro MA, Frigoletto F: The risks of lowering the cesarean-delivery rate. N Engl J Med 340:54, 1990.
49. Scott J: Mandatory trial of labor after cesarean delivery: an alternative viewpoint. Obstet Gynecol 77:811, 1991.
50. Pitkin RM: Once a cesarean? Obstet Gynecol 77:939, 1991.
51. Vaginal birth after previous cesarean delivery: clinical management guidelines for obstetricians-gynecologists. ACOG practice bulletin no. 5. Washington, DC, American College of Obstetricians and Gynecologists, July 1999.
52. Vaginal birth after previous cesarean delivery: clinical management guidelines for obstetrician-gynecologists. ACOG Practice Bulletin No. 54. Washington, DC, American College of Obstetricians and Gynecologists, July 2004.
53. National Institutes of Health Consensus Development Conference Panel: National Institutes of Health Consensus Development Conference Statement. Vaginal Birth after Cesarean: New Insights, March 8-10, 2010. Obstet Gynecol 115:1279, 2010.
54. ACOG Practice Bulletin No. 115: Vaginal birth after previous cesarean delivery. Washington, DC, American College of Obstetricians and Gynecologists, August 2010.
55. Landon MB, Leindecker S, Spong CY, for the National Institute of Child Health and Human Development Maternal-Fetal Medicine Units Network: The MFMU Cesarean Registry: factors affecting the success and trial of labor following prior cesarean delivery. Am J Obstet Gynecol 193:1016, 2005.
56. Elkousky MA, Samuel M, Stevens E, et al: The effect of birthweight on vaginal birth after cesarean delivery success rates. Am J Obstet Gynecol 188:824, 2003.
57. Grobman WA, Lai Y, Landon MB, et al: For the National Institute of Child Health and Human Development (NICHD) Maternal Fetal Medicine Units Network (MFMU). Development of a normogram for prediction of vaginal birth after cesarean delivery. Obstet Gynecol 109:806, 2007.
58. Caughey AB, Shipp TD, Repke JT, et al: Trial of labor after cesarean delivery: the effects of previous vaginal delivery. Am J Obstet Gynecol 179:938, 1998.
59. Mercer BM, Gilbert S, Landon MB, et al: For the National Institute of Child Health and Human Development (NICHD) Maternal Fetal Medicine Units Network (MFMU). Labor outcomes with increasing number of prior vaginal births after cesarean delivery. Obstet Gynecol 111:285, 2008.
60. Peaceman AM, Genoviez R, Landon MB, et al: For the National Institute of Child Health and Human Development (NICHD) Maternal Fetal Medicine Units Network (MFMU). Am J Obstet Gynecol 195:1127, 2005.
61. Flamm BL, Geiger AM: Vaginal birth after cesarean delivery: an admission scoring system. Obstet Gynecol 90:907, 1997.
62. Grobman WA, Gilbert S, Landon MB, et al: Outcome of induction of labor after one prior cesarean. Obstet Gynecol 1-0:262, 2007.
63. Grinstead J, Grobman WA: Induction of labor after one prior cesarean: predictors of vaginal delivery. Obstet Gynecol 103:534, 2004.
64. Rosen MG, Dicknson JC: Vaginal birth after cesarean: a meta-analysis of indicators for success. Obstet Gynecol 76:865, 1990.
65. Caughey AB, Shipp TD, Repke JT, et al: Rate of uterine rupture during a trial of labor in women with one or two prior cesarean deliveries. Am J Obstet Gynecol 181:872, 1999.
66. Miller DA, Diaz FG, Paul RH: Vaginal birth after cesarean: a 10 year experience. Obstet Gynecol 84:255, 1994.
67. Landon MB, Spong CY, Thom E, for the National Institute of Child Health and Human Development Maternal-Fetal Medicine Units Network: Risk of uterine rupture with a trial of labor in women with multiple and single prior cesarean delivery. Obstet Gynecol 108:12, 2006.
68. Macones GA, Cahill A, Para E, et al: Obstetric outcomes in women with two prior cesarean deliveries: is vaginal birth after cesarean delivery a viable option? Am J Obstet Gynecol 192:1223, 2005.
69. Kieser KE, Baskett TF: A 10-year population-based study of uterine rupture. Obstet Gynecol 100:749, 2002.
70. Mozurkewich EL, Hutton EK: Elective repeat cesarean delivery versus trial of labor: a meta-analysis of the literature from 1989 to 1999. Am J Obstet Gynecol 183:1187, 2000.
71. Vaginal Birth after Cesarean (VBAC). Rockville, Md.: Agency for Health Care Research and Quality. March 2003. (AHRQ publication no. 03-E018.)
72. Guise JM, Denman MA, Emis C, Marshall N, et al: Vaginal birth after cesarean. Obstet Gynecol 115:1267, 2010.
73. Landon MB, Hauth JC, Leveno KJ, et al, for the National Institute of Child Health and Human Development Maternal-Fetal Medicine Units Network: Maternal and perinatal outcomes associated with a trial of labor after prior cesarean delivery. N Engl J Med 351:2581, 2004.
74. Chauhan SP, Martin JN Jr, Henrichs CE, et al: Maternal and perinatal complications with uterine rupture in 142,075 patients who attempted vaginal birth after cesarean delivery: a review of the literature. Am J Obstet Gynecol 189:408, 2003.

75. Guise JM, McDonagh MS, Osterweil P, et al: Systematic review of the incidence and consequences of uterine rupture in women with previous cesarean section. BMJ 329:19, 2004.
76. Tahseen S, Griffiths M: Vaginal birth after two caesarean sections (VBAC-2) a systematic review with meta-analysis of success rate and adverse outcomes of VBAC-2 versus VBAC-1 and repeat (third) caesarean section. BJOG 117:5, 2010.
77. Zelop CM, Shipp TD, Repke JT, et al: Uterine rupture during induced or augmented labor in gravid women with one prior cesarean delivery. Am J Obstet Gynecol 181:882, 1999.
78. Macones G, Peipert J, Nelson D, et al: Maternal complications with vaginal birth after cesarean delivery: a multicenter study. Am J Obstet Gynecol 193:1656, 2005.
79. Chapman SJ, Owen J, Hauth JC: One-versus two-layer closure of a low transverse cesarean: the next pregnancy. Obstet Gynecol 89:16, 1997.
80. Bujold E, Bujold C, Hamilton EF, et al: The impact of a single-layer or double-layer closure on uterine rupture. Am J Obstet Gynecol 186:1326, 2002.
81. Bujold E, Goyet M, Marxouz S, et al: The role of uterine closure in the risk of uterine rupture. Obstet Gynecol 116:143, 2010.
82. Lydon-Rochelle M, Holt V, Easterling TR, Martin DP: Risk of uterine rupture during labor among women with a prior cesarean delivery. N Engl J Med 345:36, 2001.
83. Dekker GA, Chan A, Luke CG, et al: Risk of uterine rupture in Australian women attempting vaginal birth after one prior cesarean section: a retrospective population-based cohort study. BJOG 117:1358, 2010
84. Wing DA, Lovett K, Paul RH: Disruption of prior uterine incision following misoprostol for labor induction in women with previous cesarean delivery. Obstet Gynecol 91:828, 1998.
85. Smith GC, Peil JP, Pasupathy D, et al: Factors predisposing to perinatal death related to uterine rupture during attempted vaginal birth after cesarean section: retrospective cohort study. BMJ 329:359, 2004.
86. Cahill AG, Waterman BM, Stamilio DM, et al: Higher maximum doses of oxytocin are associated with an unacceptably high risk of uterine patients attempting vaginal birth after cesarean delivery. Am J Obstet Gynecol 199:41, 2008.
87. Cahill AG, Odibo AO, Allsworth JE, Macones GA. Frequent epidural dosing as marker for impending uterine rupture in patients who attempt vaginal birth after cesarean section. Am J Obstet Gynecol 202:335.e1-5, 2010.
88. Bujold E, Jastrow N, Simoneau J, et al: Prediction of complete uterine rupture of sonographic evaluation of the lower uterine segment. Am J Obstet Gynecol 201:320.e1-6, 2009.
89. McMahon MJ, Luther ER, Bowes WA, Olshan AF: Comparison of a trial of labor with an elective second cesarean section. N Engl J Med 335:689, 1996.
90. Jones R, Nagashima A, Hartnett-Goodman M, Goodlin R: Rupture of low transverse cesarean scars during trial of labor. Obstet Gynecol 77:815, 1991.
91. Rodriguez M, Masaki D, Phelan J, Diaz F: Uterine rupture: are intrauterine pressure catheters useful in the diagnosis? Am J Obstet Gynecol 161:666, 1989.
92. Clark SL, Scott JR, Porter TF, et al: Is vaginal birth after cesarean less expensive than repeat cesarean delivery? Am J Obstet Gynecol 182:599, 2000.
93. Bujold E, Gauthier RJ: Should we allow a trial of labor after a previous cesarean for dystocia in the second stage of labor? Obstet Gynecol 99:520, 2002.
94. Goetzel L, Shipp TD, Cohen A, et al: Oxytocin dose and the risk of uterine rupture in trial of labor after cesarean. Obstet Gynecol 97:381, 2001.
95. Shellhaas CS, Gilbert S, Landon MB, et al, for the Eunice Kennedy Shriver National Institutes of Health and Human Development Maternal-Fetal Medicine Units Network. The frequency and complication rates of hysterectomy accompanying cesarean delivery. Obstet Gynecol 114:224, 2009.
96. Rossi AC, Lee RH, Chmait RH: Emergency postpartum hysterectomy for uncontrolled postpartum bleeding. Obstet Gynecol 116:637, 2010.
97. Wright JD, Devine P, Shah M, et al: Morbidity and mortality of peripartum hysterectomy. Obstet Gynecol 115:1187, 2010.
98. Wright JD, Herzog TJ, Shah M, et al: Regionalization of care for obstetric hemorrhage and its effect on maternal mortality. Obstet Gynecol 115:1194, 2010.
99. Stanco LM, Schrimmer DB, Paul RH, Mischell Dr Jr: Emergency peripartum hysterectomy and associated risks. Am J Obstet Gynecol 168:879, 1993.

For full reference list, log onto www.expertconsult.com.

Section IV

Postpartum Care

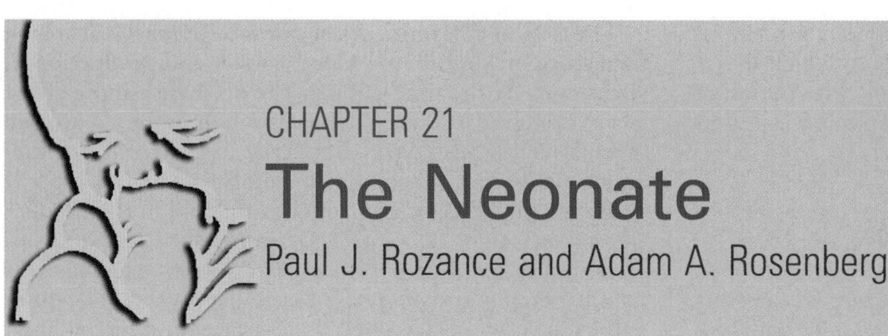

CHAPTER 21

The Neonate

Paul J. Rozance and Adam A. Rosenberg

KEY ABBREVIATIONS	
Appropriate for Gestational Age	AGA
Central Nervous System	CNS
Chronic Lung Disease	CLD
Computed Tomography	CT
Cyclic Adenosine Monophosphate	cAMP
Dipalmitoylphosphatidylcholine	DPPC
Docohexanoic Acid	DHA
Functional Residual Capacity	FRC
Glucose-6-Phosphate Dehydrogenase	G6PD
Group B Streptococcus	GBS
Hyaline Membrane Disease	HMD
Human Immunodeficiency Virus	HIV
Idiopathic Thrombocytopenic Purpura	ITP
Inferior Vena Cava	IVC
Insulin-like Growth Factor-1	IGF-1
Intrauterine Growth Restriction	IUGR
Large for Gestational Age	LGA
Magnetic Resonance Imaging	MRI
Meconium Aspiration Syndrome	MAS
Necrotizing Enterocolitis	NEC
Periventricular/Intraventricular Hemorrhage	PVH/IVH
Periventricular Leukomalacia	PVL
Persistent Pulmonary Hypertension of the Newborn	PPHN
Pulmonary Vascular Resistance	PVR
Rapid Eye Movement Sleep	REM
Respiratory Distress Syndrome	RDS
Small for Gestational Age	SGA
Surfactant Protein	SP
Thyroid-releasing Hormone	TRH
Thyroid-stimulating Hormone	TSH
Uridine Diphosphoglucuronosyl Transferase	UDPGT
Vascular Endothelial Growth Factor	VEGF

The first 4 weeks of an infant's life, the neonatal period, are marked by the highest mortality rate in all of childhood. The greatest risk occurs during the first several days after birth. Critical to survival during this period is the infant's ability to adapt successfully to extrauterine life. During the early hours after birth, the newborn must assume responsibility for thermoregulation, metabolic homeostasis, and respiratory gas exchange, as well as undergo the conversion from fetal to postnatal circulatory pathways. This chapter reviews the physiology of a successful transition as well as the implications of circumstances that disrupt this process. Implicit in these considerations is the understanding that the newborn reflects the sum total of its genetic and environmental past as well as any minor or major insults to which it was subjected during gestation and parturition. The period of neonatal adaptation is then most meaningfully viewed as continuous with fetal life.

CARDIOPULMONARY TRANSITION

Pulmonary Development

Lung development and maturation require a carefully regulated interaction of anatomic, physiologic, and biochemical processes. The outcome of these events provides an organ with adequate surface area, sufficient vascularization, and the metabolic capability to sustain oxygenation and ventilation during the neonatal period. Five stages of morphologic lung development have been identified in the human fetus[1]:

1. Embryonic period: 3 to 7 weeks postconception
2. Pseudoglandular period: 5th to 17th weeks
3. Canalicular period: 16th to 26th weeks
4. Saccular period: 24th to 38th weeks
5. Alveolar period: 36 weeks to 2 years after birth

The lung arises as a ventral diverticulum from the foregut during the fourth week of gestation. During the ensuing weeks, branching of the diverticulum occurs, leading to a tree of narrow tubes with thick epithelial walls composed of columnar-type cells. Molecular mechanisms involved in lung development include expression of transcription factors that are important for specification of the foregut endoderm, endogenous secretion of polypeptides that are important for pattern formation, growth and differentiation factors critical to cell development, and involvement of external signals such as retinoic acid. By 16 weeks, the conducting portion of the tracheobronchial tree up to and including terminal bronchioles has been established. The vasculature derived from the pulmonary circulation develops concurrently with the conducting airways, and by 16 weeks, preacinar blood vessels are formed. The canalicular stage is characterized by differentiation of the airways, with widening of the airways and thinning of epithelium. In addition, primitive respiratory bronchioles begin to form, marking the start of the gas-exchanging portion of the lung. Vascular proliferation continues, along with a relative decrease in mesenchyme, bringing the vessels closer to the airway epithelium. The saccular stage is marked by the development of the gas-exchanging portion of the tracheobronchial tree (acinus) composed of respiratory bronchioles, alveolar ducts, terminal saccules, and finally, alveoli. During this stage, the pulmonary vessels continue to proliferate with the airways and surround the developing air sacs. The final phase of prenatal lung development (alveolar) is marked by the formation of thin secondary alveolar septae and the remodeling of the capillary bed.

Throughout these periods mesenchymal and epithelial cell cross-talk directs the normal processes of lung alveolarization and vascularization.[2] Several million alveoli will form before birth, which emphasizes the importance of the last few weeks of pregnancy to pulmonary adaptation. Postnatal lung growth is characterized by generation of alveoli. At birth, there are approximately 50 million airspaces, and by 8 years of age, there are 300 million.[1]

The critical determinants of extrauterine survival are the formation of the thin air-blood barrier and production of surfactant. By the time of birth, the epithelial lining of the gas-exchanging surface is thin and continuous with two alveolar cell types (types I and II). Type I cells are thin and contain few subcellular organelles, whereas type II cells contain subcellular organelles that aid in the production of surfactant (Figure 21-1). Surfactant lipids and surfactant protein B and C are secreted by exocytosis as lamellar bodies and unravel into tubular myelin. The other surfactant proteins (A and D) are secreted independently of the lamellar bodies. Tubular myelin is a loose lattice of phospholipids and surfactant-specific proteins. The surface active component of surfactant then adsorbs at the alveolar interface between air and water in a monolayer. With repetitive expansion and compression of the surface monolayer, material is extruded that is either cleared by alveolar macrophages through endocytic pathways or taken up by the type II cell for recycling back into lamellar bodies.[3]

Because of the development of high surface forces along the respiratory epithelium when breathing begins, the availability of surfactants in terminal airspaces is critical to postnatal lung function. Just as surface tension acts to reduce the size of a bubble in water, so, too, it acts to reduce lung inflation, promoting atelectasis. This is described by the LaPlace relationship, which states that the pressure, *P,* within a sphere is directly proportional to surface tension, *T,* and inversely proportional to the radius of curvature, *r* (Figure 21-2). Surfactant has the physical property of variable surface tension dependent on the degree of surface area compression. In other words, as the radius of the alveolus decreases, surfactant serves to reduce surface tension, preventing collapse of the alveolus. If this property is extrapolated to the lung, smaller alveoli will remain stable because of lower surface tension than larger alveoli. This feature is emphasized in Figure 21-3, which compares pressure-volume curves from surfactant-deficient and surfactant-treated preterm rabbits. Surfactant deficiency is characterized by high opening pressure, low maximal lung volume, and lack of deflation stability at low pressures.

Natural surfactant contains mostly lipids, phospholipids specifically, and some protein (Figure 21-4).[3] Approximately half of the protein is specific for surfactant. The principal classes of phospholipids are:

- Saturated phosphatidylcholine compounds (the surface tension-reducing component of surfactant), 45% (more than 80% of which is dipalmitoylphosphatidylcholine [DPPC])
- Unsaturated phosphatidylcholine compounds, 25%
- Phosphatidylglycerol, phosphatidylinositol, and phosphatidylethanolamine, 10%.

Saturated phosphatidylcholine is found in lung tissue of the human fetus earlier in gestation than in other species. Surfactant is released from storage pools into fetal lung fluid at a basal rate during late gestation and is stimulated by labor and the initiation of air breathing. Four unique surfactant-associated proteins have been identified. All are synthesized and secreted by type II alveolar cells. Surfactant protein (SP)-A functions cooperatively with the other surfactant proteins and lipids to enhance the biophysical activity of surfactant, but its most

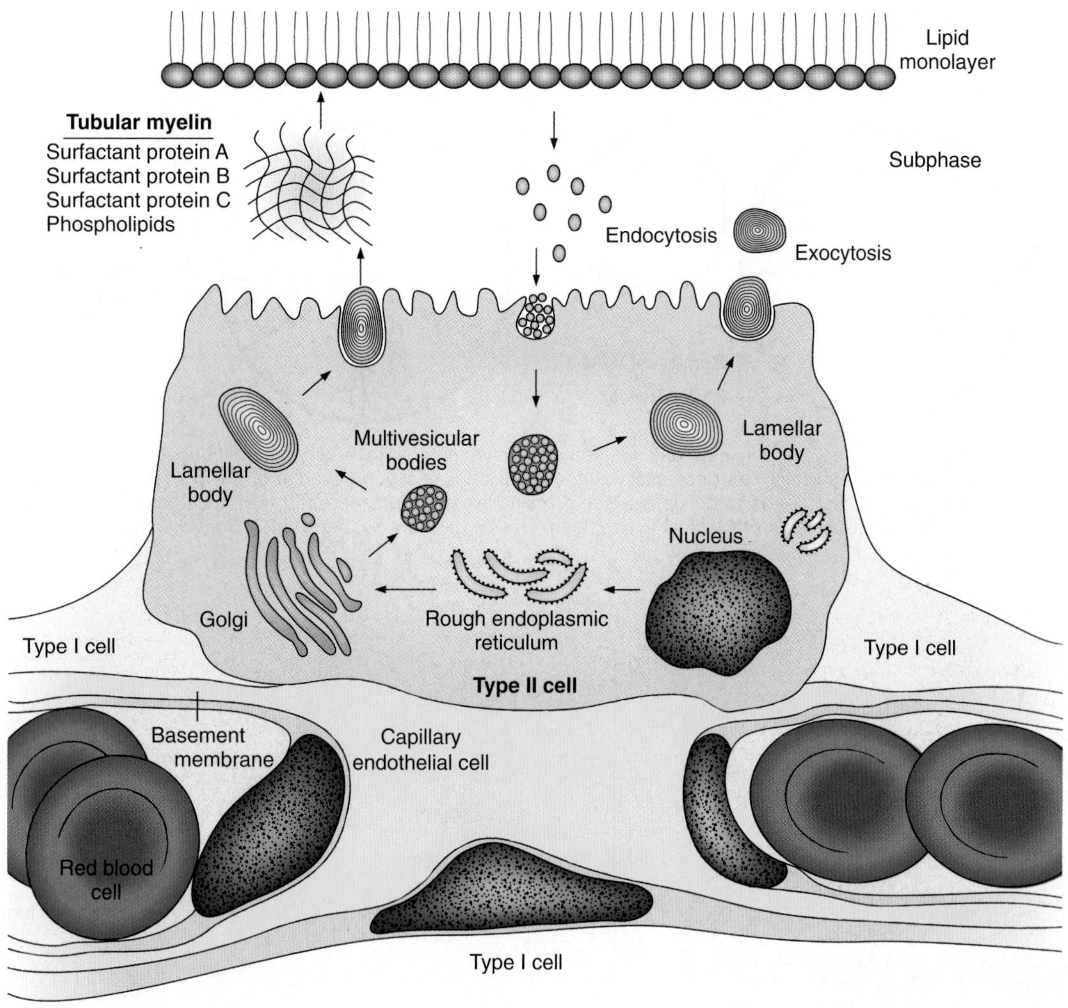

Figure 21-1. Metabolism of surfactant. Surfactant phospholipids are synthesized in the endoplasmic reticulum, transported through the Golgi apparatus to multivesicular bodies, and finally packaged in lamellar bodies. After lamellar body exocytosis, phospholipids are organized into tubular myelin before aligning in a monolayer at the air-fluid interface in the alveolus. Surfactant phospholipids and proteins are taken up by type II cells and either catabolized or reused. Surfactant proteins are synthesized in polyribosomes, modified in endoplasmic reticulum, Golgi apparatus, and multivesicular bodies. (Modified from Whitsett JA, Pryhuber GS, Rice WR, et al: Acute respiratory disorders. *In* Avery GB, Fletcher MA, MacDonald MG [eds]: Neonatology: Pathophysiology and Management of the Newborn, 5th ed. Philadelphia, Lippincott Williams & Wilkins, 1999, p 485.)

important role is in innate host defense of the lung. SP-B and SP-C are lipophilic proteins that facilitate the adsorption and spreading of lipid to form the surfactant monolayer. SP-B deficiencies are associated with neonatal pulmonary complications and death, whereas SP-C deficiencies are associated with interstitial lung disease presenting at a more variable age. SP-D plays a role in the regulation of surfactant lipid homeostasis, inflammatory responses, and host defense mechanisms.[3]

Several hormones and growth factors contribute to the regulation of pulmonary phospholipid metabolism and lung maturation: glucocorticoids, thyroid hormone, thyrotropin-releasing hormone, retinoic acid, epidermal growth factor, and others. **Glucocorticoids are the most important and are used clinically to augment the synthesis of surfactant and accelerate morphologic development.**[4] Pregnant women with anticipated preterm delivery have received corticosteroid treatment since 1972. Numerous controlled trials have since been performed. Based on a meta-analysis, a significant reduction of about 50% in the incidence of respiratory distress syndrome (RDS) is seen in infants born to mothers who received antenatal corticosteroids.[5] In secondary analysis, a 70% reduction in RDS was seen among babies born between 24 hours and 7 days after corticosteroid administration. In addition, evidence suggests a reduction in mortality and RDS even with treatment started less than 24 hours before delivery. Although most babies in the trials were between 30 and 34 weeks' gestation, clear reduction in RDS was evident when the population of babies less than 31 weeks was examined, and given the impact on neonatal morbidity and mortality, prenatal steroid use can be recommended in pregnancies as early as 23 weeks' gestation.[6] Gender and race do not influence the protective effect of corticosteroids. In the

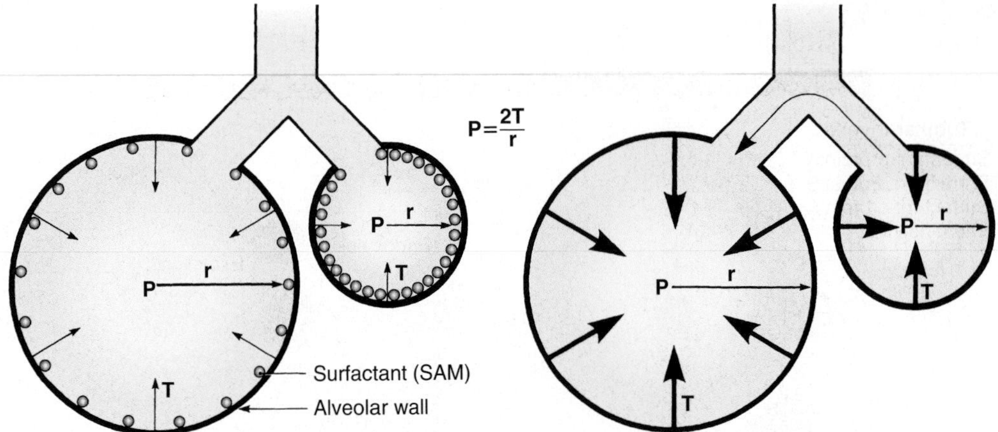

FIGURE 21-2. LaPlace's law. The pressure, *P*, within a sphere is directly proportional to surface tension, *T*, and inversely proportional to the radius of curvature, *r*. In the normal lung, as alveolar size decreases, surface tension is reduced because of the presence of surfactant. This serves to decrease the collapsing pressure that needs to be opposed and maintains equal pressures in the small and large interconnected alveoli. (Modified from Netter FH: The Ciba Collection of Medical Illustrations. The Respiratory System, Vol 7. Summit, NJ, Ciba-Geigy, 1979.)

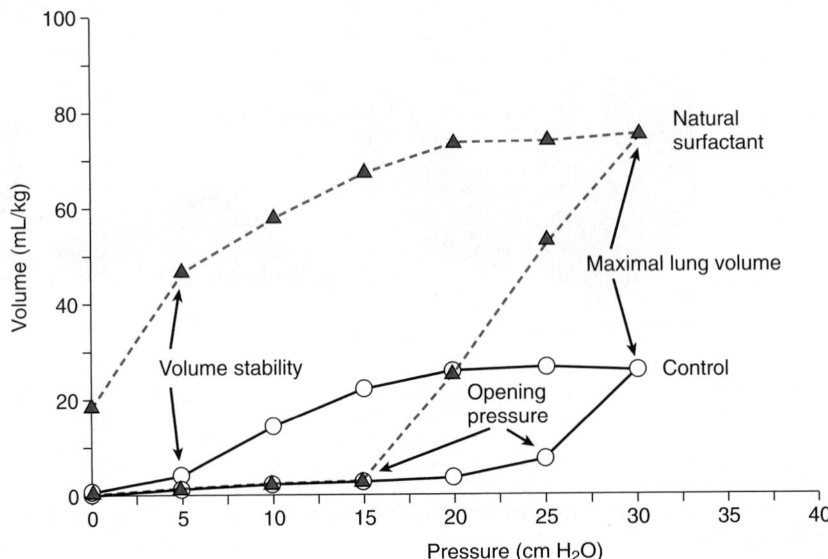

FIGURE 21-3. Pressure-volume relationships for the inflation and deflation of surfactant-deficient and surfactant-treated preterm rabbit lungs. Surfactant deficiency is indicated by high opening pressure, low maximal volume at a distending pressure of 30 cm of water, and the lack of deflation stability at low pressures on deflation. (Modified from Jobe AH: Lung development and maturation. *In* Fanaroff AA, Martin RJ [eds]: Neonatal-Perinatal Medicine: Diseases of the Fetus and Infant, 7th ed. St. Louis, Mosby, 2002, p 973.)

population of patients with preterm premature rupture of the membranes, antenatal corticosteroids also reduce the frequency of RDS.

Corticosteroids also accelerate maturation of other organs in the developing fetus, including cardiovascular, gastrointestinal, and central nervous system (CNS). Corticosteroid therapy reduces the chances of both periventricular-intraventricular hemorrhage (PVH/IVH) and necrotizing enterocolitis (NEC).[5] The significant reductions in serious neonatal morbidity are also reflected in a reduction in the risk of early neonatal mortality. The short-term beneficial effects of antenatal corticosteroids are enhanced by reassuring reports about long-term outcome. The children of mothers treated with antenatal corticosteroids show no lag in intellectual or motor development, no increase in learning disabilities or behavioral disturbances, and no effect on growth compared with untreated infants.[7,8]

Since the advent of antenatal steroids for the prevention of RDS, other therapies have been introduced that decrease mortality and morbidity. Surfactant replacement therapy to treat specifically the surfactant deficiency that is the cause of RDS has been shown to decrease mortality and the severity of RDS.[9] The effects of antenatal corticosteroids and postnatal surfactant appear to be additive in terms of decreasing the severity of and mortality caused by RDS.[10]

The First Breaths

A critical step in the transition from intrauterine to extrauterine life is the conversion of the lung from a fluid-filled organ to one capable of gas exchange. This requires

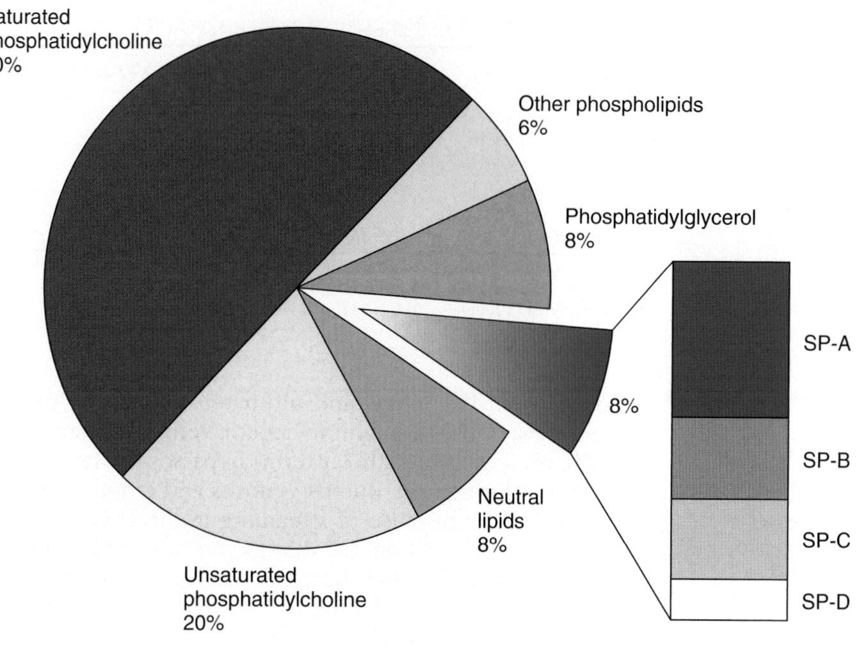

FIGURE 21-4. Composition of pulmonary surfactant. *SP,* Surfactant protein. (Modified from Jobe AH: Lung development and maturation. *In* Fanaroff AA, Martin RJ [eds]: Neonatal-Perinatal Medicine: Diseases of the Fetus and Infant, 7th ed. St Louis, Mosby, 2002, p 973.)

aeration of the lungs, establishment of an adequate pulmonary circulation, ventilation of the aerated parenchyma, and diffusion of oxygen and carbon dioxide through the alveolar-capillary membranes. This process has its origins in utero as fetal breathing.

Fetal Breathing

Fetal respiratory activity is initially detectable at 11 weeks. The most prevalent pattern is rapid, small-amplitude movements (60 to 90 per minute) present 60% to 80% of the time. Less commonly, irregular low-amplitude movements interspersed with slower larger amplitude movements are seen.[11] Initially, fetal breathing was thought to depend on behavioral influences. However, subsequent work has shown responses to chemical stimuli and other agents. Acute hypercapnea stimulates breathing. Hypoxia abolishes fetal breathing, whereas an increase in oxygen tension to levels above 200 mm Hg induces continuous fetal breathing. Although peripheral and central chemoreflexes as well as vagal afferent reflexes can be demonstrated in the fetus, their role in spontaneous fetal breathing appears minimal. The role of fetal breathing in the continuum from fetal to neonatal life is still not completely understood. Fetal respiratory activity is probably essential to the development of chest wall muscles (including diaphragm) and serves as a regulator of lung fluid volume and thus lung growth.

The mechanism responsible for the transition from intermittent fetal to continuous neonatal breathing is unknown. Prostaglandins may be involved as well as other factors surrounding birth, including blood gas changes and various sensory stimuli. Another possibility is the "release" from a placental inhibitory factor that is removed after cord occlusion.

Mechanics of the First Breath

With its first breaths, the neonate must overcome several forces resisting lung expansion: (1) viscosity of fetal lung fluid, (2) resistance provided by lung tissue itself, and (3) the forces of surface tension at the air-liquid interface.[12-14] Viscosity of fetal lung fluid is a major factor as the neonate attempts to displace fluid present in the large airways. As the passage of air moves toward small airways and alveoli, surface tension becomes more important. Resistance to expansion by the lung tissue itself is less significant. The process begins as the infant passes through the birth canal. The intrathoracic pressure caused by vaginal squeeze is up to 200 cm H_2O. With delivery of the head, approximately 5 to 28 mL of tracheal fluid is expressed. Subsequent delivery of the thorax causes an elastic recoil of the chest. With this recoil, a small passive inspiration (no more than 2 mL) occurs. This is accompanied by glossopharyngeal forcing of some air into the proximal airways (frog breathing) and the introduction of some blood into pulmonary capillaries. This pulmonary vascular pressure may have a role in producing initial continuous surfaces throughout the small airways of the lung into which surfactant can deploy.

The initial breath is characteristically a short inspiration, followed by a more prolonged expiration (Figure 21-5).[13] The initial breath begins with no air volume and no transpulmonary pressure gradient. Considerable negative intrathoracic pressure during inspiration is provided by diaphragmatic contraction and chest wall expansion. An opening pressure of about 25 cm H_2O usually is necessary to overcome surface tension in the smaller airways and alveoli before air begins to enter. The volume of this first breath varies between 30 and 67 mL and correlates with intrathoracic pressure. The expiratory phase is prolonged, because the infant's expiration is opposed by intermittent closure at the pharyngolaryngeal level with the generation of large positive intrathoracic pressure. This pressure serves to aid both in maintenance of a functional residual capacity (FRC) and with fluid removal from the air sacs. The residual volume after this first breath ranges between 4 and 30 mL, averaging 16 to 20 mL. There are really no

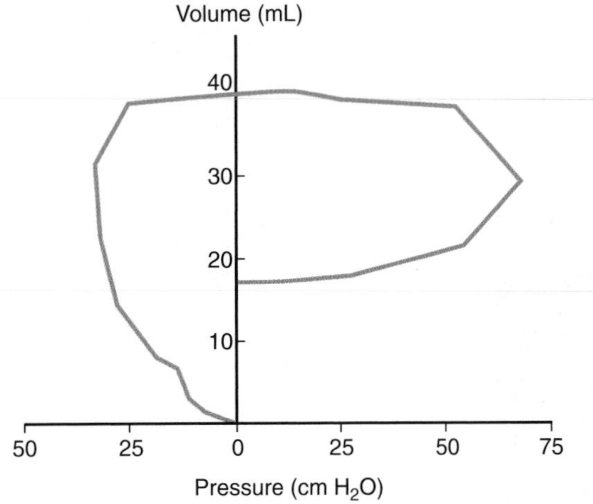

FIGURE 21-5. Pressure-volume loop of the first breath. Air enters the lung as soon as intrathoracic pressure falls and expiratory pressure greatly exceeds inspiratory pressure. (Modified from Milner AD, Vyas H: Lung expansion at birth. J Pediatr 101:879, 1982.)

major systematic differences among the first three breaths, demonstrating similar pressure patterns of decreasing magnitude. The FRC rapidly increases with the first several breaths and then more gradually. By 30 minutes of age, most infants attain a normal FRC with uniform lung expansion. The presence of functional surfactant is instrumental in the accumulation of an FRC.

In utero, alveoli are open and stable at nearly neonatal lung volume because they are filled with fetal lung liquid, probably produced by ultrafiltration of pulmonary capillary blood as well as by secretion by alveolar cells. Transepithelial chloride secretion appears to be a major factor responsible for the production of luminal liquid in the fetal lung. **Normal expansion and aeration of the neonatal lung is dependent on removal of fetal lung liquid. Liquid is removed by a combination of mechanical drainage and absorption across the lung epithelium.[15] This process begins before a normal term birth because of decreased fluid secretion and increased absorption. Once labor is initiated, there is a reversal of liquid flow across the lung epithelium.** Active transcellular sodium absorption drives liquid from the lumen to interstitial space, where it is drained through the pulmonary circulation and lymphatics.[16] In normal circumstances, the process is complete within 2 hours of birth. Cesarean-delivered infants without benefit of labor and premature infants have delayed lung fluid clearance. In both groups, the prenatal decrease in lung water does not occur. In addition, in the premature neonate, fluid clearance is diminished by increased alveolar surface tension, increased left atrial pressure, and hypoproteinemia.

Circulatory Transition

The circulation in the fetus (Figure 21-6) has been studied in a variety of species using several techniques (see Chapter 2).[17,18] Umbilical venous blood, returning from the placenta, has a Po_2 of about 30 to 35 mm Hg. Because of the left-shifted fetal hemoglobin oxyhemoglobin disassociation curve, this corresponds to a saturation of 80% to 90%. About 60% of this blood perfuses the liver (mainly to the middle and left lobes) and ultimately enters the inferior vena cava (IVC) through the hepatic veins. The remainder (40% midgestation; 20% at term) bypasses the hepatic circulation through the ductus venosus and empties directly into the IVC. Because of streaming in the IVC, the more oxygenated blood from the ductus venosus and left hepatic vein, as it enters the heart, is deflected by the crista dividens through the foramen ovale to the left atrium. The remainder of left atrial blood is the small amount of venous return from the pulmonary circulation. The less oxygenated IVC blood from the lower body, renal, mesenteric, and right hepatic veins, streams across the tricuspid valve to the right ventricle. Almost all the return from the superior vena cava (SVC) and the coronary sinus passes through the tricuspid valve to the right ventricle, with only 2% to 3% crossing the foramen ovale. In the near-term fetus, the combined ventricular output is about 450 mL/kg/min; two thirds from the right ventricle and one third from the left ventricle. The blood in the left ventricle has a Po_2 of 25 to 28 mm Hg (saturation of 60%) and is distributed to the coronary circulation, brain, head, and upper extremities, with the remainder (10% of combined output) passing into the descending aorta. The major portion of the right ventricular output (60% of combined output) is carried by the ductus arteriosus to the descending aorta, with only 7% of combined output going to the lungs. Thus, 70% of combined output passes through the descending aorta, with a Po_2 of 20 to 23 mm Hg (saturation of 55%) to supply the abdominal viscera and lower extremities. Forty-five percent of combined output goes through the umbilical arteries to the placenta. Thus, blood of a higher Po_2 supplies the critical coronary and cerebral circulations, and umbilical venous blood is diverted to where oxygenation is critical.

The diversion of right ventricular output away from the lungs through the ductus arteriosus is caused by the very high pulmonary vascular resistance (PVR) in the fetus. This high PVR is maintained by multiple mechanisms. With advancing gestational age, an increase in the number of small pulmonary vessels occurs that increases the cross-sectional area of the pulmonary vasculature. This contributes to the gradual decline in PVR that begins during later gestation (Figure 21-7). With delivery, a variety of factors interact to decrease PVR acutely including mechanical ventilation, increased oxygen tension, and the production of endothelium-derived relaxing factor or nitric oxide.[19]

With the increase in pulmonary flow, left atrial return increases with a rise in left atrial pressure (Table 21-1). In addition, with the removal of the placenta, IVC return to

TABLE 21-1 PRESSURES IN THE PERINATAL CIRCULATION

	FETAL (mm Hg)	NEONATAL (mm Hg)
Right atrium	4	5
Right ventricle	65/10	40/5
Pulmonary artery	65/40	40/25
Left atrium	3	7
Left ventricle	60/7	70/10
Aorta	60/40	70/45

Modified from Nelson NM: Respiration and circulation after birth, *In* Smith CA, Nelson NM (eds): The Physiology of the Newborn Infant, 4th ed. Springfield, IL, Charles C Thomas, 1976, p 117.

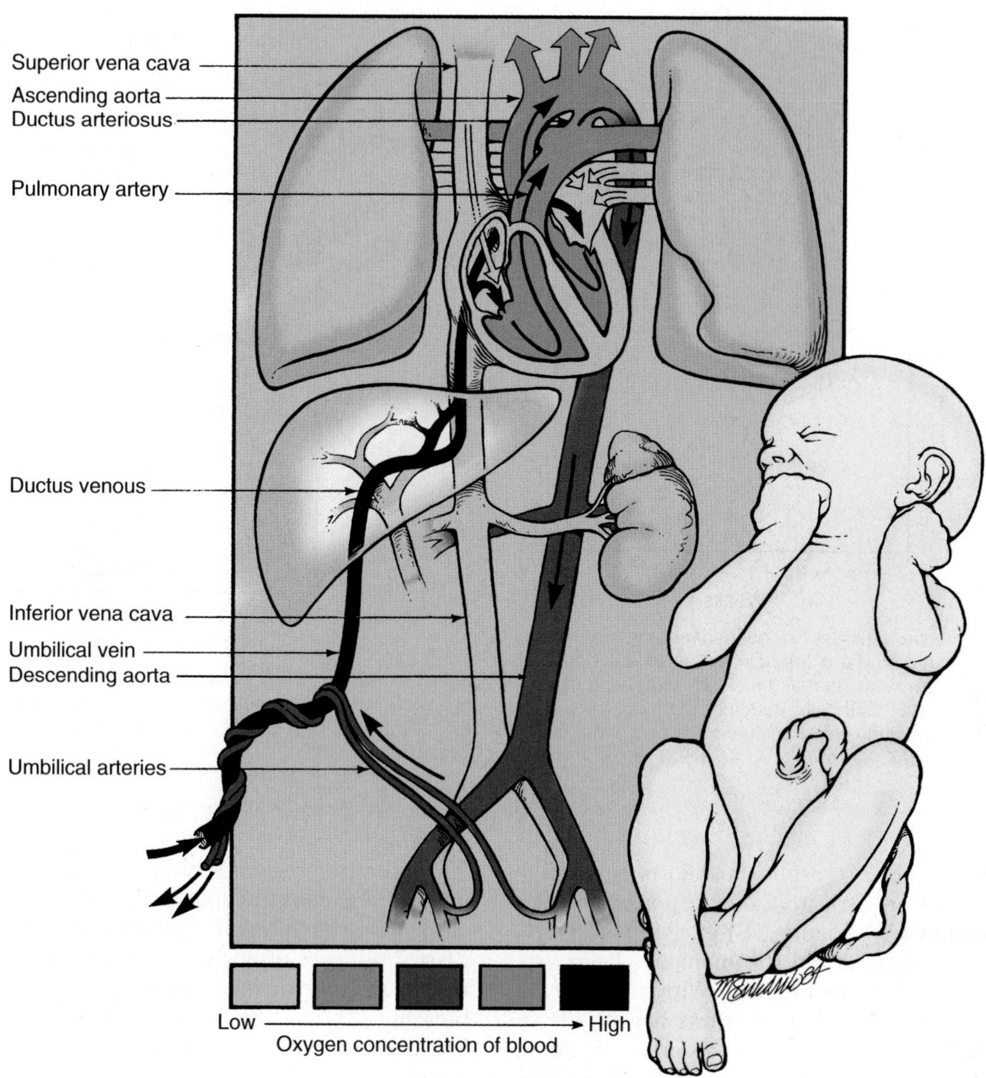

FIGURE 21-6. The fetal circulation.

the right atrium is diminished. The foramen ovale is a flap valve, and when left atrial pressure increases over that on the right side, the opening is functionally closed. It is still possible to demonstrate patency with insignificant right-to-left shunts in the first 12 hours of life in a human neonate, but in a 7- to 12-day newborn, such a shunt is rarely seen. Anatomic closure is not complete for a longer time.

With occlusion of the umbilical cord, the low-resistance placental circulation is interrupted, causing an increase in systemic pressure. This, coupled with the decrease in PVR, serves to reverse the shunt through the ductus arteriosus to a predominantly left-to-right shunt. By 15 hours of age, shunting in either direction is physiologically insignificant. Although functionally closed by 4 days of age, the ductus arteriosus is not anatomically occluded for 1 month. The role of an increased oxygen environment and prostaglandin metabolism in ductal closure is well established. Ductal closure occurs in two phases: constriction and anatomic occlusion. Initially, the muscular wall constricts, followed by permanent closure achieved by endothelial destruction, subintimal proliferation, and connective tissue formation.[20] The ductus venosus is functionally occluded shortly after the umbilical circulation is interrupted.

ABNORMALITIES OF CARDIOPULMONARY TRANSITION

Birth Asphyxia

Even normal infants may experience some limitation of oxygenation (asphyxia) during the birth process. A variety of circumstances can exaggerate this problem, resulting in respiratory depression in the infant, including (1) acute interruption of umbilical blood flow, as occurs during cord compression; (2) premature placental separation; (3) maternal hypotension or hypoxia; (4) any of the above-mentioned problems superimposed on chronic uteroplacental insufficiency; and (5) failure to execute a proper resuscitation. Other contributing factors include anesthetics and analgesics used in the mother, mode and difficulty of delivery, maternal health, and prematurity.

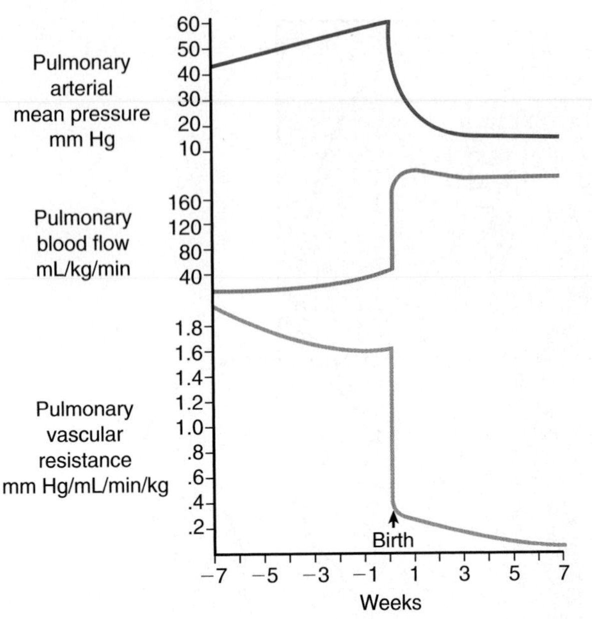

Figure 21-7. Representative changes in pulmonary hemodynamics during transition from the late-term fetal circulation to the neonatal circulation. (Modified from Rudolph AM: Fetal circulation and cardiovascular adjustments after birth. *In* Rudolph CD, Rudolph AM, Hostetter MK, et al [eds]: Rudolph's Pediatrics, 21st ed. New York, McGraw-Hill, 2003, p 1749.)

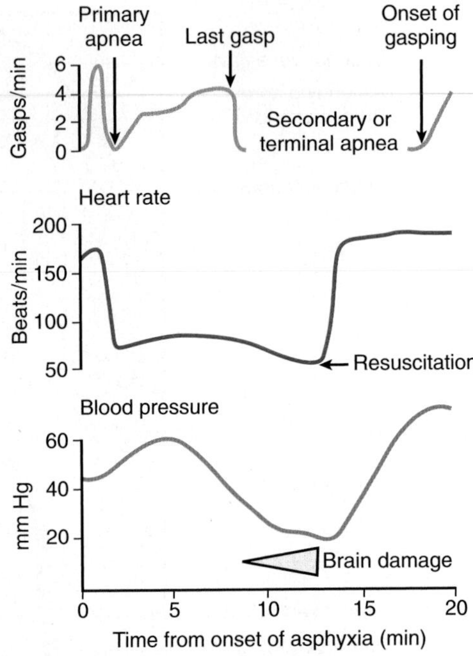

Figure 21-8. Schematic depiction of changes in rhesus monkeys during asphyxia and on resuscitation by positive-pressure ventilation. (Modified from Dawes GS: Foetal and Neonatal Physiology. Chicago, Year Book, 1968.)

The neonatal response to asphyxia follows a predictable pattern. Dawes investigated the responses of the newborn rhesus monkey (Figure 21-8).[21] After delivery, the umbilical cord was tied and the monkey's head was placed in a saline-filled plastic bag. Within about 30 seconds, a short series of respiratory efforts began. These were interrupted by a convulsion or a series of clonic movements accompanied by an abrupt fall in heart rate. The animal then lay inert with no muscle tone. Skin color became progressively cyanotic and then blotchy because of vasoconstriction in an effort to maintain systemic blood pressure. This initial period of apnea lasted about 30 to 60 seconds. The monkey then began to gasp at a rate of three to six per minute. The gasping lasted for about 8 minutes, becoming weaker terminally. The time from onset of asphyxia to last gasp could be related to postnatal age and maturity at birth; the more immature the animal, the longer the time. Secondary or terminal apnea followed and, if resuscitation was not quickly initiated, death ensued. As the animal progressed through the phase of gasping and then on to terminal apnea, heart rate and blood pressure continued to fall, indicating hypoxic depression of myocardial function. As the heart failed, blood flow to critical organs decreased, resulting in organ injury.

The response to resuscitation is qualitatively similar in many species, including humans. During the first period of apnea, almost any physical or chemical stimulus causes the animal to breathe. If gasping has already ceased, the first sign of recovery with initiation of positive-pressure ventilation is an increase in heart rate. The blood pressure then rises, rapidly if the last gasp has only just passed, but more slowly if the duration of asphyxia has been longer. The skin then becomes pink, and gasping ensues. Rhythmic spontaneous respiratory efforts become established after a further interval. For each 1 minute past the last gasp, 2 minutes of positive-pressure breathing is required before gasping begins and 4 minutes to reach rhythmic breathing. Later the spinal and corneal reflexes return. Muscle tone gradually improves over the course of several hours.

Delivery Room Management of the Newborn

A number of situations during pregnancy, labor, and delivery place the infant at increased risk for asphyxia: (1) maternal diseases, such as diabetes and hypertension, third-trimester bleeding, and prolonged rupture of membranes; (2) fetal conditions, such as prematurity, multiple births, growth restriction, fetal anomalies, and rhesus isoimmunization; and (3) conditions related to labor and delivery, including fetal distress, meconium staining, breech presentation, and administration of anesthetics and analgesics.

When an asphyxiated infant is expected, a resuscitation team should be in the delivery room. The team should have at least two persons, one to manage the airway and one to monitor heart rate and provide whatever assistance is needed. The necessary equipment for an adequate resuscitation is listed in Table 21-2. The equipment should be checked regularly and should be in a continuous state of readiness.

Steps in the resuscitation process[22] are as follows (Figure 21-9):

TABLE 21-2 EQUIPMENT FOR NEONATAL RESUSCITATION

CLINICAL NEEDS	EQUIPMENT
Thermoregulation	Radiant heat source with platform, mattress covered with warm sterile blankets, servo control heating, temperature probe
Airway management	Suction: bulb suction, meconium aspirator, wall vacuum suction with sterile catheters Ventilation: manual infant resuscitation bag connected to a pressure manometer capable of delivering 100% oxygen, appropriate masks for term and preterm infants, oral airways, stethoscope, gloves, compressed air source with oxygen blender and pulse oximeter and probe (optional) Intubation: neonatal laryngoscope with #0 and #1 blades; extra bulbs and batteries; endotracheal tubes 2.5, 3.0, 3.5, and 4.0 mm OD with stylet; scissors, tape, end tidal CO_2 detection device
Gastric decompression	Nasogastric tube, 8 Fr with 20-mL syringe
Administration of drugs/volume	Sterile gloves and sterile umbilical catheterization tray with scalpel or scissors, antiseptic prep solution, umbilical tape, three-way stopcock, umbilical catheters (3.5 and 5 Fr), volume expanders (normal saline), drug box with appropriate neonatal vials and dilutions (see Table 21-5), sterile syringes and needles
Transport	Warmed transport isolette with an oxygen source

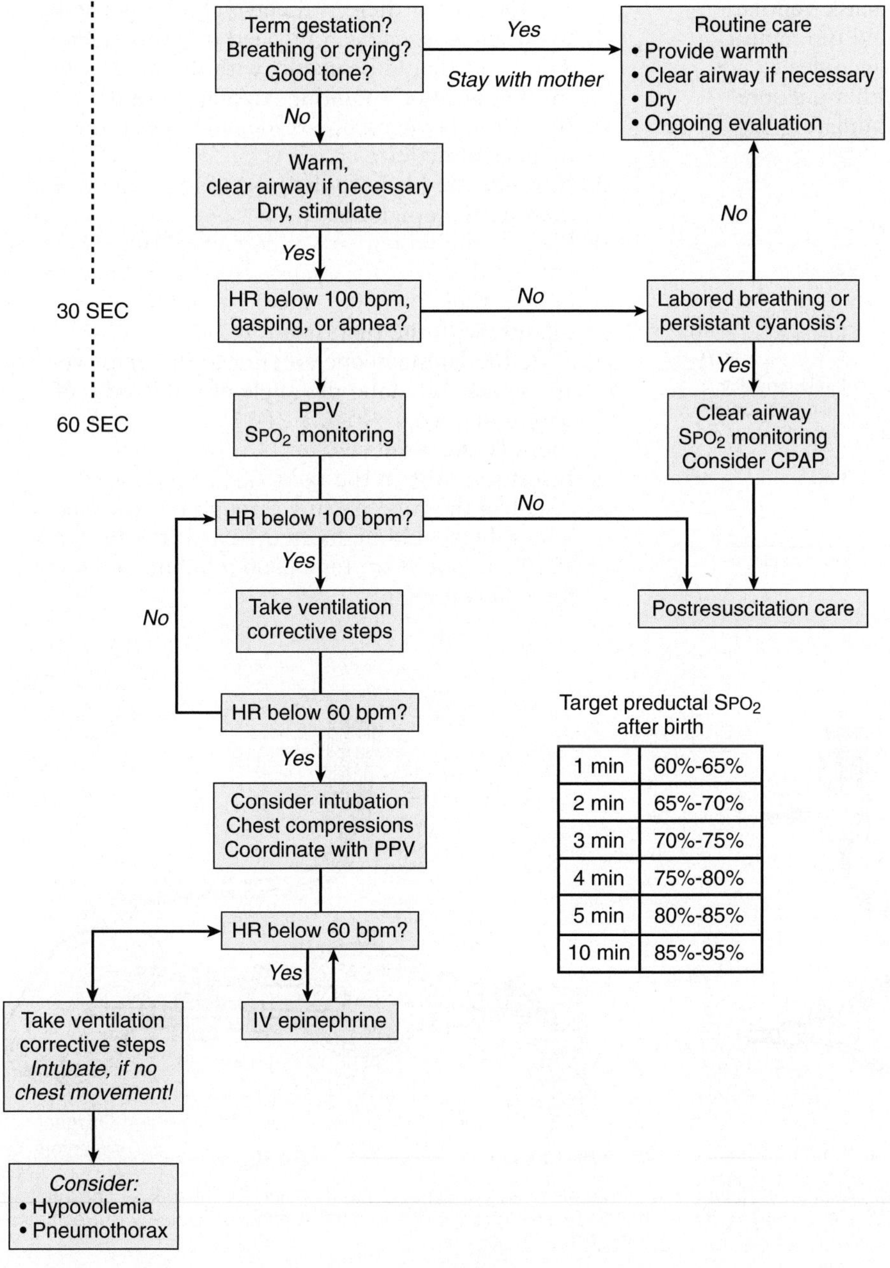

1 min	60%-65%
2 min	65%-70%
3 min	70%-75%
4 min	75%-80%
5 min	80%-85%
10 min	85%-95%

FIGURE 21-9. Delivery room management of the newborn. (From the American Heart Association and American Academy of Pediatrics: Neonatal Resuscitation Textbook, 2011.)

1. Dry the infant well and place under the radiant heat source on the back or side with the neck slightly extended. Do not allow the infant to become hyperthermic.
2. Gently suction the oropharynx and then the nose.
3. Assess the infant's condition (Table 21-3). The best criteria to assess are the infant's respiratory effort (apneic, gasping, regular) and heart rate (more or less than 100). A depressed heart rate indicative of hypoxic myocardial depression is the single most reliable indicator of the need for resuscitation.
4. Generally, infants who are breathing with heart rates over 100 bpm require no further intervention. If the infant is breathing with an adequate heart rate, but is cyanotic, provide supplemental oxygen. Infants with heart rates less than 100 bpm with apnea or irregular respiratory efforts should be gently stimulated by rubbing the baby's back with a towel.
5. If the baby fails to respond rapidly to tactile stimulation, proceed to bag and face mask ventilation using a soft mask that seals well around the mouth and nose. Choice of ventilation bags includes a flow-inflating bag (500 to 750 mL) with a pressure gauge and flow control valve or a self-inflating bag (240 to 750 mL) with an oxygen reservoir and pressure release valve (Figure 21-10). A T-piece resuscitation device may also be used. For the initial inflations, pressures of 30 to 40 cm H_2O may be necessary to overcome surface active forces in the lungs. Adequacy of ventilation is assessed by observing expansion of the infant's chest with bagging and a gradual improvement in color, perfusion, and heart rate. After the first few breaths, attempts should be made to lower the peak pressure to 15 to 20 cm H_2O. Rate of bagging should not exceed 40 to 60 bpm.
6. **Most neonates can be effectively resuscitated with a bag and face mask.** If the infant does not initially respond to bag and mask ventilation, try to reposition the head (slight extension), reapply the mask to achieve a good seal, consider suctioning the mouth and oropharynx, and try ventilating with the mouth open. It may be necessary to increase the pressure used. However, if there is no favorable response in 30 to 40 seconds, one can proceed to intubation:
   a. The head should be stable, with the nose in the sniffing position (pointing straight upward).
   b. Insert the laryngoscope blade, and sweep the tongue to the left.
   c. Advance the blade to the base of the tongue, and identify the epiglottis.
   d. Pick up the proper size endotracheal tube (2.5 mm outside diameter for infants <1000 g, 3.0 mm for infants 1000 to 2000 g, and 3.5 mm for larger infants) with the right hand.
   e. Slide the laryngoscope anterior to the epiglottis, and gently lift along the angle of the handle of the laryngoscope (Figure 21-11).
   f. Identify the vocal cords.
   g. Insert the tube in the right side of the mouth, and visualize the tube passing through the vocal cords. The tube should be located 7 cm at the lip for a 1000-g infant, 8 cm for a 2000-g infant, and 9 cm for a 3000-g infant.

TABLE 21-3 THE APGAR SCORING SYSTEM

SIGN	0	1	2
Heart rate	Absent	<100 bpm	>100 bpm
Respiratory effort	Apneic	Weak, irregular, gasping	Regular
Reflex irritability*	No response	Some response	Facial grimace, sneeze, cough
Muscle tone	Flaccid	Some flexion of arms and legs	Good flexion
Color	Blue, pale hands and feet blue	Body pink	Pink

Modified from Apgar V: A proposal for a new method of evaluation of the newborn infant. Anesth Analg 32:260, 1953.
*Elicited by suctioning the oropharynx and nose.

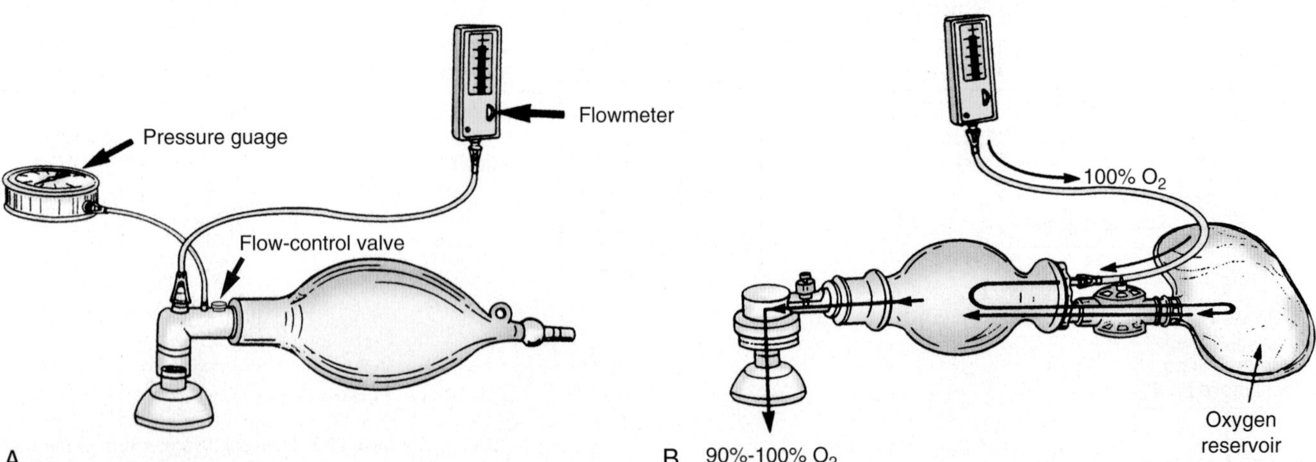

FIGURE 21-10. Bags used for neonatal resuscitation. **A,** A flow-inflating bag with a pressure manometer and flow control valve. **B,** A self-inflating bag with an oxygen reservoir to maintain 90% to 100% oxygen. (From the American Heart Association and American Academy of Pediatrics: Neonatal Resuscitation Textbook, 2000.)

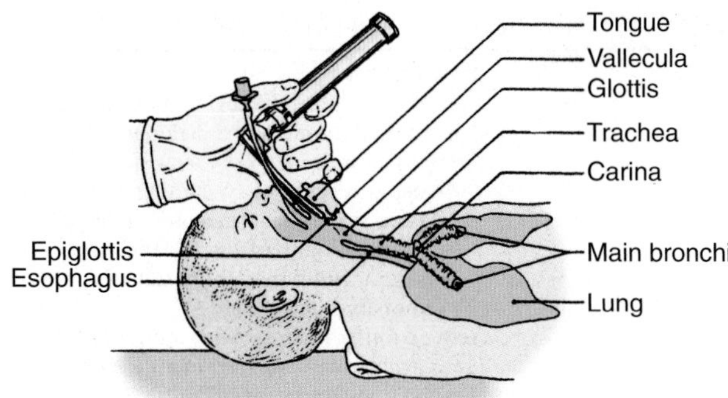

FIGURE 21-11. Anatomy of laryngoscopy for endotracheal intubation. (From the American Heart Association and American Academy of Pediatrics: Neonatal Resuscitation Textbook, 2000.)

TABLE 21-4 MECHANICAL CAUSES OF Failed RESUSCITATION

CATEGORY	EXAMPLES
Equipment failure	Malfunctioning bag, oxygen not connected or running
Endotracheal tube malposition	Esophagus, right mainstem bronchus
Occluded endotracheal tube	
Insufficient inflation pressure to expand lungs	
Space-occupying lesions in the thorax	Pneumothorax, pleural effusions, diaphragmatic hernia
Pulmonary hypoplasia	Extreme prematurity, oligohydramnios

h. Ventilate as described earlier.
i. Failure to respond to intubation and ventilation can result from mechanical causes or severe asphyxia.
j. The mechanical causes listed in Table 21-4 should be quickly ruled out. Check to be sure the endotracheal tube passes through the vocal cords. A CO_2 detector placed between the endotracheal tube and the bag can be very helpful as a rapid confirmation of tube position in the airway. Occlusion of the tube should be suspected when there is resistance to bagging and no chest wall movement. If the endotracheal tube is in place and not occluded, and the equipment is functioning, a trial of bagging with higher pressures is indicated. The other causes listed in Table 21-4 are rare compared with equipment failure or tube problems. A pneumothorax is characterized by asymmetric breath sounds not corrected by repositioning the tube above the carina. Pleural effusions usually occur with fetal hydrops, whereas a diaphragmatic hernia should be ruled out in the setting of asymmetric breath sounds and a scaphoid abdomen. Pulmonary hypoplasia should be considered if the pregnancy has been complicated by oligohydramnios. **It is very unusual for a neonatal resuscitation to require either cardiac massage or drugs.** Almost all newborns respond to ventilation with supplemental oxygen.

TABLE 21-5 NEONATAL DRUG DOSES

DRUG	DOSE	ROUTE	HOW SUPPLIED
Epinephrine	0.1-0.3 mL/kg	IV or ET	1:10,000 dilution
Sodium bicarbonate*	1-2 mEq/kg	IV	0.5 mEq/mL (4.2% solution)
Volume†	10 mL/kg	IV	Normal saline, Ringer's lactate, whole blood
Naloxone‡	0.1 mg/kg	IV, ET	1 mg/mL IM, SC

Modified from American Heart Association and American Academy of Pediatrics: Neonatal Resuscitation Textbook. American Heart Association and American Academy of Pediatrics, 2006.
*For correction of metabolic acidosis only after adequate ventilation has been achieved; give slowly over several minutes.
†Infuse slowly over 5 to 10 minutes.
‡After proceeding with proper airway management and other resuscitative techniques
IV, Intravenous; *ET,* endotracheal; *IM,* intramuscular; *SC,* subcutaneous.

7. If mechanical causes are ruled out, external cardiac massage should be performed for persistent heart rate at less than 60 bpm after intubation and positive pressure ventilation for 30 seconds. Compression of one third of the anteroposterior diameter of the chest should be performed, interposed with ventilation at a 3:1 ratio (90 compressions, 30 breaths per minute).
8. If drugs are needed for a persistent heart rate less than 60 bpm after ventilation and chest compressions (Table 21-5), the drug of choice and preferred route of delivery is 0.1 to 0.3 mL/kg of 1:10,000 epinephrine through an umbilical venous line. If intravenous access is not established, epinephrine can be given via an endotracheal tube. Higher doses (0.5 to 1 mL/kg) of a 1:10,000 formulation may be required. If volume loss is suspected (e.g., documented blood loss with clinical evidence of hypovolemia), 10 mL/kg of a volume expander (normal saline or Ringer's lactate) should be administered through an umbilical venous line. The appropriateness of continued resuscitative efforts should always be reevaluated in an infant who fails to respond to all of the previously mentioned efforts. Today, resuscitative efforts are made even in "apparent stillbirths," that is, infants whose 1-minute Apgar scores are 0 to 1. However, efforts should not be sustained in the face of little or no improvement despite an appropriate resuscitation over a reasonable period of time (i.e., 10 to 15 minutes).[22]

Data now exist to support resuscitation with room air in lieu of 100% oxygen.[23,24] Concerns have been raised about the potential harmful effects of 100% oxygen, in particular the generation of oxygen free radicals. With that in mind, room air is a more appropriate gas than 100% oxygen. For term infants, all resuscitations should begin with room air targeting normal saturations for age in minutes (Figure 21-9).[22] If resuscitation is started with room air and there is no improvement, then supplemental oxygen can be given. **Normal healthy term infants require approximately 10 to 15 minutes to achieve oxygen saturations above 90%.**[25]

A few special circumstances merit discussion at this point. Infants in whom respiratory depression secondary to narcotic administration is suspected may be given naloxone (Narcan). However, this should not be done until the airway has been managed and the infant resuscitated in the usual fashion. In addition, naloxone should not be given to the infant of an addicted mother, because it will precipitate withdrawal.

A second special group are preterm infants. Minimizing heat loss improves survival, so prewarmed towels should be available, and the environmental temperature of the delivery suite should be raised. The infant should be placed in a plastic covering after birth to minimize evaporative heat loss.[26] In the extremely-low-birthweight infant (<1000 g), proceed quickly to administration of continuous positive airway pressure (CPAP) and consider early intubation for surfactant administration. Volume expanders and sodium bicarbonate should be infused slowly to avoid rapid swings in blood pressure. Resuscitation in preterm infants also should begin with less than 100% (usually 30%-40%) oxygen.[24,27]

Finally, there is the issue of meconium-stained amniotic fluid. Meconium aspiration syndrome (MAS) is a form of aspiration pneumonia that occurs most often in term or postterm infants who have passed meconium in utero (7% to 20% of all deliveries).[28] Overall, 2% to 9% of children born through meconium-stained fluid are diagnosed with MAS.[28] Delivery room management of meconium in the amniotic fluid has been historically based on the notion that aspiration takes place with the initiation of extrauterine respiration and that the pathologic condition is related to the aspirated contents. This resulted in the practice of oropharyngeal suction on the perineum after delivery of the head, followed by airway visualization and suction by the resuscitator after delivery. Both of these assumptions are not entirely true. In utero aspiration has been induced in animal models and confirmed in autopsies of human stillbirths. In addition, the combined suction approach has not been uniformly successful in decreasing the incidence of MAS. These data have been confirmed by a large multicenter, prospective, randomized controlled trial assessing selective intubation of apparently vigorous meconium-stained infants.[29] Compared with expectant management, intubation and tracheal suction did not result in a decreased incidence of MAS or other respiratory disorders. Finally, oropharyngeal suction on the perineum before delivery of the shoulders does not prevent MAS.[30] The current recommended approach to meconium in the amniotic fluid is as follows:

1. The obstetrician carefully performs bulb suctioning of the oropharynx and nasopharynx after delivery of the baby.
2. If the baby is active and breathing and requires no resuscitation, the airway need not be inspected, thus avoiding the risk of inducing vagal bradycardia.
3. Any infant in need of resuscitation should have the airway inspected and suctioned before instituting positive-pressure ventilation.
4. Suction the stomach when airway management is complete and vital signs are stable.

Sequelae of Birth Asphyxia

The incidence of birth asphyxia is about 0.1% in term infants, with an increased incidence in infants of lower gestational age.[31] The acute sequelae that need to be managed in the neonatal period are listed in Table 21-6.

TABLE 21-6 THE ACUTE SEQUELAE OF ASPHYXIA

System	*Manifestations*
Central nervous system	Cerebral edema, seizures, hemorrhage and hypoxic-ischemic encephalopathy
Cardiac	Papillary muscle necrosis—transient tricuspid insufficiency, cardiogenic shock
Pulmonary	Aspiration syndromes (meconium, clear fluid), acquired surfactant deficiency, persistent pulmonary hypertension, pulmonary hemorrhage
Renal	Acute tubular necrosis with anuria or oliguria
Adrenal	Hemorrhage with adrenal insufficiency
Hepatic	Enzyme elevations, liver failure
Gastrointestinal	Necrotizing enterocolitis, feeding intolerance
Metabolic	Hypoglycemia, hypocalcemia
Hematologic	Coagulation disorders, thrombocytopenia

Widespread organ injury is evident. Management focuses on supportive care and treatment of specific abnormalities. This includes careful fluid management, blood pressure support, intravenous glucose, and treatment of seizures. Phenobarbital (40 mg/kg) 1 to 6 hours after the event given as neuroprotective therapy is associated with an improved neurologic outcome. **Hypothermia (selective head cooling or whole body hypothermia), especially if started within the first 6 hours of life, significantly improves outcomes at 18 to 22 months of age.**[32-34] The roles of oxygen free radical scavengers, excitatory amino acid antagonists, and calcium channel blockers in minimizing cerebral injury after asphyxia are still investigational.

If the infant survives, the major long-term concern is permanent CNS damage. The challenge is identifying criteria that can provide information about the risk of future problems for a given infant. A variety of markers have been examined to identify birth asphyxia and risk for adverse neurologic outcome. Marked fetal bradycardia is associated with increased risk, but use of electronic fetal monitoring and cesarean delivery have not altered the incidence of cerebral palsy over the last several decades. Low Apgar scores (≤3 beyond 5 minutes) at 1 and 5 minutes are not predictive, but infants with low scores that persist at 15 and 20 minutes after birth have a 50% chance of manifesting cerebral palsy if they survive. Cord pH is predictive of adverse outcome only if the pH is less than 7.00. The best predictor of outcome is the severity of the neonatal neurologic syndrome.[35] Infants with mild encephalopathy survive and are normal on follow-up examination. Moderate encephalopathy carries a 25% to 50% risk of severe handicap or death, whereas the severe syndrome carries a greater than 75% risk of death or disability. Diagnostic aids including electroencephalograms and magnetic resonance imaging (MRI) scans can also aid in predicting outcome. The circulatory response to hypoxia is to redistribute blood flow to provide adequate oxygen delivery to critical organs (e.g., brain, heart) at the expense of other organs. Thus, an insult severe enough to damage the brain should be accompanied by evidence of other organ dysfunction.

The long-term neurologic sequelae of intrapartum asphyxia are cerebral palsy with or without associated cognitive deficits and epilepsy. Although cerebral palsy can be related to intrapartum events, the large majority of cases are of unknown cause. Furthermore, cognitive deficits and epilepsy, unless associated with cerebral palsy, cannot be related to asphyxia or to other intrapartum events. **To attribute cerebral palsy to peripartum asphyxia, there must be an absence of other demonstrable causes, substantial or prolonged intrapartum asphyxia (fetal heart rate abnormalities, fetal acidosis), and clinical evidence during the first days of life of neurologic dysfunction in the infant (see box, "Relationship of Intrapartum Events and Cerebral Palsy").**[36]

Relationship of Intrapartum Events and Cerebral Palsy

Essential Criteria

Evidence of a metabolic acidosis in fetal umbilical cord arterial blood obtained at delivery (pH < 7.00 and base deficit ≥12 mmol/L)

Early onset of severe or moderate neonatal encephalopathy in infants born at 34 or more weeks' gestation

Cerebral palsy of the spastic quadriplegic or dyskinetic type

Exclusion of other identifiable etiologies such as trauma, coagulation disorders, infectious conditions, or genetic disorders

Criteria That Suggest Intrapartum Timing but Are Not Specific to Asphyxial Insults

A sentinel hypoxic event occurring immediately before or during labor

A sudden sustained fetal bradycardia or the absence of fetal heart rate variability in the presence of persistent late or variable decelerations, usually after a hypoxic sentinel event when the pattern was previously normal

Apgar scores of 0-3 beyond 5 minutes

Onset of multisystem involvement within 72 hours of birth

Early imaging study showing evidence of acute nonfocal cerebral abnormality

Modified from American College of Obstetricians and Gynecologists, American Academy of Pediatrics: Neonatal Encephalopathy and Cerebral Palsy: Defining Pathogenesis and Pathophysiology. Washington DC, ACOG, 2003.

BIRTH INJURIES

Birth injuries are defined as those sustained during labor and delivery. **Factors predisposing to birth injury include macrosomia, cephalopelvic disproportion, shoulder dystocia, prolonged or difficult labor, precipitous delivery, abnormal presentations (including breech), and use of operative vaginal delivery.**[37] Injuries range from minor (requiring no therapy) to life threatening (Table 21-7).

Soft tissue injuries are most common. Most are related to dystocia and to the use of operative vaginal delivery. Accidental lacerations of the scalp, buttocks, and thighs may be inflicted with the scalpel during cesarean delivery. Cumulatively, these injuries are of a minor nature and respond well to therapy. Hyperbilirubinemia, particularly in the premature infant, is the major neonatal complication related to soft tissue bruising.

A cephalohematoma occurs in 0.2% to 2.5% of live births. Caused by rupture of blood vessels that traverse from the skull to the periosteum, the bleeding is subperiosteal and therefore limited by suture lines, with the most common site of bleeding being over the parietal bones.

TABLE 21-7 Birth Injuries

CLASSIFICATION	EXAMPLE
Soft tissue injuries*	Lacerations, abrasions, fat necrosis
Extracranial bleeding	Cephalohematoma,* subgaleal bleed
Intracranial hemorrhage	Subarachnoid, subdural, epidural, cerebral, cerebellar
Nerve injuries	Facial nerve,* cervical nerve roots (brachial plexus palsies,* phrenic n., Horner's syndrome), recurrent laryngeal n. (vocal cord paralysis)
Fractures	Clavicle,* facial bones, humerus, femur, skull, nasal bones
Dislocations	Extremities, nasal septum
Eye injuries	Subconjunctiva* and retinal hemorrhages, orbital fracture, corneal laceration, breaks in Desçemet's membrane with corneal opacification
Torticollis†	
Spinal cord injuries	
Visceral rupture	Liver, spleen
Scalp laceration*	Fetal scalp electrode, scalpel
Scalp abscess	Fetal scalp electrode

*More common occurrences.
†Secondary to hemorrhage into the sternocleidomastoid muscle.

Associations include prolonged or difficult labor and mechanical trauma from operative vaginal delivery. Linear skull fractures beneath the hematoma have been reported in 5.4% of cases but are of no major consequence except in the unlikely event that a leptomeningeal cyst develops. Most cephalhematomas are reabsorbed in 2 weeks to 3 months. Subgaleal bleeds, which are not limited by suture lines, can occur in association with vacuum extraction alone (especially with multiple pop-offs and prolonged traction), in combination with the use of forceps, or with difficult forceps deliveries, and can result in life-threatening anemia, hypotension, or consumptive coagulopathy. Depressed skull fractures are also seen in neonates, but most do not require surgical elevations.

Intracranial hemorrhages related to trauma include epidural, subdural, subarachnoid, and intraparenchymal bleeds.[38] With improvements in obstetric care, subdural hemorrhages fortunately are now rare. Three major varieties of subdural bleeds have been described: (1) posterior fossa hematomas due to tentorial laceration with rupture of the straight sinus, vein of Galen, or transverse sinus or due to occipital osteodiastasis (a separation between the squamous and lateral portions of the occipital bone); (2) falx laceration, with rupture of the inferior sagittal sinus; and (3) rupture of the superficial cerebral veins. The clinical symptoms are related to the location of bleeding. With tentorial laceration, bleeding is infratentorial, causing brainstem signs and a rapid progression to death. Falx tears cause bilateral cerebral signs (e.g., seizures and focal weakness) until blood extends infratentorially to the brainstem. Subdural hemorrhage over the cerebral convexities can cause several clinical states, ranging from an asymptomatic newborn to one with seizures and focal neurologic findings. Infants with lacerations of the tentorium and falx have a poor outlook. In contrast, the prognosis for rupture of the superficial cerebral veins is much better, with the majority of survivors being normal. Primary subarachnoid hemorrhage is the most common variety of neonatal intracranial hemorrhage.[38] Clinically, these infants are often asymptomatic, although they may present with a characteristic seizure pattern. The seizures begin on day 2 of life, and the infants are "well" between convulsions. In general, the prognosis for subarachnoid bleeds is good.

Trauma to peripheral nerves produces another major group of birth injuries. Brachial plexus injuries are caused by stretching of the cervical roots during delivery, usually when shoulder dystocia is present. Upper arm palsy (Erb-Duchenne), the most common brachial plexus injury, is caused by injury to the fifth and sixth cervical nerves; lower arm paralysis (Klumpke) results from damage to the eighth cervical and first thoracic nerves. Damage to all four nerve roots produces paralysis of the entire arm. Outcome for these injuries is variable, with some infants left with significant residual damage. Horner syndrome due to damage to sympathetic outflow through nerve root T1 may accompany Klumpke palsy, and approximately 5% of patients with Erb palsy have an associated phrenic nerve paresis. Facial palsy is another fairly common injury caused either by pressure from the sacral promontory or fetal shoulder as the infant passes through the birth canal or by operative vaginal delivery. Most of these palsies resolve, although in some infants, paralysis is persistent.

The majority of bone fractures resulting from birth trauma involve the clavicle and result from shoulder dystocia or breech extractions that require vigorous manipulations. Clinically, many of these fractures are asymptomatic, and when present, symptoms are mild. Prognosis for clavicular as well as limb fractures is uniformly good. The most commonly fractured long bone is the humerus.

Spinal cord injuries are a relatively infrequent but often severe form of birth injury. Accurate incidence is difficult to assess, because symptoms mimic other neonatal diseases and autopsies often do not include a careful examination of the spine. Depressed tone, hyporeflexia, and respiratory failure are clues to this diagnosis. Excessive longitudinal traction and head rotation during forceps delivery predispose to spinal injury, and hyperextension of the head in a footling breech is particularly dangerous. Outcomes include death or stillbirth caused by high cervical or brainstem lesions, long-term survival of infants with paralysis from birth, and minimal neurologic symptoms or spasticity.

NEONATAL THERMAL REGULATION

Physiology

The range of environmental temperatures over which the neonate can operate is narrower than that of an adult as a result of the infant's inability to dissipate heat effectively in warm environments and, more critically, to maintain temperature in response to cold. This range narrows with decreasing gestational age.

Although some increases in activity and shivering have been observed, nonshivering thermogenesis is the most important means of increased heat production in the cold-stressed newborn.[39] Nonshivering thermogenesis can be defined as an increase in total heat production without detectable (visible or electrical) muscle activity. The site of this increased heat production is brown fat located between the scapulae; around the muscles and blood vessels of the neck, axillae, and mediastinum; between the esophagus and trachea; and around the kidneys and adrenal glands. Brown fat cells contain more mitochondria and fat vacuoles, and have a richer blood and sympathetic nerve supply compared to white fat cells.

TABLE 21-8 NEONATAL RESPONSE TO THERMAL STRESS

STRESSOR	RESPONSE	TERM	PRETERM
Cold	Vasoconstriction	++	++
	↓ Exposed surface area (posture change)	±	±
	↑Oxygen consumption	++	+
	↑Motor activity; shivering	+	–
Heat	Vasodilation	++	++
	Sweating	+	–

++, Maximum response; +, intermediate; ±, may have a role; –, no response.

Heat loss to the environment is dependent on both an internal temperature gradient (from within the body to the surface) and an external gradient (from the surface to the environment). The infant can change the internal gradient by altering vasomotor tone and, to a lesser extent, by postural changes that decrease the amount of exposed surface area. The external gradient is dependent on purely physical variables. Heat transfer from the surface to the environment involves four routes: radiation, convection, conduction, and evaporation. Radiant heat loss, heat transfer from a warmer to a cooler object that is not in contact, depends on the temperature gradient between the objects. Heat loss by convection to the surrounding gaseous environment depends on air speed and temperature. Conduction or heat loss to a contacting cooler object is minimal in most circumstances. Heat loss by evaporation is cooling secondary to water loss at the rate of 0.6 cal/g water evaporated and is affected by relative humidity, air speed, exposed surface area, and skin permeability. In infants in excessively warm environments, under overhead radiant heat sources, or in very immature infants with thin, permeable skin, evaporative losses increase considerably. Table 21-8 summarizes the neonate's efforts to maintain a stable core temperature in the face of cold or heat stress. It is advantageous to maintain an infant in a neutral thermal environment (Figure 21-12). The neutral thermal environment for a given infant depends on size, gestational age, and postnatal age.[40] In general, maintaining the abdominal skin temperature at 36.5°C minimizes energy expenditure.

CLINICAL APPLICATIONS

Delivery Room

In utero, fetal thermoregulation is the responsibility of the placenta and is dependent on maternal core temperature, with fetal temperature 0.5° C higher than maternal temperature. At birth, the infant's core temperature drops rapidly from 37.8° C because of evaporation from its wet body and radiant and convective losses to the cold air and walls of the room. Even with an increase in oxygen consumption to the maximum capability of the newborn (15 mL/kg/min), the infant can produce only 0.075 cal/kg/min and will rapidly lose heat. Measures taken to reduce heat loss after birth depend on the clinical situation. For

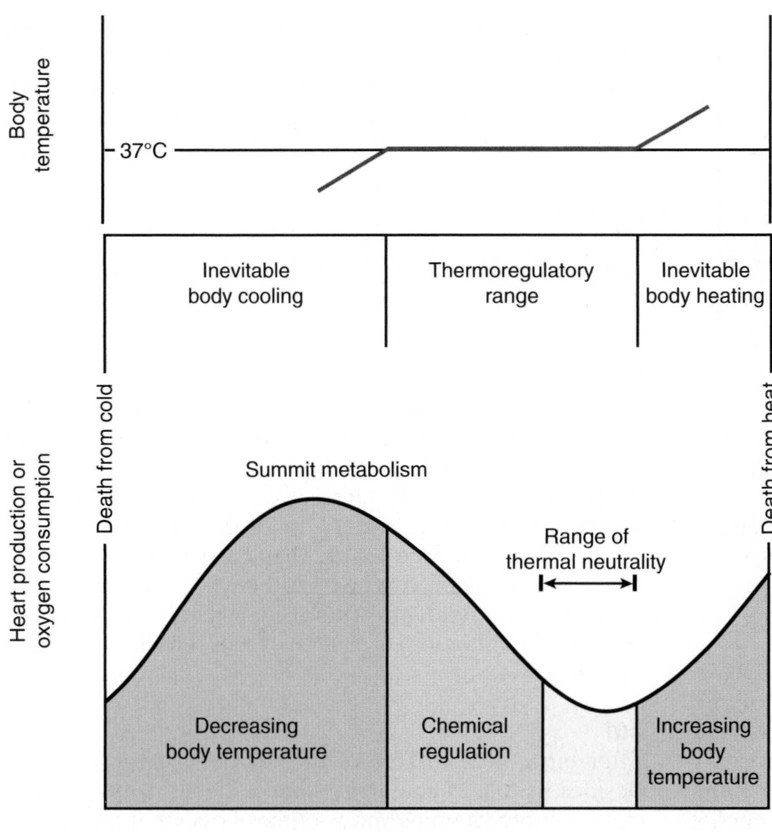

FIGURE 21-12. Effect of environmental temperature on oxygen consumption and body temperature. (Modified from Klaus MH, Fanaroff AA: The physical environment. *In* Klaus MH, Fanaroff AA [eds]: Care of the High-Risk Neonate, 5th ed. Philadelphia, WB Saunders Company, 2001, p 130.)

the well term infant, drying the skin and wrapping the baby with warm blankets is sufficient. When it is necessary to leave an infant exposed for close observation or resuscitation, the infant should be dried and placed under a radiant heat source. Room temperature can be elevated as an added precaution for the low-birthweight infant.

Nursery

Babies are cared for in the newborn nursery wrapped in blankets in bassinets (cot-nursed), in isolettes, or under a radiant heat source. Healthy full-term infants (weighing >2.5 kg) need only be clothed and placed in a bassinet under a blanket. Infants weighing 2 to 2.5 kg who are either slightly premature or growth restricted should be allowed 12 to 24 hours to stabilize in an isolette and then advanced to a bassinet. Lower birthweight babies (<2 kg) will require care in either isolettes or under radiant heat sources. **Adequate thermal protection of the low-birthweight infant is essential.** This is especially important for the very-low-birthweight infant (<1.5 kg), who often does not behave like a mature homeotherm. These neonates can react to a small change in environmental temperature with a change in body temperature rather than a change in oxygen consumption. In addition, warmer environments hasten growth of the premature infant.

The isolette, which heats by convection, is the most commonly used heating device for the low-birthweight nude infant. The major source of heat loss while in a neutral thermal environment is radiant to the walls of the isolette. The magnitude of this loss is predictable if room temperature is known. These losses can be minimized using double-walled isolettes in which the inner wall temperature is very close to the air temperature within the isolette. Once clinical status has been stabilized, the child can be dressed, which will afford increased thermal stability.

Radiant warmers can also be used to ensure thermal stability of both low-birthweight and full-sized infants. Radiant warmers are used most effectively for short-term warming during initial resuscitation and stabilization as well as for performing procedures. They provide easy access to the infant while ensuring thermal stability. The main heat losses are convection, which can be significant because of variable air speed in a room, and evaporation. Evaporative heat loss resulting in significant fluid losses is a major concern for the very-low-birthweight premature cared for under a radiant warmer. Placing a plastic shield over the infant or covering the skin with a semipermeable membrane can minimize these fluid losses.

The most economical means of thermal support for the low-birthweight infant is skin-to-skin contact with a parent. This "kangaroo" care has been shown to reduce serious illness and enhance lactation while providing adequate thermal support.

NEONATAL NUTRITION AND GASTROENTEROLOGY

At birth, the newborn infant must assume various functions performed during fetal life by the placenta.

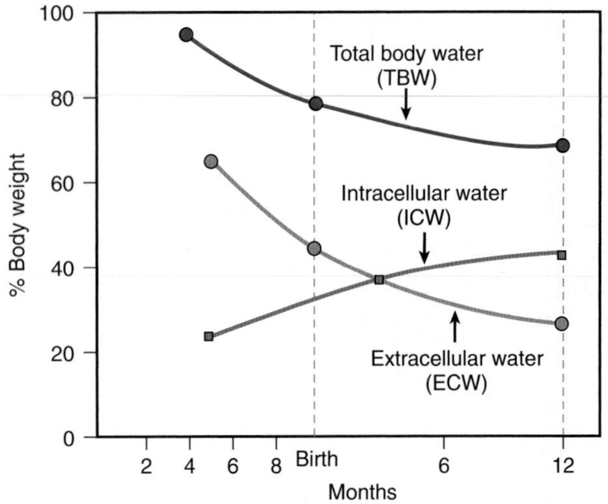

Figure 21-13. Changes in body water during gestation and infancy. (Modified from Friis-Hansen B: Water distribution in the foetus and newborn infant. Acta Paediatr Scand Suppl 305:7, 1983.)

Cardiopulmonary transition and thermoregulation have already been discussed. The final critical task for the newborn is the assimilation of calories, water, and electrolytes.

The required caloric, water, and electrolyte intake of the newborn depends on body stores and normal rate of energy expenditure. Body composition varies considerably with gestational age (Figure 21-13).[41] The average 1-kg preterm neonate consists of 85% water, 10% protein, and 3% fat as compared with 74% water, 12% protein, and 11% fat at term. Carbohydrate stores in the term infant are eight times higher. Rates of energy expenditure differ as well.

Water and Electrolytes

Maintenance water requirements are dependent on metabolic rate (evaporative losses to dissipate the heat of oxidation) and the necessary water to excrete the renal solute load. Other pertinent factors, especially for the premature infant, include environmental variation in insensible water losses and diminished ability to concentrate urine. It is normal during the first 3 to 4 postnatal days for an infant to experience a weight loss of up to 10% as the physiologic contraction of extracellular body fluid takes place. Maintenance electrolyte requirements are 2 to 3 mEq/kg/day for sodium, chloride, and bicarbonate and 1 to 2 mEq/kg/day for potassium. During periods of rapid growth, requirements will be higher.

Calories

Caloric needs are primarily dependent on oxygen consumption. The character of the feeding also affects caloric needs by altering specific dynamic action and fecal losses. The average caloric requirement for a normal full-term infant is estimated to be about 100 to 110 kcal/kg/day. The needs of the low-birthweight infant are more variable, but usually 105 to 130 kcal/kg/day is adequate.[42] Standard infant formulas and breast milk provide approximately 20 kcal/oz. Therefore, volumes of 150 to 180 mL/kg/day will provide the necessary caloric intake of 100 to 120 kcal/kg/day for the average term or preterm infant beyond 32 to 34 weeks' gestation. Infants weighing less than 1500 g should be fed with either formulas designed specifically for the premature or fortified breast milk. The goal for the growing premature is growth at a rate comparable to intrauterine growth during the third trimester.

Protein

Both the quantity and quality of protein intake are important for adequate growth, particularly for the premature infant.[42] Suggested intakes range from 2.25 to 4.0 g/kg/day (~3.5 g/kg/day for the premature infant).

Carbohydrate

Before birth, glucose is the major energy source for the human fetus. However, after birth carbohydrates are responsible for 40% to 50% of the total caloric needs. Intestinal disaccharidases develop early in fetal life, with lactase reaching mature levels at term. Both term and preterm infants can digest lactose, the major sugar in human milk and standard infant formulas. Although lactase levels are lower in preterm infants, which can lead to feeding intolerance, early initiation of enteral feeds rapidly increases lactase.

Fat

After birth, 40% to 50% of the calories oxidized are fat. Besides its role as an energy source, dietary fat is a carrier of fat-soluble vitamins and a source of essential fatty acids. Dietary fat is not completely absorbed; more so in the premature than in the term infant. For that reason, preterm formulas provide a portion of the fat energy as medium-chain triglycerides.

Infant Feeding

For the well term or slightly preterm infant, institution of oral feeds within the first 2 to 4 hours of life is reasonable practice. For infants who are SGA or large for gestational age (LGA), feeds within the first hour or two of life may be indicated to avoid hypoglycemia. Premature infants (<34 weeks' gestation) who are unable to nipple feed present a more complex set of circumstances. In addition to an inability to suck and swallow efficiently, such infants face a number of problems: (1) relatively high caloric demand; (2) small stomach capacity; (3) incompetent esophageal-cardiac sphincter, leading to gastroesophageal reflux; (4) poor gag reflex, creating a tendency for aspiration; (5) decreased digestive capability (especially for fat); and (6) slow gastric emptying and intestinal motility. These infants can initially be supported adequately with parenteral nutrition, followed by institution of nasogastric tube feedings when their cardiopulmonary status is stable.

Although a wide range of infant formulas satisfy the nutritional needs of most neonates, breast milk remains the standard on which formulas are based. The distribution of calories in human milk is 7% protein, 55% fat, and 38% carbohydrate. The whey/casein ratio is 70:30, enhancing ease of protein digestion and gastric emptying, while fat digestion is augmented by the presence of a breast milk lipase. Despite the low levels of several vitamins and minerals, bioavailability is high. In addition to the nutritional features, breast milk's immunochemical and cellular components provide protection against infection.[43]

The growth demands of the low-birthweight infant exceed what can be provided by human milk in terms of protein, calcium, phosphorus, sodium, zinc, copper, and possibly other nutrients. These shortcomings can be addressed through the addition of human milk fortifiers to mother's preterm breast milk.[44] Advantages of breast milk for the premature include its anti-infective properties, possible protection against NEC, and its role in enhancing neurodevelopmental outcome.[45]

Few contraindications to breastfeeding exist. Infants with galactosemia should not ingest lactose-containing milk. Infants with other inborn errors such as phenylketonuria may ingest some human milk, with close monitoring of the amount. The presence of environmental pollutants has been documented in breast milk, but to date no serious side effects have been reported. Most drugs do not contraindicate breastfeeding, but there are a few exceptions (see Chapter 8). Transmission of some viral infections via breast milk is a concern as well. Mothers who are human immunodeficiency virus (HIV) positive should not breastfeed if safe and effective alternatives to breast milk are available. The nursery staff must be aware of problems associated with breastfeeding and use lactation consultants to deal with poor infant latching, sore nipples, poor milk supply, and excessive hyperbilirubinemia. The obstetrician and pediatrician should serve as a source of knowledge and, most important, support. Table 21-9 illustrates what a mother can expect as she breastfeeds her infant.

Neonatal Hypoglycemia

Glucose is a major fetal fuel transported by facilitated diffusion across the placenta. After birth, before an appropriate supply of exogenous calories is provided, the newborn must maintain blood glucose through endogenous sources. Hepatic glycogen stores are almost entirely depleted within the first 12 hours after birth in the healthy term neonate and more rapidly in the preterm or stressed infant if there is no other glucose source. Fat and protein stores are then used for energy, while glucose levels are maintained by hepatic gluconeogenesis.

In the healthy unstressed neonate, glucose falls over the first 1 to 2 hours after birth, stabilizes at a minimum of about 40 mg/dL, and then rises to 50 to 80 mg/dL by 3 hours of life.[46] Low glucose concentrations can be defined as less than 45 mg/dL. **Infants at risk for low blood glucose concentrations and in whom glucose should be monitored include preterm infants, SGA infants, hyperinsulinemic (infant of a diabetic mother [IDM]), LGA infants, and infants with perinatal stress or asphyxia.** As in term babies, blood sugar drops after birth in preterm babies, but the latter are less able to mount a counterregulatory response. In addition, the presence of respiratory distress, hypothermia, and other factors can increase glucose demand, exacerbating hypoglycemia. SGA infants are at risk for hypoglycemia resulting from rapidly utilized glycogen stores as well as impaired gluconeogenesis and ketogenesis. Onset of hypoglycemia in SGA and preterm infants usually occurs at 2 to 6 hours of life. Hyperinsulinemia occurs in the infant of a diabetic mother as well as other rare conditions, including Beckwith-Weidemann syndrome and congenital hyperinsulinism. Onset of hypoglycemia in these infants can be in the first 30 to 60 minutes after birth. In the case of perinatal asphyxia, hypoglycemia is the result of excessive glucose demand and occasionally transient hyperinsulinism.[47,48] Infants with recurrent hypoglycemia over 3 to 4 days should be evaluated for endocrine (hyperinsulinism, decreased counterregulatory hormones—cortisol, growth hormone, and glucagon) and inborn errors of metabolism disorders (see box, Etiologies of Neonatal Hypoglycemia).

Etiologies of Neonatal Hypoglycemia

I. Transient neonatal hypoglycemia
   A. Preterm and IUGR infants
   B. Transient hyperinsulinism (IDM)
   C. Perinatal stress (hypoxia, RDS)
II. Persistent neonatal hypoglycemia
   A. Hyperinsulinism
      1. Potassium-ATP channel
      2. Glucokinase hyperinsulinism
      3. Glutamate dehydrogenase hyperinsulinism
      4. Beckwith-Wiedemann syndrome
   B. Counterregulatory hormone deficiency (hypopituitarism)
   C. Inborn errors of metabolism
      1. Glycogenolysis disorders
      2. Gluconeogenesis disorders
      3. Fatty acid oxidation disorders

ATP, Adenosine triphosphate; *IDM,* infant of a diabetic mother.

Symptoms of hypoglycemia include jitteriness, seizures, cyanosis, respiratory distress, apathy, hypotonia, and eye rolling.[46] However, many infants, particularly premature infants, are asymptomatic. Because of the risk of subsequent brain injury, hypoglycemia, when present, should be aggressively treated. However, the single best treatment is prevention by identifying infants at risk, including premature, SGA, IDM, LGA, and any stressed infant. These newborns should have blood glucose screened with a bedside glucose meter. All values less than or equal to 45 mg/dL should be confirmed with a laboratory measurement. Treatment is initiated by early institution of feeds or an intravenous glucose bolus (2 mL/kg of $D_{10}W$ solution) followed by a glucose infusion at a rate of 6 mg/kg/min.[49]

Congenital Gastrointestinal Surgical Conditions

Several congenital surgical conditions of the gastrointestinal tract interfere with a normal transition. Many of these conditions can be diagnosed with antenatal ultrasound, allowing transfer of the mother to a perinatal center for delivery.

Gastrointestinal Tract Obstruction

Tracheoesophageal fistula and esophageal atresia are characterized by a blind esophageal pouch and a fistulous connection between either the proximal or distal esophagus and the airway. Eighty-five percent of infants with these conditions have the fistula between the distal esophagus and the airway. Polyhydramnios is common because of the

TABLE 21-9 GUIDELINES FOR SUCCESSFUL BREAST FEEDING

	FIRST 8 HOURS	8-24 HOURS	DAY 2	DAY 3	DAY 4	DAY 5	DAY 6 ONWARD
Milk Supply	You may be able to express a few drops of milk.		Milk *should* come in between the 2nd and 4th day.			Milk should be in. Breasts may be firm and/or leak milk.	Breasts should feel softer after nursing.
Baby's activity	Baby is usually wide awake in the first hour of life. Put baby to breast within ½ hour of birth	Wake up your baby. Babies may not wake up on their own to feed.	Baby should be more cooperative and less sleepy.	Look for early feeding cues such as rooting, lip smacking, and hands to face.			Baby should appear satisfied after feedings.
Feeding routine	Baby may go into a deep sleep 2-4 hours after birth.	Use chart to write down time of each feeding. Feed your baby every 1-4 hr or as often as wanted—at least 8-12 times a day.				May go one longer interval (up to 5 hr between feeds) in a 24-hr period.	
Breastfeeding	Baby will wake up and be alert and responsive for several more hours after initial sleep.	As long as the mother is comfortable, nurse at both breasts as long as baby is actively sucking.	Try to nurse both sides each feeding, aiming at 10 min per side. Expect some nipple tenderness.	Consider hand expressing or pumping a few drops of milk to soften the nipple if the breast is too firm for the baby to latch on.	Nurse a minimum of 10-30 min per side every feeding for the first few weeks of life. Once milk supply is well established, allow baby to finish the first breast before offering the second.		Mother's nipple tenderness is improving or is gone.
Baby's urine output		Baby must have a minimum of one wet diaper in the first 24 hr.	Baby must have at least one wet diaper every 8-11 hr.	You should see an increase in wet diapers (up to four or six) in 24 hr.	Baby's urine should be light yellow.	Baby should have six to eight wet diapers per day of colorless or light yellow urine.	
Baby's stools		Baby may have a very dark (meconium) stool.	Baby may have a second very dark (meconium) stool.	Baby's stools should be in transition from black-green to yellow.		Baby should have three to four yellow, seedy stools a day.	The number of stools may decrease gradually after 4-6 wk.

Courtesy Beth Gabrielski, RN: The Children's Hospital, Denver, 1999, with permission.

high level of gastrointestinal obstruction. Infants present in the first hours of life with copious secretions, choking, cyanosis, and respiratory distress. Diagnosis can be confirmed with chest radiography after careful placement of a nasogastric tube to the point at which resistance is met. The tube will be seen in the blind esophageal pouch. If a tracheoesophageal fistula is present to the distal esophagus, gas will be present in the abdomen.[50]

Infants with high intestinal obstruction present early in life with either bilious or nonbilious vomiting. A history of polyhydramnios is common, and the amniotic fluid, if bile stained, can easily be confused with thin meconium staining. In duodenal atresia, vomitus may or may not contain bile, whereas malrotation with midgut volvulus and high jejunal atresia are characterized by bilious vomiting. Malrotation and midgut volvulus involve torsion of the intestine around the superior mesenteric artery, causing occlusion of the vascular supply to most of the small intestine. If not treated promptly, the infant can lose most of the small bowel due to ischemic injury. **Therefore, bilious vomiting in the neonate demands immediate attention and evaluation.** Diagnosis of high intestinal obstruction can be confirmed with radiographs. Duodenal atresia is characterized by a "double-bubble sign" (stomach and dilated duodenum). Diagnosis of midgut volvulus can be confirmed with an upper gastrointestinal tract series, looking for contrast not to pass the ligament of Treitz. Approximately 30% of cases of duodenal atresia are associated with Down syndrome.[51]

Low intestinal obstruction presents with increasing intolerance of feeds (spitting progressing to vomiting), abdominal distention, and decreased or absent stool.[51] Differential diagnosis of lower intestinal obstruction includes imperforate anus, Hirschsprung disease, meconium plug syndrome, small left colon, colonic and ileal atresia, and meconium ileus. Plain x-ray study of the abdomen shows gaseous distention, with air through a considerable portion of the bowel and air-fluid levels. Diagnosis of meconium ileus, meconium plug, and small left colon syndrome can be made by appearance on contrast enema. Rectal biopsy searching for absence of ganglion cells confirms the diagnosis of Hirschsprung disease. **Infants with meconium ileus and meconium plug should be screened for cystic fibrosis.**

Abdominal Wall Defects

Omphaloceles are formed by incomplete closure of the anterior abdominal wall after return of the midgut to the abdominal cavity. The size of the defect is variable, but usually the omphalocele sac contains some intestine, stomach, liver, and spleen. The abdominal cavity is small and underdeveloped. The umbilical cord can be seen to insert onto the center of the omphalocele sac. There is a high incidence of associated anomalies, including cardiac, other gastrointestinal anomalies, and chromosomal syndromes (trisomy 13). **Delivery room treatment involves covering the defect with sterile warm saline to prevent fluid loss and nasogastric tube decompression.**[52]

Gastroschisis is a defect in the anterior abdominal wall lateral to the umbilicus with no covering sac, with the herniated viscera usually limited to intestine. Furthermore, the intestine has been exposed to amniotic fluid and has a thickened, beefy red appearance. The herniation is thought to occur as a rupture through an ischemic portion of the abdominal wall. Other than intestinal atresia, associated anomalies are uncommon. Delivery room management is as described for omphalocele.[52]

Diaphragmatic Hernia

In diaphragmatic hernia, herniation of abdominal organs into the hemithorax (usually left) occurs because of a posterolateral defect in the diaphragm. Infants usually present in the delivery room with respiratory distress, cyanosis, decreased breath sounds on the side of the hernia, and shift of the mediastinum to the side opposite the hernia. The rapidity and severity of presentation with respiratory distress is dependent on the degree of associated pulmonary hypoplasia. The ipsilateral and to some extent contralateral lung are compressed in utero because of the hernia. Delivery room treatment is to intubate, ventilate, and decompress the gastrointestinal tract with a nasogastric tube. A chest radiograph confirms the diagnosis. The mortality due to diaphragmatic hernia is about 30%, with survival dependent upon the degree of lung hypoplasia and the presence of associated congenital heart disease.[53]

Necrotizing Enterocolitis

NEC is the most common acquired gastrointestinal emergency in the neonatal intensive care unit. This disorder predominantly affects premature infants, with higher incidences present with decreasing gestational age, although it is seen in term infants with polycythemia, congenital heart disease, and birth asyphyxia. The pathogenesis is multifactorial, with intestinal ischemia, infection, provision of enteral feedings, and gut maturity playing roles to varying degrees in individual patients.[54] Tocolysis with indomethacin presumably related to changes in intestinal circulation has been associated with an increased incidence of NEC and isolated intestinal perforation, whereas antenatal betamethasone may decrease the incidence.

Clinically, there is a varied spectrum of disease, from a mild gastrointestinal disturbance to a rapid fulminant course characterized by intestinal gangrene, perforation, sepsis, and shock. The hallmark symptoms are abdominal distention, ileus, delayed gastric emptying, and bloody stools. The radiographic findings are bowel wall edema, pneumatosis intestinalis, biliary free air, and free peritoneal air. Associated symptoms include apnea, bradycardia, hypotension, and temperature instability. Spontaneous intestinal perforation is a related, though likely distinct, disorder characterized by many of the same risk factors and clinical signs, but without extensive intestinal pathology.[55]

Neonatal Jaundice

The most common problem encountered in a term nursery population is jaundice. Neonatal hyperbilirubinemia occurs when the normal pathways of bilirubin metabolism and excretion are altered. Figure 21-14 demonstrates the metabolism of bilirubin. The normal destruction of circulating red cells accounts for about 75% of the newborn's

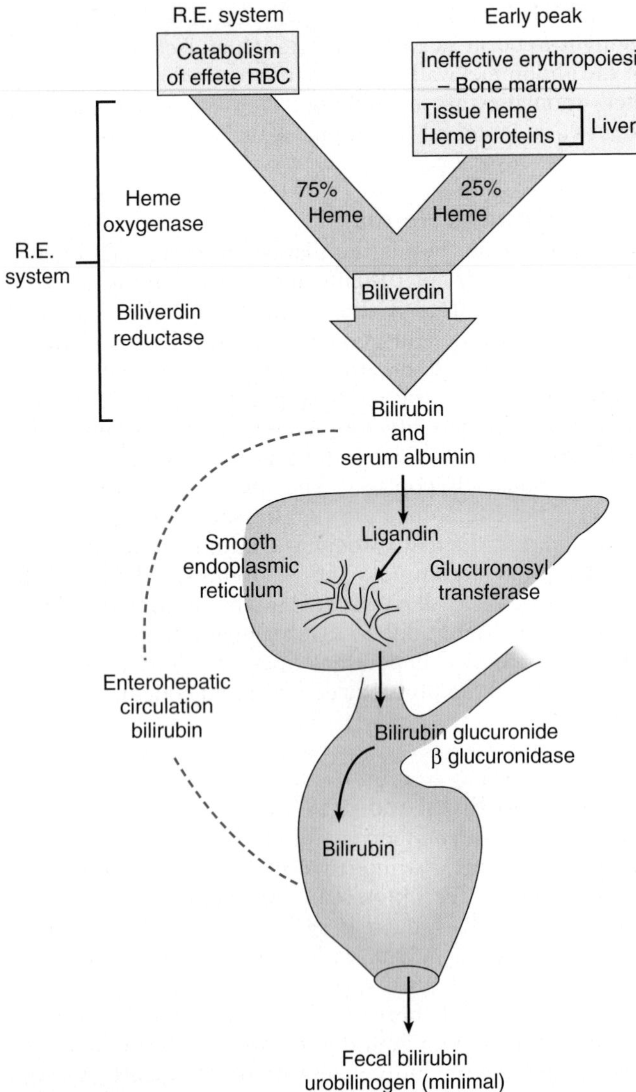

FIGURE 21-14. Neonatal bile pigment metabolism. (Modified from Maisels MJ: Jaundice. *In* Avery GB, Fletcher MA, MacDonald MG [eds]: Neonatology: Pathophysiology and Management of the Newborn, 5th ed. Philadelphia, Lippincott Williams & Wilkins, 1999, p 765.)

daily bilirubin production. The remaining sources include ineffective erythropoiesis and tissue heme proteins. Heme is converted to bilirubin in the reticuloendothelial system with carbon monoxide (CO) produced as a by-product. Unconjugated bilirubin is lipid soluble and transported in the plasma reversibly bound to albumin. Bilirubin enters the liver cells by dissociation from albumin in the hepatic sinusoids. Once in the hepatocyte, bilirubin is conjugated with glucuronic acid in a reaction catalyzed by uridine diphosphoglucuronosyl transferase (UDPGT). The water-soluble conjugated bilirubin is excreted rapidly into the bile canaliculi and into the small intestine. The enzyme β-glucuronidase is present in the small bowel and hydrolyzes some of the conjugated bilirubin. This unconjugated bilirubin can be reabsorbed into the circulation, adding to the total unconjugated bilirubin load (enterohepatic circulation). **Major predisposing factors of neonatal jaundice are (1) increased bilirubin load because of increased red cell volume with decreased cell survival, increased ineffective erythropoiesis, and the enterohepatic circulation; and (2) decreased hepatic uptake, conjugation, and excretion of bilirubin.** These factors result in the presence of clinically apparent jaundice in approximately two thirds of newborns during the first week of life and in most is considered physiologic.[56] Infants whose bilirubin levels are above the 95th percentile for age in hours and infants in high-risk groups to develop hyperbilirubinemia require close follow-up (see Figure 21-15 and the box, Risk Factors for Significant Hyperbilirubinemia).[57,58]

RISK FACTORS FOR SIGNIFICANT HYPERBILIRUBINEMIA

Jaundice observed at less than 24 hours
Blood group incompatibility with positive direct Coombs' test
Other hemolytic disease (G6PD deficiency)
Gestational age less than 35-36 weeks
Previous sibling needing phototherapy
Cephalohematoma, subgaleal blood collection, bruising
Exclusive breastfeeding, especially if nursing not going well
East Asian race

Modified from American Academy of Pediatrics Subcommittee on Hyperbilirubinemia: Management of hyperbilirubinemia in the newborn infant 35 or more weeks gestation. Pediatrics 114:297, 2004.

Pathologic jaundice during the early neonatal period is indirect hyperbilirubinemia, usually caused by overproduction of bilirubin. The leading cause in this group of patients is hemolytic disease, of which fetomaternal blood group incompatibilities (ABO, Rh, and other minor antibodies) are the most common (see Chapter 32). Other causes of hemolysis include genetic disorders such as hereditary spherocytosis and nonspherocytic hemolytic anemias, such as glucose-6-phosphate dehydrogenase (G6PD) deficiency. Other etiologies of bilirubin overproduction include extravasated blood (bruising, hemorrhage), polycythemia, and exaggerated enterohepatic circulation of bilirubin because of mechanical gastrointestinal obstruction or reduced peristalsis from inadequate oral intake. Disease states involving decreased bilirubin clearance must be considered in the patients in whom no cause of overproduction can be identified. Causes of indirect hyperbilirubinemia in this category include familial deficiency of UDPGT (Crigler-Najjar syndrome), Gilbert syndrome, breast milk jaundice, and hypothyroidism. Mixed and direct hyperbilirubinemia are rare during the first week of life.

A strong association exists between breastfeeding and neonatal hyperbilirubinemia. The syndrome of breast milk jaundice is characterized by full-term infants who have jaundice that persists into the second and third weeks of life with maximal bilirubin levels of 10 to 30 mg/dL. If breastfeeding is continued, the levels persist for 4 to 10 days and then decline to normal by 3 to 12 weeks. Interruption of breastfeeding is associated with a prompt decline in 48 hours. In addition to this syndrome, breastfed infants as a whole have higher bilirubin levels over the first 3 to 5

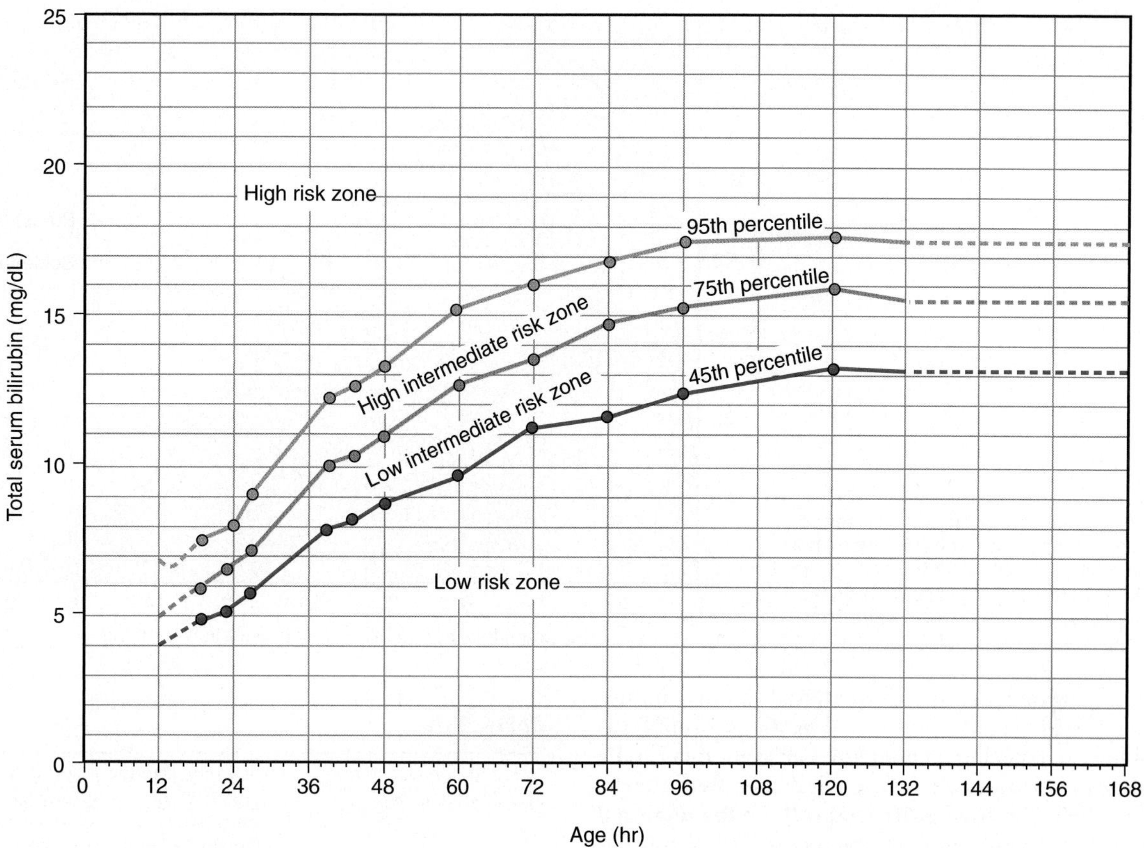

FIGURE 21-15. Risk of developing significant hyperbilirubinemia in term and near-term infants based on hour-specific bilirubin determinations. (From Bhutani VK, Johnson L, Sivieri EM: Predictive ability of a predischarge hour-specific serum bilirubin for subsequent significant hyperbilirubinemia in healthy term and near-term newborns. Pediatrics 103:6, 1999. Copyright 1999 American Academy of Pediatrics.)

days of life than their formula-fed counterparts (Figure 21-16). Rather than interrupting breastfeeding, this early jaundice is responsive to increased frequency of breastfeeding. Suggested mechanisms for breastfeeding-associated jaundice include decreased early caloric intake, inhibitors of bilirubin conjugation in breast milk, and increased intestinal reabsorption of bilirubin. In some patients, there is considerable overlap in these described syndromes.

The overriding concern with neonatal hyperbilirubinemia is the development of bilirubin toxicity causing the pathologic entity of kernicterus, the staining of certain areas of the brain (basal ganglia, hippocampus, geniculate bodies, various brainstem nuclei, and cerebellum) by bilirubin. Neuronal necrosis is the dominant histopathologic feature at 7 to 10 days of life. The early symptoms of bilirubin encephalopathy consist of lethargy, hypotonia, and poor feeding progressing to high-pitched cry, hypertonicity, and opisthotonos. Survivors usually suffer sequelae, including athetoid cerebral palsy, high-frequency hearing loss, paralysis of upward gaze, and dental dysplasia.[59] The risk of bilirubin encephalopathy is not well defined except in those infants with Rh isoimmunization in whom a level of 20 mg/dL has been associated with an increased risk of kernicterus. This observation has been extended to the management of other neonates with hemolytic disease, although no definitive data exist regarding these infants. The risk is probably small for term infants without hemolytic disease even at levels higher than 20 mg/dL. Recent descriptions of bilirubin encephalopathy in breastfed infants (in particular late preterm infants) with dehydration and hyperbilirubinemia in whom an adequate supply of breast milk has not been established mandates close follow-up of all breastfeeding mothers.[59] The true risk for nonhemolytic hyperbilirubinemia to produce brain damage in the preterm in the current era of liberal use of phototherapy that prevents marked elevation of severe bilirubin in these infants is unknown. However, most currently available data would suggest this risk is low.

NEONATAL HEMATOLOGY

Anemia

Early hematopoietic cells originate in the yolk sac. By 8 weeks' gestation, erythropoiesis is taking place in the liver, which remains the primary site of erythroid production through the early fetal period. By 6 months of gestation, the bone marrow becomes the principal site of red cell development. Normal hemoglobin levels at term range from 13.7 to 20.1 g/dL. In the very preterm infant, values as low as 12 g/dL are acceptable. Anemia at birth or appearing in the first few weeks of life is the result of blood loss, hemolysis, or underproduction of erythrocytes.[60] Blood loss resulting in anemia can occur prenatally, at the time of delivery, or postnatally. In utero blood loss can be the result of fetomaternal bleeding, twin-to-twin transfusion, or

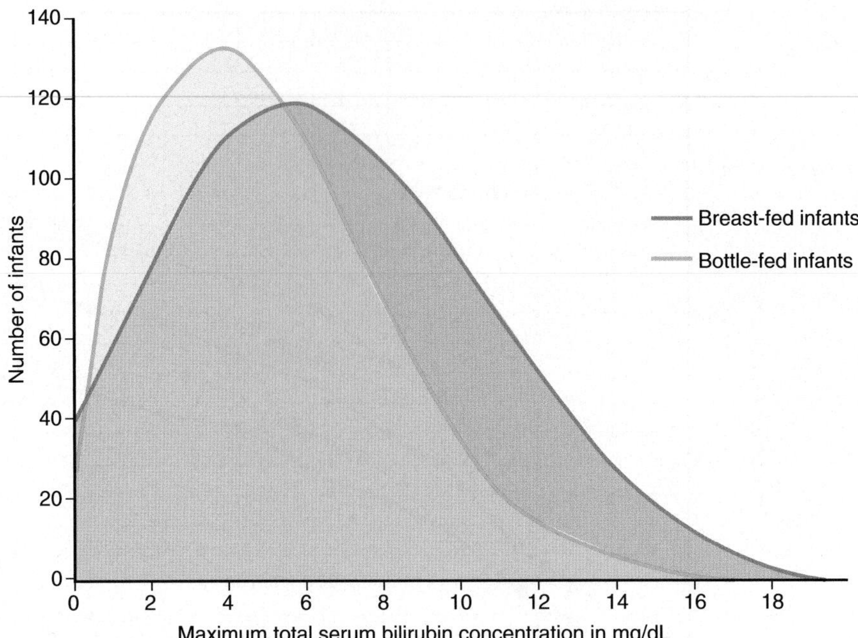

FIGURE 21-16. Distribution of maximum serum bilirubin concentrations in white infants who weigh more than 2500 g. (Modified from Maisels MJ, Gifford KL: Normal serum bilirubin levels in the newborn and the effect of breast-feeding. Pediatrics 78:837, 1986.)

blood loss resulting from trauma (maternal trauma, amniocentesis, external cephalic version). **The diagnosis of fetomaternal hemorrhage large enough to cause anemia can be made using flow cytometry or the Kleihauer-Betke technique of acid elution to identify fetal cells in the maternal circulation.** Blood loss at delivery can be caused by umbilical cord rupture, incision of the placenta during cesarean delivery, placenta previa, or abruptio placentae. Internal hemorrhage can occur in the newborn, often related to a difficult delivery. Sites include intracranial, cephalohematomas, subgaleal, retroperitoneal, liver capsule, and ruptured spleen. When blood loss has been chronic (e.g., fetomaternal), infants will be pale at birth, but well compensated and without signs of volume loss. The initial hematocrit will be low. Acute bleeding will present with signs of hypovolemia (tachycardia, poor perfusion, hypotension). The initial hematocrit can be normal or decreased, but after several hours of equilibration, it will be decreased. Anemia caused by hemolysis from blood group incompatibilities is common in the newborn period. Less common causes of hemolysis include erythrocyte membrane abnormalities, enzyme deficiencies, and disorders of hemoglobin synthesis. Impaired erythrocyte production is a rare cause of neonatal anemia.

Polycythemia

Elevated hematocrits occur in 1.5% to 4% of live births. Although 50% of polycythemic infants are appropriate for gestational age (AGA), the proportion of polycythemic infants is greater in the SGA and LGA populations. Causes of polycythemia include twin-to-twin transfusion, maternal-to-fetal transfusion, intrapartum transfusion from the placenta associated with fetal distress, chronic intrauterine hypoxia (SGA infants, LGA infants of diabetic mothers), delayed cord clamping, and chromosomal abnormalities. The consequence of polycythemia is hyperviscosity, resulting in impaired perfusion of capillary beds. Therefore, clinical symptoms can be related to any organ system (Table 21-10). Hyperviscosity is inferred from hematocrit because the major factor influencing viscosity in the newborn is red cell mass. Cord blood hematocrit greater than or equal to 57% and capillary hematocrit of at least 70% are indicative of polycythemia. Confirmation of the diagnosis is a peripheral venous hematocrit of at least 64%. Reduction of venous hematocrit to less than 60% may improve acute symptoms, but it has not been shown to improve long-term neurologic outcome.[61]

TABLE 21-10 ORGAN-RELATED SYMPTOMS OF HYPERVISCOSITY

Central nervous system	Irritability, jitteriness, seizures, lethargy
Cardiopulmonary	Respiratory distress caused by congestive heart failure or persistent pulmonary hypertension
Gastrointestinal	Vomiting, heme-positive stools, abdominal distention, necrotizing enterocolitis
Renal	Decreased urine output, renal vein thrombosis
Metabolic	Hypoglycemia
Hematologic	Hyperbilirubinemia, thrombocytopenia

Thrombocytopenia

Neonatal thrombocytopenia can be isolated or occur associated with deficiency of clotting factors. A differential diagnosis is presented in Table 21-11. The immune thrombocytopenias have implications for perinatal care. In idiopathic thrombocytopenic purpura (ITP), maternal antiplatelet antibodies that cross the placenta lead to destruction of fetal platelets. However, only 10% to 15% of infants born to mothers with ITP have platelet counts less than 100,000 and even in infants with severe thrombocytopenia, serious bleeding is rare. Alloimmune thrombocytopenia occurs when an antigen is present on fetal platelets but is not present on maternal platelets. On exposure to fetal platelets, the mother develops antiplatelet antibodies that cross the placenta causing destruction of fetal platelets. In the largest series of cases of suspected alloimmune thrombocytopenia, the majority were caused by HPA-1a alloantibodies. Because the maternal platelet count is normal, the diagnosis is suspected on the basis of a history of a previously affected pregnancy. Intracranial hemorrhage is common with this condition (10% to 20%) and can occur in the antenatal or intrapartum periods.[62] Antenatal treatment is guided by the severity of thrombocytopenia and presence of intracranial hemorrhage in the previously affected fetus. Treatment options include intravenous immunoglobulin infusions and corticosteroids given to the mother.[62]

Vitamin K Deficiency Bleeding of the Newborn

Vitamin K_1 oxide (1 mg) should be given intramuscularly to all newborns to prevent hemorrhagic disease caused by a deficiency in vitamin K–dependent clotting factors (II, VII, IX, X).[63] Babies born to mothers who are on anticonvulsant medication are particularly at risk of having vitamin K deficiency. Bleeding occurs in 0.25% to 1.4% of newborns who do not receive vitamin K prophylaxis, generally in the first 5 days to 2 weeks but as late as 12 weeks. Oral vitamin K has been shown to be effective in raising vitamin K levels, but is not as effective in preventing late hemorrhagic disease of the newborn. Late hemorrhagic disease of the newborn most commonly occurs in breastfed infants whose courses have been complicated by diarrhea.

TABLE 21-11 DIFFERENTIAL DIAGNOSIS OF NEONATAL THROMBOCYTOPENIA

DIAGNOSIS	COMMENTS
Immune	Passively acquired antibody (e.g., idiopathic thrombocytopenic purpura, systemic lupus erythematosus, drug induced) Alloimmune sensitization to HPA-1a antigen
Infections	Bacterial; congenital viral infections (e.g., cytomegalovirus, rubella)
Syndromes	Absent radii; Fanconi's anemia
Giant hemangioma	
Thrombosis	
High-risk infant with respiratory distress syndrome, pulmonary hypertension, and so forth	Disseminated intravascular coagulation Isolated thrombocytopenia

HPA-1a, Human platelet antigen-1a.

PERINATAL INFECTION

Early-Onset Bacterial Infection

The unique predisposition of the neonate to bacterial infection is related to defects in both innate and acquired immune responses.[64] The incidence of bacterial infection in infants younger than 5 days of age is 1 to 2 per 1000 live births. **Maternal colonization with group B streptococcus (GBS), rupture of membranes for more than 12 to 18 hours, and the presence of chorioamnionitis increase the risk of infection.**[65,66] Maternal fever from other etiologies (e.g., epidural anesthesia) does not increase the risk of neonatal infection and merits only close observation of the newborn. Irrespective of membrane rupture, infection rates are higher in preterm infants. The majority of early-onset bacterial infection presents on day 1 of life, with respiratory distress the most common presenting symptom. These infections are most often caused by GBS and gram-negative enteric pathogens. The algorithm for prevention of early-onset GBS infections is presented in Figure 21-17, with the approach to the newborn shown in Figure 21-18. Other etiologies of infection in the newborn are covered in Chapters 49-51.

RESPIRATORY DISTRESS

The establishment of respiratory function at birth is dependent on expansion and maintenance of air sacs, clearance of lung fluid, and adequate pulmonary perfusion. In many

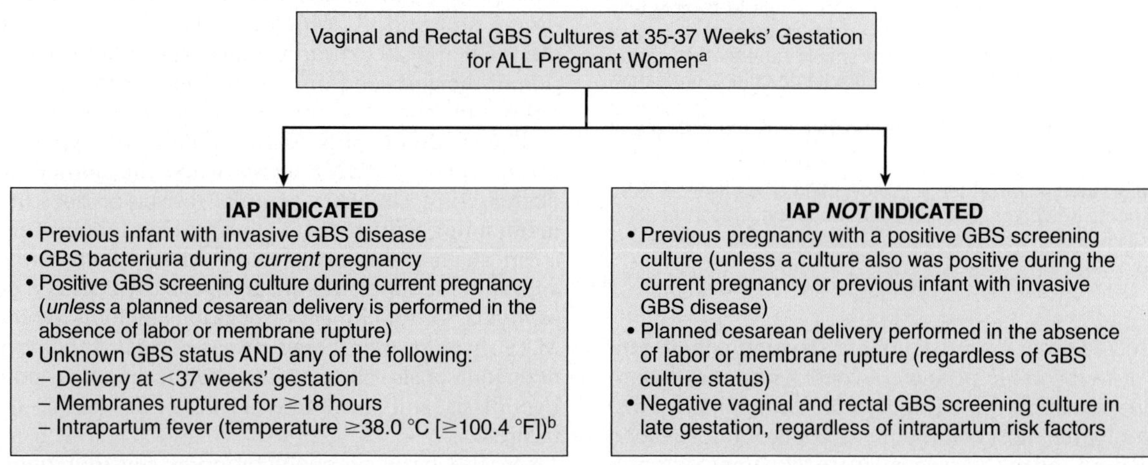

FIGURE 21-17. Indications for intrapartum antimicrobial prophylaxis to prevent early onset GBS disease using a universal prenatal culture screening strategy at 35 to 37 weeks' gestation for all pregnant women. *GBS*, Group B streptococcus; *IAP*, intrapartum anitmicribial prophylaxis. (Reproduced from the American Academy of Pediatrics: RedBook 2003 Report of the Committee on Infectious Disease, 2009.)

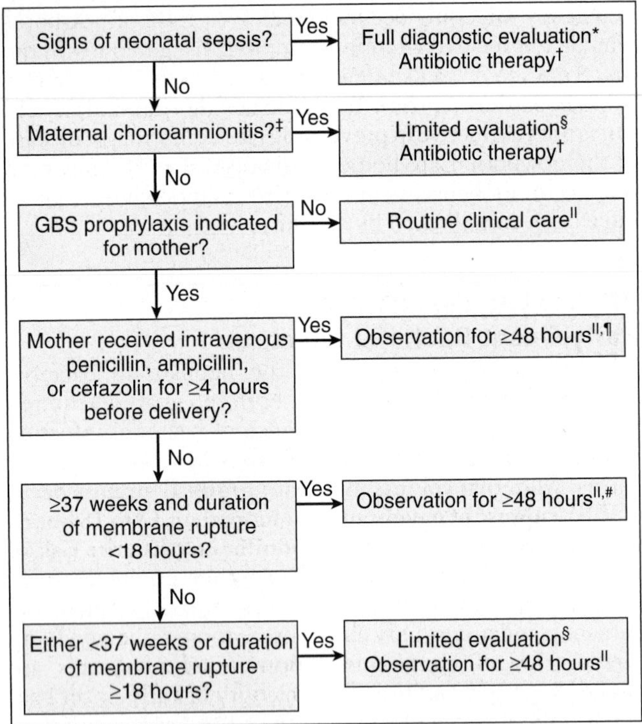

* Full diagnostic evaluation includes a blood culture, a complete blood count (CBC) including white blood cell differential and platelet counts, chest radiograph (if respiratory abnormalities are present), and lumbar puncture (if patient is stable enough to tolerate procedure and sepsis is suspected).

† Antibiotic therapy should be directed toward the most common cause of neonatal sepsis, including intravenous ampicillin for GBS and coverage for other organisms (including *Escherichia coli* and other gram-negative pathogens) and should take into account local antibiotic resistance patterns.

‡ Consultation with obstetric providers is important to determine the level of clinical suspicionn for chorioamnionitis. Chorioamnionitis is diagnosed clinically and some of the signs are nonspecific.

§ Limited evaluation includes blood culture (at birth) and CBC with differential and platelets (at birth and/or at 6–12 hours of life).

|| If signs of sepsis develop, a full diagnostic evaluation should be conducted and antibiotic therapy initiated.

¶ If ≥37 weeks'gestation, observation may occur at home after 24 hours if other discharge criteria have been met, access to medical care is readily available, and a person who is able to comply fully with instructions for home observation with be present. If any of these conditions is not met, the infant should be observed in the hospital for at least 48 hours and until discharge criteria are achieved.

\# Some experts recommend a CBC with differential and platelets at age 6–12 hours.

FIGURE 21-18. Algorithm for secondary prevention of early-onset GBS disease among newborns. (Reproduced from the Department of Health and Human Services Centers for Disease Control and Prevention. MMWR 59:RR-10, 2010.)

premature and other high-risk infants, developmental deficiencies or unfavorable perinatal events hamper a smooth respiratory transition. The presentation of respiratory distress is among the most common symptom complexes seen in the newborn and may be secondary to both noncardiopulmonary and cardiopulmonary etiologies (Table 21-12). The symptom complex includes an elevation of the respiratory rate to greater than 60 bpm with or without cyanosis, nasal flaring, intercostal and sternal retractions, and expiratory grunting. The retractions are the result of the neonate's efforts to expand a lung with poor compliance using a very compliant chest wall. The expiratory grunt is caused by closure of the glottis during expiration in an effort to increase expiratory pressure to help maintain functional residual capacity. The evaluation of such an infant requires use of history, physical examination, and laboratory data to arrive at a diagnosis. It is important to consider causes other than those related to the heart and lungs, because one's natural tendency is to focus immediately on the more common cardiopulmonary etiologies.

Cardiovascular Causes

Cardiovascular causes of respiratory distress in the neonatal period can be divided into two major groups—those with structural heart disease and those with persistent right-to-left shunting through fetal pathways and a structurally normal heart. **The two presentations of serious structural heart disease in the first week of life are cyanosis and congestive heart failure.**[67] Examples of cyanotic heart disease include transposition of the great vessels, tricuspid atresia, certain types of truncus arteriosus, total anomalous pulmonary venous return, and right-sided outflow obstruction including tetralogy of Fallot and pulmonary stenosis or atresia. Although cyanosis is the central feature in these disorders, tachypnea develops in many infants because of increased pulmonary blood flow or secondary to metabolic acidosis from hypoxia. Infants with congestive heart failure generally have some form of left-sided outflow obstruction (e.g., hypoplastic left heart syndrome, coarctation of the aorta). Left-to-right shunt lesions such as ventricular septal defect do not present with increased pulmonary blood flow and congestive heart failure until pulmonary vascular resistance is low enough to permit a significant shunt (usually 3 to 4 weeks of age at sea level). Infants with left-sided outflow obstruction generally do well the first day or so until the source of systemic flow, the ductus arteriosus, narrows. With ductal narrowing, dyspnea, tachypnea, and tachycardia develop, followed by rapid progression to congestive heart failure and metabolic acidosis. On examination, these infants have pulse abnormalities. With hypoplastic left heart syndrome and critical aortic stenosis, pulses are profoundly diminished in all extremities, whereas infants with coarctation of the aorta and interrupted aortic arch have differential pulses when the arms and legs are compared.

The syndrome of persistent pulmonary hypertension of the newborn (PPHN) occurs when the normal postnatal decrease in pulmonary vascular resistance does not occur, maintaining right-to-left shunting across the patent ductus arteriosus and foramen ovale.[19] Most infants with PPHN are full term or postmature and have experienced perinatal asphyxia. Other clinical associations include hypothermia, MAS, hyaline membrane disease (HMD), polycythemia, neonatal sepsis, chronic intrauterine hypoxia, pulmonary hypoplasia, and premature closure of the ductus arteriosus in utero.

On the basis of developmental considerations, these infants can be separated into three groups: (1) acute vasoconstriction caused by perinatal hypoxia, (2) prenatal increase in pulmonary vascular smooth muscle development, and (3) decreased cross-sectional area of the pulmonary vascular bed caused by inadequate vessel number. In

TABLE 21-12 RESPIRATORY DISTRESS IN THE NEWBORN

NONCARDIOPULMONARY	CARDIOVASCULAR	PULMONARY
Hypothermia or hyperthermia	Left-sided outflow obstruction	Upper airway obstruction
Hypoglycemia	Hypoplastic left heart	Choanal atresia
Metabolic acidosis	Aortic stenosis	Vocal cord paralysis
Drug intoxications; withdrawal	Coarctation of the aorta	Meconium aspiration
Polycythemia	Cyanotic lesions	Clear fluid aspiration
Central nervous system insult	Transposition of the great vessels	Transient tachypnea
Asphyxia	Total anomalous pulmonary venous return	Pneumonia
Hemorrhage	Tricuspid atresia	Pulmonary hypoplasia
Neuromuscular disease	Right-sided outflow obstruction	Primary
Werdnig-Hoffman disease		Secondary
Myopathies		Hyaline membrane disease
Phrenic nerve injury		Pneumothorax
Skeletal abnormalities		Pleural effusions
Asphyxiating thoracic dystrophy		Mass lesions
		Lobar emphysema
		Cystic adenomatoid malformation

the first group, an acute perinatal event leads to hypoxia and failure of pulmonary vascular resistance to drop. In the second, abnormal muscularization of the pulmonary resistance vessels results in PPHN after birth. The third circumstance includes infants with pulmonary hypoplasia (e.g., diaphragmatic hernia). Clinically, the syndrome is characterized by cyanosis, often unresponsive to increases in FIO_2, respiratory distress, an onset at less than 24 hours, evidence of right ventricular overload, systemic hypotension, acidosis, and no evidence of structural heart disease. There have been considerable advances in treatment for this condition using high-frequency ventilation, inhaled nitric oxide, and in refractory cases, extracorporeal membrane oxygenation.[19]

Pulmonary Causes

Of the causes of respiratory distress related to the airways and pulmonary parenchyma listed in Table 21-12, **the differential diagnosis in a term infant includes transient tachypnea, aspiration syndromes, congenital pneumonia, and spontaneous pneumothorax.** The syndrome of transient tachypnea presents as respiratory distress in nonasphyxiated term infants or slightly preterm infants. The clinical features include various combinations of cyanosis, grunting, nasal flaring, retracting, and tachypnea during the first hours after birth. The chest radiograph is the key to the diagnosis, with prominent perihilar streaking and fluid in the interlobar fissures. The symptoms generally subside in 12 to 24 hours, although they can persist longer. The preferred explanation for the clinical features is delayed reabsorption of fetal lung fluid. Transient tachypnea is seen more commonly in infants delivered by elective cesarean section or in the slightly preterm infant (see Mechanics of the First Breath, earlier).

At delivery, the neonate may aspirate clear amniotic fluid or fluid mixed with blood or meconium. Whether infants can aspirate a sufficient volume of clear fluid to cause symptoms is controversial. However, there are a group of infants whose clinical course is more prolonged (4 to 7 days) and severe than that of infants with transient tachypnea. These infants have a radiologic picture similar to transient tachypnea often associated with more marked hyperexpansion. Occasionally, the infiltrates are impressive, with evidence of far more fluid than is seen with transient tachypnea. MAS occurs in full-term or postmature infants. The perinatal course is often complicated by chronic intrauterine hypoxia, fetal distress, and low Apgar scores. These infants exhibit tachypnea, retractions, cyanosis, overdistended and barrel-shaped chest, and coarse breath sounds. Chest radiography reveals coarse, irregular pulmonary densities with areas of diminished aeration or consolidation. There is a high incidence of air leaks, and many of the infants exhibit persistent pulmonary hypertension.

The lungs represent the most common primary site of infection in the neonate. Both bacterial and viral infections can be acquired before, during, or after birth. The most common route of infection, particularly for bacteria, is ascending from the genital tract before or during labor. Infants with congenital pneumonia present with respiratory distress very early in life. The chest radiograph pattern is often indistinguishable from other causes of respiratory distress, particularly HMD.

Spontaneous pneumothorax occurs in 1% of all deliveries, but a much lower percentage results in symptoms. The risk is increased by manipulations such as positive-pressure ventilation. Respiratory distress is usually present from shortly after birth, and breath sounds may be diminished on the affected side. The majority of these air leaks resolve spontaneously without specific therapy.

HMD remains the most common etiology for respiratory distress in the neonatal period. It was the initial reports of Avery and Mead[68] demonstrating a high surface tension in extracts of lungs from infants dying of RDS that led to the present understanding of the role of surfactant in the pathogenesis of HMD. The deficiency of surfactant in the premature infant increases alveolar surface tension and, according to LaPlace's law (see Figure 21-2), increases the pressure necessary to maintain patent alveoli. The end result is poor lung compliance, progressive atelectasis, loss of FRC, alterations in ventilation-perfusion mismatch, and uneven distribution of ventilation. HMD is further complicated by the weak respiratory muscles and compliant chest wall of the premature infant. Hypoxemia and respiratory and metabolic acidemia contribute to increased pulmonary vascular resistance, right-to-left ductal shunting, and

TABLE 21-13 CUMULATIVE RESULTS OF PLACEBO-CONTROLLED SURFACTANT TRIALS*

	MODIFIED NATURAL† (%)		SYNTHETIC‡ (%)	
	Surfactant	**Control**	**Surfactant**	**Control**
Mortality	15	24	11	18
Patent ductus arteriosus	46	43	44	48
Severe ICH	19	19	7	8
Chronic lung disease	37	37	11	11

*Higher incidences of intracranial hemorrhage (ICH) and chronic lung disease in modified natural surfactant studies reflects the lower gestational age on average in both groups in these studies compared to the artificial surfactant studies.
†Studies with Survanta, Curosurf, and Infasurf; 2000 patients.
‡Studies with Exosurf; 4400 patients.

worsening ventilation-perfusion mismatch that exacerbate hypoxemia. Hypoxemia and hypoperfusion result in alveolar epithelial damage, with increased capillary permeability and leakage of plasma into alveolar spaces. Leakage of protein into airspaces serves to inhibit surfactant function, exacerbating the disease process. The materials in plasma and cellular debris combine to form the characteristic hyaline membrane seen pathologically. The recovery phase is characterized by regeneration of alveolar cells, including type II cells, with an increase in surfactant activity.

Clinically, neonates with HMD demonstrate tachypnea, nasal flaring, subcostal and intercostal retractions, cyanosis, and expiratory grunting. As the infant begins to tire with progressive disease, apneic episodes occur. If some intervention is not undertaken at this point, death ensues. The radiologic appearance of the lungs is consistent with an extensive atelectatic process. The infiltrate is diffuse, with a ground-glass appearance. Major airways are air filled and contrast with the atelectatic alveoli, creating the appearance of air bronchograms. The diaphragms are elevated because of profound hypoexpansion. Acute complications of HMD include infection, air leaks, and persistent patency of the ductus arteriosus.

Of more concern than acute complications are the long-term sequelae suffered by infants with HMD. The major long-term consequences are chronic lung disease (CLD) requiring prolonged ventilator and oxygen therapy, and significant neurologic impairment. In 1967, Northway et al.[69] first described the syndrome of bronchopulmonary dysplasia (BPD) in infants surviving severe HMD requiring mechanical ventilation. Today, many infants who develop CLD are extremely-low-birthweight infants who require prolonged ventilation for apnea and poor respiratory effort who initially did not have severe HMD. This is termed "new BPD" and the name differentiates this entity from that originally described by Northway, also called "old BPD." New BPD is characterized by a more uniform appearance with milder regions of injury compared to the old BPD. However, there are more prominent signs of impaired or arrested alveolarization and vascular growth, often described as alveolar simplification.[2,70] The incidence is especially high in infants born at less than 800 g. The severity is variable, ranging from very mild pulmonary insufficiency to severe disease with prolonged mechanical ventilation, frequent readmissions for respiratory exacerbations after nursery discharge, and a higher incidence of neurodevelopmental sequelae compared with very-low-birthweight controls. Although pulmonary function improves over time and most children do well, long-term pulmonary sequelae are evident. **Factors involved in the etiology of CLD are gestational age, elevated inspired oxygen concentration, ventilator volutrauma, severity of underlying disease, inflammation, and infection.**

Treatment for HMD involves supplemental oxygen, early use of nasal CPAP to maintain FRC, mechanical ventilation, and surfactant replacement therapy.[9] Modified natural surfactant, which is extracted by alveolar lavage or from lung tissue (usually bovine) and then modified by selective addition or removal of components, and true artificial surfactant, which is a mixture of synthetic compounds that may or may not be components of natural surfactant, have been used extensively. These agents (administered intratracheally) have shown efficacy in decreasing the severity of acute HMD and the frequency of air leak complications. Efficacy has been demonstrated when used in the delivery room to "prevent" or when used as a rescue treatment for established HMD. Although surfactant replacement therapy has decreased mortality and acute pulmonary morbidity, this therapy has not affected the frequency of other complications of prematurity (Table 21-13). Of note is that, despite resulting in lower ventilator settings and Fio_2 concentration over the first several days of life, the incidence of CLD has not been changed. However, the severity of long-term pulmonary complications is less. Long-term neurodevelopment follow-ups show rates of handicap similar to placebo-treated infants.

NEONATAL NEUROLOGY

Intraventricular Hemorrhage and Periventricular Leukomalacia

Periventricular/intraventricular hemorrhage (PVH/IVH) and periventricular leukomalacia (PVL) are the most common neurologic complications of prematurity. The overall incidence of PVH/IVH is 20% to 30% in infants weighing less than 1500 g or at less than 31 weeks' gestation with severe bleeds (grades 3 and 4) at 10%. The highest incidence is seen in babies of the lowest gestational age and birthweight; nearly 50% and 25%, respectively, for all IVH and severe bleeds for babies born at less than 700 g.[71] Bleeds are graded according to severity as indicated in Table 21-14. Diagnosis is confirmed with ultrasound. PVL is reported in about 2% to 4% of infants younger than 32 weeks' gestation,[71] but the cystic PVL reported likely underestimates the full spectrum of PVL (see later).

Bleeding originates in the subependymal germinal matrix located ventrolateral to the lateral ventricles in the caudothalamic groove. The germinal matrix is made up of a meshwork of thin-walled vessels in the process of remodeling into a capillary network and a mass of undifferentiated cells that are destined to become cortical neurons, astrocytes, and oligodendroglia. Rupture of a germinal matrix hemorrhage into the ventricular system leads to intraventricular hemorrhage. A proposed pathogenesis derived from a review of available information is presented in Figure 21-19. The critical predisposing event is likely an ischemia-reperfusion injury to the vessels in the germinal matrix, which is a low blood flow region prone to ischemia. Furthermore, IVH is most reliably produced by a sequence of hemorrhagic hypotension followed by hypertension.[72] The amount of bleeding is then influenced by a variety of factors that affect the pressure gradient across the injured capillary wall. Likewise, for babies who manifest parenchymal bleeding (grade 4) and PVL, the inciting event is likely ischemia with reperfusion injury. The periventricular white matter is a border zone for cerebral blood flow in the preterm infant and is vulnerable to ischemic injury. Although cystic PVL (multifocal areas of necrosis with cyst formation in deep periventricular white matter) has been well characterized by ultrasound, the expanded use of MRI scans in preterm infants has identified infants (especially among those of lower gestational age) with diffuse white matter injury often accompanied by ventricular dilation at term.

TABLE 21-14 CLASSIFICATION OF INTRAVENTRICULAR HEMORRHAGE

GRADE	DEFINITION
I	Subependymal hemorrhage
II	Intraventricular hemorrhage without ventricular dilatation
III	Intraventricular hemorrhage with ventricular dilatation
IV	Intraventricular hemorrhage with associated parenchymal hemorrhage

Modified from Papile LA, Burstein J, Burstein R, Koffler H: Incidence and evolution of subependymal and intraventricular hemorrhage: a study of infants with birth weights less than 1500 g. J Pediatr 92:529, 1978.

These findings are far more common in the preterm population than cystic PVL and represent part of the spectrum of PVL. The other important clinical correlate of PVL is maternal chorioamnionitis and neonatal infection. Infection and ischemia are additive in the pathogenesis of PVL with the critical injury to preoligodendrocytes caused by reactive oxygen and nitrogen species.

There is also emerging evidence that secondary maturational and trophic disturbances also contribute to the evolution of this brain injury in the premature.[73]

The neurodevelopmental outcome of infants with IVH is related to the severity of the original bleed, development of posthemorrhagic hydrocephalus, and the degree of associated parenchymal injury. Although cranial ultrasound is the primary modality used to diagnose IVH and PVL, it is not a sensitive predictor of outcome. In extremely low-birthweight infants with no abnormalities on cranial ultrasound, nearly one third will have some degree of neurodevelopmental handicap (cerebral palsy or cognitive delays).[74] Infants with grade I or II IVH are at slightly greater risk for handicap.[75] School-aged children who had mild IVH display a variety of neurologic and cognitive abnormalities, including motor incoordination, hyperactivity, attention and learning deficits, and visual motor difficulties.[76] Infants with progressive ventricular dilatation (grade III) or periventricular hemorrhagic infarction (grade IV) are at higher risk for major neurodevelopmental handicap as well as less severe neurologic and cognitive disabilities.[77] The presence of severe cystic PVL carries a guarded prognosis with a high risk of cerebral palsy and associated cognitive deficit.

Although the incidence and severity of intracranial hemorrhage have progressively decreased as a result of advances in both obstetric and neonatal care, the therapeutic focus continues to be on strategies to prevent this complication of prematurity. Both antenatal and postnatal approaches have been developed. For the most part, postnatal pharmacologic strategies have not had a major effect in decreasing the incidence, severity, and neurodevelopmental

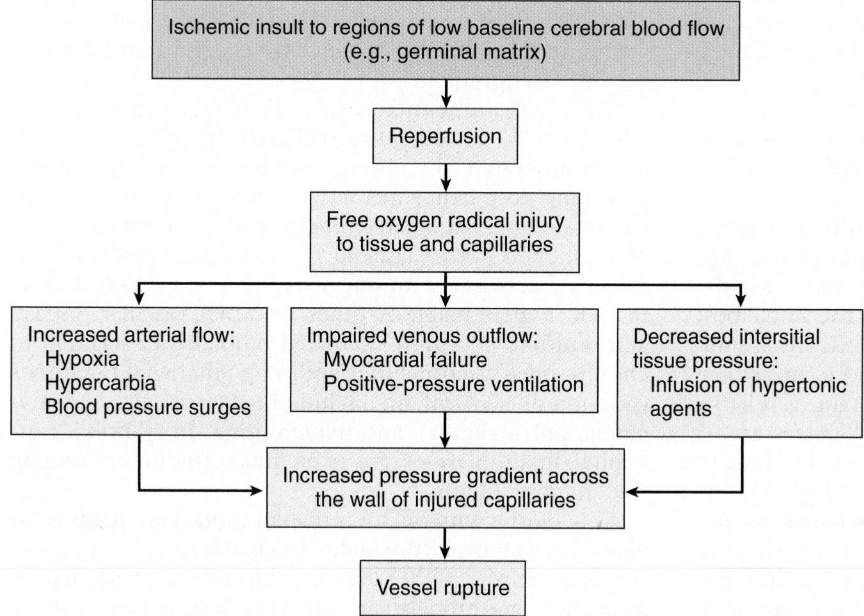

FIGURE 21-19. Pathogenesis of periventricular/intraventricular hemorrhage in the preterm infant.

outcomes of IVH. Because IVH and PVL are likely perinatal events, antenatal prevention holds the most promise. Both vitamin K and phenobarbital have been administered in this way. Antenatal phenobarbital resulted in a decrease in both frequency and severity of IVH. The proposed mechanism of action is thought to be scavenging of oxygen free radicals, although phenobarbital does decrease both brain blood flow and cerebral metabolic rate. However, two large randomized prospective studies failed to confirm the positive effects of phenobarbital shown in previous smaller studies.[78,79] One reason for the discrepancy is likely due to the widespread use of antenatal corticosteroids in the more recent studies. **Antenatal corticosteroids, although not used specifically to decrease the incidence of IVH and PVL, decrease the frequency of these complications and likely represent the most important antenatal strategy to prevent intracranial hemorrhage.**[5] Phenobarbital may still have a role in the mother who has not been "prepared" with betamethasone and is delivering at under 28 weeks' gestation.

Seizures

Newborns rarely have well-organized tonic-clonic seizures because of incomplete cortical organization and a preponderance of inhibitory synapses. Newborn seizures can be classified into four subtypes. The first is the subtle seizure characterized by ocular phenomena, oral-buccal-lingual movements, peculiar limb movements (e.g., bicycling movements), autonomic alterations, and apnea. Clonic seizures are characterized by rhythmic (one to three jerks per second) movements that can be focal or multifocal. The third seizure type is focal or generalized tonic seizures marked by extensor posturing. The fourth seizure type is myoclonic activity that is distinguished from clonic seizures by the more rapid speed of the myoclonic jerk and the predilection for flexor muscle groups. The differential diagnosis of neonatal seizures is presented in Table 21-15. The most frequent cause of neonatal seizures is hypoxic ischemic encephalopathy, with the second leading cause being intracranial hemorrhage. The prognosis for neonatal seizures depends on the cause. Difficult-to-control seizure activity, caused by hypoxic ischemic encephalopathy and hypoglycemic seizures in particular, have a high incidence of long-term sequelae.

TABLE 21-15 DIFFERENTIAL DIAGNOSIS OF NEONATAL SEIZURES

DIAGNOSIS	COMMENTS
Hypoxic-ischemic encephalopathy	Most common etiology (60%, onset first 24 hours)
Intracranial hemorrhage	≤15% of cases; PVH/IVH, subdural or subarachnoid bleeds, stroke
Infection	12% of cases
Hypoglycemia	SGA, IDM
Hypocalcemia, hypomagnesemia	Low-birthweight infant, IDM
Hyponatremia	Rare, seen with syndrome of inappropriate secretion of antidiuretic hormone (SIADH)
Disorders of amino and organic acid metabolism, hyperammonemia	Associated acidosis, altered level of consciousness
Pyridoxine deficiency	Seizures refractory to routine therapy; cessation of seizures after administration of pyridoxine
Developmental defects	Other anomalies, chromosomal syndromes
Drug withdrawal	
Benign familial neonatal seizures	
No cause found	10% of cases

IDM, Infant of diabetic mother.

CLASSIFICATION OF NEWBORNS BY GROWTH AND GESTATIONAL AGE

In assessing the risk for mortality or morbidity in a given neonate, evaluation of birthweight and gestational age together provide the clearest picture. When large populations are considered, maternal dates remain the single best determinant of gestational age. Early obstetric ultrasound is a very useful adjunct. However, in the individual neonate, especially when dates are uncertain, a reliable postnatal assessment of gestational age is necessary. A scoring system appraising gestational age on the basis of physical and neurologic criteria was developed by Dubowitz et al. and later simplified and updated by Ballard et al.[80] (Figure 21-20). The Ballard examination is less accurate before 28 weeks' gestation, but additional features can be examined to aid in the determination of an accurate gestational age. The anterior vascular capsule of the lens reveals complete coverage of the lens by vessels at 27 to 28 weeks. Foot length (from the heel to the tip of the largest toe) is 4.5 cm at 25 weeks and increases by 0.25 cm/wk. Infants can then be classified, using growth parameters and gestational age, by means of intrauterine growth curves such as those developed by Lubchenco et al.[81] (Figure 21-21). Infants born between 37 and 42 weeks are classified as term; less than 37 weeks, preterm; and greater than 42 weeks, postterm. In each grouping, infants are then identified according to growth as AGA if birthweight falls between the 10th and 90th percentiles, SGA if birthweight is below the 10th percentile, and LGA if birthweight is above the 90th percentile. Knowledge of a baby's birthweight in relation to gestational age is helpful in anticipating neonatal problems.

There are numerous causes of growth restriction (see Chapter 31). Those operative early in pregnancy such as chromosomal aberrations, congenital viral infections, and some drug exposures induce symmetric restriction of weight, length, and head circumference. In most cases, the phenomenon occurs later in gestation and leads to more selective restriction of birthweight alone. Such factors include hypertension or other maternal vascular disease and multiple gestation. Neonatal problems in addition to chromosomal abnormalities and congenital viral infections common in SGA infants include birth asphyxia, hypoglycemia, polycythemia, and hypothermia. In addition, congenital malformations are seen more frequently among undergrown infants.[82]

The most common identifiable conditions leading to excessive infant birthweight are maternal diabetes and maternal obesity. Other conditions associated with macrosomia are erythroblastosis fetalis, other causes of fetal

Neuromuscular Maturity

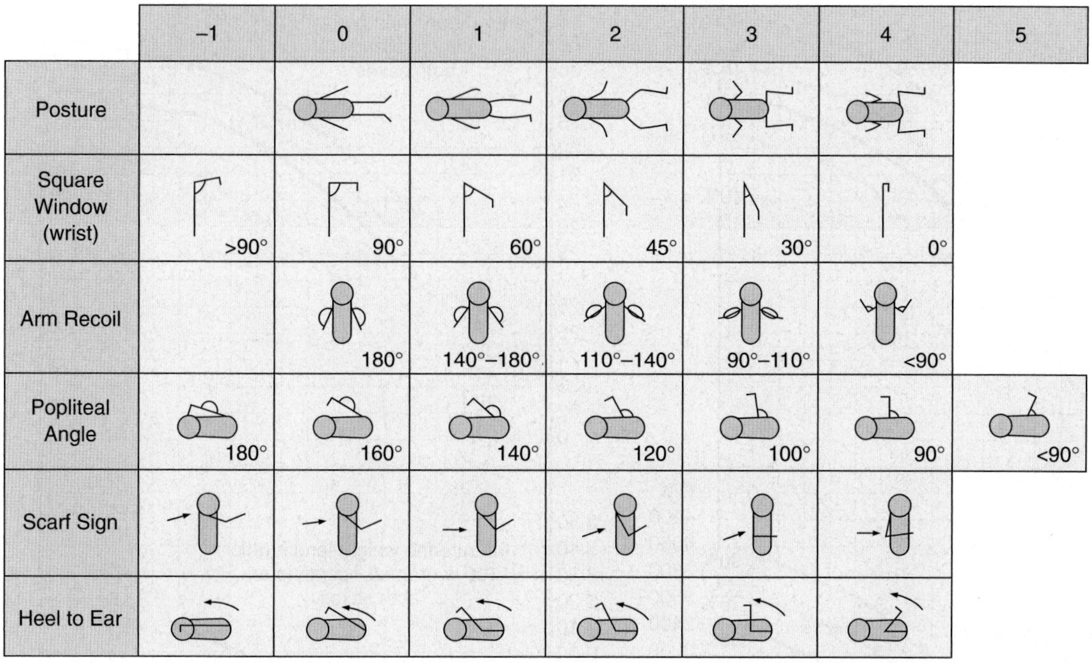

	−1	0	1	2	3	4	5
Posture							
Square Window (wrist)	>90°	90°	60°	45°	30°	0°	
Arm Recoil		180°	140°–180°	110°–140°	90°–110°	<90°	
Popliteal Angle	180°	160°	140°	120°	100°	90°	<90°
Scarf Sign							
Heel to Ear							

Physical Maturity

Skin	sticky friable transparent	gelatinous red, translucent	smooth pink, visible veins	superficial peeling &/or rash, few veins	cracking pale areas rare veins	parchment deep cracking no vessels	leathery cracked wrinkled
Lanugo	none	sparse	abundant	thinning	bald areas	mostly bald	
Plantar Surface	heel-toe 40–50 mm: −1 <40 mm: −2	>50 mm no crease	faint red marks	anterior transverse crease only	creases ant. 2/3	creases over entire sole	
Breast	imperceptible	barely perceptible	flat areola no bud	stippled areola 1-2 mm bud	raised areola 3-4 mm bud	full areola 5-10 mm bud	
Eye/Ear	lids fused loosely: −1 tightly: −2	lids open pinna flat stays folded	sl. curved pinna; soft; slow recoil	well-curved pinna; soft but ready recoil	formed & firm instant recoil	thick cartilage ear stiff	
Genitals male	scrotum flat, smooth	scrotum empty faint rugae	testes in upper canal rare rugae	testes descending few rugae	testes down good rugae	testes pendulous deep rugae	
Genitals female	clitoris prominent labia flat	prominent clitoris small labia minora	prominent clitoris enlarging minora	majora & minora equally prominent	majora large minora small	majora cover clitoris & minora	

Maturity Rating

score	weeks
−10	20
−5	22
0	24
5	26
10	28
15	30
20	32
25	34
30	36
35	38
40	40
45	42
50	44

FIGURE 21-20. Assessment of gestational age. (From Ballard JL, Khoury JC, Wedig K, et al: New Ballard Score, expanded to include extremely premature infants. J Pediatr 119:417, 1991.)

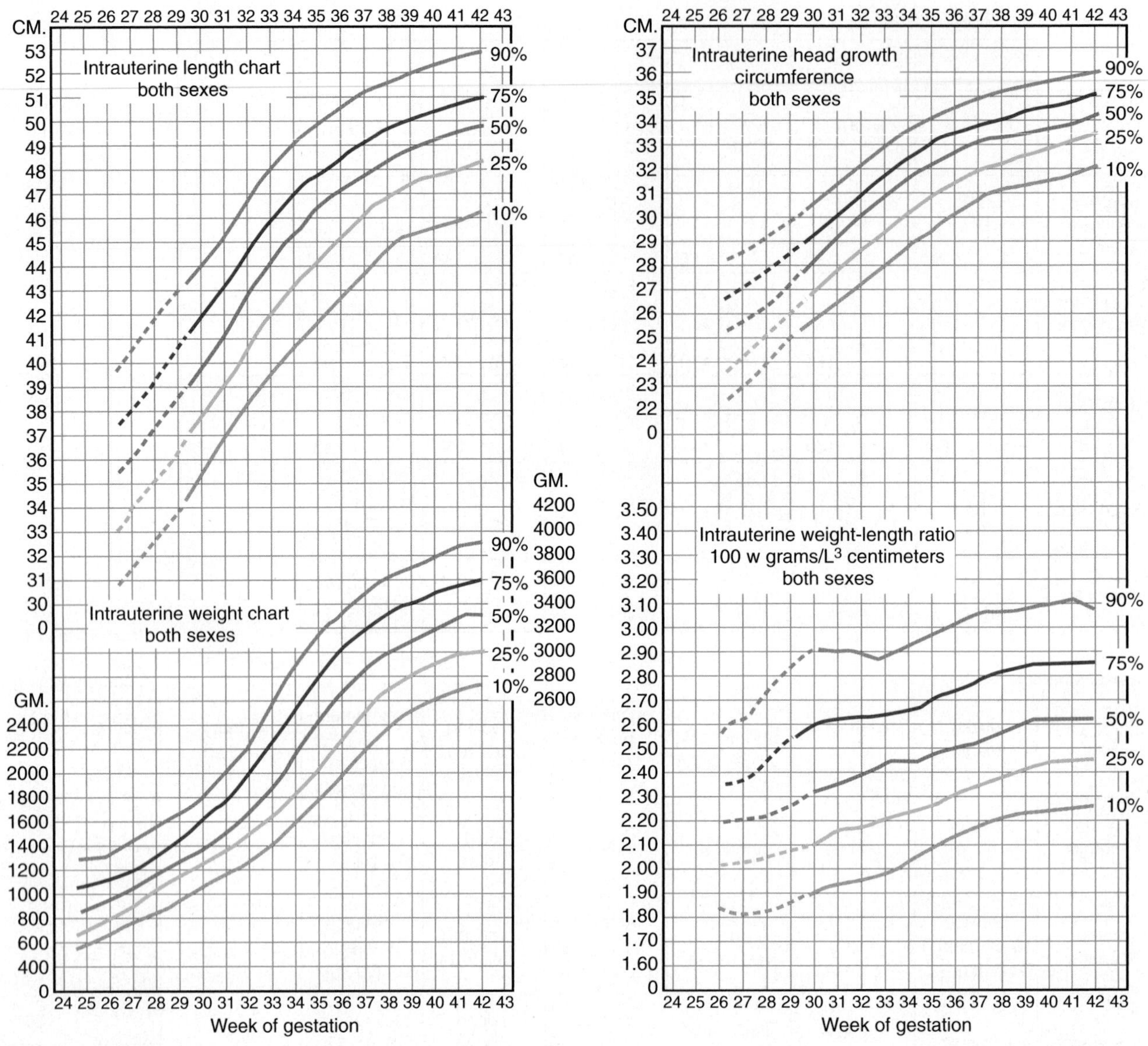

FIGURE 21-21. Intrauterine growth curves for weight, length, and head circumference for singleton births in Colorado. (From Lubchenco LO, Hansman C, Boyd E: Intrauterine growth in length and head circumference as estimated from live births at gestational ages from 26 to 42 weeks. Pediatrics 37:403, 1966.)

hydrops, and Beckwith-Wiedemann syndrome. LGA infants are at risk for hypoglycemia, polycythemia, congenital anomalies, cardiomyopathy, hyperbilirubinemia, and birth trauma.

NURSERY CARE

Nurseries are classified on the basis of level of care provided (see box, Levels of Nursery Care). Level I nurseries care for infants presumed healthy, with an emphasis on screening and surveillance. Level II nurseries can care for infants more than 32 weeks' gestation, who weigh at least 1500 g, and who require special attention, but will probably not need subspecialty services. Level III nurseries care for all newborn infants who are critically ill regardless of the level of support required.[83] A perinatal center encompasses both high-risk obstetric services and level III nursery services.

Care of the normal newborn involves observation of transition from intrauterine to extrauterine life, establishing breast- or bottle-feeds, noting normal patterns of stooling and urination, and surveillance for neonatal problems. Signs suggestive of illness include temperature instability, change in activity, refusal to feed, pallor, cyanosis, jaundice, tachypnea and respiratory distress, delayed (beyond 24 hours) passage of first stool or void, and bilious vomiting. In addition, the following laboratory screens should be performed: (1) blood type and direct and indirect Coombs' test on infants born to mothers with type O or Rh-negative blood; (2) glucose screen in infants at risk for hypoglycemia; (3) hematocrit in infants with signs and symptoms of anemia or polycythemia; and (4) mandated screening for inborn errors of metabolism, such as PKU and galactosemia, sickle cell disease, hypothyroidism, cystic fibrosis, and congenital adrenal hyperplasia. Many states now mandate or offer expanded newborn screening by tandem mass

Levels of Nursery Care

Level 1: A nursery with personnel and equipment to perform neonatal resuscitation, evaluate and provide newborn care for healthy infants, stabilize and provide care for infants born at 35-37 weeks' gestation who remain physiologically stable, and stabilize ill or less than 35 weeks' gestation infants before transport to a higher level facility.

Level 2: A facility able to provide care to infants born at more than 32 weeks' gestation weighing more than 1500 g who have physiologic immaturity; who are moderately ill with problems expected to resolve quickly; and who do not need urgent subspecialty care. Can provide convalescent care for infants after intensive care. A level 2A does not do mechanical ventilation or nasal continuous positive airway pressure, whereas a 2B can do short-term (less than 24 hours) ventilation.

Level 3: Provide care for the sickest and most complex infants.

3A: Care for infants beyond 28 weeks and 1000 g in need of conventional mechanical ventilation.

3B: Can provide care for infants less than 28 weeks and 1000 g, high-frequency ventilation, inhaled nitric oxide, on-site subspecialists, advanced imaging, on-site or nearby pediatric surgeons and anesthesiologists.

3C: Can provide ECMO and repair of complex congenital heart disease.

Modified from American Academy of Pediatrics Committee on Fetus and Newborn: Levels of neonatal care. Pediatrics 114:1341. 2004.
ECMO, Extracorporeal membrane oxygenation.

spectroscopy that looks for a variety of other inborn metabolic errors. All newborns should also have an initial hearing screen performed before discharge. Finally, babies routinely receive 1 mg intramuscular of vitamin K to prevent vitamin K–deficient hemorrhagic disease of the newborn and erythromycin ointment to prevent gonococcal ophthalmia neonatorum. Hepatitis B vaccine should be given to all newborns, and hepatitis B immunoglobulin is also administered to infants born to HB_sAg-positive mothers. Infants should be positioned supine for sleep to minimize the risk of sudden infant death syndrome.[84]

Discharge of the normal newborn is safe provided all criteria are met in the box entitled Infant Criteria for Early Discharge. The initial follow-up visit needs to occur 48 to 72 hours after discharge.[85]

Circumcision is an elective procedure to be performed only in healthy, stable infants. The procedure probably has medical benefits, including prevention of phimosis, paraphimosis, and balanoposthitis, as well as a decreased incidence of cancer of the penis, cervical cancer (in partners of circumcised men), sexually transmitted diseases (including HIV), and urinary tract infection in male infants. Most parents, however, make the decision regarding circumcision for nonmedical reasons. The risks of the procedure include local infection, bleeding, removal of too much skin, and urethral injury. The combined incidence of these complications is less than 1%. Local anesthesia (dorsal penile nerve block or circumferential ring block) with 1% lidocaine without epinephrine is safe and effective, and should always be used. Techniques that allow visualization of the glans throughout the procedure (Plastibell and Gomco clamp) are preferred to a "blind" technique (Mogen clamp) because of occasional amputation of the glans with the latter. Circumcision is contraindicated in infants with genital abnormalities. Appropriate laboratory evaluation should be performed before the procedure in infants with a family history of bleeding disorders.

Care of the Parents

Klaus and Kennell[86] outline these steps in maternal-infant attachment: (1) planning the pregnancy; (2) confirming the pregnancy; (3) accepting the pregnancy; (4) noting fetal movement; (5) accepting the fetus as an individual; (6) going through labor; (7) giving birth; (8) hearing and seeing the baby; (9) touching, smelling, and holding the baby; (10) caretaking; and (11) accepting the infant as a separate individual. Numerous influences can affect this process. A mother's and father's actions and responses are derived from their own genetic endowment, their own interfamily relationships, cultural practices, past experiences with this or previous pregnancies, and, most important, how they were raised by their parents. Also critical is the in-hospital experience surrounding the birth—how doctors and nurses act, separation from the baby, and hospital practices.

The 60- to 90-minute period after delivery is a very important time. The infant is alert, active, and able to follow with his or her eyes, allowing meaningful interaction to transpire between infant and parents. The infant's array of sensory and motor abilities evokes responses from the mother and initiates communication that may be helpful for attachment and induction of reciprocal actions. Whether a critical time period for these initial interactions exists is not clear, but improved mothering behavior does seem to occur with increased contact over the first 3 postpartum days. The practical implications of this information are that labor and delivery should pose as little anxiety as possible for the mother, and parents and baby should have time together immediately after delivery if the baby's medical condition permits.

Mothers with high-risk pregnancies are at increased risk for subsequent parenting problems. It is important for both obstetrician and pediatrician alike to be involved prenatally, allowing time to prepare the family for anticipated aspects of the baby's care as well as providing reassurance that the odds are heavily in favor of a live baby who will ultimately be healthy. If before birth one can anticipate a need for neonatal intensive care (known congenital anomaly, refractory premature labor), maternal transport to a center with a unit that can care for the baby should be planned. Before delivery, it is also very helpful to allow the parents to tour the unit their baby will occupy.

The basic principle in dealing with parents of a sick infant is to provide essential information clearly and accurately to both parents, preferably when they are together. With improved survival rates, especially in premature infants, most babies, despite early problems, will do well. Therefore, it is reasonable in most circumstances to be positive about the outcome. There is also no reason to emphasize problems that might occur in the future or to deal with individual worries of the

Infant Criteria for Early Discharge

1. Term newborn, defined as an infant born between 37 and 41 completed weeks of gestation.
2. No abnormalities that require continued hospitalization.
3. Vital signs are documented as being within normal ranges, with appropriate variations based on physiologic state, and stable for the 12 hours preceding discharge.
4. The infant has urinated regularly and passed stool spontaneously.
5. The infant has completed at least 2 successful consecutive feedings.
6. No significant bleeding at the circumcision site.
7. The clinical risk of development of subsequent hyperbilirubinemia has been assessed, and appropriate management and/or follow-up plans have been instituted.
8. The infant has been adequately evaluated and monitored for sepsis on the basis of maternal risk factors and in accordance with current guidelines for prevention of perinatal group B streptococcal disease.
9. Maternal blood test and screening results are available and have been reviewed, including maternal syphilis, hepatitis B surface antigen status; and a test for HIV in accordance with state regulations.
10. Infant blood tests are available and have been reviewed such as cord or infant blood type and direct Coombs' test results, as clinically indicated.
11. Newborn metabolic and hearing screenings have been completed per hospital protocol and state regulations.
12. The mother's knowledge, ability, and confidence to provide adequate care for her infant have been assessed for competency regarding:
    - breastfeeding or bottle feeding (the breastfeeding mother and infant should be assessed by trained staff regarding breastfeeding position, latch-on, and adequacy of swallowing).
    - the importance and benefits of breastfeeding for both mother and infant.
    - appropriate urination and defecation frequency for the infant.
    - cord, skin, and genital care, including circumcision care, for the infant.
    - the ability to recognize signs of illness and common infant problems, particularly jaundice.
    - infant safety (such as use of an appropriate car safety seat, supine positioning for sleeping, maintaining a smoke-free environment, and room sharing).
13. Family, environmental, and social risk factors have been assessed, and the mother and her other family members have been educated about safe home environment. These risk factors include but are not limited to:
    - untreated parental substance abuse or positive urine toxicology results in the mother or newborn.
    - history of child abuse or neglect.
    - mental illness in a parent who is in the home.
    - lack of social support, particularly for single, first-time mothers.
    - mothers who live in a shelter, a rehabilitation home, or on the street.
    - history of domestic violence, particularly during this pregnancy.
    - communicable illness in a parent or other members of the household.
    - adolescent mother, particularly if other above-listed conditions apply.
14. A medical home for continuing medical care for the infant has been identified and a plan for timely communication of pertinent clinical information to the medical home is in place. For newborns discharged less than 48 hours after delivery, an appointment should be made for the infant to be examined by a licensed health care professional, preferably within 48 hours of discharge based on risk factors but no later than 72 hours in most cases.
15. Barriers to adequate follow-up care for the newborn, such as lack of transportation to medical care services, lack of easy access to telephone communication, and non–English-speaking parents, have been assessed and, whenever possible, assistance has been given to the family to make suitable arrangements to address them.

physician. Questions, if asked, need to be answered honestly, but the list of parents' worries does not need to be voluntarily increased.

Before the parents' initial visit to the unit, a physician or nurse should describe what the baby and the equipment look like. When they arrive in the nursery, this can again be reviewed in detail. If a baby must be moved to another hospital, the mother should be given time to see and to touch her infant before the transfer. The father should be encouraged to meet the baby at the receiving hospital so he can become comfortable with the intensive care unit. He can serve as a link between baby and mother with information and photographs.

As a baby's course proceeds, the nursery staff can help the parents become comfortable with their infant. This can include participation in caretaking as well as skin-to-skin contact with the infant (kangaroo care). Individualized developmentally based care has also shown some benefit for high-risk infants.[87] It is also important for the staff to discuss among themselves any problems that parents may be having as well as to keep a record of visits and phone calls. This approach will allow early intervention to deal with potential problems.

The birth of an infant with a congenital malformation provides another situation in which staff support is essential. Parents' reactions to the birth of a malformed infant follow a predictable course. For most, there is initial shock and denial, a period of sadness and anger, gradual adaptation, and finally an increased satisfaction with and the ability to care for the baby. The parents must be allowed to pass through these stages and, in effect, to mourn the loss of the anticipated normal child.

The death of an infant or a stillborn is a highly stressful family event. This fact has been emphasized by Cullberg,[88] who found that psychiatric disorders developed in 19 of 56 mothers studied 1 to 2 years after the deaths of their neonates. One of the major predispositions was a breakdown of communication between parents. The

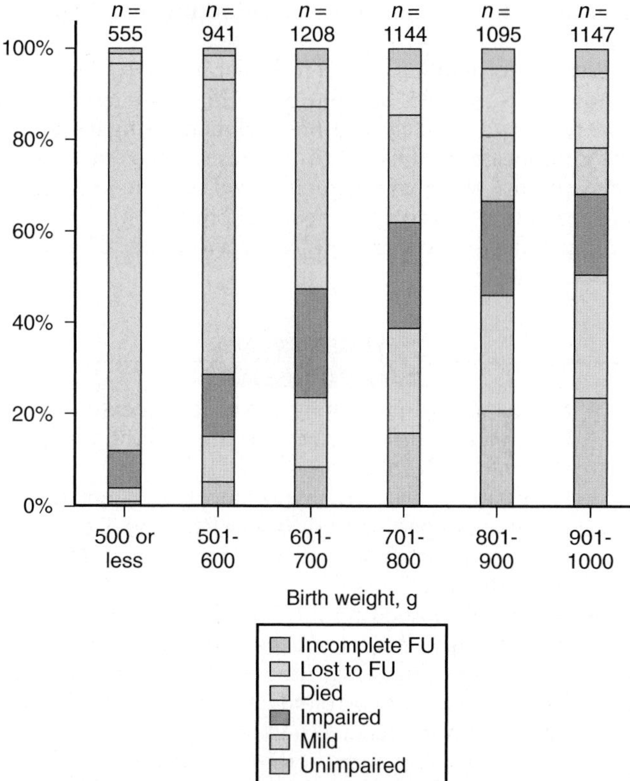

FIGURE 21-22. 18- to 22-month outcomes by birthweight in extremely-low-birthweight infants. (Reproduced with permission from Gargus RA, Vohr BR, Tyson JE, et al: Unimpaired outcomes for extremely low birth weight infants at 18-22 months. Pediatrics 124:112, 2009.)

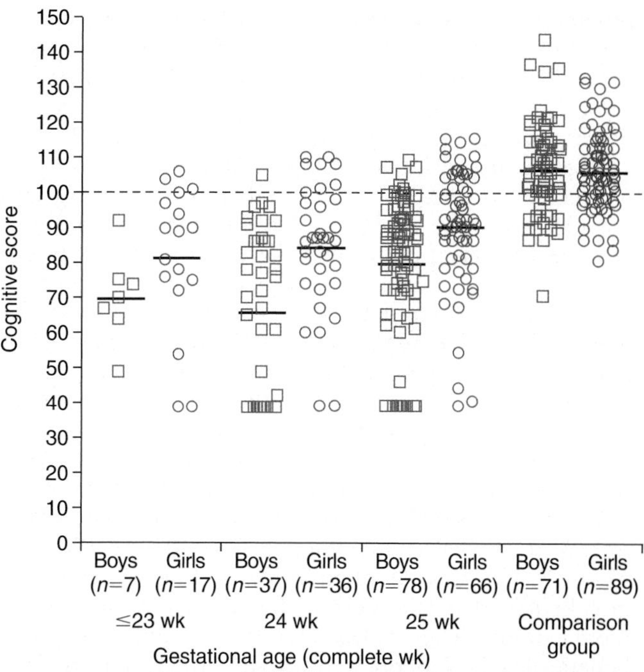

FIGURE 21-23. Cognitive scores for 241 extremely preterm children and 160 age-matched classmates who were full term at birth, according to sex and completed weeks of gestation at birth. The scores are the Kaufman Assessment Battery for Children scores for the Mental Processing Composite or developmental scores according to the Griffiths Scales of Mental Development and NEPSY. *Bars* indicate mean scores. *Dashed line* is the mean of a standardized population. (Reproduced with permission from Marlow N, Wolke D, Bracewell MA, et al: Neurologic and developmental disability at six years of age after extremely preterm birth. N Engl J Med 352:9, 2005.)

health care staff needs to encourage the parents to talk with each other, discuss their feelings, and display emotion. The staff should talk with the parents at the time of death and then several months later to review the findings of the autopsy, answer questions, and see how the family is doing.

OUTCOME OF NEONATAL INTENSIVE CARE AND THRESHOLD OF VIABILITY

More sophisticated neonatal care has resulted in improved survival of very-low-birthweight (<1500 g) infants, in particular those less than 1000 g (Figure 21-22). Current survival rates are 90% or greater for infants greater than 1000 g and 28 weeks' gestation, 85% at 800 to 1000 g and 26 to 27 weeks' gestation, and nearly 70% to 75% for infants 700 to 800 g and 25 weeks' gestation, with a considerable drop in survival below 700 g and 25 weeks.[89] **Predictions of survival can be significantly improved by consideration of clinical data in addition to birthweight and gestational age.** These data include an appropriate course of antenatal steroids, sex of the baby, and whether the pregnancy is singleton.[6] It is important to note that survival in terms of best obstetric estimate is greater at very low gestational ages than survival in terms of postnatal assessment of gestational age. The numbers in terms of best obstetric estimate based on data at the institution of birth should be referred to for antenatal counseling. This improved survival comes with a price, because a variety of morbidities are seen in these infants. The rate of severe neurologic disability is fairly constant at 10% of all very-low-birthweight survivors from 1000 to 1500 g. The number increases from 10% to 25% in infants of extremely low birthweight (<1000 g) and is particularly troubling for infants born at less than 25 weeks' gestation. In these infants, approximately half of the survivors have moderate or severe neurosensory disability (Figure 21-23).[89] In addition to the increase in severe disability, these infants have an increased rate of lesser disabilities including deficits in academic achievement, behavior and attention problems, and the need for special education in school.[90,91] Risk factors for neurologic morbidity include seizures, major intracranial hemorrhage or PVL, severe intrauterine growth restriction (IUGR), nec chorioamnionitis in the mother, neonatal infection, need for mechanical ventilation, CLD, poor early head growth, retinopathy of prematurity, and low socioeconomic class.

There are other morbidities that need to be considered as well. Because the number of survivors weighing less than 1000 g has increased, a reemergence of retinopathy of prematurity has been seen. This disorder, caused by retinal vascular proliferation leading to hemorrhage, scarring, retinal detachment, and blindness is triggered by low concentrations of insulin-like growth factor-1 (IGF-1) and relative hyperoxia in the early postnatal period leading to delayed retinal vessel growth. Later increases in IGF-1 allows a vascular endothelial growth factor (VEGF) induced angiogenesis resulting in an abnormal vascular proliferation.[92] Incidence of acute proliferative retinopathy by birthweight is less than 10% in infants weighing more than 1250 g, 20% in those 1000 to 1250 g, 50% to 60% in those 750 to 1000 g, and 70% in those less than 750 g.[71] Severe retinopathy is evident in 5% of the infants 1000 to 1250 g, in 10% of infants 750 to 1000 g, and 25% to 40% of infants less than 750 g. Of the infants with severe retinopathy, 10% (4% of the total population) will go on to have severe visual problems. The other major neurosensory morbidity is hearing loss, which occurs in 2% of neonatal intensive care unit survivors. Other sequelae of neonatal intensive care include CLD, growth failure, short gut, and need for postdischarge rehospitalization.

The information presented earlier on outcome is relevant to discussions about obstetric and neonatal intervention at the threshold of viability. If one considers the end point of survival without major disability, this occurs in 0% at 22 weeks, less than 10% at 23 weeks, approximately 20% to 25% at 24 weeks, and approximately 45% to 50% at 25 weeks.[89] With this information in mind, most neonatologists believe that care is clearly beneficial beyond 25 completed weeks, whereas less than half believe that care is beneficial at 24 to 24 6/7 weeks, and virtually none believe that care is beneficial at less than 24 completed weeks. Having said that, more than half would intervene on behalf of an infant beyond 23 weeks' gestation. These discussions need to be modified depending on circumstances. For instance, morbidity and mortality would increase in the face of overt infection or severe IUGR. A reasonable approach would seem to be to encourage interventions on behalf of the fetus or newborn beyond 25 completed weeks' gestation and not intervene at less than 23 weeks gestation. The range between 23 and 25 weeks should be evaluated on a case-by-case basis.

THE LATE PRETERM INFANT

The rate of preterm births in the United States has been increasing, especially for births between 34 0/7 and 36 6/7 weeks, which now make up 70% of all preterm births. Of these births, as many as 23% had no recorded indication for early delivery noted on birth certificates.[93] **Compared with term infants, late preterm infants have a higher mortality and prevalence of acute neonatal problems including respiratory distress, temperature instability, hypoglycemia, apnea, jaundice, and feeding difficulties.**[94] The respiratory issues are caused by delayed clearance of fetal lung fluid, surfactant deficiency, or both, and can on occasion progress to respiratory failure. Feeding issues are caused by poor coordination of suck and swallow, which can interfere with bottle feeding and cause failure to establish successful breastfeeding. This can put the infant at risk for both dehydration and excessive jaundice. Late preterm infants have at least twice the risk of an infant born at term to have significantly elevated serum bilirubin concentrations. Rehospitalizations due to jaundice, proven or suspected infection, feeding difficulties, and failure to thrive are much more common than in term infants. Long-term neurodevelopmental outcome is also compromised with reports of cognitive and emotional regulation difficulties, school problems, and slightly lower IQs.[95] There is also an increase in deficits in lung function that may persist into adulthood due to immaturity of the respiratory system at birth.[96]

Late preterm infants, even if similar in size to their term counterparts, should be considered preterm rather than near term, and need close in-hospital monitoring for potential complications. Discharge of these babies should be delayed until they have demonstrated reliable oral intake and resolution of any acute neonatal problems. Initial outpatient follow-up visit should occur within 48 to 72 hours of discharge.

KEY POINTS

- ◆ Surfactant maintains lung expansion on expiration by lowering surface tension at the air-liquid interface in the alveolus.
- ◆ Respiratory distress syndrome in premature infants is in part caused by a deficiency of surfactant and can be treated with surfactant replacement therapy.
- ◆ Antenatal corticosteroids accelerate fetal lung maturation and decrease neonatal mortality and respiratory distress syndrome in preterm infants. In addition, corticosteroids are associated with a decrease in intracranial hemorrhage and NEC.
- ◆ Transition from intrauterine to extrauterine life requires removal of fluid from the lungs, switching from a fetal to neonatal circulation, and establishment of a normal neonatal lung volume.
- ◆ The most important step in neonatal resuscitation is to achieve adequate expansion of the lungs.
- ◆ MAS likely is the result of intrauterine asphyxia with mortality related to associated persistent pulmonary hypertension.
- ◆ The best predictor of neurologic sequelae of birth asphyxia is the presence of hypoxic ischemic encephalopathy in the neonatal period. The neurologic sequelae of birth asphyxia is cerebral palsy. However, the large majority of cerebral palsy is of unknown origin or etiologies other than perinatal asphyxia.
- ◆ The major neurologic complications seen in premature infants are PVH/IVH and PVL.
- ◆ Hypoglycemia is a predictable and preventable complication in the newborn.
- ◆ Survival, in particular for infants weighing less than 1000 g, has increased with improved methods of neonatal intensive care, but comes with the price of medical and neurodevelopmental sequelae.

REFERENCES

1. Wert SE: Normal and abnormal structural development of the lung. In Polin RA, Fox WW, Abman SH (eds): Fetal and Neonatal Physiology, 3rd ed. Philadelphia, WB Saunders, 2004, p 783.
2. Stenmark KR, Abman SH: Lung vascular development: implications for the pathogenesis of bronchopulmonary dysplasia. Annu Rev Physiol 67:623, 2005.
3. Whitsett JA, Wert SE, Weaver TE: Alveolar surfactant homeostasis and the pathogenesis of pulmonary disease. Annu Rev Med 61:105, 2010.

4. Gross I, Ballard PL: Hormonal therapy for prevention of respiratory distress syndrome. In Polin RA, Fox WW, Abman SH (eds): Fetal and Neonatal Physiology, 3rd ed. Philadelphia, WB Saunders, 2004, p 1069.
5. Crowley PA: Antenatal corticosteroid therapy: a meta-analysis of the randomized trials, 1972-1994. Am J Obstet Gynecol 173:322, 1995.
6. Tyson JE, Parikh NA, Langer J, et al: Intensive care for extreme prematurity-moving beyond gestational age. N Engl J Med 358:1672, 2008.
7. Schmand B, Neuvel J, Smolders-de-Haas H, et al: Psychological development of children who were treated antenatally with corticosteroids to prevent respiratory distress syndrome. Pediatrics 86:58, 1990.
8. Smolders-de-Haas H, Neuvel J, Schmand B, et al: Physical development and medical history of children who were treated antenatally with corticosteroids to prevent respiratory distress syndrome: a 10- to 12-year follow-up. Pediatrics 86:65, 1990.
9. Engle WA, the AAP Committee on Fetus and Newborn: Surfactant-replacement therapy for respiratory distress in the preterm and term neonate. Pediatrics 121:419, 2008.
10. Jobe AH, Mitchell BR, Gunkel JH: Beneficial effects of the combined use of prenatal corticosteroids and postnatal surfactant on preterm infants. Am J Obstet Gynecol 168:508, 1993.
11. Kaplan M: Fetal breathing movements, an update for the pediatrician. Am J Dis Child 137:177, 1983.
12. Agostoni E, Taglietti A, Agostoni AF, Setnikar I: Mechanical aspects of the first breath. J Appl Physiol 13:344, 1958.
13. Milner AD, Vyas H: Lung expansion at birth. J Pediatr 101:879, 1982.
14. Arjan B, Pas TE, Davis PG, et al: From liquid to air: breathing after birth. J Pediatr 152:607, 2008.
15. Barker PM, Southern KW: Regulation of liquid secretion and absorption by the fetal and neonatal lung. In Polin RA, Fox WW, Abman SH (eds): Fetal and Neonatal Physiology, 3rd ed. Philadelphia, WB Saunders, 2004, p 822.
16. Helve O, Pitkanen O, Janer C, Andersson S: Pulmonary fluid balance in the human newborn infant. Neonatology 95:347, 2009.
17. Rudolph AM: Fetal circulation and cardiovascular adjustments after birth. In Rudolph CD, Rudolph AM, Hostetter MK, et al (eds): Rudolph's Pediatrics, 21st ed. New York, McGraw-Hill, 2003, p 1749.
18. Adamson SL, Myatt L, Byrne BMP: Regulation of umbilical flow. In Polin RA, Fox WW, Abman SH (eds): Fetal and Neonatal Physiology, 3rd ed. Philadelphia, WB Saunders, 2004, p 748.
19. Steinhorn RH: Neonatal pulmonary hypertension. Pediatr Crit Care Med 11:S79, 2010.
20. Hamrick SEG, Hansmann G: Patent ductus arteriosus of the preterm infant. Pediatrics 125:1020, 2010.
21. Dawes GS: Foetal and Neonatal Physiology. Chicago, Year Book, 1968.
22. American Heart Association and American Academy of Pediatrics: Neonatal Resuscitation Textbook. American Academy of Pediatrics and American Heart Association, 2011.
23. Saugstad OD, Ramji S, Soll RF, Vento M: Resuscitation of newborn infants with 21% or 100% oxygen: an updated systematic review and meta-analysis. Neonatology 94:176, 2008.
24. Vento M, Saugstad OD: Resuscitation of the term and preterm infant. Semin Fetal Neonatal Med 15:216, 2010.
25. Mariani G, Brener P, Ezquer A: Pre-ductal and post-ductal O_2 saturation in healthy term neonates after birth. J Pediatr 150:418, 2007.
26. Trevisanuto D, Doglioni N, Cavallin F et al: Heat loss prevention in very preterm infants in delivery rooms: a prospective, randomized trial of polyethylene caps. J Pediatr 156:914, 2010.
27. Nuntnarumit P, Rojnueangnit K, Tangnoo A: Oxygen saturation trends in preterm infants during the first 15 minutes after birth. J Perinatol 30:399, 2010.
28. Velaphi S, Vidyasagar D: Intrapartum and postdelivery management of infants born to mothers with meconium-stained amniotic fluid: evidence-based recommendations. Clin Perinatol 33:29, 2006.
29. Wiswell TE, Gannon CM, Jacob J, et al: Delivery room management of the apparently vigorous meconium-stained neonate: results of the multicenter international collaborative trial. Pediatrics 105:1, 2000.
30. Vain NE, Szyld EG, Wiswell TE, et al: Oropharyngeal and nasopharyngeal suctioning of meconium-stained neonates before delivery of their shoulders: multicentre, randomized controlled trial. Lancet 364:597, 2004.
31. Bailit JL, Gregory KD, Reddy UM, et al: Maternal and neonatal outcomes by labor onset type and gestational age. Am J Obstet Gynecol 202:245e1, 2010.
32. Gluckman PD, Wyall JS, Azzopardi D, et al: Selective head cooling with mild systemic hypothermia after neonatal encephalopathy: multicentre randomized trial. Lancet 365:663, 2005.
33. Shankaran S, Laptook AR, Ehrenkranz RA, et al: Whole-body hypothermia for neonates with hypoxic-ischemic encephalopathy. N Engl J Med 353:1574, 2005.
34. Edwards AD, Brocklehurst P, Green AJ, et al: Neurological outcomes at 18 months of age after moderate hypothermia for perinatal hypoxic ischaemic encephalopathy: synthesis and meta-analysis of trial data. BMJ 340:c363, 2010.
35. Flidel-Rimon O. Shinwell ES: Neonatal aspects of the relationship between intrapartum events and cerebral palsy. Clin Perinatol 34:439, 2007.
36. American College of Obstetricians and Gynecologists: American Academy of Pediatrics: Neonatal encephalopathy and cerebral palsy: defining pathogenesis and pathophysiology. Washington, DC, ACOG, 2003.
37. Rosenberg AA: Traumatic birth injury. Neoreviews 4:e273, 2003.
38. Volpe JJ (ed): Intracranial hemorrhage: subdural, primary subarachnoid, intracerebellar, intraventricular (term infant) and miscellaneous. In Neurology of the Newborn, 4th ed. Philadelphia, WB Saunders, 2001, p 397.
39. Sahni R, Schulze K: Temperature control in newborn infants. In Polin RA, Fox WW, Abman SH (eds): Fetal and Neonatal Physiology, 3rd ed. Philadelphia, WB Saunders, 2004, p 548.
40. Scopes JW: Metabolic rate and temperature control in the human body. Br Med Bull 22:88, 1966.
41. Friis-Hansen B: Water distribution in the foetus and newborn infant. Acta Paediatr Scand Suppl 305:7, 1983.
42. Committee on Nutrition, American Academy of Pediatrics: Nutritional needs of the preterm infant. In Kleinman RE (ed): Pediatric Nutrition Handbook, 6th ed. Elk Grove Village, IL, American Academy of Pediatrics, 2009, p 79.
43. Heinig MJ: Host defense benefits of breast feeding for the infant: effect of breast-feeding duration and exclusivity. Pediatr Clin North Am 48:105, 2001.
44. Heiman H, Schanler RJ: Enteral nutrition for premature infants: the role of human milk. Semin Fetal Neonatal Med 12:26, 2007.
45. Patel AL, Meier PP, Engstrom JL: The evidence for use of human milk in very low-birthweight preterm infants. Neoreviews 8:e459, 2007.
46. McGowan J: Neonatal hypoglycemia. NeoReviews 20:e6, 1999.
47. Collins JE, Leonard JV: Hyperinsulinins in asphyxiated and small-for-dates infants with hypoglycemia. Lancet 8398:311, 1984.
48. Hoe FM, Thornton PS, Wanner LA, et al: Clinical features and insulin regulation in infants with a syndrome of prolonged neonatal hyperinsulinism. J Pediatr 148:207, 2006.
49. Rozance P, Hay WW: Hypoglycemia in newborn infants: features associated with adverse outcomes. Biol Neon 90:74, 2006.
50. Goyal A, Jones MD, Couriel JM, Losty PD: Oesophageal atresia and trachea-oesophageal fistula. Arch Dis Child Fetal Neonatal Ed 91: F381, 2006.
51. Kays DW: Surgical conditions of the neonatal intestinal tract. Clin Perinatol 23:353, 1996.
52. Meller JL, Reyes HN, Loeff DS: Gastroschisis and omphalocoele. Clin Perinatol 16:113, 1989.
53. Kays DW: Congenital diaphragmatic hernia: real improvements in survival. Neoreviews 7:e428, 2006.
54. Caplan MS, Jilling T: The pathophysiology of necrotizing enterocolitis. Neoreviews 2:e103, 2001.
55. Gordon PV, Attridge JT: Understanding clinical literature relevant to spontaneous intestinal perforations. Am J Perinatol 26:309, 2009.
56. Cashore WJ: Bilirubin metabolism and toxicity in the newborn. In Polin RA, Fox WW, Abman SH (eds): Fetal and Neonatal Physiology, 3rd ed. Philadelphia, WB Saunders, 2004, p 1199.
57. American Academy of Pediatrics Subcommittee on Hyperbilirubinemia: Management of hyperbilirubinemia in the newborn infant 35 or more weeks of gestation. Pediatrics 114:297, 2004.
58. Maisals MJ, Bhutani VK, Bogen D: Hyperbilirubinemia in the newborn infant = 35 weeks gestation: an update with clarifications. Pediatrics 124:1193, 2009.
59. Watchko JF: Hyperbilirubinemia and bilirubin toxicity in the late preterm infant. Clin Perinatol 33:839, 2006.

60. Widness JA: Pathophysiology, diagnosis, and prevention of neonatal anemia. Neoreviews 1:e61, 2000.
61. Schimmel MS, Bromiker R, Soll RF: Neonatal polycythemia: is partial exchange transfusion justified? Clin Perinatol 31:545, 2004.
62. Bussel JB, Sola-Visner M: Current approaches to the evaluation and management of the fetus and neonate with immune thrombocytopenia. Semin Perinatol 33:35, 2009.
63. American Academy of Pediatrics Committee on the Fetus and Newborn: Controversies concerning vitamin K and the newborn. Pediatrics 112:191, 2003.
64. Wynn JL, Levy O: Role of innate host defenses in susceptibility to early-onset neonatal sepsis. Clin Perinatol 37:307, 2010.
65. Verani JR, Schrag SJ: Group B streptococcal disease in infants: progress in prevention and continued challenges. Clin Perinatol 37:375, 2010.
66. vanDyke MK, Phares CR, Lynfield R, et al: Evaluation of universal antenatal screening for group B streptococcus. N Engl J Med 360:25, 2009.
67. Silberbach M, Hannan D: Presentation of congenital heart disease in the neonate and young infant. Pediatr Rev 28:123, 2007.
68. Avery ME, Mead J: Surface properties in relation to atelectasis and hyaline membrane disease. Am J Dis Child 97:517, 1959.
69. Northway WH Jr, Rosan RC, Porter DY: Pulmonary disease following respiratory therapy of hyaline membrane disease. N Engl J Med 276:357, 1967.
70. Walsh MC, Szefler S, Davis J et al: Summary proceedings from the bronchopulmonary dysplasia group. Pediatrics 117:552, 2006.
71. Vermont Oxford Neonatal Network: Vermont Oxford Network Annual VLBW Database Summary 2003. Burlington, Vermont Oxford Network, 2004.
72. Goddard J, Lewis RM, Armstrong DL, Zeller RS: Moderate, rapidly induced hypertension as a cause of intraventricular hemorrhage in the newborn beagle model. J Pediatr 96:1057, 1980.
73. Volpe JJ: Brain injury in premature infants: a complex amalgam of destructive and developmental disturbances. Lancet Neurol 1:110, 2009.
74. Laptook AR, et al: Adverse neurodevelopmental outcome among extremely low birth weight infants with normal head ultrasound: prevalence and antecedents. Pediatrics 115:673, 2005.
75. Patra K, Wilson-Costello D, Taylor HG, et al: Grades I-II intraventricular hemorrhage in extremely low birth weight infants: effects on neurodevelopment. J Pediatr 149:169, 2006.
76. Lowe J, Papille LA: Neurodevelopmental performance of very-low-birth-weight infants with mild periventricular, intraventricular hemorrhage. Outcome at 5 to 6 years of age. Am J Dis Child 144:1242, 1990.
77. Brouwer A, et al: Neurodevelopmental outcome of preterm infants with severe intraventricular hemorrhage and therapy for post-hemorrhagic ventricular dilation. Pediatrics 152:648, 2008.
78. Thorp JA, Ferrette-Smith D, Gaston LA, et al: The effect of combined antenatal vitamin K and phenobarbital therapy for preventing intracranial hemorrhage in newborns less than 34 weeks gestation. Obstet Gynecol 86:1, 1995.
79. Shankaran S, Papile L-A, Wright LL, et al: The effect of antenatal phenobarbital therapy on neonatal intracranial hemorrhage in preterm infants. N Engl J Med 337:466, 1997.
80. Ballard JL, Khoury JC, Wedig K, et al: New Ballard Score, expanded to include extremely premature infants. J Pediatr 119:417, 1991.
81. Lubchenco LO, Hansman C, Boyd E: Intrauterine growth in length and head circumference as estimated from live births at gestational ages from 26 to 42 weeks. Pediatrics 37:403, 1966.
82. Rosenberg A: The IUGR newborn. Semin Perinatol 32:219, 2008.
83. Stark AR: American Academy of Pediatrics Committee on Fetus and Newborn: Levels of neonatal care. Pediatrics 114:1341, 2004.
84. American Academy of Pediatrics Task Force on Sudden Infant Death Syndrome: The changing concept of sudden infant death syndrome: diagnostic coding shifts, controversies regarding the sleeping environment, and new variables to consider in reducing risk. Pediatrics 116:1245, 2005.
85. American Academy of Pediatrics Committee on Fetus and Newborn: Policy statement— hospital stay for healthy term newborns. Pediatrics 125:405, 2010.
86. Klaus MH, Kennel JH: Care of the parents. In Klaus MH, Fanaroff AA (eds): Care of the High-Risk Neonate, 5th ed. Philadelphia, WB Saunders, 2001, p 195.
87. Peters KL, Rosychuk RJ, Hendson L, et al: Improvement of short- and long-term outcomes for very low birth weight infants: Edmonton NIDCAP trial. Pediatrics 124:1009, 2009.
88. Cullberg J: Mental reactions of women to perinatal death. In Morris N (ed): Psychosomatic Medicines in Obstetrics and Gynecology. New York, S Karger, 1972, p 326.
89. Gargus RA, Vohr BR, Tyson JE, et al: Unimpaired outcomes for extremely low birth weight infants at 18-22 months. Pediatrics 124:112, 2009.
90. Marlow N, Wolke D, Bracewell MA, et al: Neurologic and developmental disability at six years of age after extremely preterm birth. N Engl J Med 352:9, 2005.
91. Aarnoudse-Moens CSH, Weisglas-Kuperus N, vanGoudoever JB, et al: Meta-analysis of neurobehavioral outcomes in very preterm and/or very low birth weight children. Pediatrics 124:717, 2009.
92. Fleck BW, McIntosh N: Retinopathy of prematurity: recent developments. Neoreviews 10:e20, 2009.
93. Reddy UM, Ko C-W, Raju TNK, Willinger M: Delivery indications at late-preterm gestations and infant mortality rate in the United States. Pediatrics 124:234, 2009.
94. Engle WA, Tomashek KM, Wallman C, the Committee on Fetus and Newborn: "Late-preterm" infants: a population at risk. Pediatrics 120:1390, 2007.
95. vanBaar AL, Vermaas J, Knots E, et al: Functioning at school age of moderately preterm children born at 32 to 36 weeks gestational age. Pediatrics 124:251, 2009.
96. Colin AA, McEvoy C, Castile RG: Respiratory morbidity and lung function in preterm infants of 32 to 36 weeks gestational age. Pediatrics 126:115, 2010.

For full reference list, log onto www.expertconsult.com.

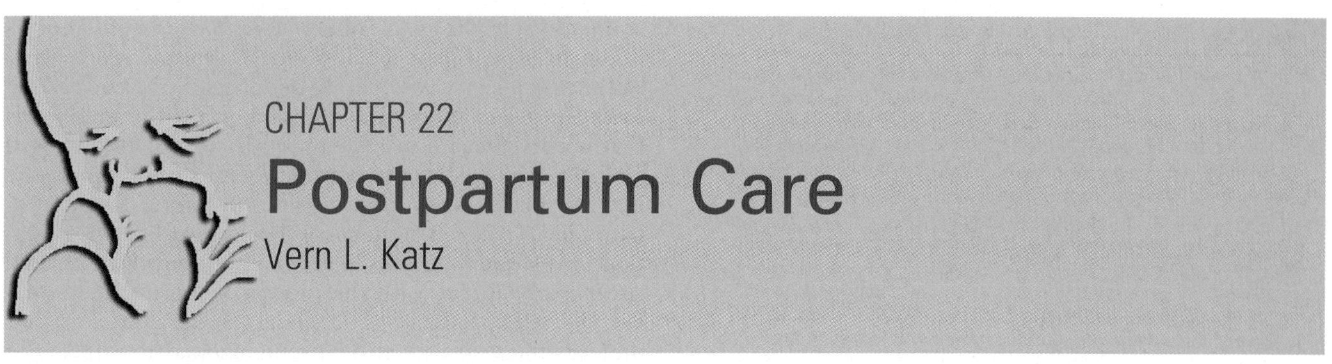

CHAPTER 22
Postpartum Care

Vern L. Katz

KEY ABBREVIATIONS	
Depot Medroxyprogesterone Acetate	DMPA
Edinburgh Postnatal Depression Scale	EPDS
Food and Drug Administration	FDA
Follicle-stimulating Hormone	FSH
Intrauterine Device	IUD
Postpartum Thyroiditis	PPT

The postpartum time period, also called the *puerperium,* lasts from delivery of the placenta until 6 to 12 weeks after delivery. Most of the physiologic changes in pregnancy will have returned to their prepregnancy state by 6 weeks.[1] However, many of the cardiovascular changes and psychological changes may persist for many more months, and some such as changes in the pelvic musculature and cardiac remodeling will last for years. This chapter examines the physiologic adjustments of the postpartum period, the return of the female genital tract to its prepregnancy state (involution), the major puerperal disease states, and the natural course of lactation.

The postpartum period is associated with as much tradition and superstition as any other rite of passage in life because the health of a new infant is so important to the survival of any family or clan. In order to support the successful recovery of the mother and the healthy transition through the neonatal period, customs, taboos, and rituals have developed in most cultures. Indeed, many of the current medical recommendations about puerperium have developed from adaptations of socially acceptable traditions, rather than science. For example, the 6-week postpartum check approximates the end of the 40 days of rest and sexual separation required in traditional societies.

Cultures throughout the world have specific postpartum traditions that include both restrictions on activity and prescribed activities, different foods for the newly delivered mother, as well as particular and unique taboos regarding postpartum care (Table 22-1). For example, bathing after delivery is a taboo in some cultures. Because women often cherish these rituals, it is essential for physicians, midwives, and nurses to be sensitive to these customs even though a woman's place of delivery may be far from her native country.

This chapter examines the normal physiologic changes of the puerperium and the transitions to prepregnancy physiology. With respect to these changes, we evaluate the principles and practices of postpartum care, the role of the provider being to help the patient through the transition. As is true of most physiologic changes, disease may occur when the change is exaggerated or insufficient.

POSTPARTUM INVOLUTION

The Uterus

The crude weight of the pregnant uterus at term (excluding the fetus, placenta, membranes, and amniotic fluid) is about 1000 g, approximately 10- to 20-fold heavier than the nonpregnant uterus.[2] The specific time course of uterine involution has not been fully elucidated, but within 2 weeks after birth, the uterus has usually returned to the pelvis, and by 6 weeks, it is usually normal size, as estimated by palpation. The gross anatomic and histologic characteristics of the involutional process are based on the study of autopsy, hysterectomy, and endometrial biopsy specimens.[3] The decrease in the size of the uterus and cervix during the puerperium has been demonstrated with serial magnetic resonance imaging.[4] The findings are consistent with those of serial sonography and computed tomography.

Immediately after delivery, rapidly decreasing endometrial surface area facilitates placental shearing at the decidual layer. The average diameter of the placenta is 18 cm;

TABLE 22-1 EXAMPLES OF POSTPARTUM RITUALS

- In the rural Philippines, the mother, who works until she goes into labor, is prohibited from working after delivery, and she is given a new name. The maternal grandmother visits daily and does the housework and cooking for 8 weeks. The mother is bathed by the grandmother daily. When the umbilical cord falls off the infant, a feast is prepared. The cord is blessed at the feast. The new father is prohibited from building stone walls and from driving nails for 6 months. For 2 months, the relatives tend the fields.
- Postpartum taboos related to *hot and cold* are found worldwide.
  - In Asian, African, and Latin American cultures, heat and cold must be maintained in balance to promote health and prevent disease. Because blood, which is "hot," is lost during delivery, the parturient must replenish her "heat" by staying bundled and drinking warm liquids.
  - Several traditional Middle Eastern areas see the bones as open after delivery, and exposure to cold creates a vulnerability to disease. Bathing is often taboo for traditional women; sponge baths may be substituted.
  - In parts of rural India, the new mother returns to her mother's house for 16 weeks. She is given a hot bath every day. Cold baths are taboo because cold water is associated with disease.
  - Many cultures have rituals regarding treatment of the placenta. It may be dried and turned to powder for its "medical" powers. The umbilical cord was hung in a nearby tree by some eastern Native American tribes. In Eastern European tradition, it was buried under certain corners of the house, to ensure prosperity.

in the immediate postpartum uterus, the average diameter of the site of placental attachment measures 9 cm. In the first 3 days after delivery the placental site is infiltrated with granulocytes and mononuclear cells, a reaction that extends into the endometrium and superficial myometrium. By the 7th day, there is evidence of the regeneration of endometrial glands, often appearing atypical, with irregular chromatin patterns, misshapen and enlarged nuclei, pleomorphism, and increased cytoplasm. By the end of the first week, there is also evidence of the regeneration of endometrial stroma, with mitotic figures noted in gland epithelium; by postpartum day 16, the endometrium is fully restored.

Decidual necrosis begins on the first day, and by the seventh day, a well-demarcated zone can be seen between necrotic and viable tissue. An area of viable decidua remains between the necrotic slough and the deeper endomyometrium. Sharman[3] described how the non-necrotic decidual cells participate in the reconstruction of the endometrium, a likely role, given their original role as endometrial connective tissue cells. By the sixth week, decidual cells are rare. The immediate inflammatory cell infiltrate of polymorphonuclear leukocytes and lymphocytes persists for about 10 days, presumably serving as an antibacterial barrier. The leukocyte response diminishes rapidly after day 10, and plasma cells are seen for the first time. The plasma cell and lymphocyte response may last as long as several months. In fact, endometrial stromal infiltrates of plasma cells and lymphocytes are a sign (and may be the only sign) of a recent pregnancy.

Hemostasis immediately after birth is accomplished by arterial smooth muscle contraction and compression of vessels by the involuting uterine muscle. Vessels in the placental site are characterized during the first 8 days by thrombosis, hyalinization, and endophlebitis in the veins, and by hyalinization and obliterative fibrinoid endarteritis in the arteries. The mechanism for hyalinization of arterial walls, which is not completely understood, may be related to the previous trophoblastic infiltration of arterial walls that occurs early in pregnancy. Many of the thrombosed and hyalinized veins are extruded with the slough of the necrotic placental site, but hyalinized arteries remain for extended periods as stigmata of the placental site. Restoration of the endometrium in areas other than the placental site occurs rapidly, with the process being completed by day 16 after delivery. The gland epithelium does not undergo the reactivity or the pseudoneoplastic appearance noted in placental site glands.

The postpartum uterine discharge or lochia begins as a flow of blood lasting several hours, rapidly diminishing to a reddish brown discharge through the third or fourth day postpartum. This is followed by a transition to a mucopurulent, somewhat malodorous discharge, called *lochia serosa,* requiring the change of several perineal pads per day. The median duration of lochia serosa is 22 to 27 days.[5,6] However, 10% to 15% of women will have lochia serosa at the time of the 6-week postpartum examination. In most patients, the lochia serosa is followed by a yellow-white discharge, called *lochia alba.* Breastfeeding or the use of oral contraceptive agents does not affect the duration of lochia. Frequently, there is a sudden but transient increase in uterine bleeding between 7 and 14 days postpartum. This corresponds to the slough of the eschar over the site of placental attachment. Myometrial vessels of greater than 5 mm in diameter are present for up to 2 weeks postpartum, which accounts for the dramatic bleeding that can occur with this phenomenon.[6] Although it can be profuse, this bleeding episode is usually self-limited, requiring nothing more than reassurance of the patient. If it does not subside within 1 or 2 hours, the patient should be evaluated for possible retained placental tissue.

Ultrasound may be helpful in the management of abnormal postpartum bleeding. The empty uterus with a clear midline echo can often be distinguished from the uterine cavity expanded by clot (sonolucent) or retained tissue (echo dense)[7] (Figure 22-1). Serial ultrasound examinations of postpartum patients showed that in 20% to 30%, there was some retained blood or tissue within 24 hours after delivery. By the fourth postpartum day, only about 8% of patients showed endometrial cavity separation, a portion of which eventually had abnormal postpartum bleeding because of retained placental tissue.[8] In cases of abnormal postpartum bleeding, ultrasound examination may be a useful adjunct in detecting patients who have retained tissue or clot and, therefore, who will benefit from uterine evacuation and curettage. Those who have an empty uterine cavity will respond to therapy with oxytocin or methylergonovine.[9]

The Cervix

During pregnancy, the cervical epithelium increases in thickness, and the cervical glands show both hyperplasia and hypertrophy. Within the stroma, a distinct decidual reaction occurs. These changes are accompanied by a substantial increase in the vascularity of the cervix. Colposcopic examination performed after delivery has

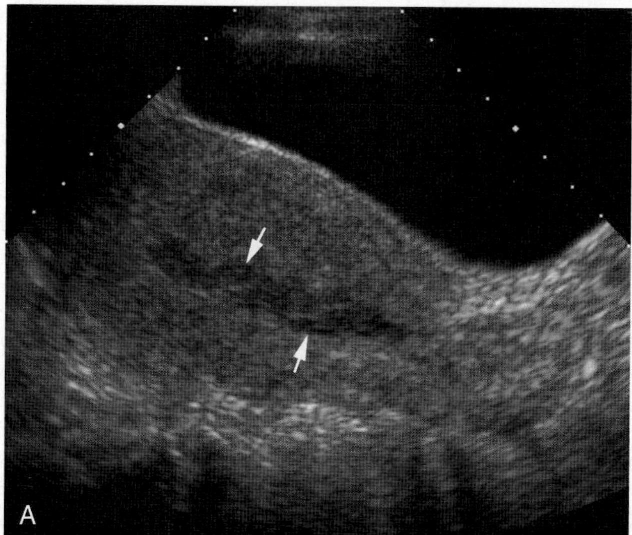

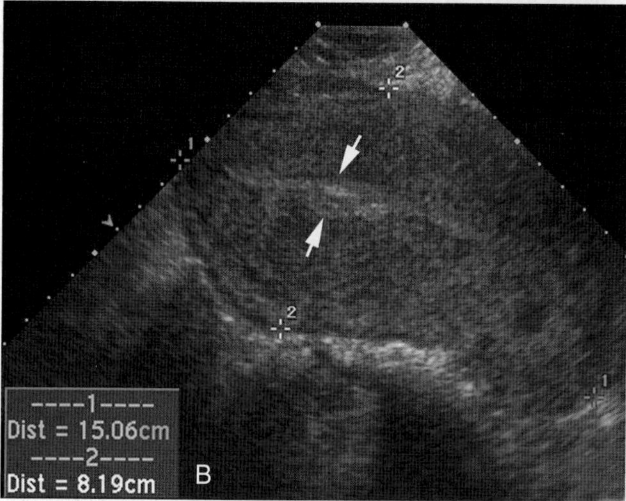

FIGURE 22-1. **A,** Sonogram of a normal postpartum uterus. **B,** Postpartum uterus with retained tissue. (From Poder L: Ultrasound evaluation of the Uterus. In Callen PW: Ultrasonography in Obstetrics and Gynecology, 5th ed. Philadelphia, Saunders, 2000, pp 939, 940.)

demonstrated ulceration, laceration, and ecchymosis of the cervix. Regression of the cervical epithelium begins within the first 4 days after delivery, and by the end of the first week, edema and hemorrhage within the cervix are minimal. Vascular hypertrophy and hyperplasia persist throughout the first week postpartum. By 6 weeks postpartum, most of the antepartum changes have resolved, although round cell infiltration and some edema may persist for several months.

The Fallopian Tube

The epithelium of the fallopian tube during pregnancy is characterized by a predominance of nonciliated cells, a phenomenon that is maintained by the balance between the high levels of progesterone and estrogen. After delivery, in the absence of progesterone and estrogen, there is further extrusion of nuclei from nonciliated cells and diminution in height of both ciliated and nonciliated cells. The number and height of ciliated cells can be increased in the puerperium by treatment with estrogen.

Fallopian tubes removed between postpartum days 5 and 15 demonstrate inflammatory changes of acute salpingitis in 38% of cases, but no bacteria are found. The specific cause of the inflammatory change is unknown. Furthermore, there is no correlation between the presence of histologic inflammation in the fallopian tubes and puerperal fever or other clinical signs of salpingitis.

Ovarian Function

Most women who breastfeed their infants are amenorrheic for extended periods of time, often until the infant is weaned. Several studies, using a variety of methods to indicate ovulation, have demonstrated that ovulation occurs as early as 27 days after delivery, with the mean time being about 70 to 75 days in nonlactating women.[10] Among women who are breastfeeding their infants, the mean time to ovulation is about 6 months.

Menstruation resumes by 12 weeks postpartum in 70% of women who are not lactating. The mean time to the first menstruation is 7 to 9 weeks. Depending on the population, as well as social and nutritional factors of the lactating women, regular menstruation may be delayed as long as 36 months. The duration of anovulation depends on the frequency of breastfeeding, the duration of each feed, and the proportion of supplementary feeds.[11] The likelihood of ovulation within the first 6 months postpartum, in a woman exclusively breastfeeding, is 1% to 5%.

The hormonal basis for puerperal ovulation suppression in lactating women appears to be the persistence of elevated serum prolactin levels. Prolactin levels fall to the normal range by the third week postpartum in nonlactating women but remain elevated into the sixth week postpartum in lactating patients. Estrogen levels fall immediately after delivery in both lactating and nonlactating women and remain depressed in lactating patients. In those who are not lactating, estrogen levels begin to rise 2 weeks after delivery and are significantly higher than in lactating women by postpartum day 17. Follicle-stimulating hormone (FSH) levels are identical in breastfeeding and nonbreastfeeding women, suggesting that the ovary does not respond to FSH stimulation in the presence of increased prolactin levels.

Weight Loss

One of the most welcome changes for most women who have recently given birth is the loss of the weight that was accumulated during pregnancy. The immediate loss of 10 to 13 lb is attributed to the delivery of the infant, placenta, and amniotic fluid and to blood loss. However, most women will not manifest that loss until 1 to 2 weeks after delivery because of fluid retention immediately after delivery. The physiologic stress of labor and delivery induces hormonal changes, including increased antidiuretic hormone, that lead to a short period of sodium and water retention. With operative birth, or epidural anesthesia with fluid boluses, the total body water increases dramatically. Women may be reassured that this temporary dependent edema is secondary to this fluid retention. For most women, weight loss postpartum does not tend to compensate for weight gain during gestation. By 6 weeks postpartum, only 28% of women will have returned to their prepregnant weight. The remainder of any weight loss occurs from 6 weeks postpartum until 6 months after delivery, with most weight loss concentrated in the first 3 months. Women with excess weight gain in pregnancy (>35 lb) are likely to have a net gain of 11 lb. Breastfeeding has relatively little effect on postpartum weight loss. With a program of diet and exercise, weight loss of about 0.5 kg/week between 4 and 14 weeks postpartum in breastfeeding, overweight women did not affect the growth of their infants.[12] Similarly, aerobic exercise has no adverse effect on lactation.[13] In a longitudinal study of pregnancy weight gain, 540 women were followed for 5 to 10 years (mean, 8.5 years) after their index pregnancy. Women who returned to prepregnancy weight by 6 months after delivery were much more likely to have gained less weight at the 5- to 10-year follow-up compared with women who retained their pregnant weight gains. In this cohort, breastfeeding and aerobic exercise were associated with a significantly lower weight gain over time.[14] A study of 1656 deliveries in a retrospective cohort found that pregnant weight gain greater than the recommended amount was directly related to the increased weight of women 1 year later.[15] Phelan[16] has emphasized that pregnancy and postpartum are "teachable moments," ideal for counseling women about weight control.

Thyroid Function

Thyroid size and function throughout pregnancy and the puerperium have been quantitated with ultrasonography and thyroid hormone levels.[17] Thyroid volume increases about 30% during pregnancy and regresses to normal gradually over a 12-week period. Thyroxine and triiodothyronine, which are both elevated throughout pregnancy, return to normal within 4 weeks postpartum. For women taking thyroid medications, it is appropriate to check thyroid levels at 6 weeks postpartum to adjust dosing. It is now recognized that the postpartum period is associated with an increased risk for the development of a transient autoimmune thyroiditis that may in some cases evolve into permanent hypothyroidism. The relationship of subclinical thyroid dysfunction and postpartum depression is controversial.[18-20] Postpartum thyroiditis (PPT), an autoimmune disease that may present with hyperthyroid or hypothyroid symptoms, occurs in 2% to 17% of women, with a mean incidence about 10%. Women with type 1 diabetes have up to a 25% risk for PPT. Women with gestational diabetes and type 2 diabetes also have a slightly increased risk. Only that subset of women who develop symptoms should be treated. Puerperal hypothyroidism often presents with symptoms that include mild dysphoria; consequently, thyroid function studies are suggested in the evaluation of patients with suspected postpartum depression that occurs 2 to 3 months after delivery. Hyperthyroid symptoms are best treated with β-blockers, and hypothyroid symptoms with thyroid supplementation. Both are acceptable with breastfeeding. Methimazole and propylthiouracil are also safe with lactation. From 5% to 30% of women with PPT eventually develop hypothyroidism. If a woman becomes symptomatic and is treated, it is reasonable to stop medications after 1 year and reevaluate thyroid status before the patient considers becoming pregnant again.[18-20]

Cardiovascular System, Immunity, and Coagulation

Blood volume increases throughout pregnancy to levels in the third trimester about 35% above nonpregnant values. The greatest proportion of this increase consists of an expansion in plasma volume that begins in the first trimester and amounts to an additional 1200 mL of plasma, representing a 50% increase by the third trimester. Red blood cell volume increases by about 250 mL.

Immediately after delivery, plasma volume is diminished by about 1000 mL secondary to blood loss. By the third postpartum day, the plasma volume is replenished by a shift of extracellular fluid into the vascular space. In contrast, the total blood volume declines by 16% of the predelivery value, suggesting a relative and transient anemia. By 8 weeks postpartum, the red cell mass has rebounded and the hematocrit is normal in most women. As total blood volume normalizes, venous tone also returns to baseline. In a prospective evaluation of 42 women, at 4 and 42 days postpartum, significant reduction in deep vein vessel size and a concomitant increase in venous flow velocity in the lower extremities were observed.[21]

Pulse rate increases throughout pregnancy, as does stroke volume and cardiac output. Immediately after delivery, these remain elevated or rise even higher for 30 to 60 minutes. Following delivery, there is a transient rise of about 5% in both diastolic and systolic blood pressures throughout the first 4 days postpartum. Data are scant regarding the rate at which cardiac hemodynamics return to prepregnancy levels. Early studies suggested cardiac output had returned to normal when measurements were made 8 to 10 weeks postpartum. Clapp and Capeless[22] performed longitudinal evaluations of cardiac function at bimonthly intervals in 30 healthy women using M-mode ultrasound before pregnancy; during gestation; and at 12, 24, and 52 weeks postpartum. Cardiac output and left ventricular volume peaked at 24 weeks' gestation. There was a slow return to prepregnancy values over the year of study. However, even 1 year after delivery, there was a significantly higher cardiac output in both nulliparous and multiparous women than prepregnancy values. The authors suggested that this "cardiac remodeling" from pregnancy may last for an extended time in healthy women. Anecdotally, elite athletes have tried to take advantage of this physiologic boost to cardiac function by planning pregnancies a year before major sporting events.

Pregnancy is known to be a time of significantly increased coagulability that persists into the postpartum period.[23] The greatest level of coagulability is observed immediately postpartum through 48 hours. Fibrinogen concentrations gradually diminish over the first 2 weeks postpartum. Compared with antepartum values, there is a rapid decrease in platelets in some patients and no change or an increase in others. Within 2 weeks after delivery, the platelet count rises, possibly as a marker of increased bone marrow output as red cell mass is replaced. Fibrinolytic activity increases in the first 1 to 4 days after delivery and returns to normal in 1 week, as measured by levels of plasminogen activation inhibitor 1. D-dimer levels are increased over pregnancy levels and are a poor marker of thrombus formation. Protein-S levels and activated protein-C resistance are decreased for up to 6 weeks or longer. In general, tests for thrombophilia and hemostasis should be delayed, if possible, for 10 to 12 weeks. The changes in the coagulation system, together with vessel trauma and immobility, account for the increased risk for thromboembolism noted in the puerperium, especially when an operative delivery has occurred.

The immune system, which is mildly suppressed during pregnancy, particularly cellular-mediated immunity, rebounds after delivery. This rebound may lead to "flare-ups" of autoimmune disease and latent infections with inflammatory reactions. The inflammatory reactions are what often produces the clinical symptoms. Autoimmune thyroiditis, multiple sclerosis, and lupus erythematosus are examples of some of the diseases that may show an increase in disease activity in the first few months postpartum.[24] Large cross-sectional studies of population databases have noted hospital admission rates after delivery to be higher than expected for age-matched controls. The readmissions are related to infections such as pneumonia, cholecystitis, and appendicitis. Postpartum admission rates vary from 0.8% to 1.5% for vaginal delivery and 1.8% to 2.7% for cesarean birth.[25-27]

The Urinary Tract and Renal Function

It is generally accepted that the urinary tract becomes dilated during pregnancy, especially the renal pelves and the ureters above the pelvic brim. These findings, demonstrated 70 years ago, affect the collecting system of the right kidney more than that of the left and are caused by compression of the ureters by the adjacent vasculature and enlarged uterus, combined with the effects of progesterone. Ultrasound studies of the urinary tract also document the enlargement of the collecting system throughout pregnancy. A study of serial ultrasound examinations of the urinary tract in 20 women throughout pregnancy included a single postpartum examination 6 weeks after delivery. The overall trend was that of dilation of the collecting system throughout pregnancy, estimated by measurements of the separation of the pelvicaliceal echo complex, from a mean of 5 mm (first trimester) to 10 mm (third trimester) in the right kidney and from 3 to 4 mm in the left collecting system. Measurements in all but two patients had returned to prepregnancy status at the time of the 6-week postpartum examination. With serial nephrosonography on 24 patients throughout pregnancy and the puerperium,[28] at 12 weeks postpartum, more than half of the patients demonstrated persistence of urinary stasis, described as a slight separation of the renal pelvis. This finding is evidence of hyperdistensibility and suggests that pregnancy has a permanent effect on the size of the upper renal tract. Intravenous urography studies also suggest that subtle anatomic changes take place in the ureters that persist long after the pregnancy has ended. Ureteral tone above the pelvic brim, which in pregnancy is higher than normal, returns to nonpregnant levels immediately after cesarean delivery.

Studies in which water cystometry and uroflowmetry were performed within 48 hours of delivery and again 4 weeks postpartum demonstrated a slight but significant decrease in bladder capacity (from 395.5 to 331 mL) and volume at first void (from 277 to 224 mL) in the study interval. Nevertheless, all the urodynamic values studied were within normal limits on both occasions. The results were not affected by the weight of the infant or by an episiotomy. However, prolonged labor and the use of epidural anesthesia appeared to diminish postpartum bladder function transiently.

The most detailed study of renal function in normal pregnancy is that of Sims and Krantz,[29] who studied 12 patients with serial renal function tests throughout pregnancy and for up to 1 year after delivery. Glomerular filtration, which increased by 50% early in pregnancy and remained elevated until delivery, returned to normal nonpregnant levels by postpartum week 8. Endogenous creatinine clearance, similarly elevated throughout pregnancy, also returned to normal by the eighth postpartum week. Renal plasma flow increased by 25% early in pregnancy, gradually diminished in the third trimester (even when measured in the lateral recumbent position), and continued to decrease to below-normal values in the postpartum period for up to 24 weeks. Normal values were finally established by 50 to 60 weeks after delivery. The reason for the prolonged postpartum depression of renal plasma flow is not clear. Because of the variable changes in renal clearance, mothers who are taking medications in which doses have been changed (because of the physiologic adaptations of pregnancy) will need to have medication levels rechecked. This should be done at 4 to 6 weeks postpartum.

Other Changes

Hair growth is altered in pregnancy and postpartum. After delivery, there is a more rapid hair turnover for up to 3 months. As a greater percentage of hair begins to undergo the growth phase, more hair falls out with combing and brushing. The loss is in a diffuse, not balding, pattern. This transient phenomenon is called *telogen effluvium,* and the patient may be reassured that her hair growth will return to normal within a few months and that the excess hair in the comb or brush will regrow.

Several investigators have reported on bone mineral changes with lactation and the associated amenorrhea. After delivery, there is a generalized decrease in bone mineralization that is temporary and resolves by 12 to 18 months postpartum in most women.[30] Bone loss appears to be greater in the femoral neck than in other areas of the skeleton.[31,32] Calcium supplementation does not seem to ameliorate the bone loss because it is not a problem of inadequate calcium stores, nor does exercise prevent it.[33] For almost all women, the bone loss is self-limited and reversible.

Management of the Puerperium

For most parturients, the immediate puerperium is spent in the hospital or birthing center. The ideal duration of hospitalization for patients with uncomplicated vaginal births has been controversial and culturally determined. During World War II, early discharge with nurse follow-up was initiated to support the "war bride" baby boom.[34] In the 1950s, the lying-in period after delivery was 8 to 14 days.[35] At present, most women stay in the hospital 24 to 48 hours after a vaginal birth. For patients with an uncomplicated postoperative course following cesarean delivery, the postpartum stay is 2 to 4 days. The optimal time is dependent on a patient's needs and home support. About 3% of women who have vaginal deliveries and 9% of women who have cesarean deliveries have at least one childbirth-related complication requiring longer hospitalization after delivery or readmission to the hospital.[36] Studies that have evaluated the safety and outcomes of discharge before 48 hours have relied on nurse or midwife home visits. Unfortunately, most insurers do not cover this service.

In one study, 1249 randomly selected patients were questioned 8 weeks after delivery about health problems that occurred during the puerperium.[37] Eighty-five percent reported at least one problem during their hospitalization, and 76% noted at least one problem that persisted for 8 weeks. A wide range of problems were reported by the patients, including a painful perineum, difficulties with breastfeeding, urinary infections, urinary and fecal incontinence, and headache. Three percent of the patients had been rehospitalized, most commonly for abnormal bleeding or infection. This study draws attention to a substantial amount of symptomatic morbidity that occurs during the puerperium. Although longer hospitalization may not improve perineal pain or incontinence, open lines of communication with patients between discharge and the 6-week visit affect patient self-care and promote a more positive patient experience. In particular, lactation consultation may help to improve effective breastfeeding, and consideration should be given to postponing discharge in primiparas until this service can be performed.

If a patient has adequate support at home (i.e., help with housekeeping and meal preparation), there is little value in an extended hospital stay, provided the mother is adequately educated about infant care and feeding and in the identification of danger signs in either the infant or herself. Except for an increased incidence of rehospitalization of some neonates for hyperbilirubinemia, there are few disadvantages to postpartum hospitalization of less than 48 hours for many patients.[38-41] For mothers who do not have adequate support at home and who are insecure about infant care and feeding, extending the hospital stay will provide time for them to gain adequate education and some measure of self-confidence. Written and video presentations are also efficient means of patient education. To be most helpful, educational material should be presented both before delivery, sometime in the late third trimester, and at the postpartum discharge. Home nursing visits can be helpful in providing support, education, and advice to mothers in selected situations. Written materials or handouts are particularly necessary because memory is temporarily affected by the sleep deprivation that is the rule in the first few days after delivery.

Before discharge, women should be offered any vaccines that may be necessary to protect immunity. MMR (measles, mumps, and rubella) vaccine is given to rubella nonimmune mothers. Hepatitis B, Tdap (tetanus, diphtheria, and pertussis), MMR, and influenza are the four most common vaccines given. All are safe with breastfeeding.[42] Tdap should be given to all women regardless of the interval since the last Td,[43] and varicella vaccine initiated in those with a negative varicella titer.[42]

The time from delivery until complete physiologic involution and psychological adjustment has been called "the fourth trimester."[44] Patients should understand that lochia will persist for 3 to 8 weeks and that on days 7 to 14, there is often an episode of heavy vaginal bleeding, which occurs when the placental eschar sloughs. Tampons are permissible if they are comfortable upon insertion and are changed frequently and if there are no perineal, vaginal, or cervical lacerations, which preclude insertion of a tampon until healing has occurred. Physical activity, including walking up and down stairs, lifting moderately heavy objects, riding in or driving a car, and performing muscle-toning exercises can be resumed without delay if the delivery has been uncomplicated. Minig and associates reviewed the scientific evidence behind many postpartum recommendations.[45] They noted that very few, if any, of the traditional recommendations are evidence based. Lifting, sexual activity, driving, and exercise do not need to be overly restricted, even for women after cesarean births. Instructions regarding exercise are patient specific. Studies have found that exercise postpartum has no affect on lactation and may decrease anxiety levels as well as decrease symptoms of postpartum depression.[46-48] As such, exercise may have benefits beyond the mother's desire to "get back into shape." The most troublesome complaint is lethargy and fatigue. Consequently, every task or activity should be a brief one in the first few days of the puerperium. Mothers whose lethargy persists beyond several weeks must be evaluated, especially for thyroid dysfunction and postpartum depression.

Sexual activity may be resumed when the perineum is comfortable and when bleeding has diminished. The desire and willingness to resume sexual activity in the puerperium varies greatly among women, depending on the site and state of healing of perineal or vaginal incisions and lacerations, the amount of vaginal atrophy secondary to breastfeeding, and the return of libido,[49] which is greatly affected by sleep patterns among other new issues. Although the median time to resuming intercourse after delivery is 6 to 7 weeks, about half of women who do so have dyspareunia. In a substantial number, dyspareunia lasts for a year or more.[50,51] Signorello and coworkers[52] noted a 2.5-fold increased risk for dyspareunia 6 months after operative vaginal delivery compared with other subsets of postpartum women. For all women, breastfeeding at 6 months is associated with a more than fourfold increase in dyspareunia. Similarly, a large review of studies examining postpartum sexuality noted the greatest incidence of sexual dysfunction to be associated with operative vaginal delivery.[53] In contrast, 25% of all women reported a heightened sexual pleasure 6 months after delivery. Postpartum dyspareunia is not always related to vulvar trauma and occurs in some women who have a cesarean delivery. Dyspareunia has also been observed in women who use oral contraceptives and do not breastfeed, suggesting that lack of estrogen effect on the vagina is not the major cause of postpartum dyspareunia. In a study of 50 parturients, Ryding[54] found that 20% had little desire for sexual activity 3 months after delivery, and an additional 21% had complete loss of desire or aversion to sexual activity. This variation in attitude, desire, and willingness must be acknowledged when counseling women about the resumption of sexual activity. Women who breastfeed tend to begin intercourse later than average, and women who deliver by cesarean section tend to begin sooner.[55] Clinicians commonly advise pregnant women on the use of vaginal lubricants for sexual activity in the first few months postpartum, because of the decreased natural lubrication with lower estrogen levels. This may be included in the written handouts given to patients when they go home. Astroglide gel and Comfort are more commonly recommended lubricants. KY Jelly is typically too dry. If patients are using barrier contraception, they should be advised against the use of petroleum-based lubricants such as Vaseline (Unilever, London, UK). If dyspareunia persists, a small amount of estrogen cream applied daily to the vagina may be helpful in breastfeeding women with atrophic changes. Clinicians may also counsel women about using different sexual positions with male partners, if deeper penetration is uncomfortable.[45]

Many patients return to work situations outside the home after their pregnancies. Frequently, the physician must complete insurance or employer forms to establish maternity leave for patients. As mentioned earlier, the 6-week return in the United States is derived from tradition, and 8 weeks are often allowed after a cesarean birth. Women will often experience discomfort, tiredness, and breast soreness well beyond 6 weeks. Similar to the return to exercise and sexual activity, the return to work should be individualized. Other nations and cultures have different standards for returning to prepregnancy routines. In China, 30 days is common, and in Western Europe and Canada, many months and even up to a year of maternity leave is offered.

HEALTH MAINTENANCE

The first follow-up visit is scheduled at the time of discharge. Many women without complications, who are multiparous, can be seen at 6 weeks. Other women, primiparous women, those with complicated labor and deliveries, those with increased pain, and those at risk for depression should be seen 2 weeks after discharge. At this visit, breastfeeding can be addressed as well as incisional checks and assessment of mood. Studies have shown that a routine postpartum visit to the physician at 1 or 2 weeks after delivery or a home visit by a nurse midwife does little to reduce maternal or infant morbidity.[56,57] However, for the patient with antepartum or intrapartum difficulties, this early postpartum visit or home visit by a nurse or nurse midwife is more productive in detecting problems and providing support for the mother. Thus, the need for this visit should be individualized.[58] Late puerperal infections, postpartum depression, and problems with infant care and feeding often occur before the 6-week postpartum visit. Open-ended questions should be asked to detect problems.

Women should also be seen about 6 weeks after delivery. At this visit, questions regarding depression, energy, sexuality, contraception, and future pregnancies should be addressed. Unfortunately, many women skip their 6-week postpartum check, deferring questions of contraception. A copy of the Edinburgh Postnatal Depression Scale (EPDS) is provided in Table 22-2. It may be used as a fast, reliable, and user-friendly tool to screen for depression. It is helpful to solicit questions about the delivery because women may be hesitant to ask them spontaneously, especially regarding sexuality and incontinence. If there are health issues that need addressing, such as glucose screens, thyroid levels, or other tests, they may be performed or scheduled at this visit.

TABLE 22-2 EDINBURGH POSTNATAL DEPRESSION SCALE

In the past 7 days:

1. I have been able to laugh and see the funny side of things:
   _ As much as I always could
   _ Not quite so much now
   _ Definitely not so much now
   _ Not at all
2. I have looked forward with enjoyment to things:
   _ As much as I ever did
   _ Rather less than I used to
   _ Definitely less than I used to
   _ Hardly at all
3. I have blamed myself unnecessarily when things went wrong:
   _ Yes, most of the time
   _ Yes, some of the time
   _ Not very often
   _ No, never
4. I have been anxious or worried for no good reason:
   _ No, not at all
   _ Hardly ever
   _ Yes, sometimes
   _ Yes, very often
5. I have felt scared or panicky for no very good reason:
   _ Yes, quite a lot
   _ Yes, sometimes
   _ No, not much
   _ No, not at all
6. Things have been getting on top of me:
   _ Yes, most of the time I haven't been able to cope at all
   _ Yes, sometimes I haven't been coping as well as usual
   _ No, most of the time I have coped quite well
   _ No, I have been coping as well as ever
7. I have been so unhappy that I have had difficulty sleeping:
   _ Yes, most of the time
   _ Yes, sometimes
   _ Not very often
   _ No, not at all
8. I have felt sad or miserable:
   _ Yes, most of the time
   _ Yes, quite often
   _ Not very often
   _ No, not at all
9. I have been so unhappy that I have been crying:
   _ Yes, most of the time
   _ Yes, quite often
   _ Only occasionally
   _ No, never
10. The thought of harming myself has occurred to me:
   _ Yes, quite often
   _ Sometimes
   _ Hardly ever
   _ Never

Response categories are scored 0, 1, 2, and 3 according to increased severity of the symptom. Items 3 and 5-10 are reverse scored (3, 2, 1, 0). The total score is calculated by adding together the scores for each of the 10 items.

From Cox JL, Holden JM, Sagovsky R: Detection of postnatal depression: development of the 10-item Edinburgh Postnatal Depression Scale. Br J Psychiatry 150:782, 1987.

Women with chronic medical diseases, such as collagen vascular disease, autoimmune disorders, and neurologic conditions, should be seen at close intervals because many patients with these disorders may experience flares of their symptoms after delivery. Ideally, these visits should be scheduled in advance with the patient's primary care or subspecialty physician. Prophylactic therapy is not recommended for women with systemic lupus erythematosus or multiple sclerosis. However, warning patients to be attuned to signs and symptoms that reflect a flare of their illness allows for early and more effective interventions. For women with epilepsy, special attention to medication doses with the changing renal clearance is necessary. Additionally, increased postpartum sleep deprivation may induce a lower seizure threshold.

Perineal Care

Many women who give birth have lacerations of the perineum or vagina. In the United States, when an episiotomy is needed, it is more often performed as midline than as a mediolateral incision. Provided that the incision or the laceration does not extend beyond the transverse perineal muscle, that there is no hematoma or extensive ecchymosis, and a satisfactory repair has been accomplished, there is little need for perineal care beyond routine cleansing with a bath or shower. Analgesia can be accomplished in most patients with nonsteroidal anti-inflammatory drugs such as ibuprofen or naproxen sodium. These drugs are superior to acetaminophen or propoxyphene for episiotomy pain and uterine cramping. Furthermore, because of a low milk-to-maternal plasma drug concentration ratio, a short half-life, and transformation into glucuronide metabolites, ibuprofen is safe for nursing mothers.

A patient who has had a mediolateral episiotomy, third- or fourth-degree perineal laceration, periurethral lacerations, or extensive perineal bruising may experience considerable perineal pain.[59] Occasionally, the pain and periurethral swelling prevent the patient from voiding, making urethral catheterization necessary. When a patient complains of inordinate perineal pain, the first and most important step is to reexamine the perineum, vagina, and rectum to detect and drain a hematoma or to identify a perineal infection. Perineal pain may be the first symptom of the rare but potentially fatal complications of angioedema, necrotizing fasciitis, or perineal cellulitis.

In cases of moderate perineal pain, sitz baths will provide additional pain relief. Although hot sitz baths have long been customary therapy for perineal pain, there is rationale for using cold or "iced" sitz baths. This therapy is similar to that for the treatment of athletic injuries, for which considerable success has been achieved with cold therapy. Cold provides immediate pain relief as a result of decreased excitability of free nerve endings and decreased nerve conduction. Further pain relief comes from local vasoconstriction, which reduces edema, inhibits hematoma formation, and decreases muscle irritability and spasm. Patients who have alternated using hot and cold sitz baths usually prefer the cold. The technique for administering a cold sitz bath is first to have the patient sit in a tub of water at room temperature to which ice cubes are then added. This avoids the sensation of sudden immersion in ice water. The patient remains in the ice water for 20 to 30 minutes. Patients with perineal incisions or lacerations should be advised to postpone sexual intercourse until there is no perineal discomfort. Tampons may be inserted whenever the patient is comfortable doing so. However, to avoid any risk for toxic shock syndrome, the use of tampons should be confined to the daytime to prevent leaving a tampon in the vagina for prolonged periods.

Frequently, what appears to be severe perineal pain is, in fact, the pain of prolapsed hemorrhoids. Witch hazel compresses, suppositories containing corticosteroids, or local anesthetic sprays or emollients may be helpful. Occasionally, a thrombus occurs in a prolapsed hemorrhoid. It is a simple task to remove the thrombus through a small scalpel incision using local anesthesia by an obstetrician trained in this procedure or a general surgeon. Dramatic relief of pain usually follows this procedure. Stool softeners, laxatives, or both should be discussed for women with hemorrhoids.

Urinary and anal incontinence is a significant problem in women after delivery. Weidner and colleagues[60] studied 58 primiparous women after delivery. They found that 14 of 58 had levator ani neuropathy at 6 weeks. Seventeen of the 58 women had the neuropathy unresolved at 6 months postpartum. Elective cesarean delivery was protective for neuropathy in this series, yet labor with subsequent cesarean delivery was not protective. About one third of women at 8 weeks and 15% of women at 12 weeks have urinary incontinence. The incontinence, as would be expected, has a very detrimental effect on quality of life.[61] A strong predictor for incontinence after delivery is a history of prior urinary incontinence or new-onset incontinence during the index pregnancy. In addition to urinary incontinence, about 5% of women have anal incontinence 3 months after vaginal birth, with most experiencing flatal rather than fecal incontinence.[62,63] Forceps-assisted, but not vacuum-assisted, vaginal delivery is associated with an twofold increased risk for fecal incontinence in primparas.[64] Similarly, anal sphincter disruption in nulliparas is associated with a 2.3-fold increase in anal incontinence 5 years after delivery.[65] Nulliparous women with sphincter disruption or operative vaginal delivery should be screened specifically for symptoms at follow-up visits.

Perineal exercises were developed by Kegel in 1948 and involve voluntary contraction of the pelvic floor. A recent meta-analysis reviewed the effectiveness of perineal exercise in treating incontinence. Harvey's review[63] found that only when the exercises are performed with a vaginal biofeedback device was there improvement in the incidence of urinary incontinence. If symptoms of either urinary or flatal incontinence persist for more than 6 months, studies should be undertaken to define the specific neuromuscular or anatomic abnormality so that the appropriate pharmacologic, biophysical, or surgical treatment can begin. Women should be counseled regarding this plan at their postpartum visit so that they can return if symptoms persist.

Delayed Postpartum Hemorrhage and Postpartum Anemia

The causes and management of immediate postpartum hemorrhage are discussed in Chapter 19. Delayed postpartum uterine bleeding of sufficient quantity to require medical attention occurs in 1% to 2% of patients. One of the most common causes of postpartum hemorrhage that occurs 2 to 5 days after delivery is von Willebrand disease. Von Willebrand factor increases in pregnancy, and thus excessive bleeding usually does not occur in the first 48 hours after birth. Women presenting with bleeding more than 48 hours after delivery should be screened for this condition.

Delayed bleeding occurs most frequently between days 8 and 14 of the puerperium.[66] Significant bleeding may require treatment with uterotonic agents or curettage. When suction evacuation and curettage are performed, retained gestational products, usually in small amounts, will be found in about 40% of cases.[67,68] Whether small placental remnants are the cause is not known. In the management of patients with heavy delayed bleeding, ultrasound examination usually determines whether there is a significant amount of retained material, although it is sometimes difficult to distinguish between blood clot and retained placental fragments (see Figure 22-1). Suction evacuation of the uterus is successful in arresting the bleeding in almost all cases whether or not there is histologic confirmation of retained gestational products. If curettage is required at this time, especially if a sharp curette is used, a course of broad-spectrum antibiotics with anaerobic coverage should be initiated before surgery, for their possible benefit in reducing the formation of uterine synechiae and the sequelae of Asherman syndrome. The curettage should be performed with care because the postpartum uterine wall is soft and easier to perforate. In those rare instances in which delayed postpartum hemorrhage does not respond to the use of oxytocic agents and curettage, selective arterial embolization may be effective in controlling the bleeding. Women with postpartum hemorrhage, and subsequent anemia, often have excessive fatigue in the postpartum period. Some investigators have advocated the use of recombinant erythropoietin as well as parenteral iron as alternatives to transfusion for symptomatic women with anemia.

Postpartum Infection

Although the standard definition of postpartum febrile morbidity is a temperature of 38° C (100.4° F) or higher on any two of the first 10 days after delivery, exclusive of the first 24 hours, most clinicians do not wait 2 full days to begin evaluation and treatment of patients who develop a fever in the puerperium. The most common cause of postpartum fever is endometritis, which occurs after vaginal delivery in about 2% of patients and after cesarean delivery in about 10% to 15%. The differential diagnosis includes urinary tract infection, lower genital tract infection, wound infections, pulmonary infections, thrombophlebitis, and mastitis. The diagnosis and management of postpartum infection are discussed in detail in Chapter 51. Almost all antibiotics are safe with lactation, and these are discussed in Chapter 8.

Maternal-Infant Attachment

Klaus and colleagues[69] were among the first investigators to study maternal-infant attachment and to bring attention to the importance of the first few hours of maternal-infant association. Their studies, as well as those of others, have contributed substantially to major changes in hospital policies dealing with patients in labor and delivery and postpartum. It is now recognized that there should be constant opportunities for parents to be with their newborns, particularly from the first few moments after birth and as frequently as possible during the first days thereafter. Immediate skin-to-skin contact is recommended. These associations are usually characterized by fondling, kissing, cuddling, and gazing at the infant, which are manifestations of maternal commitment and protectiveness toward her infant. Separation of mother and infant in the first hours after birth has been shown to diminish or delay the development of these characteristic mothering behaviors,[70] a problem that is intensified when medical, obstetrical, or newborn complications require intensive care for either the mother or her newborn infant.

Robson and Powell[71] summarized the literature on early maternal attachment and emphasized how difficult it is to perform valid research studies about this phenomenon, because of the multiple confounders. Although it is generally agreed that early association of the mother and infant is beneficial and should not be interfered with unnecessarily, there are still doubts about the long-term implications, if any, of a lack of early maternal-infant association. In their monograph summarizing their investigations about parent-infant attachment, Klaus and Kennel[72] warn against drawing far-reaching conclusions. Although favoring the theory of a "sensitive period" soon after birth, during which close parent-infant interaction facilitates subsequent attachment and beneficial parenting behavior, these investigators concur that humans are highly adaptable and state that "there are many fail-safe routes to attachment." Many hospitals and birth centers have recognized and placed emphasis on the mother-baby interactions in the first several hours after delivery. Delaying the first bath, eliminating well-baby nurseries, putting the baby onto the mother's chest in skin-to-skin contact (even during cesarean birth), and keeping the baby in the room with the mother during the first pediatric evaluation are all steps to support and promote that interaction.

The modern maternity unit should enhance and encourage parent-infant attachment by such policies as free visiting hours for the other parent and having the other parent rooming in with the mother and baby whenever possible, encouragement of the infant rooming with the mother, and strongly supportive attitudes about breastfeeding. These policies also allow the nursing staff to observe parenting behavior and to identify inept, inexperienced, or inappropriate behavior toward the infant. Some situations may call for more intensive follow-up by visiting nurses, home health visitors, or social workers to provide further support for the family during the posthospital convalescence. The role of postpartum home visits in enhancing parenting behavior is controversial. Gray and colleagues[73] found this approach beneficial. Siegel and coworkers[74] studied the effect of early and prolonged mother-infant contact in the hospital and a postpartum visitation program on attachment and parenting behavior. They found that early and prolonged maternal-infant contact in the hospital had a significant effect on enhancing subsequent parenting behavior, but the postpartum home visitations had no impact.

The development of the qualities associated with good parenting depends on many factors. Certainly, it does not depend solely on what transpires in the few hours surrounding the birth experience. There is evidence that specific identification of an infant with its mother's voice begins in utero during the third trimester. Furthermore, the parents' own experiences as children, as well as their intellectual and emotional attitudes about children, must play a large role in their own parenting behavior. Areskog and associates[75] showed that women who expressed fear of childbirth during the antenatal period had more complications and more pain in labor and also had more difficulties in attachment to their infants. Consequently, the peripartum period provides opportunities to enhance parenting behavior and to identify families for which follow-up after birth may be necessary to ensure the most favorable child development. For example, adolescents, particularly primiparous adolescents, are a particularly high-risk group. Rates of domestic abuse are especially high in adolescent mothers.

In summary, the postpartum ward should be an environment that provides parents ample opportunity to interact with their newborn infant. Personnel, including nurses, nurses' aides, and physicians caring for mothers and infants should be alert to signs of abnormal parenting (e.g., refusal of the mother to care for the infant, the use of negative or abusive names in describing or referring to the infant, inordinate delay in naming the infant, or obsessive and unrealistic concerns about the infant's health). These or other signs that maternal-infant attachment is delayed or endangered are as deserving of frequent follow-up during the postpartum period as are any of the traditional medical or obstetric complications.

Lactation and breastfeeding are reviewed in detail in Chapter 23. All cultures have emphasized the importance of breastfeeding. There are multiple steps that should be taken during the postpartum period to promote and enhance breastfeeding. The use of audiovisual aids, telephone hotlines, and in-service training for personnel have been shown to increase the incidence of successful breastfeeding (see Chapter 23).

PREGNANCY PREVENTION AND BIRTH CONTROL

The immediate postpartum period is a convenient time for a discussion of family planning with patients; however, ideally these conversations should begin during prenatal care. The period of anovulation infertility lasts from 5 weeks in nonlactating women to 8 weeks or more in women who breastfeed their infants without supplementation. With exclusive breastfeeding, the pregnancy rate during lactational amenorrhea is 1% at 1 year postpartum.[76] Exclusive breastfeeding for this period of time is uncommon, and women are unlikely to know the actual duration they will breastfeed at hospital discharge. Even for women who leave the hospital breastfeeding exclusively, most will stop breastfeeding or begin supplementation by 6 weeks postpartum, especially if they return to work. Most women have resumed intercourse by 3 months, and for some, resumption of sexual activity begins much earlier.[77] Consequently, it is important that a decision be made about pregnancy prevention before the patient leaves the hospital, even though it is usually the last thing on a new mother's mind. Part of the discussion about contraception should include recommendations about pregnancy intervals. Short pregnancy intervals (time between births of less than 16 months) are associated with poorer sibling health, higher miscarriage rates, higher stillbirth rates, and many other adverse pregnancy outcomes.[78]

A patient should be made aware of the various options of pregnancy prevention and birth control in terms that she and her partner can understand. This may be done by individual instruction from nurses, physicians, or midwives or by a variety of films or videotapes. One study found that written material, plus a discussion, given at the time of hospitalization is most helpful to mothers. The decision about family planning methods depends on the patient's motivation, number of children, state of health, whether she is breastfeeding, and the religious background of the couple. It cannot be assumed that because a woman has used a method of contraception effectively before the current pregnancy she will need no counseling thereafter. More than half of patients change contraceptive techniques between pregnancies.

Natural Methods

The natural family planning methods, which depend on predicting the time of ovulation by use of basal body temperature or assessment of cervical mucus, cannot be used until regular menstrual cycles have resumed. In the first weeks or months following birth, provided there is little or no supplemental feeding for the infant, breastfeeding will provide 98% contraceptive protection for up to 6 months. At 6 months, or if menses return, or if breastfeeding ceases to be full or nearly full before the sixth month, the risk for pregnancy increases. Once regular menses have resumed, natural family planning methods, which depend on detection of the periovulation period using changes in cervical mucus or basal body temperature, or both, can be employed. However, it is important to note that a woman will have ovulated once before the resumption of normal menses as a warning flag. In women with regular cycles, for whom periods of abstinence are acceptable to her and to her partner, natural family planning techniques are associated with pregnancy rates very close to those for barrier methods of contraception (with spermicides).

Barrier Methods

Barrier methods of contraception and vaginal spermicides were long used in Europe and England before they were manufactured in this country beginning in the 1920s. The failure rate for the diaphragm varies from 2.4 to 19.6 per 100 woman-years. Because this method of contraception requires substantial motivation, instruction, and experience, it is more effective in older women who are familiar with the technique. The failure rate was 2.4 per 100 woman-years among diaphragm users who were older than 25 years of age and who had a minimum of 5 months' experience using it. The proper size of the diaphragm should be determined at the 6-week postpartum visit, even in patients who previously used this form of contraception. In women who are breastfeeding, anovulation leads to vaginal dryness and tightness, which may make the proper fitting of a diaphragm more difficult. The diaphragm should be used with one of the spermicidal lubricants, all of which contain nonoxynol-9.

The use of condoms alone or in combination with spermicides is often advised for women who wish to postpone a decision about sterilization or oral contraceptive therapy until the postpartum visit. Pregnancy rates for the condom are reported to be from 1.6 to 21 per 100 woman-years, depending on the age and motivation of the population studied.

Hormonal Contraceptive Medications

The combined estrogen-progestin preparations have proved to be the most effective method of contraception, with pregnancy rates reported as less than 0.5 per 100 woman-years. Most compounds include 35 mcg or less of estrogen and varying amounts of progestins. Compounds containing the progestational components desogestrel, gestodene, or norgestimate appear to be less androgenic and have less impact on carbohydrate and lipid metabolism than compounds containing levonorgestrel or norethindrone. Cardiovascular complications, including hypertension, venous thrombosis, stroke, and myocardial infarction, have been substantially reduced with the reduction in estrogen content. The cardiovascular complications are found predominantly in women who smoke or have a family history of thromboembolic disease. However, all women have an increased risk for thrombosis in the early postpartum time period. In nonsmoking women, the risk-to-benefit ratio is clearly in favor of using oral contraceptive agents. This is particularly true when the additional benefits of these agents are considered, which include lowered risks for benign breast disease, ovarian and endometrial cancer, iron deficiency anemia, toxic shock syndrome, pelvic inflammatory disease, and ectopic pregnancy.

In patients who are not breastfeeding, combined hormonal contraceptive agents, oral, vaginal, or transdermal, can be taken as early as 2 to 3 weeks after delivery.[79] The effect of oral contraceptive agents on lactation is controversial. Controlled studies of the combined-type oral contraceptive agents with doses of ethinyl estradiol or mestranol of 50 mcg or more demonstrated a suppressive effect on lactation. The common contraceptives with 35 mcg or less of estrogen still have some suppressive effects. Progestin-only medications (e.g., norethindrone, 0.35 mg every day) do not diminish lactation performance and may, in fact, increase the quality and duration of lactation. There is no evidence that progestin-only contraceptive agents taken before the onset of lactation affect lactation success. A study by Halderman and Nelson[80] found that initiation of progestin-only contraception at the time of hospital discharge did not affect lactation patterns, incidence of supplementation, or discontinuation of breastfeeding. However, most clinicians begin low-dose progestin pills at 4 weeks postpartum. Depot medroxyprogesterone acetate (DMPA), 150 mg intramuscularly every 3 months, which has a contraceptive efficiency exceeding 99%, may be used with lactation as well.[81] The most troublesome side effect is unpredictable spotting and bleeding. The major advantages of this form of contraception are the ease of administration and patient convenience. Progestin-only oral contraceptives should be avoided in Hispanic women with gestational diabetes who are breastfeeding, because of an increased risk for the subsequent development of type 2 diabetes.[82]

Diaz and coworkers[83] studied the effect of a low-dose combination oral contraceptive containing 0.03 mg ethinyl estradiol and 0.15 mg levonorgestrel. The medication was begun after all women had been nursing for 1 month. Among those women taking the oral contraceptive medications, there was a small but significant decrease in lactation performance and in the weight gain of their infants compared with controls. In women whose motivation to breastfeed is marginal, the slight inhibition of lactation induced by oral contraceptive agents may be sufficient to discourage them from continuing to nurse their infants, so progestin-only preparations may be offered to these women. Combined hormonal vaginal rings begun less than 1 month after delivery may be problematic in some women, because of slower perineal and vaginal healing. However, in the nonlactating mother, use at 2 to 3 weeks is reasonable if there is no discomfort. Recent work by Espey and colleagues in a randomized controlled study showed similar effects on lactation between combined oral contraceptive and progestin only.[83a]

Levonorgestrel subdermal implants were approved by the U.S. Food and Drug Administration for contraceptive use in the United States in 1990.[84] Implants inserted 4 weeks after delivery have no effect on lactation or growth of an infant who is nursing, even though small amounts of levonorgestrel are excreted in the milk. Although the usual time of insertion is 4 to 6 weeks after delivery, the implants can be inserted in the immediate puerperium in women who are breastfeeding. Irregular uterine bleeding, expense, and the occasional difficulty in removing the implants are the major drawbacks to the use of this form of contraception. Despite the proven contraceptive effectiveness of levonorgestrel implants, there has been a decline in the perceived desirability of this method of birth control in recent years.[85] The contraceptive patch has not been well studied in the postpartum period for its effects on lactation. Many clinicians assume that it will have a lesser effect than oral contraceptives. Because it still may have some effects, it is reasonable to wait to initiate use after lactation has been established.

Intrauterine Devices

The copper-containing and progesterone-releasing intrauterine devices (IUDs) are highly effective in preventing pregnancy at rates that are comparable to tubal ligation (<1 pregnancy per 100 woman-years), yet with the added benefit of reversibility. The IUD is an ideal form of birth control in breastfeeding mothers, because of its lack of effect on milk production. Breastfeeding does not increase the risk for expulsion or other complications regardless of the time of insertion of the device. Significant complications of the IUD are infrequent and include uterine perforation (<0.7%), expulsion (5% to 10%), and discontinuation secondary to side effects (4% to 14%).[86] All women receiving an IUD should be counseled to present immediately to their physician if they suspect pregnancy so that the location of the pregnancy can be determined without delay.

Increased vaginal bleeding is noted in some women using copper-containing IUDs, but vaginal bleeding is decreased in women using progesterone-containing IUDs. Therefore, a woman's menstrual history is helpful in determining which type of IUD is ideal for her situation and decreasing copper IUD removal secondary to vaginal bleeding or dysmenorrhea.[87] Similarly, women who will be uncomfortable with amenorrhea should not be counseled for a progesterone-containing IUD. Contraindications to IUD insertion include postpartum endometritis, uterine anomalies, incomplete uterine involution, and for IUDs containing copper, Wilson disease or a known allergy to copper. Syncope as a result of the vagal response at the time of IUD insertion is uncommon with IUD insertion at 6 weeks, given that the cervix remains slightly dilated.[88,89] Insertion of the IUD immediately after delivery is an alternative strategy.[90] Surprisingly, this practice is associated with fewer perforations than are insertions between 1 and 8 weeks. Not surprising, however, is the finding of a higher expulsion rate (10% to 21%).

The investigations of Alvarez and associates[91] convincingly support the concept that the principal mode of action of IUDs is by a method other than destruction of live embryos. Both the World Health Organization and the American College of Obstetricians and Gynecologists have reviewed the evidence and concluded that the IUD is not an abortifacient.[92]

Sterilization

Tubal sterilization is the most frequently used method of contraception in the United States. The puerperium is a convenient time for tubal ligation procedures to be performed in women who desire sterilization. The procedure can be performed at the time of a cesarean delivery or within the first 24 to 48 hours after delivery. In some hospitals, the operation is performed immediately after delivery in uncomplicated patients, especially when epidural anesthesia was given for labor analgesia. With the use of small paraumbilical incision, the procedure seldom prolongs the patient's hospitalization.

The 10-year failure rate of postpartum partial salpingectomy is 0.75%. There are several modifications of this procedure: the Pomeroy, Parkland, Uchida, and Irving (see Chapter 20). Because of the relaxed abdominal wall and the easy accessibility of the fallopian tubes, the minilaparotomy has the advantages of convenience and speed without the possible risks for visceral injury that might occur with the trocar of the laparoscope. More important than the type of procedure is the discussion with the mother about the timing of the procedure. Puerperal sterilization compared with interval sterilization is associated with an increased incidence of guilt and regret. Postponing tubal ligation procedures until 6 to 8 weeks after delivery is less convenient but does provide time to ensure that the infant is healthy and to review all the implications of the decision. Importantly, interval tubal ligation may not be covered by Medicaid in some states. Laparoscopic tubal ligation can be accomplished as an outpatient procedure, with a minimum of morbidity.

The risks of tubal ligation procedures, whether performed in the puerperium or as an interval procedure, include the short-term problems of anesthetic accidents, hemorrhage, injury of the viscera, and infection. These complications are infrequent, and deaths from the procedure occur in 2 to 12 per 100,000 procedures. Long-term complications are less well defined and more controversial. About 10% to 15% of patients have irregular menses and increased menstrual pain after tubal sterilization. This so-called posttubal syndrome is sufficiently severe in some cases to require hysterectomy. Well-controlled prospective studies, however, have failed to provide convincing evidence that these symptoms occur more commonly after tubal sterilization than in control patients of the same age and previous menstrual history.[93]

There has also been concern about poststerilization depression. Because depression is common in women of childbearing age and is even more common in the puerperium, it is unlikely that sterilization procedures are independent risk factors for depression. It is obvious, however, that the loss of fertility associated with a sterilization procedure will have important conscious and subconscious implications for many women. Therefore, it is not surprising that some patients manifest transient grief reactions in response to tubal ligation. The loss of libido that may occur in such situations may be frightening to some women and equally disturbing to their partners. Reassurance that such reactions are temporary and are not necessarily symptoms of a seriously disturbed psyche is an important means of support during this crisis. Both partners must be aware of the dynamics of this situation to avoid a sense of estrangement.

Obstetricians must remember that vasectomy is often a more advisable and desirable alternative for a couple considering sterilization.[94,95] It can be performed as an outpatient procedure under local anesthesia with insignificant loss of time from work or family. Furthermore, almost all the failures (about 3 to 4 per 1000 procedures) can be detected by a postoperative semen analysis. This is a decided advantage over the tubal ligation, in which failures are discovered only when a pregnancy occurs. Furthermore, vasectomy is less expensive and overall is associated with fewer complications. In addition, women whose husbands undergo vasectomy are less likely to have hysterectomies than are women who have had tubal sterilization.[96] Studies of long-term health effects of vasectomy found no evidence of an increased risk for atherosclerotic heart disease or other chronic illnesses.[94,97]

Tubal ligation can be reversed but is expensive and often not covered by insurance. A patient should not undergo sterilization if she is contemplating reversal. Success as measured by the occurrence of pregnancy following tubal reanastomosis varies from 40% to 85%, depending on the type of tubal ligation performed and on the length of functioning tube that remains. Success rates for vas reanastomosis vary from 37% to 90%, with higher success rates being associated with shorter intervals from the time of vas ligation.

Hysterectomy has been advocated as a means of sterilization that has the advantage of protecting the patient from future uterine or cervical cancer. However, the morbidity of cesarean or puerperal hysterectomy operations is sufficiently great to preclude their consideration for elective sterilization.[98]

POSTPARTUM PSYCHOLOGICAL REACTIONS

The psychological reactions experienced following childbirth include the common, relatively mild, physiologic, and transient "maternity blues" (50% to 70% of women), true depression occurring in 8% to 20% of women, and frank puerperal psychosis occurring in 0.14% to 0.26%. These problems are discussed in Chapter 52. In patients with underlying depression, in those with a previous history of postpartum depression, and in those who report symptoms that develop during the immediate postpartum period, it is essential that a postpartum visit be scheduled sooner than the traditional 6 weeks. Other risk factors for postpartum depression include a family history of depression, a mother with postpartum depression, a poor social situation, and prolonged separation from her infant. The moderately depressed mother often experiences such guilt and embarrassment secondary to her sense of failure in her mothering role that she will be unable to call her physician or admit the symptoms of her depression. Consequently, ample time must be set aside to explore in depth even the slightest symptoms or sign of depression. Home visits in this situation may be appropriate to assess the patient. When a patient calls with a seemingly innocuous question, she should be asked two or three open-ended questions about her general status. These questions allow the patient to open up if there is an underlying depression that she is too guilty or afraid to express initially; for example:

1. How do you feel things are going?
2. How are things with the baby?
3. Are you feeling like you expected?

Because nursing staff often triage phone calls for physicians and midwives, it is important that such personnel be instructed to be alert to this protocol. Additionally, we recommend that both parents be warned before hospital discharge that if the maternity blues seem to be lasting longer than 2 weeks, or become "too tough" to handle, then either partner should call. An easy screening depression scale, the EPDS, is shown in Table 22-2. Puerperal thyroid disease will often present with symptoms that include mild dysphoria; consequently, thyroid function studies are suggested in the evaluation of patients with suspected postpartum depression that occurs 2 to 3 months after delivery.

MANAGING PERINATAL GRIEVING

For the most part, perinatal events are happy ones and are occasions for rejoicing. When a patient and her family experience a loss associated with a pregnancy, special attention must be given to the grieving patient and her family.

The most obvious cases of perinatal loss are those in which a fetal or neonatal death has occurred. Other, more subtle losses can be associated with a significant amount of grieving, such as the birth of a critically ill or malformed infant, an unexpected hysterectomy performed for intractable postpartum hemorrhage, or even a planned postpartum sterilization procedure. Grief occurs with any significant loss, whether it is the actual death of an infant or the loss of an idealized child in the case of the birth of a handicapped infant.

Mourning is as old as the human race, but the clinical signs and symptoms of grief and their psychological ramifications as they relate to loss suffered by women during their pregnancies have been given special consideration in recent years. In studying the relatives of servicemen who died in World War II, Lindemann recognized five manifestations of normal grieving. These include somatic symptoms of sleeplessness, fatigue, digestive symptoms, and sighing respirations; preoccupation with the image of the deceased; feelings of guilt; feelings of hostility and anger toward others; and disruption of the normal pattern of daily life. He also described the characteristics of what is now recognized as pathologic grief, which may occur if acute mourning is suppressed or interrupted. Some of the manifestations of this so-called morbid grief reaction are overactivity without a sense of loss; appearance or exacerbations of psychosomatic illness; alterations in relationships with friends and relatives; furious hostility toward specific persons; lasting loss of patterns of social interaction; activities detrimental to personal, social, and economic existence; and agitated depression.

Kennel and associates[99] studied the reaction of 20 mothers to the loss of their newborn infants. Characteristic signs and symptoms of mourning occurred in all the patients, even in situations in which the infant was nonviable. Similar grief reactions occurred in most of the parents of 101 critically ill infants who survived after referral to a regional neonatal intensive care unit, showing that separation from a seriously ill newborn is sufficient to provoke typical grief reaction. **Interestingly, studies over the last 15 years have found that women who do not see their stillborn infant actually have less depression; this suggests that best practice is to give mothers the choice of seeing their infant after delivery, and to hold their child, but not to necessarily encourage them to do it.**

It is important that the characteristics of the grieving patient be recognized and understood by health professionals caring for such patients; otherwise, substantial misunderstanding and mismanagement of the patient will occur. For example, if the patient's reaction of anger and hostility is not anticipated, a nurse or physician may take personally statements or actions by the patient or her family and avoid the patient at the very time she needs the most consolation and support. Because of their own discomfort with the implications of death, physicians, nurses, and others on the postpartum unit often find it uncomfortable to deal with patients whose fetus or infant has died. As a consequence, there is a reluctance to discuss the death with the patient and a tendency to rely on the use of sedatives or tranquilizers to deal with the patient's symptoms of grief. What is actually beneficial at such a time is a sympathetic listener and an opportunity to express and discuss feelings of guilt, anger, and hopelessness and the other symptoms of mourning.

It is not surprising that postpartum depression is more common and more severe in families that have suffered a perinatal loss. In one study, the prolonged grief response occurred more often in those women who became pregnant within 5 months of the death of the infant. This finding suggests that in counseling women after the loss of an infant, one should avoid the traditional advice of encouraging the family to embark soon on another pregnancy as a "replacement" for the infant who died. Just how long the normal grief reaction lasts is not known, and surely it varies with different families. Lockwood and Lewis[100] studied 26 patients who had suffered a stillbirth; they followed several patients for as long as 2 years. Their data suggest that grief in this situation is usually resolved within 18 months, invariably with a resurgence of symptoms at the first anniversary of the loss.

Somatic symptoms of grief, such as anorexia, weakness, and fatigue, are now well recognized; other psychological manifestations are also reported. Spontaneous abortion

TABLE 22-3 GUIDELINES FOR MANAGING PERINATAL LOSS

Keep parents informed; be honest and forthright.
Recognize and facilitate anticipatory grieving.
Inform parents about the grieving process.
Encourage support person to remain with the mother throughout labor.
Encourage the mother to make as many choices about her care as possible.
Support parents in seeing, touching, or holding the infant.
Describe the infant in detail, especially for couples who choose not to see the infant.
Allow photographs of the infant.
Prepare the couple for hospital paperwork, such as autopsy requests.
Discuss funeral or memorial services.
Assist the couple in how to inform siblings, relatives, and friends.
Discuss subsequent pregnancy.
Liberal use of follow-up home or office visits.

Modified from Kowalski K: Managing perinatal loss. Clin Obstet Gynecol 23:1113, 1980.

and infertility increase among couples who attempt to conceive after the loss of an infant. Physical changes that occur with grieving may account for this increase in poor reproductive success. Although the most intense suppression is noted within the first month after loss, a modified response may last for as long as 14 months.

The regionalization of perinatal health care has resulted in a large proportion of the perinatal deaths occurring in tertiary centers. In some of these centers, teams of physicians, nurses, social workers, and pastoral counselors have evolved to aid specifically in the management of families suffering a perinatal loss. Although this approach ensures an enlightened, understanding, and consistent approach to bereaved families, it suggests that the support of a grieving patient is a highly complex endeavor, to be accomplished only by a few specially trained individuals who care for postpartum patients. Enlightened and compassionate counseling of parents who have suffered a perinatal loss may be accomplished by any of the mother's health care professionals by using the guidelines listed in Table 22-3. Clearly, management of grief is not solely a postpartum responsibility. This is particularly true when a prenatal diagnosis is made of fetal death or fetal abnormality. A continuum of support is essential as the patient moves from the prenatal setting, to labor and delivery, to the postpartum ward, and finally to her home. Relaxation of many of the traditional hospital routines may be necessary to provide the type of support these families need. For example, allowing a loved one to remain past visiting hours, providing a couple a private setting to be with their deceased infant, or allowing unusually early discharge with provisions for frequent phone calls and follow-up visits often facilitates the resolution of grief.

It is also important to realize that the fathers of infants who die have somewhat different grief responses than do the mothers. In a study of 28 fathers who had lost infants, grief was primarily characterized by the necessity to keep busy with increased work, feelings of diminished self-worth, self-blame, and limited ability to ask for help. Stoic responses are typical of men and may obstruct the normal resolution of grief.

Postpartum Posttraumatic Stress Disorder

Posttraumatic stress disorder (PTSD) may occur after any physical or psychological trauma. The disorder commonly occurs after an unusual labor and delivery experience in which a woman is confronted with circumstances (pain, loss, trauma) that her defenses or sense of well-being cannot overcome. Thus, some women develop PTSD from an experience that other women will cope with easily, or that for the clinician may seem fairly unremarkable.

PTSD may lead to behavioral sequelae, including flashbacks, avoidance, and inability to function. Emergency operative deliveries, both vaginal and abdominal, and severe unexpected pain have been reported to have produced posttraumatic stress. The reaction may lead to fear of a subsequent delivery that may become incapacitating, as well as generalized symptoms of this disorder. Whenever an emergency procedure is indicated, debriefing afterward, both early and a few weeks later, may help to decrease the incidence of this problem. Women with adverse outcomes frequently experience transference of their previous experience as the next delivery approaches. One study of 1476 women who terminated pregnancies for fetal anomalies found that 46% of patients had PTSD at 4 months.[101] If anxiety is a predominant symptom at the postpartum visit, then discussions of a PTSD reaction may be indicated. The symptom complex of PTSD is less severe and sometimes eliminated with early intervention. Thus, if a woman seems to express psychological symptoms out of proportion to her labor and delivery experience, referral for further evaluation is appropriate.

KEY POINTS

- By 6 weeks postpartum, only 28% of women have returned to their prepregnant weight.
- About 50% of parturients experience diminished sexual desire during the 3 months following delivery.
- Postpartum uterine bleeding of sufficient quantity to require medical attention occurs in 1% to 2% of parturients. Of patients requiring curettage, 40% will be found to have retained placental tissue.
- Breastfeeding results in 98% contraceptive protection for up to 6 months after delivery, provided there is little or no supplemental feeding of the infant.
- Progestin-only contraceptive medication does not diminish lactation performance.
- Postpartum, major depression occurs in 8% to 20% of parturients; if possible, risk factors should be used to identify patients for increased screening and surveillance.
- Puerperal hypothyroidism often presents with symptoms that include mild dysphoria; consequently, thyroid function studies are suggested in the evaluation of patients with suspected postpartum depression that occurs 2 to 3 months after delivery.

REFERENCES

1. Williams JW: Regeneration of the uterine mucosa after delivery, with special reference to the placental site. Am J Obstet Gynecol 22:664, 1931.
2. Hytten FE, Cheyne GA: The size and composition of the human pregnant uterus. J Obstet Gynaecol Br Commonw 76:400, 1969.
3. Sharman A: Postpartum regeneration of the human endometrium. J Anat 87:1, 1953.
4. Willms AB, Brown ED, Kettritz UI, et al: Anatomic changes in the pelvis after uncomplicated vaginal delivery: evaluation with serial MR imaging. Radiology 195:91, 1995.
5. Oppenheimer LS, Sheriff EA, Goodman JDS, et al: The duration of lochia. Br J Obstet Gynaecol 93:754, 1986.
6. Visness CM, Kennedy KI, Ramos R: The duration and character of postpartum bleeding among breast-feeding women. Obstet Gynecol 89:159, 1997.
7. Poder L: Ultrasound evaluation of the uterus. In Callen PW: Ultrasonography in Obstetrics and Gynecology, 5th ed. Philadelphia, Saunders, 2000, pp 939-940.
8. Lipinski JK, Adam AH: Ultrasonic prediction of complications following normal vaginal delivery. J Clin Ultrasound 9:17, 1981.
9. Chang YL, Madrozo B, Drukker BH: Ultrasonic evaluation of the postpartum uterus in management of postpartum bleeding. Obstet Gynecol 58:227, 1981.
10. Perex A, Uela P, Masnick GS, et al: First ovulation after childbirth: the effect of breast feeding. Am J Obstet Gynecol 114:1041, 1972.
11. Gray RH, Campbell ON, Apelo R, et al: Risk of ovulation during lactation. Lancet 335:25, 1990.
12. Lovelady CA, Garner KE, Thoreno KL, et al: The effect of weight loss in overweight, lactating women on the growth of their infants. N Engl J Med 342:449, 2000.
13. Dewey KG, Lovelady CA, Nommsen-Rivers LA, et al: A randomized study of the effects of aerobic exercise by lactating women on breast-milk volume and composition. N Engl J Med 330:449, 1994.
14. Rooney BL, Schauberger CW: Excess pregnancy weight gain and long-term obesity: one decade later. Obstet Gynecol 100:245, 2002.
15. Vesco KK, Dietz PM, Rizzo J, et al: Excessive gestational weight gain and postpartum weight retention among obese women. Obstet Gynecol 114:1069, 2009.
16. Phelan S: Pregnancy: A "teachable moment" for weight control and obesity prevention. Am J Obstet Gynecol 135:e1, 2010.
17. Rasmusen NG, Hornnes PJ, Hegedus L: Ultrasonographically determined thyroid size in pregnancy and postpartum: the goitrogenic effect of pregnancy. Am J Obstet Gynecol 160:1216, 1989.
18. Kent GN, Stuckey BGA, Allen JR, et al: Post partum thyroid dysfunction: clinical assessment and relationship to psychiatric affective morbidity. Clin Endocrinol 51:429, 1999.
19. Pedersen CA, Stern RA, Pate J, et al: Thyroid and adrenal measures during late pregnancy and the puerperium in women who have been major depressed or who become dysmorphic postpartum. J Affect Disord 29:201, 1993.
20. Stagnaro-Green A: Postpartum thyroiditis. Best Prac Res Clin Endocrinol Metab 18:303, 2004.
21. Macklon NS, Greer IA: The deep venous system in the puerperium: an ultrasound study. Br J Obstet Gynaecol 104:198, 1997.
22. Clapp JF III, Capeless E: Cardiovascular function before, during, and after the first and subsequent pregnancies. Am J Cardiol 80:1469, 1997.
23. Hellgren M: Hemostasis during normal pregnancy and puerperium. Semin Thromb Hemost 29:125, 2003.
24. Singh N, Perfect JR: Immune reconstitution syndrome and exacerbation of infections after pregnancy. Clin Infect Dis 45:1192, 2007.
25. Belfort MA, Clark SL, Saade GR, et al: Hospital readmission after delivery: evidence for an increased incidence of nonurogenital infection in the immediate postpartum period. Am J Obstet Gynecol 202:35.e1, 2010.
26. Liu S, Heaman M, Joseph KS, et al: Risk of maternal postpartum readmission associated with mode of delivery. Obstet Gynecol 105:836, 2005.
27. Thung SF, Norwitz ER: Postpartum care: we can and should do better. Am J Obstet Gynecol 202:1, 2010.
28. Cietak KA, Newton JR: Serial qualitative maternal nephrosonography in pregnancy. Br J Radiol 58:399, 1985.
29. Sims EAH, Krantz KE: Serial studies of renal function during pregnancy and the puerperium in normal women. J Clin Invest 37:1764, 1958.
30. Polatti F, Capuzzo E, Viazzo F, et al: Bone mineral changes during and after lactation. Obstet Gynecol 94:52, 1999.
31. Holmberg-Marttila D, Sievanen H: Prevalence of bone mineral changes during postpartum amenorrhea and after resumption of menstruation. Am J Obstet Gynecol 180:537, 1999.
32. Lasky MA, Prentice A: Bone mineral changes during and after lactation. Obstet Gynecol 94:608, 1999.
33. Little KD, Clapp JF III: Self-selected recreational exercise has no impact on early postpartum lactation-induced bone loss. Med Sci Sports Exerc 30:831, 1998.
34. Temkin E: Driving through: postpartum care during World War II. Am J Public Health 89:587, 1999.
35. Brown S, Small R, Faber B, et al: Early postnatal discharge from hospital for healthy mothers and term infants. Cochrane Library 4:1, 2004.
36. Hebert PR, Reed G, Entman SS, et al: Serious maternal morbidity after childbirth: prolonged hospital stays and readmissions. Obstet Gynecol 94:942, 1999.
37. Glazener CMA, Abdalla M, Stroud P, et al: Postnatal maternal morbidity: extent, causes, prevention and treatment. Br J Obstet Gynaecol 102:282, 1995.
38. Liu LL, Clemens CJ, Shay DK, et al: The safety of early newborn discharge: the Washington state experience. JAMA 278:293, 1997.
39. Mandl KD, Brennan TA, Wise PH, et al: Maternal and infant health: effects of moderate reductions in postpartum length of stay. Arch Pediatr Adolesc Med 151:915, 1997.
40. Britton JR, Britton HL, Gronwaldt V: Early perinatal hospital discharge and parenting during infancy. Pediatrics 104:1070, 1999.
41. Brumfield CG: Early postpartum discharge. Clin Obstet Gynecol 41:611, 1998.
42. Bohlke K, Galil K, Jackson L, et al: Postpartum varicella vaccination: Is the vaccine virus excreted in breast milk? Obstet Gynecol 102:970, 2003.
43. Updated Tdap Vaccine Recommendations from the ACIP, 2010; Jan 14, 2011/60(01) 13-15. Accessed Jan 24, 2011 from www.cdc.gov/vaccines.
44. Jennings B, Edmundson M: The postpartum periods. After confinement: the fourth trimester. Clin Obstet Gynecol 23:1093, 1980.
45. Minig L, Trimble EL, Sarsotti C, et al: Building the evidence base for postoperative and postpartum advice. Obstet Gynecol 114:892, 2009.
46. Koltyn KF, Schultes SS: Psychological effects of an aerobic exercise session and a rest session following pregnancy. J Sports Med Phys Fitness 37:287, 1997.
47. Sampselle CM, Seng J, Yeo S, et al: Physical activity and postpartum well-being. J Obstet Gynecol Neonatal Nurs 28:41, 1999.
48. Norman E, Sherburn M, Osborne RH, et al: An exercise and education program improves well-being of new mothers: a randomized controlled trial. Phys Ther 90:348, 2010.
49. Reamy K, White SE: Sexuality in pregnancy and the puerperium: a review. Obstet Gynecol Surv 40:1, 1985.
50. Glazener CMA: Sexual function after childbirth: women's experiences, persistent morbidity and lack of professional recognition. Br J Obstet Gynaecol 104:330, 1997.
51. Goetsch MF: Postpartum dyspareunia: an unexplored problem. J Reprod Med 44:963, 1999.
52. Signorello L, Harlow B, Chekos A, et al: Postpartum sexual functioning and its relationship to perineal trauma: a retrospective cohort study of primiparous women. Am J Obstet Gynecol 184:881, 2001.
53. Hicks TL, Forester-Goodall S, Quattrone EM, et al: Postpartum sexual functioning and method of delivery: summary of the evidence. Am Coll Nurse Midwives 49:430, 2004.
54. Ryding E-L: Sexuality during and after pregnancy. Acta Obstet Gynecol Scand 63:679, 1984.
55. Byrd JE, Shibley-Hyde J, DeLamater J, et al: Sexuality during pregnancy and the year postpartum. J Family Pract 47:305, 1998.
56. Gagnon AJ, Edgar L, Kramer MS, et al: A randomized trial of a program of early postpartum discharge with nurse visitation. Am J Obstet Gynecol 176:205, 1997.
57. Gunn J, Lumley S, Chondros P, Young D: Does an early postnatal check-up improve maternal health: results from a randomized trial in Australian general practice. Br J Obstet Gynaecol 105:991, 1998.

58. Lu MC, Kotelchuck M, Culhane JF, et al: Preconception care between pregnancies: the content of internatal care. Matern Child Health J 10:S107, 2006.
59. Connolly AM, Thorp JM Jr: Childbirth-related perineal trauma: clinical significance and prevention. Clin Obstet Gynecol 42:820, 1999.
60. Weidner AC, Jamison MG, Branham V, et al: Neuropathic injury to the levator ani occurs in 1 in 4 primiparous women. Am J Obstet Gynecol 195:1851, 2006.
61. Handa VL, Zyczynski HM, Burgio KL, et al: The impact of fecal and urinary incontinence on quality of life 6 months after childbirth. Am J Obstet Gynecol 197:636.e1, 2007.
62. Chaliha C, Kalia V, Stanton S, et al: Antenatal prediction of postpartum fecal incontinence. Obstet Gynecol 94:689, 1999.
63. Harvey MA: Pelvic floor exercises during and after pregnancy: a systematic review of their role in preventing pelvic floor dysfunction. J Obstet Gynecol Can 25:487, 2003.
64. MacArthur C, Glazener C, Lancashire R, et al: Faecal incontinence and mode of first and subsequent delivery: a six-year longitudinal study. Br J Obstet Gynaecol 112:1075, 2005.
65. Pollack J, Nordenstam J, Brismar S, et al: Anal incontinence after vaginal delivery: a five-year prospective cohort study. Obstet Gynecol 104:1397, 2004.
66. King PA, Duthie SJ, Dip V, et al: Secondary postpartum hemorrhage. Aust N Z J Obstet Gynaecol 29:394, 1989.
67. Boyd BK, Katz VL, Hansen WF: Delayed postpartum hemorrhage: a retrospective analysis. J Matern Fetal Med 4:19, 1995.
68. Hoveyda F, MacKenzie IZ: Secondary postpartum haemorrhage: Incidence, morbidity and current management. Br J Obstet Gynaecol 108:927, 2001.
69. Klaus MH, Jerauld R, Kreger NC, et al: Maternal attachment: importance of the first postpartum days. N Engl J Med 286:460, 1972.
70. McClellan MS, Cabianca WC: Effects of early mother-infant contact following cesarean birth. Obstet Gynecol 56:52, 1980.
71. Robson KM, Powell E: Early maternal attachment. In Brickington IF, Kumar R: Motherhood and Mental Illness. San Diego, Academic Press, 1982, p 155.
72. Klaus M, Kennel J: Parent-Infant Bonding. St. Louis, CV Mosby, 1982.
73. Gray J, Butler C, Dean J, et al: Prediction and prevention of child abuse and neglect. Child Abuse Neglect 1:45, 1977.
74. Siegel E, Cauman KE, Schaefer ES, et al: Hospital and home support during infancy: impact on maternal attachment, child abuse and neglect and health care utilization. Pediatrics 66:183, 1980.
75. Areskog B, Uddenberg N, Kjessler B: Experience of delivery in women with and without antenatal fear of childbirth. Gynecol Obstet Invest 16:1, 1983.
76. Kazi A, Kennedy KI, Visness CM, Kahn T: Effectiveness of the lactational amenorrhea method in Pakistan. Fertil Steril 64:717, 1995.
77. Robson KM, Brant H, Kumar R: Maternal sexuality during first pregnancy after childbirth. Br J Obstet Gynaecol 88:882, 1981.
78. Klebanoff MA: The interval between pregnancies and the outcome of subsequent births. N Engl J Med 340:643, 1999.
79. Rojnik B, Kosmelj K, Andolsek-Jeras L: Initiation of contraception postpartum. Contraception 51:75, 1995.
80. Halderman LD, Nelson AL: Impact of early postpartum administration of progestin-only hormonal contraceptives compared with nonhormonal contraceptives on short-term breast-feeding patterns. Am J Obstet Gynecol 186:1250, 2002.
81. Kaunitz AM: Long-acting injectable contraception with depot medroxyprogesterone acetate. Am J Obstet Gynecol 170:1543, 1994.
82. Kjos SL, Peters RK, Xiang A, et al: Contraception and the risk of type 2 diabetes mellitus in Latina women with prior gestational diabetes mellitus. JAMA 280:533, 1998.
83. Diaz S, Peralta G, Juez C, et al: Fertility regulation in nursing women: III. Short-term influence of low-dose combined contraceptive upon lactation and infant growth. Contraception 27:1, 1983.
83a. Espey E, Ogburn T, Leeman L, et al: Effect of progestin compared with combined oral contraceptive pills on lactation: a randomized controlled trial. Obstet Gynecol 119:5, 2012.
84. Sivin I, Campodonica I, Kiriwat O, et al: The performance of levonorgestrel rod and Norplant contraceptive implants: a 5 year randomized study. Hum Reprod 13:3371, 1998.
85. Berenson AB, Wiemann CM, McCombs SL, et al: The rise and fall of levonorgestrel implants: 1992-1996. Obstet Gynecol 92:790, 1998.
86. Espy E, Ogburn T: Perpetuating negative attitudes about the intrauterine device: textbooks lag behind the evidence. Contraception 65:389, 2002.
87. Stanback J, Grimes D: Can intrauterine device removals for bleeding or pain be predicted at a one-month follow-up visit? A multivariate analysis. Contraception 58:357, 1998.
88. Farmer M, Webb A: Intrauterine device insertion-related complications: can they be predicted? J Fam Plan Reprod Health Care 29:227, 2003.
89. Mishell DR Jr, Roy S: Copper intrauterine contraceptive device event rate following insertion 4 to 8 weeks postpartum. Am J Obstet Gynecol 143:29, 1982.
90. Grimes D, Schulz K, van Vliet H, et al: Immediate post-partum insertion of intrauterine devices: a Cochrane review. Hum Reprod 17:549, 2002.
91. Alvarez T, Brache V, Fernandez E, et al: New insights on the mode of action of intrauterine contraceptive devices in women. Fertil Steril 49:768, 1988.
92. Rivera R, Yacobson I, Grimes D: The mechanism of action of hormonal contraceptives and intrauterine contraceptive devices. Am J Obstet Gynecol 181:1263, 1999.
93. Bledin KD, Brice B: Psychological conditions in pregnancy and the puerperium and their relevance to postpartum sterilization: a review. Bull WHO 61:533, 1983.
94. Peterson HB, Huber DH, Belker AM: Vasectomy: an appraisal for the obstetrician-gynecologist. Obstet Gynecol 76:568, 1990.
95. Hendrix NW, Chauhan SP, Morrison JC: Sterilization and its consequences. Obstet Gynecol Surv 54:766, 1999.
96. Hillis SD, Marchbanks PA, Taylor LR, et al: Higher hysterectomy risk for sterilized than nonsterilized women: findings from the U.S. Collaborative Review of Sterilization Working Group. Obstet Gynecol 91:241, 1998.
97. Walker MW, Jick H, Hunter JR: Vasectomy and non-fatal myocardial infarction. Lancet 1:13, 1981.
98. Haynes DM, Martin BJ: Cesarean hysterectomy: a twenty-five year review. Am J Obstet Gynecol 46:215, 1975.
99. Kennel JH, Slyter H, Claus MKH: The mourning response of parents to the death of a newborn. N Engl J Med 83:344, 1970.
100. Lockwood S, Lewis IC: Management of grieving after stillbirth. Med J Aust 2:308, 1980.
101. Korenromp MJ, Christiaens GCML, van den Bout J, et al: Adjustment to termination of pregnancy for fetal anomaly: a longitudinal study in women at 4, 8, and 16 months. Am J Obstet Gynecol 201:160.e1, 2009.

For full reference list, log onto www.expertconsult.com.

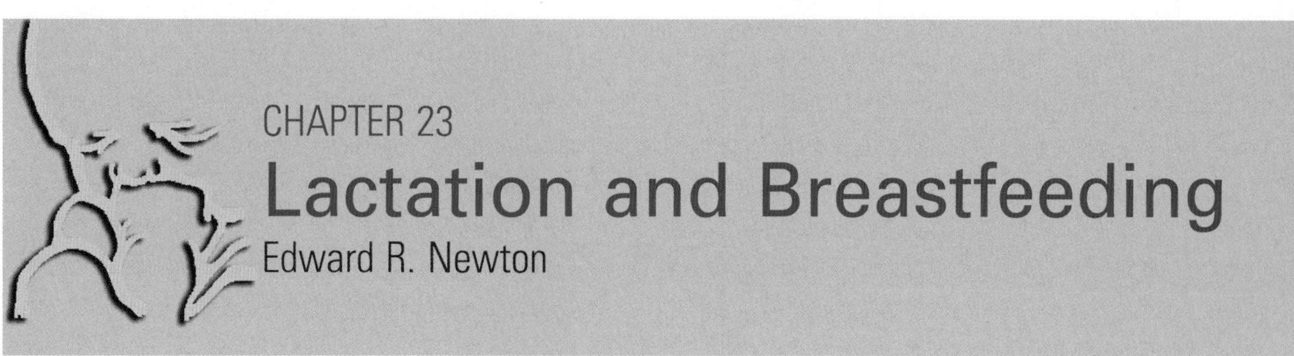

CHAPTER 23

Lactation and Breastfeeding

Edward R. Newton

KEY ABBREVIATIONS	
Confidence Interval	CI
Human Immunodeficiency Virus	HIV
Immunoglobulin A	IgA
Potassium Chloride	KOH
Luteinizing Hormone	LH
Messenger RNA	mRNA
Odds Ratio	OR
Purified Protein Derivative	PPD
Secretory Immunoglobulin A	sIgA
United Nations Children's Fund	UNICEF
World Health Organization	WHO

Breastfeeding and breast milk are the global standard for infant feeding in undeveloped and developed countries. This statement is supported by the World Health Organization, the U.S. Surgeon General, the American Academy of Pediatrics,[1] the American College of Obstetricians and Gynecologists,[2] the American Academy of Family Practice, and the Academy of Breastfeeding Medicine. **The American Academy of Pediatrics has recently published an endorsement for breastfeeding at least through the first year of life and as an exclusive method for the first 6 months.**[1] The Healthy People 2020 (www.healthypeople.gov/2020) objectives (MICH 21.1-21.5, MICH 22.2) are as follows: any breastfeeding, 81.9%; any breastfeeding at 6 months, 60.6%; any breastfeeding at 12 months, 34.1%; exclusive breastfeeding at 3 months, 46.2%; exclusive breastfeeding at 6 months, 25.5%; and reduce the number of infants who receive supplemental formula in the first 48 hours by one half to 14.2%.

Unfortunately, we have challenges to meet these objectives; the majority of American infants are not breastfed exclusively nor for an appropriate duration. Figure 23-1 and Figure 23-2 describe the trends in breastfeeding behaviors in the United States. The latest estimates of breastfeeding performance (www.healthypeople.gov/2020) are that 74% of women initiate breastfeeding in the hospital and only 43.5% of those are still breastfeeding at 6 months. Approximately 23% of American infants meet the standard of breastfeeding 1 year or more. Only 33.6% and 14% of American infants are exclusively breastfeeding at 3 and 6 months, respectively; more than 24% received supplemental formula in the first 48 hours of life.

Specific populations are at greater risk for the failure to initiate and continue breastfeeding. **Women of lower socioeconomic status, those with less education, and teenagers initiate breastfeeding at about half to two thirds the rate of mature high-school graduates of middle and upper socioeconomic statuses (Table 23-1 and 23-2).**[3,4] **Fortunately, since 1989 more women at greatest risk for feeding their infants artificial breast milk are initiating breastfeeding in the hospital.**[4] Perceived breast milk insufficiency, sore nipples and breasts, the lack of family and professional support, and the decision to return to work are the most often cited reasons for early weaning. Cultural attitudes underlie many of these risk factors for failure to breastfeed successfully.

Although dysfunctional cultural and familial attitudes are outside the direct control of medicine, these attitudes may directly affect the care delivered by physicians. The normal function of the breasts, to produce breast milk, is muted by two cultural attitudes. One cultural attitude is the association of breasts with sexual attraction. The media is replete with examples that show beautiful, well-formed breasts as a sexual ideal. A corollary of this attitude is that breastfeeding will cause the breasts to sag and lose their sex appeal. The other opposing cultural attitude is that breastfeeding restricts self-fulfillment; mothers who stay

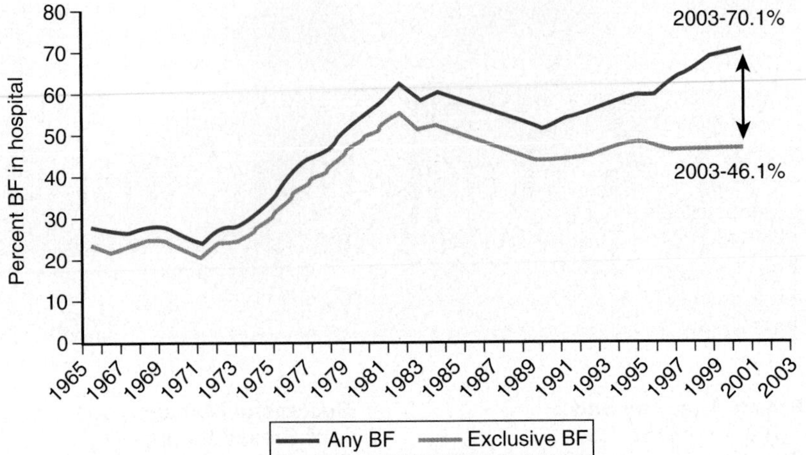

FIGURE 23-1. Incidence of breastfeeding in the hospital. (Data from American Academy of Pediatrics, Work Group on Breastfeeding: Breastfeeding and the use of human milk. Pediatr 115:625, 2005.)

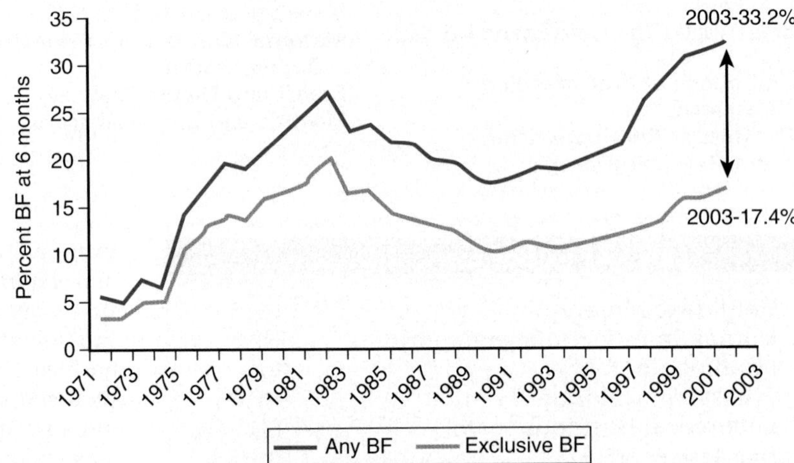

FIGURE 23-2. Incidence of breastfeeding at 6 months. (Data from American Academy of Pediatrics, Work Group on Breastfeeding: Breastfeeding and the use of human milk. Pediatr 115:625, 2005.)

TABLE 23-1 PREDICTORS OF BREASTFEEDING INITIATION

HELPFUL FACTORS	ADJUSTED OR (95% CI)
Year of birth	1.08 (1.04-1.12)
Married	1.47 (1.33-1.63)
Parity ≥1	1.48 (1.33-1.65)
Non-WIC participant	1.22 (1.10-1.35)
No prenatal discussion of nutrition	1.24 (1.09-1.42)
Normal birthweight	1.23 (1.14-1.34)
OBSTACLES	**ADJUSTED OR (95% CI)**
Black race	0.59 (0.53-0.65)
Maternal age <20	0.66 (0.57-0.77)
Maternal age 20-29	0.79 (0.77-0.86)
Maternal education: < high school	0.41 (0.36-0.46)
Maternal education: high school only	0.50 (0.46-0.54)
No prenatal discussion of breastfeeding	0.68 (0.60-0.76)
Cesarean delivery	0.71 (0.64-0.78)

Modified from Scanlon KS, Grummer-Strawn L, Chen J, Molinari N, Perrine CG: Racial and ethnic differences in breastfeeding initiation and duration, by state—national immunization survey, United States, 2004-2008. MMWR 59(11):327, 2010; and Ahluwalia I, Morrow B, Hsia J, et al: Who is breastfeeding? Recent trends from the Pregnancy Risk Assessment and Monitoring System. J Pediatr 142:486, 2003.

WIC, Federal health and nutrition program for women, infants, and children.

TABLE 23-2 PREDICTORS OF BREASTFEEDING CONTINUATION >10 WEEKS

HELPFUL FACTORS	ADJUSTED OR (95% CI)
Married	1.43 (1.26-1.63)
Non-WIC participant	1.20 (1.05-1.36)
Normal birthweight	1.37 (1.23-1.53)
OBSTACLES	**ADJUSTED OR (95% CI)**
Maternal age <20	0.50 (0.41-0.61)
Maternal age 20-29	0.72 (0.65-0.79)
Maternal education: < high school	0.64 (0.54-0.76)
Maternal education: high school only	0.68 (0.61-0.75)
Parity ≥1	0.72 (0.64-0.82)
Parity ≥2	0.79 (0.70-0.89)
Cesarean delivery	0.82 (0.72-0.93)

Modified from Scanlon KS, Grummer-Strawn L, Chen J, Molinari N, Perrine CG: Racial and ethnic differences in breastfeeding initiation and duration, by state—national immunization survey, United States, 2004-2008. MMWR 59(11):327, 2010; and Ahluwalia I, Morrow B, Hsia J, et al: Who is breastfeeding? Recent trends from the Pregnancy Risk Assessment and Monitoring System. J Pediatr 142:486, 2003.

WIC, Federal health and nutrition program for women, infants, and children.

at home to breastfeed and care for their babies are considered poor examples of the modern, independent professional woman. These attitudes are exacerbated by a lack of knowledge about breastfeeding and lactation. The normal function of the breasts is excluded from the curriculum of primary and secondary schools on the basis of the connection between breasts and sex. After completion of their education, few women experience any examples of successful breastfeeding. Only 30% of grandmothers initiated breastfeeding (1970-1980), and few of these grandmothers have breastfed more than a few weeks. The lack of exposure to successful, experienced breastfeeding mothers seriously compromises the chances of success for today's women who attempt to breastfeed.

Physicians are products of the same culture as the women they help. Unfortunately, many have the same cultural biases as their patients and the same lack of primary and secondary education regarding the normal physiology of breastfeeding. The curricula of medical school and residency training programs contribute to the problem. Most physicians reflecting on their own education on breastfeeding will identify neither a structured curriculum nor practical experiences with successfully breastfeeding mother-infant dyads. At most, he or she has experienced only one or two lectures regarding breastfeeding, often focused on breast anatomy or the endocrinology of lactation. In fact, the most commonly cited resource for physicians is another nonmedical individual or a breastfeeding spouse. On obstetric rotations, medical students and obstetrics residents rarely see normal breastfeeding dyads longer than 1 to 3 days postpartum. On pediatric rotations, learners often see the baby only in the nursery and rarely see the normal mother breastfeed as an inpatient or at newborn visits. While pediatric residents observe and support the mother who pumps or nurses her growing preterm infant, the exposure is not normal, and often is negative. As a result, there are serious gaps in physician knowledge as they attempt to serve the over 3 million newborns and mothers per year who attempt to breastfeed. **A national survey of physician knowledge revealed that 20% to 40% of physicians (obstetricians, pediatricians, and family practitioners) did not know that breastfeeding is the "gold standard" for infant feeding, and similar percentages have serious and sometimes dangerous gaps in their knowledge in the management of breastfeeding problems. A survey of fellows of the American Academy of Pediatricians revealed that only 65% recommended exclusive breastfeeding during the first month of life, and more than half agreed with or had a neutral opinion about the statement that breastfeeding and formula-feeding are equally acceptable methods for feeding infants.**

The purpose of this chapter is to begin the educational process through which obstetricians will adopt the lactating mother as their patient. **In order to support the breastfeeding mother, the obstetrician must be convinced of the biologic superiority of breastfeeding and human breast milk over formula.** This chapter reviews breast anatomy and physiology of lactation in a framework pertinent to breastfeeding management. This chapter describes the vast differences between breast milk and formula, a difference directly related to unique needs and the short- and long-term health of the infant and mother. Specific issues related to the obstetrician (or other health care provider) will be addressed and include the role of the obstetrician in preconceptional counseling, prenatal care, delivery room management, and postpartum care for the breastfeeding mother.

BREAST ANATOMY AND DEVELOPMENT

The size and shape of the breast vary greatly by stage of development, physiologic state, and phenotype. The breast is located in the superficial fascia between the second rib and sixth intercostal cartilage in the midclavicular line. There is usually a projection of the central disk into each axilla, the *tail of Spence*. The mature breast weighs about 200 g in the nonpregnant state; during pregnancy, 500 g; and during lactation, 600 to 800 g. As long as glandular tissue and the nipple are present, the size or shape of the breast has little to do with the functional success of the breast. **The adequacy of glandular tissue for breastfeeding is ascertained by inquiring whether a woman's breasts have enlarged during pregnancy. If there is failure of the breast to enlarge as the result of pregnancy, especially if associated with minimal breast tissue on examination, the clinician should be wary of primary failure of lactation.**

The nipple, or *papilla mammae,* is a conical elevation in the middle of the areola, or *areola mammae.* The areola is a circular pigmented area, which darkens during pregnancy. The contrast with the fairer skin of the body provides a visual cue for the newborn who is attempting to latch-on. The areola contains multiple small elevations, *Montgomery's tubercles,* which enlarge during pregnancy and lactation. Montgomery's tubercles contain multiple ductular openings of sebaceous and sweat glands. These glands secrete lubricating and anti-infective substances (immunoglobulin A [IgA]) that protect the nipples and areola during nursing. These substances are washed away when the breasts and nipples are washed with soap or alcohol-containing compounds, leaving the nipple prone to cracking and infection.

Unlike the dermis of the body of the breast, which includes fat, the areola and nipple contain smooth muscle and collagenous and elastic tissue. With light touch or anticipation of nursing, these muscles contract and the nipple erects to form a teat. The contraction pulls the lactiferous sinuses into the nipple-areola complex, which allows the infant to milk the breast milk from these reservoirs.

The tip of the nipple contains the openings (0.4 to 0.7 mm in diameter) of 15 to 20 milk ducts (2 to 4 mm in diameter). Each of the milk ducts empties one tubuloalveolar gland, which is embedded in the fat of the body of the breast. A sphincter mechanism at the opening of the duct limits the ejection of milk from the breast. The competency of this mechanism is variable. About 20% of women do not demonstrate milk ejection from the contralateral breast when milk ejection is stimulated. If milk leakage is demonstrated from the contralateral breast during nursing, it is indicative of an intact let-down reflex and is highly suggestive of milk transfer to the infant.

Five to 10 mm from their exit, the milk ducts widen (5 to 8 mm) into the lactiferous sinuses (Figure 23-3). When these sinuses are pulled into the teat during nursing, the infant's tongue, facial muscles, and mouth squeeze the milk from the sinuses into the infant's oropharnyx.[5] The

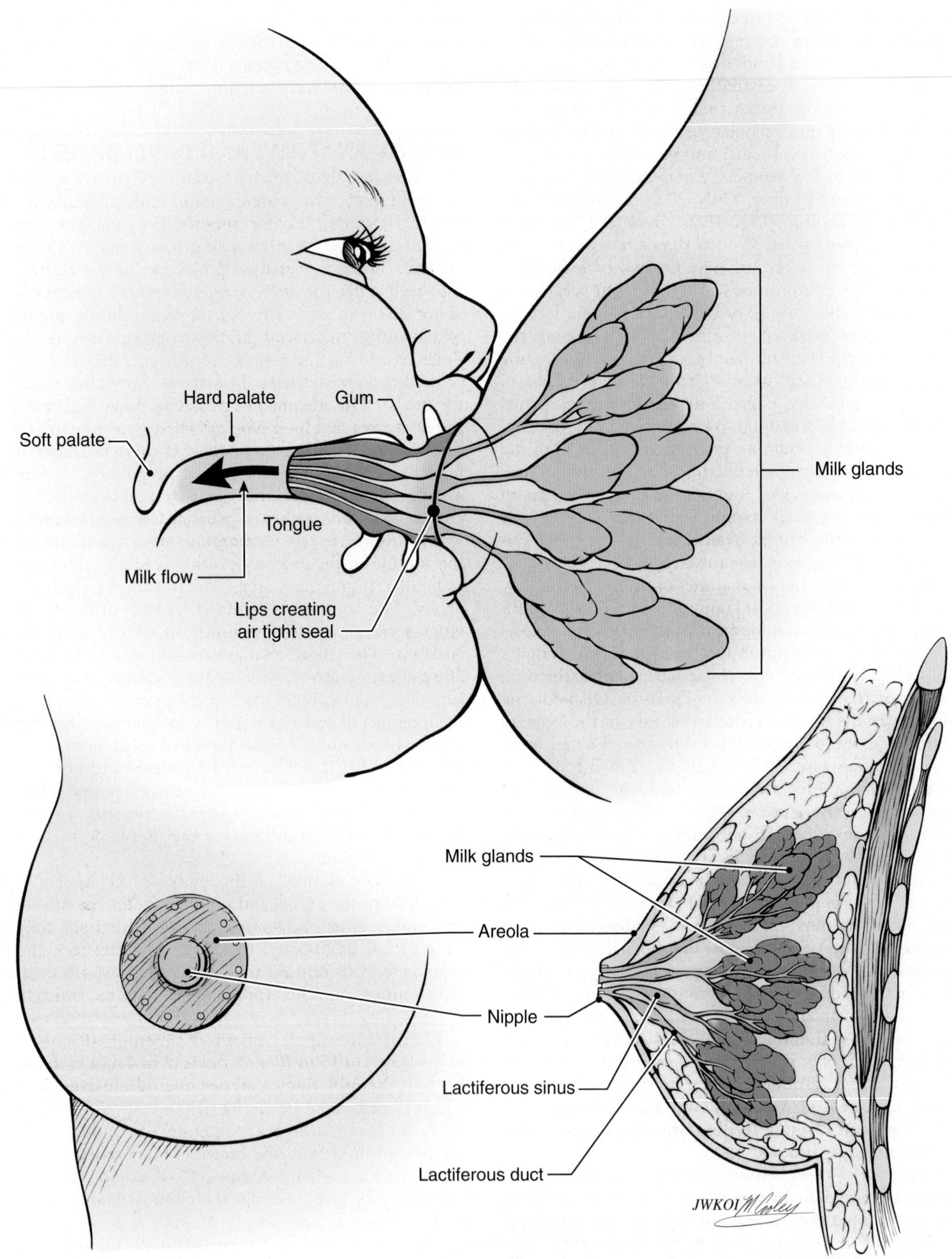

FIGURE 23-3. Anatomy of the breast.

tubuloalveolar glands (15 to 20) form lobi, which are arranged in a radial fashion from the central nipple-areola complex. The lobi and lactiferous ducts extend into the tail of Spence. Ten to 40 lactiferous ducts connect to each lactiferous sinus, each forming a lobulus. Each lobulus arborizes into 10 to 100 alveoli for tubulosaccular secretory units. The alveoli are the critical units of the production and ejection of milk. A sac of alveolar cells is surrounded by a basket of myoepithelial cells. The alveolar cells are stimulated by prolactin to produce milk. The myoepithelial cells are stimulated by oxytocin to contract and eject the recently produced milk into the lactiferous ducts, lactiferous sinuses, and beyond.

The radial projection of lactiferous ducts prompts important considerations relative to breast surgery on women who are breastfeeding or who will breastfeed. **Surgical skin incisions parallel to the circumareolar line, especially at the circumareolar line, have better cosmetic healing and are often chosen by surgeons. However, if the incision is taken deep into the parenchyma, the lactiferous ducts may be compromised; a superficial, parallel skin incision and a radial deep incision are preferred. In women who intend to breastfeed, a circumareolar incision is to be avoided. The incision compromises breastfeeding in three ways: occlusion of lactiferous ducts, restriction of the formation of a teat during nursing, and injury to the lateral cutaneous branch of the fourth intercostal nerve.**

Surgical disruption of the lateral cutaneous branch of the fourth intercostal nerve can have devastating effects on the success of breastfeeding.[6] This nerve is critical to the production and ejection of breast milk. Furthermore, the nerves provide organ-specific control of regional blood flow, and a tremendous increase in mammary blood flow occurs during a nursing episode. Disruption of this autonomic control may severely compromise lactation performance. The rate of breastfeeding failure is two to three times higher when a circumareolar incision has been performed. The obstetrician needs to be alert to old surgical incisions when a pregnant patient expresses a desire to breastfeed or when a breast biopsy is anticipated in a reproductive-aged woman.

As mammals, humans have the potential to develop mammary tissue (glandular or nipple tissue) anywhere along the milk line *(galactic band)*. The milk line extends from the axilla and inner upper arm to its current position, down the abdomen along the midclavicular line to the upper lateral mons and upper inner thigh. When accessory glands occur, this is termed hypermastia. This may involve accessory glandular tissue, supernumerary nipples, or both. Two to 6% of women have hypermastia, and the response to pregnancy and lactation is variable. **The most common site for accessory breast tissue is the axilla. These women may present at 2 to 5 days postpartum (galactogenesis) with painful enlargements in the axilla. Ice and symptomatic therapy for 24 to 48 hours is sufficient treatment. Supernumerary nipples *(polythelia)* are associated with renal abnormalities (11%).**

THE PHYSIOLOGY OF LACTATION

The best and most extensive research concerning the physiology of lactation focuses on the production of milk and has its roots in the research conducted by the multibillion-dollar dairy industry. Good milk-producing cattle, whose milk composition (i.e., milk fat percentage) can be controlled, create a competitive advantage in the marketplace. The translation of dairy research to human research plus the expected interest of pediatricians on infant nutrition has led to a preponderance of information on data on maternal milk production and delivery and its impact on neonatal and childhood outcomes. With the exception of the hypothalamic hypogonadism in the breastfeeding mother and its effect on menses and child spacing, very little is understood about the physiologic changes during the breastfeeding episode; these include vascular adaptation to the rapid production (10-30 minutes) of 100 to 200 mL of an extremely complex liquid. Most maternal benefits of breastfeeding are accrued in a dose-dependent fashion; the longer and the more intense (exclusive breastfeeding), the better the outcomes in terms of, for example, premenopausal breast cancer or cardiovascular disease. We are beginning to ask the question "why" and "how." Are the benefits of breastfeeding to the mother's health related to the duration of the hormonal changes? Is it the "antistress" effects of oxytocin? Is it the changes in gastrointestinal absorption of substrates? Is the intense pair-bonding between the mother and her breastfed children affecting allostatic load later in life? The answers to these questions will greatly improve our knowledge of the human experience.

The following sections summarize what is known about human lactation. The physiology of lactation has three major components: stages of lactogenesis, endocrinology of lactogenesis, and nursing behavior/milk transfer. Finally, the composition of mature human breast milk is summarized with a focus on the differences between breast milk and formula.

Stages of Lactogenesis

Full alveolar development and maturation of the breast must await the hormones of pregnancy (progesterone, prolactin, and human placental lactogen) for completion of the developmental process. By midpregnancy, the gland is competent to secrete milk (colostrum), although full function is not attained until the tissues are released from the inhibition of high levels of circulating progesterone. This is termed *lactogenesis stage 1*. Lactogenesis stage 2 occurs as the progesterone levels fall after delivery of the placenta, during the first 2 to 4 days after birth. Stage 2 includes dramatic increases in mammary blood flow and oxygen/glucose uptake by the breast. **At 2 to 5 days postpartum, the secretion of milk is copious and "the milk comes in." This is the most common time for engorgement if the breasts are not drained by efficient, frequent nursing.** Until lactogenesis stage 2 is developed, the breasts secrete colostrum. Colostrum is very different than mature milk in volume and constituents.[7] **Colostrum has more protein, especially secretory immunoglobulins, lactose, and lower fat content than mature milk.** Prolactin and glucocorticoids play important promoter roles in this stage of development.

After lactogenesis stage 2 (4 to 6 days postpartum) lactation enters an indefinite period of milk production formerly called galactopoiesis, now termed lactogenesis stage 3. The duration of this stage is dependent on the continued production of breast milk and the efficient transfer of the breast milk to the infant. **Prolactin appears to be the single most important galactopoietic hormone, since selective inhibition of prolactin secretion by bromocriptine disrupts lactogenesis. Oxytocin appears to be the major galactokinetic hormone.** Stimulation of the nipple and areola or behavioral cues cause a reflex contraction of the myoepithelial cells that surround the alveoli and ejection of milk from the breast.

The final stage of development is involution and cessation of breastfeeding. As the frequency of breastfeeding is reduced to less than six episodes in 24 hours and milk volume is less than 400 mL/24 hr, prolactin levels fall and a cyclic pattern ends in the total cessation of milk production. After 24 to 48 hours of no transfer of breast milk to the infant, intraductal pressure[8] and lactation inhibitory factor[9] appear to initiate apoptosis of the secretory epithelial cells and proteolytic degradation of the basement membrane. Lactation inhibitory factor is a protein secreted in the milk, whose increasing concentration in the absence of drainage appears to decrease milk production by the alveolar cells.[10,11] It counterbalances pressures to increase milk supply (increased frequency of nursing) and allows for the day-to-day adjustment in infant demands.

The Endocrinology of Lactogenesis

Prolactin is the major hormone promoting milk production. Prolactin induces the synthesis of messenger RNAs (mRNAs) for the production of enzymes and milk proteins by binding to membrane receptors of the mammary epithelial cells. Thyroid hormones selectively enhance the secretion of lactalbumin. Cortisol, insulin, parathyroid hormone, and growth hormone are supportive metabolic hormones in the production of carbohydrates and lipids in the milk. Ovarian hormones are not required for the maintenance of established milk production and are suppressed by high levels of prolactin.

The alveolar cell is the principal site for the production of milk. Neville[12] describes five pathways for milk synthesis and secretion in the mammary alveolus, including four major transcellular and one paracellular pathway. They are (1) exocytosis (merocrine secretion) of milk protein and lactose in Golgi-derived secretory vesicles, (2) milk fat secretion via milk fat globules (apocrine secretion), (3) secretion of ions and water across the apical membrane, (4) pinocytosis-exocytosis of immunoglobulins, and (5) paracellular pathway for plasma components and leukocytes. During lactation as opposed to during pregnancy, very few of the constituents of breast milk are transferred directly from maternal blood. The junctions between cells, *tight junctions*, are closed. As weaning occurs, the tight junctions are released and sodium and other minerals easily cross to the milk, changing the taste of the milk.

The substrates for milk production are primarily absorbed from the maternal gut or produced in elemental form by the maternal liver. Glucose is the major substrate for milk production. Glucose serves as the main source of energy for other reactions and is a critical source of carbon. The synthesis of fat from carbohydrates plays a predominant role in fat production in human milk. Proteins are built from free amino acids derived from the plasma.

A sizable proportion of breast milk is produced during the nursing episode. In order to supply the substrates for milk production, there is increased blood flow to the mammary glands (20%-40%), gastrointestinal tract, and liver. Cardiac output is increased by 10% to 20% during a nursing episode. The vasodilation of the regional vascular beds is under the control of the autonomic nervous system. Oxytocin may play a critical role in directing the regional distribution of maternal cardiac output through an autonomic, parasympathetic action.

Given that milk is produced during the nursing episode, variation in content during a feed is expected. During a feeding episode the lipid content of milk rises by more than two- to threefold (1%-5%) with a corresponding 5% fall in lactose concentration.[12-15] The protein content remains relatively constant. At the extreme, there can be a 30% to 40% difference in the volume obtained from each breast.[15] Likewise, there are intraindividual variations in lipid and lactose concentrations.

The rising lipid content during a feed has practical implications in breastfeeding management. **If a woman limits her feeds to less than 4 minutes, but nurses more frequently, the calorie density of the milk is lower and the infant's hunger may not be satiated.** The infant wishes to feed sooner and the frequency of nursing accelerates. This stimulates more milk production and creates a scenario of a hungry infant despite apparent good volume and milk transfer. **Lengthening the nursing episode or using one breast for each nursing episode often solves the problem.**

The volume and concentration of constituents also vary during the day. Volume per feed increases by 10% to 15% in the late afternoon and evening. Nitrogen content peaks in the late afternoon and falls to a nadir at 5:00 A.M. Fat concentrations peak in the early morning and reach a nadir at 9:00 PM. Lactose levels stay relatively stable throughout the day. The variation in milk volume and content in working women who nurse only when at home has not been studied. Presumably, the variation in volume and content is preserved if the woman pumps during the day.

Does diet affect the volume and constitution of breast milk? For the average American woman with the range of diets from teenagers to mature, health-conscious adults, the answer is "no." There is no convincing evidence that the macronutrients in breast milk—protein, fats, and carbohydrates—vary across the usual range of American diets. Volume may vary in the extremes. In developing countries where there is widespread starvation and daily calorie intake is less than 1600 kcal during prepregnancy, and pregnancy in underweight breastfeeding mothers, milk volume and calorie density are minimally decreased (5%-10%), if at all.[16] In a controlled experiment,[17] well-nourished European women reduced their calorie intake by 33% for 1 week. Milk volume was not reduced when the diet was maintained at greater than 1500 kcal/day. If the daily energy intake was less than 1500 kcal/day, milk volume was reduced 15%. **Moderate dieting and weight loss postpartum (4.5 lb/mo) are not associated with changes in milk volume,**[18,19] **nor does aerobic exercise have any adverse effect.**[18,19]

In the first year of life, the infant undergoes tremendous growth; infants double their birth weight in 180 days. Infants fed artificial breast milk lose up to 5% of their birthweight during the first week of life, while breast-milk-fed infants lose about 7% of their birthweight. A maximum weight loss of 10% of birthweight is tolerated in the first week of life in breastfed infants. If this threshold is exceeded, the breastfeeding dyad needs immediate intervention by a trained health care provider. While supplementation with donor breast milk or artificial breast milk may be a necessary part of the intervention, the key focus of intervention is establishing good breast milk transfer by ensuring adequate production, correct nursing behavior, and adequate frequency. Once stage 3 of lactogenesis occurs, "the milk has come in"; the term breastfed infant will gain about 0.75 to 1 oz/day with adequate milk transfer. **By 14 days, the breastfed infant should have returned to birthweight.**

Food intake and energy needs are not constant. The infant's need for energy and/or fluids varies by day or week with growth spurts, greater activity, fighting illness, or greater fluid losses as in hot weather. Mammals have developed an extremely efficient mechanism to adjust milk supply within 24 to 48 hours depending on demand via oxytocin and the let-down reflex (Figure 23-4), and prolactin production. The prolactin and oxytocin travel to their target cells, prolactin to the alveolar epithelium in the breast, and oxytocin to the myoepithelial cells that shroud the alveolar epithelium. In lactating women, baseline prolactin levels are 200 ng/mL at delivery, 75 ng/mL between 10 and 90 days postpartum, 50 ng/ml between 90 and 180 days postpartum, and 35 ng/mL after 180 days postpartum. Maternal serum prolactin levels rise by 80% to 150% of baseline levels within seconds of nipple stimulation. As long as nursing frequency is maintained at more than eight episodes a day for 10 to 20 minutes with each episode in 24 hours, the serum prolactin levels will suppress the luteinizing hormone (LH) surges and ovarian function.[12,20]

Serum oxytocin levels also rise with nipple stimulation. However, the oxytocin response is much more affected by operant conditioning, and its response may precede the rise in prolactin levels. The maternal cerebrum is influenced by exposure to nursing cues as well as the influences of nipple stimulation. The cerebrum either stimulates or inhibits the hypothalamus to increase or decrease the production of prolactin inhibitory factor (dopamine) and, subsequently, the release of oxytocin from the posterior pituitary. Cerebral influences have a lesser effect on the release of prolactin. Positive sights, sounds, or smells related to nursing often stimulate the production of oxytocin, which, in turn, causes the myoepithelial cells to contact and milk to leak from the breasts. This observation is a good clinical clue indicating an uninhibited *let-down reflex*.

In a classic series of experiments, Newton and Egli[21] demonstrated the power of noxious influences to inhibit the release of oxytocin and to reduce milk transfer to the infant. The baseline milk production per feed was measured in controlled situations, about 160 g per feed. During a consecutive feed, a noxious event (i.e., saline injection) was administered during the feed. The amount of milk produced was cut in half, to 80 to 100 g per feed. Subsequently, the milk production was measured in a trial in which a noxious event was administered and intranasal oxytocin was given concomitantly. The milk production was restored to almost 90% of baseline production, 130 to 140 g. A wide variety of noxious events were able to elicit the same decrease in milk production. The noxious events included placing the mother's feet in ice water, applying electric shocks to her toes, having her trace shapes while

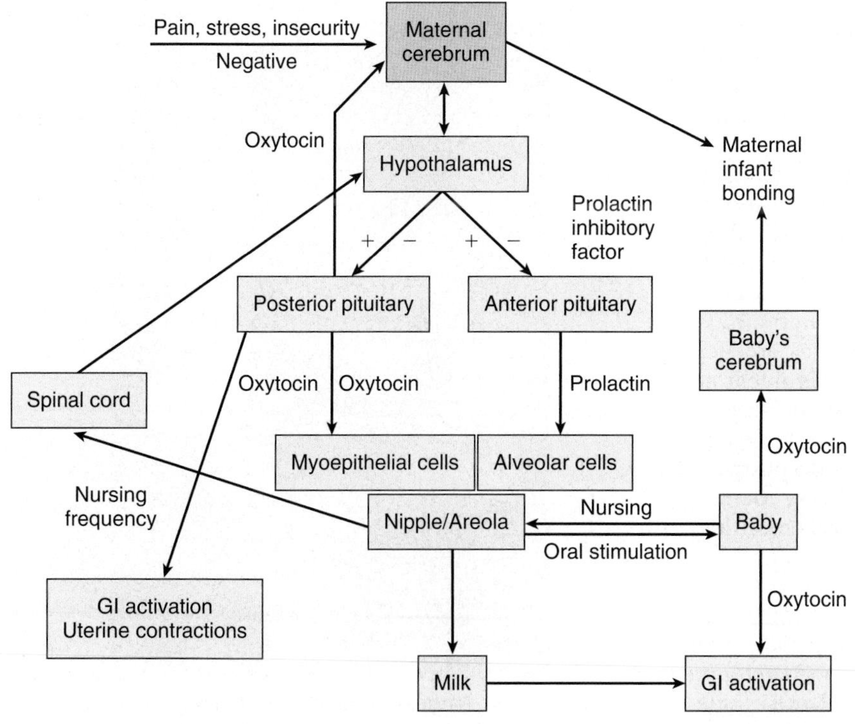

FIGURE 23-4. Oxytocin and the let-down reflex. The major reflex includes feedback stimulation from the nipple/areola to the hypothalamus to increase/decrease the release of oxytocin from the posterior pituitary and prolactin inhibitor factor (PIF-dopamine). The PIF affects the release of prolactin. Prolactin increases milk production. Oxytocin causes milk ejection. The release of both hormones is affected by positive or negative influences from the upper central nervous system. Oxytocin has three different target sites: the gastrointestinal tract (GI), uterus (contractions), and the upper CNS (mother-infant bonding). Oral stimulation in the infant initiates oxytocin release to improve GI activities and maternal-infant bonding. (From Rolland R, DeJong FJH. Schellekens LA et al: The role of prolactin in the restoration of ovarian function during the early postpartum period in the human: a study during inhibition of lactation by bromergocryptine. Clin Endocrinol 4:23, 1975.)

looking only through a mirror, or requiring her to proofread a document in a timed fashion. These observations have important implications concerning the management of breastfeeding. **Pain, anxiety, and insecurity may be hidden reasons for breastfeeding failure through the inhibitions of the let-down reflex. In contrast, the playing of a soothing motivational/educational audio tape to women who were pumping milk for their premature infants has improved milk yields.**[22] These observations have been confirmed by measuring the inhibition of oxytocin release by psychological stress.[23,24] The positive and negative influences of the cerebrum are further highlighted by the observation[25] that 75% of women who had a positive attitude during pregnancy were likely to be successful at breastfeeding. In contrast, 75% of women who had a negative attitude during pregnancy had an unsuccessful breastfeeding experience. This observation has been confirmed in more recent observations.[26] When the mother's attitude was very good or good and family was present, the exclusive breastfeeding rate was 20% at 6 months; if the mother's attitude was fair, the breastfeeding rate at 6 months was 5%.

Oxytocin has additional target cells in the mother. The effect of oxytocin on uterine activity is well known. Uterine involution is enhanced with breastfeeding. Animal and human research suggests that oxytocin is a neurohormone. Oxytocin is associated with an anti-fight/flight response in the autonomic nervous system, better toleration of stress by the mother, and improved maternal-infant bonding.[27]

In addition to the antistress effect, surges in oxytocin levels are associated with the release of gastrointestinal hormones and increased gastrointestinal motility. In the mother, these actions enhance the absorption of substrates necessary for lactogenesis. In infants, there is a growing body of knowledge that indicates similar associations with oxytocin surges. Skin-to-skin contact and the oral stimulation of nursing stimulate a parasympathetic, anti-fight/flight response in the infant. Kangaroo care of premature newborns (skin-to-skin contact) is associated with a physiologically stable state, improved stress responses, and improved weight gain.[28] Oxytocin appears to mediate this response. Breastfeeding is associated with far more skin-to-skin contact and maternal behaviors than bottle-feeding.

While the central nervous system locus for imprinting is unknown, imprinting immediately after birth is an important predictor of breastfeeding success. The survival of lambs depends on nursing within an hour after birth. If the lamb has not nursed during the critical period, maternal-infant bonding becomes dysfunctional and the lamb suffers failure to thrive. In humans, the consequences are not nearly as drastic. **Several trials with random assignment of subjects to early nursing (delivery room) or late nursing (2 hours after birth) demonstrated a 50% to 100% higher number of breastfeeding mothers at 2 to 4 months postpartum among those who had nursed in the delivery room.**[29] **One of the keys to obstetric management is have the mother nurse her newborn in the delivery room.**

Milk Transfer

Milk transfer to the infant is a key physiologic principle in lactation.[30] The initial step of this process is good latch-on. With light tactile stimulation of the cheek and lateral angle of the mouth, the infant reflexively turns its head and opens its mouth, as in a yawn (Figure 23-5). The nipple is tilted slightly downward using a "C-hold," or *palmar grasp*. In this hand position, the fingers support the breast from underneath and the thumb lightly grasps the upper surface 1 to 2 cm above the areola-breast line. The infant is brought firmly to the breast by the supporting arms while being careful to not push the back of the baby's head. The nipple and areola are drawn into the mouth as far as the areola-breast line (Figures 23-6 and 23-7). The posterior areola may be less visible than the anterior areola, and the lower lip of the infant is often curled out. The infant's lower gum lightly fixes the teat over the lactiferous sinuses. A slight negative pressure exerted by the oropharynx and mouth holds the length of the teat and breast in place and reduces the "work" to refill the lactiferous sinuses after they are drained. **The milk is extracted, not by negative pressure, but by a peristaltic wave from the tip of the tongue to the base.** There is no stroking, friction, or in-and-out motion of the teat; it is more of an undulating action. The buccal mucosa and tongue mold around the teat, leaving no space.

The peristaltic movement of the infant's tongue is most frequent in the first 3 minutes of a nursing episode; the mean latency from latch-on to milk ejection is 2.2 minutes. After milk flow is established, the frequency of sucking falls to a much slower rate. **The change in cadence is recognizable as "suck-suck-swallow-breath." Audible swallowing of milk is a good sign of milk transfer.** At the start of a feed the infant obtains 0.10 to 0.20 mL per suck. As the infant learns how to suck and as he matures he becomes more efficient at obtaining more milk in a shorter period of time. Eighty to 90% of the milk is obtained in the first 5 minutes the infant nurses on each breast, but the fat-rich and calorie-dense hind milk is obtained in the remainder

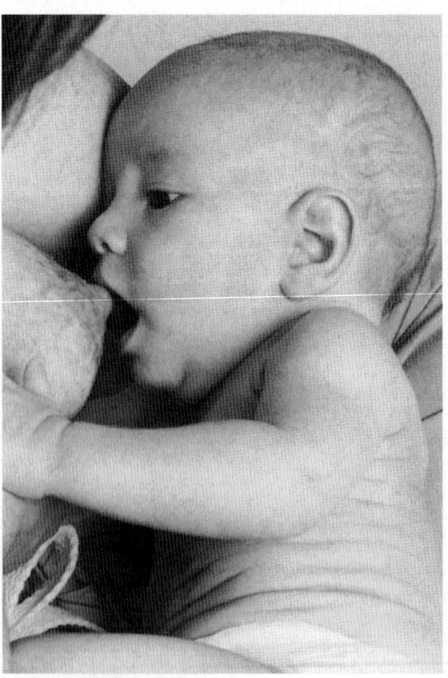

FIGURE 23-5. The latch-on reflex.

of the time sucking at each breast, usually less than 20 minutes total.[31] A bottle-feeding infant sucks steadily in a linear fashion, receiving about 80% of the artificial breast milk in the first 10 minutes.

Sucking on a bottle is mechanically very different from nursing on the human teat (Figure 23-8). The relatively

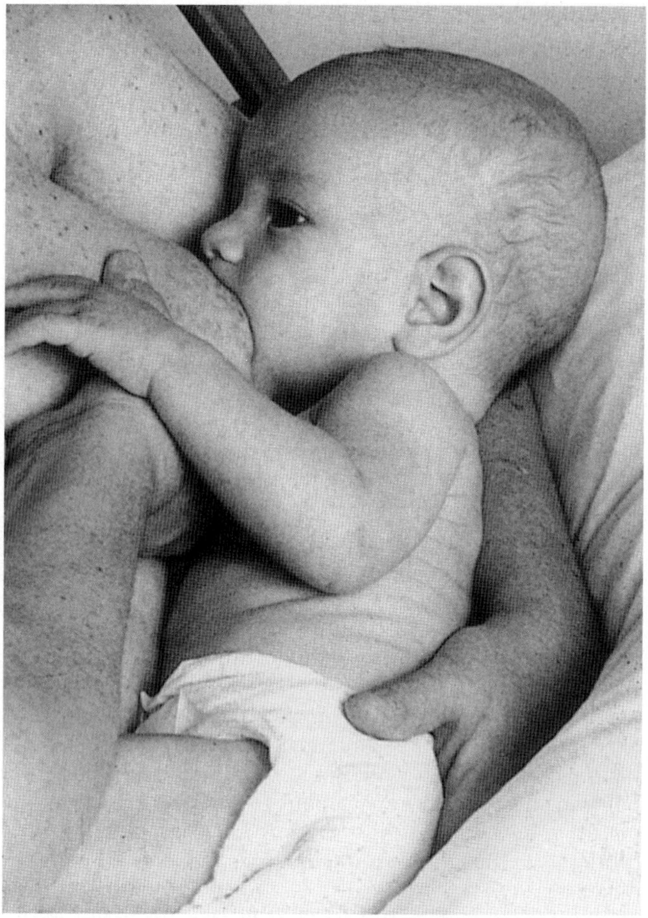

FIGURE 23-6. Appropriate latch-on.

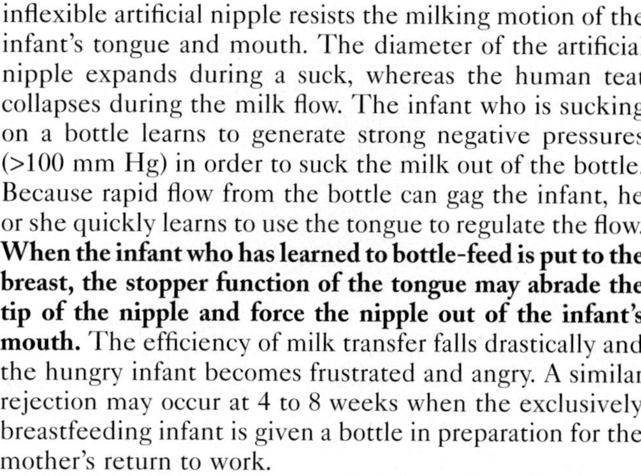

inflexible artificial nipple resists the milking motion of the infant's tongue and mouth. The diameter of the artificial nipple expands during a suck, whereas the human teat collapses during the milk flow. The infant who is sucking on a bottle learns to generate strong negative pressures (>100 mm Hg) in order to suck the milk out of the bottle. Because rapid flow from the bottle can gag the infant, he or she quickly learns to use the tongue to regulate the flow. **When the infant who has learned to bottle-feed is put to the breast, the stopper function of the tongue may abrade the tip of the nipple and force the nipple out of the infant's mouth.** The efficiency of milk transfer falls drastically and the hungry infant becomes frustrated and angry. A similar rejection may occur at 4 to 8 weeks when the exclusively breastfeeding infant is given a bottle in preparation for the mother's return to work.

Milk transfer is made more efficient by proper positioning of the infant to the breast. Proper positioning places the infant and mother chest-to-chest. The infant's ear, shoulder, and hip are in line. The three most common

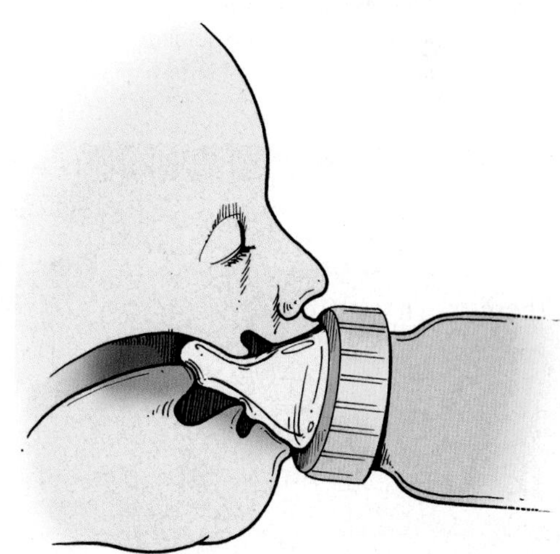

FIGURE 23-8. The mechanics of bottle feeding.

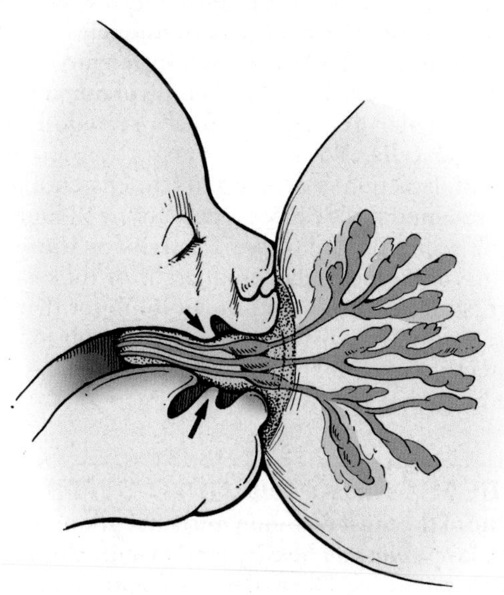

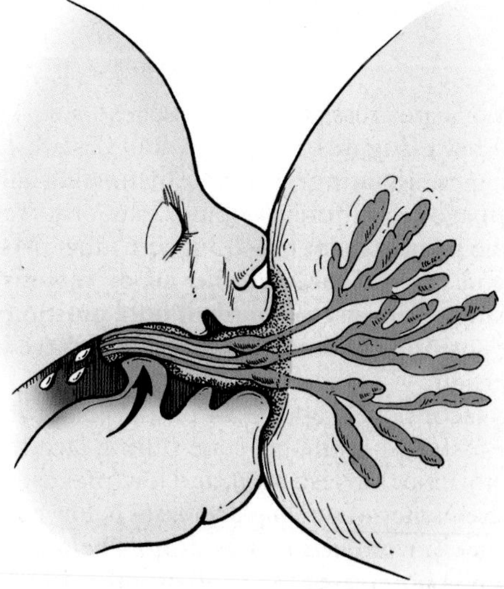

FIGURE 23-7. The mechanics of nursing.

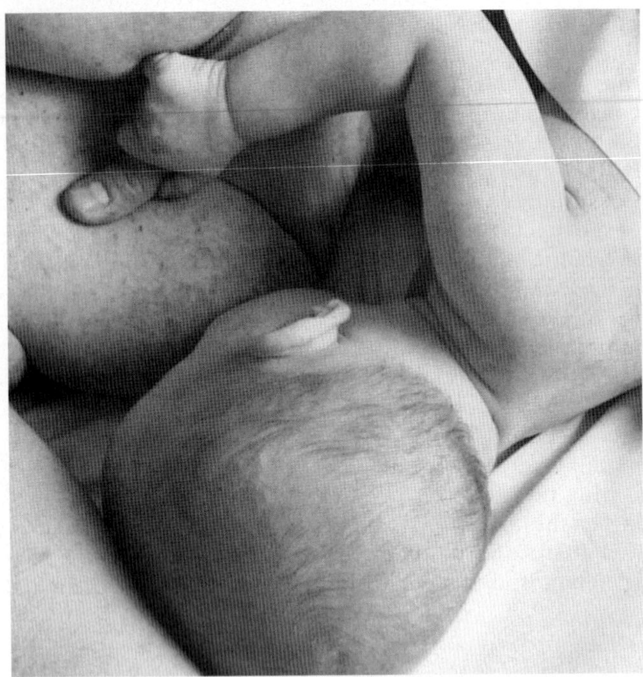

FIGURE 23-9. Side-lying nursing.

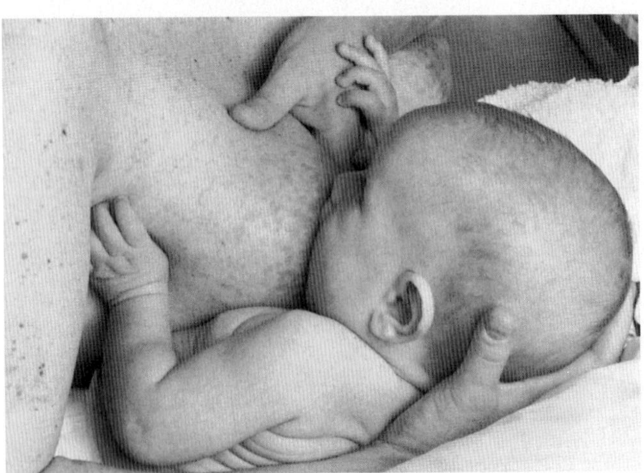

FIGURE 23-10. The football hold.

maternal positions are cross arm chest to-chest, side-lying, or the football hold (Figures 23-6, 23-9, and 23-10). Each has its advantages. Rotating positions of nursing allows improved drainage of different lobules, an observation important in the management of a "plugged" duct. **Maternal comfort and convenience are the major reasons for changing nursing positions; the football hold position and the side-lying position are more comfortable if there is an abdominal incision.**

Baseline prolactin levels appear to be the major determinant of the maternal hormonal state during lactation, a state of high-prolactin, low-estrogen, and low-progesterone levels. **As the frequency of nursing decreases below eight in 24 hours, the baseline prolactin levels drop to below a level where ovulation is suppressed (35 to 50 ng/mL), LH levels rise, and menstrual cycling is initiated.**[12] The intensity (adjusted odds ratio [OR]) of factors that initiate the onset of menses are the duration of sucking episodes less than 7 minutes (OR 2.4), night feeds less than four per 24 hours (OR 2.3), maternal age 15 to 24 years (OR 2.1), maternal age 25 to 34 years (OR 1.7), and day feeds less than seven per 24 hours (OR 1.6).[32] In women who feed their infants exclusively artificial breast milk, serum prolactin levels drop to prepregnant levels (8 to 14 ng/mL) within days. The total number of nursing episodes per day (more than eight per 24 hours) and night nursings are critical to the successful management of breastfeeding.

One of the major determinants of nursing frequency is the introduction of substitute nutriment sources for the infant, artificial breast milk or solids. **Breast milk has the nutritional content to satisfy the growth needs of the infant for at least 6 months postpartum.** In the first 6 months, feeding with artificial breast milk affects the physiology of successful lactation in three ways. Substitution with artificial breast milk reduces proportionally the nutriment requirements from breast milk, increases the gastric emptying time (slower digestion than breast milk) with a subsequent decrease in frequency of nursing episodes, and reduces the efficiency of nursing by the use of an opposing sucking technique on the artificial nipple.

Solid food (e.g., eggs, cereals, pureed food) have a similar effect on the hormonal milieu of the lactating woman. One of the errors in Western child care is the early, forced introduction of solids. In most cases, the infant's gut is filled with slowly digesting food with less nutritional quality than either artificial breast milk or breast milk. The long-term result may be childhood and adolescent obesity. The most logical time to start solid food substitution is when the infant has reached the neurologic maturity to grasp and bring food to its mouth from his or her mother's plate. The required neurologic maturity to perform this behavior usually occurs at about 6 months. As the infant matures, his or her ability to feed improves and the proportion of the diet supplied by solid food gradually increases.

The failure to develop good milk transfer is the major cause of lactational failure and breast pain, especially in the neonatal period. **Inhibition of the let-down reflex and failure to empty the breasts completely leads to ductal distention and parenchymal swelling (engorgement). Engorgement compromises the mechanics of nursing (Figure 23-11) and alveolar distention reduces secretion of milk by the alveolar cells.** Without adequate transfer of milk to the infant, lactation is doomed to fail. Distention of the alveoli by retained milk causes a rapid (6 to 12 hours) decrease in milk secretion and enzyme activity by the alveolar epithelium. The decreased production of milk is explained by pressure inhibition and by an inhibitor that is secreted in breast milk.[8,9] Distention of the alveoli inhibits secretion directly rather than indirectly by a decrease in nutriment or hormonal access.

BREAST MILK: THE GOLD STANDARD

One of the most common misconceptions by physicians and the lay public and heavily marketed by the formula industry is that modern "formulas" are equivalent to breast milk. Human breast milk is uniquely suited to our biologic needs

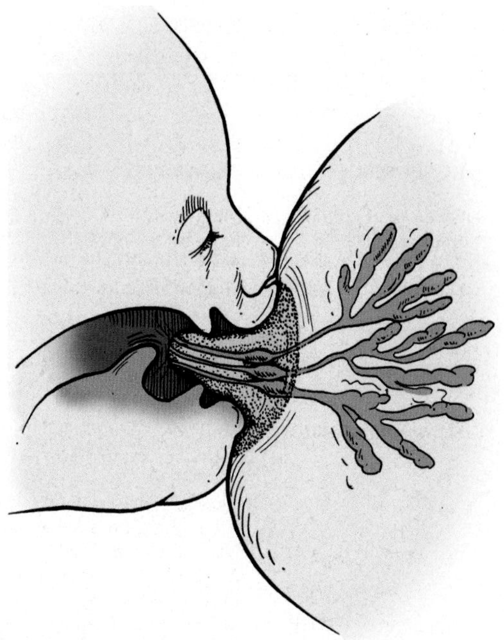

FIGURE 23-11. Breastfeeding and engorgement. The firm swollen breast parenchyma pushes the newborn's face away and she is unable to pull the teat into her mouth. Her tongue abrades the tip of the nipple.

and remains the best source of nutrition for the human infant. Human breast milk has a composition very different than that of bovine milk or soybean plants from which artificial breast milk is produced.[33] Nutritional, host-defense, hormonal, and psycho-physiological differences between human breast milk and breastfeeding versus formula and bottle feeding make the health benefits of breastfeeding understandable. This section will link the latter differences to a summary of a massive amount of basic and clinical research demonstrating the better health outcomes associated with breast milk and breastfeeding as compared to formula and bottle feeding.

The Agency for Healthcare Research and Quality (AHRQ) recently published (2007)[34] and updated (2009)[35] its analysis of the literature, "Breastfeeding and Maternal and Infant Health Outcomes in Developed Countries." The structure of the analysis is important for the reader to understand the effort and quality of the findings. Many different outcomes have been associated with a feeding method. The AHRQ used a panel of technical experts in the field of breastfeeding research to examine a specific outcome based on the following: the relevance and importance of an outcome in a developed country, date of the last systematic review on the outcome, availability or non-availability of data from a developed country, consistency or inconsistency of outcomes in previously reported studies, and consideration of the possibility that breastfeeding may have potential harms as well as benefits. All studies that were analyzed had to fulfill all the following four criteria: study designs included systematic reviews, randomized controlled trials, prospective cohort studies, and case-controlled studies; population included healthy term infants in developed countries; intervention included breastfeeding, breast milk feeding, exclusive or mixed feeding; and, the comparator was formula feeding (any type). Each primary study was graded as A (good—least bias and results are valid), B (fair—susceptible to some bias, but not sufficient to invalidate the results), or C (poor—significant biases which may invalidate the results). No conclusions were made from any Grade C studies. Prior meta-analyses were examined in a similar fashion and included sensitivity analysis in which the inclusion of poor quality studies might have affected the pooled estimates, and AHRQ tested its meta-analyses for heterogeneity.

Overview

The composition of mature human milk is very different from artificial breast milk or formula. Most artificial breast milk products use bovine milk or soybean constituents as a substrate. Minerals, vitamins, protein, carbohydrates, and fats are added to pasteurized bovine milk for perceived nutritional needs as well as marketing needs in order to make a product that will successfully compete with human breast milk. For example, human breast milk appears "thinner" than bovine milk. **Artificial breast milk manufacturers add constituents (e.g., palm- or coconut-based oils) to make artificial breast milk appear rich and creamy,** thereby creating a product that is more easily marketed to the American public.

Extensive research describes the unique composition of human milk. The infant formula industry has produced even greater volumes of data concerning their attempts to exactly reproduce human milk. In 1980, the U.S. Congress passed the Infant Formula Act (with revisions in 1985) as the result of severe health consequences when artificial breast milk failed to include key vitamins and minerals in new formula compositions. This law now requires that all formulas for artificial breast milk contain minimum amounts of essential nutrients, vitamins, and minerals. Although life-threatening omissions are unlikely, **current formulas have major differences in the total quantities and qualities of proteins, carbohydrates, minerals, vitamins, and fats when compared to human milk.** The reader is reminded that the recommended daily allowance (RDA) is the amount needed to prevent a deficiency disease, not the amount needed for the best health.

Breast milk promotes optimal somatic growth and metabolic competence. Human breast milk is designed for more efficient and better digestion by the human infant than the bovine or soybean derived formula.[33] Gastric emptying is faster in neonates fed breast milk versus formula, 1 to 2 hours versus 3 to 4 hours, respectively. The greater speed of digestion with breast milk relates to differences in casein: whey protein ratio, fatty acid content, fatty acid attachment to their glycerol backbone, and presence of gastrointestinal enzymes and gastrointestinal hormones to facilitate digestion, motility, and function. Formula contains limited and degraded hormones and enzymes appropriate for vegetarian ruminants, calves; or none in the formulas using a soybean base. In addition the bioavailability of naturally supplied vitamins and minerals in breast milk is 20% to 50% higher than the added vitamins and minerals in artificial breast milk.[33]

The nutritional differences between formula and human milk are reflected in differences in the growth patterns of infants who are exclusively breastfed for 4 to 6 months and

TABLE 23-3 THE EFFECTS OF INFANT FEEDING ON SOMATIC GROWTH AND CARDIOVASCULAR PATHOPHYSIOLOGY IN DEVELOPED COUNTRIES

	BENEFIT OF BREASTFEEDING (BF) ADJUSTED ODDS RATIO (95th CI)	RISK OF "FORMULA" ADJUSTED ODDS RATIO (95th CI)	REFERENCE	COMMENT
Childhood obesity	0.81 (0.77-0.84)	1.23 (1.14-1.3)	Owen et al (2005)[37]	Meta-analysis of 28 studies
Child developing Type 2 diabetes	0.61 (0.44-0.85)	1.64 (1.18-2.27)	Ip et al (2009)[35]	Ever BF vs. never BF AHRQ Review
Maternal cardiovascular disease (CVD)	0.72 (0.53-0.97)	1.39 (1.03-1.89)	Schwartz et al(2009)[38]	Women's Health Initiative, N = 139,681 Dose affect shown
Maternal hypertension	0.87 (0.82-0.92)	1.15 (1.09-1.22)	Schwartz et al (2009)[38]	Women's Health Initiative, N = 139,681 Dose affect shown
Maternal vascular calcifications	0.19 (0.05-0.68)	5.26 (1.47-20)	Schwarz et al (2010)[39]	Study of Women's Health Across the Nation (SWAN) N = 3302 Ages 42-52 Electron Beam Tomography
Maternal myocardial infarction	0.77 (0.62-0.94)	1.3 (1.06-1.61)	Steube et al (2009)[40]	Nurses' Health Study N = 89,329 parous women Dose effect shown
Maternal Type 2 diabetes	0.84 (0.78-0.91)	1.19 (1.10-1.28)	Steube et al (2005)[41]	Nurses' Health Study N = 89,329 parous women No gestational diabetes Dose effect shown

infants who are fed formula artificial breast milk.[36] **In general, breastfed infants have faster linear and head growth, whereas formula-fed infants tend to have greater weight gain and fat deposition.** The greater deposition in fat may relate in part to the earlier introduction of solid foods in the infants fed formula, a factor that has not been adequately controlled in current studies. **Regardless of the cause, formula has important adverse effects on the metabolic competence of the child, adolescent, and future adult (Table 23-3).**

Many clinicians feel that diet and exercise are the primary prevention intervention against obesity and cardiovascular disease. Their effect size is zero to 10%.[42] The primary prevention benefits of breastfeeding compares very well; its effect size is 15% to 560%. The alarming epidemic of obesity, especially in children and young adults, is a clarion call for breastfeeding for at least a year.

Breastfeeding enhances cognitive development. Human breast milk has superior capacity to enhance the development of the infant's brain and its integrative capacity through many defined and undefined differences between human breast milk and formula. The currently identified constituents of human breast milk that enhance integrative capacity include growth hormones, oligosaccharides, nucleotides, glycoproteins, and long-chain polyunsaturated fatty acids (LCPUFA). **In high-risk, premature neonates, human breast milk given by gavage in a dose-dependent fashion enhances the infant's later intelligence quotient (IQ) and performance on psychometric testing after controlling for maternal intelligence, family education, and socioeconomic status.**[43] While the effect is most dramatic among high-risk infants, smaller effects on IQ are seen in term infants: adjusted increment (95th CI)—3.16 points (2.35-3.98); versus low birthweight infants: 5.18 (3.59-6.77) points.[44] A recent large cohort study comparing very-low-birthweight infants[14] demonstrated that for every 10 mL/kg/day increment of breast milk fed to these high-risk neonates neurodevelopmental outcomes improved.[45] The information regarding breastfeeding, LCPUFA, and improved intelligence has been powerful enough for formula companies to change their concoctions to include more LCPUFA. However, just adding LCPUFA does not change the other deficiencies in formula. Another recent example of neurodevelopmental enhancement with breastfeeding is a strong association between breastfeeding and enhanced visual acuity: infants fed LCPUFA-enhanced formula had similar deficiencies in high-grade foveal stereoacuity—adjusted OR (95th CI) = 2.5(1.4-4.5), as infants fed standard formula.[46]

Breastfeeding enhances infant responses to infection and reduces allergic disease. At birth, the fetus enters an unsterile world with a naïve and immature immune system. Full development of the immune system may take up to 6 years. **Breast milk has a wide array of anti-infective properties that will support the developing immune system. The major mechanisms for the protective properties of breast milk include active leukocytes, antibodies, antibacterial products, competitive inhibition, enhancement of nonpathogenic commensal organisms, and suppression of proinflammatory immune responses.**[47] A critical event in host resistance is the recognition of pathogenic agents in the environment and the production of an antigen-specific adaptive immune response. Breastfeeding provides a unique system to help the infant fight infection with an adaptive antigen-specific response. Through breast milk, the neonate takes advantage of maternal recognition of these infectious agents (Figure 23-12). This important mechanism is described by Slade and Schwartz.[48] An antigen or infectious agent (virus, bacteria, fungus, and protozoa) stimulates the activity of leukocytes in the gastrointestinal or respiratory tract of

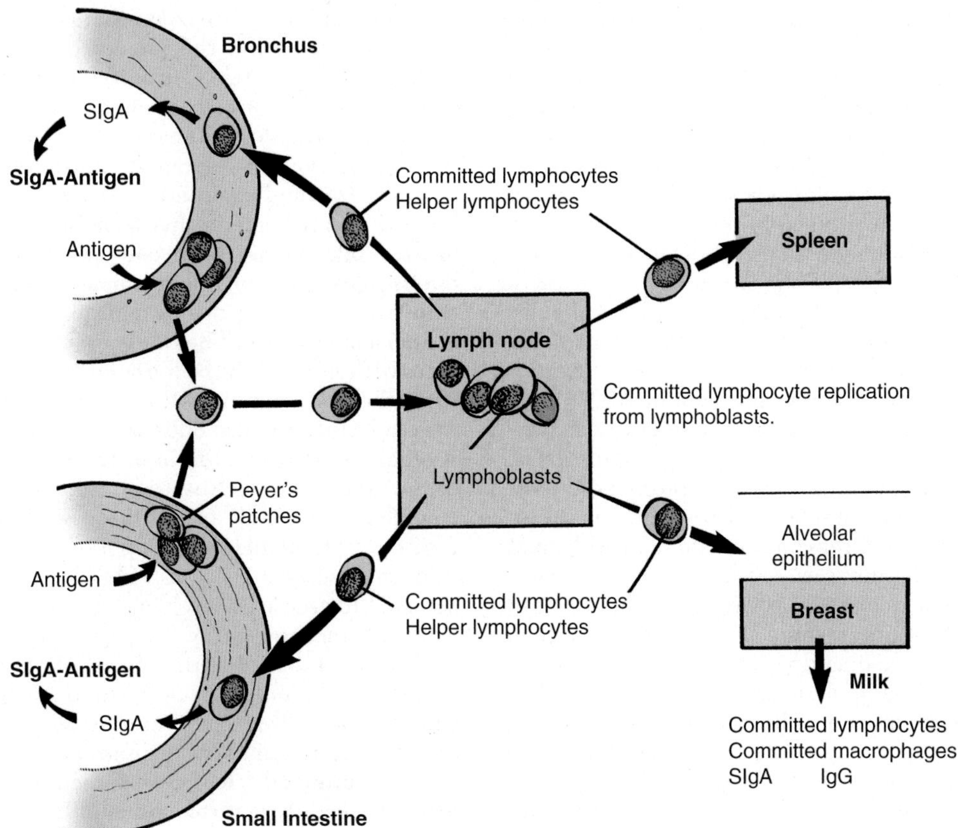

FIGURE 23-12. The immunology of the breast.

the mother. Lymphocytes, which are encoded with the antigen signature, travel to the nearest lymph node and stimulate lymphoblasts to develop cytotoxic T cells, helper T cells, and plasma cells programmed to destroy the initiating antigen through phagocytosis or complement/immunoglobulins produced by the B cells. The response is amplified by the migration of committed helper lymphocytes to other sites of white blood cell production, the spleen and bone marrow, where they stimulate the production of antigen-specific committed white blood cells. Some of the committed, antigen-specific helper lymphocytes travel to the mucosa of the breast in the lactating mother. Plasma cells, which produce secretory immunoglobulin A (sIgA), constitute 50% to 80% of the leukocytes in the breast submucosa. They may migrate into the breast milk (macrophages) or may produce immunoglobulins (sIgA, IgG—lymphocytes or plasma cells). Both are uniquely programmed to fight the specific infectious agent challenging the mother. **Active leukocytes are completely eliminated by pasteurization (formula) or freezing (stored, pumped breast milk).**

Immunoglobulins are a unique component to breast milk and absent in artificial breast milk. In contrast to monomeric serum IgA, the secretory immunoglobulin A (sIgA) in breast milk is dimeric or polymeric. Polymerization improves transport across the maternal alveolar cells into the breast milk. The sIgA is produced locally by plasma cells. The immunoglobulins in breast milk appear to be fully functional. Secretory immunoglobulin A does not activate, complement, or promote opsonic complement subfragments. As a consequence, sIgA is not bactericidal. It appears that sIgA blocks the mucosal receptors (adhesins) on the infectious agent. The virulence of pathogens is related to their ability to use adhesins capable of interacting with complementary gut epithelial cell-surface receptors. When the antigen-specific sIgA attaches, the pathogen is effectively neutralized.

In the last 5 to 10 years there has been an accelerating amount of focus and research on critically imprinting between neonatal gut flora and future immune responses. The neonate is an antigen-naïve organism and has an adaptive response that is delayed by the lack of exposure. In addition, the cytokine response to TOLL-like receptors stimulation appears to be exaggerated, especially in the preterm infant in whom damage is partly caused by cytokine-mediated injury (i.e., periventricular leukomalacia, necrotizing enterocolitis, and broncho-pulmonary dysplasia).[49] The adaptive immunologic response takes between 4 and 8 days to develop an effective defense; the neonate bombarded by new antigens/organisms during birth must rely on an innate host defense system to provide an immediate but controlled response during the first critical 0 to 7 days of breastfeeding.

Human breast milk actively limits the pathogenic microbes (e.g., *E. coli*) and promotes the growth of nonpathogenic, commensal microbes (e.g., *Bifidobacterium bifidum*).[50] The most important breast milk constituent is oligosaccharides, which are in very limited quantity in formula. Oligosaccharides are indigestible complex carbohydrate structures that have a microbe (genus)-specific ability to bind to cell-surface receptors of the microbe. The unique oligosaccharide binding to the surface receptor blocks the binding of the microbe to the infant's mucosal receptors, thereby limiting microbe virulence. On the other hand, human milk contains an oligosaccharide homologous to the infant's mucosal receptors. The oligosaccharide-mucosal receptor complex allows specific attachment of *B. bifidum* to the intestinal mucosa, further competitively inhibiting the attachment of pathogenic organisms.

A similar attachment of *B. bifidum* to dendritic cells, which interdigitate through the intestinal epithelial cells, allows for a critical modulation of the developing neonatal immune system. The interaction upregulates the anti-inflammatory cytokine system, interleukin-10, soluble IL-1 receptor antagonist, etc., and orchestrates the conversion of naive T-helper cells into a mature balanced response. These early imprinting interactions have profound effects on the incidence of inflammatory diseases in the adult, intrinsic bowel disease, asthma, rheumatoid arthritis, and perhaps cardiovascular diseases.[51]

In addition to the crosstalk between commensal gut bacteria and the immune system of the neonate, human colostrum contains large quantities of a soluble form of the bacterial pattern recognition receptor CD14 (sCD14).[52] CD14 is a known modulator of host response to bacterial lipopolysaccharides (LPS). In particular, CD14 binds to TLR-4 receptors and limits the binding of LPS from gram-negative rods. The failure to activate the TLR-4 receptor reduces the exaggerated immature cytokine response possible in neonates. Recent therapeutic interventions have used the immunomodulating qualities of the commensal bacteria–host interactions to successfully treat several important human diseases: necrotizing enterocolitis, inflammatory bowel disease, *C. difficile*-associated colitis, acute gastroenteritis, and atopic dermatitis.[50,51]

Known and unknown constituents of human breast milk (not formula) inhibit the growth of and actively destroy pathogenic organisms. Certain vitamins and minerals are essential for the growth of pathogenic bacteria. A major mechanism by which breast milk protects the infant is the competition for "essential" nutriments for pathogenic bacteria. **Iron and vitamin B_{12} are two essential nutriments for pathogenic bacteria that have been studied relative to breast milk. Breast milk contains lactoferrin, an iron-binding glycoprotein, in large quantities (5.5 mg/mL in the colostrum to 1.5 mg/mL in mature milk) and is absent in artificial breast milk. The free iron form of lactoferrin competes with siderophilic bacteria for ferric iron, and thus disrupts the proliferation of these organisms. The binding of iron to lactoferrin also enhances iron absorption; less iron is required in breast milk in order to satisfy the iron needs of the infant.** The antibacterial role of lactoferrin is more complex than simple competition for ferric iron.[53] Lactoferrin causes a release of lipopolysaccharide molecules from the bacterial cell wall. This appears to sensitize the cell wall to attack by lysozyme. Lactoferrin and lysozyme work together to destroy the pathogenic organisms.

Table 23-4 describes the effects of breastfeeding on the adaptive and innate host defenses on health. The cause of sudden infant death syndrome is not clear, but a current theory includes an aberrant immune response.

The hormonal changes of lactation—low estrogen/progesterone, hyperprolactinemic amenorrhea—favor a reduction in maternal reproductive cancers, but the relationship is undefined and the relationship between the maternal immune system and her experience with breastfeeding has not been adequately explored. However, breastfeeding in a dose-dependent fashion reduces breast cancer per year of cumulative breastfeeding by 4.3% (95th CI, 2.9%-5.8%).[34,35] Likewise, breastfeeding for greater

TABLE 23-4 BREASTFEEDING REDUCES INFECTION AND ALLERGIC DISEASE

OUTCOME	BENEFIT OF BREASTFEEDING (BF) ADJUSTED ODDS RATIO (95th CI)	RISK OF FORMULA ADJUSTED ODDS RATIO (95th CI)	REFERENCES	COMMENT
Acute otitis media	0.77 (0.64-0.94)	1.30 (1.06-1.56)	Ip et al (2009)[35]	Reduced by exclusive BF >4 months AHRQ Review
Gastrointestinal infections	0.36 (0.32-0.41) 0.54 (0.36-.80)	2.78 (2.44-3.12) 1.85 (1.25-2.78)	Ip et al (2009)[35]	Cohort studies Case-control AHRQ Review
Lower respiratory infections	0.28 (0.14-0.54)	3.57 (1.85-7.14)	Ip et al (2009)[35]	Outcome: hospitalization BF >4 months vs. "formula" only AHRQ Review
Asthma	0.73 (0.59-0.92)	1.37 (1.09-1.69)	Ip et al (2009)[35]	No family history of asthma, BF >3 months AHRQ Review
Atopic dermatitis	0.58 (0.41-0.92)	1.72 (1.09-2.44)	Ip et al (2009)[35]	Positive family history of atopy AHRQ Review
Type 1 diabetes	0.70 (0.56-0.87)	1.43 (1.15-1.77)	Gerstein et al (1994)[54]	Case-control studies, recall bias potential
Childhood leukemia	0.81 (0.71-0.91)	1.23 (1.10-1.41)	Ip et al (2009)[35]	BF >6 months vs. BF <6 months AHRQ Review
Sudden infant death syndrome	0.64 (0.51-0.81)	1.56 (1.23-1.96)	Ip et al (2009)[35]	Ever BF vs. No BF AHRQ Review

AHRQ, Agency for Healthcare Research and Quality; *BF*, breastfeeding.

than 12 months in her lifetime reduces ovarian cancer (adjusted OR [95th CI]—0.72 [0.54-0.97]); conversely, exclusive feeding with formula is associated with an enhanced risk of ovarian cancer (adjusted OR [95th CI]—1.39 [1.03-1.85]).

Breastfeeding enhances mother-infant bonding and reduces poor social adaptation. The human newborn infant is born entirely dependent on the mother for transportation, food, warmth, and social conditioning. Survival depends on a unique bond between mother and infant to enhance maternal protective behaviors. Like all other mammals, humans have a critical imprinting period (1-2 hours) for the establishment of mother-infant bonding. The most visible manifestation of the new bond is the duration of breastfeeding. Numerous studies with random assignment of breastfeeding dyads to early (<1 hr) or later initiation (>2 hrs) of breastfeeding demonstrate a significantly higher incidence of any breastfeeding or exclusive breastfeeding at 2 to 4 months after birth in those dyads who initiated breastfeeding early. A recent review by Moore et al. with Cochrane Database of Systematic Reviews (2009)[28] supports the benefits of early skin-to-skin contact. Their conclusions from the review of 30 studies involving 1925 mother-infant dyads were that early skin-to-skin contact was associated with babies who interacted more with their mothers, stayed warmer, and cried less. **Babies were more likely to be breastfed, and to breastfeed for longer, if they had early skin-to-skin contact.** More recently, a study with random assignment of subjects to immediate skin-to-skin contact or not, with timing of first feed being mother-directed and independently recorded, suggested that **early skin-to-skin contact was a better predictor of duration of exclusive breastfeeding than the timing of first sucking episode.**[55] This observation complements the success of "kangaroo mother care" in the performance of high-risk neonates in the neonatal intensive care unit.

Recent human studies based on robust animal data suggest that continued skin-to-skin contact and breastfeeding greatly affect the responsiveness to stress in the infant and mother. Experimental physiologic and psychological stressors have measured stress-induced changes in adrenocorticotropic hormone, cortisol, and autonomic responses in breastfeeding women versus women feeding their infant exclusively formula. In keeping with numerous animal studies, **the breastfeeding mothers had significantly blunted hypothalamic-pituitary-adrenal response (HPA axis), also known as "fight or flight response," to the experimental stressors.**[56] There appears to be a reciprocal relationship in the breastfeeding infant; the breastfed infant has greater parasympathetic tone and a blunted HPA-axis response than a similar infant fed formula. These observations may be partially explained by a decrease in skin-to-skin contact in infants fed formula. While "kangaroo mother care" has a salutary effect on breastfeeding incidence, the positive effects on weight gain and a blunted stress response are independently associated with the amount of skin-to-skin contact.[57,58]

The association between breastfeeding and better psychosocial outcomes has been the topic of much research over many decades. Critics have repeatedly pointed out the selection bias inherent with these studies. However, improved epidemiologic research design has confirmed the lifelong value for the breastfeeding dyad in subsequent stressful situations. Two powerful studies illustrate the risk of not breastfeeding. In the first study, **Strathearn et al. (2009)[59] explored whether breastfeeding was protective against maternal-perpetrated child maltreatment.** The study design monitored prospectively 7223 Australian mother-infant pairs (identified at first prenatal visit) and followed them over a 15-year period after birth. The outcome was substantiated maltreatment reports by a governmental child protection agency. Maternally-perpetrated substantiated abuse or neglect was identified in 313 (4.3% of cohort). The analyses adjusted for the 18 confounding variables including sociodemographic variables (5); prenatal behavior/attitudes (i.e., substance abuse, anxiety, attitude toward pregnancy) (4); infant factors, including neonatal intensive care admission (4); postnatal behaviors/attitudes (i.e., mother-infant separation, maternal stimulation/teaching of baby, maternal depression) (7). **The adjusted OR (95th CI) for maternal maltreatment cases among children fed exclusively formula was 2.2 (1.5-3.2) versus any breastfeeding, and 3.8 (2.1-7.0) versus exclusive breastfeeding for 4 months or longer.**

In the second study[1] the response of the child was measured. Montgomery et al. (2006)[60] used the data collected in the 1970 British Cohort Study. In this study the subjects were followed for 10 years; 8958 (71%) had complete data and were used in the analysis. The study analyzed childhood anxiety associated with parental divorce or separation as reported by their teachers on an analog scale of 0 to 50 related to the question, "Was (the subject) worried and anxious about many things?". Exclusive feeding with formula, after adjustment for many factors, was associated with a dramatic increase in perceived childhood anxiety, adjusted OR (95th CI) = 8.8 (5.3-12.2); whereas breastfeeding at entry had no significant effect on childhood anxiety associated with divorce, adjusted OR (95th CI) = 1.3 (−3.6-6.1).

Breastfeeding is cost-effective for the family and society. **The nonmedical costs of artificial breast milk (formula) feeding are considerably higher than for breastfeeding.**[61] The direct cost of artificial breast milk feeding includes the cost of the artificial formula (900 mL/day), bottles, and supplies. In eastern North Carolina (June 2011), the average retail cost of 900 mL of prepared formula was about $6.50 daily ($2373 yearly); of concentrate, about $4.50 daily ($1,642 yearly); and of powdered formula, about $3.65 daily ($1,332 yearly). A major indirect cost of artificial breast milk feeding is the environmental impact of large dairy herds to supply the bovine milk substrate.

Breastfeeding provides the right amount of a superior product at precisely the right time and at the right temperature. The nonmedical costs of breastfeeding include the cost of increased dietary calorie and protein needs ($1 to $2 daily), nursing bras and breast pads, and an increased number of diapers in the first 2 to 3 months. If an electric breast pump is used when the woman returns to work, the cost of breastfeeding will increase $3 to $5 per day.

Increase in acute medical diseases will manifest as increased costs of medical care for those families who choose to feed their infant artificial breast milk.[42-45] Among Medicaid populations in Colorado, California, and health

TABLE 23-5 EXCESS MEDICAL COST AMONG 1000 NEVER BREASTFED VS. 1000 EXCLUSIVE (>3 MONTHS) BREASTFED INFANTS

	EXCESS SERVICES PER YEAR/1000 NEVER BF	TOTAL EXCESS COST
Office visits	1693	$111,315
Follow-up visits	340	$22,355
Medications*	609	$7,669
Chest radiography	51	$1,836
Days of hospitalization†	212	$187,866
Total excess cost per year		$331,031

Modified from Ball TM, Wright AL: Health care costs of formula-feeding in the first year of life. Pediatrics 103:870, 1999.
*Lower respiratory infection, otitis media.
†Lower respiratory infection, gastroenteritis.

TABLE 23-6 EXCESS PEDIATRIC COSTS AND DEATHS WITH THE FAILURE TO EXCLUSIVELY BREASTFEED FOR 6 MONTHS IN 80% OF DYADS

	EXCESS COST (DEATHS) COMPARED WITH 80% COMPLIANCE*
Total	$10,491,841,489 (714)
Sudden infant death syndrome	$3,722,074,013 (352)
Necrotizing enterocolitis deaths	$2,218,109,495 (210)
Pneumonia deaths	$1,557,915,767(146)
Otitis media	$765,766,295
Atopic dermatitis	$497,497,274
Childhood obesity	$404,195,504
Pneumonia hospitalization	$381,578,219
Childhood asthma	$229,194,255
Necrotizing enterocolitis hospitalization	$219,843,084
Childhood asthma deaths	$148,022,294 (14)
Gastroenterocolitis	$162,076,307
Childhood leukemia deaths	$133,422,239 (13)
Childhood Type I diabetes deaths	$64,999,258 (6)
Type I diabetes	$5,717,067
Childhood leukemia	$1,430,416

Modified from Bartick M, Reinhold A: The burden of suboptimal breastfeeding in the United States: a pediatric cost analysis. Pediatrics 125:1048, 2010, Table 3.
*2007 $US.

maintenance organizations in Arizona, the medical cost of artificial breast milk feeding amounts to $300 to $500 dollars per year per infant. Among patients who belonged to a large health maintenance organization in Tucson, Arizona, the excess yearly medical costs of 1000 never-breastfed infants versus 1000 infants who were exclusively breastfed for at least 3 months was $331,041[62] (Table 23-5).

The health care benefits are also reflected in the reduction of medical leave taken by the working mother to care for the sick child. **The recent data demonstrate fewer days for sick leave of women who work and continue to breastfeed than working women who bottle-feed.**[61,63]

A recent cost analysis by Bartick and Reinhold (2010)[64] calculated the excess pediatric costs with current U.S. breastfeeding initiation rates in 2005 (74%) and exclusive breastfeeding rates at 6 months (12.3%) as compared to 80% exclusive breastfeeding for 6 months using the published AHRQ analysis.[34,35] The total excess cost amounted to almost $10.5 billion and 714 deaths per year (Table 23-6). Their estimates do not account for the excess burden of chronic disease in the mother and child, obesity, Type II diabetes, and cardiovascular disease. The true burden is many folds greater than just the pediatric costs.

LIMITATIONS OF BREASTFEEDING RESEARCH

In the past there have been major flaws in the designs and conclusions of epidemiologic research regarding the benefits (or lack of benefits) of breastfeeding. In the last 10 years the quality has improved, but several cautions are warranted. **A major confounder is the difference in the demographic characteristics between women who breastfeed and women who use formula. Many breastfeeding outcomes, such as infections and chronic diseases, are also more prevalent in the lower socioeconomic groups.** When comparing outcomes between breastfeeding and artificial breast milk feeding, the effect of demographic differences should be analyzed and controlled in the analysis. In addition, cultural support and demographic differences of women who breastfeed their infants have changed. In the 1950s and 1960s cultural pressures pushed better educated, wealthier middle-class women away from breastfeeding; the incidence of initiation of breastfeeding reached its nadir in the early 1970s. This change is important when considering recall data used in studies evaluating differences in chronic diseases in the older adult, especially breast cancer.

Much of the older epidemiologic research has relied on self-report and recall data, usually long after the event has occurred. Memory is not perfect and biases are often introduced, such as combining events into convenient ages or socially acceptable times of weaning. One major area of recall bias is the definition of partial breastfeeding. An example of the confounding nature of this bias is a serial survey of nurses.[65] The study showed no significant benefit of breastfeeding in the reduction of premenopausal breast cancer, which was touted by the authors as evidence of no relationship between breastfeeding and breast cancer. As this was a population of nurses, in which a significant number were working at the time they were feeding their infant (this was not measured), the definition of breastfeeding may reflect intent more than actual intensity and duration of breastfeeding.

When analyzing any article involving breastfeeding, it is important to understand the author's definition of breastfeeding. **Exclusive breastfeeding is considered when the infant does not receive any additional food or nutriment other than breast milk. Partial breastfeeding needs to be defined by the proportion of feeds that are breast milk or artificial breast milk. If an infant consumes 700 mL of formula per day, then the proportion of breast milk consumed is small regardless of the frequency of breastfeeding episodes.** Control for the "dose" effect is important in physiologic as well as epidemiologic studies. The content and character of breast milk are affected by the frequency of feeds, the duration of the feed, when in the feed the breast milk is collected, the method of breast milk collection, and the time of day of the collection.

After statistical control for demographic variables, an unavoidable bias remains self-selection. Intrinsic personality characteristics may be determinants of feeding choice; a random allocation of feeding method is not possible. The random assignment of "at risk" preterm neonates to receiving breast milk or formula designed for preterm neonates, in the evaluation of cognitive development[66] or infections[67] avoids some of the maternal self-selection. However, a well-designed prospective cohort study with a sufficient sample size remains the standard method for the design of good breastfeeding research.

Recently, newer population research designs reduce the self-selection bias. Cluster-randomized trials of breastfeeding promotion intervention modeled on the WHO/UNICEF Baby-Friendly Hospital initiative (see box, 10 Steps to Successful Breastfeeding)[68] **have been used in two separate populations.**[69,70] In these studies, maternity clinics and hospitals are assigned randomly to receive intensive educational programs to increase breastfeeding rates. The outcomes of interest are breastfeeding rates and short-term neonatal morbidities (infections, atopic dermatitis, etc.) **In both studies, breastfeeding rates were improved significantly (*P* <0.001) with exclusive breastfeeding at 3 months, 43.4% versus 6.4% in Belarus**[69] **and 79% versus 48% in India.**[70] **The interventions were associated with 30% to 50% lower prevalence of gastrointestinal infections and atopic dermatitis and better infant growth.**

10 Steps to Successful Breastfeeding

1. Have a written policy to support breastfeeding.
2. Train all health care providers.
3. Inform all pregnant women about the benefits of management of breastfeeding.
4. Initiate breastfeeding within 1 hour after birth.
5. Show mothers how to breastfeed and maintain lactation even if they are separated from their infants.
6. Give newborn infants no food or drink other than breast milk, unless medically indicated.
7. Allow mothers and infants to remain together 24 hours a day (i.e., rooming in).
8. Encourage breastfeeding on demand.
9. Give no artificial teats or pacifiers.
10. Foster the establishment of breastfeeding support groups and refer mothers to them on discharge from the hospital or clinic.

Modified from WHO/UNICEF: Protesting, promoting, and supporting breastfeeding: the special role of maternity services, a joint WHO/UNICEF statement. Geneva, World Health Organization, 1989.[68]

A potential new variable is the prevalence and intensity of breast pumping, a variable incompletely measured in breastfeeding research. **The breast pump is a critically important adaptation where breastfeeding is difficult and sometimes impossible. The availability of breast pumps have allowed women and their children to get through the difficult times and successfully feed their infant breast milk for a prolonged period.** These women will accrue much of the benefit of breastfeeding; a choice much better than formula feeding. However, the differences between exclusively breastfeeding and exclusively breast milk feeding have the potential to negatively affect some of the benefits of breastfeeding.

As many as 80% of professional women rely heavily on the breast pump. In observational surveys, many of these women will report themselves as exclusively breastfeeding when they are actually partially breastfeeding and partially feeding breast milk obtained through a breast pump, often frozen, and bottle-fed at a later time. **Pumping and bottle-feeding the breast milk later upsets the delicate supply-and-demand relationship between the dyad and reduces skin-to-skin contact, and freezing may affect the nutritional, anti-infective qualities of the stored breast milk.** The use of bottles may increase acute otitis media and negate the positive benefits seen in breastfeeding dyads, as bottle feeding is a strong predictor of acute otitis media. There is paucity of information regarding this bias and behavior; it presents a great opportunity for research.

THE ROLE OF THE OBSTETRICIAN AND GYNECOLOGIST

The gynecologist plays a primary role in the initiation of breastfeeding.[71] Between 50% and 70% of women make a decision regarding how they will feed their infants before their pregnancies. The gynecologist needs to start promotion before the first pregnancy. When the reproductive-aged woman seeks initial family planning advice and contraception, there is high likelihood she will become pregnant in the next 2 to 5 years. **The breast examination is a regular part of the family planning visit;** it is used extensively to screen for breast cancer despite its rare occurrence at the ages of usual pregnancies (less than 35 years old). **This visit is a good opportunity to reassure the woman of her normal breast anatomy and build her self-efficacy for lactation success through vocal and visible support of breastfeeding.**

The obstetrician/gynecologist amplifies support for breastfeeding by community advocacy, office environment, and personal choices. The office environment needs to be "breastfeeding friendly." **Visible, active support of breastfeeding includes the presence of breastfeeding mothers, patient educational programs on breastfeeding, a quiet area for nursing mothers, the absence of material supplied by formula companies, and visible support for office personnel who choose to breastfeed.** The physician, especially a female obstetrician/gynecologist, can be a positive role model for patients. Women will ask the female gynecologist whether and how long she breastfed her children. Her answers will have a powerful influence.

An important role of the obstetrician is to identify (early in pregnancy) those women who cannot breastfeed or who may have challenges (Table 23-7).[72] The liberal use of lactation consultants as case managers, the use of galactagogues, and tube feeding devices can mediate challenges related to breast milk production or breast milk transfer. The WHO has good guidelines regarding the use of formula in cases in which breastfeeding is contraindicated.

The obstetrician plays a major role in directing and supporting prenatal patient education about breastfeeding in the last trimester. Patient education has been shown to

TABLE 23-7 IDENTIFICATION OF WOMEN AT HIGH RISK FOR UNSUCCESSFUL BREASTFEEDING OUTCOMES

CONDITION	RISK ASSESSMENT	MANAGEMENT
HIV in United states	Contraindicated	Formula feeding
Untreated active tuberculosis	Contraindicated	Neonatal antibiotic treatment, resume breastfeeding after 2 weeks of maternal therapy if mother asymptomatic
Herpes of nipple	Contraindicated on infected side	Isolate lesions, treat mother and infant systemically
Maternal antineoplastic medications	Contraindicated	Formula feeding
Neonatal galactosemia	Breast milk and "formula" contraindicated	Lactose-free supplement
Breast reduction surgery	High risk	Prenatal consultation with lactation consultant and pediatrician
Breast augmentation	Moderate risk	Prenatal consultation with lactation consultant and pediatrician
Failure of breasts to enlarge during pregnancy, small tubular breasts	Moderate to high risk	Prenatal consultation with lactation consultant and pediatrician
Unsuccessful breastfeeding with prior child	Moderate risk	Identify issues, prenatal education, prenatal consultation with lactation consultant

increase the initiation and maintenance of breastfeeding. A recent review[73] by the U.S. Preventive Service Task Force of 38 well-conducted trials with **random assignment of subjects to primary care interventions to promote breastfeeding versus "usual care" demonstrated significantly increased rates of short-term (1 to 3 months) and long-term (6 to 8 months) exclusive breastfeeding.** In subgroup analysis a combined prenatal and postnatal intervention had a larger effect on increasing breastfeeding duration than a prenatal or postnatal intervention alone. Interventions that included individual-level professional support and lay counselors had the most impact. A similar review[74] demonstrated that a combined educational and support intervention improved breastfeeding rates (95th CI): initiation—21% (7%-35%), short-term—36% (22%-49%), and long-term—13% (1%-25%).

At the 36-week visit, the obstetrician readdresses the mother's choice and knowledge regarding breastfeeding. Simple concepts of breastfeeding physiology are reinforced: early feeds, frequent feeds (>10 per day), reinforcing environment, and no supplementation unless directed by a pediatrician. The obstetrician reinforces the appropriate way to latch the baby to the breast and ensures that the increase in her breast size reflects the hormonal readiness for breastfeeding. The patient is warned of hospital policies and attitudes that interfere with breastfeeding success. The 36-week visit is a good time to address the appropriateness of medications and breastfeeding.

In the 1980s, international professional organizations recognized that several behaviors enhance the initiation and maintenance of breastfeeding. **In 1989, the essential 10 steps (see box, 10 Steps to Successful Breast-Feeding)[68] in protecting, promoting, and supporting breastfeeding were published in a joint statement by the World Health Organization (WHO)/United Nations Children's Fund (UNICEF).[68]** These have become institutionalized in the Baby-Friendly Hospital Initiative (BFHI) and accreditation process. **These steps are well founded on evidence-based medicine that demonstrates improvement in breastfeeding success.[75-77]** Unfortunately, the United States is far behind the rest of the world in designating their maternity facilities as Baby Friendly; in 2008 only 1.93% of live births occurred in a facility designated as Baby Friendly (BFHI). In 2009, the Center for Disease Control started reporting the breastfeeding-related maternity practices and outcomes[78] (www.cdc.gov/breastfeeding/data). These data will be used to measure the quality of care given by hospitals and their providers. The obstetrician will be a key player in quality improvement related to breastfeeding and the application of the essential 10 steps, also known as the Baby-Friendly Hospital Initiative.

After postpartum discharge, the obstetrician is primarily focused on maternal concerns about breastfeeding: maternal diet, breast symptoms and signs, hormonal function postpartum, contraception, maternal medications, and as a breastfeeding advocate when the mother is referred to other specialists. A secondary but equally important focus is the growth and development of the infant. Traditionally, the obstetrician sees the mother at 4 to 6 weeks postpartum, but often the obstetrician and the mother communicate before that visit. By inquiring about the growth and feeding of her infant, the obstetrician provides an important reinforcement of the mother's decision to breastfeed and an important screen for the pediatrician regarding the growth and feeding of the infant. The obstetrician can identify critical or developing problems regarding infant growth and feeding for the pediatrician. The obstetrician must know the indicators of adequate infant growth and clinical indicators that milk is being produced and transferred. When the obstetrician remains a verbal participant in the mother's breastfeeding experience at the 4- to 6-week postpartum visit, the likelihood that the mother will continue to breastfeed at 16 weeks is almost doubled.[79] During the interpregnancy interval, the obstetrician/gynecologist identifies the challenges, myths, and obstacles in the last pregnancy and helps correct them for the subsequent lactational period.

SUCCESSFUL MANAGEMENT OF BREASTFEEDING

The successful management of breastfeeding requires the active cooperation of the mother, her support group, the obstetric care provider, and the infant care provider. In our current culture, a lactation consultant often becomes an active participant in the care of the breastfeeding dyad. There are numerous reliable resources for additional information (Table 23-8).

TABLE 23-8 RESOURCES FOR BREASTFEEDING MANAGEMENT

TYPE	RESOURCE	COMMENT
Print	Breastfeeding Handbook for Physicians, Eds, Schanler RJ, Dooley S, Gartner LM, Mass SB; AAP and ACOG Publication, 2006.	Excellent shelf resource on how to support breastfeeding as a part of a team.
	ACOG Clinical Review Breastfeeding: Maternal and Infant Aspects, 12(1 Suppl) 2007.	Succinct review of the management of breastfeeding mother for the obstetrician.
	ACOG Committee Opinion Breastfeeding: Maternal and Infant Aspects, 361, February 2007.	States the ACOG position on breastfeeding.
	Breastfeeding: A Guide for the Medical Profession, 7th ed., Lawrence RA, Lawrence RM, Mosby, 2011.	The standard textbook for physicians interested in breastfeeding.
	Infant and young child feeding: Model chapter for textbooks for medical students and allied health professionals,	www.who.int.org/child_adolescent_health World Health Organization publication.
	Drugs in Pregnancy and Lactation, 9th ed., Eds. Briggs GG, Freeman RK, Yaffe SJ.	A manual for pregnancy and lactational pharmacology.
	Medications and Mothers' Milk, 14th ed., Hale TW, Ed.	A manual of lactational pharmacology.
	Continuity of Care in Breastfeeding: Best Practice in Maternity Settings, Cadwell K, Turner-Maffei C.	Manual of application of the WHO 10 Steps.
Organizations	Academy of Breastfeeding Medicine	A physicians-only international professional organization founded by obstetricians, pediatricians, and family medicine physicians. The organization is dedicated to physician education and clinical research on breastfeeding Excellent clinical protocols on website (**www.abm.org**) Official journal: Breastfeeding Medicine (www.liebertpub.com/bfm)
	International Board of Lactation Consultants	www.ILCA.org International organization Certifying examination Official journal: Journal of Human Lactation
Online training	American Academy of Pediatrics, Breastfeeding Residency Curriculum	www.AAP.org/breastfeeding/curriculum Multidisciplinary input. Excellent.
	Well Start International	www.wellstart.org Oldest and most experienced organization in breastfeeding education.
	University of Virginia	www.breastfeedingtraining.org

ANATOMIC ABNORMALITIES OF THE BREAST

The relationship between breast anatomy and lactation should be addressed during the well-woman or family planning visits in women who anticipate future pregnancy. During pregnancy, infant feeding becomes a major focus, and the woman needs this issue addressed, as often there are hidden questions and concerns regarding her adequacy to breastfeed. The breast examination at the first prenatal visit is an excellent opportunity to address infant feeding concerns and myths relative to her breast anatomy. Self-doubt concerning the size or shape of the breasts should be addressed, and the patient should be reassured that less than 5% of lactational failures are caused by faulty anatomy.

Congenital abnormalities of the breasts (excluding inverted nipples) are rare, less than 1 in 1000 women. The most significant defect is glandular hypoplasia. These women have no development or abnormal development of one or both breasts during sexual maturation. Women with no development of the breasts often have normally shaped and sized nipples and areolas, and they may have sought consultation from a plastic surgeon. One manifestation of abnormal development is referred to as the *tubular breast.* The nipple and areola, which are often normal in size, shape, and appearance, are attached to a tube of fibrous cords. Whatever the shape or size of the breasts in a nonpregnant woman, the final evaluation of adequate glandular tissue must await the expected growth during pregnancy. The size of the average breast will grow from 200 g to 600 g during pregnancy; most women will easily recognize this growth. **A routine screening question at the 36-week prenatal visit should be, "Have your breasts grown during pregnancy?" If the response is negative in a woman with unusually small or abnormally shaped breasts, lactational failure is a possibility and prenatal consultation with a lactation expert is recommended.** Unilateral abnormalities are usually not a problem except for increased asymmetry, as the normal breast can usually produce more than enough milk for the infant. The texture of the breast and tethering of the nipple are also assessed. An inelastic breast gives the impression that the skin is fixed to dense underlying tissue, whereas the elastic breast allows elevation of the skin and subcutaneous tissue from the parenchyma. Lack of elasticity may complicate nursing because of increased rigidity with engorgement. Massage of the periareolar tissue four times a day for 10 minutes is recommended. Engorgement should be assiduously avoided in the postpartum period by early, frequent nursing.

Congenital tethering of the nipple to underlying fascia is diagnosed by squeezing the outer edge of the areola (Figure 23-13); normally, the nipple will protrude. **Severe tethering is manifested by an inverted nipple.** The most severe forms of tethering occur in less than 1% of women.

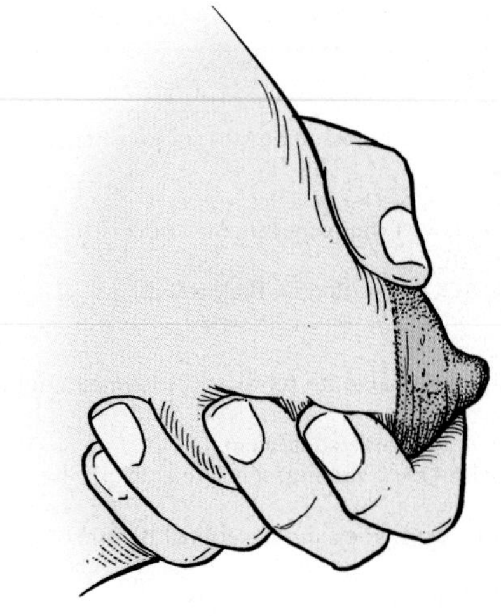

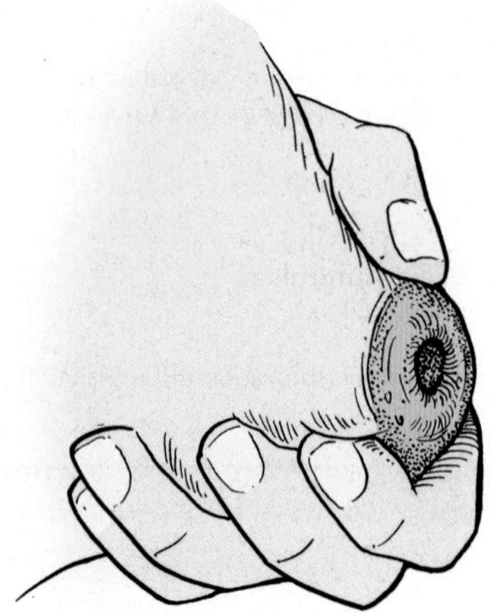

FIGURE 23-13. Assessment of nipple tethering.

While successful breastfeeding is possible in these severe cases, prenatal consultation and close follow-up are very important to identify and treat poor milk transfers. Flat or inverted nipples are much less likely to preclude successful breastfeeding. Three prenatal methods of treating tethered nipples have been described: nipple pulling, Hoffman's exercises, and nipple cups (shells). **A controlled trial failed to demonstrate efficacy**[80] **of either shells or Hoffman's exercises and recommended that these should be abandoned.**

In the early neonatal period, a breast pump may be of help in women with flat or inverted nipples. The breast is gently pumped at low settings until the teat is drawn out. The infant is immediately offered that breast. The same procedure is performed on the other side. Usually this is only required for a few days. If it is required for more than a few days, a relatively cheap alternative can be created from a 10- or 20-mL plastic syringe, the sizes depending on the size of the nipple. The end of the syringe where the needle attaches is removed and the plunger is reversed. The nipple is placed in the smooth, plunger end of the syringe and gentle traction is applied until the nipple everts. While pumping and syringe suction are practical solutions, no controlled trials have supported their efficacy.

Modern clothing (especially protective brassieres) prevents friction that toughens the skin and helps protect the nipple from cracking during early lactation. In the second half of pregnancy, nipple skin may be toughened by wearing a nursing brassiere with the flaps open. **However, washing with harsh soaps; buffing the nipple with a towel; and using alcohol, benzoin, or other drying agents are not helpful and may increase the incidence of cracking. Normally, the breast is washed with clean water and should be left to air-dry.** A cautiously used sunlamp or hair dryer may facilitate drying. Trials involving application of breast cream or expression of colostrum have not shown a reduction in nipple trauma or sensitivity when compared to those with untreated nipples.

Previous breast surgery may have significant adverse effects on breastfeeding success. The major issues are loss of sensation in the nipple or areola by nerve injury or compromise of the lactiferous ducts. Women who have had breast surgery, breast biopsy, chest surgery, or augmentation have a threefold higher incidence of unsuccessful breastfeeding.[81] Circumareolar skin incisions, which are used for cosmetic considerations in breast biopsies or breast augmentation, may compromise both the nerve and ducts.

Breast augmentation has significant potential to disrupt breastfeeding.[82] In a carefully studied, prospective series, 27 of 42 **(64%) of women who exclusively breastfed after preconceptional breast augmentation had insufficient lactation,** and the infant growth rate was less than 20 g/day. **Circumareolar incision was the dominant predictor. One half of women with a submammary or axillary incision had insufficient lactation, whereas all 11 women after a circumareolar incision for breast augmentation had lactation failure.** Compromise of the lactiferous ducts and loss of nipple sensation contribute to lactational insufficiency. Loss of nipple sensation occurs in one third to half of patients after circumareolar incision. If the woman has had a silicone implant, she can be reassured that there is no evidence that breastfeeding places her infant at risk. The concentration of silicone in artificial formula or cow's milk is 5 to 10 times higher than in breast milk from women who have silicone implants.[83] **Large epidemiologic studies of infants who have nursed from breasts with silicone implants have not shown excess adverse events.**[82]

Reduction mammoplasty is always associated with lactation insufficiency if exclusive breastfeeding is relied upon for infant nutrition. If the reduction involves the removal of greater than 500 g per breast or the procedure uses the free nipple graph technique, the production of a nominal amount of breast milk is rare. If the nipple and areola are relocated on a pedicle of vascular tissue and ducts, partial breastfeeding is a small possibility. **In any case of reconstructive surgery on the breast (i.e., reduction mammoplasty), the breastfeeding dyad is considered at high risk for lactation failure.** This observation was recently confirmed by a controlled study.[84] The control and mammoplasty reported any breastfeeding at 1 month of 94% and 58%, respectively. Similarly, the rate of exclusive breastfeeding at 1 month was 70% and 21% in the respective groups. Prenatal referral to an expert on lactation is appropriate.

LABOR AND DELIVERY MANAGEMENT

Approximately 15% of women who state they wish to breastfeed at the onset of term labor are discharged either completely feeding their infant artificial breast milk or giving the majority of the infant's feeds as artificial breast milk. A combination of obstetric management, hospital policies, and pediatric management contribute to this attrition. Obstetric interventions are often critical for the health of the mother or infant, and they may affect the success of lactation.[85] Few if any interventions directly inhibit the physiology of lactation. Most obstetric interventions reduce the success of lactation by indirect interference with physiology. Induction of labor is not associated with lactation failure, but a long, tiring induction and labor will reduce the likelihood that the mother will get appropriate amounts of infant contact in the delivery room and in the first 24 hours after birth. Cesarean delivery reduces the incidence of breastfeeding by 10% to 20% in the first week after birth. **After most cesarean sections and difficult vaginal deliveries, the infant is not put to the breast immediately after birth nor will the mother breastfeed her infant more than eight times in the first 24 hours.**[86] Well-meaning nurses become concerned for the baby's nutrition and artificial breast milk is given to the infant until the mother "recovers."

Labor analgesia (i.e., meperidine and promethazine) has long been associated with poor breastfeeding success. Intrapartum narcotics appear to adversely affect the infant's ability to nurse effectively. **Epidural anesthesia with local anesthetic agents seems to be better for breastfeeding than parenteral narcotics.** Epidural anesthesia with local anesthetics does not appear to have a major effect. The effect of epidural or intrathecal narcotics on sucking behavior and/or lactation success has been shown to be a decrease in breastfeeding success in a double-blind study with random assignment of subjects.[87] The presence of a doula, or a labor companion other than family, appears to be an effective method to reduce the need for epidural anesthesia and operative deliveries. An added benefit is earlier initiation and longer duration of breastfeeding.

Postsurgical pain control is best achieved with morphine rather than meperidine, which adversely affects neonatal behavior. Obstetric and pediatric protocols can be very effective in separating mother and baby. Several prominent examples include magnesium sulfate therapy for preeclampsia, a positive maternal group B streptococcus culture, maternal fever workup, and diabetes mellitus/hypoglycemia protocols. All of these medical interventions produce major barriers to delivery room nursing and an adequate frequency of nursing in the first 24 to 48 hours.

The peripartum period is critical for achieving successful lactation. The obstetrician must apply the five basic principles of lactation physiology: early imprinting, frequent nursing, good latch-on, a confident and comfortable mother, and no supplementation unless medically indicated. Nursing should be initiated within 30 minutes after birth, preferably in the delivery room. Contraindications include (1) a heavily medicated mother, (2) an infant with a 5-minute Apgar test result less than 7, or (3) a premature infant at less than 34 to 36 weeks' gestation.

The instructor should pay special attention to the mother's position during the first feeding; she should be in a relaxed, comfortable position. With skin-to-skin contact, the infant is presented to the breast with his ventral surface to the mother's ventral surface. A dry neonate, skin-to-skin contact, and supplemental radiant heating will prevent neonatal cold stress. Routine eye treatment should be delayed, as it may disrupt the important family bonding process.

In the recovery room and on the ward, the best place for the neonate is with the mother. This maximizes mother-infant bonding and allows "on-demand" feeding every 1 to 2 hours. Rooming-in allows the mother to participate in the care of her baby and gives her an opportunity to ask questions. **The mother should be encouraged to sleep when the neonate sleeps.** Since the hospital runs on an adult diurnal pattern, the patient should be discharged early in order to get her rest.

The frequency of early feeding is proportional to milk production and weight gain in neonates.[88] Therefore, supplementation with glucose or formula should be discouraged. Supplementation decreases milk production through a reduction in nursing frequency by satiation of the neonate and slower digestion of formula. Supplementation also undermines the mother's confidence about her lactational adequacy.[89,90] When obstetricians give information at the first prenatal visit about breastfeeding that was developed by makers of artificial breast milk, the duration of breastfeeding is significantly reduced when compared to packet information on breastfeeding developed by "breastfeeding-friendly" obstetricians and pediatricians. **A randomized trial of giving or withholding free formula samples at the time of discharge demonstrated a significantly reduced incidence of breastfeeding at 1 month and an increased likelihood of solid food introduction by the mothers given the formula samples.** This was most significant in high-risk groups: those less educated, primiparas, and those reporting illness since leaving the hospital.

Other factors influencing the success of lactation are improper positioning and nursing technique, which can lead to increased nipple trauma and incomplete emptying. In the early postpartum period, nursing technique should be evaluated in three areas: presentation and latching-on, maternal-infant positioning, and breaking of the suction. The infant should not have to turn its head to nurse. A ventral surface-to-ventral surface presentation is necessary. When latching on to the nipple, the neonate should take as much of the areola as possible into its mouth. This is facilitated by gently stimulating the baby's cheek to elicit a yawn-like opening of its mouth and rapid placement of the breast into it. A supporting hand on the breast helps; the C-hold involves four fingers cupping and supporting the weight of the breast, which is especially important in the weak or premature neonate whose lower jaw may be depressed by the weight of the breast. The thumb rests above and 1 to 2 cm away from the areolar edge and points the nipple downward. Retraction by the thumb will pull the areola away from the mouth and cause an incorrect placement. Any position that is comfortable and convenient, while allowing the appropriate mouth-areola attachment, should be encouraged; the sitting position is the most common. In cesarean section patients in whom pressure on the abdomen is uncomfortable, a side-lying or football hold may be better. **A rotation of positions is recommended to reduce focal pressure on the nipple and to**

ensure complete emptying. Removal of the nursing infant can be a problem; suction by the neonate can injure the nipple if it is not broken prior to disengagement. **A finger inserted between the baby's lips and the breast will break the suction.**

The single most difficult management issue is the control of routines and hospital attitudes detrimental to lactation. Policies that work against the physiology of lactation include formula distribution and supplementation without a medical indication, constant questioning of the mother about breastfeeding, preprinted orders for lactation suppression medication, pediatric clearance prior to the first feeding, limited maternal access to the infant, and little educational material for new mothers or staff.

When providers are not well informed or are apathetic about lactation, success of lactation is unlikely. This theme underscores the role of the obstetrician, as an opinion leader, in the education of patients, nursing staff, and support personnel about the physiology and benefits of lactation.

Breast Milk Expression

The flow of milk can be improved by placing the mother in a quiet, relaxed environment. The breast is massaged in a spiral fashion, starting at the top and moving toward the areola; the fingers are moved in a circular fashion from one spot to another, much like a breast examination. After the massage, the breast is stroked from the top of the breast to the nipple with a light stroke and shaken, while the woman leans forward. Once milk starts to flow, manual expression is begun.

Manual expression is performed by holding the thumb and first two fingers on either side of the areola, in a half circle, but the breast should not be cupped. The hand pushes the breast straight into the chest wall, as the thumb and fingers are rolled forward. Large, pendulous breasts may need lifting prior to this. The maneuver is repeated in all four quadrants of the areola to drain as many reservoirs as possible. The procedure is repeated rhythmically and gently, since squeezing, sliding, or pulling may injure the breast. The sequence of massage, stroke, shake, and express is useful in providing milk immediately for the vigorous infant, in allowing an improved latch-on by reducing periareolar engorgement, and in reducing high suction pressures on a traumatized nipple.

MATERNAL NUTRITION AND EXERCISE DURING LACTATION

The efficiency of conversion of maternal foodstuff to milk is about 80% to 90%. **If the average milk volume per day is 900 mL, and milk has an average energy content of 75 kcal/dL, the mother must consume an extra 794 kcal/day, unless stored energy is used. During pregnancy, most women store an extra 2 to 5 kg (19,000 to 48,000 kcal) in tissue, mainly as fat, in physiologic preparation for lactation.** These calories and nutrients supplement the maternal diet during lactation. As a result, the required dietary increases are easily attainable in healthy mothers and infants.

In lactation, most vitamins and minerals should be increased 20% to 30% over nonpregnant requirements. Folic acid should be doubled. Calcium, phosphorus, and magnesium should be increased by 40% to 50%, especially in the teenager who is lactating. In practical terms, these needs can be supplied by the following additions to the diet: 2 cups of milk, 2 oz of meat or peanut butter, a slice of enriched or whole wheat bread, a citrus fruit, a salad, and an extra helping (½ to ¾ cup) of a dark green or yellow vegetable. **The appropriate intake of vitamins can be ensured by continuing prenatal vitamins with 1 mg of folic acid throughout lactation.** The mother should drink at least 1 extra liter of fluid per day to make up for the fluid loss through milk.

Vegetarianism has become increasingly more common, and if the nursing mother is a vegetarian, dietary deficiencies may include B vitamins (especially B_{12}), total protein, and the full complement of essential amino acids. The recommendation should be to take a good dietary history with the focus on protein, iron, calcium, and vitamins D and B; supplement with soy flour, molasses, or nuts; use complementary vegetable protein combinations; and avoid excess phytate and bran.

Many women are concerned about losing weight postpartum.[17-19] Dewey and colleagues examined the effects of diet and exercise on maternal weight, breast milk volume, breast milk composition, and infant growth through random assignment of affluent, highly motivated, and exclusively breastfeeding women to intervention and control groups. The exercise group had training to reach a level of 45 minutes at 60% to 70% of heart rate reserve four to six times a week for 12 weeks. The target diet was individually adjusted to reduce calories and maintain protein intake. In these controlled populations, **the women lost 1.0-1.5 kg/week. There were no significant changes in the volume or composition of breast milk.** The infant grew approximately 2000 g in both the intervention and control groups. On a practical level, if 700 to 1200 kcal are used daily to nourish an infant, a mother could lose weight by not increasing her caloric intake, but a thoughtful selection of food groups and the elimination of "empty calories" are necessary. A reduction of total calories (<25 kcal/kg) and total protein (<0.6 g/kg) may reduce the daily milk volume by 20% to 30%, but not the milk quality, unless the mother is more than 10% below her ideal body weight. Because dieting mobilizes fat stores that may contain environmental toxins, women with high exposure to such toxins should not lose weight during lactation.

BREAST AND NIPPLE PAIN

Breast or nipple pain is one of the most frequent complaints of lactating mothers.[91-94] The frequency of pain is related to failure in the initial management of lactation: late first feed, decreased frequency of feedings, poor nipple grasp, and/or poor positioning. The differential diagnosis of breast pain includes problems with latching-on, engorgement, nipple trauma, mastitis and, occasionally, the let-down reflex.

Symptoms and the infant's personality help make the differential diagnosis. In some cases, the nipple and breast pain starts with latching-on and diminishes with let-down. Women describe the let-down reflex as painful; this occurs after the first minute of sucking and usually lasts only a minute or two as the ductal swelling is relieved by nursing.

Classically, the anxious, vigorous infant, who sucks strongly against empty ducts until the let-down occurs, is associated with this pain pattern. Contact pain suggests nipple trauma and may persist as long as the nipple is manipulated. The nipple-confused infant who chews on the nipple and abrades the tip with his tongue is associated with this pattern.

Engorgement causes a dull, generalized discomfort in the whole breast, worse just before a feed and relieved by it. Localized, unilateral, and continuous pain in the breast may be caused by mastitis. A physical examination and observation of nursing technique can confirm the impression left by a good history. Through observation of a nursing episode, an infant's personality and nursing technique can be assessed. The whole of the nipple and much of the areola should be included in the infant's mouth. An examination of the nipple may reveal a fissure or blood blister. Bilateral breast firmness and tenderness may indicate engorgement. Engorgement may be peripheral, periareolar, or both. Mastitis is characterized by fever, malaise, localized erythema, heat, tenderness, and induration (see below).

Infection may be a cofactor associated with the pain of nipple injury. When the microbiology of the nipple/milk of 61 lactating women with nipple pain was compared to 64 lactating women without nipple pain and 31 nonlactating women, *Candida albicans* (19%) and *Staphylococcus aureus* (30%) were more common in women with pain and nipple fissures than in controls (3%-5%).[93] The use of antibiotics is effective in treatment of nipple pain and trauma.[93]

The management of breast pain consists of general as well as specific steps. Prevention is a key component. Appropriate nursing technique and positioning will prevent, or significantly decrease, the incidence of nipple trauma, engorgement, and mastitis. Rotation of nursing position will reduce the suction pressure on the same part of the nipple, as well as ensuring complete emptying of all lobes of the breast. Frequent nursing will reduce engorgement and milk stasis. The use of soaps, alcohol, and other drying agents on the nipples tends to increase nipple trauma and pain. The nipples should be air-dried for a few minutes after each feed, and clean water is sufficient to cleanse the breast, if necessary. Some experts recommend that fresh breast milk be applied to the nipples and allowed to dry after each feed.

Stimulating a let-down and manual expression of milk is useful in the management of many breast problems. The let-down produced by manual expression is never as complete as a normally elicited one. An effective let-down can be elicited by initiating nursing on the side without nipple trauma or mastitis. This will effectively reduce breast pain.

In the first 5 days after birth, about 35% of the nipples of breastfeeding mothers show damage, and 69% of mothers have nipple pain.[92-94] The management of painful, tender, or injured nipples includes prefeeding manual expression, correction of latching-on, rotation of positions, and initiation of nursing on the less painful side first, with the affected side exposed to air. Drying is facilitated by the cautious application of dry heat (e.g., with hair dryer on low setting) for 20 minutes four times per day. Aspirin or codeine (15 to 30 mg) given half an hour before nursing, may be helpful in severe cases. Engorgement can be avoided, but if it occurs, feeding frequency should be maintained or increased by pumping. **A wide variety of preparations have been applied to traumatized nipples, including lanolin, A & D ointment, white petrolatum, antibiotics, vitamin E oil, and used tea bags, but few of these have been evaluated scientifically. Soap and alcohol have been shown to injure nipples.** Nipple shields should be used only as a last resort because of a 20% to 60% reduction in milk consumption. Thin latex shields may be better than the traditional red rubber ones, although milk flow is still reduced by 22%.

Engorgement of the breast occurs when there is inadequate drainage of milk.[92] Swollen, firm, and tender breasts are caused by distention of the ducts and increased extravascular fluid. Aside from the discomfort, engorgement leads to dysfunctional nursing behavior and nipple trauma. The firm breast tissue pushes the infant's face away from the nipple. The widened base of the nipple disrupts the attachment, and the infant's thrusting tongue abrades the tip. This leads to further engorgement, decreased milk production and, in some cases, early termination of breastfeeding.

The best treatment is prevention, but when this has not occurred, management is centered on symptomatic support and relief of distention. Proper elevation of the breasts is important. The mother should wear a firm-fitting nursing brassiere, with neither thin straps nor plastic lining. A warm shower or bath, with prefeed manual expression, is effective. Frequent suckling (every 1 to 2 hours) is the most effective mechanism to relieve engorgement; postfeed electric pumping from each breast may be helpful. In selected cases, intranasal oxytocin may be given just prior to each feed if let-down seems to be inhibited.

MASTITIS AND BREAST ABSCESS

Mastitis is an infectious process of the breast characterized by high fever (39° to 40° C), localized erythema, tenderness, induration, and palpable heat over the area.[95] Often these signs are associated with nausea, vomiting, malaise, and other flulike symptoms. Mastitis occurs most frequently in the first 2 to 4 weeks postpartum and at times of marked reduction in nursing frequency. Risk factors include maternal fatigue, poor nursing technique, nipple trauma, and epidemic *Staphylococcus aureus*. **The most common organisms associated with mastitis are *S. aureus*, *S. epidermidis*, streptococci and, occasionally, gram-negative rods.** The incidence of sporadic mastitis is 2% to 10% in lactating mothers and less than 1% in nonlactating mothers.

Until recently, the management of mastitis has been directed by retrospective clinical reviews of experience. In most cases, this consisted of bed rest, continued lactation, and antibiotics, with an 80% to 90% cure rate, a 10% abscess rate, a 10% recurrence rate, and a 50% cessation of breastfeeding. Starting in the 1980s, several important articles were published concerning pathophysiology, diagnosis, and treatment of mastitis. The diagnosis and prognosis of inflammatory symptoms of the breast could be established by counts of leukocytes and bacteria in breast milk. This is obtained after careful washing of the mother's hands and breasts with a mild soap. The milk is manually expressed, and the first 3 mL discarded. A microscopic analysis is performed on an unspun specimen. When the leukocyte count was greater than 10^6 leukocytes/mL, and the bacterial count less than 10^3 bacteria/mL, the diagnosis was noninfectious inflammation of the breast. With no treatment, the inflammatory symptoms lasted 7 days; 50% developed mastitis, and only 21% returned to normal lactation. When the breast was emptied frequently by continued lactation, the symptoms lasted 3 days, and 96% returned to normal lactation.

If the breast milk showed greater than 10^6 leukocytes/mL and greater than 10^3 bacteria/mL, the diagnosis was mastitis. Delay in therapy resulted in abscess formation in 11%, and only 15% returned to normal lactation. Frequent emptying of the infected breast by continued nursing eliminated abscess formation, but only 51% returned to normal lactation. Additional antibiotic therapy increased the return to normal lactation in 97% with resolution of symptoms in 2.1 days.

In summary, the management of mastitis includes the following: (1) breast support; (2) fluids; (3) assessment of nursing technique; (4) nursing initiated on the uninfected side first to establish let-down; (5) the infected side emptied by nursing with each feed (occasionally, a breast pump helps to ensure complete drainage); and (6) dicloxacillin, 250 mg every 6 hours for 7 days. Erythromycin may be used in patients allergic to penicillin. It is important to continue antibiotics for a full 7 days, since abscess formation is more likely with shorter courses. Maternal handwashing before each feed reduces nosocomial infection rates. Hand washing and the use of antiseptic gels by health care workers reduces nosocomial infection rates; and, more important, MRSA-associated mastitis. In the era before universal handwashing by hospital personnel, rooming-in did not reduce the acquisition of hospital strains of *S. aureus* or infection rates. In the more infection conscious environment of today, isolation (rooming-in) and early discharge may add to the benefits of handwashing by reducing the rates of MRSA-associated mastitis and abcess.[96]

Breast abscess will occur in about 10% of women who are treated for bacterial mastitis. The signs include a high fever (39° to 40° C) and a localized area of erythema, tenderness, and induration. In the center a fluctuant area may be difficult to palpate. The patient feels sick, like having the "flu." Abscesses usually occur in the upper outer quadrants and *S. aureus* is usually cultured from the abscess cavity.

The management of breast abscess is similar to that for mastitis, except that (1) drainage of the abscess is indicated and (2) breastfeeding should be limited to the uninvolved side during the initial therapy.[97] The infected breast should be mechanically pumped every 2 hours and with every let-down. Serial percutaneous needle aspiration under ultrasound guidance is the best and standard method to drain the abscess. Occasionally, surgical drainage is required. The skin incision should be made over the fluctuant area in a manner parallel to and as far as possible from the areolar edge. While the skin incision follows skin lines, the deeper extension should be made bluntly in a radial direction. Sharp dissection perpendicular to the lactational ducts increases blood loss, the risk of a fistula, and the risk of ductal occlusion. Once the abscess cavity is entered, all loculations are bluntly reduced and the cavity irrigated with saline. American surgeons pack the wound open for drainage and secondary closure. British surgeons advocate removal of the abscess wall and primary closure. In either case, wide closure sutures should be avoided, as they may compromise the ducts. Patients have a protracted recovery of 18 to 32 days and recurrent abscess formation in 9% to 15% of cases. Breastfeeding from the involved side may be resumed, if skin erythema and underlying cellulitis have resolved, which may occur in 4 to 7 days.

Candida albicans infection is considered a common cause of breast pain. **Candida infection of the breast is a commonly diagnosed by clinical presentation. Women describe severe pain when the infant nurses. She will describe the pain as "like a red hot poker being driven through my chest."** Often she has received antibiotics recently, she is a diabetic, or the infant has evidence of oral thrush or diaper rash (*C. albicans*). The areola and nipple are erythematous with a scaly sheen to the nipple. Unfortunately, the clinical presentation of candida infection of the breast is not as specific nor as accurate as a prudent clinician needs. The differential diagnosis includes let-down pain, poor latch-on, nipple trauma, allergic reaction, Raynaud's of the nipple, and early bacterial mastitis.

Often the mother is given strong antifungal agents for causes of the symptoms that are not amenable to antifungal agents. In a classic study by Hale and Berens[98] only one of 21 patients with a "classic" presentation of candida mastitis had a breast milk specimen positive for yeast. Given the nonspecificity of the clinical diagnosis, a focused physical examination and biologic confirmation of candida is prudent. Biologic confirmation is obtained through a microscopic examination and culture of a midstream sample of breast milk. The nipples and areola are gently cleaned with warm water. A letdown of breast milk is induced and a sample of breast milk is obtained after the first 5 mL have been discarded. A potassium hydroxide (KOH) smear can confirm the diagnosis. A drop of the midstream milk is combined with a drop of 10% KOH and examined under high-power light microscopy. A typical pattern of hyphae and spores will be visualized. The remainder of the sample is sent for culture and isolation of bacteria and fungus. In cases in which there have been multiple antibiotics and antifungal agents used, a sensitivity panel on the fungal isolates may be helpful. A fungal culture may take 7 to 10 days for isolation and identification, longer than for antibiotic sensitivities. Given the intensity of maternal symptoms and the risk of discontinuing breastfeeding, empiric therapy is warranted prior to the availability of culture results.

The initial treatment is to massage nystatin cream or miconazole oral gel into both nipples after each feed and in the infant's mouth three times a day for 2 weeks. Recurrent or persistent candida mastitis can be treated by swabbing the infant's mouth with gentian violet liquid (0.5%) and immediately latching the baby to the breast, twice a day for 3 days. The major disadvantage of this therapy is the permanent staining associated with gentian violet. An alternative therapy in severe cases is oral fluconazole, 200-mg loading dose followed by 100 mg/day for 14 days.

MILK TRANSFER AND INFANT GROWTH

When is an exclusive diet of breast milk insufficient to supply the nutritional needs of the growing infant? Women who wean in the first 8 weeks most often say that insufficient milk is the reason for quitting, and well-meaning family members often ask, "When are you going to start feeding your child real food?"

Correct answers are not readily available. Many nondietary factors affect the growth of infants, including high birth order, lower maternal age, low maternal weight, poor maternal nutrition during pregnancy, birth interval, birth weight less than 2.4 kg, multiple gestation, infection, death of either parent, and divorce or separation.

In addition, there are inconsistencies in the standard reference charts for growth or nutritional needs. Most growth charts are based on formula-fed infants, who often receive solid food supplementation earlier and in greater proportion than comparable breastfed infants. Reference charts with sufficiently large numbers of exclusively breastfed infants from developed countries are lacking. As milk volume is a quantitative measure of nutrition, variations in volume and concentrations of constituents caused by individual variation and different methods of collection compound the interpretation.

Despite the latter concerns, it is apparent that **a healthy and successfully breastfeeding mother can supply enough nutrition through breast milk alone for 6 months.** The clinical markers for adequate breast milk transfer include an alert, healthy appearance, good muscle tone, good skin turgor, six wet diapers per day, eight or more nursing episodes per day, three or four loose stools per day, consistent evidence of a let-down with operant conditioning, and consistent weight gain (0.75-1.0 oz/day after galatogenesis III has started, engorgement or "the milk has come in").

The term "failure to thrive" has been used loosely to include all infants who show any degree of growth failure. For the breastfeeding mother, it may just be a matter of comparing the growth of her infant to growth charts compiled from formula-fed infants. The loosely applied term can seriously undermine the mother's confidence, and ill-advised supplementation further compromises milk volume and may mask other important underlying causes. The infant should be evaluated for failure to thrive or slowed growth if (1) it continues to lose weight after 7 days of life, (2) it does not regain birthweight by 2 weeks, or (3) it gains weight at a rate below the 10th percentile beyond the first months of age. If the mother or the maternal care provider recognize jaundice after the first 7 to 10 days of life, the neonate needs to have a serum bilirubin and be seen by his care provider in an emergent fashion. If the infant is premature, ill, or small for gestational age, other growth measurements (ponderal index, height, skinfold thickness, etc.) can be used to define adequate growth. The cause of failure to thrive is often complex and is beyond the scope of this chapter.

JAUNDICE IN THE NEWBORN

Ten to 15% of breastfed neonates will have jaundice, defined by a peak serum bilirubin greater than 12 mg/dL in term infants.[99] Pediatric concerns include hemolysis, liver disease, or infection as underlying causes, and kernicterus as a consequence. **Unconjugated serum bilirubin greater than 20 mg/dL is considered the critical level for the development of kernicterus in term infants.** When the serum bilirubin is greater than 5 mg/dL in the first 24 hours, a serious disease process (hemolysis) may be present, and intervention is appropriate.

The focus on breastfeeding as related to neonatal jaundice results from the characterization of two syndromes, breastfeeding jaundice syndrome and breast milk jaundice syndrome. In the early 1960s, 5% to 10% of lactating women were found to have a steroid metabolite of progesterone, 5β-pregnane-3(α), 20(β)-diol, in their icterogenic milk, but the compound was not found in the milk of women whose infants were normal (breast milk jaundice syndrome). This metabolite is associated with an inhibition of glucosyl transferase in the liver, differences in the metabolism of long-chain unsaturated fatty acids, and/or increased resorption of bile acids in jaundiced infants.

In breast milk jaundice syndrome, the neonates are healthy and active. The hyperbilirubinemia develops after the fourth day of life and may last several months, with a gradual fall in level. When breastfeeding is stopped for 24 to 48 hours, there is a 30% to 50% decline in bilirubin levels. With resumption of nursing, serum levels will rise slightly (1 to 2 mg/dL), plateau, and then start to fall slowly, regardless of feeding method. **After excluding other causes of jaundice, and with careful monitoring of serum bilirubin, breastfeeding can continue.**

Unfortunately, the focus on rare breast milk jaundice cases, the concern about kernicterus, and the increased bilirubin in many breastfed neonates between 2 and 7 days old led to routine supplementation of infants with water, glucose, and formula, even when bilirubin concentrations were in the moderate range of 8 to 12 mg/dL. The cause of the elevated bilirubin-reduced feeding frequency or low milk transfer is often unrecognized. **It has been clearly demonstrated that feeding frequency greater than eight feedings per 24 hours is associated with lower bilirubin levels. Likewise, water supplementation studied in a controlled fashion does not decrease the peak serum bilirubin.** Management consists of prevention by improvement in the quality and frequency of nursing. Rooming-in and night feedings should be encouraged. If the mother, family, or obstetrician recognizes jaundice in an infant greater than 7 days old, an immediate referral to the child's caregiver and a serum bilirubin should be obtained; this is a pediatric emergency. The management of jaundice in the breastfeeding newborn is effectively outlined in a specific protocol produced by the Academy of Breastfeeding Medicine (www.ABM.org).

GALACTOGOGUES: DRUGS TO IMPROVE MILK PRODUCTION

Obstetricians may interface with the breastfeeding dyad when there is a question of adequate milk production and transfer by the mother. The mother and/or the pediatrician will ask for a galactogogue to be prescribed by the obstetrician.

Numerous agents have been shown to increase prolactin production; and galactorrhea is a clinical issue for women on phenothiazines or metoclopramide. It is reasonable that these drugs might be used where milk supply seems insufficient. The most understandable clinical scenarios include premature delivery requiring mechanical pumping, glandular hypoplasia, reduction mammoplasty, and relactation (nursing an adoptive child). The most common clinical presentation is perceived poor milk supply or inhibited milk let-down (oxytocin inhibition). Clinical trials with random assignment of subjects have demonstrated the effectiveness of metoclopramide, sulpiride, and nasal oxytocin for increasing milk production.

Metoclopramide (Reglan) is used to promote gastrointestinal tone; however, a secondary effect is to increase prolactin levels. Most studies demonstrate a multiple fold increase in basal prolactin levels and a 60% to 100% increase in milk volume. The effects of metoclopramide are very dose dependent; the usual dose is 10 to 15 mg three times a day. The side effects—gastric cramping, diarrhea, and depression—may limit its use. The incidence of depression increases with long-term use; treatment should be tapered over time and limited to less than 4 weeks. There appears to be little effect on the infant. The dose that the infants receive is much less than the amount used therapeutically to treat esophageal reflux, regardless of the time postpartum.

Domperidone is an agent similar to metoclopromide that blocks the dopamine receptors in the gut and brainstem but with fewer of the psycho-neurologic side-effects of metoclopromide. Domperidone is used in Canada as an antiemetic, but it is not FDA-approved in the United States. **In placebo controlled trials in mothers with decreased milk supply, domperidone increases prolactin levels and milk supply twofold- to threefold.**[100] The usual dose to improve milk supply is 10 to 20 mg, 3 to 4 times a day. Slow tapering (reduce 10 mg/week) is suggested as acute withdrawal rapidly diminishes milk supply. The relatively high protein binding in maternal serum limits transfer to the neonate, relative infant dose of 0.04%. Recently, the FDA issued a warning against its use because of a risk of cardiac arrhythmias. These potentially life-threatening reactions occurred in older patients with hypokalemia and who were receiving chemotherapy for cancer. Intravenous domperidone was used in high doses as an antiemetic in these patients.

Sulpiride is a selective dopamine antagonist used in Europe as an antidepressant and antipsychotic. Smaller doses (50 mg twice daily) do not produce neuroleptic effects in the mother, **but prolactin and milk production are increased significantly. Clinical studies suggest an increase in milk production (20%-50%) less than that seen with metoclopramide.** In a placebo-controlled study with random assignment of 130 subjects, sulpiride 50 mg twice daily for the first 7 days postpartum increased the total milk yield from 916±66 mL in the control group to 1211±65 mL in the sulpiride-treated group. The transfer of sulpiride to the breast milk was minimal and no adverse effects were seen in the infants. Sulpiride is not available in the United States.

Intranasal oxytocin substitutes for endogenous oxytocin to contract the myoepithelial cells and cause milk let-down. In theory, its use is to overcome an inhibited let-down reflex. Oxytocin is destroyed by gastrointestinal enzymes and is not given orally. Until recently, oxytocin intranasal spray was available commercially, but it has been taken off the market. A pharmacist can prepare an intranasal spray with a concentration of 2 IU per drop. The let-down dose is a spray (3 drops) to each nostril; the total let-down dose is approximately 12 IU. This is taken within 2 or 3 minutes of each nursing episode. The suggested duration of therapy is unclear. Underlying causes for an inhibited let-down reflex need to be identified and controlled.

There have been few clinical trials using oxytocin alone to improve milk production. **In a double-blind group sequential trial, intranasal oxytocin alone was used to enhance milk production in women during the first 5 days after delivery of a premature infant. The cumulative volume of breast milk obtained between the second and fifth days was 3.5 times greater in primiparas given intranasal oxytocin than in primiparas given placebo.** Because of oxytocin's complementary mechanism to prolactin-stimulating medications, they are often used in combination.

While metoclopramide, domperidone, sulpiride, and oxytocin appear to be effective and relatively safe for the mother and infant, they are only secondary support interventions. The primary focus should be to enhance prolactin and oxytocin through the natural mechanisms, appropriate and frequent stimulation of the nipple and areola. Galactagogues should only be used for a short duration (2 to 4 weeks) and in conjunction with hands-on counseling by an individual with the time, energy, and knowledge to enhance the "natural" production of breast milk.

MATERNAL DISEASE

In the vast majority of cases of lactating mothers with intercurrent disease, there is no medical reason to stop breastfeeding. However, appropriate management requires individualizing the care of the nursing dyad in order to preserve the supply-and-demand relationship of lactation. For example, a hospitalized nursing mother should have her nursing baby with her in the hospital for on-demand feedings. This situation stretches the flexibility of hospital administrators and nursing services, but the problem can be overcome by education.

The first principle is to maintain lactation. An acute hospitalization for a surgical procedure is a common complication. **If breast milk was the neonate's only source of nutrition, an acute reduction in nursing may lead to breast engorgement, confusing postoperative fever, and mastitis. The infant should be put to the breast just before premedication, and the breasts should be emptied in the recovery room. The most effective way is to have the mother nurse. Although some anesthetic may be present in the milk, most are compatible with lactation.** If there is legitimate concern or if the mother cannot communicate (on a ventilator), the breasts should be pumped mechanically and subsequently emptied every 2 to 3 hours by nursing or pumping.

The second principle is to adjust for the special nutritional requirements of nursing mothers. This principle is especially pertinent when intake is restricted postoperatively and when maternal diet must be manipulated. In the postoperative period, the surgeon must account for the calories and fluid required for lactation. **Until oral intake is established, a lactating mother needs an additional 500 to 1000 mL of fluid per day. Early return to a balanced diet is essential to offset the additional energy and protein requirements of lactation and wound healing.**

The third principle is to ensure that the maternal disease will not harm the infant. This is most pertinent with infectious disease, but it is equally important in cases in which a mother's judgment is in question, such as severe mental disease, substance abuse, or a history of physical abuse. The benefits of breastfeeding in the latter situations must be carefully evaluated, using the resources of the patient, her family, and social services.

Infection is the most common area where breastfeeding is questioned. In general, the necessary exposure of the infant to the mother in day-to-day care is such that breastfeeding does not add to the risk. This recommendation assumes that appropriate therapy is being given to both mother and infant. Isolation of infected areas should still be practiced, such as a mask in the case of respiratory infection and lesion isolation in herpes. **The three acute infections in which breastfeeding are contraindicated are herpes simplex lesions of the breast, untreated active (not just purified protein derivative [PPD]-positive) tuberculosis, and human immunodeficiency viral (HIV) disease.**

The fourth principle is to evaluate adequately the need and type of medication used for therapy (see Chapter 8). The drug management of chronic hypertension illustrates this principle. First, the need for medication must be scrutinized. There is considerable controversy in the literature as to whether or not to treat patients with mild chronic hypertension (diastolic blood pressure 90 to 100 mm Hg). The desire of a mother with mild hypertension to breastfeed may change the risk/benefit ratio so that antihypertensive drug therapy should be delayed until after lactation. Second, the medication should be evaluated for its effect on milk production. **In the first 3 to 4 months of therapy, diuretics reduce intravascular volume and, subsequently, milk volume.** On the other hand, if a patient has been on low doses of thiazide diuretics for more than 6 months, the effect on milk volume is minimal as long as adequate oral intake is maintained. Third, the medication should be evaluated for its secretion in breast milk and its possible effects on the infant. Thiazide diuretics, ethacrynic acid, and furosemide also cross into breast milk in small amounts. These agents have the potential to displace bilirubin, and their use during lactation is of concern when the infant is less than 1 month old or is jaundiced. In general, most other antihypertensive drugs are compatible with breastfeeding. Although new drugs come onto the market often, it is wise to use drugs that have had a long history of clinical use.

A fifth principle and a constant challenge is the blanket proscription by radiologists (and x-ray technicians) to "pump and dump" breast milk for 24 to 48 hours when radiocontrast agents are used. Most agents have very poor oral bioavailability and the effective infant dose is <0.1%. The guidelines of the American College of Radiology (2004) review the use of contrast media in breastfeeding mothers. On a practical level, the mother should feed her infant just before the injection of the contrast media. The delay of 2 to 3 hours until the next feed allows the mother to clear the agent before potential infant exposure; the half-life of many of these agents is less than 2 to 3 hours. If the mother is comfortable with expression or pumping, stored breast milk is an alternative for interim feeds for 2 to 3 half-lives.

DRUGS IN BREAST MILK

Most medications taken by the mother appear in the milk (see Chapter 8), but the calculated doses consumed by the nursing infant range from 0.001% to 5% of the standard therapeutic doses and are tolerated by infants without toxicity (see Table 23-8, Medications and Mother's Milk).

The following guidelines are helpful:

1. Evaluate the therapeutic benefit of medication. Diuretics given for ankle swelling provide very different benefits from those for congestive heart failure. Are drugs really necessary, and are there safer alternatives?
2. Choose drugs most widely tested and with the lowest milk/plasma ratio.
3. Choose drugs with the lowest oral bioavailability.
4. Select the least toxic drug with the shortest half-life.
5. Avoid long-acting forms. Usually, these drugs are detoxified by the liver or bound to protein.
6. Schedule doses so that the least amount gets into the milk. The rate of maternal absorption and the peak maternal serum concentration are helpful in scheduling dosage. Usually, it is best for the mother to take the medication immediately after a feeding.
7. Monitor the infant during the course of therapy. Many pharmacologic agents for maternal use are also used for infants. This implies the availability of knowledge about therapeutic doses and the signs and symptoms of toxicity.

BREAST MASSES DURING LACTATION

Breast cancer is the most common cancer of the reproductive organs of the female. While the risk of breast cancer increases tremendously after the age of 40, 1% to 3% of all breast cancers occur during pregnancy and lactation. Breast cancer diagnosed during lactation may have its origin before or during pregnancy. As a result of this assumption and small numbers of pregnant or lactating women, most studies have lumped the populations together. Recently, researchers in Japan have analyzed breast cancer in age-matched control women ($n = 192$), women who were pregnant at diagnosis ($n = 72$), and women who were lactating at diagnosis ($n = 120$). **The prognosis for breast cancer that is diagnosed during pregnancy or lactation is poorer than for breast cancer diagnosed at other times.** The 10-year survival for age-matched controls without lymph node metastasis was 93%; for women who were diagnosed during pregnancy or lactation the survival was 85%. When the lymph nodes were involved, the 10-year survival was 62% in controls and 37% in women who were diagnosed during pregnancy or lactation. The difference in survival is partially explained by a longer duration of symptoms prior to diagnosis (6.3 vs. 5.4 months), tumor size on palpation (4.6 vs. 3.0 cm), and tumor size on cut surface (4.3 vs. 2.6 cm), in lactating women versus control women, respectively. **The delay in diagnosis and the greater size at diagnosis in lactating women is a failure of the obstetric care provider and/or the lactating woman to aggressively sample a breast mass.**

The lactating woman is most likely to recognize a breast mass through her daily manipulations of her breasts. In her framework of reference, she usually considers this mass a "plugged duct." She should be encouraged to report a plugged duct that persists more than 2 weeks despite efforts to initiate drainage of that lobule. Her provider faces an expanded differential diagnosis. Fibromas and fibroadenomas are more common in young women. These solid tumors are rubbery, nodular, and mobile, and they may grow rapidly with the hormonal stimulation of pregnancy. The most common diagnosis is a dilated milk duct, a completely benign diagnosis.

A needle aspiration of the mass is the mainstay of diagnosis. **Percutaneous fine-needle aspiration is performed in the same manner as in nonpregnant women.** The use of local anesthetic is optional; infiltration of the area around a small lesion may increase the likelihood of a nondiagnostic aspiration. The area over the mass is swabbed with iodine or alcohol and, using sterile techniques, the lesion is fixed between the thumb and fingers of the nondominant hand. Using a 22-gauge needle attached to a 20-mL syringe, the center of the lesion is probed. Initial aspiration usually reveals the nature of the lesion. If milk or greenish fluid (fibrocystic disease) is found and the lesion disappears, no further diagnostic procedures need to be performed. If the tumor is solid or fails to disappear completely after aspiration, the needle is passed several times through the lesion under strong negative pressure. The aspirated tissue fluid is air-dried on a slide and sent for cytologic evaluation. The pathology requisition should note the age and lactating status. **Fine-needle aspiration biopsy appears to have the same accuracy in pregnancy and lactation as in the nonpregnant, nonlactating woman.** In a study of 214 fine-needle aspirations during pregnancy and lactation, eight (13.7%) were cancer, and the sensitivity, specificity, and positive predictive values were 100%, 81%, and 61%, respectively.

Ultrasound is an accurate method of determining the cystic nature of a breast mass in lactating women. Mammography is more difficult to interpret during lactation. Young breasts are generally more dense, and the massive increase in functioning glands may obscure small cancers. However, the accuracy is still good if the films are interpreted by experienced radiologists. In general, mammography is a secondary diagnostic modality.

A core biopsy using ultrasound or radiographic guidance is a reasonable option to avoid a surgical procedure. If a surgical biopsy is required, the surgeon will usually need guidance regarding the management of lactation. Most breast biopsies can be performed under local anesthesia. **If the mother nurses just before the procedure, she will empty the breast, which makes the surgery easier, and will allow 3 to 4 hours until the next feed.** Local anesthetics are not absorbed orally and pose no risk to the infant. The mother should be allowed to nurse on demand. Most anesthetics used for general anesthesia enter the breast milk in small amounts (1% to 3%) of the maternal dose, and minimal behavioral effects in infants have been observed. In most cases the mother can nurse within 4 hours of the anesthetic. The mother's breasts should be pumped 3 to 4 hours after the last feed regardless of the anesthetic status. She will begin to feel the discomfort of engorgement, and the fever of engorgement may confuse the postoperative picture as early as 8 or 10 hours. The failure to empty the breasts within 12 hours will begin to adversely affect milk supply.

Surgical biopsy usually has little effect on breastfeeding performance unless the procedure is done in the periareolar area or the nerves supplying the nipple are compromised. Circumareolar incisions are to be avoided if possible. Milk fistulas are an uncommon risk (5%) of central biopsy. The fistulas are usually self-limited and will spontaneously heal over several weeks. Prohibiting breastfeeding does not change the likelihood of ultimate healing.

BACK-TO-WORK ISSUES

In 2009, according to the Centers for Disease Control (CDC), about 50% of women in the workplace have a child at home less than 12 months old. One third returned to work within 3 months of birth and two thirds returned within 6 months. More than half are supplementing the feedings with formula and the duration of exclusive breastfeeding is well below the recommended duration. As a consequence, the CDC, other national organizations, and state legislatures have enhanced or initiated a major campaign to counter this challenge. The CDC has guidelines for workplace safety for working mothers who wish to express breast milk (www.cdc.gov/breastfeeding/promotion/employment.htm). **In March 2011, federal law amended Section 7 of the Fair Labor Standards Act to require employers to provide "reasonable break time for an employee to express breast milk for her nursing child for 1 year after the child's birth each time such employee has need to express the milk."**

The separation between mother and infant adversely affects the psychology and physiology of lactation through a decrease in the frequency of nursing, breast engorgement, and unsatisfied needs of the baby. The anxiety and fatigue associated with the combination of employment and lactation inhibits the let-down reflex, weakens maternal host defenses, and disrupts family dynamics. The infant must adapt to another caregiver, a new sucking technique, and unfamiliar infectious agents found in day-care settings. Therefore, it is not surprising that formula feeding is viewed as an improvement in mothers' lives, but it does create feelings of inadequacy and guilt in some women.

Breastfeeding during employment is both possible and fulfilling. Preparation, milk storage, and choice of childcare are the cornerstones to easy adaptation to employment. Preparation involves preemployment change in lifestyle to accommodate the increased stresses. **Lactation should be well established with frequent nursing (10 to 14 times per day) and no supplementation prior to return to work.** Return to full-time work prior to 4 months has a greater negative impact than return to work after 4 months. Part-time work lessens the impact. About 2 weeks prior to work, the mother should change her nursing schedule at home. During the workday, she should express or pump her breasts two or three times a day, while increasing her nursing with short, frequent feeds before and after work times. The infant is fed bottles of stored breast milk by a different person in a different place to allow it to adapt more easily.

During the 2 weeks prior to employment, the day-care arrangements should be carefully selected and observed. In addition to references, several questions are pertinent to the selection of the day-care setting. Is the sitter a mother herself, and does the sitter have experience with nursing babies? Is the mother welcome to use the child-care site for a midday nursing? Does the day-care center provide in-arm feeding, or does it use high chairs and propped bottle-feedings? Is the time and activity of the center highly structured and rigid, or is it flexible to mother or infant needs and requests? Does the staff treat the parents and children with respect? Many of these questions can be answered by an extended (1 to 2 hours) observation of the center and its children.

Fatigue is the number one enemy of the working mother. Emotional and physical support of the mother is critical. Some helpful suggestions include (1) bringing the infant's bed into the parent's room, or the construction of a temporary extension to the parents' bed; (2) use of labor-saving devices, division of domestic chores, and the elimination of less important household chores to reduce the workload; and (3) taking naps and frequent rest periods to conserve energy.

Continued stimulation of the breast during working hours is important. Pumping not only improves milk supply but it also supplies human milk for the infant. Manual expression and/or mechanical pumping should be performed more frequently (two to three times) in the first 6 months postpartum. After 6 months, the frequency can be reduced and eliminated as the infant is supplemented by fluids or solids during the day.

The collection of breast milk has become simple with the wide variety of mechanical pumps available in the market. Mechanical pumps that employ a bulb syringe produce the least amount of milk and have the highest rate of bacterial contamination. **Cyclic electric pumps produce the most milk with the least amount of nipple trauma.** Water-driven pumps are both cheap and relatively effective. The most efficient pumps are not as effective as the efficiently nursing infant in increasing milk volume and raising prolactin levels. Milk collection can be enhanced by pumping in a quiet place with soothing music in the background. Observing her infant making vocalizations can be instrumental in allowing let-down to occur.

The concern about bacterial growth in expressed and stored milk has been alleviated by recent studies showing that bacterial contamination does not increase significantly for up to 6 hours after expression, when the milk is stored at room temperature, nor were there differences in bacterial counts between specimens stored at room temperature and those stored under refrigeration for 10 hours. **Freshly refrigerated milk should be used within 2 days.** Four to 6 oz of human milk can be frozen in partially filled resealable plastic bags. When human milk is frozen, it should be cooled briefly prior to transfer to the freezer. **The milk will keep for 2 to 4 weeks in the refrigerator freezer and up to 6 months in a freezer set at 0° F.** The milk should be stored in layers and thawed quickly in warm tap water. **Frozen milk should not be thawed in the microwave, as the heating is uneven and severe oral burns have been reported. After it is thawed it should be used within 6 to 8 hours.**

WEANING

The American Academy of Pediatrics recommends exclusive breastfeeding for the first 6 months of life and continuation beyond the first 12 months of life. This recommendation in 1997 initiated a firestorm of controversy regarding "the excessive duration of breastfeeding." Breastfeeding is both a biologic process and a culturized activity. In the United States, breastfeeding has been culturized to breastfeeding for less than 6 months. From a broader biologic and historical perspective, the United States experience reflects cultural bias, not biologic reality. In a remarkable review, **Dettwyler[71] makes a very cogent argument for the "natural" age of weaning in the human to be 3 to 4 years.** She has several arguments. Traditional and prehistoric societies wean between the third and fourth year. Based on weaning when the infant weight is four times its birthweight, similar to other primates, weaning should occur between 2 and 3 years. If weaning corresponds to attainment of one third the adult weight, then weaning would occur between 3 and 4 years. If humans behaved like chimpanzees or gorillas and weaned at six times the gestational period, humans would wean at 4.5 years. The dental, neurologic, and immunologic systems are still developing until 6 years of age; breastfeeding and breast milk provide unique support for these systems up to 4 to 6 years. Developmentally, the infant is able to place solid food in its mouth at 6 months, but this intake, if left to the infant's own skills, would not reach a significant proportion of the nutritional requirements until 18 to 24 months. The ability to drink from a cup occurs close to the second year. As the infant supplements an increasing proportion of its nutritional needs with solid or liquid food, the mother will begin to ovulate. Subsequent pregnancy is increasingly more likely. **Breastfeeding, through its suppression of gonadal function, maintains a birth interval of 3 to 4 years. Clearly, breastfeeding into the third or fourth year is a cultural exception in the United States, but prolonged breastfeeding does not constitute abnormal or deviant behavior as expressed by many "modern" Americans.** As we learn more about the benefits of long-term lactation, our culture may return to more reasonable expectations for duration of breastfeeding.

KEY POINTS

- The World Health Organization, the U.S. Surgeon General, the American Academy of Pediatrics, the American Academy of Family Practice, the American College of Obstetricians and Gynecologists, and the Academy of Breastfeeding Medicine endorse breastfeeding as the gold standard for infant feeding.
- Breastfeeding accrues many health benefits for the infant, including protection against infection, less allergy, better growth, better neurodevelopment, and lower rates of chronic disease such as insulin-dependent diabetes and childhood cancer.
- Breastfeeding accrues more health benefits for the mother, including faster postpartum involution,

improved postpartum weight loss, less premenopausal breast cancer, lower rates of cardiovascular disease, and less insulin-resistant diabetes mellitus, better mother-infant bonding, and less economic burden.

- Formula lacks key components including defenses against infection, hormones and enzymes to aid digestion, polyunsaturated fatty acids, which are necessary for optimal brain growth, and adequate composition for efficient digestion.
- Prolactin is the major promoter of milk synthesis. Oxytocin is the major initiator of milk ejection. The release of prolactin and oxytocin results from the stimulation of the sensory nerves supplying the areola and nipple.
- Oxytocin released from the posterior pituitary can be operantly conditioned and is influenced negatively by pain, stress, or loss of self-esteem.
- Contact with the breast within one half hour after birth increases the duration of breast feeding. Correct positioning of the nursing infant and correct latch-on promote efficient milk transfer and reduce the incidence of breast pain and nipple injury. A frequency of nursing greater than eight per 24 hours, night nursing, and a duration of nursing longer than 15 minutes are needed to maintain adequate prolactin levels and milk supply.
- The nursing actions on a human teat versus on an artificial teat are very different. Poor lactation is the major cause of nipple injury and poor milk transfer. Perceived or real lack of milk transfer is the major reason for discontinuation of nursing.
- Milk production is reduced by an autocrine pathway through a protein that inhibits milk production by the alveolar cells, and by distention and pressure against the alveolar cells.

REFERENCES

1. American Academy of Pediatrics, Work Group on Breastfeeding: Breastfeeding and the use of human milk. Pediatr 115:625, 2005.
2. Committee on Health Care for Underserved Women, American College of Obstetricians and Gynecologists: American College of Ob/Gyn, Breastfeeding: Maternal and Infant Aspects ACOG Committee Opinion, 361, February 2007.
3. Scanlon KS, Grummer-Strawn L, Chen J, et al: Racial and ethnic differences in breastfeeding initiation and duration, by state—National immunization survey, United States, 2004-2008. MMWR 59:327, 2010.
4. Ahluwalia I, Morrow B, Hsia J, et al: Who is breastfeeding? Recent trends from the Pregnancy Risk Assessment and Monitoring System. J Pediatr 142:486, 2003.
5. Weber F, Woolridge MW, Baum JD: An ultrasonographic study of the organization of sucking and swallowing by newborn infants. Dev Med Child Neural 28:19, 1986.
6. Neifert M, DeMarzo S, Seacat J, et al: The influence of breast surgery, breast appearance, and pregnancy-induced breast changes on lactation sufficiency as measured by infant weight gain. Birth 17:31, 1990.
7. Neville MC: Determinants of milk volume and composition. In Jensen RG (ed): Handbook for Milk Composition. San Diego, Academic Press, 1995.
8. Peaker M: The effect of raised intramammary pressure on mammary function in the goat in relation to the cessation of lactation. J Physiol (Lond) 310:415, 1980.
9. Wilde CJ, Addey CVP, Boddy LM, et al: Autocrine regulation of milk secretion by a protein in milk. Biochem J 305:51, 1995.
10. Lund LR, Romer J, Thomasset N, et al: Two distinct phases of apoptosis in mammary gland involution: proteinase-independent and -dependent pathways. Development 122:181, 1996.
11. Prentice A, Addey CP, Wilde CJ: Evidence for local feedback control of human milk secretion. Biochem Soc Trans 16:122, 1989.
12. Neville MC: Physiology of lactation. Clin Perinatol 26:251, 1999.
13. Hall B: Changing composition of human milk and early development of an appetite control. Lancet 1:779, 1975.
14. Neville MC, Keller R, Seacat J, et al: Studies in human lactation: milk volumes in lactating women during the onset of lactation and full lactation. Am J Clin Nutr 48:1375, 1988.
15. Neville MC, Keller RP, Seacat J, et al: Studies on human lactation. 1. Within-feed and between-breast variation in selected components of human milk. Am J Clin Nutr 40:635, 1984.
16. Rasmussen KM: Maternal nutritional status and lactational performance. Clin Nutr 7:147, 1988.
17. Strode MA, Dewey KG, Lonnerdal B: Effects of short-term caloric restriction on lactational performance of well-nourished women. Acta Paediatr Scand 75:222, 1986.
18. McCrory MA, Nommsen-Rivers LA, Mole PA, et al: Randomized trial of the short-term effects of dieting compared with dieting plus aerobic exercise on lactation performance. Am J Clin Nutr 69:959, 1999.
19. Lovelady CA: The impact of energy restriction and exercise in lactating women. Adv Exp Med Biol 554:115, 2004.
20. Hartmann PE, Cregan MD, Ramsay DT, et al: Physiology of lactation in preterm mothers: initiation and maintenance. Pediatr Ann 32:351, 2003.
21. Newton M, Egli GE: The effect of intranasal administration of oxytocin on the let-down of milk in lactating women. Am J Obstet Gynecol 76:103, 1958.
22. Feher SDK, Berger LR, Johnson JD, et al: Increasing breast milk production for premature infants with a relaxation/imagery audiotape. Pediatrics 83:57, 1989.
23. Ueda T, Yokoyama Y, Irahara M, et al: Influence of psychological stress on suckling-induced pulsatile oxytocin release. Obstet Gynecol 84:259, 1994.
24. Dewey KG: Maternal and fetal stress are associated with impaired lactogenesis in humans. J Nutr 131:3012S, 2001.
25. Newton N, Newton M: Relationship of ability to breast-feed and maternal attitudes toward breast-feeding. Pediatr 5:869, 1950.
26. Cernadas JM, Nocess G, Barrena L, et al: Maternal and perinatal factors influence duration of exclusive breastfeeding. J Human Lact 19:136, 2003.
27. Uvnas-Moberg K: Oxytocin linked antistress effects—the relaxation and growth response. Acta Physiol Scand Suppl 640:38, 1997.
28. Moore ER, Anderson GC, Bergman N: Early skin-to-skin contact for mothers and their healthy newborn infants. Cochrane Database Sys Rev CD003519, 2007.
29. Lindenberg CS, Artola RC, Jimenez V: The effect of early postpartum mother-infant contact and breastfeeding promotion on the incidence and continuation of breastfeeding. Int J Nurs Stud 27:179, 1990.
30. Neifert M, Breastmilk Transfer: Positioning, latch-on, and screening for problems in milk transfer. Clin Obstet Gynecol 47:656, 2004.
31. Lucas A, Lucas PI, Baum JD: Differences in the pattern of milk intake between breast and bottle fed infants. Early Hum Dev 5:195, 1981.
32. Jones RE: A hazards model analysis of breastfeeding variables and maternal age on return to menses postpartum in rural Indonesian women. Hum Biol 60:853, 1988.
33. Newton ER: Breastmilk: The Gold Standard. Clin Obstet Gynecol 47:632, 2004.
34. Agency for Healthcare Research and Quality: Breastfeeding and Maternal and Infant Health Outcomes in Developed Countries—Evidence Report/Technological Assessment. AHRQ Publication No. 07-E007, 2007.
35. Ip S, Chung M, Raman G, Trikkalinos TA, Lau J: A summary of the Agency for Healthcare Research and Quality's evidence report on breastfeeding in developing countries. Breastfeeding Medicine 4:S-17, 2009.

36. Dewey KG: Growth characteristics of breast-fed compared to formula-fed infants. Bio Neonate 74:94, 1998.
37. Owen CG, Martin RM, Whincup PH, et al: Effect of infant feeding on the risk of obesity across the life course: a quantitative review of published evidence. Pediatrics 115:1367, 2005.
38. Schwartz EB, Ray RM, Steube AM, et al: Duration of lactation and risk factors for maternal cardiovascular disease. Obstet Gynecol 113:974, 2009.
39. Schwarz EB, McClure CK, Tepper PG, et al: Obstet Gynecol 115:41, 2010.
40. Steube AM, Michaels KB, Willett WC, et al: Duration of lactation and incidence of myocardial infarction in middle to late adulthood. Am J Obstet Gynecol 200:138e1, 2009.
41. Steube AM, Rich-Edwards JW, Manson JE: Duration of lactation and the incidence of Type II diabetes. JAMA 294:2601, 2005.
42. Turk MW, Yang K, Hravnak M, et al: Lifestyle interventions in primary care: a systematic review of randomized, controlled trials. Can Fam Phys 54:1706, 2008.
43. Lucas A, Morely R, Cole TJ: Randomized trial of early diet in preterm babies and later intelligence quotient. BMJ 31:1481, 1999.
44. Anderson JW, Johnstone BM, Remley DT: Breast-feeding and cognitive development: a meta-analysis. Am J Clin Nutrit 70:525, 1999.
45. Vohr BR, Poindexter BB, Dusick AM, et al: Persistent beneficial effects of breast milk ingested in the neonatal intensive care unit on outcomes of extremely low birth weight infants at 30 months of age. Pediatrics 120:e953, 2007.
46. Singhal A, Morley R, Cole T, et al: Infant nutrition and stereoacuity at age 4-6 y. Am J Clin Nutr 85:152, 2007.
47. Hanson LA: Human milk and host defense: immediate and long-term effects. Acta Paediatr Suppl 88:42, 1999.
48. Slade HB, Schwartz SA: Mucosal immunity: the immunology of breast milk. J Allergy Clin Immunol 80:346, 1987.
49. Schultz C, Temming P, Bucsky P, et al: Immature anti-inflammatory response in neonates. Clin Exp Immunol 135:130, 2004.
50. Walker WA: Mechanisms of action of probiotics. Clin Infect Dis 46:S87, 2008.
51. Broekaert IJ, Walker WA: Probiotics and chronic disease. J Clin Gastroenterol 40:270, 2006.
52. Vidal K, Donnet-Hughes A: CD14: A soluble pattern recognition receptor in milk. Adv Exp Med Biol 606:195, 2008.
53. Legrand D, Pierce A, Elass E, et al: Lactoferrin structure and functions. Adv Exp Med Biol 606:163, 2008.
54. Gerstein HC: Cow's milk exposure and Type I diabetes mellitus: a critical overview of the clinical literature. Diabetes Care 17:13, 1994.
55. Vaidya K, Sharma A, Dhungel S: Effect of early mother-baby close contact over the duration of exclusive breastfeeding. Nepal Medical College Journal 7:138, 2005.
56. Walker CD, Deschamps S, Proulx K, et al: Mother to infant or infant to mother? Reciprocal regulation of responsiveness to stress in rodents and the implications for humans. J Psychiatry Neurosci 29:364, 2004.
57. Uvnas-Moberg K: Oxytocin linked antistress effects—the relaxation and growth response. Acta Physiol Scand Suppl 640:38, 1997.
58. Mikiel-Kostyra K, Mazur J, Boltruszko I: Effect of early skin-to-skin contact after delivery on duration of breastfeeding: a prospective cohort study. Acta Paediatr 91:1301, 2002.
59. Strathearn L, Abdullah A, Mamun J, et al: Does breastfeeding protect against substantiated child abuse and neglect? A 15-year cohort study. Pediatrics 123:483, 2009.
60. Montgomery SM, Ehlin A, Sacker A: Breast-feeding and resilience against psychosocial stress. Arch Dis Child 91:990, 2006.
61. Ball TM, Bennett DM: The economic impact of breastfeeding. Ped Clin N Am 48:253, 2001.
62. Ball TM, Wright AL: Health care costs of formula-feeding in the first year of life. Pediatrics 103:870, 1999.
63. Madden JM, Soumerai SB, Lieu TA, et al: Effects on breastfeeding of changes in maternity length-of-stay policy in a large health maintenance organization. Pediatrics 111:519, 2003.
64. Bartick M, Reinhold R: The burden of suboptimal breastfeeding in the United States: A pediatric cost analysis. Pediatrics 125:e1048, 2010.
65. Michels KB, Willett WC, Rosner BA, et al: Prospective assessment of breastfeeding and breast cancer incidence among 89,887 women. Lancet 347:431, 1996.
66. Lucas A, Morley R, Cole TJ: Randomized trial of early diet in preterm babies and later intelligence quotient. BMJ 317:1481, 1998.
67. Lucas A, Cole TJ: Breast milk and neonatal necrotizing enterocolitis. Lancet 336:1519, 1990.
68. WHO/UNICEF: Protesting, promoting, and supporting breastfeeding: The special role of maternity services, a joint WHO/UNICEF statement. Geneva, World Health Organization, 1989.
69. Kramer MS, Chalmers B, Hodnett ED, et al: Promotion of Breastfeeding Intervention Trial (PROBIT): a randomized trial in the Republic of Belarus. JAMA 285:413, 2001.
70. Bhandari N, Bahl R, Mazumdar S, et al: Effect of community-based promotion of exclusive breastfeeding on diarrheal illness and growth: a cluster randomized controlled trial. Lancet 361:1418, 2003.
71. Dettwyler KA: A time to wean: the hominid blueprint for the natural age of weaning in modern human populations. In Stuart-MacAdam P, Dettwyler KA (eds): Breastfeeding: Biocultural Perspectives. New York, Aldine de Gruyter, 1995.
72. American Academy of Pediatrics, American College of Obstetricians and Gynecologists. Breastfeeding Handbook for Physicians, 2006.
73. Chung M, Rowan G, Trikalinos T, et al: Interventions in primary care to promote breastfeeding: evidence for the U.S. Preventive Task Force. Ann Intern Med 149:565, 2008.
74. Guise JM, Palda V, Westhoff C, et al: The effectiveness of primary care-based interventions to promote breastfeeding: systematic evidence review and meta-analysis for the U.S. Preventive Services Task Force. Ann Fam Med 1:70, 2003.
75. Cadwell K, Turner-Maffei C: Continuity of Care in Breastfeeding: Best Practices in Maternity Settings. Sudbury, MA, Jones & Bartlett, 2009.
76. DiGirolano AM, Grummer-Strawn LM, Fein SB: Effect of maternity care practices on breastfeeding. Pediatrics 122:s43, 2008.
77. Cramton R, Zain-Ul-Abideen M, Whalen B: Optimizing successful breastfeeding in the newborn. Current Opin in Pediatr 21:386, 2009.
78. CDC: Breastfeeding-related maternity practices at hospitals and birth centers—United States, 2007. MMWR 57:621, 2008.
79. Mansbach IK, Palti H, Pevsner B, et al: Advice from the obstetrician and other sources: do they affect women's breast feeding practices? A study among different Jewish groups in Jerusalem. Soc Sci Med 19:157, 1984.
80. Alexander JM, Grant AM, Campbell MJ: Randomized controlled trial of breast shells and Hoffman's exercises for inverted and non-protractile nipples. BMJ 304:1030, 1990.
81. Hurst NM: Lactation after augmentation mammoplasty. Obstet Gynecol 87:30, 1996.
82. Kjoller K, McLaughlin JK, Friis S, et al: Health outcomes in offspring of mothers with breast implants. Pediatrics 102:1112, 1998.
83. Semple JL, Lugowski SJ, Baines CJ, et al: Breast milk contamination and silicone implants: preliminary results using silicon as a proxy measurement for silicone. Plast Reconstr Surg 102:528, 1998.
84. Souto GC, Giugliani ER, Giugliani C, Schneider MA: The impact of breast reduction surgery on breastfeeding performance. J Hum Lact 19:43, 2003.
85. Dewey KG, Nommsen-Rivers LA, Heinig MJ, et al: Risk factors for suboptimal infant breastfeeding behavior, delayed onset of lactation, and excess neonatal weight loss. Pediatrics 112:607, 2003.
86. Patel RR, Liebling RE, Murphy DJ: Effect of operative delivery in the second stage of labor on breastfeeding success. Birth 30:255, 2003.
87. Zhang J, Bernasko JW, Leybovich E, et al: Continuous labor support from labor attendant for primiparous women: a meta-analysis. Obstet Gynecol 88:739, 1996.
88. Egli GE, Egli NS, Newton M: The influence of the number of breast-feedings on milk production. Pediatrics 27:314, 1961.
89. Howard C, Howard F, Lawrence R, et al: Office prenatal formula advertising and its effect on breast-feeding patterns. Obstet Gynecol 95:296, 2000.
90. Howard FM, Howard CR, Weitzman ML: The physician as advertiser: the unintentional discouragement of breast-feeding. Obstet Gynecol 95:296, 2000.
91. Mass S: Breast Pain: Engorgement, nipple pain and mastitis. Clin Obstet Gynecol 47:676, 2004.

92. Hill PD, Humenick SS: The occurrence of breast engorgement. J Hum Lact 10:79, 1994.
93. Livingston V, Stringer LJ: The treatment of *Staphylococcus* infected sore nipples: A randomized comparative study. J Hum Lact 15:241, 1999.
94. Morland-Schultz K., Hill P: Prevention of and therapies for nipple pain: a systematic review. JOGNN 34:428, 2005.
95. Academy of Breastfeeding Medicine Protocol Committee: ABM clinical protocol #4: Mastitis. Breastfeed Med 3:177, 2008.
96. Berens P, Swaim L, Peterson B: Incidence of methicillin-resistant *Staphylococcus aureus* in postpartum breast abscesses. Breastfeed Med 5:113, 2010.
97. Dener C, Inan A: Breast abscesses in lactating women. World J Surg 27:130, 2003.
98. Hale TW, Bateman TL, Finkelman MA, Berens PD: The absence of *Candida albicans* in milk samples of women with clinical symptoms of ductal candidiasis. Breastfeed Med 4:57, 2009.
99. Gartner LM, Herschel M: Jaundice and breastfeeding. Pediatr Clin North Am 48:389, 2001.
100. Academy of Breastfeeding Medicine Protocol Committee: ABM clinical protocol #9: Use of galactogogues in initiating or augmenting the rate of maternal milk secretion. Breastfeed Med 6:41, 2011.

For full reference list, log onto www.expertconsult.com.

Section V

Complicated Pregnancy

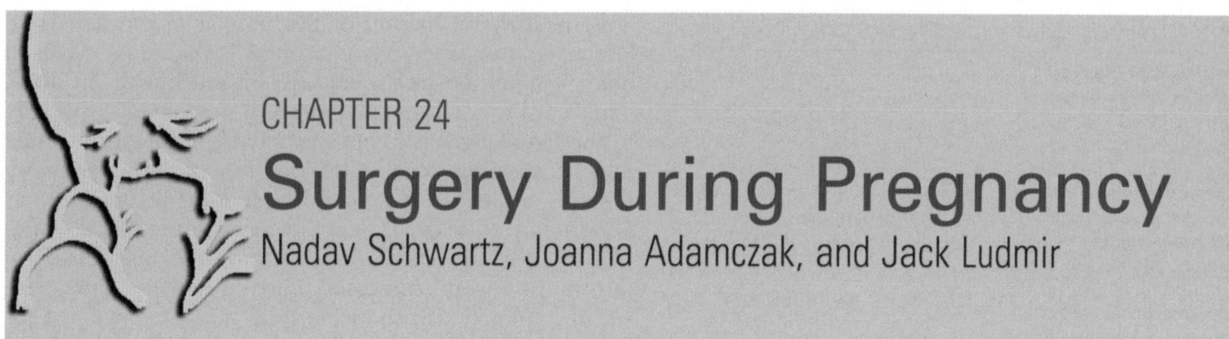

CHAPTER 24

Surgery During Pregnancy

Nadav Schwartz, Joanna Adamczak, and Jack Ludmir

KEY ABBREVIATIONS	
American Congress of Obstetricians and Gynecologists	ACOG
Association of Professors of Gynecology and Obstetrics	APGO
Computed Tomography	CT
Fetal Heart Rate	FHR
Intrauterine Growth Restriction	IUGR
Last Menstrual Period	LMP
Magnetic Resonance Imaging	MRI
Mechanical Index	MI
Society of American Gastrointestinal and Endoscopic Surgeons	SAGES
Thermal Index	TI

About 1 in 500 women will require nonobstetrical surgery during pregnancy.[1] The care of the pregnant surgical patient requires a multidisciplinary approach involving the obstetrician, surgeon, anesthesiologist, and pediatrician. There are numerous unique challenges that arise when caring for a pregnant woman presenting with symptoms that may require surgery. Evaluation of these patients is often confounded by the various changes in maternal physiology, concern for fetal well-being, and the potential risk to the continuing pregnancy. The introduction of new imaging diagnostic modalities has increased our diagnostic capabilities; however, their safety in pregnancy continues to be evaluated. In this chapter, we focus on (1) specific adaptations to pregnancy, both physiologic and anatomic, that the clinician needs to be aware of when evaluating a gravid patient; (2) the diagnostic challenges of evaluating a pregnant woman, with specific attention to radiologic studies, (3) the unique issues that arise when providing surgical anesthesia to the gravid patient; and (4) the potential risks to the pregnancy that are assumed when nonobstetrical surgery becomes necessary. Finally, although some of the more common indications for surgery in pregnancy, such as appendicitis, cholecystitis, and trauma, are addressed in more detail elsewhere, we address clinical circumstances that are being seen with increasing frequency during pregnancy, including the use of laparoscopy, the evaluation and treatment of adnexal masses, and issues related to obesity and bariatric surgery.

MATERNAL PHYSIOLOGY

Pregnancy-induced changes in maternal physiology and anatomy can confuse the clinical picture when evaluating the gravid patient presenting with abdominal complaints. Abdominal discomfort, nausea, vomiting, diarrhea, and constipation are often encountered in pregnancy in the absence of intra-abdominal pathology. Furthermore, laboratory changes that are commonly seen as abnormal in the nonpregnant surgical patient may be normal in the gravid state. Therefore, familiarity with these changes is essential when evaluating pregnant women with abdominal symptoms (Table 24-1; see Chapter 3).

Pregnancy causes profound changes in cardiovascular, hematologic, and respiratory physiology. Cardiovascular adaptations to pregnancy include a significant increase in cardiac output, heart rate, and intravascular volume.[2,3] Because the heart rate increases by up to 15 to 20 beats/minute compared with the nongravid state, it may be difficult to determine whether a mild tachycardia is physiologic or related to an underlying pathologic condition. These physiologic changes must be accounted for when evaluating a pregnant woman with a potential surgical diagnosis.

Respiratory physiology is also altered in pregnancy. The gravid uterus leads to a decrease in functional residual capacity and total lung capacity. In addition, the stimulatory effect of progesterone on respiratory drive leads to an increase in tidal volume and minute ventilation. Of note, the respiratory rate remains unchanged. As a result, pregnancy is associated with a state of relative hyperventilation and mild respiratory alkalosis.

TABLE 24-1 RELEVANT MATERNAL PHYSIOLOGIC CHANGES

I. **Cardiovascular changes**
Increased cardiac output
Increased blood volume
Increased heart rate
Decreased blood pressure
Decreased systemic vascular resistance
Decreased venous return from the lower extremities
II. **Respiratory changes**
Increased minute ventilation
Decreased functional residual capacity
III. **Gastrointestinal changes**
Decreased gastric motility
Delayed gastric emptying
IV. **Coagulation changes**
Increased clotting factors, I, VII, VIII, IX, X
Increased fibrinogen
Increased risk for thromboembolic disease
V. **Renal changes**
Increased renal plasma flow and glomerular filtration rate
Increased ureteral dilatation
VI. **Laboratory values**
Decreased serum creatinine
Decreased blood urea nitrogen (BUN)
Decreased hemoglobin and hematocrit
Increased white blood cell count
Increased alkaline phosphatase level
Increased fibrinogen levels
Increased D-dimer levels
Increased erythrocyte sedimentation rate

The physical examination of the pregnant abdomen may present a unique challenge. The enlarging gravid uterus becomes an abdominal organ after 12 weeks' gestation and may displace or compress intra-abdominal organs, making localization of pain difficult. For example, there is progressive upward displacement of the appendix, which does not return to its original position until 1 to 2 weeks postpartum.[4] However, despite the altered location, the most consistent and reliable symptom in pregnant women with appendicitis remains right lower quadrant pain.[5,6] Many other classic signs and symptoms of appendicitis, such as nausea, vomiting, and leukocytosis, may be normal findings in pregnancy. Similarly, physical examination findings of rebound and guarding may not be reliable indicators of intraperitoneal inflammation in pregnancy.[7,8] In addition, abdominal tenderness may be a sign of a pregnancy-specific complication, such as chorioamnionitis or placental abruption. Thus, the evaluation of abdominal pain in pregnancy often presents a challenging diagnostic dilemma.

The gravid uterus may also limit the ability of diagnostic imaging of abdominal organs. After the first trimester, the maternal adnexa are displaced cephalad and may be difficult to image with ultrasound. Some anatomic changes related to the growing uterus may confound the interpretation of diagnostic imaging. For example, mild to moderate hydroureter is commonly encountered in pregnancy secondary to compression of the distal ureters by the uterus, as well as progesterone-induced smooth muscle relaxation. This finding is more common on the right side and may even be associated with mild hydronephrosis. Because the incidence of both pyelonephritis and nephrolithiasis in increased in pregnancy, it is important to recognize that a degree of dilation of the upper urinary tract is often a normal finding in a pregnant patient.

Laboratory evaluation of the pregnant woman is also altered in pregnancy. Maternal blood volume is increased out of proportion to the increase in red blood cell mass. This leads to a dilutional anemia of pregnancy, especially in the later stages of pregnancy. This physiologic anemia may be mistaken for occult blood loss in the patient who is being evaluated for a surgical abdomen. Pregnancy is also associated with a progressive rise in peripheral white blood cell count, with a mean value of 14,000 cells/mm^3 during the second trimester. This physiologic leukocytosis, in conjunction with tachycardia and anemia, may confound the clinical picture and lead to an incorrect diagnosis. Other laboratory values, such as D-dimer, serum creatinine, and alkaline phosphatase, are significantly altered in pregnancy, limiting or altering their role in the diagnostic evaluation of the pregnant patient (see Table 24-1).

These significant changes in normal maternal physiology and diagnostic evaluation can complicate the diagnostic workup of the pregnant patient presenting with concerning symptoms. The utmost vigilance is necessary to rule out true pathology and arrive at the correct diagnosis in a timely fashion so that the appropriate management can be implemented and the risks to mother and fetus minimized. Familiarity with the normal pregnancy-related changes is critical to achieving optimal care.

DIAGNOSTIC IMAGING

A common concern that arises when evaluating a pregnant patient is the safety of diagnostic radiologic tests in pregnancy. When considering the potential risks related to imaging, it is important balance any small potential for harm against the significant risks associated with an erroneous or delayed diagnosis. Failure to accurately diagnose a serious condition in a timely manner can cause significant harm to the woman and her fetus.

Ionizing Radiation

The biggest concern related to diagnostic imaging is regarding the exposure of the developing fetus to ionizing radiation. The critical factors that determine the risk to the fetus are the dose of radiation to which the fetus is exposed and the gestational age of the exposure (Table 24-2). Very early in gestation, within the first 2 weeks of conception, any significant cell damage caused by radiation is believed to result in a miscarriage. This is believed to be an "all or none" phenomenon so that if the fetus remains viable after this early exposure, no adverse effects are expected. Radiation doses of greater than 50 to 100 mGy (5-10 rad; 1 mGy = 0.1 rad) are likely necessary to cause embryonic death. Postconception weeks 2 through 8 are particularly sensitive to teratogenicity because this is the period of organogenesis. At this stage, the embryo is more resistant to radiation-induced death, with doses of more than 250 to 500 mGy (25-50 rad) being necessary to cause fetal demise.[9,10]

The fetal central nervous system is the most sensitive to radiation damage during weeks 8 to 15 because this is a period of rapid neuronal development. Significant radiation exposure of 60 to 310 mGy during this period may lead to severe mental retardation and microcephaly. These risks to the fetal central nervous system persist up until about 25 weeks, although increasingly high doses of radiation are necessary to cause significant damage with

TABLE 24-2 FETAL EFFECTS OF RADIATION EXPOSURE BY GESTATIONAL AGE

GESTATIONAL AGE (FROM LMP)	ADVERSE EFFECT	ESTIMATED MINIMUM RADIATION DOSE
Weeks 3-4 (first 2 weeks postconception)	Embryonal demise ("all or none")	5-20 cGy
Weeks 4-8	Death, congenital anomalies, IUGR	20-50 cGy
Weeks 8-15*	IUGR, microcephaly, severe mental retardation†	6-50 cGy
Weeks 16-25	Mental retardation	25-150 cGy

Data from Brent RL: Saving lives and changing family histories: appropriate counseling of pregnant women and men and women of reproductive age, concerning the risk of diagnostic radiation exposures during and before pregnancy. Am J Obstet Gynecol 200:4-24, 2009; and Patel SJ, Reede DL, Katz DS, et al: Imaging the pregnant patient for nonobstetric conditions: algorithms and radiation dose considerations. Radiographics 27:1705-1722, 2007.)

*Period of neuronal development that is most sensitive to radiation damage.

†Exposure to 1 Gy of radiation during this period has been associated with a loss of 30 IQ points.

IUGR, Intrauterine growth restriction; *LMP*, last menstrual period.

TABLE 24-3 ESTIMATED FETAL EXPOSURE TO RADIATION FROM COMMON DIAGNOSTIC RADIOLOGIC STUDIES

RADIOLOGIC STUDY	ESTIMATED FETAL DOSE* (cGy)
Chest radiograph (posteroanterior, lateral)	0.0002
Abdominal radiograph	0.1-0.3
Head computed tomography (CT)	0.0005
Chest CT	0.002-0.02
Abdominal CT	0.4-0.8
Abdominopelvic CT	2.5-3.5
Abdominopelvic CT (stone protocol)	1
Ventilation scan	0.007-0.05
Perfusion scan	0.04
Intravenous pyelography	0.6-1
Bone scan	0.3-0.5
Positron emission scan	1-1.5
Thyroid scan	0.01-0.02
Mammography	0.007-0.02
Small bowel series	0.7
Barium enema	0.7

*Fetal dose can vary significantly based on a variety of patient and imaging parameters. If necessary, more precise estimates can be obtained through consultation with a radiation safety officer or radiation physicist.

increasing gestational age. After 25 weeks, the fetus is fairly resistant to radiation-induced abnormalities.[9,10]

In addition to teratogenic risk, there may be a concern for potential carcinogenic effects of ionizing radiation to the developing fetus. Some authors have estimated that the incidence of childhood leukemia and other cancers may increase by about 0.06% from baseline with each centigray of exposure.[11] Given the low background risk, diagnostic doses of radiation do not appear to significantly increase the absolute risk to the fetus.[9,12] However, the causative link between fetal exposure to diagnostic radiation and childhood leukemia has been called into question.[9]

Table 24-3 shows the estimated doses of fetal radiation exposure from various commonly used diagnostic imaging examinations that involve ionizing radiation.[12-14] It is important to note that the amount of radiation exposure from any of these diagnostic studies is well below the dose threshold for teratogenic risk. **Therefore, when evaluating a pregnant patient presenting with significant symptoms, the patient should be reassured that the radiation exposure to the fetus from a diagnostic radiologic test does not confer a significant risk for fetal harm.**[15,16] It is important for the clinician to be familiar with the relative radiation doses delivered by commonly ordered tests because this information may aid in the decision to choose one modality over another. In addition, when performing a radiologic study on a pregnant patient, the use of low-exposure techniques and abdominal lead shielding for nonpelvic studies can also help reduce the degree of fetal exposure. When clinically appropriate, consideration should be given to other diagnostic modalities, such as ultrasound or magnetic resonance imaging (MRI), that do not involve radiation.

Ultrasound

Ultrasound remains the initial imaging study of choice in the evaluation of the pregnant woman presenting with acute abdominal pain. Ultrasound involves the use of sound waves and is not a form of ionizing radiation. However, ultrasound does have the potential to transfer energy to the tissues being imaged.[17] There have been no confirmed adverse effects of diagnostic ultrasound procedures. Thus, the safety and versatility of ultrasonography has made it the first-line diagnostic tool during pregnancy whenever appropriate to address the clinical question at hand.

Magnetic Resonance Imaging

There are numerous advantages to MRI use during pregnancy. Like ultrasound, MRI does not use ionizing radiation, and there have been no reported harmful effects to the mother or fetus. In recent years, the use of MRI has expanded greatly as the image quality and availability have increased. For example, MRI has proved useful for evaluation of pathologies such as adrenal tumors, uterine and ovarian masses, gastrointestinal lesions, and retroperitoneal space evaluation, while avoiding the radiation exposure associated with computed tomography (CT) scanning.[18]

The use of diagnostic imaging in pregnant women requires adequate patient counseling to allay concerns of fetal harm and to balance any small potential risk against the need to arrive at an accurate and timely diagnosis. Although every effort should be made to minimize radiation exposure, it is widely accepted that exposure of less than 50 mGy does not confer a significant risk for fetal harm.[19,20] In fact, according to the American College of Obstetricians and Gynecologists (ACOG), "women should be counseled that x-ray exposure from a single diagnostic procedure does not result in harmful fetal effects. **Specifically, exposure to less than 50 mGy (5 rads) has not been associated with an increase in fetal anomalies or pregnancy loss.**"[12]

ANESTHESIA DURING NONOBSTETRICAL SURGERY

When anesthesia is required during pregnancy for a surgical procedure, several potential issues arise that must be addressed. From the perspective of the patient, the concern for possible adverse effects on the pregnancy is of primary importance. From the clinician's perspective, it is important to consider the physiologic changes of pregnancy that affect the delivery of safe and effective anesthesia.

Anesthesia and Teratogenicity

As is the case when examining the potential teratogenicity of any prenatal exposure, the data are limited to retrospective information emanating from case series and registries. These methods are significantly limited by a variety of potential biases that can lead to incorrect conclusions being drawn. However, because prospective research focusing on the teratogenicity of a medication is not ethically or logistically feasible, patients must be counseled based on the existing data, with acknowledgment of the inherent limitations.

Several early studies have raised the possibility that exposure to anesthesia in the first trimester may be associated with an increased risk for central nervous system malformations.[21,22] However, the methodologies used to arrive at these conclusions were particularly limited and not supported by subsequent data.[21] This example underscores the significant limitations to the data supporting a possible teratogenic risk of surgical and anesthetic exposure in the first trimester.

Most of the data have been reassuring that a significant risk for congenital malformations is unlikely when surgery occurs in the first trimester.[23,24] For example, Mazze and Kallen[24] reported on 5405 women from the Swedish Birth Registry who underwent nonobstetrical surgery during pregnancy, which included more than 720,000 deliveries between 1973 and 1981. More than 40% of these surgeries took place in the first trimester, yet there was no significant difference in the rate of congenital malformation compared with women without exposure to surgery in pregnancy. Furthermore, a recent systematic review of the literature identified more than 12,000 pregnancies exposed to nonobstetrical surgery and reported an overall 2% incidence of congenital malformation (3.9% when surgery occurred in the first trimester). Although there was no control group available in this review, the observed rate of malformation falls well within the range of expected rates of congenital malformation. Thus, the best available data appear to support the lack of a significant increased risk for malformations among pregnancies exposed to nonobstetrical surgery and anesthesia. However, unless clinically necessary, it may be preferable to defer surgical intervention until the second trimester, when the theoretical risk for teratogenicity, as well as spontaneous miscarriage, is further decreased.

Anesthesia and Pregnancy Physiology

As discussed earlier, there are many significant physiologic changes that occur in pregnancy that can have a profound impact on the delivery of safe and effective anesthesia in pregnancy (see Table 24-1). For example, several physiologic changes contribute to the increased risk for aspiration in pregnant women undergoing general anesthesia. Gastric emptying time is prolonged in pregnancy, especially in the third trimester and in obese women.[25] There is also a progesterone-mediated decreased tone at the gastroesophageal junction. Therefore, strategies to decrease the risk for aspiration, such as preoperative fasting, antacid prophylaxis (e.g., 30 mL of sodium citrate), and airway protection, are essential. In some situations, administration of histamine-2 blocker or a gastric motility agent (e.g., metoclopramide), or both, should be considered as well.

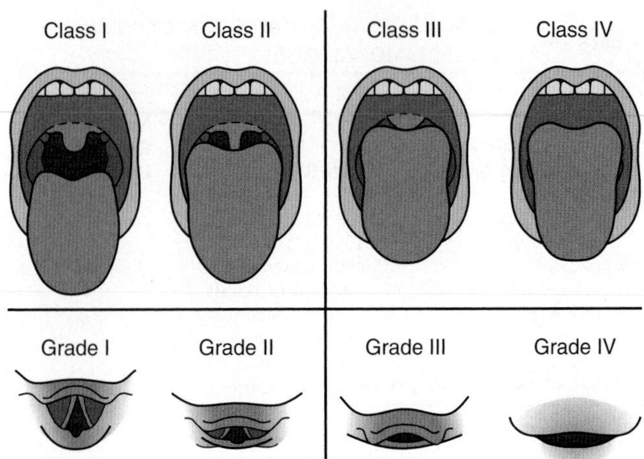

FIGURE 24-1. Mallampati airway examination with corresponding laryngoscopic view of the vocal cords. (Modified from Hughes SC, Levinson, G, Rosen MA [eds]: Shnider & Levinson's Anesthesia for Obstetrics, 4th ed. Philadelphia, Lippincott Williams & Wilkins, 2002.)

Oropharyngeal edema and narrowing of the glottis opening are common in pregnancy and can affect the safe access to the airway in a pregnant patient, especially in an emergency situation. **The Mallampati airway examination is often used to assess the airway and predict the degree of difficulty of intubation, with progression from low-risk airways (class I) to high-risk airways (class IV)** (Figure 24-1).[26] **In fact, there is a 34% increase in class IV Mallampati airways at term compared with the first trimester.**[27] **These changes are more pronounced in the third trimester, in obese women, and in patients with preeclampsia. Thus, preoperative airway examination is critical.**

One of the most significant physiologic phenomena in pregnancy is related to aortocaval compression by the gravid uterus, especially in the supine position and in the latter half of pregnancy. Compression of the inferior vena cava by the gravid uterus results in decreased preload and cardiac output with a resultant decrease in uterine and placental perfusion. In addition, venous stasis in the lower extremities increases the risk for venous thromboembolism. Thus, it is essential for the pregnant patient undergoing a surgical procedure to be positioned with a lateral tilt to relieve some of this compression by displacing the gravid uterus to the side. This can often be accomplished by placing a wedge under the right hip. Proper patient positioning, especially in the later stages of pregnancy, can help optimize cardiovascular physiology during surgery.

NONOBSTETRICAL SURGERY AND PREGNANCY OUTCOME

The largest study to explore pregnancy outcomes in women undergoing nonobstetrical surgery is based on the Swedish Birth Registry. Mazze and Kallen[24] identified 5405 nonobstetrical surgeries from more than 720,000 births between 1973 and 1981, for a prevalence of 0.75%.

The nonobstetrical surgeries included 1331 abdominal surgeries, 1008 genitourinary or gynecologic procedures, and 868 laparoscopies. Type of anesthesia was documented for only 68% of cases, but 2929 procedures (54% of all cases) were documented as being performed under general anesthesia. The authors found no difference in rate of congenital malformation or stillbirth. However, the rates of low birthweight (<2500 g) and very low birthweight (<1500 g) were significantly higher in the surgical group compared with the controls, with risk ratios of 2.0 and 2.2, respectively. The authors reported that observed reduced birthweight was due to both fetal growth restriction and prematurity. In fact, the incidence of preterm birth was increased in the surgery group (7.5% vs. 5.1%; $P < .001$). Another significant finding was an increased rate of neonatal death within 7 days of life (incidence, 1%; risk ratio, 2.1; 95% confidence interval [CI], 1.6 to 2.7). However, it is difficult to separate the multiple confounding factors that could potentially play a causative role in the development of adverse pregnancy outcomes, such as type of surgery, type of anesthesia, and underlying indication for surgery. In fact, the authors did not identify a specific type of surgical procedure or mode of anesthesia that had a significantly increased rate of adverse outcome. They conclude that the underlying illness that led to the surgery likely plays a significant role in determining the outcome.

More recently, Cohen-Kerem and coworkers[28] reviewed the literature from 1966 to 2002 and identified 12,452 pregnancies that underwent nonobstetrical surgery. The incidence of major birth defect was 2%, and the rate of prematurity was 8.2%. In addition, they found that surgical intervention led to delivery of the fetus in 3.5% of cases, although they could not differentiate whether this was caused by the procedure itself or the underlying condition that necessitated the surgical intervention. Although the lack of matched controls limits the interpretation of their data, it does support the notion that most pregnancies that undergo nonobstetrical surgery will have favorable outcomes.

Taken together, it would seem reasonable to reassure pregnant patients faced with the need for surgery in pregnancy that the rate of adverse perinatal outcome is low. In addition, although there may be an increased risk for low birthweight, preterm birth, and neonatal demise, these risks must be weighed against the potential for complications related to the underlying indication for surgery. In cases of semielective surgery, such as for an enlarged adnexal mass or refractory and severe biliary colic, it is still prudent to defer surgery until after the first trimester when the risk for spontaneous miscarriage is decreased and the theoretical concerns of teratogenicity are avoided. Similarly, surgery in the late-second and third trimesters may affect intraoperative visibility and lead to an increased risk for preterm birth. Therefore, the early second trimester is considered the optimal time for elective surgery that cannot be safely deferred until after the pregnancy.

FETAL MONITORING

The question of whether continuous intraoperative fetal monitoring should be employed when a pregnant woman requires nonobstetrical surgical intervention is a matter of debate.[29,30] Factors in favor of monitoring include the potential for changes in fetal heart rate and uterine activity during the surgery, the potential for fetal well-being to serve as an indicator of maternal status, and the potential to intervene in a case of persistently nonreassuring fetal status. On the other hand, interpretation of the fetal tracing may be unreliable in very preterm fetuses. In addition, the changes in fetal heart tracing occasionally seen, such as a decreased variability and lower baseline heart rate, are often transient and not necessarily an indication of fetal distress. Thus, continuous intraoperative fetal monitoring may lead to an unnecessary emergent cesarean delivery with significant risk for both maternal and neonatal morbidity. A recent survey of the Association of Professors of Gynecology and Obstetrics found that most respondents do not routinely perform intraoperative fetal monitoring, but simply monitor the fetus before and after the procedure.[31] **Because of the lack of data to guide management, the ACOG recommends consultation with an obstetrician who can properly counsel the pregnant women facing surgery and individualize the decision based on factors such as gestational age, type of surgery, and facilities available.**[32,33] In most cases, determining the presence of fetal heart activity before and after surgical intervention seems appropriate.

LAPAROSCOPY IN PREGNANCY

Although the safety of laparoscopy in pregnancy is widely accepted, there are several important physiologic considerations specific to pregnancy that must be considered. Pneumoperitoneum further decreases functional residual capacity and can cause ventilation-perfusion mismatch and hypercapnia. These effects can be further exacerbated by Trendelenburg positioning. Bhavani-Shanker and colleagues[34] prospectively demonstrated that end-tidal carbon dioxide pressures correlate well with arterial PCO_2 and that maintaining an end-tidal CO_2 of about 32 mm Hg and a systolic blood pressure within 20% of baseline was effective in preventing respiratory acidosis during laparoscopy. Once again, left lateral maternal position is essential to displace the gravid uterus, helping relieve aortocaval compression and optimize cardiac output.

The intra-abdominal pressure required to obtain adequate laparoscopic visualization during surgery can have significant physiologic effects for both the pregnant women and the fetus. Early animal studies showed that cardiac output decreases with increasing intraperitoneal pressure. Reedy and colleagues[35] performed laparoscopic baboon studies and compared intra-abdominal pressures of 10 and 20 mm Hg. At the higher pressure, there was a significant increase in pulmonary capillary wedge pressure, central venous pressure, pulmonary artery pressure, and peak airway pressure. In addition, a significant increase in ventilator rate was required to maintain oxygenation and end-tidal CO_2. A pressure of 20 mm Hg was also associated with an increased risk for respiratory acidosis. **Similar studies have shown significant changes in both maternal and fetal physiology at pressures greater than 15 mm Hg.**[36] **Therefore, although lower insufflation pressures may lead to limited surgical visualization, it is important to try and keep insufflation pressures below 15mm Hg.** If higher pressures are required to safely complete the procedure, it would be advisable to periodically release the pneumoperitoneum to allow for physiologic recovery. This is particularly important in obese patients, who often require higher pressures to counteract the weight of the anterior abdominal wall. Although various techniques, such as gasless laparoscopy[37,38] and mechanical lift retractors,[39] have been proposed to avoid high intra-abdominal pressures during laparoscopy, they are not widely performed.

Laparoscopic Entry Techniques in Pregnancy

Although the conventional entry approach has been using a Veress needle, a variety of other closed and open techniques have been proposed in an effort to decrease the incidence of entry complications in nonobstetrical laparoscopic procedures. However, review of the literature fails to support a significant difference in complications between the various approaches.[40,41] Nonetheless, accidental placement of a Veress needle into a 21-week uterus with subsequent pneumoamnion and pregnancy loss has been reported.[42] Thus, it may be reasonable to use an open approach in the latter half of pregnancy. Nonetheless, the Society of American Gastrointestinal and Endoscopic Surgeons (SAGES) guidelines support laparoscopic entry with any technique provided that the location of the entry is adjusted to account for the gravid uterus (Table 24-4).[43] Thus, procedures performed in the later stages of pregnancy may require a left upper quadrant insertion of the initial trocar. **The upper limit of gestational age up to which a laparoscopic approach can be performed safely in pregnancy has not be determined. Concerns related to the gravid uterus have led some to recommend that laparoscopy be avoided in the third trimester.**[44] However, current practice guidelines do not impose such a limitation.[43] Because the available evidence is insufficient to impose a definitive recommendation, the decision regarding the optimal surgical approach should be individualized.

TABLE 24-4 RELEVANT GUIDELINES FOR LAPAROSCOPY IN PREGNANCY FROM THE SOCIETY OF AMERICAN GASTROINTESTINAL AND ENDOSCOPIC SURGEONS

- Diagnostic laparoscopy is safe and effective when used selectively in the workup and treatment of acute abdominal processes in pregnancy.
- Laparoscopic treatment of acute abdominal processes has the same indications in pregnant and nonpregnant patients.
- Laparoscopy can be safely performed during any trimester of pregnancy.
- Gravid patients should be placed in the left lateral recumbent position to minimize compression of the vena cava and the aorta.
- Initial access can be safely accomplished with open (Hassan), Veress needle, or optical trocar technique if the location is adjusted according to fundal height, previous incisions, and experience of the surgeon.
- CO_2 insufflation of 10 to 15 mm Hg can be safely used for laparoscopy in the pregnant patient. Intra-abdominal pressure should be sufficient to allow for adequate visualization.
- Intraoperative CO_2 monitoring by capnography should be used during laparoscopy in the pregnant patient.
- Intraoperative and postoperative pneumatic compression devices and early postoperative ambulation are recommended prophylaxis for deep venous thrombosis in the gravid patient.
- Laparoscopic cholecystectomy is the treatment of choice in the pregnant patient with gallbladder disease regardless of trimester.
- Laparoscopic appendectomy may be performed safely in pregnant patients with suspicion of appendicitis.
- Laparoscopic adrenalectomy, nephrectomy, and splenectomy are safe procedures in pregnant patients when indicated, and standard precautions are taken.
- Laparoscopy is safe and effective treatment in gravid patients with symptomatic adnexal cystic masses. Observation is acceptable for all other adnexal cystic lesions provided ultrasound is not worrisome for malignancy and tumor markers are normal. Initial observation is warranted for most adnexal cystic lesions smaller than 6 cm.
- Laparoscopy is recommended for both diagnosis and treatment of adnexal torsion unless clinical severity warrants laparotomy.
- Fetal heart monitoring should occur before and after operation in the setting of urgent abdominal surgery during pregnancy.
- Obstetrical consultation can be obtained before and after operation based on the acuteness of the patient's disease, gestational age, and availability of the consultant.
- Tocolytics should not be used prophylactically but should be considered perioperatively when signs of preterm labor are present in coordination with obstetrical consultation.

From Yumi H: Guidelines for diagnosis, treatment, and use of laparoscopy for surgical problems during pregnancy: this statement was reviewed and approved by the Board of Governors of the Society of American Gastrointestinal and Endoscopic Surgeons (SAGES), September 2007. It was prepared by the SAGES Guidelines Committee. Surg Endosc 22:849-861, 2008.

Laparoscopy and Pregnancy Outcome

Laparoscopy has become increasingly prevalent in both pregnant and nonpregnant populations. The minimally invasive nature of laparoscopy allows for an easier recovery, with less pain, earlier return of bowel function, and shorter hospital stay. Furthermore, the quicker postoperative ambulation helps reduce the potential for venous stasis and deep venous thrombosis, which is especially important in a pregnant population that is already at increased risk for such complications.

The safety of laparoscopy in pregnancy is supported by the analysis of the Swedish Birth Registry. Reedy and coworkers[45] compared fetal outcomes of 2181 pregnancies that underwent laparoscopy between 4 and 20 weeks' gestation to 1522 pregnancies that underwent laparotomies. No differences were noted in any of the fetal outcome parameters examined. Several other series have further supported the safety of laparoscopy in pregnancy.[46-51] Nevertheless, several reports and case series have been published raising the possible increased risk for adverse outcomes. Amos and associates[52] reported a series of seven laparoscopies performed in pregnancy and found that four of the seven resulted in a fetal demise. Although this report raised a significant concern regarding the safety of laparoscopy in pregnancy, it is important to note that the four pregnancies that suffered a fetal demise were undergoing the surgery for a serious medical conditions known to be associated with intra-abdominal inflammation (three with gallstone pancreatitis and one with a perforated appendix). Therefore, it is difficult to separate the underlying indication for surgery from the surgical approach in trying to establish am etiology for these adverse outcomes.

Walsh and coworkers[53] performed a systematic review of the literature and concluded that an open appendectomy may be safer than a laparoscopic approach when managing appendicitis. This conclusion was based on the 5.8% incidence of fetal loss following a laparoscopic appendectomy compared with a 3.1% incidence reported after open appendectomy (P = .001). However, multiple potential confounders, such as severity of the appendicitis, gestational age at the time of surgery, background rate of miscarriage, and reporting bias, may have significantly affected their analysis. Furthermore, they showed a significant increase in preterm delivery in open appendectomy cases (8.1% vs. 2.1%; P < .0001). Thus, no definitive data support a significantly increased risk for adverse pregnancy outcome using the laparoscopic approach.

Similarly, McGory and colleagues[54] identified more than 3000 cases of appendectomy in pregnancy using the California Inpatient File and found that, after controlling for several potential confounders, laparoscopic appendectomy was associated with an increased risk for fetal loss compared with open appendectomy (odds ratio, 2.31; 95% CI, 1.51 to 3.55). However, the gestational age at the time of surgery was not available. Furthermore, they defined fetal loss as the presence of a diagnosis code for spontaneous abortion or intrauterine death or of a procedure code for a dilation and curettage associated with the same hospital admission as the appendectomy. The limitations and potential inaccuracies of this method of data collection are obvious. Therefore, it remains unclear whether the laparoscopic procedure itself contributed to the observed rate of fetal loss.

Overall, laparoscopy should be considered a safe option when considering surgery in a pregnant patient. In fact, the SAGES practice guidelines support laparoscopy and a safe and effective surgical approach in any trimester of pregnancy with the same indications as in nonpregnant women (see Table 24-4).[43]

ADNEXAL MASSES IN PREGNANCY

The increased use of prenatal ultrasound, the high prevalence of physiologic cysts related to ovulation, and the use of ovulation induction in the treatment of infertility make the evaluation of an adnexal mass in pregnancy a common clinic scenario. The reported prevalence of adnexal masses in pregnancy ranges from less than 1% to 25% and is dependent on a variety of factors, such as gestational age and the criteria used to characterize an adnexal finding as a mass rather than a simple follicle.[55]

Fortunately, most adnexal masses encountered in pregnancy are benign and spontaneously resolve during the course of pregnancy. In fact, rates of spontaneous resolution have been reported to be as high as 72% to 96%.[55] Most of these cysts are simple follicular cysts, which are thin-walled, unilocular cysts and contain anechoic fluid. Alternatively, a corpus luteum cyst may develop and contain varying amounts of hemorrhage within the thick-walled and unilocular cyst (Figure 24-2). These are also benign and transient findings, which generally resolve by the second trimester and rarely require further surveillance. In patients who have undergone ovulation induction for the treatment of infertility, one may encounter thin-walled, multicystic ovaries containing anechoic fluid and lacking internal septations or papillae. These usually resolve during the course of the pregnancy, although they can cause patient discomfort if they are particularly enlarged (see Figure 24-2). Theca-lutein cysts are an uncommon type of multicystic ovarian mass in pregnancy and are related to hyperelevations of β-human chorionic gonadotropin, such as in gestational trophoblastic disease and multiple gestations. They appear as thick-walled, multicystic masses with no papillae. Although they generally contain anechoic fluid, internal hemorrhage can occur, especially in large masses (see Figure 24-2).

Although most benign masses encountered in pregnancy are physiologically related to the gestation, it is not uncommon to incidentally detect other benign ovarian masses, such as mature cystic teratomas (i.e., dermoid cysts), cystadenomas, or endometriomas. *Dermoids* can contain a variety of tissue types, leading to a variable appearance on ultrasound. Often, a hyperechoic area, known as Rokitansky tubercle, can help confirm the nature of these masses. These masses are benign and persist throughout the pregnancy. Fortunately, malignant degeneration is exceedingly rare, especially in women of childbearing age. Therefore, increased surveillance and surgical intervention are rarely necessary in an asymptomatic woman. As with all sizable masses, the patient should be counseled about the risk for ovarian torsion and be educated about the typical presenting symptoms (Figure 24-3). *Cystadenomas* often contain thin internal septations and may exhibit a small mural nodule. These masses are generally hypovascular and may contain anechoic fluid (serous cystadenomas) or fluid with low-level echoes (mucinous cystadenomas) (see Figure 24-3). *Endometriomas,* benign ovarian masses containing ectopic endometrial tissue, most often display a characteristic appearance with diffuse, low-level echoes (see Figure 24-3). Affected patients often have a history of endometriosis or dysmenorrhea. These masses generally persist throughout pregnancy without significant change in size. However, occasionally, an endometrioma can undergo decidualization during pregnancy as the endometrial tissue responds to the hormonal changes. In these cases, the mass may appear heterogeneous with increased vascularization and papillary projections, sharing many of the sonographic features of an ovarian malignancy (Figure 24-4). A known history of an endometrioma before pregnancy may be helpful in differentiating this mass from a malignancy, but close surveillance and thorough patient counseling are indicated.

Although most adnexal masses encountered in pregnancy are benign, one should not discount the rare possibility of malignancy. In fact, between 1% and 3% of masses removed in pregnancy are found to be malignant.[56,57] However, these data are confounded by the indication for surgery and likely represent a high-risk group of patients. In the largest series of adnexal masses in pregnancy, Leiserowitz and coworkers[56] identified 9375 adnexal masses associated with pregnancy, 87 (0.93%) of which were found to be malignant. In their population, this translated into 1 ovarian cancer per 56,000 deliveries. An additional 115 (1.25%) cases were found to be borderline tumors. Taken together, the prevalence of clinically significant ovarian tumors was 1 in 23,800 deliveries. In addition to being extremely rare, ovarian cancer in pregnancy is associated with more favorable characteristics, such as lower stage and a higher proportion of germ cell tumors.[56,57] This is likely because of the younger patient population and the incidental

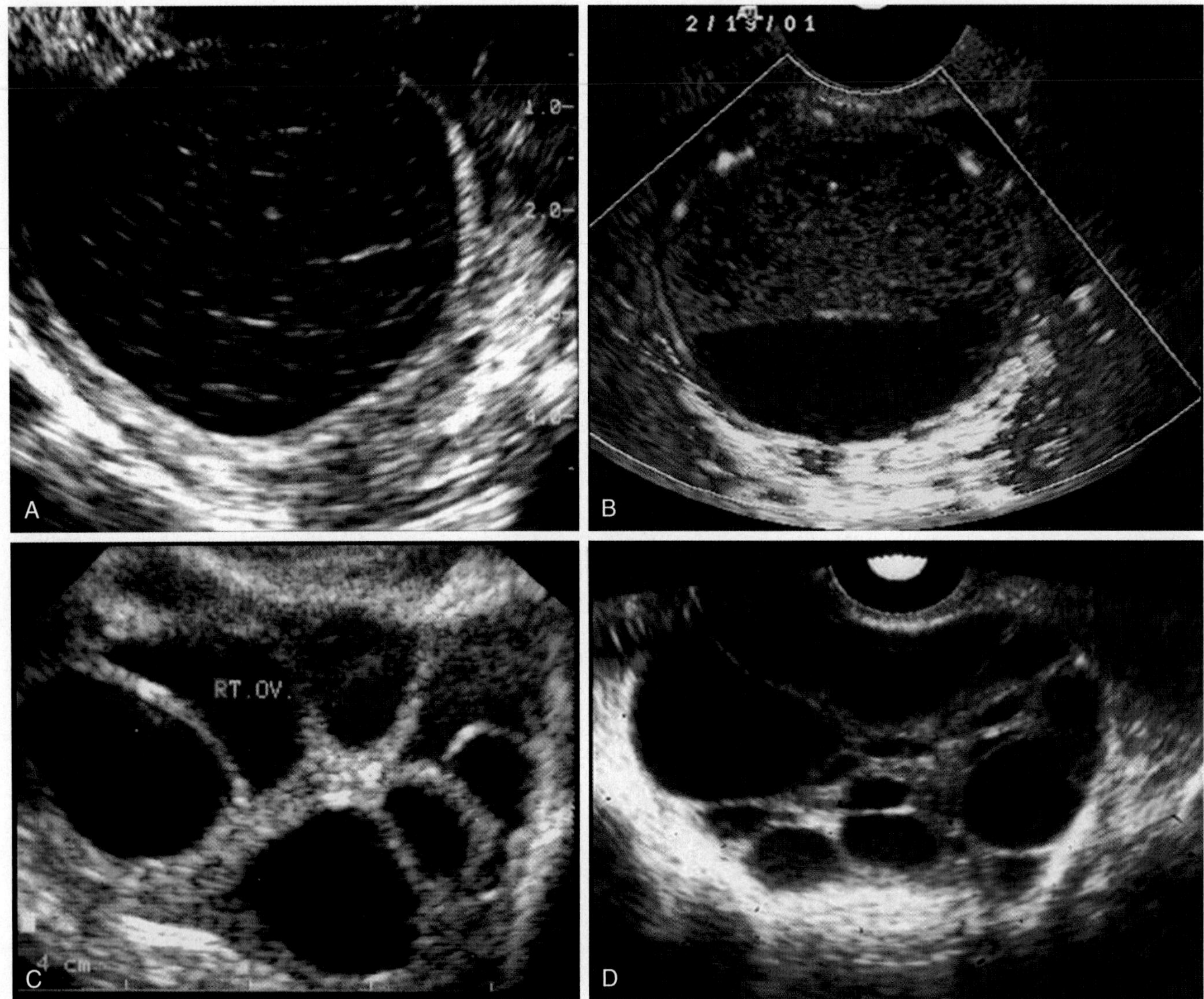

FIGURE 24-2. **A** and **B,** Variable appearance of a corpus luteum. The layered echogenicity represents hemorrhage within the cyst. Circumferential vascularity on power Doppler imaging is a typical finding. **C,** A thecal lutein cyst is seen as a thick-walled and multiloculated cyst with anechoic fluid. **D,** A typical appearance of a stimulated ovary with multiple follicular cysts after infertility treatment. (From Schwartz N, Timor-Tritsch IE, Wang E: Adnexal masses in pregnancy. Clin Obstet Gynecol 52:570-585, 2009.)

detection of these masses in asymptomatic women. Nevertheless, when a suspicious adnexal mass is encountered in pregnancy, the possibility of malignancy must be considered.

Although other imaging modalities such as MRI may be helpful in some cases in which a thorough evaluation of the mass is difficult because of the gravid uterus, ultrasound examination remains the diagnostic tool of choice when evaluating the adnexa. Several sonographic features have been associated with an increased risk for malignancy, such as size greater than 7 cm, heterogeneity with solid and cystic components, papillary excrescences or mural nodules, thick internal septations, irregular borders, increased vascularity, and low-resistance blood flow. However, the specificity of any of these findings remains limited, and no single high-risk feature is pathognomonic for malignancy. Rather, overall pattern recognition by experienced sonologists is likely the most accurate approach.[58-60] Surgical resection may become necessary when the degree of suspicion is high.

Another potential complication of an adnexal mass is ovarian torsion, which is estimated to occur in up to 7% of adnexal masses in pregnancy. Sixty percent of torsions occur in the first trimester.[61,62] Concern for this complication often leads to the recommendation to electively resect masses in pregnancy in an effort to prevent torsion. However, Lee and colleagues[61] compared 36 cases of emergency surgery for torsion in pregnancy with 53 cases of electively removed adnexal masses and found no difference in pregnancy outcomes, indicating that reserving intervention for acute torsion likely does not put the patient at increased risk for a complication. Thus, because nonobstetrical surgery in pregnancy is not without risk, preventive surgical intervention may not be appropriate. **Rather, patients with persistent adnexal masses in pregnancy should be counseled about the signs and symptoms**

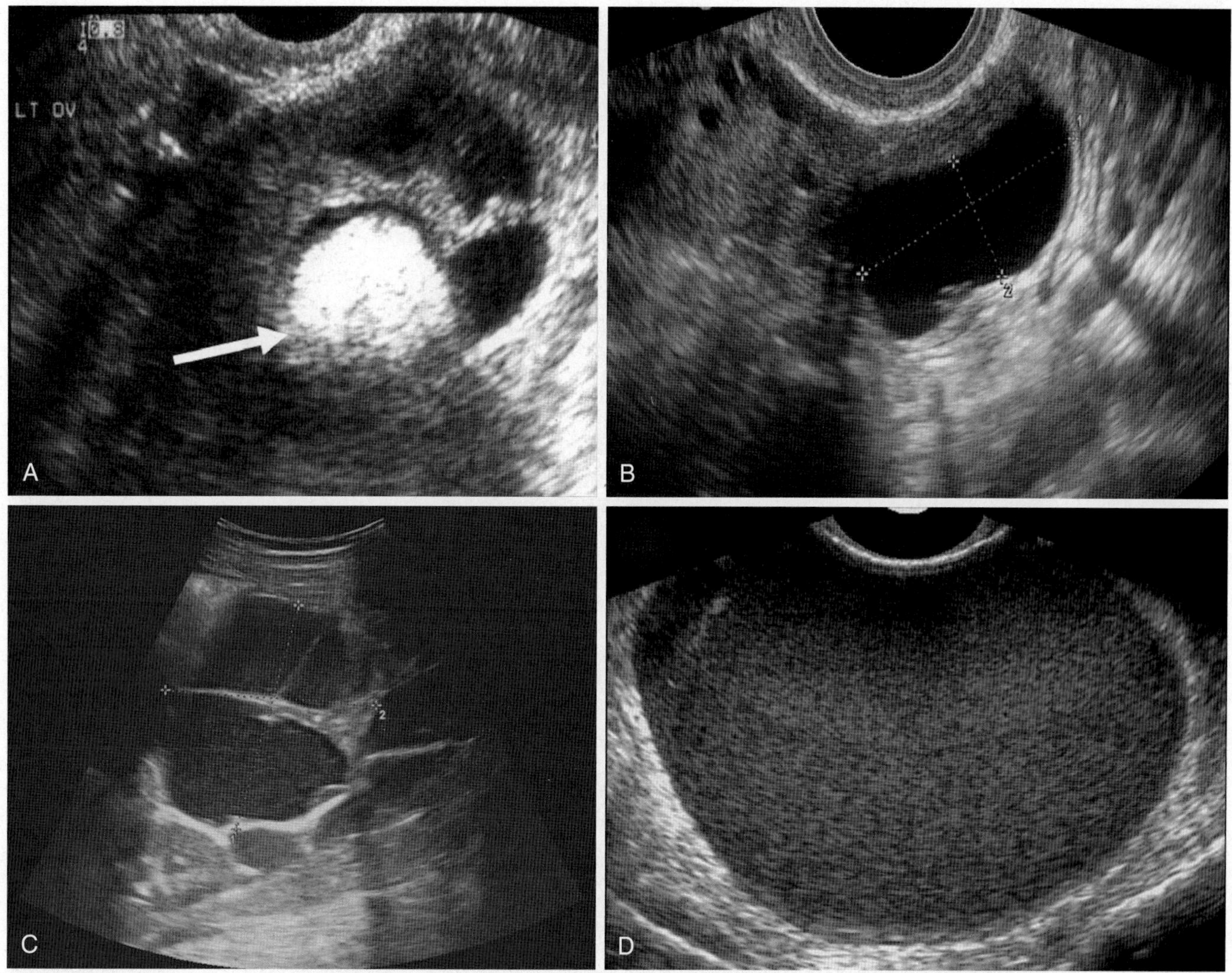

FIGURE 24-3. **A,** A dermoid cyst with heterogeneous contents and a typical Rokitansky nodule *(arrow)*. **B,** A benign, serous cystadenoma presenting as an anechoic cyst with a small mural nodule. **C,** This cystic mass with thin internal septations was shown to be a mucinous cystadenoma. **D,** Endometriomas often present as cystic masses containing homogeneous low-level echoes. (From Schwartz N, Timor-Tritsch IE, Wang E: Adnexal masses in pregnancy. Clin Obstet Gynecol 52:570-585, 2009.)

of ovarian torsion, with surgical resection reserved for symptomatic patients and for those in whom there is a suspicion of malignancy.

When ovarian torsion is confirmed during surgery, there is a question of whether there is a role for detorsion with ovarian conservation in cases in which there does not appear to be extensive necrosis (Figure 24-5). There is evidence that lends support to this approach in nonpregnant women.[63-65] **Although pregnancy data are more limited, there are several reports of successful management of ovarian torsion in pregnancy with preservation of the ovary.**[66-68] There are reports of ovarian necrosis requiring a repeat operation 2 days after a detorsion in pregnancy.[69] Therefore, the potential for recurrence must be taken into account when deciding to preserve the twisted ovary. Some authors recommend performing an oophoropexy to stabilize the ovary in the hope of minimizing recurrence, although this cannot be recommended as a routine approach. If a discrete ovarian cyst or mass is noted, excision of the mass should reduce the chance of recurrence, especially if there is any concern for potential malignancy. **Ultimately, the decision to untwist and preserve the torsed ovary should be individualized based on intraoperative findings and risk factors for recurrence.**

Overall, when presented with an adnexal mass that requires surgical resection, the decision to proceed with laparoscopy or laparotomy is based on the same approach taken outside of pregnancy. Laparoscopy has been shown to be a safe and effective method to remove adnexal masses in pregnancy,[37,51,70-72] although laparotomy may be preferred in certain scenarios, such as in patients with prior abdominal surgeries or large masses and in those who present late in pregnancy when visualization may be compromised. In general, although some have reported the safe aspiration of large simple cysts in pregnancy, this method runs the risk for leakage of cyst contents into the abdomen, which would be especially harmful if an unsuspected malignancy were present. In addition, cytologic analysis of the cyst contents may not be an accurate method to determine the pathology of the mass.[73] Therefore, cyst

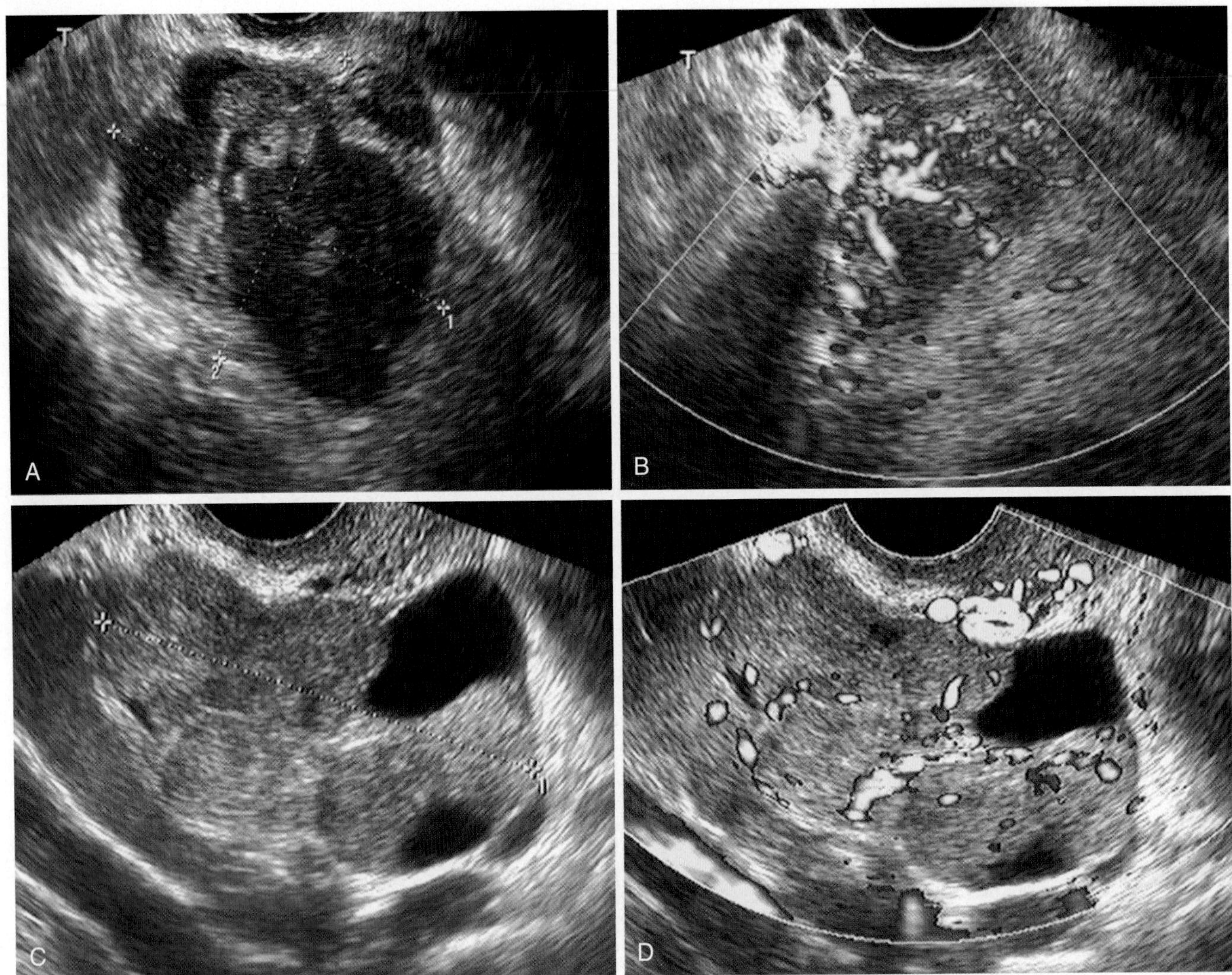

FIGURE 24-4. **A** and **B,** A complex and heterogeneous mass with thickened septations and increased vascularity in a patient with a known endometrioma. The sonographic features were suspicious for malignancy, leading to surgical excision in the middle trimester. Pathology showed it to be a decidualized endometrioma. **C** and **D,** A similar-appearing heterogeneous mass with increased vascularity. This was also excised and shown to be a stage I cystadenocarcinoma. (From Schwartz N, Timor-Tritsch IE, Wang E: Adnexal masses in pregnancy. Clin Obstet Gynecol 52:570-585, 2009.)

aspiration cannot be considered a standard approach for managing adnexal masses in pregnancy. Regardless of the surgical approach, it is important to remember that before 8 weeks' gestation, the corpus luteum is the primary source of progesterone for the pregnancy. Therefore, progesterone supplementation should be administered to patients who undergo adnexal surgery before 8 to 10 weeks' gestation.

OBESITY, BARIATRIC SURGERY, AND PREGNANCY

Maternal obesity is an increasingly common condition in pregnancy. In 2008, up to 36% of adult women in the United States were obese.[74] Obesity is associated with an increased risk for numerous significant medical comorbidities, including diabetes, hypertension, cardiac disease, and respiratory conditions. Furthermore, maternal obesity is an independent risk factor for several pregnancy-related complications, including gestational diabetes, preeclampsia, cesarean delivery, infectious morbidity, and thromboembolism. There is also an increase in fetal complications, such as congenital malformations, macrosomia, and stillbirth.[75-77] Bariatric surgery is an increasingly common and effective treatment for obesity and has been associated with a significant improvement in overall health, as well as a reduction in adverse pregnancy outcomes.[78,79] For the purposes of this chapter, it is important to review the special considerations related to surgery in the obese pregnant patient, as well as the implications of prior bariatric surgery in pregnancy.

Obesity presents unique management challenges in the perioperative period and is a risk factor for a multitude of adverse outcomes related to both general anesthesia and surgery.[80-82] Intubation is often more difficult in obese patients, and preoperative assessment of the airway using the Mallampati classification is essential.[83-85] Furthermore, gestational changes in respiratory physiology, such as a

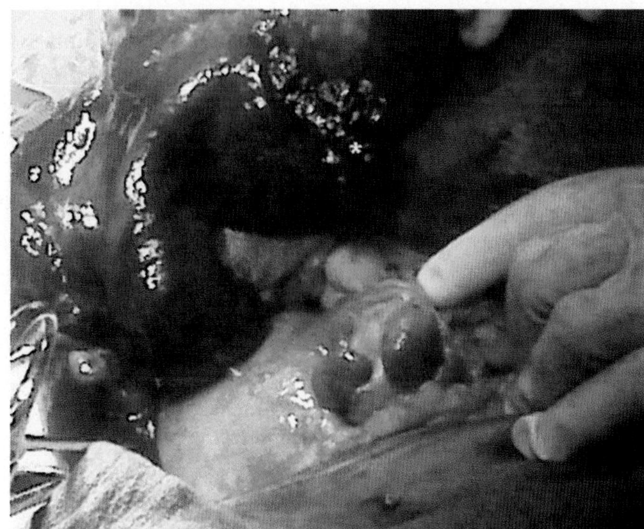

FIGURE 24-5. Intraoperative photograph of an ovarian torsion at 11 weeks' gestation. A 9-cm adnexal mass *(upper left of photograph)* was torsed around an edematous vascular pedicle. The mass was removed by laparotomy, because of concern for necrosis of the fimbria (*). The normal-appearing left ovary and tube are seen on the right, with the gravid uterus in the center. Pathology confirmed a dermoid cyst with areas of necrosis. (Courtesy Stephanie Jean, MD.)

decreased functional residual capacity and increased work of breathing, can lead to impaired ventilation and an increase in adverse respiratory events in obese pregnant patients undergoing anesthesia. In addition, the aortocaval compression seen in pregnancy may be exacerbated by maternal body habitus. For these reasons, many authors recommend various maneuvers such as adjusting patient positioning and preoperative hyperoxygenation when caring for the obese patient.

Another consideration unique to obese patients undergoing anesthesia is related to the altered pharmacokinetics of anesthetic drugs and to the volume of distribution and concentration of lipophilic drugs in the adipose tissues. Therefore, care must be taken when dosing anesthetic agents for obese patient, as well as when monitoring the recovery from anesthesia after surgery.[86,87] **Regional anesthesia should be considered if possible to avoid some of these risks, although the type of surgery and difficulty accomplishing regional anesthesia may not allow for this approach in some cases.**

Obesity is also an independent risk factor for venous thromboembolism in the postoperative period. Therefore, early ambulation should be encouraged. Prophylaxis with compression devices or with subcutaneous heparin should be considered. In addition, given the increased risk for wound infection and dehiscence in obese patients, adequate antibiotic prophylaxis is recommended.[82]

Significant weight loss before pregnancy is the most effective means of reducing the medical risks related to obesity, including pregnancy-related risks.[78,79] One of the most successful treatments for obesity is bariatric surgery, which is becoming an increasingly common procedure in the United States. Thus, it is imperative for obstetrical providers to be familiar with some of the unique concerns that arise in pregnant patients who have previously undergone bariatric surgery.

In general, bariatric surgery can be divided into restrictive procedures, such as gastric banding, and malabsorptive procedure, such as gastric bypass. Restrictive procedures are less invasive and can often be accomplished laparoscopically. These procedures do not result in the dramatic weight reduction seen with malabsorptive procedures, but they are associated with a lower risk for nutrient deficiencies and other complications related to malabsorption. The gastric band can be adjusted to lessen the degree of gastric restriction, allowing for adequate food intake in pregnancy.

The most commonly performed malabsorptive procedure is the Roux-en-Y gastric bypass, in which a proximal stomach pouch is created and the most of the stomach and proximal small bowel is bypassed. This often leads to rapid and significant weight loss, especially in the first 1 to 2 years. In fact, some recommend that pregnancy be delayed until 1 to 2 years after the procedure to avoid having rapid weight loss during pregnancy, and thorough contraception counseling is imperative.[88,89] Conception rates shortly after bariatric surgery appear to be increased,[89,90] which may be related to poor absorption of oral contraception, resumption of regular menstrual cycles, and inadequate contraceptive counseling. **The reduced absorptive capacity of the stomach and proximal small bowel often leads to deficiency in several essential nutrients, including iron, vitamin B_{12}, vitamin D, folate, and calcium. Unfortunately, long-term compliance with vitamin supplementation is poor among bariatric surgery patients.**[91,92] **Obtaining a baseline evaluation of these nutrients preconceptionally or early in pregnancy is recommended. In addition, consultation with a nutritionist should be considered.**[93]

Finally, although there is no evidence to suggest that pregnancy increases the risk for postoperative complications related to prior bariatric surgery, such complication may occur during pregnancy.[94,95] It is therefore important for obstetrical providers to be familiar with the possible complications so that the bariatric surgeon can be notified. Some known complications include anastomotic leaks, bowel obstruction, internal hernias, and erosion or migration of gastric bands. Many of these complications first manifest with symptoms commonly experienced during normal pregnancy, such as nausea, vomiting, and abdominal discomfort, so there is the potential that the accurate diagnosis of these complications can be delayed in a pregnant patient. In fact, maternal deaths have been reported.[96,97] Therefore, clinicians should have a high degree of suspicion when such patients present with significant abdominal complaints.[93]

One final complication that can be encountered in pregnant patients with a history of malabsorptive bariatric surgery is *dumping syndrome.* The consumption of simple sugars can lead to significant fluid shifts into the small intestine, causing cramping, nausea, vomiting, and diarrhea. In severe cases, the patient can become tachycardic and diaphoretic and complain of palpitations. Consideration should be given to monitoring blood glucose levels because hypoglycemia can result from hyperinsulinemia. Patients sensitive to sugar intake may not tolerate the glucose tolerance test for gestational diabetes. Having the patient monitor fasting and postprandial fingersticks for 1 to 2 weeks may be a reasonable screening approach in sensitive patients.[98]

Overall, bariatric surgery and successful weight loss can significantly improve pregnancy outcomes. With the increasing prevalence of surgical treatment of obesity among young women, clinicians should familiarize themselves with some of the unique concerns that arise when managing these patients during pregnancy.

KEY POINTS

- Care of the pregnant surgical patient requires a multidisciplinary approach with an understanding of the physiologic alterations in gestation.
- Expansion of maternal blood volume during pregnancy may mask signs of maternal hemorrhage, and clinically significant blood loss can occur before hemodynamic changes are evident.
- Delay in surgical intervention results in increased maternal and fetal morbidity and mortality, significantly increasing the risk for preterm labor and fetal loss.
- Diagnostic doses of radiation (<5 cGy) from radiographs and CT scans are unlikely to pose any significant harm to the developing fetus. MRI and ultrasound can be safely used when appropriate to further minimize radiation exposure.
- There does not appear to be a significant difference in the rate of congenital malformations in women who require nonobstetrical surgery in pregnancy. Although there may be an increased risk for preterm birth, low birthweight, and neonatal death, this may be due to the underlying illness more than the surgical procedure itself.
- Laparoscopy is a safe surgical modality in pregnancy. The use of a laparoscopic approach in the latter stages of pregnancy should be individualized based on indication and experience of the surgeon. Abdominal insufflation pressures should be kept below 15 mm Hg whenever possible.
- Adnexal masses are commonly encountered in pregnancy, although most are benign. Pregnant women diagnosed with an adnexal mass should be counseled about the signs and symptoms of ovarian torsion. Surgical resection can be reserved for symptomatic women or for masses that are suspicious for malignancy.
- There is a lack of data to guide management regarding fetal heart rate monitoring intraoperatively. In most cases, preoperative and postoperative FHR monitoring is appropriate.
- Preoperative corticosteroid administration for fetal well-being needs to be based on gestational age and nature of the planned surgery.
- Thromboembolic prophylaxis with compression devises should be considered for all gravid surgical patients.
- Obesity presents unique management challenges in the perioperative period, most notably with anesthesia-related risk, intraoperative risk, antibiotic prophylaxis, and thromboembolic prophylaxis. If early ambulation is not possible, subcutaneous heparin should be considered.
- Bariatric surgery with subsequent weight loss may reduce the risk for an adverse pregnancy outcome. The gravid patient with a history of bariatric surgery presenting with vague abdominal complaints should be critically evaluated as delay in diagnosis from internal hernias, bowel obstruction, or anastomosis leaks can often lead to catastrophic events. Such women should also be evaluated for nutritional deficiencies.

REFERENCES

1. Kilpatrick CC, Monga M: Approach to the acute abdomen in pregnancy. Obstet Gynecol Clin North Am 34:389, 2007.
2. Capeless EL, Clapp JF: Cardiovascular changes in early phase of pregnancy. Am J Obstet Gynecol 161:1449, 1989.
3. Clapp JF 3rd, Seaward BL, Sleamaker RH, Hiser J: Maternal physiologic adaptations to early human pregnancy. Am J Obstet Gynecol 159:1456, 1988.
4. Baer JL, Reis RA, Arens RA: Appendicitis in pregnancy with changes in position and axis of the normal appendix in pregnancy. JAMA 52:1359, 1932.
5. Mourad J, Elliott JP, Erickson L, Lisboa L: Appendicitis in pregnancy: new information that contradicts long-held clinical beliefs. Am J Obstet Gynecol 182:1027, 2000.
6. Yilmaz HG, Akgun Y, Bac B, Celik Y: Acute appendicitis in pregnancy. Risk factors associated with principal outcomes: a case control study. Int J Surg 5:192, 2007.
7. Sharp HT: The acute abdomen during pregnancy. Clin Obstet Gynecol 45:405, 2002.
8. Wagner JM, McKinney WP, Carpenter JL: Does this patient have appendicitis? JAMA 276:1589, 1996.
9. Brent RL: Saving lives and changing family histories: appropriate counseling of pregnant women and men and women of reproductive age, concerning the risk of diagnostic radiation exposures during and before pregnancy. Am J Obstet Gynecol 200:4, 2009.
10. Patel SJ, Reede DL, Katz DS, et al: Imaging the pregnant patient for nonobstetric conditions: algorithms and radiation dose considerations. Radiographics 27:1705, 2007.
11. Lee CI, Haims AH, Monico EP, et al: Diagnostic CT scans: assessment of patient, physician, and radiologist awareness of radiation dose and possible risks. Radiology 231:393, 2004.
12. ACOG Committee Opinion. No. 299, September 2004 (replaces No. 158, September 1995). Guidelines for diagnostic imaging during pregnancy. Obstet Gynecol 104:647, 2004.
13. Goldstone K, Yates SJ: Radiation issues governing radiation protection and patient doses in diagnostic imaging. In Adam A: Grainger & Allison's Diagnostic Radiology, 5th ed. New York, Churchill Livingstone, 2008.
14. McCollough CH, Schueler BA, Atwell TD, et al: Radiation exposure and pregnancy: when should we be concerned? Radiographics 27:909, 2007.
15. Nijkeuter M, Geleijns J, De Roos A, et al: Diagnosing pulmonary embolism in pregnancy: rationalizing fetal radiation exposure in radiological procedures. J Thromb Haemost 2:1857, 2004.
16. Winer-Muram HT, Boone JM, Brown HL, et al: Pulmonary embolism in pregnant patients: fetal radiation dose with helical CT. Radiology 224:487, 2002.
17. Nelson TR, Fowlkes JB, Abramowicz JS, Church CC: Ultrasound biosafety considerations for the practicing sonographer and sonologist. J Ultrasound Med 28:139, 2009.
18. De Wilde JP, Rivers AW, Price DL: A review of the current use of magnetic resonance imaging in pregnancy and safety implications for the fetus. Prog Biophys Mol Biol 87:335, 2005.

19. International Commission on Radiological Protection, Publication 90: Biological effects after prenatal irradiation (embryo and fetus). New York, Pergamon, Elsevier Science, 2000, no. 33.
20. American College of Radiology: Practice guideline for imaging pregnant or potentially pregnant adolescents and women with ionizing radiation. Retrieved Oct 12, 2011 from www.acr.org/SecondaryMainMenuCategories/quality_safety/guidelines/dx/Pregnancy.aspx.
21. Kallen B, Mazze RI: Neural tube defects and first trimester operations. Teratology 41:717, 1990.
22. Sylvester GC, Khoury MJ, Lu X, Erickson JD: First-trimester anesthesia exposure and the risk of central nervous system defects: a population-based case-control study. Am J Public Health 84:1757, 1994.
23. Czeizel AE, Pataki T, Rockenbauer M: Reproductive outcome after exposure to surgery under anesthesia during pregnancy. Arch Gynecol Obstet 261:193, 1998.
24. Mazze RI, Kallen B: Reproductive outcome after anesthesia and operation during pregnancy: a registry study of 5405 cases. Am J Obstet Gynecol 161:1178, 1989.
25. Chiloiro M, Darconza G, Piccioli E, et al: Gastric emptying and orocecal transit time in pregnancy. J Gastroenterol 36:538, 2001.
26. Mallampati SR, Gatt SP, Gugino LD, et al: A clinical sign to predict difficult tracheal intubation: a prospective study. Can Anaesth Soc J 32:429, 1985.
27. Pilkington S, Carli F, Dakin MJ, et al: Increase in Mallampati score during pregnancy. Br J Anaesth 74:638, 1995.
28. Cohen-Kerem R, Railton C, Oren D, et al: Pregnancy outcome following non-obstetric surgical intervention. Am J Surg 190:467, 2005.
29. Horrigan TJ, Villarreal R, Weinstein L: Are obstetrical personnel required for intraoperative fetal monitoring during nonobstetric surgery? J Perinatol 19:124, 1999.
30. Kendrick JM, Neiger R: Intraoperative fetal monitoring during non-obstetric surgery. J Perinatol 20:276, 2000.
31. Kilpatrick CC, Puig C, Chohan L, et al: Intraoperative fetal heart rate monitoring during nonobstetric surgery in pregnancy: a practice survey. South Med J 103:212, 2010.
32. ACOG: Committee opinion: nonobstetric surgery in pregnancy. No. 284, August 2003. Int J Gynaecol Obstet 83:135, 2003.
33. ACOG: Practice bulletin no. 100: critical care in pregnancy. Obstet Gynecol 113:443, 2009.
34. Bhavani-Shankar K, Steinbrook RA, Brooks DC, Datta S: Arterial to end-tidal carbon dioxide pressure difference during laparoscopic surgery in pregnancy. Anesthesiology 93:370, 2000.
35. Reedy MB, Galan HL, Bean-Lijewski JD, et al: Maternal and fetal effects of laparoscopic insufflation in the gravid baboon. J Am Assoc Gynecol Laparosc 2:399, 1995.
36. Reynolds JD, Booth JV, de la Fuente S, et al: A review of laparoscopy for non-obstetric-related surgery during pregnancy. Curr Surg 60:164, 2003.
37. Akira S, Yamanaka A, Ishihara T, et al: Gasless laparoscopic ovarian cystectomy during pregnancy: comparison with laparotomy. Am J Obstet Gynecol 180:554, 1999.
38. Schmidt T, Nawroth F, Foth D, et al: Gasless laparoscopy as an option for conservative therapy of adnexal pedicle torsion with twin pregnancy. J Am Assoc Gynecol Laparosc 8:621, 2001.
39. Stany MP, Winter WE 3rd, Dainty L, et al: Laparoscopic exposure in obese high-risk patients with mechanical displacement of the abdominal wall. Obstet Gynecol 103:383, 2004.
40. Ahmad G, Duffy JM, Phillips K, Watson A: Laparoscopic entry techniques. Cochrane Database Syst Rev 2:CD006583, 2008.
41. Vilos GA, Ternamian A, Dempster J, Laberge PY, for the Society of Obstetricians and Gynaecologists of Canada: Laparoscopic entry: a review of techniques, technologies, and complications. J Obstet Gynaecol Can 29:433, 2007.
42. Friedman JD, Ramsey PS, Ramin KD, Berry C: Pneumoamnion and pregnancy loss after second-trimester laparoscopic surgery. Obstet Gynecol 99:512, 2003.
43. Yumi H: Guidelines for diagnosis, treatment, and use of laparoscopy for surgical problems during pregnancy: this statement was reviewed and approved by the Board of Governors of the Society of American Gastrointestinal and Endoscopic Surgeons (SAGES), September 2007. It was prepared by the SAGES Guidelines Committee. Surg Endosc 22:849, 2008.
44. Fatum M, Rojansky N: Laparoscopic surgery during pregnancy. Obstet Gynecol Surv 56:50, 2001.
45. Reedy MB, Kallen B, Kuehl TJ: Laparoscopy during pregnancy: a study of five fetal outcome parameters with use of the Swedish Health Registry. Am J Obstet Gynecol 177:673, 1997.
46. Abuabara SF, Gross GW, Sirinek KR: Laparoscopic cholecystectomy during pregnancy is safe for both mother and fetus. J Gastrointest Surg 1:48; discussion, 52, 1997.
47. Barone JE, Bears S, Chen S, et al: Outcome study of cholecystectomy during pregnancy. Am J Surg 177:232, 1999.
48. Cosenza CA, Saffari B, Jabbour N, et al: Surgical management of biliary gallstone disease during pregnancy. Am J Surg 178:545, 1999.
49. Daradkeh S, Sumrein I, Daoud F, et al: Management of gallbladder stones during pregnancy: conservative treatment or laparoscopic cholecystectomy? Hepatogastroenterology 46:3074, 1999.
50. Sadot E, Telem DA, Arora M, et al: Laparoscopy: a safe approach to appendicitis during pregnancy. Surg Endosc 24:383, 2010.
51. Shalev E, Peleg D: Laparoscopic treatment of adnexal torsion. Surg Gynecol Obstet 176:448, 1993.
52. Amos JD, Schorr SJ, Norman PF, et al: Laparoscopic surgery during pregnancy. Am J Surg 171:435, 1996.
53. Walsh CA, Tang T, Walsh SR: Laparoscopic versus open appendicectomy in pregnancy: a systematic review. Int J Surg 6:339, 2008.
54. McGory ML, Zingmond DS, Tillou A, et al: Negative appendectomy in pregnant women is associated with a substantial risk of fetal loss. J Am Coll Surg 205:534, 2007.
55. Schwartz N, Timor-Tritsch IE, Wang E: Adnexal masses in pregnancy. Clin Obstet Gynecol 52:570, 2009.
56. Leiserowitz GS, Xing G, Cress R, et al: Adnexal masses in pregnancy: how often are they malignant? Gynecol Oncol 101:315, 2006.
57. Whitecar MP, Turner S, Higby MK: Adnexal masses in pregnancy: a review of 130 cases undergoing surgical management. Am J Obstet Gynecol 181:19, 1999.
58. Ameye L, Valentin L, Testa AC, et al: A scoring system to differentiate malignant from benign masses in specific ultrasound-based subgroups of adnexal tumors. Ultrasound Obstet Gynecol 33:92, 2009.
59. Bromley B, Benacerraf B: Adnexal masses during pregnancy: accuracy of sonographic diagnosis and outcome. J Ultrasound Med 16:447; quiz, 453-444, 1997.
60. Chiang G, Levine D: Imaging of adnexal masses in pregnancy. J Ultrasound Med 23:805, 2004.
61. Lee GS, Hur SY, Shin JC, et al: Elective vs. conservative management of ovarian tumors in pregnancy. Int J Gynaecol Obstet 85:250, 2004.
62. Schmeler KM, Mayo-Smith WW, Peipert JF, et al: Adnexal masses in pregnancy: surgery compared with observation. Obstet Gynecol 105:1098, 2005.
63. Cohen SB, Oelsner G, Seidman DS, et al: Laparoscopic detorsion allows sparing of the twisted ischemic adnexa. J Am Assoc Gynecol Laparosc 6:139, 1999.
64. Pansky M, Abargil A, Dreazen E, et al: Conservative management of adnexal torsion in premenarchal girls. J Am Assoc Gynecol Laparosc 7:121, 2000.
65. Wang JH, Wu DH, Jin H, Wu YZ: Predominant etiology of adnexal torsion and ovarian outcome after detorsion in premenarchal girls. Eur J Pediatr Surg 20:298, 2010.
66. Djavadian D, Braendle W, Jaenicke F: Laparoscopic oophoropexy for the treatment of recurrent torsion of the adnexa in pregnancy: case report and review. Fertil Steril 82:933, 2004.
67. Gorkemli H, Camus M, Clasen K: Adnexal torsion after gonadotrophin ovulation induction for IVF or ICSI and its conservative treatment. Arch Gynecol Obstet 267:4, 2002.
68. Rackow BW, Patrizio P: Successful pregnancy complicated by early and late adnexal torsion after in vitro fertilization. Fertil Steril 87:697, 2007.
69. Pryor RA, Wiczyk HP, O'Shea DL: Adnexal infarction after conservative surgical management of torsion of a hyperstimulated ovary. Fertil Steril 63:1344, 1995.
70. Andreoli M, Servakov M, Meyers P, Mann WJ Jr: Laparoscopic surgery during pregnancy. J Am Assoc Gynecol Laparosc 6:229, 1999.
71. Moore RD, Smith WG: Laparoscopic management of adnexal masses in pregnant women. J Reprod Med 44:97, 1999.
72. Soriano D, Yefet Y, Seidman DS, et al: Laparoscopy versus laparotomy in the management of adnexal masses during pregnancy. Fertil Steril 71:955, 1999.
73. Higgins RV, Matkins JF, Marroum MC: Comparison of fine-needle aspiration cytologic findings of ovarian cysts with ovarian histologic findings. Am J Obstet Gynecol 180:550, 1999.

74. Flegal KM, Carroll MD, Ogden CL, Curtin LR: Prevalence and trends in obesity among US adults, 1999-2008. JAMA 303:235, 2010.
75. Baeten JM, Bukusi EA, Lambe M: Pregnancy complications and outcomes among overweight and obese nulliparous women. Am J Public Health 91:436, 2001.
76. Cedergren MI: Maternal morbid obesity and the risk of adverse pregnancy outcome. Obstet Gynecol 103:219, 2004.
77. Weiss JL, Malone FD, Emig D, et al: Obesity, obstetric complications and cesarean delivery rate: a population-based screening study. Am J Obstet Gynecol 190:1091, 2004.
78. Karmon A, Sheiner E: Pregnancy after bariatric surgery: a comprehensive review. Arch Gynecol Obstet 277:381, 2008.
79. Maggard MA, Yermilov I, Li Z, et al: Pregnancy and fertility following bariatric surgery: a systematic review. JAMA 300:2286, 2008.
80. Abir F, Bell R: Assessment and management of the obese patient. Crit Care Med 32:S87, 2004.
81. Bryson GL, Chung F, Cox RG, et al: Patient selection in ambulatory anesthesia: an evidence-based review. II. Can J Anaesth 51:782, 2004.
82. King DR, Velmahos GC: Difficulties in managing the surgical patient who is morbidly obese. Crit Care Med 38:S478, 2010.
83. Juvin P, Lavaut E, Dupont H, et al: Difficult tracheal intubation is more common in obese than in lean patients. Anesth Analg 97:595, 2003.
84. Lavi R, Segal D, Ziser A: Predicting difficult airways using the intubation difficulty scale: a study comparing obese and non-obese patients. J Clin Anesth 21:264, 2009.
85. Lundstrom LH, Moller AM, Rosenstock C, et al: High body mass index is a weak predictor for difficult and failed tracheal intubation: a cohort study of 91,332 consecutive patients scheduled for direct laryngoscopy registered in the Danish Anesthesia Database. Anesthesiology 110:266, 2009.
86. Cheymol G: Effects of obesity on pharmacokinetics implications for drug therapy. Clin Pharmacokinet 39:215, 2000.
87. Servin F: Ambulatory anesthesia for the obese patient. Curr Opin Anaesthesiol 19:597, 2006.
88. Apovian CM, Baker C, Ludwig DS, et al: Best practice guidelines in pediatric/adolescent weight loss surgery. Obes Res 13:274, 2005.
89. Martin LF, Finigan KM, Nolan TE: Pregnancy after adjustable gastric banding. Obstet Gynecol 95:927, 2000.
90. Roehrig HR, Xanthakos SA, Sweeney J, et al: Pregnancy after gastric bypass surgery in adolescents. Obes Surg 17:873, 2007.
91. Dixon JB, Dixon ME, O'Brien PE: Elevated homocysteine levels with weight loss after Lap-Band surgery: higher folate and vitamin B12 levels required to maintain homocysteine level. Int J Obes Relat Metab Disord 25:219, 2001.
92. Rand CS, Macgregor AM: Adolescents having obesity surgery: a 6-year follow-up. South Med J 87:1208, 1994.
93. ACOG: Practice bulletin no. 105: bariatric surgery and pregnancy. Obstet Gynecol 113:1405, 2009.
94. Patel JA, Patel NA, Thomas RL, et al: Pregnancy outcomes after laparoscopic Roux-en-Y gastric bypass. Surg Obes Relat Dis 4:39, 2008.
95. Wax JR, Cartin A, Wolff R, et al: Pregnancy following gastric bypass surgery for morbid obesity: maternal and neonatal outcomes. Obes Surg 18:540, 2008.
96. Loar PV 3rd, Sanchez-Ramos L, Kaunitz AM, et al: Maternal death caused by midgut volvulus after bariatric surgery. Am J Obstet Gynecol 193:1748, 2005.
97. Moore KA, Ouyang DW, Whang EE: Maternal and fetal deaths after gastric bypass surgery for morbid obesity. N Engl J Med 351:721, 2004.
98. American Diabetes Association: Gestational diabetes mellitus. Diabetes Care 27:S88, 2004.

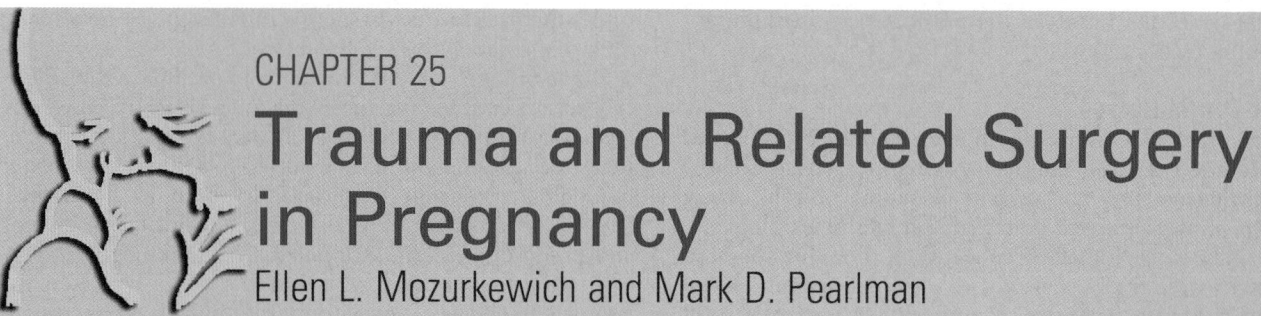

CHAPTER 25

Trauma and Related Surgery in Pregnancy

Ellen L. Mozurkewich and Mark D. Pearlman

KEY ABBREVIATIONS

1 Gray	=100 cGy or 100 rads
Computerized Tomography	CT
Focused Abdominal Sonography for Trauma	FAST
Kleihauer Betke Test	KB
Magnetic Resonance Imaging	MRI
Motor Vehicle Crashes	MVC
Radiation Absorbed Dose	Rad

INCIDENCE OF TRAUMA IN PREGNANCY

Traumatic injuries complicate 6% to 8% of all pregnancies and are the leading cause of nonobstetrical maternal death.[1-3] Approximately 30,000 pregnant women sustain treatable injuries in the United States each year as a result of trauma. Worldwide, trauma is responsible for at least 1 million deaths annually and is the leading cause of death in individuals under 40 years of age in the United States.[4] The risk of maternal death resulting from trauma is related to injury severity. In a large California database study of women hospitalized for trauma between 1991 and 1997, El Kady and colleagues found that internal injuries are the most common type of injury leading to maternal death.[5] Intracranial injury resulting from trauma was the second most common cause of maternal death.[5]

In addition to risk for maternal morbidity and mortality, traumatic injuries increase the risk for fetal death and other adverse outcomes of pregnancy.[4] Based on a review of fetal death certificates in Pennsylvania, it is estimated that motor vehicle crashes (MVCs) result in between 90 and 367 fetal deaths in the United States each year.[6] However, because of nonstandardized reporting of fetal death or injury resulting from maternal trauma, the exact magnitude of disease burden to the fetus resulting from maternal trauma is unknown, but is almost certainly underreported.[4] Risk factors for traumatic injury during pregnancy include young maternal age, African-American or Hispanic ethnicity, domestic violence, non-seatbelt use, and drug or alcohol use.[1,7] Alcohol may be involved in as many as 45% of MVCs including pregnant women, and the use of illicit substances has been implicated frequently in maternal trauma during pregnancy as well.[7]

Traumatic injuries may be categorized according to type, including blunt trauma, penetrating trauma, fractures, and thermal injuries. The most frequent causes of maternal trauma in the United States are MVCs (51%), falls (22%), and assaults (22%).[2,8] Gunshot wounds account for 4% of maternal trauma and burns account for 1%.[9] **The most common obstetrical complications following maternal trauma are abruptio placentae, preterm labor, and fetal loss.**[10]

ANATOMIC AND PHYSIOLOGIC CHANGES OF PREGNANCY

The importance of maternal physiologic changes during pregnancy and an understanding of fetal physiology are crucial to effective resuscitation of the injured pregnant woman. This is especially important relative to the maternal response to stress and hypovolemia resulting from trauma. Fundamental differences exist in the physiologic response to trauma as a result of pregnancy, and a working knowledge of the basics of these differences is important to trauma resuscitation.

Fetal Physiology

Several factors are important in determining the impact of a traumatic event on pregnancy outcome. These include gestational age, type and severity of trauma, and the extent of disruption of normal maternal and fetal physiology.[11,12] In the first week following conception, the nonimplanted embryo is relatively resistant to noxious stimuli. Even during the first trimester, the uterus resides relatively safely within the confines of the bony pelvis and is protected to a large degree from direct uterine trauma. At any gestational age after implantation, however, maternal hypovolemic shock may have a significant impact on the developing embryo/fetus. Uterine blood flow is not autoregulated and is maximally dilated in the normal physiologic state. Maternal hypovolemia may result in vasoconstriction in many vascular beds, including those of the uterus. In experimental hypovolemic shock, pregnant sheep will decrease uterine blood flow at rates greater than would be expected based on the decrease in maternal blood pressure alone. Even in the absence of uterine artery vasoconstriction, decreases in maternal blood pressure due to hypovolemia will result in decreased uterine blood flow. These facts underlie the importance of maintaining adequate maternal blood volume as an initial step in fetal resuscitation. The third-trimester fetus can adapt to decreased uterine blood flow and oxygen delivery by redistributing blood flow to the heart, brain, and adrenal glands. Furthermore, because fetal hemoglobin has a greater affinity for oxygen than adult hemoglobin, fetal oxygen consumption does not decrease until oxygen delivery is reduced by 50%.[13]

Blunt or penetrating trauma may result in rupture of the amniotic membranes. In the second trimester, rupture with oligohydramnios may result in pulmonary hypoplasia or orthopedic deformity. Injury to the placenta may precipitate placental abruption leading to fetal anemia, hypoxemia, or hypovolemia.

Maternal Anatomic and Physiologic Changes

Nearly every maternal organ system undergoes anatomic or physiologic changes during pregnancy. The description that follows emphasizes consideration of these changes that affect the usual practice of trauma management.

A major concern in the management of trauma victims is internal hemorrhage and hypovolemia. The sentinel findings on examination are vital sign abnormalities—typically, hypotension and tachycardia. Consideration should be given to the normal decrease in systemic vascular resistance resulting in a decrease in mean blood pressure of 10 to 15 mm Hg and in increased pulse of 5-15 beats per minute, particularly in the second trimester. These changes can be accentuated if the trauma victim is laid supine (e.g., strapped to a long board in order to secure the cervical spine). The resultant potential decrease in venous return from the lower extremities can reduce central venous volume and result in a diminished cardiac output by as much as 30%. Simple manual displacement of the uterus to the left, or placement of a rolled towel under the backboard while ensuring that the spine remains secure alleviates most of this effect.

Blood volume increases by a mean of 50% in the singleton gestation. This is usually maximal by 28 to 30 weeks' gestation. Red blood cell mass increases to a lesser degree than does plasma volume, resulting in a slight decrease in hemoglobin concentration and decrease in hematocrit. Iron-deficiency anemia is also common during pregnancy, and together with the normal dilution, hemoglobin concentrations may be as low as 9 to 11 g/dL. These hematologic changes have two potential implications: (1) anemia may be confused with active bleeding and hypovolemia, and (2) blood volume estimates should be adjusted upward during fluid resuscitation.

Several major pregnancy-induced changes in the gastrointestinal tract are also important for trauma management. Compartmentalization of the bowel upward serves to protect it during lower abdominal trauma, but increases the risk of injury when there is penetrating trauma to the upper abdomen in later pregnancy. Complex injuries to the small bowel can be encountered with multiple entry and exit wounds as a result of its being crowded and compacted into the upper abdomen. Decreased gastric motility results in a prolonged gastric emptying time, thereby increasing the risk of aspiration. Rebound tenderness and guarding may be less apparent in later gestation due to stretching and attenuation of the abdominal musculature and peritoneum.

The dramatic increase in uterine blood flow, up to 600 mL/minute, may result in rapid exsanguination if there is avulsion or injury to the uterine vasculature or rupture of the uterus. Retroperitoneal hemorrhage from remarkably hypertrophied pelvic vasculature is a common complication of pelvic fracture. Enlargement of the uterus makes it susceptible to direct abdominal trauma. Injury to the uterus itself (uterine laceration or rupture), or its contents (abruptio placentae or direct fetal injury), or adjacent organs (bladder rupture) are more likely during pregnancy, especially in later pregnancy. While some of these complications are associated with more direct and violent trauma, for example, direct fetal injury or uterine rupture, some injuries (e.g., abruptio placentae) can occur after relatively minor trauma.

BLUNT TRAUMA

Blunt trauma to the maternal abdomen is an important cause of abruptio placentae. This is because blunt trauma exposes the gravid uterus to acceleration-deceleration forces that have a differential effect on the uterus and the attached placenta. By changing its shape, the myometrial tissue can stretch, adapting to these forces, while the placenta is relatively inelastic. This mismatch between myometrial and placental ability to stretch creates a shearing force at the utero-placental interface that, if sufficient, can result in separation of the placenta from its myometrial attachments (i.e., placental abruption).[4,10,14] Maternal trauma may also result in intramyometrial bleeding that leads to increased uterine contractile activity through activation of thrombin, lysosomal enzymes, cytokines, and prostaglandins.[10] Severe blunt trauma may also lead to maternal splenic, hepatic, and retroperitoneal injuries that result in maternal hemorrhage and hemodynamic instability.[10] Severe injuries resulting in hypovolemia place both maternal and fetal well-being at risk.

Motor Vehicle Crashes

MVCs are the most common cause of trauma-associated fetal loss in the United States.[4,8] The likelihood that a MVC will result in fetal loss is directly related to crash severity as well as to maternal injury severity.[4,12] **For example, estimates based on case series would suggest that only about 1% of minor MVC will result in abruptio placentae, whereas as many as 40% to 50% of severe maternal trauma may result in abruptio placentae.**[10] In addition, lack of seatbelt use has been found to be associated with fetal loss, particularly if the mother has experienced ejection from the vehicle and head trauma.[12,15] However, even nonsevere MVC without substantial maternal injury may result in placental abruption and fetal loss because of exposure to the shearing acceleration-deceleration forces described earlier.[2,4,12] The forces leading to placental abruption after motor vehicle trauma are depicted in Figure 25-1.

Falls

Because pregnancy changes the center of gravity and postural stability, loss of balance is not uncommon and the likelihood of a significant fall is increased.[16-18] In fact, one retrospective study found that as many as a quarter of pregnant women experience a fall at some time during pregnancy.[16] Like MVCs falls expose the placenta to the shearing forces associated with blunt trauma. However, compared with MVCs, the likelihood that a fall may result in placental abruption and fetal death is low, accounting for only 3% of trauma-associated fetal deaths in one series.[6] In a more recent prospective cohort study involving 153 women experiencing falls during pregnancy, there were no instances of placental abruption.[19] Nonetheless, compared with pregnant women who did not experience fall-related hospitalization during their pregnancy, women hospitalized for falls remain at increased risk for adverse outcomes of pregnancy. One retrospective cohort study of 693 women hospitalized for falls during pregnancy (most of whom were in the third trimester) found that these women were at increased risk for preterm labor, placental abruption, cesarean delivery, "fetal distress," and fetal hypoxia.[18]

Domestic Violence

Pregnant women are at increased risk to suffer violent assault at home compared with nonpregnant women.[20] **The period prevalence of intimate partner violence during pregnancy has been reported to range from 6% to 22%, and up to 45% of pregnant women report a history of domestic abuse at some time during their lifetime.**[20] In one study, murder was the most frequent cause of maternal death during pregnancy and during the year subsequent to pregnancy.[21] In this study, a majority of the perpetrators of maternal homicides were found to be current or former intimate partners.[21] The analysis of pregnancy-associated homicides found that intimate partner homicides were

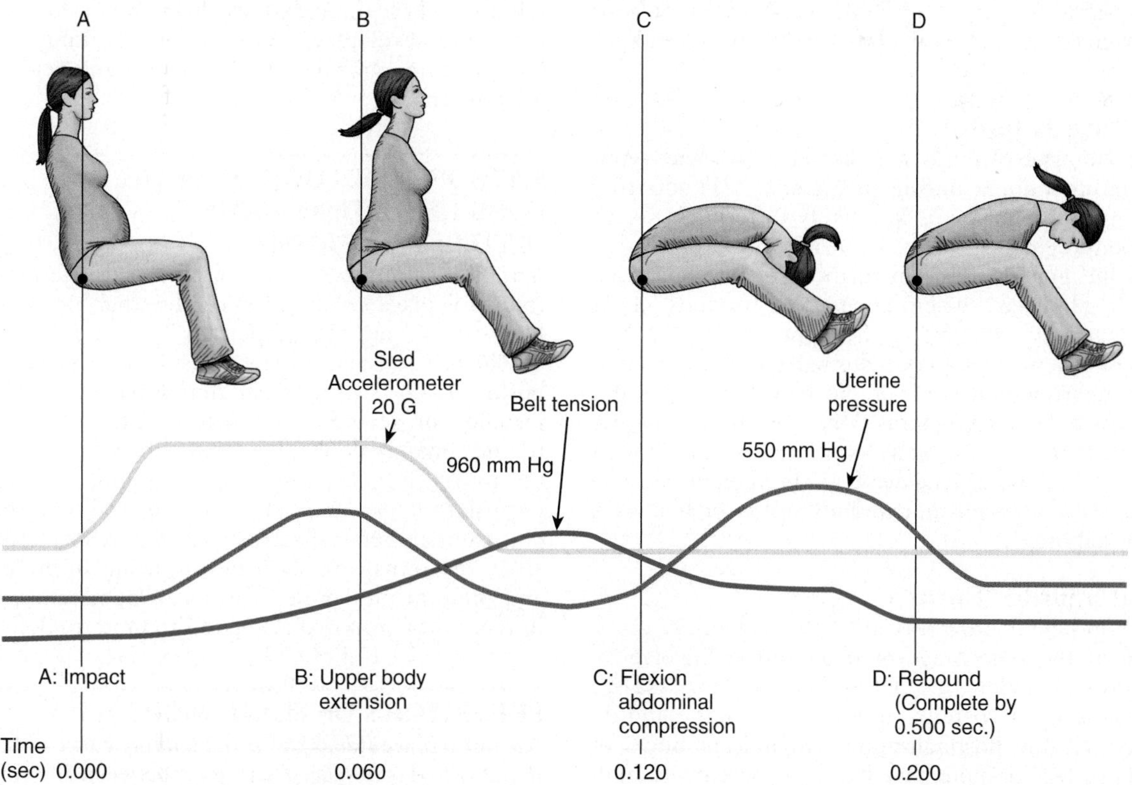

FIGURE 25-1. Impact sequence. Relationship between body motion, uterine pressure, and belt tension. (Modified from Hankins CVD: Operative Obstetrics. Stamford, CT: Appleton & Lange, 1995, Figure 35-3, p 655.)

most likely to occur during the first 3 months of pregnancy.[21] Although domestic violence occurs in all ethnic and socioeconomic groups, African-American and Native-American women and women from households with lower incomes are at increased risk for victimization by domestic violence compared with other women.[20] According to a California database study of maternal discharge records between 1991 and 1999, assaults were significantly associated with uterine rupture, and conferred significant long-term risk for placental abruption and low birthweight, even if the victim was not delivered during the initial hospitalization.[22]

SPECIFIC INJURIES

Fractures

Fractures are the most common type of maternal injury requiring hospitalization during pregnancy.[3] **The lower extremities are the most common site of fractures complicating pregnancy.**[3] **While pelvic fractures are less frequent than fractures of the extremities, pelvic fractures are most likely to result in adverse outcomes of pregnancy, including placental abruption, fetal death, neonatal death, and infant death.**[3] As such, pelvic fractures are thought to be an independent risk factor for adverse fetal outcome.[8] Pelvic fractures may also be associated with significant maternal hemorrhage and shock due to significant hypertrophy of the pelvic retroperitoneal vasculature, and subsequent laceration of these vessels due to sharp bone fragments, with resultant retroperitoneal bleeding.[23] Pelvic fractures may also be associated with bladder and urethral trauma.[1] Pelvic fractures are not a contraindication to vaginal delivery unless the fracture results in obstruction of the birth canal, or if the pelvic fracture is unstable; greater than 80% of women who have sustained pelvic fractures can deliver vaginally.[23]

Penetrating Trauma

Gunshot and stab wounds are the most frequent types of penetrating trauma during pregnancy.[4,15] Penetrating trauma during pregnancy is less likely to result in death than in nonpregnant individuals, owing to the protective effect of the gravid uterus in relation to the abdominal viscera.[14,15] However, when penetrating wounds occur during pregnancy and involve the upper abdomen, they pose major risk for complex maternal bowel injury due to the compartmentalization of the bowel in the upper abdomen by the enlarged uterus.[15] By contrast, penetrating trauma to the uterus is strongly associated with poor fetal outcome.[4,10] **The risk of fetal death has been reported to be as high as 71% after gunshot wounds and as high as 42% following stabbings.**[15]

Thermal Injuries (Burns)

Maternal and fetal prognosis after thermal injury are a reflection of the percentage of body surface involved.[23] Minor burns involving 10% or less body surface area are unlikely to result in maternal or fetal compromise and do not always require hospitalization.[10] Significant burns of 50% body surface or more have been associated with high maternal and fetal mortality. In the past, delivery of the fetus was recommended in an attempt to improve maternal prognosis.[23] More recent studies have suggested that maternal prognosis after severe thermal injury is not different between pregnant and nonpregnant individuals.[23] However, because of maternal physiologic changes associated with pregnancy, a pregnant woman with a severe burn will require more aggressive fluid resuscitation than a nonpregnant individual.

Major burns may result in maternal hypovolemia and cardiovascular instability, as well as sepsis, respiratory distress, renal failure, and liver failure.[10] Because of the decreased colloid osmotic pressure and increased body surface area associated with pregnancy, pregnant individuals who sustain burns are at risk for increased fluid loss compared with nonpregnant individuals.[24] Preterm labor may result from maternal hypovolemia, which can also result in decreased uteroplacental perfusion. Aggressive fluid resuscitation is critical to forestall this complication.[10,24]

Individuals suffering from major burns often also sustain inhalation injuries, which carry a higher maternal mortality risk and may also lead to fetal jeopardy.[10,25] In particular, carbon dioxide freely crosses the placenta and is highly bound by fetal hemoglobin, causing risk for fetal cardiac failure.[10] Administration of oxygen to the mother is recommended to reduce the half-life of carboxy-hemoglobin.[10]

Direct Fetal Injuries

Direct fetal injuries are uncommon, but are most likely to occur with both direct and severe abdominal or pelvic impact, and also in later pregnancy when the fetal head is engaged in the maternal pelvis.[4,10] Direct injury has been reported to result in rupture of the fetal spleen, fracture of the fetal skull, fetal intracranial hemorrhage, and cerebral edema.[4] These injuries have been reported to result in long-term developmental disabilities resulting from vascular infarctions, global cerebral damage, and periventricular leukomalacia.[4]

PATHOPHYSIOLOGY OF FETAL LOSS RESULTING FROM MATERNAL TRAUMA

The most frequent cause of fetal loss resulting from trauma is placental abruption.[9] Maternal hypotension and hypovolemia are also important predictors of poor fetal outcome.[6,12,15] Fetal loss may result from placental hypoperfusion due to maternal hemorrhagic shock.[9] In the instance of severe blood loss resulting from maternal trauma, maternal blood is redistributed away from the uterus via uterine artery vasoconstriction, to continue to perfuse the heart and brain. Fetal mortality in the setting of maternal hemorrhagic shock has been estimated at 80%.[26] Maternal trauma may also result in preterm labor and preterm premature rupture of membranes, resulting in morbidity or mortality related to preterm delivery.

PREDICTORS OF FETAL MORTALITY

Abruptio placentae is by far the leading cause of fetal death in published series, accounting for between 50% and 70% of all fetal losses due to trauma.[23] **Placental abruption will complicate about 1% to 2% of cases of maternal trauma with**

low injury severity scores, and up to 40% of severe maternal abdominal trauma.[15] If a placental abruption occurs, the risk of fetal mortality has been reported to be as high as 50% to 80%.[4] Maternal death has been reported as the next most frequent cause of fetal death after placental abruption, accounting for about 10% of losses.[10] In a large California database study, gestational age at delivery was the strongest predictor of fetal, neonatal, or infant death.[5] MVCs (82%) are the most frequent mechanism of injury leading to fetal death, followed by gunshot wounds (6%) and falls (3%).[4] In particular, lack of seatbelt use is a substantial risk factor for poor fetal outcome, morbidity, or mortality.[15,27,28]

Schiff and colleagues used the injury severity score to categorize the severity of maternal injuries.[29,30] The risk for adverse maternal, fetal, and neonatal outcomes was greatest among the women with severe injuries, but was also increased for women with mild injuries compared with uninjured controls. They found that injury severity scoring had limited predictive accuracy for placental abruption and fetal death and that even relatively minor injuries may result in these adverse fetal outcomes.[29,30] **Because minor injuries are much more common than severe injuries, they are responsible for 60% to 70% of fetal losses attributable to trauma, even though a severe injury is much more likely to result in loss than a nonsevere injury.**[4]

MANAGEMENT CONSIDERATIONS

Initial Approaches

Emergency personnel are often the first to evaluate and treat pregnant women experiencing trauma. The Centers for Disease Control and Prevention (CDC) has provided published guidelines for first responders and emergency medical personnel providing care in the field to injured pregnant women.[31] Guidelines for emergency medical personnel include displacing the uterus from the inferior vena cava, by positioning the mother in the lateral decubitus position.[26] During the initial evaluation, the spine immobilization board may be tilted leftward by placing a 6-inch rolled towel under the long board to achieve the same result.[26] The CDC panel recommended that, if possible, women with a pregnancy at least 20 weeks be transported to a trauma center with access to obstetrical care.

Improved outcomes can be expected by following a coordinated approach among emergency medicine physicians, trauma surgeons, and obstetricians in the evaluation of the maternal patient who has sustained traumatic injuries. All pregnant women (regardless of gestational age) who sustain or who are suspected to have sustained serious injuries should be evaluated in the emergency department first, and maternal well-being is prioritized over fetal assessment. Stabilization of the mother with identification of maternal injury is the initial priority. Fetal evaluation and interventions can be conducted in the emergency department as needed. A suggested algorithm for care of the pregnant trauma patient is presented in Figure 25-2.

Evaluation on Labor and Delivery

After clearance for severe maternal injury has been completed in the Emergency Department, we suggest that women experiencing trauma who are at or beyond 23 weeks' gestation (the threshold of fetal viability) be admitted to Labor and Delivery for observation and monitoring for signs and symptoms of placental abruption and preterm labor. Women below this threshold should have evaluation for fetal life in the Emergency Department, but do not necessarily require admission to Labor and Delivery. Based on the patient's clinical presentation and uterine contraction frequency, the patient is observed either for 4 or 24 hours prior to hospital discharge.

Fetal Monitoring

Fetal and uterine contraction monitoring is the most sensitive method for detecting abruptio placentae following trauma. Following trauma, in pregnant women who are beyond 23 to 24 weeks' gestation, frequent uterine contractions are nearly always present in women who have abruptio placentae.[32,33] **Moreover, a non-reassuring fetal heart rate pattern may reflect maternal hemorrhagic shock or hypotension.**[14] **Uterine contraction monitoring is unquestionably more sensitive than ultrasound in detecting placental abruption, with ultrasound detecting only about 40% of abruptio placentae in the setting of trauma.**[14,15,34] While several authors have recommended incorporating assessment of fetal status into the standard Focused Abdominal Sonography for Trauma (FAST) exam, it should not replace fetal monitoring.[8,10] The standard FAST exam is performed to evaluate for intraperitoneal hemorrhage and has replaced diagnostic peritoneal lavage in many centers because of its excellent sensitivity (80%-83%) for detection of intraperitoneal fluid.[8] A fetal biophysical profile test and middle cerebral artery Doppler studies may be performed at the time of the FAST exam for further information regarding fetal well-being, though its ability to predict fetal outcome in the setting of trauma has not been thoroughly assessed.[8,10] The fetal heart rate tracing has been called "the fifth vital sign," because it may provide the earliest evidence of maternal hypovolemia or hypotension.[10] Likewise, frequent uterine contractions provide the most reliable warning sign of placental abruption or preterm labor.[11,34,35] **If uterine contractions occur less frequently than every 15 minutes over 4 hours of observation, placental abruption is unlikely to occur.**[11,34,35] **Therefore, if the fetus is at or beyond 24 weeks' gestation, we recommend 4 hours of fetal monitoring. If frequent contractions are noted (every 15 minutes or more frequent), then 24 hours of monitoring is recommended because clinical identification of abruptio placentae has been reported up to 48 hours after maternal trauma.**[10,14,34]

Laboratory Testing

Laboratory tests that may be helpful in the evaluation of trauma include a complete blood count with platelets, type and Rh testing, evaluation of coagulation function if abruptio placentae is of concern, as well as a Kleihauer Betke (KB) test in the Rh-negative woman.[10] The KB test is an acid elution test designed to quantify the amount of fetal blood in the maternal circulation.[36] Published studies have demonstrated an approximate fourfold increase in the incidence of fetomaternal hemorrhage compared to uninjured controls. This increase in fetomaternal hemorrhage appears to be most important in assuring that RH-negative women are adequately protected against isoimmunization. The

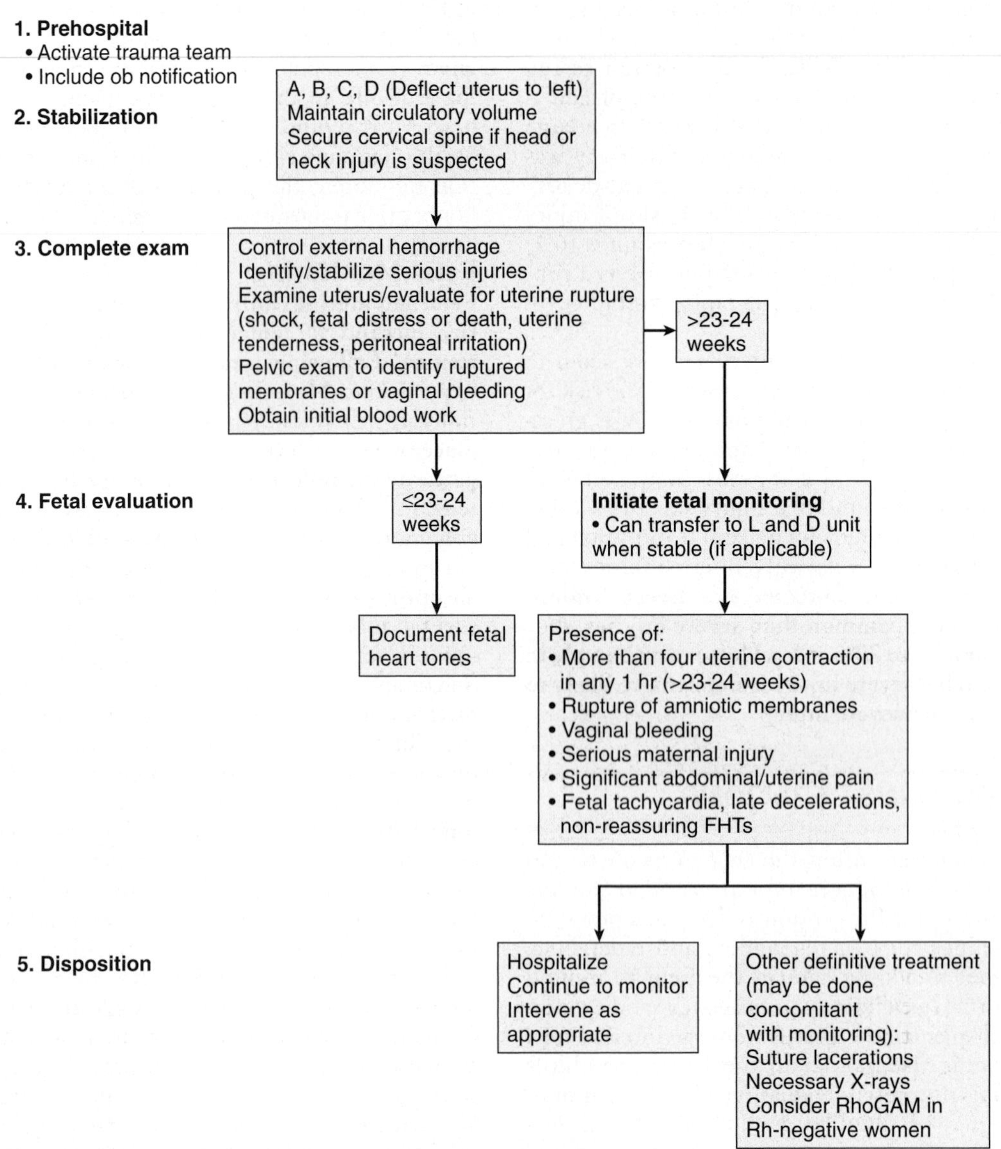
ED MANAGEMENT: TRAUMA IN PREGNANCY
1. Prehospital
• Activate trauma team
• Include ob notification
2. Stabilization
A, B, C, D (Deflect uterus to left)
Maintain circulatory volume
Secure cervical spine if head or neck injury is suspected
3. Complete exam
Control external hemorrhage
Identify/stabilize serious injuries
Examine uterus/evaluate for uterine rupture (shock, fetal distress or death, uterine tenderness, peritoneal irritation)
Pelvic exam to identify ruptured membranes or vaginal bleeding
Obtain initial blood work
>23-24 weeks
4. Fetal evaluation
≤23-24 weeks
Initiate fetal monitoring
• Can transfer to L and D unit when stable (if applicable)
Document fetal heart tones
Presence of:
• More than four uterine contraction in any 1 hr (>23-24 weeks)
• Rupture of amniotic membranes
• Vaginal bleeding
• Serious maternal injury
• Significant abdominal/uterine pain
• Fetal tachycardia, late decelerations, non-reassuring FHTs
5. Disposition
Hospitalize
Continue to monitor
Intervene as appropriate
Other definitive treatment (may be done concomitant with monitoring):
Suture lacerations
Necessary X-rays
Consider RhoGAM in Rh-negative women

FIGURE 25-2. Algorithm with suggested plan of care for pregnant women experiencing trauma.

KB test may be used to determine whether additional vials of Rh immune globulin are needed for Rh-negative women experiencing trauma.[9,34] For about 90% of pregnant women experiencing trauma, the fetal-maternal hemorrhage will be less than 30 mL and 1 vial of Rh immune globulin will be sufficient to prevent sensitization.[14] There is some controversy regarding the utility of this test among Rh-positive women. Based on a series of 71 women, Muench has recommended its use as a predictor of risk for preterm labor after trauma.[37] In that study, the authors found that the KB test had a 100% sensitivity for prediction of preterm labor.[37] Other studies have not supported the use of this test as a predictor of adverse fetal outcome.[35,38] **Our experience has been that KB testing has utility for determining those *few Rh-negative women who require additional Rh immune globulin* to protect against isoimmunization, but has little predictive value of other adverse pregnancy outcomes such as abruptio placentae, preterm birth, or fetal hypoxemia. Moreover, the use of fetal monitoring is much more likely to provide a timely diagnosis of these complications of pregnancy than KB testing.**

Coagulation studies, including PT, PTT, platelets, and fibrinogen, may be useful if there is evidence or suspicion of abruptio placentae or if the patient is experiencing massive hemorrhage that may result in dilutional coagulopathy. A urinalysis may be obtained as well. Hematuria on urinalysis may be associated with pelvic fractures or renal tract injury.[15] Given the strong association of drug and alcohol use with traumatic injuries, a urine toxicology screen is preferred if clinically indicated.[15]

DIAGNOSTIC IMAGING DURING PREGNANCY

Ultrasound

Ultrasound may be used to assess fetal well-being without exposing the fetus to ionizing radiation. Additionally, abdominal ultrasound may be a useful tool in the

TABLE 25-1 Biologic Effects of In-Utero Exposure to Ionizing Radiation

MENSTRUAL OR GESTATIONAL AGE	CONCEPTION AGE	<50 mGy (<5 rad)	50-100 mGy (5-10 rad)	>100 mGy (>10 rad)
0-2 weeks (0-14) days	Prior to conception	None	None	None
3rd and 4th weeks (15-28) days	1st and 2nd weeks (1-14) days	None	Probably none	Possible spontaneous abortion.
5th and 10th weeks (29-70) days	3rd and 8th weeks (15-56) days	None	Potential effects are scientifically uncertain and probably too subtle to be clinically detectable.	Possible malformations increasing in likelihood as dose increases.
11th and 17th weeks (71-119) days	9th and 15th weeks (57-105) days	None	Potential effects are scientifically uncertain and probably too subtle to be clinically detectable.	Increased risk of deficits in IQ or mental retardation that increase in frequency and severity with increasing dose.
18th and 27th weeks (120-189) days	16th and 25th weeks (106-175) days	None	None	IQ deficits not detectable at diagnostic doses.
>27 weeks (>189 days)	>25 weeks (>175 days)	None	None	None applicable to diagnostic medicine.

Modified from ACR Practice Guidelines for Imaging Pregnant or Potentially Pregnant Adolescents and Women with Ionizing Radiation. American College of Radiology, 2008, p 3.

evaluation of the pregnant trauma victim for free intraperitoneal fluid, with reported sensitivity between 61% and 83%, but specificity between 94% and 100%.[39] Ultrasound is not particularly sensitive for detecting abruptio placentae, with reported identification of only approximately 40%. There are no clear established guidelines whether further imaging is necessary in the event of a negative ultrasound study in a hemodynamically stable patient. The Food and Drug Administration (FDA) has arbitrarily established a safe upper limit for energy exposure during ultrasonography at 94 mW/cm^2.[40]

Ionizing Radiation

Because of concerns about fetal exposure to ionizing radiation, clinicians may be hesitant to order indicated diagnostic tests in the setting of maternal trauma. Concerns regarding exposure to ionizing radiation involve both risk for teratogenesis and risk for development of cancer in later life.[41] The most significant risk for fetal malformation involves microcephaly and mental retardation, which has been observed after human exposure to doses of 100 to 200 cGy. Exposure to ionizing radiation in utero may elevate the risk of childhood leukemia from a background of 1 in 3000 to a risk after exposure to 1 in 2000.[40,42] Similarly, exposure to 50 mGy (5 rads) ionizing during pregnancy may be associated with a 2% lifetime attributable risk for development of malignancy.[43] The risk of teratogenesis or carcinogenesis with exposure to ionizing radiation is dose-dependent.[43] Both the American College of Radiology and the American College of Obstetricians and Gynecologists have published imaging guidelines for the use of diagnostic radiologic techniques during pregnancy.[40,43] **However, in the setting of maternal trauma, the risk to the fetus for morbidity or mortality from untreated maternal injury far outweighs theoretical concerns for risks of development of malignancy in later life. Indicated diagnostic procedures should not be delayed due to concerns about fetal radiation.**[39]

Table 25-1 summarizes effects of in-uterus exposure to ionizing radiation during different stages of pregnancy. The American College or Radiology posits that "Nearly all abdominal radiographic procedures can be modified to reduce radiation exposure to a pregnant patient and her fetus."[43] For example, dose from single-phase CT study of the abdomen and pelvis would be 20 to 35 mGy. Radiation doses associated with common diagnostic tests are listed in Table 25-2.

MRI

MRI may be an attractive option because this modality does not involve the use of ionizing radiation, though there is less evidence of efficacy and safety of its use during pregnancy than other more established methods. Currently, the Food and Drug Administration states that the safety of MRI for the fetus "has not been established."[42] However, there is currently no evidence from studies of children exposed to MRI in utero of any teratogenic effects or of any long-term adverse developmental consequences.[39,42] The American College of Radiology described guidelines for the safe use of MRI, and provided support for the use of MRI during all trimesters of pregnancy if necessary for accurate diagnosis.[39,44] The precise role for the use of MRI in the management of trauma in pregnancy has not yet been clearly established.

Contrast Agents

Iodinated contrast agents cross the placenta via simple diffusion.[45] Because they are taken up by the fetal thyroid and may pose a theoretical risk for fetal hypothyroidism, iodinated contrast images are generally avoided during pregnancy, unless clearly necessary for diagnosis.[40,45] However, no cases of fetal goiter or abnormal neonatal thyroid function have been reported after clinical use of iodinated contrast agents.[45] Neonates whose mothers have received iodinated contrast media during pregnancy should be screened for hypothyroidism, an already standard practice.[42] **A recent guideline for use of CT and MRI during pregnancy has posited that the use of iodinated contrast agents during pregnancy is preferable to the patient receiving repetitive CT studies due to the suboptimal nature of studies performed without contrast agents.**[42]

The use of gadolinium for MRI in pregnancy is controversial. Gadolinium crosses the placenta and accumulates in amniotic fluid.[45] Gadolinium has not been found to be teratogenic or carcinogenic in doses that are used clinically.[15,45] However, administration of gadolinium to children and adults with underlying renal insufficiency has resulted in a syndrome known as nephrogenic systemic fibrosis in rare cases, raising theoretical concerns of toxicity after fetal exposure.[42,46] Thus, the use of gadolinium should be avoided in patients with acute or chronic renal insufficiency.

Suggested Guidelines for Radiologic Evaluation of Trauma

A recent evidence-based guideline for use of diagnostic imaging after maternal trauma has recommended the use of ultrasound as the initial modality, but recommend the use of CT as the preferred method of evaluation when visceral injuries, or injuries of the chest, aorta, mediastinum, spine, bones, bowel, or bladder are suspected.[42] Similarly, Patel has suggested an algorithm-based approach to radiologic evaluation after maternal trauma.[39] See Figure 25-3.

TABLE 25-2 RADIATION DOSES ASSOCIATED WITH COMMON DIAGNOSTIC PROCEDURES

PROCEDURE	FETAL DOSE
Single-phase CT of abdomen and pelvis, and lumbar spine	3.5 rad
Hip film (single view)	200 mrad
Chest x-ray	0.02-0.07 mrad
CT of head or chest	<1 rad
Diagnostic fluoroscopy of abdomen and pelvis	<10 rad

Modified from ACOG Committee on Obstetric Practice: ACOG Committee Opinion #299: Guidelines for Diagnostic Imaging During Pregnancy and ACR Practice Guidelines for Imaging Pregnant or Potentially Pregnant Adolescents and Women with Ionizing Radiation.

SURGERY FOR TRAUMATIC INJURIES DURING PREGNANCY

Penetrating trauma is the most common indication for nonobstetrical surgery for traumatic injuries during pregnancy.[10] Historically, surgical exploration was recommended for evaluation and repair of abdominal injuries resulting from penetrating trauma; however, given the differing pattern of abdominal injuries resulting from penetrating trauma during pregnancy, the decision for expectant management or surgery may be individualized.[10] Muench and Canterino recommend an individualized approach to penetrating trauma depending on whether the wound is in the upper or lower abdomen.[10] **Because of the significantly increased risk for bowel injury after penetrating trauma to the upper abdomen, women with penetrating wounds to the upper abdomen should undergo surgical exploration. Because the gravid uterus provides some protection from visceral injury, women sustaining penetrating wounds to the lower abdomen may be managed conservatively if they are hemodynamically stable.** Penetrating wounds to the gravid uterus increase risk for direct fetal injury, but may be managed conservatively if they do not extend past the myometrium.[10] Conservative management may include diagnostic peritoneal lavage, which may be undertaken during pregnancy through a supraumbilical incision that

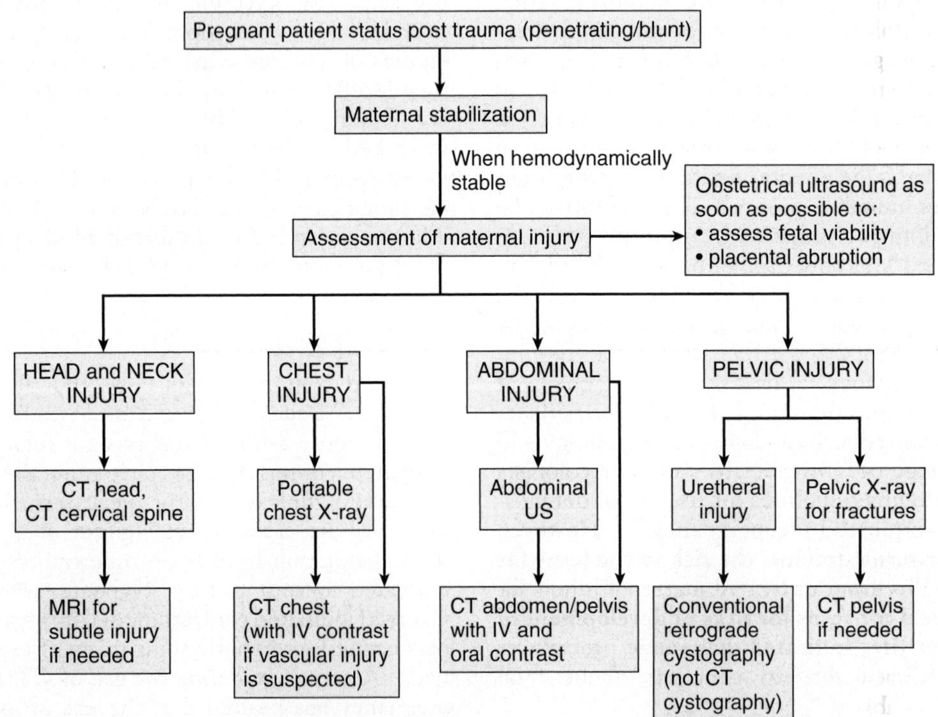

FIGURE 25-3. Algorithm with suggested plan for diagnostic imaging studies for pregnant women experiencing trauma. (Modified from: Patel SJ, Reede DL, Katz DS, et al: Imaging the pregnant patient for nonobstetric conditions: algorithms and radiation dose considerations. Radiographics 27:1719, 2007.)

may be facilitated under ultrasound guidance.[10,15] Indications for surgical exploration include penetrating trauma to the upper abdomen, gunshot wounds to the abdomen, clinical evidence of active intra-abdominal hemorrhage, or suspicion for bowel injury.

If exploratory laparatomy is undertaken, care should be taken to minimize traction on the gravid uterus and the nature and extent of any injuries should be evaluated.[10] Exploratory laparotomy does not always necessitate delivery of the fetus.[15] In the event that fetal death has occurred prior to surgical exploration, vaginal delivery after induction of labor may be a preferable approach, although Brown recommends surgical uterine evacuation if there is abruption and potential for coagulopathy.[15] In some circumstances, delivery of the fetus may be necessary to adequately explore the abdomen or to facilitate surgical repair of injured viscera.

If the pregnancy is at or beyond 24 weeks, fetal monitoring should be carried out intermittently during the surgical procedure. If non-reassuring fetal status is detected during the procedure, in most instances it can be corrected by attention to and correction of maternal hypovolemia or hypoxemia. If these supportive measures are not effective, cesarean delivery may be necessary.[15]

Uterine Rupture

Both blunt and penetrating injuries may result in uterine rupture, which occurs in approximately 0.6% to 1% of instances of maternal trauma.[15,34] **Uterine rupture most often results from direct abdominal impact, and may occur at any gestational age, although the risk for uterine rupture increases in late pregnancy.**[1,47] **The risk for uterine rupture is particularly increased for women who have experienced assaults.**[22] Most instances of uterine rupture resulting from maternal trauma are fundal in location.[34] Uterine rupture may also result in complete avulsion of the uterine arteries and massive hemorrhage.[1] Signs of uterine rupture may range from fetal heart rate abnormalities in a hemodynamically stable patient, to maternal cardiovascular instability and hypovolemic shock.[34] Uterine rupture carries a poor prognosis for the fetus and requires immediate laparotomy. Whether a hysterectomy is required depends on the extent of the myometrial and vascular injury. Uterine rupture may be associated with massive maternal hemorrhage due to the increased uterine vascularity associated with pregnancy; aggressive replacement of red cells and clotting factors is recommended.[15] Maternal mortality may be as high as 10% following traumatic uterine rupture.[4]

Perimortem Cesarean Section

In instances of severe maternal injury and maternal cardiac arrest, cardiopulmonary resuscitation may be less successful due to maternal physiologic alterations associated with pregnancy. The gravid uterus may interfere with systemic perfusion by compression of the inferior vena cava and interference with venous return. Emptying the uterus may facilitate more effective maternal resuscitation. **Long-term outcomes for children born after maternal cardiac arrest are most likely to be favorable if the child is delivered within 5 minutes of cessation of maternal circulation.**[26] Therefore we recommend that if the pregnancy is at or beyond fetal viability (23-24 weeks' gestation), perimortem cesarean delivery commence 4 minutes after maternal cardiac arrest if resuscitation has not restored maternal circulation.[10] If the maternal resuscitation is successful, we recommend that that patient be transferred to the operating theater for closure of the uterus and abdominal wound and to ensure adequate hemostasis.

OTHER CONSIDERATIONS

Long-Term Effects of Trauma

In some reports, up to 38% of women experiencing trauma during pregnancy will require delivery in the same hospitalization,[15] though in most published experiences, the great majority of pregnant women experiencing trauma will be discharged home undelivered.[4,32] Although most placental abruptions resulting from maternal trauma will occur within the first 24 hours after the event, some reports suggest that women who have experienced trauma may remain at risk for other complications including intrauterine growth restriction, intrauterine fetal demise, "fetal distress," placental abruption, and a higher risk of cesarean delivery.[3,4,48] By contrast, a prospective controlled study demonstrated that pregnancy outcomes beyond 48 hours in injured women are similar to those in the uninjured controls.[32] Suggested discharge instructions are shown in the box, Suggested Discharge Instructions for Pregnant Women Hospitalized for Observation After Trauma.

Suggested Discharge Instructions for Pregnant Women Hospitalized for Observation After Trauma

- Discharge after 24 hours of observation. Discharge may be indicated in the absence of signs or symptoms of the following: labor, abruption, rupture of membranes, fetal compromise, maternal compromise.
- Health education
  A. After discharge, woman should be instructed to call Labor and Delivery with decreased fetal movement, vaginal bleeding, rupture of membranes, abdominal pain, or uterine contractions >3 per hour.
  B. Advise fetal movement count twice daily.
  C. Advise follow-up with provider within the week.
  D. Advocate correct seatbelt use: shoulder belt between breasts and uterine fundus, lap belt under uterus and across spines of pelvis.
  E. If domestic violence is suspected, order social work consult.

Prevention of Trauma

Education and reinforcement of seatbelt use during pregnancy should be undertaken as a routine part of prenatal education and care. In a primate model of motor vehicle impact trauma and its fetal effects, three-point restraints significantly reduced fetal mortality compared with two-point restraints.[2] In a recent study of MVCs involving 43 pregnant women between 1996 and 1999, Klinich and colleagues from the University of Michigan demonstrated that proper use of seatbelts was significantly associated with good fetal outcome. The authors speculated that proper seatbelt use could prevent as many as 84% of adverse fetal outcomes.[12] **Proper counseling by the obstetrical care provider for seatbelt usage has also been shown to**

significantly improve compliance with seatbelt use during pregnancy.[49] Proper placement of seatbelts includes placing the lap belt below the lower bump of the uterus overlying the anterior superior iliac spines. The shoulder belt should be positioned off to the side of the uterus, between the breasts, and over the midportion of the clavicle.[1] Although some have expressed concern about possible harmful effects of air bag deployment in the event of a motor vehicle accident during pregnancy, the National Highway Traffic Safety Administration (NHTSA) and the American College of Obstetricians and Gynecologists do not recommend disabling air bags during pregnancy.[34,50] Indeed, a retrospective cohort study of pregnant women involved in MVCs in the state of Washington between 2002 and 2005 concluded that air bags do not increase risk for adverse outcomes of pregnancy.[51]

Screening and Identification of Women at Risk for Domestic Violence

Traumatic injuries may also be prevented by early screening and detection of intimate partner violence during pregnancy. The American College of Obstetricians and Gynecologists recommends screening all pregnant women for intimate partner violence at the first prenatal visit and at least once per trimester of pregnancy. They recommend use of a brief three-question screening tool to identify women who are at risk to experience domestic violence during pregnancy (see box, Suggested Domestic Violence Screening Questions).[52]

Suggested Domestic Violence Screening Questions

"Because violence is so common in many women's lives and because there is help available for women being abused, I now ask every patient about domestic violence:

1. Within the past year—or since you have been pregnant—have you been hit, slapped, kicked or otherwise physically hurt by someone?
2. Are you in a relationship with a person who threatens or physically hurts you?
3. Has anyone forced you to have sexual activities that made you feel uncomfortable?"

Copyright © 2011 American Congress of Obstetricians and Gynecologists. All rights reserved.

KEY POINTS

- Maternal trauma is the most frequent cause of nonobstetrical maternal death.
- Abruptio placentae complicates 1% to 2% of cases of minor blunt abdominal trauma and up to 40% of cases of severe abdominal trauma.
- Abruptio placentae is the most frequent cause of fetal death after trauma.
- Concerns about fetal effects of ionizing radiation should not delay imaging necessary to care for pregnant trauma victims.
- Seatbelt use may reduce adverse fetal outcome resulting from trauma by as much as 84%.

REFERENCES

1. Mirza FG, Devine PC, Gaddipati S: Trauma in pregnancy: a systematic approach. Am J Perinatol 27:579, 2010.
2. Pearlman MD: Motor vehicle crashes, pregnancy loss and preterm labor. Int J Gynaecol Obstet 57:127, 1997.
3. El Kady D, Gilbert WM, Xing G, et al: Association of maternal fractures with adverse perinatal outcomes. Am J Obstet Gynecol 195:711, 2006.
4. El Kady D: Perinatal outcomes of traumatic injuries during pregnancy. Clin Obstet Gynecol 50:582, 2007.
5. El Kady D, Gilbert WM, Anderson J, et al: Trauma during pregnancy: an analysis of maternal and fetal outcomes in a large population. Am J Obstet Gynecol 190:1661, 2004.
6. Weiss HB, Songer TJ, Fabio A: Fetal deaths related to maternal injury. JAMA 286:1863, 2001.
7. Oxford CM, Ludmir J: Trauma in pregnancy. Clin Obstet Gynecol 52:611, 2009.
8. Cusick SS, Tibbles CD: Trauma in pregnancy. Emerg Med Clin North Am 25:861, 2007.
9. Chames MC, Pearlman MD: Trauma during pregnancy: outcomes and clinical management. Clin Obstet Gynecol 51:398, 2008.
10. Muench MV, Canterino JC: Trauma in pregnancy. Obstet Gynecol Clin North Am 34:555, 2007.
11. Pearlman MD, Tintinalli JE, Lorenz RP: Blunt trauma during pregnancy. N Engl J Med 323:609, 1990.
12. Klinich KD, Flannagan CA, Rupp JD, et al: Fetal outcome in motor-vehicle crashes: effects of crash characteristics and maternal restraint. Am J Obstet Gynecol 198:450.e1, 2008.
13. Iwamoto HS, Kaufman T, Keil LC, et al: Responses to acute hypoxemia in fetal sheep at 0.6-0.7 gestation. Am J Physiol 256:H613, 1989.
14. Williams J, Mozurkewich E, Chilimigras J, et al: Critical care in obstetrics: pregnancy-specific conditions. Best Pract Res Clin Obstet Gynaecol 22:825, 2008.
15. Brown HL: Trauma in pregnancy. Obstet Gynecol 114:147, 2009.
16. Dunning K, LeMasters G, Levin L, et al: Falls in workers during pregnancy: risk factors, job hazards, and high risk occupations. Am J Ind Med 44:664, 2003.
17. Butler EE, Colon I, Druzin ML, et al: Postural equilibrium during pregnancy: decreased stability with an increased reliance on visual cues. Am J Obstet Gynecol 195:1104, 2006.
18. Schiff MA: Pregnancy outcomes following hospitalisation for a fall in Washington State from 1987 to 2004. BJOG 115:1648, 2008.
19. Cahill AG, Bastek JA, Stamilio DM, et al: Minor trauma in pregnancy—is the evaluation unwarranted? Am J Obstet Gynecol 198:208.e1, 2008.
20. Gunter J: Intimate partner violence. Obstet Gynecol Clin North Am 34:367, ix, 2007.
21. Cheng D, Horon IL: Intimate-partner homicide among pregnant and postpartum women. Obstet Gynecol 115:1181, 2010.
22. El Kady D, Gilbert WM, Xing G, et al: Maternal and neonatal outcomes of assaults during pregnancy. Obstet Gynecol 105:357, 2005.
23. Gunter J, Pearlman MD: Emergencies during pregnancy: trauma and nonobstetric surgical conditions. In Ling F, Duff P (eds.): Obstetrics and Gynecology: Principles for Practice. New York: McGraw-Hill, 2001, p 253.
24. Pacheco LD, Gei AF, VanHook JW, et al: Burns in pregnancy. Obstet Gynecol 106:1210, 2005.
25. Maghsoudi H, Samnia R, Garadaghi A, et al: Burns in pregnancy. Burns 32:246, 2006.
26. Tsuei BJ: Assessment of the pregnant trauma patient. Injury 37:367, 2006.
27. Curet MJ, Schermer CR, Demarest GB, et al: Predictors of outcome in trauma during pregnancy: identification of patients who can be monitored for less than 6 hours. J Trauma 49:18, 2000.
28. Pak LL, Reece EA, Chan L: Is adverse pregnancy outcome predictable after blunt abdominal trauma? Am J Obstet Gynecol 179:1140, 1998.
29. Schiff MA, Holt VL: The injury severity score in pregnant trauma patients: predicting placental abruption and fetal death. J Trauma 53:946, 2002.
30. Schiff MA, Holt VL, Daling JR: Maternal and infant outcomes after injury during pregnancy in Washington State from 1989 to 1997. J Trauma 53:939, 2002.

31. Sasser SM, Hunt RC, Faul F, et al: Guidelines for field triage of injured patients: recommendations of the National Expert Panel on Field Triage, 2011. MMWR 61:1, 2012.
32. Pearlman MD, Tintinallli JE, Lorenz RP: A prospective controlled study of outcome after trauma during pregnancy. Am J Obstet Gynecol 162:1502, 1990.
33. Williams JK, McClain L, Rosemurgy AS, et al: Evaluation of blunt abdominal trauma in the third trimester of pregnancy: maternal and fetal considerations. Obstet Gynecol 75:33, 1990.
34. ACOG Educational Bulletin: Obstetric Aspects of Trauma Management. Int J Gynaecol Obstet 64:87, 1999.
35. Dahmus MA, Sibai BM: Blunt abdominal trauma: are there any predictive factors for abruptio placentae or maternal-fetal distress? Am J Obstet Gynecol 169:1054, 1993.
36. Grossman NB: Blunt trauma in pregnancy. Am Fam Physician 70:1303, 2004.
37. Muench MV, Baschat AA, Reddy UM, et al: Kleihauer-Betke testing is important in all cases of maternal trauma. J Trauma 57:1094, 2004.
38. Goodwin TM, Breen MT: Pregnancy outcome and fetomaternal hemorrhage after noncatastrophic trauma. Am J Obstet Gynecol 162:665, 1990.
39. Patel SJ, Reede DL, Katz DS, et al: Imaging the pregnant patient for nonobstetric conditions: algorithms and radiation dose considerations. Radiographics 27:1705, 2007.
40. ACOG Committee on Obstetric Practice: ACOG Committee Opinion #299: Guidelines for Diagnostic Imaging During Pregnancy. Obstet Gynecol 104:647, 2004.
41. Gjelsteen AC, Ching BH, Meyermann MW, et al: CT, MRI, PET, PET/CT, and ultrasound in the evaluation of obstetric and gynecologic patients. Surg Clin North Am 88:361, 2008.
42. Chen MM, Coakley FV, Kaimal A, et al: Guidelines for computed tomography and magnetic resonance imaging use during pregnancy and lactation. Obstet Gynecol 112:333, 2008.
43. ACR practice guidelines for imaging pregnant or potentially pregnant adolescents and women with ionizing radiation. American College of Radiology, 2008, p 1.
44. Kanal E, Barkovich AJ, Bell C, et al: ACR Guidance Document for Safe MR Practices: 2007. Am J Roentgenol 188:1447, 2007.
45. Lee SI, Chew FS: Use of IV iodinated and gadolinium contrast media in the pregnant or lactating patient: self-assessment module. Am J Roentgenol 193:S70, 2009.
46. Marckmann P, Skov L: Nephrogenic systemic fibrosis: clinical picture and treatment. Radiol Clin North Am 47:833, 2009.
47. Augustin G, Majerovic M: Non-obstetrical acute abdomen during pregnancy. Europ J Obstet, Gynecol Reprod Biol 13:4, 2007.
48. Weiss HB, Sauber-Schatz EK, Cook LJ: The epidemiology of pregnancy-associated emergency department injury visits and their impact on birth outcomes. Accid Anal Prev 40:1088, 2008.
49. Pearlman MD, Phillips ME: Safety belt use during pregnancy. Obstet Gynecol 88:1026, 1996.
50. National Highway Transportation Safety Administration: Should Pregnant Women Wear Seat Belts? Answers to an expant mother's common questions about traffic safety. Available from: http://www.nhtsa.gov/people/injury/airbags/Internet_Services_Group/ISG-Restricted/Buckle-Up%20America/pregnancybrochure/BUA_PregnancyNHTSAchange.pdf. Accessed 9/26/2010.
51. Schiff M, Mack CD, Kaufman RP, et al: The effect of air bags on pregnancy outcomes in Washington State: 2002-2005. Obstet Gynecol 115:85, 2010.
52. ACOG: Screening tools—domestic violence. Available from: http://www.acog.org/About_ACOG/ACOG_Departments/Violence_Against_Women/Screening_Tools_Domestic_Violence.

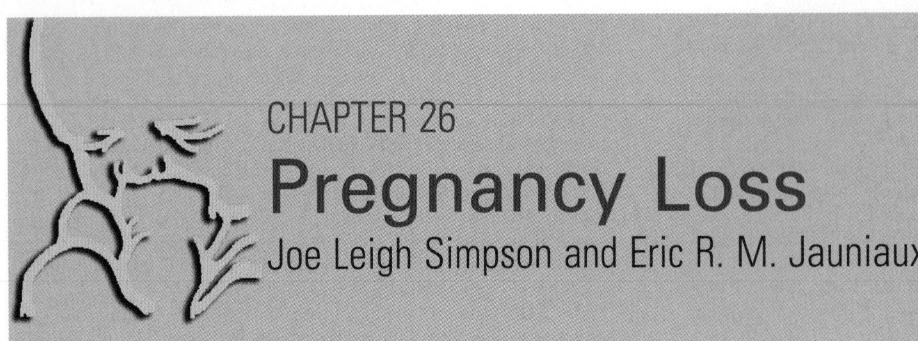

CHAPTER 26

Pregnancy Loss

Joe Leigh Simpson and Eric R. M. Jauniaux

KEY ABBREVIATIONS	
American College of Obstetricians and Gynecologists	ACOG
Anticardiolipin	aCL
Antiphospholipid Antibodies	aPL
Assisted Reproductive Technology	ART
β-Human Chorionic Gonadotropin	β-hCG
Cluster of Differentiation	CD
Confidence Interval	CI
Fluorescence in Situ Hybridization	FISH
Helper T Cell	Th cell
Human Chorionic Gonadotropin	hCG
Human Leukocyte Antigen	HLA
Immunoglobulin A	IgA
Immunoglobulin G	IgG
Interleukin	IL
Interferon	IFN
Lupus Anticoagulant	LAC
Luteinizing Hormone	LH
Luteal Phase Defect	LPD
National Institute of Child Health and Human Development	NICHD
Preimplantation Genetic Diagnosis	PGD
Rhesus (D Antigen)	Rh(D)
Royal College of Obstetricians and Gynaecologists	RCOG
Standard Deviation	SD
Three-dimensional	3D
Thyroid Receptor-β	TR-β
Thyroid-stimulating Hormone	TSH

Not all conceptions result in a live-born infant, and human reproduction is extremely inefficient compared with that of other mammal species.[1] About 50% to 70% of spontaneous conceptions are lost before completion of the first trimester, most before implantation or during the first month after the last menstrual period. These losses are often not recognized as conceptions. Of clinically recognized pregnancies, 10% to 15% are lost. Although epidemiologic data on animals living in the wild, such as monkeys, are limited, laboratory rodents are known to have postimplantation pregnancy loss rates of less than 10%.[1] Among married women in the United States, 4% have experienced two fetal losses, and 3% three or more.[2] A subset of women manifest repetitive spontaneous miscarriages, as opposed to randomly having repeated untoward events. This chapter considers the frequency and timing of pregnancy losses, the causes of fetal wastage, and the management of couples experiencing repetitive losses.

FREQUENCY AND TIMING OF PREGNANCY LOSS

Embryos implant 6 days after conception. Physical signs are not generally appreciated until 5 to 6 weeks after the last menstrual period. Fewer than half of preimplantation embryos persist, as witnessed by assisted reproductive technology (ART) success rates rarely exceeding 30% to 40% of cycles initiated. Even after implantation, judged preclinically by the presence of β-human chorionic gonadotropin (β-hCG), about 30% of pregnancies are lost.[1] After clinical recognition, 10% to 12% are lost. Most clinical pregnancy losses occur before 8 weeks. Before widespread availability of ultrasound, embryonic demise was often not appreciated until 9 to 12 weeks' gestation, at which time there was bleeding and passage of tissue (products of conception). With widespread availability of ultrasound, it has been shown that fetal demise actually occurs weeks before overt clinical signs are manifested. This conclusion was reached on the basis of cohort studies showing that only 3% of viable pregnancies are lost after 8 weeks' gestation[3]; studies involving obstetrical registrants reached similar conclusions. Fetal viability thus ceases weeks before maternal symptoms of pregnancy loss. That almost all losses are retained in utero for an interval before clinical recognition means that virtually all losses could be considered "missed abortions"; thus, this once widely used term is actually archaic.

After the first trimester, pregnancy losses occur at a slower rate. Loss rates are only 1% in women confirmed by ultrasound to have viable pregnancies at 16 weeks. Two confounding factors influencing clinical pregnancy loss rates are clinically relevant. Maternal age is positively correlated with pregnancy loss rates, a 40-year-old woman having twice the risk of a 20-year-old woman. This occurs in euploid as well as aneuploid pregnancies, as discussed later. Prior pregnancy loss also increases loss rates, but far less than once believed. Among nulliparous women who have never experienced a loss, the likelihood of pregnancy loss is low: 5% in primiparas and 4% in multiparas (Table 26-1). After one loss, the risk of another is increased but does not exceed 30% to 40% even for women with three or more losses.[4] These risks apply not only to those women whose losses were recognized at 9 to 12 weeks' gestation but also to those whose pregnancies were ascertained in the fifth week of gestation.[5] Of clinical relevance, there is no scientific evidence that women with three losses are etiologically distinct from those with two losses or even one loss. The situation may be different if, rarely, four or more losses have occurred; different etiologic factors may exist in this uncommon subgroup.

The clinical consequence of the above information is that in order to be judged efficacious in preventing recurrent first-trimester spontaneous abortions, therapeutic regimens must show success rates substantially greater than 70%. Essentially no therapeutic regimen can make this claim.

TABLE 26-1 APPROXIMATE RECURRENCE RISK FIGURES USEFUL FOR COUNSELING WOMEN WITH REPEATED SPONTANEOUS ABORTIONS*

	PRIOR ABORTIONS	RISK (%)
Women with live-born infant	0	5-10
	1	20-25
	2	25
	3	30
	4	30
Women without live-born infant	3	30-40

Data from Regan L: A prospective study on spontaneous abortion. *In* Beard RW, Sharp F (eds): Early Pregnancy Loss: Mechanisms and Treatment. London, Springer-Verlag 1988, p 22; Warburton D, Fraser FC: Spontaneous abortion risks in man: data from reproductive histories collected in a medical genetic unit. Am J Hum Genet 16:1, 1964; and Poland BJ, Miller JR, Jones DC, et al: Reproductive counseling in patients who have had a spontaneous abortion. Am J Obstet Gynecol 127:685, 1977.

*Recurrence risks are slightly higher for older women.

PLACENTAL ANATOMIC CHARACTERITICS OF SUCCESSFUL AND UNSUCCESSFUL PREGNANCIES

As judged by adult tissue criteria, the human fetus develops in a low oxygen (O_2) environment. Development of the human placenta is modulated heavily by the intrauterine environment.[6-9] During the first trimester, development takes place in a low oxygen environment supported by histotrophic nutrition from the endometrial glands. Consequently, the rate of growth of the chorionic sac is almost invariable across this period and is remarkably uniform between individuals. Toward the end of the first trimester, the intrauterine environment undergoes radical transformation in association with onset of the maternal arterial circulation and the switch to hemotrophic nutrition. The accompanying rise in intraplacental oxygen concentration poses a major challenge to placental tissues, and extensive villous remodeling takes place at this time.

The human gestational sac is designed to minimize the flux of O_2 from maternal blood to the fetal circulation.[6] In particular, the extravillous trophoblast that migrates inside the uterine tissue to anchor the pregnancy creates a cellular shell with plugs inside the tip of the uteroplacental arteries.[2,9] This additional barrier keeps most of the maternal circulation outside the placenta and thus reduces the chemical activity of free oxygen radicals inside the placenta during most of the first trimester of the human pregnancy.[6,7] In normal pregnancies, the onset of the maternal circulation is a progressive phenomenon, starting at about 9 weeks at the periphery and gradually extending toward the center of the placenta.[2,7,9] This process correlates closely with the pattern of trophoblast invasion across the placental bed (Figure 26-1).

In about two thirds of early pregnancy failures, there is anatomic evidence of defective placentation, which is mainly characterized by a thinner and fragmented trophoblast shell and reduced cytotrophoblast invasion of the lumen at the tips of the spiral arteries.[2,10-12] This is associated with premature onset of the maternal circulation throughout the placenta in most cases of miscarriages.[2,9,10-12] These defects are similar in euploid and most aneuploid miscarriages but are more pronounced in hydatidiform moles (Figure 26-2). In vivo ultrasound data and histopathologic data indicate that in most early pregnancy losses, the onset of the intervillous circulation is premature and widespread owing to incomplete transformation and plugging of the uteroplacental arteries.[7,10,11] In about 80% of missed miscarriages, the onset of the maternal placental circulation is both precocious and generalized throughout the placenta. This occurs independent of the karyotype of the conceptus,[11] leading to higher O_2 concentrations during early pregnancy, widespread trophoblastic oxidative damage, and placental degeneration. Although in vitro studies have demonstrated the ability of damaged syncytium to regenerate from the underlying cytotrophoblast, it is likely that in the face of extensive damage, this ability

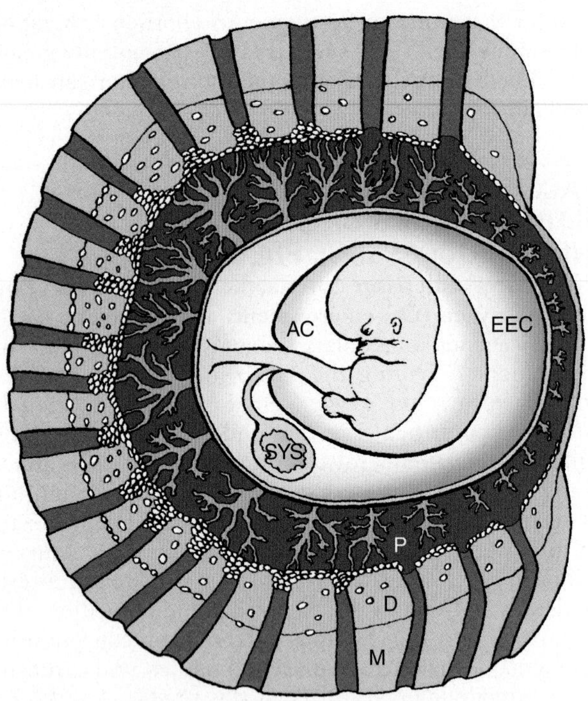

FIGURE 26-1. A gestational sac at the end of the second month (8 to 9 weeks) showing the myometrium *(M)*, the decidua *(D)*, the placenta *(P)*, the exocoelomic cavity *(ECC)*, the amniotic cavity *(AC)*, and the secondary yolk sac *(SYS)*. (From Jauniaux E, Cindrova-Davies T, Johns T, et al: Distribution and transfer pathways of antioxidant molecules inside the first trimester human gestational sac. J Clin Endocrinol Metab 89:1452, 2004.)

will be overwhelmed, leading to complete pregnancy failure.[2,12]

NUMERICAL CHROMOSOMAL ABNORMALITIES: THE MOST FREQUENT CAUSES OF EARLY PREGNANCY LOSS

Chromosomal abnormalities are the major cause of both preimplantation and clinically recognized pregnancy loss. The frequency of losses in human preimplantation embryos is very high. Of morphologically normal embryos, 25% to 50% show chromosomal abnormalities (aneuploidy or polyploidy),[13] depending on maternal age. The frequency of chromosomal abnormalities in morphologically abnormal embryos is even higher. Moreover, these data are based on studies using fluorescence in situ hybridization (FISH) with chromosome-specific probes for only seven to nine chromosomes; rates would be higher using technologies that can assess all chromosomes, for example, 24-chromosome FISH, single nucleotide polymorphism (SNP), or array comparative genome hybridization (CGH) analysis. The high aneuploidy rate in morphologically normal embryos is consistent with 5% to 10% aneuploidy in sperm of ostensibly normal men and 20% aneuploidy in oocytes (deduced from polar bodies) of women undergoing ART. Aneuploidy rates in oocytes and embryos predictably increase as maternal age increases.

At least 50% of *clinically recognized pregnancy* losses result from a chromosomal abnormality.[14] The frequency is probably higher because if one analyzes chorionic villi recovered by chorionic villus sampling (CVS) immediately after ultrasound diagnosis of fetal demise (rather than culturing spontaneously expelled products), the chromosomal abnormalities are detected in 75% to 90%.[15] In addition, CGH (microarray analysis) can detect abnormalities not evident by karyotype.

Among second-trimester losses, one observes chromosomal abnormalities more similar in type to those observed in live-born infants: trisomies 13, 18, and 21; monosomy X; and sex chromosomal polysomies. This also holds among losses after 20 gestational weeks (stillborn infants), in which the frequency of chromosomal abnormalities is about 8% to 13%, exceeding 20% of anatomic abnormalities.[16] This frequency is less than that observed in earlier abortuses but much higher than that found among live-born infants (0.6%).

Types of Numerical Chromosomal Abnormalities

Autosomal Trisomy

Autosomal trisomies represent the largest (about 50%) single class of chromosomal complements in cytogenetically abnormal spontaneous abortions. That is, 25% of all abortuses are aneuploid, given half of all abortuses have a chromosomal abnormality. Frequencies of various trisomies are listed in Table 26-2. Trisomy for every chromosome has been observed. The most common trisomy is trisomy 16. Most trisomies show a maternal age effect, but the effect varies markedly among chromosomes. The increased maternal age effect is especially impressive for double trisomies. Attempts have been made to correlate placental morphologic abnormalities with specific trisomies, but these relationships are imprecise. Comparison of ultrasound findings and placental histology indicates that villous changes following in utero fetal demise could explain the low predictive value of placental histology in identifying an aneuploidy or another nonchromosomal etiology. (By contrast, the histologic features of complete and partial hydatidiform molar gestations are so distinctive that most molar miscarriages can be correctly diagnosed by histologic examination alone.)

Trisomies incompatible with life predictably show slower growth than trisomies compatible with life (e.g., trisomies 13, 18, 21), but otherwise there are usually no features distinguishing the two groups. Abortuses from the former group may show anomalies consistent with those found in full-term live-born trisomic infants. Malformations present have been said to be more severe than those observed in induced abortuses following prenatal diagnosis.

Aneuploidy usually results from errors at meiosis I, specifically maternal meiosis I. Errors of maternal meiosis I are associated with advanced maternal age.[17-19] Once thought to involve mostly missegregation of whole chromosomes, it is now clear that chromatid errors are an equally prevalent cause of maternal meiotic errors.[20] Irrespective, the cytologic mechanism involves decreased or absent meiotic recombination.[21] In trisomy 13 and trisomy 21, 90% of these maternal cases arise at meiosis I; almost all trisomy 16 cases arise in maternal meiosis I.[18] An exception is trisomy 18, in which two thirds of the 90% of maternal meiotic cases arise at meiosis II.[18]

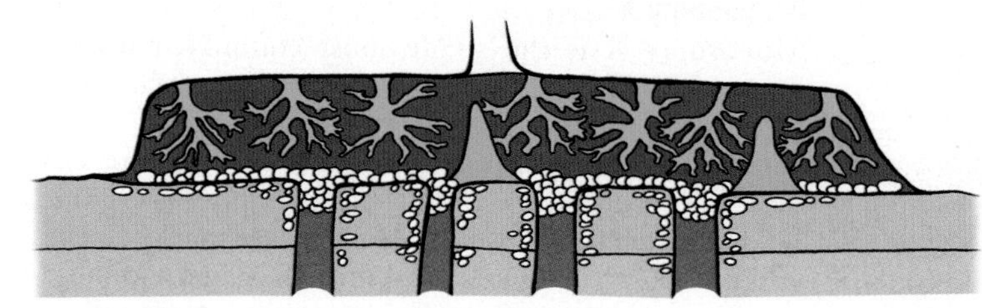

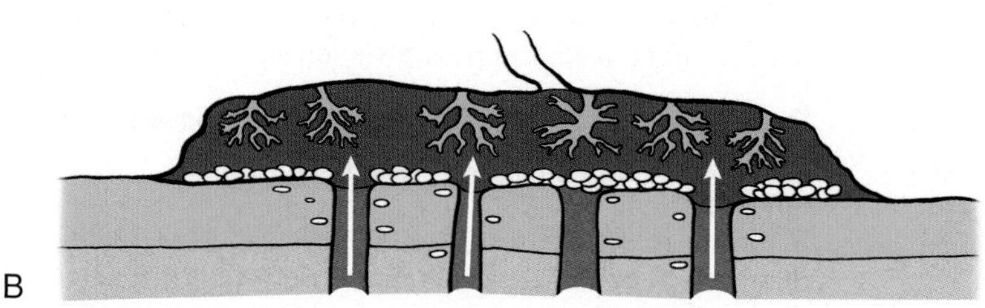

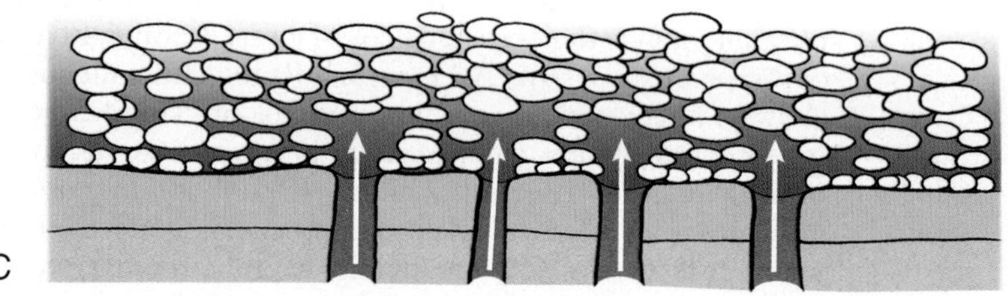

Figure 26-2. Placentation in a normal ongoing pregnancy **(A)**, in an early pregnancy failure **(B)**, and in a complete hydatidiform mole **(C)**. **A,** Note the continuous trophoblastic shell, the plugs in the lumens of the spiral arteries, and the interstitial migration of the extravillous trophoblast through the decidua down to the superficial layer of the myometrium. **B,** Note the discontinuous trophoblastic shell, the absence of plugs, and the reduced migration of extravillous trophoblastic cells. **C,** Note the absence of trophoblastic plugs and interstitial migration. (From Jauniaux E, Burton GJ: Pathophysiology of histological changes in early pregnancy loss. Placenta 26:114, 2005.)

A practical consequence of these data is that deducing chromosomal status of oocytes by analysis of polar bodies can detect 95% of more of chromosomally abnormal embryos. This is relevant because polar body analysis is a more robust predictions of embryo status than analysis of blastomere from a 3-day-old embryo. In the latter, mitotic nondisjunction can lead to spurious and unrepresentative results. Errors in *paternal* meiosis account for 10% of acrocentric (13, 14, 15, 21, and 22) trisomies.[18] In trisomy 21, paternal meiotic errors are equally likely to arise in meiosis I or II,[21] a circumstance that contrasts with the situation in maternal meiotic errors. Among nonacrocentric chromosomes, paternal contribution is uncommon. A surprising exception involves trisomy 2.

Polyploidy

In polyploidy, more than two haploid chromosomal complements are present. Nonmosaic triploidy (3n = 69) and tetraploidy (4n = 92) are common in abortuses. This phenomenon is presumably distinct from the diploid or triploid mosaicism that is found in about 30% of blastocysts.[22] Triploid abortuses are usually 69,XXY or 69,XXX, resulting from dispermy. An association exists between diandric (paternally inherited) triploidy and hydatidiform mole, a "partial" mole said to exist if molar tissue and fetal parts coexist. The more common "complete" (classic) hydatidiform mole is 46,XX, androgenetic in origin, and composed exclusively of villous tissue. Pathologic findings in diandric triploid and tetraploid placentas include a disproportionately large gestational sac, focal (partial) hydropic degeneration of placental villi, and trophoblast hyperplasia. Placental hydropic changes are progressive and may be difficult to identify in early pregnancy. By contrast, placental villi often undergo hydropic degeneration after fetal demise. This can occur in all types of miscarriage; thus, histologic and cytogenetic investigations are essential to differentiate between true mole and pseudomole because only a true mole can be associated with persistent trophoblastic disease. Fetal malformations associated with triploid miscarriage include neural tube defects and omphaloceles, anomalies reminiscent of those observed in triploid conceptuses surviving to term. Facial dysmorphia

TABLE 26-2 CHROMOSOMAL COMPLETION IN SPONTANEOUS ABORTIONS RECOGNIZED CLINICALLY IN THE FIRST TRIMESTER

CHROMOSOMAL COMPLEMENT	FREQUENCY	PERCENT
Normal 46,XX or 46,XY		54.1
Triploidy		7.7
69,XXX	2.7	
69,XYX	0.2	
69,XXY	4.0	
Other	0.8	
Tetraploidy		2.6
92,XXX	1.5	
92,XXYY	0.55	
Not stated	0.55	
Monosomy X		18.6
Structural abnormalities		1.5
Sex chromosomal polysomy		0.2
47,XXX	0.05	
47,XXY	0.15	
Autosomal monosomy (G)		0.1
Autosomal trisomy for chromosomes		22.3
1	0	
2	1.11	
3	0.25	
4	0.64	
5	0.04	
6	0.14	
7	0.89	
8	0.79	
9	0.72	
10	0.36	
11	0.04	
12	0.18	
13	1.07	
14	0.82	
15	1.68	
16	7.27	
17	0.18	
18	1.15	
19	0.01	
20	0.61	
21	2.11	
22	2.26	
Double trisomy		0.7
Mosaic trisomy		1.3
Other abnormalities or not specified		0.9
		100.0

Data from Simpson JL, Bombard AT: Chromosomal abnormalities in spontaneous abortion: frequency, pathology and genetic counseling. *In* Edmonds K (ed): Spontaneous Abortion. London, Blackwell, 1987.

and limb abnormalities have also been reported. Tetraploidy is uncommon, rarely progressing beyond 2 to 3 weeks of embryonic life. This chromosomal abnormality can also be associated with persistent trophoblastic disease and thus needs to be identified in order to offer hCG follow-up.

Sex Chromosomal Polysomy (X or Y)

The complements 47,XXY and 47,XYY each occur in about 1 per 800 live-born male births; 47,XXX occurs in 1 per 800 female births. X or Y polysomies are only slightly more common in abortuses than in live-born infants. In pregnancies conceived by intracytoplasmic sperm injection (ICSI), the frequency of 47,XXX and 47,XXY embryos and fetuses appears to be increased.[23]

Monosomy X

Monosomy X is the single most common chromosomal abnormality among spontaneous abortions, accounting for 15% to 20% of abnormal specimens. Monosomy X embryos usually consist of only an umbilical cord stump. Later in gestation, anomalies characteristic of Turner syndrome may be seen, such as cystic hygromas and generalized edema (Figure 26-3). Unlike live-born 45,X individuals, 45,X abortuses show germ cells; however, germ cells rarely develop beyond the primordial germ cell stage. The pathogenesis of 45,X germ cell failure thus involves not so much failure of germ cell development as more rapid attrition in 45,X compared with 46,XX embryos.[24,25] Monosomy X usually (80%) occurs as result of paternal sex chromosome loss. This observation is consistent with the lack of a maternal age effect in 45,X or possibly even an inverse age effect.

Relationship Between Recurrent Losses and Numerical Chromosomal Abnormalities

In both preimplantation and first-trimester abortions, recurrent aneuploidy occurs more often than expected by chance. Recurrent aneuploidy is a frequent explanation, at least until the number of losses reaches or exceeds four. In a given family, successive abortuses are likely to be either recurrently normal or recurrently abnormal. Table 26-3 shows that if the complement of the first abortus is abnormal,[26,27] recurrence usually involves aneuploidy, although not necessarily of the same chromosome.

Further supporting recurrent aneuploidy as a genuine phenomenon is the occurrence of trisomic preimplantation embryos in successive ART cycles. Rubio and collegues[28] showed increased aneuploid embryos in couples with repeated abortions compared with couples undergoing preimplantation genetic diagnosis (PGD) for mendelian indications. Frequencies of chromosomal abnormalities were 71% versus 45%, respectively. In a similar study, Munné and associates[29] found rates to be 37% versus 21% in women younger than 35 years, and 34% versus 31.5% in women older than 35 years.

Expectation of Abortus Karyotype in Recurrent Abortion

The concept of recurrent aneuploidy implies certain corollaries, one of which has often been the subject of controversy. Recurrent aneuploidy stratifies into recurrent losses in which couples have either experienced chromosomally abnormal abortuses repeatedly and recurrent losses that repeatedly show chromosomally normal abortuses. Given that 50% of all abortuses are abnormal cytogenetically, aneuploidy should be as likely to be detected in a randomly karyotyped abortus as in a sporadic abortus. This has proved to be true. Stern and coworkers[30] found a 57% prevalence of chromosomal abnormalities among abortuses of repetitively aborting women, a frequency coincidentally identical among abortuses of sporadically aborting women. Among 420 abortuses obtained from women with repeated losses, Stephenson and colleagues[31] found 46% chromosomal abnormalities; 31% of the original sample was trisomic. Their comparison was unselected pooled data, which showed 48% of abortuses to be abnormal; 27% of the original sample was trisomic.

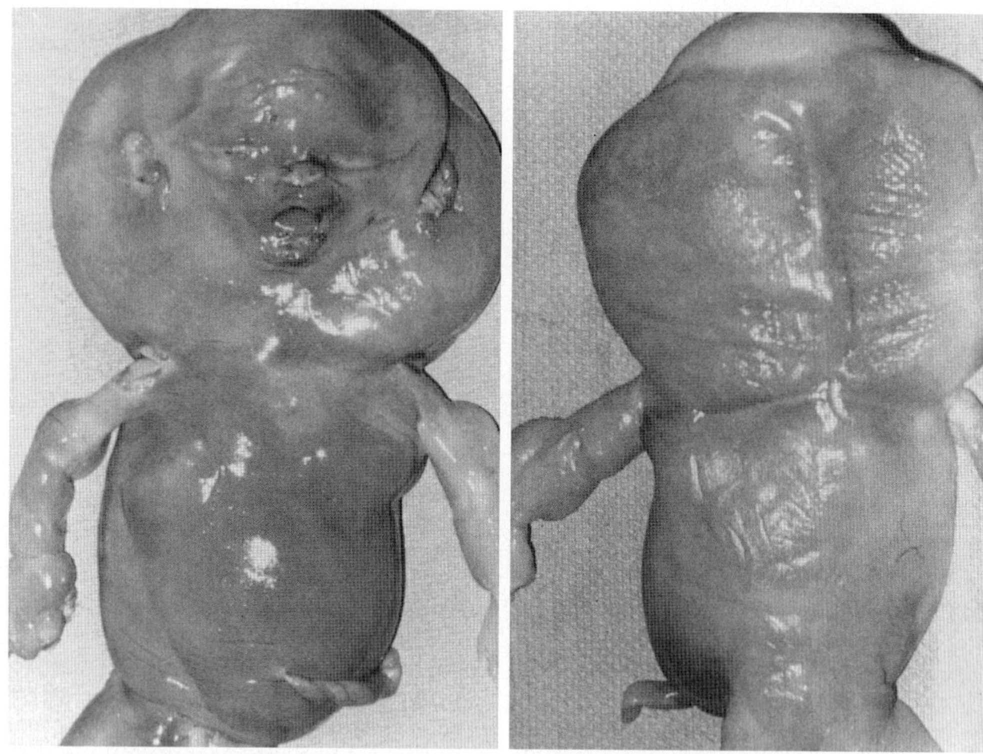

FIGURE 26-3. Photograph of a 45,X abortus. (From Simpson JL, Bombard AT: Chromosomal abnormalities in spontaneous abortion: frequency, pathology and genetic counseling. *In* Edmonds K, Bennett MJ [eds]: Spontaneous Abortion. London, Blackwell, 1987, p 51, with permission.)

TABLE 26-3 RECURRENT ANEUPLOIDY: RELATIONSHIP BETWEEN KARYOTYPES OF SUCCESSIVE ABORTUSES

COMPLEMENT OF FIRST ABORTUS	COMPLEMENT OF SECOND ABORTUS					
	Normal	Trisomy	Monosomy	Triploidy	Tetraploid	De Novo Rearrangement
Normal	142	18	5	7	3	2
Trisomy	31	30	1	4	3	1
Monosomy X	7	5	3	3	0	0
Triploidy	7	4	1	4	0	0
Tetraploidy	3	1	0	2	0	0
De novo rearrangement	1	3	0	0	0	0

From Warburton D, Kline J, Stein Z, et al: Does the karyotype of a spontaneous abortion predict the karyotype of a subsequent abortion? Evidence from 273 women with two karyotyped spontaneous abortions. Am J Hum Genet 41:465, 1987.

In contrast to these data, fetal loss—recurrent or not—are much more likely to be cytogenetically normal (85%) when occurring after the first trimester.[16] Carp and coworkers[32] found that among women having three or more abortuses, the likelihood that the abortus would have an abnormal karyotype was only 29%. In that series, inclusion criteria extended to 20 weeks' gestation, a time at which there is less reason to expect recurrent aneuploidy than recurrence of other etiologies.

Genetic Counseling for Recurrent Aneuploidy

Couples predisposed to recurrent aneuploidy are at increased risk not only for aneuploid abortuses but also for aneuploid live-born neonates. The autosome trisomic in a subsequent pregnancy might be compatible with life (e.g., trisomy 21). Indeed, the risk for live-born trisomy 21 following an aneuploid abortus has been stated to be about 1% (see Chapter 10). A meta-analysis[33] has confirmed this long-standing recurrence risk. The risk is considered similar following other aneuploides. Bianco and associates[34] provided a counseling algorithm applicable following a prior abortion of unknown karyotype. If abortions are recurrent but no information is available on the chromosomal status, the odds ratio can be used to derive a patient-specific risk. For example, if the a prior Down syndrome risk is 1 in 300 and the odds ratio is 1.5, a woman's calculated risk after three abortions would be 1/300 × 1.5, or 1/200.

Clinical Management of Recurrent Aneuploidy

If no information is available concerning the chromosomal status of prior abortuses, paraffin blocks of products of conception can be used to detect aneuploidy using FISH or array CGH. If results show a trisomy, likelihood of a live-born trisomy is increased in subsequent pregnancies. If no information can be obtained, it is unclear whether prenatal genetic diagnosis is appropriate. However, the risk for an aneuploid offspring is increased and can be calculated according to Bianco and associates.[34] The small but finite risk for amniocentesis or CVS is troublesome to couples who have had difficulty maintaining a pregnancy. Thus, noninvasive approaches (see Chapter 10) are typically the chosen option. However, the sensitivity for detecting aneuploidy by noninvasive methods is not the nearly 100% possible with CVS or amniocentesis. PGD (see Chapter 11) is another option, especially if the couple eschews clinical pregnancy termination. Selective transfer of euploid embryos clearly decreases the rate of clinical abortions in couples with repeated losses,[35,36] and live-born trisomies should be decreased.

CHROMOSOMAL REARRANGEMENTS

Translocations

Structural chromosomal abnormalities are an unequivocal explanation for repetitive abortions. The most common structural rearrangement encountered is a translocation, **found in about 5% of couples experiencing repeated losses.** Individuals with balanced translocations are phenotypically normal, but their offspring (abortuses or abnormal live-born infants) may show chromosomal duplications or deficiencies as result of normal meiotic segregation. Among couples with repetitive abortions, about 60% of translocations are reciprocal and 40% robertsonian. Women are about twice as likely as men to show a balanced translocation.[37]

The clinical consequences of a balanced translocation are illustrated in Figure 26-3. If a child has Down syndrome as result of a centric fusion (robertsonian) translocation, the rearrangement will have originated de novo in 50% to 75% of cases. That is, a balanced translocation will not exist in either parent. The likelihood of Down syndrome recurring in subsequent offspring is minimal. On the other hand, the risk is significant in the 25% to 50% of families in which individuals have Down syndrome as result of a balanced parental translocation [e.g., parental complement 45,XX,-14,-21,+t(14q;21q)]. The theoretical risk for having a child with Down syndrome is 33%, but empirical risks are considerably less. The risk is only 2% if the father carries the translocation; the risk is 10% if the mother carries the translocation.[38,39] If robertsonian (centric fusion) translocations involve other chromosomes, empirical risks are lower. In t(13q;14q), the risk for live-born trisomy 13 is 1% or less.

Reciprocal translocations do not involve centromeric fusion, but rather interchanges between two or more chromosomes. Empirical data for specific translocations are usually not available, but generalizations can be made on the basis of pooled data derived from many different translocations.[40] Again, theoretical risks for abnormal offspring (unbalanced reciprocal translocations) are far greater than empirical risks. Overall, the risk is 12% for offspring of either female heterozygotes or male heterozygotes.[38,39] Detecting a chromosomal rearrangement thus profoundly affects subsequent pregnancy management. Antenatal cytogenetic studies should be offered. The frequency of unbalanced fetuses is lower if parental balanced translocations are ascertained through repetitive abortions (3%) than through anomalous live-born infants (nearly 20%).[38] Presumably more unbalanced products are lethal.

Analysis of preimplantation embryos using PGD reveals that most embryos are unbalanced: 58% in robertsonian translocations and 76% in reciprocal translocations.[41] This means that most conceptuses would be lost, usually preclinically. When a balanced translocation is detected in a couple experiencing recurrent abortions, *cumulative* prognosis for a live-born infant is little different than if a translocation had not been detected[42]; however, the length of time to achieve pregnancy is greatly increased (mean, 4 to 6 years). Thus, a more realistic strategy is to use PGD to identify and transfer only the few balanced embryos, increasing the statistical likelihood of conception.[43] This strategy is most attractive when the prospective is relatively older and nearly imperative in the fifth decade. Using standard techniques (FISH), one can readily exclude an unbalanced embryo; however, FISH does not distinguish a balanced (translocation heterozygote) from a normal embryo lacking any translocation. Novel techniques now allow a more precise diagnosis in experienced hands.[41] This involves treating a day 3 blastomere with caffeine and colchicine, and one day later generating a metaphase that can be analyzed by fluorescent techniques (FISH) using whole chromosome painting; the "conversion" rate is about 70%.

Rarely, a translocation precludes normal live-born infants. This occurs when a translocation involves homologous, acrocentric chromosomes (e.g., t[13q13q] or t[21q21q]). If the father carries such a structural rearrangement, artificial insemination may be appropriate. If the mother carries the rearrangement, donor oocytes or donor embryos and ART should be considered.

Inversions

Inversions are uncommon parental chromosomal rearrangements but are responsible for repetitive pregnancy losses analogous to translocations. In inversions, the order of genes is reversed. Individuals heterozygous for an inversion should be normal if their genes are merely rearranged. However, individuals with inversions suffer untoward reproductive consequences as a result of normal meiotic phenomena. Crossing-over that involves the inverted segment yields unbalanced gametes (see Simpson and Elias for more details).[44] Pericentric inversions are present in perhaps 0.1% of women and 0.1% of men experiencing repeated spontaneous abortions. Paracentric inversions are even rarer.

Women with a *pericentric* inversion have a 7% risk for abnormal live-born infants; men carry a 5% risk. Pericentric inversions ascertained through phenotypically normal probands are less likely to result in abnormal live-born infants.

Inversions involving only a small portion of the total chromosomal length paradoxically are less significant clinically because large duplications or deficiencies arise following crossing-over, usually conferring lethality. By contrast, inversions involving only 30% to 60% of the total chromosomal length are relatively more likely to be characterized by duplications or deficiencies compatible with survival. Prenatal cytogenetic studies should be offered.

Paracentric inversions should carry less risk for unbalanced products than pericentric inversions because nearly all paracentric recombinants should in theory be lethal. However, abortions and abnormal live-born infants have been observed within the same kindred, and the risk for unbalanced viable offspring has been tabulated at 4%.[45] Prenatal cytogenetic studies should thus still be offered.

MENDELIAN AND POLYGENIC/ MULTIFACTORIAL ETIOLOGY

That 30% to 50% of first-trimester abortuses show no chromosomal abnormalities does not mean genetic causation is excluded. Fetal demise may have occurred as a result of other genetic etiologies. Specifically, neither mendelian nor polygenic/multifactorial disorders show chromosomal abnormalities, and yet these etiologies explain far more congenital anomalies than do chromosomal abnormalities. It would thus be naïve to assume that mendelian and polygenic/multifactorial factors do not play pivotal roles in embryonic mortality. Indeed, there are innumerable candidate genes. Especially likely to be mendelian or polygenic in etiology are abortuses that demonstrate isolated structural anomalies. Cytogenetic data are often lacking on dissected specimens, making it nearly impossible to determine the relative role of cytogenetic versus mendelian or polygenic mechanisms in early embryonic maldevelopment. Philipp and Kalousek[46] correlated cytogenetic status of missed abortuses with morphologic abnormalities at embryoscopy. Embryos with chromosomal abnormalities usually showed one or more external anomalies, but some euploid embryos also showed anatomic anomalies.

In addition to traditional single-gene perturbations (mendelian etiology), novel nonmendelian forms of inheritance probably play a greater role in embryonic loss than in live-born abnormalities. Mosaicism may be restricted to the placenta, the embryo per se being normal. This phenomenon is termed *confined placental mosaicism*. Losses caused by this mechanism may already be subsumed in extant data because most studies involved analysis only of villous material. A corollary of confined placental mosaicism is uniparental disomy, in which both homologues for a given chromosome are derived from a single parent. This presumably occurs as result of expulsion of a chromosome from a trisomic zygote ("trisomic rescue"). Although the karyotype would appear normal (46,XX or 46,XY), the product would lack a contribution from one parent.

LUTEAL PHASE DEFECTS

Implantation in an inhospitable endometrium is a plausible explanation for pregnancy loss. Progesterone deficiency in particular could result in the estrogen-primed endometrium being unable to sustain implantation. Luteal phase deficiency (LPD) has long been hypothesized, specifically caused by inadequate progesterone secreted by the corpus luteum.

Once almost universally accepted as a common cause of fetal wastage, LPD is now generally considered an uncommon explanation. One pitfall is that endometrial histology identical to that observed with luteal phase "defects" is observed in fertile women. Efficacy of treatment has also never been proved—no randomized studies exist. Indeed, meta-analysis has shown[47] no beneficial effect of progesterone treatment. The current consensus is that LPD is either an arguable entity or not proved to be treated successfully with progesterone or progestational therapy.

Luteal phase abnormalities arising during ovulation stimulation and necessitated during ART could be a different phenomenon. It is considered standard to administer progesterone until about 9 weeks' gestation. In this circumstance, the cells surrounding the oocyte, which would ordinarily contribute to the corpus luteum, may have been removed when the oocyte was aspirated.

THYROID ABNORMALITIES

Decreased conception rates and increased fetal losses are logically associated with overt hypothyroidism or hyperthyroidism. The role of subclinical thyroid dysfunction is less clear and not generally considered an explanation for repeated losses. However, Negro and colleagues[48] reported that pregnancy loss was higher in thyroid peroxidase–negative women whose thyroid-stimulating hormone (TSH) level was 2.5 to 4 mIU/L compared with those whose TSH level was less than 2.5 mIU/L (6.1% vs. 3.6%). Increased frequency of thyroid antibodies has in addition been observed in several series, and some consider autoimmune thyroid disease a significant cause.[49] However, the value of treatment in such circumstances is unproved.

Elevations of maternal thyroid hormone per se are clearly deleterious. This effect was shown by a family from the Azores in which a gene conferring resistance to thyroid hormone was segregating.[50] Family members with an autosomal dominant mutation in the thyroid receptor-β (TRβ) gene *(Arg243Gln)* secreted large amounts of TSH to compensate for end-organ resistance. During pregnancy, the fetus of such a mother becomes unavoidably exposed to high levels of maternal TSH because TSH and thyroxine readily cross the placenta. Loss rates were 22.8% in pregnancies of mothers who had the *Arg243Gln* mutation, 2% in those of normal mothers whose male partner had the mutation, and 4.4% in couples in which neither partner had the mutation.

DIABETES MELLITUS

Women whose diabetes mellitus is poorly controlled are at increased risk for fetal loss. Mills and colleagues[51] showed in a National Institute of Child Health and Human Development (NICHD) collaborative study that women whose glycosylated hemoglobin level was greater than 4 standard deviations (SD) above the mean had higher pregnancy loss rates than women with lower glycosylated hemoglobin levels. This finding is consistent with that of many retrospective studies.[52] Poorly controlled diabetes mellitus should be considered one cause for early pregnancy loss. On the other hand, well-controlled or subclinical diabetes should not be considered a cause of early miscarriage. Neither the Royal College of Obstetricians and Gynaecologists (RCOG) nor American College of Obstetricians and Gynecologists (ACOG) recommend testing for occult diabetes mellitus.

INTRAUTERINE ADHESIONS (SYNECHIAE)

Intrauterine adhesions could interfere with implantation or early embryonic development. Adhesions may follow overzealous uterine curettage during the postpartum period, intrauterine surgery (e.g., myomectomy), or endometritis. Curettage is the usual explanation, with adhesions most likely to develop when the procedure is performed 3 or 4 weeks after delivery. Individuals with uterine synechiae usually manifest hypomenorrhea or amenorrhea, but perhaps 15% to 30% have repeated abortions. If adhesions are detected in a woman experiencing repetitive losses, lysis under direct hyperoscopic visualization should be performed. Postoperatively, an intrauterine device or inflated Foley catheter temporarily placed postoperatively in the uterus discourages reapposition of healing uterine surfaces. Estrogen administration should also be initiated. About 50% of patients conceive after surgery, but the frequency of pregnancy losses remains high.

MÜLLERIAN FUSION DEFECTS

Müllerian fusion defects are an accepted cause of *second-trimester* losses and pregnancy complications. Low birthweight, breech presentation, and uterine bleeding are the most common abnormalities associated with müllerian fusion defects compared with women having hysterosalpingogram-proven normal uteri.[53] However, reports typically lack controls.

Losses are more likely to be associated with a uterine septum than a bicornuate uterus.[54] In 509 women with recurrent losses studied by three-dimensional (3D) ultrasound, Salim and associates[55] found greater uterine distortion in women recounting a history of losses. However, the major problem in attributing cause and effect for second-trimester complications and uterine anomalies is that uterine anomalies are frequent in the general population; thus, adverse outcomes could merely be coincidental. For example, in the Salim study, 23.8% of women with recurrent miscarriage had some uterine anomalies on 3D ultrasound.[55] In another study, unsuspected bicornuate uteri were found in 1.2% of 167 women undergoing laparoscopic sterilization; 3.6% had a severely septate uterus, whereas 15.3% had fundal anomalies.[56] In another series, müllerian defects were found in 3.2% (22 of 679) of fertile women; 20 of the 22 defects were septate.[57]

Treatment has traditionally involved surgical correction, namely metroplasty. Ludmir and colleagues[58] wondered whether aggressive nonsurgical treatment could be just as efficacious. A total of 101 women with an uncorrected malformation were tracked longitudinally. After first being followed without surgery and without a defined nonsurgical regimen, the same women underwent a surgically conservative but medically aggressive protocol consisting of decreased physical and tocolysis. Fetal survival rates in both bicornuate and septate groups were, however, not significantly different before (52% and 53%, respectively) or after (58% and 65%, respectively) the change in management.

In conclusion, early first-trimester abortions may be caused by müllerian fusion defects, but other explanations are more likely even when such a defect is found. Septate uteri are most plausibly causative, implantation occurring on a poorly vascularized and inhospitable surface. Abortions occurring after ultrasonographic confirmation of a viable pregnancy at, say, 8 or 9 weeks, may more properly be attributed to uterine fusion defects. Women experiencing second-trimester abortions could benefit from uterine reconstruction, but reconstructive surgery is not necessarily advisable if losses are restricted to the first trimester.

LEIOMYOMAS

Although leiomyomas are frequent, relatively few women develop symptoms requiring medical or surgical therapy. That leiomyomas cause first- or second-trimester pregnancy wastage per se, rather than obstetrical complications like prematurity, is plausible but probably uncommon. Analogous to uterine anomalies, the coexistence of two common phenomena, uterine leiomyomas and reproductive losses, need not necessarily imply a causal relationship. Hartmann and Herring[59] correlated ultrasonographically detected leiomyomas with pregnancy outcome in a cohort of North Carolina women. Of 1313 women studied early in pregnancy, the 131 with leiomyomas as ascertained by ultrasound had an increased prior spontaneous abortion rate (odds ratio [OR], 2.17). One pitfall is that uterine contractions can mimic fibroids on ultrasound.

Location of leiomyomas is probably more important than size. Submucous leiomyomas are more likely to cause abortion than subserous leiomyomas. Postulated mechanisms leading to pregnancy loss include (1) thinning of the endometrium over the surface of a submucous leiomyoma, predisposing to implantation in a poorly decidualized site; (2) rapid growth caused by the hormonal milieu of pregnancy, compromising the blood supply of the leiomyoma and resulting in necrosis ("red degeneration") that, in turn, leads to uterine contractions and eventually fetal expulsion; and (3) encroachment of leiomyomas on the space required for the developing fetus, leading to premature delivery through mechanisms presumably analogous to those operative in incomplete müllerian fusion. In pregnancies that are not lost, the relative lack of space can also lead to fetal deformations (i.e., positional abnormalities arising in a genetically normal fetus).

Surgical procedures to reduce leiomyomas may occasionally be warranted in women experiencing repetitive second-trimester abortions. More often, however, leiomyomas have no etiologic relationship to pregnancy loss. Surgery should be reserved for women whose abortuses were both phenotypically and karyotypically normal and in which viability until at least 9 to 10 weeks was documented.

CERVICAL INSUFFICIENCY

A functionally intact cervix and lower uterine cavity are obvious prerequisites for a successful pregnancy. Characterized by painless dilation and effacement, cervical incompetence (now, preferably insufficiency) usually occurs during the middle second or early third trimester. Cervical insufficiency usually followed traumatic events such as cervical amputation, cervical lacerations, forceful cervical dilation, or cervical conization. However, etiology may be genetic, for example, perturbation of a connective tissue gene (e.g., collagen, fibrillin). Indications for surgery and techniques to correct cervical incompetence are discussed in Chapter 27.

INFECTIONS

Infections are known causes of late fetal losses and logical causes of early fetal losses. Microorganisms associated with spontaneous abortion include variola, vaccinia, *Salmonella typhi*, *Vibrio fetus*, malaria, cytomegalovirus, *Brucella*, toxoplasmosis, *Mycoplasma hominis*, *Chlamydia trachomatis*, and *Ureaplasma urealyticum*. Transplacental infection occurs with each of these microorganisms, following which sporadic losses could logically result. However, infections as a cause of *repetitive* losses are much less likely.

Of the many organisms implicated in repetitive abortion, *U. urealyticum* and *M. hominis* seem most plausibly related to repetitive spontaneous abortions because they fulfill two important prerequisites: (1) the putative organism can persist in an asymptomatic state, and (2) virulence is not always so severe as to cause infertility due to fallopian tube occlusion and, hence, preclude the opportunity for pregnancy. Studies have also suggested a relationship between bacterial vaginosis, presumed to be *Gardnerella vaginalis*, and abortion. However, the latter is more typically, if not exclusively, associated with complications (premature delivery) in the second and third trimesters.

Given lack of evidence for causality for recurrent losses, one might wonder whether the infectious agents discussed previously actually cause fetal losses or merely arise after fetal demise from other causes. Cohort surveillance for infections can best shed light on the true role of infections in early pregnancy loss. The frequency of clinical infections was assessed prospectively in 386 diabetic subjects and 432 control subjects seen weekly or every other week beginning early in the first trimester.[60] Infection occurred no more often in 112 subjects experiencing pregnancy loss than in 706 experiencing successful pregnancies. This held true both for the 2-week interval in which a given loss was recognized clinically and the prior 2-week interval. Similar findings were observed in both control and diabetic subjects and were substantiated when data were stratified into ascending genital infections only versus systemic infection only.

In conclusion, infections doubtless explain some early pregnancy losses and certainly many later losses. However, in the first trimester, attributable risk is low even in sporadic cases, and in recurrent losses, infections are much less likely.

ACQUIRED THROMBOPHILIAS

An association between *second-trimester* pregnancy loss and certain autoimmune diseases is well accepted[16] (see Chapter 44). **For first-trimester losses, consensus holds that a less significant relationship exists.** The spectrum of antibodies found in women with pregnancy loss encompasses nonspecific antinuclear antibodies as well as antibodies against individual cellular components like phospholipids, histones, and double- or single-stranded DNA. The primary antigenic determinant is β_2-glycoprotein, which has an affinity for negatively charged phospholipids.[61] The antiphospholipid syndrome encompasses (1) lupus anticoagulant (LAC) antibodies, (2) anticardiolipin antibody (aCL), *or* (3) anti-β_2–glycoprotein. Values for the latter two should be greater than the 99th percentile, of moderate or higher titers, and 12 weeks apart. Descriptive studies in the 1980s initially seemed to show increased aCLs in women with first-trimester pregnancy losses. A pitfall proved to be selection bias, studying couples only following spontaneous abortions. That antibodies did not arise until *after* the pregnancy loss was also not excluded. To address this, Simpson and associates[62] analyzed sera obtained prospectively from women within 21 days of conception. A total of 93 women who later experienced pregnancy loss were matched 2 to 1 with 190 controls who subsequently had a normal live-born offspring. No association was observed between pregnancy loss and presence of either aPL or aCL. In the most recent ACOG bulletin on the topic,[61] three or more losses before the 10th week of pregnancy is considered to fulfill diagnostic criteria for antiphospholipid syndrome in the sense of justifying prophylactic heparin therapy. It was stated that this assumes "no maternal anatomic or hormonal abnormalities, and no paternal or maternal chromosomal abnormalities [are] excluded." However, ACOG provided the caveat that such an increase neither explains many losses nor confers a greatly increased risk for another loss. Given this, treatment regimens should be judicious, perhaps aspirin and heparin, if embarked on at all. Control groups of fertile women showed not dissimilar frequencies.

INHERITED THROMBOPHILIAS

Inherited maternal hypercoagulable states are unequivocally associated with increased fetal losses in the second trimester, but less convincingly in the first trimester. Postulated associations include factor V Leiden (Q1691G→A), prothrombin 2021G→A, and homozygosity for 677C→T in the methylene tetrahydrofolate reductase gene *(MTHFR)*. Meta-analysis of 31 studies published as of 2003 revealed associations between recurrent (two or more) fetal losses earlier than 13 weeks for these thrombophilias: factor V Leiden (G1691A), activated protein C resistance, prothrombin (*20210A0* gene), and protein S deficiency.[63] There were no associations between *MTHFR*, protein C, and antithrombin deficiencies and recurrent pregnancy loss. A second meta-analysis of 16 studies published by Kovalesky and coworkers[64] reported an association between recurrent pregnancy loss, defined as two or more losses in the first two trimesters, and maternal heterozygosity for either factor V Leiden or prothrombin 20210G7→A.

Evidence is less strong for an association between inherited thrombophilias and recurrent early (<10 weeks' gestation) pregnancy loss. Most authors recommend testing for factor V Leiden, activated protein C resistance, fasting homocysteine, antiphospholipid antibodies, and the prothrombin gene. Pending salutary results in randomized clinical trials, treatment for recurrent first-trimester losses with heparin or other antithrombotic or anticoagulant therapies should be initiated with caution.

EXOGENOUS AGENTS

Various exogenous agents have been implicated in fetal losses, although studies fail to stratify by sporadic and recurrent losses. Of course, every pregnant women is exposed to low doses of ubiquitous agents. Rarely are data adequate to determine with confidence the role these exogenous factors play in early pregnancy losses.

Outcomes following exposures to exogenous agents can usually be derived only on the basis of case-control studies. In such studies, women who experienced an adverse event (e.g., abortion) recalled exposure to the agent in question more often than controls. However, case-control studies have inherent biases. The primary bias is accuracy of recall, control women having less incentive to recall antecedent events than subjects experiencing an abnormal outcome. Employers also naturally attempt to limit exposure to women of reproductive age; thus, exposures to potentially dangerous chemicals are usually unwitting and, hence, poorly documented. Pregnant women are also exposed to many agents concurrently, making it nearly impossible to attribute adverse effects to a single agent. Given these caveats, **physicians should be cautious about attributing pregnancy loss to exogenous agents.** On the other hand, common sense dictates that exposure to potentially noxious agents be minimized.

X-Irradiation and Chemotherapeutic Agents

Irradiation and antineoplastic agents in high doses are acknowledged abortifacients. Of course, therapeutic radiographs or chemotherapeutic drugs are administered during pregnancy only to seriously ill women whose pregnancies often must be terminated for maternal indications. More frequently encountered, pelvic x-ray exposure of up to perhaps 10 cGy places a woman at little to no increased risk. The exposure is usually to doses that are far less (1 to 2 cGy). It is also prudent for pregnant hospital workers to avoid handling chemotherapeutic agents and to minimize exposures during diagnostic imaging.

Alcohol

Alcohol consumption should be avoided during pregnancy for reasons independent of pregnancy loss (see Chapters 6 and 8). However, alcohol probably increases pregnancy loss only slightly. Some authors found a slightly increased risk for abortion in women who drank in the first trimester, whereas others[65] found alcohol consumption to be nearly identical in women who did and did not experience an abortion: 13% of women who aborted and 11% of control women drank on average three to four drinks per week; other investigations have reached a similar conclusion. Armstrong and colleagues[66] found the odds ratio to be 1.82 with 20 drinks or more per week.

Abstinence should not be expected to prevent pregnancy loss, and evaluation for other causes is still in order. Thus, women should not attribute a loss to social alcohol exposure during early gestation.

Caffeine

In data gathered in cohort fashion, Mills and colleagues[67] showed that the odds ratio for association between pregnancy loss and caffeine (coffee and other dietary forms) was only 1.15 (95% confidence interval [CI], 0.89 to 1.49).[67] Women exposed to much higher levels may, however, be at greater risk; Klebanoff and coworkers[68] reported an association between pregnancy losses and caffeine ingestion greater than 300 mg daily (1.9-fold increase). A confounding problem with investigating caffeine is difficulty in taking into account the effects of nausea, which is believed to be more common in successful pregnancies. In general, reassurance can be given concerning moderate caffeine exposure and pregnancy loss.

Contraceptive Agents

Conception with an intrauterine device in place increases the risk for fetal loss and can rarely result in second-trimester sepsis characterized by a flulike syndrome. If the device is removed before pregnancy, there is no increased risk for spontaneous miscarriage. Oral contraceptives use before or during pregnancy is not associated with fetal loss. The same applies for injectable or implantable contraceptives. There is no evidence for increased pregnancy loss after spermicide exposure before or after conception.

Chemicals

Limiting exposure to potential toxins in the workplace is prudent for pregnant women. The difficulty lies in first defining the precise effect of lower exposures and then attributing a specific risk. False alarms concerning potential toxins are frequent. **Various chemical agents have been claimed to be associated with fetal losses, but only a few are accepted as potentially causative.**[69] These include anesthetic gases, arsenic, aniline dyes, benzene, solvents, ethylene oxide, formaldehyde, pesticides, and certain divalent cations (lead, mercury, cadmium). Workers in rubber industries, battery factories, and chemical production plants are among those at potential risk.

Cigarette Smoking

Active and passive maternal smoking has a damaging effect in every trimester of human pregnancy. Cigarette smoke contains scores of toxins that exert a direct effect on the placental and fetal cell proliferation and differentiation and can explain the increased risk for miscarriage, fetal growth restriction (FGR), stillbirth, preterm birth, and placental abruption reported by epidemiologic studies.[70] Smoking during pregnancy is often claimed to cause miscarriage, but in available studies, confounding variables are rarely excluded. Increased miscarriage rates reported in smokers do, however, appear to be independent of maternal age and alcohol consumption[71]; based on urinary cotinine levels, 400 women with spontaneous abortions were compared with 570 who experienced ongoing pregnancies. Women with urinary cotinine had increased risk for miscarriage, but the odds ratio was only 1.8 (95% CI, 1.3 to 2.6).

Smoking is associated, from early in pregnancy, with a thickening in the placenta of the trophoblastic basement membrane, an increase in collagen content of the villous mesenchyme, and a decrease in vascularization. These anatomic changes are associated with changes in placental enzymatic and synthetic functions. In particular, nicotine depresses active amino acid uptake by human placental villi and trophoblast invasion, and cadmium decreases the expression and activity of 11β-hydroxysteroid dehydrogenase type 2, which is causally linked to FGR.[70] Within this context, direct damage to placental tissue could explain the higher rate of miscarriage in heavy smokers.

TRAUMA

Women commonly attribute pregnancy losses to trauma, such as a fall or blow to the abdomen. Actually, fetuses are well protected from external trauma by intervening maternal structures and amniotic fluid. The temptation to attribute a loss to minor traumatic events should be avoided. A nested case-control study of 392 cases and 807 controls showed no relationship between physical violence and miscarriage.[72]

PSYCHOLOGICAL FACTORS

That impaired psychological well-being predisposes to early fetal losses has been claimed but never proved. Certainly, neurotic or mentally ill women experience losses, but so, too, do normal women. Whether the frequency of losses is higher in the former is less certain because potential confounding variables have not been taken into account, nor have confounding genetic factors been considered.

Investigations most frequently cited as showing a benefit of psychological well-being are those of Stray-Pedersen and Stray-Pedersen.[73] Pregnant women who previously experienced repetitive abortions received increased attention but no specific medical therapy ("tender loving care"). These women ($n = 16$) were more likely (85%) to complete their pregnancy than women ($n = 42$) not offered such close attention (36%). One pitfall was that only women living "close" to the university were eligible to be placed in the increased-attention group. Women living farther away served as "controls"; however, these women may have differed from the experimental group in other ways as well.

Other studies have also reported a beneficial effect of psychological well-being.[74,75] Again, however, pitfalls exist in study design, and the biologic explanation for this salutary effect remains obscure.

MANAGEMENT OF RECURRENT EARLY PREGNANCY LOSS

Faced with a couple having experienced a spontaneous abortion, the obstetrician has several immediate obligations: (1) provide the couple information on the overall frequency of fetal wastage (10% to 12% of clinically recognized pregnancies, and many more unrecognized) and likely etiology (genetic and especially cytogenetic); (2) provide applicable recurrence risks (see Table 26-2); and (3) determine the necessity for a formal clinical evaluation. Fulfilling responsibility to inform patients can be facilitated by summarizing the salient facts cited in this chapter, emphasizing common etiologies responsible for fetal losses covered. Explicitly worth citing is the positive correlation between loss rates and both maternal age and prior losses. The maternal age effect is not solely the result of increased trisomic abortions but is also reflective of endometrial factors.

When Is Formal Evaluation Necessary?

A couple experiencing even one loss should be counseled and provided recurrence risk rates. However, not every couple needs formal assessment and a battery of tests. Infertile couples in their fourth decade may choose to be evaluated formally after only two losses. After three losses, couples have traditionally been directed to formal evaluation. Although lacking firm scientific basis for waiting until three losses, this is the benchmark for the RCOG and the European Society of Human Reproduction and Embryology (ESHRE).[76] The ACOG defines recurrent loss as either two or three consecutive losses. This 2001 ACOG guideline[77] is perhaps more defensible scientifically, but "consecutive" is arguable.

A couple being evaluated should undergo all tests employed by a given practitioner. There is little rationale for pursuing certain studies after two losses yet deferring others until three or more losses.

Any couple having a stillborn or anomalous live-born infant should undergo cytogenetic studies unless the stillborn was known to have a normal chromosomal complement. Parental chromosomal (conventional metaphase) rearrangements (i.e., translocations or inversions) should be excluded. If chromosomal studies on the stillborn were unsuccessful, common trisomies can still be ruled out by performing FISH on stored deparaffined tissue.

Recommended Evaluation

1. Couples experiencing only one first-trimester abortion should receive relevant information, but not necessarily be evaluated formally. Provide the relatively high (10% to 15%) pregnancy loss rate in the general population and the beneficial effects of miscarriage in eliminating abnormal conceptuses. Provide relevant recurrence risks, usually 20% to 25% subsequent losses in the presence of a prior live-born infant and only slightly higher in the absence of a prior live-born infant (see Table 26-1). Risks are, however, higher for older women than younger women. If a specific medical illness exists, treatment is obviously necessary. If present, intrauterine adhesions should be performed. Otherwise, no further evaluation need be undertaken, even if uterine anomalies or leiomyomas are present.
2. Investigation may or may not be necessary after two spontaneous abortions, depending on the patient's age and personal desires. After three spontaneous abortions, evaluation is usually indicated. If not done previously, one should (a) obtain a detailed family history, (b) perform a complete physical examination, (c) discuss recurrence risks, and (d) order selected tests enumerated in this chapter. Occurrence of a stillborn or live-born infant with anomalies warrants genetic evaluation irrespective of the number of pregnancy losses.
3. Parental chromosomal studies should be undertaken on all couples having repetitive losses. Antenatal chromosomal studies should be offered if a balanced chromosomal rearrangement is detected in either

parent or if autosomal trisomy occurred in any previous abortus.

4. Although perhaps impractical to karyotype all abortuses, cytogenetic information on abortuses is valuable. Detection of a trisomic abortus suggests recurrent aneuploidy, justifying prenatal cytogenetic studies in future pregnancies. Performing invasive prenatal cytogenetic studies solely on the basis of repeated losses is more arguable, but not unreasonable among women aged 30 years and older.
5. Endocrine causes for repeated fetal losses include poorly controlled diabetes mellitus, overt thyroid dysfunction, and elevated maternal TSH levels. Subclinical diabetes or subclinical thyroid disease should not be considered firm explanations. Luteal phase defects are no longer considered a likely explanation, although luteal support is still prescribed in pregnancies achieved with in vitro fertilization.
6. Of infections agents, only *C. trachomatis* seems of equal plausibility. These two agents are more likely to cause sporadic than repetitive losses. The endometrium could be cultured for *U. urealyticum*. Alternatively, a couple could be treated empirically with doxycycline (Vibramycin).
7. If an abortion occurs after 8 to 10 weeks' gestation, a uterine anomaly or submucous leiomyoma should be considered a potential cause. The uterine cavity should be explored by hysteroscopy or hysterosalpingography. Intrauterine adhesions should be lysed. If a müllerian fusion defect (septate or bicornuate uterus) is detected in a woman experiencing one or more second-trimester spontaneous abortions, surgical correction may be warranted. A large submucous leiomyoma may also justify myomectomy. However, the same strategies do not necessarily apply following first-trimester losses. Cervical incompetence should be managed by cervical cerclage during the next pregnancy.
8. Women with either acquired or inherited thrombophilias appear to have a slightly increased risk for first-trimester pregnancy loss. Thrombophilias explain at best only a small portion of first-trimester losses. There is a much greater likelihood that thrombophilias are the cause of a second-trimester loss.
9. One should discourage exposure to cigarettes and alcohol, yet not necessarily ascribe cause and effect in an individual case. Similar counsel should apply for exposures to other potential toxins.

LATE PREGNANCY LOSS (STILLBIRTH)

***Stillbirth* is the term used to describe pregnancy loss at 20 weeks' gestation or greater.** By weight, the definition is 350 g, the 50th percentile at that week of gestation. The frequency of stillbirths in the United States is 1 in 160 deliveries, or 25,000 annually. Stillbirths are increased in a large number of conditions, whose management is discussed elsewhere in this text. These conditions include obesity, multiple gestations with or without prematurity, infections (e.g., parvovirus-B19), and a host of systemic maternal diseases that include but are not limited to diabetes mellitus, chronic and gestational hypertension, autoimmune diseases, and renal and thyroid diseases. Table 26-4 shows prevalence and estimated rates compiled by Fretts in 2005[78] and reproduced by the ACOG in 2009.[16]

TABLE 26-4 ESTIMATES OF MATERNAL RISK FACTORS AND RISK FOR STILLBIRTH

CONDITION	PREVALENCE AMONG STILLBORNS	ODDS RATIO
General population	—	1.0
Previous growth-restricted infant (<10%)	7%	2-4.6
Previous stillbirth	1%	1.4-3.2
Multiple gestation		
Twins	3%	1.0-2.8
Triplets	0.1%	2.8-3.7
Low-risk pregnancies	80%	0.86
Hypertensive disorders		
Chronic hypertension	6%-10%	1.5-2.7
Pregnancy-induced hypertension		
Mild	6%-8%	1.2-4.0
Severe	1%-3%	1.8-4.4
Diabetes		
Treated with diet	3%-5%	1.2-2.2
Treated with insulin	2.4%	1.7-7.0
Systemic lupus erythematosus	<1%	6-20
Renal disease	<1%	2.2-30
Thyroid disorders	0.2%-2%	2.2-3.0
Thrombophilia	1%-5%	2.8-5.0
Cholestasis of pregnancy	<0.1%	1.8-4.4
Smoking >10 cigarettes	10%-20%	1.7-3.0
Obesity (prepregnancy)		
BMI 25-29.9 kg/m^2	21%	1.9-2.7
BMI >30	20%	2.1-2.8
Advanced maternal age (reference <35 yr)		
35-39 yr	15%-18%	1.8-2.2
≥40 yr	2%	1.8-3.3
Black women compared with white women	15%	2.0-2.2
Low educational attainment (<12 yr vs. ≥12 yr)	30%	1.6-2.0

Modified from ACOG Practice Bulletin: Management of Stillbirth. No. 102:1, 2009.

Pregnancy loss after 20 weeks is overall higher in African Americans (11 per 1000) than in other ethnic groups (6 per 1000), which include Hispanics and Native Americans.[16]

Recurrence

Recurrence reflects disease severity and ability to treat. Thus, blended figures are not necessarily appropriate. However, a few risk factors are broadly applicable. Maternal age is positively correlated with stillborn risk. This reflects not only the predictable known fetal etiologies (e.g., chromosomal abnormalities) but also maternal complications that are simply age related.

Stillbirth occurs more often in primiparous women of a given age than in multiparous women of comparable age. This may correlate to difficulty in achieving pregnancy, which is of greatest relevance to women requiring ART. Women who are subfertile (increased time to pregnancy) but never require ART have an increased risk for birth defects compared with women who achieve pregnancy in less than 1 year.[78] **Offspring of both ART couples[79] and subfertile couples not requiring ART[80] have**

20% to 30% more birth defects (OR, 1.2 to 1.3) than those of women becoming pregnant within 12 months of attempting.

Risks for stillbirth are highest (twofold) in women delivered of a growth-restricted infant earlier than 32 weeks' gestation.[81,82] This risk is, incidentally, independent of mode of delivery (cesarean or vaginal delivery). Using Scottish Morbidity Records (1981 to 2000),[83] the odds ratio for stillbirth recurring in the *second* pregnancy was 1.94.[83]

Genetic Factors

Genetic factors for stillbirths are receiving increased recognition with ACOG, which has provided specific management recommendations. **Chromosomal abnormalities are detected in 5% to 13% of stillbirths.**[84,85] Thus, special effort should be made to determine chromosomal status of a stillborn. It is now recognized that the traditional approach of obtaining fetal tissue after a stillborn infant has been delivered is suboptimal. Cell culture often fails, leading to no results in perhaps 50% to 75% of cases. **Successful culture for chromosomal analysis occurs in 80% when amniocentesis is used to obtain cells.**[16] It is tempting to eschew an invasive procedure in an already stressed patient, but this would not be in her long-term best interest.

Detecting even trisomies clinically by examination of a stillbirth is unexpectedly difficult because maceration occurs within days of fetal demise. Thus, medical records stating lack of dysmorphia should be suspect, save for obvious structural defects (e.g. cleft lip, myelomeningocele). Ultrasound results obtained when the pregnancy was still viable are probably more reliable. If amniocentesis cannot be performed or if cultures fail, one should attempt to obtain FISH results to exclude common trisomies. This can be done on placental tissues, umbilical cord segments, or internal (noncontaminated) tissues such as connective tissue.

The major yield of autopsy for a stillborn fetus is detection of an unrecognized mendelian explanation. This obviously alters management in subsequent pregnancies, for which reason a major effort should be exerted. Whole body photographs and whole body radiographs are appropriate, as is placental examination by a physician with requisite expertise. Considerable success has been made in particular in diagnosing skeletal dysplasia, often an autosomal recessive disorder that can recur in subsequent pregnancies. Other disorders may be autosomal dominant disorders arising as a result of de novo mutations. Distinguishing between these two possibilities is important because the recurrence risk should be almost nil if the etiology is de novo autosomal dominant. If parents refuse autopsy, the provider should attempt to obtain as much information as possible: photographs, radiographs or magnetic resonance images, examination by a geneticist, ultrasound. A head-sparing autopsy is preferable to no autopsy and may be acceptable to the parents.

Polygenic/Multifactorial

The frequency of virtually any isolated birth defects is higher among stillborn fetuses than neonates. This reflects adverse selection in utero, a phenomenon recognized for years in ultrasound surveillance.

TABLE 26-5 MATERNAL LABORATORY TESTS RECOMMENDED BY THE ACOG FOLLOWING STILLBIRTH

All Mothers Having Stillbirths
- Complete blood count
- Kleihauer-Betke or other test for fetal cells in maternal circulation
- Human parvovirus-B19 immunoglobulin G; immunoglobulin M antibody
- Syphilis
- Lupus anticoagulant
- Anticardiolipin antibody
- Thyroid-stimulating hormone

Selected Mothers Having Stillbirths
- Thrombophilia
  - Factor V Leiden
  - Prothrombin gene mutation
  - Antithrombin III
  - Homocysteine (fasting)
- Protein S and protein C activity
- Parental karyotypes
- Indirect Coombs test
- Glucose screening (oral glucose tolerance test, hemoglobin A1c)
- Toxicology screen

Data from ACOG Practice Bulletin: Management of Stillbirth. No. 102:1, 2009.

If an isolated, organ-specific defect occurs (e.g., cardiac), polygenic/multifactorial etiology and recurrence risks (2% to 5%) usually apply. On the other hand, such a defect may be merely the only one evident but actually a component of a multiple malformation complex. Ability to distinguish between these possibilities is a major reason for autopsy. The multiple malformation syndrome could indicate mendelian etiology.

Maternal Evaluation

Certain maternal laboratory tests are recommended by ACOG (Table 26-5). Of course, a mother whose pregnancies has medical complications has already undergone many tests, and the cause of the stillbirth may seem obvious (e.g., diabetes mellitus). It is prudent, however, to order all these laboratory tests because the ostensible diagnosis may prove erroneous. Of note, ACOG does not recommend testing for antinuclear antibodies, for certain serologies (toxoplasmosis, rubella, cytomegalovirus, herpes simplex virus), nor at this time for genetic tests other than a karyotype. It is likely in the foreseeable future that array CGH (see Chapter 10), a panel of organ-specific mutations (e.g., skeletal dysplasias), or other genetic tests will prove practical. Caution is necessary before concluding that a stillbirth was caused by a condition signified by a positive laboratory test (e.g., thrombophilia). Such a finding does not obviate the need for fetal autopsy and fetal genetic tests.

Management in Subsequent Pregnancies

High-quality ultrasound and vigilant fetal surveillance are universally recommended. Induction is recommended at 39 weeks, but before that time, only with demonstrated fetal lung maturity.[86] Management otherwise will focus on any specific maternal factors identified (e.g., diabetes mellitus). In some pregnancies, management will differ little from that of the general obstetrical patient. In others, prenatal genetic diagnosis will be necessary.

OBSTETRICAL OUTCOME AFTER EARLY PREGNANCY COMPLICATIONS

Most early pregnancy complications occur before 12 weeks of gestation and involve placentation and early placental development. There is increasing evidence showing that many failures of placentation are associated with an imbalance of free radicals, which will further affect placental development and function and may subsequently have an influence on both the fetus and its mother[2] but are often ignored by clinicians.

Complications, including miscarriage, threatened miscarriage with or without an intrauterine hematoma, and vanishing twin, are extremely common in early pregnancy throughout the world. Very little is known about the short- and long-term consequences of these complications on ongoing and, in particular, subsequent pregnancies. Most data available are derived from small retrospective series of many different complications and pathologies or large series describing specific pathology but with wide variations in the definitions of the pathophysiology.

Recent meta-analysis and reviews have indicated an increased risk for adverse outcome in ongoing pregnancies after an early pregnancy event. Clinically relevant associations of adverse outcome in the subsequent pregnancy with an odds ratio higher than 2 after complications in a previous pregnancy are the risk for perinatal death after a single previous miscarriage, the risk for very preterm delivery (VPTD) after two or more miscarriages, and the risk for placenta previa, premature preterm rupture of membranes, VPTD, and low birthweight (LBW) after recurrent miscarriage.[87] Clinically relevant associations of adverse obstetrical outcome in the ongoing pregnancy with an odds ratio higher than 2 after complications in the index pregnancy are the risks for preterm delivery (PTD), VPTD, placental abruption, small for gestational age (SGA), LBW, and very low birthweight (VLBW) after a threatened miscarriage episode; pregnancy-induced hypertension, preeclampsia, placental abruption, PTD, SGA, and low 5-minute Apgar score following the detection of an intrauterine hematoma; and VPTD, VLBW, and perinatal death after a vanishing twin phenomenon.[88] These data indicate a link between early pregnancy complications involving the placenta and subsequent adverse obstetrical and perinatal outcomes.

There is observed heterogeneity among most studies, and many of the older controlled studies did not make adjustments for relevant confounders for adverse obstetrical outcome, such as age, ART, economic status, education level, ethnicity, height, marital status, parity, previous obstetrical outcome, prolonged infertility, smoking, and maternal weight or did not stratify for other first-trimester complications.[87,88] However, overall more recent large meta-analyses and controlled population-based prospective studies have confirmed previous data indicating a strong association between specific early pregnancy events and subsequent late obstetrical complications in the subsequent or ongoing pregnancy.[88] In particular, the risk for PTD and VPTD is increased after most first-trimester complications. This suggests that the early detection of these risk factors could improve the screening of women at high risk for specific obstetrical complications in ongoing and subsequent pregnancies. Furthermore, the antenatal identification of these parameters during the first half of pregnancy should enable better management protocols and new therapeutic guidelines aimed at improving the perinatal outcome in these groups of women at higher risk for abnormal pregnancy outcome.

KEY POINTS

- About 50% to 70% of conceptions are lost, most in the first trimester. Losses in preimplantation embryos are especially high: 25% to 50% of morphologically normal and 50% to 75% of morphologically abnormal embryos.
- Pregnancy loss is age dependent, a 40-year-old women having twice the loss rate of a 20-year-old women. Most of these pregnancies are lost before 8 weeks' gestation.
- At least 50% of clinically recognized pregnancy losses show a chromosomal abnormality. Chromosomal abnormalities in abortuses differ from those found in live-born infants, but autosomal trisomy still accounts for 50% of abnormalities. A balanced translocation is present in 5% of couples having repeated spontaneous abortions.
- Many nongenetic causes of repetitive abortions have been proposed, but few are proved. Efficacy of treatment often remains uncertain.
- Uterine anomalies are accepted causes of *second-trimester* losses, but their role in first-trimester losses is less clear. Couples experiencing a second-trimester loss may benefit from metroplasty or hysteroscopic resection of a uterine septum.
- Drugs, toxins, and physical agents are uncommon causes of spontaneous abortion, especially repetitive. One should not assume that exposures to toxicants explain repetitive losses.
- Antiphospholipid syndrome (antibodies to LAC, aPL, and anti-B1-glycoprotein) is an accepted cause of second-trimester losses; its role in first-trimester losses is arguable. Strict ACOG criteria exist for applying the diagnosis of antiphospholipid syndrome to a woman having repeated first-trimester spontaneous abortions.
- In recurrent abortions, prognosis is good even without therapy. The live-birth rate is 60% to 70% even with up to four losses and no prior live-born infants. An efficacious therapeutic regimen should show success rates greater than these expected background rates, or should be assessed in a randomized control trial. Women having greater than four losses are less likely to have a cytogenetic explanation and may have a different prognosis.
- The frequency of chromosomal abnormalities in stillbirths (losses after 20 weeks' gestation or weighing at least 350 g) is underappreciated, as are nonchromosomal genetic factors (e.g., syndromes). Tissue for cytogenetic studies should be obtained by amniocentesis or chorionic villus sampling; cultures initiated from postdelivery products often lead to unsuccessful culture.

- A major effort should be exerted to obtain full autopsy and imaging on all stillbirths because findings can alter management in future pregnancies. If a couple declines autopsy, whole body radiographs, magnetic resonance imaging, and other noninvasive imaging should be pursued.
- Adverse first-trimester events or complications in a current or in a previous pregnancy may interfere with normal placentation and increase the risks for specific later obstetrical complications.

REFERENCES

1. Jauniaux E, Poston L, Burton GJ: Placental-related diseases of pregnancy: involvement of oxidative stress and implications in human evolution. Hum Reprod Update 12:747, 2006.
2. U.S. Department of Health and Human Services: Reproductive Impairments among Married Couples. U.S. Vital and Health Statistics Series 23, No. 11, Hyattsville, MD, 1982, p 5.
3. Simpson JL, Mills JL, Holmes LB, et al: Low fetal loss rates after ultrasound-proved viability in early pregnancy. JAMA 258:2555, 1987.
4. Regan L: A prospective study on spontaneous abortion. In Beard RW, Sharp F: Early Pregnancy Loss: Mechanisms and Treatment, London, Springer-Verlag, 1988.
5. Simpson JL, Gray RH, Queenan JT, et al: Risk of recurrent spontaneous abortion for pregnancies discovered in the fifth week of gestation. Lancet 344:964, 1994.
6. Jauniaux E, Gulbis B, Burton GJ: The human first trimester gestational sac limits rather than facilitates oxygen transfer to the foetus: a review. Placenta 24:S86, 2003.
7. Jauniaux E, Hempstock J, Greenwold N, et al: Trophoblastic oxidative stress in relation to temporal and regional differences in maternal placental blood flow in normal and abnormal early pregnancies. Am J Pathol 162:115, 2003.
8. Burton GJ, Jauniaux E, Charnock-Jones DS: The influence of the intrauterine environment on human placental development. Int J Dev Biol 54:303, 2010.
9. Burton GJ, Woods AW, Jauniaux E, Kingdom JC: Rheological and physiological consequences of conversion of the maternal spiral arteries for uteroplacental blood flow during human pregnancy. Placenta 30:473, 2009.
10. Hustin J, Jauniaux E, Schaaps JP: Histological study of the materno-embryonic interface in spontaneous abortion. Placenta 11:477, 1990.
11. Jauniaux E, Greenwold N, Hempstock J, et al: Comparison of ultrasonographic and Doppler mapping of the intervillous circulation in normal and abnormal early pregnancies. Fertil Steril 79:100, 2003.
12. Hempstock J, Jauniaux E, Greenwold N, et al: The contribution of placental oxidative stress to early pregnancy failure. Hum Pathol 34:1265, 2003.
13. Munne S, Alikani M, Tomkin G, et al: Embryo morphology, development rates, and maternal age are correlated with chromosome abnormalities. Fertil Steril 64:382, 1995.
14. Simpson JL, Bombard AT: Chromosomal abnormalities in spontaneous abortion: frequency, pathology and genetic counseling. In Edmonds K: Spontaneous Abortion. London, Blackwell, 1987, p 51.
15. Sorokin Y, Johnson MP, Uhlmann WR, et al: Postmortem chorionic villus sampling: correlation of cytogenetic and ultrasound findings. Am J Med Genet 39:314, 1991.
16. ACOG Practice Bulletin: Management of stillbirth. Obstet Gynecol 102:1, 2009.
17. Hassold T, Hunt P: Maternal age and chromosomally abnormal pregnancies: what we know and what we wish we knew. Curr Opin Pediatr 21:703, 2009.
18. Hassold T, Abruzzo M, Adkins K, et al: Human aneuploidy: incidence, origin, and etiology. Environ Mol Mutagen 28:167, 1996.
19. Fragouli E, Wells D, Delhanty JDA: Chromosome abnormalities in the human oocyte. Cytogenet Genome Res 133:107, 2011.
20. Kuliev A, Zlatopolsky Z, Kirillova I, et al: Meiosis errors in over 20,000 oocytes studied in the practice of preimplantation aneuploidy testing. Reprod BioMed Online 22:2, 2011.
21. Tempest HG: Meiotic recombination errors, the origin of sperm aneuploidy and clinical recommendations. Syst Biol Reprod Med 57:93, 2011.
22. Clouston HJ, Herbert M, Fenwick J, et al: Cytogenetic analysis of human blastocysts. Prenat Diagn 22:1143, 2002.
23. Bonduelle M, Liebaers I, Deketelaere V, et al: Neonatal data on a cohort of 2889 infants born after ICSI (1991-1999) and of 2995 infants born after IVF (1983-1999). Hum Reprod 17:671, 2002.
24. Singh RP, Carr DH: The anatomy and histology of XO human embryos and fetuses. Anat Rec 155:369, 1966.
25. Jirasek JE: Principles of reproductive embryology. In Simpson JL: Disorders of Sex Differentiation: Etiology and Clinical Delineation. San Diego, Academic Press, 1976, p 51.
26. Warburton D, Kline J, Stein Z, et al: Does the karyotype of a spontaneous abortion predict the karyotype of a subsequent abortion? Evidence from 273 women with two karyotyped spontaneous abortions. Am J Hum Genet 41:465, 1987.
27. Warburton D, Dallaire L, Thangavelu M, et al: Trisomy recurrence: a reconsideration based on North American data. Am J Hum Genet 75:376, 2004.
28. Rubio C, Simon C, Vidal F, et al: Chromosomal abnormalities and embryo development in recurrent miscarriage couples. Hum Reprod 18:182, 2003.
29. Munné S, Sandalinas M, Magli C, et al: Increased rate of aneuploid embryos in young women with previous aneuploid conceptions. Prenat Diagn 24:638, 2004.
30. Stern C, Chamley L, Hale L, et al: Antibodies to beta$_2$ glycoprotein I are associated with in vitro fertilization implantation failure as well as recurrent miscarriage: results of a prevalence study. Fertil Steril 70:938, 1998.
31. Stephenson MD, Awartani KA, Robinson WP: Cytogenetic analysis of miscarriages from couples with recurrent miscarriage: a case-control study. Hum Reprod 17:446, 2002.
32. Carp H, Toder V, Aviram A, et al: Karyotype of the abortus in recurrent miscarriage. Fertil Steril 75:678, 2001.
33. Arbuzova S, Cuckle H, Mueller R, et al: Familial Down syndrome: evidence supporting cytoplasmic inheritance. Clin Genet 60:456, 2001.
34. Bianco K, Caughey AB, Shaffer BL, et al: History of miscarriage and increased incidence of fetal aneuploidy in subsequent pregnancy. Obstet Gynecol 107:1098, 2006.
35. Munne S, Fischer J, Warner A, et al: Preimplantation genetic diagnosis significantly reduces pregnancy loss in infertile couples: a multicenter study. Fertil Steril 85:326, 2006.
36. Munne S, Escudero T, Colls P, et al: Predictability of preimplantation genetic diagnosis of aneuploidy and translocations on prospective attempts. Reprod Biomed Online 9:645, 2004.
37. Simpson JL, Meyers CM, Martin AO, et al: Translocations are infrequent among couples having repeated spontaneous abortions but no other abnormal pregnancies. Fertil Steril 51:811, 1989.
38. Boué A, Gallano P: A collaborative study of the segregation of inherited chromosome structural rearrangements in 1,356 prenatal diagnoses. Prenat Diagn 4:45, 1984.
39. Daniel A, Hook EB, Wulf G: Risks of unbalanced progeny at amniocentesis to carriers of chromosome rearrangements: data from United States and Canadian laboratories. Am J Med Genet 33:14, 1989.
40. Gardner RJM, Sutherland GR, Shaffer LG: Chromosome abnormalities and genetic counseling, 4th ed. New York, Oxford, 2012.
41. Kuliev A, Janzen JC, Zlatopolsky Z, et al: Conversion and non-conversion approach to preimplantation diagnosis for chromosomal rearrangements in 475 cycles. Reprod Biomed Online 21:93, 2010.
42. Stephenson MD, Sierra S: Reproductive outcomes in recurrent pregnancy loss associated with a parental carrier of a structural chromosome rearrangement. Hum Reprod 21:1076, 2006.
43. Verlinsky Y, Tur-Kaspa I, Cieslak J, et al: Preimplantation testing for chromosomal disorders improves reproductive outcome of poor-prognosis patients. Reprod Biomed Online 11:219, 2005.
44. Simpson JL, Elias S: Genetics in Obstetrics and Gynecology, 3rd ed. Philadelphia, WB Saunders, 2003.
45. Pettenati MJ, Rao PN, Phelan MC, et al: Paracentric inversions in humans: a review of 446 paracentric inversions with presentation of 120 new cases. Am J Med Genet 55:171, 1995.
46. Philipp T, Kalousek DK: Generalized abnormal embryonic development in missed abortion: embryoscopic and cytogenetic findings. Am J Med Genet 111:43, 2002.

47. Karamardian LM, Grimes DA: Luteal phase deficiency: effect of treatment on pregnancy rates. Am J Obstet Gynecol 167:1391, 1992.
48. Negro R, Schwartz A, Gismondi R, et al: Increased pregnancy loss rate in thyroid antibody negative women with TSH levels between 2.5 and 5.0 in the first trimester of pregnancy. J Clin Endocrinol Metab 95:E44, 2010.
49. Stagnaro-Green A: Thyroid autoimmunity and the risk of miscarriage. Best Pract Res Clin Endocrinol Metab 18:167, 2004.
50. Anselmo J, Cao D, Karrison T, et al: Fetal loss associated with excess thyroid hormone exposure. JAMA 292:691, 2004.
51. Mills JL, Simpson JL, Driscoll SG, et al: Incidence of spontaneous abortion among normal women and insulin-dependent diabetic women whose pregnancies were identified within 21 days of conception. N Engl J Med 319:1617, 1988.
52. Miodovnik M, Mimouni F, Tsang RC, et al: Glycemic control and spontaneous abortion in insulin-dependent diabetic women. Obstet Gynecol 68:366, 1986.
53. Ben Rafael Z, Seidman DS, Recabi K, et al: Uterine anomalies: a retrospective, matched-control study. J Reprod Med 36:723, 1991.
54. Proctor JA, Haney AF: Recurrent first trimester pregnancy loss is associated with uterine septum but not with bicornuate uterus. Fertil Steril 80:1212, 2003.
55. Salim R, Regan L, Woelfer B, et al: A comparative study of the morphology of congenital uterine anomalies in women with and without a history of recurrent first trimester miscarriage. Hum Reprod 18:162, 2003.
56. Stampe SS: Estimated prevalence of mullerian anomalies. Acta Obstet Gynecol Scand 67:441, 1988.
57. Simon C, Martinez L, Pardo F, et al: Mullerian defects in women with normal reproductive outcome. Fertil Steril 56:1192, 1991.
58. Ludmir J, Samuels P, Brooks S, et al: Pregnancy outcome of patients with uncorrected uterine anomalies managed in a high-risk obstetric setting. Obstet Gynecol 75:906, 1990.
59. Hartmann KE, Herring AH: Predictors of the presence of uterine fibroids in the first trimester of pregnancy: A prospective cohort study. J Soc Gynecol Invest 11:340A, 2004.
60. Simpson JL, Mills JL, Kim H, et al: Infectious processes: an infrequent cause of first trimester spontaneous abortions. Hum Reprod 11:668, 1996.
61. ACOG Practice Bulletin: Antiphospholipid syndrome. Obstet Gynecol 117:192, 2011.
62. Simpson JL, Carson SA, Chesney C, et al: Lack of association between antiphospholipid antibodies and first-trimester spontaneous abortion: prospective study of pregnancies detected within 21 days of conception. Fertil Steril 69:814, 1998.
63. Rey E, Kahn SR, David M, et al. Thrombophilic disorders and fetal loss: a meta-analysis. Lancet 361:901, 2003.
64. Kovalesky G, Gracia CR, Berlin JA, et al. Evaluation of the association between hereditary thrombophilias and recurrent pregnancy loss. Arch Intern Med 164:558, 2004.
65. Halmesmaki E, Valimaki M, Roine R, et al: Maternal and paternal alcohol consumption and miscarriage. Br J Obstet Gynaecol 96:188, 1989.
66. Armstrong BG, McDonald AD, Sloan M: Cigarette, alcohol, and coffee consumption and spontaneous abortion. Am J Public Health 82:85, 1992.
67. Mills JL, Holmes LB, Aarons JH, et al: Moderate caffeine use and the risk of spontaneous abortion and intrauterine growth retardation. JAMA 269:593, 1993.
68. Klebanoff MA, Levine RJ, DerSimonian R, et al: Maternal serum paraxanthine, a caffeine metabolite, and the risk of spontaneous abortion. N Engl J Med 341:1639, 1999.
69. Savitz DA, Sonnenfeld NL, Olshan AF: Review of epidemiologic studies of paternal occupational exposure and spontaneous abortion. Am J Ind Med 25:361, 1994.
70. Jauniaux E, Burton GJ: Morphological and biological effects of maternal exposure to tobacco smoke on the feto-placental unit. Early Hum Dev 83:699, 2007.
71. Ness RB, Grisso JA, Hirschinger N, et al: Cocaine and tobacco use and the risk of spontaneous abortion. N Engl J Med 340:333, 1999.
72. Nelson DB, Grisso JA, Joffe MM, et al: Violence does not influence early pregnancy loss. Fertil Steril 80:1205, 2003.
73. Stray-Pedersen B, Stray-Pedersen S: Recurrent abortion: the role of psychotherapy. In Beard RW, Sharp F: Early Pregnancy Loss: Mechanism and Treatment. London, Royal College of Obstetricians and Gynecologists, 1988, p 433.
74. Liddell HS, Pattison NS, Zanderigo A: Recurrent miscarriage-outcome after supportive care in early pregnancy. Aust N Z J Obstet Gynaecol 31:320, 1991.
75. Clifford K, Rai R, Regan L: Future pregnancy outcome in unexplained recurrent first trimester miscarriage. Hum Reprod 12:387, 1997.
76. Jauniaux E, Farquharson RG, Christiansen OB, Exalto N: Evidence-based guidelines for the investigation and medical treatment of recurrent miscarriage. Hum Reprod 21:2216,2006.
77. ACOG: Practice bulletin: management of recurrent pregnancy loss. Number 24. Int J Gynaecol Obstet 78:179, 2002.
78. Fretts R: Etiology and prevention of stillbirth. Am J Obstet Gynecol 193:1923, 2005.
79. Hansen M, Boower C, Milne E, et al: Assisted reproductive technologies and the risk of birth defects: a systematic review. Hum Reprod 29:328, 2005.
80. Zhu JL, Basso O, Obel C, et al: Infertility, infertility treatment, and congenital malformations: Danish national birth cohort. BMJ 333:679, 2006.
81. Surkan PJ, Stephansson O, Dickman PW, Cnattingius S: Previous preterm and small-for-gestational-age births and the subsequent risk of still birth. N Engl J Med 350:777, 2004.
82. Getahum D, Ananth CV, Kinzler WL: Risk factors for antepartum and intrapartum stillbirth: a population-based study. Am J Obstet Gynecol 196:499, 2007.
83. Bhattacharya S, Prescott GJ, Black M, Shetty A: Recurrence risk of stillbirth in a second pregnancy. BJOG 117:1243, 2010.
84. Laury A, Sanchez-Lara PA, Pepkowitz S, Graham JM Fr: A study of 534 fetal pathology cases from prenatal diagnosis referrals analyzed from 1989 through 2000. Am J Med Genet 143A:3107, 2007.
85. Korteweg FJ, Bouman K, Erwich JJ, et al: Cytogenetic analysis after evaluation of 750 fetal deaths: proposal for diagnostic workup. Obstet Gynecol 111:865, 2008.
86. Reddy UM, Wapner RJ, Rebar RW, Tasca RJ: Infertility, assisted reproductive technology, and adverse pregnancy outcomes. Obstet Gynecol 109:967, 2007.
87. van Oppenraaij RH, Jauniaux E, Christiansen OB, et al: for the ESHRE Special Interest Group for Early Pregnancy (SIGEP): Predicting adverse obstetric outcome after early pregnancy events and complications: a review. Hum Reprod Update 15:409, 2009.
88. Jauniaux E, Van Oppenraaij RH, Burton GJ: Obstetric outcome after early placental complications. Curr Opin Obstet Gynecol 22:452, 2010.

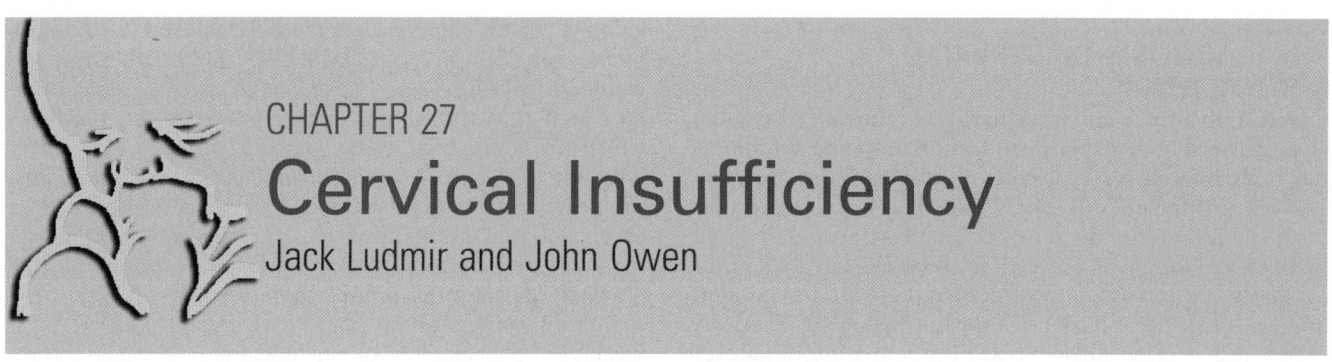

CHAPTER 27
Cervical Insufficiency

Jack Ludmir and John Owen

KEY ABBREVIATIONS	
Confidence Interval	CI
Diethylstilbestrol	DES
Loop Electrosurgical Excision Procedure	LEEP
Maternal-Fetal Medicine	MFM
National Institutes of Child Health and Human Development	NICHD

Since the initial description in 1658 of the cervix being "so slack that it cannot keep in the seed" by Cole and Culpepper,[1] few subjects in obstetrics have generated as much controversy as the term "cervical incompetence," now more correctly termed "**cervical insufficiency**." The competent or "sufficient" human uterine cervix is a complex organ that undergoes extensive changes throughout gestation and parturition. It is a key structure responsible for keeping the fetus and membranes inside the uterus until the end of gestation, and for undergoing significant changes that allow the delivery of the baby during spontaneous or induced labor.

The cervix is primarily fibrous connective tissue composed of an extracellular matrix consisting of collagen types I and II, elastin and proteoglycans, and a cellular portion consisting of smooth muscle and blood vessels. A complex remodeling process of the cervix occurs during gestation involving timed biochemical cascades, interactions between the extracellular and cellular compartments, and cervical stromal infiltration by inflammatory cells.[2] Any disarray in this timed interactions could result in early cervical ripening, cervical insufficiency, and preterm birth or miscarriage.

The incidence of cervical insufficiency in the general obstetrical population is reported to vary between approximately 1 in 100 and 1 in 2000.[3-5] Wide variation in incidence estimates is likely due to real biologic differences among study populations, the criteria used to establish the diagnosis, and reporting bias between general practitioners and referral centers.

THE SPONTANEOUS PRETERM BIRTH SYNDROME

Because spontaneous preterm birth is not a discrete, well-characterized disease process, it is best characterized as a *syndrome* comprising several anatomic and related functional components.[6] These include the uterus and its myometrial contractile function (i.e., preterm labor), decidual activation and loss of chorioamnionic integrity (i.e., preterm rupture of membranes), and finally, diminished cervical competence, either from a primary anatomic defect or from early pathologic cervical ripening (i.e., cervical insufficiency). In a particular pregnancy, a single anatomic feature may appear to predominate, even though it is more likely that most cases of spontaneous preterm birth result from the interaction of multiple stimuli and pathways that culminate in the overt clinical syndrome. Nevertheless, the relative importance of these components varies not only among different women but also in successive pregnancies for a particular patient.

Because the underlying processes (e.g., infection, inflammation) and their interactions with the anatomic components of the syndrome remain poorly characterized, the specific series of events leading to spontaneous preterm birth cannot be accurately determined, either during pregnancy, when the syndrome is recognized and managed, or by a careful retrospective analysis of the past obstetrical events. Thus, finding effective preventive management strategies has been generally unsuccessful and only empirically based.

THE DIAGNOSIS OF CERVICAL INSUFFICIENCY

Cervical insufficiency is primarily a clinical diagnosis, characterized by recurrent painless dilation and spontaneous midtrimester birth, usually of a living fetus. Because cervical insufficiency is likely part of a broader preterm birth syndrome, the diagnosis is usually retrospective and made only after poor obstetrical outcomes have occurred (or rarely, are in evolution). Because there are few proven objective criteria, and lack of a specific histologic diagnosis other than a rare, gross cervical malformation, a careful history and review of the past obstetric records are crucial to making an accurate diagnosis. Unfortunately, in many instances, the records are incomplete or unavailable, and many women cannot provide a reliable history. Even with excellent records and a complete history, clinicians might disagree on the diagnosis in all but the most classic cases. Confounding factors in the history, medical records, or current physical assessment might be used to either support or refute the diagnosis, based on their perceived importance. The physician managing a patient who experiences a spontaneous midtrimester birth is in the optimal position to assess whether the typical clinical criteria for cervical insufficiency were present. Possibly a more specific diagnosis of cervical insufficiency can be made by witnessing acute cervical insufficiency, a possible indication for *physical examination–indicated* (a.k.a. emergent) cerclage that will be covered later in the chapter. Because cervical insufficiency is generally a retrospective diagnosis and depends on a history of poor outcomes, clinicians have sought criteria that might lead to a prospective and more objective diagnosis. In women considered to be at risk for cervical insufficiency, based on an atypical history or because of other identified risk factors, serial examinations may be performed to detect progressive shortening and dilation, leading to a presumptive diagnosis of insufficiency, which may be amenable to therapeutic intervention (see box, Diagnostic Criteria for Cervical Insufficiency). Vaginal sonography as a screening and diagnostic aid will be discussed later in separate sections.

Diagnostic Criteria for Cervical Insufficiency

Historical Factors:
- History of painless cervical dilatation with preterm (midtrimester) delivery

Index Gestation:
- Painless cervical shortening and dilatation detected by serial digital evaluations
- Short cervix detected by midtrimester sonography in women with a history of spontaneous preterm birth

CERVICAL COMPETENCE AS A BIOLOGIC CONTINUUM

In 1962, Danforth and Buckingham[7] suggested that cervical incompetence was not an all or none phenomenon. Rather, it comprised degrees of insufficiency, and combinations of factors could cause "cervical failure." This concept never gained wide acceptance in spite of the obvious heterogeneity observed in clinical practice. Cervical insufficiency was generally viewed as dichotomous, possibly because available treatment strategies were similarly devised. These classic investigations demonstrated that the normal cervix is comprised predominantly of connective tissue, unlike the uterine corpus. This fibrous band is the chief mechanical barrier against the loss of the enlarging products of conception. The cervix and mucous glands also play an important immunologic role in preventing organisms from ascending into the normally sterile intrauterine environment.

In a subsequent report, these investigators analyzed cervical biopsies taken from postpartum women and compared them with hysterectomy specimens from nonpregnant patients.[8] Pregnancy was associated with increased water content, a marked decline in collagen and glycoprotein, and increased glycosaminoglycans. The cellular and biochemical changes suggested that cervical dilation in pregnancy is a dynamic process, and this might explain why a woman could have a pregnancy outcome consistent with cervical insufficiency in one pregnancy but, then without treatment, have a subsequent term birth. Presumably, the factors inciting the pathologic cervical changes might vary among pregnancies. Women with a more muscular cervix might have an unusual susceptibility or lower threshold for the effects of the factors that precipitated the clinical syndrome of preterm birth.

These earlier observations were enlarged by Leppert and colleagues,[9] who reported an absence of elastic fibers in the cervix of women with clinically well-characterized cervical insufficiency on the basis of their reproductive history. Conversely, cervical biopsy specimens from women with normal pregnancies showed normal amounts and orientation of these elastic fibers. Rechberger and colleagues[10] also compared cervical biopsy specimens among nonpregnant controls, women in the midtrimester with clinically defined cervical insufficiency, and women with normal postpartum gravidas. Compared with normal postpartum patients, they found increased collagen extractability and collagenolytic activity in women with cervical insufficiency, suggesting a high collagen turnover characterized by higher proportions of newly synthesized collagen with lower mechanical strength. It is unknown whether these microstructural and biochemical phenomena were congenital, acquired from previous trauma, or the result of other pregnancy-associated pathology. Collectively, these biochemical and ultrastructural findings support the variable, and often unpredictable, clinical course of women with a history of cervical insufficiency.[11]

Although the traditional paradigm has depicted the cervix as either competent or incompetent, both clinical data[12-15] and interpretative reviews[16-18] suggest that, as with most other biologic processes, cervical competence is rarely an all or none phenomenon and more likely functions along a continuum of reproductive performance. Although some women have tangible anatomic evidence of poor cervical integrity, most women with a clinical diagnosis of cervical insufficiency have ostensibly normal cervical anatomy. In a proposed model of cervical competence as a continuum, a poor obstetrical history results from a process of premature cervical ripening, induced by a myriad of underlying factors, including infection, inflammation, local or systemic hormonal effects, or even genetic predisposition. If and when cervical integrity is compromised, other processes may be stimulated, appearing clinically as other components of the spontaneous preterm birth syndrome (e.g., premature membrane rupture, or preterm labor). Knowing whether diminished cervical competence was due to a primary mechanical deficiency or other exogenous factors would define the optimal therapy.

TESTS FOR CERVICAL INSUFFICIENCY

Because the diagnosis of cervical insufficiency has been determined primarily from past reproductive performance and physical examination findings, the obvious limitations associated with the clinical diagnosis have prompted the search for sensitive and specific tests that could be applied in a prospective manner to women deemed at risk for cervical insufficiency, thus obviating the need for recurrent pregnancy loss. Such a test might provide a timely diagnosis and the potential for optimal therapeutic intervention.

Most of the earlier reported tests for cervical insufficiency were based on the functional anatomy of the interval os in the nonpregnant state and are of historical interest. Attempts at objective assessments include passage of a #8 Hegar dilator into the nonpregnant cervical canal without resistance[19] and traction forces required to dislodge a Foley catheter whose balloon was placed above the internal os and filled with 1 mL of saline solution.[20] Subjectively effortless passage of the dilator or removal of the Foley balloon with less than 600 g of traction force would make an objective diagnosis.

In 1988, Kiwi and colleagues[21] estimated the elastic properties of the nonpregnant cervix in two cohorts of women: 247 women with a poor obstetrical history and 42 controls. Although women in the poor obstetrical history group had significantly lower elastance values than the controls, there was significant overlap between the two groups. They reported no subsequent pregnancy outcomes, proposed no clinically useful cut-off for their evaluation, and could only suggest that such objective evaluation might ultimately prove to be clinically useful to accurately select patients for cerclage.

In 1993, Zlatnick and Burmeister[22] reported their experience with a cervical compliance score derived from the results of three other tests: hysterosalpingography, passage of a #8 Hegar dilator, and intrauterine balloon traction performed in 138 nonpregnant women. Their histories included prior delivery less than 34 weeks following clinically diagnosed preterm labor or preterm membrane rupture, with or without antecedent bleeding. A small portion of their cohort had a questionable history of cervical insufficiency. Scores could range from 0 to 5, and women with low scores of 2 or less were more likely to have been delivered at 27 to 34 weeks as compared with women with higher scores, who were more likely to have been delivered in the midtrimester at 14 to 26 weeks ($P = .01$). In subsequent pregnancies, cerclage was recommended in all women with a high score of greater than 2, and most underwent surgery. Surprisingly, in spite of surgical intervention, more women with high scores delivered at 14 to 29 weeks' gestation ($P = .07$), casting doubt on the clinical utility of this scoring system.

All such attempts at providing an objective diagnosis of cervical insufficiency failed because the tests were not evaluated with regard to standard characteristics (e.g., sensitivity, specificity) against some reference standard for the diagnosis. Moreover, none of these tests could reasonably predict pregnancy-associated conditions that would lead to premature ripening and cervical dilation (i.e., functional insufficiency). Finally, because there is no universally applicable standard for the diagnosis of insufficiency, and because the results of such tests were never evaluated and linked to a proved effective treatment, their clinical utility was, at best, theoretical. Because no test for cervical insufficiency in the nonpregnant patient has been validated, none of these tests are in common use today. **Clinical assessment of the cervix is performed in the index pregnancy when the diagnosis of cervical insufficiency is suspected.**

RISK FACTORS FOR CERVICAL INSUFFICIENCY

Based largely on the epidemiologic associations between the clinical diagnosis of cervical insufficiency and antecedent historic factors, numerous risk factors for cervical insufficiency have been recognized. These include prior cervical surgery (e.g., trachelectomy, cone biopsy), in utero diethylstilbestrol (DES) exposure, prior induced or spontaneous first- and second-trimester abortions, uterine anomalies, multiple gestations, or prior spontaneous preterm births that did not meet typical criteria for cervical insufficiency. Because DES usage was effectively curtailed in the early 1970s, this congenital risk factor should soon be of only historic interest.

Cervical damage from surgery is diminishing as indications for cone biopsy and more radical surgical procedures are diminishing. More common is the patient who has undergone a loop electrosurgical excision procedure (LEEP), usually for cervical dysplasia. These procedures are plausibly a risk factor for cervical insufficiency. Regrettably, it has not been feasible to simultaneously control for the epidemiologic risk factors that are associated with both preterm birth and dysplasia. In 1995, Ferenczy and colleagues[23] reported 574 women who had undergone LEEP and examined the reproductive performance of 55 women who conceived after the surgery. Their goal had been to obtain a nominal 7-mm thick specimen, and they cited a maximum excisional depth of 1.5 cm. In this series, there were no spontaneous preterm births before 37 weeks observed. Data from a similar series of 52 women revealed an incidence of spontaneous preterm birth of less than 10% and no midtrimester losses that might suggest a clinical diagnosis of cervical insufficiency.[24] A more recent and much larger retrospective cohort study by Sadler et al.[25] examined 652 women treated with laser conization, laser ablation, or LEEP, and compared these with a cohort of 426 untreated patients. The overall adjusted rates of preterm birth before 37 weeks' gestation were similar; however, the group with the highest tertile of cone height (≥1.7 cm) did have more than a threefold increased risk of preterm chorioamnion rupture compared with untreated women. Even considering the effect on preterm membrane rupture, the overall effect on preterm birth was not statistically significant, as the 95% confidence interval (CI) included 1.0.

Published data on cone biopsy is similarly reassuring. Weber[26] reported an incidence of preterm birth of only 7% in 577 pregnancies of women with a prior cone biopsy. Leiman[27] concluded that the risk of preterm birth was greater only when the maximum cone height was greater than 2 cm or the volume removed was greater than 4 mL. Raio and colleagues[28] performed a matched cohort study of 64 women who had undergone prior laser conization and observed no difference in the incidence of preterm birth compared with their controls (9.4% vs. 4.7%), and statistically similar gestational ages at delivery and birthweights. However, in a secondary analysis, a laser cone height greater than 10 mm was a significant independent risk factor for preterm birth. Other earlier reports have also suggested that larger cone biopsies increased the risk of preterm birth. Nevertheless, the distribution of preterm births in these populations did not confirm a disproportionate incidence of midtrimester loss consistent with a clinical diagnosis of cervical insufficiency.

Kuoppala and Saarikoski[29] retrospectively reviewed 62 women who had undergone cone biopsy and an equal number of matched control patients. The pregnancy outcomes of 22 who underwent elective cerclage were similar to those managed without cerclage, with fetal salvage rates of 97% and 100%, respectively. On the basis of their findings and review of seven other published reports, they concluded that prophylactic cerclage was not routinely indicated. Of note, in the largest published randomized trial of cerclage (summarized later), women with one or more cone biopsies *or* cervical amputations had an overall preterm birth rate of 35%. However, in this population, there was no benefit from prophylactic cerclage placement.

In summary, most women with prior LEEP or cone biopsy do not appear to have a clinically significant rate of second-trimester loss or preterm birth. However, women in whom a large cone specimen was removed or destroyed (including cervical amputations), or who have undergone multiple prior procedures, probably have an increased risk of spontaneous preterm birth. Whether prophylactic cerclage would be an effective preventive strategy in these at-risk women remains speculative. The available clinical trial data does not suggest a benefit from prophylactic cerclage, and so these women may be followed clinically for evidence of premature cervical changes. **Women with a history of prior cervical surgery and spontaneous midtrimester loss, suggesting a clinical diagnosis of insufficiency, should be considered for history-indicated (a.k.a. prophylactic) cerclage in future pregnancies.**

USE OF CERCLAGE FOR RISK FACTORS

Because of epidemiologic associations, clinicians have tried to expand the role of cerclage to include women with risk factors. To date there have been four randomized trials that included women with various risk factors for spontaneous preterm birth (and *possible* cervical insufficiency) whose managing physicians did not believe they required a prophylactic cerclage for a typical history of cervical insufficiency. Three of the trials[30-32] were relatively small and included women based on a scoring system[30]: twin gestation[31] and recurrent spontaneous preterm birth.[32] None of these trials showed a benefit to cerclage but generally confirmed a higher rate of hospitalizations and medical interventions in the cerclage groups.

The largest randomized trial of cerclage was conducted by the Royal College of Obstetricians and Gynecologists between 1981 and 1988.[33] A total of 1292 women were enrolled in 12 countries because of uncertainty on the part of their managing physicians as to whether a history-indicated cerclage was indicated. As anticipated, these patients comprised a heterogeneous group with at least six distinct risk-factor subgroups identified on the basis of their dominant history or physical examination findings. Although women assigned to cerclage had a significantly lower rate of preterm birth earlier than 33 weeks (13% vs. 17%; $P = .03$), the investigators estimated that approximately 25 cerclage procedures would be required to prevent one such birth. Moreover, women assigned to cerclage received more tocolytic medications and spent more time in the hospital. Puerperal fever was significantly more common in the cerclage group. Of interest is the finding in a secondary analysis that only the subgroup of women with multiple pregnancies affected, defined as at least three prior spontaneous preterm births including midtrimester losses, appeared to benefit from cerclage with lower rates of preterm birth (15% vs. 32%; $P = .02$). This secondary analysis confirmed the importance of assessing clinical history in considering the diagnosis and treatment of cervical insufficiency.

CAN SONOGRAPHIC EVALUATION OF THE CERVIX DIAGNOSE INSUFFICIENCY?

Over the past two decades numerous investigators have suggested that cervical insufficiency can be diagnosed by midtrimester sonographic evaluation of the cervix. Various sonographic findings, including cervical length, funneling at the internal os, and dynamic response to provocative maneuvers (e.g., fundal pressure), have been used to select women for treatment, generally cerclage (Figure 27-1). In these earlier reports, the sonographic evaluations were not blinded, leading to uncontrolled interventions and difficulty determining their value. Diagnostic criteria were disparate and, in some cases, not described in a quantitative or reproducible manner.

Later, large, blinded observational studies using reproducible methods were published.[13,34-37] These investigators reported the relationship between midtrimester cervical sonographic findings and preterm birth. The Eunice Kennedy Shriver National Institutes of Child Health and Human Development (NICHD) Maternal-Fetal Medicine (MFM) Units Network[13] completed a study of 2915 unselected women with a singleton pregnancy that underwent a blinded cervical sonographic evaluation at 24 weeks' gestation. The relative risk of spontaneous preterm birth increased inversely proportionally to cervical length. In spite of this highly significant relationship, as a test for predicting spontaneous preterm birth at less than 35 weeks, a cervical length cut-off of less than 26 mm (the

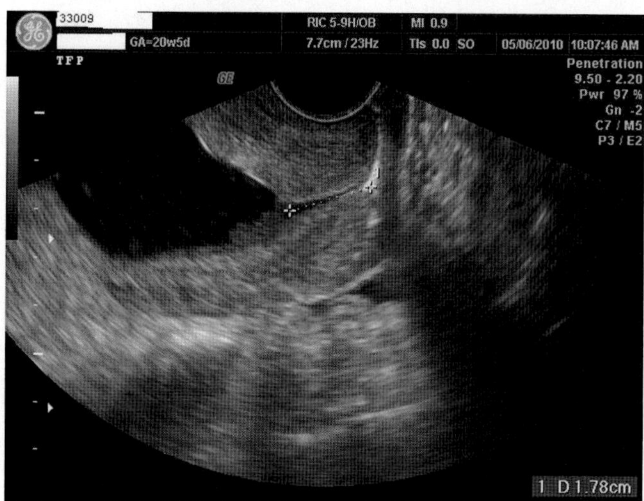

FIGURE 27-1. Short cervix *(calipers)* by transvaginal sonogram at 20 5/7 weeks' gestation. Note the presence of a biofilm (sludge) that has been associated as a potential marker for subclinical infection.[73]

population 10th percentile) had low sensitivity (37%), and poor positive predictive value (18%).

In a subsequent study, the NICHD MFM Units Network[37] examined the utility of cervical ultrasound as a predictor of spontaneous preterm birth at less than 35 weeks in high-risk women, defined as at least one prior spontaneous preterm birth at less than 32 weeks. Women believed to have cervical insufficiency (based on a clinical history) were not eligible. Beginning at 16 to 18 weeks of gestation, 183 gravidas underwent serial, biweekly sonographic evaluations until the 23rd week of gestation. The study design permitted analysis of the shortest observed cervical length over time, which also included any fundal pressure-induced (or spontaneously occurring) cervical length shortening. As in the previous study,[13] there was a highly significant inverse relationship between cervical length and spontaneous preterm birth. However, in this high-risk population, at a cervical length cut-off of less than 25 mm, the sensitivity increased to 69% and the positive predictive value to 55%. A secondary analysis of the data suggested that these high-risk women with shortened cervical length may have a clinically significant *component* of diminished cervical competence, because there was a preponderance of midtrimester births at less than 27 weeks in this group.[38]

These reports[13,37] support the concept that cervical length, as a surrogate measure of cervical competence, operates along a continuum of reproductive performance and provides prospective confirmation of an earlier published retrospective analysis.[12] Nevertheless, in spite of the consistent relationship between shortened cervical length and spontaneous preterm birth, the actual identification of an appropriate cervical length action cut-off and confirmation of the potential contribution of related cervical sonographic findings (e.g., funneling at the internal os) remains problematic. Clearly, cervical sonography performs poorly as a screening test in low-risk women,[12,13] but it appears to have significant clinical utility in high-risk women, defined as a prior early spontaneous preterm birth.[35-37] Whether cervical ultrasound has similar predictive values in other populations of at-risk women (e.g., DES, prior cervical surgery, multiple induced abortions, and so on) remains speculative, because it has not been well studied. Although some investigators have included women with these risk factors in their study populations composed primarily of women with previous spontaneous preterm birth, the results could not be subcategorized because of small sample sizes.[39] However, in a recent series of 64 women with various uterine anomalies, the authors observed an overall preterm delivery rate at less than 35 weeks of 11% and a significant relationship between cervical length of less than 25 mm and preterm birth,[40] with summary predictive values similar to other high-risk populations.[37]

Use of cervical ultrasound in twin gestations has also been reported.[41-42] However, the test characteristics, especially sensitivity and positive predictive value (<40%), appear to be generally lower than for women with a prior early spontaneous preterm birth. A systematic review[43] summarized the predictive value of vaginal sonography for preterm birth in 46 published series of both asymptomatic and symptomatic gravidas carrying singleton or twin gestations.

CERCLAGE FOR CERVICAL SONOGRAPHIC INDICATIONS

Under the presumption that shortened cervical length (with or without funneling at the internal os) is diagnostic of cervical insufficiency, several investigators have studied the effect of sonographically indicated cerclage on reproductive performance. Several investigators published retrospective analyses of uncontrolled use of cerclage in various at-risk populations with conflicting results, suggesting that cerclage was either effective[44,45] or ineffective.[46-49] In addition to the inherent biases present in these study designs and differences among study populations, small sample size, variable sonographic criteria, type of cerclage, inclusion of ancillary clinical findings, and definition of pregnancy outcome led to an inconclusive analysis.

Currently, four randomized trials of cerclage for sonographic indications have been published (Table 27-1). Althuisius and her colleagues in the Netherlands,[50,51] performed a two-tiered randomized clinical trial of high-risk patients, the majority of whom were believed to have cervical insufficiency based on their obstetrical history. In the first tier, eligible patients were randomly assigned to receive either prophylactic cerclage or to begin sonographic surveillance. Thirty-five of the patients assigned to the cervical ultrasound group were found to have a shortened cervical length less than 25 mm and underwent a second randomization to either cerclage or no cerclage. Both cerclage and no cerclage groups were instructed to use modified home rest. Of the 19 assigned to cerclage, there were no preterm births before 34 weeks versus a 44% preterm birth rate in the no cerclage–home rest group ($P = .002$). None of the women who maintained a cervical length of at least 25 mm experienced a preterm birth. Interestingly, the women who received cerclage for shortened cervical length had outcomes almost identical to women who received the earlier prophylactic cerclage. Rust and colleagues[52] enrolled 138 women who had various risk factors

TABLE 27-1 RANDOMIZED TRIALS OF CERCLAGE FOR SONOGRAPHICALLY SUSPECTED CERVICAL INSUFFICIENCY

AUTHOR, YEAR (reference)	POPULATION	*N*	SELECTION CRITERIA	GA FOR U/S EVALUATION (wk)	PRIMARY OUTCOME (wk)	CERCLAGE GROUP (%)	NO CERCLAGE GROUP (%)	BENEFIT?
Althuisius, 2001 (51)	History or symptoms suggesting CI	35	CL <25 mm	<27	PTB <34	0	44	Yes
Rust, 2001 (52)	Many had risk factors	115	CL <25 mm or >25% funnelling	16-24	PTB <34	35	36	No
To, 2004 (53)	Unselected, generally low-risk	253	CL ≤15 mm	22-24	PTB <33	22	26	No
Berghella, 2004 (54)	Most had risk factors	61	CL <25 mm or >25% funnelling	14-23	PTB <35	45	47	No
Owen, 2009 (59)	Prior spontaneous preterm birth 17-33 wk	301	CL <25 mm	16-21$\frac{6}{7}$	PTB <35	32	42	Yes*

*See text for details of reported benefit.
CI, Cervical insufficiency; *CL*, cervical length; *GA*, gestational age; *PTB*, preterm birth.

for preterm birth (including 12% with multiple gestations) and randomly assigned them to receive a McDonald cerclage or no cerclage after their cervical length shortened to less than 25 mm or they developed funneling less than 25%. Preterm birth before 34 weeks was observed in 35% of the cerclage group versus 36% of the control group.

In a multinational trial comprising 12 hospitals in six countries, To and colleagues[53] screened 47,123 unselected women at 22 to 24 weeks' gestation with vaginal ultrasound to identify 470 with a shortened cervical length of 15 mm or less. Of these 470, 253 participated in a randomized trial whose primary outcome was the intergroup rates of delivery before 33 weeks' gestation. Women assigned to the cerclage group (N = 127) underwent a Shirodkar procedure. They had a similar rate of preterm birth as the control population (N = 126), 22% versus 26%; P = .44. The authors did not specifically comment on the proportion of women in the control group who were delivered in the midtrimester after a presentation consistent with clinically defined cervical insufficiency; however, they observed four stillbirths attributed to birth at 23 to 24 weeks and five neonatal deaths in deliveries at 23 to 26 weeks. In the cerclage group, the respective counts were three and four.

Berghella and colleagues[54] screened women with various risk factors for spontaneous preterm birth (prior preterm birth, curettages, cone biopsy, DES exposure) with vaginal scans every 2 weeks from 14 to 23 weeks' gestation and randomly assigned 61 with a cervical length less than 25 mm or funneling less than 25% to a McDonald cerclage or to a no-cerclage control group. Preterm birth before 35 weeks was observed in 45% of the cerclage group and 47% of the control group.

The trial by Althuisius and colleagues[50,51] focused on women whom they believed had a clinical diagnosis of cervical insufficiency and who would have likely been candidates for history-indicated cerclage in the United States. Nevertheless, their study does suggest a potential role for cervical ultrasound in women with a clinical diagnosis of cervical insufficiency, if the intent is to *avoid* cerclage when the cervical length is maintained at 25 mm or greater.

A meta-analysis[55] of the four randomized trials[51-54] described earlier, analyzed patient-level data to estimate whether certain subgroups of women with midtrimester cervical shortening might benefit from cerclage, where benefit was defined as a reduction in the relative risk of preterm birth before 35 weeks. They observed a marginal benefit from cerclage in women with singleton gestations and especially in those who had experienced a prior spontaneous preterm birth (relative risk 0.6, 95% CI 0.4-0.9). Paradoxically, they demonstrated a significant *detriment* in women with multiple gestations (relative risk 2.15, 95% CI 1.15-4.01). Although this harmful effect has never been confirmed in a randomized trial, authors of cohort studies have not observed this relationship.[48,49]

Based on an earlier review of the utility of vaginal ultrasound for the diagnosis of cervical insufficiency,[56] the fifth randomized trial was performed by a consortium of 15 U.S. centers[57] and included only women who had had at least one prior spontaneous preterm birth at 17 to 34 weeks' gestation. They were followed with serial vaginal scans beginning at 16 weeks' gestation. As long as the cervical length was at least 30 mm, scans were scheduled every 2 weeks, but the frequency was increased to weekly if the cervical length was 25 to 29 mm. Women who developed a short cervix <25 mm between 16 and 22$\frac{6}{7}$ weeks were assigned to McDonald cerclage or no cerclage. These investigators observed a statistically significant decrease in previable births <24 weeks (6% vs. 14%), perinatal mortality (9% vs. 16%), and birth <37 weeks (45% vs. 60%), but a nonsignificant decrease in the comparative rates of preterm birth <35 weeks (32% vs. 42%). The number of patients with short cervix needed to be treated with cerclage to prevent one previable birth was 13. Of note was the observation that cerclage benefit was closely linked to cervical status and women with cervical length <15 mm at randomization accrued a much greater benefit than those who were randomized with a cervical length of 15-24 mm. This suggested that shorter lengths are more likely to be associated with a primary cervical etiology and thus more amenable to mechanical support, although the "optimal" cervical length (e.g., <25 mm, <15 mm, etc.) for recommending cerclage could not be established. Similarly the finding of a U-shaped funnel (but not a V-shaped funnel) was also a significant additional risk factor for earlier birth, even considering cervical length; in these women the beneficial effect of cerclage for prolonging gestation was also pronounced. **The results of this trial confirmed the findings of the meta-analysis[55]**

described above and established the utility of screening and ultrasound-indicated cerclage in selected women based on their *obstetrical history*.

PATIENT SELECTION FOR CERCLAGE

Most of what is known about the management of the cervical insufficiency is based on case series that reported surgical correction of the presumed underlying mechanical defect in the cervical stroma. The contemporary mainstay of treatment has been a surgical approach using one of the classic cerclage procedures, although both medical treatments and other mechanical supportive therapies have been used. Like many aspects of clinical medicine, current therapeutic standards are often based more on expert opinion and results of studies using uncontrolled interventions than the findings of randomized clinical trials.[58] This is particularly true for cervical insufficiency in which, to date, there have been no published placebo-controlled randomized trials of cerclage in women with a typical clinical history.

Branch in 1986[61] and Cousins in 1980[62] collectively tabulated over 25 case series of cerclage efficacy published between 1959 and 1981. Branch[59] estimated a precerclage survival range of 10% to 32% versus a perinatal survival range of 75% to 83% in the same cohorts of women managed with Shirodkar cerclage. Similarly, case series that used McDonald cerclage reported a cohort perinatal survival range of 7% to 50% before and 63% to 89% after cerclage. Cousins[60] estimated a "mean" survival before Shirodkar of 22% versus 82% post-therapy and 27% and 74%, respectively, for investigators who used the McDonald technique. In total, more than 2000 patients have been reported in these historic cohort comparisons. Interpretation of these series, as noted by Cousins,[60] is limited by the facts that (1) diagnostic criteria were not consistent or always reported; (2) definitions of treatment success were inconsistent (but generally recorded as perinatal survival, as opposed to a gestational age-based end point); (3) treatment approaches were not always detailed and might involve multiple combinations of surgery, medication, bed rest, and other uncontrolled therapies; and (4) cases were not subcategorized according to etiology (e.g., anatomic defects vs. a presumed functional cause). Nevertheless, based on compelling but potentially biased efficacy data, the surgical management of women with clinically defined cervical insufficiency has become standard practice, and it is unlikely that a well-designed intervention trial for classic cervical insufficiency will ever be performed if it includes a placebo or no-treatment group. Although interpretation of efficacy based on historic control groups is always problematic, collectively these reports demonstrate that even women with typical histories may have successful pregnancies without cerclage and that cerclage as a treatment is not universally effective. Both of these observations support the multiple etiologies and interactive pathways characteristic of the spontaneous preterm birth syndrome.

Because of its unproven efficacy in randomized clinical trials, and the attendant surgical risks, the recommendation for prophylactic cerclage should be limited to women with recurrent spontaneous preterm birth syndrome, when a careful history and physical examination suggest a dominant cervical component. Unless the physical examination confirms a significant cervical anatomic defect, consistent with disruption of its circumferential integrity, the clinician should assess the history for other components of the preterm birth syndrome: cervical insufficiency remains a diagnosis of exclusion.

Women with cervical insufficiency often have some premonitory symptoms such as increased pelvic pressure, vaginal discharge, and urinary frequency. These symptoms, although neither specific for cervical insufficiency nor uncommon in a normal pregnancy, should not be immediately dismissed, particularly in women with risk factors for spontaneous preterm birth. Thus, the history of rapid, relatively painless labor should perhaps better characterize the diagnosis of cervical insufficiency.

Although a history of preterm labor is generally considered to exclude the diagnosis of insufficiency, patients may develop some clinically evident uterine activity once their cervix has spontaneously dilated (Ferguson's reflex) but generally have a rapid progress in labor.

Similarly, a history of midtrimester spontaneous membrane rupture alone can neither confirm nor refute the diagnosis of cervical insufficiency, because spontaneous membrane rupture may occur after some pathologic cervical ripening and dilation has exposed the membranes to the genital tract flora. After spontaneous membrane rupture occurs, chorioamnionitis, vaginal bleeding (placental abruption), or labor may ensue, and these events may obscure the underlying etiology. However, if midtrimester membrane rupture occurs in the setting of a closed cervix on physical examination, or if it is followed by a typical course of either spontaneous or induced labor, causes other than cervical insufficiency should be emphasized. Conversely, if physical examination after membrane rupture shows marked cervical softening, effacement, and dilation with no antecedent history of painful contractions, the diagnosis of cervical insufficiency is supported, particularly if followed by a rapid and relatively painless labor.

A legitimate clinical question arises over the optimal management of a patient who has experienced one spontaneous midtrimester birth, especially when causes other than cervical insufficiency have been excluded by history and physical examination. The observation of a second similar midtrimester birth increases the specificity of the diagnosis and also the likelihood that history-indicated cerclage would be an effective treatment in the next pregnancy. Clearly, if the index midtrimester birth was associated with an identifiable anatomic defect, interval repair or prophylactic cerclage should be encouraged in the next pregnancy. However, in contemporary obstetrical practice, such anatomic defects are increasingly uncommon.

A systematic review by Blickman and colleagues addressed this issue of whether ultrasound-indicated or history-indicated cerclage was associated with better pregnancy outcomes in women at risk for cervical insufficiency.[61] They performed a thorough literature search and identified six relevant studies with varying methodologies, including cohort, case-control, and randomized trial designs. In none of these six reports was either strategy favored for preventing preterm birth. In the ultrasound-indicated groups, cerclage was avoided in 40% to 68% of women who underwent ultrasound surveillance. A more recent multicenter randomized trial of women with at least one prior spontaneous birth <34 weeks, demonstrated similar rates of preterm birth <34 weeks in the history (15%) and ultrasound (15%) groups[62]; however, in this trial fewer cerclage procedures were performed (19% vs. 32%) in the history-indicated group. Women were randomly assigned to the history or ultrasound arm prior to clinician's assessment of the history and the (clinical) diagnosis of insufficiency. While this trial confirmed the systematic review in that neither history nor ultrasound cerclage indication yields superior outcomes, the indications for cerclage in the history group were not thoroughly described (and reproducible), but rather left solely to clinician judgment. **Thus, although controlled clinical data are lacking, it seems reasonable to follow a patient with a history of suspected cervical insufficiency, using serial cervical ultrasound evaluations in the second trimester instead of empirically recommending cerclage (see box, Patient at Risk for Cervical Insufficiency: History-Indicated vs. Ultrasound-Indicated Cerclage).**

Patient at Risk for Cervical Insufficiency: History-Indicated vs. Ultrasound-Indicated Cerclage

- Preterm births will occur regardless of strategy chosen.
- Both strategies have similar rates of preterm birth.
- Fewer cerclages are performed with ultrasound-indicated cerclage strategy.
- It seems reasonable to follow patients at risk with sonography and perform cerclage based on sonographic findings.

ACUTE CERVICAL INSUFFICIENCY

Although the efficacy of cerclage for the treatment of a clinically defined history of cervical insufficiency remains unproven in controlled studies, women who present with acute cervical insufficiency, generally defined as a midtrimester cervical dilation of at least 2 cm, visible membranes, and no other predisposing cause (labor, infection, bleeding, ruptured membranes), are often considered for physical examination–indicated cerclage. Similar to case series proposing the presumed benefit of history-indicated cerclage, reports describing the outcome of women who present with acute cervical insufficiency generally have not always included a contemporary control group managed with bed rest or other intervention.

Aarts and colleagues[63] reviewed eight series published between 1980 and 1992 comprising 249 patients who received an emergent midtrimester cerclage and estimated a mean neonatal survival rate of 64% (reported range 22%-100%). Novy and colleagues[45] published 35 cases of insufficiency in evolution (cervical dilation 2-5 cm); the two cohorts included 19 women who received physical examination–indicated cerclage and 16 who were managed with bed rest. Neonatal survival was 80% in the cerclage cohort versus 75% in the bed rest group.

In a prospective, although uncontrolled, evaluation of cerclage versus bed rest (cerclage was utilized at the discretion of the attending physician), Olatunbosun and colleagues[64] studied women presenting with more advanced cervical dilation greater than 4 cm. The cerclage group comprised 22 women versus 15 in the bed-rest group. Although neonatal survival was not significantly different (17/22 with cerclage vs. 9/15 with bed rest, $P = .3$), gestational age at birth was a mean 4 weeks older in the cerclage group (33 vs. 29 weeks, $P = .001$). Rates of chorioamnionitis were similar between the two groups.

Although these reports are not of sufficient scientific quality on which to base firm management recommendations, collectively they demonstrate several important concepts. The earlier the gestational age at presentation and the more advanced the cervical dilation, the greater the risk of poor neonatal outcome. The finding of membrane prolapse into the vagina is also a significant risk factor for poor outcome.[65]

In a historical cohort study conducted by the Global Health Network for Perinatal and Reproductive Health, (women between 14 and 25$\frac{6}{7}$ weeks gestation with cervical dilatation were identified.[66] Of 225 women, 152 received a physical examination–indicated cerclage, and 73 were managed expectantly. Patients with cervical dilatation of 4 cm or more were more likely to be managed expectantly. In this study patients managed with cerclage demonstrated longer interval from presentation to delivery, improved neonatal outcome, and fewer deliveries before 28 weeks compared to expectant management.

Althuisius and colleagues[67] published a randomized clinical trial of physical exam–indicated cerclage plus bed rest versus bed rest alone in 23 women who presented with cervical dilation and membranes prolapsing to or beyond the external os before 27 weeks' gestation. Both singleton and twin gestations were eligible; however, no information on the amount of cervical dilation was reported, and so it is not known whether the groups were comparable in this important aspect. They observed a longer mean interval from presentation to delivery (54 days vs. 20 days; $P = .046$) in the cerclage group. Neonatal survival was 9/16 with cerclage and 4/14 in the bed-rest group. Although the survival differences were not statistically significant, there was significantly lower neonatal composite morbidity (which included death) in the cerclage and bed-rest group (10/16 vs. 14/14 in the bed-rest alone group; $P = .02$).

Other reports show that women who present with acute cervical insufficiency have an appreciable (nominal 50%) incidence of bacterial colonization of their amniotic fluid or other markers of subclinical chorioamnionitis[68,69] or proteomic markers of inflammation or bleeding.[70] Women with abnormal amniotic fluid markers have a much shorter presentation-to-delivery interval, regardless of whether they receive a cerclage or are managed expectantly with bed rest.

Mays and colleagues[69] performed amniocentesis in 18 women who presented with this syndrome and analyzed the amniotic fluid for glucose, lactate dehydrogenase, Gram stain, and culture; abnormal results suggested subclinical infection. Of 11 women who underwent cerclage with no evidence of subclinical infection, the neonatal survival was 100% and the mean latent phase duration from presentation to delivery was 93 days. Of the 7 women with abnormal biochemistries in whom cerclage was withheld, no neonatal survivors were observed, and the mean latent phase was 4 days. Recognizing that at least a portion

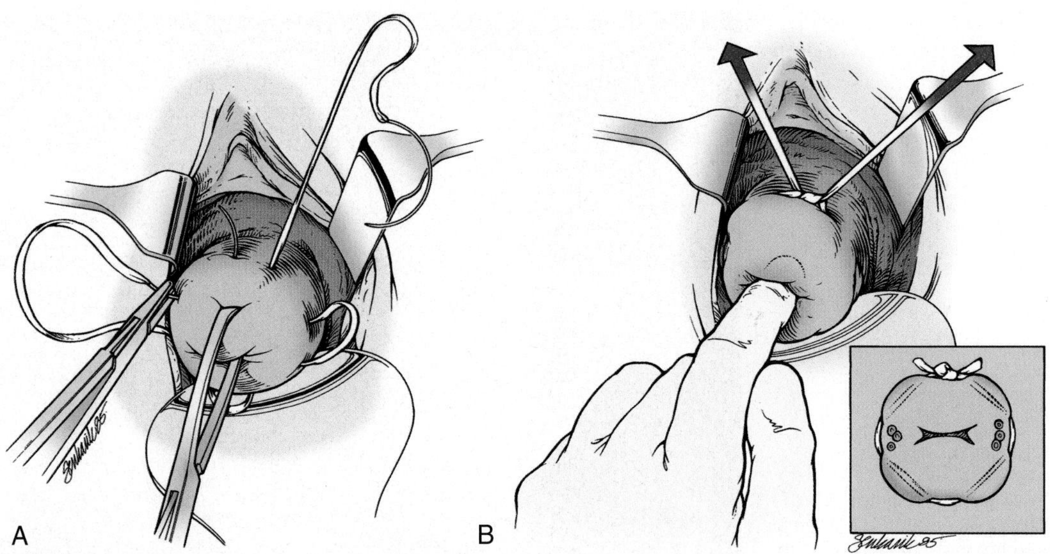

FIGURE 27-2. Placement of sutures for McDonald cerclage. *A,* We use a double-headed Mersilene band with four bites in the cervix, avoiding the vessels. *B,* The suture is placed high up in the cervix, close to the cervicovaginal junction, approximately at the level of the internal os.

of the 7 women who declined amniocentesis, but who received emergent cerclage, also had subclinical infection, it was predictable that the mean latent phase in this cohort was intermediate (17 days) as compared with the groups with amniotic fluid analyses. These investigators suggested that amniocentesis could aid in selecting candidates for emergent therapeutic cerclage. Interestingly, a sonographic marker of intrauterine subclinical infection has been reported (see Figure 27-1).[71]

In summary, the optimal management of women who present with cervical insufficiency in evolution remains indefinite. Although emergent cerclage may benefit some, patient selection remains largely empiric. Although not standard care, the evaluation of amniotic fluid makers of infection and inflammation appears to have important prognostic value, but it is still unclear whether and to what extent the results should direct patient management.

CERCLAGE TECHNIQUE

History-Indicated (a.k.a. Prophylactic) and Ultrasound-Indicated Cerclage

In 1950, Lash and Lash described repair of the cervix in the nonpregnant state involving partial excision of the cervix to remove the area of presumed weakness.[72] Unfortunately, this technique was associated with a high incidence of subsequent infertility. In 1955, Shirodkar reported successful management of cervical insufficiency with the use of a submucosal band.[73] Initially, he used cat gut as suture material, and later he used Mersilene placed at the level of the internal cervical os. The procedure required anterior displacement of the bladder in an attempt to place the suture as high as possible at the level of cervical internal os. This type of procedure resulted in a greater number of patients being delivered by cesarean delivery because of the difficulty in removing the suture buried under the cervical surface and may require leaving the suture in place postpartum. Several years later, McDonald described a suture technique in the form of a purse string, not requiring cervical dissection, which was easily placed during pregnancy.[74] This technique involves taking four or five bites as high as possible in the cervix, trying to avoid injury to the bladder or the rectum, with placement of a knot anteriorly to facilitate removal (Figure 27-2). Several types of suture material have been used.[75] We have been successful in using a Mersilene tape. However, the use of thinner suture material, such as Prolene or other synthetic nonabsorbable sutures like Ethibond, is advocated by others, with the argument that the width of the Mersilene tape places the patient at greater risk for infection.[75,76] Currently, there is no evidence that placing two sutures results in better outcomes than placing one.[77-79] Preoperative patient preparations, including the use of prophylactic antibiotics or tocolytics, have not been proven to be of benefit. We perform a culture for group B streptococcus and give preoperative penicillin to the patient with a positive culture, although the use of perioperative cultures prior to cerclage placement has not been evaluated in a proper way. History-indicated cerclage placement is performed after the first trimester, to avoid the risk of spontaneous loss most likely attributable to chromosomal abnormalities.[77,78] The choice of anesthesia for cerclage varies.[80] Chen et al.[81] did not show a difference in outcome between general versus regional anesthesia. In our experience, a short-acting regional anesthetic is sufficient. We advise patients to remain on bed rest for the first 48 hours after cerclage and to avoid intercourse until their follow-up postoperative visit. Decisions regarding physical activity and intercourse are individualized, and based on the status of the cervix as determined by outpatient digital evaluation or sonographic findings (Figure 27-3).[82] The suture is usually removed electively at 37 weeks. However, recent data suggest that removing the cerclage at the time of labor does not result in greater morbidity for the mother.[83] The mean interval between cerclage removal and spontaneous delivery is 14 days.[84]

In patients with a hypoplastic cervix, such as those exposed to DES in utero, history of a large cervical

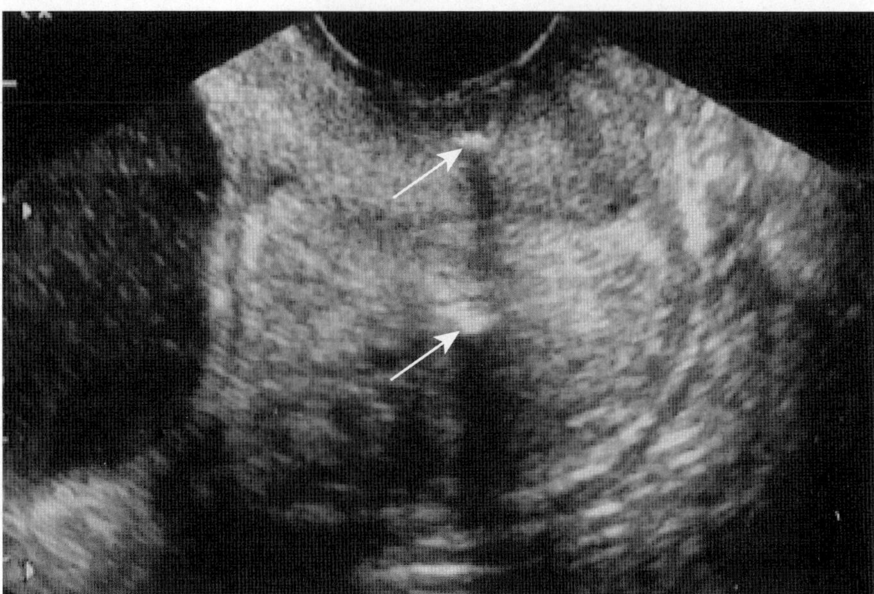

FIGURE 27-3. Transvaginal sonogram of the cervix after cerclage placement. The internal os is closed, and there is no funneling. Echogenic spots in the cervix correspond to cerclage *(arrows)*.

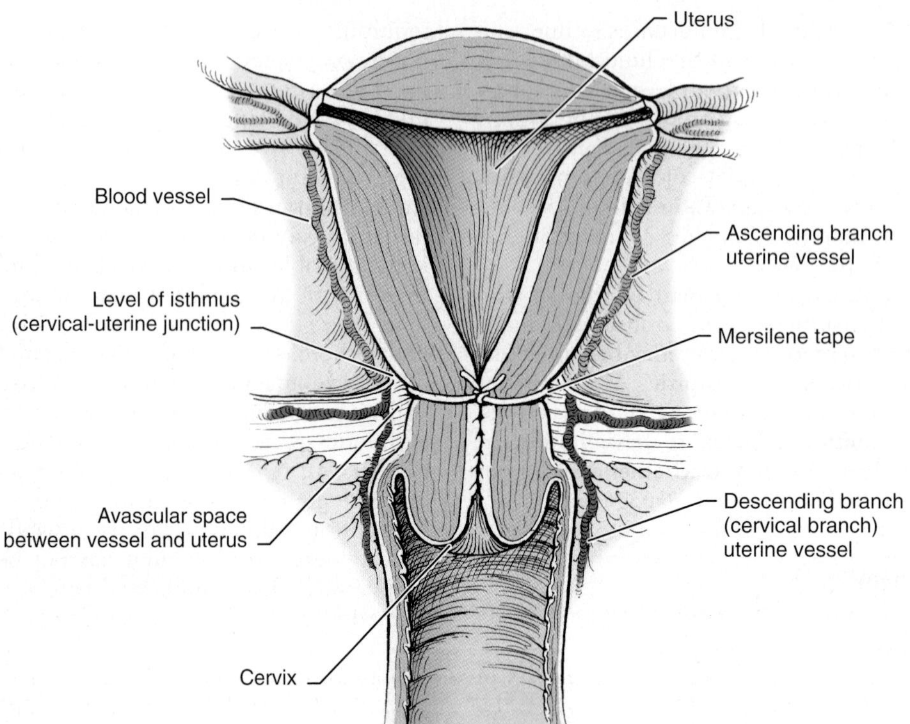

FIGURE 27-4. Abdominal cerclage. Surgical placement of circumferential Mersilene tape around uterine isthmus and median to uterine vessels. Knot is tied anteriorly.

conization, or a prior history of failed vaginal cerclage, an abdominal cerclage has been recommended.[85] This procedure is usually done between 11 and 13 weeks, and requires a laparotomy. A bladder flap is created, and a Mersilene tape is placed at the level of the junction between the lower uterine segment and the cervix, lateral to the uterus and medial to the uterine vessels (Figure 27-4). Greater morbidity, including injury to the uterine vessels, requires expertise with this procedure. In our experience with more than 60 cases, we have found it helpful to have an assistant provide fundal traction while the surgeon grasps the uterine vessels and retracts them laterally, exposing an avascular space between the artery and the cervix. A right angle clamp is passed anteriorly to posterior through this avascular space, tenting and incising the posterior leaf of the broad ligament and grasping a Mersilene tape that is brought back through the space. The same procedure is repeated on the opposite side, and the tape is tied anteriorly (Figures 27-5 to 27-8). Novy and colleagues[86] reported extensive experience with this procedure, with

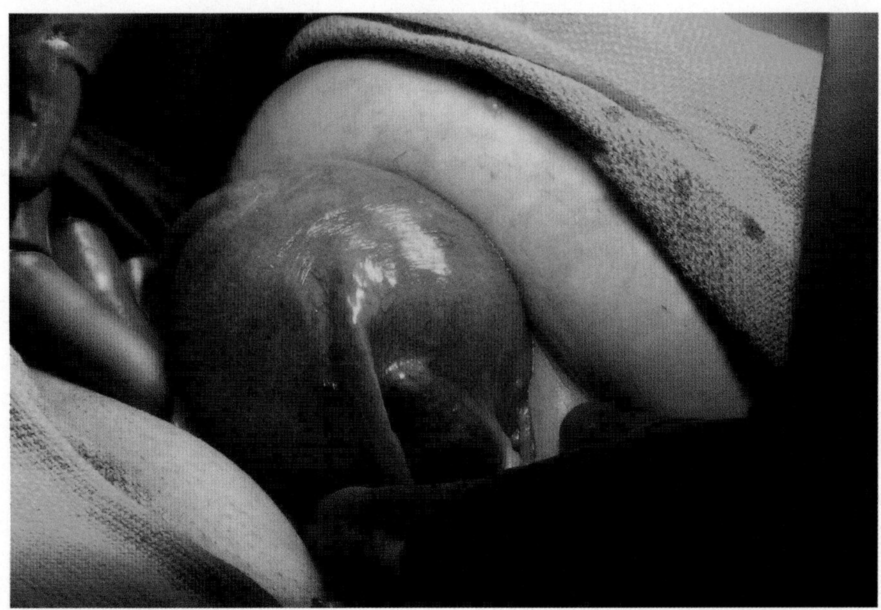

FIGURE 27-5. Abdominal cerclage at 12 weeks' gestation. Uterus is exteriorized.

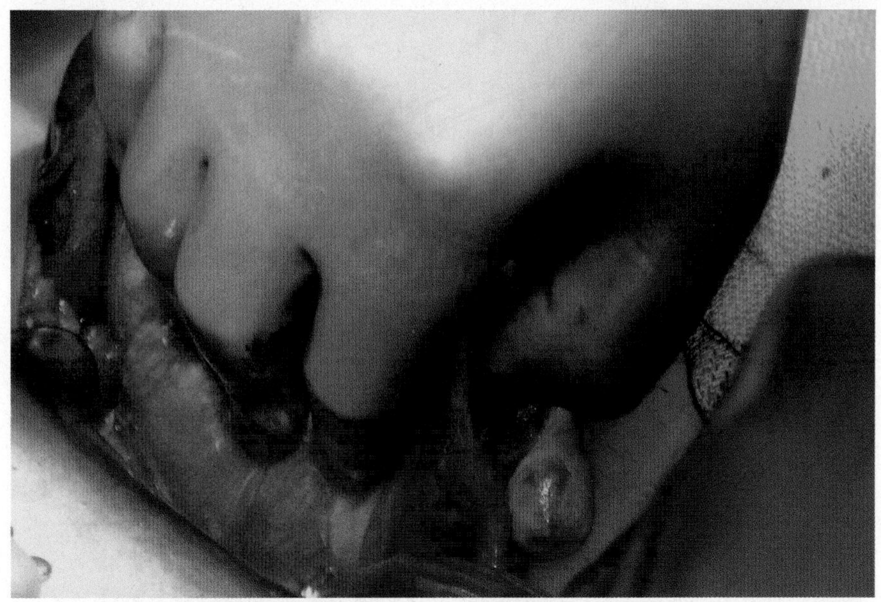

FIGURE 27-6. Abdominal cerclage. Bladder flap has been created and surgeon identifies and palpates uterine vessel.

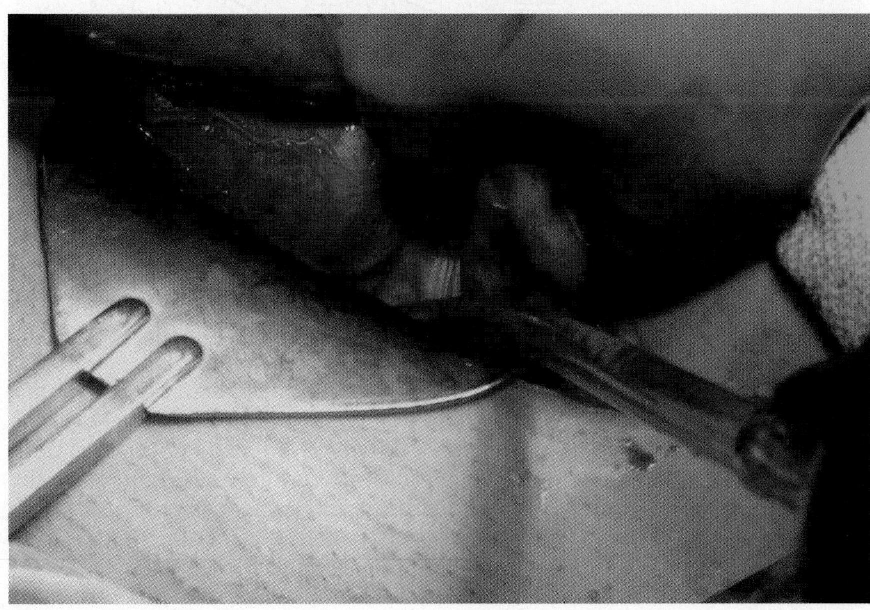

FIGURE 27-7. Abdominal cerclage. Surgeon retracts uterine vessel laterally to create an avascular space between uterus and vessel, before passing right angle clamp with Mersilene tape through this space.

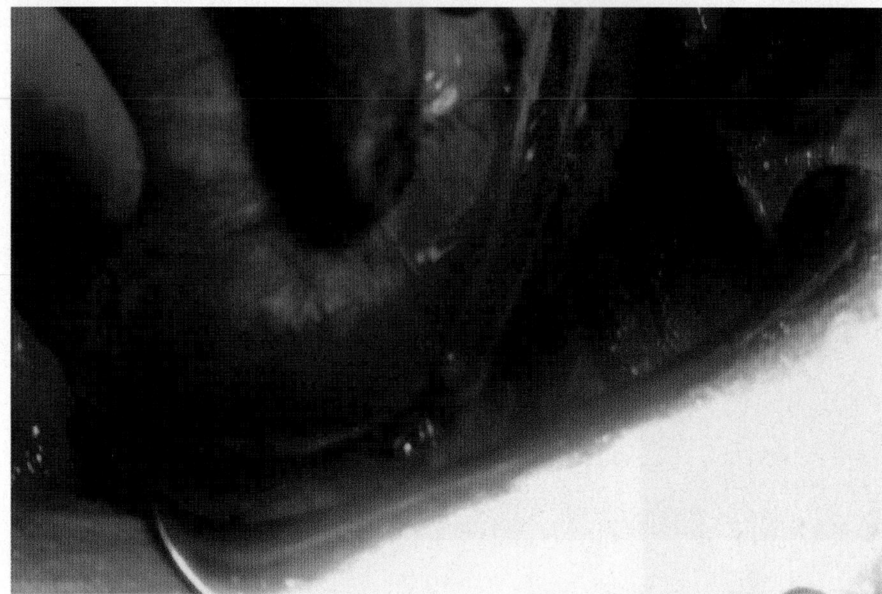

FIGURE 27-8. Abdominal cerclage. Mersilene tape has been placed circumferencially around uterine isthmus and tied anteriorly. Notice ballooning of the lower uterine segment above suture.

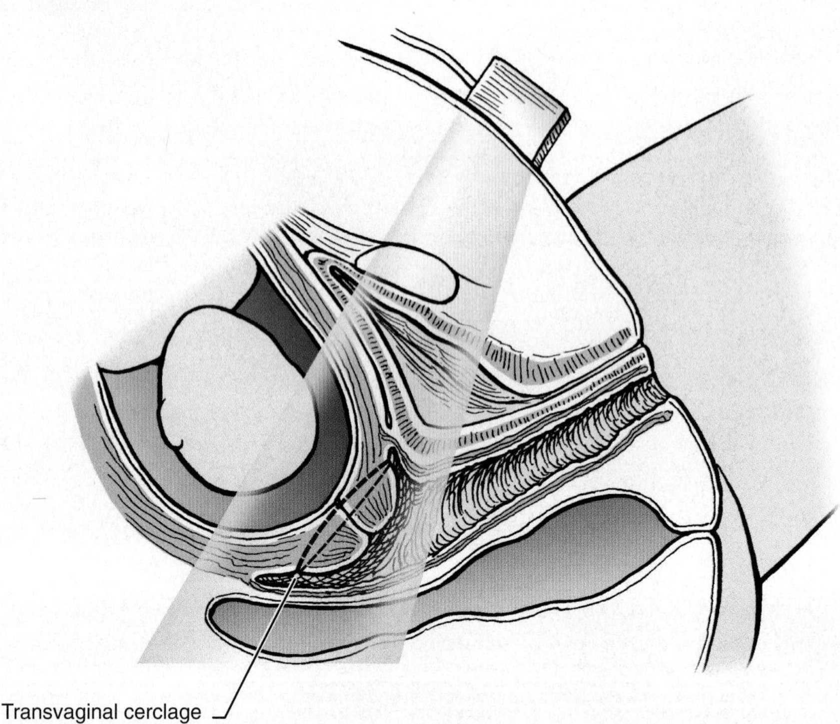

FIGURE 27-9. Transvaginal cerclage under ultrasound guidance. (Modified from Ludmir J, Jackson GM, Samuels P: Transvaginal cerclage under ultrasound guidance in cases of severe cervical hypoplasia. Obstet Gynecol 75:1067, 1991.)

low morbidity and favorable outcome. Cesarean delivery is necessary, and the suture is left in place if future fertility is desired. In cases of pregnancy complications requiring midtrimester delivery, we have either performed a posterior colpotomy, cutting the tape and allowing for vaginal delivery, or performed laparotomy and hysterotomy, leaving the suture intact. In most of the reported series of abdominal cerclage, including ours, this surgical procedure was performed during gestation.[86] However, recently Groom and colleagues[87] described this procedure as an interval cerclage in the nonpregnant state with subsequent good pregnancy outcome. Advantages of an interval procedure include avoidance of laparotomy in pregnancy and less bleeding morbidity. Disadvantages include inability to become pregnant and the difficulties of pregnancy management if the gestation results in a first-trimester miscarriage. Currently, there are no studies comparing interval versus abdominal cerclage during gestation that enable us to make specific recommendations about timing of the procedure.

To avoid an abdominal procedure in selected patients, we have described the placement of a transvaginal cerclage in cases of a hypoplastic cervix, or when the cervix is flush against the vaginal wall.[88] Under ultrasound guidance, the supravaginal portion of the cervix is dissected away from the bladder and a suture is placed either in a purse-string fashion, or in cross fashion from 12 to 6 o'clock and 3 to 9 o'clock (Figure 27-9). We have performed this procedure in 22 patients, avoiding an abdominal procedure, with successful pregnancy outcome. Fifty percent of patients had a cesarean delivery, and the rest delivered vaginally after the suture was cut through a small posterior colpotomy incision. In the last few years, a laparoscopic abdominal approach to the cervix has been described using the same principles as an abdominal cerclage.[89,90] The procedure has been described primarily in nonpregnant women with subsequent good pregnancy outcome. Cho and colleagues[91] performed laparoscopic abdominal cerclage during pregnancy in 20 patients with minimal morbidity, and reported successful outcome in 19 of them. Recently, robotic-assisted laparoscopic placement of transabdominal cerclage during pregnancy has been described by Wolfe et al.[92] and we have started to use this technique in selected cases. Because of the lack of proper evaluation of these newer modalities of cerclage placement, recommendations based on evidence cannot be made. **There is a need for randomized trials evaluating these newer techniques in the nonpregnant and pregnant state, compared with a vaginal approach to determine the best approach to patients with a history of failed cerclage or extremely short cervix that prevents a vaginal approach.**

Physical Examination–Indicated (a.k.a. Emergent) Cerclage

Patients demonstrating cervical change either by digital evaluation or transvaginal sonography may benefit from a cerclage.[93-96] However, the gestational age limit for cerclage placement is ill defined. Although some clinicians offer this therapeutic modality up to 28 weeks,[97] we do not advocate the use of cerclage beyond 24 weeks' gestation, because of fetal viability concerns and the potential to cause a preterm delivery while placing the cerclage. Some of these patients have been managed successfully with strict bed rest.[98] If the decision is made to place a cerclage, we treat preoperatively with antibiotics and nonsteroidal anti-inflammatory agents, such as indomethacin, although the perioperative management of these patients has not been subject to rigorous study. The patient is placed on strict bed rest for the first 72 hours and is advised to refrain from intercourse and strenuous physical activity for the remainder of the pregnancy. We follow these patients with frequent sonographic assessment of the cervix and recommend strict bed rest if the membranes are prolapsing to the level of the suture.[99] Prophylactic tocolytics are not used after the procedure.

In situations in which the cervix has dilated enough to allow visualization of the membranes or the membranes have prolapsed into the vagina, placing a cerclage may be difficult, but should be considered.[97,99-103] These patients are at high risk of having a subclinical infection and subsequent poor outcome, as described previously.[100,104] To rule out infection, some clinicians advocate amniocentesis before cerclage placement.[69] Several techniques have been described to reduce the prolapsing membranes, including the following: placing the patient in Trendelenburg position; the use of a pediatric Foley catheter to tease the membranes into the endocervical canal; and instilling 1 L of saline into the bladder with upper displacement of the lower uterine segment (Figure 27-10).[102-105] The efficacy of antibiotics or tocolytics has not been properly studied, but most series advocate their use. Although clinicians have been reluctant to offer cerclage in patients with protruding membranes, some reports have suggested salvage rate in excess of 70% despite advanced cervical dilatation.[106-108]

Risks of Cerclage

Cervical lacerations at the time of delivery are one of the most common complications from a cerclage, occurring in 1% to 13% of patients.[77] Three percent of patients require cesarean delivery because of the inability of the cervix to dilate secondary to cervical scarring and dystocia.[77] Although the risk of infection is minimal with a prophylactic cerclage, the risk increases significantly in cases of advanced dilatation with exposure of membranes to the birth canal.[104] However, this infectious morbidity may be the result of subclinical chorioamnionitis. Cervical cerclage displacement occurs in a small number of patients. We have not performed revision of the cerclage during the index pregnancy, although small series have reported successful surgical treatment of a failed cerclage.[79] When the clinician is faced with premature rupture of membranes distant from term in a patient with cerclage, the decision to remove or leave the suture is controversial. Our own data suggest that with suture retention, there is an increased period of latency, at the expense of an increased risk for neonatal sepsis and mortality.[109] These data have been challenged by reports from Jenkins and colleages[110] suggesting an increased latency period (244 vs. 119 hours) without an increase in neonatal morbidity, in cases of retained cerclage, and by McElrath and colleagues,[111] who did not find differences in latency or neonatal outcome in patients when the suture was left in situ after rupture of the membranes. Decisions to remove the suture at the time of ruptured membranes should be individualized until more information becomes available. Finally, even though cerclage placement is considered a benign procedure, a maternal death secondary to sepsis in a patient with retained cerclage has been reported.[112] Because of associated risks, and questionable effectiveness, the liberal use of this surgical procedure is discouraged and the decision should be carefully balanced against potential harm, in particular for patients in whom the indications for cerclage are not clear.

Alternative Treatments to Cervical Cerclage

Nonsurgical interventions have been advocated for patients with presumed cervical insufficiency. The rationale for the recommendation for bed rest alone, or in conjunction with cerclage, relies in the theoretical concept of putting less pressure on the cervix while in the recumbent position. The validity of this concept has not been scientifically proven and to date there are no proper studies evaluating this intervention alone versus cerclage, in a randomized prospective fashion. The efficacy of pharmacologic agents such as indomethacin, progesterone, antibiotics, and others remains to be elucidated. The NICHD MFM Units Network reported their results, comparing weekly injections of 17-alpha hydroxyprogesterone caproate for the prevention of preterm birth in women with a history of prior spontaneous preterm delivery. Patients receiving the progestational agent had a 33% reduction in preterm birth

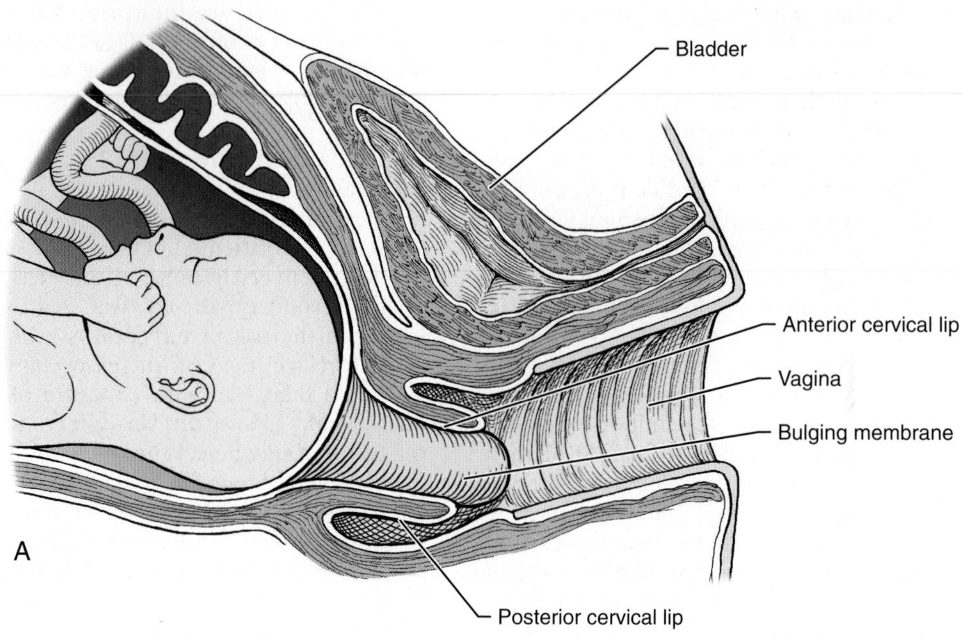

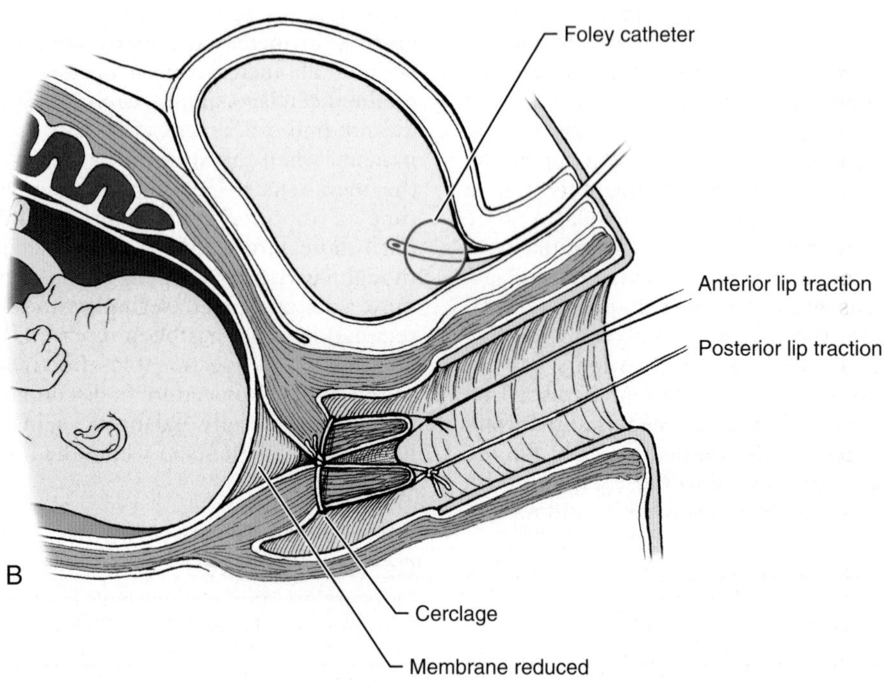

FIGURE 27-10. Emergent cerclage for bulging membranes at 23 weeks. **A,** Cervix dilated 3 cm with membranes protruding through the external cervical os into the vagina. **B,** Patient placed in Trendelenburg position, and bladder filled with saline. Stay silk sutures placed on anterior and posterior lip for traction while reducing membranes. McDonald cerclage placed distal to reduced membranes.

compared with those receiving placebo.[113] Vaginal progesterone has been associated with a reduction of preterm birth in women with a very short cervical length.[114] At this time, it is unclear how this information may be applied to patients with a clinical history of cervical insufficiency, with or without the concurrent use of cerclage, and further investigation is necessary. The authors of a recent investigation concluded that 17-alpha-hydroxyprogesterone may not confer additional benefit to ultrasound-indicated cerclage in women with prior spontaneous preterm birth.[115]

Since the description by Vitsky in 1961 of the use of a vaginal pessary instead of cerclage for patients with cervical insufficiency,[116] several studies, mainly in Europe, suggest the same outcome for patients managed with this noninvasive modality compared with a surgical intervention.[117] Recently Arabin et al.[118] studied the use of a vaginal

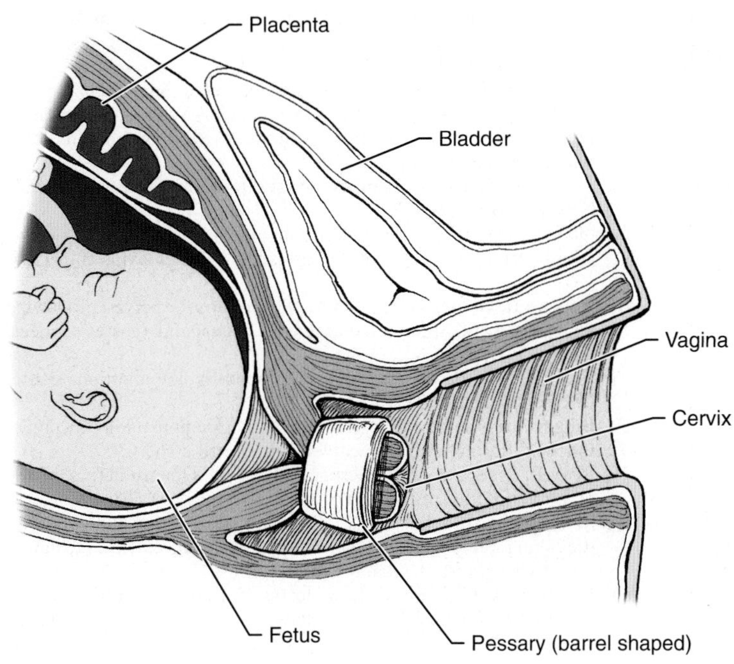

FIGURE 27-11. Vaginal pessary (Arabin type) placed at 22 weeks in patient with cervical length of 2.2 cm, funneling, and prior history of preterm delivery at 26 weeks.

pessary in patients with a sonographically detected short cervix (Figure 27-11). Patients managed with a pessary gained 99 days compared to 67 days for patients managed with bed rest alone ($P = .02$). We have reported our initial experience[119] using the same type of vaginal pessary studied by Arabin in patients with sonographic cervical shortening and a prior history of preterm delivery. When compared with bed rest alone, patients with pessaries gained significantly greater gestational age (10.0 ± 41 weeks vs. 5.1 ± 3.6 weeks; $P = .03$). Currently there are four ongoing randomized studies of pessaries in singleton and multiple gestations with short cervical length being conducted in Europe (www.clinicaltrials.gov). We are waiting for the results of these trials, and further prospective, randomized trials comparing pessary, cerclage, and bed rest are needed before conclusions regarding the efficacy of any of these interventions can be established.

SUMMARY

Cervical insufficiency is rarely a distinct and well-defined clinical entity but only one part of a larger and more complex spontaneous preterm birth syndrome. The original paradigm of obstetrical and gynecologic trauma as a common antecedent of cervical insufficiency has been replaced by the recognition of functional, as opposed to anatomic, deficits as the more prevalent origin. Cervical competence functions along a continuum, influenced by both endogenous and exogenous factors that interact through various pathways with other recognized components of the preterm birth syndrome: uterine contractions and decidual/membrane activation. Thus, the clinically convenient term, *cervical insufficiency*, may actually represent an oversimplified, incomplete version of the broader, though poorly understood, pathophysiologic process. Consequently, the continued use of traditional therapies, unsubstantiated by results of clinical trials, must be questioned. Effective, evidence-based management guidelines will stem from a more complete understanding of the preterm birth syndrome. This will improve patient selection and permit specifically tailored treatment regimens, confirmed by the results of well-designed intervention trials.

***Cervical insufficiency* remains primarily a clinical diagnosis, although cervical ultrasound has emerged as a proven, clinically useful screening and diagnostic tool in selected populations of high-risk women based on an obstetrical history of a prior (early) spontaneous preterm birth. Women with this history who then develop shortened midtrimester cervical length appear to have a treatable *component* of cervical insufficiency.** Surgical intervention in the form of prophylactic cerclage, sonographically indicated cerclage, emergent cerclage, and abdominal/laparoscopic cerclage may be reasonable in carefully selected patients. Alternative or adjunctive interventions such as bed rest and a vaginal pessary require further investigation.

KEY POINTS

- Cervical insufficiency is primarily a clinical diagnosis characterized by recurrent painless dilatation and spontaneous midtrimester loss.
- Cervical insufficiency is rarely a distinct and well-defined clinical entity, but only one component of the larger and more complex spontaneous preterm birth syndrome.
- Current evidence suggests that cervical competence functions along a continuum, influenced by both endogenous and exogenous factors, such as uterine contractions and decidual/membrane actuation.
- The traditional nomenclature of cerclage type as prophylactic, therapeutic, and emergent should

be replaced by history-indicated, ultrasound-indicated, and physical examination–indicated cerclage.

- There is no objective preconception diagnostic test for cervical insufficiency.
- History-indicated cerclage for patients with clinical history of cervical insufficiency remains a reasonable approach.
- Cervical ultrasound performs poorly as a screening test in low-risk women, but it has been proven to be a clinically useful screening and diagnostic tool in selected high-risk populations who may have a treatable *component* of cervical insufficiency.
- In women with nonclassic clinical histories of cervical insufficiency, serial sonographic evaluations of the cervix may be an acceptable alternative approach to prophylactic cerclage.
- Physical examination–indicated cerclage may be beneficial in reducing preterm birth in a subgroup of patients without markers of infection.
- Abdominal cerclage may be considered for those patients with history of failed vaginal cerclage, or for those patients with an extremely short cervix in whom a vaginal approach is not feasible.
- There is a need for randomized studies to evaluate alternative treatments for cervical insufficiency such as bed rest, pharmacologic therapy, and vaginal pessary.

REFERENCES

1. Anonymous. In Culpepper N, Cole A, Rowland W: The Practice of Physick. London, George Strawbridge, 1678, p 502.
2. Ludmir J, Sehdev HM: Anatomy and physiology of the cervix. Clin Obstet Gynecol 43:433, 2000.
3. Barter RH, Dusbabek JA, Riva HL, Parks JL: Surgical closure of the incompetent cervix during pregnancy. Am J Obstet Gyneccol 75:511, 1958.
4. Jennings CL: Temporary submucosal cerclage for cervical incompetence: report of forty-eight cases. Am J Obstet Gynecol 113:1097, 1972.
5. Kuhn R, Pepperell R: Cervical ligation: a review of 242 pregnancies. Aust N Z J Obstet Gynaecol 17:79, 1977.
6. Romero R, Espinoza J, Kusanovic JP, et al: The preterm parturition syndrome. BJOG 113:17, 2006.
7. Danforth DN, Buckingham JC: Cervical incompetence: a reevaluation. Postgrad Med 32:345, 1962.
8. Danforth DN, Veis A, Breen M, et al: The effect of pregnancy and labor on the human cervix: changes in collagen, glycoproteins and gycosaminoglycans. Am J Obstet Gynecol 120:641, 1974.
9. Leppert PC, Yu SY, Keller S, et al: Decreased elastic fibers and desmosine content in incompetent cervix. Am J Obstet Gynecol 157:1134, 1987.
10. Rechberger T, Uldbjerg N, Oxlund H: Connective tissue changes in the cervix during normal pregnancy and pregnancy complicated by cervical incompetence. Obstet Gynecol 71:563, 1988.
11. Dunn LJ, Dans P: Subsequent obstetrical performance of patients meeting the historical criteria for cervical incompetence. Bull Sloan Hosp Women 7:43, 1962.
12. Iams JD, Johnson FF, Sonek J, et al: Cervical competence as a continuum: a study of ultrasonography cervical length and obstetric performance. Am J Obstet Gynecol 172:1097, 1995.
13. Iams JD, Goldenberg RL, Meis PJ, et al: The length of the cervix and the risk of spontaneous premature delivery. N Engl J Med 334:567, 1996.
14. Buckingham JC, Buethe RA, Danforth DN: Collagen-muscle ratio in clinically normal and clinically incompetent cervixes. Am J Obstet Gynecol 91:232, 1965.
15. Ayers JWR, DeGrood RM, Compton AA, et al: Sonographic evaluation of cervical length in pregnancy: diagnosis and management of preterm cervical effacement in patients at risk for premature delivery. Obstet Gynecol 71:939, 1988.
16. Craigo SD: Cervical incompetence and preterm delivery [editorial]. N Engl J Med 334:595, 1996.
17. Olah KS, Gee H: The prevention of preterm delivery—can we afford to continue to ignore the cervix? Br J Obstet Gynaecol 99:278, 1992.
18. Romero R, Gomez R, Sepulveda W: The uterine cervix, ultrasound and prematurity [editor comments]. Ultrasound Obstet Gynecol 2:385, 1992.
19. Toaff R, Toaff ME: Diagnosis of impending late abortion. Obstet Gynecol 43:756, 1974.
20. Bergman P, Svenerund A: Traction test for demonstrating incompetence of internal os of the cervix. Int J Fertil 2:163, 1957.
21. Kiwi R, Neuman MR, Merkatz IR, et al: Determination of the elastic properties of the cervix. Obstet Gynecol 71:568, 1988.
22. Zlatnik KFJ, Burmeister LF: Interval evaluation of the cervix for predicting pregnancy outcome and diagnosing cervical incompetence. J Repro Med 38:365, 1993.
23. Ferenczy A, Choukroun D, Falcone T, Franco E: The effect of cervical loop electrosurgical excision on subsequent pregnancy outcome: North American experience. Am J Obstet Gynecol 172:1246, 1995.
24. Althuisius SM, Shornagel GA, Dekker GA, et al: Loop electrosurgical excision procedure of the cervix and time of delivery in subsequent pregnancy. Int J Gynecol Obstet 72:31, 2001.
25. Sadler L, Saftkas A, Wang W, et al: Treatment for cervical intraepithelial neoplasis and risk of preterm delivery. JAMA 29:2100, 2004.
26. Weber T, Obel E: Pregnancy complications following conization of the uterine cervix. Acta Obstet Gynecol Scand 58:259, 1979.
27. Leiman G, Harrison NA, Rubin A: Pregnancy following conization of the cervix: complications related to cone size. Am J Obstet Gynecol 136:14, 1980.
28. Raio L, Ghezzi F, Di Naro E, et al: Duration of pregnancy after carbon dioxide laser conization of the cervix: influence of cone height. Obstet Gynecol 90:978, 1997.
29. Kuoppala T, Saarikoski S: Pregnancy and delivery after cone biopsy of the cervix. Arch Gynecol 237:149, 1986.
30. Lazar P, Gueguen S, Dreyfus J, et al: Multicentred controlled trial of cervical cerclage in women at moderate risk of preterm delivery. Br J Obstet Gynaecol 91:731, 1984.
31. Dor J, Shalev J, Mashiach S, et al: Elective cervical suture of twin pregnancies diagnosed ultrasonically in the first trimester following induced ovulation. Gynecol Obstet Invest 13:55, 1982.
32. Rush RW, Isaacs S, McPherson K, et al: A randomized controlled trial of cervical cerclage in women at high risk for preterm delivery. Br J Obstet Gynaecol 91:724, 1984.
33. Final report of the Medical Research Council/Royal College of Obstetrics and Gynaecology multicentre randomized trial of cervical cerclage. Br J Obstet Gynaecol 100:516, 1993.
34. Tongsong T, Kamprapanth P, Srisomboon J, et al: Single transvaginal sonographic measurement of cervical length early in the third trimester as a predictor of preterm delivery. Obstet Gynecol 86:184, 1995.
35. Berghella V, Tolosa JE, Kuhlman K, et al: Cervical ultrasonography compared with manual examination as a predictor of preterm delivery. Am J Obstet Gynecol 177:723, 1997.
36. Andrews WW, Copper R, Hauth JC, et al: Mid-trimester cervical ultrasound findings predict recurrent early preterm birth. Obstet Gynecol 95:222, 2000.
37. Owen J, Yost N, Berghella V, et al: Mid-trimester endovaginal sonography in women at high risk for spontaneous preterm birth. JAMA 286:1340, 2001.
38. Owen J, Yost N, Berghella V, et al: Can shortened mid-trimester cervical length predict very early spontaneous preterm birth? Am J Obstet Gynecol 191:298, 2004.
39. Berghella V, Tolosa JE, Kuhlman K, et al: Cervical ultrasonography compared with manual examination as a predictor of preterm delivery. Am J Obstet Gynecol 177:723, 1997.

40. Airoldi J, Berghella V, Sehdev H, Ludmir J: Transvaginal ultrasonography of the cervix to predict preterm birth in women with uterine anomalies. Obstet Gynecol 106:553, 2005.
41. McMahon KS, Neerhof MC, Haney EI, et al: Prematurity in multiple gestations: identification of patients who are at low risk. Am J Obstet Gynecol 186:1137, 2002.
42. Imseis HM, Albert TA, Iams JD: Identifying twin gestations at low risk for preterm birth with a transvaginal ultrasonographic cervical measurement at 24 to 26 weeks' gestation. Am J Obstet Gynecol 177:1149, 1997.
43. Honest H, Bachman LM, Coomarasamy A, et al: Accuracy of cervical transvaginal sonography in predicting preterm birth; a systematic review. Ultrasound Obstet Gynecol 22:305, 2003.
44. Heath VCF, Souka AP, Erasmus I, et al: Cervical length at 23 weeks of gestation: the value of Shirodkar suture for the short cervix. Ultrasound Obstet Gynecol 12:318, 1998.
45. Novy MJ, Gupta A, Wothe DD, et al: Cervical cerclage in the second trimester of pregnancy: a historical cohort study. Am J Obstet Gynecol 184:1447, 2001.
46. Berghella V, Daly SF, Tolosa JE, et al: Prediction of preterm delivery with transvaginal ultrasonography of the cervix in patients with high-risk pregnancies: does cerclage prevent prematurity? Am J Obstet Gynecol 181:809, 1999.
47. Hassan SS, Romero R, Maymon E, et al: Does cervical cerclage prevent preterm delivery in patients with a short cervix? Am J Obstet Gynecol 184:1325, 2001.
48. Newman RB, Krombach SR, Myers MC, McGee DL: Effect of cerclage on obstetrical outcome in twin gestations with a shortened cervical length. Am J Obstet Gynecol 186:634, 2002.
49. Roman AS, Rebarber A, Pereria L, et al: The efficacy of sonographically indicated cerclage in multiple gestations. J Ultrasound Med 24:763, 2005.
50. Althuisius SM, Dekker GA, van Geijn HP, et al: Cervical Incompetence Prevention Randomized Cerclage Trial (CIPRACT): study design and preliminary results. Am J Obstet Gynecol 183:823, 2000.
51. Althuisius SM, Dekker GA, Hummel P, et al: Final results of the Cervical Incompetence Prevention Randomized Cerclage Trial (CIPRACT): therapeutic cerclage with bed rest versus bed rest alone. Am J Obstet Gynecol 185:1106, 2001.
52. Rust OA, Atlas RO, Reed J, et al: Revisiting the short cervix detected by transvaginal ultrasound in the second trimester: why cerclage may not help. Am J Obstet Gynecol 185:1098, 2001.
53. To MS, Alfirevic Z, Heath VCF, et al; on behalf of the Fetal Medicine Foundation Second Trimester Screening Group: Cervical cerclage for prevention of preterm delivery in women with short cervix: randomized controlled trial. Lancet 363:1849, 2004.
54. Berghella V, Odibo AO, Tolosa JE: Cerclage for prevention of preterm birth in women with a short cervix found on transvaginal ultrasound: a randomized trial. Am J Obstet Gynecol 191:1311, 2004.
55. Berghella V, Odibo AO, To MS, et al: Cerclage for short cervix on ultrasonography, meta-analysis of trials using individual patient-level data. Obstet Gynecol 106:181, 2005.
56. Owen J, Iams JD, Hauth JC: Vaginal sonography and cervical incompetence. Am J Obstet Gynecol 188:586, 2003.
57. Owen J, Hankins G, Iams JD, et al: Multicenter randomized trial of cerclage for preterm birth prevention in high-risk women with shortened midtrimester cervical length. Am J Obstet Gynecol 201:375.e1, 2009.
58. Romero R, Espinoza J, Erez O, Hassam S: The role of cervical cerclage in obstetric practice: can the patient who could benefit from this procedure be identified? Am J Obstet Gynecol 194:1, 2006.
59. Branch DW: Operations for cervical incompetence. Clin Obstet Gynecol 29:240, 1986.
60. Cousins JM: Cervical incompetence: 1980. A time for reappraisal. Clin Obstet Gynecol 23:467, 1980.
61. Blickman MJC, Le T, Bruinese HW, et al: Ultrasound-predicted versus history-predicated cerclage in women at risk of cervical insufficiency: a systematic review. Obstet Gynecol Surv 63:803, 2008.
62. Simcox R, Seed PT, Bennett P, et al: A randomized controlled trial of cervical scanning vs history to determine cerclage in women at high risk of preterm birth (CIRCLE trial). Am J Obstet Gynecol 200:623.e1, 2009
63. Aarts JM, Jozien T, Brons J, et al: Emergency cerclage: a review. Obstet Gynecol Survey 50:459, 1995.
64. Olatunbosun OA, Al-Nuaim L, Turnell RW: Emergency cerclage compared with bedrest for advanced cervical dilatation in pregnancy. Int Surg 80:170, 1995.
65. Kokia E, Dor J, Blankenstein J, et al: A simple scoring system for treatment of cervical incompetence diagnosed during the second trimester. Gynceol Obstet Invest 31:12, 1991.
66. Pereira L, Cotter A, Gómez R, et al: Expectant management compared with physical examination-indicated cerclage (EM-PEC) in selected women with a dilated cervix at 14(0/7)-25(6/7) weeks: results from the EM-PEC international cohort study. Am J Obstet Gynecol 197:483.e1, 2007.
67. Althuisius SM, Dekker GA, Hummel P, et al: Cervical incompetence prevention randomized cerclage trial: emergency cerclage with bedrest versus bedrest alone. Am J Obstet Gynecol 189:907, 2003.
68. Romero R, Gonzalez R, Sepulveda W, et al: Infection and Labor VIII. Microbial invasion of the amniotic cavity in patients with suspected cervical incompetence: prevalence and clinical significance. Am J Obstet Gynecol 167:1086, 1992.
69. Mays JK, Figuerioa R, Shah J, et al: Amniocentesis for selection before rescue cerclage. Obstet Gynecol 95:652, 2000.
70. Weiner CP, Lee KY, Buhimschi CS, et al: Proteomic biomarkers that predict the clinical success of rescue cerclage. Am J Obstet Gynecol 192:710, 2005.
71. Romero R, Kusamovic JP, Espinoza J, et al: What is amniotic fluid "sludge"? Ultrasound Obstet Gynecol 30:793, 2007.
72. Lash AF, Lash SR: Habitual abortion: the incompetent internal os of the cervix. Am J Obstet Gynecol 59:68, 1950.
73. Shirodkar VN: A new method of operative treatment for habitual abortions in the second trimester of pregnancy. Antiseptic 52:299, 1955.
74. McDonald IA: Suture of the cervix for inevitable miscarriage. J Obstet Gynecol Br Empire 64:346, 1957.
75. Abdelhak YE, Sheen JJ, Kuczynski E, et al: Comparison of delayed absorbable suture v. non-absorbable suture for the treatment of incompetent cervix. J Perinatal Med 27:250, 1999.
76. Aarnoudse JG, Huisjes HJ: Complications of cerclage. Acta Obstet Gynecol Scand 58:225, 1979.
77. Harger JH: Comparison of success and morbidity in cervical cerclage procedures. Obstet Gynecol 53:534, 1980.
78. McDonald IA: Incompetence of the cervix. Aust N Z J Obstet Gynaecol 18:34, 1978.
79. Schulman H, Farmakides G: Surgical approach to failed cervical cerclage: a report of three cases. J Reprod Med 30:626, 1985.
80. Steinberg ES, Santos AC: Surgical anesthesia during pregnancy. Int Anesthesiol Clin 28:58, 1980.
81. Chen L, Ludmir J, Miller FL, et al: Is regional better than general anesthesia for cervical cerclage? Nine years experience. Anesth Analg 70:SI, 1990.
82. Ludmir J, Cohen BF, Wong GP, et al: Managing the patient with cerclage: bedrest versus amulation based on sonographic findings. Presented at the 17th Annual Meeting of the Society of Perinatal Obstetricians, Anaheim, CA, 1997.
83. Abdelhak YE, Aronov R, Roque H, Young BK: Management of cervical cerclage at term: remove the suture in labor? J Perinat Med 28:453, 2000.
84. Bisulli M, Suhag A, Arvon R, et al: Interval to spontaneous delivery after elective removal of cerclage. Am J Obstet Gynecol 201:163.e1, 2009.
85. Novy MJ: Transabdominal cervicoisthmic cerclage for the management of repetitive abortion and premature delivery. Am J Obstet Gynecol 143:44, 1982.
86. Novy MJ: Transabdominal cervicoisthmic cerclage: a reappraisal 25 years after its introduction. Am J Obstet Gynecol 164:163, 1991.
87. Groom KN, Jones BA, Edmonds DK, Bennett PR: Preconception transabdominal cervicoisthmic cerclage. Am J Obstet Gynecol, 191:230, 2004.
88. Ludmir J, Jackson GM, Samuels P: Transvaginal cerclage under ultrasound guidance in cases of severe cervical hypoplasia. Obstet Gynecol 78:1067, 1991.
89. Scarantino SE, Reilly JG, Moretti ML, Pillari VT: Laparoscopic removal of a transabdominal cervical cerclage. Am J Obstet Gynecol 182:1086, 2000.
90. Gallot D, Savary D, Laurichesse H, et al: Experience with three cases of laparoscopic transabdominal cervioisthmic cerclage and two subsequent pregnancies. Br J Obstet Gynaecol 110:696, 2003.

91. Cho CH, Kim TH, Kwon SH, et al: Laparoscopic transabdominal cervicoisthmid cerclage during pregnancy. J Am Gynecol Laparosc 10:363, 2003.
92. Wolfe L, DePasquale S, Adair D, et al: Robotic-assisted laparoscopic placement of transabdominal cerclage during pregnancy. Am J Perinatol 25:653, 2008.
93. Harger JH: Cervical cerclage: patient selection, morbidity, and success rates. Clin Perinatol 10:321, 1983.
94. Cardosi RJ, Chez RA: Comparison of elective and empiric cerclage and the role of emergency cerclage. J Matern Fetal Med 7:230, 1998.
95. Ludmir J, Landon MB, Gabbe SG, et al: Management of the diethylstilbestrol-exposed pregnant patient: a prospective study. Am J Obstet Gynecol 157:665, 1987.
96. Guzman ER, Forster JK, Vintzileos AM, et al: Pregnancy outcomes in women treated with elective versus ultrasound-indicated cervical cerclage. Ultrasound Obstet Gynecol 12:323, 1998.
97. Benifla JL, Goffinet F, Darai E, et al: Emergency cervical cerclage after 20 weeks' gestation: a retrospective study of 16 years' practice in 34 cases. Fetal Diagn Ther 12:274, 1997.
98. Berghella V, Daly SF, Tolosa JE, et al: Prediction of preterm delivery with transvaginal ultrasonography of the cervix in patients with high-risk pregnancies: does cerclage prevent prematurity? Am J Obstet Gynecol 181:809, 1999.
99. Althuisius SM, Dekker GA, van Geijin HP, et al: The effect of McDonald Cerclage on cervical length as assessed by transvaginal ultrasonography. Am J Obstet Gynecol 180:366, 1999.
100. Minakami H, Matsubara S, Izumi A, et al: Emergency cervical cerclage: relation between its success, perioperative serum level of C-reactive protein and WBC count, and degree of cervical dilatation. Gynecol Obstet Invest 47:157, 1999.
101. Aarts JM, Brons JT, Bruinse HW, et al: Emergency cerclage: a review. Obstet Gynecol Surv 50:459, 1995.
102. Caruso A, Trivellini C, DeCarolis S, et al: Emergency cerclage in the presence of protruding membranes: is pregnancy outcome predictable? Acta Obstet Gynaecol Scand 79:265, 2000.
103. Barth WH Jr., Yeomans ER, Hankins GDV, et al: Emergent cerclage. Surg Gynaecol Scand 58:225, 1979.
104. Charles D, Edwards WR: Infectious complications of cerclage. Am J Obstet Gynecol 141:1065, 1981.
105. Scheerer LJ, Lam F, Bartolelucci L, et al: A new technique for reduction of prolapsed fetal membranes for emergency cervical cerclage. Obstet Gynecol 74:408, 1989.
106. Kurup M, Goldkrand JW: Cervical incompetence: elective, emergent, or urgent cerclage. Am J Obstet Gynecol 181:240, 1999.
107. Wu MY, Yang YS, Huang SC, et al: Emergent and elective cerclage for cervical incompetence. Int J Gynaecol Obstet 54:23, 1996.
108. Lipitz S, Libshsitz A, Oelsner G, et al: Outcome of second-trimester, emergency cervical cerclage in patients with no history of cervical incompetence. Am J Perinatol 13:419, 1996.
109. Ludmir J, Bader T, Chen L, et al: Poor perinatal outcome associated with retained cerclage in patients with premature rupture of membranes. Obstet Gynecol 84:823, 1994.
110. Jenkins TM, Bergehlla V, Shlossman PA, et al: Timing of cerclage removal after preterm premature rupture of membranes: maternal and neonatal outcomes. Am J Obstet Gynecol 183:847, 2000.
111. McElrath TF, Norwitz ER, Lieberman ES, et al: Management of cervical cerclage and preterm premature rupture of the membranes: should the stitch be removed? Am J Obstet Gynecol 183:840, 2000.
112. Dunn LE, Robinson JC, Steer CM: Maternal death following suture of incompetent cervix during pregnancy. Am J Obstet Gynecol 78:335, 1959.
113. Meis PJ, Klebanoff M, Thom E, et al: Prevention of recurrent preterm delivery 17 alpha-hydroxyprogesterone caproate. N Engl J Med 348:2379, 2003.
114. Fonseca C, Celik E, Parra M, et al: Progesterone and the risk of preterm birth among women with a short cervix. N Engl J Med 357:462, 2007.
115. Berghella V, Figueroa D, Szychowski JM, et al: Vaginal Ultrasound Trial Consortium: 17-alpha-hydroxyprogesterone caproate for the prevention of preterm birth in women with prior preterm birth and a short cervical length. Am J Obstet Gynecol 202:351.e1, 2010.
116. Vitsky M: Simple treatment of the incompetent cervical os. Am J Obstet Gynecol 81:1194, 1961.
117. Forster F, Dunng R, Schwartz G: Therapy of cervix insufficiency—cerclage or support pessary? Sentrablbl Gynaekol 108:230, 1986.
118. Arabin B, Halbesma JR, Vork F, et al: Is treatment with vaginal pessaries an option in patients with a sonographically detected short cervix? J Perinat Med 31:122, 2003.
119. Ludmir J, Mantione JR, Debbs RH, Sehdev HM: Is pessary a valid treatment for cervical change during the late midtrimester? J Soc Gynecol Investig 9:11, 2002.

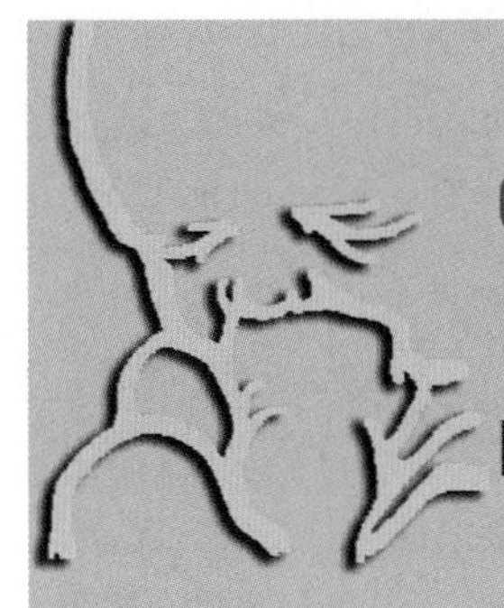

CHAPTER 28

Preterm Birth

Hyagriv N. Simhan, Jay D. Iams, and Roberto Romero

KEY ABBREVIATIONS

Adrenocorticotrophic Hormone	ACTH
Assisted Reproductive Techniques	ARTs
Bacterial Vaginosis	BV
Biophysical Profile	BPP
Bronchopulmonary Dysplasia	BPD
Confidence Interval	CI
Corticotropin-Releasing Hormone	CRH
Cyclic Adenosine Monophosphate	cAMP
Cyclo-oxygenase	COX
Estrogen Receptor	ER
Extremely Low Birth Weight	ELBW
Fetal Inflammatory Response Syndrome	FIRS
Gelatinase-B	MMP-9
Group B Streptococcus	GBS
Herpes Simplex Virus	HSV
Human Immunodeficiency Virus	HIV
In Vitro Fertilization	IVF
Inducible Form of Nitric Oxide Synthase	iNOS
Interstitial Collagenase	MMP-1
Intravenous	IV
Intraventricular Hemorrhage	IVH
Low Birth Weight	LBW
Myosin Light-chain Kinase	MLCK
National Institute of Child Health and Human Development	NICHD
Necrotizing Enterocolitis	NEC
Neutrophil Collagenase	MMP-8
Nonsteroidal Anti-inflammatory Drugs	NSAIDs
Nonstress Test	NST
Odds Ratio	OR
Patent Ductus Arteriosus	PDA
Prelabor Rupture of Membranes	PROM
Progesterone Receptor	PR
Relative Risk	RR
Respiratory Distress Syndrome	RDS
Thyrotropin-Releasing Hormone	TRH
Tumor Necrosis Factor-α	TNF-α
U.S. Food and Drug Administration	FDA
Very Low Birth Weight	VLBW
White Blood Cell	WBC

The average duration of normal human pregnancy is 267 days after conception, or 280 days (40 weeks) from the first day of the last normal menstrual period. Infants born at 39 and 40 weeks of gestation have the lowest rates of adverse outcomes. **Complications related to preterm birth account for more newborn and infant deaths than any other cause.**[1] **Although advances in neonatal care have led to increased**

survival and reduced short- and long-term morbidity for infants born preterm, surviving infants have increased risk of visual and hearing impairment, chronic lung disease, cerebral palsy, and delayed development in childhood. The causes of preterm birth are diverse, but can be usefully considered according to whether or not the parturitional process (cervical preparation, decidual-membrane activation, and/or myometrial contractions) had begun before birth occurred. Preterm births that do not follow spontaneous initiation of parturition most often are iatrogenic, when the health of the mother and/or fetus is at risk (e.g., due to major hemorrhage, hypertension, or poor fetal growth).

DEFINITIONS

A *preterm birth* is commonly defined as one that occurs after 20 weeks' gestation and before the completion of 37 menstrual weeks of gestation, regardless of birth weight. Low birth weight is defined by the size of the infant at birth, regardless of gestational age. Gestational age and birth weight are related by the terms *small for gestational age* (birth weight less than the 10th percentile for gestational age), *appropriate for gestational age* (birth weight between the 10th and 90th percentiles), *and large for gestational age* (birth weight above the 90th percentile). A **preterm** or **premature** infant is one born before 37 weeks of gestation (259 days from the first day of the mother's last normal menstrual period, or 245 days after conception). **Low birth weight** (LBW) is defined as birth weight below 2500 g, **very low birth weight** (VLBW) as birth weight below 1500 g, and **extremely low birth weight** (ELBW) as birth weight below 1000 g. The gestational boundaries of 20 and 37 weeks are historical, not scientific.[2] Infants born at 36, 37, and even 38 weeks of gestation may experience neonatal and even lifetime morbidity related to immaturity of one or more organs. The risk factors, etiologies, and recurrence risk for spontaneous births at 16 to 19 weeks do not differ from those of births at 20 to 25 weeks.[3,4] **Recognition that some infants born after 37 weeks are not fully mature, and that many births before 20 weeks arise from the same causes that lead to preterm births, has led to reevaluation of these definitions and boundaries.**[5]

FREQUENCY OF PRETERM AND LOW BIRTH WEIGHT DELIVERY

The World Health Organization has estimated **that 9.6% of all births in 2005 were preterm—almost 13 million worldwide.** Africa and Asia accounted for almost 11 million.[6] Rates are lowest in Europe (6.2%), compared to the highest rates seen in Africa (11.9%) and North America (10.6%). In the United States, the preterm birth rate rose from 10.6% in 1990 to 12.8% of all births in 2006. The rise resulted from improved pregnancy dating by ultrasound that shifted the gestational age distribution to the left, increased use of assisted reproduction techniques, and, most important, from increased willingness to choose delivery when medical or obstetrical complications occur after 34 weeks' gestation. The rate of preterm birth fell to 12.7% in 2007, 12.3% in 2008, and 12.1% in 2009 (Figure 28-1).[7] The decline has been attributed to improved fertility practices that reduce the risk of higher-order multiple

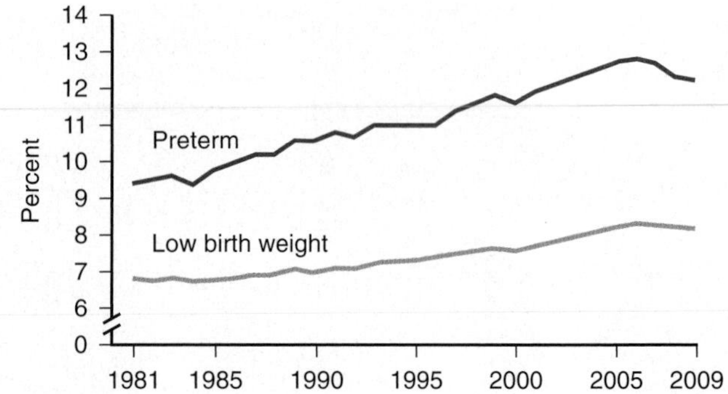

FIGURE 28-1. Preterm and low-birth-weight rates: United States, final 1981-2009, preliminary 2009. (Modified from Hamilton BE, Martin JA, Ventura SJ: Births: preliminary data for 2009. National vital statistics reports web release, vol 59, no 3, Hyattsville, MD, National Center for Health Statistics, 2010.)

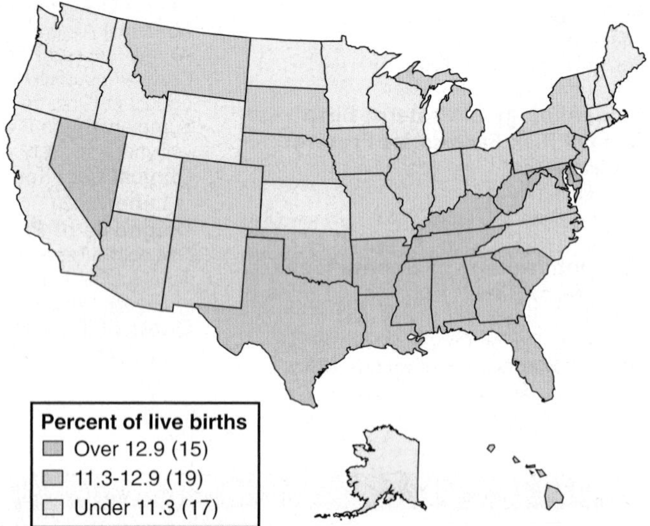

FIGURE 28-2. Percentage of live preterm births in the United States by state. (© 2011 March of Dimes Foundation. All rights reserved.)

gestation, to quality improvement programs that limited scheduled late preterm and near-term births to only those with valid indications, and to increased use of strategies to prevent recurrent preterm birth.

The rates of preterm birth vary substantially across the United States (Figure 28-2). Reasons for the geographic variation are complex but are heavily influenced by the percentage of the population that is African American. **African Americans have rates of preterm birth that are almost twofold higher than other racial/ethnic groups.** The disparity is particularly striking for births less than 32 weeks' gestation (Figure 28-3).

Outcomes for Infants Born Preterm

Gestational age at birth is strongly correlated with adverse pregnancy outcomes, including stillbirth (fetal death after 20 weeks' gestation), neonatal (less than 28 days after birth) and infant (less than 12 months after birth) death, and long-term physical and intellectual morbidities.

PERINATAL MORTALITY

Perinatal mortality is defined as the sum of stillbirths after 20 weeks' gestation + neonatal deaths through 28 days of

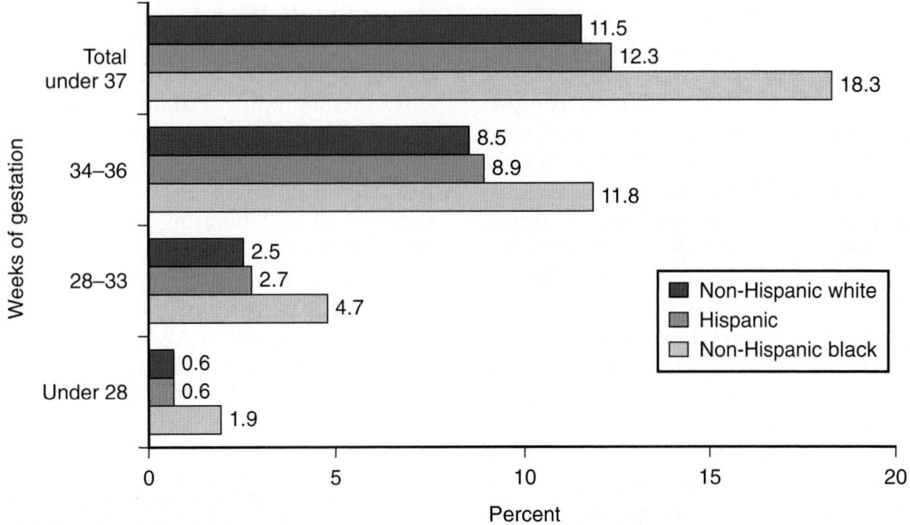

FIGURE 28-3. Percentage of live preterm births by racial group. (Data from Martin JA, Hamilton BE, et al: Births: final data for 2007. Natl Vital Stat Rep 58:1, 2010.)

life per 1000 total births (live-born + stillborn). Perinatal mortality increases markedly as gestational age and birth weight decline. Because this measure encompasses prenatal, intrapartum, and neonatal events, it reflects obstetrical and neonatal care. Stillbirth and preterm birth have a similar epidemiological profile, especially before 32 weeks. Rates of perinatal mortality declined between 1990 and 2003, mainly due to a decrease in fetal deaths after 27 weeks' gestation.[8]

Infant Mortality

The infant mortality rate is the number of deaths among live-born infants before 1 year of age per 1000 *live* births. Although congenital malformations are often listed as the leading cause of infant mortality, this ranking is achieved by separating conditions related to preterm birth into several categories. The proportion of all infant deaths in the United States in 2005 by gestational age at birth is shown in Figure 28-4.

Infant and childhood mortality and morbidity in surviving preterm infants rise as gestational age at birth declines, and vary with the level of neonatal care received. Of the estimated 8.8 million deaths in children younger than 5 years worldwide in 2008, 41% (3.6 million) occurred in neonates, and more than 1 million (12%) were attributed to preterm birth complications.

Regionalized care for high-risk mothers and preterm LBW infants, antenatal administration of corticosteroids, neonatal administration of exogenous pulmonary surfactant, and improved ventilator technology have improved outcomes for very preterm infants. Survival rates rise with gestational age at birth, from 6% for infants born at 22 weeks' gestation to more than 90% at 28 weeks' gestation for infants cared for in tertiary intensive care units.[9] Outcomes can be more accurately predicted by considering fetal number (singleton or multiple), gender, exposure or nonexposure to antenatal corticosteroids, and birth weight, in addition to gestational age.[9] Long-term survival rates by gestational age at birth in 903,402 infants born in Norway[10] are shown in Figure 28-5.

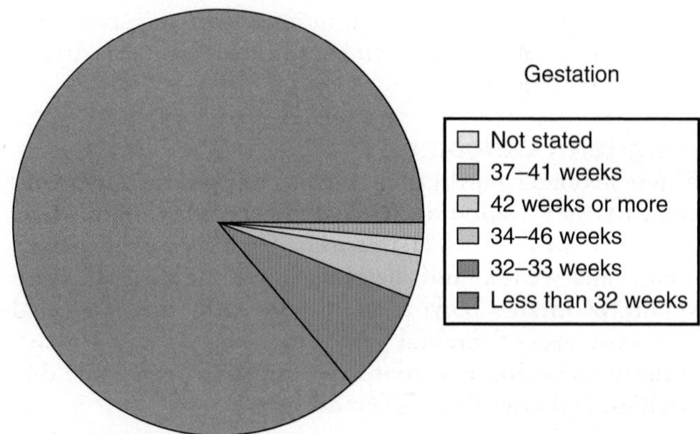

FIGURE 28-4. Proportion of all infant deaths in the United States in 2005 by gestational age at birth. (Modified from Centers for Disease Control and Prevention. National Center for Health Statistics. VitalStats. Available at www.cdc.gov/nchs/vitalstats.htm.)

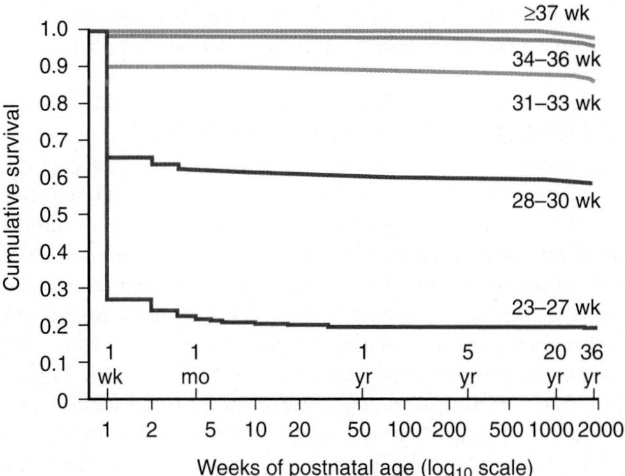

FIGURE 28-5. Cumulative long-term survival by gestational age at birth in 903,402 infants born in Norway. (Modified from Moster D, Lie RT, et al: Long-term medical and social consequences of preterm birth. N Engl J Med 359:262, 2008.)

Perinatal Morbidity

Preterm infants are at risk for specific diseases related to immaturity of various organ systems as well as to the cause and circumstances of preterm birth. **Common complications in premature infants include respiratory distress syndrome (RDS), intraventricular hemorrhage (IVH), bronchopulmonary dysplasia (BPD), patent ductus arteriosus (PDA), necrotizing enterocolitis (NEC), sepsis, apnea, and retinopathy of prematurity (ROP). Rates of morbidity also vary primarily by gestational age, but are also affected by birth weight, fetal number (singleton vs. multifetal), geographic location, proximity to neonatal intensive care, and the maternal and/or fetal condition(s) that led to preterm birth.** The frequency of major morbidity rises as gestational age decreases, especially below 30 weeks' gestation. There is wide geographic variation in the frequency of neonatal morbidities especially for VLBW infants. Reports of survival and morbidity also vary according to the denominator employed. Obstetrical datasets include all living fetuses at entry to the obstetrical suite, whereas neonatal datasets exclude intrapartum and delivery room deaths and thus report rates based on newborns admitted to the nursery. Rates of survival and morbidity at the same gestational age and/or birth weight are thus somewhat higher in neonatal datasets.

Long-term Outcomes

Major neonatal morbidities related to preterm birth that carry lifetime consequences include chronic lung disease, grades III and IV IVH (associated with cerebral palsy), NEC, and vision and hearing impairment. Follow-up studies of infants born preterm and LBW infants reveal increased rates of cerebral palsy, neurosensory impairment, reduced cognition and motor performance, academic difficulties, and attention-deficit disorders.

The incidence of long-term morbidity in survivors is especially increased for those born before 26 weeks. In a study from the United Kingdom, 78% of 308 survivors born before 25 weeks were followed and compared to classmates of normal birth weight. Almost all had some disability at age 6: 22% had severe neurocognitive disabilities (cerebral palsy, IQ greater than 3 SD below mean, blind, or deaf), 24% had moderate disability, 34% had mild disability, and 20% had no neurocognitive disability.

EPIDEMIOLOGY OF PRETERM BIRTH

The numerous maternal and fetal diagnoses that precede preterm birth may be considered according to whether parturition began spontaneously or not. **Spontaneous preterm parturition may first manifest as cervical softening and ripening, decidual activation, and/or uterine contractions. Cervical softening is the most common initial evidence that parturition has begun.** In women who later delivered spontaneously between 28 and 36 weeks' gestation, cervical length measurements at 22 to 24 weeks' gestation were significantly shorter than in women who delivered at term, indicating that cervical softening had begun before 24 weeks.[11] This same study found that more than half of women with evidence of very preterm cervical effacement delivered after 35 weeks, indicating that spontaneous preterm parturition does not always progress to preterm birth. Women with signs and symptoms of spontaneous preterm parturition often have one or more of the demographic characteristics shown in the accompanying box, Demographic Profile of Women with Spontaneous Preterm Birth, but it is important to note that approximately half of women who deliver preterm have no obvious risk factors. Among 2521 women who received prenatal care at 10 collaborating university clinics, 323 (12.8%) delivered before 37 weeks. Of these, 234 (9.3% of the total and 72% of those preterm) were born after spontaneous initiation of parturition and 89 (3.5% of the total and 27% of those preterm) were born preterm as the result of medical/obstetrical indication.[11]

DEMOGRAPHIC PROFILE OF WOMEN WITH SPONTANEOUS PRETERM BIRTH

- History of genital tract colonization, infection, or instrumentation
  - Urinary tract infection and bacteriuria
  - Sexually transmitted infections such as *Chlamydia*, gonorrhea, human papillomavirus, or *Trichomonas*
  - Bacterial vaginosis
  - Cervical dysplasia and treatment for same
  - Spontaneous or induced abortion
- African American
- Bleeding of uncertain origin in pregnancy
- History of a previous spontaneous preterm birth
- Uterine anomaly
- Assisted fertility care
- Multifetal gestation
- Cigarette smoking, substance abuse
- Poor nutrition and low prepregnancy weight (body mass index <19.6)
- Periodontal disease
- Limited education, low income, and low social status
- Late registration for prenatal care
- High levels of personal stress in one or more domains of life

Women whose preterm birth is not preceded by spontaneous parturition have medical and/or obstetrical conditions that lead to the onset of parturition or to iatrogenic intervention to benefit the mother or fetus. Their demography reflects this (see box, Demographic and Medical Profile of Women with Indicated Preterm Birth) and efforts to prolong pregnancy are primarily aimed at optimal management of their medical condition. This strategy is more successful in some, for example, in diabetes, in which maintenance of euglycemia often leads to birth at term, than in others, for example, chronic hypertension, where good blood pressure control does not prevent preeclampsia.

CLINICAL RISK FACTORS FOR SPONTANEOUS PRETERM BIRTH

Risk factors for spontaneous preterm birth arise from host factors, prior pregnancy history, and current pregnancy risks.

Demographic and Medical Profile of Women with Indicated Preterm Birth

- Diabetes, diagnosed before or during pregnancy
- Chronic or acute (preeclampsia) hypertension
- Obstetrical disorders or risk conditions in the current or previous pregnancy
  - Preeclampsia
  - Previous uterine surgery (e.g., prior cesarean birth via a vertical or T-shaped uterine incision)
  - Cholestasis
  - Placental disorders
    - Placenta previa
    - Premature separation (abruption) of the placenta
- Medical disorders
  - Seizures
  - Thromboembolism
  - Connective tissue disorders
  - Asthma and chronic bronchitis
  - Maternal HIV or HSV
  - Obesity
  - Smoking
- Advanced maternal age
- Fetal disorders
  - Fetal compromise
    - Chronic—poor fetal growth
    - Acute—fetal distress, for example, abnormal fetal testing (NST or BPP)
  - Excessive (polyhydramnios) or inadequate (oligohydramnios) amniotic fluid
  - Fetal hydrops, ascites, blood group alloimmunization
  - Birth defects
  - Fetal complications of multifetal gestation (e.g., growth deficiency, twin-to-twin transfusion syndrome)

Host Factors

Medical

Infections

Systemic and genital tract infections are associated with preterm birth. In women in spontaneous preterm labor and intact membranes, lower genital tract flora are commonly found in the amniotic fluid, placenta, and membranes. The flora include *Ureaplasma urealyticum*, *Mycoplasma hominis*, *Fusobacterium species*, *Gardnerella vaginalis*, peptostreptococci, and bacteroides species. Clinical evidence and histologic evidence of infection are more common as the gestational age at delivery decreases, especially before 30 to 32 weeks. Positive cultures of fetal membranes have been reported in 20% to 60% of women with preterm labor before 34 weeks' gestation. The frequency of positive cultures increases as gestational age decreases, from 20% to 30% after 30 weeks to 60% at 23 to 24 weeks' gestation. Evidence of infection is less common after 34 weeks.

BV is a condition in which the ecosystem of the vagina is altered so that gram-negative anaerobic bacteria (e.g., *Gardnerella vaginalis*, *Bacteroides*, *Prevotella*, *Mobiluncus*, and *Mycoplasma species*) largely replace the normally predominant lactobacilli. BV is associated with a twofold increased risk of spontaneous preterm birth. The association between BV and preterm birth is stronger when BV is detected early in pregnancy. Despite the association, antibiotic eradication of BV does not consistently reduce the risk of preterm birth. Infections outside the genital tract have also been related to preterm birth, most commonly to urinary tract and intra-abdominal infections, for example, pyelonephritis and appendicitis. The presumed mechanism of disease is inflammation of the nearby reproductive organs, but infections at remote sites, especially if they are chronic, have also been associated with increased risk of spontaneous preterm birth.

Periodontal Disease

Women with periodontal disease have an increased risk of preterm birth that is not reduced by periodontal care, suggesting shared susceptibility rather than a cause-effect relation. The genitourinary and alimentary tracts are both major sites of microbial colonization where host immune factors defend the interior of the body, so shared risk factors are not surprising.

Genitourinary Tract Factors

Cervical Length

Cervical length as measured by transvaginal ultrasound is inversely related to the risk of preterm birth in both singletons and twins. Women whose cervical length at 22 to 24 weeks' gestation was at or below the 10th percentile (25 mm by endovaginal ultrasound) had a 6.5-fold increased risk (95% CI, 4.5 to 9.3) of preterm birth before 35 weeks' gestation and a 7.7-fold increased risk (95% CI, 4.5 to 13.4) of preterm birth before 32 weeks' gestation when compared with women whose cervical length measurement was greater than the 75th percentile.[12] The explanation for the linkage between cervical length and preterm birth risk was once thought to reflect a "continuum of cervical competence" in which variable cervical resistance to uterine contractions explained the relationship. However, there is now substantial evidence that contractions do not herald the onset of preterm birth,[13] and that progesterone supplementation slows the progression of cervical shortening and reduces the risk of preterm birth when initiated before 24 weeks in women with and without a prior preterm birth.[14-18] These studies support the conclusion that preterm cervical shortening (softening and ripening) is not the passive result of tissue weakness, but instead is an active process indicating that pathologic preterm parturition has begun, regardless of its underlying cause.[11]

Cervical Procedures

A history of cervical surgery including conization and Loop electrosurgical excision procedure (LEEP) is a risk factor for preterm birth, whether by uterine colonization or cervical injury.

Congenital Abnormalities of the Uterus

Congenital structural abnormalities of the uterus, known as müllerian fusion defects, may affect the cervix, the uterine corpus, or both. The risk of preterm births in women with uterine malformations is 25% to 50% depending on the specific malformation and obstetrical history. Implantation of the placenta on a uterine septum may lead to preterm birth by means of placental separation and hemorrhage. A T-shaped uterus in women exposed in utero to diethylstilbestrol has also been associated with an increased risk of preterm labor and birth.

TABLE 28-1 RACE AND ETHNICITY

YEARS OF EDUCATION	NON-HISPANIC BLACK	NON-HISPANIC WHITE	ASIAN/PACIFIC ISLANDER	NATIVE AMERICAN	HISPANIC
<8	19.6	11.0	11.5	14.8	10.7
8-12	16.8	9.9	10.5	11.8	10.4
13-15	14.5	8.3	9.1	9.9	9.3
≥16	12.8	7.0	7.5	9.4	8.4

From Behrman RE, Stith Butler A: Committee on understanding premature birth and assuring healthy outcomes: causes, consequences, and prevention. Washington, DC, National Academies Press, 2007.

TABLE 28-2 PRETERM BIRTH RATES (PERCENT) BY MATERNAL RACE-ETHNICITY AND PRENATAL CARE USE BY TRIMESTER OF INITIATION OF PRENATAL CARE, 1998-2000

TRIMESTER	NON-HISPANIC AFRICAN AMERICAN	NON-HISPANIC WHITE	ASIAN/PACIFIC ISLANDER	AMERICAN INDIAN	HISPANIC
First	14.7	8.3	8.6	10.4	9.7
Second	17.5	10.2	10.8	12.7	11.0
Third	16.0	10.0	9.5	12.3	10.0
No prenatal care	33.4	21.7	19.4	24.0	19.8

Source: NCHS data for U.S. birth cohorts from 1998 to 2000. From Berhman RE, Butler AS: Sociodemographic and Community Factors Contributing to Preterm BirthPreterm Birth: Causes, Consequences, and Prevention. Institute of Medicine (US) Committee on Understanding Premature Birth and Assuring Healthy Outcomes. Washington, DC, National Academies Press, 2007. Copyright © 2007, National Academy of Sciences.

Behavioral

In general, studies of behavioral influences on preterm birth have, with the exception of tobacco smoking, not found a consistent relationship between maternal activities and preterm birth.

SMOKING AND SUBSTANCE ABUSE

Smoking is associated with an increased risk of preterm birth, and unlike most other risks is amenable to intervention during pregnancy.

PHYSICAL ACTIVITY

Controversy exists as to whether excessive physical activity is associated with early delivery.

NUTRITIONAL FACTORS

Low maternal prepregnancy weight (BMI <19.8 kg/m^2) has been regularly found to be associated with an increased risk of preterm birth.[19,20] Women who consume one or more servings of fish per month have lower rates of preterm birth than women who rarely or never eat fish.[21] Numerous studies of various nutritional deficiencies have been reported to be related to risk of preterm birth, but there are few if any for which supplementation has been found to reduce the incidence of prematurity.

Demography, Stress, and Social Determinants of Health

Social disadvantage is persistently associated with increased risk of preterm birth: poverty; educational attainment; geographic residence in disadvantaged neighborhoods, states, and regions; and lack of access to prenatal care are all linked to significantly higher rates of preterm birth.[22] These associations were once deemed to be social, not medical, and thus beyond the reach of medical care. The effect of the social environment on reproduction has since been examined in greater detail, revealing evidence of a causative relationship. The magnitude of the increased risk of preterm birth according to educational level is shown in Table 28-1. There is a nearly twofold difference in the rate of preterm birth for women of all racial and ethnic groups between those with the highest and lowest levels of education (Table 28-2).

Equally striking is the persistence of the disparity in rates of preterm birth in African American women regardless of their educational level, and in Table 28-2, their access to early prenatal care.

AFRICAN AMERICANS

African American women have a uniquely increased risk for preterm birth when compared to women from any other racial or ethnic background.[23] The rate of preterm birth averaged 18.4% among African American women, compared to 10.8% in Asian Americans, 11.6% in white, 12.6% in Hispanic, and 14.2% in Native American women in 2005-2007. The disparity in preterm birth rate persists after social and medical risk factors are accounted for[22,24,25] and is evident in African American but not African women. The origins of the disparity are not well understood. Regardless of the etiology, all African American women may be considered to have increased risk of preterm birth even in the absence of other risk factors.

Stress[26] and depression[27] are consistently reported to have moderate association with preterm birth, though the mechanisms again remain uncertain.

Genetic Contributors to Preterm Birth

The notion that there may be some genetic contribution to preterm birth is based on several observations. First, a woman's family history of preterm birth influences her own risk. Porter and colleagues found that a mother who was herself born preterm had an inceased risk for delivering a child preterm; the magnitude of that increased risk was inversely related to the gestational age of her own

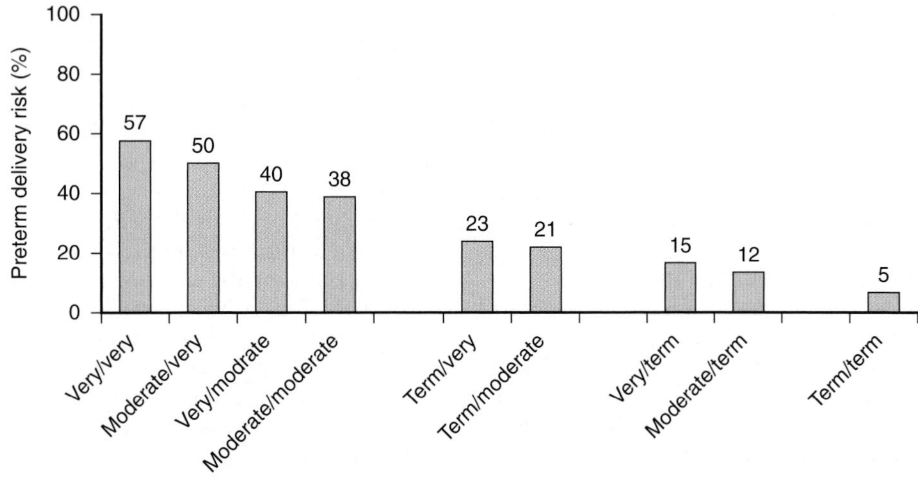

FIGURE 28-6. Risk of recurrent preterm birth in 19,025 women with two prior births according to the order and gestational age of the previous birth. (Modified from McManemy J, Cooke E, et al: Recurrence risk for preterm delivery. Am J Obstet Gynecol 196:576e1, discussion 576e6, 2007.)

birth. The odds ratio for preterm birth was 1.18 (95% CI, 1.02 to 1.37) for women who were born at 36 weeks of gestation to 2.38 (95% CI, 1.37 to 4.16) for women who were born at 30 weeks of gestation. A second set of observations supporting a genetic contribution to preterm birth are from twin studies. Treloar and colleagues[28] studied 905 female Australian twin pairs to determine whether delivery had occurred more than 2 weeks preterm. In this study, "all-cause" preterm birth was the outcome.[28,29] Twin pair correlations were higher from monozygotic twin pairs than dizygotic twin pairs ($r = 0.3 \pm 0.08$ vs. 0.03 ± 0.11 SE, respectively). Heritability was calculated at 17% for preterm delivery in the first pregnancy and 27% for preterm delivery in any pregnancy. A Scandinavian population-based twin study observed 868 monozygotic and 1141 dizygotic female twin pairs that delivered single births between 1973 and 1993.[28,29] Correlation for gestational length was higher for monozygotic compared with dizygotic twins, and heritability estimates from model fitting were approximately 30% for gestational age and 36% for preterm birth. The pattern of preterm births that occur in family pedigrees suggests the dominant form of inheritance is non-Mendelian; rather, the observed pedigrees are more consistent with the influence of many genes. There are numerous studies aimed at discovering variation in genes that contribute to preterm birth, with many associations failing to replicate across populations. **Insights into the complex genetics of preterm birth holds promise for giving insight into pathophysiology and, potentially, to risk-identification; at present, neither of these potential benefits influences clinical care.**

Past Pregnancy History

The strongest historical risk factor is a previous birth between 16 and 36 weeks' gestation. This history is often reported to confer a 1.5-fold to twofold increased risk, but varies widely according to the number, sequence, and gestational age of prior preterm births (Figure 28-6).

When the prior preterm birth occurred in a twin pregnancy, the risk of preterm birth in a subsequent singleton gestation rises as the gestational age at delivery of the twins falls below 34 weeks' gestation. There is minimal if any increased risk for women whose prior twin birth occurred after 34 weeks' gestation, but the risk of singleton preterm birth may be as much as 40% when the prior twin birth occurred before 30 weeks.

Prior stillbirth[30] and pregnancies ending between 16 and 20 weeks' gestation[3] are also associated with increased risk of preterm birth in subsequent pregnancy.

Pregnancy termination in the first and second trimesters is also associated with an increased risk of subsequent preterm birth, especially when performed with mechanical dilation or curettage, or when performed repeatedly.[31] Increased risk of preterm birth has also been found after spontaneous as well as induced abortion.[32]

Current Pregnancy Risks

Mode of conception also affects the risk of preterm birth. The increased rate of preterm birth after assisted reproduction is due not only to the increased occurrence of multiple gestations but to an increased rate of preterm births in singleton pregnancies as well. A nearly twofold increased risk of preterm birth is observed in singleton pregnancies conceived with all methods of fertility care, including ovulation promotion.[33] A meta-analysis of 15 studies that compared 12,283 IVF pregnancies with 1.9 million spontaneously conceived singleton births found approximately twofold increased rates of perinatal mortality, preterm birth, LBW and VLBW, and small for gestational age for infants born after IVF. Rates of preterm birth among multiple gestations do not appear to be increased after assisted conception relative to spontaneously conceived twins and triplets, so the explanation for the increased rates in singletons is not clear. Microbial colonization of the upper genital tract, increased stress among infertile couples, side effects of super-ovulation, and increased rates of birth defects have been proposed.

Bleeding and Vanishing Twins

Women who experience unexplained vaginal bleeding after the first trimester have an increased risk of subsequent preterm birth that increases with the number of episodes. Perhaps reflecting similar cause(s), the risk of preterm birth is also increased in women whose pregnancies are complicated by vanishing twin or by an unexplained elevation in maternal serum alpha-fetoprotein.

Multifetal Gestation and Uterine Distention

Multifetal gestation is one of the strongest risk factors for preterm birth. Rates of preterm, very preterm, LBW, and VLBW births according to fetal number are shown in Chapter 30. Slightly more than 50% of women with twins deliver before 37 weeks. The risk of early birth rises with the number of fetuses, suggesting uterine overdistention and fetal signaling as potential pathways to early initiation of labor. In addition to spontaneous preterm labor, multiple gestations are more commonly complicated by medical and obstetrical disorders that lead to indicated preterm delivery. Poor fetal growth, fetal anomalies, hypertension, abruptio placentae, and fetal compromise are more common in multiple gestation, and increase with the number of fetuses. The chorionicity of twin gestation is also an important factor in the risk of adverse pregnancy outcomes. Monochorionic twin pregnancies are more likely than dichorionic twin gestations to be complicated by stillbirth and fetal growth restriction. Newborn monochorionic twins are more likely than dichorionic twins to experience necrotizing enterocolitis and neuromorbidity. It is unclear how much of the excess rate of preterm birth among monochorionic twins is due to indicated versus spontaneous preterm birth.

Scoring Systems

Attempts to develop scoring systems based on historical and epidemiologic data plus current pregnancy risk factors have had low sensitivity to identify women who will give birth preterm, but did not include some of the historical risks listed here.

PATHOPHYSIOLOGY OF SPONTANEOUS PRETERM BIRTH

Term and preterm parturition share anatomic, physiologic, and biochemical features that are considered part of the common pathway of parturition. This pathway includes (1) increased uterine contractility, (2) cervical ripening, and (3) membrane/decidual activation. However, although spontaneous labor at term results from physiologic activation of the common pathway of parturition, preterm labor is the result of a pathologic activation of this pathway. The insult responsible for activation may lead to asynchronous recruitment of each pathway. Asynchrony is recognized clinically as (1) cervical insufficiency when the process affects predominantly the cervix; (2) preterm uterine contractions when the process affects the myometrium; or (3) preterm premature rupture of membranes if the insult targets the chorioamniotic membranes. Synchronous activation in the preterm gestation would be labeled as preterm labor with intact membranes. Whether at or before term, parturition culminates in a common pathway composed of cervical changes, persistent uterine contractions, and activation of the decidua and membranes. The fundamental difference is that labor at term is a normal physiologic activation of the common pathway, whereas preterm parturition is the result, entirely or in part, of pathologic processes that activate one or more of the components of the common pathway.

Although labor is of short duration (hours or days at the most), parturition is a longer process that includes a preparatory phase of the key organs involved in the common pathway. Thus, cervical changes occur over weeks, there is increased myometrial contractility before the onset of labor, and the appearance of fetal fibronectin in the cervicovaginal mucous can be considered to reflect extracellular matrix degradation, indicating activation of the decidua and membranes.

Normal parturition at term is currently understood as beginning several weeks before actual labor during which cervical ripening occurs as evidenced by changes in cervical consistency and effacement. A fetal maturity-based signal for labor originates in the fetal hypothalamus and leads to increased secretion of corticotropin-releasing hormone, which, in turn, stimulates adrenocorticotrophic hormone and cortisol production by the fetal adrenals, which ultimately leads to activation of the common pathway of parturition. The fetus may contribute to the onset of preterm labor in the context of the fetal inflammatory response syndrome (see later).

Spontaneous preterm birth may best be understood as a syndrome in which the clinical presentations of preterm labor, preterm ruptured membranes, and preterm cervical effacement and dilation without labor occur as the result of multiple etiologies that can occur alone or in combination. Some act to initiate preterm parturition acutely, for example, an acute posttraumatic placental abruption, but most follow a more subacute or indolent path over several weeks. It is helpful to remember that the normal process of parturition proceeds for several weeks before clinically evident labor begins. Thus, pathologic stimuli of parturition may act in concert with the normal physiologic preparation for labor, especially after 32 weeks of pregnancy. Before 30 to 32 weeks, a greater proportion of preterm labor has a pathologic stimulus.

Cervical Changes (Ripening)

The cervix is a critical structure in pregnancy and parturition; the cervix must maintain structural integrity and act as a physical barrier during pregnancy and subsequently transitions to allow passage of the fetus during delivery. This change is not acute; physiologic parturition occurs over the course of gestation, and requires evolving biochemical and biomechanical changes in the cervix that manifest as cervical ripening.[34,35] Molecular processes underlying cervical ripening are different between physiologic and pathologic parturition and may differ among etiologies of pathologic parturition. Although collagen is the main contributor to the tensile strength of the cervix, glycosaminoglycans (GAGs) are critical to determining the viscoelastic properties of the tissue. GAGs are long unbranched polysaccharides that are vital components of the extracellular matrix and serve many roles: they help to determine tissue hydration, which contributes to viscous tissue properties, and stabilize the overall architecture of the extracellular matrix. In addition, small leucine-rich proteoglycans (GAGs linked to core proteins) such as decorin have been shown to interact with soluble growth factors and mediators of inflammation. Tight junctions in the cervical epithelial cells provide structural support and regulate fluid fluxes. Cervical epithelia have numerous functions that include proliferation, differentiation, maintenance of fluid balance, protection from environmental hazards, and paracellular transport of solutes via tight junctions. Epithelial functions must be tightly regulated during pregnancy and parturition, and molecules important in epithelial integrity and function are key components of cervical changes in animal models and in women at term. Extracellular matrix turnover in the cervix is high, and thus, the mechanical properties of the cervix can change rapidly. Changes in extracellular matrix during cervical ripening include an influx of inflammatory cells (macrophages, neutrophils, mast cells, eosinophils, and so on) into the cervical stroma in a process similar to an inflammatory response. These cells produce cytokines and prostaglandins that affect extracellular matrix metabolism. Prostaglandins effect cervical ripening physiologically and have been widely used as pharmacologic agents to ripen the cervix for induction of labor. Cervical ripening is influenced by estrogen, which induces ripening by stimulating collagen degradation, and by progesterone, which blocks these estrogenic effects. Furthermore, administration of progesterone receptor antagonist can induce cervical ripening, and administration of progesterone has been reported to delay or even reverse ripening. Another mediator implicated in the mechanisms of cervical ripening is nitric oxide (NO), which can act as an inflammatory mediator.

Cervical changes normally precede the onset of labor, are gradual, and develop over several weeks. Preterm birth is often preceded by cervical ripening over a period of weeks in the second and third trimesters, evidenced in clinical examination by softening and thinning of the cervix and in ultrasound examination of the cervix by cervical "funneling" and shortening of the length of the endocervical canal.

Increased Uterine Contractility

Labor is characterized by a change in uterine contractility from episodic uncoordinated myometrial contractures that last several minutes and produce little increase in intrauterine pressure to more coordinated contractions of short duration that produce marked increases in intrauterine pressure that ultimately effect delivery. The change from the contracture to the contraction pattern typically begins at night, suggesting neural control. The transition from contractures to contractions may progress to normal labor or may occur dyssynchronously as the result of inflammation, for example, with maternal infection or abdominal surgery. Fasting may also induce the switch in humans. Oxytocin is produced by the decidua and the paraventricular nuclei of the hypothalamus, indicating both an endocrine and a paracrine role. Plasma concentrations of oxytocin mirror uterine contractility, suggesting that oxytocin may mediate the circadian rhythm in uterine contractility.

Cellular communication is another feature of labor, promulgated by formation of gap junctions that develop in the myometrium before labor and disappear after delivery. Gap junction formation and the expression of the gap junction protein connexin 43 in human myometrium is similar in term and preterm labor. These findings suggest that the appearance of gap junctions and increased expression of connexin 43 may be part of the underlying molecular and cellular events responsible for the switch from contractures to contractions before the onset of parturition. Estrogen, progesterone, and prostaglandins have been implicated in the regulation of gap junction formation, as well as in influencing the expression of connexin 43. Lye and colleagues have proposed that changes in a set of distinct proteins called "contraction-associated proteins" are characteristic of this stage of parturition.

Decidual Membrane Activation

The maternal decidua and adjacent fetal membranes undergo anatomic and biochemical changes over the final weeks of gestation that ultimately result in spontaneous rupture of membranes. Premature activation of this mechanism leads to preterm prelabor rupture of membranes (PROM), the clinical antecedent for up to 40% of all preterm deliveries. Although rupture of membranes normally occurs during the first stage of labor, histologic studies of prematurely ruptured membranes show decreased amounts of collagen types I, III, and V and an increased expression of tenascin (expressed during tissue remodeling and wound healing) and disruption of the normal wavy collagen pattern, suggesting that preterm rupture is a process that precedes the onset of labor.

Structural extracellular matrix proteins such as collagens have been implicated in the tensile strength of the membranes, whereas the viscoelastic properties were attributed to elastin. Dissolution of extracellular cements (i.e., fibronectins) is thought to be responsible for the process that allows the membranes to separate from the decidua after the birth of the infant. Degradation of the extracellular matrix, assessed by the detection of fetal fibronectin, is part of the common pathway of parturition. The presence of fetal fibronectin in cervicovaginal secretions between 22 and 37 weeks is evidence of disruption of the decidual-chorionic interface and is associated with an increased risk of preterm birth.

The precise mechanism of membrane-decidual activation is uncertain, but matrix-degrading enzymes and apoptosis (programmed cell death) have been proposed. Increased levels of matrix metalloproteinases (MMPs) and their regulators (TIMPs) have been documented in the amniotic fluid of women with preterm PROM.

Apoptosis may also play a role in the mechanism of membrane rupture, through increased expression of proapoptotic genes and decreased expression of antiapoptotic genes. MMP-9 may induce apoptosis in amnion.

Fetal Participation in the Onset of Labor

A fetal signal contributes to the onset of labor in animals and humans. Destruction of the paraventricular nucleus of the fetal hypothalamus results in prolongation of pregnancy in sheep. The human counterpart to this animal experiment is anencephaly, which is also characterized by prolonged pregnancy when women with polyhydramnios are excluded. The current paradigm is that once maturity has been reached, the fetal brain, specifically the hypothalamus, increases corticotrophin-releasing hormone (CRH) secretion, which, in turn, stimulates adrenocorticotrophic hormone (ACTH) and cortisol production by the fetal adrenals. This increase in cortisol in sheep and dehydroepiandrosterone sulfate in primates eventually leads to activation of the common pathway of parturition. A role for the human fetus in the onset of preterm labor has been proposed in the context of the fetal inflammatory response syndrome.

The Preterm Parturition Syndrome

Obstetrical taxonomy is largely based on clinical presentation, not the mechanism of disease. Preterm labor may occur as the common clinical presentation of infection, vascular insult, uterine overdistention, abnormal allogeneic recognition, stress, or other pathologic processes. Often more than one of these factors is operative in the same patient. Thus, preterm labor is a syndrome for which there is no single diagnostic test or treatment. Obstetrical syndromes share the following features:

- Multiple etiologies
- Chronicity
- Fetal involvement
- Clinical manifestations that are adaptive
- Variable susceptibility due to gene-environment interactions

Each of these features is true of preterm birth. There are clearly *multiple etiologies* for preterm labor, as listed earlier. Pathways to preterm labor are demonstrated to be *chronic*, as seen in the time interval between observation of a short cervix or increased concentrations of fetal fibronectin in vaginal fluid in the midtrimester of pregnancy and subsequent preterm labor or delivery. *Fetal involvement* has been demonstrated in women with microbial invasion of the amniotic cavity, in which fetal bacteremia and cytokine production have been detected in 30% of women with preterm PROM and a positive amniotic fluid culture for microorganisms. Similarly, neonates born after spontaneous preterm labor or preterm PROM are more likely to be small for gestational age, suggesting chronically compromised fetal supply. Preterm labor may be seen as an *adaptive* mechanism of host defense against infection that allows the mother to eliminate an infected tissue and the fetus to exit from a hostile environment. If the clinical manifestations are adaptive, it is not surprising that treatments aimed at the common terminal pathway of parturition, such as tocolysis or cerclage, and not at the fundamental mechanism of disease-inducing activation of the pathway (myometrial contractility, cervical dilation, and effacement), would not be effective. There is increasing evidence of gene-environment interaction in the steps leading to preterm labor, complicated by the presence, and even perhaps the conflicting interests, of two genomes (maternal and fetal). This is most evident in studies of the relationship between maternal genital tract colonization and preterm birth. Finally, there may be additional mechanisms not yet identified.

Pathologic processes implicated in the preterm parturition syndrome include intrauterine infection, uterine ischemia, uterine overdistention, abnormal allograft reaction, allergy-induced causes, cervical insufficiency, and endocrine disorders.

Intrauterine Infection

Systemic maternal infections such as pyelonephritis and pneumonia are frequently associated with the onset of premature labor in humans. Intrauterine infection is a frequent and important mechanism of disease leading to preterm delivery. Intrauterine infection or systemic administration of microbial products to pregnant animals can result in preterm labor and delivery, and there is substantial evidence that subclinical intrauterine infections are associated with preterm labor and delivery. Moreover, fetal infection and inflammation have been implicated in the genesis of fetal or neonatal injury leading to cerebral palsy and chronic lung disease. Microbiologic and histopathologic studies suggest that infection-related inflammation may account for 25% to 40% of cases of preterm delivery.

Frequency of Intrauterine Infection in Spontaneous Preterm Birth

The prevalence of positive amniotic fluid cultures for microorganisms in women with preterm labor and intact membranes is approximately 13%, with additional instances of infection that are identifiable using PCR techniques rather than culture. The earlier the gestational age at preterm birth, the more likely that microbial invasion of the amniotic cavity is present. In preterm PROM, the prevalence of positive amniotic fluid cultures for microorganisms is approximately 32%. Among women with a dilated cervix in the midtrimester, the prevalence of positive amniotic fluid cultures is 51%. Microbial invasion of the amniotic cavity occurs in 12% of twin gestations with preterm labor and delivering a preterm neonate. The most common microorganisms found in the amniotic cavity are genital *Mycoplasmas* and *U. urealyticum*.

Intrauterine Infection as a Chronic Process

Evidence in support of chronicity of intrauterine inflammation/infection is derived from studies of the microbiologic state of the amniotic fluid, as well as the concentration of inflammatory mediators at the time of genetic amniocentesis. Genital mycoplasmas including *M. hominis* and *U. urealyticum* have been recovered from amniotic fluid samples obtained at second-trimester genetic amniocentesis, with subsequent preterm delivery and histologic chorioamnionitis, especially in those with *U. urealyticum*. Increased levels of many inflammatory markers have been found in second-trimester amniotic fluid samples obtained from women who subsequently delivered preterm. These observations suggest that infection and inflammation in the amniotic cavity in the midtrimester of pregnancy can lead to preterm delivery weeks later. The most advanced stage of intrauterine infection is fetal infection. Fetal bacteremia has been detected in blood obtained by cordocentesis in 33% of fetuses with positive amniotic fluid culture and 4% of those with negative amniotic fluid culture.

Molecular mediators that trigger parturition (cytokines and other inflammatory mediators) are similar to those that

protect the host against infection. The onset of preterm labor in response to intrauterine infection is thus very likely a host defense mechanism with survival value for mother and, after viability, for the fetus as well.

Infection, Preterm Labor, and Neonatal Outcomes

The scenario postulated from the preceding evidence is that microorganisms that reside in or ascend to reach the decidua may, depending on host defense and environmental influences, stimulate a local inflammatory reaction, as well as the production of proinflammatory cytokines, chemokines, and inflammatory mediators. This inflammatory process, which is initially extra-amniotic, may produce cervical effacement, further inflammation of the choriodecidual interface, and uterine contractions, and may progress to the amniotic fluid and, ultimately, the fetus as well. Microorganisms are known to cross intact membranes into the amniotic cavity, where inflammatory mediators are produced by resident macrophages and other host cells within the amniotic cavity. Finally, microorganisms that gain access to the fetus may elicit a systemic inflammatory response, the fetal inflammatory response syndrome (FIRS), characterized by increased concentrations of IL-6 and other cytokines, as well as cellular evidence of neutrophil and monocyte activation. FIRS is a subclinical condition originally described in fetuses of mothers with preterm labor and intact membranes and preterm PROM. Fetuses with FIRS have a higher rate of neonatal complications and are frequently born to mothers with subclinical microbial invasion of the amniotic cavity. Evidence of multisystemic involvement in cases of FIRS includes increased concentrations of fetal plasma MMP-9, neutrophilia, a higher number of circulating nucleated red blood cells, and higher plasma concentrations of G-CSF. The histologic hallmark of FIRS is inflammation in the umbilical cord (funisitis) or chorionic vasculitis. The systemic fetal inflammatory response may result in multiple organ dysfunction, septic shock, and death in the absence of timely delivery. Newborns with funisitis are at increased risk for neonatal sepsis as well as long-term handicaps, including BPD and cerebral palsy.

When the inflammatory process does not involve the chorioamniotic membranes and decidua, systemic fetal inflammation and injury may occur in the absence of labor with eventual delivery at term. An example of this is fetal alloimmunization in which there is an elevation of fetal plasma concentrations of interleukin 6, but not preterm labor.

Gene-Environment Interactions

Gene-environment interactions underlie many complex disorders such as atherosclerosis and cancer. A gene-environment interaction is said to be present when the risk of a disease (occurrence or severity) among individuals exposed (to both genotype and an environmental factor) is greater or lower than that which is predicted from the presence of either the genotype or the environmental exposure alone. The inflammatory response to the presence of microorganisms is modulated by interactions between the host genotype and environment that determine the likelihood and course of some infectious diseases. An example of such an interaction has been reported for BV, an allele for TNF-a and preterm delivery. Maternal BV is a consistently reported risk factor for spontaneous preterm delivery, yet treatment of BV does not reliably prevent preterm birth in women with BV. One potential explanation has come from a study of preterm birth rates in women according to their carriage of BV and whether or not they had allele 2 of TNF-a known to be associated with spontaneous preterm birth. Both BV (OR 3.3; 95% CI 1.8 to 5.9) and TNF-a allele 2 (OR 2.7; 95% CI 1.7 to 4.5) were associated with increased risk for preterm delivery, but the risk of spontaneous preterm birth was substantially increased (OR 6; 95% CI 1.9 to 21.0) in women with both BV and the TNF-a allele 2. It is reasonable to assume that other gene-environment interactions may contribute to preterm birth.

Uteroplacental Ischemia/Decidual Hemorrhage

After inflammation, the most common abnormalities seen in placental pathology specimens from spontaneous preterm births are vascular lesions of the maternal and fetal circulations. Maternal lesions include failure of physiologic transformation of the spiral arteries, atherosis, and thrombosis. Fetal abnormalities include decreased number of villous arterioles and fetal arterial thrombosis.

One proposed mechanism linking vascular lesions and preterm labor/delivery is uteroplacental ischemia, evidenced in primate models and in studies that found failure of physiologic transformation in the myometrial segment of the spiral arteries, a phenomenon typical of preeclampsia and intrauterine growth restriction, in women with preterm labor and intact membranes and preterm PROM as well. Abnormal uterine artery Doppler velocimetry indicating increased impedance to flow in the uterine circulation has been reported in women with apparently idiopathic preterm labor.

The mechanisms responsible for preterm parturition in cases of ischemia have not been determined, but uterine ischemia has been postulated to lead to increased production of uterine renin from the fetal membranes. Angiotensin II can induce myometrial contractility directly or through the release of prostaglandins.

Decidual necrosis and hemorrhage can activate parturition through production of thrombin, which stimulates myometrial contractility in a dose-dependent manner. Thrombin also stimulates production of MMP-1, urokinase-type plasminogen activator (uPA), and tissue-type plasminogen activator (tPA) by endometrial stromal cells in culture. These factors can, directly or indirectly, digest important components of the extracellular matrix in the chorioamniotic membranes. Thrombin/antithrombin complexes, a marker of in vivo generation of thrombin, are increased in plasma and amniotic fluid of women with preterm labor and preterm PROM. Decidua is a rich source of tissue factor, the primary initiator of coagulation and of thrombin activation. These observations are consistent with clinical associations among vaginal bleeding, retroplacental hematomas, and preterm delivery.

Uterine ischemia should not be equated with fetal hypoxemia. Studies of fetal cord blood do not support fetal hypoxemia as a cause (or consequence) of preterm parturition.

Uterine Overdistention

The mechanisms responsible for the increased frequency of preterm birth in multiple gestations and other disorders associated with uterine overdistention are unknown. Central questions are how the uterus senses stretch, and how these mechanical forces induce biochemical changes that lead to parturition. Increased expression of oxytocin receptor, connexin 43, and the *c-fos* mRNA have been consistently demonstrated in the rat myometrium near term. Progesterone blocks stretch-induced gene expression in the myometrium. Mitogen-activated protein kinases have been proposed to mediate stretch-induced *c-fos* mRNA expression in myometrial cells. Stretch can have effects on the membranes. For example, in vitro studies have demonstrated an increase in the production of collagenase, IL-8, and prostaglandin E_2 (PGE_2), as well as the cytokine pre–B-cell colony-enhancing factor. These observations provide a possible link between the mechanical forces operating in an overdistended uterus and rupture of membranes.

Abnormal Allograft Reaction

The fetoplacental unit has been considered nature's most successful semiallograft. Abnormal recognition and adaptation to fetal antigens has been proposed as a mechanism of recurrent pregnancy loss, intrauterine growth restriction, and preeclampsia. Chronic villitis, a lesion indicative of placental rejection, has been found in the placentas of some women who deliver after spontaneous preterm labor.

Allergy-Induced Preterm Labor

Case reports indicate that preterm labor has occurred after exposure to an allergen that generates an allergic-like mechanism (type I hypersensitivity reaction) and that some women with preterm labor have eosinophils as the predominant cells in amniotic fluid, suggesting a form of uterine allergy. Mast cells in the uterus produce histamine and prostaglandins, both of which can induce myometrial contractility. Premature birth can be induced by exposure to an allergen in sensitized animals, and can be prevented by treatment with a histamine H_1 receptor antagonist.

Cervical Insufficiency

In response to cervical ultrasound measurements showing an increased risk of preterm birth in women with short cervix, the understanding of cervical function evolved from a categorical concept of cervical "incompetence" versus "competence" to one of "competence as a continuum."[12] However, subsequent analyses of this same data[11] were conducted in response to clinical trials demonstrating that preterm cervical shortening (softening and ripening) is not the passive result of tissue weakness but instead is an active process that can be slowed or prevented by progesterone supplementation in some women.[14-18] These studies have led to the conclusion that short cervix in the second trimester of pregnancy is evidence that parturition has begun, presumably in response to decidual membrane activation in response to microbial colonization and/or decidual hemorrhage, perhaps aided by cervical factors and/or subclinical myometrial activity. Figure 28-7 shows the length of the cervix at 22 to 24 weeks' gestation and the subsequent rate of cervical shortening in women who later presented after 28 weeks' gestation with preterm labor or preterm PPROM, compared to women who delivered at term or preterm due to medical indication. Significant differences in cervical length were already evident at 22 to 24 weeks, more than a month before clinical presentation, and accelerated for several weeks before clinical presentation.

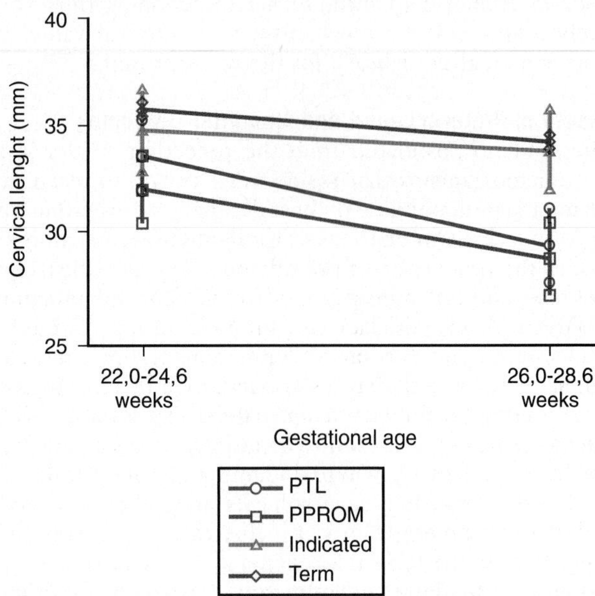

FIGURE 28-7. Length of the cervix at 22 to 24 weeks' gestation and the subsequent rate of cervical shortening in women presenting after 28 weeks with preterm labor or preterm PPROM, compared to women who delivered at term or preterm due to medical indication.

Endocrine Disorders

Estrogen and progesterone play a central role in the endocrinology of pregnancy. Progesterone is thought to maintain myometrial quiescence and inhibit cervical ripening. Estrogens have been implicated in increasing myometrial contractility and excitability, as well as in the induction of cervical ripening before the onset of labor. In many species, a fall in maternal serum progesterone concentration occurs before spontaneous parturition, but the mechanism for this progesterone withdrawal depends primarily on whether the placenta or the corpus luteum is the major source of progesterone.

A fall in serum progesterone levels has not been demonstrated before parturition in humans. Nevertheless, inhibition of progesterone action could result in parturition. Alternative mechanisms posited to explain a suspension of progesterone action without a serum progesterone withdrawal include binding of progesterone to a high-affinity protein and, thus, reduced functional active form; increased cortisol concentration that competes with progesterone for binding to the glucocorticoid receptors, resulting in functional progesterone withdrawal; and conversion of progesterone to an inactive form within the target cell before interacting with its receptor. None of these hypotheses are proven. Recent research has focused on alterations in the number and function of estrogen-progesterone receptors and progesterone binding.

The human progesterone receptor (PR) exists as two major subtypes, PR-A and PR-B. Another isoform, PR-C, has recently been described, but its function is not well understood. The human estrogen receptor (ER) also exists as two major subtypes, ERa and ERb. A functional progesterone withdrawal has been proposed in which expression of PR-A in myometrium suppresses progesterone responsiveness and that functional progesterone withdrawal occurs by increased expression of the PR-A relative to PR-B. An alternative mechanism of functional progesterone withdrawal has been proposed wherein activation of nuclear factor k B in amnion represses progesterone function. Regardless of the mechanism, there is a building consensus that a localized functional progesterone withdrawal occurs in myometrium during human parturition.

Summary of the Preterm Parturition Syndrome

Preterm parturition is a syndrome caused by multiple etiologies with several clinical presentations including uterine contractility (preterm labor), preterm cervical ripening without significant clinical contractility (cervical insufficiency or advanced cervical dilation and effacement), or rupture of the amniotic sac (preterm PROM). The clinical presentation varies with the type and timing of the insult or stimulus to the components of the common pathway of parturition, the presence or absence of environmental cofactors, and individual variations in host response by both mother and fetus. This conceptual framework has implications for the understanding of the mechanisms responsible for the initiation of preterm parturition, as well as the diagnosis, treatment, and prevention of preterm birth.

CLINICAL CARE FOR WOMEN IN PRETERM LABOR

Clinical evaluation of preterm parturition begins with assessment of potential causes of labor, looking first for conditions that threaten the health of mother and fetus. Acute maternal conditions, for example, pyelonephritis, pneumonia, asthma, peritonitis, trauma, and hypertension, or obstetrical conditions including preeclampsia, placental abruption, placenta previa, and chorioamnionitis may mandate delivery. Fetal compromise may be acute, manifested by an abnormal fetal heart rate tracing, or chronic, indicated by fetal growth restriction or oligohydramnios, and may require delivery depending on the severity and potential for in utero versus ex utero treatment. Fetal growth restriction is more common in infants delivered after preterm labor or preterm PROM, even in apparently otherwise uncomplicated pregnancies. **Conditions that suggest specific therapy such as preterm ruptured membranes or cervical insufficiency should then be sought and treated accordingly.**

The next concerns are the accuracy of preterm labor diagnosis and the balance of risks and benefits that accompany active attempts to inhibit labor versus allowing delivery. Several issues arise:

- What is the gestational age, and what is the level of confidence about the accuracy of the gestational age?
- What, in the absence of advanced labor (cervical effacement >80% with dilation >2 cm) and a clear cause of preterm labor, is the accuracy of the diagnosis of preterm labor?
- Are confirmatory diagnostic tests such as cervical sonography, fetal fibronectin, or amniocentesis for infection necessary?
- What is the anticipated neonatal morbidity and mortality at this gestational age in this clinical setting?
- Should labor be stopped?
- Is transfer to a more appropriate hospital required?
- Should fetal lung maturity be tested?
- What interventions can be applied that will reduce the risks of perinatal morbidity and mortality?
- Should drugs to arrest labor (tocolytics), glucocorticoids, and/or antibiotics be given?

DIAGNOSIS OF PRETERM LABOR

Given the pathways for preterm parturition described earlier, clinical recognition of preterm labor requires attention to the biochemical as well as the biophysical features of the onset of labor. Pathologic uterine contractility rarely occurs in isolation; cervical ripening and decidual membrane activation are almost always in progress as well, most often before uterine contractions are clinically evident. Therefore, preterm labor must be considered whenever a pregnant woman reports recurrent abdominal or pelvic symptoms that persist for more than an hour in the second half or pregnancy. Symptoms of preterm labor such as pelvic pressure, increased vaginal discharge, backache, and menstrual-like cramps occur frequently in normal pregnancy, and suggest preterm labor more by persistence than severity. **Contractions may be painful or painless, depending on the resistance offered by the cervix.** Contractions against a closed, uneffaced cervix are likely to be painful, but persistence of recurrent pressure or tightening may be the only symptoms when cervical effacement precedes the onset of contractions.

For decades, the clinical diagnosis of preterm labor has been based on the presence of regular, painful uterine contractions accompanied by cervical dilation and/or effacement. These criteria assume a crisp demarcation between "preterm parturition" and "preterm labor" that is increasingly understood as being more gradual than previously thought. If thought of as screening criteria for the outcome "preterm birth," clinical signs and symptoms demonstrate poor sensitivity and specificity. Identifying women with preterm contractions who will actually deliver preterm is an inexact process. In like fashion, identifying those women who are at increased risk of not just preterm birth, but imminent preterm birth, remains elusive. A systematic review noted that approximately 30% of preterm labor cases resolved spontaneously. In subsequent studies, 50% of patients hospitalized for preterm labor actually delivered at term. **The inability to distinguish women in "true preterm labor" from women in "false labor" accurately has greatly hampered the assessment of therapeutic interventions, since as many as 50% of untreated (or placebo treated) subjects do not actually deliver preterm. Optimal criteria**

for initiation of treatment are not clear. Contraction frequency of six or more per hour, cervical dilation of 3 cm, effacement of 80%, ruptured membranes, and bleeding are symptoms of preterm labor most often associated with preterm delivery. When lower thresholds for contraction frequency and cervical change are used, "false-positive" diagnosis (defined in randomized controlled trials as delivery at term after treatment with placebo only) occurs in nearly 40% of women, but sensitivity does not rise. Difficulty in accurate diagnosis is the product of the high prevalence of the symptoms and signs of early preterm labor in normal pregnancy, the gradual onset of preterm labor discussed earlier, and the imprecision of digital examination of the cervix below 3 cm dilation and 80% effacement. The practice of initiating tocolytic drugs for contraction frequency without additional diagnostic criteria results in unnecessary treatment of women who are not at increased risk of imminent spontaneous preterm birth.[36]

Diagnostic Tests for Preterm Labor

Women with symptoms whose cervical dilation is less than 2 cm and whose effacement is less than 80% present a diagnostic challenge. Diagnostic accuracy may be improved in these patients by testing other features of parturition, such as cervical ripening, assessed by transvaginal sonographic measurement of cervical length; and decidual activation, tested by an assay for fetal fibronectin in cervicovaginal fluid.[37,38] Both tests aid diagnosis primarily by reducing false-positive diagnosis. Transabdominal sonography has poor reproducibility for cervical measurement and should not be used clinically without confirmation by a transvaginal ultrasound. A cervical length of 30 mm or more by endovaginal sonography indicates that preterm labor is unlikely in symptomatic women if the examination is properly performed.

Similarly, a negative fibronectin test in women with symptoms before 34 weeks' gestation with cervical dilation less than 3 cm can also reduce the rate of false-positive diagnosis if the result is returned promptly and the clinician is willing to act on a negative test result by not initiating treatment. When both tests were performed in a study of 206 women with possible preterm labor, the fetal fibronectin test improved the performance of sonographic cervical length only when the sonographic cervical length was less than 30 mm (see the accompanying box, Clinical Evaluation of Patients with Possible Preterm Labor).

Clinical Evaluation of Patients with Possible Preterm Labor

1. **Patient presents with signs/symptoms of preterm labor:**
   Persistent contractions (painful or painless)
   Intermittent abdominal cramping, pelvic pressure, or backache
   Increase or change in vaginal discharge
   Vaginal spotting or bleeding
2. **General physical examination:**
   Sitting pulse and blood pressure
   Temperature
   External fetal heart rate and contraction monitor
3. **Sterile speculum examination**
   pH
   Fern
   Pooled fluid
   Fibronectin swab (posterior fornix or external cervical os, avoiding areas with bleeding)
   Cultures for chlamydia (cervix), and *Neisseria gonorrhoeae* (cervix), and group B streptococcus (outer third of vagina and perineum)
4. **Transabdominal ultrasound examination**
   Placental location
   Amniotic fluid volume
   Estimated fetal weight and presentation
   Fetal well-being
5. **Cervical examination** (after ruptured membranes excluded)
   a. **Cervix >3 cm dilation/≥80% effaced**
   Preterm labor diagnosis confirmed. Evaluate for tocolysis.
   b. **Cervix 2 to 3 cm dilation/<80% effaced**
   Preterm labor likely but not established. Monitor contraction frequency and repeat digital examination in 30-60 minutes. Diagnose preterm labor if cervical change. If not, send fibronectin or obtain transvaginal cervical ultrasound. Evaluate for tocolysis if any cervical change, cervical length <20 mm, or positive fibronectin.
   c. **Cervix <2 cm dilation and <80% effaced**
   Preterm labor diagnosis uncertain. Monitor contraction frequency, send fibronectin and/or obtain cervical sonography, and repeat digital examination in 1 to 2 hours. Evaluate for tocolysis if there is a 1 cm change in cervical dilation, effacement >80%, cervical length <20 mm, or positive fibronectin.
6. **Use of Cervical Ultrasound**
   Cervical length <20 mm *and* contraction criteria met = preterm labor
   Cervical length 20-30 mm *and* contraction criteria met = probable preterm labor
   Cervical length >30 mm = preterm labor *very unlikely* regardless of contraction frequency

Amniocentesis for Women with Preterm Labor

The goal of care for women with preterm labor is to reduce perinatal morbidity and mortality, most of which is caused by immaturity of the respiratory, gastrointestinal, coagulation, and central nervous systems of the preterm infant. Fetal pulmonary immaturity is the most frequent cause of serious newborn illness, and the fetal pulmonary system is the only organ system whose function is directly testable before delivery. If the quality of obstetrical dating is good and intrauterine fetal well-being is not compromised, the likelihood of neonatal RDS may be estimated from the gestational age.

Amniotic fluid studies may be useful in women with possible preterm labor in the following circumstances:

1. *Fetal pulmonary maturity testing.* Generally speaking, gestational age at birth is the best predictor of the frequency and severity of the consequences of prematurity to the newborn. As noted earlier, generally speaking, labor inhibition and antenatal glucocorticoid therapy are used when birth is anticipated to occur between 24 and 34 weeks' gestation. When dates are uncertain (e.g., late prenatal

Public and Professional Policies

Policies promulgated by fertility specialists intended to reduce the risk of higher-order multiple gestation have been successful in Europe, Australia, and the United States. Rates of triplet and higher-order multiple pregnancies had been rising rapidly in the United States until 1998, when the increase was arrested by voluntary adoption of limitations on the number of ova transferred. The rate of higher-order multiples fell by 50% between 1996 and 2003. A societal approach to improve pregnancy

TABLE 28-5 GUIDANCE REGARDING TIMING OF DELIVERY WHEN CONDITIONS COMPLICATE PREGNANCY AT 34 WEEKS OF GESTATION OR LATER—cont'd

CONDITION	GESTATIONAL AGE* AT DELIVERY	GRADE OF RECOMMENDATION†
Fetal congenital malformations‡	**34-39 wk:** Suspected worsening of fetal organ damage Potential for fetal intracranial hemorrhage (e.g., vein of Galen aneurysm, neonatal alloimmune thrombocytopenia) When delivery prior to labor is preferred (e.g., EXIT procedure) Previous fetal intervention Concurrent maternal disease (e.g., preeclampsia, chronic hypertension) Potential for adverse maternal effect from fetal condition	B
	Expeditious delivery regardless of gestational age: When intervention is expected to be beneficial Fetal complications develop (abnormal fetal surveillance, new-onset hydrops fetalis, progressive or new-onset organ injury) Maternal complications develop (mirror syndrome)	B
Multiple gestations: dichorionic-diamniotic‡	**38 wk**	B
Multiple gestations: monochorionic-diamniotic‡	**34-37 wk**	B
Multiple gestations: dichorionic-diamniotic or monochorionic-diamniotic with single fetal death‡	If occurs at or after 34 wk, consider delivery (recommendation limited to pregnancies at or after 34 wk; if occurs before 34 wk, individualize based on concurrent maternal or fetal conditions)	B
Multiple gestations: monochorionic-monoamniotic‡	**32-34 wk**	B
Multiple gestations: monochorionic-monoamniotic with single fetal death‡	Consider delivery; individualized according to gestational age and concurrent complications	B
Oligohydramnios—isolated and presistent‡	**36-37 wk**	B
Maternal Issues		
Chronic hypertension—no medications‡	**38-39 wk**	B
Chronic hypertension—controlled on medication‡	**37-39 wk**	B
Chronic hypertension—difficult to control (requiring frequent medication adjustments)‡	**36-37 wk**	B
Gestational hypertension§	**37-38 wk**	B
Preeclampsia—severe‡	At diagnosis (recommendation limited to pregnancies at or after 34 wk)	C
Preeclampsia—mild‡	**37 wk**	B
Diabetes—pregestational, well controlled‡	LPTB or ETB not recommended	B
Diabetes—pregestational, with vascular disease‡	**37-39 wk**	B
Diabetes—pregestational, poorly controlled‡	**34-39 wk** (individualized to situation)	B
Diabetes—gestational, well controlled on diet‡	LPTB or ETB not recommended	B
Diabetes—gestational, well controlled on medication‡	LPTB or ETB not recommended	B
Diabetes—gestational, poorly controlled on medication‡	**34-39 wk** (individualized to situation)	B
Obstetrical Issues		
Prior stillbirth—unexplained‡	LPTB or ETB not recommended	B
	Consider amniocentesis for fetal pulmonary maturity if delivery planned at less than 39 wk	C
Spontaneous preterm birth: preterm premature rupture of membranes‡	**34 wk** (recommendation limited to pregnancies at or after 34 wk)	B
Spontaneous preterm birth: active preterm labor‡	Delivery if progressive labor or additional maternal or fetal indication	B

From Spong CY, Mercer BM, D'Alton M, et al: Timing of indicated late-preterm and early-term birth. Obstet Gynecol 118(2 Pt 1):323, 2011.

*Gestational age is in completed weeks; thus, 34 weeks includes $34^{0/7}$ weeks through $34^{6/7}$ weeks.

†Grade of recommendation is based on the following: recommendations or conclusions or both are based on good and consistent scientific evidence (A); limited or inconsistent scientific evidence (B); primarily consensus and expert opinion (C). The recommendations regarding expeditious delivery for imminent fetal jeopardy were not given a grade. The recommendation regarding severe preeclampsia is based largely on expert opinion; however, higher-level evidence is not likely to be forthcoming because this condition is believed to carry significant maternal risk with limited potential fetal benefit from expectant management after 34 weeks.

‡Uncomplicated, thus no fetal growth restriction, superimposed preeclampsia, etc. If these are present, the complicating conditions take precedence and earlier delivery may be indicated

§Maintenance antihypertensive therapy should not be used to treat gestational hypertension.

ETB, Early-term birth at $37^{0/7}$ weeks through $38^{6/7}$ weeks; *LPTB*, late-preterm birth at $34^{0/7}$ weeks through $36^{6/7}$ weeks.

outcomes has been adopted in most European countries, where policies to protect pregnant women include minimum paid pregnancy leave, time off for prenatal visits, exemption from night shifts, and protection from workplace hazards. The Europop Study (European Programme of Occupational Risks and Pregnancy Outcome) of such policies found that risk of preterm birth was increased among women who worked more than 42 hours per week (OR 1.33, CI 1.1 to 1.6) and who were required to stand for more than 6 hours per day (OR 1.26, CI 1.1 to 1.5).

Social Determinants of Health

Racial disparities in health are not confined to perinatal medicine but rather are reflected throughout the life span. The increased rates of many illnesses in African Americans and other disadvantaged groups are being addressed by the public health community through the social determinants of health: promotion of school attendance and completion, food security, neighborhood nutritional programs, job fairs, and an increasing role for hospital and health providers as local leaders.[74]

SUMMARY

Preterm birth is a syndrome, the final result of several pathways that often overlap to initiate parturition. Obstetrical interventions to reduce infant morbidity such as antenatal glucocorticoids and antibiotics for group B streptococcal prophylaxis are effective tertiary therapies but have no opportunity to reduce the incidence of preterm birth. Detection of pregnancies at risk through careful review of prior pregnancies and selective or universal use of cervical ultrasound screening to identify candidates for progesterone therapy and selective use of cerclage are welcome advances. Adherence to protocols for timing of scheduled births and documentation of indications for iatrogenic preterm birth are needed to further reduce the rate of stillbirth while limiting the associated morbidity of late preterm birth.

KEY POINTS

- More than 70% of fetal, neonatal, and infant morbidity and mortality occurs in infants born preterm.
- The rate of preterm birth peaked in 2006 as the result of the increased use of assisted reproductive technology, ultrasound dating, and indicated preterm births. It has since declined largely because of the adoption of fertility practices to reduce multifetal gestations associated with infertility treatment.
- Major risk factors for preterm birth are a history of previous preterm delivery, multifetal gestation, and bleeding after the first trimester of pregnancy, but most women who deliver preterm have no apparent risk factors. Every pregnancy is potentially at risk.
- Spontaneous preterm birth is a syndrome in which the parturitional process may be initiated by one or more pathways culminating in cervical ripening, decidual activation, uterine contractions, and ruptured membranes.
- Four interventions have been shown to reduce perinatal morbidity and mortality:
  - Transfer of the mother and fetus to an appropriate hospital before preterm birth.
  - Administration of maternal antibiotics to prevent neonatal GBS infection.
  - Administration of maternal corticosteroids to reduce neonatal RDS and intraventricular hemorrhage, and neonatal mortality.
  - Administration of maternal magnesium sulfate at the time of preterm birth <32 weeks to reduce the incidence of cerebral palsy
- The risk of recurrent preterm birth may be reduced in women with a prior preterm birth and/or a short cervix <20 mm by administration of prophylactic supplemental progesterone, and by selective use of cervical cerclage.

REFERENCES

1. Callaghan WM, MacDorman MF, et al: The contribution of preterm birth to infant mortality rates in the United States. Pediatrics 118:1566, 2006.
2. Fleischman AR, Oinuma M, et al: Rethinking the definition of term pregnancy. Obstet Gynecol 116:136, 2010.
3. Edlow AG, Srinivas SK, et al: Second-trimester loss and subsequent pregnancy outcomes: what is the real risk? Am J Obstet Gynecol 197:581e1, 2007.
4. McManemy J, Cooke E, et al: Recurrence risk for preterm delivery. Am J Obstet Gynecol 196:576e1, discussion 576e6, 2007.
5. Silver RM, Branch DW, Goldenberg RL, et al: Nomenclature for pregnancy outcomes: time for a change. Obstet Gynecol 118:1402, 2011.
6. Beck S, Wojdyla D, et al: The worldwide incidence of preterm birth: a systematic review of maternal mortality and morbidity. Bull World Health Organ 88:31, 2010.
7. Hamilton BE, Martin JA, Ventura SJ: Births: Preliminary data for 2009. National vital statistics reports web release; vol 59 no 3. Hyattsville, MD, National Center for Health Statistics, 2010.
8. MacDorman MF, Kirmeyer S: Fetal and perinatal mortality, United States, 2005. Natl Vital Stat Rep 57:1, 2009.
9. Stoll BJ, Hansen NI, et al: Neonatal outcomes of extremely preterm infants from the NICHD Neonatal Research Network. Pediatrics 126:443, 2010.
10. Moster D, Lie RT, et al: Long-term medical and social consequences of preterm birth. N Engl J Med 359:262, 2008.
11. Iams JD, Cebrik D, Lynch C, et al: The rate of cervical change and the phenotype of spontaneous preterm birth. Am J Obstet Gynecol 205:130.e1, 2011.
12. Iams JD, Goldenberg RL, et al: The length of the cervix and the risk of spontaneous premature delivery. National Institute of Child Health and Human Development Maternal Fetal Medicine Unit Network. N Engl J Med 334:567, 1996.
13. Iams JD, Newman RB, et al: Frequency of uterine contractions and the risk of spontaneous preterm delivery. N Engl J Med 346:250, 2002.
14. DeFranco EA, O'Brien JM, et al: Vaginal progesterone is associated with a decrease in risk for early preterm birth and improved neonatal outcome in women with a short cervix: a secondary analysis from a randomized, double-blind, placebo-controlled trial. Ultrasound Obstet Gynecol 30:697, 2007.
15. Fonseca EB, Celik E, et al: Progesterone and the risk of preterm birth among women with a short cervix. N Engl J Med 357:462, 2007.

16. O'Brien JM, Adair CD, et al: Progesterone vaginal gel for the reduction of recurrent preterm birth: primary results from a randomized, double-blind, placebo-controlled trial. Ultrasound Obstet Gynecol 30:687, 2007.
17. O'Brien JM, Defranco EA, et al: Effect of progesterone on cervical shortening in women at risk for preterm birth: secondary analysis from a multinational, randomized, double-blind, placebo-controlled trial. Ultrasound Obstet Gynecol 34:653, 2009.
18. Hassan SS, Romero R, et al: Vaginal progesterone reduces the rate of preterm birth in women with a sonographic short cervix: a multicenter, randomized, double-blind, placebo-controlled trial. Ultrasound Obstet Gynecol 38:18, 2011.
19. Simhan HN, Bodnar LM: Prepregnancy body mass index, vaginal inflammation, and the racial disparity in preterm birth. Am J Epidemiol 163:459, 2006.
20. Zhong Y, Cahill AG, et al: The association between prepregnancy maternal body mass index and preterm delivery. Am J Perinatol 27:293, 2010.
21. Klebanoff MA, Harper M, et al: Fish consumption, erythrocyte fatty acids, and preterm birth. Obstet Gynecol 117:1071, 2011.
22. Behrman R, Stith Butler A: Preterm birth: causes, consequences, and prevention. Report of the Committee on Understanding Premature Birth and Assuring Healthy Outcomes. Institute of Medicine. National Academies Press, 2007
23. Martin JA, Hamilton BE, et al: Births: final data for 2007. Natl Vital Stat Rep 58:1, 2010.
24. Lu MC, Chen B: Racial and ethnic disparities in preterm birth: the role of stressful life events. Am J Obstet Gynecol 191:691, 2004.
25. Healy AJ, Malone FD, et al: Early access to prenatal care: implications for racial disparity in perinatal mortality. Obstet Gynecol 107:625, 2006.
26. Hobel CJ, Goldstein A, et al: Psychosocial stress and pregnancy outcome. Clin Obstet Gynecol 51:333, 2008.
27. Grote NK, Bridge JA, et al: A meta-analysis of depression during pregnancy and the risk of preterm birth, low birth weight, and intrauterine growth restriction. Arch Gen Psychiatry 67:1012, 2010.
28. Treloar SA, Macones GA, et al: Genetic influences on premature parturition in an Australian twin sample. Twin Res 3:80, 2000.
29. Clausson B, Lichtenstein P, et al: Genetic influence on birthweight and gestational length determined by studies in offspring of twins. BJOG 107:375, 2000.
30. Getahun D, Lawrence JM, et al: The association between stillbirth in the first pregnancy and subsequent adverse perinatal outcomes. Am J Obstet Gynecol 201:378e1, 2009.
31. Watson LF, Rayner JA, et al: Modelling prior reproductive history to improve prediction of risk for very preterm birth. Paediatr Perinat Epidemiol 24:402, 2010.
32. Makhlouf M: Adverse pregnancy outcomes among women with prior spontaneous or induced abortions. Am J Obstet Gynecol 205:S204, 2011.
33. Reddy UM, Wapner RJ, et al: Infertility, assisted reproductive technology, and adverse pregnancy outcomes: executive summary of a National Institute of Child Health and Human Development workshop. Obstet Gynecol 109:967, 2007.
34. Word RA, Li XH, et al: Dynamics of cervical remodeling during pregnancy and parturition: mechanisms and current concepts. Semin Reprod Med 25:69, 2007.
35. Timmons B, Akins M, et al: Cervical remodeling during pregnancy and parturition. Trends Endocrinol Metab 21:353, 2010.
36. Swamy GK, Simhan HN, et al: Clinical utility of fetal fibronectin for predicting preterm birth. J Reprod Med 50:851, 2005.
37. Berghella V, Hayes E, et al: Fetal fibronectin testing for reducing the risk of preterm birth. Cochrane Database Syst Rev CD006843, 2008.
38. Berghella V, Baxter JK, et al: Cervical assessment by ultrasound for preventing preterm delivery. Cochrane Database Syst Rev CD007235, 2009.
39. Verani JR, McGee L, et al: Prevention of perinatal group B streptococcal disease—revised guidelines from CDC, 2010. MMWR Recomm Rep 59:1, 2010.
40. Garite TJ, Kurtzman J, et al: Impact of a "rescue course" of antenatal corticosteroids: a multicenter randomized placebo-controlled trial. Am J Obstet Gynecol 200:248e1, 2009.
41. ACOG Committee Opinion No. 475: Antenatal corticosteroid therapy for fetal maturation. Obstet Gynecol 117:422, 2011.
42. Crowther CA, Hiller JE, et al: Effect of magnesium sulfate given for neuroprotection before preterm birth: a randomized controlled trial. JAMA 290:2669, 2003.
43. Marret S, Marpeau L, et al: Benefit of magnesium sulfate given before very preterm birth to protect infant brain. Pediatrics 121:225, 2008.
44. Marret S, Marpeau L, et al: Magnesium sulphate given before very-preterm birth to protect infant brain: the randomised controlled PREMAG trial. BJOG 114:310, 2007.
45. Rouse DJ, Hirtz DG, et al: A randomized, controlled trial of magnesium sulfate for the prevention of cerebral palsy. N Engl J Med 359:895, 2008.
46. American College of Obstetricians and Gynecologists Committee on Obstetric Practice, Society for Maternal-Fetal Medicine, Committee Opinion No. 455: Magnesium sulfate before anticipated preterm birth for neuroprotection. Obstet Gynecol 115:669, 2010.
47. Crowther CA, Hiller JE, et al: Magnesium sulphate for preventing preterm birth in threatened preterm labour. Cochrane Database Syst Rev CD001060, 2002.
48. Costantine MM, Weiner SJ: Effects of antenatal exposure to magnesium sulfate on neuroprotection and mortality in preterm infants: a meta-analysis. Obstet Gynecol 114:354, 2009.
49. FDA Drug Safety Communication: New warnings against use of terbutaline to treat preterm labor. Available at www.fda.gov/Drugs/DrugSafety/ucm243539.htm.
50. Food and Drug Administration, Center for Drug Evaluation and Research, Advisory Committee for Reproductive Health Drugs: Available at www.fda.gov/ohrms/dockets/ac/98/transcpt/3407t1.rtf (accessed July 11, 2011).
51. Mazaki-Tovi S, Romero R, et al: Recurrent preterm birth. Semin Perinatol 31:142, 2007.
52. Harper M, Thom E, et al: Omega-3 fatty acid supplementation to prevent recurrent preterm birth: a randomized controlled trial. Obstet Gynecol 115:234, 2010.
53. Hauth JC, Clifton RG, et al: Vitamin C and E supplementation to prevent spontaneous preterm birth: a randomized controlled trial. Obstet Gynecol 116:653, 2010.
54. Leveno KJ, McIntire DD, Bloom SL, et al: Decreased preterm births in an inner-city public hospital. Obstet Gynecol 113:578, 2009.
55. Nygren P, Fu R, Freeman M, et al: Evidence on the benefits and harms of screening and treating pregnant women who are asymptomatic for bacterial vaginosis: an update review for the U.S. Preventive Services Task Force. Ann Intern Med 148:220, 2008.
56. Keirse MJ: Progestogen administration in pregnancy may prevent preterm delivery. Br J Obstet Gynaecol 97:149, 1990.
57. da Fonseca EB, Bittar RE, Carvalho MH, et al: Prophylactic administration of progesterone by vaginal suppository to reduce the incidence of spontaneous preterm birth in women at increased risk: a randomized placebo-controlled double-blind study. Am J Obstet Gynecol 188:419, 2003.
58. Meis PJ, Klebanoff M, Thom E, et al: Prevention of recurrent preterm delivery by 17-alpha-hydroxyprogesterone caproate. N Engl J Med 348:2379, 2003.
59. Rouse DJ, Caritis SN, Peaceman AM, et al: A trial of 17 alpha-hydroxyprogesterone caproate to prevent prematurity in twins. N Engl J Med 357:454, 2007.
60. Combs CA, Garite T, Maurel K, et al: 17-hydroxyprogesterone caproate for twin pregnancy: a double-blind, randomized clinical trial. Am J Obstet Gynecol 204:e221, 2011.
61. Caritis SN, Rouse DJ, Peaceman AM, et al: Prevention of preterm birth in triplets using 17 alpha-hydroxyprogesterone caproate: a randomized controlled trial. Obstet Gynecol 113:285, 2009.
62. Combs CA, Garite T, Maurel K, et al: Failure of 17-hydroxyprogesterone to reduce neonatal morbidity or prolong triplet pregnancy: a double-blind, randomized clinical trial. Am J Obstet Gynecol 203:248.e1, 2010. Erratum in Am J Obstet Gynecol 204:166, 2011.
63. Cahill AG, Odibo AO, Caughey AB, et al: Universal cervical length screening and treatment with vaginal progesterone to prevent preterm birth: a decision and economic analysis. Am J Obstet Gynecol 202:548.e1, 2010.
64. Werner EF, Han CS, Pettker CM, et al: Universal cervical-length screening to prevent preterm birth: a cost-effectiveness analysis. Ultrasound Obstet Gynecol 38:32, 2011.
65. Campbell S: Universal cervical-length screening and vaginal progesterone prevents early preterm births, reduces neonatal morbidity and

is cost saving: doing nothing is no longer an option. Ultrasound Obstet Gynecol 38:1, 2011.
66. Owen J, Hankins G, Iams JD, et al: Multicenter randomized trial of cerclage for preterm birth prevention in high-risk women with shortened midtrimester cervical length. Am J Obstet Gynecol 201:375.e1, 2009.
67. Berghella V, Rafael TJ, Szychowski JM, et al: Cerclage for short cervix on ultrasonography in women with singleton gestations and previous preterm birth: a meta-analysis. Obstet Gynecol 117:663, 2011.
68. Berghella V, Odibo AO, To MS, et al: Cerclage for short cervix on ultrasonography: meta-analysis of trials using individual patient-level data. Obstet Gynecol 106:181, 2005.
69. Jorgensen AL, Alfirevic Z, Tudur Smith C, et al: Cervical stitch (cerclage) for preventing pregnancy loss: individual patient data meta-analysis. BJOG 114:1460, 2007.
70. Iams JD, Berghella V: Care for women with prior preterm birth. Am J Obstet Gynecol 203:89, 2010.
71. Reddy UM, Ko CW, Raju TNK, et al: Delivery indications at late-preterm gestations and infant mortality rates in the united states. Pediatrics 124:234, 2009.
72. Laughon SK, Reddy UM, Sun L, et al: Precursors for late preterm birth in singleton gestations. Obstet Gynecol 116:1047, 2010.
73. Spong CY, Mercer BM, D'Alton M, et al: Timing of indicated late-preterm and early-term birth. Obstet Gynecol 118:323, 2011.
74. Bryant AS, Worjoloh A, Caughey AB, Washington AE: Racial/ethnic disparities in obstetric outcomes and care: prevalence and determinants. Am J Obstet Gynecol 202:335, 2010.

For full reference list, log onto www.expertconsult.com.

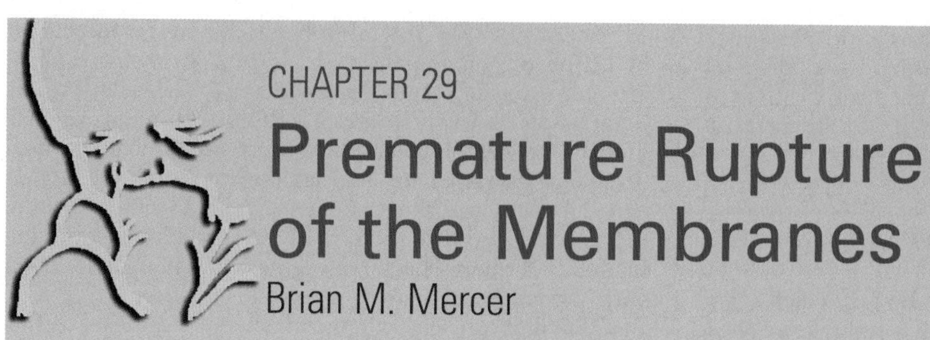

CHAPTER 29

Premature Rupture of the Membranes

Brian M. Mercer

KEY ABBREVIATIONS	
By Mouth	PO
Confidence Interval	CI
Group B Streptococcus	GBS
Herpes Simplex Virus	HSV
Human Immunodeficiency Virus	HIV
Intramuscular	IM
Intravenous	IV
Intraventricular Hemorrhage	IVH
Lamellar Body Count	LB
Lecithin-to-Sphingomyelin Ratio	L/S ratio
Maternal-Fetal Medicine Unit	MFMU
Matrix Metalloproteinase	MMP
National Institute of Child Health and Human Development	NICHD
Neonatal Intensive Care Unit	NICU
Odds Ratio	OR
Phosphatidylglycerol	PG
Premature Rupture of the Membranes	PROM
Respiratory Distress Syndrome	RDS
Surfactant-to-Albumin Ratio	S/A ratio
Tissue Inhibitors of Matrix Metalloproteinases	TIMP
U.S. Food and Drug Administration	FDA

Membrane rupture that occurs spontaneously before the onset of labor is described as premature rupture of the membranes (PROM) regardless of the gestational age at which it occurs. PROM complicates about 8% to 10% of pregnancies. Birth certificate data suggest that preterm PROM, occurring before 37 weeks' gestation, complicates about 1% of deliveries overall and is twofold more common in African Americans.[1] Like preterm labor and cervical insufficiency, PROM is considered a cause of "spontaneous preterm birth." The relative contribution of PROM to prematurity appears to vary greatly among patient populations, affecting about 10% of preterm births in national databases but 28% in certain high-risk populations, and its frequency appears to have declined during the past decade.[1,2]

PROM at any gestational age is associated with brief latency from membrane rupture to delivery and also increased risks for perinatal infection and umbilical cord compression due to oligohydramnios. Because of this, term and preterm PROM are significant causes of perinatal morbidity and mortality. When PROM occurs at term, there is a low risk for severe neonatal complications with delivery of a noninfected and nonasphyxiated infant. Clinical management should be directed toward delivery. Although complications can occur, delivery at 32 to 36 weeks' gestation is generally associated with good infant outcomes, particularly if the fetus has documented pulmonary maturity. Given the risks of continued pregnancy and anticipated brief latency, delivery of the mature fetus is generally warranted, particularly at 34 weeks' gestation or later. At 32 to 33 weeks' gestation, the immature fetus may benefit from measures to continue the pregnancy and to accelerate fetal maturation. With immediate delivery after preterm PROM at 23 to 31 weeks' gestation, there is a significant risk for newborn complications that can be reduced through delay of delivery. In the absence of contraindications, management is directed toward continuing the pregnancy, with attention to potential risks for umbilical cord compression, intrauterine infection, and abruptio placentae. When PROM occurs before the limit of viability, newborn death is inevitable with immediate delivery. Although conservative management can still lead to previable delivery, some women will benefit from extended latency with delivery of a potentially viable infant. Regardless of the gestational age, the patient should be well informed regarding the potential maternal, fetal, and neonatal complications of PROM and preterm birth. These issues are discussed in detail in this chapter.

FETAL MEMBRANE ANATOMY AND PHYSIOLOGY

The fetus develops within the amniotic sac, which is surrounded like a balloon by the fetal membranes. These membranes consist of a thin amnion layer lining the amniotic cavity and a thicker outer chorion that is directly apposed to maternal decidua. The amnion fuses to the chorion near the end of the first trimester of pregnancy, and these layers are subsequently attached by a collagen-rich connective tissue zone. For the remainder of the pregnancy, the fetal membranes include a single cuboidal amnion epithelium with subjacent compact and spongy connective tissue layers, and a thicker chorion consisting of reticular and trophoblastic layers. Together, the amnion and chorion are stronger than either layer independently; individually, the amnion has greater tensile strength than the chorion.

As the pregnancy progresses, changes in collagen content and type, intercellular matrix, and cellular apoptosis result in structural weakening of the fetal membranes. Membrane remodeling is more evident near the internal cervical os and can be stimulated by matrix metalloproteinases (e.g., MMP-1, MMP-2, MMP-9), decreased levels of tissue inhibitors of matrix metalloproteinases (e.g., TIMP-1, TIMP-3) within the membranes, and increased poly[ADP-ribose] polymerase (PARP) cleavage.[3,4] Contractions subject the amniochorionic membranes to additional physical strain that can lead to membrane rupture. Should the fetal membranes not rupture before labor, advancing cervical dilation decreases the work needed to cause membrane rupture over the internal cervical os. **Preterm PROM likely results from a variety of factors ultimately leading to accelerated membrane weakening through an increase in local cytokines and an imbalance in the interaction between MMPs and TIMPs, increased collagenase and protease activity, or other factors that cause increased intrauterine pressure (e.g., polyhydramnios).**[3-5]

ETIOLOGY OF PREMATURE RUPTURE OF THE MEMBRANES

A number of risk factors have been associated with the occurrence of preterm PROM. Among these are low socioeconomic status, uterine overdistention, second- and third-trimester bleeding, low body mass index, nutritional deficiencies of copper and ascorbic acid, maternal cigarette smoking, cervical conization or cerclage, pulmonary disease in pregnancy, connective tissue disorders (e.g., Ehlers-Danlos syndrome), and preterm labor or symptomatic contractions in the current gestation. Each risk factor, individually or in concert, could lead to PROM through the mechanisms outlined previously. However, the ultimate clinical cause of membrane rupture is often not apparent, and many at-risk patients will deliver at term without PROM.

Preterm PROM has also been linked to infections involving the urogenital tract. *Neisseria gonorrhoeae, Chlamydia trachomatis,* and *Trichomonas vaginalis* have each been associated with preterm PROM.[6] Although vaginal group B β-hemolytic streptococcus (GBS) colonization does not appear to be associated with preterm PROM, cervical colonization may be associated, and GBS bacteruria is associated with preterm PROM and low-birthweight infants.[7,8] Although bacterial vaginosis has been associated with spontaneous preterm births, including preterm PROM, it is unclear whether bacterial vaginosis is the inciting condition, facilitates ascent of other bacteria to the upper genital tract, or is simply a marker of maternal predisposition to abnormal genital tract colonization.[9,10] Bacterial invasion can facilitate membrane rupture through direct release of proteases and also through stimulation of a host inflammatory response resulting in the elaboration of local cytokines, metalloproteases, and prostaglandins. Histologic studies of the membranes after preterm PROM often demonstrate significant bacterial contamination along the choriodecidual interface with minimal involvement of the amnion.[11] Further evidence linking preterm PROM and genital tract infection is that these women have a high incidence of positive amniotic fluid cultures (25% to 35%) even in the absence of clinically suspected intrauterine infection.[12,13] Although some of these findings may reflect ascending infection subsequent to membrane rupture, it is probable that ascending colonization and infection are integral to the pathogenesis of preterm PROM in many cases.

Although the onset of vaginal fluid leakage is an acute event, there is evidence that the factors and events leading to membrane rupture are sometimes subacute or even chronic. Women with a prior preterm birth, especially because of PROM, are at increased risk for preterm birth due to PROM in future pregnancies. Studies have also suggested associations between maternal inflammatory proteins genotype and spontaneous preterm birth due to preterm labor or PROM.[14,15] Further, asymptomatic women with a short cervical length in the second trimester are at increased risk for preterm PROM occurring weeks later.[16]

PREDICTION AND PREVENTION OF PRETERM PREMATURE RUPTURE OF THE MEMBRANES

Once preterm PROM occurs, delivery is often required or inevitable. Optimally, prevention of PROM itself would offer the best opportunity to avoid its complications. **Prior preterm birth and especially prior preterm PROM have been associated with preterm PROM in a subsequent pregnancy.**[17] **The risk increases with decreasing gestational age of the index preterm birth.** Those with a prior delivery near the limit of viability (23 to 27 weeks) have a 27.1% risk of subsequent preterm birth. Those with a prior history of preterm birth due to PROM have a 3.3-fold higher risk for preterm birth due to PROM (13.5% versus 4.1%) and a 13.5-fold higher risk for preterm PROM before 28 weeks (1.8 versus 0.13%) in a subsequent gestation ($P < .01$ for each). In an analysis from a prospective evaluation of preterm birth prediction, nulliparas and women with prior deliveries were evaluated separately because those without a prior birth lacked important historical information available to those with a prior term or preterm birth.[16] In that study, multivariable analysis revealed medical complications (including pulmonary disease in pregnancy), work during pregnancy, recent symptomatic uterine contractions, and bacterial vaginosis to be significant markers for subsequent preterm birth in nulliparas, when assessed at 22 to 24 weeks' gestation (Table 29-1). Among women with prior deliveries, prior preterm birth due to preterm labor or PROM and a positive cervicovaginal fetal fibronectin screen were statistically significant clinical markers for subsequent preterm PROM after controlling for other factors. Short cervical length (<25 mm) identified by transvaginal ultrasound and low maternal body mass index (<19.8 kg/m^2) were associated with an increased risk for subsequent PROM in both nulliparas and multiparas. Nulliparas with a positive cervicovaginal fetal fibronectin and a short cervix had a 16.7% risk for preterm birth due to preterm PROM. Among multiparas, women with a prior preterm birth due to PROM, a short cervix on ultrasound, and positive cervicovaginal fetal fibronectin screen had a 10.9-fold higher risk for PROM with delivery before 35 weeks' gestation (25% versus 2.3%) than those without risk factors (Table 29-2).

TABLE 29-1 MARKERS FOR PRETERM PROM BEFORE 37 WEEKS' GESTATION*

	NULLIPARAS (*N* = 1618)	MULTIPARAS (*N* = 1711)
Medical complications	3.7 (1.5-9.0)	—
Work in pregnancy	3.0 (1.5-6.1)	—
Symptomatic contractions within 2 weeks	2.2 (1.2-7.5)	—
Bacterial vaginosis	2.1 (1.1-4.1)	—
Low body mass index (<19.8 kg/m^2)	2.0 (1.0-4.0)	1.8 (1.1-3.0)
Prior preterm birth due to PROM	—	3.1 (1.8-5.4)
Prior preterm birth due to preterm labor	—	1.8 (1.1-3.1)
Cervix <25 mm	3.7 (1.8-7.7)	2.5 (1.4-4.5)
Positive fetal fibronectin	—	2.1 (1.1-4.0)

Adapted with permission from Mercer BM, Goldenberg RL, Meis PJ, et al, for the NICHD-MFMU Network: The preterm prediction study: prediction of preterm premature rupture of the membranes using clinical findings and ancillary testing. Am J Obstet Gynecol 183:738, 2000.

*Results of multivariable analyses for nulliparas and multiparas (presented as odds ratios with 95% confidence intervals).

PROM, Premature rupture of the membranes; not significant in final model.

Unfortunately, such risk assessment systems identify only a small fraction of women who will ultimately deliver preterm. Further, although clinical and ancillary testing has increased our ability to identify women at increased risk because of potentially modifiable factors (e.g., cigarette smoking, poor nutrition, urinary tract and sexually transmitted infections, pulmonary disease, severe polyhydramnios), it is unknown whether modification of these in a given patient will reduce the risk for PROM. Regardless, women at risk for preterm birth due to PROM based on clinical findings can be counseled regarding the symptoms of membrane rupture and contractions and encouraged to seek medical care should symptoms occur.

There is current evidence to support progesterone treatment for women with a prior preterm birth due to PROM or preterm labor.[18,19] Data regarding the value of vitamin C supplementation in preventing PROM are conflicting but are not generally supportive. In one study, such treatment was associated with a lower risk (7.7% versus 24.5%; $P = .02$).[20] However, other studies have not shown a significant benefit from treatment, and review of studies in which vitamin C was given alone or in combination with other supplements suggested a negative impact on membrane strength and an increased risk for preterm birth.[21,22] Because of this, **vitamin C supplementation to prevent preterm PROM is not currently recommended.**

CLINICAL COURSE AFTER PREMATURE RUPTURE OF THE MEMBRANES

A hallmark of PROM is brief latency from membrane rupture to delivery. On average, latency increases with decreasing gestational age at membrane rupture. At term, half of expectantly managed gravidas deliver within 5 hours and 95% deliver within 28 hours of membrane rupture.[23] Of all women with PROM before 34 weeks, 93% deliver in less than 1 week. After excluding those requiring delivery soon after admission, 50% to 60% of those conservatively managed and treated with antibiotics for pregnancy prolongation will deliver within 1 week of membrane rupture.[24] A small proportion of women with membrane rupture can anticipate cessation of fluid leakage (2.6% to

TABLE 29-2 RISK FOR PRETERM BIRTH DUE TO PROM BEFORE 37 AND BEFORE 35 WEEKS' GESTATION BASED ON PARITY, CERVICAL LENGTH, FETAL FIBRONECTIN, AND PRIOR OBSTETRICAL HISTORY AMONG MULTIPARAS

	NO. OF SUBJECTS	<37 WEEKS	<35 WEEKS
All multiparas	1711	5.0	2.3
No risk factors present	1351	3.2	0.8
Prior preterm birth due to PROM only	124	10.5	4.8
Prior preterm birth due to PROM and positive FFN*	13	15.4	15.4
Prior preterm birth due to PROM and short cervix†	26	23.1	15.4
All three risk factors present	8	25.0	25.0

Adapted with permission from Mercer BM, Goldenberg RL, Meis PJ, et al, for the NICHD-MFMU Network: The preterm prediction study: prediction of preterm premature rupture of the membranes using clinical findings and ancillary testing. Am J Obstet Gynecol 183:738, 2000.

*Positive FFN, cervicovaginal fetal fibronectin screen positive (>50 ng/mL) at 22-24 weeks' gestation.

†Short cervix, cervix length <25 mm on transvaginal ultrasound at 22-24 weeks' gestation.

FFN, Fetal fibronectin; *PROM*, premature rupture of the membranes.

13%). About 86% of those with leakage after amniocentesis will reseal.[25,26]

RISKS OF PREMATURE RUPTURE OF THE MEMBRANES

Maternal Risks

Chorioamnionitis is the most common maternal complication after preterm PROM. This risk increases as the duration of membrane rupture becomes more prolonged and decreases with advancing gestational age at PROM.[27] With PROM remote from term, chorioamnionitis occurs in 13% to 60% of pregnancies and endometritis complicates 2% to 13% of cases.[28,29] **Abruptio placentae can cause PROM or occur subsequent to membrane rupture and affects 4% to 12% of these pregnancies.**[30] **Uncommon but serious complications of PROM managed conservatively near the limit of viability include retained placenta and hemorrhage requiring dilation and curettage (12%), maternal sepsis (0.8%), and maternal death (0.14%).**[31]

Fetal and Neonatal Risks

Fetal complications after membrane rupture include infection and fetal distress due to umbilical cord compression or placental abruption. Umbilical cord compression due to oligohydramnios is common after PROM.[32] Frank or occult umbilical cord prolapse can also occur, particularly with fetal malpresentation. Because of these factors, women with PROM have a higher risk for cesarean delivery for non-reassuring fetal heart rate patterns than those with isolated preterm labor (7.9% versus 1.5%). Fetal death complicates 1% to 2% of cases of conservatively managed PROM.[24]

The frequency and severity of neonatal complications after PROM vary inversely with gestational age at membrane rupture and at delivery. Respiratory distress syndrome (RDS) is the most common serious acute morbidity after preterm PROM at any gestational age. Necrotizing enterocolitis, intraventricular hemorrhage (IVH), and sepsis are common with early preterm birth but relatively uncommon near term. Serious perinatal morbidities with delivery remote from term can lead to long-term sequelae such as chronic lung disease, visual or hearing difficulties, mental retardation, developmental and motor delay, cerebral palsy, and death. Although specific data are not available for those delivering after preterm PROM, general community-based survival and morbidity data suggest that long-term morbidities and death are uncommon with delivery after about 32 weeks' gestation.[33] It is controversial whether gestational age–specific mortality is increased for preterm infants delivering after preterm PROM.[34,35]

Preterm PROM increases the risk of neonatal sepsis twofold over that seen after preterm birth due to preterm labor with intact membranes.[36] Neonatal infection can result from the same organisms present in the amniotic fluid or from others and can present as acute congenital pneumonia, sepsis, or meningitis. Late-onset bacterial or fungal infections can also occur. There is accumulating evidence that suggests fetal-neonatal infection and inflammation are associated with an increased risk for long-term neurologic complications. Cerebral palsy and cystic periventricular leukomalacia (PVL) have been linked to chorioamnionitis, which is more commonly seen after preterm PROM and is more likely with conservative management after membrane rupture.[37] Elevated amniotic fluid cytokines and fetal systemic inflammation have also been associated with preterm PROM, PVL, and cerebral palsy.[38] Although there are no data to suggest that immediate delivery on admission with PROM will avert these sequelae, these findings highlight the importance of restricting conservative management after PROM to circumstances in which there is the potential to reduce neonatal morbidity through either antenatal corticosteroid administration or extended pregnancy prolongation for fetal maturation.

Pulmonary hypoplasia is a severe complication of oligohydramnios in the second trimester that results from a lack of terminal bronchiole and alveolar development during the canalicular phase of pulmonary development.[39] It is most accurately diagnosed pathologically using radial alveolar counts and lung weights.[40] Clinical findings such as a small chest circumference with severe respiratory distress and persistent pulmonary hypertension in the newborn and radiographic findings such as small well-aerated lungs with a bell-shaped chest and elevation of the diaphragm are also supportive of the diagnosis. Whether because of fluid efflux and tracheobronchial collapse after membrane rupture or through loss of intrinsic factors within the tracheobronchial fluid, pulmonary hypoplasia develops over weeks after membrane rupture. Pulmonary hypoplasia complicates an average of about 6% of cases in series of midtrimester PROM and carries a 70% mortality rate.[41] Its incidence is inversely correlated with gestational age at membrane rupture, complicating nearly 50% of cases with membrane rupture before 19 weeks and prolonged latency.[39,42] The frequency of pulmonary hypoplasia can be as high as 74% to 82% with PROM at 15 to 16 weeks, persistent oligohydramnios, and a latency 28 days.[43] Lethal pulmonary hypoplasia rarely occurs with PROM after 26 weeks of gestation (0% to 1.4%).[44] However, other pulmonary complications such as pneumothorax and pneumomediastinum related to poor pulmonary compliance and high ventilatory pressures can occur with lesser degrees of this condition. Restriction deformities occur in about 1.5% of infants delivered after conservative management after midtrimester PROM but complicate up to 27% of fetuses with prolonged oligohydramnios.[31,45]

DIAGNOSIS OF PREMATURE RUPTURE OF THE MEMBRANES

The diagnosis of PROM involves clinical history and physical examination, as well as laboratory evaluation in some cases.

The diagnosis of membrane rupture is confirmed by the presence of the following findings:

- Visualization of evident amniotic fluid passing from the cervical canal, or
- Vaginal sidewall or posterior fornix pH of more than 6.0 to 6.5, and
- Microscopic arborized crystals ("ferning"), owing to the interaction of amniotic fluid proteins and salts, form dried vaginal secretions obtained by swabbing the posterior fornix with a sterile swab.

False-positive pH results may occur with blood or semen contamination, alkaline antiseptics, or bacterial vaginosis. Cervical mucus can yield a false-positive ferning pattern; however, the crystals appear as a more floral pattern. The fern pattern in samples heavily contaminated with blood is atypical and appears more "skeletonized." Prolonged leakage with minimal residual fluid can result in a false-negative result on visual inspection, pH, or ferning testing. If the diagnosis is equivocal after initial testing, the patient can be placed in a Trendelenburg position and reexamined after a few hours. The diagnosis of membrane rupture can be made unequivocally by ultrasound-guided dye amnioinfusion (1 mL indigo carmine plus 9 mL sterile saline), followed by observation for passage of dye onto a perineal pad. Although oligohydramnios without evident fetal urinary tract malformations or fetal growth restriction may be suggestive of membrane rupture, ultrasound alone is not definitive.

Noninvasive cervicovaginal markers such as fetal fibronectin, α-fetoprotein, prolactin, human chorionic gonadotropin, placental α-microglobulin-1 (PAMG-1), and insulin-like growth factor-binding protein-1 (IGFBP-1) have been studied for their ability to confirm or exclude membrane rupture. These have not generally been evaluated in women with an unclear diagnosis of membrane rupture after clinical examination, so their predictive value in this relevant population is uncertain. Although membrane rupture can be confirmed by the presence of PAMG-1 in cervicovaginal secretions, it has also been found to be present in nearly one third of laboring women and in 1 of 20 nonlaboring women without suspected membrane rupture.[46]

MANAGEMENT OF PREMATURE RUPTURE OF THE MEMBRANES

General Considerations

Management of PROM is based primarily on an individual assessment of the estimated risk for fetal and neonatal complications should conservative management or delivery be pursued. The risks for maternal morbidity should also be considered, particularly when PROM occurs before the limit of potential viability (currently 23 weeks' gestational age).

The diagnosis of membrane rupture is confirmed and the duration of membrane rupture determined to assist the pediatric caregivers with subsequent management decisions. The patient is assessed for fetal presentation, contractions, findings suggestive of intrauterine infection, and evidence of fetal well-being. GBS carriage is ascertained, if available, from a recent anovaginal culture performed within 5 weeks.

In general, digital cervical examinations should be avoided until it is determined that delivery is inevitable. Digital examination has been associated with a shortening of latency from membrane rupture to delivery.[47] Visualization of the cervix during a sterile speculum examination offers helpful information regarding cervical dilation and effacement. Brown and colleagues found visual estimation to be within 1 cm of digitally determined cervical dilation in 64% and within 2 cm in 84% of examinations, whereas visually estimated cervical effacement was within 1 cm in 83% of cases.[48] In addition to providing confirmatory evidence of membrane rupture, sterile speculum examination can provide the opportunity to inspect for cervicitis and to obtain appropriate cervical and vaginal cultures.

The benefit of narrow-spectrum intrapartum prophylaxis with intravenous penicillin G (5 million units intravenous [IV], then 2.5 to 3 million units IV every 4 hours) or ampicillin (2 g IV, then 1 g IV every 4 hours), to prevent vertical transmission and early-onset neonatal GBS sepsis from maternal GBS carriers has been well established, and the Centers for Disease Control and Prevention published a revised guideline for the prevention of perinatal group B streptococcal disease in November 2010.[49,50] Current indications for intrapartum GBS prophylaxis and alternative antibiotic regimens for those with a penicillin allergy are discussed in Chapter 51. Known GBS carriers with PROM at any gestation and those with preterm PROM and unknown GBS status should receive intrapartum prophylaxis regardless of prior antibiotic treatment. GBS carriers with PROM and chorioamnionitis should receive broad-spectrum intrapartum antibiotic therapy, including agents effective against GBS. Intrapartum antibiotics are not recommended if chorioamnionitis is not suspected clinically and there is a recent negative anovaginal culture for GBS because of the potential for selection of resistant organisms should neonatal sepsis occur.[51]

Although practice varies regarding the management of preterm PROM, there is general consensus regarding some issues. Gestational age should be established based on clinical history and prior ultrasound assessment, where available (Figure 29-1). Ultrasound should be performed to assess fetal growth, position, residual amniotic fluid volume, and gross fetal abnormalities that might cause polyhydramnios and PROM. Those with advanced labor, intrauterine infection, significant vaginal bleeding, or nonreassuring fetal testing are best delivered. **If conservative management of preterm PROM is to be pursued, the patient should be admitted to a facility capable of providing emergent delivery for placental abruption, fetal malpresentation in labor, and fetal distress due to umbilical cord compression or in utero infection. The facility should also be capable of providing 24-hour neonatal resuscitation and intensive care because conservative management should generally be performed only in pregnancies in which there is a significant risk for neonatal morbidity and mortality.** If the need for transfer to a tertiary care facility is anticipated, this should occur early in the course of management to avoid emergent transfer once delivery is imminent or complications arise.

Management of Premature Rupture of the Membranes at Term

Studies published in the 1970s and 1980s suggested that immediate induction after PROM at term would increase the risks for perinatal infection and cesarean delivery.[52] However, currently available data do not support these concerns. In four large studies, induction with oxytocin after PROM at term did not increase either of these complications.[23,53-55] In fact, the largest prospective study to date has found oxytocin induction in this setting to reduce the median duration of membrane rupture after PROM (17.2 versus 33.3 hours) and the frequency of

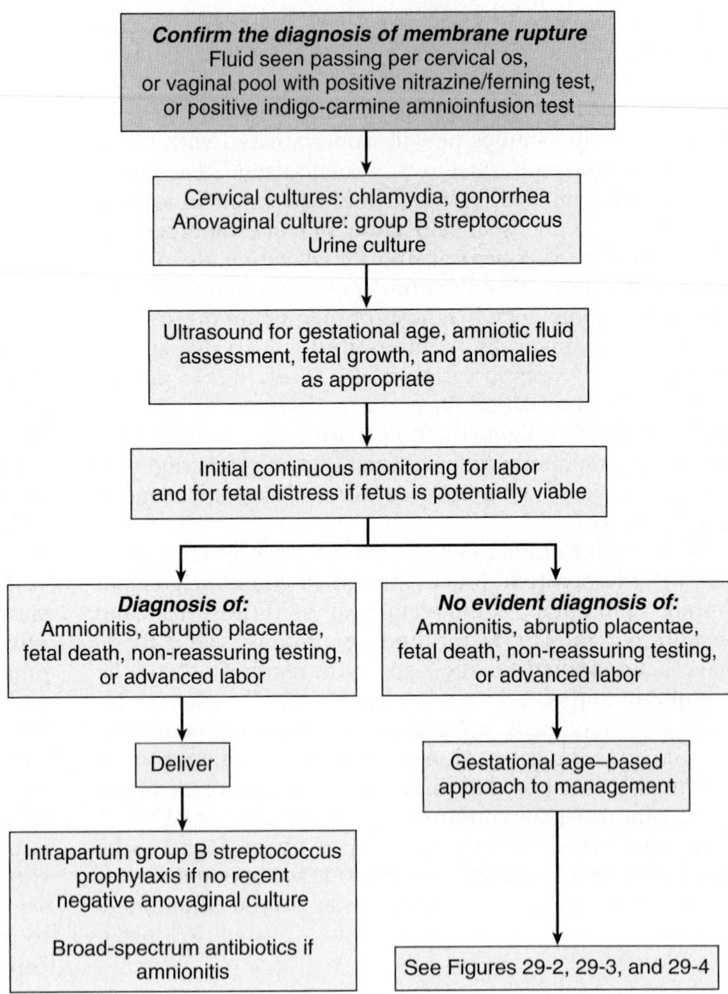
Confirm the diagnosis of membrane rupture
Fluid seen passing per cervical os, or vaginal pool with positive nitrazine/ferning test, or positive indigo-carmine amnioinfusion test
Cervical cultures: chlamydia, gonorrhea
Anovaginal culture: group B streptococcus
Urine culture
Ultrasound for gestational age, amniotic fluid assessment, fetal growth, and anomalies as appropriate
Initial continuous monitoring for labor and for fetal distress if fetus is potentially viable
Diagnosis of: Amnionitis, abruptio placentae, fetal death, non-reassuring testing, or advanced labor
No evident diagnosis of: Amnionitis, abruptio placentae, fetal death, non-reassuring testing, or advanced labor
Deliver
Gestational age–based approach to management
Intrapartum group B streptococcus prophylaxis if no recent negative anovaginal culture
Broad-spectrum antibiotics if amnionitis
See Figures 29-2, 29-3, and 29-4

FIGURE 29-1. Initial assessment and management of women with preterm premature rupture of the membranes. (From Mercer BM: Preterm premature rupture of the membranes: diagnosis and management. Clin Perinatol 31:765, 2004.)

chorioamnionitis (4% versus 8.6%) and postpartum fevers (1.9% versus 3.6%; $P \leq .008$ for each), without increasing cesarean deliveries (13.7% versus 14.1%) or neonatal infections (2% versus 2.8%).[23] An additional benefit of early oxytocin induction in this trial was a reduction in neonatal antibiotic therapy (7.5% versus 13.7%; $P < .001$). Meta-analysis of 12 studies including a total of 6814 women regarding early delivery versus expectant management for PROM at term confirmed less frequent chorioamnionitis and endometritis with planned delivery, with no increases in caesarean delivery or neonatal infection.[56] Fewer infants in the early delivery group required neonatal intensive care unit (NICU) or special care admission. Analysis of studies of prostaglandin versus oxytocin induction after PROM at or near term found increased chorioamnionitis (odds ratio [OR], 1.51; 95% confidence interval [CI], 1.07 to 2.12), neonatal infection (OR, 1.63; 95% CI, 1 to 2.66), and prolonged NICU stay (OR, 1.43; 95% CI, 1.07 to 1.91) without improvement in cesarean delivery rates (OR, 0.92; 95% CI, 0.73 to 1.16) with prostaglandin treatment.[57] This meta-analysis was dominated by the TermPROM trial, which found shorter latency from membrane rupture to delivery with oxytocin than with prostaglandin therapy (median, 17.2 versus 23 hours; $P < .001$).[23] Taken together, these data suggest that **women with PROM at term should be offered early delivery, generally with a continuous oxytocin infusion, to reduce the risk for maternal and neonatal complications.** Adequate time for latent phase of labor should be allowed. During labor, transcervical amnioinfusion of warm normal saline solution may prove useful if significant umbilical cord compression is suspected and immediate delivery is not required.[58,59]

Management of Preterm Premature Rupture of the Membranes Near Term (32 to 36 Weeks)

Severe acute newborn complications are uncommon when preterm birth occurs between 34 and 36 weeks' gestation, and antenatal corticosteroids for fetal maturation are not usually administered to accelerate fetal pulmonary maturity in this gestational age range.[33] Alternatively, **conservative management after PROM at 34 to 36 weeks' gestation only briefly prolongs pregnancy while increasing the risk for chorioamnionitis** (16% versus 2%; $P = .001$) and reducing newborn umbilical cord pH (7.35 versus 7.25; $P = .009$) without preventing neonatal complications.[60,61]

Management of the woman with PROM at 32 to 33 weeks' gestation is more controversial because pulmonary and other gestational age–dependent complications can occur, but the likelihood of survival at this gestation is high and long-term complications are uncommon. Neerhoff and colleagues found modest benefits in the duration of newborn hospital stay and the frequency of hyperbilirubinemia with conservative management at 32 to 33 weeks' gestation.[61] Alternatively, two prospective trials comparing early delivery and conservative management of PROM near term have provided useful insights. Cox and coworkers found conservative management of PROM at 30 to 33^6 weeks' gestation to increase latency only briefly (59% versus 100% delivered within 48 hours; $P < .001$).[62] Mercer and colleagues, in a study of PROM at 32 to 36^6 weeks' gestation, found a similar brief lengthening of latency with conservative management (36 hours versus 14 hours; $P < .001$).[63] However, both studies found conservative management to increase the risk for chorioamnionitis (15% versus 2%, $P = .009$, and 27.7% versus 10.9%, $P = .06$, respectively) without evident reduction in newborn complications. Secondary analysis of those with PROM at 32 to 33^6 weeks' gestation in the latter trial revealed similar trends regarding latency, infection, and infant morbidities in this subgroup.[64] The potential for umbilical cord compression during conservative management of PROM was highlighted by one stillbirth and the high incidence of non-reassuring fetal heart rate patterns found on intermittent monitoring in these studies.[62,63]

At 32 to 33 weeks' gestation, it can be helpful to assess fetal pulmonary maturity and to treat with antenatal corticosteroids those pregnancies without documented fetal maturity. Either vaginal pool or amniocentesis specimens can be used for testing. Because there is increased potential for inadvertent fetal or umbilical cord puncture during amniocentesis when the amniotic fluid volume is decreased, vaginal pool specimen collection is preferable if an adequate specimen can be obtained. If amniocentesis is required, color Doppler imaging can be helpful in differentiating umbilical cord loops from a small residual fluid pocket. Pulmonary phospholipids are not present in lavage fluid from the vagina when the membranes are intact.[65] Studies of women with ruptured membranes have found a high concordance rate (89% to 100%) between specimens collected vaginally and by amniocentesis for pulmonary phospholipids such as lecithin, phosphatidylglycerol (PG), phosphatidylinositol, phosphatidylethanolamine, and phosphatidylserine.[66] Lewis and associates found no cases of RDS among infants delivered after a mature PG result from vaginal pool fluid.[67] Similarly, in a study of vaginally collected samples, Russell and associates found no cases of RDS after a mature lecithin-to-sphingomyelin (L/S) ratio or PG result.[68] Although mature TDx-FLM and TDx-FLM II assay results are highly predictive of fetal pulmonary maturity, this platform is no longer available in the United States.[69] The presence of PG on perineal pad–collected fluid is also predictive of fetal pulmonary maturity (97.8%), and its absence is predictive of pulmonary immaturity (33.7%).[70] The lamellar body count (LBC) may also be performed from vaginally collected amniotic fluid specimens and has been shown by some to have a high predictive value for fetal pulmonary maturity.[71] Amniotic fluid pulmonary maturity testing can be confounded by the presence of contaminants such as blood and meconium (see Chapter 12). Realistically, expeditious delivery should be considered if significant blood or meconium is present in a vaginal pool or amniocentesis specimen after PROM.

Based on the available data, early delivery should be pursued when PROM occurs at 34 to 36 weeks' gestation (Figure 29-2). The infant delivered after PROM at 30 to 33 weeks' gestation is at risk for infectious and other gestational age–dependent morbidities, but the presence of fetal pulmonary maturity at 32 to 33^6 weeks' gestation suggests that there is a low risk for complications with immediate delivery. Because of the increased risk for infectious morbidity and potential for occult umbilical cord compression with conservative management, **delivery should be initiated before complications ensue if there is documented fetal pulmonary maturity after PROM at 32 to 33 weeks.** If fetal pulmonary maturity is not evident on testing, or if amniotic fluid cannot be obtained for testing, conservative management with antenatal corticosteroid administration for fetal maturation and antibiotic therapy to reduce the risk for infection (see later) is appropriate. The issue of continued conservative management versus delivery after steroid treatment is a matter of opinion. Pragmatically, if elective delivery is planned within 1 week, it is unlikely that prolonging the pregnancy further will offer significant opportunity for significant additional fetal maturation and delivery should be considered after steroids have been administered. Alternatively, if several weeks of conservative management are to be attempted, there may be benefit to continuing the pregnancy.

Management of Premature Rupture of the Membranes Remote from Term (23 to 31 weeks)

Infants born at 23 to 31 weeks' gestation are at increased risk for perinatal death, and survivors commonly suffer acute and long-term complications. Pregnancy prolongation can reduce these risks, and because of this, inpatient conservative management is generally attempted unless intrauterine infection, significant vaginal bleeding, placental abruption, and advanced labor are evident or fetal testing becomes non-reassuring. Fetal malpresentation, funic presentation, human immunodeficiency virus (HIV), primary herpes simplex virus (HSV) are examples of exceptions that might warrant expeditious delivery because of the increased potential for fetal death or infection with prolonged membrane rupture.

During conservative management, initial care generally consists of prolonged continuous fetal heart rate and maternal contraction monitoring for evidence of umbilical cord compression and occult contractions and to establish fetal well-being. If initial testing is reassuring, the patient can be transferred to an inpatient ward for modified bedrest (Figure 29-3). Because the fetus with preterm PROM remote from term is at risk for heart rate abnormalities resulting from umbilical cord compression (32% to 76%),[31] fetal assessment should be performed at least daily. More frequent or continuous monitoring may be appropriate if there are intermittent fetal heart rate decelerations but otherwise reassuring findings. Although both nonstress and biophysical profile testing have the ability to confirm fetal well-being in the setting of preterm PROM, fetal heart rate monitoring offers the opportunity to identify periodic heart rate changes and allows concurrent

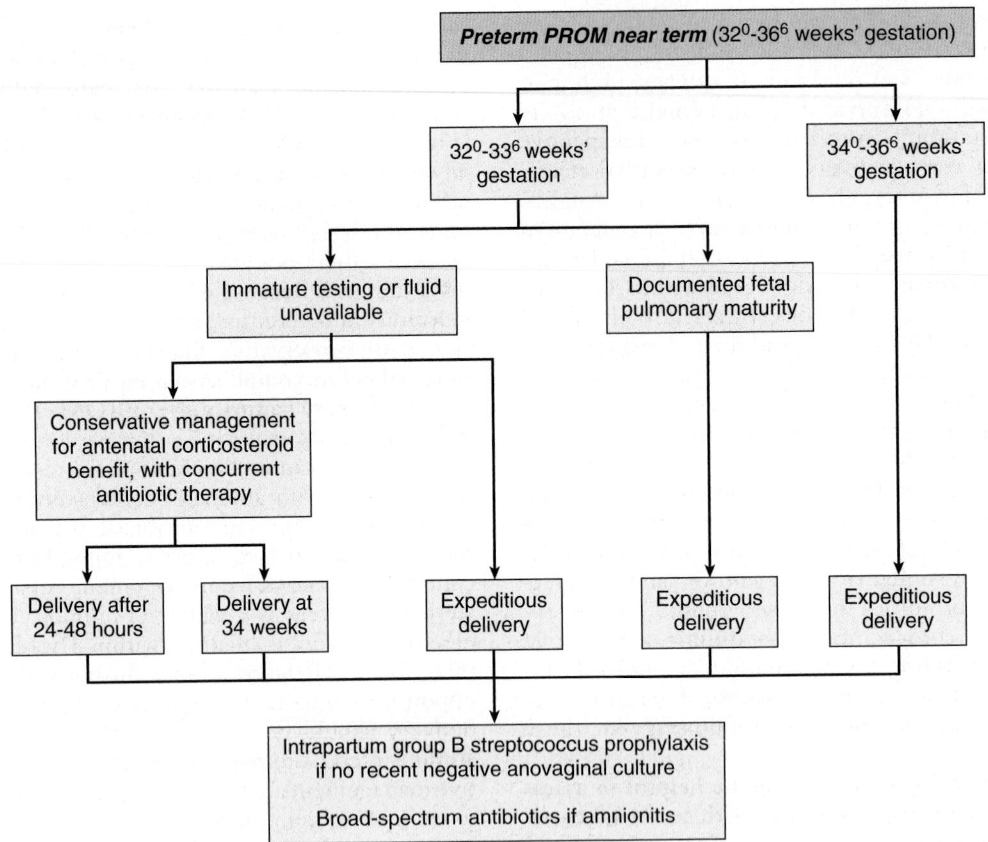
Preterm PROM near term (32⁰-36⁶ weeks' gestation)
32⁰-33⁶ weeks' gestation
34⁰-36⁶ weeks' gestation
Immature testing or fluid unavailable
Documented fetal pulmonary maturity
Conservative management for antenatal corticosteroid benefit, with concurrent antibiotic therapy
Delivery after 24-48 hours
Delivery at 34 weeks
Expeditious delivery
Expeditious delivery
Expeditious delivery
Intrapartum group B streptococcus prophylaxis if no recent negative anovaginal culture
Broad-spectrum antibiotics if amnionitis

FIGURE 29-2. Management algorithm for preterm premature rupture of the membranes (PROM) near term (32 to 36 weeks' gestation). (From Mercer BM: Preterm premature rupture of the membranes: diagnosis and management. Clin Perinatol 31:765, 2004.)

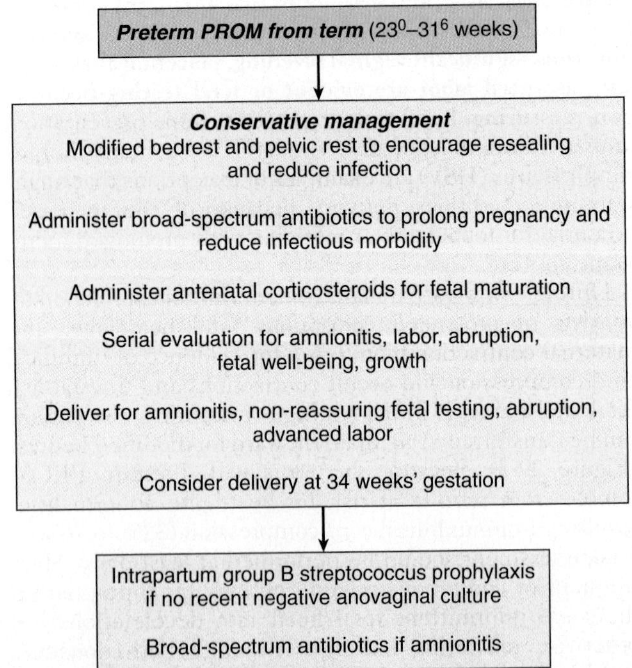
Preterm PROM from term (23⁰–31⁶ weeks)
Conservative management
Modified bedrest and pelvic rest to encourage resealing and reduce infection
Administer broad-spectrum antibiotics to prolong pregnancy and reduce infectious morbidity
Administer antenatal corticosteroids for fetal maturation
Serial evaluation for amnionitis, labor, abruption, fetal well-being, growth
Deliver for amnionitis, non-reassuring fetal testing, abruption, advanced labor
Consider delivery at 34 weeks' gestation
Intrapartum group B streptococcus prophylaxis if no recent negative anovaginal culture
Broad-spectrum antibiotics if amnionitis

FIGURE 29-3. Management algorithm for preterm premature rupture of the membranes (PROM) remote from term (23 to 31 weeks' gestation). (From Mercer BM: Preterm premature rupture of the membranes: diagnosis and management. Clin Perinatol 31:765, 2004.)

evaluation of uterine activity. Biophysical profile testing may be confounded by the presence of oligohydramnios but can be helpful should the nonstress test result be equivocal (see Chapter 12). **Although a low initial amniotic fluid index is associated with shorter latency and an increased risk for chorioamnionitis, it does not accurately predict who will ultimately develop these complications and should not be used in isolation to make management decisions.** Prolonged bedrest in pregnancy may increase the risk for deep venous thrombosis.[72] Preventive measures such as leg exercises, antiembolic stockings, and/or prophylactic doses of subcutaneous heparin may be of value during conservative management of PROM.

Twofold to fourfold increases in perinatal mortality, IVH, and neonatal sepsis have been reported in infants born after chorioamnionitis compared with gestational age–matched controls born to noninfected mothers.[28] The clinical diagnosis is made when maternal fever (temperature ≥38° C [100.4° F]) with uterine tenderness and maternal or fetal tachycardia are identified in the absence of another evident source of infection. The maternal white blood cell count can be helpful if clinical findings are equivocal. An increase in the white blood cell count from a baseline level obtained on admission is suggestive of infection but may be artificially elevated if antenatal corticosteroids have been administered within 5 to 7 days. If additional confirmation of intrauterine infection is required, amniocentesis may be helpful.[12,73] A positive amniotic fluid culture is also supportive of a clinical suspicion of clinical chorioamnionitis (sensitivity, 65% to 85%; specificity, 85%), but the clinical diagnosis will likely become clear during the 48 hours needed to achieve a culture result. An amniotic glucose concentration below 16 to 20 mg/dL (sensitivity and specificity, 80% to 90% for positive culture) or a Gram stain positive for bacteria (sensitivity, 36% to 80%; specificity, 80% to 97% for positive culture) are supportive of a clinically suspicious diagnosis of chorioamnionitis and can be rapidly obtained. However, the presence of white blood cells only in amniotic fluid is not diagnostic of intrauterine infection after PROM. Elevated amniotic fluid interleukin levels have also been associated with an increased risk for early delivery and perinatal infectious morbidity, but cytokine analyses are not readily available in most clinical laboratories,[73] limiting their utility in clinical practice. Once chorioamnionitis is diagnosed, broad-spectrum antibiotics should be initiated, and delivery should be pursued.

Corticosteroid Administration

A single course of antenatal corticosteroids, either betamethasone (12 mg intramuscularly [IM] every 24 hours for two doses) or dexamethasone (6 mg IM every 12 hours for four doses) before anticipated preterm birth has been shown to reduce the risks for RDS, IVH, necrotizing enterocolitis, perinatal death, and long-term neurologic morbidities. **Meta-analysis regarding antenatal corticosteroid administration after preterm PROM has confirmed steroid therapy to significantly reduce the risks for RDS (20% versus 35.4%), IVH (7.5% versus 15.9%), and necrotizing enterocolitis (0.8% versus 4.6%), without increasing the risks for maternal (9.2% versus 5.1%) or neonatal (7.0% versus 6.6%) infection.**[74]

Repeated courses of antenatal corticosteroids after preterm PROM have been associated with increased newborn infection in some studies and have not been consistently associated with improvements in newborn outcomes.[75] Ghidini and colleagues found less IVH and chorioamnionitis, but no reduction in the risk for RDS with repeated antenatal corticosteroid doses.[76] Alternatively, Abbassi and associates observed a lower risk for RDS with more than one course of antenatal corticosteroids after PROM (34.9% versus 45.2%).[75] Given the potential risks and the lack of clear data supporting the benefit of repeated weekly antenatal corticosteroid administration, such treatment does not appear warranted. It remains to be determined whether a single repeat "rescue" course could benefit the woman who receives an initial course of antenatal corticosteroids after PROM near the limit of viability but then remains pregnant through 30 to 33 weeks' gestation.

Antibiotic Administration

The goal of antibiotic therapy during conservative management of preterm PROM remote from term is to treat or prevent ascending infection in order to prolong pregnancy and reduce perinatal infectious and gestational age–dependent morbidity. Meta-analyses have summarized a large number of randomized controlled clinical trials in this regard.[77,78] These evaluations suggest that **antibiotic treatment significantly prolongs latency after membrane rupture, reduces chorioamnionitis and postpartum endometritis, and also prevents newborn complications including neonatal sepsis, pneumonia, and IVH.** Several published trials offer valuable insights regarding the potential role of adjunctive antibiotics in this setting. The National Institutes of Child Health and Human Development Maternal Fetal Medicine Units (NICHD-MFMU) Research Network studied women with preterm PROM remote from term (24 to 32 weeks, 0 days' gestation).[79,80] Participants received 48 hours of broad-spectrum intravenous therapy (ampicillin [2 g every 6 hours] and erythromycin [250 mg every 6 hours]), followed by 5 days of oral (PO) therapy (amoxicillin [250 mg every 8 hours] and enteric-coated erythromycin-base [333 mg every 8 hours]) or a matching placebo. GBS carriers in both study arms received ampicillin for one week and then again in labor. Antibiotic treatment doubled the likelihood of undelivered after 7 days, and this benefit persisted up to 3 weeks after randomization, suggesting that antibiotics successfully treated rather than just suppressing subclinical infection. Antibiotics improved neonatal health by reducing the number of babies with one or more major infant complication from 53% to 44% (composite morbidity: death, RDS, early sepsis, severe IVH, severe necrotizing enterocolitis; $P < .05$), and also reduced individual newborn complications including RDS (40.5% versus 48.7%), stage 3 or 4 necrotizing enterocolitis (2.3% versus 5.8%), patent ductus arteriosus (11.7% versus 20.2%), and chronic lung disease (bronchopulmonary dysplasia: 20.5% versus 13.0%) ($P < .05$ for each). Regarding individual infectious morbidities, antibiotics reduced the frequencies of chorioamnionitis overall (32.5% versus 23%), and also neonatal sepsis (8.4% versus 15.6%) and pneumonia (2.9% versus 7%), among those who were not GBS carriers ($P \leq .04$ for each). In a second multicenter placebo controlled trial, Kenyon and colleagues studied oral therapy with erythromycin, amoxicillin–clavulanic acid, or both for up to 10 days after preterm PROM before 37 weeks.[81] In summary, erythromycin prolonged latency only briefly (not significant at 7 days) but did reduce the need for supplemental oxygen (31.1% versus 35.6%) and the frequency of positive blood cultures (5.7% versus 8.2%) ($P = .02$ for both). Amoxicillin–clavulanic acid prolonged pregnancy (43.3% versus 36.7% undelivered at 7 days) and reduced the need for supplemental oxygen (30.1% versus 35.6%) but increased the risk for necrotizing enterocolitis (1.9% vs. 0.5%) ($P \leq .05$ for each). Long-term follow-up of infants delivered within this trial revealed no evident differences between antibiotic and control groups.[82] Subsequent studies have attempted to determine whether the duration of antibiotic therapy could be shortened but are of inadequate size and power to evaluate infant outcomes adequately.[83]

In summary, there appears to be a role for a 7-day course of parenteral and oral antibiotic therapy with erythromycin and amoxicillin-ampicillin during conservative management of preterm PROM remote from term, to prolong latency and to reduce infectious and gestational age–dependent neonatal complications. Extended-spectrum ampicillin–clavulanic acid treatment is not recommended because it may be harmful.

Tocolysis

There is limited evidence that prophylactic tocolysis, administered after preterm PROM and before the onset of contractions, can prolong pregnancy briefly.[84] However, therapeutic tocolysis initiated only after the onset of contractions has not been shown to prolong latency after preterm PROM. A report from the National Institutes of Health collaborative study on antenatal steroids suggested an association between tocolytic treatment after preterm PROM and subsequent neonatal RDS, but subsequent small prospective studies have found neither an increase nor decrease in neonatal complications with such tocolytic treatment.[85] Although it is plausible that tocolysis could facilitate initial uterine quiescence to allow additional time for antibiotic and corticosteroid benefits, there have been no studies of tocolytic therapy after preterm PROM in which concurrent antenatal corticosteroid and antibiotic treatments were given. In a recent small randomized controlled trial, weekly progesterone treatment did not prolong latency after PROM.[86] Pending further study, **tocolysis and progesterone therapy should not be considered expected practices after preterm PROM.**

Cervical Cerclage

After cervical cerclage, preterm PROM is a common complication, affecting about one in four elective cerclages and half of emergent procedures.[87] There are no prospective studies regarding the management of preterm PROM and a cervical cerclage in situ. Retrospective studies reveal that perinatal complications are similar to PROM without a cerclage if the stitch is removed on admission.[88] Studies comparing pregnancies in which the stitch was retained or removed after preterm PROM have been small but have yielded consistent patterns.[89,90] Each has found insignificant trends toward increased maternal infections and only brief pregnancy prolongation; one study found increased infant mortality and death due to sepsis when the cerclage was not removed.[89] **No well-controlled study has found cerclage retention to reduce the frequency or severity of newborn complications after PROM. Based on these data, early cerclage removal is recommended when PROM occurs.** The risks and benefits of short-term cerclage retention during antenatal corticosteroid treatment have not been determined.

Herpes Simplex Virus

Neonatal HSV infection most commonly results from direct maternal-fetal transmission during the delivery process, with newborn infection rates of 34% to 80% after primary and 1% to 5% after secondary maternal infection.[91] When neonatal HSV infection occurs, the mortality rate is 50% to 60%, and up to 50% of survivors will suffer serious sequelae.[92] Based on small case series of women with an active maternal genital HSV infection by Amstey ($N = 9$) and Nahmias and colleagues ($N = 26$), both in 1971, the accepted belief has been that extended latency after membrane rupture (>4 to 6 hours) is associated with an increased risk for newborn infection.[93] Major and coworkers have reported on a case series of 29 gravidas managed expectantly with PROM before 32 weeks' gestation with active *recurrent* HSV lesions.[94] Latency after membrane rupture ranged from 1 to 35 days, and cesarean delivery was performed if active lesions were present at the time of delivery. None of the infants delivered under this regimen developed neonatal herpes infection. These data are supportive of conservative management of PROM complicated by recurrent maternal HSV infection; however, such treatment should be considered only at an early gestational age when the likelihood of infant mortality and long-term complications with early delivery is high. Prophylactic treatment with antiviral agents (e.g., acyclovir) to reduce viral shedding and the frequency of recurrences is prudent under this circumstance.

Management of Previable Premature Rupture of the Membranes

The cause of PROM before the limit of viability has implications for the anticipated pregnancy outcome and can be helpful in guiding counseling and management. Previable PROM subsequent to second-trimester amniocentesis is likely related to continued leakage of fluid through a small membrane defect without concurrent infection. Under this circumstance it is likely that the membranes will reseal, and extended pregnancy can be anticipated. Alternatively, previable PROM subsequent to second-trimester bleeding, oligohydramnios, or an elevated maternal serum α-fetoprotein more likely reflects an abnormality of placentation and has a poorer prognosis. The patient with previable PROM and no indication for immediate delivery should be counseled regarding the potential risks and benefits of conservative management. Counseling should include a realistic appraisal of fetal and neonatal outcomes and the risks for maternal complications.

Most available data regarding women with preterm PROM near the limit of viability are derived from retrospective studies. **In a recent review of preterm PROM occurring at or before 24 weeks' gestation, Waters and Mercer found that median latency ranged from 6 to 13 days.**[31] Another recent evaluation found that 38% delivered within 1 week and 69% delivered within 5 weeks after periviable PROM.[95] **Other maternal risks during conservative management of PROM at 24 weeks or less include chorioamnionitis (35%), abruptio placentae (19%), retained placenta (11%), and endometritis (14%).**[31] **Maternal sepsis (0.8%) and death (1 in 619 pregnancies overall) are rare but serious complications.** Conservative management can also lead to muscle wasting, bone demineralization, and deep venous thrombosis due to prolonged bedrest. Overall infant survival after conservatively managed periviable PROM occurs in 44% of cases, but this varies with gestational age at membrane rupture (14.4% before 22 weeks versus 57.7% at 22 to 24 weeks). Stillbirth is common, complicating up to 23% to 53% of cases. Neonatal complications include pulmonary hypoplasia (19%), RDS (66%), grade III or IV IVH (5%), sepsis (19%), and necrotizing enterocolitis (4%), as well as long-term complications such as bronchopulmonary dysplasia (29%), stage III retinopathy of prematurity (5%), and contractures (3%). Prediction of individual outcomes is difficult because of the inability to predict the ultimate gestational age at delivery in any given case.

A potential management scheme for PROM before the limit of viability is presented in Figure 29-4. There is no consensus regarding the advantages of inpatient versus

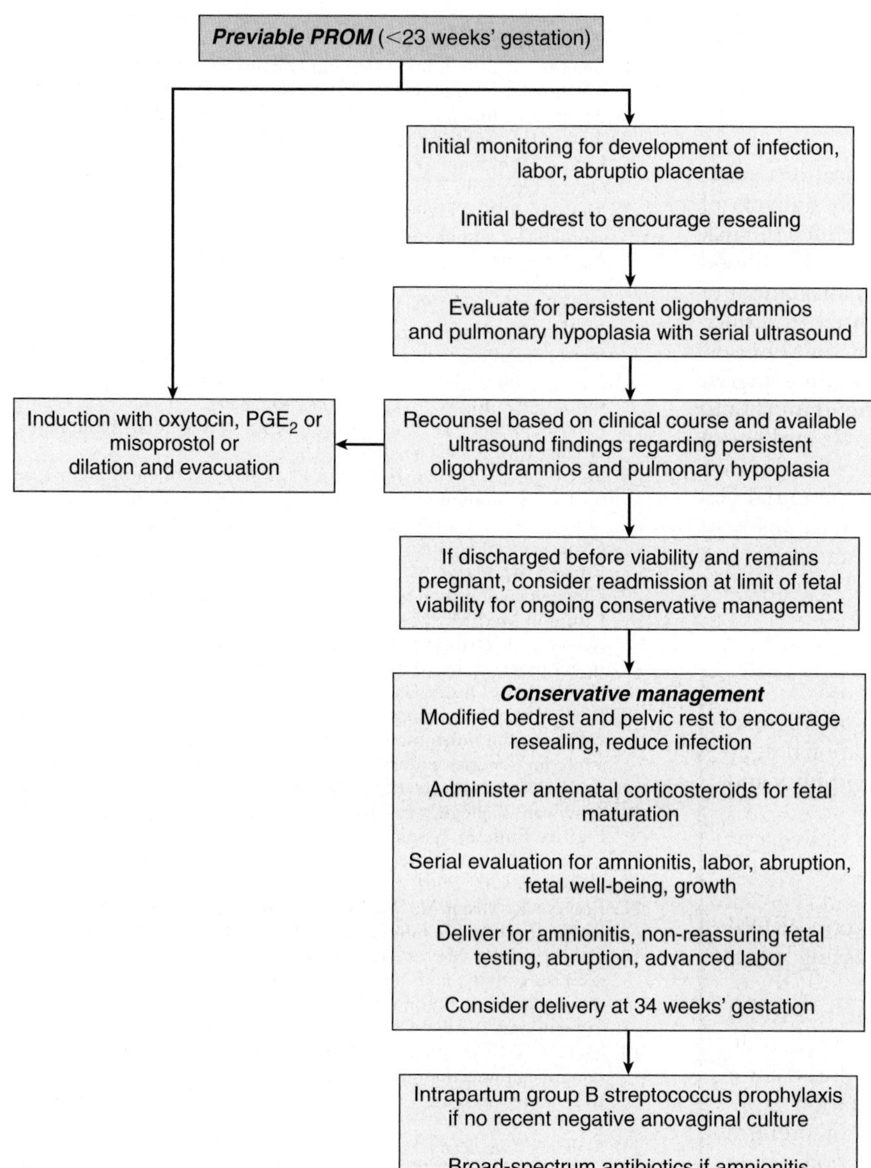

Previable PROM (<23 weeks' gestation)
Initial monitoring for development of infection, labor, abruptio placentae
Initial bedrest to encourage resealing
Evaluate for persistent oligohydramnios and pulmonary hypoplasia with serial ultrasound
Induction with oxytocin, PGE2 or misoprostol or dilation and evacuation
Recounsel based on clinical course and available ultrasound findings regarding persistent oligohydramnios and pulmonary hypoplasia
If discharged before viability and remains pregnant, consider readmission at limit of fetal viability for ongoing conservative management
Conservative management
Modified bedrest and pelvic rest to encourage resealing, reduce infection
Administer antenatal corticosteroids for fetal maturation
Serial evaluation for amnionitis, labor, abruption, fetal well-being, growth
Deliver for amnionitis, non-reassuring fetal testing, abruption, advanced labor
Consider delivery at 34 weeks' gestation
Intrapartum group B streptococcus prophylaxis if no recent negative anovaginal culture
Broad-spectrum antibiotics if amnionitis

FIGURE 29-4. Management algorithm for preterm PROM before the limit of potential viability (currently 23 weeks' gestation). *PGE_2*, prostaglandin E_2. (From Mercer BM: Preterm premature rupture of the membranes: diagnosis and management. Clin Perinatol 31:765, 2004.)

outpatient management for the patient electing conservative management after previable PROM. The benefits of an initial period of inpatient observation may include bedrest and pelvic rest to increase the opportunity for membrane resealing, as well as early identification of infection, fetal demise, and abruption. A number of novel treatments, including amnioinfusion and fibrin-platelet-cryoprecipitate or Gelfoam sealing of the membranes, have been preliminarily investigated.[96-98] The risks and benefits of these aggressive interventions have not been adequately studied to suggest that such therapy be incorporated into routine clinical practice. Typically, women with previable PROM who have been managed as outpatients are readmitted to hospital once the pregnancy reaches the limit of viability. Administration of antenatal corticosteroids for fetal maturation is appropriate at this time.

During conservative management, serial ultrasound performed every 1 to 2 weeks can evaluate for reaccumulation of amniotic fluid and interval pulmonary growth. Although persistent severe oligohydramnios is a strong marker for subsequent development of lethal pulmonary hypoplasia, serial fetal biometric evaluation (e.g., lung length, chest circumference), and ratios that adjust for overall fetal size (thoracic-abdominal circumference, thoracic circumference–femur length) can demonstrate a lack of fetal pulmonary growth over time and have a high predictive value for lethal pulmonary hypoplasia.[39,42,99,100] Studies of pulmonary artery and ductus arteriosus waveform modulation with fetal breathing movements have shown some promise but can be technically difficult to perform.

Some women will not choose to undertake the potential risks for maternal complications after previable PROM either after initial counseling or with evidence of developing pulmonary hypoplasia. Delivery can be accomplished by labor induction with vaginal prostaglandin E_2, prostaglandin E_1 (misoprostol), high-dose intravenous oxytocin, or dilation and evacuation. The optimal approach depends on patient characteristics (e.g., gestational age, evident chorioamnionitis, prior cesarean delivery), available facilities, and physician experience.

SUMMARY

The potential for significant perinatal complications exists when PROM occurs at term or preterm. Early delivery of the patient with PROM at or near term can reduce the risk for perinatal infections without increasing the likelihood of operative delivery. Careful conservative management of PROM remote from term offers the potential to reduce infectious and gestational age–dependent morbidities. Early transfer to a facility capable of providing urgent obstetrical and neonatal intensive care is important should adequate facilities not be available locally. Regardless of the management approach, infants delivering after preterm PROM and after PROM before the limit of potential viability are at high risk for perinatal complications, many of which cannot be avoided with current technology and management algorithms.

KEY POINTS

- PROM complicates about 8% to 10% of pregnancies and is a significant cause of gestational age–dependent and infectious perinatal morbidity and mortality.
- Latency from membrane rupture to delivery is typically brief and decreases with increasing gestational age at membrane rupture.
- Chorioamnionitis is common after preterm PROM and increases in frequency with decreasing gestational age at membrane rupture.
- Women with a prior preterm birth due to PROM have a 3.3-fold higher risk for subsequent preterm birth due to PROM and a 13.5-fold higher risk for preterm PROM before 28 weeks' gestation.
- Some potentially preventable causes of preterm PROM include urogenital tract infections, poor maternal nutrition with a low body mass index (<19.8 kg/m^2), and cigarette smoking.
- Vaginally collected amniotic fluid can reliably predict the presence of fetal pulmonary maturity after preterm PROM.
- Conservative management after preterm PROM with documented fetal pulmonary maturity near term (32 to 36 weeks) prolongs latency only briefly but increases the risk for perinatal infection and does not improve neonatal outcomes.
- Antenatal corticosteroid administration and limited duration broad-spectrum antibiotic administration have been shown to reduce newborn complications when given in the setting of PROM remote from term.
- Cervical cerclage retention after preterm PROM has not been shown to improve neonatal outcomes.
- Lethal pulmonary hypoplasia is common after PROM occurring before 20 weeks and can be predicted with serial ultrasound assessment of lung and chest growth.

REFERENCES

1. Ananth CV, Joseph KS, Demissie K, Vintzileos AM: Trends in twin preterm birth subtypes in the United States, 1989 through 2000: impact on perinatal mortality. Am J Obstet Gynecol 193:1076, 2005.
2. Tucker JM, Goldenberg RL, Davis RO, et al: Etiologies of preterm birth in an indigent population: is prevention a logical expectation? Obstet Gynecol 77:343, 1991.
3. McParland PC, Taylor DJ, Bell SC: Mapping of zones of altered morphology and choriodeciduaic connective tissue cellular phenotype in human fetal membranes (amnion and deciduas) overlying the lower uterine pole and cervix before labor at term. Am J Obstet Gynecol 189:1481, 2003.
4. McLaren J, Taylor DJ, Bell SC: Increased concentration of pro-matrix metalloproteinase 9 in term fetal membranes overlying the cervix before labor: implications for membrane remodeling and rupture. Am J Obstet Gynecol 182:409, 2000.
5. Parry S, Strauss JF: Premature rupture of the fetal membranes. N Engl J Med 338:663, 1998.
6. McGregor JA, French JI, Parker R, et al: Prevention of premature birth by screening and treatment for common genital tract infections: results of a prospective controlled evaluation. Am J Obstet Gynecol 173:157, 1995.
7. Romero R, Mazor M, Oyarzun E, et al: Is there an association between colonization with group B streptococcus and prematurity? J Reprod Med 34:797, 1989.
8. Regan JA, Klebanoff MA, Nugent RP, et al: Colonization with group B streptococci in pregnancy and adverse outcome. VIP Study Group. Am J Obstet Gynecol 174:1354, 1996.
9. Romero R, Chaiworapongsa T, Kuivaniemi H, Tromp G: Bacterial vaginosis, the inflammatory response and the risk of preterm birth: a role for genetic epidemiology in the prevention of preterm birth. Am J Obstet Gynecol 190:1509, 2004.
10. American College of Obstetricians and Gynecologists: ACOG Practice Bulletin. Assessment of risk factors for preterm birth: clinical management guidelines for obstetrician-gynecologists. Obstet Gynecol 98:709, 2001.
11. Romero R, Mazor M, Wu YK, et al: Infection in the pathogenesis of preterm labor. Semin Perinatol 12:262, 1988.
12. Gauthier DW, Meyer WJ: Comparison of gram stain, leukocyte esterase activity, and amniotic fluid glucose concentration in predicting amniotic fluid culture results in preterm premature rupture of membranes. Am J Obstet Gynecol 167:1092, 1992.
13. Mercer BM, Moretti ML, Prevost RR, Sibai BM: Erythromycin therapy in preterm premature rupture of the membranes: a prospective, randomized trial of 220 patients. Am J Obstet Gynecol 166:794, 1992.
14. Macones GA, Parry S, Elkousy M, et al: A polymorphism in the promoter region of TNF and bacterial vaginosis: preliminary evidence of gene-environment interaction in the etiology of spontaneous preterm birth. Am J Obstet Gynecol 190:1504, 2004.
15. Romero R, Friel LA, Velez Edwards DR, et al: A genetic association study of maternal and fetal candidate genes that predispose to preterm prelabor rupture of membranes (PROM). Am J Obstet Gynecol 203:361, 2010.
16. Mercer BM, Goldenberg RL, Meis PJ, et al, for the NICHD-MFMU Network: The preterm prediction study: prediction of preterm premature rupture of the membranes using clinical findings and ancillary testing. Am J Obstet Gynecol 183:738, 2000.
17. Mercer BM, Goldenberg RL, Moawad AH, et al, for the NICHD-MFMU Network: The preterm prediction study: effect of gestational age and cause of preterm birth on subsequent obstetric outcome. Am J Obstet Gynecol 181:1216, 1999.
18. Meis PJ, Klebanoff M, Thom E, et al, for the NICHD-MFMU Network: Prevention of recurrent preterm delivery by 17 alpha-hydroxyprogesterone caproate. N Engl J Med 348:2379, 2003.
19. da Fonseca EB, Bittar RE, Carvalho MH, Zugaib M: Prophylactic administration of progesterone by vaginal suppository to reduce the incidence of spontaneous preterm birth in women at increased risk: a randomized placebo-controlled double-blind study. Am J Obstet Gynecol 188:419, 2003.
20. Casanueva E, Ripoll C, Tolentino M, et al: Vitamin C supplementation to prevent premature rupture of the chorioamniotic membranes: a randomized trial. Am J Clin Nutr 81:859, 2005.
21. Mercer BM, Abdelrahim A, Moore RM, et al: The impact of vitamin C supplementation in pregnancy and in vitro upon fetal membrane strength and remodeling. Reprod Sci 17:685, 2010.

22. Rumbold A, Crowther CA: Vitamin C supplementation in pregnancy. Cochrane Database Syst Rev CD004072, 2005.
23. Hannah ME, Ohlsson A, Farine D, et al: Induction of labor compared with expectant management for prelabor rupture of membranes at term. N Engl J Med 334:1005, 1996.
24. Mercer B, Arheart K: Antimicrobial therapy in expectant management of preterm premature rupture of the membranes. Lancet 346:1271, 1995.
25. Gold RB, Goyer GL, Schwartz DB, et al: Conservative management of second trimester post-amniocentesis fluid leakage. Obstet Gynecol 74:745, 1989.
26. Johnson JWC, Egerman RS, Moorhead J: Cases with ruptured membranes that "reseal." Am J Obstet Gynecol 163:1024, 1990.
27. Hillier SL, Martius J, Krohn M, et al: A case-control study of chorioamnionic infection and histologic chorioamnionitis in prematurity. N Engl J Med 319:972, 1988.
28. Garite TJ, Freeman RK: Chorioamnionitis in the preterm gestation. Obstet Gynecol 59:539, 1982.
29. Simpson GF, Harbert GM Jr: Use of betamethasone in management of preterm gestation with premature rupture of membranes. Obstet Gynecol 66:168, 1985.
30. Gonen R, Hannah ME, Milligan JE: Does prolonged preterm premature rupture of the membranes predispose to abruptio placentae? Obstet Gynecol 74:347, 1989.
31. Waters TP, Mercer BM: The management of preterm premature rupture of the membranes near the limit of fetal viability. Am J Obstet Gynecol 201:230, 2009.
32. Moberg LJ, Garite TJ, Freeman RK: Fetal heart rate patterns and fetal distress in patients with preterm premature rupture of membranes. Obstet Gynecol 64:60, 1984.
33. Mercer BM: Preterm premature rupture of the membranes. Obstet Gynecol 101:178, 2003.
34. Blumenfeld YJ, Lee HC, Gould JB, et al: The effect of preterm premature rupture of membranes on neonatal mortality rates. Obstet Gynecol 116:1381, 2010.
35. Chen A, Feresu SA, Barsoom MJ: Heterogeneity of preterm birth subtypes in relation to neonatal death. Obstet Gynecol 114:516, 2009.
36. Seo K, McGregor JA, French JI: Preterm birth is associated with increased risk of maternal and neonatal infection. Obstet Gynecol 79:75, 1992.
37. Wu YW, Colford JM Jr: Chorioamnionitis as a risk factor for cerebral palsy: a meta-analysis. JAMA 284:1417, 2000.
38. Yoon BH, Romero R, Kim CJ, et al: High expression of tumor necrosis factor-alpha and interleukin-6 in periventricular leukomalacia. Am J Obstet Gynecol 177:406, 1997.
39. Lauria MR, Gonik B, Romero R: Pulmonary hypoplasia: pathogenesis, diagnosis, and antenatal prediction. Obstet Gynecol 86:466, 1995.
40. Wigglesworth JS, Desai R: Use of DNA estimation for growth assessment in normal and hypoplastic fetal lungs. Arch Dis Child 56:601, 1981.
41. Moretti M, Sibai B: Maternal and perinatal outcome of expectant management of premature rupture of the membranes in midtrimester. Am J Obstet Gynecol 159:390, 1988.
42. Rizzo G, Capponi A, Angelini E, et al: Blood flow velocity waveforms from fetal peripheral pulmonary arteries in pregnancies with preterm premature rupture of the membranes: relationship with pulmonary hypoplasia. Ultrasound Obstet Gynecol 15:98, 2000.
43. Winn HN, Chen M, Amon E, et al: Neonatal pulmonary hypoplasia and perinatal mortality in patients with midtrimester rupture of amniotic membranes: a critical analysis. Am J Obstet Gynecol 182:1638, 2000.
44. Nimrod C, Varela-Gittings F, Machin G, et al: The effect of very prolonged membrane rupture on fetal development. Am J Obstet Gynecol 148:540, 1984.
45. Blott M, Greenough A: Neonatal outcome after prolonged rupture of the membranes starting in the second trimester. Arch Dis Child 63:1146, 1988.
46. Lee SE, Park JS, Norwitz ER, et al: Measurement of placental alpha-microglobulin-1 in cervicovaginal discharge to diagnose rupture of membranes. Obstet Gynecol 109:634, 2007.
47. Alexander JM, Mercer BM, Miodovnik M, et al: The impact of digital cervical examination on expectantly managed preterm rupture of membranes. Am J Obstet Gynecol 183:1003, 2000.
48. Brown CL, Ludwiczak MH, Blanco JD, Hirsch CE: Cervical dilation: accuracy of visual and digital examinations. Obstet Gynecol 81:215, 1993.
49. Verani JR, McGee L, Schrag SJ, for the Division of Bacterial Diseases, National Center for Immunization and Respiratory Diseases, Centers for Disease Control and Prevention (CDC): Prevention of perinatal group B streptococcal disease: revised guidelines from CDC, 2010. MMWR Recomm Rep 59:1, 2010.
50. American College of Obstetricians and Gynecologists: ACOG Committee Opinion: number 279, December 2002. Prevention of early-onset group B streptococcal disease in newborns. Obstet Gynecol 100:1405, 2002.
51. Towers CV, Carr MH, Padilla G, Asrat T: Potential consequences of widespread antepartal use of ampicillin. Am J Obstet Gynecol 179:879, 1998.
52. Van der Walt D, Venter PF: Management of term pregnancy with premature rupture of the membranes and unfavourable cervix. S Afr Med J 75:54, 1989.
53. Grant JM, Serle E, Mahmood T, et al: Management of prelabour rupture of the membranes in term primigravidae: report of a randomized prospective trial. Br J Obstet Gynaecol 99:557, 1992.
54. Ladfors L, Mattsson LA, Eriksson M, Fall O: A randomised trial of two expectant managements of prelabour rupture of the membranes at 34 to 42 weeks. Br J Obstet Gynaecol 103:755, 1996.
55. Shalev E, Peleg D, Eliyahu S, Nahum Z: Comparison of 12- and 72-hour expectant management of premature rupture of membranes in term pregnancies. Obstet Gynecol 85:1, 1995.
56. Dare MR, Middleton P, Crowther CA, et al: Planned early birth versus expectant management (waiting) for prelabour rupture of membranes at term (37 weeks or more). Cochrane Database Syst Rev CD005302, 2006.
57. Tan BP, Hannah ME: Prostaglandins versus oxytocin for prelabour rupture of membranes at term. Cochrane Database Syst Rev CD000159, 2002.
58. Strong TH Jr, Hetzler G, Sarno AP, Paul RH: Prophylactic intrapartum amnioinfusion: a randomized clinical trial. Am J Obstet Gynecol 162:1370, 1990.
59. Schrimmer DB, Macri CJ, Paul RH: Prophylactic amnioinfusion as a treatment for oligohydramnios in laboring patients: a prospective randomized trial. Am J Obstet Gynecol 165:972, 1991.
60. Naef RW 3rd, Allbert JR, Ross EL, et al: Premature rupture of membranes at 34 to 37 weeks' gestation: aggressive vs. conservative management. Am J Obstet Gynecol 178:126, 1998.
61. Neerhof MG, Cravello C, Haney EI, Silver RK: Timing of labor induction after premature rupture of membranes between 32 and 36 weeks gestation. Am J Obstet Gynecol 180:349, 1999.
62. Cox SM, Leveno KJ: Intentional delivery vs. expectant management with preterm ruptured membranes at 30-34 weeks' gestation. Obstet Gynecol 86:875, 1995.
63. Mercer BM, Crocker L, Boe N, Sibai B: Induction vs. expectant management in PROM with mature amniotic fluid at 32-36 weeks: a randomized trial. Am J Obstet Gynecol 82:775, 1993.
64. Mercer BM in response to Repke JT, Berck DJ: Preterm premature rupture of membranes: a continuing dilemma. Am J Obstet Gynecol 170:1835, 1994.
65. Sbarra AJ, Blake G, Cetrulo CL, et al: The effect of cervical/vaginal secretions on measurements of lecithin/sphingomyelin ratio and optical density at 650 nm. Am J Obstet Gynecol 139:214, 1981.
66. Shaver DC, Spinnato JA, Whybrew D, et al: Comparison of phospholipids in vaginal and amniocentesis specimens of patients with premature rupture of membranes. Am J Obstet Gynecol 156:454, 1987.
67. Lewis DF, Towers CV, Major CA, et al: Use of Amniostat-FLM in detecting the presence of phosphatidylglycerol in vaginal pool samples in preterm premature rupture of membranes. Am J Obstet Gynecol 169:573, 1993.
68. Russell JC, Cooper CM, Ketchum CH, et al: Multicenter evaluation of TDx test for assessing fetal lung maturity. Clin Chem 35:1005, 1989.
69. Edwards RK, Duff P, Ross KC: Amniotic fluid indices of fetal pulmonary maturity with preterm premature rupture of membranes. Obstet Gynecol 96:102, 2000.
70. Estol PC, Poseiro JJ, Schwarcz R: Phosphatidylglycerol determination in the amniotic fluid from a PAD placed over the vulva: a method for diagnosis of fetal lung maturity in cases of premature ruptured membranes. J Perinat Med 20:65, 1992.

71. Salim R, Zafran N, Nachum Z, et al: Predicting lung maturity in preterm rupture of membranes via lamellar bodies count from a vaginal pool: a cohort study. Reprod Biol Endocrinol 7:1, 2009.
72. Kovacevich GJ, Gaich SA, Lavin JP, et al: The prevalence of thromboembolic events among women with extended bed rest prescribed as part of the treatment for premature labor or preterm premature rupture of membranes. Am J Obstet Gynecol 182:1089, 2000.
73. Romero R, Yoon BH, Mazor M, et al: A comparative study of the diagnostic performance of amniotic fluid glucose, white blood cell count, interleukin-6, and Gram stain in the detection of microbial invasion in patients with preterm premature rupture of membranes. Am J Obstet Gynecol 169:839, 1993.
74. Harding JE, Pang J, Knight DB, Liggins GC: Do antenatal corticosteroids help in the setting of preterm rupture of membranes? Am J Obstet Gynecol 184:131, 2001.
75. Abbasi S, Hirsch D, Davis J, et al: Effect of single vs. multiple courses of antenatal corticosteroids on maternal and neonatal outcome. Am J Obstet Gynecol 182:1243, 2000.
76. Ghidini A, Salafia CM, Minior VK: Repeated courses of steroids in preterm membrane rupture do not increase the risk of histologic chorioamnionitis. Am J Perinatol 14:309, 1997.
77. Egarter C, Leitich H, Karas H, et al: Antibiotic treatment in premature rupture of membranes and neonatal morbidity: a meta-analysis. Am J Obstet Gynecol 174:589, 1996.
78. Kenyon S, Boulvain M, Neilson J: Antibiotics for preterm rupture of membranes. Cochrane Database Syst Rev CD001058, 2010.
79. Mercer B, Miodovnik M, Thurnau G, et al, for the NICHD-MFMU Network: Antibiotic therapy for reduction of infant morbidity after preterm premature rupture of the membranes: a randomized controlled trial. JAMA 278:989, 1997.
80. Mercer BM, Goldenberg RL, Das AF, et al, for the NICHD-MFMU Network: What we have learned regarding antibiotic therapy for the reduction of infant morbidity. Semin Perinatol 27:217, 2003.
81. Kenyon SL, Taylor DJ, Tarnow-Mordi W, and Oracle Collaborative Group: Broad spectrum antibiotics for preterm, prelabor rupture of fetal membranes: the ORACLE I Randomized trial. Lancet 357:979, 2001.
82. Kenyon S, Pike K, Jones DR, et al: Childhood outcomes after prescription of antibiotics to pregnant women with preterm rupture of the membranes: 7-year follow-up of the ORACLE I trial. Lancet 372:1310, 2008.
83. Segel SY, Miles AM, Clothier B, et al: Duration of antibiotic therapy after preterm premature rupture of fetal membranes. Am J Obstet Gynecol 189:799, 2003.
84. Weiner CP, Renk K, Klugman M: The therapeutic efficacy and cost-effectiveness of aggressive tocolysis for premature labor associated with premature rupture of the membranes. Am J Obstet Gynecol 159:216, 1988.
85. Curet LB, Rao AV, Zachman RD, et al: Association between ruptured membranes, tocolytic therapy, and respiratory distress syndrome. Am J Obstet Gynecol 148:263, 1984.
86. Briery CM, Veillon EW, Klauser CK, et al: Women with preterm premature rupture of the membranes do not benefit from weekly progesterone. Am J Obstet Gynecol 204:54, 2011.
87. Treadwell MC, Bronsteen RA, Bottoms SF: Prognostic factors and complication rates for cervical cerclage: a review of 482 cases. Am J Obstet Gynecol 165:555, 1991.
88. Yeast JD, Garite TR: The role of cervical cerclage in the management of preterm premature rupture of the membranes. Am J Obstet Gynecol 158:106, 1988.
89. Ludmir J, Bader T, Chen L, et al: Poor perinatal outcome associated with retained cerclage in patients with premature rupture of membranes. Obstet Gynecol 84:823, 1994.
90. McElrath TF, Norwitz ER, Lieberman ES, Heffner LJ: Perinatal outcome after preterm premature rupture of membranes with in situ cervical cerclage. Am J Obstet Gynecol 187:1147, 2002.
91. Brown ZA, Vontver LA, Benedetti J, et al: Effects on infants of a first episode of genital herpes during pregnancy. N Engl J Med 317:1246, 1987.
92. Stagno S, Whitley RJ: Herpes virus infections of pregnancy. II. Herpes simplex virus and varicella zoster infections. N Engl J Med 313:1327, 1985.
93. Gibbs RS, Amstey MS, Lezotte DC: Role of cesarean delivery in preventing neonatal herpes virus infection. JAMA 270:94, 1993.
94. Major CA, Towers CV, Lewis DF, Garite TJ: Expectant management of preterm premature rupture of membranes complicated by active recurrent genital herpes. Am J Obstet Gynecol 188:1551, 2003.
95. Muris C, Girard B, Creveuil C, et al: Management of premature rupture of membranes before 25 weeks. Eur J Obstet Gynecol Reprod Biol 131:163, 2007.
96. Sciscione AC, Manley JS, Pollock M, et al: Intracervical fibrin sealants: a potential treatment for early preterm premature rupture of the membranes. Am J Obstet Gynecol 184:368, 2001.
97. Quintero RA, Morales WJ, Bornick PW, et al: Surgical treatment of spontaneous rupture of membranes: the amniograft-first experience. Am J Obstet Gynecol 186:155, 2002.
98. O'Brien JM, Barton JR, Milligan DA: An aggressive interventional protocol for early midtrimester premature rupture of the membranes using gelatin sponge for cervical plugging. Am J Obstet Gynecol 187:1143, 2002.
99. Laudy JA, Tibboel D, Robben SG, et al: Prenatal prediction of pulmonary hypoplasia: clinical, biometric, and Doppler velocity correlates. Pediatrics 109:250, 2002.
100. Yoshimura S, Masuzaki H, Gotoh H, et al: Ultrasonographic prediction of lethal pulmonary hypoplasia: comparison of eight different ultrasonographic parameters. Am J Obstet Gynecol 175:477, 1996.

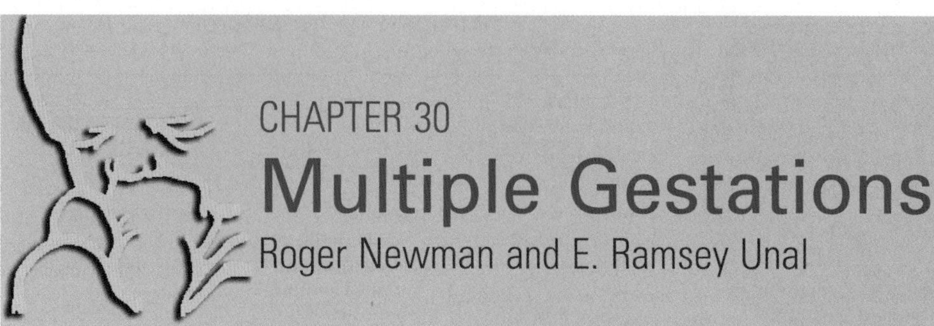

CHAPTER 30
Multiple Gestations

Roger Newman and E. Ramsey Unal

KEY ABBREVIATIONS	
Dichorionic	DC
Disseminated Intravascular Coagulation	DIC
Dizygotic	DZ
Estimated Fetal Weight	EFW
Fetal Fibronectin	FFN
Intrauterine Fetal Death	IUFD
Intrauterine Growth Restriction	IUGR
In Vitro Fertilization	IVF
Low Birthweight	LBW
Monochorionic	MC
Monozygotic	MZ
Multifetal Pregnancy Reduction	MPR
Necrotizing Enterocolitis	NEC
Neonatal Intensive Care Unit	NICU
Preterm Birth	PTB
Respiratory Distress Syndrome	RDS
Retinopathy of Prematurity	ROP
Selective Termination	ST
Transvaginal Cervical Length	TVCL
Twin–twin Transfusion Syndrome	TTTS
Twin Reversed Arterial Perfusion	TRAP
Very Low Birthweight	VLBW

The increase in multiple births during the past 30 years has been well documented, making multiple gestations one of the most common high-risk conditions encountered by obstetricians. The increase in multiples is due primarily to assisted reproduction technology but also in part to older maternal age at childbirth, which is a known risk factor for spontaneous dizygotic twinning. After years of rapidly increasing twin birth rates, the rates now seem to show signs of stabilizing. The twin birth rate rose 70% from 1980 to 2004. According to the most recent National Vital Statistics data, however, the twin rate remained stable between 2004 and 2006 at 32.1 per 1000. Likewise, rates of triplets and higher-order multiples increased by more than 400% during the 1980s and 1990s, reaching an all-time high in 1998 at a rate of 193.5 per 100,000. Since that peak, triplets and higher-order multiples have decreased by 20% to 30%, with the most recent available triplet rate at 143.4 per 100,000 and the quadruplet and higher-order birth rate at 9.89 per 100,000.[1] The apparent plateau of the twin birth rate and the decline of triplet and higher-order multiple births are likely due to refinements in assisted reproduction techniques and recommendations from the American Society for Reproductive Medicine to limit the number of embryos transferred during in vitro fertilization (IVF) procedures. Issues remain with the current use of ovulation-induction drugs.

ZYGOSITY AND CHORIONICITY

Twins can be either monozygotic (MZ) or dizygotic (DZ). Zygosity refers to the genetic makeup of the twin pregnancy, and chorionicity indicates the pregnancy's placental composition (Figure 30-1). **Chorionicity is determined by the mechanism of twinning and, in MZ twins, by the timing of embryo division. Early determination of chorionicity is vital because it is a major factor in determining obstetrical**

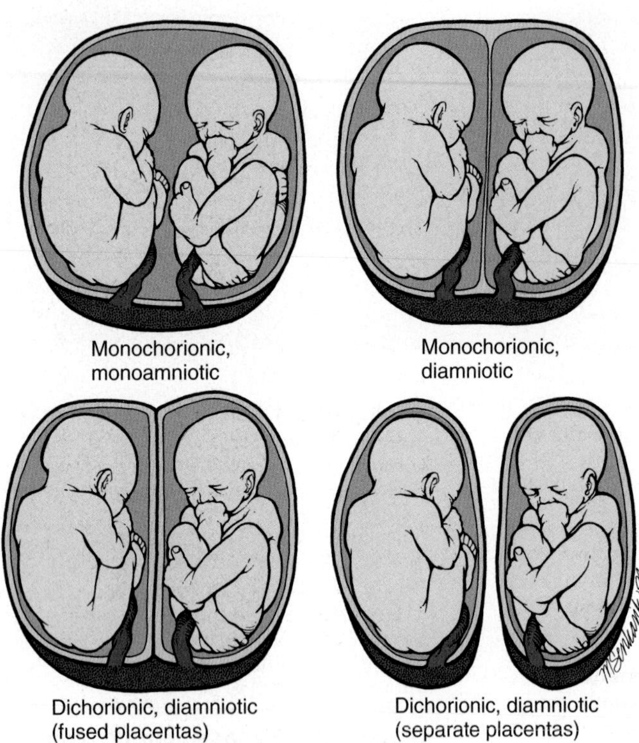

FIGURE 30-1. Placentation in twin pregnancies.

TABLE 30-1 DETERMINATION OF MONOZYGOTIC TWIN PLACENTATION

TIMING OF CLEAVAGE OF FERTILIZED OVUM	RESULTING PLACENTATION	PERCENTAGE OF MONOZYGOTIC TWINS
<72 hr	Diamniotic, dichorionic	25%-30%
Days 4-7	Diamniotic, monochorionic	70%-75%
Days 8-12	Monoamniotic, monochorionic	1%-2%
≥Day 13	Conjoined	Very rare

risks, management and outcomes. DZ twins, because they result from the fertilization of two different ova by two separate sperm, always develop a dichorionic, diamniotic placentation because each blastocyst generates its own placenta. An MZ twin pregnancy is created by the fertilization of one egg by one sperm and then subsequent spontaneous cleavage of the fertilized ovum. Thus, the type of placentation that develops is determined by the timing of this cleavage (Table 30-1).

MZ twins are at higher risk for adverse outcomes than are DZ twins. Not only do MZ twins have higher rates of anomalies than DZ twins, but they also deliver earlier, have a lower birthweight, and have higher rates of intrauterine and neonatal death. **However, several studies, including one by Carroll and colleagues using DNA analysis to confirm zygosity, have shown that monochorionicity, rather than monozygosity per se, is the determining factor.**[2] Since MZ dichorionic twins result from an earlier embryonic split, it is logical that they would have more complete separation, and thus fewer fetal anomalies and placental abnormalities, than twins in whom the embryonic split occurs later.

DISTRIBUTION AND CAUSES OF DIZYGOTIC VERSUS MONOZYGOTIC TWINNING

Among natural conceptions, DZ twins arise in about 1% to 1.5% of pregnancies and MZ twins occur in 1 in 250 pregnancies. Rates of spontaneous DZ twinning are greatly affected by maternal age, family history, and race. The risk for DZ twinning increases with maternal age, peaking at 37 years of age.[3] Maternal family history, particularly in first-degree relatives, also increases the chance of spontaneous DZ twinning; paternal family history contributes little or nothing to this risk. Finally, women of African descent have higher rates of DZ twinning than white women, who in turn have higher rates than women of Asian descent. For instance, in Japan, 1 in 250 newborns is a twin, whereas in Nigeria, 1 in 11 babies is a product of a twin gestation.[3]

The causes of DZ twinning are much better understood than the causes of MZ twinning. DZ twins result from multiple ovulation, which is associated with higher maternal follicle-stimulating hormone (FSH) levels. FSH levels, and thus rates of DZ twinning, vary with season, geography, maternal age, and body habitus. Increases in DZ twins have been reported in summer months, locations with more daylight hours, and taller, heavier, and older mothers.[3]

The causes of MZ twinning are less clear. There are no naturally occurring animal models for MZ twinning, with the exception of armadillos, which produce MZ quadruplets or octuplets. However, MZ twinning has been induced by delayed fertilization in rabbits and by iatrogenic hypoxia in mice.[3] It has been proposed that MZ twinning in humans is a teratogenic event. Theories for MZ twinning in humans include fertilization of an "old" ovum with a more fragile zona pellucida or inadequate cytoplasm and with damage to the inner cell mass leading to two separate points of regrowth and splitting of the fertilized ovum.[3] **MZ twinning rates are constant across all variables, with the exception of assisted reproduction.** IVF and ovulation induction have been shown to produce higher rates of MZ twins. Against a spontaneous rate of 0.4% in the general population, studies have reported that the rate of MZ twinning may be more than 10-fold higher in pregnancies conceived by assisted fertility. One theory to explain these increased rates of MZ twinning is that injury to the zona pellucida may be responsible for the increased tendency toward iatrogenic zygote splitting.

DIAGNOSIS OF MULTIPLE GESTATIONS

Prenatal ultrasound is invaluable in the early diagnosis of a multiple gestation. Before the advent of routine prenatal ultrasound, many twins were not diagnosed until late in gestation or at delivery. **Using transvaginal ultrasound, separate gestational sacs with individual yolk sacs can be identified as early as 5 weeks from the first day of the last menstrual period and embryos with cardiac activity can**

TABLE 30-2 DETERMINATION OF CHORIONICITY AND AMNIONICITY IN FIRST-TRIMESTER PREGNANCIES

PLACENTATION	NO. OF GESTATIONAL SACS	NO. OF YOLK SACS	NO. OF AMNIOTIC CAVITIES
Dichorionic, diamniotic	2	2	2 (thick dividing membrane)
Monochorionic, diamniotic	1	2	2 (thin dividing membrane)
Monochorionic, monoamniotic	1	1*	1

*Although this is nearly always true, there have been case reports of two yolk sacs in early pregnancy in twins later confirmed to be monoamniotic.

usually be seen by 6 weeks. Retromembranous collections of blood or fluid or a prominent fetal yolk sac should not be confused with a twin gestation. Another entity that could be confused with a multiple gestation would be a singleton pregnancy with a separate pseudosac in a bicornuate uterus (or other anomaly with a second uterine horn, such as a unicornuate uterus with a rudimentary horn or a uterine didelphys). The sonographer must be compulsive in examining the entire uterine cavity in order to avoid underdiagnosing or overdiagnosing a multiple gestation.

Determination of Chorionicity

Accurate determination of chorionicity and amnionicity early in pregnancy is vital to optimal obstetrical care. A recent editorial argued that "there is no diagnosis of twins" but rather any twin gestation must be further described as either monochorionic or dichorionic.[4] **Knowledge of chorionicity is essential in counseling patients on obstetrical and neonatal risks because chorionicity is a major determinant of pregnancy outcome.** Furthermore, in some cases, precise knowledge of chorionicity is paramount. For instance, when contemplating selective reduction of a multiple gestation, incorrectly assuming dichorionicity when the pregnancy is in fact monochorionic could have tragic consequences.

Determination of chorionicity is easiest and most reliable when assessed in the first trimester. Between 6 and 10 weeks, counting the number of gestational sacs and evaluating the thickness of the dividing membrane is the most reliable method of determining chorionicity (Table 30-2). Two separate gestational sacs, each containing a fetus, and a thick dividing membrane strongly suggest a dichorionic diamniotic pregnancy, whereas one gestational sac with a thin dividing membrane and two fetuses suggests a monochorionic diamniotic pregnancy (Figure 30-2). For monochorionic gestations, the dividing amniotic membrane may be very difficult to visualize in the first trimester. However, with rare exceptions, the number of amniotic sacs will be the same as the number of yolk sacs, which are relatively easy to count in early gestation.

After 9 weeks, the dividing membranes become progressively thinner, but in dichorionic pregnancies, they remain thicker and easy to identify. At 11 to 14 weeks' gestation, sonographic examination of the base of the intertwin membrane for the presence or absence of the lambda or twin peak sign provides reliable distinction between a fused dichorionic and a monochorionic pregnancy. The twin peak sign is a triangular projection of tissue extending beyond the chorionic surface of the placenta (Figure 30-3). This tissue is insinuated between the layers of the intertwin membrane, wider at the chorionic surface, and tapering to a point at some distance inward from that surface. This finding is produced by extension of chorionic villi into the potential interchorionic space of the twin membrane at the place where it encounters the chorion and placenta of the co-twin. This space exists only in dichorionic pregnancies. The twin peak sign cannot occur in monochorionic placentation because the single continuous chorion does not extend into the potential interamniotic space of the monochorionic, diamniotic twin membrane.

After the early second trimester, determination of chorionicity and amnionicity becomes less accurate, and different techniques are used (Figure 30-4). The sonographic prediction of chorionicity and amnionicity should be systematically approached by determining the number of placentas and the sex of each fetus, and then by assessing the membranes that divide the sacs. Scardo and associates[5] found that, using these criteria, dichorionicity could be determined with 97.3% sensitivity and 91.7% specificity and monochorionicity with 91.7% sensitivity and 97.3% specificity in twin gestations first scanned at 22.6 ± 6.9 weeks. In some pregnancies with monochorionic, diamniotic placentation, the dividing membranes may not be sonographically visualized because they are very thin. In other cases, they may not be seen because severe oligohydramnios causes them to be closely opposed to the fetus in that sac. This results in a "stuck twin" appearance, in which the trapped fetus remains firmly held against the uterine wall despite changes in maternal position. In many cases, a small portion of the dividing membrane can be seen extending from a fetal edge to the uterine wall (Figure 30-5). Diagnosis of this condition confirms the presence of a monochorionic, diamniotic gestation, which should be distinguished from a monoamniotic gestation, in which dividing membranes are absent. In the latter situation, free movement of both twins, and entanglement of their umbilical cords, can be demonstrated.

Determination of Zygosity

If a twin set is monochorionic, monozygosity can be inferred. If twins are different genders, then with very rare anecdotal exceptions, they can be assumed to be DZ. **It is estimated that based on these two findings, about 55% of all twins' zygosity can be determined by examination of the babies and placentas.** Conversely, 45% of all twins (same sex, dichorionic twins) would need further genetic testing to determine zygosity.

MATERNAL AND FETAL RISKS OF MULTIPLE GESTATION

Maternal Adaptation to Multifetal Gestation

The degree of maternal physiologic adaptation to pregnancy is exaggerated with multiple gestation.[6] Levels of maternal progesterone, estriol, and human placental

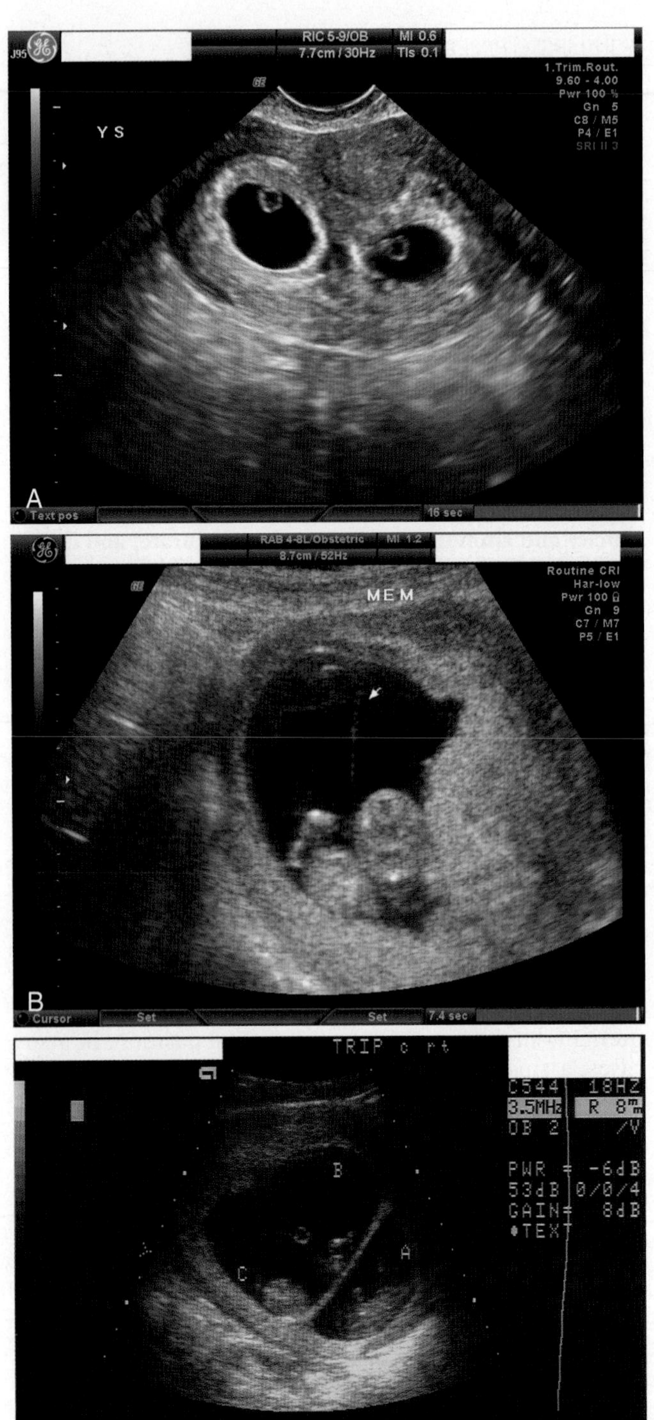

FIGURE 30-2. **A,** An early first-trimester dichorionic twin gestation. Note the clearly separate gestational sacs, each surrounded by a thick echogenic ring. **B,** A mid–first-trimester monochorionic, diamniotic twin pregnancy with a very thin, hairlike dividing membrane *(arrow)*. **C,** An early first-trimester image of a dichorionic, triamniotic triplet pregnancy. Note that monochorionic triplets B and C are separated by a very thin membrane, whereas triplet A, with its own placenta, is separated from B and C by a thick membrane.

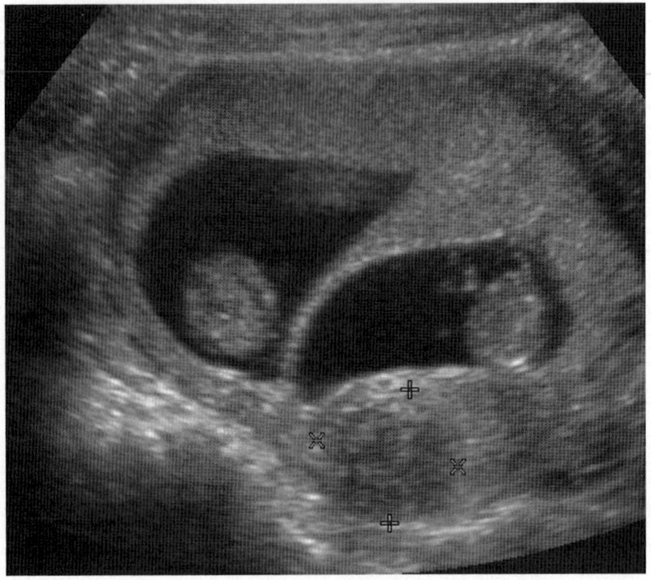

FIGURE 30-3. Twin peak sign in a dichorionic twin pregnancy with a fused anterior placenta.

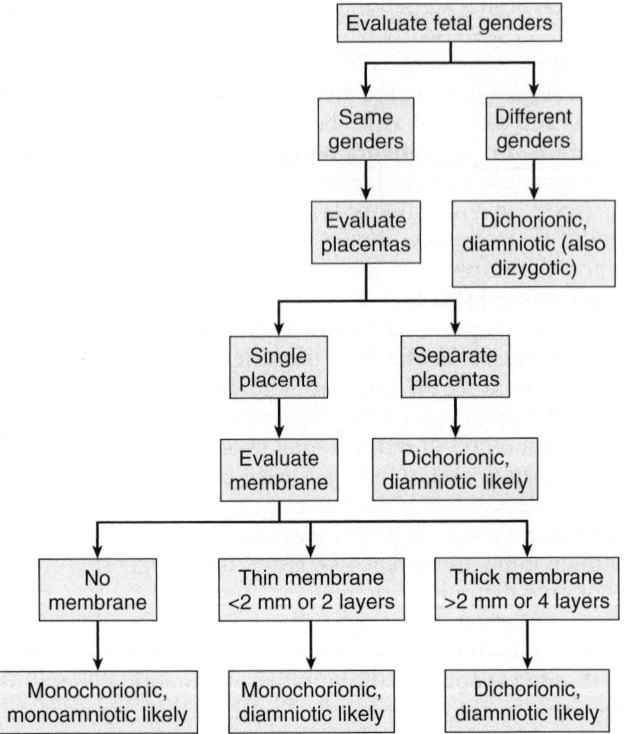

FIGURE 30-4. Algorithm for determination of chorionicity and amnionicity in the second and third trimesters.

lactogen are higher in multiple gestations than in singletons. This increase in human placental lactogen is thought to be the cause of the increased risk for gestational diabetes seen in multifetal pregnancies. Increased production of multiple placental proteins such as human chorionic gonadotropin may contribute to clinical conditions such as a greater risk for hyperemesis and complicates the interpretation of both first- and second-trimester maternal serum screening tests. Cardiovascular adaptations are also greater; both heart rate and stroke volume are increased compared with singleton gestations, resulting in increased cardiac output. In addition to these cardiac changes, plasma volume expansion and total body water are increased in twin gestations. Partially as a consequence of increased total body water, colloid osmotic pressure is reduced. Clinical effects of the decreased colloid osmotic pressure are increased dependent edema as well as a heightened sensitivity to pulmonary edema, a risk that must be considered when tocolysis of a multiple gestation is contemplated.

Studies using dye excretion have suggested that hepatic clearance capacity is reduced in pregnancy in general, and more so in twin gestation.[6] As described previously, serum protein concentrations are decreased during pregnancy. Although this is partially due to increased total body water, there is likely some degree of reduced hepatic contribution of serum proteins, again more exaggerated in multifetal gestation compared with singleton pregnancy. Most obvious to patients, marked uterine changes also occur. By 25 weeks' gestation, the average twin gestation uterine size is equal to a term singleton pregnancy. By term, the total uterine volume is often 10,000 mL, and the weight of the uterus and its contents can exceed 8 kg.

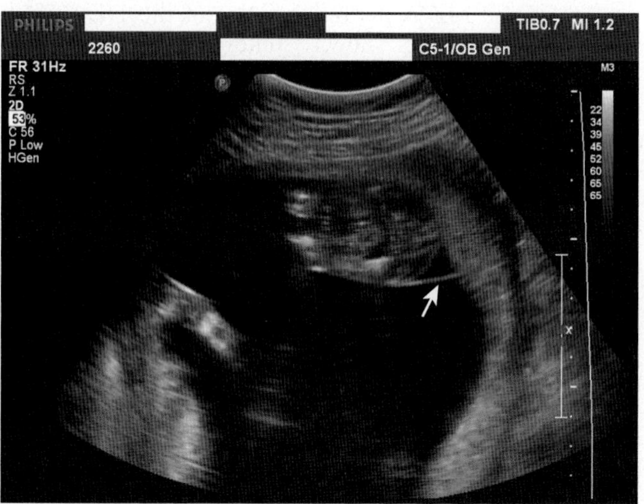

FIGURE 30-5. The donor twin "stuck" against the anterior uterine wall in a case of twin-twin transfusion syndrome. Note the small portion of membrane visible *(arrow)* extending from the edge of the fetus to the uterine wall.

Maternal Morbidity and Mortality

Rates of essentially every obstetrical complication, with the exception of macrosomia, are elevated with multiple gestations and in general rise proportionally to increasing plurality. Table 30-3 provides the relative risks for obstetrical complications in twin gestations compared with singletons.[7] In addition to the conditions listed in the table, multiples are associated with higher rates of gestational diabetes and rare but life-threatening conditions such as acute fatty liver and peripartum cardiomyopathy. **Additionally, women pregnant with multiples not only have higher risks for developing certain conditions but also are more likely to have more severe manifestations of those conditions.** For instance, Sibai and associates showed that not only are twin mothers more likely to develop preeclampsia (relative risk [RR], 2.62; 95% confidence interval [CI], 2.03 to 3.38), but also twin mothers with preeclampsia have higher rates of delivery before 37 weeks and before 35 weeks, as well as higher rates of placental abruption and small-for-gestational-age infants than singleton mothers with preeclampsia.[8] A large retrospective analysis of 24,781 singleton, 6859 twin, 2545 triplet, and 189 quadruplet pregnancies found an incidence of pregnancy-related hypertensive conditions of 6.5% in singletons, 12.7% in twins, and 20% in triplets and quadruplets. The risk for interventional delivery due to hypertensive complications also increased by plurality: about twofold higher in twins and threefold higher in triplets compared with singletons.[9] Atypical presentations of preeclampsia are also more common in multifetal gestations, especially higher-order multiples. One retrospective review of 21 triplet and 8 quadruplet pregnancies found that only half of the women who were delivered for preeclampsia had elevated blood pressures before delivery. Furthermore, proteinuria was present in only 3 of 16 women before delivery. Predominant presentations of preeclampsia in this series were laboratory abnormalities (chiefly elevated liver enzymes) and maternal symptoms.[10]

TABLE 30-3 MATERNAL COMPLICATIONS IN MULTIPLE GESTATIONS

	SINGLETON (*n* = 71,851) (%)	TWIN (*n* = 1694) (%)	RELATIVE RISK	95% CONFIDENCE INTERVAL
Hyperemesis	1.7	5.1	3.0	2.1-4.1
Threatened SAB	18.6	26.5	1.4	1.3-1.6
Anemia	16.2	27.5	1.7	1.5-1.9
Abruption	0.5	0.9	2.0	1.2-3.3
GHTN	17.8	23.8	1.3	1.2-1.5
Preeclampsia	3.4	12.5	3.7	3.3-4.3
Eclampsia	0.1	0.2	3.4	1.2-9.4
Antepartum thromboembolism	0.1	0.5	3.3	1.3-8.1
Manual placental extraction	2.5	6.7	2.7	2.2-3.2
Evacuation of retained products	0.6	2.0	3.1	2.0-4.8
Primary PPH (>1000 mL)	0.9	3.1	3.4	2.9-4.1
Secondary PPH	0.6	1.7	2.6	1.8-4.6
Postpartum thromboembolism	0.2	0.6	2.6	1.1-5.9

From Campbell DM, Templeton A: Maternal complications of twin pregnancy. Int J Gynecol Obstet 84:71, 2004.
GHTN, Gestational hypertension; *PPH*, postpartum hemorrhage; *SAB*, spontaneous abortion.

TABLE 30-4 BIRTH OUTCOMES FOR MULTIPLE GESTATIONS

	MEAN BIRTHWEIGHT (g)	GESTATIONAL AGE AT DELIVERY (wk)	DELIVERY <32 WEEKS (%)	LBW: <2500 g (%)	VLBW: <1500 g (%)
Singleton	3298	38.7	1.6	6.5	1.1
Twin	2323	35.2	12.1	57.2	10.2
Triplet	1655	32.0	36.3	95.4	34.8
Quad	1225	29.3	79.2	98	73.4

From Martin JA, Hamilton BE, Sutton PD, et al: Births: Final Data for 2006. National Vital Statistics Reports; Vol 57, No 7. Hyattsville, MD, National Center for Health Statistics, 2009.

One theory for the higher incidence of atypical preeclampsia in women with triplet and higher-order multiples is that the exaggerated hemodynamic changes found in higher-order multiples do not allow for the "typical" maternal manifestations of preeclampsia.

These increased maternal risks extend to life-threatening morbidity and even mortality. Multiple gestation has been found to be an independent risk factor for intensive care unit admission.[11] Finally, although fortunately still a very rare event, maternal death is also increased in multifetal gestations. A relative risk of 2.9 (95% CI, 1.4 to 6.1) for maternal death in women pregnant with multiples has been reported.[12]

Perinatal Morbidity and Mortality

Multifetal gestations carry significant perinatal risks. **Babies who are products of multiple gestations have higher rates of low birthweight, earlier gestational age at delivery, and higher rates of neonatal and infant death and cerebral palsy** (Table 30-4). One in eight twins and one in three triplets is born before 32 weeks' gestation, compared with only 2 in 100 singletons. Additionally, the risk for infant death is higher: 29.8 per 1000 for twins and 59.6 per 1000 for triplets, compared with 6 per 1000 for singletons.[1] Rates of cerebral palsy have been estimated as 4 to 8 times higher in twins than singletons and as much as 47 times higher in triplets.[13] Much of this increased risk is likely attributable to higher rates of preterm delivery and low birthweight in multiple gestations. Of note, although the overall rates of cerebral palsy are higher in twins than singletons, low-birthweight preterm twins do not have higher rates than like-weight, gestational age–matched singletons. Interestingly, however, most studies have demonstrated higher rates of cerebral palsy for twins born at term weighing more than 2500 g than for comparable singletons. This difference is mostly a reflection of the effect of monochorionicity on twin growth and development.

Fetal Anomalies

Fetuses in multiple gestations are known to be at increased risk for anatomic abnormalities, although the exact degree of risk is debated. The largest series available, an international study of more than 260,000 twins, found a relative risk for major anomalies of 1.25 (95% CI, 1.21 to 1.28). Anomalies were found in all organ systems.[14] This study, however, was not informed on zygosity or chorionicity, and most experts believe that much of the increased risk for structural anomalies in multiple gestation is associated with MZ twinning.

A 2009 population-based study from England found that rates of congenital anomalies were 1.7 times more frequent in twins compared with singletons (95% CI, 1.5 to 2.0) and that the relative risk for monochorionic twins was nearly twice that of dichorionic twins (RR, 1.8; 95% CI, 1.3 to 2.5).[15] A Taiwanese series of 844 twin sets compared with 4573 control singletons found a doubling of the relative risk of major congenital malformations in twins compared with singletons. When broken down by zygosity, the relative risks were 1.7 for DZ twins and 4.6 for MZ twins, with an anomaly prevalence of 0.6% for singletons, 1% for DZ twins, and 2.7% for MZ twins. Anomalies were concordant in 18% of the MZ twins but in none of the DZ twins.[16] Older studies have shown somewhat higher overall anomaly rates (both for singletons and twins) but found similar distributions. **Thus, the overall evidence supports an approximately twofold increased risk for congenital anomalies in twins versus singletons, with most of this risk occurring in MZ twins.**

There is a strong association between MZ twinning and midline defects. Nance[17] presents evidence to suggest that a group of birth defects involving midline structures, including symmelia, exstrophy of the cloaca, and midline neural tube defects, may be associated with the twinning process. Symmelia is a severe, rare defect that results from fusion of the preaxial halves of the developing hind limb buds, producing a single lower extremity with a knee that flexes in the opposite direction from normal. The incidence of this condition is 100 times higher in MZ births than in singletons. MZ twins have also been shown to have a higher frequency of neural tube defects than singletons, and they are usually discordant for the abnormality. Nance suggests that the MZ twinning process, with its attendant opportunities for asymmetry, cytoplasmic deficiency, and competition in utero, may favor the discordant expression of midline defects in these gestations.

ISSUES AND COMPLICATIONS UNIQUE TO MULTIPLE GESTATIONS

"Vanishing Twin"

The "vanishing twin" is a well-known obstetrical phenomenon. This term refers to the loss of one member of a twin (or other higher-order multiple) gestation early in pregnancy. This is typically either asymptomatic or associated with spotting or mild bleeding. Landy and colleagues reported on a series of 1000 first-trimester ultrasounds, with an incidence of twinning of just over 3%.[18] After confirming a twin gestation (two embryos with heartbeats), 21.2% ultimately delivered singletons. In general, if two gestational sacs are confirmed by the first-trimester ultrasound, the chance of delivering twins is 63% for women younger than 30 years and 52% for women 30 years or older. If two embryos with cardiac activity are seen in the first trimester, the chance of a twin birth rises to 90% for women younger than 30 years and 84% for women 30 years or older.[19] Other investigators have shown that, not unexpectedly, the earlier the initial ultrasound, the greater the chance of a vanishing twin phenomenon. Additionally, monochorionic twin gestations are at a higher risk for either a vanishing twin or a complete pregnancy loss than are dichorionic twins. Again, it is important for sonographers to identify the presence of embryonic structures before making the diagnosis of a vanishing twin.

"Appearing Twin"

Another interesting entity is that of the "appearing twin." **An appreciable percentage of cases of multiple gestations may be missed between 5 and 6 weeks' gestation.** Doubilet and Benson reported on their experiences with appearing twins in pregnancies initially diagnosed as singletons.[20] They found that 14% of pregnancies later diagnosed as multiple gestation had been initially undercounted. Monochorionic twin gestations were far more likely than dichorionic to have been undercounted (86% vs. 11%). **The authors noted that pregnancy outcomes were no different for initially undercounted pregnancies than for those pregnancies correctly diagnosed on their initial ultrasound.** The entity of an appearing twin underlines once again the importance of a thorough ultrasonographic survey of the entire uterine cavity before diagnosing any pregnancy.

First-Trimester Multifetal Pregnancy Reduction

The increasing use of ovulation induction and assisted reproduction has resulted in a growing number of multifetal pregnancies with three or more fetuses. **Because the risk for pregnancy loss, preterm delivery, and long-term morbidity for children who are products of multiple gestations is directly proportional to the number of fetuses being carried, first-trimester multifetal pregnancy reduction has been advocated as a method to reduce the risk for prematurity and associated morbidity and mortality.** Currently, the method of choice is injection of a small dose of potassium chloride into the thorax of one or more of the fetuses, either transabdominally or transvaginally, under real-time sonographic guidance. The latter approach is used less frequently because it is associated with a greater infection risk and a higher loss rate than the former. In monochorionic pregnancies, the use of these techniques is contraindicated because of the vascular communications within the placenta.

Multifetal pregnancy reduction (MPR) is an outpatient procedure. It is usually performed between 11 and 13 weeks, and chorionic villus sampling (CVS) can safely be performed on some or all of the fetuses before the procedure to confirm karyotype if desired. Ultrasound is used to map the location of each fetus, nuchal translucencies should be measured, and prophylactic antibiotics are often administered. Any fetus appearing to be anatomically abnormal or small for gestational age, or known to have a karyotypic abnormality, is included among those that are reduced. If no abnormalities can be detected, generally the fetus or fetuses that are technically most accessible are chosen for reduction. Whenever possible, the fetus whose sac overlies the cervical os is not electively reduced, in order to minimize the risk for premature rupture of the membranes. Follow-up ultrasound examinations should be performed to confirm the success of the procedure and to monitor the growth of the remaining fetuses.

Evans and colleagues[21] published a series of 3513 completed first-trimester MPR procedures from 11 centers in five countries. The overall loss rate was 9.6%, but each of the participating centers showed significant improvement in this parameter as the operators developed more experience over time. Additionally, loss rates increased steadily from 4.5% to 15.4% as the number of starting fetuses rose from three to six or more. The rate of loss for those who reduced to twins was 6%, compared with 18.4% for those who were left with triplets.

Stone and colleagues[22] reported the outcome of 1000 consecutive patients undergoing MPR at a single institution. Similar to the Evans study, these investigators also demonstrated a learning curve with fewer complications with increasing experience. The unintended pregnancy loss with the first 200 patients was 9.5% but fell to 5.4% after 1000 patients. An updated 2008 report[23] of the most recent 1000 multifetal reductions at the authors' institution found that the overall unintended pregnancy loss rate had dropped to 4.7%. This loss rate is unlikely to drop further because it approximates the baseline risk for pregnancy loss with twins in general. The rates of loss in the original report were 2.5% for those who reduced from twins to a singleton and 12.9% for those who presented with six or more fetuses, but the rate was stable at 4.7% to 5.4% for women who started with either three, four, or five fetuses. The rates of loss were 16.7%, 5.5%, and 3.5% for those who reduced to triplets, twins, and singletons, respectively. Significantly, the mean gestational ages for surviving fetuses were 35.3 weeks and 33.5 weeks for twins and triplets, respectively, which is what would be expected if these women had naturally conceived that number of fetuses.

Although perinatal morbidity and mortality are clearly improved when pregnancies with quadruplets or greater are reduced to smaller numbers, the medical advantages of reducing triplets to twins remain debatable. A 2006 meta-analysis attempted to answer this question.[24] The authors analyzed data from 893 pregnancies beginning as triplets, of which 411 were expectantly managed and 482 underwent MPR to twins. The rate of pregnancy loss before 24 weeks was higher in the MPR group (8.1% vs. 4.4%; $P = .036$). However, this risk was offset by a lower risk for delivery between 24 and 32 weeks in the MPR group (10.4% vs. 26.7%; $P < .0001$). The authors calculated that 7 reductions are needed to prevent one delivery before 32 weeks, and the number of reductions that would cause one loss before 24 weeks was 26. Thus, reducing triplets to twins may be associated with overall improvements in outcome.

Because the majority of losses occur several weeks after the procedure, the period from 18 to 24 weeks should be one of heightened surveillance. It is also recommended that these patients not undergo second-trimester aneuploidy serum screening because maternal serum α-fetoprotein (AFP) levels are often significantly elevated as a result of the retained dead fetus. Because the incidence of intrauterine growth restriction (IUGR) may be increased in the surviving fetuses after MPR procedures, serial sonographic growth assessment has been suggested. Additionally, women who have undergone MPR can have significant grief reactions, and their emotional status should be monitored carefully.

Discordance for Anomalies

When an anomaly is detected in a twin gestation, even in an MZ set, the co-twin is usually normal. The diagnosis of discordance for a major anatomic abnormality places the parents in an extremely difficult position. Management choices include the following:

1. Expectant management
2. Termination of the entire pregnancy
3. Selective termination of the anomalous fetus

Several issues should be considered when counseling patients about the management of a multiple pregnancy complicated by discordant anomalies. These include (1) severity of the anomaly, (2) chorionicity, (3) effect of the anomalous fetus on the remaining fetus or fetuses, and (4) the parents' ethical beliefs. It is important to counsel patients if conservative management could result in adverse outcomes for the healthy twin. Although not all study results are consistent, most show that in a twin pregnancy discordant for major fetal anomalies, the normal fetus is at increased risk for preterm delivery and low birthweight. Some studies have also shown a higher risk for mortality in normal co-twins of an anomalous fetus. The most recent paper, a population-based retrospective study of more than 3000 normal co-twins of fetuses with nonchromosomal structural anomalies compared with more than 12,000 control twins unaffected by structural anomalies, showed higher rates of preterm birth (both <37 and <32 weeks), low birthweight, and perinatal mortality in normal co-twins of an affected pregnancy.[25] Reasons for higher rates of preterm birth are unclear, but polyhydramnios associated with anomalies and maternal psychosocial stress from the diagnosis of a fetal anomaly are possible explanations.

Selective Termination of an Anomalous Fetus

Although multiple techniques have been used to effect selective termination (ST) of a single fetus in a multiple gestation, the most common approach in dichorionic gestations is intracardiac injection of potassium chloride.

Evans and collegues[26] reported the outcomes of 402 ST procedures from eight centers in four countries using ultrasound-guided intracardiac injection of potassium chloride. They reported successful delivery of one or more viable infants in greater than 90% of cases. There were no cases of disseminated intravascular coagulation (DIC) or serious maternal complication. Similarly, Eddleman and associates[27] reported favorable outcomes in 200 ST cases performed at one institution on 164 twins, 32 triplets, and 4 quadruplets. The median gestational age at the time of the procedure was 19 weeks, 6 days, with a range of 12 weeks to 23 weeks, 6 days. The indications included chromosomal abnormalities, structural anomalies, mendelian disorders, placental insufficiency, and cervical incompetence. The unintended pregnancy loss rate was 4%, but the losses were fivefold higher in triplets than in twins. The average gestational age at delivery was 37 weeks, 1 day, and 84% delivered after 32 weeks' gestation. Only 3.7% delivered at less than 28 weeks' gestation.

In monochorionic twins, ST is far more challenging. Ablation of the umbilical cord of the anomalous fetus is needed to avoid back-bleeding through communicating vessels, which may precipitate death or neurologic injury in the remaining normal co-twin. Furthermore, in this situation, a lethal agent injected into the anomalous twin could enter the circulation of its normal sibling. Most reported attempts at ST in monochorionic pregnancies without occlusion of all vessels in the abnormal twin's cord have resulted in the death of the second twin within a short time. The indications and technique for cord occlusion are reviewed later.

Immediate complications associated with ST procedures include selection of the wrong fetus, technical inability to accomplish the procedure, premature rupture of membranes, and infection with loss of the entire pregnancy. When the indication for ST is an abnormal karyotype diagnosed by amniocentesis or CVS, a sonographically identifiable marker may or may not be present. If the gender of the twins is different, or the affected fetus has a gross morphologic anomaly, the abnormal twin can be easily identified by sonography. However, in the absence of such visible signs, one must rely on information provided from the original diagnostic procedure, which frequently has been performed elsewhere and several days or weeks before the patient presents for ST. If accurate localizing information is lacking, fetal blood sampling with rapid karyotype determination should be performed to identify the abnormal fetus before ST is attempted. Furthermore, in all cases, a sample of aspirated fetal blood or amniotic fluid should be obtained from the terminated twin at the time of the procedure to confirm that the correct fetus has been terminated. Intracardiac potassium chloride injection without concomitant cord occlusion is contraindicated if dichorionicity cannot be confirmed.

Cord Occlusion for Selective Termination in Monochorionic Twins

Selective termination by cord occlusion can be considered in several circumstances involving monochorionic multiple gestations. **These include:**

1. **Severely discordant anomalies**
2. **Severely discordant growth with high risk for intrauterine fetal death (IUFD) at a previable or periviable gestational age**
3. **Twin reversed arterial perfusion (TRAP) sequence**
4. **Severe twin–twin transfusion syndrome (TTTS) with associated discordant anomaly or in cases in which laser ablation was precluded by position of the fetus and placenta**

Each of the above indications is discussed in more detail in corresponding sections of this chapter.

Bipolar coagulation is probably the most commonly used technique, although radiofrequency ablation, laser coagulation, and ligation of the cord have also been successful. The site for port insertion is chosen according to the position of the placenta, the amniotic sac of the target fetus, and its umbilical cord. Preferentially, the other sac is avoided. Sometimes amnioinfusion is necessary to expand the target sac. Bipolar coagulation can be accomplished with either 3-mm or 2.4-mm forceps, according to the cord diameter. Under ultrasound guidance, a portion of the umbilical cord is grasped while avoiding direct contact with the placenta, fetus, or membranes. Usually coagulation is effective at 25 watts, as demonstrated by the appearance of turbulence and steam bubbles. Limiting energy avoids tissue carbonization and cord perforation. Doppler studies can confirm arrest of flow, but many operators nonetheless coagulate three sections. In monoamniotic twins, the umbilical cord is often transected to avoid cord entanglement.

Pregnancy outcomes for the surviving co-twin are relatively favorable after selective cord occlusion. Rossi and D'Addario recently published a review of the literature regarding umbilical cord occlusion in complicated monochorionic twin pregnancies.[28] They evaluated 12 studies totaling 345 cases of cord occlusion at median gestational ages between 18 and 24 weeks. PPROM complicated 22% of pregnancies (59% of which occurred within 4 weeks), and co-twin fetal demise was a complication in 15% of cases (79% within 2 weeks of surgery). The overall survival rate for the remaining twin was 79% and was higher for cases after 18 weeks (89%) than for those undergoing the procedure earlier than 18 weeks (69%), regardless of the indication. Survival rates were 86% after radiofrequency ablation, 82% after bipolar cord coagulation, 72% after laser, and 70% after cord ligation. Long-term follow-up was not available for most studies, but in one series, the incidence of developmental delay was 8% in 67 infants older than 1 year who underwent evaluation by a pediatrician.[29]

Intrauterine Fetal Death of One Twin

IUFD of one twin occurs most commonly during the first trimester. This phenomenon is known as a vanishing twin and was discussed earlier in this chapter. Although it may be associated with vaginal spotting, the loss of one conceptus in the first trimester is often not clinically recognized, and the prognosis for the surviving twin is generally excellent. Single IUFD of one fetus in a multiple gestation in the second or third trimesters is much less common, complicating about 0.5% to 6.8% of twin pregnancies, but it can have more severe sequelae for the surviving fetus.[30] Monochorionic twins are at increased risk for a single fetal death, as are twins with a structural anomaly. In triplet pregnancies, studies have reported single IUFD rates between 4.3% and 17%.[30] In higher-order multiples, demise of a single fetus may be even more common.

The etiology of IUFD in a multiple pregnancy may be similar to that for singletons or be unique to the twinning process. Death in utero may be caused by genetic and anatomic anomalies, abruption, placental insufficiency, cord abnormalities such as a velamentous insertion, infection, and maternal diseases, including diabetes and hypertension. In diamniotic monochorionic pregnancies, IUFD may result from complications of TTTS. In addition, monoamniotic twins are at increased risk for cord entanglement and subsequent IUFD. Just as in singletons, however, the etiology of many IUFDs remains elusive.

Single IUFD in a multiple gestation can adversely affect the surviving fetus or fetuses in two ways: (1) risk for multicystic encephalomalacia and multiorgan damage in monochorionic pregnancies, and (2) preterm labor and delivery in both dichorionic and monochorionic twins.

Multicystic encephalomalacia results in cystic lesions within the cerebral white matter distributed in areas supplied by the anterior and middle cerebral arteries and is associated with profound neurologic handicap (Figure 30-6). The risk for this following single IUFD in a monochorionic pregnancy may be greater than 20% for the surviving co-twin.[31]

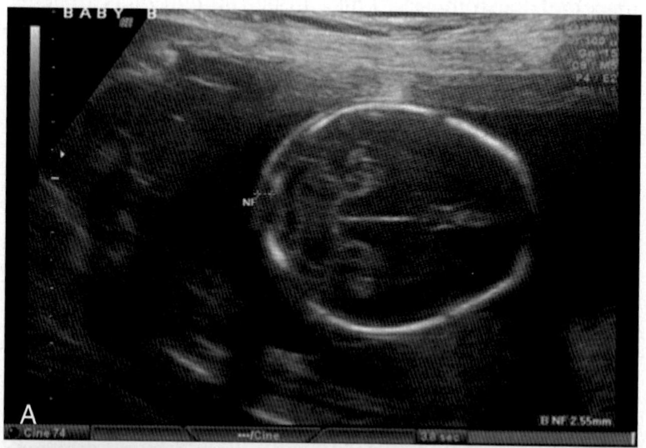

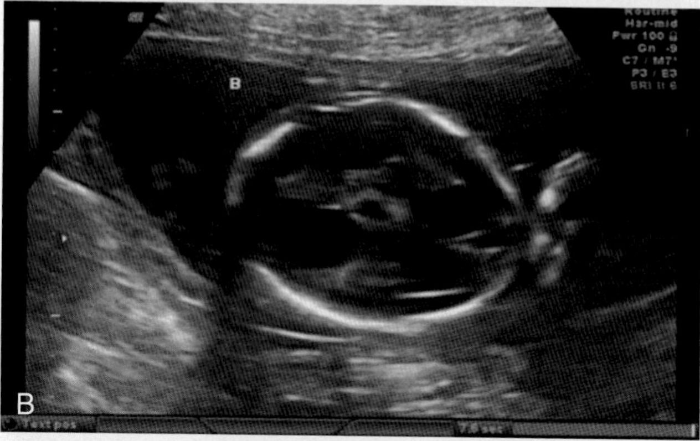

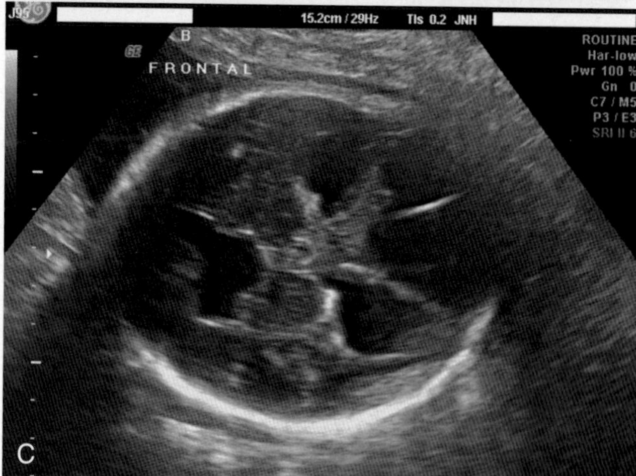

FIGURE 30-6. Ultrasound of the fetal brain of a monochorionic twin before **(A)** and after **(B, C)** intrauterine fetal death of the co-twin at 20 weeks' gestation. Note the normal brain anatomy in **A**, the dilation and cystic changes shortly after the co-twin's demise in **B**, and finally the residual irregular hydrocephalus and parenchymal loss 12 weeks later in **C**.

Two theories exist to explain this neurologic injury in the surviving co-twin in a monochorionic pregnancy. The first theory is that the deceased fetus produces thromboplastic substances, which traverse the vascular communications between the twins and cause infarcts and a DIC-like picture. The second and more widely accepted hypothesis is that significant hypotension at the time of demise of the co-twin causes neurologic injury in the surviving fetus. After death of the first twin, the resulting low pressure in that twin's circuit causes blood from the survivor to back-bleed rapidly into the demised twin through placental anastomoses. This can be thought of as an acute form of TTTS. If the resulting hypotension is severe, the surviving twin is at risk for ischemic damage to vital organs. Because the injury is coincident with the IUFD, rapid delivery of the co-twin following single IUFD in a monochorionic pregnancy will not improve the outcome.

It is unclear how early in gestation the death of one fetus in a monochorionic pregnancy can cause adverse sequelae for the surviving co-twin. Until relatively recently, it was thought that intrauterine demise in a monochorionic twin gestation could not cause neurologic injury to a co-twin until at least the mid-second trimester. However, in 2003 Weiss and coworkers reported a case of injury to a fetus after IUFD of the co-twin at about 13 weeks. Multicystic encephalomalacia was diagnosed by ultrasound and magnetic resonance imaging (MRI) in the co-twin at about 20 weeks.[32] The patient was counseled regarding the poor prognosis and opted for termination. Multicystic encephalomalacia was confirmed pathologically, although the exact timing could not be determined.

In addition, the IUFD of one twin can result in preterm delivery in both monochorionic and dichorionic pregnancies. Carlson and Towers[33] reported that 76% of 17 twin pregnancies complicated by IUFD of one fetus were delivered before 36 weeks and 41% were delivered at less than 32 weeks. The most common reason for early delivery was spontaneous labor, followed by abnormal fetal testing. The average interval from diagnosis to delivery was 16 days. Another series of 32 twin pregnancies complicated by single IUFD after 20 weeks followed by expectant management found strikingly similar numbers; the rate of delivery before 37 weeks was 81.3%, and delivery before 32 weeks occurred in 41.6% of the patients.[34] The median interval between diagnosis and delivery was 11 days. Of note, mothers with a single IUFD do not appear to be at increased risk for infection due to a retained twin demise. Cesarean delivery rates appear to be increased in these patients, often because of non-reassuring fetal status of the living twin. Dystocia caused by the dead fetus may also occasionally occur.

The determination of chorionicity is important for the counseling and management of patients with a single IUFD. Optimally, this has been established early in pregnancy. If, however, it has not been done before the IUFD, an attempt should be made to determine the chorionicity by ultrasound examination when the demise is discovered. Sonographic evaluation may not establish chorionicity with absolute certainty in some of these cases, and when the diagnosis is in doubt, DNA studies of amniocytes may be considered.

The optimal treatment for IUFD in multiples is not well established owing to the paucity of reported cases. To date, recommendations have been based on case reports, case series, and expert opinion. Referral to a tertiary care perinatal unit is advised when one fetus in a multifetal gestation has died in utero. In some of these cases, labor will already have started, and in others, coexisting maternal illness or placental abruption may make it necessary to expeditiously deliver the surviving fetus or fetuses. Clinical management depends on the gestational age, fetal lung maturity, or detection of in utero compromise of the surviving fetus or fetuses. The goal is to optimize outcome for the survivor while avoiding unnecessary or extreme prematurity and its potential adverse sequelae. It should be emphasized that close surveillance, even with reassuring antenatal testing, after the diagnosis of single IUFD in a monochorionic twin gestation cannot guarantee a good outcome for the surviving fetus.

Patients with monochorionic placentation should be counseled about the risk for multicystic encephalomalacia if an IUFD of one twin occurs after viability has been reached. It is difficult to predict which surviving monochorionic twins will develop cerebral injury. The nonstress test and biophysical profile give insight into the fetus' physiologic status but may not reflect subtle central nervous system changes. Ultrasound examination of the fetal brain may be suggestive of multicystic encephalomalacia but cannot definitively rule it out. Antenatal MRI of the fetal brain is investigational at this time but appears to be useful in detecting multicystic encephalomalacia in utero. As a consequence, we currently offer fetal MRI to all patients with monochorionic placentas approximately 2 to 3 weeks after the demise of one fetus has been detected. Although it is uncertain if normal MRI definitively rules out brain abnormalities, it is a reassuring sign. A single course of antenatal corticosteroids is recommended if premature delivery is anticipated and the gestational age is between 24 and 34 completed weeks. Surviving offspring are monitored with weekly biophysical profiles and nonstress tests.

The 2011 NICHD and SMFM workshop on timing of indicated late-preterm and early-term birth addressed the issue of single IUFD in a twin pregnancy. If the IUFD occurs at 34 weeks or beyond, delivery can be considered.[34a] Vaginal delivery is not contraindicated, and cesarean delivery is reserved for routine obstetric indications. At delivery, umbilical cord gas measurements should be performed. Autopsy should be offered for the stillborn fetus but may not be helpful if the demise has occurred several weeks earlier. Pathologic examination of the placenta is recommended. In addition, the pregnancy history should be communicated to the pediatricians caring for the neonate.

If IUFD occurs prior to 34 weeks, timing of delivery should be individualized based on other fetal or maternal issues.[34a] If, for instance, IUFD occurs at 18 weeks, delivery at term is likely the best option in the absence of any other complications, whereas a 33-week IUFD may warrant delivery between 34 and 37 weeks. Fetal surveillance should be considered once viability has been achieved. Monochorionic pregnancies complicated by IUFD before viability are more challenging. It is recommended that these patients be counseled regarding the risk of multiorgan injury, including multicystic encephalomalacia. Ultrasound imaging and fetal MRI can be helpful in making the diagnosis. Some patients may opt to terminate the entire pregnancy, whereas others will choose expectant management. Once the surviving co-twin reaches viability, these women should be managed according to the recommendations described earlier.

Besides fetal risks, there may be maternal risks associated with IUFD in a multiple pregnancy. For example, there is a theoretical possibility of maternal consumptive coagulopathy in twin pregnancies complicated by a single IUFD. It was originally estimated that there was a 25% incidence of maternal DIC when a dead fetus was retained in a multiple gestation. However, only a few isolated cases of laboratory changes consistent with a subclinical coagulopathy have been reported under these circumstances, and this 25% incidence is certainly an overestimation.[30] It is also reassuring to note that no cases of clinically significant coagulopathy have been reported in the extensive literature on ST and MPR. When IUFD occurs in a multiple pregnancy, we recommend baseline maternal hematologic studies including a prothrombin time, partial thromboplastin time, fibrinogen level, and platelet count. If these values are within normal limits, many experts do not perform serial laboratory surveillance, given the very low risk for coagulopathy.

The occurrence of IUFD causes feelings of loss, sadness, anxiety, and guilt. In women with twins and an IUFD of one of the fetuses, bereavement may be underestimated by physicians because there is a shift in focus to the living offspring. As a result, we suggest that patients with a multiple pregnancy complicated by IUFD of one fetus be offered psychological or bereavement counseling, or both.

Twin–Twin Transfusion Syndrome

Etiology

TTTS is exclusively a complication of diamniotic monochorionic pregnancies. **It occurs in about 15% of monochorionic gestations and is thus the most common severe complication specific to this type of twinning.** TTTS is characterized by an imbalance of fetal blood flow through communicating vessels across a shared placenta, leading to underperfusion of the donor twin and overperfusion of the recipient (Figure 30-7). The donor twin develops IUGR and oligohydramnios, whereas the recipient experiences volume overload with polyhydramnios and potentially cardiac failure and hydrops. On echocardiography, the recipient demonstrates decreased ventricular function, tricuspid regurgitation, and cardiomegaly.[35] These cardiac abnormalities often progress during pregnancy and persist into the neonatal period. In response to the increased blood volume, the recipient also becomes hypertensive and produces increasing amounts of atrial and brain natriuretic peptides. Resulting polyhydramnios leads to uterine overdistention and increased uterine pressure, both of which may contribute to an increased risk for preterm labor and preterm premature rupture of membranes.

The syndrome can present at any gestational age. However, earlier onset is associated with a much poorer prognosis. The transfer of blood can occur in small increments chronically over the course of the pregnancy, or it can be acute. If untreated, the reported mortality rates range from 80% to 100% (Figure 30-8). Furthermore, if one fetus dies in utero, the surviving twin is at risk for death or multiorgan damage from acute exsanguination due to back-bleeding into the demised co-twin. This organ damage frequently includes severe neurologic compromise. Even if both twins survive, the pathophysiology of TTTS can still result in adverse neurologic sequelae in one or both twins.

Although all monochorionic twins share vascular anastomoses and thus exist in a state of constant intertwin transfusion, as noted earlier, only a minority develop TTTS. The following mechanism has been proposed to explain this observation. In monochorionic placentas, there can be three types of vascular communications: arteriovenous (AV), arterioarterial (AA), and venovenous (VV). AA and VV anastomoses are typically superficial, bidirectional anastomoses on the surface of the chorionic plate. AV anastomoses, usually referred to as deep anastomoses, involve a shared cotyledon, receiving arterial supply from one twin and draining on the venous side to the other twin. All these anastomoses are identifiable at the chorionic surface, a feature that allows laser ablation of these anastomoses as a treatment of TTTS. Superficial anastomoses, especially those that are AA, are crucial for maintaining bidirectional flow. **According to this hypothesis, the absence of adequate superficial AA and VV anastomoses, which help maintain balanced blood flow, is the mechanism underlying TTTS.**

Diagnosis and Staging

The diagnosis of TTTS is made antenatally by ultrasound. Many experts recommend ultrasound examinations every 2 weeks beginning at 16 weeks' gestation in monochorionic twins in order to allow early detection of TTTS. The four requirements, none of which is pathognomonic, include (1) the presence of a single placenta, (2) same-gender fetuses, (3) significant weight discordance, and (4) significant amniotic fluid discordance, often with a "stuck twin." The most important criterion in diagnosing TTTS is disparity in the amniotic fluid volume. The maximal vertical pocket should be less than 2 cm for the donor twin and greater than 8 cm for the recipient twin. The differential diagnosis of a stuck twin includes selective uteroplacental insufficiency, structural or chromosomal abnormality (i.e., renal agenesis), abnormal placental cord insertion, intrauterine infection, and rupture of the amniotic membranes for one twin.

A staging system for TTTS was developed in 1999 by Quintero and colleagues to categorize disease severity and to standardize comparison of different treatment results.[36] The Quintero staging system is depicted in Table 30-5.

Although Quintero staging is widely used and has proved enormously useful in our evolving understanding of TTTS, many experts have noted its limitations. Stage does not always progress; nor do patients, when they do worsen, always progress sequentially through the stages. For instance, a pregnancy can become stage 5 (fetal death) without progressing through stage 4 (hydrops). Several investigators have commented on the relatively frequent

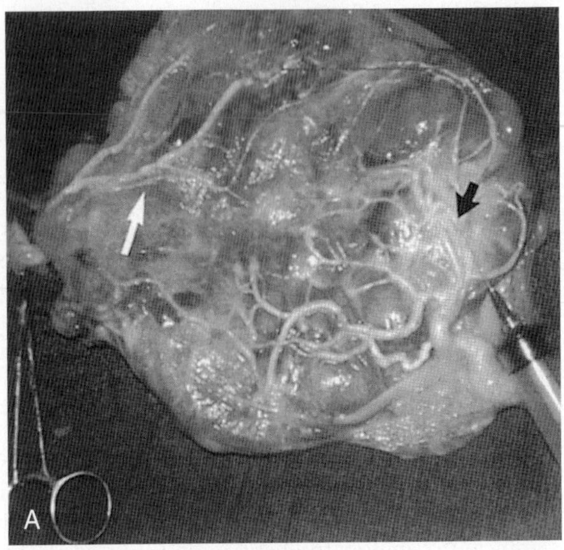

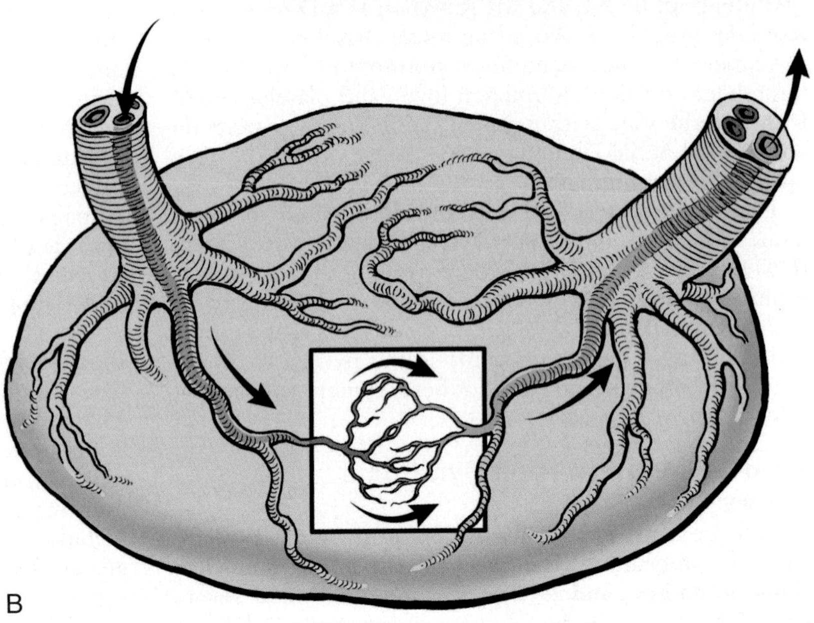

FIGURE 30-7. **A,** The placenta of a pregnancy complicated by twin-twin transfusion syndrome. Milk has been injected into an artery on the donor side of the placenta *(black arrow)*. It can be seen returning through the venous circulation on that side but is also evident in the venous circulation of the recipient *(white arrow)*. **B,** The arteriovenous shunt shown in **A.**

TABLE 30-5 QUINTERO STAGING FOR TWIN-TWIN TRANSFUSION SYNDROME

Stage I	Oligohydramnios, polyhydramnios sequence. Donor twin bladder visible.
Stage II	Oligohydramnios, polyhydramnios sequence. Donor twin bladder not visible. Doppler scan normal.
Stage III	Oligohydramnios, polyhydramnios sequence. Donor twin bladder not visible, and Doppler scans abnormal (absent or reversed end-diastolic velocity in the umbilical artery, reversed flow in the ductus venosus, or pulsatile flow in the umbilical vein).
Stage IV	One or both fetuses have hydrops.
Stage V	One or both fetuses have died.

occurrence of TTTS fetuses with Doppler abnormalities but a still visible fetal bladder in the donor. This has been referred to as an atypical stage III. Taylor and associates conducted a prospective observational study to validate the Quintero staging system's ability to predict perinatal outcomes. The study included 52 consecutive cases of TTTS that were either managed expectantly or treated with methods other than laser ablation. They found that only 45% of pregnancies progressed to a more advanced Quintero stage, and stage at presentation did not have a significant influence on survival. However, a progressive worsening of Quintero stage did predict worse outcomes. The authors concluded that Quintero staging does have a role in charting disease progress, but the stage at presentation does not accurately predict ultimate outcome.[37]

Several modifications of Quintero staging have been proposed, incorporating the differences in cardiovascular pathophysiology between donors and recipients, which is not accounted for in the Quintero staging system. None of these proposed staging alternatives, however, has been validated in prospective studies. The Cincinnati Modification categorizes all pregnancies in which the recipient exhibits cardiomyopathy (as assessed by AV valvular incompetence, ventricular wall thickness, and

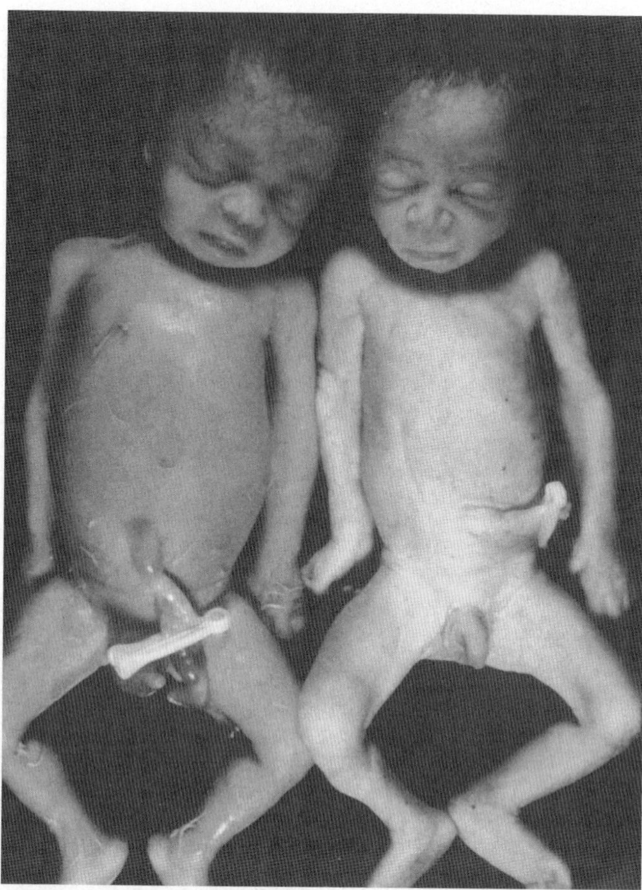

FIGURE 30-8. Stillborn male twins at 31 weeks' gestation, secondary to twin-twin transfusion syndrome. The plethoric twin on the left weighed 1670 g, and the anemic growth-restricted twin on the right weighed 1300 g.

ventricular function) as stage III. Furthermore, this modification stratifies stage III into those with abnormal Doppler scans, those with mild to moderate cardiomyopathy, and finally those with moderate to severe cardiomyopathy.[38] A 2009 meta-analysis designed to determine the efficacy of Quintero staging in patients treated with laser ablation did not find a statistically significant difference in survival by initial Quintero stage, but there was a consistent, although nonsignificant, trend toward lower survival as the stage increased. The authors proposed a new "double" staging system, one for donors and one for recipients, focused on the different pathophysiology of TTTS in donors and recipients.[39] Other parameters that have received attention as potential criteria in predicting severity and prognosis in TTTS are first-trimester discrepancy in twin nuchal translucencies (thicker in the future recipient), intertwin hemoglobin discordance (as determined by middle cerebral artery Doppler scans), amniotic fluid markers of renal and cardiac function, and presence or absence of AA anastomoses.[40]

Management

Expectant management is generally not recommended in TTTS because of the poor perinatal outcomes associated with the disorder. **However, management depends on the gestational age at diagnosis and, despite the previously mentioned limitations, on the severity of the clinical findings.** When TTTS is diagnosed after 26 to 28 weeks, conservative management may be the appropriate decision. This would include serial fetal assessment and control of polyhydramnios as needed. On the other hand, when the diagnosis is made in the early to mid-second trimester, aggressive management is generally advised. However, in patients with apparent mild stage I disease, a 1- to 2-week trial of conservative management may be warranted, mainly to confirm the correct diagnosis and assess for progression. Although medical management with digoxin and indomethacin has been attempted, there is limited evidence for success, and current treatment for severe TTTS requires physical intervention. There are three main management options: (1) serial amnioreduction, (2) amniotic septostomy, and (3) laser ablation of the anastomoses. All three options are discussed separately next.

Serial Amnioreduction

In serial reduction amniocentesis, an 18-gauge spinal needle is placed into the polyhydramniotic sac under ultrasound guidance. Amniotic fluid is withdrawn until the fluid volume returns to normal (i.e., deepest vertical pocket <8 cm). Because of the large amount of fluid to be removed, attaching the needle to a closed-system vacuum container is more practical than withdrawing fluid manually. Amnioreduction is repeated as often as necessary to maintain a near-normal amniotic fluid volume. The mechanism by which this procedure restores the amniotic fluid balance is unknown. Removing excessive fluid from the sac with polyhydramnios may result in decreased pressure on the sac with oligohydramnios. This, in turn, may result in increased placental perfusion to the stuck twin, especially through thin-walled superficial venous anastomoses with secondary improvement in its amniotic fluid volume. Additionally, normalizing the amniotic fluid may help prolong pregnancy by relieving uterine overdistention and pressure on the cervix.

Although there are no prospective studies comparing serial amnioreduction to conservative management, based on observational data amnioreduction does appear to offer a twofold to threefold increase in overall survival compared with no intervention. The exception may be late-onset (third-trimester) stage I TTTS that remains stable over a 1- to 2-week observation period. A large retrospective study using the International Amnioreduction Registry to analyze 223 sets of twins with TTTS diagnosed before 28 weeks' gestation and treated with serial amnioreduction found a live birth rate of 78%. Sixty percent of the original 446 babies were alive 4 weeks after birth. IUFD of at least one twin occurred in 31% of the pregnancies, and in 14% of cases, IUFD of both babies occurred. Of those babies alive 4 weeks after birth, 24% of the recipients and 25% of the donors had abnormal findings on cranial imaging. Poor prognostic factors for survival were earlier gestational age at diagnosis, presence of absent end-diastolic flow in the umbilical arteries, hydrops, low birthweight, and earlier gestational age at delivery. Complications within 48 hours (spontaneous rupture of the membranes, spontaneous delivery, fetal distress, fetal death, and placental abruption) occurred in 15% of patients.[41]

Septostomy

Amniotic septostomy is another management option. In this procedure, a 20-gauge spinal needle is inserted through the dividing membrane under ultrasound guidance. Amnioreduction of the polyhydramniotic sac is generally performed concomitantly. The amniotic fluid then sometimes equilibrates across the disrupted membrane. Similar to serial amnioreduction, the mechanism of action of this technique is unclear. It is possible that the defect in the membranes and reaccumulation of fluid in the donor sac allow the donor to swallow a sufficient volume of fluid to augment its circulating blood volume, secondarily increasing its urine output. The only randomized trial of amnioreduction versus septostomy for the treatment of TTTS was terminated early after enrollment of 73 women because the rate of survival of at least one infant was similar in both groups (78% vs. 80%; $P = .82$). The major advantage seen with septostomy was that women randomized to the septostomy group were more likely to require only a single procedure for treatment (64% vs. 46%; $P = .04$).[42] Because septostomy could functionally create an iatrogenic monoamniotic pregnancy with its own inherent complications and risks, the procedure has been criticized. Likewise, comparing amnioreduction to septostomy is challenging because both procedures use amnioreduction, and, alternatively, serial amnioreduction can be complicated by inadvertent septostomy.

Laser Therapy

Laser ablation of placental anastomoses is a third invasive treatment option that has been used to treat TTTS (Figure 30-9). In the United States, the use of laser therapy to treat TTTS is restricted to gestations earlier than 26 weeks. **Unlike both serial amnioreduction and septostomy, which would be considered palliative procedures, laser ablation is the only therapeutic option that aims to correct the underlying pathophysiologic aberration causing TTTS. Additionally, because laser ablation interrupts the vascular anastomoses between the fetuses, it has the advantage of being protective of the surviving twin should one twin succumb in utero.** In this procedure, first described by De Lia, the strategy is to ablate all anastomosing vessels that might connect the fetuses using either Nd:YAG, KTP, or diode laser and 400- to 600-mm fibers in a nontouch technique. The procedure is performed percutaneously under local or regional anesthesia. An endoscopic cannula is inserted into the amniotic cavity of the recipient fetus under ultrasound guidance at an angle perpendicular to the presumed vascular equator. The positions of the fetuses, umbilical cord insertions, and placenta are mapped. Initial landmarks include both umbilical cord insertions and the intertwin membrane. The operator visualizes the entire vascular equator and coagulates all visible anastomoses. Sections of about 1 to 2 cm are coagulated with pulses of 3 to 4 seconds, the duration judged by tissue response. Arteries are distinguishable from veins because they have a darker color and pass over the veins. Reduction amniocentesis is simultaneously performed. When the placenta is anterior, operative conditions are more difficult. Special instruments have been proposed, including curved sheaths, flexible endoscopes, and a double insertion technique. Most centers hospitalize patients for 1 or 2 postoperative days, and many experts use periprocedure tocolytics and antibiotics.

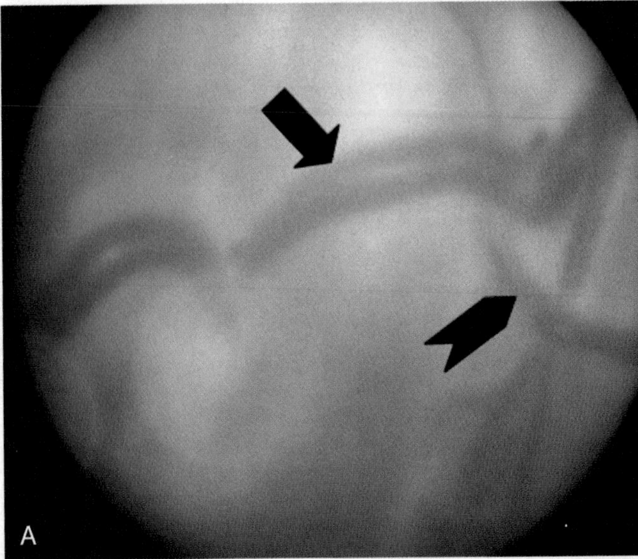

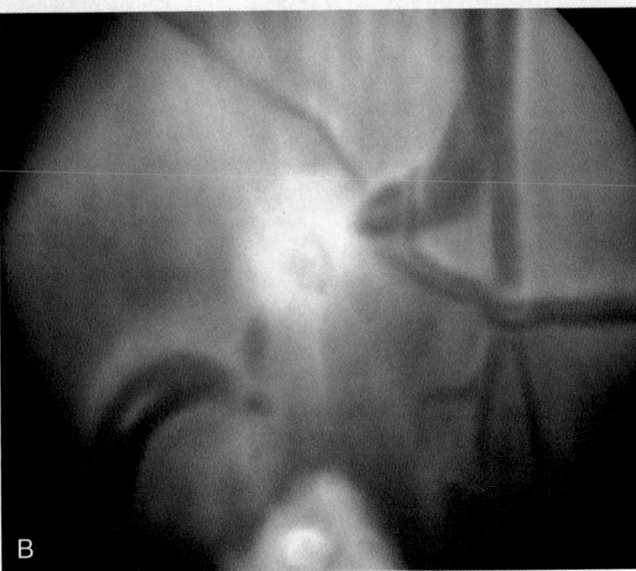

Figure 30-9. **A,** An artery from one twin going to a cotyledon, which is drained by a vein returning to the co-twin *(arrow)*. The cotyledon is also perfused by a small artery from the co-twin *(arrowhead)* and drained by a large vein going also to the co-twin. To preserve this cotyledon for the co-twin, the arterial perfusion to the cotyledon from the other twin is interrupted by laser photocoagulating the other artery. **B,** The effect of photocoagulation. (Courtesy Timothy M Crombleholme, MD, University of Cincinnati College of Medicine.)

Outcomes after Laser Therapy

In general, laser ablation has been shown to be a more effective technique than serial amnioreduction. In 2004, Senat and colleagues published the results of the European prospective multicenter randomized controlled trial of endoscopic laser (semiselective technique) versus serial amnioreduction for the treatment of severe TTTS between 15 and 26 weeks' gestation.[43] As the result of an interim analysis demonstrating a significant benefit for the laser group, the study was stopped after 142 patients had been treated. Compared with the amnioreduction group, the laser group had a higher likelihood of survival of at least one twin to 28 days of life (76% vs. 56%; $P = .009$) and 6 months of age (76% vs. 51%; $P = .002$). The median gestational age at delivery was significantly more advanced in the laser group than in the amnioreduction group (33.3 vs. 29.0 weeks; $P = .004$). Neonates from the laser group also had a lower incidence of periventricular leukomalacia and were more likely to be free of neurologic deficits at 6 months of age (52% vs. 31%; $P = .003$). The authors concluded that endoscopic laser coagulation of anastomoses is a more effective first-line treatment than serial amnioreduction for severe TTTS diagnosed before 26 weeks' gestation. Although this study did include patients in Quintero stages I to IV, most (90% of the laser group and 91% of the amnioreduction group) were stage II or III.

A National Institute of Child Health and Human Development (NICHD)-sponsored prospective randomized multicenter trial is the only other randomized clinical trial comparing amnioreduction to fetoscopic laser photocoagulation.[44] That trial, in which all patients were Quintero stages II to IV, was stopped early after only 40 patients, mainly because of recruitment difficulties but also because of concern about a trend toward adverse fetal outcomes affecting the recipient twin in the laser arm. Analysis of the 40 patients treated before termination of the study showed no difference, either for donors or recipients, in the primary outcome of 30-day neonatal survival (55% in both arms for donors, and 45% vs. 30% in the amnioreduction vs. laser arms for recipients; $P > .5$). There was an increased *fetal* mortality rate for recipients in the laser group, and this was more pronounced in Quintero stages III and IV disease. The overall conclusion of these investigators was that the trial had not conclusively demonstrated the superiority of either treatment modality, although the results were limited by the small sample size.

Subsequently, both a Cochrane review and another meta-analysis comparing laser therapy with serial amnioreduction supported the role of laser therapy in the treatment of severe TTTS. The Cochrane review found a decreased risk for perinatal and neonatal death (odds ratio [OR], 0.59; 96% CI, 0.4 to 0.87, and OR, 0.29; 95% CI, 0.14 to 0.61, respectively) as well as a higher incidence of survival without neurologic handicap at 6 months of age (OR, 1.66; 95% CI, 1.17 to 2.35) with laser therapy compared with amnioreduction. The review concluded that laser therapy should be considered in all stages, although further research is needed in stages I and II.[45] The meta-analysis by Rossi and colleagues[46] found an advantage of laser therapy in improving overall survival (OR, 2.04; 95% CI, 1.52 to 2.76), decreasing neonatal death (OR, 0.24; 95% CI, 0.15 to 0.4), and decreasing neurologic morbidity (OR, 0.2; 95% CI, 0.12 to 0.33) compared with serial amnioreduction.

Short-term complications of laser ablation include abruption, rupture of membranes, IUFD, and labor. In Senat's trial, there was a 1% to 12% risk for each of these complications in both the laser and amnioreduction groups. Rates of IUFD, pregnancy loss, and preterm premature rupture of the membranes (PPROM) within 7 days of the procedure were 1.5- to 5-fold higher in the laser group, although these differences did not reach statistical significance.[43] In the NICHD trial,[44] incidence of PPROM before 28 weeks was 4.8% in the laser arm and 0% in the amnioreduction arm. Maternal complications are not consistently reported in the literature. However, no maternal deaths have been reported in all of the TTTS laser therapy literature, and serious complications such as pulmonary edema or blood transfusion appear to be very rare.

A few papers have studied the long-term neurologic outcomes of babies treated in utero with laser ablation for TTTS. Banek and associates studied all 89 surviving infants of pregnancies treated with laser surgery at their institution between 1995 and 1997. The children underwent neurodevelopmental testing at a median age of 21 months. Normal development was seen in 78%, minor deficiencies in 11%, and major deficiencies in 11%. There was a nonsignificant trend toward normal outcome for those infants who were born as both surviving twins, as opposed to babies born following the intrauterine death of their co-twin.[47] In a more recent report, Lopriore and colleagues followed up 278 surviving babies from 212 pregnancies treated with laser ablation at three European centers between 2000 and 2005. The children underwent neurologic, mental, and psychomotor development testing at age 2 years. The overall incidence of neurodevelopmental impairment at 2 years of age was 18%, and cerebral palsy was diagnosed in 6% of the children. Risk factors associated with neurodevelopmental impairment were greater gestational age at laser surgery, lower gestational age at birth, lower birthweight, and higher Quintero stage.[48]

The current consensus is that laser ablation of vascular anastomoses is the optimal therapy for Quintero stages II to IV disease before 26 weeks' gestation. Controversy, however, exists as to the optimal management of stage I disease. This controversy is based on several observations. First, the prognosis for stage I patients can be quite good without laser surgery. In a series by Taylor and colleagues, 70% of stage I patients treated with either expectant management, amnioreduction, or septostomy remained stable or regressed.[37] O'Donoghue and colleagues reviewed all cases of TTTS at their institution between 2000 and 2006 and identified 46 cases presenting with stage I TTTS, all of which were treated either expectantly or with amnioreduction. They found that 70% either remained stable or regressed.[49] On the other hand, recent studies have shown that even in stages I and II TTTS, the recipient can suffer cardiac dysfunction, something not taken into account by the commonly used Quintero staging system. Michelfelder and associates examined echocardiographic parameters of 42 TTTS patients, of whom 14 were stage I.[50] Of the stage I patients, 57% had ventricular hypertrophy, and 14% had AV valve dysfunction. Because it has been shown that cardiac dysfunction in the recipient improves after laser therapy but not after amnioreduction, this suggests that laser therapy may be the better choice in select patients presenting with Quintero stage I TTTS.[51] A single retrospective study published in 2009 directly compared outcomes in stage I patients treated with laser surgery versus conservative management. Of 50 women presenting with stage I TTTS, 40% underwent laser surgery, and 60% were managed either expectantly, or, if maternal symptoms were present, with amnioreduction. Although short-term outcomes (gestational age at delivery and perinatal survival) were not significantly different between the two treatment groups, long-term neurodevelopmental impairment (as determined by neurologic examination and neuropsychological developmental testing at a minimum of 2 years of age) was decreased in the laser group (0/21 vs. 7/30; $P = .03$).[52] The improvement in long-term neurologic outcome in the laser-treated pregnancies in this study raises the question as to whether there is ongoing neurologic damage from mild TTTS even if the disease does not progress, and whether this damage could be prevented by interrupting the underlying cause of TTTS by laser ablation. **Synthesis of all the above information leads one to conclude that further study is needed in stage I disease, particularly focusing on echocardiographic parameters and long-term neurodevelopmental outcomes.** This sentiment was recently echoed in an excellent publication summarizing the current literature on TTTS and outlining recommendations of a scientific consensus panel convened to develop recommendations for TTTS diagnosis, therapy, and research.[40]

A wise overall approach to managing TTTS was aptly summarized in a 2005 review by Harkness and Crombleholme: "A thoughtful approach to the management of TTTS requires consideration of every aspect of the presentation, including gestational age, stage, Doppler findings, echocardiographic findings, concomitant placental insufficiency, and maternal risk factors. Until we have an effective medical therapy for TTTS, a judicious application of invasive procedures should be employed to optimize risk-to-benefit ratios for the mother and fetuses."[38]

Monoamniotic Twins

Monoamniotic twinning is an uncommon form of twinning in which both fetuses occupy a single amniotic sac. **Monoamniotic twins account for only 1% of all MZ twin pregnancies.** Historically, perinatal morbidity and mortality rates have been reported to be in excess of 50%. This has been attributed to premature delivery, growth restriction, congenital anomalies, and vascular anastomoses between twins, but mostly to umbilical cord entanglement and cord accidents (Figure 30-10). More recent reviews of prenatally diagnosed cases suggest improved perinatal outcomes, with mortality rates in the range of 10% to 20%.[53-55] This decrease is likely due to early prenatal diagnosis, the use of antenatal corticosteroids, increased fetal surveillance, and early elective delivery.

Because cord accidents are the primary cause of fetal death, most management protocols emphasize intense fetal surveillance to identify umbilical cord constriction before fetal loss. Fetal surveillance should be initiated after fetal viability has been achieved because IUFD has been documented to occur in monoamniotic twins throughout gestation.[54,56] Furthermore, this surveillance must be repeated frequently because fetal compromise and death can happen without much warning.

Many older reports on monoamniotic twins are not optimal for counseling patients because in most of those cases, the diagnosis of monoamnionicity was made postnatally. There have been several more recent series that are helpful. Rodis and coworkers reviewed 13 cases of monoamnionicity at one tertiary care center over a 10-year period.[53] All patients underwent serial ultrasound examinations and antenatal fetal surveillance two to seven times per week starting between 24 and 26 weeks' gestation. The mean gestational age at delivery was 32.9 weeks' gestation, with a mean birthweight of 1669 g. All pregnancies exhibited cord entanglement at the time of delivery, with 62% having knotted cords. Sixty-two percent of the pregnancies were delivered for abnormal fetal testing. If undelivered earlier, all patients had cesarean delivery by 35 weeks' gestation, and there were no fetal deaths. Two neonates died during the perinatal period: one from a congenital heart defect, and the other from asphyxia and sepsis. Compared with 77 sets of monoamniotic twins from the literature that had not been diagnosed prenatally, these patients had a 71% reduction in the relative risk for perinatal mortality.

A more recent study evaluated the impact of routine hospitalization for fetal monitoring on perinatal survival and neonatal morbidity in a multicenter retrospective cohort study of 96 monoamniotic twin gestations.[55] Of 87 women with both twins surviving at 24 weeks, 43 patients were admitted electively at a median gestational age of 26.5 weeks for inpatient surveillance and fetal testing two to three times daily. The remaining 44 women were followed as outpatients with fetal testing one to three times weekly. IUFD did not occur in any hospitalized patient, but 14.8% (13 of 88) of the fetuses were stillborn among those women followed as outpatients. Statistically significant improvements in birthweight, gestational age at delivery, and neonatal morbidity were also noted for the hospitalized women. This study suggests that improved neonatal survival and decreased perinatal morbidity are achievable in patients with monoamniotic twins admitted electively for daily fetal monitoring after viability.

Although the good outcomes obtained in the previously mentioned studies could be due to chance, we recommend fetal testing two to three times per day in the hospital for all patients with monoamniotic twins starting between 24 and 26 weeks' gestation. Although cord accidents cannot be predicted, daily fetal heart rate monitoring may reveal an increasing frequency of variable decelerations. If these are identified, continuous monitoring is recommended, with emergency delivery if worsening non-reassuring fetal status is encountered. Antenatal corticosteroids should be administered early because of the near certain chance of delivery at or before 34 weeks' gestation.

In the absence of non-reassuring fetal testing, the timing of elective delivery is not well established. Some authors have advocated delivery of all monoamniotic twin pregnancies as soon as fetal lung maturity has been demonstrated, whereas others have recommended elective delivery at 32 weeks' gestation.[56] Still others suggest that it is unnecessary to deliver monoamniotic twins before term. A retrospective evaluation of 24 sets of histologically confirmed monoamniotic twin pregnancies revealed no perinatal deaths after 30 weeks of gestation.[57] The authors suggested that there is no advantage to elective premature delivery of these pregnancies. Tessen and Zlatnik reviewed 20 monoamniotic twin pregnancies. In their retrospective series, there were no perinatal deaths after 32 weeks of gestation, and the authors suggested that prophylactic premature delivery of these women might not be indicated. However, in a subsequent addendum to the original paper,

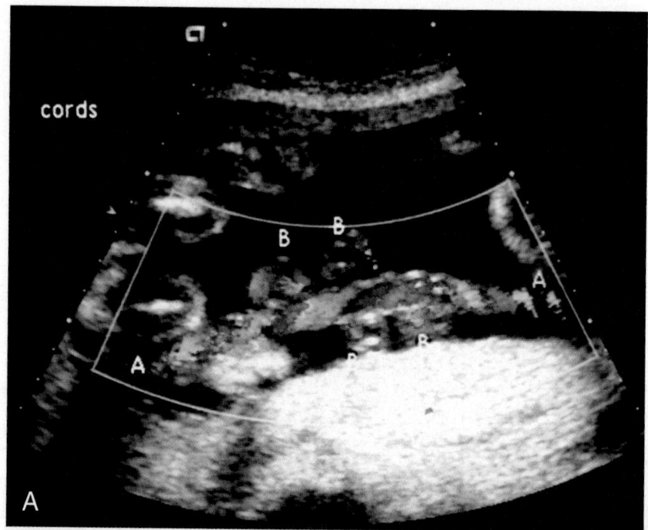

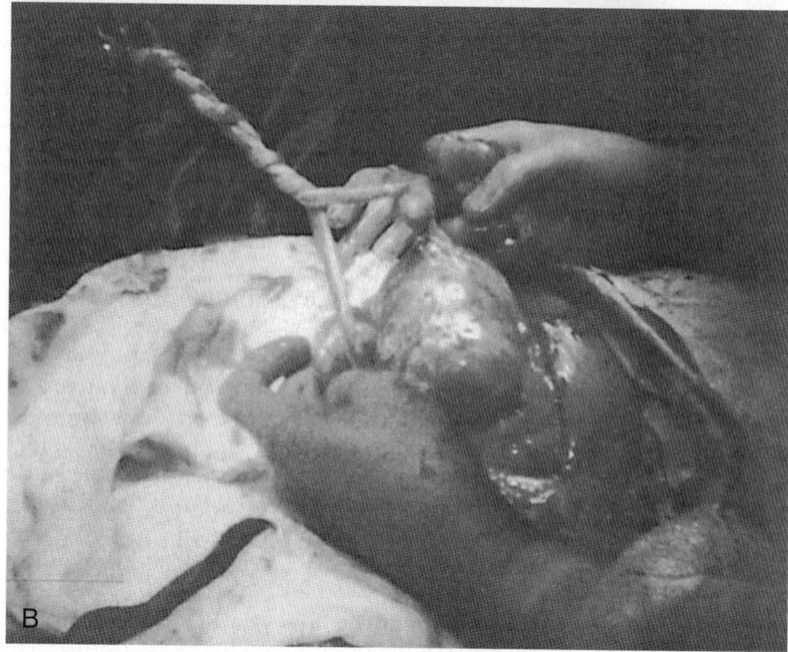

FIGURE 30-10. **A,** Cord entanglement detected by Doppler ultrasound in a monoamniotic twin gestation. **B,** Entangled cords found during cesarean delivery in a case of monochorionic monoamniotic twins.

they reported a double fetal death at 35 weeks just after publication of their report.[58] Despite these two reports suggesting a negligible risk for fetal death after 32 weeks, subsequent papers, including a 2009 study of 98 patients managed from 2000 to 2007, have confirmed the occurrence of a significant number of fetal deaths even after 32 weeks.[54,56,59]

Because of the continuing risk of fetal death, many experts perform elective delivery following the administration of antenatal corticosteroid therapy between 32 and 34 weeks' gestation. The recent 2011 NICHD and SMFM workshop addressing timing of indicated late-preterm and early-term birth also cites this gestational age interval as their recommendation.[34a] Delivery at this time is associated with a low risk of serious neonatal morbidity when weighed against the uncertain risk of continuing the pregnancy. However, it may be reasonable to manage selected cases of monoamniotic twins expectantly beyond 34 weeks' gestation, with careful ongoing fetal surveillance.

Cesarean delivery has been recommended to eliminate the risk for intrapartum cord accidents, but vaginal delivery of these patients is not entirely contraindicated if careful fetal monitoring is performed. In one series, no fetal deaths and only one case of non-reassuring fetal testing requiring emergency cesarean delivery occurred during labor in 15 monoamniotic twin pregnancies delivered vaginally.[58] On the other hand, there have been case reports of a nuchal cord affecting the first twin being cut to facilitate delivery, only to discover that the cut cord actually belonged to the second twin. Given these issues and a high incidence of intrapartum non-reassuring fetal testing, most experts recommend cesarean delivery of all monoamniotic twin pregnancies.

Twin Reversed Arterial Perfusion Sequence

The TRAP sequence, also known as acardiac twinning, is a malformation that occurs only in monochorionic

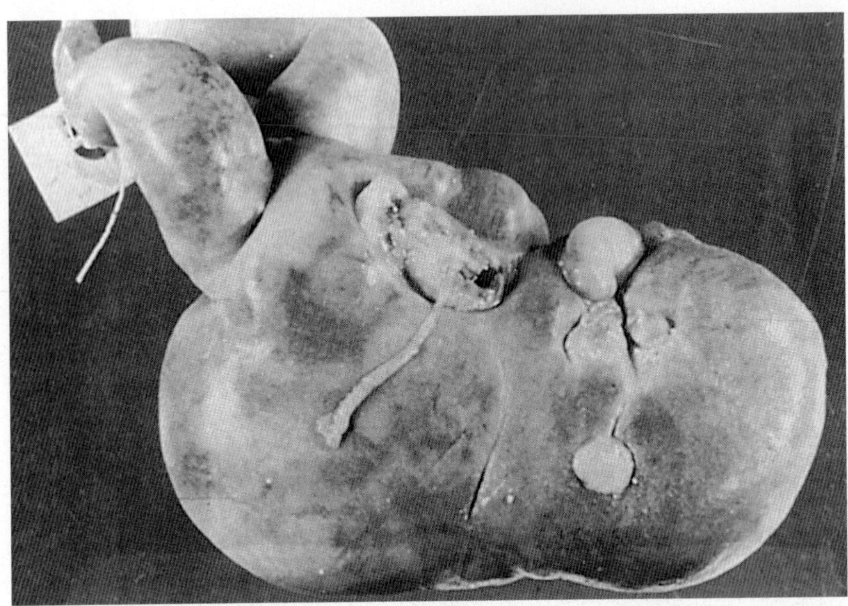

FIGURE 30-11. Acardiac twin. (Courtesy Dr. James Wheeler, Department of Surgical Pathology, Hospital of the University of Pennsylvania, Philadelphia.)

pregnancies with a frequency of about 1 per 30,000 deliveries. These extremely malformed fetuses have no heart at all (holoacardia) or only rudimentary cardiac tissue (pseudoacardia) in association with multiple other developmental abnormalities (Figure 30-11). Acardiac twins are sometimes classified by the degree of gross morphologic malformation: (1) acardius acephalus (absent head with relatively well-developed trunk and lower extremities), (2) acardius amorphous (amorphous mass of tissue, unrecognizable as a fetus), (3) acardius anceps (poorly formed head with well-developed trunk and lower extremities), and (4) acardius acormus (presence of a fetal head only, connected to the placenta by a cord). These classifications are used only as a descriptive tool because they have no clinical prognostic value.

Patients with TRAP sequence always have a monochorionic placenta with vascular anastomoses that sustain the life of the acardiac twin. Two theories exist as to the etiology of this condition. One theory holds that the TRAP anomaly is caused by an abnormal twinning event. The alternative hypothesis is that the acardia is a primary defect in cardiac development, and the acardiac twin, otherwise destined to end in an early spontaneous abortion, continues to grow because of monochorionic vascular anastomoses to a normal co-twin.

Antenatal diagnosis by ultrasound of an acardiac fetus coexisting with a normal co-twin is fairly straightforward. The only other entity in the differential diagnosis is an intrauterine fetal demise of one twin. However, continued growth of the abnormal, presumed dead twin rules this out, as can demonstration of blood flow in the presumed dead twin by color Doppler. Additionally, a retrograde pattern of fetal perfusion can be demonstrated to occur through the umbilical arteries.[60]

The acardiac twin clearly has no chance of survival, but its presence is not innocuous for the normal pump twin. The pump twin, although structurally normal, is at increased risk for in utero cardiac failure, and mortality rates of 50% or higher have been reported.[61] The estimated weight of the acardiac twin relative to the normal twin is an important prognostic factor. In the largest series of pregnancies complicated by TRAP sequence ($N = 49$), Moore and coworkers reported 90% preterm delivery, 40% polyhydramnios, and 30% cardiac failure of the normal twin when the weight ratio of acardiac to normal pump twin was more than 70%, compared with 70% preterm delivery, 30% polyhydramnios, and 10% cardiac failure for the normal pump twin when the weight ratio was less than 70%.[61]

Management of patients with pregnancies complicated by TRAP is controversial. Expectant management with serial ultrasound surveillance, including fetal echocardiography, is reasonable in the absence of the poor prognostic features outlined previously. Delivery may be indicated if signs of cardiac decompensation are noted at a viable gestational age. Maternal administration of digoxin and indomethacin have been attempted but with little evidence of benefit. In the face of previable or periviable cardiac failure in the normal pump twin or if poor prognostic features are present, another treatment option is interruption of the vascular communication between the twins. Methods of vascular interruption have included ultrasound-guided injection of thrombogenic materials into the umbilical circulation of the acardiac twin, ligation of the umbilical cord of the acardiac twin under fetoscopic guidance, and radiofrequency cord ablation.[60]

Conjoined Twins

Conjoined twins are another extremely rare complication of monochorionic twinning. They are believed to arise when an embryo incompletely divides between 13 and 15 days after fertilization. This event occurs with a frequency of about 1 per 50,000 deliveries. Most conjoined twins are female, with a reported female-to-male ratio of 2:1 or 3:1. The mortality rate is very high, as evidenced by a retrospective case series from the Children's Hospital of Philadelphia, which found an incidence of 28% intrauterine death, 54% death shortly after birth, and 18% overall survival among 14 sets of conjoined twins treated at their institution between 1996 and 2002.[62]

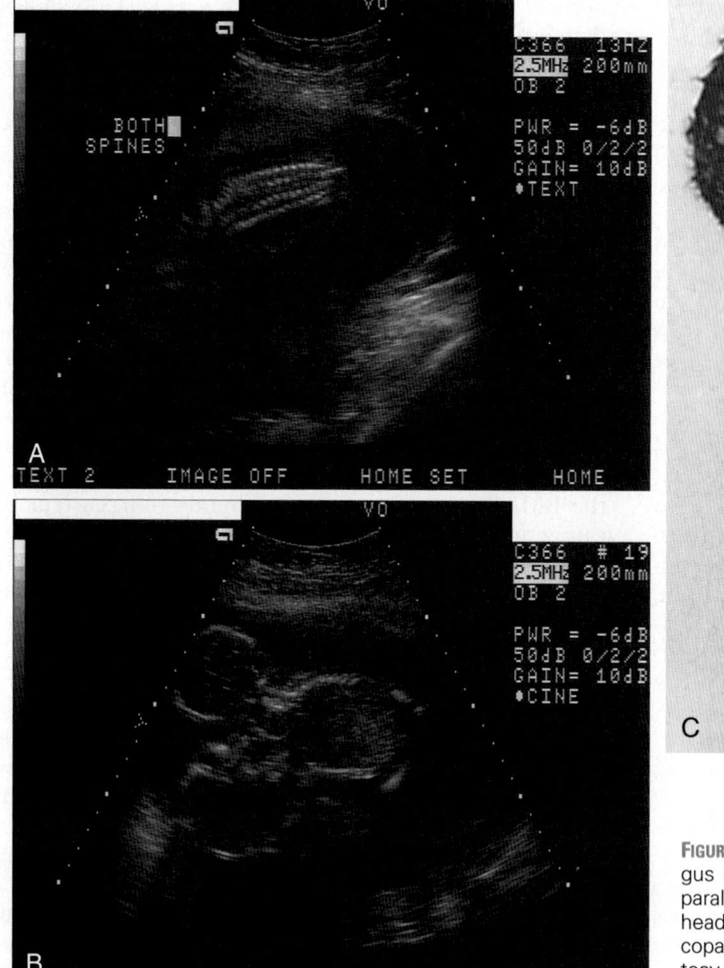

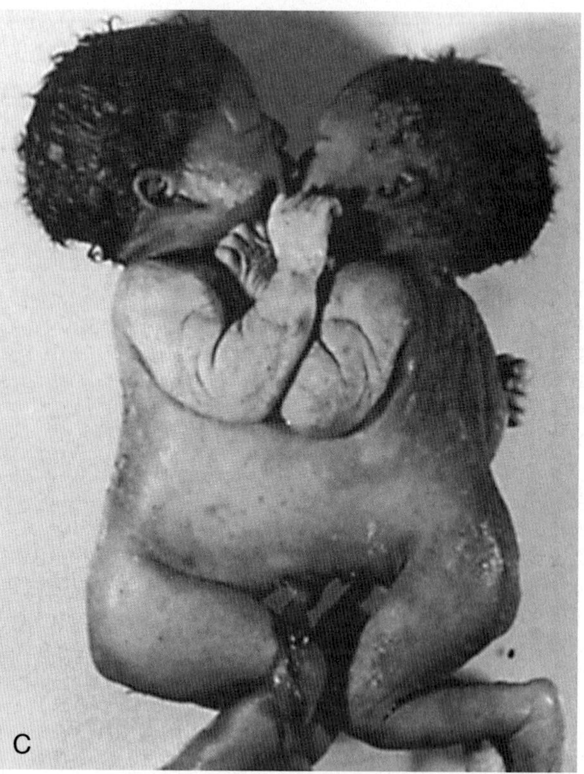

FIGURE 30-12. **A** and **B,** Late first-trimester images of thoracopagus conjoined twins. This twin set had one trunk with two parallel spinal columns **(A)**, leading to two separate necks and heads **(B)**. **C,** Conjoined twins attached at the chest or thoracopagus, the most common form of conjoined twins. (Courtesy Dr. James Wheeler, Department of Surgical Pathology, Hospital of the University of Pennsylvania, Philadelphia.)

Conjoined twins are classified according to their site of union. The most common location is the chest (thoracopagus: Figure 30-12), followed by the anterior abdominal wall (omphalopagus), the buttocks (pygopagus), the ischium (ischiopagus), and the head (craniopagus). Organs are shared to varying degrees. Major congenital anomalies of one or both twins are common, and polyhydramnios is present in almost half of the reported cases of conjoined twins.

Ultrasound can establish this diagnosis in utero, as early as the first trimester, based on visualization of a bifid fetal pole. Three-dimensional ultrasound, color Doppler, fetal echocardiography, and MRI can be used to complement two-dimensional ultrasound imaging to confirm the diagnosis, determine the extent of organ sharing, and definitively classify the type of conjoined twinning.[62,63] Once the diagnosis of conjoined twins is made, management options should be discussed with the patient. If the diagnosis is confirmed before viability, pregnancy termination should be offered. **If the patient desires expectant management, she should be counseled that the prognosis for survival and successful separation depends on the degree of organ and vascular sharing between the two fetuses, especially the heart.** Multimodality fetal evaluation as described previously should be used prenatally to carefully survey fetal anatomy. To optimize postnatal management, patients with conjoined twins should be cared for by a multidisciplinary team during the antenatal period. This team should include maternal-fetal medicine specialists, neonatologists, pediatric anesthesiologists, pediatric surgeons, and appropriate pediatric subspecialists.

Patients with conjoined twins should deliver at a tertiary care facility where neonatal and pediatric specialists are available. Cesarean delivery near term will be necessary to minimize maternal and fetal injury. If the twins are thought to have a poor chance of surviving and are believed to be small enough to pass through the birth canal without traumatizing the mother, vaginal delivery might be considered.

Of conjoined twins who undergo elective separation, survival rates approach 80%. Of conjoined twin sets who require emergent separation, however, survival rates are much lower, around 25%.[63] Although the long-term follow-up of conjoined twins who have undergone successful surgical separation is limited, the data seem favorable. Although survivors frequently require additional surgeries following the initial separation to correct urologic, orthopedic, and neurosurgical issues, many achieve educational levels similar to their singleton peers.

ANTEPARTUM MANAGEMENT OF MULTIFETAL PREGNANCY

Maternal Nutrition and Weight Gain

The two factors that most influence pregnancy outcome are gestational age at delivery and the adequacy of fetal growth. Nutritional status during gestation is linked to both these outcomes. Poor weight gain and deficient nutritional status are associated with low birthweight, preterm delivery, and higher rates of neonatal complications. **The higher baseline risk for these adverse outcomes in twin pregnancies creates a situation in which enhancement of nutrition and weight gain has the potential to provide tremendous positive impact.**

As discussed earlier in the chapter, multifetal gestation requires an exaggerated physiologic adaptation compared with singleton pregnancy. Because of these increased physiologic demands, mothers pregnant with twins have a 10% higher resting energy expenditure. Consequently, to meet the heightened metabolic expenditure, multiple gestations require modification of the current weight gain, caloric intake, and vitamin supplementation recommendations for singleton pregnancies. A recent review of nutrition in twin pregnancy outlined four goals for optimizing maternal nutrition in multifetal gestation[64]:

1. Optimize fetal growth and development
2. Reduce the incidence of obstetrical complications
3. Increase gestational age at delivery
4. Avoid excess maternal weight gain, which could result in unnecessary postpartum weight retention

Evidence demonstrates a positive relationship between maternal weight gain and infant birthweight. It also shows that poor maternal weight gain adversely affects birthweight and preterm delivery rates, mostly in women with an underweight prepregnancy body mass index (BMI). Correspondingly, poor weight gain has a lower impact on overweight and obese women, although an effect is still seen.

Both total maternal weight gain and the timing of that weight gain are critical to optimizing twin birthweight and obstetrical outcomes. Pederson and colleagues found that optimal pregnancy outcome, defined as gestational age at delivery of more than 37 weeks and both babies weighing more than 2500 g, was associated with a total weight gain of 44 lb. Furthermore, worse outcomes in general were seen with weight gain less than 37 lb.[65] Luke and colleagues have shown that weight gain before 28 weeks accounts for 80% of the maternal weight gain effect on infant birthweights.[66] Underscoring this point, Luke and colleagues demonstrated that even when there is appropriate weight gain after 24 weeks, suboptimal gain before 24 weeks is still associated with earlier delivery and poor intrauterine growth. Ideal maternal weight gain is also associated with a 1- to 2-week longer gestational period and a more than three times shorter infant length of hospital stay.[67] BMI-specific weight gain patterns associated with ideal twin birthweight, defined as 2850 to 2950 g at 36 weeks or later, are summarized in Table 30-6. Although the BMI categories used differ slightly from current BMI categories, the differences by weight status can easily be appreciated. Compared with singleton gestations, these recommended rates of weight gain are more than double early in pregnancy (0 to 20 weeks), about 50% higher during midpregnancy (20 to 28 weeks), and about 25% higher late in gestation (28 to 38 weeks).[68]

The crucial role of early weight gain and the more pronounced benefits of appropriate weight gain in underweight women suggest that early weight gain provides improved maternal nutrient stores for use later in pregnancy when fetal demands increase. Additionally, optimal maternal nutrition and weight gain early in pregnancy may enhance placental growth, thus providing a better nutrient supply to the babies. Both of these theories may explain why adequate weight gain in late pregnancy after inadequate gain in early pregnancy does not provide complete catch-up in fetal growth or outcomes.

Partially in response to evidence such as that cited previously, the Institute of Medicine issued new BMI-specific weight gain recommendations for pregnancy in 2009. These recommendations are summarized in Table 30-7. After these guidelines were published, Fox and coworkers

TABLE 30-6 Recommended Rates of Maternal Weight Gain in Twin Pregnancies

GESTATIONAL AGE PERIOD	UNDERWEIGHT (BMI <19.8)	NORMAL WEIGHT (BMI = 19.8-26)	OVERWEIGHT (BMI = 26.1-29)	OBESE (BMI >29)
Early (<20 wk)	1.25-1.75 lb/wk	1-1.5 lb/wk	1-1.25 lb/wk	0.75-1 lb/wk
Mid (21-28 wk)	1.5-1.75 lb/wk	1.25-1.75 lb/wk	1-1.5 lb/wk	0.75-1.25 lb/wk
Late (≥29 wk)	1.25 lb/wk	1 lb/wk	1 lb/wk	0.75 lb/wk

From Luke B, Hediger ML, Nugent C, et al: Body mass index-specific weight gains associated with optimal birth weights in twin pregnancies. J Reprod Med 48:217, 2003.

TABLE 30-7 2009 Institute of Medicine Recommendations for Weight Gain in Pregnancy

PREPREGNANCY BMI	BODY MASS INDEX (kg/m²) WHO CRITERIA	TOTAL WEIGHT GAIN SINGLETON (lb)	TOTAL WEIGHT GAIN TWIN (lb)
Underweight	<18.5	28-40	No recommendations made
Normal weight	18.5-24.9	25-35	37-54
Overweight	25.0-29.9	15-25	31-50
Obese	≥30.0	11-20	25-42

From Rasmussen KM, Yaktine AL (eds): Institute of Medicine (Committee to Reexamine IOM Pregnancy Weight Guidelines, Food and Nutrition Board and Board on Children, Youth, and Families). Weight Gain During Pregnancy: Reexamining the Guidelines. Washington, DC, National Academy Press, 2009.

retrospectively studied a cohort of 297 twin pregnancies from a private Maternal-Fetal Medicine practice, applying the 2009 Institute of Medicine (IOM) guidelines in order to compare pregnancy outcomes between those women who met or exceeded the weight gain guidelines and those who did not meet the recommendations.[69] They found that women with a prepregnancy BMI placing them in the normal or overweight categories who met the weight gain recommendations demonstrated improvement in outcomes. Normal-weight women who met or exceeded the weight gain recommendations had significantly larger babies and a greater likelihood of both babies weighing more than 2500 g. Overweight women meeting the weight gain recommendations had more advanced gestational ages at delivery as well as heavier weight of the larger twin. Both normal-weight and overweight women who met weight gain goals had some reduction in overall preterm birth and spontaneous preterm birth. In the obese gravidas, there were no statistically significant differences, although this group was small ($n = 29$). This study, along with the previous work cited, supports optimizing maternal weight gain in twin pregnancy in order to improve outcomes. Notably, underweight women were excluded from the study because the IOM guidelines do not provide a specific weight gain recommendation for women with an underweight prepregnancy BMI who are pregnant with twins. However, because other literature clearly demonstrates that underweight women benefit even more from optimal gestational weight gain, special attention should be given to nutritional counseling and weight gain recommendations in this population. Incorporation of formal nutritional consultation into the care of women with multiples is clinically recommended and should be cost-effective.

Although increased maternal weight gain in pregnancy is associated with improved outcomes, maternal weight retention and its long-term health effects remain of concern. There are no long-term prospective studies of weight retention in twin mothers; however, a recent abstract (using BMI-specific weight gain goals established by Luke and colleagues, which are very similar to the 2009 IOM recommendations) demonstrated higher weight retention 6 weeks postpartum in women who exceeded the recommendations compared with women who met the recommended weight gain (6 kg vs. 2 kg; $P < .001$).[70] Therefore, in the setting of multiple gestations, emphasis should be placed on appropriate weight gain, while avoiding gains exceeding the recommendations.

Just as multiple pregnancy demands higher energy expenditure, caloric intake, and weight gain compared with singleton gestation, there is likely also a greater demand for micronutrients. Some experts have suggested that supplemental calcium, magnesium, and zinc may be important to optimal fetal growth and infant and maternal outcomes, although specific evidence for individual micronutrients is generally lacking. Table 30-8 represents a reasonable protocol regarding optimal nutritional management and micronutrient intake during twin pregnancy.

Spontaneous Preterm Birth

Patients with a multiple gestation are at significant risk for preterm labor and delivery. Although this risk is an overriding concern in the antepartum care of multiple gestations, not all multiples are delivered preterm; 40% of twins are delivered at term. **Refining the risk for preterm birth in each individual patient improves pregnancy management by selecting those patients who may benefit most from increased surveillance and interventions while simultaneously minimizing unnecessary interventions in lower-risk women.**

The use of ultrasound transvaginal cervical length measurements and fetal fibronectin (FFN) sampling can help stratify preterm birth risk in multiple gestations. The NICHD Preterm Prediction Study included 147 twin

TABLE 30-8 Twin Pregnancy Nutritional Recommendations

INTERVENTION	FIRST TRIMESTER	SECOND TRIMESTER	THIRD TRIMESTER
Maternal weight gain	Assess pre-gravid BMI, determine BMI-specific weight gain goal	Assess/counsel regarding BMI-specific weight gain goal	Assess/counsel regarding BMI-specific weight gain goal
Caloric requirements by BMI category (kcal/day)			
Underweight (<18.5)	4000	Alter as necessary for weight gain goal	Alter as necessary for weight gain goal
Normal (18.5-24.9)	3000-3500		
Overweight (25-29.9)	3250		
Obese (≥30)	2700-3000		
Protein Requirements by BMI category (g/day)			
Underweight	200	Unchanged from first trimester	Unchanged
Normal	175		
Overweight	163		
Obese	150		
Micronutrient Supplementation			
MVI with iron (tablets)	1	2	2
Calcium (mg)	1500	2500	2500
Magnesium (mg)	400	800	800
Zinc (mg)	15	30	30
Folic acid (mg)	1	1	1
Nutritional Consultation	Yes	Repeat if not at weight gain goal, anemia, GDM	Repeat if not at weight gain goal, anemia, GDM
Laboratory Nutritional Assessment	HgB, ferritin, folate, B_{12}, early GDM screening if risk factors	Follow up abnormality from first trimester	HgB, ferritin, GDM screen

Modified from Goodnight W, Newman R: Optimal nutrition for improved twin pregnancy outcome. Obstet Gynecol 114:1121, 2009.

mothers screened at 24 to 28 weeks' gestation for 50 potential risk factors for preterm delivery. They found that at 24 weeks, only a short cervix (≤25 mm) was significantly associated with an elevated risk for preterm birth in twin pregnancies. The odds ratio of preterm birth before 32 weeks was 6.9 (95% CI, 2 to 24.2) in these women, corresponding to a 27% risk for spontaneous preterm birth before 32 weeks in those women with cervical length of 25 mm or less at 24 weeks compared with a 5% risk in those women with a cervical length of more than 25 mm at 24 weeks. The risk for preterm birth before 35 weeks and before 37 weeks was also significantly elevated for those women with a 24-week cervical length of 25 mm or less.

In the same study, a positive FFN at both 28 and 30 weeks was associated with preterm birth before 32 weeks (OR, 9.4 and 46.1, respectively). Specifically, a positive FFN at 28 weeks was associated with a 29% risk for spontaneous preterm birth before 32 weeks, compared with only 3.9% for those with a negative FFN at 28 weeks.[71]

The combination of cervical length and fetal fibronectin assay has been suggested as a stronger predictor of spontaneous preterm birth than either test alone. A retrospective cohort analysis was performed on 155 asymptomatic twin pregnancies evaluated with combined fetal fibronectin and cervical length testing between 22 and 32 weeks' gestation. The authors reported that they routinely performed FFN assays and measured cervical length every 2 to 3 weeks in their twin mothers. They found that the combination of a positive FFN and a cervical length less than 20 mm (at any time between 22 weeks and the gestational age endpoint in question) had a significantly higher positive predictive value for spontaneous preterm birth than either test alone. If both tests were positive, the risk for spontaneous preterm birth before 28 weeks was 50%, compared with a 13% risk if only one test was positive and only a 1.6% risk if both tests were negative. The stepwise increase in the risk for preterm birth in women with both tests negative, only one test positive, and two tests positive remained statistically significant for spontaneous preterm birth before 30, 32, 34, 35, and 37 weeks' gestation.[72]

In addition to the absolute cervical length, the degree of change in the cervical length over time may also be an important predictor of preterm birth in twins. Fox and coworkers studied a historical cohort of 121 asymptomatic twin pregnancies who had two transvaginal cervical length measurements performed 2 to 6 weeks apart between 18 and 24 weeks' gestation. They found that cervical length shortening (defined as a decrease of ≥20%) over this interval was associated with a greater risk for preterm birth before 28, 30, 32, and 34 weeks compared with women whose cervical length remained stable (15.8% vs. 1% at <28 weeks, 15.8% vs. 2% at <30 weeks, 31.6% vs. 5% at <32 weeks, and 36.8% vs. 12.9% at <34 weeks; all *P* values ≤.027). Most striking was the fact that this association with preterm birth remained even when patients with cervical length less than 25 mm were excluded. Despite the overall cervical length remaining longer than 25 mm, shortening of 20% or more was still associated with a significantly higher risk for spontaneous preterm birth before 28, 30, and 32 weeks compared with women whose cervical length remained stable (18.2% vs. 1%, 18.2% vs. 2%, and 27.3% vs. 4.1%, respectively; *P* values = 0.026, 0.049, and 0.022, respectively).[73]

The use of these tests can help guide management decisions, such as frequency of office visits or whether work or activity restriction is prudent. Identification of a patient at particularly high risk for preterm delivery based on her cervical length, fetal fibronectin, or a combination of the two can allow for heightened surveillance and may permit timely interventions such as restricted activity, tocolysis, or steroid administration. On the other hand, documentation of an above-average and stable cervical length (>35 mm) in midgestation can allow both patient and physician to feel comfortable with a patient continuing with her normal activities, avoiding the temptation to implement unnecessary interventions.

Over the years, various interventions aimed at decreasing this high rate of preterm birth have been studied, most without clear evidence of benefit in a general multiple-gestation population. Of note, very few, if any, of these studies have been carried out in the highest-risk multiple gestations based on transvaginal cervical lengths or fetal fibronectin assays. The potential value of some of these interventions in prolonging pregnancy may be quite different in a woman with a 50% risk for delivery before 28 or 30 weeks' gestation versus a 2% risk. The following section discusses the relative merits of these proposed interventions to prevent spontaneous preterm birth in multiple gestations.

Bedrest and Hospitalization

A Cochrane review analyzed six randomized trials including 600 women and 1400 babies and concluded that routine hospitalized bedrest did not provide any benefit for multiple pregnancies. A trend toward fewer low-birthweight babies was noted, although this trend did not extend to very-low-birthweight (VLBW) infants. In fact, in uncomplicated twin pregnancies, inpatient bedrest was associated with a greater chance of delivery before 34 weeks.[74] Because there is no evidence to suggest that routine hospitalization is beneficial for patients with multiples, we believe that these women should be hospitalized only for the same obstetrical indications as singletons.

There are no prospective trials of prophylactic home bedrest in multiple gestations. Older studies that suggested a benefit of bedrest were confounded by the inclusion of undiagnosed twins among the unrestricted women. Tocodynametric studies on normal uterine activity over a 24-hour period have documented that uterine contraction frequency is greater during periods of maternal activity and ambulation. However, for asymptomatic twin pregnancies in women with reassuring cervical length and no prior history of preterm birth, we do not recommend routine rest at home or cessation of work. Nonetheless, because it is difficult to refute the possibility of benefit in higher-order multiple gestations, we generally recommend rest at home starting at about 20 weeks for women carrying triplets or more.

Cerclage

Results of studies using cervical cerclage to prolong pregnancy in multiple gestations have been disappointing. Prophylactic cerclage has been studied and found to be ineffective in both twins and triplets. Even in the presence of cervical shortening, no clear benefit of cerclage placement in patients with twins has been demonstrated. Newman and coworkers[75] prospectively followed 147 twin pregnancies in women who underwent transvaginal ultrasonographic cervical length measurements between 18 and 26 weeks' gestation. Cerclage was offered to all 33 women with transvaginal cervical length of 25 mm or less and was placed in 21 women. There were no differences between the cerclage and no cerclage groups with regard to length of gestation, birthweight, delivery before 34 weeks, PPROM, or VLBW. A 2005 meta-analysis of ultrasound-indicated cerclage found that, in the subgroup with twins, cerclage placement was actually associated with a statistically significant increase in birth before 35 weeks (75% vs. 36%).[76] Because cerclage is a surgical procedure that may be associated with adverse sequelae for both the mother and her fetuses, it is recommended that cerclage placement in multiple gestations be restricted to women with either a strongly suggestive history or objectively documented cervical insufficiency rather than based on cervical length alone.

Tocolysis

Prophylactic tocolysis has been evaluated in multiple gestations and not found to be effective. In contrast, short-term use of these agents for acute tocolysis in preterm labor is helpful to gain time for administration of corticosteroids to enhance fetal lung maturity as well as to allow transport to a tertiary care facility. Tocolytic use in multiple gestations, however, must be accompanied by careful monitoring of the maternal condition. Because of the exaggerated maternal cardiovascular adaptations to a multiple gestation, women pregnant with multiples are predisposed to cardiopulmonary complications, most notably pulmonary edema. This risk is heightened with β-adrenergic agents and when tocolytics are used in combination with corticosteroids and intravenous fluids. At our institution, intravenous magnesium sulfate is used as a first-line acute tocolytic. When needed in patients before 32 weeks' gestation, we add oral indomethacin for 48 hours.

Progesterone

Weekly intramuscular administration of 17-hydroxyprogesterone caproate deserves special consideration as a unique approach to prophylactic therapy. After 17-hydroxyprogesterone caproate was shown to be effective in reducing recurrent preterm birth in singletons, there was interest in using it in populations with other risk factors for spontaneous preterm delivery, such as multiple gestation. Unfortunately, prospective randomized studies have not shown any effect of weekly 17-hydroxyprogesterone caproate in preventing preterm birth in women whose risk factor for preterm birth was twin or triplet gestation.[77,78] It should be mentioned, however, that those trials included very few women with a history of prior preterm birth. In the study of twins by Rouse and colleagues in which just over half of the participants were multiparous, only 6.1% of the treatment group and 9% of the placebo group had a history of previous preterm delivery.[78] In the triplet trial by Caritis and associates, none of the women in the treatment group and only 3% in the placebo group had a history of previous preterm birth.[77]

A 2007 trial by Fonseca and associates[79] examining the effect of nightly vaginal progesterone in women with short midgestation cervical length did include twin gestations, although twins made up only 10.4% ($N = 13$) of the placebo group and 8.8% ($N = 11$) of the treatment group. This study randomized women with a transvaginal cervical length of 15 mm or less at a median of 22 weeks' gestation to either 200 mg of vaginal progesterone nightly or placebo. They found that administration of nightly vaginal progesterone decreased spontaneous delivery before 34 weeks from 34.3% to 19.2%, which was statistically significant. In the subgroup of twin gestations, vaginal progesterone was associated with a similar reduction in preterm delivery, although the difference did not reach statistical significance because of sample size considerations.

The STOPPIT trial, published in 2009, randomized 500 women carrying twins to daily vaginal progesterone gel (90 mg) or placebo gel administered between 24 and 34 weeks' gestation.[80] The investigators did not find any difference in the primary outcome, which was intrauterine death or delivery before 34 weeks. Just less than 50% of the study participants were multiparous, but the incidence of prior preterm birth was not reported.

The results of these studies suggest that the mechanism for increased spontaneous preterm birth in multiples is likely different from the mechanism of spontaneous preterm birth in singletons. Whatever the mechanism, it appears to be less responsive to progesterone supplementation. However, this is a question deserving more study, especially for those multiples at particularly high risk for spontaneous preterm birth based on a short cervical length or positive fetal fibronectin assay.

Another population that has not been specifically studied includes women currently pregnant with multiples who have a history of spontaneous preterm birth with previous singleton gestations. These women are at very heightened risk for spontaneous preterm birth. Whatever factors put them at risk for spontaneous preterm delivery with a singleton are presumably still in effect and likely exacerbated by the additional demands of carrying twins. For these reasons, until better evidence is available, it is reasonable to use weekly 17-hydroxyprogesterone caproate for women pregnant with multiples who also have a history of a spontaneous preterm birth before 37 weeks with a prior singleton gestation. Additionally, based on the Fonseca trial, it is also reasonable to offer nightly vaginal progesterone to women carrying multiples who have a midgestation cervical length of 15 mm or less.

Antenatal Testing

Multiple gestations are at an increased risk for uteroplacental insufficiency, fetal growth restriction, and stillbirth, and for this reason many experts recommend antenatal surveillance in the form of nonstress tests or biophysical profiles. There are retrospective data showing that both nonstress tests and biophysical profiles are effective in detecting compromised twin gestations.[81] However, the optimal surveillance schedule is unknown because there are no prospective data on which to base a recommendation. The American College of Obstetricians and

Gynecologists 2004 Practice Bulletin on multiple gestation acknowledges these limitations and states that "further studies are needed to determine whether routine antepartum fetal surveillance provides objective benefit in the absence of other high-risk conditions." The 2009 NICHD reevaluation of antenatal testing also discusses the limits of the evidence regarding routine fetal surveillance in multiple gestations but lists weekly testing at 32 weeks as a reasonable strategy for twins with normal fetal growth.[82] Pregnancies complicated by growth restriction or other risk factors may require earlier and more frequent testing. Others have suggested an increased stillbirth risk even among apparently uncomplicated monochorionic, diamniotic twins and recommend twice weekly testing of these gestations after 34 weeks.

There are even fewer data for triplet and higher-order multiple gestations. However, because the stillbirth risk increases with increasing plurality, it is reasonable to begin antenatal testing earlier for triplets than for twins, acknowledging that these recommendations are based more on expert opinion and clinical practice than prospective evidence. Possibly the most compelling reason to perform routine monitoring in twins is the high incidence of both IUGR and discordant growth in the third trimester and the inability to reliably diagnose those conditions by ultrasound.

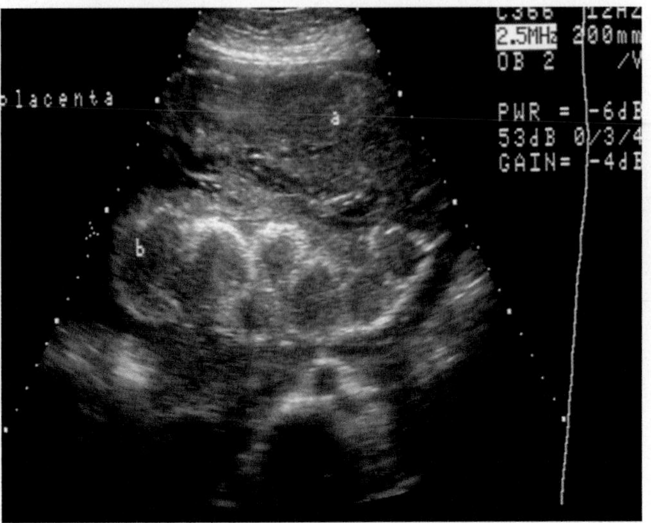

FIGURE 30-13. Normal anterior placenta of twin A and abnormal calcified grade 3 placenta of twin B in a case of selective intrauterine growth restriction of twin B. Twin B also had elevated umbilical artery S/D ratios.

Fetal Growth Surveillance

Ultrasound, although imperfect, is the only method available for assessing individual fetal growth in multiple gestations. **Normal twins grow at the same rate as singletons up to 30 to 32 weeks' gestation, after which they do not gain weight as rapidly as singletons of the same gestational age.** The restriction in each twin's somatic growth is thought to be related to "crowding" in utero and competition for nutrients. The implication of this concept is that at some point in the third trimester, the placentas can no longer keep pace with the nutrient requirements of both developing fetuses. This relative uteroplacental insufficiency occurs even earlier when more than two fetuses are present. It must, however, be cautioned that most of the studies suggesting a slowing of fetal growth after 30 weeks are based on birth weight and therefore represent size rather than growth. A retrospective longitudinal study using ultrasound to follow fetal growth velocity in 131 twin gestations found that biparietal diameter growth velocities significantly slowed between 30 and 33 weeks' gestation and that growth of the abdominal circumference was significantly slowed from 30 to 37 weeks.[83] A subsequent prospective longitudinal study of fetal growth in 162 twins was performed using ultrasound every 2 weeks from 16 weeks until delivery. Similar to the retrospective analysis, this study showed that the growth velocities for biparietal diameter, femur length, and abdominal circumference were all decreased after 32 weeks.[84] Of interest, in both of these studies, chorionicity did not significantly influence fetal growth.

Discordant Growth

Significant discordance in weights between twins is typically defined as a greater than 15% to 25% difference in actual or estimated twin weights (the difference between the weights divided by the weight of the larger twin). In a series of 1370 consecutive twin pregnancies, discordances in birthweight of 15% to 20%, 21% to 25%, 26% to 30%, 31% to 40%, and more than 40% were found in 14%, 7%, 4%, 3%, and 1% of pregnancies, respectively.[85] Because DZ twins are genetically distinct individuals, it is not surprising that they might be programmed to have very different weights at birth. There are, however, several pathologic situations in which either monochorionic or dichorionic twins may develop substantial weight differences. These include TTTS, the combination of an anomalous fetus with a normal co-twin, and selective IUGR affecting only one twin because of local placental factors (Figure 30-13) or abnormalities of the umbilical cord. IUGR can also affect both twins relatively equally, in which case they would both be small, but not discordant in size. **Although it has been argued that fetal size discrepancy is not concerning if both babies' estimated weights remain appropriate for gestational age, discordance, especially when severe, suggests clinically significant growth restriction. The exact degree of growth discordance that begins to confer increased risk is debated, but an association with increased fetal and neonatal morbidity and mortality has been demonstrated when the estimated weight discrepancy exceeds 25% to 30%.**[85]

Smaller degrees of discordance, not surprisingly, may be more worrisome in monochorionic compared with dichorionic gestations. In one study examining the significance of discordance, the risk for stillbirth, neonatal death, and preterm birth was not increased until discordance reached 30% or higher in different-sex twins, but these risks were increased with discordance of 15% or higher in same-sex twins.[86] A specific concern among monochorionic twins is the association between discordant growth and the occurrence of neurodevelopmental disability.

Ultrasound is the optimal method of assessing the progression of fetal growth in multiples. A survey of multiple biometric parameters on serial ultrasound examinations provides the most accurate assessment of the size of each individual fetus in twin gestations. No single anatomic parameter evaluated at birth adequately discriminates normal twins from those with IUGR. Consequently, multiple biometric parameters should be assessed to detect growth disorders among twins in utero, especially in the third trimester. Among individual parameters, abdominal circumference is the single most sensitive measurement in predicting both IUGR and growth discordance.

Consideration of as many biometric variables as possible will maximize the likelihood of differentiating a normally grown from a growth-restricted twin fetus. A recent prospective longitudinal study from Belgium found that ultrasound estimations of fetal weight and weight discordance among monochorionic, diamniotic twins were highly correlated with actual birthweight and the degree of weight discordance at birth.[87] The same general principles can be applied to the assessment of growth in triplets and higher-order multiple gestations. Another point that should be stressed is that growth is a dynamic process and, therefore, that patients with multifetal gestations should be followed throughout pregnancy. **It is recommended that all patients with twins undergo ultrasound testing at least every 3 to 4 weeks after 20 weeks and more frequently if IUGR or growth discordance is suspected. Additionally, many experts recommend that ultrasounds be performed every 2 weeks in monochorionic twins beginning in the mid-second trimester in order to survey for the development of TTTS or selective IUGR.**

SPECIALIZED TWIN CLINICS

The value of specialized twin clinics has been described. In these clinics, where women carrying twins are seen at regular intervals by the same obstetrical team, several advantages accrue. Patients have the opportunity to develop rapport with a small group of caregivers. This results in an increased awareness of their special problems and may increase compliance with therapeutic directives. The medical personnel become adept at detecting early signs of the specific problems associated with twin pregnancies, and special emphasis is given to nutrition, weight gain, and preterm labor surveillance. Two studies have examined the effects of such clinics and found improvements in outcomes. One study demonstrated reduced rates of VLBW babies, neonatal intensive care unit (NICU) admissions, and perinatal mortality,[88] whereas the other showed improvements in gestational age and birthweight and reduced rates of PPROM, preterm labor and delivery, preeclampsia, and low-birthweight and VLBW infants, as well as reductions in NICU admissions and individual complications such as respiratory distress syndrome, necrotizing enterocolitis, and retinopathy of prematurity. Shortened length of stay was also seen for the babies, as was a reduction in cost per twin pair.[89] These studies, although lacking a prospective randomized design, suggest that intensive education, multidisciplinary care, and surveillance, combined with careful attention to maternal nutrition and weight gain, can improve outcomes in twin pregnancies. Figure 30-14 outlines a reasonable management algorithm for antepartum care unique to twin gestations.

TIMING OF DELIVERY IN MULTIPLE GESTATIONS

Concern over preterm delivery in twin pregnancies sometimes overshadows decision making regarding timing of delivery for twin mothers who remain pregnant at or near term. Numerous population-based studies suggest that the nadir of perinatal complications occurs at earlier gestational ages in multiple gestations compared with singletons.

Unfortunately, the hypothesis that elective early delivery of twins leads to better outcomes has not been subjected to rigorous prospective study. The only randomized study of elective early delivery of twins was quite underpowered, with only 17 women in the induction group and 19 in the expectant management group. Women with uncomplicated pregnancies and a cephalic first twin were randomized at 37 weeks to either labor induction or expectant management. The study found no statistically significant differences in birthweight, Apgar score, or cesarean delivery rate. There were no fetal deaths in either group.[90]

As mentioned previously, there are numerous population-based studies that suggest early delivery of twins could be advantageous. Kahn and colleagues reviewed nearly 300,000 twin pairs and found 39 weeks to be the point of intersection that minimized both the fetal and neonatal death rates.[91] They found that the prospective risk for fetal death in twins equaled that of postterm singletons by 36 to 37 weeks' gestation. Another investigation by Sairam and associates evaluated more than 4000 multiple pregnancies (of which more than 99% were twins) and found that the stillbirth risk at 39 weeks in a twin pregnancy exceeded that of a singleton postterm pregnancy. Twins at 37 to 38 weeks had stillbirth rates equivalent to postterm singletons.[92]

Given consistent evidence of increased risk in twin pregnancies extending past 38 to 39 weeks (analogous to a postdate singleton gestation), a rational delivery approach, supported by the 2011 NICHD and SMFM workshop,[34a] is to plan elective delivery at 38 weeks in well-dated, uncomplicated dichorionic twin pregnancies. Allowing a twin gestation to go past 38 weeks requires convincing evidence of normal fetal growth, amniotic fluid, and fetal testing, as well as a strong patient desire to extend the pregnancy. Prolongation of a twin pregnancy past 39 weeks is not advisable because of clear risk without any known benefit. Figure 30-15 outlines a reasonable approach to planning delivery for uncomplicated term or near-term twin pregnancies.

Twin gestations complicated by maternal or fetal abnormalities will require individualized assessment and decision making. Figure 30-16 provides general guidelines as to how twin gestations complicated by fetal growth restriction, discordant growth, or maternal complications such as mild preeclampsia or cholestasis might be managed. Of course, the timing of delivery in the face of either maternal or fetal complications is influenced by severity and clinical judgment and may require modification of the guidelines outlined in Figure 30-16. For instance, an IUGR twin in less than the third percentile or a pregnancy with more than 35% discordance in estimated fetal weights may be an indication for delivery earlier than 37 weeks even if all other testing is normal. Additionally, twin pregnancies with

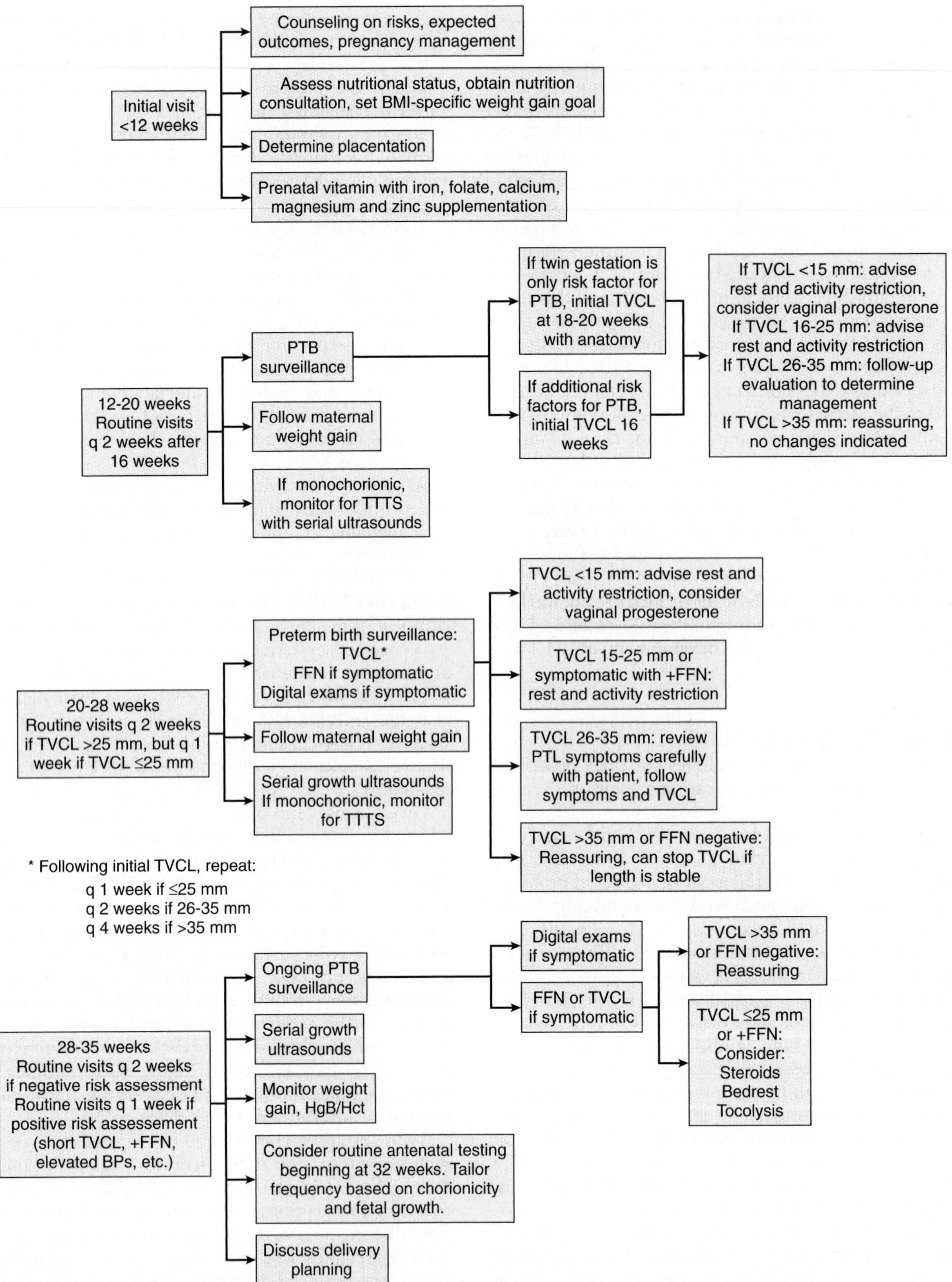

FIGURE 30-14. Suggested algorithm for antepartum management unique to twins. *BMI,* Body mass index; *BP,* Blood pressure; *FFN,* fetal fibronectin; *Hct,* hematocrit; *HgB,* hemoglobin; *PTB,* preterm birth; *TVCL,* transvaginal cervical length; *TTTS,* twin-twin transfusion syndrome.

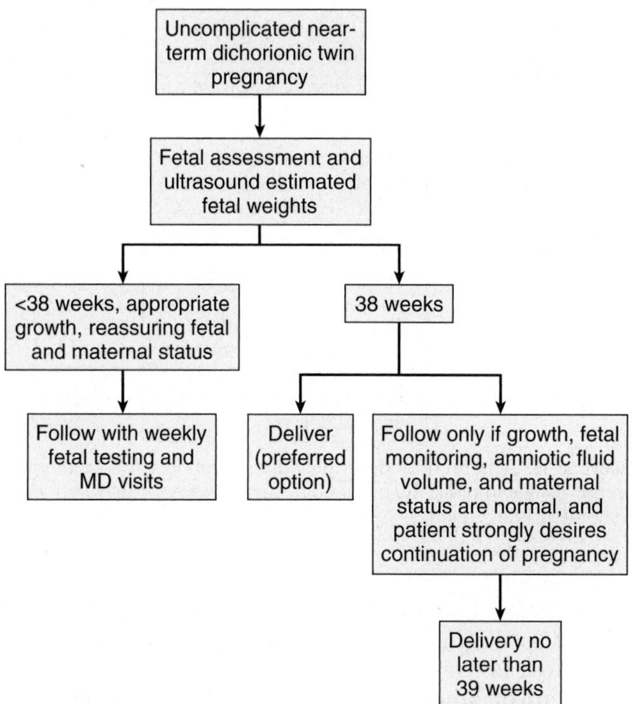

FIGURE 30-15. Timing of delivery for uncomplicated near-term twins.

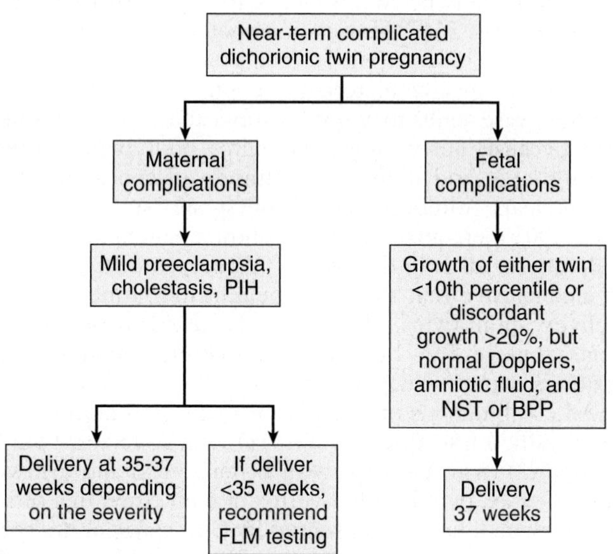

FIGURE 30-16. Timing of delivery for complicated near-term twins. *BPP*, Biophysical profile; *FLM*, fetal lung maturity; *NST*, nonstress test; *PIH*, pregnancy-induced hypertension.

more than one of the listed complications may also warrant delivery earlier than 37 weeks. Similarly, some have argued for elective early delivery of all monochorionic twins, a topic that is discussed in more detail later. Monoamniotic twins were discussed earlier in the chapter.

Monochorionic, Diamniotic Twins: Special Considerations Regarding Delivery Timing

The population-based studies outlined previously addressing the optimal timing of delivery for term and near-term twins included both dichorionic and monochorionic gestations, but they did not differentiate between the two types of placentation when evaluating outcomes. It is well established that monochorionic twins are at greater risk for a variety of pregnancy complications. **However, there is concern among some investigators that even "apparently uncomplicated" monochorionic, diamniotic twins, a term coined by D'Alton and colleagues, are at increased risk for late fetal death.** A retrospective analysis from the United Kingdom reviewed 151 uncomplicated monochorionic pregnancies in women who underwent ultrasound evaluation every 2 weeks and assessed fetal growth, amniotic fluid, and umbilical artery Doppler scans. They found that the risk for unexpected stillbirth after 32 weeks was 4.3% (1 in 23).[93] Another study of 193 monochorionic, diamniotic twin pregnancies in Portugal found that the risk for fetal death after 32 weeks in women undergoing weekly fetal testing was much lower, at 1.2%.[94] Two notable differences exist between these two studies; namely, the first study did not employ weekly fetal testing, as did the second, but rather ultrasound examination every 2 weeks. Interestingly, the authors of the second study noted that 55% of their twins were delivered preterm as a result of the surveillance program.

The latest study of "apparently uncomplicated" monochorionic, diamniotic twin pregnancies examined the records of 196 monochorionic, diamniotic and 804 dichorionic twin pregnancies. These investigators found that the monochorionic twins had higher stillbirth rates than the dichorionic twins (3.6% vs. 1.1%; P=.004), and this increased risk persisted in the "apparently normal" group and was seen at all gestational ages up to 37 weeks (P = .039).[95]

Based on these concerns, some experts recommend offering elective delivery at 34 to 35 weeks in uncomplicated monochorionic, diamniotic twins. This evidence and expert opinion were incorporated into the 2011 NICHD and SMFM workshop paper on timing of indicated late-preterm and early-term birth, which recommends delivery for monochorionic, diamniotic twins between 34 and 37 weeks. It is emphasized that this approach does not yet represent standard of care, and further data may be necessary before this more aggressive approach can be fully embraced. In the absence of early delivery for monochorionic, diamniotic twins, it would be prudent to conduct frequent antenatal testing along with periodic ultrasound assessment and fetal movement counts. Given this more intensive surveillance, it is unknown whether the stillbirth risk would be significantly different than that in uncomplicated dichorionic twins. The topic of antenatal testing for twins was discussed in more detail earlier in the chapter.

Fetal Lung Maturity in Twins

The clinical management of multiple gestations occasionally requires the assessment of fetal lung maturity. There is currently no consensus on whether pulmonary maturation differs between singletons and multiples. If elective delivery is scheduled before 37 to 38 weeks' gestation in dichorionic twins, amniocentesis for fetal lung maturity determination may be considered. Because asynchronous pulmonary maturity can occur in twins regardless of size and gender, if technically feasible, it is suggested that both gestational sacs be sampled when amniocentesis for lung maturity is required. A reasonable approach to

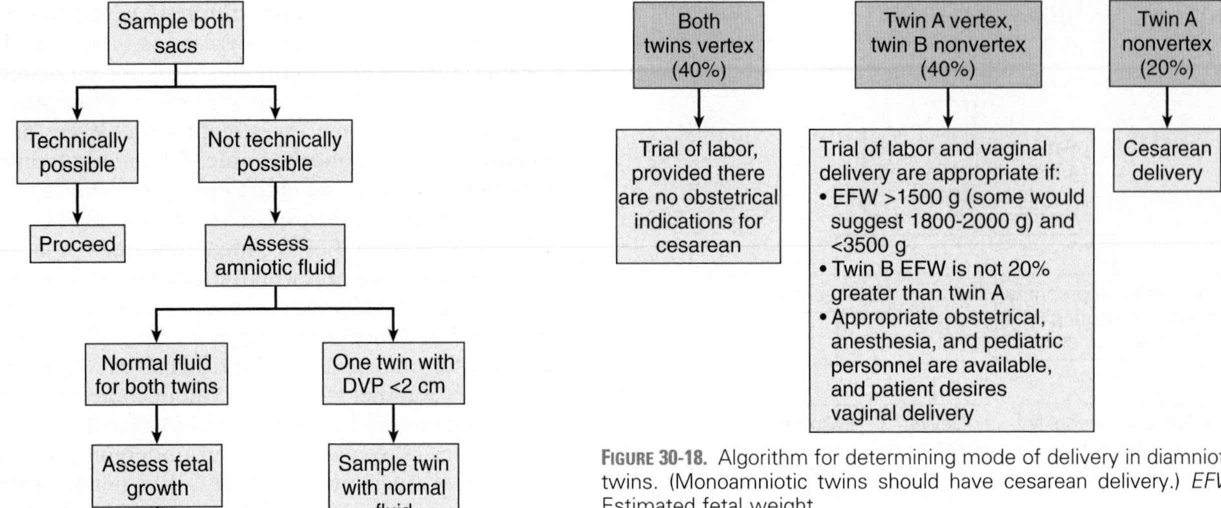

FIGURE 30-17. Assessment of fetal lung maturity in twins. *DVP,* Deepest vertical pocket.

FIGURE 30-18. Algorithm for determining mode of delivery in diamniotic twins. (Monoamniotic twins should have cesarean delivery.) *EFW,* Estimated fetal weight.

assessing fetal lung maturity in diamniotic twins is outlined in Figure 30-17. For pregnancies with triplets and higher-order multiple gestations, there are not enough data to make recommendations regarding amniocentesis for fetal lung maturity.

Timing of Delivery in Triplets

Triplets are clearly at very high risk for significant preterm birth. However, in a review of more than 15,000 triplet pregnancies, about 15% of triplets were undelivered at 36 weeks. That same study found that the point of intersection of fetal and neonatal death for triplets occurred at 36 weeks.[91] Most experts agree that if otherwise uncomplicated, well-grown triplets remain undelivered at 36 weeks, elective delivery should be undertaken.

MODE OF DELIVERY IN MULTIPLE GESTATIONS

A number of factors must be considered when determining the mode of delivery for patients with a multifetal gestation. These variables include the gestational age, estimated weights of the fetuses, their positions relative to each other, the availability of real-time ultrasound on the labor floor and in the delivery room, and the capability of monitoring each twin independently during the entire intrapartum period. Carefully considering all these variables is essential because multiple gestations are inherently at higher risk during the intrapartum period. This risk is illustrated by a large retrospective cohort study published in 2005 that examined neonatal outcomes in all twin births of 36 weeks' gestation or more in Scotland between 1985 and 2001. They found that the odds ratio for death of the second twin due to intrapartum anoxia was 21 (95% CI, 3.4 to 868.5) in twins delivered vaginally compared with those in which both twins underwent cesarean delivery. Death of either twin occurred in 0.14% (2 of 1472) with cesarean delivery compared with 0.52% (34 or 6601) with vaginal delivery ($P = .05$). The researchers calculated that the number of twins requiring cesarean delivery to prevent one death was 264.[96] However, it should be noted that the study had no information on fetal presentation, chorionicity, or other specific maternal or neonatal variables.

Older case series may not be applicable to current practice because our ability to monitor both twins closely during labor and delivery has improved considerably in recent years. Additionally, multiple smaller studies, including a 2003 meta-analysis, do not show a benefit of cesarean delivery for all twin deliveries.[97] At present, the evidence is inconclusive that there is a benefit to routine cesarean delivery of all twins. However, it is clear that twin gestations represent a high-risk intrapartum situation that requires expert management.

All combinations of intrapartum twin presentations can be classified into three groups: (1) twin A vertex, twin B vertex; (2) twin A vertex, twin B nonvertex; and (3) twin A nonvertex, twin B either vertex or nonvertex. In a series of 362 twin deliveries presented by Chervenak and associates,[98] these presentations were found in 42.5%, 38.4%, and 19.1% of cases, respectively. Each scenario is discussed separately next, and recommendations are summarized in Figure 30-18.

Vertex-Vertex Twins

A trial of labor and vaginal delivery is believed to be appropriate for all vertex-vertex twin gestations, regardless of gestational age or estimated fetal weight. No clear benefit to routine cesarean delivery of vertex-vertex twins has been found in the literature, including VLBW deliveries.[97] However, it is important to note that the presentation of the second twin may change in 10% to 20% of cases after delivery of the presenting twin. For this reason, the obstetrician should always discuss this possibility with the patient before delivery. Furthermore, when anticipating a vertex-vertex twin vaginal delivery, the obstetrical team should always have a clear plan for the management of an unexpected nonvertex second twin.

Nonvertex-Presenting Twin

Twin pregnancies with a nonvertex-presenting twin are nearly always managed by cesarean delivery. Historically, this was because of a fear of interlocking fetal heads during delivery of breech-vertex twins. Interlocking fetuses, however, are exceedingly rare. Currently, in an era in which nearly all singleton breech fetuses are delivered by elective cesarean birth, cesarean delivery is also the optimal mode of delivery for twin pregnancies with a nonvertex-presenting fetus.

Vertex-Nonvertex Twins

Although the route of delivery for the previous two scenarios is noncontroversial, the management of that subset of patients whose twins are in a vertex-breech or vertex-transverse lie is subject to significant debate. When the second twin is nonvertex after delivery of the first twin, there are two options for achievement of vaginal delivery: breech extraction or external cephalic version. Although external cephalic version is an acceptable strategy, it has been shown to be associated with more fetal distress and higher rates of cesarean delivery than breech extraction.[99] Thus, provided the obstetrician is sufficiently trained in breech extraction and the fetus is of appropriate size, this is the preferable option for achievement of vaginal delivery with a nonvertex second twin.

Some obstetricians have voiced concerns regarding the safety of breech extraction and have questioned whether it is equivalent in outcome to cesarean delivery. Chervenak and colleagues[98] cite several older references in which depressed Apgar scores and increased perinatal mortality rates were associated with vaginal breech delivery of the second twin. However, in the same report, the authors analyze their own extensive experience, along with a review of the published literature, and conclude that breech extraction of a second twin is a safe and appropriate option if the estimated fetal weight is more than 2000 g. Although the data supported the safety of breech extraction for babies weighing more than 1500 g, these investigators chose 2000 g rather than 1500 g to allow for the margin of error of an ultrasound-estimated fetal weight.

The safety of breech extraction for second twins is supported by the only randomized trial of cesarean delivery versus breech extraction. Rabinovici and associates[100] randomized 66 women with vertex-nonvertex twins of more than 35 weeks' gestation to vaginal delivery with breech extraction or cesarean delivery. They found that there were no differences in neonatal outcomes and no cases of birth trauma or neonatal death. Not surprisingly, maternal febrile morbidity was greater in the cesarean delivery group.

Several other retrospective studies also support the safety of breech extraction of second twins. Gocke and colleagues[99] analyzed 136 sets of vertex-nonvertex twins with a birthweight higher than 1500 g in whom delivery of the second twin was managed by primary cesarean delivery, external version, or primary breech extraction. No differences were noted in the incidence of neonatal mortality or morbidity among the three delivery modes, although external version was associated with a higher failure rate than breech extraction, a higher rate of non-reassuring fetal heart rate patterns, cord prolapse, and compound presentation. The authors concluded that primary breech extraction of the second nonvertex twin weighing more than 1500 g is a reasonable alternative to either cesarean delivery or external version. Fishman and coworkers[101] and Greig and colleagues[102] examined the records of more than 1200 twin gestations and concluded that there was no evidence to support cesarean delivery for nonvertex second twins weighing more than 1500 g. In fact, Greig's data did not show poorer outcomes even for babies weighing less than 1500 g delivered by breech extraction. Nonetheless, most recommend avoidance of breech extractions on second twins with estimated fetal weights of less than 1500 g.

Two recent studies on mode of delivery for twins lend further support to the safety of breech extraction for second twins. Both studies were conducted in single institutions with strict protocols for active second-stage management and breech extraction. Schmitz and colleagues[103] performed a retrospective cohort study of 758 consecutive sets of twins at more than 35 weeks' gestation with a cephalic-presenting twin A. Using a strict protocol for second-stage management in which, after delivery of the vertex-presenting twin, a nonvertex second twin was immediately delivered by total breech extraction, they found that the neonatal composite morbidity for the second twin did not differ between planned cesarean delivery and planned vaginal delivery. The second, more recent study by Fox and coworkers[104] examined a retrospective cohort of 287 twin pregnancies from a single tertiary care academic medical center. The authors described a strict protocol for second-stage management of twin vaginal delivery in which all nonvertex second twins underwent immediate breech extraction and all nonengaged vertex second twins were delivered by immediate internal podalic version and subsequent breech vaginal delivery. The study found no difference in the rates of 5-minute Apgar scores lower than 7 or a cord pH lower than 7.2 between the planned vaginal delivery group ($n = 130$) and the planned cesarean delivery group ($n = 157$).

It should be kept in mind that both of these studies were conducted in a single center by experienced obstetricians using a strict protocol for second-stage management. During the past decade, concerns about outcomes associated with singleton breech deliveries have led to virtual abandonment of vaginal delivery of breech-presenting singletons. As a consequence, fewer obstetricians are acquiring or maintaining the skills needed to safely perform vaginal breech deliveries.

Triplets

Although vaginal delivery is an option for patients with triplets, there are no large prospective studies establishing its safety. Adequate monitoring of three fetuses throughout labor and delivery is challenging. As a result, elective cesarean delivery of patients with three or more live fetuses of viable gestational age is a reasonable management strategy. Vaginal delivery of triplets should only be undertaken under optimal conditions by obstetricians experienced in such deliveries.

INTRAPARTUM MANAGEMENT OF TWIN VAGINAL DELIVERY

Safe vaginal delivery of multiples requires careful preparation and multidisciplinary cooperation between obstetrics, anesthesia, nursing, and neonatology or pediatrics. On admission to labor and delivery, both fetal presentations should be confirmed by ultrasound. If a recent (within 1 to 2 weeks) ultrasound-estimated fetal weight for both babies is not available, this should be obtained and documented. As discussed earlier, knowledge of the presentation, gestational age, and estimated weight of each twin permits the establishment of a plan regarding the anticipated route of delivery.

If a trial of labor is elected, both fetuses should be continuously monitored. Although the woman may labor in a standard room, the delivery itself is best performed in an operating room, in the event that anesthesia or cesarean delivery is emergently needed. Maternal epidural anesthesia is also advisable. The pain control afforded by an epidural enhances maternal cooperation, allows a wide range of obstetrical procedures to be performed quickly, and is available for anesthesia if emergent cesarean delivery becomes necessary. Table 30-9 provides a list of personnel and equipment that should be prepared for each planned vaginal delivery of a multiple gestation.

Time Interval Between Deliveries

A variable that many investigators have historically considered to be important in the outcome of twin pregnancies is the time interval between deliveries. After delivery of the first twin, uterine inertia may develop, the umbilical cord of the second twin can prolapse, and partial separation of its placenta may render the second twin hypoxic. In addition, the cervix can constrict, making rapid delivery of the second twin extremely difficult if non-reassuring fetal status develops. Many reports have suggested that the interval between deliveries should ideally be 15 minutes or less and certainly not more than 30 minutes. Most of the data in support of this view, however, were obtained before the advent of continuous and dual intrapartum fetal monitoring capability.

TABLE 30-9 CHECKLIST FOR MANAGEMENT OF VAGINAL DELIVERY OF TWINS

Personnel and location
Availability of a fully staffed operating room for the delivery, capable of performing an emergency cesarean delivery
Skilled obstetrical attendants present
Anesthesiologist present at delivery
Sufficient neonatal personnel for resuscitation of two infants
Supplies
Capability to continuously monitor both fetuses throughout labor and delivery
Portable ultrasound for intrapartum use
Premixed oxytocin
Methergine, 15-methyl $PGF_{2\alpha}$, misoprostol for postpartum hemorrhage
Nitroglycerin and terbutaline for uterine relaxation
Obstetrical forceps and vacuum (including Piper forceps for aftercoming head)
Blood products immediately available if needed

Rayburn and associates[105] reported the outcome of 115 second twins delivered vaginally at or beyond 34 weeks' gestation after the vertex delivery of their co-twin. Continuous monitoring of the fetal heart rate was performed in all cases. Oxytocin was used if uterine contractions subsided within 10 minutes after delivery of the first twin. In this series, 70 second twins were delivered within 15 minutes of the first twin, 28 within 16 to 30 minutes, and 17 more than 30 minutes later. The longest interval between deliveries was 134 minutes. All these infants survived, and none had a traumatic delivery. All 17 of the neonates delivered beyond 30 minutes had 5-minute Apgar scores between 8 and 10. In those cases with delivery intervals in excess of 15 minutes, the birthweight differential was not in excess of ±200 g when first and second twins were compared. In another series reported by Chervenak and colleagues,[106] when the fetal heart rate of the second twin was monitored with ultrasound visualization throughout the period between twin deliveries, no difference in the occurrence of low 5-minute Apgar scores was noted in relationship to the length of the interdelivery interval.

It appears that although some second twins may require rapid delivery, others can be safely followed with fetal heart rate surveillance and remain undelivered for substantial periods of time. This less hurried approach when the second twin is not demonstrating signs of non-reassuring fetal status may reduce the incidence of both maternal and fetal trauma associated with difficult deliveries performed to meet arbitrary deadlines.

CONCLUSION

The patient carrying more than one fetus presents a formidable challenge to the obstetrician. The elevated perinatal morbidity and mortality rates seen in multiple gestations compared with singletons are due to a variety of factors, some of which cannot currently be altered. However, extraordinary technologic advances during the past 25 years have given us new insights into problems peculiar to multifetal pregnancies as well as tools with which to detect and treat those problems. Early diagnosis of multiple gestations, determination of chorionicity, and serial follow-up studies offer the potential for administering specialized regimens to selected patients, which we hope will lead to a beneficial impact on the outcome of those pregnancies.

KEY POINTS

- Twinning is one of the most common high-risk conditions in all of obstetrics. Both maternal and perinatal morbidity and mortality are significantly higher in multifetal gestations than in singleton pregnancies.
- Chorionicity is a critical determinant of pregnancy outcome and should be ascertained by ultrasound as early in gestation as possible.
- Monochorionic pregnancies are at higher risk than dichorionic, with increased rates of spontaneous abortion, congenital structural anomalies, IUGR,

and IUFD, in addition to a 10% to 15% risk for TTTS, which is a complication unique to monochorionic pregnancies.
- Multiple gestations benefit from specialized care, including attention to maternal nutrition and weight gain, serial assessment of fetal growth by ultrasound, and careful surveillance for signs of preterm labor.
- Routine bedrest, prophylactic tocolytics, prophylactic cerclage, and prophylactic progesterone supplementation have not been shown to be effective in prolonging multiple gestations. However, none of these interventions has been studied in the highest-risk women based on prior obstetrical history, current short cervical lengths, or positive fetal fibronectin assays.
- The nadir of perinatal complications and an increase in stillbirth risk occur earlier in twin gestations than in singletons. Uncomplicated dichorionic twins appear to have the best outcomes if delivered at 38 weeks. There may be a case for earlier delivery in uncomplicated monochorionic, diamniotic twins, but this issue requires further study.
- Monoamniotic twin outcomes are best when managed with a combination of prophylactic antenatal corticosteroids, hospitalization for daily fetal assessment, and elective early cesarean delivery.
- Mode of delivery should take into account gestational age, fetal presentations, estimated weights, and the experience and skill of the obstetrician. A trial of labor is appropriate when both twins are vertex. Mode of delivery should be individualized for vertex-nonvertex twins. Cesarean delivery is optimal when the presenting twin is nonvertex.

REFERENCES

1. Martin JA, Hamilton BE, Sutton PD, et al: Births: Final Data for 2006. National Vital Statistics Reports; Vol 57, No 7. Hyattsville, MD, National Center for Health Statistics, 2009.
2. Carroll SGM, Tyfield L, Reeve L, et al: Is zygosity or chorionicity the main determinant of fetal outcome in twin pregnancies? Am J Obstet Gynecol 193:757, 2005.
3. Hall J: Twinning. Lancet 362:735, 2003.
4. Moise K, Johnson A: There is NO diagnosis of twins. Am J Obstet Gynecol 203:1, 2010.
5. Scardo JA, Ellings JM, Newman RB: Prospective determination of chorionicity, amnionicity and zygosity in twin gestations. Am J Obstet Gynecol 173:1376, 1995.
6. Yeast JD: Maternal physiologic adaptation to twin gestation. Clin Obstet Gynecol 33:10, 1990.
7. Campbell DM, Templeton A: Maternal complications of twin pregnancy. Int J Gynecol Obstet 84:71, 2004.
8. Sibai BM, Hauth J, Caritis S, et al: Hypertensive disorders in twin versus singleton gestations. Am J Obstet Gynecol 182:938, 2000.
9. Day MC, Barton JR, O'Brien JM, et al: The effect of fetal number on the development of hypertensive conditions of pregnancy. Obstet Gynecol 106:927, 2005.
10. Hardardottir H, Kelly K, Bork MD, et al: Atypical presentation of preeclampsia in high-order Multifetal gestations. Obstet Gynecol 87:370, 1996.
11. Bouvier-Colle MH, Varnoux N, Salanave B, et al: Case control study of risk factors for obstetric patients' admission to intensive care units. Eur J Obstet Gynaecol Reprod Biol 79:173, 1997.
12. Senat MV, Ancel PY, Bouvier-Colle MH, et al: How does multiple pregnancy affect maternal mortality and morbidity? Clin Obstet Gynecol 41:79, 1998.
13. Pettersen B, Nelson K, Watson L, et al: Twins, Triplets and cerebral palsy in births in western Australia in the 1980s. BMJ 307:1239, 1993.
14. Mastroiacovo P, Castilla EE, Arpino C, et al: congenital malformations in twins: an international study. Am J Med Genet 83:117, 1999.
15. Glinianaia SV, Rankin J, Wright C: congenital anomalies in twins: a register-based study. Hum Reprod 23:1306, 2008.
16. Chen CJ, Wang CJ, Yu MW, et al: perinatal mortality and prevalence of major congenital malformations of twins in Taipei City. Acta Genet Med Gemellol 41:197, 1992.
17. Nance WE: Malformations unique to the twinning process. Prog Clin Biol Res 69A:123, 1981.
18. Landy HJ, Weiner S, Corson SL, et al: The "vanishing twin:" ultrasonographic assessment of fetal disappearance in the first trimester. Am J Obstet Gynecol 155:14, 1986.
19. Dickey RP, Olar TT, Curole SN, et al: the probability of multiple births when multiple gestational sacs or viable embryos are diagnosed at first trimester ultrasound. Hum Reprod 5:880, 1990.
20. Doubilet PM, Benson CB: "Appearing twin:" undercounting of multiple gestations on early first trimester sonograms. J Ultrasound Med 17:199, 1998.
21. Evans MI, Berkowitz RL, Wapner RJ, et al: Improvement in outcomes of multifetal pregnancy reduction with increased experience. Am J Obstet Gynecol 184:97, 2001.
22. Stone J, Eddleman K, Lynch L, et al: A single center experience with 1000 consecutive cases of multifetal pregnancy reduction. Am J Obstet Gynecol 187:1163, 2002.
23. Stone J, Ferrara L, Kamrath J, et al: Contemporary outcomes with the latest 1000 cases of multifetal pregnancy reduction. Am J Obstet Gynecol 199:406.e1, 2008.
24. Papageorghiou AT, Avgidou K, Bakoulas V, et al: Risks of miscarriage and early preterm birth in trichorionic triplet pregnancies with embryo reduction versus expectant management: new data and systematic review. Hum Reprod 21:1912, 2006.
25. Sun LM, Chen XK, Wen SW, et al: Perinatal outcomes of normal cotwins in twin pregnancies with one structurally anomalous fetus: a population based retrospective study. Am J Perinatol 26:51, 2009.
26. Evans MI, Goldberg JD, Horenstein J, et al: Selective termination for structural, chromosomal, and mendelian anomalies: international experience. Am J Obstet Gynecol 181:893, 1999.
27. Eddleman KA, Stone JL, Lynch L, et al: Selective termination of anomalous fetuses in multifetal pregnancies: two hundred cases at a single center. Am J Obstet Gynecol 187:1168, 2002.
28. Rossi AC, D'Addario V: Umbilical cord occlusion for selective feticide in complicated monochorionic twins: a systematic review of the literature. Am J Obstet Gynecol 200:123, 2009.
29. Lewi L, Gratacos E, Ortibus E, et al: Pregnancy and infant outcome of 80 consecutive cord coagulations in complicated monochorionic multiple pregnancies. Am J Obstet Gynecol 194:782, 2006.
30. Cleary-Goldman J, D'Alton ME: Management of single intrauterine fetal demise in a multiple gestation. Obstet Gynecol Surv 59:285, 2004.
31. Pharoah PO, Adi Y: Consequences of in-utero death in a twin pregnancy. Lancet 355:1597, 2000.
32. Weiss JL, Cleary-Goldman J, Budorick N, et al: Multicystic encephalomalacia after first trimester intrauterine fetal demise in monochorionic twins. Am J Obstet Gynecol 190:563, 2004.
33. Carlson NJ, Towers CV: Multiple gestation complicated by the death of one fetus. Obstet Gynecol 73:685, 1989.
34. Aslan H, Gul A, Cebeci A, et al: The outcome of twin pregnancies complicated by single fetal death after 20 weeks of gestation. Twin Res 7:1, 2004.

34a. Spong CY, Mercer BM, D'Alton M, et al: Timing of Indicated Late-Preterm and Early-Term Birth. Obstet Gynecol 118:323, 2011.

35. Simpson LL, Marx GR, Elkadry EA, et al: Cardiac dysfunction in twin-twin transfusion syndrome: a prospective longitudinal study. Obstet Gynecol 92:557, 1998.
36. Quintero RA, Morales WJ, Allen MH, et al: Staging of twin-twin transfusion syndrome. J Perinatology 19:550, 1999.
37. Taylor MJO, Govender L, Jolly M, et al: Validation of the Quintero staging system for twin-twin transfusion syndrome. Obstet Gynecol 100:1257, 2002.

38. Harkness UF, Crombleholme TM: Twin-twin transfusion syndrome: where do we go from here? Semin Perinatol 29:296, 2005.
39. Rossi AC, D'Addario V: The efficacy of Quintero staging system to assess severity of twin-twin transfusion syndrome treated with laser therapy: a systematic review with meta-analysis. Am J Perinatol 26:537, 2009.
40. Stamilio DM, Fraser WD, Moore TR: Twin-twin transfusion syndrome: an ethics based and evidence-based argument for clinical research. Am J Obstet Gynecol 203:3, 2010.
41. Mari G, Roberts A, Detti L: Perinatal morbidity and mortality rates in severe twin-twin transfusion syndrome: results of the International Amnioreduction Registry. Am J Obstet Gynecol 185:708, 2001.
42. Moise KJ, Dorman K, Lamvu G, et al: A randomized trial of amnioreduction versus septostomy in the treatment of twin-twin transfusion syndrome. Am J Obstet Gynecol 193:701, 2005.
43. Senat MV, Deprest J, Boulvain M, et al: Endoscopic laser surgery versus serial amnioreduction for severe twin-to-twin transfusion syndrome. N Engl J Med 351:136, 2004.
44. Crombleholme TM, Shera D, Lee H, et al: A prospective randomized multicenter trial of amnioreduction vs. selective fetoscopic laser photocoagulation for the treatment of severe twin-twin transfusion syndrome. Am J Obstet Gynecol 197:398.e1, 2007.
45. Roberts D, Neilson JP, Kilby M, et al: Interventions for the treatment of twin-twin transfusion syndrome. Cochrane Database Syst Rev CD002073, 2008.
46. Rossi AC, D'Addario V: Laser therapy and serial amnioreduction as treatment for twin-twin transfusion syndrome: a meta-analysis and review of the literature. Am J Obstet Gynecol 198:147, 2008.
47. Banek CS, Hecher K, Hackeloer BJ, et al: Long-term neurodevelopmental outcome after intrauterine laser treatment for severe twin-twin transfusion syndrome. Am J Obstet Gynecol 188:876, 2003.
48. Lopriore E, Ortibus E, Acosta-Rojas R, et al: Risk factors for neurodevelopmental impairment in twin-twin transfusion syndrome treated with fetoscopic laser surgery. Obstet Gynecol 113:361, 2009.
49. O'Donoghue K, Cartwright E, Galea P, et al: Stage 1 twin-to-twin transfusion syndrome: rates of progression and regression in relation to outcome. Ultrasound Obstet Gynecol 30:958, 2007.
50. Michelfelder E, Gottliebson W, Border W: Early manifestations and spectrum of recipient twin cardiomyopathy in twin-twin transfusion syndrome: relation to Quintero stage. Ultrasound Obstet Gynecol 30:965, 2007.
51. Barrea C, Hornberger LK, Alkazaleh F: Impact of selective laser ablation of placental anastomoses on the cardiovascular pathology of the recipient twin in severe twin-twin transfusion syndrome. Am J Obstet Gynecol 195:1388, 2006.
52. Wagner MM, Lopriore E, Klumper FJ: Short and long-term outcomes in stage 1 twin-to-twin transfusion syndrome treated with laser surgery compared with conservative management. Am J Obstet Gynecol 201:286.e1, 2009.
53. Rodis JF, McIlveen PF, Egan JFX, et al: Monoamniotic twins: improved perinatal survival with accurate prenatal diagnosis and antenatal fetal surveillance. Am J Obstet Gynecol 177:1046, 1997.
54. Roque H, Gillen-Goldstein J, Funai E, et al: Perinatal outcomes in monoamniotic gestations. J Matern Fetal Neonatal Med 13:414, 2003.
55. Heyborne KD, Porreco RP, Garite TJ, et al: Improved perinatal survival of monamniotic twins with intensive inpatient monitoring. Am J Obstet Gynecol 192:96, 2005.
56. Beasley E, Megerian G, Gerson A, et al: Monoamniotic twins: case series and proposal for antenatal management. Obstet Gynecol 93:130, 1999.
57. Carr SR, Aronson MP, Coustan DR: Survival rates of monoamniotic twins do not decrease after 30 weeks' gestation. Am J Obstet Gynecol 163:719, 1990.
58. Tessen JA, Zlatnik FJ: Monoamniotic twins: a retrospective controlled study. Obstet Gynecol 77:832, 1991.
59. Hack KE, Derks JB, Schaap AH, et al: Perinatal outcomes of monoamniotic twin pregnancies. Obstet Gynecol 113:353, 2009.
60. Tan TYT, Sepulveda W: acardiac twin: a systematic review of minimally invasive treatment modalities. Ultrasound Obstet Gynecol 22:419, 2003.
61. Moore TR, Gale S, Benirschke K: perinatal outcome of forty-nine pregnancies complicated by acardiac twinning. Am J Obstet Gynecol 163:907, 1990.
62. MacKenzie TC, Crombleholme TM, Johnson MP, et al: Natural history of prenatally diagnosed conjoined twins. J Pediatr Surg 37:303, 2002.
63. Spitz L: Conjoined twins. Prenat Diagn 25:814, 2005.
64. Goodnight W, Newman R: Optimal nutrition for improved twin pregnancy outcome. Obstet Gynecol 114:1121, 2009.
65. Pederson A, Worthington-Roberts B, Hickok DE: Weight gain patterns during twin gestation. J Am Diet Assoc 89:642, 1989.
66. Luke B, Min SJ, Gillespie B, et al: Importance of early weight gain in the intrauterine growth and birth weight of twins. Am J Obstet Gynecol 179:1155, 1998.
67. Luke B, Minogue J, Witter FR, et al: The ideal twin pregnancy: patterns of weight gain, discordancy, and length of gestation. Am J Obstet Gynecol 169:588, 1993.
68. Luke B, Hediger ML, Nugent C, et al: Body mass index-specific weight gains associated with optimal birth weights in twin pregnancies. J Reprod Med 48:217, 2003.
69. Fox NS, Rebarber A, Roman AS, et al: Weight gain in twin pregnancies and adverse outcomes: examining the 2009 Institute of Medicine Guidelines. Obstet Gynecol 116:100, 2010.
70. Hickman MA, Rowland A, Newman R, et al: Postpartum weight retention after twin pregnancy according to attainment of weight gain goals. Am J Obstet Gynecol 201:S72, 2009.
71. Goldenberg RL, Iams JD, Miodovnik M, et al: The Preterm Prediction Study: risk factors in twin gestations. Am J Obstet Gynecol 175:1047, 1996.
72. Fox NS, Saltzman DH, Klauser CK, et al: Prediction of spontaneous preterm birth in asymptomatic twin pregnancies with the use of combined fetal fibronectin and cervical length. Am J Obstet Gynecol 201:313.e1, 2009.
73. Fox NS, Rebarber A, Klauser CK, et al: Prediction of spontaneous preterm birth in asymptomatic twin pregnancies using the change in cervical length over time. Am J Obstet Gynecol 202:155.e1, 2010.
74. Crowther CA: Hospitalisation and bed rest for multiple pregnancy. Cochrane Database Syst Rev CD000110, 2001.
75. Newman RB, Krombach S, Myers MC, et al: Effect of cerclage on obstetrical outcome in twin gestations with a shortened cervical length. Am J Obstet Gynecol 186:634, 2002.
76. Berghella V, Odibo AO, To MS, et al: Cerclage for short cervix on ultrasonography. Obstet Gynecol 106:181, 2005.
77. Caritis SN, Rouse DJ, Peaceman AM, et al: Prevention of preterm birth in triplets using 17 alpha-hydroxyprogesterone caproate: a randomized controlled trial. Obstet Gynecol 113:285, 2009.
78. Rouse DJ, Caritis SN, Peaceman AM, et al: a trial of 17 alpha-hydroxyprogesterone caproate to prevent prematurity in twins. N Engl J Med 357:454, 2007.
79. Fonseca, EB, Celik E, Parra M, et al: progesterone and the risk of preterm birth among women with a short cervix. N Engl J Med 357:462, 2007.
80. Norman, JE, Owen P, Mactier H, et al: Progesterone for the Prevention of Preterm Birth in Twin Pregnancy (STOPPIT): a randomized, double-blind, placebo-controlled study and meta-analysis. Lancet 373:2034, 2009.
81. Blake GD, Knuppel RA, Ingardia CJ, et al: evaluation of nonstress fetal heart rate testing in multiple gestations. Obstet Gynecol 63:528, 1984.
82. Signore C, Freeman RK, Spong CY: Antenatal testing: a reevaluation: executive summary of a Eunice Kennedy Shriver National Institute of Child Health and Human Development Workshop. Obstet Gynecol 113:687, 2009.
83. Smith APM, Ong S, Smith NCS, et al: A prospective longitudinal study of growth velocity in twin pregnancy. Ultrasound Obstet Gynecol 18:485, 2001.
84. Taylor GM, Owen P, Mires GJ: foetal growth velocities in twin pregnancies. Twin Res 1:9, 1998.
85. Hollier LM, McIntire DD, Leveno KJ: Outcome of twin pregnancies according to intrapair birth weight differences. Obstet Gynecol 94:1006, 1999.
86. Ananth CV, Demissie K, Hanley ML: Birth weight discordancy and adverse perinatal outcomes among twin gestations in the United States: the effect of placental abruption. Am J Obstet Gynecol 188:954, 2003.
87. Van MT, Deprest J, Klaritsch P, et al: ultrasound prediction of intertwin birth weight discordance in monochorionic diamniotic twin pregnancies. Prenat Diagn 29:240, 2009.

88. Ellings JM, Newman RB, Hulsey TC, et al: Reduction in very low birth weight deliveries and perinatal mortality in a specialized, multidisciplinary twin clinic. Obstet Gynecol 81:387, 1993.
89. Luke B, Brown MB, Misiunas R, et al: Specialized prenatal care and maternal and infant outcomes in twin pregnancy. Am J Obstet Gynecol 189:934, 2003.
90. Suzuki S, Otsubo Y, Sawa R, et al: clinical trial of induction of labor versus expectant management in twin pregnancy. Gynecol Obstet Invest 49:24, 2000.
91. Kahn B, Lumey LH, Zybert PA, et al: prospective risk of fetal death in singleton, twin, and triplet gestations: implications for practice. Obstet Gynecol 102:685, 2003.
92. Sairam S, Costeloe K, Thilaganathan B: prospective risk of stillbirth in multiple gestation pregnancies: a population-based analysis. Obstet Gynecol 100:638, 2002.
93. Barigye O, Pasquini L, Galea P, et al: High risk of unexpected late fetal death in monochorionic twins despite intensive ultrasound surveillance: a cohort study. PLoS Med 2:e172, 2005.
94. Simões T, Amaral N, Lerman R, et al: prospective risk of intrauterine death of monochorionic-diamniotic twins. Am J Obstet Gynecol 195:134, 2006.
95. Lee YM, Wylie BJ, Simpson LL, et al: Twin chorionicity and the risk of stillbirth. Obstet Gynecol 111:301, 2008.
96. Smith GCS, Shah I, White IR, et al: mode of delivery and the risk of delivery-related perinatal death among twins at term: a retrospective cohort study of 8073 births. Br J Obstet Gynaecol 112:1139, 2005.
97. Hogle KL, Hutton EK, McBrien KA, et al: Cesarean delivery for twins: a systematic review and meta-analysis. Am J Obstet Gynecol 188:220, 2003.
98. Chervenak FA, Johnson RE, Youcha S, et al: Intrapartum management of twin gestation. Obstet Gynecol 65:119, 1985.
99. Gocke SE, Nageotte MP, Garite T, et al: management of the nonvertex second twin: primary cesarean section, external version or primary breech extraction. Am J Obstet Gynecol 161:111, 1989.
100. Rabinovici J, Barkai G, Reichman B, et al: randomized management of the second nonvertex twin: vaginal delivery or cesarean section. Am J Obstet Gynecol 156:52, 1987.
101. Fishman A, Grubb DK, Kovacs BW, et al: Vaginal delivery of the nonvertex second twin. Am J Obstet Gynecol 168:861, 1993.
102. Greig PC, Veille JC, Morgan T, et al: The effect of presentation and mode of delivery on neonatal outcome in the second twin. Am J Obstet Gynecol 167:901, 1992.
103. Schmitz T, Carnavalet CDC, Azria E, et al: Neonatal outcomes of twin pregnancy according to the planned mode of delivery. Obstet Gynecol 111:695, 2008.
104. Fox NS, Silverstein M, Bender S, et al: Active second-stage management in twin pregnancies undergoing planned vaginal delivery in a U.S. population. Obstet Gynecol 115:229, 2010.
105. Rayburn WF, Lavin JP, Miodovnik M, et al: Multiple gestation: time interval between delivery of the first and second twins. Obstet Gynecol 63:502, 1984.
106. Chervenak FA, Johnson RE, Berkowitz RL, Hobbins JC: Intrapartum external version of the second twin. Obstet Gynecol 62:160, 1983.

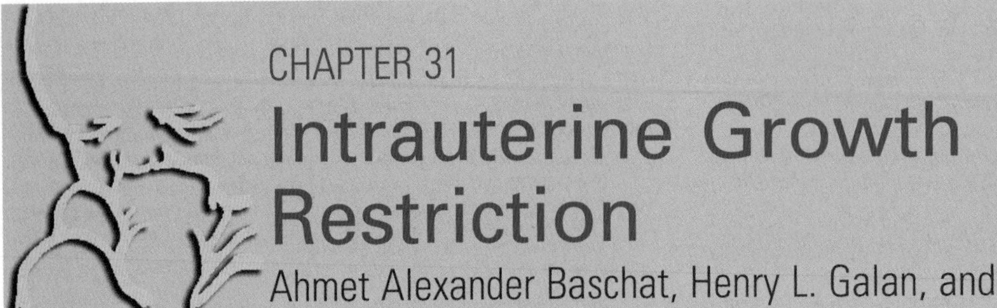

CHAPTER 31

Intrauterine Growth Restriction

Ahmet Alexander Baschat, Henry L. Galan, and Steven G. Gabbe

KEY ABBREVIATIONS	
Abdominal Circumference	AC
Absent End-Diastolic Velocity	AEDV
Amniotic Fluid Index	AFI
Amniotic Fluid Volume	AFV
Appropriate for Gestational Age	AGA
Biophysical Profile	BPS
Biparietal Diameter	BPD
Cerebroplacental Doppler Ratio	CPR
Computerized Cardiotocography	cCTG
Contraction Stress Test	CST
Femur Length	FL
Head Circumference	HC
Humerus Length	HL
Intrauterine Growth Restriction	IUGR
Low Birthweight	LBW
Neonatal Intensive Care Unit	NICU
Nonstress Test	NST
Respiratory Distress Syndrome	RDS
Reversed End-Diastolic Velocity	REDV
Small for Gestational Age	SGA
Sonographically Estimated Fetal Weight	SEFW
Systolic/Diastolic Ratio	S/D

The identification of pregnancies at risk for preventable perinatal handicap is a primary goal of the obstetric care provider. Pregnancies in which adverse intrauterine conditions result in failure of the fetus to reach its growth potential constitute such a high-risk group. Next to prematurity, intrauterine growth restriction (IUGR) is the second leading cause of perinatal mortality. **Compared to appropriately grown counterparts, perinatal mortality rates in growth-restricted neonates are 6 to 10 times greater; perinatal mortality rates as high as 120 per 1000 for all cases of IUGR and 80 per 1000 after exclusion of anomalous infants have been reported. As many as 53% of preterm stillbirths and 26% of term stillbirths are growth restricted.** In survivors, the incidence of intrapartum asphyxia may be as high as 50%.[1] Prevention of some perinatal complications that lead to adverse outcomes in growth-restricted fetuses is possible with appropriate prenatal identification and management. This chapter reviews normal and disturbed fetal growth, the definition of abnormal fetal growth, the impact of fetal growth restriction, and the incorporation of this knowledge into screening, diagnosis, and management of these high-risk pregnancies.

REGULATION OF FETAL GROWTH

Fetal growth is regulated at multiple levels and requires successful development of the placental interface between maternal and fetal compartments. In the early first trimester, anchoring villi originating from the cytotrophoblast connect the decidua to the uterus and thereby establish placental adherence. This allows formation of vascular connections between the maternal circulation and the intervillous space so that increasing quantities of placental secretory products can reach the maternal circulation. Endocrine and paracrine signaling between the placenta and maternal compartment promotes maternal metabolic and cardiovascular adaptations to pregnancy that result in greater substrate availability and enhanced placental perfusion, thereby supporting placental growth. The development of placental mass is critical for its synthetic capacity while vascular development permits nutrient and oxygen delivery to the growing trophoblast beyond the capacity of simple diffusion.

The villous trophoblast becomes the primary placental site of maternal-fetal exchange. By 16 weeks' gestation the maternal microvillous and fetal basal layer are only 4 microns apart, posing little resistance to passive diffusion. Elaboration of active transport mechanisms for three major nutrient classes (glucose, amino acids, and free fatty acids) and an increase in the villous surface area raise the capacity and efficiency of active transplacental transport. Vascular throughput across the placenta also increases in the maternal and fetal compartments. Extravillous cytotrophoblast invasion of the maternal spiral arteries results in progressive loss of the musculoelastic media, a process paralleled on the fetal side by continuous villous vascular branching. This results in significant reduction of blood flow resistance in the uterine and umbilical vessels, converting both circulations into low-resistance, high-capacitance vascular beds. The decrease in vascular resistance is related to two waves of angiogenesis within the placenta. The first is branching angiogenesis occurring at the end of the first and beginning of the second trimester, which increases the number of vascular branches. The second wave is nonbranching angiogenesis, which does not create additional branches but rather results in elongation of the existing placental vascular tree. This latter process occurs at the end of the second and beginning of the third trimester. Owing to these developments, as much as 600 mL/min of maternal cardiac output reaches a placental exchange area of up to 12 m^2 at term. In the fetal compartment this is matched with a blood flow volume of 200-300 mL/kg/min throughout gestation. This magnitude of maternal blood flow is necessary to ensure maintenance of placental function that is energy intensive and consumes as much as 40% of the oxygen and 70% of the glucose supplied. Optimal fetal growth and development depends on a magnitude of maternal nutrient and oxygen delivery to the uterus that leaves sufficient surplus for fetal substrate utilization.

Of the actively transported primary nutrients, glucose is the predominant oxidative fuel while amino acids are major contributors to protein synthesis and muscle bulk. Glucose and, to a lesser extent, amino acids drive the insulin-like growth factors axis and therefore stimulate longitudinal fetal growth. Fatty acids are necessary for the maintenance of cell membrane fluidity and permeability and also act as precursors for important bioactive compounds such as prostaglandins, thromoboxanes, and leukotrienes. Long-chain polyunsaturated fatty acids such as arachidonic acid and docosahexanoic acid are essential for normal brain and retinal development. Leptin is the hormone that co-regulates transplacental amino acid and fatty acid transport and thereby modulates fetal body fat content and proportions.

Concurrent development and maturation of the fetal circulation as a conduit for nutrient and waste delivery allows preferential partitioning of nutrients in the fetus. Nutrient- and oxygen-rich blood from the primitive villous circulation enters the fetus via the umbilical vein. The ductus venosus is the first vascular partitioning shunt encountered. Through modulation in ductus venosus shunting, the proportion of umbilical venous blood that is distributed to the liver and heart changes with advancing gestation. **Near term, 18% to 25% of umbilical venous flow shunts through the ductus venosus to reach the right atrium in this high-velocity stream, while 55% reaches the dominant left hepatic lobe and 20% the right liver lobes (Figure 31-1).** The differences in direction and velocity of blood streams entering the right atrium ensures that nutrient-rich blood is distributed to the left ventricle, myocardium, and brain while low-nutrient venous return is distributed to the placenta for reoxygenation and waste exchange. **This process of blood distribution is referred to as "preferential streaming."**[2] In addition to this overall distribution of left- and right-sided cardiac output, several organs can modify local blood flow to meet oxygen and nutrient demands by autoregulation.

When the milestones in maternal, placental, and fetal development are met, placental and fetal growth progress normally. The metabolic and vascular maternal adaptations promote a steady and enhanced nutrient delivery to the uterus, and placental transport mechanisms allow for efficient bi-directional exchange of nutrient and waste. Placental and fetal growths across the three trimesters are characterized by sequential cellular hyperplasia, hyperplasia plus hypertrophy, and, lastly, hypertrophy alone. Placental growth follows a sigmoid curve that plateaus in midgestation preceding exponential third-trimester growth of the fetus. During this exponential fetal growth phase of 1.5% per day, initial weight gain is due to longitudinal growth and muscle bulk and therefore correlates with glucose and amino acid transport. Eighty percent of fetal fat gain is accrued after 28 weeks' gestation, providing essential body stores in preparation to extrauterine life. From 32 weeks onward, fat stores increase from 3.2% of fetal body weight to 16%, accounting for the significant reduction in body water content.[3]

The ultimate growth potential of the placenta and the fetus are genetically predetermined as indicated by their relationship with the maternal body mass index and ethnicity. This genetically predetermined growth potential is probably further modified by other maternal, placental, and fetal factors that finally determine the size of the individual at birth. Several possible mechanisms may challenge compensatory capacity of the maternal-placental-fetal unit to such an extent that failure to reach the growth potential may be the end result.

DEFINITION AND PATTERNS OF FETAL GROWTH RESTRICTION

Normal fetal growth involves hyperplasia and hypertrophy on a cellular level. Disturbance of fetal growth dynamics can lead to a reduced cell number, cell size, or both, ultimately resulting in abnormal weight, body mass, or body proportion at birth. The classification of abnormal growth has evolved significantly over the last century. From its modern origins in 1919 when Ylppo was the first to label neonates with a birthweight below 2500 grams as "premature" to the description of individualized growth potential,

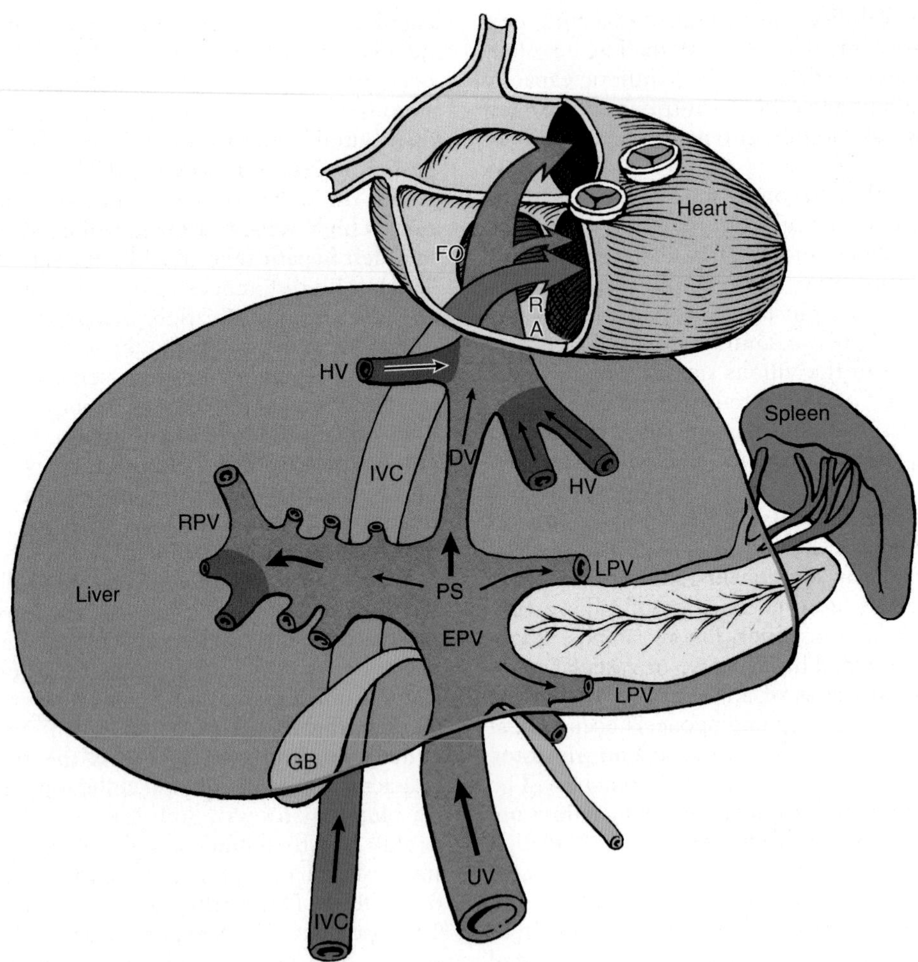

FIGURE 31-1. Fetal umbilical and hepatic venous circulation. The *arrows* indicate the direction of blood flow and the color, the degree of oxygen content (red = high, purple = medium, blue = low). The arrows indicate the direction of blood flow. *DV,* Ductus venosus; *EPV,* extrahepatic portal vein; *FO,* foramen ovale; *GB,* gall bladder *HV,* hepatic veins; *IVC,* inferior vena cava; *LPV,* left portal vein; *PS,* portal sinus; *RA,* right atrium; *RPV,* right portal vein; *UV,* umbilical vein. (Reproduced from Mavrides E, et al: The anatomy of the umbilical, portal and hepatic venous systems in the human fetus at 14-19 weeks of gestation. Ultrasound Obstet Gynecol 18:598, 2001.)

the recognition of the growth-restricted neonate has advanced significantly. With the advent of ultrasound, the recognition and study of fetal growth abnormalities extended into the prenatal period. It is important to note that several definitions describing abnormal growth are used interchangeably in the obstetric and pediatric literature, but that they do not necessarily describe the same population.

The terminology for classifying fetal growth disorders has specifically expanded over the last four decades, which has led to confusion among the various terms used. From the 1960s, growth has been classified by the absolute birthweight value as low birthweight (<2500 grams), very low birthweight (VLBW; <1500 grams), extremely low birth weight (ELBW; <1000 grams), or macrosomia (>4000 grams). Subsequently, studies by Lubchenco, Usher, Battaglia and others demonstrated that only the comparison of the actual birthweight to the expected weight in a population at the same gestational age identified small neonates at risk for adverse outcome. Adopting this concept of "light" and "heavy" for gestational age served as an introduction of population-based reference ranges for birthweight in the 1970s and allowed classification of growth by the birthweight percentile. This resulted in the currently accepted classification of birthweight as very small for gestational age (VSGA; <3rd percentile), small for gestational age (SGA; <10th percentile), appropriate for gestational age (AGA; 10th-90th percentile), or large for gestational age (LGA; >90th percentile). Although birthweight percentiles are superior in identifying the small neonate, they fail to account for proportionality of growth and the growth potential of the individual. Therefore, neonates that have a normal birthweight percentile but abnormal body proportion as a result of differential growth delay may be missed. Similarly, birthweight percentiles do not distinguish between the small neonate that is normally grown given his genetic potential, and the neonate that is growth restricted due to a disease process.

The detection of abnormal body mass, or proportions, is based on anthropometric measurements and ratios that are relatively independent of gender, race, and to a certain extent gestational age and therefore also the traditional birthweight percentiles. **The ponderal index [(birthweight (g) / crown heel length)^3 × 100] has a high accuracy for the**

identification of IUGR and macrosomia. The ponderal index correlates more closely with perinatal morbidity and mortality than traditional birthweight percentiles, but may miss the proportionally small and lean growth-restricted neonate. The classification of abnormal growth is also enhanced by adjusting birthweight reference limits for first trimester maternal height, race, birth order, and fetal/neonatal sex (growth potential). The birthweight percentile that is based on this individualized growth potential accounts for these possible sources of errors and is superior in the prediction of adverse perinatal outcome to conventional reference ranges.[4] It is anticipated that "growth potential" type curves will eventually become the primary tool in identifying the growth-restricted fetus antenatally.

The classification of abnormal growth during fetal life marks a significant advance because it opens the possibility of prenatal detection that leads to preventive or therapeutic management. The concept of percentiles has been adopted to the ultrasound biometry of the fetus. Accordingly parameters of head, abdominal, and skeletal growth are related to population-based reference ranges. The prenatal diagnosis of fetal growth restriction based on ultrasound biometry is described in detail below.

In addition to the detection of smaller individual measurements and lower weight, two principal patterns of disturbed fetal growth have been described: asymmetric and symmetric. In the asymmetric growth pattern, somatic growth (e.g., the abdominal circumference [AC] and lower body) shows a significant delay while there is relative or absolute sparing of head growth. In the symmetric form, body and head growth are similarly affected. Asymmetric growth patterns result from two processes. Firstly, liver volume is reduced due to depletion of glycogen stores as the result of limited nutrient supply, which leads to a decrease in abdominal circumference. Secondly, elevations in placental blood flow resistance increase right cardiac afterload and promote diversion of the cardiac output toward the left ventricle due to the parallel arrangement of the fetal circulation and the presence of central shunts. Blood and nutrient supply to vital structures in the upper part of the body thus increase, presumably resulting in relative "head sparing." Symmetrically restricted fetal growth typically results when interference with the growth process results in decreased cell numbers and cell size, typically resulting from a first trimester insult. As a result, all parts of the body are equally affected, producing uniformly small growth.

The pattern of fetal growth depends on the underlying cause of growth delay and on the timing and duration of the insult. Uteroplacental insufficiency is typically associated with asymmetric fetal growth delay owing to the aforementioned mechanisms. Aneuploidy, nonaneuploid syndromes, and viral infections either disrupt the regulation of growth processes, or interfere with growth at the stage of cell hyperplasia. This typically results in a symmetric growth delay. Specific conditions, such as skeletal dysplasia, may produce distinct growth patterns by their differential impacts on axial and peripheral skeletal growth. Because growth is dynamic, the pattern of growth restriction may evolve in the course of gestation. Placental disease may initially present with relative head sparing, but eventually progress to symmetrical growth delay as placental insufficiency worsens. Alternatively, the acute course of a fetal viral illness may temporarily result in arrested growth with subsequent resumption of a normal growth pattern.

While the definition and classification of fetal growth restriction has significantly evolved, research is still ongoing. Small fetal and/or neonatal size have to be considered as a physical sign rather than a specific disease warranting further investigation of underlying causes. For the purpose of this chapter, fetal growth restriction or IUGR only refers to fetuses with underlying placental pathology. Small for gestational age (SGA) refers to neonates in whom no causative pathology for the small size is evident. From the perspective of the managing obstetrician, prenatal identification of IUGR is most relevant, since it allows appropriate prospective fetal management. To formulate a uniform approach to prenatal detection and perinatal management, an understanding of the maternal and fetal impact of placental insufficiency is essential.

ETIOLOGIES OF INTRAUTERINE GROWTH RESTRICTION

The precise mechanisms by which various conditions interfere with normal placentation and culminate in either pregnancy loss or IUGR are of great importance. Conditions that result in fetal growth restriction broadly consist of maternal, uterine, placental, and fetal disorders. These conditions result in growth delay by affecting nutrient and oxygen delivery to the placenta (maternal causes), nutrient and oxygen transfer across the placenta (placental causes), and fetal nutrient uptake or regulation of growth processes (fetal causes). In clinical practice, there may be considerable overlap between the conditions that determine manifestation, progression, and outcome.

Maternal causes of fetal growth restriction include vascular disease such as hypertensive disorders of pregnancy, diabetic vasculopathy, chronic renal disease, collagen vascular disease, and thrombophilia. The associated decrease in uteroplacental blood flow is responsible for the majority of clinically recognized cases of IUGR. Poor maternal volume expansion, as may be observed in hypertensive disorders or genetic conditions such as angiotensinogen gene mutations or living at high altitude, have also been reported to compromise placental blood flow by reducing the circulating blood volume, hyperviscosity, and sludging. In addition, reduction of maternal oxygenation found in women living at high altitude, or with cyanotic heart disease, parenchymal lung disease, or reduced oxygen-carrying capacity, as observed with certain hemoglobinopathies and anemias, may be responsible for the cases of IUGR described in these conditions.

Poor maternal weight gain is a long recognized risk factor for IUGR. Studies of the offspring of pregnant women with dietary restrictions suggest that limited protein intake, especially prior to 26 weeks' gestation, can result in symmetric IUGR, while caloric restriction (maternal intake of 600 to 900 calories daily for 6 months) has only moderate effects on birthweight. The degree of malnourishment observed in the studies of Guatemalan women or during the Dutch famine would not ordinarily be found in the United States. **Nevertheless, maternal prepregnancy weight and weight gain in pregnancy are two of the most important**

variables contributing to birthweight. It is conceivable that malnutrition due to gastrointestinal syndromes such as Crohn's disease, ulcerative colitis, or bypass surgery can result in lower birthweight. However, an association with IUGR is infrequent in these conditions.

Glucose is a critical fetal nutrient driving longitudinal fetal growth. Reduced glucose supply to the fetoplacental unit can result in fetal growth restriction. This was suspected by Economides and Nicolaides, who observed significantly lower maternal and fetal glucose levels in growth-restricted fetuses. Khouzami and colleagues documented a significant association between relative maternal hypoglycemia on a 3-hour oral glucose tolerance test (GTT) and subsequent birth of non-low-birthweight but growth-restricted babies. Sokol and colleagues and Langer and colleagues have confirmed that a flat maternal response to glucose loading increased the risk for poor fetal growth as much as 20-fold.

Maternal drug ingestion may result in IUGR by a direct effect on fetal growth as well as through inadequate dietary intake. Smoking produces a symmetrically smaller fetus through reduced uterine blood flow and impaired fetal oxygenation and is a major cause of growth restriction in developed countries. The consumption of alcohol and the use of warfarin or hydantoin derivatives are now well known to produce particular dysmorphic features in association with impaired fetal growth. Mills and colleagues have demonstrated a significant increase in the risk of IUGR with the consumption of one to two drinks daily, in the absence of fetal alcohol syndrome. Maternal use of cocaine has been associated with not only IUGR but also reduced head circumference (HC) growth.

In 1971, Lobi and colleagues reported that advanced maternal age was a factor in the etiology of IUGR. Berkowitz and colleagues found no evidence that the first births of women between 30 and 34 years or those over 35 years were at increased risk for growth restriction. Chronic medical conditions of the mother do increase the risk of IUGR. **However, if one controls for underlying medical complications, maternal age is not related to restricted fetal growth.**

Multiple risk factors can act synergistically on fetal growth. For example, the adverse impact of smoking is doubled in thin Caucasian women and further potentiated by poor maternal weight gain. Similarly, the possible benefits of low-dose aspirin and the detrimental effects of excessive blood pressure reduction are also more apparent in this group of women.

Fetoplacental causes can result in fetal growth restriction due to abnormalities of the fetus and/or placenta. Chromosomal abnormalities, congenital malformations, and genetic syndromes have been associated with less than 10% of cases of IUGR.[5] Similarly, intrauterine infection, though long recognized as a cause of growth restriction, also accounts for less than 10% of all cases. However, genetic and infectious etiologies are of special importance because perinatal and long-term outcome are ultimately determined by the underlying condition, with little potential impact through perinatal interventions.

Growth restriction has been observed in 53% of cases of trisomy 13, and 64% of cases of trisomy 18, and may be manifest as early as the first trimester. Other conditions that may present with fetal growth restriction include skeletal dysplasia and Cornelia De Lange syndrome. The database of online inheritance in man lists over 100 genetic syndromes that may be associated with fetal growth restriction. Of the infectious agents, herpes, cytomegalovirus, rubella, and *Toxoplasma gondii* are well-documented causes of symmetric IUGR.

Abnormal placental development with subsequent placental insufficiency is a relatively common problem affecting about one third of cases with IUGR or about 3% of all pregnancies. Placental insufficiency accounts for the vast majority of IUGR in singleton pregnancies. An absolute or relative decrease in placental mass affects the quantity of substrate the fetus receives and antedates the development of IUGR. Thus, abnormal placental vascular development, circumvallate placenta, partial placental abruption, placenta accreta, placental infarction, or hemangioma may result in growth restriction. Intrinsic placental pathology, such as a single umbilical artery and placental mosaicism, has been identified in some cases of growth restriction.[6] Placental implantation in the lower uterine segment in placenta previa is considered suboptimal for nutrient and may therefore result in IUGR even in the absence of chronic hemorrhage.

Twin gestation is often associated with IUGR (see Chapter 30). In 1966, Gruenwald observed that the growth curve of twins deviated from that of singletons with a progressive fall of growth after 32 weeks. This finding implies relative placental insufficiency as opposed to intrinsic fetal compromise and suggests that the longer the twin pregnancy continues, the greater the delay in intrauterine growth, with "catch-up" growth observed after birth. Thus, twins represent a group of fetuses at high risk for IUGR, as confirmed by an incidence of 17.5% in one study. The appropriate growth standard to apply to twin fetuses would appear to be the same as that for singletons. Two trials demonstrate that the morbidity and mortality of fetuses from twin gestations are equivalent, or elevated when the twins are monochorionic, when compared with birthweight- and gestational age-matched singletons.[7] **Although it is beyond the scope of this chapter to discuss the spectrum of clinical consequences, it needs to be recognized that the diagnosis and prognosis of fetal growth restriction in twin pregnancies is critically determined by the chorionicity. Selective intrauterine growth restriction (sIUGR) is a specific term that is applied to fetal growth restriction occurring in monochorionic twins. The prognosis and risk profile can be determined based on the umbilical artery flow pattern.**[8]

MATERNAL AND FETAL MANIFESTATIONS OF INTRAUTERINE GROWTH RESTRICTION

The impact of placental insufficiency depends on the gestational age at onset and the severity of the placental disease. Early interference with normal placentation affects all levels of placental and fetal development and culminates in the most severe clinical picture, which may result in miscarriage, or early stillbirth. If sufficient supply to the placental mass can be established, further placental differentiation may be possible, but suboptimal maternal adaptation to pregnancy and deficient nutrient delivery pose limitations. If adaptive mechanisms permit ongoing fetal survival, early-onset growth restriction with its many fetal manifestations develops. If placental disease is mild or successful compensation has occurred, the consequences of nutrient shortage may remain largely subclinical, only to be unmasked through its restrictive effect on exponential fetal growth in the second to third trimester. In these cases, late-onset growth delay, a decrease in adipose tissue, or abnormal body proportions at birth may be the consequence.

Maternal Impacts

Placental dysfunction affects several aspects of maternal adaptation to pregnancy. Associations between poor placentation with suboptimal maternal volume expansion, increased vascular reactivity, and a "flat" glucose tolerance have been described. Abnormalities of placental vascular development are of special interest because they can be detected by Doppler ultrasound of the uterine arteries and frequently predate clinical disease (Figure 31-2). When trophoblast invasion remains confined to the decidual portion of the myometrium, maternal spiral and radial arteries fail to undergo the physiologic transformation into low-resistance vessels, which is generally expected by 22 to 24 weeks. **Maternal placental floor infarcts, fetal villous obliteration, and fibrosis each increase placental blood flow resistance, producing maternal-fetal placental perfusion mismatch that decreases the effective exchange area.** With progressive vascular occlusion fetoplacental flow resistance is increased throughout the vascular bed and eventually metabolically active placental mass is reduced. The diagnostic and screening utility of ultrasound findings that are suggestive of such pathology is discussed below.

Fetal Impacts

When placental dysfunction compromises nutrient delivery triggering fetal mobilization of hepatic glycogen stores, physical manifestation of growth delay becomes clinically apparent. In addition to the cardinal sign of fetal growth restriction, metabolic, endocrine, hematologic, cardiovascular, and behavioral manifestations of placental insufficiency have been described that relate to the severity and duration of placental dysfunction. Of these, cardiovascular and central nervous system (CNS) responses are best studied because their noninvasive assessment is readily achieved by multivessel Doppler, gray-scale ultrasound, and fetal heart rate (FHR) analysis and therefore can be utilized for fetal surveillance. Appreciating the variety of fetal manifestations helps to understand the potential limitations of antenatal surveillance and provides a basis to appreciate the possible short- and long-term impacts of placental insufficiency.

Metabolic manifestations occur early in growth-restricted fetuses. This is because with mild to moderate decline in uterine nutrient delivery, fetal supply is compromised first, while placental nutrition is preferentially maintained. With progression of placental insufficiency, nutrient deficits become universal and result in decreased fetal and placental size. Accordingly, with mild restrictions in oxygen and glucose supply, fetal demands are still met by increased fractional extraction. When uterine oxygen delivery falls below a critical value (0.6 mmol/min/kg fetal body weight in sheep), fetal oxygenation begins to fall and is eventually accompanied by fetal hypoglycemia. The initially mild hypoglycemia results in a blunted fetal pancreatic insulin response allowing gluconeogenesis from hepatic glycogen stores. The minimal hepatic glycogen stores in the fetus are quickly depleted as glucose and lactate are preferentially diverted to the placenta. An increasing nutrient deficit leads to worsening fetal hypoglycemia, decreasing the maintenance of fetal oxidative metabolism and placental nutrition. With a more significant limitation of oxidative metabolism, associated with down-regulation of placental transport mechanisms and intensifying hypoglycemia, the use of other fetal energy sources becomes necessary, and more widespread metabolic consequences ensue. Limitation of amino acid transfer and breakdown of endogenous muscle protein to obtain gluconeogenic amino acids depletes branched chain and other essential amino acids.[9] Simultaneously, lactate accumulates due to the limited capacity for oxidative metabolism. Placental transfer of fatty acids loses its selectivity, particularly for essential fatty acids. Reduced utilization leads to increased fetal free fatty acid and triglyceride levels with

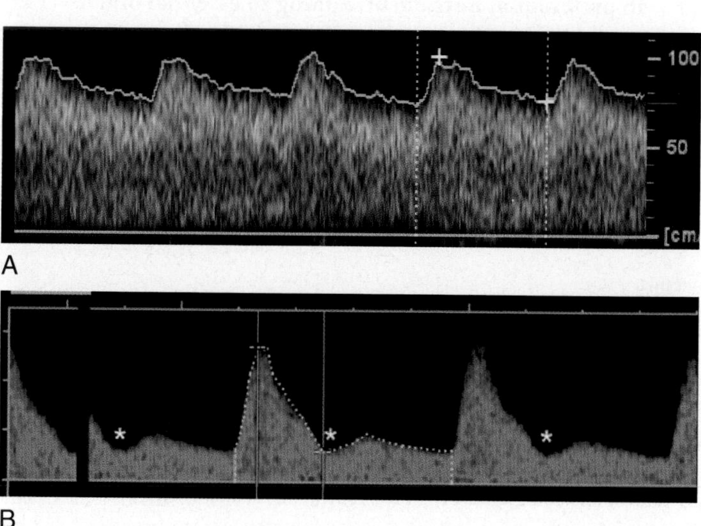

Figure 31-2. Uterine artery flow velocity waveforms. Normal trophoblast invasion results in a low-resistance, high-capacitance placental vascular circulation that can be documented with uterine artery Doppler velocimetry. The flow velocity waveform in panel **A** was obtained at 24 weeks' gestation and shows high diastolic flow velocities. Such a flow pattern indicates successful trophoblast invasion. The second waveform **(B)**, on the other hand, shows lower diastolic velocities and an early diastolic notch *(*)*. This flow pattern is reflective of increased blood flow resistance in the spiral arteries and the downstream placental vascular bed. Persistence of notching beyond 24 weeks' gestation is associated with an increased risk of fetal growth restriction and/or hypertensive disorders of pregnancy.

a subsequent failure to accumulate adipose stores. In this setting of advancing malnutrition, cerebral and cardiac metabolism of lactate and ketones is upregulated to remove these accumulating products of anaerobic metabolism. Acid–base balance can be maintained as long as acid production is met by sufficient buffering capacity of fetal hemoglobin and an equal disposition by these organs. Thus metabolic compromise progresses from simple hypoglycemia, hypoxemia, and decreased levels of essential amino acids to overt hypoaminoacidemia, hypercapnia, hypertriglyceridemia, and hyperlacticemia. The lactate production is exponentially correlated to the degree of acidemia that generally results from this metabolic state.[10] A summary of metabolic responses is provided in Table 31-1.

Fetal endocrine manifestations of placental insufficiency are of relevance because they are responsible for the downregulation of growth and developmental processes. Decrease in fetal glucose and amino acids indirectly downregulates insulin and insulin-like growth factors I and II as the principal endocrine regulators of longitudinal growth. Leptin-coordinated deposition of fat stores is similarly affected. In addition, pancreatic cellular dysfunction becomes evident through a decreased insulin/glucose ratio and impaired fetal glucose tolerance. Significant elevations of corticotrophin-releasing hormone, adreonocorticotrophic hormone, and cortisol as well as a decline in active vitamin D and osteocalcin all correlate with the severity of placental dysfunction. These hormonal imbalances are believed to have additional negative impacts on linear growth, skeletal growth, bone mineralization, and the potential for postpartum catch-up growth.

In growth-restricted fetuses, declining function at all levels of the thyroid axis correlates to the degree of hypoxemia. Thyroid gland dysfunction may develop as indicated by low levels of thyroxine and trilodothyronine despite elevated thyroid-stimulating hormone levels (TSH). In other instances, central production of TSH may be responsible for fetal hypothyroidism. Finally, downregulation of thyroid hormone receptors may limit the biologic activity of circulating thyroid hormones in specific target tissues such as the developing brain.[11]

Elevations in serum glucagon, adrenaline, noradrenaline, and stimulation of the fetal glucocorticoid axis have immediate effects in fetal life, promoting the mobilization of hepatic glycogen stores and peripheral gluconeogenesis. However, persistent alterations of these hormones may have a causative relationship with the development of diabetes and vascular complications in adult life.

Fetal hematologic responses to placental insufficiency are important because they initially provide a compensatory mechanism for hypoxemia and acidemia but eventually may become contributory to the escalation of placental vascular dysfunction. Fetal hypoxemia is a trigger for erythropoietin release and stimulation of red blood cell production through both medullary and extramedullary sites, resulting in polycythemia.[12] Oxygen-carrying capacity and the buffering capacity are thus increased through the elevation in hemoglobin count. If extramedullary hematopoiesis is increasingly induced by prolonged tissue hypoxemia and/or acidosis, the nucleated red blood cell (NRBC) count rises owing to the escape of these cells from these sites. Thus, elevated NRBC counts correlate with metabolic and cardiovascular status and are independent markers for poor perinatal outcome. In advanced placental insufficiency, more complex hematologic abnormalities supervene that may result from dysfunctional erythropoiesis, placental consumption, and vitamin and iron deficiency. Subsequently fetal anemia and thrombocytopenia are observed, particularly in fetuses with marked elevation of placental blood flow resistance and evidence of intraplacental thrombosis, suggesting a causative relationship.[13] Increase in whole blood viscosity, decrease in red blood cell membrane fluidity, and platelet aggregation may be important precursors for accelerating placental vascular occlusion and dysfunction.

Growth-restricted fetuses also show evidence of immune dysfunction at the cellular and humoral level. Decreases in immunoglobulin, absolute B-cell counts, total white blood cell counts, and neutrophil, monocyte, and lymphocyte subpopulations, as well as selective suppression of T-helper and cytotoxic T-cells, are all related to the degree of acidemia. These immune deficiencies explain the higher susceptibility of growth-restricted neonates to infection after delivery.

Fetal cardiovascular responses to placental insufficiency can be subdivided into early and late based on the degree of deterioration of cardiovascular status and the associated derangement of fetal acid-base balance (see below).[14] **Early responses are typically adaptive in nature and result in preferential nutrient streaming to essential organs.** The combination of elevated placental blood flow resistance and impaired transplacental gas transfer has several effects

TABLE 31-1 SUMMARY OF METABOLIC RESPONSES TO PLACENTAL INSUFFICIENCY

SUBSTRATE	CHANGE
Glucose	Decreased proportional to the degree of fetal hypoxemia.
Amino acids	Significant decrease in branched chain amino acids (valine, leucine, isoleucine) as well as lysine and serine. In contrast, hydroxyproline is elevated. The decrease in essential amino acids is proportional to the degree of hypoxemia. Elevated amniotic fluid glycine to valine ratio. Elevations in amniotic fluid ammonia with a significant positive correlation with the fetal ponderal index.
Fatty acids and triglycerides	Decrease in long-chain polyunsaturated fatty acids (docosahexanoic and arachidonic acids). Decrease in overall fatty acid transfer only with significant loss of placental substance. Hypertriglyceridemia due to decreased utilization. Lower cholesterol esters.
Oxygen and CO_2	Degree of hypoxemia proportional to villous damage and correlates significantly with hypercapnia, acidemia and hypoglycemia and hyperlacticemia.

on the fetal circulation. Normally nutrient-rich oxygenated blood enters the fetus via the umbilical vein, reaching the liver as the first major organ. One of the earliest cardiovascular signs of placental insufficiency is a decrease in the magnitude of umbilical venous volume flow. In response to these changes in umbilical venous nutrition content and blood flow volume, the proportion of umbilical venous blood that is diverted through the ductus venosus toward the fetal heart increases.[15] This change in venous shunting across the ductus venosus increases the proportion of nutrient-rich umbilical venous blood that bypasses the liver and reaches the left side of the heart through the foramen ovale.[16] Because of the presence of central shunts at the level of the foramen ovale and ductus arteriosus, differential changes in downstream blood flow resistance can affect the proportion of cardiac output delivered through each ventricle (Figure 31-3). Elevation of blood flow resistance in the pulmonary vascular bed and subdiaphragmatic circulation (lower body and placenta) increase right ventricular afterload. A drop in cerebral blood flow resistance decreases left ventricular afterload.[17] As a consequence, shunting of nutrient rich blood from the ductus venosus through the foramen ovale to the left side of the heart increases and left ventricular output rises in relation to the right cardiac output.[18] At the aortic isthmus, blood coming from the right ventricle through the ductus arteriosus is diverted toward the aortic arch, thereby supplementing this central shift in cardiac output from right to left. This relative shift in cardiac output toward the left ventricle that results in increased blood flow to the myocardium and brachiocephalic circulation has been termed redistribution, indicating a compensatory mechanism in response to placental insufficiency.

Late circulatory responses are associated with deterioration of cardiovascular status. Redistribution is only effective as long as adequate forward cardiac function is maintained. Marked elevations in placental blood flow resistance and progressive placental insufficiency can lead to an impairment of cardiac function. When this occurs, several aspects of cardiovascular homeostasis can be affected. Ineffective preload handling and elevation in central venous pressure may result from ineffective redistribution, a measurable decline in cardiac output, and a decline in cardiac forward function. The hallmark of this advancing deterioration in cardiovascular state is loss of diastolic forward flow in the umbilical circulation and a marked decline of forward flow in the venous system.[19] Finally, myocardial dysfunction and cardiac dilatation may result in holosystolic tricuspid insufficiency and spontaneous FHR decelerations, followed by fetal demise.[20]

In addition to the central circulatory changes that affect the distribution of cardiac output, fetal organs have the ability to regulate their individual blood flow through autoregulation. Such autoregulatory mechanisms have been identified in the myocardium, adrenal glands, spleen, liver, celiac axis, mesenteric vessels, and kidneys. These autoregulatory mechanisms are evoked at different levels of compromise and their effect is typically complementary to central blood flow redistribution by enhancing perfusion of vital organs as long as cardiovascular homeostasis is maintained. Doppler ultrasound is the fetal assessment tool to assess these cardiovascular responses to placental insufficiency (see below). A summary of Doppler findings and their physiologic significance in the context of placental insufficiency is provided in Table 31-2.

Fetal behavioral responses to placental insufficiency and characteristics of the FHR reflect developmental status and undergo significant changes with advancing gestation. Progressive sophistication of fetal behavior and increasing variation of the fetal heart rate reflect differentiation of central regulatory centers and expansion of central processing capability. Normally behavioral milestones progress from the initiation of gross body movements and fetal breathing in the first trimester to coupling of fetal behavior (e.g., heart rate reactivity) and integration of rest-activity cycles into stable behavioral states (states 1-4 F) by 28 to 32 weeks' gestation (see Chapter 12). A steady decrease in baseline heart rate reflecting increasing vagal tone accompanies these developments. In addition, short- and long-term variability and variation as well as the amplitude of accelerations increase with advancing gestation, reflecting increasing central processing. **With the completion of these milestones, heart rate reactivity by traditional criteria is present in 80% of fetuses by 32 weeks' gestation.** Differences in maturational state and behavioral state, disruption of neural pathways, and declining oxygen tension may all modulate or even abolish fetal behavior or heart rate characteristics.

Because variations of fetal behavior and the FHR rate may be due to several factors, observation of several variables over a sufficient length of time is necessary to separate physiologic from pathologic variation. Biophysical profile scoring (BPS) quantifies fetal behavior by assessing tone, movement, breathing activity, and FHR reactivity in an observation period of at least 30 minutes. Amniotic fluid volume (AFV) assessment has traditionally been a part of the BPS. From the second trimester onward, AFV is primarily related to fetal urine production and therefore renal perfusion. **Thus, AFV assessment provides an indirect assessment of renal/vascular status and constitutes the main longitudinal monitoring component of the BPS (see below). Visual FHR analysis has traditionally been the method of interobserver, posing the problems of interobserver and intraobserver variability.** These are circumvented by computerized analysis of the FHR (cCTG). The cCTG assesses short-term, long-term, and mean minute variation and periods of high variation in addition to traditional FHR parameters that also allow longitudinal observations.

In growth-restricted fetuses with chronic hypoxemia and mild placental dysfunction, the primary CNS response is a delay in all aspects of CNS maturation.[21] With the help of computerized research tools a delay of behavioral development has been documented under such circumstances. The combination of delayed central integration of FHR control, decreased fetal activity, and chronic hypoxemia results in a higher baseline heart rate with lower short- and long-term variation (on computerized analysis) and delayed development of heart rate reactivity.[22] These maturational differences in FHR parameters are particularly evident between 28 and 32 weeks.

Despite the maturational delay of some aspects of CNS function, several centrally regulated responses to

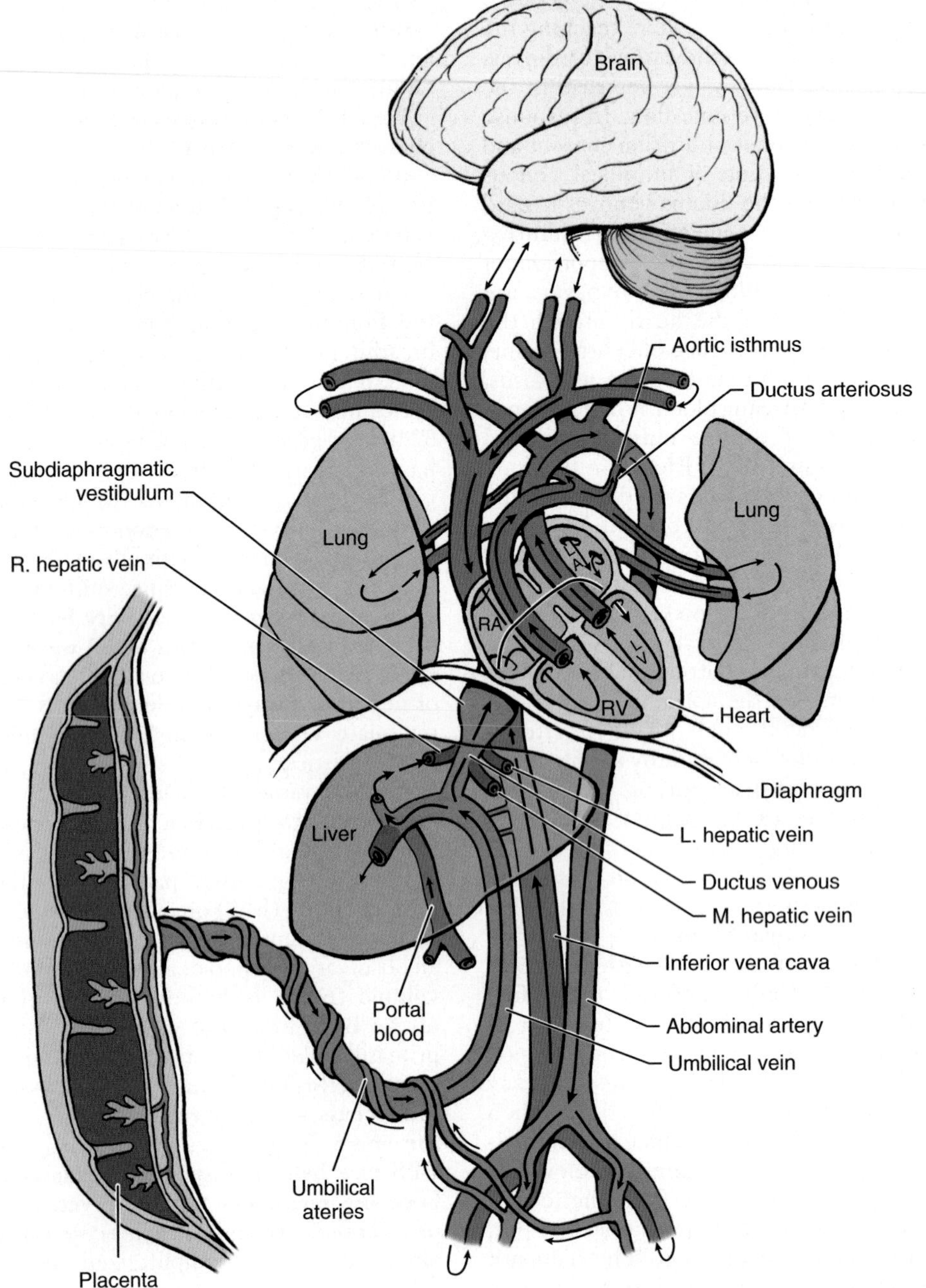

FIGURE 31-3. Schematic presentation of the fetal circulation. This figure illustrates the serial partitioning of nutrient- and oxygen-rich blood reaching the fetus via the umbilical vein. The first partition at the level of the ductus venosus distributes the majority of umbilical venous blood to the liver. Umbilical venous blood that continues toward the heart is partitioned toward the left ventricle *(LV)* at the foramen ovale. This blood supplies the brain and upper part of the body via the brachiocephalic circulation and the myocardium via the coronary circulation. A minor proportion of blood from the right ventricle *(RV)* supplies the lungs while the remainder continues through the ductus arteriosus *(DA)* toward the aorta. At the aortic isthmus bloodstreams coming from the aorta are partitioned based on the relationship of blood flow resistance in the brachiocephalic and subdiaphragmatic circulations. While net forward flow is maintained under physiologic conditions, diastolic flow reversal occurs when brachiocephalic resistance falls, and/or subdiaphragmatic (placental) resistance rises. Finally, the major proportion of descending aortic blood is partitioned at the umbilical arteries to return to the placenta for respiratory and nutrient exchange. (Reproduced from Baschat AA: The fetal circulation and essential organs—a new twist to an old tale. Ultrasound Obstet Gynecol 27:349, 2006.)

acid–base status are still preserved. Therefore, the growth-restricted fetus still maintains behavioral responses to a decline in acid–base status that are determined by the central effects of hypoxemia/acidemia independently of the cardiovascular status. **In contrast, the declining AFV that commonly accompanies the sequential loss of biophysical variables appears to be related to renal blood flow and the degree of vascular redistribution.**[23]

With worsening fetal hypoxemia a decline in global fetal activity initiates the cascade of late behavioral responses characteristic of placental insufficiency.[24] With further deepening hypoxemia, fetal breathing movement ceases.

TABLE 31-2 SUMMARY OF VASCULAR RESPONSES IN IUGR FETUSES

DOPPLER FINDING	PHYSIOLOGIC SIGNIFICANCE
Uterine artery notching	Trophoblast invasion remains limited to the myometrial portion of the spiral arteries. Subsequent failure to fully transform into a low-resistance, high-capacitance vascular bed increases risk for subsequent IUGR and/or preeclampsia.
Decreased, absent, or reversed umbilical artery end-diastolic velocity	Abnormal terminal villi and stem arteries result in increased placental vascular resistance and a proportional decrease in the umbilical artery end-diastolic velocity. Associated placental perfusion defects are responsible for impaired fetomaternal gas and nutrient exchange.
Elevation of blood flow resistance in the thoracic aorta and iliac artery	*Hind limb reflex:* Diversion of blood flow away from the carcass at the expense of the lower body. Achieved through increase in right ventricular afterload proximal to the umbilical arteries as well as increased blood flow resistance distally. In addition to centralization (see below), descending aortic blood flow is also preferentially distributed to the placenta.
1. Decrease in the cerebroplacental Doppler ratio. 2. Direct measurement of cardiac output. 3. Reversal of end-diastolic velocity in the aortic isthmus. 4. Absence or reversal of umbilical artery end-diastolic velocity.	*Centralization:* A measurable shift in the relationship between right and left ventricular afterload resulting in redistribution of cardiac output in favor of the left ventricle (i.e., the heart and brain). This can be passively mediated purely by an increase in placental blood flow resistance and therefore right ventricular afterload.
Decrease in the carotid-, or middle cerebral artery Doppler index.	*Brain sparing:* Cerebral vasodilatation in response to perceived hypoxemia.
Increased superior mesenteric artery Doppler resistance	During perceived hypoxemia and/or redistribution of cardiac output blood flow to the gut as a nonessential organ in utero is compromised.
Decrease in the splenic artery Doppler index	Splenic artery vasodilatation enhances perfusion of this important hematopoietic organ, possibly facilitating an increase in red cell mass.
Decreased Doppler resistance in the celiac axis	There may be a reflection of blood flow augmentation in the hepatic and splenic arteries, which are the main branches of this axis.
Increased Doppler resistance in peripheral pulmonary arteries	As nonessential organs in fetal life, lung perfusion may be further compromised by increased vascular resistance in the pulmonary circulation, ensuring that a greater proportion of right ventricular output bypasses the lungs to reach the placenta.
Increased Doppler resistance in the renal arteries	Redistribution and increased renal vascular tone may be the mediators of oliguria and oligohydramnios observed with chronic and/or progressive hypoxemia.
Measured dilation of the ductus venosus with elevated Doppler index accompanied by a decreased hepatic artery Doppler index	*Liver sparing:* Preferential arterial blood supply to the fetal liver invoked when increased diversion of umbilical venous blood through the ductus venosus jeopardizes hepatic perfusion.
Decreased Doppler index in the adrenal artery flow velocity waveforms	*Adrenal sparing:* Enhanced adrenal perfusion is triggered as part of the fetal stress response to chronic malnutrition or an acute worsening imposed on the chronic state.
Umbilical venous pulsations in association with elevated venous Doppler indices	Evidence of inefficient forward delivery of cardiac output with subsequent elevation of central venous pressure that is transmitted all the way back into the umbilical vein
Normalization of cerebral Doppler indices after a period of "brain sparing"	With advanced cardiovascular deterioration, brain autoregulation may become abnormal. Probably in association with a decrease in cardiac function, the interval between systolic and diastolic velocities widens, resulting in an increase (thus normalization) of the Doppler index.
Sudden ability to visualize and measure coronary Blood flow in a setting of deteriorating venous Doppler indices in a premature fetus with IUGR	*Heart sparing:* Marked augmentation of coronary blood flow in situations of acute or chronic hypoxemia that is achieved through upregulation of coronary vascular reserve and vasodilatation.

Gross body movements and tone decrease further until they are no longer observed in the traditional examination period.[25,26] **Traditional FHR variables are frequently abnormal by this time. Reduction of global fetal activity and loss of fetal coupling (absence of heart rate reactivity and fetal breathing movements) are typically observed at a mean pH of between 7.10 and 7.20.** Loss of tone and movement is characteristic as the pH drops further. Late decelerations of the FHR may develop due to a relative drop in oxygen tension that exceeds 8 torr (see Chapter 16). Spontaneous decelerations due to direct depression of cardiac contractility or "cardiac" late decelerations typically herald fetal demise.

DIAGNOSTIC TOOLS IN FETAL GROWTH RESTRICTION

Fetal growth restriction is a syndrome that is marked by failure of the fetus to reach its growth potential with consequences that are related to the underlying disorder as well as the severity of fetal disease. Because IUGR may be the consequence of many underlying etiologies, the differential diagnosis always includes maternal disease, placental insufficiency, aneuploidy, nonaneuploid syndromes, and viral infection. For appropriate patient counseling and choice of management options, comprehensive prenatal evaluation needs to go beyond the assessment of fetal size, utilizing a diagnostic approach aimed at identifying the underlying causes. After confirming small fetal size, stratification into three patient groups is of particular importance. The first group consists of constitutionally small but otherwise normal fetuses. These will not usually require any intervention and therefore do not need antenatal surveillance. The second group consists of fetuses with aneuploidy, nonaneuploid syndromes, or viral infection. In these conditions prognosis is largely determined by the underlying disease, with little potential for impact by perinatal interventions. Sensitive and knowledgeable counseling of the parents about the high likelihood of a poor prognosis is especially important in such cases. The third group consists of fetuses with placental disease. In these, progressive deterioration of the fetal condition worsens the prognosis. This subset of patients is most likely to benefit from fetal surveillance and subsequent intervention. Although gray-scale ultrasound provides important clues to the presence of IUGR, the liability of preterm delivery and iatrogenic complications is great if the diagnosis is based solely on biometry. While maternal disease is readily apparent through a history and physical examination, the accurate evaluation of the possible fetal disorder and stratification of risk requires the integration of several diagnostic modalities that evaluate fetal, placental, and amniotic fluid characteristics.[27-29]

Fetal Biometry

Ultrasound criteria have emerged as the diagnostic standard used in the identification of fetal growth restriction. For this purpose sonographic measurements of fetal bony and soft structures are related to reference ranges for gestation. In 1964, Wilcocks and colleagues first demonstrated the correlation between ultrasound measurement of the fetal head and birth weight. Campbell and Dewhurst published the first sonographic descriptions of fetal growth restriction with their analysis of the changes in biparietal diameter (BPD) over time. Two patterns of altered head growth were described: In "late flattening" (type 1, asymmetric type), the BPD increases normally until late pregnancy and then lags behind. In the "low-profile" (type 2, symmetric type), impaired head growth occurs much earlier in gestation. The asymmetric type represents approximately two thirds of cases of fetal growth restriction. The fetal AC is related to hepatic glycogen storage and liver size, therefore correlating closely with the nutritional state. Campbell and Wilkin were the first to relate combined measurements of the BPD and AC to birthweight. Additional direct measurements that are primarily utilized in clinical practice today include the HC and femur length (FL). Secondary direct measurements include the transverse cerebellar diameter (TCD) and the humerus length (HL). The most important calculated ultrasound variable of fetal growth is the sonographically estimated fetal weight (SEFW). Numerous investigators have identified distinct fetal ultrasound parameters that are useful in the calculation of the SEFW.[30] All of the techniques incorporate an index of abdominal size as a variable contributing to the estimation of fetal weight. Population-specific formulae have been derived to generate reference limits that generally have 95% confidence limits deviating approximately 15% around the actual value.

Accurate estimation of fetal growth from these fetal measurements requires knowledge of the gestational age as a reference point to calculate percentile ranks. An estimated date of confinement (EDC) should be based on the last menstrual period when the sonographic estimate of gestational age is within the predictive error (7 days in the first and 14 days in the second trimester, and 21 days in the third trimester). Once the EDC is set by this method or a first trimester ultrasound, it should not be changed because such practice interferes with the ability to diagnose IUGR.

Measurement of the BPD alone is a poor tool for the detection of IUGR. The physiologic variation in size inherent with advancing gestation is high. The majority of growth-restricted fetuses presenting with asymmetric growth restriction and delayed flattening of the cranial growth curve would be detected relatively late. Factors that interfere with a technically adequate measurement of the BPD include alterations of the cranial shape by external forces (oligohydramnios, breech presentation) and direct antero-posterior position of the fetal head.

The HC is not subject to the same extrinsic variability as the BPD. The measurement technique is important because calculated HC measurements are systematically smaller than those directly measured. Thus, the nomogram selected should be based on measurements obtained using the same methodology. As a screening tool for IUGR the HC poses a similar problem as the BPD in that two thirds of IUGR fetuses with asymmetric growth pattern would be detected late.

The TCD is one of the few soft tissue measurements that correlate well with gestational age, being relatively spared from the effects of mild to moderate uteroplacental dysfunction.[31] Whether its measurement offers any advantage over bony measurements in the assessment of compromised fetal growth is controversial.

The AC is the single best measurement for the detection of IUGR.[32] The most accurate AC is the smallest directly measured circumference obtained in a perpendicular plane of the upper abdomen at the level of the hepatic vein between fetal respirations. The AC percentile has both the highest sensitivity and negative predictive value for the sonographic diagnosis of IUGR whether defined postnatally by birthweight percentile or ponderal index. **Using the 10th percentiles as cut-offs, the AC has a higher sensitivity (98% vs. 85%) but lower positive predictive value than the SEFW (36% vs. 51%). Its sensitivity is further enhanced by serial measurements at least 14 days apart.**[33] Because of its high sensitivity, some type of abdominal measurement should be part of every sonographic growth evaluation. But because the AC reflects fetal nutrition, it should be excluded from the calculation of the composite gestational age after the early second trimester.

Calculation of the ratio between the head and abdominal circumference (HC/AC ratio) has been proposed as a tool to increase detection of the fetus with asymmetric growth restriction (Figures 31-4 and 31-5). In the normally growing fetus, the HC/AC ratio exceeds 1.0 before 32 weeks' gestation, is approximately 1.0 at 32 to 34 weeks' gestation, and

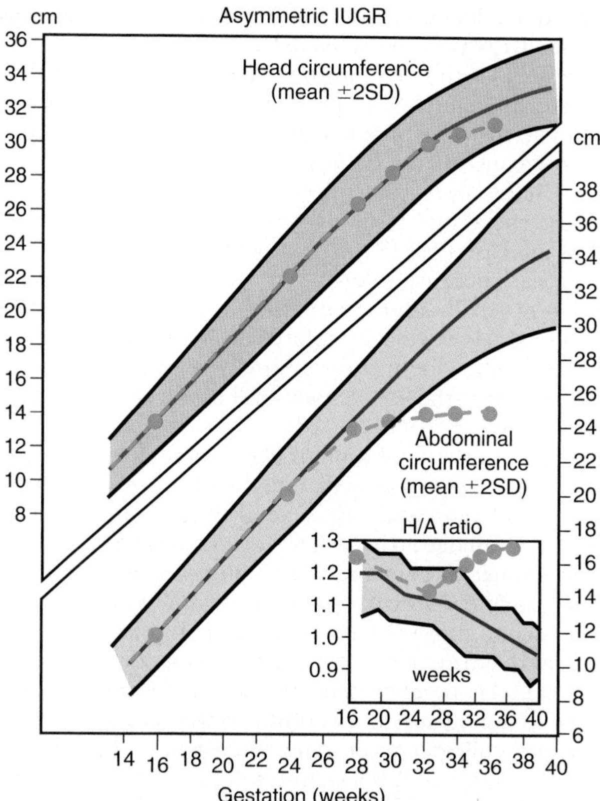

FIGURE 31-4. Growth chart in a case of asymmetric IUGR. Although head circumference is preserved, AC growth falls off early in the third trimester. For this reason, the H/A ratio shown in the lower right corner of the graph becomes elevated. (From Chudleigh P, Pearce JM: Obstetric Ultrasound. Edinburgh, Churchill Livingstone, 1986.)

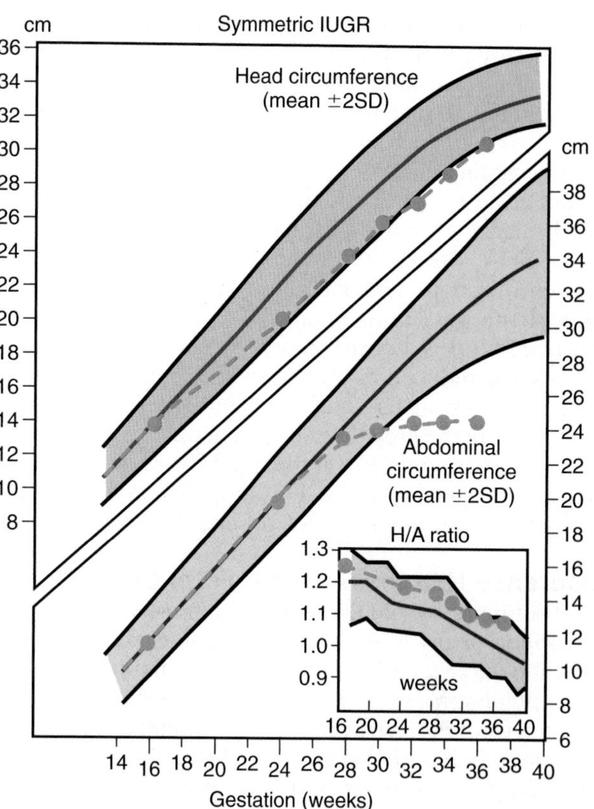

FIGURE 31-5. Growth chart in a case of symmetric IUGR. Note the early onset of both HC and AC growth restriction. For this reason, the H/A ratio shown in the lower right corner remains normal. (From Chudleigh P, Pearce JM: Obstetric Ultrasound. Edinburgh, Churchill Livingstone, 1986.)

falls below 1.0 after 34 weeks' gestation. In fetuses with asymmetric growth restriction, the HC remains larger than that of the body, resulting in an elevated HC/AC ratio,[34] while the ratio remains normal in symmetric IUGR where both direct measurements are equally affected (see Figures 31-4 and 31-5). Using the HC/AC ratio, 70% to 85% of growth-restricted fetuses are detected, with a reduction in false-negative diagnoses. Thus, a single set of measurements, even when determined in the latter part of pregnancy, can be very helpful in evaluating the status of intrauterine growth. **However, both the sensitivity and the positive predictive value of the HC/AC ratio for growth restriction does not equal either the AC percentile, or the SEFW.**[35]

In some cases, measurement of the HC may be difficult as a result of fetal position. One can then compare the FL, which is relatively spared in asymmetric IUGR, to the AC. The FL/AC ratio is 22 at all gestational ages from 21 weeks to term and so can be applied without knowledge of the gestational age. An FL/AC ratio greater than 23.5 suggests IUGR.

Several formulae have been devised to calculate a SEFW. Using a multifactorial equation and a measurement of abdominal size, a weight can be predicted and related to gestational age. Formulas that incorporate the FL may increase the accuracy of in utero weight estimation for the fetus with IUGR. Because the SEFW cannot be measured directly, but is calculated from a combination of directly measured parameters, the error in the estimate is increased. **The accuracy of most formulae (± 2SDs) is ±10%, and none has proven superior to the first devised by Warsof and reported by Sheppard.** As noted earlier, the SEFW has a lower sensitivity but higher positive predictive value than the AC and does not add to the AC percentile for the diagnosis of IUGR. However, an SEFW below the 10th percentile provides a graphic image easy for both patient and referring physician to conceptualize. Therefore use of the estimated fetal weight has become the most common method for characterizing fetal size and thereby growth abnormalities.

Fetal Body Composition

The ponderal index was first described by Rohrer in 1921 as an index of corpulence. This index of neonatal size (weight/length^3) that is normally distributed accurately reflected the nutritional state of the neonate. When compared with birthweight percentile, the ponderal index demonstrates superior ability to predict neonatal asphyxia, acidosis, hypoglycemia, and hypothermia.[36] The ponderal index also correlates with direct measures of neonatal fat as estimated by skinfold thickness. Attempts to translate the ponderal index directly to the fetus have been hampered by the difficulty in accurately assessing fetal length. Attempts to modify the ponderal index for fetal sonographic estimation have been made. Yagel and colleagues demonstrated that the addition of a fetal ponderal index improved the prediction of perinatal morbidity in fetuses already suspected of having IUGR. Alternative methods for the characterization of fetal growth by physiologic compartments have recently been attempted. Several studies have examined fetal subcutaneous fat content using ultrasound examination. Subcutaneous fat deposition has been examined in the face, abdomen, arm, and thigh.[37] Reduction in facial fat stores has been strongly associated with being SGA. Using ultrasound, Padoan and colleagues showed that both subcutaneous mass (fat mass) and lean mass (bone and muscle mass) are reduced in growth-restricted fetuses, but that proportionately, the subcutaneous mass is reduced to a greater extent than lean mass.[38] This reduction in fat content is consistent with observations made in the growth-restricted neonate and may prove to be a sensitive indicator of the small fetus at increased risk for perinatal complications. The optimal method of in utero assessment of fetal fat has not yet been determined.

Reference Ranges Defining Fetal Growth

An absolute threshold used for the definition of IUGR can be applied to any of the fetal biometric parameters evaluated. These criteria have been statistically defined rather than outcome-based and use either a threshold percentile ranking (non-normative data) or a number of standard deviations below the mean (normative data) as cut-offs. Small for gestational age is defined as a birthweight below the population 10th percentile, corrected for gestational age. However, this cut-off has also been the most widely used criterion for defining growth restriction at birth. This definition has also been adopted for the prenatal period by using a SEFW below the 10th percentile as an indicator of IUGR. Because such an approach is purely based on a weight threshold, it can only serve as a screen for the identification of the small fetus at risk for adverse outcome. **Approximately 70% of infants with a birthweight below the 10th percentile are normally grown (i.e., constitutionally small) and not at risk for adverse outcome as they present one end of the normal spectrum for neonatal size.[39] The remaining 30% consist of infants who are truly growth restricted and are at risk for increased perinatal morbidity and mortality.** When the cut-off for an abnormal birthweight is adjusted to the 3rd percentile as suggested by Usher and McLean, the proportion of truly growth-restricted infants identified increases while some with milder forms of IUGR will be missed. However, other authors have demonstrated increased mortality for birthweights through the 15th percentile with an odds ratio of 1.9 for mortality in newborns with birthweights between the 10th and 15th percentiles. As the percentile cut-offs to define abnormal growth continue to be a matter of debate, risk assessment based on weight alone is further hampered by discrepancies between the SEFW and the actual birthweight. Live birthweight criteria do not appropriately describe SEFWs, as there is a significant association of preterm birth with fetal growth restriction.[40] The weights of preterm infants are not normally distributed as they are at term, producing a significant discrepancy between birthweight-defined growth curves and SEFW-defined growth curves in preterm gestation.[41] **SEFW growth curves are generated from patient samples representing the entire obstetrical population at any gestational age. In contrast, preterm live birth normative data tables reflect only those individuals who have delivered under abnormal circumstances.** Thus, the SEFW growth curves consistently demonstrate higher fetal weights over the range of preterm gestation than do birthweight-generated growth curves. Therefore, use of an SEFW cut-off below the 10th percentile is more appropriate to define abnormal fetal growth because the ability to identify fetuses at greater perinatal risk is increased.[42] For the AC a 2.5th percentile cut-off is appropriate because reference ranges are based on a cross section of small, appropriately grown, preterm, and term newborns. However, as reference limits are based on healthy women delivering appropriately nourished neonates at term, the <10th percentile cut-off is consistent with IUGR.

Because of the limitation of population-based reference ranges to assess fetal growth, individualized growth models have been proposed by several investigators.[1,43] The obvious advantage is the lack of dependency on population-based normative data and the ability to detect a true singularly defined growth restriction even with estimated fetal weights above the 10th percentile for the population. Some of these models require three sequential sonograms. This includes baseline biometry in the second trimester, a second sonogram to establish growth potential for an individual morphometric parameter, and a third scan to identify a growth abnormality. Because this approach is cumbersome in clinical practice, other models have been developed that account for variables that contribute the majority of the variance to newborn size. These include early pregnancy weight, maternal height, ethnic group, parity, and sex.[1] Using these variables and fetal growth patterns, the estimated size of a fetus of a given mother can be projected at term and estimated at any specific point in gestation. Deviations from this projected growth pattern can then be recognized. Overall, the diagnostic advantages of these individualized growth models has been questioned when compared with the sequential comparison of the percentile ranking of individual or composite growth parameters to population-based growth curves.

Fetal growth as opposed to fetal size is a dynamic process and requires more than a single evaluation for its estimation. The appropriate observation interval for the evaluation of fetal growth has been based on the assumptions that growth is continuous rather than sporadic and that the identification of growth is limited by the technical capability of the ultrasound equipment used to measure the fetus. The recommended interval between ultrasound evaluations of fetal growth is 3 weeks, as shorter intervals increase the likelihood of a false-positive diagnosis.

In summary, the ability to correctly identify growth-restricted fetuses at risk for adverse outcome by weight estimates alone is limited. Individualized or sequential growth assessment performs better than a single measurement of fetal size. Improved stratification of risk requires the integration of additional diagnostic possibilities.

Fetal Anatomic Survey

Although the sonographic survey of fetal anatomy does not provide an assessment of fetal growth, it is the first step toward the investigation of an underlying etiology. The anatomic survey should focus on the detection of markers of aneuploidy, nonaneuploid syndromes, and fetal infection, as well as any anatomic defects. The relationship between aneuploidy and fetal anomalies such as gastroschisis, omphalocele, diaphragmatic hernia, congenital heart defects, and sonographic markers such as echogenic bowel, nuchal thickening, and abnormal hand positioning are discussed in Chapter 11. Abnormalities of skull contour, thoracic shape, or disproportional shortening of the long bones may be pointers to skeletal dysplasia or thanatophoric dwarfism. Markers for viral infection may be nonspecific, but include echogenicity and calcification in organs such as the brain and liver.[44] Identification of any of these abnormalities on ultrasound significantly affects the differential diagnosis and frequently has a decisive impact on outcome.

Amniotic Fluid Assessment

The regulation of AVF by the late second and third trimester is primarily dependent on fetal urine output, production of pulmonary fluid, and fetal swallowing. Placental dysfunction and fetal hypoxemia both may result in decreased perfusion of the fetal kidneys with subsequent oliguria and decreasing AVF.[45] Although the accuracy of ultrasound in the assessment of actual AVF is poor, two techniques are used that can provide important diagnostic and prognostic information.[46] In an early study, Manning and colleagues reported that a vertical pocket of amniotic fluid measuring 1 cm or more reflected an adequate fluid volume. Criteria for AVF assessment were subsequently broadened. A 2-cm vertical pocket was considered normal, 1 to 2 cm marginal, and less than 1 cm decreased. Alternatively, AVF may be assessed by the sum of vertical pockets from four quadrants of the uterine cavity. This four-quadrant amniotic fluid index (AFI) (nomogram by Moore T and colleagues; see Figure 33-3) is compared to reference ranges that require knowledge of the gestational age. Despite the availability of these numerical methods for semiquantification of AVF, an overall clinical impression of reduced amniotic fluid may be most important. Ultrasound criteria for a subjectively reduced AVF include a maximum vertical pocket below 3 cm, the fetus in a flexion attitude with limited room for movement, a small or empty bladder and stomach, and molding of the uterus around the fetal body. Movement of the transducer frequently generates uterine contractions, which may be associated with variable decelerations.

Overall, estimation of AVF in itself is a poor screening method for IUGR or fetal acidemia. However, in clinical practice it is an important diagnostic and prognostic tool. Oligohydramnios may be the first sign of fetal growth restriction detected on ultrasonography preceding an assessment for lagging fetal growth. If gestational age is known, ultrasound assessment of fetal growth based on the HC, AC, FL, and SEFW can be performed. If gestational age is unknown, measurements of the FL/AC ratio and single amniotic fluid pocket have to be used because they are independent of gestational age. **Up to 96% of fetuses with fluid pockets less than 1 cm may be growth restricted.**[47] In patients where growth delay is already suspected, amniotic fluid volume can be an important differential diagnostic pointer. In the setting of small fetal size, abundant AVF suggests aneuploidy or fetal infection, while normal or decreased amniotic fluid is compatible with placental insufficiency. **The volume of amniotic fluid also has prognostic significance for the course of labor. Groome et al. demonstrated that oligohydramnios associated with fetal oliguria is associated with a higher rate of intrapartum complications that may be attributed to reduced placental reserve.**[48]

TABLE 31-3 ARTERIAL AND VENOUS DOPPLER INDICES

INDEX	CALCULATION
Arterial Doppler Indices	
S/D ratio	$\frac{\text{systolic peak velocity}}{\text{diastolic peak velocity}}$
Resistance index (RI)	$\frac{\text{systolic} - \text{end-diastolic peak velocity}}{\text{systolic peak velocity}}$
Pulsatility index (PI)	$\frac{\text{systolic} - \text{end-diastolic peak velocity}}{\text{time averaged maximum velocity}}$
Venous Doppler Indices	
Inferior vena cava preload index	$\frac{\text{peak velocity during atrial contraction}}{\text{systolic peak velocity}}$
Ductus venosus preload index	$\frac{\text{systolic} - \text{diastolic peak velocity}}{\text{systolic peak velocity}}$
Inferior vena cava and ductus venosus pulsatility index for veins (PIV)	$\frac{\text{systolic} - \text{diastolic peak velocity}}{\text{time averaged maximum velocity}}$
Inferior vena cava and ductus venosus peak velocity index for veins (PVIV)	$\frac{\text{systolic} - \text{atrial contraction peak velocity}}{\text{diastolic peak velocity}}$
Percentage reverse flow	$\frac{\text{systolic time averaged velocity}}{\text{diastolic time averaged velocity}} \times 100$

Doppler Velocimetry

Similar to the assessment of AVF, the role of Doppler velocimetry in the management of fetal growth restriction is unique because it serves as a diagnostic as well as a monitoring tool. Doppler flow velocity waveforms may be obtained from arterial and venous vascular beds in the fetus. Arterial Doppler waveforms provide information on downstream vascular resistance, which may be altered due to structural changes in the vasculature or regulatory changes in vascular tone. The systolic/diastolic ratio, the resistance index, and the pulsatility index are the three Doppler indices most widely used to analyze arterial blood flow resistance (Table 31-3). An increase in blood flow resistance manifests itself with a relative decrease in end-diastolic velocity resulting in an increase in all three Doppler indices. Of these, the pulsatility index has the smallest measurement error and narrower reference limits. With extreme increase in blood flow resistance end-diastolic forward velocity may be absent (AEDV) or reversed (REDV) (Figure 31-6).

Venous Doppler parameters complement evaluation of fetal cardiovascular status by providing an assessment of cardiac forward function. Forward blood flow in the

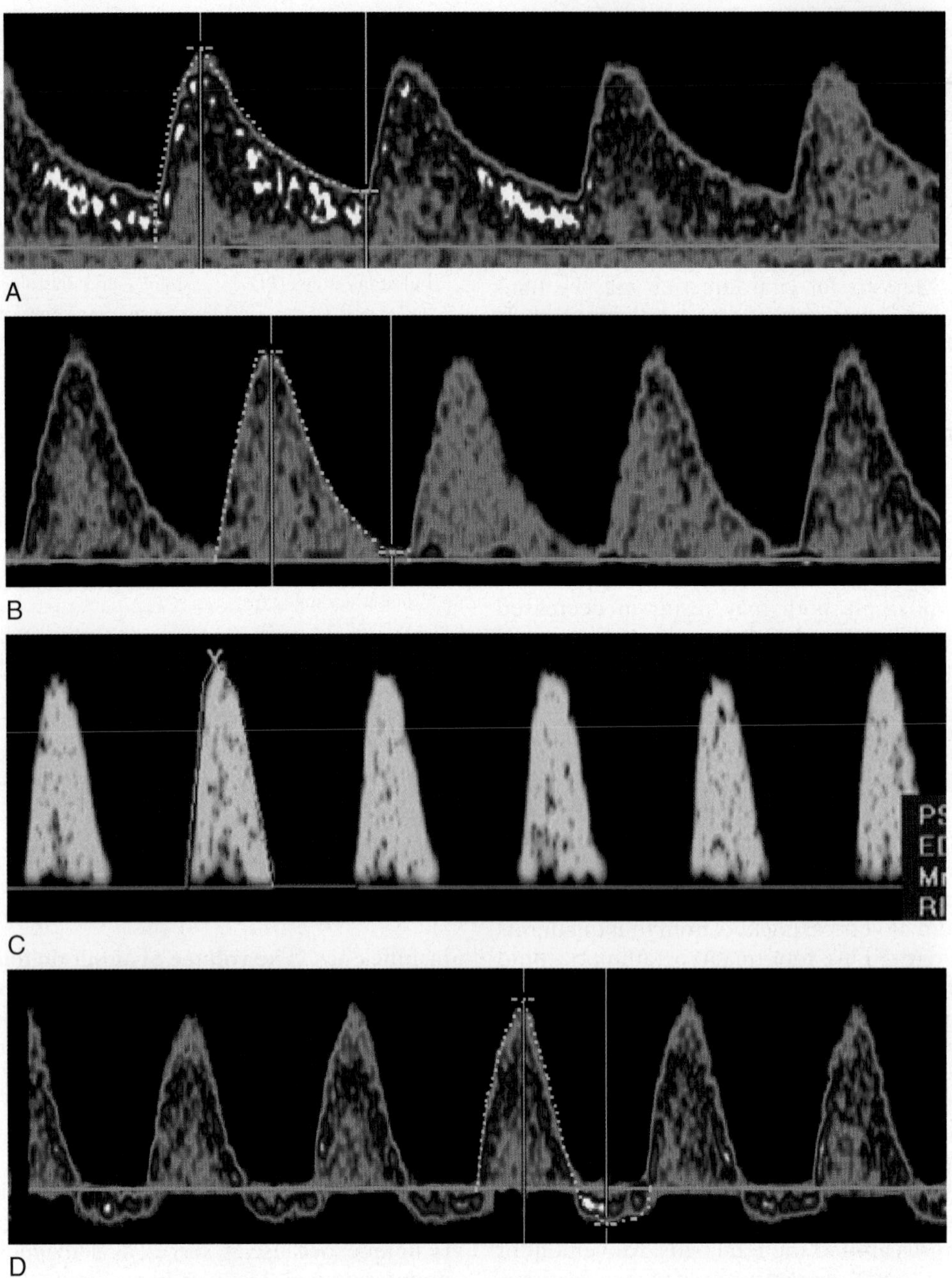

FIGURE 31-6. Umbilical artery flow velocity waveforms. The normal umbilical artery flow velocity waveform has positive end-diastolic velocities that increase toward term, reflecting a falling blood flow resistance in the villous vascular tree **(A)**. Moderate abnormalities in the villous vascular structure raise the blood flow resistance and are associated with a decline in end-diastolic velocities **(B)**. When a significant proportion of the villous vascular tree is abnormal, end-diastolic velocities may be absent **(C)** or even reversed **(D)**.

venous system is determined by cardiac compliance, contractility, and afterload and is characterized by a triphasic flow pattern that reflects pressure volume changes in the atria throughout the cardiac cycle.[49] The descent of the AV-ring during ventricular systole and passive diastolic ventricular filling generates the systolic and diastolic peaks respectively (the S-wave and the D-wave). The sudden increase in right atrial pressure with atrial contraction in late diastole causes a variable amount of reverse flow producing a second trough after the D-wave (the a-wave) (Figure 31-7). The magnitude of forward flow during the atrial systole varies considerably in individual veins and reversal may be physiologic in the inferior vena cava and hepatic veins but is always abnormal in the ductus venosus. Multiple venous Doppler indices have been described to characterize this complex waveform without any clear advantages of individual indices (see Table 31-3).

In the diagnostic assessment of the small fetus, examination of umbilical and middle cerebral artery Doppler studies are the most important to evaluate for placental dysfunction as the underlying etiology. **Randomized trials and meta-analyses confirm that the combined use of fetal biometry and umbilical artery Doppler significantly reduces perinatal mortality and iatrogenic intervention because documentation of placental vascular insufficiency effectively separates growth-restricted fetuses that require**

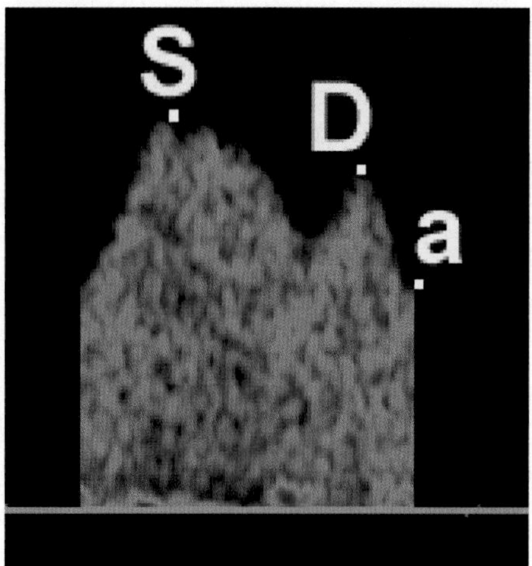

FIGURE 31-7. Venous flow velocity waveform. A typical venous flow velocity waveform is shown. The triphasic waveform (*S*, systole; *D*, diastole; *a*, atrial contraction) reflects volume flow changes during the cardiac cycle. With descent of the atrioventricular valves during ventricular systole, intra-atrial pressures fall and increased forward flow during the S-wave is observed. A temporary decrease in forward flow occurs when the atrioventricular valve ring ascends at the end of ventricular systole producing the first trough in the flow velocity waveform. When atrial pressures exceed intraventricular pressures, the atrioventricular valves open, resulting in the rapid influx of blood into the ventricles. The associated increase in venous flow results in the D-wave. With initiation of a new cardiac cycle, atrial contraction results in a sharp rise in intra-atrial pressure and decline in venous forward flow. This second trough is called the a-wave because it is produced by atrial contraction.

surveillance and possible intervention from constitutionally small fetuses.[50,51]

A free umbilical cord loop is examined with continuous or pulsed Doppler ultrasound far from the fetal and placental insertions. Most current ultrasound equipment allows concurrent use of color and pulsed Doppler with improved reproducibility of measurements. Vascular damage affecting approximately 30% of the placenta produces elevations in the Doppler index. More marked abnormalities result in umbilical artery AEDV or REDV. **Milder forms of placental vascular dysfunction, especially near term, may not produce elevation of umbilical artery blood flow resistance sufficiently to be detectable by traditional Doppler methods.**[52] If placental gas exchange is sufficiently impaired to result in perceived fetal hypoxemia, a decrease in middle cerebral artery Doppler resistance may occur (Figure 31-8). Another Doppler index frequently used clinically to detect this condition is the ratio between umbilical artery pulsatility as index of vasoconstriction in the placenta and middle cerebral artery pulsatility as index of vasodilation in the fetal brain. In milder forms of placental disease with near minimal increase in umbilical artery blood flow resistance, the cerebroplacental Doppler ratio (CPR) may decrease. Grammellini and coworkers demonstrated that a value below 1.08 identified small fetuses at risk for adverse outcome. **Subsequently Bahado-Singh and coworkers indicated that this predictive accuracy of the CPR decreased after 34 weeks' gestation.**[53]

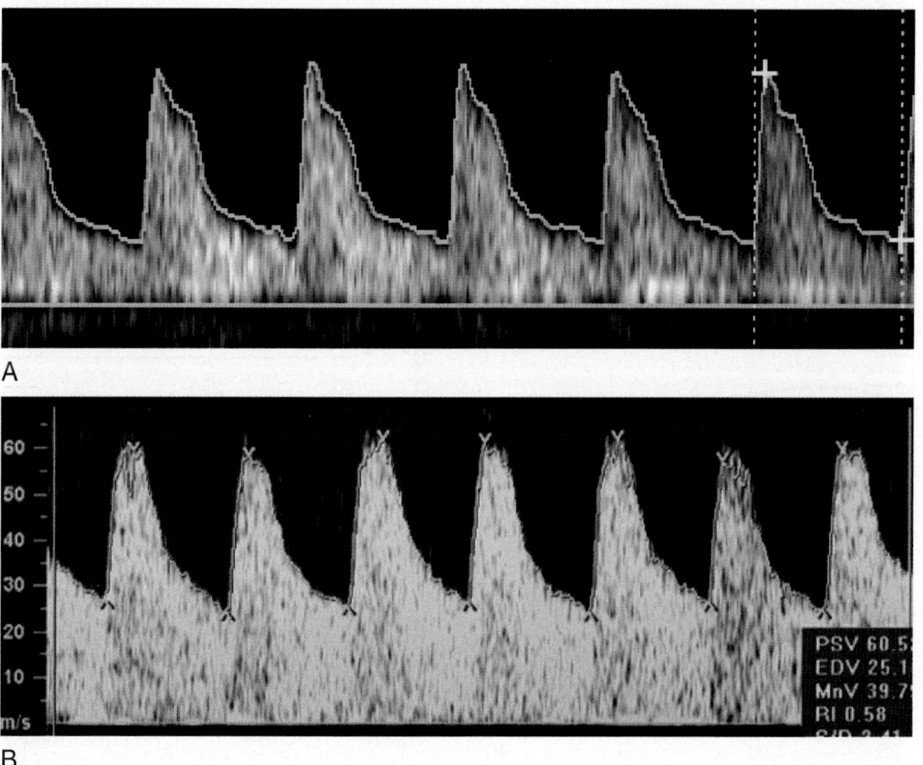

FIGURE 31-8. Middle cerebral artery flow velocity waveform. The normal middle cerebral artery flow pattern has relatively little diastolic flow **(A)**. With progressive placental dysfunction there may be an increase in the diastolic velocity resulting in a decrease in the Doppler index (brain sparing). **B,** With brain sparing, the systolic downslope of the waveform becomes smoother so that the waveform almost resembles that of the umbilical artery. The associated rise in the mean velocity results in a marked decline in the Doppler index.

This is presumably attributable to an increasing number of growth-restricted fetuses that may have normal umbilical artery blood flow resistance near term, but demonstrate isolated "brain sparing" as the only sign of placental insufficiency of oxygen transfer. These fetuses are at risk for adverse outcome.

Because of the variable presentation across gestation, comprehensive Doppler assessment of placental function should include umbilical and middle cerebral arteries. For the umbilical artery an abnormal test result is defined as a Doppler index measurement of greater than 2 SDs deviations above the gestational age mean and/or a loss of end-diastolic velocity. Like growth curves, it is best to use nomograms developed from a local or comparable population. For the CPR and also for the middle cerebral artery a greater than 2 SD decrease of the index is considered abnormal. In a setting of small fetal size, these findings identify those fetuses at greatest risk for adverse outcome (Figures 31-9 to 31-12).

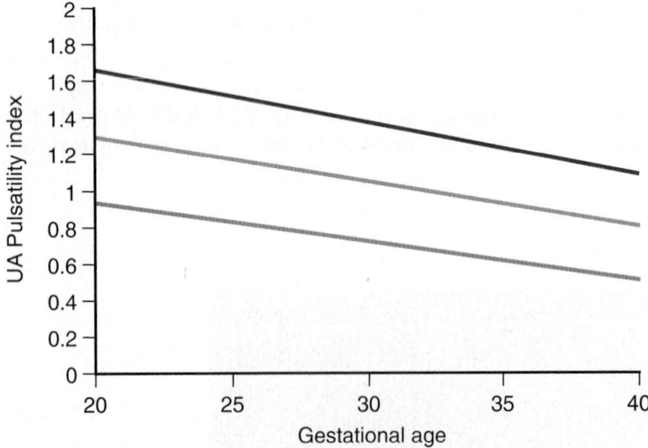

FIGURE 31-9. Umbilical artery pulsatility index with advancing gestational age. Displayed are the reference ranges (mean and 95% confidence interval) of the umbilical artery (UA) pulsatility index.

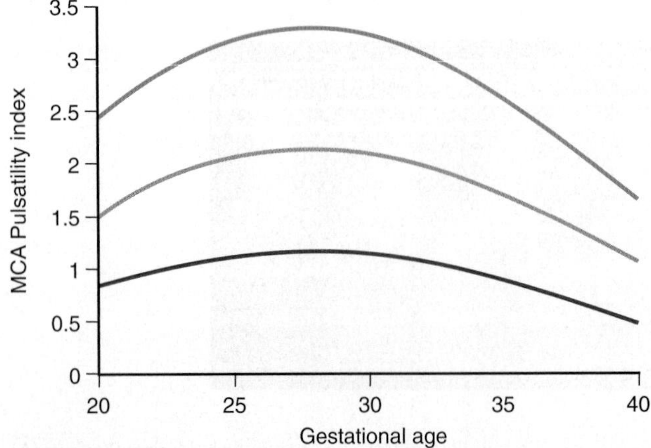

FIGURE 31-10. Middle cerebral artery pulsatility index with advancing gestational age. The graph shows the mean and 95% confidence interval of the middle cerebral artery (MCA) pulsatility index.

Invasive Testing

Several invasive tests for the evaluation of the fetus with suspected growth restriction have been described. From a clinical standpoint, only a few studies are of critical importance. These include maternal TORCH serology and invasive fetal testing to obtain amniotic fluid and/or fetal blood for karyotyping to rule out a chromosomal abnormality such as trisomy 13, 18, or 21 (Table 31-4). Trisomy 18 may present with the unusual combination of growth restriction

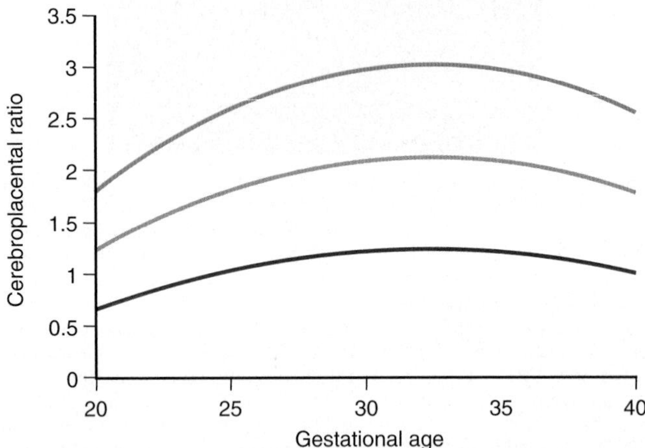

FIGURE 31-11. Cerebroplacental Doppler ratio with advancing gestational age. This graph displays the gestational reference range (mean and 95% confidence interval) of the cerebroplacental ratio based on paired measurements of the middle cerebral and umbilical artery pulsatility index.

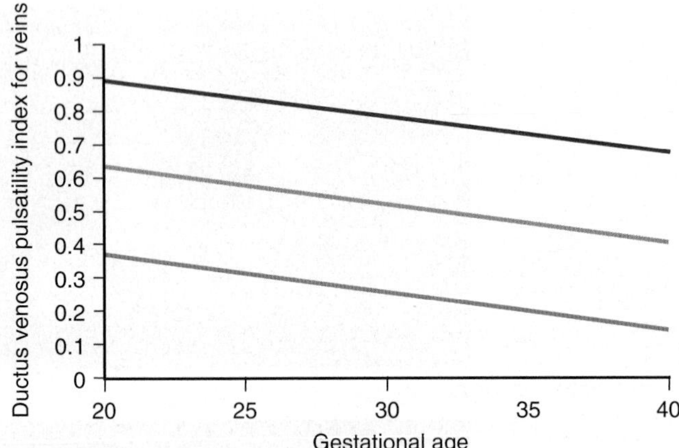

FIGURE 31-12. Ductus venosus pulsatility index for veins with advancing gestational age. This graph displays the gestational reference range (mean and 95% confidence interval) of the ductus venosus pulsatility index for veins calculated from cross-sectional data in 232 normal singleton fetuses.

TABLE 31-4 CHROMOSOMAL ABNORMALITIES AND IUGR

Ultrasound Findings Present			
IUGR	ANOMALY	HYDRAMNIOS	ABNORMAL KARYOTYPE
X			12/180 (7%)
X	X		18/57 (32%)
X		X	6/22 (27%)
X	X	X	7/15 (47%)

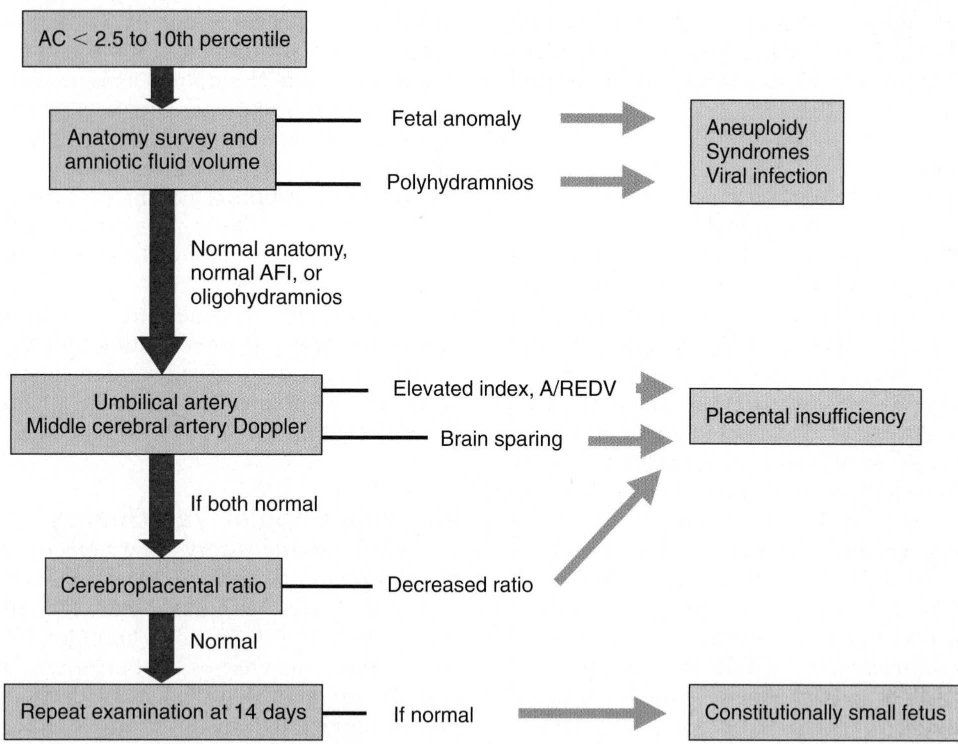

FIGURE 31-13. An integrated diagnostic approach to the fetus with suspected fetal growth restriction. This figure displays a decision tree following the evaluation of fetal anatomy, amniotic fluid volume, and umbilical and middle cerebral artery Doppler. The most likely clinical diagnosis based on the test results is presented on the right-hand side. A high index of suspicion for aneuploidy, viral, and nonaneuploid syndromes needs to be maintained at all times.

and polyhydramnios. If the diagnosis of a lethal anomaly can be made with certainty, cesarean delivery for fetal distress is unnecessary and may be prevented. Viral polymerase chain reaction (PCR) studies can be performed if there is a clinical suspicion based on the ultrasound examination or in the maternal history.

Evaluation of fetal erythropoietin and amino acid concentrations are also markers for fetal compromise with prognostic impact. Erythropoietin production in the fetus, as in the adult, is stimulated by the presence of anemia or hypoxia, and may be associated with increased red blood cell production depending on erythropoietic reserve. Elevated blood or amniotic fluid erythropoietin levels may be of help in identifying growth-restricted fetuses at risk for long-term morbidity. Ruth and colleagues identified an association between cord blood erythropoietin levels and developmental outcome including cerebral palsy and death at 2 years in offspring with evidence of acute asphyxia at birth. None of these patients had preeclampsia. Neonates from pregnancies complicated by preeclampsia had elevated cord erythropoietin levels regardless of outcome.

An increase in the cord blood glycine/valine ratio is a specific response to intrauterine starvation resulting from reduction in phosphoenolpyruvate carboxykinase activity, a rate-limiting enzyme for gluconeogenesis. Elevations of the glycine/valine ratio are observed in fetal life and have been shown to be inversely proportional to fetal arterial oxygen content. However, in contrast to the neonate where such an increased ratio is predictive of specific neonatal risks including hypoglycemia and death, such a relationship has not been demonstrated for elevations demonstrated in fetal life. Although fetal erythropoietin and amino acid levels are of academic interest, they currently add little to the contemporary clinical management of the IUGR fetus.

In summary, ultrasound examination is the primary diagnostic tool for the evaluation of fetal growth. In the presence of risk factors and clinical conditions that are associated with IUGR, a comprehensive gray-scale ultrasound examination of fetal anatomy, biometry, and amniotic fluid characteristics is required. In the absence of routine clinical indications, ultrasound screening of these high-risk pregnancies should be performed at 16 to 18 weeks for dating (if not otherwise established) and again at 32 to 34 weeks. If small fetal size is documented, Doppler ultrasound of the umbilical and middle cerebral arteries and invasive tests are of critical importance to identify fetuses most likely to benefit from antenatal surveillance and perinatal interventions. A diagnostic algorithm that utilizes this combination of test parameters is depicted in Figure 31-13.

SCREENING AND PREVENTION OF FETAL GROWTH RESTRICTION

Fetal growth restriction as a disease entity fulfills several criteria potentially justifying a screening program. It is a common clinical problem with an identifiable pre-disease state that leaves enough time for potential interventions. While treatment options in utero are limited (see below), interventions that improve outcome exist. The various screening methods that have been proposed include identification of risk factors, as well as serum and ultrasound tests.

Maternal History

A history of poor pregnancy outcome is clearly correlated with the subsequent delivery of a growth-restricted infant. Galbraith and colleagues and Tejan have shown that prior birth of a growth-restricted infant is the obstetric factor most often associated with the subsequent birth of another growth-restricted infant. These study populations did include women with underlying medical problems. Tejani and Mann in a retrospective study of 83 multigravidas who had delivered growth restricted infants noted that the perinatal wastage from their 200 prior pregnancies was 41%. This striking figure, which includes spontaneous abortions as well as neonatal and intrauterine deaths, points to the significance of poor obstetric history as a risk factor for IUGR. The history of delivery of a growth-restricted infant in the first pregnancy is associated with a 25% risk of delivering a second infant below the 10th percentile. After two pregnancies complicated by IUGR, there is a fourfold increase in the risk of a subsequent growth-restricted infant. When all indices of risk have been applied, the one third of patients considered at highest risk for delivering a growth restricted infant actually deliver over 60% of infants identified as growth restricted. The two thirds of women not considered at risk for delivering a growth-restricted infant contribute to one third of deliveries with a birthweight below the 10th percentile. The majority of these babies are considered constitutionally small.

Maternal Serum Analytes

At least four hormone/protein markers measured in the maternal sera during the early second trimester are associated with subsequent IUGR. These include serum estriol, human placental lactogen, human chorionic gonadotrophin, and α-fetoprotein (AFP). Elevated maternal serum α- fetoprotein (MSAFP) or human chorionic gonadotropin (hCG) levels in the second trimester are considered as markers of abnormal placentation and have been associated with an increased risk for IUGR.[54] Most studies conclude that a single, unexplained elevated value of 2 to 2.5 multiples of the median raises the risk of growth restriction 5- to 10-fold.

A range of first trimester serum analytes that are associated with early abnormalities in placenta angiogenesis and development have been identified in the past years. These show significant differences in their distribution among pregnancies at risk of developing early-onset preeclampsia or fetal growth restriction prior to 34 weeks' gestation. Of these markers a decrease in the pregnancy-associated protein A (PAPP-A) or the placental growth factor (PLGF) have shown the most consistent predictive performance. The advantage of PAPP-A is the current commercial availability as part of the integrated first trimester screen for aneuploidy. In this setting a decrease in the PAPP-A below 0.8 multiples of the median (MOM) is associated with an increased risk for subsequent placental dysfunction.

Clinical Examination

From the early second trimester on, each antenatal visit includes the measurement of the distance between the maternal uterine fundus and the symphysis pubis. After 20 weeks' gestation, the normal symphyseal-fundal height in centimeters approximates the weeks gestation after allowances for maternal height and fetal station. Belizan and colleagues observed that after 20 weeks' gestation a lag of the symphyseal-fundal height of 4 cm or more suggests growth restriction. The reported sensitivities of symphyseal-fundal height screening for IUGR range from 27% to 85%, and the positive predictive values range from 18% to 50%.[55] Although the measurement of the symphyseal-fundal height is a poor screening tool for the detection of IUGR, the accuracy of subsequent ultrasound prediction of IUGR is enhanced if there is a clinical suspicion of IUGR based on a lagging fundal height.

Maternal Doppler Velocimetry

Abnormal uterine artery flow velocity waveforms are a manifestation of delayed trophoblast invasion that are highly associated with gestational hypertensive disorders, IUGR, and fetal demise.[56] Therefore, Doppler velocimetry of the uterine arteries has been examined for its usefulness in predicting pregnancies destined to produce a growth-restricted fetus. Schulman and colleagues found that in women with hypertensive disorders the presence of an elevated uterine artery systolic/diastolic (S/D) ratio (>2.6) and/or diastolic notching increased the risk for IUGR and stillbirth (see Figure 31-17). They noted that the changes in uterine artery flow patterns precede those observed in the umbilical artery and antedate fetal growth restriction. Subsequent studies used various cut-offs to define an abnormal test result. These include S/D ratios above 2.18 at 18 weeks, resistance index (RI) above 0.58 at 18-24 weeks, pulsatility index (PI) above the 95th percentile (1.45) at 22-24 weeks, or the presence of notches. The screen positive rate ranges between 5% and 13% according to the gestational age and the criterion used to define an abnormal test result. In low-risk patients, a uterine artery Doppler resistance profile that is high, persistently notched, or both, identifies women at high risk for preeclampsia and IUGR, with sensitivities and positive predictive values as high as 72% and 35% when performed between 22 and 23 weeks' gestation. Uterine artery Doppler is better at predicting severe rather than mild disease. The likelihood ratio of abnormal uterine artery impedance for the development of IUGR was 3.7 with higher sensitivity for severe early-onset forms. Meta-analysis of the utility of uterine artery Doppler in the prediction of intrauterine death yields a likelihood ratio of 2.4 for patients with an abnormal result. Combining uterine artery Doppler velocimetry with other tests can improve screening sensitivities. Valensise and Romanini have demonstrated that the combination of abnormal second-trimester maternal uterine artery Doppler velocimetry and maternal glucose tolerance testing demonstrating a "flat" response results in a positive predictive value of 94% and a sensitivity of 54% for the detection of fetal growth restriction. The presence of a normal uterine artery flow velocity waveform bears a high negative predictive value, with a likelihood ratio of 0.5 and 0.8 for the development of preeclampsia and IUGR respectively.

First Trimester Integrated Screening

There are several markers that reflect early failure of normal placental development in the first trimester. One marker is abnormal maternal cardiovascular adaptation to pregnancy, resulting in a delay in the physiologic drop of mean arterial blood pressure. Deficient trophoblast invasion is associated with a slower than anticipated drop in uterine artery blood flow resistance. Placental expression of analytes relating to normal development is altered. When these markers are considered in isolation, their prediction of subsequent placental dysfunction is inaccurate. Therefore, an integrated screening algorithm using multiple independent risk factors, including a prior history of preeclampsia, maternal first trimester body mass index and blood pressure, uterine artery pulsatility index, and the PAPP-A MOM, has been developed. This combined model is capable of predicting early onset preeclampsia or fetal growth restriction with 80% to 90% sensitivity and a 5% to 10% false-positive rate. While the predictive accuracy of these algorithms needs to be confirmed in a variety of population settings, they offer the important advantage of early stratification of risk with potential for intervention.

Preventive Strategies

Efforts to prevent fetal growth restriction have been disappointing. Low-dose aspirin has been extensively evaluated as a possible preventive agent for improving placental vascular development by virtue of its inhibitory action on platelet aggregation. However, while the use of aspirin in the second trimester has been found to be safe, initiation of therapy in the second trimester improves neither placental function nor long-term outcome. Because subsets of patients with poor obstetric history appear to derive a benefit from aspirin, the utility of first trimester uterine artery screening with subsequent aspirin therapy has been investigated. The choice of target population profoundly affects the utility of this approach. While low-risk patients derive little benefit, high-risk patients (those with thrombophilia, hypertension, and/or a past history of either preeclampsia or IUGR) given low-dose aspirin because of bilateral uterine artery notching at 12 to 14 weeks experience an 80% reduction of placental disease compared to placebo-matched controls. A recent large meta-analysis found that only women who were initiated on aspirin before 16 weeks' gestation derive a 50% to 60% reduction in the relative risk for development of preeclampsia or fetal growth restriction.[57] Preliminary evidence also suggests that first trimester aspirin reduces the prevalence of preeclampsia in patients predicted to be at high risk through an integrated first trimester screen.

Presently it appears prudent to regard poor obstetric history, unexplained elevations in second trimester MSAFP, "flat" oral glucose tolerance, and abnormal second trimester uterine artery Doppler velocimetry as important risk factors for IUGR that warrant further investigation when the clinical suspicion of IUGR arises and/or maternal preeclampsia develops. Such patients should undergo ultrasound estimation of fetal size and a full diagnostic workup if these factors are confirmed.

MANAGEMENT IN CLINICAL PRACTICE

Before developing a management plan, it is important that the major underlying etiologies have been addressed by a comprehensive diagnostic workup as described above. **It is worth stressing that the majority of fetuses thought to be growth restricted are constitutionally small and require no intervention. Approximately 15% exhibit symmetrical growth restriction attributable to an early fetal insult for which there is no effective therapy. Here, an accurate diagnosis is essential. Finally, approximately 15% of small fetuses have growth restriction due to placental disease or reduced uteroplacental blood flow.** Once the diagnosis of placental insufficiency has been made, appropriate therapeutic options may be explored. However, ongoing assessment of fetal growth and parameters of fetal well-being is a more critical component of clinical management in defining the intervention thresholds when the balance of fetal versus neonatal risks favors delivery.

Therapeutic Options

Elimination of contributors such as stress, smoking, and alcohol and drug use is advocated. Tobacco smoke contains a number of substances that are vasoactive and can cause vasoconstriction. Anecdotally, the authors have observed IUGR cases with absent end-diastolic flow in the umbilical artery in which diastolic flow returned upon cessation of maternal smoking. Nonspecific therapies include bed rest in the left lateral decubitus position to increase placental blood flow. Although an inadequate diet has not been clearly established as a cause of growth restriction in this country, dietary supplementation may be helpful in those with poor weight gain or low prepregnancy weight. In patients with chronic malnutrition, improved fetal growth has been reported with total parenteral nutrition. Consideration should be given to hospitalized bed rest, which has the advantages of positive enforcement of rest and facilitation of daily fetal testing. The decision for inpatient versus outpatient management is based on the severity of the maternal and/or fetal condition and the local standard of care.

Maternal hyperoxygenation has been examined in several studies for potential benefits in the treatment of the compromised growth-restricted fetus. Studies by several groups confirm that maternal hyperoxygenation can raise the fetal cord blood pO_2.[58] Techniques used included administration of 55% oxygen by face mask or 2.5 L/min by nasal prong. Prolongation of pregnancy from the first recognition of the fetal condition ranged from 9 days to 5 weeks. However, fetal growth velocity was not improved. In addition, fetuses subjected to oxygen therapy had more hypoglycemia, thrombocytopenia, and disseminated intravascular coagulation compared to controls. The primary role of maternal hyperoxygenation lies in the safe short-term prolongation of pregnancy to allow the administration of corticosteroids to reduce the risk of neonatal respiratory distress syndrome (RDS) and intraventricular hemorrhage (IVH) in anticipation of a preterm delivery.

Maternal hyperalimentation as a means of intrauterine feeding of the growth-restricted fetus is an attractive therapeutic concept. Increasing the maternal concentration of amino acids leads to an increased umbilical uptake of some amino acids to the fetus while there is no change in the three essential amino acids: lysine, histidine, and threonine. These data further support that total parenteral nutrition can reverse abnormal fetal growth secondary to maternal nutritional deprivation. However, it does not overcome abnormal placental function. Outcomes are neither improved in animal models nor in human pregnancies. Therefore, maternal hyperalimentation only plays a role in patients where malnutrition has been established as the underlying cause of growth delay.

Maternal volume expansion as a therapeutic concept is based on the observation that poor maternal blood volume status is associated with adverse pregnancy outcome. Karsdorp and coworkers studied the effects of volume expansion on feto- and uteroplacental blood flow and neonatal outcome.[59] In a small group of centrally monitored women with abnormal placental Doppler studies, they noted that volume expansion was associated with reappearance of umbilical artery end-diastolic velocities and a significant improvement of neonatal survival. With further randomized studies pending, these data suggest that inpatient correction of maternal volume status is important in improving placental perfusion.

Low-dose aspirin in combination with dipyridamole administered from 16 weeks' gestation was first reported in 1987 by Wallenburg and Rotmans to significantly reduce the incidence of fetal growth restriction in women with a history of recurrent IUGR. Women receiving therapy had a rate of fetal growth restriction of 13%, compared with 61% in an untreated control group. No treated woman had a child with severe growth restriction (birth weight <2.3 percentile) compared with 27% in the untreated group. **In 1997, a meta-analysis of the efficacy of low-dose aspirin (50-100 mg/day) demonstrated a significant reduction in the frequency of IUGR when low-dose aspirin is used. There is a dose-dependent relationship in that higher doses (100-150 mg/day) were significantly more effective in preventing IUGR than were lower doses (50-80 mg/day).**

Two recent randomized trials illustrate important considerations regarding the use of aspirin to prevent preeclampsia and/or IUGR. In a study of patients that were randomized at 24 weeks' gestation based on the uterine artery flow velocity waveform, low-dose aspirin was not associated with any improvement in placental function or perinatal outcome. Conversely, in patients with a poor obstetric history (thrombophilia, hypertension, past history of either preeclampsia or IUGR) randomized at 12 to 14 weeks based on the uterine artery flow velocity waveforms, those receiving aspirin experienced an 80% reduction in placental disease compared to placebo matched controls. Therefore, it appears that aspirin works best in patients with significant risk factors for IUGR and that the therapeutic optimal window to commence aspirin therapy lies between 12 and 16 weeks' gestation when branching angiogenesis of the placenta is ongoing.

Although the overall safety of aspirin has been documented in a large patient population, concerns about a possible association with abdominal wall defects have been raised with administration in the early first trimester. Therefore, we suggest deferral of indicated therapy until completion of organogenesis at 12 weeks' gestation. Selected patients presenting in the second trimester may still derive benefit from aspirin, and patients should be counseled on an individualized basis. Aspirin prophylaxis can be discontinued at any point after 34 weeks' gestation because bleeding risks at delivery and during regional anesthesia outweigh the benefits of prolonging gestation.

Corticosteroids are a universally available antenatal therapeutic option that positively affects outcome by enhancing lung maturation and preventing IVH. The impact of prenatal glucocorticoid administration on neonatal complication rate in the growth-restricted newborn has recently been examined by Bernstein and coworkers in a study of 19,759 newborns between 500 and 1500 g. After controlling for a different set of confounding variables, this study demonstrated a significant reduction in neonatal RDS, IVH, and death when prenatal glucocorticoids were administered. These benefits were not qualitatively different from those observed in appropriately sized newborns. Other studies have also refuted that the "stress" of the intrauterine condition enhances maturation and protects against prematurity. In contrast, a smaller study by Elimian and colleagues demonstrated no benefits to neonatal outcome when perinatal glucocorticoids were used. While these studies indicate the need for randomized comparison of management, they also clearly show no benefit from the omission of antenatal corticosteroids. We recommend administration of a complete 48-hour course of antenatal steroids to any growth-restricted fetus when delivery is anticipated before 34 weeks' gestation, if this can be safely accomplished.

When corticosteroids are administered, it is important to account for their effect on fetal testing parameters when interpreting antenatal surveillance results. Betamethasone, for example, temporarily reduces FHR variation on day 2 and 3 after the first injection, together with a 50% decrease in fetal body movements and an almost cessation of fetal breathing movements. Subsequently the number of fetuses with an abnormal biophysical profile score increases significantly by 48 hours after steroid administration, with a return to the preadministration state at 72 hours.[60] In contrast, maternal and fetal Doppler findings are not affected to the same degree during this period. A transient decrease in the middle cerebral artery blood flow resistance has been reported 48 hours after betamethasone administration.

ASSESSMENT OF FETAL WELL-BEING (SEE CHAPTER 12)

Once the diagnosis of fetal growth restriction has been made and the differential diagnostic options have been explored, fetal assessment is instituted. Serial ultrasound evaluations of fetal growth are continued every 3 to 4 weeks and should include determinations of the BPD, HC/AC ratio, fetal weight, and AFV. The institution of antenatal surveillance is a critical component in the management of the growth-restricted fetus. Relationships between fetal testing parameters and subsequent outcome determine the balance between fetal and neonatal risks and therefore define intervention thresholds. Growth-restricted fetuses are at risk for worsening placental function, subsequent deterioration of acid–base status, decompensation, stillbirth, and adverse health effects all the way into adult life. Although prevention of long-term morbidity is an attractive goal, there is insufficient information on its relationships with prenatal variables to direct management. Of the many short-term outcomes that have been related to fetal status, only a few are presently of clinical relevance. Fetal acidemia and major neonatal complications have a significant impact on subsequent neurodevelopment while the combination of fetal and neonatal deaths determines the overall perinatal mortality.[61] The likelihood of fetal acidemia and stillbirth is therefore the strongest fetal criterion for intervention. In contrast, gestational age–specific expectations for neonatal complications and survival force conservative management. While neonatal complications are typically multifactorial and not accurately predicted prenatally, anticipation of fetal risks remains as the primary goal. Therefore, antenatal surveillance tests need to predict fetal acid–base status, rate of anticipated progression, and the resulting risk for deterioration and stillbirth. The monitoring tools that are available to achieve this include the traditional nonstress test (NST), contraction stress test, (CST), BPS profile scoring (BPS), and Doppler sonography.

Maternal Monitoring of Fetal Activity

Maternal monitoring of fetal activity has been used extensively in Great Britain, Scandinavia, and Israel for the assessment of pregnancies complicated by IUGR. In a study of 50 cases, Matthews clearly showed the predictive value of fetal activity charting for growth-restricted fetuses subsequently demonstrating distress in labor.[62] A simple technique for monitoring fetal movement is the minimum requirement of 10 movements in a 2-hour period. If this criterion is not met, additional testing is warranted. In an outpatient setting maternal kick counts or fetal activity counts (FACs) supplement medically administered antenatal surveillance. In the compliant patients with an appropriate level of awareness of fetal movements, it may also be helpful in modifying monitoring intervals as fetal deterioration occurs.

Fetal Heart Rate Analysis

The traditional NST is a visually analyzed record of the FHR baseline, variability, and episodic changes. Normal FHR characteristics are determined by gestational age, maturational and functional status of central regulatory centers, and oxygen tension. A "reactive" NST exhibits two 15-beat accelerations above the baseline maintained for 15 seconds in a 30-minute monitoring period. When the NST is analyzed as part of the five component biophysical profile score, reactivity criteria that account for gestational age are applied (see below). **Irrespective of the context, a "reactive" NST indicates absence of fetal acidemia at the moment of the FHR recording. Many growth-restricted fetuses with a normal heart rate tracing can have low-normal pO_2 values, but acidemia is virtually excluded by a reactive NST. Heart rate reactivity also correlates highly with a fetus that is not in immediate danger of intrauterine demise. Nonreactive NST results, on the other hand, are often falsely positive and require further evaluation. The development of repetitive decelerations may reflect fetal hypoxemia or cord compression due to the development of oligohydramnios and has been associated with a high perinatal mortality rate.**[63]

The CST is an additional option for testing placental respiratory reserve.[64] Positive CST results have been reported in 30% of pregnancies complicated by proven growth restriction. **In a study by Lin and colleagues,[65] 30% of growth-restricted infants had nonreactive NST results and 40% had positive CST results. Ninety-two percent of IUGR infants with a nonreactive positive pattern exhibited perinatal morbidity. However, a 25% to 50% false-positive rate has been associated with the CST by some investigators. A possible role for the CST may be evaluation of placental reserve prior to induction in IUGR fetuses in whom vaginal delivery is attempted.**

Marked intraobserver and interobserver variability of visual FHR analysis has been identified as a potential factor affecting the prediction of fetal status. Currently, traditional FHR parameters as well as short-term and long-term variation of the heart rate in milliseconds, length of episodes with low and high variation, and the rate of signal loss can be assessed by computerized analysis. The objective assessment of these variables circumvents the issue of observer variability and a direct correlation between FHR variation and pO_2 in the umbilical vein as assessed at cordocentesis prior to the onset of labor has been documented. **A computerized documentation of a mean minute variation below 3.5 milliseconds has been reported to predict an umbilical artery cord pH < 7.20 with over 90% sensitivity. In addition, FHR variation usually decreases gradually in the weeks preceding the appearance of late decelerations and fetal hypoxemia, and therefore is the most useful computerized FHR parameter for longitudinal assessment in IUGR.** As with the traditional NST, gestational age, time of day, and the presence of fetal rest-activity cycles also need to be taken into account in the interpretation of computerized results. There are wide normal ranges for FHR patterns and its variation, but the individual fetus shows a certain intrafetal consistency throughout gestation. For monitoring of trends each fetus should therefore serve as its own control, using recordings of standardized duration and appropriate reference ranges.

In summary, a visually reactive FHR provides assurance of fetal well-being at the time of analysis. While the traditional NST is most sensitive in the prediction of fetal normoxemia, computerized analysis appears superior in the prediction of hypoxemia and/or acidemia. Once traditional reactivity is lost, computerized analysis of heart rate variation is a potential tool available for ongoing longitudinal analysis. Computerized FHR analysis is more widely used in Europe and an ongoing randomized trial evaluates its utility in delivery timing of growth-restricted fetuses. FHR analysis itself does not assess the severity of disease and most importantly does not anticipate the rate of deterioration. To address these issues additional fetal tests are available.

Amniotic Fluid Volume

In the context of fetal surveillance, assessment of AFV provides an indirect measure of vascular status. A relationship between oligohydramnios and progressive deterioration of

arterial and venous Doppler studies has been documented in growth-restricted fetuses and prolonged pregnancies. Therefore, declining AFV is suggestive of ineffective downstream delivery of cardiac output, allowing some form of longitudinal monitoring even in the absence of Doppler studies. If the NST is reactive, a concurrent assessment of the AFV constitutes the "modified biophysical profile" and provides assurance of fetal well-being if both parameters are normal. Interventions based on twice weekly modified BPS result in similar perinatal outcomes as with weekly contraction stress testing and therefore have largely replaced the latter. When the fetal heart rate is nonreactive, relying on a normal AFV assessment alone is inadequate and a full biophysical profile that incorporates multiple parameters of fetal well-being should be performed because of its superior performance in identifying jeopardized fetuses.

Biophysical Parameters

The five-component fetal BPS was developed by Manning and colleagues and has been widely used in the surveillance of growth-restricted fetuses. A graded system is applied to categorize fetal tone, movement, breathing movement, heart rate reactivity, and a maximum amniotic fluid pocket as normal (2 points) or abnormal (0 points). If used in the context of the BPS, fetal heart rate reactivity criteria that account for gestational age are used. Reactivity has been defined as follows: prior to 32 weeks' gestation—greater than 10 beats/minute accelerations sustained for more than 10 seconds; between 32 to 36 weeks' gestation—greater than 15 beats/minute accelerations sustained for more than 15 seconds; and after 36 weeks' gestation—greater than 20 beats/minute accelerations sustained for more than 20 seconds. In anatomically normal fetuses, the presence of the dynamic variables is related to physiologic variations in maturation, behavioral state, as well as acid–base status. Vintzileos and coworkers have demonstrated that four components of the biophysical score are affected at different levels of hypoxemia and acidemia. The earliest manifestations of abnormal fetal biophysical activity consist of the loss of heat rate reactivity along with the absence of fetal breathing. This is followed by decreased fetal tone and movement in association with more advanced acidemia, hypoxemia, and hypercapnia. Because of amniotic fluid's relationship with vascular status, amniotic fluid assessment provides the only marker of chronic hypoxemia and is the only longitudinal monitoring component of the biophysical profile score.

Growth-restricted fetuses preserve acute central responses to acid–base status despite their maturational delay and are at risk for oligohydramnios. **The five-component BPS accounts best for physiologic and individual variations in behavior and therefore remains closely related to arterial pH in IUGR fetuses without anomalies from 20 weeks onward.[67] An abnormal score of 4 or less is associated with a mean pH of less than 7.20 and sensitivity in the prediction of acidemia is 100% for a score of 2 or less. A normal score and normal AFV indicate the absence of fetal acidemia at the time of testing. Longitudinal observations in growth-restricted fetuses have shown that the BPS deteriorates late and often rapidly.[23]** While an abnormal BPS is associated with escalating risks for stillbirth and perinatal mortality, a normal score allows no anticipation of fetal deterioration and stillbirth.

In summary, assessment of fetal biophysical variables provides an accurate measure of fetal status at the time of testing. In the patient with a nonreactive NST, a full five-component BPS needs to be performed. As a backup test for a nonreactive fetal heart rate test, the biophysical profile leads to lower rates of intervention when compared with the CST, without jeopardizing perinatal outcome. In the presence of normal AFV, a normal BPS of 8 (minus 2 for a nonreactive NST) or 10 is reassuring of fetal well-being. Nevertheless, in the absence of knowledge about placental vascular status the rate of progression cannot be anticipated and may require even daily testing in severe IUGR. The development of oligohydramnios is concerning and frequently requires modification of management or delivery. The knowledge of fetal Doppler status is complementary to BPS because it improves the anticipation of fetal deterioration and provides an additional means to assess fetal state.[66]

Doppler Ultrasound

Doppler parameters are influenced by several variables, including vascular histology, vascular tone, and fetal blood pressure. Placental respiratory function is related to the integrity of the villous vasculature, and a decrease in arterial pO_2 can trigger autoregulatory adjustments of vascular smooth muscle tone. As diagnostic tools, elevated umbilical artery blood flow resistance and/or middle cerebral artery brain sparing provide evidence of placental dysfunction. The utility of Doppler ultrasound in the assessment of fetal well-being is based on the relationship between Doppler parameters with metabolic status, rate of disease progression, and the risk for stillbirth. In this context distinction between early and late fetal vascular responses to placental insufficiency provides a useful framework within which to estimate these risks.

"Early" responses to placental insufficiency are observed in mild placental vascular disease when umbilical artery end-diastolic velocity is still present. A decrease in the cerebral/placental Doppler ratio provides an early and sensitive marker of redistribution of cardiac output, often preceding overt growth delay by up to 2 weeks. The reduction of fetal growth velocity generally mirrors the elevation in umbilical artery blood flow resistance and is followed by decreasing middle cerebral artery impedance (brain sparing). The nadir of cerebral blood flow resistance is typically reached after a median of 2 weeks and is followed by an increase in aortic blood flow impedance.[68] **Early cardiovascular responses are considered compensatory because they occur at a time when cardiac function is normal and are typically accompanied by preferential perfusion of vital organs and the placenta. While the fetus may be hypoxemic, the risk for acidemia is low.**

"Late" responses to placental insufficiency are observed when accelerating placental disease results in loss or reversal of umbilical artery end-diastolic velocity and when fetal deterioration becomes evident through parallel elevations in placental blood flow resistance and venous Doppler

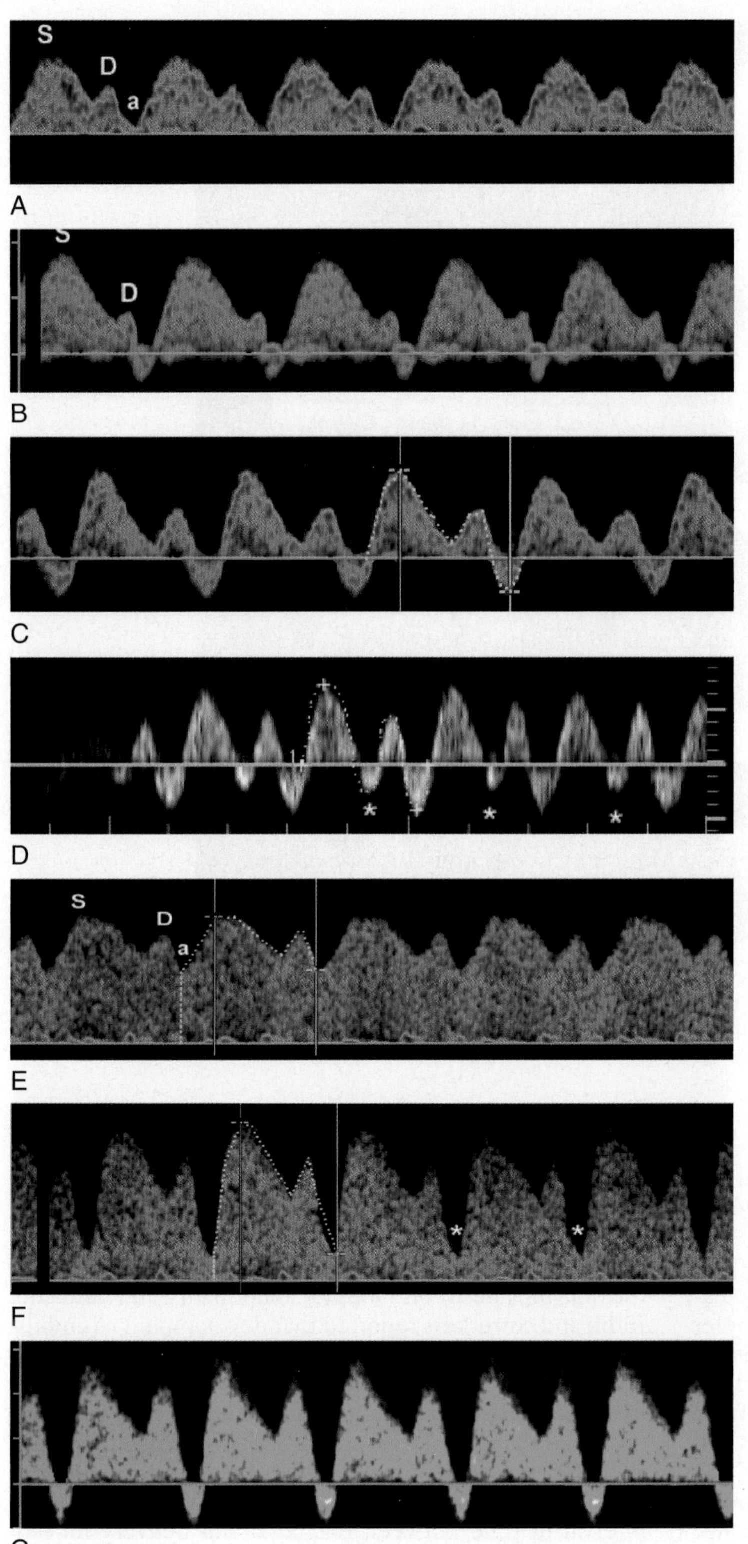

FIGURE 31-14. Normal and abnormal precordial venous flow velocity waveforms. The inferior vena cava and ductus venosus are the most commonly evaluated precordial veins, while the umbilical venous flow velocity waveform is predominantly assessed qualitatively. The inferior vena cava shows the typical triphasic pattern with systolic and diastolic peaks (*S, D,* respectively) **(A).** The a-wave may be reversed under physiologic conditions **(B).** An abnormal inferior vena cava flow velocity waveform shows a relative decrease in forward flow during the first trough, the D-wave, and the a-wave **(C).** Under extreme circumstances there may be reversed flow during the first trough (*) **(D).** In contrast to the inferior vena cava, the ductus venous has antegrade blood flow throughout the cardiac cycle with forward velocities during the S-, D-, and a-waves **(E).** A decrease in atrial systolic forward velocities (*) is the first sign of abnormality and results in an increased Doppler index **(F).** With marked elevation of central venous pressure blood flow may reverse during atrial systole **(G).**

indices. **Although the development of abnormal venous blood flows has been documented in many veins, the precordial veins, including the ductus venosus, the inferior vena cava, and the umbilical vein, are typically utilized in clinical practice (Figures 31-14 and 31-15).**[69] When fetal compromise accelerates there is a further steady rise in umbilical blood flow resistance; venous Doppler indices escalate over a wide range, and the development of oligohydramnios and metabolic acidemia is characteristic of ineffective downstream delivery of cardiac output.[70] In the final stages of compromise, cardiac dilatation with holosystolic tricuspid insufficiency, complete fetal inactivity,

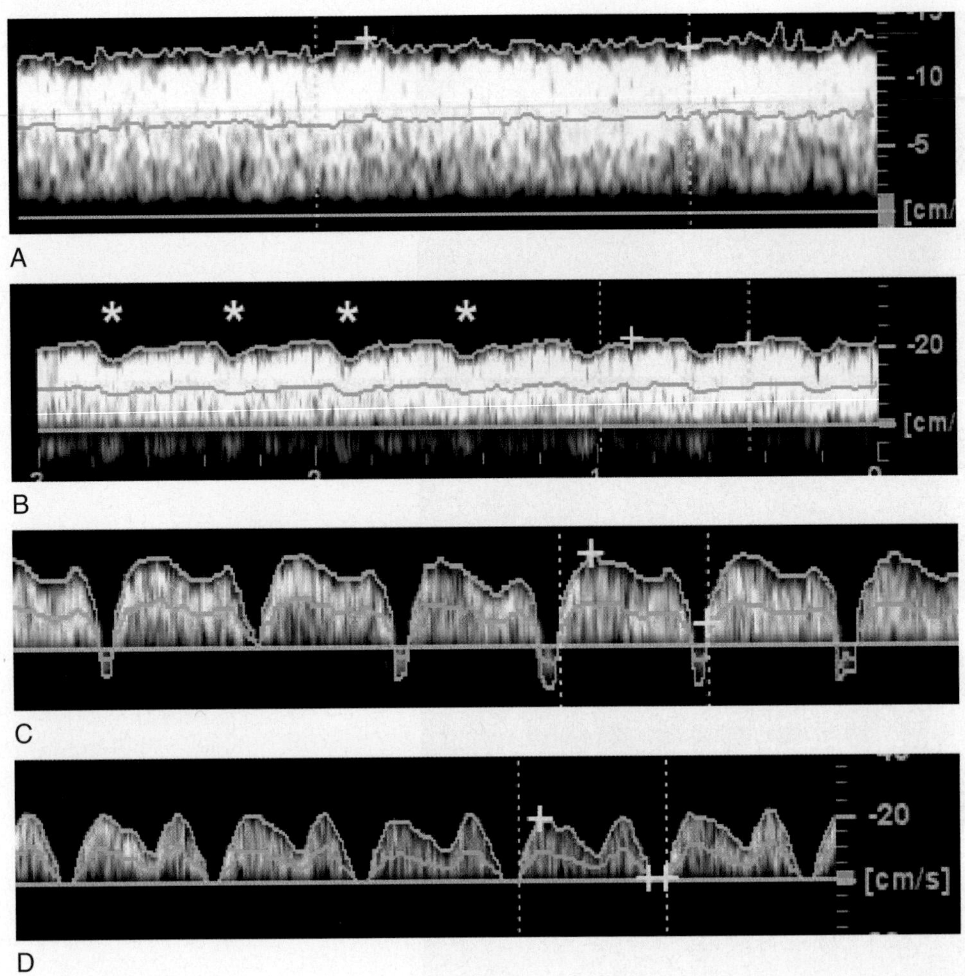

FIGURE 31-15. Normal and abnormal umbilical venous flow velocity. Umbilical venous blood flow is usually constant **(A)**. Monophasic umbilical venous pulsations (*) may be observed with moderate elevations of placental blood flow resistance and/or oligohydramnios **(B)**. Retrograde propagation of increased central venous pressure first results in biphasic and then triphasic pulsations (**C** and **D**, respectively).

short-term variation below 3.5 msec, and spontaneous "cardiac" late decelerations of the fetal heart rate can be observed as preterminal events (Figure 31-16).[71]

In the past, the major focus of Doppler studies for the assessment of fetal health has been the umbilical circulation. The association between an elevation in Doppler blood flow indices in the umbilical artery, increased disturbance of placental perfusion, and the deterioration of fetal acid–base status that is proportional to the degree of the Doppler abnormality has been demonstrated by several investigators. In the fetal compartment, elevation of the umbilical artery **Doppler index is observed when approximately 30% of the fetal villous vessels are abnormal. Absence or even reversal of umbilical artery end-diastolic velocity can occur when 60% to 70% of the villous vascular tree is damaged.**[72] **Incidences of intrauterine hypoxia ranging from 50% to 80% in fetuses with absent end-diastolic flow have been reported.** The benefit of umbilical artery Doppler in management has been documented in randomized controlled trials and meta-analyses. **In these studies, umbilical artery Doppler, when used in conjunction with standard antepartum testing, was associated with a decrease of up to 38% in perinatal mortality, antenatal admissions, inductions of labor, and cesarean deliveries for fetal distress in labor in women considered at high risk.** However, several studies that have examined the cerebral and especially the venous circulation have provided greater insight into the relationships between Doppler abnormality and outcome. Indik and coworkers reported that development of umbilical venous pulsations in fetuses with absent end-diastolic velocities in the umbilical artery was associated with a fivefold increase in mortality. Arduini and colleagues demonstrated that gestational age at onset, maternal hypertension, and the development of pulsations in the umbilical venous velocities were significantly correlated with the interval of time between diagnosis and delivery for late decelerations of the FHR.[73] Subsequently, several studies have confirmed that fetuses with abnormal arterial velocities who also developed abnormal precordial venous velocities had a higher morbidity and mortality than fetuses without abnormal venous flow.[74] These studies and subsequent analyses confirm that fetal Doppler assessment that is based on the umbilical artery alone is no longer appropriate, particularly in the setting of early onset IUGR prior to 34 weeks. Incorporation of middle cerebral artery and venous Doppler provide the best prediction of

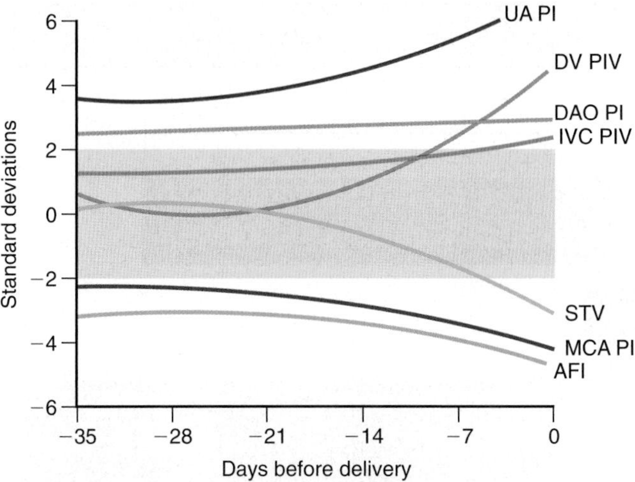

FIGURE 31-16. Longitudinal progression of antenatal testing variables. This figure displays trends in arterial and venous Doppler parameters (*DAO,* Descending aorta; *DV,* ductus venosus; *IVC,* inferior vena cava; *MCA,* middle cerebral artery; *PI,* pulsatility index; *PIV,* PI for veins, *UA,* umbilical artery), amniotic fluid index *(AFI),* and computerized fetal heart rate short-term variation *(STV)* in relation to delivery expressed as standard deviation for growth-restricted fetuses delivered before 32 weeks' gestation. The graph demonstrates that arterial Doppler parameters may be abnormal for more than 5 weeks prior to delivery, whereas venous Doppler parameters and the short-term variation deteriorate in the week prior to delivery for fetal indications. (Reproduced from Hecher K, Bilardo CM, Stigter RH, et al: Monitoring of fetuses with intrauterine growth restriction: a longitudinal study. Ultrasound Obstet Gynecol 18:564, 2001.)

acid–base status, risk of stillbirth, and the anticipated rate of progression.

In growth-restricted fetuses with an elevated Doppler index in the umbilical artery, brain sparing in the presence of normal venous Doppler parameters is typically associated with hypoxemia but a normal pH. Elevation of venous Doppler indices, either alone or in combination with umbilical venous pulsations, increases the risk for fetal acidemia. This association is strengthened by serial elevations of the ductus venosus Doppler index. Dependent on the cut-off (2 SD vs. 3 SD) and the combinations of veins examined, sensitivity for prediction of acidemia ranges from 70% to 90% and specificity from 70% to 80%. **Abnormal venous Doppler parameters are the strongest Doppler predictors of stillbirth. Even among fetuses with severe arterial Doppler abnormalities (e.g., AEDV or REDV), the risk of stillbirth is largely confined to those fetuses that have abnormal venous Dopplers.**[74] The likelihood of stillbirth increases with the degree of venous Doppler abnormality. Venous Doppler findings that are particularly ominous are absence or reversal of the ductus venous a-wave and biphasic/triphasic umbilical venous pulsations. In the setting of a 25% stillbirth rate in a preterm severe IUGR population, these Doppler findings have a 65% predictive sensitivity and 95% specificity.[75]

Although neonatal morbidity is primarily determined by gestational age at delivery and neonatal mortality is the product of several factors, both of these outcomes are also related to fetal Doppler studies. Arterial redistribution and brain sparing are not associated with a significant rise in major neonatal complications. In contrast, a 2 SD elevation of the ductus venosus Doppler index is associated with a 3-fold increase in neonatal complications, and further escalation of ductus venosus Doppler indices leads to an 11-fold increase in this relative risk. The neonatal mortality rate in fetuses with absent or reverse umbilical artery end-diastolic velocity ranges from 5% to 18% when the venous Doppler indices are normal. Elevation of the ductus venosus Doppler index greater than 2 SDs doubles this mortality rate, although predictive sensitivity is only 38% with a specificity of 98%.

In summary, Doppler evaluation of the umbilical, cerebral, and precordial vessels of the growth-restricted fetus provides important diagnostic and prognostic information. Fetal acidemia and the risk of stillbirth are high with progressive elevation of venous Doppler indices. **Advancing Doppler abnormalities indicate acceleration of disease and require increased frequency of fetal monitoring. In growth-restricted fetuses, Doppler evaluation is complementary to all other surveillance modalities.**

Invasive Fetal Testing

Direct determination of fetal acid–base status by cordocentesis was previously frequently performed during invasive karyotyping. Nicolini and colleagues examined 58 growth-restricted fetuses, using cordocentesis for acid–base evaluation in addition to karyotyping. They found significant differences in pH, pCO_2, pO_2, and the base equivalent in fetuses that had no evidence of end-diastolic flow by umbilical artery Doppler velocimetry. However, they observed no relationship between acid–base determination and perinatal outcome. Pardi and colleagues[76] examined umbilical blood acid–base status in 56 growth-restricted fetuses and demonstrated an association between acid–base status and the results of cardiotocographic and umbilical artery Doppler waveform analysis. If both FHR and Doppler studies were normal, neither hypoxemia nor acidemia was noted. When both tests were abnormal, 64% of the growth-restricted fetuses demonstrated abnormal acid–base analysis. The prognostic significance of these abnormalities remains unclear. The lack of benefit, complication rate, accuracy of noninvasive assessment of fetal acid–base status, and finally the availability for rapid karyotyping techniques from amniocytes all mean that cordocentesis is rarely necessary today.

Anticipating the Progression to Fetal Compromise

The anticipation of clinical progression is a critical component in the management of IUGR fetuses because it determines fetal surveillance intervals as well as the timing for intervention. Although deterioration of fetal status is manifested in all surveillance modalities, accelerating disease is best anticipated by AFV status and arterial and venous Doppler parameters (Figure 31-17). **However, the gestational age at onset has important impacts on the clinical presentation and, accordingly, on the diagnosis and management of FGR. In early-onset growth delay (prior to 34 weeks' gestation), the significantly decreased survival rates, as well as the higher mortality following immediate delivery, places special emphasis on safe pregnancy prolongation in these pregnancies.**[77,78] **Late onset FGR (presenting after 34 weeks' gestation) does not typically pose a dilemma for**

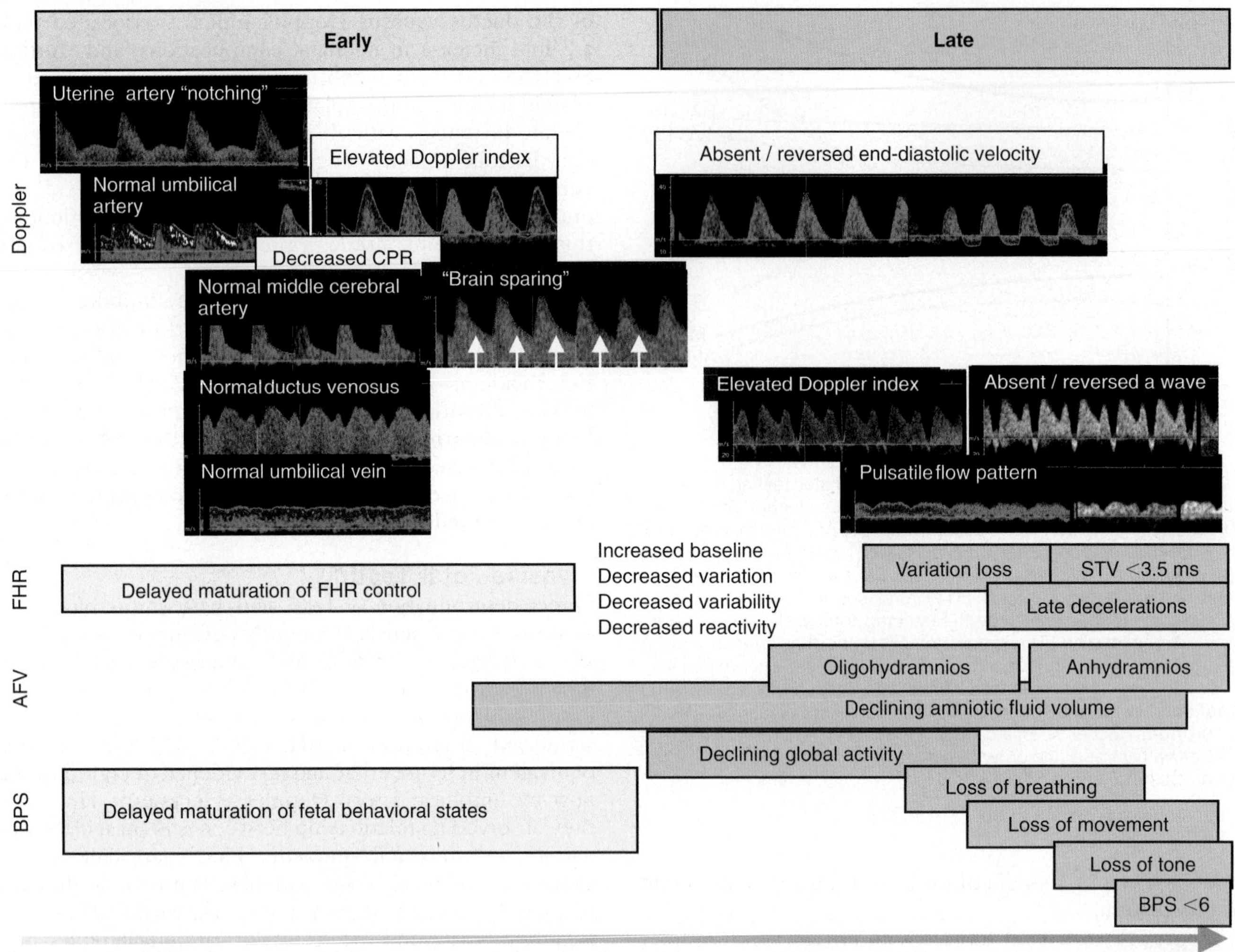

Figure 31-17. Progression of compromise in various monitoring systems. This figure summarizes the early and late responses to placental insufficiency. Doppler variables in the placental circulation precede abnormalities in the cerebral circulation. Fetal heart rate *(FHR),* amniotic fluid volume *(AFV),* and biophysical parameters *(BPS)* are still normal at this time and computerized analysis of fetal behavioral patterns is necessary to document a developmental delay. With progression to late responses, venous Doppler abnormality in the fetal circulation is characteristic, often preceding the sequential loss of fetal dynamic variables and frequently accompanying the decline in AFV. The * in the ductus venosus flow velocity waveform marks reversal of blood flow during atrial systole (a-wave). The decline in biophysical variables shows a reproducible relationship with acid–base status. Because the BPS is a composite score of five variables, an abnormal BPS less than 6 often develops late and may be sudden. Absence or reversal of the ductus venous a-wave, decrease of the short-term variation *(STV)* of the computerized fetal heart rate analysis, spontaneous late decelerations, and an abnormal biophysical profile score are the most advanced testing abnormalities. If adaptation mechanisms fail and the fetus remains undelivered, stillbirth ensues.

delivery timing because delivery thresholds can be low given the lower neonatal risks. However, late onset FGR is a significant clinical problem that contributes to over 50% of unanticipated stillbirths at term.[79] Accordingly, a more pressing issue in term pregnancies is the recognition of growth-restricted fetuses, rather than the timing of their delivery. Recognizing these important differences in management focus helps to clarify the nature of decisions that need to be based on the results of the surveillance examination. The prinicipal choices that need to be made at each monitoring visit are whether intervention is needed and the interval to the next visit. The intervention threshold is based on the balance of fetal and neonatal risks, and is high at early gestation given the high neonatal morbidity, but successively decreases as gestation advances. The monitoring interval is often empirically defined but needs to be shortened if there are fetal signs of deterioration that indicate an acceleration of the disease. This in turn requires an appreciation of the typical pattern of progression in early and late onset fetal growth restriction.[14,80]

Umbilical artery Doppler alone provides inaccurate prediction because progression to abnormal FHR parameters is highly variable and may range from 0 to 49 days, as reported in a study by Farine and coworkers. In general, early-onset IUGR presenting prior to 28 weeks is associated with more marked placental vascular problems producing marked Doppler changes. In contrast, IUGR presenting near term is typically associated with milder placental disease and therefore more subtle Doppler findings. Decreasing AFV and behavioral responses are preserved throughout gestation irrespective of Doppler status. Accordingly, longitudinal progression and clinical findings may vary based on gestational age and may be

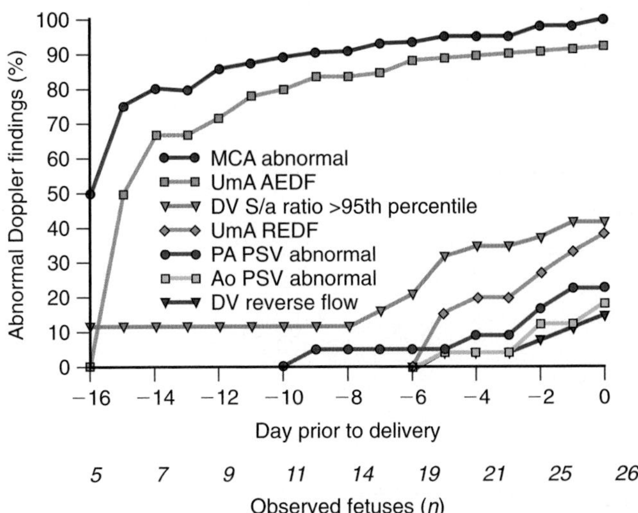

Figure 31-18. Early and late Doppler findings in growth-restricted fetuses. This figure displays cumulative onset time curves of Doppler abnormalities for each fetal vessel examined. Middle cerebral artery brain sparing and absent umbilical artery end-diastolic velocity are observed up to 16 days before delivery. *Ao PSV,* Aortic peak systolic velocity; *DV,* ductus venosus; *MCA,* middle cerebral artery; *PA PSV,* pulmonary artery peak systolic velocity; *UmA EDF,* umbilical artery absent end-diastolic flow; *UmA REDF,* umbilical artery reverse end-diastolic flow. (Modified from Ferrazzi E, Bozzo M, Rigano S, et al: Temporal sequence of abnormal Doppler changes in the peripheral and central circulatory systems of the severely growth-restricted fetus. Ultrasound Obstet Gynecol 19:140, 2002.)

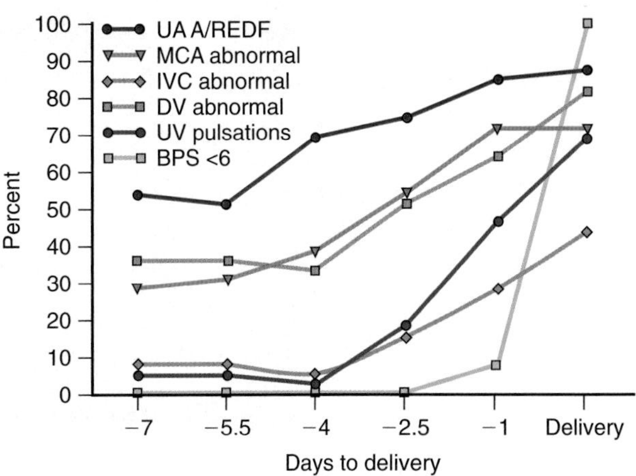

Figure 31-19. Sequential deterioration of Doppler and biophysical parameters. This figure shows the percentage of abnormal Doppler findings in individual vessels and the incidence of a biophysical profile score below 6 (BPS <6) in the last week prior to delivery represented by the lines. *A/REDF,* Absent or reversed end-diastolic flow; *DV,* ductus venosus; *IVC,* inferior vena cava; *MCA,* middle cerebral artery; *UA,* umbilical artery; *UV,* umbilical vein. Deterioration of Doppler findings precedes decline in biophysical profile score. (Reproduced from Baschat AA, Gembruch U, Harman CR: The sequence of changes in Doppler and biophysical parameters as severe fetal growth restriction worsens. Ultrasound Obstet Gynecol 18:571, 2001.)

further modulated by maternal disease.[81] Beyond 34 weeks where the umbilical artery waveform may be normal or near normal, assessment of the middle cerebral artery flow velocity waveform and/or the cerebroplacental Doppler ratio may be necessary to provide an estimate of placental disease and direct the frequency of testing.[53]

In fetuses with elevated placental blood flow resistance, onset of middle cerebral artery brain sparing and/or a decline in the AFI indicate accelerating disease. Once brain sparing is established, the next level of deterioration occurs when umbilical artery end-diastolic velocity is lost and parallel elevations in placental blood flow resistance and precordial venous Doppler indices are observed. Although this may happen after several weeks, the anticipation of such deterioration may require twice weekly rather than weekly testing. When accelerating fetal compromise occurs it is associated with a further rise in umbilical blood flow resistance (leading to REDV) whereas venous Doppler indices escalate over a wide range of distribution (see Figure 31-15). **Studies by Baschat, Ferrazzi, Hecher, and Bilardo indicate that 40% of preterm growth-restricted fetuses that deteriorate in utero have an increased ductus venosus Doppler index the week prior to delivery (Figures 31-16, 31-18, and 31-19).** On the day of delivery, an additional 20% deteriorated further. Elevations of precordial venous Doppler indices also precede sudden deterioration of the BPS by a median of 1 week in fetuses with elevated umbilical artery blood flow resistance. These findings have important impact on testing frequency. For example, in a preterm growth-restricted fetus where venous Doppler indices are elevated, a BPS of 10 does not provide assurance that fetal status will remain stable for the following week. In fact, a sizeable proportion of these fetuses may have a biophysical profile score of less than 6 after a median time of just 1 day.[23] Therefore, three-times weekly or even daily testing may be necessary in such fetuses. This is illustrated in a study by Divon and coworkers, who performed daily biophysical scoring in fetuses with absent umbilical artery end-diastolic velocity. Delivery was indicated for maternal reasons, a BPS below 6, oligohydramnios, documented lung maturity, or a gestational age beyond 36 weeks. There were no stillbirths and no cord artery pH below 7.20 using this intensive monitoring approach.

The clinical progression in Doppler and biophysical abnormalities is observed in approximately 70% to 80% of growth-restricted fetuses prior to 34 weeks' gestation.[14,23] Two rates of progression have been described by Turan and coworkers that can be anticipated based on the umbilical artery end-diastolic velocity. In pregnancies in which umbilical artery end-diastolic velocity is lost within the first 2 weeks of diagnosis, deterioration to venous Doppler and biophysical abnormalities within 4 weeks is common (Figure 31-20). If umbilical artery end-diastolic is maintained for longer periods, deterioration may not occur for 6 weeks after diagnosis. In late-onset growth restriction presenting beyond 34 weeks' gestation, several other presentations are possible. Umbilical artery blood flow resistance may be normal and brain sparing may be observed as the only Doppler sign of perceived hypoxemia. Alternatively, Doppler findings may be normal, and oligohydramnios and/or a decline of biophysical variables may be the only signs of placental insufficiency. On a similar note, the speed of progression may vary significantly in these different clinical scenarios and persistence of normal umbilical Doppler parameters for up to 9 weeks before new-onset

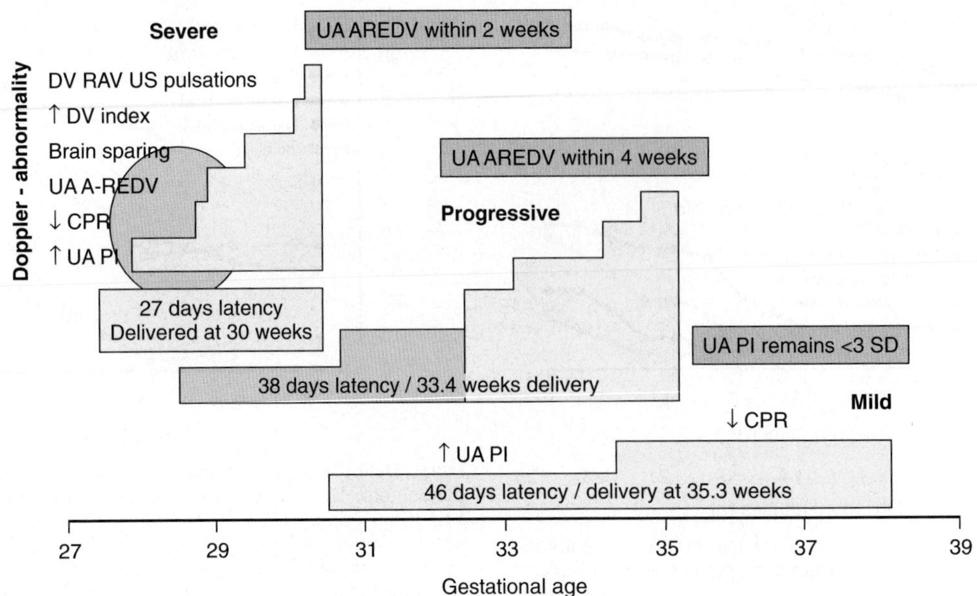

FIGURE 31-20. Two rates of progression can be anticipated based on the umbilical artery end-diastolic velocity. Losing umbilical artery end-diastolic velocity within the first 2 weeks of diagnosis commonly leads to deterioration to venous Doppler and biophysical abnormalities within 4 weeks (middle section of the figure). However, umbilical artery end-diastolic can be maintained for longer periods and deterioration may not occur for 6 weeks after diagnosis (bottom section of figure).

brain sparing is observed is not unusual. In recognition of these variable time scales and patterns of deterioration, it is evident that the combination of several testing modalities is more likely to provide evidence of deterioration. If biophysical profile scoring is used, particular attention needs to be placed to the amniotic fluid, because this is the only component reflecting longitudinal progression. The most comprehensive approach that addresses cardiovascular and behavioral responses in IUGR fetuses across all gestational ages has been described as "integrated fetal testing."

Integrated fetal testing utilizes a surveillance approach to pregnancies with IUGR that requires familiarity with the combined assessment of the five-component BPS and arterial and venous Doppler studies.[82] Doppler examination includes evaluation of the umbilical artery, middle cerebral artery, ductus venosus, and free umbilical vein flow velocity waveform. The testing is always supplemented with maternal assessment of fetal movement ("kick counts"). Surveillance is initiated no earlier than 24 weeks' gestation. In fetuses with elevated umbilical artery pulsatility, positive end-diastolic flow, and absence of any additional abnormality, weekly biophysical profile scoring and fortnightly multivessel Doppler monitoring are performed. With the onset of brain sparing, Doppler monitoring intervals are shortened to weekly visits. In fetuses with an AFI of less than 5 cm or AEDV in the umbilical artery, surveillance intervals are shortened to every 3-4 days. With elevation of the ductus venosus Doppler index to less than 2 SD, testing frequency is increased to every 2 to 3 days. Further escalation of the ductus venosus Doppler index may require daily testing, and inpatient admission may be prudent based on local practice. Any change in maternal condition, especially the development of preeclampsia, calls for reassessment of fetal status irrespective of the last examination result (Figure 31-21).

THE TIMING OF DELIVERY

In the absence of definitive fetal therapy, proper timing of delivery is often the critical management issue when dealing with the growth-restricted fetus. In principle, the decision for delivery always weighs fetal risks against risks that can be anticipated as a result of delivery. The risks of prematurity are of primary concern and make the management of the preterm growth-restricted fetus particularly challenging. Typically, the decline in neonatal mortality is greatest between 24 and 28 weeks, whereas morbidity declines progressively thereafter toward 32 weeks. Although there are surprisingly few randomized management studies that address the issue of delivery timing in IUGR, the Growth Restriction Intervention Trial (GRIT) clarifies several important points.[83] This prospective multicenter study randomized more than 500 women with complicating fetal growth restriction into immediate versus delayed delivery when their managing physicians were unsure about the timing of delivery. In the conservatively managed group, delivery was delayed until a point when their managing obstetricians were no longer unsure about the need to deliver or when fetal testing became overtly normal. With a median delay of 4.5 days, no significant differences in short-term outcome were identified between the two groups (Table 31-5). The perinatal mortality with early delivery was associated with a higher rate of neonatal deaths, whereas delaying delivery increased the risk for stillbirth. Delivery timing also had little effect on neurodevelopment at 2 years of age. However, in the subset of fetuses delivered before 32 weeks, a trend toward poor neurodevelopment was primarily attributable to neonatal complications that occurred as a result of prematurity. In 2010, Walker and colleagues reported on the 6- to 13-year GRIT study outcomes and found the two groups to be similar for cognitive, language, behavior, and motor ability (half of original cohort). This

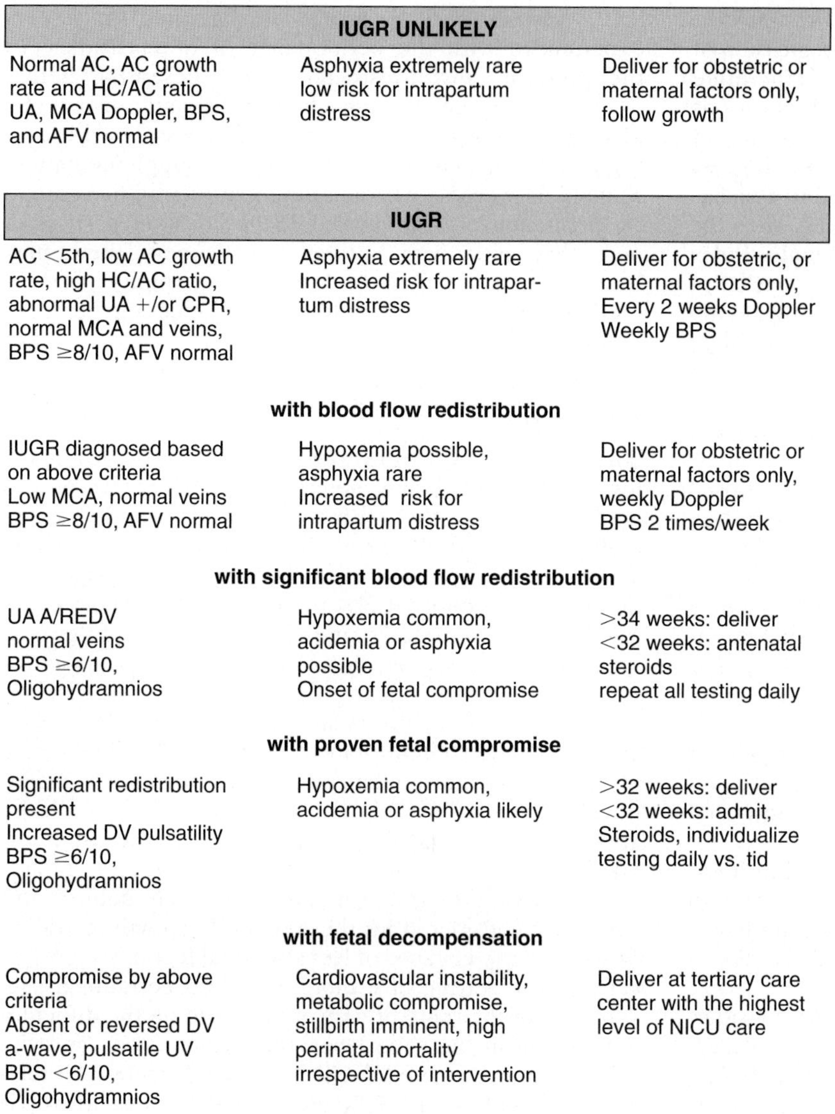

IUGR UNLIKELY

Normal AC, AC growth rate and HC/AC ratio UA, MCA Doppler, BPS, and AFV normal	Asphyxia extremely rare low risk for intrapartum distress	Deliver for obstetric or maternal factors only, follow growth

IUGR

AC <5th, low AC growth rate, high HC/AC ratio, abnormal UA +/or CPR, normal MCA and veins, BPS ≥8/10, AFV normal	Asphyxia extremely rare Increased risk for intrapartum distress	Deliver for obstetric, or maternal factors only, Every 2 weeks Doppler Weekly BPS

with blood flow redistribution

IUGR diagnosed based on above criteria Low MCA, normal veins BPS ≥8/10, AFV normal	Hypoxemia possible, asphyxia rare Increased risk for intrapartum distress	Deliver for obstetric or maternal factors only, weekly Doppler BPS 2 times/week

with significant blood flow redistribution

UA A/REDV normal veins BPS ≥6/10, Oligohydramnios	Hypoxemia common, acidemia or asphyxia possible Onset of fetal compromise	>34 weeks: deliver <32 weeks: antenatal steroids repeat all testing daily

with proven fetal compromise

Significant redistribution present Increased DV pulsatility BPS ≥6/10, Oligohydramnios	Hypoxemia common, acidemia or asphyxia likely	>32 weeks: deliver <32 weeks: admit, Steroids, individualize testing daily vs. tid

with fetal decompensation

Compromise by above criteria Absent or reversed DV a-wave, pulsatile UV BPS <6/10, Oligohydramnios	Cardiovascular instability, metabolic compromise, stillbirth imminent, high perinatal mortality irrespective of intervention	Deliver at tertiary care center with the highest level of NICU care

FIGURE 31-21. Integrated fetal testing and management protocol. The management algorithm for pregnancies complicated by fetal growth restriction is based on the ability to perform arterial and venous Doppler as well as a full five-component biophysical profile score. (From Baschat AA, Hecher K: Fetal growth restriction due to placental disease. Semin Perinatol 28:67, 2004.) *AC,* Abdominal circumference; *AFV,* amniotic fluid volume; *A/REDV,* absent/reversed end-diastolic velocity; *BPS,* biophysical profile score; *CPR,* cerebroplacental ratio; *DV,* ductus venosus; *HC,* head circumference; *MCA,* middle cerebral artery; *NST,* nonstress test; *NICU,* neonatal intensive care unit; *tid,* three times daily; *UA,* umbilical artery.

TABLE 31-5 OUTCOMES IN THE GROWTH RESTRICTION INTERVENTION TRIAL (GRIT)

	IMMEDIATE (*n* = 296)	DELAYED (*n* = 291)
GA at entry (weeks)	32 (30-34)	32 (29-34)
Steroids already given	191 (70%)	189 (69%)
Days gained in utero	0.9 (0.4-1.2)	4.9 (2-10.8)
Birthweight (g)	1200 (875-1705)	1400 (930-1940)
Apgar <7 at 5 minutes	25 (9%)	17 (6%)
Cord pH <7.0[‡]	2 (1%)	4 (2%)
Death prior to discharge	29 (10%)	27 (9%)
Stillbirth	2	9
Neonatal death	23	12
Death >28 days	4	6
Survivors after 2 years	256	251
Developmental delay at age 2 for patients delivered at 24-31 weeks	14 (13%)	5 (5%)

Data from The GRIT study group. A randomised trial of timed delivery for the compromised preterm fetus: short term outcomes and Bayesian interpretation. BJOG 110:27, 2003; Thornton JG, Hornbuckle J, Vail A, et al; The GRIT study group: Infant well-being at 2 years of age in the Growth Restriction Intervention Trial (GRIT): multicentred randomized trial. Lancet 364:513, 2004.
GA, Gestational age.

suggests that neurologic impairment may already be set by the time IUGR fetuses reach the point of delivery. Other observational studies also address the impact of gestational age on perinatal morbidity. In prenatally identified growth-restricted fetuses, the effect of gestational age overshadows all other perinatal variables. **After 27.0 weeks, when survival and intact survival first exceed 50%, a birthweight below 550 grams is associated with a high risk for neonatal death.**[84,85] **It appears that fetal deterioration of venous Doppler parameters begins to have an independent impact on neonatal survival from 28 weeks onward as postpartum morbidities become less frequent with advancing gestation.**[78] **Gestational age is also an important factor affecting perinatal mortality in patients who remain undelivered. Frigoletto has previously emphasized that the majority of fetal deaths in IUGR occur after the 36th week of gestation and before the onset of labor.**

These studies illustrate several points that are of critical importance in the management of pregnancies complicated by IUGR today. Patients need to be aware that growth-restricted fetuses have different viability thresholds and neonatal risk statistics than their appropriately grown counterparts. The major risk for the growth-restricted fetus that remains undelivered is progression of hypoxemia to acidemia and stillbirth. Delivery is therefore typically indicated when the risk for these complications is high or there is no added benefit from prolongation of pregnancy. **The risk for acidemia and stillbirth is highest when repetitive late decelerations are observed in association with oligohydramnios and/or anhydramnios, when the BPS is below 6, when the ductus venosus Doppler index elevation escalates beyond 3 SDs and/or when reversal of the ductus venosus a-wave is observed with accompanying umbilical venous pulsations.** In addition, it is helpful to consider the delivery indications according to gestational epochs.

Between 24 and 27 weeks' gestation a growth-restricted fetus is periviable, and interventions are typically undertaken for maternal conditions such as severe preeclampsia. Thresholds for fetal indications should be high, requiring strong evidence of fetal compromise and risk of stillbirth. Management is frequently individualized, and a multidisciplinary approach is helpful in stressing that outcome may be poor even with maximal support in the neonatal intensive care unit (NICU). Parents need to be aware that despite maximum management effort, perinatal mortality is in excess of 50%.[84,85]

Between 27 and 34 weeks' gestation fetal indications for delivery should be based on firm evidence of fetal compromise with an attempt to complete a course of antenatal corticosteroids whenever possible.

Beyond 34 weeks' gestation lower delivery thresholds are acceptable and may include absent fetal growth, in particular arrested head growth, documented lung maturity on amniocentesis, and Doppler evidence of accelerating disease.

In summary, surveillance and management considerations are most challenging in preterm pregnancies, placing the highest demand on the accuracy of fetal testing before 34 weeks' gestation. Once fetal growth restriction is suspected or anticipated, appropriate fetal testing and daily maternal assessment of fetal activity should be instituted. Ultrasound examinations to assess fetal growth should be scheduled every 3 to 4 weeks. As long as studies show continued fetal head growth and test results remain reassuring, no intervention is required. An understanding of the strengths and limitations of individual surveillance tests in this context is important. The NST and fetal dynamic variables (fetal breathing, movement, and tone) provide assurance of fetal well-being at the time of testing. Because the traditional NST is frequently nonreactive in preterm fetuses, it is often inadequate as a stand-alone test of fetal well-being. A combination of umbilical artery Doppler and a five-component BPS are the surveillance tests of choice in preterm growth-restricted fetuses that circumvent this limitation of the NST alone. In the presence of umbilical artery end-diastolic velocity, normal AFV, and a normal BPS, weekly testing is sufficient. Testing frequency is adjusted according to fetal status with strict criteria for delivery as indicated above. In preterm growth-restricted fetuses in which timing of delivery is most critical, the combination of multiple modalities, including arterial and venous Doppler, offers the most comprehensive approach to assess fetal well-being.[66,86] Such "integrated fetal testing" is suggested for centers experienced with the performance of these studies. In the preterm growth-restricted fetus presenting before 34 weeks' gestation, consideration should always be given to administration of steroids if necessary, with continuous FHR monitoring and oxygen supplementation. Beyond 34 weeks' gestation, lung maturity amniocentesis to direct delivery timing should be considered. It is of note that even with optimal management there may be a yet undefined background morbidity that is predetermined by the condition and not amenable to treatment.

DELIVERY

The premature growth-restricted fetus requires the highest level of NICU care and therefore predelivery transport to an appropriate institution is recommended in all cases of early onset IUGR. Because many growth-restricted infants suffer intrapartum asphyxia, intrapartum management demands continuous FHR monitoring. In principle the route of delivery is determined by the severity of the fetal and maternal condition, along with other obstetric factors. Cesarean delivery without a trial of labor is indicated when the risks of vaginal delivery are unacceptable to the mother and fetus. These circumstances include prelabor evidence of fetal acidemia, spontaneous late decelerations, or late decelerations with minimal uterine activity. In addition, absent and reversed end-diastolic flow in the umbilical artery is associated with a high incidence of fetal intolerance of labor, thus cesarean delivery is often required and should be considered for these severely growth-restricted fetuses. In the instance of less abnormal fetal testing, typically in the setting of a more advanced gestational age, selection of the route of delivery is based on the difficulty anticipated in inducing labor, the Bishop score, and the AFV. The presence of IUGR has been considered a relative contraindication to the use of prostaglandin for cervical preparation by some authors.[87] If cervical ripening is considered, preinduction oxytocin challenge testing may be helpful in determining the likelihood and safety of vaginal delivery. Pharmacologic or mechanical ripening of the cervix, coupled with labor in the left lateral decubitus position with supplemental oxygen, increases the likelihood of a successful vaginal delivery. During labor, a tracing without late decelerations is predictive of a good outcome in cases complicated by IUGR. However, with late decelerations, the incidence of asphyxia in growth-restricted infants is far greater than in normally grown infants.

OUTCOME

IUGR can transiently and/or permanently impair neonatal well-being. The potential effects of this condition at birth and from complications occurring in the neonatal period have been most extensively studied. However, additional effects of this perinatal period on intermediate and long-term health are starting to emerge. Recently, a new area of research into the fetal origin of maternal diseases has also pointed out how exposure to a hostile intrauterine environment can be a predisposing factor for the development in adulthood of cardiovascular diseases and endocrine disturbances. An understanding of these outcomes will become important when the focus of management strategies shifts from the prevention of fetal and neonatal morbidity to the improvement of intermediate- and long-term development. Studies that examine the relationship between fetal growth restriction and postdelivery outcomes are therefore best separated into those that focus on short-term outcomes and those that focus on long-term outcomes.

Short-Term Outcomes

Initial reports that evaluated the association between fetal growth restriction and neonatal morbidity suggested the possibility of a protective effect of IUGR, with reduced occurrence of RDS and IVH. Subsequent studies do not support these early assumptions. Piper and Langer found no difference in indices of fetal lung maturity comparing gestational age-matched SGA and AGA fetuses. Similarly, Thompson et al. found no difference in the frequency of ventilator support when growth-restricted and AGA infants were matched for gestational age and mode of delivery. Most recently, several large trials suggest that RDS is significantly more likely to occur in growth-restricted neonates.[88,89] Bernstein has also demonstrated a significant increase in the risk for NEC and no difference in the rates of IVH when growth-restricted newborns are evaluated. Dashe noted a significant increase in RDS in infants with asymmetric IUGR when compared with neonates with symmetric IUGR (9% vs. 4%). Other investigators have also demonstrated increased risks of multiorgan failure, intracranial hemorrhage, bronchopulmonary dysplasia, clotting disorders, and disturbed endocrine homeostasis.[90,91] Mortality rates are uniformly higher when IUGR is present. These data should put to rest the notion that fetal growth restriction is associated with any reduction in newborn illness. Additional neonatal morbidities that must be anticipated include meconium aspiration, hypoglycemia, and electrolyte abnormalities.

Meconium aspiration occurs more frequently in IUGR than appropriately grown infants and is largely a problem observed after 34 weeks. Gasping in utero in response to asphyxia appears to contribute to this problem. Historically, careful suctioning of the nasopharynx and oropharynx with the DeLee catheter at delivery has been employed to decrease the incidence of this complication; however, more recent data shows that this is not the case. Clearing of the airway can be accomplished at delivery by direct laryngoscopy and aspiration by an experienced pediatrician. To effect immediate attention to the many potential neonatal problems, appropriate pediatric support should be present in the delivery room when an infant suspected of being growth restricted is to be delivered.

Hypoglycemia is frequently observed in growth-restricted infants owing to their inadequate glycogen reserves and a gluconeogenic pathway that is less sensitive to hypoglycemia than that of the normally grown infant.[92] In anticipation of this risk for hypoglycemia, frequent blood glucose monitoring should be instituted in all growth-restricted infants. Hypocalcemia, another well-recognized problem in IUGR, may be the result of relative hypoparathyroidism, a result of intrauterine acidosis. Hyperphosphatemia secondary to tissue breakdown may also contribute. Frequent calcium monitoring is essential, as symptoms are nonspecific and similar to those associated with hypoglycemia.

Hyponatremia resulting from impaired renal function is also frequently reported in growth-restricted infants. The renal complications associated with IUGR may be attributed to asphyxia, which can produce central nervous system injury leading to inappropriate antidiuretic hormone (ADH) secretion.[92]

Neonates with growth restriction are at risk for polycythemia, anemia, thrombocytopenia, and complex hematologic derangements that may be problematic well beyond delivery.[13] Polycythemia is observed three to four times more frequently in the growth-restricted infant than in weight-matched controls. Polycythemia results from hypoxia-stimulated production of red blood cells and from transfer of blood volume from the placental to the fetal circulation in the face of intrauterine asphyxia. Thus, these infants produce more red blood cells that are shunted to them if hypoxia occurs during labor. Polycythemia leads to increased red blood cell breakdown, accounting in part for the high incidence of hyperbilirubinemia in these infants. Polycythemia is a criterion for, but does not necessarily lead to, hyperviscosity, which can result in capillary bed sludging and thrombosis. Multiple organ systems can be affected, leading to pulmonary hypertension, cerebral infarction, and NEC. Anemia can be observed in preterm IUGR fetuses with markedly abnormal placental blood flow studies. Thrombocytopenia frequently accompanies the anemia. The risk for thrombocytopenia is increased more than 10-fold if umbilical artery end-diastolic velocity (AEDV) is absent. The cause for these abnormalities could involve a combination of dysfunctional erythropoiesis coupled with placental consumption of platelets and red blood cells. Neonates with such complex hematologic abnormalities are frequently unable to sustain their blood cell counts despite repeated substitution of blood products.

Hypothermia is another common problem for the growth-restricted infant and results from decreased body fat stores secondary to intrauterine malnourishment.[92] Hypothermia, if unrecognized and untreated, can contribute to the metabolic deterioration of an already unstable growth-restricted infant.

Finally, growth-restricted neonates are at increased risk for perinatal death in light of the multiple complications that may arise in the fetal and neonatal periods. The range of reported perinatal mortality is variable but depends clearly on the level of perinatal management received: infants who received optimal intrapartum and neonatal management have a lower perinatal mortality than age-matched controls who did not have such intensive care.[93]

Long-Term Outcomes

The ultimate growth potential for growth-restricted infants appears to be good. The degree of catch-up growth observed in several longitudinal studies suggests that these infants can be expected to have normal growth curves and normal, albeit slightly reduced, size as adults. In an 8-year follow-up of children weighing less than

1500 g at birth by Kitchen and associates,[94] 75% of growth-restricted infants achieved a height and weight above the 10th percentile. Of infants whose birthweight fell below the 3rd percentile, 60% had reached the 25th percentile for weight at 8 years. In Kitchen and associates' study,[94] however, 50% of the children with small HCs still had HCs below the 10th percentile at the 8-year follow-up visit in spite of their growth in height and weight. Hediger observed that growth-restricted infants experienced a period of catch-up growth in early infancy but remained near the 25th percentile through age 47 months. Kumar and colleagues[95] noted that in infants whose birthweights were less than 1250 g, at 1 year, 46% of the growth-restricted infants remained less than the 3rd percentile for weight and 38% remained less than the 3rd percentile for height. In general, those infants suffering growth restriction near the time of delivery do tend to catch up. However, those neonates with earlier onset and more longstanding growth restriction in utero continue to lag behind.

The issue of long-term neurologic sequelae remains unresolved. In 1972, Fitzhardinge and Steven,[96] evaluating a group of 96 growth-restricted infants, noted that 50% of males and 36% of females had poor school performance and, overall, 25% had minimal cerebral dysfunction. Major neurologic deficits were much less frequent. Other studies have shown low birthweight and short gestation to be risk factors for cerebral palsy. However, the vast majority of children with cerebral palsy are not growth restricted.

The positive effect of intrapartum surveillance for the growth-restricted fetus is reflected in the data of Low and colleagues[97] In a study of 88 growth-restricted infants, they reported no severe neurologic sequelae. They did detect a lag in mental development that was significant in the growth-restricted babies when compared with appropriately grown controls, especially in the group with birthweights less than 2300 g. This study correlates well with the data of Lipper and colleagues on low-birthweight babies. They observed that growth-restricted infants with HCs below the 10th percentile have two to three times the number of serious neurologic sequelae of their normocephalic counterparts. Strauss and Dietz found that term infants with IUGR and HCs less than 2 SD below the mean had significantly poorer performance on intelligence and visual motor development testing at age 7 when compared with their control siblings.[98] Walther, in an examination of 7-year-olds who suffered no perinatal complications despite IUGR and who were matched for social class with a control group, showed an increase in teacher-identified hyperactivity, poor concentration, and clumsiness. In a study of school performance in 8-year-olds matched for socioeconomic status, Robertson and colleagues demonstrated a tendency toward hyperactivity in preterm growth-restricted children compared with control groups. Low and colleagues[99] have shown that in 9- to 11-year-olds only fetal growth restriction and socioeconomic status contributed independently to the presence of learning deficits. Intrapartum fetal asphyxia, assessed by umbilical artery base deficit, was not associated with learning deficits in this group of children. Few studies have related neurodevelopment to a full complement of antenatal surveillance parameters. A study of predominantly preterm growth-restricted pregnancies that evaluate 2-year developmental outcomes reported gestational age at delivery, birthweight, and reversal of umbilical artery end-diastolic velocity as the main determinants of motor and neurosensory morbidity. Interestingly, fetal deterioration of venous Doppler or biophysical parameters did not have a statistical impact on neurodevelopment.[100]

The pattern that emerges from evaluation of these data emphasizes that neurologic outcome depends on the degree of growth restriction, especially the impact on head growth, its time of onset, the gestational age of the infant at birth, and the postnatal environment. An early intrauterine insult, between 10 and 17 weeks' gestation, could limit neuronal cellular multiplication and would obviously have a profound effect on neurologic function. In the third trimester, brain development is characterized by glial multiplication, dendritic arborization, establishment of synaptic connections, and myelinization, all of which continue during the first 2 years of life. Recovery after a period of impaired growth in the third trimester is, therefore, more likely to occur. Thus, the preterm appropriately grown infant has more normal neurologic development and fewer severe neurologic deficits than its preterm growth-restricted counterpart. Developmental milestones and neurologic development of mature infants with IUGR and mature infants of normal birthweight are similar. Presumably, this also reflects heightened physician awareness of the growth-restricted infant that allows detection, appropriate antepartum management, intrapartum therapy, and early pediatric intervention. The premature growth-restricted infant suffers from increased susceptibility to intrauterine asphyxia and all of the neonatal complications of the premature, as well as those of the infant with IUGR. If growth restriction is associated with lagging head growth before 26 weeks, even mature infants have significant developmental delay at 4 years of age.

Recently, the long-term impacts at age 6 to 13 years of age were reported for the GRIT study. In the absence of any specific delivery triggers the cognitive development was identical in both groups. In summary, these findings are concerning that the intrauterine environment has significant impacts on neurodevelopment before delivery management issues arise and, accordingly, it is unlikely that intervention trials will demonstrate a large impact of delivery timing on neurodevelopment.[100]

Gestational programming of growth-restricted fetuses has received considerable attention over the past 10 to 15 years. Infants born growth restricted have an increased risk of metabolic syndrome, obesity, hypertension, diabetes, and stroke from coronary artery disease. For a more in-depth review of fetal programming and long-term adult outcomes from IUGR, the reader is referred to Chapter 5.

KEY POINTS

- Fetal growth restriction is a major cause of perinatal morbidity, perinatal mortality, and both short-term and lifelong morbidities.
- Although IUGR is currently defined by fetal size alone, the four primary underlying etiologies (aneuploidy, viral infection, nonaneuploid syndromes,

and placental insufficiency) produce quite different outcomes.

- Identification of growth restriction due to placental insufficiency requires a comprehensive diagnostic workup including measurement of the fetal abdominal circumference in combination with umbilical artery Doppler studies, exclusion of fetal anomalies, and possibly invasive testing to detect aneuploidy and viral infection.
- The combination of a small abdominal circumference, normal anatomy, low or normal amniotic fluid volume, and abnormal umbilical artery Doppler is strongly suggestive of placental insufficiency.
- Because mortality resulting from fetal growth restriction can be reduced with appropriate antenatal surveillance, all pregnancies at risk for IUGR should be carefully monitored.
- Deterioration of fetal biophysical and cardiovascular parameters follows a relatively predictable pattern, progressing from early to late changes that can be used for the prediction of fetal acid–base balance and the risk for stillbirth.
- Antenatal surveillance in preterm IUGR requires the combination of several testing modalities to provide fetal assessment of sufficient precision to guide intervention.
- In preterm gestations complicated by IUGR, the threshold for delivery is critically influenced by gestational age.

REFERENCES

1. Wolfe HM, Gross TL, Sokol RJ: Recurrent small for gestational age birth: perinatal risks and outcomes. Am J Obstet Gynecol 157:288, 1987.
2. Mavrides E, Moscoso G, Carvalho JS, et al: The anatomy of the umbilical, portal and hepatic venous systems in the human fetus at 14-19 weeks of gestation. Ultrasound Obstet Gynecol 18:598, 2001.
3. Sparks JW, Girard JR, Battaglia FC: An estimate of the caloric requirements of the human fetus. Biol Neonate 38:113, 1980.
4. Clausson B, Gardosi J, Francis A, et al: Perinatal outcome in SGA births defined by customised versus population-based birthweight standards. BJOG 108:830, 2001.
5. Khoury MJ, Erickson D, Cordero JE, et al: Congenital malformations and intrauterine growth retardation: a population study. Pediatrics 82:83, 1988.
6. Cowles T, Tatlor S, Zneimer S, et al: Association of confined placental mosaicism with intrauterine growth restriction [abstract]. Am J Obstet Gynecol 170:273, 1994.
7. Baker ER, Beach ML, Craigo SD, et al: A comparison of neonatal outcomes of age-matched, growth restricted twins and growth restricted singletons. Am J Perinatol 14:499, 1997.
8. Valsky DV, Eixarch E, Martinez JM, et al: Selective intrauterine growth restriction in monochorionic twins: pathophysiology, diagnostic approach and management dilemmas. Prenat Diagn 30:719, 2010.
9. Paolini CL, Marconi AM, Ronzoni S, et al: Placental transport of leucine, phenylalanine, glycine, and proline in intrauterine growth-restricted pregnancies. J Clin Endocrinol Metab 86:5427, 2001.
10. Soothill PW, Nicolaides KH, Campbell S: Prenatal asphyxia, hyperlacticaemia, hypoglycaemia, and erythroblastosis in growth retarded fetuses. Br Med J 294:1051, 1987.
11. Kilby MD, Gittoes N, McCabe C, et al: Expression of thyroid receptor isoforms in the human fetal central nervous system and the effects of intrauterine growth restriction. Clin Endocrinol (Oxf) 53:469, 2000.
12. Thilaganathan B, Athanasiou S, Ozmen S, et al: Umbilical cord blood erythroblast count as an index of intrauterine hypoxia. Arch Dis Child Fetal Neonatal Ed 70:F192, 1994.
13. Baschat AA, Gembruch U, Reiss I, et al: Absent umbilical artery end-diastolic velocity in growth-restricted fetuses: a risk factor for neonatal thrombocytopenia. Obstet Gynecol 96:162, 2000.
14. Ferrazzi E, Bozzo M, Rigano S, et al: Temporal sequence of abnormal Doppler changes in the peripheral and central circulatory systems of the severely growth-restricted fetus. Ultrasound Obstet Gynecol 19:140, 2002.
15. Bellotti M, Pennati G, De Gasperi C, et al: Simultaneous measurements of umbilical venous, fetal hepatic, and ductus venosus blood flow in growth-restricted human fetuses. Am J Obstet Gynecol 190:1347, 2004.
16. Kiserud T: The ductus venosus. Semin Perinatol 25:11, 2001.
17. Wladimiroff JW, Tonge HM, Stewart PA: Doppler ultrasound assessment of cerebral blood flow in the human fetus. Br J Obstet Gynaecol 93:471, 1986.
18. Reed KL, Anderson CF, Shenker L: Changes in intracardiac Doppler flow velocities in fetuses with absent umbilical artery diastolic flow. Am J Obstet Gynecol 157:774, 1987.
19. Hecher K, Campbell S, Doyle P, et al: Assessment of fetal compromise by Doppler ultrasound investigation of the fetal circulation. Arterial, intracardiac, and venous blood flow velocity studies. Circulation 91:129, 1995.
20. Rizzo G, Capponi A, Pietropolli A, et al: Fetal cardiac and extracardiac flows preceding intrauterine death. Ultrasound Obstet Gynecol 4:139, 1994.
21. Arduini D, Rizzo G, Caforio L, et al: Behavioural state transitions in healthy and growth retarded fetuses. Early Hum Dev 19:155, 1989.
22. Henson G, Dawes GS, Redman CW: Characterization of the reduced heart rate variation in growth-retarded fetuses. Br J Obstet Gynaecol 91:751, 1984.
23. Baschat AA, Gembruch U, Harman CR: The sequence of changes in Doppler and biophysical parameters as severe fetal growth restriction worsens. Ultrasound Obstet Gynecol 18:571, 2001.
24. Ribbert LS, Nicolaides KH, Visser GH: Prediction of fetal acidaemia in intrauterine growth retardation: comparison of quantified fetal activity with biophysical profile score. Br J Obstet Gynaecol 100:653, 1993.
25. Vintzileos AM, Fleming AD, Scorza WE, et al: Relationship between fetal biophysical activities and umbilical cord blood gas values. Am J Obstet Gynecol 165:707, 1991.
26. Manning FA, Snijders R, Harman CR, et al: Fetal biophysical profile score. VI. Correlation with antepartum umbilical venous fetal pH. Am J Obstet Gynecol 169:755, 1993.
27. Ott WJ: Intrauterine growth restriction and Doppler ultrasonography. J Ultrasound Med 19:661, 2000.
28. Hecher K, Spernol R, Stettner H, et al: Potential for diagnosing imminent risk for appropriate- and small for gestational fetuses by Doppler examination of umbilical and cerebral arterial blood flow. Ultrasound Obstet Gynecol 5:247, 1995.
29. Baschat AA: Pathophysiology of fetal growth restriction: implications for diagnosis and surveillance. Obstet Gynecol Surv 59:617, 2004.
30. Hadlock FP, Harrist RB, Sharman RS, et al: Estimation of fetal weight with the use of head, body, and femur measurements—a prospective study. Am J Obstet Gynecol 151:333, 1985.
31. Smith PA, Johansson D, Tzannatos C, et al: Prenatal measurement of the fetal cerebellum and cisterna cerebellomedullaris by ultrasound. Prenat Diagn 6:133, 1986.
32. Baschat AA, Weiner CP: Umbilical artery Doppler screening for detection of the small fetus in need of antepartum surveillance. Am J Obstet Gynecol 182:154, 2000.
33. Divon MY, Chamberlain PF, Sipos L, et al: Identification of the small for gestational age fetus with the use of gestational age-independent indices of fetal growth. Am J Obstet Gynecol 155:1197, 1986.
34. Campbell S, Thoms A: Ultrasound measurement of the fetal head to abdomen circumference ratio in the assessment of growth retardation. Br J Obstet Gynaecol 84:165, 1977.
35. Warsof SL, Cooper DJ, Little D, et al: Routine ultrasound screening for antenatal detection of intrauterine growth retardation. Obstet Gynecol 67:33, 1986.

36. Walther FJ, Ramaekers LHJ: The ponderal index as a measure of the nutritional status at birth and its relation to some aspects of neonatal morbidity. J Perinat Med 10:42, 1982.
37. Bernstein IM, Catalano PM: Ultrasonographic estimation of fetal body composition for children of diabetic mothers. Invest Radiol 26:722, 1991.
38. Padoan A, Rigano S, Ferrazzi E, et al: Differences in fat and lean mass proportions in normal and growth restricted fetuses. Am J Obstet Gynecol 191:1459, 2004.
39. Ott WJ: The diagnosis of altered fetal growth. Obstet Gynecol Clin North Am 15:237, 1988.
40. Weiner CP, Sabbagha RE, Vaisrub N, et al: A hypothetical model suggesting suboptimal intra-uterine growth in infants delivered preterm. Obstet Gynecol 65:323, 1985.
41. Bernstein IM, Meyer MC, Capeless EL: "Fetal growth charts": comparison of cross-sectional ultrasound examinations with birth-weight. Maternal Fetal Med 3:182, 1994.
42. Lackman F, Capewell V, Richardson B, et al: Fetal or neonatal growth curve: which is more appropriate in predicting the impact of fetal growth on the risk of perinatal mortality. Am J Obstet Gynecol 180:S145, 1999.
43. Rossavik IK, Deter RL: Mathematical modeling of fetal growth. I. Basic principles. J Clin Ultrasound 12:529, 1984.
44. Baschat AA, Towbin J, Bowles NE, et al: Is adenovirus a fetal pathogen? Am J Obstet Gynecol 189:758, 2003.
45. Veille JC, Kanaan C: Duplex Doppler ultrasonographic evaluation of the fetal renal artery in normal and abnormal fetuses. Am J Obstet Gynecol 161:1502, 1989.
46. Magann EF, Chauhan SP, Barrilleaux PS, et al: Amniotic fluid index and single deepest pocket: weak indicators of abnormal amniotic volumes. Obstet Gynecol 96:737, 2000.
47. Manning FA, Hill LM, Platt LD: Qualitative amniotic fluid volume determination by ultrasound: antepartum detection of intrauterine growth retardation. Am J Obstet Gynecol 193:254, 1981.
48. Groome LJ, Owen J, Neely CL, et al: Oligohydramics: antepartum fetal urine production and intrapertum fetal distress. Am J Obstet Gynecol 165:1077, 1991.
49. Hecher K, Campbell S: Characteristics of fetal venous blood flow under normal circumstances and during fetal disease. Ultrasound Obstet Gynecol 7:68, 1996.
50. Neilson JP, Alfirevic Z: Doppler ultrasound for fetal assessment in high risk pregnancies. Cochrane Database Sys Rev 1, 2002. Oxford, Update Software.
51. Westergaard HB, Langhoff-Roos J, Lingman G, et al: A critical appraisal of the use of umbilical artery Doppler ultrasound in high-risk pregnancies: use of meta-analyses in evidence-based obstetrics. Ultrasound Obstet Gynecol 17:466, 2001.
52. Yagel S, Anteby EY, Shen O, et al: Simultaneous multigate spectral Doppler imaging of the umbilical artery and placental vessels: novel ultrasound technology. Ultrasound Obstet Gynecol 14:256, 1999.
53. Bahado-Singh RO, Kovanci E, Jeffres A, et al: The Doppler cerebroplacental ratio and perinatal outcome in intrauterine growth restriction. Am J Obstet Gynecol 180:750, 1999.
54. Yaron Y, Cherry M, Kramer RL, et al: Second-trimester maternal serum marker screening: maternal serum alpha-fetoprotein, beta-human chorionic gonadotropin, estriol, and their various combinations as predictors for pregnancy outcome. Am J Obstet Gynecol 181:968, 1999.
55. Persson B, Stangenberg M, Lunell NO, et al: Prediction of size of infants at birth by measurement of symphysis fundus height. Br J Obstet Gynaecol 93:206, 1986.
56. Bower S, Kingdom J, Campbell S: Objective and subjective assessment of abnormal uterine artery Doppler flow velocity waveforms. Ultrasound Obstet Gynecol 12:260, 1998.
57. Bujold E, Roberge S, Lacasse Y, et al: Prevention of preeclampsia and intrauterine growth restriction with aspirin therapy started early in pregnancy—a meta analysis. Obstet Gynecol 116:402, 2010.
58. Battaglia C, Artini PG, D'Ambrogio G, et al: Maternal hyperoxygenation in the treatment of intrauterine growth retardation. Am J Obstet Gynecol 167:430, 1992.
59. Karsdorp VH, van Vugt JM, Dekker GA, et al: Reappearance of end-diastolic velocities in the umbilical artery following maternal volume expansion: a preliminary study. Obstet Gynecol 80:679, 1992.
60. Deren O, Karaer C, Onderoglu L, et al: The effect of steroids on the biophysical profile and Doppler indices of umbilical and middle cerebral arteries in healthy preterm fetuses. Eur J Obstet Gynecol Reprod Biol 99:72, 2001.
61. Soothill PW, Ajayi RA, Campbell S, et al: Relationship between fetal acidemia at cordocentesis and subsequent neurodevelopment. Ultrasound Obstet Gynecol 2:80, 1992.
62. Matthews DD: Maternal assessment of fetal activity in small-for-dates infants. Obstet Gynecol 45:488, 1975.
63. Pazos R, Vuolo K, Aladjem S, et al: Association of spontaneous fetal heart rate decelerations during antepartum nonstress testing and intrauterine growth retardation. Am J Obstet Gynecol 144:574, 1982.
64. Gabbe SG, Freeman RD, Goebelsmann U: Evaluation of the contraction stress test before 33 weeks' gestation. Obstet Gynecol 52:649, 1978.
65. Lin CC, Devoe LD, River P, et al: Oxytocin challenge test and intrauterine growth retardation. Am J Obstet Gynecol 140:282, 1981.
66. Baschat AA, Galan HL, Bhide A, et al: Doppler and biophysical assessment in growth restricted fetuses: distribution of test results. Ultrasound Obstet Gynecol 27:41, 2006.
67. Ribbert LS, Snijders RJ, Nicolaides KH, et al: Relationship of fetal biophysical profile and blood gas values at cordocentesis in severely growth-retarded fetuses. Am J Obstet Gynecol 163:569, 1990.
68. Harrington K, Thompson MO, Carpenter RG, et al: Doppler fetal circulation in pregnancies complicated by pre-eclampsia or delivery of a small for gestational age baby: 2. Longitudinal analysis. Br J Obstet Gynaecol 106:453, 1999.
69. Rizzo G, Capponi A, Talone PE, et al: Doppler indices from inferior vena cava and ductus venosus in predicting pH and oxygen tension in umbilical blood at cordocentesis in growth-retarded fetuses. Ultrasound Obstet Gynecol 7:401, 1996.
70. Bilardo CM, Wolf H, Stigter RH, et al: Relationship between monitoring parameters and perinatal outcome in severe, early intrauterine growth restriction. Ultrasound Obstet Gynecol 23:119, 2004.
71. Guzman ER, Vintzileos AM, Martins M, et al: The efficacy of individual computer heart rate indices in detecting acidemia at birth in growth-restricted fetuses. Obstet Gynecol 87:969, 1996.
72. Morrow RJ, Adamson SL, Bull SB, et al: Effect of placental embolization on the umbilical artery velocity waveform in fetal sheep. Am J Obstet Gynecol 161:1055, 1989.
73. Arduini D, Rizzo G, Romanini C: The development of abnormal heart rate patterns after absent end-diastolic velocity in umbilical artery: analysis of risk factors. Am J Obstet Gynecol 168:50, 1993.
74. Baschat AA: Doppler application in the delivery timing of the preterm growth-restricted fetus: another step in the right direction. Ultrasound Obstet Gynecol 23:111, 2004.
75. Baschat AA, Gembruch U, Weiner CP, et al: Qualitative venous Doppler waveform analysis improves prediction of critical perinatal outcomes in premature growth-restricted fetuses. Ultrasound Obstet Gynecol 22:240, 2003.
76. Pardi G, Cetin I, Marconi AM, et al: Diagnostic value of blood sampling in fetuses with growth retardation. N Engl J Med 328:692, 1993.
77. The GRIT study group: A randomised trial of timed delivery for the compromised preterm fetus: short term outcomes and Bayesian interpretation. BJOG 110:27, 2003.
78. Baschat AA, Cosmi E, Bilardo CM, et al: Predictors of neonatal outcome in early-onset placental dysfunction. Obstet Gynecol 109:253, 2007.
79. Froen JF, Gardosi JO, Thurmann A, et al: Restricted fetal growth in sudden intrauterine unexplained death. Acta Obstet Gynecol Scand 83:801, 2004.
80. Hecher K, Bilardo CM, Stigter RH, et al: Monitoring of fetuses with intrauterine growth restriction: a longitudinal study. Ultrasound Obstet Gynecol 18:564, 2001.
81. Hershkovitz R, Kingdom JC, Geary M, et al: Fetal cerebral blood flow redistribution in late gestation: identification of compromise in small fetuses with normal umbilical artery Doppler. Ultrasound Obstet Gynecol 15:209, 2000.
82. Baschat AA: Integrated fetal testing in growth restriction: combining multi-vessel Doppler and biophysical parameters. Ultrasound Obstet Gynecol 21:1, 2003.
83. Thornton JG, Hornbuckle J, Vail A, et al, The GRIT study group: Infant well-being at 2 years of age in the Growth Restriction Intervention Trial (GRIT): multicentred randomized trial. Lancet 364:513, 2004.

84. Baschat AA, Bilardo CM, Germer U, et al: Thresholds for intervention in severe early onset growth restriction. Am J Obstet Gynecol 191:S.143, 2004.
85. Garite TJ, Clark R, Thorp JA: Intrauterine growth restriction increases morbidity and mortality among premature neonates. Am J Obstet Gynecol 191:481, 2004.
86. Baschat AA, Gembruch U, Weiner CP, et al: Combining Doppler and biophysical assessment improves prediction of critical perinatal outcomes. Am J Obstet Gynecol 187:S147, 2002.
87. Sawai SK, Williams MC, O'Brien WF, et al: Sequential outpatient application of intravaginal prostaglandin E2 gel in the management of postdates pregnancies. Obstet Gynecol 78:19, 1991.
88. McIntire DD, Bloom SL, Casey BM, et al: Birth weight in relation to morbidity and mortality among newborn infants. N Engl J Med 340:1234, 1999.
89. Ley D, Wide-Swensson D, Lindroth M, et al: Respiratory distress syndrome in infants with impaired intrauterine growth. Acta Paediatr 10:1090, 1997.
90. Spinillo A, Capuzzo E, Piazzi G, et al: Significance of low birthweight for gestational age among very preterm infants. Br J Obstet Gynaecol 104:668, 1997.
91. Aucott SW, Donohue PK, Northington FJ: Increased morbidity in severe early intrauterine growth restriction. J Perinatol 24:435, 2004.
92. Oh W: Considerations in neonates with intrauterine growth retardation. In Frigoletto FD: Clinical Obstetrics and Gynecology. Hagerstown, MD, Harper & Row, 1977, p 989.
93. Kitchen WH, Richards A, Ryan MM, et al: A longitudinal study of very low-birthweight infants. II: Results of controlled trial of intensive care and incidence of handicaps. Dev Med Child Neurol 21:582, 1979.
94. Kitchen WH, McDougass AB, Naylor FD: A longitudinal study of very low-birthweight infants. III: Distance growth at eight years of age. Dev Med Child Neurol 22:1633, 1980.
95. Kumar SP, Anday EK, Sacks LM, et al: Follow-up studies of very low birthweight infants (1,250 grams or less) born and treated within a perinatal center. Pediatrics 66:438, 1980.
96. Fitzhardinge PM, Steven EM: The small-for-dates infant. II: Neurological and intellectual sequelae. Pediatrics 50:50, 1972.
97. Low JA, Galbraith RS, Muir D, et al: Intrauterine growth retardation: a preliminary report of long-term morbidity. Am J Obstet Gynecol 130:534, 1978.
98. Strauss R, Dietz WH: Growth and development of term children born with low birth weight: effects of genetic and environmental factors. J Pediatr 133:67, 1998.
99. Low JA, Handley-Derry MH, Burke SO, et al: Association of intrauterine fetal growth retardation and learning deficits at age 9 to 11 years. Am J Obstet Gynecol 167:1499, 1992.
100. Walker DM, Marlow N, Upstone L, et al: Long term outcomes in a randomized trial of timing of delivery in fetal growth restriction. Am J Obstet Gynecol 204:34.e1, 2011.

For full reference list, log onto www.expertconsult.com.

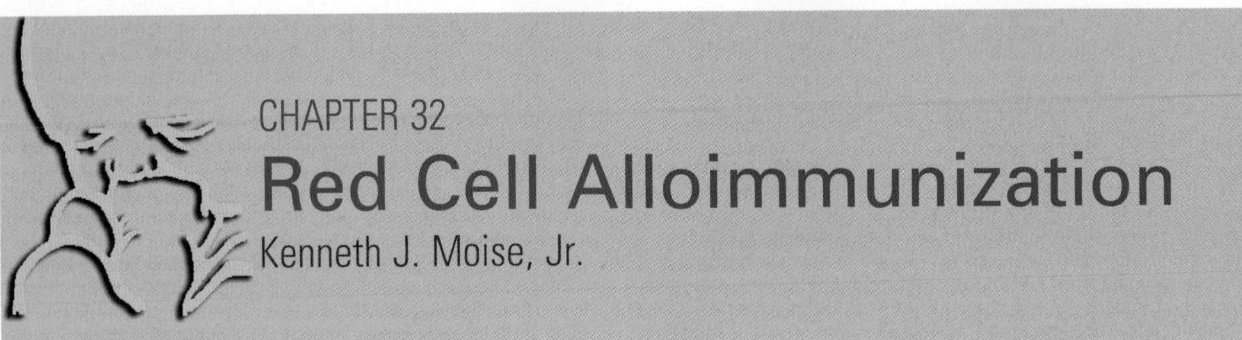

CHAPTER 32

Red Cell Alloimmunization

Kenneth J. Moise, Jr.

KEY ABBREVIATIONS	
American Association of Blood Banks	AABB
American College of Obstetricians and Gynecologists	ACOG
Cytomegalovirus	CMV
Deoxyribonucleic Acid	DNA
Diphosphotidylglycerol	DPG
Fetal Blood Sampling	FBS
Fetomaternal Hemorrhage	FMH
Grams per Deciliter	g/dL
Hemolytic Disease of the Fetus and Newborn	HDFN
Hemolytic Disease of the Newborn	HDN
Intraperitoneal Transfusion	IPT
International Units	IU
Intrauterine Transfusion	IUT
Intravascular Transfusion	IVT
Intravenous Immune Globulin	IVIG
Kleihauer-Betke	KB
Middle Cerebral Artery	MCA
Microgram	mcg
Polymerase Chain Reaction	PCR
Rhesus Immune Globulin	RhIG
Single Nucleotide Polymorphisms	SNPs

NOMENCLATURE

Exposure to foreign red cell antigens invariably results in the production of anti–red cell antibodies in a process known as *red cell alloimmunization* (formerly termed *isoimmunization*). The expression *sensitization* can be used interchangeably with *Rhesus alloimmunization*. The active transport of these antibodies across the placenta during pregnancy results in fetal anemia, hyperbilirubinemia, and ultimately, hydrops fetalis. Before the advent of obstetrical ultrasound, the perinatal effects of maternal red cell alloimmunization could be recognized only after birth in the affected neonate. Thus, the neonatal consequences of maternal red cell alloimmunization came to be known as *hemolytic disease of the newborn (HDN)*. Because the peripheral blood smear of these infants demonstrated a large percentage of circulating immature red cells known as erythroblasts, the newborn entity was also known as *erythroblastosis fetalis*. Today, ultrasound and fetal blood sampling (FBS) make the detection of the severely anemic fetus a reality. For this reason, the term *hemolytic disease of the fetus and newborn (HDFN)* would appear more appropriate to describe this disorder.

HISTORICAL PERSPECTIVES

The first case of HDFN was probably described in 1609 by a midwife in the French literature.[1] The case was a twin gestation in which the first fetus was stillborn and the second twin developed jaundice and succumbed soon after birth. In 1932, Diamond[2] proposed that the clinical entities of erythroblastosis fetalis, icterus gravis neonatorum, and hydrops fetalis represented different manifestations of the same disease. Seven years later Levine and Stetson[3] described an antibody in a woman who gave birth to a stillborn fetus. The patient experienced a severe hemolytic transfusion reaction after later receiving her husband's blood. In 1940, Landsteiner and Weiner[4] injected red blood cells from rhesus monkeys into rabbits. The antibody that was isolated from these was used to test human blood samples from caucasians, and agglutination was noted in 85% of individuals. The following year Levine and colleagues[5] were able to demonstrate a causal relationship between Rhesus D (RhD) antibodies in RhD-negative women and HDFN in their offspring.

The advent of therapy for HDFN began in 1945 with the description by Wallerstein[6] of the technique of neonatal exchange transfusion. Later Liley[7] proposed the use of amniotic fluid bilirubin assessment as an indirect measure of the degree of fetal hemolysis. Sir William Liley's major contribution to the story of rhesus disease was the introduction of the intraperitoneal fetal transfusion (IPT).[8] He learned from a visiting fellow who had returned from Africa that the infusion of red blood cells into the peritoneal cavity of children with sickle-cell disease produced normal-appearing red blood cells on peripheral blood smear. Liley realized that he had previously inadvertently entered the peritoneal cavity of fetuses at the time of amniocentesis, based on the marked contrast in the yellow hue of the ascitic fluid as compared with amniotic fluid. He postulated that purposeful entry into the fetal peritoneal cavity could be accomplished. After three unsuccessful attempts that resulted in fetal demises, the fourth fetus was delivered at 34 $\frac{4}{7}$ weeks' gestation after undergoing two successful IPTs. Early attempts at IPT used fluoroscopy for needle guidance. With the introduction of real-time ultrasound in the early 1980s, IPTs became a safer procedure as fluoroscopy was abandoned. Charles Rodeck[9] is credited with the first intravascular fetal transfusion (IVT) using a fetoscope to guide the transfusion needle into a placental plate vessel. Just 1 year later, investigators in Denmark performed the first ultrasound-guided IVT using the intrahepatic portion of the umbilical vein.[10]

The 1990s saw the introduction of genetic techniques using amniocentesis to determine fetal red cell typing.[11] The turn of the century brought the noninvasive detection of fetal anemia through Doppler ultrasound of the fetal middle cerebral artery (MCA) and the use of fetal typing through cell free DNA in maternal plasma.[12,13]

INCIDENCE

The advent of the routine administration of antenatal and postpartum rhesus immune globulin (RhIG) has resulted in a marked reduction in cases of red cell alloimmunization secondary to the RhD antigen. The Centers for Disease Control and Prevention last required the reporting of rhesus alloimmunization as a medical complication of pregnancy on U.S. birth certificates in the year 2002.[14] In that year (the most recent for which epidemiologic data are available) the incidence was reported to be 6.7 cases of Rhesus alloimmunization per 1000 live births.

Clearly, a shift to other red cell antibodies associated with HDFN has occurred as a result of the decreasing incidence of RhD alloimmunization. In one large series of women of childbearing age, a positive screen for an antibody associated with HDFN was found in 1% of samples.[15] Rhesus antibodies were the most common, accounting for more than half of significant antibodies, and with the RhD antibody accounting for almost one fourth. Kell antibodies were next most frequent, followed by Duffy, MNS, Kidd, and anti-U. In another series of more than 1000 Dutch women who screened positive for antibodies at 12 weeks of gestation, anti-E was the most common antibody that was found.[16] This was followed by anti-K then anti-D (Figure 32-1).

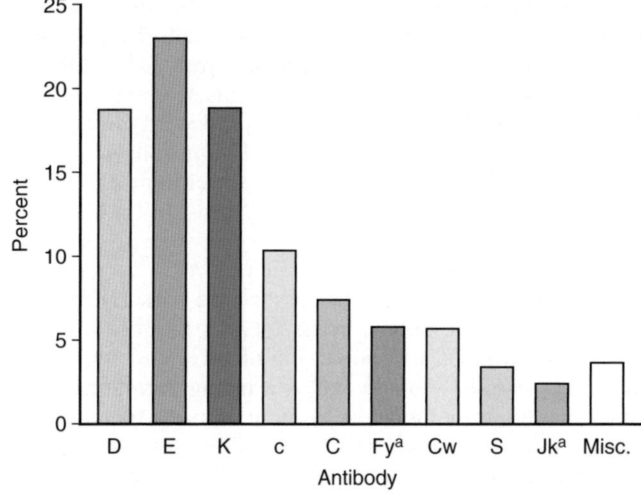

FIGURE 32-1. Incidence of maternal anti–red cell antibodies associated with hemolytic disease of the fetus and newborn (HDFN) in a Dutch population of pregnant women. (From van der Schoot CE, Tax GH, Rijnders RJP, et al: Prenatal typing of Rh and Kell blood group system antigens: the edge of the watershed. Trans Med Rev 17:31, 2003.)

PATHOPHYSIOLOGY

Although the placenta was once thought to be an absolute barrier to the transfer of cells between the maternal and fetal compartments, we now appreciate that the placental interface allows for the bidirectional movement of both intact cells and free DNA. The putative "grandmother theory" of rhesus red cell alloimmunization probably occurs more commonly than first thought. In this paradigm, maternal RhD-positive red cells gain access to the circulation of the RhD-negative fetus at the time of delivery. As many as one fourth of RhD-negative babies have been shown to be immunized in early life as a result of their delivery.[17,18] The immune response of an Rh-negative individual to RhD-positive red cells has been characterized into one of three groups: (1) Sixty to 70% of individuals are *responders* and develop an antibody to relatively small volumes of red cells. In these individuals, the probability of immunization increases with escalating volumes of cells. A small percentage of this group can be called *hyperresponders* in that they will be immunized by very small quantities of red cells. (2) The second group of individuals (10%-20%) can be immunized only by exposure to very large volumes of cells. (3) Finally, the 10% to 20% of individuals who remain appear to be *nonresponders.*

In most cases of red cell alloimmunization, a fetomaternal hemorrhage (FMH) occurs in the antenatal period or more commonly at the time of delivery. If a maternal ABO blood type incompatibility exists between the mother and her fetus, anti-A and/or anti-B antibodies lyse the fetal cells in the maternal circulation and destroy the RhD antigen.[19,20] Even if this protective effect is not present, only 13% of deliveries of RhD-positive fetuses result in RhD alloimmunization in RhD-negative women who do not receive RhIG. The vast majority of RhD-alloimmunized women produce an IgG response as their initial antibody. *Responders* may represent a group of individuals who had their initial exposure to the RhD antigen at birth due to maternofetal hemorrhage.[18] After a sensitizing event, the human antiglobulin anti-D titer can usually be detected after 5 to 16 weeks. However, approximately half of alloimmunized patients are *sensibilized.* In this scenario, an antibody screen will be negative, but memory B lymphocytes are present that can create an anti-D antibody response. When faced with the challenge of a subsequent pregnancy involving an RhD-positive fetus, the anti-D titer becomes detectable.

The anti-D immune response is the best characterized of the anti–red cell antibodies associated with HDFN. In one third of cases, only subclass IgG1 is produced; in the remainder of cases, a combination of IgG1 and IgG3 subclasses is found.[21] Anti-D IgG is a nonagglutinating antibody that does not bind complement. This results in a lack of intravascular hemolysis; sequestration and subsequent destruction of antibody-coated red cells in the fetal liver and spleen are the mechanism of fetal anemia. Most studies have not detected a relationship between a specific maternal human leukocyte antigen type and susceptibility to become alloimmunized to RhD.[22] However, sensitized women with high titers of anti-D are more likely to exhibit the DQB1*0201 and DR17 alleles as compared with women with low titers.[23] Fetal sex may also play a significant role in the fetal response to maternal antibodies. RhD-positive male fetuses are 13 times more likely than their female counterparts to become hydropic and 3 times more likely to die from their disease.[24]

Anemia results in several important physiologic changes in the fetus. Reticulocytosis from the bone marrow can be detected by FBS once the hemoglobin deficit exceeds 2 g/dL as compared to norms for gestational age; erythroblasts are released from the fetal liver once the hemoglobin deficit reaches 7 g/dL or greater.[25] In an effort to increase oxygen delivery to peripheral tissues, fetal cardiac output increases and 2-3 diphosphotidylglycerol (DPG) levels are enhanced.[26,27] Tissue hypoxia appears as anemia progresses despite these physiologic changes. An increased umbilical artery lactate level is noted when the fetal hemoglobin falls below 8 g/dL and increased venous lactate can be detected when the hemoglobin level falls below 4 g/dL.[28] **Hydrops fetalis (the accumulation of extracellular fluid in at least two body compartments) is a late finding in cases of fetal anemia. Its exact pathophysiology is unknown.** Enhanced hepatic erythropoietic function with subsequent depressed synthesis of serum proteins has been proposed as the explanation for the lower serum albumin levels that have been detected.[29] Colloid osmotic pressure appears decreased.[30] However, experimental animal models in which fetal plasma proteins have been replaced with saline did not produce hydrops.[31] An alternative hypothesis is that tissue hypoxia due to anemia enhances capillary permeability. In addition, iron overload due to ongoing hemolysis may contribute to free radical formation and endothelial cell dysfunction.[32] Central venous pressures do appear elevated in the hydropic fetus with HDFN. This may cause a functional blockage of the lymphatic system at the level of the thoracic duct as it empties into the left brachiocephalic vein.[30] This theory is supported by reports of poor absorption of donor red cells infused into the intraperitoneal cavity in cases of hydrops.[33]

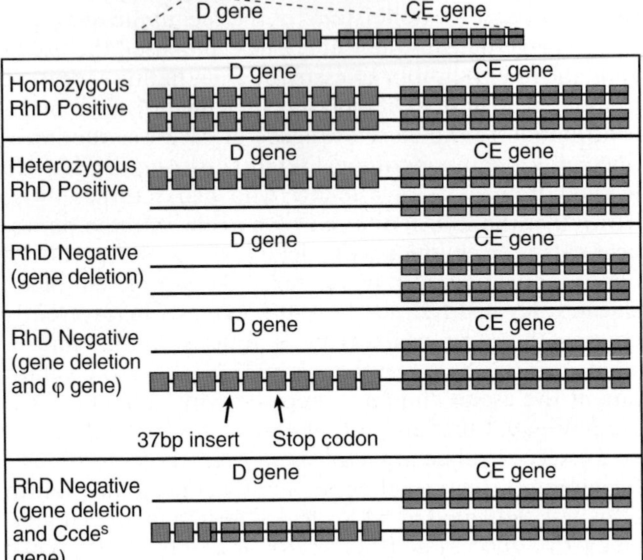

FIGURE 32-2. Schematic of Rh gene locus on chromosome 1. The homozygous RhD-positive state, heterozygous RhD-positive state, RhD-negative with heterozygosity for the RhD pseudogene, and RhD-negative with heterozygosity for the Ccde^s gene are demonstrated. (Reproduced and modified from Moise KJ: Hemolytic disease of the fetus and newborn. *In* Creasy RK, Resnik R, Iams J [eds]: Maternal-Fetal Medicine: Principles and Practice, ed 5. Philadelphia, Elsevier, Copyright © 2004.)

RHESUS ALLOIMMUNIZATION AND FETAL/NEONATAL HEMOLYTIC DISEASE OF THE NEWBORN

Genetics

Initial concepts on the genetics of the Rh antigens proposed the presence of three distinct genes.[34] Newer DNA techniques allowed for the localization of the Rh locus to the short arm of chromosome 1.[35] **Only two genes were identified—an RhD gene and an RhCE gene.** Each gene is 10 exons in length, with 96% homology. These genes presumably represent a duplication of a common ancestral gene. Production of two distinct proteins from the RhCE gene probably occurs as a result of alternative splicing of messenger RNA.[36] One nucleotide difference, cytosine to thymine, in exon 2 of the RhCE gene results in a single amino acid change of a serine to proline. This causes the expression of the *C* antigen as opposed to the *c* antigen.[37] A single cytosine-to-guanine change in exon 5 of the RhCE gene, producing a single amino acid change of a proline to alanine, results in formation of the *e* antigen instead of the *E* antigen.

The gene frequency found in different ethnic groups can be traced to the Spanish colonization in the fifteenth and sixteenth centuries. Populations native to certain land masses have a less than 1% incidence of RhD negativity—Eskimos, Native Americans, Japanese, and Chinese individuals. The Basque tribe in Spain is noted to have a 30% incidence of Rh negativity. This may well be the origin of the RhD gene deletion that is the most common genetic basis of the RhD-negative state in whites (Figure 32-2).

Whites of European descent exhibit a 15% incidence of RhD negativity, whereas an 8% incidence occurs in blacks and Hispanics of Mexico and Central America. This latter incidence probably reflects ethnic diversity secondary to Spanish colonization of the New World.

Further study of the RhD gene has revealed significant heterogeneity. Several of these genetic modifications result in a lack of expression of the RhD phenotype. Although these individuals may have an aberrant RhD gene present, serologic methods do not detect the RhD antigen on the surface of the red cells. One such example is the RhD pseudogene, which has been found in 69% of South African blacks and 24% of American blacks (see Figure 32-2).[38] In this situation, all 10 exons of the RhD gene are present. However, translation of the gene into a messenger RNA product does not occur owing to the presence of a stop codon in the intron between exons 3 and 4. Thus, no RhD protein is synthesized and the patient is serologically RhD negative. Similarly, the Ccde[s] has been detected in 22% of American blacks. It appears to contain exons 1, 2, 9, and 10 as well as a portion of exon 3 of the original RhD gene, with other exons being duplicated from the RhCE gene. In the Taiwanese population of RhD-negative individuals, five different exons of the RhD gene were evaluated.[39] Seventeen percent of individuals had all five exons detected, and an additional 135 demonstrated the presence of at least one of the five exons tested.

PREVENTION OF RhD HEMOLYTIC DISEASE IN THE FETUS AND NEWBORN

History

The history of rhesus prophylaxis can be traced to three unique individuals. Vincent Freda was an obstetrical resident who developed an interest in HDFN.[40] He was allowed to spend part of the fourth year of his residency at Columbia Presbyterian Medical Center in the laboratory of Alexander Weiner, one of the first investigators to identify the "Rh factor." When Freda returned to Columbia, he went on to establish a serology laboratory and later organized the Rh Antepartum Clinic in 1960. A seat on the hospital transfusion committee became vacant, and in an unprecedented move based on his interest, the chairman of obstetrics and gynecology, Howard C. Taylor, Jr., appointed Freda to this position even though he had not completed his residency. The chairman of pathology responded with the appointment of John Gorman to the committee, a resident in pathology with an interest in blood banking. It is here that these two individuals met and developed the collaboration that would one day end in the introduction of RhIG. In 1906, Theobald Smith[41] found that guinea pigs given excess passive antibody failed to become immunized to diphtheria toxin. Freda and Gorman proposed that anti-D could be used in a similar fashion to prevent alloimmunization after delivery. They enlisted the aid of William Pollack, a senior protein chemist at Ortho Diagnostics, who developed an IgG globulin fraction from high-titered donor plasma. An initial grant application to the National Institutes of Health was rejected. Funding was secured from the New York City Health Research Council on a second attempt. This was followed by a year's negotiations with lawyers in the state capital to allow the investigators to perform their clinical trials at the Sing Sing prison in New York beginning in 1961 (personal communication: John Gorman). Nine RhD-negative male volunteers were injected monthly with RhD-positive cells for five successive months.[42] Four of the men were immunized with intramuscular RhIG 24 hours before the injection of the red cells. Four of the five controls became alloimmunized to RhD, whereas none of the treated individuals developed anti-RhD antibodies. Their second experiment involved 27 inmates at Sing Sing, 13 controls and 14 treated. Red cells were given intravenously. However, the warden of Sing Sing would not allow the investigators to return on any fixed schedule that would enable the prisoners to know the time and day of their revisit. He was concerned that this exact foreknowledge could involve the prisoners in an escape plan. The investigators gladly accepted this limitation as they reasoned that pregnant women who delivered over a weekend would probably not receive RhIG until Monday, up to 72 hours after delivery, owing to the closure of blood banks on weekends, as was commonly practiced at the time. None of the men receiving RhIG were alloimmunized, whereas 8 of 13 controls developed anti-RhD antibodies. After two additional experiments at Sing Sing in this second group of individuals, Freda and Gorman went on to conduct a clinical trial in postpartum women at Columbia Presbyterian Medical Center starting in March of 1964.[42] In the 100 patients that received RhIG, none became sensitized, as compared with a rate of 12% sensitization to RhD in the control group. In a follow-up study in these patients in their next pregnancy, none of the treated patients developed antibodies; 5 of 10 controls were alloimmunized and delivered infants affected by HDFN.

A parallel track of investigation was being undertaken by a group of British researchers in Liverpool. This group reasoned that the natural protective effect of ABO incompatibility between a mother and her fetus in preventing the formation of anti-D antibody could be used as a preventative strategy. A preparation of plasma containing anti-D IgM was formulated and administered intravenously to male volunteers.[43] Although initial short-term antibody studies were promising, eventually 8 of 13 treated men became immunized to RhD, as compared with only 1 of 11 controls. After the publication of the initial work of Freda et al. describing the use of a gamma globulin fraction of the plasma, the British group visited the New York investigators and obtained a sample of their gamma globulin preparation. The Liverpool group began their clinical trial in postpartum women with evidence of FMH by Kleihauer-Betke (KB) stain in April 1964.[44] They are subsequently credited with the first publication of a successful clinical trial in women.

An observational trial in Canada was initiated and determined that the baseline rate of antenatal sensitization to RhD was 1.8%.[45] Between 1968 and 1974, a trial of antenatal prophylaxis using injections of 300 mcg of RhIG at 28 and 34 weeks' gestation followed.[46] As compared with the previous observational study, none of the women demonstrated the development of anti-D antibodies. In a subsequent investigation involving RhIG administered only at 28 weeks' gestation, only 0.18% of women became sensitized.

RhIG was approved by the Division of Biologics Standards of the National Institutes of Health for general clinical use in the United States as RhoGAM (Ortho-Clinical Diagnostics, Inc., Raritan, N.J.) in 1968. Recommendations for use during the immediate postpartum period were set forth by the American Congress of Obstetricians and Gynecologists (ACOG) in 1970.[47] The Food and Drug Administration approved the use of antenatal RhIG in 1981. Routine antenatal prophylaxis at 28 to 29 weeks' gestation was proposed by ACOG later that same year.[48]

Preparations

Four polyclonal products derived from human plasma are currently available in the United States for the prevention of RhD alloimmunization. Two of the products (RhoGAM, Ortho-Clinical Diagnostics, Inc., Raritan, N.J., and Hyper-Rho S/D, Talecris Biothorgenetics, Inc., Research Triangle Park, N.C.) can only be given intramuscularly because they are derived from human plasma through Cohn cold ethanol fractionation—a process that results in contamination with IgA and other plasma proteins. The remaining two products (WinRho-SDF, Cangene Corporation, Winnipeg, Manitoba; and Rhophlac, CSL Behring, L.L.C., King of Prussia, Penn.) are prepared through sepharose column and ion-exchange chromatography, respectively. At present, all available products are subject to solvent detergent treatment to inactivate enveloped viruses; many manufacturers also employ an additional micropore filtration step to further reduce the chance for viral contamination. Additionally, thimerosal, a mercury preservative used to prevent bacterial and fungal contamination, has been removed from all RhIG products used in the United States.

The dwindling resource of plasma donors for RhIG manufacture has led to the search for a synthetic product. Several monoclonal anti-D antibodies are now under study in large clinical trials. In addition a synthetic polyclonal immune globulin consisting of 25 recombinant anti-D antibodies has been developed by transfection of Chinese hamster ovary cells.[49] Clinical trials with this product are also under way. These products may soon replace the current polyclonal products derived from human plasma.

Indications

All pregnant patients should undergo determination of blood type and an antibody screen at the first prenatal visit. Patients found to be *weak Rh positive* (previously termed *Du-positive*) should be considered RhD-negative because their RhD gene encodes for an altered D protein or a reduced expression of the RhD antigen on the red cell membrane. Therefore, some of these patients can potentially be at risk for rhesus alloimmunization and do not require RhIG. **If there is no evidence of anti-D alloimmunization in the RhD-negative woman, the patient should receive 300 mcg of RhIG at 28 weeks of gestation.**[50] The 2% background incidence of RhD alloimmunization in the antenatal period can be expected to decline to 0.1%. In the United Kingdom, an antenatal protocol of administering 100 mcg (500 international units [IU]) of RhIG at 28 and 34 weeks is used in primigravida women.[51] Limited resources have not allowed for extension of this protocol to all subsequent pregnancies. The issue of repeating an antibody screen at 28 weeks before the administration of RhIG is controversial. The low incidence of a positive screen after a negative test at entry into prenatal care has resulted in the ACOG questioning the cost effectiveness of this practice.[50] Although ACOG leaves the decision to repeat the antibody screen up to the obstetrical provider, the American Association of Blood Banks (AABB) recommends that a repeat screen be obtained before antenatal RhIG.[52] If a repeat antibody screen is to be undertaken, a maternal blood sample can be drawn at the same office visit as the RhIG injection. Although the administration of the exogenous anti-D will eventually result in a weakly positive titer, this will not occur in the short interval of several hours due to the slow absorption from the intramuscular site. Some experts recommend that a second dose of RhIG be given if the patient has not delivered by 40 weeks' gestation.

Although not well studied, Level A scientific evidence has been cited by ACOG to address additional indications for the antepartum administration of RhIG.[50] **These include spontaneous abortion, elective abortion, ectopic pregnancy, genetic amniocentesis, chorion villous sampling, and FBS (see box, Indications for Administration of Rhesus Immune Globulin).** A dose of 50 mcg of RhIG is effective until 13 weeks' gestation owing to the small volume of red cells in the fetoplacental circulation. However, most hospitals and offices do not stock this dose of RhIG because the cost is equivalent to that of the standard dose of 300 mcg.

Indications for Administration of Rhesus Immune Globulin

- Spontaneous abortion*
- Elective abortion*
- Threatened abortion
- Ectopic pregnancy*
- Hydatidiform mole†
- Genetic amniocentesis*
- Chorion villus sampling*
- Fetal blood sampling*
- Placenta previa with bleeding‡
- Suspected abruption‡
- Intrauterine fetal demise‡
- Blunt trauma to the abdomen (includes motor vehicle accidents)‡
- At 28 weeks' gestation, unless father of fetus is RhD-negative*
- Amniocentesis for fetal lung maturity*
- External cephalic version‡
- Within 72 hours of delivery of an RhD-positive infant*
- After administration of RhD-positive blood components‡

*Level A evidence (good and consistent scientific evidence).[50]
†Level B evidence (at least fair scientific evidence).
‡Level C evidence (consensus and expert opinion).[50]

The use of RhIG in other scenarios involving the possibility of FMH are lacking. However, most experts (Level C scientific evidence; see box, Indications for Administration of Rhesus Immune Globulin) agree that such events as hydatidiform mole, threatened abortion, fetal death in the second or third trimester, blunt trauma to the abdomen, and external cephalic version warrant strong consideration for the use of RhIG.

The practice of evaluating a persistent maternal anti-D titer as an indication that additional RhIG is not required after an antenatal event is to be discouraged. Although the precise mechanism for the protective effect of RhIG is unknown, an excess amount of exogenous antibody in relation to the volume of RhD-positive red cells in the maternal circulation is essential for effective prophylaxis. Both animal and human studies have demonstrated that a low level of RhIG can actually enhance the chance for alloimmunization.[19] In the words of Vincent Freda, "the rule of thumb should be to administer Rh-immune globulin when in doubt, rather than to withhold it."

Because the half-life of RhIG is approximately 16 days, 15% to 20% of patients receiving it at 28 weeks have a very low anti-D titer (usually 2 or 4) at the time of admission for labor at term.[53] In North America, the current recommendation is to administer 300 mcg of RhIG within 72 hours of delivery if umbilical cord blood typing reveals an RhD-positive infant.[50] This is sufficient to protect from sensitization due to an FMH of 30 mL of fetal whole blood. In the United Kingdom, 100 mcg is given at delivery. Approximately 1 in 1000 deliveries will be associated with an excessive FMH; risk factors identify only 50% of these cases.[54] **Both ACOG and AABB now recommend routine screening of all women at the time of delivery for excessive FMH.** A qualitative yet sensitive test for FMH, the rosette test, is first performed. Results return as positive or negative. A negative result warrants administration of a standard 300 mcg dose of RhIG. If the rosette is positive, a KB stain or fetal cell stain using flow cytometry is undertaken to quantitate the amount of the FMH. The AABB then recommends that the percentage of fetal blood cells be multiplied by a factor of 50 (to account for an estimated maternal blood volume of 5000 mL) in order to calculate the volume of the FMH. This volume is divided by 30 to determine the number of vials of RhIG to be administered. A decimal point is rounded up or down for values of greater than 0.5 or less than 0.5, respectively. Because this calculation includes an inaccurate estimation of the maternal blood volume, one additional vial of RhIG is added to the calculation. As an example, a 3% KB stain is calculated to indicate a 150-mL FMH. Dividing this number by 30 yields five vials of RhIG with one additional vial added; therefore, the blood bank would prescribe six vials of RhIG (a total of 1800 mcg) for this patient. However, a recent survey by the American College of Pathologists of its member blood banks noted that even following these guidelines, an inadequate dose of RhIG was recommended in 9% of cases and an excessive dose was recommended in 12% of cases.[55] This led to the development of an online calculator that can be used to determine the correct dose of RhIG based on the percentage of fetal cells noted on KB stain or flow cytometry (www.cap.org/apps/docs/committees/transfusionmedicine/RHIGcalc.zip).

No more than five units of RhIG should be administered by the intramuscular route in one 24-hour period. Should a large dose of RhIG be necessary, an alternative method would be to give the calculated dose using one of the intravenous preparations of RhIG that are now available. Doses of up to 600 mcg (3000 IU) can be administered every 8 hours until the total dose has been achieved. **Should RhIG be inadvertently omitted after delivery, some protection has been proven with administration within 13 days; recommendations have been made to administer it as late as 28 days after delivery.**[54] If delivery is planned within 48 hours of amniocentesis for fetal lung maturity, RhIG can be deferred until after delivery. **If delivery occurs less than 3 weeks from the administration of RhIG used for antenatal indications such as external cephalic version, a repeat dose is unnecessary unless a large FMH is detected at the time of delivery.**[50]

Failed prophylaxis after the appropriate dose of RhIG is employed is rare. However, once postpartum administration is undertaken, the anti-D antibody screen may remain positive for up to 6 months. Anti-D persisting after this time is likely to be the result of sensitization.

The issue of the need for rhesus prophylaxis for the patient with a *weak Rh positive* blood type has been confusing to the clinician. Several genetic variants can account for this serologic result, some of which result in the presence of only part of the usual RhD epitope. In these cases patients can develop antibodies to the missing portion of the RhD antigen. Currently, the AABB no longer recommends routine testing for the weak D phenotype. Should this be reported as present, the patient should be considered RhD-negative and rhesus immune globulin should be administered according to standard recommendations.

Administration of RhIG after a postpartum tubal ligation is controversial. The possibility of a new partner in conjunction with the availability of in vitro fertilization would seem to make the use of RhIG in these situations prudent. In some cases, RhD-negative red cells may be in short supply if the patient presents after major trauma such as a motor vehicle accident with the need for massive transfusion. In these cases, RhD-positive blood could not be used as a life-saving alternative if the patient is alloimmunized to RhD through her previous delivery. RhIG is not effective once alloimmunization to the RhD antigen has occurred. At present, prophylactic immune globulin preparations to prevent other forms of red cell alloimmunization such as anti-K1 do not exist.

Diagnostic Methods

Maternal Antibody Determination

Once a maternal antibody screen reveals the presence of an anti-D antibody, a titer is the first step in the evaluation of the RhD-sensitized patient during the first affected pregnancy. Previous titer methodologies using albumin or saline should no longer be employed because they detect varying levels of IgM antibody. The pentamer structure of this class of antibody does not allow for transplacental passage; therefore, the contribution of IgM to the titer quantitation has no clinical relevance. The human antiglobulin titer (indirect Coombs' test) is used to determine the degree of alloimmunization as it measures the maternal IgG response. Most titer values in the obstetric literature are reported as dilutions (e.g., 1:32). By blood banking convention, however, titer values should be reported as the reciprocal of the last tube dilution that demonstrates a positive agglutination reaction, that is, a final dilution of 1:16 is equivalent to a titer of 16. Variation in results between laboratories is not uncommon because many commercial laboratories use enzymatic treatment of red cells to prevent failed detection of low titer samples.

This method causes a marked elevation in titer as compared with the use of nonenzymatic treated cells. Because standard tube methodology uses red cell agglutination as the indicator reaction, subjective interpretation of end points by the laboratory technologist accounts for the variation in results. In addition, inherent subtle differences in the indicator red cell preparations may play a role because their shelf life is only 1 month and serial titers may require the use of different reagent lots. For these reasons, serial titers should be run in tandem using stored sera from the previous draw.

In the same laboratory, the titer should not vary by more than one dilution if the two samples are run in tandem. Thus an initial titer of 8 that returns at 16 does not represent a true increase in the amount of antibody in the maternal circulation. In addition, the clinician should be aware that newer gel microcolumn assays will result in higher titers than conventional tube testing. In one study, the mean titer was 3.4-fold increased with gel technology.[56] **A critical titer is defined as the anti–red cell titer associated with a significant risk for hydrops fetalis.** When this is present, further fetal surveillance is warranted. This value will vary with institution and methodologies; however, in most centers, a critical titer for anti-D between 8 and 32 is usually used.

In the United Kingdom, quantitation of anti-D is undertaken through the use of an automated technique using a device known as the AutoAnalyzer. Red cell samples are mixed with agents to enhance agglutination by the anti-D antibodies. Agglutinated cells are separated from nonagglutinated cells and then lysed. The amount of released hemoglobin is then compared with an international standard; results are reported as international units per milliliter. Levels of less than 4 IU/mL are rarely associated with HDFN; a maternal anti-D level of less than 15 IU/mL has been associated with only mild fetal anemia.[57]

Fetal Blood Typing

Several techniques have been employed to determine the fetal blood type if the patient's partner is determined to be heterozygous for the involved red cell antigen. In 50% of cases in which the fetus is found to be antigen negative, further maternal and fetal testing is unnecessary. Historically, initial attempts at fetal testing in these cases employed serology on blood obtained by ultrasound-directed FBS. Unfortunately, this technique placed half of the antigen-negative fetuses at a 1% to 2% chance of procedure-related loss (see Chapter 11). Investigators went on to use chorion villus sampling to obtain genetic material for detection of the RhD gene. However, the major disadvantage of this method is that disruption of the chorion villi during the procedure can result in FMH and a rise in maternal titer, thereby worsening the fetal disease.[58] Therefore, this procedure should be discouraged unless the patient plans to terminate all antigen-positive fetuses that are detected. In 1990 amniocentesis was described as a reliable method for assessing the fetal blood type through DNA testing.[11] **This method has now been replaced in most situations by the use of fetal RhD typing using free fetal DNA in maternal plasma.**

The initial step in determining the fetal RhD type involves an assessment of paternity and paternal zygosity. Cases of questionable paternity may lead one to proceed with fetal RhD typing using free fetal DNA testing because this involves no risk to the fetus. Alternatively, a stepwise approach can be employed in cases of assured paternity. Once undertaken using serologic testing and population statistics, molecular techniques can now be used to accurately determine the paternal genotype at the RhD locus.[59]

Fetal RhD determination through noninvasive testing is now routine in Europe and has recently become available in the United States.[60] Free fetal DNA in the maternal serum has been used to detect RhD sequences in the case of an RhD-positive fetus. Free fetal DNA is cleared from the maternal plasma within minutes after delivery, thereby eliminating the possibility of contamination from a previous gestation. In a recent series of more than 1000 patients, free fetal DNA testing for RhD was found to be accurate in 99% of cases.[61] An RhD-positive result on free DNA testing can be considered reliable because RhD-positive genetic material cannot be from a maternal source. An RhD-negative result with free fetal DNA is more problematic. If fetal DNA fails to amplify in a background of overwhelming maternal DNA in the plasma, an RhD-negative result will be obtained. One internal control that can be used is the detection of the SRY gene found in male fetuses. The presence of this gene in free DNA indicates that fetal DNA is present, and an RhD-negative result is reliable.[62] In the case of a female fetus, the presence of single nucleotide polymorphisms (SNPs) not found in the maternal white cells can be used as an internal control.[62] If different polymorphisms than those found in the mother are noted in the plasma sample, one can be assured that these are of paternal origin; thus, fetal DNA is present. In this situation, the finding of an RhD-negative fetus can be considered reliable. **In the cases in which an inconclusive result is reported, a repeat maternal sample can be submitted or amniocentesis undertaken to determine the fetal RhD type.**

Amniocentesis to Follow the Severity of Hemolytic Disease of the Fetus and Newborn

Because it was first introduced to clinical practice, the spectral analysis of amniotic fluid has been used in alloimmunized pregnancies to determine the level of bilirubin, an indirect indicator of the degree of fetal hemolysis.[7] The peak value at 450 nm is subtracted from the baseline (a line drawn between data points at 550 and 365 nm) to determine the delta OD450 (ΔOD_{450}). A proposed management scheme using three zones based on gestational age was later introduced in 1963. The "Liley" curve has proven extremely useful in monitoring the alloimmunized pregnancy. Unfortunately, the original data were limited to 27 weeks' gestation. Despite the lack of data, later publications included extrapolated curves to earlier gestational ages.[63] The advent of FBS to determine the actual fetal hematocrit revealed that an extrapolated Liley curve back to 18 weeks' gestation failed to predict fetal anemia in as many as 70% of cases in the early second trimester.[64] For a brief period after this report, many centers used FBS exclusively in cases of severe red cell alloimmunization if fetal assessment was indicated before 27 weeks' gestation. A modified ΔOD_{450} curve (Queenan curve) for such situations was subsequently published using data from the

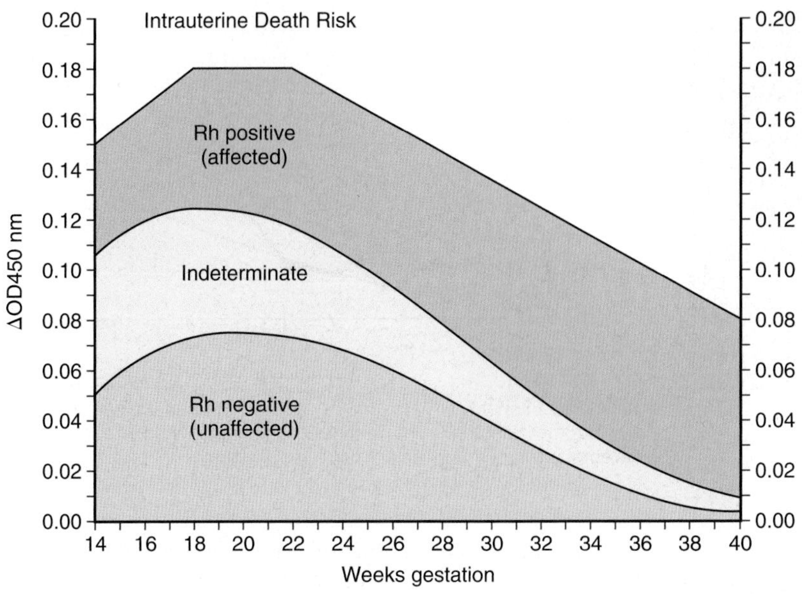

FIGURE 32-3. Queenan curve for ΔOD_{450} values. (Reproduced from Queenan JT, Tomai TP, Ural SH, King JC: Deviation in amniotic fluid optical density at a wavelength of 450 nm in Rh-immunized pregnancies from 14 to 40 weeks' gestation: a proposal for clinical management. Am J Obstet Gynecol 168:1370, 1993, Lippincott Williams and Wilkins,Copyright © 2001.)

early second trimester (Figure 32-3).[65] **The advent of noninvasive testing for fetal anemia through the use of middle cerebral artery Doppler (see below) has replaced serial amniocenteses for ΔOD_{450} except in rare circumstances where access to MCA Doppler is not available or in the management of the alloimmunized pregnancy after 35 weeks of gestation.**

Fetal Blood Sampling

Ultrasound-directed FBS (also known as *percutaneous umbilical blood sampling, cordocentesis*, and *funipuncture*) allows direct access to the fetal circulation to obtain important laboratory values such as fetal blood type, hematocrit, direct Coombs' test, reticulocyte count, and total bilirubin. Although serial FBS was once proposed as a primary method of fetal surveillance after a maternal critical titer is reached, it has been associated with a 1% to 2% rate of fetal loss, as well as up to a 50% risk for FMH with subsequent worsening of the alloimmunization.[66] For these reasons, FBS is reserved for patients with elevated peak MCA Doppler velocities.

Ultrasound

Perhaps the greatest advance in the management of the alloimmunized pregnancy has been the use of ultrasound. Gestational age can be accurately established in order to evaluate fetal parameters that vary with gestational age including hemoglobin, ΔOD_{450} levels, and peak MCA Doppler velocities. Hydrops fetalis is defined as the presence of extracellular fluid in at least two fetal compartments. Often, ascites is the first sign of impending hydrops, with scalp edema and pleural effusions noted with worsening anemia. When hydrops is present, fetal hemoglobin deficits of 7 to 10 g/dL from the mean hemoglobin value for the corresponding gestational age can be expected.[67] Unfortunately, this represents the end-stage state of fetal anemia. Survival with intrauterine transfusion (IUT) is markedly reduced in these cases. Therefore, many investigators have sought alternative ultrasound parameters that could predict the early onset of anemia. In one large series, fetal abdominal circumference, head-to-abdomen circumference ratio, intraperitoneal volume, intrahepatic and extrahepatic umbilical venous diameter, and placental thickness failed to accurately predict a fetal hemoglobin deficit of greater than 5 g/dL from the mean.[68] Because the fetal liver and spleen represent sites of extramedullary hematopoiesis and the destruction and sequestration of sensitized red cells in cases of severe HDFN, enlargement of these organs has been evaluated. Both splenic perimeter and hepatic length correlate with the degree of fetal anemia. However, neither has gained widespread acceptance for noninvasive fetal surveillance in red cell alloimmunization.

The severely anemic fetus exhibits an increased cardiac output in an effort to enhance oxygen delivery to peripheral tissues.[27] In addition, fetal anemia is associated with a lower blood viscosity that produces less shearing forces in blood vessels; this results in increased blood velocities. Using these principles, Doppler ultrasound has been employed to study the peak velocity in the fetal MCA to predict fetal anemia. A value of greater than 1.5 multiples of the median (MoMs) for the corresponding gestational age predicts moderate to severe fetal anemia with a sensitivity of 88% and a negative predictive rate of 89%.[12]

Serial MCA Doppler studies are now the mainstay of surveillance for fetal anemia in the red cell alloimmunized pregnancy. Careful attention to technique is paramount in using this method of surveillance. Because the anteroposterior axis of the fetal head typically lies in a transverse plane, the examiner can use either fetal MCA vessel for interrogation. One must first locate the anterior wing of the sphenoid bone at the base of the skull. Color or power Doppler is then used to locate the MCA (Figure 32-4). The angle of insonation is maintained as close to zero as possible by positioning the ultrasound transducer on the maternal abdomen (Figures 32-5 and 32-6). The MCA vessel closer to the maternal abdominal wall is usually studied, although the posterior vessel will give equivalent

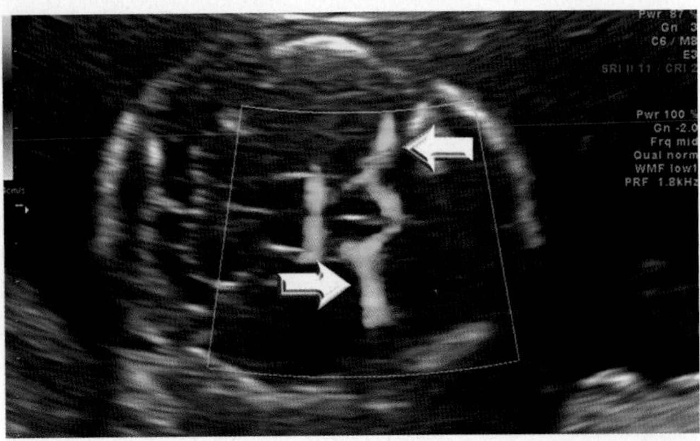

FIGURE 32-4. Power Doppler image of the fetal circle of Willis. *Arrows* point to locations where the pulsed Doppler gate should be placed for obtaining the fetal peak middle cerebral artery (MCA) Doppler velocity.

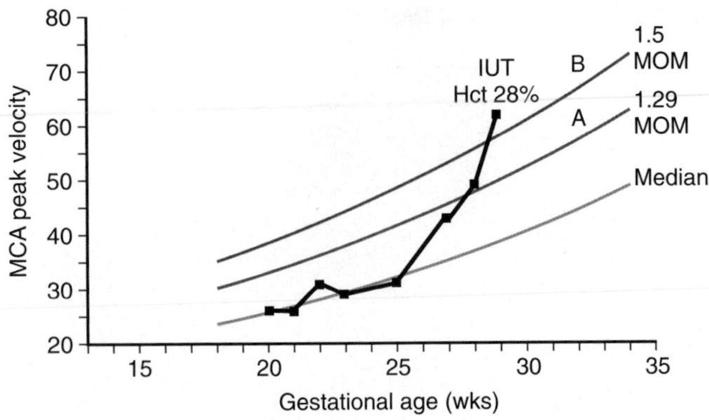

FIGURE 32-7. Serial MCA Doppler studies in one patient who required intrauterine transfusion. *IUT,* Intrauterine transfusion; *MCA,* middle cerebral artery; *MoM,* multiples of the median.

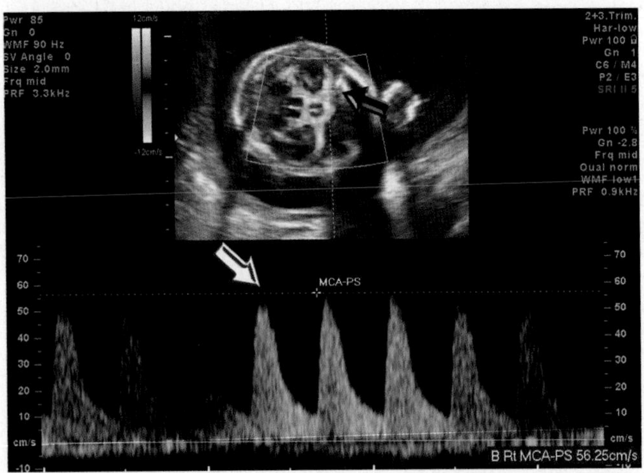

FIGURE 32-5. Pulsed Doppler of the peak systolic velocity. *Black arrow* at top of figure indicates the location of the pulsed Doppler gate; *white arrow* indicates the measurement using on-board software of a peak velocity of 56.25 cm/sec.

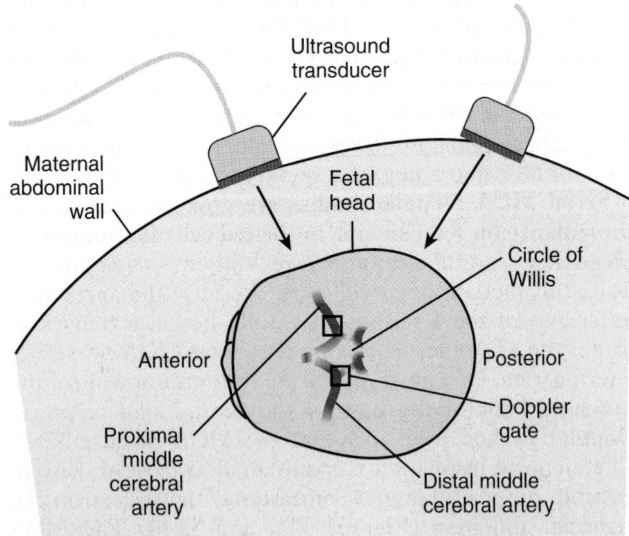

FIGURE 32-6. Correct determination of the fetal peak middle cerebral artery (MCA) Doppler velocity.

results.[69] Angle correction software is not employed. The Doppler gate is then placed in the proximal MCA because the vessel arises from the carotid siphon. Measurements in the more distal aspect of the vessel will be inaccurate because reduced peak velocities will be obtained. Finally, the fetus should be in a quiescent state during the Doppler examination because accelerations of the fetal heart rate can result in a decrease in the peak systolic velocity, especially late in the third trimester.[70]

MCA measurements can be obtained reliably as early as 18 weeks' gestation. Studies are repeated every 1 to 2 weeks depending on the trend (Figure 32-7). Values should be converted to MoMs using Internet-based calculators (e.g., www.perinatology.com). Values after 35 weeks' gestation are associated with a higher rate of false-negative results.[70]

CLINICAL MANAGEMENT

The approach using the available diagnostic tools is based on the patient's past history of fetal or neonatal manifestations of HDFN. **As a general rule, the patient's first RhD-sensitized pregnancy involves minimal fetal/neonatal disease; but subsequent gestations are associated with a worsening degree of anemia.**

First Affected Pregnancy

Once sensitization to the RhD antigen is detected, maternal titers are repeated every month until approximately 24 weeks; titers are repeated every 2 weeks thereafter (Figure 32-8). If paternity is assured, blood is drawn from the patient's partner to determine his RhD status and zygosity (DNA testing). Once a critical maternal titer is reached (usually 32), serial MCA Doppler studies are initiated at approximately 24 weeks' gestation. These are then repeated every 1 to 2 weeks depending on their trend. In cases of a heterozygous paternal phenotype or questionable paternity, free fetal DNA testing should be sent to a DNA reference laboratory to determine the fetal RhD status. In the case of an RhD-negative paternal blood type or a fetal RhD-negative genotype, further maternal and fetal monitoring is unwarranted as long as paternity is assured.

If there is evidence of an RhD-positive fetus (homozygous paternal phenotype or RhD-positive fetus by DNA

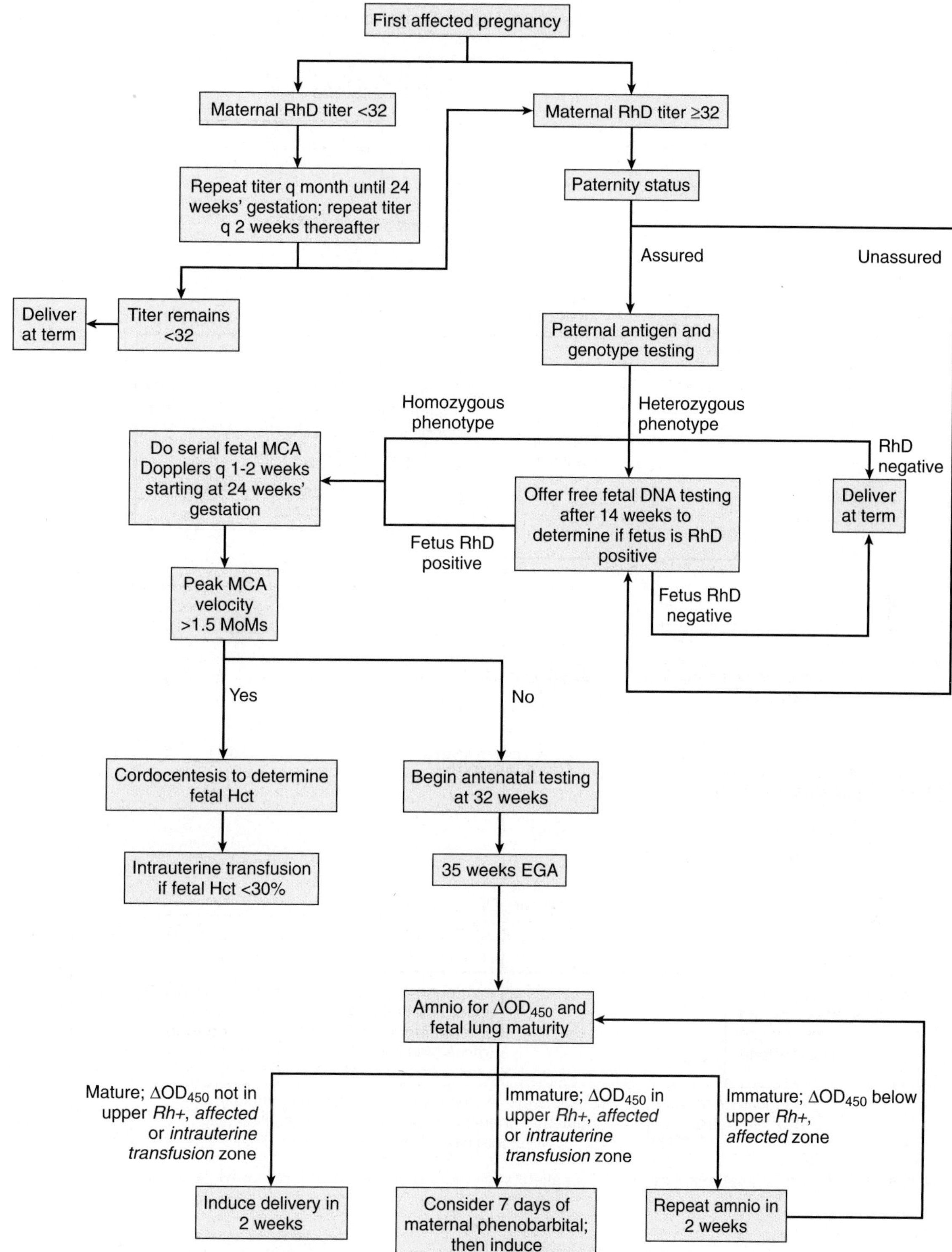

FIGURE 32-8. Algorithm for clinical management of a patient with red cell sensitization in the first affected pregnancy.

testing), serial fetal surveillance is indicated. If an MCA Doppler returns at greater than 1.5 MoM, cordocentesis should be undertaken at an experienced referral center, with blood readied for IUT if the fetal hematocrit is less than 30%.

If the peak MCA value remains at less than 1.5 MoM, amniocentesis at 35 weeks' gestation should be considered. If fetal pulmonary maturity is present and the ΔOD_{450} is not in the upper portion of the *Rh-positive, affected* zone of the Queenan curve, delivery should be induced in 2 weeks. This will enable time for fetal hepatic maturity to occur, thereby limiting the need for exchange transfusion secondary to neonatal hyperbilirubinemia. If the fetal pulmonary immaturity is noted at the time of the 35-week

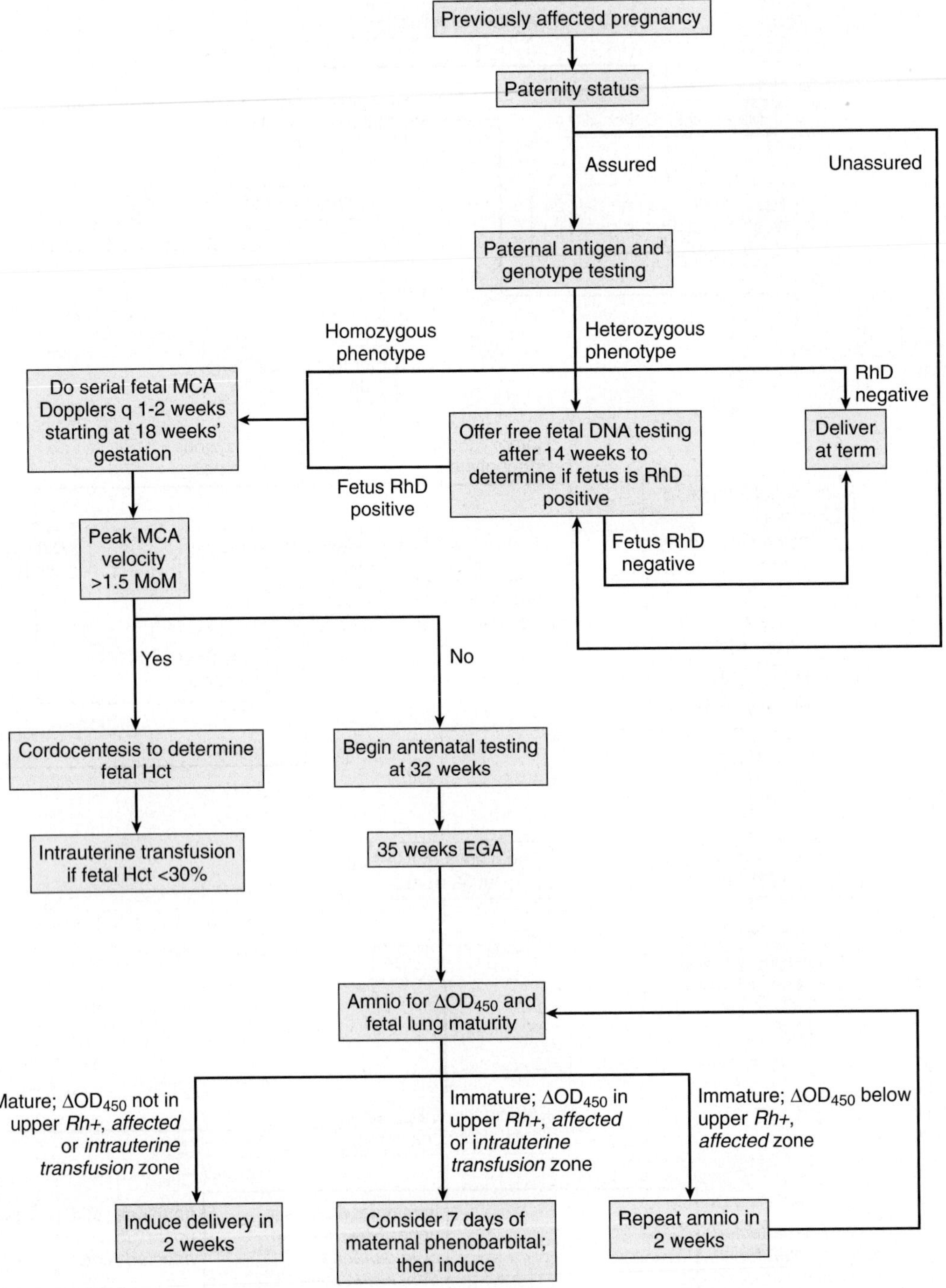

FIGURE 32-9. Algorithm for clinical management of a patient with red cell sensitization and a previously affected fetus or infant.

amniocentesis and the ΔOD_{450} is in the *Rh-positive, affected* zone of the Queenan curve, then administration of maternal phenobarbital (30 mg orally TID) with induction 1 week later will decrease the chance for neonatal exchange transfusion.[71] Finally, if results indicate fetal lung immaturity with a ΔOD_{450} that is not in the *Rh-positive, affected* zone of the Queenan curve, a repeat amniocentesis should be undertaken in 2 weeks. Surveillance with serial amniocentesis for ΔOD_{450} would follow this same management plan in the late third trimester.

Previously Affected Fetus or Infant

If there is a history of a previous perinatal loss related to HDFN, a previous need for IUT, or a previous need for neonatal exchange transfusion, the patient should be referred to a tertiary care center with experience in the management of the severely alloimmunized pregnancy (Figure 32-9). In these cases, maternal titers are *not* predictive of the degree of fetal anemia. In the case of a heterozygous paternal phenotype or questionable paternity, free fetal DNA analysis to determine the fetal RhD status is indicated. Serial MCA Doppler measurements should begin at 18 weeks' gestation and be repeated every 1 to 2 weeks.

INTRAUTERINE TRANSFUSION

Technique

IUTs today are performed under continuous ultrasound guidance with direct infusions of red blood cells into the umbilical cord vessels or into the intrahepatic portion of the umbilical vein of the fetus.[72] Some centers continue to use the intraperitoneal approach as part of a combined technique with an intravascular transfusion (IVT) in an effort to create a reservoir of red cells between procedures.[73]

Typically, a freshly donated, CMV-negative unit of type O, RhD-negative red blood cells is cross-matched to a maternal blood sample. The unit is leukoreduced and irradiated with 25 Gy to prevent graft-versus-host reaction. It is then washed and packed to a final hematocrit of approximately 75% to 80% to prevent volume overload in the fetus.

The patient is admitted to the Labor and Delivery unit as an outpatient. The procedure is typically performed in the operating room, especially when a viable gestational age had been reached should an emergency delivery be necessary. The skin is prepped with povidine-iodine and sterile drapes applied. A long-acting local anesthetic is administered; conscious sedation may also be employed for the anxious patient. A 20- or 22-gauge procedure needle is introduced into the amniotic cavity and then into the umbilical vein under continuous ultrasound guidance. In the case of an anterior placenta, the needle is passed through the placental mass into the cord root. With a posterior placentation, the cord insertion into the placenta is preferred because this represents a site of immobility as compared with a "floating" loop of cord. A sample of fetal blood is obtained for an initial hematocrit. Optimally, the sample is processed as a spun hematocrit or through the use of an automated hemocytometer located in the operating room. A short-term paralytic agent such as vecuronium is administered into the umbilical vein, causing cessation of fetal movement.[74] Paralysis is almost immediate and lasts 2 to 3 hours. The amount of packed red blood cells to be infused is based on the estimated fetal weight determined by ultrasound and standardized formulas.[75] Red cells are actively infused through the use of a syringe and sterile tubing connected to the donor unit. Once the predetermined volume of blood is infused, a small aliquot of blood is obtained to measure the hematocrit as well as the percentage of fetal versus adult hemoglobin-containing red cells through either a KB stain or flow cytometry. A final fetal hematocrit of 40% is targeted. After the first intrauterine transfusion (IUT), subsequent procedures can be empirically scheduled at 14-day intervals until suppression of fetal erythropoiesis is noted. This usually occurs by the third IUT. Thereafter, the interval for repeat procedures can be determined based on the decline in hematocrit for the individual fetus, usually a 3- to 4-week interval. The peak systolic velocity in the MCA has been shown to be useful in timing the second IUT. After the second procedure, the MCA Doppler loses its validity in predicting fetal anemia, perhaps due to the changing rheology of the transfused adult red cells that make up the majority of the fetal red mass after serial IUTs.[76] The final IUT procedure is usually not performed past 35 weeks' gestation. The patient is scheduled for delivery approximately 3 weeks later.

Severely anemic fetuses in the early second trimester do not tolerate the acute correction of their hematocrit to normal values.[77] In these situations, the initial hematocrit should not be increased by more than fourfold at the time of the first procedure. A repeat IVT is then performed within 48 hours to correct the fetal hematocrit into the normal range.[78]

Complications and Outcome

Complications from IUT are uncommon. The total procedure-related perinatal loss was 4.7% of fetuses and 1.6% of procedures in one large series.[79] Survival after IUT varies with the center, its experience, and the presence of hydrops fetalis. An overall survival rate of 85% to 90% has been reported.[80] The presence of fetal hydrops, particularly if this does not resolve after several IUTs, has been associated with a lower rate of perinatal survival.[81] Preterm premature rupture of the membranes and chorioamnionitis occur rarely. Fetal bradycardia, particularly when there is inadvertent puncture of the umbilical artery, is usually transient and responds to removal of the procedure needle. Progression to fetal distress with the need for emergency delivery increases with advancing gestation and may complicate as many as 5% of procedures after 32 weeks' gestation.[82]

Neonatal Transfusions

The practice of prolonging the gestation of the treated fetus with HDFN until near term has resulted in a virtual absence of the need for neonatal exchange transfusions. Typically, these infants are born with a virtual absence of reticulocytes with a red cell population consisting mainly of transfused red cells. The blood bank may be confused if cord blood at delivery is submitted for neonatal red cell typing—the neonate will be typed as O, RhD-negative, reflecting the antigen status of the donor blood used for the IUTs. Elevated levels of circulating maternal antibodies in the neonatal circulation in conjunction with suppression of the fetal bone marrow production of red cells often results in the need for neonatal red cell *top-up* transfusions after discharge from the nursery; this occurs in approximately 50% of infants near 1 month of age.[83] **Therefore, these children should be followed weekly with hematocrits and reticulocyte counts until there is evidence of recovery of hematopoietic function.** Typically, only one neonatal transfusion is required, although a maximum of up to three has been reported. Supplemental iron therapy in these infants is unnecessary because they have excess levels of stored iron due to previous hemolysis in utero and lysis of red cells from the IUTs. Supplemental folate therapy (0.5 mg/day) should be considered.

Neurologic Outcome

Only limited data are available for counseling the patient regarding long-term outcome because fetuses with severe anemia and hydrops are likely to survive today secondary to the use of IVTs. **Short-term studies at up to 2 years of age have revealed that more than 90% of infants are neurologically normal even in the face of hydrops fetalis.**[84] One small study of 16 neonates who presented with fetal hydrops and were subsequently treated with IUTs indicated a 12% incidence of major neurologic sequealae.[85]

Elevated levels of bilirubin have been associated with hearing loss in the neonate. Therefore, newborn screening for hearing loss would appear warranted in children with HDFN. Follow-up screening at 1 and 2 years of age should be considered.

OTHER TREATMENT MODALITIES

Before the advent of the IUT, plasmapheresis represented one of the few therapeutic modalities for severe HDFN. Most literature reports include single cases or relatively small case series. Despite these limitations, a review of the published cases reveals a perinatal survival rate of 69%.[86] Intravenous immune globulin (IVIG) has been used effectively as the sole antenatal treatment for HDFN. Hydrops fetalis was less likely to occur and the onset of anemia occurred later in pregnancies treated with IVIG. **Some experts have proposed a combined approach in patients with a previous perinatal loss in the early second trimester when technical limitations make the success of IUT unlikely.**[87] Plasmapheresis is started at 12 weeks' gestation and repeated three times in that week. The maternal titer should be expected to be reduced by 50%. IVIG is then given to replace the globulin fraction removed by plasmapheresis in the form of a 2 g/kg loading dose after the third plasmapheresis; this is followed by 1 g/kg/week of IVIG until 20 weeks' gestation.

FUTURE THERAPEUTIC OPTIONS

Patients with high anti–red cell titers and recurrent perinatal loss in the second trimester have few options other than artificial insemination with red cell antigen–negative donor semen, surrogate pregnancy, or preimplantation diagnosis (if the father is heterozygous). **Peptides associated with the proliferation of T helper cells in the development of antibody to the RhD antigen and monoclonal anti-D blocking antibodies are currently being investigated to ameliorate an established anti-D response, thereby preventing severe HDFN in a subsequent pregnancy.**[88,89]

HEMOLYTIC DISEASE OF THE FETUS AND NEWBORN DUE TO NON-RhD ANTIBODIES

Antibodies to the red cell antigens Lewis, I, and P are often encountered through antibody screening during prenatal care. Because these antibodies are typically of the IgM class, they are not associated with HDFN.[52]

However, antibodies to more than 50 other red cell antigens have been reported to be associated with HDFN (Table 32-1). **More important, only three antibodies—anti-RhD, anti-Rhc, and anti-Kell (K1)—cause significant enough fetal hemolysis that treatment with IUT is considered necessary.** In one series from a tertiary care center for IUT in the Netherlands, 85% of cases involved anti-D; 10%, anti-K1; and 3.5%, anti-c. There was also one case each of anti-E, anti-e, and anti-Fy^a.[79]

Rhc

Anti-c antibody should be considered equivalent to anti-D regarding its potential to cause HDFN. In one report, 25% of antigen-positive fetuses were noted to have severe HDFN, 7% were hydropic, and 17% required IUTs for therapy.[90]

RhC, RhE, and Rhe

RhC, RhE, and Rhe antibodies are often found in low titer in the alloimmunized patient with anti-D. Their presence may be additive to the fetal hemolytic effect of anti-D.[91] When they occur alone, mild HDFN is usually the clinical course. Only a handful of case reports have indicated the need for treatment with IUT with each of these antibodies.[79,92]

M

Anti-M is a naturally occurring IgM antibody that typically presents as a cold agglutinin. Rarely, an IgG variety has been reported to cause mild HDFN.[93] Blood bank consultation should be undertaken to determine the class of antibody present when anti-M is detected in the pregnant woman with a titer of 32 or greater.

Duffy

The Duffy antigen system consists of two antigens, Fy^a and Fy^b. Only anti-Fy^a has been associated with mild HDFN.[94]

Kidd

The Kidd antigen system consists of two antigens, Jk^a and Jk^b. Rare cases of mild HDFN have been reported.

Kell

The Kell antigen system includes 23 different members. Antibodies to at least nine of the Kell antigens have been associated with HDFN. The most common of these is Kell (also designated *K*, *K1*) and cellano (*k*, *K2*). Additional antibodies that have been reported to be causative for HDFN include -Penny (Kp^a, *K3*), -Rautenberg (Kp^b, *K4*), -Peltz (*Ku*, *K5*), -Sutter (Js^a, *K6*), -Matthews (Js^b, *K7*), -Karhula (Ul^a, *K10*) and -K22.[95] Unlike the case of other hemolytic antibodies, fetal anemia due to Kell (anti-K1) sensitization is thought to be secondary to not only hemolysis but also to suppression of fetal erythropoiesis.[96]

The majority of cases of K1 sensitization are secondary to previous maternal blood transfusion, usually as a result of postpartum hemorrhage in a previous pregnancy. Because 92% of individuals are Kell negative, the initial management of the K1-sensitized pregnancy should entail paternal red cell typing and genotype testing. If the paternal typing returns K1-negative (kk) and paternity is assured, no further maternal testing is undertaken. The majority of Kell-positive individuals will be heterozygous (Table 32-2). Amniocentesis can be used to determine the

TABLE 32-1 NON-RhD ANTIBODIES AND ASSOCIATED HDFN

ANTIGEN SYSTEM	SPECIFIC ANTIGEN	ANTIGEN SYSTEM	SPECIFIC ANTIGEN	ANTIGEN SYSTEM	SPECIFIC ANTIGEN
Frequently Associated with Severe Disease					
Kell	-K (K1)				
Rhesus	-c				
Infrequently Associated with Severe Disease					
Colton	-Co^{a}	MNS	-Mur	Scianna	-Sc2
	-Co3		-M^{V}		-Rd
Diego	-ELO		-s	Other Ags	-Bi
	-Di^{a}		-s^{D}		-Good
	-Di^{b}		-S		-
Heibel					
	-Wr^{a}		-U		-HJK
	-Wr^{b}		-Vw		-Ht^{a}
Duffy	-Fy^{a}	Rhesus	-Be^{a}		-Jones
Kell	-Js^{b}		-C		-Joslin
	-k (K2)		-Ce		-Kg
	-Kp^{a}		-C^{w}		-Kuhn
	-Kp^{b}		-ce		-Li^{a}
	-K11		-E		-MAM
	-K22		-E^{w}		-
Niemetz					
	-Ku		-Evans		-REIT
	-Ul^{a}		-G		-Reiter
Kidd	-Jk^{a}		-Go^{a}		-Rd
MNS	-En^{a}		-Hr		-Sharp
	-Far		-Hr$_{o}$		-Vel
	-Hil		-JAL		-Zd
	-Hut		-Rh32		
	-M		-Rh42		
	-Mi^{a}		-Rh46		
	-Mt^{a}		-STEM		
	-MUT		-Tar		
Associated with Mild Disease					
Duffy	-Fy^{b}	Kidd	-Jk^{b}	Rhesus	-Riv
	-Fy^{3}		-Jk^{3}		-RH29
Gerbich	-Ge^{2}	MNS	-Mit	Other	-At^{a}
	-Ge^{3}	Rhesus	-C^{X}		-JFV
	-Ge^{4}		-D^{w}		-Jr^{a}
	-Ls^{a}		-e		-Lan
Kell	-Js^{a}		-HOFM		
			-LOCR		

Reproduced with permission from Moise KJ: Hemolytic disease of the fetus and newborn. *In* Creasy RK, Resnik R, Iams J (eds): Maternal-Fetal Medicine, Principles and Practice, ed 5. Philadelphia, Elsevier, Copyright © 2004.
HDFN, Hemolytic disease of the fetus and newborn.

TABLE 32-2 GENE FREQUENCIES (%) AND ZYGOSITY (%) FOR OTHER RED CELL ANTIGENS ASSOCIATED WITH HDN

	WHITE		BLACK		HISPANIC	
	Antigen+	Heterozygous	Antigen+	Heterozygous	Antigen+	Heterozygous
C	70	50	30	32	81	51
c	80	50	96	32	76	51
E	32	29	23	21	41	36
e	97	29	98	21	95	36
K (K1)	9	97.8	2	100		
k (K2)	99.8	8.8	100	2		
M	78	64	70	63		
N	77	65	74	60		
S	55	80	31	90		
s	89	50	97	29		
U	100	—	99	—		
Fy^{a}	66	26	10	90		
Fy^{b}	83	41	23	96		
Jk^{a}	77	36	91	63		
Jk^{b}	72	32	43	21		

Reproduced with permission and modified from Moise KJ: Hemolytic disease of the fetus and newborn. *In* Creasy RK, Resnik R, Iams J (eds): Maternal-Fetal Medicine: Principles and Practice, ed 5. Philadelphia, Elsevier, Copyright © 2004.

fetal genotype in these cases as free fetal DNA typing for Kell is only available in England.[97] **A lower maternal critical antibody value of 8 has been proposed to begin fetal surviellance.[98] Serial MCA Doppler studies have proven effective in detecting fetal anemia.[99]**

KEY POINTS

- Alloimmunization to the RhD, Kell (K1), and Rhc red cell antigens is the main cause for severe HDFN.
- Despite the widespread use of RhIG, approximately six cases of RhD alloimmunization occur per 1000 live births in the United States.
- Hydrops fetalis is defined as extracellular fluid in two fetal compartments; it represents the end-stage of fetal anemia in HDFN.
- The Rh D, C, c, E, and e antigens are coded by two genes that are located on the short arm of chromosome 1.
- The rule of thumb should be to administer RhIG when in doubt, rather than to withhold it.
- A critical maternal antibody titer can be used in the first affected pregnancy to decide when to begin further fetal testing.
- The fetal peak MCA Doppler velocity can be used to determine the onset of fetal anemia.
- In the case of a heterozygous paternal phenotype for a particular red cell antigen, fetal typing can be undertaken through free fetal DNA in maternal plasma for the RHD antigen; fetal typing for other red cell antigens can be obtained through amniocentesis.
- Intravascular fetal intrauterine transfusions are the mainstay of fetal therapy with an overall perinatal survival of greater than 85%.
- Except in cases of alloimmunization to Kell antigens, irregular red cell antibodies in pregnancy should be managed in a similar fashion to RhD.

REFERENCES

1. Bowman JM: RhD hemolytic disease of the newborn. N Engl J Med 339:1775, 1998.
2. Diamond LK, Blackfan KD, Baty JM: Erythroblastosis fetalis and its association with universal edema of the fetus, icterus gravis neonatorium and anemia of the newborn. J Pediatr 1:269, 1932.
3. Levine P, Stetson R: An usual case of intragroup agglutination. JAMA 113:126, 1939.
4. Landsteiner K, Weiner AS: An agglutinable factor in human blood recognized by immune sera for rhesus blood. Proc Soc Exper Biol Med 43:223, 1940.
5. Levine P, Katzin EM, Burham L: Isoimmunzation in pregnancy: its possible bearing on etiology of erythroblastosis foetalis. JAMA 116:825, 1941.
6. Wallerstein H: Treatment of severe erythroblastosis by simultaneous removal and replacement of blood of the newborn infant. Science 103:583, 1946.
7. Liley AW: Liquor amnii analysis in the management of pregnancy complicated by rhesus sensitization. Am J Obstet Gynecol 82:1359, 1961.
8. Liley AW: Intrauterine transfusion of foetus in haemolytic disease. BMJ 2:1107, 1963.
9. Rodeck CH, Kemp JR, Holman CA, et al: Direct intravascular fetal blood transfusion by fetoscopy in severe Rhesus isoimmunisation. Lancet 1:625, 1981.
10. Bang J, Bock JE, Trolle D: Ultrasound-guided fetal intravenous transfusion for severe rhesus haemolytic disease. Br Med J (Clin Res Ed) 284:373, 1982.
11. Bennett PR, Le Van Kim C, Colin Y, et al: Prenatal determination of fetal RhD type by DNA amplification. N Engl J Med 329:607, 1993.
12. Mari G: Noninvasive diagnosis by Doppler ultrasonography of fetal anemia due to maternal red-cell alloimmunization. N Engl J Med 342:9, 2000.
13. Lo YM, Bowell PJ, Selinger M, et al: Prenatal determination of fetal RhD status by analysis of peripheral blood of rhesus negative mothers. Lancet 341:1147, 1993.
14. Martin JA, Hamilton BE, Sutton PD, et al: Births: final data for 2003. National Vital Statistics Reports 54:1, 2003.
15. Geifman-Holtzman O, Wojtowycz M, Kosmas E, Artal R: Female alloimmunization with antibodies known to cause hemolytic disease. Obstet Gynecol 89:272, 1997.
16. van der Schoot CE, Tax GH, Rijnders RJ, et al: Prenatal typing of Rh and Kell blood group system antigens: the edge of a watershed. Transfus Med Rev 17:31, 2003.
17. Carapella-de Luca E, Casadei AM, Pascone R, et al: Maternofetal transfusion during delivery and sensitization of the newborn against the rhesus D-antigen. Vox Sang 34:241, 1978.
18. Pollack W: Rh hemolytic disease of the newborn: its cause and prevention. Prog Clin Biol Res 70:185, 1981.
19. Pollack W, Gorman JG, Hager HJ, et al: Antibody-mediated immune suppression to the Rh factor: animal models suggesting mechanism of action. Transfusion 8:134, 1968.
20. Pollack W, Gorman JG, Freda VJ, et al: Results of clinical trials of RhoGAM in women. Transfusion 8:151, 1968.
21. Pollock JM, Bowman JM: Anti-Rh(D) IgG subclasses and severity of Rh hemolytic disease of the newborn. Vox Sang 59:176, 1990.
22. Kumpel BM: Monoclonal anti-D development programme. Transpl Immunol 10:199, 2002.
23. Hilden JO, Gottvall T, Lindblom B: HLA phenotypes and severe Rh(D) immunization. Tissue Antigens 46:313, 1995.
24. Ulm B, Svolba G, Ulm MR, et al: Male fetuses are particularly affected by maternal alloimmunization to D antigen. Transfusion 39:169, 1999.
25. Nicolaides KH, Thilaganathan B, Rodeck CH, Mibashan RS: Erythroblastosis and reticulocytosis in anemic fetuses. Am J Obstet Gynecol 159:1063, 1988.
26. Lestas AN, Bellingham AJ, Nicolaides KH: Red cell glycolytic intermediates in normal, anaemic and transfused human fetuses. Br J Haematol 73:387, 1989.
27. Copel JA, Grannum PA, Green JJ, et al: Fetal cardiac output in the isoimmunized pregnancy: a pulsed Doppler-echocardiographic study of patients undergoing intravascular intrauterine transfusion. Am J Obstet Gynecol 161:361, 1989.
28. Soothill PW, Nicolaides KH, Rodeck CH, et al: Relationship of fetal hemoglobin and oxygen content to lactate concentration in Rh isoimmunized pregnancies. Obstet Gynecol 69:268, 1987.
29. Nicolaides KH, Warenski JC, Rodeck CH: The relationship of fetal plasma protein concentration and hemoglobin level to the development of hydrops in rhesus isoimmunization. Am J Obstet Gynecol 152:341, 1985.
30. Moise KJ Jr, Carpenter RJ Jr, Hesketh DE: Do abnormal Starling forces cause fetal hydrops in red blood cell alloimmunization? Am J Obstet Gynecol 167:907, 1992.
31. Moise AA, Gest AL, Weickmann PH, McMicken HW: Reduction in plasma protein does not affect body water content in fetal sheep. Pediatr Res 29:623, 1991.
32. Berger HM, Lindeman JH, van Zoeren-Grobben D, et al: Iron overload, free radical damage, and rhesus haemolytic disease. Lancet 335:933, 1990.
33. Lewis M, Bowman JM, Pollock J, Lowen B: Absorption of red cells from the peritoneal cavity of an hydropic twin. Transfusion 13:37, 1973.
34. Fischer RA, Race RR: Rh gene frequencies in Britain. Nature 157:48, 1946.
35. Cherif-Zahar B, Mattei MG, Le Van Kim C, et al: Localization of the human Rh blood group gene structure to chromosome region 1p34.3-1p36.1 by in situ hybridization. Hum Genet 86:398, 1991.

36. Le Van Kim C, Cherif-Zahar B, Raynal V, et al: Multiple Rh messenger RNA isoforms are produced by alternative splicing. Blood 80:1074, 1992.
37. Carritt B, Kemp TJ, Poulter M: Evolution of the human RH (rhesus) blood group genes: a 50 year old prediction (partially) fulfilled. Hum Mol Genet 6:843, 1997.
38. Singleton BK, Green CA, Avent ND, et al: The presence of an RHD pseudogene containing a 37 base pair duplication and a nonsense mutation in Africans with the Rh D-negative blood group phenotype. Blood 95:12, 2000.
39. Lee YL, Chiou HL, Hu SN, Wang L: Analysis of RHD genes in Taiwanese RhD-negative donors by the multiplex PCR method. J Clin Lab Anal 17:80, 2003.
40. Dunn LJ: Prevention of isoimmunization in pregnancy developed by Freda and Gorman. Obstet Gynecol Surv 54:S1, 1999.
41. Smith T: Active immunity produced by so-called balanced or neutral mixtures of diptheria toxin and anti-toxin. Journal of Experimental Medicine 11:241, 1909.
42. Freda VJ, Gorman JG, Pollack W, et al: Prevention of Rh isoimmunization. Progress report of the clinical trial in mothers. JAMA 199:390, 1967.
43. Finn R, Clarke CA, Donohoe WT, et al: Experimental studies on the prevention of Rh haemolytic disease. Br Med J 5238:1486, 1961.
44. Clarke CA, Sheppard PM: Prevention of rhesus haemolytic disease. Lancet 19:343, 1965.
45. Bowman JM, Chown B, Lewis M, Pollock JM: Rh isoimmunization during pregnancy: antenatal prophylaxis. Can Med Assoc J 118:623, 1978.
46. Bowman JM, Pollock JM: Antenatal prophylaxis of Rh isoimmunization: 28-weeks'-gestation service program. Can Med Assoc J 118:627, 1978.
47. Prenatal antibody screening and use of Rho (D) immune globulin (human). American College of Obstetricians and Gynecologists Technical Bulletin 13, 1970.
48. The selective use of Rho(D) immune globulin (RhIG). American College of Obstetricians and Gynecologists Technical Bulletin Update 61, 1981.
49. Symphogen. 2010. Available at: http://www.symphogen.com/web/guest/newsarchive/. Accessed December 12, 2010.
50. Prevention of RhD alloimmunization. American College of Obstetricians and Gynecologists Practice Bulletin 4, 1999.
51. Urbaniak SJ: Consensus conference on anti-D prophylaxis, April 7 & 8, 1997: final consensus statement. Royal College of Physicians of Edinburgh/Royal College of Obstetricians and Gynaecologists. Transfusion 38:97, 1998.
52. Brecher ME: Technical Manual of the American Association of Blood Banks, 15th ed. Bethesda, Md, American Association of Blood Banks, 2005.
53. Goodrick J, Kumpel B, Pamphilon D, et al: Plasma half-lives and bioavailability of human monoclonal Rh D antibodies BRAD-3 and BRAD-5 following intramuscular injection into Rh D-negative volunteers. Clin Exp Immunol 98:17, 1994.
54. Bowman JM: Controversies in Rh prophylaxis. Who needs Rh immune globulin and when should it be given? Am J Obstet Gynecol 151:289, 1985.
55. Ramsey G: Inaccurate doses of R immune globulin after Rh-incompatible fetomaternal hemorrhage: survey of laboratory practice. Arch Pathol Lab Med 133:465, 2009.
56. Novaretti MC, Jens E, Pagliarini T, et al: Comparison of conventional tube test with diamed gel microcolumn assay for anti-D titration. Clin Lab Haematol 25:311, 2003.
57. Nicolaides KH, Rodeck CH: Maternal serum anti-D antibody concentration and assessment of rhesus isoimmunisation. BMJ 304:1155, 1992.
58. Moise KJ Jr, Carpenter RJ Jr: Chorionic villus sampling for Rh typing: clinical implications [letter; comment]. Am J Obstet Gynecol 168:1002, 1993.
59. Pirelli KJ, Pietz BC, Johnson ST, et al: Molecular determination of RHD zygosity: predicting risk of hemolytic disease of the fetus and newborn related to anti-D. Prenat Diagn 30:1207, 2010.
60. Tynan JA, Angkachatchai V, Ehrich M, et al: Multiplexed analysis of circulating cell-free fetal nucleic acids for noninvasive prenatal diagnostic RHD testing. Am J Obstet Gynecol, 2010.
61. Muller SP, Bartels I, Stein W, et al: The determination of the fetal D status from maternal plasma for decision making on Rh prophylaxis is feasible. Transfusion 48:2292, 2008.
62. Daniels G, Finning K, Martin P, Soothill P: Fetal blood group genotyping from DNA from maternal plasma: an important advance in the management and prevention of haemolytic disease of the fetus and newborn. Vox Sang 87:225, 2004.
63. Management of isoimmunization in pregnancy. American College of Obstetricians and Gynecologists Technical Bulletin 90, 1986.
64. Nicolaides KH, Rodeck CH, Mibashan RS, Kemp JR: Have Liley charts outlived their usefulness? Am J Obstet Gynecol 155:90, 1986.
65. Queenan JT, Tomai TP, Ural SH, King JC: Deviation in amniotic fluid optical density at a wavelength of 450 nm in Rh-immunized pregnancies from 14 to 40 weeks' gestation: a proposal for clinical management. Am J Obstet Gynecol 168:1370, 1993.
66. Weiner CP, Williamson RA, Wenstrom KD, et al: Management of fetal hemolytic disease by cordocentesis. II. Outcome of treatment. Am J Obstet Gynecol 165:1302, 1991.
67. Nicolaides KH, Soothill PW, Clewell WH, et al: Fetal haemoglobin measurement in the assessment of red cell isoimmunisation. Lancet 1:1073, 1988.
68. Nicolaides KH, Fontanarosa M, Gabbe SG, Rodeck CH: Failure of ultrasonographic parameters to predict the severity of fetal anemia in rhesus isoimmunization. Am J Obstet Gynecol 158:920, 1988.
69. Abel DE, Grambow SC, Brancazio LR, Hertzberg BS: Ultrasound assessment of the fetal middle cerebral artery peak systolic velocity: a comparison of the near-field versus far-field vessel. Am J Obstet Gynecol 189:986, 2003.
70. Swartz AE, Ruma MS, Kim E, et al: The effect of fetal heart rate on the peak systolic velocity of the fetal middle cerebral artery. Obstet Gynecol 113:1225, 2009.
71. Trevett TN Jr, Dorman K, Lamvu G, Moise KJ Jr: Antenatal maternal administration of phenobarbital for the prevention of exchange transfusion in neonates with hemolytic disease of the fetus and newborn. Am J Obstet Gynecol 192:478, 2005.
72. Nicolini U, Santolaya J, Ojo OE, et al: The fetal intrahepatic umbilical vein as an alternative to cord needling for prenatal diagnosis and therapy. Prenat Diagn 8:665, 1988.
73. Moise KJ Jr, Carpenter RJ Jr, Kirshon B, et al: Comparison of four types of intrauterine transfusion: effect on fetal hematocrit. Fetal Ther 4:126, 1989.
74. Daffos F, Forestier F, Mac Aleese J, et al: Fetal curarization for prenatal magnetic resonance imaging. Prenat Diagn 8:312, 1988.
75. Giannina G, Moise KJ Jr, Dorman K: A simple method to estimate the volume for fetal intravascular transfusion. Fetal Diagn Ther 13:94, 1998.
76. Scheier M, Hernandez-Andrade E, Fonseca EB, Nicolaides KH: Prediction of severe fetal anemia in red blood cell alloimmunization after previous intrauterine transfusions. Am J Obstet Gynecol 195:1550, 2006.
77. Moise KJ Jr, Mari G, Fisher DJ, et al: Acute fetal hemodynamic alterations after intrauterine transfusion for treatment of severe red blood cell alloimmunization. Am J Obstet Gynecol 163:776, 1990.
78. Radunovic N, Lockwood CJ, Alvarez M, et al: The severely anemic and hydropic isoimmune fetus: changes in fetal hematocrit associated with intrauterine death. Obstet Gynecol 79:390, 1992.
79. van Kamp IL, Klumper FJ, Oepkes D, et al: Complications of intrauterine intravascular transfusion for fetal anemia due to maternal red-cell alloimmunization. Am J Obstet Gynecol 192:171, 2005.
80. Schumacher B, Moise KJ Jr: Fetal transfusion for red blood cell alloimmunization in pregnancy. Obstet Gynecol 88:137, 1996.
81. van Kamp IL, Klumper FJ, Bakkum RS, et al: The severity of immune fetal hydrops is predictive of fetal outcome after intrauterine treatment. Am J Obstet Gynecol 185:668, 2001.
82. Klumper FJ, van Kamp IL, Vandenbussche FP, et al: Benefits and risks of fetal red-cell transfusion after 32 weeks gestation. Eur J Obstet Gynecol Reprod Biol 92:91, 2000.
83. Saade GR, Moise KJ, Belfort MA, et al: Fetal and neonatal hematologic parameters in red cell alloimmunization: predicting the need for late neonatal transfusions. Fetal Diagn Ther 8:161, 1993.
84. Hudon L, Moise KJ Jr, Hegemier SE, et al: Long-term neurodevelopmental outcome after intrauterine transfusion for the treatment of fetal hemolytic disease. Am J Obstet Gynecol 179:858, 1998.
85. Harper DC, Swingle HM, Weiner CP, et al: Long-term neurodevelopmental outcome and brain volume after treatment for hydrops fetalis by in utero intravascular transfusion. Am J Obstet Gynecol 195:192, 2006.
86. Moise KJ, Whitecar PW: Antenatal therapy for haemolytic disease of the fetus and newborn. In Hadley A, Soothill P: Alloimmune

Disorders in Pregnancy: Anaemia, Thrombocytopenia and Neutropenia in the Fetus and Newborn, 1st ed. Cambridge, UK, Cambridge University Press, 2002, p 173.

87. Ruma MS, Moise KJ Jr, Kim E, et al: Combined plasmapheresis and intravenous immune globulin for the treatment of severe maternal red cell alloimmunization. Am J Obstet Gynecol 196:138 e1, 2007.
88. Hall AM, Cairns LS, Altmann DM, et al: Immune responses and tolerance to the RhD blood group protein in HLA-transgenic mice. Blood 105:2175, 2005.
89. Nielsen LK, Green TH, Sandlie I, et al: In vitro assessment of recombinant, mutant immunoglobulin G anti-D devoid of hemolytic activity for treatment of ongoing hemolytic disease of the fetus and newborn. Transfusion 48:12, 2008.
90. Hackney DN, Knudtson EJ, Rossi KQ, et al: Management of pregnancies complicated by anti-c isoimmunization. Obstet Gynecol 103:24, 2004.
91. Spong CY, Porter AE, Queenan JT: Management of isoimmunization in the presence of multiple maternal antibodies. Am J Obstet Gynecol 185:481, 2001.
92. Joy SD, Rossi KQ, Krugh D, O'Shaughnessy RW: Management of pregnancies complicated by anti-E alloimmunization. Obstet Gynecol 105:24, 2005.
93. De Young-Owens A, Kennedy M, Rose RL, et al: Anti-M isoimmunization: management and outcome at the Ohio State University from 1969 to 1995. Obstet Gynecol 90:962, 1997.
94. Hughes L, Rossi K, Krugh D, O'Shaughnessy R: Management of pregnancies complicated by anti-Fya alloimmunization. Am J Obstet Gynecol 191:S164, 2004.
95. Daniels G: Blood group antibodies in haemolytic disease of the fetus and newborn. In Hadley A, Soothill P: Alloimmune Disorders in Pregnancy: Anaemia, Thrombocytopenia, and Neutropenia in the Fetus and Newborn. Cambridge, UK, Cambridge University Press, 2002, p 21.
96. Vaughan JI, Manning M, Warwick RM, et al: Inhibition of erythroid progenitor cells by anti-Kell antibodies in fetal alloimmune anemia [see comments]. N Engl J Med 338:798, 1998.
97. Finning K, Martin P, Summers J, Daniels G: Fetal genotyping for the K (Kell) and Rh C, c, and E blood groups on cell-free fetal DNA in maternal plasma. Transfusion 47:2126, 2007.
98. Bowman JM, Pollock JM, Manning FA, et al: Maternal Kell blood group alloimmunization. Obstet Gynecol 79:239, 1992.
99. van Dongen H, Klumper FJ, Sikkel E, et al: Non-invasive tests to predict fetal anemia in Kell-alloimmunized pregnancies. Ultrasound Obstet Gynecol 25:341, 2005.

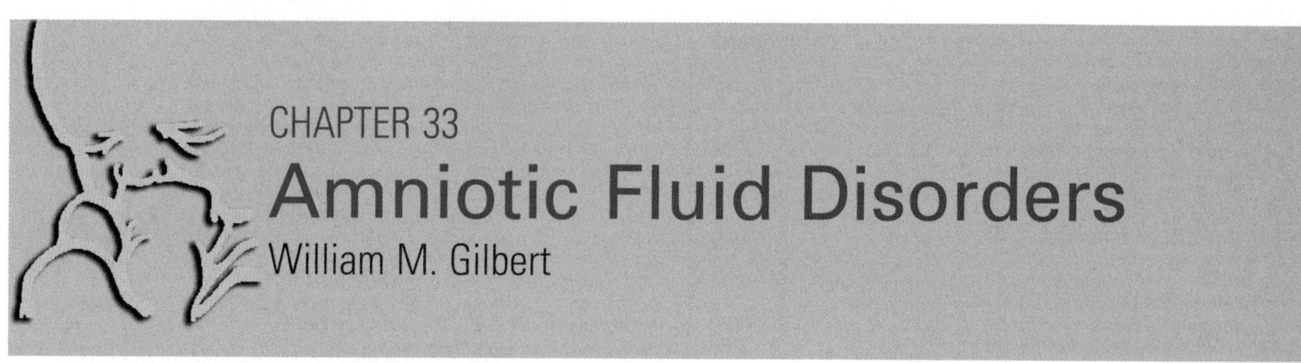

CHAPTER 33

Amniotic Fluid Disorders

William M. Gilbert

KEY ABBREVIATIONS	
Amniotic Fluid	AF
Amniotic Fluid Index	AFI
Amniotic Fluid Volume	AFV
Intrauterine Fetal Demise	IUFD
Intrauterine Growth Restriction	IUGR
Largest Vertical Pocket	LVP
Neonatal Intensive Care Unit	NICU
Perinatal Mortality Rate	PMR
Premature Rupture of the Membranes	PROM
Twin-to-twin Transfusion Syndrome	TTTS

Alterations in amniotic fluid volume (AFV) may be concerning for an underlying fetal or maternal complication during pregnancy, or fetal compromise. For example, with significant oligohydramnios in the second trimester, the perinatal mortality rate (PMR) approaches 90% to 100%.[1-3] Likewise, with marked polyhydramnios in midpregnancy, the PMR can exceed 50%.[4,5] Although these two extreme conditions are rare, other less drastic examples are more common and can affect pregnancy outcome. Efforts to study abnormalities of amniotic fluid (AF) are complicated by the fact that little is known about the processes involved in normal AFV regulation. Many of the disease states associated with the extremes of AFV are better understood than the normal physiologic state of AF.

This chapter explores what is known about the normal mechanisms affecting the formation and removal of AF, including fetal urination, swallowing, lung liquid, and intramembranous absorption.[6-8] The normal changes in AFV and composition across gestation are reviewed, as are abnormalities of AFV, including oligohydramnios and polyhydramnios, and the possible underlying causes and treatment modalities. The goal of this chapter is to offer the reader a complete understanding of normal and abnormal AFV regulation and the connection with disease states.

NORMAL AMNIOTIC FLUID VOLUME

As a result of obvious limitations, attempts to measure actual AFV are difficult. To measure the actual volume of AF, an inert dye must be injected into the amniotic cavity, and samples of AF are then obtained by amniocentesis to determine a dilution curve.[9-15] Although the dye injection technique is considered the gold standard for determining actual AFV and is compared with other methods of estimating AFV, such as ultrasound, it is impractical to use an invasive test to assess AFV in clinical practice and places the pregnancy at risk for loss and infection.

Despite these measurement limitations, Brace and Wolf identified all published measurements of AFV in 12 studies with 705 individual AFV measurements (Figure 33-1).[16] As shown in Figure 33-1, for each week of gestation, there can be wide variation in AFV. The largest variation occurs at 32 to 33 weeks of gestation; the normal range is 400 to 2100 mL (5th to 95th percentile). This represents a wide "normal range." **One of the most interesting findings of the Brace and Wolf study is that from 22 through 39 weeks' gestation, the average volume of AF (*black dots* on Figure 33-1) remained unchanged despite an increase in fetal weight from about 500 g to 3500 g, a seven-fold increase. This suggests that AFV is carefully regulated.** This concept of fluid regulation is discussed later.

ULTRASOUND MEASUREMENT OF AMNIOTIC FLUID VOLUME

Ultrasound has largely replaced the clinical assessment of AFV based on Leopold's maneuver or fundal height measurements; however, AF disorders may be suspected when the uterus measures too large or too small for gestational age. Polyhydramnios may be present if the maternal uterus is large for gestational age or if the fetus cannot be easily palpated or is ballotable. The diagnosis of oligohydramnios may be considered when the fundal height is small for gestational age or if the fetus can be easily palpated. Early ultrasound estimations of AFV were made by measuring

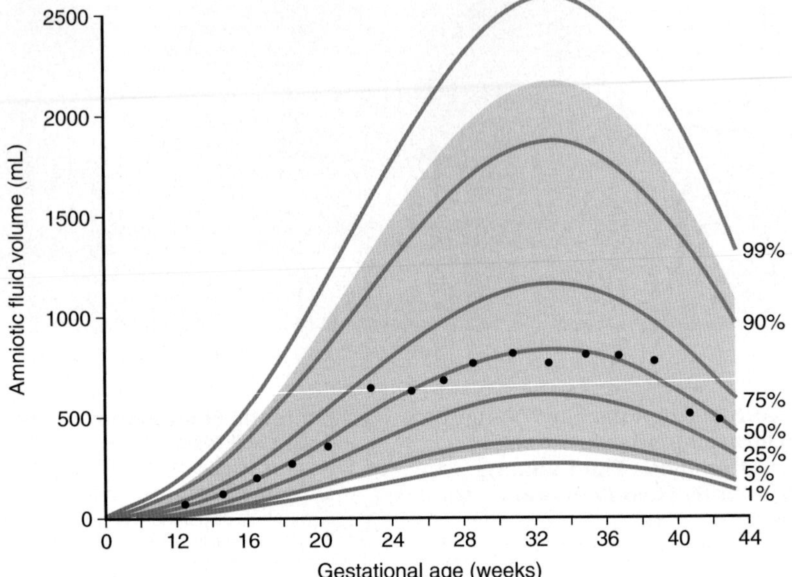

FIGURE 33-1. Nomogram showing amniotic fluid volume as a function of gestational age. The *black dots* are the mean for each 2-week interval. Percentiles calculated from polynomial regression equation and standard deviation of residuals. (From Brace RA, Wolf EJ: Normal amniotic fluid volume throughout pregnancy. Am J Obstet Gynecol 161:382, 1989.)

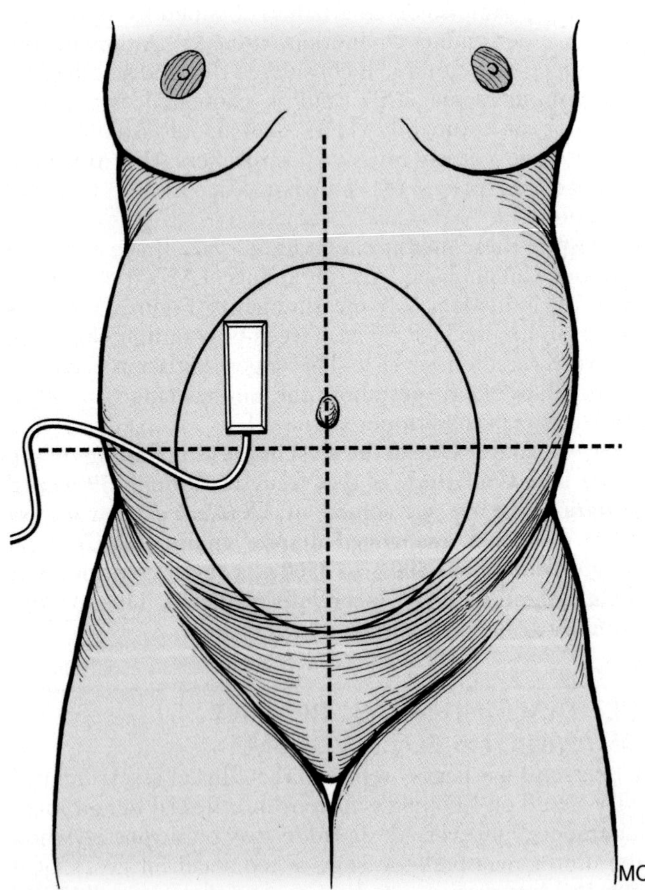

FIGURE 33-2. Schematic diagram of the technique for measuring the four-quadrant amniotic fluid index (AFI). (From Gilbert WM: Disorders of amniotic fluid. *In* Creasy RK, Resnik R [eds]: Maternal Fetal Medicine, 3rd ed. Philadelphia, WB Saunders, 1994, p 620.)

the largest vertical pocket (LVP) of AF.[17] Chamberlain and colleagues[18] and Mercer and associates[19] found that perinatal morbidity and mortality rates were increased with LVPs of less than 1 cm and 0.5 cm, respectively. These lower values of the LVP certainly identified at-risk fetuses, but the low sensitivity for identifying most pregnancy complications associated with oligohydramnios was unacceptable and prompted other investigators to select higher cut-off values.

Subsequently, Phelan and coworkers and others proposed a four-quadrant assessment of AF referred to as the *amniotic fluid index* (AFI).[20-22] After 20 weeks, the uterus is divided into four equal quadrants, as shown in Figure 33-2. The deepest clear pocket of AF is measured, making sure that the ultrasound transducer is perpendicular to the floor and that fetal body parts and umbilical cord do not interfere with the vertical measurement. The sum of the LVP in each quadrant is the AFI, shown in Figure 33-3.[22] **Moore and Cayle performed a cross-sectional study of 791 normal pregnancies; the 5th and 95th percentiles of the AFI varied for each gestational age.** For example, at the 95th percentile, the AFI at 35 to 36 weeks of gestation was 24.9 cm, whereas the AFI was 19.4 cm at 41 weeks of gestation. The variation in the AFI at the 5th percentile was less than that of the 95th percentile, but it still varied by as much as 2.5 cm. Finally, the investigators reported the interobserver and intraobserver variations to be 3.1% and 6.7%, respectively, which is acceptable for this commonly performed procedure.[22] Comparing the ultrasound estimation of the AFV by the AFI (see Figure 33-3) with the actual measured volume (see Figure 33-1) demonstrates very similar appearing curves.

Several authors have attempted to compare estimates of AFV by ultrasound (LVP and AFI) with actual measurement by the dye dilution technique, reporting that the AFI is a poor predictor of actual AFV.[9-25] Dildy and colleagues[23]

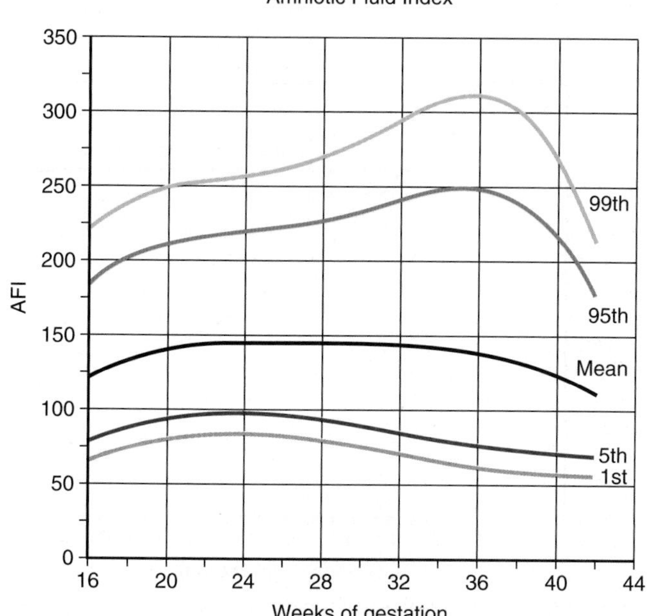

Figure 33-3. Amniotic fluid index (in millimeters) plotted with gestational age (weeks). The *solid line* denotes the 50th percentile; *dashed lines,* the 5th and 95th percentiles; and *dotted lines,* ±2 standard deviations (2.5th and 97.5th percentiles). (From Moore TR, Cayle JE: The amniotic fluid index in normal human pregnancy. Am J Obstet Gynecol 62:1168, 1990.)

found that the AFI overestimated the actual volume in 88% of cases at lower volumes and underestimated the actual volume in 54% of cases at higher volumes. The researchers concluded that the difference between actual volume and estimated volume based on the AFI should not change clinical practice.[23] Magann and coworkers have published several studies comparing the LVP, AFI, and dye dilution techniques in an effort to determine which test is superior for predicting actual AFV or perinatal morbidity and mortality.[9,11-15,24] **Consistently, they reported that both ultrasound methods (LVP and AFI) are poor predictors of actual AFV.** The sensitivity for an AFI measurement of less than 5 cm (oligohydramnios) was 10% (specificity, 96%), and the sensitivity was 5% (specificity, 98%) for LVPs up to 2 cm.[24] For cases of suspected polyhydramnios, an AFI greater than 20 cm had a sensitivity of 29% (specificity, 97%); LVPs greater than 8 cm had the same sensitivity of 29% (specificity, 94%). The LVP method had fewer false-positive results compared with the AFI.[24] More recently, the authors concluded that LVP is superior to the AFI.[25] In contrast, Moore[26] found that the AFI was superior to the LVP for identifying cases of oligohydramnios but found the two methods similar at predicting polyhydramnios.

Differences in ultrasound technique, specifically the pressure of the transducer on the maternal abdomen, can affect the accuracy of the AFI measurement. Flack and colleagues[27] reported that low pressure can result in a higher AFI (13%) compared with moderate pressure, or in a decrease in the AFI (21%) with high pressure on the maternal abdomen. Despite the fact that the actual measurement of AFV by Brace and Wolf[16] (see Figure 33-1) roughly superimposes on the graph of the normal AFI of Moore and Cayle[22] (see Figure 33-3), they will not necessarily correlate well with each other.

For many years, investigators have tried, with mixed success, to demonstrate the utility and applicability of ultrasound estimation of AFV in relation to perinatal outcome. Early work by Chamberlain and colleagues[18] showed that when the LVP was less than 1 cm, there was a marked increase in perinatal morbidity and mortality, which persisted even after correcting for birth defects. **Despite overwhelming evidence that current ultrasound methods are poor predictors of abnormal AFV, clinical practice continues to include the use of weekly or biweekly ultrasound estimates of AFV to assess fetal status.**

AMNIOTIC FLUID FORMATION

Fetal Urine

The main source of AF is fetal urination. In the human, the fetal kidneys begin to make urine before the end of the first trimester, and production of urine increases until term. Many different animal models have been used to study fetal urine production.[28-32] The fetal sheep provides an excellent model for comparative human study owing to its similar fetal weight at term, its sufficient size allowing catheter placement, and the fact that the sheep fetus has a low risk for premature labor after catheter placement. In the fetal sheep, urine production has been reported to be about 200 to 1200 mL/day in the last third of pregnancy.[28,32,33] Efforts to measure human fetal urine production have been accomplished by ultrasound measurement of the change in fetal bladder volume over time. Wladimiroff and Campbell[34] initially measured three dimensions of the fetal bladder every 15 minutes and reported a human fetal urine production rate of 230 mL/day at 36 weeks of gestation, which increased to 655 mL/day at term. Others found similar volumes using the same technique.[35-38] More recently, Rabinowitz and coworkers,[39] using the same technique as Wladimiroff and Campbell but measuring the change in volume every 2 to 5 minutes, found fetal urine production to be much greater than previously predicted, 1224 mL/day. Fetal urine production rates from several studies are shown in Figure 33-4.[34-39] **The human fetal urine production rate appears to be about 1000 to 1200 mL/day at term, suggesting that the entire AFV is replaced more frequently than every 24 hours.**

Lung Liquid

Fetal lung liquid plays an important role in AF formation. For years, it was presumed that there was actual movement of AF into the fetal lungs; however, recent data offer no support for this concept.[40,41] **In fact, throughout gestation, the fetal lungs produce fluid that exits the trachea and is either swallowed, or leaves the mouth, and enters the amniotic compartment.** In fetal sheep experiments, the lungs have been reported to produce volumes of up to 400 mL/day, with 50% being swallowed and 50% exiting through the mouth.[31,42-45] Although we do not have direct measurements in humans, the presence of surfactant in the AF near term provides evidence for the outward flow of lung liquid. During normal fetal life, fetal breathing movements provide a "to-and-fro" movement of AF into and

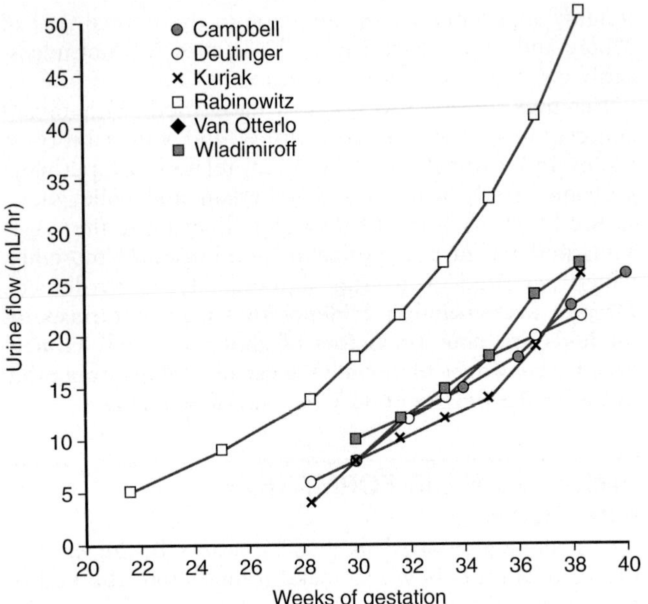

FIGURE 33-4. Normal changes in fetal urine flow rates across gestation. Lines represent mean values for six studies in the literature.[34-39] The individual first authors are shown in the figure itself. The highest line is data from Rabinowitz and colleagues and represents bladder volume measurements every 5 minutes instead of every 15 minutes, as is the case for the other five studies. (From Gilbert WM, Brace RA: Amniotic fluid volume and normal flows to and from the amniotic cavity. Semin Perinatol 7:150, 1993.)

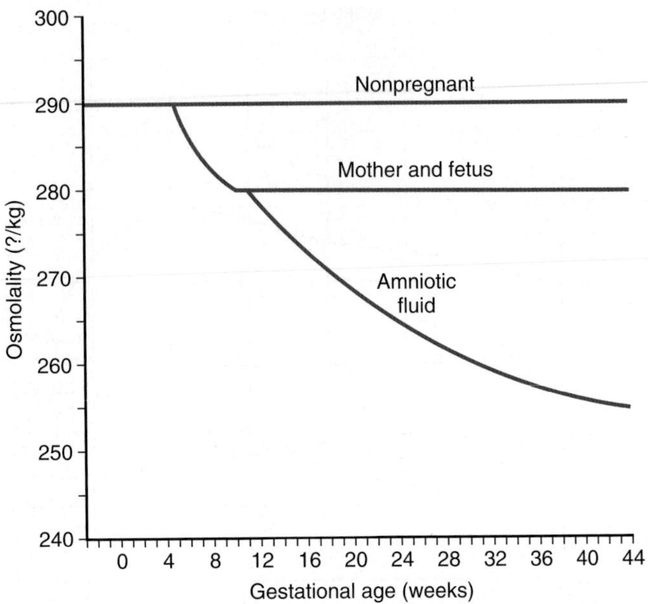

FIGURE 33-5. Change in maternal and fetal plasma and in amniotic fluid osmolality across gestation. (From Gilbert WM, Moore TR, Brace RA: Amniotic fluid volume dynamics. Fetal Med Rev 3:89, 1991.)

out of the trachea, upper lungs, and mouth.[46] Although AF may move back and forth, there is a net outward movement of fetal lung liquid into the AF.

AMNIOTIC FLUID REMOVAL

Fetal Swallowing

In the human, fetal swallowing begins early in gestation and contributes to the removal of AF. In the fetal sheep, swallowing has mostly been measured in the latter half of pregnancy and appears to increase with increasing gestational age. Sherman and associates[47] have reported that the ovine fetus swallows in episodes lasting 2 minutes and at volumes of 100 to 300 mL/kg per day. In the term ovine fetus, that volume represents a daily swallowing rate of 350 to 1000 mL/day for a 3.5-kg fetus. This is obviously more than the adult sheep, which drinks 40 to 60 mL/kg daily.[47]

Many different techniques have been used to determine swallowing rates in the animal model, including repetitive sampling of injected dye and actual flow probe measurements.[28,47] For obvious reasons, actual measurement of human fetal swallowing is much more difficult. Human fetal swallowing was studied by injecting radioactive chromium-labeled erythrocytes and Hypaque into the amniotic compartment, and swallowing rates of 72 to 262 mL/kg per day were found in early studies by Pritchard and others in the 1960s.[40,48] Abramovich[49] injected colloidal gold into the human amniotic compartment and found that fetal swallowing increased with advancing gestational age. He also found similar swallowing rates to those reported by Pritchard.[48] Obviously, similar studies could not be performed today, but the information is helpful in our understanding of human fetal swallowing. **Fetal swallowing could not remove the entire volume of fluid entering the amniotic compartment from fetal urine production and lung liquid, and therefore, other mechanisms for AF removal must occur.**

Intramembranous Absorption

One major stumbling block to the understanding of AFV regulation was the discrepancy between fetal urine and lung liquid production and its removal by swallowing. If the measurements and estimates of AF production and removal were accurate, there would be at least 500 to 750 mL/day excess fluid entering the amniotic compartment, which would result in acute polyhydramnios. This does not occur under normal conditions (see Figure 33-1), clearly demonstrating the presence of other mechanisms that remove AF in order to maintain a normal volume. A second route for AF removal has been suggested, namely the intramembranous pathway.[6-8,50,51] This process describes the movement of water and solutes between the amniotic compartment and the fetal blood, which circulates through the fetal surface of the placenta. The large osmotic gradient (Figure 33-5) between AF and fetal blood provides a substantial driving force for the movement of AF into the fetal blood. Intramembranous absorption has been described in detail in the fetal sheep and also was demonstrated to be present in the rhesus monkey fetus.[6-8,50,51] Several anecdotal studies suggest that intramembranous absorption also occurs in humans. In separate publications, Heller[52] and Renaud and associates[53] each injected labeled amino acids into the amniotic compartments of women, who were shortly thereafter delivered by cesarean section. Both groups found high levels of the amino acids concentrated in the placenta within 45 minutes of injection. They concluded that the amino acids had to be absorbed by some route other than swallowing to explain the rapid

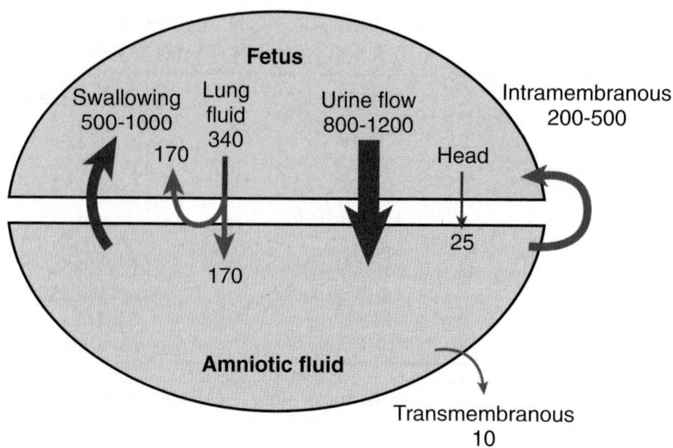

FIGURE 33-6. All known pathways for fluid and solute entry and exit from the amniotic fluid in the fetus near term. Arrow size is relative to associated flow rate. The *solid red arrows* represent directly measured flows, whereas the *blue arrows* represent estimated flows. The numbers represent volume flow in milliliters per day. The curved portion of the *double arrow* represents lung fluid that is directly swallowed after leaving the trachea, whereas the straight portion represents lung fluid that enters the amniotic cavity from the mouth and nose. (From Gilbert WM, Moore TR, Brace RA: Amniotic fluid volume dynamics. Fetal Med Rev 3:89, 1991.)

absorption into the fetal circulation within the placenta. Intramembranous absorption could easily explain this movement. **This route of absorption is now being actively investigated, and researchers have noted that 200 to 500 mL/day leaves the amniotic compartment under normal physiologic conditions.**[6,7,54] In addition, it has been reported that absorption through the intramembranous pathway can increase almost 10-fold under experimental conditions in sheep.[55] Figure 33-6 summarizes all currently identified avenues for fluid entry and exit from the amniotic compartment and measured or estimated volumes. The flow of fluid into and out of the amniotic cavity appears to be in a state of balance. Recent work on the mechanisms associated with intramembranous absorption should help clarify this final chapter in our understanding of the normal physiology associated with AFV regulation.

OLIGOHYDRAMNIOS

The incidence of oligohydramnios varies; depending on which definition is used, reported rates vary between 1% and 3%.[56] The incidence of oligohydramnios is much higher (19% to 20%) among women undergoing antepartum testing primarily because of an underlying maternal or fetal indication.[25] Three studies reported actual measured AFV with somewhat different values for oligohydramnios: Brace and Wolf, less than 318 mL; Magann and colleagues, less than 500 mL; and Horsager and associates, less than 200 mL.[9,10,16] With the advent of ultrasound estimation of AFV, multiple thresholds have been reported.[3,17,57-59] Chamberlain and colleagues[18] reported a 50-fold increase in PMR for pregnancies with an LVP of less than 1 cm. This report was instrumental in raising concern about the risk for stillbirth and neonatal mortality in the presence of oligohydramnios. A second, less-often reported finding of that study was that 40% of the cases with oligohydramnios also had other confounding factors, such as intrauterine growth restriction (IUGR), maternal hypertensive disorders, and congenital malformations.[18] **Oligohydramnios in the presence of IUGR, or preeclampsia, has markedly worse perinatal outcomes.** Other investigators have reported that oligohydramnios in the prolonged pregnancy has an increased risk for meconium staining of the AF, fetal distress in labor, and low 1-minute Apgar scores.[56] A common incidental clinical finding is the existence of a low AFI in an otherwise normal pregnancy. Because the diagnosis of oligohydramnios has been associated with poor perinatal outcomes, many women who are at or near term are sent to labor and delivery to be considered for induction, solely because of the low AFI. Frequently, their cervical examination is unfavorable for induction, and despite this, an induction is attempted. This can often result in a cesarean delivery for failed induction. **Although the evidence for induction in the prolonged pregnancy is solid, the term or preterm patient with isolated oligohydramnios may not need immediate delivery.**

Lagrew and coworkers[60] reported that 41% of women with oligohydramnios, as determined by the AFI, had a normal AFI 3 to 4 days later. They also found that a normal AFI measurement was valid for 1 week, suggesting that the test need not be repeated more often, except in certain high-risk situations. Other studies have evaluated perinatal outcomes in women with isolated oligohydramnios compared with normal AFV. Magann and colleagues[25] examined 1001 high-risk women undergoing antepartum testing. They found that those with an AFI of less than 5 cm (19% of cases) had similar outcomes to those with normal AFIs and concluded that an AFI less than 5 cm was not an indication for delivery.[25] Rainford and associates[61] examined 232 women at greater than 37 weeks of gestation who had an AFI less than 5 cm (19%). They found outcomes to be no worse compared with those with a normal AFI. In fact, the risk for meconium staining of the AF was found to be increased (35% versus 16%) in the normal group.[61] Finally, Casey and colleagues,[56] examining 6423 women at greater than 34 weeks' gestation with an AFI less than 5 cm, found an increase in intrauterine fetal death (IUFD), admissions to the neonatal intensive care unit (NICU), neonatal death, low birthweight, and meconium aspiration syndrome compared with women with an AFI greater than 5 cm. If the birth defects and IUGR were removed, there was no difference in admissions to the NICU, neonatal death, or respiratory distress syndrome. This suggests that the IUGR and birth defects contributed to the increased morbidity and mortality, not the oligohydramnios itself.

It has been clearly established that when the AFV is greatly decreased, especially in midpregnancy, the PMR approaches 100%.[1-3] The cause of the decrease or absence of AF largely determines the perinatal outcome (Table 33-1). With renal agenesis, virtually 100% of newborns die as a result of pulmonary hypoplasia. AF is required for fetal lung development during certain periods of early and midgestation, and without it, the lungs do not develop. If premature rupture of the membranes (PROM) results in a loss of all AF, neonatal survival will vary based on the gestational age when the membranes ruptured and on

TABLE 33-1 FETAL AND MATERNAL CAUSES OF OLIGOHYDRAMNIOS

Fetal Conditions
Renal agenesis
Obstructed uropathy
Spontaneous rupture of the membranes (SROM)
Premature rupture of the membranes (PROM)
Abnormal placentation—elevated MSAFP/MSHCG
Prolonged pregnancy
Severe IUGR
Maternal Conditions
Dehydration-hypovolemia
Hypertensive disorders
Uteroplacental insufficiency
Antiphospholipid syndrome
Idiopathic

MSAFP, Maternal serum α-fetoprotein; *MSHCG,* maternal serum human chorionic gonadotropin.

TABLE 33-2 CHANGE IN AMNIOTIC FLUID INDEX 4 TO 6 HOURS AFTER ORAL WATER HYDRATION

	CONTROL (*N* = 20)	HYDRATION (*N* = 20)
Pretreatment		
AFI (cm)	17.7 ± 5.0	18.4 ± 4.7
USG	1.013 ± 0.007	1.015 ± 0.008
Posttreatment		
AFI (cm)	16.2 ± 4.5*	21.4 ± 4.5†
USG	1.019 ± 0.009†	1.006 ± 0.006†
Delta AFI (cm)	−1.5 ± 2.7	3.0 ± 2.4
Intake (mL)‡	1576 ± 607	1596 ± 465

From Kilpatrick SJ, Safford KL: Maternal hydration increases amniotic fluid index in women with normal amniotic fluid. Obstet Gynecol 81:50, 1993.
*$P < .02$, paired t test, pretreatment vs. posttreatment.
†$P < .0001$, paired t test, pretreatment vs. posttreatment.
‡Intake, amount of fluid intake over the previous 24 hours other than the 2 L.
AFI, Amniotic fluid index; *delta AFI,* change in AFI from pretreatment to posttreatment; *USG,* urine specific gravity.

whether intra-amniotic infection was the cause of the membrane rupture.[62] Oligohydramnios can occur with hypertensive disorders or the antiphospholipid syndrome. In these cases, if the fetus is large enough for survival outside of the uterus, there may be little impact on perinatal outcome other than the consequences of prematurity.[62]

Evaluation and Treatment of Oligohydramnios

When the diagnosis of oligohydramnios is made in the second trimester, it is vitally important to obtain a complete history and physical examination from the patient and to perform a targeted ultrasound to help identify a cause (see Table 33-1). The patient should be questioned for any history consistent with rupture of the membranes, leakage of bloody fluid, or wetness of her underwear. If there is a question of possible rupture of the membranes, a sterile speculum examination should be performed in an attempt to obtain fluid that can be examined for evidence of rupture. Specific tests include examining for microscopic ferning, checking for a neutral pH on Nitrazine paper, and looking for pooling in the posterior vagina. The sodium chloride concentration of the AF is sufficient to cause ferning, whereas vaginal secretions usually do not fern. Determining the pH of the vaginal fluid can identify the neutral pH of AF as different from the acidic pH of normal vaginal secretions. Next, a targeted ultrasound should be performed to assess the amount of AF present, the presence of normal anatomy, including fetal kidneys and bladder, and finally, appropriate interval growth. If the fetus is normally grown with kidneys and bladder visualized, more often than not, the fetal membranes have been prematurely ruptured. If kidneys and bladder cannot be seen, then the diagnosis is most likely renal agenesis. Renal agenesis is uniformly fatal, whereas PROM can have a reasonable prognosis if it occurs after fetal viability and if infection is not present.

Although severe oligohydramnios has an increased PMR later in the third trimester, it is still not as high as earlier in pregnancy.[3,56,63] Other studies have reported similar increases in perinatal mortality associated with oligohydramnios, but most have not corrected for other underlying medical conditions.[17]

Because of the increase in perinatal morbidity and mortality associated with oligohydramnios in the prolonged pregnancy, most authors recommend delivery in these cases. As discussed earlier, however, the patient who presents with isolated oligohydramnios in the third trimester may be a candidate for continued observation.[25,56,61] Several investigators have attempted to treat oligohydramnios with the oral administration of water in the hope of "hydrating" the fetus through the mother. Animal studies have demonstrated that there is a close relationship between the hydration or dehydration of the mother and the fetus.[64,65] Attempts to dehydrate the mother have resulted in dehydration of the fetus and, in some cases, vice versa. In human pregnancies, Goodlin and colleagues[66] found that the maternal intravascular volume was low in cases of idiopathic oligohydramnios and that by increasing the intravascular volume, the oligohydramnios resolved. In a randomized study of the use of oral hydration as a treatment for women with a low AFI, Kilpatrick and coworkers[67] found that the treatment group that drank 2 L of water within 4 hours of a repeat AFI measurement had a significantly greater increase in AFI on repeat testing (6.3 cm) than the control group (5.1 cm).[67] They concluded that the oral administration of water could increase the AFI in women with oligohydramnios.[67] A follow-up study by the same group demonstrated that women with normal AFV could increase or decrease their AFI depending on the amount of water the mothers drank.[68] As illustrated in Table 33-2, the AFI significantly increased in the oral hydration group compared with the control group. The control group was given what was thought to be a "normal" volume of water to drink, but the AFI actually decreased and urine osmolality increased. This suggests that the mothers were dehydrated during the control portion of the study. **Both groups demonstrated that the AFI can be influenced by increasing or decreasing water intake orally.**

Many other studies have shown a similar improvement in AFV with either oral or intravenous administration of water or crystalloids, or both.[69,70] Several researchers have reported success in improving AFV in women with oligohydramnios by the injection of a crystalloid solution into the amniotic compartment during an amniocentesis.[71] The injection of fluid also allows for a more complete ultrasound examination of the fetus, which previously was not available owing to the lack of AF. Most of these studies, however, have been case reports, and because no large prospective studies have been performed, the routine use of amniocentesis for cases of severe oligohydramnios in midgestation cannot be justified by the literature.

Oligohydramnios in Labor

Almost 30 years ago, Gabbe and associates,[72] working with fetal monkeys, noted that when AF was removed from the amniotic compartment, variable decelerations in the fetal heart rate developed. These decelerations resolved when the AF was replaced, suggesting that cord compression was the cause of the decelerations. Since that time, multiple investigators have studied amnioinfusion as a technique by which to treat variable decelerations in labor. Although most report a decrease in the frequency of variable decelerations, few have demonstrated any decrease in perinatal morbidity or mortality, or the cesarean delivery rate.[73-76] Amnioinfusion has been studied as a possible therapy in the case of thick meconium. In several small prospective studies, it has been shown to improve neonatal outcomes, including meconium visualized below the newborn vocal cords and meconium aspiration syndrome.[77-80] Sadovsky and associates[81] found that with the randomization of women with greater than light meconium to a control or amnioinfusion treatment group, 29% of control newborns had meconium below the umbilical cords, whereas none of the treated newborns did. Two meta-analyses of the therapeutic use of amnioinfusion for thick meconium demonstrated between a 75% and 84% reduction in meconium below the vocal cords at delivery.[82,83] A more recent, multicenter, randomized trial of 1998 women in labor at 36 weeks' gestation or later with thick meconium did not find that amnioinfusion reduced the risk for moderate or severe meconium aspiration syndrome or perinatal death.[84] **Based on this large multicenter trial the American Congress of Obstetricians and Gynecologists (ACOG) recommends against routine prophylactic amnioinfusion for the dilution of meconium-stained amniotic fluid (ACOG Committee Opinion, Number 346, October 2006).**

POLYHYDRAMNIOS

The incidence of polyhydramnios has been reported to be about 1% in large population-based studies.[85-88] The earlier in gestation polyhydramnios occurs and the greater the amount of fluid, the higher the perinatal morbidity and mortality.[4] Ultrasound assessment of the LVP or AFI is used to confirm the diagnosis of polyhydramnios.

Most authors report an LVP of greater than 8 cm to define polyhydramnios.[87] Hill and colleagues divided their patients with polyhydramnios into three groups: mild (LVP 8 to 11 cm, 79% of cases), moderate (LVP 12 to 15 cm, 16.5% cases), and severe (LVP ≥16 cm, 5% of cases). Overall, the PMR was 127.5 per 1000, which corrected to 58.8 per 1000 when lethal malformations were excluded.[87] This value is markedly increased over the background rate. A specific cause was identified in only 16% of the mild cases of polyhydramnios, 90% for moderate polyhydramnios, and 100% for severe polyhydramnios.[87] Fetal and maternal conditions associated with polyhydramnios are shown in Table 33-3. In a follow-up study, Many and associates[89] examined 275 women with polyhydramnios to determine if the degree of polyhydramnios had an impact on the rate of prematurity. Although excessive amniotic fluid did not have an impact on the rate of prematurity, the presence of anomalies or diabetes mellitus was associated with an increased risk for preterm delivery.[89] Severe polyhydramnios in the second trimester has a significant PMR, which is most commonly due to prematurity or aneuploidy.[90,91] Pregnancy complications associated with polyhydramnios have been reported to increase the risk for placental abruption and postpartum hemorrhage due to overdistention (or rapid deflation) of the uterus.

TABLE 33-3 FETAL AND MATERNAL CAUSES OF POLYHYDRAMNIOS

Fetal Conditions
Congenital anomalies
Gastrointestinal obstruction
Central nervous system abnormalities
Cystic hygromas
Nonimmune hydrops
Sacrococcygeal teratoma
Cystic adenoid malformations of lung
Aneuploidy, genetic syndromes
Achondrogenesis type 1-B
Twin-to-twin transfusion syndrome
Muscular dystrophy syndromes
Infections—parvovirus B-19
Bartter syndrome
Placental abnormalities—chorioangioma
Maternal Conditions
Idiopathic
Poorly controlled diabetes mellitus
Fetal maternal hemorrhage

Using the four-quadrant AFI, Moore and Cayle[22] reported the AFI for varying gestational ages (see Figure 33-3) and concluded that one value for the AFI cannot be used throughout gestation but must be referenced to gestational age. The study found the 97.5 percentile at 35 weeks of gestation to be 27.9 cm, which represents the upper limits of normal for that gestational age. This value would clearly be abnormally increased for earlier and later measurements in gestation (see Figure 33-3).

Evaluation and Treatment of Polyhydramnios

The pregnant woman who presents with a rapidly enlarging uterus in midpregnancy, with or without preterm labor, needs to be evaluated by ultrasound examination to assess the AFV and look for a congenital malformation. Esophageal atresia with or without tracheoesophageal fistula can present with early-onset severe polyhydramnios due to an obstruction. The AFV may still be normal with some forms of tracheoesophageal fistula that allow for the movement of fluid into the stomach.[92] Other gastrointestinal obstructions, such as duodenal atresia, may result in polyhydramnios.[87] When a structural defect is seen in a fetus with polyhydramnios, consideration should be given to performing an amniocentesis (see Chapter 11).

Another common cause of acute, severe polyhydramnios in the second trimester is the condition associated with the twin-to-twin transfusion syndrome (TTTS) (see Chapter 30). The ultrasound findings associated with TTTS are marked polyhydramnios of the receiving twin and absent AFV or marked oligohydramnios of the donor twin.

When polyhydramnios occurs in the third trimester of pregnancy, it is usually mild and not associated with a structural defect.[87] Table 33-3 lists many of the causes of polyhydramnios. Although most cases in the third trimester are idiopathic, the other causes of polyhydramnios must be excluded.

In many cases, polyhydramnios may be transient. Golan and colleagues[88] examined 113 cases of polyhydramnios. On repeated examination, patients separated into two groups: cases in which the polyhydramnios worsened or the AFV remained markedly elevated, and those in which the AFV returned to normal or decreased to mild polyhydramnios. In the former group, all complications of pregnancy were greater, including preterm delivery (2.7-fold increase), preeclampsia (2.7-fold increase), IUFD (7.7-fold increase), and neonatal demise (7.7-fold increase). In the latter group, the most common diagnosis was idiopathic and showed a favorable outcome.[88] **This study suggests that if polyhydramnios is persistent, the fetus should be examined closely for congenital malformations and aneuploidy and monitored to prevent an IUFD.** In addition, the mother should be watched closely for other medical complications of pregnancy.[88]

Treatment options for patients with polyhydramnios are usually tailored to the underlying cause. With mild idiopathic polyhydramnios, in which the workup is negative and follow-up ultrasound demonstrates persistent polyhydramnios, the only possible intervention is antepartum testing with fetal kick counts, or nonstress tests. When poorly controlled diabetes mellitus is the cause of the polyhydramnios, proper glycemic control may be beneficial,[93,94] and antepartum surveillance is recommended. With the current aggressive management of diabetes in pregnancy, it is rare to see severe polyhydramnios associated with diabetes. Treatment options for TTTS are discussed in Chapter 30.

With severe polyhydramnios associated with preterm labor, one medical treatment option involves the administration of a prostaglandin inhibitor such as indomethacin, which works by decreasing fetal urine production.[95-97] This effect occurs within 5 hours of starting the medication and decreases the AFV within 24 hours.[95,96] Although indomethacin has been shown to be relatively safe when given over a short period, such as 72 hours, prolonged use may be associated with risks to the fetus such as premature closure, or narrowing, of the ductus venosus within the fetal heart and renal abnormalities in the newborn period.[96,97] Complications related to indomethacin use worsen with advancing gestational age, and such treatment beyond 31 to 32 weeks of gestation should be avoided.[98] Because of the adverse effects on the fetus associated with the long-term use of indomethacin, it probably has limited use in pregnancy for the treatment of severe polyhydramnios. The use of repetitive amino reductions, in which amniocentesis is performed and large volumes (1 to 5 L) of AF are removed through plastic tubing into a vacuum bottle, does prolong pregnancies in a number of cases but may need to be repeated on a regular basis.[5,98]

KEY POINTS

- ◆ Amniotic fluid is seldom considered important until polyhydramnios or oligohydramnios occurs, either of which may significantly impact perinatal survival.
- ◆ Amniotic fluid is dynamic, with large-volume flows into and out of the amniotic compartment each day.
- ◆ Clinical estimates of actual amniotic fluid volume through ultrasound measurements of the AFI or LVP are not very accurate at predicting true volume.
- ◆ Oligohydramnios, in the presence of IUGR or a prolonged gestation, is associated with significant increases in perinatal morbidity and mortality.
- ◆ Preterm or term isolated oligohydramnios, with an otherwise normal fetus, is not associated with an increase in perinatal morbidity or mortality.
- ◆ Early-onset or severe polyhydramnios is associated with a significant increase in aneuploidy, congenital malformations, preterm delivery, and perinatal mortality.
- ◆ The cause of mild polyhydramnios, especially in the latter part of the third trimester, is usually idiopathic, or related to diabetes mellitus, and has little positive or negative impact on perinatal survival.
- ◆ AFV, as estimated by the AFI, can be increased or decreased by the amount of water ingested orally.
- ◆ Short-term use of indomethacin decreases fetal urine production and can reduce AFV within 24 hours of administration.
- ◆ Absorption of amniotic fluid directly from the amniotic compartment into the blood vessels on the fetal surface of the placenta can explain the large differences between fetal swallowing and urine production.

REFERENCES

1. Hackett GA, Nicolaides KH, Campbell S: The value of Doppler ultrasound assessment of fetal and uteroplacental circulations when severe oligohydramnios complicates the second trimester of pregnancy. BJOG 94:1074, 1987.
2. Barss VA, Benacerraf BR, Frigoletto FD: Second trimester oligohydramnios, a predictor of poor fetal outcome. Obstet Gynecol 64:608, 1984.
3. Mercer LJ, Brown LG: Fetal outcome with oligohydramnios in the second trimester. Obstet Gynecol 67:840, 1986.
4. Wier PE, Raten G, Beisher N: Acute polyhydramnios: a complication of monozygous twin pregnancy. BJOG 86:849, 1979.
5. Reisner DP, Mahony BS, Petty CN, et al: Stuck twin syndrome: outcome in thirty-seven consecutive cases. Am J Obstet Gynecol 169:991, 1993.
6. Gilbert WM, Brace RA: The missing link in amniotic fluid volume regulation: intramembranous absorption. Obstet Gynecol 74:748, 1989.
7. Gilbert WM, Brace RA: Novel determination of filtration coefficient of ovine placenta and intramembranous pathway. Am J Physiol 259:R1281, 1990.

8. Gilbert WM, Cheung CY, Brace RA: Rapid intramembranous absorption into the fetal circulation of arginine vasopressin injected intraamniotically. Am J Obstet Gynecol 164:1013, 1991.
9. Magann EF, Nolan TE, Hess LW, et al: Measurement of amniotic fluid volume: accuracy of ultrasonography techniques. Am J Obstet Gynecol 167:1533, 1992.
10. Horsager R, Nathan L, Leveno KJ: Correlation of measured amniotic fluid volume and sonographic predictions of oligohydramnios. Obstet Gynecol 83:955, 1994.
11. Magann EF, Bass JD, Chauhan SP, et al: Amniotic fluid volume in normal singleton pregnancies. Obstet Gynecol 90:524, 1997.
12. Magann EF, Doherty DA, Field K, et al: Biophysical profile with amniotic fluid volume assessments. Obstet Gynecol 104:5, 2004. Comment in: Obstet Gynecol 104:3, 2004.
13. Magann EF, Doherty DA, Chauhan SP, et al: Dye-determined amniotic fluid volume and intrapartum/neonatal outcome. J Perinatol 24:423, 2004.
14. Magann EF, Doherty DA, Chauhan SP, et al: How well do the amniotic fluid index and single deepest pocket indices (below the 3rd and 5th and above the 95th and 97th percentiles) predict oligohydramnios and hydramnios? Am J Obstet Gynecol 190:164, 2004.
15. Magann EF, Doherty DA, Chauhan SP, et al: Is there a relationship to dye determined or ultrasound estimated amniotic fluid volume adjusted percentiles and fetal weight adjusted percentiles? Am J Obstet Gynecol 190:1610, 2004.
16. Brace RA, Wolf EJ: Characterization of normal gestational changes amniotic fluid volume. Am J Obstet Gynecol 161:382, 1989.
17. Manning FA, Hill LM, Platt LD: Qualitative amniotic fluid volume determination by ultrasound: antepartum detection of intrauterine growth retardation. Am J Obstet Gynecol 139:254, 1981.
18. Chamberlain PF, Manning FA, Morrison I, et al: Ultrasound evaluation of amniotic fluid volume. I: The relationship of marginal and decreased amniotic fluid volumes to perinatal outcome. Am J Obstet Gynecol 150:245, 1984.
19. Mercer LJ, Brown LG, Petres RE, et al: A survey of pregnancies complicated by decreased amniotic fluid. Am J Obstet Gynecol 149:355, 1984.
20. Phelan JP, Ohn MO, Smith CV, et al: Amniotic fluid index measurements during pregnancy. J Reprod Med 32:603, 1987.
21. Rutherford SE, Phelan JP, Smith CV, et al: The four quadrant assessment of amniotic fluid volume: an adjunct to antepartum fetal heart rate testing. Obstet Gynecol 70:353, 1987.
22. Moore TR, Cayle JE: The amniotic fluid index in normal human pregnancy. Am J Obstet Gynecol 162:1168, 1990.
23. Dildy GA III, Lira N, Moise KJ, et al: Amniotic fluid volume assessment: comparison of ultrasonographic estimates versus direct measurements with a dye-dilution technique in human pregnancies. Am J Obstet Gynecol 167:986, 1992.
24. Magann EF, Chauhan SP, Barrilleaux PS, et al: Amniotic fluid index and single deepest pocket: weak indicators of abnormal amniotic volumes. Obstet Gynecol 96:737, 2000.
25. Magann EF, Chauhan SP, Doherty DA, et al: The evidence for abandoning the amniotic fluid index in favor of the single deepest pocket. Am J Perinatol 24:549-555, 2007.
26. Moore TR: Superiority of the four-quadrant sum over the single-deepest-pocket technique in ultrasonographic identification of abnormal amniotic fluid volumes. Am J Obstet Gynecol 163:762, 1990.
27. Flack NJ, Dore C, Southwell D, et al: The influence of operator transducer pressure on ultrasonographic measurements of amniotic fluid volume. Am J Obstet Gynecol 171:218, 1994.
28. Tomoda S, Brace RA, Longo L: Amniotic fluid volume and fetal swallowing rate in sheep. Am J Physiol 249:R133, 1985.
29. Alexander DP, Nixon DA, Widdas WF, et al: Gestational variations in the composition in the foetal fluids and foetal urine in the sheep. J Physiol 140:1, 1958
30. Mellor DJ, Slater JS: Daily changes in foetal urine and relationships with amniotic and allantoic fluid and maternal plasma during the last two months of pregnancy in conscious, unstressed ewes with chronically implanted catheters. J Physiol 227:503, 1972
31. Adamson TM, Brodecky V, Lambert TF, et al: The production and composition of lung liquids in the in-utero foetal lamb. In Comline RS, Cross KW, Dawes GS, Nathaniel PW: Foetal and Neonatal Physiology. Cambridge, UK, Cambridge University Press, 1973, p 208.
32. Gresham EL, Rankin JHG, Makowski EL, et al: An evaluation of fetal renal function in a chronic sheep preparation. J Clin Invest 51:149, 1972.
33. Wintour EM, Barnes A, Brown EH, et al: Regulation of amniotic fluid volume and composition on the ovine fetus. Obstet Gynecol 52:689, 1978.
34. Wladimiroff JW, Campbell S: Fetal urine-production rates in normal and complicated pregnancy. Lancet 1:151, 1974.
35. Campbell S, Wladimiroff JW, Dewhurst CJ: The antenatal measurement of fetal urine production. J Obstet Gynaecol Br Commonw 80:680, 1973.
36. Van Otterlo LC, Wladimiroff JW, Wallenburg HCS: Relationship between fetal urine production and amniotic fluid volume in normal pregnancy and pregnancy complicated by diabetes. BJOG 84:205, 1977.
37. Kurjak A, Kirkinsen P, Latin V, et al: Ultrasonic assessment of fetal kidney function in normal and complicated pregnancies. Am J Obstet Gynecol 141:266, 1981.
38. Deutinger J, Bartl W, Pfersmann C, et al: Fetal kidney volume and urine production in cases of fetal growth retardation. J Perinat Med 15:307, 1987.
39. Rabinowitz R, Peters MT, Vyas S, et al: Measurement of fetal urine production in normal pregnancy by real-time ultrasonography. Am J Obstet Gynecol 161:1264, 1989.
40. Duenhoelter JH, Pritchard JA: Fetal respiration: quantitative measurements of amniotic fluid inspired near term by human and rhesus fetuses. Am J Obstet Gynecol 125:306, 1976.
41. Seeds AE: Current concepts of amniotic fluid dynamics. Am J Obstet Gynecol 138:575, 1980.
42. Mescher EJ, Platzker A, Ballard PL, et al: Ontogeny of tracheal fluid, pulmonary surfactant, and plasma corticoids in the fetal lamb. J Appl Physiol 39:1017, 1975.
43. Olver RE, Strang LB: Ion fluxes across the pulmonary epithelium and the secretion of lung liquid in the foetal lamb. J Physiol 241:327, 1974.
44. Lawson EE, Brown ER, Torday JS, et al: The effect of epinephrine on tracheal fluid flow and surfactant efflux in fetal sheep. Am Rev Respir Dis 118:1023, 1978.
45. Brace RA, Wlodek ME, Cook ML, et al: Swallowing of lung liquid and amniotic fluid by the ovine fetus under normoxic and hypoxic conditions. Am J Obstet Gynecol 171:764, 1994.
46. Patrick J, Campbell K, Carmichael L, et al: Patterns of human fetal breathing at 30-31 and 38-39 weeks' gestational age. Obstet Gynecol 56:24, 1980.
47. Sherman DJ, Ross MG, Day L, et al: Fetal swallowing: correlation of electromyography and esophageal fluid flow. Am J Physiol 258:R1386, 1990.
48. Prichard JA: Deglutition by normal and anencephalic fetuses. Obstet Gynecol 25:289, 1965.
49. Abramovich DR: Fetal factors influencing the volume and composition of liquor amnii. J Obstet Gynaecol Britt Commw 77:865, 1970.
50. Gilbert WM, Moore TR, Brace RA: Amniotic fluid volume dynamics. Fetal Med Rev 3:89, 1991.
51. Gilbert WM, Eby-Wilkens EM, Tarantal AF: The missing-link in Rhesus monkey amniotic fluid volume regulation: intramembranous absorption. Obstet Gynecol 892:462, 1997.
52. Heller L: Intrauterine amino acid feeding of the fetus. In Bode H, Warshaw J: Parenteral Nutrition in Infancy and Childhood. New York, Plenum, 1974, p 206.
53. Renaud R, Kirschtetter L, Koehl D, et al: Amino-acid intraamniotic injections. In Persianinov LS, Chervakova TV, Presl J: Recent Progress in Obstetrics and Gynaecology. Amsterdam, Excerpta Medica, 1974, p 234.
54. Jang PR, Brace RA: Amniotic fluid composition changes during urine drainage and tracheoesophageal occlusion in fetal sheep. Am J Obstet Gynecol 167:1732, 1992.
55. Faber JJ, Anderson DF: Absorption of amniotic fluid by amniochorion in sheep. Am J Physiol 282:H850, 2002.
56. Casey BM, McIntire DD, Bloom SL, et al: Pregnancy outcomes after antepartum diagnosis of oligohydramnios at or beyond 34 weeks' gestation. Am J Obstet Gynecol 182:909, 2000.
57. Manning FA, Harmon CR, Morrison I, et al: Fetal assessment based on fetal biophysical profile scoring. IV. An analysis of perinatal morbidity and mortality. Am J Obstet Gynecol 162:703, 1990.

58. Halperin ME, Fong KW, Zalev AH, et al: Reliability of amniotic fluid volume estimation from ultrasonograms: intraobserver and interobserver variation before and after the establishment of criteria. Am J Obstet Gynecol 153:264, 1985.
59. Crowley P, O'Herlihy C, Boylan P: The value of ultrasound measurement of amniotic fluid volume in the management of prolonged pregnancies. BJOG 91:444, 1984.
60. Lagrew DC, Pircon RA, Nageotte M, et al: How frequently should the amniotic fluid index be repeated? Am J Obstet Gynecol 167:1129, 1992.
61. Rainford M, Adair R, Scialli AR, et al: Amniotic fluid index in the uncomplicated term pregnancy: prediction of outcome. J Reprod Med 46:589, 2001.
62. Hill MH: Oligohydramnios: sonographic diagnosis and clinical implications. Clin Obstet Gynecol 40:314, 1997.
63. Jeng CJ, Lee JF, Wang KG, et al: Decreased amniotic fluid index in term pregnancy: clinical significance. J Reprod Med 37:789, 1992.
64. Ross MG, Ervin MG, Leake RD, et al: Bulk flow of amniotic fluid water in response to maternal osmotic challenge. Am J Obstet Gynecol 147:697, 1983.
65. Woods LL: Fetal renal contribution to amniotic fluid osmolality during maternal hypertonicity. Am J Physiol 250:R235, 1986.
66. Goodlin RC, Anderson JC, Gallagher TF: Relationship between amniotic fluid volume and maternal plasma volume expansion. Am J Obstet Gynecol 146:505, 1983.
67. Kilpatrick SJ, Safford K, Pomeroy T, et al: Maternal hydration affects amniotic fluid index (AFI). Am J Obstet Gynecol 164:361, 1991.
68. Kilpatrick SJ, Safford KL: Maternal hydration increases amniotic fluid index in women with normal amniotic fluid volumes. Obstet Gynecol 81:49,1993.
69. Flack NJ, Sepulveda W, Bower S, et al: Acute maternal hydration in third-trimester oligohydramnios: effects on amniotic fluid volume, uteroplacental perfusion, and fetal blood flow and urine output. Am J Obstet Gynecol 173:1186, 1996.
70. Doi S, Osada H, Seki K, et al: Effect of maternal hydration on oligohydramnios: a comparison of three volume expansion methods. Obstet Gynecol 92:525, 1998.
71. Sepulveda W, Flack NJ, Fisk NM: Direct volume measurement at midtrimester amnioinfusion in relation to ultrasonographic indexes of amniotic fluid volume. Am J Obstet Gynecol 170:1160, 1994.
72. Gabbe SG, Ettinger BB, Freeman RK, et al: Umbilical cord compression associated with amniotomy: laboratory observations. Am J Obstet Gynecol 126:353, 1976.
73. Nageotte MP, Bertucci L, Towers CV, et al: Prophylactic amnioinfusion in pregnancies complicated by oligohydramnios: a prospective study. Obstet Gynecol 77:677, 1991.
74. Ogundipe OA, Spong CY, Ross MG: Prophylactic amnioinfusion for oligohydramnios: a reevaluation. Obstet Gynecol 84:544, 1994.
75. Schrimmer DB, Macri CJ, Paul RH: Prophylactic amnioinfusion as a treatment for oligohydramnios I laboring patients: a prospective randomized trial. Am J Obstet Gynecol 165:972, 1991.
76. Miyazaki FS, Taylor NA: Saline amnioinfusion for relief of variable or prolonged decelerations. Am J Obstet Gynecol 146:670, 1983.
77. Chanhan SP, Rutherford SE, Hess LW, et al: Prophylactic intrapartum amnioinfusion for patients with oligohydramnios. J Reprod Med 37:817, 1992.
78. Wenstrom KD, Parsons MT: The prevention of meconium aspiration in labor using amnioinfusion. Obstet Gynecol 73:647, 1989.
79. Eriksen NL, Hostetter M, Parisi VM: Prophylactic amnioinfusion in pregnancies complicated by thick meconium. Am J Obstet Gynecol 171:1026, 1994.
80. Macri CJ, Schrimmer DB, Leung A, et al: Prophylactic amnioinfusion improves outcome of pregnancy complicated by thick meconium and oligohydramnios. Am J Obstet Gynecol 167:117, 1992.
81. Sadovsky Y, Amon E, Bade ME, et al: Prophylactic amnioinfusion during labor complicated by meconium: a preliminary report. Am J Obstet Gynecol 161:613, 1989.
82. Pierce J, Gaudier FL, Sanchez-Ramos L: Intrapartum amnioinfusion for meconium-stained fluid: meta-analysis of prospective trials. Obstet Gynecol 95:1051, 2000.
83. Glantz JC, Letteney DL: Pumps and warmers during amnioinfusion: is either necessary? Obstet Gynecol 87:150, 1996.
84. Fraser WD, Hofmeyr J, Lede R, et al: Amnioinfusion for the prevention of the meconium aspiration syndrome. N Engl J Med 353:909, 2005.
85. Chamberlain PF, Manning FA, Morrison I, et al: Ultrasound evaluation of amniotic fluid. Vol. II: the relationship of increased amniotic fluid volume to perinatal outcome. Am J Obstet Gynecol 150:250, 1984.
86. Biggio JR Jr, Wenstrom KD, Dubard MB, et al: Hydramnios prediction of adverse perinatal outcome. Obstet Gynecol 94:773, 1999.
87. Hill LM, Breckle R, Thomas ML, et al: Polyhydramnios: ultrasonically detected prevalence and neonatal outcome. Obstet Gynecol 69:21, 1987.
88. Golan A, Wolman I, Sagi J, et al: Persistence of polyhydramnios during pregnancy: its significance and correlation with maternal and fetal complications. Gynecol Obstet Invest 37:18, 1994.
89. Many A, Hill LM, Lazebnik N, et al: The association between polyhydramnios and preterm delivery. Obstet Gynecol 86:389, 1995.
90. Pauer HU, Viereck V, Krauss V, et al: Incidence of fetal malformations in pregnancies complicated by oligo- and polyhydramnios. Arch Gynecol Obstet 268:52, 2003.
91. Desmedt EJ, Henry OA, Beischer NA: Polyhydramnios and associated maternal and fetal complications in singleton pregnancies. BJOG 97:1115, 1990.
92. Lloyd JR, Clatworthy HW: Hydramnios as aid to the early diagnosis of congenital obstruction of the alimentary tract: a study of the maternal and fetal factors. Pediatrics June:903, 1958.
93. Bartha JL, Martinez-Del-Fresno P, Comino-Delgado R: Early diagnosis of gestational diabetes mellitus and prevention of diabetes-related complications. Eur J Obstet Gynecol Reprod Biol 109:41, 2003.
94. Thomas A, Kaur S, Somville T: Abnormal glucose screening test followed by normal glucose tolerance test and pregnancy outcome. Saudi Med J 23:814, 2002.
95. Stevenson KM, Lumbers ER: Effects of indomethacin on fetal renal function, renal and umbilicoplacental blood flow and lung liquid production. J Dev Physiol 17:257, 1992.
96. Kirshon B, Moise KJ, Wasserstrum N, et al: Influence of short-term indomethacin therapy on fetal urine output. Obstet Gynecol 72:51, 1988.
97. Mamopoulos M, Assimakopoulos E, Reece EA, et al: Maternal indomethacin therapy in the treatment of polyhydramnios. Am J Obstet Gynecol 162:1225, 1990.
98. Moise KJ: Polyhydramnios. Clin Obstet Gynecol 40:266, 1997.

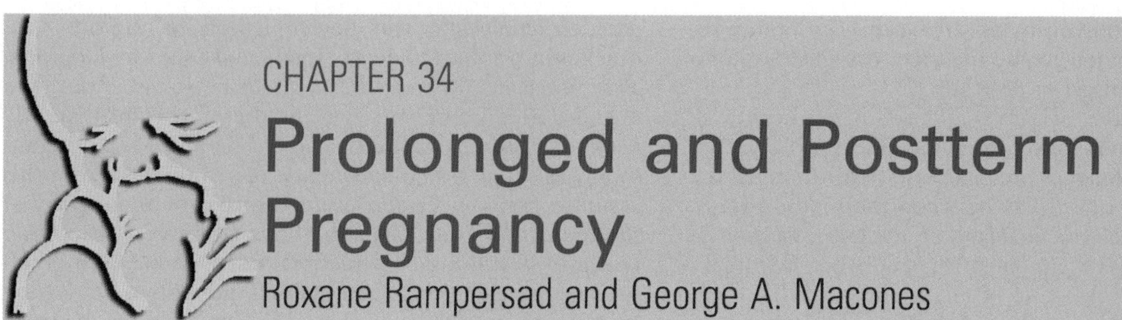

CHAPTER 34

Prolonged and Postterm Pregnancy

Roxane Rampersad and George A. Macones

KEY ABBREVIATIONS	
American College of Obstetricians and Gynecologists	ACOG
Amniotic Fluid Index	AFI
Confidence Interval	CI
Estimated Date of Delivery	EDD
Last Menstrual Period	LMP
Odds Ratio	OR
Perinatal Mortality Rate	PMR
Randomized Controlled Trial	RCT
Relative Risk	RR
World Health Organization	WHO

Obstetricians have long recognized that there can be detrimental effects of preterm delivery, but for the last century there has also been concern for pregnancies that have gone beyond the normal period of gestation. Early descriptions from prolonged pregnancies described a large fetus, resulting in a difficult delivery, with an increased risk of stillbirth.[1] Later descriptions suggested that a postterm fetus not only could be large, but also small for gestational age.[2] These concerns led some to adopt a practice of inducing labor to avoid complications in prolonged pregnancies. This practice was variable, and somewhat controversial, because the upper limit of pregnancy was not well defined and the risks were inconsistent. More recent studies show a small but significantly increased risk in perinatal morbidity and mortality in postterm pregnancies, and hence, postterm pregnancy is one of the most common reasons for induction of labor in the United States.

DEFINITION

The American College of Obstetricians and Gynecologists (ACOG) and the World Health Organization (WHO) have defined a postterm pregnancy as a gestation that has completed or gone beyond 42 weeks or 294 days from the first day of the last menstrual period (LMP).[3-5] This gestational age cut-off has been used for several decades and was first suggested based on early studies that reported an increased risk of fetal death at 42 weeks and beyond.[6] However, in view of more recent perinatal mortality data that were derived from accurately dated pregnancies, it would be reasonable to conclude that the gestational age that warrants clinical concern should be 41 weeks.

There are many terms that have been used in the literature, including postmature, postdates, prolonged, and postterm. These terms have been used with varying definitions, which has led to some confusion regarding proper terminology. For the purposes of this chapter, we use the term *postterm* to describe a pregnancy than has gone beyond 42 weeks' gestation, and the term *prolonged* for a pregnancy between 41 and 42 weeks.

INCIDENCE

According to the vital statistics reported by the Centers for Disease Control and Prevention, the overall incidence of postterm pregnancies was 6% in 2006, compared to 7% in the previous year.[7] Other published studies have shown rates between 2% and 13% depending on the population studied.[8] The incidence of prolonged pregnancies in European countries also varies widely, with rates as low as 0.6% in Austria and as high as 7% in Denmark and Sweden.[9] These differences are most likely explained by (1) different approaches for managing pregnancies beyond the estimated date of delivery (EDD) and (2) different criteria for gestational age dating.

ETIOLOGY

The etiology of the majority of pregnancies that are prolonged or postterm is unknown, but some pregnancies may be defined as prolonged or postterm as the result of an error in dating. It is common practice to assign an EDD based on the date of the last menstrual period (LMP). This practice has been proven by several studies to be unreliable and may have led to the incorrect classification of a pregnancy as prolonged or postterm.[10]

Understanding the events that lead to parturition in human gestation may help to provide clues to the pathophysiology in prolonged pregnancies. Parturition is the result of a complex interplay between the mother, fetus, and placenta.[11] The mechanism in human gestation is unknown but may be similar to that of other mammals. In sheep, the hypothalamic pituitary adrenal (HPA) axis is important in the timing of birth. The release of corticotrophin-releasing hormone from the fetal brain results in the secretion of adrenocorticotropic hormone from the pituitary gland and cortisol from the adrenal gland.[12] The increase in cortisol parallels an increase in the secretion of prostaglandin and estrogens and a fall in progesterone.[12] Decreases in progesterone and prostaglandins are known triggers uterine myometrium. Further support for the role of the HPA axis in the initiation of labor is seen in studies with hypophysectomized sheep; disruption of the HPA axis results in prolonged pregnancy.[13] More recent studies have proposed a similar involvement of the HPA axis in human gestation, and its dysregulation may play a role in prolonged pregnancies.

Early studies likened anencephaly to the hypophysectomized sheep. It is hypothesized that the absence of the fetal brain in the anencephalic fetus may result in a similar dysfunction of the HPA axis and lead to prolonged gestation. Epidemiologic studies of anencephalic pregnancies have observed prolongation of pregnancy.[14] This finding supports current thinking that the interaction between the fetal brain and placenta plays an important role in triggering labor.

Pregnancies complicated by placental sulfatase deficiency, an X-linked recessive disorder characterized by the absence of the enzyme steroid sulfatase, are marked by abnormally low estriol levels and, in general, fail to go into spontaneous labor.[15] This is an example of a genetic etiology for prolonged pregnancy and lends further support to the important role of the placenta in the initiation of labor.

A number of observational studies have identified risk factors for postterm pregnancy including primigravidity, prior postterm pregnancy, male fetus, obesity, and a genetic predisposition.[16-22] A 10-year cohort study of births in Norway failed to find a strong association of risk factors with postterm pregnancy but may have had a bias toward nondetection.[16] Intergenerational studies suggest a genetic predisposition for postterm pregnancy. Mothers who themselves were prolonged also have an increased risk of prolonged pregnancy. Twin studies have found higher rates of concordance for prolonged pregnancy among female twins as compared to male twins, implicating a maternal influence on the risk for prolonged pregnancy.[22]

DIAGNOSIS

The diagnosis of truly prolonged and postterm pregnancy is based on accurate gestational dating. The three most commonly used methods to determine the EDD are (1) knowledge of the date of the LMP, (2) timing of intercourse, and (3) early ultrasound assessment. Other methods have been described but are rarely used in contemporary practice, including the determination of uterine size, quickening, ability to detect fetal heart tones by Doptone, and fundal height measurement. In most cases, the date of conception is rarely known and therefore is infrequently used to determine gestational age. The EDD is most commonly assigned based on the first day of the LMP but this assumes that conception occurs on the fourteenth day of the menstrual cycle. This method can be very inaccurate because the timing of ovulation varies among an individual's menstrual cycles and between individuals.[23,24] Basing gestational age solely on the LMP generally results in an overestimation of gestational age, and may result in higher frequency of induction of labor for presumed postterm pregnancy.

The use of ultrasound to determine the accuracy of gestational dating based on the LMP is superior to the use of LMP alone. The EDD is most accurately determined if the crown rump length is measured in the first trimester with an error of plus or minus 5 to 7 days. Boyd and colleagues showed that the incidence of patients whose pregnancy exceeded 293 days was 7.5% based on menstrual dating and declined to 2.6% when dates were determined by early sonographic examination.[25] A similar conclusion was reached by Gardosi and colleagues, who evaluated 24,675 spontaneous, normal singleton deliveries and showed a decline in the postterm (>294 days) pregnancy rate from 7.5% when pregnancies were dated by LMP to 1.5% when ultrasound dating was used.[26] These authors also reported that about 72% of routine labor inductions at 42 weeks' gestation were not indicated because they were performed before the patients reached 42 weeks based on ultrasound assessment of gestational age. Similarly, Nguyen and colleagues evaluated 14,805 spontaneous deliveries with a reliable LMP and showed that ultrasound dating reduced the proportion of deliveries beyond 294 days of gestation by 39% (from 7.9% to 5.2%).[27] Bennett and colleagues confirmed these findings in a prospective, randomized study of 218 women and found fewer postterm inductions of labor in women dated by a first trimester sonogram when compared with women whose dates were established by second trimester sonography.[28]

PERINATAL MORBIDITY AND MORTALITY

Numerous studies have evaluated the risk to the fetus in prolonged and postterm pregnancies. Early descriptive studies found that pregnancies that continued past their EDD had an increased risk of fetal death. In 1963 McClure found a twofold increase in "fetal distress" at 42 weeks with an increase in operative deliveries and surmised that 42 weeks constituted a significant risk to the fetus, and proposed intervening with induction of labor or cesarean section to avoid the risk of fetal death.[6] Early studies were likely fraught with inaccurate dating and inconsistent definitions of postterm pregnancy. Lastly, it is important to note that these studies included pregnancies complicated by fetal anomalies, intrauterine growth restriction, and mothers with coexisting medical conditions, all of which increase the risk of fetal demise.

More recent observational studies that have evaluated the risk of perinatal mortality at each gestational week show

an increased risk as gestational age advances beyond the EDD.[29-31] Divon and colleagues evaluated fetal and neonatal mortality rates in 181,524 accurately dated term and prolonged pregnancies. A significant increase in fetal mortality was detected from 41 weeks' gestation onward (odds ratio [OR] of 1.5, 1.8, and 2.9 at 41, 42, and 43 weeks, respectively).[32] Campbell and colleagues performed a multivariate analysis of factors associated with perinatal death among 65,796 singleton postterm births (≥294 days).[16] Three variables were identified as independent predictors of perinatal mortality: (1) birthweight lower than the 10th percentile for gestational age had a relative risk (RR) of 5.7 and 95% confidence interval (CI), 4.4 to 7.4; (2) maternal age 35 years or greater had a RR of 1.88 and 95% CI, 1.2 to 2.9; (3) birthweight at the 90th percentile for gestational age or above was associated with a modest protective effect for perinatal death (RR of 0.51 with 95% CI, 0.26 to 1.0).

Many of these studies have used perinatal mortality rate, which has been suggested by Smith and others to be an inappropriate assessment of risk to the fetus.[33] The denominator in the calculation of the perinatal mortality rate is the number of deliveries.[33-36] As stated by Smith, "estimating the probability of an event requires that the number of events (numerator) be divided by the number of subjects at risk for that event (denominator)."[33] Therefore, it seems logical to calculate fetal mortality as fetal deaths per 1000 ongoing pregnancies (rather than per 1000 deliveries). When Hilder and colleagues used ongoing pregnancies in a large retrospective study that included 171,527 births, they found higher rates of stillbirth.[34] There was a nadir at 41 weeks but an eightfold increase in stillbirth at 43 weeks compared to 37 weeks' gestation (Figure 34-1).

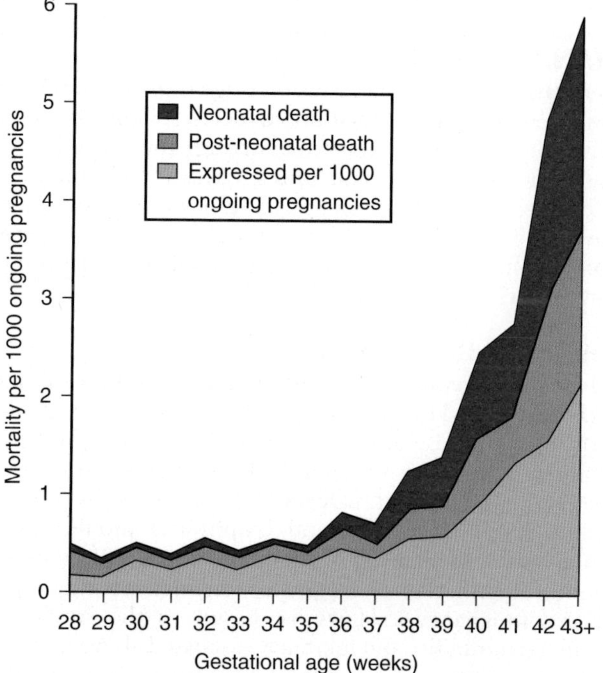

FIGURE 34-1. The summed mortality at each gestation for the rate of stillbirth (red), neonatal death (blue), and post-neonatal death (green) expressed per 1000 ongoing pregnancies. (Modified from Hilder L, Costeloe K, Thilaganathan B: Prolonged pregnancy: evaluating gestation specific risks of fetal and infant mortality. BJOG 105:169, 1998.)

Using the Scottish birth registry, Smith also found a significant increase in the risk of stillbirth from 37 weeks (0.4/1000) to 43 weeks (11.5/1000).

Several studies evaluated the association of perinatal morbidity with prolonged pregnancy. **Clausson and colleagues evaluated a large Swedish database of term and postterm (defined as ≥294 days) singleton, normal neonates, and showed that prolonged pregnancies were associated with an increased frequency of neonatal convulsions, meconium aspiration syndrome, and Apgar scores of less than 4 at 5 minutes (Table 34-1).**[37] Tunon and colleagues compared neonatal intensive care unit (NICU) admission rates among 10,048 term pregnancies and 246 prolonged pregnancies (≥296 days by both scan and LMP dates).[38] Prolonged pregnancy was associated with a significant increase in NICU admissions (OR of 2.05, 95% CI, 1.35 to 3.12).

Guidetti and colleagues reported an increased incidence of perinatal morbidity at 41 weeks' gestation or greater.[39] Maternal and fetal complications were evaluated in a large (n = 45,673) retrospective cohort study by Caughey and Musci.[40] These authors documented a significant increase in the rate of intrauterine fetal death beyond 41 weeks. They concluded that risks to both the mother and the infant increase as pregnancy progresses beyond 40 weeks' gestation.

Oligohydramnios

Oligohydramnios is a common finding in postterm pregnancies; it is presumably the result of fetal hypoxemia, which may result in altered renal perfusion and decreased urine production.[41] Doppler studies of renal blood flow are conflicting.[42,43] Thus, the etiology of oligohydramnios in postterm pregnancies is still debated.

Regardless of the pathophysiology of oligohydramnios in postterm pregnancies, there is an increased risk of perinatal morbidity and mortality in a setting of oligohydramnios.[44] The importance of oligohydramnios was identified by Leveno and colleagues, who used its presence to explain the increased incidence of abnormal antepartum

TABLE 34-1 NEONATAL MORBIDITY IN POSTTERM AGA AND SGA INFANTS

COMPLICATIONS	ODDS RATIOS AND 95% CI VERSUS TERM AGA NEONATES
Convulsions	
Term SGA	2.3 (1.6-3.4)
Postterm AGA	1.5 (1.2-2.0)
Postterm SGA	3.4 (1.5-7.6)
Meconium aspiration	
Term SGA	2.4 (1.6-3.4)
Postterm AGA	3.0 (2.6-3.7)
Postterm SGA	1.6 (0.5-5.0)
Apgar score <4 at 5 min	
Term SGA	2.2 (1.4-3.4)
Postterm AGA	2.0 (1.5-2.5)
Postterm SGA	3.6 (1.5-8.7)

Modified from Clausson B, Cnattinguis S, Axelsson O: Outcomes of post-term births: the role of fetal growth restriction and malformations. Obstet Gynecol 94:758, 1999. Copyright 1999 American College of Obstetricians and Gynecologists, with permission.

AGA, Appropriate for gestational age; *CI*, confidence interval; *SGA*, small for gestational age.

and intrapartum fetal heart rate (FHR) abnormalities seen in prolonged pregnancies.[45] These authors suggested that prolonged FHR decelerations representing cord compression preceded 75% of cesarean deliveries for fetal jeopardy. The association between a reduced amniotic fluid index (AFI) and variable decelerations is well documented, and likely related to cord compression.[46,47] Meconium passage in amniotic fluid has also been associated with oligohydramnios and it is postulated that the hypoxemia may result in rectal sphincter relaxation. Some studies have shown meconium-stained fluid as high as 29% in postterm pregnancies complicated by oligohydramnios.[48] See Chapter 33 for further discussion of oligohydramnios.

A prospective, blinded observational study of 1584 pregnancies was performed by Morris and colleagues to assess the usefulness of ultrasound assessment of amniotic fluid in the prediction of adverse outcome in prolonged pregnancies.[49] The authors demonstrated that an AFI of less than 5 cm but not a single deepest vertical pocket less than 2 cm was significantly associated with birth asphyxia or meconium aspiration. In addition, there was a significant association between an AFI less than 5 cm and fetal distress in labor, cord arterial pH less than 7.0, and low Apgar scores.

The presence of oligohydramnios is often cited as an indication for delivery of pregnancies that reach term gestation or beyond. Importantly, there are no large, prospective, randomized studies documenting the benefits of delivery in this setting. **Still, given the well-described association between oligohydramnios and adverse pregnancy outcome, at or beyond term delivery is a reasonable choice for patients with oligohydramnios.**

Fetal Growth

The risk of macrosomia has been shown to increase with advancing gestational age. Although the majority of prolonged pregnancies are appropriately grown, there is an increased risk for macrosomia. Mclean and colleagues found in a sample of 7000 pregnancies between 39 and 42 weeks that there was an increase in both fetal weight and head circumference.[50] Eden and colleagues found that, compared to term pregnancies, postterm pregnancies have a twofold increase in the risk for macrosomia.[51] Macrosomia in these pregnancies was associated with an increased risk of operative delivery and shoulder dystocia leading to fetal injury.

Chervenak and colleagues investigated the use of ultrasound to evaluate the estimated fetal weight in pregnancies that were greater than 41 weeks and also found an increased incidence of fetal weight greater than 4000 grams.[52] They also showed there was an increase in the risk of cesarean delivery (22%) because of protracted and arrested labors when compared to nonmacrosomic infants (10%; $P<.01$). The positive and negative predictive values were 70% and 87%, respectively. However, a similar study of pregnancies at 41 weeks or greater found an absolute error of approximately 8% and a positive predictive value of 64% when ultrasound was used to estimate fetal weight within 1 week of delivery.[53] The ACOG has warned that the diagnosis of fetal macrosomia by ultrasound is not precise and early induction of labor or cesarean delivery has not been shown to reduce the morbidity associated with fetal macrosomia.[54]

Postmaturity

Postmaturity, another complication of prolonged pregnancies, occurs in approximately 10% to 20% of such pregnancies.[55-57] The "postmature" infant has decreased subcutaneous fat and lacks lanugo and vernix. The features are similar to intrauterine growth restriction and some authors believe that postmaturity is really another manifestation of intrauterine growth restriction. Postmaturity is also associated with an increased incidence of meconium-stained fluid.

Meconium

Meconium-stained fluid can be seen at any gestational age, although several studies have documented a significant increased risk of meconium-stained fluid in postterm pregnancies. Meconium aspiration is a serious neonatal condition resulting in decreased lung compliance, abnormal production of surfactant, and a chemical pneumonitis.

MATERNAL COMPLICATIONS

Prolonged pregnancies are also associated with significant risk to the mother. Not only is there significant anxiety as the pregnancy advances beyond the EDD but also an increased risk of maternal morbidity during the intrapartum period. Caughey and Musci studied 119,254 women who delivered at 37 weeks and beyond and found an increased risk in significant perineal laceration (OR 1.19, 95% CI, 1.09 to 1.22), chorioamnionitis (OR 1.32, 95% CI, 1.21 to 1.44), endomyometritis (OR 1.46, 95% CI, 1.14 to 1.87), postpartum hemorrhage (OR 1.21, 95% CI, 1.10 to 1.32), and cesarean section (1.28, 95% CI, 1.20 to 1.36).[40] The indications for cesarean section in this study were nonreassuring FHR and cephalopelvic disproportion.

MANAGEMENT

Accurate assessment of gestational age is paramount in the management of prolonged pregnancies. When ultrasound is used to confirm menstrual dating, the incidence of postterm pregnancies and unnecessary interventions are decreased.[58] Because prolonged and postterm pregnancies have an increased risk of fetal mortality, modern management includes the use of antenatal fetal surveillance and carefully timed intervention.

Antenatal Surveillance

Given the increased risk of stillbirth, antenatal surveillance is recommended in the management of prolonged and postterm pregnancies. Testing options for fetal surveillance include monitoring of fetal kick counts, nonstress test (NST), contraction stress test (CST), modified biophysical profile (NST and AFI), and biophysical profile (BPP). There are few data with adequate power to assess the timing of initiation or frequency of fetal testing in prolonged pregnancies. However, based on the studies on perinatal morbidity and mortality discussed above, it would seem prudent to initiate fetal testing no later than 41 weeks of gestation. There are a number of small studies that suggest that twice weekly antepartum testing is superior to once a week in prolonged pregnancies. John and Harman reported results on twice weekly testing with BPP in 293 patients followed beyond 42 weeks. No stillbirths were observed in this small series.[59]

There are no large, randomized controlled trials comparing different modalities of fetal surveillance in prolonged pregnancies. One randomized controlled trial of 145 pregnancies beyond 42 weeks compared BPP with modified BPP.[60] This study found a significant increase in abnormal testing in the modified BPP group (42% vs. 20.5%, OR 3.5, 99% CI, 1.3 to 9.1), but no difference in cord blood gases and neonatal outcome between the two groups. Studies have not shown one modality of antepartum surveillance to be superior to another.[60]

ACOG proposed that amniotic fluid volume should be assessed when surveillance is initiated for prolonged pregnancies because oligohydramnios has been associated with abnormal fetal heart tracings, umbilical cord compression, and meconium-stained fluid. Chamberlain and colleagues studied 19,222 complicated pregnancies and found an increase in the risk of fetal demise with decreased amniotic fluid.[61]

There is a paucity of data demonstrating improved neonatal outcomes in postterm pregnancies when testing is used. Still, given the well-described increase in stillbirth in postterm pregnancies, ACOG currently recommends the initiation of fetal surveillance between 41 and 42 weeks with assessment of amniotic fluid volume.[3]

Umbilical artery Doppler measurements are sometimes used in cases of suspected placental insufficiency and hence one might imagine that this modality could be useful in postterm pregnancies. However, umbilical artery Doppler measurements have not been shown to be useful in the management of prolonged pregnancies.[62]

Expectant Management Versus Induction of Labor

Currently, ACOG does not define the gestational age at which expectant management is no longer recommended in prolonged pregnancies. Expectant management with fetal surveillance is typically advocated in pregnancies with an unfavorable cervix, whereas patients with a favorable cervix are induced presumably to decrease the risk of perinatal morbidity and mortality. There are several clinical trials that have compared induction of labor to expectant management in pregnancies that have progressed beyond their EDD. Hannah and colleagues performed one of the largest clinical trials; 3407 pregnant women were randomized at 41 weeks to induction or expectant management with fetal surveillance.[63] Delivery was indicated if the pregnancy reached 44 weeks or if there was evidence of fetal compromise. There was no difference in the perinatal mortality and neonatal morbidity, although there was an increased rate of cesarean deliveries in the expectantly managed group. There were no cases of fetal demise in the induction group and two in the expectantly managed group.

Another randomized controlled trial (RCT) of 440 uncomplicated pregnancies, performed by the National Institute of Child Health and Human Development Network of Maternal-Fetal Medicine Units, compared induction at 42 weeks versus expectant management until there was cervical effacement, dilation, or evidence of fetal compromise.[64] The primary outcome was perinatal or maternal death or a composite of variable for perinatal morbidity. Secondary outcomes for this trial included cesarean delivery, maternal infection, blood transfusion, severe variable or late deceleration, and 5-minute Apgar score less than 4. No differences were detected in primary outcome or rates of cesarean delivery. The study concluded that either induction or expectant management at 42 weeks was deemed acceptable practice.

More recently, Sanchez-Ramos published a meta-analysis that included 16 RCTs and 6588 patients, and found a 20% rate of cesarean delivery in uncomplicated pregnancies induced at 41 weeks compared to 22% in the expectantly managed group.[65] There was a nonsignificant but numerically lower perinatal mortality rate for the induction group (0.09% vs. 0.33%, OR 0.41, 95% CI, 0.14 to 1.18). They also found no differences in NICU admission and meconium aspiration.

The most recent Cochrane review, updated in 2011, is a meta-analysis of 19 RCTs.[66] The review included 7984 patients and looked at the potential benefits or harms of labor induction at or beyond 40 weeks' gestation versus expectant management. The primary outcome was perinatal mortality, which included intrauterine fetal demise and neonatal death in the first week of life. Labor induction was associated with a small but significant reduction in perinatal death (RR 0.30, 95% CI, 0.09 to 0.99), with no impact on the rate of cesarean delivery (RR 0.92, 95% CI, 0.76 to 1.12). This Cochrane meta-analysis suggests that induction may yield slightly improved perinatal outcomes, but based on the data, either approach seems reasonable.

Labor Induction

Induction of labor is discussed in Chapter 14. There are several studies that have addressed membrane sweeping as a method for labor induction in an attempt to reduce the occurrence of prolonged pregnancies. Membrane sweeping is the digital separation of the membranes from the lower uterine segment during a cervical examination. This practice is thought to increase the levels of endogenous prostaglandin, resulting in uterine contractions. A recent RCT by de Miranda and colleagues enrolled 742 patients at 41 weeks' gestation and randomized them to serial sweeping of membranes every 48 hours until 42 weeks or until labor was initiated, or to no intervention.[67] They found a decrease in the risk of postterm pregnancy in the first group; 23% were postterm (RR 0.57, 95% CI, 0.46 to 0.71) compared to 41% in the no-intervention group. The number needed to treat for this trial was six patients. Previously published trials have not shown a significant difference but these studies limited membrane sweeping to a single episode.[68,69] The most recent Cochrane review of trials that enrolled pregnant patients from 38 to 41 weeks to membrane sweeping found a reduced rate of pregnancies that continued past 41 weeks' gestation, with a number needed to treat of eight patients.[70] Although this practice may be effective in some pregnant patients, the procedure is known to cause maternal discomfort and bleeding. Thus, patients considering this option should be selected carefully and counseled appropriately.

Some have attempted to predict the likelihood of successful induction using transvaginal ultrasound of the cervix and fetal fibronectin. Pandis and colleagues compared Bishop score to ultrasound cervical assessment and found cervical length to be more predictive of a successful labor induction than Bishop score (with a sensitivity and specificity of 87% and 71%, versus 58% and 27%, respectively).[71] Although promising, the use of transvaginal ultrasound assessment of the cervix to predict induction success is not commonly used. Attempts to evaluate the role of a fetal fibronectin in cervical secretions as a predictor of the onset of spontaneous labor have been inconclusive. In fact, Rozenberg and colleagues have recently shown that the spontaneous onset of labor within 7 days of evaluation is predicted by a Bishop score greater than 7 and a cervical length less than 25 mm but not with a positive fetal fibronectin.[72]

Prostaglandins are most commonly used for labor induction in patients with an unfavorable cervix or a Bishop score that is less than 6. Studies have shown both dinoprostone (PGE1) and misoprostol (PGE2) to be efficacious in prolonged pregnancy, and either preparation is acceptable.[63,64,73]

LONG-TERM NEONATAL OUTCOMES

There is a paucity of information on neonates who are born at 42 weeks and later. Ting and colleagues evaluated a population enrolled in the Collaborative Perinatal Study in Philadelphia and found the surviving children could not be differentiated from their matched controls either physically or mentally.[74] Shime and colleagues, who followed children at 1 and 2 years of age, found similar results.[75] They assessed intelligence by the Griffiths Mental Development Scale and found no difference when these children were compared to term births. Based on these small and old studies there does not appear to be any difference in long-term neonatal outcome.

MULTIPLE GESTATION

There is no defined gestational age cut-off to define a prolonged pregnancy in twin, triplet, or higher order multiples. The average gestation lengths for twin, triplet, and quadruplet pregnancies are 36, 33, and 29 weeks, respectively. The nadir of stillbirth occurs at 38 weeks for twins, 35 week for triplets, and is unknown for quadruplets and higher order multiples.[76] Intuitively, because we use rates of perinatal mortality to define these cut-offs for singletons, we should do the same for multiple gestations. There are no current strategies recommended as these pregnancies approach the above gestational ages, though it would seem reasonable to: (1) utilize antenatal testing as these gestational ages approach and (2) accomplish delivery at the nadir of stillbirth risk.

KEY POINTS

- Establish the estimated delivery date (EDD) by use of first or second trimester ultrasound, if possible.
- There is no gestational cut-off to define a prolonged pregnancy in multiple gestations. The nadir of stillbirth risk occurs at 38 weeks for twins and 35 weeks for triplets.
- Prolonged pregnancies are associated with an increased risk for perinatal morbidity and mortality, oligohydramnios, macrosomia, postmaturity, and maternal morbidity.
- It seems prudent to initiate antenatal fetal surveillance at 41 weeks in a normal, uncomplicated pregnancy in the absence of intrauterine growth restriction.
- Antenatal fetal surveillance at 41 weeks should include a modified biophysical profile (BPP) at least once a week.
- If the cervix is favorable at 41 weeks, it may be prudent to recommend induction of labor.
- Delivery by 42 completed weeks is reasonable based on the small but increased risk of perinatal morbidity and mortality.
- Either prostaglandin preparation (PGE1 or PGE2) can be used for the induction of the postterm pregnancy.

REFERENCES

1. Ballantyne JW: The problem of the postmature infant. J Obstet Gynaecol Br Emp 2:521, 1902.
2. Clifford SH: Postmaturity with placental dysfunction, clinical syndrome and pathologic findings. J Pediatr 44:1, 1954.
3. American College of Obstetricians and Gynecologists Practice Bulletin: Management of postterm pregnancy, September 2004.
4. World Health Organization (WHO): Recommended definition terminology and format for statistical tables related to the perinatal period and rise of a new certification for cause of perinatal deaths. Modifications recommended by FIGO as amended, October 14, 1976. Acta Obstet Gynecol Scand 56:347, 1977.
5. Federation of Gynecology and Obstetrics (FIGO): Report of the FIGO Subcommittee on Perinatal Epidemiology and Health Statistics Following a Workshop in Cairo, November 11-18, 1984. London, International Federation of Gynecology and Obstetrics, 1986, p 54.
6. McClure-Brown JC: Postmaturity. JAMA 186(12):81, 1963.
7. Centers for Disease Control and Prevention. Available at: http://www.cdc.gov/nchs/datawh/vitalstats/VitalStatsbirths.htm. Accessed September 18, 2009.
8. Joseph KS, Huang L, Liu S, et al and Infant Health Study Group of the Canadian Perinatal Surveillance System: Reconciling the high rates of preterm and postterm birth in the United States. Obstet Gynecol 109(4):813, 2007.
9. Zeitlin J, Blondel B, Alexander S, Bréart G; PERISTAT Group: Variation in rates of postterm birth in Europe: reality or artefact? BJOG 114(9):1097, 2007.
10. Gardosi J: Dating of pregnancy: time to forget the last menstrual period. Ultrasound Obstet Gynecol 9:367, 1997.
11. Norwitz ER, Robinson JN, Challis JR: The control of labor. N Engl J Med 341:660, 1999.
12. Challis JR, et al: The fetal placental hypothalamic-pituitary-adrenal (HPA) axis, parturition and postnatal health. Mol Cell Endocrinol 185(1-2):135, 2001.
13. Nathanielsz, PW: Endocrine mechanisms of parturition. Annu Rev Physiol 40:411, 1978.
14. Naeye RL, Blanc WA: Organ and body growth in anencephaly: A quantitative, morphological study. Arch Pathol 91(2):140, 1971.
15. Rabe T, Hösch R, Runnebaum B: Sulfatase deficiency in the human placenta: clinical findings. Biol Res Pregnancy Perinatol 4(3):95, 1983
16. Campbell MK, Ostbye T, Irgens LM: Post-term birth: risk factors and outcomes in a 10-year cohort of Norwegian births. Obstet Gynecol 89:543, 1997.
17. Mogren I, Stenlund H, Hogberg U: Recurrence of prolonged pregnancy. Int J Epidemiol 28:253, 1999.

18. Olesen AW, Basso O, Olsen J: Risk of recurrence of prolonged pregnancy. BMJ 326:476, 2003.
19. Kistka ZA, Palomar L, Boslaugh SE, et al: Risk for postterm delivery after previous postterm delivery. Am J Obstet Gynecol 196:241, 2007.
20. Divon MY, Ferber A, Nisell H, Westgren M: Male gender predisposes to prolongation of pregnancy. Am J Obstet Gynecol 187:1081, 2002.
21. Laursen M, Billie C, Olesen AW, et al: Genetic influence on prolonged gestation: a population-based Danish twin study. Am J Obstet Gynecol 190:489, 2004.
22. Stotland NE, Washington AE, Caughey AB: Prepregnancy body mass index and the length of gestation at term. Am J Obstet Gynecol 197:378, 2007.
23. Munster K, Schmidt L, Helm P: Length and variation in the menstrual cycle: a cross-sectional study from a Danish county. Br J Obstet Gynae 99(5):422, 1992.
24. Creinin MD, Keverline S, Meyn, LA: How regular is regular? An analysis of menstrual cycle regularity. Contraception 70(4):289, 2004.
25. Boyd ME, Usher RH, McLean FH, Kramer MS: Obstetric consequences of postmaturity. Am J Obstet Gynecol 158:334, 1988.
26. Gardosi J, Vanner T, Francis A: Gestational age and induction of labor for prolonged pregnancy. Br J Obstet Gynaecol 104:792, 1997.
27. Nguyen TH, Larsen T, Engholm G, Moller H: Evaluation of ultrasound-estimated date of delivery in 17,450 spontaneous singleton births: do we need to modify Naegele's rule? Ultrasound Obstet Gynecol 14:23, 1999.
28. Bennett KA, Crane JMG, O'Shea B, et al: First trimester ultrasound screening is effective in reducing postterm labor induction rates: a randomized controlled trial. Am J Obstet Gynecol 190:1077, 2004.
29. Ingemarsson I, Kallen K: Stillbirths and rate of neonatal deaths in 76,761 postterm pregnancies in Sweden, 1982-1991: a register study. Acta Obstet Gynecol Scand 76:658, 1997.
30. Yudkin PL, Wood L, Redman CW: Risk of unexplained stillbirth at different gestational ages. Lancet 1:1192, 1987.
31. Feldman GB: Prospective risk of stillbirth. Obstet Gynecol 79:547, 1992.
32. Divon MY, Haglund B, Nisell H, et al: Fetal and neonatal mortality in the post-term pregnancy: the impact of gestational age and fetal growth restriction. Am J Obstet Gynecol 178:726, 1998.
33. Smith GCS: Estimating risks of perinatal death. Am J Obstet Gynecol 192:17, 2005.
34. Hilder L, Costeloe K, Thilaganathan B: Prolonged pregnancy: evaluating gestation-specific risks of fetal and infant mortality. Br J Obstet Gynaecol 105:169, 1998.
35. Cotzias CS, Paterson-Brown S, Fisk NM: Prospective risk of unexplained stillbirth in singleton pregnancies at term: population based analysis. BMJ 319:287, 1999.
36. Huang DY, Usher RH, Kramer MS, et al: Determinants of unexplained antepartum fetal deaths. Obstet Gynecol 95:215, 2000.
37. Clausson B, Cnattingius S, Axelsson O: Outcomes of post-term births: the role of fetal growth restriction and malformations. Obstet Gynecol 94:758, 1999.
38. Tunon K, Eik-Nes SH, Grottum P: Fetal outcome in pregnancies defined as post-term according to the last menstrual period estimate, but not according to the ultrasound estimate. Ultrasound Obstet Gynecol 14:12, 1999.
39. Guidetti DA, Divon MY, Langer O: Postdate fetal surveillance: is 41 weeks too early? Am J Obstet Gynecol 161:91, 1989.
40. Caughey AB, Musci TJ: Complications of term pregnancies beyond 37 weeks of gestation. Obstet Gynecol 103:57, 2004.
41. Nicolaides KH, Peters MT, Vyas S, et al: Relation of rate of urine production to oxygen tension in small for gestational age fetuses. Am J Obstet Gynecol 162:387, 1990.
42. Gresham EL, Rankin JHG, Makowski EL, et al: An evaluation of fetal renal function in chronic sheep preparation. J Clin Invest 51:149, 1972.
43. Bar-Hava I, Divon MY, Sardo M, Barnhard Y: Is oligohydramnios in post-term pregnancy associated with redistribution of fetal blood flow? Am J Obstet Gynecol 173:519, 1995.
44. Phelan JP, Ahn MO, Smith CV, et al: Amniotic fluid index measurements during pregnancy. J Reprod Med 32:601, 1987.
45. Leveno KJ, Quirk JG Jr, Cunningham FG, et al: Prolonged pregnancy. I. Observations concerning the causes of fetal distress. Am J Obstet Gynecol 150:465, 1984.
46. Gabbe SG, Ettinger BB, Freeman RK, Martin CB: Umbilical cord compression associated with amniotomy: laboratory observations. Am J Obstet Gynecol 126:353, 1976.
47. Miyazaki FS, Taylor NA: Saline amnioinfusion for relief of variable or prolonged decelerations. A preliminary report. Am J Obstet Gynecol 146:670, 1983.
48. Crowley P, O'Herlihy C, Boylan P: The value of ultrasound measurement of amniotic fluid volume in management of prolonged pregnancies. Br J Obstet Gynaecol 91:444, 1984.
49. Morris JM, Thompson K, Smithey J, et al: The usefulness of ultrasound assessment of amniotic fluid in predicting adverse outcome in prolonged pregnancy: a prospective blinded observational study. Br J Obstet Gynecol 110:989, 2003.
50. McLean FH, Boyd ME, Usher RH, Kramer MS: Post-term infants: too big or too small? Am J Obstet Gynecol 164:619, 1991.
51. Eden RD, Seifert LS, Winegar A, Spellacy WN: Perinatal characteristics of uncomplicated postdate pregnancies. Obstet Gynecol 69(3 Pt 1):296, 1987.
52. Chervenak LJ, Divon MY, Hirsch J, et al: Macrosomia in the postdate pregnancy: is routine sonography screening indicated? Am J Obstet Gynecol 161:753, 1989.
53. Pollack RN, Hauer-Pollack G, Divon MY: Macrosomia in postdates pregnancies: the accuracy of routine ultrasonographic screening. Am J Obstet Gynecol 167:7, 55, 1992.
54. ACOG Practice Bulletin: Fetal macrosomia, No. 22, 2000.
55. Shime J, Librach CL, Gare DJ, Cook CJ: The influence of prolonged pregnancy on infant development at one and two years of age: a prospective controlled study. Am J Obstet Gynecol 154:341, 1986.
56. Vorherr H: Placental insufficiency in relation to postterm pregnancy and fetal postmaturity. Evaluation of fetoplacental function; management of postterm gravid. Am J Obstet Gynecol 123:67, 1975.
57. Mannino F: Neonatal complications of postterm gestation. J Reprod Med 33:271, 1988.
58. Whitworth M, Bricker L, Neilson JP, Dowswell T: Ultrasound for fetal assessment in early pregnancy. Cochrane Database Sys Rev 4: CD007058, 2010.
59. John JM, Harman CR, Lange IR, Manning FA: Biophysical profile scoring in the management of the post term pregnancy: an analysis of 307 patients. Am J Obstet Gynecol 154:269, 1986.
60. Alfirevic Z, Walkinshaw SA: A randomized controlled trial of simple compared with complex antenatal fetal monitoring after 42 weeks gestation. Br J Obstet Gynaecol 102(8):638, 1995.
61. Chamberlain PF, Manning FA, Morrison I, et al: Ultrasound evaluation of amniotic fluid volume. I. The relationship of marginal and decreased amniotic fluid volumes to perinatal outcome. Am J Obstet Gynecol 150:245, 1984.
62. Zimmermann P, Alback T, Koskinen J, et al: Doppler flow velocimetry of the umbilical artery, uteroplacental arteries and fetal middle cerebral artery in prolonged pregnancy. Ultrasound Obstet Gynecol 5:189, 1995.
63. Hannah ME, Hannah WJ, Hellman J, et al: Induction of labor as compared with serial antenatal monitoring in post-term pregnancies. A randomized controlled trial. The Canadian Multicenter Post-term Pregnancy Trial Group. N Engl J Med 327:1587, 1992.
64. The National Institute of Child Health and Human Development Network of Maternal Fetal Medicine Units: A clinical trial of induction of labor versus expectant management in post term pregnancy. Am J Obstet Gynecol 170:716, 1994.
65. Sanchez-Ramos L, Olivier F, Delke I, Kaunitz AM: Labor induction versus expectant management for postterm pregnancies: a systematic review with meta-analysis. Obstet Gynecol 101:1312, 2003.
66. Gülmezoglu AM, Crowther CA, Middleton P. Induction of labour for improving birth outcomes for women at or beyond term. Cochrane Database Sys Rev 4: CD004945, 2006.
67. de Miranda E, van der Bom JG, Bonsel GJ, et al: Membrane sweeping and prevention of post-term pregnancy in low-risk pregnancies: a randomised controlled trial. BJOG 113(4):402, 2006.
68. Crane J, Bennett K, Young D, et al: The effectiveness of sweeping membranes at term: a randomized trial. Obstet Gynecol 89(4):586, 1997.
69. Wong SF, Hui SK, Choi H, Ho LC: Does sweeping of membranes beyond 40 weeks reduce the need for formal induction of labour? BJOG 109(6):632, 2002.
70. Boulvain M, Stan CM, Irion O: Membrane sweeping for induction of labour. Cochrane Database Sys Rev 1: CD000451, 2005.

71. Pandis GK, Papageorghiou AT, Ramanathan VG, et al: Preinduction sonographic measurement of cervical length in the prediction of successful induction. Ultrasound Obstet Gynecol 18:623, 2001.
72. Rozenberg P, Goffinet F, Hessabi M: Comparison of the Bishop score ultrasonographically measured cervical length, and fetal fibronectin assay in predicating time until delivery and type of delivery at term. Am J Obstet Gynecol 182:108, 2000.
73. Meydanli MM, Caliskan E, Burak F, et al: Labor induction post-term with 25 micrograms vs. 50 micrograms of intravaginal misoprostol. Int J Gynaecol Obstet 81(3):249, 2003.
74. Ting RV, Wang MH, Scott TF: The dysmature infant: associated factors and outcome at 7 years of age. J Pediatr 90:943, 1977.
75. Shime J, Librach CL, Gare DJ, Cook CJ: The influence of prolonged pregnancy on infant development at one and two years of age: a prospective controlled study. Am J Obstet Gynecol 154:341, 1986.
76. Luke B: Reducing fetal deaths in multiple births: optimal birthweights and gestational ages for infants of twin and triplet births. Acta Genet Med Gemellol (Roma) 45:333, 1996.

Section VI

Pregnancy and Coexisting Disease

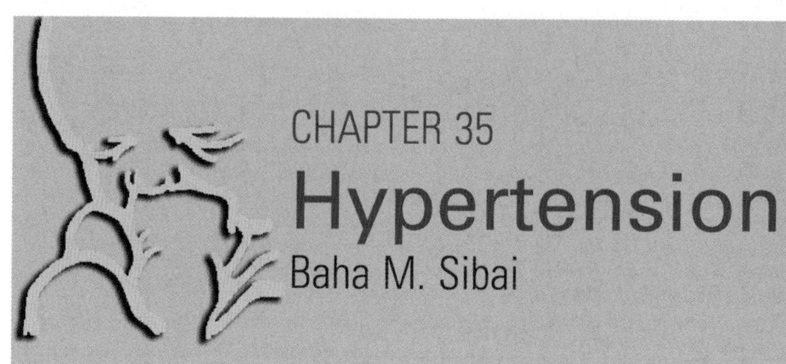

CHAPTER 35
Hypertension

Baha M. Sibai

KEY ABBREVIATIONS

Acute Fatty Liver of Pregnancy	AFLP
Acute Respiratory Distress Syndrome	ARDS
Alanine Transaminase	ALT
Angiotensin-converting Enzyme Inhibitor	ACE
Aspartate Transaminase	AST
Blood Pressure	BP
Central Venous Pressure	CVP
Computed Axial Tomography	CAT
Computed Tomography	CT
Confidence Interval	CI
Disseminated Intravascular Coagulopathy	DIC
Electrocardiogram	ECG
Electroencephalography	EEG
Glomerular Filtration Rate	GFR
Hemolysis, Elevated Liver Enzymes, and Low Platelets Syndrome	HELLP
Hemolytic Uremic Syndrome	HUS
Immune Thrombocytopenic Purpura	ITP
Intrauterine Growth Restriction	IUGR
Lactate Dehydrogenase	LDH
Magnetic Resonance Imaging	MRI
Nonstress Test	NST
Number Needed to Treat	NTT
Placental-like Growth Factor	PLGF
Prostaglandin I_2	PGI_2
Pulmonary Capillary Wedge Pressure	PCWP
Small for Gestational Age	SGA
Soluble fms-like Tyrosine Kinase 1	sFlt-1
Thrombotic Thrombocytopenic Purpura	TTP
Thromboxane A_2	TXA_2
Tumor Necrosis Factor-α	TNF-α
Vascular Endothelial Growth Factor	VEGF

Hypertensive disorders are among the most common medical complications of pregnancy, with a reported incidence between 5% and 10%.[1] The incidence varies among different hospitals, regions, and countries. These disorders are a major cause of maternal and perinatal mortality and morbidity worldwide.[2] The term *hypertension in pregnancy* is commonly used to describe a wide spectrum of patients who may have only mild elevations in blood pressure (BP) or severe hypertension with various organ dysfunctions. The clinical manifestations in these patients may be similar (e.g., hypertension, proteinuria); however, they may result from different underlying causes, such as

TABLE 35-1 HYPERTENSIVE DISORDERS OF PREGNANCY

CLINICAL FINDINGS	CHRONIC HYPERTENSION	GESTATIONAL HYPERTENSION*	PREECLAMPSIA
Time of onset of hypertension	<20 wk	>20 wk	Usually in third trimester
Degree of hypertension	Mild or severe	Mild	Mild or severe
Proteinuria*	Absent	Absent	Usually present
Cerebral symptoms	May be present	Absent	Present in 30%
Serum urate >5.5 mg/dL (0.33 mmol/L)	Rare	Absent	Usually present
Hemoconcentration	Absent	Absent	Severe disease
Thrombocytopenia	Absent	Absent	Severe disease
Hepatic dysfunction	Absent	Absent	Severe disease

*Defined as ≥1++ by dipstick testing on two occasions or ≥300 mg in a 24-hour urine collection.

chronic hypertension, renal disease, or pure preeclampsia. The three most common forms of hypertension are acute gestational hypertension complicating pregnancy, preeclampsia, and chronic essential hypertension.

DEFINITIONS

Hypertension may be present before pregnancy, or it may be diagnosed for the first time during pregnancy. In addition, in some women, hypertension may become evident only intrapartum or during the postpartum period. For clinical purposes, women with hypertension may be classified into one of three categories (Table 35-1).[1-3]

Gestational Hypertension

Gestational hypertension is the development of an elevated BP during pregnancy or in the first 24 hours postpartum without other signs or symptoms of preeclampsia or preexisting hypertension. In these women, BP returns to normal within 12 weeks after delivery. Hypertension is defined as a BP greater than or equal to 140 mm Hg systolic **or** 90 mm Hg diastolic (Table 35-2). **The hypertension should be present on at least two occasions, at least 4 hours apart, but within a maximum of a 1-week period.**[4] **It is recognized that some women with gestational hypertension may have undiagnosed chronic hypertension, whereas others will subsequently progress to develop the clinical syndrome of preeclampsia.**[5] In general, the likelihood of progression to preeclampsia depends on gestational age at time of diagnosis, with higher rates if the onset of hypertension is before 35 weeks' gestation[5-8] (Figure 35-1).

Preeclampsia and Eclampsia

The classic triad of preeclampsia includes hypertension, proteinuria, and edema. However, there is now universal agreement that edema should not be considered as part of the diagnosis of preeclampsia.[1-3,9-11] Indeed, edema is neither sufficient nor necessary to confirm the diagnosis of preeclampsia because edema is a common finding in normal pregnancy and about one third of eclamptic women never demonstrate edema[12] **In general, preeclampsia is primarily defined as gestational hypertension plus proteinuria. Proteinuria is defined as a concentration of 0.1 g/L or more in at least two random urine specimens collected 4 hours or more apart or 0.3 g (300 mg) in a 24-hour period.** In the absence of proteinuria, the syndrome of preeclampsia should be considered when gestational hypertension is present in association with persistent cerebral symptoms, epigastric or right upper quadrant pain plus nausea or vomiting, fetal growth restriction (FGR), or abnormal laboratory tests such as thrombocytopenia and elevated liver enzymes.[2,9-11] In mild preeclampsia, the diastolic BP remains below 110 mm Hg and the systolic BP remains below 160 mm Hg (see box, Criteria for Severe Preeclampsia).[2,3] Eclampsia is the occurrence of seizures during the second half of pregnancy not attributable to other causes.[12]

TABLE 35-2 CRITERIA FOR MILD GESTATIONAL HYPERTENSION IN HEALTHY PREGNANT WOMEN

Systolic blood pressure <160 mm Hg and diastolic blood pressure <110 mm Hg
Proteinuria of <300 mg per 24-hr collection
Platelet count of >100,000/mm^3
Normal liver enzymes
Absent maternal symptoms
Absent intrauterine growth restriction and oligohydramnios by ultrasound

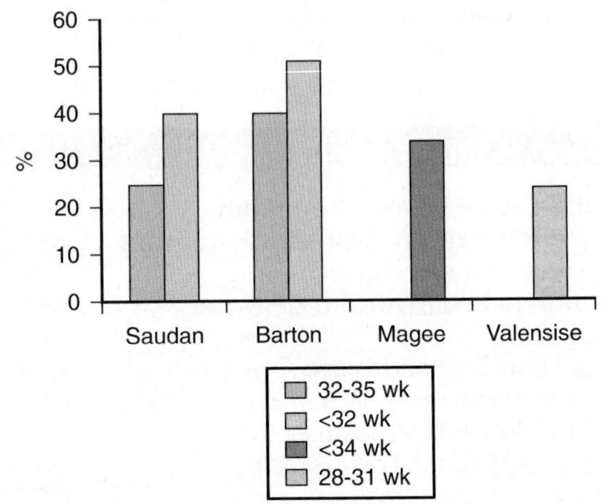

FIGURE 35-1. Rate of progression from gestational hypertension to preeclampsia by gestational age at diagnosis. *GA*, Gestational age. (Data from references 5, 6, 7, and 8.)

CRITERIA FOR SEVERE PREECLAMPSIA

1. Blood pressure of ≥160 mm Hg systolic or ≥110 mm Hg diastolic, recorded on at least two occasions at least 6 hours apart with patient on bedrest
2. Proteinuria of ≥5 g in 24 hours
3. Oliguria (<500 mL in 24 hours)
4. Cerebral visual disturbances
5. Epigastric pain, nausea, and vomiting
6. Pulmonary edema
7. Impaired liver function of unclear etiology
8. Thrombocytopenia

Chronic Hypertension

Chronic hypertension is defined as hypertension present before the pregnancy or that is diagnosed before the 20th week of gestation. Hypertension that persists for more than 3 months postpartum is also classified as chronic hypertension.[2]

Chronic Hypertension with Superimposed Preeclampsia

Women with chronic hypertension may develop superimposed preeclampsia, which increases morbidity for both the mother and fetus. The diagnosis of superimposed preeclampsia is based on one or more of the following findings: development of new-onset proteinuria, defined as the urinary excretion of 0.5 g protein or greater in a 24-hour specimen in women with hypertension; no proteinuria before 20 weeks' gestation; or, in women with hypertension and proteinuria before 20 weeks, severe exacerbation in hypertension plus development of symptoms or thrombocytopenia and abnormal liver enzymes (Table 35-3).[13,14]

Gestational Hypertension

Gestational hypertension is the most frequent cause of hypertension during pregnancy. The incidence ranges between 6% and 29% in nulliparous women[2,4,15] and between 2% and 4% in multiparous women.[2] The incidence is markedly increased in patients with multiple gestation.[13,16-18] **In general, most cases of gestational hypertension develop at or beyond 37 weeks' gestation, and thus, the overall pregnancy outcome is usually similar to that seen in women with normotensive pregnancies (Table 35-4).**[4,5,15] Both gestational age at delivery and birthweight in these pregnancies are significantly higher than in normotensive pregnancies.[2,4] However, women with mild gestational hypertension have higher rates of induction of labor and thus higher rates of cesarean delivery.[4]

Maternal and perinatal morbidities are substantially increased in women with severe gestational hypertension.[2,4,19] **Indeed, these women have increased risk for morbidity compared with women with mild preeclampsia. The rates of abruptio placentae, preterm delivery (at less than 37 and 35 weeks), and small-for-gestational-age (SGA) infants in these women are similar to those seen in women with severe preeclampsia.**[2,19] Therefore, these women should be managed as if they had severe preeclampsia. It is unclear whether this increase in preterm delivery is secondary to scheduled early delivery according to physician preference or occurs because the disease process itself remains unknown.

PREECLAMPSIA

Preeclampsia is a form of hypertension that is unique to human pregnancy. The clinical findings of preeclampsia can manifest as either a maternal syndrome (hypertension and proteinuria with or without other multisystem dysfunction) or a fetal syndrome (FGR, reduced amniotic fluid, and abnormal oxygenation).[11-20] In practice, the maternal syndrome of preeclampsia represents a clinical spectrum with major differences between near-term preeclampsia without demonstrable fetal involvement and preeclampsia that is associated with low birthweight and

TABLE 35-3 RECOMMENDED CRITERIA TO DIAGNOSE PREECLAMPSIA IN WOMEN WITH PREEXISTING MEDICAL CONDITIONS

CONDITION	CRITERIA NEEDED
Hypertension only	Proteinuria of ≥500 mg per 24 hr or thrombocytopenia
Proteinuria only	New-onset hypertension plus symptoms or thrombocytopenia or elevated liver enzymes
Hypertension plus proteinuria (renal disease or class F diabetes)	Worsening severe hypertension plus proteinuria either new onset of symptoms, thrombocytopenia, or elevated liver enzymes

TABLE 35-4 PREGNANCY OUTCOME IN WOMEN WITH MILD GESTATIONAL HYPERTENSION

	KNUIST ET AL.[15] (*n* = 396)	HAUTH ET AL.[4] (*n* = 715)	BARTON ET AL.[5] (*n* = 405)	SIBAI ET AL.[2] (*n* = 186)
Gestation at delivery (wk)*	NR	39.7	37.4†	39.1
<37 wk (%)	5.3	7.0	17.3	5.9
<34 wk (%)	1.3	1.0	4.9	1.6
Birthweight (g)*	NR	3303	3038	3217
SGA (%)	1.5‡	6.9	13.8	7.0
<2500 g (%)	7.1	7.7	23.5	NR
Abruptio placentae (%)	0.5	0.3	0.5	0.5
Perinatal deaths (%)	0.8	0.5	0	0

Modified from Sibai BM: Diagnosis and management of gestational hypertension and preeclampsia. Obstet Gynecol 102:181, 2003.
*Mean values.
†Women who developed hypertension at 24 to 35 weeks.
‡Less than the third percentile.
NR, Not reported; *SGA*, small for gestational age.

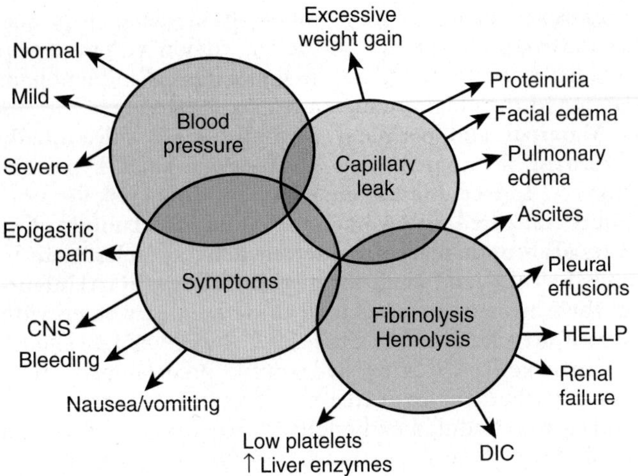

FIGURE 35-2. Various clinical and laboratory findings in women with preeclampsia or atypical preeclampsia. *CNS,* Central nervous system; *DIC,* disseminated intravascular coagulopathy; *HELLP,* hemolysis, elevated liver enzymes, and low platelets.

preterm delivery.[11,20] Preeclampsia is clearly a heterogeneous condition for which the pathogenesis could be different in women with various risk factors.[11,20,21] The pathogenesis of preeclampsia in nulliparous women may be different than that in women with preexisting vascular disease, multifetal gestation, diabetes mellitus, or previous preeclampsia. In addition, the pathophysiology of early-onset preeclampsia may be different than that of preeclampsia developing at term, during labor, or in the postpartum period.[11,20,21]

The incidence of preeclampsia ranges between 2% and 7% in healthy nulliparous women.[2,4,15] In these women, preeclampsia is generally mild, with the onset near term or intrapartum (75% of cases), and the condition conveys only a minimally increased risk for adverse fetal outcome.[2,4,15] In contrast, the incidence and severity of preeclampsia are substantially higher in women with multifetal gestation,[14,13,16,18,22] chronic hypertension,[13,14] previous preeclampsia,[23-28] pregestational diabetes mellitus,[13,29,30] or preexisting thrombophilias.[31]

Atypical Preeclampsia

The traditional criteria to confirm a diagnosis of preeclampsia include the presence of proteinuric hypertension (new onset of hypertension and new onset of proteinuria after 20 weeks' gestation). However, recent data suggest that in some women, preeclampsia and even eclampsia may develop in the absence of either hypertension or proteinuria.[10,11,32] In many of these women, there are usually other manifestations of preeclampsia, such as the presence of signs and symptoms or other laboratory abnormalities (Figure 35-2; see box, Criteria for Atypical Preeclampsia).

In the absence of proteinuria, the syndrome of preeclampsia should be considered when gestational hypertension is present in association with persistent symptoms, or with abnormal laboratory tests. It is also important to note that 25% to 50% of women with mild gestational hypertension progress to preeclampsia.[5-8] The rate of progression depends on gestational age at onset of hypertension and approaches 50% when gestational hypertension develops before 32 weeks' gestation.[5] Most of these cases result in preterm delivery or FGR, or both.[5,8] Therefore, such women require close observation for early detection of preeclampsia (frequent prenatal visits and serial evaluation of platelets and liver enzymes) and fetal growth (serial ultrasound).

Criteria for Atypical Preeclampsia

- Gestational hypertension plus one or more of the following:
  - Symptoms of preeclampsia
  - Hemolysis
  - Thrombocytopenia (<100,000/mm^3)
  - Elevated liver enzymes: two times the upper limit of the normal value for aspartate transaminase (AST) and alanine transaminase (ALT)
- Gestational proteinuria plus one or more of the following:
  - Symptoms of preeclampsia
  - Hemolysis
  - Thrombocytopenia
  - Elevated liver enzymes
- Early signs and symptoms of preeclampsia-eclampsia at <20 weeks
- Late postpartum preeclampsia-eclampsia (>48 hours postpartum)

Preeclampsia should also be considered when gestational hypertension is severe because of the associated adverse maternal-perinatal outcome reported in such women. In a secondary analysis of data from two multicenter trials, pregnancy outcomes in women with severe gestational hypertension were compared with those in women with mild or severe preeclampsia.[4,19] This analysis revealed that severe gestational hypertension is associated with higher maternal and perinatal morbidities than those found in mild preeclampsia. The results of these studies also revealed that women with severe gestational hypertension had adverse maternal or perinatal outcomes similar to those seen in women with severe preeclampsia.[4,19] **Therefore, women with severe gestational hypertension should be considered as having atypical preeclampsia and should be hospitalized.** For these patients, we recommend magnesium sulfate seizure prophylaxis, frequent laboratory follow-up, antihypertensive drugs, steroids for fetal lung maturity, and delivery beyond 34 weeks' gestation or earlier if indicated.[33]

Capillary Leak Syndrome: Facial Edema, Ascites and Pulmonary Edema, and Gestational Proteinuria

Hypertension is considered to be the hallmark for the diagnosis of preeclampsia; however, in some patients with preeclampsia, the disease may manifest as either a capillary leak (proteinuria, ascites, pulmonary edema), excessive weight gain, or a spectrum of abnormal hemostasis with multiple-organ dysfunction. These women usually present with clinical manifestations of atypical preeclampsia, such as proteinuria with or without facial edema, excessive weight gain (>5 pounds/week), ascites, or pulmonary edema, in association with abnormalities in laboratory values or presence of symptoms, but without hypertension.[32] Therefore, we recommend that women with capillary leak syndrome with or without hypertension be evaluated for platelet, liver enzyme, and renal abnormalities. Those with symptoms such as significant headache or abnormal blood tests should be considered to have preeclampsia.[32]

Gestational Proteinuria

There is general agreement that urine dipstick protein measurements should be performed at each prenatal visit after 20 weeks' gestation. Gestational proteinuria is defined as urinary protein excretion of at least 300 mg per 24-hour timed collection or persistent proteinuria (≥1+ on dipstick on at least two occasions at least 4 hours apart, but no more than 1 week apart).[34] The exact incidence of gestational proteinuria before progression to preeclampsia is not known; however, isolated gestational proteinuria was reported in 4% of women enrolled in two multicenter trials.[34,35] In addition, these studies reported that 4.3% to 7% of patients had combined gestational hypertension and gestational proteinuria. Thus, it appears that at least one third of women with gestational proteinuria may progress to preeclampsia.[34,35] Indeed, some authors suggested that gestational proteinuria alone may herald the early manifestations of impending preeclampsia.[34,36]

Women with new-onset gestational proteinuria only should be monitored very closely, at least on a twice-weekly follow-up basis, for early detection of preeclampsia because the presence of gestational proteinuria alone may signify impending preeclampsia.[32]

Preeclampsia-Eclampsia at Less Than 20 Weeks' Gestation

Preeclampsia or eclampsia, or both, occurring before the 20th week of gestation has been reported with molar or hydropic degeneration of the placenta with or without a coexistent fetus. Additionally, although exceedingly rare, preeclampsia-eclampsia can occur during the first half of pregnancy without molar degeneration of the placenta.[32] On the other hand, the presence of hypertension, proteinuria, and abnormal laboratory tests before 20 weeks' gestation may be due to lupus nephritis, hemolytic uremic syndrome (HUS), antiphospholipid antibody syndrome, or thrombotic thrombocytopenic purpura (TTP).[32] Therefore, such women should be evaluated to rule out the presence of these disorders. In the absence of other pathology, the patient should be treated as for severe preeclampsia. **In addition, women in whom convulsions develop in association with hypertension and proteinuria during the first half of pregnancy should be considered to have eclampsia until proved otherwise. These women should have ultrasound examination of the uterus to rule out molar pregnancy and hydropic or cystic degeneration of the placenta.** A diagnostic modality that is also recommended is the measurement of uterine artery Doppler flow, which shows the classic "notching" characteristic of increased resistance in the placenta of patients with preeclampsia.[32]

Risk Factors for Preeclampsia

Several factors have been identified with increased risk for preeclampsia (see box, Risk Factors for Preeclampsia). Generally, preeclampsia is considered a disease of primigravid women. The risk increases in those who have limited sperm exposure with the same partner before conception.[11,20,37] The protective effects of long-term sperm exposure with the same partner might provide an explanation for the high risk for preeclampsia in women younger than 20 years old. A previous abortion (spontaneous or induced) or a previous normal pregnancy with the same partner is associated with a lower risk for preeclampsia. However, this protective effect is lost with a change of partner.[38] Both Scandinavian and U.S. studies have confirmed the importance of paternal factors, that is, the so-called dangerous father.[39,40] Using whole population data, Lie and colleagues[40] demonstrated that men who fathered one preeclamptic pregnancy were nearly twice as likely to father a preeclamptic pregnancy in a different woman (1.8; 95% confidence interval [CI] 1.2 to 2.6; after adjustment for parity), regardless of whether the new partner had a preeclamptic pregnancy in the past or not. Thus, mothers had a substantially increased risk in their second pregnancy (2.9%) if their partner had fathered a preeclamptic first pregnancy with another woman. This risk was nearly as high as the average risk among first pregnancies.[40]

Risk Factors for Preeclampsia

- Nulliparity
- Age >40 years
- Family history of preeclampsia
- Woman born small for gestational age
- Obesity/gestational diabetes
- Multifetal gestation
- Preeclampsia in previous pregnancy
- Poor outcome in previous pregnancy
  - Fetal growth restriction, abruptio, fetal death
- Preexisting medical-genetic conditions
  - Chronic hypertension
  - Renal disease
  - Type 1 (insulin-dependent) diabetes mellitus
  - Antiphospholipid antibody syndrome, factor V Leiden mutation

Recent advances in assisted reproductive technology have introduced several challenges for the maternal immune system that also increase the risk for preeclampsia.[17,18,41] These include a greater proportion of women older than 40 years, infertile women during their first gestation, obese women with polycystic ovary syndrome, and women who become pregnant with donated gametes or embryos.[41] The use of donated gametes can influence the maternal-fetal immune interaction. In addition, many of these women have multifetal gestations.[17,18,41] In addition, infertile women with recurrent miscarriage are also reported to be at increased risk for preeclampsia.[42]

Obesity increases the risk for preeclampsia, and this risk increases with increased body mass index.[43] The worldwide increase in obesity is thus likely to lead to a rise in the frequency of preeclampsia.[44,45] Obesity has a strong link to insulin resistance, which is also a risk factor for preeclampsia. The exact mechanism by which obesity or insulin resistance is associated with preeclampsia is not well understood.

Earlier studies found an overall higher rate of thrombophilia in women with preeclampsia compared with controls.[31] Recently, a number of reports have failed to reproduce these findings.[46-48] The disparity in results can be seen to reflect the heterogeneity of the women being studied. In the largest series of preeclamptic women with thrombophilia, women had increasing risk for very-early-onset severe disease (delivery before 28 weeks) compared with those without thrombophilia.[31]

Pathophysiology

The etiology of preeclampsia remains unknown. Many theories have been suggested, but most of them have not withstood the test of time. Some of the theories still under consideration are listed in the box, Theories Associated with the Etiology of Preeclampsia.[11,21,49-51]

Theories Associated with the Etiology of Preeclampsia

- Abnormal trophoblast invasion or poor implantation
- Imbalance in angiogenesis
- Coagulation abnormalities
- Vascular endothelial damage
- Cardiovascular maladaptation
- Immunologic maladaptation
- Genetic predisposition
- Exaggerated inflammatory response
- Increased oxidative stress

During normal pregnancy, impressive physiologic changes occur in the uteroplacental vasculature in general and in the cardiovascular system in particular. These changes are most likely induced by the interaction of the fetal (parental) allograft with maternal tissue. The development of mutual immunologic tolerance in the first trimester is thought to lead to important morphologic and biochemical changes in the systemic and uteroplacental maternal circulation.

Uterine Vascular Changes

The human placenta receives its blood supply from numerous uteroplacental arteries that are developed by the action of migratory interstitial and endovascular trophoblast into the walls of the spiral arterioles. This transforms the uteroplacental arterial bed into a low-resistance, low-pressure, high-flow system. The conversion of the spiral arterioles of the nonpregnant uterus into the uteroplacental arteries has been termed *physiologic changes*.[52,53] In a normal pregnancy, these trophoblast-induced vascular changes extend all the way from the intervillous space to the origin of the spiral arterioles representing the radial arteries in the inner one third of the myometrium. It is suggested that these vascular changes are effected in two stages: "the conversion of the decidual segments of the spiral arterioles by a wave of endovascular trophoblast migration in the first trimester and the myometrial segments by a subsequent wave in the second trimester."[52,53] This process is reportedly associated with extensive fibrinoid formation and degeneration of the muscular layer in the arterial wall. These vascular changes result in the conversion of about 100 to 150 spiral arterioles into distended, tortuous, and funnel-shaped vessels that communicate through multiple openings into the intervillous space.

In contrast, pregnancies complicated by preeclampsia or by FGR demonstrate inadequate maternal vascular response to placentation. In these pregnancies, the previously mentioned vascular changes are usually found only in the decidual segments of the uteroplacental arteries. Hence, the myometrial segments of the spiral arterioles continue to exhibit their characteristic musculoelastic architecture, thereby leaving them responsive to hormonal influences.[52,53] Additionally, the number of well-developed arterioles is smaller than that found in normotensive pregnancies. It has been postulated that this defective vascular response to placentation is due to inhibition of the second wave of endovascular trophoblast migration that normally occurs from about 16 weeks' gestation onward. These pathologic changes may have the effect of curtailing the increased blood supply required by the fetoplacental unit in the later stages of pregnancy and correlate with decreased uteroplacental blood flow seen in most cases of preeclampsia.[52] Frusca and associates studied placental bed biopsy specimens obtained during cesarean delivery from normal pregnancies (n = 14), preeclamptic pregnancies (n = 24), and chronic hypertensive pregnancies only (n = 5).[54] Biopsy specimens from the preeclamptic group demonstrated abnormal vascular changes in every case, with 18 having acute atherosclerotic changes. In contrast, 13 of the 14 specimens from normotensive pregnancies had normal vascular physiologic changes, whereas specimens from hypertensive patients showed all three types of physiologic changes. In addition, they found that the mean birthweight was significantly lower in the group with atherosclerosis than it was in the other group without such findings. It is important to note that these vascular changes may also be demonstrated in a significant proportion of normotensive pregnancies complicated by FGR. Meekins and associates[55] have demonstrated that endovascular trophoblast invasion is not an all-or-none phenomenon in normal and preeclamptic pregnancies. These authors observed that morphologic features found in one spiral artery may not be representative of all vessels in a placental bed.

Vascular Endothelial Activation and Inflammation

The mechanism by which placental ischemia leads to the clinical syndrome of preeclampsia is thought to be related to the production of placental factors that enter the maternal circulation resulting in endothelial cell dysfunction.[49-51,56] **Soluble fms-like tyrosine kinase 1 (sFlt-1) is a protein that is produced by the placenta. It acts by binding to the receptor-binding domains of vascular endothelial growth factor (VEGF), and it also binds to placental like growth factor (PLGF). Increased levels of this protein in the maternal circulation results in reduced levels of free VEGF and free PLFG, with resultant endothelial cell dysfunction.**[56]

Maternal serum and placental levels of sFlt-1 are increased in pregnancies complicated by preeclampsia above values seen during normal pregnancies. Maynard and coworkers[57] demonstrated that soluble placenta-derived VEGF receptor (sFlt1), an antagonist of VEGF and PLGF, is unregulated in preeclampsia, leading to increased systemic levels of sFlt1 that fall after delivery.

Increased circulating sFlt1 in preeclampsia is associated with decreased circulating levels of free VEGF and PLGF, resulting in endothelial dysfunction. The magnitude of increase in sFlt levels correlates with disease severity,[58] lending further support to VEGF-soluble Flt balance representing one of the final common pathophysiologic pathways.

First-trimester PLGF levels are decreased in future preeclamptic pregnancies and in pregnancies complicated by FGR, whereas sFlt levels do not differ from controls.[59] Again, these data are compatible with decidual angiogenic growth factors, in particular PLGF, as being essential for early placental development (PLGF is low in both FGR and preeclampsia), with a later involvement of sFlt as a fetal rescue signal steering the maternal response, that is, the degree of maternal systemic hypertension. This hypothesis is supported by Levine and colleagues,[58] who demonstrated that during the last 2 months of pregnancy in normotensive controls, the level of sFlt-1 increased and the level of PLGF decreased.

Levine and associates[60] investigated urinary PLGF levels in pregnant women with and without preeclampsia and found that among normotensive pregnant women, urinary PLGF increased during the first two trimesters, peaked at 29 to 32 weeks, and decreased thereafter. Among women who ultimately developed preeclampsia, the pattern of urinary PLGF was similar, but levels were significantly reduced beginning at 25 to 28 weeks. There were particularly large differences among those who subsequently developed early-onset preeclampsia and in those delivering SGA infants.[60] A similar study suggested that urinary angiogenic factors can identify women with severe preeclampsia.[61]

During the past decade, our understanding of the molecular basis for the pathophysiologic abnormalities in preeclampsia has reached an unprecedented level. There is now clear appreciation for the role of cell adhesion molecules, angiogenic proteins, and activation of the inflammatory system in the pathogenesis of microvascular dysfunction in women with preeclampsia[49-52,58] There is clear evidence for an exaggerated inflammatory response (abnormal cytokine production and neutrophil activation) in women with the clinical findings of preeclampsia.[50,51] However, this enhanced inflammatory response is absent before the development of preeclampsia.[62]

Recent studies confirming increased levels of asymmetrical dimethylarginine at 23 to 25 weeks in pregnant women who develop preeclampsia have emphasized the importance of the nitric oxide–cyclic guanosine monophosphate pathway.[63,64] Endothelial dysfunction and inappropriate endothelial cell activation associated with alterations in nitric oxide levels in preeclampsia explain most typical clinical manifestations, including the increased endothelial cell permeability and increased platelet aggregation.[49,65]

Genetics and Genetic Imprinting

According to the genetic conflict theory,[11,20] fetal genes are selected to increase the transfer of nutrients to the fetus, whereas maternal genes are selected to limit transfer in excess of some optimal level. The phenomenon of genomic imprinting means that a similar conflict exists within fetal cells between genes that are maternally derived and genes that are paternally derived. The conflict hypothesis suggests that placental factors (fetal genes) act to increase maternal BP, whereas maternal factors act to reduce BP.[20] Endothelial cell dysfunction may have evolved as a fetal rescue strategy to increase nonplacental resistance when the uteroplacental blood supply is inadequate.

Nilsson and associates[66] published a model suggesting a heritability estimate of 31% for preeclampsia and 20% for gestational hypertension. It is unlikely that there will be one major preeclampsia gene because such a gene would be selected against through evolution, unless it also carried a major reproductive advantage. It is more likely that a rapidly growing number of susceptibility genes will be uncovered, many of these interacting with the maternal cardiovascular-hemostatic system or the regulation of maternal inflammatory responses.[67] These loci segregate with different populations.[68] It should be noted that these loci only explain a relatively small percentage of the overall cases of preeclampsia. In addition, although these linkage studies indicate maternal susceptibility, they do not exclude the additional involvement of fetal genes.[68] Another important consideration regarding the genetics of preeclampsia is the confounding effect of the so-called fetal origins of adult disease hypothesis suggesting that a hostile intrauterine environment for a female fetus would form the basis for the insulin resistance syndrome with its associated endothelial dysfunction and, as such, an increased risk for preeclampsia.[20]

Epigenetic features or imprinting is also involved in the pathogenesis of preeclampsia.[68,69] A direct proof of the role of imprinting was recently published by Oudejans and coworkers[68] and Nafee and associates.[69]

Changes in Prostanoids

Several investigators have described the various prostaglandins and their metabolites throughout pregnancy. They have measured the concentrations of these substances in plasma, serum, amniotic fluid, placental tissues, urine, or cord blood. The data have been inconsistent, reflecting differences in methodology.[70,71] During pregnancy, prostanoid production increases in both maternal and fetoplacental tissues. Prostacyclin is produced by the vascular endothelium as well as in the renal cortex. It is a potent vasodilator and inhibitor of platelet aggregation. Thromboxane A_2 (TXA_2) is produced by the platelets and trophoblasts. It is a potent vasoconstrictor and platelet aggregator. Hence, these eicosanoids have opposite effects and play a major role in regulating vascular tone and vascular blood flow (Figure 35-3). An imbalance in prostanoid production or catabolism has been suggested as being responsible for the pathophysiologic changes in preeclampsia. However, the precise role by which prostaglandins are involved in the etiology of preeclampsia remains unclear.[20]

Lipid Peroxide, Free Radicals, and Antioxidants

Evidence is accumulating that lipid peroxides and free radicals may be important in the pathogenesis of preeclampsia.[40,51] Superoxide ions may be cytotoxic to the cell by changing the characteristics of the cellular membrane and producing membrane lipid peroxidation. Elevated plasma concentrations of free radical oxidation products

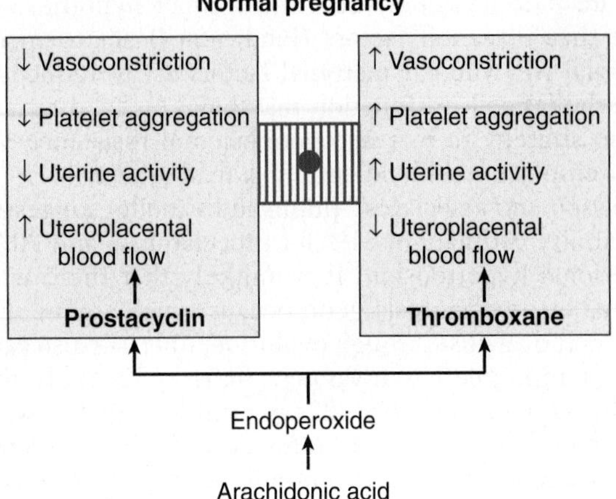

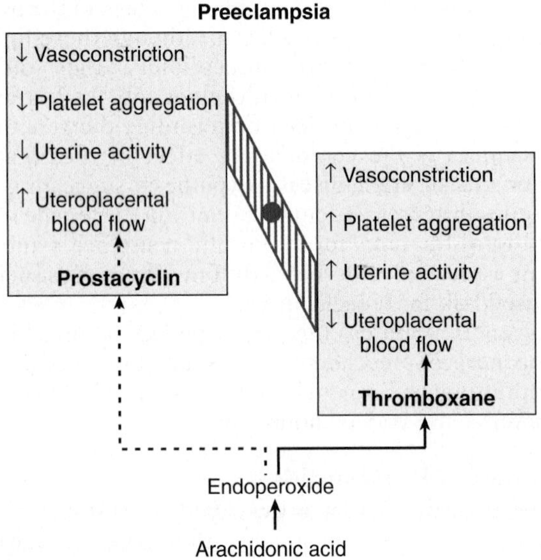

FIGURE 35-3. Comparison of the balance in the biologic actions of prostacyclin and thromboxane in normal pregnancy with the imbalance of increased thromboxane and decreased prostacyclin in pre-eclamptic pregnancy. The heavy type and box for thromboxane suggest an exacerbation of its actions in preeclampsia, whereas the lighter type and box for prostacyclin suggest a diminution of its actions. (From Walsh SW: Preeclampsia: an imbalance in placenta prostacyclin and thromboxane production. Am J Obstet Gynecol 152:335, 1985.)

precede the development of preeclampsia. In addition, some studies reported lower serum antioxidant activity in patients with preeclampsia than in normotensive pregnancies.[11,20]

Much of the controversy about oxidative stress is related to the nonspecificity of the markers. A recent study by Moretti and associates[72] measured oxidative stress "on-line" in exhaled breath (not subjective to in vitro artefacts) and confirmed greater oxidative stress in women with preeclampsia compared with uncomplicated pregnancies and nonpregnant controls.

Diagnosis of Preeclampsia

Preeclampsia is a clinical syndrome that embraces a wide spectrum of signs and symptoms that have been clinically observed to develop alone or in combination. Elevated BP is the traditional hallmark for diagnosis of the disease. The diagnosis of preeclampsia and the severity of the disease process are generally based on maternal BP. Many factors may influence the measurement of BP, including the accuracy of the equipment used, size of the sphygmomanometer cuff, duration of the rest period before recording, posture of the patient, and Korotkoff phase used (phase IV or phase V for diastolic BP measurement). **It is recommended that all BP values be recorded with the woman in a sitting position for ambulatory patients or in a semireclining position for hospitalized patients.**[2,3,9,10] The right arm should be used consistently, with the arm being in a roughly horizontal position at heart level. For diastolic BP measurements, both phases (muffling sound and disappearance sound) should be recorded. This is very important because the level measured at phase IV is about 5 to 10 mm Hg higher than that measured at phase V. A rise in BP has been used by several authors as a criterion for the diagnosis of hypertension in pregnancy. This definition is usually unreliable because a gradual increase in BP from second to third trimester is seen in most normotensive pregnancies. Villar and Sibai[74] prospectively studied BP changes during the course of pregnancy in 700 young primigravidas. One hundred thirty-seven patients (19.6%) had preeclampsia. The sensitivity and positive predictive values for preeclampsia of a threshold increase in diastolic BP of at least 15 mm Hg on two occasions were 39% and 32%, respectively. The respective values for a threshold increase in systolic pressures were 22% and 33%. Three recent studies from New Zealand,[75] the United States,[76] and Turkey[77] investigated pregnancy outcome in women with a rise in diastolic BP of more than 15 mm Hg but an absolute diastolic level below 90 mm Hg compared with gravidas who remained normotensive.[75-77] The New Zealand report[75] and Turkish study[77] included women with elevated BPs without proteinuria, whereas the American investigation[76] included women with an increased diastolic pressure by 15 mm Hg or more plus proteinuria (≥300 mg/24 hours). Overall, pregnancy outcomes were similar among women who remained normotensive and those who demonstrated a rise in diastolic pressure of 15 mm Hg or higher but did not reach 90 mm Hg. The use of an increase in BP as a diagnostic criterion is principally influenced by two factors: gestational age at time of first observation and frequency of BP measurements. Thus, these criteria are unreliable to diagnose preeclampsia as such.

The diagnosis of preeclampsia requires the presence of an elevated BP with proteinuria.[1-3] The presence of proteinuria is usually determined by the use of either dipstick or protein-to-creatinine ratio in random urine samples. The concentration of urinary protein is highly variable. It is influenced by several factors, including contamination, urine specific gravity, pH, exercise, and posture.[78] In addition, urinary protein-to-creatinine excretion is highly variable in patients with preeclampsia.[79] Moreover, urinary dipstick determinations as well as total protein-to-creatinine ratio correlate poorly with the amount of proteinuria found in 24-hour urine determinations in women with gestational hypertension.[79-82] Therefore, **the definitive test for diagnosing proteinuria should be quantitative measurement of total protein excretion over a 24-hour period.** However, the accuracy of 24-hour urine collection might not be reliable.[83] The diagnosis of severe preeclampsia requires that proteinuria of more than 5 g per 24 hours be documented. Using urine dipstick measurements (≥3+) is not adequate.[83,84]

The traditional criteria to confirm a diagnosis of preeclampsia (new onset of hypertension and proteinuria after 20 weeks' gestation) are appropriate to use in most healthy nulliparous women. However, in some women, hypertension or proteinuria may be absent in 10% to 15% of women who develop the syndrome of hemolysis, elevated liver enzymes, and low platelets (HELLP syndrome)[85] and in 20% to 25% of those who develop eclampsia.[86]

Prediction of Preeclampsia

A review of the world literature reveals that more than 100 clinical, biophysical, and biochemical tests have been recommended to predict or identify the patient at risk for the future development of the disease.[87-92] The results of the pooled data for the various tests and the lack of agreement between serial tests suggest that none of these clinical tests is sufficiently reliable for use as a screening test in clinical practice.[28]

Numerous biochemical markers have been proposed to predict which women are destined to develop preeclampsia. These biochemical markers were generally chosen on the basis of specific pathophysiologic abnormalities that have been reported in association with preeclampsia. Thus, these markers have included markers of placental dysfunction, endothelial and coagulation activation, angiogenesis, and markers of systemic inflammation. However, the results of various studies evaluating the reliability of these markers in predicting preeclampsia have been inconsistent, and many of these markers suffer from poor specificity and predictive values for routine use in clinical practice[93-100]

Doppler ultrasound is a useful method to assess uterine artery blood flow velocity in the second trimester. An abnormal uterine artery velocity waveform is characterized by a high resistance index or by the presence of an early diastolic notch (unilateral or bilateral).[88,89,92] Pregnancies complicated by abnormal uterine artery Doppler findings in the second trimester are associated with more than a sixfold increase in rate of preeclampsia.[88] However, the sensitivity of an abnormal uterine artery Doppler for predicting preeclampsia ranges from 20% to 60%, with a positive predictive value of 6% to 40%.[88,92] **Current data do not support Doppler studies for routine screening of pregnant women for preeclampsia, but uterine artery Doppler could be beneficial as a screening test in women at very high risk for preeclampsia if an effective preventive treatment becomes available.[20]**

Prevention of Preeclampsia

There are numerous clinical trials describing the use of various methods to prevent or reduce the incidence of preeclampsia.[20,100] Because the etiology of the disease is unknown, these interventions have been used in an attempt to correct theoretical abnormalities in preeclampsia. A detailed review of these trials is beyond the scope of this chapter; however, the results of these studies have been the subject of several recent systemic reviews.[100] **In short, randomized trials have evaluated protein or salt restriction; zinc, magnesium, fish oil, or vitamins C and E supplementation; the use of diuretics and other antihypertensive agents; and the use of heparin to prevent preeclampsia in women with various risk factors. These trials have had limited sample size, and results have revealed *minimal to no benefit*.** Some of the methods studied are summarized in the box, Methods Used to Prevent Preeclampsia.

Methods Used to Prevent Preeclampsia

- High-protein and low-salt diet
- Nutritional supplementation (protein)
- Calcium
- Magnesium
- Zinc
- Fish and evening primrose oil
- Antihypertensive drugs including diuretics
- Antithrombotic agents
- Low-dose aspirin
- Dipyridamole
- Heparin
- Vitamins E and C

Calcium Supplementation

The relationship between dietary calcium intake and hypertension has been the subject of several experimental and observational studies. Epidemiologic studies have documented an inverse association between calcium intake and maternal BP, and the incidences of preeclampsia and eclampsia. The BP-lowering effect of calcium is thought to be mediated by alterations in plasma renin activity and parathyroid hormone.

There are 13 clinical studies (15,730 women) comparing the use of calcium with no treatment or a placebo in pregnancy. These trials differ in the populations studied (low risk or high risk for hypertensive disorders of pregnancy), study design (randomization, double-blind, or use of a placebo), gestational age at enrollment (20 to 32 weeks' gestation), sample size in each group (range, 22 to 588), dose of elemental calcium used (156 to 2000 mg/day), and the definition of hypertensive disorders of pregnancy used.

In the Cochrane review, calcium supplementation was associated with reduced hypertension (relative risk [RR], 0.65; 95% confidence interval [CI], 0.53 to 0.81) and reduced preeclampsia (RR, 0.45; 95% CI, 0.31 to 0.65), particularly for those at high risk and with low baseline dietary calcium intake (for those with adequate calcium intake, the difference was not statistically significant). No side effects of calcium supplementation have been recorded in the trials reviewed. In contrast, a recent evidence-based review by the U.S. Food and Drug Administration concluded that "the relationship between calcium and risk of hypertension in pregnancy is inconsistent and inconclusive, and the relationship between calcium and the risk of pregnancy induced hypertension and preeclampsia is highly unlikely." At present, the benefit of calcium supplementation for preeclampsia prevention in women with low dietary calcium intake remains unclear.[28] It is also important to note that none of the published randomized trials included women with high-risk factors such as previous preeclampsia, chronic hypertension, twins, or pregestational diabetes mellitus.[28]

Antithrombotic Agents

Preeclampsia is associated with vasospasm and activation of the coagulation-hemostasis systems. Enhanced platelet activation plays a central role in the previously mentioned process and reflects abnormalities in the thromboxane-prostacyclin balance. Hence, several authors have used pharmacologic manipulation to alter the previously mentioned ratio in an attempt to prevent or ameliorate the course of preeclampsia.

Aspirin inhibits the synthesis of prostaglandins by irreversibly acetylating and inactivating cyclooxygenase. In vitro, platelet cyclooxygenase is more sensitive to inhibition by low doses of aspirin (<80 mg) than vascular endothelial cyclooxygenase. This biochemical selectivity of low-dose aspirin appears to be related to its unusual kinetics that result in presystemic acetylation of platelets exposed to higher concentrations of aspirin in the portal circulation.

Most randomized trials for the prevention of preeclampsia have used low dose of aspirin (50 to 150 mg/dL). The rationale for recommending low-dose aspirin prophylaxis is the theory that the vasospasm and coagulation abnormalities in preeclampsia are caused partly by an imbalance in the TXA_2-to-prostacyclin ratio.[20]

Recently, the Perinatal Antiplatelet Review of International Studies (PARIS) Collaborate Group performed a meta-analysis of the effectiveness and safety of antiplatelet agents (predominantly aspirin) for the prevention of preeclampsia. Thirty-one trials involving 32,217 women are included in this review. There was a 10% reduction in the risk for preeclampsia associated with the use of antiplatelet agents (RR, 0.90; 95% CI 0.84 to 0.96). For women with a previous history of hypertension or preeclampsia ($n = 6107$) who were assigned to antiplatelet agents, the RR for developing preeclampsia was 0.86 (95% CI, 0.77 to 0.97). There were no significant differences between treatment and control groups in any other measures of outcome. The reviewers concluded that antiplatelet agents, largely low-dose aspirin, have small to moderate benefits when used for prevention of preeclampsia. Low-dose aspirin was also found to be safe. However, more information is clearly required to assess which women are most likely to benefit from this therapy as well as when treatment is optimally started and what dose to use.[28] Several studies evaluated the efficacy of aspirin in the prevention of preeclampsia in high-risk pregnancies as determined by Doppler ultrasound or other risk factors when aspirin was used early in pregnancy. A meta-analysis suggested that low-dose aspirin improves pregnancy outcome in these women when aspirin is started before 16 weeks' gestation. However, this review has numerous flaws in design and data analysis. **A large multicenter National Institute of Child Health and Human Development–sponsored study that included 2539 women with pregestational insulin-treated diabetes mellitus, chronic hypertension, multifetal gestation, or preeclampsia in a previous pregnancy showed no beneficial effect from low-dose aspirin in such high-risk women** (Table 35-5).[13] **Some authors recommend that aspirin use should be based on individualized risk assessment for preeclampsia. However, the available data do not support such a recommendation.**

Vitamins C and E

Reduced antioxidant capacity, increased oxidative stress, or both in the maternal circulation and in the placenta have been proposed to play a major role in the pathogenesis of preeclampsia. Consequently, several trials were designed using vitamins C and E for the prevention of preeclampsia. The first trial suggested a beneficial effect from pharmacologic doses of vitamins E and C in women identified as being at risk for preeclampsia by means of abnormal uterine Doppler flow velocimetry. However, the study had limited sample size and must be confirmed in other populations. **In contrast, several randomized trials with large sample size in women at low risk and very high risk for preeclampsia found no reduction in the rate of preeclampsia with vitamins C and E supplementation (Table 35-6).**[29]

Laboratory Abnormalities in Preeclampsia

Women with preeclampsia may exhibit a symptom complex ranging from minimal BP elevation to derangements of multiple-organ systems. The renal, hematologic, and hepatic systems are most likely to be involved.

Renal Function

Renal plasma flow and glomerular filtration rate (GFR) increase during normal pregnancy. These changes are responsible for a fall in serum creatinine, urea, and uric acid concentrations.[78] In preeclampsia, vasospasm and glomerular capillary endothelial swelling (glomerular endotheliosis) lead to an average reduction in GFR of 25%

TABLE 35-5 LOW-DOSE ASPIRIN IN HIGH-RISK WOMEN: NICHD TRIAL

ENTRY CRITERIA	NO. OF WOMEN	ASPIRIN*	PREECLAMPSIA (%) PLACEBO*
Normotensive and no proteinuria	1613	14.5	17.7
Proteinuria and hypertension	119	31.7	22.0
Proteinuria only	48	25.0	33.3
Hypertension only	723	24.8	25.0
Insulin-dependent diabetes	462	18.3	21.6
Chronic hypertension	763	26.0	24.6
Multifetal gestation	678	11.5	15.9
Previous preeclampsia	600	16.7	19.0

Data from Caritis SN, Sibai BM, Hauth J, et al, for the National Institute of Child Health and Human Development: Low-dose aspirin therapy to prevent preeclampsia in women at high risk. N Engl J Med 338:701, 1998.

*No difference for any of the groups.

NICHD, National Institute of Child Health and Human Development.

below the rate for normal pregnancy. Serum creatinine is rarely elevated in preeclampsia, but uric acid can be increased. In a study of 95 women with severe preeclampsia, Sibai and associates reported a mean serum creatinine of 0.91 mg/dL, a mean uric acid of 6.6 mg/dL, and a mean creatinine clearance of 100 mL/minute.

The clinical significance of elevated uric acid levels in preeclampsia-eclampsia has been confusing. Hyperuricemia is associated with renal dysfunction, especially decreased renal tubular secretion, and has been consistently associated with glomerular endotheliosis. In addition, it has been linked with increased oxidative stress in preeclampsia. **Despite the fact that uric acid levels are elevated in women with preeclampsia, this test is not sensitive or specific for the diagnosis of preeclampsia or for predicting adverse perinatal outcome.**

Elevated uric acid levels above 6 mg/dL are often found in women with normotensive multifetal pregnancies. As a result, some authors suggested that to secure a diagnosis of preeclampsia based on elevated uric acid values, the upper limit should be adjusted for those with multiple gestation. Elevated uric acid values are also found in women with acute fatty liver of pregnancy and underlying renal disease. It is suggested that uric acid values not be used as an indication for delivery in women with preeclampsia.

Hepatic Function

The liver is not primarily involved in preeclampsia, and hepatic involvement is observed in only 10% of women with severe preeclampsia. Fibrin deposition has been found along the walls of hepatic sinusoids in preeclamptic patients with no laboratory or histologic evidence of liver involvement. When liver dysfunction does occur in preeclampsia, mild elevation of serum transaminases is most common. Bilirubin is rarely increased in preeclampsia, but when elevated, the indirect fraction predominates. Elevated liver enzymes are part of the of HELLP syndrome, a variant of severe preeclampsia.

Hematologic Changes

Many studies have evaluated the hematologic abnormalities in women with preeclampsia. Plasma fibrinopeptide-A, D-dimer levels, and circulating thrombin-antithrombin complexes are higher in women with preeclampsia than in normotensive gravidas. In contrast, plasma antithrombin III activity is decreased. These findings indicate enhanced thrombin generation.

Plasma fibrinogen rises progressively during normal pregnancy. In general, plasma fibrinogen levels are rarely reduced in women with preeclampsia in the absence of abruptio placentae.

Thrombocytopenia is the most common hematologic abnormality in women with severe preeclampsia. It is correlated with the severity of the disease process and the presence or absence of abruptio placentae. In a study of 1414 women with hypertension during pregnancy, Burrows and Kelton found a platelet count of less than 150,000/mm^3 in 15% of cases.

Leduc and associates studied the coagulation profile (platelet count, fibrinogen, prothrombin time, and partial thromboplastin time) in 100 consecutive women with severe preeclampsia. A platelet count lower than 150,000/mm^3 was found in 50% and a count lower than 100,000/mm^3 in 36% of the women. Thirteen women had a fibrinogen level of less than 300 mg/dL, and two had prolonged prothrombin and partial thromboplastin times as well as thrombocytopenia on admission. They found the admission platelet count to be an excellent predictor of subsequent thrombocytopenia and concluded that fibrinogen levels, prothrombin time, and partial thromboplastin time should be obtained only in women with a platelet count of less than 100,000/mm^3. A recent study by Barron confirmed these observations in more than 800 women with hypertension in pregnancy.

HELLP Syndrome

There is considerable debate regarding the definition, diagnosis, incidence, etiology, and management of HELLP syndrome.[85] Patients with such findings were previously described by many investigators. Weinstein considered it a unique variant of preeclampsia and coined the term HELLP syndrome for this entity. Barton and associates performed liver biopsies in patients with preeclampsia and HELLP syndrome. Periportal necrosis and hemorrhage were the most common histopathologic findings. In addition, they found that the extent of the laboratory abnormalities in HELLP syndrome, including the platelet count and liver enzymes, did not correlate with hepatic histopathologic findings.

Laboratory Criteria for Diagnosis

Various diagnostic criteria have been used for HELLP. Hemolysis, defined as the presence of microangiopathic hemolytic anemia, is the hallmark of the triad of HELLP syndrome.[85] The classic findings of microangiopathic

TABLE 35-6 Multicenter Trials of Vitamin C and E for the Prevention of Preeclampsia

STUDY GROUP	ENROLLMENT WOMEN	GESTATIONAL AGE (wk)	PREECLAMPSIA	
			Vitamins C and E (%)	Placebo (%)
ACTS[101]	Nulliparas	14-22	56/935 (6)	47/942 (5)
VIP[102]	High-risk	14-22	181/1196 (15)	187/1199 (16)
Global Network[103]	High-risk	12-20	49/355 (14)	55/352 (16)
WHO[104]	High-risk	14-22	164/681 (24)	157/674 (23)
NICHD[105]	Nulliparas	9-16	358/4993 (7.2)	332/4976 (6.7)
INTAPP[106]	High-risk	12-18	69/1167 (6)	68/1196 (5.7)
DAPIT[29]	Pregestational diabetes	8-22	57/375 (15)	70/3784 (19)

hemolysis include abnormal peripheral smear (schistocytes, burr cells, echinocytes), elevated serum bilirubin (indirect form), low serum haptoglobin levels, elevated lactate dehydrogenase (LDH) levels, and significant drop in hemoglobin levels. A significant percentage of published reports included patients who had no evidence of hemolysis; hence, these patients will fit the criteria for HELLP syndrome.[85] In some studies in which hemolysis is described, the diagnosis is suspect because it has been based on the presence of an abnormal peripheral smear (no description of type or degree of abnormalities) or elevated LDH levels (threshold of 180 to 600 U/L).

There is no consensus in the literature regarding the liver function test to be used or the degree of elevation in these tests to diagnose elevated liver enzymes.[85] In his original report, Weinstein mentioned abnormal serum levels of aspartate transaminase (AST), abnormal alanine transaminase (ALT), and abnormal bilirubin values; however, specific levels were not suggested. In subsequent studies in which elevated liver enzymes were described (either AST or ALT), the values considered to be abnormal ranged from 17 to 72 U/L.[85] In clinical practice, many of these values are considered normal or slightly elevated.

Low platelet count is the third abnormality required to establish the diagnosis of HELLP syndrome. There is no consensus among various published reports regarding the diagnosis of thrombocytopenia. The reported cut-off values have ranged from 75,000/mm^3 to 279,000/mm^3, with a level of less than 100,000/mm^3 being most often cited.[85]

Many authors have used elevated total LDH (usually >600 U/L) as a diagnostic criteria for hemolysis. There are five different isoforms of LDH, and only two of them, LDH_1 and LDH_2, are released from ruptured red blood cells. In most women with severe preeclampsia-eclampsia, the elevation in total LDH is probably caused mostly by liver ischemia. Therefore, many authors advocate that elevated bilirubin values (indirect form), abnormal peripheral smear, or a low serum haptoglobin level should be part of the diagnostic criteria for hemolysis.

Based on a retrospective review of 302 cases of HELLP syndrome, Martin and colleagues devised the following classification based on the nadir of the platelet count. Class I HELLP syndrome was defined as a platelet nadir below 50,000/mm^3, class 2 as a platelet nadir between 50,000 and 100,000/mm^3, and class 3 as a platelet nadir between 100,000 and 150,000/mm^3. These classes have been used to predict the rapidity of recovery postpartum, maternal-perinatal outcome, and the need for plasmapheresis.

Hemolysis, defined as the presence of microangiopathic hemolytic anemia, is the hallmark of HELLP syndrome. The role of disseminated intravascular coagulation (DIC) in preeclampsia is controversial. **Most authors do not regard HELLP syndrome to be a variant of DIC because coagulation parameters such as prothrombin time, partial thromboplastin time, and serum fibrinogen are normal.**[85] However, the diagnosis of DIC can be difficult to establish in clinical practice. When sensitive determinants of this condition are used, such as antithrombin III, fibrinopeptide-A, fibrin monomer, D-dimer, α_2-antiplasmin, plasminogen, prekallikrein, and fibronectin, many patients have laboratory values consistent with DIC. Unfortunately, these tests are time consuming and not suitable for routine monitoring. Consequently, less sensitive parameters are often employed. Sibai and associates defined DIC as the presence of thrombocytopenia, low fibrinogen levels (plasma fibrinogen <300 mg/dL), and fibrin split products above 40 mg/mL. These authors noted the presence of DIC in 21% of 442 patients with HELLP syndrome. They also found that most cases occurred in women who had antecedent abruptio placentae or peripartum hemorrhage and in all four women who had subcapsular liver hematomas. In the absence of these complications, the frequency of DIC was only 5%.

In view of the previously mentioned diagnostic problems, we recommended that uniform and standardized laboratory values be used to diagnose HELLP syndrome.[85] Plasma haptoglobin and bilirubin values should be included in the diagnosis of hemolysis. In addition, the degree of abnormality of liver enzymes should be defined as a certain number of standard deviations from the normal value for each hospital population. Our laboratory criteria to establish the diagnosis are presented in the box, Criteria to Establish the Diagnosis of HELLP Syndrome.

Criteria to Establish the Diagnosis of HELLP Syndrome

- Hemolysis (as least two of these):
  - Peripheral smear (schistocytes, burr cells)
  - Serum bilirubin (≥1.2 mg/dL)
  - Low serum haptoglobin
- Severe anemia, unrelated to blood loss
- Elevated liver enzymes
  - Aspartate transaminase (AST) or alanine transaminase (ALT) ≥ twice upper level or normal
  - Lactate dehydrogenase ≥ twice upper level or normal
- Low platelets (<100,000/mm^3)
- HELLP (hemolysis, elevated liver enzymes, and low platelets) syndrome

Clinical Findings

The reported incidence of HELLP syndrome in preeclampsia has been variable, reflecting the differences in diagnostic criteria. The syndrome appears to be more common in white women and is also more common in preeclamptic women who have been managed conservatively.[85]

Early detection of HELLP syndrome can be a challenge in that many women present with nonspecific symptoms or subtle signs of preeclampsia. The various signs and symptoms reported are not diagnostic of preeclampsia and may also be found in women with severe preeclampsia-eclampsia without HELLP syndrome.[85] Right upper quadrant or epigastric pain and nausea or vomiting have been reported with a frequency ranging from 30% to 90% (Table 35-7). Most women gave a history of malaise typical of a nonspecific viral-like syndrome for several days before presentation, which led one investigator to suggest performing laboratory investigations (completed blood count and liver enzymes) in all pregnant women with suspected preeclampsia having these symptoms during the third trimester.[85] Headaches are reported by 33% to 61% of the patients, whereas visual changes are reported in about 17%. A small subset of patients with HELLP syndrome may present with symptoms related to thrombocytopenia, such as bleeding from mucosal surfaces, hematuria, petechial hemorrhages, or ecchymosis.

TABLE 35-7 SIGNS AND SYMPTOMS IN WOMEN WITH HELLP SYNDROME

	WEINSTEIN (n = 57) (%)	SIBAI ET AL. (n = 509) (%)	MARTIN ET AL. (n = 501) (%)	RATH ET AL. (n = 50) (%)
Right upper quadrant epigastric pain	86	63	40	90
Nausea, vomiting	84	36	29	52
Headache	NR	33	61	NR
Hypertension	NR	85	82	88
Proteinuria	96	87	86	100

Modified from Sibai BM: Diagnosis, controversies, and management of HELLP syndrome. Obstet Gynecol 103:981, 2004.
HELLP, Hemolysis, elevated liver enzymes, and low platelets; *NR,* not reported.

Although most patients have hypertension (82% to 88%, see Table 35-7), it may be only mild in 15% to 50% of the cases and absent in 12% to 18%. Most of the patients (86 to 100%) have proteinuria by dipstick examination, although it has been reported to be absent in 13% of cases.

DIFFERENTIAL DIAGNOSIS

The presenting symptoms, clinical findings, and many of the laboratory findings in women with HELLP syndrome overlap with a number of medical syndromes, surgical conditions, and obstetrical complications. Therefore, the differential diagnosis of HELLP syndrome should include any of the conditions listed (see box, Medical and Surgical Disorders Often Confused with HELLP Syndrome). Because some women with HELLP syndrome may present with gastrointestinal, respiratory, or hematologic symptoms in association with elevated liver enzymes or low platelets in the absence of hypertension or proteinuria, many initially are misdiagnosed as having other conditions such as upper respiratory infection, hepatitis, cholecystitis, pancreatitis, acute fatty liver of pregnancy (AFLP), or immune thrombocytopenic purpura (ITP).[85] Conversely, some women with other conditions such as TTP, HUS, systemic lupus erythematosus, sepsis, or catastrophic antiphospholipid antibody syndrome may be erroneously diagnosed as having HELLP syndrome. In addition, preeclampsia may occasionally be superimposed on one of these disorders, further contributing to the diagnostic difficulty. Because of the remarkably similar clinical and laboratory findings of these disease processes, even the most experienced clinician can face a difficult diagnostic challenge. Therefore, efforts should be made to attempt to identify an accurate diagnosis, given that management strategies may be different among these conditions. It is important to emphasize that affected women may have a variety of unusual signs and symptoms, none of which are diagnostic of severe preeclampsia. Pregnant women with probable preeclampsia presenting with atypical symptoms should have a complete blood count, a platelet count, and liver enzyme determinations irrespective of maternal BP findings.

Occasionally, the presence of this syndrome is associated with hypoglycemia, leading to coma, severe hyponatremia, and cortical blindness. A rare but interesting complication of HELLP syndrome is transient nephrogenic diabetes insipidus. Unlike central diabetes insipidus, which results from the diminished or absent secretion of arginine vasopressin by the hypothalamus, transient nephrogenic diabetes insipidus is characterized by a resistance to arginine vasopressin mediated by excessive vasopressinase. It is postulated that elevated circulating vasopressinase may result from impaired hepatic metabolism of the enzyme.

MEDICAL AND SURGICAL DISORDERS OFTEN CONFUSED WITH HELLP SYNDROME

- Acute fatty liver of pregnancy
- Appendicitis
- Gallbladder disease
- Glomerulonephritis
- Hemolytic uremic syndrome
- Hepatic encephalopathy
- Hyperemesis gravidarum
- Idiopathic thrombocytopenia
- Pyelonephritis
- Systemic lupus erythematosus
- Antiphospholipid antibody syndrome
- Thrombotic thrombocytopenic purpura
- Viral hepatitis
- HELLP (hemolysis, elevated liver enzymes, and low platelets) syndrome

MANAGEMENT OF HELLP SYNDROME

Management of preeclamptic women presenting with HELLP syndrome is highly controversial.[85] Consequently, there are several therapeutic modalities described in the literature to treat or reverse HELLP syndrome. Most of these modalities are similar to those used in the management of severe preeclampsia remote from term (see box, Therapeutic Modalities Used to Treat or Reverse HELLP Syndrome).

THERAPEUTIC MODALITIES USED TO TREAT OR REVERSE HELLP SYNDROME

- Plasma volume expansion
  - Bedrest
  - Crystalloids
  - Albumin 5% to 25%
- Antithrombotic agents
  - Low-dose aspirin
  - Dipyridamole
  - Heparin
  - Antithrombin III
- Immunosuppressive agents
  - Steroids
- Miscellaneous
  - Fresh-frozen plasma infusions
  - Exchange plasmapheresis
  - Dialysis
- HELLP (hemolysis, elevated liver enzymes, and low platelets) syndrome

Modified from Sibai BM: The HELLP syndrome (hemolysis, elevated liver enzymes, and low platelets): much ado about nothing? Am J Obstet Gynecol 162:311, 1990.

The clinical course of women with true HELLP syndrome is usually characterized by progressive and sometimes sudden deterioration in the maternal condition.[85] Because the presence of this syndrome has been associated with increased rates of maternal morbidity and mortality, many authors consider its presence to be an indication for immediate delivery. **There is also a consensus of opinion that prompt delivery is indicated if the syndrome develops beyond 34 weeks' gestation or earlier if there is obvious multiorgan dysfunction, DIC, liver infarction or hemorrhage, renal failure, suspected abruptio placentae, or nonreassuring fetal status.**[85]

On the other hand, there is considerable disagreement about the management of women with HELLP syndrome at or before 34 weeks of gestation in whom maternal condition is stable, except for mild to moderate abnormalities in blood tests, and fetal condition is reassuring. In such patients, some authors recommend the administration of corticosteroids to accelerate fetal lung maturity followed by delivery after 24 hours,[85] whereas others recommend prolonging pregnancy until the development of maternal or fetal indications for delivery or until achievement of fetal lung maturity. Some of the measures used in these latter cases have included one or more of the following: bedrest, antihypertensive agents, antithrombotic agents (low-dose aspirin, dipyridamole), plasma volume expanders (crystalloids, albumin, fresh-frozen plasma), and steroids (prednisone, prednisolone, dexamethasone, or betamethasone).[85]

Expectant Management of HELLP Syndrome

There are few large case series describing expectant management of women with true HELLP, partial HELLP, or severe preeclampsia with isolated liver enzymes elevation. In general, these reports suggest that transient improvement in laboratory values or pregnancy prolongation from a few days to a few weeks is possible in a select group of women with HELLP syndrome. It is important to note that most of the patients included in these studies were ultimately delivered within 1 week of expectant management.[85]

Investigators from the Netherlands have reported their experience with expectant management in women with HELLP syndrome before 34 weeks' gestation. Visser and Wallenburg reported the use of plasma volume expansion using invasive hemodynamic monitoring and vasodilators in 128 women with HELLP syndrome before 34 weeks' gestation. Magnesium sulfate and steroids were not used in such women. Twenty-two of the 128 patients were delivered within 48 hours; the remaining 102 patients had pregnancy prolongation for a median of 15 days (range, 3 to 62 days). Fifty-five of these 102 women had antepartum resolution of HELLP syndrome, with a median pregnancy prolongation in these women of 21 days (range, 7 to 62 days). There were no maternal deaths or serious maternal morbidity. However, 11 (8.6%) resulted in fetal death at 25 to 34.4 weeks, and there were 7 (5.5%) neonatal deaths at 27 to 32 weeks' gestation.

Van Pampus and coworkers reported the use of bedrest, antihypertensive medication, and salt restriction in 41 women with HELLP syndrome before 35 weeks' gestation. Fourteen women (34%) were delivered within 24 hours; in the remaining 27 women, pregnancy was prolonged a median of 3 days (range, 0 to 59 days). Fifteen of these 27 women showed complete normalization of the laboratory abnormalities. There were no serious maternal morbidities; however, there were 10 fetal deaths at 27 to 35.7 weeks' gestation.

The study by Ganzevoort and colleagues included 54 women with HELLP syndrome at the time of enrollment. In a subsequent publication, the same authors compared maternal and perinatal complications in these women to the respective outcomes in women without HELLP. They found that the median days of pregnancy prolongation and maternal and perinatal complications were similar between the two groups.

There is one randomized, double-blind trial comparing prednisolone ($n = 15$) to a placebo ($n = 16$) in patients with HELLP syndrome before 30 weeks' gestation. Prednisolone was given intravenously twice a day. The primary outcome measures were the entry-to-delivery interval and the number of "recurrent HELLP" exacerbations in the antepartum period. The mean entry-to-delivery interval was similar between the two groups (6.9 days for prednisolone and 8 days for placebo). There were three cases of liver hematoma or rupture, with one maternal death in the placebo group. The perinatal mortality rate was similar between the two groups (20% in the prednisolone group and 25% in the placebo group).

The results of these studies suggest that expectant management is possible in a very select group of women with suspected HELLP syndrome before 34 weeks' gestation. However, despite pregnancy prolongation in some of these cases, the overall perinatal outcome was not improved compared with fetuses at a similar gestational age who were delivered within 48 hours after the diagnosis of HELLP syndrome.

Confounding variables make it difficult to evaluate any treatment modality proposed for this syndrome. Occasionally, some patients without true HELLP syndrome may demonstrate antepartum reversal of hematologic abnormalities following bedrest, the use of steroids, or plasma volume expansion. However, most of these patients experience deterioration in either maternal or fetal condition within 1 to 10 days after conservative management. It is doubtful that such limited pregnancy prolongation will result in improved perinatal outcome, and maternal and fetal risks are substantial.[85]

In summary, the results of these studies suggest that expectant treatment is possible in a select group of women with HELLP syndrome before 34 weeks' gestation. However, the number of women who were studied in these reports is inadequate to evaluate maternal safety. Therefore, such treatment should be considered experimental. In addition, most experts recommend delivery of such patients after completion of a course of corticosteroids for fetal lung maturity.[85]

Corticosteroids to Improve Pregnancy Outcome in Women with HELLP Syndrome

It is well established that antenatal glucocorticoid therapy reduces neonatal complications and neonatal mortality in women with severe preeclampsia at 34 weeks' gestation or less. The recommended regimens of corticosteroids for

TABLE 35-8 MATERNAL COMPLICATIONS WITH DEXAMETHASONE VERSUS PLACEBO IN HELLP SYNDROME

	NO. WITH PLACEBO (%)	NO. WITH DEXAMETHASONE (%)	CRUDE RELATIVE RISK (95% CONFIDENCE INTERVAL)
Acute renal failure*	8 (13)	6 (10)	0.8 (0.3-2.1)
Oliguria	4 (6)	5 (7.6)	1.3 (0.4-4.5)
Pulmonary edema*	1 (2)	3 (4.6)	3.1 (0.3-28)
Eclampsia	10 (15)	8 (14)	0.8 (0.3-1.9)
Infections	10 (15)	5(8)	0.5 (0.2-1.4)
Death	1 (2)	3 (5)	3.0 (0.3-28)
Platelet transfusion	10 (15)	12 (18)	1.2 (0.6-2.6)
Plasma transfusion	6 (9)	5 (8)	0.8 (0.3-2.6)

Modified from Fonseca JE, Mendez F, Catano C, Arias F: Dexamethasone treatment does not improve the outcome of women with HELLP syndrome: a double-blind, placebo-controlled, randomized clinical trial. Am J Obstet Gynecol 193:1591-1598, 2005.
*Only included patients without the event before randomization.

the enhancement of fetal maturity are betamethasone (12 mg intramuscularly every 24 hours, two doses) or dexamethasone (6 mg intramuscularly every 12 hours, four doses). These regimens have been identified as the most appropriate for this purpose because they readily cross the placenta and have minimal mineralocorticoid activity. However, it is unclear whether the same or different regimens are beneficial in women with HELLP syndrome.

Corticosteroids have been suggested as safe and effective drugs for improving maternal and neonatal outcome in women with HELLP or partial HELLP syndrome. A review of the literature reveals substantial differences in methodology, time of administration, and drug selection among investigators who advocate the use of corticosteroids in women with HELLP syndrome. Different regimens of steroids have been suggested for preventing respiratory distress syndrome (RDS) as well as to accelerate maternal recovery in the postpartum period.[85] The regimens of steroids used included intramuscular betamethasone (12 mg/12 hours or 24 hours apart on two occasions) or intravenous dexamethasone (various doses at various time intervals) or a combination of the two. Some studies used steroids only in the antepartum period (for 24 hours, 48 hours, repeat regimens, or chronically for weeks until delivery). In other studies, steroids were given for 48 hours before delivery and then continued for 24 to 48 hours postpartum, whereas others recommend their administration only in the postpartum period.[85]

There are randomized trials comparing the use of high-dose dexamethasone to either no treatment or betamethasone in women with presumed HELLP syndrome. These studies were summarized in a recent review by Sibai.[85] The results of these studies demonstrated improved laboratory values and urine output in patients receiving dexamethasone but no differences in serious maternal morbidity. In addition, the number of patients studied was limited, and neither of these small studies used a placebo.[85]

More recently, three randomized, double-blind placebo trials were conducted evaluating dexamethasone versus placebo in women with antepartum and postpartum HELLP syndrome. Two of the trials were multicenter, and one was a single center. The results of the two large multicenter trials are summarized in Tables 35-8 and 35-9. Overall, these trials revealed no maternal benefit of using dexamethasone in women with HELLP syndrome.

TABLE 35-9 MATERNAL COMPLICATIONS COMPARING DEXAMETHASONE VERSUS PLACEBO FOR POSTPARTUM HELLP SYNDROME

COMPLICATION*	DEXAMETHASONE (*n* = 56)		PLACEBO (*n* = 49)	
	n	%	*n*	%
Pulmonary edema	2	3.6	5	10.2
Hemorrhagic manifestation	20	35.7	16	32.7
Acute renal failure	9	16.1	12	24.5
Oliguria	27	48.2	22	44.9
Blood transfusion	16	28.6	19	38.6
Any complication	37	66.1	25	51
Death	2	3.6	2	4.1

Modified from Katz L, de Amorim MM, Figueiroa JN, Pinto e Silva JL: Postpartum dexamethasone for women with hemolysis, elevated liver enzymes, and low platelets (HELLP) syndrome: a double-blind, placebo-controlled, randomized clinical trial. Am J Obstet Gynecol 198:283, 2008.
*Each patient may have more than one complication.

MATERNAL AND PERINATAL OUTCOME

The presence of HELLP syndrome is associated with an increased risk for maternal death (1%)[85] and increased rates of maternal morbidities such as pulmonary edema (8%), acute renal failure (3%), DIC (15%), abruptio placentae (9%), liver hemorrhage or failure (1%), acute respiratory distress syndrome (ARDS), sepsis, and stroke (<1%).[85] Pregnancies complicated by HELLP syndrome are also associated with increased rates of wound hematomas and the need for transfusion of blood and blood products.[85] The rate of these complications depends on the population studied, the laboratory criteria used to establish the diagnosis, and the presence of associated preexisting medical conditions (chronic hypertension, lupus), or obstetrical complications (abruptio placentae, peripartum hemorrhage, fetal demise, eclampsia).[85] The development of HELLP syndrome in the postpartum period also increases the risk for renal failure and pulmonary edema. The presence of abruptio placentae increases the risk for DIC, need for blood transfusions, pulmonary edema, and renal failure. Patients who have a large volume of ascites appear to have a high rate of cardiopulmonary complications. Finally, women who meet all the criteria suggested for diagnosis will have higher rates of maternal complications than those who have partial HELLP or elevated liver enzymes only (Table 35-10).

TABLE 35-10 MATERNAL COMPLICATIONS IN 316 PREGNANCIES WITH HELLP SYNDROME, PARTIAL HELLP SYNDROME, OR SEVERE PREECLAMPSIA WITH NORMAL LABORATORY VALUES

	HELLP (*n* = 67)	PARTIAL HELLP (*n* = 71)	SEVERE (*n* = 178)
Blood products transfusion (%)	25*	4	3
Disseminated intravascular coagulation (%)	15*	0	0
Wound hematoma, infection (%)†	14‡	11§	2§
Pleural effusion (%)	6‡	0	1
Acute renal failure (%)	3‡	0	0
Eclampsia (%)	9	7	9
Abruptio placentae (%)	9	4	5
Pulmonary edema (%)	8	4	3
Subcapsular liver hematoma (%)	1.5	0	0
Intracerebral hemorrhage (%)	1.5	0	0
Death (%)	1.5	0	0

From Audibert F, Friedman SA, Frangieh AY, Sibai BM: Clinical utility of strict diagnostic criteria for the HELLP (hemolysis, elevated liver enzymes, and low platelets) syndrome. Am J Obstet Gynecol 175:460, 1996.
*P <.001, HELLP vs. partial HELLP and severe.
†Percentages of women who had cesarean delivery.
‡P <.05, HELLP vs. severe.
§P <.05, partial HELLP vs. severe.
HELLP, Hemolysis, elevated liver enzymes, and low platelets.

There is general agreement that perinatal mortality and morbidities are substantially increased in pregnancies complicated by the HELLP syndrome. The reported perinatal death rate in recent series ranged from 7.4% to 34%.[85] This high perinatal death rate is mainly experienced at very early gestational age (<28 weeks), in association with severe FGR or abruptio placentae.[85] It is important to emphasize that neonatal morbidities in these pregnancies are dependent on gestational age at time of delivery, and they are similar when corrected for gestational age to those in preeclamptic pregnancies without the HELLP syndrome. The rate of preterm delivery is about 70%, with 15% occurring before 28 weeks' gestation. As a result, these infants have a high rate of acute neonatal complications.

The HELLP syndrome may develop antepartum or postpartum. Analysis of 442 cases studied by Sibai and associates revealed that 309 (70%) had evidence of the syndrome antepartum, whereas 133 (30%) developed the condition postpartum. There were four maternal deaths, and morbidity was frequent (Table 35-11).

In the postpartum period, the time of onset of the manifestations may range from a few hours to 7 days, most developing within 48 hours postpartum. Thus, **laboratory assessment for potential HELLP syndrome should be considered during the first 48 hours postpartum in women with significant hypertension or symptoms of severe preeclampsia.** Eighty percent of the women who develop HELLP syndrome postpartum have had preeclampsia before delivery, whereas 20% had no evidence of preeclampsia either antepartum or intrapartum. It is the author's experience that patients in this group are at increased risk for the development of pulmonary edema

TABLE 35-11 SERIOUS MATERNAL COMPLICATIONS IN 442 PATIENTS WITH HELLP SYNDROME

COMPLICATION	NO.	%
Disseminated intravascular coagulopathy	92	21
Abruptio placentae	69	16
Acute renal failure	33	8
Severe ascites	32	8
Pulmonary edema	26	6
Pleural effusions	26	6
Cerebral edema	4	1
Retinal detachment	4	1
Laryngeal edema	4	1
Subcapsular liver hematoma	4	1
Adult respiratory distress syndrome	3	1
Death, maternal	4	1

From Sibai BM, Ramadan MK, Usta I, et al: Maternal morbidity and mortality in 442 pregnancies with hemolysis, elevated liver enzymes, and low platelets (HELLP syndrome). Am J Obstet Gynecol 169:1000, 1993.
HELLP, Hemolysis, elevated liver enzymes, and low platelets.

and acute renal failure (Table 35-12). The differential diagnosis should include exacerbation of systemic lupus erythematosus, TTP, and HUS.

RECOMMENDED MANAGEMENT

The clinical course of women with HELLP syndrome is usually characterized by progressive and sometimes sudden deterioration in maternal and fetal condition. Therefore, **patients with a suspected diagnosis of HELLP syndrome should be hospitalized immediately and observed in a labor and delivery unit (Figure 35-4). Such patients should be managed as if they had severe preeclampsia and should initially receive intravenous magnesium sulfate as prophylaxis against convulsions and antihypertensive medications to maintain systolic BP below 160 mm Hg or diastolic BP below 105 mm Hg.**[85] This can be achieved with a 5-mg bolus dose of hydralazine, to be repeated as needed every 15 to 20 minutes for a maximal dose of 20 mg per hour. BP is recorded every 15 minutes during therapy and every hour once the desired values are achieved. If hydralazine does not lower BP adequately or if maternal side effects such as tachycardia or headaches develop, another agent such as labetalol or nifedipine can be used.

The recommended dose of labetalol is 20 to 40 mg given intravenously every 10 to 15 minutes for a maximum of 220 mg, and the dose of nifedipine is 10 to 20 mg orally every 30 minutes for a maximum dose of 50 mg. During the observation period, maternal and fetal conditions should be followed carefully.

The recommended regimen of magnesium sulfate is a loading dose of 6 g given over 20 minutes, followed by a maintenance dose of 2 g per hour as a continuous intravenous solution. Magnesium sulfate is initiated at the beginning of the observation period and then continued during labor and for at least 24 hours postpartum. In those with abnormal renal function (oliguria or serum creatinine ≥1.2 mg/dL), the dose of magnesium sulfate should be reduced and even discontinued.

Once the diagnosis of HELLP syndrome is confirmed, a decision must be made regarding the need for delivery (see Figure 35-4). Women with HELLP syndrome at less

TABLE 35-12 OUTCOME AND COMPLICATIONS OF HELLP SYNDROME IN RELATION TO TIME OF ONSET

	ANTEPARTUM ONSET (n = 309) (%)	POSTPARTUM ONSET (n = 133) (%)	RELATIVE RISK	95% CONFIDENCE INTERVAL
Delivery at <27 wk*	15	3	4.84	2.0-11.6
Delivery at 37-42 wk†	15	25	0.61	0.41-0.91
Pulmonary edema	5	9	0.50	0.24-1.05
Acute renal failure†	5	12	0.46	0.24-0.87
Eclampsia	7	10	0.73	0.38-1.40
Abruptio placentae	16	15	1.05	0.65-1.70
Disseminated intravascular coagulation	21	20	1.09	0.73-1.64

From Sibai BM, Ramadan MK, Usta I, et al: Maternal morbidity and mortality in 442 pregnancies with hemolysis, elevated liver enzymes, and low platelets (HELLP syndrome). Am J Obstet Gynecol 169:1000, 1993.
*P <.0007.
†P <.002.
HELLP, Hemolysis, elevated liver enzymes, and low platelets.

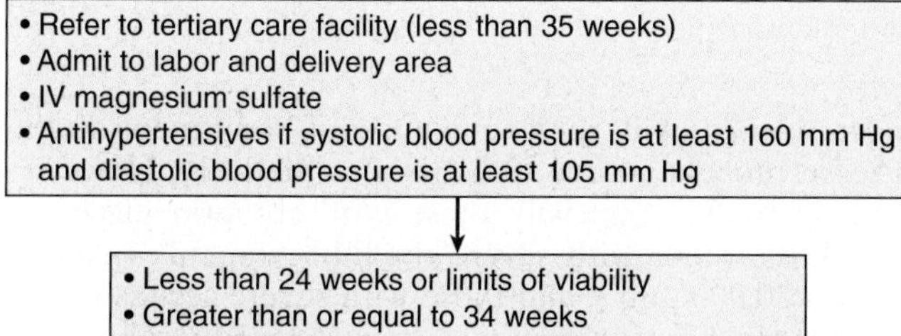

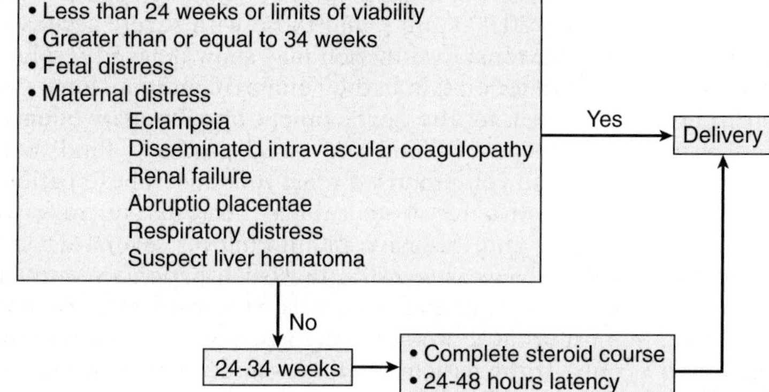

FIGURE 35-4. An algorithm for the management of HELLP syndrome.

than 35 weeks' gestation should be referred to a tertiary care facility if their condition is stable. The first priority is to assess and stabilize the maternal condition, particularly BP and coagulation abnormalities. The next step is to evaluate fetal status with the use of fetal heart rate monitoring, biophysical profile (BPP), or Doppler assessment of fetal vessels. Finally, a decision must be made as to whether delivery should be initiated or delivery could be delayed for 48 hours to allow the full benefit of corticosteroids. Thus, in practice, delivery is undertaken in all patients with true HELLP syndrome except in those with a gestational age between 24 to 34 weeks with stable maternal and fetal conditions. These latter patients are given betamethasone and are generally then delivered within 24 hours after the last dose of corticosteroids. Maternal and fetal conditions are assessed continuously during this time period. In some of these women, there may be transient improvement in maternal laboratory tests. However, delivery is still recommended despite such improvement.[85]

INTRAPARTUM MANAGEMENT

The presence of HELLP syndrome is not an indication for immediate cesarean delivery. Such an approach might prove detrimental for both mother and fetus. The decision to perform a cesarean delivery should be based on gestational age, fetal condition, the presence of labor, and the cervical Bishop score. Elective cesarean delivery is recommended for all women with HELLP syndrome before 30 weeks' gestation not in labor and with a Bishop score of less than 5. Elective cesarean delivery is also undertaken for those with HELLP syndrome complicated by FGR or oligohydramnios, particularly if the gestational age is less than 32 weeks in the presence of an unfavorable cervical Bishop score (Table 35-13).

Women having labor or rupture of membranes are allowed to deliver vaginally in the absence of obstetrical complications. When induction is indicated, it is initiated with either oxytocin infusion or prostaglandins in patients with a gestational age of more than 30 weeks, irrespective of the amount of cervical dilation or effacement. A similar approach is used for those at 30 weeks' gestation or less if the cervical Bishop score is at least 5.

Maternal pain relief during labor and delivery can be provided by intermittent use of small doses of systemic opioids. Local infiltration anesthesia can be used for all vaginal deliveries if an episiotomy or repair of a laceration is necessary. The use of a pudendal block is contraindicated in these patients because of the risk for bleeding and

TABLE 35-13 INDICATIONS AND MANAGEMENT DURING CESAREAN DELIVERY IN HELLP SYNDROME

- Indications for cesarean delivery
  - Non-reassuring fetal status
  - Abnormal fetal presentation
  - Gestation <30 weeks and Bishop score <5
  - Gestation <32 weeks with IUGR or oligohydramnios and Bishop score <5
  - Known subcapsular liver hematoma
  - Suspected abruptio placentae
- Management during cesarean delivery
  - General anesthesia for platelet count <75,000/mm^3
  - Transfuse 6 units of platelets if count <40,000/mm^3
  - Insert subfascial drain
  - Secondary skin closure or leave subcutaneous drain
- Observe for bleeding from upper abdomen before closure

HELLP, Hemolysis, elevated liver enzymes, and low platelets syndrome; IUGR, intrauterine growth restriction.

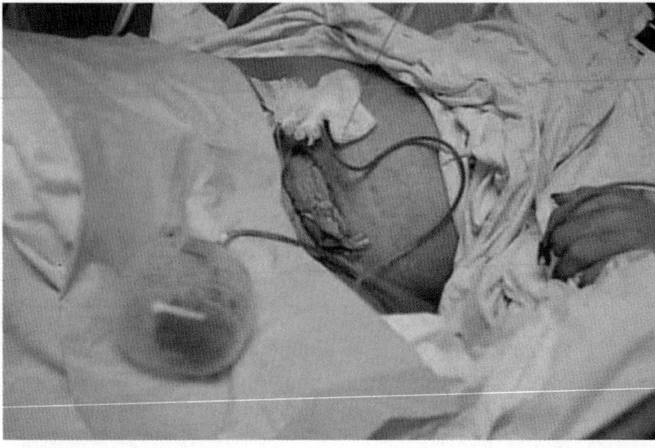

FIGURE 35-5. Subfascial drains used at time of cesarean section.

hematoma formation into this area. Epidural anesthesia is also contraindicated particularly if the platelet count is less than 75,000/mm^3. Therefore, general anesthesia is the method of choice for cesarean delivery in most thrombocytopenic women. O'Brien and coworkers assessed the impact of glucocorticoid administration on the use of epidural anesthesia in 37 women with partial HELLP syndrome who had a platelet count of less than 90,000/mm^3 before steroid administration. The authors found that administration of corticosteroids in these patients increased the use of epidural anesthesia, particularly in those who achieved a latency period of 24 hours before delivery (8 or 14 in steroid group vs. 0 or 10 in group without steroids; $P = .006$).

Platelet transfusions are indicated either before or after delivery in all patients with HELLP syndrome in the presence of significant bleeding (e.g., ecchymosis, bleeding from gums, oozing from puncture sites, wound, intraperitoneal) and in all those with a platelet count of less than 20,000/mm^3 (see Table 35-13). However, repeated platelet transfusions are not necessary because of the short half-life of the transfused platelets in such patients. Correction of thrombocytopenia is also important before any surgery. Administration of 6 units of platelets is recommended in all patients with a platelet count less than 40,000 to 50,000/mm^3 before intubation if cesarean delivery is needed. Generalized oozing from the incision site can occur during surgery or in the immediate postpartum period because of the continued drop in platelet count in some of these patients. The risk for hematoma formation at these sites is about 20%. Some individuals therefore prefer to use a vertical skin incision, whereas others employ a subfascial drain and keep the skin incision open for at least 48 hours in women requiring cesarean delivery (Figure 35-5).[85]

POSTPARTUM MANAGEMENT

After delivery, patients with HELLP syndrome should receive close monitoring of vital signs, fluid intake and output, laboratory values, and pulse oximetry for at least 48 hours. Intravenous magnesium sulfate prophylaxis is generally continued for 48 hours, and antihypertensive drugs are employed if the systolic BP is at least 155 mm Hg or if the diastolic BP is at least 105 mm Hg. In general, most women will show evidence of resolution of the disease process within 48 hours after delivery. However, some patients, especially those with abruptio placentae plus DIC, those with severe thrombocytopenia (platelet count <20,000/mm^3), and those with severe ascites or significant renal dysfunction may show delayed resolution or even deterioration in their clinical condition. Such patients are at risk for the development of pulmonary edema from transfusion of blood and blood products, fluid mobilization, and compromised renal function. These patients are also at risk for acute tubular necrosis and may require dialysis and intensive monitoring for several days. Some authors have suggested that such patients might benefit from plasmapheresis or plasma transfusions. In practice, most of these women will recover with supportive therapy only. **If the patient continues to deteriorate for more than 72 hours after delivery or shows improvement in laboratory values, and then starts to show thrombocytopenia and abnormal liver enzymes again, then a diagnosis of TTP/HUS should be considered. In such cases, plasmapheresis is indicated.**

The clinical and laboratory findings of HELLP syndrome may first appear during the postpartum period.[85] In these women, the time of onset of the manifestations ranges from a few hours to 7 days, with most developing within 48 hours postpartum.[85] Hence, all postpartum women and their health care providers should be educated and be aware of the signs and symptoms of HELLP syndrome. Management of patients with postpartum HELLP syndrome should be similar to that in the antepartum period, including the use of magnesium sulfate.

Hepatic Complications in HELLP Syndrome

Marked elevations in serum aminotransferases (>1000 to 2000 IU/L) are not typical of uncomplicated HELLP syndrome; however, when they occur, the possibility of hepatic infarction and subcapsular hematoma of the liver must be considered. The differential diagnosis should also include AFLP, abruptio placentae with DIC, acute cholecystitis with sepsis, viral hepatitis, and TTP. In addition to the signs and symptoms of preeclampsia, physical examination findings consistent with peritoneal irritation and hepatomegaly may be present.

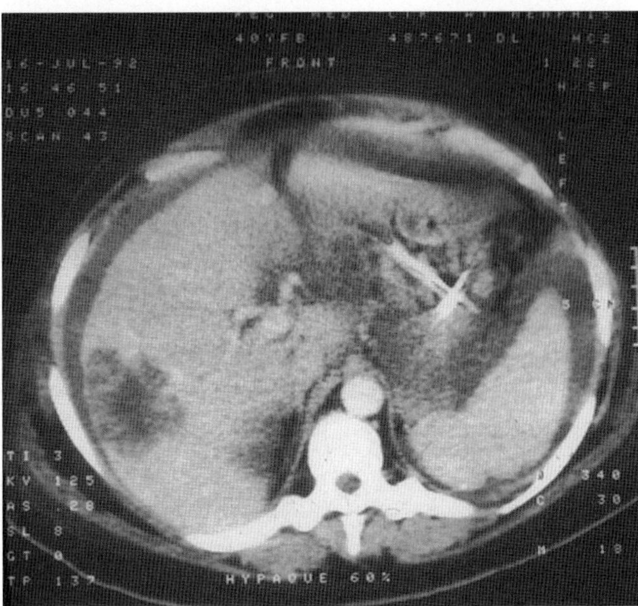

FIGURE 35-6. Computed tomography scan of the liver demonstrating hepatic infarct.

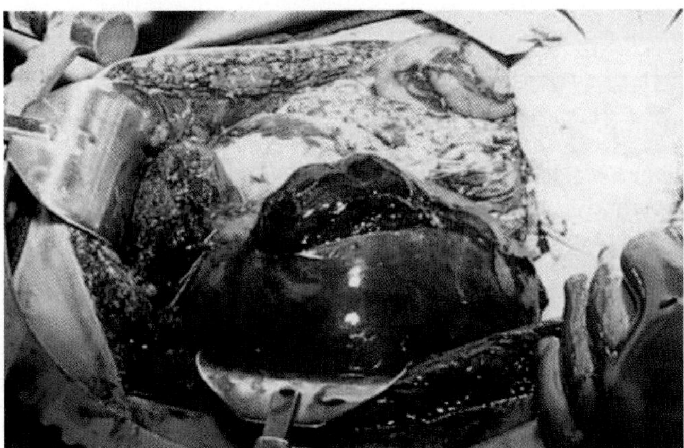

FIGURE 35-7. Subcapsular hematoma in patient with HELLP syndrome.

HEPATIC INFARCTION

Marked elevation in serum aminotransferases (usually 1000 to 2000 IU/L or higher) and LDH (usually 10,000 to 20,000 IU/L) associated with right upper quadrant pain and fever is characteristic of hepatic infarction; this diagnosis can be confirmed by hepatic imaging (Figure 35-6). Follow-up imaging after delivery typically demonstrates resolution of the infarcts. These women may have an underlying thrombophilia such as the antiphospholipid syndrome.[85]

HEPATIC HEMATOMA AND RUPTURE

HELLP syndrome may be complicated by hepatic rupture with the development of a hematoma beneath the Glisson capsule (Figure 35-7). Histology of the liver adjacent to the rupture shows periportal hemorrhage and fibrin deposition, along with a neutrophilic infiltrate suggestive of hepatic preeclampsia. The hematoma may remain contained, or rupture, with resulting hemorrhage into the peritoneal cavity. Women who develop a hepatic hematoma typically have abdominal pain and many have severe thrombocytopenia, shoulder pain, nausea, and vomiting. The aminotransferases are usually modestly elevated, but values of 4000 to 5000 IU/L can occasionally be seen. If hepatic rupture occurs, swelling of the abdomen from hemoperitoneum and shock rapidly ensue.

The management of a contained hematoma is to support the patient with volume replacement and blood transfusion, as needed, with consideration for percutaneous embolization of the hepatic arteries. If the size of the hematoma remains stable and the laboratory abnormalities are resolving, the patient may be discharged home with outpatient follow-up. It may take months for the hematoma to resolve completely.

Surgical repair has been recommended for hepatic hemorrhage without liver rupture. This complication, however, can be managed conservatively in patients who remain hemodynamically stable. Management should include close monitoring of hemodynamics and coagulation status. Serial assessment of the subcapsular hematoma with ultrasound or

Computed tomography (CT) is necessary, with immediate intervention for rupture or worsening of maternal status. It is important with conservative management to avoid exogenous sources of trauma to the liver, such as abdominal palpation, convulsions, or emesis, and to use care in transportation of the patient. Indeed, any sudden increase in intra-abdominal pressure could potentially lead to rupture of the subcapsular hematoma.

Rupture of a subcapsular hematoma of the liver is a life-threatening complication of HELLP syndrome. Profound hypovolemic shock in a previously hypertensive patient is the hallmark of rupture of hematoma. In most instances, rupture involves the right lobe and is preceded by the development of a parenchymal hematoma. Patients frequently present with shoulder pain, shock, or evidence of massive ascites, respiratory difficulty, or pleural effusions, and often with a dead fetus. Ultrasound or CT of the liver should be performed to rule out the presence of subcapsular hematoma of the liver and assess for the presence of intraperitoneal bleeding. Paracentesis can confirm intraperitoneal bleeding.

The presence of ruptured subcapsular liver hematoma resulting in shock is a surgical emergency requiring acute multidisciplinary treatment. Resuscitation should consist of massive transfusions of blood, correction of coagulopathy with fresh-frozen plasma and platelets, and immediate laparotomy.

A team experienced in liver trauma surgery should be consulted. If hepatic rupture is suspected, an incision in the upper abdomen is necessary for adequate surgical exposure. A lower abdominal midline incision can be extended superiorly. If a Pfannenstiel incision was used for operative delivery, a separate upper abdominal midline incision should be made to maximize visualization of the upper abdomen and liver. Options at laparotomy include packing and drainage, surgical ligation of the hemorrhaging hepatic segments, embolization of the hepatic artery to the involved liver segment, and loosely suturing omentum or surgical mesh to the liver to improve integrity.

Shrivastova and associates in a case report described the successful use of an argon-beam coagulator to obtain hemostasis from a ruptured liver hematoma in a patient with HELLP syndrome, although previous experience with this modality was unsuccessful. Even with appropriate treatment, maternal and fetal mortality is almost 50%. Mortality is most commonly associated with exsanguination with coagulopathy, and sepsis. Initial survivors are at increased risk for developing ARDS, pulmonary edema, liver failure, and acute renal failure in the postoperative period.

Reck and colleagues reviewed cases with HELLP syndrome–associated liver rupture (4 patients from their center in Germany and 49 identified from a MEDLINE literature search covering 1990 to 1999). Despite surgical interventions, HELLP syndrome–associated liver rupture carried a mortality rate of 39% (19 of 49) in their review. The main causes of death were hemorrhagic shock ($n = 11$) and multiorgan failure ($n = 7$). Based on their review, the authors suggested an interdisciplinary approach for patients with ruptured liver or hepatic failure, including the use of temporary packing of the liver to control bleeding. In those patients with hepatic failure or uncontrollable hepatic hemorrhage, they noted that a liver transplantation as a last resort measure must be considered.

Liver Transplantation for Intractable Hemorrhage

For women with intractable hemorrhage despite the previously described interventions and for those with necrosis with subsequent liver failure, liver transplantation has been successful in case reports and case series. Shames and colleagues queried the Organ Procurement and Transplantation Network database regarding liver transplantations performed for complications from HELLP syndrome. Eight deceased donor liver transplantations were identified in the United States with this indication between October 1987 and November 2003. At the time of their review, six of the eight patients were alive, whereas, two maternal deaths occurred within 1 month of transplantation. In addition, two patients required retransplantation. Based on the results of their review, these authors presented an algorithm in which liver transplantation is considered for patients with complicated HELLP syndrome, including ongoing, uncontrolled hemorrhage or liver necrosis and failure.

Zarrinpar and associates described eight women without a history of liver disease who underwent liver transplantation at their institution between February 1984 and December 2006 for complications of HELLP syndrome. All received cadaveric grafts with a mean interval from delivery to liver transplantation of 7 days. There were no deaths from intraoperative hematoma of the liver. There was one death from sepsis on postoperative day 19 and one death from cholangitis and sepsis more than 5 years after surgery. After liver transplantation, the Kaplan-Meier patient survival rates at 1, 5, and 10 years were 88%, 88%, and 65%, respectively; 1-, 5-, and 10-year graft survival rates were 64%, 64%, and 48%, respectively. Because of the very small number of available organs, death before transplantation is a concern. Marsh and associates suggest that potential candidates are only those in whom all other measures fail to control hemorrhage, or in whose liver has become devascularized such that there is no other alternative.

Table 35-14 Management of Patients with Documented Subcapsular Hematoma of the Liver

General Considerations

1. Inform the blood bank about the potential need for large amounts of packed red blood cells, fresh-frozen plasma, and platelet concentrate
2. Ensure consultation with a general or vascular surgeon
3. Avoid direct and indirect manipulation of the liver
4. Arrange for close monitoring of hemodynamic status
5. Intravenous magnesium sulfate to prevent seizures

Unruptured Hematoma

a. Conservative management
b. Correct coagulopathy
c. Serial computed tomography scans or ultrasound

Expanding or Ruptured Hematoma

a. Massive transfusions
b. Immediate laparotomy

Minimal Bleeding

a. Observation
b. Draining area with closed suction

Severe Bleeding

a. Application of laparotomy sponges as packs for pressure
b. Embolization of the hepatic artery to the involved liver segment
c. Surgical ligation of hemorrhaging hepatic segment
d. Loosely sutured omentum or surgical mesh to the liver to improve integrity
e. Argon beam coagulator to liver surface
f. Hepatic lobectomy
g. Hepatectomy and temporary portal caval shunt followed by liver transplantation

From our experience and review of the literature, we have developed a management plan of hepatic hematoma associated with HELLP syndrome. This plan emphasizes the potential for transfusion of large amounts of blood and blood products and the need for aggressive intervention if rupture of the hematoma is suspected (Table 35-14). We recommend 30 U of packed red blood cells, 20 U of fresh-frozen plasma, 30 to 50 U of platelets, and 20 to 30 U of cryoprecipitate be available if rupture of a subcapsular hematoma is suspected. **We agree with the observations of others that a stable patient with an unruptured subcapsular hematoma should be conservatively managed.** Constant monitoring must continue during this management, however, because patients can rapidly become unstable after rupture of the hematoma. Survival clearly is associated with rapid diagnosis and immediate medical or surgical stabilization so that these patients should be managed in an intensive care unit facility with close monitoring of hemodynamic parameters and fluid status to avoid the potential for pulmonary edema or respiratory compromise.

Postpartum follow-up for patients with subcapsular hematoma of the liver should include serial CT, magnetic resonance imaging (MRI), or ultrasonography until the defect resolves. Although the data on subsequent pregnancy outcome after a subcapsular hematoma of the liver in pregnancy are limited, we have managed three such patients who have had subsequent normal maternal and fetal outcomes, and Wust and coworkers reported the successful outcome of four subsequent pregnancies in three women with a history of hepatic rupture and preeclampsia or HELLP syndrome.

Hemodynamic Monitoring in Preeclampsia

The cardiovascular hemodynamics of preeclampsia have been investigated over the years by many authors using various techniques for measurement of BP, cardiac output, pulmonary capillary wedge pressure (PCWP), and central venous pressure (CVP).

Hemodynamic findings in women with preeclampsia remain controversial. A review of the English literature demonstrates considerable disagreement regarding one or more of the hemodynamic parameters studied. This lack of agreement has been attributed to differences in the definition of preeclampsia, variable severity and duration of the disease process, presence of underlying cardiac or renal disease, techniques used to measure cardiac output and BP, and therapeutic interventions applied before obtaining the various measurements. In addition, the dynamic minute-to-minute fluctuation of the cardiovascular parameters studied makes it difficult to standardize the conditions under which these observations are made, limiting the value of a single measurement.

Invasive techniques have been used by many authors to study the hemodynamic findings in untreated women with severe preeclampsia. The reported cardiac index ranged from a low of 2.8 to a high of 4.8 L/m^2 per minute, and the reported PCWP from a low of 3.3 to a high of 12 mm Hg. The findings suggest that cardiac index and PCWP are either low or normal in severe preeclampsia. The reported CVP values also ranged from 2 to 6 mm Hg.

The findings demonstrate that treated patients with preeclampsia have normal to high cardiac index, normal to high systemic vascular resistance index, and normal to high PCWP.

In summary, variable hemodynamic findings accompany preeclampsia. Moreover, the clinical utility of invasive hemodynamic monitoring in preeclampsia is debatable. Most of the invasive monitoring data indicate that both cardiac output and systemic vascular resistance appear to be elevated in women with severe preeclampsia. This finding suggests that the problem in preeclampsia is a systemic vascular resistance that is inappropriately high for the level of cardiac output. Both the PCWP and the CVP appear to be in the low to normal range; however, there is no correlation between the two values.

Antepartum Management of Mild Hypertension-Preeclampsia

Gestational Hypertension

Women with gestational hypertension are at risk for progression to severe hypertension, preeclampsia, or eclampsia.[5-8] The risks are increased with a lower gestational age at the time of diagnosis.[5-8] Therefore, these patients require close observation of maternal and fetal conditions. Maternal evaluations require weekly prenatal visits, education about reporting preeclamptic symptoms, and evaluation of complete blood count, platelet count, and liver enzymes.[1-3] Fetal evaluation includes ultrasound examination of fluid and estimated fetal weight at the time of diagnosis and weekly nonstress testing.[1,2] Restriction of dietary salt as well as physical activity has not proved beneficial in the management of these patients.[1,2] Additionally, **the results of several randomized trials reveal that control of maternal BP with antihypertensive drugs does not improve pregnancy outcome in women with gestational hypertension.**

In the absence of progression to severe hypertension or preeclampsia, women with gestational hypertension can continue pregnancy until 37 weeks' gestation. During labor and immediately postpartum, they do not require seizure prophylaxis because the rate of eclampsia in these women is less than 1 in 500.[2]

The HYPITAT trial was a multicenter, open-label randomized controlled trial conducted at 6 academic and 32 nonacademic hospitals in the Netherlands. It included 756 women with singleton pregnancy at a gestational age between $36^{0/7}$ weeks and $41^{0/7}$ weeks who had mild gestational hypertension (n = 496) or mild preeclampsia (n = 246); 377 were randomized to induction and 379 to expectant monitoring. The primary outcome was a composite of adverse maternal outcomes: progression to severe disease or HELLP syndrome, eclampsia, pulmonary edema, abruption placentae, postpartum hemorrhage, thromboembolic disease, or death. Secondary outcomes were a composite of adverse neonatal outcomes and rate of cesarean delivery. There were no cases of maternal, fetal, or neonatal death and no cases of eclampsia or abruption in either group. However, women randomized to the induction group had a significant reduction in the primary outcome, (31% versus 44%; RR, 0.71; 95% CI, 0.59 to 0.86). This reduction was mainly due to differences in the rates of severe hypertension. There were no differences in the overall secondary outcomes; however, subgroup analysis revealed significant differences in the primary outcomes in the group enrolled with mild preeclampsia (33% vs. 54%; RR, 0.61; 95% CI, 0.45 to 0.8), but not in those with mild gestational hypertension (31% vs. 38%; RR, 0.81; 95% CI, 0.63 to 1.03). Unfortunately, the sample size was inadequate to answer the question in those with mild gestational hypertension only. Moreover, in the induction group, the rate of cesarean delivery was lower in nulliparous women and in those with cervical Bishop score of less than 2, refuting the belief that induction of labor in these women increases the rate of cesarean delivery. Results of this trial are summarized in Tables 35-15 and 35-16.

The optimal management of women with mild gestational hypertension or preeclampsia before 37 weeks' gestation is controversial. There is disagreement regarding the benefits of hospitalization, complete bedrest, and use of antihypertensive medications.

Hospitalization

In the past, management of these women has involved hospital bedrest for the duration of pregnancy with the belief that such management diminishes the frequency of progression to severe disease and allows rapid intervention in case of sudden disease progression, including the development of abruptio placentae, eclampsia, or hypertensive crisis. However, these complications are extremely rare among compliant women with mild hypertension or mild preeclampsia and absent symptoms. In addition, the results of two randomized trials in women with gestational

TABLE 35-15 MATERNAL OUTCOME IN RANDOMIZED TRIAL COMPARING INDUCTION AND EXPECTANT MONITORING IN MILD GESTATIONAL HYPERTENSION-PREECLAMPSIA

	INDUCTION (n = 377)	EXPECTANT (n = 379)	RELATIVE RISK (95% CONFIDENCE INTERVAL)
Composite adverse outcome	117 (31)	166 (44)	0.71(0.59-0.86)
• HELLP syndrome	4 (1)	11 (3)	
• Pulmonary edema	0	2 (1)	
• Abruptio placentae	0	0	
• Eclampsia	0	0	
• Maternal intensive care unit admission	6 (2)	14 (4)	
• Cesarean delivery	54 (14)	72 (19)	0.75(0.55-1.04)

Modified from Koopmans CM, Bijlenga D, Groen H, et al: Induction of labour versus expectant monitoring for gestational hypertension or mild pre-eclampsia after 36 weeks' gestation (HYPITAT): a multicentre, open-label randomize controlled trial. Lancet 374:979-988, 2009.

TABLE 35-16 NEONATAL OUTCOME IN RANDOMIZED TRIAL COMPARING INDUCTION VERSUS EXPECTANT MANAGEMENT IN MILD HYPERTENSION-PREECLAMPSIA

Neonatal Outcome

	NO. WITH INDUCTION (%)	NO. WITH EXPECTANT (%)
Composite adverse outcome	24 (6)	32 (8)
• Perinatal deaths	0	0
• Apgar <7 at 5 min	7 (2)	9 (2)
• Cord pH <7.05	9 (3)	19 (6)
• Neonatal intensive care unit admission	10 (3)	8 (2)
• Respiratory distress syndrome	1 (0.25)	1 (0.25)

Modified from Koopmans CM, Bijlenga D, Groen H, et al: Induction of labour versus expectant monitoring for gestational hypertension or mild pre-eclampsia after 36 weeks' gestation (HYPITAT): a multicentre, open-label randomize controlled trial. Lancet 374:979-988, 2009.

hypertension and several observational studies in women with mild hypertension and mild preeclampsia suggest that most of these women can be safely managed at home or in a day-care facility provided they undergo frequent maternal and fetal evaluation.[1,2] It must be emphasized that many women included in these studies had gestational hypertension only.[2]

BEDREST

Complete or partial bed rest for the duration of pregnancy is often recommended for women with mild hypertension-preeclampsia. There is no evidence to date suggesting that this practice improves pregnancy outcome. In addition, there are no published randomized trials comparing complete bedrest and restricted activity in the management of women with mild preeclampsia. On the other hand, prolonged bedrest for the duration of pregnancy increases the risk for thromboembolism.

BLOOD PRESSURE MEDICATIONS

There are several randomized trials describing the use of antihypertensive drugs compared with no treatment or a placebo in the management of women with mild hypertension or preeclampsia remote from term. Overall, these trials revealed lower rates of progression to severe disease with no improvement in perinatal outcome.[2] Of note, the sample size of these trials is inadequate to evaluate differences in FGR, abruptio placentae, perinatal death, or maternal outcome.

FETAL AND MATERNAL SURVEILLANCE

There is universal agreement that fetal testing is indicated during expectant management of women with gestational hypertension or preeclampsia.[1-10] Most authorities in the United States recommend daily fetal movement counts in association with either nonstress testing (NST) or BPP to be performed at the time of diagnosis and serially thereafter until delivery (1 to 2 times per week).[1-3] Because uteroplacental blood flow may be reduced in some of these women, ultrasound estimation of fetal weight as well as amniotic fluid status is also recommended at the time of diagnosis and serially thereafter, with the frequency depending on findings. Doppler flow velocimetry is recommended in the presence of suspected intrauterine growth restriction (IUGR).[9-11] The frequency of these tests is usually dependent on the severity of hypertension or preeclampsia, gestational age at the time of diagnosis, and fetal growth findings. Most clinical series suggest testing once weekly in women with mild gestational hypertension or preeclampsia, twice weekly if there is suspected fetal growth delay, and daily during expectant management of women with severe preeclampsia at less than 32 weeks' gestation.[32] However, there are no large prospective studies assessing outcomes of these monitoring techniques in women with gestational hypertension or preeclampsia.

Maternal surveillance is indicated in all women with gestational hypertension and preeclampsia. The goal of monitoring in women with mild gestational hypertension is to observe progression of the condition to severe hypertension or to preeclampsia.[1-8] In women with mild preeclampsia, the goal is early detection of severe preeclampsia. In those with severe preeclampsia, the goal is to detect the development of organ dysfunction. Therefore, all such women should be evaluated for symptoms of organ dysfunction, such as severe headaches, visual changes, altered mentation, right upper quadrant or epigastric pain, nausea or vomiting, shortness of breath, and decreased urine output.[1,2,9-11] In addition, they should undergo laboratory testing for 24-hour urine protein, serum creatinine, platelet count, and liver enzymes. Coagulation function tests are not necessary in the presence of a normal platelet count and liver

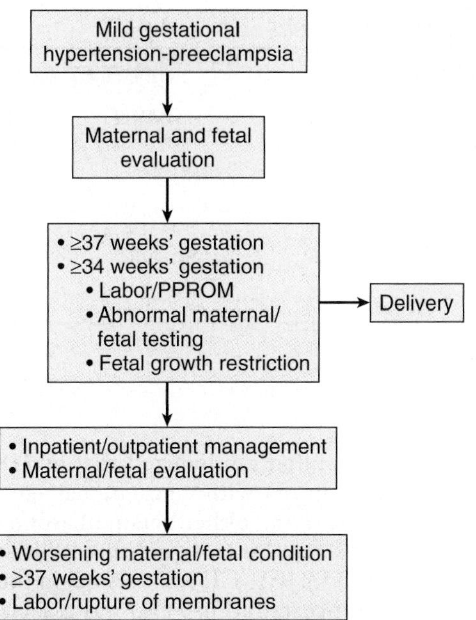

FIGURE 35-8. Management plan for patients with mild preeclampsia. *PPROM,* preterm premature rupture of the membranes.

enzymes. **The frequency of laboratory testing will depend on the initial findings, the severity of the maternal condition, and the ensuing clinical progression. Most authorities recommend evaluation and testing of platelet count, liver enzymes, and serum creatinine once weekly for women with mild gestational hypertension or mild preeclampsia, and performing these tests daily during expectant management of women with severe preeclampsia or HELLP syndrome remote from term.**[1,32]

Recommended Management

The primary objective of management in women with gestational hypertension-preeclampsia must always be safety of the mother and then delivery of a mature newborn that will not require intensive and prolonged neonatal care. This objective can be achieved by formulating a management plan that takes into consideration one or more of the following: the severity of the disease process, fetal gestational age, maternal and fetal status at time of initial evaluation, presence of labor, cervical Bishop score, and the wishes of the mother.

Mild Hypertension or Preeclampsia

Once the diagnosis of mild gestational hypertension or mild preeclampsia is made, subsequent therapy will depend on the results of maternal and fetal evaluation (Figure 35-8). **In general, women with mild disease developing at 37 weeks' gestation or later should undergo induction of labor.**

In women who remain undelivered, close maternal and fetal evaluation are essential. These women are instructed to eat a regular diet with no salt restriction and to restrict their activity but not to complete bedrest. Diuretics and antihypertensive medications are not used because of the potential to mask the diagnosis of severe disease.[1] At the time of initial and subsequent visits, the women are educated and instructed about reporting symptoms of severe preeclampsia. Those managed as outpatients are also advised to come to the hospital or outpatient facility immediately if they develop abdominal pain, uterine contractions, vaginal spotting, or decreased fetal movement.

In women with mild gestational hypertension, fetal evaluation should include an NST and an ultrasound examination of estimated fetal weight and amniotic fluid index. If the results are normal, no repeat testing is undertaken, as previously described.

Maternal evaluation includes measurements of hematocrit, platelet count, and liver function tests, once weekly. The women are usually seen twice a week for evaluation of maternal BP, urine protein by dipstick, and symptoms of impending eclampsia. This evaluation is extremely important for early detection of progression to preeclampsia or severe hypertension. The onset of maternal symptoms, a sudden increase in BP to severe values, or development of persistent proteinuria (≥2+ on dipstick) requires prompt hospitalization for close evaluation.

In women with mild preeclampsia at less than 37 weeks' gestation but at more than 32 weeks, outpatient management can be considered for reliable patients with systolic BP of 150 mm Hg or less or diastolic BP of 100 mmHg or less and no increase in proteinuria if they have no symptoms and if they have normal liver enzymes and a normal platelet count (>100,000/mm^3). Women who do not satisfy these criteria are hospitalized, particularly those with mild preeclampsia before 32 weeks. During ambulatory management, women are instructed to rest at home and perform BP measurements and urine dipstick daily, and are given instructions about prompt reporting of symptoms of severe disease. These women are then seen twice weekly, at which time a platelet count and liver enzyme test are performed. Fetal evaluation includes daily fetal movement count, twice-weekly NST, and serial ultrasound evaluation of fetal growth and amniotic fluid. If there is evidence of disease progression (significant increase in BP or proteinuria to levels above the threshold mentioned previously, new onset of symptoms, or evidence of abnormal blood tests or abnormal fetal growth), these women are hospitalized for the duration of pregnancy. Women managed in the hospital receive similar maternal and fetal evaluation. Obstetrical management is summarized in Figure 35-8.

Severe Hypertension in Preeclampsia

The incidence of severe preeclampsia ranges from 0.6% to 1%.[33] Pregnancies complicated by severe gestational hypertension or severe preeclampsia are associated with serous maternal and perinatal complications, particularly preterm delivery, fetal growth restriction, abruptio placentae, and perinatal death (Table 35-17). As a result, knowledge of the anticipated maternal, fetal, and neonatal risks is essential for appropriate counseling and management.

Expectant Management

The clinical course of severe preeclampsia may be characterized by progressive deterioration in both maternal and fetal conditions. **Because these pregnancies have been associated with increased rates of maternal morbidity and mortality and with significant risks for the fetus (growth restriction, hypoxemia, and death), there is general**

TABLE 35-17 PREGNANCY OUTCOME IN WOMEN WITH MILD AND SEVERE PREECLAMPSIA

	HAUTH ET AL.[4]		BUCHBINDER ET AL.[19]		HNAT ET AL.[23]	
	Mild (*n* = 217)	Severe (*n* = 109)	Mild (*n* = 62)*	Severe* (*n* = 45)	Mild (*n* = 86)	Severe (*n* = 70)
Delivery (wk)*						
<37 (%)	NR	NR	25.8	66.7	14.0	33.0
<35 (%)	1.9†	18.5†	9.7	35.6	2.3	18.6
SGA infant (%)*	10.2	18.5	4.8	11.4	NR	NR
Abruptio placentae (%)	0.5	3.7	3.2	6.7	0	1.4
Perinatal death (%)	1.0	1.8	0	8.9	0	1.4

*This study included women with previous preeclampsia. The other studies included only nulliparous women.
†These rates are for delivery at less than 34 weeks.

agreement that all such patients should be delivered if the disease develops after 34 weeks' gestation. Prompt delivery is also indicated when there is imminent eclampsia (persistent severe symptoms), multiorgan dysfunction, severe IUGR (<5th percentile), suspected abruptio placentae, or non-reassuring fetal testing.[33]

There is disagreement about management of patients with severe preeclampsia before 34 weeks' gestation when the maternal condition is stable and fetal condition is reassuring. Some authors consider delivery as the definitive treatment regardless of gestational age, whereas others recommend prolonging pregnancy unless maternal or fetal indications exist for delivery or fetal lung maturity is demonstrated before 34 weeks' gestation.[33]

Although delivery is beneficial to the mother, it must be weighed against the risk for prematurity. In the past, it was believed that infants born prematurely to severely preeclamptic women had lower rates of neonatal mortality and morbidity compared with infants of similar gestational age born to non-preeclamptic women. This belief was based on the clinical impression that fetuses of preeclamptic women have accelerated lung and neurologic maturation as a result of stress in utero. Reduced risk for prematurity-associated neonatal morbidity has never been documented in case-control studies. In contrast, **several recent case-control investigations have demonstrated that premature infants born after severe preeclampsia have similar neonatal complications and mortality and have higher rates of admission to neonatal intensive care units compared with other premature infants of similar gestational age. In addition, the results of case-controlled studies reveal that fetuses of preeclamptic women do not exhibit accelerated lung or neurologic maturation.**[33]

During expectant management, women should be aware that the decision to continue such management will be made on a daily basis and that the median time of pregnancy prolongation is 7 days (range, 2 to 35 days). There are only two randomized trials (133 women) that compared a policy of early elective delivery with a policy of delayed delivery.[33] Nevertheless, the results of retrospective and observational studies (more than 1000 women) suggest that expectant management is associated with reduced short-term neonatal morbidity in a select group of women with gestational age between 24 and 32 weeks.[33]

In the past, there was uncertainty regarding the efficacy and safety of corticosteroids administered to women with severe preeclampsia before 34 weeks' gestation. A prospective double-blind randomized trial of 218 women with severe preeclampsia with a gestational age between 26 and 34 weeks receiving either betamethasone (*n* = 110) or placebo (*n* = 108) reported a significant reduction in the rate of RDS (RR, 0.53; 95% CI, 0.35 to 0.82) in the steroid-treated group. Corticosteroid use also was associated with a reduction in the risks for neonatal intraventricular hemorrhage (RR, 0.35; 95% CI, 0.15 to 0.86), neonatal infection (RR, 0.39; 95% CI, 0.39 to 0.97), and neonatal death (RR, 0.5; 95% CI, 0.28 to 0.89). However, there were no differences in maternal complications between the two groups. Thus, **the data support the use of steroids to reduce neonatal complications in women with severe preeclampsia at 34 weeks' gestation or less.**

Recommended Management of Severe Hypertension-Preeclampsia

The presence of severe disease mandates immediate hospitalization in labor and delivery. Intravenous magnesium sulfate is begun to prevent convulsions, and antihypertensive medications are administered to lower severe levels of hypertension (systolic pressure ≥160 mm Hg *and/or* diastolic pressure ≥110 mm Hg). The aim of antihypertensive therapy is to keep systolic pressure between 140 and 155 mm Hg and diastolic pressure between 90 and 105 mm Hg. During the observation period, maternal and fetal conditions are assessed, and a decision is made regarding the need for delivery (Figure 35-9). Those with a gestational age of 24 to 34 weeks are given corticosteroids to accelerate fetal lung maturity. Maternal evaluation includes monitoring of BP, urine output, cerebral status, and the presence of epigastric pain, tenderness, labor, or vaginal bleeding. Laboratory evaluation includes a platelet count, liver enzymes, and serum creatinine. Fetal evaluation includes continuous fetal heart monitoring, a BPP, and ultrasonographic assessment of fetal growth and amniotic fluid. Patients with resistant severe hypertension despite maximal doses of intravenous labetalol (220 mg) plus oral nifedipine (50 mg) or persistent cerebral symptoms while on magnesium sulfate are delivered irrespective of fetal gestational age.

After the initial evaluation, the need for immediate delivery versus the potential neonatal benefit and the relative maternal and fetal risks of expectant management should be determined.[33] Women who develop eclampsia, pulmonary edema, or documented or suspected abruption placentae; those with DIC or moderate to severe renal

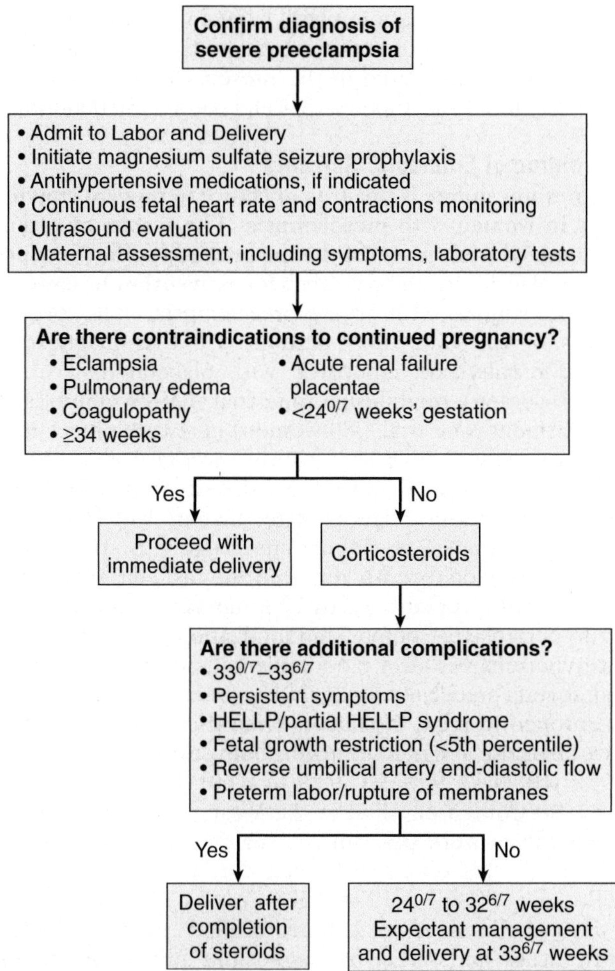
Confirm diagnosis of severe preeclampsia
• Admit to Labor and Delivery
• Initiate magnesium sulfate seizure prophylaxis
• Antihypertensive medications, if indicated
• Continuous fetal heart rate and contractions monitoring
• Ultrasound evaluation
• Maternal assessment, including symptoms, laboratory tests
Are there contraindications to continued pregnancy?
• Eclampsia
• Pulmonary edema
• Coagulopathy
• ≥34 weeks
• Acute renal failure
placentae
• <24 0/7 weeks' gestation
Yes
No
Proceed with immediate delivery
Corticosteroids
Are there additional complications?
• 33 0/7–33 6/7
• Persistent symptoms
• HELLP/partial HELLP syndrome
• Fetal growth restriction (<5th percentile)
• Reverse umbilical artery end-diastolic flow
• Preterm labor/rupture of membranes
Yes
No
Deliver after completion of steroids
24 0/7 to 32 6/7 weeks Expectant management and delivery at 33 6/7 weeks

FIGURE 35-9. Management plan for patients with severe preeclampsia.

dysfunction (serum creatinine ≥1.5 mg/dL); and those with gestational age below $23^{0/7}$ weeks' gestation should be delivered after maternal stabilization. In addition, those with non-reassuring fetal heart rate tracing (repetitive variable or late decelerations) and those with persistent BPP of 4 or lower (on two occasions at least 4 hours apart) should be delivered promptly.[33] Women with gestational age between $23^{0/7}$ and $23^{6/7}$ weeks should receive extensive counseling about the minimal neonatal benefit and high maternal complications from expectant management and they should be offered the option of pregnancy termination.

For women with gestational age of $24^{0/7}$ weeks or greater without any indication for prompt delivery, corticosteroids are administered to accelerate fetal lung maturity.[33] Patients with gestational age between $33^{0/7}$ to $34^{0/7}$ weeks, severe FGR, preterm labor or premature rupture of the membranes (PROM), reverse umbilical artery diastolic flow, HELLP syndrome or partial HELLP, or persistent symptoms (headaches, visual changes, epigastric or right upper quadrant pain, nausea or vomiting) should be delivered no later than 24 hours after the last dose of corticosteroids. These patients should remain on magnesium sulfate with continuous monitoring of uterine contractions and fetal heart rate until delivery.

Women with pregnancy between $24^{0/7}$ and $32^{6/7}$ weeks' gestation with stable maternal and fetal conditions during the initial 24-hour observation period are considered candidates for expectant management (see Figure 35-9). In these women, magnesium sulfate is generally discontinued after 24 hours with transfer to a high-risk antepartum floor for close observation. Because of the potential for rapid deterioration in maternal and fetal conditions during expectant management, these women should be managed only in a tertiary care hospital with adequate maternal and neonatal intensive care facilities. They should be managed in consultation with a maternal-fetal medicine specialist and receive counseling by a neonatologist.[33]

Oral antihypertensive medications are used as needed to keep systolic BP between 140 and 155 mm Hg and diastolic BP between 90 and 105 mm Hg.[33] Oral labetalol and oral calcium channel blockers (nifedipine or nicardipine) have been commonly used in reported studies. The author's regimen consists of an initial dose of labetalol of 200 mg every 8 hours to be increased up to 800 mg every 8 hours (600 to 2400 mg/day) as needed. If the maximal dose is inadequate to achieve the desired BP goal, short-acting oral nifedipine is added with an initial dose of 10 mg every 6 hours and subsequently increased up to 20 mg every 4 hours (40 to 120 mg/day). An alternative regimen may include the long-acting (XL) version of nifedipine (30 to 60 mg) every 8 hours. During titration of oral antihypertensive agents, if the patient has persistent severe hypertensive episodes (systolic BP ≥160 mm Hg and/or diastolic BP ≥105 mm Hg), blood pressure should be assessed every 15 minutes. If the blood pressure remains in the severe range after 60 minutes, the patient should be transferred to the labor and delivery unit for more intensive monitoring and treatment with intravenous medications such as hydralazine or labetalol. Patients with resistant severe hypertension after maximal doses of intravenous hydralazine (25 mg) or labetalol (220 mg) should receive magnesium sulfate and be delivered. In addition, patients who develop persistent severe hypertension despite combined maximal doses of oral labetalol (2400 mg/day) plus short-acting nifedipine (120 mg/day) or nifedipine XL (180 mg/day) should also be considered for delivery.

Maternal assessment includes frequent evaluation of symptoms (headaches, blurred or double vision, confusion, nausea, vomiting, epigastric or right upper quadrant pain, shortness of breath, uterine activity, and vaginal bleeding) and intake and output.[33]

Laboratory assessment includes daily testing of complete blood count with platelet count, transaminases, LDH, and serum creatinine levels.[32] Coagulation studies are obtained only if there is thrombocytopenia or suspicion of abruption placentae.

Fetal assessment includes daily fetal kick counts, at least daily NST with uterine activity monitoring with a BPP if the NST is nonreactive, and twice weekly amniotic fluid assessment.[33] Ultrasonographic assessment of fetal growth is performed every 2 weeks.[33] Severe oligohydramnios is defined as an amniotic fluid index of 2 cm or less on at least two occasions that are at least 24 hours part.[33] Severe oligohydramnios is considered an indication for delivery in women with a gestational age of more than 30 weeks, irrespective of other fetal testing results. In those at 30 weeks or less of gestation, pregnancy may be continued with a reassuring NST, BPP, and umbilical artery Doppler studies. Umbilical artery Doppler studies are performed weekly, or more often if FGR is suspected or testing reveals abnormal diastolic flow or severe oligohydramnios. If absent umbilical artery diastolic flow is present, the Doppler studies should be performed daily.

In general, most patients will require delivery within 2 weeks, but some patients may continue their pregnancies for several weeks. It is important to emphasize that this therapy is appropriate only in a select group of patients and should be practiced in a tertiary care center with adequate maternal and neonatal intensive care facilities. Once the decision is made for delivery, the patients should receive magnesium sulfate in labor and for at least 24 hours postpartum.[33]

Intrapartum Management

The goals of management of women with gestational hypertension-preeclampsia are early detection of fetal heart rate abnormalities and progression from mild to severe disease, and the prevention of maternal complications. Pregnancies complicated by preeclampsia, particularly those with severe disease or FGR, are at risk for reduced fetal reserve and abruptio placentae.[2] Therefore, women with preeclampsia should receive continuous monitoring of fetal heart rate and uterine activity. The presence of uterine tachysystole or recurrent fetal heart rate decelerations may be the first sign of abruptio placentae in these women.

Some women with mild hypertension-preeclampsia progress to severe disease as a result of changes in cardiac output and stress hormones during labor. Therefore, women with gestational hypertension-preeclampsia should have BP recordings every hour and should be assessed for symptoms suggestive of severe disease. Those who develop severe hypertension or symptoms should be managed as patients with severe preeclampsia.

Maternal pain relief during labor and delivery can be provided by either systemic opioids or segmental epidural anesthesia. Epidural analgesia is considered to be the preferred method of pain relief in women with mild gestational hypertension and mild preeclampsia. Although there is no unanimity of opinion regarding the use of epidural anesthesia in women with severe preeclampsia, evidence exists that epidural anesthesia is safe in these women. A randomized trial of 116 women with severe preeclampsia receiving either epidural analgesia or patient-controlled analgesia reported no differences in cesarean delivery rates, and the group receiving epidural had significantly better pain relief during labor.

The use of either epidural, spinal, or combined techniques of regional anesthesia is considered by most obstetrical anesthesiologists to be the method of choice during cesarean delivery. **In women with severe preeclampsia, general anesthesia carries the risk for aspiration and failed intubation owing to airway edema and is associated with marked increases in systemic and cerebral pressures during intubation and extubation.**[1] **Women with airway or laryngeal edema may require awake intubation under fiberoptic observation with the availability of immediate tracheostomy.** Changes in systemic and cerebral pressures may be attenuated by pretreatment with labetalol or nitroglycerine injections. It is important to recognize that regional anesthesia is contraindicated in the presence of coagulopathy or severe thrombocytopenia (platelet count, <50,000/mm^3).

Prevention of Eclamptic Seizures

Magnesium sulfate is the drug of choice to prevent convulsions in women with preeclampsia. The results of recent randomized trials revealed that magnesium sulfate is superior to placebo or no treatment for prevention of convulsions in women with severe preeclampsia. The overall results of the four trials demonstrate that magnesium sulfate prophylaxis, compared with placebo (two trials, 10,795 women), nimodipine (one trial, 1750 women), and no treatment (one trial, 228 women) in severe preeclampsia, is associated with a significantly lower rate of eclampsia (RR, 0.39; 95% CI, 0.28 to 0.55). Results from one of the largest randomized trials to date, that of 10,141 women with preeclampsia in 33 nations (largely in the Third World), has been recently reported. Almost all the enrolled patients had severe disease by U.S. standards: 50% received antihypertensives before randomization, 75% received antihypertensives after randomization, and the remainder had severe preeclampsia or imminent eclampsia. Among all enrolled women, the rate of eclampsia was significantly lower in those assigned to magnesium sulfate (0.8% versus 1.9%; RR, 0.42; 95% CI, 0.29 to 0.60). However, among the 1560 women enrolled in the Western world, the rates of eclampsia were 0.5% in the magnesium group versus 0.8% in the placebo, a difference that was not significant (RR, 0.67; 95% CI, 1.19 to 2.37).

Two randomized placebo-controlled trials evaluated the efficacy and safety of magnesium sulfate in women with mild preeclampsia. One of these trials included 135 women, and the other included only 222 women. There were no instances of eclampsia in either group in both of these trials. In addition, the findings of both studies revealed that magnesium sulfate does not affect either the duration of labor or the rate of cesarean delivery. However, neither of these studies had adequate sample size to address the efficacy of magnesium sulfate to prevent convulsions. Therefore, **whether there is a benefit of magnesium sulfate treatment in women with mild preeclampsia remains unclear.**

Control of Severe Hypertension

The objective of treating acute severe hypertension is to prevent cerebrovascular and cardiovascular complications such as encephalopathy, hemorrhage, and congestive heart failure.[1,2] For ethical reasons, there are no randomized trials to determine the level of hypertension to treat in order to prevent these complications. Antihypertensive therapy is recommended by some for sustained systolic BP values of 160 mm Hg or more and for sustained diastolic values of 110 mm Hg or more. Some experts recommend treating diastolic levels of 105 mm Hg, and still others use a mean arterial BP of 130 mm Hg or more.[1,2] The definition of sustained hypertension is not clear and ranges from 30 minutes to 2 hours.

Antihypertensive medications are indicated if there is sustained elevations in systolic BP to levels of 160 mm Hg or greater and/or if the diastolic BP is 105 mm Hg or

higher.[33] There are several antihypertensive medications that can be used to treat severe hypertension in severe preeclampsia. The most commonly recommended medications include intravenous bolus doses of hydralazine, bolus doses of labetalol, or oral nifedipine (rapid-acting tablets or long-acting capsules). Other antihypertensive medications recommended for treatment of severe hypertension have included intravenous ketanserin, intravenous nicardipine, and mini bolus diazoxide.

Despite the extensive literature on the subject, it remains unclear which is the ideal antihypertensive medication to use in the acute control of severe hypertension in women with severe preeclampsia. The results of a recent meta-analysis of relevant randomized trials found that parenteral hydralazine was associated with more adverse effects compared with other antihypertensives; however, such a finding was not confirmed in a recent large randomized trial. **Based on the available evidence, hydralazine, labetalol, or nifedipine can be used to treat severe hypertension in preeclampsia.**[2,3,33] **The provider should be familiar with the dosage to be used, expected response, and potential side effects of each of these drugs.** Both hydralazine and nifedipine are associated with tachycardia and headaches and thus should not be the first drug of choice in patients with heart rate above 100 beats/minute. In such case, labetalol is preferred. Labetalol, however, should be avoided in patients with moderate to severe asthma, bradycardia (heart rate <60 beats/minute) and in those with congestive heart failure. Compared with other antihypertensive medications, nifedipine has the advantage of increased renal blood flow with associated increase in urine output.[33] Thus, it may be the drug of choice in those with decreased urine output or oliguria, and for treatment of severe hypertension in the postpartum period.[33] In the past, there has been a theoretical concern that the combined use of magnesium sulfate and nifedipine in patients with severe preeclampsia can result in excessive hypotension and neuromuscular blockade. However, a recent review on this subject found that therapy with both magnesium sulfate and nifedipine does not increase the risk for the previously described complications in women with preeclampsia. Nevertheless, if neuromuscular blockage develops in these patients, this can be easily reversed by the administration of 1 g of intravenous calcium gluconate.

The recommended dose of hydralazine for the treatment of severe hypertension in pregnancy is intravenous hydralazine given as bolus injections of 5 to 10 mg every 15 to 20 minutes for a maximal dose of 20 mg. The recommended dose of labetalol is 20 to 40 mg intravenously every 10 to 15 minutes for a maximal of 220 mg, and the dose of nifedipine is 10 to 20 mg orally every 30 minutes for a maximal dose of 50 mg[33] Sustained BP values of 160 mm Hg systolic or more or 105 to 110 mm Hg diastolic or more require therapy intrapartum. For women with thrombocytopenia and those in the postpartum period, systolic values of 150 mm Hg or more or diastolic readings of 100 mm Hg or more are the recommended thresholds for therapy.[33] For this author, the first-line agent is intravenous labetalol, and if maximal doses are ineffective, oral nifedipine is added.

Mode of Delivery

There are no randomized trials comparing the optimal method of delivery in women with gestational hypertension-preeclampsia. A plan for vaginal delivery should be attempted in all women with mild disease without other indications for cesarean delivery and in most women with severe disease, particularly those beyond 30 weeks' gestation.[1,2,17] The decision to perform cesarean delivery should be based on gestational age, fetal condition, presence of labor, and cervical Bishop score. In general, the presence of severe preeclampsia is not per se an indication for cesarean delivery.

There are no randomized trials comparing the optimal methods of delivery in patients with severe hypertension or severe preeclampsia. The method for delivery will depend on gestational age, cervical Bishop score, and fetal condition. The cesarean delivery rate among reported studies in patients at before 34 weeks' gestation ranged from 66% to 96%[33] with the higher rates for patients with onset prior to 28 weeks' gestation. This high cesarean rate is expected considering that a deterioration in either fetal or maternal condition is the indication for delivery during expectant management (high rates of severe FGR, oligohydramnios, non-reassuring fetal status, abnormal presentation, high rates of maternal complications).[33] Thus, a very small percentage of these patients will be considered candidates for medical induction of labor.

There are several retrospective studies evaluating induction of labor in patients with preeclampsia before 34 weeks' gestation and absent contraindication for induction. However, most of the women included in these studies had gestational age beyond 32 weeks at the time of induction.[33] Only two of these studies included data on patients earlier than 28 weeks undergoing induction of labor.[33] Both of these studies reported a cesarean delivery rate above 95% and thus recommended elective cesarean delivery in such patients.

In general, the decision to perform cesarean delivery versus a trial of labor in such patients should be individualized and thus based on one or more of the following factors: fetal gestational age, fetal presentation, presence or absence of severe FGR, oligohydramnios, results of umbilical artery Doppler, BPP, fetal heart rate monitoring, presence of labor, and cervical Bishop score. On the basis of the available data, we recommend cesarean delivery for all women with gestational age below 28 weeks and for all those with severe FGR, severe oligohydramnios, BPP of 4 or less, or reverse umbilical artery Doppler flow at before 32 weeks of gestation.

Postpartum Management

During the immediate postpartum period, women with preeclampsia should receive close monitoring of BP and of symptoms consistent with severe disease and accurate measurements of fluid intake and urinary output.

These women often receive large amounts of intravenous fluids during labor as a result of prehydration before the administration of epidural analgesia, and intravenous fluids are given during the administration of oxytocin and magnesium sulfate in labor and postpartum. In addition, during the postpartum period, there is mobilization of extracellular fluid leading to increased intravascular volume. As a result, **women with severe preeclampsia, particularly those with abnormal renal function, those with capillary leak, and those with early-onset disease, are at increased risk for pulmonary edema and exacerbation of severe hypertension postpartum. Careful evaluation of the amount of intravenous fluids, oral intake, blood products, and urine output, as well as monitoring by pulse oximetry and chest auscultation, are advised.**[2,33]

In general, most women with gestational hypertension become normotensive during the first week postpartum.[1,2] In contrast, in women with preeclampsia, hypertension often takes longer to resolve. In addition, in some of the women with preeclampsia, there is an initial decrease in BP immediately postpartum, followed by development of hypertension again between days 3 and 6. Moreover, a recent study found that resolution of hypertension and proteinuria may take up to 1 year postpartum. Antihypertensive drug treatment should be undertaken if the systolic BP is at least 150 mm Hg or if the diastolic BP is at least 100 mm Hg. Various agents may be employed. A common regimen is to prescribe oral nifedipine, 10 mg every 6 hours, or long-acting nifedipine.[33] If the BP is well controlled and maternal symptoms are absent, the woman is discharged home with instructions for daily BP measurements by a home visiting nurse for the first week postpartum or longer if necessary. Antihypertensive medications are discontinued if the BP remains below the hypertensive levels for at least 48 hours. Recently, some authors have suggested that 5 days of oral furosemide therapy (20 mg/dL) enhances recovery and reduces the need for antihypertensive therapy in women with severe preeclampsia.

Severe hypertension or severe preeclampsia may develop for the first time during the postpartum period. Hence, all postpartum women should be educated about the signs and symptoms of severe hypertension or preeclampsia. These women are at increased risk for eclampsia, pulmonary edema, stroke, and thromboembolism. Therefore, medical providers and personnel who respond to patient phone calls should be educated and instructed about symptoms of severe postpartum hypertension. Women who have persistent severe headaches, visual changes, and epigastric pain with nausea or vomiting and those with severe hypertension require immediate evaluation and potential hospitalization. These women often require magnesium sulfate for at least 24 hours and antihypertensive therapy. If neurologic symptoms exist, brain imaging is undertaken to rule out the presence of cerebral pathology.

Maternal and Perinatal Outcome with Preeclampsia

Maternal and perinatal morbidity is substantially increased in women with severe gestational hypertension. Indeed, these women have higher morbidity rates than women with mild preeclampsia.[19] In addition, the rates of abruptio placentae, preterm delivery (at less than 37 and 35 weeks), and rates of SGA infants in these women are similar to those seen in women with severe preeclampsia. However, whether this increase in rate of preterm delivery is a result of early delivery chosen by the physician or because of the disease process itself remains unknown. Therefore, these women should be managed as if they had severe preeclampsia.[33]

Maternal and perinatal outcomes in preeclampsia are usually dependent on one or more of the following: gestational age at onset of preeclampsia as well as at time of delivery, the severity of the disease process, the presence of multifetal gestation, and the presence of preexisting medical conditions such as pregestational diabetes, renal disease, or thrombophilias.

Severe preeclampsia is also associated with an increased risk for maternal mortality (0.2%) and increased rates of maternal morbidity (5%), such as convulsions, pulmonary edema, acute renal or liver failure, liver hemorrhage, DIC, and stroke. These complications are usually seen in women who develop preeclampsia before 32 weeks' gestation and in those with preexisting medical conditions.

Counseling Women Who Have Had Preeclampsia in Prior Pregnancies

We examined the pregnancy outcomes and incidences of preeclampsia in subsequent pregnancies, as well as the frequency of chronic hypertension and diabetes mellitus in women who had severe preeclampsia (287 women) or eclampsia (119 women) in their first pregnancies (aged 11 to 25 years) compared with 409 women (aged 12 to 25 years) who remained normotensive during their first pregnancies. Each woman had at least one subsequent pregnancy (range, 1 to 11) and was followed for a minimum of 2 years (range, 2 to 24). There was no significant difference in the incidences of diabetes mellitus in the two groups (1.3% versus 1.5%). The incidence of chronic hypertension was significantly higher in the preeclampsia patients (14.8% versus 5.6%; $P < .001$). This difference became even greater for those women followed more than 10 years (51% versus 14%; $P < .001$). The incidence of severe preeclampsia was also significantly higher in the second pregnancies (25.9% to 4.6%) and in the subsequent pregnancies (12.2% to 5.0%) of women with preeclampsia.

In a later report, subsequent pregnancy outcome and long-term prognosis were studied in 108 women who had severe preeclampsia in the second trimester. These women were followed for a minimum of 2 years (range, 2 to 12 years) and had a total of 169 subsequent pregnancies. Fifty-nine (35%) subsequent pregnancies were normotensive, and 110 (65%) were complicated by preeclampsia. Overall, 21% of all subsequent pregnancies were complicated by severe preeclampsia in the second trimester. In addition, these women had a higher risk for developing chronic hypertension, with the highest incidence being in those who had recurrent severe preeclampsia in the second trimester (55%).

Hnat and associates[23] reported subsequent pregnancy outcome in women with previous preeclampsia enrolled in a multicenter trial. The rate of recurrent preeclampsia was 17%. The authors also noted that these women had a high rate of severe preeclampsia and poor perinatal outcome. In addition, even in those who remained normotensive in their subsequent pregnancy, there was a greater likelihood of adverse pregnancy outcome (preterm delivery, SGA infants, and perinatal death).

Some women with preeclampsia remote from term may have abruptio placentae. The risk for this complication is increased significantly in those with severe preeclampsia before 34 weeks' gestation and particularly in those who have severe preeclampsia in the second trimester. For women with preeclampsia complicated by abruptio placentae, the risk for abruptio in subsequent pregnancies ranges from 5% to 20%.

Pregnancy outcome and long-term prognosis were studied in 37 women with severe preeclampsia complicated by pulmonary edema, and 18 of these women had subsequent pregnancies. Ten of the 18 were normotensive, 4 were complicated by chronic hypertension, and 4 by preeclampsia; 1 of the latter women also had pulmonary edema.

Pregnancy outcome and remote prognosis were also studied in 18 women with severe preeclampsia complicated by acute renal failure. All 18 had acute tubular necrosis, 9 required dialysis, and 2 died within 8 weeks after birth. All women had serial evaluation of renal function, urine microscopic testing, and electrolyte studies at the onset of acute renal failure and during follow-up. All 16 surviving patients had normal renal function on long-term follow-up (average, 4 years). Four of the 16 women had seven subsequent pregnancies: one ended in miscarriage, one was complicated by preeclampsia at 35 weeks, and five were term pregnancies without complications.

Women with a history of HELLP syndrome are at increased risk for all forms of preeclampsia in subsequent pregnancies (Table 35-18). In general, the rate of preeclampsia in subsequent pregnancies is about 20%, with significantly higher rates if the onset of HELLP syndrome is during the second trimester. The rate of recurrent HELLP syndrome ranges from 2% to 19%, with the most reliable data suggesting a recurrence risk of less than 5%. Because of the previously mentioned risks, these women are informed that they are at increased risk for adverse pregnancy outcome (preterm delivery, FGR, abruptio placentae, and fetal death) in subsequent pregnancies. Therefore, they require close monitoring during subsequent gestations. At present, there is no preventive therapy for recurrent HELLP syndrome. There are case series describing subsequent pregnancy outcomes in women with previous ruptured liver hematomas. We have followed three women with previous ruptured liver hematomas through four subsequent pregnancies without complications. Other authors reviewed the literature and reported on several such women who had subsequent uneventful pregnancies under close maternal and fetal observation.

Liver function tests were studied in 54 women at a median of 31 months (range, 3 to 101 months) after pregnancies complicated by the HELLP syndrome. Serum levels of AST, LDH, and conjugated bilirubin were found to be normal. However, total bilirubin levels were elevated in 11 (20%) of the studied women. The authors of this report suggested the possibility that a dysfunction of the bilirubin-conjugating mechanism represents a risk factor for the development of this syndrome.

There are two reports describing long-term renal function after HELLP syndrome. One of the reports included 23 patients whose pregnancies were complicated by HELLP syndrome and acute renal failure: 8 of these women had 11 subsequent pregnancies, with 9 resulting in term gestation. All 23 women also had normal BP and renal function at an average follow-up of 4.6 years (range, 0.5 to 11 years). The other study compared renal function after at least 5 years after HELLP syndrome in 10 patients with the respective findings in 22 patients with previous normotensive gestation. There were no differences in renal function tests between the two groups. These findings suggest that the development of HELLP syndrome with or without renal failure does not affect long-term renal function.

Remote Prognosis

Women with preeclampsia should also be counseled regarding future cardiovascular risks and risks for underlying renal disease. **There is evidence that women with preeclampsia remote from term are at particular increased risk for chronic hypertension later in life.** In addition, these patients, particularly those with recurrent preeclampsia, are more likely to have underlying renal disease. In a recent report, 86 Japanese women who had severe hypertension, severe proteinuria, or both during pregnancy had a postpartum renal biopsy. The authors found that women who had gestational proteinuria or preeclampsia before 30 weeks' gestation were more likely to have had underlying renal disease.

Several recent studies suggested that women who develop preeclampsia may be at increased risk for coronary artery disease later in life. Indeed, many of the risk factors and pathophysiologic abnormalities of preeclampsia are similar to those of coronary artery disease. Ramsey and associates demonstrated for the first time, using laser Doppler imaging in vivo, impaired microvascular function in women 15 to 25 years of age following a pregnancy complicated by preeclampsia. Thus, microvascular dysfunction, which is associated with insulin resistance, may be a predisposing vascular mechanism for both coronary heart disease and preeclampsia. In addition, pregnancies complicated by preeclampsia are at increased risk for stroke later in life. Therefore, pregnancies complicated by preeclampsia may identify women at risk for vascular disease in later life and may provide the opportunity for

TABLE 35-18 PREGNANCY OUTCOME AFTER HELLP SYNDROME

	NO. OF WOMEN	NO. OF PREGNANCIES	HELLP (%)	PREECLAMPSIA (%)
Sibai et al.	139	192	3	19
Sullivan et al.	122	161	19	23
Van Pampus et al.	77	92	2	16
Chames et al.*	40	42	6	52

Modified from Sibai BM: Diagnosis, controversies, and management of HELLP syndrome. Obstet Gynecol 103:981, 2004.
*HELLP ≤28 weeks in previous pregnancy.

life style and risk factor modification to alter their risk for complications.

ECLAMPSIA

Eclampsia is the occurrence of convulsions or coma unrelated to other cerebral conditions with signs and symptoms of preeclampsia. Early writings of both the Egyptians and Chinese warned of the dangers of convulsions encountered during pregnancy. Hippocrates noted that headaches, convulsions, and drowsiness were ominous signs associated with pregnancy. The term *eclampsia* appeared in a treatise on gynecology written by Varandaeus in 1619. Clonic spasms in association with pregnancy were described by Pew in 1694. In 1772, De la Motte recognized that prompt delivery of pregnant women with convulsions favored their recovery.

Eclampsia is defined as the development of convulsions or unexplained coma during pregnancy or postpartum in patients with signs and symptoms of preeclampsia. In the Western world, the reported incidence of eclampsia ranges from 1 in 2000 to 1 in 3448 pregnancies. The reported incidence is usually higher in tertiary referral centers, in multifetal gestation, and in those without prenatal care.[12]

Pathophysiology

The pathogenesis of eclamptic convulsions continues to be the subject of extensive investigation and speculation. Several theories and pathologic mechanisms have been implicated as possible etiologic factors, but none of these has been proved conclusively. It is not clear whether the pathologic features in eclampsia are a cause or an effect of the convulsions.[86]

Diagnosis

The diagnosis of eclampsia is secure in the presence of generalized edema, hypertension, proteinuria, and convulsions. However, women in whom eclampsia develops exhibit a wide spectrum of signs, ranging from severe hypertension, severe proteinuria, and generalized edema to absent or minimal hypertension, no proteinuria, and no edema.[86] Hypertension is considered the hallmark for the diagnosis of eclampsia. The hypertension can be severe (≥160 mm Hg systolic or ≥110 mm Hg diastolic) in 20% to 54% of cases[16,86] or mild (systolic BP between 140 and 160 mm Hg or diastolic BP between 90 and 110 mm Hg) in 30% to 60% of cases.[12,86] However, in 16% of cases, hypertension may be absent.[16] In addition, severe hypertension is more common in patients who develop antepartum eclampsia (58%) and in those who develop eclampsia at 32 weeks' gestation or later (71%).[16] Moreover, hypertension is absent in only 10% of women who develop eclampsia at or before 32 weeks' gestation.[16]

The diagnosis of eclampsia is usually associated with proteinuria (at least 1+ on dipstick).[16,86] In a series of 399 women with eclampsia studied by the author, substantial proteinuria (≥3+ on dipstick) was present in only 48% of the cases, whereas proteinuria was absent in 14% of the cases.[16] Abnormal weight gain (with or without clinical edema) in excess of 2 pounds per week during the third trimester might be the first sign before the onset of eclampsia. However, edema was absent in 26% of 399 eclamptic women studied by the author.[16]

Several clinical symptoms are potentially helpful in establishing the diagnosis of eclampsia. These include persistent occipital or frontal headaches, blurred vision, photophobia, epigastric or right upper quadrant pain, and altered mental status. Women have at least one of these symptoms in 59% to 75% of the cases (Table 35-19). Headaches are reported by 50% to 75% of the patients, whereas visual changes are reported in 19% to 32% of the patients.[86] These symptoms may occur before or after the onset of convulsions.[86]

Time of Onset

The onset of eclamptic convulsions can be during the antepartum, intrapartum, or postpartum period. The reported frequency of antepartum convulsions among recent series has ranged from 38% to 53% (Table 35-20),[16] whereas the frequency of postpartum eclampsia has ranged

TABLE 35-19 SYMPTOMS IN WOMEN WITH ECLAMPSIA

	DOUGLAS & REDMAN (n = 325) (%)	KATZ ET AL. (n = 53) (%)	CHAMES ET AL. (n = 89) (%)
Headache	50	64	70
Visual changes	19	32	30
Right upper quadrant, epigastric pain	19	Not reported	12
At least one	59	Not reported	75

From Sibai BM: Diagnosis, differential diagnosis and management of eclampsia. Obstet Gynecol 105:402, 2005.

TABLE 35-20 TIME OF ONSET OF ECLAMPSIA IN RELATION TO DELIVERY

	DOUGLAS & REDMAN (n = 383) (%)	KNIGHT (n = 214) (%)	KATZ (n = 53) (%)	TUFNELL (n = 82) (%)	MATTAR & SIBAI[16] (n = 399) (%)	CHAMES ET AL. (n = 89) (%)
Antepartum	38	96	53	45	53	67*
Intrapartum	18	41	36	12	19	—
Postpartum	44	75	11	26	28	33
<48 hr	39		5	24	11	7
>48 hr	5		6	2	17	26

*Includes antepartum and intrapartum cases.

from 11% to 44%.[16] **Although most cases of postpartum eclampsia occur within the first 48 hours, some cases can develop beyond 48 hours postpartum and have been reported as late as 23 days postpartum.[16] In the latter cases, an extensive neurologic evaluation may be needed to rule out the presence of other cerebral pathology.[86]**

Almost all cases (91%) of eclampsia develop in the third trimester (≥28 weeks).[16] The remaining cases occur between 21 and 27 weeks' gestation (7.5%) or at or before 20 weeks' gestation (1.5%).[16] Eclampsia occurring before the 20th week of gestation is generally associated with molar or hydropic degeneration of the placenta with or without a coexistent fetus.[32,86] Although rare, eclampsia can occur during the first half of pregnancy without molar degeneration of the placenta.[32,86] These women may be misdiagnosed as having hypertensive encephalopathy, a seizure disorder, or TTP. Women in whom convulsions develop in association with hypertension and proteinuria during the first half of pregnancy should be considered to have eclampsia until proved otherwise.[32] These women should have an ultrasound examination to rule out molar pregnancy or hydropic degeneration of the placenta. They also should have an extensive neurologic and medical evaluation to rule out another pathologic process.

Late postpartum eclampsia is defined as eclampsia that occurs more than 48 hours but less than 4 weeks after delivery. Historically, eclampsia was believed not to occur more than 48 hours after delivery. However, several recent reports have confirmed the existence of late postpartum eclampsia.[86] These women have signs and symptoms consistent with preeclampsia in association with convulsions.[32,86] Some of these women demonstrate a clinical picture of preeclampsia during labor or immediately postpartum (56%), whereas others demonstrate these clinical findings for the first time more than 48 hours after delivery (44%). Of interest is the fact that late-postpartum eclampsia developed despite the use of prophylactic magnesium sulfate during labor and for at least 24 hours postpartum in previously diagnosed preeclamptic women.[86] Therefore, women in whom convulsions develop in association with hypertension or proteinuria or with headaches or blurred vision after 48 hours of delivery should be considered to have eclampsia and initially treated as such.[32]

Cerebral Pathology

Autoregulation of the cerebral circulation is a mechanism for the maintenance of constant cerebral blood flow during changes in BP and may be altered in eclampsia. Through active changes in cerebrovascular resistance at the arteriolar level, cerebral blood flow normally remains relatively constant when cerebral perfusion pressure ranges between 60 and 120 mm Hg. In this normal range, vasoconstriction of cerebral vessels occurs in response to elevations in BP, whereas vasodilation occurs as BP is lowered. Once cerebral perfusion pressure exceeds 130 to 150 mm Hg, however, the autoregulatory mechanism fails. In extreme hypertension, the normal compensatory vasoconstriction may become defective, and cerebral blood flow increases. As a result, segments of the vessels become dilated, ischemic, and increasingly permeable. Thus, exudation of plasma occurs, giving rise to focal cerebral edema and compression of vessels, resulting in a decreased cerebral blood flow.[86] Hypertensive encephalopathy, a possible model for eclampsia, is an acute clinical condition that results from abrupt severe hypertension and subsequent significant increases in intracranial pressure. Because this is an acute disturbance in the hemodynamics of cerebral arterioles, morphologic changes in anatomy may not be uniformly evident in pathologic material. Several autopsy findings that are relatively constant include cerebral swelling and fibrinoid necrosis of vessel walls.

The cause of eclampsia is unknown, and there are many unanswered questions regarding the pathogenesis of its cerebral manifestations. Cerebral pathology in cortical and subcortical white matter in the form of edema, infarction, and hemorrhage (microhemorrhage and intracerebral parenchymal hemorrhage) is a common autopsy finding in patients who die from eclampsia. However, although autopsy series provide information regarding the central nervous system abnormality in patients dying of eclampsia, this information is not necessarily indicative of the central nervous system abnormality present in most patients who survive this condition.[86] The diagnosis of eclampsia is not dependent on any single clinical or diagnostic neurologic findings. Focal neurologic signs such as hemiparesis or an unconscious state are rare in cases of eclampsia reported from countries in the developed world.[86] Although eclamptic patients may initially manifest a variety of neurologic abnormalities, including cortical blindness, focal motor deficits, and coma, most have no permanent neurologic deficits.[16,86] These neurologic abnormalities are probably due to a transient insult, such as hypoxia, ischemia, or edema.

Several neurodiagnostic tests, such as electroencephalography (EEG), CT, cerebral Doppler velocimetry, MRI, and cerebral angiography (both traditional and MRI angiography) have been studied in women with eclampsia. In general, the EEG is acutely abnormal in most eclamptic patients; however, these abnormalities are not pathognomonic of eclampsia. In addition, the abnormal EEG findings are not affected by the use of magnesium sulfate. Moreover, lumbar puncture is not helpful in the diagnosis and management of eclamptic women. The results of CT and MRI studies reveal the presence of edema and infarction within the subcortical white matter and adjacent gray matter mostly in the parieto-occipital lobes (see box, Reported Computed Tomography Scan and Magnetic Resonance Imaging Findings in Complicated Eclampsia). Cerebral angiography and Doppler velocimetry suggest the presence of vasospasm.

On the basis of cerebral imaging findings, attention has been directed to hypertensive encephalopathy as a model for the central nervous system abnormalities in eclampsia. The two conditions share many clinical, radiologic, and pathologic features. There is failure of normal cerebral blood flow autoregulation in patients with hypertensive encephalopathy and in some patients with eclampsia.[86] Two theories have been proposed to explain these cerebral abnormalities: forced dilation and vasospasm.[86] The forced dilation theory suggests that the lesions in eclampsia are caused by loss of cerebrovascular autoregulation.

Recently, MRI and apparent diffusion coefficient mapping were used to characterize the relative frequency

Reported Computed Tomography Scan and Magnetic Resonance Imaging Findings in Complicated Eclampsia

- Diffuse white matter low-density areas
- Patchy areas of low density
- Occipital white matter edema
- Loss of normal cortical sulci
- Reduced ventricular size
- Acute hydrocephalus
- Cerebral hemorrhage
  - Intraventricular hemorrhage
  - Parenchymal hemorrhage (high density)
- Cerebral infarction
  - Low-attenuation areas
  - Basal ganglia infarctions

of vasogenic and cytotoxic edema in two small series of eclamptic women. Cerebral edema (mostly vasogenic) was present in up to 93% to 100% of these women. However, concurrent foci of infarction evidenced by reduced apparent diffusion coefficient (restricted diffusion) were present in 6 of 27 eclamptic women studied by Zeeman and colleagues and in 3 of 17 eclamptic and preeclamptic women studied by Loureiro and associates. In addition, 5 of these 6 women reported by Zeeman and colleagues had persistent abnormalities on repeat MRI testing 6 to 8 weeks later, suggesting that these lesions might not be reversible. Moreover, 4 of the 17 women reported by Loureira and associates had persistent MRI abnormalities at a median of 8 weeks of follow-up.

In summary, cerebral imaging findings in eclampsia are similar to those found in patients with hypertensive encephalopathy. The classic findings are referred to as posterior reversible encephalopathy syndrome (PRES). Figure 35-10 demonstrates such a lesion. This syndrome is also seen in patients with reversible cerebral vasoconstriction syndrome. This syndrome is usually seen in patients who present in the postpartum period with signs and symptoms similar to eclampsia. The diagnosis is confirmed by angiogram (Figure 35-11). **Cerebral imaging is not necessary for the diagnosis and management of most women with eclampsia. Cerebral imaging is indicated for patients with focal neurologic deficits or prolonged coma. In these patients, hemorrhage and other serious abnormalities requiring specific pharmacologic therapy or surgery must be excluded. Cerebral imaging may also be helpful in patients who have an atypical presentation for eclampsia (onset before 20 weeks' gestation or more than 48 hours after delivery, and eclampsia refractory to adequate magnesium sulfate therapy).** Advances in MRI and magnetic resonance angiography, as well as in cerebral vascular Doppler velocimetry, may aid our understanding regarding the pathogenesis and improving long-term outcome of this condition.[86]

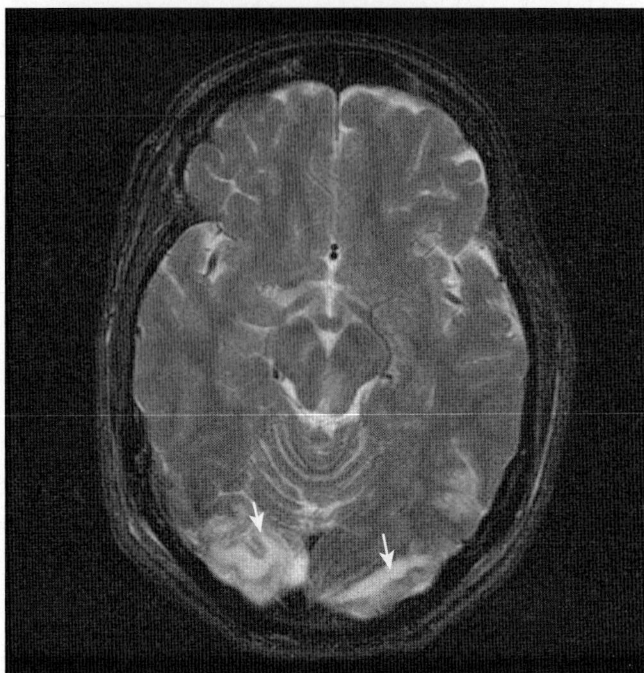

Figure 35-10. MRI of the brain revealing posterior reversible encephalopathy syndrome in patient with eclampsia. *Arrows* point at vasogenic edema that is considered reversible.

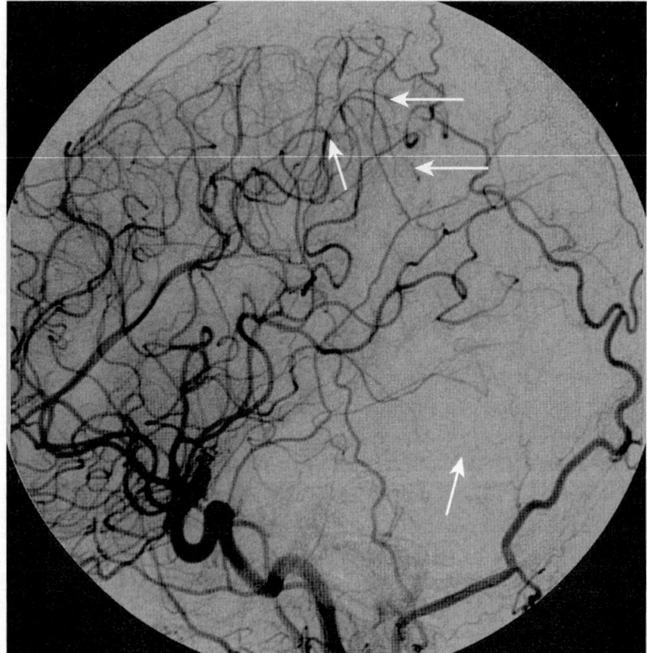

Figure 35-11. Cerebral arteriogram demonstrating cerebral vasoconstriction. *Arrows* show diffused vasoconstriction in small blood vessels.

Differential Diagnosis

The presenting symptoms, clinical findings, and many of the laboratory findings overlap with a number of medical and surgical conditions.[32] The most common cause of convulsions developing in association with hypertension or proteinuria during pregnancy or immediately postpartum is eclampsia. Rarely, other etiologies producing convulsions in pregnancy or postpartum may mimic eclampsia.[86]

These diagnoses are particularly important in the presence of focal neurologic deficits, prolonged coma, or atypical eclampsia. In addition, in some patients, gestational hypertension or preeclampsia may develop in association with these disorders (connective tissue disease, thrombophilias, seizure disorder, hypertensive encephalopathy), further contributing to the diagnostic difficulty. Therefore, an effort should be made to identify an accurate diagnosis given that management strategies may differ among these conditions.

Differential Diagnosis of Eclampsia

- Hypertensive encephalopathy
- Seizure disorder
- Hypoglycemia, hyponatremia
- Posterior reversible vasoconstriction syndrome (Figure 35-11)
- Thrombotic thrombocytopenic purpura
- Postdural puncture syndrome
- Vasculitis, angiopathy
- Amniotic fluid embolism
- Cerebrovascular accidents
- Hemorrhage
- Ruptured aneurysm or malformation
- Arterial embolism, thrombosis
- Venous thrombosis
- Hypoxic ischemic encephalopathy
- Angiomas

Maternal and Perinatal Outcome

Eclampsia is associated with a slightly increased risk for maternal death in developed countries (0% to 1.8%),[86] but the maternal mortality rate may be as high as 14% in developing countries. The high maternal mortality reported from developing countries occurs primarily among patients who have had multiple seizures outside the hospital and those without prenatal care. In addition, this high mortality rate could be attributed to the lack of resources and intensive care facilities needed to manage maternal complications from eclampsia. Of 4024 pregnancy-related deaths reported from 1979 to 1992, a total of 790 (19.6%) were considered due to preeclampsia-eclampsia, with 49% of these 790 considered related to eclampsia. In this series, the risk for death from preeclampsia or eclampsia was higher for women older than 30 years, those without prenatal care, and black women; the greatest risk for death was found among women with pregnancies at or before 28 weeks' gestation.

Pregnancies complicated by eclampsia are also associated with increased rates of maternal morbidities such as abruptio placentae (7% to 10%),[86] DIC (7% to 11%),[86] pulmonary edema (3% to 5%), acute renal failure (5% to 9%), aspiration pneumonia (2% to 3%), and cardiopulmonary arrest (2% to 5%).[86] ARDS and intracerebral hemorrhage are rare complications in series of eclamptic patients reported from the developed world. It is important to note that maternal complications are greatest among women who develop antepartum eclampsia, particularly among those who develop eclampsia remote from term.[86]

Perinatal mortality and morbidities remain high in eclamptic pregnancies. The reported perinatal death rate in recent series ranged from 5.6% to 11.8%.[86] This high perinatal death rate is related to prematurity, abruptio placentae, and severe FGR.[86] The rate of preterm delivery is about 50%, with about 25% of cases occurring before 32 weeks' gestation.[86]

Is Eclampsia Preventable?

Prevention of eclampsia requires knowledge of its etiology and pathophysiology and of methods to predict patients at high risk for development of convulsions. However, as discussed earlier, the pathogenesis of eclampsia is largely unknown. Prevention of eclampsia can be primary by preventing the development of preeclampsia or secondary by employing pharmacologic agents that prevent convulsions in women with established preeclampsia. Prevention can also be tertiary by preventing subsequent convulsions in women with established eclampsia.

Current management schemes designed to prevent eclampsia are based on early detection of gestational hypertension or preeclampsia and subsequent use of preventive therapy in such women. Some of the recommended preventive therapies have included close monitoring (in-hospital or outpatient), use of antihypertensive therapy to keep maternal BP below a certain level (less than severe range or to normal values), timely delivery, and prophylactic use of magnesium sulfate during labor and immediately postpartum in those considered to have preeclampsia. These management schemes assume that the clinical course in the development of eclampsia is characterized by a gradual process that begins with progressive weight gain, followed by hypertension (mild to severe) and proteinuria, with the subsequent onset of premonitory symptoms, and ending with the onset of generalized convulsions or coma.[86] This clinical course may be present in some women who develop eclampsia in developed countries. However, recent data from large series of eclamptic women from the United States and Europe indicate that about 20% to 40% of eclamptic women do not have any premonitory signs or symptoms before the onset of convulsions.[16] In many of these cases, the onset of convulsions is abrupt and does not follow an indolent progression from mild to severe disease before the onset of eclampsia.[86]

It is also assumed that appropriate and timely standard preventive therapy will avoid eclampsia in virtually all patients with gestational hypertension-preeclampsia.[86] The efficacy of in-hospital management of patients with gestational hypertension or preeclampsia for the prevention of eclampsia has not been evaluated in randomized trials. Moreover, data from retrospective studies from the developed countries indicate that about 50% of eclamptic women develop their first convulsion while in the hospital under "close medical supervision."[86] Thus, early and prolonged hospitalization of women with mild hypertension or preeclampsia may not prevent most cases of eclampsia.

There are several randomized trials describing the use of antihypertensive drugs versus no treatment or a placebo in the treatment of women with mild hypertension or preeclampsia. Overall, these trials revealed lower rates of progression to severe disease. However, the study design and the sample size of these trials is inadequate to evaluate potential benefits regarding prevention of eclampsia.

Prophylactic magnesium sulfate is recommended only for women who are hospitalized with the established diagnosis of preeclampsia.[1-3] Its use is recommended only during labor and for 12 to 24 hours' postpartum.[1-3] Therefore, it can be expected to have a potential effect in preventing eclampsia that develops only during this time period (40% of total).

There are several randomized trials comparing the efficacy of magnesium sulfate with other anticonvulsive agents for the prevention of recurrent seizures in women with eclampsia. In these trials, **magnesium sulfate has been compared with diazepam, phenytoin, and a lytic cocktail. Overall, these trials revealed that magnesium sulfate was associated with a significantly lower rate of recurrent seizures (9.4% versus 23.1%; RR, 0.41; 95% CI, 0.32 to 0.51) and a lower rate of maternal death (3% versus 4.8%; RR, 0.62; 95% CI, 0.39 to 0.99) than that observed with other agents.**

The low incidence of eclampsia in developed countries is probably related to prevention of cases of eclampsia in women with a classic presentation and with a classic progression from mild to severe preeclampsia.[86] As a result, most eclamptic cases described in reported series from the United States and Europe have an atypical presentation (abrupt onset, development of convulsions while receiving prophylactic magnesium sulfate, or onset of convulsions beyond 48 hours after delivery).[86] Indeed, most eclamptic convulsions in these series developed in hospitalized women, and in some of these women, the onset of convulsions was not preceded by warning signs or symptoms.[86] Overall, the percentage of eclampsia considered unpreventable in these series ranges from 31% to 87%.[86]

Maternal Transport of the Eclamptic Patient

During the past 20 years, there has been a marked reduction in the number of eclamptic patients. Consequently, most obstetricians have little or no experience in the management of eclampsia. A recent survey of a random sample of obstetricians from all 50 states indicated that about 50% of obstetricians in private practice had not seen an eclamptic patient during the past year.

Because management of the eclamptic patient requires the availability of neonatal and obstetrical intensive care units and personnel with special expertise, it is recommended that eclamptic women at term be cared for only at level II or III hospitals with adequate facilities and with consultants from other specialties. For those eclamptic patients who are remote from term, referral should be made to a tertiary care center. The following steps should be taken before transfer of these critically ill patients:

1. The referring physician or nurse should consult with the physician at the perinatal center regarding the referral and appropriate treatment. All maternal records, including prenatal data and a detailed summary of the patient's condition, should be transmitted.
2. BP should be stabilized and convulsions controlled.
3. Adequate prophylactic anticonvulsive medications should be given. An accepted regimen is 4 g intravenous magnesium sulfate as a loading dose over 20 minutes
4. Maternal laboratory assessment (complete blood count with platelet count, liver enzymes) and fetal monitoring should be undertaken.
5. Such patients should be sent in an ambulance with medical personnel in attendance for proper management in case of subsequent convulsions.

Treatment of Eclamptic Convulsions

Eclamptic convulsions are a life-threatening emergency and require proper care to minimize morbidity and mortality. The development of an eclamptic convulsion is frightening to observe. Initially, the patient's face becomes distorted with protrusion of her eyes. This is followed by a congested facial expression. Foam often exudes from the mouth. The woman usually bites her tongue unless it is protected. Respirations are absent throughout the seizure. Typically, the convulsion, which can be divided into two phases, continues for 60 to 75 seconds. The first phase, which lasts 15 to 20 seconds, begins with facial twitching, proceeding to the body becoming rigid with generalized muscular contractions. The second phase lasts about 60 seconds and consists of the muscles of the body alternately contracting and relaxing in rapid succession. This phase begins with the muscles of the jaw and rapidly involves the eyelids, other facial muscles, and then all the muscles of the body. Coma follows the convulsion, and the woman usually remembers nothing of the recent events. If she has repeated convulsions, some degree of consciousness returns after each convulsion. She may enter a combative state and be agitated and difficult to control. Rapid and deep respirations usually begin as soon as the convulsions end. Maintenance of oxygenation is usually not a problem after a single convulsion; the risk for aspiration is low in the well-managed patient.

Because eclampsia is so frightening, the natural tendency is to attempt to abolish the convulsion. Drugs such as diazepam should not be given in an attempt to stop or shorten the convulsion, especially if the patient does not have an intravenous line in place and someone skilled in intubation is not immediately available. If diazepam is used, no more than 5 mg should be given over a 60-second period. Rapid administration of diazepam may lead to apnea or cardiac arrest, or both.

Prevention of Maternal Injury During the Convulsions

The first priority in the management of eclampsia is to prevent maternal injury and to support cardiovascular functions. During or immediately after the acute convulsive episode, supportive care should be given to prevent serious maternal injury and aspiration, assess and establish airway potency, and ensure maternal oxygenation. During this time, the bed's side rails should be elevated and padded, a padded tongue blade is inserted between the teeth (avoid inducing gag reflex), and physical restraints may be needed. To minimize the risk for aspiration, the patient should lie in the lateral decubitus position, and vomitus and oral secretions are suctioned as needed.[86] Aspiration may be caused by forcing the padded tongue blade to the back of the throat, stimulating the gag reflex with resultant vomiting.

Adequate oxygenation should be maintained during the convulsive episode because hypoventilation and respiratory acidosis often occur. Although the initial seizure lasts only a few minutes, it is important to maintain oxygenation by supplemental oxygen administration through a face mask with or without an oxygen reservoir at 8 to 10 L/minute.[86] After the convulsion has ceased, the patient begins to breathe again, and oxygenation is rarely a problem. However, maternal hypoxemia and acidosis may develop in women who have had repetitive convulsions, in those with aspiration pneumonia, in those with pulmonary edema, or as a result of a combination of these factors. It is the author's policy to use transcutaneous pulse oximetry to monitor oxygenation in all eclamptic patients. Arterial blood gas analysis is required if the pulse oximetry results are abnormal (oxygen saturation ≤92%). Sodium bicarbonate is not given unless the pH is below 7.10.

Prevention of Recurrent Convulsions

The next step in the management of eclampsia is to prevent recurrent convulsions. **Magnesium sulfate is the drug of choice to treat and prevent subsequent convulsions in women with eclampsia.[86] A loading dose of 6 g over 15 to 20 minutes is recommended, followed by a maintenance dose of 2 g per hour as a continuous intravenous solution.** About 10% of eclamptic women have a second convulsion after receiving magnesium sulfate.[86] In these women, another bolus of 2 g magnesium sulfate can be given intravenously over 3 to 5 minutes. An occasional patient will have recurrent convulsions while receiving adequate and therapeutic doses of magnesium sulfate. In this patient, recurrent seizures can be treated with sodium amobarbital, 250 mg intravenously over 3 to 5 minutes.[86]

Rarely, a woman may experience an eclamptic seizure, lapse into a coma, and die. Magnesium toxicity should be considered in those women who do not regain consciousness. A case report of magnesium sulfate toxicity details the features of this serious complication. Within a few minutes of starting what was supposed to be a magnesium loading dose, 4 g magnesium sulfate in 250 mL saline, the patient went into cardiorespiratory arrest. Immediate resuscitation including intubation was performed. About half of the loading dose had been given. An intracerebral accident or eclampsia was thought to be the cause of the coma; the loading dose was continued and maintenance therapy started. Initial blood gases were normal, and the electrocardiogram (ECG) was normal 15 minutes after the arrest. Mechanical ventilatory support was required. The patient's vital signs were stable; however, her pupils were nonreactive. Serum electrolytes, glucose, blood urea nitrogen, and creatinine were normal. CT scan of the head and cerebral angiograms were normal. A magnesium level of 35 mg/dL was reported 3.5 hours later from a blood sample taken through femoral venipuncture at the time of arrest. The magnesium sulfate infusion was stopped immediately. During the first 5 hours after the cardiorespiratory arrest, 1344 mg of magnesium was excreted in the urine. Twelve hours after the arrest, an uncomplicated low vertical cesarean delivery was done for a breech presentation. The 3160-g male infant had Apgar scores of 8 and 9 at 1 and 5 minutes, respectively. Maternal and cord blood magnesium levels at delivery were 5.8 mg/dL. Both mother and baby were discharged from the hospital with no apparent sequelae. Of interest, the patient reported she could hear and see what was occurring around her, but she could not make any movements while she was intubated. Figure 35-12 presents the maternal magnesium levels in this case.

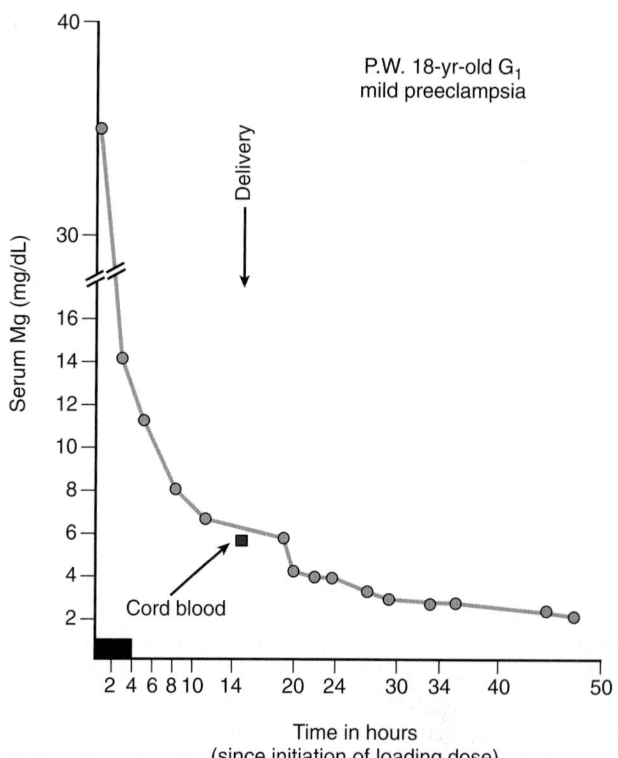

FIGURE 35-12. A patient with magnesium toxicity. (From McCubbin JH, Sibai BM, Abdella TN, et al: Cardiopulmonary arrest due to acute maternal hypermagnesemia [Letter]. Lancet 1:1058, 1981.)

Control of Severe Hypertension

The next step in the management of eclampsia is to reduce the BP to a safe range. The objectives of treating severe hypertension are to avoid loss of cerebral autoregulation and to prevent congestive heart failure without compromising cerebral perfusion or jeopardizing uteroplacental blood flow that is already reduced in many women with eclampsia.[86] Thus, **maintaining systolic BP between 140 and 160 mm Hg and diastolic BP between 90 and 105 mm Hg is a reasonable goal. This can be achieved with bolus 5 to 10 mg doses of hydralazine or labetalol (20 to 40 mg intravenously) every 15 minutes as needed.**[86] Other potent antihypertensive medications such as sodium nitroprusside or nitroglycerine are rarely needed in eclampsia. Diuretics are not used except in the presence of pulmonary edema.

Intrapartum Management

Maternal hypoxemia and hypercarbia cause fetal heart rate and uterine activity changes during and immediately after a convulsion. The fetal heart rate tracing may reveal bradycardia, transient late decelerations, decreased beat-to-beat variability, and compensatory tachycardia. Uterine contractions can increase in frequency and tone.[86] These changes usually resolve spontaneously within 3 to 10 minutes after the termination of convulsions and the correction of maternal hypoxemia. The patient should not be rushed to emergency cesarean delivery based on these findings, especially if the maternal condition remains stable.

In a review of 10 women who had undergone electronic internal fetal monitoring during an eclamptic convulsion, 6 had fetal bradycardia (fetal heart rate <120 beats/minute) that varied in duration from 30 seconds to 9 minutes. The interval from onset of the seizure to the fall in fetal heart rate was 5 minutes. Transitory fetal tachycardia occurred frequently after the prolonged bradycardia. In addition, loss of beat-to-beat variability with transitory late decelerations occurred during the recovery phase. Uterine hyperactivity demonstrated by both increased uterine tone and increased frequency of uterine contractions occurs during an eclamptic seizure. The duration of the increased uterine activity varies from 2 to 14 minutes.

Fetal outcome is generally good after an eclamptic convulsion. The mechanism for the transitory fetal bradycardia may be a decrease in uterine blood flow caused by intense vasospasm and uterine hyperactivity. The absence of maternal respiration during the convulsion may also result in fetal hypoxia and heart rate changes. Because the fetal heart rate pattern usually returns to normal after a convulsion, other conditions should be considered if an abnormal pattern persists. It may take longer for the heart rate pattern to return to baseline in an eclamptic woman whose fetus is preterm with growth restriction. Placental abruption may occur after the convulsion and should be considered if uterine hyperactivity remains or the bradycardia persists.[86]

The presence of eclampsia is not an indication for cesarean delivery. The decision to perform a cesarean delivery should be based on gestational age, fetal condition, presence of labor, and cervical Bishop score.[86] Cesarean delivery is recommended for those with eclampsia before 30 weeks' gestation who are not in labor with an unfavorable cervix (Bishop score <5). Patients having labor or rupture of membranes are allowed to deliver vaginally in the absence of obstetrical complications. When labor is indicated, it is initiated with either oxytocin infusions or prostaglandins in all patients with a gestational age at or above 30 weeks, irrespective of the Bishop score. A similar approach is used for those before 30 weeks' gestation if the cervical Bishop score is at least 5.

Maternal pain relief during labor and delivery can be provided by either systemic opioids or epidural anesthesia as recommended for women with severe preeclampsia.[2] Either epidural, spinal, or combined techniques of regional anesthesia can be used for cesarean delivery. Regional anesthesia is contraindicated in the presence of coagulopathy or severe thrombocytopenia (platelet count <50,000/mm^3). In women with eclampsia, general anesthesia increases the risk for aspiration and failed intubation due to airway edema and is associated with marked increases in systemic and cerebral pressures during intubation and extubation.[86] Women with airway or laryngeal edema may require awake intubation under fiberoptic observation with the availability of immediate tracheostomy. Changes in systemic or cerebral pressures may be attenuated by pretreatment with labetalol or nitroglycerine injections.[86]

Postpartum Management of Eclampsia

After delivery, women with eclampsia should receive close monitoring of vital signs, fluid intake and output, and symptoms for at least 48 hours. These women usually receive large amounts of intravenous fluids during labor, delivery, and postpartum. In addition, during the postpartum period, there is mobilization of extracellular fluid leading to increased intravascular volume. As a result, women with eclampsia, particularly those with abnormal renal function, those with abruptio placentae, and those with preexisting chronic hypertension are at increased risk for pulmonary edema and exacerbation of severe hypertension postpartum.[86] Careful attention to fluid status is essential.

Parenteral magnesium sulfate should be continued for at least 24 hours after delivery or for at least 24 hours after the last convulsion. If oliguria is present (<100 mL/4 hours), both the rate of fluid administration and the dose of magnesium sulfate should be reduced. Once delivery has occurred, other oral antihypertensive agents such as labetalol or nifedipine can be used to keep systolic BP below 155 mm Hg and diastolic BP below 105 mm Hg. Nifedipine offers the benefit of improved diuresis in the postpartum period.

Subsequent Pregnancy Outcome and Remote Prognosis

Women with a history of eclampsia are at increased risk for all forms of preeclampsia in subsequent pregnancies (Table 35-21). In general, the rate of preeclampsia in subsequent pregnancies is about 25%, with substantially higher rates if the onset of eclampsia was in the second trimester. The rate of recurrent eclampsia is about 2%. Because of these risks, these women should be informed that they are at increased risk for adverse pregnancy outcome in subsequent pregnancies. At present, there is no preventive therapy for recurrent antepartum eclampsia.

The long-term effects of eclampsia on maternal BP and neurologic outcome have been the subject of few reports. The findings of these studies revealed that eclampsia did not cause hypertension in women who were normotensive before the eclamptic pregnancy. Two of these studies found that the rate of chronic hypertension on follow-up was significantly higher in those who had eclampsia remote from term compared with those who had eclampsia at or beyond 37 weeks of gestation. In addition, one of these

TABLE 35-21 RECURRENT PREECLAMPSIA-ECLAMPSIA IN WOMEN WITH ECLAMPSIA

	CHESLEY	LOPEZ-LLERA & HORTON	ADELUSI & OJENGBEDE	SIBAI ET AL.
Number of women	171	110	64	182
Number of pregnancies	398	110	64	366
Eclampsia (%)	1.0	—	15.6	1.9
Preeclampsia (%)	23	35	27	22

From Sibai BM: Diagnosis, differential diagnosis and management of eclampsia. Obstet Gynecol 105:402, 2005.

reports revealed that women who had eclampsia as multiparas were at increased risk for death from cardiovascular renal disease. Moreover, these investigations revealed no evidence of neurologic deficit during the follow-up period.

INCIDENCE OF CHRONIC HYPERTENSION

The frequency of chronic hypertension in pregnancy is estimated at 1% to 5%. It is more common in older obese women and in African American women. Because of the current trend of childbearing at an older age and the obesity epidemic, it is expected that the incidence of chronic hypertension in pregnancy will continue to rise. During the new millennium, and estimating a prevalence of chronic hypertension during pregnancy of 3%, at least 120,000 pregnant women (3% of 4 million pregnancies) with chronic hypertension per year will be seen in the United States.

Definition and Diagnosis

In pregnancy, chronic hypertension is defined as elevated BP that is present and documented before conception. **In women whose prepregnancy BP is unknown, the diagnosis is based on the presence of sustained hypertension before 20 weeks of gestation, defined as either systolic BP of at least 140 mm Hg or diastolic BP of at least 90 mm Hg on at least two occasions measured at least 4 hours apart.**

The diagnosis may be difficult to establish in women with previously undiagnosed chronic hypertension who begin prenatal care after 16 weeks' gestation because physiologic decline in BP occurs at that time. An analysis of pregnancy outcome in 211 patients with mild chronic hypertension suggests that the use of antihypertensive drugs is not necessary to achieve a good pregnancy outcome. The changes in average mean arterial pressure throughout the course of pregnancy are summarized in Figure 35-13. This decrease may result in normal BP findings in the second trimester that will eventually increase again during the third trimester. These women are more likely to be erroneously diagnosed as having gestational hypertension.

Women with chronic hypertension are at increased risk for superimposed preeclampsia. The development of superimposed preeclampsia is associated with high rates of adverse maternal and perinatal outcomes.[14] The diagnosis of superimposed preeclampsia should be made as described in Table 35-3.

Etiology and Classification

The etiology and severity of chronic hypertension are important considerations in the management of pregnancy. Chronic hypertension is subdivided into primary (essential) and secondary. Primary hypertension is by far the most common cause of chronic hypertension seen during pregnancy (90%). In 10% of cases, chronic hypertension is secondary to one or more underlying disorders such as renal disease (glomerulonephritis, interstitial nephritis, polycystic kidneys, renal artery stenosis), collagen vascular disease (lupus, scleroderma), endocrine disorders (diabetes mellitus with vascular involvement, pheochromocytoma, thyrotoxicosis, Cushing disease, hyperaldosteronism), or coarctation of the aorta.

Chronic hypertension during pregnancy can be subclassified as either mild or severe, depending on the systolic and diastolic BP readings. Systolic and diastolic (Korotkoff phase V) BPs of at least 160 mm Hg or 110 mm Hg, respectively, constitute severe hypertension.

For management and counseling purposes, chronic hypertension in pregnancy is also categorized as either low risk or high risk, as described in Figure 35-13. The patient is considered to be at low risk when she has mild essential hypertension without any organ involvement. The BP criteria are based on BP measurements at the initial visit irrespective of treatment with antihypertensive medications. For example, if the patient has a BP of 140/80 mm Hg on antihypertensive drugs, she is still classified as low risk. It is important to note that a patient initially classified as low risk early in pregnancy may become high risk if she later develops severe hypertension or preeclampsia.

Maternal-Perinatal Risks

Pregnancies complicated by chronic hypertension are at increased risk for the development of superimposed preeclampsia and abruptio placentae. The reported rates of preeclampsia in the literature in mild hypertension range from 14% to 28% (Table 35-22).[14] The rate of preeclampsia in women with severe chronic hypertension ranges from 50% to 79%. Sibai and associates[14] studied the rate of superimposed preeclampsia among 763 women with

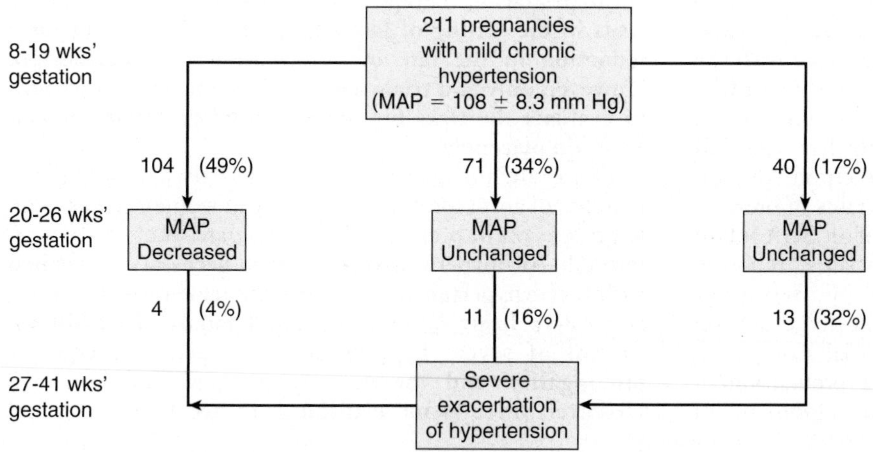

FIGURE 35-13. Mean arterial blood pressure (MAP) during pregnancy. (Modified from Sibai BM, Abdella TN, Anderson GD: Pregnancy outcome in 211 patients with mild chronic hypertension. Obstet Gynecol 61:571, 1983.)

TABLE 35-22 RATES OF ADVERSE PREGNANCY OUTCOME IN OBSERVATIONAL STUDIES DESCRIBING MILD CHRONIC HYPERTENSION IN PREGNANCY

	PREECLAMPSIA (%)	ABRUPTIO PLACENTAE (%)	DELIVERY <37 WK (%)	SGA (%)
Rey & Couturier (*n*, 337)	21	0.7	34.4	15.5
McCowan et al. (*n* = 142)	14	NR	16	11.0
Sibai et al.[14] (*n* = 763)	25	1.5	33.3	11.1
Giannubilo et al. (*n* = 233)	28	0.5	NR	16.5
Chappell et al. (*n* = 822)	22	NR	22.7	27.2
Sibai et al. (*n* = 369)	17	2.4	29.3	15.0

NR, Not reported; SGA, small for gestational age.

chronic hypertension followed prospectively at several tertiary medical centers in the United States. The overall rate of superimposed preeclampsia was 25%. The rate was not affected by maternal age, race, or presence of proteinuria early in pregnancy. However, the rate was significantly greater in women who had hypertension for at least 4 years (31% versus 22%), in those who had preeclampsia during a previous pregnancy (32% versus 23%), and in those whose diastolic BP was 100 mm Hg or higher (42% versus 24%).[14]

The reported rate of abruptio placentae in women with mild chronic hypertension has ranged from 0.7% to 2.7% (see Table 35-22). The rate in those with severe or high-risk hypertension may be 5% to 10%. In a recent multicenter study that included 763 women with chronic hypertension, the overall rate of abruptio placentae was reported at 1.5%, and the rate was significantly higher in those who developed superimposed preeclampsia than in those without this complication (3% versus 1%, $P = .04$).[14] However, the rate was not influenced by maternal age, race, or duration of hypertension.[14] In addition, the results of a systematic review of nine observational studies revealed that the rate of abruptio placentae is doubled (odds ratio [OR], 2.1; 95% CI, 1.1 to 3.9) in women with chronic hypertension compared with either normotensive patients or the general obstetrical population.

In addition to preeclampsia and abruptio placentae, women with high-risk chronic hypertension are at increased risk for life-threatening maternal complications such as pulmonary edema, hypertensive encephalopathy, retinopathy, cerebral hemorrhage, and acute renal failure. These risks are particularly increased in women with uncontrolled severe hypertension, significant renal disease early in pregnancy, or left ventricular dysfunction before conception.

Fetal and neonatal complications are also increased in women with chronic hypertension. The risk for perinatal mortality is three to four times greater compared with the general obstetrical population (OR, 3.4; 95% CI, 3.0 to 3.7). The likelihood of premature delivery and an SGA infant is also increased in women with chronic hypertension (see Table 35-22). In women with severe chronic hypertension in the first trimester, the reported rates of preterm delivery were 62% to 70% and the rates of an SGA infant were 31% to 40%. Recently, Sibai and associates[14] reported risk factors for adverse perinatal outcome in a secondary analysis of 763 women with mild chronic hypertension who were enrolled in a multicenter trial comparing low-dose aspirin with a placebo for the prevention of preeclampsia. They found that the development of superimposed preeclampsia was associated with higher rates of preterm delivery (OR, 3.9; 95% CI, 2.7 to 5.4), neonatal intraventricular hemorrhage (OR, 4.5; 95% CI, 1.5 to 14.2), and perinatal death (OR, 2.3; 95% CI, 1.4 to 4.8). In addition, the presence of proteinuria early in pregnancy was an independent risk factor associated with higher rates of preterm delivery (OR, 3.1; 95% CI, 1.8 to 5.3), an SGA infant (OR, 2.8; 95% CI, 1.6 to 5.0), and neonatal intraventricular hemorrhage (OR, 3.9; 95% CI, 1.3 to 11.6).[14]

Goals of Antihypertensive Therapy in Pregnancy

In nonpregnant individuals, long-term BP control can lead to significant reductions in the rates of stroke and cardiovascular morbidity and mortality. The side effects of therapy are, of course, restricted to the treated individual. In contrast to hypertension in pregnancy, the duration of therapy is shorter, the benefits to the mother may not be obvious during the short time of treatment, and the exposure to medication will include both mother and fetus. In this respect, one must balance the potential short-term maternal benefits against possible short-term and long-term benefits and risks to the fetus and infant.

Most women with chronic hypertension during pregnancy have mild essential uncomplicated hypertension and are at minimal risk for cardiovascular complications within the short time frame of pregnancy. Several retrospective and prospective studies have been conducted to determine whether antihypertensive therapy in these women improves pregnancy outcome. An overall summary of these studies revealed that, regardless of the antihypertensive therapy used, maternal cardiovascular and renal complications were minimal or absent. **Based on the available data, there is no compelling evidence that short-term antihypertensive therapy is beneficial for the mother or the fetus in the setting of low-risk hypertension except for a reduction in the rate of exacerbation of hypertension. However, only two trials have had a sufficient sample size to evaluate the risks for superimposed preeclampsia and abruptio placentae.**

There are no placebo-controlled trials examining the benefits of antihypertensive therapy in women with severe hypertension in pregnancy, and none are likely to be performed. **Antihypertensive therapy is necessary in women with severe hypertension to reduce the acute risks for stroke, congestive heart failure, and renal failure. In addition, control of severe hypertension may permit pregnancy prolongation and thereby improve perinatal outcome. However, there is no available evidence that control of**

severe hypertension reduces the rate of either superimposed preeclampsia or abruptio placentae.

There are no trials examining the treatment of women with chronic hypertension and other risk factors, such as preexisting renal disease, diabetes mellitus, or cardiac disease. On the other hand, there is evidence from retrospective and observational studies that uncontrolled mild to moderate hypertension may exacerbate target organ damage during pregnancy in women with renal disease, diabetes mellitus with vascular disease, or left ventricular dysfunction. Therefore, some authors recommend aggressive treatment of mild hypertension in these women because of the belief that such management may reduce both short-term and long-term cardiovascular complications.

Safety of Antihypertensive Drugs in Pregnancy

The potential adverse effects of most commonly prescribed antihypertensive agents are either poorly established or unclearly quantified. Most of the evidence on harm associated with antihypertensives in pregnancy is limited to case reports. The interpretation of these reports is difficult because it is impossible to ascertain the exact number of women exposed to antihypertensive drugs during pregnancy. Also, it is likely that the number of published case reports is an underestimate of the actual number of women experiencing the reported adverse reaction. This limitation is amplified by the fact that information related to previous exposure during pregnancy is nonexistent. Furthermore, the condition for which pregnant women are treated with antihypertensive drugs can be partially responsible for the adverse fetal and neonatal outcomes.

In general, available information about teratogenicity, except in laboratory animals, is limited and selective. All available data have been obtained from registries such as state Medicaid registry data. Because of absent multicenter randomized trials in women with chronic hypertension, there are no placebo-controlled evaluations regarding the safety of these drugs when used at the time of conception and throughout pregnancy. At the present time, there are minimal data to help the clinician evaluate the benefits or risks of most antihypertensive drugs when used in pregnancy. **Nevertheless, the limited data in the literature suggest that there are potential adverse fetal effects, such as oligohydramnios and fetal-neonatal renal failure, when angiotensin-converting enzyme (ACE) inhibitors are used in the second or third trimester.** Similar effects are to be expected with the use of angiotensin II receptor blockers. Therefore, these agents should be avoided once pregnancy is established (see Chapter 8).

The use of atenolol during the first and second trimesters has been associated with significantly reduced fetal growth along with decreased placental growth and weight. On the other hand, no such effects on fetal or placental growth have been reported with other β-blockers, such as metoprolol, pindolol, and oxprenolol, but data on the use of these agents in early pregnancy are very limited.

Prospective trials examining the effect of either methyldopa or labetalol in women with mild chronic hypertension revealed no adverse maternal or fetal outcomes with the use of these medications. In a large and unique trial in which methyldopa or labetalol was started between 6 and 13 weeks' gestation in patients with chronic hypertension, none of the exposed newborns had major congenital anomalies.

There is a large clinical experience with the use of thiazide diuretics during pregnancy. The available data suggest that treatment with diuretics in the first trimester and throughout gestation is not associated with an increased risk for major fetal anomalies or adverse fetal-neonatal events. There is little information regarding the use of calcium channel blockers in women with mild chronic hypertension. **The available evidence suggests that the use of calcium channel blockers, particularly nifedipine, in the first trimester was not associated with increased rates of major birth defects.** The effects of nifedipine on fetal-neonatal outcome were evaluated in a prospective randomized trial of 283 women with mild to moderate hypertension in pregnancy in which 47% of the participants had chronic hypertension. Sixty-six of these women were enrolled between 12 and 20 weeks' gestation. In this study, the use of slow-release nifedipine was not associated with adverse fetal-neonatal outcomes.

The long-term effects on children of mothers exposed to antihypertensive drugs during pregnancy are lacking except for limited information concerning the use of methyldopa and nifedipine. A follow-up study of infants after 7.5 years showed no long-term adverse effects on development among those exposed to methyldopa in utero compared with infants not exposed to such treatment. A similar study examining the effects of slow-release nifedipine after 1.5 years of follow-up demonstrated no adverse effects on development.

Recommended Management of Chronic Hypertension in Pregnancy

The primary objective in the management of pregnancies complicated by chronic hypertension is to reduce maternal risks and achieve optimal perinatal survival. This objective can be achieved by formulating a rational approach that includes preconceptual evaluation and counseling, early antenatal care, frequent antepartum visits to monitor both maternal and fetal well-being, timely delivery with intensive intrapartum monitoring, and proper postpartum management.

Evaluation and Classification

Women with chronic hypertension should ideally be counseled before pregnancy, when extensive evaluation and complete workup can be undertaken. Assessment of the etiology and severity of hypertension, as well as the coexistence of other medical illnesses, and ruling out the presence of target organ damage resulting from long-standing hypertension can be accomplished. An in-depth history should delineate in particular the duration of hypertension, the use of antihypertensive medications, their type, and the response to these medications. Also, attention should be given to the presence of cardiac or renal disease, diabetes mellitus, thyroid disease, and a history of cerebrovascular accident or congestive heart failure. A detailed obstetrical history should include maternal and neonatal outcomes of previous pregnancies, stressing a history of

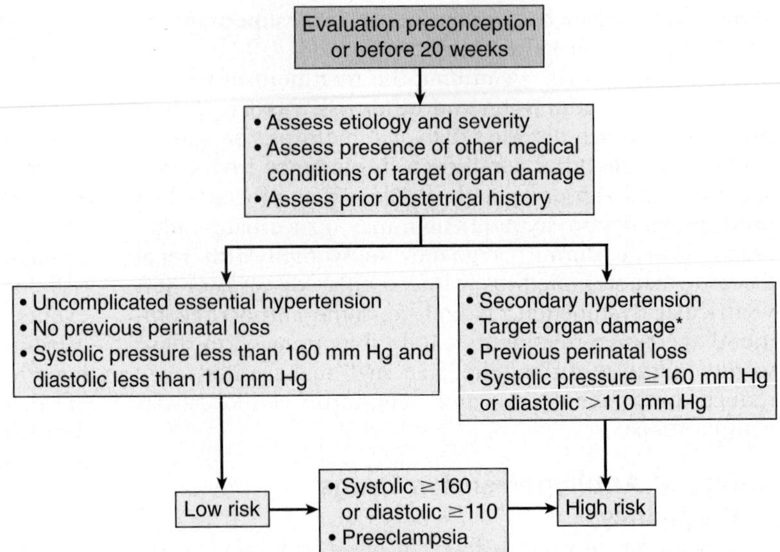

FIGURE 35-14. Initial evaluation of women with chronic hypertension. (From Sibai BM: Chronic hypertension in pregnancy. Obstet Gynecol 100:369, 2002.)

*Left ventricular dysfunction, retinopathy, dyslipidemia, maternal age above 40 years, microvascular disease, stroke.

the development of abruptio placentae, superimposed preeclampsia, preterm delivery, SGA infants, intrauterine fetal death, and neonatal morbidity and mortality.

Laboratory evaluation is obtained to assess the function of different organ systems that are likely to be affected by chronic hypertension and as a baseline for future assessments. These should include the following for all patients: urinalysis, urine culture and sensitivity, 24-hour urine evaluations for protein, electrolytes, complete blood count, and a glucose tolerance test.

Women with long-standing hypertension for several years, particularly those with a history of poor compliance or poor BP control, should be evaluated for target organ damage, including left ventricular hypertrophy, retinopathy, and renal injury. These women should undergo an ECG examination and echocardiography if the ECG is abnormal, ophthalmologic evaluation, and creatinine clearance.

Selectively, certain tests should be obtained to identify secondary causes of hypertension such as pheochromocytoma, primary hyperaldosteronism, or renal artery stenosis. These conditions require selective biochemical testing and are amenable to diagnosis with either CT or MRI. Pheochromocytoma should be suspected in women with paroxysmal severe hypertension, hyperglycemia, and sweating. Primary aldosteronism is extremely rare in pregnancy and should be considered in women with severe hypertension and marked hypokalemia. Based on this evaluation, the patient is then classified as having low-risk or high-risk chronic hypertension and managed accordingly (Figure 35-14).

Low-Risk Hypertension

Women with low-risk chronic hypertension without superimposed preeclampsia usually have a pregnancy outcome similar to that of the general obstetrical population. In addition, discontinuation of antihypertensive therapy early in pregnancy does not affect the rate of preeclampsia, abruptio placentae, or preterm delivery in these women. Many clinicians choose to discontinue antihypertensive treatment at the first prenatal visit because most of these women will experience a good pregnancy outcome without such therapy. Although many of these women will not require subsequent pharmacologic therapy, careful management is still essential (Figure 35-15). At the time of initial and subsequent visits, women are educated about nutritional requirements, weight gain, and sodium intake (maximum of 2.4 g of sodium per day). They are also counseled that consumption of alcohol and smoking during pregnancy can aggravate maternal hypertension and are associated with adverse effects on the fetus such as FGR and abruptio placentae. During each subsequent visit, they are observed closely for early signs of preeclampsia and FGR.

Fetal evaluation should include an ultrasound examination at 16 to 20 weeks' gestation, to be repeated at 30 to 32 weeks, and monthly thereafter until term. **Antihypertensive treatment with either nifedipine or labetalol is initiated if the patient develops severe hypertension before term. The development of either severe hypertension, preeclampsia, or abnormal fetal growth requires immediate fetal testing with NST or BPP. Women who develop severe hypertension and those with documented FGR by ultrasound examination require hospitalization and often delivery.** If superimposed preeclampsia is diagnosed at or beyond 37 weeks, delivery is undertaken as well. In the absence of these complications, the pregnancy may be continued until 40 weeks' gestation.

High-Risk Hypertension

Women with high-risk chronic hypertension are at increased risk for adverse maternal and perinatal complications. The likelihood and impact of these complications will depend on the etiology of the hypertension as well as the degree of target organ damage. Women with significant renal insufficiency (serum creatinine > 1.4 mg/dL), diabetes mellitus with vascular involvement (class R/F), severe collagen vascular disease, cardiomyopathy, or coarctation of the aorta should receive thorough counseling regarding the adverse effects of pregnancy before conception. These

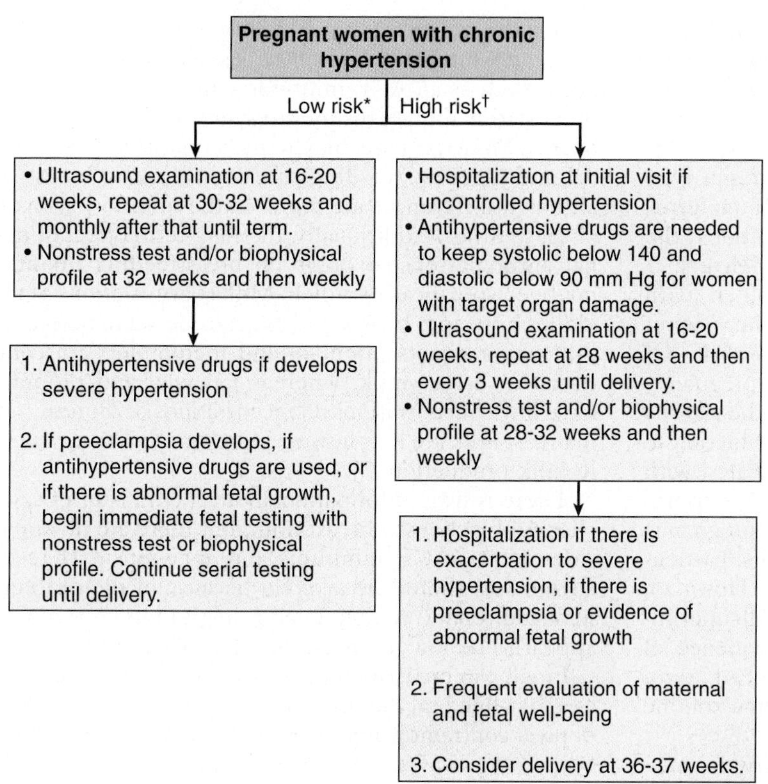

Figure 35-15. Antepartum management of chronic hypertension. (From Sibai BM: Chronic hypertension in pregnancy. Obstet Gynecol 100:369, 2002.)

women should be advised that pregnancy may exacerbate their condition, with the potential for congestive heart failure, acute renal failure requiring dialysis, and even death. In addition, perinatal loss and neonatal complications are markedly increased in these women. All such women should be managed by or in consultation with a subspecialist in maternal-fetal medicine as well as in association with other medical specialists as needed. In addition, these women must be observed and delivered at a tertiary care center with the appropriate resources for maternal and neonatal care.

Hospitalization of women with high-risk uncontrolled hypertension at the time of the first prenatal visit is recommended. This facilitates evaluation of cardiovascular and renal status and regulation of antihypertensive medications as well as other prescribed treatments (e.g., insulin, cardiac drugs, thyroid medications), if needed. Women receiving ACE inhibitors or angiotensin II receptor antagonists should have these medications discontinued under close observation. Antihypertensive therapy with one or more of the drugs listed in Table 35-23 is subsequently used in all women with systolic BP of 160 mm Hg or more, or diastolic BP of 110 mm Hg or more. In women without target organ damage, the aim of antihypertensive therapy is to keep systolic BP between 140 and 150 mm Hg and diastolic BP between 90 and 100 mm Hg. In addition, antihypertensive therapy is indicated in women with mild hypertension plus target organ damage because there are short-term maternal benefits from lowering BP in such women. In these women, maintaining systolic BP below 140 mm Hg and diastolic BP below 90 mm Hg is advised. In some women, BP may be difficult to control initially, demanding the use of intravenous therapy with hydralazine or labetalol or oral short-acting nifedipine with doses as described in Table 35-23. For maintenance therapy, one may choose either oral methyldopa, labetalol, slow-release nifedipine, or a diuretic. Methyldopa remains the drug most commonly recommended to treat hypertension during pregnancy; however, it is rarely used in nonpregnant hypertensive women. **The recommended first drug of choice for control of hypertension in pregnancy is labetalol starting at 100 mg twice daily, to be increased to a maximum of 2400 mg/day. If maternal BP is not controlled**

Table 35-23 Drugs Used to Treat Hypertension in Pregnancy

DRUG	STARTING DOSE	MAXIMUM DOSE	COMMENTS
Acute Treatment of Severe Hypertension			
Hydralazine	5-10 mg IV every 20 min	20 mg*	Avoid in cases of tachycardia and persistent headaches
Labetalol	20-40 mg IV every 10-15 min	220 mg*	Avoid in women with asthma or congestive heart failure
Nifedipine	10-20 mg oral every 30 min	50 mg*	Avoid in case of tachycardia and palpitations
Long-Term Treatment of Hypertension			
Methyldopa	250 mg bid	4 g/day	
Labetalol	100 mg bid	2400 mg/day	
Nifedipine	10 mg bid	120 mg/day	
Thiazide diuretic	12.5 mg bid	50 mg/day	

*If desired blood pressure levels are not achieved, switch to another drug.

with maximal doses of labetalol, a second drug such as a thiazide diuretic or nifedipine may be added. For women with diabetes mellitus and vascular disease, oral nifedipine is recommended. Oral nifedipine or a thiazide diuretic is the drug of choice for young black women with hypertension because these women often manifest a low-renin-type hypertension or salt-sensitive hypertension. If maternal BP is adequately controlled with these medications, the patient can continue with the same drug after delivery.

Diuretics are commonly prescribed in women with essential hypertension before conception. The use of diuretics throughout pregnancy is controversial. Of concern, women who use diuretics from early in pregnancy do not have an increase in plasma volume to the degree expected in normal pregnancy. However, this reduction in plasma volume has not been shown to be associated with an adverse effect on fetal outcome. Therefore, it is appropriate to start diuretics as a single agent during pregnancy or to use them in combination with other agents, particularly in women with excessive salt retention. However, diuretics should be discontinued immediately if superimposed preeclampsia develops or if there is evidence of suspected FGR because of the potential of reduced uteroplacental blood flow secondary to reduced plasma volume in women with these complications.

Early and frequent prenatal visits are the key for successful pregnancy outcome in women with high-risk chronic hypertension. These women need close observation throughout pregnancy and may require serial evaluation of 24-hour urine protein excretion and a complete blood count with a metabolic profile at least once every trimester. Further laboratory testing can be performed depending on the clinical progress of the pregnancy. During each visit, the woman should be advised about the adverse effects of smoking and alcohol abuse and should receive nutritional advice regarding diet and salt intake.

Fetal evaluation should include an ultrasound examination at 16 to 20 weeks' gestation, to be repeated at 28 weeks and subsequently every 3 weeks till delivery. NST or BPP testing is usually started at 28 to 32 weeks and then repeated weekly. **The development of uncontrolled severe hypertension, preeclampsia, or evidence of FGR requires maternal hospitalization for more frequent evaluation of maternal and fetal well-being. The development of any of these complications at or beyond 34 weeks' gestation should be considered an indication for delivery.** In all other women, delivery should be considered at 36 to 37 weeks' gestation after documentation of fetal lung maturity.

Postpartum Management

Women with high-risk chronic hypertension are at risk for postpartum complications such as pulmonary edema, hypertensive encephalopathy, and renal failure. These risks are particularly increased in women with target organ involvement, superimposed preeclampsia, or abruptio placentae. In these patients, BP must be closely controlled for at least 48 hours after delivery. Intravenous labetalol or hydralazine can be used as needed, and diuretics may be appropriate in women with circulatory congestion and pulmonary edema. This therapy is usually required in those who develop exaggerated and sustained severe hypertension in the first week postpartum.

Oral therapy may be needed to control BP after delivery. In some women, it is often necessary to switch to a new agent such as an ACE inhibitor, particularly in those with pregestational diabetes mellitus and those with cardiomyopathy. Some patients may wish to breastfeed their infant. All antihypertensive drugs are found in the breast milk, although differences are found in the milk-to-plasma ratio of these drugs. Additionally, the long-term effect of maternal antihypertensive drugs on breastfeeding infants has not been specifically studied. Milk concentrations of methyldopa appear to be low and are considered to be safe. The β-blocking agents (atenolol and metoprolol) are concentrated in breast milk, whereas labetalol and propranolol have low concentrations. Concentrations of diuretic agents in breast milk are low; however, they may induce a decrease in milk production.

There is little information about the transfer of calcium channel blockers to breast milk, but there are no apparent side effects. ACE inhibitors and angiotensin II receptor antagonists should be avoided because of their effects on neonatal renal function, even though their concentrations appear to be low in breast milk (see Chapter 8).

Finally, in breastfeeding women, the use of methyldopa as a first-line oral therapy is a reasonable choice. If methyldopa is contraindicated, labetalol may be used.

HYPERTENSIVE EMERGENCIES IN CHRONIC HYPERTENSION

On rare occasions, pregnant women may present with life-threatening clinical conditions that require immediate control of BP, such as hypertensive encephalopathy, acute left ventricular failure, acute aortic dissection, or increased circulating catecholamines (pheochromocytoma, clonidine withdrawal, cocaine ingestion). Patients at highest risk for these complications include those with underlying cardiac disease, chronic glomerular renal disease, multiple drugs to control their hypertension, superimposed preeclampsia in the second trimester, and abruptio placentae complicated by DIC. Although a diastolic BP of 115 mm Hg or greater is usually considered a hypertensive emergency, this level is actually arbitrary, and the rate of change of BP may be more important than its absolute level. The association of elevated BP with evidence of new or progressive end-organ damage determines the seriousness of the clinical situation.

Hypertensive Encephalopathy

Untreated essential hypertension progresses to a hypertensive crisis in up to 1% to 2% of cases for unknown reasons. Hypertensive encephalopathy is usually seen in patients with a systolic BP above 220 mm Hg or a diastolic BP above 130 mm Hg. Patients with the acute onset of hypertension may develop encephalopathy at pressure levels that are generally tolerated by those with chronic hypertension. Normally, cerebral blood flow is about 50 mL per 100 g tissue per minute. When the BP falls, cerebral arterioles normally dilate, whereas when BP increases, they constrict to maintain constant cerebral blood flow. This mechanism usually remains operative between 60 and 120 mm Hg diastolic BP. Hypertensive encephalopathy is currently considered to be a derangement of the autoregulation of cerebral arterioles, which occurs when the upper limit of autoregulation is exceeded. With severe hypertension (130 to 150 mm Hg cerebral perfusion pressure), cerebral blood vessels constrict as much as possible and then reflex cerebral vasodilatation occurs. This results in overperfusion, damage to small blood vessels, cerebral edema, and increased intracranial pressure (breakthrough theory). Others believe that hypertensive encephalopathy results from an exaggerated vasoconstrictive response of the arterioles resulting in cerebral ischemia (overregulation theory). Patients who have impaired autoregulation involving the cerebral arterioles may experience necrotizing arteriolitis, microinfarcts, petechial hemorrhages, multiple small thrombi, or cerebral edema. Typically, hypertensive encephalopathy has a subacute onset over 24 to 72 hours.

During a hypertensive crisis, other evidence for end-organ damage may be present: cardiac, renal, or retinal dysfunction secondary to impaired organ perfusion and loss of autoregulation of blood flow. Ischemia of the retina (with flame-shaped retinal hemorrhages, retinal infarcts, or papilledema) may occur, causing decreased visual acuity. Impaired regulation of coronary blood flow and marked increase in ventricular wall stress may result in angina, myocardial infarction, congestive heart failure, malignant ventricular arrhythmia, pulmonary edema, or dissecting aortic aneurysm. Necrosis of the afferent arterioles of the glomerulus results in hemorrhages of the cortex and medulla, fibrinoid necrosis, and proliferative endarteritis resulting in elevated serum creatinine (>3 mg/dL), proteinuria, oliguria, hematuria, hyaline or red blood cell casts, and progressive azotemia. Severe hypertension may result in abruptio placentae with resultant DIC. In addition, high levels of angiotensin II, norepinephrine, and vasopressin accompany ongoing vascular damage. These circulating hormones increase relative efferent arteriolar tone, resulting in sodium diuresis and hypovolemia. Because levels of renin and angiotensin II are increased, the aldosterone level is also elevated. The impact of these endocrine changes may be important in maintaining the hypertensive crisis.

Treatment of Hypertensive Encephalopathy

The ultimate goal of therapy is to prevent the occurrence of a hypertensive emergency. Patients at risk for a hypertensive crisis should receive intensive management during labor and for a minimum of 48 hours after delivery. Although pregnancy may complicate the diagnosis, once the life-threatening conditions are recognized, pregnancy should not in any way slow or alter the mode of therapy. **The only reliable clinical criterion to confirm the diagnosis of hypertensive encephalopathy is prompt response of the patient to antihypertensive therapy. The headache and sensorium often clear dramatically, sometimes within 1 to 2 hours after the treatment.** The overall recovery may be somewhat slower in patients with uremia and those in whom the symptoms have been present for a prolonged period before the therapy is given. Sustained cerebrovascular deficits should suggest other diagnoses.

Patients with hypertensive encephalopathy or other hypertensive crisis should be hospitalized for bedrest. Intravenous lines should be inserted for fluids and medications. Although there is a tendency to restrict sodium intake in patients with a hypertensive emergency, volume contraction from sodium diuresis may be present. A marked drop in diastolic BP with a rise in heart rate on standing from the supine position is evidence of volume contraction. Infusion of normal saline solution during the first 24 to 48 hours to achieve volume expansion should be considered. Saline infusion may help decrease the activity of the renin-angiotensin-aldosterone axis and result in better BP control. Simultaneous repletion of potassium losses and continuous monitoring of BP, volume status, urinary output, ECG readings, and mental status are mandatory. An intra-arterial line provides the most accurate BP information. Laboratory studies include a complete blood count with differential, reticulocyte count, platelets, and blood chemistries. A urinalysis should be obtained for protein, glucose, blood, cells, casts, and bacteria. Assessment for end-organ damage in the central nervous system, retina, kidneys, and cardiovascular system should be done periodically. Antepartum patients should have continuous fetal monitoring.

Lowering Blood Pressure in Hypertensive Encephalopathy

There are risks associated with too rapid or excessive reduction of elevated BP. The aim of therapy is to lower mean BP by no more than 15% to 25%. Small reductions in BP in the first 60 minutes, working toward a diastolic level of 100 to 110 mm Hg, have been recommended. Although cerebral blood flow is maintained constantly over a wide range of BPs, there is a lower and an upper limit to autoregulation. In chronic hypertensive women who have a rightward shift of the cerebral autoregulation curve secondary to medial hypertrophy of the cerebral vasculature, lowering BP too rapidly may produce cerebral ischemia, stroke, or coma. Coronary blood flow, renal perfusion, and uteroplacental blood flow also may deteriorate, resulting in acute renal failure, myocardial infarction, fetal distress, or death. Hypertension that proves increasingly difficult to control is an indication to terminate the pregnancy. If the patient's outcome appears to be grave, consideration of perimortem cesarean delivery should be made.

The drug of choice in a hypertensive crisis is sodium nitroprusside. Other agents such as nitroglycerin, nifedipine, trimetaphan, labetalol, and hydralazine can also be used.

Sodium Nitroprusside

Sodium nitroprusside causes arterial and venous relaxation by interfering with both influx and the intracellular activation of calcium. It is given as an intravenous infusion of 0.25 to 3 mcg/kg per minute. The onset of action is immediate, and its effect may last 3 to 5 minutes after discontinuing the infusion. Hypotension caused by nitroprusside should resolve within a few minutes of stopping the infusion because the drug's half life is so short. If it does not resolve, other causes for hypotension should be suspected. The effect of nitroprusside on uterine blood flow is controversial. Nitroprusside is metabolized into thiocyanate, which is excreted in the urine. Cyanide can accumulate if there is either increased production due to large doses (>10 mcg/kg per minute) or prolonged administration (>48 hours), or if there is renal insufficiency or decreased metabolism in the liver. Signs of toxicity include anorexia, disorientation, headache, fatigue, restlessness, tinnitus, delirium, hallucinations, nausea, vomiting, and metabolic acidosis. When it is infused at less than 2 mcg/kg per minute, cyanide toxicity is unlikely. At a maximal dose rate of 10 mcg/kg per minute, infusion should never last more than 10 minutes. Animal experiments and the few reported cases of nitroprusside use in pregnancy have revealed that thiocyanate toxicity to mother and fetus rarely occur if it is used in a regular pharmacologic dose. Tachyphylaxis to nitroprusside usually develops before toxicity occurs. Whenever toxicity is suspected, therapy should be initiated with 3% sodium nitrite at a rate not exceeding 5 mL/minute, up to a total dose of 15 mL. Then, infusion of 12.5 g of sodium thiosulfate in 50 mL of 5% dextrose in water over a 10-minute period should be started.

Nitroglycerin

Nitroglycerin is an arterial but mostly venous dilator. It is given as an intravenous infusion of 5 mcg/minute that is gradually increased every 3 to 5 minutes to titrate BP up to a maximal dose of 100 mg/minute. It is the drug of choice in preeclampsia associated with pulmonary edema and for control of hypertension associated with tracheal manipulation. Side effects such as headache, tachycardia, and methemoglobinemia may develop. It is contraindicated in hypertensive encephalopathy because it increases cerebral blood flow and intracranial pressure.

KEY POINTS

- Hypertension is the most common medical complication during pregnancy.
- Preeclampsia is a leading cause of maternal mortality and morbidity worldwide.
- The pathophysiologic abnormalities of preeclampsia are numerous, but the etiology is unknown.
- At present, there is no proven method to prevent preeclampsia.
- The HELLP syndrome may develop in the absence of maternal hypertension.
- Expectant management improves perinatal outcome in a select group of women with severe preeclampsia before 32 weeks' gestation.
- Magnesium sulfate is the preferred agent to prevent or treat eclamptic convulsions.
- Rare cases of eclampsia can develop before 20 weeks' gestation and beyond 48 hours postpartum.
- Antihypertensive agents do not improve pregnancy outcome in women with mild uncomplicated chronic hypertension.
- Labetalol is the drug of choice for the treatment of chronic hypertension; angiotensin-converting enzyme inhibitors should be avoided in pregnancy.

REFERENCES

1. Report of the National High Blood Pressure Education Program: Working group report on high blood pressure in pregnancy. Am J Obstet Gynecol 183:S1, 2000.
2. Sibai BM: Diagnosis and management of gestational hypertension and preeclampsia. Obstet Gynecol 102:181, 2003.
3. ACOG Committee on Practice Bulletins-Obstetrics: Diagnosis and management of preeclampsia and eclampsia. Obstet Gynecol 99:159, 2002.
4. Hauth JC, Ewell MG, Levine RL, et al: Pregnancy outcomes in healthy nulliparas women who subsequently developed hypertension: calcium for preeclampsia prevention study group. Obstet Gynecol 95:24, 2000.
5. Barton JR, O'Brien JM, Bergauer NK, et al: Mild gestational hypertension remote from term: progression and outcome. Am J Obstet Gynecol 184:979, 2001.
6. Saudan P, Brown MA, Buddle ML, Jones M: Does gestational hypertension become pre-eclampsia? BJOG 105:1177, 1998.
7. Magee LA, Von Dadelseen P, Bohun CM, et al: Serious perinatal complication of non-proteinuria hypertension: an international, multicenter, retrospective cohort study. J Obstet Gynecol Can 25:372, 2003.
8. Valensise H, Vasapelle B, Gagliardi G, Novelli GP: Early and late preeclampsia: two different maternal hemodynamic states in the latent phase of the disease. Hypertension 52:873, 2008.
9. Magee LA, Helewa ME, Moutquin JM, et al: SOGC guidelines; diagnosis, evaluation and management of the hypertensive disorders of pregnancy. J Obstet Gynaecol Can 30:1, 2008.
10. Lowe SA, Brown MA, Dekker GA, et al, for the Society of Obstetric Medicine of Australia and New Zealand: Guidelines for the management of hypertensive disorders of pregnancy 2008. Aust N Z J Obstet Gynaecol 49:424, 2009.
11. Steegers EAP, von Dadelszen P, Duvekot JJ, Pijnenborg R: Preeclampsia. Lancet 376:631, 2010.
12. Mattar F, Sibai BM: Eclampsia VIII risk factors for maternal morbidity. Am J Obstet Gynecol 182:307, 2000.
13. Caritis S, Sibai B, Hauth J, et al: Low-dose aspirin to prevent preeclampsia in women at high risk. N Engl J Med 338:701, 1998.
14. Sibai BM, Lindheimer M, Hauth J, et al, for the National Institute of Child Health and Human Development Network of Maternal-Fetal Medicine Units: Risk factors for preeclampsia, abruptio, and adverse neonatal outcome in women with chronic hypertension. N Engl J Med 339:667, 1998.
15. Knuist M, Bonsel GJ, Zondervan HA, Treffers PE: Intensification of fetal and maternal surveillance in pregnant women with hypertensive disorders. Int J Gynecol Obstet 61:127, 1998.
16. Sibai BM, Hauth J, Caritis S, et al, for the Network of Maternal-Fetal Medicine Units of the National Institute of Child Health and Human Development: Hypertensive disorders in twin versus singleton pregnancies. Am J Obstet Gynecol 182:938, 2000.
17. Hernández-Díaz S, Werler MM, Mitchell AA: Gestational hypertension in pregnancies supported by infertility treatments: role of infertility, treatments, and multiple gestations. Fertil Steril 88:438, 2007.
18. Erez O, Vardi IS, Hallak M, et al: Preeclampsia in twin gestations: association with IVF treatments, parity and maternal age. J Matern Fetal Neonatal Med 19:141, 2006.
19. Buchbinder A, Sibai BM, Caritis S, et al: Adverse perinatal outcomes are significantly higher in severe gestational hypertension than in mild preeclampsia. Am J Obstet Gynecol 186:66, 2002.
20. Sibai BM, Dekker G, Kupferminc M: Pre-eclampsia. Lancet 365:785, 2005.
21. Huppertz B: Placental origins of preeclampsia: challenging the current hypothesis. Hypertension 51:970, 2008.
22. Wen SW, Demissie K, Yang Q, Walker MC: Maternal morbidity and obstetric complications in triplet pregnancies and quadruplet and higher-order multiple pregnancies. Am J Obstet Gynecol 191:254, 2004.
23. Hnat MD, Sibai BM, Caritis S, et al: Perinatal outcome in women with recurrent preeclampsia compared with women who develop preeclampsia as nulliparas. Am J Obstet Gynecol 186:422, 2002.
24. Hernandez-Diaz S, Toh S, Cnattingius S: Risk of pre-eclampsia in first and subsequent pregnancies: prospective cohort study. BMJ 338:b2255, 2009.
25. Hjartardottir S, Leifsson B, Geirsson R, Steinthorsdottir V: Recurrence of hypertensive disorder in second pregnancy. Am J Obstet Gynecol 194:916, 2006.
26. Brown MA, Mackenzie C, Dunsmuir W, et al: Can we predict recurrence of pre-eclampsia or gestational hypertension? BJOG 114:984, 2007.

27. Van Rijn BB, Hoeks LB, Bots ML, et al: Outcomes of subsequent pregnancy after first pregnancy with early-onset preeclampsia. Am J Obstet Gynecol 194:723, 2006.
28. Barton JR, Sibai BM: Prediction and prevention of recurrent preeclampsia. Obstet Gynecol 112:359, 2008.
29. McCance DR, Holmes VA, Maresh MJA, et al: Vitamin C and vitamin E for the prevention of pre-eclampsia in women with type diabetes (DAPIT): a multicentre randomized placebo-controlled trial. Lancet 376:259, 2010.
30. Sibai BM: Vitamin C and E to prevent pre-eclampsia in diabetic women. Lancet 376:214, 2010.
31. Mello G, Parretti E, Marozio L: Thrombophilia is significantly associated with severe preeclampsia: results of a large scale case-controlled study. Hypertension 46:1270, 2005.
32. Sibai BM, Stella CL: Diagnosis and management of atypical preeclampsia-eclampsia. Am J Obstet Gynecol 200:481, 2009.
33. Sibai BM, Barton JR: Expectant management of severe preeclampsia remote from term: patient selection, treatment, and delivery indications. Am J Obstet Gynecol 196:514.e1, 2007.
34. Holston A, Qian C, Karumanchi A, et al: Circulating angiogenic factors in gestational proteinuria without hypertension. Am J Obstet Gynecol 200:392.e1, 2009.
35. Villar A, Abdel-Aleem H, Merialdi M, et al: Wold Health Organization trial of calcium supplementation among low calcium intake pregnant women. Am J Obstet Gynecol 194:639, 2006.
36. Morikawa M, Yamada T, Cho K, et al: Pregnancy outcome of women who developed proteinuria in the absence of hypertension after mid-gestation. J Perinat Med 36:419, 2008.
37. Einarsson JI, Sangi-Haghpeykar H, Gardner NO: Sperm exposure and development of preeclampsia. Am J Obstet Gynecol 191:254, 2004.
38. Saftlas AF, Levine RJ, Klebanoff MA, et al: Abortion, changed paternity, and the risk of preeclampsia in nulliparous women. Am J Epidemiol 157:1108, 2003.
39. Esplin MS, Fausett MB, Fraser A, et al: Paternal and maternal components of the predisposition to preeclampsia. N Engl J Med 344:867, 2001.
40. Lie RT, Rasmussen, S, Brunborg H, et al: Fetal and maternal contributions to risk of pre-eclampsia: a population based study. Br Med J 316:1343, 1998.
41. Wang JX, Knottnerus AM, Schuit G, et al: Surgically obtained sperm and risk of gestational hypertension and pre-eclampsia. Lancet 359:673, 2002.
42. Trogstad L, Magnus P, Moffett A, Stoltenberg C: The effect of recurrent miscarriage and infertility on the risk of pre-eclampsia. BJOG 116:108, 2009.
43. Catalano PM: Management of obesity in pregnancy. Obstet Gynecol 109:419, 2007.
44. Cedergren MI: Maternal morbid obesity and the risk of adverse pregnancy outcome. Obstet Gynecol 103:219, 2004.
45. Mbah AK, Kornosky JL, Kristensen S, et al: Super-obesity and risk of early and late pre-eclampsia. BJOG 117:997, 2010.
46. Said JM, Higgins JR, Moses EK, et al: Inherited thrombophilia polymorphisms and pregnancy outcomes in nulliparous women. Obstet Gynecol 115:5, 2010.
47. Silver RM, Zhao Y, Spong CY, Sibai B, et al: Prothrombin gene G20210A mutation and obstetric complications. Obstet Gynecol 115:14, 2010.
48. Kahn SR, Platt R, McNamara H, et al: Inherited thrombophilia and preeclampsia within a multicenter cohort: the Montreal Preeclampsia Study. Am J Obstet Gynecol 200:151, 2009.
49. Myatt L, Webster RP: Vascular biology of preeclampsia. J Thromb Haemost 7:375, 2009.
50. Redman CWG, Sargent IL: Immunology of pre-eclampsia. Am J Reprod Immunol 63:534, 2010.
51. Redman CS, Sargent IL: Placental stress and pre-eclampsia: a revised view. Placenta 30:38, 2009.
52. Pijnenborg R, Brosens I: Deep trophoblast invasion and spiral artery remodeling. In Pinjnenborg R, Brosens I, Romero R (eds): Placental Bed Disorders: Basic Science and Its Translation to Obstetrics. Cambridge, UK, Cambridge University Press, 2010, p 97.
53. Kong TY, DeWolf F, Robertson WB, Brosens I: Inadequate maternal vascular response to placentation in pregnancies complicated by preeclampsia and by small-for-gestational age infants. BJOG 93: 1049, 1986.
54. Frusca T, Morassi L, Pecorell S, et al: Histological features of uteroplacental vessels in normal and hypertensive patients in relation to birthweight. BJOG 96:835, 1989.
55. Meekins JW, Pijneborg R, Hanssens M, et al: A study of placental bed spiral arteries and trophoblast invasion in normal and severe preeclamptic pregnancies. BJOG 101:669, 1994.
56. Sibai BM: Discussion. Evidence supporting a role for blockade of the vascular endothelial growth factor system in the pathophysiology of preeclampsia. Am J Obstet Gynecol 190:1547, 2004.
57. Maynard SE, Min JY, Merchan J, et al: Excess placental soluble fms-like tyrosine kinase 1 (sFlt1) may contribute to endothelial dysfunction, hypertension, and proteinuria in preeclampsia. Clin Invest 111:649, 2003.
58. Levine RJ, Maynard SE, Qian C, et al: Circulating angiogenic factors and the risk of preeclampsia. N Engl J Med 350:672, 2004.
59. Thadhani R, Ecker JL, Mutter WP, et al: Insulin resistance and alterations in angiogenesis: additive insults that may lead to preeclampsia. Hypertension 43:988, 2004.
60. Levine RJ, Thadhani R, Qian C, et al: Urinary placental growth factor and risk of preeclampsia. JAMA 293:77, 2005.
61. Buhimschi CS, Norwitz ER, Funai E, et al: Urinary angiogenic factors cluster hypertensive disorders identify women with severe preeclampsia. Am J Obstet Gynecol 192:734, 2005.
62. Sibai BM: Preeclampsia: an inflammatory syndrome? Am J Obstet Gynecol 191:1061, 2004.
63. Savvidou MD, Hingorani AD, Tsikas D, et al: Endothelial dysfunction and raised plasma concentrations of asymmetric dimethylarginine in pregnant women who subsequently develop pre-eclampsia. Lancet 361:1151, 2003.
64. Speer PD, Powers RW, Frank MP, et al: Elevated asymmetric dimethylarginine concentrations precede clinical preeclampsia, but not pregnancies with small-for-gestational-age infants. Am J Obstet Gynecol 198:112.e1, 2008.
65. Wang Y, Gu Y, Zhang Y, Lewis DF: Evidence of endothelial dysfunction in preeclampsia: decreased endothelial nitric oxide synthase expression is associated with increased cell permeability in endothelial cells from preeclampsia. Am J Obstet Gynecol 190:817, 2004.
66. Nilsson E, Salonen RH, Cnattingius S, Lichtenstein P: The importance of genetic and environmental effects for pre-eclampsia and gestational hypertension: a family study. BJOG 111:200, 2004.
67. Mutze S: Rudnik-Schoneborn S, Zerresk, Rath W: Genes and the preeclampsia syndrome. J Perinat Med 36:38, 2008.
68. Oudejans CB, van Dijk M: Placental gene expression and preeclampsia. Placenta 29:78, 2008.
69. Nafee TM, Farrell WE, Carroll WD, et al: Epigenetic control of fetal gene expression. BJOG 115:158, 2008.
70. Paarlberg KM, deJong CLD, Van Geijn HP, et al: Vasoactive mediators in pregnancy-induced hypertensive disorders: a longitudinal study. Am J Obstet Gynecol 179:1559, 1998.
71. Mills JL, DerSimonian R, Raymond E, et al: Prostacyclin and thromboxane changes predating clinical onset of preeclampsia: a multicenter prospective study. JAMA 282:356, 1999.
72. Moretti M, Phillips M, Abouzeid A, et al: Increased breath markers of oxidative stress in normal pregnancy and in preeclampsia. Am J Obstet Gynecol 190:1184, 2004.
73. Khankin EV, Royle C, Karumanchi A: Placental vasculature in health and disease. Semin Thromb Hemost 36:309, 2010.
74. Villar MA, Sibai BM: Clinical significance of elevated mean arterial blood in second trimester and threshold increase in systolic or diastolic pressure during third trimester. Am J Obstet Gynecol 60:419, 1989.
75. North RA, Taylor RS, Schellenberg J-C: Evaluation of a definition of pre-eclampsia. BJOG 106:767, 1999.
76. Levine RJ, Ewell MG, Hauth JC, et al: Should the definition of preeclampsia include a rise in diastolic blood pressure of ≥15 mmHg to a level <90 mmHg in association with proteinuria? Am J Obstet Gynecol 183:787, 2000.
77. Ohkuchi A, Iwasaki R, Ojima T, et al: Increase in systolic blood pressure of > or =30 mmHg and/or diastolic blood pressure of > or =15 mmHg during pregnancy: is it pathologic? Hypertens Pregnancy 22:275, 2003.
78. Lindheimer MD, Kanter D: Interpreting abnormal proteinuria in pregnancy: the need for a more pathophysiological approach. Obstet Gynecol 115:365, 2010.

79. Wikstrom A-K, Wikstrom J, Larsson A, Olovsson M: Random albumin/creatinine ratio for quantitation of proteinuria in manifest pre-eclampsia. BJOG 113:930, 2006.
80. Gangaram R, Naicker M, Moodley J: Accuracy of the spot urinary microalbumin: creatinine ration and visual dipsticks in hypertensive pregnancy women. Eur J Obstet Gynecol Reprod Biol 144:146, 2009.
81. Cote AM, Brown MA, Lam E, et al: Diagnostic accuracy of urinary spot protein: creatinine ratio for proteinuria in hypertensive pregnant women. Systematic review. BMJ 336:1003, 2008.
82. Papanna R, Mann LK, Kouides RW, Glantz JX: Protein/creatinine ratio in preeclampsia: a systematic review. Obstet Gynecol 112:135, 2008.
83. Côté AM, Firoz T, Mattman A, et al: The 24-hour urine collection: gold standard or historical practice? Am J Obstet Gynecol 199:625.e1, 2008.
84. Meyer NL, Mercer BM, Friedman SA, Sibai BM: Urinary dipstick protein: a poor predictor of absent or severe proteinuria. Am J Obstet Gynecol 170:137, 1994.
85. Sibai BM: Diagnosis, controversies, and management of HELLP syndrome. Obstet Gynecol 103:981, 2004.
86. Sibai BM: Diagnosis, differential diagnosis, and management of eclampsia. Obstet Gynecol 105:402, 2005.
87. Conde-Agudelo A, Romero R, Lindheimer MD: Tests to predict pre-eclampsia. In Lindheimer MD, Roberts JM, Cunningham FG (eds): Chesley's Hypertensive Disorders in Pregnancy. Amsterdam, Academic Press, Elsevier, 2009, pp 189.
88. Papageorghiou AT, Leslie K: Uterine artery Doppler in the prediction of adverse pregnancy outcome. Curr Opin Obstet Gynecol 19:103, 2007.
89. Pilalis A, Souka AP, Antsaklis P, et al: Screening for pre-eclampsia and small for gestational age fetuses at the 11-14 weeks scan by uterine artery Dopplers. Acta Obstet Gynecol Scand 86:530, 2007.
90. DePaco C, Kametas N, Renceret G, et al: Maternal cardiac output between 11 and 12 weeks of gestation in the prediction of preeclampsia and small for gestational age. Obstet Gynecol 111:292, 2008.
91. Cnossen JS, Vollebregt KC, de Vrieze N, et al: Accuracy of mean arterial pressure and blood pressure measurements in predicting preeclampsia: systematic review. BMJ 336:1117, 2008.
92. Cnossen JS, Morris RK, ter Riet G, et al: Use of uterine artery Doppler ultrasonography to predict pre-eclampsia and intrauterine growth restriction: a systemic review and bivariable meta-analysis. CMAJ 178:701, 2008.
93. Poon LCY, Kametas NA, Maiz N, et al: First trimester prediction of hypertensive disorders in pregnancy. Hypertension 53:812, 2009.
94. Poon LCY, Strateiva V, Piras S, et al: Hypertensive disorders in pregnancy: combined screening by uterine artery Doppler, blood pressure and serum PAPP-A at 11-13 weeks. Ultrasound Obstet Gynecol 34:497, 2009.
95. Chaiworapongsa T, Romero R, Kusanovic JP, et al: Plasma soluble endoglin concentration in pre-eclampsia associated with an increased impedance to flow in the maternal and fetal circulations. Ultrasound Obstet Gynecol 35:155, 2010.
96. Espinoza J, Romero R, Nien JK, et al: Identification of patients at risk for early onset and/or severe preeclampsia with the use of uterine artery Doppler velocimetry and placental growth factor (published erratum appears in Am J Obstet Gynecol 2007;196:614). Am J Obstet Gynecol 196:326.e1, 2007.
97. Lapaire O, Shennan A, Stepan H: The preeclampsia biomarker soluble fms-like tyrosine kinase-1 and placental growth factor: current knowledge, clinical implications and future application. Eur J Obstet Gynaecol Reprod Biol 151:122, 2010.
98. Rana S, Karumanchi A, Levine FJ, et al: Sequential changes in antiangiogenic factors in early pregnancy and risk of developing preeclampsia. Hypertension 50:137, 2007.
99. Moore Simas TA, Crawford SL, et al: Angiogenic factors for the prediction of preeclampsia in high-risk women. Am J Obstet Gynecol 197:244.e1, 2007.
100. Bricene-Perez C, Bricene-Sanabria L, Vigil-Digracia P: Prediction and prevention of preeclampsia. Hypertens Pregnancy 28:138, 2009.
101. Rumbold AR, Cowther CA, Haslam RR, et al: Vitamins C and E and the risks of pre-eclampsia and perinatal complications. N Engl J Med 354:1796, 2006.
102. Poston L, Briley AL, Seed PT, et al: Vitamin C and E in pregnant women at risk for pre-eclampsia (VIP trial): randomised placebo-controlled trial. Lancet 367:1145, 2006.
103. Spinnato JA, Freire S, Pinto ESLJ, et al: Antioxidant therapy to prevent pre-eclampsia: a randomised controlled trial. Obstet Gynecol 110:1311, 2007.
104. Villar J, Purwar M, Meraldi M, et al: World Health Organization multicenter randomised trial of supplementation with vitamins C and E among pregnant women at high-risk for pre-eclampsia in populations of low nutritional status from developing countries. BJOG 116:780, 2009.
105. Roberts JM, Myatt L, Spong CS, et al: Vitamins C and E to prevent complications of pregnancy: associated hypertension. N Engl J Med 362:1282, 2010.
106. Xu H, Perez-Cuevas R, Xiong X, et al: An international trial of antioxidants in the prevention of pre-eclampsia (INTAPP). Am J Obstet Gynecol 202:239.e1, 2010.

For full reference list, log onto www.expertconsult.com.

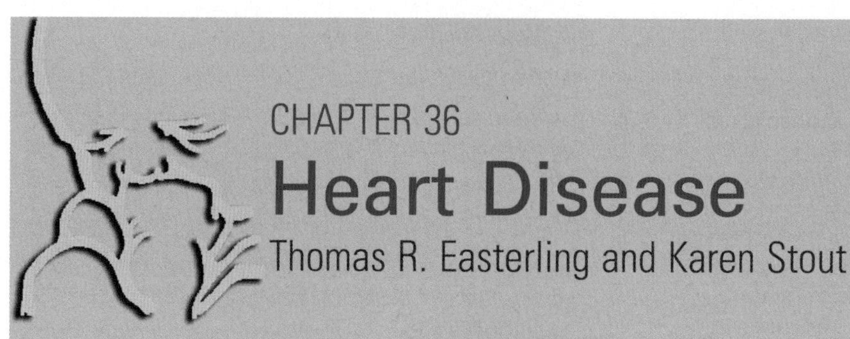

CHAPTER 36
Heart Disease

Thomas R. Easterling and Karen Stout

KEY ABBREVIATIONS	
Activated Partial Thromboplastin Time	aPTT
Acute Respiratory Distress Syndrome	ARDS
Aortic Diameter	AD
Body Surface Area	BSA
Cardiac Index	CI
Cardiac Output	CO
Central Venous Pressure	CVP
Electrocardiogram	ECG
Heart Rate	HR
Low-molecular-weight Heparin	LMWH
Mean Arterial Pressure	MAP
New York Heart Association	NYHA
Patent Ductus Arteriosus	PDA
Positive End-expiratory Pressure	PEEP
Pulmonary Artery Wedge Pressure	PAWP
Pulmonary Flow	Q_p
Pulmonary Vascular Resistance	PVR
Relative Risk	RR
Right Ventricle	RV
Stroke Volume	SV
Systemic Flow	Q_s
Systemic Vascular Resistance	SVR
Total Peripheral Resistance	TPR
Transposition of the Great Vessels	TGV
Unfractionated Heparin	UFH
Ventricular Septal Defect	VSD
Vitamin K Antagonist	VKA

Cardiovascular adaptations to pregnancy are well tolerated by healthy young women. However, these adaptations are of such magnitude that they can significantly compromise women with abnormal or damaged hearts. Without accurate diagnosis and appropriate care, heart disease in pregnancy can be a significant cause of maternal mortality and morbidity. Under more optimal conditions, many women with significant disease can experience good outcomes and should not necessarily be discouraged from becoming pregnant. This chapter develops an understanding of cardiovascular physiology as a basis for care of the pregnant woman with heart disease. Although published experience with more common conditions can be used to support these principles, information regarding many other conditions is limited to case reports. Data from case reports may, however, be biased toward more complicated cases with more adverse outcomes. The best care for women with heart disease is usually achieved from a thorough understanding of maternal cardiovascular physiology, knowledge of existing literature, and extensive clinical experience brought by a multidisciplinary team of clinicians.

MATERNAL HEMODYNAMICS

Hemodynamics refers to the relationship between blood pressure, cardiac output, and vascular resistance. Blood pressure is measured by auscultation, use of an automated cuff, or directly with an intra-arterial catheter. Cardiac output is measured by dilutional techniques requiring central venous access, by Doppler or two-dimensional echocardiographic techniques, or by electrical impedance. Peripheral resistance is calculated using Ohm's law:

$$TPR = MAP \times 80/CO$$

where TPR is total peripheral resistance (dyne · sec · cm^{-5}), MAP is mean arterial pressure (millimeters of mercury [mm Hg]), and CO is cardiac output (L/min).

Pregnancy and events unique to pregnancy, such as labor and delivery, are associated with significant and frequently predictable changes in these parameters. The hemodynamic changes of pregnancy, although well tolerated by an otherwise healthy woman, may be tolerated poorly by a woman with significant cardiac disease. Therefore, the importance of understanding these changes and placing them in the context of a specific cardiac lesion cannot be overstated.

The maternal hemodynamics of 89 nulliparous women who remained normotensive throughout pregnancy are described in Figure 36-1.[1] MAP falls sharply in the first trimester, reaching a nadir by midpregnancy. Thereafter, blood pressure increases slowly, reaching near nonpregnant levels by term. CO rises throughout the first and second trimesters, reaching a maximum by the middle of the third trimester. In the supine position, a pregnant woman in the third trimester may experience significant hypotension due to venocaval occlusion by the gravid uterus. In normal pregnancy, venocaval occlusion may produce symptoms such as diaphoresis, tachycardia, or nausea but will rarely result in significant complications. Fetal heart rate decelerations may be observed but usually resolve when the mother, often spontaneously, shifts to a more comfortable position. Women with significant right or left ventricular outflow obstruction, such as aortic stenosis, may seriously decompensate in the supine position due to poor ventricular filling.

CO is the product of heart rate (HR) and stroke volume (SV):

$$CO = HR \times SV$$

HR and SV increase as pregnancy progresses to the third trimester. After 32 weeks, SV falls, with the maintenance of CO becoming more and more dependent on HR. Vascular resistance falls in the first and early second trimesters. The magnitude of the fall is sufficient to offset the rise in CO, resulting in a net decrease in blood pressure.

Labor, delivery, and the postpartum period are times of acute hemodynamic changes that may result in maternal decompensation. Labor itself is associated with pain and anxiety. Tachycardia is a normal response. Significant catecholamine release increases afterload. Each uterine contraction acutely redistributes 400 to 500 mL of blood from the uterus to the central circulation. In Figure 36-2, Robson and colleagues[2] describe the hemodynamic changes associated with unmedicated labor. HR, blood pressure, and CO all increase with uterine contractions, with the magnitude of the change increasing as labor advances. Obstructive cardiac lesions impede the flow of blood through the heart, blunting the expected rise in CO at the expense of increasing pulmonary pressures and pulmonary congestion. In Figure 36-3, intrapartum hemodynamic changes of a patient with aortic stenosis and a peak gradient of 160 mm Hg are shown.[3] In this individual, pulmonary pressures rise in parallel with uterine contractions.

Immediately after delivery, blood from the uterus is returned to the central circulation. In normal pregnancy, this compensatory mechanism protects against the hemodynamic effects that may accompany postpartum hemorrhage. **In the context of cardiac disease, this acute centralization of blood may increase pulmonary pressures and pulmonary congestion.**[4] During the first 2 postpartum weeks, extravascular fluid is mobilized, diuresis ensues, and vascular resistance increases, returning to nonpregnant norms. Decompensation during postpartum fluid mobilization is common in women with mitral stenosis. Volume loading coupled with vasoconstriction may also unmask maternal cardiomyopathy. Unsuspected cardiac disease may be diagnosed when a woman returns to the emergency room several days postpartum with dyspnea and

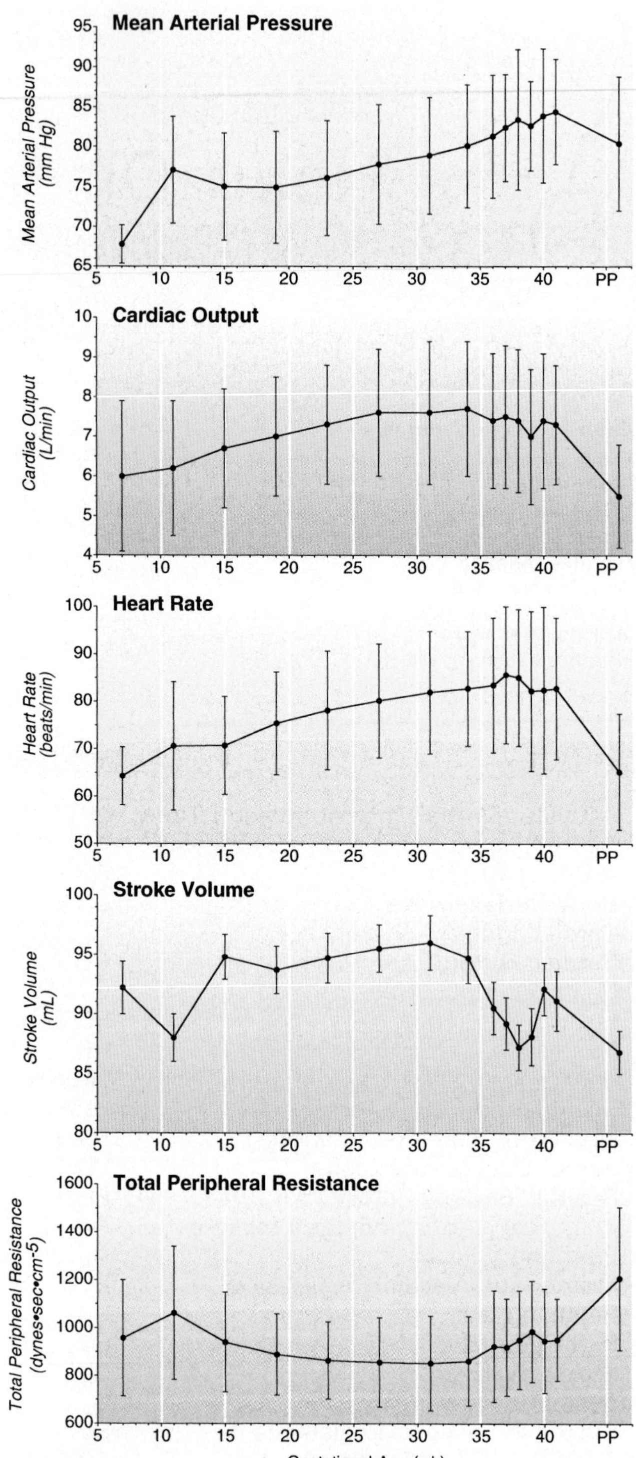

FIGURE 36-1. Changes in hemodynamic parameters throughout pregnancy (mean ± standard deviation).

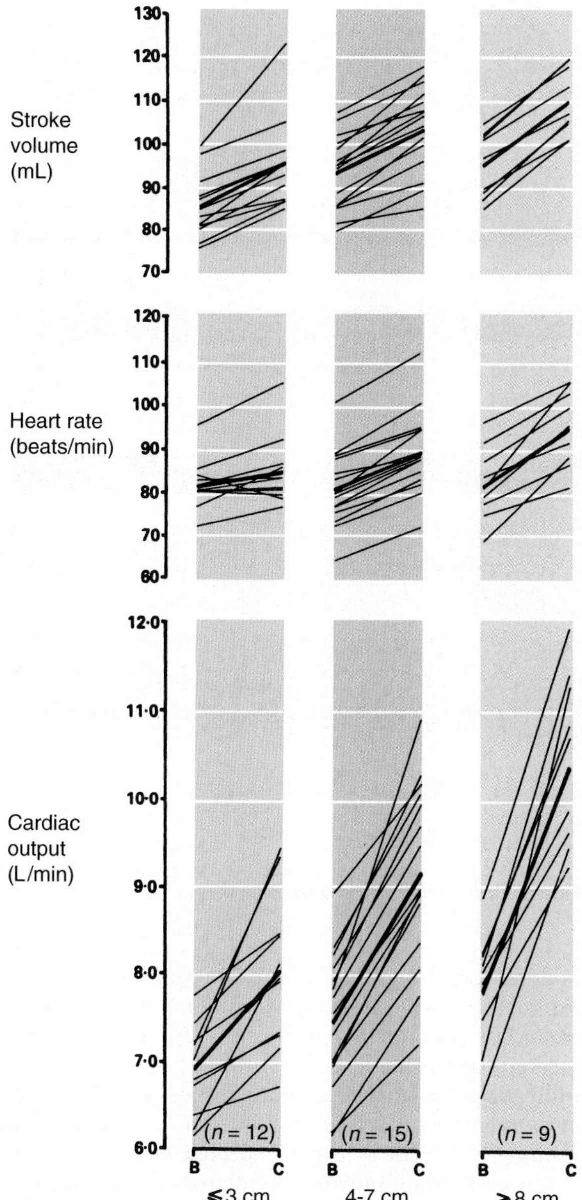

FIGURE 36-2. Changes in hemodynamic parameters at three different points during labor (≤3 cm, 4 to 7 cm, and ≥8 cm). Each line represents the change in an individual subject. *B,* Before contraction; *C,* during contraction. (From Robson S, Dunlop W, Boys R, Hunter S: Cardiac output during labour. BMJ 295:1169, 1987.)

oxygen desaturation. Maternal CO usually normalizes by 2 weeks postpartum.[5]

Three key features of the maternal hemodynamic changes in pregnancy are particularly relevant to the management of women with cardiac disease: (1) increased CO, (2) increased HR, and (3) reduced vascular resistance. In conditions such as mitral stenosis, in which CO is relatively fixed, the drive to achieve an elevated CO may result in pulmonary congestion. If a patient has an atrial septal defect, the incremental increase in systemic flow associated with pregnancy will be magnified in the pulmonary circulation to the extent that pulmonary flow exceeds systemic flow. If, for example, a shunt ratio of 3:1 is maintained in pregnancy, pulmonary flow may be as high as 20 L/min and may be associated with increasing dyspnea and potential desaturation.

Many cardiac conditions are HR dependent. Flow across a stenotic mitral valve is dependent on the proportion of time in diastole. Tachycardia reduces left ventricular filling and CO. Coronary blood flow is also dependent on the length of diastole. Patients with aortic stenosis have increased wall tension and, therefore, increased myocardial oxygen requirements. Tachycardia reduces coronary perfusion time in diastole while simultaneously further increasing myocardial oxygen requirements. The resulting imbalance between oxygen demand and supply may precipitate myocardial ischemia. Patients with complex congenital heart disease can experience significant tachyarrhythmias. The increasing HR in pregnancy may be associated with a worsening of tachyarrhythmias.

Reduction in vascular resistance may be beneficial to some patients; afterload reduction reduces cardiac work. Cardiomyopathy, aortic regurgitation, and mitral regurgitation all benefit from reduced afterload. Alternatively, patients with intracardiac shunts, in which right and left ventricular pressures are nearly equal when not pregnant, may reverse their shunt during pregnancy and desaturate because of to right to left shunting.

BLOOD VOLUME

Very early in the first trimester, pregnant women experience an expansion of renal blood flow and glomerular filtration rate. Filtered sodium increases by about 50%. Despite physiologic changes that would promote loss of salt and water and contraction of blood volume, **the pregnant woman will expand her blood volume by 40% to 50%.** In part, the stimulation to retain fluid may be a response to the fall in vascular resistance and reduction in blood pressure. The renin-angiotensin system is activated, and the plasma concentration of aldosterone is elevated. Although the simplicity of this explanation is attractive, the actual process is probably much more complicated.[6]

As plasma volume expands, the hematocrit falls, and hematopoiesis is stimulated. Red cell mass will expand from 18% to 25% depending on the status of individual iron stores. Physiologic anemia with a maternal hematocrit between 30% and 35% does not usually complicate pregnancy in the context of maternal heart disease. More significant anemia, however, may increase cardiac work and induce tachycardia. Microcytosis due to iron deficiency may impair perfusion of the microcirculation of patients who are polycythemic because of cyanotic heart disease because microcytic red blood cells are less deformable. Iron and folate supplementation may be appropriate.

In a similar fashion, serum albumin concentration falls by 22% despite an expansion of intravascular albumin mass by 20%. **As a result, serum oncotic pressure falls in parallel by 20% to about 19 mm Hg.**[7] In normal pregnancy, intravascular fluid balance is maintained by a fall in interstitial oncotic pressure. However, if left ventricular filling pressure becomes elevated or if pulmonary vascular integrity is disrupted, pulmonary edema will develop earlier in the disease process than in nonpregnant women.

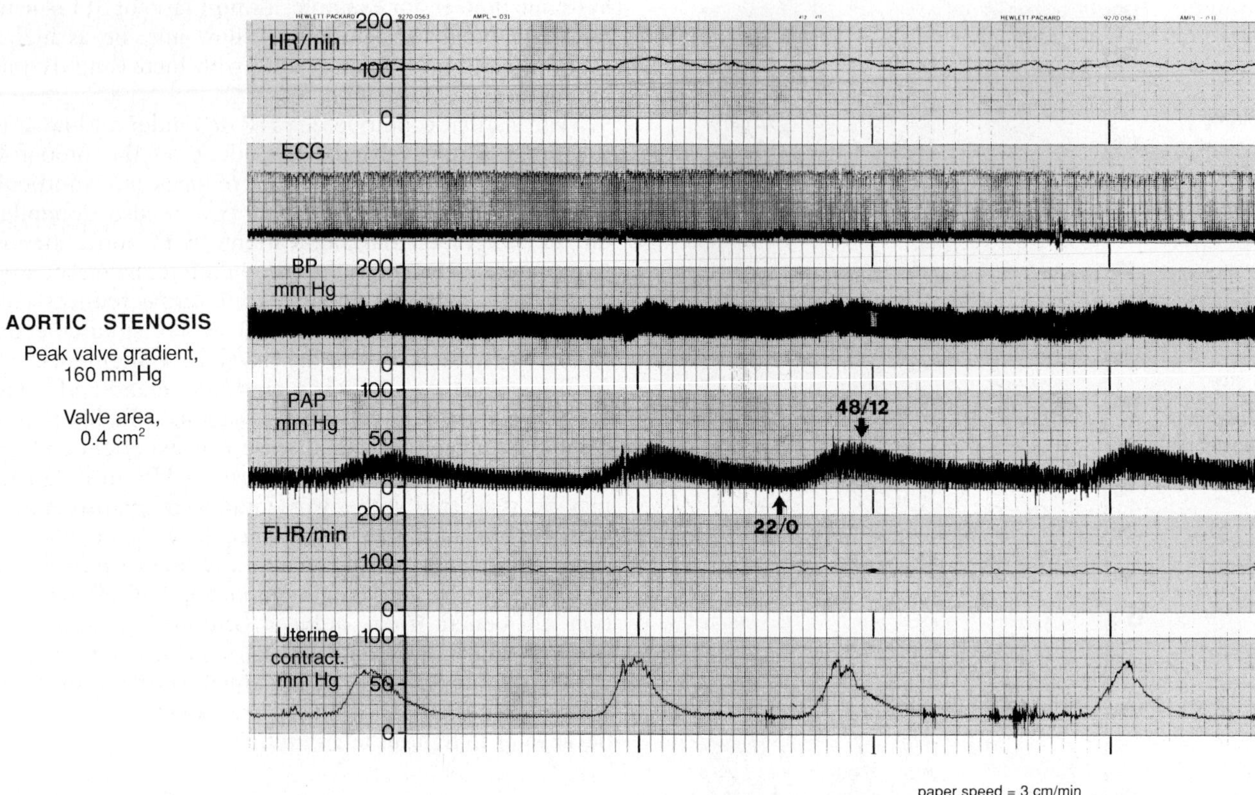

FIGURE 36-3. Hemodynamic monitoring of a patient with severe aortic stenosis in labor. *BP,* Blood pressure; *ECG,* electrocardiogram; *FHR,* fetal heart rate; *HR,* heart rate; *PAP,* pulmonary artery pressure. (From Easterling T, Chadwick H, Otto C, Benedetti T: Aortic stenosis in pregnancy. Obstet Gynecol 72:113, 1988. Reprinted with permission from American College of Obstetricians and Gynecologists.)

DIAGNOSIS AND EVALUATION OF HEART DISEASE

Many women with heart disease have been diagnosed and treated before pregnancy. For example, in women with prior surgery for congenital heart disease, detailed historical information may be available. Others report only that they have a murmur or a "hole in my heart." Alternatively, heart disease may be diagnosed for the first time during pregnancy owing to symptoms precipitated by increased cardiac demands.

The classic symptoms of cardiac disease are palpitations, shortness of breath with exertion, and chest pain. Because these symptoms also may accompany normal pregnancy, a careful history is needed to determine whether the symptoms are out of proportion to the stage of pregnancy. Symptoms are of particular concern in a patient with other reasons to suspect underlying cardiac disease, such as being native to an area where rheumatic heart disease is prevalent.

A systolic flow murmur is present in 80% of pregnant women, most likely due to the increased flow volume in the aorta and pulmonary artery. Typically, a flow murmur is grade 1 or 2, midsystolic, loudest at the cardiac base, and not associated with any other abnormal physical examination findings. A normal physiologic split second heart sound is heard in patients with a flow murmur. Any diastolic murmur and any systolic murmur that is loud (grade 3/6 or higher) or radiates to the carotids should be considered pathologic. Careful evaluation for elevation of the jugular venous pulse, for peripheral cyanosis or clubbing, and for pulmonary crackles is needed in women with suspected cardiac disease.

Indications for further cardiac diagnostic testing in pregnant women include a history of known cardiac disease, symptoms in excess of those expected in a normal pregnancy, a pathologic murmur, evidence of heart failure on physical examination, or arterial oxygen desaturation in the absence of known pulmonary disease. The preferred next step in evaluation of pregnant women with suspected heart disease is transthoracic echocardiography. A chest radiograph is helpful only if congestive heart failure is suspected. An electrocardiogram (ECG) may be nonspecific but could have changes suggestive of the underlying heart disease, such as right ventricular hypertrophy and biatrial enlargement, seen in patients with significant mitral stenosis. If symptoms are consistent with a cardiac arrhythmia, an event monitor or 24-hour ECG monitor may be indicated. Rarely, cardiac catheterization is needed for full diagnosis of valvular or congenital heart disease. The exception is an acute coronary syndrome during pregnancy in which the risk for radiation exposure with cardiac catheterization is small compared with the benefit of early diagnosis and early revascularization to prevent myocardial infarction (MI).

Echocardiography provides detailed information on cardiac anatomy and physiology that allows optimal management of women with heart disease. Basic data obtained on echocardiography include left ventricular ejection fraction, pulmonary artery systolic pressure, qualitative evaluation of right ventricular systolic function, and evaluation of valve anatomy and function. When valvular stenosis is present, the pressure gradient (ΔP) across the valve is calculated from the **Doppler-derived velocity (v) of flow across the valve: $\Delta P = 4v^2$.** Similarly, pulmonary artery systolic pressure can be calculated from the maximal Doppler velocity obtained across a tricuspid regurgitant jet.

Aortic valve area is calculated using the continuity equation. SV is calculated from the product of the cross-sectional area of the left ventricular outflow tract and the time-velocity integral derived from Doppler evaluation of the outflow tract. A time-velocity integral is then derived from the stenotic valve. Because the left ventricular outflow tract and the aortic valve are in continuity, SVs across each are equal. Therefore, valve area can be derived by dividing the stroke volume by the aortic valve time-velocity integral. Mitral valve area is measured directly by two-dimensional planimetry or by the Doppler pressure half-time method.[8] In patients with congenital disease, detailed evaluation of anatomy and previous surgical repair is possible. When complex congenital heart disease is present or when image quality is suboptimal, transesophageal imaging provides improved image quality. Cardiac magnetic resonance imaging may be used to define complex anatomy that is not well evaluated by echocardiography, but caution must be taken with magnetic resonance contrast agents such as gadolinium.

GENERAL CARE

Management of cardiac disease in pregnancy is frequently complicated by unique social and psychological concerns. Children with congenital heart disease may have experienced multiple hospitalizations and be fearful of the medical environment. Some have been cautioned against pregnancy and, therefore, have never expected to bear children. Women with rheumatic heart disease have frequently lived outside the traditional medical care system owing to conditions of poverty, immigration, and cultural differences. Care must be exercised to facilitate their access to care and their comfort with the environment of care. Their practitioner must be patient but persistent in the face of deviations from more traditional standards of compliance and medical care.

Deterioration in cardiac status during pregnancy is frequently insidious. Continuity of care with a single provider facilitates early intervention before overt decompensation. Regular visits should include particular attention to HR, weight gain, and oxygen saturation. An unexpected increase in weight may indicate the need for more aggressive outpatient therapy. A fall in oxygen saturation often precedes a clearly abnormal chest examination or radiograph. Regular use of a structured history of symptoms (see box, Structured Review of Cardiac Symptoms) alerts the physician to a change in condition. Regular review also educates the patients and reinforces their collaborative roles as "partners in care."

The physiologic changes of pregnancy are usually continuous and, therefore, offer adequate time for maternal compensation despite cardiac disease. **Intercurrent events superimposed on pregnancy in the context of maternal heart disease are usually responsible for acute decompensation.** The most common significant intercurrent events during the antepartum period are febrile episodes. Screening for bacteriuria and vaccination against influenza and pneumococcus are appropriate. Patients should be instructed to report symptoms of upper respiratory infection, particularly fever. Many women with heart disease (adolescents, recent immigrants, and those living in poverty) are also at risk for iron deficiency. Prophylaxis against anemia with iron and folate supplementation may decrease cardiac work.

A strategy of standard cardiac care for labor and delivery is described in the box. The general principles for care are similar for most cardiac diagnoses. **Physiologically, the ideal labor for a woman with heart disease is short and pain free.** Although induction of labor facilitates organization of care and early pain control, shortening the duration of pregnancy by 1 or 2 weeks at the cost of a 2- or 3-day induction of labor is not worthwhile. Induction of labor with a favorable cervix is therefore preferred. Some patients with severe cardiac disease benefit from invasive hemodynamic monitoring with an arterial catheter and a pulmonary artery catheter. These methods are discussed in detail later. Cesarean delivery is usually reserved for obstetrical indications. The American Heart Association (AHA) does not recommend routine antibiotic prophylaxis for the prevention of endocarditis, although it is optional in high-risk patients having a vaginal delivery (Table 36-1). Because bacteremia is common at the time of vaginal delivery and cesarean delivery,[9] many practitioners will provide antibiotic prophylaxis in all patients at risk. In contrast to AHA recommendations, compelling arguments supporting broad use of antibiotic prophylaxis have been

TABLE 36-1 PROPHYLACTIC REGIMENS FOR LABOR AND DELIVERY

PATIENTS	REGIMENS
High-risk patients • Prosthetic valves—both bioprosthetic and homografts • Complex cyanotic congenital heart disease (CHD) • Surgically constructed systemic pulmonic shunts or conduits • Previous bacterial endocarditis	**Ampicillin + gentamicin** In active labor: • Ampicillin 2 g IM or IV + Gentamicin 1.5 mg/kg (not to exceed 120 mg) 6 hr later: • Ampicillin 1 g IM/IV or amoxicillin 1 g PO
High-risk patients allergic to ampicillin/amoxicillin	**Vancomycin + gentamicin** • Vancomycin 1 g IV over 1-2 hr + gentamicin as above in active labor
Moderate-risk patients • Most other CHDs • Acquired valvular dysfunction (e.g., rheumatic heart disease) • Hypertrophic cardiac myopathy • Mitral valve prolapse with regurgitation	**Amoxicillin or ampicillin** In active labor • Amoxicillin 2 g PO or ampicillin 2 g IM/IV
Moderate-risk patients allergic to ampicillin/amoxicillin	**Vancomycin** In active labor • Vancomycin 1 g IV over 1-2 hr in active labor

Modified from Dajani AS, Taubert KA, Wilson W, et al: Prevention of bacterial endocarditis: recommendations by the American Heart Association. JAMA 277:1794, 1997.

IM, Intramuscularly; *IV*, intravenously; PO, by mouth.

made, citing limited large-scale studies supporting the recommendations and the high cost and risk associated with endocarditis.[10]

STRUCTURED REVIEW OF CARDIAC SYMPTOMS

"How many flights of stairs can you walk up with ease?"
"Two? One? None?"
"Can you walk a level block?"
"Can you sleep flat in bed?" "How many pillows?"
"Does your heart race?"
"Do you have chest pain?"
"With exercise?"
"When your heart races?"

STANDARD CARDIAC CARE FOR LABOR AND DELIVERY

1. Accurate diagnosis
2. Mode of delivery based on obstetrical indications
3. Medical management initiated early in labor
   - Prolonged labor avoided
   - Induction with a *favorable* cervix
4. Maintenance of hemodynamic stability
   - Invasive hemodynamic monitoring when required
   - Initial, compensated hemodynamic reference point
   - Specific emphasis based on particular cardiac condition
5. Avoidance of pain and hemodynamic responses
   - Epidural analgesia with narcotic/low-dose local technique
6. Prophylactic antibiotics when at risk for endocarditis
7. Avoidance of maternal pushing
   - Caudal for dense perineal anesthesia
   - Low forceps or vacuum delivery
8. Avoidance of maternal blood loss
   - Proactive management of the third stage
   - Early but appropriate fluid replacement
9. Early volume management postpartum
   - Often careful but aggressive diuresis

Women with significant heart disease should be counseled before pregnancy regarding the risk of pregnancy, interventions that may be required, and potential risks to the fetus. However, women with significant uncorrected disease often present with an ongoing established pregnancy. In this situation, the risks and benefits of termination of pregnancy versus those of continuing a pregnancy should be addressed. **The decision to become pregnant or carry a pregnancy in the context of maternal disease is a balance of two forces: (1) the objective medical risk, including the uncertainty of that estimate; and (2) the value of the birth of a child to an individual woman and her partner.** The first goal of counseling is to educate the patient. Only a few cardiac diseases represent an overwhelming risk for maternal mortality: Eisenmenger syndrome, pulmonary hypertension with right ventricular dysfunction, and Marfan syndrome with significant aortic dilation and severe left ventricular dysfunction. Most other conditions require aggressive management and significant disruption in lifestyle. Intercurrent events such as antepartum pneumonia or obstetrical hemorrhage pose the greatest risk for initiating life-threatening events. Fastidious care can reduce but not eliminate the risk for these events. Maternal congenital heart disease increases the risk for congenital heart disease in the fetus from 1% to about 4% to 6%.[11,12] Marfan syndrome and some forms of hypertrophic cardiomyopathy are inherited as autosomal dominant conditions; the offspring of these women carry a 50% chance of inheriting the disease. The second goal of counseling is to help each woman integrate the medical information into her individual value system and her individual desire to become a mother. Many women with significant but manageable heart disease choose to carry a pregnancy. The basis for their decisions should be individualized.

VALVULAR DISEASE

The American College of Cardiology (ACC) and the AHA have published guidelines for the management of valvular heart disease, including some guidelines for management during pregnancy.[13] These guidelines create a general framework for preconceptional care and care during pregnancy, realizing that treatment of a specific patient must be individualized.

Mitral Stenosis

Mitral stenosis is nearly always due to rheumatic heart disease. Valvular dysfunction progresses continuously throughout life. Deterioration may be accelerated by recurrent episodes of rheumatic fever. Rheumatic fever itself is an immunologic response to group A β-hemolytic streptococcus infections. The incidence of rheumatic fever in a population is heavily influenced by conditions of poverty and crowding. These same individuals are at risk for having reduced access and use of health care resources and may present undiagnosed or untreated.

Patients with asymptomatic mitral stenosis have a 10-year survival rate of greater than 80%. Once a patient is significantly symptomatic, the 10-year survival rate without treatment is less than 15%. In the presence of pulmonary hypertension, mean survival falls to less than 3 years. Death is due to progressive pulmonary edema, right-sided heart failure, systemic embolization, or pulmonary embolism.[13]

Stenosis of the mitral valve impedes the flow of blood from the left atrium to the left ventricle during diastole. The normal mitral valve area is 4 to 5 cm^2. Symptoms with exercise can be expected with valve areas less than or equal to 2.5 cm^2. Symptoms at rest are expected at less than or equal to 1.5 cm^2. The left ventricle responds with Starling mechanisms to increased venous return with increased performance, elevating CO in response to demand. The left atrium is limited in its capacity to respond. Therefore, **CO is limited by the relatively passive flow of blood through the valve during diastole; increased venous return results in pulmonary congestion rather than increased CO.** Thus, the drive for increased CO in pregnancy cannot be achieved, resulting in increased pulmonary congestion. The relative tachycardia experienced in pregnancy shortens diastole, decreases left ventricular filling, and therefore further compromises CO and increases pulmonary congestion.

The diagnosis of mitral stenosis in pregnancy before maternal decompensation is uncommon. Tiredness and dyspnea on exertion are characteristic symptoms of mitral stenosis but are also ubiquitous among pregnant women. Although the presence of a diastolic rumble or jugular venous distention may suggest mitral stenosis, these findings are subtle and may be overlooked or not appreciated. Not uncommonly, an intercurrent event such as a febrile episode will result in exaggerated symptoms and the diagnosis of pulmonary edema or oxygen desaturation. Under these circumstances, particularly in the context of a patient from an at-risk group, an echocardiogram should be performed to rule out mitral-valvular disease.

Echocardiographic diagnosis of mitral stenosis is based on the characteristic appearance of the stenotic, frequently calcified valve. Calculation of valve area from pressure half-time of the Doppler wave or by two-dimensional planimetry provides an objective measure of severity. Valve areas of 1 cm^2 or less usually require pharmacologic management during pregnancy and invasive hemodynamic monitoring during labor. Valve areas of 1.4 cm^2 or less usually require careful expectant management. Left atrial enlargement identifies a patient at risk for atrial fibrillation, subsequent atrial thrombus, and the potential for systemic embolization. Embolic complications have been reported in pregnant women with atrial enlargement without atrial fibrillation. Pulmonary hypertension, a complication of worsening mitral disease, can be diagnosed and quantified with Doppler evaluation of the regurgitant jet across the tricuspid valve. **Elevated pulmonary pressures may be due to hydrostatic forces associated with elevated left atrial pressures or, in more advanced disease, may result from pathologic elevations of pulmonary vascular resistance (PVR).** Hydrostatic pulmonary hypertension may respond to therapy that lowers left atrial pressure. Pulmonary hypertension due to elevated PVR is life threatening in pregnancy and may precipitate right-sided heart failure in the postpartum period.

Pregnancy itself does not negatively affect the natural history of mitral stenosis. Chesley[14] reviewed the medical histories of 134 women with functionally severe mitral stenosis who survived pregnancies between 1931 and 1943. These women lived before modern management of mitral stenosis and, therefore, represent the natural history of the disease. By 1974, only nine of the cohort remained alive. Their death rate was exponential; during each year of follow-up, the rate for the remaining cohort was 6.3%. Women with subsequent pregnancies had comparable survival to those who did not again become pregnant, allowing the authors to conclude that pregnancy itself did not negatively affect long-term outcome.

The goal of antepartum care in the context of mitral stenosis is to achieve a balance between the drive to increase CO and the limitations of flow across the stenotic valve. Most women with significant disease require diuresis with a drug such as furosemide. In addition, β-blockade reduces HR, improves diastolic flow across the valve, and relieves pulmonary congestion. Al Kasab and associates[15] evaluated the impact of β -blockade on 25 pregnant women with significant mitral stenosis. Figure 36-4 describes the functional status of women before pregnancy, during pregnancy before β-blockade, and after β-blockade. The deterioration associated with pregnancy and the improvement with treatment are evident. Fastidious antepartum care as described earlier should supplement pharmacologic management.

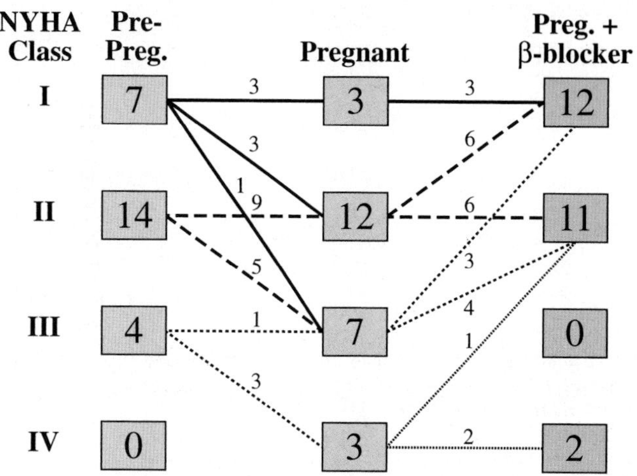

FIGURE 36-4. The effects of β-blockade on functional status of women with mitral stenosis. *NYHA*, New York Heart Association. (From Al Kasab S, Sabag T, Al Zaibag M, et al: Beta-adrenergic receptor blockade in the management of pregnant women with mitral stenosis. Am J Obstet Gynecol 163:37, 1990.)

Women with a history of rheumatic valvular disease who are at risk for contact with populations with a high prevalence of streptococcal infection should receive prophylaxis with daily oral penicillin G or monthly benzathine penicillin. Most pregnant women live in close contact with groups of children and usually are considered at risk. Atrial fibrillation is a complication associated with mitral stenosis due to left atrial enlargement. Rapid ventricular response to atrial fibrillation may result in sudden decompensation. Digoxin, β-blockers, or calcium channel blockers can be used to control ventricular response. In the context of hemodynamic decompensation, electrical cardioversion may be necessary. Anticoagulation with heparin should be used before and after cardioversion to prevent systemic embolization. Patients with chronic atrial fibrillation and a history of an embolic event should also undergo anticoagulation. Anticoagulation may be considered in women with a left atrial dimension of 55 mm Hg or greater.

Labor and delivery can frequently precipitate decompensation in patients with critical mitral stenosis. Pain induces tachycardia. Uterine contractions increase venous return and, therefore, pulmonary congestion. Women frequently cannot tolerate the work of pushing in the second stage. Clark and coworkers[4] described the abrupt elevation in pulmonary artery pressures in the immediate postpartum period associated with return of uterine blood to the general circulation (Figure 36-5). **Aggressive, anticipatory diuresis will reduce pulmonary congestion and the potential for oxygen desaturation.**

The hemodynamics of women with symptomatic stenosis or a valve area of 1 cm^2 or less may benefit from management with the aid of a pulmonary artery catheter. Ideally, hemodynamic parameters are assessed when the patient is well compensated, early in labor. These findings serve as a reference point to guide subsequent therapy. Pain control is best achieved with an epidural. HR control

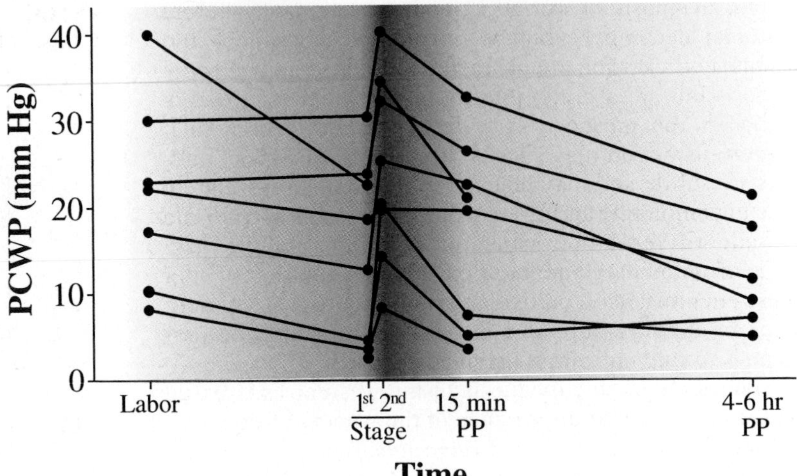

FIGURE 36-5. The changes in pulmonary capillary wedge pressure *(PCWP)* associated with delivery and subsequent diuresis in women with mitral stenosis. *PP*, postpartum. (From Clark S, Phelan J, Greenspoon J, et al: Labor and delivery in the presence of mitral stenosis: central hemodynamic observations. Am J Obstet Gynecol 152:384, 1985.)

is maintained through pain control and β-blockade. To avoid pushing, the second stage is shortened with low forceps or vacuum delivery. Aggressive diuresis is initiated immediately postpartum. Cesarean delivery is reserved for obstetrical indications. In a series of 80 pregnancies managed with a range of severity, the most common complications were pulmonary edema (31%) and arrhythmia (11%). When valve area was 1 cm^2 or less, the rate of pulmonary edema was higher (56%), as was the rate of arrhythmia (33%).[16] These rates will be dependent on the effectiveness of medical management and the timing of presentation and diagnosis.

Aggressive medical management, including hospital bedrest in selected cases, is sufficient to manage most women with mitral stenosis. The woman with uncommonly severe disease may require surgical intervention. Although successful valve replacement and open commissurotomy have been reported in pregnancy, they are now rarely needed. Two centers have reported successful balloon valvotomy in a series of 40 and 44 women with minimal complications.[17,18] Complications of balloon valvuloplasty outside of pregnancy occur at the following rates: mortality (0.5%), cerebrovascular accident (1%), and mitral regurgitation requiring surgery (2%). Mitral valvuloplasty in pregnancy has been reported with success rates between 89% and 100%. The incidence of severe mitral regurgitation requiring surgery is between 0% and 5%. The rate of fetal loss between 0% and 8%. **Medical management should be clearly exhausted before assuming these risks during pregnancy, when emergent intervention such as valve replacement is more complicated and carries a significant risk to the fetus.**

Rheumatic disease can also affect the aortic valve. Management of significant mitral stenosis, which limits ventricular filling, in the context of aortic stenosis that is critically dependent on ventricular filling, is particularly complicated.

Mitral Regurgitation

Mitral regurgitation may be due to a chronic progressive process such as rheumatic valve disease or myxomatous mitral valve disease, frequently associated with mitral valve prolapse. As regurgitation increases over time, forward flow is maintained at the expense of left ventricular dilation with eventual impaired contractility. Left atrial enlargement may be associated with atrial fibrillation that should be managed with ventricular rate control and anticoagulation. The patient with chronic mitral regurgitation may remain asymptomatic even with exercise. Preconceptional counseling should include consideration of valve replacement in consultation with a cardiologist. In general, valve replacement is recommended for (1) symptomatic patients, (2) atrial fibrillation, (3) ejection fraction less than 50% to 60%, (4) left ventricular end-diastolic dimension greater than 45 to 50 mm, or (5) pulmonary systolic pressure greater than 50 to 60 mm Hg.[13] As discussed later, the benefits of valve replacement before pregnancy must be balanced against the risks associated with a prosthetic valve in pregnancy and the potential for prosthetic valve deterioration in pregnancy. If surgery is required, valve repair rather than replacement is preferred when possible to avoid the need for anticoagulation.

Acute mitral regurgitation in young patients is uncommon and may be associated with ruptured chordae tendineae due to endocarditis or myxomatous valve disease. Without time for left ventricular compensation, forward flow may be severely compromised. Urgent valve surgery is usually required. Inotropic left ventricular support and systemic afterload reduction can be used to stabilize the patient.

The hemodynamic changes associated with pregnancy can be expected to have mixed effects. A reduction in systemic vascular resistance (SVR) tends to promote forward flow. The drive to increase CO will exacerbate left ventricular volume overload. Increased atrial dilation may initiate atrial fibrillation. Pulmonary congestion can be managed by careful diuresis with the knowledge that adequate forward flow is usually dependent on a high preload to achieve adequate left ventricular filling. Atrial fibrillation should be managed as in the nonpregnant state. An increase in SVR due to progressive hypertension secondary to advancing preeclampsia may significantly impair forward flow and should be treated. Labor and delivery should be managed with standard cardiac care. Catecholamine release due to pain or stress impairs forward flow. Particular attention should be paid to left ventricular filling. **Excessive preload results in pulmonary congestion. Insufficient preload will not fill the enlarged left ventricle and will result in insufficient forward flow.** A pulmonary artery catheter can be used to determine appropriate filling pressure in early labor or before induction. Although a large v-wave may complicate the interpretation of pulmonary artery wedge pressure, the pulmonary artery diastolic pressure can be used as a reference point. Diuresis in the early postpartum period may be required.

Myxomatous mitral valve disease or mitral valve prolapse is a common condition, affecting as many as 12% of young women. **In the absence of conditions of abnormal connective tissue such as Marfan or Ehlers-Danlos syndrome and clinically significant mitral regurgitation, women with mitral prolapse can be expected to have uncomplicated pregnancies.** They may experience an increase in tachyarrhythmias that can be treated with β-blockers. Prophylactic antibiotics are usually used at the time of delivery.

Aortic Stenosis

Most patients who develop calcific stenotic tricuspid aortic valves do so outside their childbearing years (age 70 to 80 years). Patients with bicuspid valves develop significant stenosis after the age of 50 to 60 years. Rheumatic disease can also affect the aortic valve, usually after the development of significant mitral disease. Most pregnant women with significant aortic stenosis have congenitally stenotic valves: bicuspid valves with congenitally fused leaflets, unicuspid valves, or tricuspid valves with fused leaflets.[19]

The natural history of aortic stenosis is characterized by a long, asymptomatic period. With increasing outflow obstruction, patients develop angina, syncope, and left ventricular failure. Without valve replacement, only 50% of patients will survive 5 years after the development of angina; 3 years after the development of syncope; and 2 years after the development of left ventricular failure.[20] Although valve replacement is the only definitive treatment for calcific aortic stenosis, valvuloplasty may prove beneficial in some young adults whose valves are not calcified. Medical management of symptomatic patients is not generally efficacious. Mechanical valve replacement requires anticoagulation, complicating subsequent pregnancies.

Young women with aortic stenosis are usually asymptomatic. Although they may develop increasing exercise intolerance in pregnancy, the progression is insidious and not easily distinguished from the effects of normal pregnancy. The diagnosis is usually made by the auscultation of a harsh systolic murmur. **The murmur can easily be distinguished from a physiologic murmur of pregnancy by its harshness and radiation into the carotid arteries.** Diagnosis is confirmed by echocardiography whereby the gradient across the valve can be measured by Doppler, and the valve area can be calculated with the continuity equation. Many women with significant aortic stenosis experience the expected increase in CO associated with pregnancy.[3] Increased flow across the fixed, stenotic valve results in a proportionately increased gradient across the valve. Although the pressure gradient during pregnancy may be higher than that observed postpartum, these differences are not significant.

Four series of patients with aortic stenosis in pregnancy have been reported.[3,21-23] The reports summarize experiences with wide ranges in severity of disease and management ranging from the 1960s and 1970s to the present. Arias and Pineda[21] described a series of 23 cases managed before 1978 with a maternal mortality rate of 17%. More recent series, however, do not demonstrate this high level of maternal risk.[3,22,23] The potential for serious adverse outcomes reported by Arias should, however, serve as an indication for intensive management. The rate of mortality should not necessarily be used as an indication for termination or surgical intervention. Pregnant patients have been successfully managed with aortic gradients in excess of 160 mm Hg.[3] In general, patients with a peak aortic gradient of 60 mm Hg or less have had uncomplicated courses. Those with higher gradients require increasingly intensive management.

Aortic valve replacement and balloon valvotomy have been reported during pregnancy. Balloon valvotomy in a young patient without valve calcification can provide significant long-term palliation. Valvotomy before pregnancy may provide an interval of hemodynamic stability sufficient to complete a pregnancy without the complications associated with a mechanical prosthetic valve. **Consideration for valve replacement or valvotomy during pregnancy should be reserved for patients who remain clinically symptomatic despite hospital care.** In general, intervention should not be based solely on a pressure gradient or valve area.

Aortic stenosis is a condition of excess left ventricular afterload. Ventricular hypertrophy increases cardiac oxygen requirement, whereas increased diastolic ventricular pressure impairs diastolic coronary perfusion. Each increases the potential for myocardial ischemia. The left ventricle requires adequate filling to generate sufficient systolic pressure to produce flow across the stenotic valve. **Given a hypertrophied ventricle and some degree of diastolic dysfunction, the volume-pressure relationship is very steep. A small loss of left ventricular filling results in a proportionately large fall in left ventricular pressure and, therefore, a large fall in forward flow, CO.** The pregnant patient with significant aortic stenosis is very sensitive to loss of preload associated with hemorrhage or epidural-induced hypotension. The window of appropriate filling pressure is narrow. Excess fluid may result in pulmonary edema; insufficient fluid may result in hypotension and coronary ischemia. In general, pulmonary edema associated with excess preload is much easier to manage than hypotension due to hypovolemia.

Appropriate antepartum care is described earlier. Given that most aortic stenosis in young women is congenital in origin, fetal echocardiography is indicated. Although some controversy persists, cesarean delivery is generally reserved for obstetrical indications. Pain during labor and delivery can be safely managed with regional analgesia using a low-dose bupivacaine and narcotic technique. Dense anesthesia during the second stage can be obtained with minimal hemodynamic complications using a caudal catheter. Patients with gradients above 60 to 80 mm Hg may benefit from the use of a pulmonary artery and an arterial catheter during labor. Hospital admission 1 day before planned induction of labor with a favorable cervix is preferred. A prolonged induction should be avoided. Pulmonary artery and radial artery catheters, as well as epidural and caudal catheters are placed. The patient should be gently hydrated overnight to achieve a pulmonary artery wedge pressure (PAWP) of 12 to 15 mm Hg. Some patients with milder disease spontaneously diurese in the face of a volume load such that an elevation in PAWP cannot be achieved. An elevated PAWP serves as a buffer against a loss of preload. If with bleeding or the onset of anesthesia PAWP falls, volume can be administered before a reduction in forward flow. In general, pushing is minimized, and the second stage is shortened with operative vaginal delivery. Antibiotics may be administered for the prevention of endocarditis.

Postpartum, patients should be monitored hemodynamically for 24 to 48 hours. Diuresis is usually spontaneous; the patient can be allowed to find her predelivery compensated state. When diuresis must be induced to treat pulmonary edema, it should be done gently and carefully. Predelivery hemodynamic parameters should be used as an end point. Some have found that a significant delay in valve replacement in women with quite severe disease is associated with maternal complications.[3] In a larger cohort of women with less severe disease followed for 6 years and compared with a matched cohort who did not experience a pregnancy, women who experienced a pregnancy had a reduction in event-free survival.[24] These observations may be the result of accelerated valve deterioration due to pregnancy. For this reason, valve replacement within weeks of delivery may be indicated.

Aortic Regurgitation

Aortic regurgitation is most often due to a congenitally abnormal valve. Other causes include Marfan syndrome, endocarditis, and rheumatic disease. As with mitral regurgitation, the left ventricle compensates for a loss in forward flow with an increase in left ventricular end-diastolic volume. Afterload reduction prevents progressive left ventricular dilation and is recommended for patients with left ventricular dysfunction or dilation. Valve replacement is generally recommended for (1) New York Heart Association (NYHA) functional class III and class IV symptoms, (2) an ejection fraction less than 50%, or (3) left ventricular end-systolic dimension greater than 55 mm.[13] Acute regurgitation may be due to aortic root dissection or endocarditis and usually represents a medical emergency requiring urgent valve replacement.

The reduction in vascular resistance associated with pregnancy tends to improve cardiac performance. If afterload reduction has been achieved with an angiotensin-converting enzyme (ACE) inhibitor before pregnancy, hydralazine or a calcium channel blocker such as nifedipine should be substituted. Modest elevations of HR should be tolerated. Bradycardia may be associated with increased regurgitation due to prolongation of diastole. Labor and delivery are managed with standard cardiac care. Pulmonary artery catheterization is not usually required. As the hemodynamic changes associated with pregnancy resolve, a rise in vascular resistance should be anticipated and afterload reduction maintained.

TABLE 36-2 PREGNANCY OUTCOMES WITH PROSTHETIC VALVES

	MECHANICAL	PORCINE
Women	31	57
Pregnancies	56	95
Fetal loss	27.7%	12.3%
Premature birth	5.9%	7.7%
Valve deterioration	5.3%	7.0%
Thromboembolic event	5.3%	—

Prosthetic Valves

Definitive therapy for significant valvular disease requires surgical repair, or more commonly replacement. Mechanical valves are durable but require anticoagulation. Bioprosthetic valves, when used in a young woman, usually require replacement during her lifetime. Reports of pregnancies associated with prosthetic valves suggest significant variability in outcomes. Table 36-2 summarizes a review of 151 pregnancies complicated by a prosthetic valve.[25] Mechanical valves and anticoagulation were associated with a moderate increase in miscarriage and thromboembolic events. A report from France of 55 pregnancies suggests a less favorable prognosis.[26] Mechanical valves were associated with a maternal mortality rate of 3.7% and a thromboembolic rate of 14.8%. Thromboembolism was increased fourfold with heparin use rather than warfarin. Mitral valves accounted for 81% of thrombotic complications. The impact of pregnancy on the life of a bioprosthetic valve has been studied.[25] Ten-year graft survival following two pregnancies was 16.7% compared with 54.8% following a single pregnancy, suggesting that pregnancy may adversely affect the life of a porcine valve. Accelerated deterioration of bioprosthetic valves has been suggested by some studies but not confirmed by others.[27]

The management of care with prosthetic valves outside pregnancy has been extensively reviewed. Decisions surrounding the timing and choice of valve replacement for a woman of reproductive age are complex. Managing a pregnancy with moderate valve disease may be less complicated than managing a pregnancy with a prosthetic valve. The durability of a mechanical valve has considerable advantages for a young person, but it is associated with more adverse outcomes in pregnancy. Delay in valve replacement until childbearing is completed is appropriate when the severity of heart disease is believed to be manageable in pregnancy.

Anticoagulation is required with a mechanical valve. Management of anticoagulation in pregnant women with mechanical prosthetic valves remains very controversial. Many reported clinical series are confounded by adequacy of therapeutic monitoring and heparin dosing. Oral anticoagulation with warfarin in the first trimester is associated with congenital anomalies. **Potentially serious fetal bleeding may be encountered with use during the second and third trimesters. Warfarin is clearly associated with embryopathy and increased risk for stillbirth after 20 weeks'**

these hypotheses are proven. Recent research has focused on alterations in the number and function of estrogen-progesterone receptors and progesterone binding.

The human progesterone receptor (PR) exists as two major subtypes, PR-A and PR-B. Another isoform, PR-C, has recently been described, but its function is not well understood. The human estrogen receptor (ER) also exists as two major subtypes, ERa and ERb. A functional progesterone withdrawal has been proposed in which expression of PR-A in myometrium suppresses progesterone responsiveness and that functional progesterone withdrawal occurs by increased expression of the PR-A relative to PR-B. An alternative mechanism of functional progesterone withdrawal has been proposed wherein activation of nuclear factor k B in amnion represses progesterone function. Regardless of the mechanism, there is a building consensus that a localized functional progesterone withdrawal occurs in myometrium during human parturition.

Summary of the Preterm Parturition Syndrome

Preterm parturition is a syndrome caused by multiple etiologies with several clinical presentations including uterine contractility (preterm labor), preterm cervical ripening without significant clinical contractility (cervical insufficiency or advanced cervical dilation and effacement), or rupture of the amniotic sac (preterm PROM). The clinical presentation varies with the type and timing of the insult or stimulus to the components of the common pathway of parturition, the presence or absence of environmental cofactors, and individual variations in host response by both mother and fetus. This conceptual framework has implications for the understanding of the mechanisms responsible for the initiation of preterm parturition, as well as the diagnosis, treatment, and prevention of preterm birth.

CLINICAL CARE FOR WOMEN IN PRETERM LABOR

Clinical evaluation of preterm parturition begins with assessment of potential causes of labor, looking first for conditions that threaten the health of mother and fetus. Acute maternal conditions, for example, pyelonephritis, pneumonia, asthma, peritonitis, trauma, and hypertension, or obstetrical conditions including preeclampsia, placental abruption, placenta previa, and chorioamnionitis may mandate delivery. Fetal compromise may be acute, manifested by an abnormal fetal heart rate tracing, or chronic, indicated by fetal growth restriction or oligohydramnios, and may require delivery depending on the severity and potential for in utero versus ex utero treatment. Fetal growth restriction is more common in infants delivered after preterm labor or preterm PROM, even in apparently otherwise uncomplicated pregnancies. **Conditions that suggest specific therapy such as preterm ruptured membranes or cervical insufficiency should then be sought and treated accordingly.**

The next concerns are the accuracy of preterm labor diagnosis and the balance of risks and benefits that accompany active attempts to inhibit labor versus allowing delivery. Several issues arise:

- What is the gestational age, and what is the level of confidence about the accuracy of the gestational age?
- What, in the absence of advanced labor (cervical effacement >80% with dilation >2 cm) and a clear cause of preterm labor, is the accuracy of the diagnosis of preterm labor?
- Are confirmatory diagnostic tests such as cervical sonography, fetal fibronectin, or amniocentesis for infection necessary?
- What is the anticipated neonatal morbidity and mortality at this gestational age in this clinical setting?
- Should labor be stopped?
- Is transfer to a more appropriate hospital required?
- Should fetal lung maturity be tested?
- What interventions can be applied that will reduce the risks of perinatal morbidity and mortality?
- Should drugs to arrest labor (tocolytics), glucocorticoids, and/or antibiotics be given?

DIAGNOSIS OF PRETERM LABOR

Given the pathways for preterm parturition described earlier, clinical recognition of preterm labor requires attention to the biochemical as well as the biophysical features of the onset of labor. Pathologic uterine contractility rarely occurs in isolation; cervical ripening and decidual membrane activation are almost always in progress as well, most often before uterine contractions are clinically evident. Therefore, preterm labor must be considered whenever a pregnant woman reports recurrent abdominal or pelvic symptoms that persist for more than an hour in the second half or pregnancy. Symptoms of preterm labor such as pelvic pressure, increased vaginal discharge, backache, and menstrual-like cramps occur frequently in normal pregnancy, and suggest preterm labor more by persistence than severity. **Contractions may be painful or painless, depending on the resistance offered by the cervix.** Contractions against a closed, uneffaced cervix are likely to be painful, but persistence of recurrent pressure or tightening may be the only symptoms when cervical effacement precedes the onset of contractions.

For decades, the clinical diagnosis of preterm labor has been based on the presence of regular, painful uterine contractions accompanied by cervical dilation and/or effacement. These criteria assume a crisp demarcation between "preterm parturition" and "preterm labor" that is increasingly understood as being more gradual than previously thought. If thought of as screening criteria for the outcome "preterm birth," clinical signs and symptoms demonstrate poor sensitivity and specificity. Identifying women with preterm contractions who will actually deliver preterm is an inexact process. In like fashion, identifying those women who are at increased risk of not just preterm birth, but imminent preterm birth, remains elusive. A systematic review noted that approximately 30% of preterm labor cases resolved spontaneously. In subsequent studies, 50% of patients hospitalized for preterm labor actually delivered at term. **The inability to distinguish women in "true preterm labor" from women in "false labor" accurately has greatly hampered the assessment of therapeutic interventions, since as many as 50% of untreated (or placebo treated) subjects do not actually deliver preterm. Optimal criteria**

for initiation of treatment are not clear. Contraction frequency of six or more per hour, cervical dilation of 3 cm, effacement of 80%, ruptured membranes, and bleeding are symptoms of preterm labor most often associated with preterm delivery. When lower thresholds for contraction frequency and cervical change are used, "false-positive" diagnosis (defined in randomized controlled trials as delivery at term after treatment with placebo only) occurs in nearly 40% of women, but sensitivity does not rise. Difficulty in accurate diagnosis is the product of the high prevalence of the symptoms and signs of early preterm labor in normal pregnancy, the gradual onset of preterm labor discussed earlier, and the imprecision of digital examination of the cervix below 3 cm dilation and 80% effacement. The practice of initiating tocolytic drugs for contraction frequency without additional diagnostic criteria results in unnecessary treatment of women who are not at increased risk of imminent spontaneous preterm birth.[36]

Diagnostic Tests for Preterm Labor

Women with symptoms whose cervical dilation is less than 2 cm and whose effacement is less than 80% present a diagnostic challenge. Diagnostic accuracy may be improved in these patients by testing other features of parturition, such as cervical ripening, assessed by transvaginal sonographic measurement of cervical length; and decidual activation, tested by an assay for fetal fibronectin in cervicovaginal fluid.[37,38] Both tests aid diagnosis primarily by reducing false-positive diagnosis. Transabdominal sonography has poor reproducibility for cervical measurement and should not be used clinically without confirmation by a transvaginal ultrasound. A cervical length of 30 mm or more by endovaginal sonography indicates that preterm labor is unlikely in symptomatic women if the examination is properly performed.

Similarly, a negative fibronectin test in women with symptoms before 34 weeks' gestation with cervical dilation less than 3 cm can also reduce the rate of false-positive diagnosis if the result is returned promptly and the clinician is willing to act on a negative test result by not initiating treatment. When both tests were performed in a study of 206 women with possible preterm labor, the fetal fibronectin test improved the performance of sonographic cervical length only when the sonographic cervical length was less than 30 mm (see the accompanying box, Clinical Evaluation of Patients with Possible Preterm Labor).

Amniocentesis for Women with Preterm Labor

The goal of care for women with preterm labor is to reduce perinatal morbidity and mortality, most of which is caused by immaturity of the respiratory, gastrointestinal, coagulation, and central nervous systems of the preterm infant. Fetal pulmonary immaturity is the most frequent cause of serious newborn illness, and the fetal pulmonary system is the only organ system whose function is directly testable before delivery. If the quality of obstetrical dating is good and intrauterine fetal well-being is not compromised, the likelihood of neonatal RDS may be estimated from the gestational age.

Amniotic fluid studies may be useful in women with possible preterm labor in the following circumstances:

Clinical Evaluation of Patients with Possible Preterm Labor

1. **Patient presents with signs/symptoms of preterm labor:**
   Persistent contractions (painful or painless)
   Intermittent abdominal cramping, pelvic pressure, or backache
   Increase or change in vaginal discharge
   Vaginal spotting or bleeding
2. **General physical examination:**
   Sitting pulse and blood pressure
   Temperature
   External fetal heart rate and contraction monitor
3. **Sterile speculum examination**
   pH
   Fern
   Pooled fluid
   Fibronectin swab (posterior fornix or external cervical os, avoiding areas with bleeding)
   Cultures for chlamydia (cervix), and *Neisseria gonorrhoeae* (cervix), and group B streptococcus (outer third of vagina and perineum)
4. **Transabdominal ultrasound examination**
   Placental location
   Amniotic fluid volume
   Estimated fetal weight and presentation
   Fetal well-being
5. **Cervical examination** (after ruptured membranes excluded)
   a. **Cervix >3 cm dilation/≥80% effaced**
   Preterm labor diagnosis confirmed. Evaluate for tocolysis.
   b. **Cervix 2 to 3 cm dilation/<80% effaced**
   Preterm labor likely but not established. Monitor contraction frequency and repeat digital examination in 30-60 minutes. Diagnose preterm labor if cervical change. If not, send fibronectin or obtain transvaginal cervical ultrasound. Evaluate for tocolysis if any cervical change, cervical length <20 mm, or positive fibronectin.
   c. **Cervix <2 cm dilation and <80% effaced**
   Preterm labor diagnosis uncertain. Monitor contraction frequency, send fibronectin and/or obtain cervical sonography, and repeat digital examination in 1 to 2 hours. Evaluate for tocolysis if there is a 1 cm change in cervical dilation, effacement >80%, cervical length <20 mm, or positive fibronectin.
6. **Use of Cervical Ultrasound**
   Cervical length <20 mm *and* contraction criteria met = preterm labor
   Cervical length 20-30 mm *and* contraction criteria met = probable preterm labor
   Cervical length >30 mm = preterm labor *very unlikely* regardless of contraction frequency

1. *Fetal pulmonary maturity testing.* Generally speaking, gestational age at birth is the best predictor of the frequency and severity of the consequences of prematurity to the newborn. As noted earlier, generally speaking, labor inhibition and antenatal glucocorticoid therapy are used when birth is anticipated to occur between 24 and 34 weeks' gestation. When dates are uncertain (e.g., late prenatal

care, fetal size larger than expected for dates, suggesting a more advanced gestation), it may be reasonable in some circumstances to use amniotic fluid lung maturity studies to help guide management decisions.
2. *Testing for infection.* Among women with preterm labor and intact membranes, early gestational age, short cervix, and progressive labor despite a tocolytic are all risk factor particularly increasing the probability of occult amniotic fluid infection. In this setting, amniotic fluid studies for infection may guide counseling of women and influence management decisions regarding antibiotics, labor inhibition, and delivery. In this setting, amniotic fluid glucose (amniotic fluid glucose levels less than 20 mg/dL suggest intra-amniotic infection), Gram stain for bacteria, cell count, and culture may be used.
3. *Determining fetal karyotype.* The presence of polyhydramnios or a fetal anomaly suggests that preterm labor may have occurred due to uterine distention or placental insufficiency associated with fetal aneuploidy. Fluorescence in situ hybridization studies for the most common aneuploid conditions can be available within 48 hours. In the absence of other fetal features suggestive of aneuploidy, the presence of preterm labor alone is insufficient indication for determination of fetal karyotype.

GOALS OF TREATMENT FOR WOMEN IN PRETERM LABOR

Treatment with drugs to inhibit labor after contractions and cervical change are well established or membranes have ruptured does not prolong pregnancy sufficiently to allow further intrauterine growth and maturation, but their use can often delay preterm birth long enough to permit four interventions that have been shown to reduce neonatal morbidity and mortality:

1. Antenatal transfer of the mother and fetus to the most appropriate hospital.
2. Antibiotics in labor to prevent neonatal infection with the group B streptococcus (GBS).
3. Antenatal administration of glucocorticoids to the mother to reduce neonatal morbidity and mortality due to respiratory distress, intraventricular hemorrhage, and other causes.
4. Administration of maternal magnesium sulfate at the time of preterm birth before 32 weeks to reduce the incidence of cerebral palsy.

Maternal Transfer

Many states have adopted systems of regionalized perinatal care in recognition of the advantages of concentrating care for preterm infants, especially those born before 32 weeks. Hospitals and birth centers caring for normal mothers and infants are designated as Level I. Larger hospitals that care for the majority of maternal and infant complications are designated as Level II centers; these hospitals have neonatal intensive care units staffed and equipped to care for most infants with birth weights greater than 1500 g. Level III centers typically provide care for the sickest and smallest infants, and for maternal complications requiring intensive care. This approach has been associated with improved outcomes for preterm infants.

Antibiotics

Women with preterm labor should be treated with antibiotics to prevent neonatal GBS infection (see Chapter 51). Because preterm infants have a greater risk of neonatal GBS infection than infants born at term, intrapartum prophylaxis with penicillin is recommended.[39] This policy has successfully reduced the incidence of neonatal GBS infection to such a degree that most GBS infections now occur in full-term infants. There is also evidence that infants born to women with preterm PROM have reduced perinatal morbidity when antepartum antibiotic prophylaxis has been administered for 3 to 7 days.

Antibiotic therapy in women with preterm labor and intact membranes is not effective to prolong pregnancy. The failure of antibiotics to prolong pregnancy may be attributed to treatment of women whose preterm labor did not result from infection, and to the timing of treatment relative to the infectious process. Rather than an acute infection due to the recent ascent of vaginal organisms into the uterus, the pathologic sequence in which infection-driven preterm labor occurs is often much more indolent. **Antimicrobial therapy of women in preterm labor should be limited to GBS prophylaxis, women with preterm PROM, or treatment of a specific pathogen (e.g., urinary tract infection).**

Antenatal Corticosteroids

Glucocorticoids act generally in the developing fetus to promote maturation over growth. In the lung, corticosteroids promote surfactant synthesis, increase lung compliance, reduce vascular permeability, and generate an enhanced response to postnatal surfactant treatment. Glucocorticoids have similar maturational effects on other organs including the brain, kidneys, and gut.

Studies by Liggins of mechanisms of parturition in sheep led to the discovery of the beneficial effect of antenatal glucocorticoids on the maturation and performance of the lung in prematurely born infants. Subsequent studies have shown conclusively that antepartum administration of the glucocorticoids betamethasone or dexamethasone to the mother reduces the risk of death, RDS, intraventricular hemorrhage, NEC, and PDA in the preterm neonate. Guidelines for appropriate clinical use of antenatal glucocorticoids have evolved from initial skepticism and selective use, through a period of broad and repeated treatment following the first NICHD panel report in 1994, to the practice of a single course of treatment recommended by the NICHD Consensus Panel in 2000. More recently, clinical trials support the notion that administration of a single rescue course of ACS before 33 weeks improves neonatal outcome (e.g., decreased respiratory distress syndrome, ventilator support, and surfactant use) without apparent increased short-term risk.[40] A single rescue course of antenatal corticosteroids may be considered if the antecedent treatment was given more than 2 weeks prior, the gestational age is less than $32^{6/7}$ weeks, and the women are judged by the clinician to be likely to give birth within the next week. However, regularly scheduled repeat courses or multiple courses (more

than two) are not recommended.[41] Betamethasone and dexamethasone, the only drugs found beneficial for this purpose, are potent glucocorticoids with limited if any mineralocorticoid effect. A course of treatment consists of two doses of 12 mg of betamethasone (the combination of 6 mg each of betamethasone acetate and betamethasone phosphate) administered intramuscularly twice, 24 hours apart, or four doses of 6 mg of dexamethasone given intramuscularly every 12 hours. Other corticosteroids (prednisolone, prednisone) and routes of administration (oral) are not suitable alternatives because of reduced placental transfer, lack of demonstrated benefit, and, in the case of oral dexamethasone, increased risk of adverse effects when compared with the intramuscular route.

Fetal Effects

Randomized placebo-controlled trials and meta-analyses confirm the beneficial effects of antenatal corticosteroids. Infants born to treated women were significantly less likely to experience RDS (OR 0.53), IVH (OR 0.38), and neonatal death (OR 0.60). The beneficial effects on IVH are independent of the effects on respiratory function. Other morbidities of preterm birth are also reduced by antenatal glucocorticoids, including NEC, PDA, and BPD. Although both are considered effective, betamethasone may be superior to dexamethasone with respect to reduction in morbidity and mortality to the preterm newborn.

Other Fetal Effects of Glucocorticoids

Transient reduction in fetal breathing and body movements sufficient to affect the interpretation of the biophysical profile have been described with both drugs but are more common after betamethasone, typically lasting 48 to 72 hours after the second dose. Transient suppression of neonatal cortisol levels has been reported, but neonatal response to ACTH stimulation was unimpaired.

Maternal Effects

Antenatal glucocorticoids produce a transient rise in maternal platelet and WBC count lasting 72 hours; WBC counts in excess of 20,000 are rarely due to steroids. Maternal glucose tolerance is challenged as well and often requires insulin therapy to maintain euglycemia in women with previously well-controlled gestational or pregestational diabetes. Maternal blood pressure is unaffected by antenatal steroid treatment; neither betamethasone nor dexamethasone has significant mineralocorticoid effect. Women treated with multiple courses of steroids during pregnancy had a blunted response to ACTH stimulation later in pregnancy or the puerperium.

Duration of Benefit

The duration of the beneficial fetal effects after a single course of glucocorticoids is not clear. The issue is difficult to study because the interval between treatment and delivery in clinical trials is variable, and because some effects may be transient whereas others are permanent. Neonatal benefit has been most easily observed when the interval between the first dose and delivery exceeds 48 hours, but some benefit is evident after an incomplete course. One large multicenter trial found evidence of benefit for as long as 18 days after the initial course of treatment.

Risks of Antenatal Corticosteroid Treatment

The recommendation of the 1994 NICHD Consensus Conference to increase the use of antenatal steroids, coupled with uncertainty about the duration of neonatal protection from a single course of treatment and difficulty in predicting imminent preterm delivery, resulted in increased treatment of mothers at risk. Although more women received treatment, many did not deliver within 7 days but remained at risk and were treated weekly until delivery or 34 weeks' gestation. The safety and benefit of one course of steroids has never been questioned. Long-term follow-up studies of infants in the original cohorts of infants treated with a single course of antenatal steroids have displayed no differences in physical characteristics or mental function when compared with gestational age–matched controls. The increasing use of repeated courses prompted animal and human studies that have raised concerns about the effects of prolonged exposure to steroids on fetal growth and neurologic function. The animal studies may be summarized as showing reduced fetal growth and adverse brain and neurologic development in several species.

Human studies also found reduced growth in fetuses exposed to multiple courses of antenatal steroids. An Australian study found a twofold increase in birth weights below the 10th percentile and significantly reduced head circumference in infants exposed to more than three antenatal courses of steroids. Others have also found reduced head circumference.

Other Antenatal Treatments to Reduce Fetal/Neonatal Morbidity

Respiratory Distress

The occurrence of RDS among infants born to women treated with steroid therapy has led to investigation of alternative treatment approaches to further enhance pulmonary maturation. Neonatal treatment with surfactant is an effective adjunctive therapy that adds independently and synergistically to the benefit of corticosteroids in reducing RDS-related morbidity. More than 4600 women have been enrolled into 13 trials of maternal treatment with antenatal thyrotropin-releasing hormone (TRH) to reduce neonatal lung disease. There were no benefits compared with corticosteroids alone for any neonatal outcome. Prenatal treatment with TRH actually increased risk of adverse outcomes for infants in some trials.

Neurologic Morbidity

Antenatal maternal treatment with phenobarbital, vitamin K, and magnesium sulfate has been studied to reduce or prevent neonatal neurologic morbidity. Phenobarbital was not effective in reducing intraventricular hemorrhage when given alone or in combination with vitamin K.

Antenatal maternal treatment with magnesium has been inconsistently associated with reduced rates of IVH, cerebral palsy, and perinatal mortality in premature infants. A randomized placebo-controlled trial of antenatal magnesium conducted in 1062 women delivered before 30 weeks' gestation found significantly lower rates of gross motor dysfunction and nonsignificant trends of reduced mortality and cerebral palsy in surviving infants in the treated group at 2 years of age. There were no significant adverse effects

noted in infants exposed to antenatal magnesium sulfate. In the 1990s, observational studies suggested an association between prenatal exposure to magnesium sulfate and less frequent subsequent neurologic morbidities. Subsequently, several large clinical studies have evaluated the evidence regarding magnesium sulfate, neuroprotection, and preterm births.[42-45] If tocolysis is indicated, the most effective agent with the most favorable side effect profile should be given. None of the trials demonstrated significant pregnancy prolongation when magnesium sulfate was given for neuroprotection. **However, the available evidence suggests that magnesium sulfate given before anticipated early preterm birth reduces the risk of cerebral palsy in surviving infants.**[46]

We suggest limiting magnesium sulfate for neuroprotection to women who are at least 24, but less than 32, weeks of gestation, given that the two largest trials of neuroprotective effects did not enroll women beyond this gestational age range.[45,47]

The impact of gestational age on the neuroprotective effect of antenatally administered magnesium was assessed in one meta-analysis, which included the five trials in the Cochrane review.[48] These trials were stratified by the gestational age at randomization: less than 32 to 34 weeks (5235 fetuses) or less than 30 weeks (3107 fetuses).

Major findings were similar for both gestational age ranges[48]:

- There was no significant difference in the primary outcome of "death or cerebral palsy" at 18 to 24 months of corrected age or for the outcome of perinatal/infant "death."
- The largest reduction in risk was for "moderate to severe cerebral palsy."
- Less than 32 to 34 weeks: RR 0.60 (95% CI 0.43 to 0.84).
- Less than 30 weeks: RR 0.54 (95% CI 0.36 to 0.80).
- There were statistically significant reductions in the risk of "cerebral palsy" (RR 0.7 and 0.69 at less than 32 to 34 weeks and less than 30 weeks, respectively) and for "death or moderate to severe cerebral palsy" (RR 0.85 and 0.84 at less than 32 to 34 weeks and less than 30 weeks, respectively).
- The numbers needed to treat to prevent one case of cerebral palsy in the less than 32 to 34 weeks group and the less than 30 weeks group were 56 and 46 women, respectively.

Until further data are available, a 4-g bolus of magnesium sulfate with a 1 g/hr maintenance dose is a regimen that is anticipated to have a more favorable side effect and safety profile than a higher dose regimen. Neither the neuroprotective mechanism nor the dose response to magnesium sulfate is well understood. While it seems likely that the neuroprotective effects of magnesium sulfate are secondary to residual concentrations of the drug in the neonate's circulation, there are insufficient data regarding the maternal dose that confers neonatal benefit.

Administration of magnesium sulfate is appropriate for women with preterm premature rupture of membranes or preterm labor who have a high likelihood of imminent delivery (e.g., within 24 hours), or before an indicated preterm delivery. If emergency delivery is necessary given maternal or fetal status, it should not be delayed to administer magnesium sulfate. Therapy should be reserved for women who are at high risk of imminent delivery rather than women who simply are diagnosed with preterm labor or preterm premature rupture of membranes. We do not recommend continuing the magnesium infusion for longer than 24 hours if delivery has not occurred.

Treatment Protocol

Magnesium sulfate must be given parenterally to achieve serum levels greater than the normal range. Therapeutic dosage regimens are similar to those used for intravenous seizure prophylaxis of preeclampsia. A loading dose of 4 g is given over 30 minutes, followed by an infusion of 1 g/hr.

If renal function is normal, magnesium is excreted rapidly in the urine. In patients with evidence of renal impairment, for example, oliguria or serum creatinine levels greater than 0.9 mg/dL, magnesium should be administered cautiously, followed with frequent vital signs, deep tendon reflexes and serum levels, and doses adjusted accordingly. Magnesium sulfate should not be used in patients with myasthenia gravis because the magnesium ion competes with calcium.

A clinical protocol for magnesium sulfate for fetal neuroprotection is shown here:

1. Administer loading dose of 4 g magnesium sulfate in 10% to 20% solution over 30 minutes (60 mL of 10% magnesium sulfate in 1 L D_5 0.9 normal saline).
2. Maintenance dose of 1 g/hr (40 g of magnesium sulfate added to 1 L D_5 0.9 normal saline or Ringer's lactate at 50 mL/hr).
3. Limit intravenous (IV) fluid to 125 mL/hr. Follow fluid status closely; an indwelling urinary catheter is recommended.
4. Patients treated with magnesium sulfate should be assessed with the following examinations:
   a. Deep tendon reflexes and vital signs including respiratory rate should be recorded hourly.
   b. Intake and output every 2 to 4 hours.
   c. Magnesium levels if any clinical concern about side effects.
5. Calcium gluconate should be readily available to reverse the respiratory effects of magnesium.

Tocolysis

Because the contracting uterus is the most often recognized antecedent of preterm birth, stopping contractions has been the focus of therapeutic approaches. This strategy is based on the naïve assumption that clinically apparent contractions are commensurate with the initiation of the process of parturition; by logical extension, successfully inhibiting contractions should prevent delivery. The inhibition of myometrial contractions is called tocolysis, and an agent administered to that end is referred to as a tocolytic. Although there are no medications available for use that are approved for the indication of tocolysis by the U.S. Food and Drug Administration (FDA), there are a number of classes of drugs that are used for this purpose.

Efficacy

The efficacy of tocolytic drugs has been addressed through studies that compare one tocolytic drug with another, or,

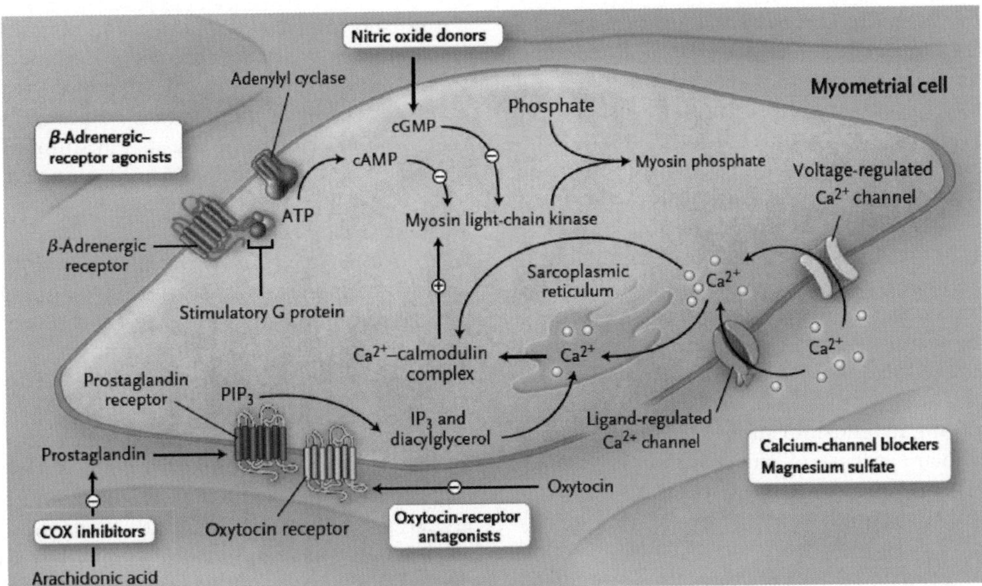

Figure 28-8. Site of action of commonly used tocolytics.

less commonly, to a placebo in their ability to prolong pregnancy for 48 hours (the time sufficient to attain the benefit of antenatal corticosteroids), or 1 week (the time considered sufficient to gain significant additional in utero fetal maturation). No studies have shown that any tocolytic can reduce the rate of preterm birth. Most are too small to allow firm conclusions so that reviews or meta-analyses, wherein several studies of similar design are combined, are the best available means to judge efficacy. The Cochrane Collaboration (www.cochrane.org/index0.htm) regularly produces meta-analyses of obstetrical interventions including tocolytic drugs. Recent Cochrane meta-analyses of tocolytic agents indicate that calcium channel blockers and oxytocin antagonists can delay delivery by 2 to 7 days with the most favorable ratio of benefit to risk, that β-mimetic drugs delay delivery by 48 hours but carry greater side effects, that there is insufficient evidence regarding cyclooxygenase (COX) inhibitors, and that magnesium sulfate is ineffective.

Meta-analyses of studies of individual tocolytic drugs typically report limited prolongation of pregnancy but no decrease in preterm birth and rarely offer information about whether prolongation of pregnancy was accompanied by improved infant outcomes. Delayed delivery for 48 hours to allow antenatal transport and corticosteroids to reduce neonatal morbidity and mortality are thus the main rationale for use of these drugs.

Choosing a Tocolytic Agent

Pharmacology

Figure 28-8 depicts a myometrial cell and the site(s) of action of commonly used tocolytic agents. The key process in actin-myosin interaction, and thus contraction, is myosin light-chain phosphorylation. This reaction is controlled by myosin light-chain kinase (MLCK). The activity of tocolytic agents can be explained by their effect on the factors regulating the activity of this enzyme, notably calcium and cyclic adenosine monophosphate (cAMP). For the myometrium to contract in a coordinated and effective manner (i.e., labor, whether term or preterm), individual smooth muscle cells must be functionally interconnected and able to communicate with adjacent cells. There are no agents used for tocolysis that influence the function or expression of gap junctions.

Contraindications to Tocolysis

Common maternal contraindications to tocolysis include severe preeclampsia or severe gestational hypertension, hemorrhage, and significant maternal cardiac disease. Preterm labor accompanied by maternal hypertension places both mother and fetus at risk of acute hypertensive crises, and may occur in response to fetal stress or distress, uterine ischemia, or occult placental abruption. Although vaginal spotting may occur in women with preterm labor because of cervical effacement or dilation, any bleeding beyond light spotting is rarely due to labor alone. Placenta previa and placental abruption must be considered, because both may be accompanied by uterine contractions. In general, both diagnoses place a woman at greater risk of hemodynamic compromise in the setting of tocolytic treatment. However, in rare instances, use of tocolysis in women with these dangerous diagnoses may be considered to achieve time for corticosteroids in the setting of extreme prematurity when the bleeding is believed to occur in response to contractions. Such treatment is fraught with difficulty, because even low doses of some tocolytic agents can be hazardous in a patient with bleeding. β-Mimetic agents and calcium channel blockers may hamper maternal cardiovascular response to hypotension, and prostaglandin inhibitors may impair platelet function. Cardiac disease is a contraindication because of the risks of tocolytic drug treatment in these patients. Fetal contraindications to tocolysis include gestational age of greater than 37 weeks, fetal demise or lethal anomaly, chorioamnionitis, and evidence of acute or chronic fetal compromise.

TABLE 28-3 SIDE EFFECT PROFILES OF TOCOLYTIC AGENTS

	SIDE EFFECTS		
AGENT OR CLASS	**MATERNAL**	**FETAL OR NEONATAL**	**CONTRAINDICATIONS**
β-Adrenergic-receptor agonists	Tachycardia and hypotension, tremor (39% vs. 4% with placebo), shortness of breath (15% vs. 1% with placebo), chest discomfort (10% vs. 1% with placebo), pulmonary edema (0.3%), hypokalemia (39% vs. 6% with placebo), hyperglycemia (30% vs. 10% with placebo)	Tachycardia	Tachycardia-sensitive maternal cardiac disease, poorly controlled diabetes mellitus
Magnesium sulfate	Flushing, diaphoresis, nausea, loss of deep-tendon reflexes (at doses of 9.6 to 12 mg/dL), respiratory paralysis (at doses of 12 to 18 mg/dL), cardiac arrest (at doses of 24 to 30 mg/dL); when used with calcium channel blockers, suppression of heart rate, contractility and left ventricular systolic pressure, and neuromuscular blockade.	Conflicting data with regard to effect on perinatal mortality	Myasthenia gravis
Calcium channel blockers	Dizziness, flushing, hypotension when used with magnesium sulfate, suppression of heart rate, contractility, and left ventricular systolic pressure and neuromuscular blockade; elevation of hepatic aminotransferase levels		Hypotension, preload-dependent cardiac lesions (e.g., aortic insufficiency)
Cyclo-oxygenase inhibitors	Nausea, esophageal reflux, gastritis, and emesis; platelet dysfunction (rarely of clinical significance in patients without underlying bleeding disorder)	In utero closure of ductus arteriosus (risk associated with use for >48 hr), patent ductus arteriosus in neonate (conflicting data)	Platelet dysfunction or bleeding disorder, hepatic or renal dysfunction, gastrointestinal or ulcerative disease, asthma (in women with hypersensitivity to aspirin)
Oxytocin-receptor antagonists	Hypersensitivity injection-site reactions	For atosiban, an increased rate of fetal or infant death (may be attributable to the lower gestational age of infants in the atosiban group)	None
Nitric oxide donors	Dizziness, flushing, hypotension		Hypotension, preload-dependent cardiac lesions (e.g., aortic insufficiency)

Tocolytic drugs may be safely used when standard protocols are followed. The choice of tocolytic requires consideration of the efficacy, risks, and side effects for each patient. Table 28-3 describes the side effect profiles of commonly used tocolytic agents.

CALCIUM CHANNEL BLOCKERS

Calcium channel blockers are used commonly for treatment of hypertension, angina, and arrhythmias and are increasingly being used as tocolytic drugs. Nifedipine is the calcium channel blocker most studied as a tocolytic agent; it more selectively inhibits uterine contractions compared with other calcium blockers such as verapamil. Calcium channel blockers directly block the influx of calcium ions through the cell membrane and also inhibit release of intracellular calcium from the sarcoplasmic reticulum, thus increasing calcium efflux from the cell. The ensuing decrease in intracellular free calcium leads to inhibition of calcium-dependent myosin light-chain kinase–mediated phosphorylation and results in myometrial relaxation. Calcium channel blockers are rapidly absorbed after oral administration. There are no placebo-controlled trials of calcium channel blockers as tocolytics. The Cochrane Collaboration meta-analyses support calcium channel blockers as short-term tocolytics compared with other available agents because of relatively greater contraction suppression and fewer side effects than other agents in 12 reported trials. Rates of birth within 7 days of treatment (RR 0.76, 95% CI 0.60 to 0.97) and before 34 weeks' gestation (RR 0.83, 95% CI 0.69 to 0.99) were significantly reduced with calcium channel blockers, as were the rates of neonatal morbidities including RDS (RR 0.63, 95% CI 0.46 to 0.88), NEC (RR 0.21, 95% CI 0.05 to 0.96), IVH (RR 0.59, 95% CI 0.36 to 0.98), and jaundice (RR 0.73, 95% CI 0.57 to 0.93) when compared with treatment with other tocolytics. Fewer women treated with calcium channel blockers ceased treatment owing to adverse drug reactions (RR 0.14, 95% CI 0.05 to 0.36).

MATERNAL EFFECTS

Nifedipine has fewer side effects when compared with β-mimetics and magnesium sulfate. Hypotension occurs frequently with nifedipine, but other side effects are more frequent with magnesium and β-mimetics. Nicardipine displayed similar advantages when compared in a randomized trial with magnesium. Pretreatment with IV fluids may reduce the frequency of maternal side effects related to hypotension such as headache (20%), flushing (8%), dizziness, and nausea (6%). Most effects are mild, but

serious complications have been reported, including a documented myocardial infarction 45 minutes after the second dose of nifedipine given to a young healthy woman. Concomitant or sequential use of calcium channel blockers with β-mimetics is not recommended, nor is concurrent administration of magnesium, owing to reports of skeletal muscle blockade when nifedipine was given with magnesium sulfate.

Fetal Effects

Initial animal studies raised questions of fetal hypotension, but a study of women treated for preterm labor revealed no changes in fetal middle cerebral artery, renal artery, ductus arteriosus, umbilical artery, or maternal vessels.

Treatment Protocol

An optimal nifedipine dosing regimen has not been defined. A common approach is to administer an initial loading dose of 20 mg orally, followed by an additional 20 mg orally in 90 minutes. An alternative regimen is to administer 10 mg orally every 20 minutes for up to four doses. If contractions persist, 20 mg can be given orally every 3 to 8 hours for up to 72 hours, with a maximum dose of 180 mg/day.The half-life of nifedipine is approximately 2 to 3 hours and the duration of action of a single orally administered dose is up to 6 hours. Plasma concentrations peak in 30 to 60 minutes. Nifedipine is almost completely metabolized in the liver and excreted by the kidney.

Summary of Treatment with Calcium Channel Blockers

Nifedipine has been used increasingly as a tocolytic because of its low incidence of significant maternal and fetal side effects and ease of administration. Nifedipine should not be combined with magnesium or β-mimetics, and should be avoided in the presence of intrauterine infection, maternal hypertension, and cardiac disease. Use should follow published dosage schedules, and the cautions noted should be kept in mind.

Magnesium Sulfate

The basis for the clinical use of magnesium sulfate as a labor-inhibiting agent is the observation from the 1960s of a reduction of human uterine contractility in vivo and in vitro. At a pharmacologic concentration (5 mmol/L), magnesium sulfate inhibits contractile response and decreases intracellular calcium concentration in pregnant human myometrial strips. Despite in vitro observations, the largest placebo-controlled randomized trial of magnesium as a tocolytic failed to demonstrate any benefit over placebo in prolongation of pregnancy. A meta-analysis that compared magnesium to controls observed no difference in the risk of birth within 48 hours of treatment for women given magnesium (RR 0.85, 95% CI 0.58 to 1.25, 11 trials, 881 women). Magnesium appeared to confer no benefit on the risk of preterm birth (less than 37 weeks) or very preterm birth (less than 34 weeks). The risk of death (fetal and pediatric) was higher for infants exposed to magnesium (RR 2.82, 95% CI 1.20 to 6.62, 7 trials, 727 infants) The body of available literature fails to support efficacy of magnesium sulfate as a tocolytic agent. Thus, in women 24 to 32 weeks of gestation who are candidates for tocolysis, we recommend that another therapy be used for labor inhibition in women also receiving magnesium sulfate for fetal neuroprotection. Because of the increased risk of maternal complications with the concomitant use of nifedipine and magnesium sulfate, an agent such as indomethacin may be a reasonable choice for tocolysis in the woman receiving magnesium sulfate for neuroprotection of the fetus.

Maternal Effects

Magnesium has a low rate of serious maternal side effects, but flushing, nausea, vomiting, headache, generalized muscle weakness, diplopia, and shortness of breath occur frequently. Chest pain and pulmonary edema have been reported with a frequency similar to that of β-mimetics.

Neonatal Effects

Magnesium crosses the placenta and achieves serum levels comparable to maternal levels, but serious short-term neonatal complications are uncommon. Lethargy, hypotonia, and respiratory depression may occur. Prolonged treatment for more than 7 days has been associated with neonatal bone abnormalities. One small trial suggested that magnesium sulfate may have adverse effects on neonatal and infant morbidity and mortality, but these observations were not confirmed by larger studies that enrolled more than 10 times as many subjects.

Summary of Treatment with Magnesium Sulfate

Magnesium sulfate has historical familiarity, but tocolytic efficacy is not supported by data. Magnesium may have a beneficial effect on the preterm newborn with respect to reducing the risk of cerebral palsy.

Cyclo-oxygenase Inhibitors

Prostaglandins are mediators of the final pathways of uterine muscle contraction. Prostaglandins cause an increase in free intracellular calcium levels in myometrial cells and increased activation of MLCK, resulting in uterine contractions. Myometrial gap junction formation, an important step in synchronized uterine activity, is enhanced by prostaglandins. Prostaglandins given to pregnant women can ripen the cervix or induce labor, depending on the dosage and route of administration. Prostaglandin synthase, also known as cyclo-oxygenase (COX), converts arachidonic acid to prostaglandin G_2. Prostaglandin synthesis is increased when the COX-2 form of this enzyme is induced by cytokines, bacterial products such as phospholipases and endotoxins, and corticosteroids, and reduced by inhibition of COX by nonsteroidal anti-inflammatory drugs (NSAIDs). The NSAID agents vary in their activity, potency, and side effect profile. Indomethacin is the NSAID most often used as a tocolytic. Indomethacin crosses the placenta. Unlike aspirin, indomethacin binds reversibly to COX, so that inhibition lasts only until the drug is cleared metabolically. Umbilical artery serum concentrations equal maternal levels within 6 hours of oral administration. The half-life in the mother is 4 to 5 hours, and in a full-term infant is 15 hours, but is significantly longer in preterm infants. The Cochrane Review concluded that indomethacin administration was associated with a significant reduction in births before the 37th week,

increased gestational age at birth, and increased birth weight.

Maternal Effects

Prostaglandin inhibition has multiple side effects because of the abundance of prostaglandin-mediated physiologic functions. Nevertheless, serious maternal side effects are uncommon when the agent is used in a brief course of tocolysis. As with any NSAID, gastrointestinal side effects such as nausea, heartburn, and vomiting are common but usually mild. Less common but more serious complications include gastrointestinal bleeding, prolonged bleeding time, thrombocytopenia, and asthma in aspirin-sensitive patients. Prolonged treatment with NSAIDs can lead to renal injury, especially when other nephrotoxic drugs are used. Hypertensive women may rarely experience acute increased blood pressure after indomethacin treatment. The antipyretic effect of an NSAID may obscure a clinically significant fever. Maternal contraindications to indomethacin tocolysis include renal or hepatic disease, active peptic ulcer disease, poorly controlled hypertension, asthma, and platelet disorders.

Fetal and Neonatal Effects

In actual practice, serious complications to the fetus/newborn with maternal administration of indomethacin have been rare, but there is risk of injury to the fetus if treatment protocols are not followed carefully. Three principal side effects raise concern: (1) in utero constriction of the ductus arteriosus, (2) oligohydramnios, and (3) neonatal pulmonary hypertension. The ductal constriction occurs because formation of prostacyclin and PGE_2, which maintain ductal vasodilation, is inhibited by indomethacin. Doppler evidence of ductal constriction was found in 7 of 14 fetuses of women treated with indomethacin between 27 and 31 weeks of pregnancy, but resolved within 24 hours after the medication was discontinued. The likelihood of ductal constriction increased from 5% to 10% before 32 weeks to 50% after 48 hours of treatment at 32 to 35 weeks. Ductal constriction is usually transient and responds to discontinuation of the drug, but persistent ductal constriction and irreversible right-sided heart failure have been reported. A review of fetal echocardiographs obtained from 61 women treated with indomethacin for preterm labor found evidence of ductal constriction in 50% of fetuses. A larger study of 124 women given indomethacin for labor inhibition for more than 48 hours revealed a 6.5% frequency of in utero ductal narrowing. In both of these studies, the ductal narrowing reversed in all fetuses after cessation of medication.

Oligohydramnios associated with indomethacin tocolysis is due to reduced fetal urine production, which is caused by indomethacin-induced reduction of normal prostaglandin inhibition of antidiuretic hormone and by direct effects on fetal renal blood flow. Prolonged treatment with indomethacin incurs a 7% frequency of oligohydramnios. These effects are reversible, but neonatal renal insufficiency and death after several weeks of unmonitored antenatal maternal treatment has been reported.

Primary pulmonary hypertension in the neonate is a potentially fatal illness that has also been associated with prolonged (greater than 48 hours) indomethacin therapy. Primary neonatal pulmonary hypertension has not been reported with 24 to 48 hours of therapy, but the incidence may be as high as 5% to 10% with long-term therapy, although more modern series of longer-term use failed to identify an increased frequency of newborn pulmonary hypertension compared with untreated gestational age–matched controls.

Other complications, including NEC, small bowel perforation, PDA, jaundice, and IVH, have been observed when indomethacin administration was outside of standardized protocols that did not limit the duration of treatment or employed the drug after 32 weeks. No association with IVH was noted in studies in which standard protocols were used. A review of outcomes of 1621 fetuses treated in utero with indomethacin found no significant differences compared with 4387 infants not exposed.

Sulindac is an NSAID that has less placental transfer than indomethacin, but tocolytic efficacy has not been studied in large numbers. Because of the effect on fetal urine production and amniotic fluid volume, indomethacin may be an appropriate tocolytic when preterm labor is associated with polyhydramnios. Indomethacin has been used to treat preterm labor in women with polyhydramnios, and for polyhydramnios without labor. Uterine activity and pain associated with degenerating uterine fibroids in pregnancy also respond well to indomethacin.

Treatment Protocol

Indomethacin is well absorbed orally. The usual regimen is a 50-mg oral loading dose followed by 25 to 50 mg by mouth every 6 hours. Therapy is limited to 2 to 3 days because of concern about side effects described earlier.

Protocol for Indomethacin Tocolysis

1. Limit use to preterm labor before 32 weeks' gestation in women with normal amniotic fluid volume and normal renal function.
2. Loading dose is 50 mg by mouth.
3. Give 25 mg orally every 6 hours for 48 hours.
4. If the drug is used beyond 48 to 72 hours, amniotic fluid volume should be monitored serially with ultrasound and ductus arteriosus flow should be evaluated with Doppler echocardiography. If amniotic fluid is significantly reduced or the ductus is narrowed, the drug should be discontinued.
5. Discontinue therapy promptly if delivery seems imminent.
6. Fetal contraindications to use of indomethacin include renal anomalies, chorioamnionitis, oligohydramnios, ductal-dependent cardiac defects, and twin-twin transfusion syndrome.

Summary of Treatment with Indomethacin

Indomethacin is an effective tocolytic agent that is generally well tolerated by the mother. Concern about fetal side effects has appropriately limited use of indomethacin to brief courses of therapy in patients with preterm labor before 32 weeks.

β-Mimetic Tocolytics

β-Sympathomimetic drugs including terbutaline, ritodrine, and others have been widely used as tocolytics for many

years. Structurally related to epinephrine and norepinephrine, these agents act to relax smooth muscle, for example, in the bronchial tree, blood vessels, and myometrium, through stimulation of the β-receptors. β-Receptors are divided into β1- and β2-subtypes. The β1-receptors are largely responsible for the cardiac effects, whereas β2-receptors mediate smooth muscle relaxation, hepatic glycogen production, and islet cell release of insulin. Stimulation of β-receptors in the heart, vascular system, and liver accounts for the side effects of these drugs. The most commonly used β-mimetic in the United States is terbutaline (marketed as a drug for asthma), but others including albuterol, fenoterol, hexoprenaline, metaproterenol, nylidrin, orciprenaline, and salbutamol are used in other countries. Ritodrine was approved by the FDA as a parenteral tocolytic in 1980, but it did not achieve wide use because of frequent maternal side effects. Ritodrine is no longer marketed in the United States. Terbutaline has a rapid effect when given subcutaneously (3 to 5 minutes). Published protocols often employ subcutaneous administration, with a usual dose of 0.25 mg (250 mg) every 4 hours. A single subcutaneous dose of terbutaline to arrest contractions during the initial evaluation of preterm contractions may aid in the diagnosis of preterm labor. In one study, women whose contractions persisted or recurred after a single dose were more likely to have true preterm labor than those whose contractions ceased. The Cochrane Database reported an analysis of 1332 women enrolled into 11 randomized placebo-controlled trials of β-mimetic drugs found that treated subjects were less likely to deliver within 48 hours (RR 0.63, 95% CI 0.53 to 0.75), but not within 7 days. Although a 48-hour delay in delivery allows sufficient time for in utero transfer and treatment with steroids, perinatal and neonatal death, and perinatal morbidity were not reduced in this analysis. Side effects requiring change or cessation of treatment were frequent.

Side Effects and Complications of β-Mimetic Tocolysis

Maternal side effects of the β-mimetic drugs are common and diverse owing to the abundance of β-receptors in the body. Maternal tachycardia, chest discomfort, palpitation, tremor, headache, nasal congestion, nausea and vomiting, hyperkalemia and hyperglycemia are significantly more common in women treated with β-mimetics. Most are mild and of limited duration, but serious maternal cardiopulmonary and metabolic complications have been reported.

Cardiopulmonary Complications of β-Mimetics. The β-mimetic agents produce a 5 to 10 mm Hg fall in diastolic blood pressure, and the extensive peripheral vasodilatation makes it difficult to mount a normal response to hypovolemia. Signs of excessive blood loss (e.g., maternal and fetal tachycardia) are masked by β-mimetics, so their use may be dangerous in women with antepartum hemorrhage. The most important steps to prevent cardiac complications are (1) excluding patients with prior cardiac disease and (2) limiting infusion rates so that maternal pulse does not exceed 130 beats/minute. Symptomatic cardiac arrhythmias and myocardial ischemia have occurred during β-agonist tocolytic therapy. Tocolysis should be discontinued and oxygen administered whenever a patient develops chest pain during β-mimetic therapy. Arrhythmias noted in association with β-mimetic therapy usually respond to discontinuation of the drug and oxygen administration. Baseline or routine electrocardiograms before or during treatment are not helpful. An electrocardiogram is indicated if there is no response to oxygen and cessation of β-mimetic therapy. Pulmonary edema has been reported with β-mimetic therapy. Restricting the duration of treatment to less than 24 hours, careful attention to fluid status, and detection of complicating conditions such as intrauterine infection may reduce this risk.

Metabolic Complications. β-Mimetic agents induce transient hyperglycemia and hypokalemia during treatment. Measurement of glucose and potassium before initiating therapy, and on occasion during the first 24 hours of treatment, is appropriate to identify significant hyperglycemia (greater than 180 mg/dL) or hypokalemia (less than 2.5 mEq/L). These metabolic changes are mild and transient, but prolonged treatment beyond 24 hours may induce significant alterations in maternal blood sugar, insulin levels, and energy expenditure. The risk of abnormal glucose metabolism is further increased by simultaneous treatment with corticosteroids, a common combination for threatened preterm labor. Other agents should be chosen for women with pregestational diabetes, and usually for those with gestational diabetes as well. β-Mimetic treatment in these women requires frequent monitoring and insulin infusion to maintain euglycemia.

Neonatal Effects. Neonatal hypoglycemia, hypocalcemia, and ileus may follow treatment with β-mimetics, and can be clinically significant if the maternal infusion is not discontinued 2 hours or more before delivery. Long-term data on neurodevelopmental outcomes in humans are lacking.

Protocols for continuous subcutaneous infusion of terbutaline have been reported to have fewer side effects than oral administration, but have had no improvement on rates of preterm birth or perinatal morbidity in randomized placebo-controlled trials. Terbutaline has been the subject of an FDA warning: "terbutaline administered by injection or through an infusion pump should not be used in pregnant women for prevention or prolonged (beyond 48-72 hours) treatment of preterm labor due to the potential for serious maternal heart problems and death. In addition, oral terbutaline tablets should not be used for prevention or treatment of preterm labor."[49] No placebo-controlled trials demonstrating effectiveness have been reported since the FDA advisory was issued.

Given their potential for clinically significant side effects and the availability of alternative choices, the β-sympathomimetic agents should not be used in women with known or suspected heart disease, severe preeclampsia or eclampsia, pregestational gestational diabetes requiring insulin, or hyperthyroidism. These drugs are contraindicated when suspected preterm labor is complicated by maternal fever, fetal tachycardia, leukocytosis, or other signs of possible chorioamnionitis.

Summary of Treatment with β-Mimetic Tocolysis

β-Mimetic drugs were once among the most commonly used tocolytics but have been replaced by agents with

better safety and side effect profiles. Terbutaline has relatively few serious side effects when used as a single subcutaneous injection of 0.25 mg to facilitate maternal transfer or to initiate tocolysis, while another agent with a slower onset of action is being given. Long-term oral or subcutaneous treatment has not been shown in controlled trials to reduce prematurity or neonatal morbidity.

Other Tocolytic Agents

Atosiban is a selective oxytocin-vasopressin receptor antagonist. Although commonly used in Europe, it is not available in the United States. In normal parturition, oxytocin stimulates contractions by inducing conversion of phosphatidylinositol to inositol triphosphate, which binds to a protein in the sarcoplasmic reticulum causing release of calcium into the cytoplasm. A Cochrane review analyzed six randomized trials (n = 1695 women) comparing the oxytocin receptor antagonist atosiban to placebo. Use of atosiban increased the risk of birth within 48 hours of initiation of treatment (RR 2.50, 95% CI 0.51 to 12.35), increased the risk of PTB at less than 28 weeks of gestation (RR 2.25, 95% CI 0.80 to 6.35), and increased the risk of PTB at less than 37 weeks (RR 1.17, 95% CI 0.99 to 1.37); however, none of these increases reached statistical significance. All neonatal morbidity and mortality outcomes evaluated were similar in both groups. There was, however, an imbalance in allocation of women with threatened PTL under 26 weeks such that significantly more women in this subgroup were allocated to the atosiban group. In addition, more women in the placebo group than the atosiban group received rescue treatment, which may have confounded the estimate of the true effects of atosiban when compared to placebo. The use of rescue tocolytics complicated analysis of these trials, since the criteria for switching therapies was not strictly defined. Last, the trial protocol did not define how glucocorticoids should be used, which resulted in a great deal of variation in use among study sites. The FDA declined to approve the use of atosiban for tocolysis because of concerns about the drug's safety when used in fetuses of less than 28 weeks' gestation.[50]

Nitric oxide donors also promote myometrial relaxation. Meta-analysis of trials comparing NO donors to other agents support the notion that NO donors do not delay delivery or improve neonatal outcome when compared with placebo, no treatment, or alternative tocolytics such as ritodrine, albuterol, and magnesium sulfate. There was, however, a reduction in number of deliveries less than 37 weeks when compared with alternative tocolytics, but the numbers of deliveries before 32 and 34 weeks were not influenced. Side effects (other than headache) were reduced in women who received nitric oxide donors rather than other tocolytics. However, women were significantly more likely to experience headache when NO donors had been used.

Clinical Use of Tocolytic Drugs

Tocolytic therapy is employed in several clinical circumstances. In a patient who is in active labor with advanced cervical effacement, the diagnosis is not in question and the goal is prompt treatment to allow maternal transfer and time for steroids and GBS prophylaxis. In this setting, initial treatment with oral indomethacin or oral nifedipine may be the best choice to stop contractions promptly. Treatment for preterm labor may be continued until contractions have stopped or occur less frequently than four times per hour without additional cervical change, or until a full course of steroid therapy is completed (48 hours).

Persistent Contractions

If contractions persist despite therapy, the wisdom of tocolytic treatment should be reevaluated. The cervix should be reexamined; if cervical dilation has progressed beyond 4 cm, and imminent delivery is thought to be inevitable, tocolytic therapy in most cases should be discontinued. In the setting of progressive preterm labor despite labor inhibition, it is critical to acknowledge the higher probability of placental abruption and/or subclinical chorioamnionitis. Clinical evaluation with focused history, physical examination, and laboratory assessment should be used to address the probability of these conditions.

Some women will have persistent uterine contractions and may exhibit a "nonthreatening" cervical examination that does not change over serial examinations. If a fibronectin swab was collected before therapy was begun, it should be sent for analysis. A positive result is not confirmatory, but a negative fibronectin, if collected before performance of a digital examination, suggests that the risk of imminent delivery is low. Alternatively, a transvaginal cervical ultrasound examination may be performed. A length of 30 mm or more substantially reduces the likelihood of imminent delivery.

Serum levels are not clinically helpful to adjust the dose of tocolytics. A change to a second agent, or combination therapy with multiple agents, may slow contractions but may result in increased risks. Combined use of β-mimetics or magnesium sulfate with calcium channel blockers should also be avoided (see the accompanying box, Management of Persistent Contractions Despite 12 to 24 Hours of Tocolysis).

Management of Persistent Contractions Despite 12 to 24 Hours of Tocolysis

1. Is subclinical amniotic fluid infection present? Repeat clinical examination, white blood cell counts, and fetal assessment. Consider amniocentesis for glucose, Gram stain, leukocyte esterase, and culture.
2. Is the fetus compromised? Review the fetal heart tracings and, if needed, do a biophysical assessment.
3. Is there evidence of abruption? Is there a suspicion of uterine anomaly with implantation of the placenta on the septum? Evaluate vitals signs for evidence of hemodynamic response to blood loss and repeat hemoglobin, hematocrit, and fibrinogen, and abdominal sonography for placental implantation site.
4. Is the diagnosis of preterm labor correct? Is the cervix changing? Do a transvaginal cervical ultrasound to measure cervical length. Send a fibronectin swab.
5. If infection, fetal compromise, and abruption can be excluded, stop parenteral tocolysis for 24 hours and observe. Most patients will stop contractions spontaneously.

Care After Acute Treatment for Preterm Labor

Maintenance Tocolytic Treatment

Continued suppression of contractions after acute tocolysis does not reduce the rate of preterm birth. Meta-analyses of these data also find no evidence of prolongation of pregnancy or decline in the frequency of preterm birth.

Posthospitalization surveillance with outpatient monitoring of uterine contractions did not improve the rate of delivery before 37 weeks, birth weight, or gestational age at delivery in any of three randomized trials or in a meta-analysis of these. A multicenter randomized trial in which uterine activity was monitored, but in which the data were masked from care providers in one group, also found no improvement in preterm birth rate when contraction data were used.

The duration of hospitalization for an episode of preterm labor varies according to several factors, including the examination of the cervix, ease of tocolysis, gestational age, obstetrical history, distance from hospital, and the availability of home and family support. Associated risk factors that may complicate or increase the risk of recurrent preterm labor, such as a positive genital culture for chlamydia or gonorrhea, urinary tract infection, and anemia, should be addressed before discharge from hospital care. Social issues such as homelessness, availability of child care, or protection from an abusive partner are important determinants of a patient's ability to adhere to recommendations for medical care, and these issues must be considered before the patient is discharged from the hospital.

CONDUCT OF LABOR AND DELIVERY FOR THE PRETERM INFANT

Intrapartum care for women in labor before term is often complicated by conditions such as malpresentation, hypertension, amnionitis, abruption, oligohydramnios, or fetal growth restriction that increase the chance of intrapartum fetal compromise. When labor is induced preterm for maternal or fetal indications, the lower uterine segment and cervix may not be well prepared for labor, leading to a prolonged latent phase.

Intrapartum Assessment of the Preterm Fetus

Intrapatrum fetal surveillance has been associated with significantly lower frequency of intrapartum death and neonatal seizures for preterm infants. Ominous heart rate tracings in preterm fetuses have the same associations with fetal acidosis as they do later in gestation. Mean fetal heart rate falls continuously, from 160 beats/minute at 22 weeks' gestation, to 140 beats/minute at term due to a gradual increase in parasympathetic tone. Fetal heart rate patterns should be considered as representative of well-being in the preterm fetus as they are at term.

Labor and Delivery

The duration of labor in preterm gestation may be shorter than that of term pregnancy. The active phase of the first stage and the second stage may be particularly brief. Care should be taken to ensure that the fetus does not have a precipitous delivery without control of the fetal head. There is no benefit for prophylactic forceps to "protect" the fetal head. The neonatal care team should be alerted to the circumstances of a preterm birth well in advance of the delivery so that appropriate personnel and equipment are available.

Cesarean Delivery

Routine cesarean delivery of all preterm or VLBW infants is not justified. Trends favoring cesarean section disappear after adjustment for confounding factors. A review of studies of neonatal and maternal morbidities after vaginal versus cesarean delivery for infants born between 24 and 36 weeks found increased maternal morbidity without clear benefit for the infant. Neonatal intracranial hemorrhage occurs as often before and after labor as it does during labor and delivery.

For infants in breech presentation, there are intuitive reasons for cesarean birth, particularly to avoid entrapment of the after-coming head and other manipulations that could lead to trauma or hypoxia. Older retrospective studies that suggested a benefit for cesarean delivery led to the current custom of cesarean delivery for preterm breech fetuses, but data in support for this practice are weak. It is illogical to perform a cesarean to avoid a traumatic vaginal delivery only to encounter a difficult cesarean birth because of an inadequate abdominal or uterine incision. The operation should be conducted to minimize the trauma of delivery through as roomy an incision as necessary. In a study of delivery mode for "high-risk" VLBW infants (e.g., preeclampsia, vaginal bleeding, abnormal heart rate tracing) versus "low-risk" VLBW infants (e.g., preterm labor, incompetent cervix), cesarean section was of no value in the low-risk group, but was associated with significantly improved survival rates in the high-risk group. Considering these factors, optimal delivery of the VLBW fetus may at times appropriately lead to a decision to perform a cesarean without labor. Generally speaking, the appropriate mode of delivery for the preterm fetus ought to be based on similar standards of obstetrical indications as at term.

PREVENTION OF PRETERM BIRTH

Care of preterm birth may be described according to the public health model as *tertiary* (treatment initiated after the parturitional process has begun to limit perinatal morbidity and mortality), *secondary* (identification and treatment for individuals with increased risk), or *primary* (prevention and reduction of risk in the population). Tertiary care described in the preceding section of this chapter has improved perinatal outcomes, but has no effect on the incidence of preterm birth. Efforts to identify women likely to deliver preterm to reduce or eliminate their risk have not achieved high sensitivity, and until recently, there were no effective interventions to reduce risk.

Prevention efforts aimed at risk factors have been undertaken with the expectation that preterm birth would decline in proportion to the contribution of that risk factor as a cause of preterm birth. The failure of this approach underlies the current understanding of preterm birth as a syndrome in which multiple factors, known and unknown, contribute to the initiation and progression of preterm parturition. Rather than a distinct entity for which there are

specific tests, preterm birth is more appropriately considered as the result of various pathologic events that affect the timing and progress of parturition. Understanding maternal risk factors, symptoms, and tests as clues to steps in a parturitional sequence that may or may not progress to early delivery, rather than "tests for preterm labor," brings some clarity to the sometimes confusing literature on this subject.

Secondary Prevention of Preterm Birth

Identification and elimination or reduction of risk may be applied before and/or after conception.

Before Pregnancy

Prepregnancy medical risk factors occur in as many as 40% of preterm births, but preconceptional medical interventions to reduce preterm birth in these women have been disappointing. A history of second trimester loss or preterm birth is most easily identified,[3,51] recalling that the risk increases as the gestational age of the previous preterm birth declines and as the number of preterm births increases. Preconceptional interventions include surgical correction of müllerian anomalies and preconceptional abdominal cerclage. A randomized trial in 1579 women of interconceptional home visits and counseling to reduce low birth weight and preterm birth reported no evidence of benefit. Another randomized placebo-controlled trial tested interconceptional antimicrobial treatment in women with a prior early preterm birth. Subjects were randomly assigned to receive metronidazole and azithromycin or placebo at 3-month intervals between pregnancies, but the recurrence risk of preterm birth was not improved.

During Pregnancy

Postconceptional prevention strategies have most often been studied in women with a prior preterm birth, with a major risk factor such as multifetal gestation or bleeding, and/or in women with a sign, symptom, or positive screening test indicating increased risk. Previous editions of this text have decried the absence of any effective interventions, but recent studies have demonstrated reduced risk in selected populations, for example, women with a prior preterm birth and with short cervix.

Modification of Maternal Activity

Despite a lack of supporting evidence, bed rest, limited work, and reduced sexual activity are often recommended to reduce the risk of preterm birth in pregnancies at risk for indicated and spontaneous births. Yost and colleagues found no relationship between coitus and risk of recurrent preterm birth.

Nutritional Supplements

Supplemental use of omega-3 polyunsaturated fatty acids (PUFA) has been recommended because populations with a high dietary intake have low rates of preterm birth, perhaps because omega-3 PUFAs reduce levels of proinflammatory cytokines. European trials of omega-3 supplements and supplemental fish oil found significant reductions preterm birth, but a placebo-controlled U.S. trial of supplemental omega-3 polyunsaturated fatty acids in women with a prior preterm birth found no benefit in women who were treated with 17 hydroxy-progesterone caproate.[52] Interestingly, women in both arms of this study who consumed more than one fish meal per month had a significantly lower rate of preterm birth than those who consumed fish once per month or less. Trials of supplemental vitamins C and E and calcium also did not reduce preterm birth risk.[53]

Enhanced Prenatal Care

Although perhaps helpful in adolescents, programs of enhanced prenatal care providing social support, home visits, and education have not reduced preterm birth. Frequent provider-initiated contact for women with a prior preterm birth also did not decrease recurrent preterm birth in randomized trials.

However, reduced rates of preterm birth have been reported for women receiving prenatal care in novel settings: Group prenatal care in Connecticut, a regional program to standardize care for an indigent population in Texas,[54] and a specialized prematurity clinic in Utah for women with a prior preterm birth have all reported lower rates of premature birth, but all are retrospective and merit confirmation.

Periodontal Care

The association of periodontal disease with increased risk of prematurity prompted intensive study of the effects of periodontal care on the rate of preterm birth. Results have been negative, suggesting shared susceptibility rather than a causal linkage.

Antibiotic Treatment

Screening and antibiotic treatment of women with abnormal genital flora has been largely ineffective to prevent preterm birth. Antibiotic treatment for women with a prior preterm birth who have bacterial vaginosis was associated with reduced risk of recurrent preterm birth in secondary analyses. Reviews and meta-analyses have also been negative, and a U.S. Preventive Services Task Force review[55] cautioned that there may be "unintended potential for harm" from screening and treatment for bacterial vaginosis in pregnancy. Antibiotic prophylaxis has also been studied in women with positive fetal fibronectin test results. Rates of preterm birth were actually increased in fibronectin-positive women who received antibiotic treatment. Similar results were reported from a trial of antibiotics in women with *Trichomonas.*

Progesterone

Progesterone supplementation for women at risk for preterm birth has been investigated based on several plausible mechanisms of action, including reduced gap junction formation and oxytocin antagonism leading to relaxation of smooth muscle, maintenance of cervical integrity, and anti-inflammatory effects. Studies performed before 1990 in women with recurrent miscarriage and preterm birth were reviewed by Keirse, who found "no support for the view that 17 alpha-hydroxy-progesterone caproate protects against miscarriage, but suggests that it does reduce the occurrence of preterm birth."[56] **Subsequent randomized trials have demonstrated an approximately 40% decrease in the rate of preterm birth in women**

TABLE 28-4 STUDIES OF PROGESTERONE TO REDUCE PRETERM BIRTH

AUTHOR	YEAR	POPULATION	EFFECT ON PTB RATE
Keirse*	1990	Meta-analysis	40% ↓
da Fonseca†	2003	Hx PTB	40% ↓
Meis*	2003	Hx PTB	35% ↓
Fonseca†	2007	Short cervix <15 mm	44% ↓
O'Brien†	2007	Hx PTB without short cervix‡	*No* ↓
DeFranco†	2007	Hx PTB with short cervix§	↓
Hassan†	2011	Short cervix 10-20 mm	45% ↓

*17 α hydroxy-progesterone caproate.
†Vaginal progesterone in various formulations.
‡Women likely to receive cerclage not enrolled. Mean cervical length at entry = 37 mm.
§Secondary analysis of O'Brien study subjects who later had short cervix <28 mm.
Hx, History; *PTB*, preterm birth variably defined.

with a prior preterm birth and/or short cervix (below 15 to 20 mm before 24 weeks' gestation) who were treated with either intramuscular 17 alpha-hydroxy-progesterone caproate 250 mg weekly, or with vaginal progesterone suppositories or cream daily between 16 and 36 weeks' gestation (Table 28-4).[14-16,18,57,58]

Several randomized placebo-controlled trials have found that progesterone supplementation does not affect the rate of preterm birth in women with multifetal gestations, indicating that the mechanism of progesterone's action to reduce risk of preterm birth in singletons is not related to uterine stretch.[59-62]

Importantly, the effect of supplemental progesterone compounds is not universally observed in women with a prior preterm birth, indicating first that some pathways to recurrent preterm birth are not influenced by this therapy, and also that many women with a preterm birth will deliver at term without treatment. The recurrence risk of spontaneous preterm birth without treatment is related to cervical length at 22 to 24 weeks, ranging from more than 35% in women whose cervical length is below 25 mm, to 15% in women with cervical lengths 25 to 35 mm, and to less than 10% in those with a cervical length above 35 mm. In the only study of women with a previous preterm birth in which supplemental progesterone did not reduce the risk of recurrent preterm birth,[16] the mean cervical length at 18 to 22 weeks' gestation was 37 mm, suggesting that women with a prior preterm birth who do not also have a short cervix will not benefit from progesterone supplementation. Indeed, a secondary analysis of this study found a reduced risk of preterm birth in women who later had short cervix.[14] Taken together, these studies indicate that *short cervix* rather than *prior preterm birth* is the most appropriate criterion for institution of progesterone therapy. However, a history of preterm birth will continue to be an indication for progesterone treatment until additional studies demonstrate that such treatment is unnecessary in women with a prior preterm birth who maintain a normal cervical length beyond 24 weeks' gestation.

Trials of progesterone in women with other risk factors, for example, a positive fetal fibronectin or bleeding, have not been reported. The mechanism of action is uncertain, but the absence of effect in multifetal gestation coupled with reductions in preterm birth in women with short cervix suggest that the pathway may be related primarily to modulation of cervical softening, a conclusion also suggested by basic studies.

The optimal strategy to identify candidates for progesterone therapy has not been determined. Universal cervical length screening of all pregnant women at 18 to 24 weeks has been proposed based on two favorable cost-effectiveness studies[63,64] and expert opinion,[65] but universal application of any screening test in obstetrical care is always accompanied by unanticipated costs and consequences, in this case likely related to reproducibility of cervical sonography and uncertain adherence to recommended treatment protocols.

An alternative list of indications for selective screening for short cervix with transvaginal ultrasound is shown in the accompanying box, Indications for Cervical Ultrasound Screening in the Second Trimester. These women are candidates for screening with the expectation that progesterone supplementation will be considered if the cervical length measurement at 16 to 24 weeks is 20 mm or less. The value and timing of repeat cervical ultrasound in women with marginal cervical length measurements is uncertain. The schema suggested is likely to be modified by broader experience with cervical sonographic screening.

INDICATIONS FOR CERVICAL ULTRASOUND SCREENING IN THE SECOND TRIMESTER

- Any previous pregnancy delivered between 16 and 36 weeks' gestation
- All pregnancies conceived after fertility care
- All women with a history of cervical instrumentation
  - Cervical cone biopsy or LEEP
  - Dilation and curettage for diagnosis or therapeutic indications, including first- and second-trimester pregnancy terminations
- All women with prior genital tract infections or persistently abnormal Pap smear
- All African Americans
- All women with depression, low body mass index (<19.6), or who smoke
- All women whose cervical length is <30 mm on a midtrimester transabdominal ultrasound examination
  - Women with signs or symptoms of preterm parturition in the current pregnancy
    - Vaginal bleeding or spotting without obvious cause
    - Persistent symptoms of pelvic pressure, cramps, change in vaginal discharge after 16 weeks' gestation

CERVICAL CERCLAGE

The link between short cervix and risk of preterm birth was initially interpreted as evidence of diminished cervical strength or competence, but subsequent clinical experience and interventional studies do not support that conclusion. Cerclage is not a uniformly effective treatment for short cervix. Although beneficial for women with a prior preterm birth whose cervical length is very short (less than 15 to 25 mm),[66,67] cerclage treatment does not reduce preterm birth risk in women with short cervix (less than 15 mm) without a history of preterm birth,[68] and actually appears to increase the risk of preterm birth in women with twins

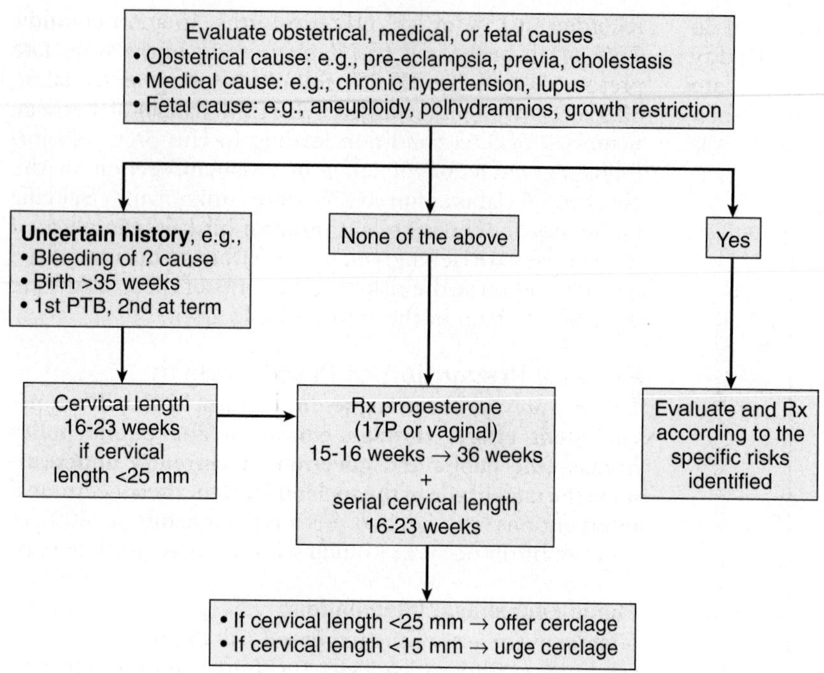
Evaluate obstetrical, medical, or fetal causes
• Obstetrical cause: e.g., pre-eclampsia, previa, cholestasis
• Medical cause: e.g., chronic hypertension, lupus
• Fetal cause: e.g., aneuploidy, polhydramnios, growth restriction
Uncertain history, e.g.,
• Bleeding of ? cause
• Birth >35 weeks
• 1st PTB, 2nd at term
None of the above
Yes
Cervical length 16-23 weeks if cervical length <25 mm
Rx progesterone (17P or vaginal) 15-16 weeks → 36 weeks + serial cervical length 16-23 weeks
Evaluate and Rx according to the specific risks identified
• If cervical length <25 mm → offer cerclage
• If cervical length <15 mm → urge cerclage
• All women receive nutritional and social work counseling at initial visit and as needed thereafter
• Smoking cessation education and program as needed
• All women receive nursing education and support at each visit and invitation to call as needed between visits

FIGURE 28-9. Care algorithm for women with a prior preterm birth at 16 to 36 weeks' gestation.

and short cervix.[68,69] In women with a prior preterm birth, cerclage is paradoxically most beneficial in women with the shortest cervical length (less than 15 mm),[66,67] suggesting that the benefit of cerclage may relate more to protection of exposed membranes than to bolstering cervical strength.

Clinical Use of Progesterone and Cerclage to Prevent Preterm Birth

The increasing evidence that progesterone is effective in reducing the risk of preterm birth in women with short cervix with or without a history of preterm birth has influenced the clinical care of women who would previously have been considered to be candidates for prophylactic cervical cerclage. Similarly, results from the NICHD Vaginal Ultrasound Cerclage Trial[66] indicate that only 30% of the more than 1000 women with a history of a preterm birth between 17 and 34 weeks displayed a cervical length of 25 mm or less before 24 weeks when followed with cervical sonography. These observations led to development of the protocol displayed in Figure 28-9 used in our clinic.[70] Cerclage is reserved for women with a history of cervical injury, uterine anomaly, and/or progressive cervical shortening to a length below 25 mm despite progesterone therapy. In these patients, cerclage is offered at 25 mm, and strongly urged if the cervical length is 15 mm or below, or membranes are visible.

Late Preterm Birth

In 2008, 12.3% of births in the United States were preterm, and 71% of these (8.8%) were *late preterm,* occurring between $34^{0/7}$ and $36^{6/7}$ weeks' gestation. Though these infants fare better than those born before 34 weeks' gestation, they experience substantially increased morbidity and mortality compared to infants born after 37 weeks' gestation and account for the overwhelming majority of admissions to neonatal intensive care. Approximately 70% of preterm births are spontaneous, but the relative percentage has declined in recent years as indicated preterm births have increased. **The rise in preterm births between 1990 and 2006 in singletons was almost entirely explained by an increased rate of indicated preterm births between 34 and 36 weeks' gestation. The principal driver of this increase was an increased willingness to consider scheduled birth as a safer option than continuing the pregnancy in women with various pregnancy complications. The rise in late preterm indicated preterm births was accompanied by a corresponding decrease in the rate of fetal deaths after 28 weeks, and a decline in overall perinatal mortality.** Figure 28-10 displays these trends, but does not show the effects of the increase in indicated preterm births on the number and rate of late preterm infants admitted to neonatal intensive care.

The decision to choose indicated preterm birth over continuation of the pregnancy at any gestational age carries great potential to create as well as to prevent or reduce perinatal morbidity and mortality. Unfortunately, the relative risks and benefits of delivery versus expectant management are difficult to weigh accurately, especially in the late preterm period. Before 34 weeks' gestation, there is clear benefit to be gained by daily increases in fetal maturity. At 34 weeks, the risks of immaturity have been considered to be acceptable in complicated pregnancies, but the

morbidity and mortality rates for infants born between 34 and 37 weeks are higher than previously realized. Reddy and colleagues[71] examined the records of 292,627 late preterm singleton births and found that 49% were associated with spontaneous labor. Remarkably, no reason was recorded in 23% of late preterm births. In another study, 7.8% of all births and 65.7% of preterm births were late preterm. Of these, 29.8% followed spontaneous labor; 32.3% followed preterm PROM; 31.8% had an obstetrical, maternal, or fetal condition leading to late preterm birth following induction of labor or cesarean section in the absence of labor; and 6.1% were unknown.[72] Specific guidelines for choosing late preterm birth in complicated pregnancies are lacking, but recent efforts to document the reasons and track the risks and benefits of these births are expected to help in the future (Table 28-5).[73]

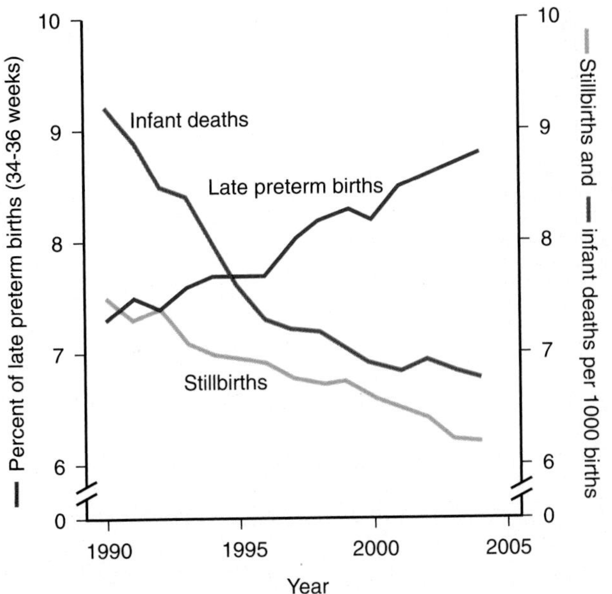

FIGURE 28-10. Trends in late preterm birth, stillbirth, and infant mortality, United States, 1990-2004. (From Ananth CV, Gyamfi C, Jain L: Characterizing risk profiles of infants who are delivered at late preterm gestations: does it matter? Am J Obstet Gynecol 199:329, 2008.)

Primary Prevention of Preterm Birth

Primary prevention strategies for preterm birth will require consistent efforts through education and public policy because the public and government currently underestimate the magnitude of the societal burden. Preconceptional interventions are needed because as many as 50% of preterm births occur in women without known risk factors.

Public Educational Interventions

Greater awareness of the increased risk of preterm birth in singleton gestations associated with assisted reproductive technology could affect attitudes and choices made in fertility care. Similar strategies to reduce the prevalence of smoking, use condoms to prevent sexually transmitted infections, and promote recognition and early treatment of depression might all have an eventual effect on preterm birth rates. Promotion of long-acting reversible contraceptives for women at risk, especially after a preterm delivery, offers a chance to reduce the risk of recurrent preterm birth.

TABLE 28-5 GUIDANCE REGARDING TIMING OF DELIVERY WHEN CONDITIONS COMPLICATE PREGNANCY AT 34 WEEKS OF GESTATION OR LATER

CONDITION	GESTATIONAL AGE* AT DELIVERY	GRADE OF RECOMMENDATION†
Placental and Uterine Issues		
Placenta previa‡	**36-37 wk**	B
Suspected placenta accrete, increta, or percreta with placenta previa‡	**34-35 wk**	B
Prior classical cesarean (upper segment uterine incision)‡	**36-37 wk**	B
Prior myomectomy necessitating cesarean delivery‡	**37-38 wk** (may require earlier delivery, similar to prior classical cesarean, in situations with more extensive or complicated myomectomy)	B
Fetal Issues		
Fetal growth restriction—singleton	**38-39 wk:**	
	Otherwise uncomplicated, no concurrent findings	B
	34-37 wk:	
	Concurrent conditions (oligohydramnios, abnormal Doppler studies, maternal risk factors, comorbidity)	B
	Expeditious delivery regardless of gestational age:	
	Persistent abnormal fetal surveillance suggesting imminent fetal jeopardy	
Fetal growth restriction—twin gestation	**36-37 wk:**	
	Dichorionic-diamniotic twins with isolated fetal growth restriction	B
	32-34 wk:	
	Monochorionic-diamniotic twins with isolated fetal growth restriction	B
	Concurrent conditions (oligohydramnios, abnormal Doppler studies, maternal risk factors, comorbidity)	B
	Expeditious delivery regardless of gestational age:	
	Persistent abnormal fetal surveillance suggesting imminent fetal jeopardy	

gestation.[28] Fetal risk appears to be dose dependent.[29] Nevertheless, less aggressive dosing will be associated with increased risk for valve thrombosis (see Chapter 43).

The ACC/AHA guidelines recommend consideration of heparin in the first trimester to avoid warfarin embryopathy, and the use of warfarin until 36 weeks, when subcutaneous heparin is substituted until after delivery.[13] These recommendations remain controversial in that they may underestimate the risk for fetal intracerebral bleeding in the absence of labor.[30] The fetus exposed to warfarin in the second and third trimesters is at risk for developmental toxicity.

The use of antithrombotic agents for prosthetic valves in pregnancy has been reviewed by the American College of Chest Surgeons (ACCS).[31] The review cites descriptive evidence regarding optimal treatment strategies in pregnancy, including no randomized trials. Cohort studies suggest an increased risk for valve thrombosis associated with use of unfractionated heparin (UFH) or low-molecular-weight heparin (LMWH). However, the cohort studies are confounded by treatment with low heparin dosing. Three possible regimens are considered:

1. Vitamin K antagonists (VKA) before 6 weeks of pregnancy; UFH or LMWH between 6 and 12 weeks of pregnancy; VKA from 12 weeks to near term; UFH or LMWH until postpartum; VKA postpartum
2. UFH throughout pregnancy
3. LMWH throughout pregnancy

If warfarin sodium (Coumadin) is used, the INR must be followed closely to maintain an INR of about 3. If UFH is used, the ACCS recommends dosing every 12 hours to achieve a therapeutic activated partial thromboplastin time (2.5 to 3 times normal) at mid-dosing interval. In our practice, we dose every 8 hours to maintain a higher trough effect. If LMWH is used, twice-daily dosing is recommended, with mid-dosing interval anti–factor Xa levels 1 to 1.2.

Before delivery, we stop heparin to permit use of regional analgesia. After delivery, we start intravenous heparin without a bolus to avoid bleeding at surgical sites and convert to oral therapy. We do not use LMWH to bridge to VKA because of excessive overlapping therapy and bleeding complications. Oral anticoagulation is consistent with breastfeeding. Individual patients should be counseled regarding the risks of either strategy and participate actively in a final choice of therapy.

Women treated for prolonged periods with heparin should be counseled regarding the risk for osteoporosis. Maternal platelet counts should be followed to screen for the development of heparin-induced thrombocytopenia (HIT). If HIT is diagnosed, heparin must be discontinued immediately and anticoagulation maintained with other agents.

When treatment with LMWH is chosen, fixed weight-based dosing is clearly inadequate and dangerous. To maintain anticoagulation in pregnancy with LMWH, anti–factor Xa levels must be monitored frequently with the expectation of increasing the dose as pregnancy advances.[32] Although monitoring of peak anti–factor Xa levels has been advocated, therapeutic trough levels are present only 15% of the time.[28] Successful treatment with LMWH has been reported when valve complications were associated uniformly with noncompliance or nontherapeutic anti–factor Xa levels.[33] Fetal survival rates were higher in women choosing LMWH (96%) than in those choosing warfarin (75%).[34] Nevertheless, lethal valve thrombosis has been reported in the face of therapeutic peak anti–factor Xa levels.

Continuous intravenous heparin infusion has been suggested. Although the incidence of line infection and subsequent endocarditis may be relatively low, the consequences are catastrophic. This choice should be made after careful counseling of the patient.

If valve thrombosis is encountered, thrombolysis can be considered. Successful thrombolytic therapy of a clotted valve in pregnancy has been reported. Although safe and effective for many patients, embolic complications, bleeding, and death have been reported in pregnancy. Surgery such as cesarean delivery cannot be performed in proximity to thrombolytic therapy.

Although clear strategies supported by randomized trials are not available and are not expected to be forthcoming, the following guidelines can be suggested:

1. Care by a team experienced with aggressive therapeutic monitoring and dose adjustment of anticoagulant medications
2. Emphasis of the need for patient compliance with frequent subcutaneous dosing
3. Monitoring of trough effect to ensure consistently adequate anticoagulation
4. Monitoring of peak dosing to assess potential for bleeding
5. Increasing dose frequency when safe peak dosing and therapeutic trough dosing cannot be achieved
6. Treatment with LMWH at a minimal dose interval of every 12 hours
7. Treatment with UFH at a minimal dose interval of every 8 hours.
8. Adjunctive treatment with aspirin
9. Avoidance of overlapping treatment with LMWH and VKA in the postpartum period

CONGENITAL HEART DISEASE

Congenital heart disease is present in 0.7% to 1% of live births, accounting for as many as 30% of infants with birth anomalies. Before the development of corrective surgery, many children died shortly after birth or in childhood. In 1939, the first patent ductus arteriosus (PDA) was ligated. In 1945, the first Blalock-Taussig shunt was performed for palliation of cyanotic heart disease. In 1953, cardiac bypass was introduced. Introduction of surgery under hypothermia in the late 1960s permitted longer and more complex repairs. Of children who survived surgery to correct tetralogy of Fallot between 1955 and 1960, the 23-year survival is 86%, approaching the expected survival rate of 96% for normal children. Before the 1960s, rheumatic heart disease was more common in pregnancy than congenital heart disease by a ratio of 4:1. By the 1980s, the ratio was 1:1. Currently, congenital disease is now estimated to exceed rheumatic disease by 4:1. Although most enter pregnancy with known heart disease, some women have their disease first recognized because of the hemodynamic demands of pregnancy.

Increased survival of children with congenital disease has created a population of young women with complex medical and psychosocial conditions entering their childbearing years. Those whose congenital heart disease was diagnosed in infancy have frequently experienced multiple cardiothoracic surgeries and extended hospitalizations. They have lived with continued concerns from parents and health care professionals regarding their ongoing health problem. Their childhood has been described as "growing up heart sick."[35] Some describe a lack of information regarding childbearing and contraception. They "seemed to believe that someone else could and would decide whether they should become pregnant." Kovacs and coworkers describe the contraception and pregnancy advice women with congenital heart disease recall receiving from their health care providers, and in many cases women received either no information or inaccurate information.[36] **Health care providers should strive to (1) objectively share information regarding reproductive health care, (2) direct decision making toward the patient rather than toward parents and health care professionals, and (3) improve self-esteem and body image.** When treating congenital heart disease during pregnancy, one must be willing to acknowledge and address the impact of the patient's disease on her life.

Table 36-3 summarizes the distribution of congenital heart disease in childhood and in pregnancy.[23,37] The spontaneous closure of lesions such as ventricular septal defect (VSD) and correction of patent ductus are reflected by reduced reporting in pregnancy. The increased reporting of aortic stenosis in pregnancy is probably due to a worsening of disease with age and the ease of recognition during pregnancy. The complexity and diversity of congenital heart disease confounds our ability to describe the prognosis or a management plan for the breadth of conditions. **Major risks in pregnancy include (1) cyanosis, (2) left (or systemic) ventricular dysfunction, and (3) pulmonary hypertension, particularly with right ventricular dysfunction.**

Outcomes have been most clearly described based on the presence or absence of maternal cyanosis. Table 36-4 is derived from a report of 482 pregnancies from 233 women with congenital heart disease who delivered between 1968 and 1982.[11] The rate of terminations was higher in the group of women with cyanotic heart disease and particularly high (42%) in those with uncorrected lesions. This reflects the anticipated poor neonatal outcome and maternal risks associated with uncorrected cyanotic disease. It is likely that patients with more severe disease are overly represented in the group of women who chose to terminate, which would bias the group who continued pregnancy toward a better outcome. Eighty-six to 90% of pregnancies without cyanosis ended in a live birth compared with 71% with an uncorrected lesion. Given an expected baseline rate of miscarriage, these outcomes are good. Corrected cyanotic disease was associated with outcomes comparable to noncyanotic disease. Table 36-5 is derived from a report of 144 pregnancies from women with congenital heart disease delivered between 1976 and 1986.[23] Adverse outcomes are again concentrated among women with uncorrected cyanotic heart disease.

Common maternal complications include congestive heart failure and pulmonary edema (4%), arrhythmia (4%), and hypertension (6%). Congestive heart failure and hypertension were commonly associated with uncorrected left ventricular outflow obstruction.[11,23] Arrhythmias were observed after surgery in and around atrial or ventricular septa. Maternal death was uncommon, 0 per 482 pregnancies in one series[11] and 1 per 144 pregnancies in a second.[23] Maternal deaths are most commonly reported in association with Eisenmenger syndrome, which is discussed more fully later.

A number of authors have recently developed criteria that predict complications in pregnancy. **A remarkable concordance in central findings are reported: impaired left ventricular function, cyanosis, impaired functional status, left ventricular outflow obstruction, and right heart dysfunction are associated with maternal complications.**[38-42]

TABLE 36-4 NEONATAL OUTCOME WITH CONGENITAL HEART DISEASE: LIVEBORN VERSUS TERMINATION

	LIVEBORN INFANT (%)	TERMINATION (%)
Noncyanotic	86	5
Cyanotic	85	26
Corrected	95	17
Palliative	87	17
Palliative	71	42

TABLE 36-3 INCIDENCE OF CONGENITAL HEART DEFECTS IN CHILDHOOD AND IN PREGNANCY

DEFECT	CHILDHOOD (%)	PREGNANCY (%)
Ventricular septal defect	35	13
Atrial septal defect	9	9
Patent ductus arteriosus	8	2.7
Pulmonary stenosis	8	8
Aortic stenosis	6	20
Coarctation of the aorta	6	8
Tetralogy of Fallot	5	12
Transposition of the great vessels	4	5.4

TABLE 36-5 NEONATAL OUTCOME WITH CONGENITAL HEART DISEASE BY SAB, SGA, PRETERM, AND BIRTHWEIGHT

	SAB (%)	SGA (%)	PRETERM (%)	BIRTH WEIGHT (g)
	(%)	(%)	(%)	
Noncyanotic	12	6	9	3,300 ± 600
Cyanotic	21	52	35	2,400 ± 800
Corrected	11	25	0	
Uncorrected/palliative	25	67	53	

Preterm, Preterm birth; *SAB*, spontaneous abortion; *SGA*, small for gestational age.

Men and women with congenital heart disease are at increased risk for having children with congenital heart disease. In a prospective study with aggressive pediatric evaluation, Whittemore and associates[11] estimated the incidence to be as high as 14.2%. In a retrospective study, Rose and coworkers found the risk to be 8.8%.[43] The rate of congenital heart disease associated with an affected mother is 2 to 3.5 times that observed with an affected father. **Specific parental defects are not generally associated with the same defect in the child. The risk for cardiac maldevelopment is inherited rather than the risk for a specific defect.** The risk for congenital heart disease and the character of the risk should be discussed with an affected mother. In Whittemore's report, 58 of 60 affected infants were diagnosed with relatively benign correctable lesions (atrial septal defect, VSD, pulmonary stenosis, aortic stenosis, patent ductus arteriosus, or mitral valve prolapse). Only two infants from 372 pregnancies (0.5%) were diagnosed with complex congenital heart disease.[11] Gill and colleagues[12] examined the recurrence pattern of congenital heart disease in 6640 pregnancies for whom fetal echocardiography was obtained due to a family history of congenital heart disease. The recurrence rate was 2.9% (95% confidence interval [CI], 2% to 4%) for mothers with congenital heart disease, a rate lower than reported by others. However, the study is limited to diagnoses established by fetal echocardiography and, therefore, may under-represent the true incidence of abnormalities. The type and severity of cardiac defect seen in the mother did not predict the type or severity of cardiac defect in the offspring, with a few exceptions. Atrioventricular canal defects, especially those associated with situs abnormalities, had a highly concordant recurrence rate.[12] Congenital heart disease–associated 22q11.2 deletion (DiGeorge syndrome, velocardiofacial syndrome) will be inherited as an autosomal dominant condition. Many parents with congenital heart disease will not have been previously screened. Referral for genetic counseling and possible screening should be considered, particularly in the context of conotruncal abnormalities and other associated anomalies. All women who have congenital heart disease should undergo fetal echocardiographic examination at midpregnancy.

Contraceptive counseling should be offered to all women with congenital heart disease. **Given the problems experienced growing up with heart disease, contraceptive education should probably be initiated as part of general health care education, before the overt need for birth control.** In the context of congenital heart disease, complications associated with pregnancy are usually greater than those associated with any form of birth control. Cyanosis, pulmonary hypertension, low CO, dilated cardiac chambers, sluggish venous conduits (e.g., Fontan), and atrial fibrillation place patients at risk for thrombosis. This small group of women should probably avoid combined estrogen-progestin oral contraceptives. Progestin-only pills are not associated with risk for thrombosis but require regular dosing to achieve optimal efficacy. Parenteral progestins are safe for women with cardiac disease and are extremely effective. They do cause irregular bleeding, which may be significant if the patient is anticoagulated. The intrauterine device may be a suitable choice for women with congenital heart lesions.

Isolated Septal Defects

Ventricular and atrial septal defects represent greater than 40% of congenital heart disease identified in childhood. Many defects identified in children close with advancing age. In adulthood, 50% of large VSDs (>1.5 cm) lead to the development of Eisenmenger syndrome. Ten percent of patients with uncorrected atrial septal defects also develop pulmonary hypertension. The management of Eisenmenger syndrome in pregnancy is discussed later.

A harsh systolic murmur that radiates to the left sternal border but not to the carotids suggests the presence of a VSD. The diagnosis can be confirmed by color-flow Doppler echocardiography demonstrating a small, high-velocity lesion. The peak velocity of the jet across the septum can be used to assess the pressure gradient between the ventricles. A high velocity between ventricles indicates a large pressure gradient and low pressure in the right ventricle (RV) and the absence of pulmonary hypertension. In the absence of associated cardiac lesions and pulmonary hypertension, the presence of a VSD does not usually complicate pregnancy. Small defects create loud murmurs but are not usually hemodynamically significant. The high-velocity jet of a small lesion does create a risk for endocarditis.

Atrial septal defects are more difficult to diagnose by auscultation. The characteristic finding, a split S_2 that is fixed with respiration, is subtle and usually not appreciated without specific attention. Increased right-sided flow secondary to shunting across the defect may create a flow murmur that will be augmented in pregnancy. Other endocardial cushion defects may be associated with ostium primum defects. In the absence of other anomalies, the significance of the atrial septal defect is related to its size rather than its etiology. Hemodynamically significant defects result in significant shunting from the systemic circulation to the pulmonary circulation. As with the VSD, Eisenmenger syndrome may develop, but usually at an older age. Increased pulmonary blood flow may result in dyspnea on exertion and restriction of activity. Atrial arrhythmias are commonly associated with atrial enlargement or intrinsic conduction abnormalities in the case of ostium primum defects.

Piesiewicz and colleagues[44] reported 54 pregnancies in women with secundum atrial septal defects. **Impaired functional status (NHYA class III or IV) increased from 5.5% in the second trimester to 11.1% in the third trimester.** Although left-to-right shunting was present in all patients in the second trimester, three patients (5.5%) developed bidirectional shunting in the third trimester. One additional patient reversed her shunt. RV diameter and systolic pulmonary artery pressure increased from the second to third trimester (34.1 ± 8.4 mm Hg to 39.1 ± 12.2 mm Hg). Over the same time frame, the pulmonary flow (Q_p): systemic flow (Q_s) ratio decreased. Increased flow associated with pregnancy appears to adversely affect right ventricular function and pulmonary pressures. The fall in Q_p/Q_s suggests that the rise in pulmonary pressure is due to increased PVR. The authors also reported supraventricular arrhythmias in 50% of women in the third trimester.

The patient with a significant pulmonary-to-systemic shunt ratio can be expected to normally expand her CO during pregnancy. However, the price of a normal systemic CO is a high pulmonary flow. The pregnant patient may begin to experience symptoms at rest that she previously noted with exercise. She may also experience an increase in tachyarrhythmias. HR control with a β-blocker may provide symptomatic relief. Early diuresis may benefit the patient postpartum. Elevated pulmonary blood flow associated with pregnancy could accelerate the progression of pulmonary vascular disease. In the absence of associated anomalies, arrhythmias, and pulmonary hypertension, the presence of an atrial septal defect does not usually complicate pregnancy.

Patent Ductus Arteriosus

The diagnosis of a PDA is suggested by the characteristic continuous murmur at the upper left sternal border. Most cases are identified and ligated in childhood. Of patients with an uncorrected patent ductus, as many as 50% develop Eisenmenger syndrome, usually in childhood. In adults with a small patent ductus, the major risk is endocarditis. **In the absence of Eisenmenger syndrome, pregnancy is not usually complicated.** As with the atrial septal defect, the increase in pulmonary blood flow associated with the increase in CO in pregnancy may result in increased dyspnea with exertion and at rest. Early diuresis may benefit the patient postpartum.

Tetralogy of Fallot

Tetralogy of Fallot is a syndrome of abnormalities due to maldevelopment of the truncus arteriosus characterized by (1) right ventricular outflow tract obstruction, (2) VSD, (3) overriding aorta, and (4) right ventricular hypertrophy. Tetralogy of Fallot is the most common cyanotic congenital heart disease, and it was among the first to be successfully surgically palliated by Blalock and Taussig in 1945 and subsequently physiologically repaired. Therefore, a significant number of adults with congenital heart disease have repaired tetralogy of Fallot. The severity of the clinical presentation in infancy is dependent on the degree of outflow tract obstruction. More severe obstruction leads to more significant cyanosis and right-to-left shunting. Surgical repair generally includes closure of a VSD and relief of right ventricular outflow tract obstruction. Some patients with repaired tetralogy of Fallot have near-normal cardiac physiology, but many have residual lesions that may complicate pregnancy.

Patients with significant cyanosis at birth often had palliative Blalock-Taussig shunts in infancy using the subclavian artery to connect the systemic circulation with the pulmonary circulation, thus increasing pulmonary blood flow and reducing cyanosis. As a consequence, blood pressures in the arm supplied by the transected artery may not be reflective of aortic pressure. Patients should be asked if one arm is unreliable for blood pressure measurements, or examined to look for evidence of a thoracotomy scar resulting from the Blalock-Taussig shunt.

Efforts to correct the right ventricular outflow tract obstruction may result in incomplete relief and persistent pulmonary stenosis. More often, significant pulmonary insufficiency is a consequence of the transannular patch approach used to enlarge the outflow tract and valve. Several studies have demonstrated that women with severe pulmonary insufficiency and right ventricular dysfunction are more likely to have complications with pregnancy. Veldtman and colleagues[45] reported a series of 43 women with tetralogy of Fallot who had 112 pregnancies. Five percent experienced cardiac complications: supraventricular tachycardia (two), heart failure (two), pulmonary embolism associated with pulmonary hypertension (one), and progressive RV dilation (one).

Tetralogy of Fallot is often well tolerated during pregnancy. Preconceptual evaluation should include assessment of right and left ventricular function, severity of pulmonary insufficiency, and stenosis, with consideration for repair of severe pulmonary insufficiency before pregnancy, if appropriate.

Transposition of the Great Vessels

Transposition of the great vessels (TGV) is present in only 5% of pregnant women with congenital heart disease but is overrepresented in the publication of case reports and case series. In complete TGV, systemic venous blood returns to the right atrium and passes through the tricuspid valve, into the RV, and directly into the transposed aorta. Although an adequate circulation for fetal life, infants decompensate at birth owing to an inadequate pulmonary circulation. Some will have a sufficiently large VSD to achieve adequate pulmonary blood flow and oxygenation; others will require an immediate palliative procedure, an atrial septostomy.

TGV was first definitively corrected in 1964 with the Mustard operation. A baffle is constructed through the left and right atria so that systemic venous return is channeled through the mitral valve into the left ventricle, and pulmonary venous return is directed through the tricuspid valve into the RV. With a modest surgical intervention, the right and left pumps are placed in series with physiologic flow of systemic venous return through the pulmonary circulation. **The RV, as the systemic ventricle, must work against systemic resistance, and the tricuspid valve is exposed to systemic pressures. Long-term complications are associated with failure of the systemic ventricle and arrhythmia.** Of patients surviving the first 30 days after repair, 90% will be alive in 10 years and 87% will be alive in 20 years. After 13 years, only 5% suffer significant disability (NYHA classes II to IV).[46] A more physiologic repair can be achieved when transposition is accompanied by a VSD. The ventricular septum is reconstructed so that the aortic outflow tract lies within the left ventricle and a conduit is constructed to connect the RV to the pulmonary artery (Rastelli repair). The pulmonary conduit is prone to stenosis and deterioration of the transplanted valve. More recently, a direct surgical switch between the pulmonary artery and the aorta has been performed. Given the time when these operations were introduced, fewer young women entering pregnancy will have a Mustard repair. Increasing numbers will have an arterial switch.

The hemodynamic changes of pregnancy will have a mixed impact on a patient with a Mustard repair. Increased

CO increases the volume load on the right heart. Decreased vascular resistance reduces afterload on the right side of the heart. The box, Pregnancy Outcomes with Transposition of the Great Vessels, summarizes nine papers reporting a total of 49 pregnancies in 36 women.[23,46-53] No maternal mortality was reported. Neonatal outcomes were generally good. Two women entered pregnancy with disability due to their heart disease (NYHA classes III to IV). One delivered at 26 weeks due to preterm labor. The other developed severe congestive heart failure near term and died 19 months postpartum. Congestive heart failure was frequently associated with uncontrolled tachyarrhythmias.

Guedes and colleagues[54] have reported echocardiographic findings of 16 women with a Mustard repair completing 28 pregnancies. Mean gestational age at delivery was 38.1 ± 1.5 weeks, with a mean birthweight of 3040 ± 540 g. In four of 21 pregnancies, right ventricular function deteriorated. In three of the four patients, function did not return to baseline conditions. Although concerning, the authors noted that the rate of deterioration was not clearly different than that of a cohort who did not get pregnant.

Canobbiio and coworkers[55] reported a series derived from a registry. Of significance, this report is derived from a diversity of practices rather than from centers with considerable experience managing congenital heart disease. Forty women carried 54 pregnancies that resulted in live births. Thirty-six had Mustard repairs; 4 had Senning repairs. In 6 pregnancies, heart failure developed in the second or third trimesters. In 5, heart failure developed postpartum. One woman required transplantation postpartum; 1 died of heart failure 1 month after delivery; 1 died 4 years later. This report clearly documents the potential for adverse outcome.

Tobler and associates[56] reported on 17 pregnancies in 9 women with an arterial switch. One developed nonsustained ventricular tachycardia; 1 developed a valve thrombosis.

Congenitally corrected TGV (ventricular inversion) is characterized by the passage of systemic venous blood into the right atrium, directly into the morphologic left ventricle, and out through the transposed pulmonary artery. Pulmonary venous return passes directly from the left atrium into the morphologic RV and out through the aorta. The RV again serves as the systemic ventricle. Congenitally corrected TGV may be an isolated anomaly but may also be associated with other anomalies that result in cyanosis. See the box for a summary of two series of pregnancies with congenitally corrected TGV.[57,58] Again, maternal and neonatal outcomes are good. Consistent with outcomes associated with other cyanotic forms of congenital heart disease, miscarriage and premature birth are concentrated among those with cyanotic lesions.

Young women with surgically or congenitally corrected TGV successfully complete pregnancy. Nevertheless, they require aggressive management by an experienced team. Women who are functionally impaired or who are cyanotic before pregnancy can expect more adverse outcomes and may deteriorate postpartum. Evaluation before pregnancy should include assessment of functional status; evaluation of right systemic heart function; and confirmation of normal oxygenation. When the right side of the heart is the systemic heart, pharmacologic afterload reduction should be maintained until pregnancy is confirmed. ACE inhibitors should be discontinued early in the first trimester. Postpartum, the systemic RV should be considered "at risk" to fail and managed with rate control (ß-blocker), afterload reduction (ACE inhibitor), and appropriate management of preload (diuresis).

Pregnancy Outcomes with Transposition of the Great Vessels	
Women	36
Pregnancies	49
Live births	41 (84%)
Miscarriages	5
Terminations	2
Fetal deaths	1
Premature birth (<35 weeks)	5 (12%)
Congenital heart disease	0 (0%)
Congestive heart failure	6 (15%)
Arrhythmia	8 (20%)

Pregnancy Outcomes with Congenitally Corrected Transposition of the Great Vessels	
Women	41
Cyanotic	4 (10%)
Pregnancies	105
Cyanotic	13 (12%)
Live births	77 (73%)
Miscarriages*	22
Terminations	6
Fetal deaths	1
Premature birth (<35 weeks*)	6 (8%)
Congenital heart disease	1 (1%)
Congestive heart failure	5 (6%)
Cerebrovascular accident	1 (1%)

*Miscarriages and premature births were concentrated among cyanotic mothers.

The reported experience with TGV is to date the most extensive for any complex defect. The conclusions drawn from this experience are probably applicable to other, less common conditions. **Functional status and cyanosis are the most reliable predictors of complicated pregnancies.** Arrhythmia is common and is frequently the cause of cardiac decompensation.

Fontan Repair

The Fontan repair was initially performed to achieve a physiologic correction of tricuspid atresia by connecting the right atrium directly to the pulmonary artery. **The Fontan repair and subsequent modifications are currently used to correct a variety of complex congenital heart conditions characterized by a single functional ventricle.** The repair achieves a noncyanotic, functional flow of systemic venous return through the lungs and a functionally systemic ventricle. Without a pulmonary pump, the cardiac price for this result is intolerance of increased intrathoracic pressure and elevated systemic and right atrial pressure if left ventricular end-diastolic or left atrial pressures increase. Experience with pregnancy in women with the Fontan repair is limited. In a survey of 76 women of reproductive age, Canobbio and associates[59] reported that 66% were counseled not to become pregnant despite a stable surgical outcome and a strong desire to have children. The remaining 34% were not counseled regarding pregnancy. Contraceptive use, despite counseling against pregnancy, was inconsistent. Although the miscarriage rate was higher than in the general population, the preterm birth rate was low. Maternal complications were limited to arrhythmia, usually atrial, and congestive heart failure in the postpartum period. Although not reported in these small series, sluggish flow through the right atrial and pulmonary circulation may increase the risk for thrombosis. The incidence of pulmonary emboli in nonpregnant patients with Fontan circulation may be as high as 17%. Another series reported 10 pregnancies in 6 women.[60] Of the 10 pregnancies, 5 ended in miscarriage before 12 weeks, and 1 was ectopic. Of the 4 completed pregnancies, 1 woman had a decline of NYHA class with both of her pregnancies, and the second pregnancy was complicated by atrial flutter. The other two women did not have maternal complications. These series remain small, and thus the ability to extrapolate to the individual with Fontan physiology is difficult, **but the uniqueness of the Fontan physiology warrants care in institutions with expertise in adult congenital heart disease.** The box, Pregnancy Outcomes with Fontan Repair, summarizes the outcomes of 43 pregnancies from 27 women reported by these groups.[59,60]

PREGNANCY OUTCOMES WITH FONTAN REPAIR	
Women	27
Pregnancies	43
Live births	19 (44%)
Miscarriages	19
Terminations	_6
Fetal deaths	_0
Premature birth (<35 weeks)	3 (15%)
Congenital heart disease	1 (5%)
Congestive heart failure	3 (15%)
Arrhythmia	3 (16%)

Eisenmenger Syndrome

Eisenmenger syndrome describes pulmonary-to-systemic shunting associated with cyanosis and increased pulmonary pressures secondary to pulmonary vascular disease. **Eisenmenger syndrome may develop from any intracardiac shunt resulting in blood from the high-pressure systemic circulation being directed into the pulmonary circulation.** Systemic pressure and excessive flow lead to microvascular injury, obliteration of pulmonary arterioles and capillaries, and in the end, elevated PVR. The time to onset of shunt reversal is variable, but most patients who have a large VSD or large PDA develop shunt reversal in infancy. Those who have an atrial septal defect are delayed until early adulthood. Survival at 10 years from diagnosis is 80%; at 25 years, it is 42%.[61]

Patients with Eisenmenger syndrome are at risk for congestive heart failure, hemoptysis due to pulmonary hemorrhage, sudden death due to arrhythmia, a cerebrovascular accident, and hyperviscosity syndrome. The diagnosis should be considered in any cyanotic patient and is confirmed by echocardiography with the demonstration of increased pulmonary pressure and an intracardiac shunt. If the shunt is due to an atrial septal defect or a PDA, transesophageal examination may be necessary to establish the diagnosis. Treatment is nonspecific and includes supportive care and avoidance of destabilizing events such as surgery and unnecessary medications. Symptomatic hyperviscosity syndrome due to an elevated hematocrit can be treated with hydration and, if necessary, phlebotomy. Iron deficiency, preexisting or secondary to phlebotomy, can exacerbate hyperviscosity; microcytic cells are less deformable and therefore more prone to occlude the microcirculation. Definitive therapy can be achieved only with heart-lung or lung transplantation. However, the 4-year survival with lung transplantation is less than 50%, a less favorable prognosis than that for many patients with Eisenmenger syndrome.

VSD, atrial septal defect, and PDA are responsible for 89% of reported cases of Eisenmenger syndrome in pregnancy.[62] Each lesion is initially associated with shunting from the systemic, oxygenated circulation to the pulmonary circulation. As PVR and pulmonary pressures increase over time and approach systemic pressures, the characteristic murmurs of a VSD or PDA diminish. Reversal of flow from the right to the left, the development of hypoxemia, and increasing hematocrit herald the development of Eisenmenger syndrome. The fall in SVR associated with pregnancy may initiate shunt reversal in a patient not previously cyanotic.

In 1979, Gleicher reviewed published cases of Eisenmenger syndrome in pregnancy.[63] Seventy pregnancies from 44 women were evaluated. Fifty-two percent of the women died during pregnancy. Thirty percent of the pregnancies resulted in maternal death. The risks for death associated with first, second, and third pregnancies were 36%, 27%, and 33%, respectively. A first successful pregnancy did not confirm the safety of subsequent pregnancies. Most deaths (70%) occurred at the time of delivery or within 1 week postpartum. Excessive blood loss was associated with 35% of deaths, whereas thromboembolic conditions were responsible for 44%. Maternal mortality associated with cesarean delivery (80%) exceeded that associated with vaginal delivery (34%). Maternal death was not reported with first-trimester termination of pregnancy. Only 26% of pregnancies resulted in a term birth. Fifty-five percent of newborns were delivered preterm, and 32% were small for gestational age.

A more modern review of cases in the United Kingdom between 1991 and 1995 confirms the poor prognosis for pregnant women with Eisenmenger syndrome despite considerable advancement in the management of cardiac disease in pregnancy.[64] Mortality remains extremely high; 40% of the women died. Most deaths (96%) occurred within the first 35 days postpartum. Late diagnosis (relative risk [RR], 5.4) and delayed hospitalization significantly increased maternal mortality.

Although the risks associated with Eisenmenger syndrome in pregnancy are clear, appropriate management is controversial. Decreased activity, hospital observation, and oxygen supplementation are usually employed. Reduction of pulmonary pressures and improved systemic oxygen saturation after oxygen supplementation indicate that PVR is not fixed and suggest a better prognosis. Intercurrent antepartum events such as pneumonia or urinary tract infection are poorly tolerated. Preventing microcytosis with iron supplementation may decrease the risk for microvascular slugging.

Cesarean delivery is reserved for obstetrical indications and is avoided whenever possible. Hemodynamic stability must be maintained during labor and the postpartum period. When PVR is not fixed, oxygen supplementation may decrease pulmonary pressures. Systemic hypotension from hemorrhage or sympathectomy from epidural analgesia results in increased right-to-left shunting, increasing hypoxemia, increasing PVR, and worsening shunt. Volume overload or excessive systemic resistance, particularly postpartum, may further tax the failing right side of the heart. A pulmonary artery catheter and a peripheral arterial catheter are usually used to guide hemodynamic management. Narcotic-based regional analgesia provides adequate pain relief without excessive hemodynamic instability. Anticoagulation remains controversial. If patients are anticoagulated, caution should be exercised to avoid excessive treatment and associated hemorrhage.

Although use of a selective pulmonary vasodilator, inhaled nitric oxide, has been reported to reduce pulmonary pressures, increase CO, and improve systemic oxygenation, maternal death was not averted. Use of sildenafil and L-arginine has been reported with apparent hemodynamic benefit and the survival of a single patient. There are other case reports using pulmonary vasodilators with improved pregnancy outcomes, but nonetheless maternal risk remains high. **Unlike many cardiac conditions in pregnancy, meticulous care frequently fails to prevent maternal death.**

Coarctation of the Aorta

Coarctation of the aorta results from a constriction of the aorta at or about the level of the ductus arteriosus or left subclavian artery. Patients have a characteristic discrepancy in blood pressure between their right arm and lower extremities. Complications include dissection at the site of coarctation, rupture of associated berry aneurysms, and cerebrovascular accidents, heart failure, and ischemic heart disease associated with cephalic hypertension.

Modern reports of uncorrected coarctation in pregnancy are limited. Historically, pregnancy was associated with a maternal mortality rate of 9% owing to aortic rupture, congestive heart failure, cerebrovascular accidents, and endocarditis. β-Blockade may serve to protect against dissection and promote diastolic flow through the aortic narrowing.

Pediatric screening identifies most significant coarctations leading to repair. After repair, systemic hypertension may persist and require treatment. In two reports of 216 pregnancies in 104 women, 41 were complicated by hypertension and 1 by a lethal dissection at 36 weeks.[65,66]

Summary

An increasing cohort of young women with corrected congenital heart disease will be presenting to their obstetricians pregnant and desiring to bear children. Some basic conclusions can be drawn from our experience with congenital heart disease to date. **First, Eisenmenger syndrome and pregnancy remain a lethal combination. New, effective strategies for therapy are not anticipated. Second, cyanotic heart disease in the absence of pulmonary hypertension is associated with increased rates of miscarriage and preterm birth. Third, mothers with cardiac disability (NYHA classes III to IV) or with evidence of right heart dilation have a more complicated course in pregnancy. Fourth, arrhythmias may become worse in pregnancy and precipitate cardiac decompensation.** Aggressive pharmacologic treatment is appropriate. Finally, many young women who are initially well compensated and acyanotic can have successful pregnancies.

CARDIOMYOPATHY

Dilated cardiomyopathy is characterized by the development of pulmonary edema in the context of left ventricular dysfunction and dilation. Patients usually present with signs and symptoms of pulmonary edema: dyspnea, cough, orthopnea, tachycardia, and occasionally, hemoptysis. These symptoms of pulmonary edema, although characteristic of heart failure, may also be due to previously undiagnosed congenital or rheumatic heart disease, preeclampsia, embolic disease, intrinsic pulmonary disease, tocolytic use, or sepsis. The diagnosis of cardiomyopathy is made in the clinical circumstances of characteristic signs and symptoms and findings of left ventricular dysfunction and dilation on echocardiographic examination. The finding of an elevated B-type natriuretic peptide (BNP) can be used to help discriminate patients who need more definitive testing such as an echocardiogram. An elevated level may also be found with women with diastolic dysfunction or other conditions in which cardiac volume loading and stretch are increased. Ventricular dysfunction may be due to conditions extrinsic to the heart such as thyrotoxicosis or hypertension or to intrinsic myocardial dysfunction. Accurate diagnosis directs appropriate therapy and permits assessment of long-term prognosis.

Peripartum cardiomyopathy is a rare syndrome of heart failure presenting in late pregnancy or postpartum. The diagnosis is made after excluding other causes of pulmonary edema and heart failure. Failure to adhere to a rigorous definition of disease in the literature confounds conclusions regarding etiology and prognosis. A definition based on criteria for idiopathic dilated cardiomyopathy has been suggested (see box, Diagnostic Criteria for Peripartum Cardiomyopathy).[67] The incidence is estimated to be between 1 in 1300 and 1 in 15,000.[68] Although some of the variability in reported incidence is due to regional and ethnic differences, much is due to the imprecise definition of the disease. The cause of peripartum cardiomyopathy is unknown. Nutritional and immunologic mechanisms have been proposed. The prevalence of antibodies to echovirus and Coxsackie virus is not higher among women with cardiomyopathy compared with controls.[69]

DIAGNOSTIC CRITERIA FOR PERIPARTUM CARDIOMYOPATHY

1. Heart failure within the last month of pregnancy or 5 months postpartum
2. Absence of prior heart disease
3. No determinable cause
4. Echocardiographic indication of left ventricular dysfunction
   - Ejection fraction of <45% or fractional shortening of <30%
   - Left ventricular end-diastolic dimension of >2.7 cm/m^2

The mortality rate for peripartum cardiomyopathy (PPCM) is reported to be 25% to 50%. Death is usually due to progressive congestive heart failure, arrhythmia, or thromboembolism.[69] Within 6 months, half of patients demonstrate resolution of left ventricular dilation. Their prognosis is very good. Of those who do not, an 85% mortality rate can be expected within the next 4 to 5 years.[70] The magnitude of risk for subsequent pregnancies after peripartum cardiomyopathy is unclear. A recent survey of 67 pregnancies in 63 women suggests a mortality rate of 8% when left ventricular dysfunction has not resolved, and 2% in patients with normal function.[70]

Women with established dilated cardiomyopathy who enter pregnancy with known disease are reported to have less severe outcomes. As might be expected, moderate to severe left ventricular dysfunction and NYHA classes III and IV symptoms are associated with worse outcomes. In a series of 36 pregnancies in 32 women, no deaths were reported. Three women developed pulmonary edema. Arrhythmia complicated 6 pregnancies. Pregnant women were much less likely to be treated with diuretic and β-blocker than nonpregnant women.[71]

Women with a diagnosis of PPCM in a previous pregnancy are at risk for heart failure in a subsequent pregnancy. If left ventricular ejection fraction (LVEF) has not normalized, the mortality rate may be as high as 19%.[72] In those in whom LVEF has normalized, a worsening of function and an increased incidence of symptoms of heart failure can be expected. Aggressive, appropriate pharmacologic management is frequently required.

Acute treatment of cardiomyopathy is directed at improving cardiac function and, when present, treating the inciting event. Diuretics are used to decrease preload and relieve pulmonary congestion. Digoxin may improve myocardial contractility and facilitate rate control when atrial fibrillation is present. Afterload reduction is achieved with ACE inhibitors postpartum or hydralazine before delivery. β-Blockade in stable, euvolemic patients has been clearly demonstrated to improve cardiac function and survival outside of pregnancy and should not be withheld from pregnant women. Significantly dilated and hypokinetic cardiac chambers pose a risk for clot formation and systemic embolization. Anticoagulation with heparin antepartum or warfarin postpartum should be considered. Implanted defibrillators have been used in pregnancy without significant complications. Arrhythmia is a common cause of death associated with cardiomyopathy outside pregnancy. Hemodynamic management during labor and delivery is frequently directed by a pulmonary artery catheter. Pain control decreases cardiac work and reduces tachycardia. A carefully dosed epidural is appropriate. Cesarean delivery is reserved for obstetrical indications.

The postpartum period represents a time of particular risk. Women have received exogenous volume loading from intravenous fluid during labor; blood volume is centralized with uterine contractions; extravascular fluid is mobilized; tachycardia persists; and SVR increases. Each physiologic change will work toward left ventricular decompensation. Preemptive HR control, diuresis, and afterload reduction should be employed.

MYOCARDIAL INFARCTION

MI is a rare event among women of reproductive age. From a population base of 3.6 million women-years, Petitti and associates[73] identified 186 cases (5 per 100,000 women-years). More recent studies suggest a rate between 2.8 and 6.2 per 100,000 deliveries.[74,75] **An increased risk for MI in pregnancy is consistently associated with maternal age greater than 40 years, chronic hypertension, diabetes, smoking, migraine headache, transfusion, and postpartum infection.**[75]

Owing to the rarity of the event, information regarding MI in pregnancy is derived from case reports and, therefore, is subject to considerable reporting bias. Roth and Elkayam have summarized information from reports of 123 pregnancies between 1922 and 1995[76] and an additional 103 cases between 1995 and 2005.[77] (see box, Myocardial Infarction in Pregnancy).[76,77] **Coronary dissection and normal coronary arteries are observed in almost 50% of cases.** Delivery within 2 weeks of infarction may be associ-

MYOCARDIAL INFARCTION IN PREGNANCY

Pregnancies	123	103
Mean age ± SD	32 ± 6 years	33 ± 5 years
Age range	16-45 years	19-44 years
Anterior infarction	73%	78%
Multiparous	84%	66%
Hypertension	19%	15%
Diabetes mellitus	5%	11%
Smoking	26%	45%
Family history of MI	8%	22%
Hyperlipidemia	2%	24%
Preeclampsia	11%	6%
CHF after MI	19%	9%
Coronary anatomy		
Stenosis	43%	40%
Thrombus	21%	8%
Dissection	16%	27%
Spasm	1%	2%
Normal	29%	13%
Death		
Maternal	21%	11%
Infant	13%*	9%

CHF, Congestive heart failure; *MI*, myocardial infarction; *SD*, standard deviation.
*Sixty-two percent of infant deaths were associated with mother's death.

ated with a maternal mortality rate as high as 50%. MI has been reported in association with diabetes mellitus, pheochromocytoma, Ehlers-Danlos type IV, antiphospholipid syndrome, multiple gestation, and sickle cell anemia. Medications such as ergot alkaloids given for bleeding, bromocriptine for lactation suppression, ritodrine and nifedipine for tocolysis, and prostaglandin E_2 in conjunction with severe hypertension have also been associated with MI.

The diagnosis of MI in pregnancy is often delayed because of the rarity of the event and common symptoms of pregnancy. During normal pregnancy, most women experience some increase in exercise intolerance and dyspnea. Chest pain due to reflux is common. ECG changes that suggest ischemia have been reported in as many as 37% of women having a repeat cesarean delivery.[76] **However, ST-segment elevation is not a normal finding and, in the context of ongoing chest pain, should markedly increase the suspicion of acute MI.** The MB fraction of creatinine kinase isoenzymes may be elevated at cesarean delivery as well. Troponin I levels are not elevated during labor and delivery. If confusion regarding the appropriate diagnosis exists in the context of a constellation of findings suggestive of MI, an echocardiogram can be used to confirm abnormal wall motion in the ischemic region.

Acute therapy is based on rapid coronary reperfusion. Coronary angioplasty and stenting have been reported in pregnancy and should not be withheld when appropriate for the mother's condition. Thrombolytic therapy has also been used in pregnancy.[76] Although effective, there may be a small but real incidence of associated maternal bleeding, preterm delivery, or fetal loss. Surgery after thrombolytic therapy is associated with significant risk for hemorrhage.

Medications commonly used in the management of MI such as morphine, organic nitrates, lidocaine, β-blockers, aspirin, magnesium sulfate, and calcium antagonists may be used in appropriate doses in pregnancy. Care should be taken to avoid the supine position and maternal hypotension during procedures. The fetus, if viable, should be monitored.

Elective delivery within 2 weeks of infarction should be avoided because it is associated with an increased risk for maternal death. Cesarean delivery is reserved for obstetrical indications. Labor and delivery are managed with standard cardiac care. Pain is controlled, usually with carefully administered regional analgesia. Tachycardia is prevented with pain control and treated with β-blockers as needed. Hemodynamic stability is maintained, frequently using information from pulmonary and peripheral arterial catheters. Maternal pushing is avoided, and the second stage of labor is shortened with low forceps or vacuum. Diuresis is gently initiated postpartum with diuretics.

The experience with pregnancy after a remote MI is limited. Of 33 reported cases, recurrent infarction and significant complications have not been reported.[78]

MARFAN SYNDROME

Marfan syndrome is an autosomal dominant genetic disorder caused by an abnormal gene for fibrillin on chromosome 15. Disease prevalence is estimated to be four to six per 10,000. Sporadic cases represent 15% of those diagnosed. The production of abnormal connective tissue results in the characteristic feature of the disease: aortic root dilation, dislocation of the optic lens, deformity of the anterior thorax, scoliosis, long limbs, joint laxity, and arachnodactyly. Diagnosis is usually based on family history and physical examination, including ocular, cardiovascular, and skeletal features.

Untreated, life expectancy is reduced by one third, with most deaths due to aortic dissection and rupture. Elective aortic repair is associated with a low mortality rate (1.5%), whereas emergent repair results in a much higher mortality rate (11.7%). Therefore, elective repair has been recommended when the aortic root diameter measures 5.5 to 6 cm. Using an absolute aortic diameter (AD) as an indication for surgery ignores relevant differences in aortic size associated with patients of different stature. These considerations are particularly important when caring for young women. An aortic ratio between measured and predicted AD can be calculated. The predicted diameter for young adults can be calculated: $AD_{predicted} = 1.02 + (0.98 \times \text{body surface area [BSA]})$. A ratio of less than 1.3 with a dilation rate of less than 5% per year suggests a low risk for a cardiovascular event.

The risk for aortic dissection is associated with the rate of change of blood pressure in the aorta over time in systole. Although simple reduction in blood pressure does not reduce the risk for dissection, β-blockade lowers the risk for reaching a clinical cardiac end point at 10 years from about 20% to 10%.

Marfan Syndrome in Pregnancy

Women	84
Pregnancies	241
Live births	181 (75%)
Miscarriages	38 (16%)
Terminations	17 (7%)
Fetal deaths	2 (0.8%)
Aortic events	8 (4.3%)
Dissection	6 (3.3%)*
Rapid dilation	2 (1.1%)*
Death	2 (1.1%)*

*Observed in patients with an aortic root diameter of less than 4 cm.

Literature surveys of case reports suggest a maternal mortality rate associated with Marfan syndrome in pregnancy in excess of 50%.[79] These case reports likely represent bias of reporting more severely affected pregnancies. Three population-based studies are summarized in the box, Marfan Syndrome in Pregnancy.[80-82] Aortic events, dissection or rapid dilation, occurred in 8% of cases. In seven of nine patients, the AD was known to be greater than 4 cm. Of the remaining two, one died due to aortic dissection and rupture without a diagnosis and without a measurement of AD; the other had a prior graft replacement. A second death was due to endocarditis associated with mitral valve prolapse.

These studies suggest that women with mild disease, an AD less than 4 cm, can attempt pregnancy with only modest risk. The risk associated with more advanced disease is certainly greater. **Given the data available, a precise risk for death from aortic dissection or rupture cannot be quantified. Women with ADs greater than 5.5 cm should certainly be counseled to have graft and valve replacement before pregnancy.** They will then assume the risk associated with an artificial valve and the risk associated with the remaining aorta. These risks may be significant; however, adequate data do not exist to quantify the risks. Women with aortic roots greater than 4 cm but less than or equal to 5.5 cm are at significant risk, but aortic replacement may be premature. Fifty percent of the offspring of women with Marfan syndrome should be expected to have the disease.

Management of pregnancies affected by Marfan syndrome should begin with an accurate assessment of the aortic root. An absolute diameter or preferably an aortic ratio can be used to assess specific risk. The aortic root should be protected from hemodynamic forces with β-blockade. A resting HR of about 70 beats/minute can usually be achieved. Although β-blockade may potentially contribute to impaired fetal growth, this risk is outweighed by the maternal risk without such treatment.

Labor and delivery are managed with standard cardiac care, with particular emphasis on the prevention of tachycardia. Patients with aortic roots less than 4 cm can be delivered vaginally, reserving cesarean delivery for obstetrical indications. Some authors have recommended cesarean delivery for women with larger roots based on concerns about increased pressure in the aorta during labor. Data do not exist to make this a firm recommendation.

PULMONARY HYPERTENSION

Although pulmonary hypertension is fundamentally a pulmonary disease, the major pathologic impact is on the right side of the heart. The incidence of primary pulmonary hypertension is 1 to 2 per 1 million, with women affected more commonly than men. Secondary pulmonary hypertension may develop as a complication of cardiac disease such as mitral stenosis or secondary to intrinsic pulmonary disease. Drugs such as cocaine or appetite suppressants may also be associated with pulmonary hypertension. If left untreated, the median survival after diagnosis is 2.5 years.[83] More recently, survival has been reported to be 68% to 77% at 1 year, 40% to 56% at 3 years, and 22% to 38% at 5 years[84] As might be expected, right heart failure and NYHA class III/IV symptoms predict adverse outcome. General therapy may include limitation of extreme exercise, supplemental oxygen, diuresis, and in some cases anticoagulation.

Pulmonary vasodilator therapy generally improves symptoms, and lifestyle changes may improve survival. About 10% of patients will respond to high-dose calcium channel blockers. Of those who initially respond to nifedipine, the 5-year survival rate is 95%. Intravenous prostacyclin is associated with a larger response rate but also is associated with side effects such as headache, jaw pain, diarrhea, flushing, and leg pain. A chronic intravenous line is required, and the dose must be increased on a regular basis. The 5-year survival rate for those who require treatment with prostacyclin is 54%. Subcutaneous and oral and inhaled prostacyclin are also available, each having limitations because of the route or timing of delivery.

Sildenafil, a cyclic guanosine monophosphate phosphodiesterase inhibitor, increases the endogenous production of nitric oxide and therefore operates as a potent vasodilator. Treatment with sildenafil improves functional status and hemodynamic profile. Ease of administration is a significant advantage. Pharmacologic management of pulmonary hypertension requires a team with considerable experience.

The maternal mortality with severe pulmonary hypertension is reported to be as high as 50%.[85] Although a review of reported cases suggests an improvement in mortality from 30% between 1978 and 1996 to 17% between 1997 and 2007, the risk remains high. The improvement may be associated with the advent of vasodilator therapy. **Sudden, irreversible deterioration in the postpartum period is common. As many as 75% of deaths will occur postpartum.**[86]

The symptoms of pulmonary hypertension are nonspecific. Increasing fatigue and shortness of breath are associated with progressive right-sided heart failure but are also ubiquitous in pregnancy. They can easily be attributed to a presumed upper respiratory infection. Hoarseness may be a result of impingement on the laryngeal nerve by an enlarged pulmonary artery. Patients may exhibit disproportionate lower extremity edema or oxygen desaturation out of proportion for a presumed illness. The diagnosis can be confirmed with echocardiography, in which the velocity of the regurgitant jet across the tricuspid valve can estimate pulmonary systolic pressure. A dilated, hypokinetic RV with displacement of the intraventricular septum into the left ventricle suggests right-sided heart failure.

Pulmonary hypertension with right ventricular dysfunction is poorly tolerated in pregnancy. A mortality rate between 17% and 30% should be expected. Antepartum management often requires hospitalization. Oxygen therapy may reduce PVR and improve right ventricular performance. Pharmacologic treatment with pulmonary vasodilators may also be effective.[84,87] Anticoagulation with heparin should be considered. Worsening disease will usually be manifest by falling CO rather than rising right ventricular pressure. Labor and delivery should be managed with standard cardiac care, with particular attention to right ventricular filling as assessed by measurement of central venous pressure (CVP). **Although the RV requires adequate filling to generate forward flow against an elevated PVR modest elevations in CVP may precipitate increasing right ventricular dysfunction.** Given fluid mobilization postpartum and the potential need to treat volume loss associated with delivery, appropriate filling may be difficult to achieve. Aggressive diuresis may be required. Modest underloading or overloading of the RV can result in rapid decompensation and death.

Women with pulmonary hypertension and right ventricular dysfunction should be strongly discouraged from becoming pregnant. Because pulmonary artery pressures fall as the RV fails, the condition of the RV may be a more important consideration than an absolute systolic pulmonary pressure. Some women may consider pregnancy after a favorable response to treatment with pulmonary vasodilators. In a small series, two women whose pulmonary pressures and right ventricular function had normalized carried three pregnancies successfully while being treated with nifedipine or prostacyclin. Neither experienced deterioration in their condition during the first year postpartum.

OTHER CONDITIONS

Young women may experience malignant ventricular arrhythmias due to idiopathic ventricular fibrillation, cardiomyopathy, long-QT syndrome, congenital heart disease, or hypertrophic cardiomyopathy. Implantable cardioverter-defibrillators (ICDs) can effectively protect them from sudden death. In a report of 44 pregnancies, no women experienced generator erosion or lead fractures due to the expanding pregnancy. Twenty-five percent experienced electrical discharges during pregnancy without complication.

Hypertrophic cardiomyopathy is a genetic condition usually inherited in an autosomal dominant pattern with variable penetrance. Although the condition can be subclassified, the physiologic impact of different forms is similar. Patients are at risk for malignant arrhythmia, diastolic dysfunction, and outflow tract obstruction. A risk for sudden death is suggested by a family history of sudden death, extreme hypertrophy (left ventricular wall $\geq$ 30 mm), a history of syncope, nonsustained ventricular tachycardia, and hypotension with exercise. Arrhythmia risk is managed with an ICD and β-blockade. Volume loading during pregnancy in the face of diastolic dysfunction may result in pulmonary edema. Serum BNP can be used to direct volume management with diuretics. Left ventricular outflow tract obstruction is uncommon in young women. Reduced ventricular filling associated with blood loss, dehydration, or tachycardia will increase the functional obstruction. Management of hypertrophic cardiomyopathy has been recently reviewed.[88]

Reviews of case reports suggest a maternal mortality rate of 1% to 2% in these cases.[89-91] Given the biases associated with case report–derived data, this estimate probably sets an upper limit of expected mortality. Thaman and colleagues[91] reported 271 pregnancies in 127 women with hypertrophic cardiomyopathy, which were only complicated by two cases of pulmonary edema postpartum that resolved with appropriate therapy. In pregnancy, increased blood volume and left ventricular dimension will tend to benefit the patient. Increased HR will not. β-Blockers are generally used to manage tachycardia and some arrhythmias. Implantable ICDs may also be used. Labor and delivery are managed with standard cardiac care, with particular emphasis to ensure generous left ventricular filling. **Excessive volume loading may reveal a stiff ventricle and diastolic dysfunction. In some patients, a relatively small increase in vascular volume results in a substantial increase in pulmonary pressure, pulmonary congestion, and desaturation.** Although diastolic dysfunction may be difficult to diagnose by echocardiography, careful attention to an O_2 saturation monitor during labor and postpartum can reveal the need for augmented diuresis. Supine hypotension must be carefully avoided, and obstetrical bleeding should be treated early and aggressively with volume replacement.

CRITICAL CARE: HEMODYNAMIC MONITORING AND MANAGEMENT

Diseases unique to pregnancy, the physiologic stresses of pregnancy, and the special conditions surrounding labor and delivery operate to create circumstances in which intensive care may be necessary more frequently than would be required among young nonpregnant individuals. Specialists in intensive care may not be familiar with the physiology of pregnancy and associated unique conditions such as preeclampsia or amniotic fluid embolus. They may also be unfamiliar with maternal-fetal physiologic relationships and decision making that must balance the needs of the mother and the fetus. **Therefore, obstetricians must be familiar with basic principles and techniques of critical care medicine in order to primarily manage critically ill pregnant women or to serve as valuable consultants to a critical care team.**

Acute indications for invasive hemodynamic monitoring can be broadly categorized based on questions of physiology (see box, Indications for Hemodynamic Monitoring). Severe preeclampsia, sepsis, acute respiratory distress syndrome (ARDS), pneumonia, previously undiagnosed heart disease, and fluid management after resuscitation from obstetrical hemorrhage are the most common conditions that require hemodynamic monitoring. Certain conditions, particularly maternal heart disease as discussed earlier, require a planned, prospective decision for invasive monitoring. In these cases, the therapeutic window for hemodynamic management is narrow, and knowledge of the patient's baseline, compensated hemodynamic status can serve as a goal for intrapartum management.

INDICATIONS FOR HEMODYNAMIC MONITORING

1. Why is the patient hypoxic?
   - Are pulmonary capillary pressures high because of relative volume overload (e.g., mitral stenosis postpartum)?
   - Are pulmonary capillary pressures high because of depressed cardiac function (e.g., cardiomyopathy)?
   - Is capillary membrane integrity intact (e.g., ARDS, pneumonia)?
2. Why is the patient persistently hypertensive?
   - Is vascular resistance elevated?
   - Is cardiac output elevated?
3. Why is the patient hypotensive?
   - Is left ventricular filling pressure low (e.g., after hemorrhage)?
   - Is vascular resistance low (e.g., septic shock)?
4. Why is the patient's urine output low?
   - Is left ventricular filling pressure low, resulting in low cardiac output?
5. Is the patient expected to be unstable in labor?
   - Is the window of left ventricular filling narrow (e.g., aortic stenosis)?
   - Will normal physiologic changes associated with delivery be tolerated poorly (e.g., volume loading postpartum, mitral stenosis, pulmonary hypertension)?

In many cases, initial therapy can and should be based empirically on an understanding of the patient's pathophysiology. If subsequent interventions are needed, specific data obtained from hemodynamic monitoring may be required. Physicians with abundant experience treating a particular disease may rely less on invasive monitoring because an improved understanding makes the clinical course more predictable. In contrast, physicians with less experience may have a lower threshold for using invasive hemodynamic monitoring. Therefore, understanding principles of management is particularly important for obstetricians who do not necessarily anticipate critically ill patients in their practice.

Hemodynamic Monitoring

The objective of hemodynamic monitoring is to provide continuous assessment of systemic and intracardiac pressures and to provide the means to determine CO and, therefore, to calculate systemic and pulmonary resistances. An arterial catheter is usually placed in the radial artery to measure systemic pressure. The diastolic pressure obtained usually correlates well with noninvasive measurements. Systolic pressure may be significantly higher than noninvasive measurements because of a very brief peak in pressure in early systole. (The spike in pressure contributes little to MAP. The noninvasive measurement is usually more clinically relevant to the patient's condition. The arterial catheter permits easy access to arterial blood sampling and relieves the patient from the discomfort of frequent blood draws.

Measurement of intracardiac pressures and CO are obtained through the insertion of a catheter into the central venous circulation and advancement into and through the right side of the heart. Venous access is most commonly obtained through the right internal jugular vein; a subclavian approach may also be employed. Traditionally, insertion is guided by using the sternocleidomastoid muscle and the clavicle as landmarks. The higher-frequency ultrasound transducer found on a vaginal probe can also be used to facilitate insertion under direct visualization. Once central venous access has been obtained and confirmed, a pulmonary artery catheter can be "floated" into the right side of the heart and pulmonary artery. Figure 36-6 demonstrates the waveforms and normal pressure values found as the catheter passes through the heart. Success in floating the catheter is initially confirmed by observation of characteristic waveforms in the RV, pulmonary artery, and wedged position, and subsequently with a radiograph. In experienced hands, complications from pulmonary artery catheterization are uncommon and include pneumothorax (<0.1%), pulmonary infarction (0 to 1.3%), pulmonary artery rupture (<0.1%), and septicemia (0.5% to 2.0%). Arrhythmias are usually transient and associated with passage of the catheter through the RV. If the patient has significant pulmonary hypertension, difficulty may be encountered maintaining placement in the pulmonary artery.

Once the catheter has been successfully placed, continuous readings of CVP and pulmonary artery pressures can be obtained. By inflating the balloon at the catheter

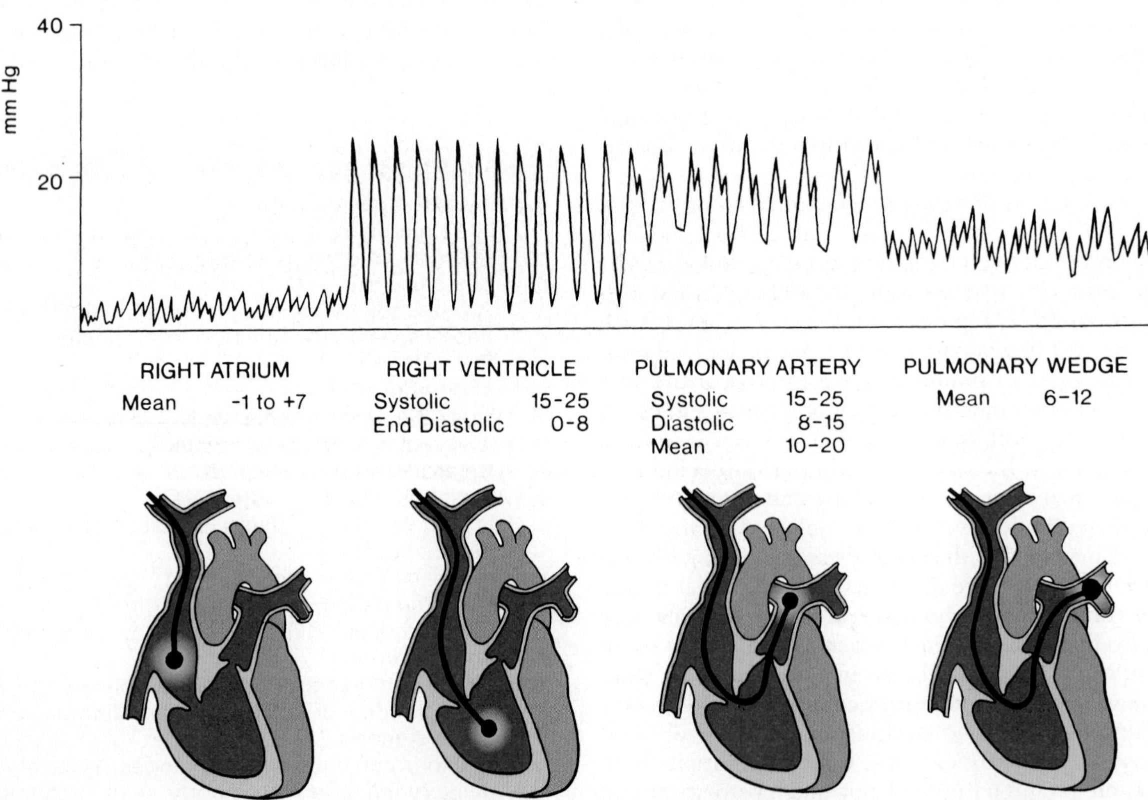

FIGURE 36-6. Hemodynamic waveforms and normal pressure values associated with catheter positions during advancement of a pulmonary artery catheter.

tip, the catheter can be wedged in the pulmonary artery to obtain a PAWP. PAWP reflects the filling pressure, preload, in the left ventricle. CVP measured in the right atrium is a measure of right ventricular filling pressure. In pregnant women, CVP cannot be assumed to accurately reflect left ventricular filling. Right atrial pressures and systolic pulmonary pressures can be measured noninvasively by echocardiography.

CO is measured by thermodilution. A bolus of cold fluid is injected into the right atrium, and a curve of temperature change over time is recorded as the bolus passes through the pulmonary artery. From the shape of the curve, CO can be calculated; when the CO is higher, the dilutional curve is shorter in time and greater in maximal temperature change. More recently, catheters have been equipped with a heating element in the right atrial segment so that continuous measurement of CO can be performed. CO can be measured noninvasively with Doppler and impedance techniques. Doppler technique has been validated under a wide range of clinical circumstances.[92-95] The impedance technique tends to underestimate CO in pregnancy but accurately reflects changes in hemodynamics in many conditions. In conditions of pathologically high flow, impedance may significantly underestimate CO.[96-98] CI can be derived from CO in order to adjust for maternal size: CI = CO/BSA. However, BSA does not seem to be related to CO in pregnancy; therefore, CO is usually preferred.[95] When CO is measured noninvasively and CVP is not available, resistance is expressed as TPR rather than SVR. In most clinical conditions, the differences between the two are not important.

Table 36-6 summarizes formulas used to calculate hemodynamic parameters not directly measured. Normal values for CO, MAP, HR, SV, and TPR are summarized in Figure 36-1. In a study of 10 normal pregnant women at term, Clark and coworkers determined that CVP, pulmonary artery pressure, PAWP, and left ventricular work index were not different from nonpregnant measurements made about 3 months postpartum.[99] The relationship between PAWP and left ventricular work index fell within the normal range for nonpregnant individuals, suggesting normal contractility in pregnancy. PVR was 34% lower, and colloid osmotic pressure was reduced by 14%.

TABLE 36-6 CALCULATED HEMODYNAMIC VARIABLES

		CALCULATION	UNITS
Mean arterial pressure	MAP	$\frac{sBP + 2(dBP)}{3}$	mm Hg
Stroke volume	SV	$\frac{CO \cdot 1000}{HR}$	mL
Systemic vascular resistance	SVR	$\frac{(MAP - CVP) \cdot 80}{CO}$	dyne · sec · cm^{-5}
Total peripheral resistance	TPR	$\frac{MAP \cdot 80}{CO}$	dyne · sec · cm^{-5}
Pulmonary vascular resistance	PVR	$\frac{80\,(mPAP - PAWP)}{CO}$	dyne · sec · cm^{-5}

CO, Cardiac output; *CVP*, central venous pressure; *dBP*, diastolic blood pressure; *mPAP*, mean pulmonary artery pressure; *PAWP*, pulmonary artery wedge pressure; *sBP*, systolic blood pressure.

Hemodynamic Management

Strategies of hemodynamic therapy that may be applicable to a variety of clinical circumstances are discussed in this section. As outlined earlier, the use of hemodynamic monitoring should be directed at answering specific questions of maternal pathophysiology. To achieve a particular goal, a number of physiologic interventions are possible. Each of these interventions will precipitate a secondary or compensatory response. The secondary response, if excessive, may adversely affect the patient. The choice of intervention from available options will often be determined by the potential for and magnitude of adverse effect. Hemodynamic monitoring permits the physician to choose an intervention and subsequently assess the positive and negative effects.

Disruption of alveolar capillary fluid dynamics is frequently associated with acute oxygen desaturation due to excess alveolar fluid. Pulmonary edema is usually due to excess hydrostatic capillary pressure (e.g., cardiomyopathy, mitral stenosis) or to a disruption of alveolar capillary membrane integrity (e.g., pneumonia, ARDS). Although a reduction in serum oncotic pressure is rarely a primary cause of pulmonary edema, the reduced serum albumin level in normal pregnancy can act in synergy with other forces, resulting in earlier or more severe pulmonary edema than would normally occur.

The use of pulse oximetry facilitates the early detection of maternal desaturation. Oxygen supplementation improves maternal saturation but does not correct the underlying cause. If desaturation is progressive, further intervention will be required. In the normal heart, diuresis to reduce preload works to decrease alveolar water in patients with elevated PAWP and in patients with capillary leak. A reduction in capillary pressure from high normal to low normal will reduce the egress of water across damaged membranes. In many circumstances, these interventions are made empirically based on a diagnosis and an understanding of maternal physiology. For example, tocolysis with β-mimetic agents can induce pulmonary edema. Timely diagnosis, discontinuation of the offending agent, oxygen supplementation, and a single diuretic dose will usually be sufficient therapy. When initial interventions do not achieve an adequate effect, invasive monitoring may be required to direct subsequent care. Maternal diuresis to improve oxygen saturation, when excessive, may lead to a reduction in CO. Fetal decompensation is usually encountered before a significant reduction in maternal perfusion and hypotension. The maternal PAWP and CO can be used to direct maternal diuresis. If desaturation continues despite hemodynamic management, intubation may be required. Positive end-expiratory pressure (PEEP) can be used to increase intra-alveolar pressure to impede the forces driving water into alveolar spaces. PEEP may impede venous return and decrease CO as a result of the effects of the associated increase in extracardiac intrathoracic pressure. A PAWP in excess of PEEP is required for adequate ventricular filling. Only in the sickest of pregnant women will PEEP have a clinically significant impact on CO.

Disorders of blood pressure and perfusion can be managed with the knowledge of maternal hemodynamics. Figure 36-7 describes the relationships between MAP, CO,

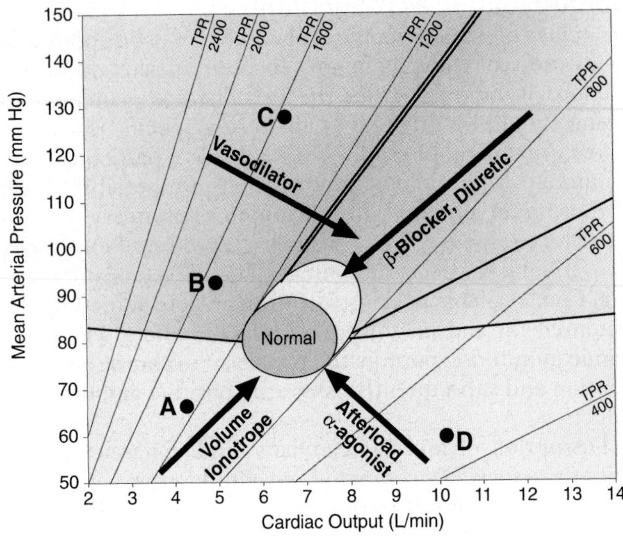

FIGURE 36-7. Hemodynamic flow chart. Cardiac output and mean arterial pressure are plotted on the *x*-axis and *y*-axis, respectively. *Diagonal lines* are isometric lines of vascular resistance. Anticipated vectors of change can be used to predict patient response to intervention. *TPR,* Total peripheral resistance.

and vascular resistance. CO and MAP are represented on the *x*-axis and *y*-axis, respectively. Resistance is represented by diagonal isometric lines. Vasodilators or vasopressors that act on resistance produce vectors of change that run perpendicular to lines of resistance. Interventions that decrease CO (β-blockers, diuresis) or increase CO (dopamine, volume) produce vectors of change that run roughly parallel to lines of resistance. The region labeled "normal" represents the goal of therapy. Plotting patient data on the chart allows one to visually determine the vector or combination of vectors that could return hemodynamics to normal.

Patient A represents a patient who is hypotensive with a low CO, as might be expected after hemorrhage or in heart failure. Given a low PAWP associated with hemorrhage, volume administration would be expected to create a vector that would return hemodynamics to normal. Alternatively, the patient could have a normal or high PAWP associated with heart failure and would need an inotropic agent such as dopamine. Patient B has a normal blood pressure but a high vascular resistance and low CO such as might be expected with a cardiomyopathy. Afterload reduction with a medication such as hydralazine will produce a vector of vasodilation and return hemodynamics to normal. Patient C is hypertensive with a mixed hemodynamic pattern. She will need a combination of vectors to approach normal hemodynamics (e.g., hydralazine and β-blocker). Patient D is hypotensive and hyperdynamic with a low vascular resistance. The hemodynamics might be found in a patient with early sepsis. Treatment with volume could increase pressure but at the expense of high filling pressures and a potentially negative impact on developing ARDS. Alternatively, a small dose of an α-adrenergic agent such as phenylephrine (Neo-Synephrine) would create a vector perpendicular to lines of resistance that return hemodynamics to normal.

KEY POINTS

- Hemodynamic changes in pregnancy may adversely affect maternal cardiac performance.
- Intercurrent events such as infection during pregnancy are usually the cause of decompensation.
- Women with heart disease in pregnancy frequently have unique psychosocial needs.
- Labor, delivery, and postpartum are periods of hemodynamic instability.
- The postpartum period can be characterized as a "perfect storm" of volume loading, tachycardia, and increased afterload—each of which may contribute to the destabilization of a pregnant woman with heart disease.
- Invasive hemodynamic monitoring should be used to address specific clinical questions.
- Many maternal heart conditions can be medically managed during pregnancy.
- Management of anticoagulation in women with mechanical valves requires an experienced team and careful consideration of the balance between maternal and fetal risk followed by appropriate counseling. Very aggressive therapeutic monitoring is required.
- Mothers with cyanotic heart disease are at particular risk for adverse fetal and neonatal outcomes.
- Eisenmenger syndrome, Marfan syndrome with a dilated aorta, and pulmonary hypertension with right heart dysfunction are associated with a very high risk for maternal mortality.
- Many women with congenital heart disease can successfully complete a pregnancy.
- Preconceptual counseling is based on achieving a balance between medical information and the patient's value system.

REFERENCES

1. Easterling T, Benedetti T, Schmucker B, et al: Maternal hemodynamics in normal and preeclamptic pregnancies: a longitudinal study. Obstet Gynecol 76:1061, 1990.
2. Robson S, Dunlop W, Boys R, et al: Cardiac output during labour. BMJ 295:1169, 1987.
3. Easterling T, Chadwick H, Otto C, et al: Aortic stenosis in pregnancy. Obstet Gynecol 72:113, 1988.
4. Clark S, Phelan J, Greenspoon J, et al: Labor and delivery in the presence of mitral stenosis: central hemodynamic observations. Am J Obstet Gynecol 152:384, 1985.
5. Robson S, Boys R, Hunter S, et al: Maternal hemodynamics after normal delivery and delivery complicated by postpartum hemorrhage. Obstet Gynecol 74:234, 1989.
6. Davison J, Lindheimer M: Volume homeostasis and osmoregulation in human pregnancy. Baillieres Clin Endocrinol Metab 3:451, 1989.
7. Whittaker P, Lind T: The intravascular mass of albumin during pregnancy: a serial study in normal and diabetic women. BJOG 100:587, 1993.
8. Otto C: Valvular stenosis: diagnosis, quantification, and clinical approach. In Textbook of Clinical Echocardiography. Philadelphia, WB Saunders, 2000, p 229.
9. Boggess K, Watts D, Hillier S, et al: Bacteremia shortly after placental separation during cesarean section. Obstet Gynecol 87:779, 1996.
10. Dhoble A, Vedre A, Abdelmoneim SS, et al: Prophylaxis to prevent infective endocarditis: to use or not to use? Clin Cardiol 32:429, 2009.

11. Whittemore R, Hobbins J, Engle M: Pregnancy and its outcome in women with and without surgical treatment of congenital heart disease. Am J Cardiol 50:641, 1982.
12. Gill H, Splitt M, Sharland G, et al: Patterns of recurrence of congenital heart disease: an analysis of 6,640 consecutive pregnancies evaluated by detailed fetal echocardiography. J Am Coll Cardiol 42:923, 2003.
13. Bonow R, Carabello B, de Leon A, et al: ACC/AGA guidelines for the management of patients with valvular heart disease. Executive summary: a report of the American College of Cardiology/American Heart Association Task Force on practice guidelines (committee on management of patients with valvular heart disease). J Heart Valve Dis 7:672, 1998.
14. Chesley L: Severe rheumatic cardiac disease and pregnancy: the ultimate prognosis. Am J Obstet Gynecol 136:552, 1980.
15. Al Kasab S, Sabag T, Al Zaibag M, et al: Beta-adrenergic receptor blockade in the management of pregnant women with mitral stenosis. Am J Obstet Gynecol 163:37, 1990.
16. Silversides CK, Colman JM, Sermer M, et al: Cardiac risk in pregnant women with rheumatic mitral stenosis. Am J Cardiol 91:1382, 2003.
17. Farhat M, Gamra H, Betbout F, et al: Percutaneous balloon mitral commissurotomy during pregnancy. Heart 77:564, 1997.
18. Gupta A, Lokhandwala Y, Satoskaar P, et al: Balloon mitral valvotomy in pregnancy: maternal and fetal outcomes. J Am Coll Surg 187:409, 1998.
19. Selzer A: Changing aspects of the natural history of valvular aortic stenosis. N Engl J Med 317:91, 1998.
20. Carabello B, Crawford F: Valvular heart disease. N Engl J Med 337:32, 1997.
21. Arias F, Pineda J: Aortic stenosis and pregnancy. J Reprod Med 20:229, 1978.
22. Lao T, Sermer M, MaGee L, et al: Congenital aortic stenosis and pregnancy: a reappraisal. Am J Obstet Gynecol 169:540, 1993.
23. Shime J, Mocarski E, Hastings D, et al: Congenital heart disease in pregnancy: short- and long-term implications. Am J Obstet Gynecol 156:313, 1987.
24. Tzemos N, Silversides CK, Colman JM, et al: Late cardiac outcomes after pregnancy in women with congenital aortic stenosis. Am Heart J 157:474, 2009.
25. Lee C, Wu C, Lin P, et al: Pregnancy following cardiac prosthetic valve replacement. Obstet Gynecol 83:353, 1994.
26. Hanania G, Thomas D, Michel P, et al: Pregnancy in patients with heart valves: a French retrospective study (155) cases. Arch Mal Coeur Vaiss 87:429, 1994.
27. Elkayam U, Bitar F: Valvular heart disease and pregnancy. Part II: prosthetic valves. J Am Coll Cardiol 46:403, 2005.
28. McLintock C, McCowan LM, North RA: Maternal complications and pregnancy outcome in women with mechanical prosthetic heart valves treated with enoxaparin. BJOG 116:1585, 2009.
29. Vitale N, De Feo M, De Santo LS, et al: Dose-dependent fetal complications of warfarin in pregnant women with mechanical heart valves. J Am Coll Cardiol 33:1637, 1999.
30. Ville Y, Jenkins E, Shearer M: Fetal intraventricular haemorrhagia and maternal warfarin. Lancet 341:1211, 1993.
31. Bates SM, Greer IA, Hirsh J, et al: Use of antithrombotic agents during pregnancy: the Seventh ACCP Conference on Antithrombotic and Thrombolytic Therapy. Chest 126:627S, 2004.
32. Barbour LA, Oja JL, Schultz LK: A prospective trial that demonstrates that dalteparin requirements increase in pregnancy to maintain therapeutic levels of anticoagulation. Am J Obstet Gynecol 191:1024, 2004.
33. McLintock C, McCowan LM, North RA: Maternal complications and pregnancy outcome in women with mechanical prosthetic heart valves treated with enoxaparin. BJOG 116:1585, 2009.
34. Yinon Y, Siu SC, Warshafsky C, et al: Use of low molecular weight heparin in pregnant women with mechanical heart valves. Am J Cardiol 104:1259, 2009.
35. Gantt L: Growing up heartsick: the experiences of young women with congenital heart disease. Health Care Women Int 13:241, 1992.
36. Kovacs AH, Harrison JL, Colman JM, et al: Pregnancy and contraception in congenital heart disease: what women are not told. J Am Coll Cardiol 12:577, 2008.
37. Findlow D, Doyle E: Congenital heart disease in adults. Br J Anaesth 78:416, 1997.
38. Zuber M, Gautschi N, Oechslin E, et al: Outcome of pregnancy in women with congenital shunt lesions. Heart 81:271, 1999.
39. Stangle V, Schad J, Gossing G, et al: Maternal heart disease and pregnancy outcome: a single-centre experience. Eur J Heart Fail 10:855-860, 2008.
40. Drenthen W, Boersma E, Balci A, et al, on behalf of the ZAHARA Investigators: Predictors of pregnancy complications in women with congenital heart disease. Eur Heart J 31:2124, 2010.
41. Siu SC, Sermer M, Colman JM, et al, on behalf of Cardiac Disease in Pregnancy (CARPREG) Investigators: Prospective multicenter study of pregnancy outcomes in women with heart disease. Circulation 104:515, 2001.
42. Khairy P, Ouyang DW, Fernandes SM, et al: Pregnancy outcomes in women with congenital heart disease. Circulation 113:517, 2006.
43. Rose V, Gold R, Lindsay G, et al: A possible increase in the incidence of congenital heart defects among the offspring of affected patients. J Am Coll Cardiol 6:376, 1985.
44. Piesiewicz W, Goch A, Binokowski Z, et al: Changes in the cardiovascular system during pregnancy in females with secundum atrial septal defect. Polish Heart J 60:218, 2004.
45. Veldtman G, Connolly H, Grogan M, et al: Outcomes of pregnancy in women with tetralogy of Fallot. J Am Coll Cardiol 44:174, 2004.
46. Genoni M, Jenni R, Hoerstrup S, et al: Pregnancy after atrial repair for transposition of the great arteries. Heart 81:276, 1999.
47. Nwosu U: Pregnancy following Mustard operation for transposition of great arteries. J Tenn Med Assoc 85:509, 1992.
48. Neukermans K, Sullivan T, Pitlick D: Successful pregnancy after the Mustard operation for transposition of the great arteries. Am J Cardiol 57:838, 1988.
49. Megerian G, Bell E, Huhta J, et al: Pregnancy outcome following Mustard procedure for transposition of the great arteries: a report of five cases and review of the literature. Obstet Gynecol 83:512, 1994.
50. Lynch-Salamond D, Maze S, Combs C: Pregnancy after Mustard repair for transposition of the great arteries. Obstet Gynecol 82:676, 1993.
51. Lao T, Sermer M, Colman J: Pregnancy following surgical correction for transposition of the great arteries. Obstet Gynecol 83:665, 1994.
52. Dellinger E, Hadi H: Maternal transposition of the great arteries in pregnancy: a case report. J Reprod Med 39:324, 1994.
53. Clarkson P, Wilson N, Neutze J, et al: Outcome of pregnancy after the Mustard operation for transposition of the great arteries with intact ventricle septum. Am Coll Cardiol 24:190, 1994.
54. Guedes A, Mercier L, Leduc L, et al: Impact of pregnancy on the systemic right ventricle after a Mustard operation for transposition of the great arteries. J Am Coll Cardiol 44:433, 2004.
55. Canobbio MM, Morris CD, Graham TP, et al: Pregnancy outcomes after atrial repair for transposition of the great arteries. Am J Cardiol 98:668, 2006.
56. Tobler D, Fernandes SM, Wald RM, et al: Pregnancy outcomes in women with transposition of the great arteries and arterial switch operation. Am J Cardiol 106:417, 2010.
57. Therrien J, Barnes I, Somerville J: Outcome of pregnancy in patients with congenitally corrected transposition of the great arteries. Am J Cardiol 84:820, 1999.
58. Connolly H, Grogan M, Warnes C: Pregnancy among women with congenitally corrected transposition of great arteries. J Am Coll Cardiol 33:1692, 1999.
59. Canobbio M, Mair D, Van der Velde M, et al: Pregnancy outcomes after the Fontan repair. J Am Coll Cardiol 28:763, 1996.
60. Drenthen W, Pieper PG, Roos-Hesselink JW, et al, on behalf of the ZAHARA investigators: Pregnancy and delivery in women after Fontan palliation. Heart 92:1290, 2006.
61. Vongpatanasin W, Brickner E, Hillis L, et al: The Eisenmenger syndrome in adults. Ann Intern Med 128:745, 1998.
62. Weiss B, Zemp L, Burkhardt S, et al: Outcome of pulmonary vascular disease in pregnancy: a systematic overview from 1978 through 1996. J Am Coll Cardiol 31:1650, 1998.
63. Gleicher N, Midwall J, Hochberger D, et al: Eisenmenger's syndrome and pregnancy. Obstet Gynecol Surv 34:721, 1979.
64. Yentis S, Steer P, Plaat F: Eisenmenger's syndrome in pregnancy: maternal and fetal mortality in the 1990's. BJOG 105:921, 1998.
65. Vriend JW, Drenthen W, Pieper PG, et al: Outcome of pregnancy in patients after repair of aortic coarctation. Eur Heart J 26:2173, 2005.
66. Beauchesne LM, Connolly HM, Ammash NM, et al: Coarctation of the aorta: outcome of pregnancy. J Am Coll Cardiol 38:1728, 2001.
67. Hibbard J, Lindheimer M, Lang R: A modified definition for peripartum cardiomyopathy and prognosis based on echocardiography. Obstet Gynecol 94:311, 1999.

68. Lampert M, Lang R: Peripartum cardiomyopathy. Am Heart J 130:860, 1995.
69. Heider A, Kuller J, Strauss R, et al: Peripartum cardiomyopathy: a review of the literature. Obstet Gynecol Sur 54:526, 1999.
70. Ostrzega E, Elkayam U: Risk of subsequent pregnancy in women with a history of peripartum cardiomyopathy: results of a survey. Circulation 92:1, 1995.
71. Sliwa K, Hilfiker-Kleiner D, Petrie MC, et al: Current state of knowledge on aetiology, diagnosis, management, and therapy of peripartum cardiomyopathy: a position statement from the Heart Failure Association of the European Society of Cardiology Working Group on peripartum cardiomyopathy. Eur J Heart Fail 12:767, 2010.
72. Elkayam U, Tummala PP, Rao K, et al: Maternal and fetal outcomes of subsequent pregnancies in women with peripartum cardiomyopathy. N Engl J Med 344:1567, 2001.
73. Petitti D, Sidney S, Queesenberry C, et al: Incidence of stroke and myocardial infarction in women of reproductive age. Stroke 28:280, 1997.
74. Ladner HE, Danielsen B, Gilbert WM: Acute myocardial infarction in pregnancy and the puerperium: a population-based study. Obstet Gynecol 105:480, 2005.
75. James AH, Jamison MG, Biswas MS, et al: Acute myocardial infarction in pregnancy: a United States population-based study. Circulation 113:1564, 2006.
76. Roth A, Elkayam U: Acute myocardial infarction associated with pregnancy. Ann Intern Med 125:751, 1996.
77. Roth A, Elkayam U: Acute myocardial infarction associated with pregnancy. J Am Coll Cardiol 52:171, 2008.
78. Dufour P, Occelli B, Puech F: Brief communication: pregnancy after myocardial infarction. Int J Obstet Gynecol 59:251, 1997.
79. Elkayam U, Ostrzega E, Shotan A, et al: Cardiovascular problems in pregnant women with the Marfan syndrome. Ann Intern Med 123:117, 1995.
80. Lipscomb K, Smith J, Clarke B, et al: Outcome of pregnancy in women with Marfan's syndrome. BJOG 104:201, 1997.
81. Pyeritz R: Maternal and fetal complications of pregnancy in the Marfan syndrome. Am J Med 71:784, 1981.
82. Rossiter J, Repke J, Morales A, et al: A prospective longitudinal evaluation of pregnancy in the Marfan syndrome. Am J Obstet Gynecol 173:1599, 1995.
83. D'Alonzo GE, Barst R, Ayres S, et al: Survival in patients with primary pulmonary hypertension. Ann Intern Med 115:343, 1991.
84. Humbert M, Sitbon O, Simonneau G: Treatment of pulmonary arterial hypertension. N Engl J Med 351:1425, 2004.
85. Martinez J, Comas C, Sala X, et al: Maternal primary pulmonary hypertension associated with pregnancy. Eur J Obstet Gynaecol Reprod Biol 54:143, 1994.
86. Branko M, Weiss MD, Lea Z, et al: Outcome of pulmonary vascular disease in pregnancy: a systematic overview from 1978 through 1996. JACC 31:1650, 1998.
87. Easterling T, Ralph D, Schmucker B: Pulmonary hypertension in pregnancy: treatment with pulmonary vasodilators. Obstet Gynecol 93:494, 1999.
88. Maron BJ: Hypertrophic cardiomyopathy: a systematic review. JAMA 287:1308, 2002.
89. Shah D, Sunderji S: Hypertrophic cardiomyopathy and pregnancy: report of a maternal mortality and review of the literature. Obstet Gynecol Surv 40:444, 1985.
90. Piacenza J, Kirkorian G, Audra P, et al: Hypertrophic cardiomyopathy and pregnancy. Eur J Obstet Gynaecol Reprod Biol 80:17, 1998.
91. Thaman R, Varnava A, Hamid MS, et al: Pregnancy related complications in women with hypertrophic cardiomyopathy. Heart 89:752, 2003.
92. Robson S, Dunlop W, Moore M, et al: Combined Doppler and echocardiographic measurement of cardiac output: theory and application in pregnancy. BJOG 94:1014, 1987.
93. Lee W, Rokey R, Cotton D: Noninvasive maternal stroke volume and cardiac output determinations by pulsed Doppler echocardiography. Am J Obstet Gynecol 158:505, 1988.
94. Easterling T, Carlson K, Schmucker B, et al: Measurement of cardiac output in pregnancy by Doppler technique. Am J Perinatol 7:220, 1990.
95. Easterling T, Watts D, Schmucker B, et al: Measurement of cardiac output during pregnancy: validation of Doppler technique and clinical observations in preeclampsia. Obstet Gynecol 69:845, 1987.
96. de Swiet M, Talbert D: The measurement of cardiac output by electrical impedance plethysmography in pregnancy: are the assumptions valid? BJOG 93:721, 1986.
97. Easterling T, Benedetti T, Carlson K, et al: Measurement of cardiac output in pregnancy: impedance versus thermodilution techniques. BJOG 96:67, 1989.
98. Masaki D, Greenspoon J, Ouzounian J: Measurement of cardiac output in pregnancy by thoracic electrical bioimpedance and thermodilution. Am J Obstet Gynecol 161:680, 1989.
99. Clark S, Cotton D, Lee W, et al: Central hemodynamic assessment of normal pregnancy. Am J Obstet Gynecol 161:1439, 1989.

For full reference list, log onto www.expertconsult.com.

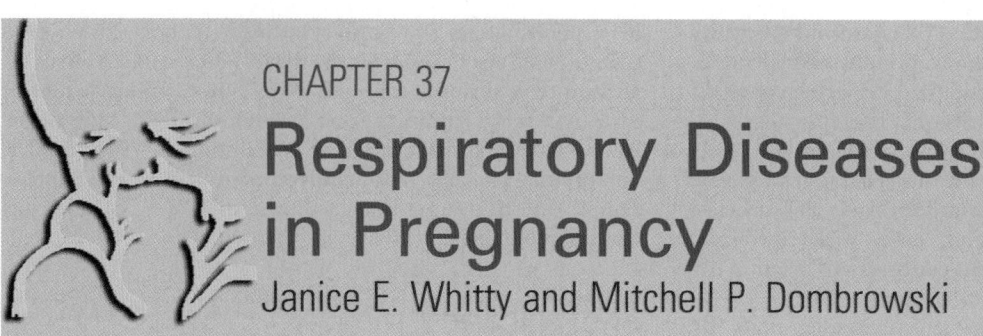

CHAPTER 37

Respiratory Diseases in Pregnancy

Janice E. Whitty and Mitchell P. Dombrowski

KEY ABBREVIATIONS

Acquired Immunodeficiency Syndrome	AIDS
Amniotic Fluid Index	AFI
Bacille Calmette-Guérin	BCG
Community-Acquired Methicillin-Resistant *Staphylococcus Aureus*	CA-MRSA
Confidence Interval	CI
Direct Amplification Tests	DATs
Dry-Powder Inhaler	DPI
Forced Expiratory Volume in 1 Second	FEV_1
Forced Vital Capacity	FVC
Highly Active Antiretroviral Therapy	HAART
Human Immunodeficiency Virus	HIV
Intrauterine Growth Restriction	IUGR
Isoniazid	INH
Long-Acting β-Agonist	LABA
Latent Tuberculosis Infection	LTBI
Leukotriene-Receptor Agonist	LTRA
Metered-Dose Inhaler	MDI
National Asthma Education and Prevention Program	NAEPP
Odds Ratio	OR
Peak Expiratory Flow Rate	PEFR
Percutaneous Needle Aspiration	PTNA
Pneumocystis Jiroveci Pneumonia	PJP
Positive End-Expiratory Pressure	PEEP
Purified Protein Derivative	PPD
Rifampin	RIF
Tuberculosis	TB
U.S. Food and Drug Administration	FDA

Pulmonary diseases are among the most common medical complications of pregnancy. The occurrence of pulmonary disease during gestation may result in increased morbidity or mortality for both the mother and her fetus. Pregnancy may have an adverse or positive impact on the pulmonary function of the gravida depending on the particular complication that is being encountered. The cardiorespiratory changes that occur in pregnancy are reviewed in Chapter 3, and the obstetrician and medical consultants should have a thorough understanding of these changes and their potential effects on the respiratory disease in question. It is also extremely important to realize that most diagnostic tests used to evaluate pulmonary function are not harmful to the fetus and, if indicated, should be performed during gestation. In this section, we discuss some of the respiratory complications that may be encountered during gestation, the impact of pregnancy on the disease, and the potential impact of the disease on pregnancy.

PNEUMONIA IN PREGNANCY

Pneumonia is an uncommon complication of pregnancy, observed in 0.78 to 2.7 per 1000 deliveries.[1,2] However,

pneumonia contributes to considerable maternal mortality and is reportedly the most common nonobstetrical infection to cause maternal mortality in the peripartum period.[3] Before the introduction of antibiotic therapy, maternal mortality was as high as 24%.[2] However, **with modern management and antibiotic therapy, the maternal mortality rate ranges from 0% to 4%.**[1,3,4] **Preterm delivery is a significant complication of pneumonia and, even with antibiotic therapy and modern management, continues to occur in 4% to 43% of affected pregnancies.**[1,3,4]

The incidence of pneumonia in pregnancy may be increasing primarily as a reflection of the declining health status of certain segments of the childbearing population.[1] In addition, the epidemic of human immunodeficiency virus (HIV) infection has increased the number of potential mothers who are at risk for opportunistic lung infections. HIV infection further predisposes the pregnant woman to the infectious complications of the acquired immunodeficiency syndrome (AIDS).[5] Reported incidence rates range from 97 to 290 cases per 1000 HIV-infected persons per year.[6] **HIV-infected persons are 7.8 times more likely to develop pneumonia** than non-HIV-infected individuals with similar risk factors.[6] Women with medical conditions that increase the risk for pulmonary infection, such as cystic fibrosis, are now living to childbearing age more frequently than in the past. This disorder also contributes to the increased incidence of pneumonia in pregnancy.

Pneumonia can complicate pregnancy at any time during gestation and may be associated with preterm birth, poor fetal growth, and perinatal loss. Benedetti and colleagues[3] described 39 cases of pneumonia in pregnancy. Sixteen gravidas presented before 24 weeks' gestation, 15 between 25 and 36 weeks' gestation, and 8 after 36 weeks' gestation. Twenty-seven patients in this series were followed to completion of pregnancy; only 2 required delivery during the acute phase of pneumonia. Of these 27 patients, 3 suffered a fetal loss, and 24 delivered live fetuses. There was one neonatal death due to prematurity.[1] Madinger and associates[4] reported 25 cases of pneumonia occurring among 32,179 deliveries and observed that fetal and obstetrical complications were much more common than in earlier studies. **Preterm labor occurred in 11 of 21 patients who had complete follow-up data. Pneumonia was present at the time of delivery in 11 patients. Preterm labor was more likely in those women who experienced bacteremia, required mechanical ventilation, or had a serious underlying maternal disease.** In addition to the complication of preterm labor, there were three perinatal deaths in this series. In Berkowitz and La Sala's report[1] of 25 patients with pneumonia complicating pregnancy, full-term delivery of normally grown infants occurred in 14 women, 1 delivered preterm, 3 had a voluntary termination of pregnancy, 3 had term deliveries of growth-restricted babies, and 4 were lost to follow-up. Birthweight was significantly lower in the study group (2770 ± 224 g versus 3173 ± 99 g in the control group; $P < .01$). In this series, pneumonia complicated 1 in 367 deliveries, and the authors attributed the increase in the incidence of pneumonia in this population to a decline in general health status, including anemia and a significant incidence of cocaine use in the study group (52 versus 10% in the general population) as well as HIV positivity in the study group (24 versus 2% in controls). **Madinger[4] reported preterm labor in 44% of cases with antepartum pneumonia, with a preterm birth rate of 36%. Maternal complications of pneumonia include respiratory failure and mechanical ventilation in 10% to 20%, bacteremia in 16%, and empyema in 8%.**[1,4] Respiratory failure due to pneumonia accounts for 12% of intubations during pregnancy.[7]

BACTERIOLOGY

Most series describing pneumonia complicating pregnancy have used incomplete methodologies to diagnose the etiologic pathogens involved, relying primarily on cultures of blood and sputum. In most cases, no identifiable pathogen is reported; however, ***Streptococcus pneumoniae* and *Haemophilus influenzae* remain the most common identifiable causes of pneumonia in pregnancy.**[1,3] Because comprehensive serologic testing has rarely been undertaken, the true incidence of viral pneumonia, *Legionella*, and *Mycoplasma* pneumonia in pregnancy is difficult to estimate. In Berkowitz and La Sala's series, one patient had *Legionella* species.[1] **Several unusual pathogens have been reported to cause pneumonia in pregnancy, including mumps, infectious mononucleosis, swine influenza, influenza A, varicella, coccidioidomycosis, and other fungi.**[8] **Varicella pneumonia complicates primary varicella infections in 9% of infections in pregnancy, compared with 0.3% to 1.8% in the nonpregnant population.**[9] Influenza A has a higher mortality in pregnant than in nonpregnant patients.[10] **The increase in virulence of viral infections reported in pregnancy may be secondary to the alterations in maternal immune status that characterize pregnancy, including reduced lymphocyte proliferative response, reduced cell-mediated cytotoxicity, and a decrease in the number of helper T lymphocytes** (see Chapter 4).[11,12] Viral pneumonias can also be complicated by superimposed bacterial infection, particularly with pneumococcus. **There are recent reports of community-acquired methicillin-resistant *Staphylococcus aureus* (CA-MRSA) causing necrotizing pneumonia in pregnancy and the postpartum period.**[11-13]

Chemical pneumonitis results after the aspiration of gastric contents. Chemical pneumonitis can be superinfected with pathogens present in the oropharynx and gastric juices, primarily anaerobes and gram-negative bacteria.[8]

Heterosexual transmission of HIV has become an increasingly important mode of transmission. Many of these women are of childbearing age. They are at risk for developing *Pneumocystis jiroveci* pneumonia (PJP) during pregnancy. The reported maternal mortality rate from PJP is as high as 50%.[14] Although the risk for maternal mortality is high with PJP infection, most HIV-infected pregnant women in the United States today are receiving prophylaxis. This practice may actually lead to a decrease in the incidence and mortality from PJP pneumonia in pregnancy.

BACTERIAL PNEUMONIA

***S. pneumoniae* (pneumococcus) is the most common bacterial pathogen to cause pneumonia in pregnancy, with**

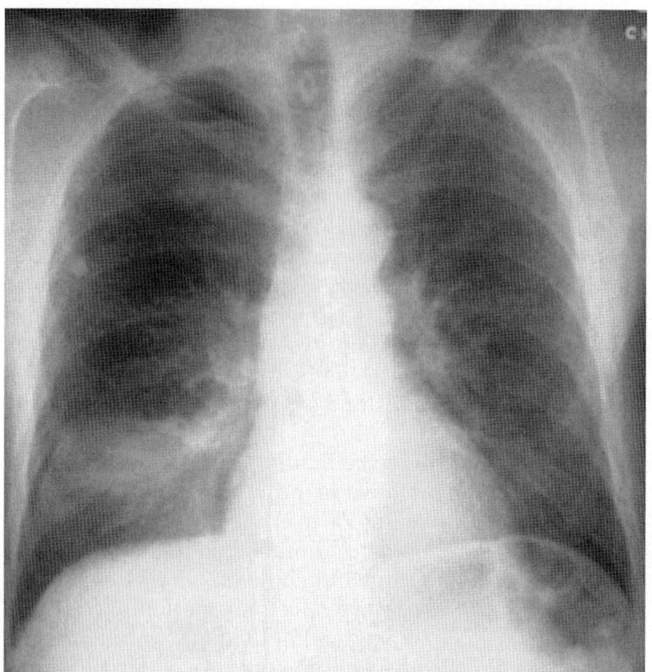

FIGURE 37-1. Right lower lobe pneumonia.

***H. influenzae* being the next most common.** These pneumonias typically present as an acute illness accompanied by fever, chills, purulent productive cough, and a lobar pattern on chest radiograph (Figure 37-1). **Streptococcal pneumonia produces a "rusty" sputum, with gram-positive diplococci on Gram stain and asymmetrical consolidation with air bronchograms on chest radiograph. *H. influenzae* is a gram-negative coccobacillus that produces consolidation with air bronchograms, often in the upper lobes. Less frequent bacterial pathogens include *Klebsiella pneumoniae*, which is a gram-negative rod that causes extensive tissue destruction, with air bronchograms, pleural effusion, and cavitation noted on chest radiograph. Patients with *S. aureus* pneumonia present with pleuritis, chest pain, purulent sputum, and consolidation without air bronchograms noted on chest radiograph. CA-MRSA can present with a viral-like prodrome that progresses to severe pneumonia with high fever, hypotension, and hemoptysis followed by septic shock and need for ventilator support.**[11] **Severe cases of CA-MRSA have been reported during influenza seasons or associated with a preceding influenza illness in 33% to 71% patients.**[11] **Leukopenia can be observed and has been found to be a predictor of poor outcome.**[11] **Patients can present with multilobar infiltrates and cavitation. Mortality from CA-MRSA pneumonia in the United States and Europe is reportedly greater than 50%.**

Patients with atypical pneumonia pathogens, such as ***Mycoplasma pneumoniae*, *Legionella pneumophila*, and *Chlamydia pneumoniae* (TWAR agent), present with gradual onset and a lower fever, appear less ill, and have a mucoid sputum and a patchy or interstitial infiltrate on chest radiograph.** The severity of the findings on chest radiograph is usually out of proportion to the mild clinical symptoms. ***M. pneumoniae* is the most common organism responsible for atypical pneumonia and is best detected by the presence of cold agglutinins, which are present in 70% of cases.**

The normal physiologic changes in the respiratory system associated with pregnancy result in a loss of ventilatory reserve. This, coupled with the relative immunosuppression that accompanies pregnancy, puts the mother and fetus at great risk from respiratory infection. **Therefore, any gravida suspected of having pneumonia should be managed aggressively. Hospital admission is generally recommended**, and an investigation should be undertaken to determine the pathologic etiology. A recent study examined 133 women admitted with pneumonia during pregnancy using protocols based on the British and American Thoracic Societies' admission guidelines for management in nonpregnant individuals.[15] The authors reported that if the American Thoracic Society guidelines were used, 25% of the pregnant women with pneumonia could have avoided admission.[16] Using the American criteria, none of the gravidas who would have been managed as an outpatient had any complications.[17] If the British Thoracic Society guidelines had been used, 66% of the pregnant women in this group would have been assigned to outpatient therapy. However, of those, 14% would have required readmission for complications. Of note, most of the 133 women who were hospitalized with pneumonia in this study did not receive a chest radiograph for confirmation of diagnosis. This limits the value of the study for use in guiding admission criteria for pneumonia in pregnancy. **Therefore, until additional information is available, admission for all pregnant women with pneumonia is prudent.**

Workup should include physical examination, arterial blood gases, chest radiograph, sputum for Gram stain and culture, as well as blood cultures. Several recently published studies have called into question the use of cultures to identify the microbiology of community-acquired pneumonia. **The successful identification of the bacterial etiology with cultures ranges from 2.1% to about 50%.**[18,19] **Review of available clinical data reflects an overall reliance on clinical judgment and the patient response to treatment to guide therapy.** There are other tests available to identify the etiology of pneumonia that do not require culture and are more sensitive and specific. **An assay approved by the U.S. Food and Drug Administration (FDA) for pneumococcal urinary antigen has been assessed in several studies.**[20] **The sensitivity for identifying pneumococcal disease in adults is reportedly 60% to 90%, with specificity close to 100%.**[20] In one study, the pneumococcal antigen was detected in 26% of patients in whom no pathogens had been identified.[21] This suggests that cases that are undiagnosed by standard testing can be identified with the assay. In this study, **10% of samples from patients with pneumonia caused by other agents were positive for the pneumococcal assay, indicating a potential problem with specificity.**[21] **Therefore, if the response to therapy directed at pneumococcus is inadequate, coverage for other potential pathogens should be added. There is a test for *Legionella* urinary antigen as well, with a sensitivity of 70% and specificity of 90% for serogroup 1.**[22] This is especially useful in the United States and Europe because about 85% of *Legionella* isolates are serogroup 1.[22] Legionella is a common cause of severe community-acquired pneumonia. Therefore, the urinary antigen for serogroup 1 should be considered for any patient requiring admission into an intensive care unit (ICU) for pneumonia.[22]

Percutaneous transthoracic needle aspiration (PTNA) has been advocated as a valuable and safe method to increase the chance of establishing a causative agent in pneumonia.[23] This test should be reserved for use in compromised individuals, suspected tuberculosis (TB) in the absence of a productive cough, selected cases of chronic pneumonia, pneumonia associated with neoplasm or foreign body, suspected PJP pneumonia, and suspected conditions that necessitate lung biopsy.[17]

When admission for pneumonia is required, there is evidence that inpatient and 30-day mortality has been reduced when antibiotics are administered in less than 8 hours. **Therefore, current U.S. federal standards require that the first dose of antibiotics be administered within 4 hours of arrival to the hospital.**[24] **Empirical antibiotic coverage should be started, usually with a macrolide for mild illness with addition of a β-lactam for severe illness.** Yost and colleagues demonstrated that monotherapy with erythromycin was adequate in 118 of 119 women with pneumonia in pregnancy.[15] **A macrolide combined with a β-lactam is safe and will provide adequate coverage for most community-acquired bacterial pneumonias, including *Legionella*.** Dual coverage has been demonstrated to improve response to therapy even for abbreviated macrolide regimens.[17] This is theoretically because of an added anti-inflammatory effect of the macrolides.[19] Azithromycin administration has been shown to be an independent predictor of positive outcome and reduced length of hospital stay in mild to moderate community-acquired pneumonia.[17] However, **the use of macrolides to treat community-acquired pneumonia should be limited when possible because their use has also been associated with increased penicillin resistance among patients with *S. pneumoniae*.**[25]

Once the results of the antigen, sputum culture, blood cultures, Gram stain, and serum studies are obtained and a pathogen has been identified, antibiotic therapy should be directed toward the identifiable pathogen. **The quinolones as a class should be avoided in pregnancy because they may damage developing fetal cartilage. However, with the emergence of highly resistant bacterial pneumonia, their use may be life-saving and therefore justified in specific circumstances.** The respiratory quinolones are not only effective against highly penicillin-resistant *S. pneumoniae* strains, but their use reportedly does not increase resistance.[25-27] **The respiratory quinolones include levofloxacin, gatifloxacin, and moxifloxacin. These are ideal agents for community-acquired pneumonia because they are highly active against penicillin-resistant strains of *S. pneumoniae*. They are also active against *Legionella* and the other atypical pulmonary pathogens.** Another advantage is a favorable pharmacokinetic profile, such that blood/lung levels are the same whether the drug is administered orally or intravenously.[28] Arguments against more extensive respiratory quinolone use are based on concerns about the potential for developing resistance, the variable incidence of *Legionella*, and cost. An additional caveat is that the respiratory quinolones are partially effective against mycobacterial TB. Therefore, evaluation for this infection should be done when considering the use of quinolones for pneumonia. **If CA-MRSA pneumonia is suspected, vancomycin or linezolid should be added to empirical therapy.**[11] Additional therapy with clindamycin can be considered in difficult-to-treat cases because it has been shown to reduce production of staphylococcal exotoxins.[26] **CA-MRSA is susceptible to fluoroquinolones and trimethoprim-sulfamethoxazole and often are only resistant to β-lactams.**[11]

In addition to antibiotic therapy, oxygen supplementation should be given. Frequent arterial blood gas measurements should be obtained. **Arterial saturation should be monitored with pulse oximetry, with a goal of maintaining the PO_2 at 70 mm Hg, a level necessary to ensure adequate fetal oxygenation. When the gravida is afebrile for 48 hours and has signs of clinical improvement, an oral cephalosporin or macrolide, or both, can be initiated and intravenous therapy discontinued. A total of 10 to 14 days of treatment should be completed.**

Pneumococcal polysaccharide vaccination prevents pneumococcal pneumonia in otherwise healthy populations, with an efficacy of 65% to 84%.[17] **The vaccine is safe in pregnancy** and should be administered to high-risk gravidas. Those at high risk include individuals with sickle cell disease secondary to autosplenectomy, patients who have had a surgical splenectomy, and individuals who are immunosuppressed. **An additional advantage to maternal immunization with the pneumococcal vaccine is that several studies have demonstrated a significant transplacental transmission of vaccine-specific antibodies.**[27] **After in utero exposure to the vaccine, there are significantly high concentrations of pneumococcal antibodies in infants at birth and at 2 months of age.**[27] **In addition, colostrum and breast milk antibodies are significantly increased in women who have received the pneumococcal vaccine.**[28]

Pneumonia in pregnancy can be complicated by respiratory failure requiring mechanical ventilation. In such cases, team management should include the obstetrician, maternal-fetal medicine specialist, and intensivist. In addition to meticulous management of the gravida's respiratory status, maintenance of the left lateral recumbent position is advocated to improve uteroplacental perfusion. **The potentially viable fetus should be monitored with continuous fetal monitoring. Serial ultrasound examinations for amniotic fluid index (AFI) and growth will help to guide clinical management. If positive end-expiratory pressure (PEEP) greater than 10 cm H_2O is required to maintain oxygenation, central monitoring with a pulmonary artery catheter should be instituted to adequately monitor volume status** and maintain maternal and uteroplacental perfusion. **There is no evidence that elective delivery results in an overall improvement in respiratory function.**[29] Therefore, elective delivery should be undertaken with caution. **However, if there is clear evidence of fetal compromise or profound maternal compromise and impending demise, delivery should be accomplished.**

VIRAL PNEUMONIAS

Influenza Virus

There are an estimated 4 million cases of pneumonia complicating influenza annually in the United States, and this is the sixth leading cause of death in this country.[30] Although three types of influenza virus can cause human disease (types A, B, and C), **most epidemic infections are due to influenza A.**[8] **Influenza A typically has an acute onset after**

a 1- to 4-day incubation period and first manifests as high fever, coryza, headache, malaise, and cough. In uncomplicated cases, the chest examination and chest radiograph remain clear.[8] **If symptoms persist longer than 5 days, especially in a pregnancy, complications should be suspected.** Pneumonia may complicate influenza as the result of either secondary bacterial infection or primary viral infection of the lung parenchyma. **In the epidemic of 1957, autopsies demonstrated that pregnant women died from fulminant viral pneumonia most commonly, whereas nonpregnant patients died most often from secondary bacterial infection.**[31] A large nested case-control study evaluated the rate of influenza-related complications over 17 influenza seasons in women enrolled in the Tennessee Medicaid system.[32] This study demonstrated a high risk for hospitalization for influenza-related reasons in low-risk pregnant women during the last trimester of pregnancy. The authors predicted that 25 of 10,000 women in the third trimester during the influenza season will be hospitalized with influenza-related complications.[32] **A more recent matched cohort study using the administrative database of pregnant women enrolled in the Tennessee Medicaid population examined pregnant women aged 25 to 44 years with respiratory hospitalization during influenza seasons in 1985 to 1993.**[33] **In this population of pregnant women, those with asthma accounted for half of all respiratory hospitalizations during influenza season. Of pregnant women with the diagnosis of asthma, 6% required respiratory hospitalization during the influenza season** (odds ratio [OR], 10.63; 95% confidence interval [CI], 8.61 to 13.83) compared with women without a medical comorbidity. This study detected no significant increases in adverse perinatal outcome associated with respiratory hospitalization during flu season.[33]

Early data on pandemic 2009 influenza A(H1N1) suggest pregnant women had an increased risk for hospitalization and death. Siston and associates identified 788 pregnant women in the United States with 2009 influenza A (H1N1).[34] Thirty died (5% of all reported 2009 influenza A [H1N1] influenza deaths in this period). Among 509 hospitalized women, 115 (22.5%) were admitted to an ICU. **Pregnant women who began treatment more than 4 days after symptom onset were more likely to be admitted to an ICU (56.9% vs. 9.4%; relative risk [RR], 6.0; 95% confidence interval [CI], 3.5 to 10.6) than those treated within 2 days after symptom onset.**[34]

Primary influenza pneumonia is characterized by rapid progression from a unilateral infiltrate to diffuse bilateral disease. The gravida may develop fulminant respiratory failure requiring mechanical ventilation and PEEP. **When pneumonia complicates influenza in pregnancy, antibiotics should be started, directed at the likely pathogens that can cause secondary infection, including *S. aureus*, pneumococcus, *H. influenza*, and certain enteric gram-negative bacteria. Antiviral agents, such as amantadine and ribavirin, can be considered. It has been recommended that the influenza vaccine be given routinely to gravidas in pregnancy during the flu season** (October to March) regardless of the trimester in order to prevent the occurrence of influenza and the development of secondary pneumonia. In addition to maternal protection, **prospective studies have demonstrated higher cord blood antibody levels to influenza in babies born to mothers who were immunized during pregnancy.** There is a delay in the onset and decrease in severity of influenza in infants who have higher antibody levels.[35]

Varicella Virus

Varicella zoster is a DNA virus that usually causes a benign self-limited illness in children but may infect up to 2% of all adults.[36] **Varicella infection occurs in 0.7 of every 1000 pregnancies.**[37] Pregnancy may increase the likelihood of varicella pneumonia complicating the primary infection.[37,38] **Varicella pneumonia occurs most often in the third trimester, and the infection is likely to be severe.**[37,38] The **maternal mortality from varicella pneumonia may be as high as 35% to 40%, compared with 11% to 17% in nonpregnant individuals. One review reported a decreased mortality with only three deaths in 28 women with varicella pneumonia.**[37] **A recent paper described 347 pregnant women with varicella-zoster viral infection. Of these, 18 (5.2%) had pneumonia treated with acyclovir. None of these women died.** The authors also noted that **women with varicella-zoster viral pneumonia were significantly more likely to be current smokers (OR, 5.1; 95% CI, 1.6 to 16) and to have 100 or more skin lesions.**[39]

Varicella pneumonia usually presents 2 to 5 days after the onset of fever, rash, and malaise and is heralded by the onset of pulmonary symptoms, including cough, dyspnea, pruritic chest pain, and hemoptysis. The severity of the illness may vary from asymptomatic radiographic abnormalities to fulminant pneumonitis and respiratory failure (Figure 37-2). **All gravidas with varicella pneumonia should**

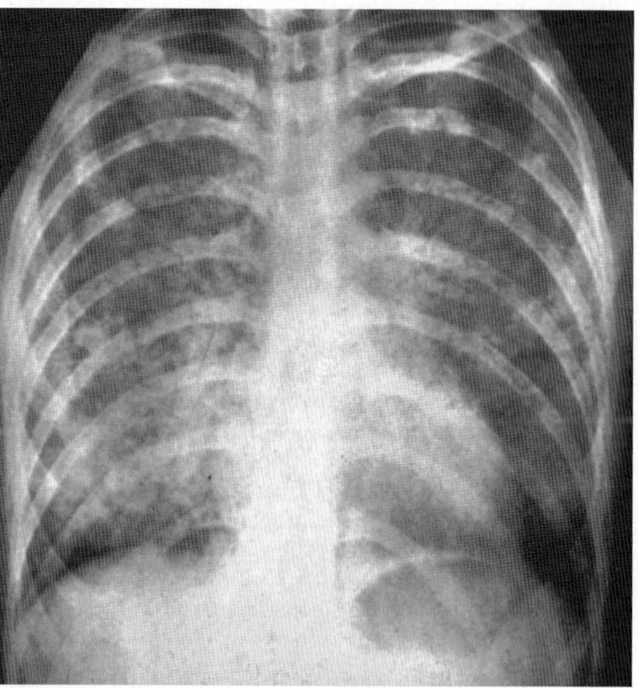

FIGURE 37-2. This chest radiograph demonstrates bilateral nodular and interstitial pneumonia characteristic of varicella pneumonia. The patient, a 27-year-old gravida 6, para 2, abortus 3 woman, was exposed to varicella infection in her two children. Characteristic skin vesicles of varicella occurred several days before the development of pulmonary symptoms. She required endotracheal intubation and mechanical ventilation for 6 days. She was treated with intravenous acyclovir and ceftazidime for possible superimposed infection. The patient recovered fully and delivered a healthy infant at term.

be aggressively treated with antiviral therapy and admitted to the ICU for close observation or intubation, if indicated. Acyclovir, a DNA polymerase inhibitor, should be started. **The early use of acyclovir has been associated with an improved hospital course after the fifth day and a lower mean temperature, lower respiratory rate, and improved oxygenation and survival.**[40] **The use of acyclovir is associated with improved survival as well.**[40] **Treatment with acyclovir is safe in pregnancy.** Among 312 exposed pregnancies, there was no increase in the number of birth defects and no consistent pattern of congenital abnormalities.[41] **A dose of 7.5 mg/kg intravenously every 8 hours has been recommended.** The use of varicella immune globulin to prevent infection in individuals exposed to varicella is not possible as it is no longer available in the United States.

Varicella vaccine is a live attenuated vaccine. It is the first vaccine against the herpesvirus. Extensive prelicensure studies have demonstrated that the **vaccine is safe and efficacious against varicella. Varicella vaccine was added to the universal childhood immunization schedule in the United States in 1995.** The program of universal childhood vaccination against varicella in the United States **has resulted in a sharp decline in the rate of death due to varicella.**[42] **This vaccine is not recommended for use in pregnancy.** However, the overall decline in the incidence of varicella secondary to vaccination will likely result in a decreased incidence of varicella infection and varicella pneumonia in pregnancy. **A recent study assessed the risk for congenital varicella syndrome and other birth defects in offspring of women who inadvertently received varicella vaccine during pregnancy or within 3 months of conception.**[43] **Fifty-eight women received their first dose of varicella vaccine during the first or second trimester. No cases of congenital varicella syndrome were identified among 56 live births** (rate, 0%; 95% CI, 0 to 15.6). Among the prospective reports of live births, five congenital anomalies were reported. No specific pattern of anomalies was identified in either the susceptible cohort or the sample population as a whole. Although the numbers in the study are small, the results should provide some reassurance to health care providers and women with inadvertent exposure before or during pregnancy.[43]

Pneumocystis jiroveci Pneumonia

PJP (formerly *Pneumocystis carinii* pneumonia, or PCP) remains the most prevalent opportunistic infection in patients infected with HIV.[44] **PJP, an AIDS-defining illness, occurs more frequently when the helper T-cell count (CD4$^+$) is less than 200 cells/mm^3.**[44] **When AIDS is complicated by PJP, the mortality rate is 10% to 20% during the initial infection, but this rate can increase substantially with the need for mechanical ventilation.** The transmission of *Pneumocystis* is not fully understood. There is some evidence that person-to-person transmission is the most likely mode; however, acquisition from environmental sources may also occur.[44]

The symptoms of PJP are nonspecific, and therefore, it may be difficult to diagnose. **Typical radiographic features of PJP are bilateral perihilar interstitial infiltrates that become increasingly homogeneous and diffuse as the disease progresses** (Figure 37-3). **The diagnosis of PJP requires microscopic examination to identify *Pneumocystis* from a clinical source such as sputum, bronchoalveolar fluid, or lung tissue** (Figure 37-4). *Pneumocystis* cannot be propagated in culture. The fungus has trophic forms as well as a cyst state. These can be detected with a modified Papanicolaou, Wright-Giemsa, or Gram-Weigert stain.[44] **Monoclonal antibodies are useful for detecting *Pneumocystis* as well.** The application of polymerase chain reaction (PCR) to detect *Pneumocystis* has been an area of active research and may be valuable for detection in sputum and bronchoalveolar lavage fluid.[44] **Trimethoprim-sulfamethoxazole is the preferred treatment for PJP. Thus far, resistance to this therapeutic agent has not been identified.**[44]

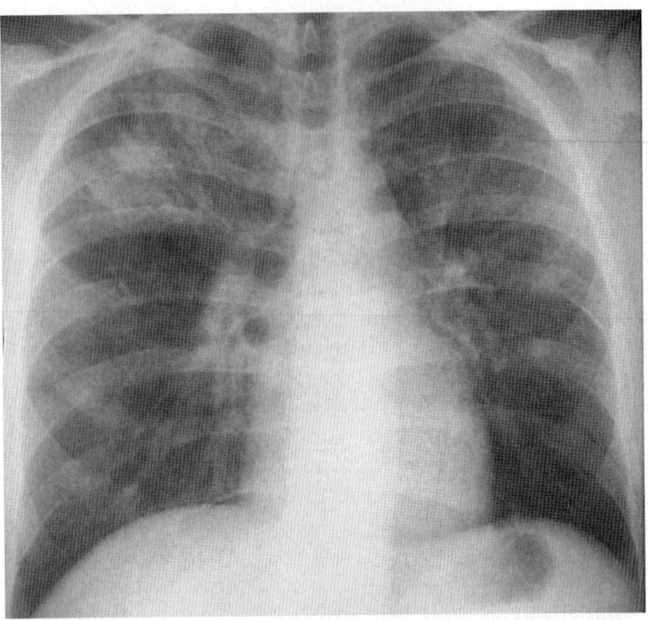

FIGURE 37-3. *Pneumocystis jiroveci (carinii)* pneumonia with mixed interstitial and alveolar opacities, ground-glass appearance.

A significant number of new infections with HIV are occurring in women of childbearing age. **As of 1995, more than 80% of women with AIDS were of reproductive age. PJP pneumonia is the most common cause of AIDS-related death in the United States.** Literature on PJP in pregnancy is scarce. A report describes five cases of PJP in pregnancy and also reviews the literature.[45] **In this series of 22 pregnant women with PJP, 11 patients (50%) died of pneumonia. The incidence of respiratory failure in this series was 59%.** In individuals who required mechanical ventilation, the survival rate was 31%. The average gestational age was 25 weeks, with a range of 6 weeks' gestation up to 1 week postpartum. Fifteen of the 22 patients had CD4$^+$ counts performed, and the mean was 93 cells/mm^3. The patients in this series were treated with a variety of regimens, including trimethoprim-sulfamethoxazole alone, trimethoprim-sulfamethoxazole and steroids, and pentamidine. Six patients received trimethoprim-sulfamethoxazole alone, and six were given trimethoprim-sulfamethoxazole and steroids; four patients (66%) survived in each group. Only 12 babies survived; there were five stillbirths, and four neonates died shortly after birth. In this series, **PJP pneumonia complicating**

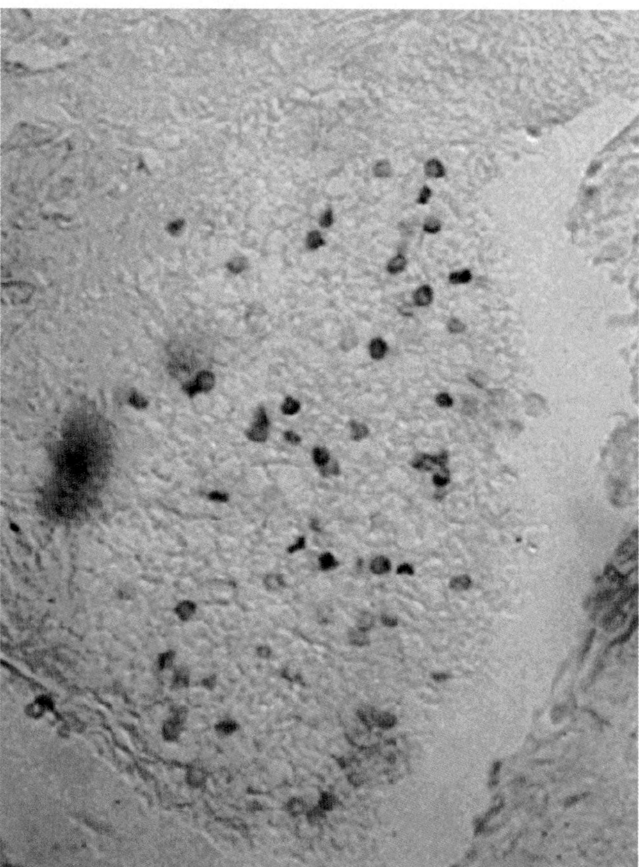

FIGURE 37-4. Wright-Giemsa stain of *Pneumocystis jiroveci (carinii)* pneumonia.

pregnancy in the third trimester had a better maternal and fetal outcome compared with disease in the first or second trimester. There was also a suggestion that treatment with trimethoprim-sulfamethoxazole with or without steroids was associated with an increased survival rate.[45]

The high mortality rate in this series may be skewed by the fact that this is a retrospective review, and severe cases are more likely to be reported than mild ones. In addition, all the women in this series were unaware of their HIV infection until the diagnosis of PJP was made. Therefore, none had received PJP prophylaxis.[45]

In summary, PJP pneumonia remains a dreaded complication of HIV infection and an AIDS-defining illness. There is a very high maternal and fetal mortality rate when PJP complicates pregnancy. **Primary prophylaxis against PJP with trimethoprim-sulfamethoxazole in HIV-infected adults, including pregnant women and patients receiving highly active antiretroviral therapy (HAART), should begin when the CD4$^+$ count is less than 200 cells/mm^3 or there is a history of oropharyngeal candidiasis**[46] (see Chapter 50). Prophylaxis should be discontinued when the CD4$^+$ cell count increases to more than 200 cells/mm^3 for a period of 3 months.[44] The use of HAART, as well as prophylaxis with trimethoprim-sulfamethoxazole, may decrease the incidence of PJP pneumonia in developed countries. However, many countries worldwide do not have the resources for HAART and, therefore, remain a reservoir for infection with PJP.

TABLE 37-1 HIGH-RISK FACTORS FOR TUBERCULOSIS

- Close contact with persons known or suspected to have tuberculosis
- Medical risk factors known to increase risk for disease if infected
- Birth in a country with a high tuberculosis prevalence
- Medically underserved status
- Low income
- Alcohol addiction
- Intravenous drug use
- Residency in a long-term care facility (e.g., correctional institution, mental institution, nursing home or facility)
- Health professionals working in high-risk health care facilities

TABLE 37-2 CLINICAL RISK FACTORS FOR DEVELOPING ACTIVE TUBERCULOSIS

- HIV infection
- Recent tuberculosis infection
- Injection drug use
- Silicosis
- Solid organ transplantation
- Chronic renal failure
- Jejunoileal bypass
- Diabetes mellitus
- Carcinoma of head or neck
- Underweight by >15%
- Human immunodeficiency virus infection

TUBERCULOSIS IN PREGNANCY

The incidence of TB in the United States began to decline in the early part of the 20th century and fell steadily until 1953, when the introduction of isoniazid led to a dramatic decrease in the number of cases, from 84,000 cases in 1953 to 22,255 cases in 1984.[47] However, since 1984, there have been significant changes in TB morbidity trends. **From 1985 through 1991, reported cases of TB increased by 18%, representing about 39,000 more cases than expected had the previous downward trend continued. This increase is due to many factors, including the HIV epidemic, deterioration in the health care infrastructure, and significantly more cases among immigrants.**[47] **The emergence of drug-resistant TB has also become a serious concern. In New York City, in 1991, 33% of TB cases were resistant to at least one drug, and 19% were resistant to both isoniazid (INH) and rifampin (RIF).**[48] Between 1985 and 1992, the number of TB cases in women of childbearing age increased by 40%.[47] One report noted TB-complicated pregnancies in 94.8 cases per 100,000 deliveries between 1991 and 1992.[49,50]

Diagnosis

Most gravidas diagnosed with TB in pregnancy are asymptomatic. The American Thoracic Society and the Centers for Disease Control and Prevention issued a statement on targeted tuberculin testing for latent tuberculosis infection (LTBI).[51] This is a strategic component of TB control that identifies persons at high risk for developing TB who would benefit by treatment of LTBI, if detected. **Persons at risk include those who have had recent infection with TB and those who have clinical conditions that are associated with an increased risk for progression of LTBI to active TB** (Tables 37-1 and 37-2).

All gravidas at high risk for TB should be screened with subcutaneous administration of intermediate-strength purified protein derivative (PPD).[52] If anergy is suspected, control antigens such as candida, mumps, or tetanus toxoids should also be placed. **The sensitivity of the PPD is 90% to 99% for exposure to TB. The tine test is not recommended for screening because of its low sensitivity.**

The onset of the recent TB epidemic stimulated the need for rapid diagnostic tests using molecular biology methods to detect *Mycobacterium tuberculosis* in clinical specimens. **Two direct amplification tests (DATs) have been approved by the FDA: the *Mycobacterium tuberculosis* Direct test (MTD; Gen-Probe, San Diego, CA) and the Amplicor *Mycobacterium tuberculosis* (Amplicor MTB) test (Roche Diagnostic Systems, Branchburg, NJ).**[53] Both tests amplify and detect *M. tuberculosis* 16S ribosomal DNA. When testing acid-fast stain smear-negative respiratory specimens, the specificity remains greater than 95%, but the sensitivity ranges from 40% to 77%.[53,54] **To date, these tests are FDA approved only for testing acid-fast stain smear-positive respiratory specimens obtained from untreated patients or those who have received no more than 7 days of anti-TB therapy.** The PPD remains the most commonly used screening test for TB. **Three cutoff levels have been recommended for defining a positive tuberculin reaction: greater than 5 mm, greater than 10 mm, and 15 mm or more induration** (Figure 37-5). **Induration of greater than 5 mm is a positive reaction in individuals with highest risk for conversion to active TB.** That includes individuals who are HIV positive, recent contacts with persons infected with TB, fibrotic changes on chest radiograph consistent with prior TB, and organ transplant recipients and other immunosuppressed persons[51] (see Table 37-2).

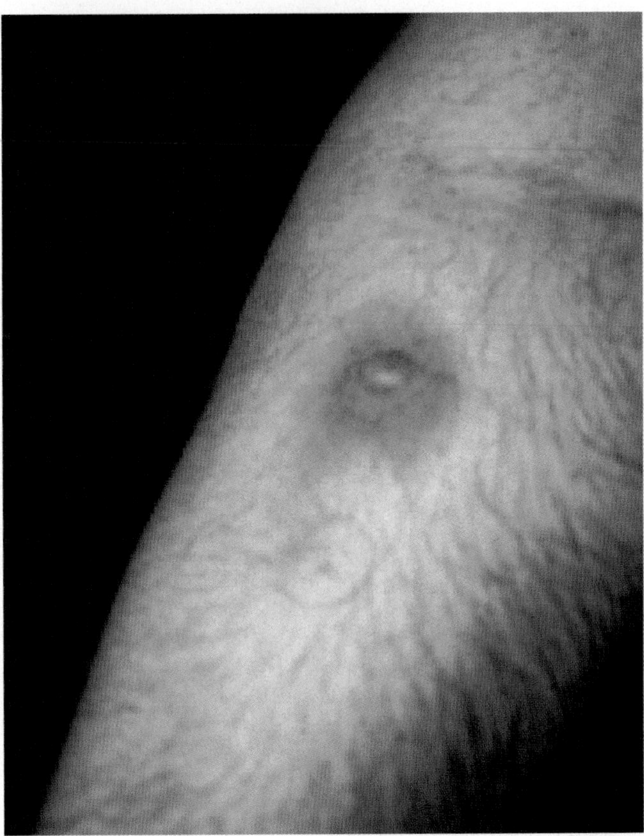

FIGURE 37-5. Positive PPD, induration greater than 10 mm. *PPD,* purified protein derivative.

Immigrants from areas where TB is endemic may have received the Bacille Calmette-Guérin (BCG) vaccine. Such individuals likely have a positive response to the PPD. However, this reactivity should wane over time. Therefore, the PPD should be used to screen these patients for TB unless their skin tests are known to be positive. **If the BCG vaccine was given 10 years earlier and the PPD is positive with a skin test reaction of 10 mm or more, that individual should be considered infected with TB and managed accordingly.**[55]

Women with a positive PPD skin test must be evaluated for active TB with a thorough physical examination for extrapulmonary disease and a chest radiograph once they are beyond the first trimester. **Symptoms of active TB include cough (74%), weight loss (41%), fever (30%), malaise and fatigue (30%), and hemoptysis (19%).**[56] Individuals with active pulmonary TB may have radiographic findings including adenopathy, multinodular infiltrates, cavitation, loss of volume in the upper lobes, and upper medial retraction of hilar markings (Figure 37-6). **The finding of acid-fast bacilli in early-morning sputum specimens confirms the diagnosis of pulmonary TB.** At least three first-morning sputum samples should be examined for the presence of acid-fast bacilli. If sputum cannot be produced, sputum-induction, gastric washings, diagnostic bronchoscopy, or PTNA may be indicated.

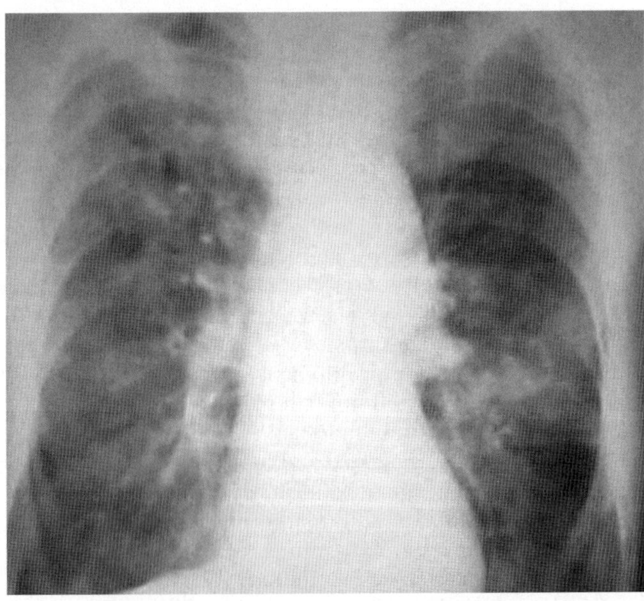

FIGURE 37-6. Pulmonary tuberculosis.

Extrapulmonary TB occurs in up to 16% of cases in the United States; however, in patients with AIDS, the pattern may occur in 60% to 70%.[57] Extrapulmonary sites include lymph nodes, bone, kidneys, and breasts. Extrapulmonary TB appears to be rare in pregnancy. **Extrapulmonary TB that is confined to the lymph nodes has no effect on obstetrical outcome, but TB at other extrapulmonary sites does adversely affect the outcome of pregnancy.**[58] Rarely, mycobacteria invade the uteroplacental circulation, and

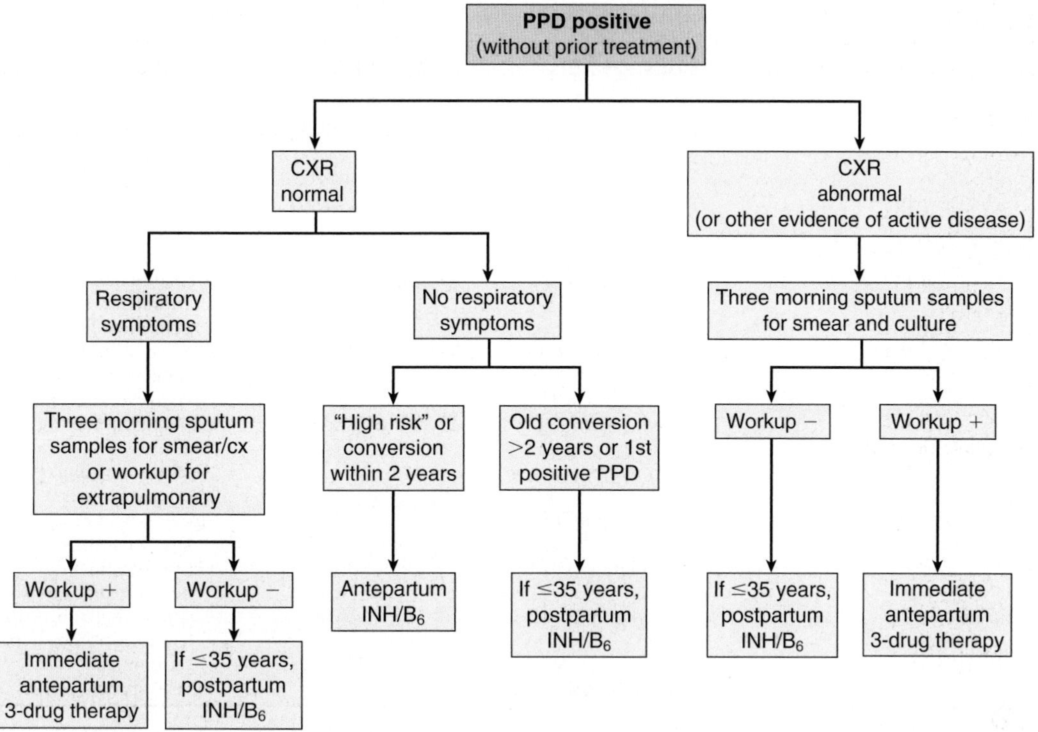

FIGURE 37-7. Algorithm for the management of positive purified protein derivative (PPD). *CX,* Culture; *CXR,* chest x-ray.

congenital TB results.[49] **The diagnosis of congenital TB is based on one of the following factors: (1) demonstration of primary hepatic complex or cavitating hepatic granuloma by percutaneous liver biopsy at birth; (2) infection of the maternal genital tract or placenta; (3) lesions noted in the first week of life; or (4) exclusion of the possibility of postnatal transmission by a thorough investigation of all contacts, including attendants.**[49]

Prevention

Most gravidas with a positive PPD in pregnancy are asymptomatic with no evidence of active disease and, therefore, are classified as having LTBI. The risk for progression to active disease is highest in the first 2 years of conversion. It is important to prevent the onset of active disease while minimizing maternal and fetal risk. An algorithm for management of the positive PPD is presented in Figure 37-7. In women with a **known recent conversion (2 years) to a positive PPD and no evidence of active disease, the recommended prophylaxis is INH, 300 mg/day, starting after the first trimester and continuing for 6 to 9 months. INH should be accompanied by pyridoxine (vitamin B_6) supplementation, 50 mg/day, to prevent the peripheral neuropathy that is associated with INH treatment.** Women with an unknown or prolonged duration of PPD positivity **(>2 years)** should receive INH, 300 mg/day, for 6 to 9 months after delivery. **INH prophylaxis is not recommended for women older than 35 years who have an unknown or prolonged PPD positivity in the absence of active disease.** The use of INH is discouraged in this group because of an **increased risk for hepatotoxicity. INH is associated with hepatitis in both pregnant and nonpregnant adults. The risk for liver inflammation in pregnancy from INH use is rare, and therefore, this therapy should be instituted when the risk for conversion to active disease is high.**[56] **Monthly monitoring of liver function tests may prevent this adverse outcome. Among individuals receiving INH, 10% to 20% develop mildly elevated liver function tests. These changes resolve once the drug is discontinued.**

Treatment

The gravida with active TB should be treated initially with INH, 300 mg/day, combined with RIF, 600 mg/day (Table 37-3).[59] Resistant disease results from initial infection with resistant strains (33%) or can develop during therapy. **If resistance to INH is identified or anticipated, ethambutol, 2.5 g/day, should be added, and the treatment period should be extended to 18 months.**[59] **Ethambutol is teratogenic in animals; however, this has not been demonstrated in humans. The most common side effect of ethambutol therapy is optic neuritis. Streptomycin should be avoided during pregnancy because it is associated with eighth nerve damage in neonates.**[60] **Antituberculous agents not recommended for use in pregnancy include ethionamide, streptomycin, capreomycin, kanamycin, cycloserine, and pyrazinamide. However, recent case reports documenting use of the above-mentioned antituberculous agents in pregnancy have revealed no adverse fetal or neonatal effects.** There were no congenital abnormalities, and pregnancy outcome in the individuals treated was good.[61,62] **Untreated TB has been associated with higher morbidity and mortality among pregnant women.** Therefore, the management of the gravida with multidrug-resistant TB should be individualized. The patient should be counseled about the small risk for teratogenicity, and the increased risk for maternal and fetal morbidity and mortality from

TABLE 37-3 ANTITUBERCULOSIS DRUGS

DRUG	DOSAGE FORM	DAILY DOSE	WEEKLY DOSE	MAJOR ADVERSE REACTIONS
First-Line Drugs (for Initial Treatment)				
Isoniazid	PO, IM	10 mg/kg up to 300 mg	15 mg/kg up to 900 mg	Hepatic enzyme elevation, peripheral neuropathy hepatitis, hypersensitivity
Rifampin	PO	10 mg/kg up to 600 mg	10 mg/kg up to 600 mg	Orange discoloration of secretions and urine, nausea, vomiting, hepatitis, febrile reaction, purpura (rare)
Pyrazinamide	PO	15-30 mg/kg up to 2 g	50-70 mg/kg	Hepatotoxicity, hyperuricemia, arthralgias, skin rash, gastrointestinal upset
Ethambutol	PO	15 mg/kg up to 2.5 g	50 mg/kg	Optic neuritis (decreased red-green color discrimination, decreased visual acuity), skin rash
Streptomycin	IM	15 mg/kg up to 1 g	25-30 mg/kg up to 1 g	Ototoxicity, nephrotoxicity
Second-Line Drugs (Daily Therapy)				
Capreomycin	IM	15-30 mg/kg up to 1 g		Auditory, vestibular, and renal toxicity
Kanamycin	IM	15-30 mg/kg up to 1 g		Auditory and renal toxicity, rare vestibular toxicity
Ethionamide	PO	15-20 mg/kg up to 1 g		Gastrointestinal disturbance, hepatotoxicity, hypersensitivity
Para-aminosalicylic acid	PO	150 mg/kg up to 1 g		Gastrointestinal disturbance, hypersensitivity, hepatotoxicity, sodium load
Cycloserine	PO	15-20 mg/kg up to 1 g		Psychosis, convulsions, rash

IM, intramuscular; *PO*, by mouth.

progression of disease when treatment is delayed. **The risk for postpartum transmission of TB to the baby may be higher among those born to patients with drug-resistant TB.[62] Therefore, in patients with active disease at the time of delivery, separation of the mother and newborn should be accomplished to prevent infection of the newborn.**

Women who are being treated with antituberculous drugs may breastfeed. Only 0.75% to 2.3% of INH and 0.05% of RIF is excreted into breast milk. Ethambutol excretion into breast milk is also minimal. However, if the infant is concurrently taking oral antituberculous therapy, excessive drug levels may be reached in the neonate, and breastfeeding should be avoided. **Breastfed infants of women taking INH therapy should receive a multivitamin supplement including pyridoxine.[13] Neonates of women taking antituberculous therapy should have a PPD skin test at birth and again at 3 months of age. Infants born to women with active TB at the time of delivery should receive INH prophylaxis (10 mg/kg per day) until maternal disease has been inactive for 3 months,** as evidenced by negative maternal sputum cultures. Active TB in the neonate should be treated appropriately with INH and RIF immediately upon diagnosis or with multiagent therapy should drug-resistant organisms be identified. **Infants and children who are at high risk for intimate and prolonged exposure to untreated or ineffectively treated persons should receive the BCG vaccine.**

Summary

In summary, high-risk gravidas should be screened for TB and treated appropriately with INH prophylaxis for infection without overt disease and with dual antituberculous therapy for active disease. In addition, the newborn should be screened for evidence of TB as well. Proper screening and therapy will result in a good outcome for mother and fetus in most cases.

ASTHMA IN PREGNANCY

About 8% of pregnancies are complicated by asthma; it may be the most common potentially serious medical condition to complicate pregnancy. In general, the prevalence and morbidity from asthma are increasing, although asthma mortality has decreased in recent years. Asthma is characterized by chronic airway inflammation with increased airway responsiveness to a variety of stimuli and airway obstruction that is partially or completely reversible. Insight into the pathogenesis of asthma has changed with the recognition that airway inflammation is present in nearly all cases. **Current medical management for asthma emphasizes treatment of airway inflammation to decrease airway responsiveness and prevent asthma symptoms. The National Asthma Education and Prevention Program (NAEPP) has found that "it is safer for pregnant women with asthma to be treated with asthma medications than it is for them to have asthma symptoms and exacerbations."[63]**

Diagnosis

The enlarging uterus elevates the diaphragm about 4 cm with a reduction of the functional residual capacity. However, there are no clinically significant alterations in forced vital capacity, peak expiratory flow rate (PEFR), or forced expiratory volume in 1 second (FEV_1) in normal pregnancy.

Diagnosis of asthma in pregnancy is no different than for a nonpregnant patient. Asthma typically includes characteristic symptoms (wheezing, chest cough, shortness of

TABLE 37-4 CLASSIFICATION OF ASTHMA SEVERITY AND CONTROL IN PREGNANT PATIENTS

ASTHMA CONTROL*	WELL CONTROLLED	NOT WELL CONTROLLED		VERY POORLY CONTROLLED
Asthma severity†	Mild intermittent	Mild persistent	Moderate persistent	Severe persistent
Symptom frequency, albuterol use	≤2 days per week	>2 days per week, but not daily	Daily symptoms	Throughout the day
Nighttime awakening	≤2 times per month	>2 times per month	>1 time per week	≥4 times per week
Interference with normal activity	None	Minor limitation	Some limitation	Extremely limited
FEV_1 or peak flow (% predicted/ personal best)	>80%	>80%	60% to 80%	<60%

*Assess in patients on long-term-control medications to determine whether step-up, step-down, or no change in therapy is indicated.
†Assess severity in patients who are not on long-term-control medications; see Table 37-5 to determine starting controller therapy based on severity.

breath, chest tightness), temporal relationships (fluctuating intensity, worse at night), and triggers (e.g., allergens, exercise, infections). Wheezing on auscultation would support the diagnosis, but its absence does not exclude the diagnosis. Ideally, the diagnosis of asthma would be confirmed by demonstrating airway obstruction on spirometry that is at least partially reversible, greater than 12% increase in FEV_1 after inhalation of albuterol.[64,65] However, reversible airway obstruction may not be demonstrable in some patients with asthma. In patients with a clinical picture consistent with asthma in whom reversible airway obstruction cannot be demonstrated, a trial of asthma therapy is reasonable. In such patients, a positive response to asthma therapy can establish the presumptive diagnosis during pregnancy. If methacholine testing is deemed necessary to confirm asthma, it should be delayed until postpartum.[64]

In patients presenting with new respiratory symptoms during pregnancy, the most common differential diagnosis would be dyspnea of pregnancy. Dyspnea (breathlessness) of pregnancy can usually be differentiated from asthma by its lack of cough, wheezing, chest tightness, or airway obstruction. Other differential diagnosis considerations include gastroesophageal reflux, chronic cough from postnasal drip, and bronchitis.

In 2004, the NAEPP defined mild intermittent, mild persistent, moderate persistent, and severe persistent asthma according to daytime and nighttime symptoms (wheezing, cough, or dyspnea) and objective tests of pulmonary function.[63] The most commonly used pulmonary function parameters are the PEFR and FEV_1. Current NAEPP guidelines suggest classifying degree of asthma *severity* in patients not on controller medication and degree of asthma *control* in patients on controller medication (Table 37-4).[65] Pregnant patients who have mild asthma by symptoms and pulmonary function, but who required regular medications to control their asthma, have been found to be similar to those with moderate asthma with respect to asthma exacerbations; those requiring regular systemic corticosteroids to control asthma symptoms were similar to severe asthma patients with respect to exacerbations.[66]

Effects of Pregnancy on Asthma

Asthma during pregnancy has been associated with considerable maternal morbidity. In a large prospective study, the effects of pregnancy on asthma were found to be variable, 23% improved and 30% become worse during pregnancy.[66] Women with mild asthma had an exacerbation rate of 12.6% and hospitalization rate of 2.3%; those with moderate asthma had an exacerbation rate of 25.7% and hospitalization rate of 6.8%; and those with severe asthma had an exacerbation rate of 51.9% and hospitalization rate of 26.9%.[66]

Effects of Asthma on Pregnancy

Compared with women without a history of asthma, women with asthma have been reported to have higher risks for several complications of pregnancy, including preeclampsia, preterm birth, low birthweight or intrauterine growth restriction, and perinatal mortality, even after adjustment for potential confounders.[67] A significant increase in congenital malformations has been associated with exacerbations during the first trimester.[68] Although residual confounding or common pathogenetic factors may explain some of these associations, observational data showing strong associations between poor asthma control (based on symptoms, pulmonary function, or exacerbations) and these increased risks suggest potential benefits of improved asthma control in pregnancy in terms of improved pregnancy outcomes.[67,69-71]

Prospective studies of the effects of asthma during pregnancy have generally had excellent perinatal outcomes.[69,72-79] Preterm birth before 37 weeks' gestation was increased among patients with asthma who had severe disease or required oral corticosteroids, preeclampsia and growth restriction was increased among those with daily symptoms, and the rate of cesarean delivery was increased among those with moderate or severe asthma.[69,77]

Although these studies show that the gravida with mild or moderate asthma can have excellent maternal and perinatal outcomes, there are important caveats when interpreting them. Prospective studies have tended to find fewer significant adverse associations, possibly because of better asthma surveillance and treatment. **The excellent maternal and perinatal outcomes were achieved at centers that tended to actively manage asthma in pregnancy.** In addition, women who enroll in research studies tend to be more compliant and better motivated than the general public. The lack of finding more adverse outcomes among women with severe asthma may also be a function of the relatively small numbers of this cohort and the resulting lack of power to find adverse outcomes that were statistically significant. Nonetheless, these prospective studies are reassuring in their consensus of good pregnancy outcomes among women with asthma. However, they do not suggest that asthma should be considered to be a benign condition because active asthma management was a part of these studies and may have positively affected outcomes.

These findings do not contradict the possibility that suboptimal control of asthma during pregnancy is associated with increased risk to the mother or baby.[77] In fact, a significant relationship has been reported between lower FEV_1 during pregnancy and increased risk for low birthweight and prematurity.[80]

ASTHMA MANAGEMENT

The ultimate goal of asthma therapy during pregnancy is to maintain adequate oxygenation of the fetus by prevention of hypoxic episodes in the mother. Other goals include achievement of minimal or no maternal symptoms day or night, minimal or no exacerbations, no limitations of activities, maintenance of normal or near-normal pulmonary function, minimal use of albuterol, and minimal or no adverse effects from medications. Consultation or comanagement with an asthma specialist is appropriate, as indicated, for evaluation of the role of allergy and irritants, complete pulmonary function studies, or evaluation of the medication plan if there are difficulties in achieving the goals of therapy or the patient has severe asthma. A team approach is helpful if more than one clinician is managing the asthma and the pregnancy. **The effective management of asthma during pregnancy relies on four integral components: objective measures for assessment and monitoring, patient education, avoidance or control of asthma triggers, and pharmacologic therapy.**

Objective Measures for Assessment and Monitoring

Subjective measures of lung function by either the patient or physician can be an insensitive and inaccurate assessment of airway hyper-responsiveness, airway obstruction, and asthma severity. **The FEV_1 following a maximal inspiration is the single best measure of pulmonary function.** When adjusted for confounders, a mean FEV_1 lower than 80% predicted has been found to be significantly associated with increased preterm delivery before 32 weeks and before 37 weeks, and birthweight less than 2500 g.[80] However, measurement of FEV_1 requires a spirometer. **The PEFR correlates well with the FEV_1 and has the advantages that it can be measured reliably with inexpensive, disposable, portable peak flow meters.**

Patient self-monitoring of PEFR provides valuable insight to the course of asthma and helps detect early signs of deterioration so that timely therapy can be instituted. Patients with persistent asthma should be evaluated at least monthly, and those with moderate to severe asthma should have daily home PEFR monitoring.[63] The typical PEFR in pregnancy should be 380 to 550 L/minute. The pregnant woman should establish her "personal best" PEFR, then calculate her individualized PEFR zones: green zone, greater than 80% of personal best; yellow zone, 50% to 80% of personal best; and red zone, less than 50% of personal best PEFR.

Patient Education

The patient should be made aware that controlling asthma during pregnancy is especially important for the well-being of the fetus. She should have a basic understanding of the medical management of asthma during pregnancy, including self-monitoring of PEFRs and the correct use of inhalers. She should be instructed on proper PEFR technique: make the measurement while standing, take a maximal inspiration, and note the reading on the peak flow meter. Women who smoke should be encouraged to quit; active smoking, but not passive smoking, has been associated with increased asthma symptoms and fetal growth abnormalities.[81] Women should also be instructed to avoid and control other asthma triggers. **The importance of adherence to treatment should be stressed.**

Avoidance or Control of Asthma Triggers

Limiting adverse environmental exposures during pregnancy is important for controlling asthma. Irritants and allergens that provoke acute symptoms also increase airway inflammation and hyper-responsiveness. Avoiding or controlling such triggers can reduce asthma symptoms, airway hyper-responsiveness, and the need for medical therapy.[65] Association of asthma with allergies is common; 75% to 85% of patients with asthma have positive skin tests to common allergens, including animal dander, house dust mites, cockroach antigens, pollens, and molds. Other common nonimmunologic triggers include tobacco smoke, strong odors, air pollutants, food additives such as sulfites, and certain drugs including aspirin and ß-blockers. Another trigger can be strenuous physical activity. For some patients, exercise-induced asthma can be avoided with inhalation of albuterol, 10 to 30 minutes before exercise.

Specific measures for avoiding asthma triggers include using allergen-impermeable mattress and pillow covers, removing carpeting, weekly washing of bedding in hot water, avoiding tobacco smoke, inhibiting mite and mold growth by reducing humidity, and leaving the house when it is vacuumed. Ideal animal dander control involves removing the pet from the home; allergic women should at least keep furry pets out of the bedroom. Cockroaches can be controlled by poison baits or traps and eliminating exposed food or garbage.

The use of allergen immunotherapy, or "allergy shots," has been shown to be effective in improving asthma in allergic patients.[65] However, anaphylaxis is a risk for allergy injections, especially early in the course of immunotherapy when the dose is being escalated, and anaphylaxis during pregnancy has been associated with fetal and maternal death. In a patient who is receiving a maintenance or near-maintenance dose, not experiencing adverse reactions to the injections, and apparently deriving clinical benefit, continuation of immunotherapy is recommended.[63] In such patients, a dose reduction may be considered to further decrease the chance of anaphylaxis. Risk-benefit considerations do not usually favor *beginning* allergy shots during pregnancy.

Pharmacologic Therapy

Medications for asthma are divided into long-term controllers that prevent asthma manifestations (inhaled corticosteroids, long-acting β-agonists, leukotriene modifiers, and theophylline) and rescue therapy to provide quick relief of symptoms, primarily albuterol.

Women who have previously been prescribed asthma medications should be asked about their use to classify their current level of therapy according to a stepped care approach (Table 37-5) and to assess potential adherence problems and barriers. Adherence to inhaled corticosteroids has been reported to be poor in many studies. For example, reported adherence rates were about 50% in one study of asthmatic adults; decreased adherence was associated with an increased frequency of asthma exacerbations in this study.[82] **Women with asthma have been reported to decrease their inhaled corticosteroid use during early pregnancy compared to their prepregnancy use, which may be due to their reported concern regarding the safety of inhaled corticosteroids during pregnancy.** Moreover, a substantial proportion of asthma exacerbations during pregnancy have been associated with nonadherence to inhaled corticosteroids.[71] In addition to assessing adherence, asking about past medications and their effectiveness and any side effects can help guide subsequent management decisions.

The goals of asthma therapy include relieving bronchospasm, protecting the airways from irritant stimuli, mitigating pulmonary and inflammatory response to an allergen exposure, and resolving the inflammatory process in the airways, leading to improved pulmonary function with reduced airway hyper-responsiveness. It is safer for pregnant women with asthma to be treated with asthma medications than it is for them to have asthma symptoms and exacerbations.[63] Current pharmacologic therapy emphasizes treatment of airway inflammation in order to decrease airway hyper-responsiveness and prevent asthma symptoms. Typical dosages of commonly used asthma medications are listed in Table 37-6. Low, medium, and high doses of inhaled corticosteroid are presented in Table 37-7. The step-care therapeutic approach uses the least amount of drug intervention necessary to control a patient's severity of asthma.

Step Therapy

The step-care therapeutic approach increases the number and frequency of medications with increasing asthma severity.[63,65] Based on clinical trials in patients of varying degrees of severity, medications (see Table 37-5) are considered to

TABLE 37-5 STEP THERAPY MEDICAL MANAGEMENT OF ASTHMA DURING PREGNANCY

STEP	ASTHMA SEVERITY AND MEDICATIONS*
1. No daily medications; albuterol as needed	Mild intermittent
2. Low-dose inhaled corticosteroid (alternative: LTRA or theophylline†)	Mild persistent
3. Medium-dose inhaled corticosteroid (alternative: low-dose inhaled corticosteroid and LABA, LTRA, or theophylline†)‡	Moderate persistent
4. Medium-dose inhaled corticosteroid and LABA (alternative: medium-dose inhaled corticosteroid plus LTRA, or theophylline†)	Moderate persistent
5. High-dose inhaled corticosteroid and LABA	Severe persistent
6. High-dose inhaled corticosteroid and LABA and oral prednisone	Severe persistent

*Starting therapy for a specific level of severity (NAEP, 2004; NAEP, 2007).
†Theophylline (serum level, 5-12 mcg/mL).
‡We have modified step 3 to reflect the choice of a medium-dose inhaled corticosteroid over a low-dose inhaled corticosteroid plus LABA because of the lack of safety data on the use of LABA during pregnancy.

TABLE 37-6 TYPICAL DOSAGES OF ASTHMA MEDICATIONS:

Albuterol MDI	2-4 puffs every 4-6 hours as needed
Salmeterol DPI	1 blister 2 times/day
Formoterol	1 capsule 2 times/day
Fluticasone/salmeterol (Advair) DPI	1 inhalation 2 times/day; strength (100, 250, 500) depends on severity of asthma
Montelukast	10-mg tablet at night
Zafirlukast	20-mg tablet twice daily
Prednisone	5-60 mg/day for active symptoms or maintenance therapy for severe asthma
Theophylline	Start 200 mg 2 times/day orally, target serum levels of 5-12 mcg/mL (decrease dosage by half if treated with erythromycin or cimetidine)
Ipratropium MDI	2-3 puffs every 6 hr

DPI, Dry-powder inhaler; *MDI*, metered-dose inhaler.

TABLE 37-7 COMPARATIVE DAILY DOSES* FOR INHALED CORTICOSTEROIDS

		LOW DOSE	MEDIUM DOSE	HIGH DOSE
Beclomethasone HFA	40 mcg/puff	2-6 puffs	>6-12 puffs	>12 puffs
	80 mcg/puff	1-3 puffs	>3-6 puffs	>6 puffs
Budesonide	180 mcg/inhalation	1-3 puffs	>3-6 puffs	>6 puffs
Flunisolide	250 mcg/puff	2-4 puffs	5-8 puffs	>8 puffs
Fluticasone HFA	44 mcg/puff	2-6 puffs		
	110 mcg/puff	2 puffs	3-4 puffs	>4 puffs
	220 mcg/puff	1 puff	2 puffs	>2 puffs
Fluticasone DPI	50 mcg/inhalation	2-6 puffs		
	100 mcg/inhalation	1-3 puffs	4-5 puffs	>5 puffs
	250 mcg/inhalation	1 puff	2 puffs	>2 puffs
Mometasone	200 mcg/inhalation	1 puff	2 puffs	>2 puffs
Triamcinolone	75 mcg/puff	4-10 puffs	11-20 puffs	>20 puffs

Modified from National Asthma Education and Prevention Program Full Report of the Expert Panel: Guidelines for the Diagnosis and Management of Asthma, 2007.
*Note that total daily puffs is usually divided as a twice-a-day regimen.
HFA, Hydrofluoroalkane.

be "preferred" or "alternative" at each step of therapy. Patients not optimally responding to treatment should be stepped up to more intensive medical therapy. Patients with not well-controlled asthma (see Table 37-4) should generally be stepped up one step, and those with very poorly controlled asthma (see Table 37-4) should be stepped up two steps. Once control is achieved and sustained for several months, a step-down approach can be considered but should be undertaken cautiously and gradually to avoid compromising the stability of the asthma control. For some patients, it may be prudent to postpone until after birth attempts to reduce therapy that is effectively controlling the patient's asthma.[63] In the case of a patient who had a favorable response to an alternative drug before becoming pregnant, it would be appropriate to maintain the therapy that successfully controlled the patient's asthma before pregnancy. However, when initiating new treatment for asthma during pregnancy, preferred medications should be considered first, rather than alternative treatment options.[63]

Patients with asthma exacerbations may require oral corticosteroids. In such cases, a short course of oral prednisone, 40 to 60 mg of prednisone per day in a single or two divided doses for 3 to 10 days, is recommended.[65]

Inhaled Corticosteroids

Inhaled corticosteroids are the preferred treatment for the management of all levels of persistent asthma during pregnancy.[63] Airway inflammation is present in nearly all cases; therefore, inhaled corticosteroids have been advocated as first-line therapy, even for patients with mild persistent asthma. The use of inhaled corticosteroids among nonpregnant asthmatic patients has been associated with a marked reduction in fatal and near-fatal asthma. Inhaled corticosteroids produce clinically important improvements in bronchial hyper-responsiveness that appear dose related, including prevention of increased bronchial hyper-responsiveness after seasonal exposure to an allergen.

In a prospective observational study of 504 pregnant subjects with asthma, 177 patients were not initially treated with inhaled corticosteroids (budesonide or beclomethasone).[75] This cohort had a 17% acute exacerbation rate compared with only a 4% rate among those treated with inhaled corticosteroids from the start of pregnancy. Randomized controlled trials with pregnant patients have shown that inhaled beclomethasone is more effective than theophylline in improving pulmonary function,[78] and that prescribing inhaled beclomethasone in addition to oral corticosteroids and inhaled β-agonists at the time of discharge after hospitalization for asthma reduces subsequent asthma readmissions compared with oral corticosteroids and inhaled β-agonists alone.[83]

The NAEPP Working Group reviewed 10 studies including 6113 patients who took inhaled corticosteroids during pregnancy for asthma.[63] **There was no evidence linking inhaled corticosteroid use to increases in congenital malformations or adverse perinatal outcomes.** Included among these studies was the Swedish Medical Birth Registry study that reported 2014 infants whose mothers had used inhaled budesonide in early pregnancy.[84] Because there are more data on using budesonide during pregnancy than on using other inhaled corticosteroids, the NAEPP considered budesonide to be the preferred inhaled corticosteroid for use during pregnancy. However, if a woman's asthma is well controlled by a different inhaled corticosteroid before pregnancy, it seems reasonable to continue that medication during pregnancy. All inhaled corticosteroids are currently labeled FDA pregnancy category C, except for budesonide, which is class B.

Inhaled β_2-Agonists

As-needed use of inhaled β_2-agonists is currently recommended for all levels of asthma during pregnancy.[63] Albuterol has a rapid onset of effect in the relief of acute bronchospasm through smooth muscle relaxation and is an excellent bronchoprotective agent for pretreatment before exercise. β_2-Agonists are associated with tremor, tachycardia, and palpitations. They do not block the development of airway hyper-responsiveness. **An increased frequency of bronchodilator use could be an indicator of the need for additional anti-inflammatory therapy.** Appropriate β_2-agonist use appears to be safe based on an NAEPP review of six published studies with 1599 women with asthma who took β_2-agonists during pregnancy.[63] Additionally, in a large prospective study, no significant relationship was found between the use of inhaled β_2-agonists (n = 1828) and adverse pregnancy outcomes.[85]

Salmeterol and formoterol are long-acting β-agonist (LABA) preparations. Data are lacking regarding the safety of LABAs during human pregnancy, although safety is considered likely based on the inhalational route and the generally reassuring data for short-acting β-agonists.[63] LABA should only be used in combination with inhaled corticosteroids during pregnancy. Long-acting β-agonists have been shown to be more effective than leukotriene receptor antagonists or theophylline as add-on therapy to inhaled corticosteroids.[65] The efficacy of these drugs during pregnancy is largely extrapolated from studies performed in nonpregnant patients.

Omalizumab

Omalizumab is a humanized monoclonal antibody to immunoglobulin E and is a Pregnancy Category B agent. An ongoing registry (sponsored by Genentech) of the use of omalizumab during pregnancy does not at this time have sufficient numbers to provide any definitive information. Because of the lack of safety data and potential risk of anaphylaxis, Omalizumab should not be initiated during pregnancy. A possible exception would be the patient who remains uncontrolled despite medical management presented in Table 37-5. However, it would seem reasonable to continue Omalizumab among women with severe asthma who become pregnant.

Theophylline

Theophylline is an alternative treatment for mild persistent asthma and an alternative add-on treatment for the step 3 or 4 management of moderate persistent asthma during pregnancy (see Table 37-5).[63] Subjective symptoms of adverse theophylline effects, including insomnia, heartburn, palpitations, and nausea, may be difficult to differentiate from typical pregnancy symptoms. High doses have been observed to cause jitteriness, tachycardia, and vomiting in mothers and neonates. **New dosing guidelines**

have recommended that serum theophylline concentrations be maintained at 5 to 12 mcg/mL during pregnancy.[63] Theophylline can have significant interactions with other drugs, which can cause decreased clearance with resultant toxicity; it may be appropriate to decrease the dosage of theophylline by half when the patient is treated with cimetidine, erythromycin, or azithromycin.[78] The main advantage of theophylline is the long duration of action, 10 to 12 hours with the use of sustained-release preparations, which is especially useful in the management of nocturnal asthma. Theophylline is only indicated for chronic therapy and is not effective for the treatment of acute exacerbations during pregnancy.

The NAEPP reviewed eight human studies that had a total of 660 women with asthma who took theophylline during pregnancy.[63] These studies and clinical experience confirm the safety of theophylline at a serum concentration of 5 to 12 mcg/mL during pregnancy. In a recent randomized controlled trial, there were no differences in asthma exacerbations or perinatal outcomes in a cohort receiving theophylline compared with the cohort receiving inhaled beclomethasone.[78] However, the theophylline cohort had significantly more reported side effects, discontinuation of study medication, and an increased proportion of those with an FEV_1 lower than 80% predicted.

Leukotriene Moderators

Leukotrienes are arachidonic acid metabolites that have been implicated in causing bronchospasm, mucous secretion, and increased vascular permeability. Bronchoconstriction associated with aspirin ingestion can be blocked by leukotriene receptor antagonists. Treatment with the leukotriene receptor antagonist montelukast has been shown to significantly improve pulmonary function as measured by FEV_1. The leukotriene receptor antagonists zafirlukast and montelukast are both pregnancy category B. Although human data are limited for leukotriene receptor antagonist use in pregnancy, their use has not been associated with an increase in congenital anomalies.[70,86] **Leukotriene modifiers are less effective as single agents than inhaled corticosteroids and less effective than LABA as add-on therapy.**[65]

Oral Corticosteroids

The NAEPP Working Group reviewed eight human studies of the use of oral corticosteroids during pregnancy, including one report of two meta-analyses.[63] Most subjects in these studies did not take oral corticosteroids for asthma, and the length, timing, and dose of exposure to the drug were not well described. The panel concluded that findings from the current evidence review were conflicting. Oral corticosteroid use during the first trimester of pregnancy was associated with a three-fold increased risk for isolated cleft lip with or without cleft palate. With a background incidence of about 0.1%, the excess risk attributable to oral steroids would thus be 0.2% to 0.3%.[87] Oral corticosteroid use during pregnancy in patients who have asthma has been associated with an increased incidence of preeclampsia, preterm delivery, and low birthweight.[69,73,85,87] A recent prospective study found that systemic corticosteroids resulted in a deficit of about 200 g in birthweight compared with nonasthmatic controls and asthmatic women exclusively treated with β_2-agonists.[70] However, it is difficult to separate the effects of the oral corticosteroids on these outcomes from the effects of severe or uncontrolled asthma.

Because of the uncertainties in these data and the definite risks of severe uncontrolled asthma to the mother and fetus, **the NAEPP Working Group recommends the use of oral corticosteroids when indicated for the long-term management of severe asthma or for exacerbations during pregnancy.**[63]

Management of Allergic Rhinitis and Gastroesophageal Reflux

Rhinitis, sinusitis, and gastroesophageal reflux may exacerbate asthma symptoms, and their management should be considered an integral aspect of asthma care. Intranasal corticosteroids are the most effective medications for control of allergic rhinitis. Loratadine (Claritin) and cetirizine (Zyrtec) are recommended second-generation antihistamines. Oral decongestant ingestion during the first trimester has been associated with gastroschisis; therefore, short-term (≤3 days) intranasal decongestants or intranasal corticosteroids should be considered before use of oral decongestants.[63] Controlling gastroesophageal reflux with acid reducers may improve asthma control.

ANTENATAL MANAGEMENT

In general, data are lacking to guide the optimal obstetrical management of the woman with asthma, and recommendations are based on extrapolation of data from other clinical settings and expert opinion. Women with asthma should be offered influenza vaccination as appropriate. Those with asthma that is not well controlled may benefit from increased fetal surveillance. Patients with moderate and severe asthma should be considered to be at risk for pregnancy complications. Adverse outcomes can be increased by underestimation of asthma severity and undertreatment of asthma. The first prenatal visit should include a detailed medical history with attention to coexisting medical conditions that could complicate the management of asthma, including rhinitis, sinusitis, reflux, or depression. The patient should be questioned about smoking history and the presence and severity of symptoms, episodes of nocturnal asthma, the number of days of work missed, and emergency care visits associated with asthma. Asthma severity or control should be determined (see Table 37-4). The type and amount of asthma medications, including the number of puffs of albuterol used each day, should be noted.

Gravidas with moderate or severe asthma should have scheduling of prenatal visits based on clinical judgment. In addition to routine care, monthly or more frequent evaluations of asthma history (emergency visits, hospital admissions, symptom frequency, symptom interference with sleep or activity, medications, dosages, and compliance) and pulmonary function (FEV_1 or PEFR) are recommended. Patients should be instructed on proper dosing and administration of their asthma medications.

Daily PEFR monitoring should be considered for patients with moderate to severe asthma, and especially for patients who have difficulty perceiving signs of worsening asthma.[63] It may be helpful to maintain an asthma diary containing daily assessment of asthma status, including peak flow measurements, symptoms and activity limitations, indication of any medical contacts initiated, and a record of regular and as-needed medications taken. Identifying and avoiding asthma triggers, especially smoking, can lead to improved maternal well-being with less need for medications. Specific recommendations can be made for appropriate environmental controls, based on the patient's history of exposure and, when available, results of blood or skin testing for immunoglobulin E–mediated sensitivity to inhalant allergen asthma triggers (see earlier).

Women with asthma that is not well controlled may benefit from additional fetal surveillance in the form of ultrasound examinations and antenatal fetal testing. Because asthma has been associated with intrauterine growth restriction (IUGR) and preterm birth, it is useful to establish pregnancy dating accurately by first-trimester ultrasound when possible. In the opinion of the Working Group,[63] the evaluation of fetal activity and growth by serial ultrasound examinations may be considered for women who have suboptimally controlled asthma, with moderate to severe asthma (starting at 32 weeks), and after recovery from a severe asthma exacerbation. The intensity of antenatal surveillance of fetal well-being should be considered on the basis of the severity of the asthma as well as any other high-risk features of the pregnancy that may be present. All patients should be instructed to be attentive to fetal activity.

Home Management of Asthma Exacerbations

An asthma exacerbation that causes minimal problems for the mother may have severe sequelae for the fetus. Therefore, asthma exacerbations in pregnancy should be optimally managed. Patients should be instructed on rescue management and educated to recognize signs and symptoms of early asthma exacerbations such as coughing, chest tightness, dyspnea, or wheezing, or by a 20% decrease in their PEFR. This is important so that prompt home rescue treatment may be instituted to avoid maternal and fetal hypoxia. In general, patients should use inhaled albuterol, 2 to 4 puffs every 20 minutes for up to 1 hour (Table 37-8). **A good response is considered if symptoms are resolved or become subjectively mild, normal activities can be resumed, and the PEFR is more than 80% of personal best.** The patient should seek further medical attention if the response is incomplete, or if fetal activity is decreased.

Hospital and Clinic Management of Asthma Exacerbations

The principal goal should be the prevention of hypoxia. Measurement of oxygenation through pulse oximetry is essential, and arterial blood gases may be obtained if oxygen saturation remains less than 95%. Chest radiographs are not commonly needed. **Continuous electronic fetal monitoring should be initiated if gestation has advanced to point of potential fetal viability. Albuterol (2.5 to 5 mg every 20 minutes for three doses, then 2.5 to 10 mg every 1 to 4 hours as needed, or 10 to 15 mg/hour continuously) should be delivered by nebulizer driven with oxygen.**[63]

TABLE 37-8 HOME MANAGEMENT OF ACUTE ASTHMA EXACERBATIONS*

Use albuterol MDI 2-4 puffs and measure PEFR.
Poor response:
PEFR is <50% predicted, or severe wheezing and shortness of breath, or decreased fetal movement, repeat albuterol 2-4 puffs by MDI and obtain emergency care.
Incomplete response:
PEFR is 50%-80% predicted or if persistent wheezing and shortness of breath, then repeat albuterol treatment 2-4 puffs MDI at 20-minute intervals up to two more times. If repeat PEFR 50%-80% predicted or if decreased fetal movement, contact caregiver or go for emergency care.
Good response:
PEFR is >80% predicted, no wheezing or shortness of breath, and fetus is moving normally. May continue inhaled albuterol 2-4 puffs MDI every 3-4 hours as needed

*Modified from NAEPP report (NAEPP, 2004).
MDI, Metered-dose inhaler; *PEFR*, peak expiratory flow rate.

Occasionally, nebulized treatment is not effective because the patient is moving air poorly; in such cases, terbutaline, 0.25 mg, can be administered subcutaneously every 20 minutes for three doses. The patient should be assessed for general level of activity, color, pulse rate, use of accessory muscles, and air flow obstruction determined by auscultation and FEV_1 or PEFR before and after each bronchodilator treatment. Guidelines for the management of asthma exacerbations are presented in Table 37-9. **For the treatment of acute exacerbations, prednisone, methylprednisolone, or prednisolone may be given, 40 to 80 mg per day in one or two divided doses.**[65] Consider adjunctive treatment such as magnesium sulfate in severe exacerbations if the patient is unresponsive to the initial treatments listed in Table 37-6.[65]

LABOR AND DELIVERY MANAGEMENT

Asthma medications should not be discontinued during labor and delivery. Although asthma is usually quiescent during labor, consideration should be given to assessing PEFR. The patient should be kept hydrated and should receive adequate analgesia to decrease the risk for bronchospasm. It is commonly recommended that women who currently or recently (during the previous 4 weeks) received systemic corticosteroids should be given intravenous corticosteroids (e.g., hydrocortisone, 100 mg every 8 hours) during labor and for the 24-hour period following delivery to prevent adrenal crisis.[63] An elective delivery should be postponed if the patient is having an exacerbation. It is rarely necessary to perform a cesarean delivery for an acute asthma exacerbation; maternal and fetal compromise usually responds to aggressive medical management.

Prostaglandin E_2 (PGE_2) or PGE_1 can be used for cervical ripening, the management of spontaneous or induced abortions, or postpartum hemorrhage, although the patient's respiratory status should be monitored.[64] **Carboprost (15-methyl $PGF_{2\alpha}$) and ergonovine and methylergonovine (Methergine) can cause bronchospasm.**[64] If tocolysis is needed, magnesium sulfate and terbutaline are preferable because they are bronchodilators; in contrast, indomethacin might induce bronchospasm in the aspirin-sensitive patient.[64] There are no reports of the use of calcium channel blockers for tocolysis among patients with

TABLE 37-9 EMERGENCY DEPARTMENT AND HOSPITAL-BASED MANAGEMENT OF ASTHMA EXACERBATION*

Initial Assessment and Treatment

History and examination (auscultation, use of accessory muscles, heart rate, respiratory rate), PEFR or FEV_1, oxygen saturation, and other tests as indicated.

- Initiate fetal assessment (consider fetal monitoring and/or BPP if fetus is potentially viable)
- **If severe exacerbation (FEV_1 or PEFR is <50% with severe symptoms at rest), then high-dose albuterol by nebulization every 20 minutes or continuously for 1 hour, and inhaled ipratropium bromide, and systemic corticosteroid**
- Albuterol by MDI or nebulizer, up to three doses in first hour
- Oral corticosteroid if no immediate response or if patient recently treated with systemic corticosteroid
- Oxygen to maintain saturation >95%
- Repeat assessment: symptoms, physical examination, PEFR, oxygen saturation
- Continue albuterol every 60 minutes for 1-3 hours provided there is improvement

Repeat Assessment

Symptoms, physical examination, PEFR, oxygen saturation, other tests as needed

Continue fetal assessment

Good Response

- FEV_1 or PEFR ≥70%
- Response sustained 60 minutes after last treatment
- No distress
- Physical examination: normal
- Reassuring fetal status
- Discharge home

Incomplete Response

- FEV_1 or PEFR ≥50% but <70%
- Mild or moderate symptoms
- Continue fetal assessment until patient stabilized
- Monitor FEV_1 or PEFR, oxygen saturation, pulse
- Continue inhaled albuterol and oxygen
- Inhaled ipratropium bromide
- Systemic (oral or intravenous) corticosteroid
- Individualize decision for hospitalization

Poor Response

- FEV1 or PEFR <50%
- PCO_2 >42 mm Hg
- Physical examination: symptoms severe, drowsiness, confusion
- Continue fetal assessment
- Admit to ICU

Impending or Actual Respiratory Arrest

- Admit to ICU
- Intubation and mechanical ventilation with 100% oxygen
- Nebulized albuterol plus inhaled ipratropium bromide
- Intravenous corticosteroid

Intensive Care Unit

- Inhaled albuterol hourly or continuously plus inhaled ipratropium bromide
- Intravenous corticosteroid
- Oxygen
- Possible intubation and mechanical ventilation
- Continue fetal assessment until patient stabilized

Discharge Home

- Continue treatment with albuterol
- Oral systemic corticosteroid if indicated
- Initiate or continue inhaled corticosteroid until review at medical follow-up
- Patient education
  - Review medicine use
  - Review/initiate action plan
  - Recommend close medical follow-up

*Modified from NAEPP report (NAEPP, 2004).

ICU, Intensive care unit; *PCO_2*, partial pressure of carbon dioxide; *PEFR*, peak expiratory flow rate.

asthma, although an association with bronchospasm has not been observed with wide clinical use. Nonselective ß-blockers may trigger bronchospasm.

Lumbar anesthesia has the benefit of reducing oxygen consumption and minute ventilation during labor. Fentanyl may be a better analgesic than meperidine, which causes histamine release, but meperidine is rarely associated with the onset of bronchospasm during labor. A 2% incidence of bronchospasm has been reported with regional anesthesia. Communication between the obstetrical, anesthetic, and pediatric caregivers is important for optimal care.

Breastfeeding

In general, only small amounts of asthma medications enter breast milk. Prednisone, theophylline, antihistamines, inhaled corticosteroids, leukotriene receptor antagonists, and β_2-agonists are not considered to be contraindications for breastfeeding.[63,64] However, among sensitive individuals, theophylline may cause neonatal vomiting, feeding difficulties, jitteriness, and cardiac arrhythmias.

Summary

Asthma is an increasingly common problem during pregnancy. Mild and moderate asthma can be associated with excellent maternal and perinatal pregnancy outcomes, especially if patients are managed according to contemporary NAEPP recommendations. Severe and poorly controlled asthma may be associated with increased prematurity, need for cesarean delivery, preeclampsia, and growth restriction. Severe asthma exacerbations can result in maternal morbidity and mortality and can have commensurate adverse pregnancy outcomes. The management of asthma during pregnancy should be based on objective assessment, trigger avoidance, patient education, and step therapy. Asthma medications should be continued during pregnancy and while breastfeeding.

RESTRICTIVE LUNG DISEASE

Restrictive ventilatory defects occur when lung expansion is limited because of alterations in the lung parenchyma or because of abnormalities in the pleura, chest wall, or the neuromuscular apparatus. These conditions are characterized by a reduction in lung volumes and an increase in the ratio of FEV_1 to forced vital capacity (FVC).[88] The interstitial lung diseases include idiopathic pulmonary fibrosis, sarcoidosis, hypersensitivity pneumonitis, pneumoconiosis, drug-induced lung disease, and connective tissue disease. **Additional conditions that cause a restrictive ventilatory defect include pleural and chest wall diseases and extrathoracic conditions such as obesity, peritonitis, and ascites.**[88] Restrictive lung disease in pregnancy has not been well studied. Consequently, little is known about the effects of restrictive lung disease on the outcome of pregnancy or the effects of pregnancy on the disease process itself. A recent study presented data on nine pregnant women who were prospectively managed with interstitial and restrictive lung disease.[89] Diagnoses included idiopathic pulmonary fibrosis, hypersensitivity pneumonitis, sarcoidosis, kyphoscoliosis, and multiple pulmonary emboli. Three of the gravidas presented in this paper had severe disease characterized by a vital capacity of 1.5 L or less (50% predicted) or a diffusing capacity less than or equal to 50% predicted. Five of the patients had exercise-induced oxygen desaturation, and four patients required supplemental oxygen. Of the group, one patient had an adverse outcome and was delivered at 31 weeks. She subsequently required mechanical ventilation for 72 hours. All other patients were delivered at or beyond 36 weeks, with no adverse intrapartum or postpartum complications. All infants were at or above the 30th percentile for growth.[89] The authors concluded that restrictive lung disease was well tolerated in pregnancy. However, exercise intolerance was common, and early oxygen supplementation may be required.[89]

Sarcoidosis

Sarcoidosis is a systemic granulomatosis disease of undetermined etiology that often affects young adults. Pregnancy outcome for most women with sarcoidosis is good.[90,91] In a study of 35 pregnancies in 18 patients with sarcoidosis, disease activity remained stable in 9 patients. During pregnancy, improvement was demonstrated in 6 patients, and in 3, there was a worsening of the disease.[90] During the postpartum period, 15 patients remained stable; however, in 3 women, a progression of the disease continued. Another retrospective study presented 15 pregnancies complicated by maternal sarcoidosis over a 10-year period.[91] **Eleven of these patients remained stable, 2 experienced disease progression, and 2 died as a result of severe complications of severe sarcoidosis. In this group, factors indicating a poor prognosis reportedly included parenchymal lesions on chest radiograph, advanced radiographic staging, advanced maternal age, low inflammatory activity, requirement for drugs other than steroids, and the presence of extrapulmonary sarcoidosis.**[91] **Both of the patients who succumbed during gestation had severe disease at the onset of pregnancy.** The overall **cesarean delivery rate was 40%;** in addition, 4 of 15 infants **(27%) weighed less than 2500 g.** None of the patients developed preeclampsia. One possible explanation for the commonly observed improvement in sarcoidosis may be the increased concentration of cortisol during pregnancy. However, because sarcoidosis improves spontaneously in many nonpregnant patients, the improvement may be coincident with but not due to pregnancy.

One study examined 17 pregnancies in 10 patients and concluded that pregnancy had no consistent effect on the course of the disease.[92] Scadding[93] separated patients into three categories based on characteristic patterns of their chest radiographs. When the chest radiograph had resolved before pregnancy, the normal radiograph persisted throughout gestation. In women with resolving radiographic changes before pregnancy, resolution continued throughout the prenatal period. Patients with inactive fibrotic residual disease had stable chest radiographs, and those with active disease tended to have partial or complete resolution of those changes during pregnancy. Most patients in this latter group, however, experienced exacerbation of the disease within 3 to 6 months after delivery.[93]

Patients with pulmonary hypertension complicating restrictive lung disease may suffer a mortality rate as high as 50% during gestation. These patients need close monitoring during labor, delivery, and the postpartum period. Invasive monitoring with a pulmonary artery catheter may be indicated to optimize cardiorespiratory function. **Gravidas with restrictive lung disease, including pulmonary sarcoidosis, may benefit from early institution of steroid therapy for evidence of worsening pulmonary status.** Individuals with evidence of severe disease need close monitoring and may require supplemental oxygen therapy during gestation as well.

During labor, consideration should be given to early use of epidural anesthesia, if it is not contraindicated. The early institution of pain management in this population will minimize pain, decrease sympathetic response, and therefore decrease oxygen consumption during labor and delivery. **The use of general anesthesia should be avoided, if possible,** because these patients may develop pulmonary complications after general anesthesia, including pneumonia and difficulty weaning from the ventilator. **In addition, close fetal surveillance throughout gestation is warranted because impaired oxygenation may compromise fetal growth.**

An additional consideration is the need to counsel all women with restrictive lung disease about the potential for continued impairment of their respiratory status during pregnancy, particularly if their respiratory disease is deteriorating at the time of conception. The individual with clinical signs consistent with pulmonary hypertension or severe restrictive disease should be cautioned about the possibility of maternal mortality resulting from worsening pulmonary function during gestation.

In summary, although the literature on restrictive lung disease in pregnancy is limited, it supports the conclusion that most patients with restrictive lung disease complicating pregnancy, including those with pulmonary sarcoidosis, will have a favorable pregnancy outcome. However, the clinician should keep in mind that a subgroup of women with restrictive lung disease can have significant worsening of their clinical condition during gestation.

Cystic Fibrosis

Cystic fibrosis involves the exocrine glands and epithelial tissues of the pancreas, sweat glands, and mucous glands in the respiratory, digestive, and reproductive tracts. **Chronic obstructive pulmonary disease, pancreatic exocrine insufficiency, and elevated sweat electrolytes are present in most patients with cystic fibrosis.** The disease is **genetically transmitted with an autosomal recessive pattern of inheritance.** The cystic fibrosis gene was identified and cloned in 1989. The gene is localized to chromosome 7, and the molecular defect accounting for the majority of cases has been identified. **In the United States, about 4% of the white population are heterozygous carriers of the cystic fibrosis gene. The disease occurs in 1 in 3000 live white births.** Morbidity and mortality in cystic fibrosis is usually secondary to progressive chronic bronchial pulmonary disease. Pregnancy and the attendant physiologic changes can stress the pulmonary, cardiovascular, and nutritional status of women with cystic fibrosis. The purpose of this section is to familiarize the obstetrician with the physiologic effects of this complex disease and the impact of the disease on pregnancy and the impact of pregnancy on the disease. Additional factors that need to be addressed are the genetics of this disorder (see Chapter 10) and the implications for the newborn, as well as social issues, including who will raise the child should the mother succumb to her disease.

Survival for patients with cystic fibrosis has increased dramatically since 1940. According to the Cystic Fibrosis Foundation's Patient Registry, mean survival in 2008 had increased to 39.6 years. Women had a slightly lower median age of survival (27.3 years) compared with men (29.6 years). The reasons for sex differences in mortality are unclear. **Today more than 45% of individuals with cystic fibrosis in the United States are older than 18 years.** This increase in survival of patients with cystic fibrosis is likely secondary to earlier diagnosis and intervention and to advances in antibiotic therapy and nutritional support. **Therefore, more women with cystic fibrosis are now entering reproductive age. In contrast to men with cystic fibrosis, who for the most part are infertile, women with cystic fibrosis are more often fertile. Infertility in women with cystic fibrosis may occasionally be due to anovulatory cycles and secondary amenorrhea, which result from significant malnutrition associated with advanced disease. A more common reason for infertility appears to result from alteration in the physiologic properties of cervical mucus.**

The first case of cystic fibrosis complicating pregnancy was reported in 1960. The annual number of cystic fibrosis pregnancies reported to the Cystic Fibrosis Foundation's Patient Registry doubled between 1986 and 1990, with 52 pregnancies reported in 1986 and 111 pregnancies reported in 1990. This same registry recently reported on a total of 680 pregnancies in 8136 women between 1985 and 1997. This documents a dramatic increase in pregnancy complicated by cystic fibrosis. Increasing numbers are reported in other countries as well. **Because the number of women with cystic fibrosis achieving pregnancy is steadily increasing, it is important that the obstetrician is familiar with the disease. Liberal consultation with a cystic fibrosis specialist should be obtained because a team effort will increase the chance for an improved pregnancy outcome.**

Effect of Pregnancy on Cystic Fibrosis

The physiologic changes associated with pregnancy (see Chapter 3) are well tolerated by healthy gravidas; however, those with cystic fibrosis may adapt poorly. During pregnancy, there is an increase in resting minute ventilation that at term may approach 150% of control values. This increase in minute ventilation is due to the increased oxygen consumption and increased carbon dioxide burden that occur during pregnancy. In addition, increased levels of circulating progesterone stimulates the respiratory drive. Enlargement of the abdominal contents and upward displacement of the diaphragm lead to a decrease in functional residual volume and a decrease in residual volume. Pregnancy is also accompanied by subtle alterations in gas exchange with widening of the alveolar-arterial oxygen gradient that is most pronounced in the supine position. These alterations in pulmonary function are of little consequence to the normal pregnant woman. However, in the gravida with cystic fibrosis, these changes may contribute to respiratory decompensation that can lead to an increase in morbidity and mortality for the mother and the fetus.

During normal pregnancy, blood volume increases by an average of 50%. Cardiac output increases as well, reaching a plateau in midpregnancy. During labor, blood volume rises acutely, in large part because of the release of blood from the contracting uterus, and is additionally increased after delivery, secondary to augmented venous return with the release of caval obstruction. **Women with cystic fibrosis and advanced lung disease may suffer from pulmonary hypertension with high pulmonary artery pressures. Regardless of the etiology, pulmonary hypertension is associated with unacceptable maternal risk during pregnancy and is considered to be a contraindication to pregnancy.** Women with significant pulmonary hypertension may develop cardiovascular collapse at the time of labor and delivery, with a maternal mortality rate exceeding 25%. Additionally, **women with pulmonary hypertension may not be able to adequately increase cardiac output during pregnancy and, therefore, suffer uteroplacental insufficiency, leading to IUGR and stillbirth.**

Nutritional requirements are increased during pregnancy, with about 300 kcal/day in additional fuel being needed to meet the requirements of mother and fetus. **Most patients with cystic fibrosis have pancreatic exocrine insufficiency. As a result, digestive enzymes and bicarbonate ions are diminished, resulting in maldigestion, malabsorption, and malnutrition.**

There are several reports suggesting that **patients with mild cystic fibrosis, good nutritional status, and less impairment of lung function tolerate pregnancy well. However, those with poor clinical status, malnutrition, hepatic dysfunction, or advanced lung disease are at increased risk from pregnancy.**[94,95] Kent and Farquharson[95] reviewed the literature and reported 217 pregnancies. In this series, the frequency of preterm delivery was 24.3% and the perinatal death rate was 7.9%. **Poor outcomes were associated with a maternal weight gain of less than 4.5 kg and an FVC less than 50% of predicted. Edenborough and colleagues[96] also reported on pregnancies in women with cystic fibrosis. There were 18 live births (81.8%), one third of which were preterm deliveries, and 18.2% of patients had abortions. There were four maternal deaths within 3.2 years after delivery.** In this series, lung function was available before delivery, immediately after delivery, and after pregnancy. Although the patients demonstrated a decline of 13% in FEV_1 and 11% in FVC during pregnancy, most returned to baseline pulmonary function after pregnancy. Although most of the women in this series tolerated pregnancy well, **those with moderate to severe lung disease, an FEV_1 less than 60% of predicted, more often had preterm infants and had increased loss of lung function compared with those with milder disease.[96] In two series, prepregnancy FEV_1 was found to be the most useful predictor of outcome in pregnant women with cystic fibrosis.[96,97] In addition, there was a positive correlation of prepregnancy FEV_1 and maternal survival.**

A more recent report examined survival in 8136 women enrolled in the U.S. Cystic Fibrosis Foundation National Patient Registry from 1985 to 1997.[98] Six hundred and eighty of these women became pregnant. The authors matched the 680 women in an index year to 3327 control women with cystic fibrosis. Women who reported a pregnancy were more likely to have had a higher percentage of predicted FEV_1 (67.5% predicted versus 67.1% predicted, respectively; $P > .001$) and a higher weight (52.9 versus 46.4 kg, respectively; $P > .001$). The 10-year survival rate in pregnant women (77%; 95% CI, 71% to 82%) was higher than in those women who did not become pregnant. A separate analysis, matching pregnant patient's FEV_1 percent of predicted, age, *Pseudomonas aeruginosa* colonization, and pancreatic function obtained similar results. In this cohort, pregnancy was not harmful in any subgroup, including patients with an FEV_1 40% of predicted or diabetes mellitus.[98] **The author concluded women with cystic fibrosis who became pregnant were initially healthier and had better 10-year survival rates than women with cystic fibrosis who did not become pregnant.**

Pulmonary involvement in cystic fibrosis includes chronic infection of the airways and bronchiectasis. There is selective infection with certain microorganisms, such as *S. aureus, H. influenzae, P. aeruginosa,* and *Burkholderia cepacia. P. aeruginosa* is the most frequent pathogen. Parenteral antibiotics are the mainstays of treatment of these acute infections. However, pregnancy- and cystic fibrosis–associated alterations in pharmacokinetics can have grave consequences for these patients. It is well known that pregnant subjects have lower serum levels and higher urine levels of antibiotics than nonpregnant subjects. The lower levels in plasma are attributed to the increase in volume of distribution and an increase in glomerular filtration and renal clearance of the drugs. Therefore, monitoring drug levels is indicated when therapeutic response is less than optimum.

Counseling Patients with Cystic Fibrosis in Pregnancy

Several factors must be considered when counseling a woman who has cystic fibrosis and is considering pregnancy, including the possibility that her fetus will have cystic fibrosis (see Chapter 10). **When the mother has cystic fibrosis and the proposed father is a white individual of unknown genotype, the risk for the fetus having cystic fibrosis is 1 in 50, compared with 1 in 3000 in the general white population. If the prospective father is a known carrier of a cystic fibrosis mutation, the risk to the fetus increases to 1 in 2.** If, however, DNA testing does not identify a cystic fibrosis mutation in the prospective father, it is still possible that the father is a carrier of an unidentified cystic fibrosis mutation, making the risk for cystic fibrosis to the offspring 1 in 492.[99]

It is important that the woman with cystic fibrosis be advised about the potential adverse effects of pregnancy on maternal health status. Factors that may predict poor outcome include prepregnancy evidence of poor nutritional status, significant pulmonary disease with hypoxemia, and pulmonary hypertension. Liver disease and diabetes mellitus are also poor prognostic factors. **Gravidas with poor nutritional status, pulmonary hypertension (cor pulmonale), and deteriorating pulmonary function early in gestation should consider therapeutic abortion because the risk for maternal mortality may be unacceptably high.**

The woman with cystic fibrosis who is considering pregnancy should also give consideration to the need for strong psychosocial and physical support after delivery. The rigors of child rearing may add to the risk for maternal deterioration during this period. Family members should also be willing to provide physical and emotional support and should be aware of the potential for deterioration in the mother's health and the potential for maternal mortality. **In addition, the need for care of a potentially preterm growth-restricted neonate with all of its attendant morbidities and potential mortality should be discussed.** Over the long term, the woman and her family should also consider the fact that her life expectancy may be shortened by cystic fibrosis. **Overall 20% of mothers with cystic fibrosis succumb to the disease before the child's 10th birthday, and this number increases to 40% if the FEV_1 is less than 40% of predicted.**[100] Plans should be made for rearing of the child in the event of maternal death.

Management of the Pregnancy Complicated by Cystic Fibrosis

Care of the gravida with cystic fibrosis should be a coordinated, team effort. Physicians familiar with cystic fibrosis, its complications, and management should be included, as well as a maternal-fetal medicine specialist and neonatal team. The gravida should be assessed for potential risk factors such as severe lung disease, pulmonary hypertension, poor nutritional status, pancreatic failure, and liver disease, preferably before attempting gestation, but certainly during the early months of pregnancy. **Gravidas should be advised to be 90% of ideal body weight before conception if possible. A weight gain in pregnancy of 11 to 12 kg is recommended.**[101] **Frequent monitoring of weight, blood glucose, hemoglobin, total protein, serum albumin, prothrombin time, and fat-soluble vitamins A and E is suggested.**[101] At each visit, the history of caloric intake and symptoms of maldigestion and malabsorption should be taken, and pancreatic enzymes should be adjusted if needed. **Patients who are unable to achieve adequate weight gain through oral nutritional supplements may be given nocturnal enteral nasogastric tube feeding. In this situation, the risk for aspiration should be considered, especially in patients with a history of gastroesophageal reflux, which is common in cystic fibrosis. If malnutrition is severe, parenteral hyperalimentation may be necessary for successful completion of the pregnancy. Baseline pulmonary function should be assessed, preferably before conception.** Assessment should include **FVC, FEV_1, lung volumes, pulse oximetry, and arterial blood gases,** if indicated. **These values should be serially monitored during gestation and deterioration in pulmonary function addressed immediately. An echocardiogram can assess the patient for pulmonary hypertension and cor pulmonale.** If pulmonary hypertension (cor pulmonale) is diagnosed, the gravida should be advised of the high maternal risk.

Early recognition and prompt treatment of pulmonary infections are important in the management of the pregnant woman with cystic fibrosis. **Treatment includes intravenous antibiotics in the appropriate dose, keeping in mind the increased clearance of these drugs secondary to pregnancy and cystic fibrosis.** Plasma levels of aminoglycosides should be monitored and adjusted as indicated. **Chest physical therapy and bronchial drainage are also important components of the management of pulmonary infections in cystic fibrosis. Because *P. aeruginosa* is the most frequently isolated bacterium associated with chronic endobronchitis**

and bronchiectasis, antibiotic regimens should include coverage for this organism.

If the patient with cystic fibrosis has pancreatic insufficiency and diabetes mellitus, careful monitoring of blood glucose and insulin therapy is indicated. As previously mentioned, pancreatic enzymes may need to be replaced in order to optimize the patient's nutritional status. **Because of malabsorption of fats and frequent use of antibiotics, the patient with cystic fibrosis is prone to vitamin K deficiency. Therefore, prothrombin time should be checked regularly, and parenteral vitamin K should be administered if the prothrombin time is elevated.**

It is imperative when managing pregnancy in a woman with cystic fibrosis to recognize that the fetus is at risk for uteroplacental insufficiency and IUGR. The maternal nutritional status and weight gain during pregnancy will likewise affect fetal growth. Therefore, **fundal height should be measured routinely, and serial ultrasound evaluations of fetal growth and amniotic fluid volume should be made.** Maternal kick counts may be useful for monitoring fetal status starting at 28 weeks. **Nonstress testing should be started at 32 weeks or sooner, if there is evidence of fetal compromise.** If there is evidence of severe fetal compromise such as no interval fetal growth, persistent decelerations, or poor biophysical profile scoring, delivery should be accomplished. Likewise, **evidence of profound maternal deterioration such as a marked and sustained decline in pulmonary function, development of right-sided heart failure, refractory hypoxemia, and progressive hypercapnia and respiratory acidosis may be maternal indications for early delivery.** If the fetus is potentially viable, the administration of betamethasone may be beneficial. Vaginal delivery should be attempted when possible.

Labor, delivery, and the postpartum period can be particularly dangerous for the patient with cystic fibrosis. The augmentation in cardiac output stresses the cardiovascular system and can lead to cardiopulmonary failure in the patient with pulmonary hypertension and cor pulmonale. These patients are also more likely to develop right-sided heart failure. **Heart failure should be treated with aggressive diuresis and supplemental oxygen. Management may be optimized by insertion of a pulmonary artery catheter to monitor right- and left-sided filling pressures. Pain control will reduce the sympathetic response to labor and tachycardia. This will benefit the patient who is demonstrating pulmonary or cardiac compromise.** In the patient with a normal partial thromboplastin time, insertion of an epidural catheter for continuous epidural analgesia may be beneficial. This is also useful in the event a cesarean delivery is indicated because general anesthesia and its possible effects on pulmonary function can be avoided. **If general anesthesia is needed, preoperative anticholinergic agents should be avoided because they tend to promote drying and inspissation of airway secretions.** Close fetal surveillance is also extremely important because the fetus who may have been suffering from uteroplacental insufficiency during gestation is more prone to develop evidence of fetal compromise during labor. **Cesarean delivery should be reserved for the usual obstetrical indications.**

In summary, more women with cystic fibrosis are living to childbearing age and are capable of conceiving. Clinical experience thus far has demonstrated that **pregnancy in women with cystic fibrosis and mild disease is well tolerated. Women with severe disease have an associated increase in maternal and fetal morbidity and mortality.** The potential risk to any individual with cystic fibrosis desirous of pregnancy should be assessed and discussed with the patient and her family in detail.

KEY POINTS

- Pneumonia is the most common nonobstetrical infection to cause maternal mortality. Preterm delivery complicates pneumonia in up to 43% of cases. *Streptococcus pneumoniae* is the most common bacterial pathogen to cause pneumonia. Empirical antibiotic coverage should be started, including a third-generation cephalosporin and a macrolide, such as azithromycin, to cover atypical pathogens. If CA-MRSA is suspected, add vancomycin or linezolid.
- The HIV-infected gravida with a $CD4^+$ count of less than 200 cells per cubic millimeter should receive prophylaxis with trimethoprim-sulfamethoxazole to prevent PJP pneumonia as well as HAART.
- High-risk gravidas should be screened for TB and treated appropriately with INH prophylaxis for infection without overt disease and with dual anti-TB therapy for active disease. If resistant TB is identified, ethambutol, 2.5 g/day, should be added to therapy, and the treatment period should be extended to 18 months.
- Asthma complicates about 8% of pregnancies.
- It is safer for pregnant women with asthma to be treated with asthma medications than it is for them to have asthma symptoms and exacerbations.
- Clinical evaluation of asthma includes subjective assessments and pulmonary function tests.
- Inhaled corticosteroids are the preferred treatment for persistent asthma in pregnancy.
- Identifying and controlling or avoiding such factors as allergens and irritants, particularly tobacco smoke, can lead to improved maternal well-being with less need for medication.
- The goal of asthma therapy during pregnancy is maintenance of near-normal pulmonary function.
- Step-care therapy uses the principle of tailoring medical therapy according to asthma severity.
- Women taking asthma medications may breastfeed.
- Asthma self-management education, including self-monitoring, correct use of inhalers, and an action plan, are part of optimal gestational asthma therapy.
- The interstitial lung diseases include idiopathic pulmonary fibrosis, sarcoidosis, hypersensitivity pneumonitis, drug-induced lung disease, and connective tissue disease. Restrictive lung disease is generally well tolerated in pregnancy; however, exercise intolerance and need for oxygen

supplementation may develop. Gravidas with pulmonary hypertension complicating restrictive lung disease may suffer a high mortality rate.

- An increasing number of women with cystic fibrosis are surviving to the reproductive years and usually maintain their fertility with meticulous management of pulmonary function, including pulmonary toilet and aggressive surveillance for signs of pulmonary infection and treatment with antibiotics in adequate doses. Close attention to nutrition is required secondary to maldigestion, malabsorption, and malnutrition, which can complicate cystic fibrosis. Gravidas with good clinical studies, good nutritional status, near-normal chest radiographs, and only mild obstructive lung disease will tolerate pregnancy well. Fetal growth should be monitored closely.

REFERENCES

1. Berkowitz K, LaSala A: Risk factors associated with the increasing prevalence of pneumonia during pregnancy. Am J Obstet Gynecol 163:981, 1990.
2. Munn MB, Groome LJ, Atterbury JL, et al: Pneumonia as a complication of pregnancy. J Matern Fetal Med 8:151, 1999.
3. Benedetti TJ, Valle R, Ledger W: Antepartum pneumonia in pregnancy. Am J Obstet Gynecol 144:413, 1982.
4. Madinger NE, Greenspoon JS, Ellrodt AG: Pneumonia during pregnancy: has modern technology improved maternal and fetal outcome? Am J Obstet Gynecol 161:657, 1989.
5. Koonin LM, Ellerbrock TV, Atrash HK, et al: Pregnancy-associated deaths due to AIDS in the United States. JAMA 261:1306, 1989.
6. Dinsmoor MJ: HIV infection and pregnancy. Med Clin North Am 73:701, 1989.
7. Jenkins TM, Troiano NH, Graves CR, et al: Mechanical ventilation in an obstetric population: characteristics and delivery rates. Am J Obstet Gynecol 188:549, 2003.
8. Rodrigues J, Niederman MS: Pneumonia complicating pregnancy. Clin Chest Med 13:679, 1992.
9. Haake DA, Zakowski PC, Haake DL, et al: Early treatment with acyclovir for varicella pneumonia in otherwise healthy adults: retrospective controlled study and review. Rev Infect Dis 12: 788, 1990.
10. McKinney WP, Volkert P, Kaufman J: Fatal swine influenza pneumonia during late pregnancy. Arch Intern Med 150:213, 1990.
11. Mercieri M, Di Rosa R, Pantosti A, et al: Critical pneumonia complicating early-stage pregnancy. Aneth Analg 110:852, 2010.
12. Rotas M, McCalla S, Liu C, Minkoff H: Methicillin-resistant *Staphylococcus aureus* necrotizing pneumonia arising from an infected episiotomy site. Obstet Gynecol 109:108, 2007.
13. Asnis D, Haralambou G, Tawiah P: Methicillin-resistant *Staphylococcus aureus* necrotizing pneumonia arising from an infected episiotomy site [letter to the editor]. Obstet Gynecol 110: 188, 2007.
14. Ahmad H, Mehta NJ, Manikal VM, et al: *Pneumocystis carinii* pneumonia in pregnancy: division of infectious disease. Chest 120:666, 2001.
15. Yost P, Bloom S, Richey S, et al: Appraisal of treatment guidelines of antepartum community acquired pneumonia. Am J Obstet Gynecol 183:131, 2000.
16. American Thoracic Society: Guidelines for the initial management of adults with community-acquired pneumonia: diagnosis assessment of severity, and initial antimicrobial therapy. Am Rev Respir Dis 148:1418, 1993.
17. Harrison BDW, Farr BM, Connolly CK, et al: The hospital management of community-acquired pneumonia: recommendation of the British Thoracic Society. J R Coll Phys 21:267, 1987.
18. Campbell SG, Marrie TJ, Anstey R, et al: Utility of blood cultures in management of adults with community acquired pneumonia discharged from the emergency department. Emerg Med J 20: 521, 2003.
19. Pimentel LP, McPherson SJ: Community-acquired pneumonia in the emergency department: a practical approach to diagnosis and management. Emerg Med Clin North Am 21:395, 2003.
20. Murdoch DR, Laing RT, Mills GD, et al: Evaluation of a rapid immunochromatographic test for detection of *Streptococcus pneumoniae* antigen in urine samples from adults with community-acquired pneumonia. J Clin Microbiol 39:3495, 2001.
21. Gutierrez F, Rodriequez JC, Ayelo A, et al: Evaluation of the immunochromatographic Binax NOW assay for detection of *Streptococcus pneumoniae* urinary antigen in a prospective study of community-acquired pneumonia in Spain. Clin Infect Dis 36:286, 1996.
22. Waterer GW, Baselski VS, Wunderink RG: Legionella and community-acquired pneumonia: a review of current diagnostic test from a clinician's viewpoint. Am J Med 110:41, 2001.
23. Niederman MS, Ahmed OA: Community-acquired pneumonia in elderly patients. Clin Geriatr Med 19:101, 2003.
24. Golden WE, Brown P, Godsey N: CMS release new standards for community acquired pneumonia. J Ark Med Soc 99:288, 2003.
25. Cunha BA: Empiric therapy of community-acquired pneumonia. Chest 125:1913, 2004.
26. Hidron A, Low C, Hoing E, Blumberg H: Emergence of community-acquired methicillin-resistant *Staphylococcus aureus* strain USA300 as a cause of necrotizing community-onset pneumonia. Lancet Infect Dis 9:384, 2009.
27. Munoz FM, Englund JA, Cheesman CC, et al: Maternal immunization with pneumococcal polysaccharide vaccine in the third trimester of gestation. Vaccine 20:826, 2001.
28. Shahid NS, Steinhoff MC, Hoque SS, et al: Serum, breast milk, and infant antibody after maternal immunization with pneumococcal vaccine. Lancet 346:1252, 1995.
29. Tomlinson MW, Caruthers TJ, Whitty JE, Gonik B: Does delivery improve maternal condition in the respiratory-compromised gravida? Obstet Gynecol 91:108, 1998.
30. National Center for Health Statistics: National hospital discharge survey: annual summary 1990. Vital Health Stat 13:1, 1992.
31. Hollingsworth HM, Pratter MR, Irwin RS: Acute respiratory failure in pregnancy. J Intensive Care Med 4:11, 1989.
32. Neuzil KM, Reed GW, Mitchel EF, et al: Impact of influenza on acute cardiopulmonary hospitalizations in pregnant women. Am J Epidemiol 148:1094, 1998.
33. Hartert TV, Neuzil KM, Shintani AK, et al: Maternal morbidity and perinatal outcome among pregnant women with respiratory hospitalizations during influenza season. Am J Obstet Gynecol 189:1705, 2003.
34. Siston AM, Rasussen SA, Honein MA, et al: Pandemic 2009 Influenza A (H1N1) virus illness among pregnant women in the United States. JAMA 303:1517, 2010.
35. Harper SA, Fukuda K, Uyeka TM, et al: Prevention and control of influenza: recommendations of the Advisory Committee on Immunization Practice (ACIP). MMWR 52:1, 2003.
36. Cox SM, Cunningham FG, Luby J: Management of varicella pneumonia complicating pregnancy. Am J Perinatol 7:300, 1990.
37. Esmonde TG, Herdman G, Anderson G: Chickenpox pneumonia: an association with pregnancy. Thorax 44:812, 1989.
38. Smego RA, Asperilla MO: Use of acyclovir for varicella pneumonia during pregnancy. Obstet Gynecol 78:1112, 1991.
39. Harger JH, Ernest JM, Thurnau GR, et al: Risk factors and outcome of varicella-zoster virus pneumonia in pregnant women. J Infect Dis 185:422, 2002.
40. Jones AM, Thomas N, Wilkins EG: Outcome of varicella pneumonitis in immunocompetent adults requiring treatment in a high dependency unit. J Infect 43:135, 2001.
41. Andrews EB, Yankaskas BC, Cordero JF, et al: Acyclovir in pregnancy registry: six years' experience. Obstet Gynecol 79:7, 1992.
42. Nguyen HQ, Jumaan AO, Seward JF: Decline in mortality due to varicella after implementation of varicella vaccination in the United States. N Engl J Med 352:450, 2005.

43. Shields KE, Galil K, Seward J, et al: Varicella vaccine exposure during pregnancy: data from the first 5 years of the pregnancy registry. Obstet Gynecol 98:14, 2001.
44. Thomas CF Jr, Limper AH: Pneumocystis pneumonia. N Engl J Med 350:2487, 2004.
45. Ahmad H, Mehta NJ, Manikal VM, et al: *Pneumocystis carinii* pneumonia in pregnancy. Chest 120:666, 2001.
46. Masur H, Kaplan JE, Holmes KK: Guidelines for preventing opportunistic infections among HIV-infected persons-2002: recommendations of the U.S. Public Health Service and the Infectious Disease Society of America. Ann Intern Med 137:435, 2002.
47. Centers for Disease Control and Prevention: Initial therapy for tuberculosis in the era of multidrug resistance-recommendations of the advisory council for the elimination of tuberculosis. MMWR 42:1, 1993.
48. Frieden TR, Sterling T, Pablos-Mendez A, et al: The emergence of drug-resistant tuberculosis in New York City. N Engl J Med 328:521, 1993.
49. Cantwell MF, Shehab AM, Costello AM: Brief report: congenital tuberculosis. N Engl J Med 330:1051, 1994.
50. Margono F, Mroveh J, Garely A, et al: Resurgence of active tuberculosis among pregnant women. Obstet Gynecol 83:911, 1994.
51. Centers for Disease Control and Prevention: The use of preventive therapy for tuberculosis infection in the United States. MMWR 39:9, 1990.
52. Griffith DE: Mycobacteria as pathogens of respiratory infection. Infect Dis Clin North Am 12:593, 1998.
53. American Thoracic Society Workshop: Rapid diagnostic tests for tuberculosis-what is the appropriate use? Am J Respir Crit Care Med 155:1804, 1997.
54. Barnes PF: Rapid diagnostic tests for tuberculosis, progress but no gold standard. Am J Respir Crit Care Med 155:1497, 1997.
55. Centers for Disease Control and Prevention: The role of BCG vaccine in the prevention and control of tuberculosis in the United States: a joint statement by the Advisory Council for the Elimination of Tuberculosis and the Advisory Committee on Immunization Practices. MMWR 45:1, 1996.
56. Good JT, Iseman MD, Davidson PT, et al: Tuberculosis in association with pregnancy. Am J Obstet Gynecol 140:492, 1081.
57. American Thoracic Society: Mycobacteriosis and the acquired immunodeficiency syndrome. Am Rev Respir Dis 136:492, 1987.
58. Jana N, Vasishta K, Saha SC, Ghosh K: Obstetrical outcomes among women with extrapulmonary tuberculosis. N Engl J Med 341: 645, 1999.
59. Fox CW, George RB: Current concepts in the management and prevention of tuberculosis in adults. J La State Med Soc 144: 363, 1992.
60. Robinson GC, Cambion K: Hearing loss in infants of tuberculosis mothers treated with streptomycin during pregnancy. N Engl J Med 271:949, 1964.
61. Lessnau KL, Qarah S: Multidrug-resistant tuberculosis in pregnancy: case report and review of the literature. Chest 123:953, 2003.
62. Shin S, Guerra D, Rich M, et al: Treatment of multidrug-resistant tuberculosis during pregnancy: a report of 7 cases. Clin Infect Dis 36:996, 2003.
63. National Asthma Education and Prevention Program Expert Panel Report: Managing asthma during pregnancy: recommendations for pharmacologic treatment-2004 update. J Allergy Clin Immunol 115:34, 2005. Available at: http://www.nhlbi.nih.gov/health/prof/lung/asthma/astpreg/astpreg_full.pdf. Accessed on January 17, 2012.
64. ACOG Practice Bulletin: Asthma in pregnancy. Obstet Gynecol 111:457, 2008.
65. National Asthma Education and Prevention Program Expert Panel Report 3: Guidelines for the diagnosis and management of asthma-Full Report 2007. Available at: http://www.nhlbi.nih.gov/guidelines/asthma/asthgdln.pdf. Accessed on January 17, 2012.
66. Schatz M, Dombrowski MP, Wise R, et al, for The NICHD Maternal-Fetal Medicine Units Network, and NHLBI: Asthma morbidity during pregnancy can be predicted by severity classification. J Allergy Clin Immunol 112:283, 2003.
67. Schatz M, Dombrowski MP: Asthma in pregnancy. N Engl J Med 360:1862, 2009.
68. Blais L, Forget A: Asthma exacerbations during the first trimester of pregnancy and the risk of congenital malformations among asthmatic women. J Allergy Clin Immunol 121:1379, 2008.
69. Bracken MB, Triche EW, Belanger K, et al: Asthma symptoms, severity, and drug therapy: a prospective study of effects on 2205 pregnancies. Obstet Gynecol 1024:739, 2003.
70. Bakhireva LN, Schatz M, Jones KL, et al: Asthma control during pregnancy and the risk of preterm delivery or impaired fetal growth. Ann Allergy Asthma Immunol 101:137, 2008.
71. Murphy VE, Clifton VL, Gibson PG: Asthma exacerbations during pregnancy: incidence and association with adverse pregnancy outcomes. Thorax 61:169, 2006.
72. Mihrshani S, Belousov E, Marks GB, Peat JK: Pregnancy and birth outcomes in families with asthma. J Asthma 40:181, 2003.
73. Schatz M, Zeiger RS, Hoffman CP, et al: Perinatal outcomes in the pregnancies of asthmatic women: a prospective controlled analysis. Am J Respir Crit Care Med 151:1170, 1995.
74. Minerbi-Codish I, Fraser D, Avnun L, et al: Influence of asthma in pregnancy on labor and the newborn. Respiration 65:130, 1998.
75. Stenius-Aarniala BSM, Hedman J, Teramo KA: Acute asthma during pregnancy. Thorax 51:411, 1996.
76. Jana N, Vasishta K, Saha SC, Khunnu B: Effect of bronchial asthma on the course of pregnancy, labour and perinatal outcome. J Obstet Gynaecol 21:227, 1995.
77. Dombrowski MP, Schatz M, Wise R, et al, for the NICHD Maternal-Fetal Medicine Units Network, and the NHLBI: Asthma during pregnancy. Obstet Gynecol 103:5, 2004.
78. Dombrowski MP, Schatz M, Wise R, et al, for the NICHD Maternal-Fetal Medicine Units Network, and the NHLBI: Randomized trial of inhaled beclomethasone dipropionate versus theophylline for moderate asthma during pregnancy. Am J Obstet Gynecol 190: 737, 2004.
79. Triche EW, Saftlas AF, Belanger D, et al: Association of asthma diagnosis, severity, symptoms, and treatment with risk of preeclampsia. Obstet Gynecol 104:585, 2004.
80. Schatz MS, Dombrowski MP, Wise R, et al, for the NICHD Maternal-Fetal Medicine Units Network, and the NHLBI: Spirometry is related to perinatal outcomes in pregnant women with asthma. Am J Obstet Gynecol 194:120, 2006.
81. Newman RB, Momirova V, Dombrowski MP, et al, for the Eunice Kennedy Shriver National Institute of Child Health and Human Development Maternal-Fetal Medicine Units (MFMU) Network: The effect of active and passive household cigarette smoke exposure on pregnant women with asthma. Chest 137: 601, 2010.
82. Williams LK, Pladevall M, Xi H, et al: Relationship between adherence to inhaled corticosteroids and poor outcomes among adults with asthma. J Allergy Clin Immunol 114:1288, 2004.
83. Wendel PJ, Ramin SM, Barnett-Hamm, et al: Asthma treatment in pregnancy: a randomized controlled trial. Am J Obstet Gynecol 175:150, 1996.
84. Kallen B, Rydhstroem H, Aberg A: Congenital malformations after use of inhaled budesonide in early pregnancy. Obstet Gynecol 93:392, 1999.
85. Schatz M, Dombrowski MP, Wise R, et al, for the NICHD Maternal-Fetal Medicine Units Network, and the NHLBI: The relationship of asthma medication use to perinatal outcomes. J Allergy Clin Immunol 113:1040, 2004.
86. Sarkar M, Koren G, Kalra S, et al: Montelukast use during pregnancy: a multicentre, prospective, comparative study of infant outcomes. Eur J Clin Pharmacol 65:1259, 2009.
87. Park-Wyllie L, Mazzotta P, Pastuszak A, et al: Birth defects after maternal exposure to corticosteroids: prospective cohort study and meta-analysis of epidemiological studies. Teratology 62: 385, 2000.
88. King TE Jr: Restrictive lung disease in pregnancy. Clin Chest Med 13:607, 1992.
89. Boggess KA, Easterling TR, Raghu G: Management and outcome of pregnant women with interstitial and restrictive lung disease. Am J Obstet Gynecol 173:1007, 1995.
90. Agha FP, Vade A, Amendola MA, Cooper RF: Effects of pregnancy on sarcoidosis. Surg Gynecol Obstet 155:817, 1982.
91. Haynes de Regt R: Sarcoidosis and pregnancy. Obstet Gynecol 70:369, 1987.
92. Reisfield DR: Boeck's sarcoid and pregnancy. Am J Obstet Gynecol 75:795, 1958.
93. Scadding JG: Sarcoidosis. London, Eyre & Spottiswoode, 1967, p 519.

94. Canny GJ, Corey M, Livingstone RA, et al: Pregnancy and cystic fibrosis. Obstet Gynecol 77:850, 1991.
95. Kent NE, Farquharson DF: Cystic fibrosis in pregnancy. Can Med Assoc J 149:809, 1993.
96. Edenborough FP, Stableforth DE, Webb AK, et al: Outcome of pregnancy in women with cystic fibrosis. Thorax 50:170, 1995.
97. Olson GL: Cystic fibrosis in pregnancy. Semin Perinatol 21: 307, 1997.
98. Goss CH, Rubenfel GD, Otto K, Aitken ML: The effect of pregnancy on survival in women with cystic fibrosis. Chest 124: 1460, 2003.
99. Lemna WK, Feldman GL, Kerem B, et al: Mutation analysis for heterozygote detection and the prenatal diagnosis of cystic fibrosis. N Engl J Med 322:291, 1990.
100. Edonborough FP, Mackenzie WE, Stableforth DE: The outcome of 72 pregnancies in 55 women with cystic fibrosis in the United kingdom 1977-1996. BJOG 107:254, 2000.
101. Cole BN, Seltzer MH, Kassabian J, et al: Parenteral nutrition in a pregnant cystic fibrosis patient. JPEN J Parenter Enteral Nutr 11:205, 1987.

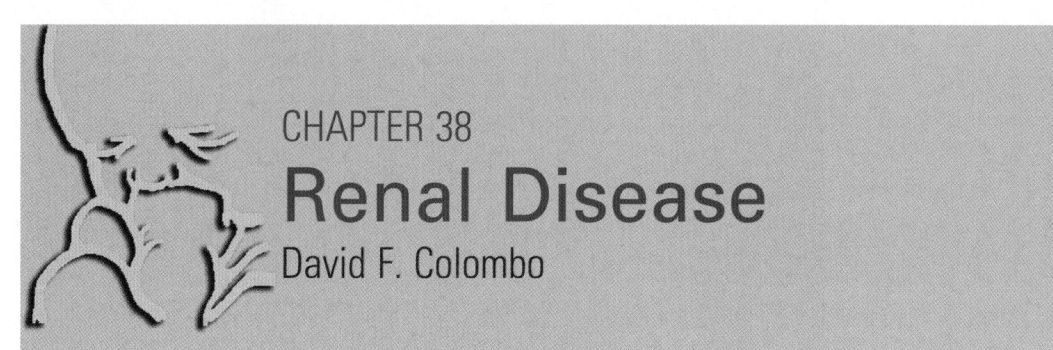

CHAPTER 38

Renal Disease

David F. Colombo

KEY ABBREVIATIONS	
American College of Obstetricians and Gynecologists	ACOG
Adult Respiratory Distress Syndrome	ARDS
Acute Renal Failure	ARF
Asymptomatic Bacteriuria	ASB
Blood Urea Nitrogen	BUN
Glomerular Filtration Rate	GFR
Intrauterine Growth Restriction	IUGR
Positive End Expiratory Pressure	PEEP
Red Blood Cell	RBC
Urinary Tract Infection	UTI

INTRODUCTION

Until relatively recently, women with preexisting renal disease were strongly discouraged from attempting pregnancy because of the expectation of poor perinatal outcome and the likelihood of renal disease progression. Currently, through better understanding of the prognosis of kidney disease during pregnancy, women with most renal conditions are no longer discouraged from attempting conception. This even holds true for women who have undergone renal transplantation.

This chapter first reviews the normal changes in the kidney and urinary collecting system in pregnancy and follows with the basic evaluation of the renal status, acute and chronic renal disorders in pregnancy, and the treatment of the post–renal transplant patient.

ALTERED RENAL PHYSIOLOGY IN PREGNANCY

Pregnancy is associated with significant anatomic changes in the kidney and its collecting system (see Chapter 3). These changes begin to occur shortly after conception and may persist for several months postpartum.[1,2] **The kidney is noted to increase in size and weight during the course of a pregnancy. Of more clinical significance is the marked dilation of the collecting system, including both the renal pelvis and ureters.** This dilation is most pronounced on the right side. This change is likely due to **hormonal changes** (i.e., progesterone, endothelin, relaxin) and as a result of mechanical obstruction by the gravid uterus (Figure 38-1).[3-5]

Renal plasma flow increases greatly during pregnancy.[6] It peaks by the end of the first trimester and, although it decreases near term, it remains higher than in the nonpregnant patient. This change is due in part to increased cardiac output and decreased renal vascular resistance. **The glomerular filtration rate (GFR) increases by 50% during a normal gestation.**[7] It rises early in pregnancy and remains elevated throughout gestation. The percentage increase in GFR is greater than the percentage increase in renal plasma flow. This elevation of the filtration fraction leads to a fall in the serum urea nitrogen (blood urea nitrogen [BUN]) and serum creatinine values.

Because GFR increases to such a great degree, electrolytes, glucose, and other filtered substances reach the renal tubules in greater amounts. The kidney handles sodium efficiently, reabsorbing most of the filtered load in the proximal convoluted tubule. Glucose reabsorption, however, does not increase proportionately during pregnancy. **The average renal threshold for glucose is reduced to 155 mg/dL from 194 mg/dL in the nonpregnant individual.**[8] **Glycosuria therefore can be a feature of normal pregnancy.**

Urate is handled by filtration and secretion. Its clearance increases early in pregnancy, leading to lower serum levels of uric acid. In late pregnancy, urate clearance and serum urate levels return to their prepregnancy values. Serum urate levels are elevated in women with preeclampsia. Whether this is due to decreased renal plasma flow,

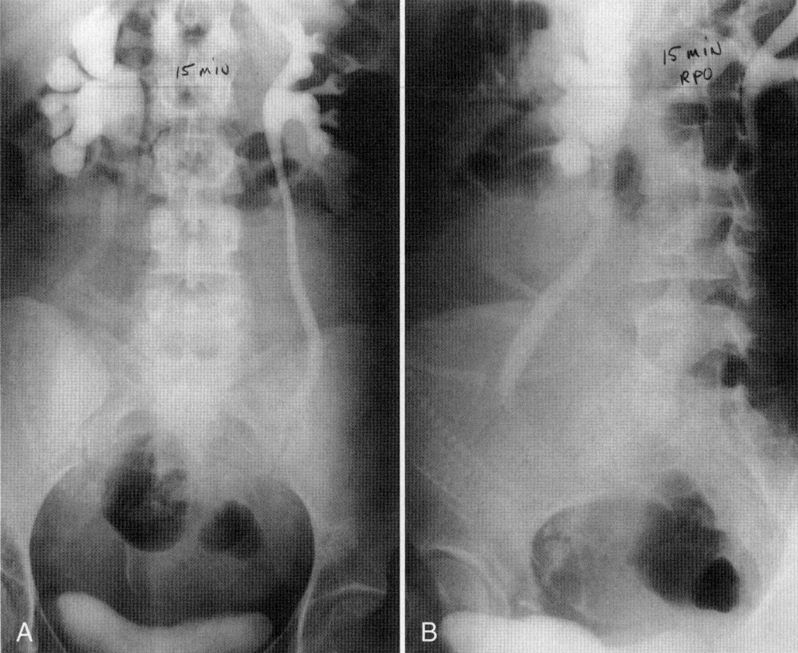

FIGURE 38-1. **A,** An intravenous pyelogram of a gravid patient in late second trimester with flank pain. The image was taken in the anteroposterior view 15 minutes after the instillation of contrast dye. Note the dilation of the renal pelves bilaterally, with the right side more dilated than the left. The fetus is seen in the vertex position. **B,** The same patient in the right lateral view.

TABLE 38-1 SUMMARY OF RENAL CHANGES IN NORMAL PREGNANCY

ALTERATION	MANIFESTATION	CLINICAL RELEVANCE
Increased renal size	Renal length about 1 cm greater on radiographs	Postpartum decreases in size should not be mistaken for parenchymal loss
Dilation of pelves, calyces, and ureters	Resembles hydronephrosis on ultrasound or IVP (usually more prominent on the right)	Not to be mistaken for obstructive uropathy Upper urinary tract infections are more virulent.
Changes in acid-base metabolism	Renal bicarbonate reabsorption threshold decreases	Serum bicarbonate is 4-5 mM/L lower in pregnancy PCO_2 is 10 mm Hg in normal pregnancy PCO_2 of 40 mm Hg actually represents retention in pregnancy
Renal water	Osmoregulation altered as the osmotic thresholds for AVP release decrease	Serum osmolarity decreased by approximately 10 mOsm/L

Modified from Lindheimer M, Grünfeld JP, Davison JM: Renal disorders. *In* Barron WM, Lindheimer M (eds): Medical Disorders during Pregnancy. St Louis, Mosby, 2000, pp 39-70.
AVP, Vasopressin; *IVP,* intravenous pyelography; PCO_2, carbon dioxide tension.

hemoconcentration, renal tubular dysfunction, or other renal circulatory changes continues to be unknown. A summary of the renal changes in normal pregnancy is shown in Table 38-1.

ASYMPTOMATIC BACTERIURIA

The diagnosis of asymptomatic bacteriuria (ASB) is based on a clean catch voided specimen. The prevalence of ASB in sexually active woman has been reported as high as 5% to 6%.[9,10] To secure a diagnosis, urine culture should reveal greater than 100,000 colonies/mL of a single organism.[11] Some investigators have suggested that two consecutively voided specimens should contain the same organism before establishing the diagnosis of bacteriuria.[12,13] Bacteriuria occurs in 2% to 7% of pregnancies, particularly in multiparous women, a prevalence similar to that seen in nonpregnant women. The pathogenic organisms are also similar in species and virulence factors to those observed in nonpregnant women. Thus, the basic mechanism of entry of bacteria into the urinary tract is likely to be the same for both groups. Bacteriuria often develops in the first month of pregnancy and is frequently associated with a reduction in concentrating ability, suggesting involvement of the kidney.[2] The smooth muscle relaxation and subsequent ureteral dilation that accompany pregnancy are believed to facilitate the ascent of bacteria from the bladder to the kidney. As a result, bacteriuria during pregnancy has a greater propensity to progress to pyelonephritis (up to 40%) than in nonpregnant women.[14] If a urine culture is negative for bacteria at the first prenatal visit, the risk of developing acute cystitis is less than 1%.[10,15]

It is important to diagnose and treat ASB in pregnancy. If left untreated, a symptomatic urinary tract infection (UTI) will develop in up to 40% of these patients.[6,10,16] **Recognition and therapy for ASB can eliminate 70% of acute UTIs in pregnancy.** Nonetheless, 2% of pregnant women with negative first trimester urine cultures develop symptomatic cystitis or pyelonephritis. This group accounts for 30% of the cases of acute UTI that develop during gestation. The American College of Obstetricians and Gynecologists (ACOG) recommends routine screening of all women for ASB at their first prenatal visit.[17] Other than progression to more serious infection, however, there is little evidence that ASB has an effect on pregnancy outcome.[9,18]

***Escherichia coli* is the organism responsible for most cases of ASB.** Women can therefore be safely treated with nitrofurantoin, ampicillin, cephalosporins, and short-acting sulfa drugs (see the accompanying box, Antimicrobial Treatment for the Pregnant Patient with Bacteriuria). Sulfa compounds should be avoided near term, as they compete for bilirubin-binding sites on albumin in the fetus and newborn and therefore pose a risk for kernicterus. Nitrofurantoin should not be used in patients with glucose-6-phosphate dehydrogenase deficiency (G6PD), as there is a risk for hemolytic crisis. If the fetus has G6PD, it may also experience hemolysis. Therapy for ASB should be continued for 7 days. A follow-up culture should be performed 1 to 2 weeks after discontinuing therapy. Approximately 15% of women will experience a reinfection and/or will not respond to initial therapy. Therapy in these cases should be reinstituted after careful microbial sensitivity testing. Women with recurrent UTI during pregnancy and those with a history of pyelonephritis should eventually undergo imaging of the upper urinary tract. This procedure should be delayed until the patient is 3 months postpartum so that the anatomic changes of pregnancy can regress.

Antimicrobial Treatment for the Pregnant Patient with Bacteriuria

- Amoxicillin 500 mg three times a day
- Ampicillin 250 mg four times a day
- Cephalosporin 250 mg four times a day
- Nitrofurantoin 100 mg four times a day
- Sustained-release nitrofurantoin 100 mg two times a day
- Trimethoprim (160 mg)/sulfamethoxazole (800 mg) two times a day

The agent of choice should be given for a 7-day course. A repeat urine culture is recommended 2 weeks after the treatment has been completed.

Occasionally it can be difficult to distinguish severe cystitis from pyelonephritis. Although the drugs used for treatment are similar, pyelonephritis treatment during pregnancy generally requires intravenous antibiotics. Sandberg and colleagues[19] studied symptomatic UTI in 174 women. They found that C-reactive protein was elevated in 91% of pregnant women with acute pyelonephritis and only 5% of women with cystitis. They also noted that the urine-concentrating ability was lower in women with acute pyelonephritis. Because the erythrocyte sedimentation rate is normally elevated in pregnancy, they found that this was not a useful parameter for distinguishing pyelonephritis from cystitis.

PYELONEPHRITIS

Pyelonephritis complicates 1% to 2% of all pregnancies, **and contributes substantially to maternal morbidity. It is among the most common nonobstetrical causes for hospitalization during pregnancy.**[20] **Recurrent pyelonephritis has been implicated as a cause of fetal death and intrauterine growth restriction (IUGR).** There also appears to be an association between acute pyelonephritis and preterm labor.[21,22] Fan and coworkers,[23] however, have shown that if pyelonephritis is aggressively treated, it does not increase the likelihood of prematurity, premature delivery, or low-birth-weight infants. Hill and colleagues,[24] reporting on 440 cases of acute pyelonephritis over a 2-year period, noted the disease to be more prevalent in younger primagravid women without racial predilection. The majority of cases (53%) presented during the second trimester. The most common pathogen was *E. coli*, accounting for 83% of cases, with gram-positive organisms accounting for another 11.6%.[24]

Acute pyelonephritis during pregnancy is most often treated on an inpatient basis, using intravenous antibiotics. Empiric therapy should be begun as soon as the presumptive diagnosis is made. Therapy can be tailored to the specific organism after sensitivities have been obtained. Because septicemia may occasionally result from pyelonephritis, blood cultures should be obtained if patients do not respond rapidly to initial antibiotic therapy. **Generally, a broad-spectrum first-generation cephalosporin is the initial therapy of choice.** Fan and colleagues[23] reviewed 107 cases of pyelonephritis in 103 pregnancies. The authors noted that 33% of the cases a decade ago were resistant to ampicillin and 13% to first-generation cephalosporins. Current rates of resistance to ampicillin and first-generation cephalosporins are likely higher. If resistance to more common therapies is encountered, a later-generation cephalosporin or an aminoglycoside can be safely administered. Peak and trough aminoglycoside levels should be measured when using aminoglycosides. Serum creatinine and BUN level should be followed as well. During the febrile period, acetaminophen treatment is advised to keep the temperature below 38° C.

Intravenous antibiotic therapy should be continued for 24 to 48 hours after the patient becomes afebrile and costovertebral angle tenderness disappears. After the cessation of intravenous therapy, treatment with appropriate oral antibiotics is recommended for 10 to 14 days. On termination of therapy, urine cultures should be obtained on each trimester for the remainder of gestation. After an episode of acute pyelonephritis, antibiotic suppression should also be implemented and continued for the remainder of the pregnancy. Nitrofurantoin 100 mg once or twice daily is an acceptable regimen for suppression. In a study by Van Dorsten and colleagues, nitrofurantoin suppression reduced the rate of subsequent positive cultures from 38% to 8%. However, nitrofurantoin did not lower the rate of positive cultures if inpatient antibiotic selection was inappropriate or if culture was positive at time of discharge.[25]

The most common maternal complications associated with pyelonepritis are anemia (23%), septicemia (17%), transient renal dysfunction (2%), and pulmonary insufficiency (7%).[24] **Pulmonary injury resembling adult respiratory distress syndrome (ARDS) can occur in pregnant women with acute pyelonephritis.**[26] Clinical manifestations of this complication usually occur 24 to 48 hours after the patient is admitted for pyelonephritis.[26,27] Some of these women will require endotracheal intubation, mechanical ventilation,[6] and positive end expiratory pressure (PEEP). **ARDS probably results from endotoxin-induced alveolar**

capillary membrane injury. Towers and colleagues[28] found evidence of pulmonary injury in 11 of 130 patients with pyelonephritis. A fever of greater than 103° F, a maternal heart rate above 110, and gestation beyond 20 weeks were factors associated with increased risk for pulmonary injury. The most predictive factors were fluid overload and tocolytic therapy.[28]

Austenfeld and Snow[29] reported 64 pregnancies in 30 women who had previously undergone ureteral reimplantation for vesicoureteral reflux. During pregnancy, 57% of these women experienced one or more UTIs, and 17% had more than one UTI or an episode of pyelonephritis.[29] More frequent urine cultures and aggressive therapy during pregnancy are recommended for this group of high-risk parturients.

ACUTE RENAL DISEASE IN PREGNANCY

Urolithiasis

Urolithiasis affects 0.03% of all pregnancies, a frequency similar to that of the general population.[30] Colicky abdominal pain, recurrent UTI, and hematuria suggest urolithiasis.[31] If the diagnosis is suspected, intravenous pyelography should be undertaken, limiting this study to the minimum number of exposures necessary to make the diagnosis. Ultrasound can often be used to establish the diagnosis without radiation exposure. Newer ultrasound flow studies can actually follow flow from the ureter to the bladder and detect obstruction without the use of ionizing radiation. If transabdominal ultrasound is not sufficient, transvaginal ultrasound can be employed to image the distal ureter.[32] Urine microscopy may detect crystals and help distinguish the type of stone before it is passed. For any women with renal calculi, serum calcium and phosphorous levels should be assayed to rule out hyperparathyroidism. Serum urate should also be determined.

Because of the physiologic hydroureter of pregnancy, 75% to 85% of women with symptomatic urolithiasis will spontaneously pass their stones.[31] Treatment should thus be conservative, consisting of hydration and narcotic analgesia.[33] Epidural anesthesia has been advocated to establish a segmental block from T11 to L2. It is unknown whether this promotes passage of the stone. Ureteral stenting to relieve obstruction is an option for managing pregnant women with renal stones. For refractory cases, nephrostomy tubes can also be employed. It should be noted that pregnancy increases the risk of stent encrustation requiring frequent stent exchange every 4 to 6 weeks until delivery.[34] Lithotripsy is contraindicated during pregnancy.[35]

Recurrent UTI with urease-containing organisms causes precipitation of calcium phosphate in the kidney that may lead to the development of staghorn calculi. Surgery is rarely indicated in these women during gestation. Individuals with staghorn calculi should have frequent urine cultures, and bacteriuria should be treated aggressively. Recurrent infections poses a risk for chronic pyelonephritis with resultant loss of kidney function.

Glomerulonephritis

Acute glomerulonephritis is an uncommon complication of pregnancy, with an estimated incidence of 1 per 40,000 pregnancies.[36] Poststreptococcal glomerulonephritis is rarely observed in the adult population. In this disorder, renal function tends to deteriorate during the acute phase of the disease, but usually later recovers.[37] **Acute glomerulonephritis can be difficult to distinguish from preeclampsia. Periorbital edema, a striking clinical feature of acute glomerulonephritis, is often seen in preeclampsia. However, hematuria, red blood cell (RBC) casts in the urine sediment, and depressed serum complement levels support glomerular disease.** Antistreptolysin O titers rise may secure the diagnosis of post-streptococcal glomerulonephritis.

Treatment of acute glomerulonephritis in pregnancy is similar to that for the nonpregnant individual. Blood pressure control is essential, and careful attention to fluid balance is imperative. Sodium intake should be restricted to 500 mg/day during the acute disease. Serum potassium levels must also be carefully monitored.

Packham and coworkers[38] extensively reviewed 395 pregnancies in 238 women with primary glomerulonephritis. Only 51% of infants were born after 36 weeks' gestation. Excluding therapeutic abortion, 20% of fetuses were lost with 15% occurring after 20 weeks' gestation. IUGR was noted in 15% of cases. Maternal renal function deteriorated in 15% of pregnancies and failed to resolve following delivery in 5% of the population.[38] Hypertension was recorded in 52% of the pregnancies and developed before 32 weeks' gestation in 26% of cases. In most cases, this blood pressure elevation was not an exacerbation of chronic hypertension. Eighteen percent of the women who developed de novo hypertension in pregnancy remained hypertensive postpartum. Increased proteinuria was recorded in 59% of these pregnancies and was irreversible in 15%.[38] The highest incidence of fetal and maternal complications occurred in patients with primary focal and segmental hyalinosis and sclerosis, whereas the lowest incidence of complications was observed in non-IgA diffuse mesangial proliferative glomerulonephritis.[38] The presence of severe vessel lesions on renal biopsy was associated with a significantly higher rate of fetal loss after 20 weeks' gestation. Packham and coworkers[39] also studied 33 pregnancies in 24 patients with biopsy-proven membranous glomerulonephritis. Fetal loss occurred in 24% of pregnancies, preterm delivery in 43%, and a term liveborn in only 33% of patients. Hypertension was noted in 46% of these pregnant women. Thirty percent of patients had proteinuria in the nephrotic range during the first trimester.[39] The presence of significant proteinuria during the first trimester correlated with poor fetal and maternal outcome.[39]

Jungers and colleagues[40] described 69 pregnancies in 34 patients with IgA glomerulonephritis. The fetal loss rate in this group was 15%. Preexisting hypertension was statistically associated with poor fetal outcome. Hypertension at the time of conception also correlated with a deterioration of maternal renal function during pregnancy. Hypertension in the first pregnancy was highly predictive of recurrence of hypertension in a subsequent pregnancy.[40] Kincaid-Smith and Fairley[41] analyzed 102 pregnancies in 65 women with IgA glomerulonephritis. They noted that hypertension occurred in 63% of pregnancies, with 18% being severe. In this subset of women, a decline in renal function was observed in 22%.[41] Abe[42] reported 240 pregnancies in 166 women with preexisting glomerular disease. Eight percent of the pregnancies resulted in a spontaneous abortion, 6% resulted in stillbirth, and 86% were liveborn. Most losses occurred in women with a GFR less than 70 mL/min and preexisting hypertension. Even though the majority of women with significant renal insufficiency had good pregnancy outcomes, the long-term prognosis for these cases was worse if the GFR was less than 50 mL/min and the serum creatinine was more than 1.5 mg/dL.[42] The histopathogenic diagnosis of membranoproliferative glomerulonephritis seemed to carry the worst prognosis with 29% developing hypertension and 33% developing a long-term decrease in renal function.

Imbasciati and Ponticelli[43] summarized six studies containing a total of 906 pregnancies in 558 women with preexisting glomerular disease. The overall perinatal mortality rate was 13%. Hypertension, azotemia, and nephrotic range proteinuria were the strongest predictive factors for a poor pregnancy outcome. In this report, the histologic type of glomerulonephritis had little correlation with pregnancy outcome. Hypertension persisted in 3% to 12% of patients who developed hypertension for the first time during pregnancy. In 25% of patients, hypertension worsened during pregnancy and normalized postpartum.[43] Some of these cases represented superimposed preeclampsia; however, this diagnosis can be difficult to establish in women with baseline hypertension and proteinuria. Remarkably, only 3% of these 166 women experienced an acceleration of their glomerular disease after pregnancy.

Acute Renal Failure in Pregnancy

Acute renal failure (ARF) is defined as a urine output of less than 400 mL in 24 hours. To establish the diagnosis, ureteral and urethral obstruction must be excluded. The incidence of ARF during pregnancy is approximately 1 per 10,000. It is seen most frequently following septic first trimester abortions and in cases of sudden severe volume depletion resulting from hemorrhage.[44] It may also be observed with marked volume contraction associated with severe preeclampsia,[45,46] dehydration from hyperemesis gravidarum,[47] and with acute fatty liver of pregnancy.[45,48]

The incidence of ARF in pregnancy has decreased over the years. Stratta and colleagues[49] reported 81 cases of pregnancy-related ARF between 1958 and 1987, accounting for 9% of the total number of ARF cases needing dialysis during that interval. In three successive 10-year periods (1958-1967, 1968-1977, and 1978-1987), the incidence of pregnancy-related ARF fell from 43% to 2.8% of the total number of cases of ARF. The incidence changed from 1 in 3,000 to 1 in 15,000 pregnancies over the study period.[49] In these 81 ARF cases, 11.6% experienced irreversible renal damage with the majority occurring in the setting of severe preeclampsia/eclampsia.[49]

Renal ischemia is the common denominator in cases of ARF. With mild ischemia, quickly reversible prerenal failure results. With more prolonged ischemia, acute tubular necrosis occurs. This process is also reversible, as glomeruli are not affected. Severe ischemia, however, may produce acute cortical necrosis. This pathology is irreversible, although on occasion a small amount of renal function is preserved.[50] Stratta and colleagues[51] have reported 17 cases of ARF complicating pregnancies over 15 years, and all were secondary to preeclampsia/eclampsia. Cortical necrosis occurred in 29.5% of the cases.[51] Progression of ARF to cortical necrosis did not appear to be related to maternal age, parity, gestational age, duration of preeclampsia before delivery, or eclamptic seizures. The only significant risk factor associated with cortical necrosis was placental abruption.[51] In another study, Turney and coworkers[16] demonstrated that acute cortical necrosis, which occurred in 12.7% of their patients with ARF, carried a 100% mortality rate within 6 years.

Sibai and colleagues[52] studied the remote prognosis in 31 consecutive cases of ARF in patients with hypertensive disorders of pregnancy. Eighteen of the 31 patients had "pure" preeclampsia, while 13 pregnancies had other hypertensive disorders and renal disease. Five percent of the 18 patients with pure preeclampsia required dialysis during hospitalization, and all 18 patients had acute tubular necrosis. Of the other 13 women, 42% required dialysis and three patients had bilateral cortical necrosis. The majority of pregnancies in both groups were complicated by placental abruption and hemorrhage.[52] All 16 surviving patients in the pure preeclampsia group recovered normal renal function on long-term follow-up. Conversely, 9 of the 11 surviving patients in the nonpreeclamptic group required long-term dialysis, and four ultimately died of end-stage renal disease.[52] Turney and colleagues[16] also performed follow-up examinations of their patients. They found that maternal survival was adversely affected by increasing age. Their 1-year maternal survival rate was 78.6%. Follow-up of survivors showed normal renal function up to 31 years after ARF.[16]

Individuals with reversible ARF experience a period of oliguria of variable duration followed by polyuria, or a high-output phase. It is important to recognize that BUN and serum creatinine levels continue to rise early in the polyuric phase. During the recovery phase, urine output approaches normal. In these patients, it is important to monitor electrolytes frequently and to carefully treat any imbalance. The urine to plasma osmolality ratio should be determined early in the course of the disease. If the ratio is 1.5 or greater, prerenal pathology is likely, and the disorder tends to be of shorter duration and less severity. A ratio near 1.0 suggests acute tubular necrosis.

The main goal of treatment is the elimination of the underlying cause. **Volume and electrolyte balance** must be evaluated frequently. To assess volume requirements, invasive hemodynamic monitoring may be useful. This is especially true during the polyuric phase. Central hyperalimentation may also be required if renal failure is prolonged.

Acidosis frequently occurs in cases of ARF. Arterial blood gases therefore should be followed regularly. Acidosis must be treated promptly as it may exacerbate hyperkalemia, which may develop rapidly and can be fatal. If hyperkalemia develops, potassium restriction should be instituted immediately. Sodium bicarbonate, used to treat acidosis, may overload the patient with sodium and water. In such cases, peritoneal or hemodialysis may be necessary. The main indications for dialysis in ARF of pregnancy are hypernatremia, hyperkalemia, severe acidosis, volume overload, and worsening uremia. There is a single report of a successful kidney transplant during pregnancy in the first trimester. Although unintentional, a patient received a kidney from her father at approximately 13 weeks' gestation and experienced a successful pregnancy.[53]

Hemolytic Uremic Syndrome

The postpartum hemolytic uremic syndrome is a rare idiopathic disorder that must be considered when a patient exhibits signs of hemolysis and decreasing renal function, particularly during in the postpartum period. This idiopathic syndrome may occur as early as the first trimester and up to 2 months postpartum.[16,54-56] In fact, it has even been reported following an ectopic pregnancy.[57] Most individuals have no predisposing factors. Prodromal symptoms include vomiting, diarrhea, and a flu-like illness. A review of forty-nine cases documented a 61% mortality rate, although with improved intensive care monitoring and treatment, the prognosis is now much improved.

Disseminated intravascular coagulation (DIC) with hemolysis usually accompanies hemolytic uremic syndrome. However, DIC is not the cause of the syndrome. Microscopically, the kidney shows thrombotic microangiopathy. The glomerular capillary wall is thick, and biopsy specimens taken later in the course of the disease show severe nephrosclerosis and deposition of the third component of complement (C_3).

Some investigators believe that this syndrome is due to decreased renal production of prostacyclin.[58,59] Prostacyclin infusions have been used to treat patients, but this therapy still remains experimental. One observer noted a decrease in antithrombin III in a woman with postpartum hemolytic uremic syndrome. This patient was successfully treated with an infusion of antithrombin III concentrate.[60]

Coratelli and coworkers[54] reported a case of hemolytic uremic syndrome that was diagnosed at 13 weeks' gestation and confirmed by renal biopsy. Circulating endotoxin was detected and was progressively reduced by hemodialysis performed daily from the third to the ninth days of the disease. Complete normalization of renal function occurred by day 34. These investigators propose that initiation of early dialysis may play an important role in supporting patients through the disease process. They also propose that endotoxins are key pathogenic factors in the disorder.[54] In contrast, Li and coworkers[61] failed to measure any endotoxin in the serum of a patient who developed hemolytic uremic syndrome after an uncomplicated cesarean delivery. This patient eventually underwent dialysis and recovered.[61] **Plasma exchange in cases of ARF caused by the postpartum hemolytic uremic syndrome can be vital to the treatment of this condition.**[62]

Polycystic Kidney Disease

Adult polycystic kidney disease is an autosomal dominant **disorder that usually begins to manifest itself in the fifth decade of life. Reproductive-age women may occasionally display symptoms. Hypertension is part of this disorder.** If a woman with adult polycystic kidney disease becomes pregnant, hypertension may be exacerbated and may not improve postpartum.[43] The overall prognosis for the disorder does not appear to worsen with an increasing number of pregnancies.

Vesicoureteral Reflux

Vesicoureteral reflux increases with pregnancy. It usually does not cause problems unless reflux becomes severe. If it is significant enough to warrant surgery, this should ideally be undertaken before pregnancy. Even with surgical correction, women with ureterovesical reflux are at increased risk for pyelonephritis and should have cultures performed frequently.[43] Antibiotic suppression, if indicated before pregnancy, should be continued.

Brandes and Fritsche[62] report a case of ARF due to ureteral obstruction by a gravid uterus. This case was complicated by a twin gestation with polyhydramnios at 34 weeks' gestation. The serum creatinine level peaked at 12.2 mg/dL, but resolved immediately after amniotomy.[62] In cases remote from term, ureteral stenting or dialysis may be necessary if significant obstruction and/or reflux is present.

Renal Artery Stenosis

Renal artery stenosis is an extremely rare complication of pregnancy.[63] This disorder may present as chronic hypertension with superimposed preeclampsia or as recurrent isolated preeclampsia. Although Doppler flow studies may be suggestive, renal angiography is the most specific and sensitive diagnostic test. Percutaneous transluminal angioplasty can be carried out at the time of angiography.[63]

Nephrotic Syndrome

The nephrotic syndrome was initially described as a 24-hour urine protein excretion of 3.5 g or more, reduced serum albumin, edema, and hyperlipidemia.[64] Currently, the syndrome is defined by massive proteinuria alone, which is often the result of glomerular damage.[64] The most common etiology of nephrotic syndrome in pregnancy (especially the third trimester) is preeclampsia. Other etiologies include membranous and mebranoproliferative glomerulpathy, minimal change disease, lupus nephropathy, hereditary nephritis, diabetic nephropathy, renal vein thrombosis, and amyloidosis.[65]

Women with newly diagnosed or persistent nephrotic syndrome need close monitoring during pregnancy. Whenever possible the etiology of the proteinuria should be determined. In some cases, steroid therapy may be employed to treat this condition; however, its use can actually aggravate the underlying disease process.[65] One common complication of nephrotic syndrome in pregnancy is profound edema secondary to protein excretion, which is further complicated by the normal decline in serum albumin associated with pregnancy.[65] A second complication is the development of a hypercoagulable state precipitated by urinary losses of antithrombin III, reduced levels of protein C and S, hyperfibrinogenemia, and enhanced platelet aggregation.[66]

CHRONIC RENAL DISEASE IN PREGNANCY

Chronic renal disease can be silent until its advanced stages. Because obstetricians routinely test a women's urine for the presence of protein, glucose, and ketones, they may be the first to detect chronic renal disease.

Any gravida with more than trace proteinuria should collect a 24-hour urine specimen for creatinine clearance and total protein excretion. Before pregnancy, 24-hour urinary protein excretion should not exceed 0.2 g. During gestation, quantities up to 0.3 g per day may be normal. Moderate proteinuria (less than 2 g per day) is often seen in glomerular disease.

Microscopic examination of the urine can reveal much about renal status. If renal disease is suspected, a catheterized specimen should be obtained. **More RBCs than one to two per high-power field or RBC casts are indicative of glomerular disease.** Less frequently, they suggest trauma or malignant hypertension. Increased numbers of white blood cells (WBCs) (more than one to two per high-power field) or the appearance of WBC casts is usually indicative of acute or chronic infection. Cellular casts are found in the presence of renal tubular dysfunction, and hyaline casts are associated with significant proteinuria.

The obstetrician can easily be misled when relying solely on BUN and serum creatinine levels to assess renal function. A 70% decline in creatinine clearance, an indirect measure of GFR, can be seen before a significant rise in serum BUN or serum creatinine occurs. Little change in serum creatinine or the BUN may be observed until the creatinine clearance falls to 50 mL/min. Below that level, small decrements in creatinine clearance can lead to large increases in the BUN and creatinine. A single creatinine clearance value less than 100 mL/min is therefore not diagnostic of renal diseases. An incomplete 24-hour urine collection is the most frequent cause of this finding. An abnormal clearance rate should therefore prompt a repeat assay.

Serum urate is an often overlooked but helpful parameter in detecting renal dysfunction. Excretion of uric acid is dependent not only on glomerular filtration but also on tubular secretion. An elevated serum urate in the presence of a normal BUN and serum creatinine may therefore implicate tubular disease. A solitary increase in uric acid may also signify impending or early preeclampsia.

Effect of Pregnancy on Renal Function

Although baseline creatinine clearance is decreased in women with chronic renal insufficiency, a physiologic rise will often occur in pregnancy. A moderate fall in creatinine clearance may then be observed during late gestation in patients with renal disease. This decline is typically more severe in women with diffuse glomerular disease and typically reverses after delivery.

The long-term effect of pregnancy on renal disease remains controversial. If the serum creatinine is less than 1.5 mg/dL, pregnancy appears to have little effect on the long-term prognosis. Pregnancy, however, is associated with an increased incidence of pyelonephritis in patients with chronic renal disease. There are few data concerning the long-term effect of pregnancy on renal disease in women with significant azotemia. Occasionally, some women with a baseline serum creatinine of more than 1.5 mg/dL will experience a significant decrease in renal function during gestation that does not improve during the postpartum period.[43,67] This deterioration occurs more frequently in women with diffuse glomerulonephritis. It is not possible, however, to predict which women with renal insufficiency will experience a permanent reduction in renal function. Moreover, if renal function significantly deteriorates during gestation, termination of pregnancy may not reverse the process. Termination therefore cannot be routinely recommended for patients who become pregnant and whose baseline serum creatinine level exceeds 1.5 mg/dL. Ideally, women with chronic renal disease should be counseled before conception about the possible deterioration in renal function.

Severe hypertension remains the greatest threat to a pregnant patient with chronic renal disease. Left uncontrolled, hypertension can lead to cerebral hemorrhage, as well as deteriorating renal function. Most pregnant women with chronic renal dysfunction also have preexisting hypertension.[11,68] Approximately 50% of these patients will have worsening hypertension as pregnancy progresses, and diastolic blood pressures of 110 mm Hg or greater will develop in about 20% of cases.[69] Those women with diffuse proliferative glomerulonephritis and nephrosclerosis are at greatest risk for the development of severe hypertension. It follows that blood pressure control is the cornerstone of successful treatment of chronic renal disease in pregnancy.

Worsening proteinuria is common during pregnancy complicated by chronic renal disease and often reaches the nephrotic range.[69] In general, massive proteinuria alone does not indicate an increased risk for mother or fetus.[70] Low serum albumin, however, has been correlated with low birth weight.[71] The development of massive proteinuria is not necessarily a harbinger of preeclampsia although such women are clearly at risk for this complication. In late pregnancy, it can be difficult to differentiate preeclampsia from worsening chronic renal disease. For this reason first trimester 24-hour urine collections to establish baselines for creatinine clearance and total protein are essential.

Effect of Chronic Renal Disease on Pregnancy

More than 85% of women with chronic renal disease will have a surviving infant if renal function is well preserved. Earlier reports were more pessimistic, citing a 6% incidence of stillbirth, a 5% incidence of neonatal deaths, and an increase risk for second trimester loss.[69] If hypertension is not controlled and if renal function is not well preserved, there is still a high likelihood of pregnancy loss.[38] Antepartum fetal surveillance and advances in neonatal care have contributed to an in improved perinatal outcome in these patients. One study reported a total fetal loss rate of 14%, including miscarriage, stillbirths, and neonatal deaths.[68]

The outlook for women with severe renal insufficiency whose baseline serum creatinine level is more than 1.5 mg/dL is less certain. This is due in part to the limited number of pregnancies in such patients. One study reported no surviving infants when the maternal BUN was greater than 60 mg/dL.[70] Other investigations, however, have found that about 80% of such pregnancies resulted in surviving infants.[68,72] **Preterm birth and IUGR remain important complications in these pregnancies. The reported incidence of preterm birth ranges from 20% to 50%.**[69,73]

Imbasciati and Ponticelli[43] summarize three studies containing 81 pregnancies in 78 women with serum creatinine concentrations greater than 1.4 mg/dL.[43] The perinatal loss rate was only 9%. However, 33% of the infants were growth restricted, and 50% were born preterm secondary to either maternal or fetal indications. Of concern, 33% of the women showed acceleration of their renal disease after delivery. Some individuals believe that growth restriction may be due to the lack of normal plasma volume increase as the pregnancy progresses. Cunningham and colleagues[74] demonstrated that women with moderate renal dysfunction exhibit increased creatinine clearance and plasma volume expansion during gestation, whereas women with severe renal dysfunction generally do not.[74]

Management of Chronic Renal Disease in Pregnancy

A 24-hour urine collection for creatinine clearance and **total protein excretion should be obtained as soon as the pregnancy is confirmed. These parameters should be monitored periodically. A general guideline is to see patients every 2 weeks until 32 weeks' gestation and weekly thereafter.**

Control of hypertension is critical in managing patients with chronic renal disease. Home blood pressure monitoring is thus advised for women with underlying hypertension. β-Blockers, calcium channel blockers, and hydralazine can be used to treat blood pressure effectively as long as the dosages are monitored carefully. Clonidine is occasionally useful in refractory patients. Doxazosin and prazosin may also be used if necessary. Angiotensin-converting enzyme inhibitors are contraindicated. These drugs have been associated with fetal and neonatal oliguria/anuria,[75,76] as well as anomalies.[77] In one study, 1 of 19 infants had anuria and required dialysis.[75,77] Congenital anomalies, including microcephaly and encephalocele,[75] have been associated with the use of angiotensin-converting enzymes inhibitors.[76]

The use of diuretics in pregnancy is controversial.[78,79] **For massive debilitating edema, a short course of diuretics can be helpful.** Electrolytes must be monitored carefully. Salt restriction does not appear to be beneficial once edema has developed. Salt restriction, however, should be instituted without hesitation in pregnant women with true renal insufficiency.

Fetal growth should be assessed with serial ultrasonography, because growth restriction is common in women with chronic renal disease. Antepartum fetal heart rate testing is often initiated at 28 to 32 weeks' gestation.[11]

The timing of delivery should be individualized. Maternal indications for delivery include uncontrollable hypertension, the development of superimposed preeclampsia, and decreasing renal function after fetal viability has been reached. Fetal indications are dictated by assessment of fetal growth and biophysical testing.

Renal biopsy is rarely indicated during pregnancy. It is not advised after 34 weeks' gestation, when delivery of the fetus and subsequent biopsy would prove a safer alternative. Excessive bleeding secondary to the greatly increased renal blood flow has been reported by some but not all observers.[80,81] If coagulation indices are normal and blood pressure is well controlled, morbidity should be no greater than that observed in the nonpregnant patient.[81] Packham and Fairley[82] report a series of 111 renal biopsies performed in 104 pregnant women over 20 years. The complication rate was 4.5%. The most likely clinical dilemma necessitating renal biopsy in a pregnant woman would be the development of nephrotic syndrome and increasing hypertension between 22 and 32 weeks' gestation. In this case, renal biopsy may distinguish chronic renal disease from preeclampsia and have a significant impact on treatment.

Hemodialysis in Pregnancy

Women with chronic hemodialysis can have successful pregnancies.[83-89] **Many women with chronic renal failure, however, experience oligomenorrhea, and their fertility is often impaired.**[90] These women commonly fail to use a method of contraception. It is therefore important that pregnancy testing be undertaken if suspected.

As in all patients with impaired renal function, the most important aspect of care is meticulous control of blood pressure. **During dialysis, wide fluctuations in blood pressure can occur.**[91] **Sudden volume shifts therefore should be avoided as they may compromise fetal well-being.**[92,93] In late pregnancy, continuous fetal heart rate monitoring should be carried out during dialysis.[92] If possible, positioning on the left side with uterine displacement from the vena cava is preferred. During dialysis, careful attention to electrolyte balance is advised. Pregnant patients are in a state of chronic compensated respiratory alkalosis, and large drops in serum bicarbonate should be avoided. Dialysates containing glucose and bicarbonate are preferred, and those containing citrates should be avoided.[89]

Women should be counseled that a successful pregnancy will often require longer and more frequent periods of dialysis.[84,89,91,93] A careful diet, ingesting at least 70 g of protein and 1.5 g of calcium daily, is proscribed. Weight gain should be limited to 0.5 kg between dialysis sessions. Chronic anemia is often a problem in hemodialysis patients. The hematocrit should be kept above 25%, and transfusion with packed RBCs or erythropoietin therapy may be necessary to accomplish this objective.[84]

Criteria for initiating hemodialysis during pregnancy are controversial.[94] **Some investigators believe that beginning of regular hemodialysis in patients with moderate renal insufficiency may improve pregnancy outcome.**[86] Redrow and coworkers[87] report 14 pregnancies in 13 women undergoing dialysis. Ten of those pregnancies were successful. Five of eight pregnancies managed with chronic ambulatory peritoneal dialysis or chronic cycling peritoneal dialysis were successful. The investigators hypothesize several advantages for peritoneal dialysis. These include a more constant chemical and extracellular environment for the fetus, higher hematocrit levels, infrequent episodes of hypotension, and no heparin requirement. They also postulate that intraperitoneal insulin facilitates the management of blood glucose in diabetic patients and that intraperitoneal magnesium used in the dialysate reduces the likelihood of preterm labor.

Preterm birth occurs more frequently in women undergoing dialysis.[95] Progesterone is removed during dialysis and at least one group has advocated that parenteral progesterone therapy should be administered to the patient undergoing dialysis.[96] In their review, Yasin and Doun[89] report a 40.7% incidence of premature labor.

Renal Transplant

Pregnancy following renal transplantation has become increasingly common.[97] **Many previously anovulatory patients begin ovulating postoperatively and regain fertility as renal function normalizes.**[98] As with women receiving hemodialysis, many transplant recipients do not recognize they are pregnant until well into the second trimester.

Many transplant recipients will discontinue all medications after discovering they are pregnant. The importance of continuing immunosuppressive therapy cannot be emphasized strongly enough to renal allograft recipients. Glucocorticoids, especially prednisone, are metabolized in the placenta by 11 β-ol-dehydrogenase, with only limited amounts reaching the fetus.[99] Azathioprine cannot be activated in the fetus because of its lack of inosinate pyrophosphorylase.[100] Azathioprine has been shown to cause decreased levels of IgG and IgM as well as a smaller thymic shadow on chest x-ray in these neonates.[101] Chromosomal aberrations, which cleared within 20 to 32 months, have also been demonstrated in lymphocytes of infants exposed to azathioprine in utero.[102] The long-term implications of this treatment are not yet known. IUGR has been reported in infants born to mothers receiving this medication.[103] These risks are outweighed, however, by the disastrous consequences of allograft rejection that may occur if medication is discontinued.

Cyclosporin A appears to be relatively safe for use during gestation, but does hold some risks. Women may develop arterial hypertension secondary to its interference with the normal hemodynamic adaptation to pregnancy.[104] Cylosporin metabolism appears to be increased during pregnancy and, as such, the dose may need to be increased to maintain therapeutic levels.[105] Cyclosporin crosses the placenta; however, there is no evidence of teratogenesis although its safety in pregnancy has not been established.[106,107] IUGR, in the absence of maternal hypertension, has been reported with cyclosporin A use during pregnancy.[108] However, most women receiving cyclosporin have had no complications attributable to the drug and the risk of allograft rejection certainly outweighs the fetal risk of the medication.

Mycophenolate mofetil (MMF) has been shown to cause adverse effects on fetal development and is associated with first trimester loss and congenital defects. These anomalies include cleft lip and palate, limb anomalies, heart defects, and renal anomalies.[109] This drug is contraindicated in pregnancy.

Sirolimus is also contraindicated in pregnancy. This medication has been shown to be embryotoxic and is associated with increased fetal mortality.[109] It is recommended that women who wish to conceive be switched from this medication before becoming pregnant.[109]

Tacrolimus has been poorly studied in pregnancy. In a study of 100 pregnancies in patients who were exposed to tacrolimus there were 68 live births with 60% being premature. There were four infants with malformations, but no consistent pattern of anomally.[110] Patients taking tacrolimus require frequent monitoring of renal function and drug levels.

Davison[111] reviewed 1569 renal transplants in 1009 women. He found that 22% of the women elected to abort their pregnancies, 16% had a spontaneous abortion, and 8% experienced perinatal deaths. Furthermore, he observed that 45% of the surviving pregnancies were delivered preterm and 22% were complicated by IUGR.[111] Three percent of the infants were born with major malformations, a rate no different from expected in the background population. Preeclampsia complicated 30% of the pregnancies, but, as previously noted, the diagnosis is difficult to make in a patient who may already have hypertension and proteinuria. The allograft rejection rate in these women was 9%, a rate no different from that expected in a nonpregnant population.[111] The long-term rejection rate was also the same as for women who had not experienced a pregnancy.

During pregnancy, renal allograft recipients must be carefully watched for signs of rejection. As previously mentioned, significant episodes of rejection may occur in as many as 9% of transplant recipients during gestation. **Unfortunately, the clinical hallmarks of rejection—fever, oliguria, tenderness, and decreasing renal function—are not always exhibited by the pregnant patient. Occasionally, rejection may mimic pyelonephritis or preeclampsia, which occurs in approximately one third of renal transplant patients.** In these cases renal biopsy is indicated to distinguish rejection from preeclampsia. Rejection has been known to occur during the puerperium, when maternal immune competence returns to its prepregnancy level.[112] Therefore, it may be advisable to increase the dose of immunosuppressive medications in the immediate postpartum period.

Infection can be disastrous for the renal allograft. Therefore, urine cultures should be obtained at least monthly during pregnancy, and any bacteriuria should be aggressively treated. It is crucial to recognize that the allograft is denervated, and pain may not accompany the pyelonephritis. The only symptoms may be fever and nausea.

Renal function, as determined by 24-hour creatinine clearance and protein excretion, should be assessed monthly. Approximately 15% of transplant recipients will exhibit a significant decrease in renal function in late pregnancy.[65] This condition usually, but not always, reverses after pregnancy. Proteinuria develops in about 40% of patients near term, but most often disappears soon after delivery unless significant hypertension is present.

Similar to women with chronic renal disease, serial ultrasonography should be used to assess fetal growth, and antepartum fetal heart rate testing should be considered at 28 to 32 weeks' gestation. Approximately 50% of renal allograft recipients will deliver preterm. Preterm labor, preterm rupture of membranes, and IUGR are common. Cesarean delivery is reserved for obstetrical indications. Allograft recipients may have an increased frequency of cephalopelvic disproportion from pelvic osteodystrophy,[113] resulting from prolonged renal disease with hypercalcemia or extended steroid use. The transplanted kidney, however, rarely obstructs vaginal delivery despite its pelvic location.

Although there have been many successful pregnancies in renal allograft recipients, there is no consensus as to when it is safe to attempt pregnancy after transplantation. Lindheimer and Katz[114] have suggested some guidelines, which are summarized in the box Guidelines for Renal Allograft Recipients Who Wish to Conceive.

Guidelines for Renal Allograft Recipients Considering Pregnancy

- Wait 2 years after cadaver transplant or 1 year after graft from living donor
- Immunosuppression should be at maintenance levels
- Plasma creatinine <1.5 mg/dL
- Absent or easily controlled hypertension
- No or minimal proteinuria
- No evidence of active graft rejection
- No pelvicalyceal distention on a recent ultrasound or intravenous pyelogram
- Prednisone dose = 15 mg/day
- Azathioprine dose = 2 mg/kg/day
- Cyclosporin A dose 2-4 mg/kg (available data on the use of this drug in pregnancy includes <150 patients)

Modified from Lindheimer M, Katz A: Pregnancy in the renal transplant patient. Am J Kidney Dis 19:173, 2000.

KEY POINTS

- ◆ Asymptomatic bacteriuria complicates 5% to 7% of pregnancies and if left untreated will result in symptomatic urinary tract infections in 40% of patients.
- ◆ Pyelonephritis complicates 1% to 2% of pregnancies, making it a frequent nonobstetrical cause of hospitalization during pregnancy.
- ◆ Women with glomerulonephritis can have successful pregnancies, but pregnancy loss rates increase greatly if the patient has preexisting hypertension.
- ◆ Creatinine clearance can decline 70% before significant increases are seen in the BUN or serum creatinine level. Therefore, a 24-hour urine specimen for creatinine clearance should be collected from any woman in whom renal disease is suspected.
- ◆ The chance of successful pregnancy is reduced if the creatinine clearance is less than 50 mL/min or if the serum creatinine level is more than 1.5 mg/dL.
- ◆ Severe hypertension poses the greatest threat to the pregnant woman with chronic renal disease.
- ◆ Growth restriction and preeclampsia are common complications in women with chronic renal disease. Frequent sonograms and antepartum fetal surveillance at 28 weeks' gestation are recommended in affected pregnancies.
- ◆ Patients with chronic renal disease are often anovulatory. Following transplantation, as renal function returns, ovulation may resume with unplanned pregnancy possible.
- ◆ Women should wait 2 years after receiving a cadaver renal allograft and 1 year after receiving a living allograft before contemplating pregnancy. Furthermore, there should be no signs of allograft rejection.
- ◆ Renal transplant patients may remain on cyclosporine throughout gestation. Levels may need to be adjusted during pregnancy. Other immunosuppressive medications such as mycophenolate and sirolimus are contraindicated.
- ◆ Renal function may decline as a result of pregnancy among patients with renal disease. Increased risk for this decline is conferred by an elevated plasma creatinine concentration (above 1.5 mg/dL or 132 micromoles/L) and hypertension.

REFERENCES

1. Cietak KA, Newton JR: Serial quantitative maternal nephrosonography in pregnancy. Br J Radiol 58:405, 1985.
2. Cietak KA, Newton JR: Serial qualitative maternal nephrosonography in pregnancy. Br J Radiol 58:399, 1985.
3. Rassmussen PE, Nielson FR: Hydronephrosis during pregnancy: a literature survey. Eur J Obstet Gynecol Reprod Biol 27:249, 1988.
4. Danielson LA, Sherwood OD, Conrad KP: Relaxin is a potent vasodilator in conscious rats. J Clin Invest 103:525, 1999.
5. Conrad KP, Gandley RE, Ogawa T, et al: Endothelin mediates renal vasodilatation and hyperfiltration during pregnancy in chronically instrumented conscious rats. Am J Physiol 276:767, 1999.
6. Davison JM, Sprott MS, Selkon JB: The effect of covert bacteriuria in schoolgirls on renal function at 18 years and during pregnancy. Lancet 2:651, 1984.
7. Davidson J: Changes in renal function and other aspects of homeostasis in early pregnancy. J Obstet Gynaecol Br Commonw 81:1003, 1974.
8. Christensen P: Tubular reabsorption of glucose during pregnancy. Scand J Clin Lab Invest 10:364, 1958.
9. Sheffield JSM, Cunningham FGM: Urinary tract infection in women. Obstet Gynecol 106:1085, 2005.
10. Hooton TM, Scholes D, Stapleton AE, et al: A prospective study of asymptomatic bacteriuria in sexually active young women. N Engl J Med 343:992, 2000.
11. Bear R: Pregnancy in patients with renal disease: a study of 44 cases. Obstet Gynecol 48:13, 1976.
12. Norden C, Kass E: Bacteriuria of pregnancy—a critical reappraisal. Annu Rev Med 19:431, 1968.
13. McFadyen I, Eykryn S, Gardner N: Bacteriuria of pregnancy. J Obstet Gynaecol Br Commonw 80:385, 1973.
14. Smaill FVJ: Antibiotics for asymptomatic bacteriuria in pregnancy. Cochrane Database Syst Rev 2007.
15. Whalley P: Bacteriuria of pregnancy. Am J Obstet Gynecol 97:723, 1967.
16. Turney JH, Ellis CM, Parsons FM: Obstetric acute renal failure 1956-1987. Br J Obstet Gynaecol 96:679, 1989.
17. American Academy of Pediatrics & American College of Gynecologists: Guidelines for Prenatal Care. Elk Grove Village, IL, American Academy of Pediatrics & American College of Obstetricians and Obstetricians and Gynecologists, 2002, p 90.
18. Smaill F: Antibiotics for asymptomatic bacteriuria in pregnancy (Cochrane Review). Oxford. Cochrane Library 2, 2001.
19. Sandberg T, Likin-Janson G, Eden CS: Host response in women with symptomatic urinary tract infection. Scand J Infect Dis 21:67, 1989.
20. Plattner MS: Pyelonephritis in pregnancy. J Perinatol Neonat Nurs 8:20, 1994.
21. Brumfitt W: The significance of symptomatic and asymptomatic infection in pregnancy. Contrib Nephrol 25:23, 1981.
22. Gilstrap L, Leveno K, Cunningham F, et al: Renal infections and pregnancy outcome. Am J Obstet Gynecol 141:709, 1981.
23. Fan YD, Pastorek JG II, Miller JM, Mulvey J: Acute pyelonephritis in pregnancy. Am J Perinatol 4:324, 1987.
24. Hill JBM, Sheffield JSM, McIntire DDP, Wendel GDJ: Acute pyelonephritis in pregnancy. Obstet Gynecol 105:18, 2005.
25. Van Dorsten JP, Lenke RR, Schifrin BS: Pyelonephritis in pregnancy: the role of in-hospital management and nitrofurantoin suppression. J Reprod Med 32:895, 1987.
26. Cunningham FG, Lucas MJ, Hankins GD: Pulmonary injury complicating antepartum pyelonephritis. Am J Obstet Gynecol 156:797, 1987.

27. Pruett K, Faro S: Pyelonephritis associated with respiratory distress. Obstet Gynecol 69:444, 1987.
28. Towers CV, Kaminskas CM, Garite CM, et al: Pulmonary injury associated with antepartum pylonephritis: can at risk patients be identified? Am J Obstet Gynecol 164:974, 1991.
29. Austenfeld MS, Snow BW: Complications of pregnancy in women after reimplantation for vesicoureteral reflux. J Urol 140:1103, 1988.
30. Harris R, Dunnihoo D: The incidence and significance of urinary calculi in pregnancy. Am J Obstet Gynecol 99:237, 1967.
31. Butler EL, Cox SM, Eberts EG, Cunningham FG: Symptomatic nephrolithiasis complicating pregnancy. Obstet Gynecol 96:753, 2000.
32. Laing FC, Benson CB, DiSalvo DN: Distal uretral calculi: detection with vaginal ultrasound. Radiology 192:545, 1994.
33. Strong D, Murchison R, Lynch D: The management of ureteral calculi during pregnancy. Obstet Gynecol Surv 146:604, 1978.
34. Parulkar BG, Hopkins TB, Wollin MR: Renal colic during pregnancy. J Urol 159:365, 1998.
35. Deliveliotis CH, Argyropoulos B, Chrisofos M, Dimopoulos CA: Shockwave lithotripsy in unrecognized pregnancy: interruption or continuation? J Endourol 15:787, 2001.
36. Nadler N, Salinas-Madrigal L, Charles A, Pollack V: Acute glomerulonephritis during late pregnancy. Obstet Gynecol 34:277, 1969.
37. Wilson C: Changes in renal function. In Morris N, Browne J: Nontoxemic Hypertension in Pregnancy. Boston, Little, Brown, 1958, p 177.
38. Packham DK, North RA, Fairly KF, et al: Primary glomerulonephritis and pregnancy. Q J Med 71:537, 1989.
39. Packham DK, North RA, Fairly KF, et al: Membranous glomerulonephritis and pregnancy. Clin Nephrol 30:487, 1988.
40. Jungers P, Forget D, Houillier P, et al: Pregnancy in IgA nephropathy, reflux nephropathy, and focal glomerular sclerosis. Am J Kidney Dis 9:334, 1987.
41. Kincaid-Smith P, Fairley KF: Renal disease in pregnancy: three controversial areas: mesangial IgA nephropathy, focal glomerular sclerosis (focal and segmental hyalinosis and sclerosis), and reflux nephropathy. Am J Kidney Dis 9:328, 1987.
42. Abe S: An overview of pregnancy in women with underlying renal disease. Am J Kidney Dis 17:112, 1991.
43. Imbasciati E, Ponticelli C: Pregnancy and renal disease: predictors for fetal and maternal outcome. Am J Nephrol 11:353, 1991.
44. Davison J: Renal disease. In deSwiet M: Medical Disorders in Obstetric Practice. Oxford, Blackwell, 1984, p 236.
45. Pertuiset N, Grunfeld JP: Acute renal failure in pregnancy. Baillieres Clin Obstet Gynaecol 1:873, 1987.
46. McDonald SD, Han Z, Walsh MW: Kidney disease after preeclampsia: a systematic review and meta-analysis. Am J Kidney Dis 55:1026, 2010.
47. Krane NK: Acute renal failure in pregnancy. Arch Intern Med 148:2347, 1988.
48. Grunfeld JP, Pertuiset N: Acute renal failure in pregnancy. Am J Kidney Dis 9:359, 1987.
49. Stratta P, Canavese C, Dogliani M, et al: Pregnancy related acute renal failure. Clin Nephrol 32:14, 1989.
50. Grunfeld JP, Ganeval D, Bournerias F: Acute renal failure in pregnancy. Kidney Int 18:179, 1980.
51. Stratta P, Canavese C, Colla L, et al: Acute renal failure in preeclampsia-eclampsia. Gynecol Obstet Invest 27:225, 1987.
52. Sibai B, Villar MA, Mabie BC: Acute renal failure in hypertensive disorders of pregnancy: pregnancy outcome and remote prognosis in thirty-one consecutive cases. Am J Obstet Gynecol 162:777, 1990.
53. Hold P, Wong C, Dhanda R, et al: Successful renal transplantation during pregnancy. Am J Transplant 5:2315, 2005.
54. Coratelli P, Buongiorno E, Passavanti G: Endotoxemia in hemolytic uremic syndrome. Nephron 50:365, 1988.
55. Robson J, Martin A, Burkley V: Irreversible postpartum renal failure: a new syndrome. Q J Med 37:423, 1968.
56. Seconds A, Louradour N, Suc J, Orfila C: Postpartum hemolytic uremic syndrome: a study of three cases with a review of the literature. Clin Nephrol 12:229, 1979.
57. Creasey GW, Morgan J: Hemolytic uremic syndrome after ectopic pregnancy: postectopic nephrosclerosis. Obstet Gynecol 69:448, 1987.
58. Remuzzi G, Misiani R, Marchesi D, et al: Treatment of hemolytic uremic syndrome with plasma. Clin Nephrol 12:279, 1979.
59. Webster J, Rees A, Lewis P, Hensby C: Prostacyclin deficiency in haemolytic uraemic syndrome. BMJ 281:271, 1980.
60. Brandt P, Jesperson J, Gregerson G: Post-partum haemolyitc-uremic syndrome successfully treated with antithrombin III. BMJ 281:449, 1980.
61. Li PK, Lai FM, Tam JS, Lai KN: Acute renal failure due to postpartum haemolytic uremic syndrome. Aust N Z J Obstet Gynaecol 28:228, 1988.
62. Brandes JC, Fritsche C: Obstructive acute renal failure by a gravid uterus: a case report and review. Am J Kidney Dis 18:398, 1991.
63. Hayborn KD, Schultz MF, Goodlin RC, Durham JD: Renal artery stenosis during pregnancy: a review. Obstet Gynecol Surv 46:509, 1991.
64. Coe FL, Brenner BM: Approach to the patient with diseases of the kidney and urinary tract. In Fauci AS, Braunwald E, Isselbacher KJ, et al: Principles of Internal Medicine. New York, McGraw-Hill, 1998, pp 1495-1498.
65. Davison J, Lindheimer M: Pregnancy in women with renal allografts. Semin Nephrol 4:240, 1984.
66. Denker BM, Brenner BM: Cardinal manifestations of renal disease. In Fauci AS, Braunwald E, Isselbacher KJ, et al: Principles of Internal Medicine. New York, McGraw-Hill, 1998, pp 258-262.
67. Hou S: Pregnancy in women with chronic renal disease. N Engl J Med 312:839, 1985.
68. Hou S, Grossman S, Madias N: Pregnancy in women with renal disease and moderate renal insufficiency. Am J Med 78:185, 1985.
69. Katz A, Davison J, Hayslett J, et al: Pregnancy in women with kidney disease. Kidney Int 18:192, 1980.
70. Mackay E: Pregnancy and renal disease: a ten-year study. Aust N Z J Obstet Gynaecol 3:21, 1963.
71. Studd J, Blainey J: Pregnancy and the nephrotic syndrome. BMJ 1:276, 1969.
72. Kinciad-Smith P, Fairley K, Bullen M: Kidney disease and pregnancy. Med J Aust 11:1155, 1967.
73. Surian M, Imbasciati E, Banfi G, et al: Glomerular disease and pregnancy. Nephron 36:101, 1984.
74. Cunningham FG, Cox SG, Harstad TW, et al: Chronic renal disease and pregnancy outcome. Am J Obstet Gynecol 163:453, 1990.
75. Piper JM, Ray WA, Rosa FW: Pregnancy outcome following exposure to angiotensin-converting enzyme inhibitors. Obstet Gynecol 80:429, 1992.
76. Hulton SA, Thompson PD, Cooper PA, Rothberg AD: Angiotensin-converting enzyme inhibitors in pregnancy may result in neonatal renal failure. S Afr Med J 78:673, 1990.
77. Cooper WO, Hernandez-Diaz S, Arbogast PG, et al: Major congenital malformations after first-trimester exposure to ACE inhibitors. N Engl J Med 354:2443, 2006.
78. Sibai B, Grossman R, Grossman H: Effects of diuretics on plasma volume in pregnancy with long term hypertension. Am J Obstet Gynecol 150:831, 1984.
79. Rodriquez S, Leikin S, Hillar M: Neonatal thrombocytopenia associated with antepartum administration of thiazide drugs. N Engl J Med 270:881, 1964.
80. Lindheimer M, Spargo B, Katz A: Renal biopsy in pregnancy-induced hypertension. J Reprod Med 15:189, 1975.
81. Lindheimer M, Fisher K, Spargo B, Katz A: Hypertension in pregnancy: a biopsy with long term follow-up. Contrib Nephrol 25:71, 1981.
82. Packham DK, Fairley K: Renal biopsy: indications and complications in pregnancy. Br J Obstet Gynaecol 94:935, 1987.
83. Ackrill P, Goodwin F, Marsh F, et al: Successful pregnancy in patient on regular dialysis. BMJ 2:172, 1975.
84. Kobayashi H, Matsumoto Y, Otsubo O, et al: Successful pregnancy in a patient undergoing chronic hemodialysis. Obstet Gynecol 57:382, 1981.
85. Savdie E, Caterson R, Mahony J, Clifton-Bligh P: Successful pregnancies treated by haemodialysis. Med J Aust 2:9, 1982.
86. Cohen D, Frenkel Y, Maschiach S, Eliahou HE: Dialysis during pregnancy in advanced chronic renal failure patients: outcome and progression. Clin Nephrol 29:144, 1988.
87. Redrow M, Cherem L, Elliott J, et al: Dialysis in the management of pregnant patients with renal insufficiency. Medicine 67:199, 1988.
88. Hou S: Pregnancy in women requiring dialysis for renal failure. Am J Kidney Dis 9:368, 1987.
89. Yasin SY, Doun SWB: Hemodialysis in pregnancy. Obstet Gynecol Surv 43:655, 1988.

90. Lim V, Henriquez C, Sievertsen G, Prohman L: Ovarian function in chronic renal failure: evidence suggesting hypothalamic anovulation. Ann Intern Med 57:7, 1980.
91. Nageotte MP, Grundy HO: Pregnancy outcome in women requiring chronic hemodialysis. Obstet Gynecol 72:456, 1988.
92. Luders C, Castro MC, Titan SM: Obstetric outcomes in pregnant women on long-term dialysis: a case series. Am J Kidney Dis 56:77, 2010.
93. EDTA Registration Committee: Successful pregnancies in women treated by dialysis and kidney transplantation. Br J Obstet Gynaecol 87:839, 1980.
94. Asamiya Y, Otsubo S, Matsuda Y: The importance of low blood urea nitrogen levels in pregnant patients undergoing hemodialysis to optimize birth weight and gestational age. Kidney Int 75:1217, 2009.
95. Fine L, Barnett E, Danovitch G, et al: Systemic lupus erythematosus in pregnancy. Ann Intern Med 94:667, 1981.
96. Johnson T, Lorenz R, Menon K, Nolan G: Successful outcome of a pregnancy requiring dialysis: effects on serum progesterone and estrogens. J Reprod Med 22:217, 1979.
97. Gill JS, Zalunardo N, Rose C, Tonelli M: The pregnancy rate and live birth rate in kidney transplant recipients. Am J Transplant 9:1541, 2009.
98. Merkatz I, Schwartz G, David D, et al: Resumption of female reproductive function following renal transplantation. JAMA 216:1749, 1971.
99. Penn I, Markowski E, Harris P: Parenthood following renal transplantation. Kidney Int 18:221, 1980.
100. Saarikoski S, Sappala M: Immunosuppression during pregnancy: transmission of azathioprine and its metabolites from mother to fetus. Am J Obstet Gynecol 115:1100, 1973.
101. Cote C, Meuwissen H, Pickering R: Effects on the neonate of prednisone and azathioprine administered to the mother during pregnancy. J Pediatr 85:324, 1974.
102. Price H, Salaman J, Laurence K, Langmaid H: Immunosuppressive drugs and the fetus. Transplantation 21:294, 1976.
103. Scott J: Fetal growth retardation associated with maternal administration of immunosuppressive drugs. Am J Obstet Gynecol 128:668, 1977.
104. Ponticelli C, Montagnino G: Causes of arterial hypertension in kidney transplantation. Contrib Nephrol 54:226, 1987.
105. McKay DB, Josephson MA: Pregnancy in recipients of solid organs—effects on the mother and child. N Engl J Med 354:1281, 2006.
106. Derfler K, Schuller A, Herold C, et al: Successful outcome of a complicated pregnancy in a renal transplant recipient taking cyclosporin A. Clin Nephrol 29:96, 1988.
107. Salamalekis EE, Mortakis AE, Phocas I, et al: Successful pregnancy in a renal transplant recipient taking cyclosporin A: hormonal and immunological studies. Int J Gynaecol Obstet 1989;30:267.
108. Pickerell MD, Sawers R, Michael J: Pregnancy after renal transplantation: severe intrauterine growth retardation during treatment with cyclosporin A. Br Med J 1:825, 1988.
109. Sifontis MN, Coscia LA, Constantinescu S: Pregnancy outcomes in solid organ transplant recipients with exposure to mycophenolate mofetil or sirolimus. Transplantation 82:1698, 2006.
110. Kainz A, Harabacz I, Cowlrick IS: Review of the course and outcome of 100 pregnancies in 84 women treated with tacrolimus. Transplantation 70:1718, 2000.
111. Davison J: Renal transplantation and pregnancy. Am J Kidney Dis 9:374, 1987.
112. Parsons V, Bewick M, Elias J, et al: Pregnancy following renal transplantation. J R Soc Med 72:815, 1979.
113. Huffer W, Kuzela D, Popovtzer M: Metabolic bone disease in chronic renal failure in renal transplant patients. Am J Pathol 78:385, 1975.
114. Lindheimer M, Katz A: Pregnancy in the renal transplant patient. Am J Kidney Dis 19:173, 2000.

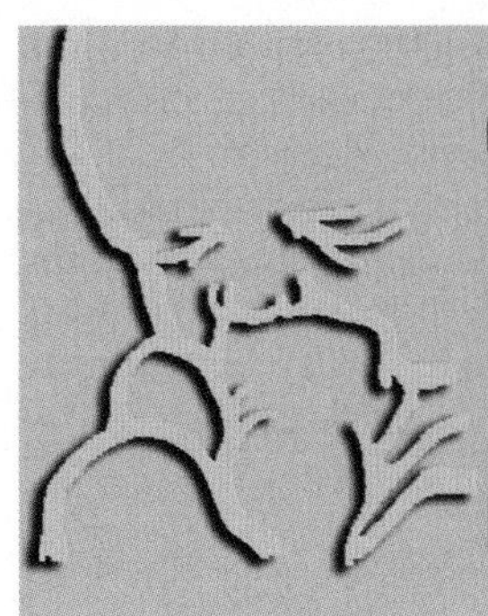

CHAPTER 39
Diabetes Mellitus Complicating Pregnancy

Mark B. Landon, Patrick M. Catalano, and Steven G. Gabbe

KEY ABBREVIATIONS

American College of Obstetricians and Gynecologists	ACOG
Biophysical Profile	BPP
Continuous Subcutaneous Insulin Infusion (pump therapy)	CSII
Depomedroxyprogesterone Acetate	DMPA
Diabetic Ketoacidosis	DKA
Disposition Index	DI
Gestational Diabetes Mellitus	GDM
Glucose Tolerance Test	GTT
Glucose Transporter	GLUT
Hemoglobin A_{1c}	HbA_{1c}
High-density Lipoprotein	HDL
Hyaline Membrane Disease	HMD
Infant of the Diabetic Mother	IDM
Insulin-dependent Diabetes Mellitus	IDDM
Insulin-like Growth Factor	IGF
Low-density Lipoprotein	LDL
Maternal Serum α-fetoprotein	MSAFP
Maturity-onset Diabetes of Youth	MODY
Nonstress Test	NST
Oral Contraceptive	OC
Phosphatidylglycerol	PG
Respiratory Distress Syndrome	RDS
Total Urinary Protein Excretion	TPE
Tumor Necrosis Factor-α	TNF-α
Urinary Albumin Excretion	UAE
Very-low-density Lipoprotein	VLDL

Insulin therapy was introduced 90 years ago and remains perhaps the important landmark in the care of pregnancy for the diabetic woman. Before insulin became available, pregnancy was not advised because it was likely to be accompanied by fetal mortality and a substantial risk for maternal death. Over the past several decades, management techniques have been developed that can prevent many complications associated with diabetic pregnancy. These advances, based on understanding of pathophysiology, now result in perinatal mortality rates in optimally managed cases that approach those of the normal population. This dramatic improvement in perinatal outcome can be largely attributed to clinical efforts to establish improved maternal glycemic control both before conception and during gestation (Figure 39-1). Excluding major congenital malformations, which continue to plague pregnancies in women with type 1 and type 2 diabetes mellitus, perinatal loss for the diabetic woman has fortunately become an uncommon event.

Although the benefit of careful regulation of maternal glucose levels is well accepted, failure to establish optimal glycemic control as well as other factors continue to result in significant perinatal morbidity. For this reason, both clinical and basic laboratory research efforts continue to focus on the etiology and prevention of congenital malformations and the pathophysiology of fetal growth abnormalities. Clinical experience has also resulted in recognition of the impact that vascular complications can have on pregnancy and the manner in which pregnancy may affect these disease processes. With modern management techniques and a skilled, organized team approach, successful pregnancies have become the norm even for women with the most complicated diabetes.

Gestational diabetes mellitus (GDM), the most common type of diabetes found in pregnancy, has represented controversy to both clinicians and investigators. After nearly 50 years since the concept of GDM was introduced, the clinical significance of this disorder is now better understood as a recent result of large-scale observational studies and treatment trials. However, controversy remains concerning screening techniques, diagnostic criteria, thresholds for insulin initiation, and whether oral hypoglycemic agents are suitable treatment.

Before considering these clinical issues, it is important to review the metabolic effects of pregnancy in relation to the pathophysiology of diabetes mellitus.

PATHOPHYSIOLOGY

Normal Glucose Tolerance

There are significant alterations in maternal metabolism during pregnancy, which provide for adequate maternal nutritional stores in early gestation in order to meet the increased maternal and fetal demands of late gestation and lactation. Although we are apt to think of diabetes mellitus as a disorder exclusively of maternal glucose metabolism, in fact **diabetes mellitus affects all aspects of nutrient metabolism.** In this section we consider maternal glucose metabolism as it relates to pancreatic β-cell production of insulin and insulin clearance, endogenous (i.e., primarily hepatic) glucose production, and suppression with insulin and peripheral glucose insulin sensitivity. We also address maternal protein and lipid insulin metabolism. Lastly, the effects of these alternations on maternal metabolism are examined as they relate to maternal energy expenditure and fetal growth.

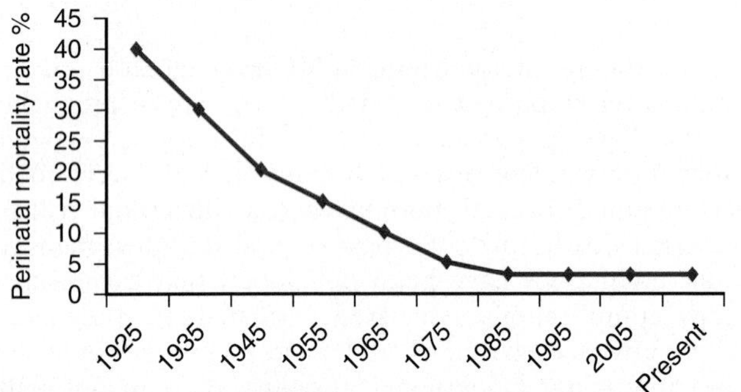

FIGURE 39-1. Perinatal mortality late in pregnancy complicated by insulin-dependent diabetes mellitus.

Glucose Metabolism

Normal pregnancy has been characterized as a "diabetogenic state" because of the progressive increase in postprandial glucose levels and increased insulin response in late gestation. **However, early gestation can be viewed as an anabolic state because of the increases in maternal fat stores and decrease in free fatty acid (FFA) concentration, particularly in non-overweight and obese women.** Garcia-Patterson and colleagues[1] have described significant decreases in maternal insulin requirements in early gestation (Figure 39-2). The mechanism for this decrease in insulin requirements has been ascribed to various factors, including increased insulin sensitivity, decreased substrate availability secondary to factors such as nausea, the fetus acting as a glucose sink, and enhanced maternal insulin secretion; however, the exact mechanism is not known. Longitudinal studies in women with normal glucose tolerance have shown significant alterations in all aspects of glucose metabolism as early as the end of the first trimester.[2]

There are progressive increases in insulin secretion in response to an intravenous glucose challenge with advancing gestation (Figure 39-3). The increases in insulin concentration are more pronounced in lean compared with obese women, most probably as a response to the greater decreases in insulin sensitivity in lean women, as described later. Data regarding insulin clearance in pregnancy are limited. In separate studies Bellman, Lind and colleagues, and Burt and Davidson reported no difference in insulin disappearance rate when insulin was infused intravenously in late gestation compared with nongravid subjects. In contrast, Goodner and Freinkel, using a radiolabeled insulin, described a 25% increase in insulin turnover in a pregnant compared with a nonpregnant rat model. Catalano and associates,[3] using the euglycemic-clamp model,

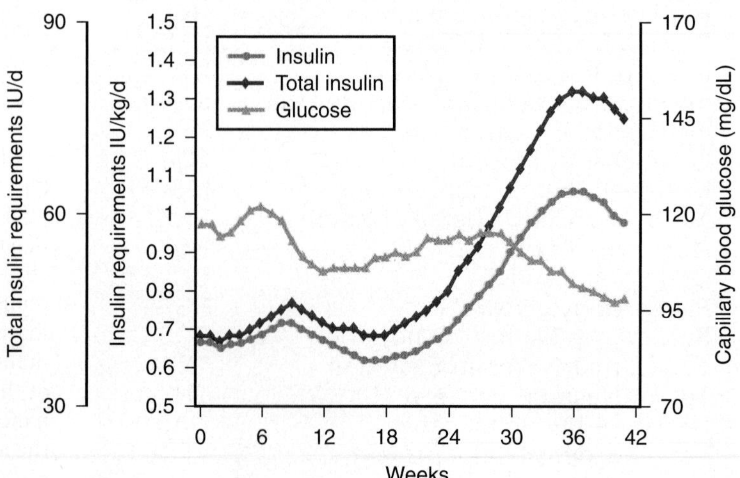

FIGURE 39-2. Mean insulin requirements and self-monitored blood glucose in women with type 1 diabetes. (Modified from Garcia-Patterson A, Gich I, Amini SB, et al: Insulin requirements throughout pregnancy in women with type 1 diabetes mellitus: three changes of direction. Diabetologia 53:446, 2010.)

reported a 20% increase in insulin clearance in lean women and a 30% increase in insulin clearance in obese women by late pregnancy (Figure 39-4). Although the placenta is rich in insulinase, the exact mechanism for the increased insulin clearance in pregnancy remains speculative.

Although there is a progressive decrease in fasting glucose with advancing gestation, the decrease is most probably a result of the increase in plasma volume in early gestation and the increase in fetoplacental glucose use in late gestation. Kalhan and Cowett, using various stable isotope methodologies in cross-sectional study designs, were the first to describe increased fasting hepatic glucose production in late pregnancy. Additionally, Catalano and coworkers,[4] using a stable isotope of glucose in a prospective longitudinal study design, reported **a 30% increase in maternal fasting hepatic glucose production with advancing gestation** (Figure 39-5), which remained significant even when adjusted for maternal weight gain. Tissue sensitivity to insulin involves both liver and peripheral tissues, primarily skeletal muscle. The increase in fasting maternal hepatic glucose production occurred despite a significant increase in fasting insulin concentration, thereby indicating a decrease in maternal hepatic glucose sensitivity in women with normal glucose tolerance. Additionally, in obese women, there was a decreased ability of infused insulin to suppress hepatic glucose production in late gestation compared with pregravid and early pregnancy measurements, thereby indicating a further decrease in hepatic insulin sensitivity in obese women.

Estimates of peripheral insulin sensitivity in pregnancy have included the measurement of insulin response to a fixed oral or intravenous glucose challenge or the ratio of

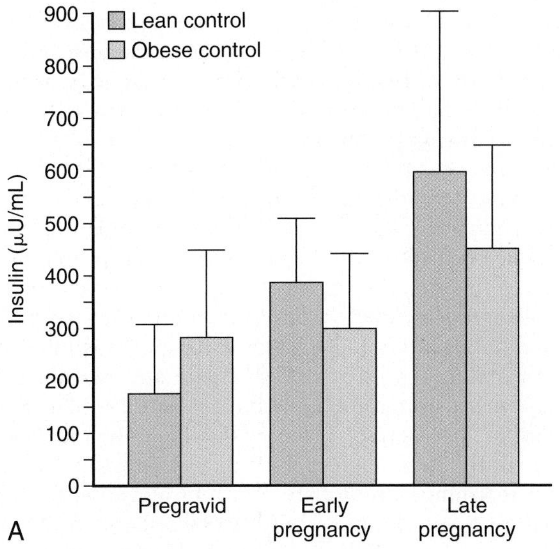

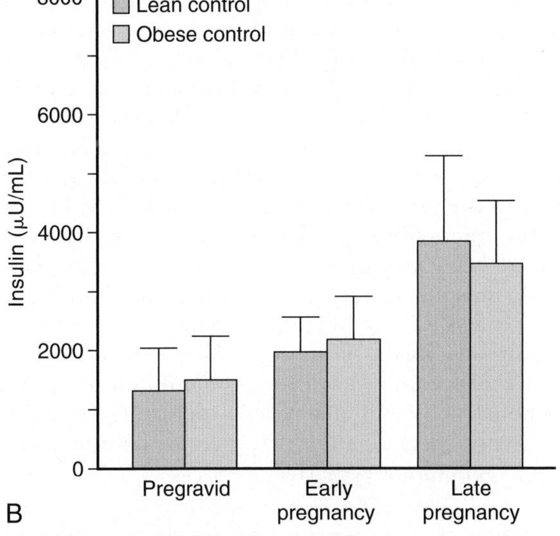

Figure 39-3. Longitudinal increase in insulin response to an intravenous glucose challenge in lean and obese women with normal glucose tolerance: pregravid, and early and late pregnancy. **A,** First phase: area under the curve from 0 to 5 minutes. **B,** Second phase: area under the curve from 5 to 60 minutes.

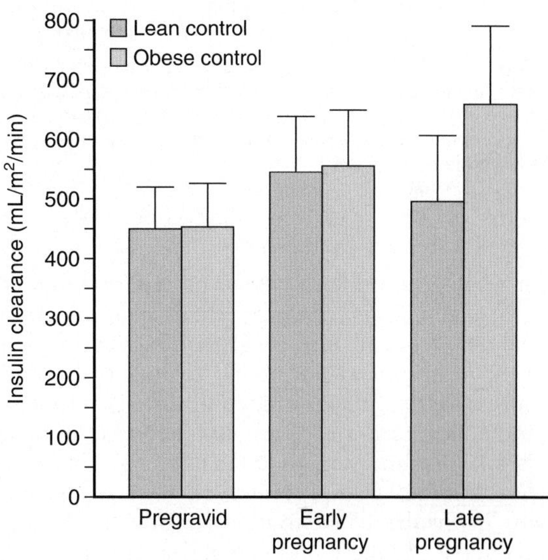

Figure 39-4. Longitudinal increases in metabolic clearance rate of insulin (mL/m^2/min) in lean and obese women with normal glucose tolerance: pregravid, and early and late pregnancy.

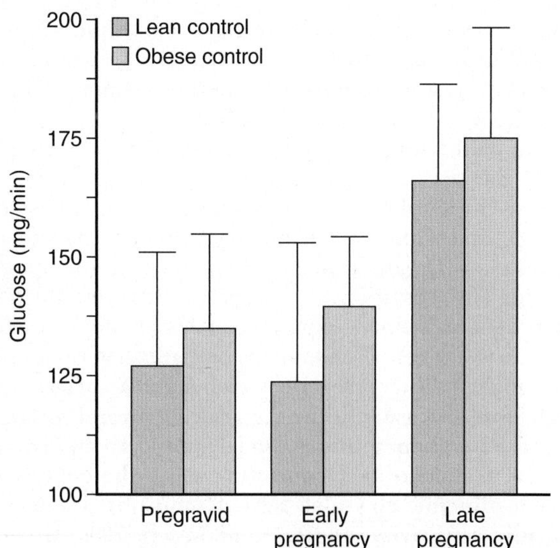

Figure 39-5. Longitudinal increase in basal endogenous (primarily hepatic) glucose production (mg/min) in lean and obese women with normal glucose tolerance: pregravid, and early and late pregnancy.

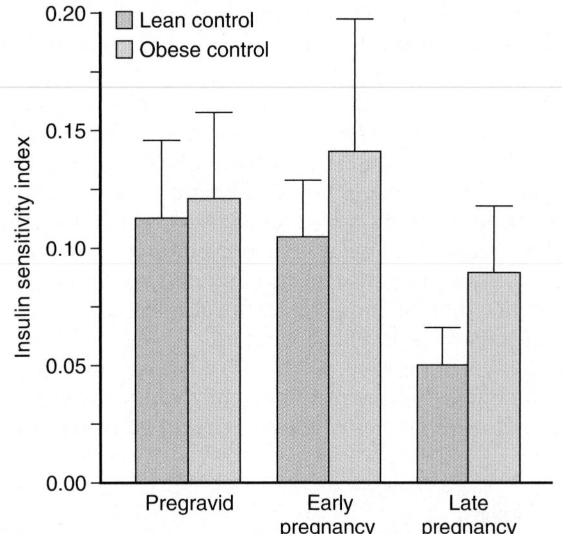

FIGURE 39-6. Longitudinal changes in the insulin sensitivity index (glucose infusion rate adjusted for residual endogenous glucose production and insulin concentrations achieved during the glucose clamp) in lean and obese women with normal glucose tolerance: pregravid and early and late gestation.

insulin to glucose under a variety of experimental conditions. In recent years, newer methodologies, such as the minimal model and the euglycemic-hyperinsulinemic clamp, have improved our ability to quantify peripheral insulin sensitivity. In lean women in early gestation, Catalano and colleagues[5] reported a 40% decrease in maternal peripheral insulin sensitivity using the euglycemic-hyperinsulinemic clamp. However, when adjusted for changes in insulin concentrations during the clamp and residual hepatic glucose production (i.e., the insulin sensitivity index) insulin sensitivity *decreased* only 10% (Figure 39-6). In contrast, there was a 15% *increase* in the insulin sensitivity index in obese women in early pregnancy compared with pregravid estimates.[6] Hence, the decrease in insulin requirements in early gestation observed in some women requiring insulin may be a consequence of an increase in insulin sensitivity, particularly in women with decreased insulin sensitivity before conception, for example, women with type 2 diabetes.

Compared with the metabolic alterations in early pregnancy, there is a uniformity of opinion regarding the decrease in peripheral insulin sensitivity in late gestation. Spellacy and Goetz were among the first investigators to report an increase in insulin response to a glucose challenge in late gestation. Additionally, Burt demonstrated that pregnant women experienced less hypoglycemia in response to exogenous insulin in comparison with nonpregnant subjects. **Later research by Fisher and associates using a high-dose glucose infusion test, Buchanan and colleagues using the Bergman minimal model, and Ryan and coworkers[7] and Catalano and associates[2] using the euglycemic-hyperinsulinemic clamp all have demonstrated a decrease in insulin sensitivity ranging from 33% to 78%.** It should be noted, however, that all these quantitative estimates of insulin sensitivity are very likely overestimates because of non-insulin-mediated glucose disposal by the fetus and placenta. Hay and colleagues reported that in the pregnant ewe model, about one third of maternal glucose use was accounted for by uterine, placental, and fetal tissue. Additionally, Marconi and coworkers reported that based on human fetal blood sampling, fetal glucose concentration was a function of fetal size and gestational age in addition to maternal glucose concentration.

Historically, the decrease in insulin sensitivity during pregnancy has been ascribed to an increased production of various placental and maternal hormones, such as human placental lactogen, progesterone, estrogen, cortisol, and prolactin. However, more recent evidence has focused on the role of several new mediators of insulin resistance such as leptin, tumor necrosis factor-α (TNF-α), and resistin. Among these factors, TNF-α and leptin are known to be produced in the placenta and therefore could play a central role in the development of insulin resistance. Kirwan and coworkers[8] reported that TNF-α was inversely correlated with the changes in insulin sensitivity from the time before conception through late gestation. In combination with other placental hormones, multivariate stepwise regression analysis revealed that **TNF-α was the strongest independent predictor of insulin sensitivity in pregnancy, accounting for about half of the variance in the decrease in insulin sensitivity during gestation.**

Pregnancy has been characterized as a chronic low-grade inflammatory condition because of the increase in activation of circulating blood leukocytes.[9] The inflammation of pregnancy is further enhanced by maternal prepregnancy obesity. This increase in low-grade inflammation, particularly observed in obese women in normal-term pregnancies, has been related to increases in macrophage infiltration in both maternal white adipose tissue and placenta. The increase in inflammation has been associated with increased circulating C-reactive protein (CRP) and interlukin-6 (IL-6). Both these factors may exacerbate the increased insulin resistance previously noted in obese women with normal glucose tolerance, because of effects on the post-receptor insulin-signaling cascade. These inflammatory factors may then relate to increased substrate availability for the developing fetus and resultant macrosomia.

Placenta glucose transport is a nonenergy process and takes place through facilitated diffusion. Glucose transport is dependent on a family of glucose transporters referred to as the GLUT glucose transporter family. **The principal glucose transporter in the placenta is GLUT1, which is located in the syncytiotrophoblast.[10] GLUT1 is located on both the microvillus and basal membranes**. Basal membrane GLUT1 may be the rate-limiting step in placental glucose transport. There is a twofold to threefold increase in the expression of syncytiotrophoblast glucose transporters with advancing gestation. Although GLUT3 and GLUT4 expression have been identified in placental endothelial cells and intervillous nontrophoblastic cells, respectively, the role they may play in placental glucose transport remains speculative.

DIABETES MELLITUS

Diabetes mellitus is a chronic metabolic disorder characterized by either absolute or relative insulin deficiency, resulting in increased glucose concentrations. Although

TABLE 39-1 MODIFIED WHITE CLASSIFICATION OF PREGNANT DIABETIC WOMEN

CLASS	DIABETES ONSET AGE (yr)	DURATION (yr)	VASCULAR DISEASE	INSULIN NEED
Gestational Diabetes				
A_1	Any	Any	0	0
A_2	Any	Any	0	+
Pregestational Diabetes				
B	>20	<10	0	+
C	10-19	or 10-19	0	+
D	<10	or >20	+	+
F	Any	Any	+	+
R	Any	Any	+	+
T	Any	Any	+	+
H	Any	Any	+	+

Modified from White P: Pregnancy complicating diabetes. Am J Med 7:609, 1949.

glucose intolerance is the common outcome of diabetes mellitus, the pathophysiology remains heterogeneous. The two major classifications of diabetes mellitus are type 1, formerly referred to as insulin-dependent or juvenile-onset diabetes, and type 2, formerly referred to as non-insulin-dependent or adult-onset diabetes. During pregnancy, classification of women with diabetes has often relied on the White classification,[11] first proposed in the 1940s. This classification is based on factors such as the age of onset of diabetes and duration as well as end-organ involvement, primarily retinal and renal (Table 39-1).

All forms of diabetes can occur during pregnancy. In addition to type 1 and type 2 diabetes, there are, however, genetic causes of diabetes, the most common of which is maturity-onset diabetes of youth (MODY). MODY is characterized by β-cell dysfunction and has an autosomal dominant mode of inheritance, usually becoming manifest in young adulthood. Mutations in the glucokinase gene are a frequent cause of MODY. Various mutations have been described, and each mutation is associated with varying degrees of disease severity. The most common of these mutations (MODY2) occurs in the European population and involves the glucokinase gene. Because the age of onset of diabetes in women with MODY coincides with the reproductive years, it may be difficult to distinguish between the two. The glucokinase gene acts as a sensor in the β cell, which leads to a secretory defect in insulin response. **Ellard and colleagues reported that 2.5% of women with GDM in the United Kingdom have the glucokinase mutation,** whereas Stoffel, in a small population in the United States, reported that 5% of patients had a glucokinase in mutation. The implication if the mother has the mutation is an increased risk for fetal macrosomia. The implications for the fetus, if inherited from the father, are a significant decrease in growth secondary to relative insulinopenia.

Type 1 Diabetes Mellitus

Type 1 diabetes mellitus is usually characterized by an abrupt onset at a young age and absolute insulinopenia with lifelong requirements for insulin replacement. Although depending on the population, the onset of type 1 diabetes may occur in individuals in their third or fourth decades of life. Patients with diabetes mellitus may have a genetic predisposition for antibodies directed against their pancreatic islet cells. The degree of concordance for the development of type 1 diabetes in monozygotic twins is 33%, suggesting that the events subsequent to the development of autoantibodies and appearance of glucose intolerance are also related to environmental factors. Because of the complete dependence on exogenous insulin, pregnant women with type 1 diabetes are at increased risk for the development of diabetic ketoacidosis. Additionally, because intensive insulin therapy is used in women with type 1 diabetes to decrease the risk for spontaneous abortion and congenital anomalies in early gestation, these women are at increased risk for hypoglycemic reactions. Studies by Diamond and Rosenn have shown that women with type 1 diabetes are at increased risk for hypoglycemic reactions during pregnancy because of diminished counterregulatory epinephrine and glucagon response to hypoglycemia. The deficiency in this counterregulatory response may be in part due to an independent effect of pregnancy.

The alterations in glucose metabolism in women with type 1 diabetes are not well characterized. Because of maternal insulinopenia, insulin response during gestation can only be estimated relative to pregravid requirements. Estimates of the change in insulin requirements are complicated by the degree of preconceptual glucose control and potential presence of insulin antibodies. Garcia-Patterson[1] reported on the change in insulin requirements in women with type 1 diabetes and strict glucose control prior to conception. In early pregnancy, both insulin requirements and total insulin peak at 9 weeks' gestation and nadir at 16 weeks to baseline prepregnancy levels. After 16 weeks, insulin requirements gradually increase through 37 weeks. This represents a total increase in insulin requirements of 5.19% per week and about a twofold increase relative to prepregnancy requirements. A 5% decrease in insulin requirements after 36 weeks' gestation was also noted by McManus and Ryan. The decrease in insulin requirements was associated with a longer duration of diabetes mellitus but not with adverse perinatal outcome. The fall in insulin requirements in early pregnancy in women with type 1 diabetes may be a reflection of increased pregravid insulin sensitivity as was described previously.

Schmitz and associates[12] have evaluated the longitudinal changes in insulin sensitivity in women with type 1 diabetes in early and late pregnancy as well as postpartum in comparison with nonpregnant women with type 1 diabetes. **In the pregnant women with type 1 diabetes, there was a 50% decrease in insulin sensitivity only in late gestation.**

There was no significant difference in insulin sensitivity in pregnant women with type 1 diabetes in early pregnancy or within 1 week of delivery compared with the nonpregnant women with type 1 diabetes. Therefore, based on the available data, women with type 1 diabetes appear to have a similar decrease in insulin sensitivity compared with women with normal glucose tolerance.

Relative to the issue of placental transporters (GLUT1), there is a report by Jansson and Powell[13] describing an increase in both basal GLUT1 expression and glucose transport activity from placental tissue in women with White class D pregnancies.

Type 2 Diabetes and Gestational Diabetes

The pathophysiology of type 2 diabetes involves abnormalities of both insulin-sensitive tissue (i.e., both a decrease in skeletal muscle and hepatic sensitivity to insulin) and β-cell response as manifested by an inadequate insulin response for a given degree of glycemia. Initially in the course of development of type 2 diabetes, the insulin response to a glucose challenge may be increased relative to that of individuals with normal glucose tolerance but is inadequate to maintain normoglycemia. Whether decreased insulin sensitivity precedes β-cell dysfunction in the development of type 2 diabetes continues to be debated. Arguments and experimental data support both hypotheses. As noted by Sims and Calles-Escadon, heterogeneity of metabolic abnormalities exists in any classification of diabetes mellitus.

Despite the limitations of any classification system, certain generalizations can be made regarding women with type 2 diabetes or GDM. These individuals are typically older and more often heavier compared with individuals with type 1 diabetes or normal glucose tolerance. The onset of the disorder is usually insidious, with few patients complaining of the classic triad of polydipsia, polyphagia, and polyuria. Individuals with type 2 diabetes are often initially recommended to lose weight, increase their activity (i.e., exercise), and follow a diet low in fats and high in complex carbohydrates. Oral agents are often used to either increase insulin response or, with newer drugs, enhance insulin sensitivity. Individuals with type 2 diabetes may eventually require insulin therapy to maintain euglycemia but are at significantly less risk for diabetic ketoacidosis. **Data from monozygotic twin studies have reported a lifetime risk for both twins developing type 2 diabetes that ranges between 58% and almost 100%, suggesting that the disorder has a strong genetic component.**

Type 2 pregestational diabetes is usually classified as class B diabetes according to the While classification system. Women developing GDM (i.e. glucose intolerance first recognized during pregnancy) share many of the metabolic characteristics of women with type 2 diabetes. Although earlier studies reported a 10% to 35% incidence of islet cell antibodies in women with GDM as measured by immunofluorescence techniques, more recent data using specific monoclonal antibodies have described a much lower incidence on the order of 1% to 2%,[14] suggesting a low risk for type 1 diabetes in women with GDM. Furthermore, postpartum studies of women with GDM have demonstrated defects in insulin secretory response and decreased insulin sensitivity, indicating that typical type 2 abnormalities in glucose metabolism are present in women with GDM. Of interest, the alterations in insulin secretory response and insulin resistance in women with a previous history of GDM compared with a weight-matched control group may differ depending on whether the women with previous GDM are lean or obese.[15] Thus, in women with GDM, the hormonal events of pregnancy may represent an unmasking of a genetic susceptibility to type 2 diabetes.

There are significant alterations in glucose metabolism in women who develop GDM relative to the changes in glucose metabolism in women with normal glucose tolerance. Decreased insulin response to a glucose challenge has been demonstrated by Yen, Fisher, and Buchanan and their colleagues in women with GDM in late gestation. In prospective longitudinal studies of both lean and obese women with GDM, Catalano and associates[5] also showed a progressive decrease in first-phase insulin response in late gestation in lean women developing GDM compared with a weight-matched control group (Figure 39-7). In contrast, in obese women developing GDM, there was no difference in first-phase insulin response, but rather a significant increase in second-phase insulin response, to an intravenous glucose challenge compared with a weight-matched control group (see Figure 39-7). These differences in insulin response may be related to the ethnicity of the various study groups. Although there is an increase in the metabolic clearance rate of insulin with advancing gestation, there is no evidence that there is a significant difference between women with normal glucose tolerance and those with GDM.[6]

There is a significant decrease in fasting glucose concentration with advancing gestation in women developing GDM. In late pregnancy, glucose and hepatic glucose production increase in women with GDM in comparison with a control group.[5,6] Whereas there was no significant difference in either fasting glucose concentration or hepatic glucose production in the longitudinal studies of Catalano and associates,[5,6] these differences may again be population specific or related to the degree of fasting hypoglycemia. However, to date all reports indicate that in late gestation, women with GDM have increased fasting insulin concentrations (Figure 39-8) and less suppression of hepatic glucose production during insulin infusion, thereby indicating decreased hepatic glucose insulin sensitivity in women with GDM compared with a weight-matched control group.[5,6,16] In the studies of Xiang and associates,[16] there was significant correlation between fasting FFA concentrations and hepatic glucose production, suggesting that increased FFA concentrations may contribute to hepatic insulin resistance.

Women with GDM have decreased insulin sensitivity in comparison with weight-matched control groups. Ryan and colleagues[7] were the first to report a 40% decrease in insulin sensitivity in women with GDM compared to a pregnant control group in late pregnancy using a hyperinsulinemic-euglycemic clamp. Xiang and associates[16] found that women with GDM who had normal glucose tolerance within 6 months of delivery had significantly decreased insulin sensitivity as estimated by the glucose clearance rate during a hyperinsulinemic-euglycemic clamp compared with a

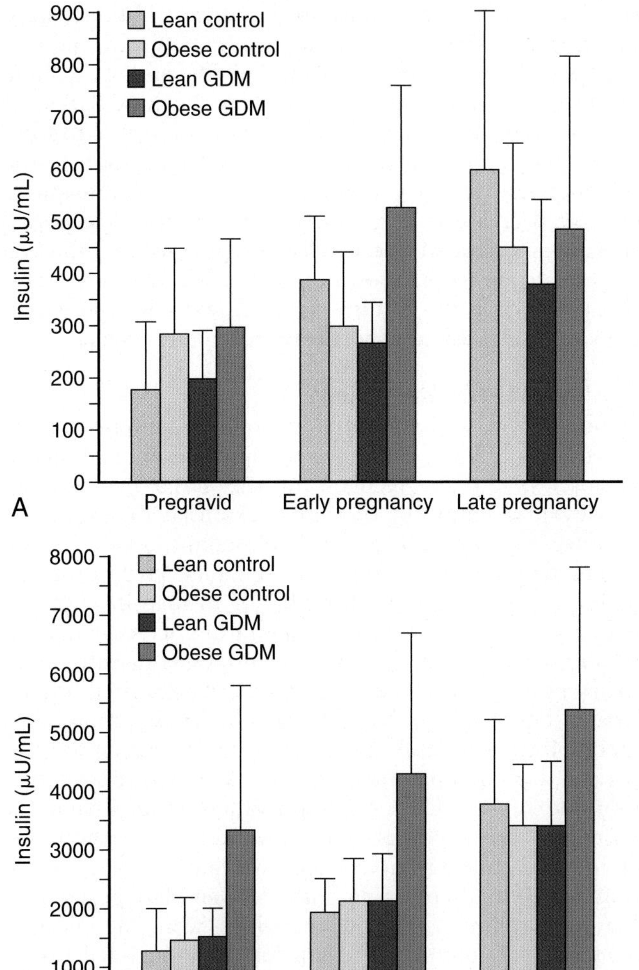

FIGURE 39-7. **A** and **B,** Longitudinal increase in insulin response to an intravenous glucose challenge in lean and obese women with normal glucose tolerance and gestational diabetes: pregravid and early and late pregnancy. **A,** First phase: area under the curve from 0 to 5 minutes. **B,** Second phase: area under the curve from 5 to 60 minutes.

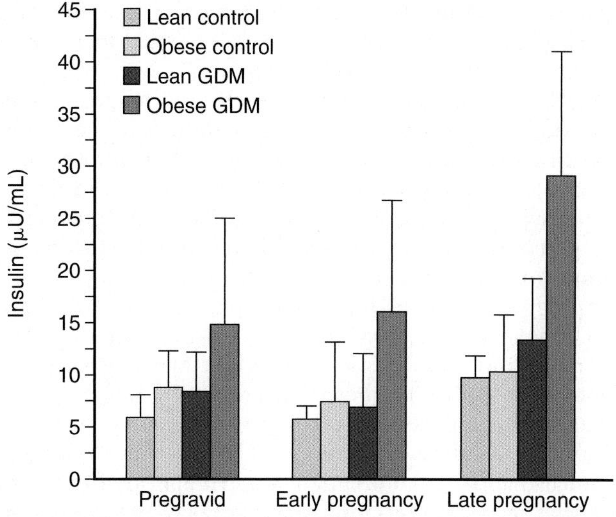

FIGURE 39-8. Longitudinal increase in basal or fasting insulin (mcg/mL) in lean and obese women with normal glucose tolerance and gestational diabetes: pregravid and early and late pregnancy.

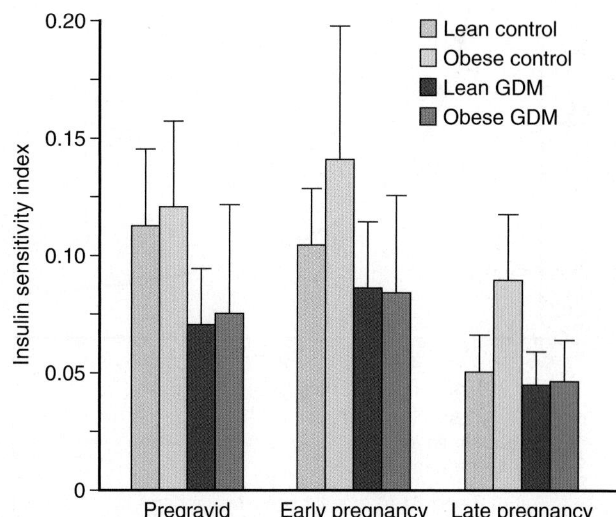

FIGURE 39-9. Longitudinal changes in the insulin sensitivity index (glucose infusion rate adjusted for residual endogenous glucose production and insulin concentrations achieved during the glucose clamp) in lean and obese women with normal glucose tolerance and gestational diabetes: pregravid and early and late pregnancy.

matched control group. Catalano and coworkers,[5,6] using similar techniques, described the longitudinal changes in insulin sensitivity in both lean and obese women developing GDM in comparison with a matched control group. Women developing GDM had decreased insulin sensitivity compared with the matched control group (Figure 39-9). The differences in insulin sensitivity were greatest before and during early gestation; by late gestation, the differences in insulin sensitivity between the groups were less pronounced but still significant. Of interest, there was an increase in insulin sensitivity from the time before conception through early pregnancy (12 to 14 weeks), particularly in those women with greatest decreases in insulin sensitivity before conception. **The changes in insulin sensitivity from the time before conception through early pregnancy were significantly correlated with changes in maternal weight gain and energy expenditure.** The relationship between these alterations in maternal glucose insulin sensitivity and weight gain and energy expenditure may help explain the decrease in maternal weight gain and insulin requirements in women with diabetes in early gestation.[1]

The interactions of ß-cell response and insulin sensitivity are hallmarks of the metabolic adaptations of pregnancy. As described by Bergman, there is a fixed relationship between insulin response and insulin resistance in nonpregnant individuals following a hyperbolic curve (i.e., the disposition index). Buchanan described a similar relationship between insulin response and insulin action during pregnancy. Indeed, when the disposition index has been compared between women with normal glucose tolerance and GDM both during and after pregnancy, the failure of the ß cell to compensate for insulin resistance in GDM has been similar to the hyperbolic changes in the control group (Figure 39-10). This relationship between insulin sensitivity and insulin resistance, however, may not hold in early pregnancy, when there is both an increase in insulin sensitivity and insulin response.

Studies in human skeletal muscle and adipose tissue have demonstrated that postreceptor defects in the insulin signaling cascade are related to decreased insulin sensitivity in pregnancy. Garvey and colleagues were the first to demonstrate that there were no significant differences in the glucose transporter (GLUT4) responsible for insulin action and skeletal muscle in pregnant compared with nonpregnant women. Based on the studies of Friedman and colleagues[17] in pregnant women with normal glucose tolerance and GDM, as well as weight-matched nonpregnant control subjects, there appeared to be defects in the insulin-signaling cascade relating to pregnancy as well as what may be additional abnormalities in women with gestational diabetes. **All pregnant women appeared to have a decrease in insulin receptor substrate-1 (IRS1) expression.** The downregulation of the IRS1 protein closely parallels the decreased ability of insulin to induce additional steps in the insulin-signaling cascade, resulting in movement of the GLUT4 to the cell surface membrane and to facilitate glucose transport into the cell. The downregulation of IRS1 protein closely parallels the ability of insulin to stimulate 2-deoxyglucose uptake in vitro. In addition to the previous mechanisms, **women with GDM demonstrate a distinct decrease in the ability of the insulin receptor-ß (that component of the insulin receptor not on the cell surface) to undergo tyrosine phosphorylation. The additional defect in the insulin-signaling cascade results in a 25% lower glucose transport activity** (Figure 39-11).

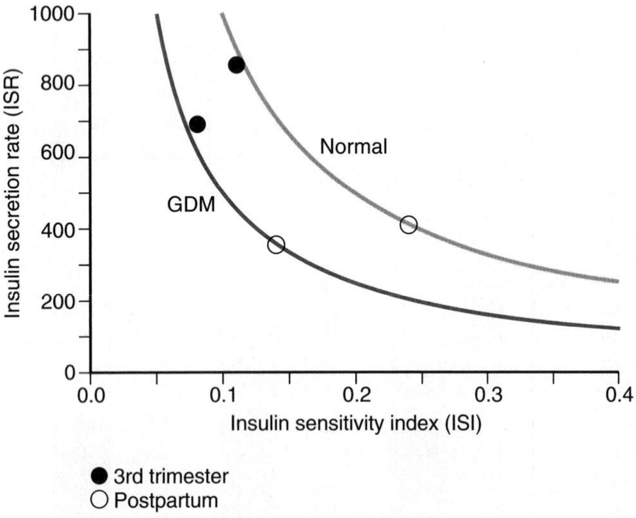

FIGURE 39-10. Insulin sensitivity index.

Amino Acid Metabolism

Although glucose is the primary source of energy for the fetus and placenta, there are no appreciable amounts of glucose stored as glycogen in the fetus or placenta. However, accretion of protein is essential for growth of fetoplacental tissue. There is increased nitrogen retention in pregnancy in both maternal and fetal compartments. There is an increase of about 0.9 kg of maternal fat-free mass by 27 weeks.[18] There is a significant decrease in most fasting maternal amino acid concentrations in early pregnancy before the accretion of significant maternal or fetal tissue. These anticipatory changes in fasting amino acid metabolism occur after a shorter period of fasting in comparison with nonpregnant women and may be another example of the accelerated starvation of pregnancy as described by Freinkel and coworkers.[19] Furthermore, amino acid concentrations such as serine correlate significantly with fetal growth in both early and late gestation.[20] Maternal amino acid concentrations were significantly decreased in mothers of small-for-gestational-age (SGA) neonates in comparison with maternal concentration in appropriately grown neonates.

Based on a review of various studies, Duggleby and Jackson have estimated that during a pregnancy, protein synthesis is similar to that in nonpregnant women in the first trimester. **However, there is a 15% increase in protein synthesis during the second trimester and a further increase**

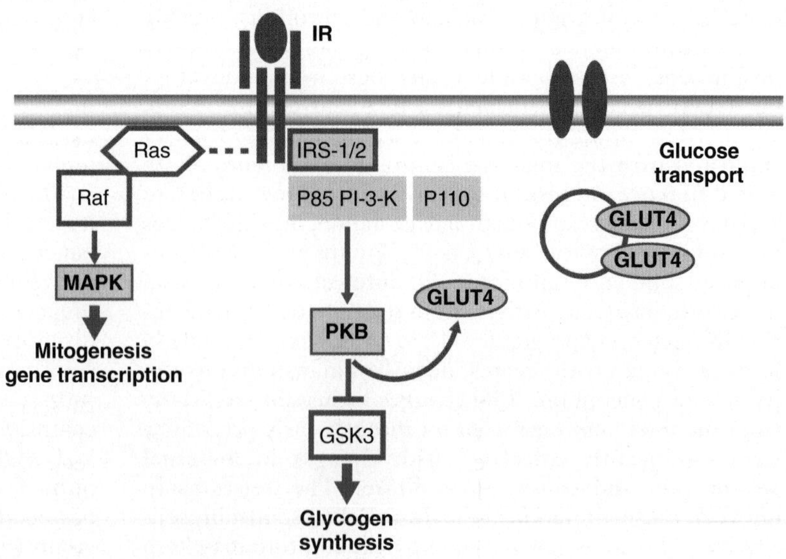

FIGURE 39-11. Schematic model of insulin signaling cascade in skeletal muscle. *GLUT,* Glucose transporter; *IR,* insulin receptor; *IRS,* insulin receptor substrate.

in the third trimester by about 25%. Additionally, there are marked interindividual differences at each time point. These differences have a strong relationship with fetal growth: mothers who had increased protein turnover in midpregnancy had babies who had increased lean body mass, after adjustment for significant covariables.

Amino acids can be used for protein accrual or oxidized as an energy source. Estimating urea synthesis using stable isotopes has been performed in a number of studies. In general, there is a modest shift in oxidation in early pregnancy with an accrual of amino acids for protein synthesis in late gestation. Furthermore, Kalhan and colleagues reported significant pregnancy-related adaptations in maternal protein metabolism early in gestation before any significant increase in fetal protein accretion. Catalano and associates have also reported decreased insulin sensitivity as manifested by a decreased suppression of leucine turnover during insulin infusion in late gestation in all pregnant women. There is evidence for an increase in basal leucine turnover in women with GDM compared with a matched control group. Whether these decreases in amino acid insulin sensitivity are related to decreased whole-body and liver protein synthesis or increased breakdown are not known at this time.

Cetin and associates reported that placental amino acid exchange is altered in pregnancies complicated by GDM. Ornithine concentrations were significantly increased in women with GDM compared with controls, and in the cord blood of infants of women with GDM, there were significant increases in multiple amino acids, including phenylalanine and leucine, but decreases in glutamate. The investigators speculate that in infants of women with GDM, the altered in utero fetal milieu affects fetal growth through multiple mechanisms affecting various nutrient compartments.

Amino acids are actively transported across the placenta from mother to fetus through energy-requiring amino acid transporters. These transporters are highly stereospecific, but they have low substrate specificity. Additionally, they may vary with location between the microvillus and basal membranes. Decreased amino acid concentrations have been reported in growth-restricted neonates in comparison with appropriately grown neonates. Decreased amino acid transporter activity has been implicated as a possible mechanism. However, the potential role, if any, of placental amino acid transporters in the development of fetal macrosomia in women with diabetes is currently unknown.

Lipid Metabolism

Although there is ample literature regarding the changes in glucose metabolism during gestation, the data regarding the alterations in lipid metabolism are meager by comparison. Darmady and Postle measured serum cholesterol and triglyceride before, during, and after pregnancy in 34 normal women.[21] There was a decrease in both cholesterol and triglyceride at about 7 weeks' gestation. Both of the levels increased progressively until term. There was then a decrease in serum triglyceride postpartum. The decrease was more rapid in women who breastfed compared with those women who bottle-fed their infants.[21] Additionally, Knopp and coworkers[22] have reported that there is a twofold to fourfold increase in total triglyceride concentration and a 25% to 50% increase in total cholesterol concentration during gestation. There is a 50% increase in low-density lipoprotein (LDL) cholesterol and a 30% increase in high-density lipoprotein (HDL) cholesterol by midgestation, which decreases slightly in the third trimester. Maternal triglyceride and very-low-density lipoprotein (VLDL) triglyceride levels in late gestation are positively correlated with maternal estriol and insulin concentrations.

A recent study by Vahratian and associates studied the changes in lipid levels during pregnancy in normal weight compared with overweight and obese women from 6 to 10 through 32 to 36 weeks' gestation. The levels of total cholesterol, triglycerides, and LDL and HDL cholesterol increased throughout gestation. Although the concentrations in the overweight and obese women were generally higher in early pregnancy, the rate of change of LDL cholesterol and total cholesterol was lower in later gestation.

FFAs have been associated with fetal overgrowth, particularly of fetal adipose tissue. There is a significant difference in the arteriovenous FFA concentration at birth, much as there is with arteriovenous glucose concentration. There are multiple clinical studies suggesting the contribution of maternal lipids to fetal growth and in particular adiposity. Knopp and coworkers[22] reported that neonatal birthweight was positively correlated with triglyceride and FFA concentration in late pregnancy. Similar conclusions were reached by Ogburn and colleagues, who showed that insulin concentrations decrease FFA concentrations, inhibit lipolysis, and result in increased fat deposition. Kleigman reported that infants of obese women had an increased birthweight and skinfold thickness and higher FFA levels compared with infants of lean women. More recently, DiCianni and associates reported that in women with a positive glucose screen but normal glucose tolerance, their serum triglycerides and prepregnancy body mass index (BMI) had a significant correlation with birthweight at term.[23] In Australia, Nolan and coworkers showed that nonfasting maternal triglycerides measured at 9 to 12 weeks' gestation were significantly correlated with neonatal birthweight ratio at term. Finally, Schaeffer-Graf and colleagues, in a well-controlled German GDM population, reported that **maternal FFA concentrations correlated with ultrasound estimates of neonatal abdominal circumference and anthropometric estimates of neonatal fat mass at delivery.**[24] Maternal FFA concentrations were positively correlated with cord FFA. Although cord FFA concentrations were higher in cord blood of large-for-gestational-age (LGA) neonates compared with either appropriate or SGA neonates, there was a paradoxical negative correlation of cord triglycerides and birthweight. The authors speculated that the SGA newborns have a lower lipoprotein lipase activity and hence were unable to hydrolyze triglycerides. In contrast, the LGA neonates have lower cord triglyceride activity because of enhanced lipoprotein lipase activity resulting from their increased number of fat cells. Similar findings were noted by Merzouk and coworkers in growth-restricted infants. In summary, in women with evidence of decreased insulin sensitivity (obesity and/or GDM) in addition to glucose, maternal lipid metabolism accounts for a significant proportion of fetal growth, particularly adiposity. These data support the original work by **Freinkel**

proposing that fetal growth or overgrowth is a function multiple nutritional factors in addition to glucose.[25]

Lipid metabolism in women with diabetes mellitus is influenced by whether the woman has type 1 or type 2 diabetes. This also applies when these women become pregnant. In women with type 2 diabetes and gestational diabetes, Knopp and coworkers[22] reported an increase in triglyceride and decrease in HDL concentration. However, Montelongo and colleagues reported little change in FFA concentrations through all three trimesters after a 12-hour fast. Koukkou and coworkers noted an increase in total triglyceride but a lower LDL cholesterol in women with GDM. Increased triglyceride concentrations during pregnancy have also been reported to be related to the development of gestational diabetes and preeclampsia in women with normal pregravid glucose tolerance, both of which are related to increased insulin resistance. In women with type 1 diabetes, there was no change in total triglyceride, but there was a lower cholesterol concentration secondary to a decrease in HDL. This is of interest because HDL acts as plasma antioxidant and thus may be related to the increase in congenital malformations in women with type 1 diabetes. Oxidative stress has been implicated as a potential factor in the incidence of anomalies in women with type 1 diabetes.

Hyperinsulinemic-euglycemic clamp studies in pregnant women with normal glucose tolerance and GDM revealed a decreased ability of insulin to suppress plasma FFAs with advancing gestation. Insulin's ability to suppress plasma FFA was lower in women with GDM compared with women with normal glucose tolerance.

Taken together, these studies demonstrate that there is decreased nutrient insulin sensitivity in all women with advancing gestation. These decreases in insulin sensitivity are further exacerbated by the presence of decreased pregravid maternal insulin sensitivity, manifesting in later pregnancy as GDM, resulting in greater nutrient availability and higher ambient insulin concentrations for the developing fetoplacental unit, which may eventually result in fetal overgrowth.

Maternal Weight Gain and Energy Expenditure

Estimates of the energy cost of pregnancy range from a cost of 80,000 kcal to a net saving of up to 10,000 kcal.[26] As a result, the recommendations for nutritional intake in pregnancy differ and depend on the population being evaluated. Furthermore, based on more recent data, recommendations for individuals within a population may be more diverse than previously believed, making general guidelines for nutritional intake difficult.

The theoretical energy cost of pregnancy was originally estimated by Hytten and Leitch[18] using a factorial method. The additional cost of pregnancy consisted of (1) the additional maternal and fetoplacental tissue accrued during pregnancy and (2) the additional "running cost" of pregnancy (e.g., the work of increased cardiac output). In Hytten's model, the greatest increases in maternal energy expenditure occur between 10 and 30 weeks' gestation, primarily because of maternal accretion of adipose tissue. However, the mean increases in maternal adipose tissue vary considerably among various ethnic groups. Forsum and associates reported a mean increase of more than 5 kg of adipose tissue in Swedish women, whereas Lawrence and colleagues found no increase in adipose tissue stores in women from the Gambia.

Basal metabolic rate accounts for 60% to 70% of total energy expenditure in individuals not engaged in competitive physical activity and correlates well with total energy expenditure. As with the changes in maternal accretion of adipose tissue, there are wide variations in the change in maternal basal metabolic rate during gestation, not only in different populations but again within relatively homogeneous groups. The cumulative energy changes in basal metabolic rate range from a high of 52,000 kcal in Swedish women to net savings of 10,700 kcal in women from the Gambia without nutritional supplementation. **The mean increase in basal metabolic rate in Western women relative to a nonpregnant, nonlactating control group averages about 20%.** However, the coefficient of variation of basal metabolic rate in these populations during gestation ranges from 93% in women in the United Kingdom to more than 200% in Swedish women.[27] When assessing energy intake in relation to energy expenditure, however, estimated energy intake remains lower than the estimates of total energy expenditure. These discrepancies have usually been explained by factors such as (1) increased metabolic efficiency during gestation, (2) decreased maternal activity, and (3) unreliable assessment of food intake.[26]

Data in nonpregnant subjects may help explain some of the wide variations in metabolic parameters during human gestation, even with homogeneous populations. Swinburn and colleagues reported that in the Pima Indian population, subjects with decreased insulin sensitivity gained less weight compared with more insulin-sensitive subjects (3.1 vs. 7.6 kg) over a period of 4 years. Furthermore, the percentage weight change per year was highly correlated with glucose disposal as estimated from clamp studies. Catalano and coworkers[28] conducted a prospective longitudinal study in early pregnancy of the changes in maternal accretion of body fat and basal metabolic rate in lean and obese women with normal GDM. Women with GDM had decreased glucose insulin sensitivity in early gestation compared with the control group and had significantly smaller increases in body fat than women with normal glucose tolerance. In these lean women, there was a significant inverse correlation between the changes in fat accretion and insulin sensitivity (i.e., women with decreased pregravid insulin sensitivity had less accretion of body fat compared with women with increased pregravid insulin sensitivity). These results are consistent with a previous report showing that total weight gain in women with GDM was 2.5 kg less compared with a weight-matched control group.

In the basal state, lean women increase the use of carbohydrate as a metabolic fuel, whereas in obese women, there is an increased use of lipids for oxidative needs. However, with the decreased in insulin sensitivity in late gestation, all women lean or obese with normal glucose tolerance or GDM have an increase in fat oxidation and decrease in nonoxidative glucose metabolism (storage). Of interest, these increases in lipid oxidation in pregnancy are positively correlated with the increases in maternal leptin concentrations, possibly accounting for a role of leptin in human pregnancy. The results of these studies show that there is a relationship between the changes in maternal insulin sensitivity and accretion of adipose tissue in early gestation. The ability of women with decreased pregravid glucose insulin sensitivity (obese women and women with GDM) to conserve energy, not significantly increase body fat, and make sufficient nutrients available to produce a healthy fetus supports the hypothesis that decreased maternal insulin sensitivity may have a reproductive metabolic advantage in women when food availability is marginal. In contrast, decreased maternal insulin sensitivity before conception in areas where food is plentiful and a sedentary lifestyle is more common may manifest as GDM and increase the long-term risk for both diabetes and obesity in the woman and her offspring.[28]

PERINATAL MORBIDITY AND MORTALITY

Fetal Death

In the past, sudden and unexplained stillbirth occurred in 10% to 30% of pregnancies complicated by type 1 diabetes mellitus, also called *insulin-dependent diabetes mellitus* (IDDM). Although relatively uncommon today, such losses still plague the pregnancies of patients who do not receive optimal care. Stillbirths have been observed most often after the 36th week of pregnancy in patients with vascular disease, poor glycemic control, hydramnios, fetal macrosomia, or preeclampsia. Women with vascular complications may develop fetal growth restriction and intrauterine demise as early as the second trimester. In the past, prevention of intrauterine death led to a strategy of scheduled preterm deliveries for type 1 diabetic women. This empirical approach reduced the number of stillbirths, but errors in estimation of fetal size and gestational age as well as the functional immaturity characteristic of the infant of the diabetic mother (IDM) contributed to many neonatal deaths from hyaline membrane disease (HMD).

Excessive stillbirth rates in pregnancies complicated by diabetes have been linked to chronic intrauterine hypoxia. Extramedullary hematopoiesis, frequently observed in stillborn IDMs, supports chronic intrauterine hypoxia as a likely cause of these intrauterine fetal deaths. Studies of fetal umbilical cord blood samples in pregnant women with type 1 diabetes have demonstrated relative fetal erythremia and lactic acidemia. Maternal diabetes may also produce alterations in red blood cell oxygen release and placental blood flow. Reduced uterine blood flow is thought to contribute to the increased incidence of intrauterine growth restriction observed in pregnancies complicated by diabetic vasculopathy. Ketoacidosis and preeclampsia, two factors known to be associated with an increased incidence of intrauterine deaths, may further decrease uterine blood flow.

Alterations in fetal carbohydrate metabolism also may contribute to intrauterine asphyxia. There is considerable evidence linking hyperinsulinemia and fetal hypoxia. Hyperinsulinemia induced in fetal lambs by an infusion of exogenous insulin produces an increase in oxygen consumption and a decrease in arterial oxygen content. Persistent maternal-fetal hyperglycemia occurs independent of maternal uterine blood flow, which may not be increased enough to allow for enhanced oxygen delivery in the face of increased metabolic demands. Thus, hyperinsulinemia in the fetus of the diabetic mother appears to increase fetal metabolic rate and oxygen requirement in the fetus. Other factors, such as hyperglycemia, ketoacidosis, preeclampsia, and maternal vasculopathy, can also reduce placental blood flow and fetal oxygenation.

Congenital Malformations

With the reduction in intrauterine deaths and a marked decrease in neonatal mortality related to HMD and traumatic delivery, **congenital malformations have emerged as the most important cause of perinatal loss in pregnancies complicated by type 1 and type 2 diabetes mellitus.** In the past, these anomalies were responsible for only 10% of all perinatal deaths. Malformations account for 30% to 50% of perinatal mortality. Neonatal deaths exceed stillbirths in pregnancies complicated by pregestational diabetes mellitus, and fatal congenital malformations account for this pattern.

Most studies have documented a twofold to sixfold increase in major malformations in infants of type 1 and type 2 diabetic mothers. At the Ohio State University Diabetes in Pregnancy Program, we observed 29 congenital anomalies in 289 (10%) diabetic woman enrolled over a 10-year period. In a prospective analysis, Simpson and associates observed an 8.5% incidence of major anomalies in the diabetic population, whereas the malformation rate in a small group of concurrently gathered control subjects was 2.4%. Similar figures were obtained in the Diabetes in Early Pregnancy Study in the United States. The incidence of major anomalies was 2.1% in 389 control patients and 9% in 279 diabetic women. A recent case-control study of 13,030 infants with congenital anomalies and 4895 controls revealed a prevalence of type 1 diabetes of 2.2% versus 0.5% and of type 2 diabetes of 5.1% versus 3.7% in controls. In general, the incidence of major malformations in worldwide studies of offspring of diabetic mothers has ranged from 5% to 10% (Table 39-2).

The insult that causes malformations in IDM affects most organ systems and must act before the seventh week of gestation. Central nervous system malformations, particularly anencephaly, open spina bifida, and holoprosencephaly, are increased 10-fold. Cardiac anomalies are the most common malformations with IDM, with ventricular septal defects and complex lesions such as transposition of the great vessels increased fivefold. The congenital defect thought to be most characteristic of diabetic embryopathy is sacral agenesis or caudal dysplasia, an anomaly found 200 to 400 times more often in offspring of diabetic

TABLE 39-2 FREQUENCY OF CONGENITAL MALFORMATIONS IN INFANTS OF DIABETIC MOTHERS

STUDY	NO.	PERCENT
Mills et al., 1988[90]	25/279	9.0
Greene, 1993[91]	35/451	7.7
Steel & Duncan, 1978[92]	12/239	7.8
Fuhrmann et al., 1983[102]	22/292	7.5
Simpson et al., 1983[94]	9/106	8.5
Albert et al., 1996[95]	29/289	10.0

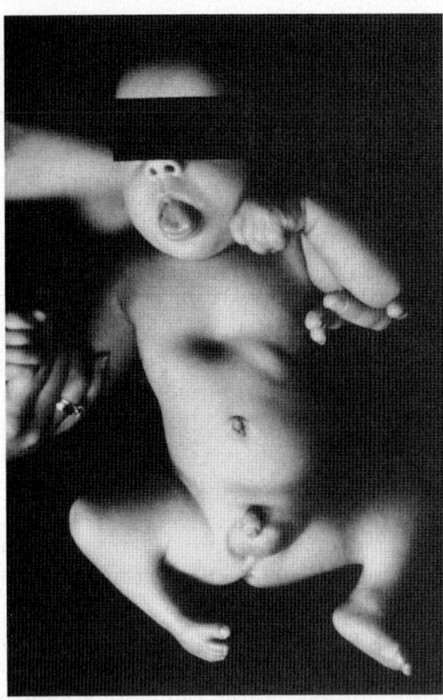

FIGURE 39-12. Infant of a diabetic mother with sacral agenesis and hypoplastic lower extremities.

women (Figure 39-12). However, this defect is not pathognomonic for diabetes because it occurs in nondiabetic pregnancies.

Impaired glycemic control and associated derangements in maternal metabolism appear to contribute to abnormal embryogenesis. Maternal hyperglycemia has been proposed by most investigators as the primary teratogenic factor, but hyperketonemia, hypoglycemia, somatomedin inhibitor excess, and excess free oxygen radicals have also been suggested (see the box, Proposed Factors Associated with Teratogenesis in Pregnancy Complicated by Diabetes Mellitus). The profile of a woman most likely to produce an anomalous infant would include a patient with poor periconceptional control, long-standing diabetes, and vascular disease. Genetic susceptibility to the teratogenic influence of diabetes may also be a factor.

Proposed Factors Associated with Teratogenesis in Pregnancy Complicated by Diabetes Mellitus

- Hyperglycemia
- Ketone body excess
- Somatomedin inhibition
- Arachidonic acid deficiency
- Free oxygen radical excess

Several mechanisms have been proposed by which the previously mentioned teratogenic factors produce malformations. Freinkel and colleagues[29] first suggested that anomalies might arise from inhibition of glycolysis, the key energy-producing process during embryogenesis. They found that the addition of D-mannose to the culture medium of rat embryos inhibited glycolysis and produced growth restriction and derangement of neural tube closure.[29] Freinkel and colleagues[29] stressed the sensitivity of normal embryogenesis to alterations in these key energy-producing pathways, a process he labeled "fuel-mediated" teratogenesis. Goldman and Baker suggested that the mechanism responsible for the increased incidence of neural tube defects in embryos cultured in a hyperglycemic medium may involve a functional deficiency of arachidonic acid because supplementation with arachidonic acid or myoinositol will reduce the frequency of neural tube defects in this experimental model. Pinter and Reece, along with Pinter and associates, confirmed these studies and demonstrated that hyperglycemia-induced alterations in neural tube closure include disordered cells, decreased mitoses, and changes indicating premature maturation. These authors further demonstrated that hyperglycemia during organogenesis has a primary deleterious effect on yolk sac function with resultant embryopathy.

Altered oxidative metabolism from maternal diabetes may cause increased production of free oxygen radicals in the developing embryo, which are likely teratogenic. Supplementation of oxygen radical-scavenging enzymes, such as superoxide dismutase, to the culture medium of rat embryos protects against growth delay and excess malformations. It has been suggested that excess free oxygen radicals may have a direct effect on embryonic prostaglandin biosynthesis. Free oxygen radical excess may enhance lipid peroxidation, and in turn, generated hydroperoxides might stimulate thromboxane biosynthesis and inhibit prostacyclin production, an imbalance that could have profound effects on embryonic development. Finally, oxidative stress on diabetic rats is associated with the accumulation of glycation products and altered vascular endothelial growth factor expression in cardiovascular regions of the developing heart associated with endocardial cushion defects.

Fetal Macrosomia

Macrosomia has been variously defined as birthweight greater than 4000 to 4500 g as well as LGA, in which birthweight is above the 90th percentile for population and sex-specific growth curves. Fetal macrosomia complicates as many as 50% of pregnancies in women with GDM and 40% of pregnancies complicated by type 1 and type 2 diabetes, including some women treated with intensive glycemic control (Figure 39-13). Delivery of an infant weighing greater than 4500 g occurs 10 times more often in women with diabetes compared with a population of women with normal glucose tolerance.

According to the Pedersen hypothesis, maternal hyperglycemia results in fetal hyperglycemia and hyperinsulinemia, resulting in excessive fetal growth. Increased fetal β-cell mass may be identified as early as the second trimester.[29] Evidence supporting the Pedersen hypothesis has come from the studies of amniotic fluid and cord blood insulin and C-peptide concentrations. Both are increased in the amniotic fluid of insulin-treated women with diabetes at term and correlate with neonatal fat mass. Lipids and amino acids, which are elevated in pregnancies complicated by GDM, may also play a role in excessive fetal growth by stimulating the release of insulin and other growth factors from the fetal pancreatic β cells and placenta. **Infants of mothers with GDM have an increase in fat mass compared with fat-free mass. Additionally, the growth is disproportionate, with chest-to-head and**

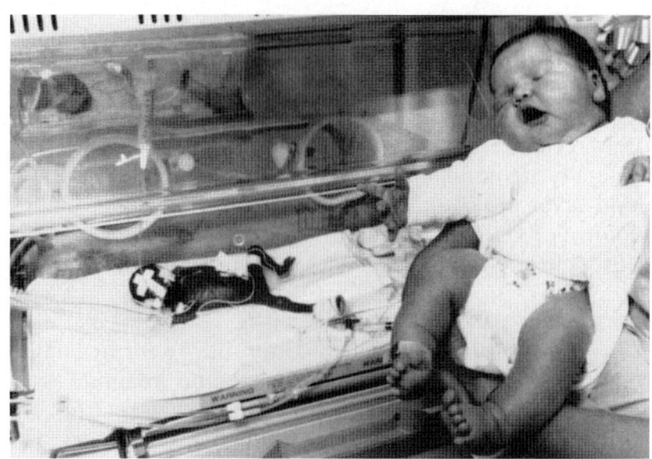

FIGURE 39-13. Two extremes of growth abnormalities in pregnancies complicated by diabetes mellitus. On the left is a severely growth-restricted infant, and on the right is a macrosomic infant.

shoulder-to-head ratios larger than those of infants of women with normal glucose tolerance. This factor may contribute to the higher rate of shoulder dystocia and birth trauma observed in these infants.

The results of several clinical series have validated the Pedersen hypothesis inasmuch as tight maternal glycemic control has been associated with a decline in the incidence of macrosomia. Landon and colleagues,[30] using daily capillary glucose values obtained during the second and third trimesters in women requiring insulin, reported a rate of 9% macrosomia when mean values were below 110 mg/dL compared with 34% when less optimal control was achieved. Jovanovic and associates have suggested that 1-hour postprandial glucose measurements correlate best with the frequency of macrosomia. After controlling for other factors, these authors noted that the strongest prediction for birthweight was third-trimester nonfasting glucose measurements.

In a series of metabolic studies, Catalano and associates[34] estimated body composition in 186 neonates using anthropometry. Fat-free mass, which represented 86% of mean birthweight, accounted for 83% of the variance in birthweight, and fat mass, which made up only 14% of birthweight, accounted for 46% of the variance in birthweight. There was also significantly greater fat-free mass in male compared with female infants. Using independent variables such as maternal height, pregravid weight, weight gain during pregnancy, parity, paternal height and weight, neonatal sex, and gestational age, the authors accounted for 29% of the variance in birth weight, 30% of the variance in fat-free mass, and 17% of the variance in fat mass. Including estimates of maternal insulin sensitivity in 16 additional subjects, they were able to explain 48% of the variance in birthweight, 53% in fat-free mass, and 46% in fat mass. Studies by Caruso and colleagues have corroborated these findings, reporting that women with unexplained fetal growth restriction had greater insulin sensitivity compared with a control group of women whose infants were appropriate weight for gestational age. The potential mechanisms for this relate to the possibility that maternal circulating nutrients for glucose, FFAs, and amino acids available for placental transport to the fetus are decreased because of the relative increase in maternal insulin sensitivity. A positive correlation between birthweight and weight gain has been observed in women with normal glucose tolerance. The correlation was strongest in women who were lean before conception and became progressively weaker as pregravid weight for height increased. In women with GDM, there were no significant correlations between maternal weight gain and birthweight, irrespective of pregravid weight for height. These studies emphasize the role of the maternal metabolic environment and fetal growth.

TABLE 39-3 NEONATAL BODY COMPOSITION

	GDM (N = 195)	NGT (N = 220)	P VALUE
Weight (g)	3398 ± 550	3337 ± 549	.26
FFM (g)	2962 ± 405	2975 ± 408	.74
Fat mass (g)	436 ± 206	362 ± 198	.0002
Body fat	12.4 ± 4.6	10.4 ± 4.6	.0001

Modified from Catalano PM, Tyzbir ED, Allen Sr, et al: Evaluation of fetal growth by estimation of body composition. Obstet Gynecol 156:1089, 1987.
FFM, Fat-free mass; *GDM,* gestational diabetes mellitus; *NGT,* normal glucose tolerance.

Normalization of birthweight in infants of women with GDM, however, may in itself not achieve optimal growth. In a study of approximately 400 infants of women with normal glucose tolerance and GDM, Catalano and coworkers[34] showed that the infants of women with GDM had increased fat mass but not lean body mass or weight compared with a control group, even after adjustment for potential confounding variables (Table 39-3). Similarly, when only infants who were appropriate size for gestational age (i.e., between the 10th and 80th percentiles) were examined, the infants of the women with GDM had significantly greater fat mass and percentage of body fat but had less lean mass compared with the control group but no difference in birthweight. Of note, in the infants of the women with GDM, the strongest correlates with fat mass were fasting glucose and gestational age. This accounted for 17% of the variance in infant fat mass.

Hypoglycemia

Neonatal hypoglycemia, a blood glucose level less than 35 to 40 mg/dL during the first 12 hours of life, results from a rapid drop in plasma glucose concentrations following clamping of the umbilical cord. Hypoglycemia, a byproduct of hyperinsulinemia, is particularly common in macrosomic newborns, in which rates exceed 50%. With near-physiologic control of maternal glucose levels during pregnancy, overall rates of 5% to 15% have been reported. The degree of hypoglycemia may be influenced by at least two factors: (1) maternal glucose control during the latter half of pregnancy and (2) control of maternal glycemia control during labor and delivery. Prior poor maternal glucose control can result in fetal β-cell hyperplasia, leading to exaggerated insulin release following delivery. IDMs exhibiting hypoglycemia have elevated cord C-peptide and free insulin levels at birth and an exaggerated pancreatic response to glucose loading.

Respiratory Distress Syndrome

Experimental animal studies have provided evidence that hyperglycemia and hyperinsulinemia can effect pulmonary surfactant biosynthesis. In vitro studies have documented that insulin can interfere with substrate availability for surfactant biosynthesis. Smith has postulated that insulin interferes with the normal timing of glucocorticoid-induced pulmonary maturation in the fetus. Cortisol apparently acts on pulmonary fibroblasts to induce synthesis of fibroblast-pneumocyte factor, which then acts on type II cells to stimulate phospholipid synthesis. Carlson and coworkers demonstrated that insulin blocks cortisol action at the level of the fibroblast by reducing the production of fibroblast-pneumocyte factor.

Clinical studies investigating the effect of maternal diabetes on fetal lung maturation have produced conflicting data. The role of amniocentesis in determining fetal lung maturity is discussed with timing and mode of delivery. **Several studies suggest that in women with well-controlled diabetes whose fetus is delivered at 38 to 39 weeks' gestation, the risk for respiratory distress syndrome (RDS) is no higher than that observed in the general population.**[32,33] Kjos and Walther[33] studied the outcome of 526 diabetic gestations delivered within 5 days of amniotic fluid fetal lung maturation testing and reported HMD in five neonates (0.95%), all of whom were delivered before 34 weeks' gestation. Mimouni and associates compared outcomes of 127 IDMs with matched controls and concluded that diabetes in pregnancy as currently managed is not a direct risk factor for the development of RDS. Yet, cesarean delivery not preceded by labor and prematurity, both of which are increased in diabetic pregnancies, clearly increase the likelihood of neonatal respiratory disease. With cesarean delivery, many of these cases represent retained lung fluid or transient tachypnea of the newborn, which usually resolves within the first days of life.

Calcium and Magnesium Metabolism

Neonatal hypocalcemia, with serum levels below 7 mg/dL or an ionized level less than 4 mg/dL, occurs at an increased rate in the IDM when controlling for predisposing factors such as prematurity and birth asphyxia. With modern management, the frequency of neonatal hypocalcemia is less than 5% in the infants of diabetic women. Hypocalcemia in the IDM has been associated with a failure to increase parathyroid hormone synthesis following birth. Decreased serum magnesium levels have also been documented in pregnant diabetic women as well as their infants. Mimouni and associates described reduced amniotic fluid magnesium concentrations in women with type 1 diabetes mellitus. These findings may be explained by a drop in fetal urinary magnesium excretion, which would accompany a relative magnesium-deficient state. Magnesium deficiency paradoxically, then, may inhibit fetal parathyroid hormone secretion.

Hyperbilirubinemia and Polycythemia

Hyperbilirubinemia is frequently observed in the IDM. Neonatal jaundice has been reported in as many as 25% to 53% of pregnancies complicated by pregestational diabetes mellitus and 38% of pregnancies in women with GDM. In the past, the jaundice observed in the IDM often was attributed to prematurity. However, jaundice is increased in macrosomic IDMs.

Although severe hyperbilirubinemia may be observed independent of polycythemia, a common pathway for these complications most likely involves increased red blood cell production, which is stimulated by increased erythropoietin in the IDM. Presumably, the major stimulus for red cell production is a state of relative hypoxia in utero, as described previously. Cord erythropoietin levels generally are normal in IDMs whose mothers demonstrate good glycemic control during gestation; however, hemoglobin A_{1c} (HbA_{1c}) values in late pregnancy are significantly elevated in mothers of hyperbilirubinemic infants.

Cardiomyopathy

A transient form of cardiomyopathy may occur in infants of diabetic mothers. Among symptomatic infants, septal hypertrophy may cause left ventricular outflow obstruction. Although most infants are asymptomatic, respiratory distress or signs of cardiac failure may arise. Cardiac hypertrophy likely results from fetal hyperinsulinemia, which leads to fat and glycogen deposition in the myocardium. Thus, cardiomyopathy generally occurs in poorly controlled pregnancies complicated by macrosomia. In most cases, symptoms do improve over several weeks with supportive care, and echocardiographic changes resolve as well.

MATERNAL CLASSIFICATION AND RISK ASSESSMENT

Priscilla White first noted that the patient's age at onset of diabetes, the duration of the disease, and the presence of vasculopathy significantly influenced perinatal outcome. Her classification system has been widely applied to pregnant women with diabetes. A modification of this scheme is presented in Table 39-1. Counseling a patient and formulating a plan of management requires assessment of both maternal and fetal risk. The White classification facilitates this evaluation.

Class A_1 diabetes mellitus includes those women who have demonstrated carbohydrate intolerance during an oral glucose tolerance test (GTT); however, their fasting and postprandial glucose levels are maintained within physiologic range by dietary regulation alone. Class A_2 includes gestational diabetic women who require insulin or oral hypoglycemic therapy in response to repetitive elevations of fasting or postpartum glucose levels following dietary intervention.

Two International Workshop Conferences on Gestational Diabetes sponsored by the American Diabetes Association in cooperation with the American College of Obstetricians and Gynecologists (ACOG) recommended that the term gestational diabetes rather than class A diabetes be used to describe women with carbohydrate intolerance of variable severity with onset or recognition during the present pregnancy. The definition applies whether insulin or only diet modification is used for treatment and whether or not the condition persists after pregnancy. It does not exclude the possibility that unrecognized glucose intolerance may have antedates or have begun with pregnancy. The term gestational diabetes fails to specify whether the patient requires dietary adjustment alone or treatment with diet and insulin. This distinction is important because those women who are normoglycemic while fasting appear to have a significantly lower perinatal mortality rate. Women with GDM who require insulin are at greater risk for a poor perinatal outcome than those whose diabetes is controlled by diet alone.

Women requiring insulin are designated by the letters B, C, D, R, F, and T. Class B patients are those whose onset of disease occurs after age 20 years. They have had diabetes for less than 10 years and have no vascular complications. Included in this subgroup of patients are those who have been previously treated with oral hypoglycemic agents.

Class C diabetes includes patients who have the onset of their disease between the ages of 10 and 19 years or have had the disease for 10 to 19 years. Vascular disease is not present.

Class D represents women whose disease is of 20 years' duration or more, or whose onset occurred before age 10 years, or who have benign retinopathy. The latter includes microaneurysms, exudates, and venous dilation.

Nephropathy

Renal disease develops in 25% to 30% of women with IDDM, with a peak incidence after 16 years of diabetes. **Overt diabetic nephropathy is diagnosed in women with type 1 or type 2 diabetes mellitus when persistent proteinuria exists in the absence of infection or other urinary tract disease.** The criteria for diagnosis in the nonpregnant state includes a total urinary protein excretion (TPE) of greater than 500 mg/24 hours or greater than 300 mg/24 hours of urinary albumin excretion (UAE).

Before the development of overt diabetic nephropathy, some individuals develop incipient diabetic nephropathy defined by repetitive increases in UAE known as *microalbuminuria*. The diagnosis is established from a 24-hour urine collection exhibiting UAE of 20 to 199 mcg/minute or 30 to 299 mg/24 hours. It is important to note that women who exhibit microalbuminuria in early pregnancy have a 35% to 60% risk for superimposed preeclampsia.[35] Without specific interventions, about 80% of individuals with type 1 diabetes who develop sustained microalbuminuria experience an increase in UAE of 10% to 20% per year to the stage of overt nephropathy. In the nonpregnant individual, improvement of glycemic and blood pressure control has been demonstrated to reduce the risk for or slow the progression of diabetic nephropathy. Renoprotective or antihypertensive therapy consisting of either angiotensin-converting enzyme (ACE) inhibitors or angiotensin II receptor blockers is indicated before pregnancy in women with microalbuminuria or overt nephropathy. **Both ACE inhibitors and angiotensin receptor blockers are contraindicated during pregnancy because they may result in fetal proximal tubal dysgenesis and oligohydramnios.** Two Israeli studies first suggested that ACE inhibitors were unlikely to be teratogenic. Thus, the practice by some has been not to discontinue such medications before conception and to discontinue use after pregnancy is confirmed. However, a population-based study has indicated potential teratogenesis in women who received ACE inhibitors in early pregnancy and thus calls into question whether such agents are advised in women attempting concraception.[36] Cooper and colleagues[36] studied a cohort of 29,507 infants enrolled in Tennessee Medicaid born between 1985 and 2000 for whom there was no evidence of maternal diabetes. A total of 209 infants with exposure to ACE inhibitors during the first trimester alone were compared with 202 infants exposed to other antihypertensives during the first trimester and to 29,096 infants with no exposure to any antihypertensive agents during pregnancy. Major congenital malformations were identified from linked vital records and hospitalization claims during the first year of life. Infants with only first-trimester exposure to ACE inhibitors had an increased risk for major congenital malformations (risk ratio, 2.71; 95% confidence interval, 1.72 to 4.27) compared with infants who had no fetal exposure to other antihypertensive medications during only the first trimester. The increased risk conferred by ACE inhibitor exposure manifested as primarily anomalies of the cardiovascular and central nervous systems. Clearly, given this information, the risk and benefits of use of ACE inhibitors in diabetic women planning pregnancy must be considered.

Women with diabetic nephropathy have a significantly reduced life expectancy. Disease progression is characterized by hypertension, declining glomerular filtration rate, and eventual end-stage renal disease requiring dialysis or transplantation. In women with overt nephropathy, end-stage renal disease occurs in 50% by 10 years and in greater than 75% by 20 years.

Class F describes the 5% to 10% of pregnant patients with underlying renal disease. This includes those with reduced creatinine clearance or proteinuria of at least 300 mg in 24 hours measured during the first 20 weeks of gestation. Two factors present before 20 weeks' gestation appear to be predictive of perinatal outcome in these women (e.g., preterm delivery, low birthweight, or preeclampsia):

1. Proteinuria greater than 3 g/24 hours
2. Serum creatinine greater than 1.5 mg/dL

In a series of 45 class F women, 12 women had such risk factors.[37] Preeclampsia developed in 92%, with a mean gestational age at delivery of 34 weeks, compared with an incidence of preeclampsia of 36% in 33 women without these risk factors who reached an average gestational age of 36 weeks. Remarkably, perinatal survival was 100% in this series, and no deliveries occurred before 30 weeks' gestation. Comparable series detailing perinatal outcomes in class F patients are presented in Table 39-4.

The management of the diabetic women with nephropathy requires great expertise. Limitation of dietary protein, which may reduce protein excretion in nonpregnant patients, has not been adequately studied during pregnancy. Although the method is controversial, some nephrologists recommend a modified reduction in protein intake for pregnant women with nephropathy. **Control of hypertension in pregnant women with diabetic nephropathy is crucial to prevent further deterioration of kidney function and to optimize pregnancy outcome.** Although debatable, some cautiously use diuretics when patients are extremely nephrotic because this group may be prone to volume-dependent forms of hypertension. Because calcium channel blockers have similar renoprotective effects as ACE inhibitors and do not appear to be teratogenic, these agents maybe a reasonable choice for treatment of hypertension in pregnant women with diabetic nephropathy. Whether such agents benefit normotensive pregnant women with microalbuminuria or nephropathy has not been determined.

TABLE 39-4 COMPARATIVE STUDIES OF OUTCOMES IN CLASS F DIABETES MELLITUS

	KITZMILLER ET AL., 1991[38]	GRENFEL ET AL., 1986[96]	REECE ET AL., 1988[97]	GORDON ET AL., 1996[98]	ROSENN ET AL, 1997[99]
No. of subjects	26	20	31	45	61
Chronic hypertension	31%	27%	22%	26%	47%
Initial creatinine >1.9 mg/dL	38%	10%	22%	11%	—
Initial proteinuria >3 g/24 hr	8.3%	—	22%	13%	—
Preeclampsia	15%	55%	35%	53%	51%
Cesarean delivery	—	72%	70%	80%	82%
Perinatal survival (%)	88.9	100	93.5	100	94%
Major anomalies	3 (11.1%)	1 (4.3%)	3 (9.7%)	2 (4%)	4 (6%)
Intrauterine growth restriction (%)	20.8	Na	19.4	11.0	11%
Delivery					
<34 wk (%)	30.8	27	22.5	15.5	25%
34-36 wk (%)	40.7	23	32.3	35.5	28%
>36 wk (%)	28.5	50	45.2	49	47%

Several studies have failed to demonstrate a permanent worsening of diabetic renal disease in women with mild to moderate renal insufficiency as a result of pregnancy. Furthermore, it has been suggested that pregnancy itself does not increase the risk for developing nephropathy, although development of proteinuria and poor glycemic control are markers for subsequent renal disease. Kitzmiller and colleagues[38] reviewed 35 pregnancies complicated by diabetic nephropathy. Proteinuria increased in 69%, and hypertension developed in 73%. After delivery, proteinuria declined in 65% of cases. In only two patients did protein excretion increase after gestation. In Gordon's series, 26 women (58%) had more than a 1-g increase in proteinuria, and by the third trimester, 25 (56%) excreted more than 3 g/24 hours. In most cases, protein excretion returned to baseline levels after gestation.

Normal pregnancy is marked by an approximate 50% increase in glomerular filtration rate and thus a rise in creatinine clearance accompanied by a modest decline in serum creatinine. Most women with diabetic nephropathy, however, do not exhibit a rise in creatinine clearance during gestation. In a study of 46 class F pregnancies, Gordon and colleagues reported a mean decrease in creatinine clearance of 7.9%. When evaluated according to initial creatinine clearance, no difference in the degree of change was noted when subjects were classified according to first trimester renal function. Whereas few patients exhibited a rise in creatinine clearance, other smaller studies have demonstrated an increase in creatinine clearance in about one third of women. Given the importance of blood pressure control in reducing cardiovascular and renal complications in the nonpregnant state, Carr and colleagues[39] studied the effect of poorly controlled hypertension in early pregnancy on renal function in 43 women with IDDM and nephropathy. Those women with mean arterial pressure exceeding 100 mm Hg demonstrated higher serum creatinine levels (1.23 vs. 0.895 mg/dL) compared with women with controlled hypertension.

With overt diabetic nephropathy, both albumin and total protein excretion may rise significantly during gestation. Importantly, a rise in total protein excretion to levels exceeding 300 mg/24 hours may also be observed in women both with and without microalbuminuria in early pregnancy. Biesenbach and Zazgornik reported an average increase by the third trimester in total protein excretion to 478 mg/24 hours in seven women with microalbuminuria in early pregnancy. This observation underscores the importance of obtaining baseline 24-hour urine measurements for total protein in all diabetic women because confusion arises as to the significance of when new-onset macroalbuminuria or proteinuria is detected during the third trimester. Despite this recommendation, it may be challenging to distinguish preeclampsia from the natural progression of diabetic nephropathy, which often manifests as progressive proteinuria during pregnancy.

Gordon and colleagues[37] have detailed the progressive rise in proteinuria during pregnancy in 46 class F pregnancies. The mean increase in proteinuria between initial values and third-trimester values was 3.08 ± 4 g/24 hours. Twenty-six women (58%) had more than 1 g increase in proteinuria, and by the third trimester, 25 (56%) excreted more than 3 g/24 hours, including 3 women exceeding 10 g/24 hours. The mean change in proteinuria was not correlated with alteration in creatinine clearance, and a similar increase in proteinuria was observed during pregnancy, regardless of the initial level present.

In summary, changes in creatinine clearance are variable during pregnancy in women with diabetic nephropathy. Most women with nephropathy will not exhibit a normal rise in creatinine clearance. Protein excretion will frequently rise during gestation to levels that can reach the nephrotic range.

With improved survival of diabetic patients after renal transplantation, a growing number of kidney recipients have now achieved pregnancy (class T). Armenti has described 28 pregnancies in diabetic renal transplant recipients. Most patients had underlying hypertension, although preeclampsia was diagnosed in only 17% of cases. Allograft rejection occurred in one case. Overall, despite an increase in deliveries before 37 weeks, perinatal survival was 100%. These excellent results have come from improvements in both perinatal management and newer immunosuppressive regimens.

Many transplantation centers strive to perform combined kidney-pancreas transplantations in diabetic individuals with end-stage renal disease. Gilbert-Hagn and colleagues reviewed pregnancy outcomes in 43 pancreas-kidney recipients, of whom 66% developed hypertension and 77% had pregnancies that resulted in preterm birth. In this series, 6% of women experienced a rejection episode during pregnancy.

Retinopathy

Class R diabetes designates women with proliferative retinopathy, representing neovascularization or growth of new retinal capillaries. These vessels may cause vitreous hemorrhage with scarring and retinal detachment, resulting in vision loss. As with nephropathy, prevalence of retinal disease is highly related to the duration of diabetes. At 20 years, nearly 80% of diabetic individuals have some element of diabetic retinopathy. There are generally background changes, whereas proliferative diabetes retinopathy complicates approximately 77% of pregnancies. Excellent glycemic control prevents retinopathy and may slow its progression. Parity is not associated with a risk for subsequent retinopathy. However, pregnancy does convey a greater than a twofold independent risk for progression of existing retinopathy.[40] Progression of diabetic retinopathy during pregnancy is associated with: (1) retinal status at inception; (2) duration and early onset of diabetes; (3) elevated first-transfer HbA_{1c} and persisting poor glycemic control or rapid normalization of blood glucose, and (4) hypertension.[41] Retinopathy may worsen significantly during pregnancy despite the major advances that have been made in diagnosis and treatment of existing retinopathy. Ideally, women planning a pregnancy should have a comprehensive eye examination and treatment before conception. For those discovered to have proliferative changes during pregnancy, laser photocoagulation therapy with careful follow-up has helped maintain many pregnancies to a gestational age at which neonatal survival is likely.

In a large series of 172 patients, including 40 cases with background retinopathy and 11 with proliferative changes, only one patient developed new-onset proliferative retinopathy during pregnancy. A review of the literature by Kitzmiller and colleagues[42] confirms the observation that progression to proliferative retinopathy during pregnancy rarely occurs in women with background retinopathy or those without any eye ground changes. Of the 561 women in these two categories, only 17 (3%) developed neovascularization during gestation. In contrast, 23 of 26 (88.5%) with untreated proliferative disease experienced worsening retinopathy during pregnancy.

Pregnancy may increase the prevalence of some background retinal changes. Characteristic streak-blob hemorrhages and soft exudates have been noted, and such retinopathy may progress despite strict metabolic control. At least two studies have related worsening retinal disease to plasma glucose at the first prenatal visit as well as the magnitude of improvement in glycemia during early pregnancy. In a subset of 140 women without proliferative retinopathy at baseline followed in the Diabetes in Early Pregnancy Study, progression of retinopathy was seen in 10.3%, 21.1%, 18.8%, and 54.8% of patients with no retinopathy, microaneurysms only, mild nonproliferative retinopathy, and moderate to severe nonproliferative retinopathy at baseline, respectively. Elevated glycosylated hemoglobin at baseline and the magnitude of improvement of glucose control through week 14 were associated with a higher risk for progression of retinopathy. Women with an initial glycohemoglobin greater than 6 standard deviations (SDs) above the control mean were nearly three times as likely to experience worsening retinopathy compared with those within 2 SDs of the mean. Whether improving control or simply suboptimal control contributes to a deterioration of background retinopathy remains uncertain. Hypertension may also be a significant risk factor for the progression of retinopathy during pregnancy. **For women with proliferative changes, laser photocoagulation is indicated, and most will respond to this therapy. However, women who demonstrate severe florid disc neovascularization that is unresponsive to laser therapy during early pregnancy may be at great risk for deterioration of their vision.** Termination of pregnancy should be considered in this group of patients.

Women with proliferative retinopathy are generally advised to avoid the Valsalva maneuver to reduce the risk for retinal hemorrhage. Shortening of the second stage or cesarean delivery has been advocated; however, studies are lacking that address this issue.

In addition to background and proliferative eye disease, vaso-occlusive lesions associated with the development of macular edema have been described during pregnancy. Cystic macular edema is most often found in patients with proteinuric nephropathy and hypertensive disease leading to retinal edema. Macular capillary permeability is a feature of this process. The degree of macular edema is directly related to the fall in plasma oncotic pressure present in these women. In one series, seven women with minimal or no retinopathy before becoming pregnant developed severe macular edema associated with preproliferative or proliferative retinopathy during the course of their pregnancies. Although proliferation was controlled with photocoagulation, the macular edema worsened until delivery in all cases and was often aggravated by photocoagulation. Although both macular edema and retinopathy regressed after delivery in some patients, in others, these pathologic processes persisted, resulting in significant visual loss.

Coronary Artery Disease

Class H diabetes refers to the presence of diabetes of any duration associated with ischemic myocardial disease. Symptomatic coronary artery disease is rare in type 1 diabetic women who are younger than 35 years. It is unknown whether the small number of women who have coronary artery disease are at an increased risk for infarction during gestation. Maternal mortality rate exceeded 50% for cases of infarction during pregnancy reported before 1980; however, all but 1 of 23 cases reported from 1980 to 2005 survived. A high index of suspicion for ischemic heart disease should be maintained in women with long-standing diabetes because anginal symptoms may be minimal and infarction may thus present as congestive heart failure. Although there are in excess of one dozen reports of successful pregnancies following myocardial infarction in diabetic women, cardiac status should be carefully assessed early in gestation or, preferably, before pregnancy. If electrocardiographic abnormalities are encountered, echocardiography may be employed to assess ventricular function, or modified stress testing may be performed. The decision to undertake a pregnancy in a woman with type 1 or type 2 diabetes mellitus and coronary artery disease needs to be made only after serious consideration. The potential for morbidity and mortality must be thoroughly reviewed with the patient and her family. The management of myocardial infarction during pregnancy is discussed in Chapter 36.

DETECTION AND SIGNIFICANCE OF GESTATIONAL DIABETES MELLITUS

It has been estimated that 6% to 7% of pregnancies are complicated by diabetes mellitus and that 90% of the cases represent women with GDM[43] (Figure 39-14). An increased prevalence of GDM is found in women of ethnic groups that have high frequencies of type 2 diabetes. These include women of Hispanic, African, Native American, Asian, and Pacific Island ancestry. Women with GDM represent a group with significant risk for developing glucose intolerance later in life. O'Sullivan projected that 50% of women with GDM would become diabetic at follow-up study of 22 to 28 years; however, Kjos and colleagues reported that 60% of Latina women will develop type 2 diabetes, and this level of risk may actually be manifest by 5 years after the GDM index pregnancy. The likelihood for subsequent diabetes increases when GDM is diagnosed in early pregnancy, and presumably some of these women with impaired β-cell function may represent cases of unidentified preexisting type 2 diabetes.

As noted earlier, GDM is a state restricted to pregnant women whose impaired glucose tolerance (IGT) is discovered during pregnancy. Because, in most cases, patients with GDM have normal fasting glucose levels, some challenge of glucose tolerance must be undertaken. Traditionally, obstetricians relied on historical and clinical risk factors to select those patients most likely to develop GDM. This group included patients with a family history of diabetes and those whose past pregnancies were marked by an unexplained stillbirth or the delivery of a malformed or macrosomic infant. Obesity, hypertension, glycosuria, and maternal age older than 25 years were other indications for screening. Interestingly, more than half of all patients who exhibit an abnormal GTT lack the risk factors mentioned earlier.

In the summary and recommendations of the Second and Third International Workshop-Conferences on GDM, screening was recommended for all pregnant women. Following the Fourth International Workshop-Conference in 1997, screening was recommended for women in ethnic groups with relatively high rates of carbohydrate intolerance during pregnancy and of diabetes later in life. It was recognized and reaffirmed at the Fifth International Workshop Conference in 2005 that certain features place women at low risk for GDM (Table 39-5), and it may not be cost-effective to screen this subgroup of women. Those at low risk include women who are not members of ethnic groups

TABLE 39-5 SCREENING STRATEGY FOR DETECTING GDM

GDM risk assessment: should be ascertained at the first prenatal visit

- Low risk: blood glucose testing not routinely required if *all* of the following characteristics are present:
  - Member of an ethnic group with a low prevalence of GDM
  - No known diabetes in first-degree relatives
  - Age <25 yr
  - Weight normal before pregnancy
  - No history of abnormal glucose metabolism
  - No history of poor obstetrical outcome
- Average risk: perform blood glucose testing at 24-28 wk using either:
  - Two-step procedure: 50-g glucose challenge test (GCT) followed by a diagnostic oral glucose tolerance test in those meeting the threshold value in the GCT
  - One-step procedure: diagnostic oral glucose tolerance test performed on all subjects
- High risk: perform blood glucose testing as soon as feasible, using the procedures described above if one or more of these are present:
  - Severe obesity
  - Strong family history of type 2 diabetes
  - Previous history of GDM, impaired glucose metabolism, or glucosuria

If GDM is not diagnosed, blood glucose testing should be repeated at 24-28 wk or at any time a patient has symptoms or signs that are suggestive of hyperglycemia.

From Metzger BE, Buchanan TA, Coustan DR, et al: Summary and recommendations of the Fifth International Workshop-Conference on Gestational Diabetes Mellitus. Diabetes Care 30:3154, 2010.

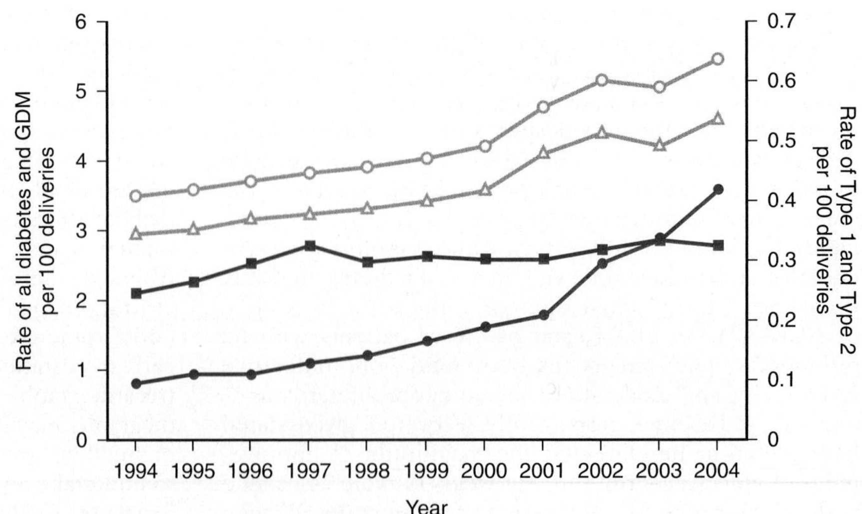

FIGURE 39-14. Trends for all diabetes *(open circle)*, gestational diabetes mellitus *(open triangle)*, type 1 diabetes *(solid square)*, and type 2 diabetes *(solid circle)* among delivery hospitalizations in the United States, 1994-2004. (Modified from Albrecht SS, Kuklina EV, Bansil P, et al: Diabetes trends among delivery hospitalizations in the U.S. 1994-2004. Diabetes Care 33:768, 2010.)

at increased risk for developing adult-onset diabetes, who have no previous history of abnormal glucose tolerance or poor obstetrical outcomes usually associated with GDM, and who have all of the following characteristics: age younger than 25 years, normal body weight, and no family history of diabetes. Danilenko-Dixon and colleagues have reported that such low-risk women represent only 10% of their population, and thus identifying such women may add complexity to screening in a busy clinic or office practice. The ACOG recognizes that although universal screening is the most sensitive approach, selective screening may be employed with the criteria cited earlier.

Despite the widespread acceptance of screening for and treating of GDM in the United States, some expert panels have questioned the benefit of GDM screening programs altogether.[44] The criteria for the diagnosis of GDM originally designated a population at increased risk for the development of type 2 diabetes in later life. The fact that O'Sullivan's original work establishing the criteria used for the diagnosis of GDM failed to evaluate an association between mild carbohydrate tolerance and perinatal outcome has led many to question the overall significance of this diagnosis. Because of the lack of high-quality evidence concerning the benefit of treatment of milder cases of GDM, it is difficult to determine the extent to which screening affects maternal and neonatal health outcomes.[45] It has been suggested that the criteria for the diagnosis of GDM are conceptually flawed in that they represent a dichotomous definition of normal and abnormal gestational glucose tolerance, when the risk for adverse maternal-fetal outcomes and later diabetes should be logically graded upward with higher values on the oral GTT and with the degree of fasting hyperglycemia.

The Hyperglycemia and Adverse Pregnancy Outcome (HAPO) study was designed to aid in the development of internationally agreed-on diagnostic criteria for GDM, based on their predictive value for pregnancy outcome.[46] This landmark multicenter international study allowed for analysis of blinded 75-g 2-hour oral GTT data in more than 25,000 nondiabetic gravidas. Glycemia was evaluated in relation to various perinatal and maternal outcomes. **Increases in each of the three values on the 75-g, 2-hour oral GTT were associated with graded increases in the likelihood of outcomes such as LGA infant, cesarean delivery, fetal insulin levels, and neonatal adiposity** (Figure 39-15). The HAPO study investigators did not offer specific recommendations for the diagnostic criteria of GDM. Because there was a continuous association between glucose values and perinatal outcome, it was apparent that any new recommended diagnostic criteria would need to be arrived at by consensus. To meet this challenge, the International Association of Diabetes and Pregnancy Study Group (ISDPGS) convened a workshop conference in 2008.[47] An odds ratio of 1.75 was selected for the outcomes of increased neonatal body fat, LGA, and cord serum C-peptide greater than the 90th percentile, which yielded the recommended diagnostic criteria for GDM (Table 39-6).

Importantly, the IADPGSG task force recommended universal 75-g, 2-hour oral GTT be performed during pregnancy and the diagnosis of GDM be made when any

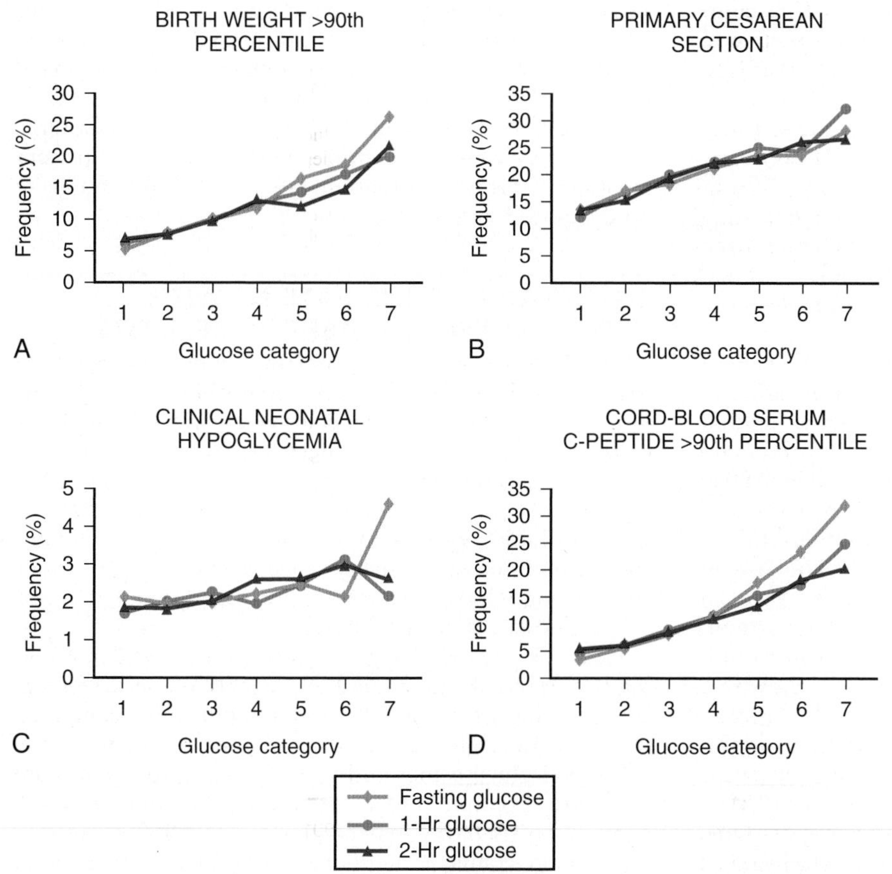

FIGURE 39-15. Frequency of perinatal and maternal outcomes in relation to maternal glycemia. (Modified from Metzger BE, Lowe LP, Dyer AR, for the HAPO Study Cooperative Research Group: Hyperglycemia and adverse pregnancy outcomes. N Engl J Med 358:1991-2001, 2008.)

TABLE 39-6 PROPOSED INTERNATIONAL ASSOCIATION OF DIABETES AND PREGNANCY STUDY GROUPS DEFINITION OF GESTATIONAL DIABETES MELLITUS (UNIVERSAL 75-g, 2-hr ORAL GLUCOSE TOLERANCE TEST)

GLUCOSE			FREQUENCY OF GESTATIONAL DIABETES (%)
Fasting	92 mg/dL	Alone	8.3
1-hr	180 mg/dL	Plus	5.7 = 14
2-hr	153 mg/dL	Plus	2.1 = 16.1*

From Metzger BE, Gabbe SG, Persson B, for the International Association of Diabetes and Pregnancy Study Groups Consensus Panel: Recommendations on the diagnosis and classification of hyperglycemia in pregnancy. Diabetes Care 33:676, 2010. Consensus Panel: Recommendations on the diagnosis and classification of hyperglycemia in pregnancy. Diabetes Care 33:676, 2010.

*1.7% of the HAPO study population were unblinded because of fasting glucose ≥105 mg/dL and/or 2-hour ≥200 mg/dL. As a result, the frequency of GDM in this population would be 17.8%.

single value on the oral GTT was met or exceeded.[47] Using the proposed criteria, 17.8% of the HAPO study population would be identified as having GDM. The resulting dramatic increase in the frequency of GDM and its consequences will now be considered by professional organizations charged with evaluating whether to endorse the proposed IADPSG criteria.

At the present time, practitioners in the United States continue to perform glucose challenge screening followed by a diagnostic 100-g oral GTT. The 50-g glucose challenge may be performed in the fasting or fed state. Sensitivity is improved if the test is performed in the fasting state. **A plasma value between 130 and 140 mg/dL is commonly used as a threshold for performing a 3-hour oral GTT.** Coustan and coworkers have demonstrated that 10% of women with GDM have screening test values between 130 and 139 mg/dL. This study indicated that the sensitivity of screening would be increased from 90% to nearly 100% if universal screening were employed using a threshold of 130 mg/dL. The prevalence of positive screening tests requiring further diagnostic testing increases from 14% (140 mg/dL) to 23% (130 mg/dL), which is accompanied by about a 12% increase in the overall cost to diagnose each case of GDM.

Whereas most women can be screened for GDM at about 24 to 28 weeks' gestation, it is advisable to screen earlier in pregnancy those with strong risk factors such as morbid obesity, a strong family history, previous GDM, prior macrosomic stillbirth, or an infant weighing more than 4500 g. If initial screening is negative, repeat testing is performed at 24 to 28 weeks. Using the plasma cut-off of 135 to 140 mg/dL, one can expect approximately 15% to 20% of patients with an abnormal screening value to have an abnormal 3-hour oral GTT. Patients whose 1-hour screening value exceeds 190 mg/dL (10.5 mmol/L) will exhibit an abnormal oral GTT in 90% of cases. In women with a screening value between 190 and 215 mg/dL, it is preferable to check a fasting blood glucose level before administering a 100-g carbohydrate load. If the fasting glucose is greater than 95 mg/dL, the patient is treated for GDM.

The criteria for establishing the diagnosis of gestational diabetes based on a 100-g, 3-hour oral GTT are listed in Table 39-7. The U.S. National Diabetes Data Group

TABLE 39-7 DETECTION OF GESTATIONAL DIABETES—UPPER LIMITS OF NORMAL (100-g ORAL GLUCOSE TOLERANCE TEST)

SCREENING TEST (50-g, 1-hr)	PLASMA (mg/dL) (130-140)	
Oral Glucose Tolerance Test*	**NDDG, 1979**[100]	**Carpenter & Coustan, 1982**[101]
Fasting	105	95
1-hr	190	180
2-hr	165	155
3-hr	145	110

*Diagnosis of gestational diabetes is made when any two values are met or exceeded.

GTT, Glucose tolerance test; *NDDG,* National Diabetes Data Group.

TABLE 39-8 TARGET PLASMA GLUCOSE LEVELS IN PREGNANCY

TIME	GLUCOSE LEVEL (mg/dL)
Before breakfast	60-90
Before lunch, supper, bedtime snack	60-105
Two hours after meals	≤120
2 AM to 6 AM	>60

criteria represent a theoretical conversion of O'Sullivan's thresholds in whole blood. Carpenter and Coustan prefer to use another modification of these data, which is supported by a comparison of the old Somogyi-Nelson method and current plasma glucose oxidase assays. Several studies have confirmed that patients diagnosed using the less stringent Carpenter criteria experience as much perinatal morbidity (macrosomia and cesarean delivery) as subjects diagnosed by the National Diabetes Data Group Criteria. Using either 100-g, 30-hour oral GTT criteria, the patient must have at least two abnormal glucose determinations to be diagnosed with GDM.

TREATMENT OF THE PATIENT WITH TYPE 1 OR TYPE 2 DIABETES MELLITUS

Clinical efforts aimed at optimizing maternal control are considered the key component responsible for the decline in perinatal death in pregnancies complicated by diabetes mellitus over the past few decades. Self-blood glucose monitoring, combined with intensive insulin therapy, has resulted in improved glycemia for many pregnant diabetic women (Table 39-8). Women with pregestational diabetes should monitor their glucose control five to seven times daily using glucose-oxidase-impregnated reagent strips and a glucose reflectance meter.

Recently, the technology of continuous glucose monitoring (CGM) has been studied in pregnant diabetic women. By providing a total of 288 measurements daily compared with six to eight blood glucose measurements using self-blood glucose monitoring, CGM can provide a more complete glycemic profile and presumably detect unrecognized postprandial hyperglycemia as well as symptomatic hypoglycemia. A randomized trial of 71 women with pregestational diabetes confirmed lower third-trimester

A1c level and reduced birthweight and macrosomia in women receiving CGM.

To achieve the best glycemic control possible for each patient, conventional insulin therapy is abandoned during pregnancy in favor of intensive therapy. An attempt is made to stimulate physiologic insulin requirements by providing basal and prandial insulin needs through three or four daily injections or continuous insulin infusion (pump therapy) (CSII). Insulin regimens have classically included multiple injections of insulin, usually before breakfast, the evening meal, and often bedtime, complemented by self-blood glucose monitoring and adjustment of insulin dose according to glucose profiles. Patients are instructed on dietary composition, insulin action, recognition and treatment of hypoglycemia, adjusting insulin dosage for exercise and sick days, as well as monitoring for hyperglycemia and potential ketosis. These principles form the foundation for intensive insulin therapy in which an attempt is made to simulate physiologic insulin requirements. Insulin administration is provided for both basal needs and meals, and rapid adjustments are made in response to glucose measurements. The treatment regimen generally involves three to four daily injections or the use of CSII devices. With either approach, frequent self-blood glucose monitoring is fundamental to achieve the therapeutic objective of physiologic glucose control. Glucose determinations are made in the fasting state and before lunch, dinner, and bedtime. Postprandial and nocturnal values are also advised. Patients are instructed on an insulin dose for each meal and at bedtime, if necessary. Mealtime insulin needs are determined by the composition of the meal, the premeal glucose measurement, and the level of activity anticipated following the meal. Basal or intermediate-acting insulin requirements are determined by periodic 2:00 AM to 4:00 AM glucose measurements, as well as late afternoon values, which reflect morning intermediate-acting insulin action.

In patients in whom diabetes is not well controlled, a brief period of hospitalization may be necessary for the initiation of therapy. Patients are encouraged to contact their physician at any time if questions should arise concerning the management of their diabetes. During pregnancy, we advise women to report their glucose values by telephone, fax, or e-mail, on an at least weekly basis.

Insulin therapy must be individualized, with dosage determinations tailored to diet and exercise. Insulin requirements during pregnancy have been reported to average 0.7 U/kg in the first trimester, increasing to 1.1 U/kg by term, although the variation in requirements is considerable. Garcia-Patterson and colleagues have noted a steady increase in insulin requirements from 16 to 37 weeks, with unstable requirements common before 16 weeks. **Semisynthetic human insulin preparations and newer insulin analogs** (Table 39-9) **are preferred for use during pregnancy. Insulin lispro and insulin aspart are rapid-acting insulin preparations that have replaced regular insulin.**[48] Insulin lispro features reversal of proline and lysine at positions B28 and B29 and remains in monomeric form and is thus rapidly absorbed. Its duration of action is shorter than that of regular insulin, so that unexpected hypoglycemia hours after injection are avoided. Insulin lispro appears to be safe for use during pregnancy and is a category B drug. Insulin aspart has also been compared

TABLE 39-9 Type of Human Insulin and Insulin Analogues

	SOURCE	ONSET (hr)	PEAK (hr)	DURATION (hr)
Short Acting				
Humulin R (Lilly)	Human	0.5	2-4	5-7
Velosulin H (Novo Nordisk)	Human	0.5	1-3	8
Novolin R (Novo Nordisk)	Human	0.5	2.5-5	6-8
Lispro	Analog	0.25	0.5-1.5	4-5
Aspart	Analog	0.25	1-3	3-5
Intermediate Acting				
Humulin Lente (Lilly)	Human	1-3	6-12	18-24
Humulin NPH (Lilly)	Human	1-2	6-12	18-24
Novolin l (Novo Nordisk)	Human	2.5	7-15	22
Novolin N (Novo Nordisk)	Human	1.5	4-20	24
Long Acting				
Humulin Ultralente (Lilly)	Human	4-6	8-20	>36
Glargine	Analogue	1	—	24
Determir	Analogue	1-2	—	24

with human insulin (Actrapid) in women with type 1 diabetes during pregnancy, with comparable fetal outcomes observed among both groups; however, limited information exists concerning glycemia in treated women.

The long-acting insulin analogs glargine and detemir have been designed to more accurately mimic basal insulin secretion, yet neither has been adequately evaluated for efficacy during pregnancy. Observational data would suggest that use of insulin glargine is safe during pregnancy. Insulin glargine has a flat profile compared with neutral protamine Hagedorn (NPH) so that when administered with short-acting insulin, unpredictable spikes in insulin levels with resulting hypoglycemia appear to be less common. **However, the flat profile of glargine may be undesirable during pregnancy when variation in basal insulin needs are likely. For this reason, we frequently suggest that women receiving glargine change to a twice-daily regimen of NPH insulin.**

Insulin is generally administered in two to three injections. We prefer a three-injection regimen, although most patients present taking a combination of intermediate-acting and short-acting insulin before dinner and breakfast. As a general rule, the amount of intermediate-acting insulin will exceed the short-acting component by a 2:1 ratio. Patients usually receive two thirds of their total dose with breakfast and the remaining third in the evening as a combined dose at dinner or split into components with short-acting or rapid-acting insulin at dinner and intermediate-acting insulin at bedtime in an effort to minimize periods of nocturnal hypoglycemia. These episodes frequently occur when the mother is in a relative fasting state, whereas placental and fetal glucose consumption continue. Finally, some women may require a small dose of short-acting insulin before lunch, thus constituting a four-injection regimen.

Open-loop CSII pump therapy is preferred by many IDDM women during pregnancy. The pump is a battery-powered unit, which may be worn during most daily activities like a beeper. These systems provide continuous short-acting insulin therapy through a subcutaneous infusion. The basal infusion rate and bolus doses to cover meals are determined by frequent self-monitoring of blood glucose. The basal infusion rate is generally close to 1 U/hour.

Pregnant women may require hospitalization before initiation of pump therapy. Women must be educated regarding the strategy of continuous infusion and have their glucose stabilized over several days. This requires that multiple blood glucose determinations be made for the prevention of periods of hyperglycemia and hypoglycemia. Glucose values may become normalized with minimal amplitude of daily excursions in most patients.

Episodes of hypoglycemia are often reduced with pump therapy. When they do occur, they are usually secondary to errors in dose selection or failure to adhere to the required diet. The risk for nocturnal hypoglycemia, which is increased in the pregnant state, necessitates that great care be undertaken in selecting patients for CSII. Patients using the pump who fail to exhibit normal counterregulatory responses to hypoglycemia should probably check their glucose values at 2:00 AM to 3:00 AM to detect nocturnal hypoglycemia.

The mechanics of the CSII systems are relatively simple. A fine-gauge butterfly needle device is attached by connecting tubing to the pump. This cannula is reimplanted every 2 to 3 days at a different site in the anterior abdominal wall. Rapid-acting insulin (usually insulin lispro) is stored in the pump syringe. Infusion occurs at a basal rate, which can be fixed or altered for specific time of day by a computer program. For example, the basal rate can be programmed for a lower dose at night. Preprandial boluses can be adjusted manually before each meal and snack. Half of the total daily insulin is usually given as the basal rate and the remainder as premeal boluses infused before each meal. The largest bolus (30% to 35%) is administered with breakfast, followed by 25% before dinner and 15% to 20% before snacks.

Patients without any pancreatic reserve may have rapid elevations of blood glucose if there is pump failure or intercurrent infection. Since the advent of buffered insulin, insulin aggregation leading to occlusion of the Silastic infusion tubing is uncommon. Failure of the pump is associated with a steady rise in ketonemia in the nonpregnant patient.

It is unclear whether CSII is superior to multiple-injection regimens. Coustan and colleagues randomized 22 patients to intensive conventional therapy with multiple injections versus pump therapy. There were no differences between the two treatment groups with respect to outpatient mean glucose levels, glycosylated hemoglobin levels, or glycemic excursions. Gabbe and colleagues reported a large retrospective cohort study of women who began pump therapy during gestation compared with a group treated with multiple-injection regimens. Women using pumps, most with insulin lispro, had fewer hypoglycemic reactions and comparable glucose control and pregnancy outcomes. Notably, **a recent systematic review comparing randomized trials of CSII versus multiple-injection regimens revealed no difference in measures of glycemic control or pregnancy outcome.**[50]

Diet therapy is critical to successful regulation of maternal diabetes. A program consisting of three meals and several snacks is employed for most patients. Dietary composition should be 40% to 60% carbohydrate, 20% protein, and 30% to 40% fat with less than 10% saturated fats, up to 10% polyunsaturated fatty acids, and the remainder derived from monosaturated sources. Caloric intake is established based on prepregnancy weight and weight gain during gestation. Weight reduction is not advised. Patients with a BMI of 22 to 27 should consume about 35 kcal/kg ideal body weight. Obese women (BMI > 30) may be managed with an intake as low as 15 kcal/kg actual weight. Any further caloric restriction resulting in ketonuria requires an increase in caloric consumption.

The presence of maternal vasculopathy should be thoroughly assessed early in pregnancy. The patient should be evaluated by an ophthalmologist familiar with diabetic retinopathy. Ophthalmologic examinations are performed during each trimester and repeated more often if retinopathy is detected. Baseline renal function is established by assaying a 24-hour urine collection for creatinine clearance and protein. An electrocardiogram and urine culture are also obtained.

Most patients with type 1 and type 2 diabetes mellitus are followed with outpatient visits at 1-to 2-week intervals. At each visit, control is assessed, and adjustments in insulin dosage are made. However, patients should be instructed to call at any time if periods of hypoglycemia (<50 mg/dL) or hyperglycemia (>200 mg/dL) occur. Ketone testing is advised for persistent glucose levels exceeding 200 mg/dL. The increased risk for hypoglycemia in pregnant individuals may be related to defective glucose counterregulatory hormone mechanisms. Both epinephrine and glucagon appear to be suppressed in pregnant diabetic women during hypoglycemia. For these reasons, patients should test glucose levels frequently, and family members should be instructed on the technique of glucagon injection for the treatment of severe reactions. Table 39-10 provides some important lessons we have learned over the years in caring for our patients.

TABLE 39-10 LESSONS LEARNED

1. Remember that the patient is more than her blood glucose.
2. Do not underestimate the patient's insight; ask for the patient's input in determining what changes to make in order to improve her glucose control.
3. Keep the insulin program simple, and make changes based on patterns.
4. Enlist the support of the patient's family.
5. Avoid hypoglycemic reactions.
6. Work closesly with the healthcare team, including the nurse educator, nutritionist, and social worker.
7. When glucose control is poor, it's often the diet.
8. Weekends are not our "friends"—especially 3-day weekends; they change the patient's daily routine, and glucose control may worsen.
9. When changing the insulin regimen, try to change just one insulin and one dose at a time.
10. Insulin analogues are valuable.
11. Respond aggressively to nausea and vomiting and fever.

Gabbe SG, Carpenter LB, Garrison EA: New strategies for glucose control in patients with type 1 and type 2 diabetes mellitus in pregnancy. Clin Obstet Gynecol 50:1014, 2007.

Ketoacidosis

With the implementation of antenatal care programs stressing strict metabolic control of blood glucose levels for women requiring insulin, diabetic ketoacidosis (DKA) has fortunately become a less common occurrence. Kilvert and colleagues reported 11 cases of ketoacidosis in 635 insulin-treated pregnancies over a 20-year period. One fetal loss and one spontaneous miscarriage complicated the pregnancies affected by DKA.

DKA can occur in the newly diagnosed diabetic patient, and the hormonal milieu of pregnancy may become the background for this phenomenon. Because pregnancy is a state of relative insulin resistance marked by enhanced lipolysis and ketogenesis, DKA may develop in a pregnant woman with glucose levels barely exceeding 200 mg/dL (11.1 mmol/L). DKA occurs in a background impaired insulin action with an increase in counterregulatory hormones such as glucagon, cortisol, and catecholamine. Thus, DKA may be diagnosed during pregnancy with minimal hyperglycemia accompanied by a fall in plasma bicarbonate (anion gap acidosis), a pH value less than 7.30, and ketonemia.

Early recognition of signs and symptoms of DKA improves both maternal and fetal outcome. As in the nonpregnant state, clinical signs of volume depletion follow the symptoms of hyperglycemia, which include polydipsia and polyuria. Malaise, headache, nausea, and vomiting are common complaints. A pregnant woman with poor fluid intake and persistent vomiting over 8 to 12 hours should be evaluated for potential DKA. A low serum bicarbonate level prompts an arterial blood gas determination to rule out this diagnosis. Occasionally, DKA may present in a woman with undiagnosed diabetes receiving β-mimetic agents such as terbutaline to arrest preterm labor.

Once the diagnosis of DKA is established and the patient is stabilized, she should be transported to a facility where tertiary care in both perinatology and neonatology is available. Therapy hinges on the meticulous correction of metabolic and fluid abnormalities. An attempt at treatment of any underlying cause for DKA, such as infection, should be instituted as well. The general management of DKA in pregnancy is outlined in Table 39-11. **Fluid resuscitation and insulin infusion should be maintained even in the face of normoglycemia until bicarbonate levels return to normal, indicating that acidemia has cleared.** DKA does represent a substantial risk for fetal compromise. However, successful fetal resuscitation often accompanies correction of maternal acidosis. Therefore, every effort should be made to correct maternal condition before intervening and delivering a preterm infant.

TABLE 39-11 MANAGEMENT OF DIABETIC KETOACIDOSIS DURING PREGNANCY

Intravenous fluids: isotonic sodium chloride; total replacement 4-6 L in first 12 hr
- Insert intravenous catheters. Maintain hourly flow sheet for fluids and electrolytes, potassium, insulin, and laboratory results.
- Administer normal saline (0.9% NaCl) at 1 to 2 L/hr for first hour.
- Infuse normal saline at 250-500 mL/hr depending on hydration state × 8 hr. If serum sodium is elevated, use half-normal saline (0.45% NaCl).
- When plasma or serum glucose reaches 200 mg/dL, change to 5% dextrose with 0.45% NaCl at 150-250 mL/hr.
- After 8 hr, use half-normal saline at 125 mL/hr.

Potassium: establish adequate renal function (urine output ~50 mL/hr).
- If serum potassium is <3.3 mEq/L, hold insulin and give 20-30 mEq K^+/hr until K^+ >3.3 mEq/L or is being corrected.
- If serum K^+ is >3.3 mEq/L but <5.3 mEq/L, give 20-30 mEq K^+ in each liter of intravenous fluid to keep serum K^+ between 4 and 5 mEq/L.
- If serum K^+ is >5.3 mEq/L, do not give K^+, but check serum K^+ every 2 hr.

Insulin: use Regular insulin intravenously.
- Consider loading dose: 0.1-0.2 U/kg intravenous bolus depending on plasma glucose.
- Begin continuous insulin infusion at 0.1 U/kg/hr.
- If plasma or serum glucose does not fall by 50-70 mg/dL in first hour, double insulin infusion every hour until a steady glucose decline is achieved.
- When plasma or serum glucose reaches 200 mg/dL, reduce insulin infusion to 0.05-0.1 U/kg/hr.
- Keep plasma or serum glucose between 100 and 150 mg/dL until resolution of diabetic ketoacidosis.

Assess need for bicarbonate:
- pH >7.0: no HCO_3
- pH = 6.9-7.0: dilute $NaHCO_3$ (50 mmol) in 200 mL H_2O with 10 mEq KCl and infuse over 1 hr. Repeat $NaHCO_3$ administration every 2 hr until pH = 7.0. Monitor serum K^+.
- pH <6.9-7.0: dilute $NaHCO_3$ (100 mmol) in 400 mL H_2O with 20 mEq KCl and infuse for 2 hr. Repeat $NaHCO_3$ administration every 2 hr until pH = 7.0. Monitor serum K^+.

ANTEPARTUM FETAL EVALUATION

Maternal diabetes may result in fetal hyperglycemia and hyperinsulinemia and thereby increase the risk for fetal hypoxia. Thus, protocols for antepartum fetal assessment in pregnancies complicated by diabetes mellitus have been incorporated into the care plan for outpatient monitoring during the third trimester. During this time period, when the risk for sudden intrauterine death increases, a program of fetal surveillance is initiated. **Because improvement in maternal control has played a major role in reducing perinatal mortality in diabetic pregnancies, antepartum fetal monitoring tests are now used primarily to reassure the obstetrician and avoid unnecessary premature intervention.** These techniques have few false-negatives results, and in a woman in whom diabetes is well controlled and who exhibits no vasculopathy or significant hypertension, reassuring antepartum testing allows the fetus to benefit from further maturation in utero.

Maternal assessment of fetal activity serves as a simple screening technique in a program of fetal surveillance. During the third trimester, women are instructed to perform daily fetal movement counting. Women with a variety of high-risk antepartum conditions, including diabetes, appear to have an increased incidence of alarming fetal activity patterns. Although the false-negative rate with maternal monitoring of fetal activity is low (~1%), the false-positive rate may be as high as 60%. Maternal hypoglycemia, although generally believed to be associated with decreased fetal movement, may actually stimulate fetal activity.

The nonstress test (NST) remains the preferred primary method to assess antepartum fetal well-being in the patient with diabetes mellitus. If the NST is nonreactive, a

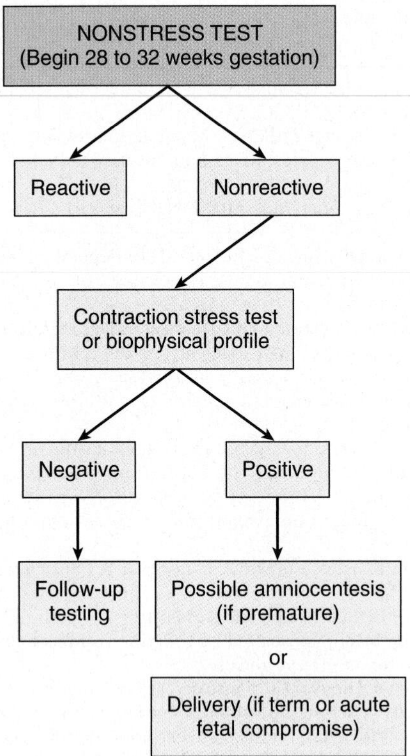

FIGURE 39-16. Scheme for antepartum fetal testing.

TABLE 39-12 ANTEPARTUM FETAL SURVEILLANCE IN LOW-RISK INSULIN-DEPENDENT DIABETES MELLITUS*

Study	Indicated
Ultrasonography at 4- to 6-week intervals	Yes
Maternal assessment of fetal activity, daily at 28 weeks	Yes
Nonstress testing at 32 weeks; contraction stress test or biophysical profile if nonstress test nonreactive	Yes
Amniocentesis for lung profile	Yes, if elective delivery planned Before 39 weeks

*Excellent control, no vasculopathy (classes B, C), no stillbirth.

TABLE 39-13 ANTEPARTUM FETAL SURVEILLANCE IN HIGH-RISK INSULIN-DEPENDENT DIABETES MELLITUS*

Study	Indicated
Ultrasonography at 4- to 6-week intervals	Yes
Maternal assessment of fetal activity, daily at 28 weeks	Yes
Nonstress testing; contraction stress test or biophysical profile if nonstress test nonreactive	Initiate at 28-30 weeks
Consider amniocentesis for lung profile prior to 38 weeks	

*Poor control (macrosomia, hydramnios), vasculopathy (classes D, F, R), prior stillbirth.

biophysical profile (BPP) or contraction stress test is then performed (Figure 39-16). Heart rate monitoring is begun early in the third trimester, usually by 32 weeks' gestation. Two studies have also demonstrated an increased fetal death rate within 1 week of a reactive NST in pregnancies complicated by IDDM compared with other high-risk gestations. **If the NST is to be used as the primary method of antepartum heart rate testing, we prefer that it be done at least twice weekly after the patient reaches 32 weeks' gestation. In patients with vascular disease or poor control, in whom the incidence of abnormal tests and intrauterine deaths is greater, testing is often initiated between 28 and 32 weeks' gestation.**

Doppler umbilical artery velocimetry has been proposed as a clinical tool for antepartum fetal surveillance in pregnancies at risk for placental vascular disease. We have found that Doppler studies of the umbilical artery may be predictive of fetal outcome in diabetic pregnancies complicated by vascular disease. Elevated placental resistance as evidenced by an increased systolic-to-diastolic ratio is associated with fetal growth restriction and preeclampsia in these high-risk patients In contrast, patients with well-controlled diabetes without vascular disease rarely demonstrate abnormal fetal umbilical artery waveforms.

It is important not only to include the results of antepartum fetal testing but also to weigh all of the clinical features involving mother and fetus before deciding to intervene for suspected fetal compromise, especially if this decision may result in a preterm delivery (Tables 39-12 and 39-13). Our review of nine series involving 993 diabetic women revealed that an abnormal test of fetal condition led to delivery 5% of the time.[51] It appears that outpatient testing protocols work well in diabetic patients requiring insulin. Whether such testing is required for all women with diabetes mellitus remains controversial.[52] Abnormal fetal testing is more common in women whose diabetes is poorly controlled, who have hypertension, or who have significant vasculopathy that may be associated with fetal growth restriction. It follows that these subgroups probably benefit most from a program of antepartum fetal surveillance.

Ultrasound can be a valuable tool in evaluating fetal growth, estimating fetal weight, and detecting hydramnios and malformations. Maternal serum α-fetoprotein (MSAFP) determination at 16 weeks' gestation is often employed in association with a detailed ultrasound study during the midtrimester in an attempt to detect neural tube defects and other anomalies. Levels of MSAFP, unconjugated estriol (uES), and inhibin A in diabetic women are lower than in the nondiabetic population. A lower threshold for the upper limit of normal MSAFP, 1.5 multiples of the median, thus may be preferable in pregnancies complicated by diabetes mellitus in order to help detect spina bifida and other major malformations that are increased in this population. **A comprehensive ultrasound examination, including fetal echocardiography, is performed at 20 to 22 weeks' gestation for the investigation of possible cardiac anomalies.** Using such an approach, Greene and Benacerraf detected 18 of 32 malformations in a series of 432 diabetic pregnancies. The specificity was in excess of 99%, and the negative predictive value was 97%. Spina bifida was identified in all cases; however, ventricular septal defects, limb abnormalities, and facial clefts were missed. A review of the prenatal diagnosis experience in 289 women with IDDM in the Ohio State University

Diabetes in Pregnancy Program revealed 29 anomalies, of which 12 were cardiac, 14 were noncardiac, and 3 were combined. Twelve of 15 (80%) cardiac and 10 of 17 (59%) noncardiac lesions were identified prenatally. When considering cardiac defects alone, we could not identify a glycosylated hemoglobin cut-off for these anomalies. Therefore, we continue to offer cardiac imaging to women with type 1 or type 2 diabetes mellitus to assist in the detection of cardiac lesions, especially those of the great vessels and cardiac septum.

Ultrasound examinations should be performed during the third trimester to assess fetal growth. The detection of fetal macrosomia, the leading risk factor for shoulder dystocia, is important in the selection of patients who are best delivered by cesarean section. **An increased rate of cephalopelvic disproportion and shoulder dystocia, accompanied by significant risk for traumatic birth injury and asphyxia, has been consistently associated with the vaginal delivery of large infants. The risk for such complications rises exponentially when birthweight exceeds 4 kg and is greater for the fetus of a diabetic mother when compared with a fetus with similar weight whose mother does not have diabetes.**[53] Sonographic measurements of the fetal abdominal circumference have proved most helpful in predicting fetal macrosomia. The abdomen is likely to be large because of increased glycogen deposition in the fetal liver and subcutaneous fat deposition. However, a single ultrasound examination may have limited accuracy in predicting macrosomia at term in women with diabetes. Using serial sonographic examinations, accelerated abdominal growth may be identified between 28 and 32 weeks' gestation in pregnancies complicated by diabetes.[54]

TIMING AND MODE OF DELIVERY

Delivery should be delayed until fetal maturation has taken place, provided that diabetes is well controlled and antepartum surveillance remains normal. In our practice, induction of labor is often planned at 38½ to 40 weeks' gestation in patients with well-controlled diabetes without vascular disease. Women with vascular disease are delivered before term only if hypertension worsens, if significant fetal growth restriction is present, or if biophysical testing mandates early delivery. Depending on clinical circumstances, antenatal steroids may be administered to accelerate fetal lung maturity. Before undertaking delivery earlier than 39 weeks' gestation, an amniocentesis may be performed to document fetal pulmonary maturity. **Tests of fetal lung maturity appear to have the same predictive value in diabetic pregnancies as in the normal population.**

The presence of the acidic phospholipid phosphatidylglycerol (PG) is the final marker of fetal pulmonary maturation. Several authors have suggested that fetal hyperinsulinemia may be associated with delayed appearance of PG and an increased incidence of RDS. Landon and coworkers have correlated the appearance of PG in amniotic fluid with maternal glycemic control during gestation. RDS may occur in the IDM with a mature lecithin-to-sphingomyelin (L/S) ratio or fetal lung maturity index but absent PG. Moore[55] compared PG production in amniotic fluid specimens from 295 diabetic women and 590 matched controls and reported that the onset of PG production was delayed in GDM from 35.9 ± 1.1 weeks to 37.3 ± 1 weeks and to 38.7 ± 0.9 weeks in pregestational diabetic pregnancies. In this study, delayed appearance of PG was not associated with level of glycemic control. Currently, the fluorescence polarization test (TDX-FLM) is commonly employed to assess amniotic fluid for lung maturity. Cut-off values of diabetic pregnancy are similar to those in the nondiabetic population.

When antepartum testing suggests fetal compromise, delivery must be considered. If amniotic fluid analysis yields a mature test result, delivery should be accomplished promptly. In the presence of presumed lung immaturity, the decision to proceed with delivery should be based on confirmation of deteriorating fetal condition by several abnormal tests. For example, if the NST and the BPP indicate fetal compromise, delivery is indicated. Finally, there are several maternal indications for delivery, including significant preeclampsia, worsening renal function, and deteriorating vision secondary to proliferative retinopathy. If a patient reaches term gestation and is at significant risk for intrauterine demise because of poor control or a history of a prior stillbirth, options for management are individualized and include delivery or amniocentesis assessment for lung maturity before delivery.

Choosing the route of delivery for the diabetic patient remains controversial. Cesarean delivery rates as high as 50% are common in series of pregestational diabetic women. This figure is likely to represent the practice trends of most U.S. obstetricians and perinatologists. Trial of labor following previous cesarean delivery may be undertaken in select cases and has a reported success rate of 64%.

The increased rate of shoulder dystocia and brachial plexus injury in the offspring of diabetic women has prompted adoption of early induction strategies as well as selection of patients for cesarean delivery based on ultrasound estimation of fetal size. Such approaches are limited by the relative inaccuracy of ultrasound prediction of birthweight. Despite the limitations, Kjos and colleagues demonstrated that induction at 38 weeks in a population of women with GDM was associated with a lower frequency of LGA and shoulder dystocia without an increased rate of cesarean delivery.[56] This is in contrast to studies of induction in nondiabetic women, in which suspected macrosomia is apparently associated with an increased rate of cesarean delivery. In a *decision tree* analysis of cost-effectiveness, Rouse and colleagues found that whereas elective cesarean delivery for macrosomia to prevent permanent brachial plexus injury was prohibitively expensive in the nondiabetic woman at a cost of several million dollars per permanent brachial plexus injury prevented, 489 cesarean deliveries at a cost per avoided birth injury of $880,000 per case for those diabetic pregnancies with an estimated fetal size greater than 4000 g seemed to be at least tenable.[57]

The overall risk for shoulder dystocia in the macrosomic fetus of an IDM is greater than in large infants of normal pregnancy. The risk for shoulder dystocia with a fetal weight greater than 4000 g in diabetic gravidae is about 30%. Somewhat less impressive, yet significantly greater frequencies of shoulder dystocia for delivery of a macrosomic fetus of IDMs compared with non-IDMs have been reported by Nesbitt and colleagues[53] (Figure 39-17). At present, the ACOG recommends consideration of cesarean delivery in diabetic women when estimated fetal weight

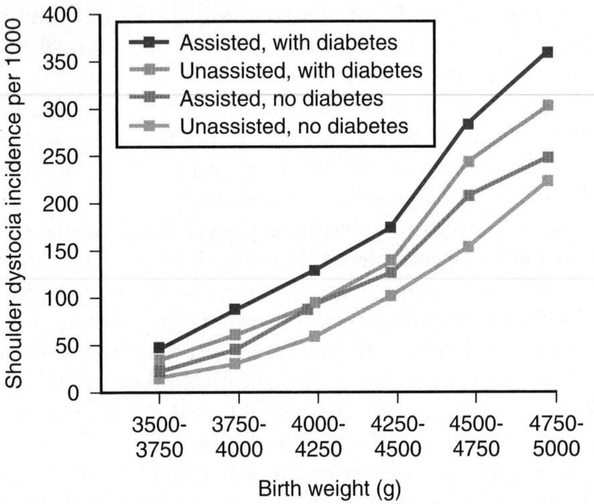

FIGURE 39-17. Frequency of shoulder dystocia for increasing birthweight by maternal diabetes status and method of vaginal delivery: spontaneous or assisted. (Modified from Nesbitt TS, Gilbert WM, Herrchen B: Shoulder dystocia and associated risk factors with macrosomic infants born in California. Am J Obstet Gynecol 17:476, 1998.)

exceeds 4500 g.[58] Our approach is to consider cesarean delivery when the estimated weight is 4000 to 4500 g, after evaluating obstetrical history and clinical pelvimetry. Despite attempts to select patients with obvious fetal macrosomia for elective cesarean delivery, arrest of dilation or descent despite adequate labor should alert the physician to the possibility of cephalopelvic disproportion. About 25% of deliveries of macrosomic infants (>4000 g) following a prolonged second stage are complicated by shoulder dystocia. It follows that cesarean delivery should be considered in a diabetic woman who demonstrates significant protracted labor or failure of descent.

GLUCOREGULATION DURING LABOR AND DELIVERY

Because neonatal hypoglycemia is in part related to maternal glucose levels during labor, it is important to maintain maternal plasma glucose levels within the physiologic normal range. The patient is given nothing by mouth after midnight of the evening before induction or elective cesarean delivery. The usual bedtime dose of insulin is administered, or for women receiving pump therapy, the infusion is continued overnight. Upon arrival to the labor and delivery department, early in the morning, the patient's capillary glucose level is assessed with a bedside reflectance meter. Continuous infusion of both insulin and glucose is then begun based on maternal glucose levels (Table 39-14). Ten units of short-acting insulin may be added to 1000 mL of solution containing 5% dextrose. An infusion rate of 100 to 125 mL/hour (1 U/hour), in most cases, will result in good glucose control. Insulin may also be infused from a syringe pump at a dose of 0.25 to 2 U/hour and adjusted to maintain normal glucose values. Glucose levels are recorded hourly, and the infusion rate is adjusted accordingly. Patients with well-controlled diabetes are often euglycemic once active labor begins and then require increased glucose infusion at a rate of 2.5 mg/kg per minute, which mimics strenuous exercise requirements. During the second stage of labor, in response to hyperglycemia associated with increased catecholamine secretion, it may be necessary to increase insulin infusion.

TABLE 39-14 INSULIN MANAGEMENT DURING LABOR AND DELIVERY

- Usual dose of intermediate-acting insulin is given at bedtime.
- Morning dose of insulin is withheld.
- Intravenous infusion of normal saline is begun.
- Once active labor begins or glucose levels fall below 70 mg/dL, the infusion is changed from saline to 5% dextrose and delivered at a rate of 2.5 mg/kg/min.
- Glucose levels are checked hourly using a portable reflectance meter allowing for adjustment in the infusion rate.
- Regular (short-acting) insulin is administered by intravenous infusion if glucose levels exceed 140 mg/dL.

From Jovanovic L, Peterson CM: Management of the pregnant, insulin-dependent diabetic woman. Diabetes Care 3:63, 1980.

When cesarean delivery is to be performed, it should be scheduled for early morning. This simplifies intrapartum glucose control and allows the neonatal team to prepare for the care of the newborn. The patient is given nothing by mouth, and her usual morning insulin dose is withheld. If her surgery is not performed early in the day, one third to one half of the patient's intermediate-acting dose of insulin may be administered. Regional anesthesia allows detection of hypoglycemia. Following surgery, glucose levels are monitored every 2 hours, and an intravenous solution of 5% dextrose is administered.

Following delivery, insulin requirements are usually significantly lower than were pregnancy or prepregnancy needs. The objective of tight control used in the antepartum period is relaxed for the first 24 to 48 hours. Patients delivered vaginally, who are able to eat a regular diet, are given one third to one half of their end of pregnancy dose of NPH insulin and short-acting or rapid-acting insulin the morning of the first postpartum day. Many women with type 2 diabetes will not require insulin for 24 to 48 hours postpartum. Frequent glucose determinations are used to guide insulin dosage. Most patients are stabilized on this regimen within a few days after delivery.

Women with diabetes are encouraged to breastfeed. The additional 500 kcal required daily are given as approximately 100 g of carbohydrate and 20 g of protein. The insulin dose may be somewhat lower in lactating diabetic women. Hypoglycemia appears to be common in the first week following delivery and immediately after nursing.

MANAGEMENT OF THE WOMAN WITH GESTATIONAL DIABETES

Is There a Benefit to the Treatment of Gestational Diabetes Mellitus?

The frequency of GDM is increasing worldwide, with 1% to 14% of pregnancies being affected.[59] The current U.S. economic burden of treatment for GDM, assuming a 4.5% incidence, translates to estimated maternal and newborn costs of $636 million annually. With both increased incidence and proposed lowering of the threshold for diagnosis, the health care cost of GDM can be expected to rise proportionately. It follows that whether a benefit exists to the treatment of GDM has assumed even greater importance now than in the past.

The 2008 guidelines of the U.S. Prevention Services Task Force concluded that there is insufficient evidence to assess the benefits and harms of screening and treatment of GDM.[60] This group, however, acknowledged that their review failed to consider intermediate outcomes such as macrosomia, cesarean delivery, and shoulder dystocia. The recent update to the Cochrane review identified eight randomized trials concerning treatment of GDM.[61] Of the 1418 women enrolled in these studies, 1000 were represented by the Australian Carbohydrate Intolerance Study in Pregnant Women (ACHOIS) study.[62] In fact, ACHOIS was the only treatment trial that included a large untreated control group because the remainder of the studies described were trials comparing various treatment modalities for GDM. The review concluded that women with GDM should only be *considered* for specific treatment in addition to routine obstetrical care.

Randomized Treatment Trials for Gestational Diabetes Mellitus

More than 40 years passed from O'Sullivan's work before the findings of the long-awaited ACHOIS study were reported.[62] The ACHOIS study was a multicenter, 10-year randomized treatment trial of 1000 women conducted at 14 sites in Australia. The study was designed to determine whether treatment of mild GDM would reduce the rate of perinatal complications.

Treatment was associated with a significant reduction in the rate of the primary outcome, a composite of serious perinatal complications (perinatal death, shoulder dystocia, birth trauma including fracture or nerve palsy) (adjusted relative risk, 0.33; 95% confidence interval, 0.14 to 0.75). Overall, 7 infants in the treatment group had a serious complication (all shoulder dystocia) compared with 23 infants in the untreated group, of whom 5 experienced perinatal death, 4 had birth trauma, and 16 had shoulder dystocia.

Among secondary neonatal outcomes, there were no significant differences in the rates of hypoglycemia requiring intravenous therapy, jaundice requiring phototherapy, respiratory disease requiring phototherapy, or respiratory disease requiring supplemental oxygen. Neonatal intensive care unit admissions were remarkably high in both groups: 71% in treated versus 61% in untreated ($P = .01$). Importantly, treatment did reduce the frequency of LGA infants from 22% to 13% and birthweight greater than 4000 g from 21% to 10%. Among maternal outcomes, preeclampsia was significantly reduced with treatment (12% vs. 18%).

The wide spectrum of views regarding the clinical significance of GDM prompted the National Institute of Child Health and Human Development (NICHD) Maternal-Fetal Medicine Unit (MFMU) Network to design a randomized controlled trial of 958 cases of mild GDM to determine whether intervention reduces perinatal mortality and obstetrical complications.[63] In this study, mild GDM was defined as a fasting glucose less than 95 mg/dL with two of the three postglucose values exceeding established thresholds.

These investigators found no significant difference in the frequency of the primary composite perinatal outcome (perinatal death, neonatal hypoglycemia, elevated cord C-peptide level, or birth trauma) in the treatment group (32.4%) compared with the usual care group (37%) ($P = .14$). Several key differences in secondary outcomes, however, were observed with treatment, including a lower frequency of LGA infants, birthweight exceeding 4000 g, and decreased neonatal fat mass.

TABLE 39-15 RESULTS OF RANDOMIZED CONTROLLED TRIALS FOR TREATMENT OF GESTATIONAL DIABETES MELLITUS

	LANDON ET AL., 2009[63]	CROWTHER ET AL., 2005[62]
Preeclampsia	↓	↓
Weight gain	↓	↓
LGA	↓	↓
Neonatal fat mass	↓	—
Shoulder dystocia	↓	Not studied

LGA, Large for gestational age.

Among maternal outcomes, rates of labor induction were similar between groups; however, cesarean delivery was less often performed in treated women (26.9% vs. 33.8). This rate remained lower after exceeding cases of abnormal presentation, prior cesarean, placenta previa, and oligohydramnios (13% vs. 19.7%) ($P = .011$). A lower rate of shoulder dystocia (1.5% vs. 4%) and preeclampsia or gestational hypertension (8.6% vs. 13.6%) was also found in the treatment group.

In summary, the NICHD MFMU trial demonstrated that although treatment of mild GDM did not reduce the frequency of several neonatal morbidities characteristic of diabetic pregnancy, it did lower the risk for fetal overgrowth, neonatal fat mass, shoulder dystocia, cesarean delivery, and hypertensive disorders of pregnancy. These findings, along with those reported in the ACHOIS study, now confirm a benefit to treatment of even mild carbohydrate intolerance of pregnancy (Table 39-15).

Treatment of the Woman with Gestational Diabetes Mellitus

The mainstay of treatment of GDM remains nutritional counseling and dietary intervention. The optimal diet should provide caloric and nutrient needs to sustain pregnancy without resulting in significant postprandial hyperglycemia. Women with GDM generally do not need hospitalization for dietary instruction and management. Once the diagnosis is established, women are begun on a dietary program of 2000 to 2500 kcal daily. This represents approximately 35 kcal/kg of present pregnancy weight. Jovanovic-Peterson and Peterson have noted that such a diet composed of 50% to 60% carbohydrate will cause excessive weight gain and postprandial hyperglycemia, and require insulin therapy in 50% of patients. For this reason, these authors have suggested limiting carbohydrates to 33% to 40% of calories. Complex carbohydrates are preferred to simple carbohydrates because they are less likely to produce significant postprandial hyperglycemia. Once the patient with GDM is placed on an appropriate diet, surveillance of blood glucose levels is necessary to be certain that glycemic control has been established. We prefer to have patients perform daily self–blood glucose monitoring, which in two retrospective studies has been associated with a decline in macrosomia at the expense of nearly half of all women requiring insulin therapy. A practical approach may be to provide women with GDM with a reflectance meter; however, if after a few weeks, both fasting and postprandial measurements are within the normal range, the frequency of testing can be reduced and tailored accordingly.

Whereas the ACOG has recommended that fasting plasma glucose levels be maintained below 105 mg/dL and 2-hour postprandial values below 120 mg/dL in women with GDM, thresholds of a fasting glucose less than 95 mg/dL and 1-hour postprandial glucose less than 140 mg/dL, as well as 2-hour postprandial glucose less than 120 mg/dL, have been suggested by the Fifth International Workshop Conference.[59] If a patient repetitively exceeds these thresholds, then insulin therapy is suggested. Approximately 25% of women with GDM require insulin therapy. Some cases are managed with a single dose of bedtime NPH insulin to treat isolated fasting hyperglycemia, whereas others require treatment of postprandial hyperglycemia with insulin lispro or aspart. Up to four injections daily may be necessary to achieve adequate control. The use of the previously mentioned cut-offs for initiating insulin are based on data regarding increased perinatal morbidity when such values are exceeded in women with preexisting diabetes. There continue to be no data from controlled trials to identify ideal glycemic targets for prevention of fetal risk for women with GDM.

Langer and colleagues have found that women with a fasting glucose between 96 and 105 mg/dL have a greater incidence of LGA infants (28.6%) when receiving diet therapy alone compared with those receiving both diet and insulin. In women with an initial fasting glucose between 95 and 104 mg/dL, 70% required insulin therapy to achieve optimal control.

Whereas Langer and coworkers have documented a relationship between maternal glycemia and macrosomia in GDM, which would establish guidelines for insulin therapy, some authors have suggested that estimation of glycemia alone may not be sufficient to optimally prescribe insulin therapy in these cases. Buchanan and colleagues have reviewed the utility of fetal ultrasound measurements to guide insulin therapy in women with GDM. In their study of diet-treated patients with GDM, ultrasound performed at 29 to 33 weeks was used to identify pregnancies with fetuses having a large abdominal circumference (>75th percentile). These patients were then randomized to diet versus diet and insulin treatment. The insulin-treated group ultimately had a frequency of LGA infants of 13%, which was far below the 45% present in the diet-treated group. Less intensified management has been suggested when normal fetal growth is apparent (fetal abdominal circumference <75th percentile for gestational age), although self-blood glucose monitoring is still advised.

During the past decade, oral hypoglycemic therapy has emerged as a suitable alternative to insulin treatment in women with GDM. Concerns with first-generation sulfonylurea agents included potential teratogenesis and increased neonatal hypoglycemia as a result of fetal β-cell stimulation. Nicholson and colleagues[64] performed **a systematic review of the evidence from randomized trials and observational studies and concluded that glycemia was equivalent in women receiving oral hypoglycemic agents compared with those receiving insulin.** Moreover, there was no evidence of increased adverse neonatal outcomes with oral hypoglycemic agent use. In a landmark study, Langer and colleagues reported results from a randomized trial of 404 women receiving insulin versus glyburide and noted similar improvement in glycemia with both regimens.[65] The frequency of macrosomia and neonatal hypoglycemia was similar in the two study groups. Only 4% of women failed glyburide therapy, requiring a change to insulin. Cord blood analysis revealed no detectable glyburide in exposed pregnancies. More recently, Hebert and colleagues reported that glyburide appears to cross the placenta in significant amounts. This observation has raised concerns regarding the safety of this agent. Importantly, clinical studies have failed to reveal increased rates of neonatal hypoglycemia with glyburide use in GDM. It is, however, unknown whether glyburide can affect progression to type 2 diabetes in treated women or whether glucose homeostasis is altered later in life in their offspring.

Following Langer's randomized trial, several smaller studies reported success in achieving good glycemic control with glyburide, but with slightly higher failure rates (15% to 20%). Jacobson and colleagues[66] recently reported on the implementation of glyburide as an alternative to insulin in a large managed care organization. These authors noted a similar frequency of LGA infants and macrosomia among 268 women treated with insulin compared with 236 receiving glyburide. In this nonrandomized study, more women in the glyburide group achieved lower mean fasting and postprandial glucose levels compared with insulin-treated subjects. Importantly, the authors noted an increased rate of preeclampsia, need for neonatal phototherapy, and birth injury in the "glyburide group," all of which point to the need for further study concerning safety.

Lain and colleagues performed a randomized trial of 99 women with GDM comparing glyburide versus insulin treatment.[67] These authors reported no increase in neonatal fat mass, body mass index, ponderal index, or anthropometric measures in glyburide-treated offspring, although a significantly greater rate of infant birthweights higher than 4000 g was observed in the glyburide treated group (22 vs. 2.4%). Similar to insulin therapy, glyburide action must be carefully balanced with meals and snacks to prevent maternal hyperglycemia. Observational data suggest that glyburide may be less successful in obese women or those marked hyperglycemia discovered early in gestation. The usual dose of glyburide is 2.5 to 20 mg daily in divided doses, although pharmacokinetic studies during pregnancy indicate daily dose as great as 30 mg may be necessary to achieve adequate control. In our experience, most women with fasting glucose levels of 115 mg/dL or higher will not be adequately controlled with glyburide and require insulin (Table 39-16).

Metformin has also been used for treatment of GDM.[68] Metformin clearly crosses the placenta; however, it does not appear to be teratogenic. Rowan and colleagues randomized 761 women with GDM at 20 to 33 weeks to metformin (and insulin as needed) versus insulin therapy. There were no differences in perinatal outcomes, and a composite of perinatal morbidity (neonatal hypoglycemia, respiratory distress, need for phototherapy, birth trauma, and prematurity) was observed in about one third of

TABLE 39-16 SUMMARY OF GLYBURIDE VERSUS INSULIN TREATMENT IN GESTATIONAL DIABETES MELLITUS

- Maternal fasting and postpartum glycemia is improved with Glyburide treatment
- Glyburide failure rate of 15%-20%
- Glyburide failures associated with earlier diagnosis of gestational diabetes, fasting >110-115 mg/dL
- Comparable neonatal outcomes
- Significant cost savings

women in each group. Metformin use was well tolerated; however, 46% of women receiving metformin required supplemental insulin to achieve glycemic control.

It appears that glyburide may be superior to metformin in achieving satisfactory control in women with GDM. A randomized trial of 149 women compared metformin to glyburide for the treatment of GDM.[69] Thirty-five percent of women randomized to metformin, compared with 16% receiving glyburide, required insulin to achieve adequate control.

Exercise may serve as a useful adjunctive treatment for women with GDM. Physical exercise may improve glycemia control because increased insulin sensitivity accompanies cardiovascular conditioning. Bung and colleagues conducted a prospective study of the utility of exercise in the treatment of GDM. These authors randomized 41 women with GDM who manifested elevated fasting glucose levels and would normally require insulin therapy. In the final analysis, 17 women completed a supervised bicycle ergometry training program compared with 17 women receiving insulin treatment. No statistical differences were observed in weekly blood glucose determinations between study groups. All fetal heart rate patterns were reactive before and after exercise. Thus, regular exercise may be an effective treatment for GDM. Brisk walking for 30 minutes at least three times each week may be recommended. Because the total number of women with GDM studied in randomized trials is limited, the role of exercise as a primary therapy in GDM remains unknown. Nonetheless, a program of moderate exercise has been advocated as part of the treatment of GDM.

Women with GDM that is well controlled are at low risk for an intrauterine death. For this reason, we do not routinely institute antepartum fetal heart rate testing in uncomplicated diet-controlled GDM patients unless the patient has a hypertensive disorder, a history of a prior stillbirth, or suspected macrosomia.[70] Women in these categories, as well as those who require insulin treatment of GDM, undergo twice-weekly heart rate testing at 32 weeks' gestation. Women with uncomplicated GDM undergo fetal heart rate testing at 40 weeks' gestation. Using such a protocol at the Ohio State University Hospital Diabetes in Pregnancy Program, only five intrauterine deaths in more than 2800 patients with uncomplicated GDM have been observed in the past 20 years. Thus, it appears that the third-trimester stillbirth rate in these patients is no higher than that of the general obstetrical population. A study of 389 women with GDM documented an antepartum stillbirth rate of 7.7 per 10,000, which was not significantly different from the rate of 4.8 per 1000 observed in nondiabetic low-risk patients. In this study, because 7% of fetuses were delivered on the basis of a low BPP score, the benefit of testing all GDM pregnancies remains in question. At present, without prospective studies comparing outcomes in monitored and nonmonitored women with GDM without other risk factors, it is not possible to determine whether any benefits exist to antepartum fetal surveillance in this population.

Because many obstetricians have extrapolated the increased risk for stillbirth in women with type 1 or type 2 diabetes to those with GDM, a remarkable number of these pregnancies are subject to scheduled delivery at term. If glycemic control is suboptimum, or maternal hypertension or a previous stillbirth exists, such an approach seems prudent. The use of amniocentesis to document fetal lung maturity in such cases should be based on clinical circumstances. As with antepartum fetal testing, in the otherwise uncomplicated group, should scheduled induction be the standard approach for these pregnancies complicated by GDM? Available observational and retrospective data do not permit an evidence-based recommendation. Lurie and coworkers have in part addressed this issue by retrospectively examining the outcomes of 124 women with GDM delivered beyond 40 weeks' gestation compared with the same number of women with GDM delivered before their expected date of confinement. Antepartum fetal surveillance was not routinely begun until 40 weeks' gestation. No significant differences in perinatal outcome, rates of cesarean delivery, or shoulder dystocia were found between study groups. A vaginal delivery rate of 75.8% was achieved in women with GDM delivering beyond 40 weeks' gestation. These authors concluded that elective induction before 40 weeks' gestation should be avoided and that every attempt should be made to allow women with GDM, both diet and insulin treated, to proceed to spontaneous labor. In contrast, a follow-up prospective study from the same institution of 96 insulin-requiring patients with GDM demonstrated that induction at 38 to 39 weeks was associated with a 1.4% shoulder dystocia rate versus 10.2% in historical controls.

Kjos and colleagues conducted a prospective randomized trial of active induction of labor at 38 weeks' gestation versus expectant management in a series that included 187 insulin-requiring women with GDM. The cesarean delivery rate was not significantly different in the expectant management group (31%) from the active induction group (25%). However, an increased prevalence of LGA infants (23% vs. 10%) was observed in the expectant management group. Moreover, the frequency of shoulder dystocia was 3% in this group, with no cases reported in those undergoing induction at 38 weeks' gestation. These data led the authors to conclude that scheduled elective induction should be considered in insulin-requiring patients with GDM because it does not increase the risk for cesarean delivery and lowers the risk for fetal death. In women managed expectantly, monitoring of fetal growth should be considered because of an apparent increasing risk for macrosomia with advancing gestational age.

POSTPARTUM FOLLOW-UP OF WOMEN WITH GESTATIONAL DIABETES MELLITUS

Women with GDM have a sevenfold increased risk for developing type 2 diabetes relative to women who do not

TABLE 39-17 DIAGNOSTIC CRITERIA FOR DIABETES MELLITUS, IMPAIRED FASTING GLUCOSE, AND IMPAIRED GLUCOSE TOLERANCE

TEST	DIABETES	IMPAIRED FASTING GLUCOSE	IMPAIRED GLUCOSE TOLERANCE
Fasting plasma glucose	Fasting plasma glucose ≥126	Fasting plasma glucose = 100-125	Not applicable
75-g 2-hr oral glucose tolerance test	Fasting plasma glucose ≥126 *or* 2-hr plasma glucose ≥200	Fasting plasma glucose = 100-226	2-hr plasma glucose = 140-199

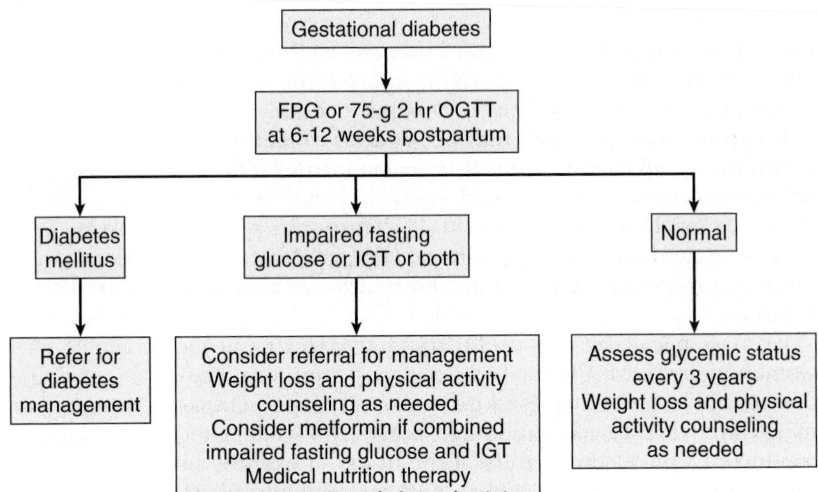

FIGURE 39-18. Management of postpartum glucose screening results. *FPG,* Fasting plasma glucose; *IGT,* impaired glucose tolerance; *OGTT,* oral glucose tolerance. (Modified from ACOG Committee Opinion No. 435, June 2009.)

have diabetes during pregnancy.[71] Follow-up studies for up to 28 years after O'Sullivan's original cohort of women indicated a prevalence of diabetes in 50% to 60% of women with former GDM. A recent follow-up study of up to 10 years in 11,270 women with GDM compared with 174,146 women without GDM revealed a 15.7% frequency of diabetes in former GDM compared with 1% in the non-GDM population.[72] Findings of abnormal carbohydrate intolerance may manifest early in the postpartum period depending on the population studied and its risk factors (Table 39-17). As many as one third of women with GDM will have overt diabetes, impaired fasting glucose, or IGT identified during postpartum testing conducted within 6 to 12 weeks of delivery.[73] Thus, both the American Diabetes Association and the ACOG (Figure 39-18) recommend postpartum glucose testing following a diagnosis of GDM.[74,75] Nevertheless, the prevalence of postpartum glucose screening with either a fasting plasma glucose or a 2-hour oral GTT has ranged from only 23% to 58% in seven reported studies.[73] A recent report of 11,825 women with GDM from a large health maintenance organization indicated that postpartum testing was performed in only 50% (n = 5939) of eligible women.[76] In this series, of 5857 women with test results, 16.3% (n = 956) had impaired fasting glucose or IGT, whereas 1.1% (n = 66) were found to have overt diabetes. After adjustment for demographic and clinical factors, abnormal postpartum test results were associated with having required insulin or oral agents during pregnancy and with a longer period from delivery to postpartum testing.

There is some debate about whether postpartum glucose testing can be limited to fasting glucose versus a 75-g 2-hour oral GTT. Whereas some have reported sufficiently high sensitivity using a fasting glucose alone (cut-off of 6 mmol/L or 108 mg/dL) to detect diabetes in prior GDM, more recent reports indicate the need for a complete 75-g 2-hour 75 oral GTT to achieve satisfactory sensitivity. McLean and colleagues reported 272 abnormal postpartum oral GTTs (27.6%), with 109 women identified as having frank diabetes. Eleven of these (10%) had fasting plasma glucose less than or equal to 6 mmol/L (<108 mg/dL), as did 62% of 114 cases of IGT. These authors concluded that a postpartum fasting plasma glucose is not sensitive enough in a high-risk population to classify glucose tolerance status accurately. However, only 5 of 109 women with overt diabetes did not require insulin during pregnancy, and of these, three had a postpartum fasting plasma glucose of less than or equal to 6 mmol/L. **Currently, the ACOG recommends using either a fasting plasma glucose or a 75-g 2-hour oral GTT at 6 to 12 weeks' postpartum. The optimal frequency of subsequent testing has not been established; however, the American Diabetes Association recommends repeat testing at least every 3 years for women with prior GDM and normal results of postpartum screening.**

Given the high risk for subsequent diabetes in women with former GDM, this population is ideally suited for preventive strategies to lower their risk for deteriorating carbohydrate tolerance.[77,78] There is substantial evidence that both lifestyle changes and pharmacotherapy can prevent or delay the progression of IGT to type 2 diabetes following GDM.[77,78] In the Diabetes Prevention Program, which compared lifestyle changes to metformin therapy, intensive lifestyle changes of diet and exercise resulted in an average weight loss of 15 pounds, most of which was sustained throughout the study. Fewer individuals randomized to lifestyle intervention developed diabetes (14%) compared with the metformin group (22%) and placebo-treated subjects (29%). Unlike the findings in the entire study group, Ratner and colleagues found that metformin and lifestyle intervention were similarly effective in reducing the incidence of diabetes in women with a history of GDM. In women with a history of GDM and IGT, the incidence of subsequent diabetes was reduced by 50% and 53% in subjects receiving metformin and lifestyle intervention, respectively, compared with placebo. It follows that women with GDM found to have IGT on postpartum glucose tolerance testing should be referred for preventive therapy.

Women with GDM are at high risk for recurrence in future pregnancies. Getahun and colleagues found a 41.3% incidence in second pregnancies of 61,462 control women.[79] These authors also documented that the risk for GDM is significantly increased in the third pregnancy if the first pregnancy was with GDM compared with a first affected pregnancy followed by an unaffected pregnancy. **Because of the high recurrence risk in former GDM, we recommend early pregnancy screening or testing, followed by screening at 24to 28 weeks or testing in those not found to have GDM earlier in pregnancy.**

Long-Term Effects of Glucose Intolerance on Mother and Fetus

The metabolic syndrome encompasses a myriad of metabolic disturbances, including core metabolic problems such as obesity, insulin resistance, and hyperinsulinemia. Related metabolic dysfunctions include hyperlipidemia, hypertension, inflammation, and atherosclerotic vascular disease. The metabolic alterations in pregnancy provide a useful paradigm for the long-term risks of both mother and her fetus relative to metabolic dysfunction.

Based on the original work of O'Sullivan and colleagues, GDM is a significant risk factor for the later development of type 2 diabetes, These findings have been replicated in a number of studies. **Kim and associates, in a review of the incidence of type 2 diabetes in women with a previous history of GDM, reported the cumulative incidence of type 2 diabetes increased markedly in the first 5 years after delivery and plateau after 10 years to about 50%. Elevated fasting glucose during pregnancy was the most common risk factor.**[80]

During pregnancy women with GDM have an increased risk for hypertensive disorders such as preeclampsia. In women with a family history of type 2 diabetes and prior history of GDM, Carr and coworkers reported that these women were at a threefold higher risk for developing the metabolic syndrome. Additionally, they were at increased risk for cardiovascular dysfunction such as coronary artery disease and stroke. Hence, not only is the diagnosis of GDM in pregnancy a harbinger of maternal chronic metabolic disease, but it also offers an opportunity for the initiation of prevention in this at risk population.

The developmental origins of health and disease (DOHAD) or perinatal programming concept has recently gained wider acceptance because of the increase in childhood and adult obesity. However, the effect of a hyperglycemic environment on long-term fetal development has been recognized for decades. On the basis of the Pima Indian studies of Pettitt and associates, children of Pima women are at increased risk for both diabetes and obesity.[81] This risk persisted when the offspring of the women with diabetes were compared with their siblings born before the mother developed glucose intolerance. These studies were later confirmed and expanded on by Dabelea and colleagues, also in a Pima Indian population.[82] **In fact, the strongest risk factor for diabetes in Pima Indian children is maternal diabetes in utero, independent of maternal obesity and birthweight.**[83] In a white population, Boney reported not only that the LGA children of the women with GDM had an increased risk for diabetes and obesity but also that 50% had evidence of the metabolic syndrome. In a recent multiethnic study, Hillier and coworkers reported that increasing levels of hyperglycemia, particularly fasting hyperglycemia less than the level diagnostic for GDM, were associated with an increased risk for childhood obesity. More recently, **Clausen and associated reported that the risk for being overweight was twofold greater in the young adults of mothers with GDM or type 1 diabetes. The risk for the metabolic syndrome was also increased fourfold in comparison with a matched cohort from the same background population.** In summary, the infants of the women with GDM are also at increased risk for childhood obesity, glucose intolerance, and associated metabolic dysregulation. The potential improvement in long-term childhood outcomes from both antepartum and postpartum interventions awaits further study.

PREPREGNANCY COUNSELING OF WOMEN WITH PREEXISTING DIABETES MELLITUS

Anomalies of the cardiac, renal, and central nervous systems arise during the first 7 weeks of gestation, a time when it is most unusual for patients to seek prenatal care. Therefore, the management and counseling of women with diabetes in the reproductive age group should begin before conception. In the United Kingdom, about 50% of diabetic women receive preconception counseling, whereas estimates as low as 20% have been reported in the United States.[84] Prepregnancy counseling includes an assessment of vascular status and glycemic control. Physicians who care for young women with diabetes must be aware of the importance of such counseling. At this time, the nonpregnant patient may learn techniques for self–blood glucose monitoring as well as the need for proper dietary management. Folic acid dietary supplementation at a dose of at least 0.4 mg daily should be prescribed to reduce the frequency of neural tube defects, although it has not specifically been studied in the diabetic population. During counseling, questions may be answered regarding risk factors for complications and the plan for general management of diabetes in pregnancy. Planning for pregnancy should optimally be accomplished over several months. Glycosylated hemoglobin measurements are performed to aid in the timing of conception.

A reduced rate of major congenital malformation in patients optimally managed before conception has been

TABLE 39-18 COMPARATIVE RATES OF MAJOR MALFORMATIONS* IN OFFSPRING OF DIABETIC WOMEN RECEIVING PRECONCEPTIONAL COUNSELING

STUDY	WITH PRECONCEPTIONAL COUNSELING	WITHOUT PRECONCEPTURAL COUNSELING
Fuhrmann et al., 1983[102]	1/128 (0.8%)	22/292 (7.5%)
Steel & Duncan, 1978[92]	2/143 (1.4%)	10/96 (10.4%)
Kitzmiller et al., 1991[85]	1/84 (1.2%)	12/110 (10.9%)
Whillhoite et al., 1993[103]	1/62 (1.6%)	8/123 (6.5%)
Tripathi et al., 2010[86]	14/240 (5.8%)	30/297 (10.1%)

*Includes adverse malformations as well as other adverse perinatal outcomes

consistently observed with special diabetes clinics (Table 39-18). Mills and associates reported that diabetic women registered before pregnancy had fewer infants with anomalies compared with late registrants (4.9% vs. 9%). Although the incidence of 4.9% remains higher than that in a normal control population (2%), normalization of glycemia was not established in the early entry group. Kitzmiller and colleagues[85] studied 84 women with pregestational diabetes mellitus who were recruited for preconception education and management during a 7-year period. A group of 110 pregnancies in women with IDDM presenting in the first trimester without preconceptional counseling served as controls in this study. One anomaly (1.2%) occurred in the preconception group compared with 12 (10.9%) malformations in the control population. Similar reductions in congenital anomalies and other adverse perinatal complications in women receiving preconceptional counseling have been reported by Tripathi and colleagues.[86]

Glycosylated hemoglobin levels obtained during the first trimester may be used to counsel diabetic women regarding the risk for an anomalous infant. Miller and colleagues[87] first observed that elevated HbA_{1c} concentrations early in pregnancy correlated with an increased incidence of malformations. In a series 58 patients with elevated glycosylated hemoglobin levels, 13 (22%) malformed infants were noted. This is in contrast to a 3.4% incidence of major malformations in 58 women whose glycosylated hemoglobin levels were in the normal range. Overall, the risk for a major fetal anomaly may be as high as 25% when the glycosylated hemoglobin level is several percent above normal values. Greene reported that 14 of 35 pregnancies with a glycosylated hemoglobin exceeding 12.8% were complicated by major malformations. In his series from the Joslin Clinic, the risk for major anomalies did not become evident until glycosylated hemoglobin values exceed 6 SD above the mean. In contrast to the investigations cited earlier is the Diabetes in Early Pregnancy study, in which malformation rates in IDMs were not correlated with first-trimester maternal glycosylated hemoglobin levels. The authors suggested that more sensitive measures are needed to identify teratogenic mechanisms or that not all malformations can be prevented by good glycemic control. Further review of these data, which included glycosylated hemoglobin levels only in the early-entry patients, demonstrates that these women were a relatively homogeneous group with respect to glycemic control; 93% had glycosylated hemoglobin levels less than 7 SD below the mean, a level of control that barely increases the risk for anomalies according to Greene's data. Regardless of the glycosylated hemoglobin value obtained, all diabetic women require a careful program of surveillance, as outlined earlier, to detect fetal malformations. The risk for spontaneous abortion also appears to be increased with marked elevations in glycosylated hemoglobin. However, for diabetic women in good control, there appears to be no greater likelihood of miscarriage. In summary, women with type 1 or type 2 diabetes mellitus should be advised to achieve an HbA_{1c} level close to the upper limit of the normal range before conceiving, to reduce the risk for a major fetal malformation or miscarriage.

CONTRACEPTION

There is no evidence that diabetes mellitus impairs fertility. Thus, family planning is an important consideration for the diabetic woman. A careful history and complete gynecologic examination and counseling are required before selecting a method of contraception. Barrier methods of birth control continue to be safe and inexpensive. The diaphragm, used correctly with a spermicide, has a failure rate of less than 10%. **Because there are no inherent risks to the diaphragm and other barrier methods, these have become the preferred interim method of contraception for women with diabetes mellitus.** The intrauterine device may also be used by diabetic women without concerns about an increased risk for infection.

Combined oral contraceptives (OCs) are the most effective reversible method of contraception with failure rates generally less than 1%. There is, however, continued controversy regarding their use in the diabetic woman. **The serious side effects of pill use, including thromboembolic disease and myocardial infarction, may be increased in diabetic women using combined oral contraceptive OCs.**[93] In a retrospective study, Steel and Duncan observed five cardiovascular complications in 136 diabetic women using primary low-dose pills. Three patients had cerebrovascular accidents; one had a myocardial infarction; and one had an axillary vein thrombosis. In a retrospective case-control study, despite diabetes increasing the risk for cerebral thromboembolism fivefold compared with controls, this risk was not enhanced by use of combined oral contraceptives.

In Steel and Duncan's report, several women exhibited rapid progression of retinopathy. Klein and colleagues[88] studied OC use in a cross-sectional study of 384 insulin-dependent women and reported no association between OCs and progression of vascular complications. For physicians who prescribe low-dose OCs to diabetic women, their use should probably be restricted to patients without serious vascular complications or additional risk factors such as a strong family history of myocardial disease or smoking. In these women, a monophasic preparation (progestin only) may be considered. In women taking OCs, the lowest dose of estrogen and progesterone should be employed. Patients should have blood pressure monitoring after the first cycle and quarterly with baseline and follow-up lipid levels as well.

Women using OCs may demonstrate increased resistance to insulin as a result of a diminished concentration of insulin receptors. Despite the fact that carbohydrate metabolism may be affected by the progestin component of the pill; disturbances in diabetic control are actually uncommon with its use. In Steel and Duncan's study, 81% of patients using the pill did not require a change in insulin dose. Triphasic OCs may also be used safely in women with a history of GDM without other risk factors. Skouby and coworkers have demonstrated that normal glucose tolerance and lipid levels can be expected in nonobese women with a history of GDM followed after 6 months of therapy. Kjos and colleagues[89] performed a prospective randomized study of 230 women with recent GDM. OC users were randomized to low-dose norethindrone or levonorgestrel preparations in combination with ethinyl estradiol. The rate of subsequent diabetes in OC users was 15% to 20%, after 1 year of follow-up. This rate was not significantly different from that in non-OC users (17%). Importantly, no adverse effects on total cholesterol, LDL, HDL, or triglycerides were found with OC use.

At present, there is little information available concerning long-acting progestins in women with diabetes or previous GDM. A statistically significant yet clinically limited deterioration in carbohydrate tolerance has been reported in healthy depomedroxyprogesterone acetate (Depo-Provera; DMPA) users. As observed with other progestins, DMPA may lower serum triglyceride and HDL cholesterol levels but not total cholesterol or LDL cholesterol. For this reason, DMPA is not recommended as a first-line method of contraception for women with diabetes. The progestin-only OC would be preferred because it does not produce significant metabolic effects in diabetic women.

KEY POINTS

- Pregnancy has been characterized as a diabetogenic state because of increased postprandial glucose levels in late gestation.
- Both hepatic and peripheral (tissue) insulin sensitivity are reduced in normal pregnancy. As a result, a progressive increase in insulin secretion follows a glucose challenge.
- In women with GDM, the hormonal milieu of pregnancy may represent an unmasking of a susceptibility to the development of type 2 diabetes mellitus.
- According to the Pedersen hypothesis, maternal hyperglycemia results in fetal hyperglycemia and hyperinsulinemia, resulting in excessive fetal growth. Tight maternal glycemic control is associated with a reduced risk for fetal macrosomia.
- Congenital malformations occur with a twofold to sixfold increased rate in offspring of women with pregestational diabetes compared with the normal population. Impaired glycemic control and associated derangement in maternal metabolism appear to contribute to abnormal embryogenesis.
- Women with class F (nephropathy) diabetes have an increased risk for preeclampsia and preterm delivery that correlates with their degree of renal impairment.
- Diabetes retinopathy may worsen during pregnancy, yet for women optimally treated with laser photocoagulation *before* pregnancy, significant deterioration of vision is uncommon.
- Screening for GDM is generally performed between 24 and 28 weeks' gestation. Screening strategies include universal screening or limiting screening to women older than 25 years with risk factors for developing adult-onset diabetes mellitus.
- Treatment of women with type 1 and type 2 diabetes mellitus during pregnancy requires intensive therapy consisting of frequent self–blood glucose monitoring and aggressive insulin dosing by multiple injections or CSII (insulin pump).
- The cornerstone of treatment for GDM is dietary therapy. Insulin and glyburide are reserved for individuals who manifest significant fasting hyperglycemia or postprandial glucose elevations despite dietary intervention.
- Antepartum fetal assessment for women with both pregestational diabetes or GDM is based on the degree of risk believed to be present in each case. Glycemic control, prior obstetrical history, and the presence of vascular disease or hypertension are important considerations.
- Delivery should be delayed until fetal maturation has occurred, provided that diabetes is well controlled and fetal surveillance remains normal. The mode of delivery for the suspected large fetus remains controversial. In cases of suspected macrosomia, a low threshold for cesarean delivery has been recommended to prevent a traumatic birth.
- Women with type 1 and type 2 diabetes mellitus should seek prepregnancy consultation. Efforts to improve glycemic control before conception have been associated with a significant reduction in the rate of congenital malformations in the offspring of such women.

REFERENCES

1. Garcia-Patterson A, Gich I, Amini SB, et al: Insulin requirements throughout pregnancy in women with type 1 diabetes mellitus: three changes of direction. Diabetologia 53:446, 2010.
2. Catalano PM, Tyzbir ED, Roman NM, et al: Longitudinal changes in insulin release and insulin resistance in non-obese pregnant women. Am J Obstet Gynecol 165:1667, 1991.
3. Catalano PM, Drago NM, Amini SB: Longitudinal changes in pancreatic b cell function and metabolic clearance rate of insulin in pregnant women with normal and abnormal glucose tolerance. Diabetes Care 21:403, 1998.
4. Catalano PM, Tyzbir ED, Wolfe RR, et al: Longitudinal changes in basal hepatic glucose production and suppression during insulin infusion in normal pregnant women. Am J Obstet Gynecol 167:913, 1992.

5. Catalano PM, Tyzbir ED, Wolfe RR, et al: Carbohydrate metabolism during pregnancy in control subjects and women with gestational diabetes. Am J Physiol 264:E60, 1993.
6. Catalano PM, Huston L, Amini SB, Kalhan SC: Longitudinal changes in glucose metabolism during pregnancy in obese women with normal glucose tolerance and gestational diabetes. Am J Obstet Gynecol 180:903, 1999.
7. Ryan EA, O'Sullivan MJ, Skyler JS: Insulin action during pregnancy: studies with the euglycemic clamp technique. Diabetes 34:380, 1985.
8. Kirwan JP, Hauguel-de Mouzon S, Lepercq J, et al: TNFα is a predictor of insulin resistance in human pregnancy. Diabetes 51:2207, 2002.
9. Sacks GP, Studena K, Sargent K, et al: Normal pregnancy and preeclampsia both produce inflammatory changes in peripheral blood leukocytes akin to those of sepsis. Am J Obstet Gynecol 180:1310, 1999.
10. Barros LF, Yudilevich DL, Jarvis SM, et al: Quantitation and immunolocalization of glucose transporters in the human placenta. Placenta 16:623, 1995.
11. White P: Pregnancy complicating diabetes. Am J Med 7:609, 1949.
12. Schmitz O, Klebe J, Moller J, et al: In vivo insulin action in type 1 (insulin-dependent) diabetic pregnant women as assessed by the insulin clamp technique. J Clin Endocrinol Metab 61:877, 1985.
13. Jansson T, Powell TL: Glucose transport and GLUT1 expression are upregulated in placentas from pregnancies complicated by severe diabetes [abstract]. Placenta 18:A30;1997.
14. Catalano PM, Tyzbir ED, Sims EAH: Incidence and significance of islet cell antibodies in women with previous gestational diabetes mellitus. Diabetes Care 13:478;1990.
15. Ryan EA, Imes S, Liu D, et al: Defects in insulin secretion and action in women with a history of gestational diabetes. Diabetes 44:506;1995.
16. Xiang AH, Peters RH, Trigo E, et al: Multiple metabolic defects during late pregnancy in women at high risk for type 2 diabetes. Diabetes 48:848, 1999.
17. Friedman JE, Ishizuka T, Shao J, et al: Impaired glucose transport and insulin receptor tyrosine phosphorylation in skeletal muscle from obese women with gestational diabetes. Diabetes 48:1807, 1999.
18. Hytten FE, Leitch I: The gross composition of the components of weight gain. In The Physiology of Human Pregnancy, 2nd ed. London, Blackwell Scientific, 1971, pp 371.
19. Freinkel N, Metzger BE, Nitzan M, et al: "Accelerated starvation" and mechanisms for the conservation of maternal nitrogen during pregnancy. Israel J Med Sci 8:426, 1972.
20. Kalkhoff RK, Kandaraki E, Morrow PG, et al: Relationship between neonatal birth weight and maternal plasma amino acids profiles in lean and obese nondiabetic women with type 1 diabetic pregnant women. Metabolism 37:234, 1988.
21. Darmady JM, Postle AD: Lipid metabolism in pregnancy. BJOG 82:211, 1982.
22. Knopp RH, Chapman M, Bergeline RO, et al: Relationship of lipoprotein lipids to mild fasting hyperglycemia and diabetes in pregnancy. Diabetes Care 3:416, 1980.
23. DiCianni G, Miccoli R, Volpe L, et al: Maternal triglyceride levels and newborn weight in pregnant women with normal glucose tolerance. Diabetes Med 22:21, 2005.
24. Schaefer-Graf UM, Graf K, Kulbacka I, et al: Maternal lipids as strong determinants of fetal environment and growth in pregnancies with gestational diabetes mellitus. Diabetes Care 31:1858, 2008.
25. Freinkel N: Banting Lecture of 1980: of pregnancy and progeny. Diabetes 29:1023, 1980.
26. Prentice AM, Poppitt SD, Goldberg CR, et al: Energy balance in pregnancy and lactation. In Allen L, King J, Lonnerdal B (eds): Nutrient Regulation During Pregnancy, Lactation and Infant Growth. New York, Plenum, 1994, pp 11.
27. Forsum E, Kabir N, Sadurskis A, Westerp K: Total energy expenditure of healthy Swedish women during pregnancy and lactation. Am J Clin Nutr 56:334, 1992.
28. Catalano PM, Thomas A, Huston-Presley L, Amini SB: Increased fetal adiposity: a very sensitive marker of abnormal in utero development. Am J Obstet Gynecol 189:1698, 2003.
29. Freinkel N, Lewis NJ, Akazawa S, et al: The honeybee syndrome: implication of the teratogenicity of mannose in rat-embryo culture. N Engl J Med 310:223, 1984.
30. Landon MB, Gabbe SG, Piana R, et al: Neonatal morbidity in pregnancy complicated by diabetes mellitus predictive value of maternal glycemic profiles. Am J Obstet Gynecol 156:1089. 1987.
31. Brans YW, Shannon DL, Hunter MA, et al: Maternal diabetes and neonatal macrosomia, II Neonatal anthropometric measurements. Early Hum Dev 8:297, 1983.
32. Dudley DKL, Black DM: Reliability of lecithin/sphingomyelin ratios in diabetic pregnancy. Obstet Gynecol 66:521, 1985.
33. Kjos SL, Walther F: Prevalence and etiology of respiratory distress in infants of diabetic mothers: predictive value of lung maturation tests. Am J Obstet Gynecol 163:898, 1990.
34. Catalano PM, Tyzbir ED, Allen SR, et al: Evaluation of fetal growth by estimation of body composition. Obstet Gynecol 79:46, 1992.
35. Ekbom P, Damn P, Feldt-Rasmussen B, et al: Pregnancy outcome in type 1 diabetic women with microalbuminuria. Diabetes Care 24:1739, 2001.
36. Cooper WO, Henandea-Diaz S, Arbogast PG, et al: Major congenital malformations after first trimester exposure to ACE inhibitors. N Engl J Med 354:2443, 2006.
37. Gordon M, Landon MB, Samuels P, et al: Perinatal outcome and long-term follow-up associated with modern management of diabetic nephropathy (class F). Obstet Gynecol 87:401, 1996.
38. Kitzmiller JL, Brown ER, Phillippe M, et al: Diabetic nephropathy and perinatal outcome. Am J Obstet Gynecol 141:741, 1981.
39. Carr DB, Koontz GL, Gardell A, et al: Diabetic nephropathy I pregnancy: suboptimal hypertensive control associated with preterm delivery. Am J Hypertens 19:513, 2006.
40. Klein BEK, Moss SE, Klein R: Effect of pregnancy on the progression of diabetic retinopathy. Diabetes Care 13:34, 1990.
41. Kitzmiller JL, Jovanovic L, Brown F, et al (eds.): Managing preexisting diabetes and pregnancy. Technical reviews and consensus. Recommendations for Care. American Diabetes Association, 2008.
42. Kitzmiller JL, Gavin LA, Gin GD, et al: Managing diabetes and pregnancy. Curr Probl Obstet Gynecol Fertil 11:113, 1988.
43. Albrecht SS, Kuklina EV, Bansil P, et al: Diabetes trends among delivery hospitalizations in the U.S. 1994-2004. Diabetes Care 33:768, 2010.
44. Periodic health examination, 1992 update: 1. Screening for gestational diabetes mellitus. Can Med Assoc J 147:435, 1992.
45. Brody SC, Harris R, Lohr K: Screening for gestational diabetes: a summary of the evidence for the U.S. Preventive Services Task Force. Obstet Gynecol 101:380, 2003.
46. The HAPO Study Cooperative Research Group: Hyperglycemia and adverse pregnancy outcome (HAPO) study: associations with neonatal anthropometrics. Diabetes 58:453, 2009.
47. Metzger BE, Gabbe SG, Persson B, for the International Association of Diabetes and Pregnancy Study Groups Consensus Panel: Recommendations on the diagnosis and classification of hyperglycemia in pregnancy. Diabetes Care 33:676, 2010.
48. Durnwald CP, Landon MB: A comparison of lispro and regular insulin for the management of type 1 and type 2 diabetes in pregnancy. J Matern Fetal Neonatal Med 21:309, 2008.
49. Landon MB, Gabbe SG: Insulin treatment of the pregnant patient with diabetes mellitus. In Reece EA, Coustan DR, Gabbe SG (eds): Diabetes Mellitus in Women. Philadelphia, Lippincott Williams & Wilkins, 2004.
50. Mukhopadhyay A, Farrell T, Fraser RB, Ola B: Continuous subcutaneous insulin infusion vs. intensive conventional insulin therapy in pregnant diabetic women: a systematic review of metaanalysis of randomized, controlled trials. Am J Obstet Gynecol 197:447, 2007.
51. Landon MB, Gabbe SG: Fetal surveillance in the pregnancy complicated by diabetes mellitus. Clin Perinatol 20:549, 1993.
52. Landon MB, Langer O, Gabbe SG, et al: Fetal surveillance in pregnancies complicated by insulin dependent diabetes mellitus. Am J Obstet Gynecol 167:617, 1992.
53. Nesbitt TS, Gilbert WM, Herrchen B: Shoulder dystocia and associated risk factors with macrosomic infants born in California. Am J Obstet Gynecol 179:476, 1998.
54. Landon MB, Mintz MG, Gabbe SG: Sonographic evaluation of fetal abdominal growth: predictor of the large-for-gestational age infant in pregnancies. Am J Obstet Gynecol 160:115, 1989.
55. Moore TR: A comparison of amniotic fluid pulmonary phospholipids in normal and diabetic pregnancy. Am J Obstet Gynecol 186:641, 2002.

56. Kjos S, Henry O, Montoro M, et al: Insulin-requiring diabetes in pregnancy: a randomized trial of active induction of labor and expectant management. Am J Obstet Gynecol 169:611, 1993.
57. Rouse DJ, Owen J, Goldenberg RL, et al: The effectiveness and costs of elective cesarean delivery for fetal macrosomia diagnosed by ultrasound. JAMA 276:1480, 1996.
58. ACOG practice bulletin: Shoulder dystocia. Number 40, November 2002.
59. Metzger BE, Buchanan TA, Coustan DR, et al: Summary and recommendations of the Fifth International Workshop-Conference on Gestational Diabetes Mellitus. Diabetes Care 30:3154, 2010.
60. U.S. Preventive Services Task Force Recommendation Statement: Screening for gestational diabetes mellitus: Ann Intern Med 148:759, 2008.
61. Alwan TN, Tuffnell DJ, West J: Treatments for gestational diabetes. Cochrane Database Syst Rev CDC003395, 2009.
62. Crowther CA, Hiller JE, Moss JR, et al: Effect of treatment of gestational diabetes mellitus on pregnancy outcomes. N Engl J Med 352:2477, 2005.
63. Landon MB, Spong CY, Thom E, et al: A multicenter, randomized trial of treatment for mild gestational diabetes. N Engl J Med 361:1339, 2009.
64. Nicholson W, Bolen S, Witkop CT, et al: Benefits and risk of oral agents compared with insulin in women with gestational diabetes: a systematic review. Obstet Gynecol 113:193, 2009.
65. Langer O, Conway DL, Berkus MD, et al: A comparison of glyburide and insulin in women with gestational diabetes mellitus. N Engl J Med 343:1134, 2000.
66. Jacobson GF, Ramos GA, Ching JY, et al: Comparison of glyburide and insulin for the management of gestational diabetes in a large managed care organization. Am J Obstet Gynecol 193:118, 2005.
67. Lain KY, Garabedian MJ, Daftary A, Jeyabalan A: Neonatal adiposity following maternal treatment of gestational diabetes with glyburide compared with insulin. Am J Obstet Gynecol 200:251, 2009.
68. Rowan JA, Hague WM, Wanzhen G, et al: Metformin versus insulin for treatment of gestational diabetes. N Engl J Med 358:208, 2008.
69. Moore LE, Clokey D, Rappaport VJ, Curet LB: Metformin compared with glyburide in gestational diabetes: a randomized trial. Obstet Gynecol 115:55, 2010.
70. Landon MB, Gabbe SG: Antepartum fetal surveillance in gestational diabetes mellitus. Diabetes 34:50, 1985.
71. Bellamy L, Casas JP, Hingorani AD, Williams D: Type 2 diabetes mellitus after gestational diabetes: a systemic review and meta-analysis. Lancet 373:1773, 2009.
72. Chodick G, Elchalal U, Sella T, et al: Epidemiology. The risk of overt diabetes mellitus among women with gestational diabetes: a population-based study. Diabetic Med 27:852, 2010.
73. Hunt KJ, Logan SL, Conway DL, Korte JE: Postpartum screening following GDM: how well are we doing? Curr Diabetes Rep 10:235, 2010.
74. Committee on Obstetric Practice: ACOG Committee Opinion No. 435: postpartum screening for abnormal glucose tolerance in women who had gestational diabetes mellitus. Obstet Gynecol 113:1419, 2009.
75. American Diabetes Association: Standards of medical care in diabetes—2009. Diabetes Care 32:S13, 2009
76. Lawrence JM, Black MH, Hsu W, et al: Prevalence and timing of postpartum glucose testing and sustained glucose dysregulation after gestational diabetes mellitus. Diabetes Care 33:569, 2009.
77. Knowler WC, Barrett-Conner E, Fowler SE, et al: Reduction in the incidence of type 2 diabetes with lifestyle intervention or metformin. N Engl J Med 346:393, 2002.
78. Ratner RE, Christophi Ca, Metzer BE, et al: Prevention of diabetes in women with a history of gestational diabetes: effects of metformin and lifestyle interventions. J Clin Endocrinol Metab Diabetes Care 93:4774, 2008.
79. Getahum D, Fassett MJ, Jacobsen SJ: Gestational diabetes: risk of recurrence in subsequent pregnancies. Am J Obstet Gynecol 203:1.e1, 2010.
80. Kim C, Newton KM, Knopp RH: Gestational diabetes and the incidence of type 2 diabetes: a systemic review. Diabetes Care 25:1862, 2002.
81. Pettitt DJ, Knowler WC, Baird HR, et al: Gestational diabetes: Infant and maternal complications of pregnancy in relation to third-trimester glucose tolerance in the Pima Indians. Diabetes Care 3:458, 1980.
82. Dabelea D, Hanson RL, Lindsay RS, et al: Intrauterine exposure to obesity conveys risks for type 2 diabetes and obesity: a study of discordant sib ships. Diabetes 49:2208, 2000.
83. Dabela D, Pettitt DJ: Intrauterine diabetic environment confers risks for type 2 diabetes mellitus and obesity in the offspring, in addition to genetic susceptibility. J Pediatr Endocrinol Metab 14:1085, 2001.
84. Clausen TD, Mathiesen ER, Hansen T, et al: Overweight and the metabolic syndrome in adult offspring of women with diet-treated gestational diabetes mellitus or type 1 diabetes. J Clin Endocrinol Metab 94:2464, 2009.
85. Kitzmiller JL, Gavin LA, Gin GD, et al: Preconception management of diabetes continued through early pregnancy prevents the excess frequency of major congenital anomalies in infants of diabetic mothers. JAMA 265:731, 1991.
86. Tripathi A, Rankin J, Aarvold J: Preconception counseling in women with diabetes: a population-based study in North of England. Diabetes Care 33:3, 2010.
87. Miller E, Hare JW, Cloherty JP, et al: Elevated maternal HbA1 in early pregnancy and major congenital anomalies in infants of diabetic mothers. N Engl J Med 304:1331, 1981.
88. Klein BEK, Moss SE, Klein R: Oral contraceptives in women with diabetes. Diabetes Care 13:895, 1990.
89. Kjos SL, Shoupe D, Dougan S, et al: Effect of low-dose oral contraceptives on carbohydrate and lipid metabolism in women with recent gestational diabetes: results of a controlled randomized prospective study. Am J Obstet Gynecol 163:1822, 1990.
90. Mills JL, Knopp RH, Simpson JP, et al: Lack of relation of increased malformation rates in infants of diabetic mothers to glycemic control during organogenesis. N Engl J Med 318:671, 1988.
91. Greene MF: Prevention and diagnosis of congenital anomalies in diabetic pregnancies. Clin Perinatol 20:533, 1993.
92. Steel JM, Duncan LJP: The effect of oral contraceptives on insulin requirements in diabetes. Br J Fam Plan 3:77, 1978.
93. Lidegard O: Oral contraceptives, pregnancy, and the risk of cerebral thromboembolism: the influence of diabetes, hypertension, migraine and previous thrombotic disease. BJOG 102:153, 1995.
94. Simpson JL, Elias S, Martin O, et al: Diabetes in pregnancy, Northwestern University Series (1977-1981). I. Prospective study of anomalies in offspring of mothers with diabetes mellitus. Am J Obstet Gynecol 146:263, 1983.
95. Albert TJ, Landon MB, Wheller JJ, et al: Prenatal detection of fetal anomalies in pregnancies complicated by insulin-dependent diabetes mellitus. Am J Obstet Gynecol 174:1424, 1996.
96. Grenfel A, Brudnell JM, Doddridge MC, Watkins PJ: Pregnancy in diabetic women who have proteinuria. Q J Med 59:379, 1986.
97. Reece EA, Coustan DR, Hayslett JP, et al: Diabetic nephropathy: pregnancy performance and fetomaternal outcome. Am J Obstet Gynecol 159:56, 1988.
98. Gordon MC, Landon MB, Boyle J, et al: Myocardial infarction during pregnancy in a patient with Class R/F diabetes mellitus: a case report and review of literature on Class H IDDM. Obstet Gynecol Surv 51:437, 1996.
99. Rosenn BM, Miodovnik M, Khoury JC, et al: Outcome of pregnancy in women with diabetic nephropathy. Am J Obstet Gynecol 176:S631, 1997.
100. National Institutes of Health Diabetes Data Group: Classification and diagnosis of diabetes mellitus and other categories of glucose intolerance. Diabetes 20:139, 1979.
101. Carpenter MW, Coustan DR: Criteria for screening tests of gestational diabetes. Am J Obstet Gynecol 144:768, 1982.
102. Fuhrmann K, Reiher H, Semmler K, et al: Prevention of congenital malformations in infants of insulin-dependent diabetic mothers. Diabetes Care 6:219, 1983.
103. Whillhoite MB, Bennert HW, Palomaki GE, et al: The impact of preconception counseling on pregnancy outcomes: the experience of the Maine Diabetes in Pregnancy Program. Diabetes Care 16:450, 1993.

For full reference list, log onto www.expertconsult.com.

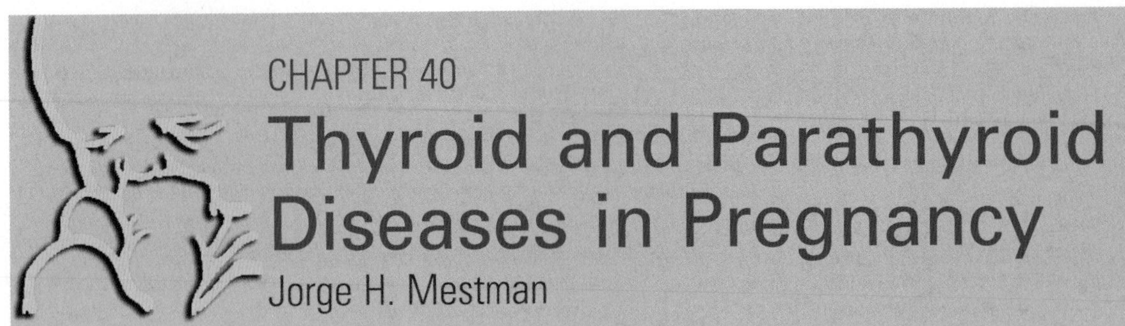

CHAPTER 40

Thyroid and Parathyroid Diseases in Pregnancy

Jorge H. Mestman

KEY ABBREVIATIONS

1,25-dihydroxyvitamin D	$1{,}25[OH]_2D_3$
American Association of Clinical Endocrinologists	AACE
American College of Obstetricians	ACOG
American Thyroid Association	ATA
Antithyroglobulin Antibodies	TGAb
Endocrine Society	ES
Familial Hypocalciuric Hypercalcemia	FHH
Fine-needle Aspiration Biopsy	FNAB
Free Thyroxine	FT_4
Free Thyroxine Index	FT_4I
Free Triiodothyronine	FT_3
Free Triiodothyronine Index	FT_3I
Human Chorionic Gonadotropin	hCG
Hyperemesis Gravidarum	HG
Immunoglobulin G	IgG
Intelligence Quotient	IQ
Intrauterine Growth Restriction	IUGR
Levothyroxine	L-thyroxine
Methimazole	MM
Parathyroid Hormone	PTH
Parathyroid Hormone–Related Protein	PTHrP
Postpartum Thyroiditis	PPT
Primary Hyperparathyroidism	PHP
Propylthiouracil	PTU
Resin Triiodothyronine Uptake	RT_3U
Thyroid-binding Inhibitor Immunoglobulin	TBII
Thyroid-blocking Antibodies	TRBAb
Thyroid Function Test	TFTs
Thyroid Hormone–Binding Ratio	THBR
Thyroid Peroxidase	TPO
Thyroid-stimulating Hormone	TSH
Thyroid-stimulating Immunoglobulin	TSI
Thyrotropin-releasing Hormone	TRH
Thyroxine	T_4
Thyroxine-binding Globulin	TBG
Total Triiodothyronine	TT_3
Total Thyroxine	TT_4
Triiodothyronine	T_3
TSH Receptor Antibody	TRAb or TSHRAb

Thyroid diseases, along with diabetes mellitus, are the most frequent endocrine pathology seen in pregnancy; parathyroid diseases, on the other hand, are rare but may present a diagnostic and therapeutic challenge to the obstetrician. The obstetrician should be aware of the symptoms and signs of the particular disease, the effect of pregnancy on the interpretation of endocrine tests, and the transfer of hormones and medications across the placenta with potential complications for the fetus and neonate. In this chapter, we present a brief description of the disease, its etiology, the interpretation of functional endocrine tests, appropriate therapy, and the potential effects of both the disease and drug therapy on the concepts. It is imperative that a team approach be used in the management of these conditions; the close cooperation of the obstetrician, endocrinologist, and anesthesiologist will offer the patient the best maternal and perinatal outcomes.

PARATHYROID DISEASES

Parathyroid diseases, uncommon in pregnancy, may produce significant perinatal and maternal morbidity and mortality if not diagnosed and properly managed. After a brief review of calcium homeostasis during pregnancy, primary hyperparathyroidism, hypoparathyroidism, osteoporosis, and vitamin D deficiency are discussed. Several reviews on these topics have been published.

Calcium Homeostasis During Pregnancy

Parathyroid hormone (PTH) and 1,25-dihydroxyvitamin D, (1,25$[OH]_2D_3$) are responsible for maintaining calcium homeostasis. **About 50% of serum calcium is protein bound (mostly to albumin), 10% is complexed to anions, and 40% circulates free as ionized calcium. During pregnancy, there is an active transfer of maternal calcium to the fetus.** A full-term infant requires 25 to 30 g of calcium during the course of pregnancy for new bone mineralization, most in the third trimester.

Total serum calcium during gestation is 8% below postpartum levels.[1] The upper limit of normal is 9.5 mg/dL. This decrease in total serum calcium is due to the physiologic hypoalbuminemia secondary to the normal expansion of the intravascular volume observed early in pregnancy. **Ionized calcium levels, however, remain unchanged throughout gestation.** Serum phosphate and renal tubular reabsorption of phosphorus also remain normal throughout pregnancy. Maternal serum PTH levels, when determined by a sensitive assay that accurately measures the levels of intact PTH, are slightly decreased in the first half of pregnancy (about 20% of the mean nonpregnant values) and return to normal by midgestation.[2]

Blood levels of 1,25$(OH)_2D_3$ (calcitriol) increase early in gestation to twice the nonpregnancy level in the third trimester. This increase is as a result of stimulation of maternal renal 1α-hydroxylase activity by estrogen, placental lactogen, and PTH, as well as synthesis of calcitriol by the placenta. Both free and total 1,25$(OH)_2D_3$ are increased in pregnancy, the total because of an increase in vitamin D–binding protein.[3]

Twenty-four-hour urinary calcium excretion also increases with each trimester of gestation and decreases in the postpartum period,[2] reflecting the increased intestinal calcium absorption induced by higher levels of 1,25-hydroxyvitamin D during gestation. Pregnancy-induced hypertension is characterized by decreased urinary calcium excretion, probably explained by a decrease in serum 1,25-vitamin D serum levels.

Parathyroid hormone-related protein (PTHrP), a peptide responsible for the hypercalcemia found in many malignant tumors, increases in early pregnancy. Hirota and colleagues[4] measured PTHrP in each trimester of human pregnancy, in umbilical venous blood and postpartum. A steady increase in plasma values was observed throughout pregnancy, with a peak in the third trimester and high values in cord blood. The plasma concentration in the postpartum period was directly related to the degree of breastfeeding. The source of maternal serum PTHrP is multiple, and both fetal and maternal sites have been postulated (placenta, myometrium, amnion, decidua, fetal parathyroid glands, breast, umbilical cord). PTHrP increases 1α-hydroxylase activity with an increase in 1,25$(OH_2)D$; PTHrP plays a role in placental calcium transport and also may have a role in protecting the maternal skeleton during pregnancy because the carboxyl-terminal portion of PTHrP ("osteocalcin") has been shown to inhibit osteoclastic bone resorption.[1] PTHrP may be involved in the transfer of maternal calcium into breast milk.

Serum calcitonin levels are higher during pregnancy and in the postpartum period, compared with nonpregnant controls. In 20% of patients, the values exceed the normal nonpregnant range. The origin of calcitonin is thyroidal C cells, breast, and placenta. Its role in pregnancy has not been elucidated, although it may protect the maternal skeleton from excessive resorption of calcium.

Osteocalcin is a bone-specific protein released by osteoblasts into the circulation proportional to the rate of new bone formation. It is slightly decreased during the second trimester of pregnancy, with an increase in the postpartum period.[2] **Markers of bone resorption increase during pregnancy, reaching values in the last trimester of pregnancy up to twice normal.** These changes are consistent with the increase in bone turnover at the time of maximal transfer of maternal calcium to the fetus.

After delivery, urinary calcium excretion is reduced; ionized serum calcium remains within normal limits; and total calcium, 1,25-hydroxyvitamin D, and serum PTH return to prepregnancy levels. Intestinal absorption of calcium decreases to the nonpregnant rate as a result of the previously mentioned return to normal levels of 1,25$(OH)_2D_3$.[1] Early concern of calcium loss in lactating mothers, with the development of osteopenia, has not been confirmed, **and extra calcium supplementation during breastfeeding appears to be unnecessary** because calcium supplementation above normal does not reduce significantly the amount of loss bone during gestation.[5] The alteration in calcium and bone metabolism that accompanies human lactation represents a physiologic response that is independent of calcium intake.

Hyperparathyroidism

Primary hyperparathyroidism (PHP) is an uncommon disease in women of childbearing age. The prevalence of PHP in women of childbearing age is about 5 per 10,000. The incidence of the disease in pregnancy is unknown, but it is definitely rare, and most of the reported cases have been single ones complemented with a review of the literature. More than 150 cases have been reported in the English literature up to 1999. With the introduction of routine automated techniques in clinical medicine and early diagnosis, most patients with PHP are symptom free, and their serum calcium elevation is mild.

The first case of PHP during pregnancy was reported in 1931. Shortly thereafter, the first case of neonatal hypocalcemia causing tetany in a mother with undiagnosed hypercalcemia due to hyperparathyroidism was described by Friderichsen. **The most common cause of PHP in pregnancy is a single parathyroid adenoma, present in about 80% of all cases.** Primary hyperplasia of the four parathyroid glands accounts for about 15% of the cases reported, 3% are due to multiple adenomas, and only a few cases due to parathyroid carcinoma have been reported in the English literature. In 1962, Ludwig reviewed the literature on the subject, describing 21 women with 40 pregnancies. The incidence of fetal wastage was 27.5%. Neonatal tetany due to hypocalcemia representing the first indication of maternal hyperparathyroidism occurred in 19% of these cases. In 1972, Johnstone and coworkers confirmed a perinatal mortality rate of 25% with a high incidence of neonatal hypocalcemia. Most of the patients reported in early years had significant metabolic complications of hyperparathyroidism, the two most common being renal and bone disease. In contrast to the previous high neonatal morbidity and mortality, Kelly,[6] reviewing the literature from 1976 to 1990, found only 2 perinatal deaths (5%) among 37 infants born of hyperparathyroid mothers. Two additional cases of perinatal deaths were reported in mothers with hypercalcemic crisis.

Currently, in the nonpregnant state, almost 70% of patients are symptom free, and the diagnosis is made through the routine use of biochemical screening. In pregnancy, because routine calcium determinations are not performed, manifestations of the disease are present in almost 70% of the diagnosed patients. In a review of 70 pregnant women, gastrointestinal symptoms such as nausea, vomiting, and anorexia were present in 36% of patients, whereas 34% presented with weakness and fatigue. In 26%, mental symptoms including headaches, lethargy, agitation, emotional lability, confusion, and inappropriate behavior were reported. Nephrolithiasis was detected in 36%, bone disease in 19%, acute pancreatitis in 13%, and hypertension in 10%. Only 24% of these patients were symptom free.

Parathyroid cancer is a rare cause of hyperparathyroidism, with very few cases documented in pregnancy. Serum calcium levels are significantly higher than in other causes of PHP. Perinatal mortality and morbidity are significant. Hypercalcemia with values above 13 mg/dL in the presence of a palpable neck mass should raise a strong suspicion of parathyroid carcinoma. On the contrary, in the presence of mild hypercalcemia and a neck mass, the most common cause of the neck lesion is a thyroid nodule. One other clinical feature of parathyroid carcinoma is poor response to the usual clinical therapeutic measures such as intensive hydration and loop diuretics. Surgery is the only effective therapy.

Hyperparathyroidism should be considered in the differential diagnosis of acute pancreatitis during pregnancy. Acute pancreatitis has been reported in 13% of women with primary hyperparathyroidism. The incidence in nonpregnant hyperparathyroid women is about 1.5% and is less than 1% in normal pregnancy. This complication is associated with significant neonatal and maternal morbidity.[7] It is more common in the primipara than in women who have had multiple pregnancies. Acute pancreatitis with PHP is mostly likely to occur during the last trimester of pregnancy or the postpartum period but has also been reported in the first trimester of pregnancy, mimicking hyperemesis gravidarum. Indeed, in two cases, hyperthyroidism was also present, which most likely represents the syndrome of transient hyperthyroidism of hyperemesis gravidarum (see Thyroid Diseases, later). **Serum calcium should be obtained in any pregnant woman with persistent significant nausea, vomiting, and abdominal pain.**

Hyperparathyroid crisis, a serious complication of PHP, has been reported during gestation and the postpartum period and is characterized by severe nausea and vomiting, generalized weakness, changes in mental status, and severe dehydration. Hypertension may be present and should be differentiated from preeclampsia. The serum calcium level is frequently higher than 14 mg/dL; hypokalemia and elevation in serum creatinine are routinely seen. If not recognized and treated promptly, hyperparathyroid crisis may progress to uremia, coma, and death. Of the 12 cases reported in the literature, 4 occurred in the postpartum period. Patients presented with severe nausea, vomiting, and elevation in serum creatinine due to dehydration. Serum calcium levels higher than 20 mg/dL were reported in 3 cases, and 3 patients died. Six cases have been associated with pancreatitis. Four fetal deaths have also been reported.

Bone disease in patients with PHP is now unusual. However, in early series, it was a common complication. Radiologic evaluation of the bones showed diffuse demineralization, subperiosteal resorption of the phalanges, and in severe cases, single or multiple cystic lesions and generalized osteoporosis. A 27-year-old woman was described with generalized musculoskeletal pain and radiographic evidence of advanced bone disease at 34 weeks' gestation.

Shani and associates reported[8] five cases of excessive amniotic fluid in mothers with PHP and serum calcium levels between 11.3 and 14 mg/dL. The mean amniotic fluid level (AFI) was 32 cm and mean gestational age nearly 30 weeks; other causes of polyhydramnios were ruled out. The authors suggested that the fetal polyuria was, similar to adult polyuria, a common symptom in patients with hyperparathyroidism.

The two most common causes of neonatal morbidity are prematurity and neonatal hypocalcemia, the latter related to levels of maternal hypercalcemia. In early reports, it was frequently the only clue of maternal hyperparathyroidism. It develops between the 2nd and 14th day of life and lasts for a few days.

Preeclampsia has been reported in some cases of PHP. Hultin and coworkers[9] recently reviewed the records of 52 women with the diagnosis of parathyroid adenoma, confirmed by surgery, and compared them with 519 women without the disease, all of whom had a subsequent singleton pregnancy between 1973 and 1997. They concluded that PHP due to a single adenoma, diagnosed before delivery, is significantly ($P < .0001$) associated with preeclampsia, with an adjusted odds ratio (OR) of 6.89 (95% confidence interval [CI], 2.30 to 20.58). Therefore, PHP should be considered a risk factor for preeclampsia.

The diagnosis of PHP is based on persistent hypercalcemia in the presence of increased serum PTH levels.[10] A persistent serum calcium value higher than 9.5 mg/dL is suspicious of hypercalcemia. Serum phosphorus is decreased in about 50% of pregnant women with PHP. A determination of 24-hour urinary calcium excretion is helpful in the diagnosis because most women with PHP have an increase in urinary calcium excretion, above the usual hypercalciuria of normal pregnancy. Urinary calcium excretion is low or low normal in the syndrome of familial hypocalciuric hypercalcemia (FHH), another cause of hypercalcemia that needs to be included in the differential diagnosis. The serum alkaline phosphatase level may be increased in PHP. However, it is also increased in normal pregnancy. High-resolution ultrasonography of the neck in expert hands is able to detect parathyroid lesions in a significant percentage of affected patients. Parathyroid imaging studies are contraindicated in pregnancy.

TABLE 40-1 CAUSE OF HYPERCALCEMIA IN PREGNANCY AND THE PUERPERIUM

Hyperparathyroidism (most common)
Rare causes related to pregnancy
Familial hypocalciuric hypercalcemia (FHH)*
Postpartum hypercalcemia in hypoparathyroidism
Parathyroid hormone–related protein (PTHrP)-induced hypercalcemia
Other causes not related to pregnancy
Malignancy
Endocrine
Thyrotoxicosis
Adrenal insufficiency
Vitamin overdose
Vitamin D
Vitamin A
Drugs
Thiazide diuretics
Lithium
Granulomatous disease
Sarcoidosis
Tuberculosis
Histoplasmosis
Coccidioidomycosis
Milk alkali syndrome
Acute and chronic renal failure
Total parenteral nutrition

From Mestman JH: Endocrine diseases in pregnancy. *In* Sciarra JJ (ed): Gynecology and Obstetrics. Philadelphia, Lippincott-Raven, 1997, p 11.
*Different expression with significant neonatal manifestations.

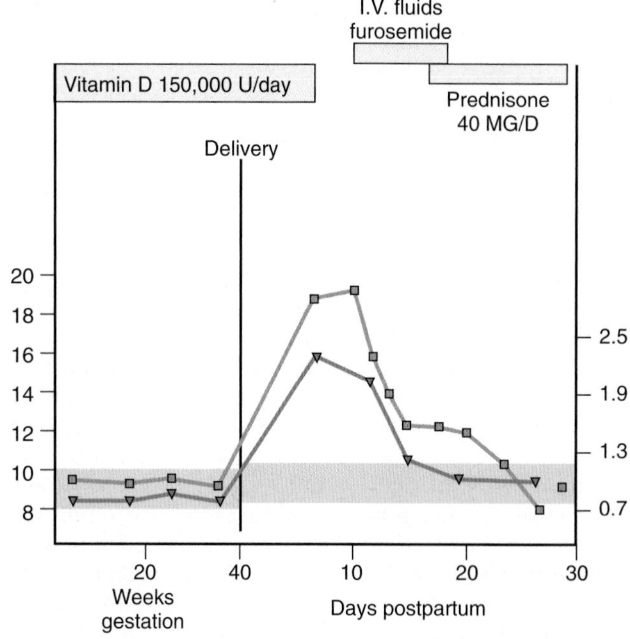

FIGURE 40-1. Serum calcium (*closed circles*) and creatinine (*closed squares*) levels during pregnancy and 1 month after delivery in a woman with hypoparathyroidism who was treated with vitamin D and calcium. *IV,* Intravenously administered; *stippled area,* normal range.

Differential Diagnosis of Hypercalcemia

Although most young women with hypercalcemia have PHP, other unusual causes should be ruled out, mainly endocrine disorders, vitamin D or A overdose, the use of thiazide diuretics, or granulomatous diseases (Table 40-1). A brief discussion of three uncommon syndromes associated with hypercalcemia during pregnancy follows.

1. FHH is an autosomal dominant condition with a high penetrance for hypercalcemia. The disorder is associated with an inactivating mutation in the gene for the calcium-sensing receptor. The main function of the receptor is in the regulation of calcium balance through changes in the parathyroid and kidneys. Mild hypercalcemia, slight elevation in serum PTH, mild hypermagnesemia, and low urinary calcium excretion are the typical findings. There is moderate hyperplasia of the four parathyroid glands. Total parathyroidectomy is seldom indicated because of the benign course of the disease. Infants born to mothers with FHH may present with different clinical manifestations. First, asymptomatic hypercalcemia can develop in an affected offspring if the mother is a carrier for FHH. In a second situation, severe neonatal hypocalcemia can occur in a mother with FHH syndrome. Although neonatal hypocalcemia could be severe, neonatal parathyroid function returns to normal a few weeks after delivery. In the third situation, severe neonatal hypercalcemia, also called neonatal severe hyperparathyroidism, occurs in infants homozygous for the FHH gene defect. Some infants require parathyroidectomy soon after birth.
2. Postpartum hypercalcemia may occur in women with treated hypoparathyroidism. The mechanism for hypercalcemia is not well understood. Nausea and vomiting develop a few days after delivery, dehydration ensues, and other manifestations of hypercalcemia develop, mainly mental changes. Serum calcium may be significantly elevated. Patients with treated hypoparathyroidism should be followed postpartum with serum calcium determinations, and vitamin D should be discontinued if hypercalcemia occurs. In severe cases, intravenous fluids and glucocorticoid therapy are required (Figure 40-1).
3. A few cases of hypercalcemia, mediated by PTHrP, during pregnancy and in the postpartum period have been reported. In one case, hypercalcemia developed in two successive pregnancies. In the second pregnancy, serum PTHrP levels were elevated to three times normal, and the infant was born with mild hypercalcemia that returned to normal within 24 hours after delivery. In a second case, a 25-year-old woman had massive bilateral breast enlargement at 24 weeks' gestation. Her serum calcium level was 14.3 mg/dL, but her serum PTH level was undetectable. She underwent bilateral mastectomy during pregnancy. The immunohistochemical studies demonstrated PTHrP antigenic activity in breast tissue. A case of hypercalcemic crisis in the first postpartum day, with serum calcium up to 19.4 mg/dL, has been reported; hypercalcemia was due to excessive amounts of serum PTHrP (28.4 pmol/L, normal <1.1 pmol/L), whereas serum PTH levels were very low. There was no evidence of other causes of low PTH hypercalcemia, and it was assumed that the

placenta was the source of the high PTHrP levels. The patient had no evidence of disease 4 years after delivery.

Therapy

Surgery is the only effective treatment for PHP. A novel oral agent that acts directly on the calcium sensor, cinacalcet, has been used in isolated cases without benefit by itself, but it reduces serum calcium in combination with calcitonin.[11] Surgery is a safe procedure when performed by a surgeon with extensive experience in neck surgery.[12] Complications due to surgery, particularly in the presence of a single lesion, are low, and the cure rate is excellent.

Although guidelines for the management of PHP in nonpregnant individuals have been suggested, the proper medical management of PHP in pregnancy has not been uniformly agreed on. For asymptomatic pregnant women in whom serum calcium is not greater than 1 mg above normal range, close follow-up with proper hydration and avoidance of medications that could elevate calcium, such as thiazide diuretics, is reasonable, although there are no studies in the literature supporting this or any other approach. Because most of the neonatal complications have been reported in patients with symptomatic disease, a surgical approach is indicated in such patients, as well as in those with complications such as nephrolithiasis and bone disease and those with persistent hypercalcemia (above 1 mg of the normal range). It is preferable to perform the surgery in the second trimester of pregnancy. In the series reported by Carella and Gossain, 38 women underwent parathyroidectomy during pregnancy, 7 during the first trimester and 18 in the second trimester. In the total group of 25, there was only 1 fetal loss. In 12 women in whom surgery was performed during the third trimester of pregnancy, the incidence of perinatal complications was 58%. For women with PHP first diagnosed after 28 weeks' gestation, the optimal treatment strategy is unclear, and the decision in such a situation should be based on the general condition of the patient, severity of hypercalcemia, and other complicating circumstances. A significantly lower incidence of complications, both maternal and fetal, was reported in a review of 16 published cases of patients operated on after 27 weeks' gestation.

Medical therapy is reserved for patients with significant hypercalcemia who are not surgical candidates. Oral phosphate therapy of 1.5 to 2.5 g/day has been shown to be effective in controlling hypercalcemia. Side effects of oral phosphate therapy include nausea, vomiting, and hypokalemia. These problems can be easily avoided by decreasing the dose of the medication. In patients in whom surgery is not advisable, it is important to prevent elevations in serum calcium. Good hydration, early treatment of urinary tract infections, and avoidance of medications known to cause elevations in serum calcium such as vitamin D, vitamin A, aminophylline, and thiazide diuretics are all important therapeutic measures. Serum calcium should be determined on a regular basis. Calcitonin in combination with oral phosphates or cinacalcet[11] was effective in controlling hypercalcemia in isolated cases.

In patients undergoing surgical treatment, hypocalcemia, albeit transient, may occur after surgery in some cases. Serum calcium should be checked every 6 hours, and if the patient develops hypocalcemic symptoms, intravenous calcium in the form of calcium gluconate, intravenous calcium (1-2 g of calcium-gluconate, equivalent to 90-180 mg elemental calcium, in 50 mL of 5% dextrose) can be infused over 10 to 20 minutes. Intermittent infusions may be repeated, or calcium gluconate can be diluted in 5% dextrose or isotonic saline and infused continuously at 1 mg/kg body weight per hour. In patients with bone disease, postsurgical hypocalcemia may be profound, and aggressive treatment is needed. These patients may benefit from vitamin D supplementation in the form of calcitriol, 0.25 to 0.5 mcg/day, for a few days before operative intervention.

Hypoparathyroidism

The most common etiology of hypoparathyroidism is damage to or removal of the parathyroid glands in the course of surgery for thyroid gland pathology. The incidence of permanent hypoparathyroidism after thyroid surgery has been estimated between 0.2% and 3.5%. In many cases, hypocalcemia in the immediate postoperative period is only transitory. Idiopathic hypoparathyroidism is a much less common cause of the disease, frequently associated with other autoimmune endocrinopathies, as part of the polyglandular autoimmune syndrome type 1. Antibodies directed against parathyroid calcium-sensing receptor have been detected in 56% of patients with idiopathic hypoparathyroidism.

The requirement for calcium supplementation and vitamin D may decrease in some women with hypoparathyroidism during the second half of pregnancy and lactation. In a few cases, hypocalcemic symptoms ameliorate with progression of pregnancy. The explanation for these findings is not clear but may be related to the increased intestinal absorption of calcium or the production of vitamin D by the placenta.

Clinical clues for the diagnosis of hypoparathyroidism include a previous history of thyroid surgery and clinical, radiologic, and laboratory information. **Typical symptoms of hypocalcemia are numbness and tingling of the fingers and toes and around the lips.** Patients may complain of carpopedal spasm, laryngeal stridor, and dyspnea. Convulsions may be a manifestation of severe hypocalcemia. Symptoms of irritability, emotional lability, impairment of memory, and depression are common. On physical examination, patients with idiopathic hypoparathyroidism demonstrate changes in the teeth, skin, nails, and hair as well as papilledema and cataracts. Chvostek sign, a twitch of the facial muscles, notably those of the upper lip, when a sharp tap is given over the facial nerve, is seen in many patients with hypocalcemia. Chvostek sign has also been described in 10% of normal adults. Trousseau sign is another sign of hypocalcemia. It is the induction of carpopedal spasm by reducing the circulation in the arm with a blood pressure cuff. The constriction should be maintained above the systolic blood pressure for 2 minutes before the test is considered negative.

The diagnosis of hypoparathyroidism is confirmed by the presence of persistent low serum calcium and high serum phosphate levels. Plasma alkaline phosphatase is usually normal. The differential diagnosis of hypocalcemia includes rickets, osteomalacia, and hypomagnesemia.

Marked hypocalcemia may occur in severely ill patients. The etiology is unclear, and a return to normal serum calcium is the rule following the recovery from the acute event.

In 1942, Anderson and Musselman published a review of the literature on hypoparathyroidism and tetany in pregnancy, collecting 240 cases. Twenty-six of the cases were due to post-thyroid surgery, and 140 were the so-called idiopathic type. It is likely that in some of these cases tetany was not due to hypoparathyroidism. Therapeutic abortion was recommended because of the high fetal and maternal mortality rates. Other reports have confirmed that hypoparathyroidism, if not properly treated, may increase perinatal loss, including spontaneous abortions, stillbirths, and neonatal deaths. **Radiologic bone changes may be present in the newborn as a consequence of intrauterine hyperparathyroidism.** They are characterized by generalized skeletal demineralization, subperiosteal bone resorption, bowing of the long bones, osteitis fibrosa cystica, and rib and limb deformities. Loughead and colleagues[13] described 16 infants of hypoparathyroid mothers. Secondary hyperparathyroidism in the infants resolved by 1 month of age.

Treatment of hypoparathyroidism in pregnancy does not differ from the nonpregnant state, including a normal high-calcium diet and vitamin D supplementation. The normal calcium supplementation of pregnancy is about 1.2 g/day. Vitamin D requirements may decrease in some patients by the second half of gestation. Calcitriol, 1 to 3 mcg/day, is used almost routinely in most patients affected with hypoparathyroidism. Calcitriol must be given in single or divided doses because its half-life is much shorter than that of vitamin D. If vitamin D is used, the dose is in the range of 50,000 to 150,000 IU/week. The importance of compliance with medications should be strongly emphasized, particularly when calcitriol is prescribed, in view of its short half-life. The major problem in the treatment of hypoparathyroidism is the recurrence of hypercalcemia and hypocalcemia. Therefore, serum calcium determinations should be performed at regular intervals. The most common symptoms of vitamin D intoxication are nausea, constipation, fatigue, headaches, and in more severe cases, vomiting and dehydration. It is important to assess serum calcium and phosphorus during pregnancy, particularly in the postpartum period, to detect the early onset of hypercalcemia (see Figure 40-1).

Lactation in mothers taking vitamin D may be contraindicated because a metabolite of vitamin D, 25-hydroxyvitamin D, has been detected in breast milk in high concentration in a mother taking 50,000 IU of vitamin D daily. Regardless of the form of vitamin D prescribed, serum calcium determinations should be done in the postpartum period, particularly in breastfeeding mothers.

Pseudohypoparathyroidism

Pseudohypoparathyroidism encompasses several different disorders, having as a common feature varying degrees of target organ resistance to PTH. Somatic changes are present in some forms of the syndrome, including short stature, obesity, round face, brachydactyly, and mental retardation, with brain calcifications. This variant is known as Albright's syndrome type 1a. Most patients suffer from hypocalcemia due to a derangement of renal 1α-hydroxylase and production of calcitriol. A few cases have been reported during pregnancy. Spontaneous normocalcemia occurred in two patients during four pregnancies. The authors provided evidence of placental synthesis of calcitriol to account for the normocalcemia. In both patients, serum PTH, which was significantly increased before pregnancy, was reduced by 50% during gestation. Serum cord calcium, phosphorus, and calcitriol concentrations were within normal limits. These infants are at risk for intrauterine fetal hyperparathyroidism, perhaps because of the relative maternal hypocalcemia during pregnancy.

Vitamin D Deficiency

Classically, vitamin D deficiency was related to the development of rickets, with its subsequent impact on obstetrical care. Deformities of weight-bearing bones, including the pelvis, prevented vaginal delivery in mothers affected by the disease.[14] In recent years, significant work has been published on the deleterious effect of vitamin D deficiency in a variety of medical problems from autoimmune disease to cancer. Several obstetrical, fetal, and neonatal complications have been reported in the last few years and have been recently reviewed.[14] The normal values for serum vitamin D 25OH (25[OH]D), the active metabolite of vitamin D, are controversial, with values varying between 20 and 40 ng/mL, equivalent to 50 to 100 nmol/L. There are barriers to the measurement of 25(OH)D in clinical practice. There are no single accepted measurements, and as a consequence, there is significant variability within and among laboratories and assays. As suggested by Barrett and McEleduff,[14] the clinician should ensure that the laboratory participates in an appropriate, validated quality control process and that the assay has been standardized against a reference method.

Vitamin D deficiency in the mother has been associated with decreased fetal growth. In 1996, Brunvand and colleagues followed 30 Pakistani women during pregnancy: 13 with elevated serum PTH levels at the time of delivery and 29 with serum levels of 25-hydroxyvitamin D below normal. There was a positive correlation between serum maternal ionized calcium levels and the crown-heel length of the newborn. The authors suggested that vitamin D deficiency could interfere with fetal growth through an effect on maternal calcium homeostasis.

Many studies in the past few years had linked low maternal 25(OH)D levels with maternal, fetal, and neonatal complications. Confirming the study done in Pakistan, in a report from Amsterdam, mothers with singleton pregnancies and serum 25(OH)D levels below 29.9 nmol/L had infants with a lower birthweight and a higher incidence of growth restriction than mothers with values of over 50 nmol/L (20 ng/mL). Low maternal 25(OH)D was associated with reduced body and lumbar spine bone mineral content in children at 9 years of age.

Other reported potential complications in infants and or mothers with vitamin D insufficiency include cardiomyopathies, immune intolerance (asthma, eczema), and an increased incidence of type 1 diabetes mellitus.

The association of vitamin D deficiency with insulin resistance and type 2 diabetes may explain the reportedly high incidence of gestational diabetes found in women with low levels of 25(OH)D. However, confounding factors have not always been considered in these studies. It was also pointed out in many of these studies that 25(OH)D was measured late in the second trimester of pregnancy. As suggested by Lewis, a randomized control trial (RCT) will be required to clarify the direction and magnitude of these effects.

The incidence of preeclampsia was higher in women with vitamin D levels lower than 37.5 nmol/L measured before 22 weeks, a fivefold increase adjusted for other cofounders such as pregnancy body mass index (BMI), ethnicity, season of the year, and gestational age. The authors reported that the risk for preeclampsia more than doubled for each 50-nmol/L decrease in maternal 25(OH) D. Calcium supplementation during pregnancy was reported to reduce the incidence of preeclampsia and its severity.[16]

Vitamin D deficiency was also reported to be an independent risk factor in the development of bacterial vaginosis in pregnancy as early as the first trimester. However, no control study is available to assess the beneficial effect of normalizing serum 25(OH)D concentration.

A inverse relationship between serum 25(OH)D and the rate of cesarean delivery in nulliparous women was recently reported.[17] It was speculated that proximal weakness and a decrease in lower extremity muscle function, an effect of 25(OH)D deficiency, contributed to the risk for cesarean delivery. The risk was fourfold higher in women with serum 25(OH)D levels below 15 ng/mL.

The information available suggests that a maternal deficiency in vitamin D could have a role in the development or progression of some maternal complications, such as gestational diabetes, preeclampsia, bacterial vaginosis, an increase in the cesarean delivery rate, and adverse fetal and neonatal outcome. It is apparent that more studies are needed, preferably an RCT to understand the interrelationship with other comorbidities such as age, ethnicity, seasonal variation, BMI, and the severity of diabetes. In the meantime, the practicing obstetrician will have to decide in a given patient if determination of 25(OH)D is indicated, what are the normal values for pregnancy, whether they are trimester-specific, what is the proper treatment, and how often the test needs to be repeated in pregnancy, also taking into consideration the cost of the tests and the possible implications for the fetus and newborn.

Just recently, a report from the Institute of Medicine (IOM)[18] became available. The committee took into account nearly 1000 published studies, including reports of protection from cancer, autoimmune disease, heart disease, and diabetes. In brief, they recommended that the lower normal limit for serum 25(OH)D should be "about" 20 ng/mL or 50 nmol/L. **The authors of the report recommended a daily vitamin D dietary allowance of 600 U, with an upper limit intake of 4000 U; for calcium, they recommended 1000 mg of dietary allowance and an upper limit intake of 2500 mg a day.**

Osteoporosis

The condition of idiopathic osteoporosis related to pregnancy was recognized in the 1950s. In the past few years, there has been increased interest in several clinical aspects of osteoporosis in pregnancy and lactation.[19] In general, osteoporosis is suspected in pregnancy when the patient presents with severe, persistent back or hip pain and radiologic examination shows signs of osteopenia. Studies measuring calciotropic hormones and biochemical markers of bone reabsorption in each trimester in pregnancy and in the postpartum period showed a slight decrease in bone mass by the third trimester, followed by recovery within the first 6 months postpartum. In a study of a group of white, upper middle class, postmenopausal women, **there was no association between the number of pregnancies and lactation as predictors of decreased bone mineral density.**

Osteoporosis may be diagnosed during pregnancy or in the postpartum period. Whether these are two different syndromes or they represent the same clinical entity is unclear because the symptoms may begin during pregnancy, but the diagnosis is made for the first time after delivery. Osteoporosis diagnosed during pregnancy may be localized in the hip or lumbar spine, or both. **Pain in one hip or back pain is the presenting symptom in most cases, usually in the second half of gestation.** Spontaneous recovery is the usual course a few months postpartum. A case has been reported of onset in the first trimester with recovery following abortion.

Although osteoporosis has been diagnosed during pregnancy, pregnancy unmasks rather than causes low bone mass. As suggested by Rizzoli and Bonjour and others, postural changes during pregnancy, including increased lordosis, when superimposed on a small and transient decrease in bone mass, may lead to pain and even fractures. In a study of 24 women with symptoms of bone pain for many years, 18 complained of back pain, 5 complained of hip pain, and 1 complained of ankle pain in late pregnancy and up to 8 months after delivery. Radiologic examination of the spine showed vertebral deformities in 17. Bone mass was measured in 21; 7 women had evidence of osteoporosis and 13 were osteopenic. The authors concluded that bone mass was probably low before pregnancy and that a transient and slight decrease in bone mass during pregnancy could have weakened the bone further. Radiologic examination of the localized painful area and studies of bone density after delivery are indicated. In some cases, a short course of calcitonin or bisphosphonate therapy plus calcium supplementation may be needed.

The impact of lactation on the progression of osteoporosis is controversial. The study by Kritz-Silverstein and associates revealed that lactation by itself was not a determinant of bone mineral density. Although one investigation reported that lactation for more than 8 months was associated with greater bone mineral at both the femoral neck and shaft, another study found that nursing for longer than 9 months produced a greater decrease in bone mass than observed during the first 6- to 9-month period of nursing. Given this controversy, the health care provider must decide whether cessation of lactation is advisable in the management of osteoporosis.

Heparin-associated osteoporosis has been reported in several cases during pregnancy. It may be related to the total dose of heparin. Treatment with calcium supplementation or calcitriol, although not proved, may be helpful in those patients receiving heparin therapy. Barbour and coworkers[20] followed 14 pregnant women requiring heparin therapy. Five of the 14 women experienced a 10% decrease from baseline proximal femur bone density measurements, compared with none in a matched control group. **The authors concluded that heparin adversely affected bone density in about one third of exposed patients.**

THYROID DISEASES

Thyroid disorders in pregnancy present a unique opportunity for health care professionals to use a similar "team approach" that has successfully improved the care of women with diabetes mellitus. Because of changes in thyroid economy occurring early in pregnancy, it is imperative to advise women with chronic thyroid diseases to plan their pregnancies and contact their health care professionals before or as soon as the diagnosis of pregnancy is confirmed. Autoimmune thyroid disease occurs five to eight times more often in women than in men, and its course could be affected by the immunologic changes occurring in pregnancy and in the postpartum period.[21,22]

In early pregnancy, the maternal thyroid gland is challenged with an increased demand for thyroid hormones secretion, due mainly to three different factors: (1) the increase in thyroxine-binding globulin (TBG) secondary to the effect of estrogens on the liver, (2) the stimulatory effect of human chorionic gonadotropin (hCG) on the thyroid-stimulating hormone (TSH) receptor, and (3) the supply of iodine available to the thyroid gland. This last factor is of importance in areas of iodine deficiency. In the United States, the iodine content in the diet, although decreased in the past decades, appears to be insufficient in only about 10% of pregnancies. **The suggested total daily iodine ingestion for pregnant women is 229 mcg/day and for lactating women 289 mcg/day; prenatal vitamins should contain at least 150 mcg of iodine in the form of potassium iodine.**[23]

The normal thyroid gland is able to compensate for the increase in thyroid hormone demands by increasing its secretion of thyroid hormones and maintaining them within normal limits throughout gestation. However, in those situations in which there is a subtle pathologic abnormality of the thyroid gland, such as chronic autoimmune thyroiditis, the normal increase in the production of thyroid hormones is not met. As a consequence, the pregnant woman could develop biochemical markers of hypothyroidism (i.e., an elevation in serum TSH and an increase in the size of the thyroid gland).

Active secretion of thyroid hormones by the fetal thyroid gland commences at about 18 weeks' gestation, although iodine uptake by the fetal gland occurs between 10 and 14 weeks.[24] **Transfer of thyroxine (T_4) from mother to embryo occurs from early pregnancy.** Maternal T_4 has been demonstrated in coelomic fluid at 6 weeks and in the fetal brain at 9 weeks. Maternal transfer continues until delivery, but only in significant amounts in the presence of fetal hypothyroidism. Thyroid hormone receptor gene expression has been shown in human fetal brain by 8 weeks' gestation, supporting the important role of maternal thyroid hormone during the first trimester of human pregnancy in fetal brain development. Several studies suggest that even mild maternal thyroid deficiency in the first trimester could result in long-term neuropsychological damage to the offspring.[25,26]

The levels of maternal thyroid hormone concentrations, both total thyroxine (TT_4) and total triiodothyronine (TT_3), increase from early pregnancy as the result of an elevation in TBG and a reduced peripheral TBG degradation rate. TBG reaches a plateau by 20 weeks' gestation and remains unchanged until delivery. Despite these acute changes in total hormone concentration, **the serum free fractions of both T_4 and T_3 remain within normal limits,** unless there is a decreased supply of iodine to the mother or in the presence of abnormalities of the thyroid gland.

Human chorionic gonadotropin is a weak thyroid stimulator, acting on the thyroid TSH receptor. It is estimated that a 10,000-IU/L increment in circulating hCG corresponds to a mean T_4 increment in serum of 0.1 ng/dL and, in turn, to a lowering of TSH of 0.1 mIU/L; the peak hCG values are reached by 9 to 12 weeks' gestation. In situations in which there is a high production of hCG, such as in cases of multiple pregnancies, hydatidiform mole, and hyperemesis gravidarum, serum free T_4 (FT_4) concentrations rise to levels seen in thyrotoxicosis, with a transient suppression in serum TSH values. In twin pregnancies, hCG levels are higher and duration of its peak longer than in singleton pregnancies, resulting in many cases with symptoms and laboratory tests compatible with gestational hyperthyroidism.

Goiter is commonly seen in pregnancy in areas of iodine deficiency. However, in the United States and other areas of the world with sufficient iodine intake, the thyroid gland does not clinically increase in size during pregnancy. **Therefore, the detection of a goiter in pregnancy is an abnormal finding that needs careful evaluation.** The most common cause of diffuse goiter is chronic autoimmune thyroiditis or Hashimoto thyroiditis. Most patients are euthyroid, and the diagnosis is made by the determination of thyroid antibodies, mainly thyroid peroxidase (TPO). Antibody concentration decreases during pregnancy and increases in the postpartum period. High values in the first trimester of pregnancy are predictors of the syndrome of postpartum thyroid dysfunction.

Thyroid Function Tests

Measurement of serum TSH is the most practical, simple, and economic screening test for thyroid dysfunction.[27] Normal TSH concentrations, as well as serum T_4 determinations, are trimester specific, dependent on iodine intake in a given population, on ethnicity, and on assay performance; serum TSH is lower in the first trimester compared with prepregnancy values and with the second and third trimester of pregnancy. An elevated serum TSH value is consistent with the diagnosis of primary hypothyroidism, whereas a low one, with few exceptions, is a normal finding in the first trimester (Figure 40-2) secondary to the stimulatory effect of hCG on the thyroid gland TSH receptor. Glinoer and Spencer[27] reviewed recent studies using a sensitive serum TSH assay, reporting a range between 0.03 and 3.67 mIU/L, (2.5th and 97.5th percentiles); different TSH reference limits will still be observed, according to the assays used. There are significant clinical data to support an upper limit of normal for serum TSH in the

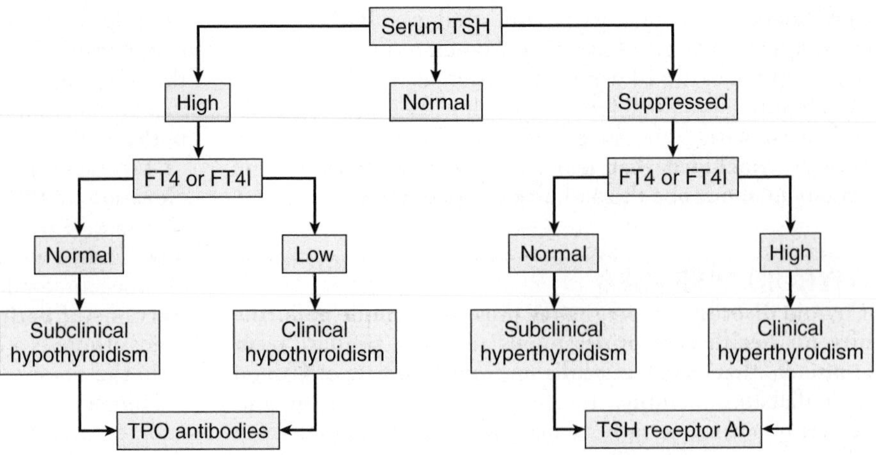

FIGURE 40-2. Algorithm for the interpretation of thyroid function test in pregnancy. Serum TSH upper limit of normal in the first trimester of pregnancy is 2.5 mIU/L; in the second and third trimesters, it is 3 mIU/L. Serum TSH lower limit of normal in the first trimester of pregnancy may be as low as 0.1 mIU/L or even undetectable. Subclinical hyperthyroidism in the absence of TSH receptor antibodies *(Ab)* is a normal first-trimester physiologic finding. Presence of serum TPO antibodies is consistent with a diagnosis of chronic thyroiditis. Presence of TSH receptor Ab is consistent with the diagnosis of Graves' disease. *FT4,* Free thyroxine; *FT4I,* free thyroxine index.

first trimester of pregnancy as a value of 2.5 to 3 mIU/L in the second and third trimesters.[28]

A word of caution is required regarding the determination of FT_4 levels in the different trimesters of pregnancy. Although discrepant findings have been reported, in most studies the free T_4 concentration increases slightly in the first trimester of pregnancy and declines with the progression of pregnancy. There is a significant inconsistency in FT_4 values in the second half of pregnancy among the different immunoassays, as reported by commercial laboratories, because of methodology used as well as variation in dietary iodine intake among the different populations studied. Currently, none of the manufactures of the automated free T_4 assays has provided trimester-specific reference ranges. Free T_4 values in the lower limits of normal and even in the hypothyroid range are not uncommonly seen in daily clinical practice, particularly in the third trimester of pregnancy. Lee and colleagues[29] compared the diagnostic performances of two different immunoassays to traditional approaches for estimating FT_4 (total T_4 and FT_4 index [FT_4I]) relative to the physiologic TSH changes that are known to occur throughout pregnancy. They studied euthyroid women who were thyroid peroxidase antibody negative in the first, second, and third trimesters of gestation. Control women were premenopausal, nonpregnant women matched for ethnicity. Serum TT_4, as expected, was elevated in all three trimesters, and serum FT_4I was elevated in the first trimester compared with controls (P <.05) and returned to the nonpregnant range in the second and third trimester; in contrast, FT_4 values, measured by two different immunoassays, were either comparable or lower than controls, and by the second and third trimesters, were about 65% of controls. The authors concluded that TT_4 and FT_4I retained an appropriate inverse relationship with serum TSH throughout pregnancy and appeared to provide a more reliable free T_4 estimate than the FT_4 test. Because the determination of FT_4 by the dialysis method, the gold standard for free T_4 assessment, or the use of tandem mass spectrometry are not routinely available because they are high-cost, cumbersome, and time-consuming procedures, the determination of total T_4 adjusted by a factor of 1.5 for pregnant patients has been suggested.[29] Therefore, it is imperative for the practicing physician to be familiar with the interpretation and significance of the thyroid tests as reported by a given commercial laboratory. The use of a limited number of thyroid function tests, properly ordered and interpreted, will allow the health care professional to assess thyroid function and make the proper therapeutic decisions.

A suppressed serum TSH value and high concentrations of FT_4 or FT_4I is diagnostic of hyperthyroidism. There are rare situations in which hyperthyroidism may be diagnosed in the presence of suppressed TSH and normal concentrations of FT_4, such as in the case of an autonomous thyroid nodule. In such cases, a serum TT_3 or free triiodothyronine index (FT_3I) determination should be obtained.

Prepregnancy Counseling

The physician may be faced with different clinical situations when counseling a woman suffering from thyroid disease contemplating pregnancy. With the advent of available information in the electronic media, it is important for the health care professional to offer the patient and her family objective and scientific data, supported by medical literature published in recognized peer-reviewed medical journals. The clinical situations may be summarized as follows:

1. *Hyperthyroidism under antithyroid drug treatment.* A choice of the three classic therapeutic options for hyperthyroidism treatment should be given: (1) long-term antithyroid drug therapy, (2) radioactive iodine-131 (^{131}I) ablation, or (3) near-total thyroidectomy. Potential side effects of antithyroid drugs on the fetus should be discussed with the future parents. If the patient opts for ^{131}I ablation therapy, there is no adverse long-term effect of ^{131}I given to the future mother or the offspring. However, it is customary to wait 3 to 6 months after the therapeutic dose is administered before pregnancy is contemplated in order to achieve target serum TSH values. Surgery is another option, selected by some physicians and patients concerned about the potential side effects of antithyroid drugs or radioactive treatment. Regardless of the form of therapy chosen, it is important for the patient to be euthyroid at the time of conception. One issue of clinical significance is the titer of maternal serum thyroid receptor antibodies (TRAbs), at the time of ablative therapy. TRAb-stimulating activity may be above normal values and does not normalize immediately after

either therapy, and may even increase after ^{131}I administration. Therefore, surgical therapy could be considered in patients contemplating pregnancy when serum TRAb titers are fivefold higher than normal and a potential risk to the fetus.[30] A high titer of TRAb in the second half of pregnancy presents a risk for fetal or neonatal hyperthyroidism. In a large series of hyperthyroid pregnant women, a doubling in incidence of congenital malformations was reported when hyperthyroidism was not controlled in the first trimester of pregnancy compared with that in women who were euthyroid early in gestation.

2. *Previous treatment with ^{131}I for thyroid carcinoma.* It is reasonable for patients treated with ablative doses of ^{131}I to wait 6 months to 1 year after completion of treatment before conception. No long-term effect on the offspring has been reported. Adjustment of the levothyroxine (L-thyroxine) dose should be done early in pregnancy and in each trimester; serum TSH should be kept in the low-normal range or undetectable, but clinical hyperthyroidism should be avoided. Data obtained from 2673 pregnancies in patients treated for thyroid carcinoma but without significant external radiation to the ovaries were analyzed by Garsi and colleagues. There was no evidence that exposure to radioiodine affects the outcome of subsequent pregnancies and offspring. The question of whether the incidences of malformations and thyroid and nonthyroid cancers are related to gonadal irradiation remains to be established.
3. *Treated hypothyroidism.* Women under treatment with thyroid hormone usually require an increase in L-thyroxine doses soon after conception.[31,32] The increase in requirements is observed as early as the first 4 to 8 weeks of gestation. As soon as the diagnosis of pregnancy is made, thyroid function tests should be performed and thyroid doses adjusted accordingly. It has been recommended to add two extra doses of L-thyroxine per week to the customary doses as soon as the diagnosis of pregnancy is confirmed until the results of thyroid function tests become available.[32] Recently, it was reported that in hypothyroid women (excluding those who underwent thyroidectomy because of thyroid cancer) on L-thyroxine replacement therapy, if the serum TSH was below 1.3 mIU/L before conception, only 17% of women needed an increase in L-thyroxine in the first trimester of pregnancy, compared with 58% of those with a serum TSH above 1.3 mIU/L.[33] After delivery, the dose should be reduced to prepregnancy levels in most women. Common medications may affect the absorption of L-thyroxine, such as ferrous sulfate and calcium, among others. Patients should take L-thyroxine at least 2 hours apart from other medications and 1 hour before or after food intake, ideally early in the morning on awakening and 1 hour before food ingestion. However, during pregnancy, in those women affected by nausea or vomiting, the dose may be taken at bedtime on an empty stomach.
4. *Euthyroid chronic thyroiditis.* Patients with Hashimoto thyroiditis are at a greater risk for developing hypothyroidism de novo early in pregnancy, spontaneous abortions, prematurity, and postpartum thyroiditis.[34]

Maternal-Placental-Fetal Interactions

Studies during the past few decades have shown an important role of maternal thyroid hormones in embryogenesis.[24,35] It is accepted that maternal T_4 crosses the placenta in the first half of pregnancy at the time when the fetal thyroid gland is not functional.

Maternal TSH does not cross the placenta. TRH does cross the placental barrier, but its physiologic significance is unknown. TRH has been given to mothers to accelerate fetal lung maturation in premature infants.

Methimazole (MM), propylthiouracil (PTU), and carbimazole (CZ), drugs used for the treatment of hyperthyroidism, do cross the placenta, and if given in inappropriate doses may produce fetal goiter and hypothyroidism. CZ is used in some European countries. Preparations containing iodine given in large doses or for prolonged periods of time are contraindicated in pregnancy because accumulation by the fetal thyroid may induce goiter and hypothyroidism.

Hyperthyroidism

Autoimmune hyperthyroidism affects pregnancy in about 0.1% to 0.4% of patients.[36] Classically, it has been stated that Graves' disease is the most common cause of hyperthyroxinemia in pregnancy, with other etiologies being uncommon (Table 40-2). As will be discussed subsequently, hyperthyroidism due to inappropriate secretion or action of hCG is recognized as the most common cause of transient hyperthyroidism in pregnancy.[37] In our experience, single toxic adenoma and multinodular toxic goiter are found in less than 10% of cases. Subacute thyroiditis is rarely seen during gestation.

Gestational Hyperthyroidism

Also known as *gestational thyrotoxicosis* or *transient gestational hyperthyroidism,* this condition is defined as transient hyperthyroidism in the first trimester of pregnancy, due, with

TABLE 40-2 CAUSES OF HYPERTHYROIDISM IN PREGNANCY

- Immune thyroid disease
  - Graves' disease
  - Chronic thyroiditis
  - Sporadic silent thyroiditis
- Non-autoimmune
  - Multinodular goiter (MNG)
  - Toxic adenoma
  - Subacute thyroiditis
- Gestational thyrotoxicosis
  - Multiple gestations
  - Nausea and vomiting
  - Hyperemesis gravidarum
    - Trophoblastic tumor
    - Hydatidiform mole
    - Choriocarcinoma
- Iatrogenic
  - Excessive levothyroxine intake
    - Overtreatment
    - Factitious
  - Iodine induced

From Patil-Sisodia K, Mestman JH: Graves hyperthyroidism and pregnancy: a clinical update. Endocr Pract 16:118-129, 2010.

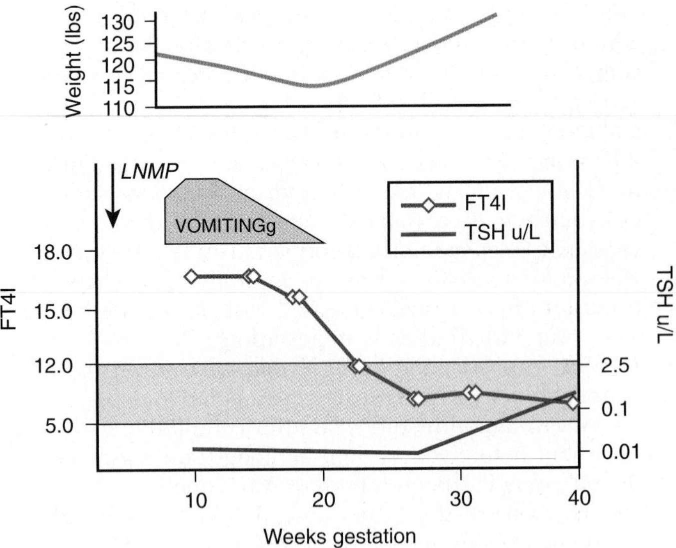

FIGURE 40-3. A representative example of transient hyperthyroidism of hyperemesis gravidarum. By week 6, vomiting begins and becomes severe by week 10. Serum free thyroxine index *(FT_4I)* is elevated, and thyrotropin is suppressed. By weeks 16 to 18, vomiting subsides, with marked improvement of the FT_4I value. During this period, the patient loses 3.6 kg. By week 18, the serum FT_4I returns to normal, but the serum thyrotropin remains suppressed until week 26. The patient regains and gains weight, with a term delivery of a healthy infant. The *gray band* indicates reference range. *LNMP,* Last normal menstrual period.

few exceptions, to high titers of hCG secretion stimulating the thyroid TSH receptor. The most common causes of gestational hyperthyroidism are hyperemesis gravidarum, multiple gestation, and hydatidiform mole. Other isolated reports included hyperplacentosis.

Transient Hyperthyroidism of Hyperemesis Gravidarum

This disorder is characterized by severe nausea and vomiting, with onset between 4 and 8 weeks' gestation, requiring frequent visits to the emergency room and sometimes repeated hospitalizations for intravenous hydration.[38] Weight loss of at least 5 kg, ketonuria, abnormal liver function tests, and hypokalemia are common findings, depending on the severity of vomiting and dehydration. FT_4 levels and TT_4 are elevated, sometimes up to four to six times the normal values, whereas TT_3 and FT_3 values are elevated in up to 40% of affected women, although FT_3 values are not as high as those of serum FT_4.[37] The T_3/T_4 ratio is less than 20, compared with Graves' hyperthyroidism, in which the ratio is more than 20. Serum TSH measured by a sensitive assay is consistently undetected or suppressed. **Despite the significant biochemical hyperthyroidism, signs and symptoms of hypermetabolism are mild or absent.** Patients may complain of mild palpitations and heat intolerance, but perspiration, proximal muscle weakness, and frequent bowel movements are rare. On physical examination, ophthalmopathy and goiter are absent, a mild tremor of the outstretched fingers is occasionally seen, and tachycardia may be present due in part to dehydration. Significant in the medical history is the lack of hyperthyroid symptoms before conception because most patients with Graves' disease diagnosed for the first time during gestation give a history of hypermetabolic symptoms antedating conception. Spontaneous normalization of hyperthyroxinemia parallels the improvement in vomiting and weight gain, with most of the cases resolving spontaneously between 14 and 20 weeks' gestation, although persistence of hyperthyroidism beyond 20 weeks' gestation has been reported in 15% to 25% of cases. Suppressed serum TSH may lag for a few more weeks after normalization of free thyroid hormone levels (Figure 40-3). **Antithyroid medications are not needed.** In one series in which antithyroid medication was used, pregnancy outcome was not significantly different in a similar group of patients receiving no therapy. Furthermore, a case has been reported in which vomiting persisted despite normalization of serum thyroid levels with antithyroid medications; vomiting subsided after termination of pregnancy. Occasionally, severe vomiting and hyperthyroidism may require parenteral nutrition.

The degree of thyroid abnormalities is directly related to the severity of vomiting and weight loss. In 67 patients studied by Goodwin and colleagues,[37] liver and electrolyte abnormalities were routinely found in women with worse symptoms, including severe vomiting, weight loss of at least 5 kg, and significant dehydration. They also presented with more significant elevations in FT_4 levels and suppression of serum TSH values; indeed, in 30% of their patients, serum TSH was undetectable (<0.04 mIU/L). Those with a lesser degree of hyperemesis had a less severe disorder of thyroid function.

Transient hyperthyroidism due to hyperemesis gravidarum should be suspected in women who present in the first few weeks after conception with sudden onset of severe nausea and vomiting and thyroid tests in the hyperthyroid range. These patients do not complain of hypermetabolic symptoms antedating pregnancy, goiter is not detected by palpation, and symptoms or signs of tissue thyrotoxicosis are mild or absent. In addition, thyroid anti-TPO antibodies and TRAb, markers of autoimmune thyroid disease, are negative. The differential diagnosis may also be difficult because vomiting may also be a presenting symptom of hyperthyroidism of Graves' disease (Table 40-3).

The cause of the elevations of thyroid hormones in patients with hyperemesis gravidarum is the endocrine effect of hCG.[39] Most likely, high levels of hCG, a known stimulator of the TSH receptor, play an important role, as well as prolongation in its biologic activity as seen in twin

TABLE 40-3 DIAGNOSIS OF GRAVES' HYPERTHYROIDISM VERSUS GESTATIONAL THYROTOXICOSIS

	GRAVES' HYPERTHYROIDISM	GESTATIONAL THYROTOXICOSIS
Symptoms before pregnancy	++	–
Symptoms during pregnancy	+/++	–/+
Nausea, vomiting	–/+	+++
Goiter, ophthalmopathy	+	–
Anti-TPO/TRAb	+	–
Thyroid ultrasound	Vascularity	Normal

From Patil-Sisodia K, Mestman JH: Graves hyperthyroidism and pregnancy: a clinical update. Endocr Pract 2010;16:118-129.
–, None; +, mild; ++, severe; *TPO,* thyroid peroxidase; *TRAb,* thyroid receptor antibodies.

pregnancies. There is a significant, albeit weak, correlation between the degree of thyroid stimulation and total hCG levels in normal women and those with hyperemesis.[39] hCG titers of more than 200,000 mIU/mL consistently bring serum TSH to undetectable values. Certain hCG fractions may have more potent biologic activity as thyroid simulators. The thyroid-stimulating activity of hCG in early pregnancy and in molar gestations correlates best with the percentage of basic, partially desialylated hCG in serum. A case has been reported in a mother and daughter with recurrent hyperemesis, in whom hCG levels were not elevated. Both were heterozygous for a missense mutation in the extracellular domain of the thyrotropin receptor. The mutant receptor was more sensitive than the wild-type receptor to hCG, accounting for the occurrence of hyperthyroidism despite the presence of normal hCG levels.

As noted previously, the diagnosis of transient hyperthyroidism of hyperemesis gravidarum should be considered in women with severe vomiting, no clinical manifestations of Graves' disease, and biochemical evidence of hyperthyroidism in early pregnancy, suppressed or undetectable serum TSH values, and elevated serum FT_4. Normal serum TSH in early pregnancy may be as low as 0.01 mIU/L; therefore, the presence of elevated serum FT_4 is required for the diagnosis. Vomiting should be persistent and severe with a significant weight loss, because most women with morning sickness of pregnancy have normal thyroid function tests. The syndrome may repeat in future pregnancies.

Hyperemesis gravidarum may also occur in women with Graves' hyperthyroidism. It may occur during remission of the disease, explained by the additional action of hCG early in gestation; the differential diagnosis between the two entities may be difficult, but the presence of TRAb favors the diagnosis of Graves' hyperthyroidism.[40]

Obstetrical outcome is not affected by gestational hyperthyroidism. Birthweight may be slightly lower, but not significantly different, compared with fetuses of control mothers and is related to maternal weight loss.

Gestational trophoblastic diseases, partial and complete hydatidiform moles, and choriocarcinoma are other causes of hyperthyroidism early in pregnancy. Patients may present without symptoms despite chemical hyperthyroidism or with various degrees of severity, including congestive heart failure. Evacuation of the mole eliminates the source of the excessive hCG and reverses the clinical and biochemical features of hyperthyroidism. Treatment with α-adrenergic blocking agents is effective in controlling the symptoms. Sodium iopanoate has been used to reduce the release of hormones by the thyroid gland and block peripheral conversion of T_4 to T_3.

TABLE 40-4 POTENTIAL MATERNAL AND FETAL COMPLICATIONS OF GRAVES' HYPERTHYROIDISM

MATERNAL	FETAL
Miscarriage	Low birthweight
Pregnancy-induced hypertension	Prematurity
Preterm delivery	Small for gestational age
Congestive heart failure	Intrauterine growth restriction
Thyroid storm	Stillbirth
Placenta abruption	Thyroid dysfunction
Infection	Fetal hyperthyroidism
	Fetal hypothyroidism
	Neonatal hyperthyroidism
	Neonatal goiter
	Neonatal central hypothyroidism

From Patil-Sisodia K, Mestman JH: Graves hyperthyroidism and pregnancy: a clinical update. Endocr Pract 2010;16:118-129.

Graves' Disease

The natural course of hyperthyroidism due to Graves' disease in pregnancy is characterized by an exacerbation of symptoms in the first trimester and during the postpartum period and an amelioration of symptoms in the second half of pregnancy. Stimulation of the thyroid gland by hCG in the first trimester and an elevation in TRAb values have been suggested as the cause of exacerbation. Immunologic responses caused by changes in lymphocyte subsets could explain spontaneous improvement in the second half of pregnancy and recurrences in the postpartum period. Kung and Jones, in a study comparing Graves' disease in pregnant and nonpregnant women, postulated that the amelioration of symptoms seen with progression of pregnancy was due to a decrease in the titers of TRAbs with stimulating activity and an increase in TRAbs with thyroid-blocking activity. The reverse was true in the postpartum period, when aggravation of Graves' hyperthyroidism usually occurs. In another study, it was suggested that the amelioration of Graves' disease in the last half of pregnancy is induced by a decrease of thyroid receptor antibodies (TRAb) (thyroid-stimulating immunoglobulins, or TSIs) but not by the appearance of thyroid stimulation–blocking antibodies (TSBAs).

When hyperthyroidism is properly managed throughout pregnancy, the outcome for mother and fetus is good; however, maternal and neonatal complications for mothers untreated or poorly controlled hypothyroidism are significantly increased (Table 40-4).[41]

In most patients in whom the diagnosis is made for the first time during pregnancy, hyperthyroid symptoms antedate conception. The clinical diagnosis of thyrotoxicosis may present difficulties during gestation because many symptoms and signs are commonly seen in normal pregnancy, such as mild palpitations, heart rate between 90 and 100 beats/minute, mild heat intolerance, shortness of breath on exercise, and warm skin. There are some clinical clues that increase the likelihood of the diagnosis of hyperthyroidism: presence of goiter, ophthalmopathy, proximal muscle weakness, tachycardia with a pulse rate of more than 100 beats/minute, and weight loss or inability to gain weight despite a good appetite. Occasionally, the patient may be seen for the first time in congestive heart failure, and the etiologic diagnosis is difficult because many of the physical findings are suggestive of cardiac valvular disease, particularly mitral insufficiency or stenosis. Hyperthyroidism under poor control is frequently complicated by preeclampsia, small-for-gestational-age (SGA) infants, and preterm delivery. The physician should suspect hyperthyroidism in the presence of systolic hypertension with an inappropriately low diastolic blood pressure and a wide pulse pressure, also seen in other conditions such as aortic insufficiency.

Classic symptoms of hyperthyroidism include nervousness, increased sweating, increased appetite, heat intolerance, insomnia, proximal muscle weakness, irritability, changes in personality, frequent bowel movements, decreased tolerance to exercise (sometimes manifested as shortness of breath), eye irritation, frequent lacrimation, pruritus, and weight loss. Not all symptoms are present in a given patient. The physician should be aware of subtle complaints, particularly in the presence of weight loss or inability to gain weight. As mentioned previously, in the first trimester of pregnancy, differentiating the diagnosis from transient hyperthyroidism of hyperemesis gravidarum presents a real challenge for the health care professional.

On physical examination, the thyroid gland is enlarged in almost every pregnant woman with Graves disease. Indeed, the absence of a goiter makes the diagnosis unlikely in young people. The gland is diffusely enlarged, between two and six times the normal size, and varies from soft to firm, sometimes being irregular to palpation, with one lobe being more prominent than the other one. A thrill may be felt or a bruit heard, indications of a hyperdynamic circulation. Examination of the eyes may reveal obvious ophthalmopathy, but in most cases, exophthalmos is absent or mild, with one eye slightly more prominent than the other. Extraocular movements may be impaired on careful eye examination. Stare is common, as is injection or edema of the conjunctiva. Severe ophthalmopathy is rare in pregnancy; glucocorticoid therapy and surgical orbital wall decompression may be required to restore visual activity. Pretibial myxedema is rare, seen in less than 10% of women. A hyperdynamic heart with a loud systolic murmur is a common finding. Proximal muscle weakness, fine tremor of the outstretched fingers, and hyperkinetic symptoms are seen frequently. The skin is warm and moist, and palmar erythema is accentuated.

As discussed previously (see Thyroid Function Tests), FT_4 determination or the calculation of FT_4I (using TT_4 levels and a test for assessment of TBG, such as resin T_3 uptake) are standard tests in most clinical laboratories, with the results available in 24 to 48 hours. Almost every patient with Graves disease will have an elevated FT_4 concentration. A undetected TSH value in the presence of a high FT_4 or TT_4 adjusted for pregnancy confirms the diagnosis of hyperthyroidism.[36] In some unusual situations, the serum FT_4 may be at the upper limit of normal or slightly elevated, in which case the determination of TT_3 or adjusted TT_3 will confirm the diagnosis of hyperthyroidism. Thyroid peroxidase antibodies (TPOAb) or thyroid antimicrosomal antibodies, markers of thyroid autoimmune disease, are elevated in most patients with Graves disease; TSHRAb, both thyroid-binding inhibitor immunoglobulin (TBII) and TSI, are elevated, and their titers have significant prognostic importance for fetal and neonatal hyperthyroidism (see later discussion).

Significant maternal and perinatal morbidity and mortality were reported in early studies of pregnancies complicated by hyperthyroidism. In the past 20 years, however, there has been a significant decrease in the incidence of maternal and fetal complications directly related to improved control of maternal hyperthyroidism (see Table 40-4).[41-43] In patients whose hypothyroidism is poorly controlled, one of the most common maternal complication is pregnancy-induced hypertension (PIH). In women with uncontrolled hyperthyroidism, the risk for severe preeclampsia was five times greater than in patients with controlled disease.[41] Other complications include preterm delivery, placental abruption, birthweight less than 2500 g, stillbirth, and miscarriage. Congestive heart failure may occur in women untreated or treated for a short period in the presence of PIH or operative delivery. Left ventricular dysfunction is usually detected by echocardiography in women with cardiovascular manifestations. Although these changes are reversible, they may persist for several weeks or months after achieving a euthyroid state. In one study, reduction in peripheral vascular resistance and higher cardiac output were still present despite normalization of T_4 levels. This is an important finding with significant clinical implications. Left ventricular decompensation in hyperthyroid pregnant women may develop in the presence of superimposed preeclampsia, at the time of delivery, or with undercurrent complications such as anemia or infection. We have seen congestive heart failure in the first half of pregnancy in women with long-standing hyperthyroidism. It is likely that the aggravation of hyperthyroidism seen in the first part of pregnancy played an important role in the development of this complication. Careful monitoring of fluid administration is imperative in these situations. Thyroid storm has been reported in pregnancy and was reported 2 weeks postpartum in a woman whose hyperthyroidism was uncontrolled during pregnancy in association with multiorgan failure.

Fetal and neonatal complications are also related to maternal control of hyperthyroidism. Intrauterine growth restriction (IUGR), prematurity, stillbirth, and neonatal morbidity are the most common complications. Millar and coworkers[41] demonstrated that uncontrolled hyperthyroidism during the entire gestation was associated with a ninefold greater incidence of low-birthweight infants compared with the control population. It was almost 2.5 times greater in those whose hyperthyroidism was treated during

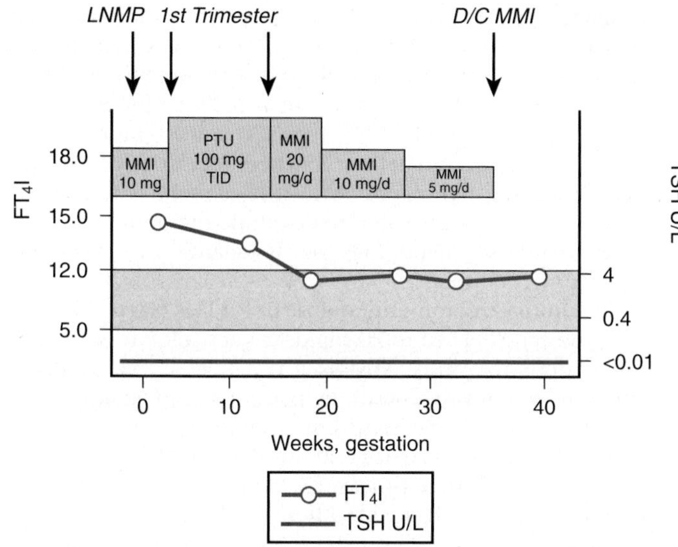

FIGURE 40-4. A representative example of management of hyperthyroidism in pregnancy. The patient is hyperthyroid at time of conception on methimazole *(MMI),* 10 mg daily. When pregnancy is diagnosed, MMI is discontinued, and propylthiouracil *(PTU)* is added at a dosage of 150 mg three times daily. By the end of the first trimester, PTU is discontinued, and MMI is given at a dosage of 20 mg daily. By week 20, the free thyroxine index *(FT_4I)* is almost normal, and the MMI dosage is reduced to 10 mg. By week 26, the FT_4I is in the upper reference range, and thyrotropin remains suppressed. The MMI dosage is reduced to 5 mg daily. The FT_4I remains in the upper reference range, and by week 34, MMI is discontinued *(D/C),* and the patient remains euthyroid until delivery. The *gray band* indicates reference range. *LNMP,* Last normal menstrual period.

pregnancy and became euthyroid at some time during gestation. In mothers achieving a euthyroid state before or early in pregnancy, the incidence of low-birthweight infants was no different from that in the control population. Mitzuda and associates correlated the risk of delivering an SGA infant to the presence of maternal thyrotoxicosis lasting more than 30 weeks of pregnancy, a duration of Graves disease for most of 10 years, and onset of Graves disease before age 20 years. Momotani and Ito reported the incidences of spontaneous abortions (25.7%) and premature delivery (14.9%) in mothers hyperthyroid at the time of conception, compared with 12.8% and 9.5%, respectively, in euthyroid mothers. Neonatal central hypothyroidism has been reported in infants whose mothers remained hyperthyroid throughout their pregnancies. Many of these infants recovered normal thyroid function in a few weeks, whereas another group have long-standing hypopituitary dysfunction.[44]

The use of ultrasonography for monitoring the size of the fetal thyroid gland as an indicator of thyroid dysfunction and possible therapeutic intervention was evaluated by Luton and associates in France.[45] In a group of hyperthyroid women considered to be at high risk (presence of TSHRAbs) and on antithyroid therapy, fetal goiter was detected in 11 of 41 patients. Four fetuses were hyperthyroid, and seven were hypothyroid secondary to high doses of maternal anti-thyroid drug treatment. All of them benefited from adjusting drug therapy. The authors concluded that ultrasonography of the fetal thyroid gland by an experienced ultrasonographer is an excellent diagnostic tool, in conjunction with close teamwork, to ensure normal fetal thyroid function.

Treatment of hyperthyroidism is essential to prevent maternal, fetal, and neonatal complications (Figure 40-4). The goal of treatment is normalization of thyroid tests as soon as possible and maintenance euthyroidism with the minimal amount of antithyroid medication. Excessive amounts of antithyroid drugs crossing the placenta may affect the fetal thyroid, with the development of fetal hypothyroidism with or without goiter. Patients should be monitored at regular intervals and the dose of their medications adjusted to keep the FT_4 or FT_4I very close to the upper limit of normal or just above it. Momotani and associates[42] showed that fetal serum TSH was elevated even in mothers with FT_4 within the normal range; furthermore, they demonstrated that normalization of serum TT_3 is a risk factor for the development of fetal hypothyroidism, supporting the recommendations that serum TT_3 determination should rarely be used to assess maternal function during gestation.

To achieved a euthyroid state and with the aim to keep the FT_4 in the upper limit of the nonpregnant reference range, and even slightly above normal, thyroid tests should be performed every 2 weeks at the beginning of treatment and every 2 to 4 weeks when euthyroidism is achieved. As mentioned earlier, because of the immunologic changes occurring with the progression of pregnancy, the requirement for antithyroid medications decreases after the second half of gestation. Some women with small goiters, short duration of symptoms, and on minimal amounts of antithyroid medication are able to discontinue antithyroid drugs by 34 weeks' gestation or beyond. It is estimated that 30% to 40% are able to remain euthyroid without therapy in the last few weeks of pregnancy.[41,43]

In a study of 44 women in 46 pregnancies, the correlation among TRAb activity, the dose of antithyroid therapy, and neonatal outcome was studied.[43] Medication was discontinued in 30 pregnancies 3 to 18 weeks before delivery. Neonatal thyrotoxicosis was seen in 4 infants whose mothers' TBII levels exceeded 70% (normal, <15%). Interestingly, of the infants born with elevated serum TSH, maternal TBII was less than 30% in most, suggesting that in Graves disease–associated hyperthyroid pregnancies, a low TBII titer is an indication to use the minimal amount of antithyroid therapy to avoid the development of fetal hypothyroidism with or without goiter.

In the United States, the two antithyroid drugs available are PTU and MM (Tapazole). Both drugs are effective in controlling symptoms. Recently, the risk for hepatic toxicity due to PTU was revisited. An alarming number of cases requiring liver transplantation and cases of death were noted (Table 40-5). MM can also induce liver toxicity, but

TABLE 40-5 SIDE-EFFECT PROFILES OF METHIMAZOLE VERSUS PROPYLTHIOURACIL

METHIMAZOLE	PROPYLTHIOURACIL
Skin rash	Skin rash
Pruritus	Pruritus
Migratory polyarthritis	Migratory polyarthritis
Lupus-like syndrome	Lupus-like syndrome
Cholestatic jaundice	Propylthiouracil hepatotoxicity:
Agranulocytosis	• Hepatitis
Methimazole embryopathy:	• Fulminant liver failure
• Choanal atresia ± esophageal atresia	
• Aplasia cutis	
• Hearing loss	
• Dysmorphic facial features	
• Developmental delay	

From Patil-Sisodia K, Mestman JH: Graves hyperthyroidism and pregnancy: a clinical update. Endocr Pract 2010;16:118-129.

these effects are milder, confined to cholestasis, not associated with liver failure, and seen more frequently in patients older than 61 years. It is estimated that about 4000 pregnant women per year in the United States would be expected to be treated with antithyroid drugs, most of them with PTU, as recommended per previous practice guidelines. Although no specific incidence of PTU-induced liver injury in pregnancy is available, it has been estimated that 4 women per year will have severe PTU-related hepatic complications.[46] Although the incidence of both liver toxicity due to PTU and embryopathy from MM are very low, a panel convened by the U.S. Food and Drug Administration (FDA) and the American Thyroid Association (ATA) recommended the use of PTU only in the first trimester of pregnancy and then a change to MM the second trimester (see Figure 40-4).[47] Other indications for the preferential use of PTU over MM are drug allergy to MM and, in thyroid storm, because of the ability of PTU to inhibit peripheral conversion of T_4 to T_3.

To our knowledge, no studies have shown PTU to be superior to MM in the management of hyperthyroidism in pregnancy; both drugs having similar placental transfer kinetics. Furthermore, when the efficacies of both drugs were compared, euthyroidism was achieved equally with equivalent amounts of drugs and at the same weeks of treatment. Neonatal outcomes were no different in both groups.

Aplasia cutis congenita, a localized lesion in the parietal area of the scalp characterized by congenital absence of the skin and a punched-out ulcer-like lesion, has occurred in a small group of infants born to mothers on MM therapy. It has never been reported with the use of PTU. However, the incidence in the general population is 0.03% of newborns. In a letter to the editor, an observation of aplasia cutis in an animal whose feed was contaminated by MM was reported. Several studies have described a specific embryopathy in infants born to mothers treated with MM in the first trimester of pregnancy.[48] This has been named *methimazole embryopathy* and includes choanal atresia or esophageal atresia, minor dysmorphic features, and developmental delay. Very few cases have been described, and none with the use of PTU. The prevalence of these malformations in the general population is 1 in 2500 for esophageal atresia and 1 in 1000 for choanal atresia. The doses of MM were 5 to 50 mg/day in one study; in the second study, both affected mothers took more than 20 mg/day. Barbero and associates,[48] in a recent epidemiologic study, reported an OR of 18 (95% CI, 3 to 121) for choanal atresia among infants whose mothers received MM in the first trimester compared with the general population; however, the authors could not exclude the possibility that hyperthyroidism itself may be associated with this and other abnormalities.

The initial recommended dose of PTU is 100 to 450 mg/day, and for MM, 10 to 20 mg/day; very seldom is a larger initial dose required. MM is given once or twice daily, allowing for improvement in patient compliance. PTU, because of its shorter half-life, should be given every 8 hours. **In our experience, 20 mg/day of MM or 100 to 150 mg of PTU three times a day is an effective initial dose in most patients.** Drug side effects are related to the antithyroid drug dose. Those with large goiters and longer duration of the disease may need higher doses at the initiation of therapy. In patients with minimal symptoms, an initial dose of 10 mg of MM daily or PTU 50 mg two or three times a day may be initiated. In most patients, clinical improvement is seen in 2 to 6 weeks, and improvement in thyroid tests occurs within the first 2 weeks of therapy, with normalization to chemical euthyroidism in 3 to 7 weeks. Resistance to drug therapy is unusual, most likely a result of poor patient compliance. **Once clinical improvement occurs, mainly weight gain and reduction in tachycardia, the dose of antithyroid medication may be reduced by half of the initial dose.** The daily dose is adjusted every few weeks according to the clinical response and the results of thyroid tests. Serum TSH remains suppressed despite the normalization of thyroid hormone levels (see Figure 33-4 in Chapter 33). Normalization of serum TSH is an indicator to reduce the dose of medication. If there is an exacerbation of symptoms or worsening of the thyroid tests, the amount of antithyroid medication is doubled.

The main concerns of maternal drug therapy are the potential side effects in the fetus, mainly, goiter and hypothyroidism—hence the importance of using the minimal dose to keep FT_4 in the upper limit of normal or just above the normal nonpregnant range. However, small elevations in serum TSH in the neonate have been reported even with lower doses of antithyroid medication. Furthermore, in one study, cord blood FT_4 values were not correlated with the antithyroid medication dose at term. As mentioned previously,[43] in the presence of maternal TBII values over 50%, the dose of MM required to control hyperthyroidism may be higher than in women with negative or low TBII titers in order to protect the fetus from hyperthyroidism. We do not recommend adding T_4 to antithyroid drug therapy in the management of Graves' disease in pregnancy. It is difficult to interpret the serum T_4 level and may require more unnecessary antithyroid medications.

Side effects of antithyroid drugs occur in 3% to 5% of treated patients (see Table 40-5). **The most common complications of both drugs are pruritus and skin rash.** These usually resolve after switching to the other antithyroid medication. In general, the rash occurs 2 to 6 weeks after initiation of therapy. Because pruritus may be an initial symptom of hyperthyroidism, it is customary to ask the patient during the first visit whether she is bothered by this. Other complications that are much less common are migratory polyarthritis, a lupus-like syndrome, and cholestatic jaundice. Agranulocytosis, a serious but unusual complication, has been reported in 1 in 300 patients receiving the drug. It manifests as fever, malaise, gingivitis, and sore throat. Agranulocytosis occurs in the first 12 weeks of therapy and appears to be related to the dose of medication. Bruner and associates reported a case of allergies to both antithyroid medications in a pregnant woman with type 1 diabetes mellitus. Patients should be made aware of the potential adverse effects of these drugs at the time the prescription is given and advised to discontinue the medication at once if these effects appear. In this setting, a leukocyte count should be obtained immediately. Although some have recommended routine white blood cell counts in patients on antithyroid therapy, such testing is not indicated because granulocytopenia or agranulocytosis may appear without warning symptoms.

β-Adrenergic blocking agents (propranolol, 20 to 40 mg every 6 hours, or atenolol, 25 to 50 mg/day) are very effective in controlling hyperdynamic symptoms and are indicated for the first few weeks in patients who have symptoms. One situation in which β-adrenergic blocking agents may be very effective is in the treatment of severe hyperthyroidism during labor. In a case reported in which both mother and fetus were affected, labetalol was infused at a rate of 2 mg/minute, controlling maternal and fetal tachycardia within 45 minutes.

Subtotal thyroidectomy in pregnancy is effective in managing the disease. However, currently, indications for surgical treatment are few and include allergy to antithyroid drugs, patients requiring large doses of medication, patient preference, and the exceptional case of resistance to drug therapy. Two issues are significant when advising surgical therapy: (1) the mother should be prepared with β-adrenergic blocking agents to render her hemodynamically stable and with Lugol's solution for at least 10 days to reduce thyroid gland vascularity (there is no contraindication to use potassium iodide for a short period of time); and (2) a determination of TRAb is of the utmost importance because a value three times greater than normal places the fetus at risk for fetal hyperthyroidism.[30]

^{131}I therapy is contraindicated in pregnancy because when given after 12 weeks' gestation, it could produce fetal hypothyroidism.[49] A pregnancy test is mandatory in any woman of childbearing age before a therapeutic or diagnostic dose of ^{131}I is administered.

Iodine crosses the placenta. If given in large amounts and for prolonged periods, it may produce a fetal goiter and hypothyroidism. Therefore, its therapeutic use is not recommended in pregnancy. However, iodine was used in small amounts, 6 to 40 mg/day, in a group of pregnant Japanese women with mild hyperthyroidism. Elevation in serum TSH was observed in 2 of 35 newborns, and the mothers were slightly hyperthyroid at the time of delivery. Despite this observation, iodine therapy is not routinely indicated in the treatment of hyperthyroidism in pregnancy.

Excessive amounts of antithyroid drugs have induced fetal hypothyroidism and goiter. The diagnosis of goiter is made by ultrasonography, which shows an increase in thyroid volume and in extreme cases hyperextension of the neck due to a large neck mass.[45] Few cases of hyperthyroidism have been confirmed by measuring serum T_4 and TSH in fetal blood obtained by cordocentesis.[50] Cordocentesis should be performed in a tertiary referral center and should be limited to the rare situations in which the diagnosis of fetal thyroid dysfunction cannot be established on clinical grounds.[51] Treatment with intra-amniotic injection of L-thyroxine, as well as discontinuation of antithyroid drugs, has resulted in resolution of the goiter.

Breastfeeding should be permitted if the daily dose of PTU or MM is less than 300 mg/day or 20 mg/day, respectively. It is prudent to give the total dose in divided doses after each feeding. Occasionally, thyroid function tests may be done in the baby.[52] In a very provocative study, PTU was given to lactating hyperthyroid mothers whose infants were born with elevated serum TSH levels. Infant TSH levels normalized even with continuation of PTU therapy by the mothers. In another study, thyroid tests were done at regular intervals in breastfed infants of mothers taking up to 20 mg of MM daily, showing no evidence of hypothyroidism. The authors followed the children up to 74 months of age, and there was no evidence of physical or intellectual developmental deficits compared with 176 controls.

Fetal surveillance with serial ultrasounds, nonstress testing, and the biophysical profile is indicated for cases with uncontrolled hyperthyroidism, in the presence of fetal tachycardia or IUGR, in pregnancies complicated by preeclampsia, or when indicated for other obstetrical or medical complications.

Treatment of Thyroid Storm

Thyroid storm is a clinical diagnosis based on severe signs of thyrotoxicosis, with significant hyperpyrexia (>103° F) and neuropsychiatric symptoms that are essential for the clinical diagnosis. Tachycardia with a pulse rate exceeding 140 beats/minute is not uncommon, and congestive heart failure is a frequent complication. Gastrointestinal symptoms such as nausea and vomiting, accompanied by liver compromise, have been reported. Burch and Wartofsky have derived a scoring system based on clinical symptoms to predict the likelihood of thyroid storm. Laboratory tests show the classic hyperthyroid changes, although the actual elevation in FT_4 values does not help in the diagnosis.

Management includes the following:

1. Admission to the intensive care unit for supportive therapy such as fluids and correction of electrolyte abnormalities, oxygen therapy as needed, and control of hyperpyrexia. Acetaminophen is the drug of choice because aspirin may increase free thyroid hormones.
2. Management of congestive heart failure, which may require large doses of digoxin.
3. Proper antibiotic therapy in case of infection.
4. β-Adrenergic blocker therapy to control hyperadrenergic symptoms, such as propranolol, 60 to 80 mg every 4 hours orally or 1 mg/minute intravenously. Esmolol, a short-acting β-acting antagonist, given intravenously with a loading dose of 250 to 500 mcg/kg of body weight followed by continuous infusion at 50 to 100 mcg/kg per minute, may be used.

5. MM, 30 mg, or PTU, 300 mg every 6 hours. If the patient is unable to take oral medications, a nasogastric tube may be needed; thioamides block the synthesis of thyroid hormones in a few hours.
6. One hour after the administration of thioamides, iodine is administered in the form of Lugol's solution, 10 drops three times a day or, if available, sodium iodide, given intravenously 1 g every 12 hours.
7. Glucocorticoids are also helpful because they reduce the peripheral conversion of serum T_4 to T_3, in the form of hydrocortisone every 8 hours; or equivalent amounts of other glucocorticoids.

In summary, thyroid storm is a life-threatening condition, with a mortality rate of 20% to 30%,[53] requiring early recognition and aggressive therapy in an intensive unit care setting.

Neonatal Hyperthyroidism

Neonatal hyperthyroidism is infrequent, with an incidence of less than 1% of infants born to mothers with Graves disease, therefore affecting 1 in 50,000 neonates. **In most cases, the disease is caused by the transfer of maternal immunoglobulin antibodies to the fetus.** These stimulating thyroid antibodies to the TSH receptor (TSIs), when present in high concentrations in maternal serum, cross the placental barrier, stimulate the TSH receptor of the fetal thyroid gland, and may produce fetal or neonatal hyperthyroidism. When the mother is treated with antithyroid medications, the fetus benefits from maternal therapy, remaining euthyroid during pregnancy despite the high circulating antibody titer. However, the protective effect of the antithyroid drug is lost after delivery, and neonatal hyperthyroidism may develop within a few days after birth. High titers of TSI receptor antibodies, a threefold to fivefold increase over baseline, in the third trimester of pregnancy are a predictor of neonatal hyperthyroidism. If neonatal hyperthyroidism is not recognized and treated properly, neonatal mortality could be as high as 30%. Because the half-life of the antibodies is only a few weeks, complete resolution of neonatal hyperthyroidism is the rule.

A few cases of familial neonatal Graves disease have been reported. The pathogenesis is not clearly understood. This condition may persist for several years.

Sporadic cases of neonatal hyperthyroidism without evidence of the presence of circulating TSI in mother or infant have been published. Activation of mutations in the TSH receptor molecule are the cause of this entity. It is inherited as an autosomal dominant trait and, in contrast to Graves neonatal hyperthyroidism, the condition persists indefinitely. Treatment with antithyroid medications followed by thyroid ablation therapy will eventually be needed.

Fetal Hyperthyroidism

In mothers with active hyperthyroidism due to Graves disease, high concentrations of TSIs crossing the placental barrier stimulate fetal T_4 receptor and may cause fetal hyperthyroidism. However, in mothers with active disease who are under treatment, the hyperactive fetal thyroid is controlled by maternal therapy, and the fetus remains euthyroid during fetal life. Within a few days after birth, when the beneficial effect of antithyroid therapy ceases, the neonate may develop neonatal hyperthyroidism (see previous section, Neonatal Hyperthyroidism). **Women at risk for fetal hyperthyroidism are those with a history of Graves disease previously treated with ablation therapy, either surgery or ^{131}I, because these immunoglobulin G (IgG) class antibodies may remain elevated after ablation therapy despite maternal euthyroidism.** The fetuses of women with Graves disease–associated hyperthyroidism who undergo therapeutic thyroidectomy in the second trimester of pregnancy are also at risk for hyperthyroidism if the mother carries high titers of TSHRAbs.[30] The fetal thyroid TSH receptor starts responding to TSI stimulation during the second trimester, and the placental transfer of IgG from mother to fetus increases by the end of the second trimester, reaching a level in the fetus similar to that of the mother at about 30 weeks' gestation. Therefore, the symptoms of fetal hyperthyroidism are not evident until 22 to 24 weeks of gestation.

Fetal hyperthyroidism is diagnosed in the presence of persistent fetal tachycardia (>160 beats/minute), IUGR, oligohydramnios, and occasionally a goiter identified on ultrasonography, sometimes manifested as hyperextension of the fetal neck.[45] The diagnosis may be confirmed by measuring thyroid hormone levels in cord blood obtained by cordocentesis. Serial cordocentesis for monitoring drug therapy has been proposed, but its value has been questioned.[51] A fetal heart monitor tracing demonstrating a sustained baseline of 170 to 180 beats/minute with moderate variability that exhibited acceleration with a lack of deceleration was present in two fetuses of hyperthyroid mothers. The authors stated that "this pattern is unique to fetal thyrotoxicosis." Heckel and associates reviewed nine cases of fetal hyperthyroidism treated by maternal administration of antithyroid medications. Fetal tachycardia was the most frequent sign, whereas oligohydramnios and IUGR were reported in only two cases. Fetal goiter was detected by ultrasonography in three cases. Treatment consisted of antithyroid medication given to the mother (MM, 10 to 20 mg/day).[54] The dose is guided by the improvement and resolution of fetal tachycardia, a decrease in the goiter size, and normalization of fetal growth. All are indicators of good therapeutic response.

Luton and associates[45] performed clinical fetal evaluation in 72 mothers with a past or present history of Graves hyperthyroidism. The main tools were the determination of maternal TSHRAbs and fetal ultrasonography. Cordocentesis was rarely indicated. In 31 mothers, TRAb titers were undetectable, and none of the patients received antithyroid medications. All infants were born euthyroid. Of 30 women positive for TRAb and on therapy, neonatal function was normal. Eleven fetuses were diagnosed with goiter by ultrasonography, and 7 of them were hypothyroid at birth. Their mothers had low TRAb titers and had received antithyroid therapy, probably in higher doses than needed. In the 4 hyperthyroid newborns, maternal TRAb titers were very high, and their mothers may not have received enough medication. The authors recommended monthly fetal ultrasonography after 20 weeks' gestation with determination of TRAbs early in gestation and again by 24 to 28 weeks' gestation.

TABLE 40-6 INDICATIONS FOR MATERNAL DETERMINATION OF THYROID-BINDING INHIBITOR IMMUNOGLOBULIN OR THYROID-STIMULATING IMMUNOGLOBULIN FOR DIAGNOSIS OF GRAVES DISEASE

- Fetal or neonatal hyperthyroidism in previous pregnancies
- Active disease or treatment with antithyroid drugs
- Thyroidectomy during pregnancy
- Euthyroid, postablation (surgery, iodine-131)
- In the presence of:
  - Fetal tachycardia
  - Intrauterine growth restriction
  - Incidental fetal goiter on ultrasound

From Mestman JH: Endocrine diseases in pregnancy. *In* Sciarra JJ (ed): Gynecology and Obstetrics. Philadelphia, Lippincott-Raven, 1997, p 27.

In summary, the diagnosis of fetal hyperthyroidism should be suspected in the presence of fetal tachycardia, IUGR, oligohydramnios or polyhydramnios, and accelerated bone maturation, with or without fetal goiter, in mothers with active hyperthyroidism or in women with a history of Graves disease treated previously by ablation therapy, and in the presence of high titers of serum TRAbs. The indications for ordering a determination of TRAbs are described in Table 40-6. This should be done in patients at risk between 22 and 28 weeks' gestation, although some investigators recommended this test early in pregnancy and late in the second trimester.[45] The diagnosis may be confirmed by the determination of fetal thyroid hormones by cordocentesis, in those centers with expertise in this technique.

Neonatal Central Hypothyroidism

Infants of untreated hyperthyroid mothers may be born with transient central hypothyroidism of pituitary or hypothalamic origin. High levels of T_4 cross the placental barrier and feed back to the fetal pituitary with suppression of fetal pituitary TSH. The diagnosis is made in the presence of a low FT_4 and a normal or low TSH level in cord blood. This complication should be avoidable with proper management of maternal hyperthyroidism.[44]

Resistance to Thyroid Hormone Syndrome

Described by Refetoff and colleagues, resistance to thyroid hormone (RTH) is a syndrome of reduced end-organ responsiveness to thyroid hormone, caused primarily by mutations in the thyroid hormone receptor β-gene. Unaffected fetuses of mothers with RTH syndrome and affected fetuses from normal mothers are at risk for poor obstetrical outcome. However, most of these pregnancies have no major consequences. Anselmo and associates reported 36 couples with 9 mothers and 9 fathers affected by the disease and 18 unaffected relatives. The rates of miscarriage were 23.7% in affected mothers, 6.7% in affected fathers, and 8.8% in unaffected first-degree relatives, with a rate of 8.1% in the general population. The birthweight of unaffected infants born to affected mothers was lower than the birthweight of affected newborns, who in addition had a lower serum TSH at birth. This finding suggests that high maternal thyroid hormone levels produced fetal thyrotoxicosis and had a direct toxic effect on the fetus. The approach to a pregnant patient with the RTH syndrome would depend on the genotype of the fetus. This requires obtaining the genotype of the fetus from DNA through amniocentesis, a history of the course and outcome of previous pregnancies, and information about other family members with RTH syndrome.[55]

Hypothyroidism

Until 1980, few cases of pregnancy in women with myxedema were published because it was believed that most hypothyroid women were infertile. Soon after the determination of serum TSH became available to establish the diagnosis of hypothyroidism, a few series of hypothyroidism in pregnancy were described.[56-58] The incidence of hypothyroidism, defined at the time of these publications as an elevation in serum TSH above 5 mIU/L, was reported to be between 2% and 4%.[59] Mild elevations in serum TSH are detected in 50% to 60% of treated hypothyroid women soon after conception as the result of the increased demand for thyroid hormones in the first weeks of gestation. There are many unresolved and controversial issues about the management of hypothyroidism, the incidence of abnormal obstetrical outcomes, universal versus selective screening, and the need for L-thyroxine therapy in subclinical hypothyroidism.[60,61] Several topics related to hypothyroidism will be discussed separately under the following headings: (1) Etiology and Classification of Hypothyroidism, Subclinical Hypothyroidism, Clinical Hypothyroidism, Isolated Hypothyroxinemia, and Universal Versus Selective Screening.

Etiology and Classification of Hypothyroidism

The two most common etiologies of primary hypothyroidism in countries with sufficient dietary iodine supply are autoimmune thyroiditis (Hashimoto thyroiditis) and post-thyroid ablation therapy, either surgical or ^{131}I induced. Other causes include congenital (about 1 in 3000 births in the United States), drug induced (lithium, amiodarone, iodine excess, antithyroid drugs), prior head and neck radiation for nonthyroid malignant disease, and congenital defects in thyroid hormone biosynthesis. Transient forms of hypothyroidism, rarely seen during pregnancy, are painful subacute thyroiditis and silent thyroiditis; the latter is observed in postpartum thyroiditis. Earlier studies in women with "hypothyroxinemia," diagnosed as a low serum protein-bound iodine (serum TSH was not available for the diagnosis of hypothyroidism), reported a high incidence of congenital malformations, perinatal mortality, and impaired mental and somatic development in infants of hypothyroid women. In contrast, recent reports showed no increase in the incidence of congenital malformations. However, there is an increased risk for adverse pregnancy complications as well as detrimental effects on neurocognitive development of the offspring.[25,26] Secondary hypothyroidism includes diseases of the pituitary gland or hypothalamus. Autoimmune hypophysitis as a cause of secondary hypothyroidism is of interest to the obstetrician for its relationship to Sheehan syndrome.

Regardless of the etiology, primary hypothyroidism is classified as subclinical hypothyroidism (normal serum T_4 and elevated serum TSH) and overt or clinical hypothyroidism (low serum T_4 and elevated TSH). The spectrum of pregnant women diagnosed with hypothyroidism includes: (1) women with subclinical and overt hypothyroidism diagnosed for the first time during pregnancy; (2) hypothyroid women who discontinue thyroid therapy before or at the time of conception because of poor medical advice or because of the misconception that thyroid medications may affect the fetus; (3) women on thyroid replacement therapy requiring larger doses in pregnancy; (4) women previously diagnosed but not consistent in taking their medication; (5) hyperthyroid patients on excessive amounts of antithyroid drug therapy; and (6) some patients on lithium or amiodarone therapy because both drugs may affect thyroid function, particularly in women affected by chronic thyroiditis.

Subclinical Hypothyroidism

Most patients with subclinical hypothyroidism do not have symptoms. Thyroid tests may be requested by the physician because of vague symptoms resembling hypothyroidism, a past history of thyroid disease, a family history of thyroid disease, or findings in the physical examination such as the presence of a goiter. As discussed later, in women presenting for preconception counseling or at the time of the first obstetrical visit, a selective list of potential risk factors should be evaluated, and if any are positive, thyroid tests should be obtained. **Laboratory tests diagnostic of subclinical hypothyroidism are an elevated serum TSH in the presence of normal trimester-specific FT_4 levels.** A determination of TPOAbs is helpful to determine the etiology of hypothyroidism because they are present in 70% to 80% of hypothyroid patients of childbearing age. As mentioned earlier under Thyroid Function Tests, normal values for serum TSH are gestation-specific reference ranges, with an upper limit of normal of 2.5 mIU/L in the first trimester and up to 3 mIU/L in the second and third trimesters.[28] A significant number of hypothyroid women on thyroid replacement therapy are euthyroid before conception but become hypothyroid, most of them subclinical, at the time of the first obstetrical visit because of the physiologic increase in the need for thyroid hormones in the first trimester of pregnancy.[31,32] In some studies, women with subclinical hypothyroidism are at risk for adverse pregnancy complications, such as miscarriage, preterm delivery, and preeclampsia.[58-63] Lower IQs in their infants and other neurocognitive deficits have been described.[25,26]

In 1993, Leung and colleagues reported on a group of 45 women diagnosed with subclinical hypothyroidism, defined at that time as a serum TSH of more than 5 mIU/L and normal FT_4I.[58] Of the 7 women developing preeclampsia, 4 had serum TSH levels between 5 and 10 mIU/L at booking.

Casey and associates[62] undertook a prospective thyroid screening study to evaluate pregnancy outcomes in women with subclinical hypothyroidism diagnosed before 20 weeks' gestation. The mean age of their patients was 26.9 years, and their ethnicity included 84% Hispanics; 7% African American, and 4% Caucasians. Their body mass index (kg/m^2) was 32.1 ± 6.3. Four hundred and four women (2.3% of the 17,298 screened) were considered to have subclinical hypothyroidism. Compared with euthyroid women, pregnancies of women with subclinical hypothyroidism were three times more likely to be complicated by placental abruption (relative risk [RR], 3.0; 95% CI, 1.1 to 8.2); preterm birth (before 34 weeks' gestation) was almost twofold higher (RR, 1.8; 95% CI, 1.1 to 2.9); and admission of their newborns to the neonatal intensive care nursery and respiratory distress was twice as likely (RR, 1.8; 95% CIs, 1.1 to 2.9 and 1.0 to 3.3, respectively).

On the contrary, Cleary-Goldman and colleagues[63] reported no adverse outcomes in a group of 247 women with subclinical hypothyroidism diagnosed on the basis of a serum TSH more than the 97.5th percentile and free T_4 between the 2.5th and 97.5th percentiles. They included 10,990 women from the FASTER Trial, a National Institute of Child Health and Human Development (NICHD)-sponsored study. They included several centers in the United States; 86% of the women were Caucasian, 1.7% African American, and 7.2 % Hispanics. Serum TSH values between 0.004 and 0.035 mIU/L represented values less than the 2.5th percentile in the first trimester, and a FT_4 less than the 2.5th percentile was reported at between 0.3 and 0.71 ng/dL. Their conclusion was that "maternal thyroid hypofunction is not associated with adverse outcomes."

In a recent randomized study by Negro and colleagues[64] in southern Italy, 4657 women were screened for serum TSH and TPOAbs within the first 11 weeks of gestation. Of this group, 642 women presented with a serum TSH between 2.5 and 5 mIU/L and negative TPOAbs. The pregnancy loss rate was 6.1%, compared with 127 of 3481 (3.6%) in women with a serum TSH below 2.5 (P = .006). All the pregnancy losses were due to miscarriages. There were no significant differences in preterm deliveries or other obstetrical outcomes between the groups. None of the patients with an elevated TSH received L-thyroxine therapy. Of note, Kuppens and coworkers[65] reported an increased risk for breech presentation in women with TSH levels above 2.5 mIU/L at the end of gestation.

There are no published randomized prospective studies at the present time on the effect of L-thyroxine treatment of subclinical hypothyroidism in women early in pregnancy, on pregnancy outcome, or on the neurodevelopment of their offspring. Two large population-based studies are underway. One of them, in the United Kingdom, includes 22,000 pregnant women recruited before 16 weeks' gestation. Mothers diagnosed with hypothyroidism or hypothyroxinemia will be randomized to L-thyroxine therapy versus placebo; the outcome end point of the study will be the percentage of children with an IQ of less than 85 at 3.5 years of age, comparing children from both groups and a control group. The second study should be completed by 2015. It is organized by the NICHD and includes a total of 120,000 pregnant women from 14 institutions in the United States. In this randomized study, women with subclinical hypothyroidism or hypothyroxinemia will receive L-thyroxine or placebo, and the obstetrical outcome and the neurocognitive function of the offspring will be evaluated.

Negro and colleagues[66] reported the results in a subset of first-trimester women recruited as part of a study evaluating universal screening versus case finding for the detection of thyroid dysfunction. Patients were grouped in a high-risk and a low-risk group according to risk factors for thyroid disease. An adverse obstetrical outcome was the end point of the study. In those women considered low risk, rates of pregnancy-related adverse events were reduced by nearly 40% after detection and treatment.[67]

Clinical Hypothyroidism

The clinical diagnosis of hypothyroidism in pregnancy is confirmed by the presence of an elevated serum TSH and an FT_4 below the trimester-specific reference range. Patients with overt hypothyroidism may complain of tiredness, cold intolerance, fatigue, muscle cramps, constipation, irregular menstrual periods, infertility, and deepening of the voice. On physical examination, the skin may be dry and cold, deep tendon reflexes may be delayed, and bradycardia may be detected as well as periorbital edema. A goiter is present in almost 80% of patients in whom the etiology is chronic thyroiditis. The characteristic goiter is a diffuse enlargement of the thyroid gland, about two to three times the normal size, firm to palpation, painless, and with a rubbery consistency. In the other 20% of women with chronic thyroiditis, no goiter is found (*atrophic thyroiditis*, also known as primary myxedema or chronic thyroiditis without goiter). A well-healed scar in the neck is seen in those patients with prior surgical thyroidectomy. The degree of severity of the clinical symptoms varies with the thyroid abnormalities on testing, although there is not always good correlation between clinical and chemical parameters. It is important to emphasize that many patients with frank hypothyroidism by laboratory tests offer no specific complaints. Spontaneous pregnancies have been reported in newly diagnosed women with a serum TSH higher than 150 mIU/L at the time of the first obstetrical visit![57]

Early studies had used a serum TSH above 5 to 6 mIU/L for diagnostic purposes, with normal values derived from a healthy nonpregnant population. In our own series,[58] the mean TSH value at the time of diagnosis of overt hypothyroidism was 89.7 + 86.2 mIU/mL (normal, 0.4 to 5.0), with a mean FT_4I of 2.1 + 1.5 (normal, 4.5 to 12). **Serum thyroid antibodies (TPOAbs, also known as antimicrosomal antibodies), are elevated in almost 95% of patients with autoimmune hypothyroidism.** Serum antithyroglobulin antibodies (TGAbs) are elevated in about 60% of patients with chronic thyroiditis; in a few patients, about 5%, TGAb is the only antibody present. The titer of antibodies does not correlate with the size of the goiter or the clinical severity of hypothyroidism but could be a predictor for the development of postpartum thyroiditis.

As in the case of hyperthyroidism, untreated overt hypothyroidism is associated with adverse neonatal outcomes, including premature birth, SGA infants, and in one study, an increased prevalence of fetal death. **One of the most common obstetrical complications is PIH, with an incidence of 21% in a combined study of 60 patients with overt hypothyroidism.**[57,58] PIH has not been reported in all series, although some of them were retrospective analyses. In some series, a higher incidence of PIH was reported in euthyroid women on thyroid replacement therapy. Low birthweight was detected in 16.6% of births, mostly related to preterm delivery. In one series,[57] 2 of 12 women with subclinical hypothyroidism developed postpartum hemorrhage. Abalovich and associates reported on 150 pregnancies in 114 hypothyroid women. Sixteen of these women were overtly hypothyroid at conception, 60% of them suffered a spontaneous abortion, and 20% of them had a premature delivery; all women properly treated carried their pregnancy to term.

The impact of maternal hypothyroidism on the intellectual development of the offspring has been the subject of several studies.[25,26] In the report by Haddow and coworkers,[25] children born to untreated mothers with elevations of serum TSH, measured between 16 and 18 weeks' gestation, were studied at age 7 to 9 years. They reported a seven-point decrease in IQ score on the Wechsler Intelligence Scale for Children and delays in motor, language, and attention. Nineteen percent of children of untreated mothers had an IQ below 75. In another study from Japan, Lui and colleagues examined a group of eight children at ages 4 and 10. IQs were compared in children whose mothers were hypothyroid in the first trimester, with their siblings when the mothers were euthyroid throughout gestation. There was no difference in the IQs of both groups of children. Mann and colleagues had reported lower IQs in children from a group of mothers considered hypothyroxinemic in pregnancy (serum TSH was not available at the time of the study). When they were studied at age 7 years, 5 of 21 (24%) had an IQ of less than 80, compared with a low IQ found in 10% of control children.

These earlier studies appear to support earlier animal research showing the importance of maternal transfer of T_4 in the first trimester of pregnancy, at a time when the fetal thyroid had not yet developed. From a practical point of view, these reports emphasize the importance of diagnosing thyroid insufficiency in women at risk for thyroid disease and promptly adjusting the dose of T_4 in women under treatment for hypothyroidism soon after conception.

Isolated Hypothyroxinemia

The term *isolated hypothyroxinemia* is reserved for those patients in areas of sufficient dietary intake with below trimester-specific FT_4 reference range in the presence of normal serum TSH values. The physiopathologic explanation for such an entity is not clear; maternal hypothyroxinemia is extremely frequent in endemic areas of iodine deficiency and is associated with increased perinatal morbidity and mortality and an increased incidence of hypothyroidism in neonates as well.[68] It is rare in nonendemic iodine-deficient areas. Pop and coworkers detected a lower Bayley Psychomotor Developmental Index at 10 months of age in a small group of children born to mothers with low FT_4 but normal TSH (hypothyroxinemia) at 12 weeks' gestation. They extended their studies to infants aged 1 to 2 years, reporting an 8 to 10 point deficit in psychomotor testing among offspring born to mothers with low FT_4 levels in the first 24 weeks of their pregnancies; babies whose mothers had a spontaneous normalization of FT_4 after 24 weeks' gestation had normal development, suggesting that prolonged hypothyroxinemia was the cause of impairment of fetal neural development. Recently, two reports from iodine-sufficient countries reaffirmed the adverse role of maternal hypothyroxinemia in neuropsychological development of children. Li and colleagues collected serum from 1268 women at 16 to 20 weeks' gestation, selected from a cohort of women who underwent screening for Down syndrome at Shenyang Maternal and Neonatal Health Clinic, in an area described as "iodine sufficient." Serum TSH, TT_4, FT_4, and TPOAb were measured. Women with other medical conditions were excluded from the study. Gestation-specific reference ranges were determined from a control group of 120 healthy pregnant women randomly selected from the enrolled cohort group; three groups of patients were identified, and intellectual and motor development scores were evaluated in the children from these pregnancies at 25 to 30 months of age, using the Bayley Scales of Infant Development. Eighteen women (1.8%) were diagnosed as having subclinical hypothyroidism; 19 women were hypothyroxinemic (1.5%), and 34 (2.6%) were euthyroid with an elevated level of TPOAbs. The authors concluded that maternal subclinical hypothyroidism, hypothyroxinemia, and euthyroidism with elevated serum TPOAb titers are all statistically significant predictors of lower motor and intellectual development at 25 to 30 months. Henrichs and colleagues,[26] in a population-based cohort study in the Netherlands, studied a group of pregnant women at about 13 weeks' gestation with severe hypothyroxinemia, defined as FT_4 concentrations below the 10th and 5th percentiles, respectively. Verbal and nonverbal cognitive development was assessed at 18 and 30 months of age in their children. Expressive vocabulary at 18 months was assessed by the MacArthur Communicative Development Inventory, and at 30 months, mothers were asked to complete the Language Development Survey. Of the mothers in this study, 1.5% had hypothyroidism, 8.5% had mild hypothyroxinemia, and 4.3% had severe hypothyroxinemia. The authors observed that mild and severe hypothyroxinemia were associated with a higher risk for expressive language delay across all ages (mild: OR = 1.44; 95% CI = 1.09 to 1.91; $P = .010$, and severe: OR = 1.8; 95% CI = 1.24 to 2.61; $P = .002$). Severe maternal hypothyroxinemia predicted a higher risk for both verbal and nonverbal cognitive delay (OR = 2.03; 95% CI = 1.22 to 3.93; $P = .007$). It is of interest in this study that a significant percentage of women had hypothyroxinemia, a total of 12.8%, compared with 1.5% with hypothyroidism. Perhaps iodine deficiency in this population could be the explanation for the high incidence of hypothyroxinemia. Hypothyroxinemia was observed in 0.9% of 2899 women tested between 4 and 12 weeks' gestation by Wang and coworkers in China, with a median urinary iodine level of 177.15 mcg/L, well within the accepted range in areas of iodine sufficiency. No adverse obstetrical outcomes were reported by Casey and associates[69] in evaluating 17,289 women before 20 weeks' gestation; the prevalence of hypothyroxinemia was 1% and subclinical hypothyroidism 3%: Cleary-Goldman and colleagues[63] reported a prevalence of hypothyroxinemia of 2.1% (232 of 10,990 women) in the first trimester and 2.3% in the second trimester of pregnancy.

Universal versus Selective Screening for Thyroid Disease

Despite the potential obstetrical and offspring complications due to maternal thyroid dysfunction reported in the past 50 years, the consistency of reports on the incidence of maternal subclinical and clinical hypothyroidism in the first trimester, and our recognized difficulty in diagnosing the disease, both by medical history and physical examination, **when and how to screen for thyroid disease in pregnant and nonpregnant individuals remains a very controversial issue, with different positions adapted by several medical organizations.** A consensus Development Conference regarding subclinical thyroid disease was sponsored by the American Association of Clinical Endocrinologist, the ATA, and the Endocrine Society. Their recommendation, based on an extensive review of the published literature available at that time, limited thyroid tests to women at high risk for thyroid disease[70]; the Committee on Obstetric Practice of the American College of Obstetricians and Gynecologists, in 2007, stated that "without evidence that identification and treatment of pregnant women with subclinical hypothyroidism improves maternal or infant outcomes, routine screening for subclinical hypothyroidism currently is not recommended." **It is reasonable to perform a determination of serum TSH at the first obstetrical visit in those women at higher risk for thyroid dysfunction** (Table 40-7). In the revised version of the Endocrine Society Guidelines (in preparation), and the ATA Clinical Guidelines for Thyroid and Pregnancy,[70a] universal screening is not recommended, but it is strongly suggested that health care professionals personally ask during preconception counseling or in the first obstetrical visit about risk factors for thyroid disease. The main barrier to universal screening is the lack of RCTs demonstrating a reversal of both obstetrical and intellectual abnormalities in the offspring after normalization of thyroid deficiency by maternal L-thyroxine replacement therapy.

Several studies have consistently demonstrated the failure to recognize women at risk for thyroid dysfunction when using a case-finding strategy, based on actual thyroid dysfunction symptoms, a personal or family history of thyroid disease, and past obstetrical history.

Vaidya and coworkers[71] offered thyroid function tests early in pregnancy to 1560 women to evaluate the effectiveness of universal screening versus case finding. They showed that targeted screening would still have missed about one third of all pregnant women with an elevated serum TSH. They divided women early in pregnancy into two groups: a low-risk group, which included 75% of the women; and a high-risk group, including the remaining

TABLE 40-7 INDICATIONS FOR THYROID TESTING IN PREGNANCY

1. History of thyroid dysfunction or prior thyroid surgery
2. Age >30 years
3. Symptoms of thyroid dysfunction or the presence of goiter
4. Thyroid peroxidase antibody positive
5. Type I diabetes or other autoimmune disorders
6. History of head/neck radiation
7. Family history of thyroid dysfunction
8. Morbid obesity (body mass index ≥40 kg/m^2)
9. Use of amiodarone or lithium, or recent administration of iodinated radiologic contrast
10. Unexplained fertility
11. Residing in an area of known moderate to severe iodine sufficiency

Stagnaro-Green A et al: Guidelines of the American Thyroid Association for the Diagnosis and Management of Thyroid Disease During Pregnancy and Postpartum. Thyroid 21:1081, 2011.

25%. The high-risk group included those with a personal and family history of thyroid disorders or other autoimmune disease and current and past treatment with antithyroid drugs, L-thyroxine, radioiodine, or thyroid surgery. Forty women, 2.6% of the total group, had an elevated serum TSH, and 70% of them were in the high-risk group.

Similar conclusions have been reported in other studies. Wang and coworkers performed thyroid tests in the first trimester of pregnancy and classified 367 (12.7%) women out of 2899 as high risk, following the recommendations of the Endocrine Society Guidelines.[28] Of the 2899, 294 had thyroid dysfunction: hypothyroidism in 7.5% (most of them with subclinical hypothyroidism); 1% hyperthyroidism, and 0.9% hypothyroxinemia. Positive antibodies were detected in 279 (9.6%), and 196 of them were euthyroid. The prevalence of thyroid dysfunction in the high-risk group was higher than in the low-risk group (15% vs. 9.4%; $P = .001$). However, of the 217 women with an elevated serum TSH, 171 (78.8%) belonged to the low-risk group. The authors concluded that a case-finding strategy for screening thyroid function in the high-risk group would miss about 81.6% of women with an elevated serum TSH and 80.4% women with hyperthyroidism. Horacek and colleagues, in a study from the Czech Republic, concluded that more than 55% of pregnant women at risk would be missed if only those with high-risk criteria were examined. The authors stated that a more extensive screening of thyroid autoimmunity and dysfunction seems warranted.

Negro and colleagues[66] reported on a prospective randomized study of 4562 women in southern Italy. Thyroid tests were done very early in pregnancy. Their conclusion was that universal screening did not affect the rate of adverse events in comparison to targeted high-risk case finding, implying a negative outcome. As discussed in the section on Subclinical Hypothyroidism, in the same article by Negro and colleagues, a subgroup of low-risk patients detected to be hypothyroid were treated with L-thyroxine and compared with a nontreated group. The rate of pregnancy-related adverse events was reduced by nearly 40% after detection and treatment.

A cost-effectiveness approach comparing universal screening and case finding was reported in two studies, both concluding that universal screening is cost-effective compared with a case-finding strategy.[72] However, Thung and colleagues added in their conclusions that a wide range of circumstances should be considered before universal screening is adapted. The same position was voiced by Stagnaro-Green and Schwartz.

There are a number of barriers before universal routine thyroid function screening can be recommended in pregnancy.[73] They include the selection of thyroid tests to be used (TSH, FT_4, TPOAb), the threshold applied to characterize an abnormality, weeks of gestation, appropriate intervention, and monitoring. The second issue still in dispute is the management of hypothyroid women in the preconceptional period. It is accepted that most of these women will need an increase in the L-thyroxine dose soon after conception.[31,32] It could be argued whether the target of serum TSH between 0.3 to 2.5 mIU/L before pregnancy is reasonable in anticipation of the increase in T_4 requirements. Abalovich and associates[74] reported that when the serum TSH is below 1.3 mIU/L before conception, only 17% of women need an increase in L-thyroxine in the first trimester. It has also been recommended that women on L-thyroxine therapy be advised at the time of confirmation of pregnancy to increase their dose empirically by two doses a week until the results of the thyroid tests are available.[32]

Therefore, until the British study and the NICHD Maternal-Fetal Medicine Units Network studies are completed, the issue of universal screening and L-thyroxine treatment for women with subclinical hypothyroidism or euthyroid chronic thyroiditis diagnosed before conception or during pregnancy is open for discussion. **The practicing physician should decide based on his or her own clinical practice whether universal screening versus case finding is warranted, and which women may benefit from T_4 therapy.**

Euthyroid Chronic or Hashimoto Thyroiditis

Chronic or Hashimoto thyroiditis[75] is a benign inflammatory disorder of the thyroid gland, the incidence depending on the definition of the entity. For example, in a long-term follow-up study in the Whickham survey, the incidence in women was 3.5 cases per 1000 per year, as contrasted with an incidence in men of 0.8 case per 1000 per year. The prevalence increases with age. In most cases, there is a family history of thyroid disease, with 18% of relatives affected in one study. **Chronic autoimmune thyroid disease is more common in women with other autoimmune diseases, particularly type 1 diabetes.**

With the advent of more sensitive assays for the determination of anti-TPO antibodies, the prevalence of chronic thyroiditis in women of childbearing age is estimated to be between 5% and 20%, depending on the type of population. The classic clinical picture is characterized by the presence of a goiter, moderate in size, bilateral in most cases, with one lobe larger than the other, with a firm, rubbery consistency, and moving freely on swallowing. It is painless, although rapid growth of the gland may elicit some tenderness on palpation. Absence of goiter (atrophic thyroiditis) may be present in 20% to 30% of patients.

On presentation, patients have no symptoms of thyroid dysfunction. A goiter is discovered on routine physical examination or detected by the patient herself or a family member or acquaintance. The diagnosis may be suggested by a hyperechoic pattern on an ultrasound of the thyroid gland. The diagnosis is confirmed by the presence of thyroid autoantibodies (anti-TPO or antithyroglobulin autoantibodies). The actual antibody titer is not correlated with the size of the goiter, symptoms, or severity of the disease. From a practical point of view, there is no need to perform a determination of TGAb if TPOAb are positive. Serum TSH should be ordered to rule out thyroid dysfunction. If the serum TSH is elevated, a serum FT_4 will determine whether the patient suffers from subclinical or clinical hypothyroidism (see earlier section, Hypothyroidism). Patients with euthyroid chronic thyroiditis may develop hypothyroidism over time. The OR was 8 over 20 years in those women with a normal serum TSH and positive antibodies.[34]

The importance of diagnosing chronic thyroiditis in women of childbearing age relates to the potential consequences in pregnancy and the postpartum period.

Women with chronic thyroiditis known to be euthyroid should be evaluated early in pregnancy because they are at risk for developing hypothyroidism de novo, miscarriages, prematurity (according to some studies), and breech presentation.[76]

In a rare situation, women with chronic thyroiditis, particularly those without a goiter, the atrophic form, may have high titers of serum TSHRAb, blocking antibodies (TRAb), compared with the stimulating antibodies present in women with Graves hyperthyroidism. These antibodies cross the placenta and, at high titers, block the fetal TSH receptor, causing transient congenital hypothyroidism.[77] The neonatal disease resolves spontaneously over 3 to 6 months as the maternal antibody is degraded. In a large population of patients screened in New York, of 788 infants with suspected congenital hypothyroidism, 9 mothers and their infants had these antibodies.[78] Therefore, in mothers who have given birth to infants with congenital hypothyroidism, thyroid tests, including TRAb, should be determined.

In 1990, Stagnaro-Green and colleagues[76] reported a twofold to threefold increased risk for spontaneous abortion in euthyroid women with positive thyroid autoantibodies, studies confirmed by later publications. One of the caveats in the early studies was that the upper normal range for serum TSH values was up to 5 mIU/L, compared with the accepted value of up to 2.5 mIU/L recommended by recent guidelines; therefore it is possible that some of the reported TPOAb-positive pregnant women had subclinical hypothyroidism. Prematurity and its relationship to thyroid autoimmunity was recently reviewed by Stagnaro-Green, who concluded that preterm delivery was associated with the presence of thyroid antibodies in three out of four reports from Belgium, Italy, Japan, and Pakistan. Haddow and coworkers[79] reported on the relationship between preterm delivery in euthyroid TPOAb-positive women studied late in the first trimester from the FASTER trial. The authors did not confirm previous studies of an association between preterm delivery and euthyroid chronic thyroiditis. They reported, however, a significant increase in preterm premature rupture of the membranes in the TPOAb-positive euthyroid group and concluded that from the six studies published, four of them reviewed by Stagnaro-Green, the evidence for a relationship between preterm delivery and chronic thyroiditis was not conclusive. The relationship was reported in three and refuted in the other three reports. Mannisto and associates,[80] in a prospective study including 9247 singleton pregnancies in Finland, found that the presence of TPOAbs in the first trimester was a risk factor for perinatal death, but not thyroid hormones status as such. In a group of 288 TPOAb-positive women, there was a twofold to threefold greater perinatal mortality than in antibody-negative mothers; four of seven perinatal deaths occurred preterm, before 28 weeks' gestation. Regarding the therapeutic use of L-thyroxine in women with euthyroid chronic thyroiditis (normal serum TSH and positive TPO antibodies), there is only one published study.[81] The authors performed thyroid tests including TPOAbs in a group of 984 women early in pregnancy; 113 (11.7%) of them were TPOAb positive, with normal serum TSH values (reference range, 0.27 to 4.2 mIU/L). Their first obstetrical visit was at 10.3 ± 3.1 weeks. Fifty-seven TPOAb-positive women were treated with L-thyroxine, with a dose between 0.5 and 1 mcg/kg per day according to TSH values and TPOAb titers. They were compared with 58 untreated TPOAb-positive women and a control group of TPOAb-negative women. Two end points were evaluated: the incidences of miscarriage and preterm delivery. The L-thyroxine-treated group had an incidence of complications similar to that of the control group, whereas the untreated chronic thyroiditis group had a threefold increase in miscarriages and preterm deliveries and in addition developed impaired thyroid function in the second half of pregnancy.

Pregnancy outcome in TPOAb-positive women was recently reported from the University of Texas Southwestern Medical Center,[82] the same population studied previously.[63] All women were screened before 20 weeks' gestation, at a mean gestational age of 11.9 weeks. Six percent of these women were TPOAb positive. As expected, the incidence in women with overt or clinical hypothyroidism was 61%, 31% in women with subclinical hypothyroidism, 5% in hypothyroxinemia, and 4% in euthyroid women. Of the entire cohort of women with positive antibodies, they were significantly older (P <.001), weighed more, and were more often parous than TPO-negative women. African American women had an incidence significantly lower than Hispanic and Caucasian women. The authors reported that the incidence of hypertensive disorders, diabetes, preterm birth, preterm premature rupture of the membranes, and cesarean delivery were not significantly different either before or after adjustment for demographic differences. The exception was the incidence of placental abruption; euthyroid TPOAb-positive women had a fourfold increased incidence compared with similar euthyroid TPOAb-negative women (OR = 4.0; 95% CI, 1.9 to 8.6). Of the 10 women with placental abruption who were TPOAb positive, 7 had euthyroid neonates. This finding and the rate of preterm birth were not significantly different between the two groups. Furthermore, they analyzed their observation of obstetrical and neonatal complications in subclinical hypothyroid women[63] and concluded that women with subclinical hypothyroidism and positive TPOAb were not at further increased risk for adverse outcomes, with the only exception being placental abruption. They recognized that their findings were not confirmed in other, similar studies.[62,81]

There is also agreement in the literature that the presence of TPOAb in the first trimester of pregnancy is a risk factor for the development of postpartum thyroiditis (see later section, Postpartum Thyroid Dysfunction).

Treatment of Hypothyroidism

L-Thyroxine is the drug of choice for the treatment of hypothyroidism. **In view of the complications mentioned previously, it is important to normalize thyroid tests as early as possible before conception or soon after the diagnosis of pregnancy.** In women on L-thyroxine replacement therapy, how much the dose will need to be increased from prepregnancy levels depends on the etiology of hypothyroidism.[83] The authors reported an increase in L-thyroxine dose of 16% by the second trimester in patients with primary hypothyroidism and a 51% increase following ablation therapy for Graves disease by surgery or ^{131}I therapy. For patients with a history of thyroid cancer, the increase was 21% by the second trimester, depending on the level of TSH suppression recommended for cancer patients. In newly diagnosed pregnant women, an initial dose of 100 mcg of L-thyroxine is well tolerated by most young hypothyroid patients. The dose may be calculated according to body weight (2 to 2.4 mcg/kg per day), a dose higher than recommended in nonpregnant patients (1.7 to 2 mcg/kg per day). In patients with severe hypothyroidism, there is a delay in the normalization of serum TSH, but normal serum FT_4 or FT_4I values are achieved in the first 2 weeks of therapy if sufficient L-thyroxine is administered. The maintenance dose required for most patients is between 75 and 250 mcg of L-thyroxine per day.

Women planning their pregnancies should have a serum TSH below 2.5 mIU/L, ideally closer to 1 mIU/L, given the greater requirements expected early in gestation. The serum TSH should be repeated every 2 to 6 weeks during the first 20 weeks' gestation and at 24 to 28 weeks' and at 32 to 34 weeks' gestation. The aim is to keep serum TSH, as well as serum FT_4 or FT_4I, within normal trimester-specific reference ranges. The T_4 dose should be adjusted. Increased thyroid requirements are seen in about 20% to 30% of patients in the second half of pregnancy. Immediately after delivery, patients should return to their prepregnancy dose. Interference in the absorption of T_4 was discussed previously.[28]

Single Nodule of the Thyroid Gland

The incidence of thyroid nodularity in pregnancy was studied by several groups using ultrasonography. The three studies available were done in Belgium, Germany, and China in areas of mild iodine deficiency, where the incidence of thyroid nodules is increased. They examined the frequency of nodules, the effect of progression of pregnancy on nodule size, and new nodule formation. Together, they showed a prevalence of 3% to 23%, the incidence higher with increasing parity. In one prospective study of 212 Chinese women, the incidence of thyroid nodules was 15.3%. None of them was malignant. The mean diameter of the nodules was 5.1 mm in the first, 5.1 mm in the second, and 5.5 mm in the third trimesters. Struve and associates in Germany showed that increasing age and parity were associated with an increase in the number of thyroid nodules. In the Belgium study, 20 women, TPOAb negative, were diagnosed with thyroid nodular disease early in pregnancy. Although it was reported that 60% of the nodules increased in size with progression of pregnancy, the final nodule size was between 5 and 12 mm, making them difficult to recognize on thyroid palpation.

It is estimated that nodular thyroid disease is clinically detectable in 10% of pregnant women. In most cases, it is discovered during the first routine clinical examination or detected by the patient herself. The probability for a single or solitary thyroid nodule to be malignant is between 5% and 10% depending on risk factors such as previous radiation therapy to the head, neck, or chest; rapid growth of a painless nodule; patient age; and family history of thyroid cancer. Papillary carcinoma accounts for almost 75% to 80% of malignant tumors, and follicular neoplasm for 15% to 20%; a few percent are represented by medullary thyroid carcinoma. Undifferentiated thyroid carcinoma is extremely rare in patients younger than 50 years.

The incidence of thyroid carcinoma in the general population has risen significantly in the past two decades, perhaps because of the increased detection of small papillary cancers, from 3.6 per 100,000 in 1973 to 8.7 per 100,000 in 2002, a 2.4-fold increase (95% CI, 2.2 to 2.6; $P < .001$ for trend). In part, this increase could be explained by the routine use of thyroid ultrasonography.

It is estimated that as many as 14 of every 100,000 pregnancies in the United States are complicated by a new diagnosis of thyroid cancer. In a retrospective study from the California Cancer Registry from 1991 to1999, 129 cases of thyroid cancer were diagnosed during pregnancy: 3.3 per 100,00 diagnosed before pregnancy; 0.3 per 100,000 at the time of delivery and 10.8 per 100,000 within 1 year after delivery. In a selective group of patients operated on during or in the few months after delivery, the incidence of thyroid cancer was reported to be near 40%. In both studies, fine-needle aspiration biopsy (FNAB) of the thyroid nodule was obtained before surgery, with findings consistent with papillary carcinoma or a highly suspicious lesion. In this and other studies, patients were referred for management of potential malignant nodules and do not represent the true incidence of malignant thyroid tumors in pregnancy.

There is a paucity of information in the literature regarding the management and timing of the workup in the presence of thyroid nodularity. The ATA management guidelines for patients with thyroid nodules and differentiated thyroid carcinoma[84] recommended a similar evaluation of thyroid nodules in pregnancy as for the nonpregnant patient, with the exception, of course, that a radionuclide scan is contraindicated. In the presence of a thyroid nodule, they stressed the importance of a careful medical history, including a family history of malignant thyroid disease. If the family history is positive for familial medullary thyroid carcinoma or multiple endocrine neoplasia type 2, the evaluation of the nodule and management requires a more aggressive approach.

Careful examination of the neck enables the physician to define and characterize the thyroid lesion (Figure 40-5). In addition to the size of the nodule, the consistency, tenderness, fixation to the skin, and presence of metastasis in the thyroid bed should be noted. A hard, painless nodule, measuring more than 2 cm in diameter, is suspicious of malignancy. Thyroid, serum TSH, and FT_4 need to be assessed. A suppressed or undetectable TSH value in the presence of a single or dominant thyroid nodule is consistent with an autonomous or "hot" thyroid nodule, rarely malignant, in which case FNAB is not indicated. Interpretation of TSH values requires caution because a low or suppressed value may be present in a number of pregnancies in the first trimester. Serum calcitonin determination is reserved for patients with a family history of medullary thyroid carcinoma.[84] High-resolution real-time ultrasound, in expert hands, is very helpful in defining the size of the lesion, characterizing the dominant nodule in a multinodular gland, and identifying characteristics of the lesion suspicious for malignancy—solid, cystic, or mixed; microcalcifications; a hypoechoic pattern; irregular margins, among other findings. If FNAB of the nodule is indicated,

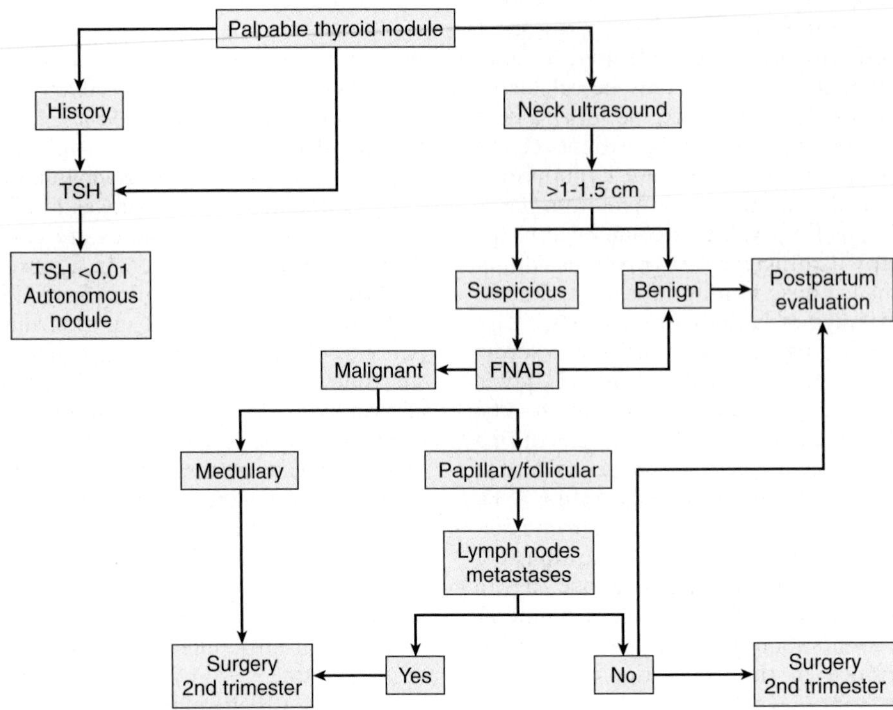

FIGURE 40-5. American Thyroid Association clinical guidelines for thyroid and pregnancy. *FNAB,* Fine-needle aspiration biopsy; *TSH,* thyroid-stimulating hormone.

pregnancy is not a contraindication and may be performed at any time during gestation, irrespective of gestational age. The importance of a competent cytopathologist in the interpretation and diagnosis of the specimens cannot be overemphasized. Radionuclide scanning is contraindicated in pregnancy, because of the risk for damaging the fetal thyroid gland, causing fetal and neonatal hypothyroidism. If performed before 12 weeks' gestation, the procedure does not affect the fetal thyroid gland because the fetal thyroid starts to incorporate iodine by 14 to 18 weeks' gestation.

In the presence of a single thyroid nodule detected on physical examination, or a dominant nodule in a multinodular gland, the following approach is recommended by the ATA Clinical Guidelines for Thyroid and Pregnancy[70a] (see Figure 40-5):

1. In the presence of a solid lesion smaller than 1 to 1.5 cm, follow up in the postpartum period is indicated.
2. Nodules larger than 1 to 1.5 cm should be considered for FNAB if there are suspicious findings on ultrasound.
3. In the presence of tracheal obstruction, immediate surgery is indicated.
4. If the FNAB is diagnostic of malignancy or it is a suspicious lesion, surgery may be postponed until after delivery, unless there are lymph node metastases or the diagnosis is a large primary lesion, or there is extensive lymph node involvement in a medullary cancer.
5. Surgery can be postponed until after delivery during the last weeks of pregnancy, and FNAB could be safely postponed until after delivery.
6. A woman with a malignant lesion or a rapidly growing lesion should be offered surgery in the second trimester of gestation.
7. Women with follicular lesions or early-stage papillary carcinoma may postpone the surgery until they are postpartum because these lesions are not expected to progress rapidly.

When advising pregnant women on the evaluation of a thyroid nodule, it has to be kept in mind that the incidence of malignancy is between 5% and 10%, and in most cases, the tumors are slow growing. As will be discussed, most published studies showed no evidence that the course of the disease or survival rate was affected when surgery was postponed until after delivery. On the other hand, knowing the result of the FNAB could be helpful to the mother in planning the postpartum course, including decisions about lactation and ^{131}I therapy if needed after the resection of the cancer.

It is generally agreed that elective surgery should be avoided in the first trimester and after 24 weeks' gestation because of the potential risks for spontaneous abortion and premature delivery, respectively. The recommendations for total thyroidectomy in the second trimester, based on clinical experience, is to avoid unnecessary exposure to the embryo to anesthetic drugs and to avoid potential prematurity due to surgery. However, there is not a well-controlled study supporting such recommendations.[85] One report showed a higher risk for complications from thyroid and parathyroid surgery during pregnancy. Thyroidectomy during pregnancy was associated with a complication rate of 21% compared with 8% for malignant lesions and of 27% compared with 14% for benign lesions. This was a retrospective, cross-sectional analysis of hospital discharge data. Complications included suspected fetal compromise, abortion, and cesarean delivery and hysterectomy. A skilled surgeon with ample experience in thyroid surgery should perform the procedure.

In the presence of papillary carcinoma without evidence of advanced disease or significant tumor growth (>50% on ultrasonography), surgical treatment may be postponed until after delivery. Follicular neoplasms or Hürthle cell neoplasms have a risk for malignancy of about 15% to 25%; in cases reported as follicular lesions or atypia, the malignancy rate is up to 10%, and surgery could be postponed safely until the postpartum period.

In one retrospective study, a conservative approach to the management of a single thyroid nodule was recommended.[86] In this report, 61 women were pregnant at the time of the diagnosis of differentiated thyroid carcinoma. The diagnoses were papillary cancer in 87% and follicular cancer in 13%. Fourteen women were operated on during pregnancy, whereas the other 47 women underwent surgical treatment 1 to 84 months after delivery. The outcome was compared with a group of 598 nonpregnant women matched for age. The median follow-up was 22.4 years, compared with 19.5 years in the nonpregnant group. Treatment and outcome were similar in both groups: those operated on during pregnancy and those in whom thyroidectomy was performed postpartum. The authors concluded that both diagnostic studies and initial therapy might be delayed until after delivery in most patients. Yasmeen and associates reviewed cancer registry data, comparing disease-related survival in 6505 women diagnosed with thyroid cancer during pregnancy or 1 year after delivery. There was no significant difference in outcome up to 11 years later compared with an age-matched nonpregnant cohort.

In a recent report, 15 women diagnosed with thyroid cancer during pregnancy or within 1 year postpartum were compared with 61 women matched for age whose cancer was treated before pregnancy. The authors reported that women diagnosed in pregnancy or in the first year postpartum are more likely to have persistent or recurrent disease and suggested that estrogen may play a role in these poorer outcomes because a higher percentage of women diagnosed during pregnancy or 1 year after delivery were estrogen receptor-α positive compared with women diagnosed 1 year after pregnancy or never pregnant.[86]

Therefore, it is imperative for the attending physician to discuss the different therapeutic options with the patient and her family. If the lesion is diagnosed before 24 weeks' gestation, they should be informed of the data showing no deleterious effect on postponing therapy until after delivery. The anxiety of the patient and her family and their wishes should be considered in making the final decision. The long-term prognosis of most thyroid cancers is good, but patients should be followed for many years. General principles of care include the determination of serum thyroglobulin before surgery and at regular intervals thereafter; the decision to use radioactive iodine, which is indicated in selective cases for completeness of thyroid ablation; and the importance of thyroid therapy to maintain serum TSH within recommended ranges in order to prevent possible recurrence of the lesion.[84]

Patients with Known Thyroid Cancer before Pregnancy

Pregnancy does not appear to be a risk factor for recurrences in women with a previous history of treated thyroid cancer. In two earlier studies, there was no evidence of recurrence or progression of the disease during pregnancy.

Recently, Leboeuf and colleagues[88] published a retrospective analysis of 36 women who became pregnant a median of 4.3 years after initial therapy for differentiated thyroid carcinoma. They were evaluated a median of 4 months after delivery (0.1 to 1.7 years). Total thyroidectomy was performed in 80% of the patients and lobectomy in 20%. Twenty-four of the 36 patients were diagnosed with papillary carcinoma, 10 with a follicular variant of poorly differentiated thyroid cancer. Twenty-three of the patients received postsurgery ^{131}I therapy. Only 1 patient had metastases at diagnosis. Serum thyroglobulin values were available before and after pregnancy. Two women treated with thyroidectomy and radioactive iodine and 1 patient treated with thyroidectomy alone, whose serum thyroglobulin values were elevated before pregnancy, had new evidence of disease with an increase in thyroglobulin values and cervical nodes detected by ultrasonography. In 8 women, the serum thyroglobulin value was higher than the prepregnancy value, and 5 of them had no evidence of metastasis by ultrasonography or clinical examination. Unfortunately, the authors did not have complete data on TSH values during pregnancy in many of their patients. The authors concluded that pregnancy "is probably a mild stimulus to cancer growth as evidenced by minor disease progression in some patients with known structural disease before pregnancy." The changes also could be explained by the lack of TSH suppression during pregnancy because the data obtained on serum TSH were retrospective.

Hirsch and associates[89] evaluated 63 consecutive women for a total of 90 births, who were followed at their institution from 1992 to 2009 and had given birth at least once after total thyroidectomy plus ^{131}I in 58 for papillary thyroid cancer. Serum thyroglobulin values and neck ultrasound were compared before and after pregnancy. In this study, levels of serum TSH during pregnancy were correlated with disease persistence before pregnancy and disease progression during pregnancy. They concluded that pregnancy does not cause thyroid cancer recurrence in survivors who have no structural or biochemical evidence of disease persistence at the time of conception. Six of the 63 women showed disease progression during the first pregnancy, and 2 had disease progression only during the second pregnancy. An interesting finding was that a nonsuppressed TSH level during pregnancy did not stimulate disease progression during pregnancy, one of the concerns in Leboufs study. The conclusions from both studies indicate no progression of the disease in women free of disease before pregnancy. However, there is possibility of progression in those patients with evidence of residual cancer at the time of conception. Further studies are needed before a firm recommendation can be offered to patients.

Women on suppressive T_4 therapy for thyroid cancer before pregnancy may continue with therapy as long as the free T_4 remains within normal limits, following the recommendations by the ATA task force, of a serum TSH value between 0.1 and 0.5 mIU/L in women free of disease and of less than 0.1 mIU/L in those with persistent disease.[84] In women treated with ^{131}I therapy after thyroidectomy for thyroid cancer, there is a potential concern for future fertility and a risk for complications, mainly birth defects. Miscarriages, preterm delivery, stillbirth, and congenital abnormalities were not reported in a systemic review of the literature by Sawka and coworkers.[90] Irregular menses in the first year after treatment occurred in 27% of women following radioactive iodine treatment, and early menopause occurred in some women. Garsi and colleagues[91] reported on 483 patients exposed to ^{131}I treatment for thyroid carcinoma. The authors concluded that there is no evidence that exposure to radioiodine affects the outcome of subsequent pregnancies and offspring, even in women receiving cumulative radiation doses to the ovaries as high as 1 Gy. The authors cautioned, however, that adverse events could occur if thyroid function tests are not normalized at the time of conception, recommending postponing conception until the thyroid hormone status has been verified.

In men, there is a transient elevation of serum follicle-stimulating hormone, luteinizing hormone, and inhibin in the months following treatment, along with a reduced sperm count.[92] It has been suggested sperm banking before radioactive iodine treatment be considered.

In a 20-year follow-up of children whose mothers were exposed during pregnancy to radiation during the Chernobyl fallout, an increase in thyroid carcinoma was observed, but it was not statistically significant.

Postpartum Thyroid Dysfunction

Postpartum thyroiditis (PPT) is defined as transient thyroid dysfunction in the first year after delivery in women who were euthyroid before pregnancy.[93,94] However, in most of the published studies, thyroid status in the first trimester of pregnancy was not reported, which could explain the discrepancies in prevalence among the publications. PPT also occurs following spontaneous or medically induced abortions.[95] The etiology in most cases is autoimmune chronic (Hashimoto) thyroiditis, with a few cases due to hypothalamic or pituitary lesions. In one study, 27% of PTT women were positive for antipituitary antibodies; in such cases, the serum TSH is normal and serum FT_4 is low, characteristic of secondary or central hypothyroidism (Table 40-8).[96]

PPT, a variant of Hashimoto or chronic thyroiditis, is the most common cause of thyroid dysfunction in the postpartum period. The prevalence is between 1.1% and 16.7% of all women,[93,94,97-99] with the difference between studies depending on the design of the study, the definition of PPT, the time of postpartum testing, genotype, the exclusion of women with preexisting thyroid dysfunction, iodine intake, and other factors. Women with type 1 diabetes mellitus and other autoimmune diseases are at higher risk for developing PPT.[100] The clinical diagnosis is not always obvious, and the clinician should be concerned about nonspecific symptoms such as tiredness, fatigue, depression, palpitations, and irritability in women following the birth of their child or a miscarriage or abortion. Fatigue is the most common complaint.[97] In some cases, the clinical symptoms resemble the syndrome of postpartum depression. Indeed, thyroid antibodies have been found more frequently in euthyroid women with postpartum depression, but this is still a controversial issue. Because the clinical symptoms are mild and many times are confused with the usual tiredness of women in the months following delivery, an argument can be made for routine screening in the postpartum period; this controversial issue has been reviewed. Several factors have been mentioned as predictors for the development of PPT, among them high titers of TPOAb in the first trimester of gestation, family or personal history of thyroid disease, presence of goiter, and smoking. In a recent study from southern Italy,[94] the best predictors of PPT were the presence of TPOAb regardless of the titer and risks factors for thyroid dysfunction, including a family history of autoimmune thyroid disease, presence of goiter, signs or symptoms of thyroid disease, personal history of autoimmune disease, neck irradiation, and prior preterm delivery or miscarriage. Previous pregnancy, age, smoking status, and week of first obstetrical visit were not significantly associated with PPT. A careful history and physical examination will allow the physician to decide whether thyroid tests are indicated in a given situation. Recognizing the mild degree of the symptoms, the presence of a goiter, the history of similar symptoms in previous pregnancies, family history of thyroid disease, and autoimmune disease in addition to type 1 diabetes mellitus, among other features, will prompt the health care professional to order serum TSH with TPOAb. Patients at risk should be evaluated in the first year postpartum at 3, 6, and 12 months after delivery.

Postpartum thyroiditis may also develop in women with negative antibodies. In a study from the Netherlands, the authors suggested two forms of PPT: an autoimmune form, which is most common and eventually will develop into chronic hypothyroidism, and a nonautoimmune form, without antibodies, that appears to be transient without progressing to permanent hypothyroidism. This has recently been confirmed.[94] The incidence of PTT in women with negative TPOAb was 1.7%.

The clinical course of PPT is not uniform in most patients (Figure 40-6). In about one third of cases, mild

TABLE 40-8 POSTPARTUM THYROID DYSFUNCTION

Chronic thyroiditis
Transient hyperthyroidism (low RAIU)
Transient hypothyroidism
Permanent hypothyroidism
Graves disease
Exacerbation of hyperthyroidism (high RAIU)
Transient hyperthyroidism of chronic thyroiditis (low RAIU)
Hypothalamic-pituitary disease
Sheehan syndrome
Lymphocytic hypophysitis

From Mestman JH: Endocrine diseases in pregnancy. *In* Sciarra JJ (ed): Gynecology and Obstetrics. Philadelphia, Lippincott-Raven, 1997, p 34.
RAIU, Radioactive iodine uptake

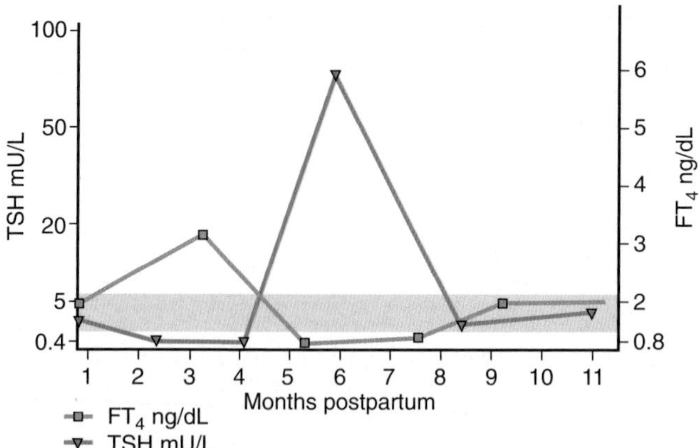

FIGURE 40-6. Clinical course of postpartum thyroiditis. *FT_4,* Free thyroxine; *TSH,* thyroid-stimulating hormone.

symptoms of hyperthyroidism may develop between 2 and 4 months postpartum. On physical examination, a goiter is felt in most cases and is firm and nontender to palpation. Tachycardia may be detected. The goiter may be discovered for the first time, or the patient may have noticed an increase in the size of a previously diagnosed goiter. Thyroid tests are in the hyperthyroid range, and thyroid antibodies (TPOAbs) are elevated in most cases. Titers of TRAb, a marker of Graves disease, are negative. Spontaneously, without specific therapy, there is a return to euthyroidism. If the symptoms are bothersome for the patients, a short course of β-adrenergic blockers is recommended. Symptoms are controlled in most patients with 20 to 40 mg of propranolol every 6 to 8 hours.

In one third of the patients, the hyperthyroid phase is followed by hypothyroidism, with spontaneous recovery and return to a euthyroid state by 7 to 12 months after delivery. Antibody titers have a tendency to increase during this process, and a change in the size of the goiter is usually noted.

In one third of patients, the course of PPT is different, characterized by an initial episode of hypothyroidism between 3 and 7 months postpartum without the initial hyperthyroid phase.

The permanent incidence of hypothyroidism 12 months after delivery ranges from 2% to 21%. However, Stagnaro-Green and colleagues found a rate of 54%, much higher than reported previously.[94] By 5 years after the diagnosis of PPT, most studies report an incidence of permanent hypothyroidism of 50%.

Graves hyperthyroidism may recur after delivery with an exacerbation in the first 3 months or between 6 and 12 months postpartum. The symptoms of hyperthyroidism are more severe than those in patients with PPT. The differential diagnosis between recurrent Graves hyperthyroidism and PPT is of clinical importance because patients with Graves' hyperthyroidism will benefit from antithyroid medications. On physical examination, women with Graves hyperthyroidism may present with ophthalmopathy, a visible goiter, and in many situations, the presence of a bruit. Titers of TRAb are positive. If not contraindicated, as in breastfeeding mothers, a 4- or 24-hour thyroid radioactive iodine uptake (RAIU) is helpful in establishing the etiology. It will be very low in patients with PPT, whereas it is high normal or elevated in patients with recurrent hyperthyroidism due to Graves disease. When hyperthyroidism is due to recurrent Graves disease, treatment with antithyroid medications is indicated, or the physician may advise ablation therapy.

Therefore, the classic presentation of PPT is characterized by symptoms of thyroid dysfunction that present in four different forms: (1) an episode of hyperthyroidism (2 to 4 months), followed by hypothyroidism (4 to 6 months) and reverting to euthyroidism (after the seventh month); (2) an episode of hyperthyroidism (3 to 4 months) reverting to euthyroidism; (3) an episode of hypothyroidism (4 to 6 months) reverting to a euthyroid state; and (4) permanent hypothyroidism after the hypothyroid phase (see Figure 40-6). However, there are exceptions to these chronologic phases. It is recommended that a diagnosis of PPT be considered for any thyroid abnormality occurring within 1 year after a delivery or miscarriages.

Although most cases of PPT recover spontaneously, treatment is indicated for symptomatic patients. In the presence of hyperthyroid symptoms, β-adrenergic blocking drugs (propranolol, 20 to 40 mg every 6 hours, or atenolol, 25 to 50 mg every 24 hours) are effective in controlling the symptoms. Antithyroid medications are not effective because the hyperthyroxinemia is secondary to the release of thyroid hormones due to the acute injury to the gland (destructive hyperthyroidism). There is no new hormone production, and therefore medications that work by blocking new thyroid hormone formation are ineffective. For hypothyroid symptoms, small amounts of L-thyroxine (50 mcg/day) will control symptoms, allowing for a spontaneous recovery of thyroid function after discontinuation of the drug. However, in women desiring future pregnancies, it has been recommended that L-thyroxine therapy be continued because these patients are at high risk for developing hypothyroidism in a future pregnancy.[98]

As noted previously, there are some features that may predict the development of PPT: presence of a goiter and high titers of thyroid antibodies in the first half of pregnancy, episodes of PPT in previous pregnancies, and a strong family history of autoimmune thyroid disease. Women with type 1 diabetes mellitus are at high risk for developing PPT. PPT may recur in future pregnancies, with a recurrence rate between 30% and 70%.[100] PPT has been reported to be associated with other autoimmune endocrine disorders, such as adrenal insufficiency and lymphocytic hypophysitis.[96]

Preventing PPT with the administration of selenium during pregnancy in women with chronic thyroiditis was evaluated by Negro and associates. They studied two groups of pregnant women: 77 received 200 mcg/day of selenium during pregnancy and postpartum, and 74 were given a placebo. There was a significant reduction in the incidence of PPT between both groups; 28.6% of women receiving selenium developed PPT compared with 48.6% of those taking placebo (P <.01). Future studies will be needed to confirm these findings.

KEY POINTS

- Hyperthyroidism due to Graves' disease needs to be differentiated in the first trimester of pregnancy from the syndrome of gestational thyrotoxicosis.
- Recent reports indicate increased for risk liver failure with the use of PTU; it is recommended that PTU be used in the first trimester of pregnancy and MM after 13 weeks' gestation. MM is not indicated in the first trimester because of the potential risk for the syndrome of methimazole embryopathy.
- The dose of antithyroid medications should be adjusted frequently, aiming to use the minimal amount of drug that will keep the FT_4 at the upper limits of normal.
- Breastfeeding is not contraindicated in women on antithyroid therapy, provided that the maximal daily dose is 200 mg of PTU and 20 mg of MM.
- Hypothyroid women on thyroid replacement therapy should have their thyroid tests checked early in pregnancy. An increase in dosage is needed in more than 50% of patients on thyroid replacement therapy.
- Women with risk factors for thyroid disease, such as a family history of thyroid disease, the presence of a goiter, a previous history of PPT, should be studied before or early in pregnancy. Determinations of serum TSH, FT_4, or FT_4I, and TPOAb are recommended in these women.
- Postpartum thyroiditis affects up to 16.7% of all women in the postpartum period. Women with chronic thyroiditis are at higher risk for developing the syndrome. Long-term follow-up is strongly advised because up to 50% of these patients will develop permanent hypothyroidism in 5 to 10 years.

Acknowledgment

The author wishes to thank Elsa C. Ahumada for her secretarial assistance.

REFERENCES

1. Kovacs CS, Kronenberg HM: Maternal fetal calcium and bone metabolism during pregnancy, puerperium and lactation. Endocr Rev 18:832, 1997.
2. Dahlman T, Sjoberg HE, Bucht E: Calcium homeostasis in normal pregnancy and puerperium: a longitudinal study. Acta Obstet Gynecol Scant 73:393, 1994.
3. Seely EW, Bron EM, DeMaggio DM, et al: A prospective study of calciotrophic hormones in pregnancy and postpartum reciprocal changes in serum intact parathyroid hormone and 1,25 dihydroxyvitamin D. Am J Obstet Gynecol 176:214, 1997.
4. Hirota Y, Anai T, Miyakawa I: Parathyroid hormone related protein levels in maternal and cord blood. Am J Obstet Gynecol 177:702, 1997.
5. Kalkwarf HJ, Specker BL, Bianchi DC, et al: The effect of calcium supplementation on bone density during lactation and after weaning. N Engl J Med 337:523, 1997.
6. Kelly T: Primary hyperparathyroidism during pregnancy. Surgery 110:1028, 1991.
7. Dahan M, Chang RJ: Pancreatitis secondary to hyperparathyroidism during pregnancy. Obstet Gynecol 98:923, 2001.
8. Shani H, Sivan E, Cassif E, et al: Maternal hypercalcemia as a possible cause of unexplained fetal polyhydramnios: a case series. Am J Obstet Gynecol 199:410.e1, 2008.
9. Hultin H, Hellman P, Lundgren E, et al: Association of parathyroid adenoma and pregnancy with preeclampsia. J Clin Endocrinol Metab 94:3394, 2009.
10. Ficinski M, Mestman JH: Primary hyperparathyroidism during pregnancy. Endocr Pract 2:362, 1996.
11. Horjus C, Groot I, Telting D, et al: Cinacalcet for hyperparathyroidism in pregnancy and puerperium. J Pediatr Endocrinol Metab 22:741, 2009.
12. Pothiwala P, Levine SN: Parathyroid surgery in pregnancy: review of the literature and localization by aspiration for parathyroid hormone levels. J Perinatol 29:779, 2009.
13. Loughead JL, Mughal Z, Mimouni F, et al: Spectrum and natural history of congenital hyperparathyroidism secondary to maternal hypocalcemia. Am J Perinatol 7:350, 1990.
14. Barrett H, McEleduff A: Vitamin D and pregnancy: an old problem revisited. Best Pract Res Clin Endocrinol Metab 24:527, 2010.
15. Leffalaar ER, Vrijkotre TG, van Eijsden M: Maternal early pregnancy vitamin D status in relation to fetal and neonatal growth: results of the multi-ethnic Amsterdam Born Children and Their Development cohort. Br J Nutr 2:1, 2010.
16. Bodnar LM, Catov JM, Simhan HN, et al: Maternal vitamin D deficiency increases the risk of preeclampsia. J Clin Endocrinol Metab 92:3517, 2007.
17. Merewood A, Mehta SD, Chen TC, et al: Association between vitamin D deficiency and primary cesarean section. J Clin Endocrinol Metab 94:940, 2009.
18. Ross CA, Abrams SA, Aloia JF, et al: Dietary reference intake for calcium and vitamin D: report at a glance. Institute of Medicine of the National Academies, released date: 11/20/2010.
19. Wiser J, Florio I, Neff M, et al: Changes in bone density and metabolism in pregnancy. Acta Obstet Gynecol Scand 94:349, 2005.
20. Barbour LA, Kick SD, Steiner JF, et al: A prospective study of heparin induced osteoporosis in pregnancy using bone densitometry. Am J Obstet Gynecol 170:862, 1994.
21. Glinoer D: The regulation of thyroid function in pregnancy: pathways of endocrine adaptation from physiology to pathology. Endocr Rev 18:404, 1997.
22. Krassas GE, Poppe K, Glineor D: Thyroid function and human reproductive health. Endocr Rev 31:702, 2010.
23. Pearce EN: Iodine in pregnancy: Is salt iodization enough? J Clin Endocrinol Metab 93:2466, 2008.
24. Kratzsch J, Pulzer F: Thyroid gland development and defects. Best Pract Res Clin Endocrinol Metab 22:57, 2008.
25. Haddow JE, Palomaki GE, Allan WC, et al: Maternal thyroid deficiency during pregnancy and subsequent neuropsychological development of the child. N Engl J Med 341:549, 1999.
26. Henrichs J, Bongers-Schokking JJ, Schenk JJ, et al: Maternal thyroid function during early pregnancy and cognitive functioning in early childhood: the generation R study. J Clin Endocrinol Meetab 95: 4227, 2010.
27. Glinoer D, Spencer CA: Serum TSH determinations in pregnancy: how, when and why? Nat Rev Endocrinol 6:526, 2010.
28. Abalovich M, Amino N, Barbour LA, et al: Management of thyroid dysfunction during pregnancy and postpartum: an Endocrine Society clinical practice guideline. J Clin Endocrinol Metab 92:S1, 2007.
29. Lee RH, Spencer CA, Mestman JH, et al: Free T4 immunoassays are flawed during pregnancy. Am J Obstet Gynecol 200:260.e1, 2009.
30. Laurberg P, Bournaud C, Karmisholt J, et al: Management of Graves' hyperthyroidism in pregnancy: focus on both maternal and foetal thyroid function, and caution against surgical thyroidectomy in pregnancy. Eur J Endocrinol 160:1, 2009.
31. Mandel SL, Larsen PR, Seely EW, et al: Increased need for thyroxine during pregnancy in women with primary hypothyroidism. N Engl J Med 323:91, 1990.
32. Yassa L, Marqusee E, Fawcett R, et al: Thyroid hormone early adjustment in pregnancy: the THERAPY trial. J Clin Endocrinol Metab 95:3234, 2010.
33. Abalovich M, Alcaraz G, Kleiman-Rubinsztein J, et al: The relationship of preconception thyrotropin levels to requirements for

increasing the levothyroxine dose during pregnancy in women with primary hypothyroidism. Thyroid 20:1175, 2010.
34. Lazarus JH, Hall R, Othman S, et al: The clinical spectrum of postpartum thyroid disease. QJM 89:429, 1996.
35. de Escobar GM, Obregon MJ, del Rey FE: Is neuropsychological development related to maternal hypothyroidism or to maternal hypothyroxinemia? J Clin Endocrinol Metab 85:3975, 2000.
36. Patil-Sisodia K, Mestman JH: Graves hyperthyroidism and pregnancy: a clinical update. Endocr Pract 16:118, 2010.
37. Goodwin TM, Montoro MN, Mestman JH: Transient hyperthyroidism and hyperemesis gravidarum: clinical aspects. Am J Obstet Gynecol 167:648, 1992.
38. Niebyl JR: Nausea and vomiting in pregnancy. N Engl J Med 363:1544, 2010.
39. Goodwin TM, Hershman JM: Hyperthyroidism due to inappropriate production of human chorionic gonadotropin. Clin Obstet Gynceol 40:32, 1997.
40. Tagami T, Hagiwara H, Kimura T, et al: The incidence of gestational hyperthyroidism and postpartum thyroiditis in treated patients with Graves' disease. Thyroid 17:767, 2007.
41. Millar LK, Wing DA, Leung AS, et al: Low birth weight and preeclampsia in pregnancies complicated by hyperthyroidism. Obstet Gynecol 84:946, 1994.
42. Momotani N, Noh J, Oyangi H, et al: Antithyroid drug therapy for Graves' disease during pregnancy: optimal regimen for fetal thyroid status. N Engl J Med 315:24, 1986.
43 Mortimer RH, Tyack SA, Galligan JP, et al: Graves' disease in pregnancy: TSH receptor binding inhibiting immunoglobulins and maternal and neonatal thyroid function. Clin Endocrinol (Oxf) 32:141, 1990.
44. Kempers MJE, van Trotsenburg ASP, van Tijn DA: Disturbance of the fetal thyroid hormone state has long-term consequences for treatment of thyroidal and central congenital hypothyroidism. J Clin Endocriol Metab 90:4094, 2005.
45. Luton D, LeGac I, Vuillard E: Management of Graves' disease during pregnancy: the key role of fetal thyroid gland monitoring. J Clin Endocrinol Metab 90:6093, 2005.
46 Copoper DS, Rivkees SA: Putting propylthiouracil in perspective. J Clin Endocriol Metab 94:1881, 2009.
47. Bahn RS, Burch HS, Cooper DS, et al: The role of propylthiouracil in the management of Graves' disease in adults: report of a meeting jointly sponsored by the American Thyroid Association and the Food and Drug Administration. Thyroid 19:673-674, 2009.
48. Barbero P, Valdez R, Rodriguez H, et al: Choanal atresia associated with maternal hyperthyroidism treated with methimazole: a case control study. Am J Med Genet 146A:2390, 2008.
49. Stoffer SS, Hamburger JI: Inadvertent 131I therapy for hyperthyroidism in the first trimester of pregnancy. J Nucl Med 17:146, 1976.
50. Polak M, Leger J, Oury JF, et al: Fetal cord blood sampling in the diagnosis and the treatment of fetal hyperthyroidism in the offspring of a euthyroid mother producing thyroid stimulating immunoglobulins. Ann Endocrinol (Paris) 58:338, 1997.
51. Kilpatrick S: Umbilical blood sampling in women with thyroid disease in pregnancy: is it necessary? Obstet Gynecol 189:1, 2003.
52. Azizi F, Khoshmiat M, Bahrainian M, et al: Thyroid function and intellectual development of infants nursed by mothers taking methimazole. J Clin Endocrinol Metab 85:3233, 2000.
53. Nayakk B, Burman K: Thyrotoxicosis and thyroid storm. Endocrinol Metab Clin North Am 35:663, 2006.
54. Van Vliet G, Polak M, Ritzen EM: Treating fetal thyroid and adrenal disorders through the mother. Nat Clin Pract 4:675, 2008.
55. Weiss RE, Dumitrescu A, Refetoff S: Approach to the patient with resistance to thyroid hormone and pregnancy. J Clin Endocrinol Metab 95:3094, 2010.
56. Davis LE, Leveno KJ, Cunningham FG: Hypothyroidism complicating pregnancy. Obstet Gynecol 72:108, 1988.
57. Leung AS, Millar LK, Koonings PP, et al: Perinatal outcome in hypothyroid pregnancies. Obstet Gynecol 81:349, 1993.
58. Klein RZ, Haddow JE, Faix JD, et al: Prevalence of thyroid deficiency in pregnant women. Clin Endocrinol (Oxf) 35:41, 1991.
59. Burman KD: Controversies surrounding pregnancy, maternal thyroid status and fetal outcome. Thyroid 19:323, 2009.
60. McClain M, Lambert-Messerlian G, Haddow JE: Sequential first- and second-trimester TSH, free thyroxine, and thyroid antibody measurements in women with known hypothyroidism: FaSTER trial study. Am J Obstet Gynecol 199:129.e1, 2008.
61. Gutenberg A, Hans V, Puchner M, et al: Primary hypophysitis: clinical-pathological correlations. Eur J Endocrinol 155:101, 2006.
62. Casey BM, Dashe JS, Wells CE, et al: Subclinical hypothyroidism and pregnancy outcome. Obstet Gynecol 105:239, 2005.
63. Cleary-Goldman J, Malone FD, Lambert-Messerlian G, et al: Maternal thyroid hypofunction and pregnancy outcome. Obstet Gynecol 112:85, 2008.
64. Negro R, Schwartz A, Gismondi R, et al: Increased pregnancy loss rate in thyroid antibody negative women with TSH levels between 2.5 and 5.0 in the first trimester of pregnancy. J Clin Endocrinol Metab 95:E44, 2010.
65. Kuppens SMI, Looirstra L, Wijnens HA, et al: Maternal thyroid function during gestation is related to breech presentation at term. Clin Endocrinol (Oxf) 72:820, 2010.
66. Negro R, Schwartz A, Gismondi R, et al: Universal screening versus case finding for detection and treatment of thyroid hormone dysfunction during pregnancy. J Clin Endocrinol Metab 95:1699, 2010.
67. Alexander EK: Here's to you, baby! A step forward in support of universal screening of thyroid function during pregnancy. J Clin Endocrinol Metab 95:1575, 2010.
68. Glinoer D: Maternal and fetal impact of chronic iodine deficiency. Clin Obstet Gynecol 40:102, 1997.
69. Casey BM, Dashe JS, Spong CY, et al: Perinatal significance of isolated maternal hypothyroxinemia identified in the first half of pregnancy. Obstet Gynecol 109:1129, 2007.
70. American Thyroid Association: Statement on early maternal thyroid insufficiency: recognition, clinical management and research direction. Thyroid 15:77, 2005.
70a. Stagnaro-Green A, et al: Guidelines of the American Throid Association for the Diagnosis and Management of Thyroid Disease During Pregnancy and Postpartum. Thyroid 21:1081, 2011.
71. Vaidya B, Anthony S, Biklous M, et al: Detection of thyroid dysfunction in early pregnancy: universal screening or targeted high-risk case finding? J Clin Endocrinol Metab 92:203, 2007.
72. Thung S, Funai EF, Grobman WA: The cost-effectiveness of universal screening in pregnancy for subclinical hypothyroidism. Am J Obstet Gynecol 200:267, 2009.
73. Brent GA: Diagnosing thyroid dysfunction in pregnant women: is case finding enough? [Editorial] J Clin Endocrinol Metab 92:39, 2007.
74. Abalovich M, Alcaraz G, Kleiman-Rubinsztein J, et al: The relationship of preconception thyrotropin levels to requirements for increasing the levothyroxine dose during pregnancy in women with primary hypothyroidism. Thyroid 20:1175, 2010.
75. Pearce EN, Farwell AP, Braverman LE: Thyroiditis. N Engl J Med 348:2646, 2003.
76. Stagnaro-Green A, Roman SH, Cobin RH, et al: Detection of at-risk pregnancy by means of highly sensitive assays for thyroid autoantibodies. JAMA 264:1422, 1990.
77. Matsuura N, Yamada Y, Nohara Y, et al: Familial neonatal transient hypothyroidism due to maternal TSH binding inhibitor immunoglobulins. N Engl J Med 303:738, 1980.
78. Brown RS, Bellasario RL, Botero D, et al: Incidence of transient congenital hypothyroidism due to maternal thyrotropin antibodies in over one million babies. J Clin Endocrinol Metab 81:1147, 1996.
79. Haddow JE, Cleary-Goldman J, McClain MR, et al: Thyroperoxidase and thyroglobulin antibodies in early pregnancy and preterm delivery. Obstet Gynecol 116:58, 2010.
80. Mannisto T, Vaarasmaki M, Pouta A, et al: Antithyroperoxidase antibody and antithyroglobulin antibody positivity during the first trimester of pregnancy is a major risk for perinatal death. J Clin Endocrinol Metab 94:772, 2009.
81. Negro R, Formoso G, Mangieri T, et al: Levothyroxine treatment in euthyroid pregnant women with autoimmune thyroid disease: effects on obstetrical complications. J Clin Endocrinol Metab 91: 2587, 2006
82. Abbassi-Ghanavati M, Casey BM, Spong C, et al: Pregnancy outcomes in women with thyroid peroxidase antibodies. Obstet Gynecol 116:381, 2010.
83. Loh JA, Wartofsky L, Jonklaas J, et al: The magnitude of increased levothyroxine requirements in hypothyroid pregnant women

depends upon the etiology of the hypothyroidism. Thyroid 19:269, 2009.
84. Cooper DS, Doherty GM, Haugen BR, et al: Revised American Thyroid Association Management Guidelines for patients with thyroid nodules and differentiated thyroid cancer. Thyroid 19:1167, 2009.
85. Sam S, Molitch ME: Timing and special concerns regarding endocrine surgery during pregnancy. Endocrinol Metab Clin North Am 32:337, 2003.
86. Moosa M, Mazzaferri EL: Outcome of differentiated thyroid cancer diagnosed in pregnant women. J Clin Endocrinol Metab 82:2862, 1997.
87. Vannucchi G, Perrino M, Rossi S, et al: Clinical and molecular features of differentiated thyroid cancer diagnosed during pregnancy. Euro J Endocrinol 162:145, 2010.
88. Leboeuf R, Emerick LE, Martorella AJ, et al: Impact of pregnancy on serum thyroglobulin and detection of recurrent disease shortly after delivery in thyroid cancer survivors. Thyroid 17:543, 2007.
89. Hrisch D, Levy S, Tsvetov G, et al: Impact of pregnancy on outcome and prognosis of survivors of papillary thyroid cancer. Thyroid 20:1179, 2010.
90. Sawka AM, Lakra DC, Lea J, et al: A systematic review examining the effects of therapeutic radioactive iodine on ovarian function and future pregnancy in female thyroid cancer survivors. Clin Endocrinol (Oxf) 69:479, 2008.
91. Garsi JP, Schlumberger M, Rubino C, et al: Therapeutic administration of I131 for differentiated thyroid cancer: Radiation dose to ovaries and outcome of pregnancy. J Nucl Med 49:845, 2008.
92. Sawka AM, Lea J, Alshehis B, et al: A systemic review of the gonadal effects of therapeutic radioactive iodine in male thyroid cancer survivors. Clin Endocrinol 68:610, 2008.
93. Nicholson WK, Robinson KA, Smallridge RC, et al: Prevalence of postpartum thyroid dysfunction: a quantitative review. Thyroid 16:573, 2006.
94. Stagnaro-Green A, Schwartz A, Gismondi R, et al: High rate of persistent hypothyroidism in a large scale prospective study in postpartum thyroiditis in Southern Italy. J Clin Endocrinol Metab 96:652-657, 2011.
95. Marqusee E, Hill JA, Mandel SJ: Thyroiditis after pregnancy loss. J Clin Endocrinol Metab 82:2455, 1997.
96. Landek-Salgado MA, Gutenberg A, Lupi I, et al: Pregnancy, postpartum autoimmune thyroiditis and autoimmune hypophysitis: intimate relationships. Autoimmun Rev 9:153, 2010.
97. Amino N, Mori H, Iwatani O, et al: High prevalence of transient postpartum thyrotoxicosis and hypothyroidism. N Engl J Med 306:849, 1982.
98. Stagnaro-Green A: Postpartum thyroiditis. Best Pract Res Clin Endocrinol Metab 18:303, 2004.
99. Muller AF, Dreshage HA, Berghout A: Postpartum thyroiditis and autoimmune thyroiditis in women of childbearing age: recent insights and consequences for antepartal and postnatal care. Endocr Rev 22:605, 2001.
100. Alvarez-Marfany M, Roman SH, Drexler AJ, et al: Long term prospective study of postpartum thyroid dysfunction in women with insulin dependent diabetes mellitus. J Clin Endocrinol Metab 79:10, 1994.

For full reference list, log onto www.expertconsult.com.

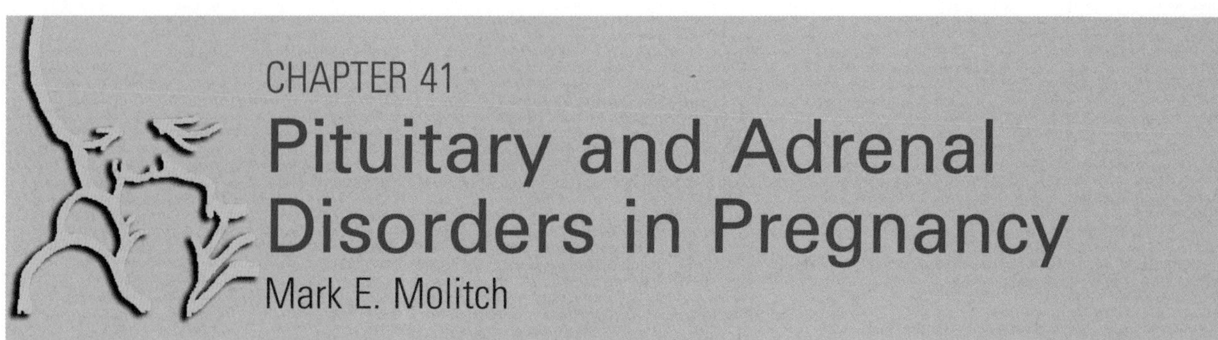

CHAPTER 41

Pituitary and Adrenal Disorders in Pregnancy

Mark E. Molitch

KEY ABBREVIATIONS	
Adrenocorticotropic Hormone	ACTH
Arginine Vasopressin	AVP
Clinically Nonfunctioning Adenoma	CNFA
Desmopressin	dDAVP
Diabetes Insipidus	DI
Follicle-stimulating Hormone	FSH
Growth Hormone	GH
Human Chorionic Gonadotropin	hCG
Insulin-like Growth Factor-1	IGF-1
Luteinizing Hormone	LH
Magnetic Resonance Imaging	MRI
Prolactin	PRL
Thyroid-stimulating Hormone	TSH

ANTERIOR PITUITARY

Anterior Pituitary Hormone Changes in Pregnancy

During pregnancy, the normal pituitary gland enlarges considerably as a result of the estrogen-stimulated lactotroph hyperplasia.[1,2] **Prolactin** (PRL) levels rise gradually throughout gestation, preparing the breast for lactation.[3] Beginning in the second half of pregnancy, circulating levels of a **growth hormone** (GH) variant made by the syncytiotrophoblastic epithelium of the placenta increase and pituitary GH secretion decreases because of negative feedback effects of insulin-like growth factor-1 (IGF-1).[4,5] In patients with **acromegaly** who have autonomous GH secretion and become pregnant, both forms of GH persist in the blood.[6] **Cortisol** levels rise progressively over the course of gestation, resulting in a twofold to threefold increase by term, as a result of both to the estrogen-induced increase in cortisol-binding globulin (CBG) levels and an increase in cortisol production, so that the bioactive "free" fraction, urinary free cortisol levels, and salivary cortisol levels are also increased.[7,8]

Pituitary Tumors

Pituitary adenomas cause problems because of hormone hypersecretion and also by causing hypopituitarism. The pregnancy-induced alterations in hormone secretion complicate the evaluation of patients with pituitary neoplasms. The influence of various types of therapy on the developing fetus may also affect therapeutic decision making.

Prolactinoma

Hyperprolactinemia commonly causes symptoms of galactorrhea, amenorrhea, and infertility.[9] The differential diagnosis of hyperprolactinemia is extensive,[9] but this discussion will focus on women with a **prolactinoma**. The choice of therapy has important consequences for decisions regarding pregnancy. Transsphenoidal surgery is curative in 50% to 60% and rarely causes hypopituitarism when it is performed on individuals with microadenomas (tumors <10 mm in diameter).[10] For patients with macroadenomas (tumors >10 mm in diameter), surgical cure rates are lower, and there is a considerably greater risk for resulting hypopituitarism.[10]

The dopamine agonists **bromocriptine** and **cabergoline** are the primary modes of therapy, restoring ovulatory menses in about 80% and 90%, respectively.[10] In addition, macroadenoma size can be reduced by 50% or more in 50% to 75% of patients with bromocriptine and in more than 90% of patients with cabergoline.[10]

The stimulatory effect of the hormonal milieu of pregnancy and the withdrawal of the dopamine agonist may result in significant prolactinoma enlargement (Figure 41-1). Tumor enlargement requiring intervention during pregnancy has been reported in 13 of 584 (2.2%) women with microadenomas, 50 of 201 (28%) with macroadenomas that had not undergone prior surgery or radiotherapy, and 7 of 161 (4.3%) with macroadenomas that had undergone prior surgery or radiotherapy.[10-12] In almost all cases, such enlargement was successfully treated with reinstitution with a dopamine agonist. If the pregnancy is sufficiently advanced, another approach is to proceed with delivery. Surgical decompression is reserved for cases in which these other approaches fail.

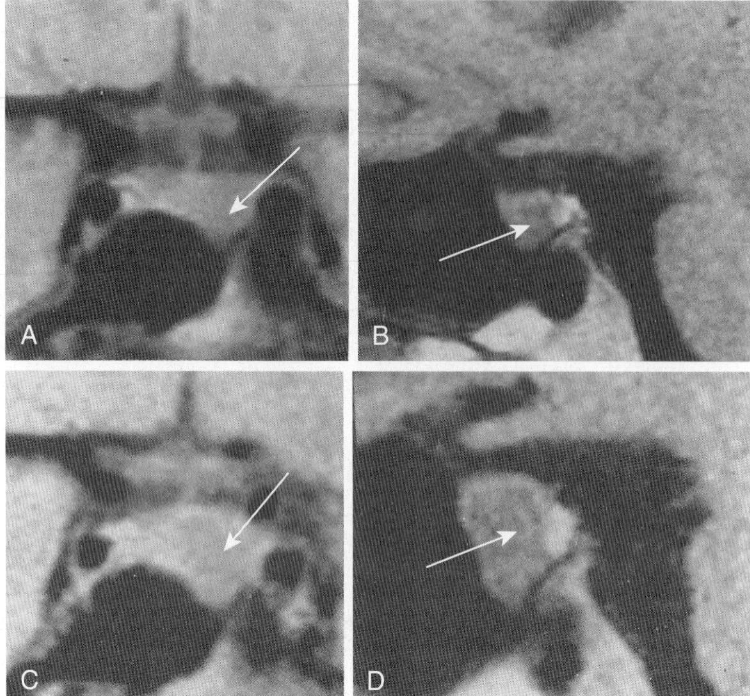

FIGURE 41-1. Coronal and sagittal magnetic resonance images of an intrasellar prolactin: secreting macroadenoma in a woman before conception **(A, B)** and at 7 months of gestation **(C, D)**. Note the marked tumor enlargement at the latter point, at which time the patient was complaining of headaches. (From Molitch ME: Medical treatment of prolactinomas. Endocrinol Metab Clin North Am 28:143, 1999.)

Usually the dopamine agonist is discontinued once pregnancy is diagnosed, in order to limit fetal exposure. When used in this fashion, no increase in spontaneous abortions, ectopic pregnancies, trophoblastic disease, multiple pregnancies, or malformations were found in more than 6000 pregnancies in which bromocriptine was used and 760 pregnancies in which cabergoline was used.[11-16] Although safety data regarding the use of continuous dopamine agonist therapy during pregnancy are scarce, the use of such medications is probably not harmful.

Patients with large macroadenomas should be assessed monthly for symptoms of tumor enlargement, and visual fields should be tested each trimester. PRL levels may rise without tumor enlargement and not rise with tumor enlargement, and therefore are often misleading[17] and are not advised.

Acromegaly

About 30% to 40% of patients with **acromegaly** have hyperprolactinemia,[18] and treatment with a dopamine agonist may be necessary to permit ovulation and conception in these patients.[19] Most patients with acromegaly are treated with surgery as primary therapy, and those not cured by surgery are usually treated medically with the **somatostatin analogs octreotide** and **lanreotide**.[20] Cabergoline may also be helpful in some cases.[20]

Conventional assays cannot distinguish between normal pituitary GH and the placental GH variant.[4] If it is critical to make a diagnosis during pregnancy, it may be possible by demonstrating GH pulsatility with frequent sampling because GH secretion in acromegaly is highly pulsatile but that of the variant is not.[6,21]

Only four patients with tumors secreting GH have been reported to have enlargement of their tumors, with a resultant visual field defect in one patient during pregnancy.[22-25] However, in one of these cases, tumor enlargement likely was due to octreotide withdrawal, and in another it was due to hemorrhage into the tumor. Therefore, as with prolactinomas, women with acromegaly and macroadenoma should be monitored for symptoms of tumor enlargement and visual field testing.

Because of the GH-induced insulin resistance, the risk for gestational diabetes is increased in acromegalic patients.[25] There is increased salt retention, and gestational hypertension is also increased.[25] Cardiac disease has not proved to be an issue in pregnant women with acromegaly.[19,24,25]

The considerations regarding the use of bromocriptine and cabergoline in women with prolactinomas also apply to those with acromegaly. Only 36 pregnant women treated with somatostatin analogs have been reported; no malformations were found in their children.[25,26] However, a decrease in uterine artery blood flow has been reported with short-acting octreotide,[26] and one fetus appeared to have intrauterine growth restriction (IUGR) that responded to a lower dose of octreotide LAR.[25] Octreotide binds to somatostatin receptors in the placenta[26] and crosses the placenta[26]; therefore, it can affect developing fetal tissues where somatostatin receptors are widespread, especially in the brain. Because of the limited data documenting safety, most authors recommend[25,27] that octreotide and other somatostatin analogs be discontinued if pregnancy is considered and that contraception be used when these drugs are administered; but not all others concur.[26] Considering the prolonged nature of the course of most cases of acromegaly, interruption of medical therapy for 9 to 12 months generally does not have a particularly adverse effect on the long-term outcome. On the other hand, these drugs can control tumor growth, and for enlarging tumors, their reintroduction during pregnancy may be warranted instead of operating. Pegvisomant, a GH receptor antagonist, has been given to a patient with acromegaly during pregnancy without harm,[28] but the safety of this medication has not been established.

Thyrotropin-Secreting Tumors

Only three cases of pregnancy occurring in women with thyroid-stimulating hormone (TSH; thyrotropin)-secreting tumors have been reported.[29-31] In one of these cases, octreotide, which had been stopped, had to be reinstituted to control tumor size[29]; in a second case, octreotide was continued during pregnancy for tumor size control.[30] The most pressing issue with such tumors is the need to control hyperthyroidism during pregnancy, which can usually be accomplished with standard antithyroid drugs.[30] However, with growing macroadenomas, octreotide may be necessary for tumor size control,[29,30] and it is possible that it may be necessary to control the hyperthyroidism if thioamides are ineffective.

Clinically Nonfunctioning Adenomas

Pregnancy would not be expected to influence tumor size in patients with clinically nonfunctioning adenomas (CNFAs), and only two cases have been reported in which tumor enlargement during pregnancy resulted in a visual field defect.[22,32] In the second case, the patient responded rapidly to bromocriptine treatment, probably because of shrinkage of the lactotroph hyperplasia with decompression of the chiasm and probably with little or no direct effect on the tumor itself.[32]

Most CNFAs are actually gonadotroph adenomas. Two patients have been reported who had gonadotroph adenomas secreting intact follicle-stimulating hormone (FSH) with a resultant ovarian hyperstimulation syndrome[33,34]; both became pregnant, one after having the FSH hypersecretion controlled by bromocriptine[33] and the second after surgical removal of the tumor.[34]

Hypopituitarism

Hypopituitarism may be partial or complete, and loss of gonadotropin secretion is common. Induction of ovulation may be difficult, and a variety of techniques have been used, including administration of human chorionic gonadotropin (hCG) and FSH,[35,36] pulsatile gonadotropin-releasing hormone,[35,36] and in vitro fertilization.[37,38] Although the malformation rate is not increased in such pregnancies, there appears to be an increased frequency of cesarean deliveries, miscarriage, and small-for-gestational-age infants.[35,36,38]

Because of increased thyroxine (T_4) turnover and volume of distribution in pregnancy, T_4 levels usually fall, and TSH levels rise with a fixed $\mathbf{T_4}$ dose over the course of gestation.[39] The average increase in T_4 need in these patients is about 0.05 mg/day. Because women with hypothalamic-pituitary dysfunction may not elevate their TSH levels normally in the face of increased need for T_4, it is reasonable to increase the T_4 supplementation by 0.025 mg after the first trimester and by additional 0.025 mg after the second trimester, also following free T_4 levels.

The dose of chronic glucocorticoid replacement usually does not need to be increased during pregnancy.[8] **Hydrocortisone** is metabolized by the placental enzyme 11β-hydroxysteroid dehydrogenase-2, so the fetus is generally protected from excess hydrocortisone; the usual dose is in the range of 12 to 15 mg/m^2 given in two or three divided doses.[8] Additional glucocorticoids are needed for the stress of labor and delivery, such as 75 mg of hydrocortisone given intravenously every 8 hours with rapid tapering postpartum.[8] Prednisolone does not cross the placenta, and prednisone crosses only minimally.[40] Suppression of neonatal adrenal function in offspring of women taking prednisone during pregnancy is very uncommon,[41] and the amounts passed in breast milk are negligible.[42]

There are few data on the use of GH during pregnancy in hypopituitary individuals, and in most series, GH therapy has been stopped at conception.[43] Because the GH variant, which is biologically active, is produced by the placenta in substantial amounts beginning in the second half of pregnancy and can access the maternal circulation (see earlier), at most the mother would be GH deficient only in the first half of pregnancy. When Curran and colleagues analyzed 25 pregnancies that occurred in 16 patients with GH deficiency during which GH therapy was not continued, they found that there was no adverse outcome of omitting GH therapy on either the fetus or mother and concluded that GH replacement therapy during pregnancy is not essential for GH-deficient women.[43]

Table 41-1 Symptoms and Signs of Sheehan Syndrome

ACUTE FORM	CHRONIC FORM
Hypotension	Light-headedness
Tachycardia	Fatigue
Failure to lactate	Failure to lactate
Hypoglycemia	Persistent amenorrhea
Extreme fatigue	Decreased body hair
Nausea and vomiting	Dry skin
	Loss of libido
	Nausea and vomiting
	Cold intolerance

Sheehan Syndrome

Sheehan syndrome consists of pituitary necrosis secondary to ischemia occurring within hours of delivery.[44] It is usually secondary to hypotension and shock from an obstetrical hemorrhage. The degree of ischemia and necrosis dictates the subsequent patient course (Table 41-1). It rarely occurs with current obstetrical practice.[45]

Acute necrosis is suspected in the setting of an obstetrical hemorrhage in which hypotension and tachycardia persist following adequate replacement of blood products. Failure to lactate and hypoglycemia may also occur.[44] Investigation should include obtaining blood samples for adrenocorticotropic hormone (ACTH), cortisol, prolactin, and free T_4. The ACTH stimulation test would be normal because the adrenal cortex would not be atrophied. Free T_4 levels might prove normal initially because the hormone has a half-life of 7 days, and an additional sample should be sent after 1 week. Prolactin levels are usually low.

Treatment with saline and stress doses of corticosteroids should be instituted immediately after drawing the blood tests. If later free T_4 levels become low, then therapy with levothyroxine is indicated. Additional pituitary testing with subsequent therapy should be delayed until recovery. Diabetes insipidus may also occur.[46]

When milder forms of infarction occur, the diagnosis may be delayed for months or years.[44] These women generally have a history of amenorrhea, decreased libido, failure to lactate, breast atrophy, loss of pubic and axillary hair, fatigue, and symptoms of secondary adrenal insufficiency with nausea, vomiting, diarrhea, and abdominal pain.[44] Rarely, some women retain gonadotropin secretion and may have normal menses and fertility.[44]

Lymphocytic Hypophysitis

Lymphocytic hypophysitis is thought to be autoimmune and is manifested by infiltration and destruction of the parenchyma of the pituitary and infundibulum by lymphocytes and plasma cells.[47-49] It generally occurs during pregnancy or the postpartum period.[47-49] It is associated with symptoms of hypopituitarism or an enlarging mass lesion with headaches and visual field defects, and is suspected based on its timing and lack of association with an obstetrical hemorrhage or prior history of menstrual difficulties or infertility.[47-49] Diabetes insipidus may also occur.[47-49] On magnetic resonance imaging (MRI), there is usually diffuse enhancement rather than a focal lesion that might indicate a tumor.[47-49] The clinical picture often allows a clinical diagnosis to be made without invasive procedures.

Treatment is generally conservative and involves identification and correction of any pituitary deficits, especially of ACTH secretion, which is particularly common in this condition.[48-49] Data regarding high-dose corticosteroid treatment are inconclusive. Surgery to debulk but not remove the gland is indicated in the presence of uncontrolled headaches, visual field defects, and progressive enlargement on scan. Spontaneous regression and resumption of partial or normal pituitary function may occur, although most patients progress to chronic panhypopituitarism.[47-49]

POSTERIOR PITUITARY

The set point for plasma osmolality at which **arginine vasopressin** (AVP) is secreted and thirst is stimulated is reduced about 5 to 10 mOsm/kg in pregnancy.[50] The placenta produces vasopressinase, an enzyme that rapidly inactivates AVP, thereby greatly increasing its clearance.[51]

Standard water deprivation tests, which require 5% weight loss, should be avoided during pregnancy because they may cause uterine irritability and alter placental perfusion. Instead, **desmopressin (dDAVP)** is used to assess urinary concentrating ability over 11 hours, with a value greater than 700 mOsm/kg considered normal.[52] Urinary concentrating ability in the pregnant patient should be determined in the seated position because the lateral recumbent position inhibits maximal urinary concentration.[50,53]

Diabetes Insipidus

Central **diabetes insipidus** (DI) may newly develop in pregnancy due to an enlarging pituitary lesion, with lymphocytic hypophysitis, or with hypothalamic disease. Because of the increased clearance of AVP by the vasopressinase, DI usually worsens during gestation, and subclinical DI may become manifest.[53-55] dDAVP is resistant to vasopressinase and provides satisfactory, safe treatment during gestation, although a higher dose may be required.[53,56] During monitoring of the clinical response, clinicians should remember that normal basal plasma osmolality and sodium concentration are 5 mEq/L lower during pregnancy.[50] dDAVP transfers minimally into breast milk.[53]

Transient AVP-resistant forms of DI secondary to placental production of vasopressinase may occur spontaneously in one pregnancy, but not in a subsequent one.[57] Some of these patients may respond to dDAVP therapy.

Acute fatty liver of pregnancy and other disturbances of hepatic function such as hepatitis may be associated with late-onset transient DI of pregnancy in some patients.[58] In some cases, this has been associated with the HELLP (*h*emolysis, *e*levated *l*iver enzymes, and *l*ow *p*latelets) syndrome.[59] It is presumed the hepatic dysfunction is associated with reduced degradation of vasopressinase, further increasing vasopressinase levels and the clearance of AVP. The polyuria may develop either before delivery or postpartum.

DI that develops postpartum may be a result of Sheehan syndrome. Transient DI of unknown etiology has been described postpartum, lasting only days to weeks.[60]

Congenital nephrogenic DI is a rare X-linked disorder caused by a mutation in the vasopressin V2 receptor gene and predominantly affects males. Female carriers of this disease may have significant polyuria during pregnancy. Treatment is with thiazide diuretics,[53] which should be used with caution in pregnant women.

ADRENALS

In addition to the changes during pregnancy in cortisol outlined previously, plasma renin activity, angiotensin II, and aldosterone increase threefold to sevenfold during pregnancy, and there is an increase in blood volume.[61]

Cushing Syndrome

Less than 150 cases of **Cushing syndrome** in pregnancy have been reported.[62-69] Less than 50% of the pregnant women described had pituitary adenomas, a similar number had **adrenal adenomas,** and more than 10% had **adrenal carcinomas.**[62-69] Pregnancies associated with the **ectopic ACTH syndrome** have been reported only rarely.[64,67,69] In many cases, the hypercortisolism first became apparent during pregnancy, with improvement and even remission after parturition.[64,66,69] Recently, cases have been reported of pregnancy-induced Cushing syndrome from hCG-induced stimulation of ectopic luteinizing hormone and hCG receptors on the adrenal.[70]

Diagnosing Cushing syndrome during pregnancy may be difficult. Both conditions may be associated with weight gain in a central distribution, fatigue, edema, emotional upset, glucose intolerance, and hypertension. The striae associated with normal pregnancy are usually pale and red or purple in Cushing syndrome. Hirsutism and acne may point to excessive androgen production. Proximal myopathy and bone fractures suggest Cushing syndrome.

The laboratory evaluation is difficult. Elevated total and free serum cortisol and ACTH levels and urinary free cortisol excretion are compatible with that of normal pregnancy. The overnight dexamethasone test usually demonstrates inadequate suppression during normal pregnancy.[8,69] ACTH levels are normal to elevated even with adrenal adenomas,[8,62,63,64] perhaps because of the production of ACTH by the placenta or from the nonsuppressible stimulation of pituitary ACTH by placental corticotropin-releasing hormone (CRH).

A persistent circadian variation in the elevated levels of total and free serum cortisol during normal pregnancy may be most helpful in distinguishing Cushing syndrome from the hypercortisolism of pregnancy because this finding is characteristically absent in all forms of Cushing syndrome.[7,8] Midnight levels of salivary cortisol during pregnancy have not yet been standardized.[66] In many cases, MRI of the pituitary (without contrast) or ultrasound of the adrenal may be helpful. Little experience has been reported with CRH stimulation testing or petrosal venous sinus sampling during pregnancy.[64,67,69]

Cushing syndrome is associated with a pregnancy loss rate of 25% due to spontaneous abortion, stillbirth, and early neonatal death because of extreme prematurity.[62,66-69] The passage of cortisol across the placenta may rarely result in suppression of the fetal adrenals.[71] Hypertension develops in most mothers with Cushing syndrome, and diabetes and myopathy are frequent. Postoperative wound infection and dehiscence are common after cesarean delivery.

In a review of 136 pregnancies collected from the literature, Lindsay and associates found that the frequency of live births increased from 76% to 89% when active treatment was instituted by a gestational age of 20 weeks.[67] Therefore, treatment during pregnancy has been advocated.[62,67,69]

Medical therapy for Cushing syndrome during pregnancy with metyrapone and ketoconazole is not very effective.[66,67,69] IUGR has been reported with ketoconoazole.[65] Aminoglutethimide and mitotane should be avoided. Transsphenoidal resection of a pituitary ACTH-secreting adenoma and laparoscopic resection of adrenal adenomas have been carried out successfully in several patients during the second trimester.[66,67,69,71] The live birth rate is about 87% after unilateral or bilateral adrenalectomy.[67,68] Although any surgery poses risks for the mother and fetus,[72] it appears that the benefit of treatment with Cushing syndrome outweighs the risks.

Adrenal Insufficiency

In developed countries, the most common etiology for primary **adrenal insufficiency** is **autoimmune adrenalitis**. Primary adrenal insufficiency from infections (**tuberculosis** or fungal), bilateral metastatic disease, hemorrhage, or infarctions is uncommon. Secondary adrenal insufficiency, from pituitary neoplasms or glucocorticoid suppression of the hypothalamic-pituitary-adrenal axis, may also occur.

Recognition of adrenal insufficiency may be difficult because many of the clinical features are found in normal pregnancies, including weakness, lightheadedness, syncope, nausea, vomiting, hyponatremia, and increased pigmentation. Addisonian hyperpigmentation may be distinguished from chloasma of pregnancy by its presence on the mucous membranes, extensor surfaces, and nonexposed areas. Weight loss, hypoglycemia, salt craving, and excessive hyponatremia should prompt a clinical evaluation. If unrecognized, adrenal crisis may ensue at times of stress, such as a urinary tract infection or labor.[73-75] The fetoplacental unit largely controls its own steroid milieu, so maternal adrenal insufficiency generally causes no problems with fetal development. Severe maternal hyponatremia or metabolic acidosis and poor maternal compliance with therapy may cause a poor fetal outcome.[73-75] Association with other autoimmune conditions such as anticardiolipin antibodies may lead to additional risks such as miscarriage.[76]

Adrenal insufficiency may be associated with laboratory findings of hyponatremia, hyperkalemia, hypoglycemia, eosinophilia, and lymphocytosis. Early morning plasma cortisol levels of 3 mcg/dL (83 nmol/L) or less confirms adrenal insufficiency, whereas a cortisol level higher than 19 mcg/dL (525 nmol/L) in the first or early second trimester excludes the diagnosis in a clinically stable patient.[77] However, plasma cortisol levels may fall in the normal nonpregnant range as a result of the increase in cortisol-binding globulin concentrations in the second and third trimesters, but will not be appropriately elevated for the stage of pregnancy.[78] Appropriate pregnancy-specific cut-offs for diagnosis with the standard cosyntropin test using a 250-mcg dose have not been established, with plasma cortisol levels 60% to 80% above nonpregnant responses in normal pregnant women tested in the second and third trimesters in one series.[78] The 1-mcg low-dose cosyntropin test has been reported to be more accurate at 24 to 34 weeks' gestation, using a cut-off of 30 mcg/dL (828 nmol/L).[77] With primary adrenal insufficiency, ACTH levels will be elevated, and a level above 100 pg/mL (22 pmol/L) is consistent with the diagnosis.[79] However, ACTH will not be low with secondary forms because of the placental production of this hormone, which is nevertheless insufficient to maintain normal maternal adrenal function.

In the unstable patient, empirical glucocorticoid therapy of hydrocortisone, 50 to 75 mg given intravenously, should be administered pending the results of diagnostic testing. Thereafter, doses of 50 to 75 mg every 6 to 8 hours should be given in the face of severe stress and during labor.[75] Despite the normal increase in plasma cortisol during pregnancy, baseline maternal replacement doses of corticosteroids usually are not different from those required in the nonpregnant state.[75] Mineralocorticoid replacement requirements usually do not change during gestation, although some clinicians have reduced doses of fludrocortisone in the third trimester in an attempt to treat addisonian patients who develop edema, exacerbation of hypertension, and preeclampsia.[73]

Patients who have received glucocorticoids as anti-inflammatory therapy are presumed to have adrenal axis suppression for at least 1 year after cessation of such therapy.[80] These patients should be treated with stress doses of glucocorticoids during labor and delivery as noted previously. They are at risk for postoperative wound infection and dehiscence, as are patients with endogenous Cushing syndrome, and their offspring are at risk for transient adrenal insufficiency.

Primary Hyperaldosteronism

Primary **hyperaldosteronism** rarely has been reported in pregnancy and is most often caused by an adrenal adenoma.[81-84] There are rare reports of glucocorticoid-remediable hyperaldosteronism in pregnancy.[85] The elevated aldosterone levels found in affected patients during pregnancy are similar to those in normal pregnant women, but the plasma renin activity is suppressed.[81] Moderate to severe **hypertension** develops in 85%, proteinuria in 52%, and hypokalemia in 55% of patients,[82] and symptoms may include headache, malaise, and muscle cramps. Placental abruption and preterm delivery are also risks.[86] Interestingly, the very high progesterone levels of pregnancy may have an antimineralocorticoid effect at the renal tubules, and thus the hypertension and hypokalemia may ameliorate during pregnancy in some women.[84]

Spironolactone, the usual nonpregnant therapy, is contraindicated in pregnancy because it crosses the placenta and is a potent antiandrogen that can cause ambiguous genitalia in a male fetus.[81] There is no published experience with the use during pregnancy of eplerenone, the new aldosterone receptor antagonist. Surgical therapy may be delayed until postpartum if hypertension can be controlled with agents safe in pregnancy, such as amiloride, methyldopa, labetalol, and calcium channel blockers.[87,88] On the other hand, laparoscopic removal of an aldosterone-producing adenoma during pregnancy has been reported.[83] Potassium supplementation may be required, but the hypokalemia may ameliorate in pregnancy because of the antikaliuretic effect of progesterone. Both hypertension and hypokalemia may exacerbate postpartum because of removal of the progesterone effect.[84]

Pheochromocytoma

Exacerbation of hypertension is a typical presentation of **pheochromocytoma** and may be frequently mistaken for pregnancy-induced hypertension or preeclampsia.[89,90] As the uterus enlarges and an actively moving fetus compresses the neoplasm, maternal complications such as severe hypertension, hemorrhage into the neoplasm, hemodynamic collapse, myocardial infarction, cardiac arrhythmias, congestive heart failure, and cerebral hemorrhage may occur. In 10% of patients, tumors may be outside of the adrenal, such as at the aortic bifurcation, and are particularly prone to hypertensive episodes with changes in position, uterine contractions, fetal movement, and Valsalva maneuver.[90] Unrecognized pheochromocytoma has been associated with a maternal mortality rate of 50%.[89,90]

There is minimal placental transfer of catecholamines,[91] likely because of high placental concentrations of catechol-O-methyltransferase and monoamine oxidase.[91] Adverse fetal effects such as hypoxia are a result of catecholamine-induced uteroplacental vasoconstriction and placental insufficiency[89,90,92] and of maternal hypertension, hypotension, or vascular collapse. Placental abruption may also occur.[89]

The diagnosis of pheochromocytoma requires a high index of suspicion. Preconception screening of families known to have multiple endocrine neoplasia type 2, von Hippel-Lindau disease, and neurofibromatosis is important.[93] The diagnosis should be considered in pregnant women with severe or paroxysmal hypertension, particularly during the first half of pregnancy or in association with orthostatic hypotension or episodic symptoms of pallor, anxiety, headaches, palpitations, chest pain, or diaphoresis.

Laboratory diagnosis of pheochromocytoma is unchanged from the nonpregnant state because catecholamine metabolism is not altered by pregnancy per se and consists of measuring urine **metanephrines** and **catecholamines** and plasma metaneprhines.[89,90] If possible, methyldopa and labetalol should be discontinued because these agents may interfere with the quantification of the catecholamines.[94] Tumor localization with MRI, with high-intensity signals noted on T2-weighted images, provides the best sensitivity without fetal exposure to ionizing radiation.[89,90]

Differentiation from preeclampsia is generally simple. The edema, proteinuria, and hyperuricemia found in women with preeclampsia are absent in those with pheochromocytomas. Plasma and urinary catecholamines may be modestly elevated in severe preeclampsia and other serious pregnancy complications requiring hospitalization, although they remain normal in mild preeclampsia or pregnancy-induced hypertension.[95] Catecholamine levels are two to four times normal after an eclamptic seizure, however.[96]

Initial medical management involves α-blockade with **phenoxybenzamine,** phentolamine, prazosin, or **labetalol.** All these agents are well-tolerated by the fetus, but phenoxybenzamine is considered the preferred agent because it provides long-acting, stable, noncompetitive blockade.[89] Phenoxybenzamine is started at a dose of 10 mg twice daily, with titration until the hypertension is controlled. Placental transfer of phenoxybenzamine occurs[97] but is generally considered safe.[89] However, two neonates of mothers treated with phenoxybenzamine have been reported with respiratory distress and hypotension requiring ventilatory and inotropic support.[98] β-Blockade is reserved for treating maternal tachycardia or arrhythmias that persist after full α-blockade and volume repletion.[90] β-Blockers may be associated with fetal bradycardia and with IUGR but generally are safe, and there is wide experience with their use.[90] All these potential fetal risks are small compared with the risk for fetal wastage from unblocked high maternal levels of catecholamines. Hypertensive emergencies should be treated with phentolamine (1 to 5 mg) or nitroprusside, although the latter should be limited because of potential fetal cyanide toxicity.

The timing of surgical excision of the neoplasm is controversial and may depend on the success of the medical management and the location of the tumor. Pressure from the uterus, motion of the fetus, and labor contractions are all stimuli that may cause an acute crisis. In the first half of pregnancy, surgical excision may proceed once adequate α-blockade is established, although there may be a higher risk for fetal loss with first trimester surgery. In the early second trimester, fetal loss is less likely with surgery compared with the first trimester, and the size of the uterus will not make excision difficult. If the pheochromocytoma is not recognized until the second half of gestation, increasing uterine size makes surgical exploration difficult. Successful laparoscopic excision of pheochromocytomas has been described in the second trimester.[89,90] Other options include combined cesarean delivery and tumor resection or delivery followed by tumor resection at a later date.

Although successful vaginal delivery has been reported,[99] it has been associated with higher rates of maternal mortality than cesarean delivery. Labor may result in uncontrolled release of catecholamines secondary to pain and uterine contractions. Severe maternal hypertension may lead to placental ischemia and fetal hypoxia. In the well-blocked patient, however, vaginal delivery may be possible with pain management with epidural anesthesia and may be facilitated by instrumental delivery.

KEY POINTS

- About 30% of prolactin-secreting macroadenomas enlarge significantly during pregnancy.
- Dopamine agonists can be used safely for the treatment of prolactinomas in women attempting conception.
- In patients with acromegaly, the risks for gestational diabetes and hypertension are increased.
- Gonadotropins, gonadotropin-releasing hormone, and in vitro fertilization techniques have been used successfully to achieve pregnancy in women with hypopituitarism.
- Sheehan syndrome is very uncommon with modern obstetrical practice but still must be considered in the postpartum unstable patient following hemorrhage.
- Lymphocytic hypophysitis occurring during pregnancy is often associated with ACTH deficiency and may be fatal.
- Subclinical diabetes insipidus may become manifest during pregnancy because of secretion of placental vasopressinase.
- Cushing syndrome is associated with adverse outcomes for mother and fetus and should be treated aggressively during pregnancy.
- Although maintenance glucocorticoid replacement does not need to be increased in pregnant women with either hypopituitarism or primary adrenal insufficiency, stress doses of hydrocortisone are required during labor and delivery and other stressful situations.
- Pheochromocytomas should be treated aggressively and usually require surgical resection during the pregnancy.

REFERENCES

1. Scheithauer BW, Sano T, Kovacs KT, et al: The pituitary gland in pregnancy: a clinicopathologic and immunohistochemical study of 69 Cases. Mayo Clin Proc 65:461, 1990.
2. Elster AD, Sanders TG, Vines FS, et al: Size and shape of the pituitary gland during pregnancy and post-partum: measurement with MR imaging. Radiology 181:531, 1991.
3. Rigg LA, Lein A, Yen SSC: Pattern of increase in circulating prolactin levels during human gestation. Am J Obstet Gynecol 129:454, 1977.
4. Frankenne F, Closset J, Gomez F, et al: The physiology of growth hormones (GHs) in pregnant women and partial characterization of the placental GH variant. J Clin Endocrinol Metab 66:1171, 1988.
5. Eriksson L, Frankenne F, Eden S, et al: Growth hormone 24-h serum profiles during pregnancy lack of pulsatility for the secretion of the placental variant. BJOG 106:949, 1989.
6. Beckers A, Stevenaert A, Foidart J-M, et al: Placental and pituitary growth hormone secretion during pregnancy in acromegalic women. J Clin Endocrinol Metab 71:725, 1990.
7. Nolten WE, Lindheimer MD, Rueckert PA, et al: Diurnal patterns and regulation of cortisol secretion in pregnancy. J Clin Endocrinol Metab 51:466, 1980.
8. Lindsay JR, Nieman LK: The hypothalamic-pituitary-adrenal axis in pregnancy: challenges in disease detection and treatment. Endocr Rev 26:775, 2005.
9. Casanueva FF, Molitch ME, Schlechte JA, et al: Guidelines of the Pituitary Society for the diagnosis and management of prolactinomas. Clin Endocrinol 65:265, 2006.
10. Gillam MP, Molitch MP, Lombardi G, et al: Advances in the treatment of prolactinomas. Endocr Rev 27:485, 2006.
11. Lebbe M, Hubinont C, Bernard P, et al: Outcome of 100 pregnancies initiated under treatment with cabergoline in hyperprolactinaemic women. Clin Endocrinol 73:230, 2010.
12. Ono M, Miki N, Amano K, et al: Individualized high-dose cabergoline therapy for hyperprolactinemic infertility in women with micro- and macroprolactinomas. J Clin Endocrinol Metab 95:2672, 2010.
13. Ricci E, Parazzini F, Motta T, et al: Pregnancy outcome after cabergoline treatment in early weeks of gestation. Reprod Toxicol 16:791, 2002.
14. Colao A, Abs R, Bárcena DG, et al: Pregnancy outcomes following cabergoline treatment: extended results from a 12-year observational study. Clin Endocrinol 68:66, 2008.
15. Molitch ME: Prolactinomas and pregnancy. Clin Endocrinol 73:147, 2010.
16. Stalldecker G, Gil MSG, Guitelman M, et al: Effects of cabergoline on pregnancy and embryo-fetal development: retrospective study on 103 pregnancies and a review of the literature. Pituitary 13:345-350, 2010.
17. Divers WA, Yen SSC. Prolactin-producing microadenomas in pregnancy. Obstet Gynecol 62:425, 1983.
18. Molitch ME. Clinical manifestations of acromegaly. Endocrinol Metab Clin North Am 21:597, 1992.
19. Herman-Bonert V, Seliverstow M, Melmed S: Pregnancy in acromegaly: successful therapeutic outcome. J Clin Endocrinol Metab 83:727, 1998.
20. Melmed S, Colao A, Barkan A, et al: Guideline for acromegaly management: an update. J Clin Endocrinol Metab 94:1509, 2009.
21. Barkan AL, Stred SE, Reno K, et al: Increased growth hormone pulse frequency in acromegaly. J Clin Endocrinol Metab 69:1225, 1989.
22. Kupersmith MJ, Rosenberg C, Kleinberg D: Visual loss in pregnant women with pituitary adenomas. Ann Intern Med 121:473, 1994.
23. Okada Y, Morimoto I, Ejima K, et al: A case of active acromegalic woman with a marked increase in serum insulin-like growth factor-1 levels after delivery. Endocr J 44:117, 1997.
24. Cozzi R, Attanasio R, Barausee M: Pregnancy in acromegaly: a one-center experience. Eur J Endocrinol 155:279, 2006.
25. Caron P, Broussaud S, Bertherat J, et al: Acromegaly and pregnancy: a retrospective multicenter study of 59 pregnancies in 46 women. J Clin Endocrinol Metab 95:4680-4687, 2010.
26. Maffei P, Tamagno G, Nardelli GB, et al: Effects of octreotide exposure during pregnancy in acromegaly. Clin Endocrinol 72:668, 2010.
27. Karaca Z, Tanriverdi F, Unluhizarci K, et al: Pregnancy and pituitary disorders. Eur J Endocrinol 162:453, 2010.
28. Brian SR, Bidlingmaier M, Wajnrajch MP, et al: Treatment of acromegaly with pegvisomant during pregnancy: maternal and fetal effects. J Clin Endocrinol Metab 92:3374, 2007.
29. Caron P, Gerbeau C, Pradayrol L, et al: Successful pregnancy in an infertile woman with a thyrotropin-secreting macroadenoma treated with the somatostatin analog (octreotide). J Clin Endocrinol Metab 81:1164, 1996.
30. Blackhurst G, Strachan MW, Collie D, et al: The treatment of a thyrotropin-secreting pituitary macroadenoma with octreotide in twin pregnancy. Clin Endocrinol 56:401, 2002.
31. Chaiamnuay S, Moster M, Katz MR, et al: Successful management of a pregnant woman with a TSH secreting pituitary adenoma with surgical and medical therapy. Pituitary 6:109, 2003.

32. Masding MG, Lees PD, Gawne-Cain ML, et al: Visual field compression by a non-secreting pituitary tumour during pregnancy. J R Soc Med 96:27, 2003.
33. Murata Y, Ando H, Nagasaka T, et al: Successful pregnancy after bromocriptine therapy in an anovulatory woman complicated with ovarian hyperstimulation caused by follicle-stimulating hormone-producing plurihormonal pituitary microadenoma. J Clin Endocrinol Metab 88:1988, 2003.
34. Sugita T, Seki K, Nagai Y, et al: Successful pregnancy and delivery after removal of gonadotrope adenoma secreting follicle-stimulating hormone in a 29-year-old amenorrheic woman. Gynecol Obstet Invest 59:138, 2005.
35. Hall R, Manski-Nankervis J, Goni N, et al: Fertility outcomes in women with hypopituitarism. Clin Endocrinol 65:71, 2006.
36. Overton CE, Davis CJ, West C, et al: High risk pregnancies in hypopituitary women. Hum Reprod 17:1464, 2002.
37. Esfandiari N, Gotlieb L, Casper RF. Live birth of healthy triplets after in vitro fertilization and embryo transfer in an acromegalic woman with elevated growth hormone. Fertil Steril 83:1041, 2005.
38. Kübler K, Klingmüller D, Gembruch U, et al: High-risk pregnancy management in women with hypopituitarism. J Perinatol 29:89, 2009.
39. Mandel SJ, Larsen PR, Seely EW, et al: Increased need for thyroxine during pregnancy in women with primary hypothyroidism. N Engl J Med 323:91, 1990.
40. Beitins IZ, Bayard F, Ances IG, et al: The transplacental passage of prednisone and prednisolone in pregnancy near term. J Pediatr 81:936, 1972.
41. Kenny FM, Preeyasombat C, Spaulding JS, et al: Cortisol production rate. IV. Infants born of steroid-treated mothers and of diabetic mothers. Infants with trisomy syndrome and with anencephaly. Pediatrics 137:960, 1966.
42. McKenzie SA, Selley JA, Agnew JE: Secretion of prednisolone into breast milk. Arch Dis Child 50:894, 1975.
43. Curran AJ, Peacey SR, Shalet SM: Is maternal growth hormone essential for a normal pregnancy? Eur J Endocrinol 139:54, 1998.
44. Kelestimur F: Sheehan's syndrome. Pituitary 6:181, 2003.
45. Feinberg E, Molitch M, Endres L, et al: The incidence of Sheehan's syndrome after obstetric hemorrhage. Fertil Steril 84:975, 2005.
46. Iwasaki Y, Oiso Y, Yamauchi K, et al: Neurohypophyseal function in post-partum hypopituitarism: impaired plasma vasopressin response to osmotic stimuli. J Clin Endocrinol Metab 68:560, 1989.
47. Caturegli P, Newschaffer C, Olivi A, et al: Autoimmune hypophysitis. Endocr Rev 26:599, 2005.
48. Rivera J-A: Lymphocytic hypophysitis: disease spectrum and approach to diagnosis and therapy. Pituitary 9:35, 2006.
49. Molitch ME, Gilliam MP: Lymphocytic hypophysitis. Horm Res 68:145, 2007.
50. Lindheimer MD, Davison JM: Osmoregulation, the secretion of arginine vasopressin and its metabolism during pregnancy. Eur J Endocrinol 132:133, 1995.
51. Davison JM, Shiells EA, Barron WM, et al: Changes in the metabolic clearance of vasopressin and of plasma vasopressinase throughout human pregnancy. J Clin Invest 83:1313, 1989.
52. Huchon DJR, Van Zijl JAWM, Campbell-Brown MB, et al: Desmopressin as a test of urinary concentrating ability in pregnancy. J Obstet Gynecol 2:206, 1982.
53. Durr JA: Diabetes insipidus in pregnancy. Am J Kidney Dis 9: 276, 1987.
54. Soule SG, Monson JP, Jacobs HS: Transient diabetes insipidus in pregnancy: a consequence of enhanced placental clearance of arginine vasopressin. Hum Reprod 10:3322, 1995.
55. Iwasaki Y, Oiso Y, Kondo K, et al: Aggravation of subclinical diabetes insipidus during pregnancy. N Engl J Med 324:522, 1991.
56. Ray JG: DDAVP use during pregnancy: an analysis of its safety for mother and child. Obstet Gynecol Surv 53:450, 1998.
57 Brewster UC, Hayslett JP: Diabetes insipidus in the third trimester of pregnancy. Obstet Gynecol 105:1173, 2005.
58. Kennedy S, Hall PM, Seymour AE, et al: Transient diabetes insipidus and acute fatty liver of pregnancy. BJOG 101:387, 1994.
59. Ellidokuz E, Uslan I, Demir S, et al: Transient postpartum diabetes insipidus associated with HELLP syndrome. J Obstet Gynaecol Res 32:602, 2006.
60. Raziel A, Rosenberg T, Schreyer P, et al: Transient postpartum diabetes insipidus. Am J Obstet Gynecol 164:616, 1991.
61. Wilson M, Morganti AA, Zervoudakis I, et al: Blood pressure, the renin-aldosterone system and sex steroids throughout normal pregnancy. Am J Med 8:97, 1980.
62. Bevan JS, Gough MH, Gillmer MD, et al: Cushing's syndrome in pregnancy: the timing of definitive treatment. Clin Endocrinol 27:225, 1987.
63. Chico A, Manzanares JM, Halperin I, et al: Cushing's disease and pregnancy. Eur J Obstet Gynecol Reprod Biol 64:143, 1996.
64. Guilhaume B, Sanson ML, Billaud L, et al: Cushing's syndrome and pregnancy: aetiologies and prognosis in twenty-two patients. Eur J Med 1:83, 1992.
65. Amado JA, Pesquera C, Gonzalez EM, et al: Successful treatment with ketoconazole of Cushing's syndrome in pregnancy. Postgrad Med J 66:221, 1990.
66. Madhun ZT, Aron DC: Cushing's disease in pregnancy. In Bronstein MD (ed): Pituitary Tumors and Pregnancy. Norwell, MA, Kluwer Academic Publishers, 2001, p 149.
67. Lindsay JR, Jonklaas J, Oldfield EH, et al: Cushing's syndrome during pregnancy: personal experience and review of the literature. J Clin Endocrinol Metab 90:3077, 2005.
68. Lindsay JR, Nieman LK: Adrenal disorders in pregnancy. Endocrinol Metab Clin North Am 35:1, 2006.
69. Vilar L, Freitas MDC, Lima LHC, et al: Cushing's syndrome in pregnancy: an overview. Arq Bras Endocrinol Metab 51:1293, 2007.
70. Chui MH, Özbey NC, Ezzat S, et al: Case report: adrenal LH/hCG receptor overexpression and gene amplification causing pregnancy-induced Cushing's syndrome. Endocr Pathol 20:256, 2009.
71. Kreines K, DeVaux WD: Neonatal adrenal insufficiency associated with maternal Cushing's syndrome. Pediatrics 47:516, 1971.
72. Cohen-Kerem R, Railton C, Orfen D, et al: Pregnancy outcome following non-obstetric surgical intervention. Am J Surg 190:467, 2005.
73. Albert E, Dalaker K, Jorde R, et al: Addison's disease and pregnancy. Acta Obstet Gynecol Scand 68:185, 1989.
74. Otta CF, de Meresian PS, Iraci GS, et al: Pregnancies associated with primary adrenal insufficiency. Fertil Steril 90:1199, 2008.
75. Ambrosi B, Barbetta L, Morricone L: Diagnosis and management of Addison's disease during pregnancy. J Endocrinol Invest 26:698, 2003.
76. Grottolo A, Ferrari V, Mariano M, et al: Primary adrenal insufficiency, circulating lupus anticoagulant and anticardiolipin antibodies in a patient with multiple abortions and recurrent thrombotic episodes. Haematologica 73:517, 1988.
77. McKenna DS, Wittber GM, Nagaraja HN, et al: The effects of repeat doses of antenatal corticosteroids on maternal adrenal function. Am J Obstet Gynecol 183:669, 2000.
78. Nolten WE, Lindheimer MD, Oparil S, et al: Desoxycorticosterone in normal pregnancy. I. sequential studies of the secretory patterns of desoxycorticosterone, aldosterone, and cortisol. Am J Obstet Gynecol 132:414, 1978.
79. Grinspoon SK, Biller BM: Clinical review 62: laboratory assessment of adrenal insufficiency. J Clin Endocrinol Metab 79:79, 1994.
80. Schlaghecke R, Kornely E, Santen RT, et al: The effect of long-term glucocorticoid therapy on pituitary-adrenal responses to exogenous corticotropin-releasing hormone. N Engl J Med 326:226, 1992.
81. Robar CA, Poremba JA, Pelton JJ, et al: Current diagnosis and management of aldosterone-producing adenomas during pregnancy. Endocrinologist 8:403, 1998.
82. Okawa T, Asano K, Hashimoto T, et al: Diagnosis and management of primary aldosteronism in pregnancy: case report and review of the literature. Am J Perinatol 19:31, 2002.
83. Nursal TZ, Caliskan K, Ertorer E, et al: Laparoscopic treatment of primary hyperaldosteronism in a pregnant patient. J Can Chir 52:E188, 2009.
84. Escher G: Hyperaldosteronism in pregnancy. Ther Adv Cardiovasc Dis 3:123, 2009.
85. Wyckoff JA, Seely EW, Hurwitz S, et al: Glucocorticoid-remediable aldosteronism and pregnancy. Hypertension 35:668, 2000.
86. Neerhof MG, Shlossman PA, Poll DS, et al: Idiopathic aldosteronism in pregnancy. Obstet Gynecol 78 489, 1991.
87. Matsumoto J, Miyake H, Isozaki T, et al: Primary aldosteronism in pregnancy. J Nippon Med Sch 67:275, 2000.
88. Deruelle P, Dufour P, Magnenant E, et al: Maternal Bartter's syndrome in pregnancy treated by amiloride. Eur J Obstet Gynecol Reprod Biol 115:106, 2004.
89. Oliva R, Angelos P, Kaplan E, et al: Pheochromocytoma in pregnancy: a case series and review. Hypertension 55:600, 2010.

90. Sarathi V, Lila AR, Bandgar TR, et al: Pheochromocytoma and pregnancy: a rare but dangerous combination. Endocr Pract 16:300, 2010.
91. Saarikoski S: Fate of noradrenaline in the human fetoplacental unit. Acta Physiol Scand 421(Suppl):1, 1984.
92. Harper MA, Murnaghan GA, Kennedy L, et al: Phaeochromocytoma in pregnancy: five cases and a review of the literature. BJOG 96:594, 1989.
93. Kolomeyevskaya N, Blazo M, van den Veyver I, et al: Pheochromocytoma and von Hippel-Lindau in pregnancy. Am J Perinatol 22:257, 2010.
94. Sheps SG, Jiang NS, Klee GC: Diagnostic evaluation of pheochromocytoma. Endocrinol Metab Clin North Am 17:397, 1988.
95. Pederson EB, Rasmussen AB, Christensen NJ, et al: Plasma noradrenaline and adrenaline in pre-eclampsia, essential hypertension in pregnancy and normotensive pregnant control subjects. Acta Endocrinol 99:594, 1982.
96. Khatun S, Kanayama N, Hossain B, et al: Increased concentrations of plasma epinephrine and norepinephrine in patients with eclampsia. Eur J Obstet Gynecol Reprod Biol 74:103, 1997.
97. Santeiro ML, Stromquist C, Wyble L: Phenoxybenzamine placental transfer during the third trimester. Ann Pharmacother 30:1249, 1996.
98. Aplin SC, Yee KF, Cole MJ: Neonatal effects of long-term maternal phenoxybenzamine therapy. Anesthesiology 100:1608, 2004.
99. Schenker JG, Granat M: Phaeochromocytoma and pregnancy: an updated appraisal. Aust N Z J Obstet Gynaecol 22:1, 1982.

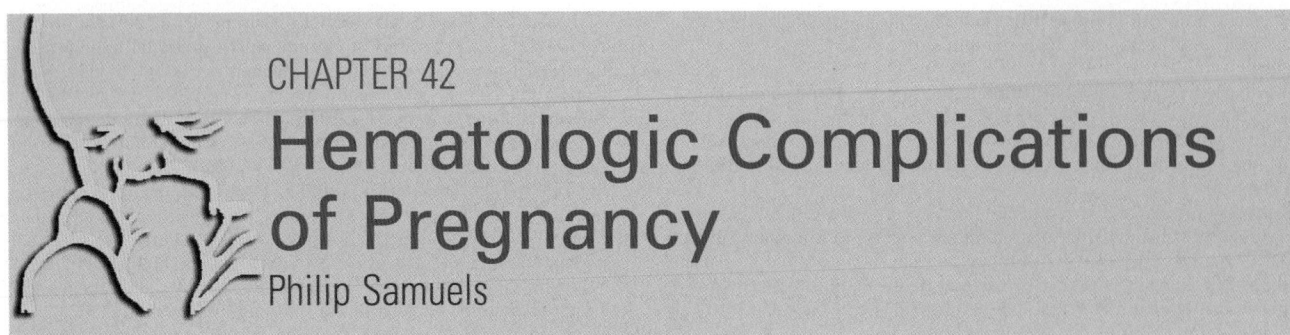

CHAPTER 42

Hematologic Complications of Pregnancy

Philip Samuels

KEY ABBREVIATIONS	
Hemolysis, Elevated Liver Enzymes, Low Platelets	HELLP
Hemolytic Uremic Syndrome	HUS
Immune Thrombocytopenic Purpura	ITP
Immunoglobulin G	IgG
Intravenous Immunoglobulin	IVIG
Polymerase Chain Reaction	PCR
Red Blood Cell	RBC
Thrombotic Thrombocytopenic Purpura	TTP
Unusually Large Multimers of von Willebrand's Factor	ULVWf
Urinary Tract Infection	UTI
von Willebrand's Cleaving Enzyme	ADAMTS-13
von Willebrand's Disease	vWD
von Willebrand's Factor	vWF

PREGNANCY-ASSOCIATED THROMBOCYTOPENIA

Affecting approximately 4% of pregnancies, thrombocytopenia is the most frequent hematologic complication of pregnancy resulting in consultation. Hospital laboratories vary on their lower limit of a normal platelet count, but it is usually between 135,000 and 150,000/mm^3. Platelet counts generally fall slightly, owing to hemodilution and increased destruction, as gestation progresses.[1] Platelet counts, however, should not fall below the normal range. **In pregnancy, the vast majority of cases of mild to moderate thrombocytopenia are caused by gestational thrombocytopenia.[2] This form of thrombocytopenia has little likelihood of causing maternal or neonatal complications.[3]** The obstetrician, however, is obliged to rule out other etiologies of thrombocytopenia that are associated with severe maternal or perinatal morbidity. The common and rare causes of thrombocytopenia in the gravida at term are shown in the box Causes of Thrombocytopenia during Pregnancy.

CAUSES OF THROMBOCYTOPENIA DURING PREGNANCY

Common Causes

- Gestational thrombocytopenia
- Severe preeclampsia
- HELLP syndrome
- Disseminated intravascular coagulation

Rare Causes

- Immune thrombocytopenic purpura
- Lupus anticoagulant/antiphospholipid antibody syndrome
- Systemic lupus erythematosus
- Thrombotic thrombocytopenic purpura
- Hemolytic uremic syndrome
- Type 2b von Willebrand's syndrome
- Hemoglobin SC crisis with splenic sequestration
- Folic acid deficiency
- Human immunodeficiency virus infection
- Hematologic malignancies
- May-Hegglin syndrome (congenital thrombocytopenia)

Gestational Thrombocytopenia

Patients with gestational thrombocytopenia generally have mild (platelet count = 100,000 to 149,000/mm^3) to moderate (platelet count = 50,000 to 99,000/mm^3) thrombocytopenia. These patients require no therapy, and the fetus appears to be at negligible risk of being born with profound thrombocytopenia (platelet count below 50,000/mm^3) or a bleeding diathesis. This distinct entity was first suggested but not specifically defined in a study published in 1986 by Hart and colleagues.[4] In this study, 28 of 116 pregnant women

(24%) who were evaluated prospectively during an 8-month period had platelet counts less than 150,000/mm^3 at least once during pregnancy. In all 17 patients who were followed after delivery, platelet counts returned to normal. Hart and colleagues[4] were actually describing gestational thrombocytopenia before the condition had been recognized as a distinct entity. Samuels and colleagues[5] also investigated 74 mothers with gestational thrombocytopenia. Regardless of platelet antibody status, none of the infants born to these mothers demonstrated thrombocytopenia. Burrows and Kelton[6] have further shown that there is little risk to the mother or neonate in cases of gestational thrombocytopenia. In their study of 1357 healthy, pregnant women, 112 (8.3%) had platelet counts less than 150,000/mm^3.[6] The lowest platelet count was 97,000/mm^3. The incidence of thrombocytopenia (platelet count less than 150,000/mm^3) in the infants of these 112 women was 4.3%, not statistically significantly different from infants born to healthy pregnant women without thrombocytopenia (1.5%).[6] None of these infants had platelet counts less than 100,000/mm^3. Indeed, the reports by Samuels and colleagues[5] and Burrows and Kelton[6] have convincingly demonstrated that gestational thrombocytopenia is an entity distinct from immune thrombocytopenic purpura (ITP).

The decrease in platelet count, occurring in gestational thrombocytopenia, is not merely due to dilution of platelets with increasing blood volume. It also appears to be due to an acceleration of the normal increase in platelet destruction that occurs during pregnancy. This is demonstrated by the fact that the mean platelet volume (MPV) is increased in patients with gestational thrombocytopenia. Pregnant women who have gestational thrombocytopenia do not require any special therapy during the puerperium. In fact, intervention, including unnecessary glucocorticoids or bone marrow aspirations, will be more harmful and confusing. However, if the platelet counts fall below 20,000/mm^3 or if there is clinical bleeding, further investigation and intervention are warranted. These complications, however, are rare, and it is difficult to determine whether these patients with profound thrombocytopenia have gestational thrombocytopenia, the new onset of ITP, or a blood dyscrasia.

Immune Thrombocytopenic Purpura

Immune thrombocytopenic purpura (ITP) affects 1 to 3 per 1000 pregnancies and rarely causes neonatal complications. Although there are rare cases of neonatal thrombocytopenia, fetal complications are almost nonexistent.[5] Therefore, the maternal-fetal medicine specialist should focus on maternal disease and well-being.

In general, **pregnancy has not been determined to cause ITP or to change its severity**, but there are rare exceptions. Harrington and colleagues[7] were the first to demonstrate that ITP was humorally mediated. Shulman and colleagues[8] showed that the mediator of this disorder was IgG. These findings were confirmed when Cines and Schreiber[9] developed the first platelet antiglobulin test, a radioimmunoassay, in 1979. Today, this test is usually performed using enzyme-linked immunosorbent assay or flow cytometry. Newer assays have shown that these autoantibodies may be directed against specific platelet surface glycoproteins, including the IIb/IIIa and Ib/IX complexes.[10] In vivo, after the platelets are coated with antibody, they are removed from circulation by binding to the Fc receptors of macrophages in the reticuloendothelial system, especially the spleen. Approximately 90% of women with ITP have platelet-associated IgG.[9] Unfortunately, this is not specific for ITP, because studies have shown that these tests are also positive in women with gestational thrombocytopenia and preeclampsia.

To make the issue more confusing, the pathogenesis of ITP in children and adults usually differs. Childhood ITP most often follows a viral infection and clinically presents with petechiae and bleeding. This form of ITP is generally self-limited and disappears over time. Conversely, adults have milder bleeding and easy bruisability, and are often diagnosed after a prolonged period of subtle symptoms. Adult ITP usually runs a chronic course, and long-term therapy is often eventually needed. Many pregnancies occur in women in their late teens and early twenties. In these women, with a history of ITP, it may be difficult to ascertain whether the patient has childhood ITP or adult ITP. The distinction is important for counseling concerning long term prognosis.

ITP has a predisposition for women ages 18 to 40, with an overall female-male ratio of 1.7.[11] It is a diagnosis of exclusion. The patient must have isolated thrombocytopenia with an unremarkable peripheral smear. She must have only bleeding clinically consistent with a depressed platelet count, such as petechiae. She must not be taking any medication, herbal compound, or illicit drug that may cause thrombocytopenia. Finally, the patient must have no other disease process than can cause thrombocytopenia, such as those listed in the box earlier in this chapter.[11,12]

Thrombotic Thrombocytopenic Purpura and Hemolytic Uremic Syndrome

These two conditions are characterized by microangiopathic hemolytic anemia and severe thrombocytopenia. Pregnancy does not predispose a patient to these conditions, but they should be considered when evaluating the gravida with severe thrombocytopenia. Thrombotic thrombocytopenic purpura (TTP) is characterized by a pentad of findings, which are shown in the box Pentad of Findings in TTP.[13,14] The complete pentad occurs only in approximately 40% of patients, but approximately 75% have a triad of microangiopathic hemolytic anemia, thrombocytopenia, and neurologic changes.[15] Pathologically, these patients have thrombotic occlusions of arterioles and capillaries.[13] These occur in multiple organs, and there is no specific clinical manifestation for the disease. The clinical picture reflects the organs that are involved.

Pentad of Findings in Thrombotic Thrombocytopenic Purpura (TTP)*

†Microangiopathic hemolytic anemia
†Thrombocytopenia
†Neurologic abnormalities, including confusion, headache, paresis, visual hallucinations, seizures
Fever
Renal dysfunction

*The classic pentad is found in only 40% of patients.
†These three findings are present in 74% of patients.[32]

TTP/HUS may mimic preeclampsia. Because preeclampsia is much more common than this disorder, it should be considered first. However, **delay in diagnosing TTP/HUS can have fatal consequences.**

To diagnose the hemolytic anemia associated with TTP, the indirect antiglobulin (Coomb's) test must be negative. This rules out an immune-mediated cause for the hemolytic anemia. Lactic dehydrogenase should be elevated, the indirect bilirubin should be increased, and haptoglobin should be decreased, indicating ongoing hemolysis. Schistocytes are usually seen on the peripheral smear, if it is carefully reviewed. To be classified as TTP, the platelet count should be less than 100,000/mm^3. In renal insufficiency associated with TTP, the urine sediment is usually normal with an occasional red blood cell (RBC). This finding helps distinguish this disorder from a lupus flare, which more often has associated hematuria and casts. The serum creatinine is usually greater than 2 mg/dL. This degree of renal dysfunction is unusual, but not rare, in preeclampsia. There is usually 1 to 2 proteinuria on urine dipstick.

The neurologic findings in TTP are usually nonspecific. They include headache, confusion, and lethargy. Infrequently tonic-clonic seizures occur, and rarely lateralizing signs are noted.

Terrell and coworkers[16] examined the epidemiology of TTP/HUS occurring in Oklahoma between 1996 and 2004. In 206 reported cases, they found that 37% were idiopathic. However, 13% were associated with an autoimmune disease, and 7% occurred in pregnancy and the postpartum period. These researchers were able to project that the incidence of suspected TTP/HUS is 11 cases/million population/year, whereas the incidence of proven cases is 4.5 cases/million population/year.[16] If this disease is so rare, why include it in a text on obstetrics? If untreated, TTP carries a 90% mortality rate, whereas treatment with plasma exchange decreases the mortality rate to 20%.[17] Therefore, obstetricians must be aware of this disease process, so it can be quickly and aggressively treated.

Recent work has helped to determine the pathophysiology of many cases of TTP. **Tsai and colleagues have found that a decrease of ADAMTS-13 activity is strongly associated with TTP.**[18,19] This metalloprotease, also known as von Willebrand's cleaving enzyme, cleaves unusually large multimers of von Willebrand factor (ULVWf). Activity can be decreased from a decrease in the metalloprotease or antibodies against it. If there is a deficiency in the activity and/or concentration of ADAMTS-13, ULVWf circulate in increased amounts, leading to increased platelet aggregation and the initiation of TTP. ADAMTS-13 can be readily assayed in commercial laboratories. Ferrari and colleagues[20] have shown all four Ig subclass of anti-ADAMTS 13 antibodies are associated with TTP, but the IgG(4) subclass is most common. Fakhouri and colleagues[21] found that there were complement gene mutations in 18 of 21 patients with TTP. These findings may lead to the development of therapies that will specifically target the etiology of TTP.

Weiner[22] has published the most extensive literature review concerning TTP. In this series of 45 patients, 40 developed the disease antepartum, with 50% occurring before 24 weeks' gestation. The mean gestational age at onset of symptoms was 23.4 weeks. This finding may be helpful when trying to distinguish TTP from other causes of thrombocytopenia and microangiopathic hemolytic anemia occurring during gestation. In Weiner's review, the fetal and maternal mortality rates were 84% and 44%, respectively. These mortality rates are overly pessimistic, because this series included many patients who contracted the disease before plasma infusion/exchange therapy was utilized to treat TTP.

However, TTP may be confused with rarely occurring early-onset severe preeclampsia. In preeclampsia, antithrombin III levels are frequently low, and this is not the case with TTP. This test, therefore, may be a useful discriminator between these two disorders.

Although the HUS has many features in common with TTP, it usually has its onset in the postpartum period. Patients with HUS display a triad of microangiopathic hemolytic anemia, acute nephropathy, and thrombocytopenia. HUS is rare in adults, and the thrombocytopenia is usually milder than that seen in TTP, with only 50% of patients having a platelet count less than 100,000/mm^3 at the time of diagnosis. The thrombocytopenia worsens as the disease progresses. A major difference between TTP and HUS is that 15% to 25% of patients with the latter develop chronic renal disease. HUS often follows infections with verotoxin-producing enteric bacteria. Cyclosporine therapy, cytotoxic drugs, and oral contraceptives may predispose adults to develop HUS. The majority of cases of HUS occurring in pregnancy develop at least 2 days after delivery. In fact, in one series, only nine of 62 cases (6.9%) of pregnancy-associated HUS occurred antepartum. Four of these nine patients developed symptoms on the day of delivery. The mean time from delivery to development of HUS in patients in this series was 26.6 days. The maternal mortality rate may exceed 50% in postpartum HUS. However, this mortality rate is based on old data. With plasmapheresis and dialysis, the likelihood of maternal death is probably much less. It is not important to make the distinction between TTP and HUS, because the initial therapy for both disorders is plasmapheresis.

EVALUATION OF THROMBOCYTOPENIA DURING PREGANCY AND THE PUERPERIUM

Before deciding on a course to follow in treating the patient with thrombocytopenia, the obstetrician must evaluate the patient and attempt to ascertain the etiology of her low platelet count. Important management decisions are dependent on arriving at an accurate diagnosis. A complete medical history, although time consuming, is critically important. It is essential to learn whether the patient has previously had a depressed platelet count or bleeding diathesis. It is also important to know whether these clinical conditions occur coincidentally with pregnancy. A complete medication history should be elicited, because certain medications, such as heparin, can result in profound maternal thrombocytopenia. The obstetrical history should focus on whether there have been any maternal or neonatal bleeding problems in the past. Excessive bleeding from an episiotomy site or cesarean delivery incision site, or bleeding from intravenous sites during labor should alert the physician to the possibility of thrombocytopenia in the previous pregnancy. The obstetrician should also question whether the infant had any bleeding diathesis or if there was any problem following a circumcision. The obstetrician should also ask pertinent questions to determine whether severe preeclampsia or HELLP (*H*emolysis, *E*levated *L*iver enzymes, *L*ow *P*latelets) syndrome is the cause of her thrombocytopenia. The treatment of preeclampsia and HELLP are discussed elsewhere in this text. All thrombocytopenic pregnant women should be carefully evaluated for the presence of risk factors for HIV infection, because this infection can cause an ITP-like syndrome. Also, a family history should be elicited, as there are familial forms of thrombocytopenia.

An accurate assessment of gestational age should also be carried out. This is important, because some of the etiologies of thrombocytopenia in pregnancy are dependent on the gestational age. A thorough physical examination of the patient should be performed. The physician should look for the presence of ecchymoses or petechiae. The conjunctivae often show petechiae, as do the nail beds. Blood pressure should be determined to ascertain whether the patient has impending preeclampsia. If the patient is developing HELLP syndrome, scleral icterus may be present. The eye grounds should be examined for evidence of arteriolar spasm or hemorrhage.

It is imperative that a peripheral blood smear be examined by an experienced hematologist or pathologist whenever a case of pregnancy-associated thrombocytopenia is diagnosed. The presence or absence of evidence of microangiopathic hemolysis on the smear will help in establishing a diagnosis. This specialist can also rule out platelet clumping, which will result in a factitious thrombocytopenia. Platelet clumping in EDTA, a lavender top tube, occurs in about 3 per 1000 individuals and may lead to a spurious diagnosis of thrombocytopenia. If platelet clumping is suspected, the physician should ask the laboratory to perform a platelet count on citrate collected blood, a blue top tube. If the count is normal, then there is probably platelet clumping, and the patient is not thrombocytopenic. Other laboratory evaluation should be performed as necessary to rule out preeclampsia and HELLP syndrome, as well as disseminated intravascular coagulopathy. If a diagnosis of ITP is entertained, appropriate platelet antibody testing may aid in the diagnosis but is of limited utility during pregnancy.

After determining the etiology of thrombocytopenia, the physician can better determine whether imminent delivery is necessary, if the thrombocytopenia should be treated before initiating delivery, or if the low platelet count should be monitored during an ongoing pregnancy.

THERAPY OF THROMBOCYTOPENIA DURING PREGNANCY

Gestational Thrombocytopenia

Gestational thrombocytopenia, the most common form of thrombocytopenia encountered in the third trimester, requires no special intervention or therapy. The most important therapeutic issue is to refrain from treatment and testing that may lead to unnecessary intervention or iatrogenic preterm delivery. In patients with mild to moderate thrombocytopenia and no antenatal or antecedent history of thrombocytopenia, the patient should be treated as a normal pregnant patient. If the maternal platelet count drops below 50,000/mm^3, the patient may still have gestational thrombocytopenia, but there are not enough data on mothers with counts this low to determine if there are any maternal or fetal risks. These patients, therefore, should be treated as if they have de novo ITP. Although approximately 4% of patients have gestational thrombocytopenia, less than 1% of uncomplicated pregnant women have gestational thrombocytopenia with platelet counts less than 100,000/mm^3.[6]

Immune Thrombocytopenic Purpura

Treatment of the gravida with ITP during pregnancy and the puerperium requires special attention to the mother, because platelet counts can drop to very low numbers during pregnancy. As in other cases of thrombocytopenia, maternal therapy needs to be instituted only if there is evidence of a bleeding diathesis or to prevent a bleeding complication if surgery is anticipated. **There is usually no spontaneous bleeding unless the platelet count falls below 20,000/mm^3.**[3,23] In a meta-analysis of 17 studies, the risk of fatal hemorrhage in an individual younger than 40 years of age with a platelet count less than 30,000/mm^3 was 0.4%. The predicted 5-year mortality rate in this setting was 2.2%.[23] Surgical bleeding does not usually occur until the platelet count is less than 50,000/mm^3.

The conventional forms of raising the platelet count in the patient with ITP include glucocorticoid therapy, intravenous gamma globulins, platelet transfusions, and splenectomy. If the patient has clinical bleeding or if the platelet count is below 20,000/mm^3, there is usually a need to raise the platelet count in a relatively short period of time. Although oral glucocorticoids can be used, intravenous glucocorticoids may work more rapidly. Any steroid with a glucocorticoid effect can be used. However, hematologists have had the most experience with methylprednisolone. This medication can be given intravenously and has very little mineralocorticoid effect. It is important to avoid steroids with strong mineralocorticoid effects because these agents can disturb electrolyte balance, cause fluid retention, and result in hypertension. The usual dose of methylprednisolone is 1.0 to 1.5 mg/kg of *total body weight* intravenously daily in divided doses. It usually takes approximately 2 days for a response, but it may take up to 10 days for a maximum response. Even though methylprednisolone has very little mineralocorticoid effect, some may be observed because of the large dose that is being administered. Therefore, it is important to follow the patient's electrolytes. There is little likelihood that methylprednisolone will cause neonatal adrenal suppression because little crosses the placenta. It is metabolized by placental 11-β-ol-dehydrogenase to an inactive 11-keto metabolite. Park-Wyllie and colleagues performed a meta-analysis, which confirmed the general safety of glucocorticoids during pregnancy.[24] They did, however, find a 3.4-fold increased risk of cleft lip and palate with first trimester exposure. The risk/benefit ratio should be discussed with the patient before initiation of therapy.

After the platelet count has risen satisfactorily using intravenous methylprednisolone, the patient can be switched to oral prednisone. The usual dose is 60 to 100 mg/day. Prednisone can be given in a single dose, but there is less gastrointestinal upset with divided doses. The physician can rapidly taper the dose to 30 to 40 mg/day and decrease it slowly thereafter. The dose should be titrated to keep the platelet count at approximately 100,000/mm^3. If therapy is initiated with oral prednisone, the usual daily dose is 1 mg/kg total body weight.

The likelihood of a favorable response to glucocorticoids is about 70%. It is important to realize that if the patient has been taking glucocorticoids for a period of at least 2 to 3 weeks, she may have adrenal suppression and should undergo increased doses of steroids during labor and delivery in order to avoid an adrenal crisis. Tapering should be slowly thereafter. Also, if the patient has been on glucocorticoids for some time, she may experience significant side effects, including fluid retention, hirsutism, acne, striae, poor wound healing, and monilia vaginitis. In rare circumstances, patients on long-term steroids during gestation can develop osteopenia or cataract formation. The chance of any fetal or neonatal side effects from the glucocorticoids, however, is remote.

Although glucocorticoids are the mainstays of treating maternal thrombocytopenia, up to 30% of patients do not respond to these medications. In such cases, intravenous immunoglobulin (IVIG) is used. This agent probably works by binding to the IgG Fc receptors on reticuloendothelial cells and preventing destruction of platelets. It may also adhere to receptors on platelets and prevent antiplatelet antibodies from binding to these sites. The usual dose is 0.4 g/kg/day for 3 to 5 days. However, it may be necessary to use as much as 1 g/kg/day. The response usually begins in 2 to 3 days and peaks in 5 days. An alternative regimen is to give 1 g/kg once and observe the patient. Often this single dose will result in an adequate increase in platelets. The length of this response is variable, and the timing of the dose is extremely important. If the obstetrician wants a peak platelet count for delivery, therapy should be instituted about 5 to 8 days before the planned delivery. The most frequent adverse reaction is postinfusion headache. This may be lessened by slowing the infusion rate.

IVIG is a blood product from many pooled donors. Early in its use, there were concerns about hepatitis C transmission. There are no recent cases of viral infection from IVIG use. This is due to careful donor screening, as well as an intensive purification process. These steps include ethanol fractionation and polyethylene glycol precipitation, as well as solvent/detergent treatments. These techniques have been tested against hepatitis B, hepatitis C, HIV, mumps, vaccinia, vesicular stomatitis, and enteric cytopathic human orphan viruses. There has been no evidence that these viruses survive the purification process.

IVG should be used before seriously contemplating splenectomy, because some patients experience long-term remission with IVIG and others have a spontaneous increase in platelet counts postpartum. In severe life-threatening hemorrhage, recombinant factor VIIa can be used in conjunction with other therapies. This is a very expensive and complicated therapy that should only be undertaken with the assistance of a physician familiar with its use.

Intravenous anti-D has been used in emergent settings in Rh-positive, direct antiglobulin–negative patients. In life-threatening situations, when other methods fail, one could consider this option. The usual dose is 50 to 75 mcg/kg.[25] Anti-D binds to IgG Fc receptors different than those bound by IVIG.

In midtrimester, splenectomy can also be used to raise the maternal platelet count. This procedure is reserved for those who do not respond to medical management, with the platelet count remaining below 20,000/mm^3 with clinical bleeding. It can also be performed postpartum if the patient does not respond to medical management. In extremely emergent cases of life-threatening bleeding or unresponsiveness to other therapies, splenectomy can be performed at the time of cesarean delivery after extending a midline incision cephalad.

Platelet transfusions are indicated when there is clinically significant bleeding, while awaiting other therapies to become effective. Platelets can be transfused during cesarean delivery if significant clinical bleeding is evident. Platelets can be transfused before a vaginal delivery if the mother's platelet count is less than 20,000/mm^3. Each "pack" of platelets increases the platelet count by approximately 10,000/mm^3. The half-life of these platelets is extremely short because the same antibodies and reticuloendothelial cell clearance rates that affect the mother's endogenous platelets also affect the transfused platelets. However, if platelets are transfused at the beginning of surgery, hemostasis adequate to carry out the surgical procedure should be provided.

If the patient with profound thrombocytopenia undergoes cesarean delivery, certain surgical precautions should be taken. The bladder flap may be left open to avoid hematoma formation. If the parietal peritoneum is closed, subfascial drains are helpful if hemostasis is imperfect. If the peritoneum is not closed, the peritoneal edges should be carefully inspected to make certain there are no bleeding vessels. If severe, life-threatening hemorrhage occurs, recombinant factor VIIa and platelet transfusion can be used.

In summary, the treatment of thrombocytopenia during gestation is dependent on its etiology. The obstetrician need not act on the mother's platelet count unless it is below 30,000/mm^3,[9] if it is below 50,000/mm^3 with evidence of clinical bleeding, or if surgery is anticipated. In these cases, the treatment depends on the diagnosis. Furthermore, whether delivery needs to be expedited or can be delayed is also dependent on the etiology of thrombocytopenia, the patient's physical health, the fetal well-being, and the gestational age.

MANAGEMENT OF THROMBOTIC THROMBOCYTOPENIC PURPURA AND HEMOLYTIC UREMIC SYNDROME

Before the use of plasma exchange, maternal and fetal outcomes in pregnancies complicated by TTP were uniformly poor.[17] The first cases treated with plasma exchange for TTP during pregnancy were reported in 1984. There are no large series of patients with TTP in pregnancy. A review of 11 patients described in case reports reveals that the prognosis has improved greatly with plasma infusion and plasma exchange.[25] These researchers also demonstrated that cyclosporin may increase the duration of remission. There is one case report where TTP relapses were prevented by using prophylactic monthly exchange throughout gestation.[26] **If TTP is suspected, plasma exchange should be initiated immediately.**

HUS has been more difficult to treat. Only a few case reports have appeared. Supportive therapy remains the mainstay in cases of HUS. Dialysis is often necessary with close attention to fluid management. Platelet function inhibitors were used in two cases during pregnancy. Plasma infusion and plasma exchange can be attempted, but the results have not been as good as observed in cases of TTP. Vincristine has been administered with some success in nonpregnant patients, but has not been tried in pregnancy. Prostacyclin infusion has been effective in children but has not been used during pregnancy.

FETAL/NEONATAL ALLOIMMUNE THROMBOCYTOPENIA

In neonatal alloimmune thrombocytopenia, a rare disorder, the mother lacks a specific platelet antigen and develops antibodies to this antigen. The disease is somewhat analogous to Rh isoimmunization, but involves platelets. If the fetus inherits an antigen from its father and the mother lacks the antigen, maternal antibody can develop and cross the placenta. This results in severe neonatal thrombocytopenia and possibly fetal intracranial hemorrhage. The mother, however, will have a normal platelet count. The most common antibodies noted in these patients is anti-PLA 1 antibodies. Several other antibodies have been identified. If this disorder is suspected, the mother's blood should be sent to a reference laboratory with experience in diagnosing neonatal alloimmune thrombocytopenia. Transfusion of maternal platelets into the neonate also improved outcome in these cases. After birth or in utero, the child can be transfused with the mother's platelets (because she lacks the antigen) or with donor platelets known to lack the antigen. Bussel and colleagues[27] have demonstrated that the antenatal use of intravenous immunoglobulin can prevent thrombocytopenia in infants at risk for neonatal alloimmune thrombocytopenia. These investigators administrated 1 g/kg per week to at-risk mothers and observed no toxicity. The concomitant use of glucocorticoids has not necessarily been shown to boost the effect of the intravenous immunoglobulin.[28] McQuilten and colleagues[29] reviewed the experience in Australia and show that cordocentesis with transfusion, IVIG administration, and corticosteroids are all used with good results. Kamphuis and Oepkes[30] reviewed the experience in the Netherlands. They demonstrate that weekly IVIG alone can virtually prevents fetal/neonatal intracranial hemorrhage in neonatal alloimmune thrombocytopenia. Therefore, they think that fetal blood sampling should be abandoned because of the risks. Rayment and coworkers[31] searched the Cochrane database and Childbirth Group's Trial Register to ascertain if they could discern the optimal management of alloimmune thrombocytopenia. They reviewed four trials involving 206 patients. Because of incomplete data and differences in interventions, they could not conclude the best treatment plan for these patients.[31] They convincingly show that more randomized studies to look at medication doses and timing need to be performed.[31] These patients should be managed in a tertiary care center where there has been experience caring for mothers and infants with this rare disorder.

IRON DEFICIENCY ANEMIA

During a singleton pregnancy, maternal plasma volume gradually expands by approximately 50% (1000 mL). The total RBC mass also increases, but only by approximately 300 mg (25%), and this starts later in pregnancy. It is not surprising, therefore, that **hemoglobin and hematocrit levels usually fall during gestation. These changes are not necessarily pathologic but usually represent a physiologic alteration of pregnancy.** By 6 weeks postpartum, in the absence of excessive blood loss during the puerperium, hemoglobin and hematocrit levels have returned to normal, if the mother has adequate iron stores.

Most researchers and clinicians diagnose anemia when the hemoglobin concentration is less than 11 g/dL or the hematocrit is less than 32%.[32] Using these criteria, 50% of pregnant women are anemic. The incidence of anemia changes depending on the population studied. It is unfortunate that this problem is often ignored. In the developing nations, iron deficiency is an overwhelming problem. Worldwide there are many maternal deaths because of excessive blood loss in women who were already anemic. Beaton[33] suggests that these numbers should be adjusted downward and different targets should be established for different times in pregnancy. As pregnancy progresses, hemoglobin levels are often in the range of 10 to 10.5 g/dL in the late second and early third trimesters. These patients, if iron stores are present, do regain their normal hemoglobin/hematocrit postpartum. Causes of anemia in pregnancy are shown in the box Causes of Anemia during Pregnancy.

Causes of Anemia During Pregnancy

Common Causes—85% of Anemia

- Physiologic anemia
- Iron deficiency

Uncommon Causes

- Folic acid deficiency
- Vitamin B_{12} deficiency(due to the rapid increase in bariatric surgery)
- Hemoglobinopathies
  - Sickle cell disease
  - Hemoglobin SC
  - β-Thalassemia minor
- Bariatric surgery
- Gastrointestinal bleeding

Rare Causes

- Hemoglobinopathies
  - β-Thalassemia major
  - α-Thalassemia
- Syndromes of chronic hemolysis
  - Hereditary spherocytosis
  - Paroxysmal nocturnal hemoglobinuria
- Hematologic malignancy

Approximately 75% of anemias that occur during pregnancy are secondary to iron deficiency. Ho and colleagues[34] performed elaborate hematologic evaluations of 221 gravidas at term in Taiwan. None of the studied patients received an added iron preparation during gestation. Of the previously nonanemic patients, 10.4% developed clinical anemia after a full-term delivery. Of these 23 patients, 11 (47.8%) developed florid iron deficiency anemia, and another 11 demonstrated moderate iron depletion.[34] The other anemic patient in the group had folate deficiency. Of the 198 nonanemic gravidas at term, 46.5% showed evidence of iron depletion even though they had a normal hematocrit.[34]

To distinguish the normal physiologic changes of pregnancy from those of pathologic iron deficiency, one must understand the normal iron requirements of pregnancy (Table 42-1) and the proper use of hematologic laboratory parameters. In adult women, iron stores are located in the bone marrow, liver, and spleen in the form of ferritin. Ferritin constitutes approximately 25% (500 mg) of the 2 g of iron stores found in the normal woman. Approximately 65% of stored iron is located in the circulating RBCs. If the dietary iron intake is poor, the interval between pregnancies is short, or the delivery is complicated by hemorrhage, iron deficiency anemia readily and rapidly develops.

The first pathologic change to occur in iron deficiency anemia is the depletion of bone marrow, liver, and spleen iron stores. The serum iron level falls, as does the percentage saturation of transferrin. The total iron-binding capacity rises, because this is a reflection of unbound transferrin. A falling hemoglobin and hematocrit follow. Microcytic hypochromic RBCs are released into the circulation. If iron deficiency is combined with folate or vitamin B_{12} deficiency, normocytic and normochromic RBCs are observed on the peripheral blood smear.

Care must be taken when using laboratory parameters to establish the diagnosis of iron deficiency anemia during gestation. A serum iron concentration less than 60 mg/dL with less than 16% saturation of transferrin is suggestive of iron deficiency. Conversely, a single normal serum iron concentration does not rule out iron deficiency. For example, a patient may take iron for several days, and this may result in a transiently normal serum iron concentration while iron stores are still negligible. An increase in iron-binding capacity is not reliable, because 15% of pregnant women without iron deficiency show an increase in this parameter.[35] If a patient has been iron deficient for an extended period of time, her serum iron level can rise before she has depleted her iron stores. The ferritin level indicates the total status of her iron stores. Serum ferritin levels normally decrease minimally during pregnancy. However, a significantly reduced ferritin concentration is indicative of iron deficiency anemia and is the best parameter to judge the degree of iron deficiency. Ferritin levels are variable and can change 25% from one day to the next.[36] Harthoorn-Lasthuizen and colleagues[37] examined erythrocyte zinc protoporphyrin testing in pregnancy. They found that serum ferritin levels did not predict the development of iron-deficient erythropoiesis. However, erythrocyte zinc protoporphyrin measurements did help determine which patients were developing iron deficiency before they developed frank anemia, and these patients benefited from iron therapy.[37] Van den Broek and colleagues[38] believed that the erythrocyte zinc protoporphyrin level was not particularly helpful and that a serum ferritin of less than 30 mcg/L was more than adequate to determine iron deficiency.

Ahluwalia[39] believes that measuring serum transferrin receptors can give a better index of true iron status. Ferritin can be elevated in acute and chronic infections, whereas transferrin receptors do not change in response to an infection. This is important in countries where chronic infection is common in pregnant women. Also receptor concentrations are not confounded by the hemodynamic changes of pregnancy. This test is not yet readily available but may help us in the future to detect iron-deficient patients.[39] Mei and colleagues,[40] working through the National Centers for Chronic Disease Prevention and Health Promotion, assessed total body iron using ferritin and soluble transferrin receptor concentrations. This was part of a large study between 1999 and 2006 and incorporated 1171 pregnant women. The found that iron deficiency increased during pregnancy from 6.9% ± 2.2% in the first trimester to 29.5% ± 2.7% in the third trimester. The prevalence of iron deficiency was highest in women with a parity of at least 2. Iron deficiency was significantly higher in Mexican American and non-Hispanic Black women. Statistical analysis showed that this difference was not due to educational level or family income.[40] Bone marrow aspiration is rarely necessary. It is reserved for persistent anemia with confusing hematologic parameters. It can be safely performed during pregnancy.

Whether all women should receive prophylactic iron in addition to that contained in prenatal vitamins during pregnancy remains controversial. In reviewing the Cochrane database, Milman and colleagues[41] found that 20% of fertile women have iron stores greater than 500 mg, which is the required minimum for pregnancy. They also noted that 40% of women have iron stores between 100 and 500 mg, and 40% have virtually no iron stores. Based on these data, most women do need some iron supplementation.[41] There was no consensus, however, on how much iron supplementation may be needed in patients with iron deficiency.

In pregnancy, iron absorption from the duodenum increases, providing 1.3 to 2.6 mg of elemental iron daily. An acid environment in the duodenum helps this absorption. Therefore, the frequent ingestion of antacid medications, commonly used by many patients, decreases the absorption of iron. Chronic use of H_2 blockers and proton pump inhibitors also diminishes iron absorption. Vitamin C, in addition to the iron, may increase the acid environment of the stomach and increase absorption. In patients

TABLE 42-1 IRON REQUIREMENTS FOR PREGNANCY AND THE PUERPERIUM

FUNCTION	REQUIREMENT
Increased red blood cell mass	450 mg
Fetus and placenta	360 mg
Vaginal delivery	190 mg
Lactation	1 mg/day

TABLE 42-2 ELEMENTAL IRON AVAILABLE FROM COMMON GENERIC IRON PREPARATIONS

PREPARATION	ELEMENTAL IRON (mg)
Ferrous gluconate 325 mg	37-39
Ferrous sulfate 325 mg	60-65
Ferrous fumarate 325 mg	107

who do not show clear signs of iron deficiency, it is uncertain whether prophylactic iron, in addition to what is in prenatal vitamins, leads to an increased hemoglobin concentration at term. Iron prophylaxis, however, is safe as only amounts that can be used are absorbed. With the exception of dyspepsia and constipation, side effects are few. One 325 mg tablet of ferrous sulfate daily provides adequate prophylaxis. It contains 60 mg of elemental iron, 10% of which is absorbed. If the iron is not needed, it will not be absorbed and will be excreted in the feces. The standard generic iron tablets and the amount of elemental iron they provide are listed in Table 42-2.

In iron-deficient patients, one iron tablet three times daily has been recommended, although the evidence-based source of this recommendation is difficult to ascertain. Most individuals can absorb as much iron as they need taking iron twice daily. Iron should be taken 30 minutes before meals to allow maximum absorption. However, when taken in this manner, dyspepsia and nausea are more common. Therapy, therefore, must be individualized to maximize patient compliance. Reveiz and colleagues[32] examined the Cochrane database to see if there is an optimal treatment for iron deficiency during pregnancy. They identified 23 trials involving 3198 women. Many of the trials were from low-income countries, were generally small, and had poor methodology. Although oral iron showed a reduction in the incidence of anemia, it was not possible to assess the effects of treatment by severity of anemia.[32] The authors conclude that despite a high incidence and large ramifications of this disease, there is a paucity of good-quality trials. These trials could be relatively easy to design and would be relatively inexpensive compared to so many other trials being carried out. There appears to be a lack of interest among researchers and funding institutions in the United States.

Young and colleagues[42] studied the effectiveness of weekly iron supplementation. They found that weekly iron supplementation was almost as effective as daily supplementation in raising the hemoglobin concentration in iron deficient patients. This approach can be used in patients with less than optimal compliance. Yakoob and Bhutta[43] systematically reviewed the Cochrane database and reviewed 31 studies to see if routine iron supplementation affected the incidence of anemia in pregnancy. They included studies that used iron alone and iron with folic acid. They showed that there was a 73% reduction in anemia with routine supplementation. There was, however, no difference in rates of anemia at term with intermittent iron-folate when compared to daily supplementation (RR, 1.61; CI, 0.82-3.14).[43]

For those patients who are noncompliant or are unable to take oral iron and are severely anemic, intravenous iron can be given. Singh and colleagues[44] found that parenteral iron can be safely given and significantly raises the hematocrit in patients. It also raises the serum ferritin. There were no adverse effects in their study of patients.[44] Hallak and colleagues[45] examined the safety and efficacy of parenteral iron administration. Of 26 patients receiving parenteral iron, only one developed signs of mild allergy during the test dose and was excluded from the study. The remaining 21 pregnant patients completed the course of therapy and received a mean of 1000 mg of elemental iron. Their hemoglobin increased an average of 1.6 g/dL from the beginning to the end of therapy and rose another 0.8 g/dL during the following 2 weeks. Ferritin levels increased from 2.9 ng/mL at the beginning of therapy to 122.8 ng/dL by the end of treatment.[45] Ferritin levels decreased to a mean of 109.4 ng/mL 2 weeks later, demonstrating that the iron was being utilized. Only mild transient side effects were noted. The authors concluded that parenteral iron therapy can be used safely during pregnancy.[45]

TABLE 42-3 PARENTERAL IRON ADMINISTRATION

MEDICATION	DOSE	PREPARATION
Iron dextran	Total dose (mL) = 0.0442 (Desired hgb − Observed hgb) × LBW + (0.26 × LBW), 100 mg/dose maximum	50 mg elemental iron/mL
Iron sucrose	100 mg/dose, usually 1 dose/day, usually 10 doses needed	20 mg elemental iron/mL
Sodium ferric gluconate complex	125 mg/dose, usually 1 dose/day, usually 8 doses needed	12.5 mg of elemental iron/mL

hgb, Hemoglobin; *LBW*, lean body weight.

Parenteral iron is indicated in those who cannot or will not take oral iron therapy and are not anemic enough to require transfusion. In fact, by building iron stores in the patients before delivery, we may be able to prevent a need for transfusion postpartum in the severely anemic patient. Iron dextran comes in a concentration of 50 mg/mL. It can be given intramuscularly or intravenously, although intramuscular injection is very painful. **Iron dextran can result in anaphylaxis,** which is caused by dissociation of the iron component and carbohydrate component. The reaction may be immediate or delayed. Therefore, a 0.5 mL test dose should be given, and epinephrine should be readily available. Anaphylaxis usually occurs within several minutes but may take 2 days to develop. In the past 3 years, our group has given iron dextran to 14 patients. Two developed a severe reaction within minutes of the test dose. Although neither patient developed shortness of breath, both exhibited severe bone pain and myalgias. The dosage for iron dextran therapy is shown in Table 42-3.

In addition to iron dextran, there are two other parenteral iron preparations. Both of these compounds have the disadvantage of requiring multiple doses to accomplish what can be done with one dose of iron dextran. However, they have the advantage of less likelihood of a severe adverse reaction. Iron sucrose complex is given intravenously with a maximum dose of 100 mg. It is usually given daily. Patients generally require 10 doses (1 g) to obtain the rise in ferritin and subsequent rise in hemoglobin concentration that are desired. Sodium ferric gluconate complex can be used similarly. The maximum dose is 125 mg. It is usually given daily, and eight doses (1 g) are most often required to obtain the desired results. Sodium ferric gluconate appears to have the least risk of adverse side effects. If the patient has concomitant renal insufficiency, subcutaneous erythropoietin can be given to help raise the hemoglobin concentration if iron stores have already been raised. These agents should be used only in patients with severe iron deficiency who cannot absorb iron or who will not or cannot take oral iron. A parenteral iron overdose can lead to hemosiderosis.

It is still not certain whether anemia results in an increased risk for poor pregnancy outcome. In their literature review, Scholl and Hediger[46] concluded that anemia diagnosed in early pregnancy is associated with preterm delivery and low birth weight. In this study, women with iron deficiency anemia had twice the risk of preterm delivery and three times the risk of delivering a low-birth-weight infant.[46] Preterm labor, however, is a multifactorial problem, and there were many confounders in this study. Yip[47] reviewed the literature concerning pregnancy outcome with anemia. He found through epidemiologic studies that there is an association between moderate anemia and poor perinatal outcome, yet he was unable to determine whether this relationship was causal. Sifakis and Pharmakides[48] observed that hemoglobin concentrations less than 6 g/dL are associated with preterm birth, spontaneous abortion, low birth weight, and fetal deaths. Nevertheless, a mild to moderate anemia did not appear to have any significant effect on fetal outcomes.[48] Hemminki and Starfield[49] reviewed controlled trials, concluding that routine iron administration did not decrease preterm labor or raise birth weight. Conversely, Stephansson and colleagues[50] found an increased risk of stillbirth and growth-restricted infants in women with hemoglobin concentrations greater than 14.6 g/dL at their prenatal visit. Demmouche and colleagues[51] found that 46.86% of 207 women were anemic, with 14.43% being severely anemic with a hemoglobin less than 9 g/dL. There was no difference in birth weight between anemic and non-anemic pregnant women.[51]

In summary, iron deficiency is very prevalent in the general pregnant population. **In developing nations, severe anemia is alarmingly common and is a major cause of maternal morbidity and mortality.** Routine iron administration like that found in prenatal vitamins should be used unless it is certain that the patient is iron replete. Iron prophylaxis can be taken as one iron tablet daily, or as one study showed, can be given on a weekly basis. There may be an association between adverse pregnancy outcome and maternal anemia, especially severe anemia. It is uncertain, however, if this is a causal relationship.

MEGALOBLASTIC ANEMIA

Folic acid, a water-soluble vitamin, is found in green vegetables, peanuts, and liver. Folate stores are located primarily in the liver and are usually sufficient for 6 weeks. After 3 weeks of a diet deficient in folate, the serum folate level falls. Two weeks later, hypersegmentation of neutrophils occurs. After 17 weeks without folic ingestion, RBC folate levels drop. In the next week a megaloblastic bone marrow develops. During pregnancy, folate deficiency is the most common cause of megaloblastic anemia. The daily folate requirement in the nonpregnant state is approximately 50 mcg, but this rises at least fourfold during gestation. Fetal demands increase the requirement, as does the decrease in the gastrointestinal absorption of folate during pregnancy.

Clinical megaloblastic anemia seldom occurs before the third trimester of pregnancy. If the patient is at risk for folate deficiency or has mild anemia, an attempt should be made to detect this disorder before megaloblastosis occurs. Serum folate and RBC folate levels are the best tests for folate deficiency. While serum folate reflects recently ingested folate, RBC folate levels give a better idea of folate status at the tissue level.

Folate deficiency rarely occurs in the fetus and is not a cause of significant perinatal morbidity. There is some evidence that fetuses that are homozygous for the C677T variant of the gene encoding for 5, 10-methylene tetrahydrofolate reductase have a 20% lower folate level and may be at risk for a neural tube defect. Because infants born to mothers with type 1 and type 2 diabetes mellitus have an increased incidence of neural tube defects, Kaplan and colleagues[52] studied 31 pregnant diabetic women and 54 controls to determine if there are aberrations in folate metabolism in patients with diabetes. They found that there were no differences in how ingested folate is processed in the pregnant patient with diabetes.[52] Prenatal vitamins that require physician prescription contain 1 mg of folic acid. Most nonprescription prenatal vitamins contain 0.8 mg of folic acid. These amounts are more than adequate to prevent and treat folate deficiency. **Women with significant hemoglobinopathies, patients taking anticonvulsant medications, women carrying a multiple gestation, and women with frequent conception may require more than 1 mg of supplemental folate daily.** If the patient is folic acid deficient, her reticulocyte count will be depressed. Within 3 days after the administration of sufficient folic acid, reticulocytosis usually occurs. In fact, folic acid deficiency should be considered when a patient has unexplained thrombocytopenia. The leukopenia and thrombocytopenia, which accompany megaloblastosis, are rapidly reversed. The hematocrit level may rise as much as 1% per day after 1 week of folate replacement.

Vollsett and colleagues[53] performed a retrospective analysis of 14,492 pregnancies in 5883 women in Norway to determine if elevated homocysteine levels were associated with pregnancy complications. An elevated homocysteine level is often found with depressed folate levels. They compared those in the upper quartile of homocysteine levels with those in the lower quartile. They noted a 32% (odds ratio 1.32) higher risk for preeclampsia, 38% (odds ratio 1.38) higher risk for prematurity, and a 10% (odds ratio 2.01) higher risk for very low birth weight. All trends were statistically significant, but the limitations inherent in retrospective epidemiologic studies apply here.[53] Munger and colleagues[54] investigated serum folate, RBC folate, active pyridoxine, and homocysteine concentrations in 347 pregnancies complicated by facial clefting and 469 controls. Low RBC and serum folate levels were significantly associated with an increased risk of clefting, whereas pyridoxine and homocysteine levels were not.[54] Therefore, homocysteine does not appear to have an etiologic role in clefting.

Iron deficiency is frequently observed in association with folic acid deficiency. If a patient with folate deficiency does not develop a significant reticulocytosis within 1 week after administration of sufficient replacement therapy, appropriate tests for iron deficiency should be performed.

Until recently, vitamin B_{12} deficiency in pregnancy was either very rare or not recognized. However, bariatric surgery has become increasingly common. Individuals who were morbidly obese and not ovulating, suddenly ovulate and become pregnant. However, **we are now regularly encountering individuals with vitamin B_{12} deficiency following bariatric surgery.** Cobalamin is found only in animal products, and the daily minimum required intake is 6 to 9 mcg. Total body stores are 2 to 5 mg, and one half of this is stored in the liver. For cobalamin to be absorbed, an individual needs the following: (1) acid-pepsin in the stomach; (2) intrinsic factor secreted by parietal cells in the stomach; (3) pancreatic proteases; and (4) an intact ileum with receptors to bind the cobalamin-intrinsic factor complex. Because of the abundant vitamin B_{12} stores in the body, it takes several years for a clinical vitamin B_{12} deficiency to develop.[94] Prolonged vitamin B_{12} deficiency can result in subacute combined degeneration, which involves the dorsal horns and lateral columns of the spinal cord. This can result in sensory and proprioception deficits, which can progress and cause serious disabilities. Fortunately, these changes are reversible when detected early.

In addition to bariatric surgery, gastrointestinal diseases such as Crohn's disease may lead to an inability to absorb vitamin B_{12}. Because of advances in medical care, more individuals with these chronic disorders are becoming pregnant. As primary care physicians for women, we must be prepared to diagnose and coordinate care in these complex patients. Furthermore, we are encountering more patients taking metformin, which is being prescribed for polycystic ovarian syndrome and other disorders in addition to type 2 diabetes mellitus. It is important to note that this medication can also result in vitamin B_{12} deficiency.[55] Approximately 10% to 30% of patients taking metformin may have depressed vitamin B_{12} levels. This can be reversed with increased calcium intake.[55] The major causes of vitamin B_{12} deficiency are listed in the box Causes of Vitamin B_{12} Deficiency That May Be Encountered in Pregnancy.

Causes Of Vitamin B_{12} Deficiency That May Be Encountered in Pregnancy

- Strict vegetarian diet
- Use of proton pump inhibitors
- Metformin
- Gastritis
- Gastrectomy
- Ileal bypass
- Crohn's disease
- Sprue
- *Helicobacter pylori* infection

Megaloblastic anemia usually leads to a suspicion of folate or vitamin B_{12} deficiency. As noted earlier, if there is an associated iron deficiency, the RBC indices may portray a normocytic, normochromic picture. Therefore, it is important to look at more specific tests for vitamin B_{12} and folate deficiencies. Vitamin B_{12} levels may fall during pregnancy, but this finding may not represent a pathologic process. Also, serum vitamin B_{12} levels may be normal in up to 5% of individuals with a true deficiency.[56]

Evaluation of methylmalonate and homocysteine levels can be used to distinguish folate deficiency from vitamin B_{12} deficiency. Vitamin B_{12} is a cofactor in the metabolism of both methylmalonic acid and homocysteine. A deficiency in vitamin B_{12}, therefore, will lead to an increased concentration of both of these compounds. Folic acid is a cofactor in the metabolism of homocysteine. A folate deficiency, therefore, will lead to an elevated homocysteine level. Savage[56] found elevated methylmalonic acid levels in 98% of individuals with a vitamin B_{12} deficiency but in only 12% of individuals with a folate deficiency. He also found elevated homocysteine levels in 96% of individuals with a vitamin B_{12} deficiency and 91% of individuals with a folate deficiency.[56] Figure 42-1 schematically shows how to incorporate methylmalonic acid and homocysteine testing into the evaluation of megaloblastic anemia.

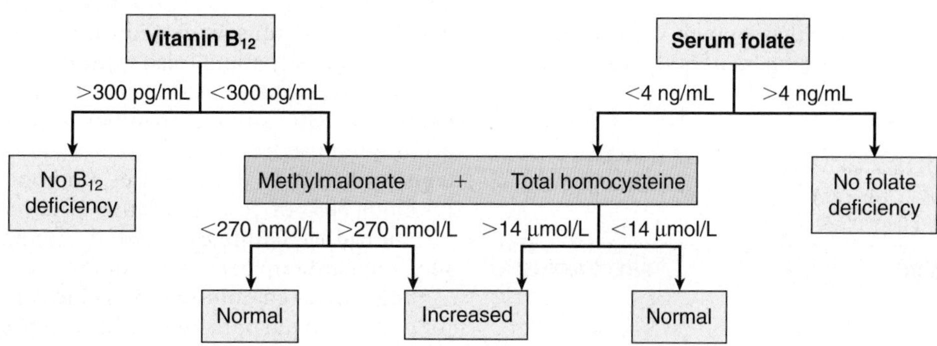

Increased methylmalonate and folate levels indicate vitamin B_{12} deficiency.
Normal methylmalonate and increased homocysteine levels indicate folate deficiency.

FIGURE 42-1. Use of methylmalonate and homocysteine levels in the workup of megaloblastic anemia.

HEMOGLOBINOPATHIES

Hemoglobin is a tetrameric protein composed of two pairs of polypeptide chains with a heme group attached to each chain. The normal adult hemoglobin A_1 comprises 95% of hemoglobin. It consists of two α-chains and two β-chains. The remaining 5% of hemoglobin usually consists of hemoglobin A_2 (containing two α-chains and two δ-chains) and hemoglobin F (with two α-chains and two γ-chains). In the fetus, hemoglobin F (fetal hemoglobin) declines during the third trimester of pregnancy, reaching its permanent nadir several months after birth. Hemoglobinopathies arise when there is a change in the structure of a peptide chain or a defect in the ability to synthesize a specific polypeptide chain. The patterns of inheritance are often straightforward. The prevalences of the most common hemoglobinopathies are listed in Table 42-4.

Hemoglobin S

Hemoglobin S, a variant form of hemoglobin, is present in patients with sickle cell disease (hemoglobin SS) and sickle cell trait (hemoglobin AS). A single substitution of valine for glutamic acid at the sixth position in the β-polypeptide chain causes a significant change in the physical characteristics of this hemoglobin. At low oxygen tensions, RBCs containing hemoglobin S assume a sickle shape. Sludging in small vessels occurs, resulting in microinfarction of the affected organs. Sickle cells have a life span of 5 to 10 days, compared with 120 days for a normal RBC. Sickling is triggered by dehydration, hypoxia, or acidosis. Infants with sickle cell anemia show no signs of the disease until the concentration of hemoglobin F falls to adult levels. Some patients do not experience symptoms until adolescence.

Approximately 1 of 12 black adults in the United States is heterozygous for hemoglobin S and, therefore, sickle cell trait (hemoglobin AS) and carries the affected gene. These individuals generally have 35% to 45% hemoglobin S and are asymptomatic. The child of two individuals with sickle cell trait has a 50% probability of inheriting the trait and a 25% probability of actually having sickle cell disease. One of every 625 black children born in the United States is homozygous for hemoglobin S, and the frequency of sickle cell disease among blacks is 1 in 708. All at-risk patients should undergo hemoglobin electrophoresis. Although it is more expensive, it will identify all patients with aberrant hemoglobin types.

The traditional teaching is that women with sickle cell trait are not at increased risk for maternal and perinatal morbidity. A report by Larrabee and Monga[57] questions this. In their study, 162 women with hemoglobin AS had a 24.7% incidence of preeclampsia compared with 10.3% of controls. Furthermore, the mean birth weight of infants born to women with hemoglobin AS was 3082 g compared with 3369 g for controls (P <0.0001). The rate of postpartum endometritis was 12.3% for sickle trait patients compared with 5.1% for controls (P <0.001) despite similar rates of cesarean delivery.[57] This study indicates that we should increase our surveillance in patients with hemoglobin AS.

If a patient has hemoglobin AS, the spouse/partner should be tested, and if both are carriers of a hemoglobinopathy, prenatal diagnosis should be offered. Prenatal diagnosis can be performed rapidly by DNA analysis with polymerase chain reaction (PCR) amplification of DNA fragments. Testing can be performed on amniocytes, and diagnosis can also be made by chorion villus sampling.

A recent study conducted on patients from Michigan highlights the possibility that adolescents with sickle cell disease may not receive adequate contraceptive counseling.[58] These researchers at Nationwide Children's Hospital found that of 250 women with sickle cell disease, only 20 had filled prescriptions for contraception. Among the 195 adolescents, 49 underwent 59 pregnancies during the study period.[58] The authors suggest that significant gaps may exist in family planning care for young women with sickle cell disease.

Painful vaso-occlusive episodes involving multiple organs are the clinical hallmark of sickle cell disease. The most common sites for these episodes are the extremities, joints, and abdomen. Vaso-occlusive episodes can also occur in the lung, resulting in pulmonary infarction. **Analgesia, oxygen, and hydration are the clinical foundations for treating these painful crises. Physicians often underestimate the pain associated with these crises.** These patients have often received many narcotics and may have a tolerance to the usual dosage of these medications. It is very important to treat this pain, no matter how much narcotic pain medication is needed. If the obstetrician is uncomfortable with these large doses, she or he should consult with a pain specialist with experience in this area.

Sickle cell disease can affect virtually all organ systems. Osteomyelitis is common, and osteomyelitis caused by salmonella is found almost exclusively in these patterns. The risk of pyelonephritis is increased, especially during pregnancy. Sickling may also occur in the renal medulla, in which oxygen tension is reduced, resulting in papillary necrosis. These patients also exhibit renal tubular dysfunction and hyposthenuria. Because of chronic hemolysis and decreased RBC survival, patients with sickle cell anemia often demonstrate some degree of jaundice. Biliary stasis commonly occurs during crises, and cholelithiasis is seen in about 30% of cases. Because of chronic anemia, high-output cardiac failure can occur. Left ventricular hypertrophy and cardiomegaly are common.

Pregnancies complicated by sickle cell disease are at risk for poor perinatal outcomes. The rate of spontaneous abortion may be as high as 25%. The perinatal mortality rate is approximately 15%. Powars and coworkers[59] studied 156 pregnancies in 79 women with sickle cell anemia. In this group, the perinatal mortality rate was 52.7% before 1972,

TABLE 42-4 FREQUENCY OF COMMON HEMOGLOBINOPATHIES IN BLACK ADULTS IN THE UNITED STATES

HEMOGLOBIN TYPE	FREQUENCY
Hemoglobin AS	1 in 12
Hemoglobin SS	1 in 708
Hemoglobin AC	1 in 41
Hemoglobin CC	1 in 4790
Hemoglobin SC	1 in 757
Hemoglobin S/β-thalassemia	1 in 1672

and 22.7% after that time. In a report by Seoud and coworkers,[60] the perinatal mortality rate was 10.5%. Much of this poor perinatal outcome is related to preterm birth. Approximately 30% of infants born to mothers with sickle cell disease have birth weights less than 2500 g. In the report by Seoud and colleagues,[60] the mean birth weight was 2443 g. In a multicenter study, Smith and colleagues[61] reported that 21% of infants born to mothers with sickle cell disease were small for gestational age. It has been hypothesized that sickling in the uterine vessels may lead to decreased fetal oxygenation and intrauterine growth restriction. Persistent hemoglobin F in the mother decreases episodes of painful crises during pregnancy and may also have a protective effect on the neonate. Morris and colleagues[62] studied 270 singleton pregnancies in 175 women with sickle cell disease. The overall rate of fetal wastage was 32.2%. Mothers with high hemoglobin F levels had a significantly lower perinatal mortality rate. Hydroxyurea reduces the incidence of painful crises and increases hemoglobin F concentration and is especially useful in children. Its safety in pregnancy has not been established. If an individual becomes pregnant while using hydroxyurea, it should be discontinued, but pregnancy termination is not justified. Parvovirus B-19 infection is usually asymptomatic in pregnant women but can cause fetal hydrops. In women with sickle cell disease, parvovirus B-19 can cause an aplastic crisis.[63]

Stillbirth rates of 8% to 10% have been described in patients with sickle cell disease. These rates include studies that took place many years ago. With the widespread use of antenatal fetal testing, the rates are significantly lower, but the rates of preterm delivery are higher. These fetal deaths happen not only during crises but also unexpectedly. Therefore, careful antepartum fetal testing must be used, including serial ultrasonography to assess fetal growth. In another study, Anyaegbunam and coworkers[64] examined Doppler flow velocimetry in patients with hemoglobinopathies. They showed abnormal systolic/diastolic ratios for the uterine or umbilical arteries in 88% of patients with hemoglobin SS compared with 7% with hemoglobin AS and 4% with hemoglobin AA. Howard and colleagues[65] observed that maternal exchange transfusions did not change uteroplacental Doppler blood flow velocimetry in these patients. These findings suggest that although maternal well-being may be improved, there is no change in uteroplacental pathology.

Although maternal mortality is rare in patients with sickle cell anemia, maternal morbidity is significant. Infections are common, occurring in 50% to 67% of women with hemoglobin SS. Most are urinary tract infections (UTIs), which can be detected by frequent urine cultures. Common infecting organisms for the bladder, kidneys, lungs, and other sites include *Streptococcus pneumoniae, Haemophilis influenzae* type B, *Escherichia coli,* salmonella, and klebsiella. Patients with hemoglobin AS are at greater risk for a UTI and should be screened as well. Pulmonary infection and infarction are also common. Patients with sickle cell anemia should receive pneumococcal vaccine before pregnancy. Maternal deaths have been reported in association with pulmonary complications in sickle cell disease. Any infection demands prompt attention, because fever, dehydration, and acidosis results in further sickling and painful crises. The incidence of pregnancy-induced hypertension is increased in patients with sickle cell anemia and may complicate almost one third of pregnancies in these patients.[61] Although painful crises appear to be more common during gestation,[66] this was not observed in one study.[61]

The care of the pregnant patient with sickle cell anemia must be individualized and meticulous. These patients benefit from care in a medical center experienced in treating the multitude of problems that can complicate such pregnancies. From early gestation, good dietary habits should be promoted. A folate supplement of at least 1 mg/day should be administered as soon as pregnancy is confirmed. Although hemoglobin and hematocrit levels are decreased, iron supplements should not be routinely given. Serum iron and ferritin levels should be checked monthly and iron supplementation started only when these levels are diminished. Often, because of ongoing hemolysis, serum ferritin values are significantly higher in pregnant women with hemoglobin SS disease than in those with hemoglobin AA. Routine iron supplementation, even that in prenatal vitamins, should not be given, because iron overload may lead to hemosiderosis and possibly hemochromatosis.

Most clinicians now feel that prophylactic exchange transfusion carry risk without benefit. This therapy, which replaces the patient's sickle cells with normal RBCs, can both improve oxygen-carrying capacity and suppress the synthesis of sickle hemoglobin. A previous study showed a sevenfold reduction in perinatal mortality in patients receiving prophylactic transfusions.[67] In the same group of patients, there was a significant decrease in fetal growth restriction and preterm births. Morrison and coworkers[68] have also previously reported reduced perinatal wastage and maternal morbidity using a regimen of exchange transfusion. Koshy and colleagues[69] followed 72 pregnant patients with sickle cell anemia, half of whom received prophylactic transfusions and one half transfusions only for medical or obstetrical emergencies. There was no significant difference in perinatal outcome between the offspring of mothers who received prophylactic transfusions and those who did not. Two risk factors were identified as harbingers of an unfavorable outcome: (1) the occurrence of a perinatal death in a previous pregnancy and (2) twins in the present pregnancy. Even though there was no difference in perinatal morbidity and mortality, prophylactic transfusion did appear to decrease significantly the incidence of painful crises.

Mahomed[70] reviewed the Cochrane database and found that there was not enough evidence to make any conclusions about the use of prophylactic RBC transfusion in patients with sickle cell disease. Many of the cited studies did not show evidence of benefit to the fetus from exchange transfusion. A review by Hassell[71] summarizes the various small studies and concludes that prophylactic transfusion does not improve fetal and neonatal outcome. He did not, however, attempt to quantify changes in maternal well-being.

In a study of 128 patients, Ngo and colleagues[72] attempted to delineate whether or not prophylactic partial exchange transfusion improved fetal/neonatal outcomes. Although their control group was patients with hemoglobin AA, they demonstrated that there were still significant perinatal/neonatal complications in patients with sickle cell disease receiving prophylactic exchange transfusions.[72] The study would have been much stronger if they had used a control group of patients with hemoglobin SS who had not received exchange transfusions. Before stating that there is no place for prophylactic exchange transfusions in patients with sickle cell disease, a study should be undertaken to look at maternal well-being during the 40 weeks of pregnancy. Very few studies have addressed this variable.

If one chooses to perform prophylactic transfusion, the goal is to maintain a percentage of hemoglobin A above 20% at all times and preferably above 40%, as well as to maintain the hematocrit above 25%. Morrison and colleagues[68] recommend that prophylactic transfusion begin at 28 weeks' gestation. Buffy-coat–poor washed RBCs are used to reduce the risk of isosensitization. Other risks of transfusion therapy include viral infection, transfusion reactions, and hemochromatosis.

Either booster or exchange transfusions can be used. Exchange transfusions are preferable. They provide more normal RBCs in less volume, therefore resulting in less stress on the cardiovascular system. This decreases the possibility of congestive heart failure. Exchange transfusions also raise the percentage of hemoglobin A more efficiently. These are usually carried out by erythrocytapheresis. If only booster transfusions are used, diuretics should probably be administered to prevent fluid overload. The patient should be positioned on her left side during the transfusion procedure to maximize uterine blood flow.

Vaginal delivery is preferred for patients with sickle cell disease, and cesarean delivery should be reserved for obstetrical indications. Patients should labor in the left lateral recumbent position and receive supplemental oxygen. Although adequate hydration should be maintained, fluid overload must be avoided. Conduction anesthesia is recommended, because it provides excellent pain relief and can be used for cesarean delivery, if necessary. Winder and colleagues[73] report a case in which epidural anesthesia was used antepartum to relieve a painful crisis. This patient's hospital stay was significantly shortened. Figure 42-2 provides a schematic presentation of the care

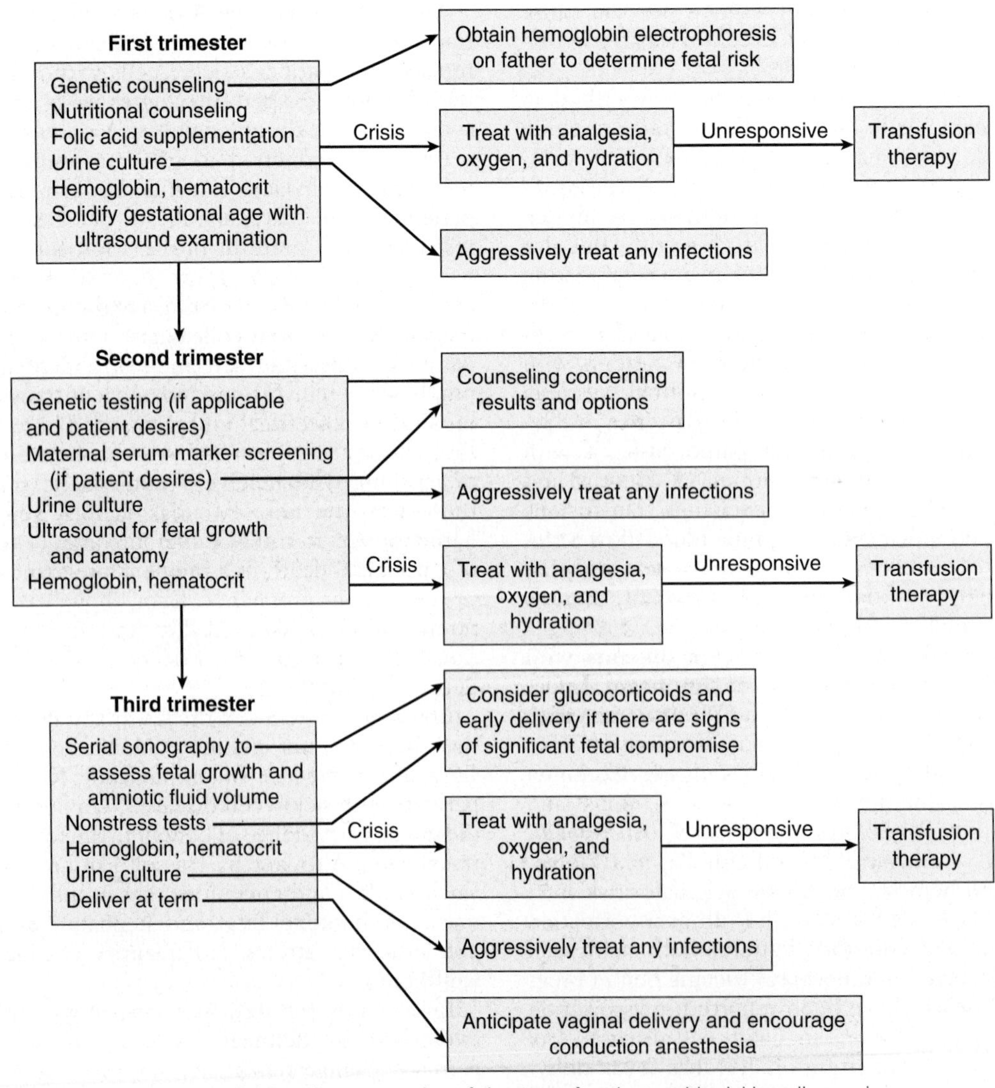

FIGURE 42-2. Schematic presentation of the care of patients with sickle cell anemia.

of patients with sickle cell anemia. It can also be adapted to patients with other hemoglobinopathies.

Hemoglobin SC Disease

Hemoglobin C is another β-chain variant. It results from a G to A point mutation in the first nucleotide of codon 6. The gene is present is 2% of blacks. Clinically significant hemoglobin SC disease occurs in 1 in 833 black adults in the United States. Women with both S and C hemoglobin suffer less morbidity in pregnancy than do patients with only hemoglobin S. As in sickle cell disease, however, there is an increased incidence of early spontaneous abortion and pregnancy-induced hypertension.

Because patients with SC disease can have only mild symptoms, this hemoglobinopathy may remain undiagnosed until a crisis occurs during pregnancy.

Whereas patients with hemoglobin SS often undergo "autosplenectomy," patients with hemoglobin SC may have an enlarged, tender spleen. **Crises in patients with hemoglobin SC may be marked by sequestration of a large volume of RBCs in the spleen accompanied by a dramatic fall in hematocrit.[74] Because these patients have increased splenic activity, they may be mildly thrombocytopenic throughout pregnancy and may become profoundly thrombocytopenic during a crisis.** During gestation, patients with hemoglobin SC should receive the same program of prenatal care outlined for women with hemoglobin SS (see Figure 42-2).

Thalassemia

Thalassemia is due to a defect in the rate of globin chain synthesis. Any of the polypeptide chains can be affected. As a result, there is production and accumulation of abnormal globin subunits, leading to ineffective erythropoiesis and a decreased life span of RBCs. The disease may range from minimal suppression of synthesis of the affected chain to its complete absence. Either α- or β-thalassemia can occur. Heterozygous patients are often asymptomatic.

Thalassemia can be detected by prenatal diagnosis. Prenatal diagnosis of β-thalassemia can be accomplished by DNA from villi or amniocytes. Because there are many beta globin mutations, it is important to report the patient's ethnicity and the geographic region of the family when submitting specimens. The laboratory can then test for specific mutations based on this information and will be able to identify β-thalassemia in 90% of cases. α-Thalassemia is also amenable to prenatal diagnosis using quantitative PCR or Southern blot analysis.[75]

Homozygous α-thalassemia results in the formation of tetramers of β-chains known as hemoglobin Bart. This hemoglobinopathy can result in hydrops fetalis. Ghosh and coinvestigators[76] reported their experience caring for 26 Chinese women who were at risk to deliver a fetus with homozygous α-thalassemia. Six of the 26 fetuses were affected. In two of the six cases, progressive fetal ascites appeared before 24 weeks' gestation. These pregnancies were terminated and the diagnoses confirmed. In the remaining four patients, there was evidence of intrauterine growth restriction by 28 weeks' gestation. At later gestational ages, an increase in the transverse cardiac diameter was seen in the affected fetuses. Woo and colleagues[77] reported that umbilical artery velocimetry reveals a hyperdynamic circulatory state in fetuses that are hydropic because of α-thalassemia. In a study from Taiwan, Hsieh and colleagues[78] demonstrated that umbilical vein blood flow measurements can help to distinguish hydrops fetalis caused by hemoglobin Bart from hydrops fetalis having other causes. The umbilical vein diameter, blood velocity, and blood flow in fetuses with hemoglobin Bart were usually higher than those in fetuses with hydrops fetalis due to other etiologies.

β-Thalassemia is the most common form of thalassemia. Patients with the heterozygous state are usually asymptomatic. They are detected by an increase in their level of both hemoglobin A_2 and hemoglobin F. Hemoglobin E is another β-chain variant found generally in patients from Southeast Asia. The clinical course is variable and similar to that described for β-thalassemia. In the homozygous state of β-thalassemia, synthesis of hemoglobin A_1 may be completely suppressed. Hemoglobin A_2 levels of greater than 50% are found in 40% of patients with β-thalassemia, and an elevated hemoglobin F level is observed in 50% of these patients. The homozygous state of β-thalassemia is known as thalassemia major, or Cooley's anemia. Patients with this disorder are transfusion dependent and have marked hepatosplenomegaly and bone changes secondary to increased hematopoiesis. These individuals usually die of infectious or cardiovascular complications before they reach childbearing age. They also have a high rate of infertility, although successful full-term pregnancies have been reported. The few patients who do become pregnant generally exhibit severe anemia and congestive heart failure.[79] Prenatal care is dependent on transfusion therapy similar to that used in the care of the patient with sickle cell disease.

Heterozygous β-thalassemia has different forms of expression. Patients with thalassemia minima have microcytosis but are asymptomatic. Those with thalassemia intermedia exhibit splenomegaly and significant anemia and may become transfusion dependent during pregnancy. Their anemia can be significant enough to produce high-output cardiac failure. If these patients have not undergone splenectomy, they are at risk for a hypersplenic crisis. Also, extramedullary hematopoiesis may impinge on the spine, resulting in neurologic symptoms.

These patients should be managed with a treatment program similar to that followed for patients with sickle cell disease (see Figure 42-2). **As in the case of sickle hemoglobinopathies, iron supplementation should be given only if necessary, because indiscriminate use of iron can lead to hemosiderosis and hemochromatosis.** White and coworkers[80] have shown that patients with a β-thalassemia usually have a much higher ferritin concentration than normal patients and those who are α-thalassemia carriers. In β-thalassemia carriers, the incidence of iron deficiency anemia is four times less common than it is in α-thalassemia carriers and normal patients.[80] Although iron is not necessary, folic acid supplementation appears important in β-thalassemia carriers. Leung and coinvestigators showed that the daily administration of folate significantly increased the predelivery hemoglobin concentration in both nulliparous and multiparous patients.

Patients who are transfusion dependent can develop iron overload. There are very little data on the safety of iron chelating agents during pregnancy. Ricchi and colleagues[81] report a case of successful pregnancy while using deferasirox in the first trimester. The pregnancy went to term and there were no fetal malformations.

As in the case of sickle cell disease, antepartum fetal evaluation is essential in patients with thalassemia who are anemic. Patients with thalassemia should undergo frequent ultrasonography to assess fetal growth, as well as nonstress testing to evaluate fetal well-being. Asymptomatic thalassemia carriers need no special testing.

Occasionally, individuals will inherit two hemoglobinopathies, such as sickle cell thalassemia (hemoglobin S thal). The prevalence of this disorder among adult blacks in the United States is 1 in 1672.[82] The clinical course is variable. If minimal suppression of β-chains occurs, patients may be free of symptoms. However, with total suppression of β-chain synthesis, a clinical picture similar to that of sickle cell disease will develop. The course of these patients during pregnancy is quite variable, and their therapy must be individualized.

In summary, Figure 42-3 presents a stepwise approach to the workup of anemia and the diagnosis of the conditions discussed in this chapter.

VON WILLEBRAND'S DISEASE

Von Willebrand's disease (vWD) is the most common congenital bleeding disorder in humans, and up to 1% of the population may have some form of the disorder. Type 1 is an autosomal dominant disorder, whereas type 3 and occasionally type 2 are autosomal recessive.[83] vWD is related to quantitative or qualitative abnormalities of von Willebrand's factor (vWF). This multimeric glycoprotein serves as carrier protein of factor VIII, prolonging its life span in plasma. It also promotes platelet adhesion to the damaged vessel and platelet aggregation. Distinct abnormalities of vWF are responsible for the three types of vWD. Types 1 and 3 are characterized by a quantitative defect of vWF, whereas type 2, comprising subtypes 2A, 2B, 2M, and 2N, refers to molecular variants with a qualitative defect of vWF. In these type s subtypes, there are various problems in binding of vWF to factor VII or platelet surface.[84] The knowledge of the structure of the vWF gene and the use of PCR have led to the identification of the molecular basis of vWD in a significant number of patients.[85] In type 2B, the only clinical symptom in pregnancy may be thrombocytopenia.[86] Therefore, this diagnosis should be considered in the gravida with isolated thrombocytopenia during pregnancy.

The clinical severity of vWD is variable. Menorrhagia, easy bruising, gingival bleeding, and epistaxis are common. Menorrhagia is most severe in patients with types 2 and 3 vWD and most common in patients with type 1 disease. In a compilation of two studies, 17% of women with severe menorrhagia had a form of vWD.[87] Some patients may be entirely asymptomatic until they have severe bleeding after surgery or trauma. Von Willebrand's disease does not appear to affect fetal growth or development.

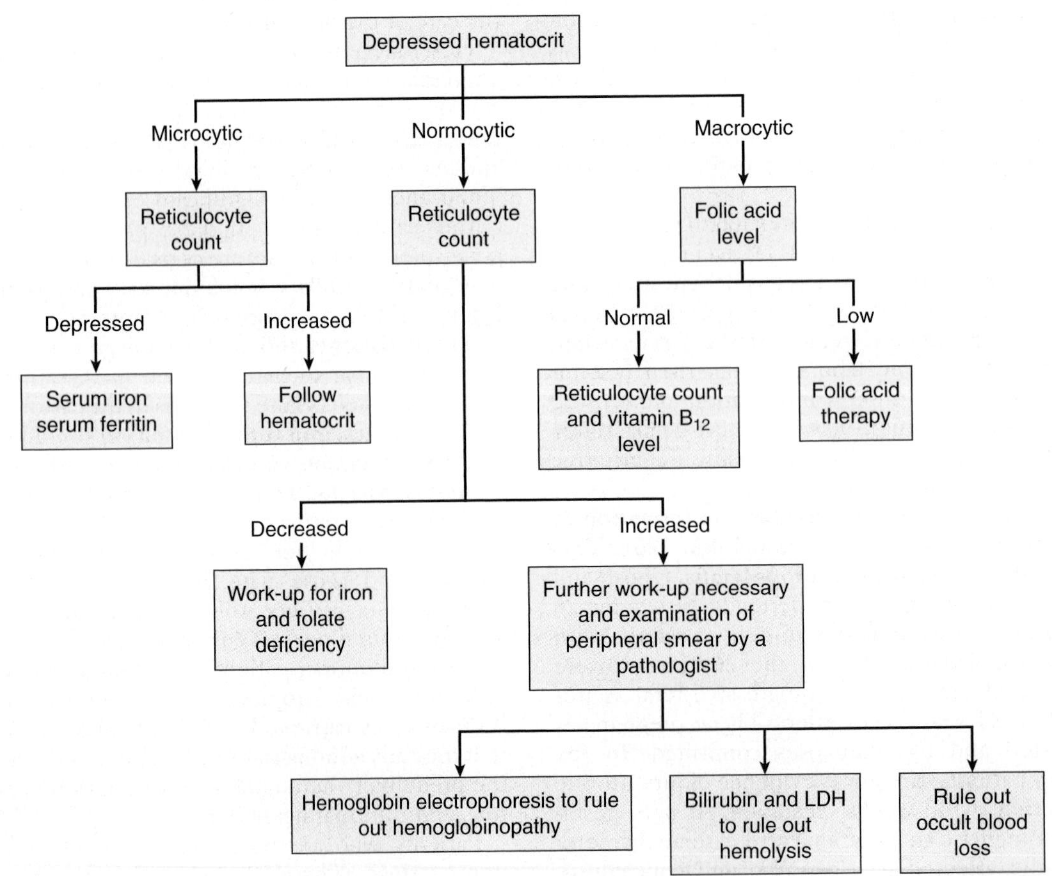

FIGURE 42-3. Evaluation of anemia.

Classically, the bleeding time is prolonged in patients with vWD as a result of diminished platelet aggregation. Occasionally, the activated partial thromboplastin time (APTT) is also abnormal. This is only seen when the factor VIII activity is extremely low.[88] In pregnancy, clotting factors including the factor VIII complex increase, and the patient's bleeding time may improve as gestation progresses.[87] This is especially true for type 1A vWD. In type 1B, the patient may not correct her bleeding time.[87] In type 2B, the platelet count decreases. This may be exacerbated in pregnancy.[88] There will, however, be an improvement in the vWF multimeric pattern.[89]

Heavy bleeding may be encountered in patients with vWD undergoing elective or spontaneous first-trimester abortion because the levels of factor VIII have not yet risen.[90] **Most important, postpartum hemorrhage may be a serious problem.** The concentration of factor VIII appears to determine the risk of hemorrhage. If the level is greater than 50% of normal and the patient has a normal bleeding time, excessive bleeding should not occur at vaginal delivery.[84] In a study by Kadir and colleagues,[90] 18.5% of patients with vWD experienced a significant postpartum hemorrhage, and 6 of 31 patients required transfusion. The clinical course during labor is variable. In a study by Chediak and colleagues,[91] bleeding complications were seen in six of eight (75%) pregnancies. Five of the newborns had vWD, one of whom was born with a scalp hematoma. Conti and associates,[92] conversely, reported no bleeding complications during the puerperium in five women with vWD. Ieko and colleagues[93] demonstrated that factor VIII concentrate could raise the platelet levels in patients with type 2B vWD. Ito and colleagues[94] followed six women with type 1 vWD in 10 term pregnancies, three induced abortions, and one spontaneous abortion. They found that bleeding complications occurred within 1 week after term delivery and immediately after both spontaneous and induced abortions.

As noted earlier, bleeding during pregnancy is rare because levels of factor VIII and vWF increase during pregnancy. However, shortly after delivery, they drop. If the factor VIII level is less than 50%, treatment during labor and delivery should be initiated. Hemorrhage can also occur several days postpartum. Therefore, factor VIII levels should be checked before the patient goes home after delivery. Desmopressin is the treatment of choice for type 1 vWD.[95] It elicits the release of vWF from endothelial cells. Intranasal preparations of 300 mcg are usually employed. The half-life of desmopressin is about 8 hours, so the dose should be repeated every 12 hours. In emergent or preoperative situations, 0.3 mcg/kg of desmopressin can be given intravenously over 30 minutes.[95] **Desmopressin can rarely cause hyponatremia and fluid retention.[96] Also, patients can develop tachyphylaxis with desmopressin, so it should not be used for prolonged periods of time.**

For those patients who do not respond to desmopressin or for those with vWD types other than 1A, Humate-P or Alphanate should be employed. These commercially available concentrates of antihemophiliac factor have been tested extensively in clinical studies. They contain 2 to 3 times more vWF than they do factor VIII concentrate.[96] The usual dose of Humate-P or Alphanate is 20 to 50 units/kg. During labor, this can be given every 12 hours. For labor and delivery, usually the lower end of the dosage range will suffice. If a cesarean delivery is needed, the upper end of the dosage range should be used.

These compounds have been heated at high temperature and treated with solvents and detergents to inactivate blood-borne viruses. It is important to note that products containing highly purified factor VIII, obtained by recombinant DNA, should not be used. They contain very little vWF and are ineffective in vWD. Therefore, the infused factor VIII has a very short half-life, because vWF is essential to prevent the degradation of factor VIII.

Bleeding during pregnancy is rare. Patients with classic type 1 vWD usually need no treatment owing to the increase in factor VIII levels during pregnancy. Those with a history of postpartum hemorrhage should be given an intravenous dose of desmopressin immediately after delivery, and the dose should be repeated 24 hours later. For those with types 2 and 3 disease, factor VIII/vWF concentrates are occasionally needed. Before a cesarean delivery, factor VIII activity should be measured. If it is less than 50% of expected, patients with type 1 vWD should be given desmopressin and patients with vWD type 2 or type 3 should receive factor VIII/vWF concentrate.[97] **If you encounter an emergent situation and the type of vWD is not known with certainty, factor VIII/vWF concentrate should be used.**

KEY POINTS

- Four percent of pregnancies will be complicated by maternal platelet counts of less than 150,000/mm^3. The vast majority of these patients have gestational thrombocytopenia with a benign course and need no intervention.
- Surgical bleeding occurs if the platelet count falls below 50,000/mm^3 and spontaneous bleeding occurs if the platelet count falls below 20,000/mm^3.
- Glucocorticoids are the first-line medication used to raise a low platelet count.
- Iron deficiency anemia is the most common cause of anemia in pregnancy, and serum ferritin is the single best test to diagnose it.
- If a patient with presumed iron deficiency does not increase her reticulocyte count with iron therapy, she may also have a concomitant folic acid deficiency.
- Patients pregnant with twins, those on anticonvulsant therapy, those with a hemoglobinopathy, and those who conceive frequently need supplemental folic acid during gestation.
- Most hereditary hemoglobinopathies can be detected in utero, and prenatal diagnosis should be offered to the patient early in pregnancy.
- As in the nonpregnant patient, analgesia, hydration, and oxygen are the key factors in treating pregnant women with sickle cell crisis.
- Patients with sickle cell disease are at high risk of having a fetus with growth restriction and adverse fetal outcomes. Therefore, they warrant frequent sonography and antepartum fetal evaluation.
- In the pregnant patient with vWD, the normal increase in the factor VIII clotting complex reduces the risk of bleeding.

REFERENCES

1. Jensen JD, Wiedmeier SE, Henry E, et al: Linking maternal platelet counts with neonatal platelet counts and outcomes using the data repositories of a multihospital health care system. Am J Perinatol 28:597, 2011.
2. McRae KR, Samuels P, Schreiber AD: Pregnancy-associated thrombocytopenia: pathogenesis and management. Blood 80:2697, 1992.
3. Aster RH: Gestational thrombocytopenia. A plea for conservative management. N Engl J Med 323:264, 1990.
4. Hart D, Dunetz C, Nardi M, et al: An epidemic of maternal thrombocytopenia associated with elevated antiplatelet antibody in 116 consecutive pregnancies: relationship to neonatal platelet count. Am J Obstet Gynecol 154:878, 1986.
5. Samuels P, Bussel JB, Braitman LE, et al: Estimation of the risk of thrombocytopenia in the offspring of pregnant women with presumed immune thrombocytopenia purpura. N Engl J Med 323:229, 1990.
6. Burrows RF, Kelton JG: Fetal thrombocytopenia and its relationship to maternal thrombocytopenia. N Engl J Med 329:1463, 1993.
7. Harrington WI, Minnich V, Arimura G: The autoimmune thrombocytopenias. In Tascantins LM: Progress in Hematology. New York, Grune Stratton, 1956, p 166.
8. Shulman MR, Marder VJ, Weinrach RS: Similarities between thrombocytopenia in idiopathic purpura. Ann N Y Acad Sci 124:449, 1965.
9. Cines DB, Schreiber AD: Immune thrombocytopenia: use of a Coombs antiglobulin test to detect IgG and C3 on platelets. N Engl J Med 300:106, 1979.
10. He R, Reid DM, Jones CE, Shulman NR: Spectrum of Ig classes, specificities, and titers of serum anti glycoproteins in chronic idiopathic thrombocytopenia purpura. Blood 83:1024, 1994.
11. Stasi R, Stipa E, Masi M, et al: Long-term observation of 208 adults with chronic idiopathic thrombocytopenic purpura. Am J Med 98:4536, 1995.
12. Cines DB, Bussell JB: How I treat idiopathic thrombocytopenic purpura (ITP). Blood 106:2244, 2005.
13. Moschcowitz E: Hyaline thrombosis of the terminal arterioles and capillaries: a hitherto undescribed disease. Proc N Y Pathol Soc 24:21, 1924.
14. Miller JM, Pastorek JG: Thrombotic thrombocytopenic purpura and the hemolytic uremic syndrome in pregnancy. Clin Obstet Gynecol 34:64, 1991.
15. Ridolfi RL, Bell WR: Thrombotic thrombocytopenic purpura: report of 25 cases and a review of the literature. Medicine 60:413, 1981.
16. Terrell DR, Williams LA, Vesely SK, et al: The incidence of thrombotic thrombocytopenic purpura-hemolytic uremic syndrome: all patients, idiopathic patients, and patients with severe ADAMTS-13 deficiency. J Thrombo Haemost 3:1432, 2005.
17. Ruggenenti P, Noris M, Remuzzi G: Thrombotic microangiopathy, hemolytic uremic syndrome, and thrombotic thrombocytopenic purpura. Kidney Int 60:831, 2001.
18. Tsai HM, Rice L, Sarode R, et al: Antibody inhibitors to von Willebrand factor metalloproteinase and increased binding of von Willebrand factor to platelets in ticlopidine-associated thrombotic thrombocytopenic purpura. Ann Intern Med 132:794, 2000.
19. Tsai HM: Advances in the pathogenesis, diagnosis and treatment of thrombotic thrombocytopenic purpura. J Am Soc Nephrol 14:1072, 2003.
20. Ferrari S, Mudde GC, Reieger M, et al: IgG subclass distribution of anti-ADAMTS13 antibodies in patients with acquired thrombotic thrombocytopenic purpura. J Thromb Hemost 7:1703, 2009.
21. Fakhouri F, Roumenina L, Provot F, et al: Pregnancy-associated hemolytic uremic syndrome revisited in the era of complement gene mutations. J Am Soc Nephrol 21:859, 2010.
22. Weiner CP: Thrombotic microangiopathy in pregnancy and the postpartum period. Semin Hematol 24:119, 1987.
23. Cohen YC, Dbulbegovic B, Shamai-Lubovitz O, Mozes B: The bleeding risk and natural history of idiopathic thrombocytopenic purpura in patients with persistent low platelet counts. Arch Intern Med 160:1630, 2000.
24. Park-Wyllie L, Mazzotta P, Pastuszak A, et al: Birth defects after maternal exposure to corticosteroids: prospective cohort study and meta-analysis of epidemiological studies. Teratology 62:385, 2000.
25. Egerman RS, Witlin AG, Friedman SA, Sibai BM: Thrombotic thrombocytopenic purpura and hemolytic uremic syndrome in pregnancy: review of 11 cases. Am J Obstet Gynecol 175:950, 1996.
26. Abou-Nassar K, Karsh J, Giulivi A, Allan D: Successful prevention of TTP relapse using monthly prophylactic plasma exchanges throughout pregnant in a patient with SLE and a prior history of refractory TTP and recurrent fetal loss. Trans Apher Sci 43:29, 2010.
27. Bussel JB, McFarland JG, Berkowitz R: Antenatal treatment of fetal alloimmune cytopenias. Blut 59:136, 1989.
28. Menell JS, Bussel JB: Antenatal management of thrombocytopenias. Clin Perinatol 21:591, 1994.
29. McQuilten ZK, Wood EM, Savoia H, Cole S: A review of pathophysiology and current treatment for neonatal alloimmune thrombocytopenia (NAIT) and introducing the Australian NAIT registry. Aust N Z J Obstet Gynecol 51:191, 2011.
30. Kamphuis MM, Oepkes D: Fetal and neonatal alloimmune thrombocytopenia: prenatal interventions. Prenat Diagn 31:712, 2011.
31. Rayment R, Brunskill SJ, Soothill PW, et al: Antenatal interventions for fetomaternal alloimmune thrombocytopenia. Cochrane Database Syst Rev CD004226, 2011.
32. Reveiz L, Gyte GM, Cuervo LG, Casasbuenas A: Treatments for iron-deficiency anaemia in pregnancy. Cochrne Database Syst Rev CD003094, 2011.
33. Beaton GH: Iron needs during pregnancy: do we need to rethink our targets? Am J Clin Nutr 72:265S, 2000.
34. Ho CH, Yuan CC, Yeh SH: Serum ferritin, folate and cobalamin levels and their correlation with anemia in normal full-term pregnant women. Eur J Obstet Gynecol Reprod Biol 26:7, 1987.
35. Carr MC: Serum iron/TIBC in the diagnosis of iron deficiency anemia during pregnancy. Obstet Gynecol 38:602, 1971.
36. Boued JL: Iron deficiency: assessment during pregnancy and its importance in pregnant adolescents. Am J Clin Nutr 59:5025, 1994.
37. Harthoorn-Lasthuizen EJ, Lindemans J, Langenhuijsen MM: Erythrocyte zinc protoporphyrin testing in pregnancy. Acta Obstet Gynecol Scand 79:660, 2000.
38. van den Broek NR, Letsky EA, White SA, Shenkin A: Iron status in pregnant women; which measurements are valid? Br J Haematol 103:817, 1998.
39. Ahluwalia N: Diagnostic utility of serum transferrin receptors measurement in assessing iron status. Nutr Rev 56:133, 1998.
40. Mei Z, Cogswell ME, Looker AC, et al: Assessment of iron status in US pregnant women from the National Health and Nutrition Examination Survey (MHANES), 1999-2006. Am J Clin Nutr 93:1312, 2011.
41. Milman N, Bergholt T, Byg KE, et al: Iron status and iron balance during pregnancy. A critical reappraisal of iron supplementation. Acta Obstet Gynecol Scand 78:749, 1999.
42. Young MW, Lupafya E, Kapenda E, Bobrow EA: The effectiveness of weekly iron supplementation in pregnant women of rural northern Malawi. Trop Doct 30:84, 2000.
43. Yakoob MY, Bhutta ZA: Effect of routine iron supplementation with or without folic acid on anemia during pregnancy. BMC Public Health 11:S21, 2011.
44. Singh K, Fong YF, Kuperan P: A comparison between intravenous iron polymaltose complex (Ferrum Hausmann) and oral ferrous fumarate in the treatment of iron deficiency anaemia in pregnancy. Eur J Haematol 60:119, 1998.
45. Hallak M, Sharon AS, Diukman R, et al: Supplementing iron intravenously in pregnancy: a way to avoid blood transfusions. J Reprod Med 42:99, 1997.
46. Scholl TO, Hediger ML: Anemia and iron-deficiency anemia: compilation of data on pregnancy outcome. Am J Clin Nutr 59:4925, 1994.
47. Yip R: Significance of abnormally low or high hemoglobin concentration during pregnancy: special consideration of iron nutrition. Am J Clin Nutr 72:272S, 2000.
48. Sifakis S, Pharmakides G: Anemia in pregnancy. Ann N Y Acad Sci 900:125, 2000.
49. Hemminki E, Starfield B: Routine administration of iron and vitamins during pregnancy: review of controlled clinical trials. Br J Obstet Gynaecol 85:404, 1978.
50. Stephansson O, Dickman PW, Johansson A, Cnattingius S: Maternal hemoglobin concentration during pregnancy and risk of stillbirth. JAMA 284:2611, 2000.
51. Demmouche A, Lazrag A, Moulessehoul S: Prevalence of anaemia in pregnant women during the last trimester: consequence for birth weight. Rev Med Pharmacol Sci 15:436, 2011.
52. Kaplan JS, Iqbal S, England BG, et al: Is pregnancy in diabetic women associated with folate deficiency? Diabetes Care 22:1017, 1999.

53. Vollsett SE, Refsum H, Irgens LM, et al: Plasma total homocysteine, pregnancy complications, and adverse pregnancy outcomes: the Hordaland homocysteine study. Am J Clin Nutr 71:962, 2000.
54. Munger RG, Tamura T, Johnston KE, et al: Oral clefts and maternal biomarkers of folate-dependent one-carbon metabolism in Utah. Birth Defects Res 91:153, 2011.
55. Bauman WA, Shaw S, Jayatilleke E, et al: Increased intake of calcium reverses vitamin B-12 malabsorption induced by metformin. Diabetes Care 23:1227, 2000.
56. Savage DG, Lindenbaum J, Stabler SP, Allen RH: Sensitivity of serum methylmalonic acid and total homocysteine determinations for diagnosing cobalamin and folate deficiencies. Am J Med 96:238, 1994.
57. Larrabee KD, Monga M: Women with sickle cell trait are at increased risk for preeclampsia. Am J Obstet Gynecol 177:425, 1997.
58. O'Brien SH, Klima J, Reed S, et al: Hormonal contraception use an pregnancy in adolescents with sickle cell diseae: analysis of Michigan Medicaid claims. Contraception 83:134, 2011.
59. Powars DR, Sandhu M, Niland-Weiss J, et al: Pregnancy in sickle cell disease. Obstet Gynecol 67:217, 1986.
60. Seoud MA, Cantwell C, Nobles G, Levy OL: Outcome of pregnancies complicated by sickle cell disease and sickle-C hemoglobinopathies. Am J Perinatol 11:187, 1994.
61. Smith JA, England M, Bellevue R, et al: Pregnancy in sickle cell disease: experience of the cooperative study of sickle cell disease. Obstet Gynecol 87:199, 1996.
62. Morris JS, Dunn DT, Poddorr D, Serjeant GR: Hematological risk factors for pregnancy outcome in Jamaican women with homozygous sickle cell disease. Br J Obstet Gynaecol 101:770, 1994.
63. Miller ST, Sleeper LA, Pegelow CH, et al: Prediction of adverse outcomes in children with sickle cell disease. N Engl J Med 342:8, 2000.
64. Anyaegbunam A, Langer O, Brustman L, et al: The application of uterine and umbilical artery velocimetry to the antenatal supervision of pregnancies complicated by maternal sickle hemoglobinopathies. Am J Obstet Gynecol 159:544, 1988.
65. Howard RJ, Tuck SM, Pearson TC: Blood transfusion in pregnancy complicated by sickle cell disease: effects on blood rheology and uteroplacental Doppler velocimetry. Clin Lab Haematol 16:253, 1994.
66. Claster S, Vichinsky EP: Managing sickle cell disease. BMJ 327:1151, 2003.
67. Cunningham FG, Pritchard JA, Mason R: Pregnancy and sickle cell hemoglobinopathies: results with and without prophylactic transfusions. Obstet Gynecol 62:419, 1983.
68. Morrison JC, Schneider JM, Whybrew WD, et al: Prophylactic transfusions in pregnant patients with sickle hemoglobinopathies: benefit versus risk. Obstet Gynecol 56:274, 1980.
69. Koshy M, Burd L, Wallace D, et al: Prophylactic red-cell transfusions in pregnant patients with sickle cell disease: a randomized cooperative study. N Engl J Med 319:1447, 1988.
70. Mahomed K: Prophylactic versus selective blood transfusion for sickle cell anaemia during pregnancy. Cochrane Database Syst Rev 2, 2000.
71. Hassell K: Pregnancy and sickle cell disease. Hematol Oncol Clin North Am 19:903, 2005.
72. Ngo C, Kayem G, Habibi A, et al: Pregnancy in sickle cell disease: maternal and fetal outcomes in a population receiving prophylactic partial exchange transfusions. Eur J Obstet Gynecol Reprod Biol 153: 138, 2010.
73. Winder AD, Johnson S, Murphy J, Ehsanipoor R: Epidural analgesia for treatment of a sickle cell crisis during pregnancy. Obstet Gynecol 118:495, 2011.
74. Solanki DL, Kletter GG, Castro O: Acute splenic sequestration crises in adults with sickle cell disease. Am J Med 80:985, 1986.
75. Rappaport VJ, Velazquez M, Williams K: Hemoglobinopathies in pregnancy. Obstet Gynecol Clin North Am 31:287, 2004.
76. Ghosh A, Tan MH, Liang ST, et al: Ultrasound evaluation of pregnancies at risk for homozygous alpha-thalassaemia-1. Prenat Diagn 7:307, 1987.
77. Woo JS, Liang ST, Lo RL, Chan FY: Doppler blood flow velocity waveforms in alpha-thalassemia hydrops fetalis. J Ultrasound Med 6:679, 1987.
78. Hsieh FJ, Chang FM, Huang HC, et al: Umbilical vein blood flow measurement in nonimmune hydrops fetalis. Obstet Gynecol 71:188, 1988.
79. Mordel N, Birkenfeld A, Goldfarb AN, Rachmilewitz EA: Successful full-term pregnancy in homozygous beta-thalassemia major: case report and review of the literature. Obstet Gynecol 73:837, 1989.
80. White JM, Richards R, Jelenski G, et al: Iron state in alpha and beta thalassaemia trait. J Clin Pathol 39:256, 1986.
81. Ricchi P, Costantini S, Spasiano A, et al: A case of well-tolerated and safe deferasirox administration during the first trimester of a spontaneous pregnancy in an advanced maternal age thalassemic patient. Acta Haematol 125:222, 2011.
82. Schmidt RM: Laboratory diagnosis of hemoglobinopathies. JAMA 224:1276, 1973.
83. Castaman G, Rodeghiero F: Current management of von Willebrand's disease. Drugs 50:602, 1995.
84. Pacheco LD, Constantine MM, Saade GR, et al: Von Willebrand disease and pregnancy: a practical approach for the diagnosis and treatment. Am J Obstet Gynecol 203:194, 2010.
85. Mazurier C, Ribba AS, Gaucher C, Meyer D: Molecular genetics of von Willebrand disease. Ann Genet 41:34, 1998.
86. Giles AR, Hoogendoorn H, Benford K: Type IIB von Willebrand's disease presenting as thrombocytopenia during pregnancy. Br J Haematol 67:349, 1987.
87. Kouides PA: Females with von Willebrand disease: 72 years as the silent majority. Haemophilia 4:665, 1998.
88. Casonato A, Sarrori MT, Bertomoro A, et al: Pregnancy-induced worsening of thrombocytopenia in a patient with type IIB von Willebrand's disease. Blood Coagul Fibrinolysis 2:33, 1991.
89. Nichols WL, Hutlin, MB, James AH, et al: Von Willebrand disease: evidence-based diagnosis and management guidelines. The National Heart, Lund and Blood Institute (NHLBI) Expert Panel report. Haemophilia 14:171, 2008.
90. Kadir RA, Lee CA, Sabin CA, et al: Pregnancy in women with von Willebrand's disease or factor XI deficiency. Br J Obstet Gynaecol 105:314, 1998.
91. Chediak JR, Alban GM, Maxey B: Von Willebrand's disease and pregnancy: management during delivery and outcome of offspring. Am J Obstet Gynecol 155:618, 1986.
92. Conti M, Mari D, Conti E, et al: Pregnancy in women with different types of von Willebrand disease. Obstet Gynecol 68:282, 1986.
93. Ieko M, Sakurama S, Sagan A, et al: Effect of factor VIII concentrate on type IIB von Willebrand's disease-associated thrombocytopenia presenting during pregnancy in identical twin mothers. Am J Hematol 35:26, 1990.
94. Ito M, Yoshimura K, Toyoda N, Wada H: Pregnancy and delivery in patient with von Willebrand's disease. J Obstet Gynaecol Res 23:37, 1997.
95. Mannucci PM: Treatment of von Willebrand's disease. N Engl J Med 351:683, 2004.
96. Bertolini DM, Butler CS: Severe hyponatremia secondary to desmopressin therapy in von Willebrand's disease. Anesth Intensive Care 28:199, 2000.
97. Nitu-Whalley IC, Griffloen A, Harrington C, Lee CA: Retrospective review of the management of elective surgery with desmopressin and clotting factor concentrates in patients with von Willebrand disease. Am J Hematol 66:280, 2001.

For full reference list, log onto www.expertconsult.com.

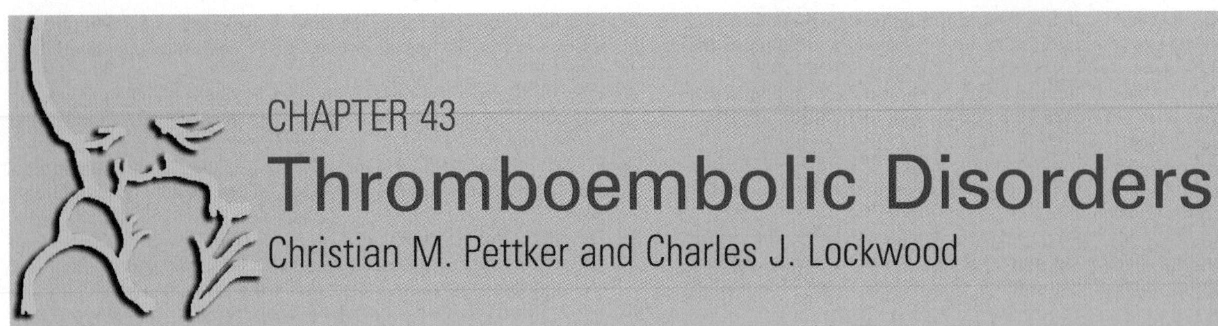

CHAPTER 43

Thromboembolic Disorders

Christian M. Pettker and Charles J. Lockwood

KEY ABBREVIATIONS	
Activated Partial Thromboplastin Time	aPTT
Activated Protein C	APC
Acute Pulmonary Embolus	APE
Adenosine Diphosphate	ADP
Antiphospholipid Antibody	APA
Antiphospholipid Antibody Syndrome	APAS
Computed Tomography	CT
Computed Tomographic Pulmonary Angiography	CTPA
Deep Venous Thrombosis	DVT
Enzyme-linked Immunosorbent Assay	ELISA
Factor V Leiden	FVL
Heparin-induced Thrombocytopenia	HIT
Inferior Vena Cava	IVC
International Normalized Ratio	INR
Low-molecular-weight Heparin	LMWH
Magnetic Resonance Angiography	MRA
Magnetic Resonance Imaging	MRI
Plasminogen Activator Inhibitor-1	PAI-1
Protein Z–Dependent Protease Inhibitor	ZPI
Pulmonary Embolus	PE
Systemic Lupus Erythematosus	SLE
Thrombin-activatable Fibrinolysis Inhibitor	TAFI
Thromboxane A_2	TXA_2
Tissue Factor	TF
Tissue Factor Pathway Inhibitor	TFPI
Venous Thromboembolism	VTE
Venous Ultrasonography	VUS
Ventilation Perfusion Scan	V/Q

Pregnancy, childbirth, and the puerperium create serious challenges to a woman's hemostatic system. The development of the high-volume, high-flow, low-resistance uteroplacental circulation requires an enhanced hemostatic response to avoid hemorrhage. The price paid for this essential hemostatic adaptation to human hemochorial placentation is an increased risk for superficial and deep venous thrombosis (DVT) and pulmonary embolus (PE). Mothers with underlying acquired or inherited thrombophilias are at particular risk. The expeditious identification and prompt treatment of such thrombotic events is critical to avoiding death and serious postphlebitic sequelae.

Epidemiology

Occurring in about in 1 in 1500 pregnancies, venous thromboembolism (VTE) is a relatively uncommon disorder but a leading cause of mortality and serious morbidity in pregnant women.[1-8] This rate represents a nearly 10-fold increase compared with nonpregnant women of comparable childbearing age. According to the most recent U.S. vital statistics, PE is the leading cause of maternal mortality, contributing to 19.6% of maternal deaths, or 2.3 pregnancy-related deaths per 100,000 live births.[9] Classic teaching viewed the postpartum period as the period of maximal thrombotic occurrence; however, management styles of prior eras (e.g., prolonged puerperal bedrest, and estrogen to suppress lactation) likely inflated this risk.[6] More recent studies have shown that most thromboembolic events happen in the antepartum period.[1,3,10-12] However, given its shorter duration and after adjusting for duration of exposure, the relative risk for VTE is about threefold to eightfold higher in the puerperium.[8]

Risk Factors

Virchow's triad—**vascular stasis, hypercoagulability, and vascular trauma**—describes the three classic antecedents to thrombosis, and many of the physiologic changes of pregnancy contribute to these criteria. Other pregnancy-specific risk factors for thrombosis include increased parity, postpartum endomyometritis, operative vaginal delivery, and cesarean delivery. The latter is associated with a substantial ninefold increase in the risk for thromboembolism compared with vaginal delivery.[10] Risk factors not unique to pregnancy include age greater than 35 years, obesity, trauma, immobility, infection, smoking, nephrotic syndrome, hyperviscosity syndromes, cancer, surgery (particularly orthopedic procedures), and a prior history of DVT or PE.

PHYSIOLOGY OF HEMOSTASIS

Vasoconstriction and Platelet Action

Vasoconstriction and platelet activity play a primary initial role in limiting blood loss following vascular disruption and endothelial damage. Vasoconstriction limits blood flow as well as the size of thrombus necessary to repair the defect. Platelet adherence to damaged vessels is mediated by the formation of von Willebrand factor "bridges" anchored at one end to subendothelial collagen and at the other to the platelet GPIb/IX/V receptor.[13] Platelet adhesion stimulates release of α-granules containing von Willebrand factor, thrombospondin, platelet factor-4, fibrinogen, β-thromboglobulin, and platelet-derived growth factor, as well as dense granules containing adenosine diphosphate (ADP) and serotonin. These latter molecules, when combined with the release of thromboxane A_2 (TXA_2), contribute to further vasoconstriction and platelet activation, and ADP causes a conformational change in the platelet GPIIb/IIa receptor that promotes aggregation by forming interplatelet fibrinogen, fibronectin, and vitronectin bridges.[14]

Coagulation Cascade

Platelet action alone is insufficient to provide adequate hemostasis in the face of a substantial vascular insult; in this setting, the coagulation cascade, with resultant fibrin-plug formation, is required to restore hemostasis. Tissue factor (TF), a cell membrane–bound glycoprotein, is the primary initiator of the coagulation cascade.[15] It is expressed constitutively by epithelial, stromal, and perivascular cells throughout the body and in abundance by endometrial stromal cells and the pregnant uterine decidua.[15,16] TF is also present in low concentrations in blood, on activated platelets, and in high levels in amniotic fluid, accounting for the coagulopathy seen in amniotic fluid embolism.[17] It is interesting to note that although intrauterine survival is possible in the absence of platelets or fibrinogen, it is not possible in the absence of TF.[18] Clotting is initiated by the binding of TF to factor VII (Figure 43-1).

After endothelial injury and in the presence of ionized calcium, perivascular cell- or platelet-bound TF comes into contact with factor VII on anionic cell membrane phospholipids. Factor VII has low intrinsic clotting activity but can be autoactivated after binding to TF or can be activated by thrombin or factors IXa, Xa, or XIIa.[15,19] The TF/FVIIa complex initiates the elements of the coagulation cascade by activating both factors X and IX. The latter (IXa) complexes with its cofactor, factor VIIIa, to indirectly activate factor X. Once generated, factor Xa binds with its

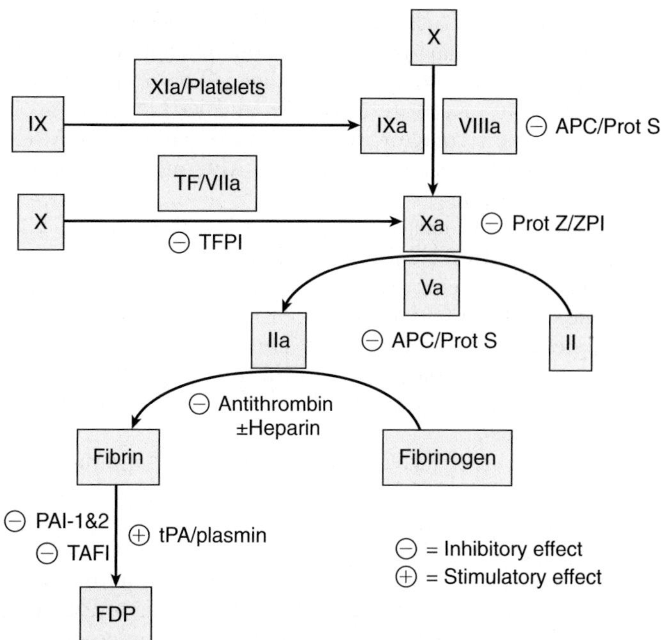

FIGURE 43-1. Hemostatic, thrombotic, and fibrinolytic pathways. *FDP,* Fibrin degradation product; *tPA,* Tissue-type plasminogen activator.

cofactor Va to convert prothrombin (factor II) to thrombin (IIa). The cofactors V and VIII can each be activated by either thrombin or factor Xa. Activated factor XII activates factor XI on the surface of activated platelets, which provides an alternative route to factor IX activation. Factor XII can be activated by kallikrein/kininogen as well as by plasmin. The key event of hemostasis occurs when thrombin cleaves fibrinogen to produce fibrin. Fibrin monomers self-polymerize and are cross-linked by thrombin-activated factor XIIIa. Although TF is the initiator of hemostasis, thrombin is the ultimate arbiter of clotting because it not only activates platelets and generates fibrin but also activates critical clotting factors and cofactors (V, VII, VIII, and XIII). Figure 43-1 provides a diagram of the interaction of the various components of the coagulation cascade.

Anticoagulant System

The risk for thrombosis, the inappropriate and excessive activation of the clotting cascade, is restrained by the anticoagulant system (see Figure 43-1). There is evidence that the coagulation system "idles" like a car engine to quickly respond to vascular injury, and, thus, the anticoagulant system performs the critical role of preventing inappropriate acceleration of clotting.[19] Tissue factor pathway inhibitor (TFPI) binds to the prothrombinase complex (factor Xa/TF/VIIa) to stop TF-mediated clotting.[20] However, as noted, factor XIa generation can bypass this block. Moreover, in the 10 to 15 seconds before TFPI-mediated prothrombinase inhibition, sufficient quantities of factors Va, VIIIa, IXa, and Xa and thrombin are generated to sustain clotting for some time. As a result, additional physiologic anticoagulant molecules are required to maintain blood fluidity.

Paradoxically, thrombin also plays a pivotal role in the anticoagulant system by binding to thrombomodulin, which causes a conformation change that allows it to activate protein C (APC). The APC molecule binds to anionic endothelial cell membrane phospholipids on damaged vessels or to the endothelial cell protein C receptor (EPCR) to inactivate factors Va and VIIIa.[21] Protein S is an important cofactor in this process, enhancing APC activity. Factor Va is also a cofactor in APC-mediated factor VIIIa inactivation.

Factor Xa can also be inhibited by the protein Z–dependent protease inhibitor (ZPI). When ZPI forms a complex with its cofactor, protein Z, its inhibitory activity is enhanced 1000-fold, although ZPI can also inhibit factor XIa independent of protein Z.[22] Deficiencies of protein Z can promote both bleeding and thrombosis, although the latter predominates particularly in the presence of other thrombophilias.

Thrombin activity is modulated by a number of serine protease inhibitors (e.g., heparin cofactor II, α_2-macroglobulin, antithrombin) that serve to inactivate thrombin and Xa. The most active inhibitor within this group is antithrombin (also known as antithrombin III). Antithrombin binds to either thrombin or factor Xa and then to heparin or other glycosaminoglycans, augmenting the antithrombin rate of thrombin inactivation 1000-fold.[23,24] The other two inhibitors work in a similar fashion.

Clot Lysis and Fibrinolysis

Fibrinolysis is a further critical element in preventing overwhelming thrombosis (see Figure 43-1). Tissue-type plasminogen activator, embedded in fibrin, cleaves plasminogen to generate plasmin, which, in turn, cleaves fibrin into fibrin degradation products. The latter are indirect measures of fibrinolysis. These fibrin degradation products can also inhibit thrombin action, a favorable effect when production is limited but a contributor to disseminated intravascular coagulation (DIC) when production is excessive. A second plasminogen activator, urokinase-type plasminogen activator (uPA), is produced by endothelial cells. There is also a series of fibrinolysis inhibitors that prevent hemorrhage from premature clot lysis. The α_2-plasmin inhibitor is bound to the fibrin clot, where it prevents premature fibrinolysis. Platelets and endothelial cells release plasminogen activator inhibitor-1 (PAI-1), an inactivator of tissue-type plasminogen activator. In pregnancy, the decidua is also a rich source of PAI-1, and the placenta produces mostly PAI-2.[25] The thrombin-activatable fibrinolysis inhibitor (TAFI) is another fibrinolytic inhibitor that is also activated by the thrombin-thrombomodulin complex.[26] TAFI modifies fibrin, rendering it resistant to inactivation by plasmin.

PATHOPHYSIOLOGY OF THROMBOSIS IN PREGNANCY

Characteristic physiologic changes in the local decidual and systemic hemostatic systems occur in pregnancy in preparation for the hemostatic challenges of implantation, placentation, and childbirth. Decidual TF and PAI-1 expression are greatly increased in response to progesterone, and levels of PAI-2, which are negligible before pregnancy, increase until term.[25,26] Pregnancy is associated with systemic changes that enhance hemostatic capability but promote thrombosis. For example, there is **a doubling in circulating concentrations of fibrinogen and 20% to 1000% increases in factors VII, VIII, IX, X, and XII, all of which peak at term in preparation for delivery.**[27] Levels of von Willebrand factor also increase up to 400% at term.[27] In contrast, levels of prothrombin and factor V remain unchanged, whereas levels of factor XIII and XI decline modestly. Concomitantly, there is a **40% decrease in the levels of free protein S, conferring an overall resistance to APC.**[27] Further reductions in free protein S concentrations are caused by cesarean delivery and infection, accounting for the high rate of PE in such patients. Coagulation parameters may normalize as early as 3 weeks postpartum, but they generally return to baseline at 6 weeks postpartum.

The risk for thrombosis in pregnancy is also related to physical changes in the gravid woman. Venous stasis in the lower extremities results from compression of the inferior vena cava and pelvic veins by the enlarging uterus.[28,29] Despite the presence of the sigmoid colon promoting uterine dextrorotation, ultrasound findings indicate lower flow velocities in the left leg veins throughout pregnancy.[30] This would explain why multiple studies have confirmed that the incidence of thrombosis is far greater in the left leg than right leg.[1,11] Hormone-mediated increases in deep vein capacitance secondary to increased circulating levels of estrogen and local production of prostacyclin and nitric oxide also contribute to the increased risk for thrombosis.

Antiphospholipid Antibody Syndrome

Overall, antiphospholipid antibody syndrome (APAS) is responsible for about 14% of thromboembolic events in pregnancy.[31,32] The diagnosis of APAS requires the presence of prior or current vascular thrombosis, or characteristic obstetrical complications, together with at least one laboratory criterion (e.g., anticardiolipin antibodies, anti-β_2-glycoprotein-I, or lupus anticoagulant).[33] The antiphospholipid antibodies (APAs) are a class of self-recognition immunoglobulins whose epitopes are proteins bound to negatively charged phospholipids. Anticardiolipin antibodies and the lupus anticoagulants represent the two most widely employed end points, but other applicable tests include anti-β_2-glycoprotein, and recently, antiprothrombin and antiannexin antibodies have been identified.[34] These antibodies must be present on two or more occasions at least 12 weeks apart for diagnosis.[33] These antibodies are present in 2.2% of the general obstetrical population, and most affected patients have uncomplicated pregnancies.[35] Thus, providers should use caution when ordering and interpreting tests in the absence of APAS-qualifying clinical criteria.

APAS has been associated with both venous (DVT, PE) and arterial (stroke) vascular events. A meta-analysis of 18 studies has shown elevated risk for DVT, PE, and recurrent VTE among patients with systemic lupus erythematous (SLE) who test positive for the APAs. Overall, when compared with SLE patients who do not test positive for either test, those with lupus anticoagulants and anticardiolipin antibodies have sixfold and twofold increased risks for venous thrombosis, respectively.[36] These antibodies pose a risk to patients without SLE as well. The lifetime prevalence of arterial or venous thrombosis in affected non-SLE patients is about 30%, with an

TABLE 43-1 INHERITED THROMBOPHILIAS AND ASSOCIATION WITH VENOUS THROMBOEMBOLISM IN PREGNANCY

RISK GROUP	THROMBOPHILIA TYPE	PREVALENCE IN THE EUROPEAN POPULATION (%)	PREVALENCE IN PATIENTS WITH VTE IN PREGNANCY (%)	RR OR OR OF VTE IN PREGNANCY (95% CI)	PROBABILITY OF VTE IN PREGNANCY (% OF PATIENTS WITH PERSONAL OR FAMILY HISTORY)	PROBABILITY OF VTE IN PREGNANCY (% OF PATIENTS WITHOUT PERSONAL OR FAMILY HISTORY)	REFERENCES
High risk	FVL homozygous	0.07*	<1*	25.4 (8.8-66)	>10	1.5	40, 42-45
	Prothrombin gene *G20210A* mutation homozygous	0.02*	<1*	N/A	>10	2.8	46, 47
	Antithrombin III deficiency	0.02-1.1	1-8	119	11-40	3.0-7.2	42, 45, 46
	Compound heterozygous (FVL/prothrombin *G20210A*)	0.17*	<1*	84 (19-369)	4.7 (overall probability of VTE in pregnancy)		40, 42, 48
Low risk	FVL heterozygous	5.3	44	6.9 (3.3-15.2)	>10	0.26	40, 42-44, 49
	Prothrombin *G20210A* mutation heterozygous	2.9	17	9.5 (2.1-66.7)	>10	0.37-0.5	40, 42, 47, 48
	Protein C deficiency	0.2-0.3	<14	13.0 (1.4-123)	†	0.8-1.7	42, 45, 46, 50
	Protein S deficiency	0.03-0.13	12.4	†	†	<1-6.6	40, 42, 46, 51

*Calculated based on a Hardy-Weinberg equilibrium.
†Data not available.
OR, Odds ratio; *RR*, relative risk.

event rate of 1% per year.[37,38] The risks for thromboembolic events are highly dependent on the presence of other predisposing factors, including pregnancy, estrogen exposure, immobility, surgery, and infection. APAS has also been associated with adverse pregnancy outcome and accounts for 14% of VTE in pregnancy.[31,32] In fact, there is a 5% risk for a thrombotic event in pregnancy, even with prophylaxis.[39]

Inherited Thrombophilias

The inherited thrombophilias are a heterogeneous group of genetic disorders associated with arterial and venous thrombosis as well as fetal loss. As with APAS, the occurrence of a thromboembolic event is highly dependent on other predisposing factors such as pregnancy, exogenous estrogens, immobility, obesity, surgery, infection, trauma, and the presence of other thrombophilias. However, the most important risk modifier is a personal or family history of venous thrombosis.[40] **Table 43-1 presents the prevalence and risk of venous thrombosis among pregnant patients with and without a personal or family history of venous thrombosis.** As noted, the thrombophilias are divided into high and low risks based on the overall risk for VTE. The screening for and management of inherited thrombophilias during and around the time of pregnancy was recently addressed by the American College of Obstetricians and Gynecologists (ACOG).[41]

Recent prospective studies have suggested that lower-risk inherited thrombophilias may have an even lower association with maternal thrombosis than observed in the retrospective studies[42-51] cited in Table 43-1. For example, a prospective study of 4885 low-risk women screened in the first trimester of pregnancy noted that 134 (2.7%) carried the factor V Leiden mutation, but none had a thromboembolic event during pregnancy or puerperium (95% confidence interval [CI], 0% to 2.7%).[52] In two other prospective studies involving 584 Irish and 4250 British pregnant women again screened for factor V Leiden early in pregnancy, no thrombotic episodes were noted among carriers.[53,54] Said and associates blindly tested 1707 Australian nulliparous women for factor V Leiden, the prothrombin gene *G20210A* mutation, and a thrombomodulin polymorphism before 22 weeks and reported expected prevalences of heterozygosity for the factor V Leiden and prothrombin *G20210A* gene mutations and homozygosity for the thrombomodulin polymorphism of 5.39%, 2.38%, and 3.51%, respectively, but again none of the patients developed venous thromboembolic events.[55] However, one prospective study of 2480 women tested for APC resistance and factor V Leiden early in pregnancy observed affected patients had an eightfold increase in VTE.[56] Thus, the true risk for thrombosis in patients with low-risk inherited thrombophilias is probably lower than suggested by retrospective case control and cohort studies and also likely dependent on the presence of concomitant risk factors such as a strong family history, obesity, and surgery.

DIAGNOSIS OF VENOUS THROMBOEMBOLISM

Deep Venous Thrombosis

Clinical Signs and Symptoms

The clinical findings typical of DVT include erythema, warmth, pain, edema, and tenderness localized to the area of the thrombosis. Occasionally, a palpable cord may correspond to a thrombosed vein, and Homans sign is the pain and tenderness elicited on compression of the calf muscles by squeezing the muscles or dorsiflexion of the foot. These are rather nonspecific signs and symptoms that involve a broad differential diagnosis, including cellulitis, ruptured or strained muscle or tendon, trauma, ruptured popliteal (Baker) cyst, cutaneous vasculitis, superficial thrombophlebitis, and lymphedema. In fact, evidence suggests that the specificities of these manifestations are less than 50%, and among patients with these signs and symptoms, the diagnosis of DVT is confirmed by objective testing in only about one third of the group.[57,58]

Risk Scoring System

Work by Chan and colleagues demonstrated that subjective assessment by "thrombosis experts" of clinical risk for DVT in symptomatic pregnant patients can categorize patients, before diagnostic testing, into two groups with low risk (1.5% prevalence, 98.5% negative predictive value) and "non-low" risk (25% prevalence).[59] Three factors **(symptoms in the left leg a leg circumference discrepancy of ≥2 cm, and first-trimester presentation)** were highly predictive of DVT. Thus, determination of prediagnostic study risk can be helpful before proceeding to the selection and interpretation of diagnostic tests.

Imaging

Contrast venography, an invasive technique involving the injection of dye into a vein distal to the site of suspected thrombosis, followed by radiographic imaging, is now rarely used for diagnosis of DVT. The risks for radiation and contrast allergy, as well as its technical difficulty, particularly preclude its use in pregnancy.[60]

The most common diagnostic modality employed in the evaluation of patients with suspected DVT is venous ultrasonography (VUS), with or without color Doppler. This modality has virtually replaced the cumbersome and less accurate impedance plethysmography technique. The ultrasound transducer is placed over the common femoral vein beginning at the inguinal ligament and then sequentially moved to image the greater saphenous vein, the superficial femoral vein, and the popliteal vein to its trifurcation with the deep veins of the calf. Compression VUS involves the application of pressure with the probe to determine whether the vein under investigation is compressible. The most accurate ultrasonic criterion for diagnosing venous thrombosis is noncompressibility of the venous lumen in a transverse plane under gentle probe pressure using duplex and color-flow Doppler imaging.[57] The overall sensitivity and specificity of VUS have been reported to be 90% to 100% for proximal vein thromboses, but traditionally have been considered lower for the detection of calf vein thromboses.[61] This is confirmed by a more recent meta-analysis demonstrating that, in nonpregnant patients, duplex ultrasound has a pooled sensitivity of 96.4% for proximal (knee or thigh) DVT, 75.2% for distal (calf) DVT, and total specificity of 94.3%.[62]

Magnetic resonance imaging (MRI) appears to have equivalent test performance characteristics to VUS. One meta-analysis demonstrated a sensitivity of 91.5% and specificity of 94.8% for diagnosis of DVT in nonpregnant patients with suspected DVT or PE.[63] Similar to VUS, there is also improved sensitivity for distal compared with proximal thrombi (93.9% versus 62.1%). The advantage of MRI may be in the ability to detect more centralized DVT, like those in the pelvic, iliac, or femoral veins.

D-Dimer Assays

Laboratory evaluation of serum concentrations of D-dimer, a product of the degradation of fibrin by plasmin, has been increasingly advocated as a helpful test in the diagnosis of DVT. Testing relies on the use of monoclonal antibodies to D-dimer fragments. The most accurate and reliable tests for D-dimers appear to be two rapid enzyme-linked immunosorbent assays (ELISAs) (Instant-IA D-dimer, Stago, Asniéres, France and VIDAS DD, bioMérieux, Marcy-l'Etoile, France) and a rapid whole blood assay (SimpliRED D-dimer, Agen Biomedical, Brisbane, Australia).

The test is limited by factors that may contribute to false-positive testing, including pregnancy, the postpartum and postoperative periods, and superficial thrombophlebitis.[64,65] In particular, normal pregnancy causes a physiologic increase in D-dimer, with levels exceeding the threshold for normal in 78% and 100% of patients in the second and third trimesters, respectively.[66]

The performance of the SimpliRED D-dimer test was evaluated in a prospective cohort of patients at risk for DVT by Chan.[66a] In this population, who had a DVT prevalence of 8.7%, sensitivity of D-dimer testing was 100%, and specificity was 60%. Utility particularly appeared to be stratified across gestation; false-positive rates were 0%, 24%, and 51% for the first, second, and third trimesters, respectively. The value of D-dimer testing in pregnancy appears to be its ability to rule-out disease because this same study showed a negative predictive value of 100%, with 95% CI interval of 95% to 100%. The value of D-dimer testing in the late-second and third trimesters is likely to be lower than in the first half of pregnancy because the former patients will likely have levels above the threshold.

Workup of Patients with Suspected Deep Venous Thrombosis

The diagnostic paradigm outlined in Figure 43-2 can be employed to diagnose DVT in pregnant patients with maximal sensitivity and specificity. A major assumption of this strategy is the availability of a sensitive assay for D-dimer. When a D-dimer test is unavailable or inappropriate (particularly in the third trimester), the testing algorithm should begin with lower extremity compression sonography. Risk may be stratified as in the section above (see Risk Scoring System).

Pulmonary Embolus

Clinical Signs and Symptoms

Tachypnea (>20 breaths/minute) and tachycardia (>100 beats/minute) are present in 90% of patients with acute PE, but these findings lack specificity and generate a broad differential diagnosis.[67] Presyncope and syncope are rarer symptoms and indicate a massive embolus.[68]

Nonspecific Studies

The classic electrocardiographic changes associated with PE are the S1, Q3, and inverted T3. Other findings include

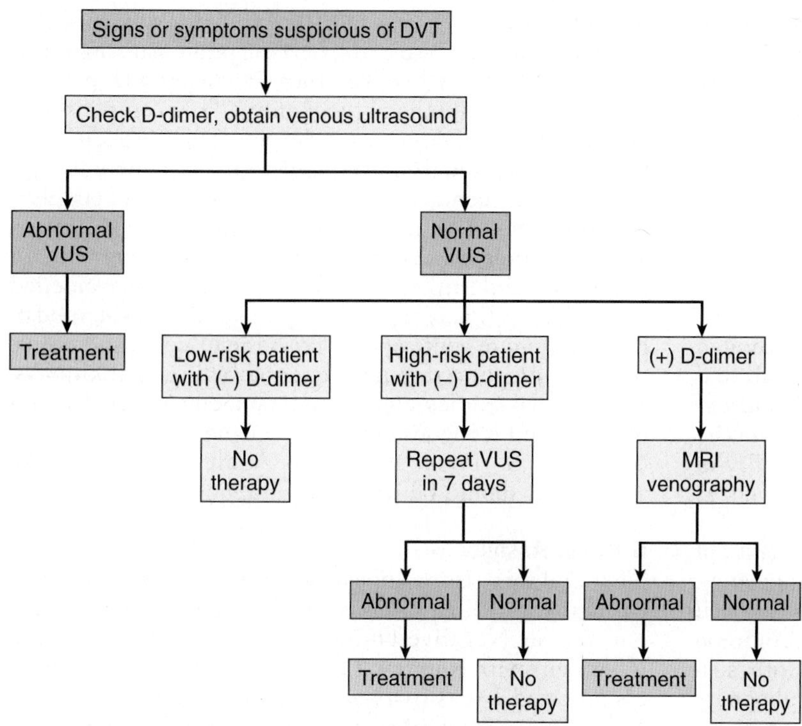

FIGURE 43-2. Diagnostic algorithm for suspected deep venous thrombosis.

nonspecific ST changes, right bundle branch block, and right axis deviation. These findings are usually associated with cor pulmonale and right-sided heart strain or overload, reflective of more serious cardiopulmonary compromise. About 26% to 32% of patients with massive PE had the previously mentioned electrocardiographic changes.[69] Arterial blood gases and oxygen saturation have limited value in the assessment of acute PE (APE), particularly in a pregnant population. Measurements of PO_2 are greater than 80 mm Hg in 29% of PE patients younger than 40 years of age.[70] In another study, up to 18% of patients with APE had PO_2 measurements of more than 85 mm Hg. The chest radiograph may be abnormal in up to 84% of affected patients.[67] The common findings on radiograph are pleural effusion, pulmonary infiltrates, atelectasis, and elevated hemidiaphragm. The eponymous findings of pulmonary infarction, such as a wedge-shaped infiltrate (Hampton hump) or decreased vascularity (Westermark sign), are rare.[71] Although a normal chest radiograph in the setting of dyspnea, tachypnea, and hypoxemia in a patient without known preexistent pulmonary or cardiovascular disease is suggestive of PE, a chest radiograph cannot be used to confirm the diagnosis.[71]

A large APE can create changes consistent with cor pulmonale and right-sided heart strain. Large emboli in the main pulmonary artery and its primary branches can result in acute right-sided heart failure, which is the ultimate cause of death in most patients with APE. Between 30% and 80% of patients with PE display echocardiographic abnormalities in right ventricular size or function.[72-74] Typical findings include a dilated and hypokinetic right ventricle, tricuspid regurgitation, and absence of preexisting pulmonary arterial or left-sided heart pathology. Transesophageal echocardiography with or without contrast appears to improve the imaging of main or right pulmonary artery emboli and, occasionally, of left pulmonary artery clots.[75] For these reasons, bedside echocardiography can be very useful for the unstable patient or the patient unable to travel for other imaging studies.

Pulmonary Arteriography

Until the advent of sensitive multidetector-row computed tomographic pulmonary angiography (CTPA, or spiral CT), intravenous contrast pulmonary arteriography or angiography was considered the gold standard for diagnosis of PE and, as such, was considered to have a sensitivity and specificity of 100%.[71] However, the sensitivity and interobserver agreement of traditional pulmonary angiography for smaller peripheral lesions decreases from 98% for lobar emboli, to 90% for segmental, and to 66% for subsegmental emboli.[76] Of all diagnostic modalities, this technique involves the highest risk, including a 0.5% mortality risk and a 3% complication rate, primarily because of the risks of contrast injection and catheter placement, including respiratory failure, renal failure, cardiac perforation, and groin hematoma requiring transfusion.[68] Furthermore, patients with evidence of cardiopulmonary compromise pose an even higher complication risk. Given its poor diagnostic efficacy and its attendant risks, pulmonary angiography is rarely used.

Ventilation-Perfusion Scanning

Perfusion scanning employs intravenously injected radioisotope-labeled albumin macroaggregates that deposit in the pulmonary capillary bed. Ventilation scanning involves the inhalation of radiolabeled aerosols whose distribution is evaluated by gamma camera. The comparison of these two images allows for interpretation of characteristic patterns that were then used to assign diagnostic probabilities (high, intermediate, or low). Greater than 90% of high-risk patients with high-probability V/Q scans have PE, whereas less than 6% of low-risk patients with low-probability scans have a PE. Given that most young healthy women have little underlying lung pulmonary pathology, the diagnostic efficacy of V/Q scanning in pregnant women is substantially higher than in older, nonpregnant patients.

Spiral Computed Tomographic Pulmonary Angiography

Spiral CT scanning requires injecting intravenous contrast while simultaneously imaging the distribution of contrast in the pulmonary vasculature with a CT scanner.[71] Although this can be an effective judge of large, segmental, and central emboli, CT is of limited value with small subsegmental vessels and horizontally oriented vessels in the right middle lobe. One strength of CTPA is its utility in diagnosing nonembolic pulmonary phenomena such as pneumonia or pulmonary edema.

In nonpregnant patients, CTPA is often the modality of choice; however, this is not likely the case in pregnancy. Several studies have shown that **CTPA performs less well in pregnant compared with nonpregnant cohorts.** Andreou demonstrated in a small study of 32 patients with suspected PE that contrast enhancement of the pulmonary arteries is less in pregnant women than nonpregnant patients, likely because of the increased cardiac output of pregnancy.[77] Another reason may be the more frequent dilution or interruption of contrast by unopacified blood from the lower vena cava in pregnancy.[78] Comparing CTPA imaging in 40 pregnant patients with 40 nonpregnant patients, U-King-Im and associates also demonstrated a threefold higher rate of suboptimal studies in the pregnant population (27.5% versus 7.5%).[79]

Ventilation-Perfusion Scanning Versus Computed Tomographic Pulmonary Angiography

V/Q scanning and CTPA have been directly compared in pregnant patients by Cahill and colleagues, who retrospectively evaluated a cohort of 304 pregnant or postpartum women evaluated for PE.[80] CTPA was performed in 108 women and V/Q in 196. In women with a normal chest radiograph, CTPA yielded nondiagnostic results 5.4 times more often than V/Q scanning (30% versus 5.4%). As would be expected, in patients with an abnormal chest radiograph, V/Q scanning was more often nondiagnostic. Ridge and colleagues evaluated these two techniques prospectively in 50 total patients.[78] Again, they found that CTPA more often gave a nondiagnostic result (35.7% versus 2.1%), and V/Q scanning was adequate for diagnosis more frequently (35.7% versus 4%). For these reasons, as well as considerations of radiation exposure (see later), **V/Q scanning is the modality of choice for patients with suspected PE and a normal chest radiograph.**

Magnetic Resonance Angiography

Magnetic resonance angiography (MRA) may be performed using MRI of a patient during intravenous injection of gadolinium. Faster image acquisition rates and improved image timing to respiratory and cardiac motion have allowed this technique to develop. Preliminary experience by Meaney and colleagues suggested a sensitivity of 100%, specificity of 95%, and positive and negative predictive values of 87% and 100%, respectively, for MRA in 30 patients also assessed by classic pulmonary angiography.[81] Another prospective study involving 141 patients showed an overall sensitivity of only 77% in comparison to pulmonary angiography, with the sensitivity broken down to 40%, 84%, and 100% for isolated subsegmental, segmental, and central pulmonary emboli, respectively.[82] Because MRA does not involve ionizing radiation, it is an appealing alternative to CT scanning and angiography for pregnancy, and further assessment in large trials is needed to prove its ultimate utility as a primary diagnostic modality. Gadolinium contrast does cross the placenta and enters the amniotic fluid through excretion by the fetal kidneys. Most animal studies suggest no teratogenic effects by gadolinium, and it is considered a pregnancy category C drug by the U.S. Food and Drug Administration (FDA), although it should be used with caution.

D-Dimer Assays

The D-dimer assay appears to have less sensitivity in patients with PE and thus is less helpful as a test for ruling out disease. Negative D-dimer testing has been observed in patients with confirmed PE.[83] Damadoram and coworkers reported a sensitivity and specificity of 73% and 15%, respectively, for D-dimer in testing for suspected PE in pregnancy.[84] The difference in D-dimer test performance for PE in pregnancy may be due to the smaller clot burden compared with DVT coupled with the increase in intravascular plasma volume of pregnancy. This unacceptably high false-negative rate indicates **no role for D-dimer testing in the workup of pregnant patients with suspected PE.**

Lower Extremity Evaluation

Most PEs (90%) arise from lower extremity DVTs, and among patients with the diagnosis of PE, half will be found to harbor a lower extremity DVT, including up to 20% of PE patients without signs or symptoms of lower extremity DVT.[85-87] In patients presenting with signs or symptoms of PE who also have left-sided lower extremity symptoms, it is reasonable to begin with lower extremity VUS to detect DVT because the need for therapeutic anticoagulation is similar. This avoids exposure to the ionizing radiation as well as the burden of more complicated testing associated with CTPA and V/Q scanning. Furthermore, in high-risk patients in whom CTPA or V/Q scanning is not diagnostic (or even negative), evaluation of the leg veins for DVT can help to reinforce results. In such cases, however, a negative VUS study is still associated with a 25% risk for PE, suggesting that further studies are generally needed.[88]

Workup of Patients with Suspected Pulmonary Embolus

Workup of patients with suspected PE should begin with evaluation of their cardiorespiratory status in order to determine whether they are critically ill. Patients who are stable hemodynamically, with favorable oxygenation status (oxygen saturation >80%), should be evaluated in a carefully ordered fashion, taking into account the possibility of lower extremity DVT and chest radiograph results (Figure 43-3).

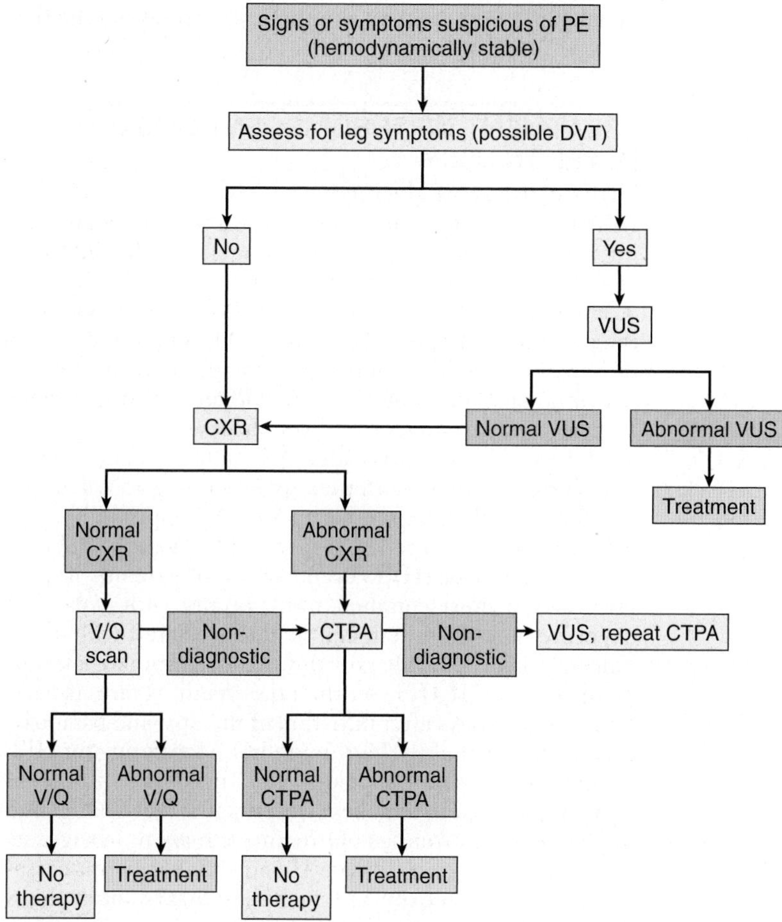

FIGURE 43-3. Diagnostic algorithm for suspected pulmonary embolus in a hemodynamically stable patient. *CXR*, Chest x-ray.

As noted previously, **D-dimer testing is no longer deemed of value in the workup in pregnant patients with suspected APE.** If lower extremity symptoms are present, particularly if left-sided, VUS is performed, and if positive, therapeutic anticoagulation should begin. **Chest radiographs should be performed for cases in which VUS is negative or in which there are no lower extremity signs or symptoms. Although the chest radiograph is not used in the actual diagnosis, it allows for proper selection of the next diagnostic test. V/Q scan is performed if the chest radiograph is normal.** A positive (high- or intermediate-probability) V/Q scan should prompt therapeutic anticoagulation. A negative test should exclude the diagnosis. A nondiagnostic result (e.g., intermediate-probability or equivocal test in any patient and a low-probability result in a high-risk patient with prior venous thrombosis, known thrombophilia, family history of thrombosis in a first-degree relative younger than 50 years, or other clinical risk factors) should trigger performance of CTPA. For such patients and those with an abnormal chest radiograph, CTPA is the diagnostic modality of choice. Positive tests prompt initiation of anticoagulation. In the patient with an abnormal chest radiograph who has a negative CTPA, the true etiology of the chest pathology is often seen on CT. Alternatively, if the CTPA is nondiagnostic, further testing is performed, such as MRA or serial lower extremity VUS.

In the critically ill patient, anticoagulation should be started, in the absence of contraindications, and a similar protocol is followed (Figure 43-4). Very unstable patients who cannot be transported safely can be evaluated with a bedside echocardiogram, which may have more test accuracy in this setting.

Radiation Exposure in Pregnancy

Fetal Exposure

The diagnosis of DVT and PE in pregnant patients poses unique challenges because of concerns about fetal radiation exposure. The ACOG advises that exposure to less than 5 cGy has not been associated with increases in pregnancy loss or fetal anomalies.[89] Exposure to ionizing radiation doses above 1 cGy, however, may create a marginally increased risk for childhood leukemia (from 1/3000 baseline to 1/2000).[90,91] Table 43-2 outlines the ***fetal*** radiation exposure of different radiation modalities. **A combination of chest radiograph, V/Q scan, and pulmonary angiography exposes the fetus to less than 0.5 cGy.**[6] CTPA is associated with only slightly lower radiation levels for the fetus compared with V/Q scanning. Although the concern for possible adverse effects should not prevent a medically important test from being performed, judicious use and selection of tests is advised.

Maternal Exposure

Radiation exposure to the maternal breast is also an important consideration when choosing tests because the increased glandularity and proliferative state of the

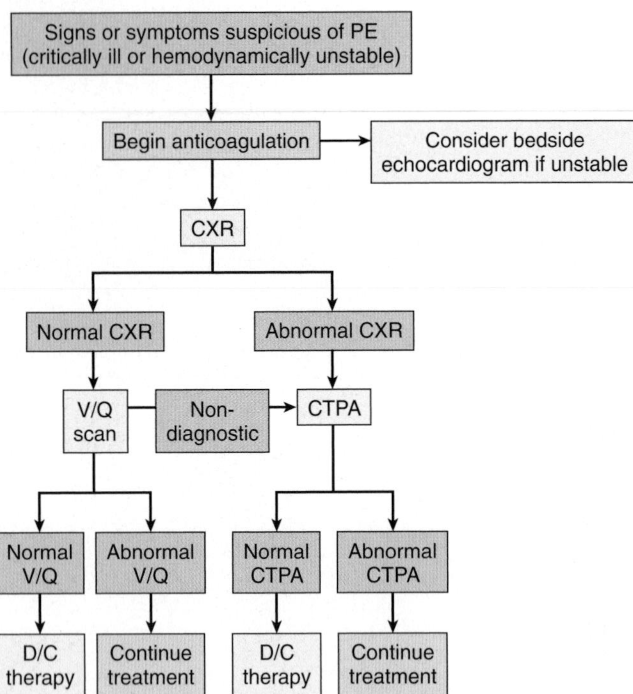

FIGURE 43-4. Diagnostic algorithm for suspected pulmonary embolism in a critically ill or hemodynamically unstable patient. *CXR,* Chest x-ray; *D/C,* discontinue.

TABLE 43-2 FETAL RADIATION EXPOSURE OF VARIOUS IONIZING MODALITIES

RADIOLOGIC MODALITY	FETAL RADIATION EXPOSURE (CGY)
Chest radiograph	<0.01
Venography	
Limited, shielded	<0.05
Full (unilateral), unshielded	0.31
Pulmonary angiography	
Brachial vein	0.05
Femoral vein	0.22-0.37
V/Q scan	0.007-0.031
Ventilation scan	0.001-0.019
Perfusion scan	0.006-0.012
CTPA (spiral CT)	0.013

Modified from Toglia M, Weg J: Venous thromboembolism during pregnancy. N Engl J Med 335:108-114, 1996.

pregnant breast presumably make it more radiosensitive. This is an important concern with respect to cumulative radiation exposure and cancer risk.[92] V/Q scanning results in substantially lower maternal breast radiation exposure. CTPA is estimated to expose maternal breast tissue to 150 times more ionizing radiation than V/Q scanning,[93] with doses estimated at 2 to 6 cGy.[94,95] This dose can be reduced about 50% to 60% with breast shielding, without significant reduction in image quality.[96]

MRI and ultrasonography have not been associated with any adverse fetal effects, and teratogenic effects have not been described after administration of gadolinium contrast media.[97] Concerns about fetal goiter following maternal radiographic contrast exposure suggest that fetal heart rates should be assessed to rule out hypothyroidism, and neonatal thyroid function should be tested during the first week of life.[97]

TREATMENT OF THROMBOEMBOLISM IN PREGNANCY

Unfractionated Heparin

Unfractionated heparin effects anticoagulation by enhancing antithrombin activity, increasing factor Xa inhibitor activity, and inhibiting platelet aggregation.[98] Unfractionated heparin (FDA pregnancy category C) does not cross the placenta and is not teratogenic.[99] The chief side effects of heparin include hemorrhage, osteoporosis, and thrombocytopenia. The former is more common with treatment coinciding with surgery or liver disease or concomitant aspirin use. Heparin-associated bone loss is usually reversible, correlates more with therapy exceeding 15,000 units/day for more than 6 months, and can be opposed by supplemental calcium use (1500 mg/day).[100] **Heparin-induced thrombocytopenia (HIT) occurs in 3% of patients.** Type I HIT is the most common form, occurs within days of exposure, is self-limited, and is not associated with a significant risk for hemorrhage or thrombosis. Immunoglobulin-mediated type II HIT, on the other hand, is rare, usually occurs 5 to 14 days after initiation of therapy, and paradoxically increases the risk for thrombosis. Monitoring for HIT should include serial platelet counts until day 14 or until heparin is stopped, whichever occurs first. A 50% decline in platelet count from its pretreatment maximum suggests immune-mediated HIT type II and should prompt cessation of all heparin exposure, including that in intravenous flushes. The diagnosis of HIT type II can be confirmed by serotonin release assays, heparin-induced platelet aggregation assays, flow cytometry, or solid-phase immunoassays.

Protamine sulfate reverses the effect of intravenously administered unfractionated heparin. It is given by low intravenous infusion of less than 20 mg/minute, with no more than 50 mg given over 10 minutes. The total dose of protamine required is calculated based on the residual amount of circulating heparin, with a ratio of 1 mg of protamine sulfate necessary for every 100 units of residual circulating heparin. Residual heparin is calculated by assuming a half-life of 30 to 60 minutes of intravenous heparin. However, repeated serial administrations of lower doses of protamine, coinciding with serial measurements of the activated partial thromboplastin time (aPTT), are required when the heparin is dosed subcutaneously.

Low-Molecular-Weight Heparin

The low-molecular-weight heparins (LMWHs; dalteparin, enoxaparin, and tinzaparin) are reliable and safe alternatives to unfractionated heparin and have fewer side effects. Enzymatic manipulation of standard heparin produces lower-molecular-weight molecules with equivalent antifactor Xa, but little or no antithrombin effects. The LMWHs have longer half-lives and a closer correlation between antifactor Xa activity and body weight than subcutaneously administered unfractionated heparin. However, we follow antifactor Xa levels in pregnant patients because there is far greater variability in binding, distribution, metabolism, and excretion. The LMWHs (pregnancy category B) do not cross the placenta and do not enter breast milk. There is a lower risk for hemorrhage associated with LMWH. **However, regional anesthesia is contraindicated within 18 to 24 hours of therapeutic LMWH administration.** Accordingly, we recommend switching to unfractionated heparin at 36 weeks' gestation or earlier if preterm delivery is expected. Protamine is not as effective in fully reversing the antifactor Xa activity of LMWH, although it may reduce bleeding. Dosing of 1 mg of protamine for every 100 antifactor Xa units of LMWH can normalize aPTT values, but antifactor Xa levels can only be reversed by 80%. The risk for HIT type II is also lower in patients receiving LMWH, but platelet counts should still be checked every 2 to 3 days from day 4 to day 14.

Fondaparinux

Fondaparinux is a synthetic heparin pentasaccharide that complexes with the antithrombin binding site for heparin to permit the selective inactivation of factor Xa, but not thrombin. A major advantage of this medication is that there does not appear to be a risk for HIT type II. It has comparable efficacy to both LMWH and unfractionated heparin in nonpregnant patients. Although it has been used in a small number of pregnant patients without complication, umbilical cord plasma concentrations at 10% of those of maternal plasma have been demonstrated, suggesting limited transplacental passage. Use of fondaparinux should be limited to women without other therapeutic alternatives, such as those with a history of HIT type II or heparin allergies or those who have failed other anticoagulants.

Coumarin

The coumarins are vitamin K antagonists that block the vitamin K–dependent, function-enhancing posttranslational modifications of prothrombin and factors VII, IX, and X, as well as the anticlotting agents proteins C and S. Coumadin (warfarin) has been shown to be effective for both the primary and secondary prevention of VTE, stroke, myocardial infarction, and systemic embolism due to artificial valves and atrial fibrillation. Coumadin is a pregnancy category X medication because fetal exposure can cause nasal and midface hypoplasia, microphthalmia, mental retardation, and other ocular, skeletal, and central nervous system malformations (see Chapter 8). Teratogenic potential is greatest between the 6th and 12th weeks of pregnancy. The risk of warfarin also includes fetal hemorrhage. As a result, warfarin is rarely employed, although the exceptional case of a patient requiring therapeutic anticoagulation, who cannot be sufficiently treated with the heparins, may require its use. Warfarin is also a favored drug for the postpartum period because it is safe to use during lactation.

Therapy is started at a dose of 5 to 10 mg for 2 days, with subsequent doses titrated to achieve an international normalized ratio (INR) of 2 to 3. Peak effects occur within 72 hours, and its half-life is from 36 to 42 hours. Warfarin metabolism is greatly affected by genetic polymorphisms, making the response to particular dosing regimens unpredictable. A pharmacogenetic approach to warfarin dosing includes testing for particular variations in vitamin K and warfarin metabolic enzymes and using this information to formulate a dosing regimen that expeditiously achieves a proper maintenance dose. A criticism of this approach is that pharmacogenetics accounts for only 30% to 50% of the variability in response because environment, diet, and comorbidities often have a significant influence as well. A nomogram for predicting warfarin dosing, based on patient-specific responses to warfarin doses as assessed by day 3 and day 5 INRs, has been proposed by Lazo-Langer. Avoiding the need for costly genetic testing, this protocol accounts for individual variation of warfarin metabolism.

Because of protein C's shorter half-life relative to the other vitamin K–dependent clotting factors, warfarin may initially create a prothrombotic state, particularly in pregnancy. Thus, patients who are initiated on warfarin postpartum should be on therapeutic doses of unfractionated or LMWH for 5 days and until the INR is therapeutic for 48 hours. Coumadin effects can be reversed by vitamin K. The INR generally normalizes within 6 hours of a 5-mg dose of vitamin K and within 4 days with cessation of warfarin therapy. Fresh-frozen plasma can be used to achieve immediate reversal of effects.

Treatment of Acute Deep Venous Thrombosis or Pulmonary Embolus

Women with new-onset VTE diagnosed during pregnancy should receive therapeutic anticoagulation. Therapeutic anticoagulation should be continued for at least 20 weeks. If this period of time expires before the end of the postpartum period, prophylactic anticoagulation should be initiated in patients without highly thrombogenic thrombophilias and continued for 6 weeks to 6 months postpartum, depending on the severity of the thrombotic event and the underlying risk factors. During pregnancy, unfractionated heparin and the LMWHs are the drugs of choice, given their efficacy and safety profile. **Therapeutic doses of the LMWH enoxaparin may start at 1 mg/kg, subcutaneously, twice daily.** Dosing should be titrated to achieve antifactor Xa levels of 0.6 to 1 U/mL when tested 4 hours after injection because of inconsistent efficacy of this weight-based regimen in pregnant patients. Unfractionated heparin for acute DVT or PE is initially given intravenously and titrated to keep the aPTT 1.5 to 2.5 times control (checked every 4 to 6 hours during the titration period), usually according to weight-based protocols (Table 43-3). Intravenous heparin should be continued for 5 to 10 days or until clinical improvement is noted. This can be changed to subcutaneous injections every 8 to 12 hours to keep the aPTT 1.5 to 2 times control, when tested 6 hours after injection.

As noted earlier, the major concerns of therapeutic anticoagulation in pregnancy are regional anesthesia use and hemorrhage risk. Regional anesthesia is contraindicated within 18 to 24 hours of therapeutic LMWH use; thus, LMWH should be converted to unfractionated heparin at 36 weeks' gestation or earlier if clinically indicated. Vaginal or cesarean delivery more than 24 hours after therapeutic LMWH dosing should not pose a risk for hemorrhage, although protamine sulfate may be necessary to partially reverse anticoagulation. Protamine sulfate may also be used to normalize completely an elevated aPTT in patients on therapeutic unfractionated heparin near the time of delivery. Heparin anticoagulation may be restarted

TABLE 43-3 WEIGHT-BASED NOMOGRAM FOR UNFRACTIONATED HEPARIN

Give a bolus of 80 U/kg, followed by a maintenance dosage of 18 U/kg/hr, following aPTT values every 6 hours and with following adjustments for aPTT values obtained:

aPTT VALUE	ADJUSTMENT
<35 sec (<1.2× control value)	Repeat full bolus (80 U/kg), then increase infusion rate by 4 U/kg/hr
35-45 sec (1.2-1.5× control)	Repeat half bolus (40 U/kg), then increase infusion rate by 2 U/kg/hr
46-70 sec (1.6-2.3× control)	No change in infusion rate
71-90 sec (2.4-3× control)	Decrease infusion rate by 2 U/kg/hr
>90 sec (>3× control)	Stop infusion for 1 hour, then decrease by 3 U/kg/hr

Modified from Raschke R, Reilly B, Guidry J, et al: The weight-based heparin dosing nomogram compared with a "standard care" nomogram: a randomized controlled trial. Ann Intern Med 119:874-881, 1993.

3 to 6 hours after vaginal delivery and 6 to 8 hours after cesarean delivery. Coumadin anticoagulation may be started on the first postpartum or postoperative day. As noted earlier, because of the paradoxical increase in APC resistance and factor VIII after starting warfarin, therapeutic doses of the heparins should be continued for 5 days and until the INR reaches therapeutic range (2 to 3) for 2 successive days.

Prophylactic Applications and Dosing

We recommend prophylactic *antepartum* and postpartum anticoagulation in patients with high-risk thrombophilias and no personal or family history of venous thrombosis, and in patients with low-risk thrombophilias but with a family (first-degree relative) or a personal history of venous thrombosis or significant other risk factor (e.g., body mass index >30, prolonged immobilization, surgery during pregnancy). Prophylactic postpartum therapy is warranted in all patients with low-risk thrombophilias without a personal or family history of thrombosis after a cesarean delivery. These issues have recently been addressed by ACOG in a 2010 Practice Bulletin (Number 283). **Prophylactic doses of the LMWH enoxaparin may start at 40 mg subcutaneously daily.** Weight-based dosing in pregnant patients may be unreliable, and some investigators recommend titrating doses to achieve antifactor Xa levels of 0.1 to 0.2 U/mL 4 hours after injection. Unfractionated heparin prophylaxis may range from 5000 to 10,000 units subcutaneously every 12 hours. Because of inconsistent efficacy in pregnant patients, this dosing should be titrated to achieve heparin levels (by protamine titration assay) of 0.1 to 0.2 U/mL.

The risk for hemorrhage or complication from regional anesthesia is minimal more than 12 hours after prophylactic LMWH. Again, given the difficulty of timing administration with the onset of labor, we recommend converting from LMWH to unfractionated heparin at 36 weeks' gestation or earlier as clinically indicated. As with therapeutic use, anticoagulation may be restarted 3 to 6 hours and 6 to 8 hours after vaginal and cesarean delivery, respectively.

Other Considerations of Therapy and Prevention

Perioperative Prevention

There is very limited evidence regarding the value of perioperative thromboprophylaxis with cesarean delivery. Perioperative administration of low-dose unfractionated heparin may be appropriate in patients undergoing cesarean delivery with clear risk factors such as obesity, malignancy, immobility, or a high-risk chronic medical disease. As noted, patients with low thrombogenic thrombophilias require postoperative prophylaxis.

Nonpharmacologic interventions aimed at preventing VTE include graduated elastic compression stockings and pneumatic compression devices. In pregnancy, a cohort study suggested that the use of graduated compression stockings reduced the prevalence of postpartum VTE from 4.3% to 0.9%. Because these stockings and pneumatic compression devices pose no hemorrhagic risk and little harm, they should be strongly considered for thromboprophylaxis in all pregnant patients. The left lateral decubitus position in the third trimester may also reduce the risk for VTE.

Inferior Vena Cava Filters

The use of inferior vena cava (IVC) filters is primarily restricted to patients with absolute contraindications to medical anticoagulation or those who have failed therapeutic anticoagulation. Pregnant patients with a history of HIT type II or with true heparin or LMWH allergies in need of prophylaxis are potential candidates for IVC filters. However, the introduction of fondaparinux may eliminate this need. The use of IVC filters is discouraged in younger patients, but newer retrievable filters may be appropriate.

KEY POINTS

- Pregnancy, childbirth, and the puerperium pose serious hemorrhagic challenges that are met by increased decidual and systemic clotting potential.
- Venous thromboembolism is a leading cause of mortality and serious morbidity in pregnant women, having a prevalence of 1 in 1000 to 2000 pregnancies, with the greatest risk for fatal PE following caesarean delivery.
- Inherited and acquired thrombophilias account for most VTEs in pregnancy.
- D-dimer testing is used in the evaluation of low-risk patients with suspected DVT because of its high negative predictive value. However, for evaluation of PE, D-dimer is associated with an intolerable rate of false-negative results and thus should not be used.
- VUS is the most common diagnostic modality employed in the evaluation of patients with suspected DVT, with an overall sensitivity and specificity of 90% to 100% for proximal vein thromboses.

- In stable patients with suspected PE and leg signs or symptoms, VUS should be performed because it may avoid the risks of radiation exposure and may detect a DVT, the cause of the PE.
- Stable patients with suspected PE should have a chest radiograph to determine the diagnostic test of choice. A normal chest radiograph should prompt performance of a V/Q scan. A patient with an abnormal chest radiograph should be evaluated with CTPA.
- Heparin remains the mainstay of therapy for patients with VTE, with its most serious but rare complication being immunoglobulin-mediated HIT type II, which usually occurs 5 to 14 days after initiation of therapy and paradoxically increases the risk for thrombosis.
- Protamine sulfate can entirely reverse the anticoagulant effect of unfractionated heparin and partially (80%) reverse the effect of LMWH.
- Graduated elastic compression stockings and pneumatic compression devices appear to reduce the likelihood of VTE in pregnancy and, at a minimum, should be used in all high-risk patients undergoing cesarean delivery.

REFERENCES

1. Ginsberg J, Brill-Edwards P, Burrows R, et al: Venous thrombosis during pregnancy: leg and trimester of presentation. Thromb Haemost 67:519, 1992.
2. Kierkegaard A: Incidence and diagnosis of deep vein thrombosis associated with pregnancy. Acta Obstet Gynecol Scand 62:239, 1983.
3. Rutherford S, Montoro M, McGehee W, Strong T: Thromboembolic disease associated with pregnancy: an 11-year review (SPO Abstract). Obstet Gynecol 164:286, 1991.
4. Simpson E, Lawrenson R, Nightingale A, Farmer R: Venous thromboembolism in pregnancy and the puerperium: incidence and additional risk factors from a London perinatal database. BJOG 108:56, 2001.
5. Stein P, Hull R, Jayali F, et al: Venous thromboembolism in pregnancy: 21-year trends. Am J Med 117:121, 2004.
6. Toglia M, Weg J: Venous thromboembolism during pregnancy. N Engl J Med 335:108, 1996.
7. Treffers P, Huidekoper B, Weenink G, Kloosterman G: Epidemiological observations of thrombo-embolic disease during pregnancy and the puerperium, in 56,022 women. Int J Obstet Gynecol 21:327, 1983.
8. McColl M, Ramsay J, Tait R, et al: Risk factors for pregnancy associated venous thromboembolism. Thromb Haemost 78:1183, 1997.
9. Chang J, Elam-Evans L, Berg C, et al: Pregnancy-related mortality surveillance: United States, 1991-1999. MMWR Surveill Stud 52:1, 2003.
10. Macklon N, Greer I. Venous thromboembolic disease in obstetrics and gynecology: the Scottish experience. Scott Med J 41:83, 1996.
11. Bergqvist A, Bergqvist D, Hallbook T. Deep vein thrombosis during pregnancy: a prospective study. Acta Obstet Gynecol Scand 62:443, 1983.
12. Bergqvist D, Hedner U. Pregnancy and venous thrombo-embolism. Acta Obstet Gynecol Scand 62:449, 1983.
13. Ruggeri Z, Dent J, Saldivar E. Contribution of distinct adhesive interactions to platelet aggregation in flowing blood. Blood 94:172, 1999.
14. Pytela R, Pierschbacher M, Ginsberg M, et al: Platelet membrane glycoprotein IIb/IIIa: member of a family of Arg-Gly-Asp-specific adhesion receptors. Science 231:1559, 1986.
15. Nemerson Y: Tissue factor and hemostasis. Blood 71:1, 1988.
16. Preissner K, de Boer H, Pannekoek H, de Groot P: Thrombin regulation by physiological inhibitors: the role of vitronectin. Semin Thromb Hemost 165:1335, 1996.
17. Lockwood C, Bach R, Guha A, et al: Amniotic fluid contains tissue factor, a potent initiator of coagulation. Am J Obstet Gynecol 165:1335, 1991.
18. Mackman N: Role of tissue factor in hemostasis, thrombosis, and vascular development. Arterioscler Thromb Vasc Biol 24:1015, 2004.
19. Mackman N: The role of tissue factor and factor VIIa in hemostasis. Anesth Analg 108:1447, 2009.
20. Broze G: The rediscovery and isolation of TFPI. J Thromb Haemost 1:1671, 2003.
21. Dahlback B: Progress in the understanding of the protein C anticoagulant pathway. Int J Hematol 79:109, 2004.
22. Broze G: Protein Z-dependent regulation of coagulation. Thromb Haemost 86:8, 2001.
23. Preissner K, Zwicker L, Muller-Berghaus G: Formation, characterization and detection of a ternary complex between protein S, thrombin and antithrombin III in serum. Biochem J 243:105, 1987.
24. Bouma B, Meijers J: New insights into factors affecting clot stability: a role for thrombin activatable fibrinolysis inhibitor. Semin Hematol 41:13, 2004.
25. Schatz F, Lockwood C: Progestin regulation of plasminogen activator inhibitor type-1 in primary cultures of endometrial stromal and decidual cells. J Clin Endocrinol Metab 77:621, 1993.
26. Lockwood C, Krikun G, Schatz F: The decidua regulates hemostasis in the human endometrium. Semin Reprod Endocrinol 17:45, 1999.
27. Bremme K: Haemostatic changes in pregnancy. Best Pract Res Clin Hematol 16:153, 2003.
28. Wright H, Osborn S, Edmunds D: Changes in the rate of flow of venous blood in the leg during pregnancy, measured with radioactive sodium. Surg Gynecol Obstet 90:481, 1950.
29. Goodrich S, Wood J: Peripheral venous distensibility and velocity of venous blood flow during pregnancy or during oral contraceptive therapy. Am J Obstet Gynecol 90:740, 1964.
30. Macklon N, Greer I, Bowman A: An ultrasound study of gestational and postural changes in the deep venous system of the leg in pregnancy. BJOG 104:191, 1997.
31. Girling J, de Swiet M: Inherited thrombophilia and pregnancy. Curr Opin Obstet Gynecol 10:135, 1998.
32. Ginsberg J, Wells P, Brill-Edwards P, et al: Antiphospholipid antibodies and venous thromboembolism. Blood 86:3685, 1995.
33. Miyakis S, Lockshin MD, Atsumi T, et al: International consensus statement on an update of the classification criteria for definite antiphospholipid syndrome (APS). J Thromb Haemost 4:295, 2006.
34. Galli M, Luciani D, Bertolini G, Barbui T: Anti-beta 2-glycoprotein I, antiprothrombin antibodies, and the risk of thrombosis in the antiphospholipid syndrome. Blood 102:2717, 2003.
35. Lockwood C, Romero R, Feinberg R, et al: The prevalence and biologic significance of lupus anticoagulant and anticardiolipin antibodies in the general obstetric population. Am J Obstet Gynecol 161:369, 1989.
36. Wahl D, Guillemin F, de Maistre E, et al: Risk for venous thrombosis related to antiphospholipid antibodies in systemic lupus erythematous: a meta-analysis. Lupus 6:646, 1997.
37. Galli M, Barbui T: Antiphospholipid antibodies and thrombosis: strength of association. Hematol J 4:180, 2003.
38. Garcia-Fuster M, Fernandez C, Forner M, Vaya A: Risk factors and clinical characteristics of thromboembolic venous disease in young patients: a prospective study. Med Clin (Barc) 123:217, 2004.
39. Branch D, Silver R, Blackwell J, et al: Outcome of treated pregnancies in women with antiphospholipid syndrome: an update of the Utah experience. Obstet Gynecol 80:612, 1992.
40. Zotz R, Gerhardt A, Scharf R: Inherited thrombophilia and gestational venous thromboembolism. Best Pract Res Clin Hematol 16:243, 2003.
41. Practice bulletin no. 113: inherited thrombophilias in pregnancy. Obstet Gynecol 116:212, 2010.
42. Gerhardt A, Scharf R, Beckmann M, et al: Prothrombin and factor V mutations in women with a history of thrombosis during pregnancy and the puerperium. N Engl J Med 342:374, 2000.
43. Juul K, Tybjaerg-Hansen A, Steffensen R, et al: Factor V Leiden: The Copenhagen City Heart Study and 2 meta-analyses. Blood 100:3, 2002.

44. Price D, Ridker P: Factor V Leiden mutation and the risks for thromboembolic disease: a clinical perspective. Ann Intern Med 127:895, 1997.
45. Franco R, Reitsma P: Genetic risk factors of venous thrombosis. Hum Genet 109:369, 2001.
46. Friedrich P, Sanson B, Simioni P, et al: Frequency of pregnancy-related venous thromboembolism in anticoagulant factor-deficient women: implications for prophylaxis. Ann Intern Med 125:955, 1996.
47. Aznar J, Vaya A, Estelles A, et al: Risk of venous thrombosis in carriers of the prothrombin G20210A variant and factor V Leiden and their interaction with oral contraceptives. Haematologica 85:1271, 2000.
48. Emmerich J, Rosendaal F, Cattaneo M, et al: Combined effect of factor V Leiden and prothrombin 20210A on the risk of venous thromboembolism-pooled analysis of 8 case-control studies including 2310 cases and 3204 controls. Study Group for Pooled-Analysis in Venous Thromboembolism. Thromb Haemost 86:809, 2001.
49. Ridker P, Miletich J, Hennekins C, Buring J: Ethnic distribution of factor V Leiden in 4047 men and women: implications for venous thromboembolism screening. JAMA 277:1305, 1997.
50. Vossen C, Conard J, Fontcuberta J, et al: Familial thrombophilia and lifetime risk of venous thrombosis. J Thromb Haemost 2:1526, 2004.
51. Goodwin A, Rosendaal F, Kottke-Marchant K, Bovill E: A review of the technical, diagnostic, and epidemiologic considerations for protein S assays. Arch Pathol Lab Med 126:1349, 2002.
52. Dizon-Townson D, Miller C, Sibai B, et al: The relationship of the factor V Leiden mutation and pregnancy outcomes for mother and fetus. Obstet Gynecol 106:517, 2005.
53. Clark P, Walker ID, Govan L, et al: The GOAL study: a prospective examination of the impact of factor V Leiden and ABO(H) blood groups on haemorrhagic and thrombotic pregnancy outcomes. Br J Haematol 140:236, 2008.
54. Murphy RP, Donoghue C, Nallen RJ, et al: Prospective evaluation of the risk conferred by factor V Leiden and thermolabile methylenetetrahydrofolate reductase polymorphisms in pregnancy. Arterioscler Thromb Vasc Biol 20:266, 2000.
55. Said JM, Higgins JR, Moses EK, et al: Inherited thrombophilia polymorphisms and pregnancy outcomes in nulliparous women. Obstet Gynecol 115:5, 2010.
56. Lindqvist PG, Svensson PJ, Marsaal K, et al: Activated protein C resistance (FV:Q506) and pregnancy. Thromb Haemost 81:532, 1999.
57. Hirsh J, Hoak J: Management of deep vein thrombosis and pulmonary embolism: a statement for healthcare professionals from the Council on Thrombosis (in consultation with the Council on Cardiovascular Radiology), American Heart Association. Circulation 93:2212, 1996.
58. Sandler D, Martin J, Duncan J, et al: Diagnosis of deep-vein thrombosis: comparison of clinical evaluation, ultrasound, plethysmography, and venoscan with X-ray venogram. Lancet 8405:716, 1984.
59. Chan WS, Lee A, Spencer FA, et al: Predicting deep venous thrombosis in pregnancy: out in "LEFt" field? Ann Intern Med 151:85, 2009.
60. Heijboer H, Cogo A, Buller H, et al: Detection of deep vein thrombosis with impedance plethysmography and real-time compression ultrasonography in hospitalized patients. Arch Intern Med 152:1901, 1992.
61. Kassai B, Boissel J, Cucherat M, et al: A systematic review of the accuracy of ultrasound in the diagnosis of deep venous thrombosis in asymptomatic patients. Thromb Haemost 91:655, 2004.
62. Goodacre S, Sampson F, Thomas S, et al: Systematic review and meta-analysis of the diagnostic accuracy of ultrasonography for deep vein thrombosis. BMC Med Imag 5:6, 2005.
63. Sampson FC, Goodacre SW, Thomas SM, van Beek EJ: The accuracy of MRI in diagnosis of suspected deep vein thrombosis: systematic review and meta-analysis. Eur Radiol 17:175, 2007.
64. Epiney M, Boehlen F, Boulvain M, et al: D-dimer levels during delivery and the postpartum. J Thromb Haemost 3:268, 2005.
65. Koh S, Pua H, Tay D, Ratnam S: The effects of gynaecological surgery on coagulation activation, fibrinolysis, and fibrinolytic inhibitor in patients with and without ketorolac infusion. Thromb Res 79:501, 1995.
66. Kline JA, Williams GW, Hernandez-Nino J: D-dimer concentrations in normal pregnancy: new diagnostic thresholds are needed. Clin Chem 51:825, 2005.
66a. Chan WS, Lee A, Spencer FA, et al: D-dimer testing in pregnant patients: towards determining the next "level" in the diagnosis of deep vein thrombosis. J Thromb Haemost 8:1004, 2010.
67. Stein P, Terrin M, Hales C, et al: Clinical, laboratory, roentgenographic, and electrocardiographic findings in patients with acute pulmonary embolism and no pre-existing cardiac or pulmonary disease. Chest 100:598, 1991.
68. Fedullo P, Tapson V: The evaluation of suspected pulmonary embolism. N Engl J Med 349:1247, 2003.
69. Junker R, Nabavi D, Wolff E, et al: Plasminogen activator inhibitor-1 4G/4G genotype is associated with cerebral sinus thrombosis in factor V Leiden carriers. Thromb Haemost 80:706, 1998.
70. Green R, Meyer T, Dunn M, Glassroth J: Pulmonary embolism in younger adults. Chest 101:1507, 1992.
71. Tapson V, Carroll B, Davidson B, et al: The diagnostic approach to acute venous thromboembolism. Clinical practice guideline. American Thoracic Society. Am J Respir Crit Care Med 160:1043, 1999.
72. Come P: Echocardiographic evaluation of pulmonary embolism and its response to therapeutic interventions. Chest 101:151S, 1992.
73. Kasper W, Meinertz T, Kersting F, et al: Echocardiography in assessing acute pulmonary hypertension due to pulmonary embolism. Am J Cardiol 45:567, 1980.
74. Gibson N, Sohne M, Buller H: Prognostic value of echocardiography and spiral computed tomography in patients with pulmonary embolism. Curr Opin Pulm Med 11:380, 2005.
75. Pruszczyk P, Torbicki A, Pacho R, et al: Noninvasive diagnosis of suspected severe pulmonary embolism: transesophageal echocardiography vs spiral CT. Chest 112:722, 1997.
76. Stein P, Athanasoulis C, Alavi A, et al: Complications and validity of pulmonary angiography in acute pulmonary embolism. Circulation 85:462, 1992.
77. Andreou AK, Curtin JJ, Wilde S, Clark A: Does pregnancy affect vascular enhancement in patients undergoing CT pulmonary angiography? Eur Radiol 18:2716, 2008.
78. Ridge CA, McDermott S, Freyne BJ, et al: Pulmonary embolism in pregnancy: comparison of pulmonary CT angiography and lung scintigraphy. AJR Am J Roentgenol 193:1223, 2009.
79. U-King-Im J, Freeman S, Boylan T, Cheow H: Quality of CT pulmonary angiography for suspected pulmonary embolus in pregnancy. Eur Radiol 18:2709, 2008.
80. Cahill AG, Stout MJ, Macones GA, Bhalla S: Diagnosing pulmonary embolism in pregnancy using computed-tomographic angiography or ventilation-perfusion. Obstet Gynecol 114:124, 2009.
81. Meaney J, Weg J, Chenevert T, et al: Diagnosis of pulmonary embolism with magnetic resonance angiography. N Engl J Med 336:1422, 1997.
82. Oudkerk M, van Beek EJ, Wielopolski P, et al: Comparison of contrast-enhanced magnetic resonance angiography and conventional pulmonary angiography for the diagnosis of pulmonary embolism: a prospective study. Lancet 359:1643, 2002.
83. To MS, Hunt BJ, Nelson-Piercy C: A negative D-dimer does not exclude venous thromboembolism (VTE) in pregnancy. J Obstet Gynaecol 28:222, 2008.
84. Damodaram M, Kaladindi M, Luckit J, Yoong W: D-dimers as a screening test for venous thromboembolism in pregnancy: is it of any use? J Obstet Gynaecol 29:101, 2009.
85. Girard P, Musset D, Parent F, et al: High prevalence of detectable deep venous thrombosis in patients with acute pulmonary embolism. Chest 116:903, 1999.
86. Girard P, Sanchez O, Leroyer C, et al: Deep venous thrombosis in patients with acute pulmonary embolism: prevalence, risk factors, and clinical significance. Chest 128:1593, 2005.
87. Yamaki T, Nozaki M, Sakurai H, et al: Presence of lower limb deep vein thrombosis and prognosis in patients with symptomatic pulmonary embolism: preliminary report. Eur J Vasc Endovasc Surg 37:225, 2009.
88. Stein P, Hull R, Saltzman H, Pineo G: Strategy for diagnosis of patients with suspected pulmonary embolism. Chest 103:1553, 1993.
89. ACOG Committee Opinion. Number 299, September 2004 (replaces No. 158, September 1995). Guidelines for diagnostic imaging during pregnancy. Obstet Gynecol 104:647, 2004.

90. Brent R: The effect of embryonic and fetal exposure to x-ray, microwaves, and ultrasound: counseling the pregnant and nonpregnant patient about these risks. Semin Oncol 16:347, 1989.
91. Stewart A, Kneale G: Radiation dose effects in relation to obstetric x-rays and childhood cancers. Lancet 1:1185, 1970.
92. Einstein AJ, Henzlova MJ, Rajagopalan S: Estimating risk of cancer associated with radiation exposure from 64-slice computed tomography coronary angiography. JAMA 298:317, 2007.
93. Bourjeily G, Paidas M, Khalil H, et al: Pulmonary embolism in pregnancy. Lancet 375:500, 2010.
94. Hopper KD, King SH, Lobell ME, et al: The breast: in-plane x-ray protection during diagnostic thoracic CT—shielding with bismuth radioprotective garments. Radiology 205:853, 1997.
95. Hurwitz LM, Yoshizumi TT, Reiman RE, et al: Radiation dose to the female breast from 16-MDCT body protocols. AJR Am J Roentgenol 186:1718, 2006.
96. Parker MS, Kelleher NM, Hoots JA, et al: Absorbed radiation dose of the female breast during diagnostic multidetector chest CT and dose reduction with a tungsten-antimony composite breast shield: preliminary results. Clin Radiol 63:278, 2008.
97. Webb J, Thomson H, Morcos S, et al: The use of iodinated and gadolinium contrast media during pregnancy and lactation. Eur Radiol 15:1234, 2005.
98. Hirsh J: Heparin. N Engl J Med 324:1565, 1991.
99. Ginsberg J, Hirsh J, Turner D, et al: Risks to the fetus of anticoagulant therapy during pregnancy. Thromb Haemost 61:197, 1989.
100. Griffith G, Nichols GJ, Asher J, Flanagan B: Heparin osteoporosis. JAMA 193:85, 1965.

For full reference list, log onto www.expertconsult.com.

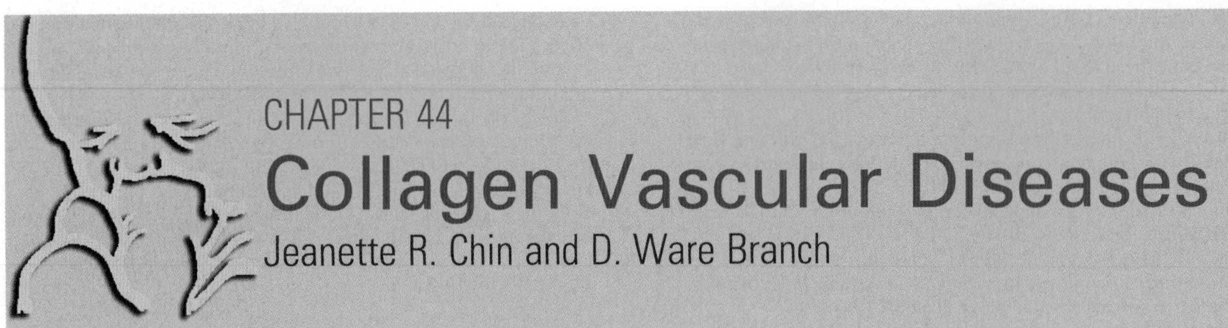

CHAPTER 44

Collagen Vascular Diseases

Jeanette R. Chin and D. Ware Branch

KEY ABBREVIATIONS

Anticentromere Antibody	ACA
Anticitrullinated Peptide Antibody	ACPA
Anti–double-stranded DNA	anti-dsDNA
Antinuclear Antibody	ANA
Antiphospholipid Antibody	aPL
Antiphospholipid Syndrome	APS
Azathioprine	AZA
β_2-Glycoprotein-I	β_2-GP-I
Congenital Heart Block	CHB
Disease-modifying Antirheumatic Drug	DMARD
Human Leukocyte Antigen	HLA
Intrauterine Growth Restriction	IUGR
Intravenous Immune Globulin	IVIG
Low-molecular-weight Heparin	LMWH
Lupus Anticoagulant	LA
Lupus Nephritis	LN
Major Histocompatability Complex	MHC
Metacarpophalangeal	MCP
Methotrexate	MTX
Mycophenolate Mofetil	MMF
Neonatal Lupus Erythematosus	NLE
Nonsteroidal Anti-inflammatory Drug	NSAID
Partial Thromboplastin Time	PTT
Preterm Birth	PTB
Preterm Premature Rupture of the Membranes	PPROM
Proximal Interphalangeal	PIP
Regulatory T Cell	Treg cell
Rheumatoid Arthritis	RA
Rheumatoid Factor	RF
Ribonucleoprotein	RNP
Single-stranded DNA	ssDNA
Systemic Lupus Erythematosus	SLE
Systemic Sclerosis	SSc
Tumor Necrosis Factor-α	TNF-α
U.S. Food and Drug Administration	FDA

Collagen vascular diseases are systemic autoimmune conditions characterized by the formation of autoantibodies directed against one's own tissues. The manifestations of these diseases range from mild and remitting to life-threatening. Reproductive-aged women are disproportionately affected by collagen vascular diseases, and frequently an initial diagnosis is made during the course of evaluation for pregnancy losses or pregnancy complications or during a postpartum flare of symptoms. With the exception of rheumatoid arthritis, most of these autoimmune conditions are associated with adverse maternal and pregnancy outcomes if there is significant multiorgan involvement or if the disease is not in remission at the onset of pregnancy. However, with appropriate pregnancy planning, close antenatal surveillance, and careful choice of medications, many women with collagen vascular diseases can achieve successful pregnancies and have healthy children.

SYSTEMIC LUPUS ERYTHEMATOSUS

Systemic lupus erythematosus (SLE) is a chronic inflammatory disorder with multisystem organ involvement, including skin, joints, kidneys, lungs, serous membranes, nervous system, liver, and heart. Similar to other autoimmune diseases, SLE is characterized by periods of increased disease activity or "flares," interspersed with periods of remission. Frequently presenting symptoms of SLE include arthralgias, fatigue, fever, malaise, weight loss, hair loss, and rash (Table 44-1).

TABLE 44-1 APPROXIMATE FREQUENCY OF CLINICAL SYMPTOMS IN SYSTEMIC LUPUS ERYTHEMATOSUS

SYMPTOMS	PATIENTS (%)
Fatigue	80-100
Fever	80-100
Arthralgia, arthritis	95
Myalgia	70
Weight loss	60
Skin	
Butterfly rash	50
Photosensitivity	60
Mucous membrane lesions	35
Renal involvement	50
Pulmonary	
Pleurisy	50
Effusion	25
Pneumonitis	5-10
Cardiac (pericarditis)	10-50
Lymphadenopathy	50
Central nervous system	
Seizures	15-20
Psychosis	25

Epidemiology and Etiology

The overall reported prevalence of SLE is 20 to 150 cases per 100,000 individuals.[1,2] More recently, the incidence of SLE has nearly tripled, most likely because of increased diagnosis. There are significant gender and racial differences in the prevalence of SLE. The disease occurs 7 to 15 times more frequently among adult women than adult men.[2] White women have a prevalence of 164 per 100,000, compared with African-American women, who have a prevalence of 406 per 100,000.[2] Most women with SLE are affected at some point during their reproductive years, with a median age at diagnosis of 30 to 50 years.

A genetic predisposition to SLE is evident in that about 5% to 12% of relatives of individuals with SLE also have the disease, and the concordance rate among monozygotic twins has been reported to be as high as 57%. Within the past several years, genome-wide association studies have allowed the identification of single nucleotide polymorphisms (SNPs) and mutations in dozens of genes that are associated with SLE.[3] Genetic factors with the most significant associations with SLE include deficiencies in complement components, particularly C1q, C2, or C4, and the presence of a mutated *TREX1* gene, which encodes a DNA-degrading enzyme.[3] The most frequent genetic predisposition, however, involves loci within the major histocompatability complex (MHC), particularly genes for human leukocyte antigens (HLA)-A1, -B8, and -DR3. The MHC contains genes that code for antigen-presenting proteins, some complement components, and cytokines.

Clinical Manifestations

Diagnosis

In 1971, the American Rheumatism Association (now the American College of Rheumatology) devised a set of diagnostic criteria for SLE, primarily to distinguish SLE from other rheumatic diseases for research purposes. These criteria were subsequently revised in 1982 and 1997 (Table 44-2) and are very sensitive and specific for SLE. To be classified as having SLE, a patient must have at least 4 of the 11 clinical and laboratory criteria, either at one time or serially. **Some patients may not meet strict criteria for SLE but still benefit from typical SLE therapies and warrant extra surveillance in pregnancy.**

TABLE 44-2 REVISED AMERICAN COLLEGE OF RHEUMATOLOGY CLASSIFICATION CRITERIA FOR SYSTEMIC LUPUS ERYTHEMATOSUS (1982 AND 1997)

CRITERION	DEFINITION
Malar rash	Fixed erythema, flat or raised, over the malar eminences, tending to spare the nasolabial folds
Discoid rash	Erythematous, raised patches with adherent keratotic scaling and follicular plugging; atrophic scarring may occur in older lesions
Photosensitivity	Skin rash as a result of unusual reaction to sunlight, by patient history or physician observation
Oral ulcers	Oral or nasopharyngeal ulceration, usually painless
Arthritis	Nonerosive arthritis involving two or more peripheral joints, characterized by tenderness, swelling, or effusion
Serositis	a. Pleuritis—convincing history of pleuritic pain or rubbing heard by a physician or evidence of pleural effusion b. Pericarditis documented by electrocardiogram or rub or evidence of effusion
Renal	a. Persistent proteinuria greater than 0.5 g/day or greater than 3+ if quantitation not performed b. Cellular casts—red cell, hemoglobin, granular, tubular, or mixed
Neurologic	a. Seizures—in the absence of offending drugs or known metabolic derangements; e.g., uremia, ketoacidosis, or electrolyte imbalance b. Psychosis—in the absence of drugs or metabolic derangements
Hematologic	a. Hemolytic anemia–with reticulocytosis b. Leukopenia—less than 4000/mm on two or more occasions c. Lymphopenia—less than 1500/mm on two or more occasions d. Thrombocytopenia—less than 100,000/mm in absence of drugs
Immunologic	a. Anti-DNA: antibody to native DNA in abnormal titer b. Anti-Sm: presence of antibody to Sm nuclear antigen c. Positive finding of antiphospholipid antibodies based on (1) an abnormal serum level of IgG or IgM anticardiolipin antibodies, (2) a positive test result for lupus anticoagulant using a standard method, or (3) a false-positive serologic test for syphilis for 6 months
Antinuclear antibody	An abnormal titer of antinuclear antibody by immunofluorescence or an equivalent assay at any point in time and in the absence of drugs known to be associated with drug-induced lupus syndrome

Clinical Features

Constitutional symptoms, such as myalgias, fatigue, weight change, and fever, occur in nearly all women with SLE at some point in the disease course. One of the most common and debilitating symptoms is generalized fatigue. Although fatigue does appear to increase with disease exacerbations, confounding factors such as sleep disturbance, anxiety, and depression are also important contributors. Although women frequently report weight loss before the diagnosis of SLE, weight gain may occur with the development of nephrotic syndrome or glucocorticoid treatment. A significant proportion of women with an SLE exacerbation also have fever that cannot be attributed to an infectious cause. **A myriad of organ-specific signs and symptoms may also be present among women with SLE, including arthritis, skin lesions, lupus nephritis (LN), pleurisy, pericarditis, and neurologic abnormalities such as seizures or psychosis.** Arthritis is one of the most common symptoms, occurring in more than 90% of patients at some point in the disease course. It is usually migratory in nature, with the most frequently affected sites being the proximal interphalangeal (PIP) and metacarpophalangeal (MCP) joints, knees, and wrists. Arthritis in SLE is typified by morning stiffness that improves as the day progresses. **Most patients also have skin manifestations at some point in the disease.** The classic skin presentation is the "butterfly rash," or erythema over the cheeks and nose, exacerbated by sun exposure. Some SLE patients may experience discoid lupus, which consists of inflammatory papules and plaques with a central depressed area that results in scarring.

Clinical evidence of renal disease is present in about 50% of patients with SLE. However, the confirmation of LN requires a renal biopsy. LN is likely the result of immune complex deposition (primarily DNA and anti-DNA antibodies) leading to complement activation and an influx of inflammatory cells in the kidneys. Multiple forms of glomerulonephritis can occur. In 2003, the International Society of Nephrology and the Renal Pathology Society published a classification system for LN aimed at standardizing definitions and resolving ambiguity.[4] The system divides LN into six classes, dependent on renal biopsy results. Class IV, diffuse LN, the most common and most severe form, is associated with hematuria and proteinuria among all patients with active disease and with nephrotic syndrome, hypertension, and renal insufficiency in a significant subset.

Laboratory Findings

Virtually all individuals with SLE have an elevated antinuclear antibody (ANA) titer. As a result, the ANA test should be ordered in all women with symptoms suspicious for SLE. The ANA staining pattern (homogenous, peripheral, speckled, nucleolar, centromeric) has traditionally been used to detect a specific antigen-antibody complex. However, interpretation of staining patterns is subjective, and the sensitivity and specificity for different autoimmune disorders are relatively poor. As a result, the interpretation of staining patterns has been largely supplanted by tests for specific antibodies. **A negative ANA test makes it very unlikely that a woman has SLE.** However, the predictive value of a positive test is relatively low because many other diseases are associated with a positive result, including rheumatoid arthritis, scleroderma, and Sjögren syndrome. Immunofluorescent assays for specific nuclear antigen-antibody reactions are more specific (albeit less sensitive) for SLE than the ANA test. Anti-double-stranded DNA (anti–dsDNA) antibodies are found in greater than 90% of patients with active disease. In a prospective study of 72 patients with SLE, 24 of 33 disease exacerbations were preceded by a significant increase in anti-dsDNA titers.[5] SLE patients may have antibodies to RNA-protein conjugates, also described as soluble or extractable antigens. These include the Sm antigen, ribonucleoprotein (RNP), and Ro/SSA and La/SSB antigens. Anti-Sm antibodies are found in 30% to 40% of SLE patients, are highly specific for the disease, and are correlated with renal involvement. Anti-RNP antibodies can be found in both SLE and systemic sclerosis and are associated with myositis and the Raynaud phenomenon. Anti-Ro/SSA and anti-La/SSB antibodies are found in the sera of both SLE and Sjögren syndrome patients and are particularly relevant to obstetrical management because of their association with neonatal lupus erythematosus (NLE) and congenital heart block (CHB).

Systemic Lupus Erythematosus and Pregnancy

Lupus frequently occurs in women of reproductive age but does not appear to impair fertility. As a result, obstetricians should be aware of the potential complications of SLE in pregnancy and be prepared to provide appropriate monitoring and treatment. They must also understand the benefits and risks of therapies most commonly used in the treatment of SLE. Maternal complications include disease exacerbation, nephritis, venous thromboembolism, and preeclampsia. Fetal and neonatal complications include miscarriage, stillbirth, intrauterine growth restriction (IUGR), preterm birth (PTB), and NLE.

Risk for Systemic Lupus Erythematosus Exacerbation (Flare)

Whether pregnancy is associated with SLE exacerbation continues to be a matter of debate. **Overall, the reported rate of flare during pregnancy or the postpartum period varies widely between 15% and 60% of women, depending mostly on how SLE flare is defined.** Studies in the 1960s and 1970s, which reported high rates of disease exacerbation as well as severe maternal morbidity and mortality, were limited by retrospective design, small sample size, the lack of a uniform definition for flare, and poor differentiation between normal pregnancy manifestations and SLE signs and symptoms.

More recent studies have produced conflicting results as to whether pregnancy is associated with SLE flare. Lockshin and colleagues matched 28 pregnant women with SLE (a total of 33 pregnancies) to nonpregnant women with SLE of similar severity and organ involvement and found no difference between the groups in terms of disease activity.[6] In a separate prospective study, Lockshin followed 80 pregnant women with SLE for manifestations of disease activity. Disease activity was scored by global assessment, prednisone therapy, total number of organ systems involved, and the presentation of abnormalities within each organ system. Disease exacerbation among this cohort occurred in less than 13% of women.[7] Meehan and Dorsey retrospectively evaluated the effect of pregnancy on SLE exacerbation among 22 pregnant patients who were all on glucocorticoids or azathioprine at conception and an equal number of nonpregnant women with

SLE, matched by disease duration and organ system involvement.[8] They found no significant difference in the number of flares between the pregnant and nonpregnant groups. Mintz and associates studied 102 pregnancies among 75 women with SLE and a control group of nonpregnant women with SLE taking oral contraceptives.[9] There was a 59.7% exacerbation rate among women who started with inactive disease, but the rate of SLE flares per month at risk was similar between cases and controls. Interestingly, among the pregnant women, about half of the flares occurred during the first trimester. Most of the exacerbations responded well to low-to-moderate doses of glucocorticoids. Urowitz and coworkers compared 79 pregnancies in women with active SLE with a matched group of 59 nonpregnant active SLE patients as well as 216 women with inactive disease.[10] Flares occurred in similar percentages of cases and controls. Importantly, inactive disease at the onset of the study was protective against flare among the pregnant patients. Georgiou and colleagues reported the results of 59 pregnancies in 47 SLE patients compared with 59 pregnancies in 57 healthy control women and 59 nonpregnant SLE patients.[11] All but one of the pregnant SLE patients had inactive disease at the onset of pregnancy and were being treated with glucocorticoids, hydroxychloroquine, or azathioprine. Using accepted clinical criteria, the authors reported SLE exacerbation in 13.5% of the pregnant SLE women and 22% of the nonpregnant SLE group.

In contrast to the studies discussed previously, two groups have reported increased SLE flares in pregnancy. Petri and associates prospectively studied 40 pregnancies in 37 women with SLE and found that they had increased rates of disease exacerbation compared with the same women outside of pregnancy and nonpregnant SLE patients.[12] Flares occurred in 60% of the pregnancies, but most were mild to moderate. Women with inactive disease at the onset of pregnancy had fewer flares (41%). Ruiz-Irastorza and coworkers studied 78 pregnancies among 68 women and a matched control group of 50 nonpregnant SLE women and found that 65% of the cases had a flare in pregnancy compared with 42% of the control group, which translated to a statistically significant difference in the flare rate per patient-month followed.[13]

Although the data on whether pregnancy increases the likelihood of flare are conflicting, it appears that disease activity at the onset of pregnancy is an important determinant of exacerbation in pregnancy.[10,11,14] Derksen and associates prospectively followed 35 pregnancies in 25 SLE patients.[14] There was sustained disease remission at the start of all but one pregnancy. In 82% of the pregnancies, the disease remained inactive, and there were no serious postpartum flares. Cortes-Hernandez and coworkers found that SLE flares in pregnancy occurred more frequently among women who had stopped maintenance therapy before pregnancy.[15] Hayslett and associates, in a review of the literature, concluded that among women with disease remission for at least 6 months before pregnancy, flare occurs in about one third of pregnancies compared with two thirds of pregnancies among women with active disease at conception.[16] **It thus appears that women with SLE should be advised to postpone pregnancy until sustained remission for at least 6 months has been achieved.** This requires not only a focus on SLE therapies but also a discussion of family planning and attention to effective contraception.

The available literature suggests that there is no more than a modest increased risk for flare among women with sustained SLE remission at the onset of pregnancy. Thus, **the prophylactic use of glucocorticoids in all women with SLE does not appear warranted.** Most flares in pregnancy appear to be mild to moderate and easily treated with glucocorticoids.

The detection of flare in pregnancy requires frequent assessment and astute clinical judgement, frequently combined with laboratory evaluation. Flare in pregnancy is most often associated with fatigue, skin and joint signs and symptoms, and renal involvement.[12] In confusing cases, serologic evaluation with anti-dsDNA and complement levels may be helpful. As mentioned previously, elevated anti-dsDNA titers are found in nearly all patients with active disease. Complement levels rise during normal pregnancy but fall with an SLE exacerbation. It has been suggested that serial evaluation of complement components is beneficial in the prediction of SLE exacerbation in pregnancy. Devoe and colleagues reported that serial assessment of C3 and C4 levels was helpful in predicting SLE flare and that levels were associated with pregnancy outcome.[17] Buyon and associates found that serum C3 and C4 levels were significantly lower among pregnant SLE patients with flare compared with normal pregnancies or those with preeclampsia.[18] In contrast, Wong and coworkers found that C3 and C4 levels were not significantly different between pregnant SLE women who had disease exacerbation and those who did not have a flare.[19] Another study found that complement activation can occur in the setting of preeclampsia, with C4 levels significantly decreased in preeclamptic women compared with normal pregnant women.[20] Furthermore, hypocomplementemia may occur in pregnancies without SLE or adverse pregnancy outcomes. Thus, the clinical utility of routinely following complement levels in otherwise asymptomatic women in pregnancy is doubtful.

Lupus Nephritis and Pregnancy

Pregnancy in women with LN is associated with significant risk, including an increased rate of preeclampsia (with attendant maternal and fetal morbidity) and a potentially permanent decline in renal function.

As with SLE flares in general, whether or not renal flares occur more commonly in pregnancy remains controversial. Two studies have reported high frequencies of renal flares (43% to 46%) during pregnancy,[19,21] whereas others have reported lower figures (9% to 28%).[9,13] Similar to the risk for SLE flare in general, it appears that disease activity at conception is an important predictor of renal flare. Jungers and associates studied 106 pregnancies in 36 women with LN and found that disease exacerbation occurred in only 9% of cases in which disease was in remission for at least 5 months before conception compared with 66% of cases in which SLE was clinically active.[22]

Data regarding the risk for permanent decline in renal function during pregnancy in LN patients are also conflicting. Fine and associates found that 9.6% of LN patients had a sustained depression in renal function for

3 to 12 months postpartum.[23] Oviasu and colleagues reviewed eight studies (151 pregnancies) published from 1973 to 1991 and found that permanent deterioration in renal function occurred in 8% of pregnancies complicated by LN.[24] In contrast, Hayslett and Lynn reported no permanent change in renal function in pregnant LN patients.[25] Petri and associates, in their experience at the Hopkins Lupus Pregnancy Center between 1987 and 1996, reported that only women with nephrotic syndrome at the onset of pregnancy went on to renal failure postpartum.[21] Given the data, the clinically prudent approach is to counsel women with SLE and a history of renal disease who are contemplating pregnancy about the potential for renal deterioration.

On occasion, it may be challenging to distinguish between a renal flare and preeclampsia. Women with LN and established proteinuria have increasing proteinuria associated with increased renal perfusion in pregnancy. Also, women without a history of significant LN may suffer the new onset of glomerulonephritis during pregnancy, presenting with proteinuria and hypertension. The distinction is important, however, particularly in significantly preterm gestations, because the treatment for preeclampsia is delivery, whereas the treatment for an SLE flare is immunosuppression. The situation may be even more confusing based on the fact that women with LN are at significantly increased risk for developing superimposed preeclampsia. Table 44-3 lists features that may be helpful in distinguishing these two entities. Examination of the urinary sediment should be performed. As mentioned previously, serologic evaluation of anti-dsDNA titers and complement levels, looking for obviously low complement levels, may be helpful. A renal biopsy should be considered in difficult cases. In practice, however, situations involving either severe SLE flare with glomerulonephritis or severe preeclampsia frequently threaten both maternal and fetal well-being and, depending on the gestational age, may prompt delivery before the establishment of a definitive diagnosis.

TABLE 44-3 DISTINGUISHING BETWEEN PREECLAMPSIA AND SYSTEMIC LUPUS ERYTHEMATOSUS OR LUPUS NEPHRITIS FLARE

TEST	PREECLAMPSIA	SLE
Serologic		
Decreased complement C3, C4	±	+++
Elevated anti-dsDNA	–	+++
Elevated Ba or Bb fragments with low CH50	±	++
Antithrombin III deficiency	++	±
Hematologic		
Microangiopathic hemolytic anemia	++	–
Coombs-positive hemolytic anemia	–	++
Thrombocytopenia	++	++
Leukopenia	–	++
Renal		
Hematuria	+	+++
Cellular casts	–	+++
Elevated serum creatinine	±	++
Elevated ratio of serum blood urea nitrogen to creatinine	++	±
Hypocalciuria	++	±
Liver		
Liver transaminases	++	±

+++, Present; ++, occasionally present; ±, may or may not be present; –, not present; SLE, systemic lupus erythematosus.

In summary, women with LN should ideally be in sustained remission for at least 6 months before attempting pregnancy. Pregnancy should be avoided in women with class IV LN, nephrotic syndrome, and severe hypertension because of the significant risk for maternal and fetal morbidity. **Moderate renal insufficiency (serum creatinine, 1.5 to 2 mg/dL) is a relative contraindication to pregnancy, and advanced renal insufficiency (creatinine > 2 mg/dL) should be considered an absolute contraindication to pregnancy.**

Pregnancy Loss

Women with SLE are at increased risk for pregnancy loss compared with the general obstetrical population. More recent reports suggest that the pregnancy loss rate associated with SLE may be declining, perhaps because of improved antenatal surveillance and treatment. Petri and Allbritton compared 481 pregnancies in 203 women with SLE with 566 pregnancies in 177 healthy relatives and 356 pregnancies in 166 healthy unrelated women and found that pregnancy loss occurred significantly more often in women with SLE (21%) compared with the healthy relatives (8%) or the unrelated controls (14%).[26] A recent smaller study of women with SLE who were all in remission at the onset of pregnancy and were maintained on low-dose glucocorticoids, hydroxychloroquine, or azathioprine found a modest, although significantly increased, rate of spontaneous abortion and stillbirth (17%) in these women compared with a control group without SLE (5%).[11]

Antiphospholipid antibodies are the most important determinant of pregnancy loss in women with SLE. Antiphospholipid syndrome (APS) is associated with an increased risk for fetal death (≥10 weeks' gestation),[27] even outside of a diagnosis of SLE. For women with SLE and a prior fetal death, the predictive value of antiphospholipid antibodies (aPL) for subsequent fetal loss has been reported at more than 85%.[28] Recurrent pre-embryonic (<6 weeks) and embryonic loss (6 to 9 weeks) also is included as an obstetrical criterion for the diagnosis of APS. In comparison with fetal loss, however, studies have generally been less consistent with regard to an association between APS and recurrent early loss.[29]

Disease activity and severity are important determinants of the risk for pregnancy loss in women with SLE. Clowse and coworkers, in a prospective study of 267 pregnancies among SLE patients between 1987 and 2002, found that only 77% of pregnancies among women with high-activity disease resulted in a live birth compared with 88% in women with low-activity SLE.[30] Furthermore, high-activity SLE in the first and second trimesters led to a three-fold increase in pregnancy loss. Pregnancy loss is also more likely if SLE is diagnosed during the index pregnancy.[22]

Preexisting renal disease appears to increase the risk for pregnancy loss among women with SLE, with higher loss rates seen among women with more severe renal impairment. One study reported a fetal loss rate of 50% in women with LN and moderate to severe renal insufficiency (serum creatinine ≥ 1.5 mg/dL).[25] Another study found that spontaneous abortions occurred in 26% of women with LN and minimally impaired renal function (serum creatinine <1 mg/dL, creatinine clearance >80 mL/minute, and proteinuria <1 g/day) compared with 36% of women with "mild" impairment (clearance, 50 to 80 mL/minute; proteinuria, 1 to 3 g/day).[23]

Preeclampsia

Hypertensive disorders, including gestational hypertension and preeclampsia, are frequent complications of pregnancies in women with SLE, occurring in 10% to 30% of cases.[7,31] Women with LN are at particular risk for developing preeclampsia. In one study, preeclampsia occurred in two thirds of pregnancies among women with LN.[32] Other risk factors for preeclampsia among SLE patients include chronic hypertension, APS, chronic glucocorticoid use, diabetes, and preeclampsia in a previous pregnancy. As mentioned earlier, it can be difficult to distinguish between preeclampsia and an SLE flare because they often have similar manifestations. Sound clinical judgment is required, but if the gestation is beyond 28 to 30 weeks, delivery after antenatal steroid administration may be the most prudent course of action. If signs and symptoms resolve relatively quickly postpartum, the diagnosis is most likely preeclampsia.

Intrauterine Growth Restriction

Lupus in pregnancy has generally been considered a significant risk factor for uteroplacental insufficiency resulting in IUGR and small-for-gestational-age neonates. Although the rate of IUGR among SLE pregnancies has been reported to be as high as 40%,[33] more recent and larger studies suggest a considerably lower rate. Clowse and coworkers, using the National Inpatient Sample, studied more than 16.7 million hospital admissions for childbirth (13,555 to women with SLE) and found that only 5.6% of SLE patients carried a diagnosis of IUGR.[31] Although this was higher than among non-SLE patients (1.5%), the difference was not statistically significant after adjusting for maternal age. Georgiou and colleagues reported no significant difference in the rate of IUGR between SLE pregnancies and healthy controls.[11] In this study, nearly all women were in remission at the onset of pregnancy. It appears less likely that SLE itself confers an increased risk for IUGR but instead that particular manifestations of the disease, such as renal impairment and chronic hypertension, play the most important roles. In addition, chronic glucocorticoid use, especially at higher doses, is a known risk factor for IUGR.

Preterm Birth

PTB is a frequent outcome among women with SLE, occurring in approximately one third of SLE pregnancies, and most PTBs in SLE pregnancies are the result of iatrogenic delivery for obstetrical or maternal medical indications.[15,26] The risk for PTB is significantly greater among women with increased SLE activity, APS, or hypertension and in those taking higher doses (>10 mg/day) of glucocorticoids.[11,15,30] In a recent study of 267 pregnancies, a full-term delivery was achieved in only 26% of women with high-activity SLE compared with 61% of those with no or mild SLE activity.[30] An association between SLE and preterm premature rupture of membranes (PPROM) has been reported; in one study, PPROM occurred in 39% of SLE pregnancies delivered between 24 and 36 weeks' gestation, and the association was independent of glucocorticoid treatment.[34] Not all studies of SLE patients indicate a particularly high frequency of PTB. In a large retrospective case-control study from the Hopkins Lupus Cohort, a 12% rate of PTB occurred among women with SLE compared with 4% among controls (relatives and nonrelatives without SLE).[26] The relatively low rate of PTB in this study may be due to the inclusion of SLE patients with quiet or less severe disease.

Neonatal Lupus Erythematosus

NLE is a transplacentally acquired autoimmune disease that occurs in a small percentage of infants born to women with SLE and is associated with the presence of maternal antibodies to the extractable nuclear antigens, Ro/SSA and La/SSB. Fortunately, the incidence of NLE is low; among all mothers with SLE, the risk for NLE is less than 5%. Of women with SLE who test positive for anti-Ro/SSA and anti-La/SSB, at most 15% to 20% will have an affected infant. Many mothers of affected neonates do not carry a current diagnosis of SLE and are unaware that they have anti-Ro/SSA and anti-La/SSB antibodies. A significant proportion of these women will develop symptomatic autoimmune disease in the future (typically Sjögren syndrome). As a result, appropriate counseling, testing, and surveillance of these mothers is important.

The most common manifestation of NLE is a lupus rash. This appears as erythematous, scaling, annular, or elliptical plaques on the face or scalp that develop in the first few weeks of life and can persist for up to 6 months. Less frequently, hematologic NLE occurs and manifests as autoimmune hemolytic anemia, leukopenia, thrombocytopenia, and hepatosplenomegaly.

The most serious manifestation of NLE is CHB. It is often diagnosed at a routine prenatal visit by detecting a fixed bradycardia of 60 to 80 beats/minute. Fetuses at 16 to 24 weeks appear to be at greatest risk; CHB rarely develops in the third trimester. CHB is caused by binding of antibodies to antigens present in the fetal cardiac tissues, with subsequent damage to the cardiac conduction system. The atrioventricular (AV) node and adjacent conduction system are particularly susceptible to damage, and the result is complete AV dissociation. In very severe cases, widespread endomyocardial damage leads to fibroelastosis, impaired myocardial contractility, hydrops fetalis, and stillbirth.

Complete CHB is irreversible, and there is no effective in utero treatment. In a report of 113 infants affected with CHB from a national NLE registry, overall mortality was 19%, with 5% of deaths occurring in utero. Sixty-three percent of the surviving infants required a pacemaker.[35]

Among women with anti-Ro/SSA and anti-La/SSB antibodies, the risk for having a fetus develop CHB is low, probably in the range of 1% to 2%. In women with a prior fetus with CHB, the risk for recurrent CHB is much higher, occurring in 15% to 20% of subsequent pregnancies.[36] The recurrence rate is unaffected by maternal health, use of steroids, antibody status, severity of disease in the first affected child, or sex of the subsequent child. Genetic factors in the fetus may play a role in determining which fetuses of antibody-positive mothers are most likely to be affected with CHB. Significant associations with NLE have been found for SNPs in the HLA region and near the tumor necrosis factor-α (TNF-α) gene.[37]

If CHB is suspected prenatally, fetal echocardiography, to rule out fetal cardiac structural abnormalities and confirm the diagnosis of CHB, and maternal testing for anti-Ro/SSA and anti-La/SSB antibodies (if not done previously) should be performed. Some experts recommend screening fetuses of antibody-positive mothers who have had a previously affected infant using weekly Doppler fetal echocardiography to measure the PR interval from 16 through at least 26 weeks. More recent experience leaves the clinical utility of this approach in doubt. Progression from first- or second-degree block to complete (third-degree) heart block can occur rapidly, and it also appears that complete block can occur without a detectable preceding prolongation of the PR interval. Moreover, the early identification of developing heart block has not been shown to alter outcome.

The optimal treatment of fetuses with CHB is somewhat uncertain. A 2004 report of 37 consecutive cases from two institutions found that a combination of dexamethasone and a β-sympathomimetic when the fetal heart rate is less than 55 beats/minute resulted in a 1-year survival rate of 95%, which is a significant improvement compared with no treatment.[38] The rationale for dexamethasone treatment is based on the belief that the etiology of CHB is an inflammatory carditis. However, results of the recently published PRIDE study are less favorable.[39] The PRIDE investigators enrolled 40 pregnant women at 33 centers with anti-Ro/SSA antibodies and a fetus with CHB. Thirty women elected to take dexamethasone, whereas 10 declined treatment. There were 31 fetuses with complete heart block, 22 treated with dexamethasone and 9 untreated. No reversals of third-degree block were seen in either group. Of the 6 fetuses who had second-degree heart block and who were treated with dexamethasone, 3 progressed to third-degree block, 2 stabilized at second degree, and only 1 reverted to normal sinus rhythm. Two fetuses with first degree heart block reverted to normal sinus rhythm with dexamethasone treatment. Premature and small-for-gestational-age infants were restricted to the dexamethasone group. Although case selection likely played a role, there were no fetal or neonatal deaths in the nondexamethasone group, but there were 6 (20%) in the dexamethasone group. And chronic steroid therapy is not without controversy, primarily because of the potential risks associated with long-term treatment, including oligohydramnios, growth restriction, and impaired neurologic development.

Heart block associated with fetal hydrops may pose a special circumstance. A retrospective analysis of 50 cases of CHB found that dexamethasone or betamethasone use was associated with improvement or resolution of hydrops, although steroid treatment had no effect on third-degree heart block.[40] Based on the available, albeit limited, data, most experts recommend a trial of dexamethasone if first- or second-degree heart block is found or in selected cases of CHB with hydrops (Table 44-4).

Intravenous immune globulin (IVIG) has the potential to lower the transplacental passage of autoantibodies against Ro/SSA and La/SSB and is being investigated as a potential treatment for high-risk women (those with antibodies and a previously affected child). The Preventive IVIG Therapy for Congenital Heart Block (PITCH) study enrolled women with positive anti-SSA/Ro or anti-SSB/La titers (or both), maternal rheumatic disease (symptomatic or not), and a previously affected child with CHB or NLE and administered IVIG every 3 weeks from 12 to 24 weeks' gestation.[41] The results were recently published. Recruitment was stopped at 20 women after three of the fetuses developed third-degree block (a predetermined stopping point of the study). One infant had a rash consistent with NLE. Sixteen infants were unaffected. Although there were no identified safety issues with IVIG therapy, there were also no significant changes in maternal anti-Ro/SSA or anti-La/SSB antibody titers with treatment. A European prospective observational study of 24 pregnancies in 22 women with a previous child affected with CHB found that IVIG was not effective at preventing third-degree block, which developed in 3 of 15 (20%) fetuses in the treatment group versus 1 of 9 (11%) in the nontreatment group.[42] These recent results strongly suggest that IVIG is not indicated for the prevention of CHB; certainly, insufficient evidence exists to recommend IVIG therapy except under an approved experimental protocol.

Fetuses with a heart rate of less than 55 beats/minute are at increased risk for hydrops and demise.[43] Case

TABLE 44-4 Management Approaches to Anti-Ro/SSA–Associated Congenital Heart Block

CLINICAL SCENARIO	MANAGEMENT
Maternal anti-Ro/SSA antibodies	Expectant management.
No previously affected fetus *or* Previous fetus with CHB	Some experts recommend serial fetal echocardiography to evaluate PR interval from 16-28 weeks, although the clinical utility of this is debated.
Fetal first-degree heart block	No management regimen has been proved effective in avoiding progression to complete heart block.
or Fetal second-degree heart block or alternating second- and third-degree block	Some experts initiate dexamethasone, 4 mg/day.* Taper and discontinue steroid treatment if there is progression to third-degree block.
Fetal third-degree (complete) heart block	No management regimen has been proved effective in reversing heart block or avoiding associated fetal or neonatal complications. Serial evaluation for hydrops. When fetal heart rate is <50-55 beats/minute, some experts initiate a trial of oral terbutaline (2.5-7.5 mg every 4-6 hours, max. 30 mg/day).†
Fetal third-degree heart block with hydrops	When fetal heart rate is <50-55 beats/minute, some experts initiate a trial of oral terbutaline (2.5-7.5 mg every 4-6 hours, max. 30 mg/day).[2] Some experts recommend a trial of dexamethasone, 4 mg/day, at least until improvement in fetal sonographic findings.

*Monitor for maternal glucose intolerance, impaired fetal growth, and oligohydramnios with chronic steroid therapy.

†Terbutaline should be used with caution or not at all in women with diabetes, hypertension, hyperthyroidism, seizures, or a history of arrhythmias.

reports and case series of maternally administered β-sympathomimetic agents suggest that these agents may increase the fetal heart rate, improve signs of cardiac insufficiency, and result in higher fetal-neonatal survival rates.[44] Jaeggi and associates compared the outcomes of fetuses diagnosed with CHB before and after 1997, when a standardized treatment protocol was initiated at the authors' institutions involving dexamethasone and β-stimulation for a fetal heart rate of less than 55 beats/minute.[43] Of those pregnancies with a fetal heart rate of less than 55 beats/minute, 9 were treated with β-sympathomimetics and 16 were not. The fetal heart rate increased spontaneously in about half of all fetuses, regardless of treatment. Although those who were treated had a lower baseline fetal heart rate, they did not have any further decrease in heart rate, in contrast to those who were untreated.

Table 44-4 details a management strategy for pregnancies at risk for CHB.

Drug Therapy and Systemic Lupus Erythematosus in Pregnancy

Nonsteroidal Anti-inflammatory Drugs

Nonsteroidal anti-inflammatory drugs (NSAIDs) are commonly used for analgesia in SLE patients outside of pregnancy. NSAIDs readily cross the placenta and block prostaglandin synthesis in a variety of fetal tissues. **The safety of NSAIDs in pregnancy is dependent on dose, timing in pregnancy, and the specific drug used.** The use of low-dose aspirin in pregnancy generally appears to be safe. First-trimester use is not associated with a significant increase in congenital anomalies. Low-dose aspirin used during pregnancy in women with APS or women at high risk for developing preeclampsia has not been associated with an increased risk for pregnancy complications.

Adult doses of aspirin near delivery have been associated with abnormal bleeding in mothers and neonates. Although short-term (≤48 hours) tocolytic therapy with indomethacin appears to be safe, chronic use has been associated with oligohydramnios and constriction of the fetal ductus arteriosus. **Given these risks, chronic use of adult dosages of NSAIDs should be avoided during pregnancy. Acetaminophen and narcotic-containing preparations are acceptable alternatives if analgesia is needed. NSAIDs are considered safe during breastfeeding.**

Glucocorticoids

Glucocorticoids are often used for the treatment of SLE in pregnancy, either as maintenance or in short courses for the treatment of disease exacerbations. Prednisone, U.S. Food and Drug Administration (FDA) category C (see Chapter 8), has been the oral glucocorticoid of choice in pregnancy secondary to its extensive metabolism by the placenta, with conversion to an inactive metabolite. The long-term use of fluorinated steroids such as dexamethasone and betamethasone should be avoided because these drugs freely cross the placenta, with fetal concentrations approximating maternal concentrations. Glucocorticoid use in pregnancy is not without risk. Multiple studies have reported an association between periconceptional glucocorticoid use and cleft lip and palate,[45] although the magnitude of risk is small. **Prolonged glucocorticoid use is associated with bone demineralization, gestational diabetes, preeclampsia, PROM, and IUGR.** Women chronically treated with glucocorticoids should be screened multiple times during pregnancy for gestational diabetes, generally around 20, 28, and 32 weeks' gestation. Chronic glucocorticoid use may also cause significant side effects in the mother, including fluid retention, weight gain, hirsutism, striae, acne, and gastrointestinal discomfort and ulceration. A low-salt diet, antacids, weight-bearing exercise, and calcium and vitamin D supplementation should be recommended to all women on chronic glucocorticoids. Women who are in sustained remission at the onset of pregnancy have been shown to have generally good maternal and fetal outcomes without prophylactic glucocorticoids.[14] The doses used in pregnancy are the same as those used in nonpregnant patients. However, carefully tapering to the lowest dose needed to manage the disease is reasonable given the potential adverse effects.

Antimalarials

Hydroxychloroquine (HCQ), an antimalarial agent, is an increasingly important treatment option for SLE in pregnancy and is an FDA category C drug (see Chapter 8). Although there were early reports of associated teratogenicity, specifically ocular toxicity and ototoxicity, more recent studies suggest that HCQ is safe at the doses typically used to treat SLE. Costedoat-Chalumeau and coworkers compared 133 pregnancies in 90 women treated with HCQ with 70 pregnancies in 53 women with similar disorders but not treated with HCQ.[46] There were no differences in the percentage of live births or congenital malformations between groups. There were also no differences in vision, hearing, growth, or development between those offspring exposed to HCQ and those unexposed (mean, 26 months of follow-up).

More recent information supports a possible salutary impact of HCQ in SLE pregnancy. In a prospective study of 257 pregnant women with SLE, disease activity was significantly higher among women who stopped taking HCQ 3 months before or during the first trimester of pregnancy.[47] Women who continued on HCQ were maintained on a lower average dose of prednisone during pregnancy. **Given the body of evidence that now indicates that HCQ is safe in pregnancy, and the known risks for chronic glucocorticoid treatment, HCQ may be the best maintenance therapy for SLE in pregnancy.** Women who become pregnant while taking HCQ should generally be continued on this medication.

Azathioprine

Azathioprine (AZA), an FDA category D drug (see Chapter 8), is metabolized to 6-mercaptopurine (6-MP) in vivo. The placenta metabolizes the majority of AZA to an inactive metabolite, thiouric acid. Studies are conflicting with regard to the fetal or neonatal risks of AZA use in pregnancy. Data have mostly come from organ transplant recipients or inflammatory bowel disease patients. Increased rates of IUGR, PTB, and impaired neonatal immunity associated with maternal AZA use have been reported.[48] However, these findings are difficult to interpret because of the use of multiple immunosuppressants among some women and difficulty in determining whether outcomes are due to drug exposure or severe illness in the mother.

TABLE 44-5 DRUGS USED IN COLLAGEN VASCULAR DISEASES

DRUG	MECHANISM OF ACTION	PREGNANCY CONCERNS
NSAIDs	Anti-inflammatory	Avoid high dose. Risk depends on timing in pregnancy. Acetaminophen preferred.
Glucocorticoids	Anti-inflammatory, immunosuppressive	Prednisone doses of ≤10 mg/day preferred. Risks for GDM, PPROM, preeclampsia, IUGR.
Acetaminophen	Analgesic	Considered safe in pregnancy. Dosages should not exceed 4 g/day.
Hydroxychloroquine	Antimalarial—exact mechanism unknown	Likely safe. Pregnant women should generally continue this medication.
Azathioprine	Inhibits purine synthesis	Possible increased risks for PTB, IUGR, impaired neonatal immunity. May be preferred over other immunosuppressants for severe SLE.
Cyclosporine	Calcineurin inhibitor	Risk for teratogenicity appears low. Possible increased risks for PTB, small-for-gestational age.
Cyclophosphamide	Alkylating agent	Teratogenic, abortifacient—avoid in pregnancy unless exceptional circumstances.
Leflunomide	Inhibits pyrimidine synthesis	Teratogenic, abortifacient—avoid in pregnancy. Extensive washout procedure recommended.
Methotrexate	Inhibits dihydrofolate reductase	Teratogenic, abortifacient—avoid in pregnancy.
Mycophenolate mofetil	Inhibits purine synthesis	Teratogenic, abortifacient—avoid in pregnancy.
TNF antagonists	Binds TNF-α and TNF-β	Alert for severe bacterial infections. Generally appear safe in pregnancy, but long-term data are lacking.

GDM, Gestational diabetes mellitus; *IUGR*, intrauterine growth restriction; *NSAIDs*, nonsteroidal anti-inflammatory drugs; *PROM*, preterm premature rupture of membranes; *PTB*, preterm birth; *SLE*, systemic lupus erythematosus; *TNF*, tumor necrosis factor.

Although AZA is an FDA category D drug in pregnancy, it may be indicated for the treatment of severe, active SLE that does not respond adequately to glucocorticoids. In these situations, it is generally preferred over other immunosuppressants in pregnancy.

Cyclosporine

Cyclosporine, a calcineurin inhibitor, selectively inhibits the transcription of interleukin-2 and several other cytokines. It may occasionally be used in more severe cases of SLE. It is an FDA category C drug (see Chapter 8). Data regarding cyclosporine use in pregnancy are mainly derived from studies of organ transplant recipients. The risk for teratogenicity with cyclosporine use in the first trimester appears to be low. An increased risk for PTB and small-for-gestational-age infants among pregnancies exposed to cyclosporine has been reported.[49] It is difficult to tell, however, whether these findings are a result of the drug itself or the mother's underlying medical condition.

Drugs with Moderate to High Risk for Fetal Harm

Cyclophosphamide, an alkylating agent, is an FDA category D drug and carries a significant risk for teratogenesis and should not be used in the first trimester (see Chapter 8). Outside of the first trimester, use should be limited to unusual circumstances, such as in women with severe, progressive proliferative glomerulonephritis. Case series of breast cancer patients treated with cyclophosphamide in the second and third trimesters have reported generally good pregnancy outcomes.

Methotrexate, a folate antagonist and FDA category X drug, is teratogenic and can induce miscarriage (see Chapter 8). Among surviving fetuses, about 10% to 20% will have anomalies that include cleft palate, hydrocephalus, anencephaly, hypertelorism, wide nasal bridge, micrognathia, ear anomalies, and delayed ossification. **Methotrexate is absolutely contraindicated in pregnancy.** Women taking methotrexate who desire to become pregnant should be advised to have several menstrual cycles off of the drug before attempting to conceive.

Mycophenolate mofetil (MMF), an inhibitor of purine biosynthesis, is sometimes used in SLE patients. It is an FDA category D drug in pregnancy because of the risk for teratogenicity and miscarriage (see Chapter 8). In a 2006 review of 119 pregnancies exposed to MMF, 31% ended in miscarriage and 15% had congenital anomalies.[49] **MMF is contraindicated in pregnancy.**

Table 44-5 lists medications used in the treatment of collagen vascular diseases and issues related to their use in pregnancy.

Obstetrical Management

Ideally, all women with SLE would have a preconceptional discussion of the complications of SLE in pregnancy with their reproductive health care provider and their rheumatologist. Women with SLE who are considering pregnancy should be advised of the risks for SLE flare, pregnancy loss, preeclampsia, IUGR, PTB, and NLE. They should also be informed of the risks of SLE drug therapies in pregnancy. **To minimize their risk, women with active SLE should be counseled to postpone pregnancy until they have been in a sustained remission for at least 6 months.** Drugs with a moderate to high risk for fetal harm should be discontinued before conception if at all possible. Every effort should be made to taper or eliminate high-dose chronic NSAID therapy. Maintenance therapy with low-dose glucocorticoids or HCQ is acceptable if deemed necessary to sustain remission. Baseline laboratory assessment should include the following:

- Evaluation for anemia and thrombocytopenia
- Assessment of renal function (urinalysis, serum creatinine, and quantification of proteinuria with a 24-hour urine collection or a spot protein-to-creatinine ratio). Women with LN should have their renal function assessed at least every trimester (more

frequently if there is suspicion of flare or preeclampsia).

- aPL (lupus anticoagulant, anticardiolipin and anti-β_2-glycoprotein-I antibodies)

Some clinicians also assess all SLE patients for anti-Ro/SSA and anti-La/SSB status before pregnancy; however, the clinical utility of this is questionable unless the patient has had an infant with CHB.

Chronic hypertension is best managed with labetalol or calcium channel blockers. Angiotensin-converting enzyme (ACE) inhibitors and receptor blockers are contraindicated in pregnancy owing to an increased risk for congenital anomalies, oligohydramnios, and neonatal renal failure.[50,51] Many experts recommend low-dose daily aspirin to decrease the risk for preeclampsia.

Because of the increased maternal and fetal risks, close antenatal surveillance is indicated. Prenatal visits should occur every 2 weeks in the first and second trimesters and weekly in the third trimester. The primary goal of those visits after 20 weeks is to detect hypertension, proteinuria, and possible IUGR. Ultrasonography to evaluate fetal growth and amniotic fluid adequacy should occur every 4 to 6 weeks after 20 weeks. Fetal surveillance for evidence of placental insufficiency should begin around 30 to 32 weeks and typically consists of daily fetal kick counts and weekly or twice-weekly nonstress tests with amniotic fluid assessment or biophysical profiles, or both. Some centers routinely include Doppler assessments of umbilical artery blood flow for fetal surveillance. In patients with disease exacerbations, hypertension, proteinuria, IUGR, or APS, earlier or more frequent maternal and fetal surveillance may be indicated.

Management of SLE during labor and delivery is a continuation of antenatal management. Any maintenance SLE medications should be continued through labor and delivery or resumed immediately postpartum at the antenatal dose. Chronic glucocorticoid therapy can suppress the hypothalamic-pituitary-adrenal (HPA) axis. Patients at greatest risk for HPA suppression are those who have been taking at least 20 mg/day of prednisone for at least 3 weeks or have a Cushingoid appearance, and such patients should receive stress-dose steroids during labor and delivery. A regimen of intravenous hydrocortisone, 100 mg every 8 to 12 hours for two or three doses, is generally sufficient. Patients who have received any dose of steroids for less than 3 weeks or have taken 5 mg/day or less of prednisone are generally considered not to be at risk for HPA axis suppression. For those taking between 5 and 20 mg/day, appropriate management is less clear, but the risk for adrenal insufficiency appears to be very low with continuation of the regular steroid dose. As a result, in the nonobstetrical fields, many have concluded that stress-dose steroids are not indicated in cases of chronic intermediate-dose steroid therapy. However, reliable data on the risk for secondary adrenal insufficiency in pregnant women taking chronic glucocorticoids are lacking.

Some women experience a postpartum SLE flare. Women who have had active disease in pregnancy or have more severe SLE manifestations are at greatest risk. Close surveillance of all women with SLE should continue postpartum, and plans for appropriate follow-up with a rheumatologist should be made.

ANTIPHOSPHOLIPID SYNDROME

The aPLs are a heterogenous group of autoantibodies directed against either negatively charged phospholipids or proteins bound to these phospholipids. **The three major aPLs are lupus anticoagulant (LA), anticardiolipin antibody (aCL), and antibody to β_2-glycoprotein-I (β_2-GP-I). The diagnosis of APS rests on the occurrence of either arterial or venous thrombosis or pregnancy morbidity and repeatedly positive testing for at least one aPL autoantibody.** Classification criteria for APS have been developed primarily for research purposes. These criteria were first published in 1999 and then revised in 2005 (Table 44-6).[52] The criteria are critical for defining relatively homogenous populations to include in research studies.

Epidemiology

APS may occur alone or in combination with another autoimmune disease, most commonly SLE. The actual prevalence and incidence of APS are not known. **aPLs are found in a small percentage (typically, <5%) of healthy controls (including healthy pregnant women) and in up to 35% of patients with SLE.**[53,54] The risks associated with an incidentally discovered positive test for aPL among otherwise healthy women are not well understood. Positive testing for aPL also may occur in association with certain bacterial or viral infections, medications, neoplasms, and advancing age. Typically, aPLs associated with these conditions occur

TABLE 44-6 REVISED CLASSIFICATION CRITERIA FOR THE ANTIPHOSPHOLIPID ANTIBODY SYNDROME*

Clinical Criteria

Vascular Thrombosis

a. One or more clinical episodes of arterial, venous, or small-vessel thrombosis in any tissue or organ, *and*
b. Thrombosis confirmed by objective, validated criteria (i.e. unequivocal findings of appropriate imaging studies or histopathology, *and*
c. For histopathologic confirmation, thrombosis should be present without significant evidence of inflammation in the vessel wall.

Pregnancy Morbidity

a. One or more unexplained deaths of a morphologically normal fetus at or beyond the 10th week of gestation, with normal fetal morphology documented by ultrasound or by direct examination of the fetus, *or*
b. One or more premature births of a morphologically normal neonate at or before the 34th week of gestation because of eclampsia or severe preeclampsia or placental insufficiency, *or*
c. Three or more unexplained consecutive spontaneous abortions before the 10th week of gestation, with maternal anatomic or hormonal abnormalities and paternal and maternal chromosomal causes excluded.

Laboratory Criteria

a. Lupus anticoagulant present in plasma, on two or more occasions at least 12 weeks apart, detected according to the guidelines of the International Society on Thrombosis and Hemostasis
b. Anticardiolipin antibody of IgG and/or IgM isotype in blood, present in medium or high titer, on at least two occasions at least 12 weeks apart, measured by standardized enzyme-linked immunosorbent assay, *or*
c. Anti-β_2-glycoprotein-I antibody of IgG and/or IgM isotype in blood, present in medium or high titer, on at least two occasions at least 12 weeks apart, measured by standardized enzyme-linked immunosorbent assay.

*Definite antiphospholipid syndrome is considered to be present if at least one of the clinical and one of the laboratory criteria are met.

in low titer and are of the immunoglobulin M (IgM) isotype.

Pathophysiology

Although still debated, it appears that aPLs, through a direct antibody-mediated effect, are the primary mediators of adverse obstetrical outcomes associated with APS. In studies using mouse models, the administration of human IgG fractions containing aPL or monoclonal aPL from mice or humans results in prolongation of the partial thromboplastin time (PTT), a prothrombotic state, and an increase in fetal loss.[55,56] aPLs have been shown to activate endothelial cells, monocytes, and platelets and to induce complement. Activated endothelial cells, in turn, express adhesion molecules such as intercellular adhesion molecule-1, vascular cell adhesion molecule-1, E-selectin, and both endothelial cells and monocytes upregulate the production of tissue factor. Activated platelets increase expression of glycoprotein 2b-3a and synthesis of thromboxane A_2.

The clinical manifestations of APS also may result from a variety of effects of aPL on phospholipids and phospholipid-binding proteins critical to coagulation pathways, including interference with the activity of protein S. In addition, aPLs may have procoagulant effects on prostacyclin, serum proteases, toll-like receptors, prothrombin, protein C, and tissue factor. Interference with annexin-A5, a natural anticoagulant, might favor placental thrombosis and fetal loss. Complex interactions of aPLs with other antibodies (including those directed against coagulation factors, annexins, tissue-type plasminogen activator, and platelet-activating factor) have been suggested to play a role in APS.

More recent work suggests that an important cause of pregnancy complications in women with APS is inflammation, not thrombosis. Complement activation is required for fetal loss and growth restriction in mouse models of APS.[57,58] Clinical studies in humans support the important role of complement in APS. Compared with a healthy control group, patients with primary APS have been found to have lower levels of CH50, C3, and C4 and increased levels of complement fragments indicative of complement activation.[59] Furthermore, placentas from women with aPLs have increased levels of complement deposition compared with controls.[60]

Regardless of the underlying mechanism, the pregnancy complications of APS appear to be tied to abnormal maternal-fetal circulation. Pathologic findings in cases of APS-associated fetal loss include narrowing of the spiral arterioles, intimal thickening, acute atherosis, fibrinoid necrosis, and placental necrosis, infarction, and thrombosis.

Clinical Manifestations

Diagnosis

The International Consensus Statement on criteria for APS is detailed in Table 44-6. **Patients with definite APS must manifest either vascular thrombosis or pregnancy morbidity.** Pregnancy morbidity is divided into three categories:

- Otherwise unexplained recurrent early miscarriages: pre-embryonic (<6 weeks' gestation) or embryonic (6 to 9 weeks' gestation) losses
- Otherwise unexplained fetal death (≥10 weeks' gestation)
- PTB occurring at less than 34 weeks' gestation secondary to severe preeclampsia or placental insufficiency

Some patients with APS have autoimmune thrombocytopenia, typically greater than 50,000 and less than 150,000. Isolated thrombocytopenia, however, is not a diagnostic criterion for APS.

Laboratory Findings

Although the diagnosis of APS rests first and foremost on clinical features, confirmation with laboratory testing for aPL is necessary. To be diagnosed with APS, a patient must have medium to high titers of aCL or anti-β_2-GP-I IgG or IgM antibodies or LA. **Because other conditions can result in transient aPLs, persistent positive testing should be present on two or more occasions at least 12 weeks apart to satisfy the laboratory criteria for APS.**

LA is reported as positive or negative and is identified by its ability to cause prolongation of in vitro clotting assays. It is critical that published laboratory criteria for the diagnosis of LA be followed because a significant number of samples thought to have LA activity are false-positive results when measured at a reference laboratory.

Both aCL and anti-β_2-GP-I antibody testing are performed using enzyme-linked immunosorbent assay (ELISA), and results are reported in international units. In the absence of a positive LA, experts agree that only repeatedly positive, medium to high titers of aCL or anti-β_2-GP-I should be used to diagnose APS. Traditionally, the cut-off for a medium to positive titer was considered 20 international units or more. However, the most recent international consensus defined medium or higher titers at more than 40 GPL or MPL units or higher than the 99th percentile of the laboratory. Clinicians should be aware that substantial variation in ELISA results from different laboratories continues to plague the field. Positive standard serum is available, and recommendations for a standardized approach to testing and reporting results have been published.[61] The standard aCL antibody assay detects β_2-GP-I-dependent aCL antibodies, those that require the presence of β_2-GP-I for binding. Notably, IgA isotypes, antiprothrombin antibodies, and antibodies directed against phosphatidylserine-prothrombin complex are not accepted as diagnostic of APS.

In general, LA and IgG anti-β_2-GP-I antibodies are more specific and aCL antibodies are more sensitive for APS. Low-positive antibody titers should be viewed with suspicion because they may be found in up to 5% of normal individuals; they therefore should not be used to make the diagnosis of APS. Isolated IgM results are also believed to have reduced specificity for APS.

Pregnancy in Women with Antiphospholipid Syndrome

As mentioned in the section on SLE, there is good evidence that aPLs are associated with an increased risk for fetal death. This association with fetal death is particularly strong in the presence of LA or medium to high titers of aCL IgG.[27,53,62] This association appears to be independent of any coexisting autoimmune disease such as SLE. In serologic evaluation of women with recurrent early miscarriage (<10 weeks), 10% to 20% are found to have detectable aPLs.[63,64]

In addition to the risk for fetal death, women with APS are at significantly increased risk for developing severe preeclampsia and IUGR. These risks are particularly elevated among women with APS and a history of SLE, prior fetal death, or thrombosis. Among such highly selected patients, hypertensive disorders complicate a median of 32% of APS pregnancies,[27,53,65] and IUGR occurs in up to 30% of births.[65] It also has been reported that women with early-onset, severe preeclampsia are more likely to test positive for aPLs compared with healthy controls.[66] Screening the general pregnant population for aPLs, however, is not recommended. Pregnancies complicated by APS are also more likely to exhibit non-reassuring antenatal and intrapartum fetal monitoring.[27,65] As a result of these pregnancy complications, it is not surprising that the rate of PTB (mostly iatrogenic) is elevated in women with APS.[65] In addition to adverse obstetrical outcomes, women with APS also appear to be at significantly increased risk for vascular thromboses during pregnancy and the puerperium.[65]

It is worth emphasizing that the risk for APS-related pregnancy complications varies with the population in which the diagnosis of APS is made. Women who meet criteria for APS because of recurrent early miscarriage, but are otherwise healthy, do not appear to be at high risk for thrombosis, fetal death, preeclampsia, or placental insufficiency.[52,63,64] However, a cautious approach and close clinical surveillance are still warranted in these women.

Treatment of Antiphospholipid Syndrome in Pregnancy

Ideally, treatment of women with APS would improve maternal, fetal, and neonatal outcomes by minimizing or eliminating the risks for the disorders discussed earlier, including maternal thrombosis, fetal loss, preeclampsia, IUGR, and the need for iatrogenic PTB. Currently, heparin and low-dose aspirin are the treatments of choice for APS in pregnancy. Heparin is usually started in the early first trimester after demonstrating either an appropriately rising human chorionic gonadotropin level or the presence of a live embryo on ultrasonography. Most investigators recommend preconceptional aspirin because of its possible beneficial effect on early stages of implantation. In the past, glucocorticoids were used to treat APS in pregnancy; however, enthusiasm for this treatment waned in the early 1990s when two small randomized trials found no benefit.[67,68] Also, results from randomized trials have shown no benefit from the use of IVIG, either when added to heparin or used alone.[69-71] A subsequent Cochrane analysis concluded that IVIG was associated with an increased risk for pregnancy loss or PTB compared with heparin and low-dose aspirin.[72]

Pregnant patients with APS diagnosed on the basis of obstetrical criteria and *who have not had a previous thrombotic event* can be classified into one of two groups for the purposes of discussing treatment: (1) patients with recurrent early (pre-embryonic or embryonic) miscarriage and no other features of APS, or (2) those with one or more previous fetal deaths (≥10 weeks' gestation) or previous early delivery (<34 weeks' gestation) because of severe preeclampsia or placental insufficiency. A third group of APS patients consists of those *with a history of thrombosis*. Recommended treatments during pregnancy for these three groups are summarized in Table 44-7.

TABLE 44-7 TREATMENT REGIMENS FOR ANTIPHOSPHOLIPID SYNDROME DURING PREGNANCY

Recurrent Pre-embryonic and Embryonic Loss; No History of Thrombotic Events

Lose-dose aspirin alone or together with unfractionated heparin:
- 5000 to 7500 U every 12 hours in the first trimester, *or*
- LMWH (usual prophylactic doses)

Prior Fetal Death or Early Delivery Because of Severe Preeclampsia or Severe Placental Insufficiency; No History of Thrombotic Events

Low-dose aspirin plus unfractionated heparin:
- 7500 to 10,000 U every 12 hours in the first trimester and 10,000 U every 12 hours in the second and third trimesters, *or*
- Administered every 8-12 hours at a dose to maintain the midinterval aPTT* 1.5 times the control mean, *or*
- LMWH (usual prophylactic doses)

Anticoagulation Regimens for Women with a History of Thrombotic Events

Low-dose aspirin plus unfractionated heparin:
- Administered every 8-12 hours to maintain the midinterval aPTT* or anti-Xa activity in the therapeutic range, *or*
- LMWH (therapeutic doses): weight-adjusted (e.g., enoxaparin, 1 mg/kg every 12 hr, or dalteparin, 200 U/kg every 12 hr)

*Women without a lupus anticoagulant in whom the aPTT is normal can be monitored with the aPTT. Women with lupus anticoagulant should be monitored with anti–factor Xa activity.

aPTT, Activated partial thromboplastin time; *LMWH,* low-molecular-weight heparin.

Heparin treatment of APS pregnancy is not without controversy. Four well-designed studies have addressed pregnancy in patients with APS who have predominantly recurrent early miscarriage.[64,73-75] In two trials, the proportion of successful pregnancies substantially improved with the addition of unfractionated heparin to low-dose aspirin.[64,73] However, the other two trials, both of which used low-molecular-weight heparin (LMWH), proved negative,[74,75] largely because the live-birth rates in the low-dose-aspirin-only patients were quite good (70% to 75%). Interestingly, two studies showed no differences in pregnancy outcomes when comparing unfractionated heparin with LMWH, both combined with aspirin.[76,77] There also are several observational studies that have reported pregnancy success rates of 79% to 100% with low-dose aspirin alone.[78,79] **Despite the obvious controversies raised by the discrepancies in these trials, a 2005 Cochrane systematic review concluded that women with APS and recurrent miscarriage should be given a combination of heparin, 5000 U subcutaneously twice daily, and low-dose aspirin.**[72] Published expert guidelines are similar and include the option of LMWH.[80]

The optimal treatment for women with APS and fetal death (≥10 weeks' gestation) or previous early delivery (<34 weeks' gestation) due to severe preeclampsia or placental insufficiency is not defined by well-designed studies. Most experts recommend low-dose aspirin and either prophylactic or intermediate-dose heparin or LMWH (see Table 44-7). The preponderance of available data show that favorable pregnancy outcomes are achieved with heparin started in the early first trimester.

Women with APS who have had a previous thrombotic event should be treated with low-dose aspirin and full anticoagulation with therapeutic doses of heparin or LMWH (see Table 44-7). Vitamin K antagonists are teratogenic and should be avoided between 6 and 12 weeks' gestation. Because of the risk for fetal bleeding, warfarin after 12 weeks' gestation should be given only in exceptional circumstances. **Antithrombotic coverage of the postpartum period is recommended in all women with APS, with or without previous thrombosis.**[80] Generally, women with previous thrombosis will need long-term anticoagulation with warfarin. In patients with no previous thrombosis, the recommendation is prophylactic-dose heparin or LMWH therapy for 4 to 6 weeks after delivery,[80] although warfarin is an option. Both heparin and warfarin are safe for breastfeeding mothers.

RHEUMATOID ARTHRITIS

Rheumatoid arthritis (RA) is a debilitating disease involving chronic symmetrical inflammatory arthritis of the synovial joints. **RA affects 1% to 2% of the U.S. adult population and, similar to other autoimmune diseases, occurs more commonly among females than males.** The incidence of RA increases steadily with age but is frequently encountered among reproductive-aged women.

Pathophysiology

The exact cause of RA is unknown. Although the diagnosis of RA is not made by histologic examination of synovial tissue, characteristic histologic features of RA have been described and include hyperplasia of the synovial lining, an inflammatory infiltrate, and the deposition of fibrin. Eventually a "pannus" is formed that degrades and destroys cartilage and bone and is responsible for much of the morbidity associated with RA.

The inflammatory damage in RA appears to be primarily mediated by $CD4^+$ T cells. These T cells are activated by as yet unknown antigens and stimulate monocytes, macrophages, and synovial fibroblasts to produce cytokines such as interleukin-1, interleukin-6, and TNF-α. These cytokines play a key role in the inflammation of RA. The activated $CD4^+$ T cells also stimulate B cells to produce immunoglobulins, including rheumatoid factor (RF). Autoantibodies alone do not cause disease but clearly play an important role. Patients with high titers of RF are more likely to manifest extra-articular disease. During inflammation, citrulline is incorporated into proteins, and anticitrullinated peptide antibodies (ACPAs) have emerged as an important diagnostic tool, particularly for early-stage RA. The presence of RF and ACPAs in the blood of asymptomatic patients represents an important risk factor for later development of disease.

A large body of evidence confirms the importance of genetic susceptibility to the development of RA. Concordance is higher among monozygotic twins than dizygotic twins (15% vs. 5%). Relatives of patients with RA have not only an increased risk for RA, but also an increased risk for other autoimmune and connective tissue disease. The HLA class II *DRB1* gene is of primary importance in RA susceptibility. Variant alleles of *DRB1* have been associated with RA and include DRB1*0401, *0404, *0405, *0101, *1402, *10, and *1001. The strength of association of these individual alleles varies with the ethnic group studied. More recently, a large number of other RA susceptibility genes have been identified.[81] One of the more significant associations (particularly among whites) is the *PTPN22* gene, which encodes a protein tyrosine phosphatase involved in the regulation of T and B cells.

Given that RA occurs two to three times more commonly in women than men, sex-specific factors likely play an important role in the pathophysiology of RA. Nulliparity is associated with an increased risk for RA. The Nurses' Health Study found a dose-dependent association between breastfeeding duration and a decreased risk for RA.[82]

Clinical Manifestations and Laboratory Findings

The onset of RA is typically insidious and involves symmetrical peripheral polyarthritis and morning stiffness. Arthritis involving the MCP and PIP joints of both hands is characteristic of RA. Fatigue, weakness, weight loss, and malaise may also frequently occur. Eventually, severe joint deformities may develop and are particularly obvious at the MCP and PIP joints of the hands. Rheumatoid nodules are composed of a local proliferation of small vessels, histiocytes, fibroblasts, and other cells and are present in 20% to 30% of patients with RA. They occur most commonly on pressure points, such as in the subcutaneous tissues of the extensor surfaces of the forearms. Nodules that become painful or interfere with joints and nerves can be treated with local injections of glucocorticoids and an anesthetic. Surgery is rarely required.

Less commonly, extra-articular tissues may be affected. These manifestations include pleuritis, pericarditis, neuropathy, vasculitis, scleritis, and renal disease. Most patients with extra-articular involvement also have classic joint symptoms.

In 2010, the American College of Rheumatology, in collaboration with the European League Against Rheumatism, released revised classification criteria for RA (Table 44-8).[83] The new criteria represent a shift in focus to features of early disease that are most likely to represent high risk for progression to erosive disease as opposed to defining the disease by its late-stage features. "Definite" RA is based on confirmed synovitis in at least one joint, absence of a better diagnosis to explain the synovitis, and a total score of at least 6 of 10 from the summation of scores in four domains: number and site of involved joints, serologic abnormality, elevated acute phase response, and symptom duration.

RFs are present in 70% to 80% of patients with RA. However, RFs may also be found in 5% to 10% of the general, healthy population, as well as in individuals with viral infections and other connective tissue diseases such as Sjögren syndrome and SLE. ACPAs have a similar diagnostic sensitivity to RF but are more specific for RA. Multiple other nonspecific laboratory abnormalities may occur in RA patients and include an elevated erythrocyte sedimentation rate (ESR) and C-reactive protein (CRP), anemia, thrombocytosis, leukocytosis, and a positive ANA.

Rheumatoid Arthritis and Pregnancy

Most women with RA, perhaps as many as 80% to 90%, experience improvement in their disease during pregnancy.

TABLE 44-8 2010 American College of Rheumatology/European League Against Rheumatism Classification Criteria for Rheumatoid Arthritis

Target Population
- Patients with at least one joint with definite clinical synovitis (swelling)
- Patients with synovitis that is not better explained by another disease

Classification Criteria	Score
• Score-based algorithm: a total score for categories A to D that is ≥6/10 is needed for classification of definite RA)	
A. Joint Involvement	
1 large joint	0
2-10 large joints	1
1-3 small joints (with or without involvement of large joints)	2
4-10 small joints (with or without involvement of large joints)	3
>10 joints (at least one small joint)	4
B. Serology (at least one test result is needed for classification)	
Negative RF *and* negative ACPA	0
Low-positive RF *or* low-positive ACPA	2
High-positive RF *or* high-positive ACPA	3
C. Acute-phase reactants (at least one test result is needed for classification)	
Normal CRP *and* normal ESR	0
Abnormal CRP *or* abnormal ESR	1
D. Duration of symptoms	
<6 weeks	0
≥6 weeks	1

ACPA, Anticitrullinated protein antibody; *CRP,* C-reactive protein; *ESR,* erythrocyte sedimentation rate; *RA,* rheumatoid arthritis; *RF,* rheumatoid factor.

Improvement in joint stiffness and pain generally begins in the first trimester and persists until several weeks postpartum. Most women who experience improvement in symptoms have a similar improvement in subsequent pregnancies. Currently, there are no laboratory or clinical characteristics that predict which patients will have the most improvement in symptoms during pregnancy.

Until recently, the reason for improvement in RA symptoms during pregnancy has been little more than speculative. However, evidence is now emerging that regulatory T cells (Treg cells), which increase in number during pregnancy, may play an important role in autoimmune conditions, including RA. Treg cells are a family of T lymphocytes that are potent suppressors of autoimmunity and function by inhibiting $CD4^+$ and $CD8^+$ T-cell proliferation and cytokine production, B-cell proliferation and immunoglobulin production, natural killer cell cytotoxicity, and maturation and function of antigen presenting cells. An expanding Treg cell population plays a critical role in the maintenance of allogeneic (but not syngeneic) murine pregnancy. RA patients have been shown to have functionally defective Treg cells, and the expansion of apparently normal Treg cells in RA patients results in improvement in disease.[84] It is reasonable to assume that Treg cell expansion in pregnancy might contribute to RA improvement. Indeed, Forger and colleagues found that among pregnant RA patients, an increased number of Treg cells inversely correlated with disease activity in the third trimester and postpartum. This effect appeared to be mediated, at least in part, by higher levels of interleukin-10 and lower levels of TNF-α and interferon-γ.[85]

A role for endogenous steroid hormones affecting RA cannot be excluded. Many women report an improvement in RA symptoms during the luteal phase of the menstrual cycle, when progesterone levels are highest. Sex hormones may play a role in immunoregulation and interactions with the cytokine system.

Nelson and coworkers reported that improvement in RA during pregnancy is associated with a greater maternal-fetal mismatch in HLA class II antigens.[86] Mismatch was noted in 75% of pregnancies with improvement in RA symptoms compared with only 25% of pregnancies with unchanged or worsened disease. A subsequent study, however, did not confirm these results.[87]

In general, there is little evidence that RA disease activity at the onset of pregnancy significantly affects pregnancy outcomes. Furthermore, the long-term prognosis of RA patients does not appear to be affected by pregnancy. Oka and Vainio compared 100 consecutive pregnant RA patients with age- and disease-matched controls and found no significant differences between the groups in terms of disease severity.[88]

Unfortunately, almost all patients who have experienced improvement in their RA symptoms during pregnancy will experience a disease flare postpartum, usually within the first 3 months. It also has been suggested that women are at increased risk for developing RA in the postpartum period, particularly after a first pregnancy.

Obstetrical Complications

Women with RA have been reported to have a slightly increased miscarriage rate compared with healthy controls. Kaplan found that women with RA had a higher frequency of miscarriage both before (25% vs. 17%) and after (27% vs. 17%) the onset of their disease compared with healthy controls.[89] Other studies, however, failed to find an increased rate of pregnancy loss among women with RA. In general, women with well-controlled RA do not appear to be at significantly increased risk for PTB, preeclampsia, IUGR, or stillbirth, and their pregnancies are typically uneventful. One recent prospective study of 152 women with RA examined the independent effects of steroid treatment and disease activity on perinatal outcomes.[90] Women who were taking steroids had a significantly lower gestational age at delivery. High-activity disease had an independent and negative affect on birthweight.

Obstetrical Management

Ideally, a woman with RA should undergo preconceptional counseling with an obstetrician and rheumatologist to discuss and possibly adjust her drug therapy in an attempt to minimize fetal harm. Given that RA typically improves in pregnancy, many women will be able to successfully discontinue some, if not all, of their antirheumatic drugs. Women with RA do not typically require increased obstetrical surveillance during pregnancy. Those with persistent or worsening symptoms will benefit from regular visits with a rheumatologist. Increased rest and visits with an experienced physical therapist may also be helpful to women with persistent symptoms. Routine antenatal testing, including serial ultrasounds, nonstress tests, and biophysical profiles, are not necessary in women with RA and should generally be reserved for typical obstetrical indications. Because of the increased incidence of disease flares postpartum, clinicians and patients should be alert to potential symptoms. Some experts recommend reinitiating RA drug therapy immediately postpartum.

Antirheumatic Medications

If at all possible, treatment of women with symptomatic RA in pregnancy should be limited to acetaminophen (FDA category A) and low-dose glucocorticoids (see Chapter 8). The use of glucocorticoids in pregnancy, including their maternal and fetal risks, is discussed in the section covering SLE. NSAIDs (also discussed previously), particularly their chronic or high-dose use, should generally be avoided in pregnancy.

However, because of changes during the past several decades in pharmacotherapy for RA, many patients present in pregnancy taking other types of medications (see Table 44-5). The obstetrician should be educated about the potential risks of these medications and be able to provide appropriate counseling. Leflunomide, a disease modifying antirheumatic drug (DMARD), is an FDA category X drug in pregnancy (see Chapter 8). It is an antimetabolite that inhibits dihydroorotate dehydrogenase, an enzyme involved in the rate-limiting step of pyrimidine biosynthesis. **Leflunomide is a teratogen and has been associated with fetal death. It is contraindicated in pregnancy.** Although the half-life of leflunomide is 15 days, its major metabolite (teriflunomide) is detectable in serum up to 2 years after discontinuing the drug. As a result, discontinuing the drug immediately before pregnancy may not be adequate to avoid embryonic exposure. The administration of cholestyramine can speed the elimination of the drug and its metabolite. Confirmation should be made by monitoring leflunomide plasma levels. Methotrexate is also considered a DMARD, is contraindicated in pregnancy, and should be discontinued for 1 to 3 months before attempting to conceive.

TNF inhibitors include the medications etanercept, infliximab, and adalimumab and the newer agents, certolizumab pegol, and golimumab. These medications are FDA category B (see Chapter 8) in pregnancy and antagonize TNF-α (an inflammatory cytokine that plays a key role in RA). TNF inhibitors have been found to increase the number of circulating Treg cells and restore the capacity of Treg cells to inhibit cytokine production.[84] An important potential side effect of these medications is an increased number of serious bacterial infections. Observational studies and case reports indicate that pregnancy complications are not significantly more common among women taking TNF inhibitors compared with women with similar diseases who are not on these medications.[49] More recently, a potential association between TNF inhibitor use in pregnancy and fetal *v*ertebral anomalies, *a*nal atresia, *c*ardiac defects, *t*racheoesophageal fistula, *e*sophageal atresia, *r*enal anomalies, and *l*imb dysplasia (VACTERL) association has been reported[91] but remains controversial. Long-term follow-up of children exposed to TNF inhibitors in utero is lacking, as are data on outcomes of pregnancies exposed to newer agents, including certolizumab pegol and golimumab.

Adequate data on the safety of more recently introduced biologic agents, including anakinra (interleukin-1 receptor antagonist), rituximab (chimeric monoclonal antibody leading to B-cell depletion), abatacept (inhibitor of T-cell co-stimulation), and tocilizumab (interleukin-6 receptor inhibitor), are generally lacking, and prudence would suggest avoiding these medications in pregnancy if possible.

TABLE 44-9 SUBSETS OF SYSTEMIC SCLEROSIS

Diffuse Cutaneous Systemic Sclerosis
- Onset of Raynaud phenomenon within 1 year of onset of skin changes
- Truncal and acral skin involvement
- Presence of tendon friction rubs
- Early and significant incidence of interstitial lung disease, oliguric renal failure, diffuse gastrointestinal disease, and myocardial involvement
- Absence of anticentromere antibodies (ACAs)
- Nailfold capillary dilation and capillary destruction
- Antitopoisomerase antibodies (30% of patients)

Limited Cutaneous Systemic Sclerosis
- Raynaud phenomenon for years (occasionally decades)
- Skin involvement limited to hands, face, feet, and forearms (acral), or absent
- Significant late incidence of pulmonary hypertension, with or without interstitial lung disease, trigeminal neuralgia, skin calcifications, telangiectasia
- High incidence of ACAs (70% to 80%)
- Dilated nailfold capillary loops, usually without capillary dropout

From LeRoy EC, Black C, Fleischmgjer R, et al: Scleroderma (systemic sclerosis): classification, subsets and pathogenesis. J Rheumatol 15:202, 1988.

SYSTEMIC SCLEROSIS

Systemic sclerosis (SSc) is an autoimmune disorder manifested by progressive fibrosis of the skin and visceral tissues and vasculopathy that includes features such as Raynaud phenomenon and renal crisis. Experts recognize two main subsets of SSc (Table 44-9): (1) diffuse cutaneous disease, usually involving cutaneous fibrosis proximal to the forearms and associated with scleroderma renal crisis and pulmonary fibrosis, and (2) limited cutaneous disease, usually involving fibrosis of the distal extremities and face and associated with digital ulcerations and pulmonary fibrosis. **SSc is relatively rare, with an annual incidence in the United States of 1 to 2 per 100,000 individuals.[1] The disease occurs about 10 times more frequently in women than men, with a peak age of onset in the fifth decade.**

Pathogenesis

The pathogenesis of SSc is complex and incompletely understood but involves an interplay between endothelial cells, monocytes, lymphocytes, fibroblasts, and noncellular matrix. Vasoconstriction, cytokine production, immunologic abnormalities, and excessive collagen synthesis are all important features of the disease. Alterations in small arteries and arterioles appear to be inciting events in SSc. The balance between endothelin-1 (a very potent vasoconstrictor as well as a promoter of fibrogenesis) and nitric oxide may be altered in SSc. These early vascular changes trigger the production of cytotoxic proteins, cytokines, growth factors, endothelial adhesion molecules, and ultimately activated fibroblasts that produce excessive amounts of collagen.

Early in the disease process, the dermis contains mononuclear cell infiltrates, edema fluid, and sometimes calcium. Collagen deposition may be subtle initially while vascular changes predominate, particularly intimal thickening, thrombosis, and occlusion of lumens by fibrosis. Remaining vessels become dilated and appear as telangiectasias.

A similar pathologic process occurs in the internal organs. Gastrointestinal tract involvement consists of gut wall fibrosis and smooth muscle cell atrophy, as well as degeneration of autonomic nerves. The kidneys demonstrate a characteristic intimal proliferation and thickening of the small arteries and glomeruli. Lung involvement mainly consists of interstitial fibrosis, capillary congestion and thickening, and occlusion of alveolar walls and arteriolar intima. Patchy fibrosis occurs in the myocardium.

Although the pathogenesis of SSc is complex and the etiology unknown, there are genetic factors that appear to influence the susceptibility of an individual to SSc. Multiple studies have focused on the Choctaw Native Americans in Oklahoma,[92,93] a group with a significantly increased rate of SSc compared with the general population. In this population, risk-associated alleles have been identified in the HLA haplotypes DRB1*1602, DQA*0501, and DQB*0301, in the fibrillin-1 gene, and at sites near the genes for SPARC (secreted protein acidic and rich in cysteine) and topoisomerase-I, a target for SSc autoantibodies. HLA has also been associated with particular SSc-specific autoantibodies.

The trigger for the development of SSc in a susceptible individual is not known, but many theories have been proposed, including viral infection, environmental exposures, organic solvents, certain drugs, and maternal microchimerism with subsequent immunologic response to circulating fetal cells associated with a prior pregnancy.

Clinical Manifestations and Diagnosis

The skin manifestations of SSc are described as either linear scleroderma or morphea. Linear scleroderma occurs more commonly in children, and skin abnormalities typically follow a dermatomal distribution. Morphea can be either localized or generalized and consists of patches of yellowish sclerotic skin, typically on the trunk. Patients with *limited* cutaneous SSc typically have skin thickening restricted to the hands and possibly the neck and face. CREST syndrome falls under the category of limited SSc and involves calcinosis of the skin, Raynaud phenomenon, esophageal dysmotility, sclerodactyly, and telangiectasias. *Diffuse* cutaneous SSc refers to skin thickening proximal to the wrists, often over the limbs and trunk. **The diffuse form of the disease is associated with a greater risk for significant and serious internal organ involvement.**

The diagnosis of SSc is based on the presence of skin thickening at more than one site in combination with internal organ manifestations. Early symptoms of the disease may be nonspecific and include subcutaneous tissue swelling and muscle and joint pain. Raynaud phenomenon occurs in more than 90% of patients with SSc and is often the first symptom. When combined with the characteristic skin changes, Raynaud phenomenon is specific for SSc. However, Raynaud phenomenon also occurs in 5% of the general population. Abnormal findings on nailfold capillaroscopy can help determine whether a patient with Raynaud phenomenon may have SSc. **The most frequent visceral complication of SSc is esophageal dysmotility resulting in heartburn and dysphagia.** The lower gastrointestinal tract may also be affected, resulting in malabsorption, diarrhea, or constipation. **Of particular concern to the obstetrician, women with long-standing or severe disease may have pulmonary hypertension.** Myocardial fibrosis is common with diffuse disease and can result in dysrhythmias. Although most patients have mild renal involvement, 10% to 20% with diffuse disease develop scleroderma renal crisis, consisting of acute-onset severe hypertension, progressive renal insufficiency, microangiopathic hemolytic anemia, and urine sediment that is either normal or shows only mild proteinuria with few cells or casts. **Scleroderma renal crisis results in progression to end-stage renal disease in a significant proportion of affected individuals and is a major cause of mortality in SSc patients.**

The diagnosis of SSc may be supported by the detection of circulating autoantibodies. ANAs are present in most patients with SSc. Antitopoisomerase-I (anti-Scl-70), anticentromere (ACA), and antiRNA polymerase III antibodies are highly specific for SSc but have moderate sensitivity. Different antibodies are associated with different clinical manifestations. For example, ACAs are more common among patients with CREST syndrome, but less so among those with diffuse disease. Anti-Scl-70 antibodies are associated with diffuse disease and a higher risk for severe interstitial pulmonary fibrosis. Both aCL and anti-β_2-GP-I antibodies also can be seen in SSc.

Systemic Sclerosis and Pregnancy

Effects of Pregnancy on Systemic Sclerosis

Pregnancy in women with SSc is uncommon. As a result, data regarding the impact of pregnancy on SSc disease activity are generally limited to case reports and case series.[94] **In general, it appears that maternal outcomes are good when SSc is clinically stable at the onset of pregnancy and the woman is without obvious renal, cardiac, or pulmonary disease.** Pregnancy has been associated with an improvement in Raynaud phenomenon. However, gastroesophageal symptoms may worsen or appear during pregnancy.

Pregnancy does not appear to increase the risk for renal crisis, a life-threatening manifestation of SSc. However, the distinction between renal crisis and preeclampsia may pose a clinical dilemma.

As mentioned earlier, some investigators have proposed that fetal microchimerism may contribute to the pathogenesis of SSc. This is based on the observation that SSc shares many features with graft-versus-host disease and that increased numbers of persistent fetal cells have been found in the circulation of affected women with a history of pregnancy (compared with women without SSc but a history of pregnancy).[95] Fetal DNA and cells also have been identified in the affected skin of SSc patients.[96] However, because this does not prove causality, the question of whether microchimerism contributes to the development of SSc remains unanswered.

Effects of Systemic Sclerosis on Pregnancy

Several studies have suggested that women with SSc have an increased risk for spontaneous abortion before, and possibly subsequent to, their diagnosis. Silman and Black mailed a questionnaire to 155 women with scleroderma and to 155 healthy controls and found that women with scleroderma had twice the rate of miscarriage before disease onset compared with controls.[97] Giordano and associates studied 299 pregnancies in 80 SSc patients and found a 17% miscarriage rate, significantly higher than among controls (10%).[98] Several other studies have not found a difference in pregnancy loss rates between women with SSc and controls.[94,99] A prospective study found that 16% of 80 SSc pregnancies ended in miscarriage compared with 14% in the control group.[94] However, the subset of women in this study with late, diffuse SSc did have a significantly increased rate of miscarriage. Thus, the available data suggest that women with SSc may be at a slightly increased risk for miscarriage compared with controls.

Although the data are generally limited to case series, it appears that up to one third of pregnancies in women with SSc will be delivered preterm.[94,98,99] In Steen's series, of 91 pregnancies in 59 women, 29% were delivered preterm.[94] PTB may be particularly prevalent among women with diffuse cutaneous disease.[94] Given the vascular pathology of SSc and the relatively frequent renal involvement, it is not surprising that these women appear to be at increased risk for preeclampsia and IUGR. A recent study using the Nationwide Inpatient Sample identified 504 deliveries (out of a total of 11.2 million) that occurred in women with SSc. SSc was significantly associated with hypertensive disorders in pregnancy (odds ratio, 3.71) and IUGR (odds ratio, 3.74).[100]

Obstetrical Management

Preconceptional counseling is important in patients with scleroderma. Women with early, progressive, diffuse SSc or significant cardiac, pulmonary, or renal disease should be appropriately counseled regarding the risks of pregnancy. Any suspicion of pulmonary hypertension should prompt appropriate diagnostic studies to exclude significant disease before recommending pregnancy.

Even in the nonpregnant state, there is no satisfactory therapy for SSc. Treatment of diffuse SSc is typically organ specific. Symptomatic relief of arthralgias and myalgias should be limited to acetaminophen if possible. Many patients take proton pump inhibitors (FDA category C) for upper gastrointestinal symptoms, and these medications may be continued in pregnancy (see Chapter 8); typical doses are unlikely to pose a substantial risk to the fetus, although data are limited. Oral vasodilators, in particular calcium channel blockers (FDA category C), may be continued in pregnancy for the treatment of Raynaud phenomenon, although definitive proof of fetal safety is also lacking (see Chapter 8). ACE inhibitors are used to treat renal crisis in nonpregnant patients. These agents should usually be avoided during pregnancy because of their known teratogenicity and adverse effects on fetal renal function (see Chapter 8). However, in pregnant women with SSc renal crisis and severe hypertension, the benefits of ACE inhibitors may outweigh the fetal risks.

Evidence-based recommendations for prenatal care are lacking. However, it seems reasonable to increase maternal surveillance with prenatal visits every 1 to 2 weeks in the first half of pregnancy and weekly thereafter. Serial laboratory evaluation is not warranted, but clinicians should have a low threshold to pursue any new and unusual symptoms. **Women should be monitored closely for preeclampsia because SSc appears to increase this risk.** Serial fetal ultrasonography to monitor for IUGR seems prudent. Most experts would recommend antenatal testing beginning at 30 to 32 weeks or earlier depending on the clinical scenario.

Among patients with mild to moderate disease, special precautions are generally not needed during labor and delivery. Women with advanced skin disease may have problems with delivery or wound healing (particularly if taking steroids). **Depending on the extent of disease, women with SSc may be at increased anesthetic risk, including problems with intravenous access, difficult intubation, and an increased risk for aspiration.** A prenatal anesthesiology consult may be indicated. For patients with significant pulmonary, cardiac, or renal involvement, intensive care management may be needed.

SJÖGREN SYNDROME

Sjögren syndrome is a chronic inflammatory disorder characterized by diminished lacrimal and salivary gland function (keratoconjunctivitis sicca). It occurs in a primary form and in a secondary form in association with other rheumatic conditions, most commonly RA. Few data exist regarding pregnancies in women with primary Sjögren syndrome. Clinicians should recognize, however, that a high proportion of women with primary Sjögren syndrome have circulating anti-Ro/SSA or anti-La/SSB antibodies, or both, and are thus at risk for a pregnancy affected by NLE and CHB. Outside of monitoring for NLE, management of Sjögren syndrome in pregnancy is usually dictated by that for any associated rheumatic disease.

KEY POINTS

- SLE is the most common, serious autoimmune disease affecting women of reproductive age.
- Overall, 15% to 60% of women with SLE have a flare during pregnancy or in the postpartum period.
- Because SLE disease activity at the onset of pregnancy is an important determinant of flare in pregnancy, women with SLE should be advised to postpone pregnancy until sustained remission for at least 6 months has been achieved.
- For women with lupus nephritis, moderate renal insufficiency (serum creatinine, 1.5 to 2 mg/dL) is a relative contraindication to pregnancy, and advanced renal insufficiency (creatinine > 2 mg/dL) should be considered an absolute contraindication to pregnancy.
- The risk for NLE, and in particular CHB, in fetuses or neonates of women with SLE is low. Among women with anti-Ro/SSA and anti-La/SSB antibodies, the risk for having an infant affected with CHB is increased if the mother had a prior affected child.

- Hydroxychloroquine may be the best maintenance therapy for SLE in pregnancy. Women who become pregnant while taking hydroxychloroquine should generally be continued on this medication.
- The diagnosis of APS rests on the occurrence of either arterial or venous thrombosis or pregnancy morbidity and repeatedly positive testing for lupus anticoagulant and/or medium to high titers of anticardiolipin or anti-β_2-GP-I IgG or IgM antibodies.
- All women with APS and a history of arterial or venous thrombosis should receive full anticoagulation during pregnancy and postpartum.
- Women with APS diagnosed on the basis of recurrent pre-embryonic and embryonic losses and without prior thrombosis should receive low-dose aspirin alone or together with prophylactic dose heparin.
- Women with APS diagnosed on the basis of fetal death, early preeclampsia, or placental insufficiency and without prior thrombosis should receive low-dose aspirin together with prophylactic or intermediate-dose heparin.
- Most women with rheumatoid arthritis will have improvement in their disease during pregnancy but will relapse in the postpartum period, usually within the first 3 months.
- Obstetrical and maternal outcomes are generally good when systemic sclerosis is clinically stable at the onset of pregnancy and the woman is without obvious renal, cardiac, or pulmonary disease.

REFERENCES

1. Lawrence RC, Helmick CG, Arnett FC, et al: Estimates of the prevalence of arthritis and selected musculoskeletal disorders in the United States. Arthritis Rheum 41:778, 1998.
2. Chakravarty EF, Bush TM, Manzi S, et al: Prevalence of adult systemic lupus erythematosus in California and Pennsylvania in 2000: estimates obtained using hospitalization data. Arthritis Rheum 56:2092, 2007.
3. Moser KL, Kelly JA, Lessard CJ, et al: Recent insights into the genetic basis of systemic lupus erythematosus. Genes Immun 10:373, 2009.
4. Weening JJ, D'Agati VD, Schwartz MM, et al: The classification of glomerulonephritis in systemic lupus erythematosus revisited. Kidney Int 65:521, 2004.
5. ter Borg EJ, Horst G, Hummel EJ, et al: Measurement of increases in anti-double-stranded DNA antibody levels as a predictor of disease exacerbation in systemic lupus erythematosus: a long-term, prospective study. Arthritis Rheum 33:634, 1990.
6. Lockshin MD, Reinitz E, Druzin ML, et al: Lupus pregnancy: case-control prospective study demonstrating absence of lupus exacerbation during or after pregnancy. Am J Med 77:893, 1984.
7. Lockshin MD: Pregnancy does not cause systemic lupus erythematosus to worsen. Arthritis Rheum 32:665, 1989.
8. Meehan RT, Dorsey JK: Pregnancy among patients with systemic lupus erythematosus receiving immunosuppressive therapy. J Rheumatol 14:252, 1987.
9. Mintz G, Niz J, Gutierrez G, et al: Prospective study of pregnancy in systemic lupus erythematosus: results of a multidisciplinary approach. J Rheumatol 13:732, 1986.
10. Urowitz MB, Gladman DD, Farewell VT, et al: Lupus and pregnancy studies. Arthritis Rheum 36:1392, 1993.
11. Georgiou PE, Politi EN, Katsimbri P, et al: Outcome of lupus pregnancy: a controlled study. Rheumatology (Oxford) 39:1014, 2000.
12. Petri M, Howard D, Repke J: Frequency of lupus flare in pregnancy. The Hopkins Lupus Pregnancy Center experience. Arthritis Rheum 34:1538, 1991.
13. Ruiz-Irastorza G, Lima F, Alves J, et al: Increased rate of lupus flare during pregnancy and the puerperium: a prospective study of 78 pregnancies. Br J Rheumatol 35:133, 1996.
14. Derksen RH, Bruinse HW, de Groot PG, et al: Pregnancy in systemic lupus erythematosus: a prospective study. Lupus 3:149, 1994.
15. Cortes-Hernandez J, Ordi-Ros J, Labrador M, et al: Predictors of poor renal outcome in patients with lupus nephritis treated with combined pulses of cyclophosphamide and methylprednisolone. Lupus 12:287, 2003.
16. Hayslett JP: Maternal and fetal complications in pregnant women with systemic lupus erythematosus. Am J Kidney Dis 17:123, 1991.
17. Devoe LD, Loy GL: Serum complement levels and perinatal outcome in pregnancies complicated by systemic lupus erythematosus. Obstet Gynecol 63:796, 1984.
18. Buyon JP, Cronstein BN, Morris M, et al: Serum complement values (C3 and C4) to differentiate between systemic lupus activity and pre-eclampsia. Am J Med 81:194, 1986.
19. Wong KL, Chan FY, Lee CP: Outcome of pregnancy in patients with systemic lupus erythematosus: a prospective study. Arch Intern Med 151:269, 1991.
20. Mellembakken JR, Hogasen K, Mollnes TE, et al: Increased systemic activation of neutrophils but not complement in preeclampsia. Obstet Gynecol 97:371, 2001.
21. Petri M: Hopkins Lupus Pregnancy Center: 1987 to 1996. Rheum Dis Clin North Am 23:1, 1997.
22. Jungers P, Dougados M, Pelissier C, et al: Lupus nephropathy and pregnancy: report of 104 cases in 36 patients. Arch Intern Med 142:771, 1982.
23. Fine LG, Barnett EV, Danovitch GM, et al: Systemic lupus erythematosus in pregnancy. Arch Intern Med 94:667, 1981.
24. Oviasu E, Hicks J, Cameron JS: The outcome of pregnancy in women with lupus nephritis. Lupus 1:19, 1999.
25. Hayslett JP, Lynn RI: Effect of pregnancy in patients with lupus nephropathy. Kidney Int 18:207, 1980.
26. Petri M, Allbritton J: Fetal outcome of lupus pregnancy: a retrospective case-control study of the Hopkins Lupus Cohort. J Rheumatol 20:650, 1993.
27. Oshiro BT, Silver RM, Scott JR, et al: Antiphospholipid antibodies and fetal death. Obstet Gynecol 87:489, 1996.
28. Englert HJ, Derue GM, Loizou S, et al: Pregnancy and lupus: prognostic indicators and response to treatment. Q J Med 66:125, 1988.
29. Roque H, Paidas MJ, Funai EF, et al: Maternal thrombophilias are not associated with early pregnancy loss. Thromb Haemost 91:290, 2004.
30. Clowse ME, Magder LS, Witter F, et al: The impact of increased lupus activity on obstetric outcomes. Arthritis Rheum 52:514, 2005.
31. Clowse ME, Jamison M, Myers E, et al: A national study of the complications of lupus in pregnancy. Am J Obstet Gynecol 199:127 e1, 2008.
32. Nossent HC, Swaak TJ: Systemic lupus erythematosus. VI. Analysis of the interrelationship with pregnancy. J Rheumatol 17:771, 1990.
33. Aggarwal N, Sawhney H, Vasishta K, et al: Pregnancy in patients with systemic lupus erythematosus. Aust N Z J Obstet Gynaecol 39:28, 1999.
34. Johnson MJ, Petri M, Witter FR, et al: Evaluation of preterm delivery in a systemic lupus erythematosus pregnancy clinic. Obstet Gynecol 86:396, 1995.
35. Buyon JP, Hiebert R, Copel J, et al: Autoimmune-associated congenital heart block: demographics, mortality, morbidity and recurrence rates obtained from a national neonatal lupus registry. J Am Coll Cardiol 31:1658, 1998.
36. Buyon JP, Clancy RM, Friedman DM: Autoimmune associated congenital heart block: integration of clinical and research clues in the management of the maternal/foetal dyad at risk. J Intern Med 265:653, 2009.
37. Clancy RM, Marion MC, Kaufman KM, et al: Genome-wide association study of cardiac manifestations of neonatal lupus identifies candidate loci at 6p21 and 21q22. Arthritis Rheum 2010.

38. Jaeggi ET, Fouron JC, Silverman ED, et al: Transplacental fetal treatment improves the outcome of prenatally diagnosed complete atrioventricular block without structural heart disease. Circulation 110:1542, 2004.
39. Friedman DM, Kim MY, Copel JA, et al: Prospective evaluation of fetuses with autoimmune-associated congenital heart block followed in the PR Interval and Dexamethasone Evaluation (PRIDE) Study. Am J Cardiol 103:1102, 2009.
40. Saleeb S, Copel J, Friedman D, et al: Comparison of treatment with fluorinated glucocorticoids to the natural history of autoantibody-associated congenital heart block: retrospective review of the research registry for neonatal lupus. Arthritis Rheum 42:2335, 1999.
41. Friedman DM, Llanos C, Izmirly PM, et al: Evaluation of fetuses in a study of intravenous immunoglobulin as preventive therapy for congenital heart block: results of a multicenter, prospective, open-label clinical trial. Arthritis Rheum 62:1138, 2010.
42. Pisoni CN, Brucato A, Ruffatti A, et al: Failure of intravenous immunoglobulin to prevent congenital heart block: findings of a multicenter, prospective, observational study. Arthritis Rheum 62:1147, 2010.
43. Jaeggi ET, Hamilton RM, Silverman ED, et al: Outcome of children with fetal, neonatal or childhood diagnosis of isolated congenital atrioventricular block: a single institution's experience of 30 years. J Am Coll Cardiol 39:130, 2002.
44. Matsubara S, Morimatsu Y, Shiraishi H, et al: Fetus with heart failure due to congenital atrioventricular block treated by maternally administered ritodrine. Arch Gynecol Obstet 278:85, 2008.
45. Carmichael SL, Shaw GM, Ma C, et al: Maternal corticosteroid use and orofacial clefts. Am J Obstet Gynecol 197:585.e1, 2007.
46. Costedoat-Chalumeau N, Amoura Z, Duhaut P, et al: Safety of hydroxychloroquine in pregnant patients with connective tissue diseases: a study of one hundred thirty-three cases compared with a control group. Arthritis Rheum 48:3207, 2003.
47. Clowse ME, Magder L, Witter F, et al: Hydroxychloroquine in lupus pregnancy. Arthritis Rheum 54:3640, 2006.
48. Goldstein LH, Dolinsky G, Greenberg R, et al: Pregnancy outcome of women exposed to azathioprine during pregnancy. Birth Defects Res A Clin Mol Teratol 79:696, 2007.
49. Ostensen M, Khamashta M, Lockshin M, et al: Anti-inflammatory and immunosuppressive drugs and reproduction. Arthritis Res Ther 8:209, 2006.
50. Cooper WO, Hernandez-Diaz S, Arbogast PG, et al: Major congenital malformations after first-trimester exposure to ACE inhibitors. N Engl J Med 354:2443, 2006.
51. Alwan S, Polifka JE, Friedman JM: Angiotensin II receptor antagonist treatment during pregnancy. Birth Defects Res A Clin Mol Teratol 73:123, 2005.
52. Miyakis S, Lockshin MD, Atsumi T, et al: International consensus statement on an update of the classification criteria for definite antiphospholipid syndrome (APS). J Thromb Haemost 4:295, 2006.
53. Lockwood CJ, Romero R, Feinberg RF, et al: The prevalence and biologic significance of lupus anticoagulant and anticardiolipin antibodies in a general obstetric population. Am J Obstet Gynecol 161:369, 1989.
54. Levine JS, Branch DW, Rauch J: The antiphospholipid syndrome. N Engl J Med 346:752, 2002.
55. Bakimer R, Fishman P, Blank M, et al: Induction of primary antiphospholipid syndrome in mice by immunization with a human monoclonal anticardiolipin antibody (H-3). J Clin Invest 89:1558, 1992.
56. Branch DW, Dudley DJ, Mitchell MD, et al: Immunoglobulin G fractions from patients with antiphospholipid antibodies cause fetal death in BALB/c mice: a model for autoimmune fetal loss. Am J Obstet Gynecol 163:210, 1990.
57. Salmon JE, Girardi G, Holers VM: Activation of complement mediates antiphospholipid antibody-induced pregnancy loss. Lupus 12:535, 2003.
58. Holers VM, Girardi G, Mo L, et al: Complement C3 activation is required for antiphospholipid antibody-induced fetal loss. J Exp Med 195:211, 2002.
59. Oku K, Atsumi T, Bohgaki M, et al: Complement activation in patients with primary antiphospholipid syndrome. Ann Rheum Dis 68:1030, 2009.
60. Shamonki JM, Salmon JE, Hyjek E, et al: Excessive complement activation is associated with placental injury in patients with antiphospholipid antibodies. Am J Obstet Gynecol 196:167.e1, 2007.
61. Tincani A, Allegri F, Sanmarco M, et al: Anticardiolipin antibody assay: a methodological analysis for a better consensus in routine determinations—a cooperative project of the European Antiphospholipid Forum. Thromb Haemost 86:575, 2001.
62. Opatrny L, David M, Kahn SR, et al: Association between antiphospholipid antibodies and recurrent fetal loss in women without autoimmune disease: a metaanalysis. J Rheumatol 33:2214, 2006.
63. Kutteh WH: Antiphospholipid antibody-associated recurrent pregnancy loss: treatment with heparin and low-dose aspirin is superior to low-dose aspirin alone. Am J Obstet Gynecol 174:1584, 1996.
64. Rai R, Cohen H, Dave M, et al: Randomised controlled trial of aspirin and aspirin plus heparin in pregnant women with recurrent miscarriage associated with phospholipid antibodies (or antiphospholipid antibodies). BMJ 314:253, 1997.
65. Branch DW, Silver RM, Blackwell JL, et al: Outcome of treated pregnancies in women with antiphospholipid syndrome: an update of the Utah experience. Obstet Gynecol 80:614, 1992.
66. Branch DW, Andres R, Digre KB, et al: The association of antiphospholipid antibodies with severe preeclampsia. Obstet Gynecol 73:541, 1989.
67. Silver RK, MacGregor SN, Sholl JS, et al: Comparative trial of prednisone plus aspirin versus aspirin alone in the treatment of anticardiolipin antibody-positive obstetric patients. Am J Obstet Gynecol 169:1411, 1993.
68. Cowchock FS, Reece EA, Balaban D, et al: Repeated fetal losses associated with antiphospholipid antibodies: a collaborative randomized trial comparing prednisone with low-dose heparin treatment. Am J Obstet Gynecol 166:1318, 1992.
69. Triolo G, Ferrante A, Ciccia F, et al: Randomized study of subcutaneous low molecular weight heparin plus aspirin versus intravenous immunoglobulin in the treatment of recurrent fetal loss associated with antiphospholipid antibodies. Arthritis Rheum 48: 728, 2003.
70. Branch DW, Peaceman AM, Druzin M, et al: A multicenter, placebo-controlled pilot study of intravenous immune globulin treatment of antiphospholipid syndrome during pregnancy. The Pregnancy Loss Study Group. Am J Obstet Gynecol 182:122, 2000.
71. Vaquero E, Lazzarin N, Valensise H, et al: Pregnancy outcome in recurrent spontaneous abortion associated with antiphospholipid antibodies: a comparative study of intravenous immunoglobulin versus prednisone plus low-dose aspirin. Am J Reprod Immunol 45:174, 2001.
72. Empson M, Lassere M, Craig J, et al: Prevention of recurrent miscarriage for women with antiphospholipid antibody or lupus anticoagulant. Cochrane Database Syst Rev CD002859, 2005.
73. Kutteh WH, Ermel LD: A clinical trial for the treatment of antiphospholipid antibody-associated recurrent pregnancy loss with lower dose heparin and aspirin. Am J Reprod Immunol 35:402, 1996.
74. Farquharson RG, Quenby S, Greaves M: Antiphospholipid syndrome in pregnancy: a randomized, controlled trial of treatment. Obstet Gynecol 100:408, 2002.
75. Laskin CA, Bombardier C, Hannah ME, et al: Prednisone and aspirin in women with autoantibodies and unexplained recurrent fetal loss. N Engl J Med 337:148, 1997.
76. Noble LS, Kutteh WH, Lashey N, et al: Antiphospholipid antibodies associated with recurrent pregnancy loss: prospective, multicenter, controlled pilot study comparing treatment with low-molecular-weight heparin versus unfractionated heparin. Fertil Steril 83:684, 2005.
77. Stephenson MD, Ballem PJ, Tsang P, et al: Treatment of antiphospholipid antibody syndrome (APS) in pregnancy: a randomized pilot trial comparing low molecular weight heparin to unfractionated heparin. J Obstet Gynaecol Can 26:729, 2004.
78. Pattison NS, Chamley LW, Birdsall M, et al: Does aspirin have a role in improving pregnancy outcome for women with the antiphospholipid syndrome? A randomized controlled trial. Am J Obstet Gynecol 183:1008, 2000.
79. Huong DL, Wechsler B, Bletry O, et al: A study of 75 pregnancies in patients with antiphospholipid syndrome. J Rheumatol 28:2025, 2001.
80. Bates SM, Greer IA, Pabinger I, et al: Venous thromboembolism, thrombophilia, antithrombotic therapy, and pregnancy: American College of Chest Physicians Evidence-Based Clinical Practice Guidelines (8th ed). Chest 133:844S, 2008.
81. Bowes J, Barton A: Recent advances in the genetics of RA susceptibility. Rheumatology (Oxford) 47:399, 2008.

82. Karlson EW, Mandl LA, Hankinson SE, et al: Do breast-feeding and other reproductive factors influence future risk of rheumatoid arthritis? Results from the Nurses' Health Study. Arthritis Rheum 50:3458, 2004.
83. Aletaha D, Neogi T, Silman AJ, et al: 2010 Rheumatoid arthritis classification criteria: an American College of Rheumatology/European League Against Rheumatism collaborative initiative. Ann Rheum Dis 69:1580, 2010.
84. Ehrenstein MR, Evans JG, Singh A, et al: Compromised function of regulatory T cells in rheumatoid arthritis and reversal by anti-TNFalpha therapy. J Exp Med 200:277, 2004.
85. Forger F, Marcoli N, Gadola S, et al: Pregnancy induces numerical and functional changes of CD4+CD25 high regulatory T cells in patients with rheumatoid arthritis. Ann Rheum Dis 67:984, 2008.
86. Nelson JL, Hughes KA, Smith AG, et al: Maternal-fetal disparity in HLA class II alloantigens and the pregnancy-induced amelioration of rheumatoid arthritis. N Engl J Med 329:466, 1993.
87. Brennan P, Barrett J, Fiddler M, et al: Maternal-fetal HLA incompatibility and the course of inflammatory arthritis during pregnancy. J Rheumatol 27:2843, 2000.
88. Oka M, Vainio U: Effect of pregnancy on the prognosis and serology of rheumatoid arthritis. Acta Rheumatol Scand 12:47, 1966.
89. Kaplan D: Fetal wastage in patients with rheumatoid arthritis. J Rheumatol 13:875, 1986.
90. de Man YA, Hazes JM, van der Heide H, et al: Association of higher rheumatoid arthritis disease activity during pregnancy with lower birth weight: results of a national prospective study. Arthritis Rheum 60:3196, 2009.
91. Carter JD, Ladhani A, Ricca LR, et al: A safety assessment of tumor necrosis factor antagonists during pregnancy: a review of the Food and Drug Administration database. J Rheumatol 36:635, 2009.
92. Tan FK, Stivers DN, Foster MW, et al: Association of microsatellite markers near the fibrillin 1 gene on human chromosome 15q with scleroderma in a Native American population. Arthritis Rheum 41: 1729, 1998.
93. Zhou X, Tan FK, Wang N, et al: Genome-wide association study for regions of systemic sclerosis susceptibility in a Choctaw Indian population with high disease prevalence. Arthritis Rheum 48:2585, 2003.
94. Steen VD: Pregnancy in women with systemic sclerosis. Obstet Gynecol 94:15, 1999.
95. Evans PC, Lambert N, Maloney S, et al: Long-term fetal microchimerism in peripheral blood mononuclear cell subsets in healthy women and women with scleroderma. Blood 93:2033, 1999.
96. Artlett CM, Smith JB, Jimenez SA: Identification of fetal DNA and cells in skin lesions from women with systemic sclerosis. N Engl J Med 338:1186, 1998.
97. Silman AJ, Black C: Increased incidence of spontaneous abortion and infertility in women with scleroderma before disease onset: a controlled study. Ann Rheum Dis 47:441, 1988.
98. Giordano M, Valentini G, Lupoli S, et al: Pregnancy and systemic sclerosis. Arthritis Rheum 28:237, 1985.
99. Steen VD, Conte C, Day N, et al: Pregnancy in women with systemic sclerosis. Arthritis Rheum 32:151, 1989.
100. Chakravarty EF, Khanna D, Chung L: Pregnancy outcomes in systemic sclerosis, primary pulmonary hypertension, and sickle cell disease. Obstet Gynecol 111:927, 2008.

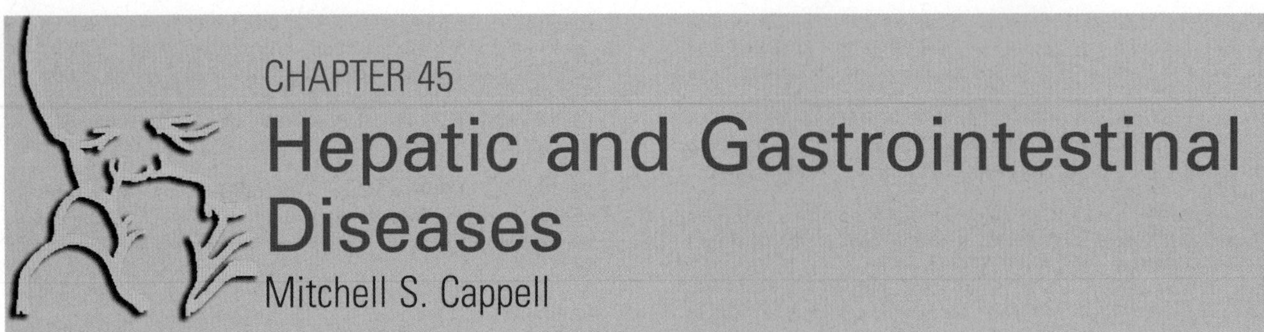

CHAPTER 45
Hepatic and Gastrointestinal Diseases

Mitchell S. Cappell

KEY ABBREVIATIONS

Acute Fatty Liver of Pregnancy	AFLP
Acute Intermittent Porphyria	AIP
Computed Tomography	CT
Disseminated Intravascular Coagulation	DIC
Endoscopic Retrograde Cholangiopancreatography	ERCP
Esophagogastroduodenoscopy	EGD
Hemolysis, Elevated Liver Enzymes, and Low Platelet Count Syndrome	HELLP
Hepatocellular Cancer	HCC
Intrahepatic Cholestasis of Pregnancy	ICP
Long-chain 3-hydroxyacyl Coenzyme A Dehydrogenase	LCHAD
Magnetic Resonance Imaging	MRI

Hepatic Disorders During Pregnancy

Hepatic, biliary, and pancreatic disorders are relatively uncommon but not rare during pregnancy. For example, about 3 per 100 women develop serum liver function test abnormalities during pregnancy, and about 1 per 500 women develop potentially life-threatening hepatic diseases during pregnancy.[1,2]

Hepatic, biliary, and pancreatic disorders are often complex and clinically challenging problems during pregnancy. First, the differential diagnosis during pregnancy is extensive. It includes both disorders related to pregnancy and disorders unrelated to pregnancy. Second, the clinical presentation and natural history of these disorders may be altered during pregnancy. Indeed, some disorders, such as intrahepatic cholestasis of pregnancy, are unique to pregnancy. Third, the diagnostic evaluation may be constrained by pregnancy. For example, radiologic tests may raise concern about fetal safety during pregnancy. Fourth, the interests of both the mother and the fetus must be considered in therapeutic decision making. Occasionally, maternal therapy must be modified to substitute alternative but safer therapy because of concerns about drug teratogenicity.[3] Rarely, maternal and fetal interests may be diametrically opposed, as in the use of certain chemotherapeutic agents or radiation for maternal cancer, in which therapy that is potentially life-saving to the mother can harm the developing fetus.[4] These conflicts raise significant medical, legal, and ethical issues.

Obstetricians, hepatologists, surgeons, and internists should be familiar with hepatic, biliary, and pancreatic disorders that can occur in pregnancy and how these conditions affect and in turn are affected by pregnancy. This chapter reviews hepatic, biliary, and pancreatic disorders during pregnancy, with a focus on features unique to pregnancy.

PHYSIOLOGIC EFFECTS OF PREGNANCY AND ASSESSMENT OF LIVER DISEASE

Assessment of the abdomen is modified during pregnancy. The expanding gravid uterus can displace abdominal viscera and may conceal an abdominal mass on physical examination.[4] During pregnancy the blood pressure normally declines modestly. A rise in blood pressure during pregnancy may, therefore, portend preeclampsia or eclampsia. Physiologic alterations of laboratory values during pregnancy include mild leukocytosis, physiologic anemia of pregnancy, and electrolyte changes, particularly mild hyponatremia.[5] The risk of thromboembolic phenomena is increased during pregnancy due to mild hypercoagulopathy (increased fibrinogen levels) from hyperestrogenemia and vascular stasis from vascular compression by the enlarged gravid uterus. The changes in serum glucose levels during pregnancy are complex. Normal pregnancy is characterized by fasting hypoglycemia despite increased hepatic insulin resistance, postprandial hyperglycemia, and hyperinsulinemia. Pregnancy does not affect the liver span. The liver may be pushed cephalad by the gravid uterus, but a liver span greater than 12 cm, when appreciated, remains a valid indicator of hepatomegaly. **Spider angiomata and palmar erythema, cutaneous lesions often associated with chronic liver disease, may appear transiently during normal pregnancy without underlying liver disease.** During pregnancy the serum alkaline phosphatase level normally increases mildly due to placental production. **The serum albumin level declines during pregnancy primarily from hemodilution and secondarily from decreased hepatic synthesis. Serum bilirubin levels tend to change little during pregnancy due to the effect of mildly impaired hepatic excretion balanced by the opposing effects of hemodilution and hypoalbuminemia.**[6] Serum bile acids tend to progressively increase during pregnancy due to impaired hepatic transport and biliary secretion. Serum levels of cholesterol, triglycerides, and phospholipids increase moderately during pregnancy due to increased hepatic synthesis. The serum aminotransferase levels are largely unaffected by pregnancy. Changes of serum levels of common blood tests during pregnancy are summarized in the box Changes in Routine Laboratory Tests and Liver Function Tests During Pregnancy.

CHANGES IN ROUTINE LABORATORY TESTS AND LIVER FUNCTION TESTS DURING PREGNANCY

Mildly Decreased Values

Sodium
Albumin

Moderately Decreased Value

Hematocrit—physiologic anemia of pregnancy

Mildly Increased Values

Leukocyte count
Alkaline phosphatase
Amylase

Moderately Increased Values

Serum bile acids
Cholesterol
Triglycerides

Other

Glucose level—fasting hypoglycemia, postprandial hyperglycemia

DIFFERENTIAL DIAGNOSIS OF HEPATOBILIARY SYMPTOMS AND CONDITIONS DURING PREGNANCY

Jaundice

As in the general population, acute viral hepatitis is the most common cause of jaundice during pregnancy.[1,2] **The differential diagnosis of jaundice during the first and second trimesters of pregnancy also includes drug hepatotoxicity and gallstone disease such as acute cholecystitis, choledocholithiasis, ascending cholangitis, or gallstone pancreatitis.** In addition to these disorders, the differential of jaundice during the third trimester includes the following pregnancy-related causes: intrahepatic cholestasis of pregnancy, acute fatty liver of pregnancy, and HELLP (hemolysis, elevated liver function tests, and low platelet count) syndrome. Moderate direct hyperbilirubinemia without jaundice during the third trimester may also be due to preeclampsia, eclampsia, and Budd-Chiari syndrome. Predominantly indirect hyperbilirubinemia during pregnancy is usually due to hemolysis (including the HELLP syndrome) or Gilbert's syndrome.

Right Upper Quadrant Abdominal Pain

As shown in the box Differential Diagnosis of Right Upper Quadrant Abdominal Pain During Pregnancy, the differential diagnosis is extensive. In addition to hepatic, biliary, gastrointestinal, and renal disorders that can occur in nonpregnant patients, the differential includes diseases related to pregnancy. Careful medical history, including the pain intensity, nature, temporal pattern, radiation pattern, exacerbating factors, and alleviating factors, helps narrow the differential diagnosis. Biliary colic produces a waxing and waning intensity of pain. Acute cholecystitis is associated with right upper quadrant pain, as well as pain referred to the right shoulder. The pain of acute pancreatitis is often boring in quality, located in the abdominal midline and radiating to the back. Physical examination of the abdomen including inspection, palpation, and auscultation can further pinpoint the cause of the pain. **Laboratory evaluation of significant abdominal pain routinely includes a hemogram, serum electrolytes, and liver function tests and often includes a leukocyte differential, coagulation profile, and serum lipase determination.** In evaluating the laboratory results, gestational changes in normative values, as mentioned, must be considered. Radiologic tests may be extremely helpful diagnostically, but the choice of radiologic imaging is constrained by the pregnancy, as discussed later. **Right upper quadrant pain and abnormal liver function tests in the setting of new-onset hypertension should strongly suggest preeclampsia with liver involvement.** Right upper quadrant pain and abnormal liver function tests in the setting of thrombocytopenia and microangiopathic hemolysis, as demonstrated by the presence of schistiocytes in a peripheral blood smear, should strongly suggest HELLP syndrome.

Occasionally, the patient is unaware of pregnancy or it is not revealed to the physician, particularly in early pregnancy, when physical findings are absent. The physician should be vigilant for possible pregnancy in a fertile woman with abdominal pain, particularly in the setting of missed menses, because pregnancy affects the differential diagnosis, clinical evaluation, and treatment. Pregnancy testing should be performed early in the evaluation of acute abdominal pain in reproductive-age women.

Differential Diagnosis of Right Upper Quadrant Abdominal Pain During Pregnancy

Hepatic Disorders

Hepatitis
Hepatic vascular engorgement
Hepatic hematoma
Hepatic malignancy

Biliary Tract Disease

Biliary colic
Choledocholithiasis
Cholangitis
Cholecystitis

Diseases Related to Pregnancy

Preeclampsia or eclampsia
Hemolysis, elevated liver enzymes, and low platelet count (HELLP) syndrome
Acute fatty liver of pregnancy
Hepatic hemorrhage or rupture

Renal Disorders

Pyelonephritis
Nephrolithiasis

Gastrointestinal Disorders

Peptic ulcer disease
Perforated duodenal ulcer

Other Conditions in RUQ

Rib fracture
Shingles

Referred Pain from Other Organ Disease

Pneumonia
Pulmonary embolus or infarct
Pleural effusion
Radiculopathy
Inferior wall myocardial infarction
Colon cancer

Nausea and Vomiting

Nausea and vomiting is ubiquitous during pregnancy. Nausea and vomiting of pregnancy is the most common cause. It typically begins at about 6 weeks of gestation and abates at about 18 weeks of gestation.[7] It is caused by the physiologic effects of the pregnancy without demonstrable mucosal or mural disease. **Hyperemesis gravidarum is a serious and potentially life-threatening form of nausea and vomiting of pregnancy associated with loss of more than 5% of the pregravid weight. Hyperemesis gravidarum is a diagnosis of exclusion, based on nausea and vomiting occurring early in pregnancy, gradually resolving during the middle second trimester, and unassociated with other symptoms.** The differential diagnosis of nausea and vomiting during pregnancy also includes hepatic disorders related to pregnancy, such as fatty liver and intrahepatic cholestasis of pregnancy. Other hepatic causes include viral hepatitis, symptomatic cholelithiasis, and acute cholecystitis. Gastrointestinal causes include gastroesophageal reflux disease (GERD), peptic ulcer disease, viral gastroenteritis, appendicitis, gastroparesis diabeticorum, and gastrointestinal obstruction. Uncommon causes include adnexal torsion, pyelonephritis, urolithiasis, and Addison's disease (glucocorticoid deficiency).

Pruritus

The differential of pruritus during pregnancy includes intrahepatic cholestasis of pregnancy, cholestatic viral hepatitis, primary sclerosing cholangitis, primary biliary cirrhosis, and mechanical choledochal obstruction from benign or malignant strictures. Pruritus sometimes occurs physiologically during pregnancy or in association with various dermatoses. It is typically mild, localized, unassociated with other symptoms, and unassociated with abnormal liver function tests.

Hepatic Lesions

Hepatic lesions identified on abdominal imaging studies are classified as cystic or solid. The differential of cystic hepatic lesion(s) includes simple hepatic cysts, hepatic cysts associated with polycystic kidney disease, Caroli's disease, bacterial abscesses, amebic abscesses, intraparenchymal hemorrhage, hemangiomas, ecchinococcal cysts, and rarely hepatic malignancies. The differential of a solid hepatic mass includes hepatic adenoma, focal nodular hyperplasia, hepatocellular carcinoma, and hepatic metastases.

Ascites

Hepatic causes of ascites during pregnancy include cirrhosis, acute fatty liver of pregnancy, Budd-Chiari syndrome, portal vein thrombosis, hepatic fibrosis, and hepatocellular carcinoma. Other causes of ascites during pregnancy include ovarian cancer, abdominal tuberculosis, cardiac failure, protein-losing nephropathy, and severe protein malnutrition (kwashiorkor).

ABDOMINAL IMAGING DURING PREGNANCY

Fetal safety of diagnostic imaging is a concern for pregnant women. Ultrasonography is considered safe and is the preferred abdominal imaging modality during pregnancy.[8] Unfortunately, test sensitivity depends on operator technique, patient cooperation, and patient anatomy. For example, test sensitivity is decreased by abdominal fat and bowel distention.[8] There are no reported harmful effects from magnetic resonance imaging (MRI) during pregnancy, but there are few data on safety during the first trimester or with use of gadolinium.[9] MRI is preferable to computed tomography (CT) scanning during pregnancy to avoid ionizing radiation, but gadolinium administration should be avoided during MRI in the first trimester.[9] Rapid-sequence MRI is preferable to conventional MRI because of briefer exposure.

Radiation can cause fetal mortality, growth restriction, genetic mutations, and neurologic abnormalities, including mental retardation. Radiation may also increase the risk of childhood leukemia.[10] Dosage is the most important risk factor, but fetal age at exposure is also important. Fetal mortality is greatest from radiation exposure during the first 2 weeks after conception, and the risk of neurologic malformations is greatest during the first trimester when organogenesis occurs.[10] Women should undergo counseling before diagnostic roentgenography. Exposure to more than 15 rads during the second and third trimesters or more than 5 rads during the first trimester should prompt consideration of elective termination of pregnancy.[10] Diagnostic studies with high radiation exposure, such as abdominal CT, typically expose the fetus to less than 1 rad and can be considered when extremely strongly indicated.

THERAPEUTIC ENDOSCOPY DURING PREGNANCY

Therapeutic Endoscopic Retrograde Cholangiopancreatography

Choledocholithiasis usually requires urgent therapy because of potentially life-threatening ascending cholangitis or gallstone pancreatitis. Symptomatic choledocholithiasis is best managed by therapeutic endoscopic retrograde cholangiopancreatography (ERCP) in the nonpregnant patient to avoid complex biliary surgery during cholecystectomy. In experienced hands, therapeutic ERCP in the general population has acceptable morbidity of about 5% and low mortality of about 0.5%.[11] Therapeutic ERCP is theoretically more attractive than biliary surgery for choledocholithiasis during pregnancy because surgery entails a significant risk of fetal loss. Aside from maternal risks, therapeutic ERCP during pregnancy entails theoretical risks to the fetus of premature labor, medication and radiation exposure, fetal hypoxia during endoscopic intubation, cardiac arrhythmias, and systemic hypotension.[11] In the largest clinical series, 68 therapeutic ERCPs were performed on 65 pregnant patients for indications including biliary pancreatitis, cholangitis, abnormal liver function tests, or choledochal dilation on abdominal ultrasonography.[12] Maternal postprocedure complications included only pancreatitis in 11 patients. Of 59 patients followed through delivery, preterm delivery occurred in 6 (10%), and low birth weight in 4 (7%). There were no fetal deaths, perinatal deaths, or fetal malformations. Jamidar and colleagues[13] analyzed 29 ERCPs performed on 23 pregnant patients, including 15 performed in the first trimester. Excluding two unknown pregnancy outcomes and two elective abortions, 17 of the 19 pregnancies (89%) resulted in healthy infants, including 16 born at term. Only 1 neonatal death was attributed to the procedure, which occurred in a mother who suffered pancreatitis after ERCP. Excluding these studies, a literature review encompassing another 95 ERCPs, including 72 endoscopic sphincterotomies, during pregnancy, revealed no maternal mortality and only 1 fetal death.[14] Maternal morbidity after ERCP included pancreatitis in four, bleeding in two, and preeclampsia in two. A total of four infants were delivered prematurely.

The accumulated data suggest that therapeutic ERCP can be performed during pregnancy for strong indications to avoid complex biliary surgery or to postpone cholecystectomy until after parturition. Special precautions to minimize fetal risks of ERCP during pregnancy include consultation with a neonatologist, radiation physicist, and anesthesiologist before ERCP; referral to a tertiary medical center for management by a team of experts; lead shielding of the mother's abdomen except for the region of the proximal pancreas and biliary tree; use of a modern fluoroscope to minimize radiation leakage; avoidance of spot radiographs for documentation because they entail considerable radiation exposure; and, if possible, delaying ERCP until the second trimester to reduce early pregnancy radiation exposure.[11]

Endoscopic Variceal Sclerotherapy or Banding

Pregnancy appears to increase the risk of variceal bleeding from portal hypertension because of the gestational increase in plasma volume. Endoscopic sclerotherapy or ligation (banding) are particularly attractive therapies for variceal bleeding during pregnancy because the radiologic alternative of transjugular intrahepatic portosystemic shunt (TIPS) requires radiation, and the surgical alternatives may be associated with fetal loss. Esophagogastroduodenoscopy (EGD) can be performed during pregnancy with relatively low fetal risks, and should be undertaken for cases of acute upper gastrointestinal hemorrhage.[11,15] Endoscopic sclerotherapy or banding raises concerns beyond that of diagnostic EGD from the additional procedure time, the typically severe underlying maternal illness, and the therapy itself. Although variceal banding is preferred over sclerotherapy in the general (nonpregnant) population, there are scant data, based on isolated case reports, on the fetal safety of variceal banding during pregnancy and more data available on sclerotherapy during pregnancy. In one clinical series, 10 women underwent a mean of three endoscopic sclerotherapy sessions during pregnancy for active variceal bleeding in five and for prophylaxis in five.[16] Hemostasis was achieved in all actively bleeding patients. One patient suffered a complication from sclerotherapy of an esophageal stricture, successfully treated using peroral esophageal dilators. All women had a normal vaginal delivery at term.[16] Nine other patients successfully underwent endoscopic sclerotherapy for actively or recently bleeding esophageal varices with delivery of healthy infants in all cases.[11] One study reported less favorable pregnancy outcomes after endoscopic sclerotherapy, attributable to the underlying maternal disease. Four of 17 pregnant patients undergoing endoscopic sclerotherapy for variceal bleeding due to noncirrhotic portal hypertension had poor pregnancy outcomes (stillbirth or neonatal death).[17] **The available data thus appear to justify endoscopic banding or sclerotherapy during pregnancy for actively bleeding esophageal varices, due to the poor outcomes associated with alternative available therapies.**

PANCREATOBILIARY DISEASE

Acute Pancreatitis

Acute pancreatitis occurs in about 1 per 3000 pregnancies, most commonly during the third trimester. Gallstones cause about 70% of cases, as alcoholism is relatively uncommon during pregnancy. The risk of cholesterol stones is increased during pregnancy because of increased cholesterol secretion into bile. Other causes include drugs, abdominal surgery, trauma, hyperlipidemia, hyperparathyroidism, vasculitis, and infections such as mumps or mononucleosis. The risk of pancreatitis from hyperlipidemia is increased during pregnancy due to significant triglyceride elevation during late pregnancy. Some cases of pancreatitis, as in nonpregnant individuals, are idiopathic.

The clinical presentation, diagnostic tests, and treatment of pancreatobiliary disorders during pregnancy are summarized in Table 45-1. **Pregnancy does not significantly alter the clinical presentation of acute pancreatitis. Epigastric pain is the most common symptom.** The pain commonly radiates to the back. Nausea, emesis, and pyrexia frequently occur. Signs include midabdominal tenderness, abdominal guarding, hypoactive bowel sounds, abdominal distention, and increased tympany. Severe cases are associated with shock and pancreatic ascites. Grey-Turner's sign or Cullen's sign suggests retroperitoneal bleeding.

Acute pancreatitis is diagnosed by the clinical presentation, laboratory tests, and radiologic examinations. Serum amylase and lipase are reliable markers of acute pancreatitis during pregnancy. Serum lipase is unchanged during normal pregnancy, and the amylase level rises only mildly during normal pregnancy.[18] Hyperamylasemia may also occur in diabetic ketoacidosis, renal failure, bowel perforation, or bowel obstruction, but the serum lipase and amylase-to-creatinine clearance ratio are normal in these conditions and are elevated in acute pancreatitis. Hypertriglyceridemia can falsely lower the serum amylase level in pancreatitis; however, the lipase level remains elevated.[3] A serum alanine aminotransferase level greater than 3 times the upper limit of normal strongly suggests biliary pancreatitis. Abdominal ultrasonography is useful in gauging pancreatic inflammation in thin patients with mild to moderate acute pancreatitis, but CT scanning is better at delineating areas of pancreatic necrosis in patients with severe pancreatitis. Abdominal ultrasonography is also useful to detect cholelithiasis and bile duct dilation, but endoscopic ultrasonography is required to reliably detect choledocholithiasis. Magnetic resonance cholangiopancreatograpy (MRCP) is preferable to ERCP as a diagnostic study to visualize the common bile duct during pregnancy, unless endoscopic therapy is contemplated, because of potential fetal risks associated with ionizing radiation with ERCP.

Acute pancreatitis during pregnancy is usually mild and usually responds to medical therapy, including discontinuing oral intake, intravenous fluid administration, gastric acid suppression, analgesia, and sometimes nasogastric suction. Meperidine is the traditional choice for analgesia because it does not cause contraction of the sphincter of Oddi. Short-term administration of meperidine appears to be relatively safe during pregnancy.[19] **Pancreatitis complicated by a pancreatic phlegmon, abscess, sepsis, or hemorrhage necessitates antibiotic therapy, total parenteral nutrition, and possible radiologic aspiration or surgical debridement, with patient monitoring in an intensive care unit.** Large and persistent pancreatic pseudocysts require endoscopic or radiologic drainage or surgery. Endoscopic sphincterotomy can be performed for gallstone pancreatitis during pregnancy with minimal fetal radiation exposure. Pregnancy should not delay these therapies. **Laparoscopic cholecystectomy can be performed during pregnancy, and**

TABLE 45-1 Clinical Presentation and Treatment During Pregnancy of Common Pancreatic Disorders Minimally Affected by Pregnancy

DISEASE OR DISORDER	SYMPTOMS AND SIGNS	LABORATORY FINDINGS	TREATMENT
Acute pancreatitis	Epigastric pain radiating to back, nausea and vomiting, pyrexia, abdominal tenderness, guarding, abdominal distention.	Increased serum lipase, leukocytosis. Abdominal ultrasound—pancreatomegaly, peripancreatic inflammation, inhomogeneous pancreas.	Discontinue oral intake, aggressive IV hydration, analgesia, nasojejunal feeding or TPN for prolonged bout of pancreatitis.
Acute cholecystitis	Epigastric or RUQ pain, nausea and vomiting, tachycardia, Murphy's sign.	Leukocytosis, variably, mildly elevated LFTs. Abdominal ultrasound—thickened gallbladder wall, pericholecystic fluid, gallstones in gallbladder.	Discontinue oral intake, IV hydration, analgesia, antibiotics. Cholecystectomy can be performed during pregnancy, particularly during second trimester.
Choledocholithiasis with ascending cholangitis	RUQ pain, pyrexia, jaundice (Charcot's triad). Epigastric tenderness.	Leukocytosis, jaundice, variably elevated other LFTs. Abdominal ultrasound—dilated choledochus, possible gallstones in gallbladder.	Discontinue oral intake, IV hydration, antibiotics. Therapeutic ERCP may be performed during pregnancy to remove CBD stones (see text).

CBD, Common bile duct; *ERCP*, endoscopic retrograde cholangiography; *IV*, intravenous; *LFTs*, liver function tests; *RUQ*, right upper quadrant; *TPN*, total parenteral nutrition.

is best performed during the second trimester after organogenesis has occurred and before the growing gravid uterus interferes with visualization of the laparoscopic field. Maternal mortality rate is low in uncomplicated pancreatitis, but may exceed 10% in complicated pancreatitis. Pancreatitis is occasionally associated with fetal death during the first trimester, and is associated with premature labor in the third trimester.

Cholelithiasis and Cholecystitis

Pregnancy promotes bile lithogenicity and sludge formation because estrogen increases cholesterol synthesis and progesterone impairs gallbladder motility. In large population surveys using abdominal ultrasonography, 12% of pregnant women in Chile had cholelithiasis[20] and 8% of pregnant women in the United States had cholelithiasis or biliary sludge detected by abdominal ultrasonography. **Most gallstones are asymptomatic during pregnancy.**[21] **Complications of cholelithiasis include biliary colic, cholecystitis, choledocholithiasis, jaundice, ascending cholangitis, hepatic abscess, and gallstone pancreatitis. Pregnancy does not increase the frequency or severity of these complications.**[21] Symptoms of gallstone disease during pregnancy are the same as in nonpregnant individuals.[20,21] The usual initial symptom is biliary colic that is located in the epigastrium or right upper quadrant and may radiate to the back or shoulders. Pain can occur spontaneously or be induced by eating a fatty meal. The pain typically lasts for several hours. Diaphoresis, nausea, and emesis are common. Physical examination is unremarkable, other than occasional right upper quadrant tenderness. About two thirds of patients with biliary colic will experience recurrent attacks during the ensuing 2 years.[3]

Acute cholecystitis is a chemical inflammation usually caused by cystic duct obstruction by a gallstone. It is the third most common nonobstetrical surgical emergency during pregnancy, with an incidence of about 4 cases per 10,000 pregnancies. As in biliary colic, the pain is located in the epigastrium and right upper quadrant, but the pain is usually more severe and prolonged. Other clinical findings include nausea, emesis, pyrexia, tachycardia, right-sided subcostal tenderness, Murphy's sign, and leukocytosis. Serum biochemical parameters of liver function and serum levels of amylase may be mildly abnormal. Jaundice suggests choledocholithiasis, and pronounced hyperamylasemia suggests gallstone pancreatitis.

Most cases of biliary colic and some cases of mild acute cholecystitis can be managed conservatively with close observation, expectant management, and deferral of surgery to immediately postpartum.[14] **However, women with recurrent biliary colic or with acute cholecystitis usually require cholecystectomy.**[20,22] Preoperative management includes discontinuing oral intake, administration of intravenous fluids, analgesia, and, usually, antibiotics. Ampicillin, cephalosporins, and clindamycin are relatively safe antibiotics during pregnancy.[23] Cholecystectomy is best performed during the second trimester. Cholecystectomy has, however, become increasingly accepted during the first and third trimesters because of improved surgical outcomes.[22] Tocolysis may be necessary during cholecystectomy performed in the third trimester. Intraoperative cholangiography is only performed during pregnancy for strong indications to avoid radiation teratogenicity. Laparoscopic cholecystectomy is safe during pregnancy and is best performed during the second trimester.[3,21]

Choledocholithiasis

Symptomatic choledocholithiasis is uncommon during pregnancy. Choledocholithiasis can produce gallstone pancreatitis, manifested by pyrexia, nausea, and severe abdominal pain; or ascending cholangitis manifested by pyrexia, right upper quadrant pain, and jaundice (Charcot's triad). Endoscopic ultrasound is relatively safe in pregnancy and is sensitive in detecting choledocholithiasis.[8] Patients with choledocholithiasis and gallstone pancreatitis should undergo endoscopic retrograde cholangiography and sphincterotomy with stone extraction, as previously described. Pancreatography can be avoided to minimize fetal radiation exposure. These women then usually undergo cholecystectomy postpartum, but can, if necessary, undergo cholecystectomy antepartum, especially during the second trimester, with acceptable maternal and fetal mortality.

Choledochal Cysts

Choledochal cysts are rare. They typically produce a diagnostic triad of abdominal pain, jaundice, and a palpable abdominal mass in nonpregnant patients. Choledochal cysts are classified as types I to V according to which segment of the biliary tree is dilated. Pregnancy can exacerbate the abdominal pain and can increase the jaundice because of choledochal compression by the enlarged gravid uterus. However, pregnancy can mask the palpable abdominal mass due to the enlarged gravid uterus.[24] Severe pain suggests cyst rupture or concomitant pancreatitis.[24] A choledochal cyst can be diagnosed by abdominal ultrasound, although cholangiography is sometimes required. MRI is preferred over abdominal CT or diagnostic ERCP. Surgical management is generally recommended for symptomatic choledocholithiasis because of the risk of recurrent cholangitis and malignant degeneration. The standard surgery is cystectomy, cholecystectomy, and reconstitution of biliary-intestinal flow by either a Roux-en-Y hepaticojejunostomy or choledochojejunostomy. Medical management, including antibiotics and temporary percutaneous or endoscopic drainage, may sometimes suffice until delivery.[24]

COMMON LIVER DISEASES INCIDENTAL TO PREGNANCY

Acute Viral Hepatitis A, B, and C

Acute viral hepatitis A, B, and C (see Chapter 50) present similarly in pregnancy as in the nonpregnant state. For example, acute hepatitis B is usually self-limited and mild during pregnancy. Typical symptoms of acute viral hepatitis include anorexia, nausea, malaise, and right upper quadrant discomfort. Patients with acute hepatitis A or hepatitis B typically have highly elevated serum aminotransferase levels. Jaundice may occur. Acute hepatitis C is frequently subclinical and typically causes only mild serum aminotransferase level elevations. Maternal mortality is rare from acute hepatitis A, B, or C during pregnancy.

Fetal mortality and neonatal morbidity are increased by acute hepatitis A or B, but are still relatively low.

Wilson's Disease

Noncirrhotic women treated for early Wilson's disease have relatively intact fertility and may therefore become pregnant. Their serum levels of copper and ceruloplasmin increase during pregnancy. They require maintenance therapy during pregnancy to prevent a flare of disease that can increase maternal morbidity and fetal mortality. Although the data are limited, trientine (triethylene tetramine dihydrochloride) or zinc therapy for Wilson's disease may be maintained during pregnancy without significant fetal toxicity.[25] D-penicillamine is regarded as potentially teratogenic, and its use during pregnancy should be discouraged when alternatives are available. Women with cirrhosis from Wilson's disease have increased risks of complications during pregnancy, including intrauterine growth retardation and preeclampsia.

Autoimmune Hepatitis

Women with autoimmune hepatitis should be maintained on immunosuppressive therapy during pregnancy. Glucocorticoids such as prednisone are relatively safe during pregnancy.[26] Patients with well-compensated and well-controlled autoimmune hepatitis tolerate pregnancy well.[26] These women typically have a reversible mild deterioration of serum parameters of liver function during pregnancy, particularly of the serum bilirubin and alkaline phosphatase, attributed to the cholestatic effects of pregnancy. Women who discontinue the immunosuppressive therapy can develop severe acute flares during pregnancy.

Hepatic Hemangiomas, Cysts, and Abscesses

Hepatic hemangiomas are the most common benign tumors of the liver in the general population. The vast majority of hepatic hemangiomas less than 5 cm are asymptomatic in the general population. Hepatic hemangiomas appear to behave similarly during pregnancy. Rare symptoms attributable to hemangiomas include right upper quadrant pain, abdominal distention, or symptoms, such as nausea, attributable to impingement of adjacent viscera. Serious complications during pregnancy include consumptive coagulopathy with hemolysis, thrombocytopenia, and hypofibrinogenemia (Kasabach-Merritt syndrome); intrahepatic hemorrhage; and spontaneous hepatic rupture. Immense hemangioma size is the major risk factor for these complications. Warning signs include progressively increasing symptoms and rapid lesion growth. These complications are rare during pregnancy. Among 20 patients with mostly very large hemangiomas, only one case of hepatic rupture and one case of intrahepatic hemorrhage occurred during 27 pregnancies.[27] Focal nodular hyperplasia is the second most common cause of a benign hepatic mass. It is usually asymptomatic during pregnancy and detected incidentally during obstetrical ultrasound.[8] This lesion occasionally grows during pregnancy, possibly because of estrogen stimulation. Most cases can be observed during pregnancy without intervention. It rarely causes hepatic hemorrhage or biliary obstruction due to compression by the enlarged gravid uterus.[27,28] Clinical findings may include abdominal pain, jaundice, or hypotension. Surgical intervention is occasionally necessary for these complications.[28]

Hepatic cysts may be isolated or associated with polycystic kidney disease, malignancy, or amebic or ecchinococcal infection.[28] Pyogenic liver abscesses during pregnancy arise from ascending cholangitis, appendicitis, or diverticulitis.[28] Both antibiotics and percutaneous drainage are usually indicated.

Hepatocellular Carcinoma and Hepatic Metastases

Hepatocellular carcinoma (HCC) usually occurs in the setting of cirrhosis secondary to chronic viral hepatitis, hemochromatosis, or alcoholism. It is rarely diagnosed during pregnancy.[28] The poor prognosis during pregnancy may result from delayed diagnosis or mild immunosuppression during pregnancy. Screening high-risk patients by serum alpha-fetoprotein determination and abdominal ultrasonography can detect HCC earlier.[28] The fibromellar variant of HCC, typically found in younger women, has a better prognosis. Hepatic metastases, particularly from colon cancer, can occur during pregnancy.[4]

LIVER DISEASES SIGNIFICANTLY AFFECTED BY PREGNANCY

Hepatitis E

Hepatitis E, although rare and sporadic in industrialized countries, is the most common epidemic water-borne form of hepatitis in developing countries. It is usually transmitted by fecal-oral transmission through a contaminated water supply. Infected patients typically have a prodrome with malaise and pyrexia, followed by an acute illness with anorexia, nausea, vomiting, abdominal pain, and jaundice. Patients often have hepatomegaly and usually have significant elevations of the serum aminotransferase levels. The infection is typically mild and self-limited without chronicity or clinical sequelae.

Pregnant patients with hepatitis E have a more severe illness, with frequent fulminant hepatitis. The mortality rate rises progressively with the term of pregnancy up to about 20% mortality rate for acute infection in the third trimester.[29] Maternal infection is likewise associated with a high risk of fetal or neonatal mortality. Medical management is supportive. Fulminant hepatitis should be managed in an intensive care unit (ICU) and may require liver transplantation. The cause of the increased severity of this hepatitis during pregnancy is unknown, but may relate to attenuated cellular immunity during pregnancy.

In the United States, this infection is rare and not routinely tested for in the evaluation of acute hepatitis, but should be tested for when patients with an acute hepatitis have recently traveled to an endemic area and have had hepatitis A, B, and C excluded by serologic tests. The infection is generally diagnosed by detecting anti-HEV antibodies in the serum. Acute infection is diagnosed by detection of IgM antibodies, whereas prior infection is

TABLE 45-2 CLINICAL PRESENTATION AND TREATMENT DURING PREGNANCY OF HEPATIC DISORDERS SIGNIFICANTLY AFFECTED BY PREGNANCY

DISEASE OR DISORDER	SYMPTOMS AND SIGNS	LABORATORY FINDINGS	TREATMENT
Hepatitis E	Anorexia, nausea and vomiting, RUQ abdominal pain, jaundice, hepatomegaly.	Significantly elevated aminotransferase levels, mild jaundice. IgM antibodies to hepatitis E. PCR for hepatitis E virus.	Supportive care. Prevention by public health measures: avoid drinking municipal water in endemic areas.
Acute intermittent porphyria	Diffuse abdominal pain, vomiting, constipation, neuropsychiatric abnormalities.	Increased porphobilinogen and delta-aminolevulinic acid levels in urine.	Hematin, parenteral glucose. Avoid precipitating drugs, avoid fasting. Narcotics or phenothiazines for symptomatic relief.
Budd-Chiari syndrome	Abdominal pain, hepatomegaly, and ascites.	Moderately elevated bilirubin and alkaline phosphatase. Relatively normal aminotransferase levels. Doppler ultrasound, hepatic venography, or MRA—no flow in hepatic vein.	Low-sodium diet and diuretics to manage ascites and fluid retention. Consider anticoagulation while balancing benefits versus risks. Consider thrombolytic therapy or angioplasty for an acute clot (but scant data on this therapy during pregnancy).

IgM, Immunoglobulin M; *MRA*, magnetic resonance angiography; *PCR*, polymerase chain reaction; *RUQ*, right upper quadrant.

diagnosed by detection of IgG antibodies. Detection of the virus in blood by PCR is more accurate than serologic tests. Tests for hepatitis E are not commercially available in the United States, but may be obtained via the Centers for Disease Control and Prevention (CDC). The infection is largely prevented by public health measures, such as a clean water supply. Pregnant women should avoid travel to endemic areas, should not drink water from the municipal water supply in endemic areas, should not consume uncooked shellfish or vegetables from endemic areas, and should wash all fruit from endemic areas using uncontaminated water. Table 45-2 summarizes the clinical presentation, diagnostic tests, and treatment during pregnancy of hepatitis E, as well as other hepatic disorders significantly affected by pregnancy.

Chronic Hepatitis B

Pregnancy does not appear to significantly affect the progression of chronic hepatitis B.[30] Maternal chronic hepatitis B infection may, however, be transmitted to the neonate, usually during delivery. The risk of vertical transmission is about 90% in mothers who are hepatitis B-e antigen positive, but is only about 25% in mothers who are hepatitis B-e antigen negative.[31] Perinatal infection is clinically important because infected neonates tend to become chronic carriers and then have a markedly increased risk of developing hepatocellular carcinoma in adulthood. All pregnant women should be tested for hepatitis BsAg in the United States.[30] Infants born to infected mothers should be passively immunized with hepatitis B hyperimmune globulin (HBIG) and actively immunized with hepatitis B vaccine immediately after birth to prevent neonatal infection from intrapartum exposure.

Chronic Hepatitis C

Women with chronic hepatitis C may exhibit transient normalization of their serum aminotransferase levels associated with an increase in the serum viral load during pregnancy, possibly due to mildly attenuated immunity. The clinical significance of this phenomenon in terms of progression of the liver disease is unclear, but chronically infected patients may develop mild progression of their liver disease, as evidenced by increased hepatic fibrosis, during pregnancy.

The risk of vertical transmission of hepatitis C from a chronically infected mother with viremia to the neonate is about 5%.[32] Viral transmission to the neonate is unlikely in mothers who have an undetectable viral load. Infants born to mothers with hepatitis C infection should undergo periodic testing for hepatitis C during the first 18 months of life to detect persistent infection.

Hepatic Adenomas

Hepatic adenomas are benign hepatic tumors that are promoted by hyperestrogenemia. They are composed of large plates of adenoma cells that are typically larger than ordinary hepatocytes. Pregnancy is associated with accelerated adenoma growth and consequent development of symptoms, such as nausea, vomiting, and right upper quadrant pain. Risks during pregnancy include adenoma hemorrhage or intraperitoneal rupture. On MRI, adenomas are typically well demarcated, hyperintense on T2-weighted images, and enhance further with gadolinium administration. Hepatic adenomas that are symptomatic or larger than 5 cm in diameter should be considered for surgical excision before conception in women contemplating pregnancy.

Acute Intermittent Porphyria

The porphyrias are rare diseases caused by deficiency of various heme biosynthetic enzymes that result in accumulation of toxic porphyrin precursors. Acute intermittent porphyria (AIP), due to porphobilinogen deaminase deficiency, is the most common hepatic porphyria, with a frequency of about 1 per 10,000 people. Acute intermittent porphyria is transmitted as an autosomal trait with incomplete penetrance and is strongly affected by environmental factors, including female sex hormone levels. Women have more severe symptoms than men, and their symptoms are exacerbated by oral contraceptive administration or during menstruation and pregnancy.[33] About one third of female patients present initially during pregnancy or immediately postpartum. Hyperemesis gravidarum is a common precipitant. Diffuse abdominal pain is common. Other symptoms include vomiting, constipation, and neuropsychiatric abnormalities. Autonomic abnormalities can cause tachycardia, hypertension, or ileus. Unlike other porphyrias, AIP lacks dermatologic manifestations.

AIP should be considered in any pregnant patient with abdominal pain and a puzzling diagnostic evaluation. Increased urinary levels of porphobilinogen and delta-aminolevulinic acid are diagnostic. Management includes avoidance of precipitating drugs, avoidance of fasting, and possible administration of hematin or parenteral glucose. Abdominal pain and nausea and vomiting should also be treated with narcotic analgesics or phenothiazines. The maternal mortality rate is less than 10%, with a fetal mortality rate of 13% and frequent low-birth-weight infants.[33] Genetic counseling is recommended.

Sickle Cell Hemoglobinopathies

The sickle hemoglobinopathies, including hemoglobin SS, hemoglobin SC, and hemoglobin S/β-thalassemia, are the most common hematologic disorders during pregnancy. They mostly occur in African Americans. Patients with these hemoglobinopathies are prone to develop preeclampsia, eclampsia, or sickle crisis during pregnancy.[34] They can develop ischemia and microinfarction of multiple organs including extremities, joints, and abdominal viscera.[34] The abdominal pain in sickle crisis can be excruciating. Hemoglobin SS patients have an increased risk of acute cholecystitis during pregnancy.[21,34]

Portal Hypertension

Pregnancy is uncommon in cirrhotic women because they frequently experience anovulation and amenorrhea secondary to abnormal estrogen and endocrine metabolism.[35] However, patients with well-compensated, early cirrhosis occasionally become pregnant. The plasma volume gradually increases during pregnancy to a maximum of about 40% above baseline.[36] The primary contributing factor is sodium retention mediated by increased serum aldosterone, estrogen, and rennin levels, but water retention is a secondary factor.[36] The maternal cardiac output increases in proportion with the plasma volume. Portal pressure appears to physiologically increase during pregnancy due to these increases in plasma volume and cardiac output, as well as increased vascular resistance due to external compression of the inferior vena cava by the gravid uterus. **Pregnancy can therefore exacerbate preexisting portal hypertension; can cause shunting of blood into portosystemic collaterals, particularly esophageal varices; can increase intravariceal pressure; and can increase the risk of variceal hemorrhage. About 30% of pregnant patients with portal hypertension develop variceal hemorrhage, and about 75% of pregnant women with preexisting esophageal varices develop variceal hemorrhage.**[36] The risk of variceal hemorrhage is highest during the second trimester when the portal hypertension peaks, and during labor when venous collateral resistance abruptly increases from use of the Valsalva maneuver to push the fetus through the birth canal. Pregnancy has variable effects on the progression of cirrhosis. **About 25% of cirrhotics experience hepatic failure during pregnancy. Others have relatively stable hepatic function during pregnancy.** Some treatments for specific liver diseases during pregnancy have to be modified during pregnancy to avoid fetal toxicity. Maternal mortality rate in cases of cirrhosis may be as high as 10%.[35]

Portal hypertension without cirrhosis is usually due to portal vein obstruction or hepatic fibrosis. Female fertility is much better preserved in portal hypertension without cirrhosis than with cirrhosis. Pregnant patients, therefore, more frequently have portal hypertension without cirrhosis than with cirrhosis. Noncirrhotic patients with portal hypertension have a much lower mortality risk from each episode of variceal hemorrhage than cirrhotic patients due to better preserved liver function, a lower incidence of coagulopathy or thrombocytopenia, and a much lower risk of hepatic failure precipitated by variceal hemorrhage.

Women with prior variceal hemorrhage or with borderline liver function contemplating pregnancy should be advised of the high risks of maternal hepatic decompensation or variceal hemorrhage during pregnancy and associated poor fetal outcomes. They should also be advised of the risk of transmitting genetic hepatic diseases, such as α_1-antitrypsin deficiency, or of transmitting hepatotropic viral infections, such as hepatitis B, to their offspring. Women with well-compensated chronic liver disease without prior variceal hemorrhage should undergo esophagogastroduodenoscopy before conception for risk stratification. Women with silent esophageal varices are at high risk of variceal hemorrhage during pregnancy, whereas patients without esophageal varices are at low risk of this complication during pregnancy. Women with esophageal varices should be informed of the benefits of β-adrenergic receptor antagonists during pregnancy to reduce portal pressure, but should also be advised of the association of fetal bradycardia and growth retardation with these medications.

About 2.5% of cirrhotics experience splenic artery rupture during pregnancy. Pregnant women with portal hypertension should undergo an ultrasound examination with Doppler studies of the upper abdomen to screen for splenic artery aneurysms at the time of their routine antenatal pelvic ultrasound. Administration of iron is contraindicated in pregnant patients with hemochromatosis and is inadvisable in pregnant patients with several other types of chronic liver disease, such as chronic hepatitis C. Routine serum parameters of liver function, including a coagulation profile, should be serially monitored during pregnancy. Variceal hemorrhage during pregnancy, like variceal hemorrhage without pregnancy, should be initially treated with endoscopic variceal banding or sclerotherapy, as mentioned. Octreotide therapy is normally administered before the endoscopic therapy and maintained for several days after the endoscopic therapy in nonpregnant patients. Several cases of prolonged administration of octreotide for pituitary tumors have been reported in pregnant patients with good pregnancy outcomes. During parturition, the second part of labor should be kept brief to minimize portal hypertension, intravenous fluids should be administered cautiously to avoid volume overload, and any coagulopathy should be corrected to minimize the risk of intrapartum variceal hemorrhage.[36]

Budd-Chiari Syndrome

The Budd-Chiari syndrome refers to hepatic vein thrombosis or occlusion that increases the hepatic sinusoidal pressure and can lead to portal hypertension or hepatic necrosis.[37] Many cases are secondary to congenital vascular anomalies or hypercoagulopathies. This syndrome is rare in pregnancy even though pregnancy tends to promote this syndrome due to pregnancy-related increases in the serum level of estrogen and pregnancy-related decreases in the serum level of antithrombin III.[38] This syndrome usually manifests in the last trimester or the puerperium. The characteristic clinical triad is abdominal pain, hepatomegaly, and ascites.[38] Acute and chronic manifestations occur. The serum bilirubin and alkaline phosphatase levels are typically moderately elevated, with normal to mildly elevated serum aminotransferase levels. This syndrome is diagnosed by pulsed Doppler ultrasound, hepatic venography, or magnetic resonance angiography.[38] Without therapy death usually occurs within one decade after diagnosis. The definitive therapy is liver transplantation. Selective thrombolytic therapy and surgical or radiologic remedy of portal hypertension for intractable ascites or variceal bleeding have also been described.[38] Anticoagulant therapy is often administered chronically during pregnancy to prevent further thrombotic events, but is associated with a moderate risk of bleeding events such as intrauterine hematomas.[39] Maternal outcome is generally good, but about 30% of pregnancies result in fetal demise.[39] Patients have had subsequent successful pregnancies after undergoing liver transplantation for Budd-Chiari syndrome manifesting during the puerperium.

Pregnancy After Liver Transplantation

Although cirrhotic women are often infertile, women often regain fertility after successful liver transplantation for cirrhosis with restoration of liver function. Immunosuppressive therapy should be maintained during pregnancy after liver transplantation even though the fetal safety of many immunosuppressive therapies is not established. **Pregnancy appears to be relatively well tolerated after liver transplantation provided the transplanted liver functions well in the recipient before conception. Maternal complications during pregnancy include hypertension, preeclampsia, infections associated with immunosuppression, and occasionally acute hepatic rejection.**[40] Chronic immunosuppression with prednisone may result in gestational diabetes.

Fetal outcome is variable following liver transplantation, with an increase in prematurity and low birth weight observed.[40]

LIVER DISEASE STRONGLY RELATED OR UNIQUE TO PREGNANCY

Alcoholism During Pregnancy

Alcoholism during pregnancy can result in the fetal alcohol syndrome characterized by facial abnormalities such as an absent philtrum, and by growth retardation and neurodevelopmental deficits. Affected infants occasionally develop hepatic dysfunction, manifested by hepatomegaly, fatty liver, or elevations of serum aminotransferase or alkaline phosphatase levels.[41]

Hepatic Involvement in Hyperemesis Gravidarum

About 15% of women with hyperemesis gravidarum experience liver dysfunction, including several-fold elevations of the serum aminotransferase levels, jaundice, or pruritus. The hepatic dysfunction may be related to dehydration, malnutrition, and electrolyte abnormalities. This dysfunction is typically mild and resolves with cessation of the vomiting and reversal of the underlying metabolic abnormalities.

Herpes Simplex Hepatitis

Herpes simplex hepatitis is uncommon during pregnancy. However, about half of all cases of this hepatitis in immunocompetent adults occur during pregnancy, possibly due to attenuated immunity during pregnancy. **Herpes simplex hepatitis has a high mortality rate during pregnancy due to a propensity for viral dissemination and delayed diagnosis.**[42] Patients typically have right upper quadrant pain, very high serum aminotransferase levels, and moderate hyperbilirubinemia after a brief viral prodrome with fever and upper respiratory tract symptoms. An oral or genital cutaneous vesicular eruption in association with highly elevated serum aminotransferase levels should suggest the diagnosis. The diagnosis may be made by viral culture or histologic analysis of infected tissue. Acyclovir therapy is recommended. Table 45-3 summarizes the clinical presentation and treatment during pregnancy of herpes simplex hepatitis and other hepatic disorders that are strongly related or unique to pregnancy.

Intrahepatic Cholestasis of Pregnancy

The incidence of intrahepatic cholestasis of pregnancy (ICP) ranges from about 2 per 10,000 in the United States to about 20 per 10,000 in Europe.[43] The cardinal symptom is pruritus resulting from cholestasis and accumulated bile salts in the dermis. The pruritus typically most severely affects the palms and soles, becomes worse at night, and begins in the third trimester. The pruritus can be intense and can cause psychologic distress. Affected women occasionally experience anorexia, nausea, and vomiting. Proposed etiologic factors include genetic predisposition, as illustrated by the extremely high rate in the Araucanian Indians in Chile, and by familial clustering; gestational hyperestrogenemia, as supported by the known cholestatic effect of estrogen; and abnormal progesterone metabolism as supported by the cholestatic effects of sulfated progesterone metabolites.[36] This syndrome is sometimes related to defects in the multidrug resistance type-3 (MDR-3) gene that encodes for the canalicular phospholipid pump protein. Aside from family history, risk factors include multiple gestations and occurrence of this syndrome during previous pregnancies. **Patients typically develop hyperbilirubinemia that is mild and predominantly conjugated. About 10% of patients develop jaundice. Typically, the serum level of alkaline phosphatase is modestly elevated, whereas the level of gamma glutamyl transpeptidase (GGTP) is normal. The serum aminotransferase levels are typically several-fold higher than normal.** Patients have elevated fasting serum levels of total bile acids, particularly conjugated bile acids, and especially cholic acid.[36] Hepatic imaging studies reveal normal hepatic parenchyma and

TABLE 45-3 Clinical Presentation and Treatment During Pregnancy of Common Hepatic Disorders Strongly Related or Unique to Pregnancy

DISEASE OR DISORDER	SYMPTOMS AND SIGNS	LABORATORY FINDINGS	TREATMENT
Herpes simplex hepatitis	RUQ abdominal pain after prodrome of upper respiratory tract symptoms and pyrexia.	Highly elevated serum aminotransferase levels, moderately increased serum bilirubin. Viral culture or histologic analysis of infected tissue—diagnostic.	Acyclovir.
Intrahepatic cholestasis of pregnancy	Intense pruritus, occasional anorexia and nausea.	Modestly elevated serum bilirubin and alkaline phosphatase. Moderately elevated aminotransferase levels. Elevated total bile acid level—diagnostic.	Ursodeoxycholic acid (also antihistamines, phenobarbitol, or cholestyramine). Parturition rapidly and completely relieves cholestasis.
Preeclampsia and eclampsia	Hypertension, peripheral edema, RUQ abdominal pain, nausea and vomiting Seizures with eclampsia.	Proteinuria. Marked serum transaminase elevations and mild bilirubin elevation.	Tight control of blood pressure, frequent nonstress testing of fetus. Magnesium to prevent seizures. Abnormalities rapidly resolve with prompt delivery after 34 weeks of gestation.
HELLP syndrome	RUQ abdominal pain, nausea, vomiting, headache, mucocutaneous bleeding, RUQ tenderness.	Hemolytic anemia, low platelet count. Mildly elevated serum AST and bilirubin levels. Often associated with preeclampsia.	Treatment of coagulopathy. Frequent nonstress testing of fetus. Abnormalities rapidly resolve with prompt delivery after 34 weeks of gestation. Occasionally requires plasmapheresis.
Hepatic hemorrhage	RUQ pain, pyrexia, hypotension, hepatic tenderness. Commonly associated with HELLP syndrome or preeclampsia with DIC.	Anemia, leukocytosis, highly elevated serum aminotransferase levels. Abdominal CT—most accurate diagnostic test.	Correct coagulopathy and hemodynamically stabilize patient. Treatments—angiography with embolization, surgical evacuation of hematoma.
Acute fatty liver of pregnancy	Anorexia, nausea and vomiting, malaise, fatigue, RUQ abdominal pain.	Variable mildly elevated LFTs. Hepatic imaging—excludes other disorders. Test for LCHAD mutation. Long-chain 3-hydoxylacyl metabolites accumulate. Liver biopsy—microsteatosis in hepatocytes (liver biopsy usually unnecessary). DIC in severely ill patients.	Specific treatments for specific complications (e.g., blood products for DIC). Prompt fetal delivery after maternal stabilization. Patients rapidly improve after fetal delivery.

AST, Aspartate aminotransferase; *CT,* computed tomography; *DIC,* disseminated intravascular coagulation; *HELLP,* hemolysis, elevated liver function tests, and low platelets; *LCHAD,* long-chain 3-hydroxyacyl coenzyme A dehydrogenase; *LFTs,* liver function tests; *RUQ,* right upper quadrant.

anatomy. Liver biopsy reveals bile staining of hepatocytes and bile plugs in biliary cannaliculi, without necroinflammatory activity, findings consistent with cholestasis. **Ursodeoxycholic acid is the generally recommended therapy. It tends to normalize the serum bile acid profile by stimulating bile acid excretion and thereby decrease the pruritus.**[44] Other treatments designed to ameliorate the pruritus and/or lower the serum bile acid concentration have included hydroxyzine, an antihistamine, phenobarbitol, cholestyramine, and, possibly, S-adenosyl methionine.[36]

Parturition results in rapid and complete relief of the cholestasis. The maternal outcome is usually good without long-term sequelae. However, gestational cholestasis increases the risk of postpartum cholesterol cholelithiasis. Vitamin K deficiency resulting from mild steatorrhea, associated with the cholestasis itself or the cholestyramine therapy for the cholestasis, increases the risk of postpartum hemorrhage. The prothrombin time should be monitored during pregnancy, especially near parturition, and vitamin K administered as necessary. ICP results in a significantly increased incidence of poor fetal outcomes such as meconium ileus, premature delivery, or stillbirth. **Fetal testing is recommended to confirm the diagnosis; testing (bile acid elevation) may require up to 1 to 2 weeks to perform. In the absence of fetal distress, the delivery should be considered at or near term or after fetal maturity has been documented.** Cholestasis recurs in about two thirds of subsequent pregnancies.

Preeclampsia and Eclampsia

Preeclampsia, defined by new onset of hypertension and proteinuria, complicates 3% to 6% of pregnancies (see Chapter 35).[45] About 10% of patients with severe preeclampsia develop hepatic dysfunction attributed to hepatic hypoperfusion from vasoconstriction.[45,46] Symptoms include nausea, emesis, and right upper quadrant pain that may radiate to the right shoulder.[1] Severe pain may herald hepatic infarction, hemorrhage, or rupture.[2]

Right upper quadrant tenderness is common. Marked serum aminotransferase elevations and minimal to mild bilirubin elevations often occur.[1,45] Pathologic examination of a liver biopsy usually demonstrates sinusoidal fibrin deposition and periportal hemorrhage, and occasionally demonstrates hepatocellular necrosis. Hepatic involvement is often accompanied by hemolysis, thrombocytopenia, renal dysfunction, altered sensorium, eclampsia, or hepatic decompensation.[37]

Patients who present near term with mild preeclampsia have minimally increased mortality risk.[37,45] Eclampsia is a severe, life-threatening form of preeclampsia characterized by seizures.[1,45] Mortality rate exceeds 20% in women without prenatal care, but is less than 1% in cases managed in tertiary hospitals.[37,45] About 15% of the maternal mortality from eclampsia is attributable to hepatic complications including hepatic failure, hemorrhage, or infarction.[2,45] Fetal mortality rate is less than 5% in deliveries performed later than 34 weeks of gestation,[45] but is much higher in deliveries occurring during the second trimester.[37]

Hemolysis, Elevated Liver Function Tests, and Low Platelet Count (HELLP) Syndrome

The HELLP syndrome occurs in about 4 per 1000 pregnancies (see Chapters 35 and 42).[1,2] Women typically present in the third trimester or occasionally present postpartum.[47] Typical clinical findings include hemolytic anemia, thrombocytopenia, and abnormal results of serum liver function tests. Laboratory criteria for this syndrome include microangiopathic hemolysis with schistocytes present on the peripheral blood smear, platelet count less than 50,000/mm^3, serum total bilirubin greater than 1.2 mg/100 mL, serum lactate dehydrogenase greater than 600 U/L, and serum aspartate aminotransferase greater than 70 U/L. Risk factors include advanced maternal age, multiparity, white ethnicity, and preeclampsia.

Women usually have epigastric or right upper quadrant pain. Other symptoms include right shoulder pain, nausea, emesis, malaise, headache, visual disturbances, mucocutaneous bleeding, and jaundice.[47] Physical examination may reveal right upper quadrant tenderness and peripheral edema.[47] Patients usually have hypertension and proteinuria. Liver injury is caused by hepatic hypoperfusion due to intravascular fibrin deposition and hypovolemia.[35] Hepatic pathologic abnormalities include periportal hemorrhage, focal parenchymal necrosis with hyaline deposition, fibrin microthrombi, and steatosis. Liver biopsy is, however, rarely performed due to the thrombocytopenia.

This syndrome is a medical emergency, with risk for both maternal and fetal mortality that depends on the gestational age at diagnosis.[2,47]

Management of Preeclampsia, Eclampsia, and HELLP Syndrome

Preeclampsia, eclampsia, and HELLP syndrome are related disorders with shared pathogenic, pathologic, and clinical features.[1] Indeed, about 15% of patients with preeclampsia or eclampsia develop the HELLP syndrome.[2] Management is tailored to the clinical manifestations as well as the clinical diagnosis. Women with severe preeclampsia, eclampsia, or HELLP syndrome should be managed at a tertiary medical center. Delivery is the definitive therapy.[2,37] If these disorders manifest after 34 weeks of gestation and after documentation of fetal lung maturity, the fetus should be promptly delivered.[2,47] Vaginal delivery can usually be performed, but cesarean section is sometimes necessary, with use of general anesthesia and preoperative transfusion of platelets. Laboratory abnormalities usually peak during the first 48 hours postpartum. During this time period the patient should remain in an ICU and receive transfusions of platelets or clotting factors as necessary for DIC.[2,47] Hypertension is managed aggressively, with parenteral agents if necessary. Plasmapheresis has been used for persistence of the HELLP syndrome beyond 72 hours postpartum.[2,47] The platelet count normalizes within 1 week after delivery.[47]

Hepatic Hemorrhage and Rupture

One percent or more of women with the HELLP syndrome have a subcapsular hepatic hematoma. Other causes of hepatic hematomas include eclampsia or preeclampsia complicated by DIC, hepatic trauma, hepatic adenoma, and hepatocellular carcinoma.[48] Pain commonly occurs in the right upper quadrant, epigastrium, or right shoulder.[49] Signs include pyrexia, hypotension, hepatomegaly, hepatic tenderness, and rebound tenderness with peritonitis.[47,49] Patients may be in shock and with acute renal failure or acute respiratory failure. Laboratory findings include leukocytosis, anemia, and highly elevated serum aminotransferase levels. Laboratory findings may reflect HELLP or DIC if they are present, but are otherwise nonspecific. Pathologic examination of the liver reveals sinusoidal fibrin deposition and extensive, primarily periportal, hepatic hemorrhage.[2] Hepatic subcapsular hematoma can be diagnosed by ultrasonography or MRI, but CT scanning is the most sensitive and specific imaging test.

Both the maternal and perinatal mortality rates from hepatic hemorrhage exceed 30%. Women should be hemodynamically stabilized, and any coagulopathy should be corrected preoperatively.[47,49] **An unruptured, contained, subcapsular hematoma may sometimes be managed medically and expectantly, with frequent serial CT scans and close clinical monitoring.**[47] **Angiography is useful to diagnose and treat ongoing active hemorrhage in situations in which it is unclear if the hemorrhage has stopped.** Invasive therapies include evacuation of the hematoma with packing and drainage, angiographic embolization, hepatic artery ligation, or hepatic resection. The mortality rate is highest with hepatic lobectomy and lowest with transarterial embolization of a bleeding hepatic artery identified at angiography.[47,49]

Hepatic rupture is a rare but catastrophic complication of pregnancy resulting from progressive hepatic bleeding and stretch of Glisson's capsule.[48] Patients are usually multiparous and older.[48,49] The rupture usually involves the right hepatic lobe and usually occurs just before or just after delivery.[49] **Hepatic rupture is a medical emergency because the fetus poorly tolerates concomitant shock. The fetus should be rapidly delivered and the liver surgically repaired.** Patients with hepatic hemorrhage rarely have recurrence during subsequent pregnancies.

Acute Fatty Liver of Pregnancy

Acute fatty liver of pregnancy (AFLP) is a rare (1 in 10,000 pregnancies) but severe disease characterized by hepatic microvesicular steatosis associated with mitochondrial dysfunction. It is related to an autosomally inherited mutation that causes deficiency of the long-chain 3-hydroxyacyl coenzyme A dehydrogenase (LCHAD), a fatty acid beta-oxidation enzyme.[3] This mutation leads to accumulation of long-chain 3-hydroxyacyl metabolites produced by the fetus and placenta that are hepatotoxic. It usually manifests in the third trimester and rarely manifests immediately postpartum.[37,50] It is more common in primiparas and twin pregnancies. About half of patients exhibit signs of preeclampsia.[50,51]

The initial symptoms, including anorexia, nausea, emesis, malaise, fatigue, and headache, are nonspecific.[37,50] **About half of women have epigastric or right upper quadrant pain, and about half have hypertension.**[51] Physical examination may reveal hepatic tenderness, usually without hepatomegaly. Serum aminotransferase and bilirubin levels are variably elevated. Jaundice usually manifests later in the course of the illness or after delivery. Characteristic laboratory abnormalities in severely affected patients include a prolonged prothrombin time, hypofibrinogenemia, and increased serum levels of fibrin-split products. Other laboratory abnormalities include increased serum levels of ammonia, uric acid, blood urea nitrogen, and creatinine.[37,51] Hepatic imaging studies primarily help to exclude other disorders or to detect hepatic hemorrhage.[50]

Liver biopsy is usually diagnostic but is not indicated for suspected AFLP unless the presentation is atypical or the postpartum jaundice is prolonged.[1,51] Hepatic pathology reveals intracytoplasmic microsteatosis in hepatocytes, preservation of hepatic architecture, and isolated foci of inflammatory and necrotic cells.[51] Sinusoidal deposition of fibrin is usually not present in AFLP, but is usually present in preeclampsia and eclampsia.[51] AFLP differs from severe acute viral hepatitis in that the serum aminotransferase levels in AFLP rarely exceed 1000 U/L, the viral serologic tests are negative, and hepatic pathologic analysis reveals much less inflammatory infiltration and hepatocytic necrosis.[37,45,51] AFLP may be difficult to distinguish from HELLP syndrome and preeclampsia or eclampsia with DIC.[47] Fortunately, the definitive treatment for all these disorders is prompt fetal delivery after maternal stabilization that may include glucose infusion, reversal of coagulopathy, and administration of albumin. Most women improve clinically, and their liver function tests normalize within several days after delivery.[50]

Complications include pulmonary edema; pancreatitis; diabetes insipidus; DIC; seizures; coma; and hepatic failure manifested by jaundice, encephalopathy, ascites, or variceal bleeding.[50] The complications may require specific therapy: hepatic encephalopathy with lactulose, renal failure with hemodialysis, gastrointestinal bleeding with blood transfusions and endoscopic therapy, DIC with blood products, and diabetes insipidus with desmopressin (DDAVP). The maternal mortality rate is very low with early diagnosis, appropriate supportive therapy, and early delivery. The fetal mortality rate of AFLP is less than 15%.[2,51] The mother, neonate, and father should be tested for LCHAD mutations. Genetic testing is available for the most common mutation leading to LCHAD deficiency (G1528C mutation), but is unavailable for the other less common mutations.[52] AFLP rarely recurs in subsequent pregnancies.

KEY POINTS

- The differential of hepatobiliary conditions complicating pregnancy is extensive in that it includes pregnancy-related as well as pregnancy-unrelated disorders. Several clinical syndromes, such as intrahepatic cholestasis of pregnancy and acute fatty liver of pregnancy, are unique to pregnancy.
- Pregnancy affects the normative values of serum parameters of liver function and pancreatic injury. During pregnancy the serum level of albumin declines, whereas the serum levels of amylase, alkaline phosphatase, bile acids, cholesterol, and triglycerides rise.
- Many causes of significant liver dysfunction during pregnancy—including preeclampsia, eclampsia, HELLP syndrome, and acute fatty liver of pregnancy—are often rapidly relieved and completely reversed by delivery. Early delivery is generally the definitive therapy for these disorders.
- Pregnancy aggravates preexisting portal hypertension and increases the risk of variceal hemorrhage. Endoscopic sclerotherapy and banding are first-line therapies for esophageal variceal bleeding in pregnant patients.
- Pregnancy greatly aggravates acute hepatitis E infection, hepatocellular adenomas, acute intermittent porphyria, and herpes simplex hepatitis.
- Neonates born to mothers who have acute or chronic hepatitis B are at high risk of vertical transmission of infection during delivery. Such infants should be passively immunized with hepatitis B hyperimmune globulin and actively immunized with hepatitis B vaccine.

REFERENCES

1. Knox TA, Olans LB: Liver disease in pregnancy. N Engl J Med 335:569, 1996.
2. Riely CA: Liver disease in the pregnant patient; American College of Gastroenterology. Am J Gastroenterol 94:1728, 1999.
3. Cappell MS, Friedel D: Abdominal pain during pregnancy. Gastroenterol Clin North Am 32:1, 2003.
4. Cappell MS: Colon cancer during pregnancy. Gastroenterol Clin North Am 32:341, 2003.
5. Delgado I, Neubert R, Dudenhauseu JW: Changes in white blood cells during parturition in mothers and newborns. Gynecol Obstet Invest 38:227, 1994.
6. Bacq Y, Zarka O, Brechot JF, et al: Liver function tests in normal pregnancy: a prospective study of 103 pregnant women and 103 matched controls. Hepatology 23:1030, 1996.
7. Niebyl JR: Nausea and vomiting in pregnancy. N Engl J Med 363:1544, 2010.

8. Derchi LE, Serafini G, Gandolfo N, et al: Ultrasound in gynecology. Eur Radiol 11:2137, 2001.
9. Shellock FG, Crues JV: MR procedures: biologic effects, safety, and patient care. Radiology 232:635, 2004.
10. Toppenberg KS, Hill DA, Miller DP: Safety of radiographic imaging during pregnancy. Am Fam Physician 59:1813, 1999.
11. Cappell MS: The fetal safety and clinical efficacy of gastrointestinal endoscopy during pregnancy. Gastroenterol Clin North Am 32:123, 2003.
12. Tang SJ, Mayo MJ, Rodriguez-Frias E, et al: Safety and utility of ERCP during pregnancy. Gastrointest Endosc 69:453, 2009.
13. Jamidar PA, Beck GJ, Hoffman BJ, et al: Endoscopic retrograde cholangiopancreatography in pregnancy. Am J Gastroenterol 90:1263, 1995.
14. Date RS, Kaushal M, Ramesh A: A review of the management of gallstone disease and its complications in pregnancy. Am J Surg 196:599, 2008.
15. Cappell MS, Colon VJ, Sidhom OA: A study of eight medical centers of the safety and clinical efficacy of esophagogastroduodenoscopy in 83 pregnant females with follow-up of fetal outcome with comparison control groups. Am J Gastroenterol 91:348, 1996.
16. Kochhar R, Kumar S, Goel RC, et al: Pregnancy and its outcome in patients with noncirrhotic portal hypertension. Dig Dis Sci 44:1356, 1999.
17. Aggarwal N, Sawhney H, Vasishta K, et al: Non-cirrhotic portal hypertension in pregnancy. Int J Gynaecol Obstet 72:1, 2001.
18. Karsenti D, Bacq Y, Brechot JF, et al: Serum amylase and lipase activities in normal pregnancy: a prospective case-control study. Am J Gastroenterol 96:697, 2001.
19. Briggs GG, Freeman RK, Yaffe SJ: Meperidine. In Drugs in Pregnancy and Lactation: A Reference Guide to Fetal and Neonatal Risk. Philadelphia, Lippincott Williams & Wilkins, 2002, p 859.
20. Valdivieso V, Covarrubias C, Siegel F, et al: Pregnancy and cholelithiasis: pathogenesis and natural course of gallstones diagnosed in early puerperium. Hepatology 17:1, 1993.
21. Davis A, Katz VL, Cox R: Gallbladder disease in pregnancy. J Reprod Med 40:759, 1995.
22. Glasgow RE, Visser BC, Harris HW, et al: Changing management of gallstone disease during pregnancy. Surg Endosc 12:241, 1998.
23. Dashe JS, Gilstrap LC III: Antibiotic use in pregnancy. Obstet Gynecol Clin North Am 24:617, 1997.
24. Hewitt PM, Krige JE, Bornman PC, Terblanche J: Choledochal cyst in pregnancy: a therapeutic dilemma. J Am Coll Surg 181:237, 1995.
25. Brewer GJ, Johnson VD, Dick RD, et al: Treatment of Wilson's disease with zinc. XVII: treatment during pregnancy. Hepatology 31:364, 2000.
26. Aggarwal N, Chopra S, Suri V, et al: Pregnancy outcome in women with autoimmune hepatitis. Arch Gynecol Obstet 284:19, 2011.
27. Cobey FC, Salem RR: A review of liver masses in pregnancy and proposed algorithm for their diagnosis and management. Am J Surg 187:181, 2004.
28. Athanassiou AM, Craigo SD: Liver masses in pregnancy. Semin Perinatol 22:166, 1998.
29. Kumar A, Beniwal B, Kar P, et al: Hepatitis E: in pregnancy. Obstet Gynecol Surv 60:7, 2005.
30. Jonas MM: Hepatitis B and pregnancy: an underestimated issue. Liver Int 29:133, 2009.
31. Tong MJ, Thursby M, Rakela J, et al: Studies on the maternal-infant transmission of the viruses which cause acute hepatitis. Gastroenterology 80:999, 1981.
32. Su GL: Hepatitis C in pregnancy. Curr Gastroenterol Rep 7:45, 2005.
33. Milo R, Neuman M, Klein C, et al: Acute intermittent porphyria in pregnancy. Obstet Gynecol 73:450, 1989.
34. Villers MS, Jamison MG, de Castro LM, James AH: Morbidity associated with sickle cell disease in pregnancy. Am J Obstet Gynecol 199:125e1, 2008.
35. Joshi D, James A, Quaglia A, et al: Liver disease in pregnancy. Lancet 375:594, 2010.
36. Sandhu BS, Sanyal AJ: Pregnancy and liver disease. Gastroenterol Clin North Am 32:407, 2003.
37. Wolf JL: Liver disease in pregnancy. Med Clin North Am 80:1167, 1996.
38. Singh V, Sinha SK, Nain CK, et al: Budd-Chiari syndrome: our experience of 71 patients. J Gastroenterol Hepatol 15:550, 2000.
39. Rautou PE, Angermayr B, Garcia-Pagan JC, et al: Pregnancy in women with known and treated Budd-Chiari syndrome: maternal and fetal outcomes. J Hepatol 51:47, 2009.
40. Nagy S, Bush MC, Berkowitz R, et al: Pregnancy outcome in liver transplant recipients. Obstet Gynecol 102:121, 2003.
41. Lefkowitch JH, Rushton AR, Feng-Chen KC: Hepatic fibrosis in fetal alcohol syndrome: pathologic similarities to adult alcoholic liver disease. Gastroenterology 85:951, 1983.
42. Kang AH, Graves CR: Herpes simplex hepatitis in pregnancy: a case report and review of the literature. Obstet Gynecol Surv 54:463, 1999.
43. Davidson KM: Intrahepatic cholestasis of pregnancy. Semin Perinatol 22:104, 1998.
44. Pathak B, Shaibani L, Lee RH: Cholestasis of pregnancy. Obstet Gynecol Clin North Am 37:269, 2010.
45. Walker JJ: Pre-eclampsia. Lancet 356:1260, 2000.
46. Rolfes DB, Ishak KG: Liver disease in toxemia of pregnancy. Am J Gastroenterol 81:1138, 1986.
47. Barton JR, Sibai BM: Care of the pregnancy complicated by HELLP syndrome. Gastroenterol Clin North Am 21:937, 1992.
48. Sheikh RA, Yasmeen S, Pauly MP, et al: Spontaneous intrahepatic hemorrhage and hepatic rupture in the HELLP syndrome: four cases and a review. J Clin Gastroenterol 28:323, 1999.
49. Sibai BM, Ramadan MK, Usta I, et al: Maternal morbidity and mortality in 442 pregnancies with hemolysis, elevated liver enzymes, and low platelets (HELLP syndrome). Am J Obstet Gynecol 169:1000, 1993.
50. Monga M, Katz AR: Acute fatty liver in the second trimester. Obstet Gynecol 93:811, 1999.
51. Castro MA, Fassett MJ, Reynolds TB, et al: Reversible peripartum liver failure: a new perspective on the diagnosis, treatment, and cause of acute fatty liver of pregnancy, based on 28 consecutive cases. Am J Obstet Gynecol 181:389, 1999.
52. Bellig LL: Maternal acute fatty liver of pregnancy and the associated risk for long-chain 3-hydroxyacyl-coenzyme a dehydrogenase (LCHAD) deficiency in infants. Adv Neonatal Care 4:26, 2004.

For full reference list, log onto www.expertconsult.com.

Gastrointestinal Disorders During Pregnancy

Mitchell S. Cappell

KEY ABBREVIATIONS	
Computed Tomography	CT
Crohn's Disease	CD
Ectopic Pregnancy	EP
Esophagogastroduodenoscopy	EGD
Hyperemesis Gravidarum	HG
Inflammatory Bowel Disease	IBD
Irritable Bowel Syndrome	IBS
Lower Esophageal Sphincter	LES
Magnetic Resonance Imaging	MRI
Nonsteroidal Anti-inflammatory Drugs	NSAIDs
Pelvic Inflammatory Disease	PID
Peptic Ulcer Disease	PUD
Small Bowel Obstruction	SBO
Ulcerative Colitis	UC

Gastrointestinal complaints and disorders are common in women of all ages, including during the childbearing years, and thus often occur during pregnancy. These complaints and disorders present unique clinical challenges during pregnancy. First, the differential diagnosis during pregnancy is extensive. Aside from gastrointestinal disorders unrelated to pregnancy, complaints may signify underlying obstetrical disorders or other intra-abdominal diseases incidental to pregnancy. Moreover, some gastrointestinal conditions, such as hyperemesis gravidarum, are unique to pregnancy. Second, the clinical presentation and natural history of gastrointestinal disorders can be altered during pregnancy. Third, the diagnostic evaluation is altered and constrained by pregnancy. For example, radiologic tests and invasive examinations may raise concern about fetal safety. Fourth, the interests of both the mother and the fetus must be considered in therapeutic decision making during pregnancy.[1,2]

The obstetrician and gynecologist, as well as the gastroenterologist and surgeon, should be familiar with the medical and surgical gastrointestinal conditions that can occur in pregnancy and how these conditions affect and are in turn influenced by pregnancy. This chapter reviews gastrointestinal symptoms and disorders during pregnancy, with a focus on aspects of these disorders unique to pregnancy.

PHYSIOLOGIC EFFECTS OF PREGNANCY ON ABDOMINAL DISORDERS

Abdominal assessment during pregnancy is modified by displacement of abdominal viscera by the expanding gravid uterus. For example, the location of maximal abdominal pain and tenderness from acute appendicitis migrates superiorly and laterally as the appendix is displaced by the growing gravid uterus.[3] A rigid abdomen with rebound tenderness remains a valid indicator of peritonitis during pregnancy, but abdominal wall laxity and the interposition of the gravid uterus between the appendix and the anterior abdominal wall in late pregnancy may mask the classical signs of peritonitis. An abdominal mass may not be palpable on physical examination due to an enlarged gravid uterus.[2]

Many extraintestinal abdominal conditions or disorders are affected by pregnancy. Mild hydronephrosis and hydroureter are common during pregnancy, particularly during the early third trimester, due to diminished muscle tone in the urinary tract from elevated progesterone levels and mechanical obstruction from fetal compression. Hydronephrosis in pregnancy is usually asymptomatic, but can cause positional abdominal discomfort. Mucosal immunity may be attenuated during pregnancy as part of physiologic immunologic tolerance of the foreign fetal antigens in the uterus. This phenomenon, as well as urinary stasis during pregnancy, contributes to an increased rate of cystitis and pyelonephritis during pregnancy. Pregnancy also promotes cholelithiasis because of increased cholesterol synthesis and gallbladder hypomotility related to gestational hormone production.

Pregnancy modifies gastrointestinal physiology. Gastroesophageal reflux is promoted by gastric compression by the enlarged gravid uterus and by decreased lower esophageal sphincter tone due to decreased serum progesterone and motilin levels during pregnancy. Pregnancy also increases the risk of aspiration of gastric contents for the same reasons. Pregnancy may decrease gastric acid secretion due to increased progesterone levels. Small bowel motility decreases during pregnancy.[4] Constipation is promoted by decreased intestinal motility, mild intestinal compression by the enlarged gravid uterus, and increased recumbency from bed rest during pregnancy.

Physiologic alterations of laboratory values during pregnancy include mild leukocytosis, physiologic anemia of pregnancy, mild dilutional hypoalbuminemia, mildly increased alkaline phosphatase level, and electrolyte changes, particularly mild hyponatremia.[3,5] The erythrocyte sedimentation rate is physiologically elevated and is a less reliable monitor of inflammatory activity during pregnancy. The fetus poorly tolerates maternal hypotension, hypovolemia, anemia, and hypoxia. This intolerance affects the type and timing of therapy for abdominal disorders during pregnancy. The gravid uterus can compress the inferior vena cava in the supine position and thereby compromise venous return, aggravating systemic hypoperfusion from hypovolemia or gastrointestinal bleeding. Simply turning the patient to the left side to displace the uterus may relieve this compression, improve venous return, and normalize the blood pressure.[5]

DIFFERENTIAL DIAGNOSIS AND EVALUATION OF GASTROINTESTINAL SYMPTOMS DURING PREGNANCY

Physiologic changes during pregnancy may cause abdominal symptoms, including nausea, emesis, early satiety, bloating, pyrosis, and abdominal discomfort. Serious disorders that produce these symptoms may, therefore, be difficult to distinguish from physiologic changes during pregnancy. Significant symptoms should not be dismissed as normal during pregnancy without a careful history, physical examination, and appropriate evaluation. Pregnancy testing should be performed early in the evaluation of significant abdominal symptoms in all reproductive-age women.

Abdominal Pain

The differential diagnosis of abdominal pain during pregnancy is extensive in that it includes obstetrical conditions as well as the usual gastrointestinal and other intra-abdominal conditions in the general population.[3] Abdominal discomfort without other symptoms or signs can be due to an enlarging uterus, fetal pressure against adjacent organs, and uterine contractions associated with normal pregnancy. The abdominal pain is typically localized to the abdominal quadrant in which the afflicted organ is located, as illustrated for pain in the right lower quadrant in the box Differential Diagnosis of Right Lower Quadrant Abdominal Pain. This general rule has occasional exceptions in nonpregnant patients due to referred pain from other nearby regions, but has more frequent exceptions during pregnancy due to displacement of viscera by the growing gravid uterus and due to referred or poorly localized pain from obstetrical conditions.In the medical history, the pain intensity, nature, temporal pattern, radiation, exacerbating factors, and alleviating factors help narrow the differential diagnosis. Abdominal pain is typically progressive in appendicitis but is nonprogressive in viral gastroenteritis. The pain from small intestinal obstruction may be intermittent but is severe. Renal colic and biliary colic also produce a waxing and waning intensity of pain. Acute cholecystitis is associated with right upper quadrant pain, as well as pain referred to the right shoulder. The pain of acute pancreatitis is often boring in quality, located in the abdominal midline, and radiating to the back. Careful physical examination of the abdomen including inspection, palpation, and auscultation can further pinpoint the etiology. Laboratory evaluation of significant abdominal pain routinely includes a hemogram, serum electrolytes, and liver function tests, and often includes a leukocyte differential, coagulation profile, and serum lipase determination. In evaluating the laboratory results, gestational changes in normative values, as mentioned, must be considered. Radiologic tests may be extremely helpful diagnostically, but the choice of radiologic imaging may be influenced by pregnancy.

When the diagnosis is uncertain, close and vigilant monitoring by a surgical team, with frequent abdominal examination and regular laboratory tests, can often clarify the diagnosis. The character, severity, localization, or instigating factors of abdominal pain often change with time. For example, acute appendicitis typically changes from a dull, poorly localized, moderate pain to an intense and focal pain as the inflammation extends from the appendiceal wall to the surrounding peritoneum. The differential diagnosis of severe abdominal pain is described in Table 45-4.

Differential Diagnosis of Right Lower Quadrant Abdominal Pain

Gastrointestinal Disorders

Appendicitis
Crohn's disease
Ruptured Meckel's diverticulum
Intestinal intussusception
Cecal perforation
Colon cancer
Ischemic colitis
Irritable bowel syndrome

Renal Diseases

Nephrolithiasis
Cystitis
Pyelonephritis

Obstetrical and Gynecologic Diseases

Ruptured ectopic pregnancy
Ovarian tumors
Ovarian cyst rupture
Ovarian torsion
Endometriosis
Uterine leiomyomas

Other

Trochanteric bursitis

TABLE 45-4 Common Causes of Acute, Severe Abdominal Pain during Pregnancy: Pain Characteristics and Diagnostic Tests

CONDITION	PAIN LOCATION	CHARACTER	RADIATION	DIAGNOSTIC TESTS
Ruptured ectopic and abdominal pregnancy	Lower abdominal or pelvic	Localized, severe	None	Serum βhCG, abdominal ultrasound
Pelvic inflammatory disease	Lower abdominal or pelvic	Gradual in onset, localized	Flanks and thighs	Abdominal ultrasound
Appendicitis	First periumbilical, later RLQ (RUQ in late pregnancy)	Gradual in onset, becomes focal	Back or flank	Abdominal ultrasound in appropriate clinical setting
Acute cholecystitis	RUQ	Focal	Right scapula, shoulder, or back	Abdominal ultrasound and serum liver function tests
Pancreatitis	Epigastric	Localized, boring	Middle of back	Serum lipase and amylase, abdominal ultrasound
Perforated peptic ulcer	Epigastric or RUQ	Burning, boring	Right back	Abdominal ultrasound, laparotomy
Urolithiasis	Abdomen or flanks	Varies from intermittent and aching to severe and unremitting	Groin	Urinalysis, abdominal ultrasound, and occasionally fluoroscopy with contrast urography

hCG, Human chorionic gonadotropin; *RLQ*, right lower quadrant, *RUQ*, right upper quadrant.

Gastrointestinal causes of abdominal pain are discussed later under their individual headings in this section, and hepatobiliary causes are discussed in the previous section of this chapter. Obstetrical causes of abdominal pain are also prominent during pregnancy. Ectopic pregnancy (EP) classically manifests with abdominopelvic pain with or without vaginal bleeding after a period of amenorrhea. The pain may initially be diffuse and vague but later becomes focal and severe.[6]

Patients typically exhibit uterine tenderness and frequent uterine contractions. Sonography may be diagnostic.[6] Uterine rupture usually occurs in laboring women with abnormal fetal heart rate recordings or fetal death, uterine tenderness, peritoneal irritation, hypotension, and vaginal bleeding.

Severe preeclampsia can cause right upper quadrant (RUQ) pain and elevated serum transaminase levels. Women exhibit hypertension and proteinuria that starts after 20 weeks of gestation. Women with the HELLP (hemolysis, elevated liver enzymes, and low platelets) syndrome often have epigastric or RUQ pain. The patients have hemolysis with a microangiopathic peripheral blood smear, elevated liver transaminase levels, and thrombocytopenia. Acute fatty liver often causes abdominal pain, as well as nausea and vomiting, anorexia, and jaundice. The definitive treatment for these three pregnancy-related conditions of preeclampsia, HELLP syndrome, and acute fatty liver of pregnancy is prompt delivery after maternal stabilization.

Adnexal torsion typically causes lower abdominal pain that is sharp and sudden in onset. Signs include unilateral lower quadrant tenderness, a palpable adnexal mass, cervical tenderness, or rebound tenderness from peritonitis. Ultrasonography, including duplex scanning, is valuable in the detection of adnexal masses, particularly cysts.

The differential of abdominal pain during pregnancy includes renal disorders.[7] Symptoms from cystitis may include suprapubic discomfort, without frank abdominal pain, but patients usually have urinary frequency, urgency, or dysuria. The diagnosis is made by urinalysis and urine culture in the appropriate clinical setting.

Upper Gastrointestinal Symptoms

Nausea and Vomiting

Nausea and vomiting during pregnancy is most commonly due to nausea and vomiting of pregnancy or hyperemesis gravidarum, idiopathic disorders without demonstrable mucosal or mural disease. See the accompanying box, Differential Diagnosis of Nausea and Vomiting During Pregnancy, for many other conditions. Nausea and vomiting of pregnancy should be diagnosed only after exclusion of organic disorders by the history, physical findings, bloods tests, and appropriate diagnostic studies. Misdiagnosis of nausea and vomiting as nausea and vomiting of pregnancy rather than more severe diseases can be catastrophic.

Dyspepsia or Pyrosis

During pregnancy, gastroesophageal reflux disease (GERD) is extremely common, whereas peptic ulcer disease (PUD) is relatively uncommon (see the accompanying box, Differential Diagnosis of Dyspepsia or Pyrosis During Pregnancy). The diagnosis of GERD rather than PUD is suggested by pain radiating substernally, with the pain exacerbated by drinking acidic citrus drinks and by recumbency; symptoms of water brash or regurgitation; and presence of extraintestinal manifestations, including nocturnal asthma, hoarseness, laryngitis, or periodontal disease.

Differential Diagnosis of Nausea and Vomiting During Pregnancy

Nausea and vomiting of pregnancy
Hyperemesis gravidarum
Pancreatitis
Symptomatic cholelithiasis
Viral hepatitis
Peptic ulcer disease
Gastric cancer
Intestinal obstruction
Intestinal pseudo-obstruction
Gastroparesis diabeticorum
Gastritis
Gastroesophageal reflux disease
Acute pyelonephritis
Drug toxicity
Vagotomy
Preeclampsia/eclampsia
Acute fatty liver of pregnancy
Hemolysis, elevated liver enzymes, and low platelets (HELLP) syndrome
Anorexia nervosa/bulimia
Other neuropsychiatric disorders

Differential Diagnosis of Dyspepsia or Pyrosis During Pregnancy

Gastroesophageal reflux disease
Peptic ulcer disease
Nausea and vomiting of pregnancy
Hyperemesis gravidarum
Pancreatitis
Biliary colic
Acute cholecystitis
Viral hepatitis
Appendicitis
Acute fatty liver of pregnancy (in late pregnancy)
Irritable bowel syndrome/nonulcer dyspepsia

Hematemesis

Upper gastrointestinal bleeding is uncommon during pregnancy. Nausea and vomiting during pregnancy increases the risk of hemorrhage from a Mallory-Weiss tear. Decreased lower esophageal sphincter (LES) pressure and increased intragastric pressure during pregnancy promote gastroesophageal reflux that can cause hemorrhage. **The most common causes of gastrointestinal hemorrhage during pregnancy are GERD, gastritis, Mallory-Weiss tears, and ulcers.**[8] Unusual causes include esophageal varices and gastric cancer. Women with upper gastrointestinal bleeding that causes hemodynamic instability are approached like nonpregnant individuals, with the following caveats. In the general population the hematocrit is not a reliable indicator of bleeding severity because of the lag between blood loss and hematocrit decline. The hematocrit may be an even less reliable indicator of bleeding severity during pregnancy because of the conflicting effects of intravascular fluid accumulation and increased erythrocyte mass.

Fluid, including transfusions of packed erythrocytes when indicated, should be aggressively administered to pregnant women with acute gastrointestinal bleeding because of the extraordinary fetal sensitivity to hypoperfusion, the difficulty in assessing volume status during pregnancy, and the usually healthy cardiac function of pregnant patients.

Dysphagia

The differential of dysphagia during pregnancy is similar to that in the general adult population, except that esophageal cancers are uncommon in these relatively young adults. Pregnant women with acquired immunodeficiency syndrome may have dysphagia or odynophagia from esophageal candidiasis or esophageal lymphoma. Dysphagia from a peptic stricture is uncommon in pregnant patients, despite their high frequency of GERD, because they typically have short-term and uncomplicated GERD. Achalasia is a motility disorder that typically manifests with a high resting LES pressure, failure of the LES to relax with swallowing, and nonperistaltic esophageal muscle contractions. Achalasia causes dysphagia and weight loss.

Definitive therapy for severe dysphagia is best performed before, rather than during, pregnancy to ensure adequate nutrition during pregnancy, a paramount concern for normal fetal development. Thus, surgery for severe achalasia or other benign esophageal diseases should be performed before contemplated pregnancy.

Lower Gastrointestinal Symptoms

Diarrhea

The pathogenesis and differential diagnosis of diarrhea in pregnant women is similar to that in the nonpregnant population.[9] Acute diarrhea is usually caused by viral, bacterial, or parasitic enteropathogens. Viral agents, such as rotavirus and Norwalk virus, typically cause an acute self-limited diarrhea, with upper gastrointestinal symptoms, and rare long-term sequelae. Bacterial causes of diarrhea include Campylobacter, Shigella, pathogenic *Escherichia coli*, and Salmonella. Pseudomembranous colitis due to *Clostridium difficile* must be considered in the differential diagnosis when the diarrhea starts after antibiotic administration. Bacterial pathogens tend to produce frequent small-volume stools, abdominal pain, and pyrexia. Inflammation of intestinal mucosa may produce fecal blood or leukocytes. Bacterial colitis is usually diagnosed by stool analysis and stool cultures. Pregnant women with advanced human immunodeficiency virus infection are prone to opportunistic enteric bacterial, fungal, parasitic, and viral infections, which often cause diarrhea. Noninfectious causes of diarrhea include medications, functional causes, food intolerances, and inflammatory bowel disease. Hyperthyroidism can cause hyperdefecation. The initial management of severe acute diarrhea includes intravenous hydration, correction of electrolyte disorders, and consideration of discontinuing oral feedings. Stool studies include bacterial culture and sensitivity, ova and parasites, *C. difficile* toxin, and fecal leukocytes. Flexible sigmoidoscopy can be considered, despite pregnancy, for persistent, refractory diarrhea if the stool studies are unrevealing.

Constipation

Constipation is common in pregnancy, affecting up to one fourth of gravidae.[10] Pregnancy tends to promote constipation from poor fluid intake due to nausea and vomiting; iron supplementation; decreased patient mobility; slowed gastrointestinal transit predominantly due to the effects of progesterone[4]; and gastrointestinal compression by the enlarged gravid uterus.[9] General measures can reverse these constipating factors during pregnancy. Adequate fluid intake and moderate exercise are important. Increased fiber intake—either by increasing dietary fiber, such as wheat bran, or by administering medications, such as methylcellulose—is recommended to promote stool bulk and softness. Patients should be advised to defecate in the morning or after meals when colonic motor activity is stimulated via the gastrocolonic reflex. Sorbitol and lactulose, poorly absorbed sugars that cause an osmotic diarrhea, may be effective for constipation during pregnancy. However, they may cause abdominal bloating and flatulence; they should be used with caution in diabetic patients; and they should be avoided in pregnant patients with nausea because they can exacerbate this symptom. Stimulant laxatives, such as senna or bisacodyl, may be considered in patients with severe constipation who fail to respond to conservative measures, bulk laxatives, or osmotic laxatives. Laxatives to be avoided during pregnancy include castor oil because it may initiate premature uterine contractions, and hypertonic saline laxatives, such as phosphosoda, because they promote sodium and water retention, which may cause renal failure in patients who are dehydrated or have preexisting renal insufficiency.[9]

Rectal Bleeding

Hemorrhoids are the most common cause of rectal bleeding during pregnancy. Other causes in the differential diagnosis of rectal bleeding during pregnancy include ulcerative colitis, Crohn's disease, rectal fissure, and infectious colitis, as well as unusual diagnoses during pregnancy, such as diverticular bleeding, bowel ischemia, or colon cancer.

DIAGNOSTIC TESTING DURING PREGNANCY

Radiologic Imaging

Fetal safety during diagnostic imaging is a concern for pregnant patients and pregnant medical personnel. Ultrasonography is considered safe during pregnancy and is the preferred imaging modality for abdominal pain during pregnancy.[6] Unfortunately, test sensitivity depends on operator technique; patient cooperation; and patient anatomy, in that sensitivity is decreased by abdominal fat and intestinal gas.[6] Magnetic resonance imaging (MRI) is preferable to computed tomography during pregnancy to avoid ionizing radiation, but gadolinium administration should be avoided during the first trimester.[11] Rapid-sequence MRI is preferable to conventional MRI because of briefer exposure. The patient should undergo counseling before diagnostic roentgenography.[11] The safety of radiologic abdominal imaging during pregnancy is briefly summarized in Table 45-5.

TABLE 45-5 GENERAL PRINCIPLES REGARDING ABDOMINAL IMAGING TESTS DURING PREGNANCY

TEST	SAFETY DURING PREGNANCY
Abdominal ultrasound	Considered safe during pregnancy and is the preferred imaging modality during pregnancy. Unfortunately, test is less sensitive and less specific than other imaging modalities for many abdominal disorders.
Magnetic resonance imaging (MRI)	Considered relatively safe based on limited clinical data. Avoid administering gadolinium, particularly during the first trimester.
Abdominal radiographs	Occasionally radiographs are required, (e.g., abdominal supine and upright radiographs for suspected intestinal obstruction). Limit fetal radiation exposure by shielding, collimation, rapid-sequence studies, and modern x-ray equipment.
Computed tomography (CT) of abdomen	Generally avoid during pregnancy, especially during first trimester. Consider MRI as alternative when abdominal ultrasound is nondiagnostic. CT may be required in rare circumstances (e.g., to avoid surgery for possible but unproven appendicitis). Consult with a radiation physicist to minimize fetal radiation exposure.

Endoscopy during Pregnancy

Endoscopy is often performed in the evaluation of abdominal symptoms in nonpregnant patients. Flexible sigmoidoscopy is performed to evaluate minor lower gastrointestinal complaints, including rectal symptoms, and esophagogastroduodenoscopy (EGD) is performed to evaluate epigastric pain, dyspepsia, or pyrosis. Although endoscopy is extremely safe in the general population, endoscopy during pregnancy raises the unique issue of fetal safety.

Sigmoidoscopy seems to be relatively safe during pregnancy. No woman suffered endoscopic complications in a study of 46 patients undergoing sigmoidoscopy during pregnancy.[12] Excluding 1 unknown pregnancy outcome and 4 voluntary abortions, 38 of 41 pregnant women delivered healthy infants, including 27 at full term. Their mean Apgar scores were not significantly different from the mean national Apgar scores. Moreover, study patients did not have a worse outcome than pregnant controls matched for sigmoidoscopy indications who did not undergo sigmoidoscopy, in terms of mean infant Apgar scores at birth and in terms of the rates of fetal or neonatal demise, premature delivery, low birthweight, and delivery by cesarean section. Additionally, no endoscopic complications were reported in 13 flexible sigmoidoscopies during pregnancy analyzed by a mailed survey of 3300 gastroenterologists. All pregnancies resulted in delivery of healthy infants at term.

Data are limited on colonoscopy during pregnancy. The two largest studies consist of 20 and 8 pregnant patients.[12,13] In the study of 20 pregnant patients, 16 colonoscopies were performed during the second trimester. Excluding one successful therapeutic colonoscopy to decompress a severely dilated colon from colonic pseudo-obstruction, colonoscopy was diagnostic in 10 of 19 cases, including diagnoses of ulcerative colitis, ischemic colitis, Crohn's colitis, and lymphocytic colitis. Colonoscopy led to therapeutic changes in 7. Two minor maternal procedural complications of mild transient hypotension occurred without clinical sequelae. Fetal outcomes were generally favorable: all infants were born relatively healthy except for one spontaneous abortion and 1 infant born with congenital defects. Colonoscopy should be considered, particularly during the second trimester, for very strong indications during pregnancy, such as suspected colon cancer, after obtaining informed consent that includes the theoretical but unsubstantiated fetal risks of colonoscopy. A polyethylene glycol (PEG) balanced electrolyte solution is generally preferred over a sodium phosphate (Fleet's phophosoda) solution to cleanse the colon for colonoscopy because sodium phosphate is associated with renal failure or electrolyte abnormalities in dehydrated or otherwise at-risk patients.

EGD is relatively safe for the fetus and the pregnant mother. In a case-controlled study of 83 EGDs during pregnancy, the mean week of gestation was 20 weeks. Indications for EGD included gastrointestinal bleeding in 37, abdominal pain in 28, vomiting in 14, and other indications in 4.[8] EGD did not cause any maternal complications. EGD did not induce labor. Excluding 6 voluntary abortions and 3 unknown pregnancy outcomes, 70 (95%) of 74 patients delivered healthy infants. In this study, the 4 bad pregnancy outcomes, including 3 stillbirths or deaths from severe prematurity and 1 involuntary abortion, occurred in high-risk pregnancies and were unrelated to EGD temporally or etiologically. This study and two other studies of 60 pregnant patients undergoing EGD during the first trimester[14] and of 30 pregnant patients undergoing EGD during pregnancy[15] suggest that EGD is at least as safe as not performing EGD in pregnant patients with a strong indication for EGD. Similar results were reported in a study of 73 pregnant patients undergoing EGD, analyzed by a mailed survey of 3300 gastroenterologists.

EGD is recommended during pregnancy for hemodynamically significant upper gastrointestinal bleeding. EGD is rarely helpful and rarely necessary for nausea and vomiting, or even hyperemesis gravidarum, during pregnancy. EGD is reserved for atypical situations, such as severe and refractory nausea and vomiting accompanied by significant abdominal pain, hematemesis, or signs of gastroduodenal obstruction. EGD is neither necessary nor indicated to evaluate typical symptoms of gastroesophageal reflux during pregnancy. EGD is useful in diagnosing complicated PUD, including gastric outlet obstruction, malignant gastric ulcer, refractory ulcer, and persistently bleeding ulcer. EGD should be performed in relatively stable patients with electrocardiographic monitoring after obstetrical consultation and after normalization of vital signs, which may require transfusion of packed erythrocytes and supplemental oxygenation. Fetal monitoring should be performed, if available, once the fetal heart sounds become detectable. General measures to increase the benefit-to-risk ratio of endoscopy during pregnancy are listed in Table 45-6.[16,17]

TABLE 45-6 GENERAL PRINCIPLES TO IMPROVE THE BENEFIT-TO-RISK RATIO OF GASTROINTESTINAL ENDOSCOPY DURING PREGNANCY

PRINCIPLE	EXAMPLE
Perform endoscopy only for strong indications.	Colonoscopy for suspected colon cancer.
Avoid endoscopy or defer it until after delivery for weak or elective indications.	Colonoscopy for routine colon cancer screening.
Use the safest drugs for sedation and analgesia (Food and Drug Administration category B preferable or at most category C) in lowest possible dosages.	Use propofol (category B) or fentanyl (category C). Avoid diazepam (category D) because of possible, albeit unlikely, association with congenital cleft palate.
Consult an anesthesiologist regarding drug safety during pregnancy.	Monitored anesthesia care (MAC) with anesthesiologist present during endoscopy.
Preferably perform endoscopy in the second trimester, if possible, to avoid potential teratogenicity during fetal organogenesis in the first trimester, and to avoid premature labor or adverse effects on the neonate after delivery in the third trimester.	Defer endoscopy during first trimester, if possible, until second trimester. Defer endoscopy during third trimester, if possible, until after delivery.
Minimize procedure time.	Performance by an individual fellow-in-training, under supervision.
Obstetrical support should be available for a pregnancy-related procedure complication.	Perform procedure in an in-hospital endoscopy suite rather than a physician's office or an ambulatory surgical center.

Based on data from references 16 and 17.

Video capsule endoscopy is routinely used for recurrent gastrointestinal bleeding after nondiagnostic EGD and colonoscopy. The most common serious complication of video capsule endoscopy in the general population is capsule retention. Pregnancy may theoretically promote capsule retention due to displacement and impingement of bowel loops by the enlarged gravid uterus. Few data exist on video capsule endoscopy safety during pregnancy.[18]

GASTROINTESTINAL DISORDERS

Key differences during pregnancy in the clinical presentation, diagnosis, and therapy of gastrointestinal disorders are summarized in Table 45-7.

Predominantly Upper Gastrointestinal Disorders

Hyperemesis Gravidarum

Nausea and vomiting occurs in more than 50% of pregnancies. It typically begins at about 5 weeks of gestation and abates by about 18 weeks of gestation. It is commonly called morning sickness but may be designated more simply as nausea and vomiting of pregnancy or *emesis gravidarum* because it occurs throughout the day. This condition should be viewed as a physiologic rather than pathologic process during early pregnancy because this condition is generally not associated with unfavorable maternal or fetal outcomes. **Hyperemesis gravidarum (HG) is a severe, pathologic form of nausea and vomiting of pregnancy characterized by greater than 5% loss of prepregnancy weight and otherwise unexplained ketonuria.** The weight loss is paradoxic because patients normally gain weight during pregnancy. HG occurs in about 0.5% of pregnancies.[19] Risk factors include primigravidas, multiple gestation, molar pregnancy, prior unsuccessful pregnancy, and prior HG.[19] Like nausea and vomiting of pregnancy, HG typically begins early in pregnancy; severe vomiting beginning after the first trimester is unlikely from HG. In other pregnancy-related conditions that cause nausea and vomiting, including acute fatty liver of pregnancy, preeclampsia, and HELLP syndrome, the nausea and vomiting typically begins in the second half of pregnancy.

Nausea and vomiting of pregnancy and HG are diagnoses of exclusion, which are diagnosed only after other conditions are excluded by appropriate tests. An abdominopelvic ultrasound is performed to exclude other causes of nausea and vomiting and to exclude gestational trophoblastic disease and multiple gestation, conditions associated with HG. Women with epigastric or right upper quadrant pain should have serum liver function tests and serum lipase determination to exclude hepatobiliary and pancreatic disease. Women with nausea and vomiting complicated by dysphagia or hematemesis may require EGD. Women with nausea and vomiting during pregnancy associated with heartburn and regurgitation should be instructed about antireflux measures of diet and lifestyle modifications and should receive mild antireflux medications, as described later.

The pathophysiology is unknown, but is believed to be multifactorial. Human chorionic gonadotropin (hCG) has been proposed as an etiologic factor because the serum hCG level peaks when HG is most severe, and the serum hCG level is higher in patients with HG than in other pregnant patients. Other postulated etiologic factors include gestational hyperestrogenemia, gastric dysrhythmias, and hyperthyroidism.[19] Aside from nausea and vomiting, symptoms of HG include xerostomia, sialorrhea, and dysgeusia. Physical findings reflective of hypovolemia include dry mucous membranes, poor skin turgor, and hypotension or orthostatic hypotension. Serum electrolyte abnormalities include hyponatremia, hypocalcemia, and hypokalemia. An increased hematocrit reflects hemoconcentration from hypovolemia. Patients with severe vomiting may develop abnormal liver function tests, particularly elevations of the serum aminotransferases. Patients may exhibit mild, transient hyperthyroidism manifesting as low thyroid-stimulating hormone levels due to elevated serum hCG levels. Chronic vomiting of gastric contents may cause hypochloremic metabolic alkalosis. Inadequate nutrition can lead to vitamin or micronutrient deficiencies.

Therapy is initially focused on aggressive intravenous rehydration and restoration of electrolyte deficiencies. Vitamins should be repleted. Thiamine should be administered before administering dextrose to prevent Wernicke's encephalopathy. After intravenous repletion, the diet is gradually advanced, initially to salty fluids and then to a bland diet, as tolerated. Nutritional consultation is recommended. Nasoenteral or nasogastric feedings are useful alternatives in patients who cannot tolerate oral

TABLE 45-7 Key Differences During Pregnancy in the Clinical Presentation and Diagnosis of Gastrointestinal Disorders

DISEASE OR DISORDER	KEY DIFFERENCES DURING PREGNANCY
Mallory-Weiss tear	Much more common cause of upper gastrointestinal bleeding during pregnancy due to mechanical trauma at the GE junction from nausea and vomiting of pregnancy or hyperemesis gravidarum.
Nausea and vomiting of pregnancy	Extremely common during pregnancy. Condition is unique to pregnancy. Begins at about 5 weeks of gestation and abates by about 18 weeks of gestation. May be related to elevated serum human chorionic gonadotropin levels during early pregnancy.
Hyperemesis gravidarum	Very severe form of nausea and vomiting during pregnancy characterized by >5% loss of prepregnancy weight, serum electrolyte disorders, and ketonuria. Condition requires aggressive therapy.
Gastroesophageal reflux	Extremely common during pregnancy due to reduced lower esophageal sphincter tone due to gestational elevation of serum progesterone level and gastric compression by the enlarged gravid uterus. Although it may produce bothersome symptoms during pregnancy, serious complications of gastroesophageal reflux are unusual during pregnancy.
Acute appendicitis	Displacement of appendix by the enlarged gravid uterus during late pregnancy may cause the point of maximal abdominal pain and tenderness to migrate several cm superiorly and laterally from McBurney's point. Rate of appendiceal perforation from appendicitis is increased during pregnancy attributed to delayed diagnosis. Ultrasound is imaging test of choice during pregnancy to diagnose appendicitis to avoid fetal exposure to ionizing radiation. Appendectomy may be performed during pregnancy, but is most safe during the second trimester.
Intestinal obstruction	More common in third trimester because of mechanical effects of enlarged gravid uterus. Can occur during parturition because of mechanical effects of fetal head descent and abrupt decrease in uterine size. Despite pregnancy, supine and upright radiographs are necessary to diagnose and monitor intestinal obstruction. Unremitting, complete intestinal obstruction generally requires surgery despite pregnancy.
Intestinal pseudo-obstruction	Although risk of intestinal pseudo-obstruction or adynamic ileus is increased after cesarean section or vaginal delivery, this complication is still uncommon. This complication is generally managed medically without surgical intervention as in nonpregnant patients.
Colonic pseudo-obstruction	Despite limited clinical data, colonoscopy can be considered for colonic decompression when the only alternative is surgery provided that colonic necrosis is not suspected. Parenteral neostigmine is often administered therapeutically in nonpregnant patients, but may be contraindicated during pregnancy.
Colon cancer	Uncommon during pregnancy because of relative youthfulness of pregnant patients. Iron deficiency anemia is common during pregnancy due to increased gestational demands and is much less frequently associated with colon cancer in pregnant patients than in the elderly. Colon cancer diagnosed during pregnancy often located in rectum or sigmoid colon. Frequently manifests at an advanced pathologic stage attributed to delayed diagnosis. Pregnant patients have a high incidence (25%) of ovarian metastases from colon cancer. Colonoscopy may be necessary during pregnancy before colon cancer surgery to obtain a pathologic diagnosis and to exclude synchronous lesions. When cancer diagnosed during first half of pregnancy, cancer surgery should be promptly performed to minimize risk of metastases. Bilateral salpingo-oophorectomy is indicated for ovarian metastases.
Inflammatory bowel disease	Ulcerative colitis does not generally affect female fertility, whereas Crohn's disease mildly decreases fertility. Patients with inactive or mild inflammatory bowel disease at conception tend to have the same disease activity during pregnancy. Patients with active disease at conception can have active disease during pregnancy with an increased risk of poor fetal outcomes, especially for Crohn's disease. Flexible sigmoidoscopy is generally well tolerated during pregnancy and can be used to help diagnose a disease flare. Corticosteroids, sulfasalazine, and 5-aminosalicylates can be administered during pregnancy. Azathioprine is classified as FDA class D during pregnancy, but gastroenterologists sometimes continue this medication during pregnancy to maintain remission. However, the tumor necrosis factor inhibitors of infliximab, adalimumab, and certolizumab are apparently safer alternatives during pregnancy and are rated as FDA category B during pregnancy. Methotrexate is contraindicated during pregnancy.
Hemorrhoids	Extremely common during pregnancy due to vascular engorgement during pregnancy, vascular compression from the enlarging gravid uterus, and increased straining at defecation because of constipation. Medical therapy is generally recommended because hemorrhoidal symptoms usually resolve spontaneously soon after delivery.
Mesenteric ischemia and infarction	Mildly increased risk of mesenteric ischemia due to mild hypercoagulability from hyperestrogenemia during pregnancy, but risk is still relatively low because mesenteric ischemia is predominantly a disease of the elderly.
Splenic artery rupture	Risk of splenic artery aneurysm rupture markedly increases during pregnancy due to estrogen weakening the elasticity of the arterial wall, but overall risk is still relatively low.

FDA, Food and Drug Administration.

feedings. Total parenteral nutrition (TPN) is rarely necessary. Patients should avoid environmental stimuli that trigger their nausea and vomiting. Patients should eat as soon as they feel hungry to avoid eating on an empty stomach, which can exacerbate nausea.

Nausea and vomiting of pregnancy differs from HG by less severe symptoms, absence of weight loss, and lack of dehydration, vitamin deficiencies, and other nutritional deficiencies. Patients with mild nausea during pregnancy typically require counseling and reassurance without treatment. Patients may benefit from a diet that emphasizes salty liquids, soups, starches, and chicken and avoids fatty foods, vegetables, and fibrous foods.[19] Bendectin (containing doxylamine, an antihistamine and vitamin B_6) was commonly administered for nausea and vomiting of pregnancy, but was withdrawn in 1983 due to unproven allegations of teratogenicity.[19] A subsequent meta-analysis reported no increase in the incidence of birth defects after in utero exposure to Bendectin.[20] Vitamin B_6 (pyridoxine), a component of Bendectin, has been used by itself to treat mild-to-moderate nausea and vomiting of pregnancy with some success.[19,20] A delayed-release form of doxylamine-pyridoxine (Diclectin) is currently approved in Canada to treat nausea and vomiting of pregnancy. Dopamine antagonists, such as promethazine, or selective serotonin antagonists, such as ondansetron, have been used as antiemetics for these conditions. Experimental therapies for HG include ginger, methylprednisone, and erythromycin.

Nausea and vomiting of pregnancy is classically associated with a favorable pregnancy outcome, but has recently been associated with possible physical and psychosocial disorders later in childhood after delivery, as well as psychologic stress in the expectant mother. The maternal and fetal prognosis of HG is relatively favorable provided that the nausea and vomiting are reversed and the mother gains adequate weight during the remainder of the pregnancy.[21]

Gastroesophageal Reflux and Peptic Ulcer Disease

The incidence of pyrosis approaches 80% during pregnancy.[3] The incidence of GERD is likewise high during pregnancy. This high incidence may relate to a hypotonic LES and delayed gastrointestinal transit, attributed to gestational hormones, especially progesterone, and gastric compression by the gravid uterus. GERD manifests in pregnancy, as in nonpregnant patients, by pyrosis, regurgitation, water brash, dyspepsia, hypersalivation, or, rarely, pulmonary symptoms. Symptoms may be exacerbated by ingesting certain foods, such as acidic drinks, or by recumbency. Complications of GERD include gastrointestinal hemorrhage from hemorrhagic esophagitis, dysphagia from a reflux-induced esophageal stricture, and Barrett's esophagus or adenocarcinoma. These complications generally relate to severe, long-standing, poorly controlled GERD. During pregnancy GERD tends to be mild and of short duration (coincident with the pregnancy), so these complications are rare. Esophagogastroduodenoscopy (EGD) is the best test to diagnose reflux esophagitis. Characteristic findings are erosions, exudates, erythema, or ulcers just above the gastroesophageal junction. EGD can be performed during pregnancy if necessary but is generally reserved for complications from GERD of gastrointestinal hemorrhage or dysphagia.

Symptomatic peptic ulcer disease (PUD) is uncommon during pregnancy, and antecedent PUD often improves during pregnancy.[22] Nausea, emesis, dyspepsia, and anorexia are so frequent during pregnancy that PUD cannot be diagnosed by symptomatology during pregnancy. The most common cause of a peptic ulcer in the duodenum is *Helicobacter pylori* infection. Nonsteroidal anti-inflammatory drugs (NSAIDs), including aspirin, can cause gastric or duodenal ulcers. These ulcers more commonly cause gastrointestinal bleeding than abdominal pain, possibly because of the analgesic properties of NSAIDs.

Although the efficacy of modern acid-suppressive drugs has rendered lifestyle modifications less important in the nonpregnant patient with GERD or PUD, lifestyle modifications remain important in the pregnant patient because of concern about potential fetal effects of medications. Pregnant patients with GERD or PUD should avoid caffeine, alcohol, smoking cigarettes, and NSAIDs, although acetaminophen is safe and the cyclo-oxygenase II (COX-II) inhibitors are less gastrotoxic than the nonselective NSAIDs. Women with GERD should elevate the head of their bed and avoid wearing tight belts. They should avoid recumbency after eating and discontinue oral intake beginning 3 hours before bedtime.

Antacids are generally safe for the fetus, but those containing sodium bicarbonate should be avoided throughout pregnancy because such antacids may cause fluid overload or metabolic alkalosis.[23] Antacids and dietary measures often suffice during the first trimester for minimally symptomatic disease.[1] Antacids must be administered frequently because of low potency, and frequent administration can cause diarrhea or constipation and electrolyte or mineral abnormalities. Sucralfate has minimal systemic absorption, and is generally believed to be safe during pregnancy, but its aluminum content is of concern to the fetus in mothers with renal insufficiency. Misoprostil is an abortifacient that is contraindicated during pregnancy. Histamine$_2$-receptor antagonists are useful in treating GERD and PUD when symptoms are more severe or occur later in pregnancy.[1] Ranitidine and famotidine are preferable, because nizatidine is possibly toxic to the fetus and cimetidine has antiandrogenic effects.[24] Proton-pump inhibitors were initially reserved for refractory, severe, or complicated GERD or PUD during pregnancy, but have recently been increasingly used due to accumulating evidence of relative fetal safety. Lansoprazole, rabeprazole, and pantoprazole (Food and Drug Administration [FDA] pregnancy category B) appear to be relatively safe and are therefore the recommended agents in this class during pregnancy.[25] Omeprazole is rated only as an FDA category C drug during pregnancy, but a study in 2001 involving 863 infants exposed to omeprazole during the first trimester revealed a rate of stillbirth and of congenital malformations comparable to that of unexposed controls. Drug therapy to eradicate *Helicobacter pylori* should be deferred until after parturition and lactation because of concern about the fetal safety of administered antibiotics.[26]

Surgery for GERD is best performed either before or after pregnancy.[1] Endoscopic therapy is the initial intervention for active bleeding from GERD or PUD,[17,22] but a hemodynamically unstable patient refractory to endoscopic therapy requires expeditious surgery, because the fetus poorly tolerates maternal hypotension. Patients in advanced pregnancy should undergo cesarean section just before gastric surgery for gastrointestinal bleeding. Pregnant PUD patients may also require surgery for gastric outlet obstruction, refractory ulcer, or malignant ulcer.

Diaphragmatic Rupture

In diaphragmatic rupture, abdominal contents herniate through a diaphragm weakened by congenital defects or abdominal or chest trauma. The risk of rupture is increased during pregnancy because of increased pressure on the diaphragm from recurrent vomiting during the first half of pregnancy, rapid growth of the gravid uterus during the second trimester, or Valsalva/Kristeller maneuvers during labor. Diaphragmatic rupture is still rare even during pregnancy. It is potentially catastrophic during pregnancy, with both maternal and fetal mortality rates from strangulation exceeding 40%.[27] Increased intra-abdominal pressure from the enlarged gravid uterus increases the risk of bowel strangulation. Herniorrhaphy is recommended during the first two trimesters for bowel penetration through a diaphragmatic hernia, even if asymptomatic, because of high mortality risk without surgery.[27] Expectant management is recommended for asymptomatic patients during the third trimester, with cesarean section and herniorrhaphy performed when the fetus is sufficiently mature. Cesarean section is performed to avoid increased abdominal pressure during active labor, which can cause bowel strangulation.

Predominantly Lower Gastrointestinal Disorders

Acute Appendicitis

Acute appendicitis is the most common nonobstetrical surgical emergency during pregnancy, with an incidence of about 1 per 1000 pregnancies.[28] Appendiceal obstruction, usually from an appendicolith, is the primary etiologic event, although stasis and other factors are also implicated. As the appendiceal lumen distends, the patient initially experiences poorly localized pain. Severe luminal distention, mural inflammation and edema, and bacterial translocation produce somatic pain that becomes severe and well-localized at McBurney's point, which is located in the right lower quadrant one third of the way from the anterior superior iliac spine to the umbilicus. Displacement of the appendix by the gravid uterus during late pregnancy may cause the point of maximal abdominal pain and tenderness to migrate superiorly and laterally from McBurney's point, but this migration is typically only a few centimeters away from McBurney's point during late pregnancy.[3] Rectal or pelvic tenderness may occur in early pregnancy but is unusual in late pregnancy as the appendix migrates from its pelvic location. Other clinical findings include anorexia, nausea, emesis, pyrexia, tachycardia, and abdominal tenderness. Periappendiceal inflammation or peritonitis causes involuntary guarding and rebound tenderness. Involuntary guarding and rebound tenderness are less reliable signs of peritonitis in late pregnancy because of abdominal wall laxity and lifting of the anterior abdominal wall away from the inflamed appendix by the growing gravid uterus. Patients may have significant leukocytosis and a predominance of neutrophils in the leukocyte differential.[29]

Radiologic imaging is indicated when the diagnosis is suspected but still ambiguous after routine laboratory studies to reduce the incidence of negative appendectomy. **Although computed tomography is the imaging test of choice in nonpregnant patients because of high diagnostic accuracy, sonography is the test of choice during pregnancy to avoid fetal exposure to radiation from CT.** In a comprehensive review, ultrasound was 86% sensitive and 81% specific in the diagnosis of appendicitis in adults or adolescents.[30] Diagnostic findings include appendiceal mural thickening, periappendiceal fluid, and a noncompressible tubular structure closed at one end and open at the other end with a 6 mm or greater diameter lumen. **Appendicitis cannot be excluded if the appendix is nonvisualized at ultrasound.**[6]

MRI is the appropriate next test in the pregnant patient if the abdominal ultrasound is inconclusive. In a study of 148 pregnant women with suspected appendicitis during pregnancy, MRI was 100% sensitive and 93% specific for the diagnosis of acute appendicitis.[31] CT can be performed with modifications to limit fetal radiation exposure to less than 300 mrad if MRI is unavailable. Abnormal CT findings with appendicitis include right lower quadrant inflammation, a nonfilling, enlarged tubular structure, and an appendicolith.

Up to one quarter of pregnant women with appendicitis develop appendiceal perforation.[3] **This high rate is attributed to delayed diagnosis during pregnancy.** The diagnosis may be missed in pregnant patients because: (1) leukocytosis, a classic sign of acute appendicitis, occurs physiologically during pregnancy; (2) nausea and emesis, common symptoms of acute appendicitis, are also common during pregnancy; and (3) the abdominal pain is sometimes atypically located.[29] Other diseases are often confused with appendicitis (see the accompanying box, Differential Diagnosis of Appendicitis During Pregnancy). Appendiceal displacement predisposes to rapid development of generalized peritonitis after perforation because the omentum may not be in close proximity to the appendix.

Differential Diagnosis of Appendicitis During Pregnancy

Gynecologic Conditions

Ruptured ovarian cyst
Adnexal torsion
Pelvic inflammatory disease or salpingitis
Endometriosis
Ovarian cancer

Obstetrical Causes

Abruptio placentae
Chorioamnionitis
Endometritis
Uterine fibroid degeneration
Labor (preterm or term)
Viscus perforation after abortion
Ruptured ectopic pregnancy

Gastrointestinal Causes

Crohn's disease
Colonic diverticulitis (right side)
Cholecystitis
Pancreatitis
Mesenteric lymphadenitis
Gastroenteritis
Colon cancer
Intestinal obstruction
Hernia (incarcerated inguinal or internal)
Colonic intussusception
Ruptured Meckel's diverticulum
Colonic perforation
Acute mesenteric ischemia

Other Causes

Pyelonephritis
Urolithiasis

Appendicitis during pregnancy mandates surgery, after intravenous hydration and correction of electrolyte abnormalities. Appendectomy is safer for the fetus during the second trimester than the first trimester. Antibiotics are usually administered for uncomplicated appendicitis and are clearly required for appendicitis complicated by perforation, abscess, or peritonitis.[3] Clindamycin is preferred over metronidazole for anaerobic coverage, even though both are category B drugs in pregnancy.[26] Clindamycin and gentamicin is a relatively inexpensive, effective, and safe antibiotic combination. **Laparoscopy may be considered during the first two trimesters for nonperforated appendicitis or when the diagnosis is uncertain.** Appendectomy is recommended even if appendicitis is not evident at surgery.[29] Maternal mortality rate from appendicitis is about 0.1% without perforation, but may exceed 4% with appendiceal perforation.[28] Fetal mortality rate is about 2% without perforation, but has been reported to exceed 30% with appendiceal perforation.[28]

Intestinal Obstruction

Acute intestinal obstruction is the second most common nonobstetrical abdominal emergency, with an incidence of 1 per 2500 pregnancies.[32] It may be incidental or secondary to pregnancy. Obstruction more commonly occurs in the third trimester because of the mechanical effects of the enlarged gravid uterus. In particular, some cases occur at term because of the mechanical effects from fetal head descent and the abrupt decrease in uterine size at delivery.[32] Adhesions, particularly from prior gynecologic surgery or appendectomy, are etiologic in 60% to 70% of small bowel obstruction (SBO) during pregnancy.[32,33] Other causes of SBO include neoplasms, particularly ovarian, endometrial, or cervical malignancy; Crohn's disease; external or internal hernias; volvulus; and intussusceptions.[32] Rare causes of SBO include EP; prior radiotherapy; and intraluminal gallstones, fecoliths, or other concretions. Colonic obstruction is caused by adhesions, colon cancer, other neoplasms, diverticulitis, and volvulus.[32]

Intestinal obstruction classically manifests with a symptomatic triad of abdominal pain, emesis, and obstipation.[32] The pain may be constant or periodic. Small bowel obstruction is more painful than colonic obstruction. The pain with SBO may be diffuse and poorly localized and may radiate to the back, flanks, or perineum. Abdominal pain is milder with volvulus and intussusception. Intestinal malrotation may produce nonspecific symptoms of mild, crampy, abdominal pain and nonbilious emesis. Intestinal strangulation, with compromised bowel perfusion, may be heralded by abdominal guarding and rebound tenderness. Emesis occurs more frequently and earlier in small bowel than colonic obstruction.[32] Constipation from complete intestinal obstruction is usually severe and unremitting and associated with abdominal pain.[32] The abdomen is typically distended and tympanitic to percussion due to inability to defecate or pass flatus. Bowel sounds are high-pitched, hypoactive, and tinkling in early intestinal obstruction and become absent in late obstruction.

The approach to intestinal obstruction is the same in pregnancy as in the general population except that decisions are more urgently required because of combined fetal and maternal risk. The diagnosis is strongly suggested by radiographic findings of distended bowel loops containing air-fluid levels, particularly with differential air-fluid levels. An abrupt transition between distended and nondistended bowel favors the diagnosis of intestinal obstruction over intestinal pseudo-obstruction. Volvulus is suspected when a single bowel loop is grossly dilated. Surgery is recommended for unremitting and complete intestinal obstruction, whereas medical management is recommended for intermittent or partial obstruction. Parenteral fluids are aggressively administered to reverse the fluid and electrolyte deficits caused by emesis and fluid sequestration. Nasogastric suction helps decompress the bowel. Maternal mortality rate is about 5%, and fetal mortality rate may range from 20% to 30%.[33]

Intestinal Pseudo-obstruction

Intestinal pseudo-obstruction (adynamic ileus) is characterized by severe abdominal distention detected on physical examination and diffuse intestinal dilation noted on abdominal roentgenogram. Intestinal pseudo-obstruction is diagnosed only after exclusion of (mechanical) intestinal obstruction by the clinical presentation, laboratory studies, and early clinical evolution. Patients with mechanical obstruction tend to be much sicker than those with pseudo-obstruction for the same degree of intestinal dilation detected by abdominal imaging and tend to progress more rapidly. **Intestinal pseudo-obstruction is a well-described, but uncommon, complication of cesarean section or vaginal delivery. Patients with pseudo-obstruction have nausea, emesis, obstipation, and diffuse abdominal pain that typically develops over several days.** Patients often have hypoperistalsis. Pyrexia, leukocytosis, and increasing abdominal tenderness may herald gastrointestinal ischemia. Treatment includes nasogastric aspiration, parenteral fluid administration, repletion of electrolytes, and rectal tube decompression. Mild pseudo-obstruction or adynamic ileus usually spontaneously resolves.

Therapeutic options for severe colonic pseudo-obstruction (Ogilvie's syndrome), manifested by a colonic luminal diameter greater than 10 cm on abdominal roentgenogram, include colonoscopic decompression or surgical therapies, including cecostomy, cecectomy with diverting ileostomy, or colonic resection when intestinal necrosis supervenes.[34] Colonoscopy can be considered for colonic pseudo-obstruction during the second trimester of pregnancy when the only alternative is surgery.[13] Parenteral neostigmine is often administered for colonic pseudo-obstruction in nonpregnant patients and may therefore be administered postpartum. Mortality rate approaches 10% with impending perforation, but can reach 70% after cecal perforation.[34]

Colon Cancer

Colon cancer is uncommon during pregnancy, with an estimated incidence of 1 per 13,000 to 1 per 50,000 pregnancies.[2,35] With approximately 4 million pregnancies per annum in the United States these incidence estimates translate into 80 to 300 colon cancers during pregnancy per annum in the United States.

The clinical presentation and evaluation of colon cancer in pregnant patients is similar to that in other patients, with notable exceptions. **Common symptoms of colon cancer in pregnant patients include abdominal pain, rectal bleeding, nausea and vomiting, and abdominal distention.**[2,36] **Colon cancer tends not to produce signs until advanced.** About one fifth of colon cancers occur in the rectum in the general population, whereas about two thirds of colon cancers occur in the rectum during pregnancy.[37] This shift during pregnancy may artifactually result from increased self-referral due to increased patient attention to rectal symptoms because of rectal compression by the gravid uterus or from increased physician detection due to frequent pelvic and rectal examinations during pregnancy.[2] Rectal examination is essential in the evaluation of suspected colon cancer during pregnancy. The cancer often arises in the rectum during pregnancy. Rectal cancer may be palpable by digital rectal examination. Stool should be tested for the presence of occult blood, even though the finding of occult blood has a low positive predictive value for colon cancer or adenomas during pregnancy because of the low disease prevalence in this rather young patient population. Iron deficiency anemia is common during pregnancy due to increased gestational demands. Iron deficiency anemia, therefore, is not nearly as strongly associated with colon cancer in the pregnant patient as it is in the elderly patient.[2] Patients with colon cancer during pregnancy are relatively young and therefore more likely than elderly patients with colon cancer to have predisposing factors, including hereditary nonpolyposis colon cancer (HNPCC), familial polyposis coli, Peutz-Jeghers syndrome, and long-standing inflammatory bowel disease.

During pregnancy, colon cancer often manifests at an advanced pathologic stage attributed to delayed diagnosis.[37] Advanced pathologic stage is highly correlated with a poor prognosis. MRI may be required to diagnose suspected hepatic metastases.[38] Complete colonoscopy is indicated preoperatively in nonpregnant patients for pathologic diagnosis and for excluding synchronous colonic lesions. Colonoscopy may, therefore, be necessary during pregnancy before colon cancer surgery for the same reasons. Colonoscopy may be technically difficult during late pregnancy because of colonic compression by the enlarged gravid uterus. If the gestation is advanced, and the fetus is viable, it may be preferable to induce labor and then perform colonoscopy and cancer surgery.

When the cancer is diagnosed during the first half of pregnancy, cancer surgery should be promptly performed to minimize the risk of metastases.[2] Such surgery can often be performed without removing the gravid uterus and disturbing the pregnancy.[37] Total abdominal hysterectomy is recommended to facilitate access to the rectum when needed for intraoperative exposure; when the mother's life expectancy is less than the time needed for the fetus to become viable; or when the cancer extends into the uterus. Otherwise, when the cancer appears resectable, curative surgery should be performed leaving the pregnancy intact.[2] When the cancer is diagnosed during the second half of pregnancy, cancer surgery should ideally be delayed until, but not beyond, the time that fetal viability is normally expected (at about 32 weeks of gestation) because further delay permits cancer growth and metastasis.[36] Bilateral salpingo-oophorectomy is indicated for ovarian metastases.[39] Colon cancer surgery is associated with a moderately increased, but still acceptable, rate of fetal death, but is associated with a high risk of preterm delivery and low birth weight. Serum carcinoembryonic antigen (CEA) levels obtained before surgery provide a baseline to monitor response to surgery and chemotherapy. Pregnancy does not significantly alter the serum CEA level.

Patients younger than 40 years old generally have a poor prognosis from colon cancer, attributed to a delayed diagnosis and an advanced pathologic stage at diagnosis. Likewise, the maternal prognosis from colon cancer, whether colonic or rectal, diagnosed during pregnancy is poor. Fetal prognosis depends on the pathologic stage of the maternal cancer, gestational age at diagnosis, and type and timing of therapy. Novel diagnostic modalities for colon cancer diagnosis with promising applications in pregnancy include video capsule endoscopy in which the colon may be imaged by a microcamera placed within a pill-sized device swallowed by the patient, and a large array of genetic markers to detect genetic abnormalities associated with colon cancer in minute quantities of DNA in stool shed from colonic mucosa.

Inflammatory Bowel Disease

The inflammatory bowel diseases (IBDs), including ulcerative colitis and Crohn's disease, are idiopathic, immunologically mediated disorders that peak in incidence during a woman's reproductive period. The incidence of UC in women less than 40 years of age is 40 to 100 per 100,000 and of CD is 2 to 4 per 100,000.[3] **Ulcerative colitis is a colonic disease manifested by bloody diarrhea, crampy abdominal pain, and pyrexia. Crohn's disease can involve any part of the gastrointestinal tract but most commonly involves the terminal ileum.** It is characterized by diarrhea, abdominal pain, anorexia, pyrexia, and malnutrition. Patients with CD may have fistulas and anorectal disease. Extraintestinal manifestations of IBD include arthritis, uveitis, sclerosing cholangitis, and cutaneous lesions.

Ulcerative colitis does not significantly affect fertility except that fertility decreases after colonic resection for ulcerative colitis.[40] Crohn's disease, however, mildly decreases fertility because of extension of ileal inflammation to the nearby oviducts or ovaries and the systemic effects of malnutrition.[41] Inflammatory bowel disease activity is mostly independent of pregnancy. Patients with inactive or mild disease before conception tend to have the same disease activity during pregnancy. Active disease at conception increases the likelihood of active disease during pregnancy and of a poor pregnancy outcome, including spontaneous abortion, miscarriage, stillbirth, or premature delivery.[42] The onset of CD, and to a lesser extent UC, during pregnancy is associated with increased fetal loss.

Differentiating the signs and symptoms of IBD from physiologic changes related to pregnancy or from other obstetrical, gynecologic, or surgical conditions may be difficult. Nausea, emesis, abdominal discomfort, and constipation may be noted during any pregnancy but may also signal a flare of IBD. The differential diagnosis of acute RLQ abdominal pain in a pregnant woman with CD includes CD exacerbation, EP, appendicitis, or adnexal disease. Pyrexia, bloody diarrhea, and weight loss suggest CD exacerbation.

The diagnostic evaluation is influenced by the pregnancy, but indicated tests should be performed. Laboratory evaluation includes a hemogram, serum chemistry profile, and electrolyte determinations, taking into account the physiologic alterations of late pregnancy including anemia, leukocytosis, and hypoalbuminemia. Flexible sigmoidoscopy is well tolerated during pregnancy without maternal complications or fetal toxicity.[17] Colonoscopy has been safely performed during pregnancy, especially during the second trimester, but the experience in the first and third trimesters is relatively limited.[13]

The beneficial effects of IBD therapy on the mother and fetus must be weighed against the potential of fetal toxicity and teratogenicity (Table 45-8). Active disease poses greater risk to the fetus than most therapies.[43] Sulfasalazine and 5-aminosalicylates seem to be safe and can be used when required during pregnancy.[42] Methotrexate, however, is an abortifacient and is associated with congenital skeletal malformations. The FDA categorizes azathioprine and 6-mercaptopurine (6-MP) as class D drugs during pregnancy. Some gastroenterologists, however, continue these medications during pregnancy if required to maintain remission.[42] Anti–tumor necrosis factor biologic therapies appear to be safer alternatives during pregnancy (see Table 45-8). Their safety during pregnancy is, however, somewhat controversial because of conflicting reports and limited data. One study noted a high rate of congenital malformations reported to the FDA associated with this drug class, but another study noted a low rate.[44] This class of drugs should generally be discontinued before contemplated pregnancy, but may be used during pregnancy to control extremely active recent disease. Metronidazole is probably best avoided during the first trimester and perhaps administered only for brief durations during the other trimesters. The antidiarrheal agent diphenoxylate should be avoided during pregnancy because of case reports of teratogenicity when administered during the first trimester.[3] Emergency surgery for toxic megacolon, intestinal obstruction, or massive bleeding should be done expeditiously, whereas elective surgery, such as fistulectomy, should be performed during the second trimester or postpartum . Severe perianal CD may necessitate cesarean section, because episiotomy during vaginal delivery can exacerbate perianal disease.

Hemorrhoids

Hemorrhoids are common in adults and are particularly common during pregnancy, with an estimated incidence of 25% during pregnancy.[45] Contributing factors during pregnancy include increased constipation resulting in increased straining at defecation, gestational increases in the circulating blood volume resulting in venous dilation and engorgement, and vascular compression from the enlarging gravid uterus resulting in venous stasis.[9] Hemorrhoids above the dentate line are internal, whereas those below the dentate line are external.

Hemorrhoids characteristically produce a clinical triad of bright red blood per rectum resembling the color of arterial blood; blood coating rather than admixed with stool; and postdefecatory bleeding, most commonly noted on the toilet paper.[46] Other clinical manifestations include anorectal discomfort, pruritus, or pain associated with prolapse, thrombosis, or incarceration of hemorrhoids.

When the pain from external hemorrhoids is mild to moderate, conservative treatment, including stool softeners, increased liquid intake, topical analgesics, and warm sitz baths, is recommended.[9] Surgical excision under local anesthesia can be performed safely during pregnancy for severely painful or acutely thrombosed external hemorrhoids. General measures for internal hemorrhoids include

Table 45-8 PHARMACOLOGIC THERAPY FOR INFLAMMATORY BOWEL DISEASE DURING PREGNANCY

DRUG	FDA CATEGORY DURING PREGNANCY	RECOMMENDATION DURING PREGNANCY
Sulfasalazine	B	Relatively safe. Concern about sulfa moiety causing neonatal jaundice.
Mesalamine	B	Relatively safe.
Infliximab (anti-TNF)	B	Not teratogenic in mice exposed to an analogous antibody. Insufficient clinical data.
Adalimumab (anti-TNF)	B	Believed to be relatively safe drug during pregnancy based on animal data. Little clinical data. Drug manufacturer is placing patients receiving this drug during pregnancy on a national registry.
Certolizumab (anti-TNF)	B	Animal studies have not revealed fetal toxicity. Few clinical data.
Loperamide	B	Relatively safe.
Metronidazole	B	Avoid during first trimester since carcinogenic in rodents.
Corticosteroids	C	Relatively safe. Concern regarding fetal adrenal function and maternal hyperglycemia. Monitor the neonates of mothers who received substantial doses of corticosteroids during pregnancy.
Ciprofloxacin	C	Use with caution, small studies show no significant risk during pregnancy.
Diphenoxylate	C	Avoid, possible teratogen.
Cyclosporine	C	Embryotoxic and fetotoxic at very high doses in rats and rabbits.
6-Mercaptopurine	D	Avoid starting after conception. Might cause IUGR.
Azathioprine	D	Avoid starting after conception. Might cause IUGR. Teratogenic in laboratory animals.
Methotrexate	X	Contraindicated. Teratogen and abortifacient.

FDA, Food and Drug Administration; *IUGR*, intrauterine growth restriction; *TNF*, tumor necrosis factor.

fiber supplements, fluids, and a high-fiber diet to decrease constipation; switching to a slow-release iron supplement to mitigate the constipating effects of iron; topical local anesthetics for anorectal discomfort; skin protectants applied after defecation to reduce anal pruritus; and avoidance of straining during bowel movements.[9] Therapies for severe or refractory symptoms from internal hemorrhoids include band ligation, injection, sclerotherapy, and coagulation. These therapies are generally safe and effective during pregnancy.[47] Invasive therapy, however, is rarely necessary for external or internal hemorrhoids as the symptoms spontaneously resolve soon after delivery.[45]

Mesenteric Ischemia and Infarction

Bowel infarction can occur during pregnancy secondary to intestinal obstruction or mesenteric venous thrombosis.[48] Digoxin, ergot alkaloids, cocaine, and other vasoconstrictors are also associated with mesenteric ischemia. Mild hypercoagulability from hyperestrogenemia during pregnancy may contribute to a mildly increased risk of mesenteric ischemia during pregnancy as compared to other middle-aged patients, but this risk is not high because mesenteric ischemia is predominantly a disease of the elderly. Patients with mesenteric venous thrombosis typically have an insidious onset of poorly localized abdominal pain, with a relatively unremarkable physical examination.[49] The thrombosis is diagnosed by the noninvasive modalities of MRI or CT scanning, and by the invasive modality of the venous phase of angiography. Hematologic evaluation for hypercoagulopathy is recommended.[48]

Irritable Bowel Syndrome

The irritable bowel syndrome (IBS) is most common in younger women. The pathogenesis is poorly defined. Both intestinal motor and sensory abnormalities, particularly hyperalgesia, have been described. IBS is diagnosed, according to the Rome III criteria, by the presence of both abdominal pain and disordered defecation for at least 6 months, with at least two of the following: pain relief by a bowel movement, onset of pain related to a change in stool frequency, and onset of pain related to a change in stool appearance. Endoscopic, radiologic, and histologic intestinal studies reveal no evident organic disease. **Young women typically have diarrhea-predominant IBS but sometimes have predominantly constipation or alternating diarrhea and constipation. Abdominal bloating and distention are common symptoms.**

Few data exist concerning the effect of pregnancy on IBS.[50] The onset of IBS typically predates the pregnancy and rarely begins during pregnancy. Gestational hormones, particularly progesterone, may exacerbate the symptoms of IBS. Presumed IBS in the absence of warning signs or symptoms (e.g., rectal bleeding, pyrexia, or weight loss) should not require invasive tests, such as sigmoidoscopy, during pregnancy. Contrariwise, signs and symptoms of organic disease, such as rectal bleeding or involuntary weight loss, should not be attributed to IBS without proper evaluation. In particular, sigmoidoscopy is indicated for significant nonhemorrhoidal rectal bleeding during pregnancy.[12] **Symptoms of IBS are best treated during pregnancy by dietary modification or behavioral therapy rather than systemic drugs.**[51] Patients with diarrhea-predominant IBS may benefit from elimination of foods from the diet that precipitate diarrhea, such as alcohol, caffeinated beverages, poorly digestible sugars, and fatty foods. Pregnant patients usually require a large amount of dairy products in their diet to ensure adequate calcium intake. Patients may benefit from lactase supplements when ingesting dairy products. Dietary fiber and fluid ingestion may improve constipation-predominant IBS. Polysaccharide bulking agents, such as methylcellulose, appear to be safe during pregnancy due to a lack of systemic absorption. IBS is not believed to affect fertility and pregnancy outcome in the absence of nutritional deficiencies or concomitant disorders.[50]

Splenic Artery Aneurysm Rupture

Splenic artery aneurysm rupture is associated with pregnancy, possibly because of the effects of gestational hormones on the elastic properties of the arterial wall. Rupture most commonly occurs in the third trimester. Patients typically are in shock with left upper quadrant abdominal pain. The diagnosis is suggested by demonstration of a calcified rim from the aneurysm on plain abdominal roentgenogram and is confirmed by abdominal CT scanning or angiography. Treatment consists of fluid resuscitation and prompt surgery, with hemostasis and splenectomy. The maternal mortality rate exceeds 75%, and the fetal mortality rate exceeds 90%.[52] Splenic artery aneurysms should therefore be surgically corrected even if asymptomatic.[52] Abdominal aortic and renal aneurysms can also rupture during pregnancy.

KEY POINTS

- Aside from gastrointestinal and other intra-abdominal disorders incidental to pregnancy, the differential of abdominal pain includes obstetrical, gynecologic, and gastrointestinal disorders related to pregnancy.
- Pregnancy can affect the clinical presentation, frequency, or severity of gastrointestinal diseases. Gastroesophageal reflux disease markedly increases in frequency, whereas peptic ulcer disease markedly decreases in frequency (or becomes inactive) during pregnancy.
- Abdominal ultrasound is the safest and most commonly used abdominal imaging modality to evaluate gastrointestinal conditions during pregnancy.
- Esophagogastroduodenoscopy and flexible sigmoidoscopy can be performed when strongly indicated during pregnancy, such as for significant acute upper and lower gastrointestinal bleeding, respectively.
- Most gastrointestinal drugs appear to be relatively safe for the fetus (FDA category B and C) and can be used when indicated during pregnancy. Gastrointestinal drugs to be avoided during pregnancy include misoprostil, which is an abortifacient (category X) and methotrexate (category X).

REFERENCES

1. Broussard CN, Richter JE: Treating gastro-esophageal reflux disease during pregnancy and lactation: what are the safest therapy options. Drug Saf 19:325, 1998.
2. Cappell MS: Colon cancer during pregnancy. Gastroenterol Clin North Am 32:341, 2003.
3. Cappell MS, Friedel D: Abdominal pain during pregnancy. Gastroenterol Clin North Am 32:1, 2003.
4. Lawson M, Kern F Jr, Everson GT: Gastrointestinal transit time in human pregnancy: prolongation in the second and third trimesters followed by postpartum normalization. Gastroenterology 89:996, 1985.
5. Martin C, Varner MW: Physiologic changes in pregnancy: surgical implications. Clin Obstet Gynecol 37:241, 1994.
6. Derchi LE, Serafini G, Gandolfo N, et al: Ultrasound in gynecology. Eur Radiol 11:2137, 2001.
7. Evans HJ, Wollin TA: The management of urinary calculi in pregnancy. Curr Opin Urol 11:379, 2001.
8. Cappell MS, Colon VJ, Sidhom OA: A study at eight medical centers of the safety and clinical efficacy of esophagogastroduodenoscopy in 83 pregnant females with follow-up of fetal outcome and with comparison to control groups. Am J Gastroenterol 91:348, 1996.
9. Wald A: Constipation, diarrhea, and symptomatic hemorrhoids during pregnancy. Gastroenterol Clin North Am 32:309, 2003.
10. Bradley CS, Kennedy CM, Turcea AM, et al: Constipation in pregnancy: prevalence, symptoms, and risk factors. Obstet Gynecol 110:1351, 2007.
11. Karam PA: Determining and reporting fetal radiation exposure from diagnostic radiation. Health Phys 79:S85, 2000.
12. Cappell MS, Colon VJ, Sidhom OA: A study at 10 medical centers of the safety and efficacy of 48 flexible sigmoidoscopies and 8 colonoscopies during pregnancy with follow-up of fetal outcome and with comparison to control groups. Dig Dis Sci 41:2353, 1996.
13. Cappell MS, Fox SR, Gorrepati N: Safety and efficacy of colonoscopy during pregnancy: an analysis of pregnancy outcome in 20 patients. J Reprod Med 55:115, 2010.
14. Debby A, Golan A, Sadan O, et al: Clinical utility of esophagogastroduodenoscopy in the management of recurrent and intractable vomiting in pregnancy. J Reprod Med 53:347, 2008.
15. Bagis T, Gumurdulu Y, Kayaselcuk F, et al: Endoscopy in hyperemesis gravidarum and *Helicobacter pylori* infection. Int J Gynaecol Obstet 79:105, 2002.
16. Cappell MS: Endoscopy in pregnancy: risks versus benefits. Nature Clin Pract Gastroenterol Hepatol 2:376, 2005.
17. Cappell MS: The fetal safety and clinical efficacy of gastrointestinal endoscopy during pregnancy. Gastroenterol Clin North Am 32:123, 2003.
18. Hogan RB, Ahmad N, Hogan RB III, et al: Video capsule endoscopy detection of jejunal carcinoid in life-threatening hemorrhage, first trimester pregnancy. Gastrointest Endosc 66:205, 2007.
19. Koch KL, Frissora CL: Nausea and vomiting during pregnancy. Gastroenterol Clin North Am 32:201, 2003.
20. McKeigue PM, Lamm SH, Linn S, Kutcher JS: Bendectin and birth defects: 1. A meta-analysis of the epidemiologic studies. Teratology 50:27, 1994.
21. Dodds L, Fell DB, Joseph KS, et al: Outcomes of pregnancies complicated by hyperemesis gravidarum. Obstet Gynecol 107:285, 2006.
22. Cappell MS: Gastric and duodenal ulcers during pregnancy. Gastroenterol Clin North Am 32:263, 2003.
23. Nakatsuka T, Fujikake N, Hasebe M, et al: Effects of sodium bicarbonate and ammonium chloride on the incidence of furosemide-induced fetal skeletal anomaly, wavy rib, in rats. Teratology 48:139, 1993.
24. Koren G, Zemlickis DM: Outcome of pregnancy after first trimester exposure to H-2 receptor antagonists. Am J Perinatol 8:37, 1991.
25. Briggs GG, Freeman RK, Yaffe SJ: Drugs in pregnancy and lactation: A Reference Guide to Fetal and Neonatal Risk, 8th ed. Philadelphia, Lippincott Williams & Wilkins, 2008.
26. Dashe JS, Gilstrap LC III: Antibiotic use in pregnancy. Obstet Gynecol Clin North Am 24:617, 1997.
27. Dumont M: Diaphragmatic hernia and pregnancy. J Gynecol Obstet Biol Reprod 19:395, 1990.
28. Mazze RI, Kallen B: Appendectomy during pregnancy: a Swedish registry of 778 cases. Obstet Gynecol 77:835, 1991.
29. Mourad J, Elliott JP, Erickson L, et al: Appendicitis in pregnancy: new information that contradicts long-held clinical beliefs. Am J Obstet Gynecol 182:1027, 2000.
30. Terasawa T, Blackmore CC, Bent S, Kohlwes RJ: Systematic review: computed tomography and ultrasonography to detect acute appendicitis in adults and adolescents. Ann Intern Med 141:537, 2004.
31. Pedrosa I, Lafornara M, Pandharipande PV, et al: Pregnant patients suspected of having acute appendicitis: effect of MR imaging on negative laparotomy rate and appendiceal perforation rate. Radiology 250:749, 2009.
32. Perdue PW, Johnson HW Jr, Stafford PW: Intestinal obstruction complicating pregnancy. Am J Surg 164:384, 1992.
33. Meyerson S, Holtz T, Ehrinpreis M, et al: Small bowel obstruction in pregnancy. Am J Gastroenterol 90:299, 1995.
34. Sharp HT: Gastrointestinal surgical conditions during pregnancy. Clin Obstet Gynecol 37:306, 1994.
35. Woods JB, Martin JN Jr, Ingram FH, et al: Pregnancy complicated by carcinoma of the colon above the rectum. Am J Perinatol 9:102, 1992.
36. Nesbitt JC, Moise KJ, Sawyers JL: Colorectal carcinoma in pregnancy. Arch Surg 120:636, 1985.
37. Bernstein MA, Madoff RD, Caushaj PF: Colon and rectal cancer in pregnancy. Dis Colon Rectum 36:172, 1993.
38. Chen MM, Coakley FV, Kaimel D, Laros RK Jr: Guidelines for computed tomography and magnetic resonance imaging use during pregnancy and lactation. Obstet Gynecol 112:333, 2008.
39. Tsukamoto N, Uchino H, Matsukuma K, Kamura T: Carcinoma of the colon presenting as bilateral ovarian tumors during pregnancy. Gynecol Oncol 24:386, 1986.
40. Ording Olsen K, Juul S, Berndtsson I, et al: Ulcerative colitis: female fecundity before diagnosis, during disease, and after surgery compared with a population sample. Gastroenterology 122:15, 2002.
41. Woolfson K, Cohen Z, McLeod RS: Crohn's disease and pregnancy. Dis Colon Rectum 33:869, 1990.
42. Friedman S: Management of inflammatory bowel disease during pregnancy and nursing. Semin Gastrointest Dis 12:245, 2001.
43. Park-Wyllie L, Mazzotta P, Pastuszak A, et al: Birth defects after maternal exposure to corticosteroids: prospective cohort study and meta-analysis of epidemiological studies. Teratology 62:385, 2000.
44. Ali YM, Kuriya B, Orozco C, et al: Can tumor necrosis factor inhibitors be safely used in pregnancy? J Rheumatol 37:9, 2010.
45. Staroselsky A, Nava-Ocampo A, Vohra S, Koren G: Hemorrhoids in pregnancy. Can Fam Physician 54:189, 2008.
46. Cappell MS, Friedel D: The role of sigmoidoscopy and colonoscopy in the diagnosis and management of lower gastrointestinal disorders: endoscopic findings, therapy, and complications. Med Clin North Am 86:1253, 2002.
47. Medich DS, Fazio VW: Hemorrhoids, anal fissure, and carcinoma of the colon, rectum, and anus during pregnancy. Surg Clin North Am 75:77, 1995.
48. Engelhardt TC, Kerstein MD: Pregnancy and mesenteric venous thrombosis. South J Med 82:1441, 1989.
49. Cappell MS: Intestinal (mesenteric) vasculopathy: I. Acute superior mesenteric arteriopathy and venopathy. Gastroenterol Clin North Am 27:783, 1998.
50. Kane SV, Sable K, Hanauer SB: The menstrual cycle and its effect on inflammatory bowel disease and irritable bowel syndrome: a prevalence study. Am J Gastroenterol 93:1867, 1998.
51. West L, Warren J, Cutts T: Diagnosis and management of irritable bowel syndrome, constipation, and diarrhea in pregnancy. Gastroenterol Clin North Am 21:793, 1992.
52. Stanley JC, Wakefield TW, Graham LM, et al: Clinical importance and management of splanchnic artery aneurysms. J Vasc Surg 3:836, 1986.

For full reference list, log onto www.expertconsult.com.

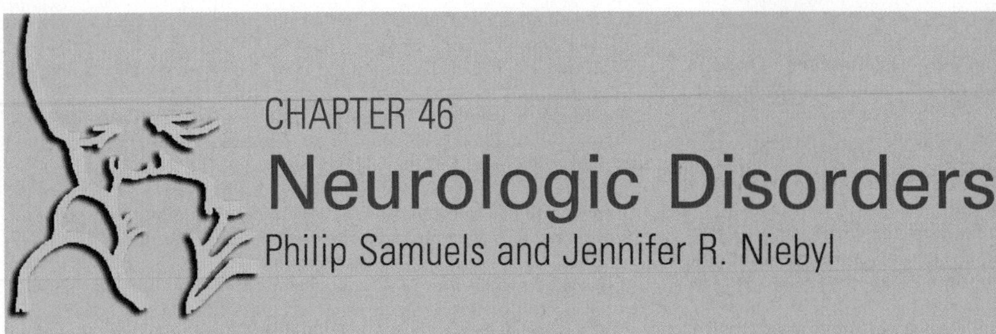

CHAPTER 46

Neurologic Disorders

Philip Samuels and Jennifer R. Niebyl

KEY ABBREVIATIONS	
Arteriovenous	AV
Blood Pressure	BP
Central Nervous System	CNS
Cerebrospinal Fluid	CSF
Computed Tomography	CT
Electroencephalogram	EEG
Hemolysis, Elevated Liver Enzymes, and Low Platelet Count	HELLP
Idiopathic Intracranial Hypertension	ICH
Intelligence Quotient	IQ
Intramuscular	IM
Intrauterine Growth Restriction	IUGR
Magnetic Resonance Imaging	MRI
Multiple Sclerosis	MS
Neural Tube Defect	NTD
Thymus Helper	Th

SEIZURE DISORDERS

Because they affect approximately 1% of the general population, seizure disorders are the most frequent major neurologic complication encountered in pregnancy. It is important that the practicing obstetrician become familiar with the basic treatment of these disorders. During pregnancy, many non-obstetricians are reticent to evaluate, much less treat, disorders that may coexist or develop during pregnancy. It is the obstetrician's duty to communicate with medical specialists and encourage them to treat the patient appropriately. The obstetrician's responsibility is to ascertain if the treatment may have a detrimental effect on the developing fetus. Together, with the patient, the physicians must establish a risk/benefit analysis and then move forward with therapy. This model not only applies to seizure disorders but to any of the myriad of medical/surgical problems that can coexist with pregnancy.

Seizure disorders may be divided into those that are acquired and those that are idiopathic. Acquired seizure disorders, which account for less than 15% of all seizures, may result from trauma, infection, space-occupying lesions, or metabolic disorders. More than 85% of seizure disorders are classified as idiopathic, meaning that no etiologic agent or inciting incident can be identified. Idiopathic seizures can be divided into types such as tonic-clonic, partial complex with or without generalization, myoclonic, focal, or absence.

In general, initial therapy is based on the type of seizure disorder experienced by the patient. There are, however, many crossovers, and patients may respond differently to each medication despite their seizure type. Therefore, it is not unusual to encounter a patient with any seizure type who may be taking any of the major antiepileptic medications. Furthermore, patients may be placed on a certain medication because they did not tolerate the side effect profile of another anticonvulsant (Table 46-1). Over the past 15 years, therapies have changed, as many new medications have been developed and marketed. Many patients with epilepsy have done very well on their medications, and have not been evaluated by a neurologist for many years. Some patients have been seizure free for many years. Often they have stopped their medications with no untoward effects. Frequently, they abruptly stop all medications as soon as they find out that they are pregnant.[1] Still others have poorly controlled seizures, and it is unclear whether this is due to noncompliance with or ineffectiveness of their medication regimen. Other patients may be taking two medications when they may need only one. **The obstetrician and neurologist must work closely together to guide the patient through her pregnancy and find the safest and most effective medical therapy for the patient.**

TABLE 46-1 COMMON SIDE EFFECTS OF ANTICONVULSANTS

DRUG	MATERNAL EFFECTS	FETAL EFFECTS
Phenytoin	Nystagmus, ataxia, hirsutism, gingival hyperplasia, megaloblastic anemia	Possible teratogenesis and carcinogenesis, coagulopathy, hypocalcemia
Carbamazepine	Drowsiness, leukopenia, ataxia, mild hepatotoxicity	Possible craniofacial and neural tube defects
Valproic acid	Ataxia, drowsiness, alopecia, hepatotoxicity, thrombocytopenia	Neural tube defects and craniofacial and skeletal defects
Lamotrigine	Rash, headache, ataxia, diplopia, blurred vision, dizziness	Possible increase in oral clefts

Through this cooperation, the majority of pregnant women with seizure disorders can have a successful pregnancy with minimal risk to mother and fetus.

Effects of Epilepsy on Reproductive Function

Women with seizure disorders should seek care from an obstetrician/gynecologist as soon as they become sexually active. Contraception may present a challenge to women with epilepsy, and the use of oral contraceptives may require special adjustments. Certain antiepileptic medications have been associated with contraceptive failure, especially the older medications. Carbamazepine, phenobarbital, and phenytoin enhance the activities of hepatic microsomal oxidative enzymes.[2] The cytochrome P450 system is shared by these medications and the steroid hormones. This increased enzymatic activity may lead to rapid clearance of these hormones, which may allow ovulation to occur. **Therefore, medicated patients taking low-dose oral contraceptives may have more breakthrough bleeding[3] and may be at increased risk for unplanned pregnancy.[4,5] This rapid clearance does not appear to be induced by valproate, benzodiazepines,[2] or the new antiepileptic medications.[6]**

Fertility rates may be lower in patients with epilepsy. A retrospective study by Webber and colleagues[3] reviewed fertility rates in individuals with epilepsy over a 50-year period. They found that fertility rates were significantly lower in both men and women with epilepsy, and that this could not be explained solely by the rate of marriage in these patients. Men appeared to be more adversely affected than women. Women with epilepsy had fertility rates 85% of the expected rate. Furthermore, in this retrospective review, women with partial seizures seemed to have lower fertility rates than those with generalized seizures. In a study by Dansky and colleagues,[4] fertility rates appeared to be lower in those women with early-onset epilepsy than those with late-onset disease. Cramer and Jones[2] also investigated the fertility rate in 263 unselected patients with epilepsy. They found that the fertility rate was half that of the general population, and 25% of married patients had no children.[2] In Finland, the birth rate was lower in patients with epilepsy than in the referenced cohort. The hazard ratio (HR), a type of relative risk (RR), was 0.58 in men and 0.88 in women. Yet, even in these studies, the majority of patients with epilepsy were able to conceive without difficulty.

Effect of Pregnancy on Epilepsy

It has been taught that between 30% and 50% of patients show an increase in seizure frequency during pregnancy. This was confirmed in the classic study of Knight and Rhind[5] of 153 pregnancies in 59 patients between 1953 and 1973. **In that study, 45% of patients showed an increase in seizure frequency during pregnancy, whereas 50% had no change and 4.8% experienced a decrease.** Anticonvulsant levels could not be readily measured until the mid-1970s. When this study was performed, anticonvulsant doses were usually only increased by physicians when patients had breakthrough seizures. An important finding from that study, however, was that patients with more frequent seizures tended to have exacerbations during pregnancy.[6] **In fact, virtually all patients who had more than one seizure each month experienced worsening of their epilepsy during pregnancy, whereas only about 25% of patients who had not had a seizure in over 9 months experienced exacerbation of epilepsy during pregnancy.**

With the introduction of new medications and the ability to monitor anticonvulsant levels, these absolute numbers are no longer true. The relationship, however, does remain. Patients with more frequent seizures tend to have exacerbations of seizures during pregnancy. In a large study by Schmidt and colleagues,[6] 63% of patients had no change or a decrease in seizure frequency during pregnancy, whereas only 37% of patients had an increase of seizures during pregnancy. Importantly, in 34 of the 50 patients who showed an increase in seizure frequency during pregnancy, the increase was associated with noncompliance with their drug regimen or sleep deprivation. Conversely, in 7 of the 18 pregnancies in which improvement of seizure frequency was shown, this was related to improved compliance with the drug regimen or a correction of sleep deprivation for the 9 months preceding pregnancy. In a study by Tanganelli and Regesta,[7] seizure frequency did not change or improved in 82.6% of pregnancies. Increases in seizure frequency were often due to noncompliance with medication regimens as well as frequent seizures in the preconception period. In contrast, Sabers and colleagues[8] summarized 151 pregnancies in 124 women with epilepsy between 1978 and 1992. They found that 21% of patients had exacerbations of their seizures during pregnancy and 71% were taking only one medication.[8] Lunardi and colleagues, via a series of interviews, examined the quality of life in women with epilepsy.[9] In this small study, pregnant women with epilepsy experienced no greater stress than those without epilepsy. However, when divided into different segments of gestation, those in late pregnancy showed more markers for stress than their nonpregnant counterparts. As stress is often associated with increased seizure frequency, the obstetrician should pay close attention to symptoms and medication dosing in late pregnancy.

In summary, we now have the means to monitor anticonvulsant levels in patients when necessary, and we have the medications to control seizures. We also understand that sleep deprivation can be a catalyst for seizures. **With patient cooperation and close surveillance, seizure frequency should remain the same or even improve in most epileptic patients during pregnancy.**

Effects of Pregnancy on the Disposition of Anticonvulsant Medications

It is well known that the levels of anticonvulsant medications can change dramatically during pregnancy. They usually decrease in total concentration as pregnancy progresses. Many factors, including altered protein binding, delayed gastric emptying, nausea and vomiting, changes in plasma volume, and changes in the volume of distribution, can affect the levels of anticonvulsant medications. Also, the addition of increased folic acid to the vitamin regimen can decrease medication levels as folic acid is a cofactor in the metabolism of many of these medications.

Phenytoin use has greatly decreased over the past 10 years, but many patients have been taking it for years and continue its use. Landon and Kirkley[10] and Kochenour and colleagues[11] showed that the serum concentration of phenytoin tends to fall during pregnancy and rise again during the puerperium and postpartum periods. Several factors can account for this. In early gestation, patients often have nausea and vomiting. Phenytoin is usually administered on a once-daily basis. If the patient vomits the medication, the drug levels will be highly variable. Furthermore, an increase in calcium intake during pregnancy, as well as the use of antacids, leads to the formation of insoluble complexes with phenytoin, resulting in lower total drug levels. Also, with delayed gastric emptying in pregnancy, the time to peak drug level is lengthened. Phenytoin is inactivated in the liver. Its rate of conversion may increase greatly during pregnancy, because the activity of oxidative enzymes increases. This is due to increased progesterone levels, which induce enzyme activity. This may also be enhanced by increased folic acid, which serves as a cofactor in these metabolic processes. Outside of pregnancy, approximately 90% of phenytoin is protein bound. Plasma albumin levels decrease during pregnancy, whereas other protein levels may rise. This process causes changes in the total phenytoin level that do not necessarily reflect the free, active phenytoin concentrations. This effect is also enhanced by free fatty acids displacing phenytoin from albumin. In a study by Yerby and colleagues,[12] free levels of phenobarbital, carbamazepine, and phenytoin rose significantly throughout pregnancy while total levels fell. Therefore, the relationship observed in nonpregnant women between total drug and free or active drug is not maintained. Although we do not advocate the routine use of anticonvulsant levels during pregnancy, some patients need to have levels checked. These include patients with frequent seizures who may have questionable compliance. **In the case of phenytoin, free phenytoin levels should be measured.** If the patient has increased seizure activity, medication doses should be increased as long as the patient is not showing signs of toxicity. Likewise, if the medication level is low but the patient is seizure free, no adjustment in dosing is necessary.

Similar pharmacokinetic changes occur with the administration of phenobarbital and carbamazepine but to different degrees. It is extremely rare to find a patient who is taking phenobarbital today, but carbamazepine is widely used. Both of these drugs also show changes in protein binding and increased hepatic clearance during pregnancy. Infants born to the rare mother who has been taking a barbiturate during pregnancy may exhibit some withdrawal symptoms that begin about 1 week after birth and usually continue for up to 2 weeks. These symptoms usually involve minor irritability but may occasionally be more serious.

Carbamazepine also has an active metabolite, carbamazepine 10,11-epoxide. This metabolite can be measured, and this measurement can be clinically useful in many instances. **Carbamazepine is not as highly protein bound as phenytoin and, therefore, is not subject to as wide a fluctuation due to changes in protein levels.** Carbamazepine also induces its own metabolic enzymes in the liver, so the half-life changes as the dose increases.[11]

Lamotrigine is used with increased frequency today. It is being used more often as a "stand-alone" anticonvulsant. In addition, it is used in the treatment of patients with bipolar disorder. **Lamotrigine (Lamictal) clearance increases more than 50% during pregnancy. This effect occurs early in pregnancy and reverts quickly after delivery. Most patients require a higher dose to maintain therapeutic levels during pregnancy.** Concomitant use of carbamazepine may also increase lamotrigine requirements.

Although levetiracetam levels are not routinely checked, pregnancy may decrease the levels of this medication, requiring increased doses. Therefore, if a previously well-controlled patient begins having breakthrough seizures, levels of levetiracetam should be obtained. Pregnancy may have similar effects on the active oxcarbazepine metabolite, the monohydroxy derivative.

All anticonvulsants interfere with folic acid metabolism. Patients on anticonvulsants may actually become folic acid deficient and develop macrocytic anemia. Folic acid deficiency has been associated with neural tube defects (NTDs) and other congenital malformations. Because organogenesis occurs during the first weeks after conception, folic acid supplementation should be begun before pregnancy if possible. A dose of 4 mg daily is recommended. As previously stated, increasing folic acid ingestion may increase the activity of hepatic microsomal enzymes and thus the clearance of anticonvulsant medications. If anticonvulsant levels are being used, they should be checked frequently after folic acid therapy is implemented. Furthermore, therapy with phenytoin may result in increased metabolism of vitamin D, leading to decreased vitamin D levels. The patient should be reminded to take her prenatal vitamins, which include an adequate amount of vitamin D. In the occasional patient on long-term phenytoin, a vitamin D_3 level may be useful in guiding the amount of vitamin D the patient should take.

Neonatal hemorrhage, due to decreased vitamin K–dependent clotting factors (II, VII, IX, X), has been reported in infants born to mothers taking phenobarbital, phenytoin, and primidone. In one series,[13] 8 of 16 infants exposed to these medications had a cord blood coagulation pattern similar to that of a vitamin K deficiency. This occurred earlier than the customary hemorrhagic disease of the newborn. These infants responded to vitamin K infusion. Bleyer and Skinner[14] reviewed a case of their own and 21 other cases of hemorrhagic disease following anticonvulsant therapy that have appeared in the literature. They reached similar conclusions that these cases are vitamin K–dependent clotting factor deficiencies and that, at birth, infants should be given 1 mg of vitamin K intramuscularly. **A more recent study did not find any increased risk of bleeding in the neonate if the infant received 1 mg of vitamin K intramuscularly (IM) at birth.**[15] This problem is rare today as most neonates are given vitamin K at birth and because phenobarbital and primidone are almost never used today and phenytoin use for epilepsy is greatly decreasing.

Effect of Epilepsy on Pregnancy

The majority of women with seizure disorders who become pregnant have an uneventful pregnancy with an excellent outcome. There appear, however, to be several pregnancy complications that are more prevalent in the mother with epilepsy than in the general population. In a review of all birth certificates for infants born in the state of Washington from 1980 to 1981, Yerby and coworkers[16] identified 200 births to mothers with seizure disorders. Although birth certificate studies are often limited, these researchers controlled for many variables including previous adverse pregnancy outcome and socioeconomic status. **They found that mothers with seizure disorders were 2.66 times more likely to have had a previous fetal death after 20 weeks' gestation than the control population.** Because of the retrospective nature of this study, the authors were unable to correlate this with intrauterine growth restriction (IUGR) or other fetal problems. This increased incidence of stillbirth is confirmed in other investigations.[5] It is unclear in any of these studies what type of fetal surveillance was used and if there were any predictors that these fetuses were at risk. With the increased use of ultrasound to identify IUGR, malformations, and oligohydramnios, many of the stillborn fetuses may have been identified as being at risk and might have undergone antepartum fetal testing and intervention before the fetal demise occurred. These studies also were not stratified by medications taken, dosages, drug levels, or seizure activity during pregnancy.

Hiilesmaa and colleagues,[17] in a study of 150 pregnant women with seizure disorders, found no difference in perinatal mortality rates between patients and controls. However, there were three third-trimester stillbirths in the epileptic group and two in the control group. **Yerby and colleagues[16] also found an increased incidence of preeclampsia in women with seizure disorders.** This finding has also been identified in other large retrospective studies.[5] In a Norwegian study, Borthen and colleagues[18] studied 205 epileptic women and found an increased risk of *severe* preeclampsia with an odds ratio (OR) of 5 and 95% confidence intervals (CIs) of 1.3 to 19.9. Even though this study can be criticized for the wide CI, the findings were statistically significant. It is the first such study to single out severe preeclampsia. Nonetheless, Hiilesmaa and colleagues[17] found no difference in the rate of preeclampsia between pregnant women with epilepsy and controls. Yerby and colleagues[16] also showed a 2.79-fold increase in low-birth-weight infants. In a carefully performed study in Italy, Mastroiacovo and coworkers[19] found that the mean birth weight in neonates born to women with epilepsy was 107 g lower than that of controls. The mean birth weight in the epilepsy group, however, still fell within the normal range for gestational age. The clinical significance of this finding, therefore, is questionable. When considering all commonly used anticonvulsants, this decrease in neonatal weight appeared to be more common in infants exposed in utero to phenobarbital, which is almost never used today.

Mastroiacovo and colleagues[19] also found a decrease in head circumference in infants of mothers with epilepsy. This effect was seen in both untreated women with epilepsy and those receiving medications. Although this change was statistically significant, the mean head circumferences of both study and control infants still fell within the normal range. These authors found no difference in neonatal length comparing groups of mothers with epilepsy and control populations. Hiilesmaa and colleagues[20] also found a decrease in head circumference in neonates born to women with epilepsy. This decrease was most marked in women taking carbamazepine both alone or in combination with phenobarbital. Again, the mean head circumferences, however, were still within the expected normal range.[20] In the follow-up of this study, head circumferences were still smaller at 18 months of age.

Along similar lines, Hvas and colleagues[21] compared pregnancy outcomes in 193 women with epilepsy with those of 24,094 women without epilepsy delivering between 1989 and 1997. They found that birth weight of infants born to women with epilepsy was 208 g less than those born to women without a seizure disorder. **The OR that a woman treated with epilepsy would give birth to an infant with IUGR was 1.9.** Head circumference and body length were also diminished in the infants born to women taking antiepileptic drugs. When smokers with and without epilepsy were compared, there was an increased risk of preterm birth in those who smoked. Battine and colleagues[22] examined anthropometrics in children born to women with epilepsy in Canada, Japan, and Italy. They found some distinct geographic differences in risk for decreased head circumference that may or may not be related to the drug regimen. The RR for small head circumference in infants exposed to more than one medication (polytherapy) was 2.7. A dose-dependent response for both head circumference and body weight was seen with the use of phenobarbital and primidone, both of which are rarely used today. The authors state that in addition to drug regimen, genetic, ethnic, and environmental effects should be taken into account when considering explanations for decreased head circumference and birth weight in infants born to women treated for epilepsy.

Hiilesmaa and colleagues[17,20] found no increase in pregnancy complications in women with epilepsy. They also observed no increase in preterm labor, bleeding, pregnancy-induced hypertension, operative vaginal delivery, or cesarean delivery rates. However, in a study from 1999 to 2006, Borthen and colleagues[18] did show an increase in labor induction and cesarean delivery in mothers being treated for seizure disorder. However, it is unknown whether the increase in induction led to the increase in cesarean deliveries.

Richmond and colleagues[23] showed increased rates of nonproteinuric hypertension, induction of labor, and fetal cardiovascular malformations in 414 women with epilepsy. Rates of other antenatal, intrapartum, and neonatal complications were similar to those in controls. They concluded that women with epilepsy are not at increased risk for obstetrical complications providing appropriate care is available.

Viinikainen[24] reviewed 179 pregnancies in women with epilepsy compared to controls. There were no significant differences in the incidences of preeclampsia, preterm labor, perinatal mortality, or low birth weight. The rate of small-for-gestational-age infants was significantly higher, and neonatal head circumferences were significantly smaller in women with epilepsy.

In summary, women with seizure disorders are at increased risk of IUGR and stillbirth. It also appears that infants born to mothers with seizure disorders, on average, are smaller than their control counterparts. Even though smaller, they are usually within the normal range for gestational age. Furthermore, the incidence of preeclampsia is probably higher in mothers with seizure disorders. **The vast majority of pregnancies, however, are uncomplicated with no increase in complications over the expected rate.** Nonetheless, because of these few potential problems, the obstetrician should be more surveillant for pregnancy-related complications in pregnant women with treated and untreated seizure disorders.

Effects of Anticonvulsant Medications on the Fetus

There is little doubt that anticonvulsant medications are associated with an increase in congenital malformations, but the magnitude of this risk and the association of certain anomalies with specific drugs remain debatable. Although there was some evidence for teratogenicity related to phenytoin in the 1960s, Hanson and Smith[25] identified a specific fetal hydantoin syndrome in 1975. They noted growth and performance delays, craniofacial abnormalities (including clefting), and limb anomalies (including hypoplasia of nails and distal phalanges). They first described this syndrome in five infants exposed to phenytoin in utero. Hanson and colleagues[26] later reported that 7% to 11% of infants exposed to phenytoin had this recognizable pattern of malformations. They furthermore found that 31% of exposed fetuses had some aspects of the syndrome. Yet in 1988 Gaily and colleagues[27] reported no evidence of the hydantoin syndrome in 82 women exposed in utero to phenytoin. Some of the patients had hypertelorism and hypoplasia of the distal phalanges, but none had the full hydantoin syndrome.

Since the original reports by Hanson and colleagues, many studies have reported congenital malformations in infants born to mothers taking both the traditional and newer anticonvulsant medications, particularly facial clefting, congenital heart disease, and NTDs.

The overall rate of anomalies is doubled, but the rate of NTDs with valproic acid is increased tenfold, from 1 to 2 per 1000 to 1% to 2%.[28] It remains of prime importance, however, to treat the patient with the medication that best controls her seizures.

It has been over three decades since Nakane and colleagues[29] published the first major, multi-institutional study investigating the teratogenicity of antiepileptic medications. This study, carried out between 1974 and 1977, examined 902 pregnancies in mothers with idiopathic epilepsy. The overall rate of congenital malformations was 7.2%. This included 8.7% in the mothers who received anticonvulsant medications during pregnancy and 1.9% in nonmedicated mothers. Looking only at live-born infants, 9.9% had malformations (11.5% in the medicated group and 2.3% in the nonmedicated group). Therefore, the incidence of malformations in mothers receiving anticonvulsant therapy was about five times that of the nonmedicated group. Interestingly, Canger and colleagues[30] began collecting data in Italy at the time Nakane's group completed their data collection. Canger and coworkers studied 517 women with epilepsy throughout pregnancy. They found a 9.7% rate of malformations, a proportion strikingly similar to that of Nakane.[29] The importance of this study was that it showed that the findings in Nakane's study were not due to something special in his geographic population but could be applied worldwide.

In Nakane's study,[29] the predominant malformations were cleft lip and palate (3.14%) and cardiovascular malformations (2.95%). Nakane's group also noted that as the number of anticonvulsant medications used in combination during pregnancy increased, the incidence of fetal malformations rose dramatically.[29] The malformation rate was less than 5% when one medication (monotherapy) was used and was greater than 20% when four medications were used. Of note, 537 patients were taking two or more medications, whereas 93 patients were taking only one medication. **This was the first study to show that the risk of anomalies was higher in those receiving polytherapy for epilepsy.**

Kaneko and colleagues[31] confirmed these findings. They performed a prospective study to determine primary factors responsible for the increased incidence of malformations in infants born to mothers being treated with anticonvulsants. They specifically looked at various drug combinations. The overall malformation rate was 14%. In the patients who were receiving a single medication, the malformation rate was 6.5%.[31] The malformation rate for those treated with multiple medications was 15.6%.

Kaneko and colleagues[32] subsequently published a follow-up study to detect malformations in infants exposed in utero to anticonvulsant medications. They compared these results with their previous investigation.[31] The first study examined infants born between 1978 and 1984, whereas the later study evaluated infants born between 1985 and 1989. Whereas 14% of infants had some malformation in the previous study, the malformation rate was only 6.3% in the second group.[32] Again, there was no relationship between the medication taken and the type of malformation found. The lower rate of malformations may be attributable to the increase in patients receiving monotherapy. In the earlier study, 16.1% of patients received a single medication, whereas 63.4% received a single medication in the later study. Jick and Terris[33] matched two nonexposed pregnant women to each of 297 pregnant women exposed to antiepileptic medication. The rate of anomalies in infants born to women with epilepsy was 3.4%,[33] a rate even lower than that found by Kaneko and colleagues in their 1992 study.[32] Nonetheless, Jick and

Terris found the RR for a woman on antiepileptic medications to give birth to an infant with an anomaly was 3.3.[33]

Most neurologists are treating patients with a single agent. **Now that blood levels of anticonvulsant medications can be easily measured, single medications can be given at higher doses to make certain that therapeutic levels are achieved.** This approach has lessened the need for multiple medications. Counseling is also more involved today because many patients are receiving the newer anticonvulsant medications with which we have less experience.

The same concept was verified in a study by Lindhout and colleagues.[34] They compared the pattern of malformations in the offspring of two cohorts of women with seizure disorders, one from 1972 to 1979 and one from 1980 to 1985. In the earlier cohort, 15 of 151 (10%) of live-born infants had at least one congenital anomaly. The most common anomalies were those most frequently reported for anticonvulsant medications: congenital heart defects, facial clefts, facial dysmorphism, and developmental delays. In the latter cohort, 13 of 172 infants (7.6%) exposed in utero to anticonvulsant medications had congenital malformations. The most frequent anomalies in this group were spinal defects and hypospadias. All of these anomalies were associated with maternal therapy with valproate, carbamazepine, or both. In the earlier cohort of patients, the mean number of drugs used during gestation was 2.2 compared with 1.7 in the later cohort. Whereas only 28% of women in the earlier cohort received only one medication, 47% of the women received monotherapy in the second group of patients. The lower overall rate of malformations in the latter cohort appeared to be due to the reduction in the number of pregnancies during which a combination of medications was used. It is also apparent in this study that neither the duration of maternal epilepsy nor maternal age was associated with malformations in the infants born to these mothers.

Dravet and colleagues[35] described the risk for malformations in the infants of 227 women participating in a prospective study between 1984 and 1988. There was a 7% malformation rate among infants born to mothers taking antiepileptic medications compared with 1.36% in the control group. Therefore, fetuses exposed in utero to anticonvulsants had an RR of 6.9 of being born with a congenital malformation. This is double the risk demonstrated by Jick and Terris.[33] In this study, the frequency of spina bifida was 17 times more than would be expected in the general population, and heart defects were 9.6 times greater than expected. Cleft lip with or without cleft palate was 8.4 times more frequent than expected in the general population. Using logistic regression, **these authors concluded that valproate and phenytoin were the two most teratogenic medications.**[35] This is important because, although phenytoin is less frequently used today, valproate is still commonly used. The cases of NTDs and congenital heart defects were studied carefully and could not be related to a familial disposition for these defects. As other studies have shown, there was a higher incidence of malformations in infants born to mothers receiving polytherapy (16%) than in those receiving monotherapy (6%). This relationship between the number of medications taken and the rate of malformations may not be as clear today, as most women taking multiple anticonvulsants are taking at least one of the newer medications. There are not a lot of data on malformations rates with combinations of these medications.

A study by Koch and colleagues,[36] however, showed no difference between the rate of malformations in mothers receiving polytherapy and mothers receiving a single medication. Furthermore, they found that the infants born to mothers with epilepsy, regardless of therapy, had only twice as many major malformations as infants born to the control population. The number of minor anomalies, however, was approximately three times greater in infants born to mothers receiving anticonvulsant medication than in the control group. **In the mothers receiving monotherapy, those taking valproate had the highest rate of minor malformations.**[36] In this study, there appeared to be a link between the dose of valproate and the rate of malformations.

Gaily and Granstrom[37] also investigated minor anomalies in children of mothers with epilepsy. These authors point out that many of the supposedly specific syndromes resulting from intrauterine exposure to certain medications have many common features. They argue that specific syndromes and their association with specific drugs, as well as the frequencies of these syndromes, have not been confirmed in epidemiologic studies. They found that many of the minor anomalies that are thought to be specific features of a medication appear to be genetically linked with epilepsy.[37] Indeed, this is in contrast to many of the other published studies. In this study only distal digital hypoplasia appeared to be a specific marker for phenytoin teratogenicity.

Yerby and colleagues[38] also looked prospectively at malformations in infants born to mothers with epilepsy. They further investigated whether pure folate deficiency might be responsible for the malformations. None of the women in their study had deficient folate levels. There was no difference in major malformations between patients and controls in this study. In fact, only 0.4 mg of folic acid supplementation is recommended preconception in a recent practice parameter update by the American Academy of Neurology. The infants born to mothers taking anticonvulsant medications, however, had a higher mean number of minor anomalies. They found no difference in the number of minor anomalies whether the child was exposed in utero to one anticonvulsant medication or to several.[38] The authors also confirm the great overlap in minor anomalies and various medications, further casting doubt on whether individual medications cause specific syndromes.[38]

Nulman and colleagues[39] examined 36 mother-child pairs exposed to carbamazepine, 34 pairs exposed to phenytoin, nine pairs of nonmedicated epileptic women, and matched each to nine mother-child pairs not exposed to teratogens. Minor anomalies were more common in offspring of mothers receiving either carbamazepine or phenytoin (RR 2.1).[39]

Valproate is still often used in in antiepileptic therapy as an anticonvulsant of choice because of its low side effect profile. It has, however, been reported to be associated with specific anomalies. DiLiberti and colleagues,[40] in 1984, reported a specific fetal valproate syndrome. This was based on seven infants. They found a consistent facial phenotype in all seven children and other birth defects in four. This syndrome phenotype was confirmed by others. Jager-Roman and colleagues,[41] in 1986, reported fetal distress in 50% of 14 infants receiving valproate. Furthermore, 28% had low Apgar scores. They also found the same craniofacial defects as reported by DiLiberti and colleagues.[40] **Lindhout and Schmidt[42] confirmed the association between NTDs and valproate exposure in utero. They contend that there is a 1.5% risk of an infant being born with an NTD if the mother took valproate in the first trimester.** Lindhout and colleagues[43] also studied 34 cases of NTDs in mothers taking anticonvulsant medications. In 33 of the 34 cases, mothers were exposed to either valproate or carbamazepine. **Most of the cases of NTDs were lumbosacral. There was only one case of anencephaly. This implies that these medications have a predisposition to cause lumbosacral defects, because in the general population, spina bifida and anencephaly are equally distributed.** In only two cases were other major malformations found. The development of NTDs in these infants of mothers taking valproate also appeared to be a dose-dependent phenomenon. In a mouse model, valproate alters folic acid metabolism in embryos. This could account for the increased risk of NTDs in infants born to mothers who have taken valproate.

The U.K. registry[44] has reported a higher malformation rate with valproate, 5.9%, than with carbamazepine, 2.3%, and lamotrigine, 2.1%. In the North American registry, the RR of having an affected offspring for the valproate-exposed woman was 7.3.[45] Valproate is associated with major malformations other than NTDs (RR 3.77). The risk is dose dependent, beginning at 600 mg/day and becoming more prominent at 1000 mg/day.[46] Polytherapy including valproate carries more risk than any other polytherapy.[47] In summary, the pattern of physical abnormalities is related to the use of anticonvulsant drugs, rather than to epilepsy itself.[48]

In 1989, Jones and colleagues[49] reported a pattern of minor craniofacial defects, fingernail hypoplasia, and developmental delay in infants exposed in utero to carbamazepine. Others have shown that there is a 1% risk of spina bifida in infants of mothers taking carbamazepine. Carbamazepine increases the incidence of NTDs, cardiovascular and urinary tract anomalies, and cleft palate. Because this spectrum of defects (except spina bifida) is similar to that in the fetal hydantoin syndrome, Jones and colleagues[49] hypothesized that, because both drugs are metabolized through an arene oxide pathway, perhaps an epoxide intermediary is the teratogenic agent. Those fetuses with low levels of epoxide hydrolase are exposed to higher levels of epoxide intermediaries, and this may lead to an increase in malformations. Conversely, fetuses with high enzyme levels clear epoxides rapidly, minimizing exposure to the potential teratogens. Phenytoin, phenobarbital, and to a lesser extent carbamazepine are metabolized through this pathway. Much work in this area is being performed by researchers who believe that low levels of epoxide hydrolase activity may be the common link explaining why only certain fetuses exposed to anticonvulsant medications in utero develop congenital malformations.

The increased risk of delivery of a child with an NTD after first trimester exposure to carbamazepine and valproate continues to be studied using epilepsy registries. Jentink and colleagues[50] showed that there was a 3.3% risk of delivering a child with a congenital malformation after first trimester carbamazepine exposure, but this is significantly higher than in the general population in their study. However, that is not significantly higher than the background risk of malformations found in most populations. However, they showed an increased risk of spina bifida (OR 2.6 with 95% confidence level of 1.2 to 5.3).[50] They found this risk, however, to be significantly lower than the risk associated with first trimester valproate exposure.

Jentink and colleagues[51] showed that after valproate exposure, there was an increase in 6 of the 14 malformations investigated. The OR for spina bifida was 12.7 (95% CI 7.7 to 20.7). However, of particular interest, the OR for craniosynostosis was 6.8 with a CI of 1.8 to 18.8. Also the OR for cleft palate was 5.2 (95% CI 2.8 to 9.9). **This study confirms that valproate exposure, even as monotherapy in the first trimester, is associated with an increased risk of major congenital malformations.[51]**

New antiepileptic drugs have been approved and have been rapidly incorporated into clinical practice in the last decade. There is a need for these medications because 25% to 30% of epileptic patients are not adequately controlled by conventional therapies. These newer medications work at the level of neurotransmitters such as gamma-aminobutyric acid and also by blockade of sodium channels. **Table 46-2 lists these drugs, with their dosages, and describes other considerations in their use.** Gabapentin and pregabalin are also used in chronic pain,

TABLE 46-2 NEWER ANTIEPILEPTIC AGENTS

MEDICATION	USUAL DOSE (mg/day)	DOSES/ DAY	SPECIAL NOTES
Gabapentin	900-3600	3	Not enzyme inducer Antacids interfere
Lamotrigine	300-500	1 or 2	Rash in 11.2% Not enzyme inducer Half-life affected by meds
Topiramate	100-400	2	May interfere with OCs Moderate enzyme inducer
Tiagabine	8-56	2 or 4	Does not interfere with OCs Not enzyme inducer
Oxcarbazepine	600-2400	2	Moderate enzyme inducer
Levetiracetam	1000-3000	2	Not enzyme inducer
Zonisamide	400-600	2	Not enzyme inducer

OCs, Oral contraceptives.

mood stabilization, and neuropathies. Lamotrigine and oxcarbazepine are commonly used to treat bipolar disorder. Therefore, the obstetrician may encounter patients other than those with epilepsy on gabapentin. At present, there are limited data on its fetal effects in pregnancy. **Patients should be warned that we do not yet know enough about the effects of the drug on the developing fetus to appropriately counsel them. Nonetheless, if this medication is necessary to keep seizures under control, it should be used.**

Lamotrigine is an adjunctive therapy for the treatment of simple and complex seizures with and without secondary generalization. Approximately 10% of patients discontinue the medication because of a rash. Severe rashes such as Stevens-Johnson syndrome and toxic epidermal necrolysis have been reported. The severe rashes have occurred with more frequency in pediatric patients. In one study, a rash necessitating discontinuation of therapy was found in only 2% of 11,316 treated patients.[52] **Cord blood levels of lamotrigine are equal to those of maternal serum. Also, the median milk/maternal plasma concentration ratio of 0.61 indicates that there are significant milk levels. In the lamotrigine pregnancy registry, of 595 exposures to date, 17 had major defects (2.9%), not significantly increased over the expected rate.[51] However, the American registry has reported an increased risk of nonsyndromic oral clefts.**

Topiramate, oxcarbazepine, and levetiracetam are also used as adjunctive therapies for epilepsy. All are effective. At this point there is limited information on the use of these medications in pregnancy. In March 2011, the FDA released an advisory that there was a 1.3% risk of oral clefts with the use of topiramate in pregnancy. This was based on findings from the North America Anti-Epilepsy Drug Registry. However, there has not yet been a major peer-reviewed publication with these data. **Molgaard-Nielsen and Hviid[53] reviewed 1532 infants who were exposed to lamotrigine, oxcarbazepine, topiramate, gabapentin, and levetiracetam in the first trimester.** They compared results with 836,263 infants that were not exposed to these medications. The rate of anomalies was 3.2% versus 2.4%, which gives an adjusted OR of 0.99. **They conclude that in Denmark these medications are not associated with an increased risk of malformations.[53]** In summary, the neurologist and obstetrician should work together and use whichever medications work best for the patient.

There has been much debate over whether epilepsy itself and the use of antiepileptic medications are associated with psychomotor delays or mental retardation. In the landmark study by Nelson and Ellenberg, an intelligence quotient (IQ) below 70 was seen in 65.2 per 1000 7-year-old children in the seizure group compared with 34 per 1000 in the age-matched control group, a statistically significant difference. Before generalizations can be made, many confounding factors must be evaluated, including other anomalies and social environment. In another review, none of the major antiepileptic medications appeared to carry special risk for mental retardation. However, polytherapy and inherited deviations in antiepileptic medication metabolism in the fetus may increase the risk for mental retardation. Other factors associated with maternal epilepsy such as seizures during pregnancy, inherited brain disorders, and a nonoptimal psychosocial environment can also affect a child's psychomotor development. These factors are hard to control in any study. In a report by Gaily and colleagues,[54] two of 48 (4.1%) infants of mothers with epilepsy had mental retardation, and two additional infants had borderline intelligence. The mean IQ of the infants exposed in utero to anticonvulsant medications was statistically lower than the control group. When these four children were excluded from the analysis, the difference in mean IQ disappeared.[54] **There was no increased risk of low intelligence attributable to fetal exposure either to antiepileptic medications below toxic levels or to brief maternal convulsions.** No particular medication appeared to be associated with a lower IQ. Social class also appeared to play a role in the differences in IQs in these patients.

Moore and colleagues[55] reviewed 57 infants with fetal anticonvulsant syndromes. Eighty-one percent reported behavioral problems, with hyperactivity being the most common (34%). Two or more autistic features were found in 34 (60%) of the 57 children. Four were diagnosed with autism and two with Asperberger's syndrome. Learning difficulties were found in 77% and speech delay in 81%. Gross and fine motor delays were identified in 60% and 42%, respectively. These percentages seem high, but it is important to remember that all of these children had already been identified as having an anticonvulsant syndrome. Meador and colleagues[56] showed that at age 3, infants with in utero exposure to valproate had a significantly lower IQ (92) when compared to exposures to carbamazepine (98), lamotrigine (101), and phenytoin (99). Even though all of these findings are statistically significant, it is unknown whether these findings are clinically significant.

In summary, there appears to be a small, undefined risk of a slightly lower IQ, psychomotor delay, and an increase in behavior problems in infants born to mothers with epilepsy. With the exception of valproate, it does not appear that any particular medication results in a higher risk of this outcome.[56]

Preconceptional Counseling for the Reproductive-Age Woman with a Seizure Disorder

Although it is not always possible, it is preferable to counsel the patient with epilepsy before she becomes pregnant. A detailed history should be taken to determine if there are any seizure disorders or congenital malformations in the family. The obstetrician must stress that the patient has greater than a 90% chance of having a successful pregnancy resulting in a normal newborn. A detailed history of medication use and seizure frequency should be obtained. The patient must be informed that if she has frequent seizures before conception, this pattern will probably continue. Furthermore, if she has frequent seizures, she should be encouraged to delay conception until control is better, even if this entails a change or an additional medication. The obstetrician must stress that controlling seizures is of primary importance and that the patient will need to take whatever medication or medications are necessary to achieve this goal throughout her pregnancy. **If the patient has had no seizures during the past 2 to 5 years, an attempt may be made to withdraw her from anticonvulsant medications.** This is usually done over a 1- to 3-month period, slowly reducing the medication. Up to 50% of patients relapse and need to start their medications again. This withdrawal should be attempted only if the patient is completely seizure free for 2 years, has a normal electroencephalogram (EEG), and only with the help of a neurologist. During the period of withdrawal from medications, patients should refrain from driving.

It is best to have the patient taking a single medication during pregnancy. If the patient is on multiple medications, the patient can be changed to monotherapy over several months. The drug of choice for the specific type of epilepsy should be the one chosen for monotherapy. As the other medications are gradually withdrawn, levels of the remaining medication should be monitored to make certain that the level remains therapeutic. Many individuals do not believe that medication levels are useful. However, when withdrawing or changing medications, any additional data available can help the physician in making decisions. The patient should refrain from conceiving until seizures have been well controlled for several months on the single medication. **The patient must also be counseled that she should get adequate rest and sleep during pregnancy, because sleep deprivation is associated with increased seizure frequency.**

The most important point is to control maternal seizures with the least side effects to the mother and fetus. There may be some additional concern for using valproate in pregnancy due to the reported increased incidence of fetal distress and malformations, including NTDs. However, if valproate is the anticonvulsant that works best for the patient, it should be used with appropriate counseling and, in pregnancy, ultrasound to detect possible fetal anomalies should be performed at the appropriate gestational age. If valproate is selected, the total dose should be divided into three to four administrations daily to avoid high peak plasma levels. As described earlier, NTDs also occur with the use of carbamazepine. There is less information concerning the newer antiepileptic drugs and teratogenesis. If they need to be used for good seizure control, they should be implemented as part of the patient's therapy.

Folic acid supplementation should be begun before pregnancy. Folic acid supplementation may help to prevent NTDs, which have been seen most commonly with carbamazepine and valproate treatment but have been reported in women taking other anticonvulsants as well. Studies have shown that folic acid may decrease the incidence of NTDs in at-risk women.[11] It is important that this be implemented before pregnancy or very early in pregnancy, because open NTDs occur by the end of the fifth week of gestation. Furthermore, low folate levels have been associated with an increase in adverse pregnancy outcomes in women taking anticonvulsants.[57] Anticonvulsant levels should be checked frequently after implementing or increasing folic acid administration, because folate leads to lower anticonvulsant levels.[57] A daily dose of folic acid of 4 mg/day is recommended. Patients should also be encouraged to take their prenatal vitamins, which contain vitamin D. This is because anticonvulsants may interfere with the conversion of 25-hydroxycholecalciferol to 1-25-dihydroxycholecalciferol, the active form of vitamin D.

Mothers with idiopathic epilepsy often ask if their child will develop epilepsy. There is a surprising paucity of studies in this area. **Children of parents without seizures have a 0.5% to 1% risk of developing epilepsy. It appears that the infant born to a mother with a seizure disorder of unknown etiology has a four times greater chance of developing idiopathic epilepsy than the general population.** Furthermore, it appears that epilepsy in the father does not increase a child's risk of developing a seizure disorder. Many of the rare seizure disorders have a stronger genetic component.[54]

Care of the Patient During Pregnancy

Once the patient becomes pregnant, it is of the utmost importance to establish accurate gestational dating. This will prevent any confusion over fetal growth in later gestation. **The patient's anticonvulsant level should be followed as needed and dosages adjusted accordingly to keep the patient seizure free.** It is a common pitfall to monitor levels too frequently and adjust dosages in a likewise frequent manner. It is important to remember that it takes several half-lives for a medication to reach a steady state (Table 46-3). Drugs such as phenobarbital have extremely long half-lives, and the levels should not be checked too frequently. If levels are measured before the drug reaches a steady state and the dosage is increased, the patient will eventually become toxic from the medication. Drug levels should be drawn immediately before the next dose (trough levels) in order to assess if dosing is adequate. If the patient is showing signs of toxicity, a peak level may be obtained.

At approximately 16 weeks' gestation, the patient should undergo blood testing for maternal serum marker screening in an attempt to detect an NTD. This, coupled with ultrasonography, gives a more than 90% detection rate for open NTDs. If the patient is difficult to scan or if she wants to be even more certain that there is no NTD, amniocentesis can be undertaken. This should be considered if the patient is taking valproate or carbamazepine,

TABLE 46-3 ANTICONVULSANTS COMMONLY USED DURING PREGNANCY

DRUG	THERAPEUTIC LEVEL (mg/L)	USUAL NONPREGNANT DOSAGE	HALF-LIFE
Carbamazepine	4-10	600-1200 mg/day in three or divided doses (two doses if extended-release forms are used)	Initially 36 hr, chronic therapy 16 hr
Phenobarbital	15-40	90-180 mg/day in two or three divided doses	100 hr
Phenytoin	10-20, total; 1-2, free	300-500 mg/day in single or divided doses*	Average 24 hr
Primidone	5-15	750-1500 mg/day in three divided doses	8 hr
Valproic acid	50-100	550-2000 mg/day in three or divided doses	Average 13 hr
Ethosuximide	40-120	1000-2000 mg/day in two divided doses	60 hr

*If a total dose of more than 300 mg is needed, dividing the dose will result in a more stable serum concentration.

because these medications appear to carry almost the same risk as if the patient had a family history of an NTD.[42,43] At 18 to 22 weeks, the patient should undergo a comprehensive, targeted ultrasound examination by an experienced obstetrical sonographer to look for congenital malformations. A fetal echocardiogram can be obtained at 20 to 22 weeks to look for cardiac malformations, which are among the more common malformations in women taking any antiepileptic medications. If fetal echocardiography is not readily available, it is reassuring to remember that an adequate four-chamber view of the heart on ultrasound will identify 68% to 95% of major cardiac anomalies.[58]

As previously noted, there appears to be an increased risk for IUGR for fetuses exposed in utero to anticonvulsant medications. If the patient's weight gain and fundal growth appear appropriate, regular ultrasound examinations for fetal weight assessment are probably unnecessary. If, however, there is a question of poor fundal growth or if the patient's habitus precludes adequate assessment of this clinical parameter, serial ultrasonography for fetal weight can be performed.

In older and retrospective studies, there appears to be an increased risk of stillbirth in mothers taking anticonvulsant medications.[5,54] In a prospective study, however, this complication was not seen.[17] As previously noted, in the studies that showed an increase in stillbirths, factors such as IUGR or oligohydramnios were not prenatally identified. With modern surveillance and the more common use of ultrasonography, many of these risk factors can be detected before the fetus faces imminent risk. Nonstress testing, therefore, is not necessary in all mothers with seizure disorders. It should be limited to those who have other medical or obstetrical complications that place the patient at an increased risk for a stillbirth. There may be an increased risk of preterm contractions and possibly preterm labor in epileptic women exposed to anticonvulsant medications.[59]

The key to managing anticonvulsants in pregnancy is individualization of therapy, ideally with a single medication. Medication levels should be used as an adjunct to following symptoms. The physician should not treat levels alone. A brief seizure during pregnancy does not appear to be deleterious to the fetus.[19] It is best to use the lowest dose of a single medication possible that will keep the patient seizure free. This, however, must be individualized. For instance, if the patient usually experiences seizures during the day and drives, it is important to make certain that the patient remains seizure free. For this type of patient, drug dosages should be increased if levels fall. If, on the other hand, the patient only has brief partial complex seizures that do not generalize and occur only during her sleep, it is optimal to keep the medications at the lowest serum concentration that will keep her seizure free. An occasional seizure of this type would not harm either the patient or her fetus.

Labor and Delivery

Vaginal delivery is the route of choice for the mother with a seizure disorder. If the mother has frequent seizures brought on by the stress of labor, she may undergo cesarean delivery after stabilization. This, however, is rare. With the use of epidural analgesia, the stress of labor can be virtually obviated in the parturient with epilepsy. Furthermore, seizures during labor may cause transient fetal bradycardia.[17] The fetal heart rate should be given time to recover. If fetal bradycardia persists, one must assume fetal compromise or placental abruption and proceed with cesarean delivery.

Management of anticonvulsant medications during a prolonged labor presents a challenge. **During labor, oral absorption of medications is erratic and, if the patient vomits, almost negligible. Phenytoin and levetiracetam are available in intravenous preparations.** Fosphenytoin, although expensive, is available and makes the administration of intravenous phenytoin much easier. If the patient's phenytoin level is normal, the usual daily dose may be administered intravenously. The medication should only be mixed in normal saline and must be administered at a rate no faster than 50 mg/min. Fosphenytoin is easier to use, as it is less likely to cause a maternal arrhythmia. It is problematic if the patient is taking carbamazepine. This medication is not manufactured in a parenteral form, although extended-release forms are now used by many patients. Oral administration may be attempted, but if the patient has seizures or a preseizure aura, she may be loaded with a therapeutic dose of phenytoin to carry her through labor. The usual loading dose is 10 to 15 mg/kg administered intravenously at a rate no faster than 50 mg/min. This should be effective in controlling seizures. Short-active benzodiazepenes may also be used for acute seizures, but one must remember that they can cause early neonatal depression as well as maternal apnea. Prenatal diagnostic techniques cannot be expected to detect all malformations. Even if the infant appears to have no anomalies, an experienced clinician should be present at the delivery of the infant born to a mother taking anticonvulsant medications.

New Onset of Seizures in Pregnancy and the Puerperium

Occasionally, seizures are diagnosed for the first time during pregnancy. This may present a diagnostic dilemma (Table 46-4). If the seizures occur in the third trimester, they are eclampsia until proven otherwise and should be treated as such until the physician can perform a proper evaluation. The treatment of eclampsia is delivery, but the patient must first be stabilized. It is often difficult, however, to distinguish eclampsia from an epileptic seizure. The patient may be hypertensive initially after an epileptic seizure and may exhibit some myoglobinuria secondary to muscle breakdown, which will test as proteinuria on a routine urinalysis. The diagnosis becomes clearer over time, but in either case, rapid, thoughtful action must be undertaken. The first physician to attend a patient after a seizure may not be an obstetrician/gynecologist, and magnesium sulfate may not be started acutely. This should be remedied as soon as possible.

If the patient develops seizures for the first time at an earlier gestational age, she should be evaluated and started on the proper medication. The physician must look for acquired causes of seizures, including trauma, infection, metabolic disorders, space-occupying lesions, central nervous system (CNS) bleeding, and ingestion of drugs such as cocaine and amphetamines. When a seizure occurs,

TABLE 46-4 DIFFERENTIAL DIAGNOSIS OF PERIPARTUM SEIZURES

	BLOOD PRESSURE	PROTEINURIA	SEIZURES	TIMING	CSF	OTHER FEATURES
Eclampsia	+++	+++	+++	Third trimester	Early: RBC, 0-1000; protein, 50-150 mg/dL Late: grossly bloody	Platelets normal or ↓ RBC normal
Epilepsy	Normal	Normal to +	+++	Any trimester	Normal	Low anticonvulsant levels
Subarachnoid hemorrhage	+ to +++ (labile)	0 to +	+	Any trimester	Grossly bloody	
Thrombotic thrombocytopenic purpura	Normal to +++	++	++	Third trimester	RBC 0-100	Platelets ↓↓ RBC fragmented
Amniotic fluid embolus	Shock	–	+	Intrapartum	Normal	Hypoxia, cyanosis Platelets ↓↓ RBC normal
Cerebral vein thrombosis	+	–	++	Postpartum	Normal (early)	Headache Occasional pelvic phlebitis
Water intoxication	Normal	–	++	Intrapartum	Normal	Oxytocin infusion rate >45 mU/min Serum na <124 mEq/L
Pheochromocytoma	+++ (labile)	+	+	Any trimester	Normal	Neurofibromatosis
Autonomic stress syndrome of high paraplegics	+++ with labor pains	–	–	Intrapartum	Normal	Cardiac arrhythmia
Toxicity of local anesthetics	Variable	–	++	Intrapartum	Normal	

Modified from Donaldson JO: Peripartum convulsion. In Donaldson JO (ed): Neurology of Pregnancy. Philadelphia, WB Saunders, 1989, p 312.

the patient must be stabilized, and the physician must make certain that an adequate airway is established for the protection of both mother and fetus. The physician should also seek focal signs that may be more suggestive of a space-occupying lesion, CNS bleeding, or an abscess. Blood samples should be obtained for electrolytes, glucose, ionized calcium, magnesium, renal function studies, and toxicologic studies while intravenous access is being established. If the patient experienced a tonic-clonic seizure, and the attending physician believes that this is probably new-onset epilepsy, she should be started on the appropriate anticonvulsant medication while awaiting results of laboratory studies. If she is not in status epilepticus and is not obtunded, this medication may be given orally.

If the patient has recurrent generalized seizures, status epilepticus, immediate therapeutic action must be taken. The drug of choice is intravenous phenytoin or fosphenytoin, because they are highly effective, have a long duration of action, and have a low incidence of serious side effects. These medications should be administered in a loading dose of 15 to 20 mg/kg at a rate not exceeding 50 mg/min. Rapid infusion of phenytoin may cause transient hypotension and heart block. Therefore, if available, fosphenytoin is a better choice. If possible, the patient should be placed on a cardiac monitor while receiving a loading dose of phenytoin. Also, this medication must be given in a glucose-free solution to avoid precipitation. If phenytoin and fosphenytoin are unavailable, a benzodiazepine may be used as a first-line drug for status epilepticus. These drugs, however, cause respiratory depression, and the physician must have the ability to intubate the patient, if necessary, when these medications are used. If these measures are ineffective, an anesthesiologist and a neurologist should be immediately consulted if they are not already involved in the patient's care.

Any patient experiencing seizures for the first time during pregnancy without a known cause should undergo an EEG and intracranial imaging. In looking only at eclamptic patients, Sibai and colleagues[60] found that EEGs were initially abnormal in 75% of patients but normalized within 6 months in all women studied. Although this group found no uniform abnormalities on computed tomography (CT) in this series of eclamptic patients, they did find that 46% and 33% had some abnormal findings on magnetic resonance imaging (MRI) and CT, respectively. Most of the findings were nonspecific and were not helpful in diagnosis or treatment. If the physician is not certain that the patient has eclampsia, an imaging study should be part of the evaluation described previously.

Postpartum Period

The levels of anticonvulsant medications must be monitored frequently during the first few weeks postpartum, because they can rise rapidly. **If the patient's medication dosages were increased during pregnancy, they will need to be decreased rather rapidly after delivery to prepregnancy levels.** All of the major anticonvulsant medications cross into breast milk. The levels vary in breast milk from 18% to 79% of the plasma levels. The use of these medications, however, is not a contraindication to breastfeeding. Topiramate has been associated with neonatal weight loss and probably should not be used if the mother is breastfeeding.

All methods of contraception are available to women with idiopathic seizure disorders. The majority of women are able to take oral contraceptives without any adverse side effects. Oral contraceptive failures are more common in women taking certain anticonvulsants, because some of the major anticonvulsant medications induce hepatic enzymes (cytochrome P 450), which metabolize estrogen faster. The enzyme-inducing drugs are phenytoin, carbamazepine, and phenobarbital. With topiramate and oxcarbazepine, the enzyme-inducing effects occur at higher doses, 200 mg and 1200 mg, respectively. This enzyme-inducing effect is not seen with lamotrigine, zonisamide, gabapentin, tiagabine, valproate, or levetiracetam (see Table 46-2).

In conclusion, the majority of women with idiopathic epilepsy have an uneventful pregnancy with an excellent outcome. To optimize neonatal outcome, the patient should take only one medication and, when possible, use the lowest dose effective in keeping her free of seizures. It is important, however, for the patient to realize that prevention of seizures is the most important goal during pregnancy. Simple interventions such as taking folic acid before conception, taking prenatal vitamins containing vitamin D, and giving the infant vitamin K at birth will help to optimize the outcome. There is an increase in congenital malformations in infants exposed to anticonvulsant medications in utero. The majority of infants exposed to these medications, however, will have no malformations. With modern techniques for prenatal diagnosis, including ultrasound and quadruple screening, many of these malformations can be detected early. The majority of women with epilepsy labor normally and have spontaneous vaginal deliveries. In short, with close cooperation and excellent communication among the obstetrician, neurologist, and pediatrician, the vast majority of these patients will have a safe pregnancy with an excellent outcome.

In 2009, the American Academy of Neurology, with some input from ACOG, made some recommendations to help guide physicians in caring for pregnant women with epilepsy.[61] **They recommend, if possible, avoiding valproate and polytherapy during the first trimester of pregnancy to help prevent anomalies. They recommend the avoidance of valproate and polytherapy throughout pregnancy to prevent reduced cognitive outcomes.** There is less evidence, but they feel that phenytoin and phenobarbital should be avoided because they may be associated with decreased cognitive outcomes. The offspring of women exposed to antiepileptic medication are probably at risk for being born small for gestational age and having a 1-minute Apgar score of less than 7.[61]

MIGRAINE

Headaches are extremely common in women, and the majority of migraine headaches occur in women of childbearing age. Migraines can be classified as those with aura (other neurologic signs and symptoms) and those without aura. Maggioni and colleagues[62] surveyed 430 women 3 days postpartum about their headache histories, and 126 (29.3%) were found to be primary headache sufferers. Of these patients, 81 suffered from migraine without aura, 12 suffered from migraine with aura, and 33 had tension-type headaches. Migraines are associated with vasodilation of the cerebral vasculature and last a variable amount of time. They are often accompanied by photosensitivity (and/or phonosensitivity) and nausea. Migraines with aura may be accompanied by sensations in the extremities and other lateralizing signs, sometimes making them difficult to distinguish from transient ischemic attacks. Migraines with these symptoms are often referred to as atypical migraines.

Migraine symptoms tend to improve during pregnancy. Maggioni and colleagues[62] found that 80% of patients experienced either complete remission or a 50% reduction in headaches during pregnancy. Improvement was more common after the first trimester. Others found that migraines disappeared during pregnancy in 67% of cases, or that 60% to 70% of women either go into remission or improve significantly, usually in the second and third trimesters. Migraine type does not seem to be a prognostic factor. Those with menstrual (catamenial) migraines showed the most improvement. However, 4% to 8% show significant worsening during pregnancy.

In 508 women with a history of migraine from the Collaborative Perinatal Project, patients with migraines smoked more heavily and had a longer smoking history than did their headache-free peers. They also found that in nonsmokers, migraine was often associated with allergies. In a study by Ertresveg and colleagues,[63] 58% of subjects with migraine reported having no headache during pregnancy. Transient neurologic symptoms were more common in patients with a history of migraine. Chen and Leviton[64] examined data from the large, prospective Collaborative Perinatal Project of 55,000 pregnancies. They found that less than 2% of women in the sample were considered to have migraines at their initial prenatal visit. Of the 484 (of 508) women with a complete data set, 17% experienced complete cessation of headache throughout pregnancy and an additional 62% had two or fewer headaches in the third trimester.[64] Only 21% of these women had no improvement in headache. They examined all available demographic and pregnancy factors and could find no factor that could be used to predict headache improvement during pregnancy.

Chancellor and colleagues[65] followed nine patients whose migraines first occurred during pregnancy at various gestational ages. They were followed for more than 4 years after pregnancy, and the prognosis for headache was excellent. Four of the nine patients developed complications of pregnancy, including preeclampsia in two. Maggioni's group found no increase in pregnancy complications in patients with migraine.[62] It is unknown if the headaches were caused by developing preeclampsia. It is important to rule out other significant complications of pregnancy before assigning a new diagnosis of migraine to a pregnant patient. Jacobson and Redman[66] reported a patient who actually lost consciousness during pregnancy because of a basilar migraine.

Using a nationwide population-based database in Taiwan, Chen and colleagues[67] identified 4911 women with migraines who delivered from 2001 to 2003. After adjusting for confounders, they found that there was an increased risk for low birth weight (OR 1.16), preterm birth (OR 1.24), cesarean delivery (OR 1.16), and preeclampsia (OR 1.34). Although these increases were not large, they were all statistically significant.[67] More research needs to be undertaken to find out if these increases apply to different populations and if they are clinically significant.

Supportive therapy is recommended for patients who experience migraine attacks during gestation. Acetaminophen is initially recommended, and narcotic analgesics can be used as necessary. The use of nonsteroidal anti-inflammatory agents should be avoided, if possible, after 24 weeks' gestation, because when used for more than 48 hours, they can cause premature closure of the ductus arteriosus and/or oligohydramnios. When pain is severe, parenteral narcotics, prochlorperazine, and other anti-emetic therapy may be used. These agents are often used in conjunction with diphenhydramine. **β-Blockers may be safely administered during pregnancy for prophylaxis,** and propranolol is probably safest. The calcium channel blockers used in the treatment of migraine can also be safely administered during gestation (see Chapter 8).

Ergotamine should be avoided during pregnancy. Previous reports have suggested that it may cause birth defects that have a vascular disruptive etiology. In addition, ergots are uterotonic and have an abortifacient potential.

Sumatriptan, a serotonin receptor agonist, is very successful in treating migraines. In a review by O'Quinn and colleagues,[68] there were no untoward effects in 76 first-trimester exposures to sumatriptan. Using logistic regression, Olesen and colleagues[69] compared 34 sumatriptan exposures with 89 migraine controls and 15,995 healthy women. They found that the risk of preterm birth was elevated (OR 6.3), as was the risk of IUGR.[69] They do state that they did not control for disease severity. A larger study by Kallen and colleagues[70] has not confirmed these findings. **In 658 infants whose mothers had used sumatriptan during pregnancy, there was no significant difference in prematurity or low birth weight.**[70] Hilaire and colleagues[71] found birth defects in 3% to 5% of infants exposed to sumatriptan in the first trimester, a rate not greater than expected.

Recent studies have demonstrated that sumatriptan can be used during pregnancy. Nezvalová-Henriksen and colleagues reviewed a large Norwegian database. They showed no increase in congenital anomalies (adjusted OR 1.0) or other adverse pregnancy outcomes. However, there was an increase in intrapartum bleeding (OR 1.5) and uterine atony (OR 1.4). Cunnington and coworkers[72] reviewed 479 first trimester exposures to sumatriptan and 50 to naratriptan. They observed an anomaly rate similar to the background population. However, this study had no control group. Evans and Lorber reviewed all available studies from 1990 through 2007 and also contacted the manufacturers of seven triptan medications. **They concluded that there are enough data to recommend the use of sumatriptan for treatment of migraine in the first trimester.** They also feel that naratriptan and rizatriptan are probably safe. Although these medications are acceptable for use in the second and third trimesters, there is little information regarding their use in late pregnancy. **Soldin and colleagues[73] confirm these findings and also stress that sumatriptan should be the triptan of choice as there are more data available concerning its use in pregnancy.** Table 46-5 lists some medications that can be used for treating migraines.

TABLE 46-5 Drug Therapy for Migraine Headaches in Pregnancy

MEDICATION	CLASS	USE	DOSAGE	ROUTE OF ADMINISTRATION	SAFE FOR PREGNANCY?
Acetaminophen	Pain reliever	Acute pain	4 g/day maximum	PO or PR	Yes
Codeine	Narcotic	Acute pain	30-90 mg q3-4hr	PO	Yes
Nalbuphine	Narcotic agonist/ antagonist	Acute pain	5-10 mg q4-6hr	IV	Yes
Prochlorperazine	Phenothiazine	Nausea	5-25 mg q2-8hr depending on route	PO, PR, IM, IV	Yes
Promethazine	Phenothiazine	Nausea	12.5-50 mg q2-8hr depending on route	PO, PR, IM, IV	Yes
Butalbital (50 mg) Acetaminophen 325 mg, caffeine 40 mg	Sedative, pain reliever, vasoconstrictor	Acute migraine	2 tablets q4hr, not to exceed 6 tablets daily	PO	Yes
Isometheptene mucate (65 mg), dichloralphenazone (100 mg), acetaminophen (325 mg)	Vasoconstrictor, sedative, pain reliever	Acute migraine reliever	2 capsules immediately followed by 1 hourly for no more than 5 capsules in 12 hours	PO	Yes
Caffeine	Vasoconstrictor	Acute pain	500 mg in 50 mL IV solution—may repeat	PO or IV	Yes
Sumatriptan	Vasoconstrictor	Acute pain relief	300 mg/day po max 6 mg sq × 2/day max	PO or SQ	Yes
Nortriptyline	TCA	Prophylaxis	25-100 mg qhs	PO	Yes
Amitriptyline	TCA	Prophylaxis	50-150 mg qhs	PO	Yes
Propranolol	Beta-blocker	Prophylaxis	80-120 mg bid	PO	Small risk for IUGR
Gabapentin	Antiepileptic treatment	Prophylaxis	300-2400 mg daily	PO	Yes Caution for IUGR
Carbamazepine	Membrane stabilizer	Prophylaxis	Up to 1200 mg/day	PO in three divided doses	Risk of NTD, other anomalies

bid, Twice daily; *hs*, bedtime; *IM*, intramuscularly; *IUGR*, intrauterine growth restriction; *IV*, intravenously; *NTD*, neural tube defect; *PO*, orally; *PR*, per rectum; *qd*, daily; *SQ*, subcutaneous; *TCA*, tricyclic antidepressant.

Dietary factors may precipitate migraine attacks. Careful history may uncover foods that should be avoided, including foods containing monosodium glutamate, red wine, cured meats, and strong cheeses containing tyramine. Relative hypoglycemia and alcohol can also trigger migraine attacks. Many individuals have recommended, without supporting evidence, dietary supplements and vitamins for migraine prevention. Maizels and colleagues,[74] in a small study, demonstrated a possible role for riboflavin and magnesium in the prevention of migraines.

CEREBROVASCULAR DISEASES

Stroke is diagnosed in 34 per 100,000 deliveries, with 1.4 deaths per 100,000. The risk of stroke increases with age older than 35 years and in African American women. Zotto and colleagues[75] reviewed multiple worldwide databases and showed that there are varied incidences between 4 and 41 per 100,000 deliveries.[75] The highest risk was in patients with preeclampsia. **It can be categorized as ischemic (arterial occlusion), cerebral venous thrombosis, intracerebral hemorrhage, and subarachnoid hemorrhage.**

Arterial Occlusion

Twelve percent of arterial occlusions occur in women between the ages of 15 and 45 years, and approximately one third of these patients may be pregnant. In a study from India, 37% of patients affected with cerebrovascular disease were younger than 40 years of age, with a significant number of thromboses occurring during pregnancy and the puerperium.[76] Overall, the incidence of cerebral arterial occlusion in pregnancy is approximately 1 per 20,000 live births. The mortality rate for pregnant women with cerebral arterial occlusion is twice that of men and three times that of nonpregnant women. **Middle cerebral artery occlusion is most common during pregnancy, whereas internal carotid artery occlusion is observed most often in the puerperium.** Hemiplegia and dysphasia are frequent findings. Predisposing factors such as preeclampsia, chronic hypertension, or hypotensive episodes can be demonstrated in about one third of these patients. Brown and colleagues[77] investigated ischemic stroke in women recruited between 1992 and 1996 and again between 2001 and 2003. They found that preeclampsia was statistically associated with an increased risk of ischemic stroke (OR 1.59, 95% CI 1.00 to 2.52). Another interesting finding was that women with a history of preeclampsia were more likely to eventually experience a nonpregnancy-related ischemic stroke.[77] Cancer has been reported as an underlying etiology. Oral contraceptives also raise the risk of ischemic cerebrovascular disease. Perhaps because of their relative frequency in the general population, the factor V Leiden mutation and other hereditary thrombophilias may be a predisposing factor in many of these patients. Half of the pregnancy-related cases occur during the immediate postpartum period and the remainder during the second and third trimesters. Lidegaard[78] concluded that pregnancy was associated with an elevated OR of only 1.3 for cerebral thromboembolism. One woman had a documented partial obstruction of the left middle cerebral artery during the third trimester of pregnancy. Following delivery, her symptoms abated, and angiography 11 weeks later revealed complete resolution of the obstruction. Embolic stroke should also be considered. In one postpartum patient, a patent foramen ovale was discovered in association with anticardiolipin antibodies.

In cases of cerebral arterial occlusion, care must be taken to avoid increased intracranial pressure. If signs of increased intracranial pressure develop, parenteral dexamethasone should be administered. Osmotic diuresis can be used if needed. Supportive measures are also necessary, including close monitoring of electrolytes to detect inappropriate secretion of antidiuretic hormone. Successful thrombolytic therapy has been reported. **A neurologic team should be immediately consulted after the event, and probably low-dose aspirin therapy will be implemented.** Physical and rehabilitative therapy should be started as soon as possible. These patients can progress normally through pregnancy and deliver vaginally.

A case of maternal death from carotid artery thrombosis associated with the HELLP syndrome (hemolysis, elevated liver enzymes, and low platelet count) has been reported and also a case of cerebellar infarction. It was proposed that the infarction occurred because the patient experienced a rebound thrombocytosis leading to a hypercoagulable state. The importance of closely following patients with HELLP syndrome was stressed so that those who develop a reactive thrombocytosis can be monitored for signs and symptoms of CNS thrombosis.

Cerebral Vein Thrombosis

The chief symptoms in patients with cerebral vein thrombosis are headache, lethargy, and vomiting. Hemiplegia has a gradual onset, and seizure activity is common (see Table **46-4).** This disorder occurs most frequently during the immediate postpartum period and may be attributed to a hypercoagulable state. An incidence of 1 in 10,000 pregnancies was suggested in one study.[79] Vora and colleagues[80] reviewed 37,420 pregnancies in a Mumbai, India hospital between 2002 and 2006, and found a 0.1% incidence of thromboembolic phenomena. Of these phenomena, 10% were documented cortical vein thromboses confirming the incidence of 1 in 10,000 pregnancies.[80] In one case in which a blood patch failed to relieve an apparent spinal headache, the ultimate diagnosis was a cerebral vein thrombosis.

Many patients with cerebral vein thrombosis show signs of seizure activity, and prophylactic anticonvulsants should be considered after neurologic consultation. Many neurologists and neurosurgeons advocate expectant management and do not routinely use anticonvulsants. Anticoagulation should be implemented as recommended by neurologic colleagues.

Subarachnoid Hemorrhage

The rate of subarachnoid hemorrhage complicating pregnancy is approximately 1 per 10,400.[81] **Because cocaine abuse is rampant in society today, the incidence may rise, as the associated increase in vasospasm associated with this drug causes bleeding from preexisting berry aneurysms and arteriovenous (AV) malformations.** Most berry aneurysms are thought to be due to a congenital defect in the elastic and smooth muscle layers of cerebral blood vessels. They are usually located in the vessels of the circle of Willis or those arising from it. Robinson and coworkers[82] evaluated 26 patients with spontaneous subarachnoid hemorrhage during pregnancy and found that approximately half were caused by berry aneurysms and half by AV malformations. They observed that AV malformations are more common in patients younger than 25 years of age and usually bleed before 20 weeks' gestation. Conversely, berry aneurysms occur in patients older than 30 years of age and usually bleed in the third trimester. Pregnancy appears to increase the risk of bleeding from an AV malformation. Stroke was hemorrhagic-arterial in 25 of 27 patients and thrombotic-arterial in two others. In the 24 patients being treated immediately before the stroke, systolic blood pressure (BP) was 160 mm Hg or higher in 96% and more than 155 mm Hg in 100%. In contrast, only 13% exhibited prestroke diastolic pressures of 110 mm Hg or higher. Only three patients received prestroke antihypertensive medications.

Diagnosis and Treatment

Any patient with localized signs of cerebral or meningeal irritation must be thoroughly evaluated. If the clinical examination dictates that further evaluation is necessary, MRI/magnetic resonance angiography or a CT scan should be performed. If necessary, contrast dyes may be used. Cerebral angiography can be safely used to pinpoint the origin of cerebral bleeding. Subarachnoid hemorrhages, whether caused by AV malformations or berry aneurysms, should be treated surgically, when possible. Surgery under hypothermia or hypotension appears to cause no adverse fetal effects. The fetal heart rate should be monitored. If fetal bradycardia occurs, BP should be raised sufficiently to normalize the fetal heart rate. Kawasaki and colleagues[83] report a case of cerebellar hemorrhage in a 32-week primigravida. She was treated conservatively until term and was delivered by elective cesarean section. Her surgery, which was delayed until after delivery, was successful. There was one case of combined cesarean delivery and clipping of an aneurysm.

If the patient has undergone corrective surgery for an aneurysm or AV malformation, she should be allowed to deliver vaginally. Because the Valsalva maneuver can increase intracranial pressure, epidural anesthesia is recommended. Moderate increases in BP do not cause spontaneous hemorrhage in nonpregnant patients with intracranial AV malformations. **If the aneurysm or AV malformation has not been surgically corrected, Robinson and colleagues[82] recommend elective cesarean delivery.** However, there are no data on which to base this decision. Therefore, the mode of delivery should be determined by the obstetrician after discussion about the individual case with neurologists, neurosurgeons, and anesthesiologists.

There are new, less invasive endovascular treatments for aneurysms and AV malformations, but there is virtually no published experience with these in pregnancy. Nonetheless, these procedures may pose less risk to the pregnancy than open neurologic surgeries. There are advantages of regional anesthesia in these patients. In one case a simultaneous cesarean delivery and ablation of a cerebral AV malformation were performed. Levy and Jaspan[84] have reviewed the anesthetic and obstetrical management of an untreated vascular anomaly that had bled earlier in pregnancy in a patient who developed severe preeclampsia.

Because pregnancy has a deleterious effect on AV malformations, those patients with inoperable lesions should be counseled about the dangers of future childbearing. The patient should be thoroughly evaluated before any recommendations are made for permanent sterilization.

Venous-venous (VV) malformations are low-pressure phenomena. Patients should progress to term and deliver vaginally without any hemorrhagic event or complications.

Women with a history of stroke have a low risk of recurrence during subsequent pregnancies, although the puerperium carries increased risk. A previous ischemic stroke is not a contraindication to a subsequent pregnancy. Studies have not addressed the role of prophylactic anticoagulation.

Reversible cerebral vasoconstriction syndrome can cause subarachnoid hemorrhage and can be confused with other causes. Thunderclap headaches occurring over a 1-week period are the hallmark symptom. Treatment with nimodipine appears to help the headaches.[85]

MULTIPLE SCLEROSIS

Multiple sclerosis (MS) is a demyelinating disease that attacks men and women equally. The onset of symptoms usually occurs between the ages of 20 and 40 years. In the United States, the disease is more common in those residing above 40 degrees north latitude. The prevalence for those living in the southern United States is 10 per 100,000, whereas it is approximately 50 per 100,000 in those living in the northern states. MS has no clear genetic predisposition.

The diagnosis of MS is often made years after the initial onset of sensory symptoms. The onset is usually subtle. Common presenting symptoms include weakness of one or both lower extremities, visual complaints, and loss of coordination. Because the disease primarily affects the white matter of the CNS, symptoms attributable to disruption of gray matter are uncommon. The disease is characterized by exacerbations and remissions. Less than one third of patients show steady progression of their disease after its onset. Because symptoms are subtle, it is often easy to attribute them to pregnancy. Many pregnant women complain of being more awkward or having some weakness. If these symptoms are persistent or progressive, they should not be ignored and the patient should be referred for neurologic consultation.

It is impossible to predict the long-range prognosis of a patient with MS. About half of patients are still able to work at their usual profession 10 years after the onset of the illness. After 20 years, however, only about one third remain employed. In a study of 185 women with MS, Weinshenker and colleagues[86] showed that there was no association between long-term disability and (1) total number of term pregnancies, (2) the timing of pregnancy relative to the onset of MS, or (3) the worsening of MS in relation to a pregnancy. The average life expectancy in patients with MS is also impossible to predict. Patients may live with the disease for more than 25 years.

The risk of onset of MS is reduced during gestation, whereas the risk of onset during the postpartum period is no different than for the nonpregnant state. There is a lower risk of onset of MS in parous than in nulliparous patients. Of 170 pregnant patients with MS studied by Millar and coworkers,[87] relapses occurred in only 45, the majority during the postpartum period. Birk and coinvestigators[88] carefully followed pregnancies in eight women with MS. None worsened during pregnancy. Six of the eight women, however, experienced relapses within the first 7 weeks after delivery. They also reported that there were differences in suppressor T-cell levels during pregnancy, but these were not predictive of changes in clinical disease. The lower rate of progression and exacerbation during pregnancy may be attributable to a pregnancy-induced shift from thymus helper (Th) 1 cytokines to Th 2 cytokines, which is reversed after delivery.

Frith and McLeod[89] studied 85 pregnancies and found no increased risk of relapse during pregnancy. They noted that most of the relapses that did occur during pregnancy took place in the third trimester, and also in the first 3 months postpartum. Nelson and colleagues[90] analyzed 191 pregnancies in women with nonprogressive MS. **The exacerbation rate during the 9-month postpartum period was 34%, three times that of the 9 months during pregnancy.** The rate was highest in the 3 months immediately following delivery and stabilized after 6 months postpartum. The exacerbation rates were the same in breastfeeding and nonbreastfeeding women. The average time to flare was also similar in both groups. **This study verifies that it is safe for women with MS to breastfeed their newborns. Breastfeeding does not protect from or cause MS exacerbations.** Relapse 1 year before pregnancy (HR = 1.5) and relapse during pregnancy (HR = 2.2) were the only factors that were related to postpartum relapse.

Bernardi and colleagues[91] showed a decreased risk of relapse during the 9 months of pregnancy and the first 6 months postpartum. In this study of 52 women, these researchers concluded that pregnancy, as a whole, is a protective event. Worthington and colleagues,[92] however, found more frequent relapses in the first 6 months postpartum, but not after that. Long-term prognosis was unaffected by pregnancy.

Verdru and colleagues[93] demonstrated that pregnancy delays the onset of long-term disability. As an index of progression, they used the length of time from onset of disease until wheelchair dependence. **In patients with at least one pregnancy after onset, the mean time to wheelchair dependence was 18.6 years compared with 12.5 years for other women.** In a study encompassing 12 European countries, Confavreux and colleagues[94] studied 269 pregnancies in 254 women with MS. They determined the relapse rate in each trimester using the Kuntzke Expanded Disability Status Scale with 0 as good function and 10 as very disabled. They found that the rate of relapse declined during pregnancy, especially in the third trimester. Relapses increased in the first 3 months postpartum before returning to prepregnancy rates. Neither breastfeeding nor epidural analgesia had an adverse effect on the rate of relapse or on the progression of disability.

Paraplegic patients with MS are more susceptible to urinary tract infections during pregnancy but may feel no symptoms. Therefore, they should be screened routinely. If the patient has become paraplegic or has lumbosacral lesions as a result of MS, there may be little pain associated with labor. It might be difficult therefore for the patient to discern when labor begins. Uterine contractions occur normally, but voluntary expulsive efforts may be hindered in the second stage of labor. Delivery by forceps or vacuum extraction therefore may be indicated. Women with MS who receive epidural anesthesia for vaginal delivery do not have a significantly higher incidence of postpartum exacerbation of their MS than those receiving only local anesthesia. In a recent study, van der Kop and coworkers[95] retrospectively analyzed 432 women with MS in British Columbia over an 11-year period ending in 2008, and compared them with 2975 controls. They looked at mode of delivery and neonatal outcomes. They found the mean just gestational age to be equivalent between the two groups. Furthermore, they found that the there was no difference between the assisted vaginal delivery rate (OR = 0.78) and the cesarean delivery rate (OR = 0.94).[95]

Corticosteroids and immunosuppressive agents are occasionally used to treat MS. There are many new agents used to treat the various symptoms and progressions of the disease. Their use in pregnancy has been limited, there are few data, and no controlled studies. **However, many are molecules that are too large to cross the placenta.**

For instance, natalizumab is a humanized monoclonal IgG4 antibody to human alpha-4 integrin. It works against many processes involved in human development. However, it is a large molecule that should not cross the placenta. Wehner and colleagues[96] looked at postnatal development in cynomolgus monkeys exposed to this medication. In the first cohort of monkeys, there was an increase in spontaneous abortions. However, the rate in the control group was very small (7%). In the second cohort studied, the spontaneous abortion rates were equivalent in both groups.[96] They found no adverse effects on the general health, survival, development, or immunologic structure or function of the newborn monkeys treated with natalizumab.

Hellwig and colleagues[97] report on 35 cases of accidental pregnancy in patients receiving natalizumab. Thirty-four of these pregnancies were followed prospectively. Twenty-nine pregnancies went to term, and there was only one anomaly, polydactyly. There were five spontaneous first trimester losses (14%) and one elective pregnancy termination.[97] **We know nothing about long-term effects, but in cases of MS relapse, natalizumab is a reasonable choice.** The patient, however, must be appropriately counseled.

Glatiramer is used to treat the frequency of relapses in those with relapsing remitting MS. It works by shifting the population of T cells from the pro-inflammatory Th1 to regulatory Th2 cells that suppress inflammation. Glatiramer is "Class B" as determined by the Food and Drug Administration. **Salminen and coworkers[98] prospectively followed 13 women who were exposed to glatiramer from preconception through pregnancy and the postpartum period. There were no congenital anomalies and treatment was well tolerated.** Fragoso and colleagues[99] retrospectively evaluated 11 women who used glatiramer continuously for at least 7 months during pregnancy. Children were followed for at least 1 year after birth. There were no congenital anomalies, neonatal complications, or developmental abnormalities in the children. Postnatal MS relapse rates remained significantly lower than antenatal rates in these women.[99]

As with the aforementioned medications, there is a paucity of information concerning the use of interferon-beta therapy in pregnancy. Sandberg-Wollheim and colleagues[100] diligently dissected data on 1022 cases of interferon-beta exposure during pregnancy. In order to avoid bias, they only included outcomes for prospective data (n = 425). There were 324 normal term live births (76.2%) and 4 infants born with malformations (0.9%). There were four third trimester stillbirths (0.9%, 1 with anomalies), 5 ectopics, 49 (11.5%) first trimester spontaneous abortions, and 39 (9.2%) elective abortions. These results are not dissimilar to the general population. The authors believe that these data will help patients with MS who are planning pregnancy or become pregnant while taking interferon-beta.[100] Amato and colleagues[101] investigated first trimester exposure to interferon-beta. They compared these patients to those who were never treated or who discontinued treatment at least 4 weeks before conception. Of the 88 exposed fetuses, there was not an increase in spontaneous abortion, malformations, or developmental abnormalities over a median follow-up of 2.1 years.[101] There was an increased incidence of low birth weight and birth length. In summary, all these data are encouraging in that there are therapeutic options available to the woman with MS who becomes pregnant.

CARPAL TUNNEL SYNDROME

The medial border of the carpal tunnel consists of the pisiform and hamate bones, and its lateral border consists of the scaphoid and trapezium bones. They are covered on the palmar surface by the flexor retinaculum. The median nerve and flexor tendons pass through this carpal tunnel, which has little room for expansion. If the wrist is extremely flexed or extended, the volume of the carpal tunnel is reduced. In pregnancy, weight gain and edema can produce the carpal tunnel syndrome that results from compression of the median nerve. The association between carpal tunnel syndrome and pregnancy was first reported in 1957. Although many pregnant women complain of pain on the palmar surface of the hand, few actually have the true carpal tunnel syndrome. Stolp-Smith and colleagues[102] found that 50 of 14,579 (0.34%) pregnant patients presenting between 1987 and 1992 actually met criteria for carpal tunnel syndrome. **Commonly, the syndrome consists of pain, numbness, and tingling in the distribution of the median nerve in the hand and wrist. This includes the thumb, index finger, long finger, and radial side of the ring finger on the palmar aspect.** These symptoms/signs are often accompanied by dysesthetic wrist pain, loss of grip strength, and problems with dexterity. Compressing the median nerve and percussing the wrist and forearm with a reflex hammer, the Tinel maneuver, often exacerbates the pain. In severe cases, weakness and decreased motor function can occur. The definitive diagnosis is made by electromyography, but this test is often unnecessary.

McLennan and coworkers[103] studied 1216 consecutive pregnancies. Of these patients, 427 (35%) reported hand symptoms. Fewer than 20% of these 427 affected women described the classic carpal tunnel syndrome. No patient required operative intervention. Most symptoms were bilateral and commenced in the third trimester of pregnancy. **Ekman-Ordeberg and colleagues[104] found a 2.3% incidence of carpal tunnel syndrome in a prospective study of 2358 pregnancies. The syndrome appeared to be more common in primigravidas with generalized edema.** Increased weight gain during pregnancy also raises the risk.[103] Padua and colleagues[105] conducted a systematic literature review concerning carpal tunnel syndrome in pregnancy. Of the 214 studied reviewed, only 6 fulfilled their criteria for inclusion. Neurophysiologically confirmed carpal tunnel syndrome ranged from 7% to 43% of those who presented with symptoms in the 6 studies. Clinically diagnosed carpal tunnel syndrome ranged from 31% to 62%. Of note in 50% of cases, symptoms persisted for more than a year and in 30% symptoms were still present 3 years postpartum.

Conservative therapy with splinting of the wrist at night completely relieved symptoms in 46 of 56 patients.[106] Of the remaining 10 women, three required surgery before delivery. In Stolp-Smith's study,[102] symptoms began with equal frequency in all trimesters, but diagnosis was delayed until the third trimester in 50% of the patients. Only four patients required surgical intervention during gestation, and three additional patients required surgery postpartum. Wand[107] retrospectively studied 40 women with carpal tunnel syndrome developing in pregnancy and 18 women with carpal tunnel syndrome that occurred in the puerperium. He confirmed that the syndrome occurs most frequently in primigravidas older than 30 years of age. All cases that developed before delivery occurred during the third trimester and resolved within 2 weeks after delivery. In those cases developing during the puerperium in women who breastfed their infants, the symptoms lasted longer, a mean of 5.8 months. In another series, 27 women developed carpal tunnel syndrome during the puerperium. The condition was associated with breastfeeding in 24 of these women. Symptoms lasted an average of 6.5 months in the breastfeeding women. Only two of these patients required surgical decompression.

Supportive and conservative therapies are usually adequate for the treatment of carpal tunnel syndrome. Symptoms usually subside in the postpartum period as total body water returns to normal. Pain scores fall by half during the first week after delivery and by half again during the next week. The reduction in score is strongly correlated with loss of the weight gained during pregnancy. However, about half of the women with carpal tunnel syndrome during pregnancy still have some symptoms 1 year later, more commonly in those whose symptoms started early in pregnancy.

Splints placed on the dorsum of the hand, which keep the wrist in a neutral position and maximize the capacity of the carpal tunnel, often provide dramatic relief. Local injections of glucocorticoids may also be used in severe cases. Although diuretics may help to control the symptoms of carpal tunnel syndrome over a short period of time, their use is not recommended because the symptoms return rather rapidly after the cessation of treatment.

Surgical correction of this syndrome should not be delayed in patients with deteriorating muscle tone and motor function. Even small changes can be documented by electromyography (EMG), which can be carried out safely during pregnancy. Decompression surgery for carpal tunnel syndrome is a simple procedure that can be safely carried out during pregnancy using local anesthesia, an axillary block, or a Bier block. With new endoscopic procedures, the procedure is even less invasive. Assmus and Hashemi[108] report 314 hands surgically treated during pregnancy or the puerperium for carpal tunnel syndrome. One hundred thirty-three cases were performed during pregnancy, most in the last trimester, including four who had both hands treated simultaneously, and 98% reported good or excellent results.[108] There were no complications, and local anesthesia was used in all cases. These authors recommend surgery if sensory loss is present or if motor latency is more than 5 msec. It is important to warn patients that carpal tunnel syndrome can persist for several years postpartum and can recur in future pregnancies.[105]

IDIOPATHIC INTRACRANIAL HYPERTENSION (PSEUDOTUMOR CEREBRI)

Idiopathic intracranial hypertension (IIH) may complicate as many as 1 in 870 births. It has been thought to be seen more frequently in pregnant women, particularly those who are obese. However, in a study by Ireland and colleagues[109] the incidences in pregnant women and in oral contraceptive users were no higher than in control groups. **More than 95% of these patients have headaches, and 15% have diplopia. Papilledema is found in virtually all patients.** In 12 women with 16 pregnancies complicated by IIH, 6 had mild and 6 had marked bilateral papilledema. There was decreased visual acuity in four of the patients. To establish the diagnosis, one must demonstrate elevated cerebrospinal fluid (CSF) pressure, normal CSF composition, and the absence of an intracranial mass on MRI or CT scan.[110]

The pathogenesis of this disorder is unknown, but CSF prolactin is markedly elevated. Prolactin appears to have an affinity for receptors in the choroid plexus, where CSF is produced. Prolactin has osmoregulatory functions and, therefore, may have a role in the increased CSF production found in IIH. Some believe that reduced CSF reabsorption is the etiology. Ahlskog and O'Neill[111] noted an association between the occurrence of IIH and the following conditions: corticosteroid therapy and its withdrawal, nalidixic acid therapy, nitrofurantoin therapy, tetracycline therapy, hypoparathyroidism, deficiencies or excesses of vitamin A, and iron deficiency anemia.

Pregnancy outcome appears to be unaffected by the illness.[110] **There is no increase in fetal wastage or congenital anomalies.** One case of IIH occurred in a 15-year-old primigravida following eclampsia, and it lasted for 3 weeks. IIH may occur in a pregnancy complicated by diabetes mellitus. **It is important to make the distinction between symptoms of IIH and visual impairment caused by diabetic retinopathy, because the treatments are different.** Thomas[112] described a case of ICH occurring in two consecutive pregnancies in a woman with hemoglobin SC. In both instances, symptoms resolved following delivery and both infants were born at term.

Most patients respond well to conservative management. **The main objectives of treatment are relief of pain and preservation of vision.** The patient should be followed closely with visual acuity and visual field determinations at intervals indicated by the clinical condition. In patients with mild disease, analgesics may be adequate. If pain persists, diuretics may be used. **Acetazolamide, a carbonic anhydrase inhibitor, will reduce CSF production in many patients.** Lee and colleagues[113] treated 12 patients with acetazolamide during pregnancy and there were no adverse fetal outcomes. They reviewed the English language literature and found nothing contradicting this assertion. The usual dose is 500 mg twice daily. In more difficult cases, prednisone in doses of 40 to 60 mg daily usually provides good results. Patients may be treated for 2 weeks, with the dose being tapered over the next month. Serial lumbar punctures to reduce CSF pressure are rarely necessary today. Surgical approaches are reserved for refractory patients in whom rapid visual deterioration occurs. The two most common procedures are optic nerve sheath fenestration and lumpoperitoneal shunt.

IIH is not an indication for cesarean delivery. A review of the literature reveals that 73% of the reported patients delivered vaginally. Cesarean delivery should be undertaken only for obstetrical indications. **Both epidural and spinal anesthesia, when expertly administered, can be safely used in patients with IIH.** Although there are no data to confirm this, the Valsalva maneuver, which can increase CSF pressure, should be minimized when possible. Therefore, the second stage of labor should be shortened by operative vaginal delivery if possible.

The recurrence rate for IIH appears to be between 10% and 12.3% in nonpregnant patients. Pregnancy does not appear to predispose to a recurrence.

KEY POINTS

- Idiopathic seizures affect approximately 1% of the general population and are the most frequent neurologic complication of pregnancy.
- Prepregnancy counseling is imperative in the patient with a seizure disorder, and preconceptional folic acid therapy, 4 mg daily, should be implemented in patients receiving anticonvulsants under the direction of an obstetrician and a neurologist.
- Those women with seizures occurring less than once each month will most likely have the best control of seizures during pregnancy.
- The anticonvulsant medication that best controls the patient's seizures should be used during pregnancy.
- Because of the changes in plasma volume, drug distribution, and metabolism that occur during

pregnancy, anticonvulsant levels should be checked and dosages adjusted when clinically indicated.

- Patients taking anticonvulsants have an increased risk of giving birth to an infant with both major and minor anomalies, but this risk is less than 10%. Therefore, the majority of patients with epilepsy give birth to healthy infants.
- Carbamazepine and valproate are associated with an increased risk of NTDs, as well as other anomalies.
- The pattern of physical abnormalities observed in the infants of patients taking anticonvulsants is related to the dose, type, and number of anticonvulsant drugs, rather than the epilepsy itself.
- Pregnancy does not hasten the onset of MS, and it decreases the onset of disability from MS. Exacerbations are decreased during pregnancy.
- Many of the newer MS medications may be acceptable for use during pregnancy. They do not appear to be associated with anomalies. The risk and benefits must be discussed with the patient. Elective abortion should not be strongly recommended to a patient who becomes pregnant while taking these medications.
- Carpal tunnel syndrome is common in pregnancy and usually responds to conservative splinting, glucocorticoid injection, or both. Surgery can be safely undertaken if indicated during pregnancy.

REFERENCES

1. Williams J, Myson V, Steward S, et al: Self-discontinuation of antiepileptic medication in pregnancy: detection by hair analysis. Epilepsia 43:824, 2002.
2. Cramer JA, Jones EE: Reproductive function in epilepsy. Epilepsia 32:S19, 1991.
3. Webber MP, Hauser WA, Ottman R, Annegers JF: Fertility in persons with epilepsy: 1935-1974. Epilepsia 27:746, 1986.
4. Dansky LV, Anderman E, Anderman F: Marriage and fertility in epileptic patients. Epilepsia 21:261, 1980.
5. Knight AH, Rhind EG: Epilepsy and pregnancy: a study of 153 pregnancies in 59 patients. Epilepsia 16:99, 1975.
6. Schmidt D, Canger R, Avanzini G, et al: Change of seizure frequency in pregnant epileptic women. J Neurol Neurosurg Psychiatry 46:751, 1983.
7. Tanganelli P, Regesta G: Epilepsy, pregnancy, and major birth anomalies: an Italian prospective, controlled study. Neurology 42:89, 1992.
8. Sabers A, Rogvi-Hansen B, Dam M, et al: Pregnancy and epilepsy: a retrospective study of 151 pregnancies. Acta Neurol Scand 97:164, 1998.
9. Lunardi LL, Costa AL, Guerreiro CA, Souza EA: Quality of life in pregnant women with epilepsy versus women without epilepsy. Arq Neuropsiquiatr 69:335, 2011.
10. Landon MJ, Kirkley M: Metabolism of diphenylhydantoin (phenytoin) during pregnancy. Br J Obstet Gynaecol 86:125, 1979.
11. Kochenour NK, Emery MG, Sawohuck RJ: Phenytoin metabolism in pregnancy. Obstet Gynecol 56:577, 1980.
12. Yerby MS, Friel PN, McCormick K, et al: Pharmacokinetics of anticonvulsants in pregnancy: alterations in plasma protein binding. Epilepsy Res 5:223, 1990.
13. Milunsky A, Jick H, Jick SS, et al: Multivitamin/folic acid supplementation in early pregnancy reduces the prevalence of neural tube defects. JAMA 262:2847, 1989.
14. Bleyer WA, Skinner AL: Fatal neonatal hemorrhage after maternal anticonvulsant therapy. JAMA 235:626, 1976.
15. Kaaja E, Kaaja R, Matila R, et al: Enzyme-inducing antiepileptic drugs in pregnancy and the risk of bleeding in the neonate. Neurology 58:549, 2002.
16. Yerby M, Koepsell T, Daling J: Pregnancy complications and outcomes in a cohort of women with epilepsy. Epilepsia 26:631, 1985.
17. Hiilesmaa VK, Bardy A, Teramo K: Obstetric outcome in women with epilepsy. Am J Obstet Gynecol 152:499, 1985.
18. Borthen I, Eide M, Dalveit A, Gilhus N: Obstetric outcome in women with epilepsy: a hospital based, retrospective study. Br J Obstet Gynaecol 118:956, 2011.
19. Mastroiacovo P, Bertollini R, Licata D: Fetal growth in the offspring of epileptic women: results of an Italian multicentric cohort study. Acta Neurol Scand 78:110, 1988.
20. Hiilesmaa VK, Teramo K, Granstrom ML: Fetal head growth retardation associated with maternal antiepileptic drugs. Lancet 1:165, 1981.
21. Hvas CL, Henriksen TB, Ostergaard JR, Dam M: Epilepsy and pregnancy: effect of antiepileptic drugs and lifestyle on birthweight. Br J Obstet Gynaecol 107:896, 2000.
22. Battine D, Keneko S, Andermann E, et al: Intrauterine growth in the offspring of epileptic women: a prospective multicenter study. Epilepsy Res 36:53, 1999.
23. Richmond JR, Krishnamoorthy P, Andermann E, et al: Epilepsy and pregnancy: an obstetric perspective. Am J Obstet Gynecol 190:371, 2004.
24. Viinikainen K, Heinonen S, Eriksson K, et al: Community-based, prospective, controlled study of obstetric and neonatal outcome of 179 pregnancies in women with epilepsy. Epilepsia 47:186, 2006.
25. Hanson JW, Smith DW: The fetal hydantoin syndrome. J Pediatr 87:285, 1975.
26. Hanson JW, Myrianthopoulos NC, Sedgwick Harvey MA, Smith DW: Risks to the offspring of women treated with hydantoin anticonvulsants, with emphasis on the fetal hydantoin syndrome. J Pediatr 89:662, 1976.
27. Gaily E, Granstrom ML, Hiilesmaa V, Bardy A: Minor anomalies in offspring of epileptic mothers. J Pediatr 112:520, 1988.
28. Rosa FW: Spina bifida in infants of women treated with carbamazepine during pregnancy. N Engl J Med 324:674, 1991.
29. Nakane Y, Okuma T, Takahashi R, et al: Multi-institutional study on the teratogenicity and fetal toxicity of antiepileptic drugs: a report of a collaborative study group in Japan. Epilepsia 21:663, 1980.
30. Canger R, Battine D, Canevini MP, et al: Malformations in offspring of women with epilepsy: a prospective study. Epilepsia 40:1231, 1999.
31. Kaneko S, Otani K, Fukushima Y, et al: Teratogenicity of antiepileptic drugs: analysis of possible risk factors. Epilepsia 29:459, 1988.
32. Kaneko S, Otani K, Kondo T, et al: Malformation in infants of mothers with epilepsy receiving antiepileptic drugs. Neurology 42:68, 1992.
33. Jick SS, Terris BZ: Anticonvulsants and congenital malformations. Pharmacotherapy 17:561, 1997.
34. Lindhout D, Meinardi H, Meijer JWA, Nau H: Antiepileptic drugs and teratogenesis in two consecutive cohorts: changes in prescription policy paralleled by changes in pattern of malformations. Neurology 42:94, 1992.
35. Dravet C, Julian C, Legras C, et al: Epilepsy, antiepileptic drugs, and malformations in children of women with epilepsy: a French prospective cohort study. Neurology 42:75, 1992.
36. Koch S, Losche G, Jager-Roman E, et al: Major and minor birth malformations and antiepileptic drugs. Neurology 42:83, 1992.
37. Gaily E, Granstrom ML: Minor anomalies in children of mothers with epilepsy. Neurology 42:128, 1992.
38. Yerby MS, Leavitt A, Erickson M, et al: Antiepileptics and the development of congenital anomalies. Neurology 42:132, 1992.
39. Nulman I, Scolnik D, Chitayat D, et al: Findings in children exposed in utero to phenytoin and carbamazepine monotherapy: independent effects of epilepsy and medications. Am J Med Genet 68:18, 1997.
40. DiLiberti JH, Farndon PA, Dennis NR, Curry CJR: The fetal valproate syndrome. Am J Med Genet 19:473, 1984.
41. Jager-Roman E, Deichl A, Jakob S, et al: Fetal growth, major malformations, and minor anomalies in infants born to women receiving valproic acid. J Pediatr 108:997, 1986.

42. Lindhout D, Schmidt D: In-utero exposure to valproate and neural tube defects. Lancet 2:1392, 1986.
43. Lindhout D, Omtzigt JGC, Cornel MC: Spectrum of neural-tube defects in 34 infants prenatally exposed to antiepileptic drugs. Neurology 42:111, 1992.
44. Tomson T, Perucca E, Battino D: Navigating toward fetal and maternal health: the challenge of treating epilepsy in pregnancy. Epilepsia 45:1171, 2004.
45. Wyszynski DF, Nambisan M, Surve T, et al: Increased rate of major malformations in offspring exposed to valproate during pregnancy. Neurology 64:961, 2005.
46. Koren G, Nava-Ocampo AA, Moretti ME, et al: Major malformations with valproic acid. Can Fam Physician 52:441, 2006.
47. Morrow J, Russell A, Guthrie E, et al: Malformation risks of antiepileptic drugs in pregnancy: a prospective study from the UK Epilepsy and Pregnancy Register. J Neurol Neurosurg Psychiatry 77:193, 2006.
48. Holmes LB, Harvey EA, Coull BA, et al: The teratogenicity of anticonvulsant drugs. N Engl J Med 344:1132, 2001.
49. Jones KL, Lacro RV, Johnson KA, Adams J: Pattern of malformations in the children of women treated with carbamazepine during pregnancy. N Engl J Med 320:1661, 1989.
50. Jentink J, Dolk H, Loane MA, et al: Intrauterine exposure to carbamazepine and specific congenital malformations: systematic review and case-control study. BMJ 341:c6581, 2010.
51. Jetink J, Loane MA, Dolk H, et al: Valproic acid monotherapy in pregnancy and major congenital malformations. N Engl J Med 362:2185, 2010.
52. Mackay FJ, Wilton LV, Pearce GL, et al: Safety of long-term lamotrigine in epilepsy. Epilepsia 38:881, 1997.
53. Molgaaard-Nielsen D, Hviid A: Newer-generation antiepileptic drugs and the risk of major birth defects. JAMA 305:1996, 2011.
54. Gaily E, Kantola-Sorsa E, Granstrom ML: Intelligence of children of epileptic mothers. J Pediatr 113:677, 1988.
55. Moore SJ, Turnpenny P, Quinn A, et al: A clinical study of 57 children with fetal anticonvulsant syndromes. J Med Genet 37:489, 2000.
56. Meador KJ, Baker GA, Browning N, et al: Cognitive function at 3 years of age after fetal exposure to antiepileptic drugs. N Engl J Med 360:1597, 2009.
57. Dansky LV, Andermann E, Rosenblatt D, et al: Anticonvulsants, folate levels, and pregnancy outcome: a prospective study. Ann Neurol 21:176, 1987.
58. Wigton TR, Sabbagha RE, Tamura RK, et al: Sonographic diagnosis of congenital heart disease: comparison between the four-chamber view and multiple cardiac views. Obstet Gynecol 82:219, 1993.
59. Rudzinski LA, Meador KJ. Epilepsy: five new things. Neurology 76:S20, 2011.
60. Sibai BM, Spinnato JA, Watson DL, et al: Eclampsia. IV. Neurological findings and future outcome. Am J Obstet Gynecol 152:184, 1985.
61. Harden CL, Meador KJ, Pennell PB, et al: Practice parameter update: management issues for women with epilepsy-focus on pregnancy (an evidence-based review): teratogenesis and perinatal outcomes. Neurology 73:133, 2009.
62. Maggioni F, Alessi C, Maggino T, Zanchin G: Headache during pregnancy. Cephalalgia 17:765, 1997.
63. Ertresvag JM, Zwart JA, Helde G, et al: Headache and transient focal neurological symptoms during pregnancy, a prospective cohort. Acta Neurol Scand 111:223, 2005.
64. Chen TC, Leviton A: Headache recurrence in pregnant women with migraine. Headache 34:104, 1994.
65. Chancellor AM, Wroe SJ, Cull RE: Migraine occurring for the first time in pregnancy. Headache 30:224, 1990.
66. Jacobson SL, Redman CW: Basilar migraine with loss of consciousness in pregnancy: case report. Br J Obstet Gynaecol 96:494, 1989.
67. Chen HM, Chen SF, Chen YH, Lin HC: Increased risk of adverse pregnancy outcomes for women with migraines: a nationwide population-based study. Cephalgia 30:443, 2010.
68. O'Quinn S, Ephross SA, Williams V, et al: Pregnancy and perinatal outcomes in migraineurs using sumatriptan: a prospective study. Arch Gynecol Obstet 263:7, 1999.
69. Olesen C, Steffensen FH, Sorensen HT, et al: Pregnancy outcome following prescription for sumatriptan. Headache 40:20, 2000.
70. Kallen B, Lygner PE: Delivery outcome in women who used drugs for migraine during pregnancy with special reference to sumatriptan. Headache 41:351, 2001.
71. Hilaire ML, Cross LB, Eichner SF: Treatment of migraine headaches with sumatriptan in pregnancy. Ann Pharmacother 38:1726, 2004.
72. Cunnington M, Ephross S, Churchill P: The safety of sumatriptan and naratriptan in pregnancy: what have we learned? Headache 49:1414, 2009.
73. Soldin OP, Dahlin J, O'Mara DM: Triptans in pregnancy. Ther Drug Monit 30:5, 2008.
74. Maizels M, Blumenfeld A, Burchette R: A combination of riboflavin, magnesium, and feverfew for migraine prophylaxis. Headache 44:885, 2004.
75. Zotto E, Giossi A, Volonghi I, et al: Ischemic stroke during pregnancy and puerperium. Stroke Res Treat 60:6780, 2011.
76. Banerjee AK, Varma M, Vasista RK, Chopra JS: Cerebrovascular disease in north-west India: a study of necropsy material. J Neurol Neurosurg Psychiatry 52:512, 1989.
77. Brown DW, Dueker N, Jamieson DJ, et al: Preeclampsia and the risk of ischemic stroke among young women: results from the stroke prevention in young women study. Stroke 37:1055, 2006.
78. Lidegaard O: Oral contraceptives, pregnancy and the risk of cerebral thromboembolism: the influence of diabetes, hypertension, migraine, and previous thrombotic disease. Br J Obstet Gynaecol 102:153, 1995.
79. Abraham J, Rios PS, Inbaraj SG, et al: An epidemiological study of hemiplegia due to stroke in south India. Stroke 1:477, 1970.
80. Vora S, Ghosh K, Shetty S, et al: Deep venous thrombosis in the antenatal period in a large cohort of pregnancies from western India. Thromb J 5:9, 2007.
81. Miller HJ, Hinkley CM: Berry aneurysms in pregnancy: a ten year report. South Med J 63:279, 1970.
82. Robinson JL, Hall CJ, Sevzimer CB: Arterial venous malformations, aneurysms, and pregnancy. J Neurosurg 41:63, 1974.
83. Kawasaki N, Uchida T, Yamada M, et al: Conservative management of cerebellar hemorrhage in pregnancy. Int J Gynaecol Obstet 31:365, 1990.
84. Levy DM, Jaspan T: Anaesthesia for caesarean section in a patient with recent subarachnoid haemorrhage and severe pre-eclampsia. Anaesthesia 54:994, 1999.
85. Ducros A, Boukobza M, Procher R, et al: The clinical and radiological spectrum of reversible cerebral vasoconstriction syndrome. A prospective series of 67 patients. Brain 130:3091, 2007.
86. Weinshenker BG, Hader W, Carriere W, et al: The influence of pregnancy on disability from multiple sclerosis: a population-based study in Middlesex County, Ontario. Neurology 39:1438, 1989.
87. Millar JHD, Allison RS, Cheeseman EA: Pregnancy as a factor influencing relapse in disseminated sclerosis. Brain 82:417, 1959.
88. Birk K, Ford C, Smeltzer S, et al: The clinical course of multiple sclerosis during pregnancy and the puerperium. Arch Neurol 47:738, 1990.
89. Frith JA, McLeod JC: Pregnancy and multiple sclerosis. J Neurol Neurosurg Psychiatry 51:495, 1988.
90. Nelson LM, Franklin GM, Jones MC: Risk of multiple sclerosis exacerbation during pregnancy and breast-feeding. JAMA 259:3441, 1988.
91. Bernardi S, Grasso MG, Bertollini R, et al: The influences of pregnancy on relapses of multiple sclerosis: a cohort study. Acta Neurol Scand 84:403, 1991.
92. Worthington J, Jones R, Crawford M, Forti A: Pregnancy and multiple sclerosis—a 3-year prospective study. J Neurol 241:228, 1994.
93. Verdru P, Theys P, D'Hooghe MB, Carton H: Pregnancy and multiple sclerosis: the influence on long-term disability. Clin Neurol Neurosurg 96:38, 1994.
94. Confavreux C, Hutchinson M, Hours MM, et al: Rate of pregnancy-related relapse in multiple sclerosis. Pregnancy in Multiple Sclerosis Group. N Engl J Med 339:285, 1998.
95. van der Kop ML, Pearce MS, Dahlgren L, et al: Neonatal and delivery outcomes in women with multiple sclerosis. Ann Neurol 22:483, 2011.
96. Wehner NG, Shopp G, Osterburg I, et al: Postnatal development in cynomolgus monkeys following prenatal exposure to natalizumab, an alpha4 integrin inhibitor. Birth Defects Res B Dev Reprod Toxicol 86:144, 2009.

97. Hellwig K, Haghikia A, Gold R: Pregnancy and natalizumab: results of an observational study in 35 accidental pregnancies during natalizumab treatment. Mult Scler 8:958, 2011.
98. Salminen HJ, Leggett, H, Boggild M: Glatiramer acetate exposure in pregnancy: preliminary safety and birth outcomes. J Neurol 257:2020, 2010.
99. Fragoso YD, Finkelsztein A, Kaimen-Maciel DR, et al: Long-term use of glatiramer acetate by 11 pregnant women with multiple sclerosis: a retrospective multicentere case series. CNS Drugs 24:969, 2010.
100. Sandberg-Wollheim M, Alteri E, Moraga MS, Kornmann G: Pregnancy outcomes in multiple sclerosis following subcutaneous interferon beta-1a therapy. Mult Scler 17:423, 2011.
101. Amato MP, Portaccio E, Ghezzi A, et al: Pregnancy and fetal outcomes after interferon-β exposure in multiple sclerosis. Neurology 75:1794, 2010.
102. Stolp-Smith KA, Pascoe MK, Ogburn PL Jr: Carpal tunnel syndrome in pregnancy: frequency severity and prognosis. Arch Phys Med Rehabil 79:1285, 1998.
103. McLennan HG, Oats JN, Walstab JE: Survey of hand symptoms in pregnancy. Med J Aust 147:542, 1987.
104. Ekman-Ordeberg G, Salgeback S, Ordeberg G: Carpal tunnel syndrome in pregnancy: a prospective study. Acta Obstet Gynecol Scand 66:233, 1987.
105. Padua L, DiPasquale A, Pazzaglia C, et al: Systematic review of pregnancy-related carpal tunnel syndrome. Muscle Nerve 429:697, 2010.
106. Turgut F, Cetinsahinahin M, Turgut M, et al: The management of carpal tunnel syndrome in pregnancy J Clin Neurosci 8:332, 2001.
107. Wand JS: Carpal tunnel syndrome in pregnancy and lactation. J Hand Surg 15:93, 1990.
108. Assmus H, Hashemi B: Surgical treatment of carpal tunnel syndrome in pregnancy: results from 314 cases. Nervenarzt 71:470, 2000.
109. Ireland B, Corbett JJ, Wallace RB: The search for causes of idiopathic intracranial hypertension: a preliminary case-control study. Arch Neurol 47:315, 1990.
110. Koontz WL, Herbert WNP, Cefalo R: Pseudotumor cerebri in pregnancy. Obstet Gynecol 62:325, 1983.
111. Ahlskog JE, O'Neill BP: Pseudotumor cerebri. Ann Intern Med 97:249, 1982.
112. Thomas E: Recurrent benign intracranial hypertension associated with hemoglobin SC disease in pregnancy. Obstet Gynecol 67:7S, 1986.
113. Lee AG, Pless M, Falardeau J, et al: The use of acetazolamide in idiopathic intracranial hypertension during pregnancy. Am J Ophthalmol 139:855, 2005.

For full reference list, log onto www.expertconsult.com.

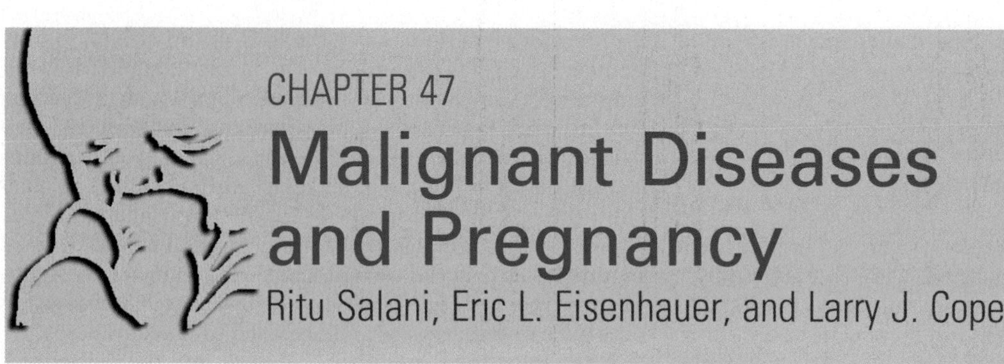

CHAPTER 47

Malignant Diseases and Pregnancy

Ritu Salani, Eric L. Eisenhauer, and Larry J. Copeland

KEY ABBREVIATIONS	
α-fetoprotein	AFP
β-human Chorionic Gonadotropin	β-hCG
Carcinoembryonic Antigen	CEA
Computed Tomography	CT
Fine Needle Aspiration	FNA
Food and Drug Administration	FDA
Gestational Trophoblastic Disease	GTD
Gray	Gy
Hodgkin's Lymphoma	HL
Magnetic Resonance Imaging	MRI
Non-Hodgkin's Lymphoma	NHL
Transverse Rectus Abdominis Myocutaneous Flap	TRAM
World Health Organization	WHO

The juxtaposition of life and death can present numerous emotional and ethical conflicts to the patient, her family, and her physicians. The diagnosis of cancer for anyone is understandably frightening. To deal with cancer in the context of pregnancy is particularly burdensome, because the patient may have to balance competing maternal and fetal interests. On occasion, a pregnant woman may be required to make decisions affecting her life or longevity versus the life or well-being of her unborn. Cancer in pregnancy complicates the management of both the cancer and the pregnancy. Diagnostic and therapeutic interventions must carefully address the associated risks to both the patient and the fetus. Informed decisions require evaluation of a number of factors, and with counseling, these considerations are the foundation on which treatment decisions are made. There has been an evolution in the philosophy of care from one of total disregard of the pregnancy with frequent immediate termination to a more thoughtful approach in which management decisions consider both maternal and fetal outcomes so as to limit risk of death or morbidity to both.

It is estimated that approximately 20% to 30% of malignancies occur in women younger than age 45 years.[1] **Although cancer is the second most common cause of death for women in their reproductive years, only about 1 in 1000 pregnancies is complicated by cancer.**[2] Because there are no large prospective studies that address cancer treatment in pregnancy, physicians tend to base treatment strategies on small retrospective studies or anecdotal reports that occasionally present conflicting information.[1,2] A successful outcome is dependent on a cooperative multidisciplinary approach. The management plan must be formulated within a medical, moral, ethical, legal, and religious framework that is acceptable to the patient and guided by communication and educational resources of the health care team.

Delays in diagnosis of the cancer during pregnancy are common for various reasons, including the following: (1) many of the presenting symptoms of cancer are often attributed to the pregnancy; (2) many of the physiologic and anatomic alterations of pregnancy can compromise physical examination; (3) serum tumor markers, such as β-human chorionic gonadotropin (β-hCG), α-fetoprotein (AFP), and CA 125, are increased during pregnancy; and (4) our ability to optimally perform either imaging studies or invasive diagnostic procedures may be altered during pregnancy. Because the gestational age is significant when evaluating the risks of treatments, it is important to determine gestational age accurately. An early ultrasound evaluation may be useful to ensure accurate dating.

The malignancies most commonly encountered in the pregnant patient are breast cancer, cervical cancer, melanoma, ovarian cancer, thyroid cancer, leukemia, lymphoma, and colorectal cancer.[2] The frequencies of these diseases complicating pregnancy may increase secondary to the trend to delay childbearing, and age is the most potent predictor of cancer. Before specific malignancies are discussed below, some general principles are reviewed.

CHEMOTHERAPY DURING PREGNANCY

Pharmacology of Chemotherapy During Pregnancy

Because pregnancy alters physiology, there is potential for altered pharmacokinetics associated with chemotherapy. Orally administered medications are subjected to altered gastrointestinal motility. Peak drug concentrations are decreased owing to the 50% expansion in plasma volume, producing a longer drug half-life unless there is a concurrent increase in metabolism or excretion. The increase in plasma proteins and fall in albumin may alter drug availability, and amniotic fluid may act as a pharmacologic third space, potentially increasing toxicity due to delayed metabolism and excretion. Hepatic oxidation and renal blood flow are both elevated during pregnancy and may influence the metabolism and excretion of most drugs.[3] However, because pharmacologic studies in the pregnant woman are lacking, we currently assume that initial drug dosages are similar to that given to the nonpregnant woman and adjustments to dose are based on toxicity on a course-by-course basis. Because most antineoplastic agents can be found in breast milk, breastfeeding is contraindicated.[3]

Drug Effects on the Fetus

All drugs undergo animal teratogenicity testing, and based on these results, the drugs are assigned risk categories (Table 47-1) by the U.S. Food and Drug Administration (FDA).[4] Based on this system, most chemotherapeutic agents are rated as C, D, or X. However, animal teratogenicity testing cannot always be reliably extrapolated to humans. For example, a drug (e.g., aspirin) may show teratogenic effects in animals and not affect humans. The opposite is also true and, as such, has serious potential to do harm; for example, a drug may show no animal teratogenicity (e.g., thalidomide) but cause serious human anomalies (see Chapter 8). Because detailed ultrasonography may fail to identify subtle anatomic but serious functional abnormalities before 20 weeks' gestation, patients should be appropriately counseled and may want to consider the option of pregnancy termination if first-trimester chemotherapy is planned or administered. **The risk of teratogenicity during the second and third trimesters is significantly reduced and is likely no different from that for pregnant woman who are not exposed to chemotherapy.**[3]

Although the literature addressing chemotherapy administration during pregnancy is somewhat limited and dated, literature reviews provide us with some information regarding the frequency of affected offspring.[3,5] Because antineoplastic agents are targeted for the rapidly dividing malignant cell, one would expect the exposed fetus to be particularly susceptible to serious toxicity. Clear documentation of such is not the case. Excluding the intentional use of abortifacients, it is difficult to clearly demonstrate that the use of chemotherapy results in an increase in the clinically recognized spontaneous abortion rate over the expected 15% to 20%. However, if continuation of the pregnancy is desired, chemotherapy is not advised in the first trimester due to an increased rate of major malformations, ranging from 10% to 17% with single agent therapy and up to 25% with combination chemotherapy.[5] Administration in the second and third trimester has been associated with intrauterine growth restriction, stillbirth, and low birthweight.[5-7] Maternal effects, such as chemotherapy-induced nausea and vomiting, may also affect fetal growth and birthweight.[8] Because early induction of labor or surgical delivery is often a component of the overall treatment plan, it has been difficult to identify premature birth as a specific result of the chemotherapy. Preterm delivery has been reported to occur in more than half of pregnancies associated with malignancies, with a majority being iatrogenically induced and associated with increased neonatal morbidity.[5] Therefore, the timing of delivery and consideration of delay of therapy, if early-stage disease, should be part of the treatment planning.

When chemotherapy is administered during the latter half of gestation, fetal organ toxicity has not been reported as a major problem, although neonatal myelosuppression and hearing loss have been reported.[5,9] Although second malignancies, impaired growth and development, intellectual impairment, and infertility have been reported after chemotherapy administration to children, the delayed effects of in utero exposure are less well documented.[5,9] Though little data is available, concerns regarding cognitive development have been evaluated and the outcomes are comparable to those not exposed to chemotherapy in utero. Growth and fertility outcomes have also been shown to be similar to those not exposed.[9]

TABLE 47-1 FDA RISK CATEGORIES FOR DRUG USE DURING PREGNANCY

CATEGORY	DEFINITION
A	Controlled studies have demonstrated no risk in first trimester, and the possibility of fetal harm appears remote.
B	*Either* animal studies have failed to identify a risk but there are no controlled studies in women, *or* animal studies have shown an adverse effect that was not confirmed.
C	*Either* animal studies have revealed adverse effects and there are no controlled studies in women, *or* studies in women and animals are not available. Use of drugs only if the potential benefit justifies the potential risks.
D	There is evidence of fetal risk, but the benefits may be acceptable despite the risk in either a life-threatening situation or a serious disease for which safer drugs are ineffective.
X	Studies in animals or humans have demonstrated fetal abnormalities and the risk of the drug clearly outweighs any possible benefit.

From Aviles A, Diaz-Maqueo JC, Talavera A, et al: Growth and development of children and mothers treated with chemotherapy during pregnancy: current status of 43 children. Am J Hematol 36:243, 1991.

Classification of Chemotherapy Agents

Antimetabolites

Historically, the antimetabolite aminopterin was used as an abortifacient, and in cases of failed abortion, the risk of fetal malformation was about 50%. Methotrexate has replaced aminopterin for chemotherapeutic purposes, and although similar types of anomalies occur, a lower overall frequency (<10%) has been reported.[8] In the first trimester, methotrexate has been associated with skeletal and central nervous system (CNS) defects. Though no anomalies were reported in the second and third trimester, methotrexate was associated with low birthweight and neonatal myelosuppresion.[9] The use of low-dose methotrexate for systemic diseases (e.g., rheumatic disease and psoriasis) does not appear to produce teratogenicity.[10] In a prospective study, 5-fluorouracil, in combination with other agents, was well tolerated and resulted in no perinatal deaths.[8]

Alkylating Agents

The alkylating agents, such as cyclophosphamide and chlorambucil, are a commonly used group of drugs for the management of malignancies. Unfortunately, most of the alkylating agents have demonstrated some teratogenic potential when administered in the first trimester, including renal agenesis, ocular abnormalities, and cleft palate.[8] In the second and third trimester, alkylating agents have been shown to be acceptably safe.[1,9]

Antitumor Antibiotics

Even when administered in early pregnancy, antitumor antibiotics (doxorubicin, idarubicin, bleomycin, daunorubicin) appear to be associated with a low risk of teratogenicity. Doxorubicin has been associated with one case of multiple anomalies; however, the patient was receiving combination chemotherapy.[9] One potential reason for the low rate of anthracycline-associated teratogenicity is its questionable ability to cross the placenta.[11]

Vinca Alkaloids

Vincristine and vinblastine, although potent teratogens in animals, do not appear to be as teratogenic in humans.[8] In limited studies, vinca alkaloids were well tolerated in both early and later stages of pregnancy.[9]

Platinum Agents

Platinum agents have been used with relatively acceptable risks. Reports of normal outcomes have been reported; however, there are cases of intrauterine growth restriction as well. Case studies have reported hearing loss and ventriculomegaly in 2.7% of cases exposed to cisplatin.[1] One case of bilateral hearing loss was noted in a woman treated with carboplatin in the second trimester of pregnancy. However, the cause cannot be fully attributed to the platinum agent, as other causes of hearing loss were also present, including prematurity and administration of gentamycin in the neonatal period.[8]

Miscellaneous

Taxane chemotherapy is used in the treatment of malignant tumors of multiple sites, and experience with this class of drugs remains limited, although a few reports to date are favorable.[8,9]

Targeted Therapies

Despite the emerging role of targeted agents in cancer treatment, they have been used only inadvertently in pregnancy. Tratuzumab has been associated with oligohydraminos and its use is not recommended in pregnancy.[1] Rituximab has been associated with transient neonatal lymphopenia, and further studies are necessary to determine an accurate safety profile. Imatinib has been associated with low birthweight and premature delivery, whereas erlotinib has showed no adverse effects in one case. The antiangiogenic agents (bevacizumab, sunitinib, and sorafenib) are not recommended for use in pregnant women.[1]

National Registry

In 1984 the National Cancer Institute established a national registry for in utero exposure to chemotherapy.[12] The registry is currently located at the University of Oklahoma, under the direction of Dr. John J. Mulvihill (jmulvihill@ouhsc.edu). Through September 2006 the registry had summaries of 720 pregnancies. The rate of anomalies following first-trimester exposure was 19%, versus 6% after later exposure (and 3% in the general population). Of 422 pregnancies with third-trimester exposure, 66 (16%) of newborns had a functional abnormality, which was primarily myelosuppression occurring in a frequency related to time between last chemotherapy and delivery.

RADIATION THERAPY

Ionizing radiation is a known teratogen and the developing embryo is particularly sensitive to its effects. Doses higher than 0.20 Gray (Gy) are considered teratogenic. Effects during early pregnancy are typically lethal or result in congenital malformations. During late gestation, radiation may cause specific organ damage, such as mental retardation, skeletal anomalies, and ophthalmologic abnormalities. Reports have indicated that radiation exposure in utero increases the risk of malignancies, such as leukemia and other childhood tumors, particularly when exposure occurred in the first trimester.[1,9] It is important to remember that these data are conflicting and data is extrapolated from data from atomic catastrosphe.[9] Regardless, recommendations for radiation exposure in pregnancy should be less than 0.05 Gy.[1,9] Radiation therapy should be postponed until the postpartum period and consideration should be given to suitable alternative therapies, such as surgery or chemotherapy. If delay of therapy is not possible, termination of the pregnancy may be required.

SURGERY AND ANESTHESIA

Aspects of surgery are addressed later in the sections on specific cancers; first, some general principles should be considered. Although complications of surgery can threaten the fetus, extraperitoneal surgery is not related to spontaneous abortion or preterm labor. **Abdominal or pelvic surgery, if flexibility in timing exists, is best performed in the second trimester to limit the risk of first-trimester spontaneous abortion or preterm labor.** In the first trimester, progesterone therapy is indicated (weeks 7 to 12) following resection of the corpus luteum. Perioperative cautions include attention to the relative safety of all drugs administered. Fever secondary to either infection or atelectasis should be treated promptly, because it may be associated with fetal abnormalities.

There is no evidence that there are significant risks of anesthesia independent of coexisting disease.[13] In the second and third trimesters, careful attention to positioning is required so as to avoid compression of the vena cava from the enlarged uterus. Use of local or regional anesthesia should be considered. Finally, continuous or intermittent fetal monitoring should be employed in cases in which extrauterine survival is possible.

PREGNANCY FOLLOWING CANCER TREATMENT

With improved survival rates for many childhood and adolescent malignancies, one must be prepared to offer prenatal counseling to the young woman who presents with a cancer history. Issues worthy of review and in need of clarification for the obstetrician and the patient are listed in the box, Counseling Issues for Pregnancy Following Cancer Treatment.

Counseling Issues for Pregnancy Following Cancer Treatment

1. What is the risk of recurrence of the malignancy?
2. If a recurrence was diagnosed, depending on the most likely sites, what would be the nature of the probable treatment? How would such treatment compromise both the patient and the fetus?
3. Will prior treatments—pelvic surgery, radiation to pelvis or abdomen, or chemotherapy—affect fertility or reproductive outcome?
4. Will the hormonal milieu of pregnancy adversely affect an estrogen receptor–positive tumor?

Previous abdominal irradiation for a Wilms' tumor appears to adversely affect the risk of pregnancy complications, including increased perinatal mortality, low birthweight, and abnormal pregnancy. In contrast, a review of pregnancies following treatment for Hodgkin's lymphoma revealed no increase in poor pregnancy outcome.[14] However, the rate of ovarian failure following the multiple drug combinations is greater than 50% in some reports.[15] Also, a combination of pelvic irradiation and chemotherapy for Hodgkin's disease results in an even higher rate of ovarian failure. Over recent years, a number of women with early cervical cancer have received fertility preservation surgery with radical trachelectomy and regional lymphadenectomy. The preliminary fertility and pregnancy outcomes have been favorable.[16]

Will pregnancy increase the risk of recurrence or accelerate recurrence? Even in women with estrogen receptor–positive breast cancer, there is no evidence that subsequent pregnancy adversely affects survival. In addition to the altered hormonal milieu, concern is also directed toward the potential for accelerated tumor activity associated with alterations in the pregnant patient's immune system. There are no data to support this concern. However, it has been recommended that after a cancer diagnosis, pregnancy should be delayed for at least 2 years (during which recurrence risk is highest).

CANCER DURING PREGNANCY

Breast Cancer

The predicted number of breast cancer cases in women in the United States for the year 2010 was 207,090, and the predicted number of related deaths was 39,840.[17] Though the lifetime risk of developing breast cancer is 1 in 8, the risk is 1 in 206 for women 40 years or younger. Each year, this results in approximately 7% to 15% of premenopausal breast cancers being diagnosed in women who are pregnant or lactating.[8,18] Although it has been predicted that there may be an increase in the frequency of breast cancer complicating pregnancy due to delayed childbearing, recent publications are consistent with a frequency of breast cancer concurrent with pregnancy of 1.3 per 10,000 live births.[1,2,8]

In general, the risk of breast cancer is directly related to the duration of ovarian function. Therefore, both early menarche and late menopause appear to increase the likelihood of developing breast cancer. However, interruption of the normal cyclic ovarian function by pregnancy appears protective. This apparent protective effect may be secondary to the normal hormonal milieu of pregnancy that produces epithelial proliferation, followed by marked differentiation and mitotic rest. Multiparous women, particularly those who breastfeed, have a lower risk of developing breast cancer than do nulliparous women. However, based on one study of almost 90,000 women, breastfeeding may not be an independent protective factor.[19] Paradoxically, carriers of BRCA1 and BRCA2 mutations may have an increased risk of developing breast cancer by having children.[20]

Diagnosis and Staging

Breast abnormalities should be evaluated in the same manner as if the patient were not pregnant. The most common presentation of breast cancer in pregnancy is a painless lump discovered by the patient. Because the breast changes become more pronounced in later pregnancy, it is important to perform a thorough breast examination at the initial visit. Despite the striking physiologic breast changes of pregnancy, including nipple enlargement and increases in glandular tissue resulting in engorgement and tenderness, a newly found breast mass should be evaluated promptly. Diagnostic delays, which may increase the risk of nodal involvement, are often attributed to physician reluctance to evaluate breast complaints or abnormal findings in pregnancy.[21] Although bilateral serosanguinous discharge may be normal in late pregnancy, masses require prompt and definitive evaluation. The lengths of delays in diagnosis of breast cancer in pregnancy are commonly 3 to 7 months or longer.[21,22] A case-control study from Princess Margaret Hospital suggested that pregnant patients are at higher risk of presenting with advanced disease because pregnancy impedes early detection.[23]

Less common presentations may include bloody nipple discharge, which should be evaluated with mammography and ultrasound.[18] In cases of mastitis or breast abscesses, or evaluation of breast edema or inflammation, a skin biopsy should be considered to evaluate for inflammatory breast cancer.

Mammography in pregnancy is controversial. Although the radiation exposure to the fetus is negligible, the hyperproliferative changes in the breast during pregnancy are characterized by increased tissue density, making interpretation more difficult.[9,18] Breast ultrasound has a high sensitivity and specificity and can distinguish between solid and cystic masses, making it the preferred imaging modality for pregnant women. Magnetic resonance imaging (MRI), without gadolinium, has also been used; however, there is limited data on its accuracy in this population. Fine needle aspiration (FNA) of a mass for cytologic study may be used, but is often misleading due to changes in the breast during pregnancy. For breast masses, a core needle biopsy is the preferred method for histologic diagnosis.[9,21]

Before proceeding with treatment, staging should be undertaken. All draining lymph nodes should be evaluated. Sentinel lymph node biopsy techniques appear safe in pregnancy.[24] The contralateral breast must be carefully assessed. Laboratory tests should include baseline liver function tests and serum tumor markers, carcinoembryonic antigen (CEA), and CA 15-3. CA 15-3 appears to be a useful tumor marker for monitoring breast cancer in pregnancy.[25] A chest radiograph is indicated, and if the liver function tests are abnormal, the liver can be evaluated by ultrasound. If bone metastases are suspected, a bone scan can be performed in pregnancy. In a symptomatic patient, radiographs of the specific symptomatic bones are advised. However, in an asymptomatic patient with normal blood tests, because the yield is low, bone scanning is usually not performed.

Treatment

The treatment of breast carcinoma at any time is often overshadowed by psychological and emotional factors. Because of potential risks to the developing fetus, treatment decisions carry an additional burden. Therapy must be individualized in accordance with present knowledge and with the specific desires of the patient, and maternal treatment should adhere to standard recommendations.

Local Therapy

The usual criteria for breast-preserving therapy versus modified radical mastectomy pertain to the patient with breast cancer, stages I to III.[2,18] Though breast surgery can be safely performed in all trimesters with minimal fetal risks, the use of radiation is complicated by the presence of the pregnancy.[21,26] One publication presents a mathematical model suggesting that the risk of axillary metastases due to treatment delay is minimal and may be acceptable to some third-trimester patients with early breast cancer who prefer lumpectomy with radiation postpartum.[27] Consideration should be given to the delay of irradiation until after delivery. Experimental calculations suggest that a tumor dose of 5 Gy will expose the fetus to 0.010 to 0.015 Gy while the fetus is within the true pelvis. Later in pregnancy, parts of the fetus may receive as much as 0.200 Gy.[28] Because these levels exceed the upper limit of safety, alternative approaches should be considered. Reports have shown that in the late second or third trimester, delaying treatment without impacting maternal outcome may be reasonable.

Pregnancy Termination

Because early studies suggested more unfavorable outcomes in pregnant women, it was assumed that the hormonal changes of pregnancy contributed to rapid tumor growth. Therefore, therapeutic abortion was frequently advised. At present, a harmful effect of continuing pregnancy has not been demonstrated in most published series.[2] A series of 130 women with breast cancer diagnosed during pregnancy reported equivalent outcomes whether the pregnancy was terminated, spontaneous miscarriage occurred, or the pregnancy continued.[8] However, it is difficult to evaluate potential selection bias toward performing an abortion in patients with advanced disease. Because young women tend to have hormone receptor–negative tumors, it is difficult to make an argument, based on hormonal concerns, for either termination of pregnancy or oophorectomy as an adjunct to therapy.[18]

Chemotherapy

In general, women who present with either metastatic breast carcinoma or rapidly progressive inflammatory carcinoma should avoid any delays in therapy. Immediate initiation of chemotherapy is critical to providing the patient with inflammatory carcinoma with any chance for long-term survival. In the patient with a clinical indication for adjuvant chemotherapy other than inflammatory carcinoma, the delay of instituting chemotherapy and awaiting fetal pulmonary maturity should be considered in select third-trimester situations. Current literature shows that the use of cytotoxic agents for breast cancer in pregnancy is relatively safe, and includes the use of 5-fluorouracil, doxorubicin, cyclophosphamide, epirubicin, and taxanes.[21] Others concur with the use of chemotherapy in the second and third trimesters in the management of breast cancer.[18,29] Pregnancy is a contraindication to the use of tamoxifen due to the risk of adverse fetal outcomes, including oculoauriculovertebral dysplasia and ambiguous genitalia. Data regarding the safety of trastuzumab in pregnancy are limited, and currently it is not recommended due to reports of oligohydramios and deaths due to respiratory and renal failure.[21]

Prognosis

As with any malignant disease, prognosis best correlates with the anatomic extent of disease at the time of diagnosis. Outcomes in stage I and II disease are favorable, with survival rates approaching 86% to 100%; however, the presence and extent of nodal involvement is especially predictive of prognosis in both nonpregnant and pregnant patients.[8] Table 47-2 provides 5- and 10-year survival data by nodal status.[30-37] Although nodal status is of prognostic significance, the number of positive nodes is also important. In the pregnant patient, the 5-year survival rate is 82% for patients with three or fewer positive nodes, and 27% if greater than three nodes contain tumor.[36] Pregnancy, probably due to the associated delays in diagnosis, appears to increase the frequency of nodal disease, with 60% to 85% of patients exhibiting axillary nodal disease at diagnosis.[36]

Reports have demonstrated that up to 60% to 80% of breast cancer cases in the pregnant population are estrogen receptor negative and have a rate of HER2 positivity between 38% and 58%.[18] Additionally, breast tumors in pregnant women are more frequently reported to be larger, to be higher grade, and to have a higher rate of pathologic lymph node involvement compared to nonpregnant counterparts.[18] Thus, some reports concluded that breast cancer in pregnancy was associated with a worse prognosis.

TABLE 47-2 5- AND 10-YEAR SURVIVAL RATES, BY NODAL STATUS, OF PREGNANT OR LACTATING PATIENTS TREATED FOR BREAST CANCER

		OVERALL		NODE NEGATIVE		NODE POSITIVE	
Investigators	**No. of Patients**	**5-Yr (%)**	**10-Yr (%)**	**5-Yr (%)**	**10-Yr (%)**	**5-Yr (%)**	**10-Yr (%)**
White and White[30]	806	13	9	21	13	7	6
Holleb and Farrow[31]	117	31	—	65	—	17	—
Byrd et al.[32]	29	55	—	100	80	28	6
Applewhite et al.[33]	48	25	15	56	22	18	13
Riberio and Palmer[34]	59	31	24	90	90	37	21
Clark and Reid[35]							
Pregnant	121	—	22	—	35	—	22
Lactating	80	—	32	—	69	—	18
King et al.[36]	63	53	49	82	71	36	36
Petrek et al.[37]	56	61	45	82	77	47	25

However, these rates are histologically identical to the nonpregnant patient of similar age and, when controlled for age and stage, pregnancy does not seem to affect prognosis adversely.[23,37]

Subsequent Pregnancy

The risk of pregnancy after breast cancer has been a focus of a number of studies.[38,39] Although the consensus is that subsequent pregnancies do not adversely affect survival, there are recommendations regarding the timing of a subsequent pregnancy.[40] It is generally advised that women with node-negative disease wait for 2 to 3 years, and this interval should be extended to 5 years for patients with positive nodes. Others have advised that no delay is indicated for the patient with good prognostic disease who does not receive postoperative adjuvant chemotherapy.[40] It has been advised that patients should undergo a complete metastatic workup before a subsequent pregnancy.

Although no studies indicate that subsequent pregnancy adversely affects survival, the retrospective reports that suggest a potential favorable effect of subsequent pregnancy are too small to draw firm conclusions.[41] A trend toward better survival is also noted in patients who received adjuvant chemotherapy and subsequently became pregnant.[42]

Lactation and Breast Reconstruction

Lactation is possible in a small percentage of patients after breast-conserving therapy for early-stage breast cancer.[43] Lumpectomy using a radial incision rather than the cosmetically preferred circumareolar incision is less likely to disrupt ductal anatomy. Disruption of the ductal system may increase the rate of mastitis. Breastfeeding is contraindicated in women receiving chemotherapy, because significant levels of the drug can be found in breast milk.

Breast reconstruction with the use of autologous tissue has increased secondary to questions about the use of silicone-filled implants. The transverse rectus abdominis myocutaneous flap (TRAM) is one popular method of breast reconstruction. Because the donor site is a portion of the anterior abdominal wall, there is potential concern when the patient develops abdominal distention from pregnancy. In one case report and review of the literature, nine women who became pregnant following breast reconstruction experienced no problem with anterior abdominal wall integrity.[44] However, because data are limited, it may be best to address reconstruction in the postpartum period.

Lymphoma

Hodgkin's Lymphoma

Approximately 33,980 cases of lymphoma were expected to be diagnosed in women in the United States in the year 2010, and only about 11% of these would be Hodgkin's lymphoma (HL).[17] **Hodgkin's lymphoma is the second most commonly diagnosed cancer in women aged 15 to 29 years, and presents at a mean age of 32 years. It is therefore more commonly associated with pregnancy than non-Hodgkin's lymphoma (NHL), where the peak age incidence is 42 years.** Lymphomas complicate approximately 1 in 6000 pregnancies, and there are few large series to evaluate the many issues affecting these women. However, spontaneous abortion, stillbirth rates, and preterm births do not appear to be increased. Pregnancy does not appear to adversely affect the course of the disease.[45] **Termination of pregnancy should not be routinely advised.** Although some advocate therapeutic abortion for the patient with a first-trimester pregnancy and HL to allow complete staging, others limit therapeutic abortion to those women requiring infradiaphragmatic irradiation or those with systemic symptoms or visceral disease, which are best managed with multiagent chemotherapy.

Women with HL frequently present with enlarged cervical or axillary lymph nodes. The diagnosis is established by biopsy of the suspicious nodes. The presence of systemic symptoms, such as night sweats, pruritus, or weight loss, suggests more extensive disease. In a series of 17 women diagnosed with HL during pregnancy, the average time of diagnosis was 22 weeks of gestation and systemic symptoms were uncommon.[45] Two histologic variants, nodular sclerosis and lymphocyte predominant, have a better prognosis than mixed-cellularity and lymphocyte-depleted tumors. Nodular sclerosis type has been reported in approximately 75% of the cases diagnosed during pregnancy.[45] Clinical staging for lymphoma requires systemic evaluation by history, laboratory findings, bone marrow, and radiographic imaging. Clinical treatment and staging are individualized. Although pathologic staging for HL in the nonpregnant patient may involve laparotomy and splenectomy, these are not generally performed in pregnancy. The routine evaluation for HL during pregnancy includes

TABLE 47-3 STAGING CLASSIFICATION OF HODGKIN'S DISEASE*

STAGE	DESCRIPTION
I	Involvement of a single lymph node region (I) or of a single extralymphatic organ site (I_E)
II	Involvement of two or more lymph node regions on the same side of the diaphragm (II) or localized involvement of an extralymphatic organ site and of one or more lymph node regions on the same side of the diaphragm (II_E)
III	Involvement of lymph node regions on both sides of the diaphragm (III), which also may be accompanied by localized involvement of an extralymphatic organ or site (III_E), of the spleen (III_S), or of both (III_{SE})
IV	Diffuse or disseminated involvement of an extralymphatic organ with or without localized lymph node involvement (liver, bone marrow, lung, skin)

*Symptoms of unexplained fever, night sweats, and unexplained weight loss of 10% of normal body weight result in classification of patients as B; absence of these symptoms is denoted as A.

a single anterior/posterior view chest x-ray, liver function tests, serum creatinine clearance, complete blood count, erythrocyte sedimentation rate, and bone marrow biopsy. **Evaluation of the abdomen is compromised by the gravid uterus, and MRI is preferred, because it can accurately assess nodes, liver, and spleen.** Chest tomography or computed tomographic (CT) scan of the mediastinum may be necessary to evaluate nodal enlargement in the chest. Isotope scans of the liver and bone are best avoided during pregnancy. A single-shot lymphangiogram results in an exposure of less than 1 cGy to the fetus and is probably safe after the first trimester, but has become less available and may have limited accuracy.[46] Ultrasonography is safe and may provide useful information.

Disease stage (Table 47-3) is the most important factor in treatment planning and prognosis. The survival rate for early-stage HL exceeds 90%, whereas patients with disseminated nodal disease have a 5-year survival rate of about 50%. As expected, patients with stage IV disease have poor survival rates. Radiation therapy is the mainstay of treatment for early-stage HL, and combination chemotherapy is employed for the treatment of advanced-stage disease with organ involvement. **Most investigators agree that treatment should not be withheld during pregnancy except in early-stage disease, particularly if the diagnosis is made in late gestation.**

Radiotherapy to the supradiaphragmatic regions may be performed with abdominal shielding after the first trimester. When this approach is chosen, irradiation should be delayed until after the first trimester, total fetal dose should be limited to 10 cGy or less, and the goal is partial therapy with completion therapy after delivery. Thomas and Peckham reported three cases of mantle field irradiation with abdominal shielding for supradiaphragmatic disease. The estimated radiation exposures to the fetus for these patients at 10, 15, and 16 weeks were 2.5, 4.4, and 10.4 cGy, respectively.[46] Although these pregnancies went to term with apparent normal outcomes, long-term follow-up on these infants was not presented. Spontaneous abortion has been reported with an estimated first-trimester fetal dose of 9 cGy secondary to scatter from delivering 4400 cGy to the chest of a patient receiving treatment for a recurrence.[47] In general, if the estimated exposure to a first-trimester fetus is expected to exceed 10 cGy or if combination chemotherapy is planned for the first trimester, therapeutic abortion should be considered because of an increased risk of fetal malformations.[48] Asymptomatic early-stage disease presenting in the second half of pregnancy may be followed closely while preparations are made for early delivery.[47] The use of corticosteroids and single-agent chemotherapy has been proposed for the patient with systemic symptoms.

Subdiaphragmatic or advanced disease requires chemotherapy. ABVD (doxorubicin, bleomycin, vinblastine, dacarbazine) is considered the standard-of-care regimen, with MOPP (mechloretamine, vincristine, procarbazine, prednisone) also reported with the second most frequency.[49] Because many of these chemotherapeutic agents are known teratogens, such treatment is best avoided in the first trimester. A recent systematic review found 42 pregnancies in which HL was treated with chemotherapy.[50] Seventeen were exposed to chemotherapy in the first trimester, resulting in six congenital anomalies and three spontaneous abortions. Similar treatments should also be approached with caution later in pregnancy, although most case reports have documented only intrauterine growth restriction and neonatal neutropenia as complications. The aforementioned systematic review found normal pregnancy outcomes in women treated after the first trimester, with the exception of a single third-trimester intrauterine fetal demise (IUFD). Long-term follow-up toxicity studies are lacking.

Following therapy for HL, it has been suggested that pregnancy planning should take into consideration that about 80% of recurrences manifest within 2 years. Treatments for HL may compromise the reproductive potential of young patients.[15,51] As reflected in Figure 47-1, ovarian failure is more likely to occur in older patients, even if treated with fewer courses of chemotherapy.[51] Early studies reported normal ovarian function in only 12% of women following therapy for HL. Combined treatment with radiation and chemotherapy lead to the highest risk of ovarian failure. **More recent series have shown the pregnancy rate among reproductive-age HL survivors to be similar to the normal female population.**[52] Regimen changes that have occurred since the earlier reports include improved pelvic shielding during primary irradiation, ovarian transposition when pelvic radiation is required, and the more frequent use of the ABVD regimen instead of MOPP. Whereas combined oral contraceptives have been advocated to preserve ovarian function, there is no evidence of efficacy. Depending on their availability, new reproductive technologies, including oocyte donation and embryo cryopreservation, can be considered for select situations.

Patients who become pregnant after treatment for HL do not demonstrate increased adverse perinatal outcomes such as fetal wastage, preterm birth, and birth defects when compared with sibling controls.[53] Although fetal anomalies have occurred after treatment for HL, chromosomal abnormalities or a new gene mutation have not been diagnosed.[51] The absence of a repetitive pattern of malformations makes it difficult to imply a causal relationship

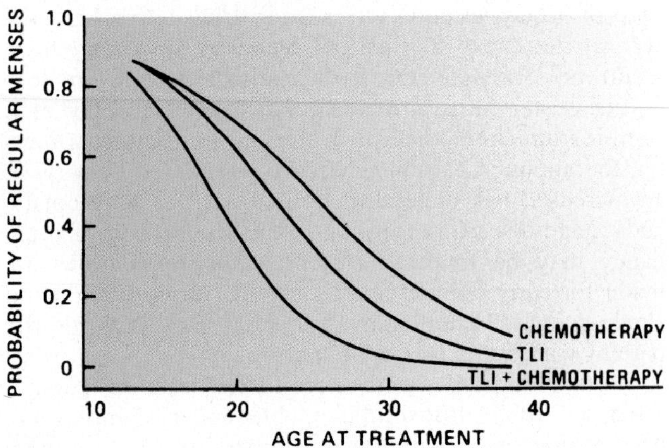

FIGURE 47-1. Probability of regular menses after chemotherapy, total lymphoid irradiation (TLI), and TLI and chemotherapy in patients with Hodgkin's disease. The synergistic effect is more apparent in younger women. (From Horning SJ, Hoppe RT, Kaplan HS: Female reproduction after treatment for Hodgkin's disease. N Engl J Med 304:1377, 1981.)

between any birth defects observed and previous therapy for Hodgkin's disease.

General recommendations, therefore, include delaying therapy until at least the second trimester due to the increased first-trimester fetal risk. **After the first trimester, therapy should not be delayed for patients with symptomatic, subdiaphragmatic or progressive HL.** Treatment options include supradiaphragmatic radiation therapy for early-stage disease, and combination chemotherapy for bulky, subdiaphragmatic, progressive, or advanced disease. Radiation fields should be tailored to limit fetal dose, and a maximal fetal dose calculation should be performed prior to treatment. Pregnant women with HL should be managed by a maternal-fetal medicine specialist, and whether pregnancy termination should be pursued will depend on the clinical situation.

Non-Hodgkin's Lymphoma

Non-Hodgkin's lymphoma (NHL) occurs at a mean age of 42 years and, therefore, is reported less frequently than Hodgkin's lymphoma in association with pregnancy. **In general, NHL is more likely to complicate pregnancy because more patients have an aggressive histology and advanced-stage disease.** Indolent lymphomas are less common in younger patients and are rarely described in pregnancy. Up to 70% of NHL in pregnancy is diffuse large B-cell lymphoma.[54] Burkitt's lymphoma is usually rapidly progressive and may involve the breast and ovary. Lymphoma of the breast has a particularly poor prognosis, and it has been speculated that there may be a hormonal influence on this malignancy in pregnant patients.

A recent systematic review identified 75 women with NHL treated with systemic therapy in pregnancy.[50] CHOP (cyclophosphamide, doxorubicin, vincristine, prednisone) is the most widely used regimen for aggressive NHL, and CHOP or CHOP-B (plus bleomycin) was the most common regimen in the above series. Overall, CHOP/CHOP-B did not have a clear adverse effect on pregnancy outcomes. Approximately 25% of these patients received chemotherapy in the first trimester, with no congenital anomalies reported. Two miscarriages were reported in patients treated with non–CHOP-based regimens. In patients treated after the first trimester, there was one IUFD and one stillborn infant, both with non-CHOP-based regimens, as well as a 33-week infant with transient leukopenia. The anti-CD20 antibody rituximab was incorporated into the regimen of seven patients. Adverse events in these seven infants included one episode of transient pulmonary insufficiency, and one episode of premature B-cell depletion that resolved at 12 weeks.[55]

Adult T-cell leukemia/lymphoma, caused by the human T-cell lymphotropic virus type I, is found in Japan, the Caribbean, and the southern United States. The virus is present in familial clusters and is transmitted by sexual intercourse, blood transfusions, and breast milk. Infants seroconvert between 12 and 19 months of age at a rate of 20% to 25%.[56]

Acute Leukemia

Although the incidence of leukemia in pregnancy is not specifically known, it is estimated to occur in fewer than 1 in 75,000 pregnancies. **Acute leukemia represents about 90% of leukemias coexisting with pregnancy.** Acute myeloid leukemia (AML) accounts for about 60% and acute lymphoblastic leukemia (ALL) for about 30% of cases. More than three fourths of the cases are diagnosed after the first trimester.[11] The prognosis for acute leukemia in pregnancy is guarded.[57] Although there is no evidence that pregnancy adversely affects the prognosis of acute leukemia, a study in 1988 reported a median survival of 27.5 months in a nonpregnant population.[58] However, the differences in patients and the varied treatments preclude any reliable comparison.[59] Optimal care of the pregnant patient with acute leukemia necessitates a team effort and is best achieved in a cancer referral center.

The diagnosis of acute leukemia is rarely difficult. The signs and symptoms of anemia, granulocytopenia, and thrombocytopenia, including fatigue, fever, infection, and easy bleeding or petechiae, usually prompt a complete blood count. A normal or elevated white blood cell count (WBC) is present in up to 90% of patients with ALL. A WBC in excess of 50,000 is found in only one fourth of patients. In contrast, patients with acute nonlymphocytic leukemia (ANLL) may present with markedly elevated WBC, although one third present with leukopenia. The diagnosis of leukemia should be confirmed by bone marrow biopsy and aspirate. The biopsy material is usually hypercellular with leukemic cells. The smear of the aspirate reveals decreased erythocyte and granulocytic precursors as well as megakaryocytes. Leukemic cells comprise greater than half of the marrow's cellular elements in most patients. The morphology of the marrow and the peripheral leukemic cells help to distinguish between lymphocytic and nonlymphocytic leukemias. This latter group includes acute myelocytic (granulocytic), promyelocytic, monocytic, and myelomonocytic leukemias and erythroleukemia. Acute myelocytic leukemia is the most common form of ANLL. Patients who develop ANLL as a result of previous chemotherapy have a particularly poor response to treatment.

There are numerous reports of successful pregnancies in patients aggressively treated with combination

chemotherapy for acute leukemia. Acute leukemia and its therapy are associated with an increase in stillbirths (approximately 15%), prematurity (approximately 50%), and fetal growth restriction.[59] In 1988 and 1991 reports by Aviles and colleagues showed no serious long-term effects of in utero exposure to chemotherapy.[60] The first report included 17 children, aged 4 to 22, whose mothers received treatment for acute leukemia.[60] In the second report, 43 children who were born to mothers with a variety of hematologic malignancies were examined at 3 to 19 years of age.[60] In both studies, greater than 40% of the cases involved exposure during the first trimester. Anthracyclines (daunorubicin, idarubicin, doxorubicin) are important components of acute leukemia therapy; daunorubicin and idarubicin in particular are associated with a high rate of congenital defects. Although doxorubicin is no longer generally included in leukemia induction regimens, it appears to have comparable efficacy and a more favorable side-effect profile in pregnancy.[61] In patients with breast cancer treated during pregnancy, doxorubicin has been used effectively with a favorable toxicity profile.[8] It may be rational to favor doxorubicin for anthracycline-based regimens in pregnancy.

If the mother is exposed to cytotoxic drugs within 1 month of delivery, the newborn should be monitored closely for evidence of granulocytopenia or thrombocytopenia.

Chronic Leukemia

Chronic leukemia accounts for approximately 10% of cases of leukemia during pregnancy, with the majority of these being patients with chronic myelocytic leukemia (CML).[59] Chronic lymphocytic leukemia has a median age of onset of about 60 years, making cases during pregnancy rare. The median age of patients with CML is 35 years. CML is characterized by excessive production of mature myeloid cell elements, with granulocyte counts averaging 200,000/dL. Most patients have thrombocytosis and a mild normochromic normocytic anemia. Platelet function is often abnormal, although hemorrhage is usually limited to patients with marked thrombocytopenia. CML tends to be indolent, and normal hematopoiesis is only mildly affected in the early stages of disease. Therefore, delay of aggressive treatment is more feasible than with acute leukemia. Unless complications such as severe systemic symptoms, autoimmune hemolytic anemia, recurrent infection, or symptomatic lymphatic enlargement occur, treatment for chronic leukemia should be withheld until after delivery. Therapy, when necessary, has included prednisone and an alkylating agent such as chlorambucil or cyclophosphamide. High-dose steroids alone may be used to treat autoimmune hemolytic anemia. Targeting the BCR/ABL fusion gene with imatinib, however, has caused a shift in the treatment paradigm for this disease. Due to the high rate of teratogenicity, however, imatinib is not labeled for use in pregnancy. Currently, the median survival time for CML is more than 60 months, with survivals up to 10 years common.

Often, the diagnosis of CML antedates the pregnancy. **Although pregnancy does not appear to affect CML adversely, therapy does increase the frequency of preterm birth and low birthweight.** Information about contemporary management and prognosis is scarce secondary to the fact that few recent cases of CML during pregnancy have been reported. There are reports of CML treatment with leukapheresis during pregnancy. This treatment appears to be both safe and effective. Leukapheresis results in improvement of blood counts, systemic symptoms, and splenomegaly. This treatment, although costly and involved, has less risk of teratogenesis than cytotoxic treatments.[57,62] Although allogeneic stem cell transplants offer the highest cure rates, such therapy is hazardous during pregnancy. Interferon (IFN) therapy has been reported in a limited number of pregnancies with good outcomes. In 2001 the FDA gave accelerated approval to imatinib mesylate (Gleevec), a synthetic inhibitor of the BCR/ABL kinase, STI571, for (1) treatment of patients in the chronic phase after failure of IFN therapy, (2) accelerated phase, and (3) blast crisis. This drug carries a category D warning in pregnancy.[63] Pye and colleagues reported the largest clinical report on the safety of imatinib in pregnancy in 2008.[64] A total of 180 pregnant women were exposed to imatinib (80% CML), but after excluding patients with unknown outcomes and those who underwent therapeutic abortion, 55 patients were remaining for evaluation. While 40 women delivered live infants without anomalies, there were eight spontaneous abortions and seven congenital anomalies (plus one termination for anomaly). **Although flawed by the limited data available in this series, it does appear that early exposure to imatinib is associated with a high rate of congenital anomalies and miscarriage.** Imatinib therapy initiated in the second and third trimester may not add significant additional risk, but better outcome data are necessary to determine.

Hairy cell leukemia during pregnancy is rare, with only six reported cases. A predilection for men and the older age groups is the reason for the infrequency. IFN treatment has been used in two cases with no adverse fetal effects.[62]

Melanoma

The incidence of malignant melanoma is increasing in the childbearing years, with reports of melanoma ranging from 1% to 3.3% in pregnant or lactating women and accounting for 8% of malignancies diagnosed in gestation.[1,2,65] The understanding of the natural history of melanoma has been advanced by the identification of prognostic variables.[65] Prognostic features of the primary tumor include tumor thickness, ulceration, and body location.[66] The methods used to describe the depth of invasion for melanoma are depicted in Figure 47-2.

A topic of continued debate is whether pregnancy exerts a negative effect on the course of malignant melanoma. Reports have suggested that melanoma arising during pregnancy is associated with an aggressive clinical course, more likely to be diagnosed at an advanced stage, and associated with a shorter disease-free interval.[9,65,66] Although many studies suggest that melanoma developing during pregnancy is more likely to appear in locations associated with a poor prognosis,[67-70] others show no increase in poor prognostic location of lesions in the pregnant patient and comparable survival outcomes to nonpregnant cohorts.[65,66]

The World Health Organization (WHO) 1991 study examined the relevant prognostic features of melanoma in

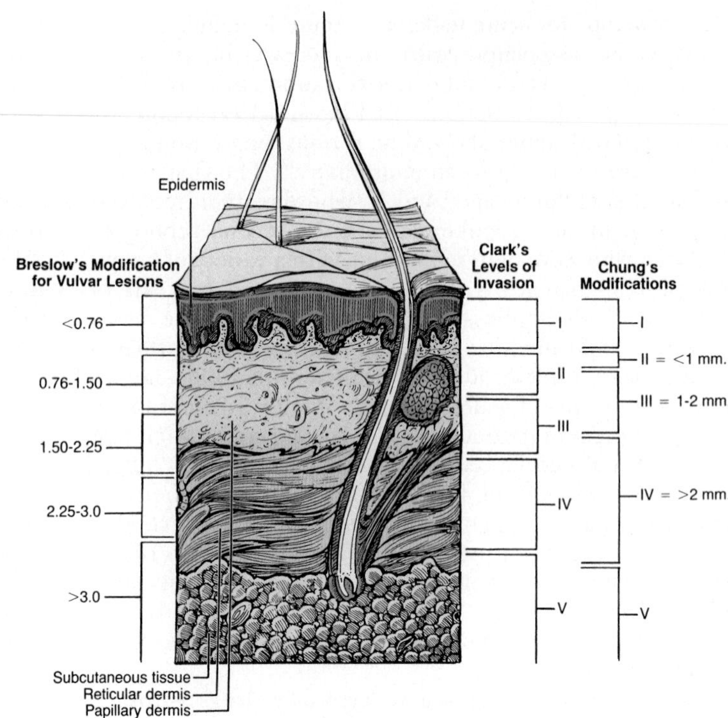

FIGURE 47-2. Schematic comparison of the different levels of invasion for melanoma. (From Gordon AN: Vulvar tumors. *In* Copeland LJ [ed]: Textbook of Gynecology, ed 2. Philadelphia, WB Saunders, 2000, p 1202.)

TABLE 47-4 WHO STAGES I AND II STUDY OF MALIGNANT MELANOMA

RELATIONSHIP TO TIME OF PREGNANCY	NO. OF PATIENTS	MEAN TUMOR THICKNESS (mm)
Before	85	1.29
During	92	2.38*
After all	143	1.96
Between	68	1.78

From MacKie RM, Bufalino R, Morabito A, et al: Lack of effect on pregnancy outcome of melanoma. Lancet 337:653, 1991.
*$P = .004$. When corrected for tumor thickness, survival rates were not different. Multivariate analysis identified tumor thickness as an independent prognostic variable, not pregnancy.

TABLE 47-5 PRIMARY MELANOMA TUMOR THICKNESS IN PREGNANT AND NONPREGNANT PATIENTS

	TUMOR THICKNESS (mm)		
Study	Pregnant	Nonpregnant	*P* Value
MacKie et al.[67]	2.3	1.7	.002
Slingluft et al.[68]	2.7	1.5	.052
Travers et al.[69]	2.3	1.2	.0001

the childbearing years and in pregnancy.[67] This report suggested that patients who were diagnosed during pregnancy had tumors demonstrating significantly greater tumor thickness, which has been confirmed by other studies as well (Tables 47-4 and 47-5).[67-69] However, after correcting for tumor thickness, survival rates were similar. Other investigators have found no difference in lesion thickness in pregnancy.[70] The issue remains unsettled, and explanations for the increased tumor thickness in pregnancy include hormonal stimulation, growth factor stimulation, immunologic alterations of pregnancy, and delays in diagnosis, secondary to pigmentation changes during pregnancy.[69] Once diagnosis is suspected, biopsy is recommended. Wide surgical excision with appropriate margins remains the most effective modality for the treatment of melanoma. For patients with stage I or II tumors, the standard surgical excision with margins appropriate for tumor thickness should be performed. Lymph node dissection is undertaken in the patient with regional disease, and more recently, sentinel node evaluation and biopsy has been used successfully.[9] Because adjuvant chemotherapy is experimental and has not demonstrated improved survival, it is not recommended for the pregnant patient because of the potential risk to the fetus. Because chemotherapy results in a clinical response, usually of short duration, it is usually most appropriate to plan for early delivery in cases of disseminated disease presenting late in pregnancy.

Despite rare reports of regression after delivery, no studies support any therapeutic benefit associated with therapeutic abortion.[71] However, given the aggressive nature of the current therapies available for metastatic disease, it is appropriate to consider termination when managing advanced disease presenting in the first trimester.[71]

The patient who has undergone apparent successful treatment for a malignant melanoma may express concern about the safety of a future pregnancy. No adverse impact on recurrence or survival has been identified in most studies addressing this issue.[67] However, the timing of subsequent pregnancy deserves some consideration. The probability of survival of a specific cancer should be evaluated based on the known prognostic variables. The 5-year survival rate for the patient with a melanoma less than 1.5 mm thick is 90%. For a tumor of intermediate thickness (1.5 to 4 mm), the 5-year survival rate is 50% to 75%, and for a more deeply invasive tumor, survival is less than

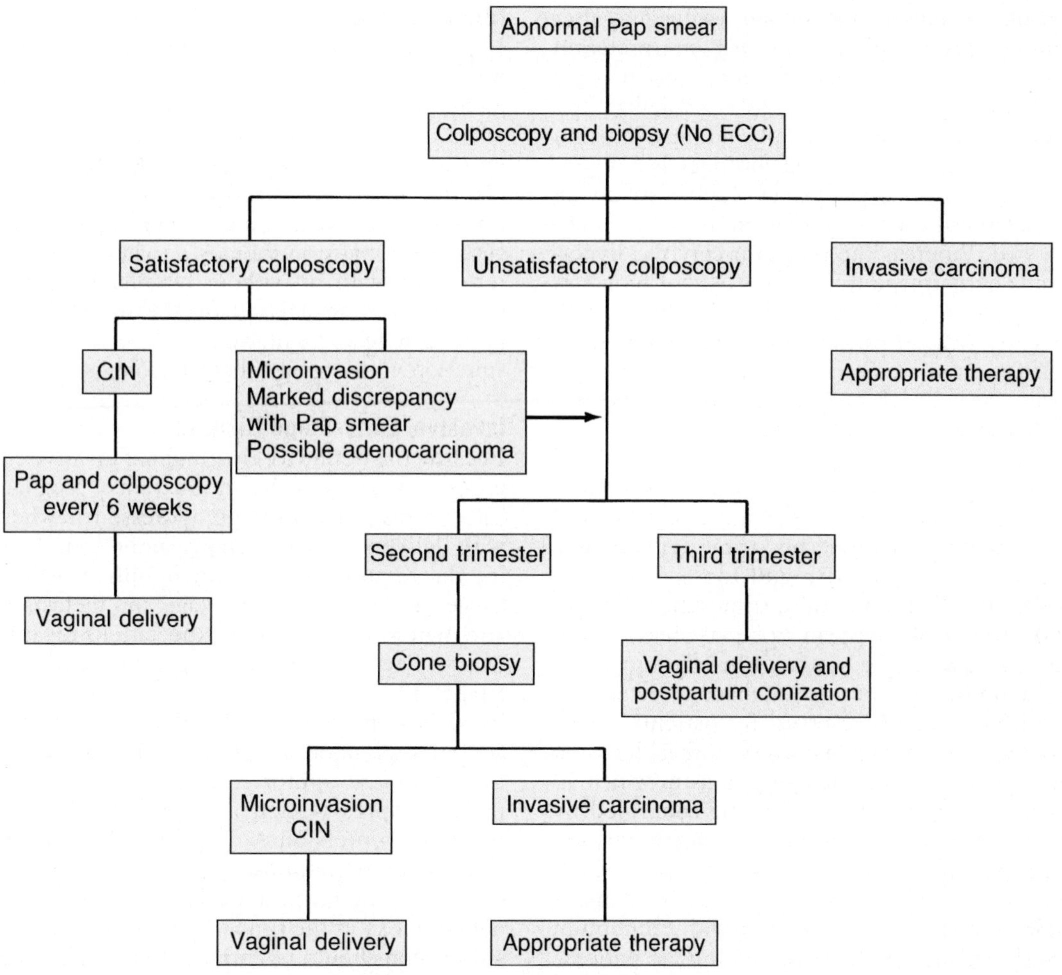

FIGURE 47-3. Suggested protocol for evaluation of abnormal cervical cytology in pregnancy. *ECC,* Endocervical curettage; *CIN,* cervical intraepithelial neoplasia. (From Hacker NF, Berek JS, Lagasse LD, et al: Carcinoma of the cervix associated with pregnancy. Obstet Gynecol 59:735, 1982.)

50%. Although some report that approximately 60% to 70% of patients develop their recurrence within 2 years and 80% to 90% within 5 years, the WHO study claimed that 83% of recurrences develop within the first 2 years.[71] Based on this information, it is generally recommended that patients wait 2 to 3 years before attempting another pregnancy, especially with nodal disease.[67] Furthermore, the use of hormonal agents, such as oral contraceptives, has not been demonstrated to adversely affect previously treated melanoma and recommendations for their use should be individualized.[72]

Cervical Cancer

Cervical cancer is the most common gynecologic malignancy associated with pregnancy, occurring in approximately 1 per 2200 pregnancies, and approximately 3%, or 1 in 34 cases, of all invasive cervical cancers occur during pregnancy.[1,2] Though it is the only cancer whose screening is part of the prenatal evaluation, the true incidence is difficult to ascertain due to the reporting biases associated with the reports originating from large referral centers. Also, various reports may include patients who have preinvasive lesions as well as those who are diagnosed in the postpartum period.

The initial obstetrical visit should include visualization of the cervix and cervical cytology, including an endocervical brush. The general principles of screening for cervical neoplasia apply during pregnancy. If the cervix appears friable, cervical cytology alone may not be sufficient to alert the physician to the presence of a malignant tumor. False-negative cervical cytology is at increased risk in pregnancy owing to excess mucus and bleeding from cervical eversion. Therefore, it is necessary to obtain a biopsy to ensure that tissue friability is not secondary to tumor. Also, an ulcerative or exophytic lesion must have histologic sampling performed. Although approximately one third of pregnant patients with cervical cancer are asymptomatic at the time of diagnosis, the most common symptoms are vaginal bleeding or discharge. Though these complaints are common and usually attributed to pregnancy-related conditions, it is important to evaluate for the possibility of neoplastic disease of the lower genital tract in pregnant women with these symptoms.

Cervical cytology suggestive of a squamous intraepithelial lesion or a report of atypical glandular cells during pregnancy requires appropriate clinical evaluation (Figure 47-3). Colposcopy during pregnancy is usually enhanced by the physiologic eversion of the lower endocervical canal.

However, vascular changes and redundant vagina may alter or obscure normal visualization, rendering interpretation difficult, and referral to a gynecologic oncologist may be appropriate. During pregnancy, failure to visualize the entire transformation zone and squamocolumnar junction is uncommon. Although endocervical curettage is not generally recommended during pregnancy, lesions involving the lower endocervical canal can often be directly visualized and biopsied. Whereas the pregnant cervix is hypervascular, serious hemorrhage from an outpatient biopsy is uncommon, and the risk of bleeding is offset by the risk of missing an early invasive cancer. Following a colposcopy evaluation with appropriate tissue sampling, most patients with preinvasive lesions can be followed with repeat colposcopy at 6- to 8-week intervals to delivery.[73]

Patients with cervical neoplasia will require a careful and complete colposcopic evaluation 6 weeks postpartum. Cone biopsy during pregnancy, when necessary, should ideally be performed during the second trimester to reduce the risks of first-trimester abortion and rupture of membranes or premature labor in the third trimester.[74] Complications from conization of the pregnant cervix are common. Therapeutic conization for intraepithelial squamous lesions is contraindicated during pregnancy. Diagnostic cone biopsy in pregnancy is reserved for patients whose colposcopic-directed biopsy has shown superficial invasion (suspect microinvasion) or in other situations in which an invasive lesion is suspected but cannot be confirmed by biopsy. When a cone biopsy is necessary during pregnancy, one should keep in mind the anatomic alteration of the cervix secondary to pregnancy. A shallow disk-like cone is usually satisfactory to clarify the diagnosis with a minimum of morbidity. It should be kept in mind that patients who have had a conization during pregnancy are at higher risk for residual disease. Therefore, close follow-up is essential.

Considering the routine practice of performing cervical cytology in early pregnancy, one would expect there to be a preponderance of early-stage disease diagnosed in the first trimester. Surprisingly, this is not the situation. The diagnosis of cervical cancer is commonly made postpartum rather than during pregnancy, and although stage IB disease is the most common stage found, all stages are represented in significant numbers. Both patient and physician factors, including lack of prenatal care, failure to obtain cervical cytology or to biopsy gross cervical abnormalities, false-negative cytology, and failure to evaluate abnormal cytology or vaginal bleeding properly, contribute to the delays in diagnosis.

Following the diagnosis of invasive cervical cancer, a staging evaluation is indicated. The standard cervical staging is clinical and usually based on the results of physical examination, cystoscopy, proctoscopy, chest radiograph, and intravenous pyelogram. A CT scan or, in some centers, lymphangiography is often performed to identify lymph node metastasis; however, in the pregnant patient, the standard staging evaluation is modified. The chest radiograph is performed with abdominal shielding. Sonography is used to detect hydronephrosis and, if additional retroperitoneal imaging is desired for the evaluation of lymphadenopathy, consideration should be given to employing MRI because it does not involve ionizing radiation.

Microinvasion

In patients with a microinvasive squamous carcinoma with negative margins on cone biopsy, consideration can be given to conservative management until delivery. The risk of occult metastatic disease is predominantly dependent on two pathologic features: (1) the depth of invasion and (2) the presence or absence of lymph-vascular space involvement.[75] Whether the cone biopsy can be considered sufficient long-term therapy or whether a postpartum hysterectomy with or without lymphadenectomy should be performed is also based on the detailed analysis of the pathologic features of the cone biopsy. In these cases, consultation with a gynecologic oncologist is appropriate.

Invasive, Early-Stage Disease

Because the definitive treatment of invasive cervical cancer is not compatible with continuation of pregnancy, the clinical question that must be addressed is when to proceed with delivery so that therapy can be completed. Considering this requirement, treatment options will be influenced by gestational age, tumor stage and metastatic evaluation, and maternal desires and expectations regarding the pregnancy. The management of early invasive cervical cancer (stages IA2, IB, and IIA) in the young patient is usually by radical hysterectomy, pelvic lymphadenectomy, and aortic lymph node sampling.[76,77] The primary advantage of this treatment approach over radiation therapy for these patients is preservation of ovarian function. For the woman with a high probability of having a poor prognostic lesion and, therefore, requiring postoperative irradiation, consideration can be given to performing a unilateral or bilateral oophoropexy at the time of the hysterectomy. The ovarian suspension should be intraperitoneal, because retroperitoneal placement seems to predispose to subsequent ovarian cyst formation. In the first trimester, this surgery is usually carried out with the fetus in utero. In the third trimester, the radical hysterectomy and pelvic +/− para-aortic lymphadenectomy are performed after completion of a high classic cesarean delivery. Delays in therapeutic intervention have not been reported to increase recurrence rates for patients with small-volume stage I disease.[76] Although the pelvic vessels are large, the dissection is enhanced by more easily defined tissue planes.[77]

Second-trimester situations are more problematic. Studies have supported delay in management of early-stage disease until after fetal viability in women diagnosed after 20 weeks' gestation.[76] Other reports have suggested the administration of one to three cycles of platinum-based chemotherapy, allowing an additional 7 to 15 weeks of fetal maturation. In one study, maturation from 26 to 27 weeks' gestation compared with 34 to 35 weeks increased neonatal survival from 67% to 97%.[78] The neoadjuvant chemotherapy approach (chemotherapy before either surgery or irradiation) has been reported in nine cases of cervical cancer diagnosed during pregnancy. Three patients, all with advanced disease, ultimately died of disease, but all neonatal outcomes were normal.[79] Certainly in terms of general fetal salvage and outcome, the risk of extreme prematurity would far outweigh the risk of the chemotherapy exposure. Although this management of second-trimester cervical cancer presentations seems logical, there is scant information about this treatment approach. In cases diagnosed remote from fetal maturity, between 20 and 30 weeks of gestation, assessment of nodal involvement should be considered and will dictate further recommendations for management.[79]

Invasive, Locally Advanced Disease

The management of the patient with more advanced, local disease is based on treatment with chemotherapy and irradiation, both external beam to treat the regional nodes and shrink the central tumor and brachytherapy to complete the delivery of a tumoricidal dose to the cervix and adjacent tissues.[79] Coordinating a chemoradiation treatment plan for pregnant patients with stage IIB, stage III, and stage IVA is challenging. The patient with a first-trimester pregnancy can usually be treated in the standard fashion with initiation of chemotherapy and external therapy to the pelvis or extended field, as dictated by standard treatment guidelines. Most of these patients proceed to abort spontaneously within 2 to 5 weeks of initiating the radiation. Patients in the late first trimester are least likely to abort spontaneously, and it may be necessary to perform a uterine evacuation on the completion of external therapy in some patients. Following either spontaneous abortion or uterine evacuation, the brachytherapy component of the radiation therapy can proceed in the standard fashion. Patients in either their second or third trimester should have a high classic cesarean delivery before starting standard chemotherapy and irradiation. Again, it would seem appropriate to strongly consider neoadjuvant chemotherapy for this group of patients, especially the patient with a second-trimester or early third-trimester presentation, when the opportunity for further fetal maturation can be provided.

Invasive, Distant Metastasis

Metastatic disease to extrapelvic sites carries a poor prognosis. Although a select few patients with aortic node metastasis may receive curative therapy, it is unlikely for the patient with pulmonary metastasis, bone metastasis, or supraclavicular lymph node metastasis to be cured. Personal patient choices and ethical considerations are the major factors guiding treatment in these situations.

Small cell neuroendocrine tumors of the cervix associated with pregnancy are rare. Neoadjuvant or adjuvant chemotherapy with cisplatin, etoposide, and doxorubicin is recommended, and long-term survivors have been reported.[80] These tumors are considered to be histologically aggressive, and pregnancy preservation is not recommended. However, each case should be individualized.[79,80]

Method of Delivery

Controversy continues to surround the issue of the method of delivery for the term patient with cervical cancer. It seems heroic and unjustifiably risky to encourage vaginal delivery of a patient with a large, firm, barrel-shaped tumor or a large friable and hemorrhagic exophytic tumor. However, many small-volume stage IB, IIA, and early IIB tumors are potential candidates for vaginal delivery. Whether vaginal delivery promotes systemic dissemination of tumor cells is unknown, although the general opinion is that survival rates are not influenced by the mode of delivery.

Although systemic tumor dissemination secondary to vaginal delivery has not been documented, there are reports of episiotomy implants for both squamous carcinoma and adenocarcinoma following vaginal delivery.[81] Episiotomy implants are sufficiently rare that the risk should not be a determining factor for a given patient. However, the episiotomy should be carefully followed in a cervical cancer patient who delivers vaginally. Episiotomy nodules in these patients must be promptly evaluated by biopsy, because an early diagnosis may permit curative therapy.[81] Diagnostic delays secondary to suspicion of the nodules representing stitch abscess should be avoided.

Survival

Although some authors have suggested that the survival of patients with cervical cancer associated with pregnancy is compromised, most reports indicate that the prognosis is not altered.[75-78]

Ovarian Cancer

Although adnexal masses are often observed in pregnancy, only 2% to 5% are malignant ovarian tumors.[82] Ovarian cancer occurs in approximately 1 in 18,000 to 1 in 56,000 pregnancies.[82] With the increased use of diagnostic ultrasound, ovarian cysts and neoplasms are more frequently encountered in early pregnancy.[82,83] Ultrasonic features that are associated with an increased risk of malignancy include the presence of excrescences/papillary structures, irregular borders, septations/complex appearance, and presence of ascites, and these features should prompt further evaluation.[83]

Whereas the three major categories of ovarian tumors (epithelial, including borderline tumors, germ cell, and sex-cord stromal) occur during pregnancy, the majority of cases are diagnosed in early stages, resulting in favorable outcomes.[82] Germ cell tumors account for 30% to 50% (Figure 47-4), 37.5% to 50% are epithelial tumors, and the remainder are sex-cord stromal tumors or metastatic tumors to the

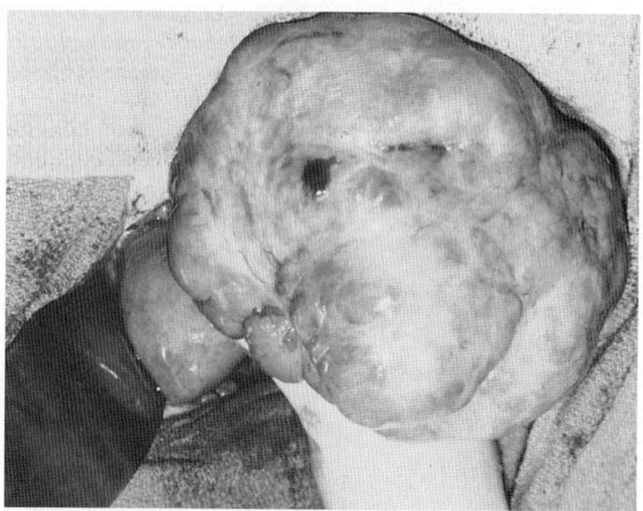

FIGURE 47-4. Dysgerminoma, the most common malignant ovarian neoplasm found in pregnancy, characterized by a lobulated solid gross appearance. (From Copeland LJ: Gestational trophoblastic neoplasia. *In* Copeland LJ [ed]: Textbook of Gynecology, ed 2. Philadelphia, WB Saunders, 2000, p 1391.)

ovary.[82] This distribution is undoubtedly skewed by the reporting bias associated with rare tumors. Characteristic of epithelial tumors in young patients who are not pregnant, the majority of epithelial ovarian tumors complicating pregnancy are of low grade (grade 1 or low malignant potential) or early stage, and not uncommonly these tumors are both low grade and stage I.

Management of the adnexal mass in pregnancy is controversial. The risks of surgical intervention may favor a conservative approach.[82,83] Serial sonograms may be of some value in determining the nature and biologic potential of the tumor. A number of opposing risks require consideration before following a conservative approach. The risk of greatest concern is that a delay of surgical intervention could permit a malignant ovarian tumor to spread, resulting in a decreased opportunity for cure. However, considering the rarity of advanced-stage poorly differentiated epithelial tumors in this age group, this risk is relatively small. Although ovarian tumors may be the cause of obstructed labor, this is uncommon.[82] Skilled sonographic examination is essential to determining the potential for malignancy based on size and imaging characteristics. Serial sonographic evaluations will also identify the rare tumor that remains in the pelvis as the gestation progresses. Because most ovarian masses relocate to the abdomen as the pregnancy advances, other explanations should be considered for persistent pelvic masses, including pelvic kidney, uterine fibroids, and colorectal or bladder tumors.

There does appear to be an increased probability that an adnexal mass during pregnancy will undergo torsion or rupture, and surgical intervention for these events is associated with higher fetal loss than an elective procedure.[84] Prompt surgical exploration is also performed for the mass associated with ascites or when there is evidence of metastatic disease. Because surgical exploration during pregnancy is associated with an increase in pregnancy loss and neonatal morbidity, it is ideal to delay surgical intervention until term or after delivery. However, if intervention is required during pregnancy, surgery should be performed after 16 weeks of gestation to reduce the risk of spontaneous abortion and allow the resolution of functional cysts.[84]

When a malignant ovarian tumor is encountered at laparotomy, surgical intervention should be similar to that for the nonpregnant patient. If the patient is preterm and the tumor appears confined to one ovary, consideration should be given to limiting the staging to removal of the involved ovary, cytologic washings, omentectomy, pelvic and para-aortic lymph node dissection, and a thorough manual exploration of the abdomen and pelvis.[85] The potential benefit of more extensive staging may be offset by higher pregnancy loss or neonatal morbidity. Before surgery, a comprehensive discussion with the patient should guide the extent of surgery if metastatic disease, especially a high-grade epithelial lesion, is encountered. Depending on the gestational age and the patient's desires, limited surgery followed by chemotherapy and additional extirpative surgery following delivery may be offered in select cases.[85]

Preoperative serum tumor markers are of limited value during pregnancy secondary to the physiologic increases in β-hCG, AFP, and CA 125. Kobayashi and colleagues have reported the mean CA 125 level during the first trimester is 72 units/mL and then normalizes during the second trimester.[86] However, following diagnostic confirmation of a malignant ovarian tumor, the appropriate serum markers may be useful to monitor the course of the disease.

Virilizing ovarian tumors during pregnancy are most commonly secondary to theca-lutein cysts, and their evaluation and management should be conservative. These benign exaggerated physiologic "tumors" may redevelop with subsequent pregnancies.[82,83]

Postoperative Adjuvant Therapy

Postoperative adjuvant therapy should follow the treatment guidelines for the nonpregnant patient. Though it may be reasonable for patients with low-risk, low-stage tumors to have adjuvant therapy delayed until after delivery, patients with advanced epithelial tumors should receive combination chemotherapy. Until 1995 the standard therapy was a platinum agent and an alkylating agent, which were well tolerated in pregnancy. With the superior effectiveness of the combination of a platinum agent and paclitaxel, these agents offer the patient a better survival. There are few reports that suggests tolerability of this regimen when used in the second and third trimester, including favorable case reports on the treatment of stage III serous ovarian carcinoma with postoperative platinum-based chemotherapy.[85] There also have been a number of favorable treatment outcomes reported in patients who have malignant germ cell tumors and are pregnant.[87]

Young and colleagues reviewed their collective experience with stromal ovarian tumors in pregnancy.[88] One third of the patients presented with tumor rupture. Despite reports of successful use of bleomycin, etoposide, and platinum in pregnancy, the role of adjuvant chemotherapy for stromal tumors is complex and controversial, and consultation with a gynecologic oncologist is recommended.

Vulvar and Vaginal Cancer

Because vulvar and vaginal cancers usually occur after age 40, the diagnosis of either disease concurrent with pregnancy is rare. Fewer than 30 cases of vulvar carcinoma diagnosed and treated during pregnancy have been reported.[85,89]

Vulvar carcinoma in pregnancy is usually stage I or II disease. The diagnosis is based on biopsy, and neither pregnancy nor the young age of a patient should discourage the biopsy of a vulvar mass. Because verrucous squamous carcinoma tends to be misdiagnosed as condyloma, it is important to inform the pathologist of the clinical characteristics of unusually large or aggressive condyloma-like lesions. Surgical management is similar to that used in the nonpregnant patient, with the preference being to perform surgery in the second trimester to avoid the fetal risks of exposure to anesthesia in the first trimester and the maternal risks associated with operating on the hypervascular vulva in the third trimester. If vulvar carcinoma is diagnosed after 36 weeks' gestation, treatment is generally deferred until the postpartum period.[85] The surgical management of vulvar carcinoma is trending to more conservative procedures.[85] Vaginal delivery has been reported following surgical resection of vulvar cancers during pregnancy.[85]

Vaginal carcinoma is less common than vulvar carcinoma. The same limitations apply to vaginal cancer as apply to locally advanced cervical cancer in pregnancy. The cornerstone of treatment is irradiation therapy. Clear cell adenocarcinoma of the vagina has been reported in 16 pregnant patients, and 13 were long-term survivors.[90]

Endometrial Cancer

Approximately 35 cases of endometrial cancer associated with pregnancy have been reported in the literature. Although more than half of these cases were diagnosed in the first trimester, abnormal bleeding later in pregnancy or postpartum may be the presenting symptom of this tumor. Only about 30% of these cases are associated with a viable fetus.[91] Fortunately, a majority of cases of endometrial cancer in pregnancy are diagnosed with stage I disease (88%) and grade 1 tumors (80%). With a thorough evaluation excluding metastatic disease and extensive counseling, these patients may be candidates for conservative treatment with hormonal manipulation, repeat endometrial evaluation, and modifications of risk factors, in order to preserve fertility.[91]

Gastrointestinal Cancers

Upper Gastrointestinal Cancers

The diagnostic delay in detecting pregnancy-related upper gastrointestinal (GI) cancers is often attributable to the frequency and duration of GI symptoms in pregnancy. In the United States, stomach cancer is rarely diagnosed in women during the reproductive years. During pregnancy, persistent severe upper GI symptoms are best evaluated by gastroduodenoscopy rather than radiologic studies. Because curative resection of localized stomach cancer is possible in only approximately 30% of patients, it is imperative that treatment not be delayed.

Malignant hepatic tumors are rare during the reproductive years. Hepatocellular tumors detected during pregnancy should be resected, because the maternal and fetal mortality associated with subcapsular hemorrhage and liver rupture during pregnancy is high. Elevated steroid levels may predispose the tumor to rupture during pregnancy. There is no increase in the vascularity of the liver during pregnancy. In patients with unresectable hepatomas, therapeutic abortion can be considered to decrease the risk of subsequent rupture and bleeding.

Colon and Rectal Cancer

The incidence of colon cancer during pregnancy is about 1 in 13,000 live-born deliveries.[92] Colorectal carcinoma is usually found in women beyond childbearing age, with only 8% of patients diagnosed before age 40.

Because pregnancy is often accompanied by constipation and exacerbations of hemorrhoids and anal fissures, the symptoms of colorectal carcinoma, namely, rectal bleeding, constipation, pain, and backache, tend to be attributed to the pregnancy, and diagnostic delay is common. **The majority of colorectal carcinomas during pregnancy are rectal and palpable on rectal examination, in contrast to more proximal lesions found in the nonpregnant patient (Table 47-6).**[92] Patients with unexplained hypochromic microcytic anemia should be evaluated with stool guaiac testing. If a colorectal lesion is suspected, endoscopic methods of evaluation are preferred to radiologic imaging studies. Unfortunately, most cases of colorectal cancer are not diagnosed until late pregnancy or at the time of delivery. Delays in diagnosis are probably responsible for a higher likelihood of advanced-stage colorectal cancer in pregnancy and an associated poor prognosis. The hormonal effect of pregnancy on tumor development is unknown. A report by Woods and colleagues suggests that colorectal carcinoma in pregnancy adversely affects the pregnancy.[92] Only 78% of their cases resulted in healthy live-born infants.

TABLE 47-6 DISTRIBUTION OF COLON AND RECTAL CARCINOMAS IN NONPREGNANT AND PREGNANT POPULATIONS

PATIENT GROUP	TOTAL	COLON	RECTUM
General population	1704	1244 (73%)	460 (27%)
Age under 40 years	186	127 (68%)	59 (32%)
Pregnant	244	41 (17%)	203 (83%)

From Medich DS, Fazio VW: Hemorrhoids, anal fissure, and carcinoma of the colon, rectum, and anus during pregnancy. Surg Clin North Am 75:77, 1995.

Management of colon cancer is determined by gestational age at diagnosis and tumor stage. During the first half of pregnancy, colon resection with anastomosis is indicated for colon or appendiceal cancers.[93] Abdominoperineal resection or low anterior resection has been accomplished up to 20 weeks' gestation without disturbing the gravid uterus. In some cases, access to the rectum may not be possible without a hysterectomy or uterine evacuation.

In late pregnancy, a diverting colostomy may be necessary to relieve a colonic obstruction and allow the development of fetal maturity before instituting definitive therapy. Some patients with a diagnosis after 20 weeks may opt to continue the pregnancy to fetal viability. Vaginal delivery is planned unless the tumor is obstructing the pelvis or is located on the anterior rectum. If cesarean delivery is performed, tumor resection can be accomplished immediately. Neoadjuvant chemotherapy or radiation therapy for colorectal carcinoma in the pregnant patient has not demonstrated sufficient response to risk fetal exposure.

There are two reports of pregnant patients with metastatic colorectal cancer treated with combination chemotherapy.[94] Both received FOLFOX6 (oxaliplatin, 5-FU, leucovorin). After diagnosis at 20 and 23 weeks' gestation, they were treated and delivered at 33 and 31 weeks, respectively. Normal development was reported at 1 and 3 years.

In one report, the stage-specific survival rates for pregnant patients with rectal cancer were 83%, 27%, and 0% for stages B, C, and D, respectively.[95] The corresponding survival rates for the same stages of colon cancer were 75%, 33%, and 0%. No Dukes' A classification rectal or colon cancer was reported, consistent with the frequency of diagnostic delays.[95]

Urinary Tract Cancers

Fewer than 50 cases of renal cell carcinoma and fewer than 10 cases of bladder cancer have been reported during pregnancy. Urethral carcinoma during pregnancy is also rare.

The hallmark of urinary tract cancers is hematuria. The initial evaluation of hematuria in pregnancy should be urethrocystoscopy, urinary cytology, and renal ultrasonography. The primary therapy for renal cell carcinoma is surgery, and the survival rate for localized disease may exceed 50%. Although preoperative arterial embolization may facilitate surgery on hypervascular tumors, improved survival rates have not been conclusively demonstrated. Adjuvant radiotherapy or chemotherapy tends to have minimal impact on long-term outcomes.

Transitional carcinoma of the bladder can be managed by local fulguration or resection if it is well differentiated and superficial. Less-differentiated, deeply invasive, and recurrent tumors may require a partial or complete cystectomy. Treatment of urethral carcinoma varies with the size and location. Distal urethral tumors are usually treated with excision and interstitial brachytherapy implants.

CENTRAL NERVOUS SYSTEM TUMORS

The spectrum of CNS tumors found in pregnant patients is similar to that of the nonpregnant patient. In pregnancy, 32% of brain tumors are gliomas, 29% meningiomas, 15% acoustic neuromas, and the other 24% are divided among other more rare subtypes. Spinal tumors account for only one eighth of the central nervous system tumors. Vertebral hemangiomas comprise 61% of the spinal tumors and 18% of meningiomas. Unfortunately, the presenting symptoms of headache and nausea and vomiting are often attributed to normal complaints of pregnancy, and delays in diagnosis result. Meningiomas, pituitary adenomas, acoustic neuromas, and vertebral hemangiomas may demonstrate rapid enlargement during pregnancy. This may be secondary to fluid retention, increase in blood volume, or hormonal stimulation. MRI is the preferred imaging technique used to diagnose intracranial neoplasms.

Because painful contractions and pushing increase intracranial pressure, it is recommended that labor be as pain free as possible, and the second stage of labor should be assisted with forceps to reduce the risk of herniation. The anesthetic management of labor and delivery for patients with intracranial neoplasms has been reviewed by Finfer.[95]

Whereas high-grade glial tumors should undergo prompt diagnosis and treatment, low-grade glial tumors such as astrocytomas and oligodendrogliomas do not usually require immediate intervention. Adjuvant cranial radiotherapy with abdominal shielding should be considered for patients with high-grade tumors. Adjuvant chemotherapy is not usually effective and, therefore, should probably be delayed until after delivery. A single series of six patients with malignant gliomas treated during pregnancy has been reported.[96] Three patients received procarbazine, lomustine, and vincristine, and three received temozolomide; all were unintentionally exposed during the first 4 weeks of pregnancy. Chemotherapy was stopped in all cases, and all patients delivered without immediate or remote fetal adverse events.

Successful surgical removal of a variety of CNS tumors has been reported.[95,96] Corticosteroids are recommended to reduce the surrounding edema of intracranial masses.

Bromocriptine may be used during pregnancy if a prolactin-secreting adenoma enlarges, causing symptoms. The safety of this medication is supported by a report of no adverse fetal effects in more than 1400 pregnancies following first-trimester exposure.

MISCELLANEOUS TUMORS

Similar to the management for small cell neuroendocrine tumors of the cervix,[80] neuroendocrine tumors or neuroblastomas of other primary sites tend to demonstrate excellent response to surgery or chemotherapy. Pheochromocytoma during pregnancy is rare and may mimic hypertensive disorders of pregnancy (see Chapter 41).

FETAL-PLACENTAL METASTASIS

Metastatic spread of a maternal primary tumor to the placenta or fetus is rare. In general, the biologically aggressive spectrum of malignancies seem to carry the highest risk for fetal metastases. One review identified 45 cases of placental metastases and seven cases of fetal metastases.[97] **Malignant melanoma is the most frequently reported tumor metastatic to the placenta.** Hematologic malignancies are the second most common tumor to spread to the placenta. Placental and fetal dissemination of lymphomas, leukemias, lung cancer, and CNS tumors have been reported.[97,98] Choriocarcinoma metastatic to a fetus usually results in death within a few months of age.[99] Therefore, in pregnant women with a concurrent malignancy, in addition to notifying the neonatology service, a thorough visual and histologic inspection of the placenta is recommended to assess for metastatic disease.[99]

GESTATIONAL TROPHOBLASTIC DISEASE AND PREGNANCY-RELATED ISSUES

It is uncommon for a normal viable pregnancy to be complicated by gestational trophoblastic disease (GTD). A comprehensive summary of the evaluation and management of the complete spectrum of GTD is beyond the scope of this chapter. However, the aspects of GTD related to the general obstetric and postpartum care are reviewed.

Hydatidiform Mole (Complete Mole)

The incidence of hydatidiform mole has great geographic variability. In the United States it occurs in approximately 1 in 1000 to 1 in 1500 pregnancies. The two clinical risk factors that carry the highest risk of a molar pregnancy are (1) the extremes of the reproductive years (age 50 or older carries a relative risk of over 500) and (2) the history of a prior hydatidiform mole (the risk for development of a second molar pregnancy is 1% to 2%, and the risk of a third after two is approximately 25%).[100,101] Patients with these risk factors should have an ultrasound evaluation of uterine contents in the first trimester. Although historically approximately 50% of patients were not diagnosed with a molar pregnancy before vaginal expulsion of molar tissue, currently in developed countries, most patients are diagnosed either by ultrasound while asymptomatic or by ultrasound for the evaluation of vaginal spotting or cramping

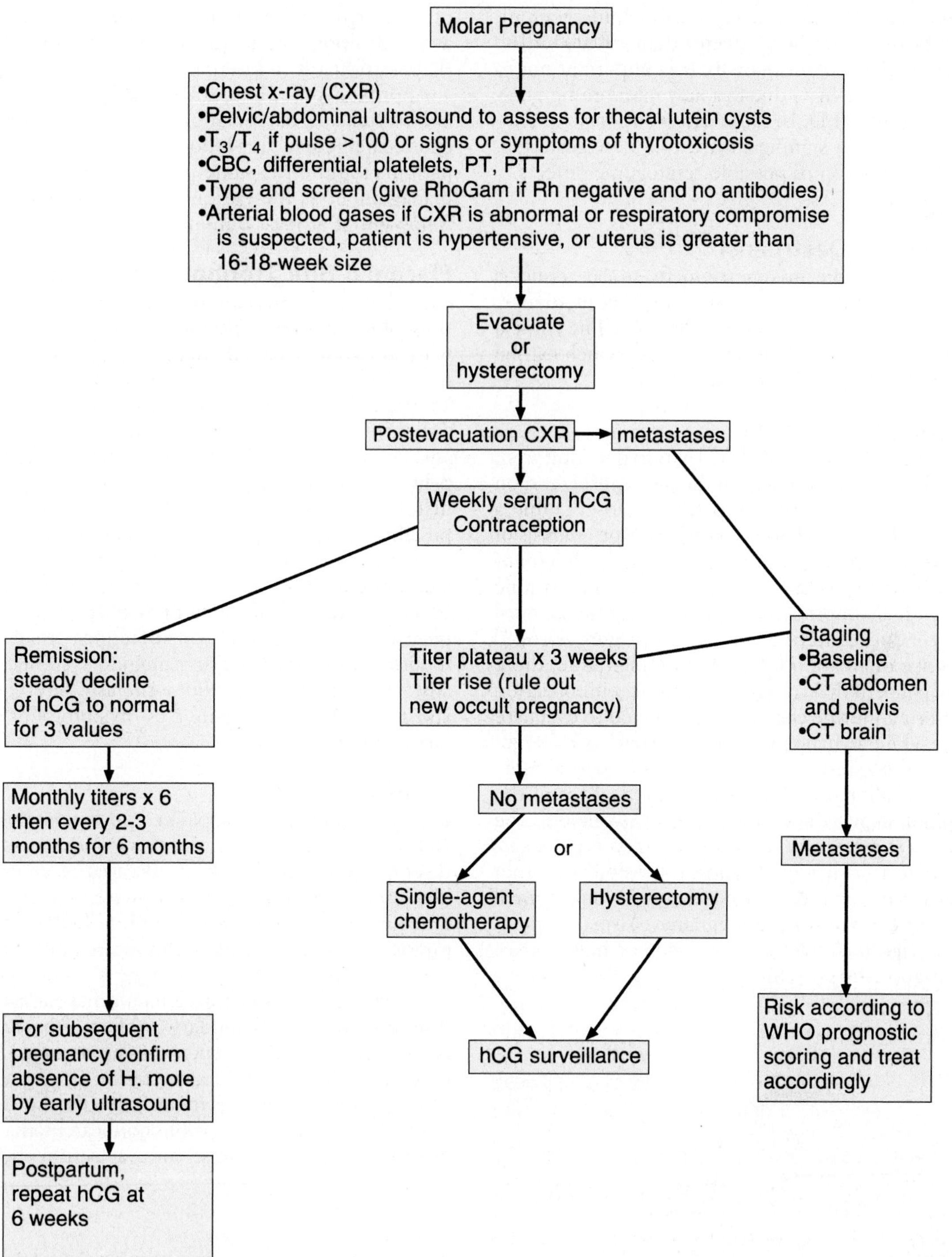

FIGURE 47-5. Algorithm for the management of molar pregnancy. (From Copeland LJ: Gestational trophoblastic neoplasia. *In* Copeland LJ [ed]: Textbook of Gynecology, ed 2. Philadelphia, WB Saunders, 2000, p 1414.)

symptoms. Approximately 95% of complete hydatidiform moles have a 46,XX paternal homologous chromosomal pattern.

The safest technique of evacuating a hydatidiform mole is with the suction aspiration technique. Oxytocin should not be initiated until the patient is in the operating room and evacuation is imminent in order to minimize the risk of embolization of trophoblastic tissue. The alternative management for the elderly patient who requests concurrent sterilization is hysterectomy. Following either evacuation or hysterectomy, weekly β-hCG is drawn until the hCG titer is within normal limits for 3 weeks. The titers are then observed at monthly intervals for 6 to 12 months. Figure 47-5 illustrates an algorithm for molar pregnancy management.[102]

For the patient with a complete molar pregnancy, the risk of requiring chemotherapy for persistent GTD is approximately 20%. Clinical features that increase this risk include delayed hemorrhage, excessive uterine enlargement, theca-lutein cysts, serum hCG greater than 100,000 mIU/mL, and maternal age older than 40. It is important not to misinterpret a rising β-hCG due to a new intervening pregnancy as persistent GTD, because intervention with chemotherapy would be a significant risk to a new gestation, inducing either abortion or possible teratogenic defects.

Invasive Mole (Chorioadenoma Destruens)

Because invasion of the myometrium by molar tissue is clinically occult, it is difficult to assess the true incidence, and it is estimated to be between 5% and 10%. The clinical hallmark of an invasive mole is hemorrhage, which can be severe, and either vaginal or intraperitoneal.

Partial Hydatidiform Mole

Most partial moles have a triploid (paternally inherited, diandric, triploidies) karyotype, and the next most common are tetraploidies. A minority of partial moles exhibit a mosaic or partially diploid karyotype. Karyotype analysis of the accompanying fetus is important in planning therapeutic intervention. A partial mole associated with a nonviable fetal chromosomal abnormality requires either mechanical or medically induced uterine evacuation (Figure 47-6).[102] In the presence of an abundance of hydropic tissue, there is always the concern that trophoblastic tissue embolization may occur during uterine contractions induced to evacuate molar tissue. The management of a patient with sonographic findings suggestive of a diagnosis of a partial mole is particularly challenging if the karyotype analysis of the fetus is diploid, especially if the diagnosis is made in the second or third trimester. When a normal karyotype exists, it is appropriate to consider diagnostic possibilities other than partial mole, such as a twin gestation—one normal developing fetus and one molar pregnancy. Also, degenerative changes (hydropic villi), retroplacental hematomas, placental abnormalities (chorioangiomas), degenerative uterine myomas, and aborted tissue, sometimes referred to as a "transitional mole," may lead to imaging abnormalities that are difficult to interpret.

Approximately 2% to 6% of patients develop persistent GTD after a partial molar pregnancy.[103] Therefore, because choriocarcinoma can follow a true partial mole, these patients require the same postevacuation surveillance and management as the patient with a complete mole, with a follow-up of at least 6 months.[104]

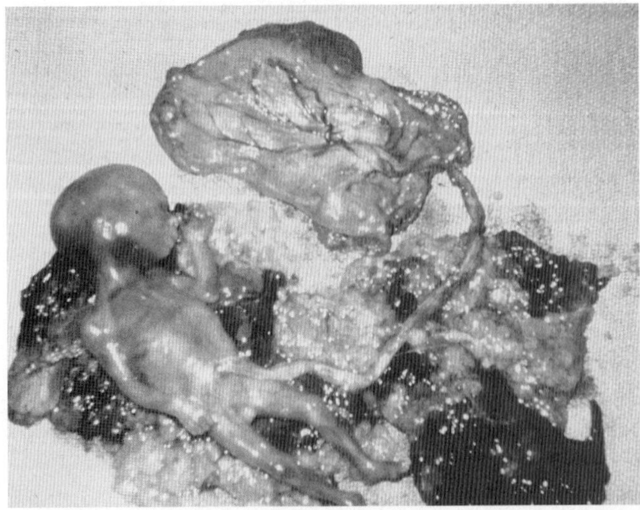

FIGURE 47-6. Partial mole with dead fetus of abnormal karyotype. (From Copeland LJ: Gestational trophoblastic neoplasia. *In* Copeland LJ [ed]: Textbook of Gynecology, ed 2. Philadelphia, WB Saunders, 2000, p 1416.)

Placental Site Trophoblastic Tumor

Less than 1% of all patients with GTD have placental site trophoblastic tumor. Although this tumor usually presents with abnormal vaginal bleeding following a term pregnancy, it can also be a sequela to a molar pregnancy or abortion. The postpartum presentation is characterized by a slightly enlarged uterus, persistent bleeding or, occasionally, amenorrhea, and a slightly elevated β-hCG level. **The β-hCG may not reliably reflect disease progression.** The histologic diagnosis may be obtained by uterine curettage, possibly hysteroscopically directed. Because this disease tends to metastasize late and be somewhat resistant to chemotherapy, surgical excision (hysterectomy) should be considered. If the patient is desirous of future childbearing, management considerations that have been reported with some success include systemic chemotherapy, regional infusion chemotherapy, uterine curettage, and local excision of tumor by hysterotomy and uterine reconstruction.[105]

Choriocarcinoma

Choriocarcinoma develops in approximately 1 in every 40,000 term pregnancies, and this clinical presentation represents about one fourth of all cases of choriocarcinoma. The other cases follow molar disease or an abortion (spontaneous, therapeutic, or ectopic). GTD following a term pregnancy is always either choriocarcinoma or a placental site trophoblastic tumor, assuming a singleton pregnancy.

Choriocarcinoma is notorious for masquerading as other diseases. This is secondary to hemorrhagic metastases producing symptoms such as hematuria, hemoptysis, hematemesis, hematochezia, stroke, or vaginal bleeding. The common sites for metastatic disease are listed in Table 47-7. The diagnosis of choriocarcinoma is based on history, imaging studies, and a serum β-hCG level.

TABLE 47-7 COMMON SITES FOR METASTATIC CHORIOCARCINOMA*

SITE	PERCENT
Lung	60-95
Vagina	40-50
Vulva/cervix	10-15
Brain	5-15
Liver	5-15
Kidney	0-5
Spleen	0-5
Gastrointestinal	0-5

From Copeland LJ: Gestational trophoblastic neoplasia. *In* Copeland LJ (ed): Textbook of Gynecology, ed 2. Philadelphia, WB Saunders, 2000, p 1391.

*Frequencies vary, depending on whether data are based on autopsy studies or are obtained from pretreatment imaging.

Histologic confirmation is neither necessary for the diagnosis nor a prerequisite to initiate therapy. Again, it is necessary to exclude the presence of a new gestation as the source of a rising β-hCG level before extensive diagnostic imaging or therapeutic intervention. **It is also important to rule out phantom β-hCG production if the clinical scenario warrants, such as situations with low titers and no histologic or convincing imaging evidence of GTD.**

The complexities of the general treatment approach or treatment for special situations is beyond the scope of this chapter. It is recommended that the reader refer to a gynecology or gynecologic oncology resource for discussions of the therapeutic subtleties and pitfalls. Choriocarcinoma should be managed by a gynecologic oncologist, preferably one with a special interest in the disease.

KEY POINTS

- Because many of the common complaints of pregnancy are also early symptoms of metastatic cancer, pregnant women with cancer are at risk for delays in diagnosis and therapeutic intervention.
- The safest interval for most cancer therapies in pregnancy is the second and third trimesters, thereby avoiding induction of teratogenic risks or miscarriage in the first trimester. For most malignancies diagnosed during the second trimester, chemotherapy should be undertaken as indicated because fetal risk is generally lower than the risk of delaying treatment or proceeding with preterm delivery.
- Antimetabolites and alkylating agents present the greatest hazard to the developing fetus.
- Diagnostic delays of breast cancer in pregnancy are often attributed to physician reluctance to properly evaluate breast complaints or abnormal findings in pregnancy.
- Treatment for Hodgkin's disease may compromise the reproductive potential, and combined treatment with irradiation and chemotherapy provides the highest risk of ovarian failure.
- If a mother is exposed to cytotoxic drugs within 1 month of delivery, the newborn should be monitored closely for evidence of granulocytopenia or thrombocytopenia.
- The effect of pregnancy on the clinical course of melanoma has been the subject of debate. When corrected for tumor thickness, pregnancy does not appear to be an independent prognostic variable for survival.
- After stratifying for stage and age, patients with pregnancy-associated cervical carcinoma have survival rates similar to the nonpregnant patient.
- Because most malignant ovarian tumors found in pregnancy are either germ cell tumors or low-grade, early-stage epithelial tumors, the therapeutic plan will usually permit continuation of the pregnancy and preservation of fertility.
- Although rare, most colorectal carcinomas in pregnancy are detectable on rectal examination, underscoring the need for a rectal examination at the patient's first prenatal visit.
- Phantom β-hCG should be ruled out in patients suspected of having gestational trophoblastic disease when not documented by other clear clinical evidence (histology, imaging, and clinical history), especially when β-hCG titers are low.

REFERENCES

1. Pentheroudakis G, Orecchia R, Hoekstra HJ, Pavlidis N: Cancer, fertility and pregnancy: ESMO clinical practice guidelines for diagnosis, treatment and follow-up. Ann Oncol 21:V226, 2010.
2. Pavlidis NA: Coexistence of pregnancy and malignancy. The Oncologist 7:279, 2002.
3. Doll DC, Ringenberg QS, Yarbro JW: Antineoplastic agents and pregnancy. Semin Oncol 16:337, 1989.
4. Briggs GG, Freeman RK, Yaffe SJ: Drugs in pregnancy and lactation: a reference guide to fetal and neonatal risk, 8th ed. Philadelphia, Lippincott, Williams & Wilkins, 2008.
5. Van Calseteren K, Hyens L, De Smet F, et al. Cancer during pregnancy: ana analysis of 215 patients emphasizing the obstetrical and the neonatal outcomes. J Clin Oncol 28:683, 2009.
6. Zemlickis D, Lishner M, Degendorfer P, et al: Fetal outcome after in utero exposure to cancer chemotherapy. Arch Intern Med 152:573, 1992.
7. Aviles A, Diaz-Maqueo JC, Talavera A, et al: Growth and development of children and mothers treated with chemotherapy during pregnancy: current status of 43 children. Am J Hematol 36:243, 1991.
8. Cardonick E, Iacobucci A: Use of chemotherapy during human pregnancy. Lancet Oncol 5:283, 2004.
9. Weisz B, Meirow D, Schiff E, Lishner M: Impact and treatment of cancer during pregnancy. Exper Rev Anticancer Ther 4:889, 2004.
10. Schardein JL: Cancer chemotherapeutic agents. In Schardein JL: Chemically Induced Birth Defects, 2nd ed. New York, Marcel Dekker, 1993.
11. Roboz J, Gleichner N, Wu K, et al: Does doxorubicin cross the placenta? Lancet 2:2691, 1979.
12. Mulvihill JJ, Stewart KR: A registry of pregnancies exposed to chemotherapeutic agents. Teratology 33:80, 1986.
13. Mazze RI, Kallen B: Reproductive outcome after anesthesia and operation during pregnancy: a registry study of 5405 cases. Am J Obstet Gynecol 161:1178, 1989.
14. Aisner J, Weirnik PH, Pearl P: Pregnancy outcome in patients treated for Hodgkin's disease. J Clin Oncol 11:507, 1993.
15. Clark ST, Radford JA, Crowther D, et al: Gonadal function following chemotherapy for Hodgkin disease: a comparative study of MVPP and a seven-drug hybrid regimen. J Clin Oncol 13:134, 1995.
16. Plante M, Renaud MC, Francoid H, Roy M: Vaginal radical trachelectomy: an oncologically safe fertility-preserving surgery. An updated series of 72 cases and review of the literature. Gynecol Oncol 94:614, 2004.
17. Jemal A, Siegel R, Xu J, Ward E: Cancer statistics, 2010. CA Cancer J Clin 60:277, 2010.
18. Ring A: Breast cancer and pregnancy. Breast 16:S155, 2007.
19. Michels KB, Willett WC, Rosner BA, et al: Prospective assessment of breastfeeding and breast cancer incidence among 89,877 women. Lancet 347:431, 1996.
20. Jernstrom H, Lerman C, Ghadirian P, et al: Pregnancy and risk of early breast cancer in carriers of BRCA1 and BRCA2. Lancet 354:1846, 1999.
21. Amant F, Deckers S, Van Calsteren K, et al: Breast cancer in pregnancy: recommendations of an international consensus meeting. Eur J Cancer doi:10.10/j.ejca.2010.09.010, 2010.
22. Pereg D, Koren G, Lishner M: Cancer in pregnancy: gaps, challenges and solutions. Cancer Treat Rev 34:302, 2008.
23. Zemlickis D, Lishner M, Degendorfer P, et al: Maternal and fetal outcomes after breast cancer in pregnancy. Am J Obstet Gynecol 166:781, 1992.

24. Gentilini O, Cremonesi M, Trifiro G, et al: Safety of sentinel node biopsy in pregnant patients with breast cancer. Ann Oncol 15:1348, 2004.
25. Botsis D, Sarandakou A, Kassanos D, et al: Breast cancer markers during normal pregnancy. Anticancer Res 19:3539, 1999.
26. Kuerer HM, Gwyn K, Ames FC, et al: Conservative surgery and chemotherapy for breast carcinoma during pregnancy. Surgery 131:108, 2002.
27. Nettleton J, Long J, Kuban D, et al: Breast cancer during pregnancy: quantifying the risk of treatment delay. Obstet Gynecol 87:414, 1996.
28. van der Vange N, van Donegan JA: Breast cancer and pregnancy. Eur J Surg Oncol 17:1, 1991.
29. Ring AE, Smith IE, Jones A, et al: Chemotherapy for breast cancer during pregnancy: 18-year experience from five London teaching hospitals. J Clin Oncol 23:4192, 2005.
30. White TT, White WC: Breast cancer and pregnancy: report of 49 cases followed five years. Ann Surg 144:384, 1956.
31. Holleb AI, Farrow JH: The relationship of carcinoma of the breast and pregnancy in 283 patients. Surg Gynecol Obstet 115:65, 1962.
32. Byrd BF Jr, Bayer DS, Robertson JC, Stephenson SE: Treatment of breast tumors associated with pregnancy and lactation. Ann Surg 155:940, 1962.
33. Applewhite RR, Smith LR, DiVincenti F: Carcinoma of the breast associated with pregnancy and lactation. Ann Surg 39:101, 1973.
34. Riberio GG, Palmer MK: Breast carcinoma associated with pregnancy: a clinician's dilemma. BMJ 2:1524, 1977.
35. Clark RM, Reid J: Carcinoma of the breast in pregnancy and lactation. Int Radiat Oncol Biol Phys 4:693, 1978.
36. King RM, Welch JS, Martin JK Jr, Coul CB: Carcinoma of the breast associated with pregnancy. Surg Gynecol Obstet 160:228, 1985.
37. Petrek JA, Dukoff R, Rogatko A: Prognosis of pregnancy-associated breast cancer. Cancer 67:869, 1991.
38. Mueller BA, Simon MS, Deapen D, et al: Childbearing and survival after breast carcinoma in young women. Cancer 98:1131, 2003.
39. Blakely LJ, Buzdar AU, Lozada JA, et al: Effects of pregnancy after treatment for breast carcinoma on survival and risk of recurrence. Cancer 100:465, 2004.
40. Velentgas P, Daling JR, Malone KE, et al: Pregnancy after breast carcinoma: outcomes and influence on mortality. Cancer 85:2424, 1999.
41. Partridge A, Schapira L: Pregnancy and breast cancer: epidemiology, treatment, and safety issues. Oncology 19:693, 2005.
42. Sutton R, Buzdar AU, Hortobagyi GN: Pregnancy and offspring after adjuvant chemotherapy in breast cancer patients. Cancer 71:2499, 1990.
43. Higgins S, Haffty B: Pregnancy and lactation after breast-conserving therapy for early-stage breast cancer. Cancer 73:2175, 1994.
44. Miller MJ, Ross ME: Case report: pregnancy following breast reconstruction with autologous tissue. Cancer Bull 45:546, 1993.
45. Gelb AB, van de Rijn M, Warnke RA: Pregnancy-associated lymphomas. A clinicopathologic study. Cancer 78:304, 1996.
46. Thomas PRM, Peckham MJ: The investigation and management of Hodgkin's disease in the pregnant patient. Cancer 38:1443, 1976.
47. Jacobs C, Donaldson SS, Rosenberg SA, Kaplan HS: Management of the pregnant patient with Hodgkin's disease. Ann Intern Med 95:649, 1981.
48. Friedman E, Jones GW: Fetal outcome after maternal radiation treatment of supradiaphragmatic Hodgkin's disease. Can Med Assoc J 149:1281, 1993.
49. Connors JM: State-of-the-art therapeutics: Hodgkin's lymphoma. J Clin Oncol 23:6400, 2005.
50. Azim HA, Pavlidis N, Peccatori FA: Treatment of the pregnant mother with cancer: a systematic review on the use of cytotoxic, endocrine, targeted agents and immunotherapy during pregnancy. Part II: Hematological tumors. Cancer Treat Rev 36:110, 2010.
51. Dein RA, Mennuti MT, Kovach P, Gabbe SG: The reproductive potential of young men and women with Hodgkin's disease. Obstet Gynecol Surv 39:474, 1984.
52. Ortin TT, Shostak CA, Donaldson SS: Gonadal status and reproductive function following treatment for Hodgkin's disease in childhood: the Stanford experience. Int J Radiat Oncol Biol Phys 19:873, 1990.
53. Janov AJ, Anderson J, Cella DF, et al: Pregnancy outcome in survivors of advanced Hodgkin's disease. Cancer 70:688, 1992.
54. Aviles A, Neri N: Hematological malignancies and pregnancy: a final report of 84 children who received chemotherapy in utero. Clin Lymphoma 2:173, 2001.
55. Ward FT, Weiss RB: Lymphoma and pregnancy. Semin Oncol 16:397, 1989.
56. Manns A, Blattner WA: The epidemiology of the human T-cell lymphotropic virus type I and type II: etiologic role in human disease. Transfusion 31:67, 1991.
57. Caligiuri MA, Mayer RJ: Pregnancy and leukemia. Semin Oncol 16:338, 1989.
58. Hoelzer D, Thiel E, Loffler H, et al: Prognostic factors in a multicenter study for treatment of acute lymphoblastic leukemia in adults. Blood 71:123, 1988.
59. Antonelli NM, Dotters DJ, Katz VL, Kuller JA: Cancer in pregnancy: a review of the literature. Part II. Obstet Gynecol Surv 51:135, 1996.
60. Aviles A, Niz J: Long-term follow-up of children born to mothers with acute leukemia during pregnancy. Med Pediatr Oncol 16:3, 1988.
61. AML Collaborative Group: A systematic collaborative overview of randomized trials comparing idarubicin with daunorubicin (or other anthracyclines) as induction therapy for acute myeloid leukaemia. Br J Haematol 103:100, 1998.
62. Bazarbashi MS, Smith MR, Karanes C, et al: Successful management of Ph chromosome chronic myelogenous leukemia with leukapheresis during pregnancy. Am J Hematol 38:235, 1991.
63. Cohen MH, Johnson JR, Pazdur R: U.S. Food and Drug Administration Approval Summary: conversion of imatinib mesylate (STI571; Gleevec) tablets from accelerated approval to full approval. Clin Cancer Res 11:12, 2005.
64. Pye SM, Cortes J, Ault P, et al: The effects of imatinib on pregnancy outcome. Blood 111:5505, 2008.
65. Stensheim H, Møller B, van Dijk T, et al: Cause-specific survival for women diagnosed with cancer during pregnancy or lactation: a registry-based cohort study. J Clin Oncol 27:45, 2009.
66. Houghton AN, Flannery J, Viola MV: Malignant melanoma of the skin occurring during pregnancy. Cancer 48:407, 1981.
67. MacKie RM, Bufalino R, Morabito A, et al: Lack of effect on pregnancy outcome of melanoma. Lancet 337:653, 1991.
68. Slingluff CL Jr, Reintgen D, Vollmer RT, et al: Malignant melanoma arising during pregnancy: a study of 100 patients. Ann Surg 211:552, 1990.
69. Travers R, Sober A, Barnhill R, et al: Increased thickness of pregnancy-associated melanoma: a study of the MGH pigmented lesion clinic. Melanoma Res 3:44, 1993.
70. Lederman JS, Sober AJ: Effect of prior pregnancy on melanoma survival. Arch Dermatol 121:716, 1985.
71. Ross MI: Melanoma and pregnancy: prognostic and therapeutic considerations. Cancer Bull 46:412, 1994.
72. Lederman JS, Lew RA, Koh HK, Sober AJ: Influence of estrogen administration on tumor characteristics and survival in women with cutaneous melanoma. J Natl Cancer Inst 74:981, 1985.
73. Economos K, Perez Veridiano N, Delke I, et al: Abnormal cervical cytology in pregnancy: a 17-year experience. Obstet Gynecol 81:915, 1993.
74. Hannigan EV: Cervical cancer in pregnancy. Clin Obstet Gynecol 33:837, 1990.
75. Copeland LJ, Silva EG, Gershenson DM, et al: Superficially invasive squamous cell carcinoma of the cervix. Gynecol Oncol 45:307, 1992.
76. Sorosky JI, Squatrito R, Ndubisi BU, et al: Stage I squamous cell cervical carcinoma in pregnancy: planned delay in therapy awaiting fetal maturity. Gynecol Oncol 59:207, 1995.
77. Sood AK, Sorosky JL, Krogman S, et al: Surgical management of cervical cancer complicating pregnancy: a case-control study. Gynecol Oncol 63:294, 1996.
78. Greer BE, Easterling TR, McLennan DA, et al: Fetal and maternal considerations in the management of stage IB cervical during pregnancy. Gynecol Oncol 34:61, 1989.
79. Amant F, Van Calsteren K, Halaska M, et al: Gynecologic cancers in pregnancy: guidelines of an international consensus meeting. Int J Gynecol Cancer 19:S1, 2009.
80. Balderston KD, Tewari K, Gregory WT, et al: Neuroendocrine small cell cervix cancer in pregnancy: long-term survivor following combined therapy. Gynecol Oncol 71:128, 1998.

81. Cliby WA, Dodson WA, Podratz KC: Cervical cancer complicated by pregnancy: episiotomy site recurrences following vaginal delivery. Obstet Gynecol 84:179, 1994.
82. Leiserowitz GS, Xing G, Cress R, et al: Adnexal masses in pregnancy: how often are they malignant. Gynecol Oncol 101:315, 2006.
83. Schwartz N, Timor-Tritsch IE, Wang E. Adnexal masses in pregnancy. Clin Obstet and Gynecol 52:570, 2009.
84. Katz VL, Watson WJ, Hansen WF, et al: Massive ovarian tumor complicating pregnancy: a case report. J Reprod Med 38:907, 1993.
85. Latimer J: Gynaecological malignancies in pregnancy. Curr Opin Obstet Gynecol 19:140, 2007.
86. Kobayashi F, Sagawa N, Nakamura K, et al: Mechanism and clinical significance of elevated CA 125 levels in the sera of pregnant women. Am J Obstet Gynecol 160:563, 1989.
87. Horbelt D, Delmore J, Meisel R, et al: Mixed germ cell malignancy of the ovary concurrent with pregnancy. Obstet Gynecol 84:662, 1994.
88. Young RH, Dudley AG, Scully RE: Granulosa cell, Sertoli-Leydig cell and unclassified sex-cord stromal tumors associated with pregnancy: a clinical pathological analysis of 36 cases. Gynecol Oncol 18:181, 1984.
89. Bakour SH, Jaleel H, Weaver JB, et al: Vulvar carcinoma presenting during pregnancy, associated with recurrent bone marrow hypoplasia: a case report and literature review. Gynecol Oncol 87:207, 2002.
90. Senekjian EK, Hubby M, Bell DA, et al: Clear cell adenocarcinoma of the vagina and cervix in association with pregnancy. Gynecol Oncol 24:207, 1986.
91. Yael HK, Lorenza P, Evelina S, et al: Incidental endometrial adenocarcinoma in early pregnancy: a case report and review of the literature. Int J Gynecol Cancer 19:1580, 2009.
92. Woods JB, Martin JN Jr, Ingram FH, et al: Pregnancy complicated by carcinoma of the colon above the rectum. Am J Perinatol 9:102, 1992.
93. Nesbitt JC, Moise KJ, Sawyers JL: Colorectal carcinoma in pregnancy. Arch Surg 120:636, 1985.
94. Gensheimer M, Jones CA, Graves CR, et al: Administration of oxaliplatin to pregnant patients with rectal cancer. Cancer Chemother Pharmacol 63:371, 2009.
95. Finfer SR: Management of labor and delivery in patients with intracranial neoplasms. Br J Anaesth 67:784, 1991.
96. Blumenthal DT, Parreno MG, Batten J, et al: Management of malignant gliomas during pregnancy: a case series. Cancer 113:3349, 2008.
97. Dildy GA III, Moise KJ Jr, Carpenter RJ Jr, et al: Maternal malignancy metastatic to the products of conception: a review. Obstet Gynecol Surv 44:535, 1989.
98. Rothman LA, Cohen CJ, Astarola J: Placental and fetal involvement by maternal malignancy: a report of rectal carcinoma and a review of the literature. Am J Obstet Gynecol 116:1023, 1973.
99. Andreitchouk AE, Takahashi O, Kedama H, et al: Choriocarcinoma in infant and mother: a case report. J Obstet Gynaecol Res 22:585, 1996.
100. Bandy LC, Clarke-Pearson DL, Hammond CB: Malignant potential of gestational trophoblastic disease at the extreme age of reproductive life. Obstet Gynecol 64:395, 1984.
101. Berkowitz RS, Goldstein DP, Bernstein MR, Sablinska B: Subsequent pregnancy outcomes in patients with molar pregnancies and gestational trophoblastic tumors. J Reprod Med 32:680, 1987.
102. Copeland LJ: Gestational trophoblastic neoplasia. In Copeland LJ: Textbook of Gynecology, 2nd ed. Philadelphia, WB Saunders, 2000, p 1414.
103. Rice LW, Berkowitz RS, Lage JM, Goldstein DP: Persistent gestational trophoblastic tumor after partial molar pregnancy. Gynecol Oncol 48:165, 1993.
104. Seckl MH, Fisher RA, Salerno G, et al: Choriocarcinoma and partial hydatidiform moles. Lancet 356:36, 2000.
105. Leiserowitz GS, Webb MJ: Treatment of placental site trophoblastic tumor with hysterotomy and uterine reconstruction. Obstet Gynecol 88:696, 1996.

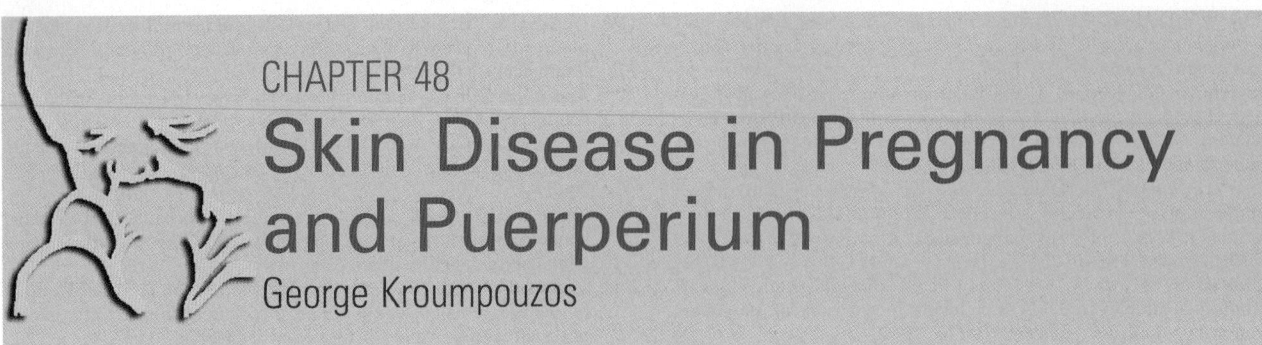

CHAPTER 48

Skin Disease in Pregnancy and Puerperium

George Kroumpouzos

KEY ABBREVIATIONS	
Atopic Dermatitis	AD
Herpes Gestationis	HG
Intrahepatic Cholestasis of Pregnancy	ICP
Pruritic Urticarial Papules and Plaques of Pregnancy	PUPPP
Prurigo of Pregnancy	PP
Pruritic Folliculitis of Pregnancy	PFP
Psoralen with Ultraviolet Light A	PUVA
Ultraviolet Light B	UVB

This chapter reviews both the physiologic skin changes induced by pregnancy and the following categories of skin problems that can occur during pregnancy:

- Preexisting skin diseases and tumors
- Diagnosis and treatment of melanoma
- Pruritus
- Specific dermatoses of pregnancy

Common skin conditions that are discussed in the text are defined (Table 48-1).

PHYSIOLOGIC SKIN CHANGES INDUCED BY PREGNANCY

The human skin undergoes substantial changes during pregnancy induced by the combined effect of endocrine, metabolic, mechanical, and blood flow alterations. **Physiologic changes, while they may prompt cosmetic complaints, are not associated with risks to the mother or fetus and can be expected to resolve or improve postpartum** (Table 48-2).[1-3]

Pigmentary Changes

Mild forms of localized or generalized hyperpigmentation occur to some extent in up to 90% of pregnant women and are most noticeable in the areolae, nipples, genital skin, axillae and inner thighs. Familiar examples include the darkening of the *linea alba (linea nigra)* and periareolar skin. Melasma *(chloasma or "mask of pregnancy")* refers to the facial hyperpigmentation reported in up to 70% of pregnant women.[2] Hyperpigmented, symmetric, poorly demarcated patches are commonly seen on the malar areas (malar pattern) and are often distributed over the entire central face (centrofacial pattern) (Figure 48-1). In 16% of cases, hyperpigmentation occurs on the ramus of the mandible (mandibular pattern).[4,5] Melasma results from melanin deposition in the epidermis (70%), dermal macrophages (10 to 15%), or both (20%). It is likely secondary to the hormonal changes of gestation with increased expression of alpha-melanocyte-stimulating hormone. Melasma typically is exacerbated by exposure to ultraviolet and visible light.[5,6] Hyperpigmentation is often more pronounced in brunettes and women with more melanocytes than in women with lighter baseline skin tone; the use of a broad-spectrum sunscreen with high sun protection factor during pregnancy may decrease the severity of hyperpigmentation.

Melasma usually resolves postpartum but may recur in subsequent pregnancies or with the use of oral contraceptives.[4] Troublesome persistent melasma can be treated postpartum with topical hydroquinone 2% to 4% and sunscreen, with or without a topical retinoid and mild topical steroid.[7] Despite treatment postpartum melasma persists in approximately 30% of patients, especially in women with the dermal or mixed subtypes in which the deeper level of pigmentation results in decreased efficacy of topical agents. Combination therapies including laser treatment[8,9] and chemical peels[10] may be effective in resistant cases. There have been no reports of adverse fetal

TABLE 48-1 COMMON SKIN CHANGES AND DISEASES WITH BRIEF DESCRIPTIONS

Pseudoacanthosis nigricans	Hyperpigmentation of the skin folds and neck mimicking acanthosis nigricans
Dermal melanocytosis	Clusters of melanocytes abnormally located in the dermis and resulting in ill-defined bluish-gray patches
Vulvar melanosis	Irregularly distributed patches of pigmentation on the vulva
Verrucous areolar hyperpigmentation	Pigmented wartlike papules on the areolae
Miliaria	Sweat retention reflecting obstruction of eccrine sweat ducts
Hyperhidrosis	Skin disorder characterized by increased sweat secretion
Dyshidrosis	Recurrent vesicular eruption of palms and soles
Fox-Fordyce disease	Chronic pruritic disorder of the apocrine glands characterized by blockage of the apocrine duct and sweat retention
Onycholysis	Detachment of nail plate from nail bed
Subungual hyperkeratosis	Deposition of keratinous material on the distal nail beds
Palmoplantar pompholyx eczema	See dyshidrosis above (synonyms)
Acne conglobata	Variant of acne vulgaris characterized by severe eruptive nodulocystic lesions without systemic manifestations
Pemphigus vulgaris	Autoimmune bullous disorder of the skin and oral mucosa produced by antidesmoglein-3 antibodies that cause intraepidermal acantholysis
Pemphigus vegetans	Variant of pemphigus vulgaris characterized by pustules that form fungoid vegetations or papillomatous proliferations
Pemphigus foliaceus	Autoimmune bullous skin disorder produced by antidesmoglein-3 antibodies that cause subcorneal acantholysis
Spitz nevi	Seen predominantly in children or young adults and characterized by prominent epithelioid and/or spindled melanocytes that can have atypical features

effects from laser skin treatment during pregnancy. Most laser experts agree that laser radiation does not penetrate through the skin into deeper soft tissues and, therefore, should not affect the fetus or the placenta. Still, because of potential liability issues, most dermatologists and plastic surgeons prefer not to perform laser procedures during gestation.

Uncommon pigmentary patterns, such as pseudoacanthosis nigricans,[11] dermal melanocytosis, vulvar melanosis and verrucous areolar hyperpigmentation can also be seen in pregnancy (see Table 48-2).[12] Postinflammatory hyperpigmentation secondary to specific dermatoses of pregnancy (see section "Specific Dermatoses of Pregnancy") is also common in women with more highly pigmented skin types.

Vascular Changes

As a result of the combination of rising estrogen levels and increased blood volume in pregnancy, blood flow to the skin increases (4 to 16 times in the first 2 months of

TABLE 48-2 PHYSIOLOGIC SKIN CHANGES IN PREGNANCY

Pigmentary
Common
Hyperpigmentation
Melasma
Uncommon
Jaundice
Pseudoacanthotic changes
Dermal melanocytosis
Verrucous areolar pigmentation
Vulvar melanosis
Hair Cycle and Growth
Hirsutism
Postpartum telogen effluvium
Postpartum male-pattern alopecia
Diffuse hair thinning (late pregnancy)
Nail
Subungual hyperkeratosis
Distal onycholysis
Transverse grooving
Brittleness and softening
Glandular
Increased eccrine function
Increased sebaceous function
Decreased apocrine function
Connective Tissue
Striae
Skin tags *(molluscum fibrosum gravidarum)*
Vascular
Spider telangiectasias
Pyogenic granuloma *(granuloma gravidarum)*
Palmar erythema
Nonpitting edema
Severe labial edema
Varicosities
Vasomotor instability
Gingival hyperemia
Hemorrhoids
Mucous Membrane
Gingivitis
Jacquemier-Chadwick sign
Goodell sign

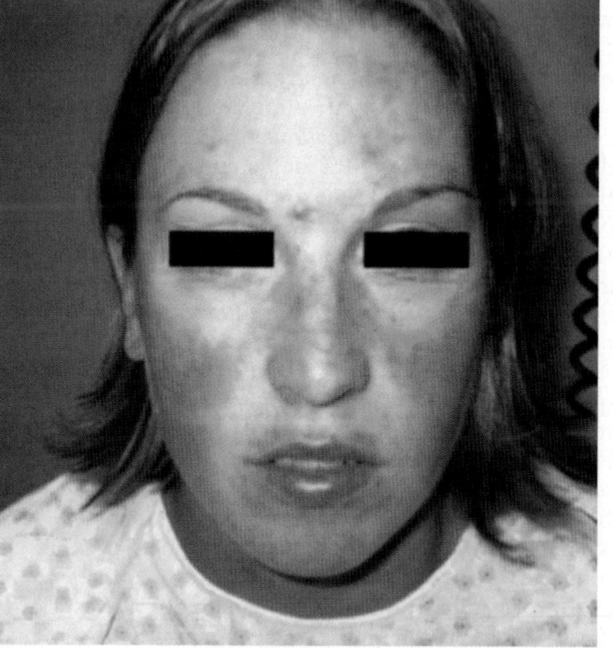

FIGURE 48-1. Centrofacial type of melasma involving the cheeks, nose, upper lip, and forehead.

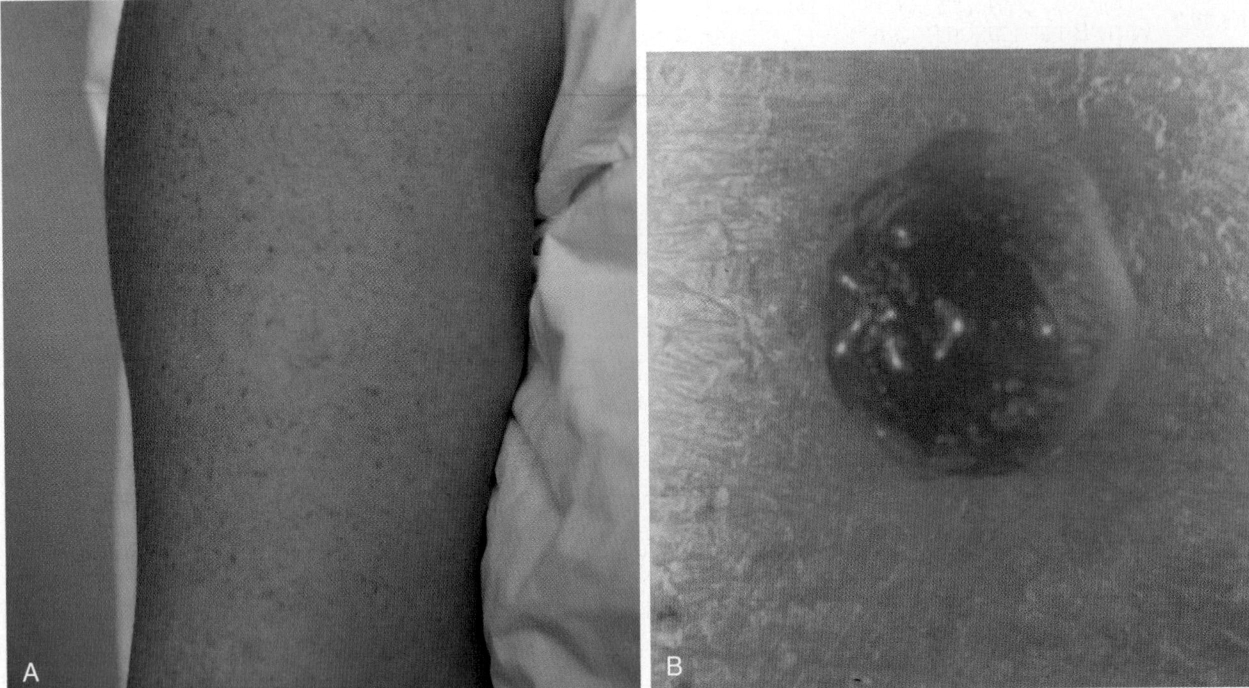

FIGURE 48-2. **A,** Numerous telangiectasias and spider angiomas on the arm of a pregnant female. **B,** Pyogenic granuloma of pregnancy *(granuloma gravidarum)*, a benign vascular proliferation, is typically seen as a nodule on the gingivae and is shown here at a less common extramucosal site.

pregnancy and doubles again during the third month) resulting in significant vascular sequelae (see Table 48-2). Spider nevi (spider angiomas) and telangiectasias develop in approximately two thirds of Caucasian women and 10% of African American women between the second and fifth months of pregnancy, and usually resolve within 3 months postpartum[1,4] (Figure 48-2*A*). Approximately 10% of women have persistent spider nevi; treatment with electrodessication or pulsed dye laser is effective in women who find these cosmetically troubling.

Palmar erythema, likely secondary to capillary engorgement, is also very common, occurring in up to 70% of Caucasian and 30% of African American women. While varicosities of the distal leg veins and hemorrhodial veins develop in more than 40% of women, thrombosis within these superficial varicosities occurs infrequently (<10%). Nonpitting edema can be seen on the ankles (70%) and face (50%) and is most pronounced in the early months of gestation. Varicosities may regress postpartum but usually not completely; varicosities are likely to recur in subsequent pregnancies.

Gum hyperemia and gingivitis are common and frequently result in mild bleeding from the gums during routine oral hygiene. This is most prominent during the third trimester and resolves postpartum. Good dental hygiene will minimize symptoms. Periodontal disease has been associated with adverse pregnancy outcomes and so women without a recent dental examination should be referred.[13]

The pyogenic granuloma of pregnancy (*granuloma gravidarum* or pregnancy epulis) is a benign proliferation of capillaries that usually occurs in the gingiva but can occasionally be identified on the lip or extramucosal sites (Figure 48-2*B*). Pyogenic granulomas commonly appear between the second and fifth months of pregnancy and affect up to 2% of pregnancies.[4] Presenting as a vascular, deep-red or purple, exuberant, often pedunculated nodule between the teeth or on the buccal or lingual surface of the marginal gingival, a pyogenic granuloma may be more likely after mucosal trauma. Spontaneous shrinkage of the tumor usually occurs postpartum, and most cases do not require treatment. Surgical excision or electrosurgical destruction should be reserved for cases complicated by excessive bleeding or severe discomfort.

Connective Tissue Changes

***Striae gravidarum* (*striae distensae* or "stretch marks") develop in up to 90% of Caucasians between the sixth and seventh months of gestation** and less commonly in Asians and African Americans.[4] Risk factors include younger maternal age, excessive pregnancy weight gain, and concomitant use of corticosteroids; however genetic susceptibility likely plays a key role. Striae are most prominent on the abdomen, breasts, buttocks, groin and axillae; while usually asymptomatic, a proportion of patients complain of mild to moderate pruritus. The treatment of striae gravidarum is a challenge; at present there is no optimal treatment. The erythema (red color) of early striae responds well to various pulsed-dye lasers or intense pulsed light. The red color tends to become pale over time (with or without treatment), but the atrophic lines never disappear completely and do not respond to laser treatment. Topical tretinoin 0.1% cream has been shown to improve the appearance of the striae (decreased their length by 20%) and is occasionally used in combination with topical glycolic acid (up to 20%) in an effort to increase elastin content of the affected areas.[14] Nevertheless, tretinoin can be very irritating to the skin and does not make striae completely disappear. No topical therapy prevents or affects the course of striae. They are less apparent postpartum but may never disappear.

Skin tags *(molluscum fibrosum gravidarum)* present as 1- to 5-mm fleshy, pedunculated, exophytic growths on the neck, axillae, inframammary region or groin, and usually appear during the later months of gestation. Treatment can be postponed until completion of the pregnancy as lesions may regress postpartum. Cryotherapy with liquid nitrogen or shave removal is effective for persistent or enlarging lesions. Skin tags do not have malignant potential, and treatment is unnecessary unless inflammation or ulceration develops.

Glandular Changes

Increased eccrine function has been reported during pregnancy and may account for the increased prevalence of miliaria, hyperhidrosis, and dyshidrosis.[4,12] **Conversely, apocrine activity may decrease** during gestation contributing to the decreased prevalence of Fox-Fordyce disease and possibly hidradenitis suppurativa in pregnancy.[2] Changes in sebaceous function are variable, and the effects of pregnancy on acne vulgaris are unpredictable. Treatment for acne vulgaris during pregnancy is discussed below. During pregnancy, the sebaceous glands on the areolae enlarge *(Montgomery's glands or tubercles)*.

Hair and Nail Changes

Most pregnant women develop mild hirsutism affecting their face, trunk and extremities that commonly regresses within 6 months postpartum. In addition, **postpartum hair shedding *(telogen effluvium)* may be noted as a greater proportion of hairs enter the telogen phase,** and this can cause distress (Figure 48-3). The severity of *telogen effluvium* varies considerably, and the hair loss becomes noticeable when more than 40% to 50% of hairs become affected. Recovery is spontaneous, and there are no effective treatments. Patients can be counseled that hair thinning usually resolves within 1 to 5 months but that complete resolution may occasionally take up to 15 months.[1,4] Frontoparietal hair recession and diffuse hair thinning in the later months of pregnancy have been noted in some women. Nail changes can be seen as early as the first trimester of gestation. These changes include brittleness, onycholysis, subungual hyperkeratosis, and transverse grooving. There is no specific treatment for nail changes during pregnancy, and most are expected to resolve postpartum. An attempt should be made to eliminate external sensitizers, such as nail polish removers, and infections. The nails should be kept short if they are brittle or prone to onycholysis.[6]

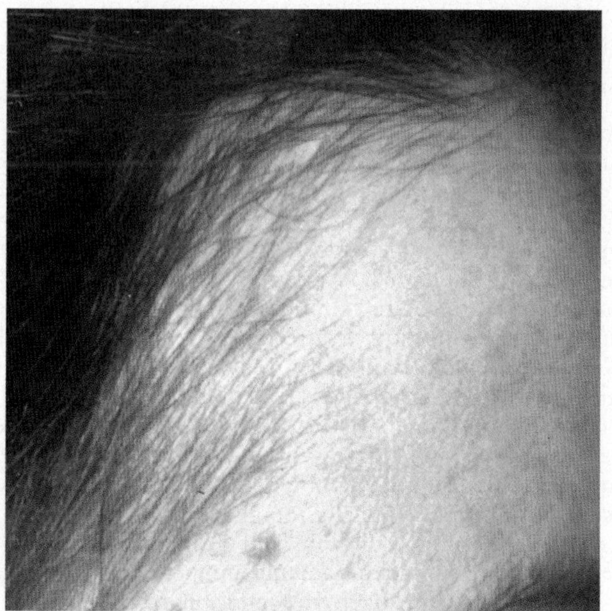

FIGURE 48-3. *Telogen effluvium* that develops within 5 months postpartum typically presents with temporal recession and hair thinning.

PREEXISTING SKIN DISEASES AND TUMORS AFFECTED BY PREGNANCY

Pregnancy can aggravate or, less often, improve many skin conditions and primary skin tumors.[15] Diseases that may improve during pregnancy include atopic eczema, acne, some subtypes of psoriasis, Fox-Fordyce disease, hidradenitis suppurativa, linear IgA dermatosis, sarcoidosis and autoimmune progesterone dermatitis (see Table 48-1).

Atopic Eczema and Dermatitis

Atopic dermatitis (AD) (atopic eczema) is a very common skin condition and is often exacerbated by pregnancy, although remission has been noted in up to 24% of cases.[16] Two large studies, using diagnostic criteria established in pediatric populations, indicated a high prevalence of AD in gestation, including "new AD" (AD presenting during gestation for the first time); however, the true prevalence may be revised as the criteria for gestational AD are refined.[16-20] Risk factors include a history of prior atopy (27%), family history of atopy (50%), and offspring with infantile AD (19%). Other risk factors for AD include African American or Asian race and tobacco use.[21,22] The prevalence of intrinsic ("nonallergic") versus extrinsic (IgE-associated) type of AD[23] during gestation is unknown, although a small study showed that intrinsic AD that is more affected by pregnancy.[24]

Most patients present with lesions in the flexural surfaces of the extremities, occasionally with concomitant lesions on the trunk. Less common presentations are palmoplantar pompholyx eczema, follicular and facial eczema. Eczematous lesions can develop bacterial or viral (i.e. *eczema herpeticum* secondary to herpes simplex virus) superinfection in pregnancy; treatment with dicloxacillin or a first-generation cephalosporin should be used as necessary in these cases. *Eczema herpeticum* should be promptly treated with intravenous acyclovir in order to minimize maternal and fetal risks.

AD is not associated with an increased risk of adverse fetal outcomes. The effects of breastfeeding and maternal food antigen avoidance during pregnancy on AD in the offspring are controversial. Treatment for gestational exacerbations of AD is primarily symptomatic. Using a moisturizer and low- to mid-potent topical steroid is the first-line treatment. Systemic antihistamines, such as chlorpheniramine or diphenhydramine, can also be used as necessary for relief of pruritus. A short course of oral steroids may be required for severe AD. Ultraviolet light B (UVB) is a safe second-line treatment for eczema in pregnancy. There is less experience with the newer topical immunomodulators (pimecrolimus, tacrolimus).[25] Although their bioavailability is limited (<5%) and no pattern of anomalies has been reported after exposure to these drugs in utero, several infants have had neonatal hyperkalemia.[26] Therefore, these immunomodulators should be used as third-line treatment for refractory AD that has not responded to UVB. If systemic agents are needed for refractory AD, cyclosporine is the safest option.

The course of gestational AD in the postpartum period has not been studied. Irritant hand dermatitis and nipple eczema are often seen postpartum.[1] Irritant hand dermatitis is treated with emollients and hand protection. Nipple eczema can evolve into painful fissures and be complicated with bacterial superinfection, most commonly with *Staphylococcus aureus*. Superinfected nipple eczema should be treated with a topical steroid combined with a topical or systemic antibiotic.

Acne Vulgaris

The effects of pregnancy on acne vulgaris are unpredictable. **In one study, pregnancy affected acne in approximately 70% of women, with 41% reporting improvement and 29% worsening with pregnancy.**[27] Two patients had improvement and exacerbations with two different pregnancies. Some patients may develop acne for the first time during pregnancy or in the postpartum period ("postgestational acne"). Comedonal acne should be treated with topical keratolytic agents, such as benzoyl peroxide, whereas inflammatory acne should be treated with azelaic acid, topical erythromycin, topical clindamycin, or oral erythromycin base. Although first trimester use of topical tretinoin has not been associated with an increased rate of malformations in controlled studies, the number of reported exposures is too small to exclude a small increased risk. A theoretical concern remains as the percutaneous absorption is 5 to 30% and use of tretinoin is not recommended during pregnancy (see Chapter 8).

Other Inflammatory Skin Conditions

Recurrent flares of urticaria may worsen in pregnancy. Of interest, these flares show common features with hereditary angioedema and may have been exacerbated in the past by oral contraceptive use or prior to menses. Chronic plaque psoriasis may develop for the first time during pregnancy. **Women with existing chronic psoriasis can be counseled that between 40% and 63% of women have symptomatic improvement, compared to only 14% of women with symptomatic deterioration**; postpartum flares are common (80%).[28] Topical steroids and topical calcipotriene are relatively safe treatment options for localized psoriasis in pregnancy.[29] For severe psoriasis that has not responded to topical medications, UVB and/or a short course of cyclosporine are considered second-line treatment options.

Autoimmune Progesterone Dermatitis

Autoimmune progesterone dermatitis is caused by hypersensitivity to progesterone through autoimmune or nonimmune mechanisms. Although this rare dermatosis can take various forms (urticarial, papular, vesicular or pustular) the hallmark is recurrent cyclic lesions that usually appear during the luteal phase of the menstrual cycle. Limited information is available regarding the effects of pregnancy on autoimmune progesterone dermatitis. Case series report instances of both improvement and exacerbation.[30] Increased cortisol levels and/or the gradual increase in the sex hormone levels during pregnancy with subsequent hormonal desensitization in some patients are both possible mechanisms for observed improvement. Diagnosis is based on either an immediate local urticarial reaction or more frequently a delayed hypersensitivity reaction following intradermal challenge with synthetic progesterone. Intramuscular administration of progesterone should be avoided in these patients as it has been associated with angioedema. Circulating antibodies to progesterone or the *corpus luteum* have been detected by indirect immunofluorescence in several patients. The sensitivity of this test seems to be lower than that of the intradermal progesterone challenge; therefore, these antibodies are not widely used to confirm this diagnosis. No specific therapy for the condition during pregnancy has been proposed. Autoimmune estrogen dermatitis has also been reported in a patient presenting with urticaria in early pregnancy.[31]

Impetigo Herpetiformis

Impetigo herpetiformis is a rare variant of generalized pustular psoriasis that develops primarily during pregnancy, often in association with hypocalcemia[32] **or low serum levels of vitamin D.**[33] Although familial occurrence has been reported, more commonly a personal or family history of psoriasis is absent. The eruption usually develops in the third trimester but can also start in earlier trimesters and postpartum. While the overwhelming majority of cases resolve postpartum, persistent cases have been reported, and can be associated with oral contraceptive use.[34] Various infections during pregnancy may also trigger a flare of pustular psoriasis in a genetically predisposed individual.[35]

Impetigo herpetiformis is characterized by numerous grouped discrete sterile pustules at the periphery of erythematous patches (Figure 48-4*A*). Lesions typically originate in the major flexures (axillae, inframammary areas, groin, and gluteal fold) and progress onto the trunk, usually sparing the face, hands, and feet. Painful mucosal erosions may also develop. Onycholysis or complete nail shedding secondary to subungual lesions has been reported. Constitutional symptoms are common including fever, malaise, diarrhea, and vomiting with resultant dehydration. Rarely patients develop complications secondary to hypocalcemia including tetany, convulsions, and delirium. Common laboratory findings are leukocytosis and elevated erythrocyte sedimentation rate; rarer perturbations include hypocalcemia, decreased serum vitamin D levels, and signs of hypoparathyroidism. Historically reported maternal risks, such as tetany, seizures, delirium, and death from cardiac or renal failure or septicemia are uncommon. Fetal risks, such as stillbirth, neonatal birth, and fetal abnormalities secondary to placental insufficiency,[33] have been reported even when the condition was well controlled.[36] While maternal

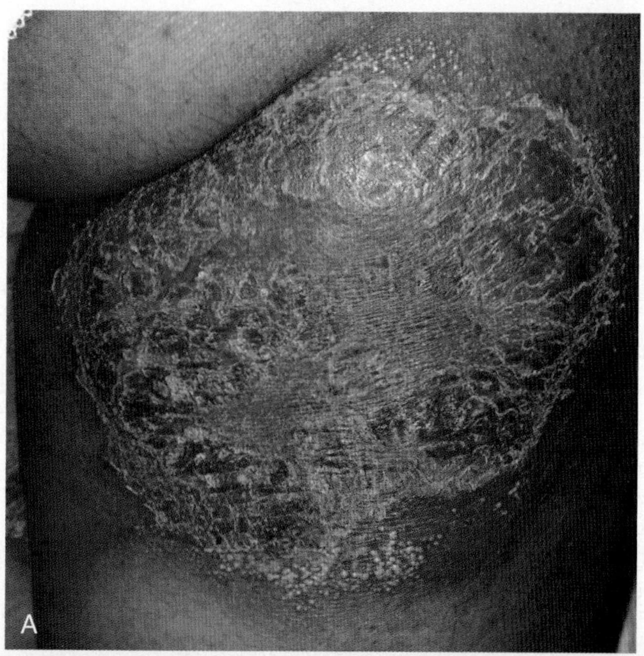

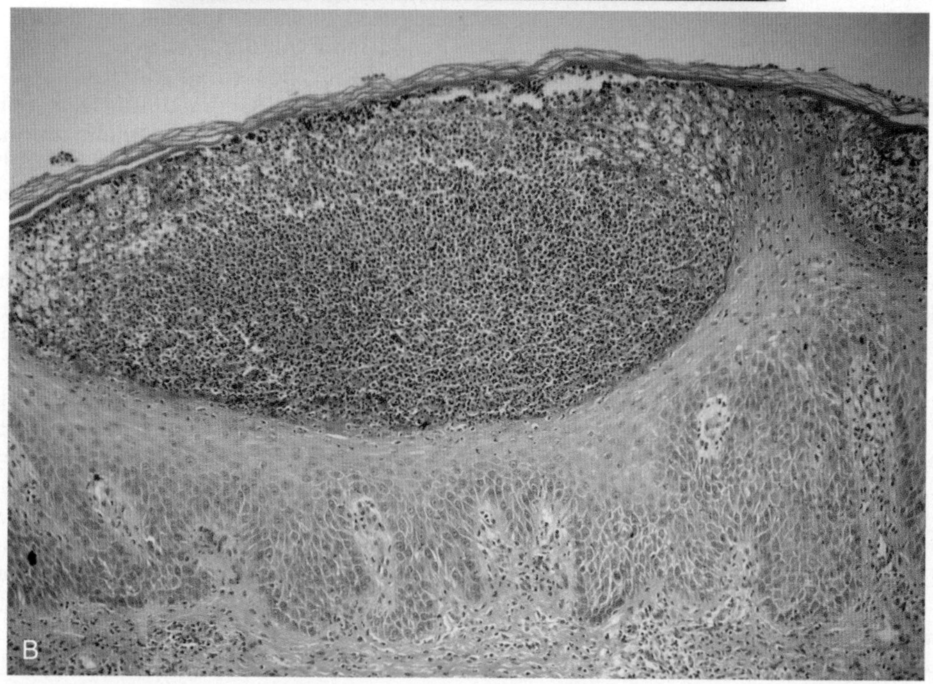

FIGURE 48-4. **A,** Impetigo herpetiformis: discrete grouped sterile pustules at the periphery of an erythematous crusted plaque. **B,** Histopathology of impetigo herpetiformis shows the characteristic spongiform pustule of Kogoj, which is formed of neutrophils in the uppermost portion of the spinous layer (hematoxylin-eosin stain). (Photograph courtesy Aleksandr Itkin, MD.)

prognosis is excellent with early diagnosis, aggressive treatment, and supportive care, an increased risk of perinatal mortality may persist despite maternal treatment.[37] The risk is difficult to quantify as it is based on sparse case reports that span decades. Intensive fetal monitoring should be considered until the mother is stabilized. After acute treatment the appropriate degree of fetal surveillance is not known, however periodic assessment of fetal well being is likely prudent after viability.

Definite diagnosis of impetigo herpetiformis is based on histopathology that shows typical features of pustular psoriasis (see Figure 48-4*B*). Direct and indirect skin immunofluorescence is negative. Systemic steroids are first-line therapy for impetigo herpetiformis; 20 to 40 mg/day of prednisone is usually effective. Cases of pustular psoriasis exacerbated by pregnancy have been treated with cyclosporine.[37] Calcium and vitamin D replacement therapy should be undertaken if necessary, and can lead to remission of the eruption.[25] Systemic antibiotics should be administered if bacterial superinfection is suspected. Postinflammatory hyperpigmentation may develop, but scarring is usually absent. Impetigo herpetiformis has been treated postpartum with oral steroids, oral retinoids[38] or photochemotherapy (psoralen with ultraviolet light A

[PUVA])[39] as single agents or in combination. Resistant cases can be treated with a combination of PUVA and clofazimine or methotrexate.

Cutaneous Manifestations of Autoimmune Disorders

Cutaneous lesions may be prominent in some individuals affected by autoimmune disorders, and these patients often have questions regarding how pregnancy will affect the appearance of these lesions. The cutaneous manifestations of chronic discoid lupus are not affected by pregnancy. Cutaneous flares of systemic lupus erythematosus can usually be managed with oral steroid treatment. Dermatomyositis/polymyositis may show exacerbation of the characteristic heliotrope rash in approximately half of affected individuals.[40] The cutaneous progression of scleroderma is not significantly altered by pregnancy, and symptoms of Raynaud's phenomenon may improve. Pregnant women with limited skin disease do significantly better than those with diffuse scleroderma.[41] The medical and obstetric management of pregnancies complicated by collagen vascular disease is discussed in detail in Chapter 44.

Bullous Disorders

Bullous dermatologic disorders develop secondary to autoantibodies that target constituents of the skin and/or oral mucosa. **Pemphigus vulgaris,[42] vegetans or foliaceus may develop or worsen during pregnancy** whereas linear IgA disease may improve.[43] In more than 50% of cases of pemphigus vulgaris, lesions may initially appear within the oral cavity. Diffuse skin involvement with multiple flaccid vesicles follows, with confluence of vesicles forming large eroded areas. Skin biopsy with immunofluorescence studies are needed for a definitive diagnosis. Biopsy for routine histopathology and immunofluorescence is indicated in patients with new-onset lesions, most critically to differentiate pemphigus from herpes gestationis (see section IV below). In cases of pemphigus, fetal and neonatal skin lesions can occur secondary to transplacental transfer of IgG antibodies but resolve spontaneously within 2 to 3 weeks after birth. Pemphigus should be treated with oral corticosteroids, and high doses may be required. A recent study of 49 pregnancies complicated by pemphigus vulgaris showed 12% perinatal mortality. Forty-five percent of live neonates had pemphigus lesions at birth.[44] Increased fetal surveillance is prudent in pregnancies affected by active pemphigus, although the effectiveness of this surveillance in preventing morbidity and fetal loss is not known.

Acrodermatitis enteropathica is a rare autosomal recessive disorder of zinc deficiency characterized by dermatitis, diarrhea, and alopecia. Vesiculobullous and/or eczematous skin lesions can develop on the extremities and periorificial sites, such as the mouth, perianal, and genital areas. The disease usually flares early in gestation[45] as serum zinc levels decrease, but may also flare with oral contraceptives.

Skin Tumors

Most skin neoplasms that present or enlarge during pregnancy (pyogenic granuloma, hemangioma, hemangioendothelioma, glomus tumor, glomangioma, dermatofibroma, dermatofibrosarcoma protuberans, leiomyoma, keloid, desmoid tumor and neurofibroma) are benign. **Melanocytic nevi may develop, enlarge or darken during pregnancy but these changes seem to be less dramatic than previously thought.** A mild degree of histopathologic atypia has been reported in a few studies. Pennoyer et al[46] compared photographs of moles taken during the first trimester and again in the third trimester. Only 3% of nevi enlarged during pregnancy, and another 3% regressed. In contrast, dysplastic nevi in women with familial dysplastic nevus syndrome do have a tendency to increase in size and undergo color change during pregnancy.[47] Spitz nevi, another class of common pigmented benign neoplasms, may also increase in size or erupt during pregnancy.[48] Studies that used dermoscopy showed that the pigment network of nevi becomes thicker and more prominent, and the globules darker during pregnancy; these features, however, return to their original condition within 1 year after delivery.[49] Any suspicious pigmented skin lesion should prompt a dermatologic referral. The "ABCDE" clinical criteria for pigmented lesions are helpful in determining which lesions are of higher malignant potential: Asymmetry, Border irregularity, Color variegation, Diameter greater than 6 mm, and Evolution (i.e. an enlarging or otherwise changing lesion).[50] Seborrheic keratoses are also common and may enlarge or darken during gestation. None of these benign lesions require treatment during pregnancy; the pregnant woman should be reassured that these changes are benign and may improve postpartum.

Malignant Melanoma

Malignant melanoma accounts for approximately 8% of malignant tumors during pregnancy with an overall incidence of approximately 2.8 cases per 1000 births.[51] Melanomas that develop during pregnancy are thicker than melanomas in non-pregnant women[52] possibly due to a delayed diagnosis because of a shared misconception by the patient and/or her physician that darkening and changing of a nevus is normal in pregnancy. Despite initial concerns, **several epidemiologic studies evaluating the effect of pregnancy status at diagnosis suggest that the 5-year survival rate is not affected after controlling for confounding factors.**[53-55] In the largest study to date,[55] Lens compared 185 women diagnosed with melanoma during pregnancy with over 5000 women of childbearing age who developed melanoma while not pregnant. Pregnancy status at the time of diagnosis was associated with a hazard ratio for death of 1.08 (95% CI 0.0-1.9). **The major prognostic determinants of survival in pregnant women with localized melanoma are tumor thickness (Breslow scale) and ulceration status,**[56] with level of invasion only significant in women with tumors more than 1 mm in thickness.

Surgery is the treatment of choice in patients presenting with early melanoma in pregnancy.[57] Sentinel lymph node biopsy using a combination of isosulfan blue dye and tenetium should be performed as indicated and is not contraindicated in pregnancy.[58] For pregnant women with advanced disease, the prognosis, risks, and benefits of systemic therapy should be discussed. The decision to administer systemic therapy should be determined based on the gestational age at presentation with consideration given to the potential consequence of delayed treatment on ultimate survival. In early gestation, the option of termination of pregnancy should also be considered. Melanoma is the most common type of malignancy to metastasize to the placenta and fetus, representing 31% of such metastases.[59] However, it should be emphasized that placental and/or fetal metastases are extraordinarily rare (27 cases) and that even in the setting of placental metastasis, fetal metastasis only occurs in 17% of cases. Histologic evaluation of the placenta should be performed because of the association between melanoma and placental metastasis. The presence of placental metastases is associated with widespread disease and dismal maternal survival. The role of systemic therapy in preventing metastases to the placenta and fetus has not been adequately studied.

There are currently no standard guidelines for patients who desire to become pregnant after the diagnosis and treatment of melanoma, although in a recent study pregnancy subsequent to a diagnosis of melanoma was associated with nonsignificant decrease in mortality.[55] Similarly, most studies did not show an increased risk of melanoma recurrence with oral contraceptive or hormone replacement therapy use.[60,61] In most cases, melanoma cell lines lack type I estrogen receptors.[62,63] In contrast, there appears to be some evidence for an inhibitory effect of estrogens on melanoma cell lines through type II estrogen receptors.[61] These findings may indicate a protective effect of female gender on the prognosis of melanoma.[64,65] The primary reason to delay pregnancy following a recent diagnosis of melanoma is the time-dependent risk of tumor recurrence and subsequent maternal mortality. Patients should be counseled on a case-by-case basis depending primarily on risk of recurrence, taking into account the thickness of their original tumor and other prognostic factors. Women with a significant risk of recurrence may want to delay pregnancy until they can be assured of a low recurrence risk. In women with a thin tumor with a low risk of recurrence, no delay may be necessary.

PRURITUS IN PREGNANCY

Itching is the most common dermatologic symptom of pregnancy. Mild pruritus attributed to pregnancy *(pruritus gravidarum)* is common, occurring most frequently over the abdomen. Pruritus has been reported in up to 17% of pregnancies,[66] but a more recent report suggests that significant pruritus requiring a more thorough evaluation occurs in only 1.6% of patients.[67] **A broad differential diagnosis needs to be considered; the constellation of clinical and laboratory findings will help establish a diagnosis and guide management decisions.** Pruritic skin diseases that are not specifically related to pregnancy, such as AD and scabies, should be considered. In cases of pruritus without eruption, systemic diseases are more likely. Intrahepatic cholestasis of pregnancy (ICP) is a common etiology (see Chapter 45 for diagnosis and management); however other conditions such as lymphoma, liver, renal, and thyroid disease should be considered.[12] In the patient with pruritus and skin lesions other than excoriations, referral to a dermatologist for evaluation of a specific dermatosis of pregnancy (see section "Specific Dermatoses of Pregnancy") is appropriate unless a clear etiologic agent for a systemic or topical allergic reaction can be elucidated.

SPECIFIC DERMATOSES OF PREGNANCY

Specific dermatoses of pregnancy refer to a group of skin diseases that are encountered predominantly during or immediately following pregnancy and **include only those skin diseases which result directly from the state of gestation or the products of conception.**[16] Included in this definition are: herpes gestationis (HG), pruritic urticarial papules and plaques of pregnancy (PUPPP), prurigo of pregnancy (PP), and pruritic folliculitis of pregnancy (PFP) (Table 48-3). A recent reclassification[17] that included ICP in the specific dermatoses of pregnancy and grouped AD, PP, and PFP under "atopic eruption of pregnancy" has been debated.[18]

Herpes (Pemphigoid) Gestationis

HG is a rare autoimmune skin disease affecting between 1 in 7,000 and 1 in 50,000 pregnancies.[20] While HG and bullous pemphigoid recognize the same antigen[68] and share certain features, HG is confined to pregnant women or women affected by gestational trophoblastic disease. Some authors[69] have suggested that exposure to paternal antigens may play a critical role in disease initiation but "skip pregnancies" while having the same partner have been reported and would argue against this association. Of interest, expression of the HG antigen in the placenta begins in the midtrimester correlating with the timing of clinical symptoms. The antibody that incites the pathology in HG belongs to the IgG1 subclass and recognizes the NC16A2 (MCW-1) epitope in the noncollagenous domain (NC16A) of the transmembrane 180-kd antigen (bullous pemphigoid antigen 2).[70] HG primarily affects Caucasians with only scattered case reports in African Americans[71]; this observation is consistent with the association between HG and the human leukocyte antigens (HLA) DR3 (61%-80%), DR4 (52%), or both (43%-50%), which are less frequent in the African American population.

Clinically, **HG usually presents in the second or third trimester of pregnancy, with extremely pruritic urticarial lesions that typically begin on the abdomen and trunk, commonly involving the umbilicus** (Figure 48-5*A*). These urticarial plaques rapidly progress to widespread bullous lesions (Figure 48-5*B*) that may affect the palms and soles but rarely the face and mucous membranes. Tense bullous lesions arise in both inflamed and clinically normal skin and usually heal without scarring. Up to 25% of cases can present in the postpartum period, although these may represent recrudescences of previously undiagnosed mild HG. The most important clinical and laboratory features of HG are summarized in Table 48-3.

Although the differential diagnosis of HG includes drug eruption, erythema multiforme and allergic contact dermatitis, the most common diagnosis to exclude is the far more common pruritic papules and plaques of pregnancy (PUPPP, see below). PUPPP can manifest with urticarial and/or vesicular lesions almost indistinguishable from those of HG, although PUPPP classically begins in the abdominal striae and spares the umbilicus. Definitive diagnosis should be based on immunofluorescence of perilesional skin demonstrating the hallmark finding of HG, linear C3 deposition along the basement membrane zone.[1]

TABLE 48-3 OVERVIEW OF SPECIFIC DERMATOSES OF PREGNANCY

	PREVALENCE (UNITED STATES)	CLINICAL DATA	LESION MORPHOLOGY AND DISTRIBUTION	IMPORTANT LABORATORY FINDINGS	FETAL RISKS
Herpes gestationis (HG)	1:50,000	Second or third trimester or postpartum Flare at delivery (75%) Resolution postpartum +++ recurrence in future pregnancies	Abdominal urticarial lesions progress into a generalized bullous eruption	Skin immunofluorescence shows linear deposition of C3 along basement membrane	Neonatal HG Small-for-gestational age infants Preterm delivery
Pruritic urticarial papules and plaques of pregnancy (PUPPP)	1:130 to 1:300	Third trimester or postpartum Primigravidas Resolution postpartum Association with multiple gestation No recurrence in future pregnancies	Polymorphous eruption starts in the abdominal striae and shows periumbilical sparing	None	None
Prurigo of pregnancy (PP)	1:300 to 1:450	Second or third trimester Resolution postpartum + recurrence in future pregnancies	Grouped excoriated papules over the extensor extremities and occasionally abdomen	None	None
Pruritic folliculitis of pregnancy (PFP)	Approximately 30 cases	Second or third trimester Resolution postpartum ± recurrence in future pregnancies	Follicular papules and pustules	Biopsy: sterile folliculitis	None

Modified from Kroumpouzos, G, Cohen LM: Specific dermatoses of pregnancy: an evidence-based systematic review. Am J Obstet Gynecol 18:1083, 2003.

In addition, skin histopathology shows a spongiotic epidermis, marked papillary dermal edema, and an eosinophilic infiltrate. Serum antibody titers with conventional indirect immunofluorescence do not correlate with the course of disease but parallel disease activity when BP-180 NC16A-ELISA was used.[72]

Oral corticosteroids remain the cornerstone of treatment in HG. The majority of patients will respond rapidly to relatively low-dose treatment with prednisone (20 to 40 mg/day). In resistant cases, doses as high as 180 mg/day have been tried. Once new blister formation has been suppressed, prednisone should be tapered to 5 to 10 mg/day. Typically, up to 75% of patients will experience spontaneously resolution or improvement in the late third trimester and steroid treatment can often be discontinued. However, since HG typically flares at delivery or within the days following delivery, steroid doses can be increased in anticipation. A subset of patients will have persistent HG or recurrent flares lasting weeks or months. Patients at risk for prolonged or chronic HG tend to be older with higher parity, more widespread lesions and a history of HG in prior pregnancies.[73] Oral contraceptive use has been implicated in postpartum flares; 20% to 50% of patients using oral contraceptives within 6 months of delivery have associated flares. This association should be considered when counseling patients on their contraceptive options. Breast feeding was associated with a significantly shorter duration of active lesions in one study,[74] but this has been debated. HG recurs in 95% of future pregnancies, and lesions may be more severe, appear earlier in gestation, and persist longer postpartum. Treatment for chronic, recalcitrant HG is generally unsatisfactory, although case reports have described successful treatment with plasmapheresis, immunoapheresis, chemical oophorectomy with goserelin, ritodrine, rituximab, high-dose intravenous immunoglobulin combined with cyclosporine or other immunosuppressant medications, and minocycline or doxycycline combined with nicotinamide, immunosuppressive and anti-inflammatory agents, such as cyclophosphamide, azathioprine, rituximab, pyridoxine, sulfapyridine, gold, methotrexate or dapsone, have been used postpartum in refractory cases with some success but their use is limited to nonlactating patients.[20]

The maternal effects of HG are largely limited to symptomatic pruritus and a small risk of lesion superinfection. An association between HG and Grave's disease has been reported and HG[75] is an indication for performing both immediate and periodic screening tests of thyroid function. **An association with small-for-gestational age infants and preterm delivery has been reported** but the effect of HG on the fetus remains difficult to estimate from the small study cohorts due to the rarity of the disease. The largest cohort to date compared fetal outcome between the affected and unaffected pregnancies of 74 women; a 16% versus 2% rate of delivery at less than 32 weeks complicated pregnancies with active HG.[76] Mild placental insufficiency has been postulated as a mechanism; therefore sonographic evaluation of fetal interval growth and third-trimester fetal surveillance is appropriate. Finally, **approximately 5% to 10% of neonates will manifest bullous skin lesions (neonatal HG) secondary to passive transplacental transfer of HG antibody.**[77] Parents should be reassured that these lesions will resolve spontaneously without scarring over a period of a few weeks as the maternal antibodies clear from the infant's blood. However, parents should be counseled about the signs and symptoms of

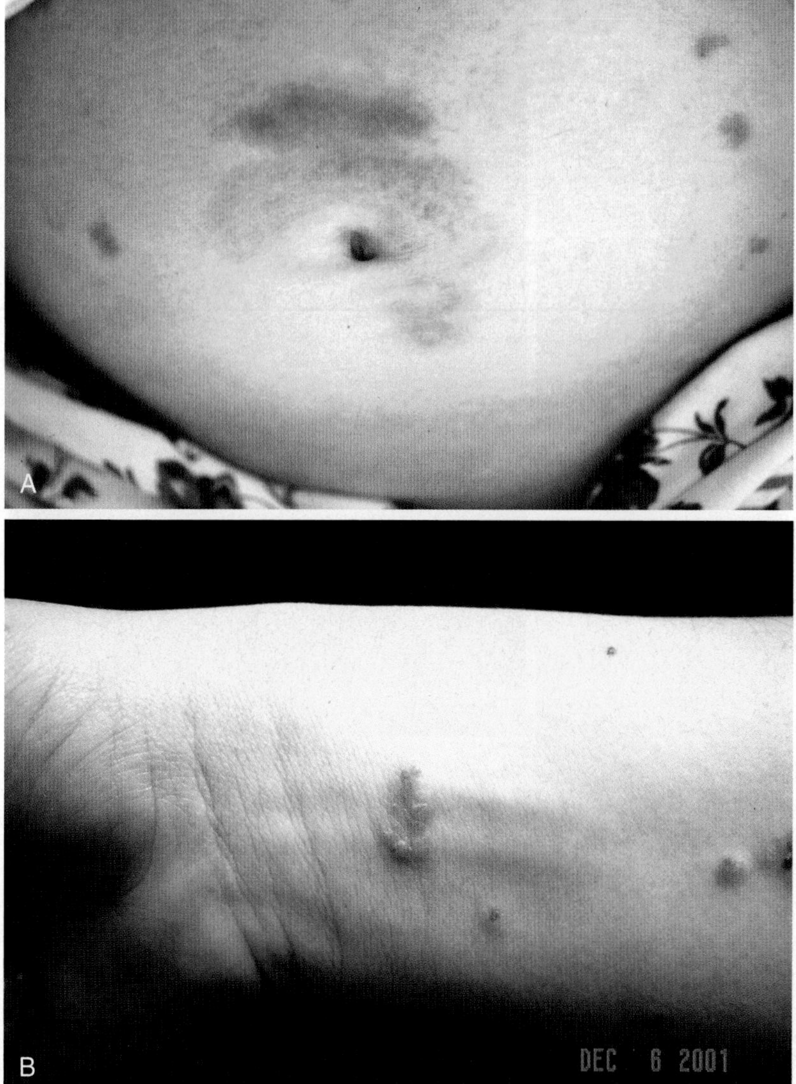

FIGURE 48-5. **A,** Pruritic abdominal urticarial plaques develop in the early phase of herpes gestationis and typically involve the umbilicus. (Photograph courtesy Helen Raynham, MD.) **B,** Characteristic tense vesicles on an erythematous base on the forearm in a patient with herpes gestationis. (Photograph courtesy Jeffrey Callen, MD.) (From Kroumpouzos G, Cohen LM: Skin disease. *In* James DK, Steer PJ, Weiner CP, Gonik B (eds): High-Risk Pregnancy: Management Options, 3rd ed. Philadelphia, Elsevier, 2005.)

bacterial superinfection so that timely treatment can prevent progression to systemic infection.

Pruritic Urticarial Papules and Plaques of Pregnancy

PUPPP, also known as "polymorphic eruption of pregnancy," is the most common specific dermatosis of pregnancy, affecting between 1 in 130 and 1 in 300 pregnancies. It occurs classically in primigravidas in the mid to late third trimester, and has been associated with a slight predominance of male babies (55%).[20,78,79] **Lesions typically begin in the abdominal striae and spare the periumbilical region** (Figure 48-6*A*).[1,80] PUPPP can be difficult to characterize as the eruption is polymorphous and can include urticarial and occasionally vesicular, purpuric, polycyclic or targetoid lesions, reminiscent of erythema multiforme or herpes gestationis (Figure 48-6*B*).[79] Although lesions can spread over the trunk and extremities they usually spare the palms and soles, and involvement of the face is very unusual. Generalized PUPPP may resemble a toxic erythema or atopic dermatitis (Figure 48-6*C*).

Skin histopathology is often nonspecific, showing spongiotic dermatitis with variable numbers of eosinophils. In contrast to HG, immunofluorescence studies and serologic tests are typically negative. IgE elevation (uncontrolled) was reported in 28% of PUPPP cases in a recent study[81] but the significance and specificity of IgE elevations in pregnancy remain unclear.[18] The high prevalence (55%) of personal and/or family history of atopy[81] has not been confirmed by other studies. The pathogenesis of PUPPP has not been established, but the immunohistologic profile (T helper lymphocytes, dermal dendritic cells, and epidermal Langerhans cells)[82] suggests a delayed hypersensitivity reaction to an unknown antigen. Some authors have proposed that rapid abdominal wall distention in primigravidas may trigger an inflammatory process; this has been supported by the association between PUPPP and multiple-gestation pregnancy, excess maternal weight gain, and

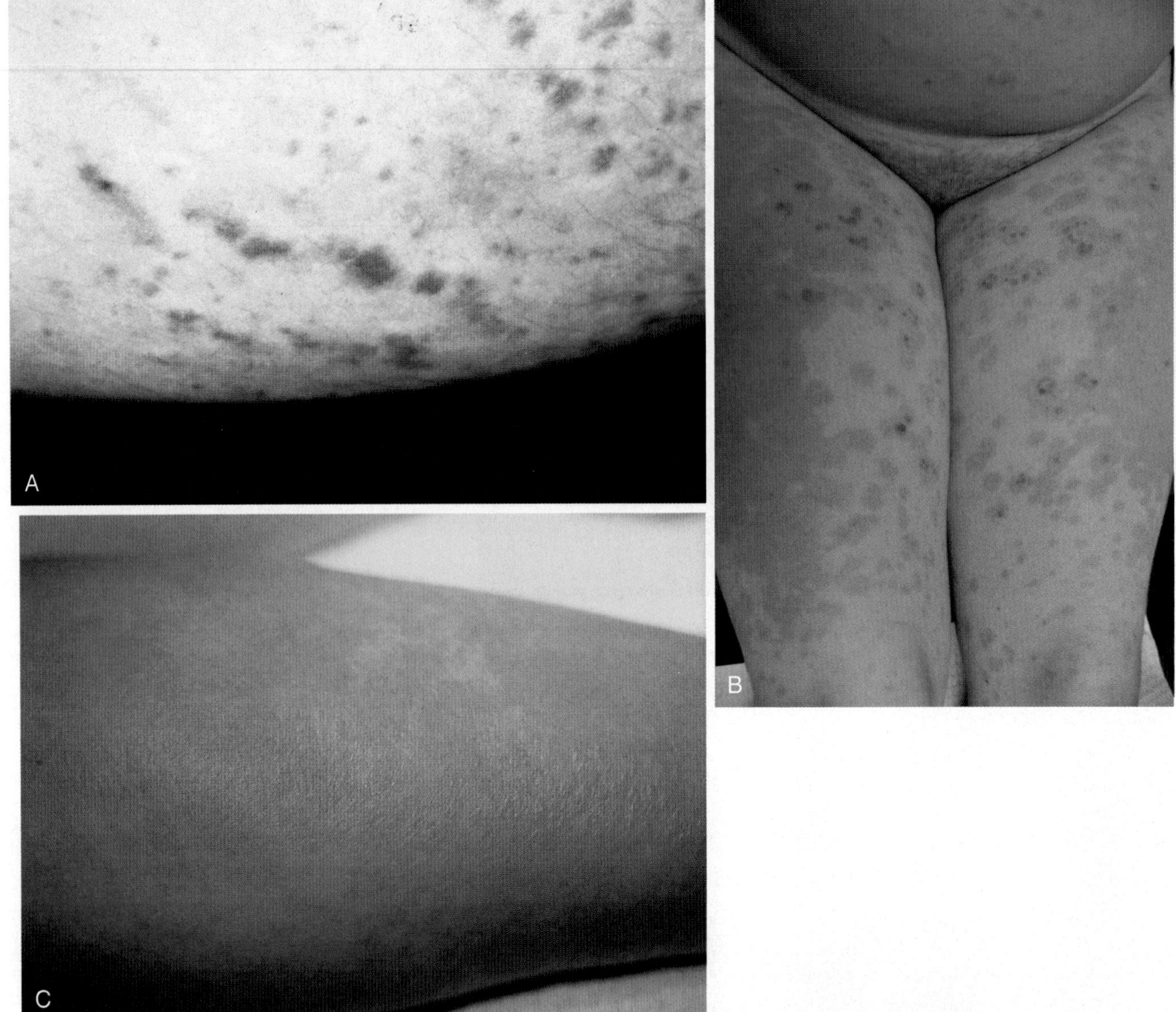

FIGURE 48-6. **A,** Pruritic urticarial papules and plaques of pregnancy (PUPPP) include urticarial lesions that typically start in the abdominal striae. **B,** Vesicular lesions superimposed on urticarial plaques and targetoid lesions reminiscent of erythema multiforme or herpes gestationis. **C,** Widespread PUPPP may resemble a toxic erythema or atopic dermatitis. (Photograph courtesy Helen Raynham, MD.)

fetal macrosomia.[83,84] **A meta-analysis revealed a 10-fold higher prevalence of multiple gestation in pregnancies affected by PUPPP.**[80] Multiple-gestation pregnancy is associated with higher estrogen/progesterone levels, and progesterone has been shown to aggravate the inflammatory process at the tissue level. Interestingly, increased progesterone receptor levels have been detected in skin lesions of PUPPP.[85] Finally, fetal DNA has been detected in PUPPP lesions[86]; still, the importance of microchimerism in the pathogenesis of PUPPP remains uncertain.

PUPPP is not associated with adverse maternal or fetal outcomes. The association with cesarean section in two recent studies needs to be clarified.[87] The goal of therapy is the relief of maternal discomfort. Mild PUPPP can be treated with antipruritic topical medications, topical steroids, and oral antihistamines. In cases of severe itching a short course of oral prednisone may be necessary. UVB has been used anecdotally.[80]

Prurigo of Pregnancy

PP affects between 1 in 300 and 1 in 450 pregnancies. It manifests itself with grouped excoriated or crusted pruritic papules over the extensor surfaces of the extremities, and occasionally on the trunk and elsewhere[1] (see Table 48-3). The condition lacks pathognomonic histopathologic features, and skin immunofluorescence is negative. Serologic tests may show elevated IgE levels.[16] Early reports[88] of a dismal fetal outcome in patients with PP have not been confirmed by subsequent studies, and **PP has not been associated with increased maternal risk.** PP should be differentiated from pruritic dermatoses unrelated to pregnancy, other specific dermatoses of pregnancy, drug eruptions, arthropod bites, and infestations such as scabies. PP is treated with moderately potent topical steroids, if necessary intralesional or under occlusion, and oral antihistamines.[80] A short course of oral steroid is rarely required.

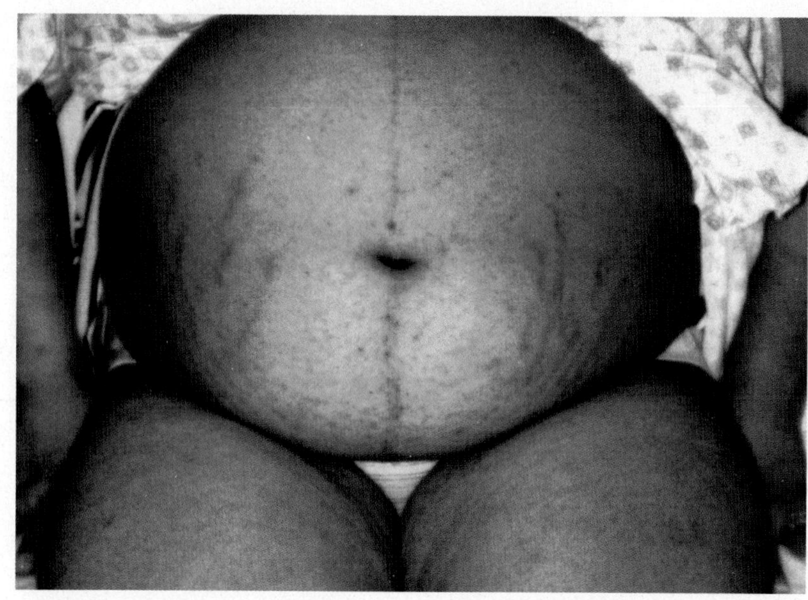

FIGURE 48-7. Pruritic folliculitis of pregnancy: discrete follicular erythematous or pigmented papules on the abdomen.

PP has been associated with a family history of ICP (see Chapter 45). It has been proposed that PP and ICP are closely related conditions, distinguished only by the absence of primary lesions in ICP.[16] These authors reported an association with a personal or family history of AD and elevation of serum IgE (uncontrolled), and suggested that PP may be the result of ICP in women with an atopic predisposition. A reclassification of PP under "atopic eruption of pregnancy" by the same group[17] has been debated[18] because there has been no history of AD or established atopic background in some PP patients and several PP patients fulfill only minor criteria of atopy.[17] Furthermore, the association with atopy has not been confirmed by other groups, and the importance of mild serum IgE elevations in pregnancy has been controversial.[18,20]

Pruritic Folliculitis of Pregnancy

PFP is a rare specific dermatosis of pregnancy the exact prevalence of which remains unknown (see Table 48-3). Approximately 30 cases have been reported.[20] **PFP presents with pruritic follicular erythematous papules and pustules that affect primarily the trunk** (Figure 48-7).[89] PFP resolves spontaneously at delivery or postpartum, but may recur in subsequent pregnancies.[67] The histopathology is that of folliculitis and special stains for microorganisms are negative. Skin immunofluorescence studies and serology are negative. The differential diagnosis of PFP includes an infectious folliculitis and specific dermatoses of pregnancy. An infectious folliculitis can be ruled out with stains for microorganisms and cultures from the pustular lesions. PFP was associated with decreased birth weight and a male to female ratio of 2:1 in one study.[16] Preterm delivery was reported in one case but no other maternal or fetal risks have been noted.

The pregnant patient should be reassured that **PFP resolves postpartum and has not been associated with substantial risks for the fetus.** PFP has been treated with low- or mid-potent topical steroids, benzoyl peroxide, and UVB.[90] The etiology of PFP remains unknown. Increased serum androgen levels in PFP or association with ICP have been reported but were probably coincidental. It has been postulated that PFP may be a form of hormonally induced acne, based on clinical similarities with the acne that develops after the administration of systemic steroids or progestogens.[91] Other authors[67] have considered PFP to be a variant of PUPPP based on reports of follicular lesions in some PUPPP patients. Nevertheless, the clinical presentation and histopathology of PFP differ overall from those of PUPPP. An association with *Pityrosporum* has been debated.[92] A reclassification[17] of PFP under "atopic eruption of pregnancy" on the basis of personal and family history of eczema in a patient with PFP has been debated[18] because, among other factors, history of atopy has not been reported in other PFP cases. Further studies will be required to define whether PFP is a distinct specific dermatosis of pregnancy.

KEY POINTS

- With the physiologic skin changes of pregnancy, there are no risks for the mother or fetus. The changes should be expected to resolve postpartum.
- Preexisting melanocytic nevi may show mild changes in pregnancy but no increased risk for malignant transformation.
- Preexisting skin disorders are more likely to worsen than improve in pregnancy; atopic dermatitis (eczema) is the most common dermatosis in pregnancy.
- Prognosis of melanoma is not adversely affected by pregnancy.
- Pruritus occurs in up to 3% to 14% of pregnancies. A constellation of clinical and laboratory findings is crucial to establishing etiology.
- Impetigo herpetiformis (pustular psoriasis of pregnancy) is often associated with reduced

calcium or vitamin D. There are serious maternal and fetal risks with this disease.

- Herpes gestationis typically flares at delivery. Treatment is with oral steroids. Fetal risks, such as small-for-gestational-age infants, preterm delivery, and neonatal herpes gestationis, have been associated with this disease.
- PUPPP starts in the abdominal striae and spares the periumbilical area. There is an association with multiple-gestation pregnancy, but there are no maternal or fetal risks.
- Prurigo and pruritic folliculitis of pregnancy carry no maternal or fetal risks.

REFERENCES

1. Kroumpouzos G, Cohen LM: Dermatoses of pregnancy. J Am Acad Dermatol 45:1, 2001.
2. Winton GB, Lewis CW: Dermatoses of pregnancy. J Am Acad Dermatol 6:977, 1982.
3. McKay M: Physiologic skin changes of pregnancy. In Black M, McKay M, Braude P, et al: Obstetric and Gynecologic Dermatology, 5th ed. London, Mosby, 2002, p 17.
4. Wong RC, Ellis CN: Physiologic skin changes in pregnancy. J Am Acad Dermatol 10:929, 1984.
5. Sanchez NP, Pathak MA, Sato S, et al: Melasma: a clinical, light microscopic, ultrastructural, and immunofluorescence study. J Am Acad Dermatol 4:698, 1981.
6. Snell RS, Bischitz PG: The effects of large doses of estrogen and progesterone on melanin pigmentation. J Invest Dermatol 35:73, 1960.
7. Kligman AM, Willis I: A new formula for depigmenting human skin. Arch Dermatol 111:40, 1975.
8. Angsuwarangsee S, Polnikorn N: Combined ultrapulse CO_2 laser and Q-switched alexandrite laser compared with Q-switched alexandrite laser alone for refractory melasma: split-face design. Dermatol Surg 29:59, 2003.
9. Tse Y, Levine VJ, McClain SA, et al: The removal of cutaneous pigmented lesions with the Q-switched ruby laser and the Q-switched neodymium:yttritium-aluminum-garnet laser: a comparative study. J Dermatol Surgery Oncol 20:795, 1994.
10. Lee GY, Kim HJ, Whang KK: The effect of combination treatment of the recalcitrant pigmentary disorders with pigmented laser and chemical peeling. Dermatol Surg 28:1120, 2002.
11. Kroumpouzos G, Avgerinou G, Granter S: Acanthosis nigricans without diabetes during pregnancy. Br J Dermatol 146:925, 2002.
12. Kroumpouzos G, Cohen LM: Skin disease. In James DK, Steer PJ, Weiner CP, Gonik B: High-Risk Pregnancy: Management Options, 3rd ed Philadelphia, Elsevier, 2005, p 1138.
13. Khader YS, Ta'ani Q: Peridontal diseases and the risk of preterm birth and low birth weight: a meta-analysis. J Periodontol 76:161, 2005.
14. Rangel O, Arias I, Garcia E, Lopez-Padilla S: Topical tretinoin 0.1% for pregnancy-related abdominal striae: an open-label, multicenter, prospective study. Adv Ther 18:181, 2001.
15. Winton GB: Skin diseases aggravated by pregnancy. J Am Acad Dermatol 20:1, 1989.
16. Vaughan Jones SA, Hern S, Nelson-Piercy C, et al: A prospective study of 200 women with dermatoses of pregnancy correlating the clinical findings with hormonal and immunopathological profiles. Br J Dermatol 141:71, 1999.
17. Ambros-Rudolph CM, Müllegger RR, Vaughan-Jones SA, et al: The specific dermatoses of pregnancy revisited and reclassified: results of a retrospective two-center study on 505 pregnant patients. J Am Acad Dermatol 54:395, 2006.
18. Cohen LM, Kroumpouzos G: Pruritic dermatoses of pregnancy: to lump or to split? J Am Acad Dermatol 56:708, 2007.
19. Hanifin JM, Rajka G: Diagnostic features of atopic eczema. Acta Derm Venereol 92(Suppl):44, 1980.
20. Kroumpouzos G: Specific dermatoses of pregnancy: advances and controversies. Expert Rev Dermatol 5:633, 2010.
21. Moore MM, Rifas-Shiman, SL, Rich-Edwards JW, et al: Perinatal predictors of atopic dermatitis occurring in the first six months of life. Pediatrics 113:468, 2004.
22. Schafer T, Dirschedl P, Kunz B: Maternal smoking during pregnancy and lactation increases the risk for atopic eczema in the offspring. J Am Acad Dermatol 36:550, 1997.
23. Wuthrich B, Schmid-Grendelmeier P: The atopic eczema/dermatitis syndrome. Epidemiology, natural course, and immunology of the IgE-associated ("extrinsic") and the nonallergic ("intrinsic") AEDS. J Investig Allergol Clin Immunol 13:1, 2003.
24. Cho S, Kim HJ, Oh SH, et al: The influence of pregnancy and menstruation on the deterioration of atopic dermatitis symptoms. Ann Dematol 22:180, 2010.
25. Hale EK, Pomeranz MK: Dermatologic agents during pregnancy and lactation: an update and clinical review. Int J Dermatol 41:197, 2002.
26. Kainz A, Harabacz I, Cowlrick IS, et al: Review of the course and outcome of 100 pregnancies in 84 women treated with tacrolimus. Transplantation 70:1718, 2000.
27. Shaw JC, White LE: Persistent acne in adult women. Arch Dermatol 137:1252, 2001.
28. Boyd AS, Morris LF, Phillips CM, et al: Psoriasis and pregnancy: hormone and immune system interaction. Int J Dermatol 35:169, 1996.
29. Tauscher AE, Fleischer AB Jr, Phelps KC, et al: Psoriasis and pregnancy. J Cutan Med Surg 6:561, 2002.
30. Bierman SM: Autoimmune progesterone dermatitis of pregnancy. Arch Dermatol 107:896, 1973.
31. Lee AY, Lee KH, Lim YG: Oestrogen urticaria associated with pregnancy. Br J Dermatol 1999;141:774.
32. Bajaj AK, Swarup V, Gupta OP, et al: Impetigo herpetiformis. Dermatologica 155:292, 1977.
33. Ott F, Krakowski A, Tur E, et al: Impetigo herpetiformis with lowered serum level of vitamin D and its diminished intestinal absorption. Dermatologica 164:360, 1982.
34. Oumeish OY, Farraj SE, Bataineh AS: Some aspects of impetigo herpetiformis. Arch Dermatol 118:103, 1982.
35. Rackett SC, Baughman RD: Impetigo herpetiformis and *Staphylococcus aureus* lymphadenitis in a pregnant adolescent. Pediatric Dermatol 14:387, 1997.
36. Beveridge GW, Harkness RA, Livingston JRB: Impetigo herpetiformis in two successive pregnancies. Br J Dermatol 78:106, 1966.
37. Finch TM, Tan CY: Pustular psoriasis exacerbated by pregnancy and controlled by cyclosporin A [Letter]. Br J Dermatol 142:582, 2000.
38. Gimenez-Garcia R, Gimenez Garcia MC, Llorente de la Fuente A: Impetigo herpetiformis: response to steroids and etretinate. Int J Dermatol 28:551, 1989.
39. Breier-Maly J, Ortel B, Breier F, et al: Generalized pustular psoriasis of pregnancy (impetigo herpetiformis). Dermatology 198:61, 1999.
40. Gutierrez G, Dagnino R, Mintz G: Polymyositis/dermatomyositis and pregnancy. Arthritis Rheum 27:291, 1984.
41. Steen VD: Scleroderma and pregnancy. Rheum Dis Clin North Am 23:133, 1997.
42. Yair D, Shenhav M, Botchan A, et al: Pregnancy associated with pemphigus. Br J Obstet Gynecol 102:667, 1995.
43. Collier PM, Kelly SE, Wojnarowska FW: Linear IgA disease and pregnancy. J Am Acad Dermatol 30:407, 1994.
44. Kardos M, Levine D, Gürkan HM, et al: Pemphigus vulgaris in pregnancy: analysis of current data on the management and outcomes. Obstet Gynecol Surv 64:739, 2009.
45. Bronson DM, Barsky R, Barsky S: Acrodermatitis enteropathica: recognition at long last during a recurrence in pregnancy. J Am Acad Dermatol 9:140, 1983.
46. Pennoyer JM, Grin CM, Driscoll MS: Changes in size of melanocytic nevi during pregnancy. J Am Acad Dermatol 36:378, 1997.
47. Ellis DL: Pregnancy and sex steroid hormone effects on nevi of patients with dysplastic nevus syndrome. J Am Acad Dermatol 25:467, 1991.
48. Onsun N, Saracoglu S, Demirkesen C, et al: Eruptive widespread Spitz nevi: can pregnancy be a stimulating factor? J Am Acad Dermatol 40:866, 1999.

49. Rubegni P, Sbano P, Burroni M, et al: Melanocytic skin lesions and pregnancy: digital dermoscopy analysis. Skin Res Technol 13:143, 2007.
50. Brodell RT, Helms SE: The changing mole: additional warning signs of malignant melanoma. Postgrad Med 104:145, 1998.
51. Slingluff CL Jr, Reintgen DS, Vollmer RT, et al: Malignant melanoma arising during pregnancy: a study of 100 patients. Ann Surg 211:552, 1990.
52. Travers RL, Sober AJ, Berwick M, et al: Increased thickness of pregnancy-associated melanoma. Br J Dermatol 132:876, 1995.
53. Mackie RM, Bufalino R, Morabito A, et al: Lack of effect of pregnancy on outcome of melanoma. Lancet 337:653, 1991.
54. Wong JH, Sterns EE, Kopald KH, et al: Prognostic significance of pregnancy in stage I melanoma. Arch Surg 124:1227,1989.
55. Lens MB, Rosdahl I, Ahlbom A, et al: Effect of pregnancy on survival in women with cutaneous malignant melanoma. J Clin Oncol 22:4369, 2004.
56. Balch CM: Prognostic factors analysis of 17,600 melanoma patients: validation of the American Joint Committee on Cancer melanoma staging system. J Clin Oncol 19:3622, 2001.
57. Schwartz JL, Mozurkewich EL, Johnson TM: Current management of patients with melanoma who are pregnant, want to get pregnant, or do not want to get pregnant [editorial]. Cancer 97:2130, 2003.
58. Nicklas AH, Baker ME: Imaging strategies in the pregnant cancer patient. Semin Oncol 27:623, 2000.
59. Alexander A, Samlowski WE, Grossman D, et al: Metastatic melanoma in pregnancy: risk of transplacental metastases in the infant. J Clin Oncol 21:2179, 2003.
60. Smith M, Fine JA, Barnhill RL, Berwick M: Hormonal and reproductive influences and risk of melanoma in women. Int J Epidemiol 27:751, 1998.
61. Lama G, Angelucci C, Bruzzese N, et al: Sensitivity of human melanoma cells to oestrogens, tamoxifen and quercetin: is there any relationship with type I and II oestrogen binding site expression? Melanoma Res 9:530, 1999.
62. Flowers JL, Seigler HF, McCarty KS, et al: Absence of estrogen receptors in human melanoma as evaluated by monoclonal antiestrogen receptor antibody. Arch Dermatol 123:764, 1987.
63. Lecavalier MA, From L, Gaid N: Absence of estrogen receptors in dysplastic nevi and malignant melanoma. J Am Acad Dermatol 23:242, 1990.
64. Thorn M, Adam HO, Ringborg U, et al: Long-term survival in malignant melanoma with special reference to age and sex as prognostic factors. J Natl Cancer Inst 79:969, 1987.
65. Ries LG, Pollack ES, Young JL: Cancer patient survival: surveillance, epidemiology and end results program, 1973-79. J Natl Cancer Inst 70:693, 1983.
66. Furhoff A: Itching in pregnancy. Acta Med Scand 196:403, 1974.
67. Roger D, Vaillant L, Fignon A, et al: Specific pruritic diseases of pregnancy: a prospective study of 3192 pregnancy women. Arch Dermatol 130:734, 1994.
68. Morrison LH, Labib RS, Zone JJ, et al: Herpes gestationis autoantibodies recognize a 180-kd human epidermal antigen. J Clin Invest 81:2023, 1988.
69. Kelly SE, Black MM: Pemphigoid gestationis: placental interactions. Semin Dermatol 8:12, 1989.
70. Engineer L, Bhol K, Ahmed AR: Pemphigoid gestationis: a review. Am J Obstet Gynecol 183:483, 2000.
71. Shornick JK, Meek TJ, Nesbitt LT, Gilliam JN: Herpes gestationalis in blacks. Arch Dermatol 120:511, 1984.
72. Sitaru C, Powell J, Messer G, et al: Immunoblotting and enzyme-linked immunosorbent assay for the diagnosis of pemphigoid gestationis. Obstet Gynecol 103:757, 2004.
73. Boulinguez S, Bedane C, Prost C, et al: Chronic pemphigoid gestationis: comparative clinical and immunopathological study of 10 patients. Dermatology 206:113, 2003.
74. Holmes RC, Black MM, Jurecka W, et al: Clues to the etiology and pathogenesis of herpes gestationis. Br J Dermatol 109:131, 1983.
75. Shornick JK, Black MM: Secondary autoimmune diseases in herpes gestationis (pemphigoid gestationis). J Am Acad Dermatol 26:563, 1992.
76. Shornick JK, Black MM: Fetal risks in herpes gestationis. J Am Acad Dermatol 26:63, 1992.
77. Karna P, Broecker AH: Neonatal herpes gestationis. J Pediatr 119:299, 1991.
78. Lawley TJ, Hertz KC, Wade TR, et al: Pruritic urticarial papules and plaques of pregnancy. JAMA 241:1696, 1979.
79. Aronson IK, Bond S, Fiedler VC, et al: Pruritic urticarial papules and plaques of pregnancy: clinical and immunopathologic observations in 57 patients. J Am Acad Dermatol 39:933, 1998.
80. Kroumpouzos G, Cohen LM: Specific dermatoses of pregnancy: an evidence-based systematic review. Am J Obstet Gynecol 188:1083, 2003.
81. Rudolph CM, Al-Fares S, Vaughan-Jones SA, et al: Polymorphic eruption of pregnancy: clinicopathology and potential risk factors in 181 patients. Br J Dermatol 154:54, 2006.
82. Carli P, Tarocchi S, Mello G, et al: Skin immune system activation in pruritic urticarial papules and plaques of pregnancy. Int J Dermatol 33:884, 1994.
83. Cohen LM, Capeless EL, Krusinski PA, et al: Pruritic urticarial papules and plaques of pregnancy and its relationship to maternal-fetal weight gain and twin pregnancy. Arch Dermatol 125:1534, 1989.
84. Elling SV, McKenna P, Powell FC: Pruritic urticarial papules and plaques of pregnancy in twin and triplet pregnancies. J Eur Acad Dermatol Venereol 14:378, 2000.
85. Im S, Lee E-S, Kim W, et al: Expression of progesterone receptor in human keratinocytes. J Korean Med Sci 15:647, 2000.
86. Aractingi S, Bertheau P, Le Goue C, et al: Fetal DNA in skin of polymorphic eruptions of pregnancy. Lancet 352:1898, 1998.
87. Regnier S, Fermand V, Levy P, Uzan S, et al: A case-control study of polymorphic eruption of pregnancy. J Am Acad Dermatol 58:63, 2008.
88. Spangler AS, Reddy W, Bardawil WA, et al: Papular dermatitis of pregnancy: a new clinical entity? JAMA 181:577, 1962.
89. Zoberman E, Farmer ER: Prutitic folliculitis of pregnancy. Arch Dermatol 117:20, 1981.
90. Kroumpouzos G, Cohen LM: Pruritic folliculitis of pregnancy. J Am Acad Dermatol 43:132, 2000.
91. Kroumpouzos G, Cohen LM: Diseases of pregnancy and their treatment. In Krieg T, Bickers D, Miyachi Y: Therapy of Skin Diseases. Berlin, Springer Verlag, 2010, p 677.
92. Kroumpouzos G: Pityosporum folliculitis during pregnancy is not pruritic folliculitis of pregnancy. J Am Acad Dematol 53:1098, 2005.

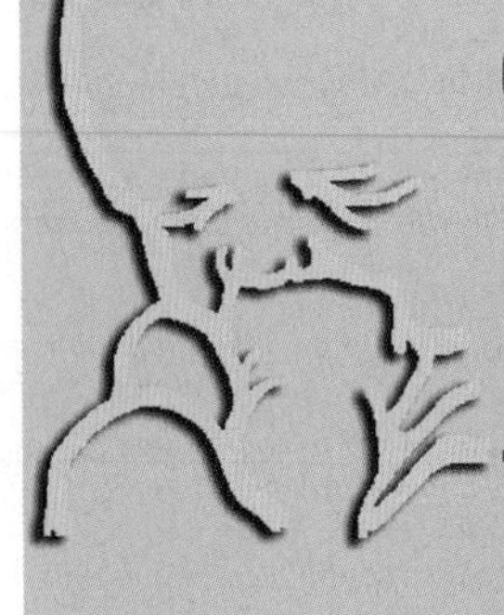

CHAPTER 49

Maternal and Perinatal Infection: The Sexually Transmitted Diseases Chlamydia, Gonorrhea, and Syphilis

Kirk D. Ramin and Daniel V. Landers

KEY ABBREVIATIONS	
By Mouth	PO
Centers for Disease Control and Prevention	CDC
Central Nervous System	CNS
Cerebrospinal Fluid	CSF
Direct Fluorescence Assays	DFA
Elementary Bodies	EB
Enzyme Immunoassays	EIA
Human Immunodeficiency Virus	HIV
Human Papillomavirus	HPV
Institute of Medicine	IOM
Intramuscular	IM
Intravenous	IV
Lipopolysaccharide	LPS
Major Outer Membrane Protein	MOMP
Microhemagglutination *Treponema pallidum*	MHA-TP
Morbidity and Mortality Weekly Report	MMWR
Nucleic Acid Amplification Tests	NAATS
Polymerase Chain Reaction	PCR
Rapid Plasma Reagin	RPR
Reticulate Body	RB
Ribonucleic Acid	RNA
Sexually Transmitted Disease	STD
Venereal Disease Research Laboratories	VDRL
World Health Organization	WHO
World War II	WWII

Maternal and perinatal infections represent common complications of the peripartum interval. In many industrialized nations, the role of sexually transmitted pathogens is declining in its relative contribution to infections in women; however, in the United States and developing nations, the epidemic persists. Many of these pathogens are either proved or presumed to play an integral role in infectious morbidities of pregnancy and the neonatal period, and thus, understanding the social, economic, and pathophysiologic burden is essential. Indeed, as our ability to readily screen the population as a whole for the most prevalent or malignant of these infectious agents (e.g., chlamydia, gonorrhea, and syphilis) has improved, epidemiologic statistics have provided evidence for their implied role in preterm labor, preterm premature rupture of the membranes, intrauterine growth restriction, neonatal conjunctivitis, neonatal pneumonia, and congenital syphilis. Thus, a greater understanding of the role of these prevalent pathogens in mediating disease pathogenesis has mandated that the obstetrician be well versed in the identification and management of these organisms. In this chapter, we review current trends in epidemiology, diagnosis, treatment, and prevention.

EPIDEMIOLOGY

The two most valuable sources of incidence and prevalence data on the sexually transmitted pathogens are provided by the Centers for Disease Control and Prevention (CDC) and the World Health Organization (WHO). The CDC reports sexually transmitted disease (STD) estimates for the United States using reported cases and estimates after accounting for underreporting. The Institute of Medicine (IOM) provides WHO estimates on worldwide incidences and prevalence of the four curable sexually transmitted infections (chlamydia, gonorrhea, syphilis, and *Trichomonas*). **Overall, the WHO places annual estimates of worldwide incidence at 89.1 million new cases of chlamydia infection, 62.6 million new cases of gonorrhea, and 12.2 million new cases of syphilis among persons aged 15 to 49 years.** In addition, epidemiologic studies have revealed a number of basic truths regarding STDs: (1) sexually active adolescents have the highest rates of STDs of any age group[1]; (2) gender differences are observed in the transmission of the most prevalent STDs, with more efficient transmission from men to women; (3) curable STDs (i.e., not human immunodeficiency virus [HIV], human papillomavirus [HPV], or chronic recurrent herpes simplex virus) are associated with more serious long-term consequences in women than in men; (4) having one or more STDs predisposes an individual to acquisition and transmission of other STDs; (5) STDs in developing nations are both hyperendemic and epidemic; and (6) there exists marked racial disparity.

Chlamydia

Genital tract chlamydial infections are generally ascribed to *Chlamydia trachomatis* and account for the most prevalent reported infectious disease in the United States annually. More than 1.2 million cases are reported to the CDC annually, with an actual presumed number of new cases (accounting for estimates of underreporting) of 3 million annually.[1] **These infections present unique problems for public health control programs because 50% to 70% of infections in women are clinically silent.** Unrecognized and untreated, the bacteria may remain infectious in the host for months and be readily transmitted to sex partners. Furthermore, most reported infections occur in the 15- to 24-year-old age group, individuals who do not partake in preventive health care programs. Estimates on worldwide exposure approximate that 90 million new cases of *C. trachomatis* infection occur on an annual basis, accounting for a rising majority of perinatal and neonatal complications.[2-5] Of note, a primary goal of *Healthy People 2010* is the elimination of racial disparities among multiple sexually transmitted pathogens. An assessment of the racial disparities of nationally notifiable disease for the year 2002 revealed a nearly 10-fold increase rate for chlamydia in blacks compared with whites (805.9 versus 90.2 per 100,000).[6]

The cost of treatment, prevention, and management of complications of chlamydial infections is estimated at $2.4 billion in health care costs annually.[3-5] Taken together, these factors have resulted in the endorsement of a nationwide broad-based screening program by both the CDC and IOM. Specific recommendations regarding population-based screening and prevention programs are reviewed later in this chapter.

Gonorrhea

The reported incidence of *Neisseria gonorrhoeae* infection is just over 300,000 cases in the United States annually.[1] However, the actual number of reported cases may be underrepresented by as much as 40%, yielding a U.S. estimate of 700,000 cases annually.[7] In contrast to chlamydia, the worldwide prevalence of gonorrhea may be significantly less than that observed in the United States, as supported by epidemiologic data from Canada and Western Europe.[8]

Historically, review of trends in incidence of reported gonorrhea in the United States from 1941 to 1997 reveal peak increases among both men and women in the interval around World War II (WWII), and again in 1975, peaking at 473 cases per 100,000.[7] The steady decline since 1975 has been accompanied by three interesting observations. First, the male-to-female ratio of reported cases has declined from a high of 3:1 to its current gender equivalence of 1:1.[7] Second, racial disparity is noted, with a 24-fold higher rate among blacks compared with whites (570.4 versus 23.6 per 100,000).[6] **Third, the single greatest determinant of gonorrhea incidence since 1975 is age: annual reported cases are twice as high in adolescents (aged 15 to 19 years) than in women aged 20 to 24 years.**[8,9]

Syphilis

Historically, syphilis has long been recognized as a chronic systemic infectious process secondary to infection with the spirochete *Treponema pallidum*. Throughout the centuries, epidemics of syphilis have been periodically reported. In the United States, the observed incidence of primary and secondary syphilis initially mirrored that of gonorrhea (reflecting the principle that epidemiologic synergy among the STDs occurs), with a rising peak during and shortly after WWII to 76 per 100,000 population to its reported nadir of 4 per 100,000 in 1955 to 1957.[10] Since the mid-1950s, recurrent epidemics have occurred, the most recent in 1985 to 1990, with a peak incidence of 23.5 cases per 100,000.[11] **Beginning in 2001 syphilis has increased each year to 13,997 cases in 2009.**[1]

Of concern are observations from both the WHO and CDC that the prevalence of syphilis in both the United States and developing nations has fluctuated over the past two decades. Again noted are elements of racial disparity, with a disproportionate number of cases in blacks compared with whites (9.4 versus 1.1 per 100,000),[6] as well as gender disparity, with a predilection in women aged 15 to 24 years.[7]

Congenital Syphilis

As might be expected, the trend toward increasing prevalence in reproductive-aged women is accompanied by fluctuations in the incidence of congenital syphilis. Thus, there existed an epidemic of congenital syphilis from 1986 to 1992.[10] Fortunately, 2002 congenital syphilis surveillance data from the CDC report that provisional cases are at 348 per 100,000 births.[1] Of concern, however, is the observation that the rates of congenital syphilis remain disproportionately high in black and southern U.S. populations.[1,6,7] In their most recent report, the CDC summarized 2002 congenital syphilis surveillance data, which indicated that congenital syphilis rates decreased among all racial and ethnic minority populations, as well as in all regions of the United States, except the Northeast. Thus, rates of congenital syphilis per 100,000 live-born infants were determined from U.S. natality data and demonstrated a 21.1% decrease, from 14.2 to 11.2 cases per 100,000 live births, reflecting that primary and secondary syphilis rates among reproductive-aged women declined 35.3%, from 1.7 to 1.1 cases per 100,000 women.[12] The rate of congenital syphilis fell 50.6% among American Indian/Alaska Native infants, 22.4% among Hispanic infants, 21.4% among Asian/Pacific Islander infants, and 19.8% among non-Hispanic black infants; the rate remained unchanged among non-Hispanic white infants.[12] **Of concern is a recent rise in the number of congenital syphilis cases from 339 in 2005 to 437 in 2008 according to the CDC.**[1]

Review of the data involved in recent trends in congenital syphilis demonstrate one of the successes of STD prevention and therapy and is worth mentioning at this juncture. To summarize the report of the CDC,[12] among the 451 cases of congenital syphilis reported in 2002, a total of 333 (73.8%) occurred because the mother had no documented treatment or received inadequate treatment of syphilis before or during pregnancy; **many of these cases occurred among infants born to women who had no prenatal care or no documented prenatal care.** In 63 (14.0%) cases, the mother was treated adequately but did not have an adequate serologic response to therapy, and the infant was evaluated inadequately for congenital disease. In 39 (8.6%) cases, the mother was treated adequately but did not have an adequate serologic response to therapy, and the infant's evaluation revealed laboratory or clinical signs of congenital syphilis. A total of 16 (3.6%) cases were reported for other reasons. In 288 (63.9%) of the cases reported in 2002, the mother received prenatal care; the mother did not receive prenatal care in 130 (28.8%) cases; and no information on prenatal care was reported for 33 (7.3%) cases. When examined for trimester of pregnancy in which prenatal care occurred, in 86 instances care was initiated during the first trimester of pregnancy, 93 during the second trimester, and 59 during the third trimester. A total of 18 (30.5%) mothers who initiated prenatal care during the third trimester did so less than 30 days before delivery. In 2002, among those infants with congenital syphilis, 18 (4.0%) were stillborn, and 8 (1.8%) died within 30 days of delivery. Taken together, these findings highlight that decreases in incidence of congenital syphilis closely parallel decreases in prevalence of primary and secondary syphilis among women, and interventions designed to prevent, detect, and treat syphilis among women of reproductive age have likely played an important role in the eventual decline of congenital disease. Indeed, following the epidemic of 1985 to 1990, efforts to eliminate syphilis were initiated with the implementation of a "National Plan to Eliminate Syphilis" in 1998.[13] Elimination efforts initially focused on syphilis among racial and ethnic minority populations and persons living in the South and employed the following three methods: enhanced screening of women at high risk for acquiring syphilis; increased provider awareness, education, and training regarding syphilis; and increased awareness of the disease among communities with high rates of infection. However, it is important to note that although the incidence of congenital syphilis decreased with the implementation of the aforementioned initiative, most congenital syphilis cases reported were preventable.[9,12,13]

PATHOGENESIS

Endocervical Infections

Chlamydia and gonorrhea are the sexually transmitted pathogens generally associated with endocervical infections and have been noted to bear resemblance in their profile of observed maternal and perinatal clinical syndromes.[14,15] Although they are common in their association with increased cervical discharge, they are unique in almost every other aspect of their pathogenesis.

Chlamydia

Species of *Chlamydia* were initially serotyped according to their biologic and biochemical properties, and a greater than 95% homology in their 16s ribosomal ribonucleic acid (RNA) sequences was observed. Subsequent molecular analyses led to the reclassification of some *Chlamydia psittaci* strains as *Chlamydia pneumoniae*, a human pathogen, and *Chlamydia pecorum*, a pathogen of ruminants. Nevertheless, of the four species of chlamydiae (*C. trachomatis, psittaci, pneumoniae,* and *pecorum*), only *C. trachomatis* and *C. pneumoniae* claim primates as their endogenous hosts. Each of the species bears multiple strains based on serotype, which, in turn, are associated with distinct clinical entities. These are as summarized in Table 49-1.

Chlamydiae are obligate intracellular bacteria that grow in eukaryotic epithelial cells, and they employ a growth cycle unique to that from all other pathogens. During the

TABLE 49-1 SPECTRUM OF HUMAN AND MAMMALIAN DISEASES CAUSED BY *CHLAMYDIAE* SEROTYPES

SPECIES SEROTYPE	ACUTE DISEASES	CLINICAL SEQUELAE
Chlamydia trachomatis	Conjunctivitis	Trachoma
A, B, Ba, C	Acute urethral syndrome cervicitis, endometritis, salpingitis,	Proctitis, epididymitis, Reiter syndrome
D-K	inclusion conjunctivitis, neonatal pneumonia	Pelvic inflammatory disease, ectopic pregnancy
		Tubal infertility, Fitz-Hugh–Curtis syndrome
L1, 12, 13	Lymphogranuloma venereum	Reactive airway disease
Chlamydia pneumoniae	Pharyngitis	
	Sinusitis	
	Bronchitis	
	Community acquired	
	Pneumonia	
Chlamydia psittaci	Atypical pneumonia	
Parrot	Conjunctivitis	
Cats	Abortion	
Ewes		

1970s, the infectivity and growth cycle of chlamydiae was initially characterized.[16-20] Known to specifically infect the cuboidal or nonciliated columnar epithelial cells common to the endocervix, urethra, and conjunctiva, this growth cycle involves infection of a susceptible host cell through a receptor-specific phagocytic process. This phagocytic process involves chlamydiae *elementary bodies* (EBs) binding to the host cell through a heparin sulfate–like molecule to glycosaminoglycan receptors, and these subsequently are phagocytosed into cytoplasmic vacuoles termed *phagosomes*.[21] In this fashion, chlamydiae may be considered to have a unique biphasic life cycle with dimorphic forms that are functionally and morphologically distinct. Once endocytosed, the EB differentiates into a larger pleomorphic form called the *reticulate body* (RB), which replicates by binary fission. The chlamydiae remain in the phagosome throughout their growth cycle, presumptively as an acquired means of escaping host lysosomes.[18-21] The endosome is transported to the distal region of the Golgi apparatus and incorporates host-derived sphingolipids into the inclusion membrane. Thus, it appears that chlamydiae are able to intercept host vesicular traffic bound for the plasma membrane to sequester lipids and possibly other host substances synthesized in the Golgi. Subversion of host vesicular traffic may represent a dual advantage for chlamydiae in obtaining materials from the host for its metabolism as well as in modifying the inclusion membrane to evade lysosomal fusion and immune detection.

Because chlamydiae depend on their host cell for the generation of adenosine triphosphate (ATP), they require viable cells for survival.[22] Chlamydiae are incapable of de novo nucleotide biosynthesis and thus are dependent on host nucleotide pools. In this manner, one may consider this unique pathogen to be virus like. On the other hand, chlamydiae resemble a bacterial pathogen in that they contain both DNA and RNA, have a modified rigid cell wall with a lipopolysaccharide similar to that in the outer membrane of gram-negative bacteria (albeit lacking the intervening peptidoglycan layer), and multiply by binary fission.[18-22]

Some interesting insights into the interaction of chlamydiae and its host immune system have emerged in the past decade. These new observations include the extensive but unexpected polymorphism of the major outer membrane protein (MOMP), the evidence for genetic susceptibility to disease, and the association of antibody response to the 60-kDa heat shock protein (CHSP60) with the development of adverse sequelae following ocular and genital infections. By way of summary, MOMP is a major target for protective host immune responses, such as neutralizing antibodies and possibly protective T-cell responses.[23,24] The basis for MOMP antigenic variation is allelic polymorphism at the omp-1 locus, and immune selection appears to be occurring in host populations frequently exposed to *C. trachomatis*.[25] Combined with the observations that there appears to be a clear genetic susceptibility to disease, because only a subset of infected persons appear to have long-term complications after acute or repeated chlamydial infections, it is now believed that chronic immune activation plays a role in propagating clinical disease.[26] Thus, susceptibility to chlamydial pelvic inflammatory disease in a study of sex workers in Nairobi, Kenya has been associated with an HLA class I allele, HLA-A31.[27,28] Similarly, allelic variation in the class II allele (DQ) have been shown to be positively associated with *C. trachomatis* tubal infertility.[29,30]

In addition to host genotype playing a role in determining the severity of chlamydia-mediated disease, aberrations in humoral immunity also appear to modulate clinical disease. Antibody response to a 57-kDa chlamydial protein was initially observed more frequently in women with tubal infertility than in controls.[15,26] This protein was subsequently identified as a heat shock protein of the GroEL family of stress proteins. The association between antibody response to CHSP60 and pelvic inflammatory disease, ectopic pregnancy, tubal infertility, and trachoma has been subsequently observed in a number of population-based serotype studies.[15,16] Suffice it to say, although it remains unclear whether antibody to CHSP60 is causally involved in chlamydial immunopathogenesis or is merely a marker of persistent chlamydial infection, in cells persistently infected with *C. trachomatis*, the constitutive expression of CHSP60 may provide continued antigenic stimulation for the CHSP60 antibody response observed in persons with long-term sequelae. Moreover, observed immunopathology may also result from aberrations in self-tolerance mediated by shared and similar epitopes between CHSP60 and endogenous HSP60, which, in turn, results in a classic immune cascade resulting in tissue damage.

Gonorrhea

In contrast to chlamydiae species, the pathogenesis of *N. gonorrhoeae* and human disease is more straightforward and reflects classic bacterial pathogenesis. *N. gonorrhoeae* is a gram-negative diplococcus for which humans are the only natural hosts. Like the other endocervical infectious pathogens, gonorrhea also bears a predilection for the columnar epithelium, which lines the mucous membranes of the anogenital tract.[7,31] Gonococcal pathogens adhere to these mucosal cells through attachment of pili and other surface proteins, resulting in the release of lipopolysaccharide, which likely instigates mucosal damage. Following adherence, *N. gonorrhoeae* is pinocytosed and thereby transported into epithelial cells. Unlike chlamydiae, the gonococcus does not replicate in the phagosome and, hence, evades lysosomal degradation. **Rather, gonococci persist in the host by virtue of their ability to alter the host environment.** In sum, multiple structures of *N. gonorrhoeae* enable pathogenesis by a variety of immune evasive mechanisms, including immunoglobulin A (IgA) proteases, iron repression, and cell-adherence mechanisms.[7,31]

Systemic Infection

Syphilis is a chronic disease caused by the spirochete *Treponema* subspecies *pallidum*. *T. pallidum* belongs to the order Spirochaetales, characterized by slender, nonflagellated, flexuous, tightly spiraled protozoa-like organisms. Motility is attained by the flexuous bending of this long slender body. This motility is responsible for the attainment of access through disrupted integument (mostly mucous membranous) primarily during sexual contact. This anaerobic and obligate human parasite is acquired by 50% of individuals having sexual contact with an infected partner.[7] Following mucosal invasion, an incubation period of about 1 week to 3 months ensues until the chancre appears, heralding primary infection. The chancre arises at the point of entry by the spirochetes. The chancre is a broad-based, typically nontender ulcerated lesion that gives a characteristic "woody" or "rubbery" feel on palpation. It is seldom secondarily infected, and it resolves without medical treatment in 3 to 6 weeks. The organism then hematogenously spreads through the body during the period in which the immune system has responded, about 4 to 10 weeks.[7] Secondary syphilis is characterized by a generalized maculopapular eruption, constitutional symptoms, major organ involvement, and lymphadenopathy. Like the other major organ systems, the central nervous system (CNS) is invaded in about 40% of individuals during this hematogenous phase.[32,33] Secondary syphilis resolves over 2 to 6 weeks as the patient enters the latent phase of the disease.[7] The latent phase is divided into early latent (<1 year) and late latent (>1 year) disease in which no symptoms or signs of clinical disease are noted. If left untreated, progress to tertiary disease with cardiovascular system, CNS, and musculoskeletal system involvement occurs. The organism has an affinity for the arterioles, and the inflammatory response that follows results in obliterative endarteritis.[34] Subsequent end-organ destruction then occurs. In immunocompromised individuals (e.g., immune-suppressive medications, HIV infection), the progression to tertiary disease, especially CNS, is known to occur early after the onset of disease. **Congenital infection results from transplacental migration of the organism to the fetus. Congenital disease occurs with all stages of maternal infection as well as at any gestational age.**[35] Past theories of a placental impasse during the first half of gestation were disproved by pathologic examination of infected first-trimester abortuses and by the demonstration of living organisms in amniotic fluid obtained by amniocentesis in the early second trimester.[35,36] It is now believed that transplacental infection must be close to 100% during the early stages of maternal disease because of the known hematogenous spread, with lower rates of transmission, falling to 10%, as bacteremia abates with the subsequent mounting of the maternal immunologic response during late latent disease.[37-39] Like chlamydia, *T. pallidum* invades the host and evades the host defense mechanisms while being completely dependent on the host for survival. It lacks the fundamental biosynthetic machinery to create complex molecules and fatty acids.[40,41] The ability to evade the host defense mechanisms stems from its basic construct of an inner membrane with few integral membrane proteins protruding through the surface gaining exposure through the outer membrane.[42] Berman concluded that this construct "may provide some understanding of how the organism elicits such a vigorous inflammatory and immunological response, but manages to evade immunological clearance, although a paucity of surface proteins means that its surface presents few targets for a host immune response."[43] Of paramount importance in the pathogenesis of fetal disease is knowledge of fetal immunologic development. Disease early in gestation incites little response because the immune system functions little until midgestation. Following this period, the fetus is able to mount a vigorous response with marked endarteritis and end-organ involvement. Characteristics of subsequent fetal damage and loss are covered further in the section on diagnosis.

DIAGNOSIS

Chlamydia and Gonorrhea

In women, the gold standard for diagnosis of gonorrhea infection requires isolation of the organism by culture. Traditionally, specimens are streaked on a selective (Thayer-Martin or Martin-Lewis) or nonselective (chocolate agar) medium. Inoculated media are incubated at 35° to 36.5° C in an atmosphere supplemented with 5% CO_2 and examined at 24-hour intervals for 72 hours. Subsequent diagnosis is made by identification of the organism with growth on this selective media, with a Gram stain and oxidase test on colonies identifying gram-negative, oxidase-positive diplococci morphology. A confirmed laboratory diagnosis of *N. gonorrhoeae* cannot be made on the basis of these tests alone. A presumptive test result is sufficient to initiate antimicrobial therapy, but additional tests must be performed to confirm the identity of an isolate as *N. gonorrhoeae.* Culture isolation is also suitable for non–genital tract specimens. Using selective media is necessary if the anatomic source of the specimen normally contains other bacterial species. Given ongoing concerns by the CDC regarding resistant species,[44] all gonorrhea cases in the United States are confirmed by culture to allow for antimicrobial susceptibility testing. In women, a single endocervical culture on selective media detects 80% to 90% of uncomplicated gonorrhea.[31,44] Thus, it is recommended that for optimal yield, two consecutive endocervical specimens or a combination of an endocervical and rectal-vaginal swab should be obtained.[7]

The advantages of gonorrheal culture are high sensitivity and specificity, low cost, suitability for use with different types of specimens, and the ability to retain the isolate for additional testing. The major disadvantage of culture for *N. gonorrhoeae* is that specimens must be transported under conditions adequate to maintain the viability of organisms. Another disadvantage is that a minimum of 24 to 72 hours is required from specimen collection to the report of a presumptive culture result.[44]

Because curative antibiotic therapies for chlamydial infections are available and inexpensive, early diagnosis is an essential component of management and prevention. Historically, isolation of chlamydia in cell culture had been the traditional method for laboratory diagnosis and has remained the gold standard in diagnoses because of its specificity. However, culture requires expensive equipment, technical expertise, and stringent transport conditions to preserve specimen viability. **Thus, chlamydial culture is being replaced by antigen-detection methods, such as enzyme immunoassay (EIA) and direct fluorescence assay (DFA), which have less demanding transport requirements and can provide results on the same day.** Assays are typically based on the capture of the chlamydial lipopolysaccharide using monoclonal or polyclonal antibodies linked to a solid-phase support. Early problems with low specificity because of cross-reactivity between the chlamydial lipopolysaccharide (LPS) and that of other gram-negative bacteria have been largely overcome by confirmation with DFA or a blocking antibody assay.

A substantial number of EIA tests have been marketed for detecting *C. trachomatis* infection. By contrast, the performance and cost characteristics of EIA tests for *N. gonorrhoeae* infection have not made them competitive with culture.[44] *C. trachomatis* EIA tests detect chlamydial LPS with a monoclonal or polyclonal antibody that has been labeled with an enzyme. The enzyme converts a colorless substrate into a colored product, which is detected by a spectrophotometer. Specimens can be stored and transported without refrigeration and should be processed within the time indicated by the manufacturer.

The DFA procedure identifies either the MOMP or LPS as its antigen, and staining consists of coincubation with a fluorescein-labeled monoclonal antibody that binds to *C. trachomatis* elementary bodies. DFA with a *C. trachomatis*–specific anti-MOMP monoclonal antibody is considered to be highly specific. Similar to EIAs, DFA is not appropriate as a diagnostic test for the direct detection of *N. gonorrhoeae* in clinical specimens.[44]

Nucleic acid–based hybridization probes and nucleic acid amplification tests (NAATs) based on polymerase chain reaction (PCR), ligase chain reaction, and transcription-mediated amplification technology are now commercially available.[16,44] The common characteristic among NAATs is that they are designed to amplify nucleic acid sequences that are specific for the organism being detected and thus do not require viable organisms. The increased sensitivity of NAATs is attributable to their ability to produce a positive signal from as little as a single copy of the target DNA or RNA. Most commercial NAATs have been cleared by the U.S. Food and Drug Administration to detect *C. trachomatis* and *N. gonorrhoeae* in endocervical swabs from women, urethral swabs from men, and urine from both men and women.[44] The ability of NAATs to detect *C. trachomatis* and *N. gonorrhoeae* without a pelvic examination is a key advantage of NAATs, and this ability facilitates screening men and women in other nontraditional screening venues. A disadvantage of NAATs is that specimens can contain amplification inhibitors that result in false-negative results.

In addition to the NAATs, nucleic acid hybridization assays are now available to detect *C. trachomatis* or *N. gonorrhoeae*. Both the PACE and Hybrid Capture assays can detect *C. trachomatis* or *N. gonorrhoeae* in a single specimen. In the Gen-Probe hybridization assays, a DNA probe that is complementary to a specific sequence of *C. trachomatis* or *N. gonorrhoeae* ribosomal RNA hybridizes with any complementary ribosomal RNA that is present in the specimen.[44] RNA hybridization probes in the Digene assay are specific for DNA sequences of *C. trachomatis* and *N. gonorrhoeae*, including both genomic DNA and cryptic plasmid DNA.[44] One of the advantages of the nucleic acid hybridization tests is the ability to store and transport specimens for up to 7 days at ambient temperatures.

Duplex testing for the simultaneous detection of chlamydial and gonococcal DNA from a single specimen is also commercially available in some markets.[44] However, it bears mention that inherent in the increased sensitivity of these molecular techniques is the potential for false-positive results due to cross-contamination between specimens as well as contamination from equipment, reagents, and supplies.

Serology screening has no or limited value in testing for uncomplicated genital *C. trachomatis* infection and should not be used for screening because previous chlamydial infection frequently elicits long-lasting antibodies that cannot be easily distinguished from the antibodies produced in a current infection. A serologic screening or diagnostic assay is not available for *N. gonorrhoeae*.

Syphilis

The ability to diagnose infection with the organism *T. pallidum* has been problematic for two primary reasons. The first is the failure of the organism, as of yet, to be cultured on an artificial medium. The second lies in the long-recognized tendency of clinical manifestations to mimic or imitate a variety of other diseases. Reports continue to surface touting the difficulty with which syphilis is recognized at any stage.[45] Although the primary genital lesion of syphilis, the chancre, is commonly recognized by affected males, women more often than not fail to identify this lesion. As reviewed earlier in this chapter, the chancre is a painless, sharply demarcated, woody-based (induration), 1- to 2-cm erosion of the mucosal surface at the site of the organism's entrance. It occurs typically without constitutional symptoms and is seldom secondarily infected. Examination of the serous exudates from the chancre under dark-field microscopy definitively diagnoses the condition by identification of the flexuous (spiraled) bodied organism. Unfortunately, dark-field microscopy lacks sensitivity, owing in part to specimen collection technique. The lesion must be abraded with a gauze sponge or cotton-tip application until bleeding ensues. The lesion is then squeezed to express clear serum, which is pressed onto a microscope slide. Direct fluorescent-antibody tests have the advantage that they can be performed on slides that are air-dried as well as on stored paraffin-embedded tissue.[46] PCR has increased the sensitivity for detection in samples obtained from genital lesions, cerebrospinal fluid (CSF), amniotic fluid, serum, and paraffin-embedded tissue.[47] Great difficulty in the diagnosis of syphilis lies in the fact that primary syphilis often goes unrecognized by the infected individual, as eluded to earlier.

Because most individuals infected with *T. pallidum* are in the asymptomatic latent phase of the disease, serologic testing is the primary means of diagnosis. Historically, reliance has been placed on two nonspecific antibody tests: the rapid plasma reagin (RPR) and the Venereal Disease Research Laboratories (VDRL) tests. Both pregnant and nonpregnant women are primarily screened using one of these two tests. **In an effort to reduce the incidence of congenital syphilis, the WHO and the CDC recommend at a minimum screening all pregnant women in the first trimester.**[48,49] It would be ideal if pregnant women were additionally screened at the start of the third trimester to enhance the detection of newly acquired infection after first-trimester screening as well as reinfection.[50] If prenatal screening is not available, then screening at the time of delivery should be performed.[46] Once appropriately treated, most individuals (pregnant or not) lose reactivity to these nontreponemal serologic tests.[49] **Confirmation that the infection is indeed due to *T. pallidum* is made by the *Treponema*-specific microhemagglutination–*Treponema pallidum* (MHA-TP) and fluorescent treponemal antibody**

absorbed (FTA-ABS) tests. For most individuals, the MHA-TP and FTA-ABS tests remain positive lifelong.[51] False-positive reactions occur with both nonspecific antibody tests (RPR, VDRL) because of viral infections and autoimmune disease. Although most HIV-infected individuals exhibit normal serologic testing, occasionally one encounters patients with expressed lesion exudates or biopsy-proven disease, and serologic testing is negative.[51] The following recommendations for diagnosing syphilis in HIV-infected individuals have been made by the CDC.[52] First, individuals with HIV should be screened for syphilis, and all sexually active individuals with syphilis should be screened for HIV. If clinical examination and findings suggest syphilis in the presence of negative serologic testing, then DFA for *T. pallidum* staining of lesion exudates and biopsy or dark-field microscopic examination should be performed. In these individuals, all laboratories should titrate the nontreponemal tests (RPR, VDRL) to the exact final end point to better guide response to therapy. Finally, neurosyphilis must be entertained as a diagnosis in the HIV-infected individuals and appropriate consultations obtained to better interpret serologic results. Neurosyphilis is diagnosed in non–HIV-infected and HIV-infected patients by examination of CSF through spinal tap.

Spinal tap and examination of CSF is not currently recommended in non–HIV-infected individuals who have early asymptomatic syphilis.[49] Individuals in whom CSF testing should be considered include those with neurologic or ophthalmologic symptoms, active tertiary disease, or treatment failure and HIV-positive individuals.[49]

Nonimmune fetal hydrops, polyhydramnios, and intrauterine fetal demise have long been associated with congenital syphilis. Recent reports confirm the constellation of nonimmune hydrops (ascites, pleural effusion, scalp or skin edema), hepatomegaly, polyhydramnios, and placentomegaly as markers for congenital syphilis.[53,54] Hollier and colleagues prospectively identified and followed 24 women with untreated syphilis to better define the pathophysiology of fetal disease.[55] Ultrasound examination with amniocentesis and funipuncture was performed. Maternal treatment was with benzathine penicillin G given intramuscularly (IM) as per current CDC guidelines (Table 49-2). Six women had primary, 12 secondary, and 6 early latent disease. Ultrasound examination was abnormal in 16 (66%) of the 24 fetuses. Thirteen of these fetuses had hepatomegaly, 3 had hepatomegaly and ascites, and 1 had nonimmune hydrops. Increased placental thickness was seen in 17 (71%) and hydramnios in only 1 fetus with abnormal ultrasound. Sixteen (66%) of these fetuses had either congenital syphilis or *T. pallidum* identified in the amniotic fluid specimens. Maternal stage of disease (primary, secondary, early latent) correlated with fetal infection rates of 50%, 67%, and 83%, respectively. γ-Glutamyl transpeptidase was elevated in 79% of fetuses compared with aspartate aminotransferase elevation in only 58% of cases. The authors recommend ultrasound examination as an important tool in the diagnosis and management of the syphilis-infected gravida and her unborn child. The authors conclude that the pathophysiologic disease process begins with hepatic and placental involvement, followed by amniotic fluid infection and the development of hematologic abnormalities. The intrauterine fetal demise of 1 of the 24 fetuses serves as a chilling reminder of the severity of devastation following infection with this relatively simple organism.

TABLE 49-2 RECOMMENDED TREATMENT REGIMENS* FOR *TREPONEMA PALLIDUM* INFECTIONS

Primary, Secondary, Early Latent Disease

Benzathine penicillin G, 2.4 million U IM as a single dose

Children: 50,000 U/kg IM (maximum, 2.4 million U) as a single dose

Late Latent and Latent Disease of Unknown Duration

Benzathine penicillin G, 2.4 million U IM weekly for 3 doses (7.2 million U total)

Children: 50,000 U/kg IM weekly for 3 doses (maximum, 150,000 U/kg or 7.2 million U)

Penicillin Allergy (Documented)

Pregnancy: desensitization and penicillin therapy as above

Nonpregnant:

- Doxycycline, 100 mg PO twice daily for 2 weeks, or tetracycline, 500 mg PO four times a day for 2 weeks†
- Ceftriaxone, 1 g IM or IV daily for 8-10 days†
- Azithromycin, 2 g PO as a single dose†

Tertiary Disease

Neurosyphilis: aqueous crystalline penicillin G, 18-24 million U IV daily (3-4 million U every 4 hours or continuous infusion) for 10-14 days

Alternative: procaine penicillin, 2.4 million U IM once daily, with probenecid, 500 mg PO four times a day for 10-14 days

No neurosyphilis: benzathine penicillin G, 2.4 million U IM weekly for 3 weeks (7.2 million U total)

From Centers for Disease Control and Prevention: Sexually transmitted diseases treatment guidelines 2006. MMWR Morb Mortal Wkly Rep 55:1, 2006.

*The Centers for Disease Control and Prevention recommend penicillin as the treatment of choice in individuals with syphilis.

†Efficacy data are limited.

TABLE 49-3 RECOMMENDED TREATMENT REGIMENS* FOR *CHLAMYDIA TRACHOMATIS* INFECTIONS

Recommended Regimen

Azithromycin, 1 g orally in a single dose, *or*

Doxycycline, 100 mg orally twice a day for 7 days

Alternative Regimens

Erythromycin base, 500 mg orally four times a day for 7 days, *or*

Erythromycin ethylsuccinate, 800 mg orally four times a day for 7 days, *or*

Ofloxacin, 300 mg orally twice a day for 7 days, *or*

Levofloxacin, 500 mg orally for 7 days

Modified from the Centers for Disease Control and Prevention: Sexually transmitted diseases treatment guidelines 2002. MMWR Morb Mortal Wkly Rep 51:1, 2002.

*The Centers for Disease Control and Prevention recommend treating persons with a positive sensitive nucleic acid amplification chlamydia test. Although tetracycline and doxycycline have the greatest activity against *Chlamydia trachomatis*, these drugs should not be used in pregnancy because of their enamel effects. Owing to gastrointestinal side effects with erythromycin, azithromycin is the drug of choice in pregnancy.

TREATMENT

Chlamydia

The recommended treatment regimen for uncomplicated genital chlamydia infection has remained unchanged since 1998. **The CDC recommends either azithromycin, 1 g in a single oral dose, or doxycycline, 100 mg orally twice a day for 7 days** (Table 49-3). Although the results of clinical trials indicate that azithromycin and doxycycline are equally efficacious, single-dose treatment maximizes compliance.[56] To minimize transmission and reinfection, patients should be instructed to abstain from sexual intercourse for 7 days after single-dose therapy or until completion of a 7-day regimen and should also be instructed to abstain from sexual intercourse until all of their sex partners have been treated. Longitudinal studies of chlamydia-infected adolescent female patients demonstrate a high risk for chlamydia reinfection and other STD infections within a few months of initial diagnosis. Because of the high incidence of chlamydia infection that can occur in the months following a treated infection, CDC guidelines suggest that providers consider the repeat screening of chlamydia-infected female patients 3 to 4 months after treatment.

Gonorrhea

Although uncomplicated genital gonorrhea infections can be treated with single-dose therapy, there are fewer oral treatment options compared with efficacious therapy in chlamydial infections (Table 49-4). Moreover, recent emergence of quinolone-resistant *N. gonorrhoeae* in California, Hawaii, Asia, and the Pacific Islands has led to the generalized recommendation that these agents should not be used to treat gonorrhea infections acquired in these areas or in areas with an increased prevalence of quinolone resistance.[44] The CDC recommendations became somewhat complicated in July 2002, when Wyeth Pharmaceuticals (Collegeville, PA) discontinued cefixime. In the absence of cefixime, the primary recommended treatment option for gonorrhea in Hawaii and California is ceftriaxone.[44] In addition, because of the risk for coinfectivity with *N. gonorrhoeae* and *C. trachomatis*, the CDC recommends empirically treating patients with positive gonorrhea test results for both gonorrhea and chlamydia.[44]

In 2007 the Gonococcal Isolate Surveillance Project (GISP) found 27% of *N. gonorrhoeae* infections were resistant to penicillin, tetracycline, ciprofloxacin, or a combination of these antibiotics. In 2009, a CDC Working Group for Cephalosporin-Resistant Gonorrhea Outbreak Response Plan was convened to address the growing resistance to these antibiotics by *N. gonorrhoeae*.[57] The CDC in their *Morbidity and Mortality Weekly Report* dated May 13, 2011 reviewed five cases of urethral gonorrhea with high mean inhibitory capacities (9.1%) of azithromycin representing 10% of those treated for *N. gonorrhoeae* in San Diego County August to October 2009.[58] In this monograph they reinforce the 2010 STD Treatment Guidelines recommending dual therapy with 250 mg ceftriaxone and either 1 g of azithromycin orally or 100 mg of doxycycline twice daily for 7 days for uncomplicated urogenital, rectal, and pharyngeal gonorrhea. The CDC does not recommend azithromycin as monotherapy in the treatment of gonorrhea. If azithromycin is prescribed because of cephalosporin allergy, a 2-g oral dose is recommended, with a test of cure performed 1 week after treatment. Culture is recommended, and if not available, a NAAT should be performed. If the NAAT is positive, a culture should be obtained.

TABLE 49-4 RECOMMENDED TREATMENT REGIMEN* FOR UNCOMPLICATED GENITAL *NEISSERIA GONORRHOEAE* INFECTIONS

Ceftriaxone, 250 mg IM in a single dose, *plus*
Azithromycin, 1 g orally in a single dose, *or*
Doxycycline, 100 mg orally twice a day for 7 days

Modified from the Centers for Disease Control and Prevention: Sexually transmitted diseases treatment guidelines 2002. MMWR Morb Mortal Wkly Rep 51:1, 2002.

*The Centers for Disease Control and Prevention recommend treating persons with a positive gonorrhea test result for both gonorrhea and chlamydia unless a negative result has been obtained with a sensitive nucleic acid amplification chlamydia test.

Syphilis

It was not long after the introduction of penicillin about the time of WWII that it became recognized as the primary antimicrobial for the treatment of syphilis. **Penicillin has been effective in the treatment of disease and in the prevention of disease progression in both nonpregnant and pregnant women as well as in the prevention and treatment of congenital syphilis** (see Table 49-2).[49,56] CDC 2006 treatment guidelines recommend benzathine penicillin G, 2.4 million U IM as a single dose, for primary, secondary, and early latent syphilis in both pregnant and nonpregnant women.[51] Likewise, children are treated with benzathine penicillin G, 50,000 U/kg IM (maximum dose, 2.4 million U as a single dose). Late latent syphilis and latent syphilis of unknown duration are treated with 2.4 million U IM benzathine penicillin G weekly for three doses (7.2 million U total).[49] Children, in turn, are treated with 50,000 U/kg weekly for 3 doses (150,000 U/kg or 7.2 million U maximum) for late latent and latent syphilis of unknown duration.

Individuals with documented allergies to penicillin present a particular treatment problem. Treatment recommendations differ as to whether the individual is pregnant or not. For early disease in nonpregnant women, doxycycline, 100 mg by mouth (PO) twice daily for 2 weeks (tetracycline, 500 mg four times daily) has been used with little available data. Alternatively, ceftriaxone, 1 g IM or intravenously (IV) daily for 8 to 10 days, or azithromycin, 2 g PO as a single dose may be effective. These alternatives should not be considered in individuals who are HIV positive, noncompliant, or pregnant. These aforementioned individuals should undergo penicillin desensitization and penicillin therapy.

Therapy for tertiary syphilis is dependent on the presence or absence of neurosyphilis. Provided CSF examination is negative, individuals are treated with benzathine penicillin G, 2.4 million U IM weekly for 3 weeks (7.2 million U total).[49] If neurosyphilis has been diagnosed, then aqueous crystalline penicillin G, 18 to 24 million U IV daily (3 to 4 million U every 4 hours or continuous infusion) for 10 to 14 days is given. An alternative therapy in compliant individuals is procaine penicillin, 2.4 million U IM once daily, with probenecid, 500 mg orally four times a day for 10 to 14 days. Follow-up CSF evaluation is recommended to assess response to therapy. Attempts at targeted mass treatment for syphilis in populations at risk to reduce outbreaks and ultimately congenital syphilis have met with failure.[59]

The implementation of appropriate screening and treatment of pregnant women should theoretically result in the elimination of congenital syphilis.[37,43] Unfortunately, children continue to be born with increased prematurity, low birthweight, hepatomegaly, and cutaneous and bone lesions in developed as well as developing nations.[48] Almost 90% of stillbirths attributed to congenital syphilis occur among women who are never treated or inappropriately treated.[60] Alexander and colleagues examined the CDC guidelines for the treatment of maternal syphilis among 340 gravidas and found better than 95% success for all stages of clinical disease in preventing congenital disease.[61] Sheffield and associates[62] evaluated 43 women who received antepartum therapy with treatment failure. Her work revealed that preterm delivery (<36 weeks), short interval between treatment and delivery, higher VDRL titer at time of treatment and delivery, and early stage of maternal disease were associated with treatment failure. The optimal management (transplacental vs. neonatal) of the fetus with severe or advanced clinical disease remains unknown and requires consultation with experienced clinicians.[63]

KEY POINTS

- Sexually active adolescents have higher rates of sexually transmitted diseases than any other age groups.
- Marked racial disparity exists in the rates of chlamydia, gonorrhea, and syphilis, with the highest rates found among minority populations.
- Transmission and long-term sequelae of sexually transmitted diseases are greater in women than in men.
- Much of the end-organ damage seen with sexually transmitted disease is a result of the host's immune response and to a lesser extent is due to the invading organism itself.
- Even though *Treponema pallidum* and *Chlamydia trachomatis* lack the biosynthetic machinery necessary for life and thus are dependent on the host, they are masters at evading the host's immune system.
- Most cases of congenital syphilis in the United States should be preventable.
- *Neisseria gonorrhoeae* is a gram-negative diplococcus for which humans are the only natural hosts.
- Given concerns for antibiotic resistance, all cases of gonorrhea in the United States are confirmed by culture to allow susceptibility testing.
- Serologic testing for uncomplicated genital *C. trachomatis* infection has little or no value because previous infection elicits long-lasting antibody response.
- Penicillin is the antimicrobial of choice in treating syphilis among pregnant women and reducing the incidence of congenital syphilis.

REFERENCES

1. Wall KM, Khosropour CM, Sullivan PS: Centers for Disease Control and Prevention. Sexually Transmitted Disease Surveillance 2009. Atlanta, U.S. Department of Health and Human Services, 2010.
2. Hammerschlag MR, Anderka M, Semine DZ, et al: Prospective study of maternal and infantile infection with *Chlamydia trachomatis*. Pediatrics 64:142, 1979.
3. Mangione-Smith R, O'Leary J, McGlynn EA: Health and cost-benefits of Chlamydia screening in young women. Sex Transm Dis 26:309, 1999.
4. Sweet RL, Landers DV, Walker C, et al: *Chlamydia trachomatis* infection and pregnancy outcome. Am J Obstet Gynecol 156:824, 1987.
5. Schachter J, Grossman M, Sweet RL, et al: Prospective study of perinatal transmission of *Chlamydia trachomatis*. JAMA 255:3374, 1986.
6. Centers for Disease Control and Prevention: Racial Disparities in Nationally Notifiable Diseases-United States, 2002. MMWR Morb Mortal Wkly Rep 54:9, 2005.
7. Sweet RL, Gibbs R: Sexually transmitted diseases. In Sweet R, Gibbs R (eds): Infectious Diseases of the Female Reproductive Tract, 4th ed. Philadelphia, Lippincott Williams & Wilkins, 2002, p 118.
8. Hook EW, Handsfield HA: Gonococcal infections in adults. In Holmes KK, Sparling PF, Mardh P-A, et al (eds): Sexually Transmitted Diseases. New York, McGraw-Hill, 1999, p 451.
9. Ickovics JR, Niccolai LM, Lewis JB, et al: High postpartum rates of sexually transmitted infections among teens: pregnancy as a window of opportunity for prevention. Sex Transm Infect 79:469, 2003.
10. Centers for Disease Control and Prevention: Summary of notifiable diseases, United States 1992. MMWR Morb Mortal Wkly Rep 41:1, 1993.
11. Aral SO, Holmes KK: Social and behavioral determinants of the epidemiology of STDs: industrialized and developing countries. In Holmes KK, Sparling PF, Mardh P-A, et al (eds): Sexually Transmitted Diseases. New York, McGraw-Hill, 1999, p 39.
12. Centers for Disease Control and Prevention: Primary and secondary syphilis: United States 2002. MMWR Morb Mortal Wkly Rep 52:1117, 2003.
13. Kaplan J: National syphilis elimination launch: Nashville, Tennessee, Oct 7, 1999: Syphilis elimination: History in the making-opening remarks (From the CDC). Sex Transm Dis 27:63, 2000.
14. Stamm WE: *Chlamydia trachomatis* infections of the adult. In Holmes KK, Sparling PF, Mardh P-A, et al (eds): Sexually Transmitted Diseases. New York, McGraw-Hill, 1999, p 407.
15. Sweet RS, Gibbs R: Chlamydial Infections. In Sweet R, Gibbs R (eds): Infectious Diseases of the Female Reproductive Tract, ed 4. Philadelphia, Lippincott Williams & Wilkins, 2002, p 57.
16. Schachter J: Chlamydial infections. N Engl J Med 298:428, 1978.
17. Sweet RS, Schachter J, Landers DV: Chlamydial infections in obstetrics and gynecology. Clin Obstet Gynecol 26:143, 1983.
18. Friis RR: Interaction of L cells and *Chlamydia psittaci:* entry of the parasite and host responses to its development. J Bacteriol 110:706, 1972.
19. Kuo CC, Wang SP, Grayson JT: Effect of polycations, polyanions, and neuraminidase on the infectivity of trachoma-inclusion conjunctivitis and LGV organisms in HeLa cells: sialic acid residues as possible receptors for trachoma-inclusion conjunctivitis. Infect Immun 8:74, 1973.
20. Nurminen M, Leinonen M, Saikku P, et al: The genus-specific antigen of chlamydias resembles to the lipopolysaccharide of enteric bacteria. Science 220:1279, 1983.
21. Bavoil PH, Ohlin A, Schachter J: Role of disulfide bonding in outer membrane structure and permeability in *Chlamydia trachomatis*. Infect Immun 44:479, 1984.
22. Schachter J: Biology of *Chlamydia trachomatis*. In Holmes KK, Sparling PF, Mardh P-A, et al (eds): Sexually Transmitted Diseases. New York, McGraw-Hill, 1999, p 391.
23. Brunham RC, Peeling RW: *Chlamydia trachomatis* antigens: role in immunity and pathogenesis. Infect Agents Dis 3:218, 1994.
24. Brunham RC, Plummer F, Stephens RS: Bacterial antigenic variation, host immune response and pathogen-host co-evolution. Infect Immun 61:2273, 1994.
25. Brunham R, Yang C, Maclean I, et al: *Chlamydia trachomatis* from individuals in a sexually transmitted disease core group exhibit frequent sequence variation in the major outer membrane protein (omp1) gene. J Clin Invest 94:458, 1994.
26. Morrison RP, Manning DS, Caldwell HD: Immunology of *Chlamydia trachomatis* infections: immunoprotective and immunopathologic responses. In Gallin JI, Fauci AS, Quinn TC (eds): Advances in Host Defense Mechanisms, Vol. 8: Sexually Transmitted Diseases. New York, Raven Press, 1992, p 57.
27. Hayes LJ, Bailey RL, Mabey DCW, et al: Genotyping of *Chlamydia trachomatis* from a trachoma endemic village in the Gambia by a

nested polymerase chain reaction: identification of strain variants. J Infect Dis 166:1173, 1992.

28. Conway DJ, Holland MJ, Campbell AE, et al: HLA class I and class II polymorphism and trachomatous scarring in a *Chlamydia trachomatis*-endemic population. J Infect Dis 174:643, 1996.
29. Kimani J, Maclean IW, Bwayo JJ, et al: Risk factors for *Chlamydia trachomatis* pelvic inflammatory disease among sex workers in Nairobi, Kenya. J Infect Dis 173:1437, 1996.
30. Brunham RC, Maclean IW, Binns B, Peeling RW: *Chlamydia trachomatis:* its role in tubal infertility. J Infect Dis 152:1275, 1985.
31. Sparling PF: Biology of *Neisseria gonorrhoeae*. In Holmes KK, Sparling PF, Mardh P-A, et al (eds): Sexually Transmitted Diseases. New York, McGraw-Hill, 1999, p 433.
32. Stokes JH, Beerman H, Ingraham NR: Modern Clinical Syphilology, Diagnosis and Treatment: Case Study, 3rd ed. Philadelphia, WB Saunders, 1945.
33. Lukehart SA, Hook EW III, Baker-Zander SA, et al: Invasion of central nervous system by *Treponema pallidum:* implications for diagnosis and treatment. Ann Intern Med 109:855, 1988.
34. Tranont EC: Syphilis in adults: from Christopher Columbus to Sir Alexander Flemming to AIDS. Clin Infect Dis 21:1361, 1995.
35. Harter CA, Bernirsche K: Fetal syphilis in the first trimester. Am J Obstet Gynecol 124:705, 1976.
36. Nathan L, Bohman VR, Sanchez PJ, et al: In utero infection with *Treponema pallidum* in early pregnancy. Prenat Diagn 17:119, 1997.
37. Ingraham NR: The value of penicillin alone in the prevention and treatment of congenital syphilis. Acta Derm Venereol 31:60, 1951.
38. Zenker PN, Berman SM: Congenital syphilis: trends and recommendations for evaluation and management. Pediatr Infect Dis J 10:516, 1991.
39. Fiumara NJ, Flemming WL, Downing JG, et al: The incidence of prenatal syphilis at the Boston City Hospital. N Engl J Med 247:48, 1952.
40. Radolf JD, Steiner B, Shevchenko D: *Treponema pallidum:* doing a remarkable job with what it's got. Trends Microbiol 7:7, 1999.
41. Pennisi E: Genome reveals wiles and weak points of syphilis. Science 281:324, 1998.
42. Weinstock GM, Hardham JM, McLeod MP, et al: The genome of *Treponema pallidum:* new light on the agent of syphilis. FEMS Microbiol Rev 22:323, 1998.
43. Berman SM: Maternal syphilis: pathophysiology and treatment. Bull World Health Org 82:1, 2004.
44. Johnson RE, Newhall WJ, Papp JR, et al: Centers for Disease Control and Prevention. Screening tests to detect *Chlamydia trachomatis* and *Neisseria gonorrhea* infections—2002. MMWR Morb Mortal Wkly Rep 51:1, 2002.
45. Baum EW, Bernhardt M, Sams WM Jr, et al: Secondary syphilis. Still the great imitator. JAMA 249:3069, 1983.
46. Larsen SA, Hunter EF, Creighton ET: Syphilis. In Holmes KK, Mardh P-A, Sparling PF, et al (eds): Sexually Transmitted Diseases. New York, McGraw-Hill, 1990, p 927.
47. Burstain JM, Grimprel E, Lukehart SA, et al: Sensitive detection of *Treponema pallidum* by using the polymerase chain reaction. J Clin Microbiol 29:62, 1991.
48. Saloojee H, Velaphi S, Goga Y, et al: The prevention and management of congenital syphilis: an overview and recommendations. Bull World Health Org 82:424, 2004.
49. Centers for Disease Control and Prevention: Sexually transmitted diseases treatment guidelines. MMWR Morb Mortal Wkly Rep 55:1, 2006.
50. Lubiganon P, Piaggio G, Villar J, et al: The epidemiology of syphilis in pregnancy. Int J STD AIDS 13:486, 2002.
51. Hicks CB, Benson PM, Lupton, GP, Tramont EC: Seronegative secondary syphilis in a patient infected with the human immunodeficiency (HIV) with Kaposi sarcoma: a diagnostic dilemma. Ann Intern Med 107:492, 1987.
52. Centers for Disease Control: Current trends: recommendations for diagnosing and treating syphilis in HIV-infected patients. MMWR Morb Mortal Wkly Rep 37:600, 1988.
53. Burton JR, Thorpe EM Jr, Shaver DC, et al: Nonimmune hydrops fetalis associated with maternal infection with syphilis. Am J Obstet Gynecol 167:56, 1992.
54. Jacobs A, Rotenberg O: Nonimmune hydrops fetalis due to congenital syphilis associated with negative intrapartum maternal serology screening. Am J Perinatol 15:233, 1998.
55. Hollier LM, Harstad TW, Sanchez PJ, et al: Fetal syphilis: clinical and laboratory characteristics. Obstet Gynecol 97:947, 2001.
56. Ingraham NR: The value of penicillin alone in the prevention and treatment of congenital syphilis. Acta Derm Venereol Suppl (Stock) 31:60, 1951.
57. Consultation Meeting on Cephalosporin-Resistant Gonorrhea Outbreak Response Plan. Report of an external consultants' meeting convened by the Division of STD Prevention, National Center for HIV, STD, and TB Prevention, Centers for Disease Control and Prevention (CDC), September 14-15, 2009:1-12.
58. Centers for Disease Control and Prevention: *Neisseria gonorrhoeae* with reduced susceptibility to azithromycin—San Diego County, California, 2009. MMWR Morb Mortal Wkly Rep 60:579, 2011.
59. Rekart ML, Patrick DM, Chakraborty B, et al: Targeted mass treatment for syphilis with oral azithromycin. Lancet 361:313, 2003.
60. Gust DA, Levine WC, St Louis ME, et al: Mortality associated with congenital syphilis in the United State, 1992-1998. Pediatrics 109:E79, 2002.
61. Alexander JM, Sheffield JS, Sanchez PJ, et al: Efficacy of treatment for syphilis in pregnancy. Obstet Gynecol 93:5, 1999.
62. Sheffield JS, Sanchez PJ, Morris G, et al: Congenital syphilis after maternal treatment for syphilis during pregnancy. Am J Obstet Gynecol 186:569, 2002.
63. Wendel GD Jr, Sheffield JS, Hollier LM, et al: Treatment of syphilis in pregnancy and prevention of congenital syphilis. Clin Infect Dis 35:S200, 2002.

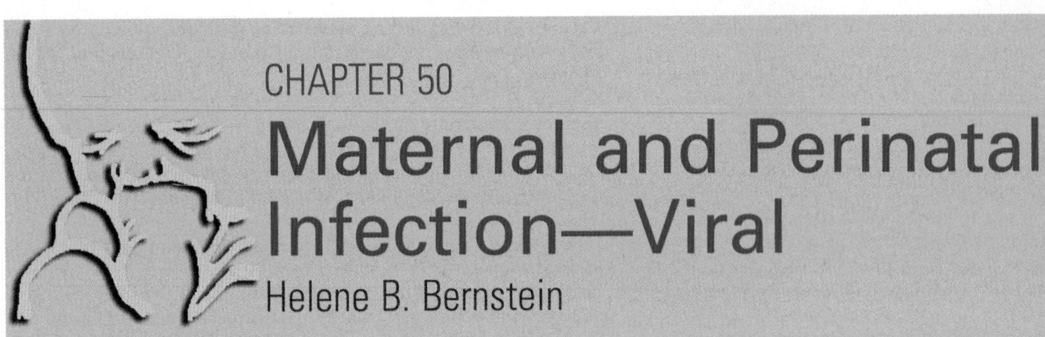

CHAPTER 50

Maternal and Perinatal Infection—Viral

Helene B. Bernstein

KEY ABBREVIATIONS

Acquired Immunodeficiency Syndrome	AIDS
AIDS Clinical Trials Group	ACTG
Antiretroviral	ARV
Antiretroviral Therapy	ART
American Congress of Obstetricians and Gynecologists	ACOG
CC-Chemokine Receptor Type 5	CCR5
Centers for Disease Control and Prevention	CDC
Central Nervous System	CNS
Chorionic Villous Sampling	CVS
Congenital Rubella Syndrome	CRS
Congenital Varicella Syndrome	CVS
C-X-C Chemokine Receptor Type 4	CXCR4
Cytomegalovirus	CMV
Deoxyribonucleic Acid	DNA
Disseminated Intravascular Coagulopathy	DIC
Efavirenz	EFV
Enzyme-Linked Immunosorbent Assay	ELISA
Epstein-Barr Virus	EBV
Erythema Infectiosum	EI
Glycoprotein	gp
Hemagglutinin	HA or H
Hepatitis A Virus	HAV
Hepatitis B Core Antigen	HBcAg
Hepatitis B Immune Globulin	HBIg
Hepatitis B Surface Antigen	HBsAg
Hepatitis B Virus	HBV
Hepatitis C Virus	HCV
Hepatitis Delta Antigen	HDAg
Hepatitis Delta Virus	HDV
Herpes Simplex Virus	HSV
Human Immunodeficiency Virus	HIV
Human Papillomavirus	HPV
Immune Reconstitution Inflammatory Syndromes	IRIS
Immunoglobulin	Ig
Intrauterine Growth Restriction	IUGR
Intravenous	IV
Lamivudine	3TC
Long Terminal Repeat	LTR
Measles, Mumps, Rubella	MMR
Mother to Child Transmission	MTCT
Mycobacterium Avium Complex	MAC
Neuraminidase	N or NA

Nevirapine	NVP
Non-nucleoside Reverse Transcriptase Inhibitors	NNRTIs
Nucleic Acid Test	NAT
Nucleoside Reverse Transcriptase Inhibitors	NRTIs
Opportunistic Infections	OI
Papanicolaou Smear	Pap Smear
Polymerase Chain Reaction	PCR
Protease Inhibitors	PIs
Rapid Influenza Diagnostic Tests	RIDTs
Recombinant Immunoblot Assay	RIBA
Reverse Transcriptase	RT
Ribonucleic Acid	RNA
Sexually Transmitted Diseases	STDs
Subacute Sclerosing Panencephalitis	SSPE
Tuberculin Skin Test	PPD
Tuberculosis	TB
Varicella Zoster Immune Globulin	VZIG
Varicella Zoster Virus	VZV
West Nile Virus	WNV
Zidovudine	AZT

Viruses have been identified in virtually all living organisms. They are among the simplest of living organisms, yet they have significantly shaped our history and remain an important causative factor for infectious disease. Viruses are obligate intracellular parasites, utilizing the host cell's structural and functional components for replication, while exhibiting remarkably diverse strategies for gene expression and replication. Viral infection ranges from asymptomatic and/or subclinical to overwhelming and highly lethal, with findings such as meningoencephalitis or hemorrhagic fever with shock. The duration of viral infection is also highly variable; many viruses are limited to acute infection, whereas some viruses can establish chronic and/or latent infection. Latent viruses can reactivate their gene expression many years after acute infection. Retroviruses can integrate into the host cell genome; and some viruses have demonstrated oncogenic potential.

Virus particles contain nucleic acid and structural proteins which together are referred to as a nucleocapsid. Viral nucleic acid is composed of either deoxyribonucleic acid (DNA) or ribonucleic acid (RNA), which may be single or double stranded. Viral genomes can be linear or circular, existing in multiple segments or as a single segment. Viral genome size ranges from two genes in parvovirus B19 to more than 200 genes in cytomegalovirus. Some viruses have lipid bilayer envelopes external to the nucleocapsid; these envelopes are derived from the host cell and contain viral proteins. Herpesviruses have an additional layer, called a tegument, between the nucleocapsid and envelope.

Viruses are classified by the International Committee on Taxonomy of Viruses into Orders, Families, Subfamilies, Genera, and Species. Classification is based on morphology, nucleic acid type, the presence or absence of an envelope, genome replication strategy, and homology to other identified viruses.

Infection is typically initiated by the virus binding to a specific host cell receptor. These receptors are normally functional host cell membrane proteins, but are also recognized by a viral protein ligand within the viral envelope or nucleocapsid. The viral protein and cellular receptor interaction defines, in part, the host-range of the virus; limiting infection to cells displaying the appropriate receptor. Virus then penetrates the host cell via translocation of the virion across the plasma membrane, involving endocytosis or fusion of the viral envelope with the cell membrane. The virus then uncoats its nucleic acid for replication, ultimately leading to viral gene expression and replication. This may occur in either the cytoplasm or nucleus of the cell and may involve integration into the host genome, in the case of retroviruses. Intracellular assembly of progeny virions occurs, followed by release of newly formed virions by cell lysis or by budding from the cell surface, in the case of most enveloped viruses.

Despite their inability to replicate independently, viruses play an important role in infectious disease. For productive infection to occur, viruses must enter cells, replicate their genome, and release infectious virions. The inability of a virus to complete any of these required steps results in a "nonproductive infection"; by default most viruses alter the structure and/or function of the host cell. Viral pathogenesis does not require productive infection and is mediated via several mechanisms. These include direct effects on infected host cells, which may result in cell death via lysis or apoptosis. Infected cells can also be killed by antiviral antibody and complement or by cell-mediated immune mechanisms. In addition, some viral genomes encode oncogenes that can mediate transformation of infected host cells. Viral proteins can also affect the function of uninfected cells, including the immune system. Finally, the host immune response to viral infection encompasses both local and systemic effects via activation of immune cells, the induction of an adaptive immune response, and the release of cytokines, chemokines, and antibodies. Thus the immune response contributes to or causes the signs and symptoms associated with viral infections, including fever, rash, arthralgias, and myalgias. The outcome of viral infection is dependent on host factors including immune status, age, nutritional status, and genetic background. Genetic factors can alter susceptibility to viral infection, the immune response generated following infection, and the long-term consequences of viral infection.

This chapter discusses many of the viral infections relevant to pregnancy (i.e., those that can have significant impact on maternal health and/or pregnancy outcome). The virology, epidemiology, diagnosis, clinical manifestations, management during pregnancy, and impact on the fetus/neonate are detailed for the viruses listed in Table 50-1.

HUMAN IMMUNODEFICIENCY VIRUS

Virology

Human immunodeficiency virus (HIV) is a member of the Retroviridae family, which is characterized by spherical, enveloped viruses. The virus envelope surrounds an icosahedral capsid containing the viral genome, consisting of

TABLE 50-1 SUMMARY OF ETIOLOGY, DIAGNOSIS, AND MANAGEMENT OF MAJOR PERINATAL VIRAL INFECTIONS

	COMPLICATIONS		DIAGNOSIS		TREATMENT/MANAGEMENT	
Virus	**Maternal**	**Fetal/ Neonatal**	**Maternal**	**Fetal/ Neonatal**	**Maternal**	**Fetal/Neonatal**
HIV	Opportunistic infection	Perinatal infection	Antibody detection	PCR	Combination ART*	ART to prevent perinatal transmission*
Influenza	Pneumonia, increased maternal mortality	N/A	RIPT screening, RT-PCR or immunofluorescence for diagnosis	N/A	Osteltamivir for prophylaxis and treatment, supportive care, vaccinate annually	None
Parvovirus B19	Rare	Anemia/hydrops/ death	PCR or antibody detection	PCR, ultrasound for anemia	Supportive care	Intrauterine transfusion for severe anemia
Rubeola measles	Otitis media, pneumonia, encephalitis	Abortion, preterm delivery	RT-PCR or antibody detection	N/A	Supportive care, prevention-vaccinate prior to pregnancy	N/A
Rubella	Rare	Congenital infection	Antibody detection or RT-PCR	RT-PCR, ultrasound for congenital rubella syndrome	Supportive care, prevention-vaccinate prior to pregnancy	Consider pregnancy termination for fetus with CRS*
CMV	Chorioretinitis	Congenital infection	PCR	PCR, ultrasound for detection of sequelae	Ganciclovir for severe infection	Consider pregnancy termination for infected fetus with primary maternal infection*
HSV	Disseminated infection, primarily in immunocompromised patients	Neonatal infection, intrauterine infection is extremely rare	Examination, PCR, antibody detection	Examination, PCR, antibody detection	Antiviral Tx for infection and prophylaxis against recurrent outbreaks*	Cesarean delivery when mother has active genital lesions
Varicella	Pneumonia, encephalitis, zoster	Congenital or perinatal infection	History, PCR, antibody detection	Ultrasound	VZIG, antivirals for prophylaxis and/or treatment	VZIG, antivirals for prophylaxis and/or treatment
Hepatitis A	Rare	None	RT-PCR or antibody detection	N/A	Supportive care, prevention-hepatitis A vaccine	Immune globulin to neonate if mother acutely infected at delivery
Hepatitis B	Chronic liver disease	Neonatal infection	Surface antigen detection, PCR	N/A	Supportive care, prevention-hepatitis B vaccine, HBIg for exposed, susceptible individuals	HBIg+ hepatitis B vaccine immediately following delivery
Hepatitis C	Chronic liver disease	Neonatal infection	ELISA screen followed by RIBA, PCR	N/A	Supportive care	None
Hepatitis D	Chronic liver disease	Neonatal infection	Antigen and antibody detection		Supportive care	HBIg+ hepatitis B vaccine immediately following delivery
Hepatitis E	Increased mortality	Neonatal infection	RT-PCR, antibody detection	N/A	Supportive care	None

*See text for detailed discussion of patient management.

ART, Antiretroviral therapy; *CMV,* cytomegalovirus; *CNS,* central nervous system; *HBIg,* hepatitis B immune globulin; *HIV,* human immunodeficiency virus; *HSV,* herpes simplex virus; *PCR,* polymerase chain reaction; *RT-PCR,* reverse transcriptase PCR; *VZIG,* varicella zoster immune globulin.

two identical pieces of positive sense, single-stranded RNA, about 9.2 kb long. HIV has three main genes: gag, pol, and env, which are surrounded by long terminal repeat (LTR) regions, and a total of nine genes. The gag gene encodes the precursor for the virion capsid proteins, which include the full-length p55 polyprotein precursor and its cleavage products: p17 matrix, p24 capsid, p9 nucleocapsid, and p7. The pol gene encodes the precursor polyprotein for several viral enzymes including protease, reverse transcriptase, RNase H, and integrase. The env gene encodes the envelope glycoprotein (gp160), which is cleaved to the surface unit (gp120) and the transmembrane protein (gp41) that is necessary for fusion. Retroviruses are unique because the viral genome is transcribed into DNA via the viral enzyme reverse transcriptase, followed by integration into the host cell genome via the viral enzyme integrase. HIV also has the capacity to become latent within quiescent infected cells, making eradication of the virus thus far impossible.

The HIV envelope glycoprotein (gp120) is a ligand for CD4, the cellular HIV receptor; thus HIV predominantly infects CD4$^+$ cells, including T cells, monocytes, and macrophages. Coreceptors required for viral entry and infection have also been identified. The two primary HIV coreceptors are the chemokine receptors CXCR4 and CCR5.[1] New infections almost always occur with an HIV strain utilizing the CCR5 coreceptor,[2] potentially reflecting viral fitness. Individuals homozygous for a 32-base pair deletion within the CCR5 gene are much less likely to become HIV-infected, even following significant exposure; moreover, some CCR5 polymorphisms correlate with disease progression of HIV in perinatally infected children and adults.[3,4]

Epidemiology

The CDC estimates that more than 1 million people in the United States are HIV infected, with 21% of infected individuals undiagnosed (or unaware of their infection).[5] Approximately 56,300 Americans are diagnosed with HIV infection annually; women account for 27% of new HIV infections and 25% of existing infections. Women typically acquire their HIV infection by heterosexual contact. Caucasian women have the highest percentage of HIV infections attributable to injection drug use (24%), whereas injection drug use accounts for 15% of HIV infections in Hispanic/Latinas and 13% in African American women. African American women have an HIV incidence rate approximately 15 times greater than that of Caucasian women and almost 4 times that of Hispanic women. Factors associated with an increased prevalence of HIV infection (and HIV transmission risk) include the following: a high number of sexual contacts, high-risk sexual exposure, receptive anal intercourse, sexual contact with an uncircumcised male, intravenous (IV) drug and/or crack cocaine use, residing in the "inner city," and the presence of other STDs, particularly those which cause genital ulcers (herpes, syphilis, chancroid).[6]

HIV infection is limited to humans and chimpanzees and most infections in the United States are caused by HIV-1. HIV-1 is divided into three groups: M, N, and O. More than 95% of HIV-1 infections are caused by group M, which is divided into subtypes (or clades) A to K. The predominant type of HIV within the United States is clade B, whereas other clades predominate in other regions of the world. HIV-2, a related strain of HIV, is endemic in Africa, Portugal, and France and appears to have a lower vertical transmission rate compared to HIV-1.[7] Much less is known about the treatment of these related viruses given their prevalence in areas of the world where antiretroviral (ARV) treatment is not readily available.

Screening, Diagnosis, and Staging

Chronic HIV infection is diagnosed via detection of virus-specific antibody; diagnostic algorithms employ an initial screening assay followed by an antigen-specific confirmatory assay. The most commonly utilized serologic screen is the enzyme-linked immunosorbent assay (ELISA), which is highly sensitive, inexpensive, and well suited for large sample numbers. Positive ELISAs are repeated for verification, followed by Western blot confirmation or immunofluorescent antibody assay. The Western blot identifies antibodies recognizing specific viral antigens and is considered positive when any two of the following three antigens are identified: p24 (capsid), gp41 (envelope), and gp120/160 (envelope). Most serologic tests in use detect either HIV-1– or HIV-2–specific antibodies, and several salivary and/or rapid blood tests are available with efficacy comparable to ELISA.[8] Patients with early, acute HIV infection may not yet have detectable HIV-specific antibodies; therefore HIV viral load determination should be used for diagnosing acute HIV infection.[9] Any patient suspected of having the acute retroviral syndrome should have a repeat viral load and serologic assessment in 2 weeks. Although clinicians in the United States infrequently encounter patients infected with HIV-2 or a non–clade-B HIV-1 subtype, accurate diagnosis and plasma HIV RNA (viral load) assessment require assays capable of detecting the virus carried by the patient. Thus, consultation with an expert familiar with "atypical" HIV infection is warranted when caring for patients with an indeterminate HIV diagnosis and untreated patients with an undetectable viral load, particularly if HIV infection was acquired outside the United States or there is possible HIV-2 or nonclade-B HIV-1 infection.

Given the increasing prevalence of HIV infection and studies demonstrating that identification and early ARV treatment of HIV-infected pregnant women most effectively prevents perinatal HIV transmission, both the American Congress of Obstetricians and Gynecologists (ACOG) and the CDC recommend an "opt out" approach ensuring routine HIV screening for all pregnant women, ideally performed at the first prenatal visit. The CDC also advocates for repeat testing in the third trimester, citing its cost effectiveness even in areas of low prevalence.[10] A second HIV test in the third trimester is recommended for women at increased risk of HIV infection and women living in areas of elevated HIV incidence including residents of Alabama, Connecticut, Delaware, the District of Columbia, Florida, Georgia, Illinois, Louisiana, Maryland, Massachusetts, Mississippi, Nevada, New Jersey, New York, North Carolina, Pennsylvania, Puerto Rico, Rhode Island, South Carolina, Tennessee, Texas, and Virginia, as well as women receiving health care in facilities in which

TABLE 50-2 STAGES OF HIV INFECTION

CDC STAGE	CD4+ T-LYMPHOCYTE COUNT AND PERCENTAGES
Stage 1 (HIV infection)	CD4+ T-lymphocyte count of ≥500 cells/μL or % of ≥29
Stage 2 (HIV infection)	CD4+ T-lymphocyte count of 200-499 cells/μL or % of 14-29
Stage 3 (AIDS)	CD4+ T-lymphocyte count of <200 cells/μL or % of <14

prenatal screening identifies at least one HIV-infected pregnant woman per 1000 women screened.[10]

Clinical Manifestations and Staging

The clinical presentation of HIV infection and/or acquired immunodeficiency syndrome (AIDS) depends on when infection occurred and whether there is a resulting immunodeficiency. Following exposure and primary infection, 50% to 70% of individuals infected with HIV develop the acute retroviral syndrome. At this time patients may have "mononucleosis-like" symptoms, including fever, rigors, pharyngitis, arthralgias, myalgias, maculopapular rash, urticaria, abdominal cramps, diarrhea, headache, and lymphocytic meningitis. The acute phase of infection usually occurs 4 to 6 weeks following HIV exposure and can last several weeks; however, it is uncommon for individuals to be diagnosed during acute infection. Following primary HIV infection, patients enter the latent phase of illness, which can last approximately 5 to 10 years in untreated patients and comprises stages 1 and 2 of infection (Table 50-2). During this asymptomatic phase of infection, in the absence of antiretroviral therapy (ART) there is chronic immune activation and progressive destruction of lymphatic tissue.[11] If untreated, most patients will develop stage 3 infection, AIDS, typically including one or more of the conditions listed in the box, AIDS-Defining Conditions in Adults.

AIDS-DEFINING CONDITIONS IN ADULTS

Candidiasis of bronchi, trachea, or lungs
Candidiasis of esophagus*
Cervical cancer, invasive†
Coccidioidomycosis, disseminated or extrapulmonary
Cryptococcosis, extrapulmonary
Cryptosporidiosis, chronic intestinal (>1 month's duration)
Cytomegalovirus disease (other than liver, spleen, or nodes), onset at age >1 month
Cytomegalovirus retinitis (with loss of vision)*
Encephalopathy, HIV related
Herpes simplex: chronic ulcers (>1 month's duration) or bronchitis, pneumonitis, or esophagitis (onset at age >1 month)
Histoplasmosis, disseminated or extrapulmonary
Isosporiasis, chronic intestinal (>1 month's duration)
Kaposi sarcoma*
Lymphoid interstitial pneumonia or pulmonary lymphoid hyperplasia complex*
Lymphoma, Burkitt's (or equivalent term)
Lymphoma, immunoblastic (or equivalent term)
Lymphoma, primary, of brain
Mycobacterium avium complex or *Mycobacterium kansasii,* disseminated or extrapulmonary*
Mycobacterium tuberculosis of any site, pulmonary,*† disseminated,* or extrapulmonary*
Mycobacterium, other species or unidentified species, disseminated,* or extrapulmonary*
Pneumocystis jirovecii pneumonia*
Pneumonia, recurrent*†
Progressive multifocal leukoencephalopathy
Salmonella septicemia, recurrent
Toxoplasmosis of brain, onset at age >1 month*
Wasting syndrome attributed to HIV

*Condition that might be diagnosed presumptively.
†Only among adults and adolescents 13 years or older. (CDC: 1993 Revised classification system for HIV infection and expanded surveillance case definition for AIDS among adolescents and adults. MMWR 41[No. RR-17], 1992.)

Management During Pregnancy

Initial Evaluation

Beyond the standard initial antenatal assessment for all pregnant women, including a first trimester ultrasound to confirm gestational age, evaluation of an HIV-infected pregnant woman should include a status assessment as described in the box, Assessment of HIV Disease Status. Viral loads are typically determined using the Roche COBAS Amplicor Monitor, using reverse transcriptase polymerase chain reaction (RT-PCR) technology.[12] If the patient's HIV viral load is undetectable in the absence of treatment, retesting and/or using an alternative assay is recommended (bDNA signal amplification or a NASBA-based technique).[13] Some patients may have an undetectable viral load; however, the patient could be infected with a non–clade B HIV-1 isolate or HIV-2. None of the previously mentioned assays detect HIV-2 plasma RNA. Consultation with an infectious disease physician with experience in the management of HIV disease can be helpful in these cases or when the woman's genotype and phenotype assay demonstrate significant resistance to ART. Following complete evaluation, recommendations for a plan of HIV-related medical care, including antepartum, intrapartum, and postpartum care, should be provided, taking into account issues described in the following sections.

Ethical Considerations

Patients should be offered ART based on the same principles used for nonpregnant individuals, taking into account pregnancy-specific maternal or fetal safety issues. When caring for HIV-infected pregnant women, there are two separate but related goals: (1) treatment of maternal infection and (2) chemoprophylaxis to reduce the risk of perinatal HIV transmission. Providers caring for HIV-infected women may encounter patients declining to start or continue ART. For guidance, the author supports the recommendations of the Panel on Treatment of HIV-Infected Pregnant Women and Prevention of Perinatal Transmission.[14] In summary, the provider is responsible for providing information to enable the woman to make an informed choice regarding this and other medical recommendations (including elective cesarean delivery). Coercive and punitive policies potentially undermine trust and

Assessment of HIV Disease Status

1. HIV History Review:
   a. Duration of HIV infection, transmission route (if known), prior HIV-related illnesses and hospitalizations (including opportunistic infections), and immunization history.
   b. Prior and/or ongoing use, duration, and tolerance of ARV, including whether treatment was given for maternal benefit, and/or to prevent perinatal HIV transmission, and history of adherence issues.
   c. Outcome of HIV-affected pregnancies.
   d. Past CD4 cell counts and plasma HIV viral loads (plasma HIV RNA copy number/mL of plasma) and their relationship to ARV, and results of prior and current HIV ARV drug-resistance studies.
   e. Immunization/infection/serology status with attention to hepatitis B, hepatitis C, tuberculosis, and pneumococcus.
2. Laboratory Assessment:
   a. CD4 count and HIV viral load.
   b. ARV drug-resistance studies (genotype preferred), indicated prior to starting or modifying ARV regimens in patients with HIV RNA levels above the threshold for resistance testing (e.g., >500 to 1000 copies/mL).
   c. Baseline complete blood cell count with platelets, renal and liver function testing.
   d. Serologic assessment as indicated by history.
   e. HLA-B*5701 testing, if abacavir use is anticipated.
   f. In PPD positive patients, a chest x-ray should be performed to rule out active pulmonary disease.
   g. If CD4 count is <200, serology for cytomegalovirus and *Toxoplasma gondii*.
   h. If abnormal Pap smear—HPV testing and colposcopy as indicated.

the provider/patient relationship. Results can include the discontinuation of prenatal care or refusal (or failure) to disclose her HIV status to other health care providers, preventing the adoption of behaviors to enhance maternal and fetal well-being. Out of respect for patient autonomy, we consider it unethical to consider punitive actions against a patient secondary to her decisions regarding her HIV treatment or disclosure of her HIV status. Moreover, disclosure carries risks ranging from discrimination to intimate partner violence, making it critical to respect the patient's decision. Clinicians should be aware of local legal requirements regarding confidentiality and disclosure of HIV-related health information.

Treatment of HIV Infection During Pregnancy

Historically, the PACTG 076 study first showed that ART reduces perinatal HIV transmission.[15] This randomized, placebo-controlled study included treatment naïve, HIV-infected women with a CD4 count above 200/mm^3 beyond the first trimester of pregnancy. Treatment included prenatal oral zidovudine (AZT), IV AZT during labor, and following delivery infants within the treatment arm received oral AZT for 6 weeks; randomization was ethical secondary to the unknown safety (within pregnancy) and efficacy of AZT at the time the study was initiated. Interim data analysis revealed a substantially reduced risk of vertical HIV transmission (8.3% vs. 25.5% in placebo arm); subsequent studies have confirmed the efficacy of oral AZT and other nucleoside analog drugs in preventing perinatal HIV transmission.

Combination care with at least three drugs from at least two classes of ARV is the standard of care for HIV infection in the United States. Considerations include the following: timing of therapy initiation, dosing changes secondary to pregnancy-associated physiologic changes, side effects, drug interactions, teratogenicity, comorbidities, convenience and adherence potential, the results of genotypic resistance testing, and the pharmacokinetics and toxicity of transplacentally transferred drugs. Regimens containing antepartum and intrapartum maternal treatment and postpartum infant treatment provide the best protection against perinatal HIV transmission. This three-part regimen is superior to regimens not containing all three components. Maternal ART should be started as soon as feasible, following review of ARV resistance panel results, preferably prior to the second trimester. The European National Study of HIV in Pregnancy and Childhood demonstrated that with longer duration of antenatal ARV prophylaxis (starting prior to 28 weeks' gestation), each additional week of therapy corresponds to a 10% reduced risk of HIV transmission after adjusting for viral load, mode of delivery, and sex of the infant.[16] Moreover, expanding infant postexposure prophylaxis does not fully substitute for the protective effect of increased maternal ART duration. Women with undetectable viral loads should also receive combination ART because their risk of perinatal transmission is 9.8% if untreated.[17] ART-treated women who become pregnant should continue their medications; if a component of their regimen is contraindicated in pregnancy the regimen should be altered without therapy interruption. If pregnancy-associated vomiting interferes with ongoing adherence to therapy, antiemetics should be aggressively used prior to discontinuing therapy.

The most commonly used ARTs in pregnancy are described in Table 50-3; classes include nucleoside (and nucleotide) reverse transcriptase inhibitors (NRTIs), nonnucleoside reverse transcriptase inhibitors (NNRTIs), and protease inhibitors (PIs). The ideal regimen demonstrates durable virologic suppression with immunologic and clinical improvement, is well tolerated with a simple dosage regimen, and has been shown to be effective in pregnancy in terms of reducing perinatal HIV transmission. ARV drug combinations used today are more convenient and better tolerated than previously utilized regimens, resulting in greater efficacy and improved adherence. Up-to-date U.S. treatment recommendations are available at www.AIDSinfo.nih.gov, and the National Perinatal HIV Hotline (1-888-448-8765) provides free clinical consultation on all aspects of perinatal HIV care.[14]

Nuceloside Reverse Transcriptase Inhibitors

These drugs are used within combination regimens, usually including two NRTIs with either an NNRTI or a PI. Lamivudine (3TC) and AZT are preferred agents; together they comprise the dual-NRTI backbone recommended in pregnancy secondary to extensive experience. AZT should be included in pregnancy-based regimens whenever possible, because of its proven efficacy in

Table 50-3 Commonly Used Antiretroviral Drugs in Pregnancy[14]

ARV DRUG DOSAGE RECOMMENDATIONS	FDA PREGNANCY CATEGORY	ANIMAL STUDIES CARCINOGEN/ TERATOGEN	PHARMACOKINETICS IN PREGNANCY	CONCERNS IN PREGNANCY	RECOMMENDED USE IN PREGNANCY
NRTIs					
Preferred Agents					
Lamivudine (3TC) (Epivir) • 150 mg BID or 300 mg once daily	C	*Carcinogen:* Negative *Teratogen:* Negative	Pharmacokinetics not significantly altered in pregnancy; no change in dose indicated. High placental transfer to fetus.	No evidence of human teratogenicity (1.5-fold increase in birth defects ruled out). Well-tolerated, short-term safety demonstrated for mother and infant. If HBV co-infected, possible HBV flare if drug is stopped postpartum.	Because of extensive experience, 3TC and ZDV are the recommended dual NRTI backbone for pregnant women. Has antiviral activity against HBV.
Zidovudine (ZDV) (Retrovir) (AZT) • 300 mg BID	C	*Carcinogen:* Vaginal neoplasms in rodents. *Teratogen:* Increased resorption at extremely high dosage.	Not significantly altered in pregnancy; no change in dose indicated. High placental transfer to fetus.	No evidence of human teratogenicity (1.5-fold increase in birth defects ruled out). Well tolerated, short-term safety demonstrated for mother and infant. Associated with macrocytic anemia.	**Preferred** NRTI for use in combination ARV regimens in pregnancy based on efficacy studies and extensive experience; should be included in regimen unless significant toxicity, d4T use, resistance, or the women is already on a fully suppressive regimen.
Alternative Agents					
Abacavir (ABC) (Ziagen) • 300 mg BID or 600 mg once daily	C	*Carcinogen:* Thyroid tumors in female rats, and liver, preputial, and clitoral gland tumors of mice and rats. *Teratogen:* Developmental toxicity, anasarca and skeletal malformations at 35× human exposure during organogenesis.	Pharmacokinetics not significantly altered in pregnancy; no change in dose indicated. High placental transfer to fetus.	No evidence of human teratogenicity (2-fold increase in birth defects ruled out). Hypersensitivity reactions occur in ~5%-8% of nonpregnant persons; a much smaller percentage are fatal and are usually associated with rechallenge. Rate in pregnancy unknown. Patient should be educated regarding symptoms of hypersensitivity reaction; HLA-B*5701 testing identifies patients at risk.	Alternative NRTI for dual nucleoside backbone of combination regimens. Part of a triple NRTI regimen; however, this is less potent virologically and should only be used when NNRTI- or PI-based combination regimens cannot be used.
Didanosine (ddI) (Videx) • ≥60 kg: 400 mg once daily; *with TDF* 250 mg once daily • <60 kg: 250 mg daily; *with TDF* 200 mg once daily	B	*Carcinogen:* Negative *Teratogen:* Negative	Pharmacokinetics not significantly altered in pregnancy; no change in dose indicated. Moderate placental transfer to fetus.	Human birth defect rate was 4.7% (19 of 406), compared to 2.7% in the general population; no pattern of defects was discovered. Cases of lactic acidosis, some fatal, have been reported in pregnant women receiving ddI and d4T together.	Alternative NRTI for dual nucleoside backbone of combination regimens. ddI should be used with D4T only if no other alternatives are available.
Emtricitabine (FTC) (Emtriva) • Biologically active form of 3TC • 200 mg capsule once daily	B	*Carcinogen:* Negative *Teratogen:* Negative	Pharmacokinetic study shows slightly lower levels in third trimester compared to postpartum. No clear need to increase dose. High placental transfer to fetus.	No evidence of human teratogenicity (2-fold increase in birth defects ruled out). If HBV co-infected, possible HBV flare if drug is stopped postpartum.	Alternative NRTI for dual nucleoside backbone of combination regimens. Has antiviral activity against HBV.
Stavudine (d4T) (Zerit) • ≥60 kg: 40 mg BID • <60 kg: 30 mg BID	C	*Carcinogen:* Liver tumors in mice and bladder tumors in rats at very high doses. *Teratogen:* Negative, however incomplete ossification of sternebra at very high exposure.	Pharmacokinetics not significantly altered in pregnancy; no change in dose indicated. High placental transfer to fetus.	No evidence of human teratogenicity (2-fold increase in birth defects ruled out). Cases of lactic acidosis, some fatal, have been reported in pregnant women receiving ddI and d4T together.	Alternative NRTI for dual nucleoside backbone of combination regimens. d4T should not be used with ddI or AZT.

Tenofovir Disoproxil Fumarate (TDF) (Viread) • 300 mg once daily	B	*Carcinogen:* Liver adenomas in female mice at 16× human exposure. *Teratogen:* Negative, however primate exposure equivalent to 25× the human AUC show reduced fetal growth and bone porosity within 2 months of starting maternal therapy.	Limited studies in human pregnancy; data indicate AUC lower in third trimester than postpartum but trough levels adequate. High placental transfer to fetus.	No evidence of human teratogenicity (2-fold increase in birth defects ruled out). Clinical studies in humans (particularly children) show bone demineralization with chronic use; clinical significance unknown. If HBV co-infected, possible HBV flare is drug is stopped postpartum.	Alternative NRTI for dual-NRTI backbone of combination regimens. TDF would be a preferred NRTI in combination with 3TC or FTC in women with chronic HBV infection. Because of potential renal toxicity, renal function should be monitored.
NNRTIs					
Preferred Agent					
Nevirapine (NVP) (Viramune) • 200 mg once daily for 14 days, then 200 mg BID	C	*Carcinogen:* Hepatocellular adenomas and carcinomas in mice and rats. *Teratogen:* Negative	Pharmacokinetics not significantly altered in pregnancy; no change in dose indicated. High placental transfer to fetus.	No evidence of human teratogenicity (2-fold increase in birth defects ruled out). Increased risk of symptomatic, often rash-associated, and potentially fatal liver toxicity among women with $CD4^+$ counts >250/mm^3 when first initiating therapy, pregnancy not thus far found to increase risk.	NVP should be initiated in pregnant women with $CD4^+$ counts >250 cells/mm^3 only if benefit clearly outweighs risk due to the increased risk of potentially life-threatening hepatotoxicity in women with high $CD4^+$ counts. Women who become pregnant while taking NVP-containing regimens and are tolerating them well should continue therapy regardless of $CD4^+$ count.
Special Circumstances					
Efavirenz (EFV) (Sustiva) • 600 mg once daily at or before bedtime	D	*Carcinogen:* Hepatocellular adenomas and carcinomas, pulmonary alveolar/bronchiolar adenomas in female mice at 1.7× human exposure. *Teratogen:* Increased fetal resorption, anencephaly, anophthalmia, microphthalmia, and cleft palate in cynomolgus monkey at exposures comparable to humans.	AUC decreased during third trimester, compared with postpartum, but nearly all third-trimester subjects exceeded target exposure and no change in dose is indicated. Moderate placental transfer to fetus.	Prospective data from the Antiretroviral Pregnancy Registry documents birth defects in 17 of 623 live births following first trimester EFV exposure, including a single case of neural tube defect with fetal alcohol syndrome and a single case of bilateral facial clefts, anopthalmia and amniotic band, (2.7%, 2-fold increase in overall birth defects ruled out). (REF) Risk of EFV is unclear, given the low prevalence of neural tube defects (0.1%-0.4%) in the general population. Retrospective data includes 6 case reports of central nervous system defects following EFV exposure. Meta-analysis of 1437 first trimester EFV-exposed live births showed no increase in overall birth defects (2.0%) and 1 neural tube defect overall incidence 0.07%).(Ford, 2011)	EFV should be avoided in the first trimester. After the first trimester, EFV can be considered if this is the best patient choice. If EFV is continued postpartum, adequate contraception must be ensured. Women of childbearing age must be counseled regarding the teratogenic potential of EFV and avoid pregnancy while using this drug. Because no contraceptive method is 100% effective, alternative ARV regimens should be strongly considered in women of childbearing potential.
Insufficient Data to Recommend Use					
Etravirine (ETR) (Intelence) • 200 mg BID	B	*Carcinogen:* Negative *Teratogen:* Negative	Limited PK data in human pregnancy, but is comparable to nonpregnant adults. Limited data suggests high placental transfer to fetus.	No experience in human pregnancy.	Safety and pharmacokinetic data are insufficient to recommend use during pregnancy.

Continued

TABLE 50-3 COMMONLY USED ANTIRETROVIRAL DRUGS IN PREGNANCY—cont'd

ARV DRUG DOSAGE RECOMMENDATIONS	FDA PREGNANCY CATEGORY	ANIMAL STUDIES CARCINOGEN/ TERATOGEN	PHARMACOKINETICS IN PREGNANCY	CONCERNS IN PREGNANCY	RECOMMENDED USE IN PREGNANCY
Rilpivirine (RPV) (Endurant) • 25 mg once daily		*Carcinogen:* Hepatocellular neoplasms at 21× human exposure. *Teratogen:* Negative	No pharmacokinetic studies in human pregnancy. Placental transfer unknown.	No experience in human pregnancy.	Safety and pharmacokinetic data are insufficient to recommend use during pregnancy.
Protease Inhibitors					
Recommended Agent					
Lopinavir/ Ritonavir (LPV/r) (Kaletra) • Built-in low-dose ritonavir boosting: 400/100 mg BID • In third (and second) trimester: 600/150 mg BID	C	*Carcinogen:* Hepatocellular adenomas and carcinomas in rodents at 1.6-2.2× (mice) and 0.5× (rats) human exposure. *Teratogen:* No teratogenicity, but fetal developmental toxicity observed at a maternally toxic dose.	AUC decreased in second and third trimester with standard dosing. LPV/r 600 mg/150 mg twice daily resulted in AUC similar to nonpregnant adults receiving LPV/r 400 mg/100 mg twice daily. Low placental transfer to fetus.	No evidence of human teratogenicity (2-fold increase in birth defect ruled out). Well-tolerated, short-term safety demonstrated in Phase I/II studies.	PK studies support increasing LPV/r to 600/150 mg BID in the third trimester, and considering this increased dose in the second trimester, especially in PI experienced patients. An alternative strategy is adding a pediatric LPV/r tablet (100/25 mg) to the standard adult dose. If standard dosing is used, monitor virologic response and LPV drug levels. Once-daily dosing is not recommended in pregnancy, as no data exist to evaluate the adequacy of drug levels with this administration.
Alternative Agents					
Atazanavir (ATV) (Reyataz) • Combined with low-dose ritonavir boosting (ATV 300 mg + RTV 100 mg once daily; adjust dose for TDV, EFV, or H_2 blocker)	B	*Carcinogen:* Benign hepatocellular adenomas in female mice at 2.8× human exposure. *Teratogen:* Negative	PK studies of ATV with RTV boosting during pregnancy suggests that standard dosing yields decreased AUC; however, for most pregnant women no dose adjustment was needed. TDF reduces ATV AUC in all patients 25%. Low placental transfer to fetus.	No evidence of human teratogenicity (2-fold increase in birth defects ruled out). Adults treated with ATV frequently have elevated indirect bilirubin levels; increased bilirubin has been reported in some infants born to mothers receiving ATV and is associated with uridine diphosphate glucuronosyltransferase 1 (UGT1A1) genotypes linked to decreased UGT function. Neonatal hypoglycemia has been reported in 3 of 38 ATV-exposed infants.	Alternative PI for use in combination regimens in pregnancy. Should give as low-dose RTV-boosted regimen, may use once-daily dosing. A study of 41 pregnant women concluded that no dose adjustment was needed for the majority of pregnant women infected with HIV strains susceptible to ATV. ART-experienced pregnant women on either TDV or an H_2 blocker (not both) should increase ATV dose to 400 mg (with RTV 100 mg).
Ritonavir (RTV) (Norvir) • 100-400 mg per day in 1-2 divided doses as booster	B	*Carcinogen:* Hepatocellular adenomas and carcinomas in male mice. *Teratogen:* No teratogenicity, but fetal developmental toxicity observed at maternally toxic dose.	RTV levels are reduced in pregnancy, including low-dose RTV regimens used to boost the concentrations of other PIs. Minimal placental transfer to fetus.	Limited experience at full dose in human pregnancy; is currently used as low-dose RTV boosting with other PIs. No evidence of human teratogenicity (2-fold increase in birth defects ruled out).	Given low levels in pregnant women when used alone, should only be used in combination with second PI (dual PI treatment) or as low-dose RTV "boost" to increase levels of another PI.
Saquinavir HGC (hard-gel capsule) (SQV) (Invirase) • Combined with low-dose ritonavir boosting (SQV 1000 mg + RTV 100 mg) BID	B	*Carcinogen:* Negative *Teratogen:* Negative	Limited PK data suggests that 1000 mg SQV HGC/100 mg RTV twice daily achieves adequate SQV drug levels in pregnant women. Minimal placental transfer to fetus.	Well-tolerated, short-term safety demonstrated for mother and infant for SQV in combination with low-dose RTV boosting. Baseline ECG recommended before starting because PR and/or QT interval prolongations have been observed.	PK data on SQV in pregnancy is limited; however the HGC and tablets both appear to achieve adequate drug levels. RTV-boosted SQV is an alternative PI for combination ARV regimens in pregnancy and are alternative, initial ARV recommendations for nonpregnant adults. Data are too limited to recommend once daily dosing within pregnancy at present.

Continued

Use in Special Circumstances					
Indinavir (IDV) (Crixivan) • Combined with low-dose ritonavir boosting (IDV 800 mg + RTV 100-200 mg) BID	C	*Carcinogen:* Thyroid adenomas in male rats at 1.3× human exposure. *Teratogen:* Negative	Limited studies using IDV showed markedly lower pregnancy levels, compared to postpartum, although HIV RNA suppression was seen. Minimal placental transfer to fetus.	No evidence of human teratogenicity (2-fold increase in birth defects ruled out). Pill burden and potential for renal stones are concerns. In rhesus monkeys neonatal IDV exacerbated transient physiologic hyperbilirubinemia; this was not seen following in utero exposure.	Given limited data regarding dosing, trough drug levels should be monitored during IDV use in pregnancy. IDV should only be used when preferred and alternative agents cannot be used, and this PI must be given as part of a low-dose RTV-boosted regimen. Furthermore, IDV as the sole "therapeutic" PI is not recommended in HIV-infected pregnant patients.
Nelfinavir (NFV) (Viracept) • 1250 mg BID	B	*Carcinogen:* Thyroid follicular adenomas and carcinomas in rats. *Teratogen:* Negative	Using the new 625-mg tablet formulation and 1250 mg BID dosing, lower AUC and peak levels were seen in the third trimester versus postpartum; however, viral load was suppressed in most women. Minimal to low placental transfer to the fetus.	No evidence of human teratogenicity (can rule out 2-fold increase in overall birth defects). Well-tolerated, short-term safety demonstrated for mother and infant.	Given extensive experience with use in pregnancy, NFV might be considered in special circumstances to reduce perinatal HIV transmission in women for whom therapy would not otherwise be indicated and/or when alternative agents are not tolerated. In clinical trials of initial therapy in nonpregnant adults, NFV based regimens had a lower rate of viral response compared with LPV/r or EFV-based regimens, but similar viral response to ATV or NVP-based regimens.
Insufficient Data to Recommend Use					
Darunavir (DRV) (Prezista) • Must be combined with low-dose RTV boosting • ARV-naïve (DRV 800 mg + RTV100 mg) once daily • ARV exp, with mutations: (DRV 600 mg + RTV 100 mg) BID	C	*Carcinogen:* Hepatic adenomas and carcinomas, thyroid neoplasms (male rats) at 0.4-0.7× (mice) and 0.7-1× (rats) human exposure. *Teratogen:* Negative	No PK studies in human pregnancy. Low to moderate placental transfer to fetus.	Very limited experience in human pregnancy.	Safety and PK data in pregnancy are insufficient to recommend use in ARV-naïve patients. Must give as low-dose RTV-boosted regimen.
Fosamprenavir (FPV) (Lexiva) • A prodrug of amprenavir, recommended to be combined with low-dose RTV boosting (FPV 1400 mg + RTV 100-200 mg) once daily or FPV 700 mg + RTV 100 mg BID)	C	*Carcinogen:* Interstitial cell hyperplasia and uterine endometrial adenocarcinoma in rats. In all rodents hepatic adenomas and carcinomas, thyroid adenomas, at 0.1-0.7× (mice) and 0.3-1.4× (rats) human exposure. *Teratogen:* Increased abortion in rabbits, decreased fertility and gestational body weights in rats.	With RTV boosting, AUC is reduced in the third trimester; however, levels appear adequate for patients without PI resistance mutations. Low placental transfer to fetus.	Limited experience in human pregnancy.	Safety and PK data in pregnancy are insufficient to recommend use in ARV-naïve patients. Recommended to be given as low-dose RTV-boosted regimen.
Tipranavir (TPV) (Aptivus) • Must be combined with low-dose RTV boosting • (TPV 500 mg + RTV 200 mg) BID	C	*Carcinogen:* Hepatic adenomas and carcinomas in mice below human exposure levels; benign thyroid adenomas in female rats at human exposure levels. *Teratogen:* Negative	Ongoing study in human pregnancy. Unknown rate of placental transfer to fetus.	Ongoing study in human pregnancy.	Safety and PK data in pregnancy are insufficient to recommend use in ARV-naïve patients. Must give as low-dose RTV-boosted regimen.

TABLE 50-4 PROPHYLACTIC ANTIBIOTIC REGIMENS FOR COMMON OPPORTUNISTIC INFECTIONS*

CONDITION	INDICATION FOR PROPHYLAXIS	ANTIBIOTIC REGIMEN
Pneumocystis jiroveci pneumonia	Prior infection or CD4 <200/mm^3	TMP-SMX 1 DS tablet qd indefinitely
Toxoplasmic encephalitis	CD4 <100/mm^3, serology	TMP-SMX 1 DS tablet qd indefinitely
Tuberculosis	+PPD >5 mm No active disease on chest radiograph	300 mg INH and 50 mg pyridoxine qd ×12 mo
Disseminated infection with *Mycobacterium avium* complex (MAC)	CD4 <50/mm^3	1200 mg azithromycin weekly
Cryptococcosis	CD4 <50/mm^3	Prophylaxis not recommended Patients treated for acute cryptococcal infection should receive 200 mg fluconazole qd indefinitely

*Recommendations in this table are based on guidelines from the CDC, NIH, and IDSA.[23]
INH, Isoniazid; TMP-SMX, trimethoprim-sulfamethoxazole.

preventing perinatal HIV transmission. Commonly encountered alternative agents include abacavir, which is associated with hypersensitivity reactions. HLA-B*5701 testing identifies patients at risk; testing should be performed and documented prior to initiating this therapy.[14] Tenofovir is a preferred NRTI for HIV-infected adults; however, it is an alternative agent in pregnancy secondary to concerns regarding fetal and postnatal growth and bone mineralization. All NRTIs bind to mitochondrial γ-DNA polymerase, potentially causing dysfunction manifesting as clinically significant myopathy, cardiomyopathy, neuropathy, lactic acidosis, or fatty liver, resembling HELLP syndrome. Lactic acidosis and hepatic failure have been noted with long-term, combined stavudine and didanosine use, linked to a genetic defect in mitochondrial fatty acid metabolism, so this regimen should not be used in pregnancy.[14] Mitochondrial toxicity has been observed in children born to HIV-infected mothers treated with NRTIs,[18,19] although no increase in mortality was observed[20]; long-term follow-up is ongoing.

NON-NUCLEOSIDE REVERSE TRANSCRIPTASE INHIBITORS

NNRTIs are typically used in combination regimens with two NRTI drugs. Nevirapine (NVP), the preferred agent in pregnancy, is associated with rash-associated hepatotoxicity. This drug should not be used for initial treatment in ART-naïve pregnant women with CD4$^+$ cell counts greater than 250 cells/mm^3; however it is safe to continue this drug in women becoming pregnant while taking NVP-containing regimens. Efavirenz (EFV), the preferred NNRTI for nonpregnant adults, is associated with central nervous system (CNS) defects. Although the relative risk is unclear, this drug should not be used in the first trimester of pregnancy.[21]

PROTEASE INHIBITORS

PIs are typically paired with two NRTI drugs and are characterized by minimal transplacental passage and few adverse side effects. Low-dose ritonavir boosting improves the pharmacokinetics of several of these drugs in all patients. PIs are associated with hyperglycemia in adults, but it is unclear if pregnancy increases the risk[22]; an early glucose challenge test followed by repeat testing after 28 weeks is reasonable in "high-risk" patients. Conflicting data exists regarding preterm delivery in women receiving PIs (discussed in counseling section). Lower serum concentrations of lopinovir/ritonavir, atazanavir, and nefinavir have been reported in pregnant women; adjusted dosage regimens are detailed in Table 50-3.[14]

OPPORTUNISTIC INFECTION PROPHYLAXIS

Patients with a CD4 count below 200 cells/mm^3 should also receive prophylaxis against opportunistic infections (OIs). Transient CD4 count decreases may occur secondary to pregnancy-associated hemodilution; in these cases the relative percentage of CD4$^+$ cells (Table 50-2) can be used to guide decisions regarding OI prophylaxis. Prophylaxis regimens for *Pneumocystis jiroveci* pneumonia, toxoplasmosis, tuberculosis (TB), *Mycobacterium avium* complex (MAC), and cryptococcosis are listed in Table 50-4. When HIV-untreated patients are diagnosed with a treatable OI, including TB, MAC, PCP, toxoplasmosis, histoplasmosis, HBV, CMV, VZV, or cryptococcal meningitis, consideration should be given to initiating OI treatment prior to starting ART to avoid immune reconstitution inflammatory syndromes (IRIS). At advanced gestational age or when diagnosed with an OI without specific treatment, ART may be started prior to or concurrent with treatment.[23]

SUMMARY

The preferred regimen for ART-naïve patients is AZT, 3TC, and lopinavir/ritonavir. Patients entering pregnancy on ART with complete viral suppression should continue their current therapy, unless a component of their regimen is contraindicated in pregnancy. Recommendations for ARV drug regimens during pregnancy should be individualized according to the woman's specific ARV history and the presence of comorbidities; incorporating the use of one or more NRTIs with good placental passage is recommended. The NRTIs lamivudine, emtricitabine, and tenofovir have antiviral activity against hepatitis B, therefore tenofovir in combination with emtricitabine or 3TC is the preferred NRTI backbone for HBV/HIV co-infected women. As needed, consultation with specialists in the treatment of HIV infection is advised for women with previous ARV use for maternal indications, who demonstrate significant ARV resistance upon testing, or when there is a suboptimal response to ART.[14] When a patient presents late in pregnancy, ARV therapy should be started immediately and not delayed for resistance testing results. Testing should still be performed because the information is important for ongoing patient care and can be used to modify treatment if needed.

Ongoing Management

In addition to routine prenatal care and evaluation, viral load and CD4 count assessment should be performed monthly when starting a new medication regimen or a change in viral load is detected. Patients on stable ART regimens and suppressed viremia can have viral loads and CD4 counts checked in each trimester. Vaccinations (as needed) should include the following: pneumococcus, influenza, hepatitis B (for women $HBsAg^-$, $HBcAb^-$, $HBsAb^-$), and hepatitis A (for women with chronic HBV infection). Women with HBV co-infection should have liver transaminase testing 1 month after initiating ARV and every 3 months thereafter. Coordination of services among prenatal care providers, primary care and HIV specialty care providers, mental health and drug abuse treatment services, and public assistance programs are essential to ensure that infected women remain active participants in their care and adhere to their ARV drug regimens.

Antenatal Karyotype Determination

In patients desiring fetal karyotype determination, the risks and benefits of amniocentesis or chorionic villous sampling (CVS) should be discussed and referral to a genetic counselor made. One study assessed vertical HIV transmission following amniocentesis; 1 of 61 infants was infected, which was not significantly different than the transmission rate in women deferring amniocentesis.[24] A second prospective cohort study reported no increase in mother-to child transmission rates in the 162 women undergoing amniocentesis (of 9302 HIV-infected pregnancies); moreover, no cases of MTCT were identified in 81 women receiving ART at the time of amniocentesis.[25] Larger studies are needed to better estimate the risk of HIV transmission following amniocentesis or CVS; however, published reports suggest that there is no increased risk of HIV transmission.[14]

Intrapartum Management of HIV

Every effort should be made to avoid instrumentation increasing the neonate's exposure to infected maternal blood and secretions. Recommendations include leaving the fetal membranes intact as long as possible, avoiding fetal scalp sampling and fetal scalp electrode placement, and reserving episiotomy and assisted vaginal delivery for select circumstances. If spontaneous rupture of membranes (SROM) has occurred, augmentation and/or induction of labor with pitocin should not be delayed for AZT administration. Intrapartum maternal IV AZT is given as a loading dose of 2 mg/kg administered over 1 hour and a maintenance dose of 1 mg/kg/hr.[15] Other ART should be taken with a sip of water, with the exception of stavudine, which is antagonistic to AZT and should be withheld. AZT is given intrapartum to all women, even those with AZT resistance, as wild type virus is most often transmitted. AZT is metabolized to its active form within the placenta and has good CNS penetration. If elective cesarean section is planned, patients should receive IV AZT for 3 hours prior to the procedure. However, if operative delivery is indicated for obstetric reasons, delivery must not be delayed for AZT administration. In cases of uterine atony, methergine should be avoided if possible in patients receiving a PI or efavirenz. These drugs are CYP3A4 inhibitors and concomitant ergotamine use is associated with exaggerated vasoconstrictive responses.

Intrapartum Testing

Rapid HIV testing should be performed for all women in labor without a documented HIV test during pregnancy unless the patient declines intrapartum testing, because 40% to 85% of HIV-infected infants in the United States are born to women whose HIV status is unknown prior to delivery.[26] Women who are found to be HIV seropositive upon rapid testing should be given intrapartum and postpartum ARV prophylaxis to limit perinatal HIV transmission without waiting for confirmatory testing.[14]

Spontaneous Rupture of Membranes (SROM)

Increasing duration of ruptured membranes is associated with perinatal HIV transmission; however, the incremental increased risk of transmission is not clinically significant. Meta-analysis of 4721 deliveries determined that the risk of HIV transmission increases by 2% over the baseline transmission risk (after adjusting for all other factors influencing transmission) for each hour increment following rupture of membranes.[27] Presuming a patient on ART with an undetectable viral load has a baseline perinatal HIV transmission rate of 2%, the risk of transmission after 1 hour of ruptured membranes would be 2.04%, and after 8 hours the risk of HIV transmission would be 2.32%. Given that prolonged SROM does not appreciably increase HIV transmission risk in term patients, we do not recommend elective cesarean delivery, as it is unlikely to reduce perinatal HIV transmission risk in patients being actively managed using oxytocin for augmentation or induction.

Untreated Women

For HIV-infected women who have not received ART before labor, IV AZT should be given during labor. Maternal single-dose NVP is not recommended; there is no added efficacy and a high likelihood of maternal harm, specifically the emergence of resistant virus. The safest, most effective option to reduce perinatal HIV transmission in this setting is expanded infant prophylaxis, consisting of AZT for 6 weeks with the addition of three doses of NVP in the first week of life (at birth, 48 hours post birth, and 96 hours after the second dose).[14] Providers should also evaluate whether the patient is a candidate for initiation of maternal therapy postpartum.

Elective Cesarean Delivery

Scheduled cesarean delivery at 38 weeks' gestation, documented by last menstrual period and ultrasonography, is recommended for women with HIV RNA levels >1000 copies/mL near the time of delivery, irrespective of ART, and for women with unknown HIV RNA levels near the time of delivery. These recommendations are based on studies conducted when the majority of HIV-infected women received AZT monotherapy or no ART, whereas a more recent study of 4864 European women showed that the perinatal HIV transmission rate in women receiving at least 14 days of ARV was 0.8%, regardless of the mode of delivery.[16] At this gestation the risk of any neonatal adverse event, including death, respiratory complications, hypoglycemia, sepsis, or NICU admission is 11%, as compared to 8% at 39 weeks. HIV-infected women have increased morbidity and mortality following cesarean delivery, and the risk of complications is related to the degree of immunosuppression. Therefore, the patient's autonomy in decision-making regarding the route of delivery should be respected and prophylactic antibiotics should be administered.

Cesarean delivery after the onset of labor or SROM does not protect against HIV transmission, so in this setting we recommend delivery for obstetrical indications, irrespective of viral load. Scheduled cesarean delivery is not recommended for preventing perinatal HIV transmission in women receiving combination ART who have plasma HIV RNA levels <1000 copies/mL near the time of delivery. Data are insufficient to evaluate the potential benefit of cesarean delivery in this group, and given the low rate of transmission in these patients, it is unclear whether scheduled cesarean delivery would confer additional benefit in reducing HIV transmission. Delivery decisions should be individualized based on discussion between the obstetrician and the mother.

Postpartum Care of the HIV-Infected Woman

One of the primary issues following delivery is managing the woman's HIV infection outside of pregnancy. Women who have not received antepartum ART therapy can be started on ART postpartum, if indicated for their health as discussed later. For women receiving ART during pregnancy, they should establish a relationship with an HIV-medicine provider during the latter part of pregnancy, to transition into ongoing care. The guidelines for managing HIV infection in adults recommend treatment for individuals with a CD4 count below 350 cells/mm^3 or an HIV RNA level greater than 55,000 copies/mm^3, based on randomized, controlled clinical trial data demonstrating reduced morbidity and mortality.[12] The HIV treatment guidelines also make a moderate-to-strong recommendation for initiating lifelong ART in individuals with CD4 cell counts between 350 and 500 cells/mm^3, based on observational studies suggesting a relative decrease in mortality and possibly a decrease in complications such as cardiovascular events with initiation of ART in this setting compared with waiting until CD4 cell counts drop below 350 cells/mm^3. For individuals with CD4 counts >500 cells/mm^3, some experts would recommend initiating lifelong therapy, whereas other experts view this as optional, given that data are inconclusive on the clinical benefit of starting treatment at higher CD4 cell counts (>500 cells/mm^3). The adult HIV treatment guidelines discourage interruption of therapy; however, no increased risk of disease progression has been shown in studies of pregnant women with relatively high CD4 counts who stop ARV drugs after delivery. The potential benefits of early, continued therapy, including decreased HIV transmission risk to an uninfected partner, and consideration of future childbearing plans (to avoid episodic receipt of ART), must be weighed against possible drug toxicity, cost, and the risk of development of viral resistance with suboptimal adherence, which may be more likely during the postpartum period. Given the complexity of this decision, the risks and benefits of continuing or stopping ART postpartum should be discussed with women prior to delivery in consultation with the provider assuming responsibility for the woman's HIV care following the postpartum period.

If the patient continues ART postpartum, standard medication doses can be used immediately following delivery, predominantly affecting PIs. If ART is discontinued following delivery, all drugs should be stopped simultaneously, unless the patient is on an NNRTI-containing regimen. For women receiving NNRTI-based regimens, continuing the dual-NRTI backbone for at least 7 days after stopping the NNRTI is recommended to reduce the development of NNRTI resistance. An alternative, more conservative strategy is to replace the NNRTI with a PI while continuing the NRTIs, then to discontinue all the drugs at the same time. The optimal interval between stopping an NNRTI and stopping the other ARV drugs is unknown, but at least 7 days is recommended. Drug concentrations may be detectable for more than 3 weeks after EFV discontinuation; therefore some experts recommend continuing the other ARV agents, or substituting a PI for EFV in addition to the other agents for up to 30 days.[14]

Infant and maternal postpartum ARV prophylaxis significantly lowers, but does not completely eliminate, the risk of postnatal HIV transmission through breast milk. Studies showing this were performed in areas of the world where formula feeding is not a viable alternative. Because the benefits of breastfeeding in the United States do not outweigh the risk of HIV transmission, breastfeeding is not recommended for HIV-infected women in the United States. Women should also be counseled about the availability of highly effective contraceptives, including long-term reversible methods (implants, injectables, and IUDs) to be used in conjunction with condoms, to prevent unintended pregnancy. Finally, women should be counseled regarding the potential that the demands of caring for a new baby could make adherence to ART more difficult; nonetheless, maintaining adherence can prolong the effectiveness of ART.[14]

Infant Screening and Diagnosis

Because the fetus receives maternal immunoglobulin G (IgG) by transplacental passage, serologic tests of the HIV-exposed neonate will almost always be positive. In infants the diagnosis of HIV infection is made via PCR amplification of HIV DNA (more sensitive for the neonatal period) or RNA assays. Virologic tests to diagnose HIV infection should be performed within the first 14 to 21 days of life, at 1 to 2 months, and at 4 to 6 months of age. Two positive tests (on different specimens, excluding cord blood) are required to diagnose HIV infection; one positive test is a presumptive diagnosis. HIV is presumptively excluded with two or more negative tests, one at age 14 days or older and the second at age 1 month of older; definitive exclusion in a nonbreastfed infant is based on two negative tests at age 1 month or older and at age 4 months or older. Further details on case definitions for HIV infection are available from the CDC at www.cdc.gov.[9]

Factors Influencing Transmission

Perinatal HIV transmission risk is associated with cigarette smoking, illicit drug use, genital tract infections, and unprotected sexual intercourse with multiple partners during pregnancy. Eliminating these modifiable risk factors not only reduces perinatal HIV transmission but improves maternal health. Other key factors influencing HIV transmission are listed in the box, Factors Increasing the Risk of Perinatal HIV Transmission. Most perinatal HIV transmission occurs within the intrapartum period and effective ART, or elective cesarean delivery in patients without viral suppression, substantially reduces transmission. A minority of infected infants acquire HIV in utero, as characterized by an infant who is PCR positive at birth. Most studies were not designed or powered to prevent in utero HIV transmission; however, newly reported data suggest that early, sustained control of viral replication may prevent in utero HIV transmission. The study evaluated perinatal transmission risk factors in women with HIV RNA <500 copies/mL at delivery; the overall HIV transmission rate was 0.5% in this population. HIV transmitters were less likely to have received ARV drugs at the time of conception than nontransmitters; moreover, HIV transmitters were less likely to have HIV RNA <500 copies/mL at 14, 28, and 32 weeks of gestation. Among women starting ARV during pregnancy, viral load decreased earlier in nontransmitting women, with both groups initiating therapy at the same gestational age (30 weeks). **This suggests that early and sustained control of viral replication is associated with decreased HIV transmission (including starting therapy prior to conception), and supports initiating ARV drugs as early in pregnancy as possible for all women.**[14,16]

Factors Increasing the Risk of Perinatal HIV Transmission

- History of previous child with HIV infection
- Mother with AIDS
- Preterm delivery
- Decreased maternal CD4 count
- High viral load
- Firstborn twin
- Chorioamnionitis
- Modifiable factors (cigarette smoking, illicit drug use, STDs, unprotected sexual intercourse with multiple partners during pregnancy)
- Intrapartum blood exposure (e.g., episiotomy, vaginal laceration, forceps delivery)
- Delivery following prolonged rupture of membranes
- Breastfeeding

ART and viral load at delivery are independent risk factors for HIV transmission; therefore ART is recommended for all women regardless of whether complete viral load suppression can be achieved. Moreover, this strategy protects neonates born following SROM or spontaneous labor occurring prior to a "planned elective cesarean delivery." Mechanisms of protection include the following: using ARVs with good placental transfer, and permitting adequate systemic drug levels in infants at birth. This is likely important when the fetus is exposed to virus within the birth canal, and when the fetus is the recipient of maternal-fetal blood transfusion during uterine contractions. ARVs can also decrease genital tract viral load and be excreted into genital tract secretions; AZT and 3TC are present at high concentrations within genital secretions, another potential mechanism of protection against HIV transmission. Most perinatal HIV transmission in the United States occurs in women who are not known to be HIV-infected prior to the birth of their child. Given this knowledge it is critical to emphasize the importance of prenatal care, universal HIV testing, and strategies to diagnose acute HIV infection in late pregnancy and during breastfeeding.

Preconception Counseling for HIV-Infected Women

Health care providers should discuss childbearing intentions, including preconception counseling and care, with all of their patients in a nonjudgmental manner as recommended by the ACOG and the CDC. Issues relevant to HIV-infected women include HIV disease status assessment, hepatitis B status assessment, the need for prophylaxis or treatment of opportunistic infections, and evaluating and potentially changing therapy based on the effectiveness and teratogenic potential of drugs within the ARV regimen. As approximately half of all pregnancies in the United States are unintended, avoiding drugs of teratogenic potential in women of reproductive age should be considered. It is also recommended that HIV-infected women attain a stable, maximally suppressed viral load prior to conception, because early and sustained control of HIV replication may be associated with maximally decreasing perinatal transmission. Counseling should also include discussing the influence of HIV on pregnancy, appropriate contraceptive choices to reduce the likelihood of unintended pregnancy and account for the fact that ART (predominantly NNRTIs and PIs) reduces hormonal contraceptive efficacy, and safe sexual practices to minimize the risk of acquiring sexually transmitted infections or acquiring more virulent or resistant HIV strains.[14]

HIV Discordant Couples

HIV-uninfected pregnant women with HIV-infected partners may seek consultation. Recommendations are to review and encourage safe sexual practices, including consistent use of barrier contraception, and establish a plan for HIV screening. As a high-risk patient, first and third trimester serum screening is appropriate; routine screening should not include viral load determination, because serology is sufficiently sensitive with a lower false-positive rate. If women present to labor and delivery without documented negative serology at 36 weeks, rapid intrapartum testing should be performed. Women should also be counseled to recognize the signs and symptoms of acute HIV infection and advised to seek immediate care if they experience these symptoms (diagnosis of acute HIV infection is discussed in the section on screening).

Consultation in the preconception period should include screening and treatment of genital tract infections in both partners, because inflammation is associated with viral shedding and increased HIV acquisition in both partners. This is also an opportunity to ensure that the HIV-infected partner is on an ARV regimen with maximal or complete suppression of viral load. Methods of safe conception depend on which partner is HIV infected. For the HIV-infected woman the safest method of conception is via artificial insemination. This can be accomplished by the patient at home using a syringe. If the HIV-infected partner is male, the goal is to achieve pregnancy with as few sperm exposures as possible. The possibility of using donor sperm should be considered; if this is not an option sperm analysis should be performed because HIV and ARV may reduce sperm count and quality, raising the possibility that attempting conception is futile. Sperm preparation techniques coupled with intrauterine insemination (potentially with ovulation induction), in vitro fertilization, or intracytoplasmic sperm injection have been reported to be effective in avoiding seroconversion in uninfected women and offspring. The National Perinatal HIV Hotline (1-888-448-8765) is a resource for a list of institutions offering reproductive services for HIV-serodiscordant couples. In patients without resources enabling assisted reproductive technology, timed periovulatory unprotected intercourse (condoms all other times) with a maximally suppressed partner is probably the safest way to facilitate conception. Oral embtricitabine/tenofovir postexposure treatment prevented HIV transmission to males; however, this regimen did not protect women from HIV acquisition. Tenofovir gel prevented HIV acquisition in women, but it is not yet commercially available.[14]

Counseling

Ongoing care of the HIV-infected pregnant woman is enhanced by having a multidisciplinary team, which may include the physician(s), social workers, nutritionist, psychologists, and peer counselors. Management should include frequent visits and ongoing discussion regarding adherence to medication regimens to reduce perinatal HIV transmission and prevent the development of resistance to ART. Patients should be counseled about the impact of HIV infection on pregnancy, including the risk of perinatal transmission, side effects of medications, potential methods of delivery, and treatment options. Studies have shown that pregnancy does not affect the progression of HIV disease. It is unclear whether ART influences preterm delivery. Some studies have shown an increased risk; however, a recent prospective cohort study enrolling more than 800 patients between 2002 and 2008, in which all patients received combination ART, did not find an increased incidence of preterm birth in women receiving PIs.[28] Although a potential increased risk of preterm birth with ART cannot be fully ruled out, the clear maternal health benefits and reduced perinatal HIV transmission support the use of ART during pregnancy. Ascertaining whether the patient has disclosed her HIV serostatus to sex partners and needle sharing partners is appropriate. Addressing barriers preventing disclosure, including recommendations and/or referral for assistance regarding how to safely disclose HIV serostatus, is warranted. Some state and local governments require that clinicians report any known partners of HIV-infected patients to the local health department; thus providers should be aware of regulations that will influence their practice.

For both HIV-infected and exposed women, HIV prevention should be discussed using a straightforward, nonjudgmental approach. Identification of ongoing risks should be performed, including sexual behaviors, IV drug use, sexually transmitted diseases, and untreated psychiatric issues, which could increase a person's likelihood of engaging in risk behavior. Behavior interventions, treatment, and avoidance or risk factors should be discussed, emphasizing the importance of consistent condom use even though ART decreases the risk of HIV transmission. Although no reliable data on HIV serodiscordance rates in the United States exist, data on women from sub-Saharan Africa show that women in serodiscordant relationships may be particularly vulnerable to HIV infection; thus HIV testing of sexual partners should be encouraged.[14]

INFLUENZA

Virology/Epidemiology

Influenza is part of the Orthomyxoviridae family, containing the genera influenza A, B, and C. Influenza B is restricted to humans, whereas influenza A and C infect humans in addition to mammalian and avian species. Influenza virus has a negative-stranded, segmented RNA genome enabling reassortment, the rearrangement of viral gene segments in cells infected with two different influenza viruses. This results in the rapid generation of new influenza virus strains (recombinants), which have been responsible for pandemic outbreaks; this process is termed "antigenic shift." Point mutations within the viral genome result in minor, gradual antigenic changes defined as "antigenic drift." These genetic strategies, combined with a wide host range and our inability to generate a protective immune response against the entire genera, enable influenza virus to remain an important pathogen.

Influenza viruses are enveloped, hemagglutinin (H or HA) and neuraminidase (N or NA) viral glycoproteins are present on the surface, and the virus capsid proteins are M1 and M2. HA binds the cell surface receptor (neuraminic acid), is highly antigenic, and is the target of neutralizing antibodies protecting against infection. NA does not induce neutralizing antibodies; however, antibodies recognizing NA are disease suppressive while permitting infection. NA cleaves sialic acid from the infected cell surface, facilitating virus release (budding) from these cells, and may remove sialic acid from mucin, enabling cell-free virus to reach epithelial cells. Viral entry begins when HA binds the cell receptor, followed by endocytosis of the viral particle. Within the endocytic compartment, low pH triggers conformational changes in HA, which are required for fusion. Viral uncoating also requires M2, an ion channel protein permitting influx of H^+ ions into the virus particle, enabling the viral nucleoprotein to enter the cytoplasm.

Influenza strains are named according to their genus (type), the species from which the virus was isolated (omitted if human), and the H and N subtypes. H subtypes confer species specificity and there is only a single NA subtype for influenza B. Influenza is spread by respiratory droplets, is highly contagious, and occurs as an epidemic typically during the winter months. Approximately 50 million cases occur annually in the United States; children younger than 2 years old and the elderly have the highest hospitalization rates. In 2009 a novel influenza A, H1N1, emerged secondary to complex genetic reassortment. A unique pandemic ensued: 90% of hospitalizations and 87% of deaths occurred in people <65 years old, and 788 pregnant women with confirmed or probable H1N1, resulting in 280 ICU admissions and 56 deaths, were documented. The documented case reports potentially underreport infection and overestimate the prevalence of severe illness; however, the influence of this pandemic can be extrapolated from the mortality rate. Five percent of H1N1-related deaths occurred in pregnant women (representing 1% of the population), suggesting that pregnant women infected with influenza had an elevated risk of serious illness and death, in accordance with previously published studies.[29]

Clinical Manifestations

Influenza virus causes acute upper respiratory tract illness, characterized by the abrupt onset of fever, chills, headache, myalgias, malaise, a dry cough, and nasal discharge. GI manifestations and conjunctivitis can also be present. The incubation period ranges from 1 to 5 days. Most cases of influenza are self-limited. Complications include pneumonia, occurring in up to 12% of influenza-infected pregnant women,[30] Reye's syndrome, and disseminated intravascular coagulation (DIC). Changes in the immune, cardiac, and respiratory systems likely increase the risk of severe illness in pregnant women infected with influenza.

Diagnosis

Rapid influenza diagnostic tests (RIDTs) are immunoassays identifying influenza A and B viral nucleoproteins in 15 minutes or less. RIDTs are very specific (90%-95%); however, sensitivity is limited (10%-70%), with the potential for false-negative results during periods of high influenza incidence. False-positive results occur when influenza is at low prevalence. Some RIDTs distinguish between influenza A and B, but they cannot determine viral subtype. The optimal time of specimen collection is within 48 to 72 hours of illness onset.[31] Confirmation is via RT-PCR, culture, ELISA, or immunofluorescence of respiratory secretions; immunofluorescence and RT-PCR have the most rapid turnaround.

Management of Influenza During Pregnancy

Pregnant women suspected to be infected with influenza should be treated immediately, without delay for diagnostic confirmation. The recommended treatment for both seasonal and pandemic influenza infection is osteltamivir (dosages are shown in Table 50-5); acetaminophen should be used as an antipyretic and additional recommendations regarding adjunctive therapy are presented in Chapter 37. The preterm birth rate following pandemic H1N1 infection was 30%, and increased preterm parturition also occurs following seasonal influenza infection; so appropriate monitoring should be undertaken, particularly in women with respiratory compromise.[29,32,33] Early antiviral treatment reduces illness duration, secondary complications, and hospitalizations; however, initiating treatment up to 5 days after symptom onset still confers benefit. The risk of severe illness and death is highest in the latter part of pregnancy, compared to the first trimester; other risk factors are described in the box, Risk Factors for Severe Illness and Death in Influenza Virus–Infected Pregnant Women.[29,32] The pregnancy-associated risk of illness persists for 2 weeks postpartum.

RISK FACTORS FOR SEVERE ILLNESS AND DEATH IN INFLUENZA VIRUS–INFECTED PREGNANT WOMEN

Asthma
Smoking
Obesity
Chronic hypertension
Delayed treatment

Chemoprophylaxis can be given to high risk, unvaccinated women exposed within 48 hours of presentation (see Table 50-5); alternative therapy for infection includes amantadine or rimantidine, which block M2 channel activity in influenza A. However, there is significant viral resistance to these drugs.[34] **ACOG and the CDC recommend vaccination of all pregnant women during influenza season (October-May) using the intramuscular, inactivated vaccine.**[35] The World Health Organization (WHO) and U.S. Public Health Service recommend the strains to be included in the annual vaccine based on recent prevalence; the vaccine is produced in eggs, which should be taken into account for patients with allergies. The optimal time to vaccinate patients is in October and November to minimize the risk of acquiring influenza; however, vaccination is safe and effective at any time of the year or gestational age. A study of 2000 pregnant women receiving the inactivated vaccine demonstrated no adverse fetal effects and safety in breastfeeding women; moreover, maternal vaccination also protects infants up to 6 months of age.[36] The intranasal vaccine contains live virus and should not be used during pregnancy.

PARVOVIRUS

Virology/Epidemiology

Parvoviruses are small, nonenveloped viruses containing negative-stranded DNA encoding two major genes: the REP or NS gene encoding functions required for transcription and DNA replication, and the CAP or S gene encoding the coat proteins VP1 and VP2. Parvovirus B19 was identified in the 1970s within blood bank specimens, and was first linked to sickle cell disease patients with transient aplastic crisis. Parvovirus B19 was then associated with

TABLE 50-5 ANTIVIRAL MEDICATION DOSING RECOMMENDATIONS FOR INFLUENZA

ANTIVIRAL AGENT	ACTIVITY	ACTION	USE	DOSAGE	DURATION	CONTRAINDICATIONS
Osteltamivir	Influenza A and B	NA inhibitor	Treatment Prophylaxis	75 mg BID 75 mg daily	5 days 7-10 days	None
Zanamivir	Influenza A and B	NA inhibitor	Treatment prophylaxis	10 mg BID inhaled 10 mg daily, inhaled	5 days 7-10 days	Underlying respiratory disease

Fifth's disease, or erythema infectiosum (EI), and later linked to hydrops fetalis.[37] Parvoviruses preferentially infect rapidly dividing cells, explaining the observed fetal and neonatal susceptibility. Parvovirus B19 infection is restricted to humans; the cellular receptor is erythrocyte P antigen, explaining the propensity of this virus to infect red blood cells and their precursors. P antigen is also expressed on megakaryocytes, endothelial cells, placenta, fetal liver, and fetal heart.[37] Parvovirus B19 is spread via respiratory droplets, infected blood products, perinatally, and with hand to mouth contact. The incubation period ranges from 4 to 20 days following exposure. Seroprevalence increases with age and 65% of pregnant women have evidence of prior infection and are immune. Conversely, susceptible women have approximately a 50% risk of seroconversion following exposure to parvovirus B19. Daycare workers, teachers, and parents have all been shown to be at increased risk of seroconversion.[38]

Clinical Manifestations

The most common presentation of B19 parvovirus infection is EI, which is characterized by a facial rash consistent with a slapped cheek appearance and a reticulated or lace-like rash on the trunk and extremities (Figure 50-1). The rash is immune-complex-mediated and may reappear secondary to temperature changes, sunlight exposure, and stress for several weeks. Infection can also be accompanied by fever, malaise, lymphadenopathy, and symmetrical peripheral arthropathy. The hands are most frequently affected followed by the knees and wrists. Symptoms are typically self-limiting, but may last for several months.[39] Asymptomatic infection occurs 20% of the time. Persistent parvovirus infection is rare and presents as pure red cell aplasia in patients failing to mount a neutralizing antibody response.[40] Fetal infection can be asymptomatic or characterized by aplastic anemia of varying severity. Severe anemia can lead to high-output congestive heart failure and non-immune hydrops. Direct infection of the myocardium may also contribute to fetal heart failure.

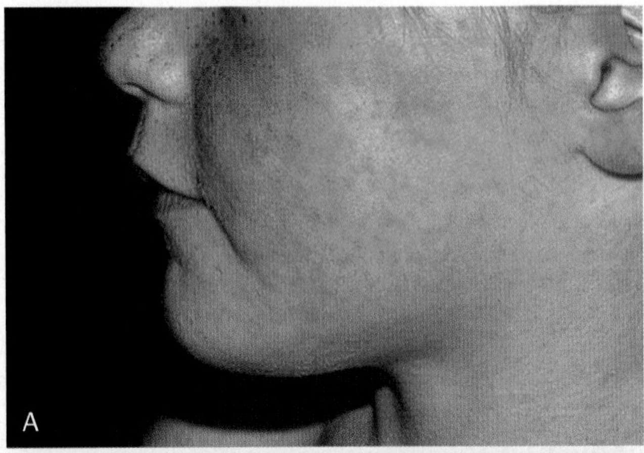

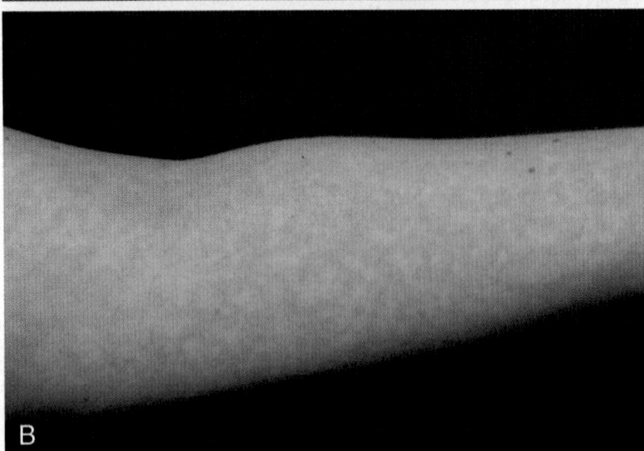

Figure 50-1. **A,** Characteristic "slapped cheek" rash of erythema infectiosum. (From Ferri F, et al: Ferri's Fast Facts in Dermatology. Philadelphia, Saunders, 2011.) **B,** Note lace-like rash on upper extremity.

Diagnosis

Serologic testing via ELISA detects IgG and IgM against B19 parvovirus. However, PCR amplification of viral DNA from maternal or fetal blood is a more sensitive method to confirm acute parvovirus infection, because viremia occurs prior to the development of specific antibodies and viral protein/antibody complexes can result in false-negative serology.[41] Maximum sensitivity is achieved with concurrent serologic and nucleic acid testing.[42]

Management of Parvovirus During Pregnancy

Following exposure to B19 parvovirus in a presumed seronegative woman, serologic and DNA testing should be performed. The presence of IgG antibody is consistent with prior exposure and/or infection, and no further workup is needed. Susceptible women should have repeat testing performed in about 3 weeks. Pregnant women with confirmed infection should be treated with supportive care because maternal B19 parvovirus infection is usually self-limited. The relationship between the gestational age at the time of exposure to B19 parvovirus and the risk of fetal parvovirus infection resulting in a severely affected fetus is shown in Table 50-6. Serial ultrasounds to evaluate the fetus for hydrops should be performed for 8 to 10 weeks after maternal illness. If no signs of hydrops are seen during this period, further evaluation is unnecessary. Recent studies have shown that measurement of the fetal middle cerebral artery peak systolic velocity can be useful in documenting fetal anemia prior to the development of hydrops in cases of congenital B19 parvovirus infection.[43]

Fetal infection occurs following approximately 33% of maternal infections.[44] However, the rate of fetal death secondary to intrauterine B19 parvovirus infection is dependent on when maternal infection occurs. Fetal death is rare when maternal infection occurs beyond 20 weeks of gestation, but fetal mortality associated with fetal hydrops is

Table 50-6 Association Between Gestational Age at Time of Exposure and Risk of Fetal Parvovirus Infection

TIME OF EXPOSURE (WEEKS' GESTATION)	FREQUENCY OF SEVERELY AFFECTED FETUSES (%)
1-12	19
13-20	15
>20	6

approximately 11% when maternal B19 infection occurs during the first 20 weeks of pregnancy.[45] Although 33% of fetal hydrops will resolve without treatment,[46] there are no reliable predictors for the resolution of hydrops versus fetal death. Thus, cordocentesis and intrauterine transfusion are recommended when fetal hydrops is present.[47] Recent studies have documented thrombocytopenia in parvovirus B19–infected fetuses at the time of cordocentesis;[48] however, it is unclear whether there is benefit to providing platelets at the time of RBC transfusion. The majority of fetuses infected with parvovirus B19 demonstrate normal long-term development.[49-51] Rare cases of neurologic morbidity, persistent infection with severe anemia, and other sequelae have been reported following fetal infection.

MEASLES

Virology/Epidemiology

Measles, or rubeola, is an enveloped, negative-stranded RNA virus, part of the Paramyxoviridae family, which includes respiratory syncytial virus, canine distemper virus, mumps virus, and parainfluenza viruses. Measles host range is limited to humans. The envelope of this virus contains fusion and hemagglutinin (HA) proteins; HA binds the cellular receptor, which is a complement regulatory protein, and the fusion protein permits viral entry into the cell. **Rubeola (measles) is one of the most infectious viruses, spread primarily via respiratory droplets; with exposure 75% to 90% of susceptible contacts become infected.** A live, attenuated vaccine is readily available, resulting in three major patterns of measles outbreaks in the United States: unvaccinated preschoolers (including those <15 months of age), previously vaccinated school-age children and college students, **and persons originating from outside the United States.** The incidence of outbreaks in previously vaccinated individuals has been reduced since implementation of a two-dose vaccination strategy. Between 2001 and 2003, 44% of the measles cases reported in the United States occurred in an immigrant population.[52]

Clinical Manifestations

Rubeola has an incubation period of 10 to 14 days. Infected individuals first manifest prodromal symptoms, which may include fever, malaise, myalgias, and headache. These are followed by ocular symptoms including photophobia and a nonexudative conjunctivitis. Koplik spots, tiny white spots on a red base on the buccal mucosa lateral to the molar teeth, may appear during the prodrome and are pathognomonic for measles infection. If Koplik spots are visualized, they typically appear a day or so prior to the rash and disappear within 2 days of its appearance. The rash of measles appears between 2 and 7 days following the prodrome and is initially present behind the ears or on the face as a blotchy erythema. The rash then spreads to the trunk, followed by the extremities; the hands and feet may be spared. The rash is initially macular and blanches with pressure, but becomes papular and coalescent with a red, nonblanching component (Figure 50-2). The rash tends to fade after about 5 days. Fever can persist for up to 6 days and may reach 41° C; a productive cough may develop, which can persist after defervescence. Lymphadenopathy accompanies the fever and can persist for several weeks.

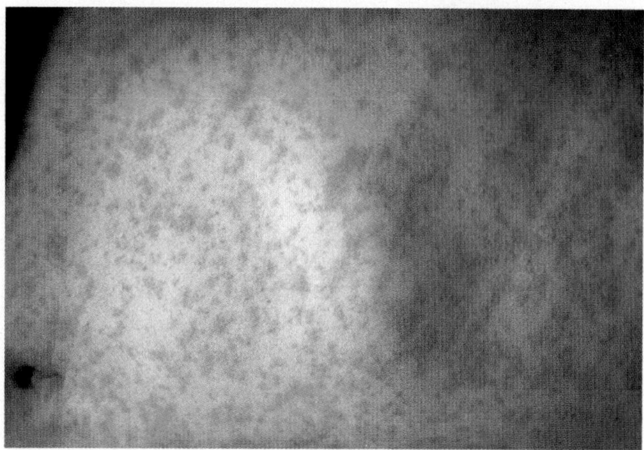

FIGURE 50-2. Maculopapapular rash of measles or rubeola showing coalescence of lesions. (Courtesy CDC/Dr. Heinz F. Eichenwald.)

Complications can include laryngitis, bronchiolitis, pneumonia, and otitis media due to secondary bacterial infections. Rare complications include hepatitis, encephalitis, atypical measles, and acute encephalitis. Encephalitis occurs in about 1 in 1000 cases of measles, resulting from either viral infection of the CNS or a hypersensitivity reaction to systemic viral infection. Symptoms include recurrence of fever and headache, vomiting, and a stiff neck followed by stupor and convulsions. The mortality is 10% and permanent neurologic sequelae, including mental retardation, develop in 50% of individuals. Atypical measles, which occurs in adults vaccinated with the formalin-inactivated measles vaccine, is characterized by high fever, pneumonia with pleural effusions, obtundation, and a hemorrhagic exanthema. These patients usually have high antibody titers to measles but lack antibodies to the fusion protein. Atypical measles is usually self-limiting, and patients are not contagious to others. A rare complication of measles infection is subacute sclerosing panencephalitis (SSPE), which occurs in 0.5 to 2 per 1000 cases of measles years after the acute infection. SSPE is most common in children who contracted measles prior to 2 years of age and is characterized by progressive neurologic debilitation and a virtually uniformly fatal outcome.

Diagnosis

Clinical features are usually used to diagnose infection; Koplik spots are pathognomonic for measles infection. In their absence diagnosis is based on a history of recent exposure and/or the presence of a rash. An increase in antibody titer may be detected as early as the first or second day of the rash; assays for detection of IgM and viral RNA are also available. Differential diagnoses include rubella, scarlet fever, infectious mononucleosis, secondary syphilis, toxic shock syndrome, Kawasaki's disease, erythema infectiosum, and drug rash. A guide to differentiating these illnesses is shown in Table 50-7.[53]

Management of Measles During Pregnancy

Pregnant women with rubeola infection should receive supportive care and undergo careful observation for

TABLE 50-7 A GUIDE TO THE DIFFERENTIAL DIAGNOSIS OF MEASLES

	CONJUNCTIVITIS	RHINITIS	SORE THROAT	EXANTHEM	LEUKOCYTOSIS	SPECIFIC LABORATORY TESTS
Measles	++	++	0	+	0	+
Rubella	0	±	±	0	0	+
Exanthem subitum	0	±	0	0	0	+
Enterovirus infection	0	±	±	0	0	+
Adenovirus infection	+	+	+	0	0	+
Scarlet fever	±	±	++	0	+	+
Infectious mononucleosis	0	0	++	±	±	
Drug rash	0	0	0	0	0	0

evidence of complications. The largest, most recently reported study of measles in pregnancy revealed that pregnant women with measles were twice as likely to require hospitalization (60%), three times as likely to acquire pneumonia (26%), and six times as likely to die from complications (3%) compared to nonpregnant adults.[54] Given the higher rate of maternal morbidity and mortality in the setting of measles infection, secondary bacterial infections should be treated promptly with antibiotics. Ribavirin can be considered for cases of viral pneumonia; however, it has not been conclusively shown to be of benefit.

There is a 20% to 60% risk of spontaneous abortion and preterm delivery following measles infection during pregnancy.[54] If miscarriage does not occur, patients should be counseled that measles does not appear to be associated with an increased risk of fetal malformations and that the risk of congenital measles infection appears to be well below 25%; two recent studies assessing a total of 98 maternal measles infections showed an absence of congenital measles infections.[54,55] Detailed serial ultrasounds may be performed. Evidence of in utero infection includes microcephaly, growth restriction, and oligohydramnios. There have been conflicting reports regarding whether an association exists between measles infection in pregnancy and Crohn's disease in offspring.[56,57] Others have reported an association between measles exposure at the time of birth and the development of Hodgkin's disease in children.[58]

The most effective way to prevent measles infection in pregnancy is to ensure vaccination prior to pregnancy using a two-dose series, which usually includes the trivalent MMR (measles, mumps, and rubella) vaccine. This live, attenuated vaccine should not be given to pregnant women, and patients are recommended to use effective contraception for 3 months postvaccination, although no cases of congenital measles infection have been reported secondary to the measles vaccine.[59] Although most pregnant women will have been previously vaccinated against measles, between 3.2% and 20.5% of pregnant women have either absent or low antibody titers, which would classify them as seronegative.[60] Any pregnant women exposed to measles should have an IgG titer drawn. Seronegative (susceptible) women should be treated with 0.25 mL/kg of immune globulin intramuscularly within 6 days of exposure (maximum dose of 15 mL).[59] Neonates delivered to a parturient who developed measles within 7 to 10 days of delivery should receive intramuscular immune globulin at a dose of 0.25 mg/kg. These children should also receive the MMR vaccine at 12 to 15 months of age.[59]

RUBELLA

Virology/Epidemiology

Rubella is a small, spherical, enveloped single-stranded RNA virus that is part of the Togavirus family. Transmission occurs via respiratory droplets and close personal contact. Following infection of respiratory mucosa, virus is found within cervical lymph nodes and disseminates hematogenously. Rubella outbreaks occur in school-aged children and in settings where crowded conditions exist, such as military bases, religious communities, college campuses, and prisons. No recent, major outbreaks have occurred in the United States secondary to routine vaccination. Elimination of endemic rubella is a national health objective; there were only seven reported rubella cases in the United States in 2009.[61] Most infections occur in foreign-born, unvaccinated individuals.

Clinical Manifestations

The incubation period following exposure is 12 to 19 days; however, acute rubella infection is not always diagnosed because 20% to 50% of infections are asymptomatic and there is no associated prodromal illness. Symptomatic, infected patients present with a rash, malaise, fever, conjunctivitis, and generalized lymphadenopathy. The rash is nonpruritic, begins on the face and neck as a faint macular erythema, and spreads rapidly to the trunk and extremities (Figure 50-3). The rash lasts approximately 3 days and blanches with pressure. Transient polyarthralgias and/or polyarthritis lasting 5 to 10 days may appear in adolescents and adults following the rash. Rare complications include thrombocytopenic purpura, encephalitis, neuritis, and orchitis.

Diagnosis

Serology is most commonly used to document exposure and/or infection with rubella. IgM specific for rubella is detectable prior to the onset of the rash.[62] Isolation and culture of the virus is possible as is detection of viral RNA by RT-PCR. In cases of suspected congenital rubella infection, RT-PCR can be used to detect viral RNA within chorionic villi, fetal blood, and amniotic fluid specimens.[63]

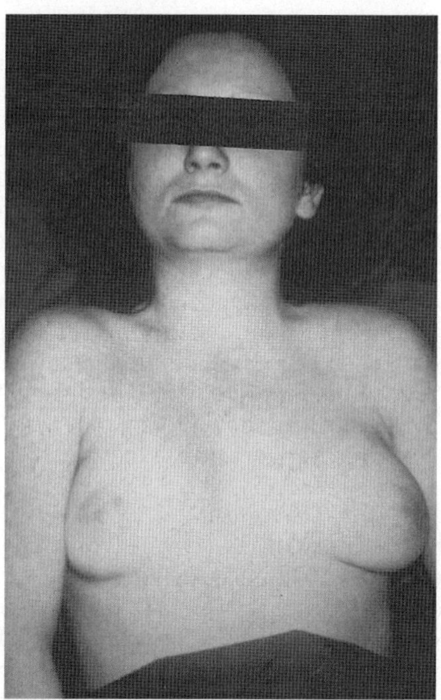

FIGURE 50-3. Photograph shows typical erythematous, maculopapular rash of rubella.

Management of Rubella Infection During Pregnancy

Maternal rubella infection is usually self-limited. However, congenital rubella infection is associated with miscarriage and/or stillbirth and can have significant deleterious effects on the fetus. IVIG administration does not prevent congenital rubella infection. The primary purpose of the rubella vaccine is to prevent congenital rubella infection; however, this live attenuated vaccine is contraindicated during pregnancy. Rubella vaccine is available as a monovalent form, a bivalent form (measles-rubella), or a trivalent form (MMR). The CDC has followed 500 cases of congenital rubella infection occurring from the vaccine strain, with no reported congenital malformations,[64] and smaller studies report similar findings. These observational studies demonstrate that rubella vaccination during pregnancy does not carry a significant risk of birth defects secondary to congenital rubella infection; therefore, therapeutic termination of pregnancy is not recommended in these cases.[64] Rubella serology is typically performed on obstetrical intake to identify women with inadequate levels of antibody. These women should receive rubella vaccine in the postpartum period.

Congenital Infection

There were 26 cases of congenital rubella infection documented in the United States from 1997 to 1999, and 92% of these infants were born to foreign-born mothers.[64] Because rubella cases have markedly declined in the past decade we have currently eliminated congenital rubella syndrome (CRS).[61] Several studies have established relationships between the frequency and severity of CRS and the timing of rubella infection in pregnancy. In general, infection in early pregnancy is associated with increased CRS severity. When maternal infection occurs within the first 12 weeks of pregnancy and is accompanied by a rash, more than 80% of fetuses become infected with rubella.[65] Of these infants, 67% will have findings consistent with CRS.[66] First-trimester infection with rubella is also associated with miscarriage, although some of the women in these studies terminated their pregnancy secondary to exposure. As the pregnancy progresses the risk of congenital rubella infection decreases; risk is 54% at 13 to 14 weeks, and 25% at the end of the second trimester.[65] The association of congenital rubella infection with CRS also decreases with increasing gestational age, with fetal defects being rare in fetuses infected beyond the 16th week of pregnancy.[65,66] Given that the association of congenital rubella infection and CRS is not absolute at any gestational age, ultrasound may be a useful adjunct in determining whether a fetus is affected, although this technique cannot detect many of the associated abnormalities.

The most common manifestation of congenital rubella infection is growth retardation. Sensorineural hearing loss is the most common single defect associated with CRS, affecting up to 90% of congenitally infected infants, and the rate of hearing loss is inversely related to the gestational age of congenital rubella infection.[64] When infection occurs prior to 12 weeks' gestation, other common defects include cardiac lesions (13%), most commonly patent ductus arteriosus, and eye defects (13%) such as cataracts, glaucoma, or retinitis.[66] Other findings consistent with CRS include micropthalmia, microcephaly, cerebral palsy, mental retardation, and intrauterine growth restriction (IUGR). Most of these findings are seen only in fetuses infected within the first 12 weeks of gestation; however, virtually all fetuses infected prior to the 11th week of gestation have CRS.[65] Severe disease can also include thrombocytopenic purpura or hepatosplenomegaly. Fetuses infected between 13 and 16 weeks of gestation have up to a 35% risk of being affected by CRS[65] and typically have hearing loss as their principal manifestation of CRS. Fetuses infected at more advanced gestational ages rarely have sequelae associated with CRS. Following congenital rubella infection, infants may shed virus for up to 1 year after birth. Even in neonates who are asymptomatic at birth, up to one third can manifest long-term complications, including type 1 diabetes mellitus and progressive panencephalitis in the second decade of life.[67,68]

CYTOMEGALOVIRUS INFECTION

Virology/Epidemiology

Cytomegalovirus (CMV) is a large, double-stranded DNA, enveloped virus that is a β-herpesvirus. Herpesviruses have large, complex genomes, replicating in the nucleus of infected cells, enabling these viruses to establish acute, persistent, and latent infection. Recurrent CMV infection occurs following reactivation from latently infected cells or by superinfection with a different strain or serotype of virus. CMV is not highly contagious; transmission primarily occurs by contact with infected saliva or urine, and CMV can also be transmitted via blood or by sexual contact. The incubation period is about 40 days following exposure. Within the United States, the rate of primary CMV infection in pregnant women ranges from 0.7% to 4%, and recurrent infection can be as high at 13.5%. Young infants and children with subclinical infection are a major source of infectious CMV; approximately 50% of children attending day care actively shed CMV virus in their saliva and/or urine and fomites within day-care centers are potential sources of CMV infection. Thus day-care workers are at high risk for infection. Small children pose an infection risk to family members, with annual seroconversion rates of approximately 10% for parents and uninfected siblings.[69] CMV seropositivity correlates with lower socioeconomic status, birth outside North America, increasing parity and age, abnormal Pap smears, infection with *Trichomonas*, and the number of sex partners.[70] CMV infection is also increased in immunocompromised patients. Between 0.2% and 2.2% of infants born in the United States become infected with CMV in utero secondary to maternal infection, and congenital CMV is the leading cause of hearing loss in children. Another 6% to 60% of children become infected within the first 6 months of life secondary to intrapartum transmission, environmental exposure, and/or breastfeeding; however, peripartum-infected infants rarely demonstrate serious sequelae of CMV infection.[71]

Clinical Manifestations

Infected patients may be asymptomatic or have a mononucleosis-like syndrome with fever, malaise, myalgias, chills, and cervical lymphadenopathy. Infrequent complications include pneumonia, hepatitis, Guillain-Barré syndrome, and aseptic meningitis. Laboratory abnormalities include atypical lymphocytosis, elevated hepatic transaminases, and a negative heterophile antibody response (distinguishing CMV from Epstein-Barr virus infection).

Diagnosis

Active, maternal CMV infection is best diagnosed by culture, detection of CMV antigens, or DNA PCR of blood, urine, saliva, amniotic fluid, or cervical secretions. Serologic tests are available, but antibody levels may not be detectable for up to 4 weeks after primary infection and titers can remain elevated, making a serologic diagnosis of reinfection difficult. A fourfold increase in IgG titers within multiple specimens suggests active infection. IgM is used to diagnose recent or active infection, but both false-positive and false-negative results can occur. **Routine screening for CMV infection during pregnancy is not recommended given the prevalence of seropositivity.** Fetal infection is documented by culture or PCR of amniotic fluid; the sensitivity of PCR approaches 100% in gestations beyond 21 weeks.[72] Fetal serology and culture of fetal blood are much less sensitive. Fetal CMV infection can occur weeks to months following maternal infection; thus repeat testing may be warranted at 7-week intervals.[72] Antepartum CMV detection does not predict the severity of congenital CMV infection, and 80% to 90% of children with congenital CMV infection have no neurologic sequelae.

Management of Cytomegalovirus During Pregnancy

Pregnant women should be counseled regarding preventive measures: careful handling of potentially infected articles such as diapers, clothing, and toys; avoiding sharing food and utensils; and frequent handwashing. Antiviral therapy is not indicated in immunocompetent, infected individuals and ganciclovir is not effective for intrauterine treatment of congenital CMV infection. Passive maternal immunization of pregnant women with primary CMV infection with CMV-specific hyperimmune globulin was associated with a decreased incidence of congenital CMV infection and the number of infants born with symptomatic CMV disease[73]; however, as discussed in a recent Cochrane review no randomized controlled trials exist examining interventions for preventing antepartum CMV transmission and adverse outcomes in congenitally infected infants.[74] A recombinant protein vaccine against CMV glycoprotein B was recently shown to prevent maternal CMV infection; however, this vaccine is not yet commercially available.[75]

Congenital Infection

Congenital CMV infection is diagnosed by detection of virus or viral nucleic acid within the first 2 weeks of life. The risk of intrauterine **CMV transmission is highest in the third trimester and the overall risk of fetal transmission is 30% to 40%.**[76] **Serious sequelae occur most commonly after first-trimester infection; 24% of these infected fetuses have sensorineural hearing loss and 32% have other CNS sequelae.** For fetuses infected after the second trimester, 2.5% demonstrated sensorineural hearing loss and 15% had CNS sequelae.[77] Congenital CMV infection may occur following primary or recurrent CMV infection of pregnant women, but the incidence of serious sequelae is lower following recurrent infection.[78] Most infants with congenital CMV infection exhibit no obvious clinical findings at birth. However, subclinical, congenital CMV infection is associated with hearing loss in 15% of cases.[78]

After primary, maternal CMV infection, approximately 5% to 18% of infants exhibit serious sequelae, typically following infection during the first half of pregnancy. Clinical findings in these infected infants may include jaundice, petechiae, thrombocytopenia, hepatosplenomegaly, growth restriction, and nonimmune hydrops. Long-term neurologic sequelae include developmental delays, seizure activity, and gross neurologic impairment, including sensorineural hearing loss.[78] Ultrasound can be useful in identifying a congenitally infected infant with likely impairment. Findings consistent with fetal injury include microcephaly, ventriculomegaly, intracerebral calcifications, ascites, hydrops, echogenic bowel, IUGR, and oligohydramnios. Unusual findings include fetal heart block and meconium peritonitis.[79,80] In the setting of confirmed fetal infection with serial normal ultrasounds, the risk of clinical symptoms of congenital CMV infection following birth is approximately 10%. Thus, ultrasound findings (or a lack thereof) are an important part of counseling.

HERPESVIRUS

Virology/Epidemiology

Herpes simplex virus (HSV) is another large, enveloped, double-stranded DNA virus, replicating in the host cell nucleus. Epithelial cells are the primary targets; however, HSV can disseminate via hematogenous spread or its capacity to form latent infections within dorsal root ganglia. Latent viral infection can be associated with integration of the viral genome into the host cell DNA. The HSV genome is complex, encoding more than 80 polypeptides, including several glycoproteins present on the envelope of the virus. Glycoprotein g permits differentiation of two well-defined antigenic and biologic viruses, HSV-1 and HSV-2. HSV-1 is typically associated with nongenital infection. The mouth and lips are the most common sites of viral replication; infection with this virus is most prevalent in lower socioeconomic populations, where 75% to 90% of individuals have antibodies against HSV-1 by 10 years of age. HSV-2 infection is usually acquired via sexual contact and is also related to socioeconomic factors. In the United States, 25% to 65% of individuals have antibodies to HSV-2, and seroprevalence risk correlates with the number of sexual partners. Some individuals have asymptomatic or subclinical primary HSV infections, accounting for seropositive patients in the absence of a clinical history of infection.

Clinical Manifestations

HSV-1 infection is normally evidenced by herpes simplex labialis (cold sores), whereas HSV-2 infection customarily involves the genital area and may affect the vulva, vagina, and/or cervix. Painful vesicles appear 2 to 14 days after viral exposure; the vesicles undergo spontaneous rupture, leaving lesions appearing as shallow eroded ulcers (Figure 50-4). Later in infection, a dry crust forms and lesions heal without scarring. Primary infection can be associated with fever, malaise, anorexia, bilateral inguinal lymphadenopathy, and is infrequently associated with aseptic meningitis. Women may also have dysuria and urinary retention secondary to urethral involvement. Rates of symptomatic and subclinical HSV shedding from the cervix and vulva during the first 3 months following primary infection are 1% to 3%.[81]

Healing of primary HSV-2 infection may take several weeks and primary symptoms are less severe in individuals with prior HSV-1 infection. Nonprimary, first episodes of genital HSV occur when a second HSV strain (either HSV-1 or HSV-2) establishes infection in the presence of preexisting antibodies from previous infection at a nongenital site (usually oral). Secondary or recurrent HSV infections usually represent viral reactivation and vary in frequency and intensity. Recurrent infections are usually less severe than primary infection, and associated with fewer lesions and a shorter period of viral shedding. One third of HSV-infected individuals have no recurrences, one third have approximately three recurrences per year, and another third have more than three recurrences per year. Table 50-8 compares clinical findings during primary and recurrent HSV infection. Disseminated HSV infection is rare, arising primarily in immunocompromised individuals, but it can also occur in pregnancy. Disseminated infection is characterized by skin, mucous membrane, and visceral organ involvement, and may include ocular involvement, meningitis, encephalitis, and ascending myelitis. Treatment with IV acyclovir should be initiated promptly in suspected cases of disseminated HSV.

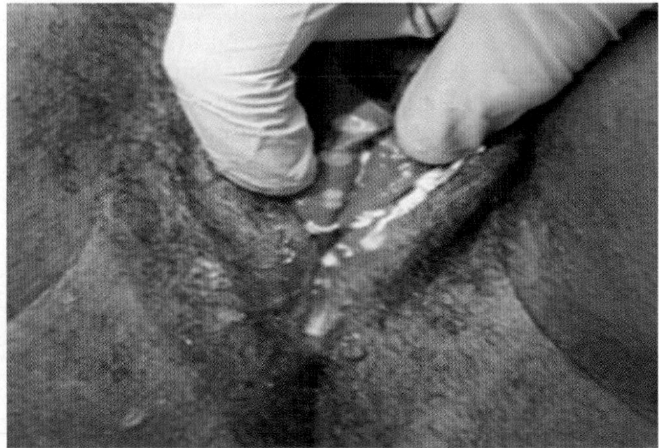

Figure 50-4. Ulcerated lesions characteristic of herpes simplex infection. (From Ferri F, et al: Ferri's Fast Facts in Dermatology. Philadelphia, Saunders, 2011.)

Diagnosis

Definitive diagnosis of active HSV infection is made by viral culture or by nucleic acid detection of HSV DNA, which provides a more rapid and sensitive diagnosis. Both methods can differentiate between HSV-1 and HSV-2. Culture specimens should be collected from fresh vesicles or pustules, because viral recovery from crusted lesions is poor; this is not as critical for PCR-based assays. Serology can be useful to assess and differentiate primary infection from secondary infection, via IgM detection. Cytologic preparations (Tzanck test) show characteristic multinucleated giant cells and intranuclear inclusions; however, this is rarely performed given the enhanced sensitivity and specificity of the above methods.

Management of Herpesvirus During Pregnancy

Maternal primary infection with HSV prior to labor does not usually affect the fetus; increased rates of miscarriage following primary HSV infection have been reported, but a recent prospective study showed no increase in spontaneous pregnancy loss.[82] In addition, intrauterine HSV infection is rare, occurring in approximately 1 in 200,000 deliveries. Sequelae in such cases include skin vesicles and/or scarring, eye disease, microcephaly, or hydranencephaly.[83] An association between HSV infection in the

Table 50-8 Comparison of Primary Versus Recurrent Herpes Simplex Virus Infection

	Type of Infection	
Stage of Illness	**Primary (Days)**	**Recurrent (Days)**
Incubation period and/or prodrome	2-10	1-2
Vesicle, pustule	6	2
Wet ulcer	6	3
Dry crust	8	7
Total	22-30	13-14

TABLE 50-9 HERPESVIRUS TREATMENT

DRUG	PRIMARY INFECTION	RECURRENT INFECTION	PROPHYLAXIS
Acyclovir	400 mg TID for 7-10 days	800 mg BID for 5 days or 800 mg TID for 2 days	400 mg BID
Valacyclovir	1 g BID for 7-10 days	500 mg BID for 3 days or 1 g daily for 5 days	500-1000 mg once daily
Famciclovir	250 mg TID for 7-10 days	500 mg followed by 250 g BID for 2 days or 1 g BID for 1 day	250 mg BID

third trimester of pregnancy and IUGR has also been reported. However, this observation was based on five patients.[84] Birthweight of infants born to asymptomatic HSV shedding mothers is lower than those of nonshedding mothers, but this small observed effect may be due to differences in gestational age at birth.[85] Treatment regimens are described in Table 50-9; women with more than two HSV recurrences per year are candidates for prophylaxis to decrease the frequency and severity of recurrences.

The greatest risk associated with intrapartum HSV exposure is that of developing neonatal herpes infection. Neonatal HSV infection complicates approximately 1 in 3500 deliveries in the United States; 70% of cases are caused by HSV-2, and significant neonatal morbidity and mortality follows neonatal infection. The estimated risk of neonatal HSV during primary maternal infection is 50%, whereas with recurrent HSV infection the neonatal HSV incidence ranges from 0% to 3%.[86] Thus, primary maternal HSV infection, rather than recurrent infection, accounts for the vast majority of neonatal HSV infections.[87] The ACOG recommends elective cesarean delivery for women with demonstrable genital herpes lesions or prodromal symptoms in labor to reduce the incidence of neonatal HSV infection.[86] Unfortunately, 60% to 80% of neonatal HSV infection cases occur following asymptomatic, primary maternal infection, limiting our ability to prevent neonatal HSV infection by performing cesarean delivery. A recent cost/benefit analysis of the current guidelines for the prevention of neonatal HSV infection found that given the low risk of neonatal HSV transmission with recurrent maternal infection, it takes 1580 elective cesarean sections to prevent one case of neonatal HSV.[88]

The risk of neonatal HSV infection in cases of active, nongenital maternal HSV lesions (i.e., thigh, buttock, mouth) is low. Therefore cesarean delivery is not recommended for these women. The duration of ruptured membranes prior to delivery increases the risk of neonatal HSV infection. However, there is no evidence that there is a period of time beyond which cesarean delivery is no longer beneficial. In the case of premature rupture of membranes, acyclovir or other antivirals should be considered in women with active HSV lesions being managed expectantly and given steroids to enhance fetal lung maturity.[86]

Various studies have investigated strategies to limit neonatal HSV transmission and reduce the number of cesarean deliveries performed prophylactically to limit neonatal HSV transmission.[89] Positive HSV cultures in the antepartum period are not associated with a positive culture at the time of delivery.[89] Prophylactic acyclovir or valacyclovir decreases the incidence of HSV shedding and reduces the number of cesarean deliveries performed to prevent neonatal HSV infection.[90] This strategy may be considered for women who have experienced a recurrence of HSV at some point during their pregnancy.

Neonatal Herpes Infection

Approximately 70% of neonatal HSV infections are caused by HSV-2. Factors predicting neonatal HSV transmission include cervical HSV shedding, invasive monitoring, preterm delivery, maternal age less than 21 years of age, and HSV viral load.[91] Neonatal HSV infection is treated with IV acyclovir. There are three patterns of neonatal HSV infections occurring with equal frequency: (1) Local or skin, eyes, and mouth (SEM) disease, limited to the skin, eyes, and mouth; this pattern has limited morbidity. (2) Disseminated infection involving multiple visceral organs including lungs, liver, adrenal glands, skin, eyes, and brain. Both SEM and disseminated disease present early, at 10 to 12 days of life. (3) CNS disease, occurring in the presence or absence of skin involvement, occurs later, during the second or third week of life. Using high-dose neonatal acyclovir, the 1-year mortality is 29% for disseminated disease and 4% for CNS disease; moreover, 83% of disseminated disease survivors have normal neurologic development and 31% of CNS disease survivors are neurologically intact.[92] Complications of neonatal HSV infection also include DIC and hemorrhagic pneumonitis.

VARICELLA

Virology/Epidemiology

Varicella, or chickenpox, is caused by the varicella zoster virus (VZV), a member of the α-herpesvirus subfamily. This enveloped virus contains double-stranded DNA and has at least 69 genes. Viral replication initially occurs within respiratory epithelial cells and is followed by systemic viremia. Long-term, latent infection occurs within the non-neuronal cells of the dorsal root ganglia. Humans are the only known host for varicella, a highly contagious disease transmitted by respiratory droplets or close contact. Approximately 95% of susceptible household contacts will become infected following exposure. The incubation period is about 14 days. Patients are infectious from 1 day prior to the rash until lesions are crusted. Immunity is usually lifelong. Prior to the advent of the VZV vaccine, most natural varicella infections occurred in early childhood, a time when VZV infection is usually self-limited. More than 50% of varicella-associated mortality occurs in adults, who represent less than 10% of all varicella infections.[93] Most adults (>90%) are immune to VZV, even in the absence of a clinical history of chickenpox.[94]

Clinical Manifestations

Infected patients classically present with a centripetal rash characterized by erythematous macules, papules, and vesicles that are highly pruritic, appearing in crops. The rash spreads to the extremities, and evidence of excoriation and scabbed lesions is typically seen. Fever is common and infected adults frequently present with malaise, myalgias, arthralgias, and headache. Bacterial superinfection of skin lesions can occur. Patients should be carefully observed for the development of varicella pneumonia because the rate of this complication approaches 20% in pregnancy.[95,96] Cough and dyspnea usually occur about 3 days after the appearance of the first skin lesions. Cyanosis, hemoptysis, and pleuritic chest pain are common. Encephalitis is a rare complication of adult VZV infection. Reactivation of latent VZV infection causes herpes zoster or shingles, occurring primarily in the elderly and immunocompromised. Shingles is characterized by a rash within a segmental distribution correlating with specific dermatomes. Pain, itching, and/or paresthesias can occur as a prodrome or with the appearance of the rash. Although zoster is usually self-limited, patients are infectious and can transmit VZV to susceptible individuals.

Diagnosis

Diagnosis is usually made based on a history of exposure and the presence of a rash. Rapid diagnosis of acute infection can be obtained by PCR amplification of VZV-specific DNA from vesicular fluid, and/or throat swabs. Serologic confirmation of infection can be made by ELISA, which can quantitate VZV-specific IgG and IgM; this method is most useful to diagnose prior exposure. The Tzanck stain can also be used to identify multinucleated giant cells present within lesions, and varicella can be cultured.

Management of Varicella During Pregnancy

Pregnant women infected with VZV should be offered supportive care including calamine lotion, antipyretics, and if necessary, systemic antipruritics. Oral acyclovir (800 mg by mouth 5 times per day) or valacyclovir (1 g by mouth 3 times a day) are safe in pregnancy, decrease the duration of illness if instituted within 24 hours of the rash, and should be given to all infected women. Maternal varicella pneumonia usually presents 3 to 5 days following the rash and has a 5% mortality rate; patients should be treated with IV acyclovir upon diagnosis, 10 to 15 mg/kg every 8 hours. If maternal varicella occurs within 5 days before and 2 days following delivery, varicella zoster immune globulin (VZIG) should be given to the newborn to reduce the incidence of neonatal varicella. The infant should also be isolated from the mother until all vesicles have crusted over to prevent VZV transmission. If possible, delivery should be delayed 5 to 7 days following the onset of maternal illness to potentially prevent neonatal VZV, which has a 20% to 30% mortality rate.[96]

Prevention includes ascertaining VZV status prior to pregnancy in women without a clinical history of infection and offering the live, attenuated VZV vaccine (Varivax, Merck) to susceptible women. Adults should receive two subcutaneous doses of vaccine 4 to 8 weeks apart. The vaccine is 70% to 80% effective at preventing natural infection. This live vaccine is contraindicated during pregnancy, and pregnancy should be deferred for 3 months following vaccination, although there is no evidence of congenital VZV infection following vaccination during pregnancy.[97] If a pregnant woman without a clinical history of VZV infection or vaccination is exposed to varicella, serology should be performed within 96 hours of exposure. Most patients will be seropositive for varicella IgG, and not at risk for acute infection. If VZV susceptibility is confirmed or serology cannot be obtained in a timely fashion, the preferred prophylaxis is high-titer varicella zoster immune globulin (VZIG). VariZIG is given by intramuscular injections and can be obtained 24 hr a day from the sole authorized U.S. distributor (FFF Enterprises, Temecula, CA, tel. 1-800-843-7477; or online at www.fffenterprises.com); the recommended dose is 125 units/10 kg of body weight, up to a maximum of 625 units. In the absence of VariZIG, IV immune globulin (IVIG) can be substituted if necessary at a dose of 400 mg/kg.[98] Prophylactic acyclovir, 800 mg PO 5 times daily for 5 to 7 days, beginning within 9 days of exposure, is effective at preventing VZV infection in children, with an 85% reduction in infection.[99] These two therapies can be combined, potentially further reducing the risk of maternal varicella infection; a small study comparing varicella postexposure prophylaxis in children found that acyclovir and VZIG together are more efficacious than VZIG alone.[100] Given the time constraints for prophylactic treatment following exposure, consider varicella serologic assessment at the first prenatal visit for women denying a history of VZV infection/vaccination. Results can be useful during pregnancy, and can be used to plan vaccination of susceptible patients in the postpartum period.

Congenital Infection

Congenital varicella infection can lead to spontaneous abortion, intrauterine fetal demise, and varicella embryopathy. Congenital varicella syndrome (CVS) is characterized by cutaneous scars, limb hypoplasia, muscle atrophy, malformed digits, psychomotor retardation, microcephaly, cortical atrophy, cataracts, chorioretinitis, and microophthalmia. There is a low frequency of anomalies following exposure before 13 weeks; in a study of 472 women, only 0.4% of neonates were born with features of CVS. The highest risk occurs with maternal infection between 13 and 20 weeks' gestation; CVS incidence in this group is 2%.[101] No congenital malformations have been observed following maternal infection beyond 20 weeks' gestation, but neonatal skin lesions or scarring can be seen after birth. Ultrasound examination is the preferred assessment tool, because serology and the presence of VZV DNA do not predict fetal injury.[102] Ultrasound findings suggestive of CVS can include polyhydramnios, hydrops, echogenic foci within abdominal organs, cardiac malformations, limb deformities, microcephaly, and IUGR.[103]

HEPATITIS

Viral hepatitis comprises a spectrum of syndromes ranging from subclinical to fulminant disease, and is caused by several different viruses. Symptoms of acute viral hepatitis infection may include jaundice, malaise, fatigue, anorexia, nausea, vomiting, and right upper quadrant pain. Hepatic transaminases and bilirubin are moderately to markedly elevated and liver biopsy shows extensive hepatocellular injury with a prominent inflammatory infiltrate (Figure 50-5). Most cases of viral hepatitis are self-limited and resolve without treatment, but certain types of viruses can cause

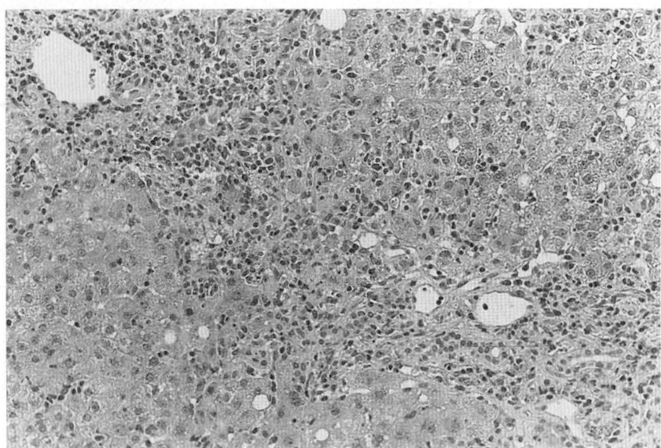

FIGURE 50-5. Photomicrograph of liver biopsy showing characteristic histologic changes of acute viral hepatitis. Note the intense inflammatory infiltrate.

persistent infection leading to chronic liver disease (see Chapter 45). The majority of hepatitis infections in the United States are caused by hepatitis viruses A, B, C, and D, whereas hepatitis E is endemic to Asia, Africa, and Mexico. Other viruses causing liver infection and inflammation (hepatitis) include cytomegalovirus, herpes simplex virus, Epstein-Barr virus, rubella, and yellow fever.[104]

Hepatitis A

Hepatitis A (HAV) is a small, single-stranded RNA virus that is part of the picornavirus family. HAV is transmitted primarily via oral-fecal contact and is responsible for approximately one third of acute hepatitis cases in the United States. The incidence of HAV in pregnancy is approximately 1 in 1000, and diagnosis is based on HAV IgM and IgG serology or detection of viral nucleic acid. The incubation period is approximately 28 to 30 days following exposure. Risk factors for HAV infection include exposure to contaminated food or water, recent travel outside the United States, illicit drug use, and having a child in day care. HAV infection is usually self-limited. Fewer than 0.5% of patients require hospitalization. HAV does not cause chronic infection. Physical activity should be limited to prevent hepatic trauma, and drugs with potential hepatotoxicity should be avoided. Sexual and household contacts of infected individuals should receive immunoprophylaxis with a single dose of HAV immune globulin and with HAV vaccine, an inactive vaccine that is safe for use in pregnancy.[105] Perinatal transmission has not been documented. However, infants delivered to an acutely infected mother should receive HAV immune globulin to prevent horizontal transmission following delivery.[106] HAV infection may be complicated by cholestatic hepatitis, characterized by pruritus, dark urine, direct hyperbilirubinemia, and elevated alkaline phosphatase. The duration of this syndrome can span several months, prognosis is good, and corticosteroid therapy is effective at alleviating symptoms.[104]

Hepatitis B

Virology/Epidemiology

Hepatitis B (HBV) is caused by a small, enveloped double-stranded DNA virus. The intact virus is called the Dane particle. There are three antigens of clinical importance associated with HBV. They are the surface antigen (HBsAg) or viral envelope glycoprotein, the core antigen (HBcAg), associated with viral nucleic acid, and HBeAg, a protein secreted from infected cells that is not a part of an infectious virus particle. HBV is transmitted primarily via parenteral routes, sexual transmission, and perinatal exposure. The incubation period is 4 weeks to 6 months following exposure, depending on viral inoculum; the clinical course is shown in Figure 50-6.[104] Eighty-five percent to 90% of patients acutely infected with HBV clear their infection. Fewer than 1% of infected patients develop fulminant hepatitis, characterized by massive hepatic necrosis and potentially accompanied by pancreatitis. Fifteen percent of patients become chronically infected with HBV, and 15% to 30% of these patients will develop liver cirrhosis and are at substantially increased risk for hepatocellular carcinoma.[104] HBV is the etiologic agent of 40% to 45% of all hepatitis infections and it is estimated that 1 million individuals in the United States are chronic viral carriers. The incidence of acute HBV infection in pregnancy is 1 to 2 per 1000, and 5 to 15 per 1000 pregnant women have chronic HBV infection.[107] Populations with increased HBV prevalence include Asians, Eskimos, drug addicts, dialysis patients, prisoners, and residents and employees of chronic care facilities.[104]

Diagnosis

Acute HBV infection is diagnosed by detection of HBsAg and IgM to the core antigen (HBc) or by viral load determination. Women with positive HBsAg serology greater than 6 months following acute HBV infection have chronic hepatitis; serologic findings are reviewed in Figure 50-6. Further testing is warranted to determine their level of viremia and assess ongoing liver injury manifested by elevated liver function tests. Chronic HBV infection has three forms. Typical chronic HBV (formerly described as chronic active) is characterized by positive HBsAg and HBeAg, an HBV DNA titer ranging from 10^7 to 10^{11}, and positive hepatic nuclear HBcAg. HBeAg-negative chronic HBV is characterized by positive HBsAg, negative HBeAg, an HBV DNA titer ranging from 10^5 to 10^9, and positive hepatic cytoplasmic HBcAg. Inactive HBV carrier state (formerly described as chronic persistent hepatitis) is characterized by positive HBsAg, negative HBeAg, an HBV DNA titer ranging from 10^1 to 10^5, and negative hepatic HBcAg.[108] In regard to other serologic markers, anti-HBs is present following hepatitis infection or vaccination, whereas antibody-recognizing core, or e antigen, is present only in patients who have been infected with hepatitis. Interpretation of serologic tests specific for hepatitis B are reviewed in Table 50-10.

Management of HBV Infection during Pregnancy

HBV infection is prevented by vaccination using a recombinant vaccine that is safe in pregnancy and should be offered to patients with significant risk factors, including a history of STDs, health care workers, and those with infected household or sexual contacts.[109] Lamivudine has been used to treat acute and chronic HBV infection in pregnancy and should be considered for maternal benefit in consultation with a hepatologist.[110] Pregnant women

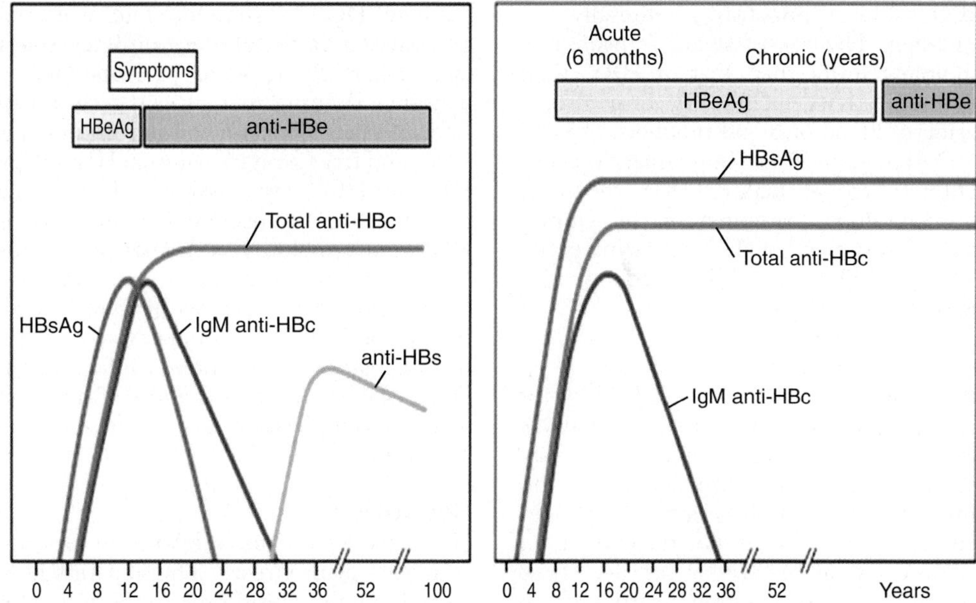

FIGURE 50-6. Typical course of hepatitis B. Timeline in weeks of acute hepatitis B infection is shown on the left and of chronic hepatitis B on the right. HBc, hepatitis B core; Hbe, hepatitis B early; HBsAg, hepatitis B surface antigen; IgM, immunoglobulin M. (From Mandell G, et al: Mandell, Douglas, and Bennett's Principles and Practice of Infectious Disease, ed 7. Philadelphia: Churchill-Livingstone, p 2066.)

TABLE 50-10 INTERPRETATION OF SEROLOGIC TESTS IN HEPATITIS B

TEST	ACUTE HEPATITIS B	IMMUNITY THROUGH INFECTION*	IMMUNITY THROUGH VACCINATION	CHRONIC HEPATITIS B†	HEALTHY CARRIER
HBsAg	+	–	–	+	+
Anti-HBs	–	+	+	–	–
HBeAg	+	–	–	+/–	–
Anti-HBe	–	+/–	–	+/–	+
Anti-HBc	+	+	–	+	+
IgM anti-HBc	+	–	–	–	–
HBV DNA‡	+	–	–	+	+ (low)
ALT	Elevated	Normal	Normal	Elevated	Normal

Reproduced from Mandell G, et al: Mandell, Douglas, and Bennett's Principles and Practice of Infectious Disease, ed 7. Philadelphia: Churchill-Livingstone, p 2073.
*Isolated anti-HBc IgG occurs during the window period of acute infection or can indicate remote prior infection with loss of HBsAg or anti-HBs. HBV DNA test and hepatology consult is indicated for these patients.
†The presence of HBeAg and anti-HBe together is considered a sign of high-titer virus production and increased infectivity. Individuals infected with HBeAg$^-$ HBV will have negative HBeAg and anti-HBe on serologic assessment.
‡Presence of HBV DNA depends on the sensitivity of the test used.
ALT, Alanine aminotransferase; *HBc,* hepatitis B core; *HBe,* hepatitis B e antigen; *HBsAg,* hepatitis B surface antigen; *HBV,* hepatitis B virus; *IgM,* immunoglobulin M.

with known hepatitis B should be vaccinated against hepatitis A to prevent further liver injury. Amniocentesis is safe in chronically infected women.[111] There is no contraindication to HBV-infected women breastfeeding, because perinatal transmission is not increased in these patients.[112]

In the United States, all newborns receive HBV vaccine as part of the CDC's recommendations to decrease HBV prevalence.[113] Infants born to mothers who are HBsAg seropositive should receive the hepatitis B vaccine series and hepatitis B immune globulin (HBIg).[109] The combination of HBV vaccine and HBIg is 85% to 95% effective at preventing perinatal HBV transmission. Similar to HIV, the rate of perinatal HBV transmission correlates with maternal viral load.[114] It is reasonable to measure maternal viral load between 30 and 34 weeks, permitting counseling regarding the risk of perinatal transmission. Lamivudine and HBIg limit intrauterine HBV transmission in viremic pregnant women better than HBIg alone.[115] Lamivudine is administered orally at a dose of 150 mg daily starting at 34 weeks to reduce perinatal HBV transmission in high-risk patients (i.e., those with a viral load $>10^7$); consultation with a hepatologist is recommended. Up to 80% to 90% of the infants of women acutely infected with HBV in the third trimester of pregnancy will be HBsAg positive at birth[105]; however, it is not known whether antiviral treatment during acute HBV infection lowers this risk.

Hepatitis C

Virology/Epidemiology

Hepatitis C virus (HCV) is an enveloped, single-stranded RNA virus that is part of the Flaviviridae family. Prior to its identification in the 1980s it was known as non-A non-B hepatitis. HCV is transmitted primarily parenterally and via vertical transmission. The risk of sexual transmission of HCV is substantially lower than that of HBV. Risk factors for HCV seropositivity include IV drug use, a history of transfusion of blood or blood products, obesity, and high gravidity.[116] More than 50% of individuals infected with HCV are chronic carriers, making HCV the most common chronic blood-borne pathogen in the United States.[117] The incubation period for HCV following exposure is 5 to 10 weeks, and 75% of acutely infected individuals are asymptomatic.

Diagnosis

The recommended initial screening test is ELISA for HCV-specific antibodies; for screen positive individuals the CDC recommends a more specific supplemental assay to verify serologic evidence of HCV infection, either the recombinant immunoblot assay (RIBA) or a nucleic acid test (NAT).[118] Universal screening is not recommended but individuals at risk should be tested (see box, Risk Factors for Hepatitis C). To assess chronic carrier status HCV viral loads are quantitated via PCR,[119] recognizing that there can be significant viral load and hepatic transaminase level variation over time. Thus, a single negative HCV viral load or normal hepatic transaminase level does not rule out chronic carrier status.[117]

RISK FACTORS FOR HEPATITIS C

Definite Indications for Screening

- History of injection of illegal drugs (even once, many years prior)
- Known HIV positive
- Persistently abnormal liver function tests
- History of long-term hemodialysis
- History of blood transfusion or organ transplant prior to July 1992
- History of clotting factor concentrates before 1987
- History of exposure to blood from an individual known to have HCV
- History of incarceration

Consider Screening (Need Uncertain)

- In-vitro fertilization from anonymous donors
- History of intranasal cocaine or other non-injectable illegal drug use
- History of tattooing or body piercing
- Known sexually transmitted disease or multiple partners
- Steady sex-partner of known HCV-positive individual
- Steady sex-partner of individual with history of injection drug use

HCV in Pregnancy

There is no effective vaccine against HCV. Interferon and ribavirin therapy is used in adults, but these drugs are contraindicated in pregnancy,[117] resulting in expectant management of HCV-infected pregnant women. A ribavirin registry reported no increased incidence of birth defects in 49 direct exposures and 69 indirect exposures.[120] Perinatal HCV transmission correlates with maternal HCV viral load; detectable HCV viremia has a 4% to 7% perinatal HCV transmission rate, whereas perinatal HCV transmission in the absence of detectable HCV viremia is rare. Other risk factors for perinatal HCV transmission are maternal IV drug use and HIV co-infection. The HCV infection prevalence in children co-infected with HIV was 1.5%, and treatment of maternal HIV infection lowers both HIV and HCV transmission.[121] The strongest predictor of perinatal HCV transmission is maternal HCV viral load. HCV transmission risk is increased with invasive fetal monitoring and rupture of membranes greater than 6 hours[14]; however, elective cesarean delivery does not reduce perinatal HCV transmission.[122] Pregnant women with a history of hepatitis C infection should be immunized against hepatitis A and B if not immune, and there is no contraindication to breastfeeding in women chronically infected with HCV.

Hepatitis D

Hepatitis delta virus (HDV) is an incomplete RNA virus related to plant viruses. The hepatitis D genome encodes a single nucleocapsid protein, HDAg, which is present as two peptides. The short form is required for RNA replication and the long form is packaged with HDV RNA and the HBsAg envelope glycoprotein. Because hepatitis D virus utilizes HBV as a helper virus (providing envelope glycoprotein), simultaneous or chronic HBV infection is required for viral replication. HDV is present worldwide, with a high prevalence in the Mediterranean basin, Middle East, Central Asia, West Africa, and the Amazon basin. Risk factors include IV drug use and exposure to infected blood products. Chronic HDV infection occurs at a rate of 1% to 3% when acquired as an HBV co-infection; the chronic infection rate is 70% to 80% when HDV superinfection occurs in an individual chronically infected with HBV. Patients chronically co-infected with HBV and HDV have a 70% to 80% risk for developing cirrhosis and portal hypertension, and 25% die of hepatic failure. Acute infection with HDV is characterized by HDV antigen positivity in the absence of HDV antibody. Individuals chronically infected with HDV will have detectable HDV antigen and HDV antibody. Acute hepatitis D infection is associated with an increased incidence of fulminant hepatic failure, which has a mortality rate of 2% to 20%. HDV can be perinatally transmitted,[123] although perinatal HBV prophylaxis is also effective at preventing perinatal HDV transmission in patients co-infected with HBV.[105]

Hepatitis E

Hepatitis E virus is an enveloped, RNA virus that is most closely related to the togavirus family, which also includes rubella. Hepatitis E is transmitted by oral-fecal contact and is endemic outside of the United States in regions such as Africa, Asia, and Latin America. Similar to hepatitis A, hepatitis E infection causes only acute disease. Diagnosis can be made by the presence of a specific IgM or of viral nucleic acid (RT-PCR). There are 4 genotypes; genotypes 1 and 2 are non-zoonotic and present in developing countries, and genotypes 3 and 4 are zoonotic and present in industrialized countries. The mortality rate following acute hepatitis E infection in the general population is 1%. Significantly higher mortality (up to 20%) has been observed in pregnant women infected with hepatitis E. Most of these women were infected with genotypes 1 and 2.[124] The preterm delivery rate in patients with hepatitis E is estimated as high as 66%,[125] and maternal morbidity and mortality escalates with increasing gestational age.[105,125] Hepatitis E virus can also be perinatally transmitted and it has been associated with significant perinatal morbidity and mortality.[126]

WEST NILE VIRUS

West Nile virus (WNV) is a flavivirus transmitted by mosquitoes that infects a variety of birds and mammals, including humans. Most infections are subclinical (80%) and most symptomatic infections present with "West Nile fever" consisting of fever, headache, fatigue, rash, lymphadenopathy, and eye pain. Much less common is severe disease, which includes gastrointestinal symptoms, ataxia, extrapyramidal signs, seizures, weakness, mental status changes, and other neurologic findings. Severe disease is associated with aseptic meningitis, encephalitis, and flaccid paralysis. No specific treatment is available for WNV infection; supportive care should be provided. Diagnosis of WNV infection is based on the presence of specific IgM antibody and by neutralization assays; PCR is of limited usefulness because of transient and low viremia. Overall outcome in pregnant women infected with WNV is good, although some infections result in severe disease or encephalitis.[127] Outcome is good for the majority of exposed infants; there have been rare cases of encephalitis, and no reports of congenital malformations.[128] There is one documented case of WNV transmission during breastfeeding; no adverse outcome was noted, leading the CDC to recommend that women infected with WNV continue breastfeeding.[127] Prevention of potential maternal WNV infection includes avoiding the outdoors during peak mosquito feeding times, wearing protective clothing, and using insect repellants containing DEET.

COXSACKIE VIRUS

Coxsackie virus is the causative agent of hand, foot, and mouth disease; it is an enterovirus transmitted through the fecal-oral route. Several serotypes exist, and adult infection typically results in a self-limited febrile illness requiring no treatment.[129] There is one reported case of coxsackie B virus infection in pregnancy leading to acute liver failure that resolved following expectant management.[130] Coxsackie virus infection during pregnancy has also been associated in several studies with an increased rate of miscarriage[129,131] and an increased rate of insulin-dependent diabetes in offspring,[129,132] although a causative relationship has not been established.

HUMAN PAPILLOMAVIRUS

Human papillomaviruses HPVs are a group of small DNA viruses. Some types cause warts (HPV types 6, 11), whereas other types do not cause warts and are instead highly associated with the development of cervical and oral cancer (HPV types 16, 18, 31, 33, 52b, 58). Infections are sexually and/or vertically transmitted and the incidence of infection in college-aged women is nearly 50%. Therefore, it is not uncommon for pregnant women to have evidence of HPV infection. A recent study found that 37% of pregnant women without evidence of infection had detectable HPV DNA in the cervix, demonstrating an unexpectedly high rate of HPV infection in asymptomatic women.[133] Anogenital warts, caused by non-oncogenic HPV types, are one presentation of HPV infection and may be managed expectantly. However, hormonal effects can cause rapid proliferation and growth of warts necessitating treatment. Trichloroacetic acid and/or cryotherapy are used to treat anogenital warts in pregnancy, as podophyllin is contraindicated and little is known regarding the safety of imiquimod in pregnancy. Vaginal delivery is not contraindicated, unless the wart burden and position would result in dystocia. Maternal HPV infection with HPV types 6 and 11 is associated with pediatric laryngeal papillomatosis. However, given the high prevalence of maternal HPV infection and the rarity of laryngeal papillomatosis, prophylactic cesarean delivery is not recommended.[133,134] Cervical dysplasia is another consequence of HPV infection; appropriate management of abnormal Pap smears should be undertaken independent of pregnancy.

EPSTEIN-BARR VIRUS

The causative agent of infectious mononucleosis is Epstein-Barr Virus (EBV), a member of the herpesvirus family. Clinical presentation includes malaise, headache, fever, pharyngitis, lymphadenopathy, atypical lymphocytosis, heterophile antibody, and transient mild hepatitis. Infection is typically self-limited. EBV establishes latent infection in B lymphocytes; EBV can be reactivated, and is associated with the development of Hodgkin's and non-Hodgkin's lymphoma. Most adults (>95%) are seropositive for EBV; thus primary EBV infection in pregnancy is rare. Primary infection and/or reactivation of EBV is not associated with significant adverse pregnancy outcome.[135] There is an association between EBV reactivation in pregnancy and the development of childhood acute lymphoblastic leukemia,[136] and in utero EBV transmission has been demonstrated by detection of EBV DNA in neonatal lymphocytes.[137] However, in utero infection has not been associated with adverse outcome. Routine testing is not indicated given the extremely high prevalence of seropositivity and the lack of impact on pregnancy.

SMALLPOX

Variola virus is the causative agent of smallpox. Variola virus infection is restricted to humans and is highly transmissible via inhalation of airborne droplets or by direct contact with smallpox lesions on an infected individual.[138] Secondary to widespread vaccination, the last case of reported smallpox in the United States was in 1949; the World Health Organization declared smallpox's global eradication in 1980. Recent concerns regarding the potential use of variola virus as a bioterrorism agent has led to renewed interest in the clinical presentation and treatment of smallpox disease.

Patients with smallpox infection first experience high fever, chills, headache, backache, and vomiting; these

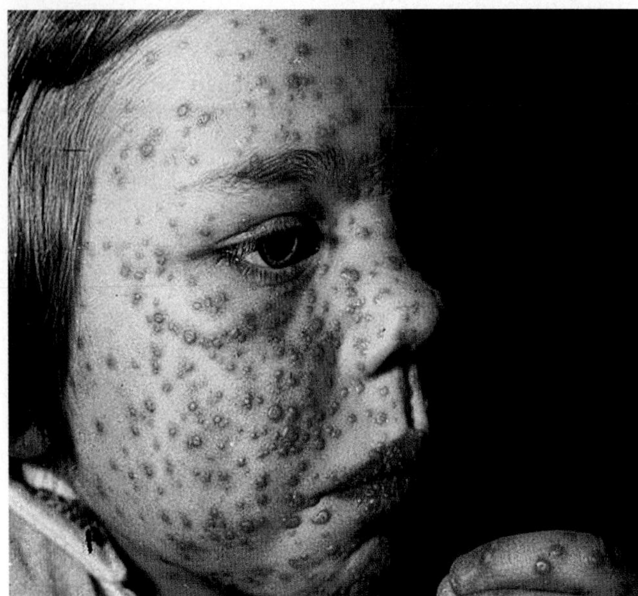

Figure 50-7. Smallpox vesicles, day 3 of clinical infection. (From Tyring S, et al: Tropical Dermatology. Edinburgh, Saunders, 2005.)

symptoms differentiate smallpox from chickenpox (varicella virus), which has a minimal prodrome.[138] Delirium is present in 15% of cases, and some infections progress to encephalitis. Skin lesions appear 2 to 3 days following the onset of symptoms, and progress from macula to papule to vesicle (Figure 50-7), vesicle to pustule to scabs, which then form pitted scars. Smallpox lesions appear in a centrifugal distribution and affect the soles and palms, in contrast to varicella infection, which exhibits a centripetal distribution of lesions and spares the palms and soles. Diagnosis should be confirmed by PCR reaction of pustular fluid and/or scabs in a biocontainment facility.

Maternal treatment is supportive; vaccination and containment are critical. The maternal mortality rate of unvaccinated women is more than 60%.[138] Death usually occurs secondary to viral pneumonitis, bacterial pneumonia, or cardiovascular collapse; moreover, pregnant women are at increased risk for hemorrhagic smallpox, a more severe and lethal manifestation of infection. When infection occurs prior to 24 weeks, 75% of pregnancies end in loss or premature delivery. During the latter half of pregnancy, smallpox infection is associated with a 55% rate of subsequent preterm delivery. Variola virus crosses the placenta, leading to intrauterine infection. During epidemics of the disease, the reported incidence of congenital variola (infection) ranges from 9% to 60%.

Vaccination within 2 to 3 days of initial exposure affords almost complete protection against disease.[138,139] The currently available vaccine, Dryvax, is composed of live, attenuated vaccinia virus. This vaccine has a higher risk of complications than other viral vaccines, including postvaccinal encephalitis (incidence 12 per million vaccines, 40% mortality rate), mild generalized vaccinia, and eczema vaccinatum. Smallpox vaccination is currently restricted to women in military service and researchers utilizing related viruses. Data on women vaccinated during pregnancy are being compiled in the National Smallpox Vaccine in Pregnancy Registry.[139] Fetal infection following maternal vaccination (fetal vaccinia) is rare, and is characterized by skin lesions and internal organ involvement but is not associated with fetal malformations. Therefore, vaccination is not considered an indication for pregnancy termination. The CDC recommends deferring elective smallpox vaccination while pregnant; however, immediate vaccination is indicated following smallpox exposure, independent of pregnancy, secondary to the risk of clinical smallpox infection to the mother and fetus.[139]

KEY POINTS

- All pregnant women should be offered HIV screening, using an "opt out" approach. In areas of high seroprevalence, repeat screening in the third trimester may be warranted.
- Rapid HIV testing should be offered in early labor to women without documented HIV status, because most perinatally infected infants are born to women who do not know their HIV status.
- Combination care with at least three drugs from at least two classes of ARV is the standard of care for HIV infection in the United States.
- Early and sustained control of viral replication is associated with decreased HIV transmission (including starting therapy prior to conception). ART should be started as early in pregnancy as possible for all women.
- Pregnant women suspected to be infected with influenza should be treated immediately, without delay for diagnostic confirmation.
- The ACOG and the CDC recommend vaccination of all pregnant women during the influenza season (October-May) using the intramuscular, inactivated vaccine.
- Fetal parvovirus infection may result in fetal anemia and hydrops. Women with documented infection should be screened serially with ultrasound and middle cerebral artery Doppler studies.
- Rubeola (measles) is one of the most infectious viruses; 75% to 90% of exposed, susceptible contacts become infected. Outbreaks often originate in individuals born outside the United States.
- Preconceptual vaccination with live attenuated viral vaccines can prevent antenatal rubeola, rubella, and varicella infection but should be avoided in pregnancy.
- Routine screening for CMV infection during pregnancy is not recommended given the prevalence of seropositivity.
- CMV transmission is highest in the third trimester and the overall risk of fetal transmission is 30% to 40%. Serious sequelae occur most commonly after first-trimester infection; 24% of these infected fetuses have sensorineural hearing loss and 32% have other CNS sequelae.
- Women without a history of varicella should be considered for serum testing. Susceptible women exposed to varicella should be treated with VZIG to reduce the risk of transmission.

- All pregnant women should be screened for hepatitis B infection. Infants delivered to seropositive mothers should receive both hepatitis B immune globulin (HBIg) and hepatitis B vaccine shortly after birth.
- Hepatitis A and B vaccination is safe in pregnancy and should be offered to susceptible women at risk.

REFERENCES

1. Berger EA, Murphy PM, Farber JM: Chemokine receptors as HIV-1 coreceptors: roles in viral entry, tropism, and disease. Annu Rev Immunol 17:657, 1999.
2. Ometto L, Zanchetta M, Mainardi M, et al: Co-receptor usage of HIV-1 primary isolates, viral burden, and CCR5 genotype in mother-to-child HIV-1 transmission. AIDS 14:1721, 2000.
3. Mangano A, Gonzalez E, Dhanda R, et al: Concordance between the CC chemokine receptor 5 genetic determinants that alter risks of transmission and disease progression in children exposed perinatally to human immunodeficiency virus. J Infect Dis 183:1574, 2001.
4. Ometto L, Bertorelle R, Mainardi M, et al: Analysis of the CC chemokine receptor 5 m303 mutation in infants born to HIV-1-seropositive mothers. Aids 13:871, 1999.
5. Centers for Disease Control and Prevention: HIV Surveillance Report, 2009. Available at http://www.cdc.gov/hiv/topics/surveillance/resources/reports/. Accessed March 13, 2011.
6. Alpert PL, Shuter J, DeShaw MG, et al: Factors associated with unrecognized HIV-1 infection in an inner-city emergency department. Ann Emerg Med 28:159, 1996.
7. Cavaco-Silva P, Taveira NC, Lourenco MH, et al: Vertical transmission of HIV-2. Lancet 349:177, 1997.
8. Martinez P, Ortiz de Lejarazu R, Eiros JM, et al: Usefulness of oral mucosal transudate for HIV antibody testing. Jama 277:1592, 1997.
9. Schneider E, Whitmore S, Glynn KM, et al: Revised surveillance case definitions for HIV infection among adults, adolescents, and children aged <18 months and for HIV infection and AIDS among children aged 18 months to <13 years—United States, 2008. MMWR Recomm Rep 57:1, 2008.
10. Branson BM, Handsfield HH, Lampe MA, et al: Revised recommendations for HIV testing of adults, adolescents, and pregnant women in health-care settings. MMWR Recomm Rep 55:1, 2006.
11. Pantaleo G, Fauci AS: New concepts in the immunopathogenesis of HIV infection. Annu Rev Immunol 13:487, 1995.
12. Panel on Antiretroviral Guidelines for Adults and Adolescents. Guidelines for the use of antiretroviral agents in HIV-1-infected adults and adolescents. Department of Health and Human Services. January 10, 2011; 1-166. Available at http://www.aidsinfo.nih.gov/ContentFiles/AdultandAdolescentGL.pdf. Accessed Sept. 22, 2011.
13. Pas S, Rossen JWA, Schoener D, et al: Performance evaluation of the new Roche Cobas AmpliPrep/Cobas TaqMan HIV-1 test version 2.0 for quantification of human immunodeficiency virus type 1 RNA. J Clin Microbiol 48:1195, 2010.
14. Panel on Treatment of HIV-Infected Pregnant Women and Prevention of Perinatal Transmission. Recommendations for Use of Antiretroviral Drugs in Pregnant HIV-1-Infected Women for Maternal Health and Interventions to Reduce Perinatal HIV Transmission in the United States. Department of Health and Human Services, 1-207. Available at http://aidsinfo.nih.gov/contentfiles/PerinatalGL.pdf. Accessed September 18, 2011.
15. Connor EM, Sperling RS, Gelber R, et al: Reduction of maternal-infant transmission of human immunodeficiency virus type 1 with zidovudine treatment. Pediatric AIDS Clinical Trials Group Protocol 076 Study Group. N Engl J Med 331:1173, 1994.
16. Townsend CL, Cortina-Borja M, Peckham CS, et al: Low rates of mother-to-child transmission of HIV following effective pregnancy interventions in the United Kingdom and Ireland, 2000-2006. AIDS 22:973, 2008.
17. Ioannidis JP, Abrams EJ, Ammann A, et al: Perinatal transmission of human immunodeficiency virus type 1 by pregnant women with RNA virus loads <1000 copies/ml. J Infect Dis 183:539, 2001.
18. Blanche S, Tardieu M, Rustin P, et al: Persistent mitochondrial dysfunction and perinatal exposure to antiretroviral nucleoside analogues. Lancet 354:1084, 1999.
19. Mandelbrot L, Landreau-Mascaro A, Rekacewicz C, et al: Lamivudine-zidovudine combination for prevention of maternal-infant transmission of HIV-1. Jama 285:2083, 2001.
20. Nucleoside exposure in the children of HIV-infected women receiving antiretroviral drugs: absence of clear evidence for mitochondrial disease in children who died before 5 years of age in five United States cohorts. J Acquir Immune Defic Syndr 25:261, 2000.
21. Ford N, Calmy A, Mofenson L: Safety of efavirenz in first-trimester of pregnancy: an updated systematic review and meta-analysis. AIDS 25:2301, 2001.
22. Hitti J, Andersen J, McComsey G, et al: Protease inhibitor-based antiretroviral therapy and glucose tolerance in pregnancy: AIDS Clinical Trials Group A5084. Am J Obstet Gynecol 196:331 e1, 2007.
23. Kaplan JE, Benson C, Holmes KH, et al: Guidelines for prevention and treatment of opportunistic infections in HIV-infected adults and adolescents: recommendations from CDC, the National Institutes of Health, and the HIV Medicine Association of the Infectious Diseases Society of America. MMWR Recomm Rep 58:1, 2009.
24. Somigliana E, Bucceri AM, Tibaldi C, et al: Early invasive diagnostic techniques in pregnant women who are infected with the HIV: a multicenter case series. Am J Obstet Gynecol 193:437, 2005.
25. Mandelbrot L, Jasseron C, Ekoukou D, et al: Amniocentesis and mother-to-child human immunodeficiency virus transmission in the Agence Nationale de Recherches sur le SIDA et les Hepatites Virales French Perinatal Cohort. Am J Obstet Gynecol 200:160 e1, 2009.
26. Peters V, Liu KL, Dominguez K, et al: Missed opportunities for perinatal HIV prevention among HIV-exposed infants born 1996-2000, pediatric spectrum of HIV disease cohort. Pediatrics 111:1186, 2003.
27. International Perinatal HIV Group: Duration of ruptured membranes and vertical transmission of HIV-1: a meta-analysis from 15 prospective cohort studies. AIDS 15:357, 2001.
28. Patel K, Shapiro DE, Brogly SB, et al: Prenatal protease inhibitor use and risk of preterm birth among HIV-infected women initiating antiretroviral drugs during pregnancy. J Infect Dis 201:1035, 2010.
29. Siston AM, Rasmussen SA, Honein MA, et al: Pandemic 2009 influenza A(H1N1) virus illness among pregnant women in the United States. JAMA 303:1517, 2010.
30. Goodnight WH, Soper DE: Pneumonia in pregnancy. Crit Care Med 33:S390, 2005.
31. Centers for Disease Control and Prevention (CDC): Evaluation of rapid influenza diagnostic tests for detection of novel influenza A (H1N1) Virus—United States, 2009. MMWR Morb Mortal Wkly Rep 58:826, 2009.
32. Varner MW, Rice MM, Anderson B, et al: Influenza-like illness in hospitalized pregnant and postpartum women during the 2009-2010 H1N1 pandemic. Obstet Gynecol 118:593, 2011.
33. Centers for Disease Control and Prevention (CDC): Maternal and infant outcomes among severely ill pregnant and postpartum women with 2009 pandemic influenza A (H1N1)—United States, April 2009—August 2010. MMWR Morb Mortal Wkly Rep 60:1193, 2011.
34. Fiore AE, Fry A, Shay D, et al: Antiviral agents for the treatment and chemoprophylaxis of influenza—recommendations of the Advisory Committee on Immunization Practices (ACIP). MMWR Recomm Rep 60:1, 2011.
35. ACOG Committee on Obstetric Practice: ACOG committee opinion number 305, November 2004. Influenza vaccination and treatment during pregnancy. Obstet Gynecol 104:1125, 2004.
36. Centers for Disease Control and Prevention (CDC): Influenza vaccination coverage among pregnant women—United States, 2010-11 influenza season. MMWR Morb Mortal Wkly Rep 60:1078, 2011.
37. Berns K, Parrish C: Parvoviruses. In Knipe P, Howley P: Fields Virology, vol 2, 5th ed. Philadelphia, Lippincott-Raven, 2007, p 2437.
38. Valeur-Jensen AK, Pedersen CB, Westergaard T, et al: Risk factors for parvovirus B19 infection in pregnancy. Jama 281:1099, 1999.
39. Centers for Disease Control (CDC): Risks associated with human parvovirus B19 infection. MMWR Morb Mortal Wkly Rep 38:81, 1989.
40. Thurn J: Human parvovirus B19: historical and clinical review. Rev Infect Dis 10:1005, 1988.

41. Bredl S, Plentz A, Wenzel JJ, et al: False-negative serology in patients with acute parvovirus B19 infection. J Clin Virol 51:115, 2011.
42. Bonvicini F, Puccetti C, Salfi NC, et al: Gestational and fetal outcomes in b19 maternal infection: a problem of diagnosis. J Clin Microbiol 49:3514, 2011.
43. Cosmi E, Mari G, Delle Chiaie L, et al: Noninvasive diagnosis by Doppler ultrasonography of fetal anemia resulting from parvovirus infection. Am J Obstet Gynecol 187:1290, 2002.
44. Prospective study of human parvovirus (B19) infection in pregnancy. Public Health Laboratory Service Working Party on Fifth Disease. BMJ 300:1166, 1990.
45. Enders M, Weidner A, Zoellner I, et al: Fetal morbidity and mortality after acute human parvovirus B19 infection in pregnancy: prospective evaluation of 1018 cases. Prenat Diagn 24:513, 2004.
46. Rodis JF, Borgida AF, Wilson M, et al: Management of parvovirus infection in pregnancy and outcomes of hydrops: a survey of members of the Society of Perinatal Obstetricians. Am J Obstet Gynecol 179:985, 1998.
47. Sahakian V, Weiner CP, Naides SJ, et al: Intrauterine transfusion treatment of nonimmune hydrops fetalis secondary to human parvovirus B19 infection. Am J Obstet Gynecol 164:1090, 1991.
48. de Haan TR, van den Akker ESA, Porcelijn L, et al: Thrombocytopenia in hydropic fetuses with parvovirus B19 infection: incidence, treatment and correlation with fetal B19 viral load. Br J Obstet Gynaecol 115:76, 2008.
49. Miller E, Fairley CK, Cohen BJ, et al: Immediate and long term outcome of human parvovirus B19 infection in pregnancy. Br J Obstet Gynaecol 105:174, 1998.
50. Perkin MA, English PM: Immediate and long term outcome of human parvovirus B19 infection in pregnancy. Br J Obstet Gynaecol 105:1337, 1998.
51. Rodis JF, Rodner C, Hansen AA, et al: Long-term outcome of children following maternal human parvovirus B19 infection. Obstet Gynecol 91:125, 1998.
52. Epidemiology of measles—United States, 2001-2003. MMWR Morb Mortal Wkly Rep 53:713, 2004.
53. Brunell PA: Measles. In Bennett J, Plum F: Cecil Textbook of Medicine, 20th ed. Philadelphia, W. B. Saunders, 1996, p 1758.
54. Eberhart-Phillips JE, Frederick PD, Baron RC, et al: Measles in pregnancy: a descriptive study of 58 cases. Obstet Gynecol 82:797, 1993.
55. Ali ME, Albar HM: Measles in pregnancy: maternal morbidity and perinatal outcome. Int J Gynaecol Obstet 59:109, 1997.
56. Ekbom A, Wakefield AJ, Zack M, et al: Perinatal measles infection and subsequent Crohn's disease. Lancet 344:508, 1994.
57. Pardi DS, Tremaine WJ, Sandborn WJ, et al: Perinatal exposure to measles virus is not associated with the development of inflammatory bowel disease. Inflamm Bowel Dis 5:104, 1999.
58. Nyari TA, Dickinson HO, Parker L: Childhood cancer in relation to infections in the community during pregnancy and around the time of birth. Int J Cancer 104:772, 2003.
59. Measles prevention. MMWR Morb Mortal Wkly Rep 38:1, 1989.
60. Neubert AG, Samuels P, Goodman DB, et al: The seroprevalence of the rubeola antibody in a prenatal screening program. Obstet Gynecol 90:507, 1997.
61. Centers for Disease Control and Prevention (CDC): Progress toward control of rubella and prevention of congenital rubella syndrome—worldwide, 2009. MMWR Morb Mortal Wkly Rep 59:1307, 2010.
62. Tookey P: Congenital rubella: down but not out. Lancet 360:803, 2002.
63. Tanemura M, Suzumori K, Yagami Y, et al: Diagnosis of fetal rubella infection with reverse transcription and nested polymerase chain reaction: a study of 34 cases diagnosed in fetuses. Am J Obstet Gynecol 174:578, 1996.
64. Control and prevention of rubella: evaluation and management of suspected outbreaks, rubella in pregnant women, and surveillance for congenital rubella syndrome. MMWR Recomm Rep 50:1, 2001.
65. Miller E, Cradock-Watson JE, Pollock TM: Consequences of confirmed maternal rubella at successive stages of pregnancy. Lancet 2:781, 1982.
66. Munro ND, Sheppard S, Smithells RW, et al: Temporal relations between maternal rubella and congenital defects. Lancet 2:201, 1987.
67. McIntosh ED, Menser MA: A fifty-year follow-up of congenital rubella. Lancet 340:414, 1992.
68. Townsend JJ, Baringer JR, Wolinsky JS, et al: Progressive rubella panencephalitis. Late onset after congenital rubella. N Engl J Med 292:990, 1975.
69. Taber LH, Frank AL, Yow MD, et al: Acquisition of cytomegaloviral infections in families with young children: a serological study. J Infect Dis 151:948, 1985.
70. Chandler SH, Alexander ER, Holmes KK: Epidemiology of cytomegaloviral infection in a heterogeneous population of pregnant women. J Infect Dis 152:249, 1985.
71. Stagno S, Pass RF, Dworsky ME, et al: Maternal cytomegalovirus infection and perinatal transmission. Clin Obstet Gynecol 25:563, 1982.
72. Stagno S, Britt W: Cytomegalovirus Infections, 6th ed. Philadelphia, Elsevier, 2006.
73. Nigro G, Adler SP, La Torre R, et al: Passive immunization during pregnancy for congenital cytomegalovirus infection. N Engl J Med 353:1350, 2005.
74. McCarthy FP, Giles ML, Rowlands S, et al: Antenatal interventions for preventing the transmission of cytomegalovirus (CMV) from the mother to fetus during pregnancy and adverse outcomes in the congenitally infected infant. Cochrane Database Sys Rev CD008371, 2011.
75. Pass RF, Zhang C, Evans A, et al: Vaccine prevention of maternal cytomegalovirus infection. N Engl J Med 360:1191, 2009.
76. Stagno S, Pass RF, Cloud G, et al: Primary cytomegalovirus infection in pregnancy. Incidence, transmission to fetus, and clinical outcome. JAMA 256:1904, 1986.
77. Pass RF, Fowler KB, Boppana SB, et al: Congenital cytomegalovirus infection following first trimester maternal infection: symptoms at birth and outcome. J Clin Virol 35:216, 2006.
78. Fowler KB, Stagno S, Pass RF, et al: The outcome of congenital cytomegalovirus infection in relation to maternal antibody status. N Engl J Med 326:663, 1992.
79. Lewis PE 2nd, Cefalo RC, Zaritsky AL: Fetal heart block caused by cytomegalovirus. Am J Obstet Gynecol 136:967, 1980.
80. Pletcher BA, Williams MK, Mulivor RA, et al: Intrauterine cytomegalovirus infection presenting as fetal meconium peritonitis. Obstet Gynecol 78:903, 1991.
81. Koelle DM, Benedetti J, Langenberg A, et al: Asymptomatic reactivation of herpes simplex virus in women after the first episode of genital herpes. Ann Intern Med 116:433, 1992.
82. Brown ZA, Selke S, Zeh J, et al: The acquisition of herpes simplex virus during pregnancy. N Engl J Med 337:509, 1997.
83. Baldwin S, Whitley RJ: Intrauterine herpes simplex virus infection. Teratology 39:1, 1989.
84. Brown ZA, Vontver LA, Benedetti J, et al: Effects on infants of a first episode of genital herpes during pregnancy. N Engl J Med 317:1246, 1987.
85. Brown ZA, Benedetti J, Selke S, et al: Asymptomatic maternal shedding of herpes simplex virus at the onset of labor: relationship to preterm labor. Obstet Gynecol 87:483, 1996.
86. ACOG Practice Bulletin: Clinical management guidelines for obstetrician-gynecologists. No. 82 June 2007. Management of herpes in pregnancy. Obstet Gynecol 109:1489, 2007.
87. Prober CG, Sullender WM, Yasukawa LL, et al: Low risk of herpes simplex virus infections in neonates exposed to the virus at the time of vaginal delivery to mothers with recurrent genital herpes simplex virus infections. N Engl J Med 316:240, 1987.
88. Randolph AG, Washington AE, Prober CG: Cesarean delivery for women presenting with genital herpes lesions: efficacy, risks, and costs. JAMA 270:77, 1993.
89. Arvin AM, Hensleigh PA, Prober CG, et al: Failure of antepartum maternal cultures to predict the infant's risk of exposure to herpes simplex virus at delivery. N Engl J Med 315:796, 1986.
90. Andrews WW, Kimberlin DF, Whitley R, et al: Valacyclovir therapy to reduce recurrent genital herpes in pregnant women. Am J Obstet Gynecol 194:774, 2006.
91. Brown ZA, Wald A, Morrow RA, et al: Effect of serologic status and cesarean delivery on transmission rates of herpes simplex virus from mother to infant. JAMA 289:203, 2003.
92. Thompson C, Whitley R: Neonatal herpes simplex virus infections: where are we now? In Curtis N, Finn A, Pollard AJ: Hot topics in infection and immunity in children VII, vol 697. New York, Springer, 2011, p 221.

93. Centers for Disease Control and Prevention (CDC): Varicella-related deaths among adults—United States, 1997. MMWR Morb Mortal Wkly Rep 46:409, 1997.
94. Wharton M: The epidemiology of varicella-zoster virus infections. Infect Dis Clin North Am 10:571, 1996.
95. Brunell PA: Varicella in pregnancy, the fetus, and the newborn: problems in management. J Infect Dis 166:S42, 1992.
96. Chapman S, Duff P: Varicella in pregnancy. Semin Perinatol 17:403, 1993.
97. Wald ER: Transmission of varicella-vaccine virus: what is the risk? J Pediatr 133:310, 1998.
98. Smith CK, Arvin AM: Varicella in the fetus and newborn. Sem Fetal Neonatal Med 14:209, 2009.
99. Asano Y, Yoshikawa T, Suga S, et al: Postexposure prophylaxis of varicella in family contact by oral acyclovir. Pediatrics 92:219, 1993.
100. Goldstein SL, Somers MJ, Lande MB, et al: Acyclovir prophylaxis of varicella in children with renal disease receiving steroids. Pediatr Nephrol 14:305, 2000.
101. Enders G, Miller E, Cradock-Watson J, et al: Consequences of varicella and herpes zoster in pregnancy: prospective study of 1739 cases. Lancet 343:1548, 1994.
102. Isada NB, Paar DP, Johnson MP, et al: In utero diagnosis of congenital varicella zoster virus infection by chorionic villus sampling and polymerase chain reaction. Am J Obstet Gynecol 165:1727, 1991.
103. Pretorius DH, Hayward I, Jones KL, et al: Sonographic evaluation of pregnancies with maternal varicella infection. J Ultrasound Med 11:459, 1992.
104. Wedemeyer H, Pawlotsky JM: Acute viral hepatitis. In Goldman L, Schafer AI: Goldman's Cecil Medicine, 24th ed. Philadelphia, Elsevier Saunders, 2012, p 966.
105. ACOG Practice Bulletin No. 86: Viral hepatitis in pregnancy. Obstet Gynecol 110:941, 2007.
106. Protection against viral hepatitis. Recommendations of the Immunization Practices Advisory Committee (ACIP). MMWR Recomm Rep 39:1, 1990.
107. Snydman DR: Hepatitis in pregnancy. N Engl J Med 313:1398, 1985.
108. Kao JH, Chen DS: Global control of hepatitis B virus infection. Lancet Infect Dis 2:395, 2002.
109. Centers for Disease Control and Prevention (CDC): Hepatitis B vaccination—United States, 1982-2002. MMWR Morb Mortal Wkly Rep 51:549, 2002.
110. Potthoff A, Rifai K, Wedemeyer H, et al: Successful treatment of fulminant hepatitis B during pregnancy. Z Gastroenterol 47:667, 2009.
111. Davies G, Wilson RD, Desilets V, et al: Amniocentesis and women with hepatitis B, hepatitis C, or human immunodeficiency virus. J Obstet Gynaecol Can 25:145, 2003.
112. Hill JB, Sheffield JS, Kim MJ, et al: Risk of hepatitis B transmission in breast-fed infants of chronic hepatitis B carriers. Obstet Gynecol 99:1049, 2002.
113. Hepatitis B: Virus: a comprehensive strategy for eliminating transmission in the United States through universal childhood vaccination. Recommendations of the Immunization Practices Advisory Committee (ACIP). MMWR Recomm Rep 40:1, 1991.
114. Wang Z, Zhang J, Yang H, et al: Quantitative analysis of HBV DNA level and HBeAg titer in hepatitis B surface antigen positive mothers and their babies: HBeAg passage through the placenta and the rate of decay in babies. J Med Virol 71:360, 2003.
115. Mast EE, Margolis HS, Fiore AE, et al: A comprehensive immunization strategy to eliminate transmission of hepatitis B virus infection in the United States: recommendations of the Advisory Committee on Immunization Practices (ACIP) part 1: immunization of infants, children, and adolescents. MMWR Recomm Rep 54:1, 2005.
116. Murphy EL, Fang J, Tu Y, et al: Hepatitis C virus prevalence and clearance among US blood donors, 2006-2007: associations with birth cohort, multiple pregnancies, and body mass index. J Infect Dis 202:576, 2010.
117. Centers for Disease Control and Prevention: Recommendations for prevention and control of hepatitis C virus (HCV) infection and HCV-related chronic disease. MMWR Recomm Rep 47:1, 1998.
118. Alter MJ, Kuhnert WL, Finelli L: Guidelines for laboratory testing and result reporting of antibody to hepatitis C virus. Centers for Disease Control and Prevention. MMWR Recomm Rep 52:1, 2003.
119. Alter HJ, Sanchez-Pescador R, Urdea MS, et al: Evaluation of branched DNA signal amplification for the detection of hepatitis C virus RNA. J Viral Hepat 2:121, 1995.
120. Roberts SS, Miller RK, Jones JK, et al: The Ribavirin Pregnancy Registry: Findings after 5 years of enrollment, 2003-2009. Birth Defects Res A Clin Mol Teratol 88:551, 2010.
121. Schuval S, Van Dyke RB, Lindsey JC, et al: Hepatitis C prevalence in children with perinatal human immunodeficiency virus infection enrolled in a long-term follow-up protocol. Arch Pediatr Adolesc Med 158:1007, 2004.
122. A significant sex—but not elective cesarean section—effect on mother-to-child transmission of hepatitis C virus infection. J Infect Dis 192:1872, 2005.
123. Ramia S, Bahakim H: Perinatal transmission of hepatitis B virus-associated hepatitis D virus. Ann Inst Pasteur Virol 139:285, 1988.
124. Renou C, Pariente A, Nicand E, et al: Pathogenesis of hepatitis E in pregnancy. Liver Int 28:1465; author reply 1466, 2008.
125. Kumar A, Beniwal M, Kar P, et al: Hepatitis E in pregnancy. Int J Gynaecol Obstet 85:240, 2004.
126. Khuroo MS, Kamili S, Jameel S: Vertical transmission of hepatitis E virus. Lancet 345:1025, 1995.
127. Centers for Disease Control and Prevention (CDC): Interim guidelines for the evaluation of infants born to mothers infected with West Nile virus during pregnancy. MMWR Morb Mortal Wkly Rep 53:154, 2004.
128. O'Leary DR, Kuhn S, Kniss KL, et al: Birth outcomes following West Nile Virus infection of pregnant women in the United States: 2003-2004. Pediatrics 117:e537, 2006.
129. Ornoy A, Tenenbaum A: Pregnancy outcome following infections by coxsackie, echo, measles, mumps, hepatitis, polio and encephalitis viruses. Reprod Toxicol 21:446, 2006.
130. Archer JS: Acute liver failure in pregnancy: a case report. J Reprod Med 46:137, 2001.
131. Axelsson C, Bondestam K, Frisk G, et al: Coxsackie B virus infections in women with miscarriage. J Med Virol 39:282, 1993.
132. Dahlquist GG, Ivarsson S, Lindberg B, et al: Maternal enteroviral infection during pregnancy as a risk factor for childhood IDDM. A population-based case-control study. Diabetes 44:408, 1995.
133. Worda C, Huber A, Hudelist G, et al: Prevalence of cervical and intrauterine human papillomavirus infection in the third trimester in asymptomatic women. J Soc Gynecol Investig 12:440, 2005.
134. Lacey CJ: Therapy for genital human papillomavirus-related disease. J Clin Virol 32:S82, 2005.
135. Eskild A, Bruu AL, Stray-Pedersen B, et al: Epstein-Barr virus infection during pregnancy and the risk of adverse pregnancy outcome. BJOG 112:1620, 2005.
136. Lehtinen M, Koskela P, Ogmundsdottir HM, et al: Maternal herpesvirus infections and risk of acute lymphoblastic leukemia in the offspring. Am J Epidemiol 158:207, 2003.
137. Meyohas MC, Marechal V, Desire N, et al: Study of mother-to-child Epstein-Barr virus transmission by means of nested PCRs. J Virol 70:6816, 1996.
138. Suarez VR, Hankins GD: Smallpox and pregnancy: from eradicated disease to bioterrorist threat. Obstet Gynecol 100:87, 2002.
139. Centers for Disease Control and Prevention (CDC): Women with smallpox vaccine exposure during pregnancy reported to the National Smallpox Vaccine in Pregnancy Registry—United States, 2003. MMWR Morb Mortal Wkly Rep 52:386, 2003.

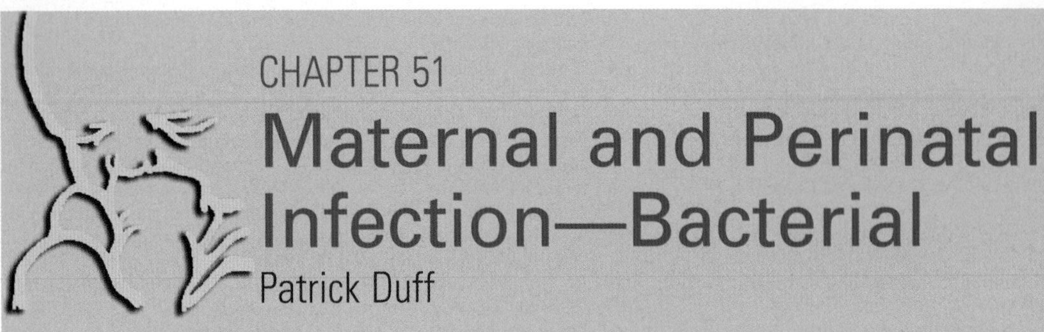

CHAPTER 51

Maternal and Perinatal Infection—Bacterial

Patrick Duff

KEY ABBREVIATIONS

Activated Partial Thromboplastin Time	aPTT
Acute Respiratory Distress Syndrome	ARDS
Centers for Disease Control and Prevention	CDC
Computed Tomography	CT
Group B Streptococcus	GBS
Listeria monocytogenes	LM
Magnetic Resonance Imaging	MRI
Polymerase Chain Reaction	PCR
Premature Rupture of the Membranes	PROM

Bacterial infections are the single most common complication encountered by the obstetrician. Some infections, such as puerperal endometritis and lower urinary tract infection, are of principal concern to the mother and pose little or no risk to the fetus or neonate. Others, such as listeriosis and toxoplasmosis, are of greatest threat to the fetus. Still others, such as group B streptococcal infection (GBS), pyelonephritis, and chorioamnionitis, may cause serious morbidity, even life-threatening complications, for both the mother and baby. The purpose of this chapter is to review in detail the major bacterial infections and the key protozoan infection (toxoplasmosis) that the obstetrician confronts in daily clinical practice.

GROUP B STREPTOCOCCAL INFECTION

Epidemiology

Streptococcus agalactiae is a gram-positive encapsulated coccus that produces β-hemolysis when grown on blood agar. **On average, about 20% to 25% of pregnant women harbor GBS in their lower genital tract and rectum.** The GBS is one of the most important causes of early-onset neonatal infection. The prevalence of neonatal GBS infection now is about 0.5 per 1000 live births, and about 10,000 cases of neonatal streptococcal septicemia occur each year in the United States.[1]

Neonatal GBS infection can be divided into early-onset and late-onset infection. **About 80% to 85% of cases of neonatal GBS infection are early in onset and result almost exclusively from vertical transmission from a colonized mother.** Early-onset infection presents primarily as a severe pneumonia and overwhelming septicemia. In preterm infants, the mortality rate from early-onset GBS infection may approach 25%. In term infants, the mortality rate is lower, averaging about 5%.[2] Late-onset neonatal GBS infection occurs as a result of both vertical and horizontal transmission. It is typically manifested by bacteremia, meningitis, and pneumonia. The mortality rate from late-onset infection is about 5% for both preterm and term infants.[1]

Unfortunately, obstetrical interventions have proved ineffective in preventing late-onset neonatal infection. Therefore, the remainder of this discussion focuses on early-onset infection.

Major risk factors for early-onset infection include preterm labor, especially when complicated by preterm premature rupture of the membranes (PROM); intrapartum maternal fever (chorioamnionitis); prolonged rupture of membranes, defined as greater than 18 hours; previous delivery of an infected infant; young age; and black and Hispanic ethnicity.[1] About 25% of pregnant women have at least one risk factor for GBS infection. The neonatal attack rate in colonized patients is 40% to 50% in the presence of a risk factor and less than 5% in the absence of a risk factor. In infected infants, neonatal mortality approaches 30% to 35% when a maternal risk factor is present but is less than 5% when a risk factor is absent.[2,3]

Maternal Complications

Several obstetrical complications occur with increased frequency in pregnant women who are colonized with GBS. The organism is one of the major causes of chorioamnionitis and postpartum endometritis. It may cause postcesarean delivery wound infection, usually in conjunction with other aerobic and anaerobic bacilli and staphylococci. The organism also is responsible for about 2% to 3% of lower urinary tract infections in pregnant women.[1] GBS urinary

TABLE 51-1 RELIABILITY OF RAPID DIAGNOSTIC TESTS FOR GROUP B STREPTOCOCCI

	TEST PERFORMANCE			
TEST	**SENSITIVITY (%)**	**SPECIFICITY (%)**	**PV⁺ (%)**	**PV⁻ (%)**
Gram stain	34-100	60-70	13-33	86-100
Growth in starch medium	93-98	98-99	65-98	89-99
Antigen detection (coagglutination, latex particle agglutination, enzyme immunoassay)	4-88*	92-100	15-100	76-99
DNA probe†	71	90	61	94

Data based on Romero R, Jimenez C, Lohda AK, et al: Amniotic fluid glucose concentration: a rapid and simple method for the detection of intraamniotic infection in preterm labor. Am J Obstet Gynecol 163:968, 1990.
*Sensitivities for identification of heavily colonized women ranged from 29% to 100%.
†Specimens were grown in culture for 3.5 hr before DNA probe was used.

tract infection, in turn, is a risk factor for preterm PROM and preterm labor. For example, Thomsen and colleagues[4] reported a study of 69 women at 27 to 31 weeks' gestation who had streptococcal urinary tract infections. Patients were assigned to treatment with either penicillin or placebo. Treated patients had a significant reduction in the frequency of both preterm PROM and preterm labor.

Other investigations have confirmed the association between GBS colonization and preterm labor and preterm PROM. Women with the latter complication who are colonized with GBS tend to have a shorter latent period and higher frequency of chorioamnionitis and puerperal endometritis compared with noncolonized women.[5]

Diagnosis

The gold standard for the diagnosis of GBS infection is bacteriologic culture. Todd-Hewitt broth or selective blood agar is the preferred medium. **Specimens for culture should be obtained from the lower vagina, perineum, and perianal area, using a simple cotton swab.** In recent years, considerable research has been devoted to assessment of rapid diagnostic tests for the identification of colonized women. Table 51-1 summarizes the results of several investigations of rapid diagnostic tests. The information in this table is based on the review by Yancey and associates.[6] These authors noted that, although the rapid diagnostic tests had reasonable sensitivity in identifying heavily colonized patients, they had poor sensitivity in identifying lightly and moderately colonized patients.

Although the first-generation rapid diagnostic tests were not as valuable as originally hoped, Bergeron and colleagues[7] recently reported exceptionally favorable results with a new polymerase chain reaction (PCR) assay for GBS. In a series of 112 patients, the authors documented a sensitivity of 97%, specificity of 100%, positive predictive value of 100%, and negative predictive value of 99%. This PCR assay now is commercially available and offers clear promise as a rapid test for screening patients at the time of admission for labor.

Prevention of Group B Streptococcal Infection

In the past 20 years, several different strategies have been proposed for the prevention of neonatal GBS infection.[2,3,8-10] Each strategy has had major imperfections. In 1996, however, the Centers for Disease Control and Prevention (CDC) published a series of recommendations that incorporated the major advantages of previous protocols and minimized some of the more problematic aspects of selected strategies.[11] The initial CDC guidelines recommended either universal culturing of all patients at 35 to 37 weeks and intrapartum treatment of all colonized women or selective treatment on the basis of identified risk factors. Subsequently, in a large population-based survey, Rosenstein and Schuchat[12] assessed the theoretical impact of the CDC recommendations and showed that a strategy of universal culturing and treatment of all colonized patients would prevent 78% of cases of neonatal infection. In contrast, only 41% of cases were prevented when patients were targeted for prophylaxis just on the basis of risk factors. In addition, Locksmith and colleagues[13] confirmed that universal culturing also was of value in decreasing the rate of maternal infection compared with a strategy of only treating on the basis of risk factors.

In 2002, the CDC issued revised guidelines for prevention of early-onset GBS infection.[1] **The newest guidelines recommend universal cultures in all patients as the optimal method of prevention. Cultures should be performed at 35 to 37 weeks. All patients who test positive should receive intrapartum antibiotic prophylaxis with one of the regimens outlined in Table 51-2. Ideally, antibiotics should be administered at least 4 hours before delivery.** DeCueto and coworkers[14] demonstrated that the rate of neonatal GBS infection was reduced significantly when patients were treated for at least this period of time. In a subsequent investigation assessing timing of antibiotic prophylaxis, McNanley and associates[15] showed that mean vaginal GBS counts decreased 5-fold within 2 hours of antibiotic administration, 50-fold within 4 hours, and almost 1000-fold within 6 hours.

The new CDC guidelines also addressed issues that previously had been imprecisely defined.[1] Colonized patients scheduled for an elective cesarean delivery do not require intrapartum prophylaxis. Patients who tested positive for GBS in a previous pregnancy should not be assumed to be colonized and should be retested in the present pregnancy. This recommendation is supported by a later report from Edwards and coworkers.[16] These authors noted that only 59% of patients who were culture positive in a previous pregnancy were positive in the present pregnancy. Conversely, however, patients who have GBS bacteriuria in pregnancy, even if treated, should be considered heavily colonized and should be targeted for intrapartum prophylaxis. Moreover, patients who had a previous infant with GBS infection also should be considered colonized and treated during labor.

TABLE 51-2 ANTIBIOTICS WITH ACTIVITY AGAINST GROUP B STREPTOCOCCI

DRUG	DOSE FOR INTRAPARTUM PROPHYLAXIS
Ampicillin	2 g initially, then 1 g q4h
Penicillin	5 million units initially, then 2.5 to 3 million units q4h
Cefazolin*	1 g q8h
Clindamycin†	900 mg q8h
Vancomycin†	1000 mg q12h

Recommendations based on Prevention of perinatal group B streptococcal disease: revised guidelines from the CDC. MMWR Morb Mortal Wkly Rep 51(Suppl):1, 2002.
*Cefazolin should be used in patients who have a history of a non-life-threatening allergy to penicillin.
†Clindamycin or vancomycin should be used in patients who have a history of a life-threatening allergy to penicillin. Clindamycin should be used only if sensitivity testing confirms that the organism is sensitive (up to 10% of strains of GBS may be resistant). Vancomycin should be used if the organism is resistant to clindamycin or sensitivity tests are not available.

URINARY TRACT INFECTIONS

Acute Urethritis

Acute urethritis (acute urethral syndrome) is usually caused by one of three organisms: coliforms (principally *Escherichia coli*), *Neisseria gonorrhoeae*, and *Chlamydia trachomatis*. Coliform organisms are part of the normal vaginal and perineal flora and may be introduced into the urethra during intercourse or when wiping after defecation. *N. gonorrhoeae* and *C. trachomatis* are sexually transmitted pathogens.[17] Affected patients typically experience frequency, urgency, and dysuria. Hesitancy, dribbling, and a mucopurulent urethral discharge also may be present. On microscopic examination, the urine usually has white blood cells, but bacteria may not be consistently present. Urine cultures may have low colony counts of coliform organisms, and cultures of the urethral discharge may be positive for gonorrhea and chlamydia. A rapid diagnostic test, such as a nucleic acid probe, may be used in lieu of culture for gonorrhea and chlamydia.[17]

Most patients with acute urethritis warrant empirical treatment before the results of laboratory tests are available. Infections caused by coliforms usually respond to the antibiotics described later for treatment of asymptomatic bacteriuria and cystitis. **If gonococcal infection is suspected, the patient should be treated with intramuscular ceftriaxone (250 mg in a single dose).**[18] If the patient is allergic to β-lactam antibiotics, an effective alternative is azithromycin, 2000 mg orally in a single dose. This high dose of azithromycin is more likely to be associated with gastrointestinal side effects than more conventional lower doses. An alternative choice in the penicillin-allergic patient is ciprofloxacin 500 mg orally in a single dose. **If chlamydial infection is suspected or confirmed, the patient should be treated with azithromycin (1000 mg) in a single dose.**[18] The powder formulation of azithromycin is less expensive than the tablet formulation.

Asymptomatic Bacteriuria and Acute Cystitis

The prevalence of asymptomatic bacteriuria in pregnancy is 5% to 10%, and most cases antedate the onset of pregnancy. The frequency of acute cystitis in pregnancy is 1% to 3%. Some cases of cystitis arise de novo; others develop as a result of failure to identify and treat asymptomatic bacteriuria.[19]

***E. coli* is responsible for at least 80% of cases of initial infections and about 70% of recurrent cases. *Klebsiella pneumoniae* and *Proteus* species also are important pathogens, particularly in patients who have a history of recurrent infection. Up to 10% of infections are caused by gram-positive organisms such as GBS, enterococci, and staphylococci.**[17,19]

All pregnant women should have a urine culture at their first prenatal appointment to detect preexisting asymptomatic bacteriuria. If the culture is negative, the likelihood of the patient subsequently developing an asymptomatic infection is less than 5%. If the culture is positive (defined as greater than 10^5 colonies/mL urine from a midstream, clean-catch specimen), prompt treatment is necessary to prevent ascending infection. In the absence of effective treatment, about one third of pregnant women with asymptomatic bacteriuria will develop acute pyelonephritis.

Patients with acute cystitis usually have symptoms of frequency, dysuria, urgency, suprapubic pain, hesitancy, and dribbling. Gross hematuria may be present, but high fever and systemic symptoms are uncommon. In symptomatic patients, the leukocyte esterase and nitrate tests are usually positive. When a urine culture is obtained, a catheterized sample is preferred because it minimizes the probability that urine will be contaminated by vaginal flora. With a catheterized specimen, a colony count greater than 10^2/mL is considered indicative of infection.[20]

Asymptomatic bacteriuria and acute cystitis characteristically respond well to short courses of oral antibiotics. Single-dose therapy is not as effective in pregnant women as in nonpregnant patients. However, a 3-day course of treatment appears to be comparable to a 7- to 10-day regimen for an initial infection.[17] Longer courses of therapy are more appropriate for patients with recurrent infections. Table 51-3 lists several antibiotics of value for treatment of asymptomatic bacteriuria and cystitis.

When sensitivity tests are available, for example, for patients with asymptomatic bacteriuria, they may be used to guide antibiotic selection. When empirical treatment is indicated, the choice of antibiotics must be based on established patterns of susceptibility. In recent years, 20% to 30% of strains of *E. coli* have developed resistance to ampicillin. Thus, this drug should not be used when the results of sensitivity tests are unknown unless the suspected pathogen is enterococci.[18,21] When enterococcus is the offending pathogen, ampicillin or amoxicillin is the drug of choice.

When choosing among the drugs listed in Table 51-3, the clinician should consider the following factors. First, the sensitivity patterns of ampicillin, amoxicillin, and cephalexin are the most variable. Second, these drugs, along with amoxicillin-clavulanic acid, also have the most pronounced effect on normal bowel and vaginal flora and, thus, are the most likely to cause diarrhea or monilial vulvovaginitis. In contrast, nitrofurantoin monohydrate has only minimal effect on vaginal or bowel flora. Moreover, it is more uniformly effective against the common

TABLE 51-3 ANTIBIOTICS FOR TREATMENT OF ASYMPTOMATIC BACTERIURIA AND ACUTE CYSTITIS

DRUG (TRADE NAME)	STRENGTH OF ACTIVITY	ORAL DOSE	RELATIVE COST
Amoxicillin	Some *Escherichia coli*, most *Proteus* species, group B streptococci, enterococci, some staphylococci	500 mg tid or 875 mg bid	Low
Amoxicillin-clavulanic acid (Augmentin)	Most gram-negative aerobic bacilli and gram-positive cocci	875 mg bid	High
Ampicillin	Some *E. coli*, most *Proteus* species, group B streptococci, enterococci, some staphylococci	250 mg four times daily	Low
Cephalexin (Keflex)	Most *E. coli*, most *Klebsiella* and *Proteus* species, group B streptococci, staphylococci	250 mg four times daily	Low
Nitrofurantoin monohydrate macrocrystals—sustained-release preparation (Macrobid)	Most uropathogens except enterococci and *Proteus* species	100 mg bid	Moderate
Sulfisoxazole (Gantrisin)	Most gram-negative aerobic bacilli	2 g × 1 dose, then 1 g four times daily	Low
Trimethoprim-sulfamethoxazole double-strength (Bactrim-DS, or Septra-DS)	Most uropathogens except some strains of *E. coli*	800 mg/160 mg bid	Low

uropathogens, except for *Proteus* species, than trimethoprim-sulfamethoxazole. Third, amoxicillin-clavulanic acid and trimethoprim-sulfamethoxazole usually are the best empirical agents for treatment of patients with suspected drug-resistant pathogens.[22] In this situation, the latter drug offers a major cost advantage over the former. Finally, because of theoretical concerns about their effect on protein binding of bilirubin, sulfonamide drugs should be avoided near the time of delivery.

For patients who have an initial infection and experience a prompt response to treatment, a urine culture for test of cure may not be clinically necessary or cost-effective.[17,22] Cultures during, or immediately after, treatment are indicated for patients who have a poor response to therapy or who have a history of recurrent infection. During subsequent clinic appointments, the patient's urine should be screened for nitrites and leukocyte esterase. If either of these tests is positive, repeat urine culture and retreatment are indicated.

Acute Pyelonephritis

The incidence of pyelonephritis in pregnancy is 1% to 2%.[19] Most cases develop as a consequence of undiagnosed or inadequately treated lower urinary tract infection. Two major physiologic changes occur during pregnancy that predispose to ascending infection of the urinary tract. First, the high concentration of progesterone secreted by the placenta has an inhibitory effect on ureteral peristalsis. Second, the enlarging gravid uterus often compresses the ureters, particularly the right, at the pelvic brim, thus creating additional stasis. Stasis, in turn, facilitates migration of bacteria from the bladder into the ureters and renal parenchyma (Figure 51-1).

About 75% to 80% of cases of pyelonephritis occur on the right side. Ten to 15% are left sided, and a slightly smaller percentage are bilateral.[19] ***E. coli* is again the principal pathogen.**[19,21] ***K. pneumoniae* and *Proteus* species also are important causes of infection, particularly in women with recurrent episodes of pyelonephritis.** Highly virulent gram-negative bacilli, such as *Pseudomonas*, *Enterobacter*, and *Serratia*, are unusual isolates except in immunocompromised patients. Gram-positive cocci do not frequently cause upper tract infection. Anaerobes also are unlikely pathogens unless the patient is chronically obstructed or instrumented.

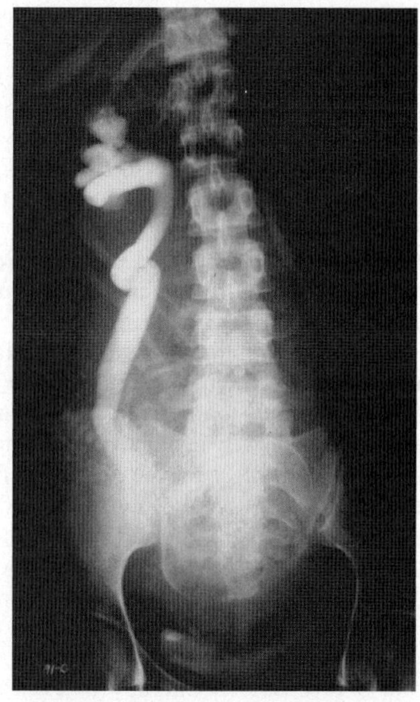

FIGURE 51-1. Intravenous pyelogram in a pregnant woman shows marked dilation of the right ureter and mild dilation of renal collecting system.

The usual clinical manifestations of acute pyelonephritis in pregnancy are fever, chills, flank pain and tenderness, frequency, urgency, hematuria, and dysuria. Patients also may have signs of preterm labor, septic shock, and acute respiratory distress syndrome (ARDS). Urinalysis is usually positive for white blood cell casts, red blood cells, and bacteria. Urine colony counts greater than 10^2 colonies/mL, in samples collected by catheterization, confirm the diagnosis of infection.

Pregnant patients with pyelonephritis may be considered for outpatient therapy if their disease manifestations are mild, they are hemodynamically stable, and they have no evidence of preterm labor.[23] If an outpatient approach is adopted, the patient should be treated with agents that have a high level of activity against the common uropathogens. Acceptable oral agents include amoxicillin-clavulanic acid, 875 mg twice daily, or trimethoprim-sulfamethoxazole-DS, twice daily for 7 to 10 days. Alternatively, a visiting home nurse may be contracted to administer a parenteral agent, such as ceftriaxone, 2 g intramuscularly or intravenously (IV), once daily. Although an excellent drug for lower tract infections, nitrofurantoin monohydrate does not consistently achieve the serum and renal parenchymal concentrations necessary for successful treatment of more serious infections.

Pregnant patients who appear to be moderately to severely ill or who show any signs of preterm labor should be hospitalized for intravenous antibiotic therapy. They should receive appropriate supportive treatment and be monitored closely for complications such as sepsis, ARDS, and preterm labor. One reasonable choice for empirical intravenous antibiotic therapy is ceftriaxone, 2 g every 24 hours. Compared with a first-generation cephalosporin like cefazolin, ceftriaxone has expanded coverage against aerobic gram-negative bacilli and has the advantage of once-daily dosing.[18] If the patient is critically ill or is at high risk for a resistant organism, a second antibiotic, such as gentamicin (7 mg/kg/ideal body weight every 24 hours) or aztreonam (500 mg to 1 g every 8 to 12 hours) should be administered, along with ceftriaxone, until the results of susceptibility tests are available.

Once antibiotic therapy is initiated, about 75% of patients defervesce within 48 hours. By the end of 72 hours, almost 95% of patients are afebrile and asymptomatic.[19] The two most likely causes of treatment failure are a resistant microorganism and obstruction. The latter condition is best diagnosed with computed tomography (CT) scan or renal ultrasonography and typically results from a stone or physical compression of the ureter by the gravid uterus.

Once the patient has begun to defervesce and her clinical examination has improved, she may be discharged from the hospital. Oral antibiotics should be prescribed to complete a total of 7 to 10 days of therapy. Selection of a specific oral agent should be based on considerations of efficacy, toxicity, and expense. A repeat urine culture should be obtained after 5 to 7 days of therapy to ensure that the urine is sterile before antibiotics are discontinued.

About 20% to 30% of pregnant patients with acute pyelonephritis develop a recurrent urinary tract infection later in pregnancy. The most cost-effective way to reduce the frequency of recurrence is to administer a daily prophylactic dose of an antibiotic, such as sulfisoxazole, 1 g, or nitrofurantoin monohydrate, 100 mg. Patients receiving prophylaxis should have their urine screened for bacteria at each subsequent clinic appointment. They also should be questioned about recurrence of symptoms. If symptoms recur, or the dipstick test for nitrite or leukocyte esterase is positive, a urine culture should be obtained to determine whether retreatment is necessary.

UPPER GENITAL TRACT INFECTIONS

Chorioamnionitis

Epidemiology

Chorioamnionitis (amnionitis, intra-amniotic infection) occurs in about 1% to 5% of term pregnancies.[24] In patients with preterm delivery, the frequency of clinical or subclinical infection may approach 25%.[25] Although chorioamnionitis may result from hematogenous dissemination of microorganisms, it more commonly is an ascending infection caused by organisms that are part of the normal vaginal flora. **The principal pathogens are *Bacteroides* and *Prevotella* species, *E. coli*, anaerobic gram-positive cocci, GBS, and genital mycoplasmas.**

Several clinical risk factors for chorioamnionitis have been identified. The most important are young age, low socioeconomic status, nulliparity, extended duration of labor and ruptured membranes, multiple vaginal examinations, and preexisting infections of the lower genital tract (e.g., bacterial vaginosis).[24]

Diagnosis

In most situations, the diagnosis of chorioamnionitis can be established on the basis of the clinical findings of maternal fever and maternal and fetal tachycardia, in the absence of other localizing signs of infection. In more severely ill patients, uterine tenderness and purulent amniotic fluid may be identified. The disorders that should be considered in the differential diagnosis of chorioamnionitis include respiratory tract infection, pyelonephritis, viral syndrome, and appendicitis.[24]

Laboratory confirmation of the diagnosis of chorioamnionitis is not routinely necessary in term patients who are progressing to delivery. However, in preterm patients who are being evaluated for tocolysis or corticosteroids, laboratory assessment may be of value in establishing the diagnosis of intrauterine infection. In this clinical context, amniotic fluid should be obtained by transabdominal amniocentesis. Table 51-4 summarizes the abnormal laboratory findings that may be present in infected patients.[24-29]

Management

Both the mother and infant may experience serious complications when chorioamnionitis is present. Bacteremia occurs in 3% to 12% of infected women. When cesarean delivery is required, up to 8% of women develop a wound infection, and about 1% develop a pelvic abscess. Fortunately, maternal death due to infection is exceedingly rare.[24]

Five to 10% of neonates delivered to mothers with chorioamnionitis have pneumonia or bacteremia. The predominant organisms responsible for these infections are GBS and *E. coli*. Meningitis occurs in less than 1% of term infants and in a slightly higher percentage of preterm infants. Mortality due to infection ranges from 1% to 4% in term neonates but may approach 15% in preterm infants because of the confounding effects of other complications such as hyaline membrane disease and intraventricular hemorrhage.[24]

To prevent maternal and neonatal complications, parenteral antibiotic therapy should be initiated as soon as the diagnosis of chorioamnionitis is made, unless delivery is imminent. Three separate investigations have demonstrated that mother-infant pairs who receive prompt intrapartum treatment have better outcomes than patients treated after delivery.[30-32] The principal benefits of early treatment include decreased frequency of neonatal

TABLE 51-4 DIAGNOSTIC TESTS FOR CHORIOAMNIONITIS

TEST	ABNORMAL FINDING	COMMENT
Maternal white blood cell count (WBC)	≥15,000 cells/mm^3 with preponderance of leukocytes	Labor and/or corticosteroids also may result in elevation of WBC
Amniotic fluid glucose	≤10 to 15 mg%	Excellent correlation with positive amniotic fluid culture and clinical infection
Amniotic fluid interleukin-6	≥7.9 ng/mL	Excellent correlation with positive amniotic fluid culture and clinical infection
Amniotic fluid leukocyte esterase	≥1$^+$ reaction	Good correlation with positive amniotic fluid culture and clinical infection
Amniotic fluid gram stain	Any organism in an oil immersion field	Allows identification of particularly virulent organism such as group B streptococci. However, the test is very sensitive to inoculum effect. In addition, it cannot identify pathogens such as mycoplasmas.
Amniotic fluid culture	Growth of aerobic or anaerobic microorganism	Results are not immediately available for clinical management
Blood cultures	Growth of aerobic or anaerobic microorganism	Will be positive in 5% to 10% of patients; however, will usually not be of value in making clinical decisions unless patient is seriously ill or is at increased risk for bacterial endocarditis, is immunocompromised, or has a poor response to initial treatment

bacteremia and pneumonia and decreased duration of maternal fever and hospitalization.

The most extensively tested intravenous antibiotic regimen for treatment of chorioamnionitis is the combination of ampicillin (2 g every 6 hours) or penicillin (5 million units every 6 hours) plus gentamicin (1.5 mg/kg every 8 hours or 7 mg/kg/ideal body weight every 24 hours). The latter regimen of gentamicin is the most cost-effective.[18,24] These antibiotics specifically target the two organisms most likely to cause neonatal infection: GBS and *E. coli.* With rare exceptions, gentamicin is preferred to tobramycin or amikacin because it is available in an inexpensive generic formulation. Amikacin should be reserved for immunocompromised patients who are particularly likely to be infected by highly virulent, drug-resistant aerobic gram-negative bacilli. In patients who are allergic to β-lactam antibiotics, clindamycin (900 mg every 8 hours) should be substituted for ampicillin.

If a patient with chorioamnionitis requires cesarean delivery, a drug with activity against anaerobic organisms should be added to the antibiotic regimen. Either clindamycin (900 mg) or metronidazole (500 mg) is an excellent choice for this purpose. Failure to provide effective coverage of anaerobes may result in treatment failures in 20% to 30% of patients.[18]

Extended-spectrum cephalosporins, penicillins, and carbapenems also provide excellent coverage against the bacteria that cause chorioamnionitis. Dosages and dose intervals for several of these agents are listed in Table 51-5.[18] As a general rule, these drugs are more expensive than the generic combination regimens outlined earlier.

Antibiotics usually can be discontinued soon after delivery. Edwards and Duff[33] recently reported a randomized clinical trial in which patients were treated intrapartum with ampicillin plus gentamicin. In one group of patients, treatment was discontinued after the first postpartum dose of each antibiotic. In the second group, patients were treated until they had been afebrile and asymptomatic for 24 hours. Patients in both groups received at least one dose of clindamycin if they delivered by cesarean. There were

TABLE 51-5 SINGLE AGENTS OF VALUE IN TREATMENT OF CHORIOAMNIONITIS AND PUERPERAL ENDOMETRITIS

DRUG	DOSAGE AND DOSE INTERVAL	RELATIVE COST TO THE PHARMACY*
Extended-Spectrum Cephalosporins		
Cefepime	2 g q12h	Intermediate
Cefotaxime	2 g q8-12h	Intermediate
Cefotetan	2 g q12h	Low
Cefoxitin	2 g q6h	High
Ceftizoxime	2 g q12h	Intermediate
Extended-Spectrum Penicillins		
Ampicillin-sulbactam	3 g q6h	Low
Mezlocillin	3-4 g q6h	Intermediate
Piperacillin	3-4 g q6h	Intermediate
Piperacillin-tazobactam	3.375 g q6h	Intermediate
Ticarcillin-clavulanic acid	3.1 g q6h	Low
Carbapenem		
Ertapenem	1 g q24h	High
Imipenem-cilastatin	500 mg q6h	High
Meropenem	1 g q8h	High

*Cost estimates do not include dose preparation fees and administration charges.

no significant differences in treatment outcome in the two groups.

Patients with chorioamnionitis are at increased risk for dysfunctional labor. About 75% require oxytocin for augmentation of labor, and up to 30% to 40% require cesarean delivery, usually for failure to progress in labor. Although chorioamnionitis by itself should not be considered an indication for cesarean delivery, affected patients need close monitoring during labor to ensure that uterine contractility is optimized. In addition, the fetus also needs close surveillance. Fetal heart rate abnormalities such as tachycardia and decreased variability (Figure 51-2) occur in more than three fourths of cases, and additional tests such as scalp stimulation may be necessary to evaluate fetal well-being.[34]

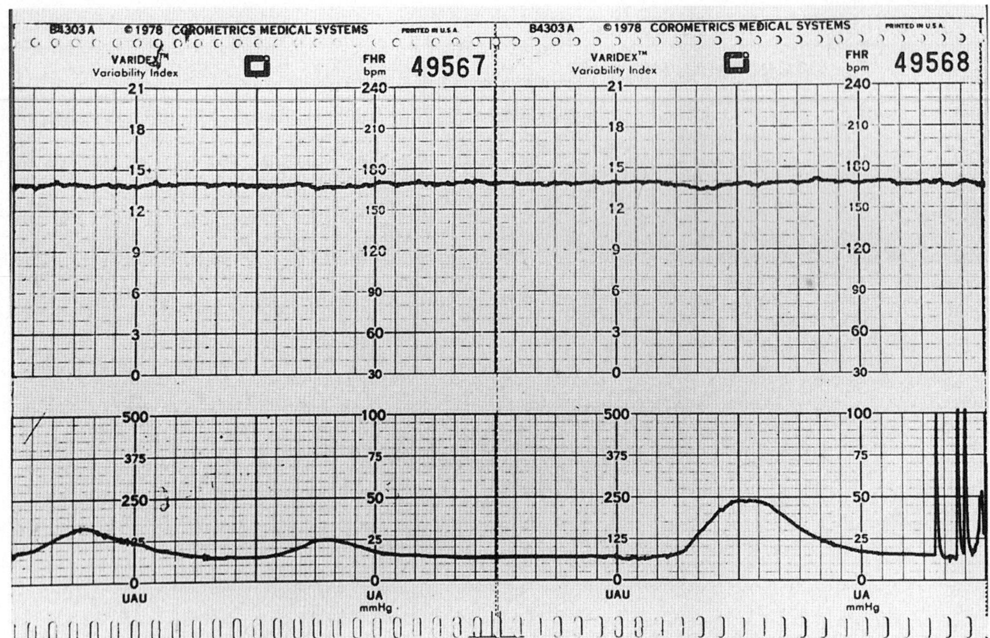

FIGURE 51-2. Fetal heart tracing from a patient with chorioamnionitis. Note the tachycardia of 170 beats/minute and the decrease in both short- and long-term variability.

Puerperal Endometritis

Epidemiology

The frequency of puerperal endometritis in women having vaginal delivery is about 1% to 3%. In women having a scheduled cesarean delivery before the onset of labor and rupture of membranes, the frequency of endometritis ranges from 5% to 15%. When cesarean delivery is performed after an extended period of labor and ruptured membranes, the incidence of infection is 30% to 35% without antibiotic prophylaxis and about 60% less with prophylaxis. In highly indigent patient populations, the frequency of infection may be even higher.[35]

Similarly to chorioamnionitis, endometritis is a polymicrobial infection caused by microorganisms that are part of the normal vaginal flora. These bacteria gain access to the upper genital tract, peritoneal cavity, and occasionally the bloodstream as a result of vaginal examinations during labor and manipulations during surgery. **The most common pathogens are GBS, anaerobic gram-positive cocci, aerobic gram-negative bacilli (predominantly *E. coli, K. pneumoniae,* and *Proteus* species), and anaerobic gram-negative bacilli (principally *Bacteroides* and *Prevotella* species).** *C. trachomatis* is not a common cause of early-onset puerperal endometritis but has been implicated in late-onset infection. The genital mycoplasmas may be pathogens in some patients, but they usually are present in association with more highly virulent bacteria.[35]

The principal risk factors for endometritis are cesarean delivery, young age, low socioeconomic status, extended duration of labor and ruptured membranes, and multiple vaginal examinations. In addition, preexisting infection or colonization of the lower genital tract (gonorrhea, GBS, bacterial vaginosis) also predisposes to ascending infection.

Clinical Presentation and Diagnosis

Affected patients typically have a fever of 38° C or higher within 36 hours of delivery. Associated findings include malaise, tachycardia, lower abdominal pain and tenderness, uterine tenderness, and discolored, malodorous lochia. A small number of patients also may have a tender, indurated inflammatory mass in the broad ligament, posterior cul de sac, or retrovesical space.

The initial differential diagnosis of puerperal fever should include endometritis, atelectasis, pneumonia, viral syndrome, pyelonephritis, and appendicitis. Distinction among these disorders usually can be made on the basis of physical examination and a limited number of laboratory tests such as white blood cell count, urinalysis and culture, and in select patients, chest radiograph. Blood cultures should not be done *routinely* because of their expense and their lack of impact on clinical decision making. However, they are indicated in patients who have a poor initial response to therapy and in those who seem seriously ill, are immunocompromised, or are at increased risk for bacterial endocarditis.

Management

Patients who have mild to moderately severe infections, particularly after vaginal delivery, can be treated with short intravenous courses of single agents such as the extended-spectrum cephalosporins and penicillins or carbapenem antibiotics such as imipenem-cilastatin, meropenem, and ertapenem. Table 51-5 lists several antibiotics that have acceptable breadth of coverage against the polymicrobial genital tract flora. Combination antibiotic regimens should be considered for more severely ill patients, particularly those who are indigent and in poor general health. Table 51-6 lists several antibiotic combinations of proven value in treatment of puerperal endometritis. As a general rule, the combination generic drug regimens are less expensive than the single agents whose brand-name patents still are intact.

Once antibiotics are begun, about 90% of patients defervesce within 48 to 72 hours. When the patient has been afebrile and asymptomatic for about 24 hours, parenteral antibiotics should be discontinued, and the patient should be discharged. As a general rule, an extended course of oral antibiotics is not necessary after discharge.[18,36] There are at least two notable exceptions to this rule. First, patients who have had a vaginal delivery and who defervesce within 24 hours are candidates for early discharge. In these individuals, a short course of an oral antibiotic such as amoxicillin-clavulanate (875 mg every 12 hours) may be substituted for continued parenteral therapy. Second, patients who have had staphylococcal bacteremia may require a more extended period of administration of parenteral and oral antibiotics with specific antistaphylococcal activity.[37]

Patients who fail to respond to the antibiotic therapy outlined earlier usually have one of two problems. The first is a resistant organism. Table 51-7 lists possible weaknesses in coverage of selected antibiotics and indicates the appropriate change in treatment. **The second major cause of treatment failure is a wound infection.** Wound infections may take the form of an incisional abscess or a cellulitis with no actual purulent collection. Incisional abscesses should be opened completely to provide drainage, and a specific antistaphylococcal antibiotic should be added to the treatment regimen. If extensive cellulitis at the margin of the incision is present, an antibiotic with specific coverage against staphylococci should be added, but the wound should not be opened. Vancomycin (1 g IV every 12 hours) is an excellent antistaphylococcal antibiotic, particularly against methicillin-resistant *Staphylococcus aureus* (MRSA).[18]

When changes in antibiotic therapy do not result in clinical improvement and no evidence of wound infection is present, several unusual disorders should be considered. The differential diagnosis of persistent puerperal fever is summarized in Table 51-8.[35]

TABLE 51-6 COMBINATION ANTIBIOTIC REGIMENS FOR TREATMENT OF PUERPERAL ENDOMETRITIS

ANTIBIOTICS	INTRAVENOUS DOSE	RELATIVE COST TO THE PHARMACY*
Regimen 1		
Clindamycin plus	900 mg q8h	Intermediate
Gentamicin	7 mg/kg ideal body weight q24h†	Low
Regimen 2		
Clindamycin plus	900 mg q8h	Intermediate
Aztreonam	1-2 g q8h	High
Regimen 3		
Metronidazole plus	500 mg q12h	Low
Penicillin or	5 million units q6h	Low
Ampicillin plus	2 g q6h	Low
Gentamicin	7 mg/kg ideal body weight q24h†	Low

*Cost estimate does not include dose preparation fees and administration charges.
†Single daily dosing of aminoglycoside antibiotics is more effective and less expensive than multidose treatment. In addition, it is less likely to cause toxicity.

TABLE 51-7 TREATMENT OF RESISTANT MICROORGANISMS IN PATIENTS WITH PUERPERAL ENDOMETRITIS

INITIAL ANTIBIOTICS	PRINCIPAL WEAKNESS IN COVERAGE	MODIFICATION OF THERAPY
Extended-spectrum cephalosporins	Some aerobic and anaerobic gram-negative bacilli Enterococci	Change treatment to clindamycin or metronidazole plus penicillin or ampicillin plus gentamicin
Extended-spectrum penicillins	Some aerobic and anaerobic gram-negative bacilli	As above
Clindamycin plus gentamicin or aztreonam	Enterococci Some anaerobic gram-negative bacilli	Add ampicillin or penicillin* Consider substitution of metronidazole for clindamycin

*Ampicillin alone is highly active against enterococci. Penicillin *plus* gentamicin works synergistically to provide excellent coverage against this organism.

TABLE 51-8 DIFFERENTIAL DIAGNOSIS OF PERSISTENT PUERPERAL FEVER

CONDITION	DIAGNOSTIC TESTS	TREATMENT
Resistant microorganism	Blood culture	Combination antibiotics to cover all possible pelvic pathogens
Wound infection	Physical examination Needle aspiration Ultrasound	Incision and drainage if abscess is present Add antibiotic to cover staphylococci
Pelvic abscess	Physical examination Ultrasound Computed tomography Magnetic resonance imaging	Drainage Combination antibiotics to cover all possible pelvic pathogens
Septic pelvic vein thrombophlebitis	Ultrasound Computed tomography Magnetic resonance imaging	Heparin anticoagulation Combination antibiotics to cover all possible pelvic pathogens
Recrudescence of connective tissue disease	Serology	Corticosteroids
Drug fever	Inspection of temperature graph White blood cell count—identify eosinophilia	Discontinue antibiotics
Mastitis	Physical examination	Add antibiotic to cover staphylococci

Prevention of Puerperal Endometritis

Prophylactic antibiotics clearly are of value in reducing the frequency of postcesarean delivery endometritis, particularly in women having surgery after an extended period of labor and ruptured membranes.[38] For many years, the standard of care was to administer one dose of a relatively limited-spectrum antibiotic immediately after the baby's umbilical cord was clamped.[39] This practice was based primarily on two older studies, one prospective[40] and one retrospective,[41] that showed that delay in administration of antibiotics did not compromise the effectiveness of prophylaxis. Moreover, when compared with the effects of preoperative antibiotics, the delay in drug administration decreased the probability that neonates would require evaluations for sepsis.

Recently, however, several investigators have challenged the assumptions inherent in this standard. In 2007, Sullivan and colleagues[42] observed a significant reduction in the rate of endometritis and wound infection when intravenous cefazolin (1 g) was administered before surgery rather than after cord clamping. In patients who received antibiotics before the surgical incision, the relative risk for endometritis was 0.2; the 95% confidence interval [CI] was 0.15 to 0.94. The authors noted no increase in the rate of infection or the need for sepsis evaluations in the neonates exposed to preoperative antibiotics (level I evidence).

In a retrospective cohort study (level II evidence) using historical controls, Kaimal and coworkers[43] also noted a significant reduction in the overall rate of surgical site infection (adjusted odds ratio [AOR], 0.33) and endometritis (AOR, 0.34) when antibiotics were administered before surgery. Similarly, Owens and coworkers[44] conducted a retrospective study (level II evidence) comparing 4229 patients who received cefazolin after cord clamping with 4781 patients who received antibiotics before surgery. In patients who received antibiotics preoperatively, the authors noted a 50% reduction in the rate of endometritis and a 30% reduction in the rate of wound infection. There was no difference in the rate of culture-proven early-onset neonatal infection. In fact, there was actually a decreased rate of late-onset neonatal infection in the group that received antibiotics preoperatively. Finally, in a recent meta-analysis, Costantine and associates[45] reviewed five well-designed studies and concluded that administration of antibiotics before the skin incision, rather than after cord clamping, was more effective in reducing the frequency of endometritis (relative risk [RR], 0.47) and composite infection-related morbidity (RR, 0.50).

In another interesting departure from the previous standard of care, Tita and associates[46,47] showed that extending the spectrum of antibiotic activity by adding azithromycin (500 mg) to cefazolin (1 g) further reduced the risk for endometritis (RR, 0.41). The use of the broader-spectrum regimen also significantly decreased the rate of wound infection (1.3% vs. 3.1%; P <.002).

Dinsmoor and coworkers[48] recently reexamined the issue of whether the benefits of prophylaxis extended to seemingly low-risk women having cesarean delivery before the onset of labor. They conducted a secondary analysis of a previously reported observational study of cesarean delivery performed at 13 centers from 1999 to 2000 (level II evidence). The study included 9432 patients. Low-risk women who received antibiotic prophylaxis were less likely to develop postpartum endometritis (2% vs. 2.6%; AOR, 0.40; 95% CI, 0.28 to 0.59) and wound infection (0.52% vs. 0.96%; AOR, 0.49, 95% CI, 0.28 to 0.86).

Another important step in prevention of endometritis relates to the method of placental delivery. In 1997, Lasley and colleagues[49] conducted a prospective randomized trial (level I evidence) comparing manual removal of the placenta with removal by gentle traction on the umbilical cord. One hundred sixty-five women were randomized to the manual removal arm of the study, and 168 had spontaneous removal of the placenta. All patients in this study received prophylactic antibiotics, usually cefazolin, after the umbilical cord was clamped. In the patients whose placenta was removed by traction on the cord, the rate of endometritis was reduced from 27% to 15% (RR, 0.6; 95% CI, 0.4 to 0.9; P = .01).

Subsequently, the Cochrane database[50] evaluated 15 randomized trials (N = 4694 patients) comparing different methods of removing the placenta. A consistent finding in these trials was decreased blood loss, a decreased rate of endometritis, and, subsequently, a shorter duration of hospitalization in women whose placenta was removed by gentle traction on the umbilical cord.

A previous report by Yancey and associates[51] provides a logical explanation for why manual removal of the placenta is associated with an increased risk for infection. In that study, the authors specifically evaluated the contamination of the surgeon's dominant hand as a result of delivering the infant's head from the lower uterine segment. After this step of the operation, the bacterial contamination of the surgeon's glove was markedly increased. When the surgeon then places this hand behind the placenta and manually extracts the placenta, he or she inevitably introduces many microorganisms into the raw vascular bed beneath the placenta.

Based on the studies outlined earlier, I recommend that both low- and high-risk patients having cesarean delivery receive antibiotics 30 to 60 minutes before the start of surgery. I recommend use of cefazolin, 1 g, given as a rapid intravenous infusion, plus azithromycin, 500 mg administered IV over 1 hour. I also recommend that, whenever possible, the placenta be removed by traction on the umbilical cord, rather than by manual extraction.

Patients who have an immediate hypersensitivity to β-lactam antibiotics pose a special problem. The best alternative is to administer a single dose of clindamycin (900 mg) plus gentamicin (1.5 mg/kg) before surgery. Although these antibiotics commonly are used for treatment of overt infections, their administration still is warranted in penicillin-allergic patients who are at high risk for postoperative infection.[18]

Serious Sequelae of Puerperal Infection

Wound Infection

Wound infection after cesarean delivery may occur in association with endometritis or as an isolated infection. About 3% to 5% of patients who have a cesarean delivery develop a wound infection. The major risk factors for wound infection are listed in the box, Principal Risk Factors for Postcesarean Wound Infection. **The principal causative**

organisms are *S. aureus*, aerobic streptococci, and aerobic and anaerobic bacilli.[52]

Principal Risk Factors for Postcesarean Wound Infection

- Poor surgical technique—failure to close the bottom half of the subcutaneous layer, incorrect suture, or gauge of suture.
- Low socioeconomic status
- Extended duration of labor and ruptured membranes
- Preexisting infection, such as chorioamnionitis
- Obesity
- Insulin-dependent diabetes
- Immunodeficiency disorder
- Corticosteroid therapy
- Immunosuppressive therapy
- Connective tissue disorder
- Smoking

The diagnosis of wound infection always should be considered in patients who have a poor clinical response to antibiotic therapy for endometritis. Clinical examination characteristically shows erythema, induration, and tenderness at the margins of the abdominal incision. When the wound is probed with either a cotton-tipped applicator or fine needle, pus usually exudes. Some patients, however, may have an extensive cellulitis without harboring frank pus in the incision. Clinical examination should be sufficient to establish the correct diagnosis. Nevertheless, culture of the wound exudate is indicated to identify particularly virulent microorganisms such as MRSA.

When pus is present in the incision, the wound must be opened and drained completely. Antibiotic therapy should be modified to provide coverage against staphylococci because some regimens for endometritis may not specifically target this organism. Vancomycin, 1 g IV every 12 hours, is an excellent choice to cover MRSA.

Once the wound is opened, a careful inspection should be made to be certain that the fascial layer is intact. If it is disrupted, surgical intervention is necessary to reapproximate the fascia. Otherwise, the wound should be irrigated two to three times daily with a solution such as warm saline, a clean dressing should be applied, and the incision should be allowed to heal by secondary intention. Antibiotics should be continued until the base of the wound is clean and all signs of cellulitis have resolved. Patients usually can be treated at home once the acute signs of infection have subsided.

***Necrotizing fasciitis* is an uncommon but extremely serious complication of abdominal wound infection.** It also has been reported in association with infection of the episiotomy site.[53] This condition is most likely to occur in patients with type 1 diabetes mellitus, cancer, or an immunodeficiency disorder. Multiple bacterial pathogens, particularly anaerobes, have been isolated from patients with necrotizing fasciitis.

Necrotizing fasciitis should be suspected when the margins of the wound become discolored, cyanotic, and devoid of sensation. When the wound is opened, the subcutaneous tissue is easily dissected free of the underlying fascia, but muscle tissue is not affected. If the diagnosis is uncertain, a tissue biopsy should be performed and examined by frozen section.

Necrotizing fasciitis is a life-threatening condition and requires aggressive medical and surgical management. Broad-spectrum antibiotics with activity against all potential aerobic and anaerobic pathogens should be administered. Intravascular volume should be maintained with infusions of crystalloid, and electrolyte abnormalities should be corrected. Finally, and most importantly, the wound must be débrided and all necrotic tissue removed. In many instances, the required dissection is extensive and may best be managed in consultation with an experienced general or plastic surgeon.[54]

Pelvic Abscess

With the advent of modern antibiotics, pelvic abscesses after cesarean or vaginal delivery have become extremely rare. **Less than 1% of patients with puerperal endometritis develop a pelvic abscess.**[35] **When present, abscesses typically are located in the anterior or posterior cul de sac, most commonly the latter, or within the broad ligament.** The usual bacteria isolated from abscess cavities are coliforms and anaerobic gram-negative bacilli, particularly *Bacteroides* and *Prevotella* species.[55]

Patients with an abscess typically experience persistent fever despite initial therapy for endometritis. In addition, they usually have malaise, tachycardia, lower abdominal pain and tenderness, and a palpable pelvic mass anterior, posterior, or lateral to the uterus. The peripheral white blood cell count usually is elevated, and there is a shift toward neutrophils and bands. Ultrasound, CT scan, and magnetic resonance imaging (MRI) may be used to confirm the diagnosis of pelvic abscess.[56] Although CT and MRI may be slightly more sensitive, ultrasound offers the advantages of decreased expense and ready availability.

Patients with a pelvic abscess require surgical intervention to drain the purulent collection. When the abscess is in the posterior cul de sac, colpotomy drainage may be possible. For abscesses located anterior or lateral to the uterus, drainage may be accomplished by CT- or ultrasound-guided placement of a catheter drain.[57] When access is limited or the abscess is extensive, open laparotomy is indicated.

Patients with a pelvic abscess must receive antibiotics with excellent activity against coliform organisms and anaerobes.[18,55] One regimen that has been tested extensively in obstetrical patients with serious infections is the combination of penicillin (5 million units IV every 6 hours) or ampicillin (2 g IV every 6 hours) plus gentamicin (7 mg/kg of ideal body weight every 24 hours) plus clindamycin (900 mg IV every 8 hours) or metronidazole (500 mg IV every 12 hours). If a patient is allergic to β-lactam antibiotics, vancomycin (1 g IV every 12 hours) can be substituted for penicillin or ampicillin. Aztreonam (1 g IV every 8 hours) can be used instead of gentamicin when the patient is at risk for nephrotoxicity. Alternatively, the single agents imipenem-cilastatin (500 mg IV every 6 hours), meropenem (1 g every 8 hours), and ertapenem (1 g every 24 hours) provide excellent coverage against the usual pathogens responsible for an abscess. Antibiotics should be discontinued until the patient has been afebrile and asymptomatic for a minimum of 24 to 48 hours.

Septic Pelvic Thrombophlebitis

Like pelvic abscess, septic pelvic thrombophlebitis is extremely rare, occurring in 1 in 2000 pregnancies overall and in less than 1% of patients who have puerperal endometritis.[58] Intrauterine infection may cause seeding of pathogenic microorganisms into the venous circulation; in turn, these organisms may damage the vascular endothelium and initiate thrombosis.

Septic pelvic thrombophlebitis occurs in two distinct forms.[58] **The most commonly described disorder is acute thrombosis of one (usually the right), or both, ovarian veins (ovarian vein syndrome).**[59] Affected patients typically develop a moderate temperature elevation in association with lower abdominal pain in the first 48 to 96 hours postpartum. Pain usually localizes to the side of the affected vein but may radiate into the groin, upper abdomen, or flank. Nausea, vomiting, and abdominal bloating may be present.

On physical examination, the patient's pulse usually is elevated. Tachypnea, stridor, and dyspnea may be evident in pulmonary embolization has occurred. The abdomen is tender, and bowel sounds often are decreased or absent. Most patients demonstrate voluntary and involuntary guarding, and 50% to 70% have a tender, ropelike mass originating near one cornua and extending laterally and cephalad toward the upper abdomen. The principal conditions that should be considered in the differential diagnosis of ovarian vein syndrome are pyelonephritis, nephrolithiasis, appendicitis, broad ligament hematoma, adnexal torsion, and pelvic abscess.

The second presentation of septic pelvic vein thrombophlebitis is termed *enigmatic fever*.[60] Initially, affected patients have clinical findings suggestive of endometritis and receive systemic antibiotics. Subsequently, they experience subjective improvement, with the exception of temperature instability. They do not appear to be seriously ill, and positive findings are limited to persistent fever and tachycardia. Disorders that should be considered in the differential diagnosis of enigmatic fever are drug fever, viral syndrome, collagen vascular disease, and pelvic abscess.

The diagnostic tests of greatest value in evaluating patient with suspected septic pelvic vein thrombophlebitis are CT scan and MRI (Figure 51-3).[61] These tests are most sensitive in detecting large thrombi in the major pelvic vessels. They are not as useful in identifying thrombi in smaller vessels. In such cases, the ultimate diagnosis may depend on the patient's response to an empirical trial of heparin.[58,62]

Patients with septic pelvic vein thrombophlebitis should be treated with therapeutic doses of either intravenous unfractionated heparin or low-molecular-weight heparin. Therapy should be continued for 7 to 10 days. Long-term anticoagulation with oral agents probably is unnecessary unless the patient has massive clotting throughout the pelvic venous plexus or has sustained a pulmonary embolism. Patients should be maintained on broad-spectrum antibiotics throughout the period of heparin administration.

Once medical therapy is initiated, the patient should have objective evidence of a response within 48 to 72 hours. If no improvement is noted, surgical intervention may be necessary.[58,62] The decision to perform surgery should be based on clinical assessment and the relative certainty of the diagnosis. The surgical approach, in turn, should be tailored to the specific intraoperative findings. In most instances, treatment requires only ligation of the affected vessels. Extension of the thrombosis along the vena cava to the point of origin of the renal veins may necessitate embolectomy or placement of an umbrella filter. Excision of the infected vessel and removal of the ipsilateral adnexa and uterus is indicated only in the presence of a well-defined abscess. Whenever any of the previously mentioned procedures are being considered, consultation with an experienced vascular surgeon or interventional radiologist is imperative.

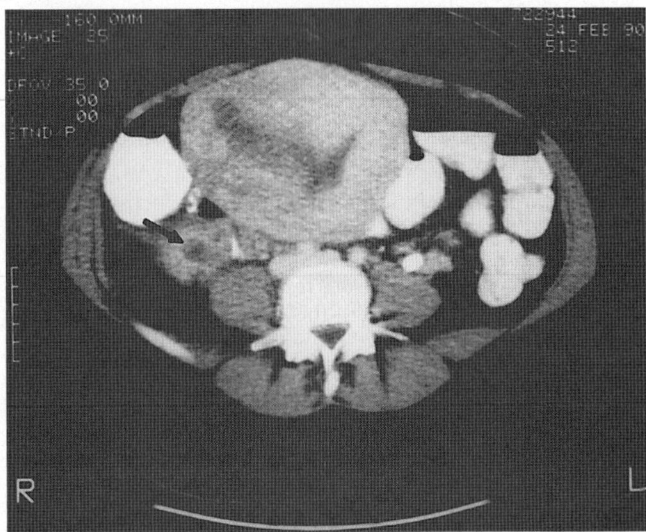

FIGURE 51-3. Computed tomography scan shows a thrombus *(arrow)* in the right ovarian vein.

Septic Shock

Septic shock in obstetrical patients usually is associated with four specific infections: septic abortion, acute pyelonephritis, chorioamnionitis, or endometritis. Fortunately, fewer than 5% of patients with any of these infections develop septic shock. **The most common organisms responsible for septic shock are the aerobic gram-negative bacilli, principally *E. coli, K. pneumoniae,* and *Proteus* species.** Highly virulent, drug-resistant coliforms such as *Pseudomonas, Enterobacter,* and *Serratia* species are uncommon except in immunosuppressed patients.[63]

Aerobic gram-negative bacilli have a complex lipopolysaccharide in their cell wall, which is termed *endotoxin.* When released into the systemic circulation, endotoxin is capable of causing a variety of immunologic, hematologic, neurohormonal, and hemodynamic derangements that ultimately result in multiorgan dysfunction.

In the early stages of septic shock, patients usually are restless, disoriented, tachycardic, and hypotensive. Although hypothermia is occasionally present, most patients have a relatively high fever (39° to 40° C). Their skin may be warm and flushed owing to an initial phase of vasodilation (warm shock). Subsequently, as extensive vasoconstriction occurs, the skin becomes cool and clammy.

Cardiac arrhythmias may be present, and signs of myocardial ischemia may occur. Jaundice, often due to hemolysis, may be evident. Urinary output typically decreases, and frank anuria may develop. Spontaneous bleeding from the genitourinary tract or venipuncture sites may occur as a result of disseminated intramuscular coagulation. ARDS is a common complication of severe sepsis and is associated with manifestations such as dyspnea, stridor, cough, tachypnea, and bilateral rales and wheezing.[64] In addition to these systemic signs and symptoms, affected patients also may have findings related to their primary site of infection such as purulent lochia, uterine tenderness, peritonitis, or flank tenderness.

The differential diagnosis of septic shock in obstetrical patients includes hypovolemic and cardiogenic shock, diabetic ketoacidosis, anaphylactic reaction, anesthetic reaction, and amniotic fluid or venous embolism. Distinction among these disorders usually can be made on the basis of a thorough history and physical examination and a limited number of laboratory studies. The white blood cell count initially may be decreased but, subsequently, is elevated in most patients. A large percentage of bands is usually evident. The hematocrit may be decreased if blood loss has occurred. Tests of coagulation such as platelet count, serum fibrinogen concentration, serum concentration of fibrin degradation products, prothrombin time, and activated partial thromboplastin time are frequently abnormal. Serum concentrations of the transaminase enzymes and bilirubin often are increased. Similarly, increased concentrations of blood urea nitrogen and creatinine reflect deterioration of renal function. Chest radiograph in patients with septic shock is indicated to determine whether pneumonia or ARDS is present. In addition, CT scan, MRI, and ultrasound may be of value in localizing an abscess.[57] Affected patients also require electrocardiographic monitoring to detect arrhythmias or signs of ischemic injury.

The first goal of treatment of septic shock is to correct the hemodynamic derangements precipitated by endotoxin. Two large-bore intravenous catheters and a urinary catheter should be inserted. Isotonic crystalloid such as Ringer lactate solution or normal saline should be administered and the infusion titrated in accordance with the patient's pulse, blood pressure, and urine output. If the patient is bleeding, packed red cells should be administered, and the goal is to maintain a hemoglobin concentration of 9 g/dL.

If the initial fluid infusion is not successful in restoring hemodynamic stability, a right-sided heart catheter should be inserted to monitor pulmonary artery wedge pressure. The "7-3" rule is helpful in gauging the volume of fluid replacement. An increment of 150 to 200 mL of isotonic crystalloid should be administered over 10 to 15 minutes. If the pulmonary capillary wedge pressure (PCWP) rises by more than 7 mm Hg, the fluid infusion shall be temporarily discontinued. If the PCWP increase is less than 3 mm Hg, additional increments of fluid should be given. The goals of fluid resuscitation are to achieve the following:

- Central venous pressure = 8 to 12 mm Hg
- Mean arterial pressure ≥65 mm Hg
- Urine output ≥0.5 mL/kg per hour
- Central venous oxygen or mixed venous oxygen saturation ≥70%

In addition, dopamine (starting dose, 1 to 3 mcg/kg per minute) should be administered. In low doses, this vasopressor stimulates myocardial contractility and improves perfusion of central organs. In higher doses, the drug has primarily vasoconstrictive effects and may actually compromise tissue perfusion. Norepinephrine (5 to 15 mcg/minute), vasopressin (0.01 to 0.03 U/minute), and dobutamine (0.5 to 1 mcg/kg per minute, maximum 40 mcg/kg per minute) also may be used as pressor agents.[65]

Hydrocortisone (200 to 300 mg/day for 7 days in three or four divided doses or by continuous infusion) should be administered early in the course of septic shock. Although ultimate mortality is not improved, patients who receive corticosteroids have a more rapid reversal of the shock state than those who are not treated.[66,67]

The second objective of treatment is to administer broad-spectrum antibiotics targeted against the most likely pathogens.[18] For genital tract infections, the combination of penicillin (5 million units IV every 6 hours) or ampicillin (2 g IV every 6 hours) plus clindamycin (900 mg IV every 8 hours) or metronidazole (500 mg IV every 8 hours) plus gentamicin (7 mg/kg ideal body weight IV every 24 hours) or aztreonam (1 to 2 g IV every 8 hours) is an appropriate regimen. Alternatively, imipenem-cilastatin (500 mg IV every 6 hours), meropenem (1 g every 8 hours), or ertapenem (1 g IV every 24 hours) can be administered as single agents. Patients also may require surgery, for example, to evacuate infected products of conception, drain a pelvic abscess, or remove badly infected pelvic organs. Indicated surgery never should be delayed because a patient is unstable; operative intervention may be precisely the step necessary to reverse the hemodynamic derangements of septic shock.

Patients with septic shock require meticulous supportive care. Core temperature should be maintained as close to normal as possible by use of antipyretics and a cooling blanket. Coagulation abnormalities should be identified promptly and treated by infusion of platelets and coagulation factors, as indicated. Finally, patients should be given oxygen supplementation and observed closely for evidence of ARDS, one of the major causes of mortality in cases of severe sepsis.[64] Oxygenation should be monitored by means of a pulse oximeter or radial artery catheter. If evidence of respiratory failure develops, the patient should be intubated and supported with mechanical ventilation.

The prognosis in patients with septic shock clearly depends on the severity of the patient's underlying illness. In previously healthy patients, mortality should not exceed 15%.[68] Fortunately, most obstetrical patients are in the latter category. Therefore, the prognosis for complete recovery is excellent provided that the patient receives competent, timely intervention.

Toxoplasmosis

Epidemiology

Toxoplasma gondii is a protozoan that has three distinct forms: trophozoite, cyst, and oocyst. The life cycle of *T. gondii* is dependent on wild and domestic cats, which are the only host for the oocyst. The oocyst is formed in the cat intestine and subsequently excreted in the feces. Mammals, such as cows, ingest the oocyst, which is disrupted in the animal's intestine, releasing the invasive trophozoite. The trophozoite then is disseminated throughout the body, ultimately forming cysts in brain and muscle.[69]

Human infection occurs when infected meat is ingested or when food is contaminated by cat feces through flies, cockroaches, or fingers. Infection rates are highest in areas of poor sanitation and crowded living conditions. Stray cats and domestic cats that eat raw meat are most likely to carry the parasite. The cyst is destroyed by heat.[69]

About 40% to 50% of adults in the United States have antibody to this organism, and the prevalence of antibody is highest in lower socioeconomic populations. The frequency of seroconversion during pregnancy is 5%, and about 3 in 1000 infants show evidence of congenital infection. Clinically significant congenital toxoplasmosis occurs in about 1 in 8000 pregnancies. Toxoplasmosis is more common in western Europe, particularly France, most likely because of the practice in that country of eating rare or raw meat. More than 80% of women of childbearing age in Paris have antibody to *T. gondii*, and the incidence of congenital toxoplasmosis is about twice as frequent as that in the United States.[70]

Clinical Manifestations

The ingested organism invades across the intestinal epithelium and spreads hematogenously throughout the body. Intracellular replication leads to cell destruction. Clinical manifestations of infection are the result of direct organ damage and the subsequent immunologic response to parasitemia and cell death. Host immunity is mediated primarily through T lymphocytes.[69]

Most infections in humans are asymptomatic. Even in the absence of symptoms, however, patients may have evidence of multiorgan involvement, and clinical disease can follow a long period of asymptomatic infection. Symptomatic toxoplasmosis usually presents as an illness similar to mononucleosis.

In contrast to infection in the immunocompetent host, toxoplasmosis can be a devastating infection in the immunosuppressed patient. Because immunity to *T. gondii* is cell mediated, patients with human immunodeficiency virus infection and those treated with chronic immunosuppressive therapy after organ transplantation are particularly susceptible to new or reactivated infection. In these patients, dysfunction of the central nervous system is the most common manifestation of infection. Findings typically include encephalitis, meningoencephalitis and intracerebral mass lesions. Pneumonitis, myocarditis, and generalized lymphadenopathy also occur commonly.[69]

Diagnosis

The diagnosis of toxoplasmosis in the mother can be confirmed by serologic and histologic methods. Serologic tests that suggest an acute infection include detection of immunoglobulin M (IgM)-specific antibody, demonstration of an extremely high IgG antibody titer, and documentation of IgG seroconversion from negative to positive. Clinicians should be aware that serologic assays for toxoplasmosis are not well standardized. When initial laboratory tests appear to indicate that an acute infection has occurred, repeat serology should be performed in a well-respected reference laboratory. In addition, toxoplasmic DNA can be identified in the patient's serum using the PCR test.

T. gondii is most easily identified in lymphatic or brain tissues. Histologic preparations can be examined by light and electron microscopy. For light microscopy, specimens should be stained with either Giemsa or Wright stain.[70,71]

Congenital Toxoplasmosis

Congenital infection can occur if a woman develops acute primary toxoplasmosis during pregnancy. Chronic or latent infection is unlikely to cause fetal injury except perhaps in an immunosuppressed patient. **About 40% of neonates born to mothers with acute toxoplasmosis show evidence of infection.** Congenital infection is most likely to occur when maternal infection develops in the third trimester. However, fetal injury is most likely to be severe when maternal infection occurs in the first half of pregnancy. Less than half of affected infants are symptomatic at birth (see box, Clinical Manifestations of Congenital Toxoplasmosis).[70-72]

Clinical Manifestations of Congenital Toxoplasmosis

- Rash
- Hepatosplenomegaly
- Ascites
- Fever
- Chorioretinitis
- Periventricular calcifications
- Ventriculomegaly
- Seizures
- Mental retardation
- Uveitis

The most valuable tests for antenatal diagnosis of congenital toxoplasmosis are ultrasound, cordocentesis, and amniocentesis.[70-72] Ultrasound findings suggestive of infection include ventriculomegaly, intracranial calcifications, microcephaly, ascites, hepatosplenomegaly, and growth restriction. Fetal blood samples can be tested for IgM-specific antibody after 20 to 22 weeks' gestation. Fetal blood and amniotic fluid can be inoculated into mice, and the organism can subsequently be recovered from the blood of infected animals. In addition, Hohlfeld and coworkers[73] have now identified a specific gene of *T. gondii* in amniotic fluid using PCR. In this investigation, 34 of 339 infants had congenital toxoplasmosis confirmed by serologic testing or autopsy. All amniotic fluid specimens from affected pregnancies were positive by PCR, and test results were available within 1 day of specimen collection.

In a subsequent investigation, Romand and colleagues[74] reported that the PCR test had an overall sensitivity of 64% (95% CI, 53% to 75%) for diagnosing congenital toxoplasmosis. No false-positive results were noted, and the positive predictive value was 100%.

Management

Toxoplasmosis in the immunocompetent adult is usually an asymptomatic or self-limited illness and does not require treatment. Immunocompromised patients, however, should be treated, and the regimen of choice is a combination of oral sulfadiazine (4 g loading dose, then 1 g four times daily) plus pyrimethamine (50 to 100 mg initially, then 25 mg daily). In such patients, extended courses of treatment may be necessary to cure the infection.[71]

Treatment also is indicated when acute toxoplasmosis occurs during pregnancy. **Treatment of the mother reduces the risk for congenital infection and decreases the late sequelae of infection.[70,72,75] Pyrimethamine is not recommended for use during the first trimester of pregnancy because of possible teratogenicity, although specific adverse fetal effects have not been documented to date. Sulfonamides can be used alone, but single-agent therapy appears to be less effective than combination therapy. In Europe, spiramycin has been used extensively in pregnancy with excellent success. It is available for treatment in the United States through the CDC.**

Aggressive early treatment of infants with congenital toxoplasmosis is indicated and consists of combination therapy with pyrimethamine, sulfadiazine, and leucovorin for 1 year. Early treatment reduces, but does not eliminate, the late sequelae of toxoplasmosis, such as chorioretinitis.[76]

In the management of the pregnant patient, prevention of acute toxoplasmosis is of paramount importance. Pregnant women should be advised to avoid contact with cat litter if at all possible. If they must change the litter, they should do so daily, wear gloves, and wash their hands afterward. They should always wash their hands after preparing meat for cooking and should never eat raw or rare meat. Meat should be cooked thoroughly until the juices are clear. Fruits and vegetables also should be washed carefully to remove possible contamination by oocysts.

Listeriosis

Listeria monocytogenes (LM) is a gram-positive bacillus responsible for severe infections in humans and a large variety of animal species. It is a facultative intracellular pathogen that invades macrophages and most tissue cells of infected hosts, where it can proliferate. **LM can cause meningitis, encephalitis, bacteremia, and febrile gastroenteritis.** In infected hosts, the bacteria cross the intestinal wall at Peyer patches to invade the mesenteric lymph nodes and blood. The main target organ is the liver, where the bacteria multiply inside hepatocytes. Most disease occurs in patients with impaired cell-mediated immunity, and, therefore, LM is an important cause of severe infections in neonates, pregnant women, elderly people, and transplant recipients. Although dramatic epidemics have received the most publicity, most cases of perinatal listeriosis are isolated.

LM is naturally widespread in nature and can be readily found in soil and vegetation. Recent seroepidemiologic studies show that the infection is foodborne. Heightened surveillance and quality control by the food industry have been instituted (see box, U.S. Department of Agriculture's Food Safety and Inspection Service and U.S. Food and Drug Administration's Advice for Pregnant Women to Prevent Listeriosis during Pregnancy), leading to a reduction in the number of cases and deaths from this infection in the past decade. However, most parents are still not aware of the risks of listeriosis and recommended practices for listeriosis prevention; thus, they are not taking precautions during their pregnancy to prevent listeriosis.[77] **Because LM can grow and multiply at temperatures as low as 0.5° C (or 32.9° F), refrigerating contaminated foods does not always prevent infection, but cooking contaminated foods at high temperatures consistently destroys the bacteria.** LM can also be contracted through the handling of the products of conception of animals, when the miscarriage is due to listeriosis. Therefore, it is important for pregnant women working with animals not to touch these tissues, if possible, or to wear gloves if contact cannot be avoided. Owing to the ubiquity of the organism in the environment, outbreaks and sporadic disease continue to occur.[78]

U.S. Department of Agriculture's Food Safety and Inspection Service and U.S. Food and Drug Administration's Advice for Pregnant Women to Prevent Listeriosis During Pregnancy

- Do not eat hot dogs, luncheon meats, or deli meats unless they are reheated until steaming hot.
- Do not eat soft cheeses such as feta, Brie, Camembert, blue-veined cheeses, or Mexican-style cheeses such as *queso blanco fresco.* Hard cheeses, semisoft cheeses such as mozzarella, pasteurized processed cheese slices and spreads, cream cheese, and cottage cheese can be safely consumed.
- Do not eat refrigerated paté or meat spreads. Canned or shelf-stable paté and meat spreads can be eaten.
- Do not eat refrigerated smoked seafood unless it is an ingredient in a cooked dish such as a casserole. Examples of refrigerated smoked seafood include salmon, trout, whitefish, cod, tuna, and mackerel, which are most often labeled as "nova style," "lox," "kippered," "smoked," or "jerky." This fish is found in the refrigerated section or sold at deli counters of grocery stores and delicatessens. Canned fish such as salmon and tuna or shelf-stable smoked seafood may be safely eaten.
- Do not drink raw (unpasteurized) milk or eat foods that contain unpasteurized milk.

The incubation period of LM ranges from as little as 1 day to as long as 90 days, making identification of the food or activity that caused the listeriosis extremely difficult. **Maternal symptoms can vary from "flu-like" or "food poisoning" to septicemia, meningitis, or pneumonia.** Because there is no reliable serologic evaluation, listeriosis is a difficult infection to test for outside the septic peak when it can be demonstrated in blood cultures. An overall perinatal mortality rate of 50% due to late miscarriage, premature delivery, and stillbirth was recorded before the use of modern therapies.[79] The clinical characteristics of neonatal listeriosis are similar to neonatal GBS sepsis, with early- and late-onset forms of disease. The mortality rate among liveborn infants is about 10%.[80]

The standard therapy for listeriosis is a combination of ampicillin and gentamicin or, for patients who are intolerant of β-lactam agents, trimethoprim-sulfamethoxazole. If LM chorioamnionitis is diagnosed preterm, in contrast to other types of chorioamnionitis, in utero therapy with high-dose penicillin or trimethoprim-sulfamethoxazole is possible, and preterm delivery may be avoided.

KEY POINTS

- Overall, 85% of neonatal GBS infections are early in onset and result from transmission from a colonized mother.
- All pregnant women should be cultured for GBS at 35 to 37 weeks. Culture-positive patients should receive intrapartum antibiotic prophylaxis to prevent early-onset neonatal infection.
- Patients with GBS bacteriuria should be considered heavily colonized and be targeted for intrapartum prophylaxis.
- All pregnant women should have a urine culture at their first prenatal appointment to detect asymptomatic bacteriuria.
- Most cases of pyelonephritis occur as a consequence of undiagnosed or inadequately treated lower urinary tract infections.
- The organisms most likely to cause chorioamnionitis and puerperal endometritis are GBS, *E. coli*, and gram-positive and gram-negative anaerobes.
- Prophylactic antibiotics are highly effective in preventing postcesarean endometritis. They should be administered before the surgical incision.
- Resistant organisms and wound infection are the most common causes of persistent fever in patients who are being treated for puerperal endometritis.
- Septic pelvic thrombophlebitis is another important cause of refractory postoperative fever. This condition is best diagnosed by CT or MRI and is treated with broad-spectrum antibiotics and intravenous heparin.
- The most common causes of septic shock in obstetrical patients are septic abortion, pyelonephritis, chorioamnionitis, and endometritis.
- The two most common methods of transmission of toxoplasmosis are consumption of undercooked beef and contact with cat litter.
- The best diagnostic tests for congenital toxoplasmosis are identification of toxoplasmic DNA in amniotic fluid by PCR and identification of specific fetal injury by ultrasound.
- Pregnant women and immunocompromised patients may reduce their risk for contracting listeriosis by avoiding unpasteurized dairy products.

REFERENCES

1. Prevention of perinatal group B streptococcal disease: revised guidelines from the CDC. MMWR Morb Mortal Wkly Rep 51:1, 2002.
2. Yancey MK, Duff P: An analysis of the cost-effectiveness of selected protocols for the prevention of neonatal group B streptococcal infection. Obstet Gynecol 83:367, 1994.
3. Boyer KM, Gotoff SP: Prevention of early-onset neonatal group B streptococcal disease with selective intrapartum chemoprophylaxis. N Engl J Med 314:1665, 1986.
4. Thomsen AC, Morup L, Hansen KB: Antibiotic elimination of group B streptococci in urine in prevention of preterm labor. Lancet 1:591, 1987.
5. Newton ER, Clark M: Group B streptococcus and preterm rupture of membranes. Obstet Gynecol 71:198, 1988.
6. Yancey MK, Armer T, Clark P, Duff P: Assessment of rapid identification tests for genital carriage of group B streptococci. Obstet Gynecol 80:1038, 1992.
7. Bergeron MG, Ke D, Menard C, et al: Rapid detection of group B streptococci in pregnant women at delivery. N Engl J Med 343:175, 2000.
8. Siegel JD, McCracken GH, Threlkeld N, et al: Single-dose penicillin prophylaxis against neonatal group B streptococcal infections. N Engl J Med 303:769, 1980.
9. Yow MD, Mason EO, Leeds LJ, et al: Ampicillin prevents intrapartum transmission of group B streptococcus. JAMA 241:1245, 1979.
10. Boyer KM, Gadzala CA, Kelly PD, Gotoff SP: Selective intrapartum chemoprophylaxis of neonatal group B streptococcal early-onset disease. III. Interruption of mother-to-infant transmission. J Infect Dis 148:810, 1983.
11. Prevention of perinatal group B streptococcal disease: a public health perspective. MMWR Morb Mortal Wkly Rep 45:1, 1996.
12. Rosenstein NE, Schuchat A: Opportunities for prevention of perinatal group B streptococcal disease: a multistate surveillance analysis. Obstet Gynecol 90:901, 1997.
13. Locksmith GJ, Clark P, Duff P: Maternal and neonatal infection rates with three different protocols for prevention of group B streptococcal disease. Am J Obstet Gynecol 180:416, 1999.
14. DeCueto M, Sanchez M-J, Sanpedro A, et al: Timing of intrapartum ampicillin and prevention of vertical transmission of group B streptococcus. Obstet Gynecol 91:112, 1998.
15. McNanley AR, Glantz C, Hardy DJ, et al: The effect of intrapartum penicillin on vaginal group B streptococcus colony counts. Am J Obstet Gynecol 197:583e1, 2007.
16. Edwards RK, Clark P, Duff P: Intrapartum antibiotic prophylaxis 2: positive predictive value of antenatal group B streptococci cultures and antibiotic susceptibility of clinical isolates. Obstet Gynecol 100: 540, 2002.
17. Duff P: Urinary tract infections. Prim Care Update Ob/Gyn 1:12, 1994.
18. Duff P: Antibiotic selection in obstetrics: making cost-effective choices. Clin Obstet Gynecol 45:59, 2002.
19. Duff P: Pyelonephritis in pregnancy. Clin Obstet Gynecol 27:17, 1984.
20. Stamm WE, Counts GW, Running KR, et al: Diagnosis of coliform infection in acutely dysuric women. N Engl J Med 307:463, 1982.
21. Dunlow S, Duff P: Prevalence of antibiotic-resistant uropathogens in obstetric patients with acute pyelonephritis. Obstet Gynecol 76:241, 1990.
22. Stamm, WE, Hooton TM: Management of urinary tract infections in adults. N Engl J Med 329:1328, 1993.
23. MacMillan MC, Grimes DA: The limited usefulness of urine and blood cultures in treating pyelonephritis in pregnancy. Obstet Gynecol 78:745, 1991.
24. Gibbs RS, Duff P: Progress in pathogenesis and management of clinical intraamniotic infection. Am J Obstet Gynecol 164:1317, 1991.
25. Armer TL, Duff P: Intraamniotic infection in patients with intact membranes and preterm labor. Obstet Gynecol Surv 46:589, 1991.
26. Romero R, Jimenez C, Lohda AK, et al: Amniotic fluid glucose concentration: a rapid and simple method for the detection of intraamniotic infection in preterm labor. Am J Obstet Gynecol 163:968, 1990.
27. Kirshon B, Rosenfeld B, Mari G, Belfort M: Amniotic fluid glucose and intraamniotic infection. Am J Obstet Gynecol 164:818, 1991.
28. Gauthier DW, Meyer WJ, Bieniarz A: Correlation of amniotic fluid glucose concentration and intraamniotic infection in patients with preterm labor or premature rupture of membranes. Am J Obstet Gynecol 165:1105, 1991.
29. Romero R, Yoon BH, Mazor M, et al: The diagnostic and prognostic value of amniotic fluid white blood cell count, glucose, interleukin-6, and Gram stain in patients with preterm labor and intact membranes. Am J Obstet Gynecol 169:805, 1993.
30. Sperling RS, Ramamurthy RS, Gibbs RS: A comparison of intrapartum versus immediate postpartum treatment of intra-amniotic infection. Obstet Gynecol 70:861, 1987.
31. Gilstrap LC, Leveno KJ, Cox SM, et al: Intrapartum treatment of acute chorioamnionitis: impact on neonatal sepsis. Am J Obstet Gynecol 159:579, 1988.
32. Gibbs RS, Dinsmoor MJ, Newton ER, et al: A randomized trial of intrapartum versus immediate postpartum treatment of women with intra-amniotic infection. Obstet Gynecol 72:823, 1988.

33. Edwards RK, Duff P: Single additional dose postpartum therapy for women with chorioamnionitis. Obstet Gynecol 102:957, 2003.
34. Duff P, Sanders R, Gibbs RS: The course of labor in term patients with chorioamnionitis. Am J Obstet Gynecol 147:391, 1983.
35. Duff P: Pathophysiology and management of postcesarean endomyometritis. Obstet Gynecol 67:269, 1986.
36. Milligan DA, Brady K, Duff P: Short-term parenteral antibiotic therapy for puerperal endometritis. J Matern Fetal Med 1:60, 1992.
37. Duff P: Staphylococcal infections. In Gleicher N (ed): Principles and Practice of Medical Therapy in Pregnancy, 2nd ed. New York, Appleton & Lange, 1992, p 518.
38. Duff P: Prophylactic antibiotics for cesarean delivery: a simple cost-effective strategy for prevention of postoperative morbidity. Am J Obstet Gynecol 157:794, 1987.
39. Duff P: A simple checklist for preventing serious complications after cesarean delivery. Obstet Gynecol 116:1393, 2010.
40. Howard HR, Phelps D, Blanchard K: Prophylactic cesarean section antibiotics: maternal and neonatal morbidity before or after cord clamping. Obstet Gynecol 53:151, 1979.
41. Cunningham FG, Leveno KJ, DePalma RT, et al: Perioperative antimicrobials for cesarean delivery: before or after cord clamping? Obstet Gynecol 62:151, 1983.
42. Sullivan SA, Smith T, Chang E, et al: Administration of cefazolin prior to skin incision is superior to cefazolin at cord clamping in preventing postcesarean infectious morbidity: a randomized controlled trial. Am J Obstet Gynecol 196:455.e1, 2007.
43. Kaimal AJ, Zlatnick MG, Chang YW, et al: Effect of a change in policy regarding the timing of prophylactic antibiotics on the rate of postcesarean delivery surgical-site infections. Am J Obstet Gynecol 199:310.e1, 2008.
44. Owens SM, Brozanski BS, Meyn LA, et al: Antimicrobial prophylaxis for cesarean delivery before skin incision. Obstet Gynecol 114:573, 2009.
45. Costantine MM, Rahman M, Ghulmiyah L, et al: Timing of perioperative antibiotics for cesarean delivery: a metaanalysis. Am J Obstet Gynecol 199:301.e1, 2008.
46. Tita ATN, Hauth JC, Grimes A, et al: Decreasing incidence of postcesarean endometritis with extended-spectrum antibiotic prophylaxis. Obstet Gynecol 111:51, 2008.
47. Tita AT, Owen J, Stamm AM, et al: Impact of extended-spectrum antibiotic prophylaxis on incidence of postcesarean surgical wound infection. Am J Obstet Gynecol 199:303e1, 2008.
48. Dinsmoor MJ, Gilbert S, Landon MB, et al: Perioperative antibiotic prophylaxis for non-laboring cesarean delivery. Obstet Gynecol 114:752, 2008.
49. Lasley D, Eblen A, Yancey MK, et al: The effect of placental removal method on the incidence of postcesarean infections. Am J Obstet Gynecol 176:1250, 1997.
50. Anorlu RI, Maholwana B, Hofmeyr JG: Methods of delivering the placenta at cesarean section. Cochran Database Syst Rev 3:CD004737, 2008.
51. Yancey MK, Duff P, Clark P: The frequency of glove contamination during cesarean delivery. Obstet Gynecol 83:538, 1994.
52. Gibbs RS, Blanco JD, St. Clair PJ: A case-control study of wound abscess after cesarean delivery. Obstet Gynecol 62:498, 1983.
53. Shy KK, Eschenbach DA: Fatal perineal cellulitis from an episiotomy site. Obstet Gynecol 54:292, 1979.
54. Golde S, Ledger WJ: Necrotizing fasciitis in postpartum patients. Obstet Gynecol 50:670, 1977.
55. Weinstein WM, Onderdonk AB, Bartlett JG, Gorbach SL: Experimental intra-abdominal abscesses in rats: development of an experimental model. Infect Immun 10:1250,1974.
56. Knochel JQ, Koehler PR, Lee TG, Welch DM: Diagnosis of abdominal abscesses with computed tomography, ultrasound, and ^{111}In leukocyte scans. Radiology 137:425, 1980.
57. Gerzof SG, Robbins AH, Johnson WC, et al: Percutaneous catheter drainage of abdominal abscesses: a five-year experience. N Engl J Med 305:653, 1981.
58. Duff P, Gibbs RS: Pelvic vein thrombophlebitis: diagnostic dilemma and therapeutic challenge. Obstet Gynecol Surv 38:365,1983.
59. Brown TK, Munsick RA: Puerperal ovarian vein thrombophlebitis: a syndrome. Am J Obstet Gynecol 109:263, 1971.
60. Dunn LJ, Van Voorhis LW: Enigmatic fever and pelvic thrombophlebitis. N Engl J Med 276:265, 1967.
61. Brown CEL, Lowe TE, Cunningham, FG, Weinreb JC: Puerperal pelvic vein thrombophlebitis: impact on diagnosis and treatment using x-ray computed tomography and magnetic resonance imaging. Obstet Gynecol 68:789, 1986.
62. Duff P: Septic pelvic-vein thrombophlebitis. In Pastorek JG (ed): Obstetric and Gynecologic Infectious Disease. New York, Raven Press, 1994, p 165.
63. Duff P, Gibbs RS: Maternal sepsis. In Berkowitz RL (ed): Critical Care of the Obstetric Patient. New York, Churchill Livingstone, 1983, p 189.
64. Kaplan RL, Sahn SA, Petty TL: Incidence and outcome of the respiratory distress syndrome in gram-negative sepsis. Arch Intern Med 139:867, 1979.
65. DeBacker D, Biston P, Devriendt J, et al: Comparison of dopamine and norepinephrine in the treatment of shock. N Engl J Med 362:779, 2010.
66. Dellinger RP, Carlet JM, Masur H, et al: Surviving sepsis campaign guidelines for management of severe sepsis and septic shock. Crit Care Med 32:858, 2004.
67. Sprung CL, Annane D, Keh D, et al: Hydrocortisone therapy for patients with septic shock. N Engl J Med 358:111, 2008.
68. Freid MA, Vosti KL: The importance of underlying disease in patients with gram-negative bacteremia. Arch Intern Med 121:418, 1968.
69. Krick JA, Remington JS: Toxoplasmosis in the adult: an overview. N Engl J Med 298:550, 1978.
70. Daffos F: Prenatal management of 746 pregnancies at risk for congenital toxoplasmosis. N Engl J Med 318:271, 1988.
71. Egerman RS, Beazley D: Toxoplasmosis. Semin Perinatol 22:332, 1998.
72. Desmonts G, Couvreur J: Congenital toxoplasmosis: a prospective study of 378 pregnancies. N Engl J Med 290:1110, 1974.
73. Hohlfeld P, Daffos F, Costa JM, et al: Prenatal diagnosis of congenital toxoplasmosis with a polymerase-chain reaction test on amniotic fluid. N Engl J Med 331:695,1994.
74. Romand S, Wallon M, Franck J, et al: Prenatal diagnosis using polymerase chain reaction on amniotic fluid for congenital toxoplasmosis. Obstet Gynecol 97:296, 2001.
75. Foulon W, Villena I, Stray-Pedersen B, et al: Treatment of toxoplasmosis during pregnancy: a multicenter study of impact on fetal transmission and children's sequelae at age 1year. Am J Obstet Gynecol 180:410,1999.
76. Guerina NG, Hsu HW, Meissner HC, et al: Neonatal serologic screening and early treatment for congenital *Toxoplasma gondii* infection. N Engl J Med 330:1858, 1994.
77. Cates SC, Carter-Young HL, Conley S, O'Brien B: Pregnant women and listeriosis: preferred educational messages and delivery mechanisms. J Nutr Educ Behav 36:121, 2004.
78. MacDonald PD, Whitwam RE, Boggs JD, et al: Outbreak of listeriosis among Mexican immigrants as a result of consumption of illicitly produced Mexican-style cheese. Clin Infect Dis 40:677, 2005.
79. McLauchlin J: Human listeriosis in Britain, 1967-85, a summary of 722 cases. 1. Listeriosis during pregnancy and in the newborn. Epidemiol Infect 104:181, 1990.
80. Frederiksen B, Samuelsson S: Feto-maternal listeriosis in Denmark 1981-1988. J Infect 24:277, 1992.

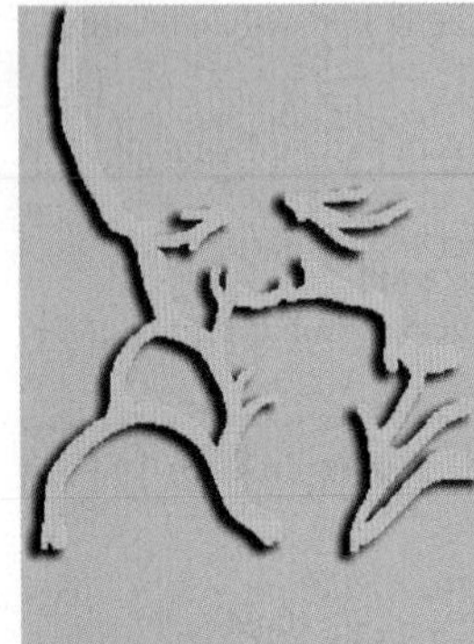

CHAPTER 52

Mental Health and Behavioral Disorders in Pregnancy

Katherine L. Wisner, Dorothy K. Y. Sit, Margaret Altemus, Debra L. Bogen, Christopher S. Famy, Teri B. Pearlstein, Dawn P. Misra, Sarah K. Reynolds, and James M. Perel

KEY ABBREVIATIONS

American Academy of Pediatrics	AAP
American Academy of Neurology	AAN
American College of Obstetricians and Gynecologists	ACOG
American Psychiatric Association	APA
Anorexia Nervosa	AN
Antiepileptic Drugs	AED
Bipolar Disorder	BD
Body Mass Index	BMI
Bulimia Nervosa	BN
Carbamazepine	CBZ
Cognitive Behavioral Therapy	CBT
Confidence Interval	CI
Diagnostic and Statistical Manual of Mental Disorders	DSM-IV
Docosahexaenoic Acid	DHA
Edinburgh Postnatal Depression Scale	EPDS
Electroconvulsive Therapy	ECT
Food and Drug Administration	FDA
Interpersonal Psychotherapy	IPT
Intrauterine Growth Restriction	IUGR
Lamotrigine	LTG
Major Depressive Episode	MDE
Methadone Maintenance Treatment	MMT
Neonatal Abstinence Syndrome	NAS
Neonatal Intensive Care Unit	NICU
Olanzapine	OLZ
Omega-3 Fatty Acids	O-3 FAs
Odds Ratio	OR
Personality Disorder	PD
Preterm Birth	PTB
Randomized Controlled Trial	RCT
Selective-Serotonin Reuptake Inhibitor	SSRI
Small for Gestational Age	SGA
Thyroid-Stimulating Hormone	TSH
Tricyclic Antidepressant	TCA
Valproic Acid	VPA

Mental health is fundamental to health. This statement, made by Surgeon General David Satcher, emphasized the foundation that emotional well-being provides for health. In medical practice, we compartmentalize symptoms and diseases into manageable units; however, the patient comes as an integrated whole. The effect of pathology in any part of the body affects the entire patient. Psychiatric disorders are defined in the *Diagnostic and Statistical Manual of Mental Disorders* (DSM-IV),[1] a categorical classification that divides mental disorders into types based on criteria sets with defining features. This chapter covers the major

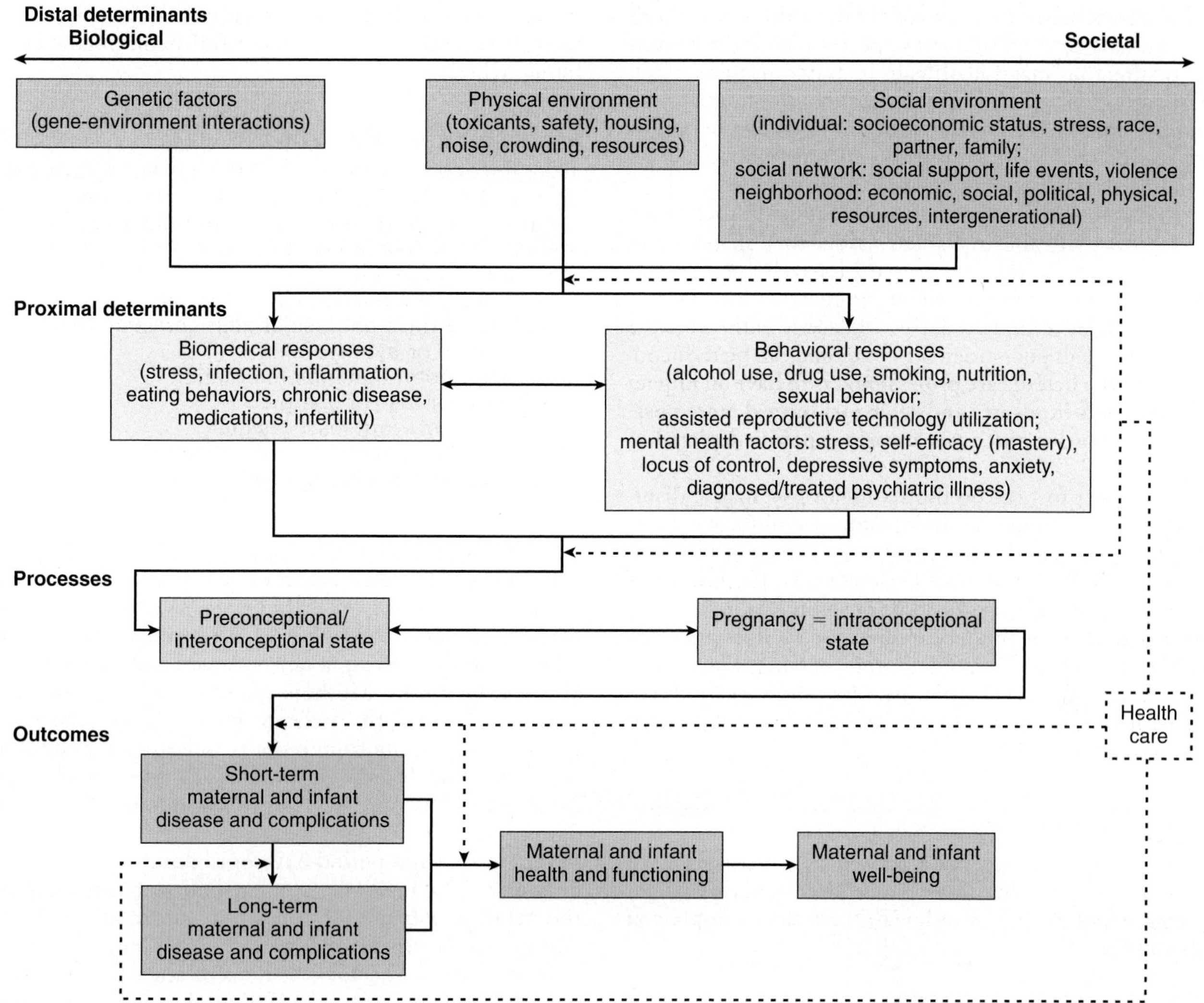

FIGURE 52-1. Integrated perinatal health framework: a multiple determinants model with a life span approach. (From Misra DP, Guyer B, Allston A: Integrated perinatal health framework. A multiple determinants model with a life span approach. Am J Prev Med 25:65, 2003. Included here with adaptations] with permission from Dawn P. Misra, Ph.D. [03/07/05]. [Illustrative examples are in brackets.])

classifications of disorders that affect women of childbearing age as well as the tragedies of suicide and infanticide. For the pregnant woman and her family, the capacity to function optimally, enjoy relationships, manage the pregnancy, and prepare for the infant's birth is critical.

Perinatal health can be conceptualized within a model that integrates the complex social, psychological, behavioral, environmental, and biologic forces that shape pregnancy. Misra and colleagues[2] presented a comprehensive perinatal framework that integrates a life span approach with a multiple determinants model (Figure 52-1). The model contains four hierarchical levels that provide a paradigm for considering the determinants of perinatal health outcomes. The first level in the model is *Distal Determinants,* which brings focus to *distal* (in time) risk factors that place a woman at greater susceptibility to *proximal* (current) risk factors. Distal determinants derive from biologic, physical, and social domains. Although they have the potential to directly influence health status, distal factors typically increase or decrease a woman's likelihood of developing health problems, engaging in high-risk behaviors, or being exposed to potential toxins. Some of the most powerful influences on pregnancy outcome are related to these *distal* women's health factors that occur long before pregnancy. At the next level, *proximal determinants,* risk factors that have a direct impact on a woman's health status, are represented by biomedical and behavioral responses. The interaction between *distal* and *proximal* risk factors determines an individual's overall health status. The relationship between a woman's health status directly before conception and the demands of pregnancy affect perinatal health outcomes. For example, a woman who is told that her infant has spina bifida after an ultrasound examination (due to long-term low folate intake, a distal risk resulting in a negative outcome) develops a recurrence of a major depressive episode (proximal risk) that further affects maternal and fetal health. The third level, *processes,* is presented to emphasize the dynamic interaction of pre-, inter- and intraconceptional factors (as time variables in the women's health life course) on perinatal outcomes. At the fourth level, *outcomes,* the model includes constructs of disease, functioning, and well-being, which together provide a comprehensive assessment of health status (both short and long term). Potential opportunities for interventions to affect perinatal health are included in this model. Childbearing is an opportune health promotion time because women have contact with professionals, access to health coverage, and are motivated toward positive behaviors to invest in the welfare of their offspring.

Each patient can be understood as coming to pregnancy with sets of malleable risks and assets that shape pregnancy outcome. To the extent that biopsychosocial exposures with negative impact upon pregnancy outcome can be diminished, eliminated, or replaced with positive factors, the risk of poor pregnancy outcome can be reduced. **The role of the health care professional is to have an impact on the patient's exposures and behaviors toward more positive comprehensive outcomes at various points depicted in Figure 52-1.**

This chapter focuses on the six major psychiatric disorders that occur commonly in women of childbearing age and their courses during pregnancy, postpartum, and breastfeeding. Within the life cycle context, the impact of childbearing on existing disorders or vulnerabilities in the female patient is of primary interest, as well as episodes that are etiologically related to childbearing. Treatment considerations for psychiatric disorders during childbearing invoke special modifications of the risk/benefit decision-making process.

MOOD DISORDERS

The mood disorders are characterized by a disturbance of affective state as the most prominent feature. Major depression and bipolar disorder (BD) are the exemplars of this category.

Major Depressive Episode

Diagnosis and Prevalence During Pregnancy and Postpartum

In the DSM-IV,[1] a major depressive episode (MDE) is defined as at least a 2-week period of either persistent depressed mood or loss of interest or pleasure in daily activities (the "gatekeeper" symptoms) plus four associated symptoms (or three if both gatekeeper symptoms are present) (see box, DSM-IV Criteria). *Persistent* is operationalized as meaning the symptom must be present for most of the day nearly every day. The patient also must have impairment of function in interpersonal relationships or work. Note that it is possible to have a *diagnosis* of MDE without the *symptom* of depression. A woman could have persistent loss of interest or pleasure but no depressed mood and four other symptoms from the following: appetite disturbance or significant weight change, sleep loss/excess, psychomotor agitation/retardation, fatigue or energy loss, feelings of worthlessness or guilt, impaired thinking or concentration, and suicidal ideation. Appetite, sleep, and motor activity can be either decreased or increased. For example, a fatigued woman who derives no pleasure from previously enjoyable activities, sleeps 15 hours per day, sits for long periods when awake, and is gaining weight has MDE. A guilt-ridden woman with depressed mood and 4 hours per day of sleep, weight loss of 15 pounds, and pacing at night also has MDE. Another mood disorder, dysthymia, is chronic depression (for at least 2 years) that does not meet full symptomatic criteria for an MDE.

DSM-IV Criteria

Over the last 2 weeks, most of the day nearly every day, five of the following (one symptom must be mood or interest), which must cause marked distress or impairment in important areas of functioning:

- Depressed mood
- Markedly diminished interest or pleasure
- Significant weight loss or gain unrelated to dieting
- Insomnia or hypersomnia
- Psychomotor agitation/retardation
- Fatigue or loss of energy
- Feelings of worthlessness/guilt
- Diminished ability to concentrate
- Recurrent thoughts of death

Nearly twice as many women (12%) as men (6.6%) suffer from a depressive disorder each year.[3] Women are at the greatest risk for MDE between 25 and 44 years. **The period prevalence of MDE is 12.7% during pregnancy (with 7.5% of women having a new episode) and 21.9% the year after parturition.**[4] Mothers at high risk are inner-city women, those with preterm infants, and adolescents. Depression persists from months to years after childbirth, with lingering limitations in physical and psychological functioning following recovery from depressive episodes. Twenty-five to 50% of women who experience depression in the postpartum period have episodes that last 7 months or longer.[5] The major factor contributing to the duration of the MDE is delay in identification and treatment.

Based on a prospective study of 680 female twins the strongest predictors for MDE were stressful life events, genetic factors, history of MDE, and excessive emotional sensitivity.[6] Other authors have identified stressful life events and history of MDE in the patient and her family[5] as predictors of MDE with postpartum onset. Women who have suffered one episode of postpartum onset MDE are at increased risk (25%-33%) for another episode after a subsequent birth, and more than 40% have later episodes of non-postpartum MDE.[7]

The most commonly used measure to screen for MDE is the Edinburgh Postnatal Depression Scale (EPDS; Figure 52-2), which has been validated for use both during and after pregnancy. This brief self-report instrument contains 10 items ranked from 0 to 3. The EPDS is scored by simple addition and is free to health care professionals. It is the most commonly used screening measure worldwide and is available in 23 languages. The recommended cut-off score is 15 or higher during pregnancy. Cox and Holden[8] suggested a cut-off score of 13 or higher (sensitivity for identifying MDE = 86%, specificity = 78%, positive predictive value = 73%) for postpartum depression (PPD) screening in clinical settings. As with any screening tool, positive scores on the EPDS must be followed with diagnostic assessment.

Natural History Across Childbearing

Consistently, specific female life-cycle periods of hormonal fluctuation (i.e., menstrual cycle, pregnancy, postpartum,

How are you feeling?
As you have recently had a baby, we would like to know how you are feeling now. Please check the answer which comes closest to how you have felt in the past 7 days, not just how you feel today.

1.	I have been able to laugh and see the funny side of things:	Score
	As much as I always could	0
	Not quite so much now	1
	Definitely not so much now	2
	Not at all	3
2.	I have looked forward with enjoyment to things:	
	As much as I ever did	0
	Rather less than I used to	1
	Definitely less than I used to	2
	Hardly at all	3
3.	I have blamed myself unnecessarily when things went wrong:	
	Yes, most of the time	3
	Yes, some of the time	2
	Not very often	1
	No, never	0
4.	I have been anxious or worried for no good reason:	
	No, not at all	0
	Hardly ever	1
	Yes, sometimes	2
	Yes, very often	3
5.	I have felt scared or panicky for no very good reason:	
	Yes, quite a lot	3
	Yes, sometimes	2
	No, not much	1
	No, not at all	0
6.	Things have been getting on top of me:	
	Yes, most of the time I haven't been able to cope at all	3
	Yes, sometimes I haven't been coping as well as usual	2
	No, most of the time I have coped quite well	1
	No, I have been coping as well as ever	0
7.	I have been so unhappy that I have had difficulty sleeping:	
	Yes, most of the time	3
	Yes, sometimes	2
	Not very often	1
	No, not at all	0
8.	I have felt sad or miserable:	
	Yes, most of the time	3
	Yes, quite often	2
	Not very often	1
	No, not at all	0
9.	I have been so unhappy that I have been crying:	
	Yes, most of the time	3
	Yes, quite often	2
	Only occasionally	1
	No, never	0
10.	The thought of harming myself has occurred to me:	
	Yes, quite often	3
	Sometimes	2
	Hardly ever	1
	Never	0

FIGURE 52-2. Edinburgh Postnatal Depression Scale. © 1987 The Royal College of Psychiatrists. The Edinburgh Postnatal Depression Scale may be photocopied by individual researchers or clinicians for their own use without seeking permission from the publishers. The scale must be copied in full and all copies must acknowledge the following source: Cox, J.L., Holden, J.M., & Sagovsky, R. (1987). Detection of postnatal depression. Development of the 10-item Edinburgh Postnatal Depression Scale. British Journal of Psychiatry, 150, 782-786. Written permission must be obtained from the Royal College of Psychiatrists for copying and distribution to others or for republication (in print, online, or by any other medium).

and perimenopause) are associated with MDE. During pregnancy, the brain is exposed to a 100-fold increase in estradiol levels, which abruptly decreases in the first postpartum week. Investigators have suggested that the rapid change in gonadal steroid levels is involved in the etiology of postpartum-onset MDE.[9] Although all women experience this phenomenon, the neurobiology of women who develop postpartum depression appears differentially sensitive to the mood-destabilizing effects of withdrawal from gonadal steroids.

Postpartum MDE does not differ from MDE at other periods during the childbearing years with respect to clinical presentation and duration of untreated episodes. However, aggressive obsessional thoughts (see Anxiety Disorders section) occur more commonly in women who have postpartum-onset MDE. **The differential diagnosis of depressed mood in the early postpartum period includes the maternity blues, a transient syndrome experienced by up to 80% of new mothers, which resolves by 10 days after birth. Usually a manifestation of BD, postpartum psychosis occurs in 1 to 2 per 1000 mothers within the first 8 weeks after delivery and represents a psychiatric emergency.**

The physiologic milieu created by MDE adversely affects maternal function and outcomes in offspring. Gestational MDE is associated with lack of prenatal care, poor nutrition, smoking, alcohol and drug use, and suicide. A recent meta-analysis affirmed that gestational MDE was associated with both low birthweight and preterm birth (PTB).[10] Offspring of women with MDE during pregnancy are at risk for insecure attachment, poor cognitive performance, sleep and eating disorders, and depression at age 16 years. Finally, gestational MDE is the strongest predictor of postpartum MDE.

Other serious sequelae of maternal mental illness are increased rates of accidental injury, child abuse, neglect, and infanticide. Early identification and intervention for postpartum MDE has the potential to prevent negative sequelae for women and families.

Treatment of MDE During Pregnancy

The emergence of an episode of mood disorder during childbearing compels a complete medical and family history, review of systems, and focused physical examination to assess for organic contributions to the mood disorder. The use of prescribed and over-the-counter medication as well as drugs and alcohol must be assessed. Thyroid abnormalities and anemia, which are common in childbearing women, should be ruled out; however, our experience is that the full depressive syndrome seldom remits with correction of hypothyroidism alone.[11]

Although MDE is a common condition, only 1 in 5 Americans receive any guideline-concordant intervention[12] and the rate is even lower in pregnant women.[13] In nearly 6500 Medicaid recipients with established MDE treatment, women who became pregnant had a significantly greater drop in both outpatient visits and antidepressant prescription claims compared with matched nonpregnant women, and did not resume care after birth.[14]

Evidence-based treatments for MDE are psychotherapy and antidepressant medications.[1] Interpersonal psychotherapy and pharmacotherapy during pregnancy both reduce depressive symptoms and improve maternal function. Psychotherapy is the preferred treatment[12]; however, it is not readily available in all practice settings nor is it feasible for many mothers. Barriers to clinic-based depression care include the physical demands of pregnancy, transportation, and childcare for other children. Adult mental health settings do not typically offer flexible appointment schedules or allow children on site. If psychotherapy is not feasible, or the woman prefers pharmacotherapy, decision making tends to focus on the potential adverse effects of medication rather than the adverse effects of the depressive disorder. Many physicians avoid drug treatment of pregnant women because of lack of expertise or medicolegal liability. The result is often the choice by the woman or her physician to avoid or stop drug treatment to obviate fetal exposure without equal consideration of the risks of MDE to both the mother and fetus. **For most pregnant women, the reality is that accessible and acceptable mental health treatment is very limited.** However, many federally funded programs provide home visitation to disadvantaged pregnant women, and program staff are potential partners for collaborative care with obstetricians and mental health professionals to improve rates of depression treatment.

Individually tailored interventions for the treatment of MDE are considered in view of their capacity to maximize maternal wellness while minimizing toxicity for the maternal-fetal pair. The patient and physician each contribute expertise to the process, because the patient's assignment of her own values dictates her choice. For example, some women will not consent to pharmacotherapy during pregnancy regardless of the degree of impairment related to the depressive episode. Others choose pharmacotherapy because they are not confident that other treatments will be efficacious, or because discontinuing medication invariably has been followed by recurrence with major psychosocial consequences. The verbal informed consent process promotes the treatment alliance, recognizes the patient's responsibility to make choices for herself and her baby, and provides an opportunity for ongoing assessment of the woman's competence to make decisions.

Although used commonly, the word *safe* has no operational definition in this context and its use implies a clear boundary between safe and unsafe. Confirming any exposure as harmless presents the impossible task of proving no effect on a number of reproductive and developmental outcomes such as intrauterine fetal demise, physical malformations, growth effects, neurobehavioral teratogenicity, and neonatal effects. What can be estimated from available studies is the magnitude of a subset of reproductive risks in women treated with selective-serotonin reuptake inhibitors (SSRI).[15] A prominent conclusion from published papers is the dearth of data to separate the impact of the drug exposure from the sequelae, both physiologic and psychosocial, of the underlying MDE.

Intrauterine Fetal Demise and Miscarriage. Studies to support an association between miscarriage rates and antidepressant use have inadequate control for confounding variables related to the depressive disorder.[16] There is no evidence that the rate of stillbirths is increased during antidepressant treatment.

Physical Malformations. The majority of studies do not demonstrate an association between tricyclic antidepressants (TCA) and birth defects. Similarly, studies of first-trimester SSRI exposure do not demonstrate consistent data to support a risk for structural malformations. **Two large-scale case-control studies revealed no increased risk for overall rates of malformations, including cardiac anomalies, for grouped SSRI exposure.** Louik and colleagues (2007)[17] compared the rates of malformation among 9849 case and 5860 control infants from the Slone Epidemiology Center Birth Defects Study. Analyses of the associations between individual SSRIs and specific defects showed significant associations between the use of sertraline and omphalocele (odds ratio 5.7, 95% CI, 1.6 to 20.7; 3 exposed subjects) and septal defects (odds ratio 2.0, 95% CI, 1.2 to 4.0; 13 exposed) and between the use of paroxetine and right ventricular outflow tract obstruction defects (odds ratio 3.3, 95% CI, 1.3 to 8.8; 6 exposed). Alwan et al[18] studied outcomes from 9622 infants with major birth defects and 4092 control infants from the National Birth Defects Prevention Study. Maternal SSRI use was associated with anencephaly (odds ratio 2.4, 95% CI, 1.1 to 5.1; 9 exposed); craniosynostosis (odds ratio 2.5, 95% CI, 1.5 to 4.0; 24 exposed), and omphalocele (odds ratio 2.8, 95% CI, 1.3 to 5.7; 11 exposed). In an editorial, Greene[19] observed that the malformations reported by each group were different, and that most had not been previously associated with SSRI exposure. These findings support associations by chance due to multiple comparisons. In individual drug analyses, both groups found a significant relationship between paroxetine and right ventricular outflow tract abnormalities; however, the specific defects were very rare and the absolute risks are small.

Agents released more recently, such as bupropion, venlafaxine, duloxetine, and mirtazepine, have been studied less rigorously. None of the investigations have demonstrated a significant difference in the rate of congenital anomalies compared to unexposed populations.[16]

Growth Effects. **In an elegant meta-analysis, Grote and colleagues found that maternal MDE or depressive symptoms during pregnancy increases the risk of PTB and low birthweight (LBW).**[10] Twenty studies assessed the association between antenatal depression and PTB (relative risk [RR] 1.13, 95% CI, 1.06 to 1.21). Eleven studies evaluated the association between antenatal depression and LBW (RR 1.18, 95% CI, 1.07 to 1.30). Twelve studies evaluated the association between antenatal depression and intrauterine growth restriction (IUGR), and with only 2 showing a significant association, the summary RR was not significant. In a prospective study (of 238 pregnant women with MDE, MDE with SSRI treatment, and controls with neither exposure), more than 20% of women who were either continuously treated with an SSRI (23%) or continuously exposed to MDE (21%) experienced PTB.[20] The rates of late and early PTB were similar. Therefore, avoiding SSRI treatment does not reduce the risk for PTB if the woman relapses.

Behavioral teratogenicity refers to long-term postnatal effects on offspring behavior due to prenatal exposure to agents that affect the central nervous system. Cognitive function, temperament, and general behavior were similar in children who were exposed prenatally to tricyclics or fluoxetine compared with controls. There are limited data about the postbirth development of individuals exposed to SSRI in utero; however, all converge on the finding that mental development as assessed by the Bayley Scales of Infant Development is similar in exposed compared to nonexposed children. Pedersen and colleagues reported a slight delay (within normal limits) to achievement of motor milestones in children exposed to SSRIs, but no differences were observed between the exposed and control groups at 19 months.[21]

Neonatal Effects. Both direct pharmacologic effects and withdrawal signs can occur in neonates after prenatal exposure to any antidepressant. Compared with early gestational SSRI exposure or no exposure, late SSRI exposure incurs an overall risk ratio of 3.0 (95% CI, 2.0 to 4.4) for a neonatal behavioral syndrome.[20] The most SSRI-related neonatal case reports specifically involved paroxetine and fluoxetine exposures.[20,23] Neonatal signs include central nervous system, motor, respiratory, and gastrointestinal signs that are usually mild and transient with resolution by 2 weeks of age. A severe syndrome that consists of seizures, dehydration, excessive weight loss, hyperpyrexia, or intubation is rare in full-term infants (1 in 313 quantifiable cases).[23] Based on the premise that neonatal signs are due to direct pharmacologic effects, tapering and discontinuation of the antidepressant over 10 to 14 days before the estimated delivery date, with reintroduction of the drug immediately after birth, has been suggested.[23] However, if a woman has a history of rapid decompensation during antidepressant taper or discontinuation, this strategy is likely to carry more risk to the maternal-fetal pair than continued treatment.

Antidepressant Treatment Modifications During Pregnancy. To review and guide the process of antidepressant treatment during pregnancy, members of the American College of Obstetricians and Gynecologists (ACOG) and the American Psychiatric Association (APA) developed a consensus document.[16] For mild cases of depression in pregnant women, psychotherapy is the treatment of choice as the initial intervention. Interpersonal psychotherapy (IPT) is a brief treatment to address relationship problems in the context of an MDE. It is delivered across 8 to 16 weekly sessions that focus on grief, interpersonal role disputes, role transitions, or interpersonal problems. Depressed pregnant women treated with IPT had a significant symptomatic improvement compared with a parenting education control group, and 60% of women who received IPT achieved recovery criteria.[24] However, IPT is not widely available outside academic settings. Other focused short-term therapies, such as cognitive behavioral therapy, are attractive options for MDE during childbearing and may be delivered by psychiatrists and nonphysician professionals such as psychologists, psychiatric nurse clinical specialists, or licensed clinical social workers.

For moderate to severe MDE with marked functional impairment, antidepressant pharmacotherapy should be considered. **Established efficacy and tolerability of any antidepressant for the individual woman is a strong consideration in drug choice during the risk/benefit decision-making process.** Women with chronic or highly recurrent MDE may already be taking maintenance antidepressant medication when pregnancy occurs. The risk of relapse in pregnant women who discontinued medication proximate to conception was significantly greater compared to women who maintained antidepressant treatment.[25] Among 82 women who continued their medication, 26% relapsed compared with 68% of the 65 women who discontinued medication.

For pregnant women who have not been previously treated with an antidepressant, results from a large-scale meta-anlysis[26] are available to guide the selection of specific agents. Sertraline, escitalopram, venlafaxine, and mirtazepine were significantly more efficacious than duloxetine, fluoxetine, fluvoxamine, paroxetine, and reboxetine (not available in the United States). Sertraline and escitalopram had the most favorable profile of acceptability as assessed by significantly fewer discontinuations. The authors concluded that sertraline was the best choice when starting treatment for moderate to severe MDE in adults because it has the most favorable balance among efficacy, acceptability, and cost. This agent is a reasonable choice for pregnant women as well.

Dosage Changes Across Pregnancy. In a publication about the management of TCA dosage across pregnancy that included serum drug levels,[27] a strategy to determine the minimum *effective* dose of any antidepressant across gestation was presented. The mothers selected a target depressive symptom that was most disturbing (e.g., insomnia or irritability toward other children). Women were asked to contact the physician each time the symptom emerged, and a small incremental dose was added. The dosages increased during the second half of pregnancy and rapidly accelerated during the third trimester. The final dose achieved during gestation was an average of 1.6 times the nonpregnant dose for TCA.

Sit and colleagues examined the dose requirements and level-to-dose (L/D) ratios of citalopram, escitalopram, and sertraline during pregnancy and postpartum.[28] In the majority of women, the L/D ratios for the parent compound and primary metabolites decreased between 20 weeks' gestation and delivery, which reflects increased drug metabolism. By 12 weeks postpartum the L/D ratios were similar to those detected at 20 weeks' gestation. **These cases illustrate that dose requirements frequently increase during the second half of pregnancy to offset greater drug metabolism and maintain optimal pharmacotherapy.**

Integrative Treatments. Bright light therapy, delivered as an early morning bolus of 10,000 lux illuminance with commercially available boxes, is an efficacious treatment for MDE (Figure 52-3). Widely recognized as a treatment for seasonal (winter) MDE, light therapy is also efficacious for nonseasonal MDE. The responsivity of depressed pregnant women to bright light therapy was explored in three small studies, including a randomized controlled trial (RCT)[29] with 16 patients in the bright white (active) and 11 in the dim (placebo) arms. The response rates were significantly greater for bright white than dim light after 5 weeks of 1 hour early morning light therapy, and comparable to antidepressant drug treatment. An excellent clinician's guide is available.[30]

Manber and colleagues[31] performed a novel RCT (N = 150) of acupuncture treatment specific to MDE, acupuncture treatment targeted to a condition other than MDE, and a massage control group over 8 weeks (12 sessions). Women who received acupuncture specific for MDE had a significantly greater response rate than the control conditions, comparable to standard MDE treatments.

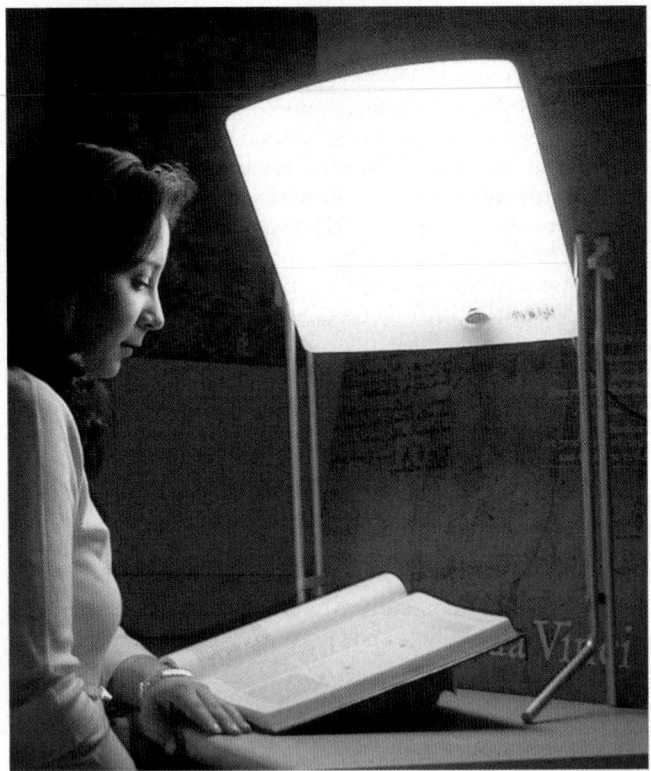

FIGURE 52-3. Light therapy. (From the Center for Environmental Therapeutics.)

Overall nutritional status plays an important role in mental health, and poor nutrition may contribute to the pathogenesis of MDE. Folate and vitamin B_{12} are needed for single-carbon metabolism involved in the synthesis of serotonin and other monoamine neurotransmitters and catecholamines. Deficiencies of folate, vitamin B_{12}, iron, zinc, and selenium are more common among depressed than nondepressed persons.[32] The depletion of nutrient reserves throughout pregnancy and lactation may increase a woman's risk for MDE. Marginal or low folate status also increases the likelihood of nonresponse to antidepressant medication as well as the probability of relapse in initial responders. Several RCTs have demonstrated that folic acid is an efficacious augmentation strategy for antidepressant medications.[32] Omega-3 fatty acid (O-3 FA) deficiency during pregnancy may potentially increase the risk of depression. In cross-national studies, an inverse relationship has been shown between per capita fish intake and prevalence rates of MDE, postpartum MDE, and BD.[33] O-3 FAs have received specific study in perinatal MDE in small RCTs; however, efficacy against placebo controls has not been convincingly demonstrated.[33]

Treatment of MDE in the Postpartum Period

Because of the dearth of treatment studies specifically in women with postpartum MDE, the assumption is that medications effective for MDE in women outside of childbearing are effective during childbearing. Evidence from

DOSES OF SUBJECTS WHO ACHIEVED REMISSION AT WEEK 8 IN AN RCT

SERTRALINE mg/day	<100	100	125 or 150	200
N (% remitted)	1 (4%)	12 (50%)	4 (17%)	7 (29%)

NORTRIPTYLINE mg/day	<100	100	125 or 150
N (% remitted)	15 (58%)	7 (27%)	4 (15%)

Start with half of the usual starting dose of any antidepressant (e.g., 25 mg of sertraline) for at least 2 days, then increase as tolerated to usual starting dose. Increase every 2 weeks as tolerated until full remission or the maximum recommended dose is achieved (e.g., 200 mg of sertraline or about 150 mg/day of nortriptyline (note: the dose is driven by serum levels for nortriptyline).

FIGURE 52-4. Treating postpartum depression: dose ranges for sertraline and nortripyline.

the few available RCTs support this contention.[34] Agents studied for postpartum MDE in RCTs include fluoxetine and paroxetine, both of which were efficacious compared to placebo. In a randomized comparative efficacy trial with no placebo, the TCA nortriptyline ($N = 54$) was compared to sertraline ($N = 55$).[35] The proportion of women who responded was equal; however, the majority of women required higher doses of sertraline than the usual starting dose and require dose adjustment approximately 2 weeks after treatment initiation (Figure 52-4). The total side effect burden for each drug was similar, although the side effect profiles differed for each drug.

In a novel study of the efficacy of estradiol treatment, Gregoire et al[36] randomized women with severe postpartum MDE to placebo ($N = 27$) or estradiol ($N = 34$) (200 mcg/day) delivered by transdermal patch for 6 months. By 3 months of treatment, 80% of the estradiol-treated and 31% of the placebo-treated group responded. Because assessments were done monthly, the time course of response in the early weeks of treatment is unknown. Estradiol treatment was well-tolerated as judged by low attrition. Endometrial changes were found in 3 participants at the study conclusion (6 months), despite co-administration of progesterone (10 mg/day, 12 days per month in the final 3 months of the trial); however, these changes resolved at follow-up. The inclusion of women who took concurrent antidepressant medications limits the ability to separate an estradiol-specific treatment effect. Further studies are needed to evaluate the potential of estradiol as a therapy for postpartum MDE. Little is known about estradiol secretion into breast milk; however, estradiol was not detected in the breast milk of 18 lactating women who used transdermal estradiol at doses of 50 to 100 mcg/day for 12 weeks.[37]

Prevention of Postpartum-Onset MDE. Studies of the efficacy of antidepressants or hormonal supplements for the *prevention* of postpartum MDE are limited to three RCTs.[34] The one positive placebo-controlled pharmacologic prevention study demonstrated the efficacy of sertraline.[38] Women with any history of MDE (not only postpartum) are candidates for the initiation of sertraline immediately following birth to prevent the emergence of episodes. The physician has the option of following the dosing protocol utilized in the original study as well as more flexible dosing for individual patients. For example, doses higher than the maximum used in that protocol (75 mg/day) could be prescribed for women who had previously responded to and tolerated higher doses. The duration of preventive treatment should be a minimum of 6 months. Although other serotonergic antidepressants have not been evaluated for preventive efficacy, the explanation for the efficacy of sertraline is based upon its serotonergic impact. Therefore, use of another serotonergic agent, particularly one to which the woman has responded in the past, is also a reasonable intervention.

Although open label studies supported that progesterone prevented recurrence, a placebo-controlled RCT of synthetic progesterone increased the risk of depressive symptoms at 6 weeks after birth. Estrogen was efficacious in preventing postpartum MDE recurrence in a small open study, which was not replicated in an RCT.

Treatment During Breastfeeding. The magnitude of antidepressant exposure through breast milk is substantially lower than during pregnancy. The approach to studying risk to infants when lactating mothers take antidepressants has been mother and nursing infant serum level monitoring. Comprehensive reviews of antidepressants in maternal serum, breast milk, and infant serum have been published.[34] SSRIs (sertraline or paroxetine) and TCAs (nortriptyline) are the drugs of first choice for the breastfeeding woman because they are the most evidence-based medications (similar findings across multiple laboratories, usually undetectable infant serum levels, and no reports of short-term adverse events). However, established efficacy of another drug for the individual woman must be considered strongly in the decision-making process (Table 52-1). Although TCAs are reasonable treatment options for PPD, they remain second-line drugs due to their toxicity in overdose. The more recently released antidepressants (escitalopram, duloxetine, bupropion) are second-line choices in breastfeeding women unless demonstrated efficacy in past episodes is clear and no new contraindications exist for their use in the individual woman.

Nursing infants' clinical conditions, particularly for sick or low-birthweight infants, should be monitored to detect initial adverse effects that may be attributed to the maternal drug (behavioral activation or sedation; new-onset feeding or sleeping problems). Routine laboratory measurement of serum drug levels in healthy full-term infants is not warranted. Serum level monitoring in premature and sick infants has not been described in the literature.

Bipolar Disorder

Diagnosis and Prevalence

Bipolar disorder (BD) includes normal, depressed, and elevated mood states (mania or its less intense form, hypomania); depression is the predominant mood state in many bipolar patients and is mistaken for unipolar depression in 30% of cases. Mania is a persistent, abnormally elevated, expansive or irritable mood state with inflated self-esteem, excessive physical goal-directed activity, agitation, distractibility, and poor judgment, for a minimum of 1 week. Impairment in function at work or in relationships must be present. Hypomania is defined by a minimum of 4 continuous days of persistent increased creativity,

TABLE 52-1 SELECTED ANTIDEPRESSANT LEVELS IN BREASTFED INFANTS' SERA

ANTIDEPRESSANT DRUG	SERUM LEVEL RANGE IN BREASTFED INFANTS	TYPICAL MATERNAL DOSE RANGE, MG/DAY
Nortriptyline*	Nortriptyline, below limit of quantifiability to 10 ng/mL	50-150; maternal therapeutic serum levels = 50-150 ng/mL
Nortriptyline metabolites	E-10-OH- Nortriptyline = <4-16 ng/mL Z-10-OH- Nortriptyline = <4-17 ng/mL	
Sertraline	Sertraline, below limit of quantifiability to 8 ng/mL	50-200
Sertraline metabolites	Norsertraline, = below limit of quantifiability to 26 ng/mL	
Paroxetine	Paroxetine, below limit of quantifiability	10-60
No active metabolites		
Other Antidepressants[†]		
Fluoxetine	Fluoxetine, below quantifiability to 340 ng/mL	20-60
Fluoxetine metabolite[‡]	Norfluoxetine, below quantifiability to 265 ng/mL	
Citalopram	Citalopram, below quantifiability to 12.7 ng/mL	20-40
Citalopram metabolite	Desmethylcitalopram, below quantifiability to 3.1 ng/mL	
Venlafaxine	Venlafaxine, below quantifiability to 5	75-300
Venlafaxine metabolite	O-desmethylvenlafaxine, below quantifiability to 38 ng/mL	
Bupropion Multiple metabolites	Average infant exposure expected to be 2% of the standard maternal dose on a molar basis; infant serum levels not measured in largest series of $N = 10$[§]	300

*The most-studied tricyclic antidepressant during breastfeeding; minimal use of this drug class currently.
[†]Established efficacy of an antidepressant in a woman is a strong consideration in drug selection.
[‡]As active as fluoxetine and has a longer half-life than parent drug.
[§]Haas et al.[130]

productivity, and sociability, or increased irritability that family or coworkers notice. The woman's function may be enhanced by creativity and increased energy. Women also experience mixed states in which symptoms of depression and hypomania/mania occur within the same day. During a mixed episode, patients may experience bouts of low mood, loss of interest, tearfulness and hyperphagia (depressive symptoms) that are intermingled with periods of elation or intense irritability, decreased need for sleep, heightened energy, pressured speech, excessive spending, and risky behaviors (hypomanic symptoms).

BD is divided into two major types. BD I is characterized by the presence of depression and mania. This illness affects women and men equally, and the lifetime prevalence is estimated at 1.3%. Much higher prevalence rates (3.7%-6.4%) have been reported for BD II (depression plus hypomania rather than full-blown mania) and bipolar spectrum disorders. Several bipolar variants occur more commonly in women, such as BD II, mixed states, and rapid cycling BD (four or more episodes yearly).

Conditions that frequently co-occur with BD include panic disorder, agoraphobia, social phobia, marijuana use, and bulimia nervosa (BN). Women with BD more commonly have a history of past sexual abuse, alcohol abuse/dependence, migraines, drug-induced metabolic syndrome, pain disorders, and hypothyroidism compared to men. A seasonal pattern of mood episodes, with winter depression characterized by atypical symptoms like weight gain, hypersomnia, and extremely low energy, is also more common in women. In contrast, spring and summer are associated with hypomania or mania.

Inadequate screening for bipolarity contributes to the significant delay in diagnosis from illness onset to the confirmation of BD of about 11 years. In addition, antidepressant medication without an anti-manic agent increases the risk for cycle acceleration, mania, or a mixed state. The mood criterion symptoms for hypomania (high mood and/or irritability) can be used as a simple screen (because formal measures have low predictive value in general populations): "Have you ever had 4 continuous days in which you felt so good, high, excited, or "hyper" that other people thought you were not your usual self or you got into trouble? Have you ever had 4 continuous days when you were so irritable you found yourself shouting at people, or starting fights or arguments?"

Natural History Across Childbearing

The course of bipolar symptoms during pregnancy is unpredictable. Some researchers have described a benign course or mood stabilization for women with BD during gestation, whereas others have observed that patients are at high risk for another episode. Viguera and colleagues[39] reported that 71% of pregnant women with BD had at least one episode of major depression, mixed state, hypomania, or mania. Patients who discontinued mood stabilizer treatment proximal to conception had higher rates of recurrence (86%) compared to patients who continued treatment (37%).[39] **Because abrupt discontinuation of mood stabilizers increases the risk for a recurrent episode, drug tapering is advisable.** The overall risk of a new episode of mania was significantly greater after rapid (less than 2 weeks) than gradual (2 to 4 weeks) lithium discontinuation.

Women with BD have a high risk for both recurrence and first admission in the immediate period after birth (within 10 to 19 days).[40] Recent psychiatric hospitalization (in the past 3 years), hospitalization during the pregnancy, and frequent past hospitalizations (>4) are risk factors for severe postpartum episodes that require hospital care. Postpartum psychosis is typically a manifestation of BD,[41] which presents as a manic, depressive, or mixed state episode of BD with psychosis. It occurs in 1 to 2 per 1000 births within 2 weeks of delivery. Women develop mood lability, confusion, delusional thinking, hallucinations, poor concentration, and impaired judgment and insight. Acute-onset postpartum psychosis is an emergency, and women must be screened for thoughts of harming themselves or others, especially the newborn.[41]

Women with mental illness have an overall higher risk for adverse pregnancy outcome than the general population. Jablensky and colleagues[42] determined the rate of complications during pregnancy in women with BD, schizophrenia, or MDE in a population-based cohort (N = 3174 children born from 1980 to 1992). A comparison sample of 3129 births to women without a psychiatric diagnosis was randomly selected from women who gave birth during the same time. Women with bipolar illness or MDE did not have elevated risk for placental complications; however, the rate of antepartum hemorrhage was significantly higher in mothers with bipolar illness (OR 1.66, 95 percent CI, 1.15 to 2.39). Separating adverse pregnancy outcomes related to the underlying disorder versus the medication treatments is an even greater challenge than for MDE.

Treatment of Bipolar Disorder During Childbearing

Although medication maintenance is the mainstay of treatment for BD, psychotherapy and educational interventions are critical adjuncts to pharmacotherapy. The physician has a major role in providing educational support and promoting treatment adherence. Early treatment for low-grade symptoms results in lower rates of relapse, increased time to recurrence, improved medication adherence, and better functioning.

Several classes of drugs are indicated for the treatment of mania. Lithium, some antiepileptic drugs (AEDs), and several newer atypical antipsychotic medications are efficacious; however, these agents result in a treatment response in only 36% to 50% of cases.[1] Therefore, patients often receive more than one drug to manage their mood symptoms. Strategies to minimize fetal exposure include the following: (1) use the lowest *effective* dose(s), (2) minimize the number of drugs to achieve response, and (3) divide daily doses to avoid high peak serum concentrations.

Lithium. Lithium is the standard drug for acute and maintenance therapy for BD. Before initiating lithium treatment, renal and thyroid function should be assessed, and gestational age considered. The starting dose is 300 mg twice daily. Serum drug levels and renal function tests should be repeated after 5 to 7 days of treatment. The target serum level is 0.4 to 1.0 mEq/L, measured at 12 hours post-dose. The dose can be increased by 300 mg every 5 to 7 days as tolerated with re-evaluation of the serum level. Treatment response is usually achieved at 900 to 1200 mg daily.

Patients are encouraged to have their lithium level monitored every 4 weeks throughout pregnancy to monitor for declining serum levels; the level should be checked weekly in the last month, and every few days shortly after delivery.[41] Typical side effects of lithium include sedation, tremor, renal dysfunction, weight gain, nausea, and vomiting. Lithium has a relatively narrow window between therapeutic and toxic serum levels. Toxicity is associated with excessive sedation, severe tremors, acute renal dysfunction, and intractable vomiting. Women who are dehydrated from hyperemesis are especially vulnerable. Lithium toxicity must be managed immediately with drug discontinuation, rehydration therapy, and monitoring of fluid and electrolyte balance and renal function. Diuretics and nonsteroidal anti-inflammatory drugs should be avoided in lithium-treated patients because these drugs may decrease the renal clearance of lithium and increase the risk for toxicity.

Lithium exposure during the first trimester was linked with Ebstein's anomaly in the past but subsequent prospective studies demonstrated that the risk was overestimated due to voluntary reporting to a registry, which inflates the number of cases (numerator) while underestimating the magnitude of population exposed (denominator).[41] **The absolute risk of Ebstein's anomaly after first-trimester exposure is 1 in 1000 to 2000** (20 to 40 times higher than the general population).[41] Lithium-exposed neonates are at risk for large for gestational age, hypotonia, feeding difficulties, depressed reflexes, cyanosis, apnea, bradycardia, hypothyroidism, and diabetes insipidus.[41] The neonatal symptoms appear to be temporary and may be linked with higher maternal serum concentrations at delivery (>0.64 mEq/L).[43] The suspension of lithium 24 to 48 hours before a scheduled delivery or at the onset of labor reduces the likelihood for perinatal complications.[43] Developmental milestones are normal in infants exposed prenatally to lithium.[41]

Valproic Acid (VPA). VPA was the first FDA-indicated AED for the treatment of BD (specifically for mania). The starting dose is 500 to 750 mg daily in divided doses. Therapeutic levels range from 50 to 125 mcg/mL. Side effects include nausea, weight gain, fatigue, tremor, ataxia, diarrhea, abdominal pain, alopecia, hepatitis, thrombocytopenia, and rarely pancreatitis.

VPA increases the rates of birth defects including neural tube defects in offspring exposed during pregnancy. Because more than half of pregnancies in America are unplanned and the impact on neural tube development occurs 17 to 30 days postconception, **the use of valproate as a first-line treatment for BD in childbearing-aged women should be avoided.** VPA is associated with the highest rate of birth defects (10.7%; 95% CI, 8.2 to 13.3) compared to other anticonvulsants: lamotrigine 1%, carbamazepine 8.2%, phenytoin 10.7%, and VPA 20.3%.[44,45] Women treated with AED polytherapy have 2 to 5 times the risk for major malformations compared to monotherapy. The rates of malformations with polytherapy were 6% (N = 770) versus monotherapy 3.7% (N = 2598).[46] Although registry data suggest the hazard of AED polytherapy is from the exposure to valproate,[47] the American Academy of Neurology (AAN) consensus statement concluded that AED polytherapy probably contributes to the development of major malformations and impaired cognition compared to monotherapy. The relationship between the AED dose or serum level and risk for malformation needs to be clarified for all AEDs.

Complications associated with VPA use near delivery include fetal decelerations, and infant irritability, jitteriness, feeding difficulties, abnormal tone, hepatic toxicity, hypoglycemia, and reduction in neonatal fibrinogen levels. Because VPA is concentrated in the fetal compartment, the lowest effective dose in divided doses is recommended to avoid high single peak levels.[41] Postnatal studies suggest that VPA exposure is associated with slightly lower IQ scores at 3 years of age.[48]

Carbamazepine (CBZ) and Oxcarbazepine. CBZ is prescribed at doses between 400 and 1600 mg daily for BD to achieve a target range of 4 to 12 mcg/mL. Drug-induced toxicity is usually detectable from clinical symptoms, and the serum level provides objective evidence. During pregnancy, the total AED levels drop, but the amount of unbound bioavailable drug remains unchanged. Serum levels are useful in the assessment of patients with exacerbation of mood symptoms, serious side effects, and questionable treatment adherence. Hepatitis, leukopenia, thrombocytopenia, rash, sedation, and ataxia are CBZ side effects. Due to the potential for bone marrow suppression, combining CBZ and the antipsychotic clozapine is contraindicated.

The AAN committee found no increased risk of major malformations in the offspring of women who received CBZ for epilepsy. However, infants exposed to CBZ had twice the risk for being small for gestational age (SGA) and an increased risk for low Apgar scores (less than 7) but not for perinatal death. The exposed children do not have reduced cognitive function or developmental delays compared to children without AED exposure.

Fetal serum levels of CBZ are 50% to 80% of maternal levels.[49] Because adequate levels of vitamin K are necessary for normal midfacial growth and for the functioning of clotting factors, CBZ exposure in utero could increase the risk of neonatal bleeding.[41] Some experts recommend administering vitamin K 20 mg daily throughout pregnancy and 1 mg intramuscularly to neonates.[41]

Oxcarbazepine is a newer AED that has been used to treat mania despite minimal efficacy data and without an FDA indication. It is prescribed in divided doses (total dose, 600 to 1200 mg/day). The parent compound is rapidly and almost completely metabolized to an active hydroxy metabolite. The metabolite undergoes hepatic glucuronidation, and the conjugate product is excreted by the kidneys. Adverse effects include hyponatremia, hypersensitivity reactions, and decreased thyroxine levels (without altered triiodothyronine or TSH). Side effects include headaches, dizziness, gait disturbance, fatigue, and concentration and memory changes. In 55 babies exposed in utero to oxcarbazepine (20 combination therapy, 35 monotherapy), one cardiac malformation was reported in an infant also exposed to phenobarbital.[50]

Lamotrigine (LTG) is indicated for bipolar depression maintenance therapy at doses of 50 to 200 mg/day.[51] Higher doses (up to 500 mg/day) have been used for long-term treatment of patients with BD. Reported side effects include headaches, rash, dizziness, diarrhea, abnormal dreams, and pruritus, which did not differ from the rates of placebo-treated patients.[52] Aseptic meningitis is a rare but serious potential complication of treatment with LTG. A maculopapular or erythematous rash is most likely to occur with rapid dose escalation, when combined with VPA, and among adolescents.[53] In controlled studies, the rates of benign rash were 8.3% in LTG-treated and 6.4% in placebo-treated patients.[54] One case of Stevens-Johnson syndrome that did not require hospitalization occurred in a patient treated with LTG. Although the condition is potentially life-threatening, the very low risk of serious rash must be weighed against the much more common risks associated with BD.[54]

Continuing LTG may prevent recurrent illness in pregnant women with BD. Thirty percent of women who continued versus all who stopped LTG relapsed during pregnancy (P <0.0001; OR 23.2, 95% CI, 1.5 to 366).[55] Patients who stopped treatment suffered relapses rapidly (within 2 weeks) compared to patients who continued treatment. In the second and third trimesters LTG clearance increases by 65% to more than 90% compared to preconception; therefore, patients need higher doses to prevent recurrent symptoms.[56] After delivery, LTG metabolism reverts to the prepregnancy rate within 2 weeks.

The rate of congenital malformations is similar in infants exposed in utero to LTG monotherapy compared to the general population; however, the malformation rates may increase when LTG is combined with other AEDs.

Contrary to earlier reports of an increased risk for isolated clefts with LTG exposure, more recent findings indicate the odds for orofacial cleft malformations is not increased with LTG monotherapy compared to nonexposed controls.[57] No evidence of growth problems, postnatal occult malformations, neonatal seizures, or deviations in psychomotor development up to 1 year of age were observed in 62 infants exposed to LTG in utero.[58]

Atypical Antipsychotics. Antipsychotic medications are efficacious treatments for BD (and also schizophrenia). Antipsychotic medications are classified into first-generation (also called "typical," e.g., haloperidol) and second-generation ("atypical," e.g., olanzapine) agents. Antipsychotic drugs block dopamine-2 receptors and reduce symptoms such as hallucinations, but substantial variability in the response of individuals to antipsychotics is the rule. The atypical agents are associated with fewer extrapyramidal side effects such as tardive dyskinesia, tremor, rigidity, akathisia, bradykinesia, and dystonia compared to the older typical antipsychotic drugs. Other side effects include somnolence, dry mouth, akathisia (internal sense of restlessness), and increased hepatic transaminases. A marked and sustained hyperprolactinemia is frequently associated with risperidone (88% of patients), compared with conventional antipsychotics like haloperidol (48%) or olanzapine (minimal, if any).[59]

More recent indications for these medications include bipolar maintenance therapy, bipolar depression (quetiapine and olanzapine-fluoxetine combined therapy), and treatment-resistant depression. The usual daily maintenance dose ranges for these drugs are: olanzapine (5 to 20 mg), risperidone (1 to 6 mg), quetiapine (100 to 400 mg, maximum 800 mg), ziprasidone (80 to 160 mg), and aripiprazole (15 to 30 mg). The initial treatment is started at a lower dose and titrated against tolerance. Standard clinical practice does not include serum level monitoring of these drugs.

The metabolic side effects of atypical agents are a public health concern. Patients are at risk for significant weight gain, elevated triglycerides, and new-onset metabolic syndrome or insulin intolerance, particularly with olanzapine. Mothers treated with antipsychotics had increased risk for gestational diabetes and surgical delivery compared to all mothers who gave birth.[60] **Use of an atypical antipsychotic agent should prompt close monitoring of gestational weight gain and glucose tolerance throughout pregnancy.**

The reproductive risks of atypical antipsychotics have received minimal research attention. Pregnant women who received either typical or atypical drugs had increased risks for PTB, LBW, and major malformations compared to the general population. The malformations (mainly atrial and ventricular septal defects) affected only infants with exposure to first-generation (typical) antipsychotic agents.[60] The rates of PTB were similar among patients who received typical or atypical agents. Although genetic liability and gene-environment interactions contribute to these outcomes, maternal risk factors, substance abuse, nutritional status, and biological and behavioral concomitants of severe mental illness are likely to be the major determinants of increases in reproductive pathology in this cohort.

Infants of mothers who received typical antipsychotic drugs weighed less (3158 g ± 440) than infants of mothers who received atypical (3391 g ± 446) or non-antipsychotic (3382 g ± 384) drugs.[61] Significantly more large-for-gestational-age babies were born to mothers who received atypical agents (20%) compared to mothers who received typical agents (2%) or non-antipsychotic treated women (3%).[61]

Alternative or Supplemental Treatment Options. Some patients do not respond, have prohibitive side effects, or have medical disorders that complicate the use of lithium, anticonvulsants, and antipsychotics. Additional therapies are being evaluated to expand the therapeutic armamentarium during childbearing. An inverse correlation between O-3 FA dietary consumption and the population prevalence of BD has been demonstrated.[62] Increased duration of remission of episodes of BD occurred in subjects who were randomized to fish oil versus placebo supplementation.[33] Sporadic reports of the use of calcium channel blockers for BD have been published. Verapamil (VPM) possesses clinically relevant dopamine antagonist properties, as evidenced by its ability to increase prolactin release, as well as antiepileptic activity.[63] Although open case series data showed reduction of manic symptoms,[63] results of controlled studies have been less encouraging. The efficacy of VPM (or any other calcium channel blocker) has never been explored in randomized acute treatment trials with adequate power.

Electroconvulsive therapy (ECT) is highly effective for the management of treatment-resistant depression, acute mania, and severe mixed episodes.[41] ECT involves the delivery of an electrical stimulus with a brief pulse device to generate a brief grand mal seizure blocked from peripheral expression by succinylcholine. During ECT, the patient receives short-acting anesthetic agents, which are not likely to cause adverse impact on the mother-infant pair.[41]

Prevention of Bipolar Episode Recurrence After Delivery

The risk for recurrence of mania, depression, or mixed states after delivery is the highest at any point in a woman's life, and breakthrough episodes even with continued medication treatment are common. Viguera and colleagues[64] retrospectively compared recurrence rates in childbearing compared with non-childbearing women who discontinued lithium treatment. In the year before lithium discontinuation, the rate of recurrence was 21%. After lithium discontinuation, the rates of recurrence over the first 40 weeks were similar in pregnant (52%) and nonpregnant (58%) women. In the postpartum period, recurrences occurred at three times the rate observed in the nonpregnant women during the same time frame (70% vs. 24%). Nine women who continued lithium and remained well during pregnancy were also observed, and three suffered rapid postpartum recurrences despite continued lithium treatment. In a prospective trial, VPA did not reduce the number or time to episode recurrence in postpartum women with BD compared with nonmedicated women.[65]

In the clinical management of women with BD, educating partners to observe for manic and depressive symptoms and communicate with the treatment team is the most important strategy at this point in our knowledge of prophylactic approaches. The most prudent pharmacologic plan is to use the drug(s) to which the individual woman has responded and prepare a plan for rapid additional intervention if a breakthrough episode occurs.[41]

Breastfeeding for Women with Bipolar Disorder

The mother's commitment to breastfeeding is an important consideration in the postpartum management of women with BD. Sleep deprivation, which is often unavoidable in the postpartum period, is a major precipitant of mania and hypomania. If a partner can feed the baby at night, sleep can be preserved in vulnerable women; however, this level of support is not always available. Lactation success also may be compromised by not breastfeeding through the night early in the postbirth period.

Lithium is in the category of drugs that have been associated with significant effects in some nursing infants and should be given to nursing mothers with caution.[66] Viguera and colleagues examined 10 pairs of lithium-treated mothers and their breastfeeding babies 4 to 12 weeks after delivery.[66] They measured maternal and infant serum, breast milk lithium concentrations, and renal and thyroid function in the infants. One infant had an elevated thyroid-stimulating hormone (TSH) that resolved by 2 weeks after discontinuation of lithium exposure. Infant serum lithium levels were 25% of maternal levels. The investigators recommended clinical monitoring of breastfed infants for signs of toxicity or dehydration, such as poor feeding, lethargy, and hypotonia, and serum levels of lithium, TSH, blood urea nitrogen, and creatinine every 8 to 12 weeks while breastfeeding.[66] Mothers must be educated to observe for the evidence of dehydration in infants due to poor intake, excessive fluid loss, or fever, which increases the risk for lithium toxicity, and to seek pediatric evaluation for behavioral changes in their infants.[41] To avoid spuriously high levels of lithium, infant blood samples must be collected in tubes that do not contain lithium heparin as the stabilizing agent.

The American Academy of Pediatrics (AAP) Committee on Drugs and the AAN concluded that CBZ and VPA are compatible with breastfeeding because they are transferred into the breast milk in small amounts that are not likely to be clinically relevant. The outcomes of 25 breastfed infants whose mothers were treated with LTG revealed no adverse effects.[67] The ratio of infant to maternal concentrations was 18.3%; the ratio of free to maternal concentration was 1.7 times greater at 30.9%. LTG undergoes glucuronidation and renal excretion, which is substantially lower in infants than adults. The risk for toxicity may be increased in the breastfeeding infants of women who receive additional similarly metabolized agents (e.g., lorazepam, aspirin, olanzapine, acetaminophen, VPA); however, we were unable to locate any published reports of LTG toxicity during breastfeeding.

ANXIETY DISORDERS

Diagnosis and Prevalence

Anxiety disorders are characterized by prominent symptoms of anxiety that impair functioning. Examples are obsessive-compulsive disorder (OCD), posttraumatic stress disorder (PTSD), generalized anxiety disorder, panic disorder, agoraphobia, and other phobias. Each of these disorders is distinct and defined by specific diagnostic criteria according to DSM-IV.[1] In women, the lifetime prevalence of anxiety disorders is 5% for panic disorder, 5% for generalized anxiety disorder, 3% for OCD, 6% for social phobia, 13% for other specific phobias, and 10% for PTSD. However, the rule rather than the exception is for multiple anxiety disorders to occur in an individual. Without treatment, anxiety disorders usually have a chronic course. Although rates of OCD are similar in men and women, all other anxiety disorders are 1.5 to 2 times more common in women. In addition, women with anxiety disorders have an increased risk for development of comorbid MDE.

Panic attacks are characterized by brief (5 to 15 minutes), intense episodes of fear or discomfort. Panic attacks occur in a variety of anxiety disorders, as well as in healthy individuals exposed to acute stress. Symptoms include palpitations, sweating, shortness of breath, choking, nausea, abdominal discomfort, dizziness, unsteadiness, numbness or tingling, chills, hot flashes, or a fear of dying or losing control. Panic disorder is diagnosed if panic attacks are recurrent or associated with a continuing fear of future attacks, which result in anxiety between attacks. The most disabling consequence of panic disorder, agoraphobia, occurs in 30% to 40% of women with untreated panic disorder. Individuals with agoraphobia restrict their activities outside the home or insist on being accompanied by another individual due to fear of having a panic attack where help is unavailable.

Generalized anxiety disorder is characterized by excessive worrying about multiple problems. The issues of concern to persons with generalized anxiety disorder are realistic but the level of worry is much more intense than appropriate. For example, a woman might worry for hours about whether a friend received a thank-you note for a baby shower gift. Individuals with generalized anxiety disorder often have physical symptoms associated with worrying, such as muscle tension, fatigue, headache, nausea, diarrhea, or abdominal pain. To meet criteria for the disorder, individuals must have significant impairment of functioning and anxiety for at least 6 months.

In contrast to generalized anxiety disorder, women with OCD focus on more idiosyncratic and often unrealistic concerns. OCD is characterized by disturbing intrusive thoughts and performance of compulsions to temporarily relieve the distress generated by the intrusive thoughts. Intrusive thoughts usually center on a few key themes: contamination, causing harm, offensive violent or sexual images, religious preoccupations, and urges for symmetry or ordering. Compulsions performed to relieve these intrusive worries include cleaning or washing, checking, repeating, ordering, hoarding, and mental rituals like counting and praying. To meet criteria for the disorder, the symptoms must interfere with functioning and last at least 1 hour per day. During pregnancy and postpartum, contamination concerns are particularly common. **New mothers with OCD can experience repeated disturbing mental images of harming their infant, but, in contrast to women with acute psychosis, they are not at increased risk of actually causing any harm.**

Exposure to trauma in which a woman experienced or witnessed an event that involved actual or threatened death or serious injury (such as rape or military combat) is required for a diagnosis of posttraumatic stress disorder. The traumatic event is persistently re-experienced in one or more of the following ways: recurrent and intrusive distressing recollections of the event, recurrent distressing dreams, acting or feeling as if the event were recurring (flashbacks), intense distress at cues that remind her of the event, physiologic hyperarousal, and exaggerated startle responses. Symptoms usually begin within 3 months of the trauma and they must persist for at least 1 month to meet diagnostic criteria for posttraumatic stress disorder. There has been little study of whether birth trauma can result in new onset or a recurrence of PTSD. Preliminary estimates suggest an incidence of 1% to 2%.[68]

Finally, excessive fear of a discrete object or situation constitutes a phobia. Social phobia refers to fears of speaking or eating in public and fears of humiliation in social interactions. These fears must be excessive and significantly impair an individual's social or occupational functioning for the diagnosis to be made. Other common specific phobias are body injury phobia (blood drawing or medical procedures), acrophobia (heights), arachnophobia (spiders), and claustrophobia (enclosed spaces). Even the possibility of confronting the feared object or situation stimulates anxiety, which is described as anticipatory anxiety, which can be a feature of any anxiety disorder. Individuals with panic disorder often have fear of situations from which they could not escape if they had a panic attack, including airplanes, bridges, and subways. These fears are considered to be a feature of panic disorder and agoraphobia, and would not warrant an additional diagnosis of simple phobia.

Fear of Labor and Delivery. In modern obstetric practice, perinatal morbidity and mortality of mother and neonate are rare; however, some women have intense fear about childbearing. Approximately 5% to 10% of pregnant women develop extreme fear of delivery, which may be considered a type of phobia. These women often request a surgical delivery to avoid labor. Risk factors for intense fear of delivery and requesting cesarean section include prior emotional problems, abuse, less social support, unemployment, and prior complicated deliveries. Referral for focused, short-term psychotherapy can often enable these women to proceed with a vaginal delivery and can reduce the likelihood of having a subjectively negative birth experience.

Natural History Across Childbearing

Pregnancy, delivery, and lactation produce profound changes in physiology, including changes in multiple hormonal and neurotransmitter systems that modulate anxiety symptoms. Although pregnancy and the postpartum period have been identified as times of increased risk for relapse of depressive disorders, the course of anxiety disorders has not been as carefully studied. Most of the available data was collected retrospectively, which limits reliability of the information. In one large prospective study, more women scored above threshold on an anxiety scale during weeks 18 and 32 of pregnancy compared with 8 weeks and 8 months postpartum, suggesting that nonspecific anxiety symptoms worsen during pregnancy. Antenatal anxiety was associated with an increased risk of postpartum depression, even after controlling for antenatal depression.[69] Anxiety disorders seem to be as common as MDE in the postpartum period. With respect to specific anxiety disorders, there is preliminary evidence that panic disorder can improve during pregnancy, but recur postpartum. Weaning also may precipitate relapse of panic disorder.[70] Pregnancy and childbirth can trigger the onset of OCD and the exacerbation of preexisting OCD. In addition, obsessive-compulsive symptoms are very common in postpartum depression, and intrusive violent thoughts and contamination concerns are quite common in new mothers without psychiatric disorders. There is no information on the effects of pregnancy on the course of generalized anxiety disorder, phobias, or PTSD.

Beta-adrenergic agonists (e.g. terbutaline) may precipitate panic attacks and other anxiety symptoms during the treatment of premature labor. **Hyperthyroidism is associated with panic attacks and anxiety symptoms, and should be considered in the differential diagnosis of postpartum-onset anxiety episodes.**

Effects of Anxiety During Childbearing

Anxiety disorders are associated with an increased risk of preeclampsia, but less is known about any relationship with other delivery complications. Psychosocial stress has been linked to higher rates of PTB and several physiological pathways have been proposed to mediate the association. However, not all women who experience high levels of stress have anxiety disorders or symptoms.

In contrast, perinatal anxiety has been associated with adverse effects on offspring. The offspring of highly anxious women are exposed to an altered physiologic milieu during pregnancy and maternal anxiety-related behaviors postpartum. High levels of anxiety symptoms have been linked to increased uterine artery resistance, which potentially compromises blood supply to the fetus.[71] Fetuses of anxious women show increased heart rate reactivity to maternal stressors, and newborns of highly anxious mothers have reduced heart rate variability and poor autonomic regulation.[72,73] Poor autonomic regulation of heart rate has been linked to impaired emotional regulation in older children and adults. In utero and as newborns, offspring of anxious women spend more time in deep sleep.[72,73]

Maternal anxiety during pregnancy is associated with attention deficits, motor immaturity, and difficult temperament in offspring. In two large prospective, longitudinal studies, anxiety during pregnancy increased the risk for hyperactivity and anxiety in childhood, after controlling for obstetrical and sociodemographic risks as well as maternal depression. Further research is needed to determine whether developmental and psychiatric problems in offspring of anxious mothers are due to genetic risk factors or to an altered in utero environment.

Treatment of Anxiety Disorders

The boundary between normal and pathologic anxiety cannot be drawn with great precision. When anxiety substantially impairs work, family, or social adjustment, mental health evaluation is indicated and treatment is appropriate. Panic disorder responds to most antidepressant medications, which are first-line therapies for this disorder. Benzodiazepines are also effective but are associated with abuse and physical dependence in a subset of patients. Cognitive therapy, a time-limited, structured psychotherapy, also is efficacious for panic disorder. In contrast, OCD is effectively treated specifically with SSRIs. A specific behavioral therapy technique, exposure and response prevention, is also effective for OCD. Generalized anxiety disorder responds to a variety of antidepressant medications as well as cognitive therapy. Posttraumatic stress disorder is partially responsive to antidepressant medication, but cognitive therapy with exposure is more effective. The first-line medication treatment for social phobia is SSRIs, and cognitive therapy can also be very helpful. Specific phobias are most effectively treated with focused desensitization psychotherapy rather than medication.

A risk/benefit evaluation for treatments during pregnancy must be individualized for the pregnant woman with anxiety disorder, which, like MDE, can have a negative impact on pregnancy outcome. If psychotherapy treatment is refused, not available, or ineffective, pharmacologic treatment should be considered. The use of antidepressants in pregnancy and lactation has been reviewed in the section on major depression. Evidence from the available studies indicates that teratogenic risk from benzodiazepine exposure, if any, is very small. However, less is known about the effect of benzodiazepines on neurodevelopment. At delivery, neonates exposed to higher doses can have withdrawal seizures or "floppy baby" syndrome. There is also little known about the degree to which benzodiazepines are absorbed into the circulation of breastfed infants. Because alternative treatments are available for anxiety disorders, benzodiazepines often can be avoided or used to treat targeted symptoms for limited time periods during pregnancy and lactation. A useful handout for patients entitled "Benzodiazepines during Pregnancy" can be downloaded from the Organization of Teratology Information Specialists: www.otispregnancy.org/files/benzodiazepines.pdf. An excellent educational program and workbook on anxiety disorders is available (see Additional Resources list at the end of this chapter).

EATING DISORDERS

Eating disorders are characterized by serious disturbances in eating behavior and are 10 times more common in women. The most familiar and well described are anorexia nervosa (AN) and bulimia nervosa (BN). Binge-eating disorder and subclinical forms of AN and BN also occur.

Eating disorders are particularly relevant during pregnancy and lactation, when the increased requirement for nutritional intake is directly affected by disordered eating (see Chapter 7).

Diagnosis and Prevalence

AN is characterized by the woman's refusal to maintain a minimally normal body weight, defined as less than 85% of that expected for age and height. Amenorrhea (absence of at least three menstrual cycles) is required for the diagnosis of AN.[1] The prevalence of AN in adolescents and young women is 0.5% to 1%, and the mean age of onset is 17 years of age. The course of AN is highly variable, with a range of outcomes that include recovery, residual partial symptomatology, and a fluctuating or chronic course. Remission rates approximate 50% at 10 or more years after initial diagnosis. AN is associated with both elevated mortality rates and suicide rates.

BN occurs in 1% to 3% of young adult women. Women with BN maintain body weight at or above a minimally normal range but use binge eating plus compensatory methods to prevent weight gain. A binge is excess eating in a discrete period of time (within 2 hours) of an amount of food that is decisively larger than most people would eat during a similar period of time. The binge eating and inappropriate compensatory behaviors must occur at least twice a week for 3 months.[1] Inappropriate compensatory behaviors that occur in both AN and BN are self-induced vomiting; laxative, diuretic, or other medication (such as ipecac) abuse; fasting; and excessive exercise. A disturbance in the perception of body shape and weight that leads to negative self-evaluation is an essential feature of both disorders. Remission rates of BN are reported to be 75% at 10 or more years after intake, but the longitudinal course of BN may be chronic or intermittently recurrent. In women with BN, menstrual irregularities are common, but they have minimal impact on later ability to achieve pregnancy.[75] Follow-up of women 11.5 years after initial evaluation for BN revealed that 74.6% had been able to achieve pregnancy and only 1.7% reported an inability to conceive.

The etiology of eating disorders has contributions from multiple domains: the societal ideal of thinness and encouragement of women to define themselves by the way others perceive them; families that demand conformity and high achievement; genetic susceptibility (50% to 80% of the variance in liability to AN and BN is accounted for by genetic factors); personality traits that include low self-esteem, impulsivity, obsessionality, perfectionism, and affective dysregulation; and life events, such as chronic disease (e.g., diabetes mellitus). Dysregulation of neurotransmitters, neuropeptides, and endocrine factors also likely contribute to etiology. Dieting frequently triggers the onset of eating disorder in vulnerable individuals.

Women with eating disorders rarely voluntarily disclose their maladaptive eating behaviors, but they may present to their obstetrician-gynecologist with complaints of irregular menses or secondary amenorrhea, infertility, sexual dysfunction, unexplained vomiting, fatigue, or palpitations. However, fewer than half of obstetrician-gynecologists screen patients for eating disorders. The obstetrician-gynecologist or primary care clinician can screen for eating disorders with questions about restricted eating, binge eating, purging behavior, and compulsive exercise. Medical examination should include weight, loss of dental enamel, and abrasions on the hands from self-induced vomiting. Laboratory investigations may disclose abnormalities of electrolytes, blood urea nitrogen, creatinine, amylase, and thyroid indices. There are many medical consequences of AN and BN, and the medical complications of AN may be life threatening (see box, Physical and Laboratory Findings in Women with Eating Disorders).[76] Arrhythmias are common in AN and are typically reversible with improvement in nutritional status. Irreversible cardiomyopathy may occur due to chronic ipecac (emetine) abuse.[76] Osteopenia and osteoporosis of the lumbar spine occurs in women with active AN (54%) compared with recovered women (21%); in contrast, patients with BN typically have bone mineral densities within the normal range.[77] Weight restoration and nutritional replenishment are the ideal treatments for osteopenia and to prevent osteoporosis, whereas estrogen replacement and other medications demonstrate minimal benefit.[78]

Physical and Laboratory Findings in Women with Eating Disorders

Common in Women with Eating Disorders

Bradycardia
Hypotension and orthostasis
Hypothermia
Cardiac murmur (mitral valve prolapse)
Dry skin

More Common in Anorexia Nervosa Due to Severe Calorie Restriction

Emaciated, may wear oversized clothes
Sunken cheeks, sallow skin
Lanugo (fine downy body hair)
Atrophic breasts/atrophic vaginitis
Pitting edema of extremities
Dull, thinning scalp hair
Cold extremities, acrocyanosis
Fluid retention after laxative or diuretic withdrawal
Laboratory: Anemia, ↑BUN, ↑cholesterol, ↑liver function studies, ↑amylase; ↓platelets, ↓magnesium, ↓zinc, ↓phosphates, ↓thyroid. With laxative abuse: metabolic acidosis

More Common in Women Who Purge

Parotitis
Calluses on dorsal hand surface from self-induced emesis
Oral mucosal abrasions
Dental enamel erosion, tooth chipping, extensive cosmetic dental work
Cardiac and skeletal myopathies from ipecac abuse
Laboratory: metabolic alkalosis; ↓sodium, ↓chloride, ↓potassium, ↑bicarbonate from purging

Data from American Psychiatric Association: American Psychiatric Association: Diagnostic and Statistical Manual for Psychiatric Disorders, ed 4, Text Revision. Washington, DC, American Psychiatric Association, 2000; Mitchell-Gieleghem A, Mittelstaedt ME, and Bulik CM: Eating disorders and childbearing: concealment and consequences. Birth 29:182, 2002; Rome ES, et al: Children and adolescents with eating disorders: the state of the art. Pediatrics 111:e98, 2003.

Natural History Across Childbearing

Pregnancy can be a stimulus that moves a woman through the continuum from sub-threshold symptoms to frank eating disorder. Changing body shape and loss of control of weight gain may reactivate deviant eating patterns and concerns about body shape in women with a history of an eating disorder. Persistence of active eating disorder symptoms and the development of binge eating during pregnancy have been reported. However, several studies have suggested that many pregnant women with BN have a decrease in binge eating and purging. Some women with active eating disorders "allow" themselves to eat nutritiously and do not purge, with motivation derived from promoting the health of the growing baby. The optimal treatment of pregnant women with a prior or active eating disorder includes a multidisciplinary team of the obstetrician-gynecologist and/or primary care clinician, a nutritionist, and a mental health clinician. Frequent prenatal visits, regular weighing, and enhanced support are necessary to encourage recommended weight gain and nutrition to ensure fetal well-being. Women with past or current eating disorders have been reported to have a significantly higher risk of hyperemesis during pregnancy compared to controls, and women with hyperemesis gravidarum should be screened for BN.

Adverse birth outcomes in women with eating disorders include higher rates of miscarriage, low birthweight, PTB, congenital malformations, and cesarean sections. Sollid and colleagues[79] performed a follow-up study of 302 women who were hospitalized with an eating disorder before pregnancy and their 504 children. Outcomes were compared with 900 control subjects and their 1552 children. The risk of a low-birthweight infant was twice as high in women with a history of eating disorder. Weight-controlling behaviors (strict dieting, vomiting, and excessive physical exercise) that lead to undernutrition may contribute to impaired fetal growth. The undernutrition may also impact fetal brain development and fetal stress responses.

Maternal dieting behaviors are associated with an increased risk of neural tube defects (NTD).[80] In an analysis of 538 cases of NTD and 539 controls between 1989 and 1991, dieting to lose weight (OR 2.1, 95% CI, 1.1 to 4.1) and fasting diets (OR 5.8, 95% CI, 1.7 to 20.0) were associated with increased risk for NTD, presumably secondary to altered folate intake and absorption.

Mothers with a history of eating disorders are at equal or greater risk of developing postpartum MDE than women with a history of MDE. The risk of perinatal depression is three times higher in women with a history of BN or binge-eating disorder compared to women without an eating disorder.[81] Increased stress with a new infant, feelings of lack of control, and desire to lose pregnancy weight may precipitate recurrence of AN or BN even if the symptoms were in good control during pregnancy. The postpartum period is another critical time for a woman with an eating disorder to receive enhanced support and treatment from a multidisciplinary team.

Treatment of Eating Disorders

Treatment needs to address both the eating disorder symptoms and the underlying issues. Central to all eating disorders is that self-evaluation is unduly influenced by body shape and weight.[1] Specific treatment goals for patients with eating disorders include the following: (1) Address dysfunctional attitudes about self, weight and shape, and relationships with others. Alternatives to the patient's perfectionism, low self-esteem, pursuit of thinness, mood lability and poor coping skills must be developed through psychotherapy and experience to promote recovery. (2) Establish healthy eating behaviors. (3) Weight and nutritional stabilization are essential for recovery. Normalization of nutritional status improves physical and mental well-being. (4) Treat comorbid conditions such as depression and anxiety. Treatments targeted to these disorders may improve adherence to healthy behaviors. A nonconfrontational educational approach is used to engage the woman with an eating disorder.

Treatment of Anorexia Nervosa

Women with AN may require hospitalization because of emaciation, severe electrolyte disturbances, severe depression, suicidality, or failure of outpatient treatment. A structured behavioral inpatient program involves a multidisciplinary treatment that includes individual and group psychotherapy, meal planning and supervision, nutritionist consultation, psychiatric consultation, and medical monitoring. Caloric intake that increases too rapidly may lead to the re-feeding syndrome, a potentially serious condition characterized by electrolyte and mineral abnormalities and shifts in fluids. Length of inpatient hospitalization and weight achieved at discharge may be favorable prognostic predictors, yet 50% of weight-restored women with AN have a relapse in the first posthospitalization year.[82]

Psychotherapies that have been studied for anorexia nervosa include cognitive behavioral therapy (CBT), interpersonal psychotherapy (IPT), insight-oriented psychotherapy, supportive psychotherapy, and family therapy. Current research is evaluating the role of "enhanced" CBT in underweight women with AN, which involves the treatment of core eating disorder psychopathology in addition to eating disorder symptoms.[83] Following successful weight restoration, CBT may have a role in relapse prevention.[84]

No medications are approved by the FDA for the treatment of AN nor recommended by treatment guidelines. Although few randomized clinical trials are available to guide treatment, pharmacotherapy in AN is usually instituted to treat depression, obsessive perfectionism, and cognitive disturbances; to target potential neurotransmitter disturbances; or to treat psychiatric or medical comorbidities. The core symptoms of AN are relatively refractory to psychotropic agents. Older antipsychotics (haloperidol, chlorpromazine, amisulpride), TCAs (amitriptyline), SSRIs (fluoxetine, citalopram), and hormones have been studied. Recent studies have evaluated newer atypical antipsychotic medications such as olanzapine (OLZ), which may decrease anxiety with eating and increase weight.[85] Although initial studies were promising, there are concerns about the use of OLZ and other atypical antipsychotics during pregnancy, including weight gain, risk of metabolic syndrome, and insufficient data to inform use in pregnancy and lactation.

Relapse prevention is the most challenging clinical problem in the treatment of AN. Although initial reports suggested that fluoxetine might be helpful after weight restoration, a controlled study reported that fluoxetine was not superior to placebo in weight-restored women also receiving CBT.[86] As mentioned earlier, CBT may help prevent a relapse in weight-restored women.

Treatment of Bulimia Nervosa

CBT is considered the first-line therapy for BN.[87] In CBT, the therapist identifies the stimuli to thought processes and emotions that maintain the binge-purge-starve cycle. The woman develops strategies to manage the disturbed eating, change the dysfunctional cognitions, and build alternative ways to manage distress. CBT is a time-limited individual or group psychotherapy. "Enhanced" CBT that also targets core psychopathology may be superior for marked mood intolerance, clinical perfectionism, low self-esteem, and interpersonal difficulties.[83] In locations where a CBT therapist is not available, self-help manuals and web-based programs utilizing the principles of CBT have wide appeal. *Overcoming Binge Eating*[88] is readable and provides a clear discussion of the implementation of self-help strategies. CBT appears to have both short- and long-term efficacy for BN.[87,88]

IPT has been less studied than CBT; it appears to have comparable recovery rates but may take longer to be effective. IPT involves evaluation of patient's significant life events, relationship between psychological symptoms and interpersonal processes, and the identification of areas of interpersonal difficulty such as role transitions, role disputes, grief, and interpersonal deficits. In IPT for eating disorders, the relationship between eating disorder symptoms and negative social evaluation and low self-esteem are explored.

Placebo-controlled studies with antidepressant medications have been far more promising for the acute treatment of BN than AN.[87] The first-line medication most commonly used is an SSRI, usually fluoxetine, which is FDA approved for BN at a dose of 60 mg/day. Efficacy has also been reported with TCA and monoamine oxidase inhibitors. Bupropion is contraindicated due to reduced seizure threshold in patients with eating disorders. Antidepressants reduce both binge eating and purging frequency, and the symptom relief is independent of comorbid depression. Many studies of antidepressants also demonstrate reduction of core eating disorder psychopathology such as weight and food preoccupation.[87] Although antidepressants may be as effective as CBT in the short-term, their long-term efficacy is less promising. Symptomatic improvement and sustained remission may be enhanced with combined CBT and antidepressant medication.[89] In general, a combination of CBT and an antidepressant drug is a prudent clinical strategy.

Other medications that hold promise for reducing binge eating and purging frequency include ondansetron and AED. Ondansetron is a 5-HT_3 antagonist that reduced symptoms compared to placebo, possibly due to regulation of vagal activity.[90] Topiramate has been reported to reduce the number of binge-purge days and improve self-esteem, eating attitudes, anxiety, and body image in short-term RCTs.[91] The dose may be limited by side effects (memory impairment, paresthesias, fatigue).[91] Medications reported to be helpful for reducing binge eating frequency in binge-eating disorder, such as lamotrigine, zonisamide, and sibutramine, may have a role in the treatment of BN and deserve further study, but there are limited data on reproductive side effects.[91]

SCHIZOPHRENIA

Diagnosis and Prevalence

Schizophrenia is a disabling disease that affects 1% of the population. The defining feature of schizophrenia is psychosis, which does not refer to the *severity* of the episode but to specific symptoms. Schizophrenia is characterized by the presence (for at least 6 months) of symptoms from three clusters[1]: (1) positive symptoms (delusions or fixed false beliefs; hallucinations or distortions of reality), (2) negative symptoms (decrease or loss of normal functions: lack of pleasure, social withdrawal, minimal speech production), and (3) cognitive impairment (inattention, poor working memory, and executive function deficits). The etiology of schizophrenia is unknown, but proposed mechanisms are: (1) excessive dopamine transmission, (2) in utero exposure to influenza or other viral agents, which results in neurobiologic disruptions, and (3) altered neuroplasticity or neurodevelopmental trajectories. Schizophrenia is distinguished from mood disorders, which may also present with psychosis, by the persistence of hallucinations or delusions even when mood symptoms have remitted. The mortality and morbidity of schizophrenia is high, and 10% of patients complete suicide.

Women are more likely to have a later onset, prominent mood symptoms, and a better prognosis than men. The median age of onset is in the late 20s for women. Women have lower symptom severity, fewer hospitalizations, a higher likelihood to return to work and more social support than males.[92] About 67% of women compared with 29% of men with schizophrenia are married, and women are twice as likely to have children.[92]

Natural History of Schizophrenia Across Childbearing

Women with schizophrenia have lower fertility rates compared with healthy women despite less frequent use of contraception and higher rates of irreversible causes of infertility (hysterectomy, menopause, sterilization).[93] Pregnant women are less likely to obtain prenatal care and have an increased risk for interventions during labor and delivery than unaffected women. They have a high frequency of recurrence of psychosis (27%) or depression (38%) in the first postpartum year.[94]

Children born to women with schizophrenia are susceptible to subtle problems in neurodevelopment but the origins (genetic, environment, psychosocial) are complex. Data on the mothers' nutritional status, exposures to psychotropic medications, other prescription or over-the-counter drugs that impact reproductive outcomes, violence, and comorbid medical disease are usually lacking.[42] Concurrent maternal smoking, substance use, and socioeconomic problems increase the risk for less optimal outcomes.

The data on relapse risk for schizophrenia in the general population must be extrapolated to pregnant patients because no specific data exist. A meta-analysis of 66 studies and more than 4000 patients indicated that individuals with chronic schizophrenia who stop treatment have a cumulative relapse rate of 53%, compared with 16% among patients who remain on antipsychotic therapy over a 10-month period.[95] The highest rate of relapse occurred within the first 3 months of treatment discontinuation. Sudden cessation of antipsychotic medication, younger age, early age of illness onset, need for high doses of antipsychotic therapy, and recent psychiatric admission predicted recurrence. Patients with severe and persistent symptoms of schizophrenia, frequent relapses, dangerous behavior, poor self-care, and hospitalization often reasonably choose to remain on antipsychotic treatment throughout pregnancy. Very few women with schizophrenia achieve a sustained symptom-free period and good function without antipsychotic medications before pregnancy. If a woman elects to remain monitored without medication, a plan should be developed for reinstituting medication rapidly if prodromal symptoms occur. The antipsychotic agent that achieved the greatest symptom reduction and the least side effects for the individual patient balanced against its side effects is the preferred drug.

In a population-based cohort of more than 3000 children born from 1980 to 1992, Jablensky and colleagues[42] reported that women with schizophrenia had more than twice the risk for placental abruption compared to healthy controls (OR 2.75, 95% CI, 1.32 to 5.74). Rates of antepartum hemorrhage were significantly higher in mothers with schizophrenia (OR 1.65, 95% CI, 1.02 to 2.69) compared to women without psychiatric illness.

Treatment Interventions for Women with Schizophrenia

Mothers with schizophrenia often struggle with poverty, poor housing, social isolation, and difficulty obtaining basic services for their offspring. Comprehensive clinical services that offer case-integrated obstetrical and psychiatric management, consultation, pharmacotherapy, parent education groups, and family programs are optimal for promoting positive outcomes. Optimal maternal and infant outcomes are achieved through individualized treatment planning by a mental health team in collaboration with community programs. The antipsychotic agent associated with the greatest symptom reduction, balanced against its side effects, is the preferred drug for the individual pregnant woman. An additional consideration in risk/benefit discussions is whether that preferred drug could be replaced by one with a more favorable reproductive risk profile *without* compromising efficacy and tolerability, but no antipsychotic has emerged as definitively more efficacious or having less adverse reproductive effects than any other. Several factors affect the choice of a medication change, including patient and physician concern about the lack of data for the preferred drug, particularly for newer agents, and prior treatment experience with a drug that has less impact on a medical condition that existed before or developing during pregnancy. A factor in every risk benefit decision is the fact that pregnancy outcome data for drug exposure is inextricably tied to outcomes related to the underlying illness for which the drug is being prescribed.

In a double-blind controlled trial of 1500 nonpregnant patients with schizophrenia sponsored by the National Institute of Mental Health (NIMH), subjects were randomized to one of four atypical antipsychotics (OLZ, quetiapine, risperidone, ziprasidone) or an older typical antipsychotic (perphenazine) and followed for 18 months (Clinical Antipsychotic Trials of Intervention Effectiveness trial).[96] Few differences in outcome were observed among groups treated with the various medications. The typical antipsychotic perphenazine was as well tolerated as the newer compounds and as effective as three of the four newer agents. OLZ was slightly better than all the others in terms of lower drug discontinuation and hospitalization rates, but it was associated with higher rates of weight gain and metabolic side effects. Although this NIMH study excluded pregnant women, the results have implications for their treatment. Significantly more data about use during pregnancy are available for the older typical antipsychotics, and exposure for the period limited to pregnancy can be favorable in the risk/benefit analysis for some women, particularly women with insulin resistance, hypertension, and obesity. For the atypical antipsychotics, blood pressure, heart rate, and appropriate weight gain should be monitored. **Control of the disorder (which usually requires medication continuation) is paramount for maternal and fetal health.**

Antipsychotic Drugs During Pregnancy

Data on the use of atypical antipsychotics during gestation largely originate from case studies (which cannot establish etiological association), case series (which do not produce risk estimates), and rare controlled, prospective designs without long-term outcomes. However, data on the effects of these drugs during pregnancy are emerging as their duration of time on the market increases. Clozapine was the first atypical agent to be released; burdensome side effects (weight gain, lowered seizure threshold, tachycardia, dyslipidemia, sedation, drooling) and mandatory periodic monitoring for agranulocytosis create significant barriers to use. Clozapine is reserved for patients whose illness is nonresponsive to treatment with less toxic drugs. Clozapine use in pregnancy has been associated with normal deliveries as well as gestational diabetes, shoulder dystocia, hypotonia, and neonatal convulsions.[97]

The most reproductive data is available for OLZ. Goldstein and colleagues[98] prospectively identified 37 pregnancies with OLZ exposure at doses of 5 to 25 mg daily. One woman experienced an ectopic pregnancy, and 13 women underwent elective abortions unrelated to fetal anomalies. Of the remaining 23 pregnancies, 3 resulted in miscarriage. No major malformations were associated with the remaining 20 pregnancies, but 4 had adverse outcomes that included stillbirth, gestational diabetes, premature birth, and postdates birth.

Risperidone is an atypical agent with diverse receptor-blocking activities. At doses above 6 mg daily, hyperprolactinemia and motor side effects may emerge. A postmarketing survey provided 68 prospective and 197 retrospective reports of outcomes following treatment during pregnancy.[99] In the prospective group, tricuspid atresia occurred in one infant and multiple deformities in two infants; however, all infants were exposed to other drugs. From the retrospective group, 12 infants had malformations; 9 were exposed to multiple agents in the first trimester.

Quetiapine is an atypical antipsychotic with a wide dose range that allows for easy titration. Side effects include sedation, weight gain, and headache. The few published cases of in utero exposure to quetiapine resulted in normal intrauterine growth, full-term deliveries, and favorable Apgar scores. Yaeger and colleagues presented a sophisticated case discussion of quetiapine treatment of a pregnant woman[100] that provides an interesting clinical review.

Ziprasidone is a suitable choice for managing psychosis, with its neutral effects on weight and lipid and glucose metabolism[101]; however, its use may be associated with prolonged QTc syndrome. Limited information on perinatal exposures with ziprasidone is available. Among 57 in utero exposed cases with known outcomes, one malformation was observed.[102]

Aripiprazole has novel dopamine antagonist and partial agonist activity. It is indicated for schizophrenia, bipolar mania, mixed episodes, and severe MDE (combined with an antidepressant). One mother who received aripiprazole during the latter half of pregnancy required surgical delivery for fetal tachycardia.[103] Breastfeeding could not be established, which could be related to the partial dopamine-2 receptor agonist effect of this agent. At 6 months, the infant had normal developmental milestones.

Asenapine is a new atypical antipsychotic drug for the treatment of patients with acute schizophrenia and acute manic or mixed episodes of BD type I. Asenapine is contraindicated for patients with hepatic impairment. Common side effects include somnolence, extrapyramidal effects, akathisia, weight gain, dizziness, headache, and oral hypoesthesia after 6 weeks of treatment. As with newly released drugs, meaningful pregnancy exposure data is lacking.

Antipsychotic Drugs During Breastfeeding

Breast milk has a high concentration of clozapine attributed to its lipophilicity, and breastfed infants have developed sedation, agranulocytosis, and cardiovascular effects.[104] The excretion of OLZ, a highly protein-bound agent, in breast milk has been assessed in small case series. The median estimated dose in infants was 1.6% to 4.0% of the maternal dose.[105] Three breastfed infants of mothers who were treated with risperidone had undetectable serum drug metabolite levels and no adverse reactions.[106] A mother who was treated with risperidone (6 mg/day) provided serial samples of plasma and breast milk every 4 hours over a 24-hour period. The infant drug intake was estimated to be 0.84% of the maternal dose for risperidone, 3.5% for its metabolite, and 4.3% of the weight-adjusted maternal dose.[107] Six breastfeeding women who received treatment with quetiapine[108] provided breast milk; the total daily infant exposure was less than 0.01 mg/kg for five infants and less than 0.10 mg/kg for one infant. The only report on ziprasidone in human milk was obtained from a mother who began treatment 9 days after delivery; the investigators collected milk and maternal plasma samples daily from 9 to 25 days postpartum.[109] Breast milk drug levels were detectable only after 10 days of treatment; the milk (11 ng/mL) to plasma (170 ng/mL) ratio was 0.06; the estimated relative dose received by the infant was 1.2%. A woman who was treated with aripiprazole throughout pregnancy breastfed her full-term infant; at 27 days, no detectable levels of aripiprazole and its metabolite were found in milk samples.[110]

SUBSTANCE-RELATED DISORDERS

Diagnosis and Prevalence

Substance-related disorders among pregnant women comprise a public health problem associated with major individual and societal costs, yet women who abuse substances rarely are identified by health care professionals. The most objective picture of pregnant women who use drugs was derived from blinded urine toxicology screens conducted at representative hospitals nationally.[111] **The study revealed that the common perception of substance abuse as an affliction of poor, minority, and young women was erroneous. Similar rates of substance use during pregnancy occurred in women of different ages, races, and social classes.** The specific substances used differed by race and social class, with African American and poor women more likely to use illicit substances, particularly cocaine, and white and educated women more likely to use alcohol, although polysubstance use was common.

The National Pregnancy and Health Survey was the first national survey of drug use among pregnant women in the United States. A representative sample of the 4 million women who delivered during 1992 was obtained. Illicit drugs (marijuana, cocaine, methamphetamine, heroin, methadone, inhalants, hallucinogens, or nonmedical use of psychotropics during pregnancy) were used by 5.5% of pregnant women.[112] In a national survey done in 2002 to 2003 of pregnant women aged 15 to 44 years, 9.8% reported drinking alcohol during the past month, 4.1% reported binge alcohol use, and less than 1% reported heavy alcohol use.[113] In the year after pregnancy, women increased their substance use, although not to the level of nonpregnant women who were not recent mothers[113] (Figure 52-5).

Obstetricians are in a unique position to identify women with substance use disorders and to encourage treatment.

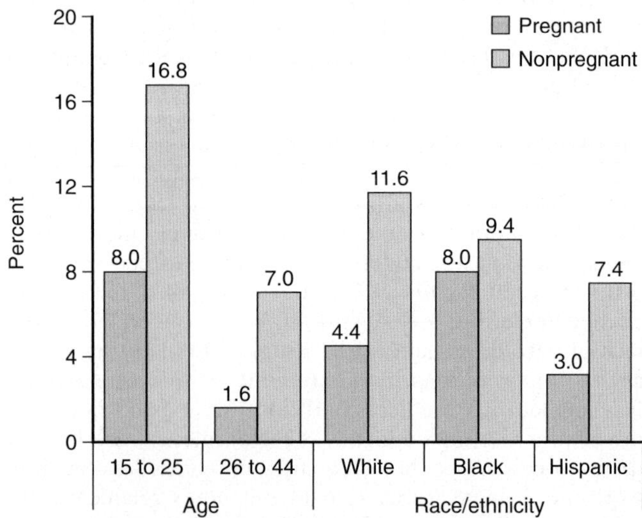

FIGURE 52-5. Drug and alcohol use during pregnancy. (From National Survey on Drug Abuse and Health: Substance Use During Pregnancy: 2002 and 2003 Update, http://oas.samhsa.gov/2k5/pregnancy/pregnancy.htm.)

Pregnancy is a strong motivator for change because most women want to protect their baby; however, women do not volunteer information about substance abuse unless asked. They fear stigma, being judged, or legal and custody concerns. For example, they worry that they will be reported to a child welfare agency or that their employer will learn about their drug use. Universal screening improves detection and has the potential to improve pregnancy and infant outcomes.

In the DSM-IV,[1] psychoactive substance use disorders are classified into two categories, abuse and dependence. The diagnosis of abuse is established if at least one of the following criteria is fulfilled in the past 12 months: (1) recurrent use resulted in failure to fulfill major role obligation at work, home, or school; (2) recurrent use in physically hazardous situations; (3) legal problems result from use; and (4) continued use despite persistent or recurrent social or interpersonal problems caused or exacerbated by substance use. Substance abuse is distinguished from dependence. At least three of the following criteria must be met in the past 12 months for substance dependence: (1) tolerance (marked increase in amount; marked decrease in effect); (2) characteristic withdrawal symptoms and substance is taken to relieve withdrawal; (3) substance is taken in larger amount and for longer period than intended; (4) persistent desire or repeated unsuccessful attempt to quit; (5) significant time and activity are spent to obtain, use, and recover from use; (6) given up or reduced important social, occupational, or recreational activities; and (7) use continues despite knowledge of adverse consequences. Although physiologic tolerance and withdrawal are not essential diagnostic criteria for dependence, they often occur. Abuse is often a precursor to dependence, or a category for those who do not fulfill the criteria for dependence but use substances in maladaptive ways that are harmful to themselves or others.

Comorbidity, or co-occurrence, of substance use with psychiatric illness is the rule rather than the exception. The neurobiologic sequelae of chronic stress may affect brain reward and other pathways to predispose or unmask vulnerability to psychiatric disorders, substance use disorders, or both. In a general population of women who were seeking treatment for cocaine and alcohol abuse, the co-occurring psychiatric disorders were: any mood or anxiety disorder, 70%; posttraumatic stress disorder, 46%; major depression, 40%; panic disorder, 18%; social phobia, 10%; and BD, 4%. For women, the co-occurring condition usually precedes the onset of substance use. One third to one half of substance-abusing women experienced sexual abuse during childhood,[111] and they are frequently involved with drug-using partners. Interpersonal violence is common in the lives of substance-abusing women.[111] Obstetricians provide potentially life-saving interventions for these women by monitoring for domestic violence, offering emergency resources to mothers, identifying children at risk, and reporting to child protective services as mandated by state law.

Obtaining a Substance Use History

Substance use information can be obtained by interview or with a screening tool. The overall approach and emotional tone of the clinician is more important than the specific wording or content. Women are more likely to divulge substance use when asked in a nonjudgmental manner by an empathetic interviewer and within the context of general health questions. Similar to obtaining a sexual history, the questions should be sequenced from least to most personal for the patient. In addition, questions should be open-ended.

Physicians and other health care providers, like all people, have developed personal beliefs and biases over their lifetime that can influence their approach to the issue of substance use. It is challenging but important for physicians to recognize and confront their personal biases in order to keep them from interfering with the care they provide. Helping women with substance use disorders challenges physicians to go beyond the traditional medical care paradigm to an expanded model of psychosocial care, which includes social services and establishing collaboration with addictions and psychiatric professionals (see section on Personality Disorders for other management strategies).

A general screening measure for substances in pregnancy is the *4 P's Plus* (Table 52-2), which was designed to identify obstetrical patients who need in-depth assessment. The *4 P's Plus* has been validated in multiple obstetric populations. This five-question screen is administered during a prenatal visit and takes less than 1 minute to complete.[114] The first *P* is for *Parents*, and the query is about family use of substances. A positive response does not predict the woman's substance use but allows the physician to introduce the issue in a nonthreatening manner. The second question, about the *Partner*, pertains to the partner's substance use. The partner's use does not predict the woman's substance use in pregnancy, but it is correlated with risk for domestic violence, a common psychosocial problem in women with substance use. The third *P*, for the woman's *Past* use of alcohol, places her at risk for use during pregnancy and can be coupled with prevention education as part of prenatal care. The fourth *P*, for *Pregnancy*, contains an open-ended question about cigarette use in the month before pregnancy. The fifth *P* is the amount of wine/beer/liquor consumed in the month before pregnancy. The authors observed that substance use *during* pregnancy was not as effective a screen as asking about a woman's use of substances *before* pregnancy. Women often use substances at prepregnancy levels until the pregnancy is confirmed after early first-trimester exposure has occurred. They often decrease, or report less use, of drugs during gestation. In administering the

TABLE 52-2 SCREENING WITH THE 4 P'S PLUS

- Parents Did either of your parents ever have a problem with alcohol or drugs?
- Partner Does your partner have a problem with alcohol or drugs?
- Past Have you ever had any beer or wine or liquor?
- Pregnancy
  - In the month before you knew you were pregnant, how many *cigarettes* did you smoke?
  - In the month before you knew you were pregnant, how much *beer/wine/liquor* did you drink?

Copyright NTI, 1998. Chasnoff IJ, Hung WC: The 4P's Plus. Chicago, NTI Publishing, 1999.

4Ps Plus, it is preferable to use the terms beer and wine (and liquor) because some women do not recognize beer to be alcohol.

Laboratory screening is another approach to substance use detection but it must be negotiated with the pregnant woman. In general, laboratory measures detect current exposure but do not reflect the historic pattern of use. Because pregnant women with substance use disorders are at increased risk for a variety of infections and medical conditions, a comprehensive medical history, examination, and laboratory studies are indicated. The studies should include a complete blood count, syphilis and hepatitis B and C serology, tuberculosis test, assessment of common sexually transmitted diseases, and confidential human immunodeficiency virus screening.

Specific Drugs of Abuse: Impact and Treatment Approaches

The impact of maternal substance use on pregnancy and infant outcomes is influenced by a variety of factors, such as the specific exposures, gestational timing, duration of exposure, and nutritional status. Disentangling the effects of substance use, co-occurring mental disorders, and the biopsychosocial milieu on pregnancy and infant outcomes is a challenging task (see Figure 52-1).[2] The following sections provide an overview of specific classes of drugs and their use during pregnancy.

Alcohol and Sedative Hypnotics

Most women who drink before becoming pregnant either reduce their intake or stop drinking during pregnancy. However, findings from the 2008-2009 National Survey on Drug Use and Health indicated that a minority of women continue alcohol use during pregnancy. Among pregnant women ages 15 to 44 years, 10% reported current alcohol use, 4.4% reported binge drinking in the past 30 days (5 or more drinks at least once in the past 30 days), and 0.8% reported heavy drinking.[115]

During pregnancy, the dose of alcohol at which no negative offspring outcomes occur has not been defined. Women who consumed more than three drinks per week had a significantly increased risk for miscarriage.[116] Women who consumed five or more drinks per week increased their risk for intrauterine fetal death by two to three times compared with nondrinkers.[117] Consumption of one or more drinks per day was associated with reduced birth weight and IUGR.[118]

Prenatal exposure to alcohol is probably the most common preventable cause of mental retardation in the United States. Children exposed to binge drinking are 1.7 times more likely to have mental retardation and 2.5 times more likely to demonstrate delinquent behavior than unexposed children.[119] Young adult offspring of binge drinkers also have increased odds of developing somatoform disorders, alcohol/drug abuse or dependence, and paranoid, antisocial, and passive aggressive personality disorder.[120] Neonatal effects of alcohol exposure can be subtle, such as slower habituation (attenuation of response to repetitive stimuli) and longer reaction times.[120] Moderate prenatal alcohol exposure is associated with learning problems, memory deficits, and mood disorders in school-aged children.[121]

Fetal alcohol spectrum disorders encompass the array of physical, cognitive, and behavioral deficits found in children born to mothers who consume alcohol during pregnancy. The incidence of fetal alcohol syndrome, the most severe manifestation of exposure, is approximately 1 in 100 births. The characteristic facial dysmorphology is midfacial hypoplasia, flat philtrum, low nasal bridge, epicanthal folds, shortened palpebral fissure, low-set ears, and microcephaly. Affected children may have visual, skeletal, and cardiac anomalies.

Detecting alcohol use among pregnant women is an important step toward preventing alcohol-related birth defects. Several short screening tools to detect pregnancy risk drinking are available. In a critical review, Chang[122] identified the T-ACE[123] (see Chapter 6) as a valuable and efficient tool for identifying alcohol use specifically in pregnant women. This brief tool was developed for detection of risk drinking (defined as 1 ounce or more of absolute alcohol per day). The four questions of the T-ACE reliably differentiated risk from nonrisk drinkers. The T-ACE questions take about 1 minute to ask. A positive screen indicates the need for education about the risks of alcohol use during pregnancy. Such brief interventions promote harm reduction, facilitate antenatal visit compliance, promote healthier choices during pregnancy, and support patients in making lifestyle changes. Screening is also useful to identify women who require referral to substance use treatment programs for alcohol intoxication and withdrawal during pregnancy.

Pregnant women requiring withdrawal from alcohol should be admitted for acute inpatient management. Clinical manifestations occur 6 to 24 hours after the last drink with early withdrawal signs including anxiety, sleep disturbance, vivid dreams, anorexia, nausea, and headache. Physical signs include tachycardia, elevation of blood pressure, hyperactive reflexes, diaphoresis, hyperthermia, and tremor in extended hands or tongue. Alcohol withdrawal seizures (generalized major motor seizures) peak 24 hours after the last drink and are preceded by hyperactive reflexes at biceps and knees. Alcohol withdrawal can progress within 72 to 96 hours to delirium tremens (DTs), characterized by extreme agitation, hallucinations, and autonomic hyperactivity that can be fatal to mother and infant. Benzodiazepines are effective for alcohol withdrawal symptoms and prevention of seizures. Treatment schedules may be "fixed dose" or "symptom based" using an alcohol withdrawal severity scale. The Clinical Institute Withdrawal Assessment of Alcohol Scale, Revised (CIWA-Ar) is a withdrawal severity scale, not copyright protected, available free online, and designed to be administered within 2 to 5 minutes. Symptom-guided withdrawal results in more rapid detoxification and lower total doses of benzodiazepine treatment but requires trained staff to implement. Chlordiazepoxide, diazepam, lorazepam, and oxazepam are common detoxification agents. These benzodiazepines have differing onset and duration of action, and are available in intravenous formulation. A typical fixed dose taper starts with chlordiazepoxide, 50 mg every 6 hours, or lorazepam, 2 mg every 6 hours, adjusting the dosing until symptoms are controlled. The dose is then tapered by 10% to 25% per day as tolerated. Acute management also requires thiamine replacement and maintaining adequate hydration and electrolyte balance. A patient can be safely discharged to outpatient treatment when benzodiazepine treatment is no longer required to control symptoms for more than 24 hours.

Although, there are four FDA-approved medications for the treatment of alcohol dependence, there is little clinical data and experience with their use during pregnancy. Naltrexone is available in both oral and depot forms as an opioid antagonist that decreases the reinforcing effects of alcohol to prevent relapse to heavy drinking. Naltrexone's opioid antagonist activity blocks opioid analgesia with parturition and complicates pain control postoperatively. Naltrexone is not appropriate for use in patients on chronic opiate therapy. Acamprosate is a GABA receptor agonist and NMDA receptor modulator with more limited data showing modest improvement in maintaining abstinence and reducing drinking. These medications have modest efficacy and unknown reproductive risks, which must be weighed against the significant risk of continued alcohol consumption. Disulfram is an aversive medication to reduce alcohol intake. It has modest efficacy but potentiates the teratogenic effects of alcohol; therefore, it is contraindicated during pregnancy.

Long-term use of sedative-hypnotics, such as benzodiazepines, can result in dependence and addiction. **Withdrawal from benzodiazepines is similar to that with alcohol, with significant morbidity and potential mortality if untreated.** Women treated with benzodiazepine drugs that have a short half-life, such as alprazolam, will develop withdrawal symptoms upon discontinuation more rapidly than agents with longer half-lives. Clinically significant withdrawal symptoms occur with adherence to recommended dosing after 4 to 6 months of use and within 6 to 12 weeks for dosing above the recommended upper limits. Acute inpatient withdrawal is often accomplished by a fixed-dose drug taper with substitution of a long-acting benzodiazepine with provision of doses as needed to treat breakthrough symptoms. Once the patient has achieved a comfortable level of symptom control, the dose is tapered by 10% daily as tolerated. Close monitoring is needed for the patient tapering from benzodiazepines while on opioid medications because the risk of respiratory depression is additive. There is increasing evidence that adjunctive use of carbamazepine or valproate can be used in conjunction with a shorter inpatient benzodiazpine taper and be continued for up to 1 month to treat protracted sedative hypnotic withdrawal. However, polypharmacy in pregnant women, and particularly exposure to valproate, should be avoided.

Smoking

Women are more likely to attempt to stop smoking during pregnancy than at any other point in their lives, but only one third stop successfully and many relapse after birth. An office-based intervention for pregnant smokers called the 5 A's (*Ask* about tobacco use, *Advise* to quit, *Assess* willingness to make a quit attempt, *Assist* in quit attempt, and *Arrange* follow-up) was endorsed by the ACOG. The approach involves providing patients with a brief counseling session and pregnancy-specific self-help materials, and increases quit rates among pregnant smokers by a factor of 2 to 3. Web-based tools are also available for education and support for smoking cessation (www.cdc.gov/tobacco/how2quit.htm).

Carbon monoxide and nicotine from inhaled tobacco smoke interfere with oxygen supply to the fetus. Smoking is associated with increased risk for miscarriage, intrauterine and perinatal fetal death, PTB, and IUGR. Paradoxically, smoking appears to reduce the risk of preeclampsia, probably by inhibition of thromboxane A2 production or suppression of the immune system.[124] Newborns with in utero exposure to maternal smoking experienced poorer autonomic regulation and decreased auditory responsiveness compared to nonexposed infants.[125] **Infants of smokers have more than three times the risk of sudden infant death syndrome compared with infants of nonsmokers.**[126]

A negative dose-response relationship between maternal smoking and offspring intelligence was demonstrated across all social classes.[127] An analysis of nearly 3000 subjects who participated in an 11-year community cohort study in western Norway was performed to examine the impact of passive smoking exposure on risk of respiratory disease in adulthood.[128] After adjustment for multiple confounders, 17.3% of the adult incidence of asthma was attributable to maternal smoking, whereas 9.3% was due to exposure from other household smokers. Findings from the Maternal Lifestyles Study also found that maternal smoking during pregnancy is associated with sleep problems through age 12.[128]

Behavioral therapy is the first-line choice to support smoking cessation in pregnant women; however, pharmacologic approaches may be necessary, particularly in heavy smokers. Nicotine replacement therapy during pregnancy has been shown to improve smoking cessation in heavy smokers during pregnancy and 1-year postpartum.[129] Nicotine patch use in the second and third trimesters was not associated with maternal or fetal compromise.

The antidepressants bupropion and nortriptyline offer another pharmacologic approach to smoking cessation. Bupropion and nortriptyline double the likelihood of smoking cessation. A large retrospective epidemiologic study examined 1213 infants exposed to bupropion in the first trimester of pregnancy. The prevalence of congenital malformations was not increased in exposed infants.[129] Limited data show that bupropion doses up to 300 mg/day produce low levels in breast milk.[130] In a study of 10 healthy postpartum volunteers taking 150 mg of bupropion for 3 days and then 300 mg for 4 days, the mean infant exposure was 2% of the standard maternal dose, and no adverse effects in the infants were observed. Motivation to breastfeed is an opportunity to support continued cessation or reduction of smoking beyond that achieved during pregnancy. Breastfeeding is not contraindicated in mothers who smoke.[131] The most recent AAP Policy Statement from the Section on Breastfeeding concludes: "Tobacco smoking by mothers is not a contraindication to breastfeeding, but health care professionals should advise all tobacco-using mothers to avoid smoking within the home and to make every effort to wean themselves from tobacco as rapidly as possible."

Cannabis

During pregnancy, the most frequently used illicit drug was cannabis (2.9% of women).[112] Prenatal cannabis use is not associated with increased rates of major birth defects, stillbirth, or spontaneous abortions.[132] Infants born to women who used cannabis during their pregnancies displayed altered responses to visual stimuli, increased tremulousness, exaggerated startle response, and high-pitched cries, which may indicate neurologic impairment. Deficits in sustained attention, memory, and cognitive function (e.g., problem-solving skills) in both preschool and school-aged children have been demonstrated in marijuana-exposed children.[124]

Continued exposure to cannabis through breastfeeding was associated with decreased motor capability in infants at 1 year of age.[133] The finding persisted after adjusting for the effects of prenatal and lactational exposure to nicotine, alcohol, and cocaine. However, none of the variance in infant mental scores was explained by maternal pre- or postpartum use of cannabis. Nonetheless, the AAP lists cannabis as contraindicated during breastfeeding.[131]

Certainly smoking, whether tobacco or cannabis, carries risks during pregnancy and should be discouraged to promote overall health. Numerous studies have associated regular cannabis use with psychotic symptoms in the cannabis user. Counseling and brief interventions that target lifestyle changes and provide support toward abstinence are primary goals of treatment.

Cocaine

About 1% of women used cocaine at some time during their pregnancy.[112] Cocaine can be snorted, injected, or smoked in the form of crack cocaine. Crack and injected cocaine reach the brain quickly and bring an intense and immediate high.

In a prospective, large, blinded, systematic investigation of prenatally cocaine-exposed children, no increase or consistent pattern of abnormalities was found, although significantly more cocaine-exposed infants were premature and had lower birthweight, length, and head circumference compared with unexposed matched for race, parity, level of pregnancy risk, and socioeconomic status.[134]

The risk of spontaneous abortion, abruptio placentae, premature rupture of membranes, and meconium-stained amniotic fluid are all associated with cocaine use. A pooled odds ratio of 33.92 was shown for abruptio placentae and cocaine use in a meta-analysis.[135]

Frank and colleagues[136] reviewed outcomes in early childhood after prenatal cocaine exposure. After controlling for confounders, there was no consistent association between prenatal cocaine exposure and physical growth, developmental test scores, or receptive or expressive language. Differences in neurophysiologic testing and short-term lag in motor scores were found. However, outcomes thought to be specific effects of in utero cocaine exposure were correlated with other factors, such as prenatal exposure to tobacco and other drugs, as well as the child's environment.

The pregnant woman using cocaine should be referred for psychosocial treatment. There are currently no effective medications for treatment of cocaine addiction. Acute cocaine intoxication and withdrawal can be treated with supportive measures. Women with a history of cocaine use should be counseled not to breastfeed their infants if they use cocaine due to the risk of tremulousness, hypertension, tachycardia, and lethargy.

Methamphetamine

Methamphetamine use has been called the twenty-first century's first drug "epidemic" but there are limited national data regarding prenatal methamphetamine prevalence. Data obtained from admissions to federally funded treatment centers in the United States showed that methamphetamine use accounted for 8% of pregnant women admitted in 1994 and 24% by 2006. The majority of methamphetamine admissions during pregnancy occurred in western states among white unemployed women.[137] As with cocaine dependence, lifestyle risk factors confound interpretation of studies of prenatal exposure to the fetus. Maternal adverse effects of methamphetamine include mood disturbance, psychotic symptoms, cardiovascular problems, hyperthermia, and convulsions. Long-term use is associated with exacerbation of psychiatric symptoms (especially psychotic disorders), cognitive deficits, dependent living, risky sexual behaviors, and criminal justice involvement.

For acute methamphetamine intoxication, judicious use of benzodiazepines and antipsychotic medications can be used to calm the agitated, combative, or psychotic patient. There is no effective treatment other than supportive care for methamphetamine withdrawal. As with cocaine, the AAP[131] lists amphetamines as contraindicated during breastfeeding.

Opioids

During pregnancy, 1% of women report opiate use and as many as 4% test positive for opiates.[138] Because there is no known teratogenic effect of maternal opiates on the fetus, the goals of treating opiate dependence during pregnancy are to minimize maternal and neonatal morbidity. **For women abusing heroin and prescription narcotics, therapy with methadone or buprenorphine decreases opioid and other drug abuse, reduces criminal activity, improves individual functioning, and decreases rates of infections such as hepatitis B and C, human immunodeficiency infection, sexually transmitted diseases, cellulitis, bacterial endocarditis, and tuberculosis.** Opioid replacement therapy is associated with superior relapse prevention, reduced fetal exposure to illicit drug use, improved adherence to obstetrical care, and enhanced neonatal outcomes.

Methadone has been the gold standard of treatment since the 1970s to treat opioid addiction during pregnancy. The methadone doses used to treat pregnant women have increased across time. Higher doses of methadone were not associated with an increased risk of neonatal withdrawal but did have a positive effect on decreasing maternal drug abuse. Methadone has direct effects upon fetal neurobehavioral functions. At peak methadone levels, the fetal heart rate was slower and less variable, and displayed fewer accelerations. Fetuses displayed less motor activity, and the integration between heart rate and motor activity was attenuated.[139] Between 34 and 37 weeks a slower rate of and fewer fetal breathing movements were observed on ultrasound for the methadone-treated group regardless of time since the mothers' daily dose compared to untreated women.[132]

Conversion to methadone during pregnancy has been outlined in the box entitled Initiation of Methadone Maintenance Treatment in Pregnancy. Between 30% and 80%[140] of infants exposed to opioids in utero require treatment for neonatal abstinence syndrome (NAS). NAS is characterized by irritability, tremulousness, sweating, nasal stuffiness, poor suckling, diarrhea, vomiting, and seizures. NAS can occur with any prolonged fetal opiate exposure, but the incidence of NAS is higher with methadone exposure than with shorter-acting opiates. NAS can begin as early as 24 hours and as late as 14 days, depending on the specific opioid. Short-acting opiates have earlier onset of NAS symptoms, whereas long-acting opiates, such as methadone, have later onset of NAS.

Initiation of Methadone Maintenance Treatment in Pregnancy

- Medical and substance abuse history.
- Physical examination to evaluate stigmata of IV opioid use (needle scars, phlebitis, and skin abscesses).
- Laboratory tests: Urine drug testing to document opioid and other drug use. Serum infection screening and baseline liver function if known hepatitis C infection.
- Quantify withdrawal symptoms with a standardized assessment such as Clinical Opioid Withdrawal Scale—COWS[165] (www.csam-asam.org/pdf/misc/COWS_induction_flow_sheet.doc).
- Initial dose of methadone 10-30 mg with additional dosing of 5-10 mg every 4 to 6 hours while patient is awake for breakthrough withdrawal symptoms.
- Titrate dose up to relieve withdrawal symptoms for 24 hours with minimal or no craving.
- Methadone has been associated with rate-corrected QTc prolongation and possible consequent cardiac arrhythmia. Review personal and family history for risk factors. Consider screening ECG and follow-up evaluation in collaboration with outpatient methadone clinic.
- Discharge, when stable, to methadone clinic to monitor subsequent dosing.
- Evaluate for methadone drug-drug interactions (tricyclic antidepressants, antipsychotic medications, and certain antiemetics and antibiotics are also associated with prolonged QT interval).
- As pregnancy progresses, the same methadone dosage produces lower blood methadone levels, so higher dosing may be required to control symptoms.
- After birth, monitor for signs of overmedication and adjust dosing as needed.

Neither the incidence nor severity of NAS correlate directly with maternal methadone dose at delivery, and NAS can occur in infants with maternal methadone doses as low as 10 mg per day. Babies born to mothers who reported smoking 20 or more cigarettes per day had significantly higher NAS peak scores and took longer to reach peak scores than lighter smokers. Methadone doses less than 90 mg were not significantly associated with PTB or low birthweight.[134] Arbitrarily limiting methadone dose as a way of minimizing the risk of NAS is not warranted. In an investigation of high-dose (>100 mg/day) and low-dose (<100 mg/day) administration, no difference in the rate of medication treatment for NAS or days of infant hospitalization between the high-dose (mean 132 mg) and low-dose (mean 62 mg) groups was observed. The group of mothers who received high-dose medication had less illicit drug use at delivery.[141] However, we do not yet have a method to determine which infants will develop NAS that requires treatment. Because methadone has a very long half-life in infants, methadone-exposed neonates should be observed for at least 7 days for onset of NAS.

To minimize the fetal load of methadone at birth, some investigators have suggested tapering the dose during pregnancy. Luty and colleagues[142] investigated the safety of methadone detoxification in pregnancy in a retrospective case series of 101 pregnant opiate-dependent women who underwent a 21-day methadone taper during hospitalization. One miscarriage occurred with detoxification in the first trimester. No miscarriages occurred in the second trimester, and no increase in PTB was observed. Dashe and colleagues[143] observed outcomes during tapering of methadone in 34 women at an average of 24 weeks' gestation. In opiate-using women not on methadone maintenance treatment (MMT), methadone was commenced at 20 mg daily and increased by 5 to 10 mg every 6 hours as needed to alleviate withdrawal symptoms. After reaching a stable dose, the methadone was tapered by 20% or less of the stable dose every 3 days. Each woman was observed in the hospital for several days after methadone was discontinued. Daily qualitative assessments of fetal activity were augmented with semiweekly fetal heart rate monitoring with gestations at or more than 24 weeks. Mild maternal symptoms of withdrawal that included cravings or restlessness were managed with supportive care, counseling, or both. Withdrawal signs that included nausea, vomiting, abdominal discomfort, or a concerning fetal heart rate tracing were managed with clonidine (38%) or methadone (62%). A 0.2-mg transdermal dose of clonidine was supplemented by 0.1 mg orally every 4 to 6 hours to decrease physiologic symptoms. Newborns were kept in the hospital nursery for 3 to 7 days to observe for NAS. The median time to detoxification in the mother was 12 days, and there were no observed fetal deaths, PTB, IUGR, or other perinatal complications. Fifteen percent of neonates needed treatment for NAS. Overall, 20 (59%) women successfully completed detoxification and did not relapse, whereas 10 (29%) resumed prenatal opioid use and 4 (12%) did not complete detoxification and elected methadone maintenance. The decision to opt for methadone detoxification compared with MMT during pregnancy involves consideration of the risks of obstetrical and neonatal complications produced by methadone dependence at delivery versus the risks of relapse and continued intravenous drug use after detoxification. If a woman declines MMT, plans to move to an area where MMT is unavailable, or plans to detoxify in a structured treatment program, a carefully individualized tapering regimen managed closely by a multidisciplinary team provides a viable treatment option.

Buprenorphine is a partial agonist-partial antagonist synthetic opioid with a long duration of action (72 hours). Buprenorphine has been used to treat opioid dependence both in Europe and in the United States. There is increasing evidence to support its use as an alternative to methadone. Because methadone is the standard of care, buprenorphine should be prescribed only if the woman does not tolerate methadone, if she is already on buprenorphine therapy, or if she refuses methadone. Buprenorphine has more complex pharmacology and should be prescribed by an experienced physician with a special federal waiver to treat patients.

Buprenorphine is equally effective as moderate dosing of methadone and has the benefit of a "ceiling effect" as a partial opioid agonist that limits risk of respiratory depression at higher dosing and results in milder withdrawal symptoms upon discontinuation. Study findings to date suggest that infants exposed to buprenorphine compared to methadone have less severe NAS, lower medication doses, and shorter lengths of hospital stay.[144]

The AAP supports the use of methadone (without dose limitation) during breastfeeding. On average, infants receive 2% to 3% of the weight-adjusted maternal dose via breast milk. The doses of methadone received through milk are unlikely to fully prevent NAS but may be beneficial. Findings from four studies suggest that breastfeeding reduces the severity of NAS and shortens length of hospital stay. However, two infants who abruptly discontinued breastfeeding by mothers on methadone (70 mg and 130 mg/day) developed withdrawal symptoms.[145]

Infants of mothers on MMT are at risk for feeding problems, which may be due to altered sucking patterns. Opiate-exposed infants showed prolonged sucking, fewer pauses, more feeding problems, and increased arousal. Intrauterine drug exposure may adversely affect development of brainstem respiratory and swallow centers, which dysregulate the underlying biorhythms of feeding. Apnea and sudden infant death syndrome occur with increased incidence in infants born to opiate-addicted mothers, which may be due to respiratory abnormalities. In utero drug exposure may result in delayed maturation of the neurorespiratory axis.[146] Infants with NAS who experience excess weight loss (>8%-10%) or slow weight gain (not back to birth weight by 10 days) may benefit from caloric supplementation through the addition of breast milk fortifier or 24 kcal/oz infant formula.

Acute Pain Management for Women on Maintenance Opioids

Treatment of acute pain in labor and post-delivery is challenging in women on MMT. Common misconceptions about patients who receive maintenance treatment with methadone (or buprenorphine) include the following: (1) The maintenance opioid agonist provides analgesia; (2) the use of opioids for analgesia may result in addiction relapse; (3) the additive effects of opioid analgesics and maintenance therapy may cause respiratory and central nervous system depression; and (4) complaints of pain demonstrate drug seeking secondary to opioid addiction. Alford[147] also provided recommendations for acute pain management in patients who take maintenance opioids. Uninterrupted maintenance treatment (after verification of the daily dose) is imperative. Undertreating acute pain may lead to decreased responsiveness to opioid analgesics, which renders subsequent pain control more difficult. Multimodal analgesia (e.g., nonsteroidal anti-inflammatory drugs and acetaminophen) and adjuvant drugs that enhance opioid effects (e.g., TCAs) may be coadministered. Analgesic dosing should be continuous or scheduled rather than as needed. Mixed agonist and antagonist opioid analgesics, such as pentazocine, nalbuphine, and butorphanol, must be avoided because they may displace the maintenance opioid from receptors and precipitate acute opioid withdrawal.

PERSONALITY DISORDERS

Personality disorders (PDs) are a heterogeneous group of disorders that arise when an individual's personality traits are maladaptive and inflexible. The person's rigid belief systems and behaviors prevent adaptability of thinking, and limit use of problem-solving skills with effective coping strategies when confronted with new or stressful events. Coping with medical illness or a high-risk pregnancy creates a major challenge for these individuals. Most patients with PD have significant difficulty in interpersonal relationships[142] and are emotionally sensitive. They may react strongly to a long clinic wait or terse office staff.

Diagnosis and Prevalence

Unlike many of the disorders described in this chapter, there is no acute stressor or even a clear onset for PDs. Such traits develop gradually in adolescence or early adulthood and persist throughout life. Although the clinical features of a PD sound similar to characteristics that anyone could display occasionally, an actual PD is defined by exhibiting extremes on various traits and would not be diagnosed unless the patterns of behavior were chronic, pervasive, and dysfunctional.[1] The personality difficulty must lead to emotional distress and/or significantly impaired functioning across several domains. Within the health care system, women with a PD or PD-related traits (such as hostility or anxiety) often use medical resources extensively.

Although we were unable to locate any epidemiologic data on PDs specifically in obstetrical settings, information is available from primary care and internal medicine settings. Prevalence rates vary from 24% with interview-based diagnoses of PD[148] to 32% based on a questionnaire that indicated that the person was at high risk for PD.[149] Some investigators have suggested a much greater prevalence of PD among certain patient groups. Between 47% and 60% of chronic pain patients meet criteria for a PD,[150] and an association also has been found between PD and fibromyalgia.[151] The relationship of PD with medically unexplained symptoms is particularly strong,[147] and one investigator[152] demonstrated that an increasing number of medically unexplained symptoms among patients in primary care was positively correlated with PD-relevant traits (neuroticism, harm avoidance) and with the degree of functional impairment. Patients with an Axis I disorder, such as depression, also are more likely to have a comorbid PD, which typically interferes with their successful treatment. A common clinical perception is that dependent (anxious/fearful cluster), histrionic, and borderline PDs are more often diagnosed in women. Although there is some empirical support for borderline PD being more common in women, when population sex-ratios are controlled, these gender differences tend to attenuate or disappear.

Clinical Implications

Mental health treatments for patients with PD tend to be long-term with slow progress, particularly in severe forms of the disorder. Available treatments include both psychotherapy and pharmacotherapy, although it is generally agreed that medication alone cannot fully treat the multidimensional problems associated with PD. Limited data have been published on the efficacy of different treatments; however, for severe PD, dialectical behavior therapy has the greatest amount of empirical support. Obstetricians generally do not have the time or training to provide formal psychotherapy to patients with PD. However, physicians can develop rapport, feel less frustrated, and develop better clinical recognition skills. This can help the physician make the decision to refer a patient to a mental health specialist for screening and treatment recommendations if PD is suspected. Physicians also will be in a better position to develop and coordinate effective treatment strategies for other disorders in the context of a PD. There are a number of strategies that can be used to interact with persons who have PDs.

Build a Working Alliance

One of the most important ways to begin to develop an alliance is to initiate eye contact with the patient, and maintain it while shaking her hand and introducing yourself. Second, use reflective listening in which you simply restate to the patient what she has said, perhaps by paraphrasing. This conveys that you listened and understood what she was telling you, which will facilitate the communication. For example, if a patient with gestational diabetes defensively explains that she did not check her glucose levels as prescribed because she kept forgetting to take her glucometer to work, a reflective statement such as "It sounds like you've had a hard time checking it four times daily" is neutral yet communicates interest and attentiveness.

Structure the Relationship

A common feature of many patients with PD is difficulty in conforming to the expectations or "script" of their current context. In the medical setting, they may make unreasonable demands for special treatment from the physician or clinic. They may become dependent and begin calling the physician excessively at the clinic or at home. Other patients with PD are mistrustful of authority figures, and may infer dishonesty or hostile intent on the part of the physician and clinic staff when there is any minor inconsistency in clinic procedure.

For these reasons, it is useful to make clear the procedures and respective roles of the doctor-patient relationship from the outset (e.g., appointments, emergencies, prescriptions, other aspects of clinic procedure). Doing so is to the benefit of the patient because it reduces the possibility of misunderstanding and promises that cannot be kept. The rules should be presented in a frank, nonjudgmental way, and it is useful to elicit some form of verbal agreement from the patient to these rules. The rules should be delivered in an emotionally neutral, matter-of-fact presentation as non-negotiable, with the option to seek another physician or clinic if she cannot agree to them. Allowing her to air concerns and discuss any pitfalls can both heighten adherence to the rules and reduce the likelihood of future problems. An important caveat is to keep the number of such rules to the minimum necessary and avoid listing numerous potential egregious behaviors and appearing as though you have negative expectations of the patient.

On the other hand, the moment it appears that a problem behavior is arising, swift and clear communication of the unacceptability of the behavior is needed. For example, the patient who becomes angry and begins shouting in the waiting area should be calmly told, "We don't tolerate shouting in the clinic; you'll have to calm down or leave immediately and reschedule your appointment." This conveys that the behavior (not the patient) is entirely unacceptable and yet the physician-patient relationship is reparable: the patient may reschedule her appointment. Finally, to reduce the frequency and disruptiveness of unscheduled phone contacts and requests for visits, it can be useful to schedule brief, frequent visits that follow a structured format.

Respect Patient Autonomy

Patients with PD may behave in a passive manner regarding their medical care and fail to adhere to the medical regimen, yet become angry when the physician cannot "fix" the problem for them. Other patients may feel very uncomfortable in a "one-down" role and may chafe at the notion that they are being "told what to do." To guard against these problems, it is advisable to encourage the most collaborative relationship possible. The most useful approach is: "How can we work this out together?" A physician's willingness to take this approach can be severely tested if the patient has serious medical problems or is engaging in egregious behaviors (drug abuse, consistent nonadherence with diabetes therapy) that could produce poor birth outcomes. A useful approach is to make statements that highlight the patient's freedom to choose, such as "I can't force you to do anything; I can only tell you the consequences of your behavior, but ultimately it's up to you to make the decision." Give these patients as much choice as possible; for example, ask them about their medication preferences and allow them to regulate medication within prescribed limits.

Find Something to Validate in the Patient's Response

Validation is a key technique to reduce conflict, strengthen the alliance, and promote change. Validation requires the physician to communicate to the patient, in word or action, that her response makes sense and is understandable within the current context. In the face of a great deal of problematic behavior, a physician may have to search for the "kernel of truth" and reflect this back to the patient. The physician may acknowledge, "I understand how hard it has been for you to get to your appointments." Or, "A lot of women would be very stressed by all the things you have going on in your home." Or "I know you are angry about this; you have a reason to be mad."

Physician Self-Regulation

When faced with a hostile, antagonistic patient, or one who is sobbing and demanding, it can be difficult for a physician to manage his or her own emotional reaction. Indeed, many physicians may disavow their strong feelings of irritation at a patient because they think they are unprofessional or uncompassionate. Managing emotional reactions requires that they be recognized and discussed with a colleague on a regular basis. Peer support is vital for maintaining morale, warding off burnout, and providing an objective viewpoint. Physicians need not necessarily like the patient nor condone her behavior. Nonetheless, making a conscious effort to strive for empathy and a nonjudgmental stance toward the patient can greatly reduce physician frustration and increase effectiveness. Likewise, physicians must bear in mind that behavior change typically occurs slowly, and patience is required to develop some sense of acceptance of the patient-physician relationship.

SUICIDE

Suicide is a tragic outcome associated with psychiatric illness. Oates[153] performed an evaluation of the Confidential Enquiry into Maternal Deaths in the late 1990s from the United Kingdom. Psychiatric disorder, and suicide in particular, was the leading cause of mortality and accounted for 28% of maternal deaths. Women also died from other complications related to psychiatric disorder and a significant minority from problems related to substance abuse. The suicide rate following delivery was not significantly different to other times in women's lives and for the first 6 weeks following delivery may be elevated.[153] The overwhelming majority of the women died violently, which contrasts with the usual observation that women are more likely to die from an overdose of medication.

Suicide assessment requires direct questioning of the patient about her desire to live or die, specific thoughts about killing herself, plans for carrying out the act, and access to and lethality of means. The APA practice guidelines for the assessment of suicidal behaviors provide a comprehensive list of more than 40 questions that can help clinicians assess suicidal thoughts, plans, and behaviors.[153] Initial questions address patients' feelings about living ("Have you ever thought that life was not worth living?" "Did you ever wish you could go to sleep and just not wake up?"). These are followed by questions that address specific thoughts about death, self-harm, and suicide ("Have things ever reached the point that you've thought of harming yourself?"). If thoughts of self-harm are endorsed, physicians should evaluate the details of the thoughts including the nature, intensity, frequency, timing, persistence, and circumstances. Physicians must also ask whether the patient has made a specific plan. Routinely asking about pills, household poisons, firearms, or access to dangerous settings as part of the suicide assessment is critical. Has the patient made preparations for the plan or for after her death (i.e., purchasing the means, writing a will, arranging for childcare)? Answers to each of these questions inform evaluation of the immediate safety of the patient. If screening elucidates a significant potential risk, immediate emergency psychiatric consultation or involuntary commitment to a psychiatric facility is indicated.

The practice guidelines also identify situations in which a suicide assessment is clinically appropriate; these include emergency room evaluations, an abrupt change in clinical symptoms, lack of improvement or gradual worsening despite treatment, anticipation or experience of a significant interpersonal loss or stressor (divorce, loss of custody of children, financial loss, legal problems, personal humiliation), or onset of a physical illness associated with a threat to life, disfigurement, severe pain, or loss of function. Patients with increased risk are those with previous suicide attempts, major mood disorders (especially BD), schizophrenia, and substance use.

A potential association between antidepressant use and emergent suicidal behavior was the subject of an FDA black box warning for the use of antidepressants for children and adolescents, as well as considerable debate. Although 60% of suicides occur in persons with mood disorders (the majority untreated), little is known about the relationship between antidepressant drug use and the rate of suicide. Data from all Americans who committed suicide between 1996 and 1998 were analyzed for associations between prescriptions and suicide rate at the county level. The overall relationship between antidepressant prescription and suicide rate was not significant.[154]

INFANTICIDE AND NEONATICIDE

Resnick[155] differentiated filicide (murder of a child) from neonaticide (killing within 24 hours of birth) and infanticide (killing after the first day). In further elaboration of this conceptual framework, Oberman[156] defined four subtypes of infanticide that provide a model for a "differential diagnosis" of infanticide (Table 52-3). The total dependence of the newborn on the caretaker creates a number of risks. Direct killing of an infant by poisoning, traumatic injury, or starvation has been described. The serious cognitive disorganization in women with postpartum psychosis also can lead to failure to provide the vulnerable newborn with life-sustaining needs, such as adequate fluid and nutritional intake, appropriate environmental temperatures, safety, and emergency medical care. Environmental factors that are correlated with parental psychiatric illness, such as violence, hostility, irritability, and involvement in parental delusions, are also important predictors of poor infant outcomes.

TABLE 52-3 CATEGORIES OF INFANTICIDE

CATEGORY	DESCRIPTION
Neonaticide	Unaware of pregnancy, no prenatal care, unassisted birth (often into toilet), family/friends unaware of pregnancy, minimal physical signs of pregnancy
Assisted/Coerced	Killing is done in conjunction with violent, abusive, usually male partner
Neglect	Caretaker distraction results in accidental death, such as baby left in care of young siblings, limited resources, overwhelmed by economic obligations
Abuse	Chronic child abuse, marked irritability, poor caretaker impulse control, efforts to discipline result in unintentional death (most frequently at mealtime and bedtime)
Overt mental illness	Acute-onset postpartum psychosis with altruistic homicide delusions that involve the infant; chronic schizophrenia, social isolation, incapable of parenting without assistance

Postpartum Psychosis

The tragic case of Andrea Yates, who drowned her five children, resulted in discussions about the current conceptualization of postpartum psychosis juxtaposed against legal criteria that involve only tests of the cognitive capacity to acknowledge actions.[157] Women are more vulnerable to psychosis in the postbirth period than at any other time during their lives. In the first 30 days after birth, a woman is 21.7 times more likely to develop psychosis than in the 2-year period prior to childbirth. If she has not had a child before, she is 35 times more likely to suffer psychosis than women who have children.[158] **The magnitude of these relative risks demonstrates that postpartum psychiatric morbidity is a major public health problem.** The reasons for the vulnerability of postpartum women to psychosis and the high risk for postbirth decompensation in women with BD have not been elucidated. Sleep deprivation and marked interference with circadian rhythms related to labor are likely contributors to mood instability.[41] Hormone elevations near the end of gestation and massive postbirth withdrawal also contribute to the risk.[9]

Specific types of delusional thoughts are related to risk for infanticide. Delusional altruistic homicide (often associated with maternal suicide) to save them both "from a fate worse than death" was described in a review of filicides.[155] This type of delusion was present in the clinical symptoms of Andrea Yates. In his classic paper, Resnick[155] observed that 40% of the perpetrators of filicide had seen physicians shortly before the tragedy. Sensitive, direct questions about thoughts of harm to the infant, as well as harm to the self, are imperative in the examination. Nonjudgmental inquiry can be made as follows: "Some new mothers have thoughts such as wishing the baby were dead or about harming the baby; has this happened to you?"

The clinical picture of postpartum psychosis is characterized by rapid onset of hectic mood fluctuation, marked cognitive impairment suggestive of delirium, bizarre behavior, insomnia, visual and auditory hallucinations, and unusual hallucinations (tactile and olfactory). Women with acute-onset psychoses related to childbearing usually had recurrence of previously undiagnosed cyclic mood disorders rather than the triggering of a new disorder. **As discussed in the section on BD, postpartum psychosis is frequently a manifestation of bipolar illness: mania or depression with psychotic features.** In a historical cohort design, our group[159] studied mothers who presented to a psychiatric evaluation center. Half of the group with at least one child under the age of 3 years presented with episodes that began during pregnancy or postpartum. Women who presented with psychoses during childbearing had symptom patterns that differed from those of women who presented with non-childbearing related psychoses. **Particularly prominent was cognitive disorganization, which mimicked a delirium and often resulted in an extensive medical assessment.**

Delusions must be differentiated from the far more common occurrence of obsessional thoughts in the context of depression. Many depressed women have obsessional thoughts. Obsessions are recurrent and persistent thoughts, impulses, or images that are experienced as intrusive and inappropriate and cause marked anxiety or distress. For example, some mothers have obsessional thoughts about drowning their baby and refuse to bathe the child. Women often have "what if" questions such as: "What if I throw the baby over the banister?" Obsessions differ from psychotic symptoms because the patient recognizes that the thoughts, impulses, or images are a product of her own mind (not imposed by an external force as might occur in psychosis). Additionally, obsessional visual images also may occur but are brief and perceived as being in the "mind's eye" as opposed to an external hallucination. For example, a woman might have frightening images of her dead baby in a bathtub, but she is aware that the image was not actually present in the real world. The distinction is important clinically because women with obsessional thoughts are vigilant about preventing any action they might take in response to obsessional thoughts (such as asking that all knives be locked away), whereas women with psychosis are at risk for taking action. Although these symptom sets are not mutually exclusive, co-occurrence is very rare.

Prevention of infanticide involves increased *awareness* and a heightened index of suspicion by physicians, midwives, obstetric nurses, other health care professionals, patients, and families. Women with a previous episode of postpartum psychosis and women with BD are at high risk for the onset of postpartum psychosis. At a minimum, postpartum *monitoring* for the emergence of symptoms should be a collaborative plan between the physician and the patient's family. Because postpartum disorders are common in the general population of new mothers, *screening* (such as with the EPDS, see Figure 52-2), to identify cases for *early intervention* is an important public health goal. Aggressive *treatment* for women who develop the disorder with a thoughtful plan for family monitoring of the infant for safety or alternative care while the mother recovers is imperative.[41]

Neonaticide

Neonaticide refers to the death of a newborn within the first 24 hours of life. A striking consistency in the clinical presentations of neonaticides occurs. The adolescent or adult woman has minimal weight gain during pregnancy, perceives birth as the need to have a bowel movement, and secretly delivers into a toilet. She puts the baby in a bag, abandons or hides it, and continues her usual activities. If not rescued, the infant may suffocate or die from exposure. Affected women vary in terms of age, race, and demographics, and may have other children. Family members, friends, and boyfriends usually were not aware of their pregnancies, and the father is rarely identified. Childhood sexual trauma, physical abuse, and emotional abuse are common in women who commit neonaticide.

A common element in these cases is the psychophysiologic denial of pregnancy; that is, the conscious awareness of the pregnancy is suppressed. This is classic denial, in that the woman behaves in a way that demonstrates failure to accept either an obvious fact (pregnancy) or its significance. A fragmentation of perceptions (no pregnancy, delivery, or pain) and memory (no sexual encounter and continued menses) occurs to suppress painful emotional awareness. The woman denies somatic symptoms of pregnancy, perceives no fetal movements, claims to have menstrual cycles, and recognizes impending birth only as a bowel movement. Essentially, the pregnancy is *not there, not real* for these patients in both mind and body. Most of these patients will not be seen by an obstetrician unless they present for another problem and the pregnancy is discovered, or if the baby is recovered and the mother is presented for pelvic examination, often due to legal intervention.

Neonaticide is the polar opposite of a desired but unachievable pregnancy, which in extreme cases results in pseudocyesis (see next section). Psychophysiologic mechanisms are common to both states, and both have neurohormonal underpinnings but opposite somatic manifestations.

PSEUDOCYESIS

Pseudocyesis is a condition in which the woman believes that she is pregnant but no conceptus exists. Pseudocyesis is characterized by an increase in body weight, enlargement of the mammary glands, and milk production. In animal models, it is associated with the abnormal persistence of the corpus luteum. Spontaneous cases of pseudocyesis have been reported in a number of mammalian species, including dogs, cats, bears, rodents, and humans; curiously, it occurs rarely in nonhuman primates.[160]

Women with pseudocyesis have amenorrhea, lactation, colostrum secretion, increased abdominal girth, and subjective experiences of fetal movement. Physical changes consistent with pregnancy have been detected upon examination, such as an enlarged uterus and softened, congested cervix. Women with pseudocyesis present with behaviors and somatic symptoms consistent with pregnancy, and they may be admitted to the delivery suite. Psychophysiologic mechanisms are common to both pseudocyesis and denial of pregnancy, which have neurohormonal underpinnings but opposite somatic manifestations. A psychiatric diagnostic assessment is crucial, because pseudocyesis must be differentiated from psychosis, in which a fixed conviction of pregnancy persists despite evidence to the contrary and other psychotic symptoms are present. Delusions of pregnancy also have been described in patients with schizophrenia.[161] Gentle and supportive provision of information to challenge the belief of pregnancy with referral for psychotherapy is an appropriate intervention strategy.[162]

FINAL COMMENT

We ended where we began; this is, with the powerful mind-body connections that impact the entire spectrum of outcomes for childbearing women. The biopsychosocial forces that affect women at the time of pregnancy create a plethora of childbearing experiences for our patients. **As health care professionals, we influence the trajectory of these forces to promote the well-being of the mother, her newborn, and her family, at a time when motivation for positive health behaviors to promote the offspring's well-being is maximal.**

ADDITIONAL RESOURCES

- National Library of Medicine, free search for reproductive and developmental toxicity of drugs during pregnancy and lactation: www.toxnet.nlm.nih.gov
- Physician and patient information (fact sheets for multiple drugs and conditions during pregnancy) is available from the Organization of Teratology Information Services: www.otispregnancy.org
- National Institute of Mental Health booklet on depression in women: www.nimh.nih.gov/health/publications/depression-in-women/index.shtml
- Society for Women's Health Research: www.womenshealthresearch.org/index.htm
- The Depression and Bipolar Support Alliance, a patient-directed organization: www.dbsalliance.org
- National Alliance on Mental Illness (NAMI), a nonprofit, grass roots, self-help, support, and advocacy organization of consumers, families, and friends of people with severe mental illnesses, such as schizophrenia, major depression, bipolar disorders, obsessive-compulsive disorder, and anxiety disorders: www.nami.org
- The National Depressive and Manic Depressive Association educates patients, families, professionals and the public concerning the nature of depressive and manic-depressive illness as treatable medical diseases: www.ndmda.org
- Postpartum Depression Website for Primary Care Physicians and Patients: www.MedEdPPD.org
- Postpartum Support International: www.postpartum.net
- The Marcé Society for Perinatal Mental Health, an international society for the understanding, prevention, and treatment of mental illness related to childbearing: www.marcesociety.com
- Anxiety Disorders Association of America: www.adaa.org
- *The Anxiety and Phobia Workbook*, Fourth Edition. Edmund J. Bourne, Ph.D., Oakland, CA, New Harbinger Publications, 2005
- Suicide Prevention Resource Center: www.sprc.org
- *Beyond the Blues: Prenatal and Postpartum Depression, A Treatment Manual.* S.S. Bennett and P. Indman, San Jose, CA, Moodswings Press, 2002
- Patty Duke has bipolar disorder and an educational website: www.officialpattyduke.com/polar.htm
- Center for environmental therapeutics, for comprehensive light therapy information: www.cet.org
- *Down Came the Rain: My Journey Through Postpartum Depression.* Brooke Shields, New York, Hyperion, 2005.
- National Eating Disorders Association, toll-free: 800-931-2237; www.NationalEatingDisorders.org
- National Association of Anorexia Nervosa and Associated Disorders, telephone: 847-831-3438; www.anad.org
- Academy for Eating Disorders: www.aedweb.org
- National Institutes of Health, alcohol and substance use information: www.niaaa.nih.gov or www.drugabuse.gov
- National Partnership to Help Pregnant Smokers Quit: www.helppregnantsmokersquit.org
- Community-based advocacy groups that support efforts to reduce and prevent substance abuse: www.jointogether.org

KEY POINTS

- Mental health is fundamental to health. To the extent that maternal biopsychosocial exposures with negative impact on pregnancy outcomes can be diminished, eliminated, or replaced with positive factors, the risk of poor pregnancy outcome can be reduced.
- Major depression is a treatable illness that is the leading cause of disease burden among girls age 5 years and older worldwide. The period prevalence of depression during pregnancy is 12.7% during pregnancy, with 7.5% of women having a new (incident) episode.
- A brief and efficient 10-item self-report screening instrument, the Edinburgh Postnatal Depression Scale, is available to screen for perinatal depression. For clinical practice screening, the cutoff score for probable major depression in postpartum women is 13 or more and for pregnant women 15 or more.
- Women who present with depression should be evaluated for bipolar disorder, which is characterized by not only depression but also episodes of hypomania, mania, or mixed states, before prescribing antidepressant treatment because the pharmacologic intervention differs.
- The first-line medications for treatment of a breastfeeding woman are sertraline, paroxetine, and nortriptyline; however, established efficacy of another drug in the individual woman must be considered strongly in the decision-making process for drug choice.
- Abrupt discontinuation of any psychotropic medication creates a higher risk for recurrence than does gradual tapering and discontinuation (over at least 2 weeks).
- Cognitive behavioral psychotherapy or behavioral therapy and antidepressants are the first-line treatments for anxiety disorders and bulimia nervosa.
- Antipsychotic drug maintenance treatment and psychosocial support interventions aimed at maximizing function are the mainstays of treatment for schizophrenia. Concurrent maternal smoking, substance use, poor nutrition, and socioeconomic problems increase the risk for less optimal pregnancy outcomes.
- The perception of substance use disorders as afflictions solely of poor, minority, and young women is erroneous. Screening measures are available and easy to use, and multidisciplinary treatment intervention results in improved reproductive outcomes.
- Postpartum psychosis is characterized by rapid onset of hectic mood fluctuation, marked cognitive impairment suggestive of delirium, bizarre behavior, insomnia, visual and auditory hallucinations, and often, unusual hallucinations (tactile and olfactory). Women with acute onset postpartum psychosis usually have recurrences of previously undiagnosed bipolar disorder.

REFERENCES

1. American Psychiatric Association: American Psychiatric Association: Diagnostic and Statistical Manual for Psychiatric Disorders, 4th ed, text revision. Washington DC, American Psychiatric Association, 2000.
2. Misra DP, Guyer B, Allston A: Integrated perinatal health framework: A multiple determinants model with a life span approach. Am J Prev Med 25:65, 2003.
3. Murray C, Lopez A: A comprehensive assessment of mortality and disability from diseases, injuries, and risk factors in 1990 and projected to 2020. In Cambridge M: The global burden of disease and injury series, vol 1. Boston, Harvard University Press, Harvard School of Public Health on behalf of the World Health Organization and the World Bank, 1996.
4. Gaynes BN, et al: Perinatal depression: prevalence, screening accuracy, and screening outcomes. Evidence Report/Technology Assessment (summary) 119:1, 2005.
5. O'Hara MW, Neunaber DJ, Zekoski EM: Prospective study of postpartum depression: prevalence, course, and predictive factors. J Abnormal Psych 93:158, 1984.
6. Kendler KS, et al: The lifetime history of major depression in women: reliability of diagnosis and heritability. Arch Gen Psych 50:863, 1993.
7. Davidson J, Robertson E: A follow-up study of post partum illness, 1946-1978. Acta Psych Scand 71:451, 1985.
8. Cox J, Holden J: Perinatal Mental Health: A Guide to the Edinburgh Postnatal Depression Screening Scale. London, RC Psych Publications, 2003.
9. Bloch M, et al: Effects of gonadal steroids in women with a history of postpartum depression. Am J Psych 157:924, 2000.
10. Grote NK, et al: A meta-analysis of depression during pregnancy and the risk of preterm birth, low birth weight, and intrauterine growth restriction. Arch Gen Psychiatry 67:1012, 2010.
11. Wisner KL, Stowe ZN: Psychobiology of postpartum mood disorders. Seminars in Reprod Endocrinol 15:77, 1997.
12. Gonzalez HM, et al: Depression care in the United States: too little for too few. Arch Gen Psychiatry 67:37, 2010.
13. Vesga-Lopez O, et al: Psychiatric disorders in pregnant and postpartum women in the United States. Arch Gen Psychiatry 65:805, 2008.
14. Bennett IM, et al: Pregnancy-related discontinuation of antidepressants and depression care visits among Medicaid recipients. Psychiatr Serv 61:386, 2010.
15. Wisner KL: SSRI treatment during pregnancy: are we asking the right questions? Depress Anxiety 27:695, 2010.
16. Yonkers KA, et al: The management of depression during pregnancy: a report from the American Psychiatric Association and the American College of Obstetricians and Gynecologists. Obstet Gynecol 114:703, 2009.
17. Louik C, et al: First-trimester use of selective serotonin-reuptake inhibitors and the risk of birth defects. N Engl J Med 356:2675, 2007.
18. Alwan S, et al: Use of selective serotonin-reuptake inhibitors in pregnancy and the risk of birth defects. N Engl J Med 356:2684, 2007.
19. Greene MF: Teratogenicity of SSRIs—serious concern or much ado about little? N Engl J Med 356:2732, 2007.
20. Wisner KL, et al: Major depression and antidepressant treatment: impact on pregnancy and neonatal outcomes. Am J Psychiatry 166:557, 2009.
21. Pedersen LH, Henriksen TB, Olsen J: Fetal exposure to antidepressants and normal milestone development at 6 and 19 months of age. Pediatrics 125:e600, 2010.
22. Reference deleted in proofs.
23. Moses-Kolko EL, et al: Neonatal signs after late in utero exposure to serotonin reuptake inhibitors: literature review and implications for clinical applications. JAMA 293:2372, 2005.
24. Spinelli MG, Endicott J: Controlled clinical trial of interpersonal psychotherapy versus parenting education program for depressed pregnant women. Am J Psychiatry 160:555, 2003.
25. Cohen LS, et al: Relapse of major depression during pregnancy in women who maintain or discontinue antidepressant treatment. JAMA 295:499, 2006.
26. Cipriani A, et al: Comparative efficacy and acceptability of 12 new-generation antidepressants: a multiple-treatments meta-analysis. Lancet 373:746, 2009.

27. Wisner K, Peindl K, Gigliotti T: Tricyclics vs SSRIs for postpartum depression. Arch Women Ment Health 1:189, 1999.
28. Sit DK, et al: Changes in antidepressant metabolism and dosing across pregnancy and early postpartum. J Clin Psychiatry 69:652, 2008.
29. Wirz-Justice A, et al: A randomized, double-blind, placebo-controlled study of light therapy for antepartum depression. J Clin Psych, in press.
30. Wirz-Justice A, Benedetti F, Terman M: Chronotherapeutics for affective disorders: a clinician's manual for light and wake therapy. Basel/New York, Karger, 2009, p xii, 116.
31. Manber R, et al: Acupuncture for depression during pregnancy: a randomized controlled trial. Obstet Gynecol 115:511, 2010.
32. Bodnar LM, Wisner KL: Nutrition and depression: implications for improving mental health among childbearing-aged women. Biol Psychiatry 58:679, 2005.
33. Freeman MP, et al: Complementary and alternative medicine in major depressive disorder: the American Psychiatric Association Task Force report. J Clin Psychiatry 71:669, 2010.
34. Lanza di Scalea T, Wisner KL: Antidepressant medication use during breastfeeding. Clin Obstet Gynecol 52:483, 2009.
35. Wisner KL, et al: Postpartum depression: a randomized trial of sertraline versus nortriptyline. J Clin Psychopharmacol 26:353, 2006.
36. Gregoire AJ, et al: Transdermal oestrogen for treatment of severe postnatal depression. Lancet 347:930, 1996.
37. Perheentupa A, Ruokonen A, Tapanainen JS: Transdermal estradiol treatment suppresses serum gonadotropins during lactation without transfer into breast milk. Fertil Steril 82:903, 2004.
38. Wisner KL, et al: Prevention of postpartum depression: a pilot randomized clinical trial. Am J Psychiatry 161:1290, 2004.
39. Viguera AC, et al: Risk of recurrence in women with bipolar disorder during pregnancy: prospective study of mood stabilizer discontinuation. Am J Psychiatry 164:1817, 2007.
40. Munk-Olsen T, et al: Risks and predictors of readmission for a mental disorder during the postpartum period. Arch Gen Psychiatry 66:189, 2009.
41. Yonkers KA, et al: Management of bipolar disorder during pregnancy and the postpartum period. Am J Psychiatry 161:608, 2004.
42. Jablensky AV, et al: Pregnancy, delivery, and neonatal complications in a population cohort of women with schizophrenia and major affective disorders. Am J Psychiatry 162:79, 2005.
43. Newport DJ, et al: Lithium placental passage and obstetrical outcome: implications for clinical management during late pregnancy. Am J Psychiatry 162:2162, 2005.
44. Meador KJ, et al: In utero antiepileptic drug exposure: fetal death and malformations. Neurology 67:407, 2006.
45. Meador K, et al: Pregnancy outcomes in women with epilepsy: a systematic review and meta-analysis of published pregnancy registries and cohorts. Epilepsy Res 81:1, 2008.
46. Montouris G: Importance of monotherapy in women across the reproductive cycle. Neurology 69:S10, 2007.
47. Vajda FJ, et al: The teratogenic risk of antiepileptic drug polytherapy. Epilepsia 51:805, 2010.
48. Meador KJ, et al: Cognitive function at 3 years of age after fetal exposure to antiepileptic drugs. N Engl J Med 360:1597, 2009.
49. Nau H, et al: Anticonvulsants during pregnancy and lactation. Transplacental, maternal and neonatal pharmacokinetics. Clin Pharmacokinet 7:508, 1982.
50. Meischenguiser R, D'Giano CH, Ferraro SM: Oxcarbazepine in pregnancy: clinical experience in Argentina. Epilepsy Behav 5:163, 2004.
51. Calabrese JR, et al: A double-blind placebo-controlled study of lamotrigine monotherapy in outpatients with bipolar I depression. Lamictal 602 Study Group. J Clin Psychiatry 60:79, 1999.
52. Bowden CL, et al: Safety and tolerability of lamotrigine for bipolar disorder. Drug Saf 27:173, 2004.
53. Calabrese JR, et al: Rash in multicenter trials of lamotrigine in mood disorders: clinical relevance and management. J Clin Psychiatry 63:1012, 2002.
54. Ketter TA, et al: Metabolism and excretion of mood stabilizers and new anticonvulsants. Cellular and Molecular Neurobiology 19:511, 1999.
55. Newport DJ, et al: Lamotrigine in bipolar disorder: efficacy during pregnancy. Bipolar Disorders 10:432, 2008.
56. Pennell PB, et al: Lamotrigine in pregnancy: clearance, therapeutic drug monitoring, and seizure frequency. Neurology 70:2130, 2008.
57. Dolk H, et al: EUROCAT Antiepileptic Drug Working Group. Does lamotrigine use in pregnancy increase orofacial cleft risk relative to other malformations? Neurology 71:714, 2008.
58. Dominguez-Salgado M, Morales A, et al: Gestational lamotrigine monotherapy: congential malformations and psychomotor development. Epilepsia 45:229, 2004.
59. Kinon BJ, et al: Hyperprolactinemia in response to antipsychotic drugs: characterization across comparative clinical trials. Psychoneuroendocrinology 28:69, 2003.
60. Reis M, Kallen B: Maternal use of antipsychotics in early pregnancy and delivery outcome. J Clin Psychopharmacol 28:279, 2008.
61. Newham JJ, et al: Birth weight of infants after maternal exposure to typical and atypical antipsychotics: prospective comparison study. Br J Psychiatry 192:333, 2008.
62. Noaghiul S, Hibbeln JR: Cross-national comparisons of seafood consumption and rates of bipolar disorders. Am J Psychiatry 160:2222, 2003.
63. Wisner KL, et al: Verapamil treatment for women with bipolar disorder. Biol Psychiatry 51:745, 2002.
64. Viguera AC, et al: Risk of recurrence of bipolar disorder in pregnant and nonpregnant women after discontinuing lithium maintenance. Am J Psychiatry 157:179, 2000.
65. Wisner KL, et al: Prevention of postpartum episodes in women with bipolar disorder. Biol Psychiatry 56:592, 2004.
66. Viguera A, et al: Lithium and Lactation. NIMH/NCDEU Annual Meeting, 2004.
67. Newport DJ, et al: Lamotrigine in breast milk and nursing infants: determination of exposure. Pediatrics 122:e223, 2008.
68. Ayers S, et al: Post-traumatic stress disorder following childbirth: current issues and recommendations for future research. J Psychosom Obstet Gynaecol 29:240, 2008.
69. Heron J, et al: The course of anxiety and depression through pregnancy and the postpartum in a community sample. J Affect Disord 80:65. 2004.
70. Bandelow B, et al: Panic disorder during pregnancy and postpartum period. Eur Psychiatry 21:495, 2006.
71. Teixeira JM, Fisk NM, Glover V: Association between maternal anxiety in pregnancy and increased uterine artery resistance index: cohort based study. Br Med J 318:153, 1999.
72. Field T, et al: Pregnancy anxiety and comorbid depression and anger: effects on the fetus and neonate. Depress Anxiety 17:140, 2003.
73. Kinsella MT, Monk C: Impact of maternal stress, depression and anxiety on fetal neurobehavioral development. Clin Obstet Gynecol 52:425, 2009.
74. Reference deleted in proofs.
75. Crow SJ, et al: Long-term menstrual and reproductive function in patients with bulimia nervosa. Am J Psychiatry 159:1048, 2002.
76. Hsu LK: Eating disorders: practical interventions. J Am Med Women's Assoc 59:113, 2004.
77. Zipfel S, et al: Osteoporosis in eating disorders: a follow-up study of patients with anorexia and bulimia nervosa. J Clin Endocrinol Metab 86:5227, 2001.
78. Mehler PS, MacKenzie TD: Treatment of osteopenia and osteoporosis in anorexia nervosa: a systematic review of the literature. Int J Eat Disord 42:195, 2009.
79. Sollid CP, et al: Eating disorder that was diagnosed before pregnancy and pregnancy outcome. Am J Obstet Gynecol 190:206, 2004.
80. Carmichael SL, et al: Dieting behaviors and risk of neural tube defects. Am J Epidemiol 158:1127, 2003.
81. Mazzeo SE, et al: Associations among postpartum depression, eating disorders, and perfectionism in a population-based sample of adult women. Int J Eat Disord 39:202, 2006.
82. Attia E, Walsh BT: Behavioral management for anorexia nervosa. N Engl J Med 360:500, 2009.
83. Murphy R, et al: Cognitive behavioral therapy for eating disorders. Psych Clin N Am 33:611, 2010.
84. Carter JC, et al: Maintenance treatment for anorexia nervosa: a comparison of cognitive behavior therapy and treatment as usual. Int J Eat Disord 42:202, 2009.
85. McKnight RF, Park RJ: Atypical antipsychotics and anorexia nervosa: a review. Eur Eat Disord Rev 18:10, 2010.

86. Walsh BT, et al: Fluoxetine after weight restoration in anorexia nervosa: a randomized controlled trial. JAMA 295:2605, 2006.
87. Shapiro JR, et al: Bulimia nervosa treatment: a systematic review of randomized controlled trials. Int J Eat Disord 40:321, 2007.
88. Fairburn CG: Overcoming Binge Eating. New York, Guilford Press, 1995.
89. American Psychiatric Association: Treatment of patients with eating disorders. Am J Psychiatry 163:4, 2006.
90. Faris PL, et al: De-stabilization of the positive vago-vagal reflex in bulimia nervosa. Physiol Behav 94:136, 2008.
91. McElroy SL, et al: Role of antiepileptic drugs in the management of eating disorders. CNS Drugs 23:139, 2009.
92. Hafner H: Gender differences in schizophrenia. Psychoneuroendocrinology 28:17, 2003.
93. Howard LM, et al: The general fertility rate in women with psychotic disorders. Am J Psychiatry 159:991, 2002.
94. Howard LM, et al: The psychosocial outcome of pregnancy in women with psychotic disorders. Schizophr Res 71:49, 2004.
95. Gilbert PL, et al: Neuroleptic withdrawal in schizophrenic patients. A review of the literature. Arch Gen Psychiatry 52:173, 1995.
96. Lieberman JA, et al: Effectiveness of antipsychotic drugs in patients with chronic schizophrenia. N Engl J Med 353:1209, 2005.
97. Waldman MD, Safferman AZ: Pregnancy and clozapine. Am J Psychiatry 150:168, 1993.
98. Goldstein DJ, Corbin LA, Fung MC: Olanzapine-exposed pregnancies and lactation: early experience. J Clin Psychopharmacol 20:399, 2000.
99. Coppola D, et al: Evaluating the postmarketing experience of risperidone use during pregnancy: pregnancy and neonatal outcomes. Drug Safety 30:247, 2007.
100. Yaeger D, Smith HG, Altshuler LL: Atypical antipsychotics in the treatment of schizophrenia during pregnancy and the postpartum. Am J Psychiatry 163:2064, 2006.
101. Simpson GM, et al: Randomized, controlled, double-blind multicenter comparison of the efficacy and tolerability of ziprasidone and olanzapine in acutely ill inpatients with schizophrenia or schizoaffective disorder. Am J Psychiatry 161:1837, 2004.
102. Einarson A, Boskovic R: Use and safety of antipsychotic drugs during pregnancy. J Psychiatric Pract 15:183, 2009.
103. Mendhekar DN, Sunder KR, Andrade C: Aripiprazole use in a pregnant schizoaffective woman. Bipolar Disorders 8:299, 2006.
104. Barnas C, et al: Clozapine concentrations in maternal and fetal plasma, amniotic fluid, and breast milk. Am J Psychiatry 151:945, 1994.
105. Ambresin G, et al: Olanzapine excretion into breast milk: a case report. J Clin Psychopharmacol 24:93, 2004.
106. Wisner KL, Sit DK, Moses-Kolko E: Antipsychotic treatment during pregnancy: a model for decision making. Adv Schizophr Clin Psychiatry 3:48, 2007.
107. Hill RC, et al: Risperidone distribution and excretion into human milk: case report and estimated infant exposure during breastfeeding. J Clin Psychopharmacol 20:285, 2000.
108. Misri S, et al: Quetiapine augmentation in lactation: a series of case reports. J Clin Psychopharmacol 26:508, 2006.
109. Schlotterbeck P, et al: Low concentration of ziprasidone in human milk: a case report. Int J Neuropsychopharmacology 12:437, 2009.
110. Lutz UC, et al: Aripiprazole in pregnancy and lactation: a case report. J Clin Psychopharmacol 30:204, 2010.
111. Hans SL: Demographic and psychosocial characteristics of substance-abusing pregnant women. Clin Perinatol 26:55, 1999.
112. National Institute on Drug Abuse: National Pregnancy and Health Survey: Drug use among women delivering live births. National Institutes of Health Publication No. 96-3819, NIH, Rockville, Md., 1996.
113. Substance Abuse and Mental Health Services Administration: National Survey on Drug Abuse and Health: Substance Use During Pregnancy. 2002 and 2003 update.
114. Chasnoff IJ, et al: The 4P's Plus screen for substance use in pregnancy: clinical application and outcomes. J Perinatol 25:368, 2005.
115. Ebrahim SH, et al: Alcohol consumption by pregnant women in the United States during 1988-1995. Obstet Gynecol 92:187, 1998.
116. Windham GC, et al: Moderate maternal alcohol consumption and risk of spontaneous abortion. Epidemiology 8:509, 1997.
117. Kesmodel U, et al: Moderate alcohol intake during pregnancy and the risk of stillbirth and death in the first year of life. Am J Epidemiol 155:305, 2002.
118. Passaro KT, et al: The effect of maternal drinking before conception and in early pregnancy on infant birthweight. The ALSPAC Study Team. Avon Longitudinal Study of Pregnancy and Childhood. Epidemiology 7:377, 1996.
119. Bailey BN, et al: Prenatal exposure to binge drinking and cognitive and behavioral outcomes at age 7 years. Am J Obstet Gynecol 191:1037, 2004.
120. Jacobson SW, Jacobson JL, Sokol RJ: Effects of fetal alcohol exposure on infant reaction time. Alcohol Clin Exp Res 18:1125, 1994.
121. Streissguth AP, Barr HM, Sampson PD: Moderate prenatal alcohol exposure: effects on child IQ and learning problems at age 7 1/2 years. Alcohol Clin Exp Res 14:662, 1990.
122. Chang G: Alcohol-screening instruments for pregnant women. Alcohol Res Health 25:204, 2001.
123. Sokol RJ, Martier SS, Ager JW: The T-ACE questions: practical prenatal detection of risk-drinking. Am J Obstet Gynecol 160:863, 1989.
124. Conde-Agudelo A, et al: Cigarette smoking during pregnancy and risk of preeclampsia: a systematic review. Am J Obstet Gynecol 181:1026, 1999.
125. Fried PA, Makin JE: Neonatal behavioural correlates of prenatal exposure to marihuana, cigarettes and alcohol in a low risk population. Neurotoxicology and Teratology 9:1, 1987.
126. Wisborg K, et al: A prospective study of smoking during pregnancy and SIDS. Arch Disease in Childhood 83:203, 2000.
127. Mortensen EL, et al: A dose-response relationship between maternal smoking during late pregnancy and adult intelligence in male offspring. Paediatr Perinat Epidemiol 19:4, 2005.
128. Skorge D, et al: The adult incidence of asthma and respiratory symptoms by passive smoking in utero or in childhood. Am J Resp Crit Care 172:61, 2005.
129. Cole JA, et al: Bupropion in pregnancy and the prevalence of congenital malformations. Pharmacoepidemiol Drug Saf 16:474, 2007.
130. Haas JS, et al: Bupropion in breast milk: an exposure assessment for potential treatment to prevent post-partum tobacco use. Tobacco Control 13:52, 2004.
131. American Academy of Pediatrics Committee on Drugs: The transfer of drugs and other chemicals into human milk. Pediatrics 108:776, 2001.
132. Tennes K, et al: Marijuana: prenatal and postnatal exposure in the human. NIDA Research Monograph 59:48, 1985.
133. Astley S, Little S: Maternal marijuana use during lactation and infant development at one year. Am J Epidemiol 130:804, 1989.
134. Behnke M, et al: The search for congenital malformations in newborns with fetal cocaine exposure. Pediatrics 107:E74, 2001.
135. Hulse GK, et al: Assessing the relationship between maternal cocaine use and abruptio placentae. Addiction 92:1547, 1997.
136. Frank DA, et al: Growth, development, and behavior in early childhood following prenatal cocaine exposure: a systematic review. JAMA 285:1613, 2001.
137. Terplan M, et al: Methamphetamine use among pregnant women. Obstet Gynecol 113:1285, 2009.
138. Lester BM, et al: The Maternal Lifestyle Study: drug use by meconium toxicology and maternal self-report. Pediatrics 107:309, 2001.
139. Jansson LM, Dipietro J, Elko A: Fetal response to maternal methadone administration. Am J Obstet Gynecol 193:611, 2005.
140. van Baar AL, et al: Neonatal behavior after drug dependent pregnancy. Arch Dis Childhood 64:235, 1989.
141. Reference deleted in proofs.
142. Luty J, Nikolaou V, Bearn J: Is opiate detoxification unsafe in pregnancy? J Subst Abuse Treat 24:363, 2003.
143. Dashe JS, et al: Opioid detoxification in pregnancy. Obstet Gynecol 92:854, 1998.
144. Jones HE, Kaltenbach K, Heil SH, et al: Neonatal abstinence syndrome after methadone or buprenorphine exposure. New Engl J Med 363:2320, 2010.
145. Malpas TJ, Darlow BA: Neonatal abstinence syndrome following abrupt cessation of breastfeeding. NZ Med J 112:12, 1999.
146. Gibson E, et al: Increased incidence of apnea in infants born to both cocaine and opiate addicted mothers. Pediatr Res 27:10A, 1990.
147. Alford DP, Compton P, Samet JH: Acute pain management for patients receiving maintenance methadone or buprenorphine therapy. Ann Intern Med 144:127, 2006.

148. Rendu A, et al: Economic impact of personality disorders in UK primary care attenders. Brit J Psychiatry 181:62, 2002.
149. Hueston WJ, Werth J, Mainous AG 3rd: Personality disorder traits: prevalence and effects on health status in primary care patients. Int J Psychiatry Med 29:63, 1999.
150. Monti DA, et al: Personality assessment of patients with complex regional pain syndrome type I. Clin J Pain 14:295, 1998.
151. Epstein SA, et al: Psychiatric disorders in patients with fibromyalgia. A multicenter investigation. Psychosomatics 40:57, 1999.
152. Katon WJ, Walker EA: Medically unexplained symptoms in primary care. J Clin Psychiatry 59:15, 1998.
153. Oates M: Perinatal psychiatric disorders: a leading cause of maternal morbidity and mortality. Br Med Bull 67:219, 2003.
154. Gibbons RD, et al: The relationship between antidepressant medication use and rate of suicide. Arch Gen Psychiatry 62:165, 2005.
155. Resnick PJ: Child murder by parents: a psychiatric review of filicide. Am J Psychiatry 126:325, 1969.
156. Oberman M: A brief history of infanticide and the law. In Spinelli M: Infanticide: Psychosocial and Legal Perspectives on Mothers Who Kill. Washington, DC, American Psychiatric Publishing, 2003, p 3.
157. McFarlane J: Criminal defense in cases of infanticide and neonaticide. In Spinelli M: Infanticide: Psychosocial and Legal Perspectives on Mothers Who Kill. Washington, DC, American Psychiatric Publishing, 2003, p 133.
158. Kendell RE, Chalmers JC, Platz C: Epidemiology of puerperal psychoses. British J Psychiatry 150:662, 1987.
159. Wisner KL, Peindl KS, Hanusa BH: Psychiatric episodes in women with young children. J Affect Disord 34:1, 1995.
160. Guedes D, Young RJ: A case of pseudo-pregnancy in captive brown howler monkeys (Alouatta guariba). Folia Primatol (Basel) 75:335, 2004.
161. Shiwach RS, Dudley AF: Delusional pregnancy with polydipsia: a case report. J Psychosom Res 42:477, 1997.
162. Bianchi-Demicheli F, Ludicke F, Chardonnens D: Imaginary pregnancy 10 years after abortion and sterilization in a menopausal woman: a case report. Maturitas 48:479, 2004.
163. Mitchell-Gieleghem A, Mittelstaedt ME, Bulik CM: Eating disorders and childbearing: concealment and consequences. Birth 29:182, 2002.

For full reference list, log onto www.expertconsult.com.

Section VII

Legal and Ethical Issues in Perinatology

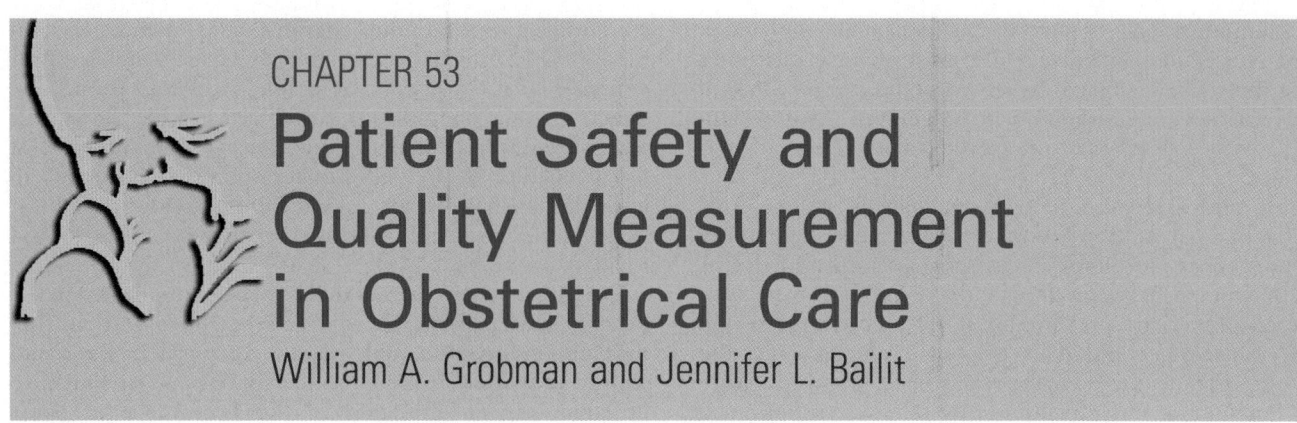

CHAPTER 53

Patient Safety and Quality Measurement in Obstetrical Care

William A. Grobman and Jennifer L. Bailit

KEY ABBREVIATIONS	
Catholic Healthcare Partners	CHP
Crew Resource Management	CRM
Hospital Corporation of America	HCA
Hypoxic-ischemic Encephalopathy	HIE
Intensive Care Unit	ICU
Institute of Medicine	IOM
Nulliparous Term Singleton Vertex	NTSV
Situation, Background, assessment, Recommendation	SBAR

Health care quality has been defined by the Institute of Medicine (IOM) as "the degree to which health services for individuals and populations increase the likelihood of desired health outcomes and are consistent with current professional knowledge."[1] Under the IOM framework, safety is part of the larger concept of health care quality.[1] The intent of this chapter is to describe methods to enhance patient safety and to measure and achieve high-quality care in obstetrics.

PATIENT SAFETY

Overview

Patient safety has become an increasing focus of the attention of the medical community. Although the reasons for the increased focus are multifactorial, one important contributor has been the recognition of significant numbers of preventable adverse events that commonly occur. The relatively high number of medical errors has been documented in the IOM report, *To Err is Human*. That report, published in 1998, suggested that between 44,000 and 98,000 mortalities occur in hospitals each year as the result of medical errors.[2] This report, correspondingly, noted the importance of error reduction as a means to improve health care and patient outcomes.

Because obstetrical admissions are the leading cause of hospitalization for women in the United States, accounting for more than 4 million hospital discharges each year,[3] pregnant women are at particular risk for encountering a medical error. Emphasizing the importance of obstetrical safety further is the fact that each obstetrical admission has the potential to affect the health not only of a single individual but of both a mother and her infant.

Frequency of Preventable Obstetrical Adverse Events

Many studies that have sought to determine the frequency of preventable obstetrical adverse events have used retrospective designs and studied in detail cases in which *adverse outcomes* have occurred. The overall frequency of preventable *adverse events* on a given obstetrical unit cannot be determined from these studies. This is particularly true given that adverse events may occur (e.g., administration of a medication to which the patient is stated to be allergic) that do not result in an actual adverse outcome (e.g., anaphylactic shock). However, these studies do give insight into the frequency with which, when an adverse outcome occurs, that adverse outcome may have been preventable.

Geller and colleagues analyzed cases of morbidity and mortality that occurred at their institution.[4] These cases included those with severe morbidity and with "near-miss" morbidity. It should be emphasized that their near-miss morbidity is not so named because a woman nearly misses having morbidity but because she nearly misses a mortal event.[5] Thus, in their framework, maternal morbidity has a spectrum of severity, and there is none that is more severe than near-miss morbidity. In their study, morbid and mortal events were often found to be preventable, with "preventable" being defined as an event that could have been avoided by any action or inaction on the part of the health care provider (e.g., clinical mismanagement, failure or delay in diagnosis), the system (e.g., failure in communication), or the patient (e.g., noncompliance). Moreover, women who had the most adverse outcomes were more likely to have had preventable events: 16% of cases with severe morbidity were judged preventable compared with 46% of near-miss events and 41% of mortal events.

Berg and associates focused exclusively on maternal deaths that occurred in North Carolina.[6] They studied the circumstances surrounding the pregnancy-related deaths of 108 women between 1995 and 1999. Death were considered potentially preventable if (1) preconception care and counseling could have improved outcome; (2) the patient had not adhered to medical advice; (3) the structure and functioning of the health care system were suboptimal; or (4) clinical care was not satisfactory. In their study, 40% of deaths were considered preventable, although this frequency significantly differed on the basis of the primary underlying cause of death. For example, 93% of deaths related to hemorrhage but only 22% of deaths related to cardiomyopathy were thought to be preventable.

White and coworkers examined 90 cases that had resulted in litigation and in which the claims had been closed.[7] It should be noted that these cases included both gynecology and obstetrics cases, although most were related to obstetrics. In their study, 78% of these cases were thought to have had a contributing factor that was potentially avoidable. Clark and colleagues also analyzed claims data and focused only on those claims related to perinatal care.[8] Their findings were quite similar to those of White and coworkers; specifically, they noted that 70% of cases were potentially preventable and related to the care the patient received in the hospital.

Forster and associates did attempt to prospectively quantify the frequency of adverse events that occur on an obstetrical unit.[9] These investigators placed an observer in the labor and delivery unit during the weekday hours of a 6-week period. This observer was trained to ascertain poor patient outcomes, procedural errors, and unsafe working conditions. Cases of concern that were ascertained by the observer were then further evaluated by a multidisciplinary team. The primary outcome of the study was the occurrence of a "quality problem," defined as the occurrence of either an adverse event (i.e., "an adverse outcome due to health care management as opposed to progression of natural disease") or a potential adverse event (i.e., "defective processes that have a high likelihood of causing harm"). Of the more than 400 patients who were cared for during the study period, 5% had a quality problem occur (2% had an adverse event, and 3% had a potential adverse event). Sixty-six percent of the adverse events that occurred were judged to be due to errors in health care delivery.

Factors Contributing to Preventable Adverse Events

The literature that exists would suggest that there are multiple factors that contribute to the occurrence of adverse obstetrical events. Data from The Joint Commission illustrate how multiple factors can precipitate major adverse maternal and perinatal outcomes. For example, their analysis of major maternal adverse events revealed multiple root causes, including the lack of adequate communication, training, staffing, and patient assessment.[10] Other investigators similarly have found that preventable adverse events or potential events cannot be traced to one simple and easily remediable cause but rather are multifactorial and due to a complex interplay of factors. Geller, White, and Forster and their colleagues all have demonstrated the many different factors present at both the provider and systems level that have contributed to adverse events.[5,7,9]

Despite the many factors that have been implicated in the occurrence of preventable adverse events, it is worth noting that communication and systems issues that transcend simple individual error consistently have been found to be predominant etiologies in the occurrence of these events.[5,7,9-11] *Systems issues* is a term that refers to problems that stem not from an individual's actions but from the interconnected relationships of people, institutional policies, and the physical environment. **With regard to the sentinel events in maternal care that were analyzed by The Joint Commission, a communications issue was judged to be present in more than 80% of cases.**[10] This frequency far outstripped the next most frequent factors—competency and patient assessment—which were present in fewer than 40% of cases. In their review of closed claims, White and coworkers noted that inadequate communication among providers was the single most common preventable factor associated with the claim.[7] Similarly, in their prospective study, Foster and associates noted that systems issues were the most common reason that their trained observer was alerted to further assess the possibility of a quality problem.[9]

Approaches to Improve Obstetrical Safety

The previous discussion highlighting the different factors that contribute to patient safety suggests that efforts to improve safety may require multiple different approaches. The potential need for a multifaceted approach is further suggested by the different levels within an organization at which these factors can manifest. **Specifically, key components required for the prevention of adverse events occur at (1) the individual level (e.g., the level of education or training provided to workers); (2) the group level (e.g., team effectiveness and communication); and (3) the structural level (e.g., standardization of processes within an organization).**[11] Correspondingly, attempts to enhance patient safety within obstetrics have used several different types of modalities. The theoretical underpinning to believe that these modalities should be effective, as well as the evidence supporting their use, with a focus on obstetrics, is discussed in the following sections.

Checklists and Protocols

Because of the complexity of health care processes and the corresponding potential for errors in communication, one approach to improve patient safety has been the introduction of standardized approaches to patient care. These approaches have taken the form of protocols (i.e., mandatory items for completion to lead the user to a predetermined outcome) and checklists (i.e., a list of action items or criteria arranged in a systematic manner, allowing the user to record the presence or absence of the individual items listed to ensure that all are considered or completed). Although both are concerned with standardization, checklists provide explicit lists of items, an action thought to be a cognitive aid because of grouping of relational items in an organized fashion in order to improve recall performance.[12]

Pronovost and coworkers have demonstrated the potential utility of checklists in their study regarding catheter-related bloodstream infections in the intensive care unit (ICU).[13] In this study, checklists detailing five key actions that were required during any central catheter placement were introduced in 108 ICUs throughout the state of Michigan. Of note, these key actions were evidence based. Also, the checklists were not merely posted, but were supported by local leaders versed in the supporting evidence who provided feedback with regard to optimal methods for implementation. Not only did the incidence of catheter-related bloodstream infections significantly decline by 3 months after implementation (incidence rate ratio [IRR], 0.62; 95% confidence interval [CI], 0.47 to 0.81), but this incidence also continued to decline until 18 months (IRR, 0.34; 95% CI, 0.23 to 0.50) after implementation, which was the end point of data collection.

A checklist to guide the administration of oxytocin was developed by Clark and colleagues, who then implemented this checklist in a private hospital setting.[14] The outcomes of the 100 women before checklist implementation were then compared with those of the 100 women receiving oxytocin after the implementation. After implementation, there was no difference in duration of labor, duration of oxytocin administration, or frequency of operative delivery, although the maximal dose of oxytocin used was significantly lower, as was the frequency of newborns with one or more complications ($P = .049$).

The potential benefits of a standardized approach to the evaluation and management of preeclampsia has been demonstrated by Menzies and associates.[15] After establishing a set of best practices, this group of investigators introduced these practices for preeclampsia management at British Columbia Women's Hospital. Among women with preeclampsia who were managed after the standardized approach was put into place, 0.7% experienced the composite end point of maternal adverse outcomes, which was an 86% reduction compared with the preintervention frequency of 5.1% ($P < .001$). Adverse perinatal outcomes also were reduced, although this finding did not reach statistical significance (odds ratio [OR], 0.65; 95% CI, 0.37 to 1.16).

Simulation

Simulation refers to the re-creation of an actual event that has previously occurred or could potentially occur.[16] **Simulation may be used to enhance patient safety in that an action or procedure can be repeated, thereby improving the execution of that action or procedure, without ever exposing providers or patients to harm.** Essentially, simulation of events is an opportunity for health care workers to prepare and train for interventions. Although simulation may have benefits for any type of obstetrical procedure (e.g., vaginal delivery), it has often been studied in the context of events such as shoulder dystocia and eclampsia. In these occurrences, simulation may be particularly helpful not only for the novice but also for experienced professionals, who can maintain skills in unpredictable and uncommon events.

Shoulder Dystocia

Data from multiple studies suggest that simulation may enhance several aspects of shoulder dystocia management, including performance of the maneuvers, communication among the team members, and documentation of the event. Moreover, these enhancements have been demonstrated for providers during both their residency training and postresidency experiences.

Deering and colleagues have demonstrated, in a randomized trial, that those residents who were assigned to train for a shoulder dystocia using an obstetrical birth simulator were significantly more likely to use maneuvers in a timely and correct fashion in a subsequent simulation when compared with those residents who did not undergo initial simulation training.[17] Furthermore, when judged by a blinded observer, those residents who had undergone simulation training scored higher on measures of overall performance and preparedness.

A study examining presimulation and postsimulation training outcomes among both residents and attending physicians was performed by Goffman and colleagues.[18] In this study, participants underwent a simulation of a shoulder dystocia event followed by a debriefing that included (1) a brief lecture about shoulder dystocia, (2) a review of the basic maneuvers and a basic algorithm for management of shoulder dystocia, (3) a discussion of optimizing team performance during an obstetrical emergency, (4) a review of the key components of documentation, and (5) a review of the digital recording of the simulations and discussion of provider performance. During a second, unanticipated, shoulder dystocia simulation, providers demonstrated significant improvements in use of maneuvers, communication, and overall performance.

Similar results were obtained by Crofts and coworkers in their multicenter comparison of presimulation and postsimulation outcomes.[19] This study additionally attempted to ascertain whether high-fidelity simulation (i.e., using a mannequin with a high degree of biofidelity) would enhance performance to a greater extent than low-fidelity simulation (e.g., using a simple doll-like mannequin) by randomizing participants to one of these options. Regardless of randomized group, performance during a simulated shoulder dystocia was improved subsequent to simulation training. Although some measures of performance (e.g., total applied force) were improved to a greater extent in those participants who had undergone high-fidelity training, many other measures (e.g., peak force, use of maneuvers) were no different between the high- and low-fidelity groups. Improvement in performance of simulated shoulder dystocia events has been demonstrated to persist up to12 months after training.[20]

The previous studies have examined outcomes during simulation events but have not demonstrated improvements in actual clinical outcomes related to simulation training. One observational study has assessed these clinical outcomes. In that study, investigators examined outcomes both before and after a shoulder dystocia training program was initiated at a single institution.[21] After the training program, there was a significant increase in the frequency with which appropriate maneuvers were used during shoulder dystocias and a significant reduction in neonatal injury at birth after shoulder dystocia (9.3% to 2.3%; relative risk [RR], 0.25; 95% CI, 0.11 to 0.57).

Eclampsia

Studies that have evaluated simulation training for eclamptic seizure management have demonstrated improvements in response as measured during additional simulations. For example, after having staff in a single center participate in simulated eclamptic events with a debriefing session, Thompson and colleagues found that subsequent simulations of eclampsia were associated with patient resuscitations that were better managed.[22] Of note, these authors conducted their simulations on the actual delivery unit (as opposed to a separate simulation laboratory) and used their initial simulations not only for training but also for elucidating site-specific barriers (e.g., efficient paging system) to an optimal response. This ability of simulation to identify systems-level barriers to best practice has been noted by others as well.[23]

Ellis and associates also examined pretraining and posttraining outcomes during eclampsia simulations.[24] In their study, training was associated with an increase in the appropriate and timely completion of desired tasks (e.g., magnesium sulfate administration). Of note, although all participants underwent simulation training, they also were randomized to different training sites (i.e., simulation center vs. hospital unit) and to inclusion of teamwork training in their educational process. Neither site nor additional teamwork education was associated with additional improvement in performance.

Other Obstetrical Events

Other obstetrical events that have been examined in the context of simulation include breech delivery, postpartum hemorrhage, and cord prolapse. In one study that focused on breech delivery, residents, after undergoing a simulation of an imminent term vaginal breech, took part in a training session with the simulator on the proper techniques for vaginal breech delivery.[25] After this training, residents repeated the standardized simulation. Simulations both before and after training were videotaped and judged by an investigator who was blinded to whether the simulation occurred before or after training. Scores for skill and safety were significantly greater for residents participating in the simulated breech delivery after the training. With regard to postpartum hemorrhage, Toledo and colleagues used simulated examples of blood loss volumes to improve care providers' accuracy with regard to blood loss estimation.[26]

Siassakos and colleagues assessed whether clinical outcomes associated with cord prolapse improved after introduction of an obstetrical emergency training program that included cord prolapse drills.[27] They found that after these drills, there was a significant reduction in diagnosis to delivery interval (25 to 14.5 minutes; P <.001), although no significant difference in low Apgar scores or rate of admission to the neonatal ICU could be found.

Draycott and colleagues also examined clinical outcomes after introduction of a training session that included fetal heart tracing education and drills in shoulder dystocia, postpartum hemorrhage, eclampsia, twin deliveries, breech deliveries, adult resuscitation (including cardiopulmonary resuscitation), and neonatal resuscitation.[28] After this training, the frequency of hypoxic-ischemic encephalopathy (HIE) decreased by about half at their institution (27.3 to 13.6 per 10,000 births; P = .03). This decrease did not appear to be related to other preexisting trends in the frequency of HIE or changes in the population during the period of study.

Enhancement of Communication in General

Rather than focus on simulation of specific obstetrical events, some investigators have focused on improvement of communication processes and teamwork in general. One approach to this is through the establishment of a specific team that is trained to function and be engaged specifically at the time of obstetrical emergencies. **One institution, for example, created a "Condition O" team, according the precepts outlined for rapid-response systems.[29] These precepts include (1) case detection that triggers a medical crisis team response, (2) a medical crisis team response available at all times, (3) an evaluation and process improvement system, and (4) an administrative structure to support the system.** After implementation of this system, the investigators reported several quality improvement interventions that were able to be introduced because of case reviews associated with Condition O being invoked, although improvements in particular outcomes were not yet demonstrated.

A different approach is the training for and implementation of standardized communication processes throughout a unit or institution. **One often-cited approach to this type of intervention is Crew Resource Management (CRM). CRM training has been used extensively within the airline industry, where it was noted that accidents were primarily related to lack of coordination and poor teamwork.[30] CRM seeks to engender effective communication through standardized language, situational awareness, briefing and debriefing, and a leveling of hierarchy, allowing all team members to voice concerns about safety.** There is some evidence both from observational longitudinal studies and randomized trials that communication training can improve teamwork and communication among providers.[31,32]

In one longitudinal observational study, the introduction of a CRM course at a single institution was noted to be associated with a 62% reduction in "law suits, claims, and observation" of cases (i.e., those cases in which the insurance carrier reserves money) that were of high severity.[33] However, in the one randomized trial that was performed, and in which this CRM course (i.e., the MedTeams Labor and Delivery Team Coordination Course) was evaluated, investigators reported that institutions that were randomized to the intervention were no more likely to reduce the primary measure of obstetrical adverse outcomes (i.e., mean Adverse Outcome Index) than institutions that received no intervention at all.[34]

Multifaceted Approaches

Some have asserted that the complexity of obstetrical care is such that improvements in safety will come not through the use of one particular intervention but from a multifaceted approach that ultimately results in a fundamental

culture change within an institution. Correspondence with principles of high-reliability organizations have helped to guide some of these efforts. Longitudinal observational studies have suggested that the introduction of such programs is associated with outcome improvements. Examples of such programs have been reported by the following organizations:

- *Catholic Healthcare Partners* (CHP).[35] CHP instituted a program at 16 sites that included interdisciplinary education, routine medical record reviews to monitor ongoing adherence to appropriate practice, and standardization of forms to encourage adherence with best practices. After introduction of this program, birth trauma rates decreased from 5.0 to 0.17 per 1000 births, and the number of adverse obstetrical occurrences (specified as a birth-related event or injury that may lead to a claim) decreased by 65%, from 7.2 to 2.5 per 1000 births.
- *Seton Family Hospitals.*[36] At four sites, this organization began a program that included standardization of forms and care processes, introduction of routine communication processes such as SBAR (situation, background, assessment, recommendation), active surveillance of adverse outcomes with temporally proximate feedback, and interdisciplinary obstetrical crisis simulation with high-fidelity mannequins. Subsequent to the introduction of this program, birth injury rates declined from a 2-year average of 0.3% to 0.08%, and the average length of stay for infants admitted to the neonatal ICU for birth injury declined by 80%.
- *Yale–New Haven Hospital.*[37] This obstetrical department began a program of outside expert review of adverse events, anonymous event reporting, protocol standardization, the creation of a patient safety nurse position and patient safety committee, and training in team skills and fetal heart monitoring interpretation. Introduction of this program was associated with a significant reduction ($P = .01$) in their outcome of choice, the mean quarterly Adverse Outcome Index.
- *Hospital Corporation of America* (HCA).[38] HCA instituted a program including standardized processes, active peer review and feedback, and the empowerment of any member of the health care team to halt care considered possibly dangerous. Subsequent to this program's initiation, there was a significant reduction ($P < .001$) in the number of professional liability claims per 10,000 deliveries.

Summary

It seems clear that at least some of the adverse outcomes that occur in obstetrics are preventable and that the root causes of these preventable events, although many, often involve communication and teamwork. Theory supports several different approaches to error reduction, many of which have been used in obstetrics. **Although some studies have documented improvements in outcomes related to patient safety initiatives, these studies have been predominantly observational and have used different outcomes (e.g., provider satisfaction and perception, demonstration of skill acquisition in simulated scenarios, actual care processes, actual patient outcomes) to assess improvement.** Further work will be necessary to understand best the combination of practices and practice methodologies (e.g., simulation on site versus simulation in a laboratory) that most effectively improves care.

MEASUREMENT OF OBSTETRICAL QUALITY OF CARE

Understanding whether safe care is being provided and whether changes in approaches to patient safety are actually improving the quality of care requires measurement. Examples of patient safety measures include "retained surgical sponge" or "wrong site surgery" rates. In contrast, a quality measure assesses the degree to which maternal and neonatal care is optimized. This section details different approaches to measurement that have been used in an effort to optimize obstetrical care.

Overview

Many types of stakeholders have an interest in high-quality obstetrical care. Patients, physicians, and insurers desire high obstetrical quality at an affordable cost. However, each of these groups may perceive quality differently. Patients want to feel that their physicians are caring individuals and produce good outcomes. Physicians want to be sure that they have the best possible outcome for the patient but also, regardless of outcome, that they are employing best practices. Insurers are primarily concerned with whether the care given is cost effective. Each of these groups wants and needs access to quality measures that reflect their own interests. Thus, one of the first steps in measuring quality is to understand how and by whom the measure will be used.

Type of Quality Measures

There are three major categories of quality measures: structure, outcome, and process.[39] **Structural measures** assume that if the hospital contains high-quality components, the product (medical care) will be of high quality as well. Examples of structural measures include board certification, physician licensure, and hospital accreditation. Structural measures are appealing because they are easy to measure and reproduce. However, although structural measures may reflect that optimal structures are present, these measures do not guarantee that the different components of the hospital will work well together.

Outcome measures, as indicated by their name, reflect patient outcomes. Examples of outcome measures are "the frequency of maternal mortality" and "the frequency of neonatal hypoglycemia." **Because obstetricians generally treat healthy women, adverse outcomes in obstetrics are relatively uncommon. Consequently, the usefulness of many outcome measures (e.g., maternal mortality) may be limited because most hospitals may have none or few of these outcomes to measure.** Furthermore, if outcome measures are to be maximally useful and reflective of the actual care provided at a given institution, they need to reflect outcomes that the institution can actually affect and be **risk-adjusted** in order to account for differences in patient populations that may materially affect the outcome of interest. For example, although "preterm birth" is an adverse outcome, "frequency of preterm birth" may not be a good measure to reflect a hospital's quality of care given the lack of useful interventions to prevent this adverse outcome. Also, a comparison of hospitals according to their frequency of peripartum hysterectomies may not reflect comparative quality of care if one hospital is much more likely to care for women with abnormal placentation. Finally, outcome measures may pose distinct challenges in obstetrics, when outcomes of two patients, the mother and the baby, occur. Thus, although a hospital may have comparatively good maternal outcomes, it also may have comparatively poor neonatal outcomes, and examination of only one of these sets of outcomes would not fully convey the care environment.

Process measures reflect practices that physicians or hospitals actually employ in their care of patients. An example of a process measure is "the frequency with which known GBS positive women receive appropriate antibiotics." **If a process measure were to conceivably be an adequate reflection of care quality, there should be evidence that the process is related to improved outcomes.** The most central advantage of a process measure is that it gives direct insight into desired actions within the health care system. Correspondingly, these measures give immediately insight into the processes that need to be attended to in order to enhance patient care. Conversely, one of the disadvantages of process measures is that outcomes are often due to the interplay of many different factors and processes, and improvements in these process measures may give false reassurance that improvements in quality of care have been fully realized.

With these considerations in mind, several criteria should be considered in whether a measure meets criteria for a good measure. **A good measures should (1) balance maternal and neonatal outcomes (e.g., not reflect improved care for one member of the mother-child dyad while embodying markedly worse care for the other), (2) have the potential to be altered by behaviors within the health care system of interest, (3) be affordable and applicable for use on a large scale, (4) be acceptable to stakeholders as a meaningful marker of quality, and (5) be reliable and reproducible.**[40]

Attempts to Establish Quality Measures

Because measuring the quality of care is a seminal step in improving patient safety and achieving enhanced quality care, there have been many attempts by a multitude of different organizations to determine quality measures in obstetrics. In lieu of reviewing all current quality measures, we have chosen to present some examples of measures to illustrate the strengths and weaknesses of different choices. The examples include traditional measures as well as those more recently suggested.

Traditional Measures

The more traditional measures often have been raw frequencies of selected adverse outcomes. One example of this type of measure is maternal mortality. It has been used because it is clearly a catastrophic bad outcome and there is little potential for misascertainment. However, in the modern era within developed countries, maternal mortality is so relatively uncommon that it is difficult to use within a hospital or health care system to reflect quality of health care. Many hospitals will have no maternal mortality even over a period of many years, and few hospitals will have a sufficient number of cases to enable them to use this measure to track their adequacy of care delivery. Furthermore, the absence of this outcome does not mandate that good-quality care is being provided; lack of quality care may still exist, and poor outcomes, short of death, may still be present. This does not suggest that any maternal mortality should not be fully investigated as a critical part of quality assurance and improvement efforts, but only that maternal mortality is unlikely to be useful as a quality marker for intrainstitutional quality tracking and interinstitutional comparisons.

Neonatal mortality has also been used as a marker of obstetrical quality. Neonatal mortality may be problematic as a marker for obstetrical quality for several reasons. First, when a neonate dies, it is unclear to what extent obstetrical care, pediatric care, or both may have contributed. Second, a large proportion of mortality is due to prematurity and lethal birth defects, neither of which can be materially affected by obstetrical care.[41] Thus, the residual fraction of obstetrics-related mortality is relatively small and once again may be so uncommon as to limit its use for evaluation of trends or institutional comparisons.

The cesarean delivery rate has been a common measure employed to reflect obstetrical quality of care. Although there is debate about whether cesarean delivery is a process measure or an outcome measure, it is regardless a flawed measure. First, because of perinatal regionalization, women with greater obstetrical complications are concentrated at particular hospitals best suited to providing specialized care. Thus, a comparison of cesarean rates among hospitals without accounting for the differences in patient populations among these hospitals may be misleading. Hospitals with the highest cesarean rates may be giving high-quality care but have high rates because of their patient population. Conversely, a hospital may be giving poor care and have an average rate of cesarean delivery when in fact the cesarean rate should be much lower for their low-risk population.

Newer Approaches to Measures

Although the use of "raw" cesarean rates to measure quality is not ideal, cesarean delivery rates are appealing as a measure because cesarean is an event that is easy to ascertain and is meaningful to multiple stakeholders. One approach to try and account for population differences among institutions is to calculate and use a "risk-adjusted" cesarean rate. **Many different techniques for risk adjustment for cesarean delivery, as well as other obstetrical outcomes, have been described.**[42-47] **Fundamentally, risk adjustment creates a model that predicts what the cesarean rate should be for the particular patient population and allows comparison with the actual rate.** By taking account of differences (such as parity, plurality, and comorbidities) among populations, risk-adjustment seeks to reflect differences in outcomes related to the health care system and not the patients contained within it.

Another approach to determining an outcome measure that is dependent on the health care system rather than the differences in patient populations is to determine an outcome frequency not for all women under care but for a more homogeneous group. Main and colleagues have suggested, for example, the use of a cesarean rate only among nulliparous women who have a term singleton fetus in the vertex (NTSV) presentation.[48] Using data from the Sutter Health Care network of 20 birthing units, in which more than 40,000 women each year deliver, Main and colleagues determined age-adjusted NTSV cesarean rates. They found that 53% of the variation in NTSV cesarean rates was associated with differences in frequency of labor induction and early admission in labor. This finding suggests that some health care practices are associated with the NTSV cesarean rate. The disadvantage of the NTSV cesarean rate is that it excludes women having preterm deliveries and those who are multiparous, and thus gives no insight into their care.

One process measure that has recently gained attention is a "scheduled elective delivery prior to 39 weeks of gestation." This measure has gained popularity as the risks of early term birth have become better known.[49,50] This process measure has the advantage of being well supported by evidence, reflects a practice under the control of the health care system, and does not require risk adjustment. The difficulty with this measure is the lack of consensus for several indications as to whether or not they are indeed elective.

The frequency with which antenatal corticosteroids are administered to infants who are delivered at less than 34 weeks is another measure that has become widely used. This process measure is appealing because of the data showing that antenatal corticosteroids improve outcomes for premature infants. Nevertheless, this measure does have its disadvantages. Ascertainment of steroid administration, especially in a health care setting without electronic medical records, can be difficult. Steroids given during the pregnancy, but not during the delivery hospitalization, are time intensive to ascertain because inpatient and outpatient records may need to be reviewed. And, although 100% administration is the goal, it is not possible to administer corticosteroids to all women before premature delivery because of late patient arrival or emergent circumstances, such as a maternal trauma.

The frequency of neonates with a birthweight of less than 1500 g born outside of a tertiary care center is one recently suggested process measure that is appealing because it may reflect adequacy of coordination of an entire health care system. Although there are data that very-low-birthweight neonates have worse outcomes when delivered outside of a tertiary care center, many incentives may work against delivery at such a location.[51-53] This measure is easy to calculate from birth certificates, and the items from the birth certificate that are needed to calculate the measure are reliable.[43]

The quality measures discussed thus far have represented inpatient care. Outpatient quality measures do exist, although they are often process measures. An example of such a measure is the frequency with which pregnant women receive HIV screening early in their antepartum care.[54] One difficulty with these measures has to do with accurate ascertainment because prenatal care happens in many different settings and outpatient medical records data are often not in electronic form. Furthermore, although hospitals are required to generate administrative data that can be helpful for measuring inpatient quality, outpatient clinics are not required to generate the same kind of data.

Data Sources

Administrative data (i.e., data collected primarily for billing or nonmedical purposes) are a rich source of information. Administrative data have the advantages of being complete for the population and relatively cheap to use. **Unfortunately, administrative data often lack the clinical detail needed to make meaningful quality judgments.**[55] Paper-based medical records contain clinical detail but are hard to obtain in a uniform manner for a population and are expensive to collect.

Increasingly, electronic medical records have been used to provide the basis for quality measures. These data are easy to collect within an institution and have clinical detail. However, because there are many different types of electronic medical records systems, collating medical records information from many sources can be time intensive. **Electronic medical records also can have the advantage of linking outpatient and inpatient information, something that is very difficult to do with administrative data or paper-based medical records.** The types of information that are available from electronic medical records will increase and improve with time, and there is hope that eventually vital statistics records will be based on actual medical records rather than data extraction, thereby making birth certificate data a richer, more accurate source of medical data.

Quality Improvement

The main point of measuring quality of care is to use the measurements to improve care. Quality measurement tools allow stakeholders to assess the effects of changes in the system. **There are many ways to accomplish improved quality of care with measurement, but one of the most effective is benchmarking.**[56] **Benchmarking, also known as audit and feedback, is a technique whereby quality is measured, compared with like entities, and then shared back with the participants, often in a blinded manner.** For example, NTSV rates for all the hospitals in a city would be calculated. Each hospital would then receive a graph showing their rate (unblinded) compared with the rates of all the other hospitals (blinded) in the city.

One example in which this technique has been used and believed to be helpful was in the Ohio Perinatal Quality Collaborative.[57] This was a group of 20 hospitals in Ohio that came together to share data and compare techniques on how to lower the frequency of scheduled deliveries before 39 weeks' gestation without documentation of a medical indication. Each hospital collected data on the scheduled deliveries 36 0/7 to 38 6/7 weeks in their own institution and submitted the data to a central location for data collation. This data center then created reports that showed each hospital their own rate compared with the rates of all the other hospitals. Each hospital took that information and designed their own program to lower their frequency. There were monthly phone calls for hospitals to share their designs and progress. At the initiation of the project, 25% of scheduled deliveries between 36 and 38 6/7 weeks did not have a documented medical indications; this frequency was lowered to less than 5% ($P < .05$) after 1 year. It was estimated that approximately 1000 births were moved from between 36 0/7 and 38 6/7 to over 39 weeks' gestation in the state of Ohio during the 12 months of this effort.

Summary

No one measure of quality is perfect, and a variety of quality measures will be needed to give a complete picture of the quality of obstetrical care.[58] Structure, process, and outcomes measures all have a role in measuring quality of care and moving toward optimal health care delivery. Hospitals, providers, patients, and insurers can use these different types of measures to help track the care being provided and better understand the areas that need to be targeted for improvement.

KEY POINTS

- A proportion of adverse obstetrical events have been shown to be preventable; this proportion varies with the clinical circumstances.
- Although multiple factors have been associated with the occurrence of adverse obstetrical events, issues with communication have been implicated as a frequent contributor.
- Because different factors contribute to patient safety, efforts to improve safety may require multiple different approaches.
- Specific approaches that have been considered to enhance obstetrical patient safety include checklists and protocols, simulation, and teamwork training.
- Further investigation is required to understand what approaches, and combinations of approaches, most improve clinical care and outcomes.
- Quality measure assesses the degree to which maternal and neonatal care is optimized.
- Major categories of quality measures include structural, process, and outcome measures.

REFERENCES

1. Lohr KN, Schroeder SA: A strategy for quality assurance in Medicare. N Engl J Med 322:707, 1990.
2. Institute of Medicine: To Err Is Human: Building a Safer Health Care System. Washington, DC, National Academy Press, 1999.
3. DeFrances C, Hall M, Podgornik M: 2003 National Hospital Discharge Survey. Advance Data from Vital and Health Statistics; no. 359. Hyattsville, MD, National Center for Health Statistics, 2005.
4. Geller SE, Rosenberg D, Cox SM, et al: The continuum of maternal morbidity and mortality: factors associated with severity. Am J Obstet Gynecol 191:939, 2004.
5. Geller SE, Rosenberg D, Cox S, et al: A scoring system identified near-miss maternal morbidity during pregnancy. J Clin Epidemiol 57:716, 2004.
6. Berg CJ, Harper MA, Atkinson S, et al: Preventability of pregnancy-related deaths. Obstet Gynecol 106:1228, 2005.
7. White AA, Pichert JW, Bledsoe SH, et al: Cause and effect analysis of closed claims in obstetrics and gynecology. Obstet Gynecol 105:1031, 2005.
8. Clark SL, Belfort MA, Dildy GA, Meyers JA: Reducing obstetric litigation through alterations in practice patterns. Am J Obstet 112:1279, 2010.
9. Forster AJ, Fung I, Caughey S, et al: Adverse events detected by clinical surveillance on an obstetric service. Obstet Gynecol 108:1073, 2006.
10. The Joint Commission: Sentinel Event Alert. Available at: http://www.jointcommission.org/SentinelEvents/SentinelEventAlert/sea_30.htm. Accessed May 10, 2010.
11. Hoff T, Jameson L, Hannan E, Fink E: A Review of the Literature Examining Linkages between Organizational Factors, Medical Errors, and Patient Safety. Med Care Res Rev 61:3, 2004.
12. Hales BM, Pronovost PJ: The checklist: a tool for error management and performance improvement. J Crit Care 21:231, 2006.
13. Pronovost P, Needham D, Berenholtz S: An intervention to decrease catheter-related bloodstream infections in the ICU. N Engl J Med 355:2725, 2006.
14. Clark S, Belfort M, Saade G, et al: Implementation of a conservative checklist-based protocol for oxytocin administration: maternal and newborn outcomes. Am J Obstet Gynecol 197:480.e1, 2007.
15. Menzies J, Magee LA, Li J, et al: Instituting surveillance guidelines and adverse outcomes in preeclampsia. Obstet Gynecol 110:121, 2007.
16. Hunt EA, Shilkofski NA, Atavroudis TA, Nelson KL: Simulation: translation to improved team performance. Anesthesiol Clin 25:301, 2007.
17. Deering S, Poggi S, Macedonia C, et al: Improving resident competency in the management of shoulder dystocia with simulation training. Obstet Gynecol 103:1224, 2004.
18. Goffman D, Heo H, Pardanani S, et al: Improving shoulder dystocia management among resident and attending physicians using simulations. Am J Obstet Gynecol 199:294.e1, 2008.
19. Crofts JF, Bartlett C, Ellis D, et al: Training for shoulder dystocia: a trial of simulation using low-fidelity and high-fidelity mannequins. Obstet Gynecol 108:1477, 2006.
20. Crofts JF, Bartlett C, Ellis D, et al: Management of shoulder dystocia: skill retention 6 and 12 months after training. Obstet Gynecol 110:1069, 2007.
21. Draycott TJ, Crofts JF, Ash JP, et al: Improving neonatal outcome through practical shoulder dystocia training. Obstet Gynecol 112:14, 2008.
22. Thompson S, Neal S, Clark V: Clinical risk management in obstetrics: eclampsia drills. Qual Safety Health Care 13:127, 2004.
23. Osman H, Campbell OMR, Nass AH: Using emergency obstetric drills in maternity units as a performance improvement tool. Birth 36:43, 2009.
24. Ellis D, Crofts JF, Hunt LP, et al: Hospital, simulation center and teamwork training for eclampsia management. Obstet Gynecol 111:723, 2008.
25. Deering S, Brown J, Hodor J, Satin AJ: Simulation training and resident performance of singleton vaginal breech delivery. Obstet Gynecol 107:86, 2006.
26. Toledo P, McCarthy RJ, Burke CA, et al: The effect of live and web-based education on the accuracy of blood loss estimation in simulated obstetric scenarios. Am J Obstet Gynecol 202:400.e1, 2010.
27. Siassakos D, Hasafa Z, Sibanda T, et al: Retrospective cohort study of diagnosis-delivery interval with umbilical cord prolapse: the effect of team training. BJOG 116:1089, 2009.
28. Draycott T, Sibanda T, Owen L: Does training in obstetric emergencies improve neonatal outcome? BJOG 113:177, 2006.
29. Gosman GG Baldisseri MR, Stein KL: Introduction of an obstetric-specific medical emergency team for obstetric crises: implementation and experience. Am J Obstet Gynecol 198:367.e1, 2008.
30. Helmreich RL, Merritt AC, Wilhelm JA: The evolution of Crew Resource Management training in commercial aviation. Int J Aviat Psychol 9:19, 1999.
31. Alder, JR, Christen R, Zemp E, Bitzer J: Communication skills training in obstetrics and gynaecology: whom should we train? A randomized controlled trial. Arch Gynecol Obstet 276:605, 2007.
32. Haller G, Garnerin P, Morales M, et al: Effect of crew resource management training in a multidisciplinary obstetrical setting. Int J Qual Health Care 20:254, 2008.
33. Pratt, SD, Mann S, Salisburty M, et al: Impact of CRM-based training on obstetric outcomes and clinicians' patient safety attitudes. Jt Comm J Qual Patient Saf 33:720, 2007.
34. Nielsen, PE, Goldman MB, Mann S, et al: Effects of teamwork training on adverse outcomes and process of care in labor and delivery: a randomized controlled trial. Obstet Gynecol 109:48, 2007.
35. Simpson KR, Kort CC, Knox GE: A comprehensive perinatal patient safety program to reduce preventable adverse outcomes and costs of liability claims. Jt Comm J Qual Patient Saf 35:565, 2009.
36. Mazza F, Kitchens J, Akin M: The road to zero preventable birth injuries. Jt Comm J Qual Patient Saf 34:201, 2008.

37. Pettker CM, Thung SF, Norwitz ER, et al: Impact of a comprehensive patient safety strategy on obstetric adverse events. Am J Obstet Gynecol 200:492.e1, 2009.
38. Clark SL, Belfort MA, Byrum SL, et al: Improved outcomes, fewer cesarean deliveries, and reduced litigation: results of a new paradigm in patient safety. Am J Obstet Gynecol 199:105.e1, 2008.
39. Donabedian A: Evaluating the quality of medical care. Milbank Mem Fund 44:166, 1966.
40. Bailit JL, Love TE, Dawson NV: Quality of obstetric care and risk-adjusted primary cesarean delivery rates. Am J Obstet Gynecol 194:402, 2006.
41. Hein H, Lofgren M: The changing pattern of neonatal mortality in a regionalized system of perinatal care: a current update. Pediatrics 104:1064, 1999.
42. Keeler E, Park R, Bell R, et al: Adjusting cesarean delivery rates for case mix. Health Serv Res 32:511, 1997.
43. Bailit J, Garrett J: Comparison of risk-adjustment methodologies. Obstet Gynecol 102:45, 2003.
44. Aron D, Harper D, Shepardson L, Rosenthal G: Impact of risk-adjusting cesarean delivery rates when reporting hospital performance. JAMA 279:1968, 1998.
45. Glantz JC: Cesarean delivery risk adjustment for regional interhospital comparisons. Am J Obstet Gynecol 181:1425, 1999.
46. Gregory KD, Korst LM, Platt LD: Variation in elective primary cesarean delivery by patient and hospital factors. Am J Obstet Gynecol 184:1521, 2001.
47. Grobman WA, Feinglass J, Murthy S: Are the Agency for Healthcare Research and Quality obstetric trauma indicators valid measures of hospital safety? Am J Obstet Gynecol 195:868, 2006.
48. Main EK, Moore D, Farrell B, et al: Is there a useful cesarean birth measure? Assessment of the nulliparous term singleton vertex cesarean birth rate as a tool for obstetric quality improvement. Am J Obstet Gynecol 194:1644, 2006.
49. Tita AT, Landon MB, Spong CY, et al: Timing of elective repeat cesarean delivery at term and neonatal outcomes. N Engl J Med 360:111, 2009.
50. Bailit J, Gregory K, Reddy U, et al: Maternal and neonatal outcomes by labor onset type and gestational age. Am J Obstet Gynecol 202:243, 2010.
51. Warner B, Musial J, Chenier T, Donovan D: The effect of birth hospital type on the outcomes of very low birth weight infants. Pediatrics 113:35, 2004.
52. Chien L, Whyte R, Aziz K, et al: Improved outcome of preterm infants when delivered in tertiary care center. Obstet Gynecol 98:247, 2001.
53. Phibbs C, Bronstein J, Buxton E, Phibbs R: The effect of patient volume and level of care at the hospital of birth and neonatal mortality. JAMA 276:1054, 1996.
54. Agency for Health Care Research and Quality: Prenatal care: percentage of patients, regardless of age, who gave birth during a 12-month period who were screened for HIV infection during the first or second prenatal care visit. National Quality Measures Clearinghouse. Available at: http://qualitymeasures.ahrq.gov/content.aspx?id=11683. Accessed September 23, 2010.
55. Bailit J: Rates of labor induction without medical indication are overestimated when derived from birth certificate data. Am J Obstet Gynecol 203:269.e1, 2010.
56. Jamtvedt G, Young JM, Kristoffersen DT, et al: Audit and feedback: effects on professional practice and health are outcomes. Cochrane Database Syst Rev 2:2, 2004.
57. Iams J, for the Ohio Perinatal Quality Collaborative: A statewide initiative to reduce inappropriate scheduled births at 36 0/7 to 38 6/7 weeks' gestation. Am J Obstet Gynecol 202:243.e1, 2010.
58. Pronovost PJ, Thompson DA, Holzmueller CG, et al: Defining and measuring patient safety. Crit Care Clin 21:1, 2005.

CHAPTER 54

Legal and Ethical Issues in Obstetrical Practice

George J. Annas and Sherman Elias

Society has great expectations that modern medical technologies will improve longevity and quality of human life, and nowhere are these expectations higher than in the practice of obstetrics and the desire and expectation of having a healthy child. Along with the rapidly expanding capabilities in diagnosis and treatment, physicians find themselves facing numerous ethical dilemmas while practicing in a legal and social climate in which malpractice suits can threaten even the most competent and conscientious practitioner.

We cannot address in a single chapter the wide variety of ethical and legal controversies facing contemporary obstetrical practice and research. Instead, we focus on selected topics of particular relevance to the practicing obstetrician.

REPRODUCTIVE LIBERTY*

Although only about one in four pregnancies ends in elective abortion, abortion has been the most controversial and political medical procedure in the United States for the past four decades. The political debate over abortion has shifted among various dichotomous views of the world: life versus choice, fetus versus woman, fetus versus baby, constitutional rights versus states' rights, government versus physician, physician and patient versus state legislature. Most recently, in 2010, the abortion debate came close to derailing the Affordable Care Act, and was also the basis for an injunction temporarily halting National Institutes of Health (NIH) funding of human embryonic stem cell research. Because the 1973 U.S. Supreme Court opinion of *Roe v. Wade* remains so central to the law (and ethics) regarding the physician-patient relationship, as well as federal financing and regulation of clinical medicine and research, it is essential that obstetricians have a clear understanding of *Roe* and its enduring influence on patient rights—especially reproductive liberty, medical practice, and politics.[1]

Hundreds of statutes (including relatively new ones requiring ultrasound images of the fetus be made available to pregnant women before abortion, and suggesting that 20-week-old fetuses feel pain), and almost two dozen Supreme Court decisions on abortion later, the core legal aspects of *Roe v. Wade*,[2] the most controversial health-related decision by the Court ever, remain substantially the same as they were in 1973. Attempts to overturn *Roe* in both the courtroom and the legislature have failed, although they continue. **Pregnant women still have a constitutional right to abortion. The fetus is still not a person under the Constitution.** States still cannot make abortion a crime (either for the woman or the physician) before the fetus becomes viable (with the exception of the use of a specific procedure labeled "partial-birth abortion" by Congress). States still can outlaw abortion after the fetus becomes viable only if there is an exception that permits abortion to protect the life or health of the pregnant woman. And states still can impose restrictions on abortion before fetal viability only if those restrictions do not actually create a substantial obstacle to a pregnant woman's obtaining an abortion.

The first case to embrace the concept of reproductive liberty was *Griswold v. Connecticut*, in which the Court ruled in 1965 that a Connecticut statute criminalizing the use of contraceptives violated the constitutional right to privacy that married couples had in sexual relations.[3] Later, in 1972, the Court found that even outside marriage, a person had a "right to privacy…to be free from unwarranted governmental intrusion into matters so fundamentally affecting a person as the decision to bear or beget a child."[4] The following year, in *Roe*, the Court struck down a Texas law that made it a crime for physicians to perform an abortion unless it was necessary to save the life of the patient; there were no exceptions for the woman's health. The Court held that women have a constitutional right of privacy that is fundamental and "broad enough to encompass a woman's decision…to terminate her pregnancy."[2] Because the right is fundamental, states that wish to restrict abortion rights were required to demonstrate a compelling interest to restrict the exercise of this right. The Court ruled that the

*This section is adapted from Annas,[1] with permission.

state's interest in the life of the fetus became compelling only at the point of viability, defined as the point at which the fetus can survive independently of its mother. Even after the point of viability, the state cannot favor the life of the fetus over the life or health of the pregnant woman. Under the right of privacy, physicians must be free to use their "medical judgment for the preservation of the life or health of the mother."[2] On the same day that the Court decided *Roe*, it also decided *Doe v. Bolton*,[5] in which the Court defined health very broadly: "The medical judgment may be exercised in the light of all factors—physical, emotional, psychological, familial, and the woman's age—relevant to the well-being of the patient. All these factors may relate to health. This allows the attending physician the room he needs to make his best medical judgment."[5]

Roe and *Doe* together established that both physician and patient were protected by the constitutional right of privacy. In later cases, the Court continued to defer to the medical judgment of the attending physician. For example, in 1976 in *Planned Parenthood of Central Missouri v. Danforth*, the Court concluded that state legislatures could not determine when viability occurred; rather this "essentially medical concept…is, and must be, a matter for the judgment of the responsible attending physician."[6] This remains the case today; even as viability in general moves earlier in the pregnancy, it is not up to legislatures or courts to determine when an individual fetus is viable by drawing a line based on the age of the fetus—the viability of a specific fetus remains a matter of medical judgment to be determined by the attending physicians in a manner consistent with good and accepted obstetrical practice. **By the end of the 1980s, a pattern in Court decisions could be discerned in which abortion regulations that significantly burdened a woman's decision, treated abortion differently from other similar medical or surgical procedures, interfered with the exercise of professional judgment by the attending physician, or were stricter than accepted medical standards were struck down by the Court.**[7] Privacy as a constitutional right became a one-word description of liberty to make decisions regarding marriage, procreation, contraception, sterilization, abortion, family relationships, child rearing, and sexual relationships free of governmental interference.

One strategy to change *Roe* was to change the composition of the Supreme Court by appointing anti-*Roe* justices. Because of new justices on the Court in 1992, in *Casey*, the Court had its first real opportunity to overturn *Roe v. Wade*. Many Court observers thought it would. Instead, in an unusual procedure for the Court, three potentially anti-*Roe* justices, Justices Sandra Day O'Connor, David Souter, and Anthony Kennedy, joined together to write a joint opinion confirming the "core holding" of *Roe*. (They were joined in most of their opinion by two justices who would have simply upheld *Roe*, making this a 5-to-4 decision.) Most centrally, the authors of the joint opinion believed that although the pressure to overrule *Roe* had grown "more intense," doing so would severely and unnecessary damage the Court's legitimacy by undermining "the Nation's commitment to the rule of law."[8] Specifically, the three justices wrote that they were reaffirming "*Roe*'s essential holding" that before the point of viability a woman has a right to choose abortion without undue state interference, that after the point of viability the state can restrict abortion "if the law contains exceptions for pregnancies which endanger the woman's life or health," and that "the state has legitimate interests from the outset of the pregnancy in protecting the health of the woman and the life of the fetus that may become a child." The Court applied these principles to uphold laws mandating much more detailed requirements for abortion, as well as a mandatory 24-hour waiting period, but struck down a spousal-notification requirement as an "undue burden." Thus, **after *Casey*, *Roe* stood for the proposition that pregnant women have a "personal liberty" right ("privacy" went unmentioned) to choose to terminate their pregnancies before the point of viability and that the state cannot "unduly burden" such a right by erecting barriers that effectively prevent the exercise of that choice.**[9] Of course, a major problem was definitional: burdensome regulations were acceptable, "unduly burdensome" ones were not—but it was not clear what qualified as which. Put another way, the state could demonstrate its concern for fetal life by requiring that physicians make women seeking abortions jump through new and burdensome hoops (including offers of detailed and accurate information on abortion, the status of the fetus, adoption, sources of help for childbirth, and a 24-hour waiting period), as long as doing so did not "unduly burden" women by actually preventing them from being able to make a decision to have an abortion. With the loss of a realistic expectation in 1992 that the Court would overrule *Roe* wholesale without significant changes in the Court's membership, **anti-*Roe* advocates switched strategies dramatically, focusing on criminalizing a specific procedure that they believed would horrify most Americans and that they labeled "partial-birth abortion."** The first such bill passed Congress in 1996 and was vetoed by President Bill Clinton because the prohibition did not contain an exception for the health of the woman, as required by *Roe* and *Casey*. In 1997, this time with the support of the American Medical Association, the bill passed Congress again. President Clinton vetoed it, again for failure to contain a health exception.[10]

Proponents of the ban took their cause to the individual states, most of which enacted substantially identical laws. In 2000, Nebraska's partial-birth abortion law reached the Supreme Court. The Nebraska law carried a penalty of up to 20 years in prison for physicians who performed the procedure. The law reads in relevant part:

> No partial-birth abortion shall be performed in this state, unless such a procedure is necessary to save the life of the mother whose life is endangered by a physical disorder, physical illness, or physical injury, including a life-endangering physical condition caused by or arising from the pregnancy itself.
>
> [A "partial-birth abortion" is] an abortion procedure in which the person performing the abortion partially delivers vaginally a living unborn child before killing the unborn child and completing the delivery….[The statute further defines the phrase "partially delivers vaginally a living unborn child before killing the unborn child" as] deliberately and intentionally delivering into the vagina a living unborn child, or a substantial portion thereof, for the purpose of performing a procedure that the person performing such procedure knows will kill the unborn child and does kill the unborn child.

This ban applies throughout pregnancy and has no exception to protect the woman's health, only to save her life. In a 5-to-4 opinion in *Stenberg v. Carhart*,[11] the Court found this law unconstitutional for two reasons. First, the description of the banned procedure was too close to dilation and evacuation (D&E), another procedure that was permitted by the law and widely used for second-trimester abortions. Therefore, this law would discourage physicians from using the lawful procedure, which would place an undue burden on their patients. Second, the law failed to provide an exception for instances in which the procedure was deemed necessary by the physician to protect the woman's health, as required by *Roe* and *Casey*. Justice John Paul Stevens, in his concurring opinion, noted that the extreme anti-*Roe* rhetoric as exemplified in the partial-birth abortion debate obscured the fact that during the 27-year period since *Roe* was decided, the core holding of *Roe* "has been endorsed by all but 4 of the 17 Justices who have addressed the issue."

A notable dissenting opinion was written by Justice Kennedy, who had specifically endorsed the core of *Roe* in *Casey*. Kennedy argued that the outlawing of "partial-birth abortion" was consistent with *Casey* because of the interest the state has throughout pregnancy in protecting the life of the fetus that may become a child. In his view, the banned procedure conflates abortion and childbirth in a way that "might cause the medical profession or society as a whole to become insensitive, even disdainful, to life, including life of the human fetus." He also argued that such a ban was not unduly burdensome to women because state legislatures can determine that specific medical procedures, like this one, are not medically necessary.[11]

Justice Stephen Breyer, the author of the *Stenberg* majority opinion, stated that a more precise law, with a health exception, could be constitutional.[11] In 2003, Congress passed a slightly revised law. It did not contain a health exception, but its preface did contain a declaration that the outlawed procedure was never medically necessary for the health of the woman. President Bush signed it into law on November 5, 2003. By the time the Court ruled on the constitutionality of this law in April 2007, in *Gonzales v. Carhart*,[12] there were two important changes in the composition of the Court: a new chief justice, John Roberts, who replaced the consistently anti-*Roe* Chief William Rehnquist, and Justice Samuel Alito, who replaced Justice Sandra Day O'Connor, who was consistently pro-*Roe* (as interpreted in *Casey*). The federal law provides that

> (a) Any physician who, in or affecting interstate or foreign commerce, knowingly performs a partial birth abortion and thereby kills a human fetus shall be fined under this title or imprisoned not more than 2 years, or both. This subsection does not apply to a partial birth abortion that is *necessary to save the life of a mother* whose life is endangered by a physical disorder, physical illness, or physical injury, including a life-endangering physical condition caused by or arising from the pregnancy itself....
>
> (b) (1) The term "partial-birth" abortion means an abortion in which the person performing the abortion
>
> (A) *Deliberately and intentionally* vaginally delivers a living fetus until, in the case of a head-first presentation, the *entire fetal head is outside* the body of the mother, *or*, in the case of breech presentation, *any part of the fetal trunk past the navel is outside* the body of the mother, for the purpose of performing an overt act that the person knows will kill the partially delivered living fetus; and
>
> (B) Performs the overt act, other than completion of delivery, that kills the partially delivered living fetus [emphasis added].

The Court decided, 5 to 4, that this law was constitutional.[12] Justice Kennedy wrote the majority opinion for himself, Justices Antonin Scalia and Clarence Thomas, and the two new justices. In it he substantially adopts his dissenting opinion in *Stenberg* as the Court's new majority opinion. Although he concludes that his decision is consistent with *Stenberg*, all three U.S. District courts and all three Courts of Appeal that had examined this federal law found it unconstitutional under the principles in *Casey* and *Stenberg*, primarily because of the vagueness of the definition and the lack of a health exception. As to the vagueness argument, Kennedy writes that the new law is no longer vague because it clarifies the distinction between the prohibited procedure (which he calls "intact D&E") and standard D&E abortions because the former requires the delivery of an intact fetus, whereas the latter requires "the removal of fetal parts that are ripped from the fetus as they are pulled through the cervix." In addition, the new federal law specifies fetal landmarks (e.g., the "navel") instead of the vague description of a "substantial portion" of the "unborn child."

Because the law applies to fetuses both before and after the point of viability, Kennedy concedes that under *Casey* the law would be unconstitutional "if its purpose or effect is to place a substantial obstacle in the path of a woman seeking an abortion before the fetus attains viability." Kennedy finds Congress's purpose is twofold: first, lawmakers wanted to "express respect for the dignity of human life" by outlawing "a method of abortion in which a fetus is killed just inches before completion of the birth process," because use of this procedure "will further coarsen society to the humanity of not only newborns, but of all vulnerable and innocent human life...." Second, Congress wanted to protect medical ethics, finding that this procedure "confuses the medical, legal and ethical duties of physicians to preserve and promote life...."

The key to Kennedy's legal analysis is his conclusion that these reasons are constitutionally sufficient to justify the ban because under *Casey*, "the State, from the inception of pregnancy, maintains its own regulatory interest in protecting the life of the fetus that may become a child [and this interest] cannot be set at naught by interpreting *Casey's* requirement of a health exception so it becomes tantamount to allowing the doctor to choose the abortion method he or she might prefer." Kennedy then goes on to write that "respect for human life finds an ultimate expression in the bond of love the mother has for her child," and that "while no reliable data" exist on the subject, "it seems unexceptionable to conclude some women come to regret their choice to abort the infant life they once created and sustained.... Severe depression and loss of esteem can follow." Such regret, Justice Kennedy believes, can be caused or exacerbated if women later learn what the procedure entails, suggesting that physicians fail to describe it to patients because they "may prefer not to disclose precise details of the means [of abortion] that will be used...."

The final, critical issue is whether the prohibition would "ever impose significant health risks on women" and whether physicians or Congress should make this determination. Kennedy picks Congress: "The law need not give abortion doctors unfettered choice in the course of their medical practice, nor should it elevate their status above other physicians in the medical community....Medical uncertainty does not foreclose the exercise of legislative power in the abortion context any more than it does in other contexts." Furthermore, Kennedy argues, the law does not impose an "undue burden" on women for another reason: alternative ways of killing a fetus have not been prohibited. In his words, "If the intact D&E procedure is truly necessary in some circumstances, it appears likely an injection that kills the fetus is an alternative under the Act that allows the doctor to perform the procedure."[12]

Writing for the four justices in the minority, Justice Ruth Bader Ginsburg observes, "Today's decision is alarming. It refuses to take *Casey* and *Stenberg* seriously. It tolerates, indeed applauds, federal intervention to ban nationwide a procedure found necessary and proper in certain cases by the American College of Obstetricians [and Gynecologists] (ACOG). It blurs the line, firmly drawn in *Casey*, between previability and postviability abortions. And, for the first time since *Roe*, the Court blesses a prohibition with no exception safeguarding a woman's health." Ginsburg argues that the majority of the Court has overruled the conclusion in *Stenberg* that a health exception is required when "substantial medical authority supports the proposition that banning a particular abortion procedure could endanger women's health...." This conclusion, bolstered by evidence presented by nine professional organizations, including the ACOG, and conclusions by all three U.S. District Courts that heard evidence concerning the Act and its effects, directly contradicted the congressional declaration that "there is no credible medical evidence that partial-birth abortions are safe or are safer than other abortion procedures." Even Justice Kennedy agreed that Congress's finding was untenable.

Justice Ginsburg concludes that this leaves only "flimsy and transparent justifications" for upholding the ban. She rejects those justifications, arguing that the state's interest in "preserving and promoting fetal life" cannot be furthered by a ban that targets only a method of abortion and that cannot save "a single fetus from destruction" by its own terms but may put women's health at risk. Ultimately, she believes that the decision rests entirely on the proposition, never before enshrined in a majority opinion and explicitly repudiated in *Casey*, that "ethical and moral concerns" unrelated to the government's interest in "preserving life" can overcome what had been considered fundamental rights of citizens. The majority seeks to bolster its conclusion by describing pregnant women as in a fragile emotional state that physicians may take advantage of by withholding information about abortion procedures. Justice Ginsburg concludes that the majority's solution to this hypothetical problem is to "deprive women of the right to make an autonomous choice, even at the expense of their safety." She continues, "This way of thinking [that men must protect women by restricting their choices] reflects ancient notions about women's place in the family and under the Constitution—ideas that have long since been discredited." Ginsburg further notes that the majority simply cannot contain its hostility to reproductive rights as articulated in *Roe* and *Casey*, calling physicians "abortion doctors," describing the fetus as an "unborn child" and as a "baby," labeling second-trimester abortions as "late term," and dismissing "the reasoned medical judgments of highly trained doctors...as 'preferences' motivated by 'mere convenience.'"[12]

Ginsburg makes two final points. First, although the Court invites a lawsuit to challenge the Act "as applied," it gives "no clue" as to how such a lawsuit should be brought. Surely, she asks, "the Court cannot mean that no suit to challenge the ban [based on how it affects an actual woman or her physician] may be brought until a woman's health is immediately jeopardized." Second, she argues that the opinion threatens to undercut the "rule of law" and the "principle of stare decisis," both of which the Court affirmed in *Casey*, concluding that, "A decision so at odds with our jurisprudence should not have staying power." As described in *Casey*, stare decisis is a doctrine that obligates courts to follow the principles set forth in prior cases, called precedents, to assure continuity in the law, and precedents should not be abandoned under "political pressure" or as an "unprincipled emotional reaction."

The major change in the law this opinion brings with it is the new willingness of Congress and the Court to discount the health of pregnant women and the medical judgment of their physicians.[13] This departure from precedent was made possible by categorizing physicians as unprincipled "abortion doctors" and infantilizing pregnant women as incapable of making serious decisions about their lives and health. The majority opinion ignores or marginalizes long-standing principles of constitutional law, substituting the personal morality of Justice Kennedy and four of his colleagues.

The majority asserts that giving Congress constitutional authority to regulate medical practice is not new but identifies no case in which Congress had ever outlawed a medical procedure. Its reliance on the more than 100-year-old case of *Jacobson v. Massachusetts* is especially inapt.[14] *Jacobson* was about mandatory smallpox vaccination during an epidemic. Refusal was punishable by a fine. The statute had an exception for "children who present a certificate, signed by a registered physician, that they are unfit subjects for vaccination," and the Court implied that a similar medical exception would be constitutionally required for adults. It is not just abortion regulations that have had a health exception for physicians and their patients—all health regulations have.[15]

On the other hand, **those who expect *Roe* to be overturned by this Court may be disappointed.** Although Justice Alito has replaced Justice O'Connor and is likely to vote in the opposite direction on *Roe*-related issues, Justice Kennedy is the new swing vote on the Court, and he insists that he is upholding the principles of *Roe v. Wade* as reaffirmed in *Casey*. Just as the question of whether a specific abortion regulation was an "undue burden" was once a determination Justice O'Connor could effectively make for the Court, the meaning of *Roe v. Wade* is, at least for now, up to Justice Kennedy. The replacement of two Pro-*Roe* Justices (Souter and Stevens) with Sonia Sotomayor and Elena Kagan during the first 2 years of the Obama administration has made no change in this balance. On the other hand, the Court has become so political in the past decade that the replacement of any one of the five justices who currently support the "core" of *Roe* with an anti-*Roe* justice (which is very unlikely to happen during Obama's presidency) could result in *Roe* being overturned, and the contours of abortion law would then be returned to the individual states—some of which would outlaw abortion, but most of which would retain the law substantially as it now is.

ABORTION POLITICS AND NATIONAL HEALTH INSURANCE REFORM*

President Barack Obama made it clear during the great debate on health insurance reform that he did not want abortion politics to sabotage his legislation. In his September 10, 2009 speech about health insurance reform to a joint session of Congress, he said, "Under our plan, no federal dollars will be used to fund abortions." Nonetheless, the centrality of abortion in U.S. politics made it inevitable that abortion funding would play a major role in determining whether there was any health insurance reform law at all. The debate revolved around the Stupak amendment in the House of Representatives, which provided that "No funds authorized or appropriated by this Act…may be used *to pay for any abortion or to cover any part of the costs of any health plan that includes coverage of abortion*, except in the case where a woman suffers from a physical disorder, physical injury, or physical illness that would, as certified by a physician, place the woman in danger of death unless an abortion is performed, including a life-endangering physical condition caused by or arising from the pregnancy itself, or unless the pregnancy is the result of rape or incest" (italics added). The House passed this amendment by a vote of 240 to 194, with 64 Democrats voting in favor (the House health care bill itself passed 220 to 215). Many thought that the Catholic bishops who lobbied fervently for passage of the Stupak amendment were the most influential in supporting it. More influential, however, were the previously secret fundamentalist Christian political leadership group known variously as the Family or the Fellowship, which includes among its members both of the amendment's main sponsors, Bart Stupak (D-MI) and Joe Pitts (R-PA).[16]

The Stupak amendment was defended as merely continuing the practice created by the Hyde amendment. That amendment, named after the late Congressman Henry Hyde (R-IL), which has been attached to every Health and Human Services Appropriations Act passed since 1976 (and has also been added to appropriations legislation for the Defense Department, the Indian Health Service, and federal employees' health insurance plans) prohibits the use of federal funding for "any abortion" or for any "health benefits coverage that includes abortion," unless the pregnancy is the result of "rape or incest" or "would, as certified by a physician, place the woman in danger of death unless an abortion is performed." Under the Hyde amendment, states may use their own funds to finance abortion services through their Medicaid programs, and 17 states currently do so.

The U.S. Supreme Court has ruled on the constitutionality of limiting government funding for abortion twice. The first case, in 1977, involved a Connecticut regulation that limited state Medicaid funding to "medically necessary" abortions, thus excluding those not necessary to preserve a woman's life or health. The Court ruled that women have a constitutional right to choose to have an abortion, but the state has no obligation to pay for the exercise of this right and may constitutionally encourage women to continue their pregnancies to term by providing funding for childbirth and not abortion. The state may not constitutionally create obstacles to abortion, but it has no obligation to remove obstacles, such as poverty, that are not of its own making.[17]

Three years after the Connecticut decision, **the Court upheld the Hyde amendment, which prohibited federal funding for medically necessary abortions.[18] Under this ruling, even low-income women who would have devastating health outcomes if they continued a pregnancy could not have an abortion paid for by Medicaid.** In both cases, the Court ruled that the government could make "a value judgment favoring childbirth over abortion and [implement] that judgment by the allocation of public funds." There is no constitutional requirement for the federal government to fund any abortion. Federal funding is a political question to be decided by Congress.

The U.S. Senate bill on health insurance reform, which Majority Leader Harry Reid (D-NV) created by blending bills from two committees, did not contain the Stupak amendment but specifically excluded federal funding for abortions as prohibited by any federal law (including the Hyde amendment) that was in effect "6 months before the beginning of the plan year involved." States must also ensure that "no federal funds pay or defray the cost" of abortion services in new health plans that cover abortion. Moreover, states are required to offer at least two plans in the proposed health insurance exchanges (where most people who currently lack coverage will purchase insurance): one that covers abortion services and one that does not. Nonfederal funds for abortion coverage in any plan must be segregated, and payment must be made separately, in an amount estimated by the secretary of health and human services, to cover this benefit.

Three major questions were raised about the differences between the House and Senate approaches: Did they fulfill Obama's no-federal-funding promise? Did they follow the Hyde amendment "tradition"? And did they represent good health insurance policy? As for the first question, the Senate version fulfilled the President's promise by requiring abortion funding to come from sources other than federal tax dollars. This aspect of the provision was denigrated as a "bookkeeping trick," but all payments involve bookkeeping. Even federal employees who pay for abortions with their government salaries are using funds that came from federal tax dollars. As for the second question, the Stupak amendment goes far beyond the Hyde amendment by prohibiting the use of federal tax

*This section is adapted from Annas,[16] with permission.

dollars not only for abortion itself but also for any health plan available on the proposed exchanges that covers abortion. The goal is to limit access to abortion, even when no federal funds are being used for it. The third question relates to public health policy. The Hyde amendment institutionalizes the moral view of some members of Congress that even medically necessary abortions should not be considered health care. This view, for example, led Congress to criminalize an abortion procedure (designated "partial-birth abortion," discussed previously) without an exception for the health of the pregnant woman. These are the types of federal government intrusions into health care that opponents of public insurance plans usually decry.

After the Democrats lost Ted Kennedy's Senate seat in a special election in Massachusetts (and with it the 60 votes needed to end a filibuster), the bill previously passed by the Senate became the vehicle for health insurance reform, and a budget "reconciliation" measure (requiring only 51 votes for Senate passage), negotiated by Democratic House and Senate leaders, was used to make modifications to the Senate bill to make it acceptable to the House.

Because the Stupak-Pitts abortion language was not in the Senate bill, it was uncertain whether the 216 House votes needed for passage could be found. **Stupak himself ultimately agreed to vote for the Senate bill as long as President Obama signed an executive order agreeing not to use any aspect of the legislation to fund abortions.** The bill ultimately passed 219 to 212, which suggests that the votes of Stupak and his colleagues were essential. President Barack Obama signed the order on March 24, at a private White House event.

The order aims to "establish an adequate enforcement mechanism to ensure that Federal funds are not used for abortion services (except in cases of rape or incest, or when the life of the woman would be endangered), consistent with a longstanding Federal statutory restriction that is commonly known as the Hyde Amendment." In addition to this general language, the order contains specific language on the two areas of the health care bill that have continued to foster controversy: abortion coverage by insurance policies to be offered on the future health insurance exchanges, and the possibility that community health centers will use new funds provided under the act to offer abortion services. As to the former, the order requires, as in the Senate bill, that any payment for abortion coverage not consistent with the Hyde Amendment be made with private segregated funds. To clarify how that can be done, the executive order requires the director of the Office of Management and Budget and the secretary of health and human services "to develop, within 180 days…a model set of segregation guidelines for State health insurance commissioners to use" to determine whether exchange plans are in compliance with the act. These guidelines will then go through the process of becoming federal regulations with the force of law.

Conservative critics of the executive order argued that to be upheld in the courts it must be consistent with current law. It is, so that's not an issue. They also argued that the President could rescind it at any time. Although this is true as a matter of law, it is not as a matter of politics. If Obama did not intend to follow the law, he would have issued a "signing statement" (as president George W. Bush did for almost every portion of every bill he signed into law to which he objected), not a pledge to enforce it. The executive order will be in place as long as President Obama is in office, and no Republican president is likely to change it. Barring some extraordinary event, the order and its resulting regulations will be the rule for federal funding of abortion services for the foreseeable future. The National Organization for Women has indicated that it will campaign for the repeal of the Hyde Amendment. It seems unlikely that such a campaign could succeed, although a more modest one, aimed at expanding the exceptions permitted to include, for example, serious fetal disorders, might. Soon after the passage of the Affordable Care Act, abortion politics shifted to stem cell research and a "companion" funding restriction amendment to the Hyde Amendment: the Dicky-Wicker Amendment.

HUMAN EMBRYONIC STEM CELL RESEARCH FUNDING*

Embryo research was born political. Expressions of shock and surprise at the August 23, 2010 ruling of federal district court judge Royce Lamberth enjoining federal funding of stem cell research—which was based largely on his reading of an amendment to an appropriations bill—were thus not terribly persuasive.[19,20] The amendment, known as the **Dickey-Wicker amendment, provides that no federal funds can be expended by the NIH for "(1) the creation of a human embryo or embryos for research purposes; or (2) research in which a human embryo or embryos are destroyed, discarded, or knowingly subjected to risks of injury or death."** The creation and destruction of human embryos for research are deeply tied not only to political and religious debates concerning abortion but also to in vitro fertilization (IVF). In 1979, during the Carter administration, the Ethics Advisory Board of the Department of Health, Education, and Welfare (forerunner of the Department of Health and Human Services) recommended that the government support research on embryos in order to study and improve IVF. Federal research funding was never authorized, and IVF was introduced to clinical medicine without a research phase. The Reagan administration dissolved the ethics board and ignored its recommendations. The issue was next taken up during the Clinton administration by an NIH Human Embryo Research Panel, which voted on 27 goals of embryo research and recommended 7 as "acceptable for federal funding" —but failed to produce a credible ethical justification for its recommendations, which were widely ignored.[21] Congress, however, responded to the report, and in 1996 President Clinton signed the first appropriations bill containing the Dickey-Wicker amendment, named for its sponsors, Representatives Jay Dickey (R-AR) and Roger Wicker (R-MS). It has been added to NIH appropriations bills every subsequent year, just as the Hyde Amendment restricting abortion funding is added.

*This section is adapted from Annas,[20] with permission.

The derivation of stem cells from embryos involves destroying the embryo. In 2001, President George W. Bush authorized federal funding for human embryonic stem cell (ESC) research but limited it to cell lines that had been derived before his August 9, 2001 speech—and specifically to cell lines from surplus IVF embryos used with the consent of the couple whose egg and sperm were used to create them. No one challenged this policy as a violation of Dickey-Wicker, perhaps because, as Bush said, the "life and death decision" for these embryos had already been made.

President Barack Obama was well aware that federal funding of ESC research represents a political flash point, but he had promised to rescind the Bush policy, and there is wide support for expanded federal funding of ESC research. When Obama announced his new policy authorizing funding for cell lines derived after August 2001 (if derived from surplus IVF embryos, without the use of federal funds), he knew he could be reawakening the funding debate. He expressed his hope that "Congress will act on a bipartisan basis to provide further support for this research."

Congress did not act. Instead, the debate shifted to the courts, where the core question is whether the new Obama guidelines are consistent with Dickey-Wicker. Although he has not (as of this writing) decided this question, Lamberth has said he believes Dickey-Wicker is "unambiguous" and does not permit the NIH "to separate the derivation of ESCs from research on the ESCs," because "derivation of ESCs from an embryo is an integral step in conducting ESC research."[19] Whether he will change his mind after briefing, argument, and perhaps testimony—or whether the Court of Appeals will rule otherwise—remains to be seen. **The Obama administration's new guidelines are based on the political compromise of deriving ESCs only from surplus IVF embryos, and as part of this compromise, the NIH seemed to have conceded that derivation is an integral part of stem cell research, which is why it sets strict limits on the source of the embryos used and the quality of consent obtained.** The political argument for permitting the use of surplus IVF embryos is that these embryos were created for a legitimate reproductive purpose, and when they're no longer wanted for that purpose, their donation for research is ethically preferable to their destruction without any potential societal benefit.[21] Of course, anyone who objects to the creation of embryos for IVF would also object to this compromise. Does Dickey-Wicker permit this political compromise as a matter of law?

President Clinton's National Bioethics Advisory Commission argued in 1999 that it was not ethically reasonable to separate the derivation of stem cells for research from their use in research. The commission believed that the federal government should fund both, for at least as long as the embryos used were those "remaining after infertility treatments."[21] Their reasons were "the close connection in practical and ethical terms between derivation and use of the cells" and the hope that permitting funding for cell derivation could advance science in this area. Lawyers asked by the commission to examine the meaning of Dickey-Wicker concluded that the NIH's distinction between derivation and use of human ESCs was a "reasonable" interpretation of the amendment—but that "there is no indication that either proponents or opponents [of ESC research] contemplated the situation...in which research that destroyed the embryo was separately conducted from research using the cells derived from the embryo."[22]

The Clinton panel's report got less attention than it deserved because at that time the national debate was focused on creating research embryos through cloning (somatic cell nuclear transfer). Bush's Council on Bioethics concentrated on cloning, but it was also the only national ethics panel ever to discuss federal funding as an ethical (rather than political) issue. It concluded that "the decision to fund an activity is...a declaration of official national support and endorsement, a positive assertion that the activity in question is deemed by the nation as a whole...to be good and worthy." Such rhetoric seems disconnected from special-interest legislation[23]; a more honest statement regarding federal funding is that since *Roe v. Wade,* funding for anything remotely related to abortion (and since no one is pregnant, embryo research is only remotely related) has become a potent political liability in Congress. Obama's own ethics panel has sensibly stayed out of this political funding debate.

Three paths are open to proponents of federal funding for human ESC research. The first is to mount a vigorous defense in the ongoing lawsuit, aiming to persuade the courts that the Obama administration's interpretation of Dickey-Wicker is correct. As of July 2011 this strategy is succeeding, with the federal Court of Appeals ruling 2 to 1 in 2011 that Dickey-Wicker permitted the funding of research on human ESCs that had been derived from leftover IVF embryos by nonfederal employees who did not use federal money. I think this opinion is solid and will prevail. But because ultimate court victory remains at least somewhat uncertain, the Obama administration could also seek congressional authorization for its current regulations. The vehicle could be a bill proposed by Representative Diana DeGette (D-CO), which authorizes research on stem cells derived from surplus IVF embryos; it has been passed twice (and vetoed by Bush) and would certainly be signed by Obama. Because this approach would retain Dickey-Wicker, however, and could thus lead to more legal challenges, it would be preferable (and probably more politically feasible) to amend Dickey-Wicker by adding language such as the following: "Nothing in part (2) prohibits the NIH from funding research using embryos created for procreation, including the derivation of stem cells, when the couple no longer wants to use them for procreation and has provided their informed authorization for them to be used in NIH-funded research." Doing so would legislatively adopt the ethics position of the Clinton bioethics commission. The third path is continued reliance on private and state funding until sufficient scientific progress is made that the public demands federal funding for this research.

NIH Director Francis Collins has said that this issue "goes beyond politics...to patients and their families who are counting on us to do everything in our power, ethically and responsibly, to learn how to transform these cells into entirely new therapies." This argument, of course, is itself political, and if Collins is right, **the only place to ultimately resolve the funding issue is in Congress.**

GENETIC COUNSELING, SCREENING, AND PRENATAL DIAGNOSIS

All women who rely on a physician for prenatal care should have the right to have the physician fully inform her of any reason the physician has to believe that her fetus might have a disability and to inform her further of the existence of diagnostic tests that might identify the precise condition. The physician incurs this duty to disclose because it is this type of information that the pregnant woman seeks prenatal care to discover (i.e., to learn all she can to help her have a healthy child). It is therefore entirely reasonable for the pregnant woman to expect her physician to apprise her of any relevant information regarding her fetus and options she might have so that she and the child's father can determine what action to take.[24]

If relevant information is not provided to the pregnant woman, and if a child with a serious disability is born, there are two potential types of lawsuits that could be brought against the physician. A wrongful birth suit must allege and prove not only that the physician was negligent in the care of the pregnant woman, but also that had the negligent act not been done the child would not have been born (e.g., had the woman been properly informed that she was at risk to have a child with Down syndrome, she could have sought amniocentesis or chorionic villus sampling and had an abortion if her fetus were so affected). A related but far more controversial lawsuit is brought by the child (through its parents or guardian) against the physician because it was born, a so-called wrongful life suit. Most courts have rejected lawsuits by the child because they thought it was impossible to put a monetary value on life in an impaired condition compared with nonexistence. The choice for these children is *never* to be born healthy, but only to be born with a handicap (such as Down syndrome or Tay-Sachs disease) or not to be born at all. We think that future courts are likely to limit such actions to *serious* handicaps, those in which fetuses, if they could speak to us (which, of course, they can only do through their parents), would agree with an "objective societal consensus" that their own best interest would be served if they were aborted. Put another way, they would be better off *from their own perspective* if they never existed. Conditions like deafness and Down syndrome would not qualify, whereas conditions like Tay-Sachs would. Measuring damages *is* problematic, but courts are likely to award at least the added medical costs caused by the handicap itself. However, because medical costs can be recovered in a wrongful birth case directly, wrongful life cases are only likely to be brought in those rare instances in which for some reason (e.g., the child has been given up for adoption) the parents have lost the right to sue on their own behalf.[25]

The following conclusions may be drawn regarding the legal and ethical obligations of the obstetrician in relationship to genetic counseling and prenatal diagnosis:

- **First, the law requires physicians to give accurate information to the parents and forbids the withholding of vital information from them.** These principles are consistent with the doctrine of informed consent and the reasonable expectations of pregnant women under a physician's care. The physician does not guarantee a healthy child, but the reasonable expectation of the patient is that she will be apprised of any information the physician has that the child might be seriously disabled and of the alternative ways to proceed so that the patient can determine what action to take.[26]
- Second, no obstetrician can be required to perform chorionic villus sampling, genetic amniocentesis, or fetal DNA analysis. Indeed, many are not qualified to perform these procedures and for them to do so may itself be malpractice.
- Third, genetic counseling should be morally nondirective (to the extent possible); that is, the counselor should remain impartial and objective in providing information that will allow competent counselees to make their own informed decision. The Judicial Council of the American Medical Association[27] has given the following opinion:

> Physicians, whether they oppose or do not oppose contraception, sterilization, or abortion, may decide that they can engage in genetic counseling and screening, but should avoid the imposition of their personal moral values and the substitution of their own moral judgment for that of the prospective parents. The ethical and moral decisions have to be made by the family and should not be imposed by the physician.

- **Fourth, to ensure the patient's interest in both autonomy and privacy, no information obtained in genetic counseling or screening should be disclosed to any third party, including insurers and employers (now prohibited by federal law), without the patient's informed consent.**[28,29] Such strict nondisclosure policies should be maintained unless and until specific state legislation is enacted that would clearly delineate the circumstance in which confidentiality must be breached, analogous to certain contagious diseases, gunshot wounds, and child abuse. On the other hand, counselors should be permitted to attempt to persuade patients to make disclosures of important information to potentially affected relatives if there is a high probability of serious harm and if the disclosure is limited to pertinent genetic information. We recommend that the genetic counselor make clear, both verbally and in writing, the policy that he or she follows so that the patient can refuse to be screened or counseled if he or she is not in agreement with the disclosure policy. Such agreements will serve to heighten the public's confidence in genetic counseling and will encourage people to participate voluntarily in both screening and counseling.

Genetic Screening*

Our ability to translate our expanding genetic knowledge into usable information for individual patients is at best uncertain, as is the future of "personalized medicine." Taking a family history and, when indicated, recommending certain tests to identify carriers of genetic diseases are standard in obstetrical care. Today's screening tests usually focus on conditions that occur either in the family or in the racial or ethnic group of one or both prospective

*This section has been adapted from Elias and Annas,[30] with permission.

parents. As our ability to identify genes associated with particular diseases increases, a panel of screening tests to identify carriers of numerous genes will be offered more routinely. It will then become increasingly difficult, if not impossible, to inform those offered screening or testing for reproductive purposes about all the genetic information that can be obtained and the implications of that information.

Our current model for screening and testing requires pretest counseling.[30] Such counseling is a method of obtaining informed consent, and the obligation to counsel can be seen as inherent in the fiduciary nature of the doctor-patient relationship.[31] For ordinary medical procedures, the physical risks and treatment alternatives are the chief items of information that must be disclosed. There are few physical risks in genetic screening. What must be conveyed in counseling regarding genetic screening is that the tests may yield new information that may ultimately force some unwelcome choices (such as whether to marry, abort, or adopt). **Self-determination and rational decision making are the central values protected by informed consent.**[32] In the setting of reproductive genetics, what is at stake is the right to decide whether or not to have a genetic test, with emphasis on the right to refuse if the potential harm (in terms of stigma or unacceptable choices) outweighs, for the individual person or family, the potential benefit.

As the Human Genome Project bears fruit, hundreds of new genetic screening tests, and even full genome screening, will compete for introduction into routine clinical practice. Already some researchers have suggested population-based screening to identify carriers of the genes for such conditions as the fragile X syndrome and myotonic dystrophy. Each new screening test presents the same questions: What information should be given to which patients, when should it be presented, who should present it, and how and by whom should the results be conveyed? It will soon be impossible to do meaningful prescreening counseling about all available carrier tests. Giving too much information ("information overload") can amount to misinformation and make the entire counseling process either misleading or meaningless. **To prevent disclosure from being pointless or counterproductive, we believe that strategies based on general or "generic" consent should be developed for genetic screening. Their aim would be to provide sufficient information to permit patients to make informed decisions about carrier screening, yet avoid the information overload that could lead to "misinformed" consent.**

Traditionally, goals of reproductive genetic counseling, including counseling about screening carrier status, involve helping the person or family to (1) comprehend the medical fact, including the diagnosis, the probable course of the disorder, and the available management; (2) appreciate the way heredity contributes to the disorder, and the risk for recurrence in specified relatives; (3) understand the options for dealing with the risk for recurrence; (4) choose the course of action that seems appropriate to them in view of their risk and their family goals and act in accordance with that decision; and (5) make the best possible adjustment to the disorder in an affected family member or to the risk for recurrence of that disorder.

For example, in the current context of counseling a couple at least one of whom is of Italian ancestry, each of these issues would be discussed as it relates specifically to α-thalassemia, with explanation of the use of hemoglobin electrophoresis as a screening test to determine carrier status. If consideration of another prenatal test were appropriate—as in the case of screening of maternal serum for α-fetoprotein, human chorionic gonadotropin, and unconjugated estriol to detect fetal aneuploidy, open neural tube defects, and other abnormalities—a separate discussion about these tests, including information on their sensitivity and specificity, and of each of the possible associated fetal disorders would also be required. Even knowledgeable couples could become confused, frustrated, and anxious if faced with scores of such options for genetic screening.

By contrast, **an approach based on generic consent would emphasize broader concepts and common denominator issues in genetic screening.** We envision a situation in which patients would be told of the availability of a panel of screening tests that can be performed on a single blood sample. They would be told that these tests could determine whether they carry genes that put them at increased risk for having a child with a birth defect that could involve serious physical abnormalities, mental disabilities, or both. Several common examples could be given to indicate the frequency and spectrum of severity of each type or category of condition for which screening was being offered. For example, prenatal screening could include tests for fetal conditions such as neural tube defects and chromosome abnormalities such as cystic fibrosis and fragile X syndrome. In the near future, a sample of fetal blood cells may be retrievable from maternal blood to be used not only for estimation of risks but also perhaps for definitive diagnosis.

In the course of such counseling, **important factors common to all genetic screening tests would be highlighted.** Among these are the limitations of screening tests, especially the fact that negative results cannot guarantee a healthy infant; the possible need for additional, invasive tests, such as chorionic villus sampling or amniocentesis, to establish a definitive diagnosis; the reproductive options that might have to be considered, such as prenatal diagnosis, adoption, gamete donation, abortion, or acceptance of risks; the costs of screening; issues of confidentiality, including potential disclosure to other family members; and the possibility of social stigmatization, including discrimination in health insurance and employment. If carrier status is detected in the woman, it must be emphasized that the partner should also be screened. Before prenatal testing was agreed to in such cases, the woman would need to be told that she would be advised to consider abortion if the fetus was found to be affected with a nontreatable condition.

This type of generic consent to genetic screening can be compared with obtaining consent to perform a physical examination. Patients know that the purpose of the examination is to locate potential problems that are likely to require additional follow-up and that could present them with choices they would rather not have to make. The patient is not generally told, however, about all the possible abnormalities that can be detected by a routine physical examination or routine blood work, but only the general purpose of each. On the other hand, tests that may produce especially sensitive and stigmatizing information, such as screening of blood for the human immunodeficiency virus, should not be performed without specific consent. Similarly, because of its reproductive implications, genetic testing has not traditionally been carried out without specific consent. Even in a generic model, **tests for untreatable fatal diseases such as Huntington disease should not be combined with other tests or performed without specific consent.**[33]

What is central in the concept of generic consent for genetic screening is not a waiver of the individual patient's right to information. Rather, it would reflect a decision by the genetics community **that the most reasonable way to conduct a panel of screening tests to identify carriers of serious conditions is to provide basic, general information to obtain consent for the screening and much more detailed information on specific conditions only after they have been detected.** Since, in most cases, no such conditions will in fact be found, this method is also the most efficient and cost-effective. Some patients require more specific and in-depth information on which to base their decision regarding screening. It is therefore essential to build into the screening program ample opportunity for patients to obtain all the additional information they need to help them make decisions. Clinicians, of course, must be open and responsive to the concerns and questions of patients. Counseling could be provided in person by a physician or other health professional. Alternatively, audiovisual aids could be used, which would help ensure consistency in the information provided, be more efficient, and respond to the shortage of genetic counselors.

Generic consent for genetic screening should help prevent information overload and wasting time on useless information. It would not, however, solve what is likely to be an even more central problem in genetic screening: are there genetic conditions for which screening should not be offered to prospective parents? Examples might include genes that predispose a person to a particular disease late in life (such as Alzheimer disease, Parkinson disease, or breast cancer). From the perspective of the fetus, life with the possibility—or even the high probability—of developing these diseases in late adulthood is much to be preferred to no life at all. Thus, in this case, unlike that of the fetus with anencephaly, for example, no reasonable argument could be made that precluding abortion by denying this information could amount to forcing a "wrongful life" on the child.[31] Because of a personal experience with a friend or family member who suffered from one of these diseases, however, the couple might see abortion as a reasonable choice under such circumstances.

We must address this question directly and publicly. Are there genetic diseases and predispositions for which screening of prospective parents and testing of fetuses should not be offered as a matter of good medical practice and public policy, regardless of the technical ability to screen and the wishes of the couple? Offering carrier screening to assist couples in making reproductive decisions is not a neutral activity but, rather, implies that some action should be taken on the basis of the results of the test. Thus, for example, merely offering screening for a breast cancer or colon cancer gene suggests to couples that artificial insemination, adoption, and abortion are all reasonable choices if they are found to be carriers of such a gene.[34] In general, we do not believe that pregnancies in women who want to have a child should be terminated for this reason, and thus we believe carrier screening for the breast cancer gene should not be offered in the context of reproductive planning, at least outside of preimplantation genetic diagnosis in cases in which a woman is a known carrier and has had personal experience with a strong family history of breast or ovarian cancer. In the absence of an effective way to set the standard of care for carrier screening, however, we recognize that prenatal screening tests for these and similar genes will inevitably be offered by at least some commercial companies and private physicians.

A standard of care for genetic screening and consent in the face of hundreds or thousands of available genetic tests will inevitably be set. We believe the medical profession should take the lead in setting such standards and that, with public input, the model of generic consent for genetic screening will ultimately be accepted.

FORCED CESAREAN DELIVERY

Almost 25 years ago, Kolder and colleagues[35] reported a U.S. national survey revealing that court orders had been obtained for cesarean deliveries in 11 states, for hospital detentions in 2 states, and for intrauterine transfusions in 1 state. Among 21 cases in which court orders were sought, the orders were obtained in 86%; in 88% of those cases, the orders were received within 6 hours. Most of the women involved were black, Asian, or Hispanic, and all were poor. Nearly half were unmarried, and one fourth did not speak English as their primary language. In the survey, they also found that 46% of the heads of fellowship programs in fetomaternal medicine thought that women who refused medical advice and thereby endangered the life of the fetus should be detained. Forty-seven percent supported court orders for procedures such as intrauterine transfusions. Until 1990, with the exception of one case in the Georgia State Supreme Court, all cases had been decided by lower courts and therefore had little precedential importance.[36] In most cases, judges were called on an emergency basis and ordered interventions within hours. The judge usually went to the hospital. Physicians should know what most lawyers and almost all judges know: when a judge arrives at the hospital in response to an emergency call, he or she is acting much more like a lay person than a jurist. Without time to analyze the issues, without representation for the pregnant woman, without briefing or thoughtful reflection on the situation, in almost total ignorance of the relevant law, and in an unfamiliar setting faced by a relatively calm physician and a woman who can easily be labeled "hysterical," the judge will almost always order whatever the doctor advises.

There is nothing in *Roe v. Wade,*[2] or any other appellate decision, that gives either physicians or judges the right to favor the life or well-being of the fetus over that of the pregnant woman. Nor is there legal precedent for a mother being ordered to undergo surgery (e.g., kidney or partial liver transplantation) to save the life of her dying child. It would be ironic and inconsistent if a woman could be forced to submit to more invasive surgical procedures for the sake of a fetus than a child. Forcing pregnant women to follow medical advice also places unwarranted faith in that advice. Physicians often disagree about the appropriateness of obstetrical interventions, and they can be mistaken.[37] In three of the first five cases in which court-ordered cesarean delivery was sought, the women ultimately delivered vaginally and uneventfully. In the face of such uncertainty—uncertainty compounded by decades of changing and conflicting expert opinion on the management of pregnancy and childbirth—the moral and legal primacy of the competent, informed pregnant woman in decision making is overwhelming.[38]

Physicians may feel better after being "blessed" by the judge, but they should not. First, the appearance of legitimacy is deceptive; the judge has acted injudiciously, and there is no opportunity for meaningful appeal. Second, the medical situation has not changed, except that more time has been lost that should have been used to continue discussion with the woman directly. And, finally, the physician has now helped to transform himself or herself into an agent of the state's authority.[38]

The question of how to deal with a woman who continues to refuse intervention in the face of a court order remains. Do we really want to attempt to restrain and forcibly medicate and operate on a competent, refusing adult? Although such a procedure may be "legal," it is hardly humane. It is not what one generally associates with modern obstetrical care and may cause harm. It also encourages an adversarial relationship between the obstetrician and the patient. Moreover, even from a strictly utilitarian perspective, this marriage of the state and medicine is likely to harm more fetuses than it helps because many women will quite reasonably avoid physicians altogether during pregnancy if failure to follow medical advice can result in forced treatment, involuntary confinement, or criminal charges.

Extending notions of child abuse to "fetal abuse" simply brings government into pregnancy with few, if any, benefits and with great potential for invasions of privacy and deprivations of liberty. It is not helpful to use the law to convert a woman's and society's moral responsibility to her fetus into the woman's legal responsibility alone.[35] After birth, the fetus becomes a child and can and should thereafter be treated in its own right. Before birth, however, we can obtain access to the fetus only through its mother and, in the absence of her informed consent, can do so only by treating her as a fetal container, a nonperson without rights to bodily integrity.

In 2005, the ACOG revised and updated its 1987 Ethics Committee report on "Patient Choice: Maternal Fetal Conflict," now titled "Maternal Decision Making, Ethics, and the Law"[39] that we believe provides thoughtful and useful guidance for the medical practitioner. The statement highlighted six considerations, which we combine into three:

1. Coercive and punitive legal approaches to pregnant women who refuse medical advice fail to recognize that all competent adults are entitled to informed consent and bodily integrity.
2. Court-ordered interventions in cases of informed refusal, as well as punishment of pregnant women for their behavior that may put a fetus at risk, neglect the fact that medical knowledge and predictions of outcomes in obstetrics have limitations...[and treat medical problems] as if they were moral failings.
3. Coercive and punitive policies are potentially counterproductive in that they are likely to discourage prenatal care and successful treatment, adversely affect infant mortality rates, and undermine the physician-patient relationship...[and] unjustly single out the most vulnerable women...and create the potential for criminalization of many types of otherwise legal maternal behavior.

Based on these, the Committee on Ethics made four recommendations, the most central of which are:

1. Pregnant women's autonomous decisions should be respected....In the absence of extraordinary circumstances, circumstances that, in fact, the Committee cannot currently imagine, judicial authority should not be used to implement treatment regimens aimed at protecting the fetus, for such actions violate the pregnant woman's autonomy.
2. Pregnant women should not be punished for adverse perinatal outcomes.
3. Policy makers, legislators, and physicians should work together to find constructive and evidence-based ways to address the needs of women with alcohol and other substance abuse problems.

This 2005 statement is even stronger than a 1990 opinion by the District of Columbia Court of Appeals, which ruled that the decision of the pregnant woman must be honored in all but "extremely rare and truly exceptional" cases.[40] ACOG's Ethics Committee "cannot currently imagine" what that "rare and truly exceptional" case might look like,

KEY POINTS

- In *Roe v. Wade* (1973), the U.S. Supreme Court determined that a fundamental "right to privacy existed in the Fourteenth Amendment's concept of personal liberty" that is "broad enough to encompass a woman's decision whether or not to terminate a pregnancy" before fetal viability without state interference.
- In *Planned Parenthood of Southeastern Pennsylvania v. Casey* (1992), the U.S. Supreme Court reaffirmed the "core" of *Roe v. Wade* and ruled that, before fetal viability, states cannot "unduly burden" a woman's decision to terminate a pregnancy (i.e., although consent and waiting periods may be constitutionally acceptable, states cannot regulate abortion in ways that will actually prevent women from obtaining them).
- *Roe* and *Casey* are critical to understanding the rights of obstetricians (which are derived from the rights of their patients) because they are the major sources of law regarding how far states can go to regulate decisions made in the obstetrician-patient relationship.
- With the exception of a procedure Congress has labeled "partial birth abortions," unless they contain an exception for the health of the pregnant

woman, laws that criminalize abortions are unconstitutional because they are inconsistent with *Roe* and *Casey*.

- *Roe* has been the source of political controversy since it was decided in 1973. Congress has enacted the "Hyde Amendment" every year since the mid-1970s, prohibiting the use of federal funds for almost all abortions, and its constitutionality has been upheld by the U.S. Supreme Court.
- The Hyde Amendment was the basis for another similar amendment, the Dickey-Wicker Amendment, which prohibited the use of federal funds for human embryonic stem cell research, and was the basis for a temporary injunction prohibiting the NIH from funding such research in 2010 (overturned in 2011) under the Obama administration's changed rules.
- The legal and ethical obligations of an obstetrician in relationship to genetic counseling and prenatal diagnosis can be summarized as follows: (1) the physician must give accurate information to the parents and cannot withhold vital information from them; (2) no obstetrician can be required to perform prenatal diagnostic procedures; (3) prenatal genetic counseling should be morally nondirective; and (4) to protect patient privacy and autonomy, no information obtained in genetic counseling or screening should be disclosed to any third party without the patient's authorization.
- "Generic" consent for genetic *screening* that emphasizes broad concepts and common denominator issues should help maximize rational decision making by preventing information overload and wasting time on useless information.
- Self-determination and rational decision making are the central purposes of informed consent, and information on recommended procedures, risks, benefits, and alternatives should be presented in a way that furthers these purposes.
- Consent of the pregnant woman is a mandatory prerequisite for both investigative procedures and therapy. Her consent must be informed, and she should be told as clearly as possible about the proposed experimental procedures or therapy, its risks to herself and her fetus, and alternatives, success rates, and the likely problems of recuperation.
- The fetomaternal relationship is a unique one that requires physicians to promote a balance of maternal health and fetal welfare while respecting maternal autonomy. Obstetricians should not perform procedures that are refused by pregnant women, although reasonable steps to persuade a woman to change her mind are appropriate.

REFERENCES

1. Annas GJ: The Supreme Court and abortion rights. N Engl J Med 356:2201, 2007.
2. *Roe v. Wade*, 410 U.S. 113 (1973).
3. *Griswold v. Connecticut*, 381 U.S. 479 (1965).
4. *Eisenstadt v. Baird*, 405 U.S. 438 (1972).
5. *Doe v. Bolton*, 410 U.S. 179 (1973).
6. *Planned Parenthood of Central Missouri v. Danforth*, 428 U.S. 52 (1976).
7. Elias S, Annas GJ: Reproductive genetics and the law. Chicago, Year Book Medical, 1987, pp 145-162.
8. *Planned Parenthood of Southeastern Pennsylvania v. Casey*, 505 U.S. 833 (1992).
9. Annas GJ: The Supreme Court, liberty, and abortion. N Engl J Med 327:651, 1992.
10. Annas GJ. Partial-birth abortion, Congress, and the Constitution. N Engl J Med 339:279, 1998.
11. *Stenberg v. Carhart*, 530 U.S. 914 (2000).
12. *Gonzales v. Carhart*, 2007 U.S. LEXIS 4338 (2007).
13. Greene MF, Ecker JL: Abortion, health, and the law. N Engl J Med 350:184, 2004.
14. *Jacobson v. Massachusetts*, 197 U.S. 11 (1905).
15. Mariner WK, Annas GJ, Glantz LH: *Jacobson v Massachusetts:* it's not your great-great-grandfather's public health law. Am J Public Health 95:581, 2005.
16. Annas GJ: Abortion politics and health insurance reform. N Engl J Med 361:2589, 2009.
17. *Maher v. Roe*, 432 U.S. 464 (1977).
18. *Harris v. McRae*, 448 U.S. 297 (1980).
19. *Sherley v. Sebelius*, 2010 U.S. Dist. LEXIS 86441 (Aug. 23, 2010).
20. Annas GJ: Resurrection of a stem cell funding barrier: Dickey-Wicker in court. N Engl J Med 362:1259, 2010.
21. Annas GJ, Caplan A, Elias S: The politics of human-embryo research: avoiding ethical gridlock. N Engl J Med 334:1329, 1996.
22. Ethical Issues in Human Stem Cell Research. Vol. 1. Report and Recommendations of the National Bioethics Advisory Commission. Rockville, MD, National Bioethics Advisory Commission, 1999.
23. Annas GJ, Elias S: Politics, moral and embryos: can bioethics in the United State rise above politics? Nature 431:19, 2004.
24. Annas GJ, Coyne B: "Fitness" for birth and reproduction: legal implication of genetic screening. Family Law Q 9:463, 1975.
25. Annas GJ, Elias S: Legal and ethical implications of fetal diagnosis and gene therapy. Am J Med Genet 35:215, 1990.
26. Annas GJ: Medical paternity and "wrongful life." Hastings Center Rep 11:8, 1981.
27. Recent opinions of the Judicial Council of the American Medical Association. JAMA 251:278, 1984.
28. Annas GJ, Roche P, Green RC: Gina, genism, and civil rights. Bioethics 22:7, 2008.
29. President's Commissions for the Study of Ethical Problems in Medicine and Biomedical and Behavioral Research: Screening and Counseling for Genetic Conditions, February 1983. Library of Congress No. 83-600502. Washington, DC, U.S. Government Printing Office, 1983.
30. Elias S, Annas GJ: Generic consent for genetic screening. N Engl J Med 330:1611, 1994.
31. Elias S, Annas GJ: Reproductive genetics and the law. Chicago, Yearbook, 1987.
32. Annas GJ: The rights of patients, 3rd ed. New York, New York University Press, 2004.
33. Andrews LB, Fullarton JE, Holtsman NA, Motulsky AG: Assessing genetic risks: implications for health and social policy. Washington, DC, National Academy Press, 1994.
34. Biesecker BB, Boehnke M, Calzone K, et al: Genetic counseling for families with inherited susceptibility to breast and ovarian cancer. JAMA 269:1970, 1993.
35. Kolder VEB, Gallagher J, Parsons MT: Court-ordered obstetrical interventions. N Engl J Med 316:1192, 1987.
36. Nelson LJ, Milliken N: Compelled medical treatment of pregnant women. JAMA 259:1060, 1988.
37. Notzon FC, Placek PJ, Taffel SM: Comparisons of national cesarean-section rates. N Engl J Med 316:386, 1987.
38. Annas GJ: Protecting the liberty of pregnant patients. N Engl J Med 316:1213, 1987.
39. ACOG Committee Opinion: Maternal Decision Making, Ethics, and the Law, No. 321. Washington DC, American College of Obstetricians and Gynecologist, October 1987.
40. *In Re A.C.*, 573 A 2d 1235 (DC App 1990).

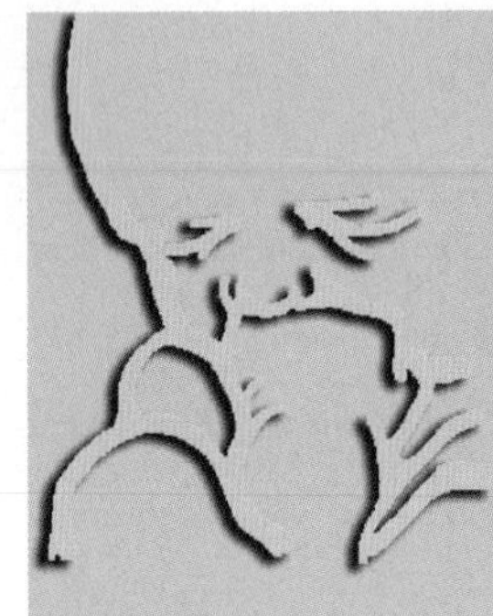

APPENDIX I

Normal Values in Pregnancy

Henry L. Galan and Laura Goetzl

Invasive Cardiac Monitoring

MEASURE	VALUE (36-38 WEEKS)	UNITS
Cardiac output	6.2 ± 1.0	liters/minute
Systemic vascular resistance	1210 ± 266	dyne cm second^{-5}
Heart rate	83 ± 10	beats/minute
Pulmonary vascular resistance	78 ± 22	dyne cm second^{-5}
Colloid oncotic pressure	18.0 ± 1.5	mm Hg
Mean arterial pressure (MAP)	90.3 ± 5.8	mm Hg
Pulmonary capillary wedge pressure (PCWP)	7.5 ± 1.8	mm Hg
Central venous pressure (CVP)	3.6 ± 2.5	mm Hg
Left ventricular stroke work index	48 ± 6	g mm^{-2}

Modified from Clark SL, Cotton DB, Lee W, et al: Central hemodynamic assessment of normal term pregnancy. Am J Obstet Gynecol 161:1439, 1989; Spatling L, Fallenstein F, Huch A, et al: The variability of cardiopulmonary adaptation to pregnancy at rest and during exercise. Br J Obstet Gynaecol 99(Suppl 8):1, 1992.

Cardiac output is increased in pregnancy but is essentially unchanged over the course of pregnancy.

Heart rate gradually rises 5 to 10 bpm over the course of pregnancy.

Noninvasive Cardiac Monitoring

MEASURE	10-18 WEEKS	18-26 WEEKS	26-34 WEEKS	34-42 WEEKS
Cardiac output (L/min)	7.26 ± 1.56	7.60 ± 1.63	7.38 ± 1.63	6.37 ± 1.48
Stroke volume (mL)	85 ± 21	85 ± 21	82 ± 21	70 ± 14
SVR (dyne cm second^{-5})	966 ± 226	901 ± 224	932 ± 240	1118 ± 325
Heart rate (beats/min)	87 ± 14	90 ± 14	92 ± 14	92 ± 7
Mean arterial pressure (mm Hg)	87 ± 7	84 ± 7	84 ± 7	86 ± 7

Modified from Van Oppen CA, Van Der Tweel I, Alsbach JGP, et al: A longitudinal study of maternal hemodynamics during normal pregnancy. Obstet Gynecol 88:40, 1996.

SVR, Systemic vascular resistance.

Arterial Blood Gas Values (Third Trimester)

	NORMAL ALTITUDE	MODERATE ALTITUDE (1388 M, PROVO, UT)
Arterial pH	7.40-7.48	7.44-7.48
Arterial P_{O_2} (mm Hg)	80-90	78.9-93.5
Arterial P_{CO_2} (mm Hg)	26.9-32.5	23.9-29.3
Sodium bicarbonate (mEq/L)	19.9-24.1	16.7-20.5

Modified from Hankins GD, Clark SL, Harvey CJ, et al: Third trimester arterial blood gas and acid base values in normal pregnancy at moderate altitude. Obstet Gynecol 88:347, 1996; Eng M, Butler J, Bonica JJ: Respiratory function in pregnant obese women. Am J Obstet Gynecol 123:241, 1975.

Pulmonary Function Tests

	8-11 WEEKS	20-23 WEEKS	28-31 WEEKS	36-40 WEEKS
Respiratory Rate (br/min)	15 (14-20)	16 (15-18)	18 (15-20)	17 (16-18)
Tidal Volume (mL)	640 (550-710)	650 (625-725)	650 (575-720)	700 (660-755)

(Median, 25th-75th Percentile)

Modified from Spatling L, Fallenstein F, Huch A, et al: The variability of cardiopulmonary adaptation to pregnancy at rest and during exercise. Br J Obstet Gynaecol 99:1, 1992.

Mean Values

	FIRST TRI	SEC TRI	THIRD TRI
Mean Vital Capacity (L)	3.8	3.9	4.1
Mean Inspiratory Capacity (L)	2.6	2.7	2.9
Mean Expiratory Reserve Volume (L)	1.2	1.2	1.2
Mean Residual Volume (L)	1.2	1.1	1.0

Modified from Gazioglu K, Kaltreider NL, Rosen M, Yu PN: Pulmonary function during pregnancy in normal women and in patients with cardiopulmonary disease. Thorax 25:445, 1920; Puranik BM, Kaore SB, Kurhade GA, et al: A longitudinal study of pulmonary function tests during pregnancy. Indian J Physiol Pharmacol 38:129, 1994.

Peak Flows (5th% Shown as Lower Limit of Normal) Stable Over Gestation

	PEAK FLOW (L/min)
Standing	>320
Sitting	>310
Supine	>300

Modified from Harirah HM, Donia SE, Nasrallah FK, et al: Effect of gestational age and position on peak expiratory flow rate: a longitudinal study. Obstet Gynecol 105:372, 2005.

Liver/Pancreatic Function Tests

	FIRST TRIMESTER	SEC TRIMESTER	THIRD TRIMESTER	TERM
Total alkaline phosphatase (IU/L)	17-88	39-105	46-228	48-249
Gamma glutamyl transferase (IU/L)	2-34	2-31	4-32	5-79
Aspartate transaminase (AST, IU/L)	4-40	10-33	4-32	5-103
Alanine transaminase (ALT, IU/L)	1-30	2-34	2-26	5-115
Total bilirubin (mg/dL)	0.05-1.3	0.1-1.0	0.1-1.2	0.1-1.1
Unconjugated bilirubin (mg/dL)	0.1-0.5	0.1-0.4	0.1-0.5	0.2-0.6
Conjugated bilirubin (mg/dL)	0-0.1	0-0.1	0-0.1	—
Lactate dehydrogenase (U/L)	78-433	80-447	82-524	—
Amylase (IU/L)	11-97	14-92	14-97	10-82
Lipase (IU/L)	5-109	8-157	21-169	—

Modified from Bacq Y, Zarka O, Brechot JF, Mariotte N, Vol S, Tichet J, Weill J: Liver function tests in normal pregnancy: a prospective study of 103 pregnant women and 103 matched controls. Hepatol 23:1030, 1996; Karensenti D, Bacq Y, Brechot JF, Mariotte N, Vol S, Tichet J: Serum Amylase and lipase activities in normal pregnancy: a prospective case-control study. Am J Gastroenterol 96:697, 2001; Larsson A, Palm M, Hansson L-O, Axelsson O: Reference values for clinical chemistry tests during normal pregnancy. BJOG 15:874, 2008; Lockitch G: Handbook of Diagnostic Biochemistry and Hematology in Normal Pregnancy. Boca Raton, FL, CRC Press, 1993; van Buul EJA, Steegers EAP, Jongsma HW, et al: Haematological and biochemical profile of uncomplicated pregnancy in nulliparous women: a longitudinal study. Neth J Med 46:73, 1995.

Electrolytes, Osmolality, and Renal Function

	FIRST TRIMESTER	SECOND TRIMESTER	THIRD TRIMESTER	TERM
Total osmolality (mOsm/kg)	267-280	269-289	273-283	271-289
Sodium (mEq/L)	131-139	129-142	127-143	124-141
Potassium (mEq/L)	3.2-4.9	3.3-4.9	3.3-5.2	3.4-5.5
Chloride (mEq/L)	99-108	97-111	97-112	95-111
Bicarbonate (meq/L)	18-26	18-26	17-27	17-25
Urea nitrogen (BUN, mg/dL)	5-14	4-13	3-13	4-15
Creatinine (mg/dL)	0.33-0.80	0.33-0.97	0.3-0.9	0.85-1.1
Serum albumin (g/dL)	3.2-4.7	2.7-4.2	2.3-4.2	2.4-3.9
Uric Acid (mg/dL)	1.3-4.2	1.6-5.4	2.0-6.3	2.4-7.2
Urine volume (mL/24 hours)	750-2500	850-2,400	750-2700	550-3900
Creatinine clearance (mL/min)	69-188	55-168	40-192	52-208
Urine protein (mg/24 hours)	19-141	47-186	46-185	—

Modified from Ezimokhai M, Davison JM, Philips PR, Dunlop W: Non-postural serial changes in renal function during the third trimester of normal human pregnancy. Br J Obstet Gynaecol 88:465, 1981; Higby K, Suiter J, Phelps JY, et al: Normal values of urinary albumin and total protein excretion during pregnancy. Am J Obstet Gynecol 171:984, 1994; Larsson A, Palm M, Hansson L-O, Axelsson O: Reference values for clinical chemistry tests during normal pregnancy. BJOG 15:874, 2008; Lockitch G: Handbook of Diagnostic Biochemistry and Hematology in Normal Pregnancy. Boca Raton, FL, CRC Press, 1993; Milman N, Bergholt T, Byg KE, Eriksen L, Hvas AM: Reference intervals for haematologic variables during normal pregnancy and postpartum in 434 healthy Danish women. Eur J Haematol 79:39, 2007; van Buul EJA, Steegers EAP, Jongsma HW, et al: Haematological and biochemical profile of uncomplicated pregnancy in nulliparous women: a longitudinal study. Neth J Med 46:73, 1995.

Cholesterol and Lipids

	FIRST TRI	SECOND TRI	THIRD TRI	TERM
Total cholesterol (mg/dL)	117-229	136-299	161-349	198-341
High density (HDL)(mg/dL)	40-86	48-95	43-92	44-98
Low density (LDL)(mg/dL)	39-153	41-184	42-224	86-227
Very low density (VLDL)(mg/dL)	10-18	13-23	15-36	25-51
Triglycerides (mg/dL)	11-209	20-293	65-464	103-440

Modified from Belo L, Caslake M, Gaffney D, Santos-Silva A, Pereira-Leite L, Quintanilha A, et al: Changes in LDL size and HDL concentration in normal and preeclamptic pregnancie. Atherosclerois 162:425, 2002; Desoye G, Schweditsch MO, Pfeiffer KP, Zechner R, Kostner GM: Correlation of hormones with lipid and lipoprotein levels during normal pregnancy and postpartum. J Clin Endocrinol Metab 64:704, 1987; Jimenez DM, Pocovi M, Ramon-Cajal J, Romero MA, Martinez H, Grande H: Longitudinal study of plasma lipids and lipoprotein cholesterol in normal pregnancy and puerperium. Gynecol Obstet Invest 25:158, 1988; Lain KY, Markovic N, Ness RB, Roberts JM: Effect of smoking on uric acid and other metabolic markers throughout normal pregnancy. J Clin Endocrinol Metab 90:5743, 2005; Lockitch G: Handbook of diagnostic biochemistry and hematology in normal pregnancy. Boca Raton, FL, CRC Press, 1993.

Hematologic Indices, Iron and B12

	FIRST TRIMESTER	SECOND TRIMESTER	THIRD TRIMESTER	TERM
White blood cells (10^3/mm^3)	3.9-13.8	4.5-14.8	5.3-16.9	4.2-22.2
Neutrophils (10^3/mm^3)	2.2-8.8	2.9-10.1	3.8-13.1	4.8-12.9
Lymphocytes (10^3/mm^3)	0.4-3.5	0.7-3.9	0.7-3.6	0.9-2.5
Monocytes (10^3/mm^3)	0-1.1	0-1.1	0-1.4	0-0.8
Eosinophils (10^3/mm^3)	0-0.6	0-0.6	0-0.6	—
Basophils (10^3/mm^3)	0-0.1	0-0.1	0-0.1	—
Platelet count (10^9/L)	149-433	135-391	121-429	121-397
Hemoglobin (g/dL)	11.0-14.3	10.5-13.7	11.0-13.8	11.0-14.6
Hematocrit (%)	33-41	32-38	33-40	33-42
Mean cell volume (MCV, fL)	81-96	82-97	81-99	82-100
Mean corpuscular hemoglobin (pg)	27-33	—	28-33	28-34
Free erythrocyte propoporphyrin (mcg/g)	<3	<3	<3	<3
Ferritin (serum, ng/mL)	10-123	10-101	10-48	10-64
Total iron binding capacity (mcg/dL)	246-400	216-400	354-400	317-400
Iron (mcg/dL)	40-215	40-220	40-193	40-193
Folate (Serum, ng/mL)	2.3-39.3	2.6-15	1.6-40.2	1.7-19.3
Transferrin saturation (%)	>16	>16	>16	>16
B_{12} (pg/mL)	118-438	130-656	99-526	—

Modified from American College of Obstetricians and Gynecologists: Anemia in Pregnancy. ACOG Practice Bulletin No. 95. Obstet Gynecol 112:201, 2008; Balloch AJ, Cauchi MN: Reference ranges in haematology parameters in pregnancy derived from patient populations. Clin Lab Haemetol 15:7, 1993; Lockitch G: Handbook of diagnostic biochemistry and hematology in normal pregnancy. Boca Raton, FL, CRC Press, 1993; Malkasian GD, Tauxe WN, Hagedom AB: Total iron binding capacity in normal pregnancy. J Nuclear Med 5:243, 1964; Milman N, Agger OA, Nielsen OJ: Iron supplementation during pregnancy. Effect on iron status markers, serum erythropoietin and human placental lactogen. A placebo controlled study in 207 Danish women. Dan Med Bull 38:471, 1991; Milman N, Bergholt T, Byg KE, Eriksen L, Hvas AM: Reference intervals for haematologic variables during normal pregnancy and postpartum in 434 healthy Danish women. Eur J Haematol 79:39, 2007; Romslo I, Haram K, Sagen N, Augensen K: Iron requirements in normal pregnancy as assessed by serum ferritin, serum transferring saturation and erythrocyte protoporphryin determinations. Br J Obstet Gynaecol 90:101, 1983; Tamura T, Goldenberg RL, Freeberg LE, Cliver SP, Cutter GR, Hoffman HJ: Maternal serum folate and zinc concentrations and their relationship to pregnancy outcome. Am J Clin Nutr 56:365, 1992; van Buul EJA, Steegers EAP, Jongsma HW, et al: Haematological and biochemical profile of uncomplicated pregnancy in nulliparous women; a longitudinal study. Neth J Med 46:73, 1995; Walker MC, Smith GN, Perkins SL, Keely EJ, Garner PR: Changes in homocysteine levels during normal pregnancy. Am J Obstet Gynecol 180:660, 1999.

Homocysteine, Vitamin, and Mineral Levels

	FIRST TRIMESTER	SECOND TRIMESTER	THIRD TRIMESTER	TERM
Homocysteine (μmol/L)	4.1-7.7	3.3-11.0	3.9-11.1	4.7-12.8
Homocysteine (μmol/L), on folate	5.0-7.6	2.9-5.5	3.1-5.8	—
Vitamin D 25(OH)D (ng/mL)	>30	>30	>30	>30
Copper (mcg/dL)	69-241	117-253	127-274	163-283
Selenium (mcg/L)	98-160	85-164	84-162	84-144
Zinc (mcg/dL)	51-101	43-93	41-88	39-71

Modified from Alvarez SI, Castanon SG, Ruata MLC: Updating of normal levels of copper, zinc and selenium in serum of pregnant women. J Trace Elem Med Biol 21:49, 2007; Ardawi MSM, Nasrat HAN, BA'Aqueel HS: Calcium-regulating hormones and parathyroid hormone-related peptide in normal human pregnancy and postpartum: a longitudinal study. Eur J Endocrinol 137:402, 1997; Dawson-Hughes B, Heany RP, Holick MF, Lips P, et al: Estimates of optimal vitamin D status. Osteopor Int 16:713, 2005; Lockitch G: Handbook of diagnostic biochemistry and hematology in normal pregnancy. Boca Raton, FL, CRC Press, 1993; Milman N, Bergholt T, Byg KE, Eriksen L, Hvas AM: Reference intervals for haematologic variables during normal pregnancy and postpartum in 434 healthy Danish women. Eur J Haematol 79:39, 2007; Mimouni F, Tsang RC, Hertzberg VS, Neumann V, Ellis K: Parathyroid hormone and calcitor: changes in normal and insulin dependent diabetic pregnancies. Obstet Gynecol 74:49, 1989; Murphy MM, Scott JM, McPartlin JM, Fernandez-Ballart JD: The pregnancy-related decrease in fasting plasma homocysteine is not explained by folic acid supplementation, hemodilution, or a decrease in albumin in a longitudinal study. Am J Clin Nutr 76:614, 2002; Qvist I, Abdulla M, Jagerstad M, Svensson S: Iron, zinc and folate status during pregnancy and two months after delivery. Acta Obstet Gynecol Scand 65:15, 1986; Walker MC, Smith GN, Perkins SL, Keely EJ, Garner PR. Changes in homocysteine levels during normal pregnancy. Am J Obstet Gynecol 180:660, 1999.

CALCIUM METABOLISM

	FIRST TRIMESTER	SECOND TRIMESTER	THIRD TRIMESTER	TERM
Total calcium (mg/dL)	8.5-10.6	7.8-9.4	7.8-9.7	8.1-9.8
Ionized calcium (mg/dL)	4.4-5.3	4.2-5.2	4.4-5.5	4.2-5.4
Parathyroid hormone (pg/mL)	7-15	5-25	5-26	10-17

Modified from Ardawi MSM, Nasrat HAN, BA'Aqueel HS: Calcium-regulating hormones and parathyroid hormone-related peptide in normal human pregnancy and postpartum: a longitudinal study. Eur J Endocrinol 137:402, 1997; Lockitch G: Handbook of diagnostic biochemistry and hematology in normal pregnancy. Boca Raton, FL, CRC Press, 1993; Mimouni F, Tsang RC, Hertzberg VS, Neumann V, Ellis K: Parathyroid hormone and calcitorl changes in normal and insulin dependant diabetic pregnancies. Obstet Gynecol 74:49, 1989; Pitkin RM, Reynolds WA, Williams GA, Hargis GK: Calcium metabolism in normal pregnancy: a longitudinal study. Am J Obstet Gynecol 133:781, 1979; Seki K, Makimura N, Mitsui C, et al: Calcium-regulating hormones and osteocalcin levels during pregnancy: a longitudinal study. Am J Obstet Gynecol 164:1248, 1991.

COAGULATION

	FIRST TRIMESTER	SECOND TRIMESTER	THIRD TRIMESTER	TERM
PT (sec)	8.9-12.2	8.6-13.4	8.3-12.9	7.9-12.7
INR	0.89-1.05	0.85-0.97	0.81-0.95	0.80-0.94
PTT (sec)	24.3-38.9	24.2-38.1	23.9-35.0	23.0-34.9
Fibrinogen (mg/dL)	278-676	258-612	276-857	444-670
D-dimer (mcg/mL)	0.04-0.50	0.05-2.21	0.16-2.8	—
Antithrombin III (%)	89-112	88-112	81-135	82-138
Protein C, FA(%)	78-121	83-132	73-125	67-120
Protein S, total(%)	39-105	27-101	33-101	—
Protein S, free (%)	34-133	19-113	20-69	37-70
Protein S, FA (%)	57-95	42-68	16-42	—
Factor II (%)	70-224	73-214	74-179	68-194
Factor V (%)	46-188	66-185	34-195	39-184
Factor VII (%)	60-206	80-280	84-312	87-336
Factor X (%)	62-169	74-177	78-194	72-208
Von Willebrand factor (%)	—	—	121-258	132-260

Modified from Cerneca F, Ricci G, Someone R, et al: Coagulation and fibrinolysis changes in normal pregnancy. Increased levels of procoagulants and reduced levels of inhibitors during pregnancy induce a hypercoagulable state, combined with a reactive fibrinolysis. Eur J Obstet Gynecol Reprod Biol 73:31, 1997; Choi JW, Pai SH: Tissue plasminogen activator levels change with plasma fibrinogen concentrations during pregnancy. Ann Hematol 81:611, 1997; Faught W, Garner P, Jones G, Ivey B: Changes in protein C and protein S levels in normal pregnancy. Am J Obstet Gynecol 172:147, 1995; Francalanci I, Comeglio P, Liotta AA, Cellai AP, Fedi S, Parretti E: D-dimer concentrations during normal pregnancy, as measured by ELISA. Thromb Res 78:399, 1995; Lefkowitz JB, Clarke SH, Barbour LA: Comparison of protein S functional and antigenic assays in normal pregnancy. Am J Obstet Gynecol 175:657, 1996; Lockitch G: Handbook of diagnostic biochemistry and hematology in normal pregnancy. Boca Raton, FL, CRC Press, 1993; Morse M: Establishing a normal range for d-dimer levels through pregnancy to aid in the diagnosis of pulmonary embolism and deep vein thrombosis. J Thromb Haemost 2:1202, 2004; Stirling Y, Woolf L, North WRS, et al: Haemostasis in normal pregnancy. Thromb Haemost 52:176, 1984; Wickstrom K, Edelstam G, Lowbeer CH, Hansson LO, Siegbahn A: Reference intervals for plasma levels of fibroenectin, von Willebrand factor, free protein S and antithrombin during third trimester pregnancy. Scand J Clin Lab Invest 64:31, 2004.

FA, Functional activity; *INR*, international normalized ratio; *PAI*, plasminogen activator inhibitor; *PT*, prothrombin time; *PTT*, partial thromboplastin time (activated).

INFLAMMATION AND IMMUNE FUNCTION

	FIRST TRIMESTER	SECOND TRIMESTER	THIRD TRIMESTER	TERM
C-Reactive Protein (mg/L)	0.52-15.5	0.78-16.9	0.44-19.7	—
C3 Complement (mg/dL)	44-116	51-119	60-126	64-131
C4 Complement (mg/dL)	9-45	10-42	11-43	16-44
ESR (mm/h)	4-57	7-83	12-90.5	—
Immunoglobulin A (mg/dL)	21-317	23-343	12-364	14-338
Immunoglobulin G (mg/dL)	838-1410	654-1330	481-1273	554-1162
Immunoglobulin M (mg/dL)	10-309	20-306	0-361	0-320

Modified from Saarelainen H, Valtonen P, Punnonen K, et al: Flow mediated vasoldilation and circulationg concentrations of high sensitive C-reactive protein, interleukin-6 and tumor necrosis factor-α in normal pregnancy—the cardiovascular risk in young Finns study. Clin Physiol Funct Imaging 29:347, 2009; Van den Brock NR, Letsky EA: Pregnancy and the erythrocyte sedimentation rate BJOG 108:1164, 2001; Lockitch G: Handbook of diagnostic biochemistry and hematology in normal pregnancy. Boca Raton, FL, CRC Press, 1993.

ESR, Erythrocyte sedimentation rate.

ENDOCRINE TESTS

	FIRST TRI	SECOND TRI	THIRD TRI	TERM
Cortisol (mcg/dL)	7-23	6-51	12-60	21-64
Aldosterone (ng/dL)	6-104	9-104	15-101	—
TSH (μIU/mL)	0.1-4.4	0.4-5.0	0.23-4.4	0.0-5.3
Thyroxine, free (ng/dL)	0.7-1.3	0.4-1.2	0.3-1.0	0.3-1.2
Thyroxine, total (mcg/dL)	3.6-9.0	4.0-8.9	3.5-8.6	3.9-8.3
Triiodothyronine, free (pg/mL)	4.1-44	4.0-4.2	—	—
Triiodothyronine, total (ng/dL)	71-175	84-195	97-182	84-214

Modified from Goland R, Jozak S, Conwell I: Placental corticotropin-releasing hormone and the hypercortisolism of pregnancy. Am J Obstet Gynecol 171:1287, 1994; Larsson A, Palm M, Hansson L-O, Axelsson O: Reference values for clinical chemistry tests during normal pregnancy. BJOG 15:874, 2008; Lockitch G: Handbook of diagnostic biochemistry and hematology in normal pregnancy. Boca Raton, FL, CRC Press, 1993; Mandel SJ, Spencer CA, Hollowell JG: Are detection and treatment of thyroid insufficiency in pregnancy feasible? Thyroid 15:44, 2005; Price A, Obel O, Cresswell J, Catch I, Rutter S, Barik S, et al: Comparison of thyroid function in pregnant and non-pregnant Asian and western Caucasian women. Clin Chim Acta 308:91, 2001.
TSH, Thyroid-stimulating hormone.

UMBILICAL CORD BLOOD GAS VALUES AND HEMATOLOGIC PARAMETERS*

	ARTERY	VEIN
pH	7.06-7.36	7.14-7.45
P_{CO_2} (mm Hg)	27.8-68.3	24.0-56.3
P_{O_2} (mm Hg)	9.8-41.2	12.3-45.0
Base deficit (mmol/L)	0.5-15.3	0.7-12.6
White blood cell count (10^9/L)		11.1-16.2
Red cell count (10^{12}/L)		4.13-4.62
Hemoglobin (g/dL)		15.3-17.2
Hematocrit (%)		45.2-50.9
MCV (fl)		107.4-113.3
Platelet count (10^9/L)		237-321
Reticulocyte count (10^9/L)		145.8-192.6

Modified from Eskes TKAB, Jongsma HW, Houx PCW: Percentiles for gas values in human umbilical cord blood. Eur J Obstet Gynecol Reprod Biol 14:341, 1983; Mercelina-Roumans P, Breukers R, Ubachs, J, Van Wersch J: Hematological variables in cord blood of neonates of smoking and non-smoking mothers. J Clin Epidemiol 49:449, 1996.
Ranges represent 25th to 75th percentile.

CROWN-RUMP LENGTH (6-18 WEEKS)

Crown Rump Length (mm)	Menstrual Age (wk)	Crown Rump Length (mm)	Menstrual Age (wk)	Crown Rump Length (mm)	Menstrual Age (wk)
.	.	30	10.0	61	12.6
.	.	32	10.1	62	12.6
3	5.9	33	10.2	63	12.7
4	6.1	34	10.3	64	12.8
5	6.2	35	10.4	65	12.8
6	6.4	36	10.5	66	12.9
7	6.6	37	10.6	67	13.0
8	6.7	38	10.7	68	13.1
9	6.9	39	10.8	69	13.1
10	7.1	40	10.9	70	13.2
11	7.2	41	11.0	71	13.3
12	7.4	42	11.1	72	13.4
13	7.5	43	11.2	73	13.4
14	7.7	44	11.2	74	13.5
15	7.9	45	11.3	75	13.6
16	8.0	46	11.4	76	13.7
17	8.1	47	11.5	77	13.7
18	8.3	48	11.6	78	13.8
19	8.4	49	11.7	79	13.9
20	8.6	50	11.7	80	14.0
21	8.7	51	11.8	81	14.1
22	8.9	52	11.9	82	14.2
23	9.0	53	12.0	83	14.2
24	9.1	54	12.0	84	14.3
25	9.2	55	12.1	85	14.4
26	9.4	56	12.2	86	14.5
27	9.5	57	12.3	87	14.6
28	9.6	58	12.3	88	14.7
29	9.7	59	12.4	89	14.8
30	9.9	60	12.5	90	14.9

From Hadlock FP, Shah YP, Kanon DJ, Lindsey JV: Fetal crown-rump length: reevaluation of relation to menstrual age (5-18 weeks) with high-resolution real-time US. Radiology, 182:501, 1992.

Head Circumference (Percentile Values)

Menstrual Age (wk)	HEAD CIRCUMFERENCE (cm)				
	3rd	10th	50th	90th	97th
14.0	8.8	9.1	9.7	10.3	10.6
15.0	10.0	10.4	11.0	11.6	12.0
16.0	11.3	11.7	12.4	13.1	13.5
17.0	12.6	13.0	13.8	14.6	15.0
18.0	13.7	14.2	15.1	16.0	16.5
19.0	14.9	15.5	16.4	17.4	17.9
20.0	16.1	16.7	17.7	18.7	19.3
21.0	17.2	17.8	18.9	20.0	20.6
22.0	18.3	18.9	20.12	21.3	21.9
23.0	19.4	20.1	21.3	22.5	23.2
24.0	20.4	21.1	22.4	23.7	24.3
25.0	21.4	22.2	23.5	24.9	25.6
26.0	22.4	23.2	24.6	26.0	26.8
27.0	23.3	24.1	25.6	27.0	27.9
28.0	24.2	25.1	26.6	28.1	29.0
29.0	25.0	25.9	27.5	29.1	30.0
30.0	25.8	26.8	28.4	30.0	31.0
31.0	26.7	27.6	29.3	31.0	31.9
32.0	27.4	28.4	30.1	31.8	32.8
33.0	28.0	29.0	30.8	32.6	33.6
34.0	28.7	29.7	31.5	33.3	34.3
35.0	29.3	30.4	32.2	34.1	35.1
36.0	29.9	30.9	32.8	34.7	35.8
37.0	30.3	31.4	33.3	35.2	36.3
38.0	30.8	31.9	33.8	35.8	36.8
39.0	31.1	32.2	34.2	36.2	37.3
40.0	31.5	32.6	34.6	36.6	37.7

From Hadlock FP, Deter RL, Harrist RB, Park SK: Estimating fetal age: computer-assisted analysis of multiple fetal growth parameters. Radiology 152:497, 1984.

Abdominal Circumference (Percentile Values)

Menstrual Age (wk)	ABDOMINAL CIRCUMFERENCE (cm)				
	3rd	10th	50th	90th	97th
14.0	6.4	6.7	7.3	7.9	8.3
15.0	7.5	7.9	8.6	9.3	9.7
16.0	8.6	9.1	9.9	10.7	11.2
17.0	9.7	10.3	11.2	12.1	12.7
18.0	10.9	11.5	12.5	13.5	14.1
19.0	11.9	12.6	13.7	14.8	15.5
20.0	13.1	13.8	15.0	16.3	17.0
21.0	14.1	14.9	16.2	17.6	18.3
22.0	15.1	16.0	17.4	18.8	19.7
23.0	16.1	17.0	18.5	20.0	20.9
24.0	17.1	18.1	19.7	21.3	22.3
25.0	18.1	19.1	20.8	22.5	23.5
26.0	19.1	20.1	21.9	23.87	24.8
27.0	20.0	21.1	23.0	24.9	26.0
28.0	20.9	22.0	24.0	26.0	27.1
29.0	21.8	23.0	25.1	27.2	28.4
30.0	22.7	23.9	26.1	28.3	29.5
31.0	23.6	24.9	27.1	29.4	30.6
32.0	24.5	25.8	28.1	30.4	31.8
33.0	25.3	26.7	29.1	31.5	32.9
34.0	26.1	27.5	30.0	32.5	33.9
35.0	26.9	28.3	30.9	33.5	34.9
36.0	27.7	29.2	31.8	34.4	35.9
37.0	28.5	30.0	32.7	35.4	37.0
38.0	29.2	30.8	33.6	36.4	38.0
39.0	29.9	31.6	34.4	37.3	38.9
40.0	30.7	32.4	35.3	38.2	39.9

From Hadlock FP, Deter RL, Harrist RB, Park SK: Estimating fetal age: computer-assisted analysis of multiple fetal growth parameters. Radiology 152:497, 1984.

Femur Length (Percentile Values)

Gestational Age (wk)	FEMUR (mm)		
	5th	50th	95th
12	3.9	8.1	12.3
13	6.8	11.0	15.2
14	9.7	13.9	18.1
15	12.6	16.8	21.0
16	15.4	19.7	23.9
17	18.3	22.5	26.8
18	21.1	25.4	29.7
19	23.9	28.2	32.6
20	26.7	31.0	35.4
21	29.4	33.8	38.2
22	32.1	36.5	40.9
23	34.7	39.2	43.6
24	37.4	41.8	46.3
25	39.9	44.4	48.9
26	42.4	46.9	51.4
27	44.9	49.4	53.9
28	47.3	51.8	56.4
29	49.6	54.2	58.7
30	51.8	56.4	61.0
31	54.0	58.6	63.2
32	56.1	60.7	65.4
33	58.1	62.7	67.4
34	60.0	64.7	69.4
35	61.8	66.5	71.2
36	63.5	68.3	73.0
37	65.1	69.9	74.7
38	66.6	71.4	76.2
39	68.0	72.8	77.7
40	69.3	74.2	79.0

From Jeanty P, Cousaert E, Cantaine F, Hobbins JC, Tack B, et al: A longitudinal study of fetal limb growth. Am J Perinatol 1:136, 1984.

Humerus Length (Percentile Values)

Gestational Age (wk)	HUMERUS (mm)		
	5th	50th	95th
12	4.8	8.6	12.3
13	7.6	11.4	15.1
14	10.3	14.1	17.9
15	13.1	16.9	20.7
16	15.8	19.7	23.5
17	21.2	22.4	26.3
18	23.8	25.1	29.0
19	26.3	27.7	31.6
20	28.8	30.3	34.2
21	31.2	32.8	36.7
22	33.5	35.2	39.2
23	33.5	37.5	41.6
24	35.7	39.8	43.8
25	37.9	41.9	46.0
26	39.9	44.0	48.1
27	41.9	46.0	50.1
28	43.7	47.9	52.0
29	45.5	49.7	53.9
30	47.2	51.4	55.6
31	48.9	53.1	57.3
32	50.4	54.7	58.9
33	52.0	56.2	60.5
34	53.4	57.7	62.0
35	54.8	59.2	63.5
36	56.2	60.6	64.9
37	57.6	62.0	66.4
38	59.0	63.4	67.8
39	60.4	64.8	69.3
40	61.9	66.3	70.8

From Jeanty P, Cousaert E, Cantaine F, Hobbins JC, Tack B, et al: A longitudinal study of fetal limb growth. Am J Perinatol 1:136, 1984.

Tibia Length (Percentile Values)

Gestational Age (wk)	TIBIA (mm)		
	5th	50th	95th
12	3.3	8.2	11.2
13	5.6	9.6	13.6
14	8.1	12.0	16.0
15	10.6	14.6	18.6
16	13.1	17.1	21.2
17	15.6	19.7	23.8
18	18.2	22.3	26.4
19	20.8	24.9	29.0
20	23.3	27.5	31.6
21	25.8	30.0	34.2
22	28.3	32.5	36.7
23	30.7	34.9	39.1
24	33.1	37.3	41.6
25	35.4	39.7	43.9
26	37.6	41.9	46.2
27	39.8	44.1	48.4
28	41.9	46.2	50.5
29	43.9	48.2	52.6
30	45.8	50.1	54.5
31	47.6	52.0	56.4
32	49.4	53.8	58.2
33	51.1	55.5	60.0
34	52.7	57.2	61.6
35	54.2	58.7	63.2
36	41.2	60.3	64.8
37	55.8	61.8	66.3
38	58.7	63.2	67.8
39	60.1	64.7	69.3
40	61.5	66.1	70.7

From Jeanty P, Cousaert E, Cantaine F, Hobbins JC, Tack B, et al: A longitudinal study of fetal limb growth. Am J Perinatol 1:136, 1984

Fibula Length (Percentile Values)

Gestational Age (wk)	FIBULA (mm)		
	5th	50th	95th
12	1.7	5.7	9.6
13	4.7	8.7	12.7
14	7.7	11.7	15.6
15	10.6	14.6	18.6
16	13.3	17.4	21.4
17	16.1	20.1	24.2
18	18.7	22.8	26.9
19	21.3	25.4	29.5
20	23.8	27.9	32.0
21	26.2	30.3	34.5
22	28.5	32.7	36.9
23	30.8	35.0	39.2
24	33.0	37.2	41.5
25	35.1	39.4	43.6
26	37.2	41.5	45.7
27	39.2	43.5	47.8
28	41.1	45.4	49.7
29	42.9	47.2	51.6
30	44.7	49.0	53.4
31	46.3	50.7	55.1
32	47.9	52.4	56.8
33	49.5	53.9	58.4
34	50.9	55.4	59.9
35	52.3	56.8	61.3
36	53.6	58.2	62.7
37	54.9	59.4	64.0
38	56.0	60.6	65.2
39	57.1	61.7	66.3
40	58.1	62.8	67.4

From Exacoustos C, Rosati P, Rizzo G, Arduini D: Ultrasound measurements of fetal limb bones. Ultrasound Obstet Gynecol 1:325, 1991.

Radius Length (Percentile Values)

Gestational Age (wk)	RADIUS (mm)		
	5th	50th	95th
12	3.0	6.9	10.8
13	5.6	9.5	13.4
14	8.1	12.0	16.0
15	10.5	14.5	18.5
16	12.9	16.9	20.9
17	15.2	19.3	23.3
18	17.5	21.5	25.6
19	19.7	23.8	27.9
20	21.8	25.9	30.0
21	23.9	28.0	32.2
22	25.9	30.1	34.2
23	27.9	32.0	36.2
24	29.7	34.0	38.2
25	31.6	35.8	40.0
26	33.3	37.6	41.9
27	35.0	39.3	43.6
28	36.7	41.0	45.3
29	38.3	42.6	46.9
30	39.8	44.1	48.5
31	41.2	45.6	50.0
32	42.6	47.0	51.4
33	44.0	48.4	52.8
34	45.2	49.7	54.1
35	46.4	50.9	55.4
36	47.6	52.1	56.6
37	48.7	53.2	57.7
38	49.7	54.2	58.8
39	50.6	55.2	59.8
40	51.5	56.2	60.8

From Exacoustos C, Rosati P, Rizzo G, Arduini D: Ultrasound measurements of fetal limb bones. Ultrasound Obstet Gynecol 1:325, 1991.

Ulna Length (Percentile Values)

Gestational Age (wk)	ULNA (mm)		
	5th	50th	95th
12	2.9	6.8	10.7
13	5.8	9.7	13.7
14	8.6	12.6	16.6
15	11.4	15.4	19.4
16	14.1	18.1	22.1
17	16.7	20.8	24.8
18	19.3	23.3	27.4
19	21.8	25.8	29.9
20	24.2	28.3	32.4
21	26.5	30.6	34.8
22	28.7	32.9	37.1
23	30.9	35.1	39.3
24	33.0	37.2	41.5
25	35.1	39.3	43.5
26	37.0	41.3	45.6
27	38.9	43.2	47.5
28	40.7	45.0	49.3
29	42.5	46.8	51.1
30	44.1	48.5	52.8
31	45.7	50.1	54.5
32	47.2	51.6	56.1
33	48.7	53.1	57.5
34	50.0	54.5	59.0
35	51.3	55.8	60.3
36	52.6	57.1	61.6
37	53.7	58.2	62.8
38	54.8	59.3	63.9
39	55.8	60.4	64.9
40	56.7	61.3	65.9

From Jeanty P, Cousaert E, Cantaine F, Hobbins JC, Tack B, et al: A longitudinal study of fetal limb growth. Am J Perinatol 1:136, 1984.

Foot Length (mm; Mean and SD)

Gestational Age Weeks	−2 SD mm	Mean (Predicted) mm	+2 SD mm
12	77	8	9
13	10	11	12
14	13	15	16
15	16	18	20
16	19	21	23
17	22	24	27
18	24	27	30
19	27	30	34
20	30	33	37
21	32	36	40
22	35	39	43
23	37	42	46
24	40	45	50
25	42	47	53
26	45	50	55
27	47	53	58
28	49	55	61
29	51	58	64
30	54	60	67
31	56	62	68
32	58	65	72
33	60	67	74
34	62	69	77
35	64	71	79
36	66	74	82
37	67	76	84
38	69	78	86
39	71	80	88
40	72	81	90

From Mercer BM, et al: Am J Obstet Gynecol, 156:350, 1987.

Transcerebellar Diameter (Percentile Values and Mean ± SD)

	TCD Percentile Values (mm)						
Age (Weeks)	**5th**	**10th**	**50th**	**90th**	**95th**	**Mean**	**SD**
15	14.2	14.5	15.8	17.1	17.4	14.6	1.4
16	14.6	15.0	16.5	17.9	18.3	16.1	1.0
17	15.2	15.6	17.3	18.9	19.3	17.1	1.0
18	15.9	16.4	18.2	19.9	20.5	18.3	1.2
19	16.8	17.3	19.2	21.1	21.7	19.4	1.1
20	17.7	18.3	20.4	22.4	23.0	20.3	1.2
21	18.8	19.4	21.6	23.8	24.5	21.4	1.3
22	19.9	20.5	23.0	25.3	26.0	22.8	1.8
23	21.2	21.8	24.4	26.8	27.6	24.3	1.6
24	22.5	23.2	25.9	28.5	29.3	25.9	1.7
25	23.9	24.6	27.4	30.2	31.0	27.6	1.6
26	25.3	26.0	29.1	31.9	32.8	29.1	1.8
27	26.7	27.6	30.7	33.8	34.7	30.8	1.7
28	28.2	29.1	32.4	35.6	36.6	32.5	1.8
29	29.8	30.7	34.2	35.6	36.6	32.5	1.7
30	31.3	32.2	35.9	39.5	40.6	36.0	2.2
31	32.8	33.8	37.7	41.5	42.6	37.8	2.4
32	34.4	35.4	39.5	43.4	44.7	39.2	2.4
33	35.9	37.0	41.3	45.4	46.7	41.4	2.6
34	37.3	38.5	43.1	47.4	48.8	42.9	2.7
35	38.8	40.0	44.8	49.5	50.9	44.7	3.0
36	40.1	41.4	46.5	51.4	53.0	46.6	3.4
37	41.4	42.8	48.2	53.4	55.0	48.0	3.2
38	42.7	44.1	49.9	55.4	57.1	49.8	3.3

From Chavez MR, et al: Am J Obstet Gynecol 189:1021, 2003.

Amniotic Fluid Index (Percentile Values)

Gestational Age (wk)	Amniotic Fluid Index (mm)				
	2.5th	5th	50th	95th	97.5th
16	73	79	121	185	201
17	77	83	128	194	211
18	80	87	133	202	220
19	83	90	138	207	225
20	86	93	141	212	230
21	88	95	144	214	233
22	89	97	146	216	235
23	90	98	147	218	237
24	90	98	148	219	238
25	89	97	148	221	240
26	89	97	148	223	242
27	85	95	148	226	245
28	86	94	148	228	249
29	84	92	147	231	254
30	82	90	147	234	258
31	79	88	146	238	263
32	77	86	146	242	269
33	64	83	145	245	274
34	72	81	144	248	278
35	70	79	142	249	279
36	68	77	140	249	279
37	66	75	138	244	275
38	65	73	134	239	269
39	64	72	130	226	255
40	63	71	125	214	240
41	63	70	119	194	216
42	63	69	112	175	192

From Moore TR, Gayle JE: The amniotic fluid index in normal human pregnancy. Am J Obstet Gynecol 162:1168, 1990.

Small Head Circumference Measurements (SD)

Age (wk)	Small Head Circumference Measurements (mm)			
	–2 SD	–3 SD	–4 SD	–5 SD
20	145	131	116	101
21	157	143	128	113
22	169	154	140	125
23	180	166	151	136
24	191	177	162	147
25	202	188	173	158
26	213	198	183	169
27	223	208	194	179
28	233	218	203	189
29	242	227	213	198
30	251	236	222	207
31	260	245	230	216
32	268	253	239	224
33	276	261	246	232
34	283	268	253	239
35	289	275	260	245
36	295	281	266	251
37	301	286	272	257
38	306	291	276	262
39	310	295	281	266
40	314	299	284	270

Reproduced with permission from Chervenak FA, Jeanty P, Cantraine F, et al: Am J Obstet Gynecol 149:512, 1984.

Umbilical Artery Resistance Index (RI) and Systolic-to-Diastolic (S/D) Ratio

Age (Weeks)	5th Percentile		50th Percentile		95th Percentile	
	RI	S/D	RI	S/D	RI	S/D
16	0.70	3.33	0.80	5.00	0.90	10.00
17	0.69	3.23	0.79	4.76	0.89	9.09
18	0.68	3.13	0.78	4.55	0.88	8.33
19	0.67	3.03	0.77	4.35	0.87	7.69
20	0.66	2.94	0.76	4.17	0.86	7.14
21	0.65	2.86	0.75	4.00	0.85	6.67
22	0.64	2.78	0.74	3.85	0.84	6.25
23	0.63	2.70	0.73	3.70	0.83	5.88
24	0.62	2.63	0.72	3.57	0.82	5.56
25	0.61	2.56	0.71	3.45	0.81	5.26
26	0.60	2.50	0.70	3.33	0.80	5.00
27	0.59	2.44	0.69	3.23	0.79	4.76
28	0.58	2.38	0.68	3.13	0.78	4.55
29	0.57	2.33	0.67	3.03	0.77	4.35
30	0.56	2.27	0.66	2.94	0.76	4.17
31	0.55	2.22	0.65	2.86	0.75	4.00
32	0.54	2.17	0.64	2.78	0.74	3.85
33	0.53	2.13	0.63	2.70	0.73	3.70
34	0.52	2.08	0.62	2.63	0.72	3.57
35	0.51	2.04	0.61	2.56	0.71	3.45
36	0.50	2.00	0.60	2.50	0.70	3.33
37	0.49	1.96	0.59	2.44	0.69	3.23
38	0.47	1.89	0.57	2.33	0.67	3.03
39	0.46	1.85	0.56	2.27	0.66	2.94
40	0.45	1.82	0.55	2.22	0.65	2.86
41	0.44	1.79	0.54	2.17	0.64	2.78
42	0.43	1.75	0.53	2.13	0.63	2.70

From Kofinas AD, Espeland MA, Penry M, Hatjis C: Utero-placental Doppler flow velocity wave-form indices in normal pregnancy: a statistical exercise and the development of appropriate reference values. Am J Perinat 9:94, 1992.

Middle Cerebral Artery Pulsatility Index (Percentile Values)

Age (Weeks)	Middle Cerebral Artery Pulsatility Index				
	5th	10th	50th	90th	95th
21	1.18	1.26	1.6	2.04	2.19
22	1.25	1.33	1.69	0.15	2.30
23	1.32	1.41	1.78	2.25	2.41
24	1.38	1.47	1.86	2.36	2.52
25	1.44	1.54	1.94	2.45	2.62
26	1.50	1.6	2.01	2.53	2.71
27	1.55	1.65	2.06	2.60	2.78
28	1.58	1.69	2.11	2.66	2.84
29	1.61	1.71	2.15	2.70	2.88
30	1.62	1.73	2.16	2.72	2.90
31	1.62	1.73	2.16	2.71	2.90
32	1.61	1.71	2.14	2.69	2.87
33	1.58	1.68	2.10	2.64	2.82
34	1.53	1.63	2.04	2.57	2.74
35	1.47	1.56	1.96	2.47	2.64
36	1.39	1.48	1.86	2.36	2.52
37	1.30	1.39	1.75	2.22	2.38
38	1.20	1.29	1.63	2.07	2.22
39	1.1	1.18	1.49	1.91	2.05

From Ebbing C, Rasmussen S, Kiserud T: Ultrasound Obstet Gynecol 30:287, 2007.

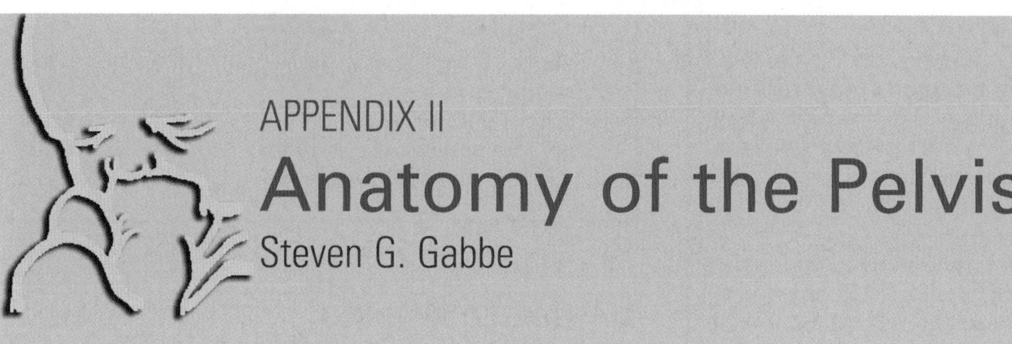

APPENDIX II

Anatomy of the Pelvis

Steven G. Gabbe

***The illustrations for the Anatomy of the Pelvis Appendix can be found online at *www.expertconsult.com*.**

KEY POINTS

- To facilitate childbearing, the female pelvis—as opposed to the male pelvis—is characterized by a wider subpubic angle, increased width of the sciatic notch, and greater distance from the symphysis pubis to the anterior edge of the acetabulum.
- The levator ani, the major supporting structure for the pelvic viscera, is a tripartite muscle mass composed of the iliococcygeus, pubococcygeus, and puborectalis; the iliococcygeus is the broadest and most posterior portion.
- Innervation of the levator ani is through the third and fourth sacral nerves.
- The major nerve supply of the perineum is derived from the pudendal. However, the ilioinguinal, genitofemoral, perineal branch of the posterior femoral cutaneous, coccygeal, and last sacral nerve also contribute; thus, a pudendal nerve block anesthetizes only a portion of the perineum.
- The internal iliac (hypogastric) artery arises at the level of lumbosacral articulation. It can be distinguished from the external iliac by its smaller size and by its more medial and more posterior position.
- The ureter lies more superficially and is either medial or slightly anterior to the internal iliac artery.
- The cardinal ligaments are located at the base of the broad ligament, are continuous with the connective tissue of the parametrium, and are attached to the pelvic diaphragm through continuity with the superficial superior fascia of the levator ani.

- Because the origin of the uterine artery is variable, its isolation and ligation for control of postpartum bleeding are often fruitless. The uterine artery usually arises as an independent vessel from the internal iliac artery, but it may also arise from the inferior gluteal, internal pudendal, umbilical, or obturator arteries.
- Afferent pain fibers for the uterus, tubes, and ovary enter the cord at T10, T11, T12; thus, spinal or epidural anesthesia must extend to these levels. Fortunately, efferent fibers to the uterus enter above these levels, thus not interfering with contractions.
- The body of the nonpregnant uterus weighs approximately 70 g, whereas at term it weighs approximately 1100 g.

SUGGESTED READING

Moore KL, Dalley AF II: Pelvis and perineum. *In* Clinically Oriented Anatomy, ed 5. Baltimore, Lippincott Williams & Wilkins, 2006, p 357.

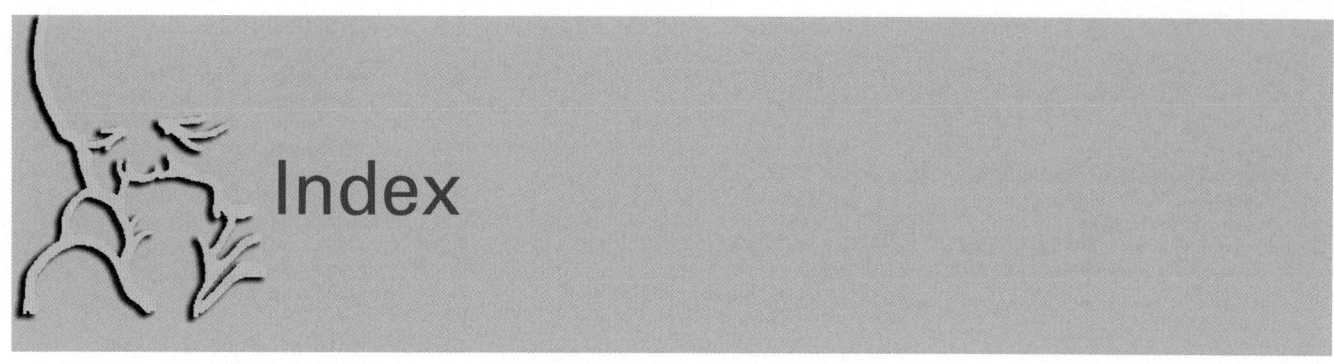

Index

Note: Page numbers followed by b indicate boxes. Page numbers followed by f indicate figures. Page numbers followed by t indicate tables.

N

P

S